CONN'S
Current Therapy 2009

CONN'S Current Therapy 2009

Robert E. Rakel, MD
Professor, Department of Family and
 Community Medicine
Baylor College of Medicine
Houston, Texas

Edward T. Bope, MD
Director, Riverside Family Practice
 Residency Program
Clinical Professor, Department of Family Medicine
The Ohio State University College of Medicine
Columbus, Ohio

LATEST APPROVED METHODS
OF TREATMENT FOR THE
PRACTICING PHYSICIAN

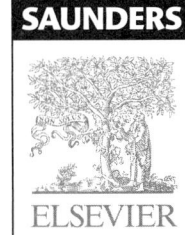

South University Library
Richmond Campus
2151 Old Brick Road
Glen Allen, Va 23060

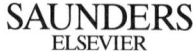

1600 John F. Kennedy Blvd.
Ste 1800
Philadelphia, PA 19103-2899

CONN'S CURRENT THERAPY 2009   ISBN: 978-1-4160-5974-5

Copyright © 2009, 2008 by Saunders, an imprint of Elsevier Inc.

All rights reserved. No part of this publication may be reproduced or transmitted in any form or by any means, electronic or mechanical, including photocopying, recording, or any information storage and retrieval system, without permission in writing from the publisher. Permissions may be sought directly from Elsevier's Rights Department: phone: (+1)215 239 3804 (US) or (+44) 1865 843830 (UK); fax: (+44) 1865 853333; e-mail: healthpermissions@elsevier.com. You may also complete your request on-line via the Elsevier website at http://www.elsevier.com/permissions.

Notice

Knowledge and best practice in this field are constantly changing. As new research and experience broaden our knowledge, changes in practice, treatment, and drug therapy may become necessary or appropriate. Readers are advised to check the most current information provided (i) on procedures featured or (ii) by the manufacturer of each product to be administered, to verify the recommended dose or formula, the method and duration of administration, and contraindications. It is the responsibility of the practitioner, relying on his or her experience and knowledge of the patient, to make diagnoses, to determine dosages and the best treatment for each individual patient, and to take all appropriate safety precautions. To the fullest extent of the law, neither the Publisher nor the Editors assume any liability for any injury and/or damage to persons or property arising out of or related to any use of the material contained in this book.

The Publisher

Library of Congress Cataloging-in-Publication Data
Current therapy; latest approved methods of treatment for the practicing physician.
Editors: H. F. Conn and others
    v. 28 cm. annual
    ISBN 978-1-4160-5974-5
    1. Therapeutics. 2. Therapeutics, Surgical. 3. Medicine—Practice.
    I. Conn, Howard Franklin, 1908–1982 ed.

RM101.C87 616.058 49–8328 rev*

Acquisitions Editor: Druanne Martin
Developmental Editor: Lucia Gunzel
Publishing Services Manager: Frank Polizzano
Project Manager: Jeff Gunning
Design Direction: Steve Stave

Working together to grow
libraries in developing countries

www.elsevier.com | www.bookaid.org | www.sabre.org

ELSEVIER   BOOK AID International   Sabre Foundation

Printed in the United States of America

Last digit is the print number: 9 8 7 6 5 4 3 2 1

Contributors

Charles S. Abrams, MD
Associate Professor of Medicine, Division of Hematology-Oncology, University of Pennsylvania School of Medicine; Staff Physician, Division of Hematology-Oncology, University of Pennsylvania Medical Center, Philadelphia, Pennsylvania
Platelet-Mediated Bleeding Disorders

Mark J. Abzug, MD
Professor of Pediatrics (Infectious Diseases), University of Colorado–Denver School of Medicine; Medical Director, The Children's Hospital Clinical Trials Organization, The Children's Hospital, Denver, Colorado
Viral Meningitis and Encephalitis

Sujeet S. Acharya, MD
Resident Physician, The University of Chicago Medical Center, Chicago, Illinois
Renal Calculi

Tod C. Aeby, MD
Residency Program Director, Department of Obstetrics, Gynecology, and Women's Health, University of Hawaii John A. Burns School of Medicine, Honolulu, Hawaii
Uterine Leiomyomas

Gorav Ailawadi, MD
Assistant Professor of Surgery, University of Virginia School of Medicine, Charlottesville, Virginia
Acquired Diseases of the Aorta

Murad Alam, MD
Chief of Cutaneous and Aesthetic Surgery; Associate Professor of Dermatology, Otolaryngology, and Surgery, Northwestern University, Chicago, Illinois
Cancer of the Skin

Daniel Albo, MD, PhD
Associate Professor of Surgery, Baylor College of Medicine; Chief, General Surgery and Surgical Oncology, and Associate Operative Care Line Executive for Operating Room Affairs, Michael E. DeBakey VA Medical Center, Houston, Texas
Tumors of the Colon and Rectum

Carl M. Allen, DDS, MSD
Professor, Department of Oral Pathology, The Ohio State University College of Dentistry; Director, Oral & Maxillofacial Surgery and Pathology, University Hospital; Professor, Department of Pathology, The Ohio State University College of Medicine and Public Health, Columbus, Ohio
Diseases of the Mouth

Navin M. Amin, MD
Professor of Family Medicine, University of California, Irvine, School of Medicine, Irvine; Associate Professor of Medicine, David Geffen School of Medicine at UCLA, Los Angeles; and Associate Professor of Medicine, Stanford University School of Medicine, Stanford, California
Infective Endocarditis

Girish Anand, MD
Fellow in Gastroenterology, Albert Einstein Medical Center, Philadelphia, Pennsylvania
Dysphagia and Esophageal Obstruction

Deverick J. Anderson, MD
Clinical Associate, Duke University Medical Center, Durham, North Carolina
Rickettsial and Ehrlichial Infections

Kelly P. Anderson, MD
Clinical Associate Professor of Medicine, University of Wisconsin School of Medicine and Public Health–Marshfield Clinic Campus, Marshfield, Wisconsin
Heart Block

Karim Aoun, MD
Associate Professor, University of Tunis Faculty of Medicine; Attending Physician, Pasteur Institute of Tunis, Tunis, Tunisia
Leishmaniasis

Paul M. Arguin, MD
Captain, U.S. Public Health Service; Chief, Domestic Malaria Unit, Centers for Disease Control and Prevention, Atlanta, Georgia
Malaria

Aydin Arici, MD
Professor, Department of Obstetrics, Gynecology and Reproductive Sciences, Yale University School of Medicine, New Haven, Connecticut
Dysfunctional Uterine Bleeding

Ann M. Aring, MD
Assistant Program Director, Family Medicine Residency, Riverside Methodist Hospital; Assistant Clinical Professor, Department of Family Medicine, The Ohio State University College of Medicine, Columbus, Ohio
Fever

Isao Arita, MD
Chairman, Agency for Cooperation in International Health, Kumamoto, Kumamoto City, Japan
Smallpox

Anthony C. Arnold, MD
Professor of Neuro-Ophthalmology, David Geffen School of Medicine at UCLA; Chief, Neuro-Ophthalmology Division, Jules Stein Eye Institute, Los Angeles, California
Optic Neuritis

Ashok Attaluri, MD
Attending, University of Iowa Hospitals and Clinics, Iowa City, Iowa
Gaseousness and Indigestion

Claus Bachert, MD, PhD
Professor, University of Ghent Faculty of Medicine; Chief of Clinics, Ear-Nose-Throat Department, University Hospital of Ghent, Ghent, Belgium
Nonallergic Perennial Rhinitis

James F. King, MD
Endowed Chair in Gastroenterology and Professor of Internal Medicine, Saint Louis University School of Medicine; Director, Division of Gastroenterology, Saint Louis University Hospital, St. Louis, Missouri
Hemochromatosis

Gopal H. Badlani, MD
Vice Chairman, Department of Urology, Long Island Jewish Medical Center, New Hyde Park, New York
Benign Prostatic Hyperplasia

Adrianne Williams Bagley, MD
Clinical Associate Professor, Johns Hopkins University School of Medicine; Associate Staff, Johns Hopkins Hospital, Baltimore, Maryland
Pelvic Inflammatory Disease

Jeffrey L. Ballard, MD
Clinical Professor of Surgery, University of California, Irvine, School of Medicine, Irvine; Staff Vascular Surgeon, St. Joseph Hospital, Orange, California
Peripheral Arterial Disease

Theodore Barber, MD
Fellow, Department of Pediatric Urology, University of Texas Southwestern; Fellow, Department of Pediatric Urology, Children's Medical Center, Dallas, Texas
Trauma to the Genitourinary Tract

Philip S. Barie, MD, MBA
Professor of Surgery and Public Health and Chief, Division of Critical Care and Trauma, Weill Cornell Medical College; Director, Trauma Services, and Director, Anne and Max A. Cohen Surgical Intensive Care Unit, NewYork–Presbyterian Hospital/Weill Cornell Medical Center, New York, New York
Bacterial Infections of the Skin

Brenda L. Bartlett, MD
Clinical Research Fellow, Center for Clinical Studies, Houston, Texas
Pruritus Ani and Vulvae

James C. Barton, MD
Clinical Professor, Department of Medicine, University of Alabama at Birmingham School of Medicine; Medical Director, Southern Iron Disorders Center, Birmingham, Alabama
Iron Deficiency

Nurcan Baykam, MD
Associate Professor of Infectious Diseases, University of Ankara Faculty of Medicine; Staff, Infectious Diseases and Clinical Microbiology Clinic, Ankara Numune Education and Research Hospital, Ankara, Turkey
Brucellosis

Carolyn E. Beck, MD, MSc
Assistant Professor, University of Toronto Faculty of Medicine; Staff Paediatrician, Division of Paediatric Medicine, The Hospital for Sick Children, Toronto, Ontario, Canada
Parenteral Fluid Therapy for Infants and Children

Meg Begany, RD, CSP, LDN
Clinical Neonatal Dietitian, The Children's Hospital of Philadelphia, Philadelphia, Pennsylvania
Normal Infant Feeding

Jerome Belinson, MD
Staff, Department of Obstetrics and Gynecology, Taussig Cancer Institute; Director, Gynecologic Oncology Fellowship Program, Cleveland Clinic, Cleveland, Ohio
Ovarian Cancer

Nicholas P. Bell, MD
Clinical Assistant Professor, Department of Ophthalmology and Visual Science, University of Texas Medical School at Houston, Houston, Texas
Glaucoma

Pelayo C. Besa, MD
Adjunct Professor of Radiation Oncology, Department of Radiology; Program Head, Radiation Oncology, Hospital Clinico, Pontificia Universidad Católica de Chile, Santiago, Chile
Hodgkin's Disease: Radiation Therapy

Karl R. Beutner, MD, PhD
Associate Clinical Professor of Dermatology, University of California, San Francisco, School of Medicine, San Francisco, California
Condyloma Acuminatum (Genital Warts)

Zulfiqar A. Bhutta, MB, BS, PhD
Husein Lalji Dewraj Professor of Pediatrics, Aga Khan University and Medical Center, Karachi, Pakistan
Typhoid Fever

John P. Bilezikian, MD
Professor, Department of Medicine, Columbia University College of Physicians and Surgeons; Attending Physician, NewYork–Presbyterian Hospital, New York, New York
Primary Hyperparathyroidism and Hypoparathyroidism

Beverly M. K. Biller, MD
Professor of Medicine, Harvard Medical School; Physician in Medicine, Massachusetts General Hospital, Boston, Massachusetts
Hyperprolactinemia

Mark Boguniewicz, MD
Professor; Department of Pediatrics, Division of Allergy-Immunology, National Jewish Health and University of Colorado School of Medicine, Denver, Colorado
Atopic Dermatitis

Herbert L. Bonkovsky, MD
Professor, University of Connecticut School of Medicine, Farmington, Connecticut; Professor, University of North Carolina College of Medicine; Vice President for Research, Carolinas Health Care System, Charlotte, North Carolina
Porphyria

Patrick Borgen, MD
Chief, Breast Service, Department of Surgery, Memorial Sloan-Kettering Cancer Center, New York, New York
Diseases of the Breast

Harisios Boudoulas, MD, PhD
Professor of Medicine and Pharmacy Emeritus, The Ohio State University College of Medicine and Public Health, Columbus, Ohio; Director, Center of Clinical Research, Academy of Athens, Athens, Greece
Mitral Valve Prolapse: The Floppy Mitral Valve, Mitral Valve Prolapse, and Mitral Valvular Regurgitation

Aida Bouratbine, MD
Professor, University of Tunis Faculty of Medicine; Head, Laboratory of Parasitology, Pasteur Institute of Tunis, Tunis, Tunisia
Leishmaniasis

Krystene I. Boyle, MD
Clinical Instructor, Department of Obstetrics and Gynecology, University of Cincinnati College of Medicine; Clinical Fellow, Department of OB/GYN, Division of Reproductive Endocrinology, University of Cincinnati Medical Center, Cincinnati, Ohio
Menopause

Robert Bradsher, MD
Richard V. Ebert Professor of Medicine, University of Arkansas College of Medicine; Program Director, Internal Medicine Residency and Infectious Diseases Fellowship Training Program; Vice-Chairman, Department of Internal Medicine; Director, Division of Infectious Diseases, University of Arkansas for Medical Sciences, Little Rock, Arkansas
Blastomycosis

Daniel M. Brailita, MD
Fellow in Gastroenterology, University of Texas Southwestern Medical Center, Dallas, Texas
Acute and Chronic Hepatitis

Chad M. Braun, MD
Program Director, Family Medicine Residency, Mount Carmel Hospital; Assistant Clinical Professor, Ohio State University College of Medicine, Columbus, Ohio
Nausea and Vomiting

Mark E. Brecher, MD
Professor and Vice Chair, Department of Pathology and Laboratory Medicine, University of North Carolina at Chapel Hill School of Medicine; Director, McLendon Clinical Laboratories, Chapel Hill, North Carolina
Therapeutic Use of Blood Components

Patricia D. Brown, MD
Associate Professor of Medicine, Division of Infectious Diseases, Wayne State University School of Medicine; Chief of Medicine, Detroit Receiving Hospital, Detroit, Michigan
Pyelonephritis

Patrick Brown, MD
Assistant Professor of Oncology and Pediatrics, Johns Hopkins University School of Medicine; Director, Pediatric Leukemia and Lymphoma Program, Sidney Kimmel Comprehensive Cancer Center at Johns Hopkins, Baltimore, Maryland
Acute Leukemia in Children

John Brusch, MD
Assistant Professor of Medicine, Harvard Medical School, Boston; Associate Chief of Medicine, Cambridge Health Alliance, Cambridge, Massachusetts
Streptococcal Pharyngitis

Cathy L. Budman, MD
Associate Professor of Psychiatry, New York University School of Medicine, New York; Director, Movement Disorders Program in Psychiatry, North Shore–Long Island Jewish Health System, Manhassett, New York
Gilles de la Tourette Syndrome

Irina Burd, MD, PhD
Instructor, Department of Obstetrics and Gynecology, University of Pennsylvania School of Medicine; Staff, Hospital of the University of Pennsylvania, Philadelphia, Pennsylvania
Menopause

Jeffrey Burgess, DDS, MSD
Director, Oral Care Research Associates, Seattle, Washington
Temporomandibular Disorders and Orofacial Pain

Craig N. Burkhart, MD, MS
Assistant Professor (Clinical) of Dermatology, University of North Carolina at Chapel Hill School of Medicine; Staff, Department of Dermatology, University of North Carolina Hospitals, Chapel Hill, North Carolina
Bullous Diseases

John J. Byrnes, MD
Professor of Medicine, University of Miami Miller School of Medicine; Chief of Hematology and Medical Oncology, Miami VA Medical Center, Miami, Florida
Disseminated Intravascular Coagulation

Diego Cadavid, MD
Associate Professor, Department of Neurology and Neuroscience, UMDNJ–New Jersey Medical School, Newark, New Jersey
Relapsing Fever

Grant R. Caddy, MD
Consultant Physician and Gastroenterologist, Ulster Hospital, Belfast, Northern Ireland
Cholelithiasis and Cholecystitis

Umberto Capitanio, MD
Resident in Training, Vita-Salute University, Milan, Italy
Prostatitis

Thomas R. Caraccio, PharmD
Associate Professor of Emergency Medicine, Stony Brook University School of Medicine, Stony Brook; Assistant Professor of Pharmacology and Toxicology, New York College of Osteopathic Medicine, Old Westbury, New York
Medical Toxicology: Ingestions, Inhalations, and Dermal and Ocular Absorptions

Enrique V. Carbajal, MD
Associate Clinical Professor of Medicine, University of California, San Francisco, School of Medicine, San Fancisco; Staff Physician–Cardiology, VA Central California Health Care System, Fresno, California
Premature Beats

Miriam M. Chan, BSc, PharmD
Clinical Assistant Professor of Family Medicine, College of Medicine and Public Health, and Clinical Assistant Professor of Pharmacy, College of Pharmacy, The Ohio State University, Columbus, Ohio; Adjunct Assistant Professor of Pharmacy, Ohio Northern University, Ada, Ohio; Affiliate Faculty of Pharmacy Practice, Idaho State University, Pocatello, Idaho; Director of Pharmacy Education, Riverside Family Medicine Residency, Riverside Methodist Hospital, Columbus, Ohio
Some Popular Herbs and Nutritional Supplements; New Drugs in 2008 and Agents Pending FDA Approval

Sam S. Chang, MD
Associate Professor of Urologic Surgery, Vanderbilt University School of Medicine, Nashville, Tennessee
Malignant Tumors of the Urogenital Tract

Charles W. Chappuis, MD
Professor of Clinical Surgery, Department of Surgery, Louisiana State University School of Medicine, New Orleans; Chief of Surgery, University Medical Center, Lafayette, Louisiana
Diverticula of the Alimentary Tract

Emery Chen, MD
Endocrine Surgeon, Woodland Clinic, Woodland, California
Thyroid Cancer

Meera Chitlur, MD
Assistant Professor of Pediatrics, Wayne State University School of Medicine; Staff Physician, Carman and Ann Adams Department of Pediatrics, Division of Hematology/Oncology, Children's Hospital of Michigan, Detroit, Michigan
Hemophilia and Related Bleeding Disorders

Stella T. Chou, MD
Instructor in Pediatrics, University of Pennsylvania School of Medicine; Attending Physician, The Children's Hospital of Philadelphia, Philadelphia Pennsylvania
Nonimmune Hemolytic Anemia

Gary S. Chuang, MD
Department of Dermatology, Columbia University College of Physicians and Surgeons, New York, New York
Papulosquamous Eruptions

Bart L. Clarke, MD
Associate Professor of Medicine, Mayo Clinic College of Medicine, Rochester, Minnesota
Osteoporosis

Claus-Frenz Claussen, MD
Julius-Maximilians-Universität Würzburg, Würzburg; Head, 4-G Research Institute, Neurootologisches Forschungsinstitut, Bad Kissingen, Germany
Tinnitus

Donald Clemons, MD
Clinical Assistant Professor, Department of Family Practice, Quillen School of Medicine, Johnson City, Tennessee
Premalignant Lesions

Michael S. Cookson, MD
Associate Professor of Urologic Surgery, Vanderbilt University School of Medicine, Nashville, Tennessee
Malignant Tumors of the Urogenital Tract

Robert A. Copeland, Jr., MD
Department of Ophthalmology, Howard University Hospital, Washington, DC
Conjunctivitis

Yvon Cormier, MD
Professor of Medicine, Laval University Faculty of Medicine; Respirologist, Hôpital Laval, Quebec City, Quebec, Canada
Hypersensitivity Pneumonitis

Jorge E. Cortes, MD
Professor of Medicine and Deputy Chair, Department of Leukemia, The University of Texas M.D. Anderson Cancer Center, Houston, Texas
Chronic Leukemias

Linda Cox, MD
Assistant Clinical Professor of Medicine, NOVA Southeastern College of Osteopathic Medicine, Davie, Florida; Member, Board of Directors, and Chair of Immunotherapy and Allergy Diagnostics Committee, and Chair of Practice and Policy Division, American Academy of Allergy, Asthma and Immunology, Milwaukee, Wisconsin
Allergic Rhinitis

John F. Coyle II, MD
Clinical Professor, Department of Medicine, University of Oklahoma College of Medicine–Tulsa, Tulsa, Oklahoma
Disturbances Caused by Heat

Michael A. Crouch, MD, MSPH
Virginia Commonwealth University Medical College of Virginia, Richmond, Virginia
Management of Patients with Dyslipoproteinemias (Cholesterol and Triglyceride Disorders)

Lester M. Crawford, PhD
Formerly Research Professor, Georgetown University School of Medicine, Washington, DC, and Head, Department of Physiology, University of Georgia College of Medicine, Athens, Georgia
Foodborne Illness

Michael A. Crouch, MD, MSPH
Memorial Family Medicine Residency Program, Sugar Land; Memorial Hermann Southwest Hospital, Houston, Texas
Management of Patients with Dyslipoproteinemias (Cholesterol and Triglyceride Disorders)

Michael D. Crowell, PhD
Professor of Medicine, Mayo Clinic College of Medicine, Rochester, Minnesota; Co-Director, GI Physiology and Motility, and Consultant, Division of Gastroenterology and Hepatology, Mayo Clinic, Scottsdale, Arizona
Irritable Bowel Syndrome

Burke A. Cunha, MD
Professor of Medicine, Stony Brook University School of Medicine, Stony Brook; Chief, Infectious Disease Division, Winthrop-University Hospital, Mineola, New York
Viral and Mycoplasmal Pneumonias; Urinary Tract Infections in Women

Anne B. Curtis, MD
Division of Cardiovascular Disease, University of South Florida, Tampa, Florida
Atrial Fibrillation

Craig E. Daniels, MD
Assistant Professor of Medicine, Mayo Clinic Graduate School of Medicine; Attending, Mayo Clinic, Rochester, Minnesota
Pleural Effusion and Empyema Thoracis

Stella Dantas, MD
Physician, Department of Obstetrics and Gynecology, Beaverton Medical Office, Northwest Permanente PC Physicians and Surgeons, Beaverton, Oregon
Uterine Leiomyomas

Andre Dascal, MD, FRCPC
Associate Professor, Departments of Medicine, Microbiology, and Immunology, McGill University Faculty of Medicine; Senior Infectious Disease Physician, Sir Mortimer B. Davis–Jewish General Hospital, Montreal, Quebec, Canada
Acute Infectious Diarrhea; Toxic Shock Syndrome

Susan Davids, MD, MPH
Assistant Professor of Medicine, Medical College of Wisconsin; Associate Program Director, Internal Medicine Residency, Clement J. Zablocki VA Medical Center, Milwaukee, Wisconsin
Acute Bronchitis

Susan A. Davidson, MD
Associate Professor, University of Colorado School of Medicine; Chief, Gynecologic Oncology, University of Colorado Hospital, Denver, Colorado
Neoplasms of the Vulva

Terry F. Davies, MD
Baumritter Professor of Medicine, Mount Sinai School of Medicine, New York; Director, Division of Endocrinology and Metabolism, James J. Peters VA Medical Center, Bronx, New York
Hypothyroidism

Kevin Deane, MD
Assistant Professor of Medicine, University of Colorado–Denver School of Medicine, Aurora, Colorado
Bursitis, Tendinitis, Myofascial Pain, and Fibromyalgia

Prakash C. Deedwania, MD
Professor of Medicine, University of California, San Francisco, School of Medicine, San Francisco; Chief, Cardiology Section, VA Central California Health Care System, Fresno, California
Premature Beats

Jennifer L. DeFazio, MD
Clinical Assistant Professor, Department of Dermatology, Stony Brook University School of Medicine, Stony Brook; Clinical Assistant, Department of Medicine, Division of Dermatology, Memorial Sloan-Kettering Cancer Center, Hauppauge, New York
Melanoma

Stephen R. Deputy, MD
Assistant Professor of Neurology, Louisiana State University School of Medicine; Staff Neurologist, Children's Hospital, New Orleans, Louisiana
Traumatic Brain Injury in Children

Richard D. deShazo, MD
Professor of Medicine and Pediatrics and Billy S. Guyton Distinguished Professor, University of Mississippi College of Medicine; Chair, Department of Medicine, University of Mississippi Medical Center, Jackson, Mississippi
Pneumoconiosis

Kenneth R. DeVault, MD
Professor of Medicine, Mayo Clinic Education; Chair, Division of Gastroenterology and Hepatology, Mayo Clinic, Jacksonville, Florida
Gastroesophageal Reflux Disease

Luis A. Diaz, MD
Professor and Chair of Dermatology, University of North Carolina at Chapel Hill School of Medicine; Staff, Department of Dermatology, University of North Carolina Hospitals, Chapel Hill, North Carolina
Bullous Diseases

John K. DiBaise, MD
Professor of Medicine, Mayo Clinic College of Medicine, Rochester, Minnesota; Consultant, Division of Gastroenterology and Hepatology, Mayo Clinic, Scottsdale, Arizona
Irritable Bowel Syndrome

Hans-Christoph Diener, MD
Chairman and Professor, Department of Neurology and Essen Headache Center, University Hospital Essen Medical School, Essen, Germany
Ischemic Cerebrovascular Disease

José G. Díez, MD
Assistant Professor of Medicine, Baylor College of Medicine; Staff, Interventional Cardiology, St. Luke's Episcopal Hospital/Texas Heart Institute, Houston, Texas
Acute Pericarditis

Alice N. Do, DO
Research Fellow, Solano Clinical Research, Division Dow Pharmaceutical Sciences, Vallejo, California
Condyloma Acuminatum (Genital Warts)

Sunil Dogra, MD, DNB, MNAMS
Assistant Professor, Department of Dermatology, Venereology and Leprology, Postgraduate Institute of Medical Education and Research, Chandigarh, India
Leprosy

Basak Dokuzoguz, MD
Chief, Infectious Diseases and Clinical Microbiology Clinic, Ankara Numune Education and Research Hospital, Ankara, Turkey
Brucellosis

Douglas A. Drevets, MD, DTM&H
Professor and Interim Chief, Section of Infectious Diseases, University of Oklahoma Health Sciences Center School of Medicine; Staff Physician, VA Medical Center, Oklahoma City, Oklahoma
Plague

Carol Drucker, MD
Associate Professor, Department of Dermatology, and Associate Medical Director, Cancer Prevention Center, The University of Texas M.D. Anderson Cancer Center, Houston, Texas
Keloids; Verrucae (Warts)

Jean Dudler, MD
Associate Professor of Medicine, Division of Rheumatology, Centre Hospitalier Universitaire Vaudois and University of Lausanne, Lausanne, Switzerland
Rat-Bite Fever

Soumitra R. Eachempati, MD
Associate Professor of Surgery and Public Health, Weill Cornell Medical College; Associate Attending Surgeon, NewYork–Presbyterian Hospital/Weill Cornell Medical Center, New York, New York
Bacterial Infections of the Skin

Julian Elliott, MB, BS, FRACP
Conjoint Senior Lecturer, National Centre in HIV Epidemiology and Clinical Research, University of New South Wales, Sydney; Infectious Diseases Physician, Alfred Hospital, Melbourne; HIV Clinical Advisor, International Health Research Group, Macfarlane Burnet Institute for Medical Research and Public Health, Melbourne, New South Wales, Australia
Psittacosis

John M. Embil, MD, FRCP(C), FACP
Associate Professor, Department of Medicine and Medical Microbiology, Section of Infectious Diseases, University of Manitoba Faculty of Medicine; Director, Infection Prevention and Control Unit, Health Science Centre, Winnipeg, Manitoba, Canada
Necrotizing Skin and Soft Tissue Infections

Scott K. Epstein, MD
Dean for Educational Affairs and Professor of Medicine, Tufts University School of Medicine, Boston, Massachusetts
Acute Respiratory Failure

Amanda Nickles Fader, MD
Clinical Fellow in Gynecologic Oncology, Cleveland Clinic, Cleveland, Ohio
Ovarian Cancer

Vincent Falanga, MD
Professor of Dermatology and Biochemistry, Boston University School of Medicine, Boston, Massachusetts; Chairman, Department of Dermatology, Roger Williams Medical Center, Providence, Rhode Island
Venous Leg Ulcers

Fred G. Fedok, MD, FACS
Professor, Department of Surgery, Pennsylvania State University School of Medicine, University Park; Chief, Division of Otolaryngology–Head and Neck Surgery, Penn State Hershey Medical Center, Hershey, Pennsylvania
Bell's Palsy (Idiopathic Acute Peripheral Facial Paralysis)

Steven R. Feldman, MD, PhD
Professor of Dermatology, Wake Forest University School of Medicine, Winston-Salem, North Carolina
Acne Vulgaris and Rosacea

Eve S. Ferdman, BA
Managing Editor, *Brachytherapy*, Memorial Sloan-Kettering Cancer Center, New York, New York
Brain Tumors

Terry D. Fife, MD
Associate Professor of Clinical Neurology, University of Arizona College of Medicine; Director, Balance Center, Barrow Neurological Institute; Teaching Faculty, Barrow Neurological Institute and St. Joseph's Hospital, Phoenix, Arizona
Episodic Vertigo

Robert Fisher, MD
Professor of Medicine, Temple University School of Medicine; Chief, Gastroenterology Section, Temple University Hospital, Philadelphia, Pennsylvania
Constipation

L. Jaime Fitten, MDS
Professor of Psychiatry and Biobehavioral Sciences, David Geffen School of Medicine at UCLA; Director, Geriatric Psychiatry, Greater Los Angeles Veterans Administration, Sepulveda Campus, Los Angeles, California
Alzheimer's Disease

Jonathan M. Flacker, MD
Assistant Professor of Medicine, Emory University School of Medicine; Medical Director, The Emory Clinic at Wesley, Atlanta, Georgia
Delirium

Alan B. Fleischer, Jr., MD
Professor and Chair, Department of Dermatology, Wake Forest University School of Medicine, Winston-Salem, North Carolina
Acne Vulgaris and Rosacea

Robert J. Fox, MD
Assistant Professor of Neurology, Cleveland Clinic Lerner College of Medicine; Staff Neurologist and Medical Director, Mellen Center for Multiple Sclerosis, Cleveland Clinic Foundation, Cleveland, Ohio
Multiple Sclerosis

Ellen W. Freeman, PhD
Research Professor, Departments of Obstetrics/Gynecology and Department of Psychiatry, University of Pennsylvania School of Medicine, Philadelphia, Pennsylvania
Premenstrual Syndrome

Eugene P. Frenkel, MD
Professor of Internal Medicine and Radiology, University of Texas Southwestern Medical School at Dallas; Patsy R. & Raymond D. Nasher Distinguished Chair in Cancer Research; Elaine Dewey Sammons Distinguished Chair in Cancer Research in honor of Eugene P. Frenkel, M.D.; and A. Kenneth Pye Professorship in Cancer Research, Harold C. Simmons Comprehensive Cancer Center, Southwestern Medical Center, Dallas, Texas
Pernicious Anemia and Other Megaloblastic Anemias

Jeremy N. Friedman, MB, ChB
Associate Professor, Department of Paediatrics, University of Toronto Faculty of Medicine; Head, Division of Paediatric Medicine, The Hospital for Sick Children, Toronto, Ontario, Canada
Parenteral Fluid Therapy for Infants and Children

R. Michael Gallagher, DO
Director, Headache Center of Central Florida, Melbourne, Florida
Headache

Andrea Gallina, MD
Resident in Training, Vita-Salute University–San Raffaele Hospital, Milan, Italy
Prostatitis

Juan Armando Garcia, MD
Staff-Intensivist, Cardiovascular ICU, The Methodist Hospital, Houston, Texas
Management of Chronic Obstructive Pulmonary Disease

Christine Geers, MSN, CPNP
Pediatric Nurse Practitioner, Children's Healthcare of Atlanta, Georgia Urology Pediatrics, Atlanta, Georgia
Childhood Incontinence

Glenn S. Gerber, MD
Associate Professor of Surgery/Urology, Director of Endourology, and Director of Residency Program and Student Clerkship, University of Chicago Pritzker School of Medicine, Chicago, Illinois
Renal Calculi

Aron J. Gewirtzman, MD
Dermatopharmacology Fellow, Albert Einstein College of Medicine, Bronx, New York
Urticaria and Angioedema

Khalil Ghanem, MD, PhD
Assistant Professor of Medicine, Division of Infectious Diseases, Johns Hopkins University School of Medicine, Baltimore, Maryland
Gonorrhea

Paul L. F. Giangrande, MD
Senior Lecturer in Haematology, University of Oxford; Consultant Haematologist, Oxford Haemophilia Centre and Thrombosis Unit, Churchill Hospital, Oxford, United Kingdom
Venous Thrombosis

Robert Giusti, MD
Assistant Professor of Pediatrics, SUNY Downstate Medical Center College of Medicine; Director, Cystic Fibrosis Center; Vice Chairman, Department of Pediatrics, Long Island College Hospital, Brooklyn, New York
Cystic Fibrosis

David B. K. Golden, MD
Associate Professor of Medicine, Johns Hopkins University School of Medicine; Chief of Allergy Services, Sinai Hospital and Franklin Square Hospital, Baltimore, Maryland
Allergic Reactions to Insect Stings

Monica Peterson Gordon, MD
Geriatric Psychiatry Fellow, David Geffen School of Medicine at UCLA, Los Angeles, California
Alzheimer's Disease

E. Ann Gormley, MD
Professor of Surgery (Urology), Dartmouth Medical School, Hanover; Staff Urologist, Dartmouth-Hitchcock Medical Center, Lebanon, New Hampshire
Urinary Incontinence

Alice Gottlieb, MD, PhD
Department of Dermatology, Tufts Medical Center, Boston, Massachusetts
Papulosquamous Eruptions

Eduardo Gotuzzo, MD
Principal Professor of Medicine, Universidad Peruana Cayetano Heredia; Chief, Department of Infectious, Tropical, and Dermatologic Diseases, Hospital National Cayetano Heredia, Lima, Peru
Cholera

Mark A. Granner, MD
Associate Professor of Neurology, University of Iowa Carver College of Medicine; Director, Iowa Comprehensive Epilepsy Program, University of Iowa Hospitals and Clinics, Iowa City, Iowa
Seizures and Epilepsy in Adolescents and Adults

Jane M. Grant-Kels, MD
Professor and Chair, Department of Dermatology; Dermatology Residency Director; and Assistant Dean of Clinical Affairs, University of Connecticut School of Medicine; Director of Dermatopathology and Director of Melanoma Program and Cutaneous Oncology Center, University of Connecticut Health Center, Connecticut.
Melanocytic Nevi

Joseph Greensher, MD
Professor of Pediatrics, Stony Brook University School of Medicine, Stony Brook; Medical Director and Associate Chair, Department of Pediatrics, Long Island Regional Poison and Drug Information Center, Winthrop-University Hospital, Mineola, New York
Medical Toxicology: Ingestions, Inhalations, and Dermal and Ocular Absorptions

Tamsin J. Greenwell, MD
Consultant Urologist, University College Hospital, London, United Kingdom
Urethral Stricture Disease

Charles Grose, MD
Professor of Pediatrics, University of Iowa Carver College of Medicine; Director of Infectious Diseases Division, Children's Hospital of Iowa, Iowa City, Iowa
Varicella (Chickenpox)

Eva C. Guinan, MD
Associate Professor of Pediatrics, Harvard Medical School; Associate Director, Center for Clinical and Translational Research, Dana-Farber Cancer Institute, Boston, Massachusetts
Aplastic Anemia

Rashidul Haque, MB, PhD
Scientist, Laboratory Sciences Division, International Centre for Diarrhoea Disease Research, Bangladesh (ICDDR, B), Dhaka, Bangladesh
Amebiasis

Rachel Haroz, MD
Assistant Professor of Emergency Medicine, UMDNJ-Robert Wood Johnson Medical School at Camden; Attending Physician, Department of Emergency Medicine, Cooper University Hospital, Camden, New Jersey
Spider Bites and Scorpion Stings

Lucinda A. Harris, MD
Assistant Professor of Medicine, Mayo Clinic College of Medicine, Rochester, Minnesota; Consultant, Division of Gastroenterology and Hepatology, Mayo Clinic, Scottsdale, Arizona
Irritable Bowel Syndrome

Thomas N. Helm, MD
Clinical Associate Professor of Dermatology and Pathology, University at Buffalo School of Medicine and Biomedical Sciences, Buffalo; Director of Dermatopathology, Buffalo Medical Group, Williamsville, New York
Hair Disorders

J. Claude Hemphill III, MD, MAS
Associate Professor of Clinical Neurology and Neurological Surgery, University of California, San Francisco, School of Medicine; Director, Neurocritical Care, San Francisco General Hospital, San Francisco, California
Intracerebral Hemorrhage

David G. Hill, MD
Waterbury Pulmonary Associates, Waterbury; Yale University School of Medicine, New Haven, Connecticut
Cough

Christopher D. Hillyer, MD
Transfusion Medicine Program, Department of Pathology and Laboratory Medicine, Emory University School of Medicine, Atlanta, Georgia
Adverse Effects of Blood Transfusion

David C. Hodgson, MD, MPH
Associate Professor, Department of Radiation Oncology, University of Toronto Faculty of Medicine; Radiation Oncologist, Princess Margaret Hospital, Toronto, Ontario, Canada
Hodgkin's Lymphoma

E. Ekramul Hoque, MBBS, MPH (Hons), PhD
Lecturer, Viral Hepatitis Epidemiology and Prevention Program, National Centre in HIV Epidemiology and Clinical Research, University of New South Wales Faculty of Medicine, St Vincent's Hospital Medical Centre, Darlinghurst, New South Wales, Australia
Giardiasis

Lynn L. Horvath, MD
Associate Professor of Medicine, University of Texas Health Science Center–Tyler, Tyler; Clinical Assistant Professor of Medicine, University of Texas Health Science Center–San Antonio School of Medicine, San Antonio; Staff, Infectious Disease, Texas Center for Infectious Diseases, San Antonio, Texas
Coccidioidomycosis

Brenda Horwitz, MD
Associate Professor of Medicine, Temple University School of Medicine; Gastroenterology Fellowship Director, Temple University Hospital, Philadelphia, Pennsylvania
Constipation

Duane R. Hospenthal, MD, PhD
Professor of Medicine, Uniformed Services University of Health Sciences F. Edward Hébert School of Medicine, Bethesda, Maryland; Clinical Professor of Medicine, Department of Medicine, University of Texas Health Science Center–San Antonio School of Medicine, San Antonio, Texas; Chief, Infectious Disease Service, San Antonio Military Medical Center (Brooke Army Medical Center), Fort Sam Houston, Texas
Coccidioidomycosis

Lewis L. Hsu, MD, PhD
Associate Professor and Interim Chief, Pediatric Hematology, Drexel University College of Medicine; Interim Director, Marian Anderson Comprehensive Sickle Cell Center, St. Christopher's Hospital for Children, Philadelphia, Pennsylvania
Sickle Cell Disease

Samuel S. Hsu, MD
Assistant Professor, University of Maryland School of Medicine, Baltimore, Maryland
Tetanus

Christine Hudak, MD
Summa Health System, Akron, Ohio
Vulvovaginitis

Scott A. Hundahl, MD
Professor of Clinical Surgery, University of California, Davis, School of Medicine, Sacramento; Chief of Surgery, VA Northern California Health Care System, Mather, California
Tumours of the Stomach

Stephen P. Hunger, MD
Professor of Pediatrics, University of Colorado–Denver School of Medicine; Section Chief, Center for Cancer and Blood Disorders, and Ergen Family Chair in Pediatric Cancer, The Children's Hospital, Aurora, Colorado
Acute Leukemia in Children

Mahreen Hussain, BSc (Hons), MRCS
Specialist Registrar in Urology, The Royal Free Hospital, London, United Kingdom
Urethral Stricture Disease

Nader Husseinzadeh, MD
Professor, University of Cincinnati School of Medicine, Cincinnati, Ohio
Cancer of the Uterine Cervix

Neil H. Hyman, MD
Samuel B. and Michelle D. Labow Professor of Surgery and Chief, Division of General Surgery, University of Vermont College of Medicine, Burlington, Vermont
Hemorrhoids, Anal Fissure, and Anorectal Abscess and Fistula

Robert D. Inman, MD
Professor of Medicine and Immunology, University of Toronto Faculty of Medicine; Director, Arthritis Center of Excellence, University Health Network, Toronto, Ontario, Canada
Ankylosing Spondylitis

Jon E. Isaacson, MD
Division of Otolaryngology, Head and Neck Surgery, Department of Surgery, Pennsylvania State University College of Medicine, University Park, Pennsylvania
Bell's Palsy (Idiopathic Acute Peripheral Facial Paralysis)

Sei Iwai, MD
Associate Professor of Clinical Medicine, Department of Medicine, Division of Cardiology, Cornell Weill Medical College; Associate Attending Physician, NewYork–Presbyterian Hospital, New York, New York
Tachycardias

Alan C. Jackson, MD, FRCPC
Professor of Medicine (Neurology) and Medical Microbiology, University of Manitoba Faculty of Medicine; Head, Section of Neurology, Winnipeg Regional Health Authority, Winnipeg, Manitoba, Canada
Rabies

Robert M. Jacobson, MD
Professor of Pediatrics, Mayo Clinic College of Medicine; Chair, Department of Pediatric and Adolescent Medicine, and Consultant in Pediatric and Adolescent Medicine, Mayo Clinic, Rochester, Minnesota
Office-Based Immunization Practices

Mamta K. Jain, MD, MPH
Assistant Professor, University of Texas Southwestern Medical School at Dallas, Dallas, Texas
Acute and Chronic Hepatitis

James J. James, MD, DrPH, MHA
Director, Center for Disaster Preparedness and Emergency Response, American Medical Association, Chicago, Illinois
Toxic Chemical Agents Reference Chart: Symptoms and Treatment; Biologic Agents Reference Chart–Symptoms, Tests, and Treatment

Philip G. Janicak, MD
Professor of Psychiatry, Rush Medical College; Medical Director, Psychiatric Clinical Research Center, Rush University Medical Center, Chicago, Illinois
Schizophrenia

Camila K. Janniger, MD
Clinical Professor and Chief, Pediatric and Geriatric Dermatology, UMDNJ–New Jersey Medical School, Newark, New Jersey
Pigmentary Disorders

Nathaniel Jellinek, MD
Department of Dermatology, Brown Medical School, Providence, Rhode Island
Diseases of the Nails

Stephen G. Jenkinson, MD
Chief, Pulmonary Diseases Section, Audie Murphy VA Medical Center, San Antonio, Texas
Management of Chronic Obstructive Pulmonary Disease

Gordon L. Jensen, MD, PhD
Professor of Medicine and Head, Department of Nutritional Sciences, College of Health and Human Development, Pennsylvania State University, University Park; Penn State Hershey Medical Center, Hershey, Pennsylvania
Obesity

Candice E. Johnson, MD, PhD
Clinical Professor of Pediatrics, University of Colorado School of Medicine; Volunteer Faculty, The Children's Hospital, Denver, Colorado
Bacterial Infections of the Urinary Tract in Girls

David R. Jones, MD
Professor of Surgery, University of Virginia School of Medicine; Division Chief, Thoracic and Cardiovascular Surgery, and Chief, General Thoracic Surgery, University of Virginia Medical Center, Charlottesville, Virginia
Atelectasis

James F. Jones, MD
Research Medical Officer, Chronic Viral Diseases Branch, National Center for Zoonotic, Vector-Borne, and Enteric Diseases, Centers for Disease Control and Prevention, Atlanta, Georgia
Chronic Fatigue Syndrome

Joseph L. Jorizzo, MD
Professor, Founder, and *formerly* Chair, Department of Dermatology, Wake Forest University School of Medicine, Winston-Salem, North Carolina
Cutaneous Vasculitis

Marc A. Judson, MD
Professor of Medicine, Division of Pulmonary and Critical Care Medicine, Department of Medicine, Medical University of South Carolina, Charleston, South Carolina
Sarcoidosis

S. Patrick Kachur, MD
Commander, U.S. Public Health Service; Chief, Malaria Strategic Applied Science Unit, Centers for Disease Control and Prevention, Atlanta, Georgia
Malaria

Tamilarasu Kadhiravan, MD
Senior Research Associate, Department of Medicine, All India Institute of Medical Sciences, New Delhi, India
Management of the Patient with HIV Disease

Patrick S. Kamath, MD
Professor of Medicine, Mayo Clinic College of Medicine, Rochester, Minnesota
Bleeding Esophageal Varices

Hagop M. Kantarjian, MD
Professor and Chair, Department of Leukemia, The University of Texas M.D. Anderson Cancer Center, Houston, Texas
Chronic Leukemias

Pierre I. Karakiewicz, MD
Associate Professor, Department of Urology, University of Montreal Faculty of Medicine; Urologic Oncologist and Director, Cancer Prognostics and Health Outcomes Unit, University of Montreal Health Center, Montreal, Quebec, Canada
Prostatitis

Matthew E. Karlovsky, MD
Staff Urologist (Voiding Dysfunction/Female Urology), Private Practice, Center for Urological Services, PC, Phoenix, Arizona
Benign Prostatic Hyperplasia

Philip O. Katz, MD
Clinical Professor of Medicine, Jefferson Medical College of Thomas Jefferson University; Chairman, Division of Gastroenterology, Albert Einstein Medical Center, Philadelphia, Pennsylvania
Dysphagia and Esophageal Obstruction

Jennifer Kelly, DO
Assistant Professor of Medicine, Division of Endocrinology, Diabetes and Metabolism, SUNY Upstate Medical University College of Medicine, Syracuse, New York
Diabetes Insipidus

Rebecca Lewis Kelso, MD
Assistant Professor, Department of Dermatology, University of Texas Medical Branch School of Medicine, Galveston, Texas
Fungal Diseases of the Skin

Stephen F. Kemp, MD
Professor of Medicine and Associate Professor of Pediatrics, University of Mississippi College of Medicine; Director, Allergy and Immunology Fellowship Program, Departments of Medicine and Pediatrics, University of Mississippi Medical Center, Jackson, Mississippi
Anaphylaxis and Serum Sickness

Sripathi R. Kethu, MD
Digestive Health Associates of Texas, Richardson Regional Medical Center, Richardson, Texas
Gastritis and Peptic Ulcer Disease

Sundeep Khosla, MD
Professor of Medicine, Mayo Clinic College of Medicine; Consultant, Mayo Clinic, Rochester, Minnesota
Osteoporosis

Andrew Kirsch, MD
Clinical Professor of Urology, Emory University School of Medicine; Academic Director, Emory University, Atlanta, Georgia
Childhood Incontinence

Joseph E. Kiss, MD
Associate Professor of Medicine, Division of Hematology-Oncology, University of Pittsburgh School of Medicine; Medical Director, Hemapheresis and Blood Services, The Institute for Transfusion Medicine, Pittsburgh, Pennsylvania
Thrombotic Thrombocytopenic Purpura

Craig S. Kitchens, MD
Professor of Medicine, University of Florida College of Medicine; Consultant, Malcom Randall VA Medical Center, Gainesville, Florida
Snakebite

Joel D. Klein, MD, FAAP
Professor of Pediatrics, Jefferson Medical College of Thomas Jefferson University, Philadelphia, Pennsylvania; Division of Pediatric Infectious Diseases, Alfred I. duPont Hospital for Children, Wilmington, Delaware
Mumps

Jonathan E. Kolitz, MD
Associate Professor of Medicine, New York University School of Medicine, New York; Director, Leukemia Service, Monter Cancer Center, North Shore University Hospital, Lake Success, New York
Acute Leukemias in Adults

Luciano Kolodny, MD
Endocrinologist, HealthPartners Medical Group, Woodbury, Minnesota
Erectile Dysfunction

Gerald B. Kolski, MD, PhD
Clinical Professor of Pediatrics, Temple University School of Medicine; Adjunct Clinical Professor of Pediatrics, Drexel University College of Medicine, Philadelphia; Attending Physician, Crozer Chester Medical Center, Upland, Pennsylvania
Asthma in Children

Frederick K. Korley, MD
Robert E. Meyerhoff Assistant Professor of Emergency Medicine, Johns Hopkins University School of Medicine; Staff, Johns Hopkins Medical Institutions, Baltimore, Maryland
Disturbances Due to Cold

Milind J. Kothari, DO
Professor of Neurology and Vice Chair of Education and Training, Pennsylvania State College of Medicine, University Park, Pennsylvania
Myasthenia Gravis and Related Disorders

Mark Krasna, MD
St. Joseph Cancer Institute, Towson, Maryland
Primary Lung Abscess

Christopher Kratochvil, MD
Professor of Psychiatry and Pediatrics, University of Nebraska College of Medicine, Omaha, Nebraska
Attention-Deficit/Hyperactivity Disorder

Jeffrey A. Kraut, MD
Chief of Dialysis, VA Greater Los Angeles Healthcare System; Professor of Medicine, David Geffen School of Medicine at UCLA, Los Angeles, California
Chronic Renal Failure

Jacques Kremer, PhD
Post-Doctoral Program, Institute of Immunology, National Laboratory of Health, Luxembourg, Luxembourg
Measles (Rubeola)

John N. Krieger, MD
Professor of Urology, University of Washington School of Medicine; Chief of Urology, VA Puget Sound Health Care System, Seattle, Washington
Bacterial Infections of the Male Urinary Tract; Epididymitis; Nongonococcal Urethritis

Leonard R. Krilov, MD
Professor of Pediatrics, Stony Brook University School of Medicine, Stony Brook; Chief, Pediatric Infectious Disease, and Vice-Chairman of Pediatrics, Winthrop-University Hospital, Mineola, New York
Infectious Mononucleosis

Michael Kroll, MD
Professor of Medicine, The University of Texas M.D. Anderson Cancer Center, Houston, Texas
Polycythemia Vera

Irving L. Kron, MD
S. Huet Watts Professor and Chairman, Department of Surgery, Medical College of Wisconsin, Madison, Wisconsin, and University of Virginia Health System, Charlottesville, Virginia
Acquired Diseases of the Aorta

Roshni Kulkarni, MD
Professor, Department of Pediatrics and Human Development, Michigan State University College of Medicine, East Lansing, Michigan
Hemophilia and Related Bleeding Disorders

Bhushan Kumar, MD, MNAMS
Former Professor and Head, Department of Dermatology, Post-Graduate Institute of Medical Education and Research, Chandigarh, India
Leprosy

Timothy M. Kuzel, MD
Professor, Department of Medicine, Division of Hematology/Oncology, Northwestern University Feinberg School of Medicine; Attending Physician, Robert H. Lurie Comprehensive Cancer Center of Northwestern University, Chicago, Illinois
Cutaneous T-Cell Lymphomas (Mycosis Fungoides and Sézary's Syndrome)

Paul Y. Kwo, MD
Associate Professor of Medicine, Division of Gastroenterology/Hepatology, Indiana University School of Medicine, Indianapolis, Indiana
Cirrhosis

Yves Lacasse, MD
Professor of Medicine, Laval University Faculty of Medicine; Respirologist, Hôpital Laval, Quebec City, Quebec, Canada
Hypersensitivity Pneumonitis

Lori M. B. Laffel, MD, MPH
Associate Professor of Pediatrics, Harvard Medical School; Chief, Pediatric, Adolescent, and Young Adult Section, and Investigator, Section on Genetics and Epidemiology, Joslin Diabetes Center, Boston, Massachusetts
Diabetes Mellitus in Children and Adolescents

Gabriella Lakos, MD, PhD
Visiting Assistant Professor of Medicine, Northwestern University Feinberg School of Medicine, Chicago, Illinois
Connective Tissue Disorders

Ashutosh Lal, MD
Associate Hematologist/Oncologist, Children's Hospital and Research Center Oakland, Oakland, California
Thalassemia

Paul R. Lambert, MD
Professor and Chairman, Department of Otolaryngology, Medical University of South Carolina, Charleston, South Carolina
Ménière's Disease

Stephen R. Larsen, MB, BS
Gene and Stem Cell Therapy Program, Centenary Institute, University of Sydney, New South Wales, Australia
Autoimmune Hemolytic Anemia

Barbara A. Latenser, MD
Clara L. Smith Professor of Burn Treatment and Clinical Professor of Surgery, University of Iowa Carver College of Medicine; Medical Director, Burn Treatment Center, University of Iowa Hospitals and Clinics, Iowa City, Iowa
Burn Treatment Guidelines

Yung R. Lau, MD
Professor of Pediatric Cardiology, University of Alabama at Birmingham School of Medicine, Birmingham, Alabama
Congenital Heart Disease

Luca Lazzarini, MD
Department of Infectious Diseases and Tropical Medicine, San Bortolo Hospital, Vicenza, Italy
Osteomyelitis

Jerrold B. Leikin, MD
Professor of Emergency Medicine, Northwestern University Feinberg School of Medicine; Professor of Medicine, Rush Medical College, Chicago; Director of Medical Toxicology, Evanston Northwestern Healthcare–Omega, Glenbrook Hospital, Glenview, Illinois
Disturbance Due to Cold

Bruce B. Lerman, MD
H. Altschul Professor of Medicine, Weill Cornell Medical College; Chief, Division of Cardiology, NewYork–Presbyterian Hospital, New York, New York
Tachycardias

Moshe Levi, MD
Professor of Medicine, University of Colorado School of Medicine; Nephrology Fellow, University of Colorado Hospital, Aurora, Colorado
Hyponatremia

Jeffrey A. Linder, MD, MPH
Assistant Professor of Medicine, Harvard Medical School; Associate Physician, Brigham and Women's Hospital, Boston, Massachusetts
Influenza

Gary H. Lipscomb, MD
Professor and Director, Division of General Obstetrics and Gynecology, Department of Obstetrics and Gynecology, Northwestern University Feinberg School of Medicine, Chicago, Illinois
Ectopic Pregnancy

James A. Litch, MD, DTMH
Clinical Assistant Professor, University of Washington School of Medicine and School of Public Health and Community Medicine, Seattle, Washington
High-Altitude Illness

Kelly E. Lyons, PhD
Research Associate Professor, Department of Neurology, University of Kansas School of Medicine, Kansas City, Kansas
Parkinsonism

James M. Lyznicki, MS, MPH
Senior Scientist, Center for Disaster Preparedness and Emergency Response, American Medical Association, Chicago, Illinois
Toxic Chemical Agents Reference Chart: Symptoms and Treatment; Biologic Agents Reference Chart—Symptoms, Tests, and Treatment

Carl D. Malchoff, MD, PhD
Professor of Internal Medicine, University of Connecticut School of Medicine, Farmington, Connecticut
Adrenocortical Insufficiency

Susan Manzi, MD, MPH
Associate Professor of Medicine and Epidemiology and Co-Director, Lupus Center of Excellence, University of Pittsburgh School of Medicine; Attending, UPMC Magee and UPMC Presbyterian, Pittsburgh, Pennsylvania
Connective Tissue Disorders

Ashfaq A. Marghoob, MD
Associate Professor of Dermatology, Stony Brook University School of Medicine, Stony Brook; Associate Member, Memorial Sloan-Kettering Cancer Center, Hauppauge, New York
Melanoma

Ali J. Marian, MD
Center for Cardiovascular Genetic Research and Brown Foundation Institute of Molecular Medicine, University of Texas Health Science Center; Staff Cardiologist, The Methodist Hospital; Professional Staff, St. Luke's Episcopal Hospital/Texas Heart Institute, Houston, Texas
Hypertrophic Cardiomyopathy

Peter Mariuz, MD
Associate Professor of Medicine, Division of Infectious Diseases, University of Rochester School of Medicine and Dentistry; Attending Physician, Department of Medicine, Strong Memorial Hospital, Rochester, New York
Toxoplasmosis

Vickie Martin, MD
Resident, Department of Obstetrics and Gynecology, Kingston General Hospital, Kingston, Ontario, Canada
Amenorrhea

Maria Mascarenhas, MBBS
Associate Professor of Pediatrics, University of Pennsylvania School of Medicine; Section Chief, Nutrition Division of Gastroenterology and Nutrition; Director, Nutrition Support Service, The Children's Hospital of Philadelphia, Philadelphia, Pennsylvania
Normal Infant Feeding

Wissam E. Mattar, MD
Indiana University School of Medicine, Indianapolis, Indiana
Cirrhosis

Eric L. Matteson, MD, MPH
Professor of Medicine, Mayo Clinic College of Medicine; Consultant in Rheumatology, Mayo Clinic, Rochester, Minnesota
Rheumatoid Arthritis

Pinckney J. Maxwell IV, MD
Assistant Professor of Surgery, Division of Colon and Rectal Surgery, Jefferson Medical College of Thomas Jefferson University; Attending Surgeon, Thomas Jefferson University Hospital, Philadelphia, Pennsylvania
Diverticula of the Alimentary Tract

Anthony L. McCall, MD, PhD
James M. Moss Professor of Diabetes, University of Virginia School of Medicine; Endocrinologist, University of Virginia Health Care System, Charlottesville, Virginia
Diabetes Mellitus in Adults

Michael T. McCann, MD
Clinical Assistant Professor, Baylor College of Medicine, Houston, Texas
Spine Pain

Laura J. McCloskey, PhD
Assistant Professor of Pathology, Anatomy, and Cell Biology, Jefferson Medical College of Thomas Jefferson University; Associate Director, Clinical Laboratories; Director, Clinical Immunology Laboratory and Jefferson Hospital for Neuroscience Laboratory, Thomas Jefferson University Hospitals, Philadelphia, Pennsylvania
Reference Intervals for the Interpretation of Laboratory Tests

Jacqueline Carinhas McGregor, MD
Director, Baylor Child Psychiatry Clinic; Associate Professor, Menninger Department of Psychiatry and Behavioral Sciences, Baylor College of Medicine, Houston, Texas
Anxiety Disorders

Michael McGuigan, MD
Medical Director, Long Island Regional Poison and Drug Information Center, Winthrop-University Hospital, Mineola, New York
Medical Toxicology: Ingestions, Inhalations, and Dermal and Ocular Absorptions

Dilcia McLenan, MD
Assistant Professor of Pediatrics, Baylor College of Medicine, Pearland, Texas
Care of the High-Risk Neonate

D. Scott McMeekin, MD
Presbyterian Foundation Presidential Professor, University of Oklahoma College of Medicine; Section Chief, Gynecologic Oncology, University of Oklahoma Health Sciences Center, Oklahoma City, Oklahoma
Cancer of the Endometrium

J. Scott McMurray, MD
Associate Professor of Pediatric Otolaryngology, Department of Surgery, University of Wisconsin School of Medicine and Public Health, Madison, Wisconsin
Otitis Media

Donald McNeil, MD
Associate Professor of Clinical Medicine, Department of Immunology, The Ohio State University College of Medicine and Public Health, Columbus, Ohio
Allergic Reactions to Drugs

Anupama Menon, MD, MPH
Assistant Professor of Medicine, Division of Infectious Diseases, University of Arkansas for Medical Sciences College of Medicine; Staff Physician, Central Arkansas Veterans Healthcare System, Little Rock, Arkansas
Blastomycosis

Moises Mercado, MD
Professor of Medicine, Faculty of Medicine, Universidad Nacional Autónoma de México; Head, Endocrine Service, and Experimental Endocrinology Unit, Hospital de Especialidades, Centro Médico Nacional Siglo XXI, Instituto Mexicano del Segero Social, Mexico City, Mexico
Acromegaly

Ralph M. Meyer, MD
Edith Eisenhauer Chair in Clinical Oncology and Professor, Departments of Oncology, Medicine, and Community Health and Epidemiology, Queen's University Faculty of Medicine; Director, Institute of Canada Clinical Trials Group at Queen's University, Kingston, Ontario, Canada
Hodgkin's Lymphoma

Ted A. Meyer, MD, PhD
Assistant Professor, Department of Otolaryngology, Medical University of South Carolina College of Medicine, Charleston, South Carolina
Ménière's Disease

Norman S. Miller, MD
Department of Medicine, Michigan State University, East Lansing, Michigan
Drug Abuse

Paul D. Miller, MD
Distinguished Clinical Professor of Medicine, University of Colorado School of Medicine, Aurora; Medical Director, Colorado Center for Bone Research, Lakewood, Colorado
Paget's Disease of Bone

Peter A. Millward, MD
Assistant Professor of Pathology, Pennsylvania State College of Medicine University Park; Medical Director, Blood Bank and Apheresis Service, Penn State Hershey Medical Center, Hershey, Pennsylvania
Therapeutic Use of Blood Components

Howard C. Mofenson, MD
Professor of Pediatrics and Emergency Medicine, Stony Brook University School of Medicine, Stony Brook; Professor of Pharmacology and Toxicology, New York College of Osteopathic Medicine, Old Westbury, New York
Medical Toxicology: Ingestions, Inhalations, and Dermal and Ocular Absorptions

Alladi Mohan, MD
Professor and Chairman, Department of Medicine, Sri Venkateswara Institute of Medical Sciences, Andhra Pradesh, India
Tuberculosis and Other Mycobacterial Diseases

Terry L. Moore, MD
Professor of Internal Medicine, Pediatrics, and Molecular Microbiology and Immunology, Saint Louis University School of Medicine; Director, Division of Rheumatology and Pediatric Rheumatology, Saint Louis University Medical Center, St. Louis, Missouri
Juvenile Idiopathic Arthritis

Enrique Morales, MD
Attending Nephrologist, Hospital 12 de Octubre, Madrid, Spain
Primary Glomerular Diseases

John F. Moran, MD
Professor of Medicine, Loyola University Stritch School of Medicine, Maywood, Illinois
Angina Pectoris

Rita Moretti, MD
Head Researcher, Neurodegenerative Disorders, Department of Clinical Medicine and Neurology, University of Trieste, Trieste, Italy
Hiccups

Warwick L. Morison, MD
Professor of Dermatology, Johns Hopkins University School of Medicine, Baltimore, Maryland
Sunburn

Arnold M. Moses, MD
SUNY Distinguished Service Professor of Medicine, SUNY Upstate Medical University College of Medicine; Attending, University Hospital, Syracuse, New York
Diabetes Insipidus

Scott Moses, MD
Medical Staff, Fairview Lakes Regional Medical Center, Wyoming, Minnesota
Pruritus

Alan C. Moss, MD
Instructor in Medicine, Harvard Medical School; Director of Translational Research, Center for Inflammatory Bowel Disease, Beth Israel Deaconess Medical Center, Boston, Massachusetts
Inflammatory Bowel Disease

Steven F. Moss, MD
Associate Professor of Medicine, The Warren Alpert Medical School of Brown University; Director, Gastroenterology Fellowship Training Program, Rhode Island Hospital, Providence, Rhode Island
Gastritis and Peptic Ulcer Disease

Claude P. Muller, MD
Immunology, University of Trier Faculty of Medicine, Trier; Experimental Medicine, University of Saarland Faculty of Medicine, Homburg, Germany; HOD Institute of Immunology, National Laboratory of Health, Luxembourg, Luxembourg
Measles (Rubeola)

Michael Murphy, MD
Associate Professor, Department of Dermatology, University of Connecticut School of Medicine, Farmington, Connecticut
Melanocytic Nevi

Tashanna K. N. Myers, MD
Fellow in Gynecologic Oncology, University of Oklahoma Health Sciences Center, Oklahoma City, Oklahoma
Cancer of the Endometrium

Lisa B. Nachtigall, MD
Assistant Professor of Medicine, Harvard Medical School; Co-Director, Neuroendocrine Clinical Center, Massachusetts General Hospital, Boston, Massachusetts
Hyperprolactinemia

Ashwatha Narayana, MD
Associate Professor of Radiation Oncology, New York University School of Medicine; Residency Program Director and Associate Chair of Clinical Research, Department of Radiation Oncology, New York University Medical Center, New York, New York
Brain Tumors

Laeth S. Nasir, MBBS
Professor, Department of Family Medicine, University of Nebraska College of Medicine; Staff Physician, University of Nebraska Medical Center, Omaha, Nebraska
Dysmenorrhea

Gideon Nesher, MD
Clinical Associate Professor of Medicine, The Hebrew University Medical School; Head, Department of Internal Medicine A, Shaare-Zedek Medical Center, Jerusalem, Israel
Polymyalgia Rheumatica and Giant Cell Arteritis

David N. Neubauer, MD
Assistant Professor, Johns Hopkins University School of Medicine; Associate Director, Johns Hopkins Sleep Disorders Center, Baltimore, Maryland
Sleep Disorders

David H. Neustadt, MD
Clinical Professor of Medicine, University of Louisville School of Medicine; Senior Attending, Jewish Hospital, Louisville, Kentucky
Osteoarthritis

Peter E. Newburger, MD
Ali and John Pierce Professor of Pediatric Hematology/Oncology, University of Massachusetts Medical School; Director, Pediatric Hematology/Oncology, UMass/Memorial Medical Center, Worcester, Massachusetts
Neutropenia

Richard Ohrbach, DDS, PhD
Department of Oral Diagnostic Sciences, State University of New York at Buffalo School of Dental Medicine, Buffalo, New York
Temporomandibular Disorders and Orofacial Pain

David L. Olive, MD
Professor of Obstetrics and Gynecology, University of Wisconsin School of Medicine and Public Health, Madison, Wisconsin
Endometriosis

Steven M. Opal, MD
Professor of Medicine, The Warren Alpert Medical School of Brown University, Providence; Director, Infectious Disease Service, Memorial Hospital of Rhode Island, Pawtucket, Rhode Island
Severe Sepsis and Septic Shock

Richard R. Orlandi, MD
Associate Professor, Division of Otolaryngology–Head and Neck Surgery, University of Utah School of Medicine; Associate Director, Center for Therapeutic Biomaterials, University of Utah Health Sciences Center, Salt Lake City, Utah
Sinusitis

Finbar D. O'Shea, MB, MRCPI
Spondylitis Fellow, Arthritis Center of Excellence, Toronto Western Hospital, Toronto, Ontario, Canada
Ankylosing Spondylitis

Gregory A. Otterson, MD
Associate Professor of Internal Medicine, Division of Hematology/Oncology, The Ohio State University College of Medicine and Public Health; Staff, James Cancer Hospital/Solove Research Institute, Columbus, Ohio
Lung Cancer

Matthew T. Oughton, MD, FRCPC
Assistant Professor, Department of Medicine, McGill University Faculty of Medicine; Infectious Disease Physician, Sir Mortimer B. Davis–Jewish General Hospital, Montreal, Quebec, Canada
Acute Infectious Diarrhea

Gary D. Overturf, MD
Professor of Pediatrics and Pathology, University of New Mexico College of Medicine; Medical Director, Infectious Diseases, TriCore Reference Laboratories, Albuquerque, New Mexico
Bacterial Meningitis

Rajesh Pahwa, MD
Professor of Neurology, University of Kansas School of Medicine, Kansas City, Kansas
Parkinsonism

Trish Palmer, MD
Assistant Professor, Departments of Family Medicine and Orthopedic Surgery, Rush Medical College, Chicago, Illinois
Pain

Jaymie Panuncialman, MD
Attending, Roger Williams Medical Center, Providence, Rhode Island
Venous Leg Ulcers

Manisha J. Patel, MD
Assistant Professor, Johns Hopkins University School of Medicine, Baltimore, Maryland
Cutaneous Vasculitis

Eleni Patrozou, MD
Teaching Fellow in Medicine–Infectious Diseases, The Warren Alpert Medical School of Brown University, Providence; Infectious Disease Fellow, Memorial Hospital of Rhode Island, Pawtucket, Rhode Island
Severe Sepsis and Septic Shock

Mark A. Peppercorn, MD
Professor of Medicine, Harvard Medical School; Senior Consultant, Center for Inflammatory Bowel Disease, Beth Israel Deaconess Medical Center, Boston, Massachusetts
Inflammatory Bowel Disease

Allen Perkins, MD, MPH
Professor and Chairman, Department of Family Medicine, University of South Alabama College of Medicine, Mobile, Alabama
Marine Poisonings, Envenomations, and Trauma

Jay Peters, MD
Professor of Medicine, University of Texas Health Science Center at San Antonio School of Medicine; Interim Chief, Pulmonary Division, Department of Medicine, University of Texas Health Science Center at San Antonio, San Antonio, Texas
Management of Chronic Obstructive Pulmonary Disease

William A. Petri, Jr., MD, PhD
Chief, Division of Infectious Disease and International Health, University of Virginia Medical Center, Charlottesville, Virginia
Amebiasis; Travel Medicine

Michael E. Pichichero, MD
Professor of Microbiology and Immunology, Pediatrics, and Medicine, Department of Microbiology and Immunology, University of Rochester School of Medicine and Dentistry, Rochester, New York
Pertussis

Pierre-François Plouin, MD
Professor of Cardiovascular Medicine, Université Paris-Descartes; Head, Hypertension Unit, Hôpital Emopeen G. Pompladh, Paris, France
Pheochromocytomas

Uday Popat, MD
Associate Professor of Medicine, The University of Texas M.D. Anderson Cancer Center, Houston, Texas
Non-Hodgkin's Lymphoma

Pauline S. Powers, MD
Professor of Psychiatry and Behavioral Medicine, University of South Florida College of Medicine, Tampa; Director, Eating Disorder Program, Fairwinds Treatment Center, Clearwater, Florida
Bulimia Nervosa

Manuel Praga, MD
Associate Professor of Medicine, Universidad Complutense; Head, Nephrology Department, Hospital 12 de Octubre, Madrid, Spain
Primary Glomerular Diseases

Abhiram Prasad, MD
Associate Professor of Medicine, Mayo Clinic College of Medicine, Rochester, Minnesota
Acute Myocardial Infarction

Richard A. Prinz, MD
Helen Shedd Keith Professor and Chairman, Department of General Surgery, Rush Medical College; Chairman, Department of General Surgery, Rush University Medical Center, Chicago, Illinois
Acute and Chronic Pancreatitis; Thyroid Cancer

L. Michael Prisant, MD
Professor of Medicine and Director of Hypertension and Clinical Pharmacology, Department of Medicine, Medical College of Georgia, Augusta, Georgia
Hypertension

Gregory Proctor, MD
Nephrology Fellow, University of Colorado School of Medicine/University of Colorado Hospital, Aurora, Colorado
Hyponatremia

Christiane Querfeld, MD
Robert H. Lurie Comprehensive Cancer Center of Northwestern University; Section of Dermatology, University of Chicago Medical Center, Chicago, Illinois
Cutaneous T-Cell Lymphomas (Mycosis Fungoides and Sézary's Syndrome)

Beth W. Rackow, MD
Assistant Professor, Department of Obstetrics, Gynecology and Reproductive Sciences, Yale University School of Medicine, New Haven, Connecticut
Dysfunctional Uterine Bleeding

Jeffrey Rado, MD, MPH
Assistant Professor of Psychiatry and Internal Medicine, Rush Medical College, Chicago, Illinois
Schizophrenia

Sharon S. Raimer, MD
Professor and Chair, Department of Dermatology, University of Texas Medical Branch School of Medicine, Galveston, Texas
Fungal Diseases of the Skin

Sumanth Rajagopal, MD
Assistant Professor of Medicine, University of Rochester School of Medicine and Dentistry; Attending Physician, Division of Infectious Disease, Strong Memorial Hospital/University of Rochester Medical Center, Rochester, New York
Toxoplasmosis

Kirk D. Ramin, MD
Associate Professor and Director, Maternal-Fetal Medicine Fellowship Program, Department of Obstetrics and Gynecology, University of Minnesota Medical School, Minneapolis, Minnesota
Antepartum Care

Julio A. Ramirez, MD
Professor of Medicine, University of Louisville School of Medicine; Chief, Division of Infectious Diseases, Department of Veterans Affairs Medical Center, Louisville, Kentucky
Legionellosis

Satish S.C. Rao, MD, PhD
Professor of Medicine, University of Iowa Carver College of Medicine; Director, Neurogastroenterology/GI Motility, University of Iowa Hospitals and Clinics, Iowa City, Iowa
Gaseousness and Indigestion

Didier Raoult, MD, PhD
Professor, Faculty of Medicine–Marseille, Université de la Méditerranée, Marseille, France
Q Fever

Shahzad Raza, MD
Research Associate, Division of Radiation Oncology, New York University Medical Center, New York, New York
Brain Tumors

Elizabeth Reddy, MD
Fellow, Department of Medicine, Division of Infectious Disease, Duke University, Durham, North Carolina
Intestinal Parasites

Guy S. Reeder, MD
Professor of Medicine, Mayo Clinic College of Medicine, Rochester, Minnesota
Acute Myocardial Infarction

Susan E. Reef, MD
Medical Epidemiologist, Centers for Disease Control and Prevention, Atlanta, Georgia
Rubella and Congenital Rubella Syndrome

Robert L. Reid, MD
Professor, Department of Obstetrics and Gynecology, Queen's University Faculty of Medicine; Chair, Division of Reproductive Endocrinology and Infertility, Kingston General Hospital, Kingston, Ontario, Canada
Amenorrhea

Robert W. Rho, MD
Assistant Professor of Medicine, Division of Cardiology, University of Washington School of Medicine, Seattle, Washington
Cardiac Arrest: Sudden Cardiac Death

Lawrence Rice, MD
Professor of Medicine and Professor of Thrombosis Research, Baylor College of Medicine; Staff Physician, The Methodist Hospital, Houston, Texas
Non-Hodgkin's Lymphoma

Douglas S. Richards, MD
Professor, Department of Obstetrics and Gynecology and Director, Obstetric and Gynecologic Ultrasound, University of Florida College of Medicine, Gainesville, Florida
Hemolytic Disease of the Fetus and Newborn

James R. Roberts, MD
Professor of Emergency Medicine and Senior Consultant in Medical Toxicology, Drexel University College of Medicine; Chairman of Emergency Medicine and Director, Division of Toxicology, Mercy Hospital of Philadelphia, Philadelphia, Pennsylvania
Spider Bites and Scorpion Stings

Jenice Robinson, MD
Assistant Professor of Neurology, Pennsylvania State College of Medicine, Hershey, Pennsylvania
Myasthenia Gravis and Related Disorders

Malcolm K. Robinson, MD
Assistant Professor of Surgery, Harvard Medical School; Metabolic Support Service, Department of Surgery, Brigham and Women's Hospital, Boston, Massachusetts
Parenteral Nutrition in Adults

Griffin P. Rodgers, MD
Director, National Institute of Diabetes, Digestive and Kidney Disorders; Chief, Molecular and Clinical Hematology Branch, National Institutes of Health, Bethesda, Maryland
Sickle Cell Disease

Linda Roethel, MD
Adjunct Clinical Assistant Professor of Family Medicine, Stony Brook University School of Medicine, Stony Brook and College of Osteopathic Medicine, Old Westbury; Faculty/Attending Physician in Family Medicine and Coordinator of Women's Health, South Nassau Communities Hospital, Oceanside, New York
Contraception

Robb L. Romp, MD
Assistant Professor of Pediatric Cardiology, University of Alabama at Birmingham School of Medicine, Birmingham, Alabama
Congenital Heart Disease

Steven P. Roose, MD
Columbia University College of Physicians and Surgeons; New York State Psychiatric Institute, New York, New York
Mood Disorders

Steven T. Rosen, MD
Genevieve Teuton Professor, Department of Medicine, Northwestern University Feinberg School of Medicine; Director, Robert H. Lurie Comprehensive Cancer Center of Northwestern University, Chicago, Illinois
Cutaneous T-Cell Lymphomas (Mycosis Fungoides and Sézary's Syndrome)

Leon Rosenthal, MD
Sleep Medicine Associates of Texas, Dallas, Texas
Sleep Apnea

Richard N. Rosenthal, MD
Professor of Clinical Psychiatry, Columbia University College of Physician and Surgeons; Chairman, Department of Psychiatry, St. Luke's–Roosevelt Hospital Center, New York, New York
Alcoholism

David S. Rubenstein, MD, PhD
Professor of Dermatology, University of North Carolina at Chapel Hill School of Medicine; Staff, Department of Dermatology, University of North Carolina Hospitals, Chapel Hill, North Carolina
Bullous Diseases

Beth K. Rubinstein, MD
Assistant Professor of Medicine, Division of Rheumatology, Allergy, and Immunology, Virginia Commonwealth University School of Medicine, Richmond, Virginia
Hyperuricemia and Gout

Bret R. Rutherford, MD
Columbia University College of Physicians and Surgeons; New York State Psychiatric Institute, New York, New York
Mood Disorders

Silonie Sachdeva
Department of Dermatology, Venereology and Leprosy, Dayanand Medical College and Hospital, Ludhiana, Punjab, India
Herpes Simplex Virus Types 1 and 2

Samuel A. Sandowski, MD
Adjunct Clinical Associate Professor, New York College of Osteopathic Medicine, Old Westbury, and Stonybrook University School of Medicine, Stonybrook; Director, Family Medicine Residency Program, South Nassau Communities Hospital, Oceanside, New York
Contraception

Linus H. Santo Tomas, MD, MS
Assistant Professor of Pulmonary Critical Care Medicine, Medical College of Wisconsin, Milwaukee, Wisconsin
Histoplasmosis

Richard Santucci, MD
Professor, Michigan State University College of Medicine, East Lansing; Specialist-in-Chief, Urology, The Detroit Medical Center, Detroit, Michigan
Trauma to the Genitourinary Tract

O. D. Saugstad, MD, PhD
Professor, Faculty of Medicine, University of Oslo; Director, Department of Pediatric Research, Rikshospitalet, Olso, Norway
Resuscitation of the Newborn

J. Terry Saunders, PhD
Assistant Professor of Medical Education in Internal Medicine, University of Virginia School of Medicine, Charlottesville, Virginia
Diabetes Mellitus in Adults

Peter C. Schalock, MD
Instructor in Dermatology, Harvard Medical School; Assistant in Dermatology, Massachusetts General Hospital, Boston, Massachusetts
Contact Dermatitis

Ralph M. Schapira, MD
Professor and Vice Chair, Department of Medicine, Medical College of Wisconsin; Staff Physician, Milwaukee VA Medical Center, Milwaukee, Wisconsin
Histoplasmosis; Acute Bronchitis

Michael Schatz, MD, MS
Clinical Professor, Department of Medicine, University of California, San Diego, School of Medicine, La Jolla; Chief, Department of Allergy, Kaiser Permanente, San Diego, California
Asthma in Adolescents and Adults

Stacey A. Scheib, MD
Resident Physician, Department of Obstetrics and Gynecology, Thomas Jefferson University Hospital, Philadelphia, Pennsylvania
Menopause

Lawrence R. Schiller, MD
Clinical Professor of Internal Medicine, University of Texas Southwestern College of Medicine at Dallas; Attending Physician, Digestive Health Associates of Texas; Program Director, Gastroenterology Fellowship, Baylor University Medical Center, Dallas, Texas
Malabsorption

Kerrie Schoffer, MD, FRCPC
Assistant Professor in Neurology, Dalhousie University Faculty of Medicine; Neurologist, QEII Health Sciences Centre, Halifax, Nova Scotia
Peripheral Neuropathies

Kevin Schroeder, MD
Program Director, Transitional Year, and Medical Director of Acute Dialysis, Riverside Methodist Hospital, Columbus, Ohio
Acute Renal Failure

Kathryn G. Schuff, MD
Associate Professor of Endocrinology and Clinical Research Compliance Manager, General Clinical Research Center, Oregon Health and Science University School of Medicine, Portland, Oregon
Cushing's Syndrome

Robert A. Schwartz, MD, MPH
Professor and Head of Dermatology, UMDNJ–New Jersey Medical School, Newark, New Jersey
Pigmentary Disorders

W. Cooper Scurry, Jr., MD
Fellow, McCollough Plastic Surgery Clinic, Gulf Shores, Alabama
Bell's Palsy (Idiopathic Acute Peripheral Facial Paralysis)

Carlos Seas, MD
Associate Professor of Medicine, Universidad Peruana Cayetano Heredia; Chief, Inservice Department, Hospital National Cayetano Heredia, Lima, Peru
Cholera

Edward Septimus, MD
Clinical Professor of Medicine, University of Texas Medical School at Houston, Houston, Texas; Medical Director, Infection Prevention, HCA Healthcare System, Nashville, Tennessee
Bacterial Pneumonia

Daniel J. Sexton, MD
Professor, Duke University School of Medicine, Durham, North Carolina
Rickettsial and Ehrlichial Infections

Mrunal Shah, MD
Clinical Assistant Professor of Family Medicine, The Ohio State University College of Medicine and Public Health; Assistant Program Director, Riverside Family Practice Residency Program, Riverside Methodist Hospital, Columbus, Ohio
Syphilis

Vijay H. Shah, MD
Professor of Medicine, Mayo Clinic College of Medicine, Rochester, Minnesota
Bleeding Esophageal Varices

Surendra Kumar Sharma, MD, PhD
Chief, Division of Pulmonary, Critical Care and Sleep Medicine; Professor and Chair, Department of Medicine, All India Institute of Medical Sciences, New Delhi, India
Management of the Patient with HIV Disease; Tuberculosis and Other Mycobacterial Diseases

Philip D. Shenefelt, MD, MS
Associate Professor, Department of Dermatology and Cutaneous Surgery, University of South Florida College of Medicine, Tampa, Florida
Parasitic Diseases of the Skin

Chelsea A. Sheppard, MD
Transfusion Medicine Program, Department of Pathology and Laboratory Medicine, Emory University School of Medicine, Atlanta, Georgia
Adverse Effects of Blood Transfusion

Mona Shimshi, MD
Assistant Professor, Mount Sinai School of Medicine, New York; Staff Physician, James J. Peters VA Medical Center, Bronx, New York
Hypothyroidism

Baha M. Sibai, MD
Professor, Department of Obstetrics and Gynecology, University of Cincinnati College of Medicine, Cincinnati, Ohio
Hypertensive Disorders of Pregnancy

Marc A. Silver, MD
Clinical Professor of Medicine, University of Illinois at Chicago College of Medicine, Chicago; Adjunct Professor, Department of Biomedical Engineering, Illinois Institute of Technology, Chicago; Chairman, Department of Medicine, and Director, Heart Failure Institute, Advocate Christ Medical Center, Oak Lawn, Illinois
Heart Failure

Tamara Simpson, MD
Assistant Professor of Medicine, University of Texas Health Science Center at San Antonio School of Medicine; Staff, Pulmonary Division, University of Texas Health Science Center at San Antonio, San Antonio, Texas
Management of Chronic Obstructive Pulmonary Disease

Peter A. Singer, MD
Professor of Clinical Medicine, Keck School of Medicine of USC; Chief, Clinical Endocrinology, Department of Medicine, LAC–USC Medical Center, Los Angeles, California
Hyperthyroidism

Sylvia T. Singer, MD
Associate Physician, Division of Hematology/Oncology, Children's Hospital and Research Center Oakland, Oakland, California
Thalassemia

Michael J. Smith, MD, MSCE
Assistant Professor, Department of Pediatrics, University of Louisville School of Medicine; Attending Physician, Division of Pediatric Infectious Diseases, Kosair Children's Hospital, Louisville, Kentucky
Cat-Scratch Disease

Cynthia B. Snider, MD, MPH
Department of Medicine, University of Virginia School of Medicine, Charlottesville, Virginia
Travel Medicine

Carmen C. Solorzano, MD
Assistant Professor of Surgery, University of Miami Miller School of Medicine; Chief, Endocrine Surgery, University of Miami/Sylvester Cancer Center, Miami, Florida
Acute and Chronic Pancreatitis

Suman Sood, MD
Instructor of Medicine, Division of Hematology–Oncology, University of Pennsylvania School of Medicine; Staff Physician, Division of Hematology–Oncology, Hospital of the University of Pennsylvania, Philadelphia, Pennsylvania
Platelet-Mediated Bleeding Disorders

Richard K. Sterling, MD, MSc
Professor of Medicine, Division of Gastroenterology, Hepatology, and Nutrition, Virginia Commonwealth University School of Medicine, Richmond, Virginia
Cirrhosis

Catherine Stevens-Simon, MD[†]
Formerly Associate Professor of Pediatrics, Division of Adolescent Medicine, University of Colorado School of Medicine; Staff Physician, Children's Hospital–Denver, Colorado
Chlamydia trachomatis

A. Keith Stewart, MB, ChB
Senior Associate Consultant, Mayo Clinic, Scottsdale, Arizona
Multiple Myeloma

Christopher D. Still, DO
Medical Director, Center for Nutrition and Weight Management, Department of Gastroenterology and Nutrition, Geisinger Health Care System, Danville, Pennsylvania
Obesity

Erik K. St. Louis, MD
Senior Associate Consultant, Department of Neurology, Mayo Clinic and Foundation, Rochester, Minnesota
Seizures and Epilepsy in Adolescents and Adults

Brenda Stokes, MD
Clinical Assistant Professor of Family Medicine, University of Virginia School of Medicine, Charlottesville; Assistant Clinical Professor, Department of Family Medicine, Virginia Commonwealth University School of Medicine, Richmond; Medical Staff, Centra Health–Lynchburg General and Virginia Baptist Hospitals, Lynchburg, Virginia
Postpartum Care

[†]*Deceased*

Paniti Sukumvanich, MD
Fellow, Breast Service, Department of Surgery, Memorial Sloan-Kettering Cancer Center, New York, New York
Diseases of the Breast

Jessica P. Swartout, MD
Fellow in Maternal-Fetal Medicine, Department of Obstetrics and Gynecology, University of Minnesota Medical School, Minneapolis, Minnesota
Antepartum Care

Misha F. Syed, MD
Assistant Professor, Department of Ophthalmology and Visual Sciences, University of Texas Medical Branch School of Medicine, Galveston, Texas
Glaucoma

Manuel E. Tancer, MD
Professor, Department of Psychiatry and Behavioral Neurosciences, Wayne State University School of Medicine; Specialist-in-Chief, Department of Psychiatry, Detroit Medical Center; Service Chief, Psychiatry, Detroit Receiving Hospital, Detroit, Michigan
Panic Disorder

Matthew D. Taylor, MD
Surgical Resident/Thoracic Research Fellow, University of Virginia Medical Center, Charlottesville, Virginia
Atelectasis

Marty S. Teltscher, MD, CM
Infections Diseases and Medical Microbiology Fellow, McGill University Faculty of Medicine/Sir Mortimer B. Davis–Jewish General Hospital, Montreal, Quebec, Canada
Toxic Shock Syndrome

Victor J. Test, MD, FCCP
Assistant Professor of Clinical Medicine, Division of Pulmonary, Medicine and Critical Care, University of California, San Diego, School of Medicine, La Jolla, California
Pulmonary Embolism

Manish Thapar, MD
Instructor, University of Missouri College of Medicine; Attending Physician, University Hospital, Columbia, Missouri
Porphyria

Nathan Thielman, MD, MPH
Duke Global Health Institute, Duke University, Durham, North Carolina
Intestinal Parasites

David R. Thomas, MD
Professor of Medicine, Division of Geriatric Medicine, Saint Louis University School of Medicine, St. Louis, Missouri
Pressure Ulcers

Rodger E. Tiedemann, MB, ChB, PhD
Clinical Senior Lecturer in Medicine, University of Auckland Faculty of Medicine, School of Medicine, Auckland, New Zealand; Research Associate, Mayo Clinic, Scottsdale, Arizona
Multiple Myeloma

Paola Torre, MD
Head Researcher, Neurodegenerative Disorders, Department of Clinical Medicine and Neurology, University of Trieste, Trieste, Italy
Hiccups

Anne Marie Tremaine, MD
Clinical Research Fellow, University of California, Irvine, School of Medicine, Irvine, California
Erythema Multiforme, Stevens-Johnson Syndrome, and Toxic Epidermal Necrolysis

Maria Trent, MD, MPH
Assistant Professor of Pediatrics, Johns Hopkins University School of Medicine; Active Staff, Johns Hopkins Hospital Children's Center, Baltimore, Maryland
Pelvic Inflammatory Disease

Elaine B. Trujillo, MS, RD
Nutritionist, National Cancer Institute, National Institutes of Health, Bethesda, Maryland
Parenteral Nutrition in Adults

Mark W. Tyndall, BSc, MD, DSc, FRCPC
Associate Professor of Medicine, University of British Columbia Faculty of Medicine; Head, Division of Infectious Diseases, Providence Health Care, Vancouver, British Columbia, Canada
Chancroid and Granuloma Inguinale

Stephen K. Tyring, MD, PhD
Clinical Professor of Dermatology, University of Texas Medical School at Houston; Director, Center for Clinical Studies, Houston, Texas
Erythema Multiforme, Stevens-Johnson Syndrome, and Toxic Epidermal Necrolysis

Arvid E. Underman, MD, FACP, DTMH
Clinical Professor of Medicine and Microbiology, Keck School of Medicine of USC, Los Angeles; Director of Graduate Medical Education, Huntington Hospital, Pasadena, California
Salmonellosis

Nicholas Van Bruaene, MD
ENT in Training, Department of Oto-Rhino-Laryngology, University Hospital Ghent, Ghent, Belgium
Nonallergic Perennial Rhinitis

Mary Lee Vance, MD
Professor of Medicine and Neurosurgery, University of Virginia School of Medicine; Attending Physician, University of Virginia Hospital, Charlottesville, Virginia
Hypopituitarism

John Varga, MD
Gallagher Professor of Medicine, Northwestern University Feinberg School of Medicine, Chicago, Illinois
Connective Tissue Disorders

Donald C. Vinh, MD, FRCP(C), Dip(ABIM)
Division of Infectious Diseases, Department of Medicine, and Department of Medical Microbiology, McGill University Health Center, Montreal General Hospital, Montreal, Quebec, Canada
Necrotizing Skin and Soft Tissue Infections

Todd W. Vitaz, MD
Assistant Professor, Department of Neurological Surgery, University of Louisville School of Medicine; Director of Neurosurgical Oncology; Co-Director, Neurosciences ICU, Norton Hospital, Louisville, Kentucky
Management of Head Injuries

Jeffery T. Vrabec, MD
Associate Professor, Department of Otolaryngology–Head and Neck Surgery, Baylor College of Medicine; Clinical Associate Professor, Department of Head and Neck Surgery, The University of Texas M.D. Anderson Cancer Center; Active Staff, Otolaryngology–Head and Neck Surgery, The Methodist Hospital; Courtesy Staff, Otolaryngology Service, Texas Children's Hospital, and Head and Neck Surgery, M.D. Anderson Cancer Center, Houston, Texas; Chair, Facial Nerve Disorders Committee, and Member, SIPac Committee, American Academy of Otolaryngology–Head and Neck Surgery; Chair, ByLaws Committee, American Neurotology Society Membership Committee
Otitis Externa

Shobha Wani, MD
Fellow, Section of Rheumatology, Washington Hospital Center, Washington, DC
Lyme Disease

Anthony P. Weetman, MD, DSc
Pro Vice-Chancellor and Professor of Medicine, The Medical School, University of Sheffield; Honorary Consultant Endocrinologist, Sheffield Teaching Hospitals, Sheffield, United Kingdom
Thyroiditis

Mitchell P. Weikert, MD, MS
Assistant Professor of Ophthalmology, Baylor College of Medicine; Staff Physician, Michael E. DeBakey VA Medical Center and Texas Children's Hospital, Houston, Texas
Laser Vision Correction

Arthur Weinstein, MD, FACP, FACR
Professor of Medicine, Georgetown University School of Medicine; Associate Chairman, Department of Medicine, and Director, Section of Rheumatology, Washington Hospital Center, Washington, DC
Lyme Disease

Mitchell J. Weiss, MD, PhD
Associate Professor of Pediatrics, University of Pennsylvania School of Medicine; Attending, The Children's Hospital of Philadelphia, Philadelphia, Pennsylvania
Nonimmune Hemolytic Anemia

David N. Weissman, MD
Adjunct Professor of Medicine and Microbiology (Immunology), West Virginia University School of Medicine; Director, Division of Respiratory Disease Studies, National Institute for Occupational Safety and Health, Morgantown, West Virginia
Pneumoconiosis

Robert C. Welliver, Sr., MD
Professor, University at Buffalo State University of New York School of Medicine; Co-Director, Division of Infectious Diseases, Women and Children's Hospital of Buffalo, Buffalo, New York
Viral Respiratory Infections

Dennis Y. Wen, MD
Associate Professor of Family and Community Medicine, University of Missouri–Columbia School of Medicine, Columbia, Missouri
Common Sports Injuries

Martin Wetzel, MD
Assistant Professor of Psychiatry, University of Nebraska College of Medicine, Omaha, Nebraska
Attention-Deficit/Hyperactivity Disorder

Isaiah D. Wexler, MD, PhD
Department of Pediatrics and CF Center, Hadassah University Hospital-Mount Scopus Campus, Hadassah Hebrew University Medical Center, Jerusalem, Israel
Diabetic Ketoacidosis

Lucile E. White, MD
Private Practice, DermSurgery Associates, Houston, Texas
Cancer of the Skin

William Wierda, MD, PhD
Associate Professor of Medicine, University of Texas Medical School at Houston/M.D. Anderson Cancer Center, Houston, Texas
Chronic Leukemias

Dennis A. Wigle, MD, PhD
Mayo Clinic, General Thoracic Surgery, Rochester, Minnesota
Pleural Effusion and Empyema Thoracis

Steven R. Williams, MD
Clinical Assistant Professor, Department of Obstetrics and Gynecology, The Ohio State University College of Medicine and Public Health, Columbus, Ohio
Infertility

Nathaniel Winer, MD
Professor of Medicine, SUNY Downstate Medical Center College of Medicine; Attending Physician, Department of Medicine, Division of Endocrinology, Diabetes, and Hypertension, University Hospital of Brooklyn; Director, Thyroid Clinic and Diabetes Clinic, King's County Hospital Center, Brooklyn, New York
Primary Aldosteronism

Christopher Wise, MD
W. Robert Irby Professor of Medicine, Department of Medicine, Division of Rheumatology, Allergy, and Immunology, Virginia Commonwealth University School of Medicine, Richmond, Virginia
Hyperuricemia and Gout

Jamie R. S. Wood, MD
Instructor in Pediatrics, Harvard Medical School; Research Associate, Sections on Genetics and Epidemiology and Vascular Cell Biology, and Staff Physician, Pediatric, Adolescent, and Young Adult Section, Joslin Diabetes Center, Boston, Massachusetts
Diabetes Mellitus in Children and Adolescents

Jon B. Woods, MD
Associate Professor of Pediatrics, Uniformed Services University of the Health Sciences F. Edward Hébert School of Medicine, Bethesda, Maryland; Pediatric Infectious Diseases, Wilford Hall Medical Center, Lackland Air Force Base, San Antonio, Texas
Anthrax

Gayle Woodson, MD
Professor and Chair, Division of Otolaryngology, Southern Illinois University School of Medicine, Springfield, Illinois
Hoarseness and Laryngitis

Charles F. Wooley, MD[†]
Formerly Professor of Medicine Emeritus, Division of Cardiology, Heart and Lung Research Institute/The Ohio State University School of Medicine and Public Health, Columbus, Ohio
Mitral Valve Prolapse: The Floppy Mitral Valve, Mitral Valve Prolapse, and Mitral Valvular Regurgitation

---

[†]*(Deceased)*

Jennifer Wright, MD
Fellow, Hematology/Oncology, Baylor College of Medicine, Houston, Texas
Polycythemia Vera

Angela Yen
Arlington Center for Dermatology, Arlington, Texas
Herpes Simplex Virus Types 1 and 2

Ronald F. Young, MD
Director of Neurosurgery, California Neuroscience Institute, St. John's Regional Medical Center, Oxnard, California
Trigeminal Neuralgia

Lei Yu, MD
Thoracic Surgeon, Beijing Tongren Hospital, Beijing City, China
Primary Lung Abscess

Jami Star Zeltzer, MD
Associate Professor, Department of Obstetrics and Gynecology, Division of Maternal-Fetal Medicine, University of Massachusetts Medical School, Worcester, Massachusetts
Vaginal Bleeding in Late Pregnancy

Richard D. Zorowitz, MD
Associate Professor of Physical Medicine and Rehabilitation, Johns Hopkins University School of Medicine; Chairman, Department of Physical Medicine and Rehabilitation, Johns Hopkins Bayview Medical Center, Baltimore, Maryland
Rehabilitation of the Stroke Survivor

Kathryn A. Zug, MD
Associate Professor of Medicine (Dermatology), Dartmouth Medical School, Hanover; Staff Physician, Dartmouth Hitchcock Medical Center, Lebanon, New Hampshire
Contact Dermatitis

Mary Zupanc, MD
Heidi Marie Bauman Chair of Epilepsy and Professor, Departments of Neurology and Pediatrics; Chief, Division of Pediatric Neurology, Medical College of Wisconsin; Director, Pediatric Comprehensive Epilepsy Program, and Director, Pediatric Neurology, Children's Hospital of Wisconsin, Milwaukee, Wisconsin
Epilepsy in Infants and Children

Preface

Since 1949, *Conn's Current Therapy* has provided a yearly update on the practical treatment of nearly 400 diseases and disorders. Howard Conn was the initial developer and author, who set out to provide a concise and up-to-date reference on the most recent advances in therapy for conditions most commonly encountered in practice. Some less common conditions also are included, because certain disorders can have serious consequences if not diagnosed early and managed appropriately. Well-known scholar and clinician Robert Rakel, MD, took over editorship in 1984 after Dr. Conn's death and remains today as the editor. Edward Bope, MD, joined him in 2001 to share the editor responsibilities.

Each year, new experts are chosen to write on the topics. They are selected on the basis of recommendations from other authorities, or scholarly activity and/or research. Changing authors with each edition keeps the book crisp in coverage, fresh in tone, and brimming with the latest practical advice. The authors give references for their discussions but also tell you how they manage the problem in their own clinical practice. Such practical wisdom is of immense value to today's physician, who typically is inundated with sometimes conflicting information from multiple sources. New topics are included every year, so the book remains current with the problems likely to be encountered in practice.

Now with the purchase of *Conn's Current Therapy 2009* you also can have your favorite or commonly referenced topics available on your computer. In fact, you will have access to the 2007, 2008, and 2009 editions for downloading your favorite articles from the book. Readers are encouraged to compare the treatments presented in these editions to see how different experts manage the same problem.

Conn's Current Therapy is indeed an international book. Contributing authors from around the world offer advice about the diagnosis and management of conditions not common to the United States. The contribution of these international experts adds greatly to the comprehensive nature of the book, and given the amount of international travel, it is quite possible to see unusual disorders far from the homeland of their origin.

Each chapter includes Key Diagnostic and Key Therapeutic boxes for quick reference. As always, tables, graphs, and figures are used when possible to present in-depth data in a convenient format. References for further reading provide some options for additional information if needed. In keeping with today's emphasis on evidence-based medicine, the clinician is pointed toward good evidence, when available, for treatment success. Careful attention is given to ensuring that the information included is correct and up-to-date. All of the material is reviewed by a pharmacist, Dr. Rakel or Dr. Bope, and multiple copy editors for accuracy and readability. Trade names are included alongside the generic drug names to help the clinician identify the medicines by whatever name is most familiar. The treatments recommended are those found to work best in the experience of the author. When a drug is not FDA approved for that use, this is indicated by a footnote; such notations may merely reflect that approval for that indication was never requested.

We greatly appreciate the assistance of the very capable editorial staff at Elsevier and particularly the contribution of our pharmacist reviewers, Miriam Chan, RPH, PharmD, and Grace Kuo, PharmD.

Robert E. Rakel, MD

Edward T. Bope, MD

Contents

SECTION 1
Symptomatic Care Pending Diagnosis

Pain 1
Trish Palmer, MD

Nausea and Vomiting 5
Chad M. Braun, MD

Gaseousness and Indigestion 9
Satish S. C. Rao, MD, PhD, and Ashok Attaluri, MD

Hiccups 12
Rita Moretti, MD, and Paola Torre, MD

Acute Infectious Diarrhea 13
Matthew T. Oughton, MD, FRCPC, and
Andre Dascal, MD, FRCPC

Constipation 20
Robert Fisher, MD, and Brenda Horwitz, MD

Fever 23
Ann M. Aring, MD

Cough 25
David G. Hill, MD

Pruritus 29
Scott Moses, MD

Tinnitus 35
Claus-Frenz Claussen, MD

Spine Pain 39
Michael T. McCann, MD

SECTION 2
The Infectious Diseases

Management of the Patient with
HIV Disease 45
Surendra Kumar Sharma, MD, PhD, and
Tamilarasu Kadhiravan, MD

Amebiasis 59
Rashidul Haque, MB, PhD, and
William A. Petri, Jr., MD, PhD

Giardiasis 61
M. Ekramul Hoque, MBBS, MPH (Hons), PhD

Severe Sepsis and Septic Shock 65
Eleni Patrozou, MD, and Steven M. Opal, MD

Brucellosis 72
Basak Dokuzoguz, MD, and Nurcan Baykam, MD

Varicella (Chickenpox) 76
Charles Grose, MD

Cholera 78
Carlos Seas, MD, and Eduardo Gotuzzo, MD

Foodborne Illness 81
Lester M. Crawford, PhD

Necrotizing Skin and Soft Tissue Infections 83
John M. Embil, MD, FRCP(C), FACP, and
Donald C. Vinh, MD, FRCP(C), Dip(ABIM)

Toxic Shock Syndrome 86
Marty S. Teltscher, MD, CM, and
Andre Dascal, MD, FRCPC

Influenza 90
Jeffrey A. Linder, MD, MPH

Leishmaniasis 93
Karim Aoun, MD, and Aida Bouratbine, MD

Leprosy 97
Bhushan Kumar, MD, MNAMS, and
Sunil Dogra, MD, DNB, MNAMS

Malaria 103
Paul M. Arguin, MD, and S. Patrick Kachur, MD

Bacterial Meningitis 112
Gary D. Overturf, MD

Infectious Mononucleosis 116
Leonard R. Krilov, MD

Chronic Fatigue Syndrome 117
James F. Jones, MD

Mumps 121
Joel D. Klein, MD, FAAP

Plague 122
Douglas A. Drevets, MD, DTM&H

Anthrax 123
Jon B. Woods, MD

Psittacosis ... 127
Julian Elliott, MB, BS, FRACP

Q Fever ... 128
Didier Raoult, MD, PhD

Rabies ... 130
Alan C. Jackson, MD, FRCPC

Rat-Bite Fever ... 131
Jean Dudler, MD

Relapsing Fever ... 133
Diego Cadavid, MD

Lyme Disease ... 136
Arthur Weinstein, MD, FACP, FACR, and
Shobha Wani, MD

Rubella and Congenital Rubella Syndrome ... 140
Susan E. Reef, MD

Measles (Rubeola) ... 141
Claude P. Muller, MD, and Jacques Kremer, PhD

Tetanus ... 143
Samuel S. Hsu, MD

Pertussis ... 146
Michael E. Pichichero, MD

Office-Based Immunization Practices ... 147
Robert M. Jacobson, MD

Travel Medicine ... 155
Cynthia B. Snider, MD, MPH, and
William A. Petri, Jr., MD, PhD

Toxoplasmosis ... 163
Peter Mariuz, MD, and Sumanth Rajagopal, MD

Cat-Scratch Disease ... 169
Michael J. Smith, MD, MSCE

Salmonellosis ... 170
Arvid E. Underman, MD, FACP, DTMH

Typhoid Fever ... 174
Zulfiqar A. Bhutta, MB, BS, PhD

Rickettsial and Ehrlichial Infections ... 176
Deverick J. Anderson, MD, and Daniel J. Sexton, MD

Smallpox ... 179
Isao Arita, MD

SECTION 3
Diseases of the Head and Neck

Laser Vision Correction ... 187
Mitchell P. Weikert, MD, MS

Conjunctivitis ... 193
Robert A. Copeland, Jr., MD

Optic Neuritis ... 196
Anthony C. Arnold, MD

Glaucoma ... 198
Misha F. Syed, MD, and Nicolas P. Bell, MD

Otitis Externa ... 201
Jeffrey T. Vrabec, MD

Otitis Media ... 203
J. Scott McMurray, MD

Episodic Vertigo ... 204
Terry D. Fife, MD

Ménière's Disease ... 210
Ted A. Meyer, MD, PhD, and Paul R. Lambert, MD

Sinusitis ... 212
Richard R. Orlandi, MD

Nonallergic Perennial Rhinitis ... 214
Claus Bachert, MD, PhD, and
Nicholas Van Bruaene, MD

Hoarseness and Laryngitis ... 218
Gayle Woodson, MD

Streptococcal Pharyngitis ... 220
John Brusch, MD

SECTION 4
The Respiratory System

Acute Respiratory Failure ... 225
Scott K. Epstein, MD

Atelectasis ... 230
David R. Jones, MD, and Matthew D. Taylor

Management of Chronic Obstructive
Pulmonary Disease ... 231
Tamara Simpson, MD, Juan Armando Garcia, MD,
Stephen G. Jenkinson, MD, and Jay Peters, MD

Cystic Fibrosis ... 236
Robert Giusti, MD

Sleep Apnea ... 239
Leon Rosenthal, MD

Lung Cancer ... 242
Gregory A. Otterson, MD

Coccidioidomycosis ... 248
Lynn L. Horvath, MD, and
Duane R. Hospenthal, MD, PhD

Histoplasmosis ... 251
Linus H. Santo Tomas, MD, MS, and
Ralph M. Schapira, MD

Blastomycosis ... 254
Robert Bradsher, MD, and Anupama Menon, MD, MPH

Pleural Effusion and Empyema Thoracis............256
Craig E. Daniels, MD, and Dennis A. Wigle, MD, PhD

Primary Lung Abscess.................................258
Mark Krasna, MD, and Lei Yu, MD

Acute Bronchitis......................................259
Susan Davids, MD, MPH, and Ralph M. Schapira, MD

Bacterial Pneumonia..................................261
Edward Septimus, MD

Viral Respiratory Infections..........................264
Robert C. Welliver, Sr., MD

Viral and Mycoplasmal Pneumonias.................266
Burke A. Cunha, MD

Legionellosis..270
Julio A. Ramirez, MD

Pulmonary Embolism.................................271
Victor J. Test, MD, FCCP

Sarcoidosis...274
Marc A. Judson, MD

Pneumoconiosis......................................278
Richard D. deShazo, MD, and David N. Weissman, MD

Hypersensitivity Pneumonitis.......................280
Yvon Cormier, MD, and Yves Lacasse, MD

Tuberculosis and Other Mycobacterial
Diseases..282
Surendra Kumar Sharma, MD, PhD, and
Alladi Mohan, MD

SECTION 5
The Cardiovascular System

Acquired Diseases of the Aorta......................291
Gorav Ailawadi, MD, and Irving L. Kron, MD

Angina Pectoris......................................295
John F. Moran, MD

Cardiac Arrest: Sudden Cardiac Death..............302
Robert W. Rho, MD

Atrial Fibrillation.....................................308
Anne B. Curtis, MD

Premature Beats.....................................312
Prakash C. Deedwania, MD, and Enrique V. Carbajal, MD

Heart Block..315
Kelley P. Anderson, MD

Tachycardias...320
Sei Iwai, MD, and Bruce B. Lerman, MD

Congenital Heart Disease............................326
Robb L. Romp, MD, and Yung R. Lau, MD

Hypertrophic Cardiomyopathy......................331
Ali J. Marian, MD

Mitral Valve Prolapse: The Floppy
Mitral Valve, Mitral Valve Prolapse,
and Mitral Valvular Regurgitation..................334
Charles F. Wooley, MD, and
Harisios Boudoulas, MD, PhD

Heart Failure...338
Marc A. Silver, MD

Infective Endocarditis...............................342
Navin M. Amin, MD

Hypertension..349
L. Michael Prisant, MD

Acute Myocardial Infarction........................360
Guy S. Reeder, MD, and Abhiram Prasad, MD

Acute Pericarditis....................................367
José G. Díez, MD

Peripheral Arterial Disease..........................373
Jeffrey L. Ballard, MD

Venous Thrombosis.................................375
Paul L. F. Giangrande, MD

SECTION 6
The Blood and Spleen

Aplastic Anemia.....................................379
Eva C. Guinan, MD

Iron Deficiency......................................383
James C. Barton, MD

Autoimmune Hemolytic Anemia...................387
Stephen R. Larsen, MB, BS

Nonimmune Hemolytic Anemia....................390
Stella T. Chou, MD, and Mitchell J. Weiss, MD, PhD

Pernicious Anemia and Other Megaloblastic
Anemias..394
Eugene P. Frenkel, MD

Thalassemia...397
Ashutosh Lal, MD, and Sylvia T. Singer, MD

Sickle Cell Disease...................................404
Lewis L. Hsu, MD, PhD, and Griffin P. Rodgers, MD

Neutropenia...413
Peter E. Newburger, MD

Hemolytic Disease of the Fetus
and Newborn..416
Douglas S. Richards, MD

Hemophilia and Related Bleeding Disorders.......419
Meera Chitlur, MD, and Roshni Kulkarni, MD

Platelet-Mediated Bleeding Disorders.............425
Suman Sood, MD, and Charles S. Abrams, MD

Disseminated Intravascular Coagulation............428
John J. Byrnes, MD

Thrombotic Thrombocytopenic Purpura............430
Joseph E. Kiss, MD

Hemochromatosis.............432
Bruce R. Bacon, MD

Hodgkin's Lymphoma.............434
Ralph M. Meyer, MD, and David C. Hodgson, MD, MPH

Hodgkin's Disease: Radiation Therapy.............439
Pelayo C. Besa, MD

Acute Leukemias in Adults.............444
Jonathan E. Kolitz, MD

Acute Leukemia in Children.............450
Patrick Brown, MD, and Stephen P. Hunger, MD

Chronic Leukemias.............456
Jorge E. Cortes, MD, Hagop M. Kantarjian, MD, and William Wierda, MD, PhD

Non-Hodgkin's Lymphoma.............464
Lawrence Rice, MD, and Uday Popat, MD

Multiple Myeloma.............467
Rodger E. Tiedemann, MB, ChB, PhD, and A. Keith Stewart, MB, ChB

Polycythemia Vera.............472
Michael Kroll, MD, and Jennifer Wright, MD

Porphyrias.............475
Herbert L. Bonkovsky, MD, and Manish Thapar, MD

Therapeutic Use of Blood Components.............480
Peter A. Millward, MD, and Mark E. Brecher, MD

Adverse Effects of Blood Transfusion.............484
Chelsea A. Sheppard, MD, and Christopher D. Hillyer, MD

SECTION 7
The Digestive System

Cholelithiasis and Cholecystitis.............493
Grant R. Caddy, MD

Cirrhosis.............496
Richard K. Sterling, MD, MSc, Wissam E. Mattar, MD, and Paul Y. Kwo, MD

Bleeding Esophageal Varices.............504
Vijay H. Shah, MD, and Patrick S. Kamath, MD

Dysphagia and Esophageal Obstruction.............508
Philip O. Katz, MD, and Girish Anand, MD

Diverticula of the Alimentary Tract.............511
Pinckney J. Maxwell IV, MD, and Charles W. Chappuis, MD

Inflammatory Bowel Disease.............514
Mark A. Peppercorn, MD, and Alan C. Moss, MD

Irritable Bowel Syndrome.............521
Michael D. Crowell, PhD, John K. DiBaise, MD, and Lucinda A. Harris, MD

Hemorrhoids, Anal Fissure, and Anorectal Abscess and Fistula.............525
Neil H. Hyman, MD

Gastritis and Peptic Ulcer Disease.............527
Sripathi R. Kethu, MD, and Steven F. Moss, MD

Acute and Chronic Hepatitis.............533
Mamta K. Jain, MD, MPH, and Daniel M. Brailita, MD

Malabsorption.............539
Lawrence R. Schiller, MD

Acute and Chronic Pancreatitis.............545
Carmen C. Solorzano, MD, and Richard A. Prinz, MD

Gastroesophageal Reflux Disease.............552
Kenneth R. DeVault, MD

Tumors of the Stomach.............556
Scott A. Hundahl, MD

Tumors of the Colon and Rectum.............558
Daniel Albo, MD, PhD

Intestinal Parasites.............563
Nathan Thielman, MD, MPH, and Elizabeth Reddy, MD

SECTION 8
Metabolic Disorders

Diabetes Mellitus in Adults.............575
Anthony L. McCall, MD, PhD, and J. Terry Saunders, PhD

Diabetes Mellitus in Children and Adolescents.............583
Lori M. B. Laffel, MD, MPH, and Jamie R. S. Wood, MD

Diabetic Ketoacidosis.............590
Isaiah Wexler, MD, PhD

Hyponatremia.............595
Gregory Proctor, MD, and Moshe Levi, MD

Hyperuricemia and Gout 599
Beth K. Rubinstein, MD, and Christopher M. Wise, MD

Management of Patients with
Dyslipoproteinemias (Cholesterol
and Triglyceride Disorders) 601
Michael A. Crouch, MD, MSPH

Obesity 606
Christopher D. Still, DO, and Gordon L. Jensen, MD, PhD

Osteoporosis 612
Barte L. Clarke, MD, and Sundeep Khosla, MD

Paget's Disease of Bone 615
Paul D. Miller, MD

Parenteral Nutrition in Adults 618
Elaine B. Trujillo, MS, RD, and Malcolm K. Robinson, MD

Parenteral Fluid Therapy for Infants
and Children 626
Jeremy N. Friedman, MB, ChB, and
Carolyn E. Beck, MD, MSc

SECTION 9
The Endocrine System

Acromegaly 633
Moises Mercado, MD

Adrenocortical Insufficiency 637
Carl D. Malchoff, MD, PhD

Cushing's Syndrome 640
Kathryn G. Schuff, MD

Diabetes Insipidus 646
Jennifer Kelly, DO, and
Arnold M. Moses, MD, FACP, FACE

Primary Hyperparathyroidism and
Hypoparathyroidism 649
John P. Bilezikian, MD

Primary Aldosteronism 653
Nathaniel Winer, MD

Hypopituitarism 656
Mary Lee Vance, MD

Hyperprolactinemia 659
Lisa B. Nachtigall, MD, and
Beverly M. K. Biller, MD

Hypothyroidism 661
Mona Shimshi, MD, and Terry F. Davies, MD

Hyperthyroidism 665
Peter A. Singer, MD

Thyroid Cancer 670
Richard A. Prinz, MD, and Emery Chen, MD

Pheochromocytomas 673
Pierre-François Plouin, MD

Thyroiditis 676
Anthony P. Weetman, MD, DSc

SECTION 10
The Urogenital Tract

Bacterial Infections of the Male
Urinary Tract 679
John N. Krieger, MD

Urinary Tract Infections in Women 682
Burke A. Cunha, MD

Bacterial Infections of the Urinary
Tract in Girls 686
Candice E. Johnson, MD, PhD

Childhood Incontinence 689
Christine Geers, MSN, CPNP, and Andrew Kirsch, MD

Urinary Incontinence 693
E. Ann Gormley, MD

Epididymitis 696
John N. Krieger, MD

Primary Glomerular Diseases 699
Manuel Praga, MD, and Enrique Morales, MD

Pyelonephritis 704
Patricia D. Brown, MD

Trauma to the Genitourinary Tract 706
Richard Santucci, MD, and Theodore Barber, MD

Prostatitis 709
Andrea Gallina, MD, Umberto Capitanio, MD, and
Pierre I. Karakiewicz, MD

Benign Prostatic Hyperplasia 712
Gopal H. Badlani, MD, and
Matthew E. Karlovsky, MD

Erectile Dysfunction 715
Luciano Kolodny, MD

Acute Renal Failure 721
Kevin Schroeder, MD

Chronic Renal Failure 725
Jeffrey A. Kraut, MD

Malignant Tumors of the Urogenital Tract 731
Michael S. Cookson, MD, and Sam S. Chang, MD

Urethral Stricture Disease...................740
Mahreen Hussain, BSc (Hons), MRCS, and
Tamsin J. Greenwell, MD

Renal Calculi...................742
Sujeet S. Acharya, MD, and Glenn S. Gerber, MD

SECTION 11
The Sexually Transmitted Diseases

Chancroid and Granuloma Inguinale...................749
Mark Tyndall, MD

Gonorrhea...................750
Khalil Ghanem, MD, PhD

Nongonococcal Urethritis...................752
John N. Krieger, MD

Syphilis...................754
Mrunal Shah, MD

Contraception...................755
Linda Roethel, MD, and Samuel Sandowski, MD

SECTION 12
Diseases of Allergy

Anaphylaxis and Serum Sickness...................759
Stephen F. Kemp, MD

Asthma in Adolescents and Adults...................762
Michael Schatz, MD, MS

Asthma in Children...................770
Gerald B. Kolski

Allergic Rhinitis...................776
Linda Cox, MD

Allergic Reactions to Drugs...................781
Donald McNeil, MD

Allergic Reactions to Insect Stings...................784
David B. K. Golden, MD

SECTION 13
Diseases of the Skin

Acne Vulgaris and Rosacea...................787
Steven R. Feldman, MD, PhD, and
Alan B. Fleischer, Jr., MD

Hair Disorders...................790
Thomas N. Helm, MD

Cancer of the Skin...................793
Lucile E. White, MD, and Murad Alam, MD

Cutaneous T-Cell Lymphomas
(Mycosis Fungoides and Sézary's
Syndrome)...................795
Christiane Querfeld, MD, Timothy M. Kuzel, MD, and
Steven T. Rosen, MD

Papulosquamous Eruptions...................801
Gary S. Chuang, MD, and Alice Gottlieb, MD, PhD

Connective Tissue Disorders...................805
John Varga, MD, Susan Manzi, MD, MPH, and
Gabriella Lakos, MD, PhD

Cutaneous Vasculitis...................813
Manisha J. Patel, MD, and Joseph L. Jorizzo, MD

Diseases of the Nails...................816
Nathaniel Jellinek, MD

Keloids...................820
Carol Drucker, MD

Verrucae (Warts)...................822
Carol Drucker, MD

Condyloma Acuminatum
(Genital Warts)...................824
Karl R. Beutner, MD, PhD, and Alice N. Do, DO

Melanocytic Nevi...................827
Jane M. Grant-Kels, MD, and Michael Murphy, MD

Melanoma...................830
Jennifer L. DeFazio, MD, and Ashfaq A. Marghoob, MD

Premalignant Lesions...................833
Donald Clemons, MD

Bacterial Infections of the Skin...................835
Philip S. Barie, MD, MBA, and
Soumitra R. Eachempati, MD

Herpes Simplex Virus Types 1 and 2...................839
Angela Yen, MD, and Silonie Sachdeva, MD

Parasitic Diseases of the Skin...................843
Philip D. Shenefelt, MD, MS

Fungal Diseases of the Skin...................846
Rebecca Lewis Kelso, MD, and
Sharon S. Raimer, MD

Diseases of the Mouth...................849
Carl M. Allen, DDS, MSD

Venous Leg Ulcers...................855
Jaymie Panuncialman, MD, and
Vincent Falanga, MD

Pressure Ulcers...................857
David R. Thomas, MD

Atopic Dermatitis...................859
Mark Boguniewicz, MD

Erythema Multiforme, Stevens-Johnson
Syndrome, and Toxic Epidermal Necrolysis........862
  Anne Marie Tremaine, MD, and
  Stephen K. Tyring, MD, PhD

Bullous Diseases...866
  Craig N. Burkhart, MD, MS, David S. Rubenstein, MD, PhD,
  and Luis A. Diaz, MD

Contact Dermatitis.......................................870
  Peter C. Schalock, MD, and Kathryn A. Zug, MD

Pruritus Ani and Vulvae...............................871
  Brenda L. Bartlett, MD

Urticaria and Angioedema...........................873
  Aron J. Gewirtzman, MD

Pigmentary Disorders..................................876
  Robert A. Schwartz, MD, MPH, and
  Camila K. Janniger, MD

Sunburn..879
  Warwick L. Morison, MD

SECTION 14
The Nervous System

Alzheimer's Disease.....................................881
  Monica Peterson Gordon, MD, and
  L. Jaime Fitten, MD

Sleep Disorders...887
  David N. Neubauer, MD

Intracerebral Hemorrhage............................890
  J. Claude Hemphill III, MD, MAS

Ischemic Cerebrovascular Disease................893
  Hans-Christoph Diener, MD

Rehabilitation of the Stroke Survivor.............895
  Richard D. Zorowitz, MD

Seizures and Epilepsy in Adolescents
and Adults...898
  Erik K. St. Louis, MD, and Mark A. Granner, MD

Epilepsy in Infants and Children...................907
  Mary Zupanc, MD

Attention-Deficit/Hyperactivity
Disorder..916
  Christopher Kratochvil, MD, and
  Martin Wetzel, MD

Gilles de la Tourette Syndrome....................918
  Cathy L. Budman, MD

Headache...921
  R. Michael Gallagher, DO

Viral Meningitis and Encephalitis..................927
  Mark J. Abzug, MD

Multiple Sclerosis..932
  Robert J. Fox, MD

Myasthenia Gravis and Related Disorders....940
  Jenice Robinson, MD, and Milind J. Kothari, DO

Trigeminal Neuralgia...................................947
  Ronald F. Young, MD

Bell's Palsy (Idiopathic Acute Peripheral
Facial Paralysis)..949
  W. Cooper Scurry, Jr., MD, Jon E. Isaacson, MD, and
  Fred G. Fedok, MD, FACS

Parkinsonism..952
  Rajesh Pahwa, MD, and Kelly E. Lyons, PhD

Peripheral Neuropathies..............................958
  Kerrie Schoffer, MD, FRCPC

Management of Head Injuries......................965
  Todd W. Vitaz, MD

Traumatic Brain Injury in Children...............969
  Stephen R. Deputy, MD

Brain Tumors..972
  Ashwatha Narayana, MD, Eve S. Ferdman, BA, and
  Shahzad Raza, MD

SECTION 15
The Locomotor System

Rheumatoid Arthritis...................................977
  Eric L. Matteson, MD, MPH

Juvenile Idiopathic Arthritis.........................983
  Terry L. Moore, MD

Ankylosing Spondylitis................................986
  Finbar D. O'Shea, MB, MRCPI, and
  Robert D. Inman, MD

Temporomandibular Disorders and
Orofacial Pain...988
  Richard Ohrbach, DDS, PhD, and
  Jeffrey Burgess, DDS, MSD

Bursitis, Tendinitis, Myofascial Pain,
and Fibromyalgia..994
  Kevin Deane, MD

Osteoarthritis..998
  David H. Neustadt, MD

Polymyalgia Rheumatica and Giant
Cell Arteritis...1002
  Gideon Nesher, MD

Osteomyelitis...1005
Luca Lazzarini, MD

Common Sports Injuries..............................1007
Dennis Y. Wen, MD

SECTION 16
Obstetrics and Gynecology

Antepartum Care..1011
Kirk D. Ramin, MD, and Jessica P. Swartout, MD

Ectopic Pregnancy..1017
Gary H. Lipscomb, MD

Vaginal Bleeding in Late Pregnancy..............1019
Jami Star Zeltzer, MD

Hypertensive Disorders of Pregnancy............1021
Baha M. Sibai, MD

Postpartum Care...1027
Brenda Stokes, MD

Resuscitation of the Newborn.......................1029
O. D. Saugstad, MD, PhD

Care of the High-Risk Neonate.....................1033
Dilcia McLenan, MD

Normal Infant Feeding..................................1041
Meg Begany, RD, CSP, LDN, and
Maria Mascarenhas, MBBS

Diseases of the Breast..................................1045
Panitil Sukumvanich, MD, and Patrick Borgen, MD

Endometriosis...1054
David L. Olive, MD

Dysfunctional Uterine Bleeding....................1058
Beth W. Rackow, MD, and Aydin Arici, MD

Infertility..1060
Steven R. Williams, MD

Amenorrhea...1062
Vicky Martin, MD, and Robert L. Reid, MD

Dysmenorrhea..1065
Laeth S. Nasir, MBBS

Premenstrual Syndrome...............................1066
Ellen W. Freeman, PhD

Menopause..1070
Irina Burd, MD, PhD, Stacey A. Scheib, MD, and
Krystene I. Boyle, MD

Vulvovaginitis...1074
Christine Hudak, MD

Chlamydia trachomatis................................1076
Catherine Stevens-Simon, MD

Pelvic Inflammatory Disease.........................1079
Adrianne Williams Bagley, MD, and
Maria Trent, MD, MPH

Uterine Leiomyomas.....................................1081
Tod C. Aeby, MD, and Stella Dantas, MD

Cancer of the Endometrium.........................1083
D. Scott McMeekin, MD, and
Tashanna K. N. Myers, MD

Cancer of the Uterine Cervix........................1086
Nader Husseinzadeh, MD

Neoplasms of the Vulva................................1091
Susan A. Davidson, MD

Ovarian Cancer...1094
Amanda Nickles Fader, MD, and
Jerome Belinson, MD

SECTION 17
Psychiatric Disorders

Alcoholism...1097
Richard N. Rosenthal, MD

Drug Abuse..1104
Norman S. Miller, MD

Anxiety Disorders...1111
Jacqueline Carinhas McGregor, MD

Bulimia Nervosa...1115
Pauline S. Powers, MD

Delirium..1118
Jonathan M. Flacker, MD

Mood Disorders..1120
Bret R. Rutherford, MD, and Steven P. Roose, MD

Schizophrenia..1128
Jeffrey Rado, MD, MPH, and Philip G. Janicak, MD

Panic Disorder...1131
Manuel E. Tancer, MD

SECTION 18
Physical and Chemical Injuries

Burn Treatment Guidelines..........................1135
Barbara A. Latenser, MD

High-Altitude Illness....................................1140
James A. Litch, MD, DTMH

Disturbances Due to Cold 1143
Frederick K. Korley, MD, and Jerrold B. Leikin, MD

Disturbances Caused by Heat 1148
John F. Coyle II, MD

Spider Bites and Scorpion Stings 1150
Rachel Haroz, MD, and James R. Roberts, MD

Snakebite 1152
Craig S. Kitchens, MD

Marine Poisonings, Envenomations,
and Trauma 1155
Allen Perkins, MD, MPH

Medical Toxicology: Ingestions,
Inhalations, and Dermal and Ocular
Absorptions 1160
Howard C. Mofenson, MD, Thomas R. Caraccio, PharmD,
Michael McGuigan, MD, and Joseph Greensher, MD

SECTION 19
Appendices and Index

Reference Intervals for the Interpretation of
Laboratory Tests 1217
Laura J. McCloskey, PhD

Toxic Chemical Agents Reference Chart:
Symptoms and Treatment 1226
James J. James, MD, DrPH, MHA, and
James M. Lyznicki, MS, MPH

Biologic Agents Reference Chart—Symptoms,
Tests, and Treatment 1229
James J. James, MD, DrPH, MHA, and
James M. Lyznicki, MS, MPH

Some Popular Herbs and Nutritional
Supplements 1234
Miriam M. Chan, BSc, PharmD

New Drugs in 2008 and Agents Pending FDA
Approval 1243
Miriam M. Chan, BSc, PharmD

Index 1251

SECTION 1

Symptomatic Care Pending Diagnosis

Pain

Method of
Trish Palmer, MD

Pain is one of the major determinants of quality of life. To this extent, it is imperative to assess and manage pain, regardless of the diagnosis. The patient experiences pain physically, psychologically, and psychosocially, especially when it is chronic. All of these aspects of pain must be taken into account for effective pain management.

According to the National Center for Health Statistics, one in four adults suffered a day-long bout of pain within the last month, and 1 in 10 adults reports pain lasting longer than 1 year. Low back pain is the most common, followed by headache and joint pain (usually at the knee).

Classification

Definitions of acute and chronic pain vary. Acute pain has a definite start date, is abrupt in onset, and lasts less than 6 weeks, whereas chronic pain is more gradual in onset and lasts for more than 6 weeks. Acute pain in general is expected to resolve; with chronic pain, the expectation is to use long-term tools to manage the pain.

Pain is also commonly classified as nociceptive, neuropathic, or a mixture of both. Nociceptive pain results from irritated musculoskeletal tissue (somatic) or organ tissue (visceral). Neuropathic pain involves irritation of nerves. Some painful problems (cancer, back pain) can have a mixed origin. Although not always possible, it is quite helpful to localize the pain generator or to narrow the diagnosis to the most specific cause possible, because this opens up many disease-specific management options. Migraines can respond to triptans, diabetic peripheral neuropathy can respond to pregabalin (Lyrica), and rheumatoid arthritis can respond to disease-modifying antirheumatic drugs (DMARDs) or biologicals (Box 1).

Pain as a Vital Sign

It is important to assess pain at every medical visit when pain is a complaint. Think of pain as a vital sign. Ask about the level of pain at every visit, and attach a number to it. Use a numerical rating scale, with a rating of 0 to 10, 0 representing the absence of pain and 10 representing the worst pain imaginable. The validity of this approach is well documented. This helps the physician, as well as the patient, to follow the pain level to assess the effectiveness of different interventions. Try to avoid making your own assumptions about the severity of pain, which can lead to undertreatment of pain and underdiagnosis of pain-related urgencies. It is often surprising how well different people deal with pain and a change in their abilities. Ask about current function. This may be the most telling aspect of your conversation and helps to drive disease-specific interventions.

Treatment

Pain is an individual experience. The treatment plan should be tailored to the patient with options for self-management. The objective is to empower the patient as much as possible. What is appealing or acceptable differs from one person to another. Try to understand what your patient is willing to try to decrease the pain, and remember that some of these preferences might stem from their culture or gender. Keep an open mind about how to work within the patient's own framework of dealing with pain. The goal is to decrease pain with methods that the patient understands and accepts, otherwise the pain will not be decreased.

The overriding goals of pain management should be established early on in management. At times it is not realistic to expect to completely alleviate pain, as with some cancers and arthritides. The goal may be to make the pain tolerable enough to permit a desired activity level. This often requires a team approach and creativity. Pain should be treated from a multimodal approach, involving a variety of medications, medication vehicles, nondrug approaches, and complementary methods.

Treatment of acute pain often involves the use of short-acting medications on an as-needed basis. Short-acting medications induce a peak–trough phenomenon: The medication takes a certain amount of time to reach peak effectiveness, and after several hours the effect wears off. This is acceptable for treating short-term or milder pain. There is good patient acceptance of these medications due to experience with these medications, especially because some are available over the counter.

For chronic pain, long-acting preparations are more effective for pain control and less likely to cause problems (e.g., confusion about appropriate use, overdosing). Use of long-acting or extended-release formulations avoids the peak–trough effect of short-acting preparations by providing more constant levels of pain medication and therefore a more constant level of pain control. It is imperative to address patient acceptance and concerns of chronic pain management. Many people are concerned about becoming dependent on medications, especially opioids. Most of these patients are ideal candidates for opioids because they are less likely to misuse these medications.

BOX 1 Disease-Specific Medications

Diabetic Neuropathic Pain
First-Line Medications
Duloxetine (Cymbalta)
Oxycodone (OxyContin)[1]
Pregabalin (Lyrica)
Tricyclic antidepressants[1]

Second-Line Medications
Carbamazepine (Tegretol)[1]
Gabapentin (Neurontin)[1]
Lamotrigine (Lamictal)[1]
Tramadol (Ultram)[1]
Venlafaxine ER (Effexor XR)[1]

Fibromyalgia
Pregabalin (Lyrica)

Gout
Allopurinol (Zyloprim)
Colchicine

Migraine
Triptans

Muscle Spasm
Muscle relaxants

Neuropathic Pain
Anticonvulsants
Gabapentin (Neurontin)[1]
Pregabalin (Lyrica)
Tricyclic antidepressants

Rheumatic Process
Biologicals
Disease-modifying antirheumatic drugs

Swelling
Cyclooxygenase 2 inhibitors
Nonsteroidal antiinflammatory drugs
Steroids

Adapted from Argoff CE, Backonja MM, Belgrade MJ, et al: Consensus guidelines: Treatment planning and options. Diabetic peripheral neuropathic pain. Mayo Clin Proc 2006;81:S12-S25.
[1]Not FDA approved for this indication.

Situations that bode poorly for obtaining good pain relief include older patients, patients receiving worker's compensation, disability, or personal injury claims; and drug abusers or diverters. Depression or other psychopathology can make pain more difficult to manage due to the patient's enhanced perception of pain.

The process of addressing concerns proactively may include a pain contract. A pain contract should define the behavior expected of both the patient and physician and should address all aspects of care, goals of treatment, measures of outcome, and consequences for violating the contract (e.g., lost prescriptions, drug testing, failure to complete recommended testing). The patient should also agree to random drug screens as a part of the monitoring process.

PHARMACOLOGIC TREATMENT

There are three general rules for managing pain: Choose medication to fit the pain; start low and titrate up; and reevaluate the pain at intervals.

Determine whether the pain is likely to be short term or long term, and choose medications specific to the situation. For long-term pain management, I use methods that have the least risk of misuse (side effects, interactions, confusion). In this situation, I use long-acting (twice-daily at maximum) regimens.

Start a single medication at a low dose and titrate up to either side effects or reduction of pain. This helps to determine if a medication is causing a side effect, helps to avoid side effects, and helps to avoid confusion. Add in other medications and nondrug therapies one at a time to be able to assess effectiveness.

Reevaluate the treatment frequently (every 1-2 weeks) until pain is well controlled. Also assess for side effects that can limit use of a medication or modality. The objective is to work with the patient to use methods of pain control that are effective for the individual patient and to introduce them in a stepwise manner.

Medications

Acetaminophen

Acetaminophen (Tylenol, 500-1000 mg PO q6h) is commonly considered to have the least risk, and it is therefore commonly recommended as first-line treatment for many types of pain. It is very effective and often overlooked as a treatment for acute pain and as an adjunct to potentially decrease the dosing of other pain medications.

Many prescription and nonprescription medications contain acetaminophen, and for this reason accidental overdose is a common cause of drug-induced liver failure. Patients at increased risk for liver toxicity include those who fast or have inadequate protein intake (eating disorder) and those who use alcohol on a regular basis.

Nonsteroidal Antiinflammatory Drugs

Nonsteroidal antiinflamatory drugs (NSAIDs) include traditional NSAIDs such as ibuprofen, cyclooxygenase 2 (COX-2) inhibitors, and salicylates (Table 1). These medications are commonly used and are effective for many types of pain. One advantage is that they can decrease swelling, which by itself causes pain and needs to be treated directly. These medications are also used as adjuncts to decrease the dosing of other pain medications. They are relatively safe to use in the short term. Long-term use requires periodic monitoring of complete blood count (CBC) and kidney and liver function.

Celecoxib (Celebrex) is safer for those with a history of peptic ulcer, who are older than 65 years, or who use warfarin (Coumadin) or steroids. For protection against drug-induced peptic ulcer, nonacetylated salicylates or NSAIDs (prefereably etodolac [Lodine] or meloxicam [Mobic]) combined with a proton pump

TABLE 1 Nonopioid Pain Medications

Drug	Dose Range	Frequency
Cyclooxygenase 2 Inhibitor		
Celecoxib (Celebrex)	100-400 mg	Daily
Nonsteroidal Antiinflammatory Drugs		
Diclofenac (Cataflam, Voltaren)	50-100 mg[3]	q8h
Etodolac (Lodine)	200-300 mg	q8h
Mefenamic acid (Ponstel)	250 mg	q6h
Ibuprofen (Motrin)	400-800 mg	q8h
Ketorolac (Toradol)	15-30 mg	xxx
Naproxen (Anaprox, Naprelan, Naprosyn)	250-550 mg	q12h
Salicylates		
Choline magnesium trisalicylate (Trilisate)	500-1000 mg	q8h
Diflunisal (Dolobid)	250-500 mg	q8-12h

Data from Monthly Prescribing Reference. Available at http://www.prescribingreference.com/(accessed April 24, 2008).
[3]Exceeds dosage recommended by the manufacturer.

inhibitor or misoprostol (Cytotec) are recommended. Peptic ulcer occurs without warning symptoms, and it is not related to the dyspepsia also potentially caused by these medications. Heart issues are a recent concern, and the U.S. Food and Drug Administration (FDA) recommends all NSAIDs and COX-2 medications be given "at the lowest dose and for the shortest time needed."

NSAIDs and COX-2 medications increase the risk of myocardial infarction or cerebral vascular accident in those who take these medications for longer periods and in those who have heart disease, although details are not clear at this point. These drugs should never be used just before or after heart surgery, especially coronary artery bypass graft.

Aspirin for cardioprotection should be taken 2 hours before ibuprofen because of the potential for competition for the same binding sites.

Because several NSAIDs are available in a nonprescription strength, it is imperative to know what over-the-counter medications the patient is taking.

Steroids

Steroid (prednisone, Medrol dose pack[1]) medication can be particularly effective for treating pain and swelling. I prescribe prednisone 50 mg PO daily for 5 days, as is commonly done for asthma exacerbations, for acute treatment of severe inflammatory pain. Long-term use of steroids is associated with avascular necrosis, osteoporosis, and adrenal suppression and therefore is avoided.

Tramadol

Tramadol (Ultram 50-100 mg PO q6h or Ultram ER 100-300 mg PO qd) is considered a non-narcotic opioid. It can potentiate seizures in those who are epileptic or who take selective serotonin reuptake inhibitors (SSRIs), tricyclic antidepressants, or opioids. Tramadol can also potentiate serotonin syndrome if taken concomitantly with SSRIs (documented cases), and caution is also recommended if it is taken with monoamine oxidase inhibitors, other antidepressants, or opioids. Symptoms include nausea, tachycardia, agitation, seizure, coma, and hypertension.

Opioids

Opioid medications may be effective in several ways. Short-acting opioids, especially in combination with adjuvants (acetaminophen or NSAIDs) work well on an as needed or short-term scheduled basis for acute pain and as-needed for breakthroughs of chronic pain or exacerbations of pain. Long-acting preparations on a scheduled basis are especially useful for managing chronic pain. The advantage is that these medications have no maximum dose, and dosing is only limited by side effects (Table 2).

Dose-limiting side effects include constipation, nausea and vomiting, sedation, cognitive impairment, and pruritus. I specifically ask about each of these side effects at each visit, because they can occur at any time with opioid use and are easier to manage if treated early. Most side effects decrease over 2 to 3 days after starting the medication or changing the dosing, except for constipation. Constipation is almost universal, and I recommend when starting an opioid medication to begin a bowel regimen with stimulant or emollient laxatives. It is reasonable to give 100-200 mg daily of docusate with senna, 2 pills bid.

Opioid intolerance often results from pseudoallergy due to histamine release causing pruritus. This is most likely with use of codeine, morphine, and meperidine (Demerol); using other opioids often avoids this side effect. Combination products (with acetaminophen, NSAIDs) potentially decreases the amount of opioid necessary to decrease pain and are considered opioid sparing. However, there is a ceiling on dosing these products, usually because of the adjunct.

---

[1]Not FDA approved for this indication.

CURRENT DIAGNOSIS

- Associated constitutional symptoms should prompt a timely work-up for infection and malignancy.
- Bowel or bladder changes associated with back or neck pain should prompt an immediate work-up for cauda equina syndrome.
- Pain that does not follow a typical course deserves a further work-up: blood testing to look for metabolic causes, a second type of imaging, and specialist referral.

Chronic pain should be treated with long-acting medications on a scheduled basis to avoid the rollercoaster phenomenon. Change in activity amount or type, changes in weather, and progression of disease can worsen chronic pain, causing breakthrough pain. Making a plan for treating breakthrough pain, with a prescription for acetaminophen, an NSAID, or a short-acting opioid is effective and lessens anxiety.

Routes of Administration

Typically, pain medication is given by pill, but other methods exist. Many are available in oral liquid, nasal spray, rectal, injectable, transdermal, epidural, or intrathecal forms. These routes minimize gastrointestinal side effects and drug interactions at times. Direct introduction of pain-decreasing modalities to the pain generator can also be more effective than oral dosing.

Topical agents commonly used include capsaicin (Capsin, Zostrix) and lidocaine (Lidoderm). Capsaicin tends to burn initially and needs to be applied several times per day. Lidocaine 5% patch (Lidoderm) is applied for 12 hours per day. Topical NSAIDs are available as Flector Patch and Voltaren Gel. Intraspinal administration tends to avoid gastrointestinal, skin, and sedation problems. Injectables commonly used for osteoarthritis include cortisone and viscosupplementation into the joint. American patients often prefer pills, but these other routes may be more effective and safer for the patient with multiple medical problems.

NONPHARMACOLOGIC TREATMENT

Pay attention to the whole patient. Depression is a common comorbid condition in patients with chronic pain. Try to elicit their concerns because they may be afraid they have cancer, will be debilitated, or will die as a result of their pain. Allaying fears is a powerful method of decreasing pain.

Formal education and support groups can empower the patient to learn to self-administer methods to decrease the pain. The Arthritis Foundation has a self-help course for managing arthritis pain. Some counselors and psychologists specialize in pain control and can help decrease pain and increase functionality. A pain clinic can combine several drug and nondrug aspects of pain control.

For many types of pain (osteoarthritis, low back pain, any source of lower extremity pain), more weight causes more pain. I initially approach the overweight patient with the idea of weight maintenance. I explain that gaining weight will likely make the problem worse. This is a nice introduction for most patients to the idea of trying to lose weight through dietary modification and daily exercise.

Bracing is effective for many types of musculoskeletal pain. There are braces built to offload the medial or lateral joint compartment of the knee to decrease pain due to osteoarthritis and for the lower back to decrease low back pain. Splints and braces are available for almost every joint in the body, some off the shelf, some custom made. Crutches and walkers can offload a lower extremity joint for pain control.

Physical and occupational therapy might help the patient to regain range of motion, decrease swelling, restore better biomechanics,

TABLE 2 Opioid-Based Medications

Drug	Availability	Formulation	Frequency
Butorphanol (Stadol)	IR	1 mg nasal spray	q1-4h
Codeine + acetaminophen	IR	30-60/300 mg tab Liquid	q4h
Dihydrocodeine + acetaminophen + caffeine (Panlor DC, Panlor SS)	IR	16/356.4/30 mg tab 32/712.8/60 mg tab	q4h
Dihydrocodeine + aspirin + caffeine (Synalgos-DC)	IR	16/356.4 mg tab	q4h
Fentanyl (Fentora)	IR	100-800 µg buccal tab	q30min Max: 4 doses
Fentanyl (Duragesic)	ER	12-100 µg/h patch	q3d
Hydrocodone + acetaminophen (Lortab, Maxidone, Norco, Vicodin, Xodol, Zydone)	IR	2.5-10/300-750 mg tab Exilir (Lortab)	q6h
Hydrocodone + ibuprofen (Vicoprofen)	IR	7.5/200 mg	q6h
Hydromorphone (Dilaudid)	IR	2-8 mg tab Liquid Rectal suppository Injection	q4h
Meperidine (Demerol)	IR	50-100 mg tab Liquid	q4h
Morphine sulfate (Avinza)	IR and ER	15-200 mg cap, tab	qd
Morphine sulfate (Kadian, MS Contin, Oramorph SR)	ER	15-200 mg cap, tab	qd
Morphine sulfate (MSIR)	IR	15-30 mg tab, cap Oral sol'n	q4h
Nalbuphine (Nubain)	IR	10-20 mg injection (SC, IM, IV)	q3-6h
Oxycodone (OxyIR)	IR	5 mg cap Liquid	q6h
Oxycodone (OxyContin)	ER	10-80 mg tab	Q12h
Oxycodone + acetaminophen (Percocet, Tylox)	IR	2.5-10/325-650 mg tab	q6h
Oxycodone + acetaminophen (Roxicet)	IR	Liquid	q6h
Oxycodone + aspirin (Percodan)	IR	4.8/325 mg	q6h
Oxycodone + ibuprofen (Combunox)	IR	5/400 mg tab	q6h
Oxymorphone (Opana)	IR	5-10 mg tab	q4h
Oxymorphone (Opana ER)	ER	20-40 mg tab	q12h
Pentazocine + acetaminophen (Talacen)	IR	25/650 mg tab	q4h
Pentazocine + naloxone (Talwin-NX)	IR	50/0.5 mg tab	q3-4h
Propoxyphene (Darvon, Darvon N)	IR	65-100 mg tab	q4h
Propoxyphene + acetaminophen (Balacet, Darvocet N50, Darvocet N100, Darvocet A500)	IR	50-100/325-650 mg tab	q4h
Propoxyphene + aspirin + caffeine (Darvon Compound 32, Darvon Compound 65)	IR	32-65/389/32.4 mg tab	q4h

Data from Monthly Prescribing Reference. Available at http://www.prescribingreference.com/ (accessed April 24, 2008).
cap = capsule; ER = extended release; IR = immediate release; max = maximum; sol'n = solution.

and learn positioning to protect the body part(s). Modalities such as electrical stimulation, ultrasound, iontophoresis, and phonophoresis can decrease swelling and pain. Assistive devices can help the patient to attend to activities of daily living that have become difficult.

Interruption of neural pathways can decrease pain. This is accomplished by injection of alcohol[1] or phenol[1] or by radiofrequency, cryoanalgesia, or surgery. When specific bone or soft tissue structures are the cause of pain, surgery may be effective.

Osteoarthritis of the knee is managed effectively with several nondrug treatments. Acupuncture has been shown to be effective to decrease pain due to osteoarthritis of the knee. Supplements such as glucosamine,[1,7] methylsulfonylmethane (MSM),[1,7] and S-adenosylmethionine (SAM-e)[1,7] are proven effective to decrease joint pain due to osteoarthritis. Fish oil supplements[1,7] are likely beneficial in decreasing pain because of their omega-3 fatty acid content. Supplements are not regulated by the FDA, and patients should be advised to use those that have the USP label (which decreases product variability). Avocado and soybeans might slow progression of osteoarthritis of the hip. Steroid or hyaluronic acid (Orthovisc, Synvisc, Hyalgan, Euflexxa, Supartz) injection into the joint might decrease pain. Specific braces to offload the medial or lateral joint space can decrease pain. Joint replacement surgery can decrease pain and improve mobility.

Issues in Pain Management

Understanding the issues of addiction, dependence, and tolerance is essential for those who are involved in any type of pain management. There is no validated method to predict patient misuse of opioid medication. Published rates of abuse and addiction in chronic pain populations are approximately 10%. A personal or family history of substance abuse and comorbid psychiatric disorders put a patient at risk for misuse of pain medication.

Addiction is a craving for or excessive or persistent use despite adverse consequences. In patients with pain, addiction is rare, especially with long-term use of the medication. Look for the three Cs of addiction: consequences, control, and craving. Consequences of personal harm resulting from use or misuse include intoxication, somnolence, sedation, declining activity level, labile mood, increasing sleep disturbance, increasing pain complaints, and increasing relationship dysfunction. Impaired control over use can be indicated

---
[1]Not FDA approved for this indication.
[7]Available as dietary supplement.

CURRENT THERAPY

- Pain management is individual.
- Use a stepwise approach to pain medications.
- Drug and nondrug therapies are effective and should be used concomitantly.
- Combinations of medications can decrease total dose and side effects.

by reports of lost or stolen prescription or medications, frequent early renewal requests, urgent calls or unscheduled visits, abusing other drugs or alcohol, not being able to produce other medications on request, withdrawal noted on clinic visits, and reports of overuse or sporadic use by observers. Signs of craving include frequently missed appointments unless opioid renewal is expected, avoidance of nonopioid treatments, inability to tolerate multiple medications, and failure to improve.

Undertreatment of pain often leads to patients exhibiting drug-seeking behavior, which for the patient is actually an appropriate response. To prevent this, it is important to educate the patient on realistic expectations (pain might not be eliminated) and to see the patient frequently until pain is well controlled.

Dependence is a normal physiologic response to regular use of opioids for more than a few days. Dependence leads to withdrawal on abrupt cessation of the medication. Fear of dependence often leads both patients and physicians to avoid opioid medication, thereby potentially precluding adequate pain relief.

Tolerance is a condition in which progressively larger doses of opioid are needed to produce the same level of analgesia; it is usually limited to the initial phase of drug titration and rarely seen afterward. What seems to be tolerance after pain control is achieved may be a worsening of the underlying condition causing the pain.

Fear of litigation should not limit use of opioids in appropriate patients. All of the legal cases have been based on inappropriate behavior by physicians, consisting of prescribing for themselves or for those who are not their patients, prescribing without a reasonable indication for opioids, failure to address addictive behavior, and lack of documentation of history or physical examination.

Often, patients taking opioids desire to stop the medication. Although this may be understandable, it is often an unrealistic goal. If the pain is not resolvable, it is more realistic to continue medication to maintain pain control. This should not induce fear or concern on the part of the physician or patient, because some types of pain are not resolvable. Just as diabetic patients need to continue insulin, or they will develop symptoms and complications of diabetes, patients with chronic pain need to continue pain medication. Many medical problems are not curable, yet they can be effectively managed.

Pain Emergencies

Any type of pain that is associated with constitutional symptoms such as fevers, chills, night sweats, or weight loss should prompt an investigation looking for infection and malignancy. Back or neck pain associated with bowel or bladder changes indicates possible cauda equina syndrome, which requires immediate surgical evaluation. Any pain that does not follow a typical course deserves a further work-up, including blood testing to look for metabolic causes, a second type of imaging, or specialist referral. A patient with known cancer and an acute pain increase or a new pain should be urgently evaluated.

REFERENCES

Agency for Healthcare Research and Quality: Assessment and management of chronic pain. Available at http://www.guidelines.gov/summary/summary.aspx?doc_id=10724&nbr=005586&string=chronic+AND+pain (accessed April 24, 2008).
American Society of Addiction Medicine, American Academy of Pain Medicine, American Pain Society: Definitions related to the use of opioids for the treatment of pain. Consensus statement, 2001. Available at http://www.ampainsoc.org/advocacy/opioids2.htm (accessed April 24, 2008).
Bope ET, Douglass AB, Gibovsky A, et al: Pain management by the family physician: The Family Practice Pain Education Project. J Am Board Fam Pract 2004;17:S1-S12.
Berman BM, Lao L, Langenberg P, et al: Effectiveness of acupuncture as adjunctive therapy in osteoarthritis of the knee: A randomized controlled trial. Ann Intern Med 2004;141(12):901-910.
Catella-Lawson F, Reilly MP, Kapoor SC, et al: Cyclooxygenase inhibitors and the antiplatelet effects of aspirin. N Engl J Med 2001;345:1809-1817.
Federal Drug Administration: Medication guide for non-steroidal anti-inflammatory drugs (NSAIDs). Available at www.fda.gov/cder/drug/infopage/COX2/NSAIDmedguide.htm (accessed April 24, 2008).
Hardy M, Coulter I, Morton SC, et al: S-Adenosyl-L-methionine (SAMe) for depression, osteoarthritis, and liver disease. Evidence Report/Technology Assessment Number 64, 2002. Rockville, Md: Agency for Healthcare Research and Quality, US Department of Health and Human Services. AHRQ publication 02-E033. Available at http://www.ahrq.gov/clinic/tp/sametp.htm (accessed April 24, 2008).
Jensen MP, Karoly P: Self-report scales and procedures for assessing pain in adults. In Turk DC and Melzack R (eds): Handbook of Pain Assessment, 2nd ed, New York: Guilford Press, 1991, pp 15-35.
Lequesne M, Maheu E, Cadet C, Dreiser RL: Structural effect of avocado/soybean unsaponifiables on joint space loss in osteoarthritis of the hip. Arthritis Rheum 2002;47:50-58.
Richard J, Reidenberg MM: The risk of disciplinary action by state medical boards against physicians prescribing opioids. J Pain Symptom Manage 2005;29(2):206-212.
Spiller H, Gorman S, Villalobos D, et al: Prospective multicenter evaluation of tramadol exposure. J Toxicol Clin Toxicol 1997;35:361-364.
Usha PR, Naidu MUR: Randomised, double-blind, parallel, placebo-controlled study of oral glucosamine, MSM, and their combinations. Clin Drug Invest 2004;24:353-364.

Nausea and Vomiting

Method of
Chad M. Braun, MD

Nausea and vomiting are protective reflexes caused by a wide range of etiologies spanning from benign conditions to emergent disorders. Nausea and vomiting can occur independently but most often are associated. Usually nausea precedes vomiting and is often accompanied by skin pallor, increased sweating, and feeling flushed. It is also described as the urge to vomit. Vomiting (emesis) is the forceful oral expulsion of the contents of the stomach. Retching is the repetitive contraction of the muscles of the diaphragm and abdominal wall that often precede or accompany vomiting. Nausea and vomiting are mediated by efferent stimuli from the vomiting center in the brain to the musculature in the abdomen and chest. The neurotransmitters commonly associated with nausea and vomiting are acetylcholine, histamine, serotonin, and dopamine. These neurotransmitters are important in the treatment of persistent or severe nausea and vomiting. Most episodes of nausea and vomiting are acute, self-limited, and easily diagnosed based on the clinical picture. Chronic nausea and vomiting (1 month or more) is a diagnostic and therapeutic challenge for the clinician.

TABLE 1 Differential Diagnosis of Nausea and Vomiting

Medications
Analgesics—acetaminophen, aspirin, nonsteroidal anti-inflammatory drugs (NSAIDs), rheumatologic and antigout drugs, opioids (codeine, morphine, oxycodone [Roxicodone])
Anesthetic agents—halothane, fentanyl (Sublimaze)
Antiasthmatics—theophylline
Anticonvulsants—phenobarbital, phenytoin (Dilantin)
Antidepressants—selective serotonin reuptake inhibitors (SSRIs)
Antimicrobials—acyclovir (Zovirax), erythromycin, itraconazole (Sporanox), metronidazole (Flagyl), sulfonamides, tetracycline
Antiparkinsonian drugs—levodopa (Dopar), carbidopa (Lodosyn)
Cancer chemotherapy—cisplatin (Platinol-AQ), cyclophosphamide (Cytoxan), dacarbazine (DTIC-Dome), nitrogen mustard
Cardiovascular agents—antiarrhythmics, antihypertensives, β-blockers, calcium channel antagonists, digoxin, diuretics
Corticosteroids—prednisone
Diabetic drugs—sulfonylureas, metformin (Glucophage)
Ergot alkaloids—dihydroergotamine (Migranal), ergotamine (Ergomar), methysergide (Sansert)
Gastrointestinal agents—azathioprine (Imuran), sulfasalazine (Azulfidine)
Hormonal agents—estrogen, progesterone, oral contraceptives
Iron replacement—ferrous sulfate
Substance abuse—alcohol, nicotine

Infectious Causes
Gastroenteritis—viral, bacterial, parasitic
Other—otitis media, systemic sepsis

Gastrointestinal Disorders
Functional disorders—chronic intestinal pseudoobstruction, gastroparesis, irritable bowel syndrome, nonulcer dyspepsia
Mechanical obstruction—gastric outlet obstruction, small bowel obstruction
Organic gastrointestinal disorders
Appendicitis
Hepatobiliary disease—biliary colic, cholecystitis, hepatitis, neoplasia
Inflammatory bowel disease—Crohn's disease
Mesenteric ischemia
Peptic diseases—esophagitis, *Helicobacter pylori*, nonulcer dyspepsia, peptic ulcer disease

Pancreatic disease—pancreatitis, pancreatic adenocarcinoma
Paralytic ileus
Peritoneal irritation—peritonitis, metastases
Postoperative gastric surgery
Retroperitoneal fibrosis

Central Nervous System (CNS) Disorders
Increased intracranial pressure—abscess, hemorrhage, hydrocephalus, infarction, malignancy, meningitis, pseudotumor cerebri
Demyelinating disorders
Labyrinthine disorders—labyrinthitis, Méniére's disease, motion sickness
Migraine headaches
Parkinsonian disorders
Seizures—complex partial

Psychologic/Psychiatric Disorders
Anxiety
Depression
Eating disorders—anorexia nervosa, bulimia nervosa
Pain
Psychogenic vomiting

Medical Conditions
Cardiac—acute myocardial infarction, congestive heart failure
Genitourinary—acute nephritis, nephrolithiasis, ovarian torsion, pyelonephritis, testicular torsion
Endocrinologic and metabolic conditions—acute intermittent porphyria, Addison's disease, diabetic ketoacidosis, hypercalcemia, hyperparathyroidism, hyperthyroidism, hypoparathyroidism, uremia
Pregnancy—hyperemesis gravidarum, morning sickness

Postoperative Nausea and Vomiting

Radiation Therapy

Idiopathic Conditions
Cyclic vomiting syndrome
Gastric dysrhythmias

Differential Diagnosis

Causes of nausea and vomiting are numerous and varied (Table 1). Of these causes, one of the most common is an adverse reaction to a medication. Nonsteroidal anti-inflammatories, chemotherapeutic agents, antidepressants, narcotics, antibiotics, and oral contraceptives are all commonly associated with nausea and vomiting. It is important to note, however, that almost any medication can cause nausea. An accurate medication history thus is very important.

Viral and bacterial infections are another common cause of nausea and vomiting. This manifestation is often as an acute syndrome with fever and diarrhea. Common viral agents are rotavirus, enterovirus, and adenovirus. Bacterial causes such as *Salmonella*, *Campylobacter*, and *Shigella* are usually seen with the consumption of tainted food or water and can be associated with bloody diarrhea.

CURRENT DIAGNOSIS

- Acute and chronic nausea and vomiting must be differentiated.
- Nausea and vomiting have a wide range of possible causes.
- Control patient symptoms and then look for an underlying etiology.
- Few evidence-based therapy guidelines exist outside of postchemotherapy and postoperative nausea and vomiting.

Disorders of the gastrointestinal tract can cause nausea and vomiting. Common examples of this are peptic ulcer disease, gastroparesis, dyspepsia, and irritable bowel disease. In addition, gastrointestinal emergencies such as acute appendicitis, acute cholecystitis, mesenteric ischemia, and intestinal obstruction can be associated with nausea and vomiting.

Nausea and vomiting are also exhibited during pregnancy. This is usually most frequent in the first trimester and manifested as "morning sickness." It is most common in the first pregnancy and is usually self-limited. Rarely seen is hyperemesis gravidarum, a condition characterized by intractable vomiting and weight loss that is often accompanied by fluid and electrolyte abnormalities.

Psychological disorders are also associated with nausea and vomiting. These can be seen in anxiety, depression, eating disorders such as anorexia and bulimia, and in psychogenic vomiting. Note that patients with psychogenic vomiting usually maintain a normal level of nutrition because they vomit only a small amount of the ingested food.

Other causes of nausea and vomiting not to be overlooked include central nervous system (CNS) disorders such as acute labyrinthitis, Méniére's disease, and motion sickness. In addition, any condition that causes increased intracranial pressure can cause nausea and vomiting. Further, approximately three fourths of all surgical procedures are complicated by postoperative nausea and vomiting. Most of this is thought to be anesthesia related.

Clinical Assessment

To narrow the wide differential associated with nausea and vomiting, it is important for the clinician to use a thoughtful approach to determine the underlying cause. Assessment begins with the differentiation of these symptoms from regurgitation (passive retrograde flow of gastric or esophageal contents into the mouth) and rumination (an effortless regurgitation of recently digested food into the mouth followed by spitting or reswallowing). With a thorough history and physical examination, the clinician can determine whether the patient can be effectively treated as an outpatient or requires hospitalization for treatment and further evaluation. To do this, the clinician must effectively characterize the patient's symptoms with special attention to the onset, duration, frequency, and severity of the symptoms. Some sample questions and scenarios follow.

When did the symptoms begin? How long have they been present? Acute causes of nausea and vomiting such as gastroenteritis or an adverse reaction to a medication has a much different course than chronic causes such as gastroparesis or irritable bowel syndrome. When does the vomiting occur? Is it in the morning or after meals? The temporal course is important. Early morning vomiting is often associated with pregnancy and uremia, whereas nausea and vomiting after meals can be seen with a motility disorder or an obstruction. It is also important to explore the character of the vomitus, specifically if it contains food, bile, or blood. In addition, the clinician should query the patient about any exacerbating or alleviating factors and whether or not the patient has experienced any weight loss or recently traveled.

After completing the history, the clinician should perform a focused physical examination. Here the key is to search for any consequences or complications of vomiting and to identify any signs that may point to the cause of the symptoms. Areas to be highlighted would be as follows. Vital signs, mucous membranes, and skin turgor should be examined for signs of dehydration. Bowel sounds should be quantified as normal, hyperactive, or hypoactive. The abdomen should be evaluated for distention and tenderness because specific sites of discomfort can give a clue to a diagnosis. Any visible hernias, surgical scars, or peristalsis should be noted. A neurologic exam should also be performed, including an assessment of the patient's optic fundus and gait. The teeth should be inspected for signs of enamel breakdown. A brief screening for any signs of psychological disease such as anxiety or depression should also be undertaken.

Diagnostic Testing

The history and physical examination guides the clinician to any further diagnostic testing that is required. Many cases of nausea and vomiting do not require any further testing. If necessary, screening laboratory testing should include serum chemistries, which may detect electrolyte abnormalities, dehydration or uremia, and a complete blood count, which may detect signs of infection. Depending on the clinical picture, an erythrocyte sedimentation rate (ESR), thyroid-stimulating hormone, and liver and pancreatic function testing can be considered. All women of childbearing age should have a pregnancy test. Stool studies can also be considered (e.g., giardiasis). Serum drug levels for toxicity should be considered in appropriate patients.

Further diagnostic testing is dictated by the patient presentation. If any obstruction or perforation is suspected, flat and upright abdominal radiographs can be obtained. Note that these can be normal in early or intermittent obstruction. Further studies such as an upper gastrointestinal barium study or a small bowel followthrough can be helpful if obstruction is considered. Esophagogastroduodenoscopy (EGD) is used to evaluate the mucosa of the esophagus, stomach, and duodenum for signs of inflammation. Additional testing that may be helpful depending on symptomatology includes an abdominal ultrasound, abdominal computed tomography (CT) scan, enteroclysis, and electrogastrography. For hypothesized gastric motility disorders, a gastric emptying study and antroduodenal manometry can be pursued.

If nausea and vomiting are persistent or severe and a gastrointestinal cause is not found, other etiologies such as systemic disease, CNS disorders, and psychological causes must be considered. CNS causes are best evaluated by head CT or magnetic resonance imaging (MRI). MRI provides better visibility of a posterior fossa lesion if that is of concern. Patients with chronic unexplained nausea and vomiting should also be screened for psychiatric disorders. If the clinician has pursued this diagnostic evaluation and is still unsure of the cause of persistent symptoms, consultation with a specialist should be obtained. Most often this would begin with a gastroenterologist but would depend on the symptom picture.

CURRENT THERAPY

- Most cases of nausea and vomiting do not require any therapy except dietary change.
- Hydration status must be monitored.
- Depending on symptom severity, antiemetics can be given by a variety of routes: oral, intravenous, and rectal.
- Use of medications is often limited by adverse effects.

Treatment

Effective treatment of nausea and vomiting depends on identification and correction of the underlying cause. Most cases of nausea and vomiting require no specific treatment. However, patients may require evaluation for fluid and electrolyte disorders associated with nausea and vomiting. Symptomatic therapy should be based on symptom severity and the clinical presentation. Except in the case of pregnancy or drug overdose, antiemetic agents are often used empirically for relief. Oral rehydration, or intravenous if necessary, can then be pursued. If abdominal pain is also present, surgical consultation may be warranted.

With mild nausea and vomiting, dietary changes may be sufficient. Patients should be counseled to try small amounts (1-4 ounces/serving) of cool, clear liquids and advance as tolerated. A goal of 1 to 2 liters of fluid a day is a good one. If the patient successfully tolerates clear liquids, addition of small portions of easily digested foods such as bananas, rice, bouillon, and toast are in order. Dietary fat content should be reduced. Dairy products should be avoided. The diet can gradually be advanced with easily tolerated foods such as plain chicken or turkey and vegetables, bland soups, and fruit. Food should be consumed deliberately, and the patient should take care not to overeat. Increased physical activity around times of eating should be avoided. Note that nausea and vomiting associated with pregnancy can very often be treated with dietary changes alone.

With persistent or severe nausea and vomiting, antiemetic agents may be warranted. Most of these agents are centrally acting and can be divided into nine families (Table 2). By using medications from different families as needed or in combination, the likelihood of adverse drug reactions can be lessened. Because these agents work in the CNS, most adverse effects are also central, such as sedation, lethargy, and extrapyramidal effects. Outside of postoperative and postchemotherapy nausea and vomiting, there are few trials that identify an antiemetic of choice. Commonly used antiemetics are prochlorperazine (Compazine), promethazine (Phenergan), metoclopramide (Reglan), and trimethobenzamide (Tigan).

Antiemetic Drugs

SEROTONIN ANTAGONISTS

Ondansetron (Zofran), granisetron (Kytril), and dolasetron (Anzemet), especially when introduced prior to treatment, are effective in the prevention of chemotherapy- and radiation-associated emesis. They are also effective in postoperative nausea and vomiting, but less expensive options (e.g., droperidol [Inapsine] and dexamethasone [Decadron][1]) are equally effective. The serotonin antagonists are usually well tolerated.

---

[1]Not FDA approved for this indication.

TABLE 2 Commonly Used Medications for Nausea and Vomiting

Class/Medication	Usual Dosage	Route(s)	Adverse Effects
Anticholinergic			
Scopolamine (Transderm Scop)	1 patch every 3 d	Transdermal	Dry mouth, drowsiness, impaired eye accommodation; rare: disorientation, memory disturbance, dizziness, hallucinations
Antihistamines			
Diphenhydramine (Benadryl)	25-50 mg q4-6h	IM, IV, PO	Sedation, dry mouth, constipation, confusion, blurred vision, urinary retention
Hydroxyzine (Atarax, Vistaril)	25-100 mg q6h	IM, PO	
Meclizine (Antivert)	25-50 mg q6h	PO	
Promethazine (Phenergan)	12.5-25 mg q4-6h	IM, IV, PO, PR	
Benzamides			
Metoclopramide (Reglan)	5-15 mg q6h	IM, IV, PO	Sedation, restlessness, diarrhea, agitation, central nervous depression, extrapyramidal effects, hypotension, neuroleptic syndrome, supraventricular tachycardia
Trimethobenzamide (Tigan)	250 mg q6-8h	IM, PO, PR	
Benzodiazepines			
Lorazepam (Ativan)[1]	0.5-2.5 mg q8-12h	IM, IV, PO	Sedation, amnesia, respiratory depression, ataxia, blurred vision, hallucinations, emotional reactions
Butyrophenones			
Droperidol (Inapsine)	0.625-1.25 mg q3-4h[3]	IM, IV	Sedation, hypotension, tachycardia, extrapyramidal effects, dizziness, blood pressure increase, hallu-cinations, chills, QT prolongation, torsade de pointes
Haloperidol (Haldol)[1]	0.5-5 mg q8h	IM, IV, PO	
Cannabinoids			
Dronabinol (Marinol)	2.5-5 mg q8h	PO	Drowsiness, euphoria, vision difficulties, somnolence, vasodilation, abnormal thinking, dysphoria, diarrhea, flushing, tremor, myalgias
Corticosteroids			
Dexamethasone (Decadron)[1]	4 mg q6h	IM, IV, PO	Gastrointestinal upset, anxiety, insomnia, hyperglycemia, facial flushing, euphoria, peritoneal itching
Phenothiazines			
Chlorpromazine (Thorazine)	10-25 mg q4-6h	IM, PO, PR	Sedation, lethargy, skin irritation, cardiovascular effects, extrapyramidal effects, cholestatic jaundice, hyperprolactinemia, neuroleptic malignant syndrome, blood abnormalities
Prochlorperazine (Compazine)	5-10 (25PR) mg q6h	IM, IV, PO, PR	
Thiethylperazine (Torecan)	10-20 mg q6h[3]	IM, IV, PO	
5-HT3 Serotonin Antagonists			
Ondansetron (Zofran)	8 mg q8h	IV, PO	Headache, constipation, fever, asthenia, arrhythmias, diarrhea, dizziness, ataxia, tremor, somnolence, thirst, nervousness, elevated hepatic transaminases
Granisetron (Kytril)	2 mg per 24 h	IV, PO	
Dolasetron (Anzemet)	100 mg per 24 h	IV, PO	

[1]Not FDA approved for this indication.
[3]Exceeds dosage recommended by manufacturer.
Abbreviations: IM = intramuscular; IV = intravenous; PO = orally; PR = per rectum.

DOPAMINE ANTAGONISTS

The phenothiazines, butyrophenones, and substituted benzamides are all examples of antiemetics that work through dopaminergic blockade. Phenothiazines are often not effective for severe vomiting and have a high incidence of side effects including sedation, hypotension, and extrapyramidal effects. Metoclopramide (Reglan) is more effective for severe nausea and vomiting but again has a high incidence of adverse effects. This agent has been especially effective in treating gastroparesis. It should be noted that droperidol (Inapsine) has been associated with QT prolongation and electrocardiogram (EKG) monitoring is recommended with administration.

ANTIHISTAMINES AND ANTICHOLINERGICS

Antihistamines and anticholinergics are of value in the prevention of nausea and vomiting associated with inner ear disturbances, motion sickness, vertigo, and migraines. They often cause drowsiness.

BENZODIAZEPINES

These medications can be helpful in psychogenic and anticipatory vomiting.

CORTICOSTEROIDS

Dexamethasone (Decadron)[1] is commonly used in combination with other antiemetics. Use of steroids and serotonin antagonists is effective in chemotherapy-associated nausea and vomiting, and steroids and low-dose droperidol (Inapsine) is useful in postoperative nausea and vomiting.

CANNABINOIDS

Marijuana is used as an antiemetic and an appetite stimulant. Its efficacy is increased when combined with prochlorperazine (Compazine). Dronabinol (Marinol) is a synthetic cannabinoid available by prescription. CNS side effects are very common with these drugs.

NONPHARMACOLOGIC OPTIONS

Note that both ginger and acupressure are effective in the treatment of nausea and vomiting.

Special Circumstances

CHEMOTHERAPY INDUCED

Attempt to treat patients prophylactically to avoid nausea and vomiting. Use combination therapy. Try to avoid using medications from the same family to decrease the chance of adverse reactions. Note that chemotherapy-induced emesis may begin as long as 24 hours post treatment and may require therapy for 4 to 7 days.

DIABETES

Use promotility agents such as metoclopramide (Reglan) for gastroparesis-associated nausea and vomiting.

PREGNANCY

Morning sickness is common in the first trimester of pregnancy but usually resolves by the second. Reassurance, frequent small meals, and dietary changes are usually sufficient. For some patients, pyridoxine (vitamin B_6)[1] is helpful. In most cases, antiemetics are avoided in pregnancy. In severe cases involving protracted symptoms and fluid and electrolyte abnormalities (hyperemesis gravidarum), hospitalization and intravenous hydration may be required. No antiemetics are approved for use in pregnancy. Selection of any medication to be used in pregnancy should be with careful consideration of the severity of symptoms and potential risk to the fetus. Meclizine (Antivert) and promethazine (Phenergan) are used in pregnancy but neither is FDA-approved for this indication.

MOTION SICKNESS

Anticholinergics and antihistamines are effective here. Transdermal scopolamine patches (Transderm Scop) are convenient for those exposed to motion for long periods (cruise ships).

POSTOPERATIVE

Approximately 80% of patients who undergo anesthesia experience nausea and vomiting in the perioperative or postoperative period. Serotonin antagonists or combination therapy with dexamethasone (Decadron)[1] and droperidol (Inapsine) are effective here.

REFERENCES

American Gastroenterological Association: Medical position statement: Nausea and vomiting. Gastroenterology 2001;120(1):261-262.
Anthony L: Nausea and vomiting. *Conn's Current Therapy*, 2004.
Hasler WL, Chung O: Approach to the patient with gastrointestinal disease. *Harrison's Principles of Internal Medicine*, 16th ed. 2005.
McQuaid KR: Nausea and vomiting. *Current Medical Diagnosis and Treatment*. 2006.
Miser WF: Nausea and vomiting. *Conn's Current Therapy*. 2005.
Pasricha PJ: Treatment of disorders of bowel motility and water flux; antiemetics; agents used in biliary and pancreatic disease. *Goodman and Gilman's The Pharmacological Basis of Therapeutics*, 11th ed. 2005.

Gaseousness and Indigestion

Method of
*Satish S. C. Rao, MD, PhD, and
Ashok Attaluri, MD*

Gaseousness and indigestion are common symptoms and usually represent benign illnesses. However, they can cause significant distress, impair quality of life, and lead to loss of time at work. Today, it is possible to diagnose and treat most disorders that cause these symptoms. The key is to identify the underlying pathophysiology and use an evidence-based approach for their management.

Gaseousness

ETIOLOGY

Intestinal gas arises from four sources: swallowed air; CO_2 produced by chemical interaction of gastric acid, food or alkaline secretions; bacterial fermentation; and diffusion of gas from blood supplying the gut. Mostly, intestinal gas consists of H_2, CH_4, CO_2, N_2, O_2, H_2S, and other trace gases. Symptoms arise from an imbalance in production, transit, and expulsion of gas.

PATHOPHYSIOLOGY

Excessive swallowing of air (aerophagia) leads to belching, eructation, or bloating. Fermentation of unabsorbed carbohydrate residues, malabsorption, or bacterial overgrowth causes excessive gas production. Impaired clearance (excess retention) of intestinal gas or gut hypersensitivity has been demonstrated in patients with unexplained bloating. Common conditions that cause gaseousness are shown in Table 1. Gaseousness commonly manifests as belching, bloating, or flatulence.

Belching

Belching refers to the act of bringing up and expelling air from the stomach and through the mouth. Although occasional postprandial belching is normal, excessive belching represents an underlying disorder. Meal-related belching is usually from aerophagia or consumption of carbonated beverages. Hence, further evaluation is not needed. Symptoms unrelated to meals are due to gastroesophageal reflux disease (GERD), achalasia, or peptic ulcer disease. Based on clinical suspicion, these patients might need further testing (see Table 1).

Bloating

Bloating refers to the sensation of fullness in the abdomen, with or without physical distension. Bloating occurs in many functional gastrointestinal disorders, including irritable bowel syndrome (IBS), constipation, and functional dyspepsia. Functional bloating is defined as a recurrent feeling of bloating or visible distention for at least 3 days per month for 3 months *and* insufficient criteria for diagnosis of functional dyspepsia, IBS, or other functional GI disorder (Rome III criteria).

When persistent bloating is associated with abdominal pain, weight loss, or steatorrhea, one should suspect malabsorption, small intestinal bacterial overgrowth, or carbohydrate intolerance. Consumption of nonabsorbable sugars called *fructans* that are present in wheat, onions, and other foods can cause gaseousness. A dietary history, assessed through a prospective 1-week food and symptom diary, is useful. Breath hydrogen and methane testing can facilitate the diagnosis of small intestinal bacterial overgrowth and lactose or fructose malabsorption.

TABLE 1 Causes And Management Options For Gaseousness

Condition	Cause(s)	Diagnosis	Treatment(s)
Mechanical obstruction	Neoplasm, adhesion, stricture, volvulus, intussusception, perforation	Plain abdomen x-ray, barium follow-through or barium enema, upper endoscopy (EGD), colonoscopy, CT scan	Treat underlying disease Surgery
Aerophagia	Anxiety, GERD, smoking, chewing gum, sucking, drinking soda	History, plain abdomen x-ray	Behavioral modification Stop smoking, chewing gum, or drinking soda
Malabsorption	Lactose, fructose, sorbitol, beans, legumes, fats, gluten, fructans	History, food diary, hydrogen breath test, 3-day fecal fat, stool elastase, anti-tTG	Withdrawal of the offending agent (gluten, lactose, fructose), enzyme supplements such as lactase and pancreatic enzymes
Motility disorder	Gastroparesis, dumping syndrome, gas–bloat syndrome hepatic–splenic flexure syndrome, constipation, dyssynergic defecation	History, abdomen x-ray, gastric emptying study, colon transit study, anorectal manometry	Gastroparesis: Prokinetics: erythromycin[1] 125 mg tid, metoclopramide (Reglan)[1] 10 mg tid, domperidone (Motilium)[5] 10-20 mg tid Constipation: Laxatives: PEG (Miralax) 17 g qd, milk of magnesia 10-30 mL bid, bisacodyl (Dulcolax) 5-10 mg qd; chloride channel activators: lubiprostone (Amitiza) 24 µg bid Dyssynergic defecation: biofeedback therapy Gas–bloat syndrome: Small meals, prokinetics, dilation, reversal of Nissen fundoplication
Bacterial overgrowth	Diabetes, chronic PPI use, gastrectomy, Nissen fundoplication, scleroderma	Hydrogen breath test, EGD with small bowel aspirate and culture	Antibiotics for 2 weeks: amoxicillin[1] 500 mg tid, metronidazole (Flagyl)[1] 500 mg tid, levofloxacin (Levaquin)[1] 500 mg qd, rifaximin (Xifaxan)[1] 400 mg bid-tid
Chronic cholecystitis	Gallstones	Ultrasound, CT scan, HIDA scan	Cholecystectomy
Functional gas and bloating	Irritable bowel syndrome, visceral hyperalgesia	History, Rome criteria, limited tests to exclude organic disease	Low dose antidepressants: amitriptyline (Elavil)[1] 25 mg qhs, nortriptyline (Pamelor)[1] 25 mg qhs, citalopram (Celexa)[1] 20 mg qd, trazodone (Desyrel)[1] 50 mg qhs, sertraline (Zoloft)[1] 50 mg qd, paroxetine (Paxil)[1] 20 mg qd Antispasmodics: dicyclomine (Bentyl) 10-20 mg bid

[1]Not FDA approved for this indication.
[5]Investigational drug in the United States.
CT = computed tomography; EGD = esophagogastroduodenoscopy; GERD = gastroesophageal reflux disease; HIDA = hydroxyiminodiacetic acid; PEG = polyethylene glycol; PPI = proton pump inhibitor; tTG = tissue transglutaminase.

Chronic cholecystitis, pancreatitis, obstruction from intestinal stricture, or inflammatory bowel disease affecting the small bowel or colon also cause bloating. If clinical suspicion is high, patients require a colonoscopy, capsule endoscopy, or barium follow-through studies. If celiac disease is suspected, serologic testing, tissue transglutaminase (tTG) antibody, and endoscopy and small bowel biopsy are useful. Children in daycare and persons who consume well water are susceptible to giardiasis. A stool examination for ova and parasites can be diagnostic. Following Nissen fundoplication, 10% to 20% of patients report postprandial bloating (gas–bloat syndrome) from their inability to belch air.

Flatulence

Flatulence is the act of passing intestinal gas from the anus. New onset of excessive flatulence, especially when associated with pain, weight loss, or steatorrhea, suggests malabsorption. Persistent or intermittent symptoms without weight loss can result from carbohydrate malabsorption (see Table 1) or motility disorders such as slow-transit constipation, dyssynergic defecation, gastroparesis, or pseudo-obstruction syndromes. Rarely, functional disorders such as hepatic–splenic flexure syndrome cause symptoms because of prolonged entrapment of colonic gas from anatomic aberrations. Recently, altered fecal microbiota has been shown in IBS, suggesting an imbalance of colonic flora.

TREATMENT

Treatment depends on the underlying etiology (see Table 1). Mechanical obstruction that does not respond to conservative management is best treated by surgery. Aerophagia requires behavioral modification. The cornerstone for treating carbohydrate malabsorption is withdrawal of the offending agent. Lactose-free milk or cheese and lactase enzyme supplements are helpful. Dietary fructose intolerance is best treated by decreasing fructose consumption; 70% of patients can improve. Adding dextrose powder to fructose products can facilitate fructose absorption. Products such as Beano or Fiberase[2] can help patients with maldigestion of beans or legumes. Bacterial overgrowth is best treated with a 2-week course of antibiotics, and celiac disease requires a gluten-free diet (see Table 1).

---

[2]Not available in the United States.

TABLE 2 Causes and Management Options for Indigestion

Condition	Diagnosis	Medication
Drug-induced dyspepsia (NSAIDs, theophylline, bisphosphonates, KCl)	History, EGD with biopsy	Withdrawal of drug PPI (see Table 3) H₂ blockers (see Table 3) Sucralfate (Carafate)[1] 1000 mg bid-tid
Helicobacter pylori gastritis	H. pylori serum antibody or breath test or stool antigen Rapid urease test Gastric biopsy	Triple therapy: Metronidazole (Flagyl) 500 mg PO tid or amoxicillin 500 mg tid plus Clarithromycin (Biaxin) 500 mg tid plus PPI (see Table 3) Bismuth subsalicylate (Pepto-Bismol) 262 mg, 2 tabs bid*
Bile reflux gastritis	Endoscopy Antral biopsy	Sucralfate[1] 1000 mg bid-tid Metoclopramide (Reglan)[1] 10 mg tid Alginate antacids
Gastroesophageal reflux disease	History 24-hour pH study Endoscopy	PPI (see Table 3) H₂ blocker (see Table 3) Sucralfate[1] 1000 mg bid-tid
Peptic ulcer disease	Endoscopy, biopsy Barium study	PPI (see Table 3) H₂ blocker (see Table 3) Sucralfate[1] 1000 mg bid-tid
Functional or nonulcer dyspepsia	History Rome criteria EGD	PPI (see Table 3) Low-dose antidepressants Prokinetics (see Table 1)
Cholelithiasis	Ultrasound, CT scan	Cholecystectomy

[1]Not FDA approved for this indication.
*May be used alone or in combination with triple therapy.
CT = computed tomography; EGD = esophagogastroduodenoscopy; NSAID = nonsteroidal antiinflammatory drug; PPI = proton pump inhibitor.

The management of patients with functional bloating or IBS is less satisfactory. Low-dose antidepressants or antispasmodics might help. A subset of patients with IBS symptoms have small intestinal bacterial overgrowth and might benefit from antibiotics.

Osmotic laxatives (magnesium hydroxide [milk of magnesia], polyethylene glycol [Miralax]), bisacodyl (Dulcolax), or lubiprostone (Amitiza), a chloride channel activator can help constipation. Fiber supplements and lactulose (Cephulac) increase gaseousness and must be avoided. Likewise, sorbitol products, artificial sweeteners, carbonated beverages, and chewing gum should be discontinued.

Indigestion

Indigestion or dyspepsia is defined as persistent or recurrent epigastric discomfort or pain, often following meals. Dyspepsia manifests with a constellation of symptoms, including pain or discomfort, postprandial fullness, bloating, early satiety, nausea, vomiting, heartburn, and acid regurgitation. The prevalence of dyspepsia is estimated at 5% to 20% and is more common in women. Functional dyspepsia has been defined (Rome III) as persistent or recurrent epigastric discomfort or pain, without evidence of organic disease, relief by defecation, or altered bowel function, over at least 12 weeks over the preceding 12 months.

PATHOPHYSIOLOGY

The pathophysiology of dyspepsia is complex and incompletely understood. Organic diseases including GERD, peptic ulcer disease, and *Helicobacter pylori* infection are common, but most patients with dyspepsia have no identifiable organic disease, and their symptoms are therefore classified as functional dyspepsia (Tables 2 and 3). Visceral hypersensitivity, delayed or accelerated gastric emptying, impaired gastric accommodation, or small bowel dysmotility can cause functional dyspepsia. Anxiety and depression are also common and might play a role.

EVALUATION

Diagnostic testing is only indicated when alarm symptoms such as dysphagia, nocturnal symptoms, weight loss, or atypical GERD are present. If so, an upper endoscopy, pH testing, *H. pylori* testing or, specialized testing with gastric emptying, or balloon distention studies or small bowel manometry may be useful (see Tables 2 and 3).

TABLE 3 H₂ Blocker and Proton Pump Inhibitor Dosing

Drug	Dose
H₂ Blockers	
Famotidine (Pepcid)	20 mg qd-bid
Ranitidine (Zantac)	150-300 mg qd-bid
Proton Pump Inhibitors	
Esomeprazole (Nexium)	40 mg qd-bid
Lansoprazole (Prevacid)	30 mg qd-bid
Omeprazole (Prilosec)	20-40 mg qd-bid
Pantoprazole (Protonix)	40 mg qd-bid
Rabeprazole (Aciphex)	20 mg qd-bid

TREATMENT

In younger patients with mild or occasional GERD and no alarm features, empiric treatment with H_2 blockers or proton pump inhibitors is sufficient. If *H. pylori* is present, eradication can improve symptoms. A recent Cochrane Database[1] review found good evidence to support the empiric use of H_2 blockers or proton pump inhibitors and prokinetic agents (cisapride [Propulsid],[5] domperidone [Motilium][5]). However, cisapride is only available through an investigational limited-access program. There is little evidence to support the use of metoclopramide (Reglan),[1] misoprostol (Cytotec),[1] sucralfate (Carafate),[1] and antacids.

There is good evidence for the use of antianxiety and antidepressant medications (selective serotonin reuptake inhibitors and tricyclic antidepressants). In selects patients, cognitive behavior therapy and hypnotherapy may be useful. Generous and repeated reassurance, follow-up, and supportive therapy remain the mainstays of treatment.

REFERENCES

Bharucha AE, Wald A, Enck P, Rao S: Functional anorectal disorders. Gastroenterology 2006;130:1510-1518.
Choi YK, Kraft N, Zimmerman B, et al: Fructose intolerance in IBS and utility of fructose-restricted diet. J Clin Gastroenterol 2008;42(3):233-238.
Longstreth GF, Thompson WG, Chey WD, et al: Functional bowel disorders. Gastroenterology 2006;130:1480-1491.
Moayyedi P, Soo S, Deeks J, et al: Pharmacological interventions for non-ulcer dyspepsia. Cochrane Database Syst Rev 2006;(4):CD001960.
Pimentel M, Chow EJ, Lin HC: Eradication of small intestinal bacterial overgrowth reduces symptoms of irritable bowel syndrome. Am J Gastroenterol 2000;95:3503-3506.
Ramkumar D, Rao SSC: Efficacy and safety of traditional medical therapies for chronic constipation: Systematic review. Am J Gastroenterol 2005; 100:936-971.
Saad RJ, Chey WD: Review: Prokinetics, histamine H2 receptor antagonists, antimuscarinics, and proton pump inhibitors improve global symptoms in non-ulcer dyspepsia. Evid Based Med 2007;12(3):79.

Hiccups

Method of
Rita Moretti, MD, and Paola Torre, MD

Hiccup is a distinctive sound caused by contractions of the inspiratory muscles and terminated abruptly by the closure of the glottis. The closure occurs almost immediately after the onset of diaphragmatic contraction, minimizing the ventilatory effect. The frequency of hiccupping is modulated by arterial P_{CO_2}. Accordingly, hiccups are most common at maximal inspiration, because the vagal afferents are inhibited by maximal lung inflation.

The real nature of hiccups is not perfectly clear; it has been proposed that hiccups are an abnormal reflex, or myoclonus, generated by repetitive activity of the inspiratory solitary nucleus due to release of higher nervous system inhibitory-regulatory control.

Etiology

Hiccup, therefore, may be due to a persistent disturbance of one of its reflex arc components, which include vagal and phrenic sensory afferents, medullary respiratory center, descending fibers to the C3 to C5

---

[1]Not FDA approved for this indication.
[5]Investigational drug in the United States.

CURRENT DIAGNOSIS

- Hiccup is a distinctive sound caused by contractions of the inspiratory muscles terminated abruptly by the closure of the glottis. The closure occurs almost immediately after the onset of diaphragmatic contraction, minimizing the ventilatory effect.
- It has been proposed that hiccups are an abnormal reflex, or myoclonus, generated by repetitive activity of the inspiratory solitary nucleus due to release of higher nervous system inhibitory-regulatory control.
- Chronic hiccup is defined as persisting symptoms for more than 24 hours or recurring as repetitive attacks.
- Hiccup is typically defined as of peripheral or central origin.
- Intractable hiccups can be associated with potentially fatal consequences, and safe management can require inpatient rehabilitation.

spinal region, and the efferent motor phrenic fibers to the diaphragm. Recent reports hypothesized that a hiccup-like reflex can be elicited by electrical stimulation to a limited area within the medullary reticular formation, the hiccup-evoking site (HES), and hiccups are rapidly suppressed after microinjection of baclofen (Lioresal)[1] into the HES. Following injections of cholera toxin subunit B into the HES, retrograde-labeled cells were found distributed in the lower brainstem and, in particular, in the nucleus raphe magnus, which contains γ-aminobutyric acid (GABA) cells. It is hypothesized that the nucleus raphe magnus is most likely to be the source of the GABAergic inhibitory inputs to the hiccup reflex arc.

Chronic hiccup is defined as persisting symptoms for more than 24 hours or recurring as repetitive attacks.

Hiccup is typically defined as of peripheral or central origin. In the first case, it has been described as due to gastric distension, sudden changes in temperature, and rapid and abundant ingestion of alcohol. Often it has been observed that gastroesophageal reflux, achalasia, and esophageal or small bowel obstruction can cause hiccups. By irritation of the thoracic afferent fibers, mediastinal diseases and thoracic aortic aneurysms can cause hiccups. Many other causes, such as irritation of the efferent phrenic nerve fibers, subphrenic and hepatic disease, pleural effusion, and lateral myocardial infarction determine hiccups. The involvement of the auricular branch of the vagus nerve might explain the association of hiccups with a foreign body in the external auditory meatus. Systemic disorders such as uremia, diabetes mellitus, hyponatremia or hypocalcaemia, and Addison's disease can cause intractable hiccups. Many drugs, such as doxycycline (Doryx), ceftriaxone (Rocephin), imipenem and cilastatin (Primaxin)) dopamine agonists, and chemotherapeutics in general, somehow cause intractable hiccups.

The origin of central hiccups is tightly related to structural or functional pathologies of the medullary region of the vagal nuclei and of the nucleus tractus solitarius. An occlusion in the territory of the posterior inferior cerebellar artery, brainstem tumors, tuberculoma of the brain, sarcoidosis, infections (such as viral encephalitis, HIV encephalopathy), and demyelination of various origins (multiple sclerosis, lupus erythematosus, vasculitis) of the medullary region can produce intractable hiccups.

Treatment

Treatment of hiccups is sometimes unsatisfactory, and it is still debated. Reversing or treating any underlying causative factors may be useful. A beneficial effect can be derived from stimulation of the pharynx opposite C2 and C3, but this is not easy to perform. Some benefits

---

[1]Not FDA approved for this indication.

CURRENT THERAPY

- Reversing or treating any underlying causative factors may be useful.
- Some benefits have been reported from drugs such as chlorpromazine[1], droperidol,[1] olanzapine,[1] intravenous midazolam,[1] baclofen,[1] dexamethasone[1] alone or plus metoclopramide[1] or plus mycophenolate mofetil,[1] amitriptyline,[1] intravenous high-dose methylprednisolone,[1] high-dose nifedipine[1] and fludrocortisone,[1] amantadine,[1] and various antiepileptic drugs.
- One promising treatment is 3 mL of 4% topical lidocaine.[1] The patient must be instructed to avoid eating or drinking 30 minutes before and 2 hours after taking the drug to decrease the risk of aspiration due to a short-term loss of the gag reflex.
- Many reports show good and persistent results using gabapentin[1] for chronic hiccups. An α2δ ligand, pregabalin,[1] has been employed with good results.

[1] Not FDA approved for this indication.

have been reported from different drugs, such as chlorpromazine (Thorazine),[1] haloperidol (Haldol),[1] droperidol (Inapsine),[1] olanzapine (Zyprexa),[1] intravenous midazolam (Versed),[1] baclofen (Lioresal),[1] dexamethasone (Decadron)[1] alone or plus metoclopramide (Reglan)[1] or plus mycophenolate mofetil (Cellcept),[1] amitriptyline (Elavil),[1] intravenous high-dose methylprednisolone (Solu-Medrol),[1] high-dose nifedipine (Procardia)[1] and fludrocortisone (Florinef),[1] amantadine (Symmetrel)[1], and various antiepileptic drugs. Currently, 3 mL of 4% topical lidocaine (Xylocaine)[1] in a small-particle nebulizer seems to be a promising treatment, but the patient must be instructed to avoid eating or drinking 30 minutes before and 2 hours after administration to decrease the risk of aspiration due to a short-term loss of the gag reflex.

Benefits have been reported from these treatments, but because of the low number of treated patients, the short time of follow-up, and mainly the potentially dangerous long-term side effects of the suggested therapies, none has been uniformly recommended to treat hiccups.

Many reports show good results using gabapentin for the persistent treatment of chronic hiccups. Gabapentin (Neurontin)[1] is a novel amino acid derived by the addition of a cyclohexyl group to the chemical backbone of GABA, the major inhibitory neurotransmitter in the mammalian brain. Gabapentin possesses low inherent toxicity; it is not metabolized and does not affect hematologic or biochemical variables to any significant degree. Recent studies with ^{3}H-gabapentin reveal a specific site of binding in brain but not in other organs. Some electrophysiologic studies suggest that gabapentin acts as a partial agonist at the glycine modulatory site of the N-methyl-D-aspartate (NMDA) receptor. More recently, an α2δ ligand, pregabalin (Lyrica),[1] has been employed with good results.

Intractable hiccups' impact on quality of life has been evaluated, and hiccups are related to other significant complications, including aspiration pneumonia, respiratory arrest, and nutritional depletion. Intractable hiccups can have potentially fatal consequences, and safe management can require inpatient rehabilitation.

It is widely demonstrated that there is a direct GABAergic modulation of the hiccup reflex arc. GABA is an inhibitory neurotransmitter that decreases the transmission of monosynaptic extensor and polysynaptic flexor reflexes at the spinal cord level. Gabapentin[1] causes an enhancement of GABA-mediated inhibition or a modulation of voltage-dependent ion channels involved in action potential propagation or burst generation. Pregabalin[1] is a lipophilic analogue of GABA that can diffuse over the blood–brain barrier; however, it is not pharmacologically active at GABA receptors. It exerts it actions at the α2δ binding site that is located on voltage-gated Ca^{2+} channels in the central nervous system. Binding at calcium-ion channels causes a decreased depolarization-induced calcium influx, resulting in a reduction in the release of excitatory neurotransmitters.

It has been reported that gabapentin causes an elevation of central nervous system serononin, which plays an important role in the inhibition of pain via the raphe–spinal descending control system. This system carries signals from the raphe magnus to inhibit nociception in the substantia gelatinosa of the spinal cord, which contains a high density of projections from the raphe magnus and substance P terminals, opiate receptors, and serotonin terminals. Interestingly, the nucleus raphe magnus is most likely the source of the GABAergic inhibitory inputs to the hiccup reflex arc.

REFERENCES

Brown J, Boden P, Singh L, Gee N: mechanism of action of gabapentin. Rev Contempo Pharmacother 1996;7:203-214.
Fodstad H, Nilson S: Intractable singultus: A diagnostic and therapeutic challenge. Br J Neurosurg 1993;7(3):255-260.
Howard R: Persistent hiccups. BMJ 1992;305(6864):1237-1238.
Jatzko A, Stegmeier-Petroianu A, Petroianu GA: Alpha-2-delta ligands for singultus (hiccup) treatment: Three reports. J Pain Symptom Manage 2007;33(6):756-760.
Kumar A, Droemrick A: Intractable hiccups during stroke rehabilitation. Arch Phys Med Rehabil 1998;79(6):697-699.
Moretti R, Torre P, Antonello RM, et al: Gabapentin as a drug therapy of intractable hiccup because of vascular lesion: A three year follow-up. Neurologist 2004;10(2):102-105.
Oshima T, Sakamoto M, Tatsuta H, Arita H: GABAergic inhibition of hiccup-like reflex induced by electrical stimulation in medulla of cats. Neurosci Res 1998;30(4):287-293.
Rao M, Clarenbach P, Valensieck M, Krätzschmar S: Gabapentin augments whole blood serotonin in healthy young men. J Neural Transm 1988;73:129-134.
Samuels L: Hiccup: A ten years review of anatomy, etiology and treatment. Can Med Assoc J 1952;67:315-322.

Acute Infectious Diarrhea

Method of
Matthew T. Oughton, MD, FRCPC, and Andre Dascal, MD, FRCPC

Diarrhea is defined as production of at least 200 g of stool per day. However, accurate measurement of stool mass is impractical and is most often used only in clinical trials. A more functional definition of diarrhea is an increase in stool frequency and liquidity compared to the patient's usual bowel habit. Diarrhea is generally classified as acute if it lasts no more than 14 days, persistent if longer than 14 days, and chronic if longer than 30 days.

Clinically, there are two major types of diarrhea. Secretory diarrhea is watery, usually produced in large volumes, and contains little or no blood or leukocytes. Inflammatory diarrhea is bloody, usually has leukocytes, and is produced in smaller volumes. Recognizing the class of diarrhea can be useful in suggesting etiologies and in managing the diarrhea.

The precise cause of a case of diarrhea is usually difficult to ascertain, because diarrhea is a nonspecific reaction by the intestine to numerous insults, including infections, toxins, and autoimmune disorders. Acute infectious diarrhea, by definition, is caused by a microbial pathogen. Although infections are the leading cause of diarrhea, many different pathogens cause acute infectious diarrhea, and the likelihood of any particular agent depends on the patient's age, symptoms, and epidemiologic risk factors.

[1] Not FDA approved for this indication.

> **BOX 1 Clinical History for Acute Infectious Diarrhea**
>
> - Description of diarrhea
>   - Duration
>   - Frequency
>   - Presence of blood, pus, "grease" in stool
>   - Symptoms of fever, tenesmus, dehydration
>   - Weight loss
> - Other GI symptoms
>   - Anorexia
>   - Cramping
>   - Emesis
>   - Nausea
> - Previous episodes with similar symptoms
> - Ill contacts with similar symptoms
> - Recent antibiotic exposure
> - Other medication exposure
>   - Anticholinergics
>   - Antimotility agents
>   - Aspirin (ASA)
>   - Proton pump inhibitors (PPIs)
> - Recent dietary history
>   - Shellfish
>   - Undercooked meat (chicken)
>   - Unsanitary water
> - Animal contacts
>   - Turtles
>   - Other reptiles
> - Travel history
>   - Travel to endemic or epidemic areas
> - Sexual history
> - Vaccination history
> - Contact with institutions, e.g., hospitals, nursing homes, daycare facilities
> - Employment history
> - Immune status
>   - Presence of HIV
>   - Presence of other congenital or acquired immunodeficiencies

In immunocompetent adults in the developed world, acute infectious diarrhea is most often a minor and self-resolving ailment. Recent data for the United States estimate an annual burden of between 211 million and 375 million cases, with more than 900,000 hospitalizations and 6000 deaths. However, acute infectious diarrhea can cause severe illness in infants, immunocompromised patients, and malnourished patients; it remains a major cause of global morbidity and mortality. The World Health Organization (WHO) estimates that more than 4 billion cases of acute infectious diarrhea occur each year worldwide and attributes 2 million deaths (5% of all deaths) to diarrheal diseases annually. Most of these deaths are in children who are younger than 5 years and live in developing countries.

Thorough investigation of a patient with acute diarrhea should include a detailed history, physical examination, and laboratory tests (Boxes 1 and 2). In general, clinical investigation of an individual case of acute infectious diarrhea is more useful in identifying sequelae of diarrhea, such as dehydration, than it is in revealing the exact etiologic agent. However, identification of the causative organism can sometimes reveal the existence of a common-source outbreak. One well-known example occurred in 1994, when the state public health laboratory in Minnesota noted an increase in *Salmonella* serotype enteritidis detected in submitted samples; this ultimately led to the recognition of a multistate *Salmonella* outbreak related to improperly cleaned ice cream trucks.

Etiology

It is uncommon to identify the exact etiologic agent in a case of acute infectious diarrhea. However, in some clinical situations, exact identification is important for determining optimal management or possible sequelae. The treatment of inflammatory diarrhea varies depending on the causative organism, and some diseases require alterations in therapy (e.g., suspected *Campylobacter* resistance to fluoroquinolones) or even avoidance of antibiotic therapy (e.g., enterohemorrhagic *Escherichia coli*, in which antibiotic therapy has been associated with more frequent adverse outcomes) (Boxes 3 and 4).

BACTERIA

Escherichia coli

E. coli is a versatile pathogen that causes a wide spectrum of disease affecting numerous organ systems. This is illustrated by the wide variety of diarrheagenic *E. coli*, including enterotoxigenic (ETEC),

> **BOX 2 Physical Examination for Acute Infectious Diarrhea**
>
> - Vital signs
>   - Blood pressure (look for postural changes)
>   - Heart rate (look for postural changes)
>   - Respiratory rate
>   - Temperature
>   - Weight (particularly useful to assess effects of rehydration)
> - Cardiovascular examination
>   - Volume status (jugular venous pressure)
> - Respiratory examination
>   - Rule out hyperventilation (compensatory respiratory alkalosis for metabolic acidosis due to dehydration and loss of bicarbonate)
> - Abdominal examination
>   - Focal tenderness
>   - Guarding
>   - Hepatosplenomegaly
>   - Consider rectal examination (look for bloody stool)
> - Integument examination
>   - Lymphadenopathy
>   - Rashes (rose spots)

> **BOX 3 Etiologic Agents of Predominantly Secretory Diarrhea**
>
> **Bacterial**
> - Enteroaggregative *Escherichia coli* (EAEC)
> - Enterotoxigenic *E. coli* (ETEC)
> - *Vibrio cholerae*
>
> **Viral**
> - Adenovirus (types 40 and 41)
> - Astrovirus
> - Caliciviruses (Norwalk, Sapporo)
> - Rotavirus
>
> **Protozoal**
> - *Cryptosporidium*
> - *Cyclospora*
> - *Dientamoeba fragilis*
> - *Giardia lamblia*
> - *Isospora belli*
> - Microspora species (especially *Enterocytozoon bieneusi*)

> **BOX 4 Etiologic Agents of Predominantly Inflammatory Diarrhea**
>
> **Bacterial**
> - *Aeromonas* sp.
> - *Bacteroides fragilis* (enterotoxigenic strains)
> - *Campylobacter* sp. (particularly FQ-resistant strains)
> - *Clostridium difficile* (toxigenic strains)
> - *Escherichia coli* (enterohemorrhagic, enteroinvasive)
> - *Pleisomonas* sp.
> - *Shigella* sp.
> - *Salmonella enterica* serotypes *typhi* and *paratyphi*
> - Nontyphoid *Salmonella* species
> - Noncholera *Vibrio* species
> - *Yersinia*
>
> **Protozoal**
> - *Entamoeba histolytica*

enteroaggregative (EAEC), enterohemorrhagic (EHEC), enteropathogenic (EPEC), and enteroinvasive (EIEC) strains. In general, people are exposed to diarrheagenic *E. coli* by consuming contaminated food and water.

ETEC is a major cause of infantile diarrhea and traveler's diarrhea. Infantile diarrhea affects infants usually in developing countries, particularly during warm and wet conditions, and traveler's diarrhea affects the immunologically naive tourist under similar conditions. In both cases, a large inoculum is required to cause disease. Major virulence factors of ETEC strains include species-specific fimbriae for enterocyte adherence, as well as heat-stable and heat-labile plasmid-encoded enterotoxins. After a relatively brief incubation period of 1 to 2 days, the infected patient develops a secretory diarrhea that lasts up to 5 days. The cornerstones of management are prevention (through dietary hygiene) and adequate rehydration. Antibiotics use is controversial and usually reserved for moderate to severe disease.

EAEC is recognized as a major cause of children's and traveler's diarrhea. Since the initial identification of EAEC in 1985, studies have identified numerous putative virulence factors, including specific aggregative adherence fimbriae. However, no one factor has been identified in all EAEC strains. This suggests that apart from their aggregative adherence to enterocytes, EAEC strains are probably a heterogeneous collection. However, the clinical disease caused by EAEC is relatively consistent and includes persistent secretory diarrhea with low-grade fever. Management of disease from EAEC requires adequate rehydration; the role of antibiotics remains controversial.

The notorious virulence of EHEC (also known as Shiga-like toxin–producing *E. coli*) has led to frequent media reports of "hamburger disease." *E. coli* O157:H7 is the most common strain of EHEC, although several others have been documented. Unlike most other categories of diarrheagenic *E. coli*, EHEC can cause disease with an infectious dose as low as 10 to 100 organisms. Sequelae of EHEC infection include hemorrhagic diarrhea, hemolytic-uremic syndrome, and thrombotic thrombocytopenic purpura. The primary virulence factor is Shiga-like toxin, which damages ribosomes. The gene for Shiga-like toxin is transmitted between EHEC strains by a bacteriophage vector. A separate virulence plasmid has been identified in certain strains of EHEC, but its significance is uncertain. Management of EHEC disease is supportive, because some evidence suggests that antibiotics can enhance the release of Shiga-like toxin and increase the risk of developing hemolytic-uremic syndrome.

EPEC has been associated most strongly with pediatric diarrhea in both epidemic and sporadic forms. EPEC adheres to enterocytes, causing the pathognomic attaching and effacing lesion seen on pathologic section. It then secretes proteins that initiate signal transduction within the enterocyte, ultimately resulting in secretory diarrhea. Because EPEC causes persistent diarrhea that can lead to significant dehydration, rehydration and antibiotic therapy are usually indicated.

As its name implies, EIEC invades enterocytes, where it then replicates and spreads to adjacent cells. The resulting diarrhea may be secretory or inflammatory and lasts up to 7 days. EIEC is closely related to *Shigella* genetically and in the clinical disease that they both cause. As with *Shigella*, antibiotic treatment reduces duration of symptomatic illness.

Shigella Species

The genus *Shigella* consists of four serovars pathogenic to humans: *Shigella sonnei* (Group A), *Shigella flexneri* (Group B), *Shigella boydii* (Group C), and *Shigella dysenteriae* (Group D). *S. sonnei*, the most commonly isolated species, typically causes secretory diarrhea, and the remaining *Shigella* species cause bacillary dysentery with fever, bloody diarrhea, cramping, and tenesmus. As with the typhoid group of *Salmonella*, humans are the sole host for *Shigella* species; however, the low infectious dose required by *Shigella* species to cause disease is more similar to the nontyphoid *Salmonella* species.

Salmonella Species

For clinical purposes, the genus *Salmonella* can be divided into two broad groups: typhoid and nontyphoid.

The typhoid group, consisting of *Salmonella enterica* serotypes *typhi* and *paratyphi*, causes typhoid (enteric) fever. These organisms exclusively infect human hosts and are transmitted via contaminated food or water. A large inoculum of typhoid group bacteria is required to experimentally produce infection. Some infected persons become chronic carriers who can transmit infection to others, such as the infamous Typhoid Mary. Typhoid fever is endemic in the developing world. The classic presentation of typhoid fever evolves over 3 weeks: a stepwise fever with temperature-pulse dissociation in the first week, abdominal pain and rose spots on the trunk in the second week, and hepatosplenomegaly with intestinal bleeding in the third week. Because these species are only transmitted between human hosts, identification of one case of typhoid fever becomes a public health issue that mandates contact tracing. Possible complications include bacteremia, gastrointestinal bleeding or perforation, cholangitis, pneumonia, and osteomyelitis.

The nontyphoid group consists of all *Salmonella* species except *S. enterica* serotypes *typhi* and *paratyphi*. These species generally incubate in animals and are transmitted to humans through consumption of contaminated food or water; direct human-to-human transmission is exceedingly rare. In contrast to the typhoid group, nontyphoid *Salmonella* species can cause disease with inocula as low as 10 to 100 organisms. The disease that results is most often a gastroenteritis with fever, emesis, and diarrhea that can be secretory or inflammatory, lasting up to 7 days. Possible complications include bacteremia, endovascular infection from seeding of atherosclerotic plaques or prosthetic grafts, and Reiter's syndrome

Campylobacter Species

Campylobacter species are common bacterial causes of acute infectious diarrhea; *Campylobacter jejuni* is the major species that causes human disease. Infection is contracted through consumption of contaminated poultry, milk, or water. After an incubation period of 2 to 7 days, the patient develops bloody diarrhea. *Campylobacter* diarrhea is also notable for its manifold extraintestinal complications, including autoimmune phenomena such as reactive arthritis and Guillain-Barré syndrome. Antibiotic therapy is usually reserved for severe disease or immunocompromised patients, in whom recurrent disease is more frequent.

Vibrio cholerae

Vibrio cholerae is the prototype of an enterotoxic bacterium that causes secretory diarrhea. It is almost exclusively a disease of developing countries with poor sanitation. There have been several pandemics in the last century, with the most recent affecting South America and Central America as well the more typical regions in Africa and Asia. The only two serotypes to cause human disease are O1 and O139; serotype O1 is divided into biotypes *cholerae* and *eltor*. Cholera toxin affects enterocytes to produce a secretory diarrhea described as *rice-water stools*. Disease severity ranges from mild to severe with profound dehydration. Rehydration is the cornerstone of treatment, via oral or intravenous routes as dictated by clinical severity.

Clostridium difficile

Clostridium difficile has been recognized as one cause of antibiotic-associated diarrhea and the leading cause of pseudomembranous colitis since the late 1970s. *C. difficile*–associated diarrhea was conventionally thought to only be a health issue for institutionalized patients who have had recent exposure to antibiotics or chemotherapy. In the last 5 years, however, significant expansions in *C. difficile*–associated diarrhea disease severity and host range have been described by researchers in North America and Europe. Disease severity ranges from asymptomatic colonization to mild diarrhea to fulminant pseudomembranous colitis resulting in colectomy, need for intensive care, and high attributable mortality rate.

Other Bacteria

Several other bacteria are less-common causes of acute infectious diarrhea. They merit some discussion because of their specific clinical presentations or potential for causing severe disease.

Vibrio parahemolyticus

Vibrio parahemolyticus causes gastrointestinal illness associated with consumption of raw or undercooked oysters and other seafood. The spectrum of illness varies widely. Immunocompetent patients usually develop self-limited secretory diarrhea or gastroenteritis with fever lasting from 1 to 3 days, and immunocompromised patients present with severe diarrhea, septicemia, and a profound hemolytic anemia.

Staphylococcus aureus

Staphylococcus aureus causes a variety of gastrointestinal illnesses. It is a common cause of enterotoxin-mediated foodborne illness, manifesting with emesis, watery diarrhea, and cramping after a brief incubation period of 1 to 6 hours. *S. aureus*, particularly methicillin-resistant *S. aureus* (MRSA), is also an uncommon but recognized cause of pseudomembranous colitis.

Bacteroides fragilis

Although *Bacteroides fragilis* is recognized as part of the normal flora of the large intestine, certain strains produce a metalloprotease that has been associated with diarrhea in several studies of human and animal populations. Some studies have suggested that these enterotoxigenic *B. fragilis* strains may be more likely than nontoxigenic strains to cause blood infections.

Clostridium perfringens

Clostridium perfringens is a ubiquitous pathogen that is a common cause of enterotoxin-mediated secretory diarrhea. Its specific enterotoxin (CPE) has been found in all five toxinotypes of *C. perfringens*. Gastrointestinal disease can result from ingestion of preformed toxin, with a short incubation period before clinical disease, or ingestion of a large bacterial inoculum, requiring a longer incubation before disease. Treatment is usually supportive.

PROTOZOA

Giardia lamblia

Giardia lamblia is a protozoan pathogen that causes diarrhea that can be chronic and refractory to treatment. The infectious cyst form is ingested in contaminated food or water, and the trophozoite then attaches to the intestinal wall. *Giardia* has expanded its environmental niche in recent years from the beaver fever endemic to isolated rivers and lakes, becoming a global pathogen.

Entamoeba histolytica

Entamoeba histolytica can cause amoebic dysentery, which can manifest as acute, subacute, or chronic diarrhea. Diagnosis of *E. histolytica* is complicated by the highly similar but nonpathogenic *Entamoeba dispar*. Other than the rare situation where microscopy of stool detects ingested erythrocytes (pathognomic of *E. histolytica*), the two species are morphologically identical and can only be distinguished by methodologies such as serology, antigen detection, or nucleic acid testing.

VIRUSES

Rotavirus

Rotavirus primarily affects infants and children from 3 to 36 months of age, resulting in a spectrum of disease from asymptomatic shedding to severe gastroenteritis with dehydration. Globally, it is the leading viral cause of severe gastroenteritis. Other groups affected include travelers, the immunocompromised, and patients in hospitals or other institutions.

Calicivirus

Norwalk virus is the most well-known member of the calicivirus family. Outbreaks of Norwalk often occur in long-term care facilities, cruise ships, and hospitals. It is highly contagious, with attack rates often greater than 10%. The clinical syndrome of Norwalk infection usually features rapid onset of severe nausea and emesis along with varying degrees of diarrhea.

Differential Diagnosis

OTHER INFECTIONS

Infections that cause diarrhea are not necessarily primarily gastrointestinal (Box 5). Systemic infections that result in diarrhea are probably underrecognized as a distinct etiology; however, the astute clinician should usually be able to recognize a systemic infection after a proper history, physical examination, and appropriate

---

BOX 5 Diseases That Can Mimic Acute Infectious Diarrhea

Infectious Etiologies
- Dengue fever
- *Francisella* sp.
- Hantavirus
- *Legionella* sp.
- Leptospirosis
- Lyme borreliosis
- Malaria
- SARS

Noninfectious Etiologies
- Antibiotic-associated diarrhea
- Bacterial overgrowth
- Brainerd diarrhea (infectious etiology suspected but unproved)
- Endocrinopathies (e.g., VIPoma)
- Inflammatory bowel disease
- Irritable bowel syndrome
- Other medications

Abbreviations: SARS = severe acute respiratory syndrome; VIP = vasoactive intestinal peptide.

laboratory tests. Bacterial infections such as Group A streptococcosis, legionellosis, leptospirosis, and some tick-borne infections (including borreliosis, ehrlichosis, tularemia, and Rocky Mountain spotted fever) can manifest with diarrhea as an initial symptom. Septicemia, caused by a variety of pathogens such as gram-negative enteric organisms, can also cause diarrhea and other gastrointestinal symptoms. Viremia is another cause of diarrhea; the most common cause is probably influenza, but other viruses including severe acute respiratory syndrome–associated coronavirus (SARS-CoV), hantaviruses, dengue virus (*Flavivirus* sp.), and hemorrhagic fever viruses should be considered in the presence of correlating exposures. *Plasmodium falciparum* malaria can result in diarrhea severe enough to mimic bacillary dysentery, particularly in children, and severe diarrhea has been associated with poor outcome.

OTHER NONINFECTIOUS ETIOLOGIES

A variety of noninfectious causes can result in acute diarrhea (see Box 5). For instance, diarrhea is a common adverse effect of antimicrobial agents and other medications. The mechanism varies by antibiotic, but common reasons include direct stimulation of gut motility, increased gut osmolality, and disruption of the normal gut flora.

Although not strictly an infection, diarrhea is one of the most common symptoms of bacterial overgrowth. This disease occurs after disruption of host mechanisms that normally regulate bacterial intestinal colonization, such as pancreatitis or intestinal dysmotility. Definitive treatment should address the underlying condition, but broad-spectrum antibiotics can result in a long-lasting cure.

Brainerd diarrhea was initially described after an outbreak in Brainerd, Minnesota, in 1983. It manifests as an acute secretory diarrhea that can last for several months. Its etiology remains unknown, but several outbreaks have demonstrated epidemiologic links to consumption of unpasteurized milk and undertreated water.

Some endocrinopathies, such as VIPoma, can cause profuse diarrhea. Inflammatory bowel diseases (e.g., Crohn's disease, ulcerative colitis) can manifest with an inflammatory diarrhea and constitutional symptoms. Irritable bowel syndrome can result in periods of diarrhea; however, there are alternating periods of constipation and a lack of constitutional symptoms.

Special Cases

TRAVELER'S DIARRHEA

According to the Centers for Disease Control and Prevention (CDC), 20% to 50% of international travelers develop diarrhea related to their travels. The etiologic agents vary by exposure, geographic region, and local outbreaks. Bacteria are the most commonly implicated pathogens, with ETEC being the most commonly identified cause. Other etiologic agents include the other common bacterial, viral, and protozoal enteric pathogens described earlier. Diarrhea is usually mild to moderate and self-limited; 90% of patients report resolution of symptoms after 1 week, and 98% after 4 weeks. Although it is usually a nuisance rather than a severe threat to health, diarrhea can significantly limit the traveler's activities.

Because traveler's diarrhea is self-limited, investigations of the cause are usually reserved for diarrhea that is prolonged or manifests with higher-risk features such as fever or bloody stool. Stool should be examined for ova and parasites (O&P) if the travel history is supportive.

The focus for management should be supportive care. People seen for travel medicine advice should be counseled to avoid consuming water or food not known to be safe. The safest diet for travelers consists of freshly prepared foods served thoroughly heated, fruits and vegetables that are peeled or are washed with safe water, and beverages that are bottled or boiled before consumption. Ice and tap water should be considered contaminated. Patients for whom diarrhea could be catastrophic should be advised to avoid traveling unless it is strictly necessary.

After the traveler has developed diarrhea, a variety of medications are available for treatment (Box 7). One review determined that antibiotics shorten the duration of traveler's diarrhea but had higher rates of adverse effects compared with placebo.

IMMUNOCOMPROMISED STATES

Gastrointestinal illness is a common problem in immunocompromised patients. Apart from the infectious etiologies of diarrhea described earlier, other causes found in immunocompromised patients include the agent causing the immunocompromised state (such as HIV or chemotherapeutic agents), opportunistic organisms, adverse effects of medications, dysfunction of intestinal absorption, and idiopathic enteropathies.

Opportunistic organisms that can cause diarrhea include parasites (e.g., *Cryptosporidium parvum*, *Cyclospora cayetanensis*, *Isospora belli*, microsporidia), fungi (e.g., disseminated fungal infections from *Histoplasma capsulatum* and *Cryptococcus neoformans*), bacteria (e.g., *Mycobacterium avium-intracellulare* complex), and viruses (e.g., cytomegalovirus, herpes simplex virus). In general, treatment requires prolonged courses of antimicrobial agents and can be complicated by concomitant medications or diseases; consultation with an appropriate specialist is suggested.

Prevention

Methods of prevention are listed in Box 6.

AVOIDANCE

An effective method for preventing acute infectious diarrhea is to eliminate exposures that put one at risk. This applies particularly to patients who would be at high risk for contracting acute infectious diarrhea or having adverse outcomes, for example, patients who are immunocompromised or physically debilitated. Exposure avoidance is usually situational and patient-specific, such as suggesting that travel be postponed to a region currently undergoing a cholera epidemic or cautioning against consumption of raw seafood.

HYGIENE

Proper handwashing by health care workers caring for patients with acute diarrhea is essential to prevent institutional transmission, and its importance cannot be overstated. Barrier precautions are also commonly implemented, particularly if the patient is incontinent of stool. Other precautions, such as tailoring environmental cleaning practices to specific pathogens during outbreaks, are also proven effective.

PROPHYLACTIC ANTIBIOTICS

There is a limited role for antibiotics in preventing acute infectious diarrhea, particularly traveler's diarrhea. The normally mild severity and self-limited nature of the disease, along with the risk of adverse effects from antibiotics, means that prophylactic antibiotics are most often reserved for brief durations in patients at high risk for contracting acute infectious diarrhea or for experiencing adverse outcomes.

BOX 6 Prevention of Acute Infectious Diarrhea

- Avoidance
- Hygiene
- Prophylactic antibiotics
- Probiotics
- Vaccines
  - Cholera/ETEC (Dukoral)[2]
  - Rotavirus (RotaTeq)
  - *Salmonella typhi* (Vivotif Berna, Typhim Vi)

[2]Not available in the United States.
Abbreviation: ETEC = enterotoxigenic *Escherichia coli*.

PROBIOTICS

There has been a surge of publications concerning the role of probiotics in preventing diarrhea of varying etiologies. Although individual studies have produced varied results for diarrhea caused by *C. difficile*–associated diarrhea and traveler's diarrhea, one meta-analysis of 34 studies supported a role for probiotics in preventing diarrhea, with an overall risk reduction of at least 21%. Stratification by type of diarrhea found a much larger reduction in antibiotic-associated (52%) than traveler's (8%) diarrhea. However, these findings were challenged due to the variety of organisms and treatment regimens between different studies, and the low proportion of adult patients in those studies reporting reductions in antibiotic-associated diarrhea.

VACCINES

Rotavirus

A live human-bovine reassortant rotavirus oral vaccine (RotaTeq) has been licensed since February 2006 in the United States for infants 6 to 32 weeks of age. The vaccine appears efficacious in preventing rotaviral gastroenteritis, and consequently it reduces the need for outpatient and inpatient assessment. A large phase III trial demonstrated no increased risk over placebo of intussusception, an adverse effect that led to the withdrawal of a previous rotavirus vaccine. An attenuated human rotavirus vaccine (RotaRix) is licensed in countries throughout Europe, Asia, and Africa, but not North America.

Vibrio cholerae and ETEC

An oral inactivated cholera vaccine (Dukoral), available in Canada but not in the United States, has demonstrated some efficacy in preventing traveler's diarrhea. The B subunit of *V. cholerae* toxin used in this vaccine has sufficient structural homology with ETEC heat-labile toxin to provide moderate short-term protection against this common cause of traveler's diarrhea, lasting up to 3 months.

Salmonella typhi

Enteral and parenteral vaccines are available to prevent typhoid. The enteral form (Vivotif Berna) is a live attenuated strain of *S. typhi*,

CURRENT DIAGNOSIS

History
- Duration and frequency of diarrhea
- Other gastrointestinal symptoms (emesis, tenesmus, abdominal pain)
- Presence of bloody stool, fever
- Medication use, including recent antibiotic use
- Recent contact with ill persons, travel, and animal contact
- Consumption of raw or undercooked poultry or seafood
- Immunocompromised state (rule out)

Physical Examination
- Hydration status
- Gastrointestinal examination
- Other systems as indicated by symptoms

Laboratory Tests
- For limited secretory diarrhea: usually none
- For bloody diarrhea: complete blood count (CBC), stool for culture (rule out O157:H7); consider ova and parasites test (O&P)
- For chronic diarrhea: consider *C. difficile* assay, O&P
- For traveler's diarrhea: CBC, stool for culture and O&P
- For immunocompromised patients: CBC, stool for culture and O&P

BOX 7 Management of Acute Infectious Diarrhea

Rehydration
- Enteral
  - World Health Organization formulation
  - Commercially available rehydration solutions
  - Home remedies
- Parenteral
  - Intravenous
  - Intraosseus
  - Enteroclysis

Medications
- Antidiarrheals
  - Bismuth subsalicylate
  - Morphine derivatives
- Antibiotics
- Probiotics

---

which is taken as four capsules over 7 days and confers immunity for approximately 5 years. The parenteral form (Typhim Vi) is purified capsular polysaccharide that is given as a single intramuscular injection. This is the preferred route for patients with contraindications to live attenuated vaccines, such as immunocompromised status. Neither vaccine is completely protective, and neither provides protection against *S. paratyphi*.

Treatment

Management of acute infectious diarrhea is listed in Box 7.

CURRENT THERAPY

- Supportive care
- Rehydration (always replace previous losses and provide maintenance)
  - Enteral
  - Parenteral (intravenous, intraosseus, enteroclytic)
- Antidiarrheal medications (only if patient is afebrile and stools are not bloody)
  - Morphine derivatives
  - Bismuth subsalicylate (Pepto-Bismol)
- Antibiotics (only if necessary as indicated by symptoms, severity, and risk factors)
  - Empiric therapy
    - Adults
      - Ciprofloxacin (Cipro) 500 mg PO bid for 3-5 d
      - Levofloxacin (Levaquin)[1] 500 mg PO qd for 3-5 d
    - Children
      - Azithromycin (Zithromax)[1] 5-10 mg/kg PO qd for 3-5 d
      - Trimethoprim-sulfamethoxazole (Septra) 5-25 mg/kg/d PO in two equally divided doses for 3-5 d *plus*
      - Erythromycin 10 mg/kg/d PO qid for 5 d
  - Specific therapy as directed by pathogen identification and susceptibilities
- Probiotics

---

[1]Not FDA approved for this indication.

TABLE 1 Empiric Therapy of Diarrheal Disease

Clinical Syndrome	Adult Patients	Pediatric Patients
Febrile dysenteric diarrhea in industrialized regions, or moderate to severe traveler's diarrhea	Ciprofloxacin (Cipro) 500 mg PO bid or levofloxacin (Levaquin)[1] 500 mg PO qd for 3-5 d	Azithromycin (Zithromax)[1] 5-10 mg/kg PO qd for 3-5 d or trimethoprim-sulfamethoxazole (Septra) 5-25 mg/kg/d PO in two divided doses for 3-5 d plus erythromycin[1] 10 mg/kg PO qid for 5 d
Persistent diarrhea (≥14 d in duration) in industrialized countries	Consider anti-*Giardia* therapy: metronidazole (Flagyl)[1] 250 mg PO tid for 7 d	Consider anti-*Giardia* therapy: metronidazole (Flagyl)[1] 20 mg/kg/d PO in three divided doses for 7 d

Adapted from Montes M, DuPont HL: Enteritis, enterocolitis and infectious diarrhea syndromes. In Cohen J, Powderly WD: Infectious Diseases, 2nd ed. St Louis: Mosby, 2004, pp 477-489.

REHYDRATION

Maintaining adequate hydration is usually the cornerstone of management for acute diarrhea. The route of administration depends on the patient's hydration status and disease severity; enteral hydration is preferred to parenteral, if possible.

In 2003 the WHO reformulated their well-known oral rehydration solution (ORS). The new lower-osmolarity formula has been found to reduce stool volume, emesis, and the need for switching to intravenous therapy in children with diarrhea. This new formulation has 75 mmol/L sodium, 75 mmol/L glucose, and a total osmolarity 245 mOsm/L, which can be achieved with a recipe of 2.6 g sodium chloride, 13.5 g anhydrous glucose, 1.5 g potassium chloride, 2.5 g sodium bicarbonate and 1.5 g trisodium citrate dihydrate per liter of water.

A homemade solution can be prepared with 40 mL sugar and 5 mL table salt per liter of clean water; however, this preparation lacks potassium. Furthermore, commercially prepared rehydration solutions should be preferred to homemade in order to minimize the chance of errors in preparing the solution. Most sports drinks are not equivalent to actual rehydration solutions, because sports drinks often have higher carbohydrate and lower electrolyte loads.

Parenteral rehydration is usually intravenous, although intraosseus administration can be used for infants in whom intravenous access cannot be obtained and enteroclysis can be used in adult patients with difficult vascular access who do not require large volumes of replacement fluid. Sufficient volumes of fluid should be given to replace preexisting fluid deficits as well as ongoing losses and maintenance requirements.

ANTIDIARRHEAL MEDICATIONS

Some medications reduce intestinal motility by affecting the myenteric motor plexus to inhibit peristalsis. Opioid derivatives, such as loperamide (Imodium), are the class of medications most commonly used for this purpose. Although licensed for use with acute, chronic, and traveler's diarrhea, loperamide is contraindicated in the presence of fever or bloody stool or in situations where inhibition of peristalsis is otherwise undesirable or potentially harmful.

Other medications are classified as antidiarrheal but have different mechanisms of action. Bismuth subsalicylate (Pepto-Bismol) appears to function by multiple mechanisms including intestinal secretion reduction, intestinal reabsorption of fluids and electrolytes, toxin binding, and direct antimicrobial effects. It has proven efficacy in the management of traveler's diarrhea, although its dosing frequency may be difficult for some patients. Racecadotril (or acetorphan)[2] is a new synthetic enkephalinase inhibitor that acts by the same mechanism as the opioid derivatives and has been studied for its antidiarrheal effect in pediatric patients.

ANTIBIOTICS

Antibiotics should be used cautiously in the treatment of acute infectious diarrhea. Most clinical cases adequately resolve without antibiotic therapy. Furthermore, their use may lead to further diarrhea (including antibiotic-associated diarrhea), contribute to selective pressures favoring development of antibiotic-resistant organisms, and prolong the carriage of certain pathogens. Recommendations in the empiric and pathogen-specific treatment of acute infectious diarrhea are given in Tables 1 and 2.

PROBIOTICS

As with the prevention of diarrhea, a growing body of evidence has yet to provide definite conclusions on the use of probiotics for treating acute infectious diarrhea. One of the major limitations to using probiotics is the variation in species and doses used in different

[2]Not available in the United States.

TABLE 2 Pathogen-Specific Therapy of Diarrheal Disease

Pathogen	Adult Patients	Pediatric Patients
Campylobacter jejuni	Azithromycin (Zithromax)[1] 500 mg PO qd for 3 d	Erythromycin stearate[1] 40 mg/kg/d in four divided doses for 5 d or azithromycin[1] 10 mg/kg/d
Clostridium difficile	Initial disease: metronidazole (Flagyl) 250 mg PO qid for 10-14 d or vancomycin (Vancocin) 125-500 mg PO qid for 10-14 d	Initial disease: metronidazole 20 mg/kg/d in three divided doses for 10-14 d or vancomycin 125-500 mg PO qid for 10-14 d
EAEC, EIEC, EPEC, ETEC	Same as empiric therapy for febrile dysentery and traveler's diarrhea (see Table 1)	Azithromycin[1] 10 mg/kg/d. If resistance is suspected, use ceftriaxone (Rocephin),[1] cefixime (Suprax),[1] or cefotaxime (Claforan)[1]
EHEC*	No antimicrobial therapy (increased risk of increasing toxin release and hemolytic-uremic syndrome)	No antimicrobial therapy (increased risk of increasing toxin release and hemolytic-uremic syndrome)

Continued

TABLE 2 Pathogen-Specific Therapy of Diarrheal Disease—cont'd

Pathogen	Adult Patients	Pediatric Patients
Entamoeba histolytica	Metronidazole 500 mg PO tid for 10 d or tinidazole (Tindamax) 1 g PO bid for 3 d Follow with paromomycin (Humatin) 500 mg PO tid for 7 d	Metronidazole 50 mg/kg/d IV in three divided doses plus diiodohydroxyquin (Yodoxin) 40 mg/kg/d in three divided doses for 20 d
Giardia lamblia	Metronidazole[1] 250 mg PO tid for 7 d or albendazole (Albenza)[1] 400 mg PO qd for 5 d or tinidazole 2 g PO in one dose	Metronidazole[1] 20 mg/kg/d in three divided doses for 7 d or furazolidone (Furoxone) 6 mg/kg/d divided in four doses for 7 d
Shigella sp.	Ciprofloxacin (Cipro) 500 mg PO bid for 3-5 d or levofloxacin (Levaquin)[1] 500 mg PO qd for 3-5 d	Azithromycin[1] 10 mg/kg/d If resistance is suspected, use ceftriaxone,[1] cefixime,[1] or cefotaxime[1]
Salmonella sp. non-typhoid group	Asymptomatic or mild: no antimicrobial therapy At risk for complications: ciprofloxacin[1] 500 mg PO bid or levofloxacin[1] 500 mg PO qd for 5-7 d Alternatives: azithromycin[1] or erythromycin stearate (Erythrocin stearate)[1] 500 mg PO bid for 5 d	≤6 mo old: ceftriaxone[1] 50 mg/kg IV qd >6 mo old and healthy, and asymptomatic or with mild illness: no antimicrobial therapy At risk for complications: ceftriaxone[1] 50 mg/kg IV qd (not to exceed 2 g/d)
typhoid group	Ciprofloxacin (Cipro) 500 mg PO bid for 7-10 d or levofloxacin (Levaquin)[1] 500 mg PO OD for 7-10 d or ceftriaxone 2 g IV q 24h for 14 d	Ceftriaxone 75-100 mg/kg IVq24h for 14 d (not to exceed 4 g/d) or azithromycin 20 mg/kg PO OD for 5-7 d (not to exceed 1 g/d)
Vibrio cholerae	Doxycycline 300 mg PO for one dose or ciprofloxacin[1] 1 g PO for one dose Recurrent disease can require prolonged courses of antibiotics or adjunctive therapy (e.g., IVIG,[1] resins[1])	TMP-SMX (Septra)[1] 1 DS tab PO bid for 3 d or azithromycin[1] 20 mg/kg PO for one dose (not to exceed 1 g)

Adapted from Montes M, DuPont HL: Enteritis, enterocolitis and infectious diarrhea syndromes. In Cohen J, Powderly WD: Infectious Diseases, 2nd ed. St Louis: Mosby, 2004, pp 477-489.
[1]Not FDA approved for this indication.
[2]Not available in the United States.
*Shiga toxin and Shiga-like toxin–producing E. coli.
Abbreviations: DS = double strength; EAEC = enteroaggregative E. coli; EHEC = enterohemorrhagic E. coli; EIEC = enteroinvasive E. coli. EPEC = enteropathogenic E. coli; ETEC = enterotoxigenic E. coli; IVIG = intravenous immunoglobulin; TMP-SMX = trimethoprim-sulfamethoxazole.

---

clinical trials. However, there may be a class effect that is most likely a combination of competition for intestinal binding sites or nutritional resources, elaboration of antibacterial compounds, and immune stimulation. Another recognized limitation is the rare but serious case of blood infection from the probiotic organism; documented cases have occurred not only in recipients but also in other patients being cared for in close proximity to the recipient.

REFERENCES

Aranda-Michel J, Giannella RA: Acute diarrhea: A practical review. Am J Med 1999;106:670-676.
DuPont HL: What's new in enteric infectious diseases at home and abroad. Curr Opin Infect Dis 2005;18:407-412.
Dupont HL, and the Practice Parameters Committee of the American College of Gastroenterology: Guidelines on acute infectious diarrhea in adults. Am J Gastroenterol 1997;92(11):1962-1975.
Guerrant RL, Van Gilder T, Stiner TS, et al: Practice guidelines for the management of infectious diarrhea. Clin Infect Dis 2001;32:331-350.
Hahn S, Kim Y, Garner P: Reduced osmolarity oral rehydration solution for treating dehydration due to diarrhea in children: Systematic review. Br Med J 2001;323:81-85.
Helton T, Rolson DD: Which adults with acute diarrhea should be evaluated? What is the best diagnostic approach? Cleve Clin J Med 2004;71(10):778-785.
Musher DM, Musher BL: Contagious acute gastrointestinal infections. N Engl J Med 2004;351(23):2417-2427.
Reisinger EC, Fritzsche C, Krause R, Krejs GJ: Diarrhea caused by primarily non-gastrointestinal infections. Nat Clin Practice Gastroenterol Hepatol 2005;2(5):216-222.
Sazawal S, Hiremath G, Dhingra U, et al: Efficacy of probiotics in prevention of acute diarrhoea: A meta-analysis of masked, randomised, placebo-controlled trials. Lancet Infect Dis 2006;6:374-382.
Thielman NM, Guerrant RL: Acute infectious diarrhea. N Engl J Med 2004;350:38-47.
World Health Organization: Oral rehydration salts: Production of the new ORS. 2006. PDF available at http://www.who.int/child-adolescent-health/New_Publications/CHILD_HEALTH/WHO_FCH_CAH_06.1.pdf (accessed April 5, 2007).

Constipation

Method of
Robert Fisher, MD, and Brenda Horwitz, MD

Epidemiology and Pathophysiology

Chronic constipation is a common disorder affecting approximately 15% (2%-28%) of the U.S. population, nearly 40 million Americans.

> **BOX 1 Rome III Criteria for Functional Constipation**
>
> Must include 2 or more of the following:
> - Straining during at least 25% of defecations
> - Lumpy or hard stools in at least 25% of defecations
> - Sensation of incomplete evacuation for at least 25% of defecations
> - Sensation of anorectal obstruction or blockage for at least 25% of defecations
> - Manual maneuvers to facilitate at least 25% of defecations (e.g., digital evacuation, support of the pelvic floor)
> - Fewer than three defecations per week
>
> Loose stools are rarely present without the use of laxatives.
> There are insufficient criteria for irritable bowel syndrome.
> ___
> *Note:* Criteria must be fulfilled for the last 3 months, with symptom onset at least 6 months before diagnosis.

> **BOX 3 Medications as a Cause of Chronic Constipation**
>
> Antacids: Calcium-containing antacids and supplements
> Anticholinergics
> Antihypertensives: calcium channel blockers, α-agonists
> Cation-containing agents (e.g., aluminum)
> Iron salts
> Nonsteroidal antiinflammatory drugs
> Opioids
> Resins
> Others

The prevalence of constipation is higher in women than in men, in persons of color, and in the elderly. Studies have shown that quality of life is diminished by the presence of chronic constipation. The overall economic burden of constipation in the United States is estimated to be several billion dollars each year.

The term *constipation* most accurately describes a symptom with a variety of definitions. When polled, physicians use frequency of bowel movements to define constipation. Patients however, are more likely to define constipation as straining to have a bowel movement, a sensation of incomplete evacuation, hard stools, or the need for digital maneuvers. By broadening the definition of constipation, more patients will be identified and treated. The recently revised Rome III criteria address these issues (Box 1).

Constipation can be either a primary disorder or secondary to an underlying disease state (Box 2) or medications (Box 3). A careful history and physical examination is of paramount importance in identifying and excluding these possible secondary causes, although discontinuing causative medications is usually not a practical option.

Once secondary causes have been excluded, primary constipation can be classified as normal transit, slow transit, pelvic floor dyssynergia or dysfunction, and irritable bowel syndrome (IBS) with constipation.

Clinical Features and Diagnosis

A complete history and physical examination including a careful rectal examination are the first steps in the evaluation process. Blood work should be ordered to exclude metabolic causes (calcium, phosphorus, thyroid-stimulating hormone, blood urea nitrogen and creatinine, and glucose). A colonoscopy should then be performed in all patients ages 50 years and older. If the patient lacks alarm symptoms (rectal bleeding, unintentional weight loss, anemia, family history of colon cancer, or inflammatory bowel disease) and is younger than 50 years, then the decision to perform colonoscopy is at the discretion of the clinician.

Once the colon examination is found to be normal and secondary causes have been excluded, it is useful to define the type of primary constipation. This can be suggested by the patient's history, although symptoms alone cannot make this determination with complete accuracy.

In normal transit constipation the patient complains of infrequent stools and perhaps bloating and abdominal distension; however, colonic transit time is normal if testing is performed. This is the most common type of constipation and typically responds to lifestyle modifications, addition of dietary fiber, and osmotic laxatives. IBS with constipation is also characterized by normal colonic transit; however, lower abdominal pain or discomfort is the more prevalent complaint along with infrequent passage of stools.

Pelvic floor dyssynergia or dysfunction (also known as functional rectosigmoid obstruction) occurs when pelvic floor muscles fail to relax appropriately during defecation or the muscles contract inappropriately. Pelvic floor dyssynergia is suggested by feelings of incomplete evacuation of the rectum, straining, the passage of small stools, the need to apply pressure on the perineum in order to pass stool or the need to digitally extract stool. Pelvic floor dyssynergia can be diagnosed with anal manometry demonstrating inappropriate contraction of the anal sphincter during straining. An abnormal balloon expulsion test with the inability to expel the balloon within 1 minute also suggests this disorder. In some cases, defecography is also performed to evaluate the pelvic floor muscles as well as exclude obstruction by a rectocele or rectal prolapse. Alternatively, dynamic MRI of the pelvis is now available at some tertiary centers. If the diagnosis of pelvic floor dyssynergia is confirmed, then a program of biofeedback with retraining of the anal sphincter and pelvic floor muscles can be undertaken.

Slow-transit constipation, also known as colonic inertia, is a severe colonic motor disorder characterized by markedly delayed colonic transit times. This disorder is suggested by a history of bowel movements occurring less than once per week. In clinical practice, the Sitz marker study is used to screen for slow-transit constipation. The patient ingests a capsule containing 24 radiopaque markers, and

> **BOX 2 Medical Causes of Chronic Constipation**
>
> Advanced renal disease
> Central nervous system disorders
> Endocrine disorders
> Infiltrative disorders: Amyloidosis, scleroderma
> Metabolic disorders
> Neuromuscular disorders
> Obstructing lesions: Strictures, tumors (benign and malignant)

CURRENT DIAGNOSIS

- Careful history and physical examination are needed to exclude secondary causes.
- Full colon examination should be performed in patients older than 50 years (possibly younger) if clinically indicated by family history of colon cancer or presence of alarm symptoms.
- Perform motility studies in patients refractory to conventional therapy.

abdominal films are taken on days 1 and 5. A normal result is the expulsion of 80% of the markers by day 5. In slow-transit constipation, 20 or more markers remain by day 5 and are distributed throughout the colon. In tertiary referral centers, nuclear transit scans may be available to evaluate gastric emptying along with both small intestinal and colonic transit and are indicated in severe and refractory cases of constipation. Given the severity of slow-transit constipation, symptoms are often refractory to usual measures including fiber and laxatives, and subtotal colectomy may be indicated. The exclusion of concommitent gastric and small bowel dysfunction is imperative in patients in whom surgery is being considered.

Treatment

Historically, the initial treatment of constipation has included an increase of dietary and supplemental fiber, adherence to an exercise program, increased fluid intake, and allowance of enough time for defecation. However, these measures have rarely been proved effective in clinical trials.

FIBER

Patients should be instructed to increase fiber intake to 20 to 30 g daily. Because this is hard to accomplish on a Western diet, a fiber supplement is generally added (Box 4). Patients should increase the dose of fiber slowly over several weeks to prevent gas and bloating.

LAXATIVE THERAPY

Laxative therapy (see Box 4) is initiated if lifestyle changes and fiber supplementation are ineffective. Stool softeners work by increasing stool water, thereby softening stools. Lubricants such as mineral oil should be used with caution in the elderly and in patients with neurologic impairment due to the pulmonary risks of aspiration. Stimulant laxatives enhance motility and alter electrolyte transport across intestinal mucosa and should be reserved for the short-term treatment of constipation. Patients may experience intestinal cramping and discomfort. Osmotic laxatives are nonabsorbable molecules that exert their effects by promoting the excretion of water into the intestinal lumen to maintain osmotic balance. Long-term treatment of chronic constipation with osmotic laxatives is probably safe, and doses can be increased until the desired effect is obtained.

The serotonin agonist tegaserod (Zelnorm) was proved in clinical trials to improve constipation and reduce bloating and abdominal pain in women with IBS with constipation. In March 2007, the marketing of tegaserod was suspended due to an increase in cardiovascular events reported in 11 clinical trials of tegaserod-treated patients compared with the placebo arm of the trials.

CURRENT THERAPY

- Treat secondary causes of constipation and adjust constipation-causing medications, if possible.
- Advise lifestyle modifications and increasing dietary or supplemental fiber.
- Begin a trial of laxatives with possible combination therapy.
- Refer patients to a tertiary referral center in refractory cases.
- Surgery may be needed for slow-transit constipation after an extensive evaluation that excludes gastric and small bowel motility disorders.

BOX 4 Treatment Options for Chronic Constipation

Fiber
Guar gum (Benefiber)
Methylcellulose (Citrucel)
Polycarbophil (FiberCon)
Psyllium (Metamucil, Konsyl); titrate up to 20 g/day

Stool Softeners
Docusate calcium (Surfak), 240 mg qd
Docusate sodium (Colace, others), 100 mg bid

Lubricants
Mineral oil, 15-45 mL PO daily

Stimulant Laxatives (dose as directed on package)
Aloe[7]
Bisacodyl (Dulcolax, Correctol, others)
Cascara
Castor oil
Senna (Senokot)
Sennosides (Ex-lax)
Teas

Suppositories
Bisacodyl, 10 mg qd
Glycerin

Osmotic Laxatives
Lactulose (Cephulac, Enulose, Kristalose)
Magnesium-containing (magnesium citrate, milk of magnesia), 1-3 tablets qd or bid
Polyethylene glycol (MiraLax, Glycolax), 17-36 g qd or bid
Sorbitol, 15-30 mL qd or bid

Prokinetics
Tegaserod (Zelnorm), marketing suspended March 2007

Bicyclic Fatty Acids
Lubiprostone (Amitiza), 24 μg bid with food

[7]Available as dietary supplement

Lubiprostone (Amitiza), an intestinal chloride channel activator, works by promoting the secretion of chloride into the intestinal lumen. Chloride is then followed by sodium and water to maintain chemical and osmotic neutrality. This action increases intestinal secretions, thereby enhancing motility and reducing constipation. This agent has no restrictions on age, gender, or duration of therapy. Nausea has been reported in up to 30% of treated patients but can be reduced by the administration of lubiprostone with food. A negative pregnancy test should be documented in women of childbearing potential due to the report of fetal demise in guinea pigs given lubiprostone.

Combination therapy with fiber plus laxatives or prescribing multiple laxatives with different mechanisms of action can be used in patients refractory to monotherapy.

SURGERY

For patients with well-documented slow-transit constipation without small bowel delay or pelvic floor dysfunction who have failed all of the above treatments, surgery may be considered. Subtotal colectomy with ileorectal anastomosis or total colectomy with Brooke ileostomy have been performed with relief of the incapacitating symptoms.

REFERENCES

Chiaroni G, Salandini L, Whitehead WE: Biofeedback benefits only patients with outlet dysfunction, not patients with isolated slow transit constipation. Gastroenterology 2003;125:19-31.
Dennison C, Prasad M, Lloyd A, et al: The health-related quality of life and economic burden of constipation. Pharmacoeconomics 2005;23:461-476.
Higgins PD, Johanson JF: Epidemiology of constipation in North America: A systematic review. Am J Gastroenterol 2004;99:750-759.
Irvine EJ, Ferrazi S, Pare P, et al: Health-related quality of life in functional GI disorders: Focus on constipation and resource utilization. Am J Gastroenterol. 2002;97:1986-1993.
Longstreth GF, Thompson WG, Chey WD, et al: Functional bowel disorders. Gastroenterology 2006;130:1480-1491.
Minguez M, Herreros B, Sanchiz V, et al: Predictive value of the balloon expulsion test for excluding the diagnosis of pelvic floor dyssynergia in constipation. Gastroenterology 2004;126:57-62.
Mollen RM, Kuijpers JC, Claassen AT: Colectomy for slow transit constipation: Preoperative functional evaluation is important but not a guarantee for a successful outcome. Dis Colon Rectum. 2001;44:577-580.

Fever

Method of
Ann M. Aring, MD

Patients often come to the physician's office with a fever. Fever can be present in a wide variety of clinical presentations ranging from self-limited viral illnesses to serious bacterial infections. Most febrile conditions can be easily diagnosed with other presenting symptoms and a problem-focused physical examination. However, fever produces anxiety for patients, parents, and health care providers, which can lead to overtreatment. Typically, fever is transient and only requires treatment to provide patient comfort.

Definitions

The definition of fever is arbitrary, because temperature varies daily within individual persons. The hypothalamic thermostat maintains core body temperature at about 37°C (98.6°F). Normal body temperature varies in a regular pattern each day. This circadian temperature rhythm, or diurnal variation, results in lower body temperatures in the early morning and temperatures approximately 1°C higher in the late afternoon or early evening.

The word *fever* is derived from the Latin *fovere* (to warm). In adults and children older than 12 years, fever is generally accepted as a rectal temperature higher than 38°C (100.4°F), an oral temperature higher than 37.5°C (99.5°F), or an axillary temperature higher than 37°C (98.6°F).

The methods of determining body temperature are oral, rectal, and axillary. The oral route of determining temperature is preferred in children older than 5 years and in adults. Typically, rectal temperatures are obtained in infants by placing a lubricated thermometer in the rectum. In general, axillary temperatures are inaccurate and should not be used. Liquid crystal strips applied to the forehead and temperature-sensitive pacifiers are popular with parents but are inaccurate and miss fevers in many children.

The temperature considered to be the physiologic limit to febrile illness is 41.1°C (106°F). Hyperthermia is characterized by a temperature higher than this hypothalamic set point. Hyperthermia is due to an interference within the normal mechanisms that balance heat production and dissipation or an insult to the hypothalamus.

CURRENT DIAGNOSIS

- The definition of fever is arbitrary, because temperature varies within individual persons daily. Oral temperatures of 37.5°C (99.5°F) or rectal temperatures of 100.4°F (38°C) are consistent with fever.
- Temperature accuracy depends on the measurement technique. Oral temperatures are preferred in patients older than 5 years. Rectal temperatures are preferred in infants.
- Fever in infants younger than 3 months or in neutropenic patients is considered a medical emergency that warrants immediate further evaluation.
- Fever is beneficial but is associated with increased cardiac demand and increased metabolic needs. Benign febrile seizures can occur in young children with a fever.
- Fever of unknown origin (FUO) in children merits a thorough evaluation based on the age of the child. FUO in adults is defined as a temperature higher than 101°F that is of at least 3 weeks' duration and whose cause remains undiagnosed after 3 days in the hospital or after three outpatient visits.
- Hyperthermia is characterized by a temperature above the upper limit of the hypothalamic set point of 41.1°C (106°F).

When the cause of a fever is unknown, two terms may be used: fever of unknown origin (FUO) and fever of unknown source. The definition of FUO in adults includes a temperature higher than 101°F that is of at least 3 weeks' duration and whose source remains undiagnosed after 3 days in the hospital or after three outpatient visits. FUO is also used to define a fever that occurs at different periods over weeks or months. Fever of unknown source is defined as a fever in the first week of an illness.

Pathogenesis and Physiology

Fever is a physiologic mechanism that occurs when an inciting stimulus causes an inflammatory response. Fever may be caused by infections, vaccines, tissue injury, malignancy, drugs, collagen vascular diseases, granulomatous disease, inflammatory bowel disease, endocrine disorders such as thyrotoxicosis and pheochromocytoma, and central nervous system abnormalities. Dehydration, increased physical activity, and heat exposure can all cause an elevation in temperature. Infections cause most fevers in all age groups.

Monocytes or tissue macrophages are activated by the microbial or nonmicrobial stimuli to produce various cytokines with pyrogenic activity. The list of currently recognized pyrogenic cytokines includes interleukin-1 (IL-1), tumor necrosis factor α (TNF-α), IL-6, interferon-β (IFN-β), and interferon-γ (IFN-γ). These cytokines activate the arachadonic acid cascade and increase production of prostaglandin E_2 (PGE$_2$). PGE$_2$ then resets the thermoregulatory set point in the hypothalamus at a higher level.

Thermoregulatory responses include redirecting blood to or from cutaneous vascular beds, increased or decreased sweating, and behavioral responses such as seeking warmer or cooler environmental temperatures. The body dissipates heat via evaporation of water from the body surface and lungs through radiation (60%), convection (12%), and conduction (3%).

Risks and Benefits of Fever

Fever is beneficial and not usually harmful to the host, with a few exceptions. Fever is associated with increased cardiac demand and increased metabolic needs. In pregnancy, fever is associated with harmful clinical effects. Many animal studies have shown that fever enhances the immunologic response to infectious agents. Use of antipyretic medications to lower fever increases both morbidity and mortality in infected laboratory animals and prolongs varicella infections in humans.

Febrile seizures are usually benign but can cause considerable parental anxiety. Febrile seizures are divided into two types: simple (generalized, last <15 minutes, and do not recur within 24 hours) and complex (prolonged, recur more than once in 24 hours, or are focal). Recent studies have shown that in previously normal children, most simple febrile seizures are not associated with recurrent seizures or brain damage.

Fever of Unknown Origin

ADULTS

The evaluation of FUO remains among the most challenging problems facing the clinician. There are four categories. Classic FUO is commonly caused by infections, drug fever, malignancy, and inflammatory diseases. Neutropenic FUO (neutrophils <500/mm^3) is seen in periodontal and perianal infections; candidemia and aspergillosis are major causes. Nosocomial FUO is commonly caused by septic thrombophlebitis, drug fever, and *Clostridium difficile* colitis. In HIV-associated FUO, *Mycobacterium avium* complex infections, tuberculosis, non-Hodgkin's lymphoma, cytomegalovirus, and drug fever are important etiologies.

CHILDREN

Febrile illness in infants and young children is common. A complete history and physical examination, including vital signs, skin color and exanthems, behavior state, and hydration status, do not reveal a source of infection in 20% of febrile children. The child's age determines the need for further investigation. Febrile infants younger than 28 days should have a complete blood count (CBC) with differential; electrolytes; serum glucose; cerebrospinal fluid (CSF) Gram stain and cell count; cultures from blood, CSF, and urine; group B streptococcal antigen from urine and CSF; and a chest x-ray. Management requires hospitalization and empiric parenteral antibiotics.

For children 28 to 90 days old, obtain a CBC with differential and urinalysis with culture. A low-risk child is defined as a previously healthy term infant who has no focal bacterial infection on examination. If the white blood cell count (WBC) is greater than 15,000/mm^3, blood cultures should be obtained, as well as CSF Gram stain, culture, cell count, glucose, and protein. For a positive CSF Gram stain or abnormal CSF count, the patient should be admitted and parenteral antibiotics should be given. For negative CSF Gram stain, normal CSF cell count, and negative urinalysis, the child should be given ceftriaxone (Rocephin) 50 mg/kg (maximum dose, 1 g) and reevaluated in 24 hours. For a positive urinalysis or urine culture, the patient may be given oral antibiotics as an outpatient and reexamined in 24 hours. If the child cannot take oral antibiotics, he or she must be admitted for parenteral antibiotics. For a WBC less than 15,000 mm^3 with a negative urinalysis and CSF Gram stain, the child may be followed closely as an outpatient. The child should be reevaluated in 24 hours. High-risk infants are toxic appearing with lethargy, signs of poor perfusion, hypoventilation, hyperventilation, or cyanosis. High-risk infants need to be admitted to the hospital with parental antibiotics.

For children 3 to 36 months old who have a fever without a source, no diagnostic tests or antibiotics are needed if the child appears well and the fever is less than 39°C (102.2°F) (low risk). Acetaminophen (Tylenol) 10 mg/kg may be given with instructions

CURRENT THERAPY

- Antipyretic therapy for children includes acetaminophen 10 to 15 mg/kg every 4 to 6 hours for children older than 3 months or ibuprofen 10 mg/kg every 6 hours for children older than 6 months.
- Antipyretic therapy for adults and adolescents includes acetaminophen 650 mg to 1000 mg every 6 hours to a maximum of 4000 mg per day, or ibuprofen 200 to 400 mg every 6 hours.
- Aspirin (salicylic acid) should not be used in children due to the risk of Reye's syndrome. In adults, the dose is 325 to 650 mg every 6 hours as needed for fever.
- Combining two antipyretics for fever, such as ibuprofen and acetaminophen, has not been proved to produce quicker or longer-lasting responses.
- Sponge bathing should be done with tepid water and no alcohol.

to give every 6 hours as needed. The child's caregiver should also be instructed to return to the clinician if the fever persists longer than 48 hours or if the patient's condition worsens. If the temperature is greater than 39°C, obtain a CBC with differential. In addition, a boy younger than 6 months or a girl younger than 2 years should have a urine culture. Blood cultures are indicated if the WBC is greater than 15,000/mm^3 and the fever is higher than 39°C. CSF cultures are indicated when the diagnosis of sepsis or meningitis is suspected based on history, observation, and physical examination. Empiric antibiotic therapy with ceftriaxone 50 mg/kg (maximum dose, 1g) should be given if the temperature is higher than 39°C and the WBC is greater than 15,000/mm^3. The child needs to be followed up in 24 to 48 hours. High-risk children in this age group should be admitted to the hospital for broad-spectrum parenteral antibiotics.

Treatment

Antipyretic medications are commonly used for the symptomatic relief of fever. Acetaminophen, ibuprofen (Advil, Motrin), and aspirin are inhibitors of hypothalamic cyclooxygenase, thus inhibiting PGE$_2$ synthesis. These drugs are all equally effective antipyretic agents. Ibuprofen and aspirin are also antiinflammatory agents; acetaminophen does not have any antiinflammatory properties.

Acetaminophen is available in a wide variety of dosage forms including drops, elixir, syrup, capsule, tablet, chewable tablet, and suppository. Dosing is generally 10 to 15 mg/kg every 4 to 6 hours in children older than 3 months. For adults, acetaminophen dosing is 650 to 1000 mg every 6 hours. Maximum daily dose of acetaminophen is 75 mg/kg (or 720 mg) in children and 4000 mg in adolescents and adults.

Ibuprofen is a nonsteroidal antiinflammatory (NSAID) drug that may be given to febrile children 6 months or older. Ibuprofen is quickly absorbed and produces a more rapid temperature fall and longer duration of action than acetaminophen. This advantage might not be maintained after the first dose is given. Dosing in children is 10 mg/kg every 6 to 8 hours. Adults and adolescents may take doses of 200 to 400 mg every 6 hours. Ibuprofen is also available in a wide variety of dosage forms including drops, elixir, syrup, capsule, tablet, and chewable tablet.

Aspirin (salicylic acid) remains an effective treatment for fever in adults. Because aspirin is associated with Reye's syndrome in children, aspirin is not recommended for treating fever in children. Adult dosing is 325 to 650 mg every 4 to 6 hours as needed.

Combining two antipyretics for fever, such as ibuprofen and acetaminophen, is common clinical practice. Combinations have not been proved to produce quicker or longer-lasting responses. The American Academy of Pediatrics (AAP) cautions against using multiple antipyretics because of an increase in the likelihood of dosing errors. Combining drugs is more expensive and could also delay proper diagnosis or therapy.

Nonpharmacologic treatment can also provide relief from the discomfort of fever. Extra oral fluids should be encouraged to prevent dehydration. Sponge bathing with tepid water may be used. Alcohol or ice water should not be used for sponge bathing. Alcohol is absorbed through the skin and can cause hypoglycemia or dehydration. Both alcohol and ice water increase shivering and can cause more discomfort.

REFERENCES

Aronoff DM, Neilson EG: Antipyretics: Mechanisms of action and clinical use in fever suppression. Am J Med 2001;111(4):304-315.
Baraff LJ: Management of fever without source in infants and children. Ann Emerg Med 2000;36:602-614.
Crocetti M, Moghbeli N, Serwint J: Fever phobia revisited: Have parental misconceptions about fever changed in 20 years? Pediatrics 2001; 107(6):1241-1246.
Finkelstein JA: Fever in pediatric primary care: Occurrence, management, and outcomes. Pediatrics 2000;105:260-266.
Greisman LA, Mackowiak PA: Fever: Beneficial and detrimental effects of antipyretics. Curr Opin Infect Dis 2002;15(3):241-245.
Kourtis AP, Sullivan DT, Sathian U: Practice guidelines for the management of febrile infants less than 90 days of age at the ambulatory network of a large pediatric health care system in the United States: Summary of new evidence. Clin Pediatr 2004;43(1):11-16.
Knockaert DC, Vanderschueren S, Blockmans D: Fever of unknown origin in adults: 40 years on. J Intern Med 2003;253:263-275.
Mackowiak PA: Temperature regulation and the pathogenesis of fever. In Mandell GL, Bennett JE, Donlin R (eds): Principles and Practices of Infectious Diseases, vol 1. Philadelphia: Churchill Livingstone, 2000, pp 604-622.
McCarthy PL: Fever without apparent source on clinical examination. Curr Opin Pediatr 2004;16(1):94-106.
Mourad O, Palda V, Detsky A: A comprehensive evidence-based approach to fever of unknown origin. Arch Intern Med 2003;163:545-551.
Roth AR, Basello GM: Approach to the adult patient with fever of unknown origin. Am Fam Phys 2003;68(11):2223-2228.

Cough

Method of
David G. Hill, MD

Cough is among the most common presenting complaints of outpatients in the United States. It serves as a protective reflex against foreign material and as a method to clear secretions from the airway. The cough center is located in the medulla, and the cough reflex is mediated by way of multiple nervous system pathways including the trigeminal, glossopharyngeal, vagus, and phrenic nerves. Cough is mediated by separate neural pathways from bronchoconstriction. When cough occurs there is a synchronized activation of muscles, the glottis opens, and the lungs expand. At the peak of inspiration the glottis closes and expiratory muscles contract. This results in increased intrathoracic pressure; when the glottis opens airflow can reach 500 miles per hour. The cough reflex varies in different patient populations. Women have a more sensitive cough reflex than men. Smokers' cough reflexes are depressed despite the increased frequency of cough in this population. Patients who have a decreased cough sensitivity following cerebral vascular accidents have an increased incidence of pneumonia. Angiotensin-converting enzyme (ACE) inhibitors increase cough reflex sensitivity and have been shown to decrease the risk of pneumonia in patients with cerebrovascular accidents. The evaluation of cough as a patient complaint may best be pursued by examining the duration of the symptoms. Cough can be subcategorized into acute and chronic cough. Cough that occurs following an acute respiratory infection may narrow the differential diagnosis and is addressed separately.

BOX 1 Causes of Acute Cough

- Viral upper respiratory infections (the common cold)
- Acute sinusitis (usually viral, occasionally bacterial)
- Exacerbation of chronic obstructive pulmonary disease
- Allergic rhinitis
- *Bordetella pertussis* infection

Acute Cough

Acute cough may be defined as cough that has been present for less than 8 weeks. Because all causes of chronic coughs initially cause acute symptoms, patients with acute cough may actually have cough caused by one of the etiologies discussed later in this section; however, acute cough more commonly is the result of a less indolent process (Box 1). Infectious etiologies are a frequent cause of acute cough. Most acute cough is the result of viral infections, specifically the common cold. Most cough resulting from the common cold is self-limited and lasts less than 3 weeks. Most episodes of sinusitis are of viral etiology; however, bacterial sinusitis can also result in acute cough. The presence of a significant smoking history raises the possibility of an acute exacerbation of chronic obstructive pulmonary disease (COPD) as the cause of acute cough, especially in patients with previously documented COPD. *Bordetella pertussis* infection may also be the etiology of an acute episode of cough. Noninfectious processes that lead to acute cough include allergic rhinitis, congestive heart failure, asthma, and aspiration. The clinical history, physical examination, and diagnostic testing are of particular importance in differentiating these disease states and often point to the diagnosis.

Postinfectious Cough

Postinfectious cough begins with an acute upper respiratory tract infection but persists following the resolution of the other acute symptoms (Box 2). Postnasal drip syndrome may present following the common cold or sinusitis. Bronchospasm may lead to postinfectious cough either as a result of a single episode of postinfectious wheezing or an exacerbation of underlying asthma. Postinfectious cough may be the initial presentation of asthma. Recurrent episodes of airflow obstruction are required to confirm the diagnosis of this chronic illness. Because *B. pertussis* can present with an indolent course, this infection can be confused with a postinfectious cough. Similarly, bacterial sinusitis can be confused with postinfectious cough. Both of these etiologies of cough are the result of ongoing infection rather than true postinfectious cough. *Mycoplasma*

BOX 2 Causes of Postinfectious Cough

- Postnasal drip syndrome
- Bronchospasm
- *Bordetella pertussis* infection
- Bacterial sinusitis
- *Mycoplasma pneumoniae/Chlamydia pneumoniae* infection

BOX 3 Causes of Chronic Cough
• Postnasal drip syndrome • Asthma • Gastroesophageal reflux disease (GERD) • Eosinophilic bronchitis • Angiotensin-converting enzyme inhibitors

pneumoniae and *Chlamydia pneumoniae* infections may also result in postinfectious cough likely because of persistent airway inflammation and increases in cough reflex sensitivity.

Chronic Cough

Chronic cough presents the most difficult diagnostic dilemma for the health care practitioner. Cough of greater than 8 weeks' duration can be considered chronic. Lesser duration of symptoms may still be indicative of one of the etiologies discussed in this section, but such cough is more likely the result of one of the infectious or postinfectious etiologies described previously. In patients who have never smoked, chronic cough is most likely the result of asthma, postnasal drip syndrome, or gastroesophageal reflux. These three etiologies are the most common cause of chronic cough regardless of patient age. In nonsmokers with a normal chest radiograph who are not taking an ACE inhibitor, these three etiologies alone or in combination are the cause of more than 85% of chronic cough (Box 3). Postnasal drip syndrome is the most common of these etiologies. Cough may be the sole presenting symptom of any of these conditions; they are not mutually exclusive and may coexist, particularly in the patient with troublesome, persistent symptoms. Most patients with problematic, persistent cough have multiple etiologies contributing to their symptoms. COPD must be considered in current smokers and in those patients with a significant smoking history. Smokers can have a cough of any etiology, however, and it should not be assumed that their cough is the result of smoking or COPD. Although smokers frequently admit to cough when a history is taken, they infrequently seek medical attention for this symptom. Cough resulting from the use of ACE inhibitors must be considered in all patients being treated with these medications. Less common, yet frequent causes of cough include chronic bronchitis from irritants other than tobacco smoke and eosinophilic bronchitis. Occasionally, chronic cough may be the result of:

- Bronchogenic carcinoma
- Metastatic carcinoma
- Bronchiectasis
- Sarcoidosis
- Pulmonary fibrosis
- Pneumoconiosis
- Hypersensitivity pneumonitis
- Congestive heart failure
- Chronic infection, such as tuberculosis or *Mycobacterium avium* complex
- Recurrent aspiration because of pharyngeal or esophageal abnormalities

Key Diagnostic Points

The evaluation of acute cough should focus on the history and physical examination. Most acute cough will be the result of self-limited viral upper respiratory infections. More thorough evaluation is necessary in the workup of cough of longer duration particularly if the cough has been present for more than 2 months. The history of onset of the cough and whether it was associated with an acute infectious episode should be elicited. Exposure to sick contacts particularly to a known case of *B. pertussis* are important historic

CURRENT DIAGNOSIS

All Patients Presenting With Cough

- Perform thorough history and physical examination.
- Review timing and nature of cough along with exacerbating or mitigating factors.
- Review prior history of cough, allergies, asthma, or gastroesophageal reflux.
- Take medication history, particularly use of ACE inhibitors.
- Focus physical examination on head, neck, and thorax.

Patients With Postinfectious or Chronic Cough

- Obtain chest radiograph, particularly in patients with an abnormal respiratory examination.
- Evaluate airflow obstruction with spirometry.
- Stop ACE inhibitors and assess for improvement.
- Administer empiric therapy for postnasal drip, asthma, or gastroesophageal reflux.
- Consider methacholine challenge testing to evaluate for airway hyperreactivity.
- Induce sputum for eosinophils or empiric trial of corticosteroids for eosinophilic bronchitis.
- If cough persists, consider esophagoscopy, 24-hour pH probe monitoring, high-resolution chest CT, or bronchoscopy.

Abbreviations: ACE = angiotensin-converting enzyme; CT = computed tomography.

considerations. The timing and nature of the cough and any associated sputum must be described. Factors that mitigate or worsen the cough should be examined, and prior history of episodic cough, allergies, wheezing, asthma, and gastroesophageal reflux should be questioned. A thorough medication history particularly regarding use of ACE inhibitors must be obtained. Environmental factors both at home and in the work place should be reviewed. Although smoking history is important, it is again noted that smoking-related cough is an infrequent reason for a patient to seek medical attention. The physical examination should focus most on the head, neck, and thorax with a thorough examination of the upper respiratory tract including the auditory canal, nose, and oropharynx. The cardiopulmonary examination should also be thorough to elicit signs of less common illnesses.

Acute cough associated with an acute respiratory illness and prominent upper airway symptoms can be assumed to be secondary to the common cold. Diagnostic testing is not indicated in such patients; a chest radiograph would be normal and is thus not recommended. Patients who have abnormal sinus transillumination, purulent nasal secretions, sinus pain or tenderness, or maxillary toothache could possibly have bacterial sinusitis. Again, a viral etiology of sinusitis is more likely than bacterial sinusitis, and antibiotic therapy should be initiated only in patients with persistent symptoms despite symptomatic therapy. Patients with documented COPD who present with acute cough, purulent sputum, dyspnea, and wheezing have an exacerbation of their underlying COPD and should be treated appropriately. Allergic rhinitis usually presents with a clear clinical history of episodic nasal and other allergy symptoms, and allergen avoidance can be initiated. It is important to note that allergic rhinitis can present with perennial symptoms.

Postinfectious cough should be evaluated with thorough history and physical examinations followed by limited diagnostic evaluation and empiric therapies. Patients should be treated for postnasal drip syndrome, particularly in the setting of described rhinitis, postnasal drip, or frequent throat clearing. The presence of nasal inflammation and congestion, cobblestoning of the pharyngeal mucosa, or mucus in the oropharynx should also lead to empiric therapy for postnasal drip syndrome. If cough persists in the patients with suspected postnasal drip syndrome, evaluation of the sinuses with imaging and treatment of those patients with evidence of bacterial sinusitis should be pursued. Computed tomography (CT) imaging of the sinuses is the gold standard for diagnosing bacterial sinusitis. Patients with postinfectious cough and an abnormal respiratory examination should have a chest radiograph. Patients with a normal radiograph and evidence of bronchospasm can be empirically treated for airway hyperreactivity. Again, the diagnosis of asthma requires recurrent airflow obstruction and cannot be made on the basis of a single episode of postinfectious wheezing or airway hyperreactivity. In subjects with cough and vomiting, known exposure to a case of B. pertussis, or in the presence of a B. pertussis epidemic in the community, empiric therapy for this illness should be pursued.

Before the vaccine era, B. pertussis was an endemic disease, which occurred in cyclic epidemics. It has been documented that B. pertussis continues to circulate in the adult population despite control of the disease in the pediatric population by vaccination. Immunity to B. pertussis, whether as a result of primary infection or immunization, is shortlived. The longer the elapsed interval since prior infection or immunization and repeat infection, the more likely repeat infection will be symptomatic. Perhaps repeat adolescent and adult booster immunization programs should be implemented to effectively control or eliminate this infection.

History and physical examinations remain paramount in the patient presenting with chronic cough. The majority of patients should have a chest radiograph obtained as part of their evaluation. If the history and physical examination suggest that postnasal drip, asthma, or gastroesophageal reflux is the etiology of a patient's symptoms, empiric therapy for these conditions should be initiated. Cough triggered by environmental factors or changes may be secondary to rhinitis and postnasal drip or airway hyperreactivity and asthma. Substernal burning or a sour taste in the mouth, particularly when triggered by supine positioning or bending, should increase the suspicion of gastroesophageal reflux.

If asthma is suspected, spirometry should be performed to document whether airflow obstruction is present. Response to inhaled bronchodilator with normal spirometry is indicative of airway hyperreactivity. Improvement in symptoms and spirometry with empiric asthma therapy even in the setting of normal baseline flow rates also confirms an asthmatic etiology. A methacholine challenge can be performed to confirm airway hyperreactivity. If cough in the setting of a positive methacholine challenge shows absolutely no response to empiric asthma therapy with inhaled corticosteroids and bronchodilators, consider a trial of systemic steroids. If the cough does not respond to aggressive asthma therapy, the methacholine challenge test results were probably false positive; asthma therapy can be discontinued and diagnostic efforts focused elsewhere.

Cough patients being treated with ACE inhibitors should cease these medications. Up to 30% of patients treated with ACE inhibitors will develop a persistent cough, more commonly in women, nonsmokers, and patients of Chinese ancestry. It may take 4 weeks or more for cough caused by ACE inhibitors to resolve following cessation of these medications. In the presence of ACE inhibitor use, further evaluation of dry cough should not be pursued until the patient has been withdrawn from these medications for 1 month.

An abnormal chest radiograph can direct further diagnostic studies and therapies, whereas a normal chest radiograph makes less common etiologies of chronic cough such as carcinoma, congestive heart failure, sarcoidosis, or interstitial lung disease unlikely. Evidence of basilar infiltrates or fibrosis may suggest interstitial lung disease or chronic aspiration. Severe gastroesophageal reflux must be considered in those patients with radiographic evidence of chronic aspiration.

Chronic cough without a definitive etiology can be troubling to both patient and health care provider. A systematic approach can simplify both diagnosis and treatment (Figure 1). It is again stressed that such a cough may be the result of multiple etiologic factors.

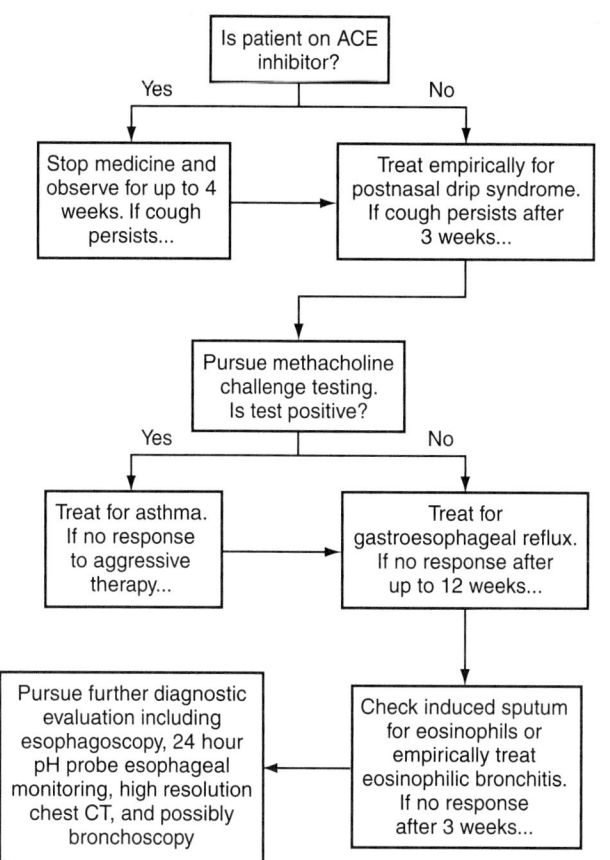

FIGURE 1. Approach to chronic cough of uncertain origin. ACE = angiotensin-converting enzyme; CT = computed tomography

In the absence of specific factors that help to point to an etiology of chronic cough, empiric treatment for postnasal drip syndrome should be pursued. Methacholine challenge testing will rule out asthma if it is negative and should also be performed early in the evaluation of chronic cough. Cough may be the sole manifestation of asthma in nearly 60% of patients presenting with chronic cough. A positive methacholine challenge does not have 100% predictive value but should lead to empiric asthma therapy.

Empiric therapy for silent gastroesophageal reflux should be initiated in those who do not respond to treatment for postnasal drip syndrome and do not have evidence of or respond to treatment for asthma. Cough may be the only manifestation of gastroesophageal reflux up to 30% of the time. Definitive diagnosis of gastroesophageal reflux requires invasive testing and may require more than one testing modality. Therefore it is recommended that empiric therapy for reflux be pursued before diagnostic testing. Reflux therapy should include conservative approaches such as dietary and lifestyle changes, bed positioning, and pharmacologic treatment. Gastroesophageal reflux–related cough can be particularly troublesome and persistent and may take weeks or months to respond to appropriate and intensive antireflux therapy. This may include higher-than-normal doses of proton pump inhibitors and promotility agents. Surgical treatment of reflux may be necessary to effectively treat reflux related cough in some patients. In patients with persistent cough, the common etiologies of cough often coexist and exacerbate one another. Therapy should often be additive, for instance treating both asthma and reflux, rather than mutually exclusive. Persistent cough should result in further diagnostic evaluation including sputum studies, esophagoscopy, 24-hour pH probe esophageal monitoring, high-resolution chest CT, and possibly bronchoscopy. In the presence of normal chest imaging, bronchoscopy is unlikely to yield beneficial diagnostic information in the patient with chronic cough.

CURRENT THERAPY

Treatment of Acute Cough

- Common cold: Supportive care with dexbrompheniramine, 6 mg, and pseudoephedrine, 120 mg (Drixoral Cold and Allergy Tablets); or ipratropium nasal spray (Atrovent, 0.06%), two 42-mcg sprays in each nostril 3 times daily for 4 to 7 d depending on duration of symptoms.
- Acute sinusitis: Treat as a common cold. Add oxymetazoline (Afrin), two sprays twice daily for three days. If symptoms persist, consider antibiotic therapy directed against *Haemophilus influenzae* and *Streptococcus pneumoniae* such as azithromycin (Zithromax), 500 mg daily for 3 d.
- Exacerbation of chronic obstructive pulmonary disease: Antibiotics directed against *H. influenzae* and *S. pneumoniae* for 3 to 7 d such as clarithromycin (Biaxin), 500 mg twice daily for 7 d; systemic corticosteroids such as prednisone (Deltasone), 40 mg tapered over 10 d; inhaled anticholinergics such as tiotropium (Spiriva), one inhalation daily; and short-acting β-agonists such as albuterol (Proventil), two inhalations every 4 h as needed; smoking cessation.
- Allergic rhinitis: Nasal corticosteroids such as mometasone (Nasonex), two sprays in each nostril daily; nonsedating antihistamines such as fexofenadine (Allegra), 180 mg daily; allergen avoidance if possible.
- *Bordetella pertussis*: Erythromycin 500 mg four times daily for 14 d or trimethoprim 160 mg/sulfamethoxazole (Bactrim DS),[1] 800 mg twice daily for 14 d. Other macrolide antibiotics such as azithromycin (Zithromax)[1] or clarithromycin (Biaxin)[1] are likely effective and may be better tolerated.

Treatment of Postinfectious Cough

- Postnasal drip syndrome: Dexbrompheniramine, 6 mg, and pseudoephedrine (Drixoral Cold and Allergy Tablets), 120 mg for up to 3 wk; ipratropium (Atrovent), 0.06% nasal spray for up to 3 wk; azelastine (Astelin) nasal spray (137 mcg), two sprays each nostril twice daily for up to 3 wk.
- Bronchospasm: Inhaled corticosteroid such as budesonide (Pulmicort),[1] two inhalations daily with or without inhaled long-acting β-agonist such as formoterol (Foradil), two inhalations twice daily; short-acting β-agonist such as albuterol (Ventolin), two puffs every 4 h as needed. Oral steroids such as prednisone (Deltasone), 40 mg tapered over 10 d.
- *Bordetella pertussis*: Erythromycin, 500 mg four times daily for 14 d, or trimethoprim 160 mg/sulfamethoxazole, 800 mg (Bactrim DS)[1] twice daily for 14 d. Other macrolide antibiotics such as azithromycin (Zithromax)[1] or clarithromycin (Biaxin)[1] are likely effective and may be better tolerated.
- Bacterial sinusitis: Dexbrompheniramine, 6 mg, and pseudoephedrine (Drixoral Cold and Allergy Tablets), 120 mg for up to 3 wk; oxymetazoline (Afrin), two sprays twice daily for 3 d; azithromycin (Zithromax), 500 mg daily for 3 d.
- Chlamydia/mycoplasma: Clarithromycin (Biaxin), 500 mg twice daily for 14 d.

Treatment of Chronic Cough

- Postnasal drip syndrome
    Nonallergic: Dexbrompheniramine, 6 mg, and pseudoephedrine (Drixoral Cold and Allergy Tablets), 120 mg for up to 3 wk; ipratropium (Atrovent), 0.06% nasal spray for up to 3 wk; azelastine (Astelin) nasal spray (137 mcg), two sprays each nostril twice daily for up to 3 wk.
    Allergic: Fluticasone (Flonase) (50 mcg), two sprays each nostril daily; fexofenadine (Allegra), 180 mg daily; allergen avoidance.
- Asthma: Albuterol (Proventil), two puffs every 4 hours as needed; inhaled corticosteroid such as budesonide (Pulmicort), two inhalations daily with or without inhaled long-acting β-agonist such as formoterol (Foradil), two inhalations twice daily; combination of long-acting β-agonist and inhaled steroid such as fluticasone/salmeterol (Advair) (100/50 mcg), inhaled twice daily; montelukast (Singulair), 10 mg daily; prednisone (Deltasone), 40 mg daily with tapering dose over 10 d.
- Gastroesophageal reflux: Dietary and lifestyle modifications, lansoprazole (Prevacid), 30 mg daily for up to 3 mo; metoclopramide (Reglan), 10 mg before meals and sleep.
- Eosinophilic bronchitis: Fluticasone (Flovent)[1] (110 mcg), two inhalations twice daily; prednisone (Deltasone), 30 mg daily for 3 wk.
- ACE inhibitor: Discontinue medication.

[1]Not FDA approved for this indication.

Eosinophilic bronchitis in the absence of asthma is also a frequent cause (up to 13% of cases) of chronic cough. Patients with eosinophilic bronchitis will have normal spirometry and a negative methacholine challenge. The disease may be diagnosed by appropriate induced sputum analysis showing at least 3% eosinophils. Alternatively it can be empirically treated with a course of inhaled corticosteroids. Most patients appear to respond to inhaled corticosteroids within 3 weeks. Systemic corticosteroids may be required to improve the symptoms in some cases. There may be an association of gastroesophageal reflux with eosinophilic bronchitis. Patients with gastroesophageal reflux have been found to have increased sputum eosinophilia.

Bronchiectasis may infrequently result in chronic cough. Bronchiectasis is characterized by the abnormal dilatation of one or more branches of the bronchial tree. It can effectively be diagnosed by high resolution CT scan of the thorax. Bronchiectasis may occur following a severe infection, distal to an area of airway obstruction, congenitally, from chronic inflammatory processes, and as a result of chronic parenchymal scarring and traction. Patients with bronchiectasis may present with productive or nonproductive coughs.

They may have recurrent episodes of infection resulting from persistent colonization of the abnormal bronchial segment. Infectious agents may include routine bacterial organisms and typical or atypical myco-bacterium. Bronchiectasis may be seen in a variety of chronic illnesses. The presence of bronchiectasis in a patient without a known predisposing cause should prompt the clinician to look for appropriate clinical states. such as:

- Primary or acquired immunodeficiencies
- Abnormalities of ciliary function, such as ciliary dyskinesia or cystic fibrosis
- Postinfectious inflammatory processes, such as allergic bronchopulmonary aspergillosis
- Collagen vascular diseases
- Inflammatory bowel disease
- Sarcoidosis
- Yellow nail syndrome

The presence of localized bronchiectasis may be an indication to pursue flexible fiberoptic bronchoscopy to rule out an obstructing lesion and to obtain appropriate culture specimens. Treatment of bronchiectasis is aimed at the underlying disease state if one can be identified. Infections should be treated with appropriate antibiotics. Clearance of bronchial secretions can be aided with mucolytics and chest physiotherapy including use of percussive devices. In some cases surgical therapy to remove the bronchiectatic segment can be considered.

Treatment

The key treatments for cough are best described based on the suspected etiology. Acute cough therapy should focus on supportive treatment of the underlying suspected etiology, which will likely be a viral upper respiratory infection. Therapy for exacerbation of chronic obstructive pulmonary disease, allergic rhinitis, bacterial sinusitis, or B. pertussis infection is more specific. Postinfectious cough should focus on therapy for postnasal drip syndrome or airways reactivity if suspected. In chronic cough of uncertain etiology (see Figure 1), cough therapy should begin with empiric treatment of postnasal drip syndrome, evaluation and treatment of asthma, empiric treatment of gastroesophageal reflux syndrome, and finally evaluation or empiric therapy for eosinophilic bronchitis.

Cough is a frequent and troublesome symptom for both patient and health care provider. Acute cough although at times troubling is usually self-limiting. Postinfectious cough and chronic cough are more problematic, but can effectively be evaluated and treated by performing a thorough history and physical examination and pursuing a systematic approach to diagnostic evaluation and both empiric and guided therapies. The resolution of chronic troubling cough is a therapeutic relief for the patient and a gratifying experience for the caregiver.

REFERENCES

Barnes TW, Afessa B, Swanson KL, Lim KG: The clinical utility of flexible bronchoscopy in the evaluation of chronic cough. Chest 2004;126:268-272.
Breitling CE, Ward R, Goh KL: Eosinophilic bronchitis is an important cause of chronic cough. Am J Respir Crit Care Med 1999;160:406-410.
Cherry JD: Epidemiological, clinical, and laboratory aspects of pertussis in adults. Clin Infect Dis 1999;28(suppl2):S112-S117.
Cohen M, Sahn SA: Bronchiectasis in systemic diseases. Chest 1999; 116:1063-1074.
Irwin RS, Madison JM: Symptom research on chronic cough: A historical perspective. Ann Intern Med 2001;134:809-814.
Irwin RS, Madison JM: The diagnosis and treatment of cough. N Engl J Med 2000;343:1715-1721.
Irwin RS, Madison JM: The persistently troublesome cough. Am J Respir Crit Care Med 2002;165:1469-1474.
Kiljander TO: The role of proton pump inhibitors in the management of gastroesophageal reflux disease-related asthma and chronic cough. Am J Med 2003;115(3A):S65-S71.

Pruritus

Method of
Scott Moses, MD

Because pruritus is the most common symptom in dermatology, clinicians are often asked to reduce its distressing effect on comfort and sleep. Left untreated, itch and its associated persistent scratching increases risk of chronic skin changes and secondary infection. Although pruritus is most often caused by a dermatologic condition, it can also be a symptom of underlying systemic disease.

The sensation of itch starts in the skin's free nerve endings, travels via unmyelinated C-fibers to the spine, and finally travels via the spinothalamic tract to the brain. Histamine, commonly associated with allergic rhinitis and urticaria, is only one of several chemical mediators of pruritus. Serotonin is integral to the pruritus of uremia, cholestasis, polycythemia vera, lymphoma, and morphine-associated pruritus. In atopic dermatitis, proinflammatory mediators (e.g., cytokines) are released in an immune-mediated response. Pruritus has been attributed to neuropathy in a wide variety of conditions including herpes zoster, brachioradial pruritus, notalgia paresthetica, spinal tumors, and multiple sclerosis.

Diagnosis

History is the key to identifying the cause of pruritus. Most causes are evident from the associated dermatitis (Box 1), distribution (Figure 1), or exogenous exposure history (Box 2). Clinicians should focus on the timing of pruritus and associated rash development, food and medication exposures, possible allergen and irritant exposures, pet exposure, and travel history.

In children, pruritus rarely has a systemic cause. However, clinicians should be alert for children who demonstrate red flag symptoms such as growth failure, anorexia, fatigue, associated bowel or bladder changes, and nighttime awakenings due to pruritus.

Underlying systemic disease is responsible for up to 50% of pruritus in older adults and should be considered in refractory cases and where skin findings are absent. Reassuring findings that suggest a non-systemic cause include recent onset, localized itch, pruritus limited to exposed skin, household members also with pruritus, and recent travel history.

Dermatitis distribution and appearance often indicate the cause. The examination can also reveal the chronicity of pruritus.

CURRENT DIAGNOSIS

- Reassuring findings that suggest a nonorganic cause include recent onset, localized itch, pruritus limited to exposed skin, household members also with pruritus, and recent travel history.
- Underlying systemic disease is responsible for up to 50% of pruritus in older adults and is uncommon in children.
- Laboratory testing to consider in atypical cases includes a complete blood count, ferritin, thyroid-stimulating hormone, serum bilirubin, alkaline phosphatase, serum creatinine, blood urea nitrogen, HIV test, and skin scrapings, biopsy, and culture.

BOX 1 Dermatitis-Associated Causes of Pruritus

Allergic Contact Dermatitis
- Sharply demarcated erythematous lesion with overlying vesicles
- Reaction within 2-7 d of exposure (see Box 4)

Atopic Dermatitis
- Atopic patients (allergic rhinitis, asthma) with the itch that rashes
- Affects flexor wrists and ankles, antecubital and popliteal fossa

Bullous Pemphigoid
- Initially pruritic urticarial lesions, often in intertriginous areas
- Tense blisters form after urticaria

Cutaneous T-Cell Lymphoma (Mycosis Fungoides)
- Oval eczematous patch on non–sun-exposed skin (e.g., buttocks)
- Can also manifest as erythroderma (exfoliative dermatitis)
- Can also manifest as a new eczematous disorder in older adults

Dermatitis Herpetiformis
- Rare vesicular dermatitis affects lumbosacral spine, elbows, knees

Folliculitis
- Pruritus out of proportion to appearance of dermatitis
- Papules and pustules at follicular sites on chest, back, or thighs

Lichen Planus
- Lesions often on the flexor wrists
- 6 Ps: pruritus, polygonal, planar, purple papules and plaques

Lichen Simplex Chronicus
- Complication of chronic scratching (e.g., atopic dermatitis)
- Thickened plaques over lower legs, posterior neck, and groin

Parasitic Skin Infections
Insects
- Chigger bites (harvest mite): Southeastern United States
- Cutaneous myiasis (bot fly): Central and South America, Africa
- Leishmaniasis (sand fly): Central and South America, Africa, Asia

Pediculosis (lice)
- Occiput of school-aged child
- Genitalia affected in adults (STD)

Scabies
- Burrows at hand web spaces, axillae, and genitalia
- Hyperkeratotic plaques, pruritic papules or scale present
- Face and scalp affected in children but not adults

Prurigo nodularis
- Complication of chronic scratching (variant of lichen simplex)
- 1-2 cm nodules on extensor arms and legs

Psoriasis
- Plaques on extensor extremities, low back, palms, soles, and scalp

Sunburn
- Consider photosensitizing causes (e.g., NSAIDs, cosmetics)

Xerotic Eczema
- Intense itching during winter in northern climates
- Involves back, flanks, abdomen, waist, and distal extremities

Abbreviations: NSAIDs = nonsteroidal anti-inflammatory drugs; STD = sexually transmitted disease.

CURRENT THERAPY

- Pruritus is usually self-limited and responds well to nonspecific measures such as liberal use of skin lubricants and avoidance of provocative factors.
- Antihistamines are not uniformly effective in reducing itch.
- Left untreated, itch and its associated persistent scratching increases risk of impetigo and cellulitis in the short term and lichen simplex chronicus and prurigo nodularis in chronic cases.

Excoriations and impetigo are seen acutely, and postinflammatory pigment changes and lichenification are seen with chronic scratching. Clinicians should be alert for findings consistent with thyroid disease, renal disease, liver disease, anemia, and hematologic malignancy. Examination should include careful palpation of the lymph nodes, liver, and spleen. Systemic causes of pruritus are listed in Box 3. Pruritic conditions specific to pregnancy are summarized in Box 4.

In cases refractory to 2 weeks of symptomatic therapy or in which an underlying systemic cause is considered, a limited laboratory evaluation is indicated and is summarized in Table 1. When itch persists or is refractory to general measures, remember that up to one half of older adults have pruritus caused by an underlying systemic problem.

CAUSES OF PRURITUS

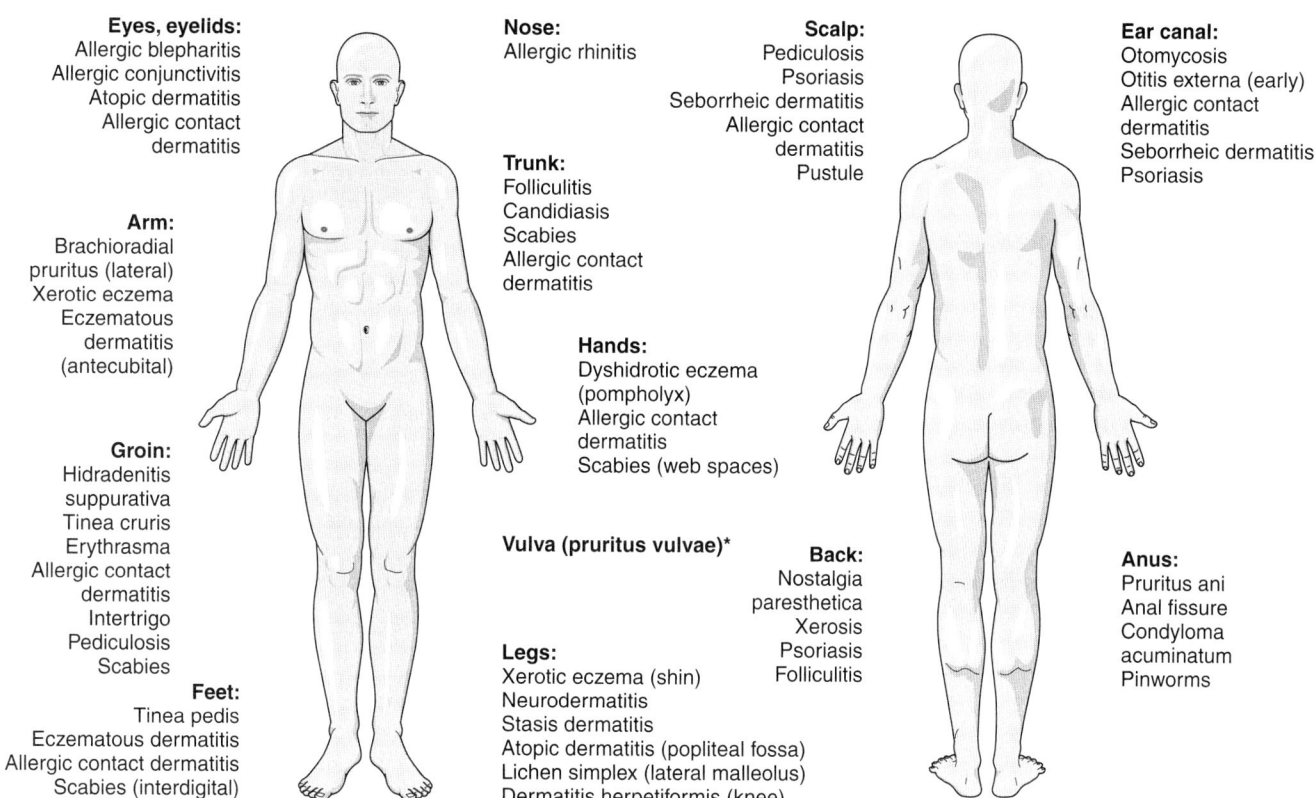

Eyes, eyelids:
Allergic blepharitis
Allergic conjunctivitis
Atopic dermatitis
Allergic contact dermatitis

Arm:
Brachioradial pruritus (lateral)
Xerotic eczema
Eczematous dermatitis (antecubital)

Groin:
Hidradenitis suppurativa
Tinea cruris
Erythrasma
Allergic contact dermatitis
Intertrigo
Pediculosis
Scabies

Feet:
Tinea pedis
Eczematous dermatitis
Allergic contact dermatitis
Scabies (interdigital)

Nose:
Allergic rhinitis

Trunk:
Folliculitis
Candidiasis
Scabies
Allergic contact dermatitis

Hands:
Dyshidrotic eczema (pompholyx)
Allergic contact dermatitis
Scabies (web spaces)

Vulva (pruritus vulvae)*

Legs:
Xerotic eczema (shin)
Neurodermatitis
Stasis dermatitis
Atopic dermatitis (popliteal fossa)
Lichen simplex (lateral malleolus)
Dermatitis herpetiformis (knee)

Scalp:
Pediculosis
Psoriasis
Seborrheic dermatitis
Allergic contact dermatitis
Pustule

Back:
Nostalgia paresthetica
Xerosis
Psoriasis
Folliculitis

Ear canal:
Otomycosis
Otitis externa (early)
Allergic contact dermatitis
Seborrheic dermatitis
Psoriasis

Anus:
Pruritus ani
Anal fissure
Condyloma acuminatum
Pinworms

*—Causes of pruritus vulvae: prepubertal girls—poor hygiene, streptococcal infection, Escherichia coli infection, pinworms, scabies, allergic contact dermatitis; young women—vaginitis, allergic contact dermatitis, hidradenitis suppurativa, lichen simplex chronicus; postmenopausal women—atrophic vaginitus, lichen sclerosus, vulvar cancer, Paget's disease; females with diabetes mellitus—candidiasis, other dermatophyte infections.

FIGURE 1. Causes of pruritus (by distribution). (Adapted from Moses S: Pruritus. Am Fam Physician 2003;68:1135-1146.)

BOX 2 Exposure-Related Pruritus

Allergic Contact Dermatitis
- Topical medications: Neomycin, benzocaine (Americaine)
- Nickel, latex, cosmetics, black hair dye
- Laundry detergents or fabric softeners
- Paint-on tattoos (paraphenylenediamine)
- Tattoo dye: cadmium yellow, mercuric sulfide (red)
- Ointments highly concentrated in inert oil

Heat Exposure
- Miliaria rubra (prickly heat)
- Cholinergic urticaria (response to hot bath, fever, exercise)

Occupational Exposure
- Dyes (e.g., glyceryl monothioglycolate)
- Potassium dichromate in cements and dyes
- Rosins or epoxy resins in adhesives
- Rubber, methyl methacrylate, fiberglass

Systemic Medications
- Drug hypersensitivity (rifampin [Rifadin], vancomycin [Vancocin])
- Itraconazole (Sporanox), fluconazole, ketoconazole (Nizoral)
- Niacinamide (niacin), B vitamins, aspirin, quinidine (Quinidex)
- Nitrates (food preservatives)
- Spinal narcotics (pruritus affects face, neck, and upper chest)

Water Exposure
- Aquagenic pruritus (associated with polycythemia vera)
- Cholinergic urticaria (response to warm water)
- Itching within 15 min of any water contact
- Polycythemia vera
- Swimmer's itch (7-d eruption after freshwater swimming)

BOX 3 Systemic Causes of Pruritus

Cholestasis
- Intense itching, worse at night
- Affects hands, feet, and pressure sites
- Reactive hyperpigmentation spares midback (butterfly appearance)

Chronic Renal Failure
- Severe paroxysms of generalized itching
- Worse in summer

Delusions of parasitosis
- Focal erosions on exposed areas of arms and legs

Human Immunodeficiency Virus
- Pruritus is a common presenting symptom due to secondary causes
- Causes: Eczema, drug reaction, eosinophilic folliculitis, seborrhea

Hodgkin's Lymphoma
- Prolonged generalized pruritus often precedes diagnosis

Hyperthyroidism
- Skin is warm and moist
- Pretibial edema may be present
- Onycholysis, hyperpigmentation, and vitiligo have been associated

Iron-Deficiency Anemia
- Other dermatologic signs include glossitis and angular cheilitis

Malignant Carcinoid
- Intermittent head and neck flushing
- Explosive diarrhea

Multiple Myeloma
- Affects elderly with bone pain, headache, cachexia, anemia, and renal failure

Neurodermatitis or Neurotic Excoriations
- Bouts of intense itching that can awaken the patient from a sound sleep
- Affects scalp, neck, wrist, extensor elbow, outer leg, ankle, perineum

Parasitic Infection (usually in returning travelers or immigrants)
- Filariasis: Tropical parasite responsible for lymphedema
- Onchocerciasis: Transmitted by black fly in Africa, Latin America
- Schistosomiasis: Fresh water exposure in Africa, Mediterranean, South America
- Trichinosis: Undercooked pork, bear, wild boar, or walrus meat

Parvovirus B19
- Slapped cheek appearance in children
- Arthritis in some adults

Peripheral Neuropathy
- Brachioradial pruritus: Affects lateral arms of white patients in the tropics
- Notalgia paresthetica: Midback pruritus with hyperpigmented patch
- Herpes zoster: Accompanies painful prodrome 2 d before rash

Polycythemia Rubra Vera
- Pricking-type itch persists for hours after hot shower or bath

Scleroderma
- Nonpitting extremity edema, erythema, and intense pruritus
- Edema phase with pruritus precedes fibrosis of the skin

Urticaria
- Response to allergen, cold, heat, exercise, sunlight, or direct pressure

Weight Loss (Rapid) in Eating Disorders
- Other signs include hair loss or fine lanugo hair on back and cheeks
- Also yellow skin discoloration and petechiae

BOX 4 Causes of Pruritus in Pregnancy

Pruritic Urticarial Papules and Plaques of Pregnancy
- Common in the third trimester
- Intense pruritus involves abdomen
- Spreads to thighs, buttocks, breasts, and arms

Prurigo of Pregnancy
- Common in second half of pregnancy
- Extensor arms and abdomen with excoriated papules and nodules
- Associated with atopic dermatitis

Herpes Gestationis or Pemphigoid Gestationis
- Uncommon
- Autoimmune condition associated with Graves' disease
- Vesicles and bullae on abdomen and extremities in second half of pregnancy
- Responds to prednisone[1] 0.5 mg/kg (Level A)

Intrahepatic Cholestasis of Pregnancy
- Uncommon
- Trunk and extremity itching without rash in late pregnancy
- Jaundice not present in the mild form (prurigo gravidarum)
- Responds to cholestyramine (Questran) and Vitamin K_1 (Aquamephyton)[1] (Level B)

Pruritic Folliculitis of Pregnancy
- Uncommon, occurs in second half of pregnancy
- Erythematous follicular papules over trunk, with spread to extremities
- May be a variant of prurigo of pregnancy

Other Common Pruritic Conditions Exacerbated in Pregnancy
- Atopic dermatitis
- Contact dermatitis

---

[1] Not FDA approved for this indication.
Levels of evidence: Level A: Evidence from high-quality randomized controlled clinical trials or meta-analyses; Level B: Evidence from nonrandomized clinical studies or nonquantitative systematic reviews.

TABLE 1 Diagnostic Evaluation of Pruritus for Atypical, Persistent, or Refractory Cases

Tests	Findings
Complete blood count,* serum ferritin*	Iron deficiency anemia, polycythemia rubra vera, Hodgkin's lymphoma, multiple myeloma, parasitic infection
Serum bilirubin, alkaline phosphatase*	Cholestasis (e.g., cirrhosis)
Serum creatinine, blood urea nitrogen*	Uremia (e.g., chronic renal failure)
Thyroid stimulating hormone*	Hyperthyroidism
Microscopy of skin scrapings, skin culture, skin biopsy	Dermatophytes, scabies; skin bacterial, fungal or viral infection; mastocytosis, mycosis fungoides, bullous pemphigoid
HIV test	HIV infection
Chest radiograph	Hodgkin's lymphoma, multiple myeloma
Stool tests	Parasites, *Helicobacter pylori*
	Children: pinworms, perianal streptococcus

*Denotes a first-line test. Unmarked tests are performed if history indicates.

Treatment

Pruritus is usually self-limited and responds well to nonspecific measures such as liberal use of skin lubricants and avoidance of provocative factors (Box 5). Oral antihistamines are not uniformly effective in all causes of pruritus. Specific management of dermatitis, as with atopic dermatitis, scabies, and contact dermatitis, can relieve symptoms.

In the atypical case, where these measures fail, a systemic condition may be uncovered. In these patients, the itch should be alleviated by treating the underlying condition, as with thyroid replacement in hypothyroidism or iron supplementation in iron deficiency anemia. Uremia and cholestasis-related pruritus have established effective therapies beyond treating the causative chronic renal or hepatic insufficiency (Box 6).

Complications

Itch and the scratch it induces are not benign. When scratching is left unchecked, fingernails introduce bacteria into abraded skin, and impetigo or cellulitis can ensue. Lichen simplex chronicus and prurigo nodularis are chronic skin changes seen with long-term scratching and in particular with atopic dermatitis.

BOX 5 Nonspecific Management of Pruritus

- Use skin lubricants liberally
  - Petrolatum or skin lubricant cream at bedtime
  - Apply alcohol-free, hypoallergenic lotions frequently during day
- Avoid excessive bathing
  - Briefly pat dry after bath and immediately apply skin lubricants
  - Decrease bathing frequency
  - Limit bathing to brief exposure to tepid water
- Limit soap use
  - Use mild, unscented, hypoallergenic soap 2 or 3 times per wk
  - Daily use of soap only in groin and axillae; spare legs, arms, and torso
- Minimize dryness
  - Humidify dry indoor environment (especially in winter)
- Choose clothing that does not irritate the skin
  - Doubly rinsed cotton clothes and silk are best
  - Add bath oil (e.g., Alpha Keri) to rinse cycle when washing sheets
  - Avoid heat-retaining fabrics (synthetics)
  - Avoid wool and smooth-textured cotton clothes
- Avoid vasodilators
  - Avoid caffeine, alcohol, spices, hot water, and excessive sweating
- Avoid provocative topical medications
  - Avoid prolonged topical corticosteroids (risk of skin atrophy)
- Avoid topical anesthetics and antihistamines
  - May sensitize exposed skin and risk contact dermatitis
- Standard antipruritic topical agents
  - Menthol and camphor (e.g., Sarna Lotion)
  - Oatmeal baths (e.g., Aveeno)
  - Pramoxine[1] (e.g., PrameGel [pramoxine + menthol], Pramosone [pramoxine + hydrocortisone])
  - Calamine lotion (Use on weeping lesions only, not on dry skin)
- Antipruritic topical agents for refractory cases (used in severe atopic dermatitis)
  - Doxepin 5% cream (Zonalon)
  - Burow's solution (wet dressings with aluminum acetate 5% in water)
  - Unna's boot[1] (zinc oxide paste bandages)
  - Coal tar emulsion[1] (Zetar)
- Systemic antipruritic agents (used in allergic and urticarial disease)
  - Doxepin (Sinequan)[1] 1 mg/kg up to 25 mg at bedtime (Level A)
  - Hydroxyzine (Atarax) 0.5 mg/kg up to 25-50 mg at bedtime
  - Nonsedating antihistamines (e.g., Fexofenadine [Allegra], Level A)
- Prevent complications of scratching
  - Keep fingernails short and clean
  - Rub skin with palms if urge to scratch is irresistible

[1]Not FDA approved for this indication.
Level A: Evidence from high-quality randomized controlled clinical trials or meta-analyses.

BOX 6 Specific Management of Pruritic Conditions

Cholestasis
- Cholestyramine (Questran) (Level B)
  - Adult: 4 g 30 min before meals
  - Child: 240 mg/kg/d divided tid (up to 6 g/d)
- Ursodiol (Actigall)[1] 15 mg/kg/d divided before meals
- Ondansetron (Zofran)[1] 4-8 mg IV, then 4 mg PO q8h (Level B)
- Opioid receptor antagonist (Level A)
  - Naloxone (Narcan)[1] 0.002 mcg/kg/h IV, titrate to max 0.25 mcg/kg/h
  - Naltrexone (Revia)[1] 12.5 mg PO qd (advance to 50 mg PO qd)
- Rifampin (Rifadin)[1] 10 mg/kg/d divided bid (max: 300 mg bid) (Level B)
- Bile duct stenting from extrahepatic cholestasis (Level A)
- Lidocaine (Xylocaine)[1] IV has been used
- Bright light therapy (Level B)
- Plasmapheresis

Neurotic Excoriation
- Pimozide (Orap)[1] for delusions of parasitosis
- Selective serotonin reuptake inhibitor (SSRI)

Notalgia Paresthetica
- Topical capsaicin (Zostrix)[1] applied 4-6 times per d for several wk (Level B)

Polycythemia Vera
- Aspirin[1] 500 mg PO q8-24h (Level B)
- Paroxetine (Paxil)[1] 10-20 mg PO qd (Level B)
- Interferon-α (Intron A)[1] 3-35 million IU/wk (Level B)

Spinal Opioid–Induced Pruritus
- Ondansetron (Zofran)[1] 8 mg IV concurrent with opioid (Level A)
- Nalbuphine (Nubain)[1] 5 mg IV concurrent with opioid (Level B)

Uremia
- UV B phototherapy twice weekly for 1 mo (Level A)
- Activated charcoal[1] 6 g/d (Level A)
- Topical capsaicin[1] 0.025% cream to localized areas (Level A)
- Ondansetron and naltrexone are not efficacious in uremia (Level A)

[1]Not FDA approved for this indication.
Level A: Evidence from high-quality randomized controlled clinical trials or meta-analyses; Level B: Evidence from nonrandomized clinical studies or nonquantitative systematic reviews.

Medications to treat pruritus are also not without adverse effects. Antihistamines can affect alertness and learning if used during the day, and with chronic use, the associated dry mouth can predispose to tooth decay.

Follow-Up

General measures to treat pruritus should be reviewed at each visit. Consistent practice of these simple home strategies can prevent sleepless nights, frequent evaluations, unnecessary medications, and the complications of scratching.

REFERENCES

Belsito DV: The diagnostic evaluation, treatment and prevention of allergic contact dermatitis in the new millennium. J Allergy Clin Immunol 2000;105:409-420.

Bender BG: Sedation and performance impairment of diphenhydramine and second-generation antihistamines: A meta-analysis. J Allergy Clin Immunol 2003;111:770-776.

Bergasa NV: An approach to the management of the pruritus of cholestasis. Clin Liver Dis 2004;8:55-66.

Berger R, Gilchrest BA. Skin disorders. In Duthie EH, Katz PR (eds): Practice of Geriatrics, 3rd ed. Philadelphia: WB Saunders, 1998, pp 467-472.

Boiko S, Zeiger R: Diagnosis and treatment of atopic dermatitis, urticaria, and angioedema during pregnancy. Immunol Allergy Clin North Am 2000;20:839.

Callen JP, Bernardi DM, Clark RAF, Weber DA: Adult-onset recalcitrant eczema: A marker of noncutaneous lymphoma or leukemia. J Am Acad Dermatol 2000;43:207-210.

Correale CE, Walker C, Lydia M, Craig TJ: Atopic dermatitis: A review of diagnosis and treatment. Am Fam Physician 1999;60:1191-1210.

Cyr PR, Dreher GK: Neurotic excoriations. Am Fam Physician 2001;64:1981-1984.

Diehn F, Tefferi A: Pruritus in polychaemia vera: Prevalence, laboratory correlates and management. 2001;115:619-621.

Fagan EA: Intrahepatic cholestasis of pregnancy. Clin Liver Dis 1999;3:603-632.

Finn AF, Kaplan AP, Fretwell R, et al: A double-blind, placebo-controlled trial of fexofenadine HCl in the treatment of chronic idiopathic urticaria. J Allergy Clin Immunol 1999;103:1071-1078.

Fisher AA: Aquagenic pruritus. Cutis 1993;51:146-147.

Gelfand JM, Rudikoff D: Evaluation and treatment of itching in HIV-infected patients. Mt Sinai J Med 2001;68:298-308.

Ghent CN: The pruritus of cholestasis. Hepatology 1999;29:1003-1006.

Gupta MA, Gupta AK, Voorhees JJ: Starvation-associated pruritus: A clinical feature of eating disorders. J Am Acad Dermatol 1992;27:118-120.

Habif TP. Clinical Dermatology 3rd ed. Chicago: Mosby–Year Book, 1996.

Harrigan E, Rabinowitz LG: Atopic dermatitis. Immunol Allergy Clin North Am 1999;19:383-396.

Heymann WR: Chronic urticaria and angioedema associated with thyroid autoimmunity: Review and therapeutic implications. J Am Acad Dermatol 1999;40:229-232.

Koblenzer CS: Itching and atopic skin. J Allergy Clin Immunol 1999;104:S109-S113.

Krajnik M, Zylicz Z: Understanding pruritus in systemic disease. J Pain Symptom Manage 2001;21:151-168.

Kroumpouzos G, Cohen LM: Dermatoses of pregnancy. J Am Acad Dermatol 2001;45:1-19.

Leung AKC: Pruritus in children, J Roy Soc Health 1998;118:280-286.

Lidofsky S, Scharschmidt BF: Jaundice. In Feldman M, Scharschmidt BF, Sleisenger MH, Fordtran JS (eds): Sleisenger and Fordtran's Gastrointestinal and Liver Disease, 6th ed. Philadelphia: WB Saunders, 1998, pp 230-231.

Moses S: Pruritus, Am Fam Physician 2003;68:1135-1146.

Parker F. Structure and function of skin. In Goldman L, Bennett JC (eds): Cecil Textbook of Medicine, 21st ed. Philadelphia: WB Saunders, 2000, p 2266.

Paus R, Schmeiz M, Biró T, Steinhoff M: Frontiers in pruritus research: Scratching the brain for more effective itch therapy. J Clin Invest 2006;116:1174-1185.

Robinson-Bostom L, DiGiovanna JJ: Cutaneous manifestations of end-stage renal disease. J Am Acad Dermatol 2000;43:975-986.

Shellow WVR: Evaluation of pruritus. In Goroll AH, Mulley AG (eds): Primary Care Medicine, 4th ed, Philadelphia: Lippincott Williams & Wilkins, 2000, pp 1001-1004.

Stambuk R, Colvin R: Dermatologic disorders. In Gabbe SG, Niebyl JR, Simpson JL (eds): Obstetrics: Normal and Problem Pregnancies, 4th ed. New York: Churchill Livingstone, 2002, pp 1283-1290.

Tennyson H: Neurotropic and psychotropic drugs in dermatology. Dermatol Clin 2001;19:179-197.
Tormey WP, Chambers JPM: Pruritus as the presenting symptom in hyperthyroidism. Br J Clin Pract 1994;48:224.
Valsecchi R, Cainelli T: Generalized pruritus: A manifestation of iron deficiency. Arch Dermatol 1983;119:630.
Veien NK, Hattel T, Laurberg G. Spaun E: Brachioradial pruritus. J Am Acad Dermatol 2001;44:704-705.
Villamil AG, Bandi JC, Galdame OA, et al: Efficacy of lidocaine in the treatment of pruritus in patients with chronic cholestatic liver disease. Am J Med 2005;118:1160-1163.
Waxler B, Dadabhoy Z, Stojiljkovic L, Rabito SF: Primer of postoperative pruritus for anesthesiologists. Anesthesiology 2005;103:168-178.
Zirwas MJ, Seraly MP: Pruritus of unknown origin: A retrospective study. J Am Acad Dermatol 2001;45:892-896.

Tinnitus

Method of
Claus-Frenz Claussen, MD

Tinnitus is noise(s) in the ear, which is usually subjective and can be extremely disturbing and frustrating to those affected. According to studies of the American Tinnitus Association, approximately 36 million Americans older than 40 years suffer from tinnitus.

Tinnitus has been regarded as a disease entity for many centuries. During the second half of the 20th century, physicians were able to discriminate among several different kinds of tinnitus including bruits, maskable tinnitus, and nonmaskable tinnitus. Under the influence of Shulman and his team, the term *tinnitology* was coined.

The present interest of researchers in the field of tinnitology is split into two fields of action: suggestions for improvement of objective and quantitative differential diagnostics in tinnitus and research and development to improve various types of treatment for different kinds of tinnitus.

General Phenomena of Tinnitus

A noise without any human information function, a tinnitus, can be a normal as well as a pathologic function of human hearing. On the one hand, tinnitus can be regarded as a problem of acoustic resolution of the inner ear microphone, that is, the cochlear noise-to-signal ratio. In a well-dampened soundproof chamber, most normal-hearing persons experience a sizzling sound in their ears because of their perception of molecular vibrations from inner ear fluids (as known from thermodynamics). Yet this underlying percept is masked in everyday life by normal environmental noise.

CURRENT DIAGNOSIS

Irritating subjective or objective perception of irritating acoustic noise or sound in the ear, head, or body that may be described, for example, as:
- Pulsating
- Humming
- Roaring
- Whistling
- Hissing

On the other hand, tinnitus patients regularly tell their physicians about subjective ear noises that they describe, for example, as pulsating, humming, roaring, whistling, hissing, fullness of the ear, and pressure and/or pain in the ear.

Table 1 presents the subjective sensational qualities of tinnitus in 823 tinnitus patients (77.52% male and 22.48% female with a mean age of 50.87 years ± 8.68 years) from Bad Kissingen, Germany, who underwent clinical inpatient rehabilitation therapy for several weeks for severe disabling tinnitus.

In these same patients, we looked for descriptions of different time/intensity patterns of their tinnitus (Table 2), and the subjective background of discomfort was investigated as shown in Table 3. Additionally, the patients named the most irritating factors related to their tinnitus (Table 4).

Sleep disturbance is a common and frequent complaint. Scientific studies report decreased tolerance and increased discomfort when insomnia and depression are associated with tinnitus.

In 1991, a sample of 338 New Zealanders regularly experiencing tinnitus completed and returned questionnaires to associations for people with tinnitus or hearing impairment. Nearly half the sample was sometimes depressed because of tinnitus. Those reporting depression and those reporting more severe problems as a consequence of the tinnitus saw more health care professionals and used more coping strategies. Most respondents did not remember exactly when they first noticed the tinnitus.

A questionnaire investigation comprising 1091 patients from Bispebjerg Hospital, Copenhagen (1993), concerning "tinnitus-incidence and handicap," was conducted at a hearing center. A majority of patients, 59%, claimed that they were troubled by tinnitus. Neither a greater degree of hearing loss nor a longer duration of tinnitus was associated with more severe tinnitus. Among patients with both subjective hearing loss and tinnitus, 23% stated that tinnitus was the greater problem, and 38% said that tinnitus and hearing loss were equally troublesome. The corresponding figures for patients with hearing impairment of such a degree that a hearing aid was deemed necessary were 9% and 41%, respectively. Stress symptoms such as headache, tension of facial muscles, and sleep disturbances were correlated to tinnitus. Of patients with tinnitus, 83% were interested in obtaining treatment for it.

The so-called Copenhagen Male Study reported on the results from a 10-year follow-up examination concerning hearing and factors known to cause hearing problems. The original sample comprised 5050 subjects, and at the present examination, 3387 (67%)

TABLE 1 Subjective Classification of Ear Noises in 823 (= 100%) Tinnitus Patients

Complaints	Right Ear (%)	Left Ear (%)
Pulsating	1.94	1.94
Humming	7.41	6.93
Roaring	14.10	14.22
Whistling	50.67	51.76
Hissing	9.96	10.81
Pressure in the ear	6.32	5.83
Pain in the ear	14.10	14.22

TABLE 2 Subjective Classification of Different Time/Intensity Patterns of Tinnitus in 823 (= 100%) Patients

Time/Intensity Patterns	%
Permanent	59.17
Intermittent	19.97
Swelling up and going down	43.26

TABLE 3 Subjective Classification of Subjective Background of Discomfort in 823 (= 100%) Patients

Subjective Complaints About Factors of Discomfort	%
Headache	69.02
Migraine	4.13
Exhaustion	59.99
Lacking in drive	42.16
Feeling of weakness	55.29
Forgetfulness	68.41
Disorientation	0.49
Daze	44.84
Tiredness	63.91
Insomnia	69.50

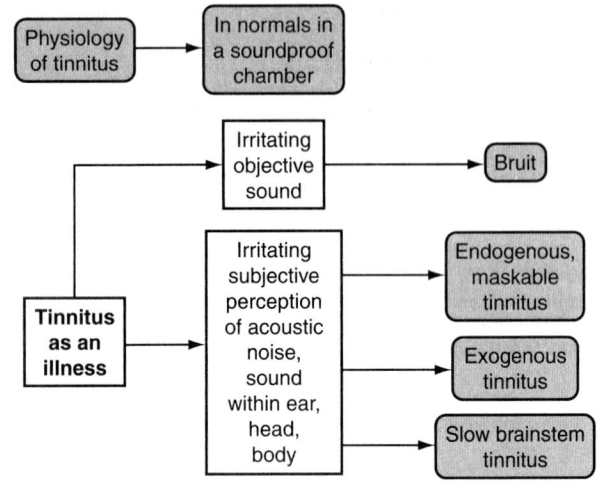

FIGURE 1. Categories of physiologic and clinical types of tinnitus.

men at a median of 63 years of age (range, 53 to 75 years) participated. An increasing prevalence of 30% to 40% of hearing problems was demonstrated with increasing age. A prevalence of 17% of tinnitus of more than 5 minutes' duration was found; 3% indicated that tinnitus was so annoying that it interfered with sleep, reading, and/or concentration. The prevalence of tinnitus increased up to 70 years of age and seemed to remain constant thereafter.

In Norway, 15% of the adult population has experienced shorter or longer periods of tinnitus. Three percent of these, in total approximately 7000 to 10,000 persons, suffer from continuous tinnitus followed by symptoms that represent a handicap or occupational disability. Similar observations were reported from many other countries.

Clinical Types

Tinnitus is no longer considered to be a syndrome or a single disease. Because of improvements in neuro-otometry, several different types of tinnitus can be differentiated.

By means of modern audiometry, the framework for normal hearing can be described objectively and quantitatively. Therefore, in any tinnitus case, a thorough analysis of the hearing function and pathways needs to be performed including threshold audiometry, audiometric tinnitus masking (if possible), acoustic dynamics between the measurable thresholds of hearing and acoustic discomfort, speech audiometry, otoacoustic emissions, acoustic brainstem-evoked potentials, and acoustic late-evoked potentials. Thereby signs of pathology within the hearing pathways between the ear and the human brain cortex can be measured.

Thus, we know from thorough neuro-otologic studies that approximately 24% of cases of disabling tinnitus have their source within the otoacoustic periphery (i.e., inner ear and the eighth cranial nerve). Approximately 35% originate from the acoustic pathways within the brainstem. Approximately 41% have their cause within supratentorial structures and/or functions. These pathologies also should serve as basic information for planning systematic pharmacotherapy directed to the central nervous system (CNS) focus of dysfunction.

At least four different kinds of tinnitus (Figure 1) can be discriminated, which can be determined by the physician using a simple question-and-answer procedure as follows.

BRUITS

Q: Has someone informed you that he or she could hear a noise coming from your head?
A: Yes. Their description of what they heard listening from outside my head is similar to what I perceive.

By means of auscultation through a stethoscope or a microphone, a real sound can be objectively heard emanating from the patient's skull. Patients frequently report, for example, a bubbling, hissing, or pulsating sound.

The cause can be vascular in origin, that is, abnormal curling of blood caused by atheromas, vascular dissections, scars, compressions, or high blood pressure amplitudes, for example.

Bruits also can originate from the middle ear and its connections toward the epipharynx: middle ear inflammaitons with bubbling sounds of gas from within the effusions, whizzing middle ear muscles, or an open eustachian tube.

Cracking sounds, which are misinterpreted as tinnitus, are reported from arthritic and other mandibular joint disorders. Also, sounds can be transferred from the cervical spine and its joints as well as its vessels into the cranial structures so that they become misinterpreted as tinnitus.

ENDOGENOUS TINNITUS

Q: Where is your feeling of well-being better, in a busy and noisy environment or in cavelike silence?
A: I much prefer a busy and noisy environment.

The patient with a maskable or endogenous tinnitus prefers covering it with external sounds. When using masking procedures, easily three zones of tinnitus can be discriminated within the hearing field:
1. Low-tone tinnitus (at and below 750 Hz)
2. Middle-frequency tinnitus (1 to 2 kHz)
3. High-frequency tinnitus (above 2 kHz until 10 kHz or even 12 kHz)

Low-tone tinnitus is more frequently found in Ménière's disease and some other cochlear-apical disorders, and middle-tone tinnitus is more frequently found in diseases such as otosclerosis. Most frequently tinnitus is matched in the high-tone range and is related, for example, to noise trauma, whiplash, head and skull trauma, cardiovascular failure, stress, acoustic neuromas, and toxic events including those associated with pharmaceutical, nicotine, or drug abuse. Also, several masking points may exist simultaneously.

TABLE 4 Subjective Classification of Most Irritating Factors Related to Their Tinnitus in 823 (= 100%) Patients

Most Irritating Factors Related to Tinnitus	%
All patients with specific additional statements	25.76
Difficulties in going to sleep	10.69
Difficulties in sleeping through the night	11.06
Depression	0.24
Abnormal sounds (also hallucinations)	2.67
Acute hearing loss	8.38

Dysfunctions of the inner ear contribute to the development of tinnitus. But tinnitus by itself depends on a cortical process of the human brain. A sleeping patient does not suffer from any kind of tinnitus.

Since approximately 1985, the Würzburg neuro-otology group of Claussen et al. has been able to detect by means of vestibular evoked potentials (VestEP) and brain electrical activity mapping (BEAM) groups of patients suffering from a maskable or endogenous tinnitus that respond cortically in a typical, reproducible, and measurable manner:

1. Location of the site of the potentials around the upper gyrus of the temporal lobe (Brodmann's area 41)
2. Typical shortening of the latencies of evoked quantitative electroencephalograms (QEEGs) (i.e., VestEP waves I, II, III)
3. Enlarged DC shift of the evoked QEEGs (i.e., difference between VestEP waves III and IV)
4. Typical cortical electrical burst expansion in three phases on the brain surface

Since approximately 1990, the New York group of Shulman, Strashun, and Goldstein has followed a neuroradiologic path for deciphering the cortical modalities in tinnitus patients by using single-photon emission computer tomography (SPECT). They discovered remarkably elevated metabolic processes in the temporal lobes of patients suffering from a maskable tinnitus.

Thereafter we were able to prove in therapeutic trials with pharmacotherapy (e.g., extractum ginkgo biloba [EGB 761]*), as well as with physiotherapy (competitive kinesthetic interaction therapy [KKIT]), that the subjective reduction or abolition of tinnitus goes together with an electrophysiologic measurable normalization of the VestEP with BEAM or QEEG. So the endogenous tinnitus could be proven to be a CNS network phenomenon.

EXOGENOUS TINNITUS

Q: Where is your feeling of well-being better, in a busy and noisy environment or in cavelike silence?
A: I much prefer a cavelike silence because noise and/or a group of people speaking at the same time are most confusing. It provokes ringing and shrieking sounds within my ears.

Unlike endogenous tinnitus, patients suffering from exogenous tinnitus cannot benefit from masking noises from their surroundings. Some physicians wrongly call this condition *hyperacusis*, but these patients do not hear better as this term suggests. Seemingly better is the named syndrome of the hypersensitive ear.

In exogenous tinnitus, pure-tone audiometry may be normal or exhibit regular deficits of the hearing threshold, but there is no maskable tinnitus. However, when measuring the acoustic dynamics by adding the audiometrically recorded discomfort threshold, the discomfort level, which is usually between 1 and 8 kHz below 95 dB, rises below this level to values of 90 to 60 dB or even 50 dB. The person being exposed to sound exceeding the level of his low discomfort threshold experiences a loss of understanding together with subjective pain and noise in the ears accompanied by possible vegetative reactions.

Hearing aids can adjust the incoming sounds by filtering, peak clipping, and cleaning of the sound signals so they fit optimally into the remaining acoustic dynamics of the individually existing hearing field. Thus, hearing aids are the first choice for treating exogenous tinnitus. Some other methods for treating this type of tinnitus are physiotherapy, psychotherapy, stress reduction, and supportive pharmacotherapy.

TINNITUS IN SLOW BRAINSTEM SYNDROME (CLAUSSEN)

Q: How would you best describe your tinnitus?
A: I am becoming increasingly more in a daze and more disoriented and hear ringing and other sounds, which I cannot really localize in my ears or my head. The noise disturbs me as much as my mental instability.

We regularly see older patients who complain about a hazy tinnitus in combination with vertigo, giddiness, and dizziness and also report a reduced state of alertness. These patients have a connected statoacoustic problem. Objectively, affected patients exhibit an increase in the latencies of the experimentally provoked vestibular nystagmus as well as of the acoustically evoked brainstem potentials.

Especially in this group, we have noted by evaluating our therapeutic responses that a combination of cocculus† (picrotoxin), conium† (coneine), amber and petrol oil (Vertigoheel†) has a so-called tuning-up effect on the brainstem. Then the typical symptoms also disappear.

COMBINED ENDOGENOUS AND EXOGENOUS TINNITUS

A combination of both types of subjective tinnitus, endogenous and exogenous, is also found in tinnitus patients. Affected patients report that the noise they hear is present during both the day and night; however, the noise fluctuates. Especially the intensity of the noise can be very increased, for example when the patient is in a noisy environment or busy place or in a conversation with several participants.

Even though patients with combined endogenous and exogenous tinnitus have maskable tinnitus, they report that therapeutic acoustic maskers do not reduce their symptoms. They need a thorough audiometric and neuro-otologic workup.

Contemporary and Practical Treatment

Modern therapy of tinnitus appears to be complex and sometimes incomprehensible. But when talking about therapy of disabling tinnitus, we emphasize a main therapeutic approach in the sense that we have to break and inhibit the psychosomatic cycle of deterioration from tinnitus to stress, to insomnia, to panic. Some aspects of this reactional behavior are similar to pain.

The steps for individual tinnitus therapy must be chosen according to the kind of tinnitus diagnosed. Tinnitus is frequently associated with conditions such as stress, hearing loss, noise trauma, otorhinolaryngologic disorders (e.g., Ménière's disease, otosclerosis, perilymphatic fistula, acoustic neuroma), high blood pressure, metabolic disorders, allergy, intoxications, whiplash and other head and neck traumas, functional disorders of the neck, burnout syndrome, mandibular joint problems, and extracranial and intracranial vascular problems.

The Current Therapy box lists different therapeutic approaches to tinnitus. These ten therapies must be individually interrelated with the different types of tinnitus (see Figure 1). Besides the severe disabling types of tinnitus, minor forms of tinnitus also occasionally occur that may be event related or may be time limited.

NOISE AVOIDANCE AND BASICS OF THERAPY

Avoidance can help in noise-related tinnitus by the prevention of noise exposure or at least by wearing ear protection. The use of ototoxic drugs must be controlled and limited. Inflammatory ear disease needs specific treatment of the external and the middle ear with antibiotics and anti-inflammatory drugs. Control and maintenance of a satisfactory degree of aeration of the middle ear is necessary. Acoustic neuroma calls for surgical removal of the tumor. Surgery is also necessary in otosclerosis and perilymphatic fistula. Specific gnatholic therapy by a dentist is recommended in a temporomandibular joint syndrome.

INSTRUMENTATIONS FOR THERAPY

Instrumentations currently available and frequently used according to the type and the chronicity of tinnitus are as follows:
1. Tinnitus maskers/tinnitus instruments, tapes/CDs for masking and relaxation

---

†Available as homeopathic remedy.

CURRENT THERAPY

- Avoidance of noise, ototoxic drugs, allergens
- Treatment of bruits by medical or surgical measures
- Instrumental therapy
- Tinnitus maskers
- Hearing aids
- Electrostimulation
- Specific pharmacotherapy
  - Lidocaine (Xylocaine)[1]
  - Carbamazepine (Tegretol)[1]
- Calming pharmacotherapy
  - Diazepam (Valium)[1]
  - Amitriptyline (Elavil)[1]
- Nontropic pharmacotherapy
- Gingko*
- Flunarizine[2]
- Neurotransmitter-directed pharmacotherapy
  - Betahistine*
  - Gabapentin (Neurontin)
- Psychotherapy
  - Retraining therapy (TRT)
- Physiotherapy
  - Competitive kinesthetic interaction therapy (KKIT)
- Other therapies
  - Hypnotherapy
  - Counseling
  - Acupuncture

[1]Not FDA approved for this indication.
[2]Not available in the United States.
*Available as dietary supplement.

2. Acoustic ultra-high-frequency stimulation
3. Hearing aids
4. External electrical stimulations
5. External magnetic stimulation

PHARMACOTHERAPY

Pharmacotherapy, that is, treatment with pharmaceutical agents, is important in the management of tinnitus. It may be the main therapy or may play only a supportive, palliative, or intermittent role. The four lines of therapeutic agents used in the treatment of tinnitus may overlap and may be combined.

First-Line Agents

First-line therapeutic agents can relieve tinnitus either slowly or quickly. Lidocaine (Xylocaine),[1] a local anesthetic drug, only has a temporary effect in suppressing tinnitus. It is an aminoethylamide, which is well soluble in water.

A daily intravenous dose of lidocaine of 1 mg per kg of body weight can temporarily alleviate the phenomenon of endogenous tinnitus. The duration, however, depends on the blood level. As soon as the level of lidocaine in the blood is lowered below a threshold, tinnitus returns.

In tinnitus, lidocaine is best applied by iontophoresis through an electrical field with an active electrode in the external ear and a passive electrode at an arm, after instillation of a solution of lidocaine (1:100,000) into the external meatus.

[1]Not FDA approved for this indication.

This therapy temporarily relieves the disturbing tinnitus, so that the patients at least get some hours of rest and sleep. However, the untoward side effects of lidocaine also have to be taken into consideration.

Some forms of tinnitus also have an acoustic hallucinatory component, as in epilepsy. Therefore, carbamazepine (Tegretol),[1] which is an important antiepileptic agent used for bipolar affective disorders, is also used in tinnitus with a supratentorial focus. We have seen beneficial effects in very specific cases of endogenous tinnitus. Chemically, carbamazepine belongs to the tricyclic antidepressants. In adults, we give a daily dose of 200 mg. However, renal, hepatic, and hematologic parameters have to be monitored thoroughly.

Second-Line Agents

This group of drugs is especially used to treat the emotional effects seen in endogenous tinnitus, exogenous tinnitus, and combined endogenous and exogenous tinnitus, which can lead via sleeplessness to anxiety and panic. Here we see an indication for alprazolam (Xanax)[1] and similar substances. Alprazolam is administered to tinnitus patients in a daily dosage of 0.75 to 1.5 mg. Also chlordiazepoxide (Librium)[1] can alternatively be applied in a daily dosage of 15 to 30 mg. Even diazepam (Valium)[1] is used in a daily dosage of 4 to 30 mg.

The mood changes associated with tinnitus can lead to psychosis and insomnia. Here a tricyclic antidepressant such as amitriptyline (Elavil)[1] in a daily dosage of 75 to 150 mg can be helpful.

Additionally, this agent has a desired sedative component. Other sedatives and psychotropic drugs are also used to treat the psychologic effects associated with tinnitus, but they must be applied very carefully.

Third-Line Agents

Third-line therapeutic agents comprise the so-called nootropic drugs. These are pharmacologic agents that activate brain function through improved metabolism, leading to a better adaptation and interconnection. They were originally developed to treat senile dementia. Within this group, in Germany, we use piracetam (Nootrop, Normabraïn) in a daily dosage of 800 to 1200 mg.

We have seen very beneficial effects from extract of ginkgo biloba (EGB 761*) (Tebonin, Rökan), which is administered in a daily dosage of 120 mg.

We also use calcium channel antagonists, among which flunarizine (Sibelium),[2] in a daily dosage of 15 to 30 mg, is effective in tinnitus with irritative foci, especially in mesencephalic and diencephalic areas. Cinnarizin[2] was the predecessor. This holds especially for the endogenous tinnitus group.

Fourth-Line Agents

The fourth line of therapy involves neurotransmitter-directed pharmacotherapy. According to the chemical structures of the neurotransmitters, we mainly use one system of the amines (i.e., the histamine mechanism) and one system of amino acids (i.e., γ-aminobutyric acid [GABA]).

Because it is known that inner ear functions are regulated at the neurotransmission level of the histaminergic H_1, H_2, and H_3 receptors, betahistine (Serc)[2] plays an important role in inner ear receptor-targeted therapy. The daily dosage that we administer in peripheral cochlear tinnitus is 16 to 48 mg.

The inhibitory neurotransmitter GABA is extremely potent in its ability to alter neuronal discharges because of failures in the supratentorial CNS neurotransmission. According to recent findings, endogenous tinnitus with a supratentorial dysregulation can be influenced by gabapentin (Neurontin).[1] It is used in dosages starting with 300 mg daily and can be increased to 900 mg daily. Originally

[1]Not FDA approved for this indication.
*Available as dietary supplement.
[2]Not available in the United States.

gabapentin was used as an additional therapy in partial epilepsia without secondary generalized seizures. Like with other antiepileptic drugs, the parameters from kidney, liver, and blood have to be supervised.

ADAPTED PSYCHOTHERAPY

Nowadays so-called tinnitus retraining therapy (TRT) is widely applied. It includes a therapeutic wide-band low-level noise generator. It is based on habituation, which is defined as a reduced response to a stimulus after repeated exposure. It is a state in which the tinnitus signal no longer elicits any response. Resetting or reprogramming neuronal networks involved in subcortical signal detection brings about habituation.

Also, in cases with a known interrelation of stress and tinnitus, a stress–diathesis model for tinnitus was proposed by Shulman et al. Stress management techniques require a counselor and the close cooperation of the patient, physician, biofeedback therapist, and psychologist.

A cognitive therapy that provides significant support to the patient with severe disabling tinnitus, particularly for control of the effect, is strongly recommended and encouraged.

ADAPTED PHYSIOTHERAPY

A specific program of physiotherapy successfully applied in endogenous tinnitus is KKIT. This therapy uses expressive movements of body language. In a special rehabilitation program, different groups of muscles in the hand, arm, leg, foot, and body, rising from the feet up to the face, are activated, which guides the tinnitus patient into a situation of peaceful resting, reduction of tension, and finally into relaxation. This scheme was adapted from a program of treating pain. KKIT points toward mechanisms of interference of expressive gestural movements with facilitating tinnitus from around the basal ganglia of the brain.

OTHER METHODS OF THERAPY

Other methods of tinnitus therapy recommended in the literature include acupuncture, counseling, group therapy, and hypnotherapy.

REFERENCES

Alster J, Shemesh Z, Ornan M, Attias J: Sleep disturbance associated with chronic tinnitus. Biol Psychiatry 1993;34:84-90.
Arnesen AR, Engdahl B: Tinnitus—etiology, diagnosis and treatment. Tidsskr Nor Laegeforen 1996;116:2009-2012.
Bergmann JM, Bertora GO: Cortical and brainstem topodiagnostic testing in tinnitus patients—a preliminary report. Int Tinnitus J 1996;2:151-158.
Bertora GO, Bergmann JM: Tinnitus: Supratentorial areas study through brain electric tomography (LORETA). ASN 2004;2:2, ISSN 1612-3352. Available at http://www.neurootology.org
Claussen CF: Treatment of the slow brainstem syndrome with Vertigoheel. Biol Med 1985;3:447-470, 4:510-514.
Claussen CF: Medical classification of tinnitus between bruits: Exogenous and endogenous tinnitus and other types of tinnitus. ASN 2004;2, (ISSN)1612-3352. Available at http://www.neurootology.org
Claussen CF, Kolchev C, Schneider D, Hahn A: Neurootological brain electrical activity mapping in tinnitus patients. Proceedings of the 4th International Tinnitus Seminar, Bordeaux, 1991;1092:351-355.
Claussen CF, Schneider D, Koltchev C: On the functional state of central vestibular structures in monaural symptomatic tinnitus patients. Int Tinnitus J 1995:1:5-12.
George RN, Kemp S: A survey of New Zealanders with tinnitus. Br J Audiol 1991;25:331-336.
Jastreboff PJ, Hazell JWP: A neurophysiological approach to tinnitus: Clinical implications. Br J Audiol 1993;27:1-11.
Parving A, Hein HO, Suadicani P, et al: Epidemiology of hearing disorders. Some factors affecting hearing. The Copenhagen Male Study. Scand Audiol 1993;22:101-107.
Quaranta A, Assennato G, Sallustio V: Epidemiology of hearing problems among adults in Italy. Scand Audiol Suppl 1996;42:9-13.
Shulman A: A final common pathway for tinnitus—the medial temporal lobe system. Tinnitus J 1996;2:115-126.
Shulman A, Aran JM, Feldmann H, et al: Tinnitus diagnosis/treatment. Philadelphia, Lea & Febiger, 1991.
Shulman A, Strashun AM, Afriyie M, et al: SPECT imaging of brain and tinnitus—neurotologic/neurologic implications. Int Tinnitus J 1995: 1:13-29.

ACKNOWLEDGMENT

Sponsored by grant Projekt D. 1417, durch die LVA Baden-Württemberg, Stuttgart, Germany.

Spine Pain

Method of
Michael T. McCann, MD

Back pain is one of the most common musculoskeletal complaints seen in primary care practices; empirical treatment is frequently based on conjecture. Our understanding of the pathophysiology of spine and radicular pain has increased dramatically over the last decade as a result of new technology and more advanced diagnostic testing. Early and accurate diagnosis is imperative if we are to provide specific lesion-based treatment to optimize patient outcomes and health care spending.

Although patients are satisfied with their care for most major illnesses, 20% to 25% of surveyed patients were dissatisfied with their care for back pain. Only headache treatment also received such poor scores. The top reason patients listed for dissatisfaction with their physician's care was inadequate explanation of why they hurt.

Although muscle strain is the most common reason given to patients as the cause of their back pain, it is actually highly unlikely to be the etiology for back pain severe enough for a patient to seek medical care or for pain that lasts more than 2 weeks. An underlying spinal disorder is usually present, leading to overlying myofascial tenderness and tightness. Isolated back pain is not a neurologic problem. Rather, it is an orthopedic problem, as will be evident from the following discussion.

Epidemiology

Eighty percent of the U.S. population develops back pain, limiting day-to-day activities, at some time in their lives. The peak incidence of such pain is between 35 and 65 years of age, declining thereafter. Based on radiographic degeneration alone, we would expect the incidence to increase linearly with age. In 80% of patients, episodes are self-limited, but in 15% to 20%, the pain chronically restricts function. Direct and indirect economical costs are estimated to be between $80 and $100 billion per year in the United States and, from an insurer's standpoint, costs may exceed expenditures on pediatric and obstetrical care combined. The majority of treatment expenditures are on the 20% of patients whose pain does not resolve spontaneously: recurrent or chronic back pain sufferers. To limit expenditures and optimize patient outcomes, it is vital that we prevent progression to a chronic state. Such prevention can best be achieved by early and accurate diagnosis and treatment.

Pathophysiology

Somatic (nociceptive) pain is caused by noxious stimulation of nerve endings in the vertebrae, joints, ligaments and disks, whereas

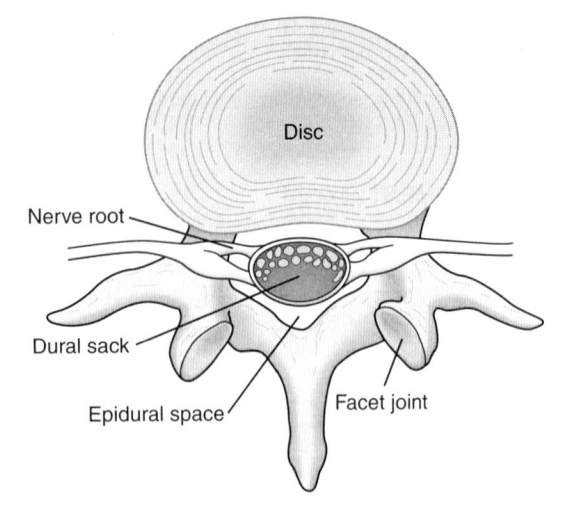

FIGURE 1. Spine cross section.

radicular (neuropathic) pain is produced by evoked ectopic impulses in the dorsal root ganglia (Figure 1).

Somatic Pain

In primary somatic back pain, we try diagnostically to separate the pain generators into two anatomic categories based on their relation to the spinal canal. Treatment is significantly different based on the site of the lesions. Note that primary spinal nerve or cord pathology does not in and of itself produce axial back pain.

Pain generators in the anterior column are the disks and vertebral bodies. Only the outer third of a disk's annulus is innervated. Tears of these outer annular fibers produce exquisite pain and back spasm even without complete disruption of the disk. This is a frequent missed cause of nonspecific back pain because these internal disk disruptions are rarely visualized on routine spine magnetic resonance imaging (MRI) or computer tomography (CT) scans. If noted on MRI, a high-intensity zone (HIZ) finding in a disk is highly suggestive of a painful internal annular tear. Definitive diagnosis is established with manometric provocative CT diskography. Diskitis, although rare, is also suggested by MRI findings, although aspiration may be necessary to establish an inflammatory or infectious etiology definitively.

Vertebral compression fractures, whether osteoporotic, traumatic, or pathologic, also contribute to anterior column primary axial pain. CT scanning or plain radiographs generally confirm the diagnosis; however, bone scanning may be necessary to confirm acuteness of a finding and to help rule out metastatic foci. Osteomyelitis should also be considered in any fracture with associated fever or a recent septic source.

The posterior column sources of back pain include the facet joints from the atlanto-occipital articulation caudad to the sacroiliac joints. All are true diarthrodial joints. The surfaces are capped with articular cartilage and lined with a synovial membrane. These paired innervated structures are subject to degeneration and painful traumatic injuries. In double-blind placebo controlled studies, the cervical facets appear to be the source of pain in 59% of patients with post-whiplash cervicalgia. Estimates regarding the lumbar spine place the incidence of facet-based low back pain between 15% and 40%, and the incidence increases significantly after 65 years of age.

Spondylolisthesis refers to a shift in the alignment between two vertebrae. With associated stress fractures of the pars interarticularis (spondylolysis), it is another posterior column source of pain. In chronic cases, instability leads to associated fibrosis under the pars fractures that produce radicular compression and neuropathic extremity pain. The slippage may also lead to central and foraminal stenosis with neurogenic claudication.

Neuropathic Pain

The most common cause of lumbar radicular pain in young patients is disk herniation (98%). Nerve compression alone, however, does not offer a satisfactory explanation for the pain produced. In human studies, root compression alone produces distal extremity paresthesias and numbness but no pain. Isolated lumbar radiculopathy does not cause significant back pain, and disk herniation size does not correlate with severity of pain on straight leg raise testing. Nucleus pulposus placed within the epidural space produces extreme inflammation with a 100,000-fold increase in phospholipase-A_2 immunoreactivity that can be directly correlated with mechanical hyperalgesia. In the complete absence of root compression, nucleus pulposus stimulates sustained discharges of $A\delta$ and $A\beta$ pain fibers in the dorsal root ganglia and causes a conduction delay in the roots. Intravenous methylprednisolone (Solu-Medrol)[1] prevents this conduction delay. Radicular pain appears to be caused by a combination of mechanical irritation in an otherwise chemically sensitized root.

Other sources of radicular pain include central spinal and lateral recess stenosis caused by facet arthropathies, ligamentous hypertrophy, and spondylolisthesis. Even more etiologies include neuromeningeal anomalies, neoplasms, infections, and vascular malformations. Peripheral neuropathies, including thoracic outlet, cubital and carpal tunnel syndromes, piriformis syndrome, tarsal tunnel, and other primary mononeuropathies, may also mimic or exist in conjunction with radiculopathies.

Assessment

The goal of the initial assessment is to screen for emergent causes of back or radicular pain including aneurysms, infections, segmental instability, fractures, tumors, and myelopathy. A careful history and examination should help delineate referred cardiac, pulmonary, gastrointestinal, urologic, gynecologic, and vascular sources.

History

For all patients presenting with back or radicular pain, the screening history should include weight loss, recent fevers or infections, and significant change in bowel or bladder function, including incontinence. For patients with cervicothoracic or upper extremity radicular pain, a cardiac history should be added. Abdominal symptoms, hematuria, dysuria, or vaginal discharge should be included for lumbar pain.

Radicular pain is lancinating with superficial and deep components that extend in distinct, but not necessarily dermatomal, distributions. Pain may extend partially or entirely in the distribution of the affected spinal nerve. Somatic referred pain is deep, aching, and diffuse. It can overlap with radicular symptoms in the proximal extremities. Proximal extremity pain can be radicular, whereas distal extremity pain is not necessarily always radicular.

Diffuse distal symptoms with dysesthesia, complaints of bowel or bladder urgency or incontinence, and a history of balance difficulties are red flags for myelopathy. Most patients also give a history of cervicothoracic or associated radicular pain. If accompanied by severe low back pain and complaints of saddle numbness, consider cauda equina syndrome, a surgical emergency.

Claudication symptoms are suggestive of spinal stenosis and usually there is little pain at rest. Differentiation from vascular claudication is sometimes difficult, but pain with neurogenic claudication is usually not worsened with supine positioning and leg elevation.

---

[1] Not FDA approved for this indication.

CURRENT DIAGNOSIS

Emergent or Urgent Conditions Associated with Back Pain (Red Flags)

Associated Symptoms	Condition
New onset bowel or bladder incontinence	Myelopathy
Balance difficulties	Myelopathy
Diffuse distal weakness or immobility	Myelopathy
Recent weight loss	Tumor
Severe chest or abdominal pain	Aortic aneurysm

History	Condition
Osteoporosis	Fracture
Recent trauma	Fracture
Intravenous drug use	Infection
Recent infection	Infection
Immunosuppressed state	Infection

Age	Condition
<15 y or >60 y	Tumor suspicion
Male >55 y (M:F 4:1)	Aortic aneurysm

Associated Signs	Condition
Tender abdomen	Aortic aneurysm
Saddle sensory loss	Cauda equina syndrome
Hyperreflexia with positive clonus, Babinski's sign, and Hoffmann's sign	Myelopathy

Examination

Although clinical exam may establish the presence of a radiculopathy or localize the segmental pain level, etiology must be established by other means. Tumors, cysts, stenosis spondylolisthesis, and disk herniations may all cause very similar clinical signs.

Muscle pain and spasm should not be considered the primary source of the patient's back pain unless all other potential sources are ruled out or an objective rheumatologic etiology is identified pointing to a myositis. An antalgic gait from distal degenerative joint disease may cause lumbar muscular aching, but rarely is the back the site of greatest pain. This is not to say that muscles cannot be painful, but rather that in the majority of primary back pain cases, the muscles are simply reacting to an underlying derangement in the spine itself.

More specifically, examination should note hyperreflexia and clonus and test for Babinski's and Hoffmann's signs to note upper motor neuron irritability. Screening cardiovascular and abdominal examination helps rule out other sources of back pain.

Natural Course of the Disease

For lumbar radicular pain in patients treated conservatively, 50% of patients can expect to have resolution of radicular symptoms after 4 weeks. At 12 months, in 49% of males and 33% of females, radicular pain remains improved. Unfortunately, 60% to 70% of these patients developed back pain by 4 weeks that persisted at 12 months regardless of the radicular pain improvement.

For patients treated surgically versus conservatively, at 10 years there appears to be little statistically significant difference in outcome for radicular pain, with both groups achieving approximately 60% good results and poor results in 7% to 8%. This only holds true if surgery is not applied randomly, but as a last resort for patients who fail to respond to conservative care.

For cervical radiculopathic symptoms, 70% can be expected to improve with time and 20% become asymptomatic. In patients for whom surgery was an option, 90% are improved or only mildly incapacitated at long-term follow-up. Isolated recurrences are seen in 32% of cases, whereas 10% have moderate to severe persistent disability.

Although studies exist detailing favorable outcomes overall for radicular symptoms, the same does not necessarily hold true for mechanical back pain. Although 80% of patients appear to have resolution of initial symptoms independent of their course of care, 20% develop progressive or unrelenting pain. It appears that approximately 35% of persons have intermittent recurrences that limit their activities.

Management

Take an algorithmic approach to the patient presenting with back and/or radicular symptoms of new onset. If initial history and examination suggest an emergent cause for these symptoms, appropriate additional diagnostic testing and referral should be made. Indications for urgent surgical interventions are few but include progressive motor deficit and cauda equina syndrome—progressive neurologic deterioration with loss of bowel and bladder function.

Once an emergent source of pain is ruled out, studies show that primary care physicians who prescribe the least amount of analgesics and place the fewest restrictions on activities have the best patient outcomes. In many cases, a more aggressive approach may reinforce illness behavior and foster a fear of future debilitation.

Radicular Pain Predominating

If radicular pain predominates in a minimally distressed patient, simple reassurance and an explanation of the natural course of recovery may suffice. Avoiding bed rest and activity modification to prevent axial loading should be discussed (no lifting in a forward flexed position and no repetitive flexion activities). A 2-week reassessment allows any insidious red flag conditions to be picked up, provides reassurance, and allows adjustment of treatment.

For more significantly distressed patients with acute radicular pain, additional analgesics and more frequent follow-up may be required. Although no analgesic regimen alters the natural course of recovery, based on the inflammatory pathogenesis of radicular pain a pulse dose of prednisone or methylprednisolone with a taper can be considered over a week. However, in randomized controlled trials, the nonsteroidal anti-inflammatory drugs (NSAIDs) piroxicam (Feldene) and indomethacin (Indocin) did not offer any greater analgesia or enhance recovery more than placebo. A limited course of muscle relaxants and opioid analgesics may be prescribed but often provide little relief in cases of true neuropathic pain. The limited duration of these prescriptions should be explained to the patient at the outset. Despite ongoing pain, the goal is to avoid dependency and reliance on these medications for activities that may be detrimental to the natural course of the disorder.

Currently, greater success may be found with early initiation and titration of gabapentin (Neurontin)[1] for radicular pain. With low toxicity and few side effects, tolerance is usually good. Initiate dosing at night with 100 to 300 mg (lower dosing in patients <65 years old), escalating every 1 to 3 days as tolerated up to 1200 mg three times daily. If improvement is not obtained by 600 mg three times daily, further escalation is unlikely to be efficacious.

For distressed patients, duloxetine (Cymbalta)[1] may be efficacious while providing additional anxiolysis and antidepressive effects. Because nausea is a frequent side effect for the first few days upon

---

[1]Not FDA approved for this indication.

CURRENT THERAPY

Acute Presentation without Red Flags: Treatment Ladders (Frequent Reassessment as Indicated)

BACK OR NECK PAIN PREDOMINATING

- Education, activity modification, and reassurance
- Limited course of analgesics dependent on stress
    - NSAIDs
    - Opioids
    - Muscle relaxants
    - Consider steroid taper regimen
- Physical therapy with spinal stabilization regimen
- Screening radiographs with flexion and extension views (rule out gross instability)
- Referral for spinal diagnostic assessment or orthopedic spine evaluation
- Fusion or disk replacement as indicated

RADICULAR PAIN PREDOMINATING

- Education, activity modification, and reassurance
- Early treatment of inflammation with steroid taper regimen
- Limited course of analgesics and muscle relaxants
- Early initiation of neuropathic pain medications
    - Gabapentin (Neurontin)[1]
    - Duloxetine (Cymbalta)[1]
    - Pregabalin (Lyrica)[1]
- Physical therapy guided by McKenzie assessment
- MRI (with gadolinium contrast for cancer, spinal cord pathology, and postoperative spine cases)
- Selective transforaminal steroid injection
- Surgical assessment for decompression

[1]Not FDA approved for this indication.
Abbreviations: NSAIDs = nonsteroidal anti-inflammatory drugs.

---

initiation of dosing, we start with 30 mg every morning and advance to 60 mg every morning after 1 week. If sedation occurs, change to every-evening dosing. Symptomatic improvement is often seen by 7 to 10 days.

If at follow-up significant progress is not made and reassessment still lacks red flags, physical therapy with instructions for a McKenzie assessment and therapy over 2 weeks is indicated, with a home program to follow. Again, no scientific studies validate any particular regimen of therapy. However, from a spinal education standpoint, and as an impetus to maintaining function, an empirical recommendation can be made. Follow-up should be scheduled and if progress is partial, another 2 weeks of therapy could be considered.

Failure to improve or deterioration of function at any point would be an indication for additional imaging studies. An MRI provides the most comprehensive survey of causes for radicular symptoms. It does not, however, guarantee that anatomic changes are definitively the source for a patient's symptoms. In asymptomatic patients younger than 40 years, 30% had abnormal spine MRIs, whereas 60% to 70% of patients older than 40 years had abnormal MRIs. The prevalence of asymptomatic disk herniations alone ranged between 20% and 40% in patients between 40 and 60 years of age.

Evidence-based review of the literature currently does not support the use of electromyogram and nerve conduction velocity (EMG/NCV) studies) for diagnosis in cases of radiculopathic pain. Pain is mediated through Aδ and C fibers, and an EMG tests activity in Aα motor fibers. H and F reflexes similarly lack specificity in clinical trials with radiculopathy, despite proposed theoretical foundations. EMG/NCV testing would be indicated in cases where peripheral neuropathy or nerve entrapment is suspected and when objective muscle strength testing is suspect or primary myopathy may be present.

Recent prospective randomized blinded studies support selective nerve root injection (i.e., fluoroscopically guided transforaminal epidural steroid or epiradicular injections) as the next line of treatment. This highly selective procedure may reduce the need for surgical intervention in up to 59% of radicular cases and should be considered in cases where lack of improvement is noted as soon as 2 weeks. Serial MRI studies in humans show statistically significant improvement in the rate of disk reabsorption and symptoms in patients treated with transforaminal injections as compared to controls. The older regimen of translaminar epidural steroid injections is not nearly as efficacious and in some studies appears no more effective than placebo. Partial improvement at 10- to 14-day follow-up would be an indication for repeat injection. An automatic series of three injections is no longer considered standard of care, and response to a single transforaminal injection should guide additional treatment. Lack of improvement or further functional decline would lead to surgical assessment.

Long-term management of a patient with radicular pain either unrelieved with surgery or in the patient for whom surgical options do not exist falls into the realm of neuropathic pain control. Narcotic regimens should be avoided because long-term efficacy has never been demonstrated. Medication options are limited, but gabapentin (Neurontin)[1] and duloxetine (Cymbalta)[1] are efficacious in reducing pain for a large number of patients with both radicular and other sources of neuropathic pain. The newest drug with indications for neuropathic pain is pregabalin (Lyrica)[1]. Efficacy for radicular pain is as yet undetermined but is expected to approximate gabapentin with fewer dose-related side effects. Other drugs to be considered include mexiletine (Mexitil)[1], tricyclic antidepressants,[1] and some of the newer anticonvulsants including levetiracetam (Keppra),[1] oxcarbazepine (Trileptal),[1] zonisamide (Zonegran),[1] and tiagabine (Gabitril).[1] All modify neuropathic pain in the presence and absence of associated depression.

For patients in whom neuropathic extremity pain far exceeds any mechanical back pain, despite optimization of all conservative treatment and surgical options, spinal cord stimulation may be considered. This modality is efficacious in between 60% and 70% of patients with neuropathic extremity pain predominating. It is not indicated for mechanical back pain. For permanently implanted patients, 70% continue to have approximately 50% improvement in neuropathic pain at 5-year follow-up.

Axial Pain Predominating

For patients with nonurgent acute back or neck pain, again the level of distress helps guide care. Studies regarding early treatment and analgesic regimens for nociceptive back pain lack validity and specificity because early diagnosis is not usually sought because of the high incidence of spontaneous improvement. Early treatment thus remains empirical.

In a minimally distressed patient, supportive education and activity modification support the natural course of recovery. For an initial episode, physical therapy with spinal stabilization exercises, followed by a home program, is recommended to provide back education and to help reduce recurrences.

For the more distressed patient, oral analgesics may be indicated. Because the source of axial pain is nociceptive, NSAIDs should be considered as a first-line analgesic, with opioids reserved for very severe pain and again only for a limited duration. Failure to improve is not an indication for continued daily use of opioids. For moderate to severe pain where a significant inflammatory component is suspected, a bolus/taper dose of steroids over 1 week is often efficacious, and risks are low with this regimen. Muscle spasms are best managed with gradual stretching and paced activities. In severe cases, however,

[1]Not FDA approved for this indication.

muscle relaxants may be beneficial, and even a limited course of benzodiazepines can be considered.

If at 2-week reassessment progress is not seen, physical therapy over 1 month (usually 3 to 4 times per week) for range of motion and stabilization exercise should be considered. Partial improvement would be an indication for another month of therapy or, in the motivated patient, another month of a home exercise program.

The goal of therapy is to maintain range of motion, strengthen supportive musculature, and maintain activities of daily living without additional injury. To this end, almost all exercise regimens claim efficacy, although no valid studies as yet show that any specific therapy actually alters the natural history.

Should a patient with primary back or neck pain fail to improve with therapy, screening radiographs may be indicated. Plain radiographs for mechanical back pain should always be obtained with flexion and extension views to rule out gross instability as well as other mechanical derangements, including spondylolisthesis, spondylolysis, and compression fractures.

Unfortunately, although all radiographic studies of the spine demonstrate anatomic abnormalities, they cannot show whether these abnormalities are painful. With physical examination also notoriously unreliable for making a definitive diagnosis, referral for more advanced spinal diagnostic assessment may often be indicated in patients who fail to improve or who have frequent recurrences.

For the 20% of patients whose function remains limited by back pain despite maximized conservative care, identification of the exact pain source is imperative to improving outcomes. These patients are prone to seek numerous opinions, undergo fruitless operations, and pay for unproven modality-based treatments. Physicians tend toward making diagnoses based on response to treatment as opposed to the other way around. An early definitive diagnosis allows realistic treatment options and prognosis to be given. Patients can thus adjust their lifestyle to function within the limits imposed by their spinal condition.

Significant advances are being made in the field of diagnosing back pain. Select spinal injection techniques are refined to isolate the exact source of a patient's pain in the majority of cases. Validity testing can also determine if a patient's complaint has an anatomic basis or if symptom magnification is present.

CT-provocative diskography is the only test available to document internal disk anatomy precisely and to determine if a disk is the source of a patient's back pain. Studies show that compared with surgical findings, its anatomic accuracy exceeds MRI and CT myelography. With the use of manometry, intradiskal symptomatic pressures help determine the proper surgical technique to optimize patient outcomes. Diagnostic facet injections can also identify a symptomatic joint precisely, further helping determine options for treatment.

New nonsurgical or minimally invasive treatments are now validated, including radiofrequency thermocoagulation (RFTC) lesioning for desensitization of painful facet joint arthropathies, intradiskal electrothermal therapy (IDET) for treatment of painful disk lesions, and percutaneous disk decompression by both mechanical and laser techniques. For vertebral compression fracture, vertebroplasty and kyphoplasty may offer remarkable and rapid relief of associated fracture pain but do carry a risk of severe neurologic injury and embolism. Treatment outcomes for all of these procedures rely heavily on obtaining an exact diagnosis using the preceding tests.

Surgical assessment for nonemergent back pain should be reserved for those patients who fail conservative management and are not candidates for minimally invasive treatment or who have identifiable gross segmental spinal instability. Unlike radicular pain, decompression alone does not improve primary back pain. For mechanical back pain from segmental instability, the only surgical option is fusion. Poor pain relief is seen most frequently in patients who undergo fusion procedures for back pain based on radiographic findings alone. Provocative testing to isolate the actual pain generators and to determine the integrity of surrounding support structures

TABLE 1 Clinical Pearls

Muscle strain is a very unusual cause of back pain severe enough to seek medical attention.
For back pain, think facets, disks, and vertebrae.
Referred back and neck pain can extend into the extremities and mimic radicular patterns.
Radicular pain does not always extend into the distal extremities (L5 radiculopathy can mimic hip trochanteric bursitis).
Magnetic resonance imaging (MRI) cannot tell you what hurts, only what might be causing pain.
MRI does not rule out all spinal pathology that can cause pain.
Order MRI with gadolinium contrast only if:
    You suspect cancer.
    You suspect a primary spinal cord lesion.
    Spine surgery was performed in the suspect region.
Laminectomy alone should not be used to treat predominant back pain (only radicular pain).
Fusions and disk replacements are for predominant back pain.
Only spinal diagnostic testing (selective computer tomography [CT] diskography, facet blocks, and transforaminal injections) can isolate the source of pain in refractory cases.
Electromyogram and nerve conduction velocity (EMG/NCV) studies should be used only if you:
    Suspect an underlying peripheral neuropathic process (double crush).
    Suspect lack of effort on motor testing.
    Suspect a primary myopathy.
Early referral for accurate diagnostic testing is the key to optimizing care: the more accurate the diagnosis, the more accurate the care.

maximizes the chances for success. For patients with isolated diskogenic pain, validated with manometric CT diskography, newer disk replacement techniques hold promise. Fusions cause a load shift to adjacent spinal motion segments causing degeneration. This leads to a 30% reoperation rate for fusion patients within 10 years. The hope is that disk replacements will prevent this transitional zone degeneration and lower the reoperation rate.

Not all patients are candidates for surgical reconstruction. In many cases, surgical intervention may only serve to worsen a patient's state. Tolerance of symptoms with acceptance of functional limitations is the preferred course.

To conclude, patients presenting with pain of spinal origin should be divided into those with predominantly radicular symptoms and those with primarily mechanical back or neck pain. In the vast majority of cases, back and neck pain originates from derangements of the facets, disks, or vertebrae, not the muscles. Radicular pain is most likely secondary to a compressive lesion with associated underlying inflammation.

Proper diagnosis is paramount to optimizing patient treatment (both conservative and surgical) and to prevention of progress to a chronic dysfunctional state. MRIs have limitations in what they are able to visualize and do not guarantee that anatomic derangements are actually the source of the patient's pain. For an accurate diagnosis in a patient who fails to respond to initial conservative care, more specialized interventional spinal diagnostic testing is indicated (Table 1).

Identification and isolation of specific spinal pain generators has allowed for the development of specific lesion-based minimally invasive treatments. These include transforaminal injections for radiculopathy, RFTC desensitization for facet-based pain, and percutaneous decompression for disk displacement pain. Decompressive surgery is very effective at relieving severe radicular pain unresponsive to conservative care and injections, but it is complicated by postlaminectomy spinal instability. Spinal fusion surgery for well-diagnosed painful segmental instability remains the definitive treatment for this disorder; newer disk replacement surgery may offer an alternative to fusion for primary diskogenic back or neck pain.

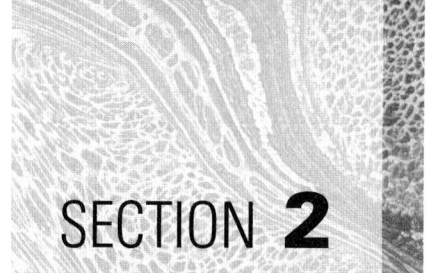

SECTION 2

The Infectious Diseases

Management of the Patient with HIV Disease

Method of
Surendra Kumar Sharma, MD, PhD, and Tamilarasu Kadhiravan, MD

AIDS was described initially in the United States in 1981 among several case clusters of previously healthy young men who had sex with men, presenting with unusual infections such as *Pneumocystis jiroveci* pneumonia (PCP), mucosal candidiasis, disseminated cytomegalovirus (CMV) disease, and Kaposi's sarcoma. The cause of AIDS remained elusive then, leading to several speculations. A few years later, amid much controversy, the causative agent was established as HIV, which has a predilection to infect and destroy the immune effector cells, primarily the CD4+ T lymphocytes. The discovery of HIV led to the development of definitive diagnostic tests that unearthed, to everyone's dismay, a widespread, hitherto invisible, smoldering pandemic in evolution.

Epidemiology

Since the beginning of the epidemic, approximately 25 million people have died of AIDS worldwide, making it one of the most devastating epidemics of all times. An estimated 33.2 million people are living with HIV/AIDS globally, including 15.4 million women and 2.5 million children younger than 15 years. In 2007 alone, an estimated 2.5 million people got newly infected, and approximately 2.1 million people died because of AIDS. More than two-thirds of the burden of HIV/AIDS is borne by sub-Saharan Africa, particularly the southern African nations. In countries such as Botswana, South Africa, Zimbabwe, Swaziland, and Namibia, the prevalence of HIV infection among expectant mothers is consistently in excess of 20%.

North America accounts for approximately 1.3 million people living with HIV/AIDS, most of them in the United States. Every year, more than 35,000 new cases are reported in the United States. Blacks and Hispanics are disproportionately represented among them, and pediatric AIDS accounts for approximately 1% of the cases. With the widespread implementation of preventive measures, a marginal but significant fall in HIV infection rates was observed for the first time among non-Hispanic blacks and injection drug users.

The Causative Agent

HIV is an enveloped single-stranded RNA virus (family: Retroviridae; subfamily: Lentivirinae). Embedded in its envelope are glycoprotein spikes (gp120, gp41) that are crucial for binding with the host cell surface receptors such as CD4, CCR5, and CXCR4 and subsequent entry into the host cell. HIV is a retrovirus that elaborates the enzyme reverse transcriptase. It enables transcription of genomic RNA to proviral DNA for integration into the host cell DNA. Host cells that bear CD4+ (helper T cells, macrophages, etc.) are the main targets of HIV infection. There are two human immunodeficiency viruses, HIV-1 and HIV-2. Compelling genetic evidence suggests that they originated from the simian immunodeficiency viruses, of the chimpanzee (SIVcpz) and the sooty mangabey monkeys (SIVsm), respectively, in Africa several decades back. HIV-1 is global in distribution, whereas HIV-2 is confined mainly to western Africa. HIV-2 infection is less effectively transmitted and results in lower levels of viremia and slower disease progression compared to HIV-1.

Isolates of HIV-1 across the globe exhibit marked genetic heterogeneity and are classified into three groups (M, O, and N) and several clades. Clade C is the most common form worldwide. In North America and Europe, clade B is the predominant subtype. Genetic recombination among co-circulating clades often occurs, and such a recombinant subtype AE is the most prevalent form in Southeast Asia. Clade AE viruses are transmitted more effectively by the heterosexual route than the clade B virus. The genetic heterogeneity of HIV has to be taken into consideration in the development and evaluation of HIV vaccines.

Modes of Transmission

Transmission of HIV occurs through contact with the body fluids of a HIV-infected person. The routes of transmission are sexual, both male to male as well as heterosexual contact; mother to child; transfusion of HIV-tainted blood and blood products; injection drug use; and occupational exposure in health care and laboratory workers. No evidence suggests that HIV is transmitted by casual contact and insect bites. Heterosexual transmission is the most prevalent route of HIV transmission worldwide, especially in developing countries. In the United States, male-to-male sexual contact is the most common route of transmission; however, the proportion of cases caused by heterosexual transmission is steadily increasing.

The average risk of HIV transmission per coital act in sero-discordant heterosexual couples is approximately 0.1%. Several factors, such as the presence of other sexually transmitted infections (ulcerative as well as nonulcerative) and higher viral load, increase the risk of transmission; condom use and male circumcision considerably reduce the risk. Female-to-male transmission is less effective than male-to-female transmission. Commercial sex is associated with a higher risk of transmission of approximately 5% to 10%. Receptive anal intercourse is associated with a higher risk of transmission as compared to vaginal intercourse. Even though the risk of transmission by oral sex is very low, it should not be considered completely safe.

Mother-to-child transmission of infection can occur during pregnancy, during delivery, or by breast-feeding. More than half of the transmissions occur intrapartum, mediated by direct contact of infant mucosa with HIV-laden maternal blood, amniotic fluid, and cervical/vaginal secretions. Placental microtransfusion also plays a role. High maternal plasma viremia, prolonged rupture of membranes, and chorioamnionitis increase the risk of mother-to-child transmission, whereas cesarean delivery and use of peripartum antiretroviral prophylaxis decrease the risk markedly.

With the implementation of mandatory testing practices, transmission through infected blood and blood products is almost eliminated in the developed world. However, despite using the highly sensitive nucleic acid-based tests, given the enormous number of transfusions in clinical practice, the risk of transfusion-transmitted HIV infection cannot be overlooked. It is estimated that each year 16 infectious donations are available for transfusion in the United States.

Although injection drug use is responsible for approximately 20% of HIV transmission in the United States, it is the driving force behind the HIV epidemic in Southeast Asian countries and China. Apart from direct transmission through sharing of contaminated needles and other paraphernalia, injection drug use also promotes risk-taking behavior and unsafe sexual practices. In developing countries, unsafe injections administered at health care facilities are a potential, but underappreciated, route of HIV transmission. Occupational transmission occurs through percutaneous needle stick injuries and after mucous membrane or nonintact skin exposure to infected body fluids. The risk of HIV infection following a contaminated needle stick injury is approximately 0.3% and is approximately 0.09% following mucous membrane exposure.

Pathogenesis and Natural History of HIV Infection

Following infection, HIV localizes to the lymphoid organs of the body where it productively infects the CD4+ helper T lymphocytes in the milieu provided by the dendritic cells and subsequently spills over into the circulation. In the absence of an immune response, this results in intense viremia in the early weeks following primary infection. During this phase, extensive dissemination of the virus occurs throughout the body. In approximately 50% to 70% of individuals, this might become clinically manifest as a self-limited, mononucleosis-like illness known as "acute HIV syndrome" (Table 1). Soon, with the elaboration of HIV-specific cell-mediated as well as humoral immune responses, viremia is brought under control albeit incompletely. A balance thus is struck between the opposing influences of viremia and the host immune response, establishing the viral load around a relatively low, stable level known as the virologic setpoint. The virologic setpoint is one of the important determinants of the pace of subsequent disease progression. Even if the viremia gets suppressed to below-detectable limits, despite the disease being clinically silent, active viral replication occurs throughout the course of HIV disease.

Some aspects of viral dynamics in vivo are important from a therapeutic point of view. An enormously large amount of virions (10^{10} to 10^{11}) are produced and cleared every day. Thus, the chances of a drug-resistant strain emerging under the selection pressure exerted by antiretroviral therapy are very high. Even in patients who achieve undetectable viral loads for prolonged periods of time following treatment, ongoing active viral replication occurs. If therapy is stopped in these patients, viral load promptly bounces back. Further, antiretroviral therapy does not eliminate the large reservoir of latently infected cells that are capable of giving rise to replication-competent virus. Theoretically, it would take several decades of uninterrupted viral suppression for this reservoir to get depleted on its own.

During the phase of clinical latency, continuous viral replication leads to progressive depletion of CD4+ helper T cells, resulting from direct cytopathicity as well as by diverse indirect mechanisms. When the CD4+ cell count falls below 200 cells/μL, the risk of opportunistic infections (OIs) increases greatly, culminating in AIDS. The CD4+ cell count, as an index of immunosuppression because of HIV infection, predicts strongly the risk of OIs and thereby the risk of progression to AIDS and subsequent death (Table 2). However, when the CD4+ counts are above 350 cells/μL, their usefulness in predicting the risk of disease progression is limited. Conversely, the plasma viral load is a more robust predictor of the risk of AIDS, independent of the CD4+ count at all levels (Table 2). The rate of decline in CD4+ count is highly variable among individuals. Some progress very rapidly, whereas a few others maintain normal levels of CD4+ counts and immunocompetence for prolonged periods without treatment. In Western populations, the median time to development of AIDS is approximately 10 years, and approximately 10% of patients remain asymptomatic beyond 20 years. The latter are known as long-term nonprogressors.

Apart from the viral load, several host-related factors also influence the rate of disease progression. It is well known that people who are homozygous for the deletion mutation *CCR5-Δ 32*, which codes for a nonfunctional CCR5, are highly resistant to HIV infection despite repeated exposure. HIV-infected individuals who are heterozygous for this allele have comparatively lower plasma viral loads and slower rate of progression to AIDS. Likewise, homo/heterozygosity for the mutant allele *CCR2 64I*, the product of which dimerizes with and decreases the expression of CXCR4 on the cell surface, results in slower disease progression. HLA alleles B*5701 and B*2705 also are

TABLE 1 Acute HIV Syndrome*

Clinical Features	Differential Diagnosis
Common (>50%)	
Fever	Infectious mononucleosis
Malaise	Acute cytomegalovirus
Lymphadenopathy	infection
Pharyngitis	Secondary syphilis
Rash—erythematous,	Acute toxoplasmosis
maculopapular; urticarial;	Rickettsial infections
mucocutaneous ulcers	Rubella
Myalgia and arthralgia	Systemic lupus
	erythematosus
	Still's disease
Frequent (10%–50%)	
Diarrhea	
Headache	
Nausea and vomiting	
Hepatosplenomegaly	
Oral thrush	
Anorexia and weight loss	
Occasional (< 10%)	
Aseptic meningitis	
Acute meningoencephalitis	
Guillain-Barré syndrome	
Myelopathy	
Brachial neuritis	
Facial palsy	
Peripheral neuropathy	
Opportunistic infections	

*Occurs approximately 3–6 wk following primary infection; symptoms last for 1 to several weeks, followed by gradual, spontaneous resolution; in a small proportion (approximately 10%), despite resolution of initial symptoms, rapid immunologic deterioration follows.

TABLE 2 Predicted 6-Month Risk of AIDS in the CASCADE Project, Based on Age, Current CD4+ Count, and Plasma Viral Load

Viral Load (copies/mL)	Predicted Risk at Current CD4+ Cell Count (cells/μL)									
	50	100	150	200	250	300	350	400	450	500
Age 25 y										
3,000	6.8	3.7	2.3	1.6	1.1	0.8	0.6	0.5	0.4	0.3
10,000	9.6	5.3	3.4	2.3	1.6	1.2	0.9	0.7	0.5	0.4
30,000	13.3	7.4	4.7	3.2	2.2	1.6	1.2	0.9	0.7	0.6
100,000	18.6	10.6	6.7	4.6	3.2	2.4	1.8	1.4	1.1	0.8
300,000	25.1	14.5	9.3	6.3	4.5	3.3	2.5	1.9	1.5	1.2
Age 35 y										
3,000	8.5	4.7	3.0	2.0	1.4	1.0	0.8	0.6	0.5	0.4
10,000	12.1	6.7	4.3	2.9	2.0	1.5	1.1	0.9	0.7	0.5
30,000	16.6	9.3	5.9	4.0	2.8	2.1	1.6	1.2	0.9	0.7
100,000	23.1	13.2	8.5	5.8	4.1	3.0	2.3	1.7	1.3	1.1
300,000	30.8	18.0	11.7	8.0	5.7	4.2	3.1	2.4	1.9	1.5
Age 45 y										
3,000	10.7	5.9	3.7	2.5	1.8	1.3	1.0	0.7	0.6	0.5
10,000	15.1	8.5	5.4	3.6	2.6	1.9	1.4	1.1	0.8	0.7
30,000	20.6	11.7	7.5	5.1	3.6	2.6	2.0	1.5	1.2	0.9
100,000	28.4	16.5	10.6	7.3	5.2	3.8	2.9	2.2	1.7	1.3
300,000	37.4	22.4	14.6	10.1	7.2	5.3	4.0	3.1	2.4	1.9
Age 55 y										
3,000	13.4	7.5	4.7	3.2	2.3	1.7	1.2	0.9	0.7	0.6
10,000	18.8	10.7	6.8	4.6	3.3	2.4	1.8	1.4	1.1	0.8
30,000	25.4	14.6	9.4	6.4	4.6	3.3	2.5	1.9	1.5	1.2
100,000	34.6	20.5	13.3	9.2	6.5	4.8	3.6	2.8	2.2	1.7
300,000	44.8	27.5	18.2	12.6	9.1	6.7	5.0	3.9	3.0	2.4

Abbreviation: CASCADE = Concerted Action on Seroconversion to AIDS and Death in Europe.
Reproduced with permission from Phillips A; CASCADE collaboration: Short-term risk of AIDS according to current CD4 cell count and viral load in antiretroviral drug-naïve individuals and those treated in the monotherapy era. AIDS 2004;18(1):51-58.

strongly associated with long-term nonprogressor status. Conversely, individuals having the single nucleotide polymorphism at the promoter site of the inhibitory cytokine IL-10 (IL-10-5′-592A) are at a higher risk for HIV infection upon exposure, and they progress to AIDS more rapidly once infected. Certain exogenous factors might also influence the course of HIV infection. The orphan virus GB virus C slows down disease progression and is associated with better survival in patients dually infected with HIV and GB virus C. CMV coinfection possibly augments the rate of HIV disease progression. Incident OIs, especially tuberculosis and deficiency of micronutrients, also accelerate disease progression.

Changing Face of HIV/AIDS

Highly active antiretroviral therapy (HAART) has dramatically changed the long-term outcome of patients with HIV/AIDS, which once was a rapidly fatal illness. HAART not only improves the CD4+ counts but also decreases the risk of OIs and reduces the mortality substantially. The benefit of HAART is evident even in those patients with advanced immunosuppression. From a public health perspective, HAART is a cost-effective intervention, in the developed world and the developing nations alike. In fact, HAART is comparatively more cost-effective than some of the widely accepted therapies for certain non-HIV diseases.

Since the introduction of HAART in 1995, AIDS-related mortality has declined considerably in the United States. With improved survival of patients with AIDS, noninfectious complications of AIDS such as AIDS-related malignancies and chronic renal failure are increasingly seen. Similarly, some novel problems of long-term antiretroviral therapy, such as lipodystrophy, insulin resistance syndrome, increased risk of cardiovascular events, and osteoporosis, are also being recognized. However, the changing face of AIDS is not a global phenomenon; paradoxically, the populations that need it the most are the ones with poor access to HAART.

Whom to Test for HIV Infection

HIV testing should be offered to all persons reporting any of the known risk factors for HIV acquisition and those requesting a HIV test on their own, irrespective of their risk behavior. Patients presenting with OIs and noninfectious illnesses possibly related to HIV, such as lymphoma, cervical cancer, and anal cancer, should also be tested for HIV infection. Subtle clinical clues of immunocompromise, such as oral thrush, herpes zoster in a young person, or failure to thrive in children, should alert the physician to the possibility of HIV infection. In developing nations, it is not uncommon for a young child to be the index case of a HIV-infected family. All women who are receiving antenatal care and, in underdeveloped nations, antenatal cases coming into contact with the health care system for the first time while in labor should be screened for HIV infection. In addition, patients seen in certain high-risk settings in which the prevalence of HIV infection is known to be high, such as sexually transmitted disease clinics, tuberculosis clinics, detoxification clinics, and correctional facilities, should also be offered HIV testing. HIV infection should be systematically excluded by testing while evaluating patients presenting with fever of unknown origin, autoimmune disorders such as Sjögren's syndrome, systemic lupus erythematosus, Reiter's syndrome, and polymyositis, and neurologic illnesses such as young-onset dementia and unexplained peripheral neuropathy. To say there are no contraindications for offering HIV testing to a patient is no overstatement.

It is estimated that every fourth HIV-infected person in the United States is not aware of his or her serostatus. This not only jeopardizes their own care but also places others at risk of potential transmission, which could be prevented if they are detected early. In recent times, the current trend of "HIV exceptionalism" has come under considerable criticism. This calls for a public health approach, based on standard principles of epidemic control, which encompasses a nonselective HIV testing strategy instead of the targeted-testing practices in vogue. Recent evidence suggests that nonselective HIV testing, in health care settings and possibly in the general population also, could be cost effective.

Diagnosis of HIV Infection

All persons who are offered HIV testing should receive appropriate pretest counseling, and their explicit consent must be obtained. The CDC-recommended "opt-out" HIV screening strategy for health care settings, however, does not require pre-test counseling, and a general consent for medical care would suffice for HIV testing. Notification of the result must be confidential and has to be accompanied by post-test counseling. Post-test counseling should focus on behavior modification for persons who test negative and for persons who test positive as well.

Laboratory diagnosis of HIV infection is based on a sequential testing strategy for the detection of antibodies to HIV-specific antigens. The first test is a highly sensitive enzyme immunoassay (EIA) that contains antigens of both HIV-1 and HIV-2. If the test is negative, further testing is not warranted, unless the exposure was within the past 3 months, in which case it has to be repeated in 3 months. If the first test returns positive or indeterminate, the test is repeated in duplicate. If the repeat EIA tests are positive or indeterminate, the HIV-1 Western blot assay is needed for confirmation. A Western blot demonstrating antibodies to products of all three major genes of HIV (*gag*, *pol*, and *env*) is conclusive evidence of HIV infection (rare false-positives can occur with the conventional Centers for Disease Control and Prevention criterion that does not require reactivity to products of *pol*); a negative assay shows no bands. Patterns that fall in between are considered indeterminate and must be repeated after an interval of 1 month. Alternatively, one may proceed to a specific test such as the p24 antigen capture assay or HIV-1 RNA assay. If the HIV-1 Western blot result is discordant with that of EIA, the possibility of HIV-2 infection should be considered, and HIV-2-specific testing is warranted.

Six rapid tests—OraQuick Advance, Uni-Gold Recombigen, Reveal G3, Clearview HIV 1/2 STAT-PAK, Clearview Complete HIV 1/2, and Multispot HIV-1/HIV-2—are approved by the U.S. Food and Drug Administration for point-of-care testing in acute care settings and for on-site testing at outreach testing sites. A positive result by any of these tests should be considered only as "preliminary positive," and further confirmatory testing is essential.

Management of the HIV-Infected Patient

Similar to any other disease, there seems to be a learning curve in the case of HIV care as well. It is well known that the outcome of patients with HIV/AIDS receiving treatment, at least to a certain extent, depends on the expertise of the care provider. However, this does not mean that all HIV-infected patients should be treated only by a specialist, which is not a feasible proposition. The sheer magnitude of the problem calls for greater participation on the part of the primary care physician. The U.S. Department of Health and Human Services panel recommends care by a physician with at least 20, preferably 50, HIV-infected patients. It is essential for a primary care physician to be familiar with the initial care of patients with HIV/AIDS. Primary care physicians who have not cared for a considerable number of patients with HIV/AIDS should liaise with a specialist in the field. Referral to a specialist is warranted in cases of treatment-failure and for the management of complications. Care of HIV-infected patients is multifaceted, and it needs a multidisciplinary approach. Such a comprehensive care is delivered better by the primary care physician.

CURRENT DIAGNOSIS

- Threshold to offer HIV testing to a patient should be low; nonselective "opt-out" HIV testing in health care settings is recommended.
- A repeatedly reactive enzyme immunoassay, rapid test, or nucleic acid-based test for HIV infection needs confirmation with a Western blot assay.
- Estimation of CD4+ count and plasma viral load should be performed to assess the need for antiretroviral therapy and the risk of opportunistic infections.

INITIAL EVALUATION

Evaluation of the HIV-infected patient is carried out in several stages: assessment of the stage of disease and the need for antiretroviral therapy; symptom-oriented evaluation for opportunistic conditions; screening to assess the risk of opportunistic infections (OIs) in the future; screening for diseases that are co-transmitted, such as sexually transmitted infections and viral hepatitis; and prevention of further transmission of HIV infection.

History should be elicited with reference to the route and time of HIV acquisition. Time of exposure and earlier negative HIV tests are useful to assess reasonably the latter but may not be available in every case. More often than not, patients have multiple risk factors, and some patients may not report any of the known risk factors. A non-judgmental approach is important while taking a sexual history. In addition, questions should focus on symptoms of other sexually transmitted infections such as urethral/vaginal discharge, genital ulcers, dysuria, dyspareunia in females, and perianal/oral ulcers and sore throat in those who report anal/oral sex. It is also important to elicit how the patient is coping with the diagnosis of HIV infection and the social and family support available to the patient. All patients have to be screened for depression and the presence of suicidal ideations, and they should be encouraged to inform their spouse/sexual partner of their HIV status. The physician has to be aware of the legal obligations regarding partner notification because they vary from place to place.

History should focus also on symptoms such as unexplained weight loss, prolonged fever, chronic diarrhea, recurrent oral ulcers, dysphagia, shortness of breath, cognitive decline, and new-onset seizures pointing toward the presence of opportunistic conditions that need further diagnostic evaluation. In treatment-experienced patients, details of previous antiretroviral treatment and the response to it should be meticulously looked into and properly recorded. This can be invaluable while changing the therapy in cases of treatment failure. Medication history should include details of allergic reaction to drugs such as cotrimoxazole (Bactrim), nevirapine (Viramune), and abacavir (Ziagen), and details of other drug-related adverse effects, such as pancreatitis, peripheral neuropathy, and hepatitis too. Details of past illnesses like tuberculosis and viral hepatitis, contact with cases of tuberculosis, and travel to areas endemic for certain infections such as histoplasmosis (Ohio and Mississippi river valleys), coccidioidomycosis (southwestern United States, northern Mexico), penicilliosis (Southeast Asia), and leishmaniasis (tropics, subtropics, and southern Europe) should be elicited.

A complete physical examination has to be performed at the time of initial evaluation and at subsequent visits. Attention should be paid to the presence of lymphadenopathy, hepatomegaly/splenomegaly, serosal effusions, and features of wasting or lipodystrophy. Examination of the nervous system should focus on possible peripheral neuropathy, proximal myopathy, focal neurologic signs, meningism, and cognitive impairment. If the latter is suspected, further neuropsychological testing is required. In patients presenting with OIs, skin lesions often hold the clue. Funduscopic examination should be done, and in patients with CD4+ less than 50 cells/μL, detailed examination by an ophthalmologist is needed to screen for

TABLE 3 Initial and Subsequent Laboratory Evaluation of the HIV-Infected Patient

Baseline Testing	Follow-up Testing[a]
CD4+ count[b]	Once in 3–6 mo
Plasma HIV RNA load[c]	Once in 3–4 mo if not on treatment; at 2–8 wk after initiating/changing treatment, then q3–4 mo
Viral resistance testing[d]	Recommended in virologic failure
Complete blood count	q3 mo, especially in patients taking zidovudine (Retrovir)
Blood urea, creatinine, electrolytes	q3–6 mo, especially in patients taking indinavir (Crixivan) or other nephrotoxic drugs
Transaminases, alkaline phosphatase, bilirubin, albumin	q2 wk in first month, monthly for next 3 mo, then once in 3 mo
Fasting blood glucose	If on PIs, at 1–3 mo after initiation, then q3–6 mo
Fasting serum lipids	If on PIs, at 3–6 mo, then annually
Urinalysis—proteinuria, sediments	q3–6 mo, especially in patients taking indinavir (Crixivan)
Chest radiograph	As clinically indicated
Electrocardiogram	As clinically indicated
Serologic Screening	
Antitoxoplasma IgG[e]	If seronegative, when CD4+ < 100/µL and unable to take cotrimoxazole (Bactrim)
Syphilis serology (VDRL or RPR)	Annually, if sexually active[f]
Anticytomegalovirus IgG[g]	As clinically indicated
HBsAg, HBsAb, HCV-Ab, HAV-Ab[h]	As clinically indicated
Antivaricella IgG[i]	Not indicated
Tuberculin skin test or IGRA[j]	If negative at baseline, repeat once CD4+ > 200/µL
Urine-based (first-void) NAAT for *Chlamydia* species, *Neisseria gonorrhoeae*[k]	Annually, if sexually active[f]
In Women	
Cervical Papanicolaou smear	Annually, if sexually active[f]
Vaginal secretions for *Trichomonas* species	Annually, if sexually active[f]
Cervical specimen for NAAT for *Chlamydia* species (if sexually active)	Annually, if sexually active[f]

Note: In addition, HLA-B*5701 status to be tested, if avaliable, before starting abacavir; contraindicated if positive.
[a] May be repeated more frequently if clinically indicated
[b] Preferably 2 baseline values measured 1–4 wk apart; if discordant, repeat third time.
[c] Preferably 2 baseline values measured 1–4 wk apart.
[d] Recommended regardless of whether treatment will be initiated.
[e] Seronegative patients should be counseled regarding proper preparation of meat and appropriate handling of cat feces.
[f] q3–6 mo in asymptomatic persons at higher risk.
[g] Seronegative patients should be transfused CMV-negative or leukocyte-depleted blood products only.
[h] Vaccination recommended for hepatitis B and hepatitis A, if found susceptible; testing for antibody to hepatitis B core antigen is optional.
[i] May be tested if no history of chickenpox or shingles; if seronegative, postexposure prophylaxis with varicella zoster immune globulin is indicated.
[j] Unless a history of tuberculosis or positive test earlier.
[k] In men and women reporting receptive anal sex, culture rectal sample for *Chlamydia* species, and *N. gonorrhoeae*, and in those reporting receptive oral sex, culture pharyngeal sample for *N. gonorrhoeae*.
Abbreviations: HAV-Ab = hepatitis A antibody; HBsAb = hepatitis B surface antibody; HBsAg = hepatitis B surface antigen; HCV-Ab = hepatitis C antibody; IGRA = interferon-γ release assay; NAAT = nucleic acid amplification test; PI = protease inhibitor; RPR = rapid plasma reagin test; VDRL = venereal diseases research laboratory test.

cytomegalovirus (CMV) retinitis and other ocular manifestations of HIV. One should look for thrush, hairy leukoplakia, mucosal lesions of Kaposi's sarcoma, and aphthous ulcerations while examining the oral cavity. Diligent examination of the anogenital area for urethral discharge, genital/perianal ulcerations, condylomata, and adnexal tenderness in females is needed. Table 3 describes the laboratory evaluation of HIV-infected patients.

ANTIRETROVIRAL THERAPY

Antiretroviral drugs fall into five classes: nucleoside/nucleotide reverse transcriptase inhibitors (NRTIs), non-nucleoside reverse transcriptase inhibitors (NNRTIs), protease inhibitors (PIs), entry and fusion inhibitors; and integrase inhibitors (Table 4). HAART is a combination of at least three potent antiretroviral drugs, typically a combination of two NRTIs as the backbone, along with either a PI or an NNRTI. Antiretroviral drugs act by inhibiting the enzyme reverse transcriptase either competitively (NRTIs) or noncompetitively (NNRTIs) or by inhibiting the viral protease that is essential for virion assembly (PIs), or by causing functional inhibition of gp41 that is important for entry into the host cell (enfuviritide) or by blocking the CCRs (maraviroc), or by preventing the integration of proviral DNA into host cell genome (raltegravir). NNRTIs are specific for the HIV-1 reverse transcriptase and have no activity against HIV-2. HIV-2 carries, constitutively, many of the mutations associated with PI resistance that might limit the activity of PIs against HIV-2.

The goal of treatment is to achieve maximal and sustained suppression of plasma viremia to undetectable levels (less than 50 to 80 copies/mL for currently available tests). In this regard, HAART is far superior to dual and monotherapies and is the standard of care. Table 5 presents the regimens recommended currently for use in treatment-naïve HIV-1-infected patients. Selection among these regimens is made individually, taking into consideration factors such as pill burden, co-morbidities, potential drug interactions, and pregnancy. Triple NRTI regimens are inferior to PI- and NNRTI-based regimens in achieving durable viral suppression, and hence triple NRTI regimens are to be used only when PI/NNRTI-based regimens cannot be given. NNRTI-based regimens containing nevirapine (Viramune) should be avoided in females with CD4+ more than 250 cells/µL and in males with CD4+ more than 400 cells/µL because of the high risk of serious hepatotoxicity. Efavirenz (Sustiva) is the

TABLE 4 Currently Approved Antiretroviral Drugs

Drug	Dosage	Food/Fasting Requirement
Nucleoside/Nucleotide Reverse Transcriptase Inhibitors (NRTIs)		
Abacavir (Ziagen)	300 mg bid or 600 mg qd	No effect of meals
Didanosine (Videx)	400 mg qd or 200 mg bid ($\geq$60 kg); 250 mg qd or 125 mg bid (<60 kg)	½ hr before or 2 hr after meals
Emtricitabine (Emtriva)	200 mg qd	No effect of meals
Lamivudine (Epivir)	150 mg bid or 300 mg qd	No effect of meals
Stavudine (Zerit)	40 mg bid ($\geq$60 kg); 30 mg bid (<60 kg)	No effect of meals
Tenofovir (Viread)	300 mg qd	No effect of meals
Zalcitabine (Hivid)	0.75 mg tid	No effect of meals
Zidovudine (Retrovir)	300 mg bid or 200 mg tid	No effect of meals
Non-Nucleoside Reverse Transcriptase Inhibitors (NNRTIs)		
Delavirdine (Rescriptor)	400 mg tid	No effect of meals
Efavirenz (Sustiva)	600 mg qd	At or before bedtime; empty stomach
Etravirine (Intelence)	200 mg bid	With meals
Nevirapine (Viramune)	200 mg qd for 14 d; then 200 mg bid	No effect of meals
Protease Inhibitors (PIs)		
Amprenavir (Agenerase)	1400 mg bid	No effect of meals; avoid high-fat meals[a]
Atazanavir (Reyataz)	400 mg qd	With meal[b]
Darunavir (Prezista)/rtv	600/100 mg bid	With meals
Fosamprenavir (Lexiva)	1400 mg bid; 1400/rtv 200 mg qd[c]	No effect of meals
Indinavir (Crixivan)/rtv	800/100–200 mg q12h[d]	No effect of meals; if given unboosted, 1 hr before or 2 hr after meals
Lopinavir/rtv (Kaletra)	400/100 mg bid or 800/200 mg qd[e]	With meals
Nelfinavir (Viracept)	1250 mg bid or 750 mg tid[f]	With meal or snack
Ritonavir (Norvir)	100–400 mg/d[g]	With meals
Saquinavir hard gel (Invirase)/rtv	1000/100 mg bid	Within 2 hr of meals
Saquinavir soft gel (Fortovase)/rtv	1000/100 mg bid	With or up to 2 hr after meals
Tipranavir (Aptivus)/rtv	500/200 mg bid	With meals
Entry and Fusion Inhibitors		
Enfuvirtide (Fuzeon)	90 mg SC bid	Injectable only
Maraviroc (Selzntry)	300 mg bid	No effect of meals
Integrase Inhibitor		
Raltegravir (Isentress)	400 mg bid	No effect of meals

Note: Fixed-dose combinations of various NRTIs with or without an NNRTI are also commercially available.
[a]Ritonavir, if given for boosting, should not be administered simultaneously.
[b]Not to be taken with antacids.
[c]Should be given only as 2 equally divided doses in PI-experienced patients.
[d]800 mg q8h if given unboosted.
[e]533/133 mg bid in patients taking nevirapine or efavirenz.
[f]In pregnant patients, 750 mg tid should not be used.
[g]Doses given for pharmacokinetic boosting.
Abbreviations: rtv = ritonavir-boosted; SC = subcutaneous.

CURRENT THERAPY

- History of any AIDS-defining illness, CD4+ count < 200 cells/μL, and symptomatic HIV disease warrant initiation of highly active antiretroviral therapy (HAART).
- HAART should be initiated also in patients with CD4+ counts 200-350 cells/μL, irrespective of viral load and symptoms.
- HAART is indicated in patients with HIV nephropathy and HBV co-infection requiring treatment.
- Once initiated, HAART has to be continued lifelong without interruption.
- Adherence is a very important determinant of virologic outcome.
- Regular monitoring of viral load should be done to diagnose treatment failure early.
- At least two fully active drugs, based on treatment history and resistance testing, should be included in the salvage regimen.

preferred NNRTI in such situations. Efavirenz-based regimens are equivalent to PI-based regimens in terms of efficacy and durability and have the advantage of low pill burden and limited long-term toxicity. Once initiated, for reasons mentioned earlier, HAART has to be continued lifelong. Structured treatment interruptions, aimed at preventing drug resistance, place the patient unduly at risk of disease progression and death during the period of interruption and are not recommended. Similarly, the strategy of withholding HAART once CD4+ counts improve following treatment (CD4+-guided therapy) is also inferior to uninterrupted treatment.

WHEN TO INITIATE HAART?

The decision to start HAART is a fine balance between the potential benefits of delaying the treatment and the risk of progression to AIDS and death. The patient has to be fully apprised of the benefits as well as the risks involved, and he or she has to play an active role in decision making. Initiation of HAART is warranted in patients with history of any of the AIDS-defining illnesses (irrespective of CD4+ count and viral load) and in those with advanced immunosuppression (CD4+ less than 200 cells/μL, irrespective of viral load and symptoms). Conversely, initiation of HAART can be delayed safely in patients with CD4+ counts more than 350 cells/μL and plasma

TABLE 5 First-Line Antiretroviral Regimens for Treatment-Naïve HIV-1-Infected Patients

Recommendation	Regimen Class		
	NNRTI-based	PI-based	Dual NRTI Backbone
Preferred	Efavirenz (Sustiva)*	Atazanavir (Reyataz)/rtv[†] -or- Fosamprenavir (Lexiva)/rtv (bid) -or- Lopinavir/rtv (Kaletra) (bid)	Abacavir + Lamivudine (Epzicom) -or- Tenofovir + Emtricitabine (Truvada)
Alternative	Nevirapine (Viramune)[‡]	Atazanavir (Reyataz) -or- Fosamprenavir (Lexiva) -or- Fosamprenavir (Lexiva)/rtv (qd) -or- Lopinavir/rtv (Kaletra) (qd) -or- Saquinavir (Invirase)/rtv	**First Choice:** Zidovudine + Lamivudine (Combivir) **Second choice:** Didanosine (Videx EC) + (Lamivudine [Epivir] or Emtricitabine [Emtriva])

Note: For a first-line regimen, combine either an NNRTI or a PI with a dual NRTI backbone; once daily regimens can be tailored by selecting the appropriate drug among the interchangeable choices presented here.
NRTI = nucleoside reverse transcriptase inhibitor; NNRTI = non-nucleoside reverse transcriptase inhibitor; PI = protease inhibitor; rtv = low-dose ritonavir (Norvir) 100-400 mg/day for pharmacokinetic boosting, not considered as fourth drug in the regimen; ritonavir (Norvir) alone should not be used as the sole PI.
*Contraindicated in women who are pregnant, plan to conceive, or not using effective contraception.
[†]If combined with efavirenz (Sustiva) or tenofovir (Viread; Truvada), atazanavir (Reyataz) should be boosted with rtv.
[‡]Avoid in women with CD4+ > 250/µL and men with CD4+ > 400/µL (see text).
Based on Guidelines for the use of antiretroviral agents in HIV-1-infected adults and adolescents, U.S. Department of Health and Human Services, January 2008.

---

viral load less than 100,000 copies/mL. HAART is also indicated irrespective of CD4+ cell count in patients with HIV-associated nephropathy, HBV co-infection (if HBV treatment is indicated), and in pregnancy. Data from randomized, controlled trials are lacking regarding the optimal time of initiating HAART in patients with CD4+ counts of 200 to 350 cells/µL. Observational data suggest that it is desirable to initiate HAART in these patients before their CD4+ counts drop below 200 cells/µL. Current consensus is that these patients should be initiated on treatment. Treatment of patients having CD4+ more than 350 cells/µL with high viral loads (more than 100,000 copies/mL) is considered optional, and if treatment is deferred, CD4+ count and viral load should be monitored closely (every 3 months). Likewise, in the absence of supporting evidence, treatment of patients with acute HIV infection and those in whom seroconversion occurred within the past 6 months is considered optional.

MONITORING RESPONSE TO ANTIRETROVIRAL THERAPY

In a patient on treatment, CD4+ counts have to be monitored every 3 to 6 months and the viral load every 3 to 4 months. A reproducible change in absolute CD4+ count of at least 30% and/or 3 percentage point change in the CD4+ percentage are considered significant. Similarly, for viral load, a threefold or 0.5 $\log_{10}$ copies/mL change is deemed significant. It is important that these estimations are not performed during an episode of intercurrent infection or vaccination because transient fluctuations in viremia and CD4+ counts can occur during such episodes. Because of large variations in absolute CD4+ count estimations and interassay differences in estimating viral load, serial evaluations should be obtained from the same laboratory using the same assay. Before making any treatment change based on the laboratory results, they should be repeated and reconfirmed.

Following the initiation of effective antiretroviral therapy, CD4+ counts rapidly improve within a few weeks, largely as a result of redistribution of cells, and they subsequently improve at the rate of approximately 100 cells/µL per year over the subsequent years until a plateau is reached. Plasma viral load rapidly falls in the initial weeks and becomes undetectable in approximately 4 to 6 months. The rate of initial decline in viral load depends on the potency of the HAART regimen, and it predicts the durability of viral suppression. Determination of viral load at 2 to 8 weeks after the initiation or change in treatment thus is also recommended. An adequate response is defined as a decrease of at least 1.0 $\log_{10}$ copies/mL at 2 to 8 weeks after starting treatment; plasma viral load should become undetectable by 16 to 24 weeks.

DRUG RESISTANCE AND RESISTANCE TESTING

A patient may be infected with a drug-resistant virus to begin with (primary resistance) or else resistance can emerge as a result of treatment (secondary). The latter is more common. With widespread use of antiretrovirals, primary resistance is increasing. Most NNRTI-associated resistance mutations confer cross-resistance to all other NNRTIs as well. Among NRTIs, cross-resistance is common but varies by drug. Paradoxically, lamivudine(Epivir) resistance related to the M184V mutation enhances the susceptibility to zidovudine (Retrovir). With PIs, initial mutations might confer limited resistance only; however, accumulation of sequential mutations leads to broad cross-resistance. Tipranavir (Aptivus)/ritonavir (Norvir) is active against such strains of HIV-1 resistant to multiple PIs.

Drug-resistance testing is done by either genotypic or phenotypic assays. Overall, the resistance tests have a limited sensitivity. Resistance may not be detected if viremia is less than 1000 copies/mL or the frequency of resistant quasispecies is less than 10% to 20%. These tests are to be performed while the patient is still taking the failing regimen or within 4 weeks after discontinuation to avoid overgrowth of the resistant quasispecies by the wild strain. The exact role of resistance testing in clinical practice is not yet clear. In patients receiving tailored regimens based on resistance testing, benefit in terms of improved virologic outcome is modest only. However, testing for drug resistance is indicated in patients failing treatment, those having suboptimal virologic response, and in those with acute HIV infection. Routine resistance testing in drug-naïve patients with chronic HIV infection should also be considered, especially if the prevalence of primary resistance is more than 4%.

TABLE 6 Salvage Therapy in Patients with Treatment Failure (Virologic Failure)

Initial Regimen	First Virologic Failure — Resistance Identified	First Virologic Failure — No Resistance Identified	Subsequent Virologic Failures
NNRTI-based (2 NRTIs + NNRTI)	2 NRTIs (based on resistance testing) + PI (unboosted or rtv-boosted)	Check adherence to treatment; if poor, address compliance. Was the resistance testing properly timed? (see text); if not properly timed, continue same regimen; repeat genotypic testing in 2–4 wk or start a new regimen; repeat genotypic testing in 2–4 wk. If adherence and timing of testing are acceptable, start a new regimen; repeat genotypic testing in 2–4 wk or intensify by adding 1 NRTI (tenofovir [Viread]) or boost the PI with rtv.	Include at least 2, preferably 3, fully active drugs (see text); add a drug from new class, if available. If 3-class virologic failure, start > 1 NRTI (based on resistance testing) + a new boosted-PI (based on resistance testing) ± enfuvirtide (Fuzeon). If only 1 fully active agent available, add to failing regimen only if CD4+ < 100/µL; otherwise, continue failing regimen. If no fully active agent available, continue failing regimen; do not interrupt.
PI-based (2 NRTIs + PI [unboosted or rtv-boosted])	2 NRTIs (based on resistance testing) + NNRTI or 2 NRTIs (based on resistance testing) + a new boosted PI (based on resistance testing) or 1 or more NRTI(s) (based on resistance testing) + NNRTI + a new boosted PI (based on resistance testing)		
Triple NRTI (3 NRTIs)	2 NRTIs (based on resistance testing) + NNRTI or PI (unboosted or rtv-boosted) or 1 or more NRTI(s) (based on resistance testing) + NNRTI + PI (unboosted or rtv-boosted) or NNRTI + PI (unboosted or rtv-boosted)		

Based on Guidelines for the use of antiretroviral agents in HIV-1-infected adults and adolescents, U.S. Department of Health and Human Services, January 2008.
Abbreviations: NNRTI = non-nucleoside reverse transcriptase inhibitor; NRTI = nucleoside reverse transcriptase inhibitor; PI = protease inhibitor; rtv = ritonavir (Norvir).

Failure to identify any resistance in a patient failing treatment points toward poor adherence.

TREATMENT FAILURE

Failure of treatment can be classified into virologic failure, immunologic failure, and clinical progression. Virologic failure is evidenced by repeated detection of viremia more than 400 copies/mL after 24 weeks or more than 50 copies/mL after 48 weeks of treatment in a drug-naïve patient or by persistent viremia after achieving complete suppression (virologic rebound). Inadequate CD4+ response (improvement of fewer than 25 to 50 cells/µL in the first year) or a fall below the pretreatment CD4+ level constitutes immunologic failure. Occurrence or recurrence of HIV-related events after the third month of HAART, in the absence of an alternative explanation, is considered indicative of clinical progression. Usually virologic failure is the first to occur, to be followed months to years later by immunologic failure, and finally by clinical progression. Sometimes discordant responses (i.e., immunologic failure and clinical progression despite suppressed viremia) may occur. Provided that viremia is well suppressed, changing the regimen may not be warranted in such settings.

In a patient with virologic failure, although drug resistance is the proximate cause of failure, one must carefully look for factors that contributed to the emergence of drug resistance in that particular patient and try to address them. Otherwise, the new regimen is also bound to fail. Such factors include inadequate regimen potency, high baseline viral load, poor adherence, drug intolerance, preexisting resistance, and suboptimal pharmacokinetics because of malabsorption, noncompliance with food/fasting requirements, and drug interactions. Past-treatment experience of the patient should also be evaluated to inform them about further treatment choices (Table 6). In general, the new regimen should include at least two, preferably three, fully active drugs. A fully active drug is one that is likely to be effective based on both the treatment history and susceptibility on resistance testing. Addition of a single drug may be justified if substitution is being made to manage toxicity in a patient with otherwise good response or in a patient failing treatment where no resistance is identified, after ruling out poor adherence and improperly timed resistance testing. Although the goal of treatment remains complete suppression of viremia below detectable limits, in treatment-experienced patients with resistance to multiple drugs, this may not always be feasible. In such patients with limited options, even a 0.5 to 1.0 $\log_{10}$ reduction in viral load may be acceptable. In patients failing treatment with extensive prior treatment, if no fully active drug is available, continuing with the failing regimen might decrease the risk of clinical progression.

ADHERENCE TO TREATMENT

Adherence to prescribed treatment is a complex issue but of utmost importance. Antiretroviral treatment is very exacting in terms of adherence when compared to other chronic diseases; missing as little as 5% to 10% of doses is known to affect virologic outcome adversely. The natural tendency is to miss a few doses, and physician estimates of adherence are known to be unreliable. It is thus important to suspect noncompliance in every patient. Before initiating treatment, the patient must be counseled regarding medication requirements, and readiness to take the treatment has to be ensured. It has to be impressed on the patient that the first regimen has the best chance for long-term success. Adherence counseling and assessment of adherence should be done at each clinical encounter. Adherence is conventionally assessed by patient self-reports, pill counting, and a patient-recorded medication diary. Microelectronic monitoring systems like Medication Event Monitoring System (MEMS Track Cap) and therapeutic drug monitoring could provide more objective assessment of adherence. However, all these methods have their limitations, and it is preferable to use more than one method simultaneously.

Noncompliance with treatment has many causes. Patient-related factors, such as substance abuse, depression, lack of social support, and age; medication-related factors, such as dosing frequency, pill burden, food/fasting requirements, and adverse effects; and health care system–related factors, such as attitude of staff, communication, and accessibility, all operate in tandem to influence the adherence. Adherence can be improved by simplifying the dosage schedules, providing pillboxes, tailoring to suit the lifestyle, entrusting medication intake to a family member, using reminder calls and alarms and community-based case managers, alerting to adverse effects, providing patient education materials, making the clinic appointments convenient, and making the health system encounter pleasant. In patients found nonadherent, enough time should be spent to identify the responsible factors and to find acceptable solutions while involving the patient actively in the process.

ADVERSE DRUG REACTIONS AND DRUG INTERACTIONS

Adverse drug reactions (ADRs) are common with antiretroviral therapy and an important cause of nonadherence. They also contribute to a significant proportion of clinic visits and mortality. ADRs can be idiosyncratic, dose related, time related (delayed), or dose and time related (cumulative). A particular ADR may be common to all drugs of the same class (e.g., lactic acidosis and fatty liver because of NRTIs, lipodystrophy because of PIs), or it might be drug specific (e.g., hypersensitivity to abacavir [Ziagen], nephrolithiasis because of indinavir [Crixivan]). The patient often is on other drugs as well, with overlapping ADR profiles, apart from antiretrovirals. A symptom-based approach is useful from a practical point of view (Table 7). Although many of the ADRs can be managed conservatively, some, such as symptomatic lactic acidosis, systemic hypersensitivity reactions, Stevens-Johnson syndrome, acute pancreatitis, and severe hepatotoxicity, are potentially life threatening. Serious ADRs necessitate withdrawal of the offending drug, and rechallenge of the drug should not be attempted in these situations.

Drug interactions are often the underlying cause of ADRs. PIs are metabolized by the hepatic cytochrome P450 (CYP) enzymes. At the same time, PIs are potent inhibitors of CYP. Conversely, NNRTIs, especially efavirenz (Sustiva), are a potent inducer of CYP. When antiretrovirals are co-administered with other drugs metabolized by or affecting CYP (antihistamines, prokinetics, lipid-lowering agents, antifungals, antitubercular drugs, anticonvulsants, etc.), complex pharmacokinetic interactions occur; this can lead to potentially toxic or subtherapeutic drug levels. In a patient on HAART, unnecessary prescriptions are to be avoided, and it is prudent always to check the compatibility and the dose modifications needed before prescribing.

Management of Opportunistic Conditions

GENERAL CONSIDERATIONS

OIs are the most common cause of disability and death in HIV-infected patients who are not receiving treatment. Hence, it is important that OIs are promptly recognized and treated. Different pathogens may cause similar disease patterns, and multiple OIs may occur concurrently. Although it is important to make a definitive diagnosis in these patients, diagnostic workup should not delay unduly the initiation of appropriate treatment. Empirical treatment based on clinical suspicion may be justified in acutely ill patients. In a patient with a severe OI as the initial manifestation of HIV disease, management of the OI takes precedence over immediate initiation of HAART. This avoids potential drug interactions and possibly decreases the occurrence of immune reconstitution inflammatory syndrome (IRIS). However, in patients with OIs for which no effective treatment is available (cryptosporidiosis, microsporidiosis, progressive multifocal leukoencephalopathy, and Kaposi's sarcoma), HAART itself can result in improvement and hence should be initiated as soon as possible.

IRIS manifests as the occurrence of a new OI or worsening of a preexisting OI following initiation of HAART, usually in the first 3 months. Symptoms include fever, lymphadenopathy, serosal effusions, worsening or fresh pulmonary infiltrates, vitreitis, uveitis, and intracranial lesions. Occasionally life-threatening complications like acute respiratory distress syndrome (ARDS) and acute renal failure develop. Most instances of IRIS respond well to nonsteroidal anti-inflammatory drugs. HAART and OI-specific treatment need to be continued without interruption. Steroids may be useful in patients with life-threatening complications.

OIs can be prevented by timely initiation of primary chemoprophylaxis (Table 8). It has to be stressed that OIs listed in the table can also occur, albeit less often, in patients with CD4+ counts above the cutoffs for initiation of prophylaxis. Following treatment for an episode of OI, lifelong secondary prophylaxis is needed to prevent relapse. However, if a sustained improvement in CD4+ count is achieved following HAART, secondary prophylaxis for most of the OIs and primary prophylaxis can be withdrawn safely. Table 9 presents the possible etiology of opportunistic conditions. Management of common potentially life-threatening OIs is presented next.

PNEUMOCYSTIS JIROVECI PNEUMONIA (PCP)

PCP is the most common OI in HIV-infected patients. Approximately 90% of cases occur among patients with CD4+ less than 200 cells/µL. Although the overall mortality is approximately 10% to 20%, it exceeds 50% in those requiring mechanical ventilation for respiratory failure. PCP manifests as a subacute febrile illness accompanied by nonproductive cough and progressive exertional dyspnea. In patients with mild disease, physical findings are often scanty, barring tachypnea and scattered so-called cellophane crackles. Hypoxemia is useful to assess the severity of disease, and moderate to severe hypoxemia (PaO_2 less than 70 mm Hg or [A-a]DO_2 more than 35 mm Hg while breathing ambient air) indicates severe disease. Chest radiograph demonstrates diffuse, bilateral, interstitial infiltrates in a perihilar distribution. Atypical radiographic appearances like upper lobe predominance (in patients on inhaled pentamidine [NebuPent] prophylaxis), nodular infiltrates, cysts, and pneumothorax are also seen. An apparently normal-looking radiograph in a patient with compatible clinical presentation does not rule out a diagnosis of PCP. Diagnosis is established by the demonstration of cysts and trophozoites of *Pneumocystis* in induced sputum (sensitivity, 50% to 90%), bronchoalveolar lavage (90% to 99%), and transbronchial lung biopsy (95% to 100%) specimens by Gomori methenamine silver, Giemsa, or calcofluor staining. Immunofluorescent staining has better sensitivity and specificity than the tinctorial stains. rRNA-PCR techniques are currently being evaluated and can be used on oral washings.

TABLE 7 Approach to Adverse Drug Reactions in the HIV-Infected Patient[a]

Adverse Effect	Manifestations	Causative Drug(s) Antiretroviral(s)	Causative Drug(s) Other Drugs	Stepwise Action
Stevens-Johnson syndrome/toxic epidermal necrolysis[b]	Rash, mucosal ulcerations, fever, hepatic dysfunction	NNRTIs most commonly NVP; rarely APV, LPV/r, ATV, ABC, ZDV, ddI	Cotrimoxazole, sulfadiazine, dapsone, atovaquone, voriconazole	Discontinue all ARVs and any other possible drug; manage like severe burns; do not rechallenge offending drug.
Hypersensitivity reaction[c]	Fever, diffuse rash, malaise, arthralgia, respiratory and GI symptoms, circulatory collapse	ABC, enfuvirtide (Fuzeon)	Cotrimoxazole, sulfadiazine, dapsone	Discontinue all ARVs and any other possible drug; rule out other causes; do not rechallenge ABC/enfuvirtide.
Skin rash	Maculopapular rash only; no blisters, skin tenderness, mucosal ulceration, or fever	DLV >EFV >APV, fAPV = ATV > NVP > ABC, TPV[d]	Cotrimoxazole, sulfadiazine, dapsone, atovaquone, voriconazole	Antihistamines; continue offending drug; watch for progression of rash; if so, discontinue.
GI intolerance[e]	Anorexia, nausea, vomiting, epigastric pain	PIs, ddI, ZDV	Isoniazid, rifamycins, pyrazinamide	Administer with food (not for ddI, unboosted IDV); antiemetics; switch to less emetogenic ARV.
	Diarrhea	PIs, especially NFV, LPV/r, and buffered ddI formulations	Clindamycin, atovaquone	Rule out OIs; antimotility agents, calcium salts, bulk forming agents; rehydration, if needed.
Hepatotoxicity[f]	Jaundice, fever, vomiting, hepatic necrosis, encephalopathy	NVP	Isoniazid, rifamycins, pyrazinamide	Discontinue all ARVs and any other possible drug; rule out viral hepatitis; supportive management; do not rechallenge NVP.
	Symptomatic or subclinical hepatic enzyme elevations	NNRTIs, d4T, ddI, ZDV, PIs, especially TPV	Isoniazid, rifamycins, pyrazinamide, azithromycin, clarithromycin, all azole antifungals	If symptomatic, discontinue all ARVs and switch to nonhepatotoxic ARVs after normalization; if asymptomatic, monitor closely.
Lactic acidosis, fatty liver[g]	Nonspecific GI symptoms, tachypnea, tachycardia, hepatomegaly, hyperlactatemia, multiorgan failure	NRTIs especially d4T, ddI, ZDV	Metformin	Discontinue all ARVs; hydration; supportive treatment; IV thiamine/riboflavin; switch to ABC/3TC/TDF or NRTI-sparing regimens.
Pancreatitis[g]	Epigastric pain-postprandial, vomiting, fever, elevated amylase, lipase	ddI, d4T, ddC, RTV; 3TC (in children)	Alcohol, cotrimoxazole, pentamidine	Discontinue offending drugs; manage like acute pancreatitis related to any other cause; do not rechallenge.
Peripheral neuropathy[g]	Numbness, paresthesia–often painful; recovery possibly incomplete	ddI, d4T, ddC	Isoniazid	Switch to ABC/3TC/TDF; gabapentin, tricyclic antidepressants, narcotic analgesics.
Myopathy[g]	Myalgia, muscle tenderness, proximal weakness, elevated creatine kinase	ZDV	Statins, fibrates, steroids	Switch to another NRTI; improves in 3–4 wk after discontinuation; coenzyme-Q, L-carnitine (unproven).
Nephrolithiasis, crystalluria[h]	Flank pain, nondescript abdominal pain, dysuria, hematuria, renal dysfunction	IDV, ATV	Cotrimoxazole, sulfadiazine, acyclovir	Discontinue IDV; hydration and analgesics; IDV can be resumed with plenty of oral fluids; if recurs, consider switching.

[a]Only common and serious side effects are dealt with; side effects such as osteoporosis, avascular osteonecrosis (PIs), unconjugated hyperbilirubinemia, retinoid-like effects (IDV) and cranial malformations (EFV) are also known to occur.
[b]Approximately 0.3%–1% with NVP; a low dose, lead-in period for NVP (see Table 4) may decrease the risk; less common (0.1%) with DLV and EFV; occurs in the initial weeks after initiation; safety of replacing NVP with another NNRTI is unknown.
[c]Approximately 5% with ABC; once daily dosing possibly increases the risk; If ABC-related, symptoms resolve within 48 hrs after discontinuation of ABC.
[d]APV, fAPV, and TPV are sulfonamide derivatives; potential cross-hypersensitivity with sulfonamides.
[e]Symptoms begin with first doses; might abate with time.
[f]Low-dose, lead-in period for NVP might reduce the risk; monitoring: see Table 3; onset within the first few weeks with NNRTIs, after weeks to months with PIs, and after months to years with NRTIs; discontinuation of 3TC, FTC, or TDF in HBV co-infected patients might cause acute flare-up of hepatitis; safety of replacing NVP with another NNRTI is unknown.
[g]Class-specific adverse effect of NRTIs, because of mitochondrial toxicity; do not combine ddI/d4T/ddC; ABC, 3TC, and TDF are less prone; all 4 syndromes can occur in variable combinations; symptomatic lactic acidosis is rare but is associated with high mortality.
[h]Approximately 10% of patients taking IDV experience at least 1 episode of colic; monitoring: see Table 3; recurrence is seen in only 50%, if fluid intake is improved (at least 1.5–2 L of noncaffeinated fluid; water preferably).

TABLE 7 Approach to Adverse Drug Reactions in the HIV-Infected Patient—cont'd

Adverse Effect	Manifestations	Causative Drug(s) Antiretroviral(s)	Other Drugs	Stepwise Action
Nephrotoxicity	Renal dysfunction; nephrogenic diabetes insipidus; Fanconi syndrome	IDV, TDF	Acyclovir, amphotericin B, cotrimoxazole, pentamidine	Discontinue offending drug; hydration; generally reversible.
Hematologic	Anemia, neutropenia[i]	ZDV	Cotrimoxazole, dapsone, sulfadiazine, pyrimethamine, flucytosine, trimetrexate, amphotericin B, ganciclovir, valganciclovir, rifabutin	Discontinue concomitant marrow suppressant, if any; exclude marrow involvement by OIs/malignancy; erythropoietin or filgrastim; switch to another NRTI.
	Bleeding tendency in hemophiliacs	PIs		Factor VIII infusion; consider NNRTI-based regimens.
	Eosinophilia	Enfuvirtide (Fuzeon)	Cotrimoxazole, dapsone, sulfadiazine	Exclude disseminated strongyloidiasis, malignancy; watch for hypersensitivity.
CNS symptoms[j]	Drowsiness, insomnia, vivid dreams, nightmares, hallucination, worsening of psychiatric disorders, suicidal ideation	EFV	Isoniazid, dapsone, steroids	Usually resolve in 2–4 wk; consider discontinuation, if persistent or exacerbates psychiatric illness.
Lipodystrophy	Loss of subcutaneous fat, buffalo hump, double chin, dyslipidemia, insulin resistance, diabetes mellitus	PIs (except ATV); NRTIs, especially d4T	Steroids	Assess cardiac risk factors; lifestyle modification; metformin, glitazones, statins, fibrates[k]; consider early switching to ATV- or NNRTI-based regimens.

[i]Almost all ZDV-treated patients have isolated macrocytosis; anemia and neutropenia occur in approximately 1%-4% and 2%-8% respectively; monitoring: see Table 3.
[j]Occurs during initial weeks of treatment; patients are to be warned to restrict risky activities.
[k]Only atorvastatin (Lipitor) and pravastatin (Pravachol) among statins, and gemfibrozil (Lopid) and fenofibrate (Triglide) among fibrates, can be co-administered with PIs.
Abbreviations: 3TC = lamivudine (Epivir); ABC = abacavir (Ziagen); APV = amprenavir (Agenerase); ATV = atazanavir (Reyataz); CNS = central nervous system; d4T = stavudine (Zerit); ddC = zalcitabine (Hivid); ddI = didanosine (Videx); DLV = delavirdine (Rescriptor); EFV = efavirenz (Sustiva); fAPV = fosamprenavir (Lexiva); FTC = emtricitabine (Emtriva); GI = gastrointestinal; IDV = indinavir (Crixivan); LPV/r = lopinavir/ritonavir (Kaletra); NFV = nelfinavir (Viracept); NNRTI = non-nucleoside reverse transcriptase inhibitor; NRTI = nucleoside reverse transcriptase inhibitor; NVP = nevirapine (Viramune), OI = opportunistic infection; PI = protease inhibitor; RTV = ritonavir (Norvir); TDF = tenofovir (Viread); TPV = tipranavir (Aptivus); ZDV = zidovudine (Retrovir).
Based on Guidelines for the use of antiretroviral agents in HIV-1-infected adults and adolescents, U.S. Department of Health and Human Services, January 2008.

Cotrimoxazole (TMP-SMX, Bactrim) is the drug of choice. Mild to moderately severe cases can be managed with oral TMP-SMX (two double-strength tablets [Bactrim DS] three times daily for 21 days) on an ambulatory basis. Patients developing PCP despite TMP-SMX (Bactrim) prophylaxis can also be effectively treated with standard doses of TMP-SMX. Intravenous therapy (15-20 [TMP]/75-100 [SMX] mg/kg/day every 6 to 8 hours for 21 days) is indicated for patients with severe hypoxemia. In addition, steroids (prednisone,[1] 40 mg orally twice daily for days 1 to 5, 40 mg every day for days 6 to 10, and 20 mg every day for days 11 to 21) improve the mortality and reduce the need for mechanical ventilation in severe cases and should be started within 72 hours of starting anti-PCP treatment. Lack of clinical improvement or worsening hypoxemia after at least 4 to 8 days of anti-PCP treatment indicates failure and warrants changing of treatment. Serious ADRs related to TMP-SMX (Bactrim) also often necessitate a treatment change. The preferred alternative treatments are pentamidine (Pentam, 4 mg/kg intravenously [IV] every day) or clindamycin (Cleocin, 600 to 900 mg IV every 6 to 8 hours) plus primaquine[1] (15 to 30 mg [base] orally every day). Dapsone (100 mg orally every day) plus trimethoprim (Trimpex,[1] 15 mg/kg/day orally thrice daily), atovaquone (Mepron, 750 mg orally twice daily), or trimetrexate (Neutrexin, 1.2 mg/kg IV every day with leucovorin, 0.5 mg/kg IV every 6 hours) can be used also as alternatives in mild to moderately severe PCP. Following treatment, patients should be administered secondary prophylaxis, which has to be discontinued if the CD4+ counts improve to more than 200 cells/µL for 3 months after initiating HAART. However, in those who develop PCP while their CD4+ counts were more than 200 cells/µL, it is prudent to continue the secondary prophylaxis lifelong.

CRYPTOCOCCOSIS

Cryptococcosis occurs mostly among patients with CD4+ less than 50 cells/µL. Although the route of infection is via the lungs, most

---
[1]Not FDA approved for this indication.

TABLE 8 Primary Chemoprophylaxis for Opportunistic Infections in the HIV-Infected Patient*,†

Opportunistic Pathogen	Criteria for Initiation	Preferred Regimen	Alternative Regimens	Criteria for Discontinuation[‡]
Pneumocystis jiroveci	CD4+ < 200/µL; oropharyngeal candidiasis	TMP-SMX (Bactrim), 960 mg qd or 480 mg qd	TMP-SMX (Bactrim), 960 mg tiw, or dapsone, 100 mg qd, or aerosolized pentamidine (NebuPent), 300 mg monthly, or atovaquone (Mepron), 1500 mg qd	CD4+ >200/µL for ≥ 3 mo
Toxoplasma gondii	CD4+ ≤ 100/µL in IgG toxoplasma antibody-positive patients	TMP-SMX (Bactrim), 960 mg qd	TMP-SMX (Bactrim), 480 mg qd, or dapsone, 50 mg qd, + pyrimethamine, 50 mg qw, + leucovorin, 25 mg qw, or atovaquone (Mepron), 1500 mg qd	CD4+ >200/µL for ≥ 3 mo
Mycobacterium avium-intracellulare	CD4+ < 50/µL	Azithromycin (Zithromax), 1200 mg qw, or clarithromycin (Biaxin), 500 mg bid	Rifabutin (Mycobutin), 300 mg qd	CD4+ >100/µL for ≥ 3 mo
Mycobacterium tuberculosis[§]	TST ≥ 5 mm; positive TST in past without treatment; contact with active case, irrespective of TST	Isoniazid (Laniazid) + pyridoxine, 300 + 50 mg qd or 900 + 100 mg biw, for 9 mo	Rifampicin (Rifadin), 600 mg qd for 4 mo	Not applicable

*Apart from chemoprophylaxis, annual influenza immunization in all, pneumococcal vaccination in those with CD4+ ≥ 200/µL, and hepatitis A and hepatitis B vaccinations in susceptible patients are recommended.
†Primary chemoprophylaxis not recommended for cytomegalovirus, *Cryptococcus neoformans*, *Histoplasmsa capsulatum*, *Coccidioides immitis*, *Salmonella* species, herpes simplex, and *Candida* species
‡Primary prophylaxis to be restarted if CD4+ falls again below levels recommended for initiation.
§Not prophylaxis in strict sense. For isoniazid-susceptible *M. tuberculosis* only; if probability of exposure to isoniazid-resistant *M. tuberculosis* is high, rifampicin (Rifadin), 600 mg qd, or rifabutin (Mycobutin), 300 mg qd, for 4 mo.
Abbreviations: biw = twice weekly; TMP-SMX = cotrimoxazole (Bactrim); TST = tuberculin skin test; qw = once a week; tiw = 3 times a week.
Based on USPHA/IDSA guidlines for the prevention of opportunistic infection in persons infected with HIV, 2001.

---

often the disease manifests as meningitis. Disseminated infection is common in HIV-infected patients, and in fact approximately 60% of patients with AIDS-associated cryptococcal meningitis have fungemia. Pulmonary involvement occurs either as a part of disseminated disease or as primary pneumonia. Molluscoid skin lesions with central hemorrhagic crust may be seen. Patients typically present with subacute onset of fever, prominent headache, and vomiting. The classical signs of meningeal inflammation are often absent. Occasionally, cognitive decline and personality changes might be the only presenting symptoms. Cryptococcomas may present as a focal neurologic deficit.

Diagnosis is readily established by the demonstration of yeast cells by India ink staining of cerebrospinal fluid (CSF). Fungal culture and latex agglutination for cryptococcal antigen have better sensitivity than the India ink stain. The antigen can also be detected in the blood in most patients with meningitis. Untreated disease is uniformly fatal. Amphotericin B deoxycholate (Fungizone, 0.7 mg/kg IV every day for 2 weeks) is the preferred treatment. Infusion-related ADRs such as chills, rigors, and fever are common and can be reduced by premedicating with acetaminophen (Tylenol). Liposomal preparations of amphotericin B (AmBisome, 4 mg/kg/day) can be used also to reduce nephrotoxicity. Addition of flucytosine (Ancobon, 25 mg/kg orally four times a day for 2 weeks) sterilizes the CSF faster and reduces the rate of relapse but not mortality. Amphotericin B is to be followed by fluconazole (Diflucan, 400 mg orally every day) for at least 8 weeks or until the CSF cultures become sterile and then lifelong (200 mg every day) for secondary prophylaxis. In patients with immune recovery following HAART, secondary prophylaxis can be discontinued if the CD4+ count is more than 100 to 200 cells/µL for 6 months. Raised intracranial pressure is very common and associated with early deaths. If symptomatic, daily lumbar punctures to reduce the pressure are needed, and in refractory cases, CSF shunting should be performed.

DISSEMINATED *MYCOBACTERIUM AVIUM* INFECTION

Like cryptococcosis and CMV disease, disseminated atypical mycobacterial infections occur more commonly in patients with CD4+ less than 50 cells/µL. Most infections are caused by *Mycobacterium avium-intracellulare*. Infections by *Mycobacterium kansasii* and *Mycobacterium haemophilum* are also known to occur. Symptoms are nonspecific and include fever, weight loss, diarrhea, and abdominal pain. Peripheral and axial lymphadenopathy, hepatosplenomegaly, anemia, elevated alkaline phosphatase, and bone marrow infiltration are common features. Localized manifestations occur commonly as a manifestation of IRIS. Pulmonary lesions in the form of miliary nodules and air-space infiltrates may be seen. Diagnosis is established by demonstrating mycobacteremia or by isolating the organism from involved tissue specimens.

Treatment should include at least two effective drugs, usually clarithromycin (Biaxin, 500 mg orally twice daily) and ethambutol (Myambutol,[1] 15 mg/kg orally every day). Addition of a third drug should be considered, especially when CD4+ is less than 50 cells/µL, effective HAART is unavailable, or the mycobacterial load is high (more than 2.0 $\log_{10}$ colony-forming units/mL of blood). Rifabutin (Mycobutin,[1] 300 mg orally every day) is the preferred third drug. Fluoroquinolones and amikacin (Amikin)[1] can be used as alternative agents. Generally, if possible, HAART should be initiated within 1 to 2 weeks after initiating antimycobacterial therapy. Lack of clinical improvement accompanied by persisting mycobacteremia after 4 to 8 weeks of treatment indicates failure, and further selection of drugs should be guided by susceptibility testing. Treatment has to be continued lifelong for secondary prophylaxis. However, if the CD4+

---

[1]Not FDA approved for this indication.

TABLE 9 Etiology of Opportunistic Conditions in the HIV-Infected Patient

System Affected	Very common	Somewhat common	Rare
Pulmonary	PCP *Streptococcus pneumoniae* *Haemophilus influenzae* *Myobacterium tuberculosis*[a]	*Pseudomonas aeruginosa* *Staphylococcus aureus* Enteric GNB *Histoplasma* species *Cryptococcus* species Cytomegalovirus Kaposi's sarcoma *Aspergillus* species Pulmonary lymphoma Heart failure	*Nocardia* species *Legionella* species *Myobacterium avium* complex *Toxoplasma gondii* *Cryptosporidium* *Rhodococcus equi* *Strongyloides* Primary pulmonary hypertension DILS
Central nervous system (CNS)	*Cryptococcus* species Toxoplasmosis ADRs Psychiatric illness HIV dementia PMLE CNS lymphoma	*M. tuberculosis*[a] Cytomegalovirus Bacterial brain abscess	*Nocardia* species *Histoplasma* species *Coccidioides immitis* *Aspergillus* species *Listeria monocytogenes* Varicella-zoster virus Herpes simplex virus *Treponema pallidum* *Acanthamoeba* species *Trypanosoma cruzi* DILS
Gastrointestinal (GI)	Cytomegalovirus *Clostridium difficile* *Salmonella* species *M. avium* complex *Giardia lamblia* ADRs	*Shigella* species *Campylobacter* species *Microsporum* *Cryptosporidium Isospora* *Cyclospora* *Cryptococcus* species *Histoplasma* species	Amebiasis *Strongyloides* GI lymphoma Kaposi's sarcoma Enteroaggregative *Escherichia coli* DILS
Undifferentiated fever	*M. avium* complex *M. tuberculosis** Cytomegalovirus ADRs Sinusitis Catheter-related Early PCP Acute HIV syndrome	Endocarditis Lymphoma	Extrapulmonary *Pneumocystis* *Bartonella henselae* *Coccidioides immitis* *Mycobacterium kansasii* *Penicillium marneffei* *Leishmania* species *Toxoplasma gondii*

*Incidence of tuberculosis varies greatly depending on the local prevalence.
Abbreviations: ADR = adverse drug reaction; DILS = diffuse infiltrative lymphocytosis syndrome; GNB = gram-negative bacilli; PCP = *Pneumocystis jiroveci* pneumonia; PMLE = progressive multifocal leukoencephalopathy.
Adapted from Sax PE: Opportunistic infections in HIV disease: Down but not out. Infect Dis Clin North Am 2001;15:433-455.

---

count improves to more than 100 cells/μL for 6 months, it can be discontinued, provided the patient is asymptomatic and treatment has been given for at least 12 months.

CYTOMEGALOVIRUS DISEASE

Retinitis is the most common manifestation of CMV disease. It presents as progressive painless loss of vision, and patients often experience floaters. Funduscopy reveals focal necrotizing retinitis, characterized by perivascular fluffy infiltrates with hemorrhages. Lesions spread centrifugally from the periphery, and those adjacent to the macula are sight threatening. Visual loss, if it occurs, is irreversible. Other manifestations include colitis, esophagitis, meningoencephalitis, and pneumonitis. Colitis causes persistent diarrhea and may result in extensive hemorrhage, perforation, and bacterial sepsis. CNS disease presents as dementia, ventriculoencephalitis, or ascending polyradiculomyelopathy. Viremia in the absence of end-organ disease may be seen but does not warrant immediate therapy.

Sight-threatening retinitis is treated with an intraocular ganciclovir implant (Vitrasert) along with valganciclovir (Valcyte, 900 mg orally every day) lifelong. For peripheral lesions, valganciclovir (Valcyte), 900 mg orally twice daily for 2 to 3 weeks is to be followed by 900 mg every day for life. Ganciclovir (Cytovene, 5 mg/kg IV every 12 hours), foscarnet (Foscavir, 60 mg/kg IV every 8 hours), or cidofovir (Vistide, 5 mg/kg IV every day) for 2 to 3 weeks can be used as alternatives. Colitis and esophagitis are treated with ganciclovir (Cytovene) or foscarnet (Foscavir) for at least 3 to 4 weeks or until symptoms resolve. A combination of ganciclovir (Cytovene) and foscarnet (Foscavir) until symptoms resolve is required for the treatment of neurologic disease. Secondary prophylaxis can be discontinued if CD4+ is more than 100 to 150 cells/μL for 6 months. However, regular ophthalmologic monitoring should be done to detect relapse early. IRIS occurs in most of the patients with CMV retinitis following initiation of HAART, resulting in vitreitis or uveitis. Periocular steroids or short courses of oral steroids often control the symptoms.

TUBERCULOSIS IN HIV-INFECTED PATIENTS

Tuberculosis is the most common OI in HIV-infected patients from developing countries. In contrast to other OIs, tuberculosis can occur at any level of CD4+ count. Extrapulmonary and disseminated forms become more common as the immunosuppression worsens. Meningeal and miliary dissemination often occurs. In advanced immunosuppression, typical cavitary and sputum-smear-positive pulmonary disease are seldom seen. Diagnostic and therapeutic approaches to tuberculosis remain the same as in a HIV-negative

TABLE 10 Pharmacokinetic Interactions between Antiretrovirals and Rifamycins

Antiretroviral Drug	Compatibility with Rifampicin (Rifadin) — Antiretroviral dose change	Rifampicin (Rifadin) dose change	Compatibility with Rifabutin (Mycobutin) — Antiretroviral dose change	Rifabutin (Mycobutin) dose change
Saquinavir (Invirase, Fortovase)	Should not be used together		Should not be used together	
Saquinavir/ritonavir (Invirase Fortovase/Norvir)	(↓ 400/↑ 400) mg bid	None	None	↓ 150 mg qod*
Indinavir (Crixivan)	Should not be used together		↑ 1000 mg tid	↓ 150 mg qd†
Nelfinavir (Viracept)	Should not be used together		↑ 1000 mg tid	↓ 150 mg qd†
Amprenavir (Agenerase)	Should not be used together		None	↓ 150 mg qd†
Atazanavir (Reyataz)	Should not be used together		None	↓ 150 mg qod*
Lopinavir/ritonavir (Kaletra)	(400/↑ 400) mg bid	None	None	↓ 150 mg qod*
Efavirenz (Sustiva)	↑ 800 mg qd	None	None	↑ 450 mg qd‡
Nevirapine (Viramune)	None	None	None	None
Delavirdine (Rescriptor)	Should not be used together		Should not be used together	

Note: Increase or decrease in the doses are indicated with appropriately directed arrows.
*Can be administered as 150 mg tiw.
†Can be administered as 300 mg tiw.
‡Can be administered as 600 mg tiw.
Based on Centers for Disease Control and Prevention: Updated guidelines for the use of rifamycins for the treatment of tuberculosis among HIV-infected patients, 2004.

patient, except that once-weekly rifapentine (Priftin) and if CD4+ counts are less than 100 cells/μL, twice-weekly rifabutin (Mycobutin)[1] should not be used. Standard four-drug short-course regimens (see chapter on tuberculosis) are equally effective in HIV-infected patients with drug-susceptible tuberculosis. All patients should receive directly observed treatment, and thrice-weekly intermittent regimens can be used. Extensive interactions occur between rifamycins, PIs, and NNRTIs. If the patient is already on HAART, rifabutin (Mycobutin) is the preferred rifamycin, and HAART has to be continued with appropriate changes (Table 10). If the patient is not on HAART, it is better started after the completion of the intensive phase in those with CD4+ more than 200 cells/μL. In those with CD4+ less than 200 cells/μL, it is preferable to initiate HAART early, after approximately 2 weeks of intensive-phase treatment.

Management of the Pregnant HIV-Infected Woman

Apart from the usual indications for initiating HAART, in a pregnant HIV-infected woman, an additional aim is to prevent perinatal transmission. This is most effectively achieved by suppressing viremia to undetectable levels with HAART. From this perspective, all pregnant HIV-infected women should be initiated on HAART, irrespective of the viral load, CD4+ count, and symptoms. Efavirenz (Sustiva), a combination of didanosine (Videx) and stavudine (Zerit), nevirapine (Viramune) in those with CD4+ more than 250 cells/μL, and oral liquid formulations of amprenavir (Agenerase) should be avoided. Although NRTIs and nevirapine (Viramune) can be administered in the usual adult doses, nelfinavir (Viracept) has to be given only twice daily (Table 4). Initiation is better timed at the second trimester, to improve the tolerability and to avoid early fetal exposure to antiretrovirals. A detailed second-trimester fetal survey is indicated.

The goal of treatment, follow-up assessment, and indications for resistance testing all remain the same as in a nonpregnant patient. HAART has to be continued without interruption through delivery. Intrapartum, zidovudine (Retrovir) has to be administered IV until the umbilical cord is clamped and other drugs can be continued by oral route. The option of elective cesarean delivery should be offered to patients with viral loads higher than 1000 copies/mL despite HAART. If opted for, elective cesarean delivery is performed at 38 weeks' gestation, avoiding an amniocentesis to document fetal lung maturity. Following delivery, the infant should receive zidovudine (Retrovir) for 6 weeks. To avoid transmission through breast milk, nursing the infant should be avoided completely, if resources permit. Where the sole indication for initiating HAART was the prevention of perinatal transmission, HAART may be discontinued (in a staggered fashion, if nevirapine [Viramune] was included) after delivery. All infants exposed to antiretrovirals in utero should be followed up for possible adverse effects, regardless of the HIV status. Combined together, these interventions, namely HAART, cesarean delivery, and avoidance of breast-feeding, have brought down the risk of mother-to-child HIV transmission from approximately 25% to 1% to 2% in developed countries. In resource-limited settings and for HIV-infected women without prior HAART presenting in labor, peripartum prophylaxis with zidovudine (Retrovir), zidovudine with lamivudine (Combivir), nevirapine (Viramune), or zidovudine with nevirapine are acceptable alternatives.

Postexposure Prophylaxis of HIV Infection

The importance of adhering to universal precautions in preventing occupational transmission of HIV cannot be overstated.

---
[1]Not FDA approved for this indication.

Administration of postexposure prophylaxis (PEP) can substantially reduce the risk of HIV transmission following accidental occupational exposure in the health care setting. However, PEP is associated with significant morbidity and potentially serious side effects. HIV testing of the health care personnel should be done at the time of exposure, at 6 weeks, 12 weeks, and 6 months after exposure. Generally, all grades of percutaneous, mucous membrane, and nonintact skin exposure to a known HIV-infected source warrant administration of PEP. In the case of mucosal or nonintact skin exposure to a small volume (a few drops) of body fluid from a known HIV-infected source, the decision to initiate PEP should be made on a case-to-case basis, after discussing with the exposed person the benefits as well as the risks of PEP.

PEP should be initiated as soon as possible, preferably within hours following the exposure. The basic prophylaxis is with a two-drug regimen, usually a combination of two NRTIs (zidovudine + lamivudine [Combivir] or emtricitabine + tenofovir [Truvada]). If the exposure is more severe, three-drug regimens containing a PI are recommended. PEP is to be given for 4 weeks. If the source serostatus is unknown, administration of basic prophylaxis should be considered if the source is likely to be HIV infected and the exposure was percutaneous or involved a large volume of potentially infectious body fluid. The recommendations for PEP were extended recently to include nonoccupational exposures also (e.g., those reporting within 72 hours following an unanticipated sexual or injection drug use exposure to a known HIV-infected source).

REFERENCES

Aberg JA, Gallant JE, Anderson J, et al: Primary care guidelines for the management of persons infected with human immunodeficiency virus: Recommendations of the HIV Medicine Association of the Infectious Diseases Society of America. Clin Infect Dis 2004;39:609-629.

Carr A, Cooper DA: Adverse effects of antiretroviral therapy. Lancet 2000;356:1423-1430.

Centers for Disease Control and Prevention: Treating opportunistic infections among HIV-infected adults and adolescents: Recommendations from CDC, the National Institutes of Health, and the HIV Medicine Association/Infectious Diseases Society of America. MMWR Morb Mortal Wkly Rep 2004;53(No. RR-15):1-112.

Centers for Disease Control and Prevention: Antiretroviral postexposure prophylaxis after sexual, injection-drug use, or other nonoccupational exposures to HIV in the United States: Recommendations from the U.S. Department of Health and Human Services. MMWR Morb Mortal Wkly Rep 2005;54(No. RR-2):1-19.

Centers for Disease Control and Prevention: Updated U.S. Public Health Service guidelines for the management of occupational exposures to HIV and recommendations for postexposure prophylaxis. MMWR Morb Mortal Wkly Rep 2005;54(No. RR-9):1-17.

Chesney MA: Factors affecting adherence to antiretroviral therapy. Clin Infect Dis 2000;30(Suppl 2):S171-S176.

Grinspoon S, Carr A: Cardiovascular risk and body fat abnormalities in HIV-infected adults. N Engl J Med 2005;352:48-62.

Hammer SM: Management of newly diagnosed HIV infection. N Engl J Med 2005;353:1702-1710.

Panel on antiretroviral guidelines for adults and adolescents, U. S. Department of Health and Human Services: Guidelines for the use of antiretroviral agents in HIV-1-infected adults and adolescents. January 29, 2008. Available at http://AIDSinfo.nih.gov (accessed April 27, 2008).

Sax PE: Opportunistic infections in HIV disease: Down but not out. Infect Dis Clin North Am 2001;15:433-455.

Yeni PG, Hammer SM, Hirsch MS, et al: Treatment of adult HIV infection. 2004 recommendations of the International AIDS Society—USA panel. JAMA 2004;292:251-265.

Amebiasis

Method of
*Rashidul Haque, MB, PhD, and
William A. Petri, Jr., MD, PhD*

Amebiasis, a disease caused by the protozoan parasite *Entamoeba histolytica*, is estimated to be the third leading parasitic cause of deaths worldwide in humans. There are noninvasive species of ameba including *Entamoeba dispar* and *Entamoeba moshkovskii* that are morphologically indistinguishable from *E. histolytica* by traditional light microscopy. Amebiasis is distributed worldwide, but the majority of cases are found in developing countries. The World Health Organization estimates that approximately 50 million people suffer from invasive amebiasis each year, resulting in 40,000 to 100,000 deaths annually. For example, a prospective study of preschool children in an urban slum of Dhaka, Bangladesh, demonstrated a 39% incidence of *E. histolytica* infection during the first year of observation.

Human beings are the only known host of the parasite *E. histolytica*. Individuals become infected with *E. histolytica* when they ingest cysts in fecally contaminated food or water. When these cysts reach the intestine, they swell and release the motile, symptom-inducing form of *E. histolytica*, called the trophozoite. Trophozoites can remain in the intestine and even form new cysts without causing disease symptoms. They colonize the large intestine by adhering to colonic mucins via a galactose and N-acetyl-d-galactosamine (Gal/GalNAc)–specific lectin. Reproduction of trophozoites is without a recognized sexual cycle, and the overall population structure of *E. histolytica* appears to be clonal. Aggregation of amebae in the mucin layer likely signals encystation via the Gal/GalNAc lectin. Cysts excreted in stool perpetuate the life cycle by further fecal–oral spread. Invasive disease results when the trophozoite penetrates the intestinal mucus layer, which acts as barrier to invasion by inhibiting amebic adherence to the underlying epithelium and by slowing trophozoite motility. In addition, trophozoites can be carried through the blood to other organs, most commonly the liver, where they form life-threatening abscesses.

Intestinal Amebiasis

There are several clinical classifications of amebiasis based on the invasiveness and site of infection with different treatments. Intestinal amebiasis is a term that encompasses the entire spectrum of clinical intestinal disease, including amebic colitis. Patients with amebic colitis typically present with a several week history of cramping abdominal pain, weight loss, and watery or, less commonly, bloody diarrhea. The insidious onset and variable signs and symptoms make diagnosis difficult, with fever and grossly bloody stool absent in most cases. Differential diagnosis of a diarrheal illness with occult or grossly bloody stools should include *Shigella, Salmonella, Campylobacter*, and enteroinvasive and enterohemorrhagic *Escherichia coli*. Noninfectious causes include inflammatory bowel disease, ischemic colitis, diverticulitis, and arteriovenous malformation.

Unusual manifestations of amebic colitis include acute necrotizing colitis, toxic megacolon, ameboma, and perianal ulceration with potential fistula formation. Acute necrotizing colitis is rare (<0.5% of cases) and is associated with a greater than 40% mortality. Patients with acute necrotizing colitis are typically very ill-appearing with fever, bloody mucoid diarrhea, abdominal pain with rebound tenderness, and peritoneal signs of irritation. Surgical intervention is indicated if there is bowel perforation or if the patient fails to improve on antiamebic therapy. Toxic megacolon is rare (approximately 0.5% of cases) and typically is associated with corticosteroid use.

Amebic Liver Abscess

Amebic liver abscess is 10 times more common in men than women and is a rare disease in children. Approximately 80% of patients with amebic liver abscess present with symptoms that develop relatively acutely (typically < 2 to 4 weeks in duration) with fever, cough, and a constant, dull, aching abdominal pain in the right upper quadrant or epigastrium. Involvement of the diaphragmatic surface of the liver may lead to right pleural pain or referred shoulder pain. Associated gastrointestinal symptoms occur in up to 10% to 35% of cases and include nausea, vomiting, abdominal cramping, abdominal distention, diarrhea, or constipation. Hepatomegaly with point tenderness over the liver, below the ribs, or in the intercostal spaces is a typical finding. Complications from amebic liver abscess may arise from rupture of the abscess with extension into the peritoneum, pleural cavity, or pericardium. Extrahepatic amebic abscesses have occasionally been described in the lung, brain, and skin, and presumably reach these sites hematogenously.

Diagnosis

Historically, diagnosis of amebiasis was complicated and often unreliable for various reasons. The signs and symptoms of amebiasis can provide means to obtain clinical diagnosis. However, the confirmation of an amebic infection rests with laboratory identification. Over the last 25 years, various molecular diagnostic tests have been developed to diagnose E. histolytica. The diagnosis of intestinal amebiasis must be based on tests that distinguish E. histolytica from E. dispar. E. histolytica-specific antigen detection test and polymerase chain reaction (PCR) tests are now available for specific diagnosis of E. histolytica (Table 1). Enzyme-linked immunoabsorbent assay–based antigen detection kits are now commercially available. Field studies that directly compared PCR to stool culture or antigen-detection tests for the diagnosis of E. histolytica infection suggest that these three different methods perform equally well. An important aid to antigen detection and PCR-based tests is the detection of serum antibodies to amebae, which are present in 70% to 90% of patients with symptomatic E. histolytica infection. A drawback of current serologic tests is that patients remain positive for years after infection, making it difficult to distinguish new from past infection in regions of the world where amebiasis is endemic. Colonic mucosal biopsies and exudates can reveal a range in histopathologic appearance and severity of intestinal lesions associated with amebic colitis.

Amebic liver abscess patients may reveal a mild to moderate leukocytosis and anemia. Patients with an acute presentation of amebic liver abscess tend to have a normal alkaline phosphatase and elevated aspartate transaminase with the opposite true for patients with a chronic presentation. Ultrasound, abdominal computed tomography scan, and magnetic resonance imaging of the liver are all excellent imaging modalities for detecting liver lesions (most commonly single and in the right lobe) but are not specific for amebic liver abscess. The differential diagnosis of a liver mass should include pyogenic liver abscess, necrotic hepatoma, and echinococcal cyst (usually an incidental finding that would not be the cause of fever and abdominal pain). Patients with amebic abscess are more likely than patients with pyogenic liver abscesses to be male and younger than age 50 years; have immigrated from or traveled to an endemic country; and lack jaundice, biliary disease, or diabetes mellitus. Fewer than half of patients with amebic liver abscess have parasites detected in their stool by antigen detection. Helpful clues to the diagnosis include the presence of epidemiologic risk factors for amebiasis and the presence of serum antiamebic antibodies (present in 70% to 80% of patients at the time of presentation; see Table 1). Occasionally, aspiration of the abscess is required to rule out a pyogenic abscess. Amebae are visualized in the abscess pus in a minority of patients with amebic liver abscess. Traditional PCR and real-time PCR tests can be used for the detection of E. histolytica DNA in the stool and liver abscess pus samples and have been found to be sensitive and specific (see Table 1).

Therapy

Therapy differs for invasive versus noninvasive infections (Table 2). Noninvasive infections can be treated with lumen active agents such as paromomycin (Humatin) to eradicate cysts and lumen-dwelling trophozoites. Nitroimidazoles, particularly metronidazole (Flagyl), are the mainstay of therapy for invasive amebiasis (see Table 2). Nitroimidazoles with longer half-lives (namely tinidazole [Tindamax], secnidazole,[2] and ornidazole[2]) are better tolerated and allow shorter duration of treatment; they are recently available in the United States. Approximately 90% of patients presenting with mild to moderate amebic colitis or dysentery respond to nitroimidazole treatment. In the rare case of fulminant amebic colitis, it is prudent to add broad-spectrum antibiotics to treat intestinal bacteria that may spill into the peritoneum, with patients occasionally requiring surgical intervention for acute abdomen, gastrointestinal bleeding, or toxic megacolon. Parasites persist in the intestine in as many as 40% to 60% of metronidazole (Flagyl)-treated patients. Therefore, metronidazole (Flagyl) treatment should be followed with paromomycin (Humatin) or the second-line agent diloxanide furoate (Furamide)[2] to cure luminal infection (see Table 2). Do not treat with

---

[2]Not available in the United States.

TABLE 1 Sensitivity of Laboratory Tests for the Diagnosis of Amebiasis

Laboratory Tests	Amebic Colitis	Amebic Liver Abscess
Microscopy (stool)*	25%–60%	8%–44%
Microscopy (abscess fluid)	N/A	<20%
Stool antigen detection[†]	>90%	40%
Serum antigen detection[†]	<65%	>90% (before therapy)
PCR/real-time PCR (stool)	>90%	>40%
PCR/real-time PCR (abscess fluid)	N/A	90%–100% (before therapy)
Serology		
Acute	50%–70%	70%–90%
Convalescent	>90%	>90%

*Does not distinguish Entamoeba histolytica from the commensal parasites Entamoeba dispar and Entamoeba moshkovskii.
[†]TechLab E. histolytica II antigen detection test.
Abbreviation: PCR = polymerase chain reaction.

TABLE 2 Drug Therapy for the Treatment of Amebiasis*

Type of Infection	Drug	Adult Dosage	Pediatric Dosage
Asymptomatic intestinal colonization	Paromomycin (Humatin) or	25–35 mg/kg/d in 3 doses × 7 d	25–35 mg/kg/d in 3 doses × 7 d
	Diloxanide furoate (Furamide)*	500 mg tid × 10 d	20 mg/kg/d in 3 doses × 10 d
Amebic liver abscess[†]	Metronidazole (Flagyl) or	750 mg tid × 7–10 d in 3 doses × 7–10 d	35–50 mg/kg/d
	Tinidazole (Tindamax) followed by luminal agent	800 mg tid × 5 d[3] in 3 doses × 5 d	60 mg/kg/d[3]
	Paromomycin (Humatin)	25–35 mg/kg/d in 3 doses × 7 d	25–35 mg/kg/d in 3 doses × 7 d
	Diloxanide furoate (Furamide)[5] or	500 mg tid × 10 d in 3 doses × 10 d	20 mg/kg/d
Amebic colitis[†]	Metronidazole (Flagyl) followed by luminal agent (similar to amebic liver abscess)	500–750 mg tid × 7–10 d in 3 doses × 7–10 d	35–50 mg/kg/d

*The information is updated annually by the Medical Letter on Drugs and Therapeutics at http://www.medletter.com/htmlprm.htm#Parasitic.
[†]Treatment of amebic liver abscess and amebic colitis should be followed by a treatment with a luminal agent.
[3]Exceeds dosage recommended by the manufacturer.
[5]Investigational drug in the United States.

metronidazole (Flagyl) and paromomycin (Humatin) at the same time because the diarrhea, a common side effect of paromomycin, (Humatin) may make it difficult to assess response to therapy.

Therapeutic aspiration of an amebic liver abscess is occasionally required as adjunctive treatment to antiparasitic therapy. Abscess drainage should be considered in patients who fail to clinically respond to drug therapy within 5 to 7 days or those with high risk of abscess rupture as defined by cavity size greater than 5 cm or location in the left lobe. Bacterial coinfection of amebic liver abscess has been occasionally observed (both prior to and as a complication of drainage), and it is reasonable to add antibiotics or drainage, or both, to the treatment regimen if a prompt response to nitroimidazole therapy is not observed. Imaging-guided percutaneous treatment (needle aspiration or catheter drainage) has replaced surgical intervention over more recent years as the procedure of choice for therapeutically reducing abscess size.

REFERENCES

Diamond LS, Clark CG: A redescription of *Entamoeba histolytica* Schaudin 1903 (amended Walker 1911) separating it from *Entamoeba dispar* (Brumpt 1925). J Eukaryot Microbiol 1993;40:340-344.

Haque R, Mollah NU, Ali IKM, et al: Diagnosis of amebic liver abscess and intestinal infection with the TechLab *Entamoeba histolytica* II antigen detection and antibody tests. J Clin Microbiol 2000;38:3235-3239.

Haque R, Ali IKM, Akther S, Petri WA Jr: Comparison of PCR, isoenzyme analysis, and antigen detection for diagnosis of *Entamoeba histolytica* infection. J Clin Microbio 1998;36:449-452.

Haque R, Ali IKM, Sack RB, et al: Amebiasis and mucosal IgA antibody against the *Entamoeba histolytica* adherence lectin in Bangladeshi children. J Infect Dis 2001;183:1787-1793.

Haque R, Huston CD, Hughes M, et al: Current concepts: Amebiasis. N Engl J Med 2003;348:1565-1573.

Petri WA Jr, Haque R, Lyerly D, Vine RR: Estimating the impact of amebiasis on health. Parasitol Today 2000;16:320-321.

Petri, WA Jr, Singh U: State of the art: Diagnosis and management of amebiasis. Clin Infect Dis 1999;29:1117-1125.

Stanley SL Jr: Amoebiasis. Lancet 2003;22;361(9362):1025-1034.

MTanyuksel SL, PetriJr: Laboratory diagnosis of amebiasis. Clin Microbiol Rev 2003;16:713-729.

World Health Organization WA: Amoebiasis. Wkly Epidemiol Rec 1997;72: 97-100.

Giardiasis

Method of
M. Ekramul Hoque, MBBS, MPH (Hons), PhD

Background

Giardiasis is a parasitic infection of the upper small intestine caused by a flagellated protozoan, *Giardia lamblia* (also called *Giardia intestinalis* and *Giardia duodenalis*). This ubiquitous parasite is a major cause of intestinal infection among adults and children in developing and developed countries. The existence of this parasite was reported in the prehistoric era across the continents. However, pathogenicity of the organism among humans was known only in the latter part of the last century.

Organism

Giardia is a microscopic organism that exists in two life forms. The trophozoite, which is environmentally unstable, causes clinical illness, and the resistant cysts are responsible for the transmission of infection. Trophozoites are binucleated, flagellated, and pear shaped, measuring 12 to 15 µm long and 6 to 8 µm wide. They have a pair of claw-shaped median bodies and a concave ventral disk used for nourishment and attachment on the wall of the small intestine of vertebrate hosts. Cysts are smaller and oval, usually 8 to 12 µm long and 7 to 10 µm wide, and contain four nuclei.

Epidemiology

Giardiasis is one of the most common intestinal infections in the world. More than 200 million people are reported to have symptoms of giardiasis, and some 500,000 new cases are reported annually. Some estimates suggest the worldwide prevalence of giardiasis is 20% to 60%. Others report from 2% to 7% in industrialized countries and 20% to 30% in developing countries. In the United States, giardiasis became nationally notifiable in 2002. In 2005, there were 20,075 giardiasis cases reported from 49 states, with an incidence rate

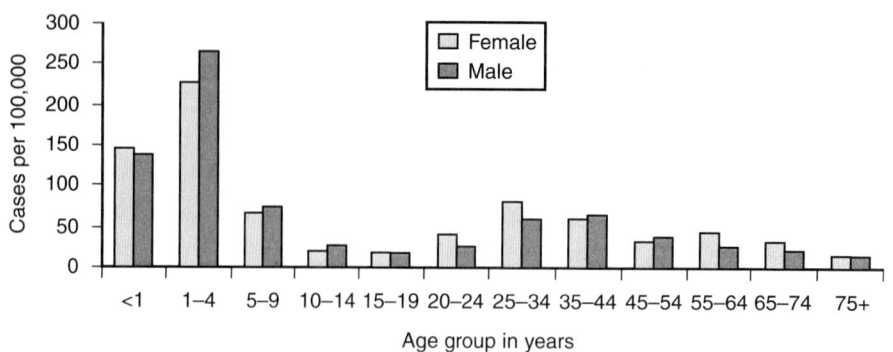

FIGURE 1. Notification rate of giardiasis in New Zealand by age and gender.

of 6.8 cases per 100,000 population. The incidence varied by state from 1.4 to 30 cases per 100,000 population; rates were higher in the northern states than the southern states. *Giardia* infection is highly underreported, and therefore the true burden of giardiasis in the United States is probably underestimated. An estimate suggests there are 2 million giardiasis cases in the United States annually, and 5000 people are hospitalized due to severe infection. New Zealand reports nearly 30 cases of giardiasis per 100,000 population every year, which is one of the highest among the industrialized countries. *Giardia* infection is reported to be more prevalent in urban areas than in rural populations.

Humans are the primary reservoir of the parasite. Other possible hosts are farm, wild, and domestic animals. Polymerase chain reaction (PCR) testing of samples of human feces from different geographic locations has so far associated *G. intestinalis* genotypes (assemblages) A and B with human infections. The role of animals in transmitting *G. intestinalis* to humans and the most likely routes of infection remain unclear.

Transmission of the *Giardia* infection is through the fecal-oral route following direct or indirect contact with cysts of *Giardia*. Cysts are infectious immediately after being excreted in feces. An infected person can excrete a maximum of 10^9 cysts per day for several months. Cysts may be killed by simple drying and heat, but they can survive for several weeks in cool and wet environments. Infectious dose is low; ingestion of as few as 10 cysts can cause infection. Commonly, the organism spreads by water or food or directly through person-to-person contact. Outbreaks of waterborne giardiasis have been reported year round, suggesting frequent contamination of water sources and longer survival of cysts in water.

Giardiasis shows a bimodal pattern of age distribution, peaking in children younger than 5 years and in adults 25 to 44 years (Figure 1). Incidence of infection varies by season, peaking in late summer and early autumn and dropping in winter. Persons at increased risk for infection include (among others) children of diaper age, children attending daycare centers, daycare workers, immunocompromised persons, pregnant women, institutionalized persons, travelers to endemic regions, people drinking contaminated water during outdoor activities, sewage and irrigation workers, and men who have sex with men.

It is not clear whether giardiasis causes malnutrition or malnutrition predisposes to *Giardia* infection. However, nutritional insufficiency can contribute to chronicity of the disease. Repeated exposure to the parasite can elicit an immune response, which might explain asymptomatic giardiasis cases. Breast-fed infants of immune mothers might acquire temporary protection against giardiasis, but this is not conclusive.

Pathogenesis

Clinical illness results from the interaction of *Giardia* organisms with the human host and the host's subsequent response to the parasite. *Giardia* isolates can vary in virulence, which might further explain the intensity of the symptoms.

After a person ingests *Giarda* cysts, excystation begins in the duodenum in the presence of gastric acid, pancreatic enzymes, and parasite-derived cysteine protease. Two tropozoites are formed from each cyst by binary fission (miotic division). The motility of parasites and the inflammatory cytokine response to parasitic attachment on the mucosal brush borders results in secretion of fluid and electrolytes, hence diarrhea and malabsorption. Trophozoites frequently slough off villi, which are swept into the fecal stream and replaced by new sets. After 4 to 15 days of colonization, some trophozoites encyst in the jejunum under an alkaline environment of bile secretion. Immotile cysts undergo a single cell division to form four nuclei, which are then passed intermittently in the feces.

Giardia trophozoites remain adherent to the intestinal mucosa but are not invasive. This close association might directly affect the brush border and its enzyme system. Hospital-based investigation observed partial villous atrophy in up to 25% of patients. Malabsorption of vitamin B_{12} occurs in 20% to 40% cases. Parasites are also found in extraintestinal sites such as the gallbladder and the urinary tract.

Clinical Features

Clinical manifestations of giardiasis vary from asymptomatic infection to severe diarrhea. The incubation period for *Giardia* infection varies from 1 week to several weeks. However, a period of 5 to 25 days is average.

Freshly exposed persons in an endemic area can present with acute symptoms that usually begin about 15 days (range, 1-46 days) following exposure. The symptoms include nausea, anorexia, upper abdominal discomfort, malaise, low-grade fever, and chills followed by the sudden onset of explosive, watery, foul-smelling diarrhea associated with foul flatulence and abdominal distention. Generally, the acute stage resolves spontaneously within 2 to 4 weeks. Some patients become asymptomatic passers of cysts for a period. Others have periodic brief recurrences of acute symptoms.

About 30% to 50% of infected patients go on to a subacute or chronic stage. Overseas travelers to *Giardia*-endemic areas often do not recognize or remember the infection during their travel and subsequently present periodically with persistent or recurrent mild to moderate symptoms. Features of subacute to chronic *Giardia* infection include flatulence, mushy foul stools, upper abdominal cramps, abdominal distention, steatorrhea, marked weight loss, and fatigue. Uncommon manifestations are cholecystitis, pancreatitis, immunologic reactions (including arthritis, retinal arteritis, and iridocyclitis), and occasionally rash and urticaria, mostly in adults. In rare cases, symptoms persist for years, but most cases resolve spontaneously after a variable period of weeks or months.

Generally, 10% to 30% of infected people remain symptom free, but the true percentage may be as high as 60%. The prevalence of asymptomatic infection is higher among children than among adults, especially among those in daycare. The duration of the asymptomatic cyst-passing state is not determined.

Diagnosis

Clinical signs and symptoms along with the history of risk behavior and exposure to *Giardia* risk factors can lead to a preliminary diagnosis of the disease. Laboratory diagnostic procedures are then applied to confirm the infection (Figure 2)

Traditionally, diagnosis is based on microscopic detection of *Giardia* cysts or trophozoites in the fecal specimens. At least three specimens of feces collected on consecutive days may be required to recover the parasite. The sensitivity of parasite detection is 50% to 70% in one specimen and 90% in three specimens.

Immunologic methods for detecting *Giardia* have superior sensitivity and specificity compared with other conventional methods of diagnosis. Widely used methods are enzyme immunoassay (EIA) detecting soluble antigens, direct fluorescent antibody (DFA) detecting intact organisms, and immunochromatographic lateral-flow immunoassays or rapid assay. Sensitivity of immunoassay varies between 94% and 97%, and specificity varies between 99% and 100%. EIA and rapid assay can pick up antigens of recently cured cases; DFA detects *Giardia* cysts. Immunoassay tests are quick and costs are reasonable.

Serologic tests do not have great diagnostic value in clinical practice because immunoglobulin G (IgG) persists even after infection; IgM, however, can indicate active infection. Negative serology does not exclude infection.

Duodenal aspirates or string test and duodenal mucosal biopsy are costly and invasive. They should be reserved for situations when giardiasis is strongly suspected despite persistent negative feces tests. PCR is used mostly in epidemiologic studies.

Treatment

Giardiasis, if diagnosed, should be treated. There are unresolved debates on the significance of treatment of asymptomatic cases.

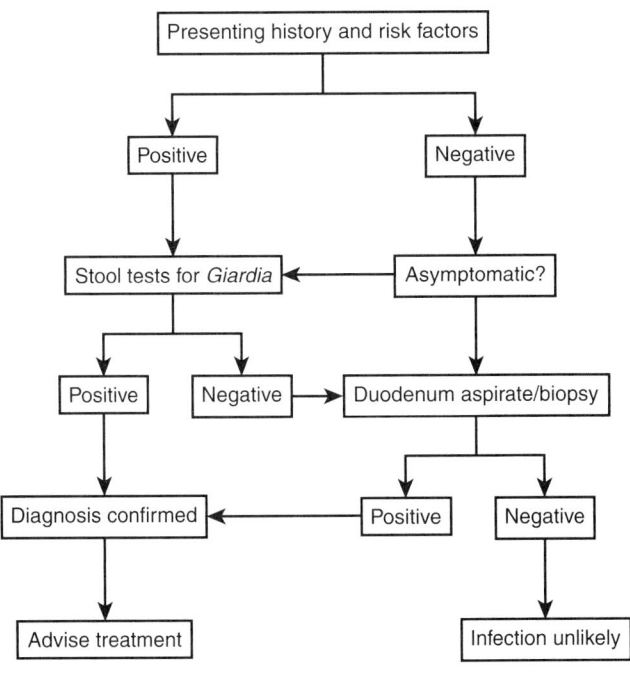

FIGURE 2. Diagnostic algorithm for giardiasis.

CURRENT DIAGNOSIS

- Giardiasis is a common parasitic infection of the small intestine.
- Children, caregivers, travelers, and persons exposed to contaminated water are at greater risk for infection.
- Clinical manifestations vary widely.
- A large fraction of infected persons remain asymptomatic.
- Infective cysts pass intermittently with patients' feces.
- Diagnosis is by detection of *Giardia* parasites in feces by repeated microscopy or by immunologic assays.
- Assays can give false positives in recently cured persons.
- Infection can resolve spontaneously or can go into a chronic stage lasting for months with marked weight loss.

However, asymptomatic cases can remain a potential source of infection and can turn symptomatic at any moment.

PHARMACOLOGIC THERAPY

A number of effective antigiardial drugs are available (Table 1).

Metronidazole (Flagyl)[1] is preferred and widely used because of its broad-spectrum coverage. It is not approved by the FDA for routine treatment of giardiasis in the United States. Metronidazole is effective and well tolerated and has a cure rate of 80% to 95%. The common side effects are gastrointestinal upset, headache, nausea, leukopenia, and metallic taste in the mouth. It is contraindicated in the first trimester of pregnancy due to its suspected carcinogenic, teratogenic, and mutagenic effects. Although the drug on therapeutic doses has shown no significant increased risk of cancer in humans. Other minor side effects are peripheral neuropathy, seizures, depression, irritability, restlessness, and insomnia. Drug resistance is not yet widespread.

Furazolidone (Furoxone)[2] is the primary drug of choice in the United States. It is available in liquid form and is widely used to treat children. Cure rates are between 80% and 89%. It is not recommended in pregnancy. Side effects include gastrointestinal disturbances, hemolytic anemia, disulfiram-like reactions with alcohol, hypersensitivity reactions, brown discoloration of the urine, orthostatic hypotension, and hypoglycemia.

Albendazole (Albenza)[1] is an anthelminthic whose efficacy is equal to that of metronidazole and with cure rates of 62% to 95%. Absence of anorexia in using this drug is an advantage for treating children. Notable side effects are gastrointestinal upset, abdominal pain, nausea, vomiting, diarrhea, dizziness, vertigo, fever, increased intracranial pressure, alopecia, and (reversible) increase in serum transaminases after prolonged use. Albendazole is contraindicated in pregnancy due to teratogenicity. Paromomycin (Humatin)[1] is a poorly absorbed aminoglycoside that is excreted in the feces without being metabolized. Its efficacy rate is between 60% and 70%. It is recommended for giardial infection in pregnant patients. Common side effects are nausea, increased gastrointestinal motility, abdominal pain, and diarrhea. 5-Nitroimidazole compounds, tinidazole (Tindamax) ornidazole (Tiberal), and secnidazole (Noameba-DS, Secnil)[1,2] are effective as first-line agents and have a cure rate of 90%. They have longer serum half-lives than metronidazole and are effective in single doses. Common side effects are gastrointestinal upset, vertigo, and bitter taste. They need caution to use in pregnant

---
[1]Not FDA approved for this indication.
[2]Not available in the United States.

TABLE 1 Therapeutic Doses of Antigiardial Drugs

Drugs	Adult Dose	Pediatric Dose
Metronidazole (Flagyl)[a]	250 mg tid x 5-7 d	5 mg/kg tid x 5-7 d
Tinidazole (Tindamax)[b]	2 g single dose	50 mg/kg single dose (max, 2 g)
Ornidazole (Tiberal)[c]	2 g single dose	40-50 mg/kg single dose (max, 2 g)
Secnidazole (Noameba-DS, Secnil)[b]	2 g single dose	30 mg/kg single dose
Quinacrine (Atabrine)[c]	100 mg tid x 5-7 d[e]	2 mg/kg tid x 5-7 d (max 300mg/d)[e]
Furazolidone[d]	100 mg qid x 7-10 d	1.5 mg/kg qid x 10 d
Paromomycin[a]	500 mg tid x 10 d[f]	8-10 mg/kg tid x 5-10 d[f]
Albendazole	400 mg qd x 5 d	15 mg/kg/day x 5-7 d (max 400 mg/d)
Nitrazoxanide	500 mg bid x 3 d	7.5 mg/kg bid x 3 d

[a]Not a U.S. FDA approved indication; [b]Not available in the U.S.; [c]No longer produced in the U.S.; [d]Available in liquid formulation; [e]After meal; [f]With meal
qd, once a day; bid, twice a day; tid, three times a day; qid, four times a day

patients. Quinacrine[2] was one of the most effective drugs against giardial infection, with a cure rate of 92% to 95%. This drug is no longer produced in the United States and elsewhere in the world due to a number of pharmacokinetic issues and adverse effects. Other potential drugs include benzimidazole derivatives such as mebendazole (Vermox)[1] and a 5-nitrothiazole derivative (Nitazoxanide), which are not used widely. Nitazoxanide (Alinia) has been used successfully in France in resistant giardiasis patients infected with HIV.

OTHER MEASURES

Diet modification can reduce acute symptoms, improve host defense mechanisms, and inhibit growth and replication of *Giardia* trophozoites in the lumen of the intestine. General advice is to consume a diet of whole foods that is high in fiber, low in simple carbohydrates, and low in fat.

---

[1]Not FDA approved for this indication.
[2]Not available in the United States.

CURRENT THERAPY

- Metronidazole (Flagyl)[1] is widely used because of its broad-spectrum coverage, but it is contraindicated in the first trimester of pregnancy.
- Furazolidone (Furoxone)[2] is available in liquid form to treat children.
- Absence of anorexia with albendazole (Albenza)[1] is an advantage for treating children.
- Paromomycin (Humatin)[1] is recommended in pregnancy due to its poor absorption rate.
- Tinidazole (Tindamax), ornidazole (Tiberal); and secnidazole (Noameba-DS, Secnil)[2] are effective in single doses.
- Nitazoxanide (Alinia) is used in drug-resistant giardiasis.
- Some diet modifications can reduce acute symptoms, improve host defense, and inhibit trophozoite replications.

---

[1]Not FDA approved for this indication.
[2]Not available in the United States.

Follow-up

Follow-up stool tests are advised to ensure resolution of infection. Hygiene practices should be enhanced during outbreaks. Symptomatic persons should be kept away from public contact.

Prognosis

Giardiasis is usually a self-limited intestinal infection. Effective antigiardial agents shorten the infection period. If untreated, giardiasis often resolves spontaneously in a few weeks. Prognosis is, therefore, generally excellent.

Prevention

Eradication of giardiasis is not possible because the disease is endemic in the human population, animal population, and environment. Prevention and control methods are the way forward. Health departments in all countries, including the Centers for Disease Control and Prevention in the United States, publish recommendations for prevention and control of giardiasis. These include decontamination of water supplies and sanitary and hygiene practices. Potentially contaminated water may be treated by boiling for more than 1 minute or filtering through a pore size of 1 μm or smaller. Chlorination and iodination are unreliable. Laws and regulations to protect provisions of safe water should be enforced and monitored. Regular surveillance and reviews of sanitation can ensure quality.

People involved in recreational water activities and persons traveling overseas must be informed about the possibility of exposure to the parasite. Persons with symptomatic infection should not swim in a pool until 2 weeks after the treatment. Other occupational groups (e.g., daycare workers, medical personnel, irrigation and sewage workers) need to be cautioned. In daycare centers, hand washing with soap after changing diapers and a separate diaper-changing area should be implemented. All symptomatic family members, daycare center teachers, and children in daycare should be treated for giardiasis. Treatment of asymptomatic cases should be considered if the infected person is suspected to be a potential source of transmission of the disease.

REFERENCES

Cacciò SM, Thompson RCA, McLauchlin J, Smith HV: Unravelling *Cryptosporidium* and *Giardia* epidemiology. Trends Parasitol 2005;21(9):430-437.

Centers for Disease Control and Prevention: Parasitic disease information: Giardiasis fact sheet. Available at http://www.cdc.gov/ncidod/dpd/parasites/giardiasis/factsht_giardia.htm (accessed April 5, 2007).
Escobedo AA, Cimerman S: Giardiasis: a pharmacotheraphy review. Expert Opin Pharmacother 2007;8(12):1885-1902.
Falagas ME, Walker AM, Jick H: Late incidence of cancer after metronidazole use: a matched metronidazole user/nonuser study. Clin Infect Dis 1998;26(2):384-388.
Gardner TB, Hill DR: Treatment of giardiasis. Clin Microbiol Rev 2001;14(1):114-128.
Hanson KL, Cartwright CP: Use of an enzyme immunoassay does not eliminate the need to analyze multiple stool specimens for sensitive detection of *Giardia lamblia*. J Clin Microbiol 2001;39(2):474-477.
Hetsko ML, McCaffery JM, Svard SG, et al: Cellular and transcriptional changes during excystation of *Giardia lamblia* in vitro. Exp Parasitol 1998;88(3):172-183.
Hlavsa MC, Watson JC, Beach MJ: Giardiasis surveillance—United States, 1998-2002. MMWR Surveill Summ 2005;54(SS01):9-16.
Hoque ME, Hope VT, Scragg R: *Giardia* infection in Auckland and New Zealand: Trends and international comparison. The N Z Med J 2002;115(1150):121-123.
Institute of Environmental Science and Research Limited: Notifiable and other diseases in New Zealand: Annual report 2006. Available at http://www.surv.esr.cri.nz/PDFsurveillance/AnnSurvRpt/2006AnnualSurvRpt.pdf (accessed May 14, 2008).
Islam A, Stoll BJ, Ljungstrom I, et al: *Giardia lamblia* infections in a cohort of Bangladeshi mothers and infants followed for one year. J Pediatr 1983;103(6):996-1000.
Kulda J, Nohynkova E: Flagellates of the human intestine and of intestines of other species. In Kreier JP (ed). Protozoa of Veterinary and Medical Interest. Vol. II. New York: Academic Press, 1978, pp 69-104.
Lebwohl B, Deckelbaum RJ, Green PHR: Giardiasis. Gastrointest Endosc 2003;57(7):906-913.
Mineno T, Avery MA: Giardiasis: Recent progress in chemotherapy and drug development. Curr Pharm Des 2003;9:841-855.
New Zealand Ministry of Health: Communicable disease control manual. Wellington: New Zealand Ministry of Health, 1998.
Yoder JS, Beach MJ: Giardiasis surveillance – United States, 2003-2005. MMWR 2007;56(SS07):11-18.

Severe Sepsis and Septic Shock

Method of
Eleni Patrozou, MD, and Steven M. Opal, MD

Sepsis is defined as a deleterious systemic inflammatory response to an infection. The precise incidence of sepsis is unknown, owing to the lack of a readily available and consistently applied definition, but a variety of epidemiologic studies indicate that it is increasing in incidence. The Centers for Disease Control and Prevention (CDC) has reported a threefold increase in the incidence of sepsis since the 1990s. Using hospital discharge coding data, it is estimated that there are between 660,000 and 750,000 episodes of severe sepsis each year in the United States. Severe sepsis accounts for 1 of every 10 intensive care unit (ICU) admissions and represents 2% to 3% of all hospital admissions.

Incidence of sepsis in the United States is projected to rise at a rate of 1.5% per year. The rising incidence of sepsis is primarily related to the aging of the population in developed countries, but the increased number of immunocompromised patients, the increased use of implantable devices in patient care, and the growing problem of antibiotic-resistant microorganisms probably contribute as well. Male patients are consistently and significantly more likely to develop sepsis than female patients.

Since the late 1980s, gram-positive organisms have surpassed gram-negative bacterial pathogens as the predominant causative organisms that lead to sepsis. There has also been a remarkable increase in the number of episodes of fungal sepsis. This is an unfavorable trend because fungal sepsis is associated with a worse outcome than bacterial sepsis.

Sepsis is now reported to be the tenth most common cause of death in the United States and is one of the most common causes of death in the noncoronary ICU.

Systemic Inflammatory Response Syndrome and Sepsis

A major clinical issue in the recognition and early management of sepsis is the imprecise definitions and vague terminology used to describe the septic process. There is no single clinical or laboratory test that verifies the diagnosis of sepsis, severe sepsis, and septic shock. A constellation of physiologic and laboratory studies are employed in concert to make a diagnosis of sepsis (see the Current Diagnosis box).

The term *systemic inflammatory response syndrome* (SIRS) implies early evidence of an acute physiologic insult that may be induced by an infection. SIRS can result from a diverse group of insults such as trauma, severe drug reactions, burns, and pancreatitis. The term *sepsis* is used to define the SIRS response to a documented infection and generally implies a deleterious state in which the septic patient is at risk from both the infecting organism and the systemic host response itself. The lack of specificity in the clinical presentation of SIRS is problematic because the initial manifestations of sepsis mimic many other inflammatory states.

SIRS is operationally defined as the presence of two or more of the following:

- Temperature >38°C (100.4°F) or <36°C (96.8°F)
- Heart rate >90 beats per minute
- Respiratory rate >20 breaths per minute or Paco$_2$ <32 mm Hg
- White blood cell count (WBC) >12,000 cells/mm^3, <4000 cells/mm^3, or >10% immature band forms

Sepsis is the systemic inflammatory response to a documented infection. The diagnosis of sepsis requires the presence of at least two of the SIRS criteria as a response to an invasive infection in a normally sterile space (e.g., blood, lung parenchyma, renal interstitial space, cerebrospinal fluid). Uncomplicated sepsis can progress in a continuum of disease severity to severe sepsis and septic shock. *Severe sepsis* is defined as the presence of organ dysfunction or tissue hypoperfusion from the septic response. Perfusion abnormalities can include lactic acidosis, oliguria, or an acute alteration in mental status.

Sepsis-induced hypotension occurs when the systolic blood pressure falls to less than 90 mm Hg or falls more than 40 mm Hg from baseline systolic blood pressure. Septic shock is a subset of severe sepsis with hypotension despite adequate fluid resuscitation, along with the presence of perfusion abnormalities. Patients who require vasopressor agents to maintain blood pressure yet continue to present with hypoperfusion abnormalities or organ dysfunction are still considered to be in septic shock.

Multiple Organ Dysfunction Syndrome (MODS) is sepsis-induced alteration of organ function. A gradation of organ dysfunction from mild biochemical abnormalities to complete organ failure necessitating interventional support exists in sepsis-related MODS.

In 2001, the International Sepsis Definitions Conference reaffirmed the basic usefulness of these clinical definitions originally proposed in 1991 by the American College of Chest Physicians and Society of Critical Care Medicine. The consensus conference generated a series of common signs and symptoms of sepsis (see the Current Diagnosis box). The conference participants also proposed a new classification scheme called the *PIRO system* (Box 1) to stratify septic patients on the basis of *p*redisposing factors, the nature of the *i*nfection, the host *r*esponse, and the pattern of *o*rgan dysfunction.

BOX 1 PIRO Staging of Sepsis

Predisposition
Premorbid conditions that influence likelihood of infection, sepsis, morbidity, survival (age, gender, hormonal state, genetic polymorphisms for immune response and coagulation proteins)

Infection
Organism associated with the sepsis response (type of organism, virulence potential, toxins, community or nosocomial acquisition)

Response
Clinical and immunologic manifestations of the septic response (either hyperinflammation or hypoinflammation) (e.g., procalcitonin, IL-6, HLA-DR, TNF, PAF)

Organ Dysfunction
Type and number of dysfunctional organs (reversible versus irreversible dysfunction), severity of dysfunction

Abbreviations: HLA-DR = human leukocyte antigen-D related; IL = interleukin; PAF = platelet activating factor; TNF = tumor necrosis factor.
From Levy MM, Fink MP, Marshall JE et al: 2001 SCCM/ESICM/ACCP/ATS/SIS International Sepsis Definitions Conference. Crit Care Med 2003;31:1250-1256.

The validity and practical usefulness of this proposed staging system to further the understanding of sepsis remain to be demonstrated.

Pathogenesis

Sepsis often begins as a physiologic host response as the microbial clearance mechanisms of the innate immune system are called into play to eliminate a microbial invader. Sepsis becomes evident as the host response becomes excessive or dysfunctional, culminating in diffuse endothelial injury, MODS, and septic shock. The molecular pathogenesis of sepsis begins when the host response becomes a disadvantageous process in which host-derived mediators and coagulation factors induce damage to tissues remote from the site of the initiating infectious process. Generalized release of a network of proinflammatory and anti-inflammatory molecules and mediators produce a maladaptive state leading to dysfunctional cellular, tissue, and organ system injury. A complex and dynamic web of interacting inhibitors and activators of cell signaling events ensues, and these can deteriorate over time to refractory organ failure and shock unless appropriate interventions are instituted.

As the process unfolds, anti-inflammatory events dominate and an immune refractory state evolves. This immunodepressed state is now well recognized in the later stages of sepsis, and it is characterized by excess anti-inflammatory mediators and cytokine inhibitors, cellular apoptosis of CD4+ lymphocytes, follicular dendritic cells, and tissue refractoriness to endotoxin or other inflammatory signals. This paradoxically renders the patient susceptible to a variety of secondary infections by intrinsically less virulent pathogens such as fungal organisms, enterococcal pathogens, and a variety of antibiotic-resistant nosocomial pathogens.

Host factors responsible for the important first line of defense against the infectious insult include epithelial barriers, antimicrobial peptides, mucociliary flow, pH of body fluids, urine volume, and secretory immunoglobulins. Once the integument and mucosal barriers are breached, the innate immune system of the host (neutrophils, monocytes, macrophages, dendritic cells, natural killer [NK] cells, alternate complement, and mannose-binding lectin pathways) provide key defenses against infectious insults. The adaptive arm of host immunity, composed of highly specific and clonal B cells and T cells, plays primarily a support role in sepsis. This adaptive response becomes more relevant to host defenses in repeated infection from the same or similar pathogens or as the septic process persists over days to weeks.

The innate immune system recognizes highly conserved, essential, and unique structures found only in microbial pathogens. These

 CURRENT DIAGNOSIS

- Infection (documented or suspected) plus some of the following.

General Variables

- Fever (core temperature >38.3°C [101°F])
- Hypothermia (core temperature <36°C [96.8°F])
- Heart rate >90 bpm or >2 SD above the normal value for age
- Tachypnea
- Altered mental status
- Significant edema or positive fluid balance (>20 mL/kg for longer than 24 h)
- Hyperglycemia (plasma glucose >120 mg/dL or 7.7 mmol/L in absence of diabetes)

Inflammatory Variables

- Leukocytosis (WBC count >12,000/μL)
- Leukopenia (WBC count <4000/μL)
- Normal WBC count with 10% immature forms (bands)
- Plasma C-reactive protein >2 SD above the normal value
- Plasma procalcitonin >2 SD above the normal value

Hemodynamic Variables

- Arterial hypotension (systolic BP <90 mm Hg, MAP <70 mm Hg, or a systolic BP decrease >40 mm Hg in adults or <2 SD below normal for age)
- Svo_2 >70%
- Cardiac index >3.5 L/min/m^2
- Organ dysfunction variables
- Arterial hypoxemia (Pao_2/Fio_2 <300)
- Acute oliguria (urine output <0.5 mL/kg/h or <45 mmol/L for at least 2 h
- Creatinine increase >0.5 mg/dL
- Coagulation abnormalities (INR >1.5 or aPTT >60 sec)
- Ileus (absent bowel sounds)
- Thrombocytopenia (platelet count <100,000/μL)
- Hyperbilirubinemia (plasma total bilirubin >4 mg/dL or >70 mmol/L)

Tissue Perfusion Variables

- Hyperlactatemia (>1 mmol/L)
- Decreased capillary refill or mottling

Abbreviations: aPTT = activated partial thromboplastin time; bpm = beats per minute; INR = international normalized ratio; MAP = mean arterial pressure; SD = standard deviation; WBC = white blood cell.
From Levy MM, Fink MP, Marshall JC, et al: 2001 SCCM/ESICM/ACCP/ATS/SIS International Sepsis Definitions Conference. Crit Care Med 2003;31:1250-1256.

> **BOX 2** **Potential Molecules Involved in the Pathogenesis of Severe Sepsis and Septic Shock**
>
> **Proinflammatory Molecules**
> - Arachidonic acid metabolites: Prostaglandins, prostacyclin, thromboxane, leukotrienes
> - CD14, MD2
> - Clotting factors, PAI-1
> - Complement and activation of the complement cascade
> - Cytokines and chemokines (ILs-1, -2, -6, -8, -12, TNF, IFN-γ, G-CSF, MCP-1)
> - Elastase and lysosomal enzymes
> - Endorphins
> - Endotoxin and other microbial toxins and mediators
> - High mobility group box 1 (HMGB1)
> - Histamine and serotonin
> - Kinases: Protein kinases, tyrosine kinases, serine/theonine kinases
> - Kinins (e.g., bradykinin)
> - Mannose-binding lectin
> - Monocyte migration inhibitory factor (MIF)
> - Neopterin
> - NF-κB
> - PAF, oxidized phospholipids
> - Proteolytic enzymes
> - Reactive nitrogen intermediates: Nitric oxide, peroxynitrite
> - Soluble adhesion molecules
> - Toll-like receptors (1-10)
> - Toxic oxygen metabolites: Superoxide, hydroxyl radical, hydrogen peroxide
> - Vasoactive neuropeptides
>
> **Potential Anti-inflammatory Molecules**
> - BPI
> - Epinephrine
> - Glucocorticoids and glucocorticoid receptors
> - IL-1ra
> - IL-1 receptor type II
> - IL-4, IL-10, IL-13
> - IκB
> - Leukotriene B$_4$ receptor antagonist
> - Soluble CD14
> - sTNFr type 1 and type 2
> - TGF-β
>
> ---
> *Abbreviations:* BPI = bactericidal/permeability increasing protein; G-CSF = granulocyte colony-stimulating factor; IFN-γ = interferon-γ IκB = inhibitor of NFκB; IL = interleukin; IL-ra = interleukin-1 receptor antagonist; MCP = monocyte chemoattractant protein; NFκB = nuclear factor κB; PAF = platelet-activating factor; PAI-1 = plasminogen activator inhibitor-1; sTNFr = soluble TNF receptor; TGF-β = transforming growth factor-β TNF = tumor necrosis factor.

PAMPs (pathogen-associated molecular patterns) are detected by cognate pattern-recognition receptors. These receptors include CD14, complement receptors for C3b, and a remarkable group of 10 human transmembrane receptors known as the *Toll-like receptors* (TLR). TLR4 is the recognition receptor of bacterial endotoxin from gram-negative bacteria. TLR2 partners with TLR1 or TLR6 to recognize a variety of microbial structures including bacterial lipopeptides, peptidoglycans, outer membrane proteins, and mycobacterial antigens. TLR5 detects bacterial flagella, and TLR9, TLR8, and TLR3 recognize prokaryotic DNA sequences, single-stranded RNA, and double-stranded RNA, respectively. Engagement of the TLRs initiates a series of intracellular phosphorylation events that terminate as transcriptional activation for a large number of genetic programs for inflammation, coagulation, and other acute-phase responses.

Gram-positive organisms produce an array of potent exotoxins, some of which function as superantigens. Superantigens induce massive activation of mononuclear cells, macrophages, and T cells, leading to overproduction of inflammatory cytokines. The prototypic superantigenic disease entity is staphylococcal toxic shock syndrome caused by release of TSST-1 (toxic shock syndrome toxin-1). Streptococcal toxic shock from invasive group A streptococcal infections has now supplanted *Staphylococcus aureus* as the predominant superantigen-mediated form of toxic shock today.

Some of the more commonly recognized primary pro- and anti-inflammatory molecules and mediators are listed in Box 2. Included in the list of proinflammatory cytokines are tumor necrosis factor (TNF)-α, interleukin (IL)-1, IL-6, and interferon-γ (IFN-γ).

An overwhelming systemic inflammatory response results when the host is unable to contain the proinflammatory response locally at the site of microbial invasion. The massive, uncontrolled production of inflammatory signals induces diffuse endothelial dysfunction and systemic activation of the coagulation system. The result is microvascular thrombi and up-regulation of endothelial adhesion molecules, causing increased microvascular permeability, vasodilation, organ dysfunction, and shock.

Treatment

In 2003, critical care and infectious disease experts representing 11 international organizations developed management guidelines for severe sepsis and septic shock based on the best available published evidence. These guidelines, produced by the Surviving Sepsis Campaign (SSC), were published in 2004 and updated in 2006 and 2008 as new clinical trial data has became available.

Management of sepsis and septic shock begins with prompt recognition of the process. Along with determination of the probable site of infection and causative microorganism, the initial management begins with an assessment of physiologic derangements. The general management strategy involves source control, restoration and maintenance of normal hemodynamic function, adequate oxygenation, ventilation, tissue oxygen delivery, and prevention of complications. The Current Therapy box outlines the general management principles.

SOURCE CONTROL

Prompt and effective management of the source of the infection is the cornerstone of sepsis management. Necessary specimens should be sent for culture and susceptibility testing as early as possible and before antimicrobial therapy is initiated. This information will guide subsequent antimicrobial therapy to eradicate the causative pathogen(s). Recommendations for the initial antimicrobial regimen based on the source and likely pathogen are given in Table 1.

Intravenous antibiotic therapy should be started within an hour of recognizing severe sepsis. Effective antimicrobial administration within the first hour of documented hypotension has been associated with increased survival to hospital discharge in adult patients with septic shock. For every additional hour to effective antimicrobial initiation in the first 6 hours after onset of hypotension, survival drops an average 7.6%.

After the likely pathogen is identified, antibiotic selection should be guided by the susceptibility patterns of the causative microorganisms. The antimicrobial therapy should then be appropriately tailored with the aim of using a narrow-spectrum antibiotic to prevent the development of resistance, reduce toxicity, and reduce costs. Once a causative agent is identified, there is no evidence that combination therapy is more effective than monotherapy. However, most experts recommend combination therapy for patients with *Pseudomonas*

CURRENT THERAPY

Identify the Cause and Source of Infection
- Obtain suitable material for cultures, Gram stains, serologies, antigenic assays, and other diagnostic studies.
- Implement percutaneous or surgical drainage where appropriate.

Initiate Appropriate Antibiotic Therapy
- Initial therapy is empiric, but tailored therapy should begin as soon as microbiological data are available.
- Survival is improved when the initial antibiotic therapy is effective against the isolated organism(s) and started early.

Restore and Maintain Hemodynamic Function
- Implement an early goal-directed therapeutic approach.
- Fluids are the initial choice for volume resuscitation and may include crystalloids, colloids, volume expanders, or blood products.
- If hypotension and poor perfusion persist, then vasoactive agents should be used as necessary to ensure adequate hemodynamic function.
- Hemodynamic monitoring is often used to ensure the adequacy and effectiveness of therapy (arterial line, CVP, PA catheter).
- Hydrocortisone could be considered only for adult sepsis shock when hypotension remains poorly responsive to adequate fluid resuscitation and vasopressors.

Provide Antithrombotic, Profibrinolytic, Anti-inflammatory Therapy
- Use drotrecogin alfa (activated) (Xigris) per package insert recommendations.

Provide Metabolic Support
- Maintain early nutritional support.
- Maintain intestinal mucosa barrier function by the enteral route, the preferred method.
- Maintain tight glycemic control to decrease infectious complications; patient might need IV insulin therapy.

Prevent Complications of Critical Illness
- Provide DVT prophylaxis.
- Prevent stress-related gastrointestinal bleeding.
- Prevent organ system dysfunction.
- Prevent nosocomial and secondary infections.
- Recognize critical illness polyneuropathy and myopathy.
- Anticipate anemia of critical illness.

Abbreviations: CVP = central venous pressure; DVT = deep vein thrombosis; PA = pulmonary artery.

TABLE 1 Suggested Empiric Antibiotic Choices in Severe Sepsis

Likely Source of Infection	Antimicrobial Choice
Community-acquired pneumonia	Third-generation cephalosporin with a macrolide Alternative: fluoroquinolones
Hospital-acquired pneumonia	Third- or fourth-generation cephalosporins, extended-spectrum penicillins ± an aminoglycoside Alternatives: fluoroquinolones, carbapenems, β-lactam–β-lactamase inhibitors
Urinary tract infections	Extended-spectrum β-lactam agent ± an aminoglycoside Add vancomycin (Vancocin) if MRSA is suspected Add linezolid (Zyvox) if VRE is suspected
Intraabdominal infections	Third- or fourth-generation cephalosporins with metronidazole (Flagyl) or clindamycin (Cleocin) *or* Extended-spectrum penicillins or β-lactam–β-lactamase inhibitor ± an aminoglycoside or fluoroquinolones and metronidazole
Biliary tract infections	Extended-spectrum penicillin ± an aminoglycoside or fluoroquinolones
Neutropenic patients	Extended-spectrum β-lactam agent Add vancomycin if MRSA is suspected Add aminoglycoside or fluoroquinolone if *Pseudomonas aeruginosa* is suspected Add a triazole antifungal or a β-glucan inhibitor if candidemia is suspected

Abbreviations: MRSA = methicillin-resistant *Staphylococcus aureus*; VRE = vancomycin-resistant enterococci.

infections and for neutropenic patients with severe sepsis or septic shock. The duration of therapy should typically be 7 to 10 days and guided by clinical response.

All patients with severe sepsis should be evaluated for the presence of a focus of infection amenable to source-control measures, specifically drainage of an abscess or local focus of infection, débridement of necrotic tissue, removal of a potentially infected device, or definite control of a source of ongoing microbial contamination. The source-control objective should be accomplished with the least invasive method; for example, percutaneous rather than surgical drainage should be used for abscess drainage, if possible.

HEMODYNAMIC MANAGEMENT

Sepsis is characterized by vasodilative or distributive shock, and there is an increase in vascular capacitance along with the decrease in the systemic vascular resistance. Septic patients are functionally volume depleted in the intravascular space from increased permeability as a result of endothelial cell injury. Early recognition of significant hemodynamic derangements and restoration of normal tissue perfusion are vital to prevent organ dysfunction and failure. The goal of hemodynamic resuscitation should be to raise the mean arterial pressure above 65 mm Hg. The resuscitative efforts and the adequacy of tissue perfusion can be assessed at the bedside by monitoring heart rate, BP, orthostatic BP changes, mental status, hourly urine output, and skin perfusion.

The initial hemodynamic resuscitation should take the form of fluid for volume replacement. Debate continues regarding the appropriateness of colloid versus crystalloid fluids. Because the volume of distribution is much larger for crystalloids than for colloids, resuscitation with crystalloids requires about three times more fluid to achieve the same endpoints, and it results in more edema. The SAFE (Saline versus Albumin Fluid Evaluation) study indicated that albumin administration was indeed safe and as effective as crystalloid fluids. However, there was a nonsignificant decrease in mortality rates in a subset analysis of septic patients ($P = 0.09$). Meta-analyses of small studies of ICU patients have demonstrated no difference between crystalloid and colloid resuscitation. The lack of clear evidence of benefit of colloid agents (albumin, dextran, and plasma expanders) and their high cost have generally resulted in the use of saline solutions for volume expansion. More recently, Brunkhost and colleagues found an increased rate of acute renal failure in patients with sepsis treated with low-molecular-weight hydroxyethyl starch (HES200/0.5) and the toxicity increased with accumulating doses. Furthermore, patients in the HES group had a lower median platelet count and received more units of packed red cells than did those in the Ringer's lactate group. Notably, there were no significant differences in the hemodynamic effects between HES and Ringer's lactate. Based on the above study, fluid resuscitation with 10% HES 200/0.5 is shown to be harmful in patients with severe sepsis and should be avoided.

A delicate balance is required between maintaining tissue perfusion and preventing fluid overload, with its attendant risk of lung injury. Bolus infusions are typically administered using the clinical response or measurements of central venous pressure (CVP) or pulmonary capillary wedge pressure (PCWP) as a guide. A CVP of 8 to 12 mm Hg or a PCWP of 12 mm Hg is generally considered a reasonable resuscitation target.

Optimal fluid management in patients with acute lung injury is unknown. A large prospective, randomized study was performed to determine whether a liberal or a conservative strategy of fluid management was more effective in patients with established lung injury. Although there was no difference in 60-day mortality between the two treatment groups, patients in the group treated according to a conservative strategy of fluid management had significantly improved lung function and central nervous system function and a decreased need for sedation, mechanical ventilation, and intensive care.

Invasive vascular monitoring may be used to aid in determining adequate hemodynamic resuscitation. If a central venous catheter is present, the CVP can be measured to assess the adequacy of the intravascular volume status. In select patients with hemodynamic insufficiency, insertion of pulmonary artery catheters to measure the left-sided and right-sided filling pressures and the various hemodynamic parameters may be beneficial. The use of pulmonary artery catheters has declined because multiple randomized trials now indicate that pulmonary artery catheters are not useful for routine hemodynamic monitoring in critically ill patients and are associated with more complications than the CVC.

In shock states, estimation of blood pressure using a sphygmomanometer is commonly inaccurate. Insertion of an arterial line may be required, especially if the patient is unresponsive to initial volume resuscitation and requires the addition of vasopressor therapy for hemodynamic resuscitation.

VASOPRESSOR MANAGEMENT

If adequate fluid resuscitation is insufficient to restore adequate hemodynamic function, then vasopressor or inotropic therapy, or both, will be necessary. There are a wide variety of vasoactive medications that are useful in the hemodynamic resuscitation of septic shock. Table 2 highlights the differences and advantages of some of the more commonly used agents. Despite a wide range of possible agents, dopamine (Intropin) and norepinephrine (Levophed) are typically used in most clinical units. Some centers prefer to use phenylephrine (Neo-Synephrine) in patients with tachycardia or a history of arrhythmias because this pure α-adrenergic agent causes less tachycardia and arrhythmias.

Unfortunately, there is a lack of large, prospective, randomized, protocol-controlled clinical trials that have compared dopamine and norepinephrine for managing patients who have septic shock. Dopamine has been the preferred agent in many units, in part because of its ease of use, the concept that it improves splanchnic and renal perfusion, and its safety record. Notably, recent clinical trial results have revealed that there is no specific beneficial effect of renal dose dopamine in preventing the development of renal failure and its use is not recommended by the SCC guidelines. Another European observational study suggested that dopamine administration might actually be associated with increased mortality rates. Norepinephrine is a potent vasoconstrictor that also has some increased inotropic and chronotropic effects on the heart. A large observational study of French septic shock patients who required high doses of vasopressor therapy demonstrated a significant improvement in survival with the use of norepinephrine as compared with high doses of dopamine with or without the addition of epinephrine.

TABLE 2 Vasoactive Agents Commonly Used in Managing Severe Sepsis[1]

Vasoactive Agent/ Receptor Activity	α₁	α₂	β₁	β₂	V₁	V₂			
Dopamine (Intropin)	3+	3+	3+	2+			<5 µg/kg/min	Vasodilation	Dopaminergic effects predominate Dilation of renal and mesenteric arteries Increased GFR and sodium excretion
							5–10 µg/kg/min	↑Inotropy and chronotropy	β-Adrenergic effects predominate Increased CI, increased stroke volume
							>10 µg/kg/min	Vasoconstriction	α-Adrenergic effects predominate
Dobutamine (Dobutrex)	1+		3+	2+	1+		2–20 µg/kg/min	↑Inotropy and chronotropy	25% increase in CI decreases PAOP
Epinephrine	3+	3+	3+	2+	1+		0.1–0.5 µg/kg/min	↑Stroke volume and CI	Decrease splanchnic blood flow Increase oxygen consumption
Norepinephrine (Levophed)	3+	2+	2+				0.03–1.5 µg/kg/min	Vasoconstriction	Minimal change in heart rate or CI Can decrease lactate
Phenylephrine (Neo-Synephrine)	3+						0.5–8 µg/kg/min	Vasoconstriction	Increases MAP CI can decrease
Vasopressin					1+		0.01–0.04	Vasoconstriction	Vasoconstrictor effect on the up-regulated V₁, splanchnic vasoconstriction
(Pitressin)[1]							U/min		

[1]Not FDA approved for this indication.
Abbreviations: CI = cardiac index; GFR = glomerular filtration rate; MAP = mean aortic pressure; PAOP = pulmonary artery occluded pressure.

There has been renewed interest in the use of vasopressin (Pitressin)[1] in patients with vasodilative shock. The initial release of stored vasopressin from the posterior pituitary during hypotension depletes the body's store of the hormone. Unlike dopamine and epinephrine, vasopressin is a direct vasoconstrictor without inotropic or chronotropic effects and can lead to decreased cardiac output and hepatosplenic flow. Most published reports exclude patients from vasopressin treatment if the cardiac index is less than 2 to 2.5 L/min/m^2. Vasopressin should be used with caution in patients with cardiac dysfunction.

The 2008 SCC guidelines recommend either norepinephrine or dopamine as the first choice vasopressor agents and discourage the use of epinephrine, phenylephrine, or vasopressin as initial vasopressors. In septic shock that is poorly responsive to norepinephrine or dopamine, epinephrine is recommended as a first alternative agent.

Some patients with severe sepsis and septic shock have a reversible biventricular myocardial dysfunction, which has been attributed to circulating TNF-α, IL-1, or nitric oxide that are elaborated as part of the SIRS response. Ventricular dilation and a reduced ejection fraction are the components of this myocardial depression. Inotropic agents such as dobutamine (Dobutrex) or epinephrine can improve the myocardial contractility and hemodynamic function in these patients. By increasing stroke volume and heart rate, dobutamine increases the cardiac index. Although epinephrine can also increase the cardiac index, its use should be limited in the septic patient because it can impair splanchnic blood flow and increase systemic and regional lactate concentrations.

SUPPORT OXYGENATION AND VENTILATION

Abnormalities of the respiratory system are some of the most common evidence of organ system involvement in sepsis. Septic patients should be assessed for adequacy of oxygenation, oxygen delivery, ventilation, and the ability to protect the airway. Septic patients commonly have abnormalities of oxygenation and increased work of breathing. Patients who are hypoxemic should be given supplemental oxygen with a goal of achieving arterial oxygen saturation of at least 90%.

Another decision to make in caring for the septic patient is the need and timing for endotracheal intubation and ventilatory support. Acute lung injury (ALI) and acute respiratory distress syndrome (ARDS) are relatively common manifestations of pulmonary dysfunction in the patient with severe sepsis and septic shock. Up to 35% of septic patients present with ARDS. The goal of mechanical ventilation is to maintain the Pao_2 in the 55 to 70 mm Hg range while keeping the inspired oxygen concentration (Fio_2) below 60%. The traditional approach to mechanically ventilating patients who have ALI and ARDS has been to employ tidal volumes in the 10 to 15 mL/kg range. The Acute Respiratory Distress Syndrome Network (ARDSNet) trial used low tidal volume ventilation of 6 mL/kg ideal body weight, coupled with maintaining an end-inspiratory plateau pressure up to 30 cm H_2O and a nomogram for positive end-expiratory pressure (PEEP) titration based on Fio_2 and oxygenation goals. This combination demonstrated an overall decrease in hospital mortality along with an increase in ventilator-free and organ failure–free days.

The risk of infection and ventilator-associated complications increases with the duration of ventilatory support. Patients should be removed from the ventilator as soon as they no longer need mechanical ventilatory support. The use of weaning protocols implemented by trained ICU support staff have been shown to speed the weaning process and improve the overall process of extubating the critically ill patient. It is also important to use sedation and analgesia appropriately in this critically ill population. Excessive sedation and analgesia have been linked to prolonged stays on mechanical ventilatory support and increased complications.

In a large multicenter controlled trial conducted in critically ill patients without ischemic cardiac disease or acute blood loss, the restrictive practice of packed red blood cell (RBC) transfusions in the management of anemia and low hemoglobin levels (7.0-9.0 g/dL) was shown to provide adequate oxygen delivery to the tissues. In a subgroup of younger patients and less ill patients, it was found to be associated with a lower mortality rate compared with a more liberal transfusion policy with hemoglobin levels maintained between 10.0 and 12.0 g/dL. Banked, stored RBCs are less deformable, are less efficient at releasing oxygen from their 2,3-diphosphoglycerate–depleted hemoglobin stores, and might have immunosuppressive effects. Aggressive use of packed RBC transfusions in an effort to achieve supernormal oxygen delivery states should be discouraged. Furthermore, the use of weekly recombinant erythropoietin (Epogen)[1] reduces the need for transfusions in critically ill patients but with no effect on clinical outcome, and therefore erythropoietin is not recommended as a standard treatment for anemia associated with severe sepsis.

SUPPORTIVE CARE FOR THE CRITICALLY ILL PATIENT

Patients with severe sepsis and septic shock are critically ill and susceptible to the multiple complications common in the critically ill population. These complications include deep venous thrombosis (DVT) and pulmonary emboli, stress-related gastrointestinal bleeding, nosocomial infections, MODS, and critical illness polyneuropathy and myopathy.

Patients in the ICU who have sepsis or septic shock should receive prophylaxis for DVT with unfractionated heparin or low-molecular-weight heparin, unless they have contraindications to their use. Pneumatic compression devices may be used in patients who have a coagulopathy or increased risk of bleeding. In patients at high risk, such as those with severe sepsis and a history of DVT, trauma, or orthopedic surgery, a combination of pharmacologic and mechanical therapies is recommended unless contraindicated.

Prophylaxis for stress-related GI bleeding may be accomplished with H_2-receptor blockers,[1] proton pump inhibitors,[1] sucralfate (Carafate),[1] or early enteral feeding. Proper nutrition is important for maintaining the necessary immune function during the septic metabolic process. Enteral administration of nutrition can prevent stress-related GI bleeding and might prevent the translocation of bowel organisms or endotoxin by maintaining the integrity of the GI tract's mucosal barrier function.

Adequate nutrition is responsible for improved wound healing, decreased susceptibility of critically ill patients to infection, and optimized immune function. The following nutritional guidelines have been recommended for patients with sepsis:

- Daily caloric intake: 25 to 30 kcal/kg of usual body weight per day
- Protein: 1.3 to 2.0 g/kg per day
- Glucose: 30% to 70% of total nonprotein calories to maintain serum glucose lower than 150 mg/dL
- Lipids: 15% to 30% of total nonprotein calories
- Omega-6 polyunsaturated fatty acids: Reduce in septic patients, maintaining a level that prevents deficiency of essential fatty acids (7% of total calories)—generally 1 g/kg/day

Metabolic management also includes correction of electrolyte abnormalities as well as tight control of blood sugar, which might require constant insulin infusion. In initial studies in medical and surgical ICU patients, tight glucose control aimed at keeping the blood sugar between 80 and 110 mg/dL was associated with a significant improvement in ICU and hospital survival. However, a recent multicenter randomized control trial of intensive insulin therapy failed to demonstrate improvement in mortality and was stopped early because of high rates of hypoglycemia and adverse events in

---

[1]Not FDA approved for this indication.

the intensive insulin therapy group. A large randomized controlled trial is ongoing to compare targeting 80 to 110 mg/dL versus 140 to 180 mg/dL and recruit >6000 patients. Pending these results, the SCC guidelines recommend intravenous insulin therapy targeting glucose levels <150 mg/dL range.

INNOVATIVE THERAPIES

Corticosteroid Therapy

The use of corticosteroids as an adjunctive therapy in septic shock has been controversial for decades. Experimental studies in animal models of sepsis and septic shock have demonstrated improved survival using pretreatment or early treatment with high doses of corticosteroids. However, trials of high-dose steroids in patients with severe sepsis failed to improve survival and this treatment practice was abandoned.

More recently, the observation that basal cortisol levels and the cortisol response to the administration of adrenocorticotropic hormone (ACTH)[1] could predict survival in patients with severe sepsis and septic shock renewed interest in steroid therapy. In a French study, patients who had septic shock and an intact pituitary-adrenal axis had a 74% survival rate. In comparison, patients who had impaired adrenal function, had a basal cortisol level of more than 34 μg/dL, and were unable to increase their cortisol level by at least 9 μg/dL had an 18% survival rate. Researchers hypothesized that patients with septic shock have a state of relative adrenal insufficiency and would benefit from the use of more physiologic corticosteroid replacement therapy.

Annane and colleagues performed a multicenter, prospective, randomized, controlled trial of 299 patients with vasopressor-dependent septic shock that demonstrated an improved survival rate in patients with impaired adrenal function who were given physiologic corticosteroid replacement therapy. Subjects were given a stress dose of 50 mg of hydrocortisone (Solu-Cortef)[1] intravenously every 6 hours for 7 days combined with a once-daily oral dose of 50 μg of fludrocortisone (Florinef).

More recently, a large multicenter randomized, placebo-controlled, double blind clinical trial (CORTICUS) found no significant effect of hydrocortisone therapy on the rate of death at 28 days, regardless of the patients' adrenal responsiveness to corticotropin. Unlike the trial performed by Annane and colleagues, which only enrolled shock patients with blood pressure unresponsive to vasopressors, the CORTICUS study included patients with septic shock regardless of how the blood pressure responded to vasopressors. Although corticosteroids did appear to promote shock reversal, the lack of mortality improvement generally tempered the enthusiasm about steroids. The revised Surviving Sepsis Guidelines published in 2008 suggest use of hydrocortisone *only* for adult sepsis shock when hypotension remains poorly responsive to adequate fluid resuscitation and vasopressors. ACTH simulation testing was not recommended to identify the subset of adults with impaired adrenal function.

High-Volume Continuous Venovenous Hemofiltration Therapy

The use of high-volume, continuous hemofiltration (either continuous arteriovenous or venovenous) benefits the hemodynamic course and outcome in patients with intractable circulatory failure resulting from septic shock. This form of management is expensive, requires defined expertise, and may be associated with metabolic and coagulation abnormalities. Further studies are needed to determine if this mode of therapy improves outcome in septic patients. Its use should probably be limited to patients with renal indications for hemofiltration.

Antithrombotic Therapy

New therapies have been directed toward inhibitors of the coagulation system as a potential therapeutic strategy for patients with severe sepsis and septic shock. Among the therapies currently in use or under investigation are antithrombin tissue factor pathway inhibitor and recombinant human activated protein C.

The protein C system is one of the endogenous antithrombotic agents. Drotrecogin alfa (activated) (Xigris) is the recombinant form of human activated protein C. Two international multicenter controlled trials of drotrecogin alfa, the Recombinant Human Activated Protein C Worldwide Evaluation of Severe Sepsis (PROWESS) and Administration of Drotrecogin alfa (activated) in Early Stage Severe Sepsis (ADDRESS) trials, have produced inconsistent results. Drotrecogin alfa was approved on the basis of the favorable results of the PROWESS study, a phase III trial that demonstrated a significant survival benefit in 1690 patients with severe sepsis and septic shock. Treatment with a 96-hour infusion of drotrecogin alfa produced a 6.1% absolute risk reduction and a 19.4% relative risk reduction in the 28-day all-cause mortality in patients with severe sepsis ($P = 0.005$). The drotrecogin alfa–treated population experienced more serious bleeding complications (3.5%) compared with the placebo group (2.0%). The number needed to treat to save an additional life was 16.

The U.S. Food and Drug Administration (FDA) and 19 other regulatory bodies in other countries (including the European Union) have approved drotrecogin alfa to treat severe sepsis in adult patients with a high risk of mortality. The FDA gives the example of using the Acute Physiology and Chronic Health Evaluation (APACHE) II to estimate the risk of death (APACHE II score 25), and other regulatory agencies use sepsis-induced multiorgan failure as an indication for its use. Drotrecogin alfa is contraindicated in patients with known sensitivity to drotrecogin alfa and in patients with a high risk of death from or significant morbidity associated with bleeding.

However, the recently published ADDRESS trial demonstrated no evidence of benefit of drotrecogin alfa in patients with severe sepsis and at low risk of death. The results of the ADDRESS trial also failed to confirm the observation made in the PROWESS trial of a large reduction in mortality among patients with APACHE II scores of 25 or higher, although the number of patients (324) in this group was too small for a meaningful statistic comparison. Further trials of drotrecogin alfa in prospectively defined high-risk patients are required to clarify its optimal role in management of severe sepsis.

Intensive Care of Patients with HIV Infection

Antiretroviral therapy has increased the life expectancy of patients who are infected with HIV and has reduced the incidence of illnesses associated with AIDS. However, the incidence of pulmonary, cardiac, gastrointestinal, and renal diseases that are often not directly related to underlying HIV disease has increased. Although the guiding principles of management in the ICU pertain to critically ill patients with HIV infection, antiretroviral therapy and unresolved questions regarding its use in the ICU add an additional level of complexity to already complicated cases.

Patients who are receiving antiretroviral therapy with evidence of virologic suppression (plasma HIV RNA below the limit of detection) before admission to the ICU should continue their antiretroviral regimen, if possible. Patients who continue to receive treatment should have no contraindications to continuation of treatment, such as major interactions between drugs used in the ICU and antiretroviral therapy. Drug interactions are particularly common and can be severe with hepatically metabolized agents via cytochrome P-450 3A (CYP 3A). In contrast, the benefits of continued antiretroviral therapy in the ICU are less clear for patients with detectable

---

[1]Not FDA approved for this indication.

plasma HIV RNA. For these patients, practitioners should consult with an HIV expert.

Patients who did not receive antiretroviral therapy before ICU admission are the largest subgroup of patients with HIV infection admitted to the ICU. Initiation of antiretroviral therapy should be deferred in patients admitted to the ICU who have a condition that is not associated with AIDS. In these patients, the immediate prognosis is generally better than in those who have an AIDS-associated diagnosis, and the short-term outcome is most likely related to successful treatment of the underlying non-AIDS condition. However, antiretroviral therapy should be considered in patients whose CD4 cell count is less than 200 cells/mm^3 and whose stay in the ICU is prolonged. For such patients, prophylaxis against opportunistic infections should also be prescribed (e.g., trimethoprim-sulfamethoxazole for *Pneumocystis* pneumonia), as recommended in current guidelines.

In contrast, antiretroviral therapy should be considered for patients who are admitted to the ICU with an AIDS-associated diagnosis. This recommendation especially applies to patients whose physiologic condition is worsening despite optimal ICU management and treatment for the AIDS-associated condition. Moreover, patients who receive antiretroviral therapy should be followed for development of the immune reconstitution syndrome.

Prognosis

Despite the tremendous advances in the care of septic patients, the mortality rate for patients with severe sepsis and septic shock remains high. Mortality rates attributable to severe sepsis and septic shock remain in the 20% to 50% range. Factors associated with adverse outcome include advanced age, comorbid conditions, respiratory site of infection, virulent organisms, severity of illness, the number of organ system failures, and specific organ systems failing. In addition, a patient's genetic makeup or gender can have a dramatic impact on whether the patient develops sepsis as well as on the severity, clinical manifestations, and outcome of the sepsis. Survivors of sepsis have increased 6- and 12-month mortality rates compared with critically ill patients who do not have sepsis. Patients who have survived an episode of sepsis have a reduced quality of life and more health-related issues. These observations underscore the importance of early aggressive management of the septic patient and suggest that our future focus should also be directed toward prevention of sepsis.

REFERENCES

Annane D, Sebille V, Charpentier C, et al: Effect of treatment with low doses of hydrocortisone and fludrocortisone on mortality on patients with septic shock. JAMA 2002;288:862-871.
Brunkhorst FM, Engel C, Bloos F, et al: Intensive insulin therapy and pentastarch resuscitation in severe sepsis. N Engl J Med 2008; 358(2):125-139.
Dellinger RP, Levy MM, Carlet JM, et al: Surviving sepsis campaign guidelines for management of severe sepsis and septic shock. Crit Care Med 2008;36(1):296-327.
Friedrich JO, Adhikari NK, Meade MO: Drotrecogin alfa (activated) (Xigris)(activated): does current evidence support treatment for any patients with severe sepsis? Crit Care 2006;10(3):145.
Huang L, Quartin A, Jones D, Havlir DV: Intensive care of patients with HIV infection. N Engl J Med 2006;355(2):173-181.
Kumar A, Roberts D, Wood KE, et al: Duration of hypotension before initiation of effective antimicrobial therapy is the critical determinant of survival in human septic shock. Crit Care Med 2006;34(6):1589-1596.
Martin GS, Mannino DM, Eaton S, et al: The epidemiology of sepsis in the United States from 1979 through 2000. N Engl J Med 2003; 348:1546-1554.
Sakr Y, Reinhart K, Vincent JL, et al: Does dopamine (Intropin) administration in shock influence outcome? Results of the Sepsis Occurrence in Acutely Ill Patients (SOAP) Study. Crit Care Med 2006;34(3):589-597.
Sprung CL, Annane D, Keh D, et al: Hydrocortisone therapy for patients with septic shock. N Engl J Med 2008;358(2):111-124.
Van den Burghe G, Wilmer A, Hermans G, et al: Intensive insulin therapy in the medical ICU. N Engl J Med 2006;354:449-461.
Wheeler AP, Bernard GR, Thompson BT, et al: Pulmonary-artery versus central venous catheter to guide treatment of acute lung injury. N Engl J Med 2006;354(21):2213-2224.
Wiedemann HP, Wheeler AP, Bernard GR, et al: Comparison of two fluid-management strategies in acute lung injury. N Engl J Med 2006; 354(24):2564-2575.

Brucellosis

Method of
Basak Dokuzoguz, MD, and
Nurcan Baykam, MD

Brucellosis is a common bacterial zoonotic disease. It has become more significant in recent years as a bioterrorism agent. Brucellosis is known as a historic disease, and the sequencing of the *Brucella melitensis* genome was completed in 2002.

Etiology

The disease is caused by bacteria of the genus *Brucella*, which are nonmotile, gram-negative, aerobic, unencapsulated cocci or short rods. *Brucella* species are divided into six subtypes based on the main host animals (Table 1). Of these, *B. abortus*, *B. melitensis*, *B. suis*, and *B. canis* are known human pathogens. Two new species, provisionally called *B. pinnipediae* and *B. cetaceae*, have been shown to cause human diseases.

Epidemiology

Brucellosis is one of the major zoonotic diseases and occurs all over the world. Some countries in Europe and North America have achieved control and prevention of the disease based on vaccination programs. However, brucellosis remains endemic in other parts of the world, especially in the Mediterranean, the Middle East, Central Asia, Africa, and Latin America. The real incidence of the disease is not known because underreporting of the disease is believed to be common.

The most common causes of human brucellosis are reported as *B. melitensis* followed by *B. abortus*. The biotypes of *Brucella* species vary by geographic region.

The disease is transmitted to humans by direct contact with infected animals, by ingestion of raw or unpasteurized milk and

TABLE 1 Subtypes and Hosts of *Brucella* Species

Species	Host Animal	Human
B. abortus	Cows, camels, yaks, buffalo	+
B. melitensis	Goats, sheep, camels	+
B. suis	Pigs, wild hares, caribou, reindeer, wild rodents	+
B. canis	Canines	+
B. neotomae	Rodents	−
B. ovis	Sheep	−
B. pinnipediae	Minke whales, dolphins	+
B. cetaceae	Seals	+

milk products, through cuts and abrasions, or by inhalation of aerosols. It is an occupational disease of farmers, veterinarians, slaughterhouse workers, and health care workers, especially laboratory staff. Some individual cases occur as a result of ingesting contaminated dairy products, handling infected animal tissue or body fluids, or handling aborted animal fetuses and placentas. However, the transmission route for outbreaks is usually inhalation of aerosols. Human-to-human transmission of brucellosis is very rare, but there are a few case reports of humans infected through sexual contact, transplacental transmission, or transplantation.

Pathogenesis

The *Brucella* species are pathogenic for humans and animals. *Brucella* species prefer to survive and multiply within phagocytic cells of the host. Unlike other pathogenic bacteria, they do not have classic virulence factors such as exotoxins, cytolysins, capsules, fimbria, plasmids, and endotoxic lipopolysaccharides. Instead of these factors, the bacteria have molecular determinants that are necessary for cell invasion and survival in the cellular compartment. The major one of these molecular determinants is S lipopolysaccharide (S LPS).

The bacteria are phagocytosed by M cells, macrophages, and neutrophils after invasion of mucosa. Fc receptors, complement, lectin, and fibronectin receptors mediate the bacteria for internalization. Most intracellular *Brucella* species are eliminated in phagolysosomes, but some of them reproduce in the acidic compartment. The intracellular mechanism of the organism is not completely described, but intracellular replication of bacteria does not destroy the cell or the cell's function.

After they are taken up by local tissue lymphocytes, the bacteria disseminate into the circulation, and with tropism to the reticuloendothelial system, they become localized within bone marrow, liver, spleen, and lymph nodes. The characteristic feature of the disease is the formation of granulomas in these tissues.

As a host humoral immune response to the disease, the titers of IgM antibodies increase within the first week of infection, and IgG synthesis follows after the second week. Cell-mediated immunity is probably the main mechanism for recovery from the infection.

Clinical Features

Human brucellosis is a multisystem disease that can manifest with a broad spectrum of clinical features. The musculoskeletal, genital, cardiac, respiratory, and nervous systems are involved. The definition and the classification of cases recommended by the World Health Organization (WHO) is presented in Box 1. Some authors classify the disease course as acute, subacute, or chronic, but such a classification has no clinical significance.

The onset of symptoms can be insidious or acute after the incubation period, which is 2 to 8 weeks. A broad spectrum of symptoms such as fever, headache, back pain, weakness, profuse sweating, chills, depression, and joint pain can be observed. These symptoms can also mimic various infectious and noninfectious diseases. Usually an undulant fever pattern is accompanied by so much sweating that the patient needs to change clothes frequently. On the other hand, the physical examination might not reveal any specific finding (Table 2). In children, the range of clinical signs and symptoms may be different than in adults, because children have fewer constitutional symptoms but more hepatic and splenic involvement.

Hepatomegaly, elevated transaminase levels, and granulomatous lesions are the presentations of hepatic involvement in brucellosis. The most common complication of brucellosis is osteoarticular disease, which occurs as peripheral arthritis, sacroiliitis, and spondylitis. This complication is reported in 10% to 80% of cases, and this range may be related to the age and genetic predisposition

---

BOX 1 Recommended Case Definitions and Classifications by the World Health Organization

Clinical Description

An illness characterized by acute or insidious onset, with continued, intermittent, or irregular fever of variable duration; profuse sweating, particularly at night; fatigue; anorexia; weight loss; headache; arthralgia and generalized aching. Local infection of various organs can occur.

Laboratory Criteria for Diagnosis

- Isolation of *Brucella* spp. from clinical specimen *or*
- Brucella agglutination titer (e.g., standard tube agglutination tests: STA> 160) in one or more serum specimens obtained after onset of symptoms *or*
- ELISA (IgA, IgG, IgM), 2-mercaptoethanol test, complement fixation test, Coombs' test, fluorescent antibody test (FAB), radioimmunoassay for detecting antilipopolysaccharide antibodies, counterimmunoelectrophoresis (CIE)

Case Classification

Suspected

A case that is compatible with the clinical description and is epidemiologically linked to suspected or confirmed animal cases or contaminated animal products.

Probable

A suspected case that has a positive rose bengal test.

Confirmed

A suspected or probable case that is laboratory confirmed.

Abbreviations: ELISA = enzyme-linked immunosorbent assay; Ig = immunoglobulin.

(HLA-B39) of patients and the infecting *Brucella* species. Genitourinary system involvements exist in 2% to 20% of patients with brucellosis. Prostatitis, epididymo-orchitis, cystitis, pyelonephritis, interstitial nephritis, exudative glomerulonephritis, and renal abscess are the clinical manifestations of this complication. Neurobrucellosis can develop at any stage of disease and can have widely variable manifestations, including encephalitis, meningoencephalitis, radiculitis, myelitis, peripheral and cranial neuropathies, subarachnoid hemorrhage, and psychiatric manifestations. Brucellosis can cause a variety of ocular lesions and different types of skin rash that are nonspecific and reported rarely. Another rare (<2%) but severe complication of brucellosis is endocarditis, which most often involves the aortic valve and requires surgery. Mortality from brucellosis is rare and is usually related to endocarditis.

Diagnosis

The absolute diagnosis of brucellosis is based on identification of bacteria from blood, bone marrow, and materials from affected organs such as cerebrospinal fluid, liver, lymph nodes, synovial fluid, or prostatic fluid by culture. The rate of bacteria isolation from the blood is between 15% and 70%. Lysis centrifugation technique and automated systems improve the range of culture positivity.

TABLE 2 Clinical Presentation and Laboratory Findings of Human Brucellosis

Feature	Percentage
Signs and Symptoms	
Fever	72–91
Constitutive symptoms (e.g., malaise, arthralgias)	26–90
Hepatic involvement	17–31
Splenomegaly	14–16
Osteoarticular involvement	9–22
CNS disorder	3–13
Lymphadenopathy	2–7
Genitourinary involvement	1–5.7
Respiratory disorders	0.2–6
Cardiovascular disorders	0.4–1.8
Skin rashes	0.4–3
Laboratory Findings	
Hematologic	
Relative lymphocytosis	40
Anemia	31
Leukopenia	2–27
Thrombocytopenia	5–15
Pancytopenia	2
Biochemistry	
Elevated transaminase	24–31

Abbreviation: CNS, central nervous system.
Data derived from Aygen B, Doganay M, Sümerkan B, et al: Clinical manifestations, complications and treatment of brucellosis: An evaluation of 480 patients. Med Mal Infect 2002;32:485-493; Dokuzoguz B, Ergonul O, Baykam N, et al: Characteristics of *B. melitensis* versus *B. abortus* bacteremias. J Infect 2005;50(1):1-5; Pappas G, Akritidis N, Bosilkovski M, Tsianos E: Brucellosis. N Engl J Med 2005;352:2325-2336.

CURRENT THERAPY

- The treatment requires combined regimens for their synergistic effect plus agents with good penetration capacity into the macrophages.
- At least 6 weeks of therapy may be extended to 6 months, according to the complications of the disease.
- Rifampin (Rifadin)[1] plus doxycycline (Vibramycin) treatment is a favorable regimen and the most synergistic one.
- Rifampin may be replaced by streptomycin or gentamycin (Garamycin)[1] as the first-line therapy choice.
- Combinations with trimethoprim-sulfamethoxazole (TMP-SMX; Bactrim)[1] is usually recommended in the second-line treatment regimens.
- Quinolones[1] are alternative drugs in cases with side effects due to first-line drugs and relapses.
- Rifampin in a combination with TMP-SMX[1] or an aminoglycoside are the main regimens for children younger than 8 years.
- Rifampin and TMP-SMX[1] combination is preferred in pregnancy
- Although the use of ceftriaxone (Rocephin)[1] is controversial in brucellosis, it could be preferred in the treatment of central nervous system involvement.
- Rifampin[1] (600-900 mg qd) plus doxycycline (100 mg bid) regimen for 2-3 weeks is recommended as postexposure prophylaxis.

[1]Not FDA approved for this indication.

Compatible clinical findings with a serum agglutinin titer of at least 1/160 in the standard tube agglutination test (STA) have diagnostic value. In endemic areas, the titer of at least 1/320 is recommended in the diagnosis. False-negative results of STA may be attributed to blocking antibodies; results can be improved by testing with 2-mercaptoethanol or antihuman immunoglobulin. Negative results in the early phase of the disease can be overcome by repeating the test after 2 weeks. Diagnosis of *B. canis* infection is unavailable with routine STA. False-positive results may be related to cross-reactions of some gram-negative bacterial infections.

Enzyme-linked immunosorbent assay (ELISA) is another serologic test that has higher specificity and sensitivity compared with STA. Although it is not used in current clinical practice because of standardization problems, polymerase chain reaction (PCR) is a promising diagnostic tool in brucellosis. Duration of diagnosis can be shortened by automated culture systems and PCR techniques. Rose bengal and a new dipstick test are also rapid tests useful for early diagnosis, but positive results should be confirmed by STA.

CURRENT DIAGNOSIS

- The common symptoms of brucellosis, which can also mimic various infectious and noninfectious diseases, are fever, headache, back pain, weakness, profuse sweating, chills, depression, and joint pain.
- The absolute diagnosis of brucellosis is based on identification of bacteria from blood, bone marrow, and materials of affected organs such as cerebrospinal fluid, liver, lymph nodes, synovial fluid, and prostatic fluid by culture.
- Compatible clinical findings with a serum agglutinin titer of ≥ 1/160 in the standard tube agglutination test (STA) have diagnostic value.

Treatment

Because the *Brucella* species are intracellular pathogens, treatment requires not only combined regimens for their synergistic effect but also agents with good penetration into the macrophages. For success of the therapy, adequate duration of drug therapy is another important factor. At least 6 weeks of drug therapy is recommended by the WHO. This duration may be extended to 6 months, depending on such complicatiorns of the disease as neurobrucellosis, spondylodiskitis, and abscessers.

The drug combinations listed in Table 3 are widely used in brucellosis. Rifampin (Rifadin)[1] plus doxycycline (Vibramycin) treatment for human brucellosis was recommended by WHO two decades ago; it is still a favorable regimen and was found to be the most synergistic one. Rifampin may be replaced by streptomycin or gentamycin (Garamycin)[1] as first-line therapy choices. Combinations with trimethoprim-sulfamethoxazole (TMP-SMX, Bactrim)[1] is usually recommended in second-line treatment regimens. Combination rifampin plus a quinolone[1] is not preferred in

[1]Not FDA approved for this indication.

TABLE 3 Drug Combinations Used to Treat Brucellosis

Generic Name (Trade Name)	Adult Dose	Pediatric Dose	Renal Failure	Hepatic Insufficiency	Adverse Effects
Ciprofloxacin[1] (Cipro)	500-750 mg PO q12h *or* 400 mg IV q8-12h	Not suggested	Necessary	No change	Drug fever, rash, seizures, Achilles tendon rupture or tendinitis
Doxycycline (Vibramycin, Vibra-tabs)	100 mg PO q12h	2.2-4.4 mg/kg[3] PO div. q12h (≥ 8 y)	No change	No change	Nausea, vomiting, eosinophilia, photosensitivity
Gentamicin[1] (Garamycin)	2 mg/kg IM/IV q8h *or* 5 mg/kg IM/IV q24h[1] *or* 240 mg q24h	2.5 mg/kg q8-12h IM/IV	Necessary	No change blockade (rapid infusion)	Ototoxicity, nephrotoxicity, neuromuscular
Ofloxacin[1] (Floxin, Oflox)	400 mg PO bid	Not suggested	Necessary	Moderate: no change Severe: necessary	Drug fever, rash, mild neuroexcitatory symptoms
Rifampin[1] (Rifadin, Rimactane)	600-900 mg PO qd	20 mg/kg PO qd Do not exceed 600 mg qd	No change	Moderate: caution Severe: avoid	Red/orange discoloration of body secretions, flu-like symptoms, elevated AST/ALT, drug fever, rash, thrombocytopenia
Streptomycin	15 mg/kg IM q24h *or* 1 g IM qd for 2-3 wk	20-40 mg/kg IM qd	Necessary	No change	Ototoxic, nephrotoxic
TMP-SMX[1] (Bactrim, Septra)	1 DS tab PO q12h (160 mg TMP/800 mg SMX)	Do not exceed 1 g qd 8-12 mg/kg TMP PO q12h	Necessary; avoid use	No change	Folate deficiency, hyperkalemia, leukopenia, thrombocytopenia, hemolytic anemia ± G6PD, aplastic anemia, elevated AST/ALT, hypersensitivity reactions (Stevens-Johnson syndrome, erythema multiforme)

[1] Not FDA approved for this indication.
[3] Exceeds dosage recommended by the manufacturer.
Abbreviations: ALT = alanine aminotransferase; AST = aspartate aminotransferase; DS = double strength; G6PD = glucose-6-phosphate dehydrogenase; TMP-SMX = trimethoprim-sulfamethoxazole.

the initial therapeutic regimen because of the reported decreased activity in pH 5 and lack of synergism between quinolones and other antibiotics that are used in brucellosis. Quinolones are alternative drugs for patients who have relapses or who have side effects from first-line drugs.

Rifampin[1] in combination with TMP-SMX[1] or an aminoglycoside are the main regimens for children younger than 8 years. The rifampin and TMP-SMX combination may be prescribed for pregnant patients.

Although the use of ceftriaxone (Rocephin)[1] is controversial in brucellosis, it may be preferred for treating central nervous system involvement. Because their activity is decreased in an acidic environment, macrolides are not used in brucellosis treatment.

Because there are no significantly important resistance problems for antibiotics targeted to *Brucella* species, susceptibility tests are not recommended routinely except in epidemiologic studies and for some rare recurrent cases. Most of the recurrences are related to noncompliance or to short duration of therapy. In tuberculosis-endemic populations, community-acquired rifampin resistance should be taken into consideration in treating brucellosis.

Supportive therapy might be useful depending on the clinical situation. The cognitive and emotional disturbances in neurobrucellosis can be improved by antibiotics without any antidepressant or antipsychotic therapy.

In the management of *Brucella* endocarditis, medical treatment alone is often effective in patients with early diagnosis and no cardiac failure. However, in most cases, surgery is required in addition to medical treatment.

---

[1] Not FDA approved for this indication.

Prevention

Various vaccines have been applied to humans in some countries in the 20th century, but an acceptable vaccine has not yet been developed for humans. Although investigations of the *B. melitensis* outer membrane protein 25 and cytoplasmic protein BP26 are promising for future vaccine development, prevention of the disease in humans is related to controlling and eliminating animal brucellosis. In this respect, vaccination and slaughter programs of animals, pasteurization of milk and milk products, and education programs about contact precautions for persons at risk must be emphasized.

Because *Brucella* bacteria can be transmitted via the inhalational route, laboratory workers should be warned about the risk, and biosafety level 2 prevention measures should be applied.

Because of laboratory accidents and biological warfare, rifampin[1] (600-900 mg qd) plus doxycycline (100 mg bid) for 2 to 3 weeks is recommended as postexposure prophylaxis.

---

[1] Not FDA approved for this indication.

REFERENCES

Aygen B, Doganay M, Sümerkan B, et al: Clinical manifestations, complications and treatment of brucellosis: An evaluation of 480 patients. Med Mal Infect 2002;32:485-493.

Baykam N, Esener H, Ergonul O, et al: In vitro antimicrobial susceptibility of *Brucella* species. Int J Antimicrob Agents 2004;23(4):405-407.

Bossi P, Tegnell A, Baka A, et al: Bichat guidelines for the clinical management of brucellosis and bioterrorism-related brucellosis. Euro Surveill 2004;9(12):E15-E16.

Dokuzoguz B, Ergonul O, Baykam N, et al: Characteristics of *B. melitensis* versus *B. abortus* bacteremias. J Infect 2005;50:(1):1-5.

Eren S, Bayam G, Ergonul O, et al: Cognitive and emotional changes in neurobrucellosis. J Infect 2006;53:184-189.

Ergonul O, Celikbas A, Tezeren D, et al: Analysis of risk factors for laboratory-acquired *Brucella* infections. J Hosp Infect 2004;56:223-227

Falagas ME. Bliziotis IA: Quinolones for treatment of human brucellosis: Critical review of the evidence from microbiological and clinical studies. Antimicrob Agents Chemother 2006;50(1):22-33.

Giannacopoulos I, Nikolakopoulou NM, Eliopoulou M, et al: Presentation of childhood brucellosis in Western Greece. Jpn J Infect Dis 2006;59:160-163.

Joint Food and Agriculture Organization/World Health Organization: FAO-WHO Expert Committee on Brucellosis (sixth report). WHO Technical Report Series No. 740. Geneva: World Health Organization, 1986, pp 56-57.

Pan American Health Organization: Case definition: Brucellosis. Epidemiol Bull 2000;21(3):13. PDF available at http://www.paho.org/english/dd/ais/EB_v21n3.pdf (Accessed April 27, 2007).

Pappas G, Akritidis N, Bosilkovski M, Tsianos E: Brucellosis. N Engl J Med 2005;352:2325-2336.

Young EJ: *Brucella* species. In Mandel GL, Bennett JE, Dolin R (eds): Mandell, Douglas and Bennett's Principles and Practice of Infectious Diseases, 6th ed. Philadelphia: Churchill Livingstone, 2005, pp 2669-2672.

Varicella (Chickenpox)

Method of
Charles Grose, MD

Chickenpox is caused by varicella zoster virus (VZV). After chickenpox occurs, VZV enters the sensory nerve and establishes latency in the dorsal root ganglia along the spinal cord. When VZV reactivates in late adulthood, the virus causes the disease known as shingles (herpes zoster).

Pathogenesis of Chickenpox

Chickenpox is an airborne infection. The virus first infects the mucosa tissues of the nose and subsequently establishes an infection in the tonsils or lymph nodes around the neck. After 4 to 6 cycles of replication, the primary viremia occurs (Figure 1). The virus then disperses to multiple organs in the body. After a second period of replication, the second viremia occurs. The virus is carried within lymphocytes in the bloodstream. The vesicular lesions occur after the virus exits the capillaries and enters the epidermis.

Epidemiology after Approval of the Vaccine

The varicella vaccine was approved for administration to children in the United States in 1995, and the vast majority of states have approved the administration of varicella vaccine to all young children. Approximately 4 million cases of chickenpox occurred annually in the United States prior to 1995. There were also approximately 100 deaths annually, the vast majority in otherwise healthy children, and more than 14,000 hospitalizations per year.

CURRENT DIAGNOSIS

- Diagnosis of chickenpox is usually made by observation or rash.
- Diagnosis is confirmed by a rapid viral diagnosis kit performed on a vesicle smear.
- Diagnosis of past varicella infection is made by serology.
- Commercial antibody kits may not be sensitive enough to detect serum antibody after varicella vaccination.

More than 10 years later, the effect of universal varicella immunization in the United States is dramatic. The number of hospitalizations and deaths was reduced by 75%. Similarly, the total number of cases of chickenpox in the United States has also decreased dramatically. Nevertheless, more than one half million cases of chickenpox will probably continue to occur annually. These cases will include many immunocompromised children who remain unimmunized.

ADMINISTRATION OF VARICELLA VACCINE

Varicella vaccine is a live attenuated virus. Each dose of vaccine (0.5 mL) is administered subcutaneously. The virus must replicate in the infected child for an immune response to occur (Figure 2). The initial virus replication can cause a few vesicles near the site of infection. The replication can also lead to a viremia with a short-lived rash anywhere on the body. The vaccine virus can, in very few cases, replicate to a sufficient extent that the infection transfers to another person who will subsequently develop a mild case of vaccine-related chickenpox. In 1995, a single dose of varicella vaccine was originally recommended. As of 2007, two doses of varicella vaccine are recommended for every child. The first dose is given between 12 and 15 months. The second dose is routinely recommended between 4 and 6 years. Instead of single-dose vials of vaccine (Varivax), the vaccine can also be administered as a component of the 4-in-1 vials of measles-mumps-rubella-varicella vaccine (Pro Quad). This approach reduces the number of injections given to a child. Children 13 years and above, who have never received varicella vaccine, should be given 2 doses of vaccine (Varivax), separated by a 4-week interval.

RISK FACTORS FOR BREAKTHROUGH CHICKENPOX

Breakthrough chickenpox refers to a wild-type chickenpox that is usually a mild illness with less than 50 vesicles that occurs in children given varicella vaccine at least 42 days previously. Thus, breakthrough chickenpox is a form of vaccine failure. Breakthrough chickenpox was believed to be relatively uncommon during the prelicensure clinical studies. However, by 2000 it was apparent that breakthrough chickenpox was not a rare event. Several reports documented large outbreaks of wild-type chickenpox in immunized children who were attending large daycare facilities or grade schools.

A major risk factor is believed to be immunization with one dose of vaccine. The 2-dose regimen of varicella vaccine should eliminate most cases of breakthrough chickenpox.

Treatment

TREATMENT OF SEVERE CHICKENPOX IN HEALTHY CHILDREN

Chickenpox is considered a more severe disease in children younger than 1 year and in postpubertal adolescents. VZV is highly susceptible

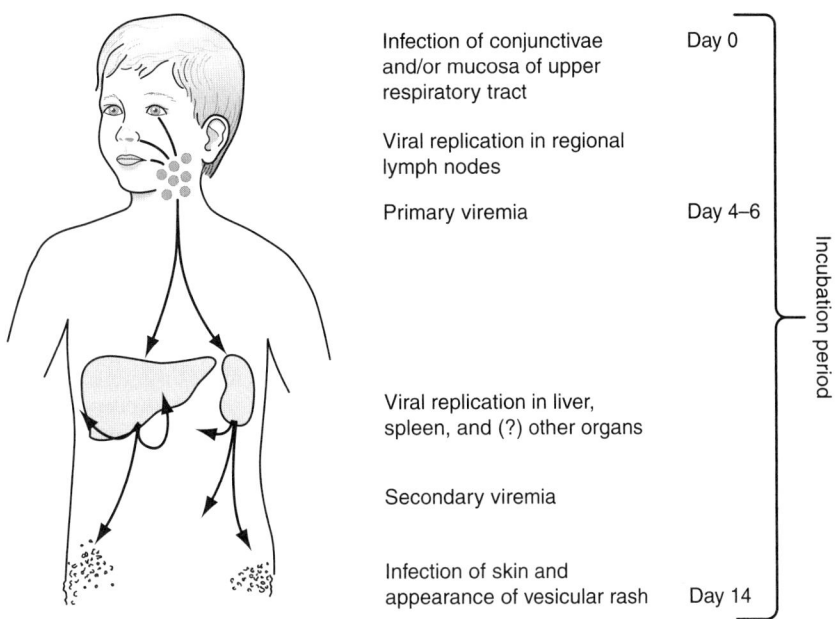

FIGURE 1. Diagrammatic representation of the pathogenesis of acute varicella infection. There are two viremias during the 14-day incubation period. The first viremia occurs after local replication at the site of infection. The typical chickenpox rash appears at the end of the second viremia. See Grose (2005) for a more detailed description.

to acyclovir and two second-generation antiviral agents: famciclovir (Famvir) and valacyclovir (Valtrex). Acyclovir is now a generic drug and very economic. Every case of chickenpox in a child younger than 1 year should be treated with acyclovir. The oral dosage is 20 mg/kg four times a day for 5 to 7 days. Chickenpox in children older than 1 year can also be treated with acyclovir to reduce the severity and duration of disease. The maximum dosage is 800 mg four times a day. Acyclovir is available in a liquid suspension and tablets containing 200, 400, or 800 mg. The 800-mg tablet is very large and may be difficult for some children to swallow.

Famciclovir (Famvir) or valacyclovir (Valtrex) are the preferred antiviral agents for adolescents because these are better adsorbed than acyclovir. However, they are much more expensive. The dosage of famciclovir (Famvir) is 500 mg orally three times a day. The dosage of valacyclovir (Valtrex) is 1 g three times a day. For most adolescents, a 5-day regimen should be sufficient treatment.

TREATMENT OF CHICKENPOX IN CHILDREN WITH AN UNDERLYING IMMUNODEFICIENCY

Children with HIV infection who contract chickenpox can usually be managed with oral acyclovir treatment as long as their HIV is under control. The majority of children diagnosed with acute chickenpox who have cancer or have undergone organ transplantation should be considered for admission to the hospital and begin immediate treatment with intravenous (IV) acyclovir. The dosage of IV acyclovir is 10 mg/kg every 8 hours. The dosage can be raised to 15 mg/kg every 8 hours in patients presenting varicella pneumonia or varicella encephalitis. The serum creatinine level should be

CURRENT THERAPY

- Severe chickenpox in infants and immunosuppressed children is treated with intravenous acyclovir (30 mg/kg/d).
- Severe chickenpox in healthy children is treated with oral acyclovir (80 mg/kg/d).
- Severe chickenpox in adolescents is treated with either famciclovir (Famvir) (500 mg tid) or valacyclovir (Valtrex) (1 g tid).
- Prophylaxis following exposure to chickenpox can be managed with a course of oral acyclovir (40 mg/kg/d).

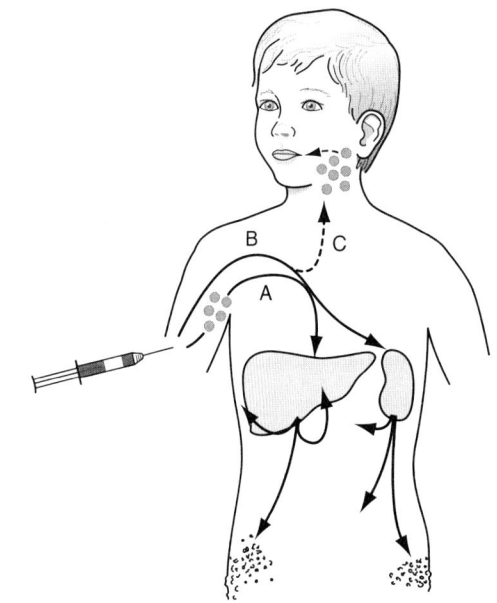

FIGURE 2. Pathways of infection following administration of varicella vaccine. Pathway A shows a rash that sometimes appears at the site of injection after local replication of the virus. Pathway B shows a viremia with appearance of a few small papulovesicular lesions on the skin distant from the site of injection. Pathway C shows the virus as it travels to the respiratory tract where infection can be spread on rare occasions to other individuals. See Grose (2005) for a more detailed description.

monitored daily and the acyclovir dosage adjusted downward if the serum creatinine reaches 1 mg/dL.

The efficacy of oral famciclovir or valacyclovir is better than oral acyclovir, allowing older children with chickenpox and an immunosuppressive condition to be discharged more quickly from the hospital. Discharge is generally considered after no new vesicle formation is noted for 24 hours. Antiviral therapy (combined IV and oral) for 10 to 14 days is usually suggested, although each case must be assessed individually. Children who have varicella encephalitis or varicella pneumonia may require more than 2 weeks of antiviral therapy.

TREATMENT OF CHICKENPOX IN CHILDREN RECEIVING CORTICOSTEROIDS

Children receiving high-dose oral corticosteroid treatment for conditions such as acute asthma are also at high risk of severe chickenpox. These children should be treated with antivirals just as aggressively as those with cancer. Children receiving only intermittent inhaled corticosteroids do not appear to be at high risk of severe chickenpox.

TREATMENT OF ZOSTER IN CHILDREN

Zoster in otherwise healthy children is usually a benign illness. The disease is normally improving by the time the diagnosis is made. However, zoster in immunocompromised children may persist for 2 weeks or longer, requiring immediate treatment with one of the oral antiviral drugs recommended. The dosage is the same as for severe chickenpox.

ALTERNATIVES TO VARICELLA-ZOSTER IMMUNE GLOBULIN

Varicella-zoster immune globulin (VZIG) has been given in the past to infants and children with cancer who were exposed to chickenpox. VZIG has been discontinued after 2005. Physicians can consider the administration of IV gammaglobulin as a single infusion of 500 mg/kg for infants who are exposed to varicella shortly after birth. An alternative regimen is oral acyclovir suspension at 40 mg/kg per day divided every 6 hours. Acyclovir should be initiated on the day of exposure and continued for 10 days.

Prophylaxis with oral acyclovir also can be considered for VZV-nonimmune children with cancer after an exposure to chickenpox. The recommended dosage is one half of the therapeutic dosage, meaning oral acyclovir can be given at 40 mg/kg per day. The daily dosage for children who can swallow tablets can be divided three times a day rather than four times a day during the 10-day therapy period. Children who develop chickenpox despite oral acyclovir treatment should be admitted to the hospital for treatment with IV acyclovir at 10 mg/kg every 8 hours. There are extremely few examples of true acyclovir-resistant VZV; most failures are caused by inadequate absorption of the oral formulation.

REFERENCES

Davis MM, Patel MS, Gebremariam A: Decline in varicella-related hospitalizations and expenditures for children and adults after introduction of varicella vaccine in the United States, Pediatrics 2004;114:786-792.
Grose C: Varicella vaccination of children in the United States: Assessment after the first decade, 1995-2005, J Clin Virol 2005;33:89-95.
Grose C, Widerman J: Generic acyclovir vs. famciclovir and valacyclovir. Pediatr Infect Dis J 1997;16:838-841.
Hay M, Kimura H, Oshiro M, et al: Varicella exposure in a neonatal medical center: Successful prophylaxis with oral acyclovir. J Hosp Infect 2003;54:212-215.
Nguyen HQ, Jumaan AO, Seward JF: Decline in mortality due to varicella after implementation of varicella vaccination in the United States. N Engl J Med 2005;352:450-458.
Takahashi M: Effectiveness of live varicella vaccine. Expert Opin Biol Ther 2004;4:199-216.

Cholera

Method of
Carlos Seas, MD, and Eduardo Gotuzzo, MD

Cholera is an ancient scourge recognized since the time of Hippocrates. More accurate descriptions of the disease began approximately in 1817. Since then, cholera has caused seven pandemics, affecting all continents, and it remains endemic in almost all affected areas. Recent examples of severe epidemics are the Latin American extension of the seventh pandemic in Peru in 1991, explosive epidemics among refugees in Africa, and unexpected epidemics of cholera due to a new serogroup in Asia since 1992. We can conclude from these epidemics that it is very difficult to predict when a new epidemic will start, that appropriate treatment reduces the mortality to values less than 1%, and that the pathogen continues to evolve in the environment despite interventions to control its spread.

Etiology

Cholera is caused by a curved gram-negative bacillus that belongs to the family Vibrionaceae. Two serogroups, O1 and O139, are associated with clinical cholera, and both cause the same clinical entity. These serogroups have shown both regional and pandemic potential. *Vibrio cholerae* is a natural inhabitant of certain aquatic environments, where it lives attached to copepods, algae, and crustacean shells in a symbiotic association. If conditions are not favorable for growth, *V. cholerae* adopts a dormant state. In this state it remains metabolically inactive for long periods. The switch to a metabolically active state occurs when conditions become suitable for division. Humans get the infection by consuming contaminated water, beverages, or food. During epidemics, a single source can be identified, but usually multiple routes of transmission play a role simultaneously. Epidemics tend to occur during the warmest months of the year, and association with climate variability and El Niño southern oscillation has been recently documented.

V. cholerae O1 and O139 secrete a number of potent exotoxins that induce the characteristic isotonic dehydration of cholera. The better studied toxin is the cholera toxin, which has two subunits, A and B. The B subunit allows the toxin to attach to a specific receptor present along the small intestine of humans, and the A subunit activates the adenylate cyclase enzyme. The chain of events that follows this enzymatic activation is mediated by cyclic adenosine

CURRENT DIAGNOSIS

- History of travel to an endemic area.
- Acute voluminous watery diarrhea with rice-water appearance, leading to severe dehydration in a matter of hours.
- Muscle cramps, vomiting, and signs of severe dehydration such as loss of skin elasticity (slow skin-pinch retraction), hoarse voice, sunken eyes, and wrinkled hands and feet (washerwoman hands).
- Fever is absent in most patients.
- Milder forms of dehydration cannot be distinguished from other common causes of acute diarrhea.
- Stool culture using proper media is positive for *V. cholerae* O1 or O139. Dark field microscopy of a fresh stool sample can detect the presence of vibrio; specific antisera confirm the serogroup.

TABLE 1 Electrolyte Concentrations (mmol/L)

Substance	Sodium	Chloride	Potassium	Bicarbonate	Osmolality
Cholera Stool					
Adults		130	100	20	44
Children		100	90	33	30
Rehydration Solution					
Ringer's lactate*	130	109	4	28*	271
Normal saline	154	154	0	0	308
Rice-based ORS	75	65	20	10	180
WHO ORS[‡]	75	65	20	10[†]	245

*Ringer's lactate contains lactate instead of bicarbonate.
[†]Bicarbonate is replaced with trisodium citrate, which stays fresh longer than bicarbonate in sachets.
[‡]Reduced osmolality formula.
Abbreviations: ORS = oral rehydration solution; WHO = World Health Organization.

monophosphate (cAMP) and includes blockage of the absorption of sodium and chloride by the microvillus and promotion of secretion of chloride and water by crypt cells. The result of these events is the massive liberation of water and electrolytes into the intestinal lumen, as shown in Table 1.

Treatment

The objectives of therapy are to replace the fluid and electrolyte losses caused by diarrhea and vomiting, to maintain hydration, and to reduce the volume of diarrhea and excretion of vibrios to the environment. The treatment is divided into two phases: the rehydration phase and the maintenance phase.

REHYDRATION PHASE

The objective of the rehydration phase is to replace the losses that occurred before the patient was admitted. This phase begins with a thorough evaluation of the degree of dehydration. Table 2 shows the clinical signs according to the degree of dehydration.

Patients with severe dehydration present with a constellation of signs that reflect a deficit of at least 10% of body weight. The pulse is feeble and very rapid, the blood pressure is not measurable, the skin elasticity is lost, the eyes are sunken, and the voice is inaudible or hoarse. The intravenous route is recommended for rehydrating all patients with severe dehydration. The rate and speed of the infusion is recommended at 50 to 100 mL/kg/hour for the first 2 to 4 hours. After this time, the patient must be fully rehydrated to begin the maintenance phase. The preferred intravenous solution is Ringer's lactate solution. If this solution is not available, normal saline may be used, but the recovery from metabolic acidosis is less efficient. Oral rehydration solutions (ORS) should be started as soon a possible in these patients.

Milder forms of dehydration due to cholera cannot be clinically distinguished from other common causes of acute diarrhea. Symptoms due to some degree of dehydration are seen when water deficit is greater than 5% of body weight. The intravenous route may be used in these patients if the stool output is high (<10-20 mL/kg/hour) or if the patient does not tolerate the oral route. The great majority of patients with milder forms of dehydration can be rehydrated by the oral route.

Laboratory abnormalities in patients with severe cholera reflect hemoconcentration and include a high hematocrit, increase in white blood cell count, azotemia, and elevation of specific gravity and total proteins. These laboratory parameters are good indicators of the degree of dehydration on admission, but they are not useful for following the rehydration status. Metabolic acidosis with a high anion gap is typically seen in patients with severe cholera. Hypokalemia or normal values (due to acidosis) and normal or low serum sodium and chloride are also observed in these patients. Hyperglycemia results from high levels of epinephrine, glucagon, and cortisol stimulated by hypovolemia. Hypoglycemia is rare but carries a poor prognosis, particularly in children.

MAINTENANCE PHASE

The maintenance phase begins when the patient has been fully rehydrated. A good indicator of the recovery of the normal hydration status is not only the absence of clinical signs of dehydration but also the volume of urine output. Urine outputs greater than 0.5 mL/kg/hour are expected in fully hydrated patients. The maintenance phase has the objective of preserving the normal hydration status, and it lasts until the diarrhea abates.

The oral route is advised for the maintenance phase, and the ORS recommended by the World Health Organization (WHO) is the preferred oral solution. Recently, WHO has promoted the use of ORS with lower osmolality (75 mmol/L of sodium and total osmolality of 245 mOsm/L vs. the former solution containing 90 mmol/L of sodium and total osmolality of 311 mOsm/L) to treat all kinds of acute diarrheal diseases. Adults should be observed for hyponatremia when using this reduced-osmolality ORS. ORS uses the principle of common transportation of solutes, electrolytes, and water not affected by cholera in the intestine. ORS containing rice instead of glucose is also preferred, because the purging rate is lower with solutions containing rice than with glucose-based solutions. If ORS in packets is not available, a solution can be made with 2.6 g sodium chloride, 2.9 g sodium citrate, 1.5 g potassium chloride, and 13.5 g glucose or 50 g rice powder to 1 L of boiled water.

TABLE 2 Clinical Findings by Degree of Dehydration

Clinical Finding	Degree of Dehydration	
	Some	Severe
Loss of fluid (% of body weight)	5%-10%	>10%
Mentation	Restless	Drowsy or comatose
Radial pulse rate	Rapid	Very rapid
Radial pulse intensity	Weak	Feeble or impalpable
Respiration	Normal or deep	Deep and rapid
Systolic blood pressure	Low	Very low or undetectable
Skin elasticity	Retracts slowly	Retracts very slowly
Eyes	Sunken	Very sunken
Voice	Hoarse	Not audible
Urine production	Scant	Oliguria

CURRENT THERAPY

- Identify the degree of dehydration on admission.
- Register the intake and output regularly in predesigned charts.
- Rehydrate the patient in two phases. The rehydration phase lasts 2-4 hours. The maintenance phase lasts until diarrhea abates.
- Use the intravenous route for patients who have severe dehydration during the rehydration phase, those who purge more than 10-20 mL/kg/h, and those who do not tolerate the oral route during the maintenance phase. The amount and speed of the intravenous infusion vary between 50 and 100 mL/kg/h.
- The preferred intravenous solution is Ringer's lactate solution. Normal saline may be used, but the acidosis resolves less efficiently.
- Use the oral rehydration solution advised by the World Health Organization during the maintenance phase for severely dehydrated patients and for milder forms of dehydration in the rehydration phase. The amount of oral fluids advised is 500-1000 mL/h.
- Start antibiotics once the patient can tolerate the oral route. Doxycycline (Vibramycin) in a single dose of 300 mg, is the preferred regimen, given with a light meal.
- Start a normal diet as soon as the patient tolerates anything by mouth.
- Discharge patients when all the following criteria are fulfilled: oral tolerance <600-800 mL/h, stool output >400 mL/h, urine output <30-40 mL/h.

TABLE 3 Antimicrobial Regimens for the Treatment of Cholera

Drug	Adult	Children
Preferred Regimen		
Doxycycline (Vibramycin)	300 mg with food	
Alternative Regimens		
Azithromycin (Zithromax)[1]	1 g as a single dose	20 mg/kg as a single dose
Ciprofloxacin (Cipro)[1]	1 g single-dose or 250 mg qd for 3 d or 500 mg bid for 3 d	Not recommended
Cotrimoxazole (Bactrim)[1]	TMP 160 mg and SMX 800 mg bid for 3 d	TMP 8 mg/kg and SMX 40 mg/kg divided in 2 doses for 3 d
Doxycycline (Vibramycin)	300 mg as a single dose	Not evaluated
Erythromycin[1]	250 mg qid for 3 d	12.5 mg/kg q6h for 3 d
Furazolidone (Furoxone)	100 mg qid for 3 d	5 mg/kg qid for 3 d or 7 mg/kg as a single dose
Norfloxacin (Noroxin)[1]	400 mg bid for 3 d	Not recommended
Tetracycline	500 mg qid for 3 d	50 mg/kg body weight qid for 3 d*

[1]Not FDA approved for this indication.
*Only for children older than 8 years.
Abbreviations: SMX = sulfamethoxazole; TMP = trimethoprim.

The amount of oral fluids should match the ongoing losses to prevent dehydration during this phase. Periodic review of the patient's chart is advised for this purpose. Predesigned forms to register intake and output and vital signs should be available to monitor the hydration status regularly. Cholera cots or cholera chairs facilitate the collection and measurement of stools and urine during treatment.

Discharging patients from the hospital is a critical issue, particularly when health centers are overloaded with patients with varying degrees of dehydration. Patients can be safely discharged if all the following criteria are met: oral intake between 600 and 800 mL/hour, urine output between 30 and 40 mL/hour, and stool output lower than 400 mL/hour. Case fatality rates in centers with experience in the treatment of cholera are extremely low, about 0.14%.

PHARMACOLOGIC THERAPY

An oral antibiotic is advised to reduce the volume of diarrhea, the requirement for intravenous fluids, and the hospital stay. Antibiotics are not lifesaving and should not be offered if the patient cannot tolerate the oral route. A reduction in almost 50% of the volume and duration of diarrhea and a reduction in the excretion of vibrios to 1 to 2 days have been documented with the use of effective antimicrobials. Single-dose regimens are preferred over multiple-dose regimens. A single dose of doxycycline (Vibramycin) 300 mg, given with a light meal, is the preferred regimen. Alternative regimens are listed in Table 3.

The quinolones are the group of antimicrobials more extensively studied to date, and excellent results in both clinical and bacteriologic parameters have been reported in clinical trials. Quinolones should not be used in children or pregnant women. Resistance to the quinolones has emerged in endemic areas of India and Bangladesh. Oral azithromycin (Zithromax)[1] (1 g in a single dose) is an alternative to treat infections by quinolone-resistant strains in both children and adults. Chemoprophylaxis with antimicrobials to prevent transmission of cholera is not recommended.

Complications and Prognosis

The most severe complication of cholera is acute renal failure. A careful evaluation of the medical charts of these patients disclosed improper replacement of fluids during the rehydration or maintenance phases. The nonoliguric form predominates. All age groups are affected, and the mortality rate is very high.

The presentation of cholera in children is similar to that in adults. Certain features are distinctive in children, however, such as fever, seizures, mental alteration, and hypoglycemia.

Cholera in the elderly carries a bad prognosis. The common presence of comorbidities, the difficulties in properly evaluating the hydration status, and the higher incidences of acute renal failure and pulmonary edema account for the higher mortality observed in this population.

Cholera in pregnant women is associated with more severe illness and with fetal losses.

REFERENCES

Griffith DC, Kelly-Hope LA, Miller MA: Review of reported cholera outbreaks worldwide, 1995-2005. Am J Trop Med Hyg 2006;75:973-977.
Khan WA, Bennish ML, Seas C, et al: Randomized controlled comparison of single-dose ciprofloxacin and doxycycline for cholera caused by *Vibrio cholerae* O1 or O139. Lancet 1996;348:296-300.
Khan WA, Saha D, Rahman A, et al: Comparison of single-dose azithromycin and 12-dose, 3-day erythromycin for childhood cholera: A randomized, double-blind trial. Lancet 2002;360(9347):1722-1727.

[1]Not FDA approved for this indication.

Nalin DR, Hirschhorn N, Greenough W III, et al: Clinical concerns about reduced-osmolarity oral rehydration solution. JAMA 2004;291:2632-2635.

Sack DA, W, Sack RB, Nair GB, Siddique AK: Cholera. Lancet 2004;363:223-233.

Saha D, Karim MM, Khan WA, et al: Single-dose azithromycin for the treatment of cholera in adults. N Engl J Med 2006;354:2452-2462.

Seas C, Gotuzzo E: Cholera. In Mandell GL, Bennett JE, Dolin R (eds): Principles and Practice of Infectious Diseases. Philadelphia: Churchill-Livingstone, 2005, pp 2536-2544.

Foodborne Illness

Method of
Lester M. Crawford, PhD

History

In the 1920 edition of *Principles and Practice of Medicine*, Sir William Osler devoted three of the 1168 pages to food poisoning. He got virtually everything right, even by today's standards. He just had very little to report on a disease complex that was vitally important in his time. Today, the Centers for Disease Control and Prevention (CDC) estimates approximately 76 million illnesses, 325,000 hospitalizations, and 5000 deaths from foodborne disease each year in the United States. Viruses account for 67% of these infections, bacteria for 30%, and parasites for 2%.

Therapy of foodborne disease has passed through a variety of stages. In Osler's time, treatment primarily consisted of stomach lavage and enemas. After World War II, antibiotics were freely used. By the 1980s, competitive exclusion by antibiotic-resistant bacteria had dictated a more conservative approach that relied on supportive therapy including fluids. In severe cases, selective use of specific targeted antibacterials remained necessary. The remarkable success rate of oral rehydration therapy under primitive conditions in developing countries underscored the critical importance of maintaining fluid balance. Today, fluid therapy has become the cornerstone of the treatment of foodborne disease.

Etiology, Diagnosis, and Treatment

There are 30 principal foodborne diseases. Waterborne diseases are classified as foodborne diseases. Six of the 30 diseases are dealt with in other chapters. These are hepatitis, salmonellosis, typhoid, cholera, giardiasis, and toxoplasmosis. This chapter deals with the remaining major causes of this group of diseases.

AEROMONAS SPECIES

Although the role of *Aeromonas* in foodborne disease was elucidated in the 1890s, it has only recently been appreciated as the ubiquitous pathogenic organism that it is. These are, in fact, aquatic organisms, but *Aeromonas* has been isolated from a variety of plants, animals, and foodstuffs. *Aeromonas* has also been found in stool cultures, skin, and sputum samples from healthy persons. Gastrointestinal infections caused by this organism are characterized by mucoid, bloody stools, watery diarrhea typical of dysentery, and low-grade fever. This syndrome can progress to pneumonia, arthritis, osteomyelitis, endocarditis, and urinary tract infections, particularly in children, the elderly, and immunocompromised patients. *Aeromonas* can affect virtually any organ system and can cause hemolytic uremic syndrome.

The organism is amenable to antibiotic therapy and may be successfully treated with trimethoprim-sulfamethoxazole (Bactrim),[1] aminoglycosides, tetracyclines, cephalosporins, and the quinolones. Antibiotic resistance has now become a problem; it has been demonstrated that *Aeromonas* spp. can produce β-lactamases and transferable tetracycline R-plasmids. Therefore, it may be preferable to initiate therapy with trimethoprim-sulfamethoxazole or one of the fluoroquinolones when *Aeromonas* is isolated.

BACILLUS CEREUS

Bacillus cereus was not recognized as a significant foodborne pathogen until the 1950s, and the first major outbreak was not until 1971 in England. This organism is ubiquitous in the environment but is not pathogenic until conditions favor its growth. Pathogenesis is accomplished through a wide variety of extracellular toxins and enzymes. There is a diarrheagenic toxin and an emetic toxin.

Foods become toxic when the levels of *B. cereus* approach millions of organisms per gram. The usual syndrome involves nausea (but not vomiting), watery diarrhea, rectal straining, and abdominal pain. There is an incubation period of 8 to 19 hours; the duration of illness is usually 12 to 24 hours. In some cases, an emetic syndrome occurs that is more severe and acute than the diarrheal syndrome. The emetic syndrome is characterized by an incubation period of approximately 3 hours and is typified by severe vomiting. Diarrhea is generally not present in the emetic syndrome. The emetic syndrome closely mirrors staphylococcal food poisoning.

The diarrheal syndrome generally requires minimal therapeutic intervention other than monitoring of fluid and food intake. The emetic syndrome, although brief, can require intravenous fluids and medication such as phenobarbital[1] to moderate the frequency of vomiting.

CALICIVIRUSES

Caliciviruses cause the majority of foodborne illness in the United States and, most likely, the rest of the world. Indeed, without the cases caused by norovirus, cases of foodborne disease would be reduced by approximately two thirds according to some estimates, and there would likely be little need for or interest in this chapter.

Norwalk, Ohio, was the site of the first reported outbreak (1968) of this disease complex. The virus was therefore named *Norwalk virus*. The name was later changed to *Norwalk-like virus* (NLV), and the current name is *norovirus*.

There are three genotypes of enteric caliciviruses. In addition to norovirus, the calicivirus family includes Desert Shield virus, Hawaii virus, Mexico virus, Snow Mountain virus, and others.

Etiology

Fecal-oral transmission is the most common route of infection, but vomitus can also transmit infectious doses of the agent. Although swimming pools and uncooked or partially cooked food can transmit the infection, the primary source is drinking water. The recent spate of cruise ship infections has generally been traced to drinking water. Properly chlorinated water is generally safe, but nonchlorinated water is problematic. Inadequately chlorinated or brominated water can transmit norovirus, as can chlorinated water that comes from an overwhelmingly contaminated source. Leakage of sewage into treated water can result in individual cases or outbreaks.

Diagnosis

The disease entity is characterized by epidemic diarrhea. Symptoms include gastroenteritis, vomiting, diarrhea, headache, and 2 to 3 days of low-grade fever. People of all ages are affected. In the United States, older children and adults are more likely to be infected, and in the Third World, young children are more often involved. Diagnosis may

---
[1]Not FDA approved for this indication.

be by isolation of the virus from feces and confirmation by radioimmunoassay (RIA) or enzyme-linked immunosorbent assay (ELISA), or both.

Treatment

There is no specific treatment for norovirus infection. Supportive therapy, especially including fluids, is generally adequate for most patients. For patients in developing countries, oral rehydration therapy is generally the treatment of choice.

A specific vaccine for norovirus is being developed. The virus has been isolated, cloned, and sequenced, and an experimental vaccine is in clinical trials.

CAMPYLOBACTER SPECIES

Campylobacter has gone from not being recognized as a human pathogen to being the leading cause of bacterial diarrhea in just over 25 years. The agent is estimated to cause about 2.5 million illnesses, which is 12% of all foodborne disease in the United States. Moreover, serious sequelae such as Guillain-Barré syndrome (1:1000 cases) and Reiter's syndrome (1:100 cases) infrequently supervene.

Diagnosis

Difficulty in culturing *Campylobacter* prevented isolation and characterization of the organism until the early 1970s. *Campylobacter jejuni* is the species most associated with foodborne illness. Campylobacteriosis is characterized by abdominal pain, diarrhea, and fever lasting 2 to 5 days. Longer durations of illness and relapses are not uncommon. Diagnosis is confirmed by direct microscopic examination of the stool or through the use of selective media.

Treatment

Seriously ill patients should be treated with antibiotics, as should infants, older people, and the immunosuppressed. Seriously ill patients are defined as those with persistent high fever or refractory or bloody diarrhea. Clarithromycin (Biaxin)[1] is generally accepted as the antibiotic of choice, and fluoroquinolones such as ciprofloxacin (Cipro)[1] are the first alternative. The tetracyclines are also useful. Campylobacteriosis is resistant to the cephalosporins, vancomycin (Vancocin), and rifampin (Rifadin). Supportive therapy aimed at electrolyte replacement and hydration is also important.

CLOSTRIDIUM BOTULINUM

Clostridium botulinum elaborates one of the most potent substances in nature. One nanogram per kilogram of body weight is sufficient to paralyze an otherwise healthy person. When the toxin is ingested in food in sufficient quantities to cause illness, near total paralysis occurs in humans, often requiring artificial ventilation for extended periods. Mild botulism can consist of nothing more than double vision or a few days of dysphagia.

The mechanism of action of botulism is to block release of acetylcholine at the neuromuscular junction by attaching to specific receptors on the nerve terminal side of the junction. Nerve conduction restores activity at the neuromuscular junction.

Any food can contain botulinum toxin, but the most common vehicles in the United States are fruits and vegetables. Infant botulism is usually associated with consumption of honey.

Diagnosis

Diagnosis is confirmed by isolation of botulinum toxin either from the suspect food or from the patient's blood serum or feces. Resorting to symptomatic diagnosis can lead to confusing botulism with Guillain-Barré syndrome or even stroke.

---

[1]Not FDA approved for this indication.

Treatment

Therapy must center around the management of respiratory impairment. This requires accessibility to an intensive care unit. The Centers for Disease Control and Prevention (CDC) can provide polyvalent vaccines[5,10] that are effective against the six botulism toxins (A, B, C, D, E, F). The toxin can persist in the patient's serum for as much as a month after ingestion, and relapses and exacerbations are possible. The toxicity to the neuromuscular junctions can continue for months and, in rare cases, for as long as a year. Careful management and diagnostic advances have reduced mortality to well under 10%.

CLOSTRIDIUM PERFRINGENS

McClane has written, "*Clostridium perfringens* is ideally suited for its role as a major foodborne pathogen." He was referring to its ubiquity in soil and in human and animal feces; moreover, the organism has a doubling time of less than 10 minutes once established in foods. Finally, *C. perfringens* is heat resistant and it elaborates two toxins that can induce specific pathology in the human intestinal tract. Indeed, *C. perfringens* is the third leading cause of foodborne illness in the United States, after norovirus and *B. cereus*.

Diagnosis

The two forms of human disease caused by this organism are *C. perfringens* type A food poisoning and *C. perfringens* type C food poisoning, better known as necrotic enteritis. The type A syndrome is much more common but type C is a more serious disease.

Abdominal cramps and diarrhea typify the type A disease. These symptoms develop 8 to 16 hours after ingestion of contaminated food and persist for 12 to 24 hours, with a complete recovery in most patients. However, severe illness and even death can supervene in older or debilitated patients.

The necrotic enteritis form of the disease is characterized by vomiting, intense abdominal pain, bloody diarrhea, and severe gastroenteritis. The incubation period is 1 to 5 days after exposure. The more advanced cases can progress to jejunal necrosis and death if not managed well.

Treatment

Treatment for the type A disease is supportive therapy. Necrotic enteritis can require surgical repair of the small intestine, including removal of the affected area. *C. perfringens* is quite susceptible to penicillin, and some authorities report that the antibiotic may be useful in the management of severe cases of type C.

ENTEROBACTER SAKAZAKII

Enterobacter sakazakii causes meningitis or necrotizing enterocolitis in neonates, which results in a mortality rate of 40% to 80%. Surviving patients sometimes develop hydrocephalus, paralysis, or neurologic deficits. *E. sakazakii* has been isolated from dry infant formulas. The natural source of the organism is not well known.

Enterobacters are generally resistant to the cephalosporins but are responsive to medium-spectrum penicillins, such as carbenicillin (Geocillin),[1] piperacillin (Pipracil),[1] and ticarcillin (Ticar).[1] The aminoglycosides and the fluoroquinolones are also indicated.

ESCHERICHIA COLI O157:H7

This variant of *Escherichia coli* burst on the scene in North America in the late 1970s, and now it can be found in practically every country in the world. The reservoir for the disease is believed to be cattle, but

---

[1]Not FDA approved for this indication.
[5]Investigational drug in the United States.
[10]Available in the United States from the Centers for Disease Control.

wildlife of various kinds can likewise harbor the organism. In cattle, the disease is silent, causing no overt signs.

In humans, the verocytotoxin, a Shiga-like toxin that has been genetically incorporated into the organism, can cause hemorrhagic colitis and hemolytic-uremic syndrome, which leads, in some cases, to disseminated intravascular coagulation (DIC). DIC can result in a layer of fibrin forming in the glomerular capillary bed and acute renal failure. These sequelae are most likely to occur in children and older persons and in pregnant women. The young patients generally fully recover but sometimes require dialysis.

The number of cases is low and the fatality rate is small, but the severity and permanence of some of the sequelae have given great prominence to the disease. Major outbreaks such as the Jack-in-the-Box event of 1993 and the 2006 spinach outbreak have focused public attention on *E. coli* 0157:H7. Control of this organism depends on proper cooking and handling of food, assiduous hand washing, and effective water-treatment programs. There is much interest in a vaccine for cattle or humans for *E. coli* 0157:H7.

Diagnosis

Diagnosis is made by serotyping for specific antibodies to *E. coli* 0157:H7. Transmission of the organism generally occurs from ingesting contaminated food but can occur from direct contact. The incubation period is 12 to 60 hours.

Treatment

Therapy consists of fluid replacement. Antibiotics are of no use because the lesional insult is caused by a combination of toxins that continue to be pathogenic for a period of time after the elaborating organism is no longer active. In fact, the U.S. Food and Drug Administration (FDA) has issued (January 2007) a warning against the use of antibiotics in enterohemorrhagic *E. coli* cases because such therapy could adversely affect the outcome. Dialysis is indicated in cases that progress to kidney failure. In the more severe cases of intestinal hemorrhage, blood transfusion may be necessary.

LISTERIA MONOCYTOGENES

Although *Listeria monocytogenes* infects a relatively small number of patients, listeriosis results in a 25% to 40% fatality rate, and severe aftereffects are relatively common in affected patients. It is extremely difficult to identify the specific food responsible because of the highly variable incubation period, which ranges from 3 to 70 days.

There are three modes of transmission: contaminated food, direct contact with the organism or with contaminated soil, and inhalation of the organism. Initial symptoms include fever, headache, and vomiting, but these may be followed by endocarditis, meningoencephalitis, and septicemia. These later symptoms can lead to hemorrhagic shock, disorientation, and coma. Listeriosis is a leading cause of stillbirth and miscarriage and must be handled aggressively in pregnant women. Neonatal cases likewise must be managed with care. Almost one half of all listeriosis cases are in neonates.

Confirmation of the diagnosis is accomplished by isolation of the organism from blood or cerebrospinal fluid. Virtually all β-lactam antibiotics are effective against *L. monocytogenes* including potassium penicillin G (Pfizerpen). Erythromycin (Ery-Tab),[1] tobramycin (Nebcin),[1] and other antibiotics in the macrolide and aminoglycoside families also are effective against *L. monocytogenes*.

STAPHYLOCOCCUS AUREUS

Whereas most food borne illnesses have incubation periods of days and even weeks, *Staphylococcus aureus* infections usually trigger symptoms in 2 to 6 hours. The organism elaborates a complex system of toxins in food under certain conditions that results in nausea, vomiting, retching, and abdominal cramping. Severe cases result in muscle cramping,

---

[1]Not FDA approved for this indication.

vacillations in blood pressure and heart rate, and severe headaches. The disease usually runs its course in 2 days, but some cases last longer. Death can occur in the young, the elderly, and the debilitated.

Incriminated foods in *Staphylococcal* outbreaks are generally those that require a great deal of human handling such as salads and various meats, although canned foods have caused clusters of infection. The usual inciting factor is not keeping the prepared foods hot enough or cold enough to prevent the proliferation of organisms and the formation of the causative toxins. Stored foods should be maintained at temperatures of 45°F (7.2°C) or kept warm at 140°F (60°C). Foods should be brought to these temperatures as rapidly as technologically possible.

Supportive therapy is indicated. Antibiotic therapy is not useful because the causative agent, the toxin, is not affected by antibiotics. Persistent vomiting or dehydration can indicate fluid therapy, such as 5% dextrose, together with electrolyte replacement, particularly potassium.

REFERENCES

Allos BM, Blaster MJ: *Campylobacter jejuni* and the expanding spectrum of related infections. Clin Infect Dis 1995;20:1092-1101.
Ball JM, Graham DY, Opekum AR, et al: Recombinant Norwalk-like particles given orally to volunteers: Phase I study. Gastroenterology 1999;117:40-48.
Bennett RW: *Bacillus cereus*. In Labbé RG, García S (eds): Guide to Foodborne Pathogens. New York: John Wiley and Sons, 2001, pp 51-60.
Gill DM: Bacterial toxins: A table of lethal amounts. Microbiol Rev 1982;46:86-94.
Greatorex JS, Thorne GM: Humoral immune response to Shiga-like toxins and *Escherichia coli* O157:H7 lipopolysaccharide in hemolytic-uremic syndrome patients and healthy subjects. J Clin Microbiol 1994;32:1172-1178.
Lawrence GW: The pathogenesis of enteritis necroticans. In Rood JA, McClane, Songer JG, et al (eds): The Clostridia: Molecular Genetics and Pathogenesis. London: Academic Press, 1997, pp 198-207.
Lederberg J, Shope RE, Oaks SC (eds): Emerging Infections: Microbial Threats to Health in the United States. Washington, DC: National Academies Press, 1992.
Miliotis MD, Bier JW (eds): International Handbook of Foodborne Pathogens. New York: Marcel Dekker, 2003.
Olsen SJ, MacKinnon LC, Goulding JS, et al: Surveillance for foodborne-disease outbreaks—United States, 1993-1997. MMWR CDC Surveill Summ 2000;49(1):1-62.
Schlech WF: Foodborne listeriosis. Clin Infec Dis 2000;31:770-775.

Necrotizing Skin and Soft Tissue Infections

Method of
John M. Embil, MD, FRCP(C), FACP, and Donald C. Vinh, MD, FRCP(C), Dip(ABIM)

Necrotizing skin and soft tissue infections (SSTIs) are a heterogeneous group of infections that progress unimpeded across anatomic boundaries, producing destruction of the subcutaneous, fascial, or muscle layers of the integument, resulting in gangrenous cellulitis, necrotizing fasciitis, or myonecrosis, respectively. These infections have an acute onset, usually the patient appears toxic, and the infection is potentially limb- or life-threatening. Although necrotizing SSTIs are relatively uncommon, early recognition and appropriate interventions are crucial for optimal outcome. Thus, clinicians assessing a patient presenting with an SSTI should always consider the possibility of an underlying necrotizing process that would require consultation with a surgeon and infectious disease specialist.

Etiology

Necrotizing SSTIs are most often bacterial in origin and can be either monomicrobial (type II) or polymicrobial (type I). Much less often, fungal pathogens cause such infections.

TABLE 1 Causes and Risk Factors for Monomicrobial Acute Necrotizing Skin and Soft Tissue Infections

Pathogen	Risk Factors
Aeromonas hydrophila	Wounds contaminated by freshwater (e.g., lakes, rivers, streams)
Clostridium perfringens (gas gangrene)	Contamination of traumatic wounds (e.g., by soil) Deterioration in a postsurgical wound (e.g., dehiscence, duskiness, bullae)
Clostridium septicum	Malignancy (e.g., colon cancer, hematologic malignancy)
Community-acquired methicillin-resistant Staphylococcus aureus	No established regular risk factors Close contacts who have a recent history of furuncles or difficult-to-treat skin abscesses may be suggestive
Group A streptococci (S. pyogenes)	Breaks in integrity of skin Impaired lymphatic or venous circulation Diabetes mellitus Superinfection of chickenpox
Pseudomonas aeruginosa	Ecthyma gangrenosum: Immunocompromise (hematologic malignancy, neutropenia) Malignant otitis externa: Diabetes mellitus
Vibrio vulnificus	Wounds contaminated by saltwater (e.g., Atlantic Gulf Coast) Wounds exposed to saltwater crustaceans and other seafood Chronic liver disease or cirrhosis Chronic renal failure or dialysis

Polymicrobial necrotizing SSTIs are, by far, most common. These infections are caused by the synergistic interaction between mixed facultative anaerobic and obligate anaerobic gram-positive and gram-negative bacteria, such as *Escherichia coli*, *Klebsiella spp*, *Proteus spp*, the staphylococci, the streptococci, and *Bacteroides spp*. On average, 4 or 5 different organisms are involved. The polymicrobial nature can be suggested by the location of the infected site; most commonly, they occur in the head and neck area (especially if odontogenic), the abdominal area (e.g., postsurgical sites), the pelvic, genital, and perineal areas (e.g., Fournier's gangrene, infections following gynecologic procedures, and infections originating from sacral decubitus ulcers), and extremities with neglected care (especially diabetic foot infections). Culture and susceptibility testing (C&S) should be performed on any discharge or deep tissue to guide therapy.

Monomicrobial necrotizing SSTIs occur less often (Table 1). These pathogens should be especially considered among patients with certain risk factors (see Table 1) who present with community-acquired infections. By far the most common isolate responsible for this condition is group A streptococcus (*Streptococcus pyogenes*), which might or might not cause concomitant streptococcal toxic shock syndrome and which can have devastating consequences. Because no clinical features are absolutely diagnostic for a specific pathogen, cultures should be obtained.

Fungal pathogens are emerging as an important cause of acute necrotizing SSTIs. Most commonly, these are due to saprophytic septated molds (e.g., *Aspergillus spp*, *Fusarium spp*, *Paecilomyces spp*) and to the aseptated zygomycetes producing mucormycosis. Major risk factors include diabetic ketoacidosis, iron overload states and deferoxamine (Desferal) therapy, immunocompromised states (prolonged neutropenia, hematologic malignancy, corticosteroid therapy, solid organ or stem cell transplant), and soft tissue trauma (e.g., burns, contaminated wounds).

Clinical Features

The distinction between necrotizing SSTIs and uncomplicated SSTIs (e.g., cellulitis) may be difficult. Both usually manifest with erythema, edema, and tenderness of a localized area of skin. A systematic approach for clinical features favoring the presence of a necrotizing SSTI should be undertaken, including a systemic evaluation of the patient, a focused assessment of the involved region, and laboratory investigations (Table 2).

TABLE 2 Clinical Clues to the Presence of Acute Necrotizing Skin and Soft Tissue Infections

Systemic Features	Local Features	Laboratory Investigations
Altered mental status (e.g., delirious, stuporous, obtunded)	Anesthesia of the affected area	Myonecrosis (e.g., increased creatine kinase, increased myoglobin)
	Crepitus	Radiography: Gas in the soft tissues
Hypotension (systolic BP < 90 mm Hg or < 5th percentile by age for children < 16 years)	Rapidly progressive spread of erythema or pain	WBC ≥ 12,000 cells/μL or ≤ 4000 cells/μL or > 10% immature granulocytes
	Focal areas of dermal necrosis	
Hypothermia or fever (temperature ≤ 36 C or ≥ 38° C)	Foul smell	Acidosis
Hypoxia	Purulent discharge, particularly if grayish or blackish or with gas bubbles	Electrolyte derangements (e.g., hyponatremia, hypocalcemia)
Tachycardia (heart rate ≥ 90 bpm)	Dusky, violaceous, or brownish discoloration Bullae (serum filled or blood filled)	Anemia
Tachypnea (respiratory rate ≥ 20 breaths/min)	Generalized erythematous macular rash with or without desquamation	Thrombocytopenia with or without DIC
Toxic appearance	Exquisite tenderness out of proportion to the appearance of the affected area	Organ dysfunction (e.g., increased serum creatinine, increased hepatic transaminase)

Note: A patient who has a necrotizing soft tissue infection might also have limited clinical findings, and thus the history and clinical acumen will be of great value in helping to guide therapeutic interventions.
Abbreviations: DIC = disseminated intravascular coagulation; WBC = white blood cell count.

TABLE 3 Empiric Antimicrobial Therapy for Necrotizing Skin and Soft Tissue Infections

Pathogen(s)	Empiric Antimicrobial Therapy* First Line	Alternative[†]
Polymicrobial Aerobic or anaerobic gram-negative or gram-positive bacteria	Ticarcillin-clavulanate (Timentin) 3.1 g IV q6h or Piperacillin/tazobactam (Tazocin, Zosyn) 3.375 g IV q6h or Meropenem (Merrem) 1 g IV q8h or Imipenem-cilastatin (Primaxin) 500 mg IV q6h	Vancomycin (Vancocin) 1 g IV q12h plus a fluoroquinolone plus metronidazole (Flagyl) 500 mg IV q8h or Vancomycin 1 g IV q12h plus aztreonam (Azactam) 1 g IV q8h plus metronidazole 500 mg IV q8h or Ceftriaxone (Rocephin) 1 g IV q24h plus clindamycin (Dalacin, Cleocin) 600 mg q8h
Monomicrobial Group A streptococcus (S. pyogenes)	Penicillin G 4 million units IV q4h plus clindamycin 600-900 q4h plus mg IV q8h	Clindamycin 600-900 mg IV q8h
Clostridium perfringens, Clostridium septicum	Penicillin G 4 million units IV q4h plus clindamycin 600-900 mg IV q8h	Clindamycin 600-900 mg IV q8h or Metronidazole 500 mg PO or IV q8h
Aeromonas hydrophila	Ciprofloxacin (Cipro) 400 mg IV q12h or levofloxacin (Levaquin) 750 mg IV q24h	Trimethoprim-sulfamethoxazole (TMP/SMX, Septra, Bactrim)[1] 10 mg/kg/d (based on TMP) IV divided q6h or Ceftriaxone[1] 1 g IV q12h or Cefotaxime (Claforan)[1] 1 g IV q8h
Vibrio vulnificus	Minocycline (Minocin, Dynacin)[1] 100 mg IV q12h plus either ceftriaxone[1] 1 g IV q12h or cefotaxime[1] 1 g IV q8h	Ciprofloxacin (Cipro)1 400 mg IV q12h
Pseudomonas aeruginosa	Ciprofloxacin 400 mg IV q12h or Ceftazidime (Fortaz, Tazicef) 1 g IV q8h or Piperacillin-tazobactam 4.5 g IV q8h or Meropenem 1 g IV q8h	
Community-acquired methicillin-resistant Staphylococcus aureus	Vancomycin 1 g IV q12h	TMP/SMX[1] 10 mg/kg/d (based on TMP) IV divided q6h or Linezolid (Zyvox) 600 mg PO/IV q12h or Daptomycin (Cubicin) 4 mg/kg IV qd[‡]
Fungal Septated molds (e.g., Aspergillus spp, Fusarium spp, Scedosporium spp)	Amphotericin B deoxycholate (Fungizone) 1-1.5 mg/kg/d or Amphotericin B lipid-based formulations: Amphotericin B lipid complex (ABLC, Abelcet)[1] 5 mg/kg IV qd or Liposomal amphotericin B (L-AmB, AmBisome)[1] 5 mg/kg IV qd	Voriconazole (Vfend) 6 mg/kg IV q12h × 1 d, then 4 mg/kg IV q12h[‡]
Zygomycetes or mucormycosis	Amphotericin B deoxycholate 1-1.5 mg/kg/d or Amphotericin B lipid-based formulations: Amphotericin B lipid complex[1] 5 mg/kg IV qd or Liposomal amphotericin B[1] 5 mg/kg IV qd	Posaconazole (Noxafil) 200 mg PO qid[1,‡,§]

[1]Not FDA approved for this indication.
*The dosages of antimicrobial agents provided are based on normal renal function in adults weighing ≥70 kg and may need to be modified in patients with renal insufficiency. Drug serum levels should be monitored where appropriate.
[†]Alternative recommended regimens may be used in patients with a history of type 1 hypersensitivity reaction (anaphylaxis) to penicillin or other β-lactams. Other regimens with equivalent coverage are also appropriate.
[‡]Currently, there is a paucity of published clinical experience with these agents for necrotizing SSTIs.
[§]Posaconazole is available only orally.

Diagnosis

A key component in diagnosing a necrotizing SSTI is to clinically suspect it. Imaging modalities (e.g., plain radiographs, computed tomographic [CT] scans, magnetic resonance image [MRI] scans) may be useful to delineate the depth and extent of infection. However, the time required to obtain such investigations can lead to inappropriate delays in diagnostic and life-saving interventions. The most important diagnostic procedure in suspected cases is surgical exploration to determine the gross and microscopic appearance of the subcutaneous, fascial, and muscle layers. Hence, early surgical consultation is necessary. Specimens of the tissue itself (rather than a swab) should be sent for Gram stain and microbiological culture and susceptibility testing; these results will help in guiding management.

Treatment

Effective management of all forms of necrotizing SSTIs requires a combined surgical and medical approach. Early and aggressive débridement of gangrenous tissue is crucial. Repeated exploration

CURRENT DIAGNOSIS

- Appropriate diagnosis and management of a necrotizing skin and soft tissue infection (SSTI) require early clinical suspicion and a prompt comprehensive examination. Focus on the following:
  - Systemic evaluation: Presence of certain risk factors, hemodynamic instability, respiratory distress, toxic appearance, delirium
  - Local features: Rapidly progressive erythema or pain, pain out of proportion to appearance of infection, dermal necrosis, bullae, crepitus, undermining of the skin, and tissue planes that separate when a blunt probe is passed through openings in the skin
  - Key laboratory investigations: Hematologic derangement, organ failure, gas in the soft tissues
- Diagnosis is best established by prompt surgical assessment of the involved soft tissue for gross and microscopic evaluation. Tissue specimens should be sent for immediate Gram stain, culture, and susceptibility testing.

CURRENT THERAPY

- Expeditious and aggressive surgical débridement is mandatory; second look surgeries with repeated débridements are usually required.
- Broad-spectrum antimicrobial therapy covering aerobic and anaerobic gram-positive and gram-negative organisms should be initiated empirically. Once culture results are available, the antimicrobial regimen can be tailored.

and débridements are commonly necessary. Amputation is required in some cases.

Medical therapy consists of early initiation of appropriate antimicrobial therapy and supportive care (usually in an intensive care unit) (Table 3). In the case of STSIs, adjunctive therapy with intravenous immunoglobulin (IVIG, Baygam)[1] may be used. Because these infections may be difficult to treat, consultation with an infectious disease specialist is encouraged.

Because most necrotizing SSTIs are polymicrobial, it is usually most prudent to initiate broad-spectrum empiric antimicrobial therapy that covers the typical mixed aerobic and anaerobic flora of such infections. No single regimen is superior to others. Given the usual toxicity of such patients, intravenous therapy should be used, at least initially. In patients with a history of penicillin allergy, alternative regimens must be created that cover the same spectrum of pathogens (gram-positive, gram-negative, and anaerobic bacteria). Examples of recommended regimens are provided in the Current Therapy box.

Monomicrobial necrotizing SSTIs do not, in theory, require empiric broad-spectrum therapy. However, because it may be difficult to confidently predict either the monomicrobial nature of the infection on initial presentation or the specific single pathogen involved, it may be most prudent to administer broad-spectrum antibiotic coverage empirically. Once results of cultures and susceptibilities become available, the regimen can be focused on the isolated pathogen.

Fungal necrotizing SSTIs should be empirically treated with amphotericin B (either deoxycholate [Fungizone] or lipid-based formulation [Abelcet, AmBisome]), because this is currently the only antifungal agent with generally reliable coverage against septated molds and zygomycetes (although exceptions do occur). In addition, the underlying immunocompromised state, if possible, should be reversed (e.g., discontinue or decrease steroids and other immunosuppressive therapies).

Once the results of cultures and susceptibilities are available, the antimicrobial regimen can be tailored. The duration of antimicrobial therapy should be individualized.

REFERENCES

Bisno AL, Stevens DL: Streptococcal infections of skin and soft tissues. N Engl J Med 1996;334:240-245.
DiNubile MJ, Lipsky BA: Complicated infections of skin and skin structures: When the infection is more than skin deep. J Antimicrob Chemother 2004;53:37-50.
Ellis MW, JSLewis2nd: Treatment approaches for community-acquired methicillin-resistant *Staphylococcus aureus* infections. Curr Opin Infect Dis 2005;18:496-501.
Eron LJ, Lipsky BA, Low DE, et al: Managing skin and soft tissue infections: Expert panel recommendations on key decision points. J Antimicrob Chemother 2003;52:3-17.
Nichols RL, Florman S: Clinical presentations of soft-tissue infections and surgical site infections. Clin Infect Dis 2001;33(suppl 2):S84-S93.
Lipsky BA, Berendt AR, Deery HG, et al for the Infectious Disease Society of America: Diagnosis and treatment of diabetic foot infections. Clin Infect Dis 2004;39:885-910.
Stevens DL, Bisno AL, Chambers HF, et al for the Infectious Disease Society of America: Practice guidelines for the diagnosis and management of skin and soft-tissue infections. Clin Infect Dis 2005;41:1373-1406.
Vinh DC, Embil JM: Rapidly progressive soft tissue infections. Lancet Infect Dis 2005;5:501-513.
Vinh DC, Embil JM: Rapidly progressive soft tissue infections—Authors' reply. Lancet Infect Dis 2006;6:66-67.

Toxic Shock Syndrome

Method of
*Marty S. Teltscher, MD, CM, and
Andre Dascal, MD, FRCPC*

Initially reported as early as 1927 as *staphylococcal scarlet fever*, toxic shock syndrome (TSS) was defined by Todd and colleagues in 1978, and it was brought to the forefront of public concern in the early 1980s when healthy young women were contracting severe systemic illness associated with use of highly absorbent tampons. Reports of a similar syndrome involving invasive streptococcal disease soon followed in the late 1980s.

TSS is a rapidly progressive, potentially lethal toxin-mediated syndrome characterized by hyperpyrexia, erythrodermic rash, and multiorgan dysfunction. Original descriptions were attributed to toxin-producing strains of *Staphylococcus aureus* (SA-TSS) and the invasive group A β-hemolytic streptococcus *Streptococcus pyogenes* (GAS-TSS). There have been case reports of TSS associated with infection by groups B, C, and G β-hemolytic streptococci and with *Clostridium sordellii*.

---
[1]Not FDA approved for this indication.

Epidemiology

SA-TSS is categorized as either menstrual or nonmenstrual. Menstrual cases are defined as TSS occurring 2 days before menses or 2 days after menstruation. The vast majority of cases of menstrual SA-TSS were associated with tampon use, but it can occur during menses without tampon use. These cases demonstrate how noninvasive colonization by toxin-producing *S. aureus* can produce toxin-mediated disease. Nonmenstrual SA-TSS is associated with wound infections (surgical and nonsurgical), recalcitrant erythematous desquamating syndrome (mainly in the HIV/AIDS population), presence of foreign bodies (including intrauterine devices, diaphragms, tampons, nasal packing), burns, osteomyelitis, septic arthritis, post-influenza superinfection, and, increasingly, community-acquired methicillin-resistant *S. aureus* (CA-MRSA) infection.

Both forms of SA-TSS occur overwhelmingly in young women. Between 1979 and 1980, menstrual SA-TSS accounted for 91% of all TSS cases; surveillance through 1987 to 1996 noted a decline to 58% of cases. By the end of the 1980s, with change of tampon materials, removal of certain products from the market, and changes in patterns of tampon use, the incidence of SA-TSS diminished from 10 cases per 100,000 women of menstrual age to 1 case per 100,000 women.

In 2004, Schlievert and colleagues published data suggesting a reemergence of both menstrual and nonmenstrual cases of TSS, having observed the rate of 1 per 100,000 (in 2000) jump to nearly 4 per 100,000 by 2003. There was a concomitant 18% increase of all TSS reported by the Centers for Disease Control and Prevention (CDC). The reemergence of TSS is hypothesized to be associated with increased prevalence of CA-MRSA infection, earlier menarche, and a larger population of nonimmune menstruating women.

The case-fatality rate overall for SA-TSS was 3% between 1979 and 1980 and 5% between 1987 and 1996. Over the same time periods there was a marked decrease between case-fatality rates of menstrual cases from 5.5% to 1.8%; nonmenstrual rates remained relatively constant, diminishing only from 8.6% to 6%.

GAS-TSS most commonly occurs with GAS soft tissue infections such as cellulitis, necrotizing fasciitis, and myonecrosis. In up to 50% of cases, there is no identifiable portal of entry for GAS infection. Patients who develop GAS-TSS in the absence of invasive disease often develop an invasive infection over time. Because of the increasing frequency of invasive GAS infections, there are increased reports of GAS-TSS. GAS-TSS is estimated to have a prevalence of 1 to 5 cases per 100,000 persons. Risk factors include disruption of skin or mucosal barriers, diabetes, alcoholism, varicella infection, pregnancy, use of nonsteroidal anti-inflammatory medications (NSAIDs), immunocompromised state, recent surgery, and nonsurgical trauma. The morbidity and mortality rates for GAS-TSS are estimated at 30% to 80%.

Pathogenesis

Toxic shock syndrome is the culmination of an exaggerated inflammatory immune response by bacterial endotoxins and exotoxins belonging to the superantigen (SAG) superfamily. Biochemical and genetic analyses demonstrate that SAG proteins likely have common ancestry and are homologous in structure and function. SAGs complex with the class II major histocompatibility molecule on antigen-presenting cells and facilitate the cross-linking with the variable β region on the T cell αβ receptor without normal antigen processing and outside of the standard antigen-presenting groove. A normal T-cell response recruits 1 in 10,000 T lymphocytes, but a SAG can activate up to 20% of all T lymphocytes. The end result is a rapid cytokine storm from T lymphocytes, macrophages, and other immune cells involving release of tumor necrosis factor α (TNF-α), interleukin-1 (IL-1), IL-2, and interferon-γ (INF-γ). Clinical manifestations of this immunologic process include hyperpyrexia, capillary leak syndrome, vasodilation, myocardial suppression, hypotension, erythroderma, coagulopathy, acute renal failure, and ultimately multisystem organ failure and death.

The host's immune system and ability to respond to the infectious agent are also implicated in disease severity. Immunocompromised patients and persons with low antibody titers to the offending toxin are likely to develop more severe disease. Superantigens contribute to further immune dysfunction by disrupting the reticuloendothelial system; increasing host susceptibility to endotoxin, causing shock; deleting T-lymphocyte populations mediating humoral immunity; and disrupting cellular immunity through T-cell anergy and accelerated apoptosis.

SA-TSS was initially associated with toxic shock syndrome toxin-1 (TSST-1). Ninety percent of strains isolated from menstrual cases produce TSST-1. Highly absorbent tampons facilitated toxin production by optimizing conditions for *S. aureus* toxin production, namely elevated Po_2, elevated Pco_2, neutral pH, and elevated protein levels. TSST-1 easily crosses mucosal barriers. In nonmenstrual SA-TSS, TSST-1 is only implicated in 50% of cases; the culprit toxins in the other half of these cases are staphylococcal enterotoxins (SEs), most commonly SEB and SEC.

GAS-TSS is mediated by streptococcal pyrogenic exotoxins (SPEs) and streptococcal mitogenic exotoxin Z. In addition, the cell surface M protein, a filamentous protein conveying antiphagocytic properties, is a contributing virulence factor. M serotypes 1 and 3 are associated with invasive streptococcal disease; these, in addition to serotypes 12 and 28, are associated with GAS-TSS.

Diagnosis

Cases of TSS should be suspected in otherwise healthy persons presenting with rapidly progressing symptoms featuring fever,

---

CURRENT DIAGNOSIS

Common Clinical Features

- Fever, hypotension, and shock
- Multiorgan system dysfunction
- Diffuse macular erythroderma including the soles and palms
- Desquamation of soles and palms can occur in convalescent stages

Type-Specific Clinical Features

STAPHYLOCOCCAL TOXIC SHOCK SYNDROME

- History of current or recent menstruation
- Influenza-like prodrome
- Bacteremia in 5% of cases
- Microbiology: *Staphylococcus aureus* is isolated from the patient in 80% to 90% of cases but is not mandatory for diagnosis
- Serology: Lack of antibody to toxin at onset of illness is associated with severe illness
- Case fatality rate is 5%

STREPTOCOCCAL TOXIC SHOCK SYNDROME

- Presence of surgical or nonsurgical wound or foreign body
- Soft tissue infection, often invasive, including cellulitis, necrotizing fasciitis, or myonecrosis
- Dusky or gangrenous tissue carries a poor prognosis
- Bacteremia in 30%-60% cases
- Microbiology: Isolation of group A β-hemolytic streptococci
- Serology: Presence of antibody to toxin in convalescent stage confirmatory if initially absent
- Presence of anti-DNase B antibody and antistreptolysin O antibody are supportive
- Case fatality rate is 30%-80%

> **BOX 1 Case Definitions for *Staphylococcus aureus* Toxic Shock Syndrome**
>
> **Standard Definition**
>
> A definite case is an illness that meets 6 out of 6 original criteria. A probable case is an illness that meets 5 out of 6 criteria.
> - Fever: Temperature >38.9°C
> - Hypotension
>   - Systolic blood pressure <90 mm Hg
>   - Orthostatic drop in diastolic blood pressure >15 mm Hg
>   - Orthostatic syncope or dizziness
> - Rash: Diffuse macular erythroderma, often involving palms and soles
> - Desquamation 1-2 wk after onset, particularly on the palms and soles
> - Multisystem organ involvement (≥3)
>   - CNS: Disorientation or altered level of consciousness without focal neurologic signs when fever and hypotension are absent
>   - GI: Vomiting or diarrhea at onset of illness
>   - Hematologic: Platelet count <100,000/mm^3)
>   - Hepatic: Total bilirubin, ALT, or AST > twice the upper limit of normal
>   - Mucous membranes: Vaginal, oropharyngeal, or conjunctival hyperemia
>   - Muscular: Severe myalgia or CK > twice the upper limit of normal
>   - Renal: BUN or creatinine > twice the upper limit of normal or pyuria in the absence of UTI
> - Negative results of
>   - Blood, throat, or CSF cultures (blood cultures may be positive for *S. aureus*)
>   - Serologic tests for Rocky Mountain spotted fever, leptospirosis, or measles
>
> **Revised Definition**
>
> A revised definition seeks to incorporate laboratory findings confirming presence of an agent and susceptibility of the host.
> - Any of the following laboratory findings†
>   - Isolation of *S. aureus* from a mucosal or normally sterile site
>   - Production of TSS-associated SAG by isolate
>   - Lack of antibody to the implicated toxin at the time of acute illness
>   - Development of antibody to the toxin during convalescence
>
> *Abbreviations*: ALT = alanine aminotransferase; AST = aspartate aminotransferase; BUN = blood urea nitrogen; CK = creatine phosphokinase; CNS = central nervous system; CSF = cerebrospinal fluid; GI = gastrointestinal; SAG = superantigen; TSS = toxic shock syndrome; UTI = urinary tract infection.
> Standard definition adapted from Reingold AL, Hargrett NT, Shands KN, et al: Toxic shock syndrome surveillance in the United States, 1980 to 1981. Ann Intern Med 1982;96:875-880.
> Revised definition from Parsonnet J: Case definition of staphylococcal TSS: A proposed revision incorporating laboratory findings. In Arbuthnott J, Furman B (eds). European Conference on Toxic Shock Syndrome. International Congress and Symposium Series 229. London: Royal Society of Medicine Press, 1997.

> **BOX 2 Case Definitions for Group A Streptococcal Toxic Shock Syndrome**
>
> A definite case is an illness that meets criteria IA and IIA.
> A probable case is an illness that meets criteria IB and IIB.
>   I. Isolation of group A streptococcus
>   A. From a normally sterile site
>   B. From a nonsterile site
>   II. Clinical signs of severity
>   A. Systolic blood pressure <90 mm Hg
>   B. Multisystem organ involvement (2 of the following):
>   - Renal impairment: Creatinine >177 μmol/L or elevation > twice over baseline
>   - Coagulopathy: Platelets <100,000/mm^3 or DIC
>   - Liver involvement: Total bilirubin, AST, ALT > twice elevation or > twice upper limit of normal
>   - ARDS
>   - Generalized erythematous, macular rash that might desquamate
>   - Soft tissue necrosis, including necrotizing fasciitis, myositis, or gangrene
>
> *Abbreviations:* ALT= alanine aminotransferase; ARDS= acute respiratory distress syntrome; AST= aspartate aminotransferase; DIC= disseminated intravascular coagulation.
> Adapted from the Working Group on Severe GAS Infections: Defining the group A streptococcal toxic shock syndrome. JAMA 1993;269:390-391.

erythroderma, hypotension, and multiorgan dysfunction. Case definitions for SA-TSS and GAS-TSS are presented in Boxes 1 and 2, respectively.

Onset of SA-TSS occurs 2 to 3 days after surgery or onset of menses. Early manifestations include a diffuse red, macular rash that does not spare soles or palms. The rash might involve the mucosa. In some severe cases petechiae, ulcerations, vesicles, and bullae occur. During the convalescent phase of the illness, 1 to 2 weeks after onset of symptoms, a nonspecific maculopapular rash with desquamation of the palms and soles can occur.

A major review on the subject of TSS and superantigens in 2001 by McCormick and colleagues urges revision and modernization of the case definition by incorporating specific laboratory findings. The isolation of *S. aureus* from a mucosal or normally sterile site, production of TSS-associated SAG by isolated strains, lack of antibody to the implicated toxin at the time of acute illness, and development of antibody to the toxin during convalescence should contribute to the diagnosis of a likely case of SA-TSS. Although isolation of *S. aureus* from wounds and mucosal sites occurs in up to 90% of cases of SA-TSS, it is not required for the diagnosis. Bacteremia is present in only about 5% of cases.

In GAS-TSS, infection can begin within 1 to 3 days after a minor local trauma. Suspicions should be raised in cases with rapidly progressive localized or diffuse pain that might indicate invasive streptococcal soft tissue infection. Soft tissue disease is present in 80% of cases. Invasive disease is present in 50% of cases. Repeated meticulous physical examination is necessary to detect the manifestation of initially unidentified invasive soft tissue disease. An influenza-like prodrome occurs before toxic presentation in 20% of cases. Bacteremia is present in 60% of patients with GAS-TSS. Titers of antibody to DNase B and antistreptolysin O can be measured to confirm exposure to GAS.

The differential diagnosis of TSS includes septic shock, meningococcemia, Rocky Mountain spotted fever, scarlet fever, leptospirosis, ehrlichiosis, Kawasaki's disease, lupus erythematosus, measles, dengue fever, other viral exanthema, and adverse cutaneous drug eruption.

Treatment

Management of TSS requires early and definitive treatment. Critical care expertise early in the presentation of these patients is desirable. Treatment focuses on stabilizing the patient, eradicating the culprit organism, minimizing the toxin-mediated effects, and modulating the inflammatory immune response. Initial therapy includes large volumes of crystalloid intravenous fluids and vasopressor support to minimize hypotension-induced end-organ damage. Blood products may be required to reverse coagulopathies and anemia. Surgical intervention in both GAS-TSS and SA-TSS should not be overlooked because it may be critical for exploration of affected tissues, débridement of necrotic tissues, and removal of foreign bodies. Antibiotics contribute to the management by reducing the number of toxin-producing organisms (β-lactams and vancomycin [Vancocin]), as well as reducing production of toxin (clindamycin [Cleocin]) and possibly by modulating immune response (clindamycin).

ANTIBIOTICS

Antibiotics must be selected empirically, initially, and thereafter tailored to the specific resistance patterns of the organism. Penicillins and vancomycin should be appropriately adjusted for the degree of renal insufficiency. Patients who have allergies to β-lactams and therefore cannot take penicillins and cephalosporins should be treated with vancomycin. Macrolides are not recommended due to resistance patterns, despite their superiority to penicillin in vitro and in animal studies. Minimal data are available about the use of fluoroquinolones, quinpristin-dalfopristin (Synercid), and linezolide (Zyvox) in TSS.

Current recommendations for the treatment of SA-TSS include combination of a penicillinase-resistant penicillin such as oxacillin (Bactocill), nafcillin (Unipen), or cloxacillin (Cloxapen) (2 g IV q4h) and high-dose clindamycin (900 mg IV q8h). Due to increasing rates of toxin-producing CA-MRSA, the addition of vancomycin (2 g/day IV in divided doses) is advised until sensitivity to penicillinase-resistant penicillins is confirmed.

Current recommendations for the treatment of GAS-TSS include a combination of penicillin (4 million U q4h) and clindamycin (900 mg IV q8h). In severe GAS infections, ceftriaxone (Rocephin) (2 g IV q12h) should be considered. Although GAS is susceptible to penicillin, in large numbers of organisms the efficacy is reduced, likely due to reduction in the penicillin-targeted penicillin-binding proteins (PBPs) when GAS enters the stationary phase of growth. Ceftriaxone may have preferred activity, likely due to the increased expression of PBPs that it targets. Clindamycin affects protein synthesis rather than structural cell wall building factors, and the number of organisms has no bearing on efficacy.

ADJUNCTIVE THERAPY

Immunomodulatory Therapy

Adjunctive therapies include intravenous immunoglobulin (IVIg)[1] and other immunomodulators of the exaggerated inflammatory reaction initiated by toxic superantigens.

Although there are minimal clinical trial data available on the use of IVIg in TSS, there is anecdotal and in vitro evidence supporting its early administration. It has been shown that polyclonal commercially available IVIg binds and inactivates toxins that mediate TSS; however, there is variability in efficacy from brand to brand, as well as between batches within brands. In vitro studies have demonstrated increased potency of IVIg against GAS toxins as compared with *S. aureus* toxins, raising doubt about appropriate protective doses of IVIg. In a 2003 survey of infectious disease and critical care specialists across Canada, 76% of respondents reported that they would use IVIg in GAS-TSS, but only 26% would add it to therapy for SA-TSS.

In a recent clinical trial, a trend toward a protective effect of IVIg (Endobulin) (1.0 g/kg on day 1, 0.5 g/kg on days 2 and 3) was elucidated. However, this trial was underpowered and halted prior to completion due to lack of enrollment. It is theorized that IVIg is particularly useful early in disease manifestation to minimize the inflammatory reaction until definitive antibiotic therapy is initiated.

The use of IVIg is not without risk. There have been case reports of acute tubular necrosis, aseptic meningitis syndrome, central retinal vein obstruction, myocardial infarction, and thromboembolic diseases associated with IVIG use. Furthermore, patients with immunoglobulin A (IgA) deficiency can have severe anaphylactic reactions to IVIg infusion.

In summary, due to lack of unequivocal objective data, IVIg therapy remains controversial, but it may be reasonable for treating TSS, especially GAS-TSS. Further research and well-formulated large-scale clinical trials are necessary.

Immunomodulatory therapy focuses on inhibiting the signaling cascades induced by superantigens as well as the cytokines that are

---

CURRENT THERAPY

Initial Management

- Volume and crystalloid resuscitation
- Vasopressors and inotropic agents to support blood pressure as needed
- Correction of coagulopathy and anemia (frozen plasma, cryoprecipitate, and packed red blood cells)
- Initiation of appropriate antibiotic therapy
- Surgical consultation should be considered early in manifestation
- Critical care and infectious disease consultation

Staphylococcal Toxic Shock Syndrome

- Antibiotics
  - One penicillinase-resistant penicillin:
  - Oxacillin (Bactocill) 2 g IV q4h
  - Nafcillin (Unipen) 2 g IV q4h
  - Cloxacillin (Cloxapen) 2 g IV q4h*

plus

- Clindamycin (Cleocin) 900 mg IV q8h

plus

- Vancomycin (Vancocin) 2 g IV q12h†
- Adjust dose of penicillins and vancomycin for degree of renal dysfunction

Streptococcal Toxic Shock Syndrome

ANTIBIOTICS

- Penicillin 4 million U IV q4h

with or without

- Ceftriaxone (Rocephin) 2 g IV q12h

plus

- Clindamycin (Cleocin) 900 mg IV q8h
- Adjust dose of penicillins and vancomycin for degree of renal dysfunction

INTRAVENOUS IMMUNOGLOBULIN[1] (IVIG)

- 1.0 g/kg d 1, 0.5 g/kg d 2 and 3 of treatment
- Data are not sufficient to recommend IVIG in all cases
- May be beneficial in streptococcal toxic shock
- Reasonable in some severe cases of staphylococcal toxic shock
- Staphylococcal toxic shock may require higher doses

---

*Intravenous cloxacillin formulation is available only in Canada.
†The addition of vancomycin should be based on prevalence of community-acquired methicillin-resistant *S. aureus* in the patient's population. Discontinue if appropriate when sensitivities are known.
[1]Not FDA approved for this indication.

ultimately expressed. A combination of in vivo and in vitro data has been reported using a variety of agents demonstrating the effectiveness of suppressing SEB-mediated effects of TSS. Pentoxifylline (Trental)[1] is a TNF-α inhibitor that has been shown to dampen the inflammatory reaction, as has the corticosteroid dexamethasone (Decadron).[1] Other synthetic compounds and antibiotics have also been proposed. These therapies have not yet been approved for use in TSS, and inadequate data are available to recommend their use at this time.

Chemoprophylaxis

Chemoprophylaxis remains a controversial issue. The rate of secondary cases among close contacts of patients with invasive GAS disease is 200 times that of the general population. *Close contact* has been defined as persons spending more than 4 hours a day or 20 hours a week together, sharing sleeping arrangements, or having direct mucous membrane contact within 7 days of illness of the index patient.

In 1998, The CDC did not recommend antibiotic prophylaxis for all close contacts but rather individualization of prophylaxis for those exposed to patients with invasive GAS infection. The matter was revisited in a review in 2005 with a similar conclusion, stating that chemoprophylaxis was not warranted and that close contacts should be notified and urged to present for examination at the first signs of suspicious symptoms. Some public health authorities in Canada agree that close contacts should receive chemoprophylaxis with penicillin, first-generation cephalosporins, clindamycin, or erythromycin for 10 days. The official recommendations vary from province to province and depend on the type of invasive streptococcal disease.

The theoretical risks of empiric antibiotic use in the select few exposed to patients with this rare disease are probably negligible in the face of potentially new invasive GAS infections. Possible risks include antibiotic-associated diarrhea and *C. difficile* colitis.

REFERENCES

Darenberg J, Ihendyane N, Sjolin J, et al; the StreptIg Study Group: Intravenous immunoglobulin G therapy in streptococcal toxic shock syndrome: A European randomized, double-blind, placebo-controlled trial. Clin Infect Dis 2003;37:333-340.
Davies DH: Flesh-eating disease: A note on necrotizing fasciitis. Can J Infect Dis 2001;12:136-140.
Durand G, Bes M, Meugnier H, et al: Detection of new methicillin-resistant *Staphylococcus aureus* clones containing the toxic shock syndrome toxin 1 gene responsible for hospital- and community-acquired infections in France. J Clin Mircobiol 2006;44:847-853.
Gosbell IB: Epidemiology, clinical features and management of infections due to community methicillin-resistant *Staphylococcus aureus* (cMRSA). Intern Med J 2005;35:S120-S135.
Krakauer T: Chemotherapeutics targeting immune activation by staphylococcal superantigens. Med Sci Monit 2005;11(9):RA290-RA295.
Llewelyn M, Cohen J: Superantigens: Microbial agents that corrupt immunity. Lancet Infect Dis 2002;2:156-162.
McCormick JK, Yarwood JM, Schlievert PM: Toxic shock syndrome and bacterial superantigens: An update. Annu Rev Microbiol 2001;55:77-104.
Reingold AL, Hargrett NT, Shands KN, et al: Toxic shock syndrome surveillance in the United States, 1980 to 1981. Ann Intern Med 1982;96:875-880.
Schlievert PM: Use of intravenous immunoglobulin in the treatment of staphylococcal and streptococcal toxic shock syndromes and related illnesses. J Allergy Clin Immunol 2001;108:S107-S110.
Schlievert PM, Tripp TJ, Peterson ML: Reemergence of staphylococcal toxic shock syndrome in Minneapolis–St. Paul, Minnesota, during 2000-2003 surveillance period. J Clin Microbiol 2004;42:2875-2876. Correspondence and reply: Tierno PM: Reemergence of staphylococcal toxic shock syndrome in the United States since 2000. J Clin Microbiol 2005;43:2032-2033.
Smith A, Lamagni TL, Olivier I, et al: Invasive group A streptococcal disease: Should close contacts routinely receive antibiotic prophylaxis? Lancet Infect Dis 2005;5:494-500.
Stevens DL: The flesh-eating bacterium: What's next? J Infect Dis 1999;179:S366-S374.
Todd J, Fishaut M, Kapral F, Welch T: Toxic-shock syndrome associated with phage-group-I Staphylococci. Lancet 1978;2(8100):1116-1118.

---

[1]Not FDA for this indication.

Influenza

Method of
Jeffrey A. Linder, MD, MPH

Influenza is a highly contagious viral infection that should be considered in any patient with respiratory symptoms between October and May in North America. Influenza infects 5% to 20% of the population of the United States in a typical year and is responsible for up to 226,000 hospitalizations and 36,000 deaths per year. Influenza can range in severity from mild illness to life-threatening disease. Those at highest risk of hospitalization, death, or complications from influenza are children younger than 5 years, adults older than 65 years, adults older than 50 years who have underlying medical conditions, those infected with HIV, and pregnant women.

Information about influenza changes rapidly. To optimally care for patients with influenza-like illness during the influenza season, clinicians need to keep abreast of updated recommendations and the current prevalence of influenza in their community. The influenza vaccine remains the best means of reducing the incidence, severity, and complications from influenza, but antiviral medications and symptomatic treatments have an important role in the prevention and treatment of influenza as well (Box 1).

Microbiology

There are two types of influenza viruses, A and B. Influenza A is separated into subtypes based on two surface antigens: hemagglutinin (H) and neuraminidase (N). The predominant circulating strains of influenza in recent decades have been influenza A (H1N1), influenza A (H3N2), and influenza B. Influenza A (H3N2) subtypes generally cause more severe influenza and are associated with higher mortality than other types. Influenza viruses undergo slight genetic changes from year to year, termed *antigenic drift*. Major changes in surface glycoproteins are termed *antigenic shift* and can result in severe pandemic influenza in a nonimmune population. Because of antigenic drift and because immunity to a given type or subtype of influenza provides limited cross-immunity to other types and subtypes, the influenza vaccine needs to be reformulated and administered each year.

Patients contract influenza by being exposed to large-sized respiratory droplets from an infected person or contact with surfaces harboring influenza virus. Influenza has a latency of 1 to 4 days before the onset of symptoms. Adults are infectious from the day before symptom onset through about day 5 of illness, but immunosuppressed adults and children shed virus for longer periods. Symptoms generally last from 7 to 14 days.

Highly pathogenic influenza A (H5N1), also called *avian influenza*, spreads rapidly among birds and has very high mortality. To date, there have been several hundred cases of influenza A (H5N1) among humans, with about 60% mortality. Influenza A (H5N1), if it acquires the ability to be highly transmissible among humans, is a threat to cause pandemic influenza.

Prevention

Influenza vaccination is between 30% and 90% effective in preventing influenza or complications of influenza. Influenza vaccination is highly cost-effective and can even be cost-saving in high-risk groups. Influenza vaccination is less effective in younger children, in adults older than 65 years, in adults with comorbid conditions, and if there is a poor match between the influenza vaccine and circulating influenza. The Centers for Disease Control and Prevention's (CDC) Advisory Committee on Immunization Practices puts out annual recommendations and supplementary updates on the prevention and treatment of influenza (www.cdc.gov/flu). At present, there are two types of influenza

> **BOX 1 Persons for Whom Annual Influenza Vaccination Is Recommended**
>
> All persons who want to reduce the risk of becoming ill with influenza or of transmitting influenza to others
> All children aged 6 months to 18 years—especially 6 months to 4 years old—and adults 50 years old and older
> Children and adolescents receiving long-term aspirin therapy who might therefore be at risk for experiencing Reye's syndrome after influenza virus infection
> Women who will be pregnant during the influenza season
> Adults and children who have chronic pulmonary (including asthma), cardiovascular (except hypertension), renal, hepatic, hematologic, or metabolic disorders (including diabetes)
> Adults and children who have immunosuppression (e.g., from medications or HIV)
> Adults and children who have any condition that can compromise respiratory function or the handling of secretions or that can increase the risk of aspiration
> Residents of nursing homes and other chronic-care facilities
> Health care workers
> Healthy household contacts and caregivers of children ages 0 to 4 years and adults aged 50 years and older, with particular emphasis on vaccinating contacts of children younger than 6 months old
> Healthy household contacts and caregivers of persons with medical conditions that put them at higher risk for severe complications from influenza
>
> ---
>
> Adapted from Centers for Disease Control and Prevention: Prevention and control of influenza: Recommendations of the Advisory Committee on Immunization Practices (ACIP), 2008. MMWR 2008;57(RR-7):1-60.

vaccine: the trivalent inactivated vaccine (TIV) and the live, attenuated influenza vaccine (LAIV).

The TIV (Fluzone, Fluvirin, Fluarix, FluLaval, Afluria) is administered as an intramuscular injection. The main adverse effect of the TIV is soreness at the injection site. Patients often report a mild immune response of fever, malaise, myalgia, and headache that can last for 1 to 2 days, but rates of most of these symptoms are no different from those who receive placebo injection. The TIV should not be administered to patients with egg allergies. Allergic reactions to egg proteins or other vaccine components (e.g., antibiotics and inactivating compounds) include angioedema, hives, asthma, and anaphylaxis. Vaccination should be deferred in patients with acute febrile illness, but patients with more moderate illness can be vaccinated. Guillain–Barré syndrome was associated with the 1976 swine flu vaccine, but there is no consistent evidence that modern influenza vaccines are associated with Guillain–Barré syndrome.

The LAIV (FluMist) is administered as a nasal spray and is approved for patients ages 2 to 49 years. The LAIV is contraindicated in children with recurrent wheezing, in patients with comorbid conditions, in pregnant women, and in family members or close contacts of severely immunosuppressed patients who require a protected environment (e.g., hematopoetic stem cell transplant recipients). The LAIV should not be administered to those with severe nasal congestion. Adverse effects of the LAIV include runny nose, nasal congestion, headache, sore throat, chills, and tiredness, although these are only slightly more common than in patients receiving placebo. Those receiving the LAIV should avoid contact with severely immunosuppressed persons for 7 days.

Patients should begin to be vaccinated in the fall when the seasonal vaccine becomes available, generally starting in October. In the event of vaccine shortages, higher-risk patients should receive priority. Patients should continue to be vaccinated until February and beyond because in the majority of recent influenza seasons, the peak has been February or later. Children 6 months to 8 years of age who have not been previously immunized against influenza should be given two doses separated by at least 4 weeks for both vaccines.

Evaluation

COMMUNITY PREVALENCE OF INFLUENZA

In caring for a patient with suspected influenza, the single most important piece of data is the community prevalence of influenza among patients with influenza-like illness. This ranges from near 0% during summer months to about 30% during a typical influenza seasonal peak. The prevalence may be higher during a particularly severe outbreak. Clinicians can check the local prevalence of influenza among patients with influenza-like illness through the CDC (www.cdc.gov/flu) and their state department of public health.

HISTORY AND PHYSICAL EXAMINATION

Beyond the local prevalence of influenza, the diagnosis of influenza rests on the patient's history. All methods of diagnosing influenza—symptom complexes, clinician judgment, and testing—generally are highly specific but have poor sensitivity. Thus, it is important to consider a diagnosis of influenza in any patient with respiratory symptoms during influenza season. Influenza is classically described as the very sudden onset of fever, headache, sore throat, myalgias, cough, and nasal symptoms. Children can also have otitis media, nausea, and vomiting. In differentiating influenza from nonspecific upper respiratory tract infections, it is most useful to consider the circulating prevalence of influenza, the abruptness of onset, and the severity of symptoms.

Certain symptom complexes have been shown in trials of antiviral treatment to strongly suggest influenza. For example, in an area with circulating influenza, the acute onset of cough and fever can have a positive predictive value as high as 85%. Similarly, several clinical trials found patients likely to have influenza while influenza was circulating if patients had symptoms for 48 hours or less, subjective fevers, or a measured temperature of at least 100.5°F, and any two symptoms of headache, cough, sore throat, or myalgias. Other studies, outside of clinical trials, have shown that clinician judgment performed as well as or better than hard-and-fast symptom complexes or rapid testing.

The physical examination in influenza primarily serves to identify the severity of influenza, complications, and worsening of underlying medical conditions. Clinicians should record vital signs and perform examinations of the ears, nose, sinuses, throat, neck, lungs, and heart for all patients suspected to have influenza.

TESTING

Rapid influenza test kits can provide a point-of-care result in about 30 minutes and are available as nasopharyngeal swabs, nasal washes, and nasal aspirates. All forms of rapid testing have a sensitivity of about 70% and are more than 90% specific. Testing is likely most useful when there is an intermediate probability of influenza (e.g., a community prevalence of influenza among patients with influenza-like illness of 10%-30%), and patients have an intermediate probability of complications from influenza. If circulating prevalence of influenza is low (e.g., <10%), testing is unlikely to be positive and is not necessary. If the circulating prevalence of influenza is high (e.g., <30%), the relatively low sensitivity of rapid tests makes the risk of a false-negative test unacceptably high. In the event of a high prevalence of influenza or a high risk of complications from influenza, empiric antiviral treatment is indicated. Testing may be particularly helpful for hospitalized patients to rule out a need for antibiotics. Chest radiography, cultures, and blood tests are not routinely indicated, but they should be obtained for patients with suspected pneumonia or to identify other suspected complications.

Complications

Complications of influenza include primary complications, suppurative complications, and worsening of comorbid conditions. Primary complications of influenza include viral pneumonia, which is a feared complication and is likely a main cause of mortality in pandemic influenza. Other, less common primary complications of influenza include myositis and rhabdomyolysis, Reye's syndrome, myocarditis, pericarditis, toxic shock syndrome, and central nervous system disease (e.g., encephalitis, transverse myelitis, and aseptic meningitis). Children can have a severe course with influenza, including signs and symptoms of sepsis along with febrile seizures. Suppurative complications of influenza include bacterial pneumonia, otitis media, and sinusitis. Influenza can cause worsening of comorbid conditions like asthma, chronic obstructive pulmonary disease, congestive heart failure, and chronic kidney disease.

Chemoprophylaxis

Antiviral medications can be used to prevent influenza in patients who did not receive the influenza vaccine, cannot receive the influenza vaccine, received the vaccine in the prior 2 weeks (before reliable immunity develops) or in the event of poor matching between vaccine and circulating influenza strains (Table 1). Chemoprophylaxis should also be considered for close contacts of patients with confirmed influenza or for patients with immune deficiency who are unlikely to respond to the influenza vaccine but who are at high risk for having complications from influenza.

Amantadine (Symmetrel) and rimantadine (Flumadine) are no longer recommended for chemoprophylaxis or treatment because of a high prevalence of resistant influenza A strains. The neuraminidase inhibitors oseltamivir (Tamiflu) and zanamivir (Relenza) are about 80% effective in preventing influenza in household contacts of persons with influenza and more than 90% effective in preventing influenza in institutional settings. Chemoprophylaxis should be taken for a minimum of 2 weeks or until 1 week after the end of an outbreak. For patients allergic to or unable to respond to the vaccine, chemoprophylaxis should be used for the duration of circulating influenza. The TIV can be given to patients receiving chemoprophylaxis. The LAIV should not be given from 2 days before to 14 days after taking an antiviral medication. Patients

CURRENT DIAGNOSIS

- Influenza should be considered in any patient with respiratory symptoms between October and May in North America.
- The single most important piece of information when considering a diagnosis of influenza is the community prevalence of influenza.
- During outbreaks, sudden onset of fever and cough has a positive predictive value of about 85%.
- Rapid testing should be used when the community prevalence of influenza among patients with influenza-like illness is between 10% and 30%.

who receive the LAIV in this window should be revaccinated at a later date.

Treatment

The influenza vaccine is the best means of reducing influenza-related morbidity and mortality, but its limitations include production problems, low vaccination rates, and the variable effectiveness of the vaccine itself. Given these limitations, there is an important role in management for influenza-specific antiviral medications (see Table 1). Antiviral medications reduce the duration of influenza symptoms by 1 to 2 days, reduce complications requiring antibiotics by 30% to 40%, might decrease hospitalizations and mortality, and are cost-effective.

The neuraminidase inhibitors zanamivir and oseltamivir are recommended for treating influenza. Again, amantadine and rimantadine are no longer recommended for the treatment of influenza because of a high prevalence of resistant of influenza A strains. Zanamivir is taken as an oral inhaled powder and is not recommended for patients with underlying lung or heart disease. Adverse effects of zanamivir include worsening of underlying lung disease and allergic reactions. Oseltamivir is taken as a capsule or oral suspension. The dose of oseltamivir should be reduced in patients with renal disease. Adverse effects of oseltamivir include nausea, vomiting, and, extremely rarely, behavioral changes.

Antibiotics are generally not necessary, but they should be prescribed to treat suppurative complications of influenza. Antitussives such as guaifenesin with codeine (Robitussin AC) help coughing

TABLE 1 Antiviral Agents for the Treatment and Prophylaxis of Influenza

Antiviral Agent	Treatment* Children	Treatment* Adults	Prophylaxis† Children	Prophylaxis† Adults	Comments
Oseltamivir (Tamiflu)	Approved for children ≥ 1 y Dose for 5 d bid: ≤ 15 kg: 30 mg 16-23 kg: 45 mg 24-40 kg: 60 mg > 40: 75 mg	75 mg bid for 5 d	Approved for children ≥ 1 y Dose qd: ≤ 15 kg: 30 mg 16-23 kg: 45 mg 24-40 kg: 60 mg > 40: 75 mg	75 mg qd	For patients with creatinine clearance < 30 mL/min, oseltamivir dosing should be reduced to qd for treatment and to qod for prophylaxis
Zanamivir (Relenza)	Approved for children ≥ 7 y 10 mg (2 inhalations) bid for 5 d	10 mg (2 inhalations) bid for 5 d	Approved for children ≥ 5 y 10 mg (2 inhalations) qd	10 mg (2 inhalations) qd	

*Treatment must be started within the first 48 hours of symptoms.
†Prophylaxis should be given for at least 2 weeks or until 1 week after the end of an outbreak.
Adapted from Centers for Disease Control and Prevention: Prevention and control of influenza: Recommendations of the Advisory Committee on Immunization Practices (ACIP), 2008. MMWR 2008;57(RR-7):1-60.

CURRENT THERAPY

- The influenza vaccine is the best means of preventing influenza. The trivalent inactivated influenza vaccine is recommended for health care workers, children aged 6 months to 4 years, all persons 50 years old and older, and patients with chronic conditions.
- The antivirals zanamivir (Relenza) and oseltamivir (Tamiflu) can be used for prophylaxis of influenza in unimmunized patients, in close contacts of infected patients, and during institutional outbreaks of influenza.
- Zanamivir and oseltamivir can be used to treat influenza, but they must be started within 48 hours of onset of symptoms.

patients sleep at night. β-Agonists, such as albuterol (Proventil),[1] can help patients with cough, especially if there is wheezing on examination. Analgesics and antipyretics like acetaminophen (Tylenol) and ibuprofen (Motrin) reduce fever and generally help patients feel better. Patients should be encouraged to rest and drink plenty of fluids. Patients with suspected influenza should minimize contact with others to avoid spreading the infection.

[1]Not FDA approved for this indication.

REFERENCES

Centers for Disease Control and Prevention: Prevention and control of influenza: Recommendations of the Advisory Committee on Immunization Practices (ACIP), 2008. MMWR 2008;57(RR-7):1-60.
Cooper NJ, Sutton AJ, Abrams KR, et al: Effectiveness of neuraminidase inhibitors in treatment and prevention of influenza A and B: Systematic review and meta-analyses of randomised controlled trials. BMJ 2003;326(7401):1235.
Falsey AR, Murata Y, Walsh EE: Impact of rapid diagnosis on management of adults hospitalized with influenza. Arch Intern Med 2007;167(4):354-360.
Rothberg MB, Bellantonio S, Rose DN: Management of influenza in adults older than 65 years of age: Cost-effectiveness of rapid testing and antiviral therapy. Ann Intern Med 2003;139:321-329.
Stein J, Louie J, Flanders S, et al: Performance characteristics of clinical diagnosis, a clinical decision rule, and a rapid influenza test in the detection of influenza infection in a community sample of adults. Ann Emerg Med 2005;46(5):412-419.

Leishmaniasis

Method of
Karim Aoun, MD, and Aida Bouratbine, MD

Leishmaniasis is a worldwide vector-borne disease caused by protozoan flagellates of the genus *Leishmania*. Metacyclic infective stages of these parasites are transmitted to humans and other mammalian hosts through the bites of sand flies belonging to the genus *Phlebotomus* in the Old World and *Lutzomyia* in the New World. Around 20 *Leishmania* species are anthropophilic and responsible for pathologic disorders ranging from localized cutaneous lesions to disseminated visceral leishmaniasis. The species is identified by parasite isoenzyme analysis or polymerase chain reaction (PCR) amplification of *Leishmania* DNA. Because no vaccine is available, many treatments are suggested for leishmaniasis without any definitive evidence. Treatment methods depend mainly on the clinical features, the involved species, the patient's immune status, the availability of effective drugs, and patients' access to health care.

Pathogenesis

After a person is inoculated by sand fly bites, metacyclic promastigotes enter dermal mononuclear phagocytes and change into intracellular amastigotes. According to their tropism and their interaction with the host immune response, species can disseminate to different organs and determine the clinical expression of the infection. In cases of localized cutaneous lesions, parasites remain restricted to the initial injection sites by a strong cell-mediated inflammatory reaction.

Diffuse cutaneous leishmaniasis results from a large dissemination from the initial lesion to other skin sites because of the motility of the infected dermal macrophages. The parasite's spread is related to an insufficient cell-mediated immune response that is observed with *L. aethiopica*, *L. mexicana*, and *L. amazonensis* and in immunocompromised patients.

Visceral leishmaniasis is caused by *L. donovani* and *L. infantum*, which can induce spread of the parasites following the mononuclear phagocyte system route. All viscera are invaded, but spread is mainly to the spleen, the bone marrow, and the lymph nodes.

Mucocutaneous leishmaniasis is the result of an oronasal mucosa metastasis of some New World species, mainly *L. braziliensis*. The secondary local lesions can be delayed for a long time after the primary cutaneous ones, even if these original lesions are cured. The factors enabling that dissemination are not yet well understood.

Epidemiology

Leishmaniasis is observed in tropical and temperate-climate regions where the weather is optimal for the life cycle of sand flies. More than 350 million people are exposed in endemic areas. Because of their high incidence and large geographic distribution, visceral leishmaniasis and localized cutaneous lesions are the most relevant forms. The estimated incidence of all forms of leishmaniasis is 2 million new cases per year, of which about 0.5 million are visceral leishmaniasis and about 1.5 million are localized cutaneous. Mucocutaneous and diffuse cutaneous leishmaniasis are more rarely observed.

VISCERAL LEISHMANIASIS

Visceral leishmaniasis, also called *kala-azar*, is endemic in the Indian subcontinent, East Africa, the Mediterranean basin, the Middle East, and South America. Ninety percent of new cases are identified in just five countries: India, Bangladesh, Nepal, Sudan, and Brazil. India harbors the highest burden of leishmaniasis in the world, and around 90% of reported cases occur in Bihar.

In the Indian subcontinent and East Africa, visceral leishmaniasis is caused by *L. donovani*. The predominant mode of transmission is anthroponotic, and the major reservoir for ongoing transmission is constituted by humans with kala-azar or post–kala-azar dermal leishmanoid. In these areas, poverty, poor health care, military conflicts, and population movements contribute to irregular and incomplete treatment courses of visceral leishmaniasis, leading to rapid development of drug-resistant parasites.

In the Mediterranean, the Middle East, and Brazil, the disease caused by *L. infantum* is zoonotic. The domestic dog is the reservoir host, and human cases occur mostly in children or immunocompromised adults.

CUTANEOUS LEISHMANIASIS

Based on its geographic distribution, cutaneous leishmaniasis can be divided into Old World (including southern Europe, the Middle East, parts of southwest Asia, and Africa) and New World (Central and South America) leishmaniasis. Afghanistan, Algeria, Brazil, Iran, Peru, Saudi Arabia, and Sudan account for 90% of cutaneous leishmaniasis cases.

Cutaneous leishmaniasis is caused by various *Leishmania* species and involves a broad spectrum of reservoir hosts. In the Old World, *L. tropica* and *L. major* are the most common species.

Mucocutaneous leishmaniasis is restricted to South America. It is sporadic and is subject to variation according to the region. Mucocutaneous leishmaniasis is mainly attributed to *L. braziliensis*, but cases caused by *L. panamensis*, *L. guyanensis*, and *L. amazonensis* have been described.

Most of the exceptional cases of diffuse cutaneous leishmaniasis are observed in East Africa and Central and South America, where *L. aethiopica*, *L. mexicana*, and *L. amazonensis* are endemic. Diffuse cutaneous leishmaniasis occurs elsewhere with other dermotropic species in immunocompromised patients.

Clinical Features

Clinical symptoms of leishmaniasis appear following an incubation period varying from weeks to months after the infective sand fly bite. The common symptoms of visceral leishmaniasis, either in children or in adults, are fever, hepatosplenic enlargement, anemia, weight loss, and blood cytopenia. Unusual involvement of the lung or the digestive tract is reported in immunocompromised patients. If diagnosis is not established early and appropriate treatment is not given, the infection is uniformly fatal. The mortality number for visceral leishmaniasis is about 60,000 each year.

The typical localized cutaneous lesion starts as an erythematous papule of few millimeters in diameter that gradually expands and ulcerates. The lesions are single or multiple and affect uncovered parts of the body. Both wet and dry types are observed. Regression of localized cutaneous lesions is spontaneous within months to years, leaving depressed and usually disfiguring scars.

Old World species mostly cause benign and often self-limited cutaneous disease, but New World species cause a broad spectrum of conditions from benign to severe manifestations, including mucosal involvement. Tissues of the nose and the mouth are the most invaded during mucocutaneous leishmaniasis. Lesions consist of a long-lasting infiltration and erosion of mucosa that are not self-healing. Bacterial superinfection or obstruction of the airways or the digestive tract can complicate the course and cause death. Lesions of diffuse cutaneous leishmaniasis are disseminated and remain for a long time. They are nodular and nonulcerative, resembling those in lepromatous leprosy.

Treatment

PHARMACOLOGIC THERAPY

Pentavalent Antimonials

Pentavalent antimonials (Sb) meglumine antimoniate (Glucantime, Prostib)[2] for IM administration and sodium stibogluconate (Pentostam, Solustibosan, Stibanate)[10] for IV or IM administration have been the first-line drugs for treating all forms of leishmaniasis since 1940. Their respective Sb contents are 85 mg/mL and 100 mg/mL. Recently, studies comparing efficiency of generics with branded products established the worth of generics in terms of efficacy and safety in visceral leishmaniasis and cutaneous leishmaniasis.

The main target for Sb is the alteration of the bioenergetics mechanisms of the parasites. Pentavalent antimonials have many side effects, which include intolerance (fever, myalgias, arthralgias,

---
[2]Not available in the United States.
[10]Available in the United States from the Centers for Disease Control and Prevention.

 CURRENT THERAPY

Visceral Leishmaniasis
- Pentavalent antimonials (Glucantime,[2] Pentostam[10]): 20 mg Sb/kg/d for 28 d
- Amphotericin B (Fungizone): 0.75-1 mg/kg/d IV for 15-20 d
- Liposomal amphotericin B (AmBisome): Total dose of 18-20 mg (2 × 10 mg/kg/d or 3 mg × 6 (d 1 to 5 and d 10)
- Immunocompromised (HIV) patients: Secondary prophylaxis every 2-4 wk after cure

Mucocutaneous Leishmaniasis
- Pentavalent antimonials: 20 mg Sb/kg/d for 28 d
- Amphotericin B: 0.75-1 mg/kg/d IV for 15-20 d

Cutaneous Leishmaniasis

NEW WORLD
- Pentavalent antimonials: 20 mg Sb/kg/d IM for 20 d
- Pentamidine (Pentacarinat):[1] 3 mg/d IM for four injections (infection from French Guyana)

OLD WORLD
- 15% Paromomycin ointment (Humatin):[1,5-6] twice daily for 2-4 wk
- Pentavalent antimonials: 2 to 10 local infiltrations or 20 mg Sb/kg/d IM for 20 d
- Therapeutic abstention

OTHER
- Ketoconazole (Nizoral):[1] 600 mg/d for 28 d (*L. mexicana*)
- Fluconazole (Diflucan):[1] 200 mg/d for 6 wk (*L. major*)

---
[1]Not FDA approved for this indication.
[2]Not available in the United States.
[5]Investigational drug in the United States.
[6]May be compounded by pharmacists.
[10]Available in the United States from the Centers for Disease Control and Prevention.

---

abdominal pain) and toxic disorders that could be cardiac, renal, hematologic, or pancreatic.

The dose of Sb recommended by the World Health Organization (WHO) is 20 mg/kg/day for 28 days in fresh cases of visceral leishmaniasis, double duration (40-60 days) in relapse cases, and 20 mg/kg/day for 20 days for cutaneous leishmaniasis.

Resistance is still observed, mainly in Bihar, where leishmaniasis is hyperendemic; in Bihar, 40% to 60% of visceral leishmaniasis cases are unresponsive to Sb. In vitro studies conducted there have shown that *L. donovani* strains from nonresponder patients required five times the concentration of Sb as responders required to kill parasites.

The optimal duration of treatment with the dose of 20 mg/kg/day in cutaneous leishmaniasis is still debated. Some authors consider a 10-day course of treatment sufficient, but some studies indicate a clear positive correlation between treatment duration and efficacy.

Intralesional treatment of cutaneous leishmaniasis with Sb produces the maximum concentration in the lesions and has fewer side effects, but it does not reach metastatic localizations caused by New World species. The basic aim is to fill the infected part of the dermis. This requires carefully infiltrating the area around the lesion, including the base of the lesion, until the surface has blanched. Treatment should be given every 5 to 7 days for a total of two to ten treatments.

Amphotericin B

Amphotericin B (AmpB) was originally developed as a systemic antifungal. Amphotericin B deoxycholate (Fungizone) has proven antileishmanial activity. Its activity was attributed to its selective affinity for ergosterol-like sterols, which are abundant in the membranes of *Leishmania* species. To address the increasing Sb unresponsiveness of visceral leishmaniasis in India, AmpB has been used successfully at a dosage of 0.75 to 1 mg/kg for 15 to 20 infusions administered either daily or on alternate days. However, the major limiting factors include an almost universal occurrence of infusion-based reactions including high fever with rigor and chills, thrombophlebitis, and occasional serious toxicities such as myocarditis, severe hypokalemia, renal dysfunction, and death.

Lipid Formulations of Amphotericin B

Toxic effects of AmpB deoxycholate have been largely reduced with the advent of lipid formulations. In these compounds, deoxycholate has been replaced by lipids that mask AmpB from susceptible tissues, targeting its delivery to parasitized cells. This minimizes toxicity and emphasizes activity.

Three formulations are commercially available: liposomal AmpB (AmBisome); AmpB lipid complex (Abelcet), and AmpB colloidal dispersion (Amphocil, Amphotec).[1] Liposomal AmpB was the first one evaluated and is licensed in several European countries and the United States for treating visceral leishmaniasis. A total dose of 20 mg/kg is adequate to treat immunocompetent children and adults. The exact dosage schedule can be flexible and divided into doses of 10 mg/kg on two consecutive days or in smaller doses (3 mg/kg from the first to the fifth days then 3 mg/kg on the 10th day). However, liposomal AmpB pharmacokinetics suggests that an initial dose of at least 5 mg/kg will provide a better tissue level. The high cost of liposomal AmpB is the principal dose-limiting factor. Thus, the main purpose of recent clinical trials in India was to determine its lowest total dose with acceptable efficacy for Indian visceral leishmaniasis.

In patients with severe immunosuppression, relapse rates after treatment with Sb or liposomal AmpB are extremely high. However, because liposomal AmpB is less toxic, most clinicians consider it the antileishmanial drug of choice in patients coinfected with visceral leishmaniasis and HIV. Lipid AmpB has also been used successfully to treat cutaneous leishmaniasis in immunocompromised patients and children. However, because cutaneous leishmaniasis is usually a self-limited infection, the treatment cost appears to be disproportionate.

Miltefosine

Miltefosine (Miltex, Impavido),[5] a phospholipid-derived hexadecyl-phosphocholine, was initially developed as an anticancer drug and is the first effective oral treatment for visceral leishmaniasis. Miltefosine induces modulation of cell surface receptors, inositol metabolism, phospholipase activation, and protein kinase C and other mitogenic pathways, culminating in apoptosis.

Its use is limited by gastrointestinal disturbances and renal toxicity, which are fortunately reversible. It is also teratogenic, so it is contraindicated in pregnancy.

Its prolonged half-life (6-7 days) might allow the emergence of resistance and relapses when it is used as monotherapy. In vitro studies have shown that miltefosine-resistant lines of *L. donovani* promastigotes can be selected.

In many trials, miltefosine firmly established itself as a clinically effective antileishmanial compound in India. The recommended dose in India is 2.5 mg/kg/day for 28 days for patients 2 years and older. Concerning cutaneous leishmaniasis, the results of an uncontrolled trial in Colombia (phase I/II) are promising. However, further controlled studies with various species are needed before miltefosine can be proposed as a routine treatment for cutaneous leishmaniasis.

Paromomycin (Humatin)

Paromomycin (identical to aminosidine) is an aminoglycoside that possesses antibacterial and antiprotozoal activity. It remained neglected until the 1980s, when topical formulations[6] were found to be effective in cutaneous leishmaniasis and a parenteral formulation[5] for visceral leishmaniasis was developed.

Action of paromomycin has been linked to the inhibition of cytochrome C reduction. However, mechanisms specific to *Leishmania* require further elucidation.

A resistance to paromomycin has been induced experimentally in vitro in *L. donovani* promastigotes. Development of the parenteral formulation of paromomycin for visceral leishmaniasis was slow, but phase III trials are currently under way in India. Preliminary analysis suggested an efficacy equal to that of other licensed drugs and an excellent tolerability.

As an ointment for topical use,[6] paromomycin has been tested in different formulations. The combination of paromomycin with methylbenzethonium appears to be more effective, but it causes local inflammatory reactions. A 15% paromomycin–methylbenzethonium chloride ointment[6] was applied with success in New World cutaneous leishmaniasis caused by *L. mexicana* and *L. panamensis* and Old World cutaneous leishmaniasis caused by *L. major*. A lack of efficacy is related to a variability of the response depending on the species involved (*L. tropica* in the Old World) and the type of lesion being treated (lesions with epithelial thickness). Topical formulations offer significant advantages over systemic therapy, such as easier drug use, fewer adverse effects, and lower cost.

Azoles

Azoles, including ketoconazole (Nizoral),[1] fluconazole (Diflucan),[1] and itraconazole (Sporanox),[1] are essentially sterol biosynthesis inhibitors. They specifically block ergosterol synthesis, a membrane component of fungi and *Leishmania* species. They have the advantage of oral administration and few adverse effects, but they are only effective against some species. Most trials were conducted on cutaneous leishmaniasis.

Ketoconazole 600 mg daily for 28 days is effective against *L. mexicana* leishmaniasis. Fluconazole 200 mg daily for 6 weeks shows promising results in *L. major* leishmaniasis.

Pentamidine (Pentacarinat)

Pentamidine is an aromatic diamidine. Its leishmanicidal activity has not been yet assessed. It might act on polyamine biosynthesis and mitochondrial potential.

Pentamidine was extensively used as a second-line drug for Sb-unresponsive visceral leishmaniasis in Bihar from the 1970s until 2003. Because of its declining efficacy and its unacceptable toxicity, including irreversible insulin-dependent diabetes mellitus, its use has been abandoned.

The isothionate salt of pentamidine (Pentacarinat) is the only formulation available for cutaneous leishmaniasis. It is used as the first-line treatment for cutaneous leishmaniasis in French Guyana, where *L. guyanensis* is responsible for more than 90% of the cases. Pentamidine is recommended as a short-course, low-dose regimen of four injections containing 3 mg/kg/day every other day. At this dosage, no cases of new diabetes mellitus were observed.

Sitamaquine (WR 6026)

Another oral drug that might be effective against visceral leishmaniasis is the 8-aminoquinoline derivative sitamaquine, which is currently in development. The common adverse events observed were vomiting, dyspepsia, cyanosis, and nephrotoxicity. Further clinical trials need to be done to assess its safety before it can be used in combination therapy with other antileishmanial agents.

---

[1] Not FDA approved for this indication.
[5] Investigational drug in the United States.

[1] Not FDA approved for this indication.
[5] Investigational drug in the United States.
[6] May be compounded by pharmacists.

Imiquimod (Aldara)

Imiquimod is an antiviral compound used extensively for the topical treatment of genital warts caused by human papillomavirus. Imiqimod induces the production of cytokines and nitric oxide in infected macrophages. It has been used successfully in conjunction with standard antimonial chemotherapy to treat patients with cutaneous leishmaniasis whose lesions did not respond to antimonial therapy alone.

PHYSICAL TREATMENTS

Cutaneous leishmaniasis has been treated in patients of all ages with a wide range of physical methods including cauterization, surgical excision, cryotherapy, local heat, and CO$_2$ laser. Cryotherapy is the most promising method. It is performed by repeated topical applications of liquid nitrogen with a cotton-tipped applicator or a cotton swab with moderate pressure to the lesion. The freezing time per application is 15 to 20 seconds. The procedure is repeated two or three times at short intervals.

COMBINATION THERAPY

To solve the problems of resistance and relapse and to reduce the length of monotherapy regimens, combination of at least two antileishmanial drugs is the preferred option in visceral leishmaniasis. Miltefosine and paromomycin, which are potent antileishmanial drugs, must be reserved for combined therapy to prevent the emergence of resistance. Liposomal AmpB plus miltefosine or paromomycin should be tested.

Sb in a standard dose has already been combined with allopurinol (Zyloprim), which is an analogue of hypoxanthine. In visceral leishmaniasis patients, the association was found superior to Sb as monotherapy. In a prospective trial, Sb plus paromomycin for 21 days at 12 to 18 mg/kg/day was significantly more effective than Sb alone. However, an expert committee convened by WHO in 2005 recommended a combination regimen that does not include Sb when unresponsiveness to antimonial drugs exceeds a threshold of 10% to 20%.

Combination therapy has also been tested in cutaneous leishmaniasis. Cryotherapy plus Sb has shown better results than cryotherapy or Sb alone. Sb with allopurinol was more effective in *L. panamensis* infection than Sb alone. However, the addition of allopurinol to Sb provided no clinical benefit in mucocutaneous leishmaniasis cases.

SPECIFIC RECOMMENDATIONS

Anthroponotic Visceral Leishmaniasis (South Asia and East Africa)

Sb remains the treatment of choice in areas with a low rate of Sb resistance. When unresponsiveness to Sb exceeds a threshold of 10% to 20%, the WHO expert committee recommends that policymakers should strongly consider a shift to an alternative first-line regimen. AmpB deoxycholate has demonstrated a cure rate of nearly 100% in Sb-resistant areas. However, its use at peripheral health posts was prevented by frequent adverse events, the need for prolonged hospitalization, and close monitoring.

A possible alternative regimen is liposomal AmpB. However, its current price tends to be prohibitively expensive for poor countries. Funding sources and the public health community should work in concert with governments and drug companies to provide it at the lowest possible price.

Despite its proven efficacy, no consensus has been reached about the use of oral miltefosine as a first-line drug.

Zoonotic Visceral Leishmaniasis

In the Mediterranean basin, the Middle East, and Brazil, visceral leishmaniasis burdens are lower than in Asia and East Africa, and access to treatment is generally much better. Liposomal AmpB is the first-line drug in Europe. Elsewhere, because of cost constraints, Sb compounds are still used in WHO guidelines. However, in patients coinfected with visceral leishmaniasis and HIV, liposomal AmpB is considered the antileishmanial drug of choice. Secondary prophylaxis with doses of liposomal AmpB[1] every 2 to 4 weeks after initial clinical cure of visceral leishmaniasis is now the standard of care in Europe. However, data are insufficient to recommend a specific regimen.

Cutaneous Leishmaniasis

To manage cutaneous leishmaniasis cases, three options involving systemic treatment, local treatment, or therapeutic abstention may be adopted.

Because of the risk of developing mucosal disease, systemic treatment is obvious for all New World species, except for *L. mexicana* infection, for which there is no risk. In fact, there is evidence that early and complete systemic treatment can prevent mucosal metastasis.

Parenteral Sb is still considered the gold standard treatment. A 20-day course of Sb 20 mg/kg is the most common schedule. Because the cure rate of Sb is low in patients infected with *L. guyanensis*, a short-course regimen of pentamidine[1] is recommended. Ketoconazole[1] may be used as the first choice for uncomplicated lesions caused by *L. panamensis*.

Local treatment should be used in self-limited cutaneous leishmaniasis caused by Old World species and *L. mexicana*. Treatment involves intralesional injections of Sb, application of paromomycin ointments,[6] or cryotherapy. The choice depends on the physician's experience and the availability of the method.

Based on expert opinion, systemic treatment is used in patients with multiple lesions (>5), large lesions (>5 cm) and para-articular or periorificial lesions. Systemic treatment is also recommended in patients with metastatic spread and in lesions not responsive to local treatment. If systemic treatment is indicated, ketoconazole[1] is an option for *L. mexicana*. Ketoconazole[1] and fluconazole[1] may be used for *L. major*. A recent study, using PCR for species-specific diagnosis, showed recurrent failure of local paromomycin and intralesional Sb treatment against *L. tropica*. Otherwise, it demonstrated a good response to a 10-day Sb systemic regimen. *L. tropica* appeared also to be less responsive to ketoconazole[1] than *L. major* is. However, local treatment is essential in patients with contraindications to systemic treatment, such as pregnant women or cardiac patients.

Mucocutaneous Leishmaniasis

Sb given IM for 28 days is the first-line drug for mucosal infection. In cases of poor response or large tissue destruction, AmpB deoxycholate could be prescribed; 3 g of the product is sometimes necessary to achieve a total cure. To reduce side effects and the duration of treatment, liposomal AmpB is recommended when it is available. Pentamidine[1] at a tolerable dose of 2 mg/kg for seven injections every other day does not seem sufficiently effective against *L. brazilensis*. Surgery is sometimes necessary to repair deep mutilations.

Diffuse Cutaneous Leishmaniasis

Diffuse cutaneous leishmaniasis is characterized by a lower sensitivity to classic drugs that are used in localized cutaneous lesions. Sb, pentamidine,[1] or AmpB should be used at the higher recommended doses, with close observation for side effects. To help therapeutic decision-making, clinical trials, which are constrained by the low number and the broad dispersion of cases, must be conducted with new and old drugs.

---

[1] Not FDA approved for this indication.
[6] May be compounded by pharmacists.

REFERENCES

Alvar J, Croft S, Olliaro P: Chemotherapy in the treatment and control of leishmaniasis. Adv Parasitol 2006;61:223-274.

Bern C, Adler-Moore J, Berenguer J, et al: Liposomal amphotericin B for the treatment of visceral leishmaniasis. Clin Infect Dis 2006;43:917-924.

Blum J, Desjeux P, Schwartz E, et al: Treatment of cutaneous leishmaniasis among travellers. J Antimicrob Chemother 2004;53:158-166.

Croft SL, Seifert K, Yardley V: Current scenario of drug development for leishmaniasis. Indian J Med Res 2006;123:399-410.

Desjeux P: Therapeutic options for visceral leishmaniasis. Med Mal Infect 2005;35:S74-S76.

Jha TK: Drug unresponsiveness and combination therapy for kala-azar. Indian J Med Res 2006;123:389-398.

Sundar S, Chatterjee M: Visceral leishmaniasis: Current therapeutic modalities. Indian J Med Res 2006;123:345-352.

Leprosy

Method of
*Bhushan Kumar, MD, MNAMS, and
Sunil Dogra, MD, DNB, MNAMS*

Leprosy is a chronic, very mildly infectious disease of the skin and peripheral nerves caused by *Mycobacterium leprae*. The first historical descriptions of leprosy came from India in about 600 BC when it was called *kushta*. Leprosy is also known as *Hansen's disease* after the demonstration of *M. leprae* by Gerhard Armauer Hansen in 1873. The damage to peripheral nerves results in sensory and motor impairment with the characteristic hideous deformities and disabilities so deeply associated with the disease. Leprosy was once widely distributed in Europe and Asia but now occurs mainly in resource-poor countries in tropical and warm temperate regions. Stigma remains a major obstacle to leprosy control, despite advances in bacteriology, chemotherapy, and epidemiology.

Epidemiology

As of August 2006, leprosy remained a public health problem in six countries: Brazil, Congo, Madagascar, Mozambique, Nepal, and Tanzania. Global registered prevalence of leprosy at the beginning of 2006 was 219,826 cases. The number of new cases reported during 2005 was 296,499. The global detection of new cases continues to show a sharp decline; the number of new cases reported fell by more than 110,000 cases (27%) during 2005 compared with the number of new cases reported during 2004. India, which has the highest number of leprosy cases in the world, achieved national-level elimination of leprosy in December 2005. *Elimination* is defined as less than one case per 10,000 population, and the prevalence in India was 0.84 per 10,000 population as of the end of March 2006.

After the successful implementation of and subsequently very encouraging results reported with multidrug therapy (MDT), a highly effective treatment regimen, in 1991 the World Health Assembly developed the global strategy for eliminating leprosy as a public health problem by 2000. The goal to reduce the prevalence of leprosy to less than one case per 10,000 population at the global level by 2000 was achieved; however, several countries had not done so at the national level. Therefore, the deadline for achieving the goal for these countries was extended to the end of 2005.

Major achievements of the leprosy elimination strategy have included achieving elimination in more than 120 countries (including cure of more than 18 million patients), free supply of MDT drugs, increased coverage of leprosy services, and integration of the leprosy elimination strategy within general health services.

However, reaching a prevalence level of less than one per 10,000 population is not the end of leprosy or leprosy work. The new challenge is to build on the success of the leprosy campaign and deliver sustainable care for leprosy patients who have been treated successfully or who are likely to trickle in because of the long incubation of the disease.

Etiopathogenesis

Modern-day leprosy dates from 1873 following the discovery of *M. leprae* (the first bacillus to be associated with a human disease). *M. leprae* is an acid- and alcohol-fast, gram-positive, obligate intracellular, noncultivable bacterium, which has been successfully inoculated and has multiplied in the nine-banded armadillo and nude mouse.

The principal means of transmission of *M. leprae* is probably through nasal or respiratory mucosa and skin-to-skin transmission in contacts of heavily infected multibacillary (MB) patients. The incubation period varies widely from months to 30 years, and the average time is usually 5 to 7 years. Apart from humans, nine-banded armadillos and, very rarely, sooty mangabey monkeys are the only known reservoir of infection.

More than 95% of adults are resistant to the infection. Subclinical infections occur more commonly in endemic areas, but clinical disease manifests in only a small fraction having specific impairment of cell-mediated immunity (CMI) to *M. leprae*.

The disease presents a broad spectrum of clinical and histopathologic manifestations ranging from bacteriologically scanty tuberculoid to highly bacilliferous lepromatous leprosy. The clinicopathologic bipolarity stems from the immunologic status, which guides the dual response of monocytes and macrophages to *M. leprae*. In cases located at the tuberculoid pole, these cells can destroy and eliminate all the bacilli; in cases near the lepromatous pole, the bacilli proliferate and persist in these cells and can be also partially killed simultaneously.

Clinical Features

The clinical features of leprosy reflect the pathology, which in turn depends on the balance between bacillary multiplication and the host cell–mediated immune response (Table 1). Leprosy affects skin and nerves and produces systemic involvement in lepromatous disease. Patients commonly present with skin lesions, weakness or numbness caused by involvement of a peripheral nerve trunk, deformities, resorption of fingers and toes, or a burn or ulcer in an anesthetic hand or foot. Sometimes patients present with nerve pain, sudden palsy, new skin lesions, painful red eye, or a systemic febrile illness.

Inspection of the whole body in good light is important because otherwise lesions with faint erythema or slight hypopigmentation (more often on covered areas in borderline disease) might be missed. Skin lesions should be examined for hypoesthesia to light touch and temperature and for anhidrosis.

TYPES OF LEPROSY

Indeterminate Leprosy

The classic skin lesion of indeterminate leprosy is most commonly found on the face, the extensors of the limbs, the buttocks, or the trunk. There may be one or more slightly hypopigmented or erythematous macules, a few centimeters in diameter, with poorly defined margins (Figure 1). Hair growth and nerve function are usually not affected. A biopsy might show perineurovascular infiltrate; however, acid-fast bacilli (AFB) are mostly not demonstrable. Many patients do not notice such lesions and present only with characteristic determinant lesions at some point. Perhaps three out of four indeterminate lesions heal spontaneously and the rest become determinate and enter the clinical spectrum.

TABLE 1 Characteristics of the Ridley-Jopling Classification*

Observation	TT	BT	BB	BL	LL
Number of lesions	Usually 1 (up to 3)	Single, few (up to 10)	Several (10-30)	Many, asymmetric (>30)	Multiple, symmetric
Size of lesions	Variable, usually large	Variable, some are large	Variable	Variable, not very large†	Small
Surface	Very dry, scaly, lesions look turgid	Dry	Dull, slightly shiny	Shiny	Shiny
Sensations in lesions	Absent	Markedly diminished	Moderately diminished	Slightly diminished	Minimally diminished or not affected
Hair growth in lesions	Absent	Markedly diminished	Moderately diminished	Slightly diminished	Not affected
AFB in lesions	Nil	Nil or scanty	Moderate number	Many	Very many (globi)
Lepromin	Strongly positive (++++)	Weakly positive (+ or ++)	Negative	Negative	Negative

*Compartmentalization of the features is not very stringent. All these features occur in various combinations as the disease progresses.
†Presence of large lesions indicates downgrading of the disease from a higher spectrum.
Abbreviations: AFB = acid fast bacilli; BB = borderline borderline leprosy; BL = borderline lepromatous leprosy; BT = borderline tuberculoid leprosy; LL = lepromatous leprosy; TT = tuberculoid leprosy.

Tuberculoid Leprosy

Tuberculoid leprosy (TT) often has one or few skin lesions, and lesions seldom measure more than 10 cm in diameter. The typical lesion is a well-defined erythematous plaque with a raised and clear-cut edge sloping toward a rather flattened and usually hypopigmented center, acquiring an annular configuration. Erythema might not be apparent on dark skin. The surface is dry, hairless, anesthetic, and sometimes scaly. Sensory impairment may be difficult to demonstrate on the face because of the generous supply of sensory nerve endings. Less commonly, the lesion is a dry, anesthetic macule with sparse hair; the lesion appears erythematous on light skin and hypopigmented (never depigmented) on dark skin. Usually, a solitary peripheral nerve trunk is thickened in the vicinity of a TT lesion—for example, a thickened ulnar nerve if the lesion is on the arm.

Borderline Tuberculoid Leprosy

The skin lesions of borderline tuberculoid (BT) leprosy resemble those of tuberculoid leprosy, but there is evidence that the disease is not contained. Individual lesions do not show the well-defined margins, and the edge in part might fade imperceptibly into normal skin (Figure 2). There may be satellite lesions. The number of lesions can vary from three to ten and show variation in size and contour. Loss of sensation is less intense than in the lesions of tuberculoid leprosy. Xerosis, scaling, and erythema or hypopigmentation are also less conspicuous than in the TL form.

Several of the peripheral nerves are likely to be enlarged irregularly and in an asymmetric pattern. Nerve damage is an important characteristic of BT leprosy, and anesthesia or motor deficit is often found at the time of presentation.

Borderline Borderline Leprosy

Borderline borderline (BB) disease is unstable and mostly downgrades toward the lepromatous pole, especially when it is untreated. There are many skin lesions of all shapes and sizes including papules, nodules, plaques, and circinate lesions. Characteristic skin lesions are annular or dimorphic. In annular lesions, the inner edge is abrupt, and the outer edge slopes toward normal skin and has islands of clinically normal-looking skin within the plaque, giving a Swiss cheese appearance. The classic dimorphic lesion is shown in Figure 3.

The face might show infiltration, with occasional nodules over the ears and chin. Because of immunologic instability, the BB state is short-lived, and such patients are evidently rarely seen; the disease usually changes rapidly to borderline lepromatous (BL) or

FIGURE 1. Indeterminate leprosy.

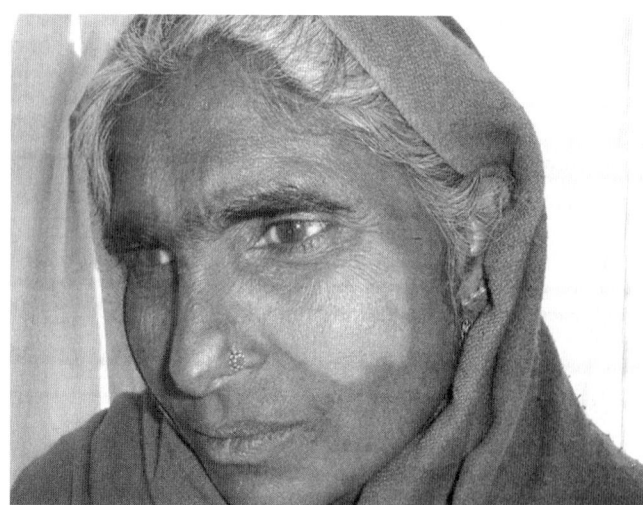

FIGURE 2. Borderline tuberculoid leprosy.

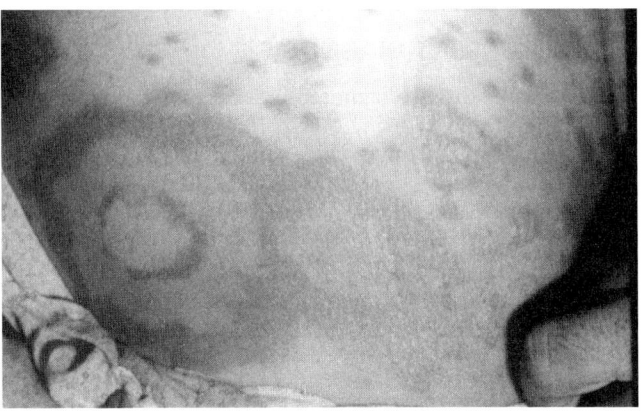

FIGURE 3. Borderline borderline leprosy.

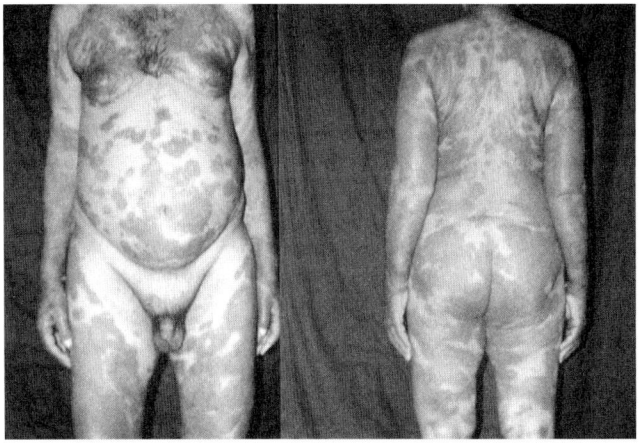

FIGURE 4. Borderline lepromatous leprosy.

BT leprosy. Many nerves are involved, although not symmetrically as in lepromatous leprosy.

Borderline Lepromatous Leprosy

There are numerous skin lesions in BL, and they are classically distinct but not so well defined. There occur slightly infiltrated macules variable in shapes in not so symmetric distribution, with areas of apparently normal skin in between. With disease progression, papules, nodules, and plaques can develop, although they usually have sloping margins that merge imperceptibly into normal skin (Figure 4). Associated large lesions and of variable morphology indicate downgrading of disease from a higher spectrum. Eyebrows are not completely lost. Peripheral nerve trunks become thickened and develop corresponding anesthesia and paresis but lack symmetry. Nerves are, however, unlikely to be damaged as quickly as in BB and BT leprosy.

Lepromatous Leprosy

The early lesions of lepromatous leprosy (LL) are minimally infiltrated macules that are innumerable, widely disseminated, and symmetrically distributed. The edges are indistinct, and their surface is shiny and erythematous rather than hypopigmented. In rapidly progressive cases, they coalesce so that the skin is diffusely involved. The early macules of LL are not anesthetic.

If the disease is untreated and allowed to progress, the affected skin takes on a waxy appearance and feels full. Thickness of skin is most marked over the face, especially the forehead, earlobes, eyebrows, nose, and malar surfaces (Figure 5). The eyebrows and, ultimately, the eyelashes are lost. The thickened skin accentuates into folds, producing the classic leonine facies. Nodules and even plaques on the face and other areas of the body can follow. By this time, peripheral anesthesia is extensive and is accompanied by anhidrosis, with compensatory hyperhidrosis of the trunk and axillae.

The sensory loss is symmetric and is first detected over the extensors of forearms, legs, hands, and feet, which gradually results in the typical glove-and-stocking distribution. Weakness usually starts in the intrinsic muscles of the hands and feet.

EXTENT OF INVOLVEMENT

Nerve Involvement

Nerve damage occurs in two settings: peripheral nerve trunks and small dermal nerves. Small dermal sensory and autonomic nerves are affected in the early part of disease establishment, producing hypoesthesia and anhidrosis within skin lesions. The posterior tibial is the most commonly affected nerve trunk, followed by the ulnar, median, lateral popliteal, and facial nerves. Involvement of these nerves produces enlargement, with or without tenderness, and regional sensory and motor loss. Thickening of the greater auricular nerve is better seen than felt (Figure 6). Rarely, nerve abscess is encountered in peripheral nerve trunks, mostly in the ulnar and lateral popliteal nerves.

The morbidity and disability associated with leprosy are secondary to nerve damage. About 25% of leprosy patients have some degree of disability, which is greatest in patients with BL and LL disease. Early recognition and treatment are crucial to prevention of deformities.

Systemic Involvement

Features of systemic involvement occur usually in longstanding disease and are mainly seen in patients near the lepromatous pole because of bacillary infiltration and the associated granulomatous infiltration that affects various organs, especially the nasal mucosa, eyes, bones, testes, kidneys, lymph nodes, liver, and spleen. Besides the disease, systemic manifestations in the form of such constitutional symptoms as fever, malaise, joint pains, and acute inflammation of eyes, joints, and the reticuloendothelial system (among others) can occur as a part of a type 2 lepra reaction.

Diagnosis

CLINICAL DIAGNOSIS

The diagnosis and classification of leprosy have been based on clinical features and skin smears when facilities are available. Clinical diagnosis of leprosy is based on patients having one or more of the three cardinal signs. The cardinal signs are hypopigmented or erythematous skin lesion(s), with definite loss of or impairment of sensations; involvement of the peripheral nerves, as demonstrated by definite

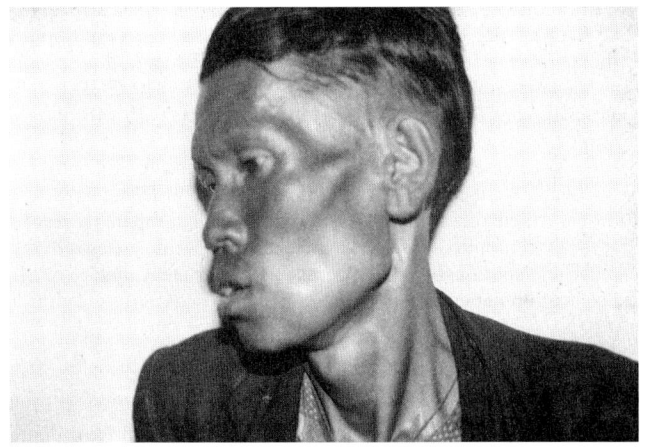

FIGURE 5. Lepromatous leprosy (diffuse infiltration).

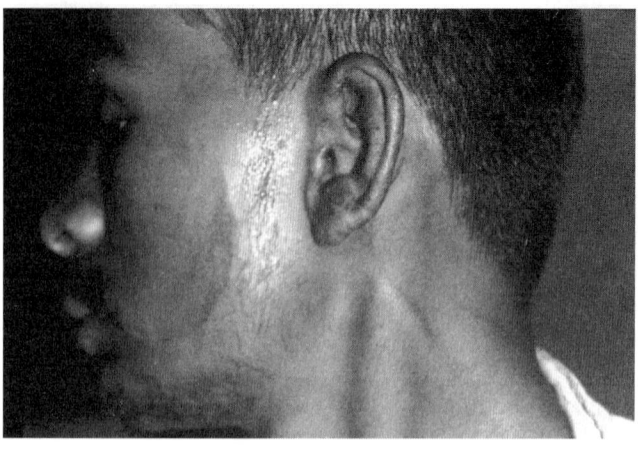

FIGURE 6. Nerve involvement (greater auricular nerve thickening).

thickening, with sensory impairment; and skin smear positive for AFB.

LABORATORY DIAGNOSIS

Laboratory diagnostic tests such as slit skin smears, histologic examination of involved tissues, serology, and polymerase chain reaction (PCR) studies have been confined to areas where such facilities are available and in academic and research centers.

Slit Skin Smears

The diagnostic specificity of skin smears is almost 100%; however, the sensitivity is rarely more than 50% because smear-positive patients represent only 10% to 50% of cases. The inherent problems of skin smears are the logistics and the reliability of the technique of taking, staining, and interpreting the smears. Skin smears help identify patients with MB disease and patients who are experiencing clinical relapse.

Skin Biopsies

The biopsy helps to confirm the clinical diagnosis and classification of disease, but it cannot be regarded as the diagnostic gold standard because a number of the histologic features can be nondiagnostic or doubtful. In practice, a clinical and histopathologic correlation may be necessary for resolving a diagnostic difficulty.

Serology and Polymerase Chain Reaction

Serology and PCR are rarely used in endemic countries because of their limited availability and lack of uniform diagnostic values across the disease spectrum. The basis of serologic tests is to determine the presence of anti–phenolic glycolipid-1 (PGL-1) antibodies by the *M. leprae* particle agglutination assay (MLPA) and the enzyme-linked immunosorbent assay (ELISA) techniques. The PGL-1 antibody test is specific and more sensitive in patients with MB disease, but unfortunately it is not very helpful in the diagnosis of paucibacillary (PB) disease, and it has low predictive value for diagnosis of early disease. Antibodies to the 35-kD protein of *M. leprae* have been studied for their role in diagnosis of disease with comparable results. PCR for detection of *M. leprae* DNA encoding specific genes is highly sensitive and specific, because it detects *M. leprae* DNA in 95% of MB and 55% of PB patients. Currently, PCR is not used in routine clinical practice.

Lepromin Test

The lepromin test is not a diagnostic test, but it is helpful for identifying the level of CMI against *M. leprae* in a given patient. It is a nonspecific test of some value in classifying a case of leprosy. It is strongly positive in TL; weakly positive in BT; negative in BB, BL, and LL; and unpredictable in indeterminate leprosy. Lepromin (lepromin A, 160 million bacilli/mL) 0.1 mL is injected intradermally, and the reaction is read at 48 hours (Fernandez reaction) and at 3 to 4 weeks (Mitsuda reaction). Neither test is diagnostic, because both may be positive in persons with no evidence of leprosy. However, close contacts of an MB patient who have negative lepromin tests have a greater risk of developing disease.

Classification Of Disease

Ridley and Jopling (1966) defined five groups on the basis of clinical, bacteriologic, histologic, and immunologic features. These groups are tuberculoid, borderline tuberculoid, midborderline (borderline borderline), borderline lepromatous, and lepromatous leprosy. This is a very useful classification for research purposes, but it is often not feasible in field conditions and primary health centers. This classification does not include the indeterminate and pure neuritic type of leprosy. In general, PB disease is equivalent to indeterminate, tuberculoid, and BT leprosy, and MB disease is equated with BB, BL, and LL disease.

In 1998, the WHO Expert Committee on Leprosy declared skin-slit smears as not essential for institution of MDT. This was necessitated by the unavailability or unreliability of technical expertise for the skin smear in many leprosy-control programs and the potential for transmitting HIV and hepatitis by nonsterile techniques.

Recently, for field workers, WHO has classified leprosy based on the number of skin lesions for treatment purposes. PB leprosy is leprosy with one to five skin lesions. MB leprosy includes more than five skin lesions. If facilities are available, any patient with a positive slit-skin smear should be considered to have MB leprosy.

CURRENT DIAGNOSIS

A case of leprosy is diagnosed in a person who has one or more of the following cardinal signs and who has yet to complete a full course of treatment:
- Hypopigmented or erythematous skin lesion(s) with definite loss or impairment of sensations
- Involvement of the peripheral nerves, as demonstrated by definite thickening with sensory impairment
- Skin smear positive for acid-fast bacilli

Rare Variants

Lucio Leprosy

Lucio leprosy (LuLp) is a diffuse form of LL. It is common in Mexico and Costa Rica and less common in the Gulf Coast, but it is quite rare in the rest of the world. It manifests as slowly progressive, diffuse, shiny infiltration of skin of the face and most of the body (*lepra bonita*, "beautiful leprosy"). There is loss of eyebrows, hoarseness of voice, and numbness and edema of hands and feet that mimic myxedema. This form of the disease is liable to the most severe of all reactional states, the Lucio phenomenon, in which destructive vasculitis leads to skin necrosis and ulcers.

Pure Neuritic Leprosy

Pure neuritic leprosy is characterized in the absence of any skin patch by an area of sensory loss along the distribution of a thickened nerve trunk with or without motor deficit. This form is seen most often, but not exclusively, in India and Nepal, where it accounts for 5% to 10% of leprosy cases. Histology of a cutaneous nerve might reveal an infiltrate that is characteristic of any type of leprosy.

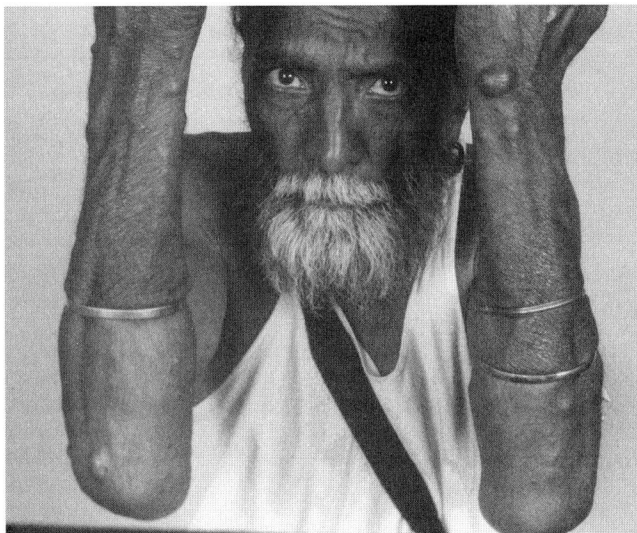

FIGURE 7. Histoid leprosy.

Histoid Leprosy

Histoid leprosy, first described in 1960, is now a well-recognized but rarely reported entity. Controversy still remains whether to consider histoid leprosy as a separate entity. It usually occurs in patients who had received irregular or inadequate treatment or dapsone monotherapy or as a spectrum under lepromatous leprosy. It manifests as superficially or deeply fixed cutaneous nodules, plaques, or pads (Figure 7). In a given patient, the number of lesions can vary from a few to a hundred. Histopathologically, the striking feature is predominance of spindle-shaped cells and unusually large numbers of AFB.

Treatment

The concept of chemotherapy for leprosy has undergone a phenomenal change over the last two decades. The WHO MDT has been successful in eliminating leprosy in many countries. However, the search for new drugs and new drug regimens continues. The goals of advanced therapy include improved patient compliance, alternative agents against clofazimine- and rifampin-resistant bacilli, more efficient killing of persistent bacteria, uniform MDT for all types of leprosy, and supervised short regimens for preventing drug resistance.

WHO MULTIDRUG THERAPY

The MDT introduced in 1982 has proved to be the most effective tool in controlling leprosy. More than 18 million patients have been cured of the disease, with acceptable cumulative relapse rates of 0.77% for MB and 1.07% for PB disease. MDT as recommended by WHO remains the current and most accepted treatment by all countries with endemic leprosy. A single dose of rifampin (Rifadin)[1] 600 mg plus ofloxacin (Floxin)[1] 400 mg and minocycline (Minocin)[1] 100 mg (ROM therapy) is an acceptable and cost-effective alternative regimen for PB leprosy with one skin lesion, although most still favor the conventional WHO MDT PB regimen.

OTHER REGIMENS FOR SPECIAL SITUATIONS

Drug Substitutions

For adult MB patients who cannot take rifampin, the Seventh WHO Expert Committee on Leprosy recommended daily administration of 50 mg of clofazimine (Lamprene), together with two of the following three drugs: 400 mg ofloxacin,[1] 100 mg minocycline,[1] or 500 mg

---

[1]Not FDA approved for this indication.

 CURRENT THERAPY

Multidrug Therapy Regimen for Paucibacillary Leprosy (6 months)

ADULT (50-70 KG)

- Dapsone: 100 mg daily
- Rifampin (Rifadin)[1]: 600 mg once a mo under supervision

CHILD (10-14 Y)

- Dapsone: 50 mg daily
- Rifampin: 450 mg once a mo under supervision

Adjust dose appropriately for a child younger than 10 y. For example, dapsone 25 mg daily and rifampicin 300 mg given once a mo under supervision.

Multidrug Therapy Regimen for Multibacillary Leprosy (12 months)

ADULT (50-70 KG)

- Dapsone: 100 mg daily
- Rifampin:[1] 600 mg once a mo under supervision
- Clofazimine (Lamprene): 50 mg daily and 300 mg once a mo under supervision

CHILD (10-14 Y)

- Dapsone: 50 mg daily
- Rifampin[1]: 450 mg once a mo under supervision
- Clofazimine: 50 mg daily and 150 mg once a mo under supervision

Adjust dose appropriately for a child less than 10 y. For example, dapsone 25 mg daily and rifampin 300 mg given once a mo under supervision, clofazimine 50 mg given twice a wk, and clofazimine 100 mg given once a mo under supervision.

---

[1]Not FDA approved for this indication.

clarithromycin (Biaxin)[1] once daily for 6 months, followed by daily administration of 50 mg clofazimine plus 100 mg minocycline or 400 mg ofloxacin for at least an additional 18 months. For MB patients who cannot take clofazimine, clofazimine should be replaced with ofloxacin 400 mg daily or minocycline 100 mg daily. Alternatively, the patient may be treated with a monthly administration of a combination consisting of rifampin[1] 600 mg, ofloxacin 400 mg, and minocycline 100 mg (ROM therapy) for 24 months. MB patients who cannot tolerate dapsone should receive only daily clofazimine with no substitution; in PB cases dapsone should be replaced with clofazimine.

Accompanied Multidrug Therapy

Accompanied MDT (A-MDT) recommended by WHO is an essential element of the "flexible and patient friendly MDT delivery system" suitable to migrant populations, patients living in remote areas, and patients living in areas of civil war. In this policy, the patient is provided the entire supply of MDT drugs at the time of diagnosis: 6 months of medication for a PB patient and 12 months for an MB patient, while asking "someone close or important to the patient" to assume the responsibility of helping the patient complete the full course of treatment. However, poor adherence to self-administration of treatment, a common phenomenon in tuberculosis and leprosy patients, and the associated risk of drug resistance and relapses are to be expected.

---

[1]Not FDA approved for this indication.

Pregnancy and Lactation

Leprosy is exacerbated during pregnancy, so it is important that the standard multidrug therapy be continued during pregnancy. The standard MDT regimens are safe, both for the mother and the child, and therefore should be continued unchanged during pregnancy and lactation.

Concomitant Active Tuberculosis

If the patient has both leprosy and active tuberculosis, it is necessary to treat both infections at the same time. Give appropriate antituberculosis therapy in addition to the MDT appropriate to the type of leprosy. Rifampin is common to both regimens, and it must be given in the doses required for tuberculosis.

Concomitant HIV Infection

The management of a leprosy patient infected with HIV is the same as that of any other leprosy patient without infection with HIV.

NEWER DRUGS

A few new drugs are available to complement or replace the currently used MDT (Box 1). The objective of the new drugs is not to induce quick clinical regression but to minimize relapses or to address special situations like drug resistance or drug intolerance. Promising bactericidal activity of ofloxacin,[1] clarithromycin,[1] and minocycline[1] against *M. leprae* has been demonstrated in the mouse foot-pad system and then confirmed in clinical trials. Strong bactericidal effects against *M. leprae* of moxifloxacin (Avelox),[1] rifapentine (Priftin),[1] and other derivatives have been identified in in vitro studies. However, no precise recommendation of their use is available yet.

Reactions

During the course of leprosy, immunologically mediated episodes of acute or subacute inflammation known as *reactions* can occur. Most reactions belong to one of the two major types; reversal reaction (RR or type 1) or erythema nodosum leprosum (ENL or type 2). Reversal reactions can occur throughout the spectrum of leprosy but are more common in patients with borderline leprosy. On the other hand, ENL occurs exclusively in patients with MB disease, especially lepromatous and borderline lepromatous leprosy. Reactions can be disastrous; they cause acute nerve damage resulting in deformities. Almost 30% of MB patients develop reactions during the course of their disease. Reactions may be seen at presentation, during treatment, and even after treatment.

The principles of treatment of reactions are to control the acute inflammation in skin and nerves, ease the pain, halt eye damage, and prevent spread of the disease. Standard antileprosy chemotherapy should be started or continued along with antireaction treatment. Clinical evidence of ongoing neuritis (nerve tenderness, new anesthesia, motor loss) should be carefully sought and, if neuritis is present, corticosteroid treatment should be started immediately.

TYPE 1 REACTIONS

The type 1 reaction is a type IV hypersensitivity (delayed-type hypersensitivity) reaction, and it typically occurs in borderline disease. It is characterized by acutely inflamed skin lesions or acute neuritis, or both. Existing skin lesions become erythematous or edematous and can desquamate or, rarely, ulcerate. Often, new small lesions also appear at distant sites (Figure 8). Occasionally, edema of face, hands, or feet is the presenting symptom; however, constitutional symptoms are unusual. Although type 1 reactions can occur

---

[1]Not FDA approved for this indication.

BOX 1 Newer Drugs and Alternate Drugs

Quinolones
- Clinafloxacin[5]
- Moxifloxacin (Avelox)[1]
- Ofloxacin (Floxin)[1]
- Pefloxacin (Pefocin)[2]
- Sparfloxacin (Zagam)[2]
- Temafloxacin (Omniflox)[2]

Macrolides
- Clarithromycin (Biaxin)[1]

Tetracyclines
- Minocycline (Minocin)[1]

Ansamycins
- KRM-1648[5]
- KRM-1657[5]
- KRM-1668[5]
- Rifabutin (Mycobutin)[1]
- Rifapentine (Priftin)[1]

[1]Not FDA approved for this indication.
[2]Not available in the United States.
[5]Investigational drug in the United States.

---

spontaneously and at any time during the course of the disease, the usual times are after starting treatment and during the puerperium.

Because of the high risk of permanent damage to peripheral nerve trunks, RR needs to be diagnosed as soon as possible and managed adequately. The drug of choice is prednisolone (Delta-Cortef). The usual course begins with 40 to 60 mg daily (up to a maximum of 1 mg/kg), gradually reducing the dose weekly or biweekly and eventually stopping in about 12 weeks. Neural impairment of up to 6 months' duration may be helped by systemic corticosteroid therapy tapered over a period of 4 to 6 months. Adverse effects associated with long-term corticosteroid therapy must be kept in mind.

TYPE 2 REACTIONS

The type 2 reaction, a type III hypersensitivity reaction (immune-complex mediated) occurs in patients with LL and BL disease. Attacks are often acute in onset but can become chronic or recur over several years. ENL typically manifests as painful, red evanescent nodules on the face and extensor surfaces of the limbs. Rarely, they appear as bullous, pustular, necrotic forms. ENL is often accompanied by systemic symptoms producing fever and malaise, and in severe form it may be complicated by uveitis, dactylitis, arthritis, neuritis, lymphadenitis, myositis, and orchitis.

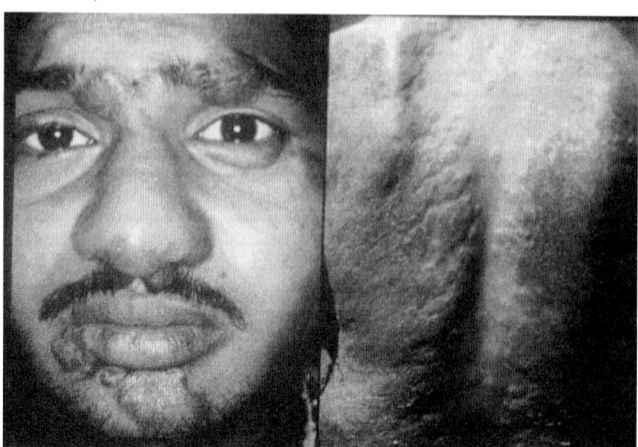

FIGURE 8. Borderline tuberculoid leprosy with type 1 reaction.

Acute or subacute neuritis with or without nerve function impairment is one of the major criteria for distinguishing mild and severe ENL. The treatment of ENL should start with general measures as in type 1 reaction. Mild ENL can be treated with analgesics like aspirin. In moderate and severe ENL, corticosteroids or thalidomide (Thalomid) are more useful and may be life saving. Thalidomide (100 mg q8h) has a dramatic effect in controlling ENL, and it may be useful in preventing recurrent ENL, but its teratogenic effects preclude its use in women of childbearing age. Clofazimine (Lamprene) has a useful anti-inflammatory effect in ENL and can be used at 300 mg daily in divided doses as an adjuvant to prednisolone and tapered over several months. Injectable antimonials are often used by Indian leprologists.

LUCIO'S PHENOMENON

The Lucio phenomenon occurs only in patients with Lucio leprosy. It results from infarction consequent on deep cutaneous vasculitis, causing the appearance of irregularly shaped erythematous patches. The patches sometimes darken and heal, but sometimes they form bullae that necrose, leaving deep, painful ulcers that are slow to heal. The systemic features are severe and can be fatal. Treatment with glucocorticoids (prednisolone) should be instituted at doses of 60 to 80 mg in two equal daily doses supplemented preferably with an augmented daily dose (200-300 mg) of clofazimine.

Prevention Of Disabilities and Rehabilitation

The socioeconomic impact resulting from the physical and psychological disabilities of leprosy continues to be a burden in endemic countries. Approximately 25% of leprosy patients have some degree of disability, which is greatest in patients with long-standing BL and LL disease.

Preventing patients with nerve damage from progressing to disability and deformity is a challenge that will last for the patient's lifetime. Among the important efforts for prevention are periodic measurement of neural impairment, early and adequate management of reactions, and advice for care of eyes, hands, and feet. Special footwear needs to be provided for patients with foot deformities to prevent ulceration. Early detection and treatment of reactions significantly reduce and prevent such complications as nerve damage with its resultant impairment, eye involvement, and loss of vision. Socioeconomic rehabilitation is another important component of caring for patients.

Prevention

Large population-based trials in different countries suggest that bacille Calmette-Guérin (BCG) vaccine[1] gives variable protection against leprosy, ranging from 34% to 80%. Therefore, BCG immunization of children for tuberculosis can contribute to leprosy control.

In a recently published large study from India, vaccine containing cultivable mycobacterium, ICRC,[5] provided a protective efficacy of 65% (heat-killed *M. leprae* BCG provided 64% protective efficacy). The role of chemoprophylaxis with bactericidal drugs in contacts of leprosy patients is still debated.

WHO Strategy For 2006 Through 2010

The WHO Technical Advisory Group (TAG) recognizes that new cases will continue to appear in most of the currently endemic countries, and therefore, expertise will have to be maintained at the appropriate level even within an integrated system. The main aim of the strategy is to sustain antileprosy services and the gains made so far. It is expected that by 2010 the disease burden will be further reduced to very low levels through services that would ensure enhancing community awareness, quality diagnosis, adequate management of patients including referral facilities, reduction of stigma, prevention of disabilities, rehabilitation, long-term care of the disabled, and effective partnerships among all stake holders.

REFERENCES

Abulafia J, Vignale RIA: Leprosy: Pathogenesis updated. Int J Dermatol 1999;38:321-334.
Bhattacharya SN, Sehgal VN: Reappraisal of the drifting scenario of leprosy multi-drug therapy: New approach proposed for the new millennium. Int J Dermatol 2002;41:321-326.
Britton WJ, Lockwood DN: Leprosy. Lancet 2004;363:1209-1219.
Grosset JH: Newer drugs in leprosy. Int J Lepr Other Mycobact Dis 2001;69(2 suppl):S14-S18.
Gupte MD: South India immunoprophylaxis trial against leprosy: Relevance of the findings in the context of trends in leprosy. Lepr Rev 2000;71(suppl):S43-S47; discussion S47-S49.
Kumar B, Dogra S, Kaur I: Epidemiological characteristics of leprosy reactions: 15 years experience from North India. Int J Lepr Other Mycobact Dis 2004;72:125-133.
Kumar B, Kaur I, Dogra S, Kumaran MS: Pure neuritic leprosy in India: An appraisal. Int J Lepr Other Mycobact Dis 2004;72:284-290.
Lockwood DN, Kumar B: Treatment of leprosy. BMJ 2004;328:1447-1448.
Naafs B: Current views on reactions in leprosy. Indian J Lepr 2000;72:97-122.
Noordeen SK: Vision beyond 2005. Indian J Lepr 2004;76:171-172.
Pfaltzgraff RE, Bryceson A: Clinical leprosy. In Hastings RC (ed): Leprosy. New York: Churchill Livingstone, 1989, pp 134-176.
WHO Expert Committee on Leprosy: Seventh Report. WHO Technical Report Series No. 874. Geneva: World Health Organization, 1998.
World Health Organization: The Weekly Epidemiological Record 2006; 81(32):309-316. PDF available for download at http://www.who.int/wer/2006/wer8132/en/index.html (accessed May 15, 2007).

Malaria

Method of
Paul M. Arguin, MD, and S. Patrick Kachur, MD*

Malaria is caused by infection with protozoa of the genus *Plasmodium*; it is transmitted by the bite of a female *Anopheles* mosquito, which serves as the vector and definitive host for plasmodia. Rarely, malaria can be transmitted through exposure to infected blood and blood products, injection equipment, or organ transplantation (induced malaria) or by vertical transmission (congenital malaria).

Malaria remains one of the most prevalent infectious diseases in the world. There are an estimated 350 million to 500 million cases every year, and more than 1 million deaths, mostly in children younger than 5 years of age, attributable to this disease. Precise estimates of the burden of the disease are hampered by both massive under-reporting from areas lacking adequate health infrastructure and overestimation when liberal case definitions are employed that are not based on laboratory confirmation.

In nonendemic countries, imported malaria (malaria acquired while traveling in an endemic area) is also a significant public health concern. Each year there are about 235 million trips to malaria-endemic countries; about 25 million of these travelers are residents of the United States. As a result, health care providers in

---

[1]Not FDA approved for this indication.
[5]Investigational drug in the United States.

*The findings and conclusions in this chapter are those of the authors and do not necessarily represent the views of the Centers for Disease Control and Prevention.

nonendemic areas such as the United States must be able to adequately prepare these travelers to help reduce their risk of becoming infected with malaria while traveling and must be alert for the diagnosis in returning ill travelers. In addition, blood banks must also be aware of the travel history of potential donors who may be harboring malaria parasites at the time of donation in order to prevent cases of transfusion-transmitted malaria.

The Centers for Disease Control and Prevention (CDC) receives reports of, on average, 1400 cases of imported malaria and six malaria deaths in the United States each year. Each year there are about four cases of malaria reported in persons who do not have a travel history, including cases of congenitally acquired infection, transfusion-transmitted infection, cryptic infection, and occasional instances of locally acquired mosquito-borne infection.

In areas where malaria is not endemic, such as the United States, locally acquired mosquito-borne transmission of malaria (introduced malaria) can occur when a local mosquito acquires the parasite by biting an infected person and then transmits that infection to another person. There have been 11 outbreaks of locally acquired mosquito-borne malaria transmission in the United States since 1992, with the most recent one involving eight cases of *Plasmodium vivax* infection in Florida in 2003. Although the United States was officially recognized as malaria-free in 1970, competent malaria vectors continue to exist in the 48 continental states, Puerto Rico, the Virgin Islands, and Guam. Local transmission can occur whenever infectious persons, competent vectors, conducive environmental conditions, and opportunities for exposure of susceptible persons to mosquitoes come together.

Etiology

Infection with protozoa of the genus *Plasmodium* causes malaria. Four species of *Plasmodium* typically cause clinical disease in humans: *P. falciparum*, *P. vivax*, *P. ovale*, and *P. malariae*. Recently, *P. knowlesi*, a parasite of Old World monkeys, has been documented as a cause of human infections and some fatalities in Southeast Asia. Investigations are ongoing to determine the extent of its transmission to humans. The life cycle of malaria starts with inoculation of sporozoites into humans from the salivary glands of a female *Anopheles* mosquito during a blood meal (Figure 1) and progresses through an exoerythrocytic phase (tissue schizogany) and an erythrocytic phase (blood schizogany). The development of gametocytes that can be ingested by a subsequent female *Anopheles* mosquito allow the completion of the life cycle.

In *P. vivax* and *P. ovale* infections, some sporozoites might not enter exoerythrocytic schizogony but instead develop into latent hepatic forms, or hypnozoites. These forms can reactivate later and cause acute illness. The resulting infection, which is termed *relapse*, can occur months to years after the initial infection. Persons with *P. vivax* or *P. ovale* infection can have several relapses for up to 4 years and occasionally longer after the primary infection. However, if *P. vivax* or *P. ovale* infections are acquired congenitally or through exposure to blood or blood products, no liver phase occurs and therefore relapses cannot occur. Neither *P. falciparum* nor *P. malariae* has a hypnozoite form. However, if *P. malariae* infection is not treated, symptomatic recrudescences, often associated with splenectomy or immunosuppression, can occur decades after the primary infection.

The incubation period, or the period from infection to the appearance of symptoms, is species dependent. The incubation period is usually 9 to 14 days for *P. falciparum*, 12 to 17 days for *P. vivax*, 16 to 18 days for *P. ovale*, and 18 to 40 days (or longer) for *P. malariae*. Persons taking chemoprophylaxis and those who have acquired partial immunity from repeated exposure to malaria infection can experience a prolonged incubation period.

Epidemiology

Malaria is endemic to Africa, South Asia, Southeast Asia, parts of Central Asia and the Caucasus, Oceania, Central America, parts of South America, parts of the Caribbean, and parts of Turkey and the Middle East. The species-specific geographic distribution is presented in Table 1. *P. falciparum* is the most common species in the tropics and subtropics. *P. vivax* is prevalent in many temperate zones as well as in the tropics and subtropics, making it the species with the widest geographic distribution. Together, *P. falciparum* and *P. vivax* account for more than 90% of clinical malaria illnesses worldwide.

The development of resistance to antimalarial drugs has complicated malaria prophylaxis and treatment. Species-specific resistance patterns are presented in Table 1. Knowledge of species-specific resistance patterns is essential to making appropriate decisions about chemoprophylaxis and treatment. The most up-to-date information about this rapidly evolving process can usually be found on the CDC Web site (www.cdc.gov/malaria) and the World Health Organization (WHO) Web site (www.who/int/topics/malaria).

Among U.S. travelers, the majority of cases of malaria diagnosed each year are acquired in sub-Saharan Africa. Most of these patients report not taking any or one of the recommended drugs for malaria chemoprophylaxis. Also, the most common subgroup of travelers who become infected with malaria are first- and second-generation immigrants who return to their countries of origin to *visit friends and relatives* (VFR travelers).

Clinical Features

The clinical presentation of malaria is nonspecific; therefore, clinicians must maintain a high index of suspicion of malaria and routinely elicit a travel history from febrile patients. The clinical presentation of malaria can vary substantially, depending on the infecting species, the level of parasitemia, and the immune status of the patient. The initial clinical symptoms usually include a flu-like prodrome with headache, malaise, and myalgias that is followed by fever. In travelers with these symptoms, the differential diagnosis should include influenza, meningitis, typhoid fever, dengue fever and other arboviral infections, leptospirosis, typhus, and hepatitis.

Malaria paroxysms are produced when infected red blood cells rupture and release merozoites. After a number of cycles of erythrocytic schizogony, the release of merozoites can become synchronized, resulting in classic cyclic fevers. With *P. falciparum*, *P. vivax*, and *P. ovale* infections (tertian malaria), the paroxysms occur in 48-hour cycles, whereas with *P. malariae* infections (quartan malaria), the cycles are 72 hours. However, patients, particularly those with *P. falciparum*, might not develop cyclic paroxysms at all, and so a lack of cyclic fevers should not rule out a diagnosis of malaria.

Other symptoms include headache, chills, rigors, myalgias and arthralgias, and abdominal pain. Patients also might complain of diarrhea, vomiting, chest pain, and cough. The presence of gastrointestinal and respiratory symptoms should not lead the physician to exclude malaria as a potential diagnosis. On physical examination, a patient might have jaundice, tachycardia, hypotension (usually secondary to dehydration), and splenomegaly. Laboratory abnormalities in cases of uncomplicated malaria can include mild anemia, an elevated reticulocyte count, thrombocytopenia, lymphopenia, hyperbilirubinemia, and mildly elevated transaminases.

An uncomplicated malaria infection can progress to severe disease or death within hours. Risk factors for severe malaria include delays in treatment, inadequate or inappropriate treatment, a high parasite burden, and lack of acquired immunity. *P. falciparum*, more than any other species of *Plasmodium*, is responsible for the severe disease and death associated with malaria. This tendency has been linked to several features of this species. The tissue and blood schizonts in *P. falciparum* release a larger number of merozoites when they rupture, resulting in a more rapid rise in parasitemia. *P. falciparum*, unlike the other species, can infect both reticulocytes and mature erythrocytes. This destruction of large numbers of red blood cells and suppression of erythropoiesis can produce devastating anemia. In addition, *P. falciparum*–infected erythrocytes adhere to the vascular endothelium of postcapillary venules. It is believed that cytoadherence and severe anemia contribute to tissue hypoxia and

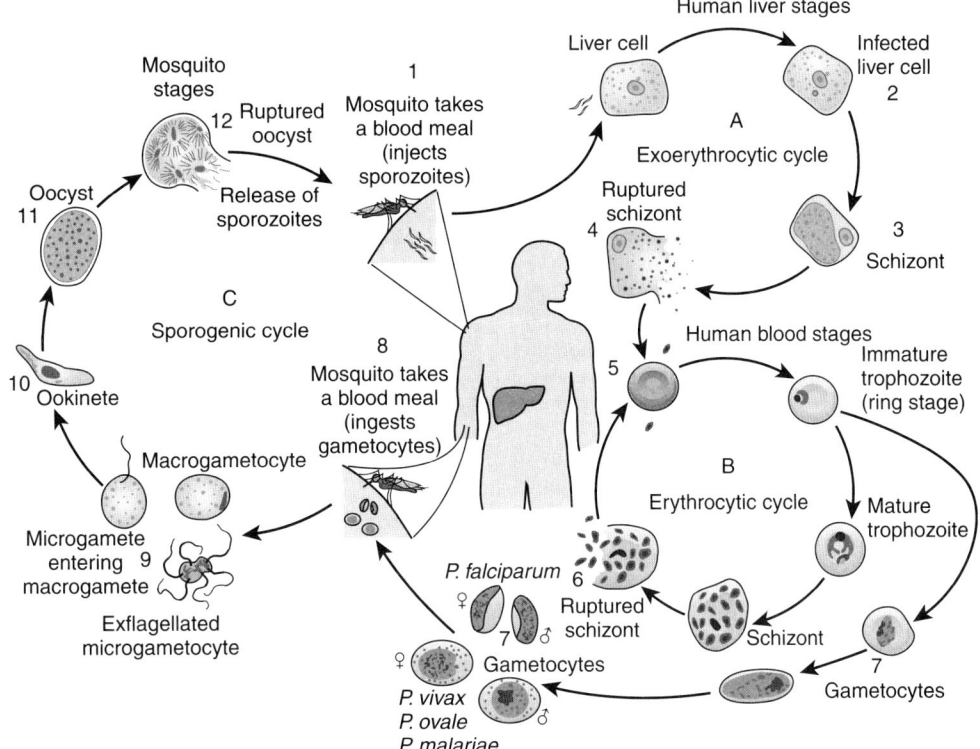

FIGURE 1. The malaria parasite life cycle involves two hosts. During a blood meal, a malaria-infected female *Anopheles* mosquito inoculates sporozoites into the human host *(1)*. Sporozoites infect liver cells *(2)* and mature into schizonts *(3)*, which rupture and release merozoites *(4)*. (In *P. vivax* and *P. ovale*, a dormant stage [hypnozoites] can persist in the liver and cause relapses by invading the bloodstream weeks or even years later.) After this initial replication in the liver (exo-erythrocytic cycle or tissue schizogony A), the parasites undergo asexual multiplication in the erythrocytes (erythrocytic cycle or blood schizogony B). Merozoites infect red blood cells *(5)*. The ring stage trophozoites mature into schizonts, which rupture, releasing merozoites *(6)*. Some parasites differentiate into sexual erythrocytic stages (gametocytes) *(7)*. Blood-stage parasites are responsible for the clinical manifestations of the disease.

The gametocytes, male (microgametocytes) and female (macrogametocytes), are ingested by an Anopheles mosquito during a blood meal *(8)*. The parasites' multiplication in the mosquito is known as the sporogonic cycle *(C)*. While in the mosquito's stomach, the microgametes penetrate the macrogametes, generating zygotes *(9)*. The zygotes in turn become motile and elongated (ookinetes) *(10)*, which invade the midgut wall of the mosquito, where they develop into oocysts *(11)*. The oocysts grow, rupture, and release sporozoites *(12)*, which make their way to the

TABLE 1 Malaria Species Distribution and Drug-Resistance Pattern

Species	Known Geographic Distribution	Drug-Resistance Pattern
Plasmodium falciparum	Most malaria-endemic areas except Republic of Korea, China north of Yunnan Province, and some areas of Central Asia and the Caucasus	Chloroquine (Aralen) resistance in nearly all endemic countries with the exception of Haiti, the Dominican Republic, Central America west of the Panama canal, and parts of the Middle East (resistance identified in Oman, Saudi Arabia, and Yemen) Sulfadoxine/pyrimethamine (Fansidar) resistance widespread in South America, Southeast Asia, and Africa Mefloquine (Lariam) resistance in parts of Southeast Asia Reduced susceptibility to quinine and artemisinin drugs has been documented in parts of Southeast Asia; combination therapies and a longer course of treatment are required
Plasmodium malariae	Same as for *P. falciparum*	No chloroquine resistance is documented
Plasmodium ovale	Sub-Saharan Africa Reported sporadically in Southern China, Burma, and Southeast Asia	No chloroquine resistance is documented
Plasmodium vivax	Central and South America, South Asia, Southeast Asia, Oceania, parts of the Middle East, Mexico, North Africa, and Horn of Africa Not common to absent in sub-Saharan Africa, and the Caribbean	Chloroquine resistance in Papua New Guinea, Indonesia and East Timor Rare instances of chloroquine-resistant *P. vivax* have been reported in Myanmar, India, and Central and South America

end-organ dysfunction. Even the immune response itself contributes to many of the cellular and humoral processes that manifest in severe malaria illness.

Severe malaria caused by *P. falciparum* and occasionally *P. vivax*, is associated with a 15% to 20% mortality rate. Signs and symptoms of severe malaria can include impaired consciousness, coma (cerebral malaria), generalized seizures, severe anemia, acute renal failure, pulmonary edema, acute respiratory distress syndrome, hypotension and circulatory collapse, disseminated intravascular coagulation, spontaneous bleeding, metabolic (lactic) acidosis, hypoglycemia, hemoglobinuria, jaundice, and a parasitemia greater than 5%.

Cerebral malaria is characterized by coma that is not attributable to any other cause in a patient infected with *P. falciparum*. It is a life-threatening complication with an estimated 10% to 40% mortality rate. Coma or impaired mental status caused by malaria has to be distinguished from other causes of neurologic symptoms, including hyperpyrexia, hypoglycemia, and concurrent infections. Signs of cerebral malaria range from disorientation to focal neurologic signs to coma with extensor posturing (including decorticate or decerebrate rigidity) or opisthotonos.

Complications with other species are rare. Splenic rupture has been described in patients who, because of long-standing untreated *P. vivax* infection, have developed massive splenomegaly. With effective chemotherapy, this complication is unusual. Nephritis is a rare complication of persistent *P. malariae* infection but occurs more commonly in children.

Diagnosis

To provide appropriate therapy, it is essential to identify the infecting malaria species, determine where the infection was acquired, and determine the parasite density. Health care providers evaluating patients for possible malaria must get the results of their malaria smears immediately. Sending these diagnostic tests to offsite laboratories where results are not available for extended periods of time is an unacceptable practice that can result in increased morbidity and mortality from delayed diagnosis and delayed recognition of hyperparasitemia. Initial evaluation of patients with slide-confirmed malaria ideally also should include glucose, a complete blood count, electrolytes, creatinine, urea, and liver function tests. In patients with severe disease or respiratory symptoms, lactate level and arterial blood gases to determine acid-base status should also be obtained.

Malaria should be considered in any febrile patient with a history of travel to an area of malaria transmission regardless of whether the patient gives a history of taking prophylaxis. Information on the location and duration of the trip, the date of return, the history of prophylaxis, and the date of symptom onset enables the physician to assess the risk of malaria and, if necessary, to choose an appropriate course of treatment. Rapid diagnosis and institution of antimalarial treatment can prevent the development of severe morbidity and mortality. A list of key diagnostic points, including elements of the history, physical examination, and laboratory investigations, is presented in the Current Diagnosis box.

A thick and a thin blood smear should be obtained from any patient suspected of having malaria. Blood smears can be used to detect the presence of parasites, identify the species, and determine the parasite density. Initial blood smears may be negative, particularly in symptomatic semi-immune persons and those taking prophylaxis. Consequently, a diagnosis of malaria cannot be dismissed on the basis of a single negative smear. Blood smears should be repeated every 12 to 24 hours for a total of 48 to 72 hours before the diagnosis of malaria is excluded. Nearly all patients with clinical symptoms caused by malaria have detectable parasites on well-stained thick blood smears within 48 hours of symptom onset.

Blood smears should he prepared with Giemsa stain and examined under a light microscope. Thick blood smears are more sensitive in detecting malaria parasites, and thin smears are more reliable for identifying species. Both thick and thin smears should be scanned at low magnification and then examined using the

CURRENT DIAGNOSIS

History

- Did the patient travel to a malaria-endemic area? (including duration of journey and date of return)
- Which medicine (if any) was prescribed for prophylaxis?
- Was the patient fully compliant with the malaria prophylaxis regimen?
- Is there a history of blood transfusion, organ transplant, intravenous drug use?
- Is there a history of previous malaria infection?
- Has the patient been exposed to mosquitoes?
- Has the patient been around recent visitors from malaria-endemic areas?

Signs and Symptoms

- Prodrome with headaches, myalgias, and malaise
- Fever
- Chills
- Abdominal pain, nausea, vomiting, diarrhea
- Respiratory distress
- Splenomegaly
- Tachycardia
- Hypotension
- Jaundice
- Seizures
- Altered consciousness, coma

Initial Laboratory Investigations

- Thick and thin blood smears required for diagnosis; results must be available immediately
  - Thick smear used for parasite detection
  - Thin smear used for species identification and determination of parasite density
- Complete blood count
- Electrolytes
- Blood urea nitrogen and creatinine
- Hepatic transaminases

---

100 × oil-immersion lens. The easiest way to determine the percent parasitemia using the thin smear is to count the parasitized erythrocytes among 500 to 2000 erythrocytes, divide the number of parasitized erythrocytes by the total number of erythrocytes counted, and multiply by 100.

To avoid missing low-density infections, at least 300 high-power fields should be examined before a slide is considered negative. Further details about preparation and interpretation of smears can be found at the CDC Division of Parasitic Diseases diagnostic Internet site (www.dpd.cdc.gov/dpdx).

The severity of malaria can vary with the percent parasitemia. Persons with parasitemia lower than 1% usually have mild disease. Those with 1% to 5% parasitemia can have manifestations of more moderate disease. Although severe malaria can occur even with apparently low parasitemia, persons with greater than 5% parasitemia are at high risk for severe malaria. Thus, it is essential to determine the parasite burden at the time of diagnosis as an assessment of disease severity.

If malaria parasites are detected, blood smears should he repeated every 12 to 24 hours, depending on the severity of illness, until the smears are negative. Sequential smears are useful for monitoring the response to treatment and detecting potential drug failure. Although gametocytes can persist much longer, blood smears should be negative for asexual parasites within 48 to 72 hours after the completion of therapy.

Alternative methods for diagnosis are available. Rapid diagnostic tests (RDTs) detect the presence of parasite antigens by measuring either histidine-rich protein-2 (HRP-2) or parasite enzymes like aldolase and lactate dehydrogenase (pLDH). Determination of parasite density is not possible with these methods. The polymerase chain reaction (PCR) method may be more sensitive for detecting parasites than is microscopy. PCR is particularly valuable for identifying the species of a parasite when species cannot be determined by morphology alone. Currently, PCR is used mostly as a research tool and is available only in reference laboratories. Malaria serology detects antibodies to all four species but cannot be used to diagnose current infections. However, it may be useful for identifying an infective donor in cases of transfusion-related malaria, investigating congenital malaria, assessing the validity of clinical malaria diagnoses in empirically treated nonimmune travelers, and diagnosing tropical splenomegaly syndrome.

Treatment

GENERAL INFORMATION

Ideally, treatment for malaria should not be initiated until the diagnosis has been confirmed by laboratory investigations. However, health care providers should not delay treatment when malaria is strongly suspected but the health care system fails to meet the standard of care and provide smear results in a timely manner. Once the diagnosis is confirmed, appropriate antimalarial therapy must be initiated immediately. The choice of treatment should he guided by the degree of parasitemia and the species of *Plasmodium* found, the clinical status of the patient, and the likely drug susceptibility of the infecting species as determined by where the infection was acquired. Although all four species require treatment with a rapidly acting blood schizonticide, patients with *P. vivax* or *P. ovale* also require treatment with primaquine phosphate to decrease the likelihood of a relapse.

Species identification is necessary to distinguish falciparum malaria from nonfalciparum malaria. *P. falciparum* can cause rapid progression of disease and death. Patients with *P. falciparum*, mixed infections with *P. falciparum*, or infections in which the species cannot be identified immediately should he hospitalized and monitored closely to assess for the development of severe malaria and subsequent complications. If the infecting species or probable origin of infection cannot be determined, patients should be treated for multidrug–resistant *P. falciparum* until another species is identified. All patients should have repeat blood smears 12 to 24 hours after initiating treatment to assess for appropriate response.

Using available clinical and laboratory data, physicians must determine whether a patient has uncomplicated or severe malaria. Patients with uncomplicated malaria typically can be treated with oral therapy but might need parenteral therapy if they are unable to take oral medication because of nausea, vomiting, or other reasons. Patients with severe malaria should be immediately started on parenteral malaria therapy.

For detailed treatment information, including doses and frequency of therapy, refer to Table 2.

ANTIMALARIAL DRUGS

Because of the emergence and spread of drug-resistant strains, the slow rate of development of new antimalarial drugs, and the infrequency with which new drugs that are developed are submitted for FDA approval, relatively few drugs are available for prophylaxis and treatment of malaria infections in the United States. For example, resistance to sulfadoxine-pyrimethamine (Fansidar) is widespread in the Amazon River basin area of South America, much of Southeast Asia, other parts of Asia, and, increasingly, in large parts of Africa, rendering this medication largely ineffective for nonimmune travelers. The choice of antimalarial drugs used

CURRENT THERAPY

Recommended Drugs for Treatment of Specific Types of Malaria*

UNCOMPLICATED CHLOROQUINE-SENSITIVE *P. FALCIPARUM*

- Chloroquine phosphate (Aralen) *or*
- Regimen given for unknown resistance or species

RESISTANCE UNKNOWN OR SPECIES UNKNOWN

- Quinine sulfate* *plus one of the following:*
  - Doxycycline[†] (Vibramycin)[1]
  - Tetracycline[†],[1]
  - Clindamycin (Cleocin)[1]
- Atovaquone/proguanil (Malarone)
- Mefloquine[‡] (Lariam)

UNCOMPLICATED *P. MALARIAE*

- Chloroquine phosphate

UNCOMPLICATED *P. VIVAX* OR *P. OVALE* (EXCEPT CHLOROQUINE-RESISTANT *P. VIVAX*)

- Chloroquine phosphate *plus*
- Primaquine phosphate[§]

UNCOMPLICATED CHLOROQUINE-RESISTANT *P. VIVAX*

- Quinine sulfate* *plus one of the following:*
  - Doxycycline[†],[1] plus primaquine phosphate[§]
  - Tetracycline[†],[1] plus primaquine phosphate[§]
- Mefloquine[‡] plus primaquine phosphate[§]

CHLOROQUINE-SENSITIVE MALARIA DURING PREGNANCY

- Chloroquine phosphate

CHLOROQUINE-RESISTANT *P. FALCIPARUM* DURING PREGNANCY

- Quinine sulfate* *plus* clindamycin[1]

CHLOROQUINE-RESISTANT *P. VIVAX* DURING PREGNANCY

- Quinine sulfate*

SEVERE MALARIA

- Qunindine gluconate *plus one of the following:*
  - Doxycycline[†, 1]
  - Tetracycline[†,1]
  - Clindamycin[1]
- Artesunate *followed by either:*[1,**]
  - Atovaquone/proguanil
  - Doxycycline[†,1]
  - Clindamycin[†,1]
  - Mefloquine

---

[1]Not FDA approved for this indication.
*For dosing, see Table 2.
[†]Not indicated for use in children younger than 8 years.
[‡]Because of resistant strains, treatment with mefloquine is not recommended in persons who have acquired infections in parts of Thailand, Burma, Cambodia, Laos, China, and Vietnam.
[§]All persons who take primaquine should have a documented normal glucose-6-phosphate dehydrogenase (G6PD) level before starting the medication.
**Available via Investigational New Drug protocol at the U.S. Centers for Disease Control and Prevention.

for treatment should be guided by several factors: the infecting species, where it was acquired (or at least a travel history), drug-resistance patterns, severity of symptoms, and percent parasitemia. The options for antimalarial drugs that can be used for prevention are based on the drug-resistance patterns at the traveler's destination. Additional factors are discussed in more detail in the prevention section.

Antimalarial drugs can be categorized by their ability to kill the organism at various stages in its life cycle (see Figure 1). Drugs that kill malaria parasites infecting liver cells during the exoerythrocytic cycle are referred to as *tissue schizonticides*. Drugs with high levels of tissue schizonticidal activity are useful in preventing relapses from infection with *P. vivax* and *P. ovale*. Drugs that kill malaria parasites that have been released into the bloodstream and are asexually replicating in the erythrocytic cycle are collectively referred to as *blood schizonticides*. Rapidly acting blood schizonticides are the essential components of acute malaria treatment regimens. Drugs can also have activity against the gametocytes, or *gametocytocidal activity*. This activity does not affect a patient's clinical response but can reduce the patient's infectiousness. Currently no medications are available that have activity against malaria sporozoites. Such a drug would have potential usefulness as a chemoprophylactic agent.

Quinine sulfate (oral) (Qualaquin) and its dextroisomer, quinidine gluconate (intravenous), are used to treat malaria. They are blood schizonticides that are effective against the erythrocytic stages of all four species of *Plasmodium* and are also active against the gametocytes of *P. vivax*, *P. ovale*, and *P. malariae*. Common side effects include cinchonism, a syndrome of tinnitus, deafness, headache, nausea, and visual disturbance, as well as hyperinsulinemic hypoglycemia. The longer the duration of therapy, the higher the

TABLE 2 Malaria Treatment Recommendations

Drug	Adult Dose	Pediatric Dose
Atovaquone-proguanil (Malarone)	Adult tab contains 250 mg atovaquone and 100 mg proguanil 4 adult tabs PO as a single daily dose for 3 consecutive d	Pediatric tab contains 62.5 mg atovaquone and 25 mg proguanil Daily dose taken for 3 consecutive d: 5-8 kg: 2 pediatric tabs 9-10 kg: 3 pediatric tabs 11-20 kg: 1 adult tab 21-30 kg: 2 adult tabs 31-40 kg: 3 adult tabs $\geq$ 41 kg: 4 adult tabs
Chloroquine phosphate (Aralen and generic)	600 mg base (=1 g salt) PO, then 300 mg base (=500 mg salt) at 6, 24, and 48 h	10 mg base/kg PO, then 5 mg base/kg at 6, 24, and 48 h
Clindamycin oral (Cleocin)[1]	20 mg base/kg/d PO divided tid for 7 d	20 mg base/kg/d PO divided tid for 7 d
Clindamycin parenteral (Cleocin)[1]	10 mg base/kg IV followed by 5 mg base/kg IV q8h Switch to oral clindamycin as soon as the patient is able, to complete a 7-d course	10 mg base/kg IV followed by 5 mg base/kg IV q8h Switch to oral clindamycin as soon as the patient is able to complete a 7-d course
Doxycycline* (Vibramycin and generic)[1]	100 mg PO or IV bid for 7 d	2.2 mg/kg PO or IV bid for 7 d*
Mefloquine (Lariam and generic)[†]	750 mg salt (=684 mg base) PO followed by 500 mg salt (=456 mg base) PO 6-12 h after the initial dose	15 mg salt/kg (=13.7 mg base/kg) PO followed by 10 mg salt/kg (=9.1 mg base/kg) PO 6-12 h after the initial dose
Primaquine[‡]	30 mg base PO qd for 14 d[3]	0.6 mg base/kg PO qd for 14 d[3]
Quinidine gluconate	6.25 mg base/kg (=10 mg salt/kg) loading dose[§] IV over 1-2 h, then 0.0125 mg base/kg/min (=0.02 mg salt/kg/min) continuous infusion for $\geq$ 24 h Alternative regimen: 15 mg base/kg (=24 mg salt/kg) loading dose IV infused over 4 h, followed by 7.5 mg base/kg (=12 mg salt/kg) infused over 4 h q8h, starting 8 h after the loading dose Once parasite density is < 1% and the patient can take oral medication, complete treatment with oral quinine	6.25 mg base/kg (=10 mg salt/kg) loading dose[§] IV over 1-2 h, then 0.0125 mg base/kg/min (=0.02 mg salt/kg/min) continuous infusion for $\geq$ 24 h Alternative regimen: 15 mg base/kg (=24 mg salt/kg) loading dose IV infused over 4 h, followed by 7.5 mg base/kg (=12 mg salt/kg) infused over 4 h q8h, starting 8 h after the loading dose Once parasite density is < 1% and the patient can take oral medication, complete treatment with oral quinine
Quinine sulfate (Qualaquin)**	650 mg salt (=542 mg base) PO tid for 3-7 d[¶]	10 mg salt/kg (=8.3 mg base/kg) PO tid for 3-7 d[¶]
Tetracycline[1],*	250 mg PO qid for 7 d	25 mg/kg/d PO divided qid for 7 d*
Artesunate[1],††	2.4 mg/kg IV at 0 h, 12 h, 24 h, and 48 h.	2.4 mg/kg IV at 0 h, 12 h, 24 h, and 48 h.

[1]Not FDA approved for this indication.
[3]Exceeds dosage recommended by the manufacturer.
*Not indicated for children younger than 8 years.
[†]Because of resistant strains, treatment with mefloquine is not recommended in persons who have acquired infections in parts of Thailand, Burma, Cambodia, Laos, China, and Vietnam.
[‡]All persons who take primaquine should have a documented normal glucose-6-phosphate dehydrogenase (G6PD) level before starting the medication.
[§]Patients should be given a loading dose of quinidine unless they have received more than 40 mg/kg of quinine in the preceding 48 hours or if they received mefloquine treatment within the preceding 12 hours.
[¶]Treat for 7 days if infection was acquired in Southeast Asia; treat for 3 days if infection was acquired in Africa or South America.
**U.S. manufactured quinine sulfate capsule is in a 324 mg dosage; therefore, 2 capsules should be sufficient for adult dosing. Pediatric dosing may be difficult due to unavailability of non-capsule forms of quinine.
[††]Available via an Investigational New Drug protocol at the U.S. Centers for Disease Control and Prevention.
Abbreviations: tab = tablet.

risk of adverse events. To shorten the course of therapy, quinine and intravenous quinidine often can be combined with doxycycline (Vibramycin)[1], tetracycline[1], or clindamycin (Cleocin)[1] (see Table 2 for details).

Chloroquine phosphate (Aralen) is approved for preventing and treating malaria, but hydroxychloroquine sulfate (Plaquanil) is approved only for treating malaria. These drugs are blood schizonticides that are active against the erythrocytic stages of all four *Plasmodium* species. They also have gametocytocidal activity against *P. vivax*, *P. ovale*, and *P. malariae*. Chloroquine is the treatment of choice for susceptible strains of *P. falciparum* and *P. vivax*, although chloroquine-resistant forms of both species of malaria have become major public health concerns. Chloroquine is also effective for the treatment of *P. ovale* or *P. malariae* infections. Chloroquine can be taken safely by pregnant women and children. Side effects include gastrointestinal disturbance, dizziness, blurred vision, insomnia, headache, and pruritus. Overdose (ingestion of more than 25 mg base/kg at one time) can lead to acute toxic effects. The toxic effects are predominantly cardiac, leading to cardiac arrest and respiratory failure, usually within 1 to 3 hours after an overdose. For adults, 2.5 to 3 g base may be a fatal dose; for children, 30 to 50 mg base/kg may be fatal.

Atovaquone-proguanil (Malarone), a fixed combination antimalarial drug that is both a blood and tissue schizonticide, can be used for general malaria prophylaxis and for treatment of chloroquine-resistant *P. falciparum*. The tissue schizonticide activity is not sufficient to prevent relapses of *P. vivax* and *P. ovale*. Side effects are rare, but abdominal pain, nausea, vomiting, and headache have been reported. Treatment efficacy, safety, and pharmacokinetic data in children who weigh 5 to 11 kg have recently been extrapolated, allowing prophylaxis doses in these children. Providers should note that this prophylactic dosing for children weighing less than 11 kg constitutes off-label use in the United States. Atovaquone-proguanil should not he used for prophylaxis and treatment in children who weigh less than 5 kg. It is contraindicated in pregnant women, women who are breast-feeding infants who weigh less than 5 kg, and persons with severe renal impairment.

Mefloquine (Lariam) is a long-acting blood schizonticide that is used for preventing and treating malaria. It is effective against the erythrocytic stages of all four species. Side effects include nausea, vomiting, diarrhea, abdominal pain, mild neuropsychiatric complaints (dizziness, headache, somnolence, sleep disorders), myalgia, a mild skin rash, and fatigue. Mefloquine has been associated with rare serious adverse reactions such as seizures and psychoses at prophylactic doses. Although mefloquine can be used to treat chloroquine-resistant *P. falciparum*, adverse reactions are more common at the higher doses used for treatment. Because other options that have fewer adverse events are available for treatment, mefloquine normally is not recommended. Mefloquine is contraindicated in patients with known hypersensitivity to the drug and persons with a history of psychiatric disease. Mefloquine also is contraindicated in persons with a history of seizures (not including febrile seizures in childhood). It should be avoided in patients with cardiac conduction disorders because it prolongs the QTc interval and should be used with caution in persons taking β-blockers. Concomitant administration of mefloquine and quinine or quinidine can produce arrhythmias and increase the risk of seizures. Mefloquine prophylaxis in the second and third trimesters is not associated with an adverse fetal or pregnancy outcome. More limited data suggest that it is probably safe in the first trimester.

Tetracyclines are blood schizonticides that are effective against the erythrocytic stages of all four species of *Plasmodium*. They have some activity against liver schizonts, but not enough to prevent relapses. Because of their relatively slow onset of action, tetracyclines should never be used alone for treatment. Combined with quinine or quinidine, they are effective against chloroquine-resistant *P. falciparum* and *P. vivax*. Doxycycline alone is effective as prophylaxis against chloroquine-resistant and mefloquine-resistant *P. falciparum*. Side effects include gastrointestinal symptoms, *Candida* vaginitis or stomatitis, and idiosyncratic photosensitivity reactions. Tetracyclines should not be used in pregnant women or in children younger than 8 years.

Clindamycin[1] is active against blood schizonts of all four species of *Plasmodium*. Clindamycin can be used in combination with quinine to treat chloroquine-resistant *P. falciparum* infections in people who are not able to take doxycycline. Side effects include diarrhea, nausea, and skin rashes.

Derivatives of artemisinin (such as artesunate,[2] artemether,[2] and dihydroartemisinin[2]) are compounds derived from the Chinese medicinal plant quinghaosu (*Artemisia annua*) that are active against blood schizonts and gametocytes. Artemisinin and its derivatives are short-acting, highly effective antimalarial drugs for the treatment of uncomplicated multidrug–resistant *P. falciparum* and severe *P. falciparum* infection. These drugs are available in oral, rectal, and intravenous formulations. Although they can be used alone for at least 7 days, combining them with other antimalarial drugs can treat malaria infection effectively and decrease the length of treatment to as little as 3 days. Therefore, using these drugs as a component of combination therapy is recommended for the added efficacy and to safeguard against selecting for drug-resistant parasites. Commonly used artemisinin-based combination therapies (ACTs) include artesunate copackaged with mefloquine (Artequin)[1] and artemether coformulated with lumefantrine (Coartem or Riamet).[1] Intravenous artesunate is now available for the treatment of severe malaria via an Investigational New Drug Protocol. To enroll a patient with severe malaria in this treatment protocol, contact the CDC Malaria Hotline: 770-488-7788 (M-F, 8 AM-4:30 PM, eastern time) or after hours, call 770-488-7100, and request to speak with a CDC Malaria Branch clinician.

Primaquine phosphate, a tissue schizonticide with gametocytocidal activity, is the only drug available to prevent relapse of *P. vivax* and *P. ovale* infections. Primaquine may be used for primary prophylaxis in areas where principally *P. vivax* is present or when other prophylactic agents are contraindicated or unavailable. In parts of Southeast Asia and Latin America, short doses of primaquine are used to eliminate gametocyte carriage in patients treated for malaria. Primaquine can cause hemolysis and methemoglobinemia in glucose-6-phosphate dehydrogenase (G6PD)-deficient persons. Before primaquine is used, G6PD deficiency must be ruled out by appropriate laboratory testing. The most common side effect is abdominal pain. Primaquine is contraindicated in pregnant and breast-feeding women.

DRUG-RESISTANT *P. FALCIPARUM*

For *P. falciparum* infections acquired in chloroquine-resistant areas, there are three treatment options: quinine sulfate plus doxycycline,[1] tetracycline[1], or clindamycin[1]; atovaquone-proguanil alone; and mefloquine alone. Because mefloquine has a higher rate of severe neuropsychiatric reactions at treatment doses, it is not recommended unless the other two options are not available. Also, mefloquine is not recommended for the treatment of *P. falciparum* malaria in persons who acquired the infection in the borders of Thailand with Myanmar and Cambodia, in the western provinces of Cambodia, in the eastern states of Myanmar, on the border between Myanmar and China, in Laos along the borders of Laos and Myanmar, in the adjacent parts of the Thailand-Cambodia border, and in southern Vietnam because of the potential for mefloquine-resistant strains.

CHLOROQUINE-SENSITIVE *PLASMODIUM* SPECIES

For *P. malariae*, *P. ovale*, chloroquine-sensitive *P. vivax*, and chloroquine-sensitive *P. falciparum* infection, prompt treatment with oral chloroquine phosphate is recommended. In addition, infections with

---

[1] Not FDA approved for this indication.

[1] Not FDA approved for this indication.
[2] Not available in the United States.

P. vivax and *P. ovale* require primaquine to reduce the likelihood of a relapse. Before starting primaquine treatment, patients must be screened for G6PD deficiency.

DRUG-RESISTANT *P. VIVAX*

Chloroquine-resistant *P. vivax* should he treated with either quinine sulfate plus doxycycline[1] or tetracycline[1] or with mefloquine alone. In addition to either of those regimens, after screening for G6PD deficiency, persons infected with chloroquine-resistant *P. vivax* should be treated with primaquine phosphate to prevent relapse.

SEVERE MALARIA

Patients with severe malaria and those who are unable to take oral medications because of depressed sensorium, vomiting, or other reasons should be treated with parenteral antimalarial therapy. Severe malaria is a medical emergency, and treatment with intravenous medication should be initiated immediately (see Current Therapy box and Table 2). However, intravenous artesunate is now available for the treatment of severe malaria via an Investigational New Drug Protocol. To enroll a patient with severe malaria in this treatment protocol, contact the CDC Malaria Hotline: 770-488-7788 (M-F, 8 AM-4:30 PM, eastern time) or after hours, call 770-488-7100 and request to speak with a CDC Malaria Branch clinician.

If possible, the patient should be admitted to an intensive care unit. Continuous blood pressure and cardiac monitoring (to assess the QTc interval) and regular measurements of blood glucose are strongly recommended for patients who receive quinidine therapy. In addition to antimalarial therapy, patients should receive the necessary supportive care. If there is impaired consciousness, the airway should be secured, and breathing and circulation should be assessed. Fluid status, level of consciousness, and vital signs including blood pressure, temperature, and respiratory status should be monitored closely.

Because these patients are at risk for hypoglycemia, severe anemia, renal failure, and acidosis, regular assessment of blood glucose, hemoglobin and hematocrit, creatinine, urea, electrolytes, and acid-base status also is required. Severe anemia requires blood transfusion with packed red blood cells. One should consider exchange transfusion if parasitemia is greater than 10% or if the patient has altered mental status, noncardiogenic pulmonary edema, or renal complications. Dialysis is usually necessary in patients with acute renal failure. Oxygen and other respiratory support may be required in patients with noncardiogenic pulmonary edema.

Corticosteroids should not be used because they have not been shown to provide benefit and have been associated with increased mortality in this setting. Blood smears should be repeated every 12 hours to monitor the therapeutic response. Once parasite density is lower than 1% and the patient is able to eat and drink, the treatment course can be completed with oral medications.

CONGENITAL AND PREGNANCY-ASSOCIATED MALARIA

Malaria in pregnancy affects both the mother and her fetus. Infection with *P. falciparum* during pregnancy can increase the mother's risk of developing severe disease and anemia and can increase the risk of stillbirth, prematurity, and low birth weight. Babies born to non-immune mothers with acute malaria are at risk for congenital malaria. If a mother is parasitemic at the time of delivery, blood smears should be performed on the infant. If the blood smears demonstrate malaria parasites, the infant should be treated according to the species present. Primaquine treatment of infants is unnecessary because there is no liver phase with congenital infections. If the infant's blood smear is negative at the time of delivery, health care providers should remain alert for the development of signs and symptoms consistent with malaria and initiate a prompt diagnostic evaluation. Congenital malaria often manifests as fever, anemia, or failure to thrive at 1 to 2 months of age and can be difficult for an unsuspecting clinician to detect.

For pregnant women with uncomplicated malaria caused by *P. malariae*, *P. ovale*, chloroquine-sensitive *P. vivax*, and chloroquine-sensitive *P. falciparum*, prompt treatment with chloroquine is recommended. For pregnant women with chloroquine-resistant *P. vivax*, treatment with quinine for 7 days is recommended. After treatment, all pregnant women with *P. vivax* and *P. ovale* should be given chloroquine prophylaxis for the duration of the pregnancy to prevent relapses; women can be treated with primaquine after delivery if they have a normal G6PD screening test. For pregnant women with uncomplicated chloroquine-resistant *P. falciparum* malaria, prompt treatment with quinine and clindamycin[1] is recommended.

MALARIA IN CHILDREN

For pediatric patients, treatment options are the same as those for adults except that the drug dose is adjusted by patient weight. The pediatric dose should not exceed the recommended adult dose. To treat chloroquine-resistant *P. falciparum* in children younger than 8 years, doxycycline and tetracycline should not be used; quinine sulfate given in combination with clindamycin[1] or atovaquone-proguanil alone are the recommended treatment options. Mefloquine can be considered if these options are not available. In rare instances, doxycycline[1] or tetracycline[1] can be used in combination with quinine in children younger than 8 years if other treatment options are not available or are not tolerated and the benefit of adding doxycycline or tetracycline is judged to outweigh the risk.

Prevention

A combination of personal protective measures and chemoprophylaxis can be highly effective in preventing malaria. Travelers should avoid being outdoors during the peak *Anopheles* biting period between dusk and dawn. When outdoors, travelers should wear clothing that minimizes the amount of exposed skin and apply insect repellents that contain DEET (*N,N*-diethyl-m-toluamide). DEET may be used on adults and children and on infants older than 2 months. Higher concentrations of DEET can have a longer repellent effect, but concentrations greater than 50% provide no added protection. Travelers who are not staying in well-screened or air-conditioned rooms should sleep under insecticide-treated bed nets.

The choice of prophylactic medication should be made in light of the traveler's destination, length of stay, the presence of resistant strains, and the traveler's age, drug allergies, other medications, and medical history. Health care providers should help travelers make informed decisions about the available chemoprophylaxis options to improve compliance. Often, potential side effects, convenience of the dosing regimen, and cost affect patients' choices of medications. Detailed prophylaxis recommendations are presented in Table 3.

Malaria infection in pregnant women can be more severe than it is in nonpregnant women. Women who are pregnant or likely to become pregnant should be advised to avoid travel to malaria-risk areas. However, pregnant women who choose to travel to these areas should take appropriate antimalarial prophylaxis and use personal protective measures.

Long-term travelers to parts of the world where relapsing forms of malaria (*P. vivax* and *P. ovale*) are present can benefit from presumptive antirelapse therapy, also known as terminal prophylaxis. After returning and completing their standard chemoprophylaxis, persons who are not G6PD deficient can take a 14-day course of primaquine as described in Table 3 to decrease the chance of developing malaria later.

---

[1]Not FDA approved for this indication.

TABLE 3 Malaria Chemoprophylaxis Recommendations

Drug	Use	Adult Dose	Pediatric Dose	Comments
Atovaquone-proguanil (Malarone)	Prophylaxis in areas with chloroquine-resistant or mefloquine-resistant P. falciparum	Adult tab contains 250 mg atovaquone and 100 mg proguanil HCl 1 adult tab PO qd	Pediatric tab contains 62.5 mg atovaquone and 25 mg proguanil HCl 5-8 kg:[1] ½ tab qd 9-10 kg:[1] ¾ tab qd 11-20 kg: 1 tab qd 21-30 kg: 2 tabs qd 31-40 kg: 3 tabs qd ≥ 41 kg: 1 adult tab qd	Begin 1-2 d before travel to malaria-endemic areas. Take daily at the same time each d while in the area and for 7 d after leaving such areas Contraindicated in persons with severe renal impairment (creatinine clearance < 30 mL/min) Take with food Not recommended for prophylaxis for children < 5 kg or pregnant women. Partial-tab dosages may need to be prepared by a pharmacist and dispensed in individual capsules
Chloroquine phosphate* (Aralen and generic)	Prophylaxis only in areas with chloroquine-sensitive P. falciparum	300 mg base (500 mg salt) PO once/wk	5 mg/kg base (8.3 mg/kg salt) PO once/wk, up to max adult dose of 300 mg base	Begin 1-2 wk before travel to malaria-endemic areas. Take weekly on the same d of the wk while in the area and for 4 wk after leaving such areas. Can exacerbate psoriasis
Doxycycline[†] (Vibramycin and generic)	Prophylaxis in areas with chloroquine-resistant or mefloquine-resistant P. falciparum	100 mg PO qd	≥ 8 y: 2 mg/kg up to adult dose of 100 mg/d[†]	Begin 1-2 d before travel to malaria-endemic areas. Take daily at the same time each d while in the area and for 4 wk after leaving such areas. Contraindicated in children < 8 y and pregnant women
Hydroxychloroquine sulfate (Plaquenil)[1]	Alternative to chloroquine for prophylaxis only in areas with chloroquine-sensitive P. falciparum	310 mg base (400 mg salt) PO once/wk	5 mg/kg base (6.5 mg/kg salt) PO once/wk, up to max adult dose of 310 mg base	Begin 1-2 wk before travel to malaria-endemic areas. Take weekly on the same d of the wk while in the area and for 4 wk after leaving such areas
Mefloquine (Lariam and generic)[‡]	Prophylaxis in areas with chloroquine-resistant P. falciparum	228 mg base (250 mg salt) PO once/wk	≤ 9 kg: 4.6 mg/kg base (5 mg/kg salt) PO once/wk 10-19 kg: ¼ tab once/wk 20-30 kg: ½ tab once/wk 31-45 kg: ¾ tab once/wk ≥ 46 kg: 1 tab once/wk	Begin 1-2 wk before travel to malaria-endemic areas. Take weekly on the same d of the wk while in the area and for 4 wk after leaving such areas. Contraindicated in persons allergic to mefloquine or related compounds (e.g., quinine and quinidine) and in persons with active depression, a recent history of depression, generalized anxiety disorder, psychosis, schizophrenia, other major psychiatric disorders, or seizures. Use with caution in persons with psychiatric disturbances or a previous history of depression. Not recommended for persons with cardiac conduction abnormalities.
Primaquine[§]	An option for prophylaxis in special circumstances	30 mg base (52.6 mg salt) PO qd[3]	0.6 mg/kg base (1.0 mg/kg salt) up to adult dose PO qd[3]	Begin 1-2 d before travel to malaria-endemic areas. Take daily at the same time each d while in the area and for 7 d after leaving such areas. Contraindicated in persons with G6PD[§] deficiency Contraindicated during pregnancy and lactation unless the infant being breast-fed has a documented normal G6PD level Use in consultation with malaria experts

[1] Not FDA approved for this indication.
[3] Exceeds dosage recommended by the manufacturer.
*All pregnant women with P. vivax and P. ovale should be given chloroquine prophylaxis for the duration of the pregnancy to prevent relapses. They can be treated with primaquine after delivery.
[†] Not indicated for children younger than 8 years.
[‡] Because of resistant strains, treatment with mefloquine is not recommended in persons who have acquired infections in parts of Thailand, Burma, Cambodia, Laos, China, and Vietnam.
[§] All persons who take primaquine should have a documented normal G6PD level before starting the medication.

TABLE 3 Malaria Chemoprophylaxis Recommendations—cont'd

Drug	Use	Adult Dose	Pediatric Dose	Comments
Primaquine	Used for presumptive antirelapse therapy (terminal prophylaxis) to decrease the risk of relapses of *P. vivax* and *P. ovale*	30 mg base (52.6 mg salt) PO qd, for 14 d after departure from the malaria-endemic area[3]	0.6 mg/kg base (1.0 mg/kg salt) up to adult dose PO qd for 14 d after departure from the malaria-endemic area[3]	Indicated for persons who have had prolonged exposure to *P. vivax* and *P. ovale* or both Contraindicated in persons with G6PD[§] deficiency Contraindicated during pregnancy and lactation unless the infant being breast-fed has a documented normal G6PD level

Abbreviations: G6PD = glucose-6-phosphate dehydrogenase; max = maximum; tab = tablet.

Travelers should be advised that they can contract malaria despite the use of prophylaxis and personal protective measures. Travelers should be aware of the signs and symptoms of malaria and should urgently seek medical care if they develop fever or experience flu-like symptoms. Because many health care providers do not always ask about a history of recent travel, travelers should be advised to specifically inform them of their recent travel to a malaria-endemic country so that the appropriate diagnostic evaluation can be initiated.

REFERENCES

Baird JK: Effectiveness of antimalarial drugs. N Engl J Med 2005;352:1565-1577.
Centers for Disease Control and Prevention: Guidelines for treatment of malaria in the United States. Available at http://www.cdc.gov/malaria/pdf/treatmenttable.pdf (accessed May 15, 2007).
Chen LH, Keystone JS: New strategies for the prevention of malaria in travelers. Infect Dis Clin N Amer 2005;19:185-210.
Guinovart C, Navia MM, Tanner M, et al: Malaria: Burden of disease. Curr Mol Med 2006;6:137-140.
Kitchen AD, Chiodini PL: Malaria and blood transfusion. Vox Sang 2006;90:77-84.
Leder K, Black J, O'Brien D, et al: Malaria in travelers: A review of the GeoSentinel surveillance network. Clin Infect Dis 2004;39:1104-1112.
Magill AJ: The prevention of malaria. Prim Care 2002;29:815-842.
Newman RD, Parise ME, Barber AM, et al: Malaria-related deaths among U.S. travelers, 1963-2001. Ann Intern Med 2004;141:547-555.
Parise ME, Lewis LS: Severe malaria: North American perspective. In CFeldman, GASarosi, editors): Tropical and Parasitic Infections in the ICU. New York: Springer Science, 2005, pp 17-38.
Skarbinski J, James EM, Causer LM, et al: Malaria surveillance—United States, 2004. MMWR Surveill Summ 2006;55:23-37.
White NJ: The treatment of malaria. N Engl J Med 1996;335(11):800-806.
Whitty CJM, Edmonds S, Mutabingwa TK: Malaria in pregnancy. BJOG 2005;112:1189-1195.

Bacterial Meningitis

Method of
Gary D. Overturf, MD

Acute bacterial meningitis occurs in all age groups, but predominantly in children younger than 2 years and the elderly (older than 60 years). With the introduction of effective protein conjugate vaccines for *Haemophilus* and pneumococcal infection, the incidence of bacterial meningitis is rapidly declining in children, and adults are now the major population affected. Bacterial meningitis is a medical emergency requiring rapid and decisive action to prevent death or neurologic sequelae. Since the introduction of chloramphenicol (Chloromycetin) in the early 1950s, the mortality has remained between 5% and 40% depending on the age of the patient and the etiology. Of the survivors, 10% to 30% suffer permanent neurologic deficits. Prognosis is affected by the timeliness of therapy, the age of the patient, and the etiology. Presumptive diagnosis and administration of therapy are critical.

Diagnosis

Acute bacterial meningitis must be considered in the differential diagnosis of persons of any age presenting with fever and headache or signs of meningeal irritation or acute central nervous system dysfunction. Presentations can be subtle at the extremes of age or in patients who have received partially effective antibiotic therapy. The diagnosis of bacterial meningitis requires the examination of the cerebrospinal fluid (CSF), which must be performed as expeditiously as possible. Studies indicate that lumbar puncture may be safely performed on patients who have normal mental status or are without focal neurologic signs or papilledema; clinical impression are predictive of the computed tomography (CT) findings. If there are signs or symptoms suggesting the presence of an intracranial mass (e.g., tumor, cerebral hematoma, or brain abscess), blood cultures should be obtained and empirical antibiotics should be administered prior to the performance of a CT scan.

The CSF findings in bacterial meningitis include a cell count of greater than 500 to 1000 white blood cells (WBC) per mm^3 with a predominance of neutrophils, a protein concentration of greater than 150 mg/mL, and a low glucose (e.g., less than 35 to 40 mg/dL). No single value is absolute, and a single value may be normal in up to a third of the cases. The Gram-stained sediment of centrifuged CSF is the critical examination leading to a specific diagnosis. In patients who have not received antibiotics capable of reaching the CSF, the

---

CURRENT DIAGNOSIS

- Patient age and epidemiology:
  - Clinical symptoms: Fever, headache, meningeal signs
  - CSF examination: High opening pressure >300 mm Hg
  - Elevated white blood cell count (>10 –>5000)
  - >60% polymorphonuclear cells
- Low CSF glucose (<40 mg/dL or <50% serum glucose)
- High CSF protein (>50 –>1.0 g/dL)
- Bacteria present on Gram stain of CSF

Abbreviation: CSF = cerebrospinal fluid.

TABLE 1 Cerebrospinal Fluid Gram Stain Morphology and Antibiotic Recommendations

Morphology	Possible or Probable Pathogens	Treatment Options	Alternative Therapies
Gram-positive cocci, short chains or pairs	Streptococcus pneumoniae, Streptococcus agalactiae (group B streptococci)	Ceftriaxone (Rocephin) or cefotaxime (Claforan) plus vancomycin (Vancocin)	Chloramphenicol (Chloromycetin)
Gram-positive cocci, clusters; or gram-positive bacilli	Staphylococcus aureus, Listeria monocytogenes	Vancomycin, ampicillin plus gentamicin (Garamycin)	Nafcillin (Unipen) or Oxacillin, trimethoprim-sulfamethoxazole (Bactrim)
Gram-negative diplococci	Neisseria meningitidis	Ceftriaxone or cefotaxime	Ampicillin, Penicillin G, or chloramphenicol
Gram-negative coccobacilli	Haemophilus influenzae	Ceftriaxone or cefotaxime	Chloramphenicol
Gram-negative bacilli	Escherichia coli, Klebsiella species, Pseudomonas aeruginosa	Cefepime (Maxipime) or ceftazidime (Fortaz)	Imipenem (Primaxin) or meropenem (Merrem)

Gram stain is positive in 80% to 90% of culture-confirmed cases. In persons previously treated with antibiotics (e.g., beta-lactam antibiotics, tetracycline, fluoroquinolones), the frequency of positive Gram stains is much reduced (e.g., 60% to 70%), but the cells, cell type, protein, and glucose concentrations are not significantly affected. CSF antigen tests are not reliable, and high false-positive and false-negative rates direct against relying on the use of such tests. Clinical judgment is paramount, and antibiotics should be given in situations of ambiguous results of the CSF examination.

Antibiotic Selection

The outcome of bacterial meningitis is closely related to the timely use of antibiotics. Hypotension, seizures, an altered mental status, and hypoglycorrhachia at the time of initial antibiotic administration are predictive of higher case fatality and neurologic sequelae. Because prompt administration of antibiotics is critical, the choice of antibiotics usually is made before results of the CSF cultures are known. If organisms are seen on Gram stain, therapy may be directed by the probable bacterial etiology (Table 1). In the event the CSF Gram stain fails to reveal a possible pathogen, empirical antibiotic therapy should be begun based on the age of the patient for those persons who have acquired their infection in the community (Table 2). For those persons who are members of special risk groups, empirical therapy should be based on the likely etiology (Table 3). Once the CSF cultures are completed, therapy can be modified according to results of the culture and sensitivity data.

Antibiotics used in bacterial meningitis should be rapidly bactericidal and achieve high concentrations in the CSF. Antibiotics should be given in maximal doses (Table 4). Because the bactericidal activity of antibiotics in CSF is dose dependent, the fractional CSF-to-serum ratio is very small. Finally, the use of combinations of antibiotics should be minimized to avoid antagonizing the bactericidal activity.

Special Considerations for Antibiotic Therapy

During the past two decades, resistance to penicillin and some third-generation cephalosporins (e.g., ceftriaxone [Rocephin], cefotaxime [Claforan]) has steadily increased among strains of Streptococcus pneumoniae. Currently, approximately 30% to 50% of isolates are either intermediately (inhibitory concentration, 0.1 to 1.0 µg/mL) or fully (inhibitory concentration more than 2.0 µg/mL) resistant to Penicillin G and ampicillin. Resistance to ceftriaxone (Rocephin) and cefotaxime (Claforan) may occur as well in 10% to 15% of strains. Vancomycin (Vancocin) is recommended in those regimens for meningitis when pneumococci are considered. However, higher maximal doses are required for vancomycin because of its relatively poor penetration into the CSF. In general, lumbar puncture with CSF culture should be repeated in 48 hours in those cases where vancomycin therapy is the primary drug because of demonstrated penicillin or cephalosporin resistance.

Meningitis caused by gram-negative bacilli such as Pseudomonas aeruginosa, Escherichia coli, or Enterobacter cloacae should be treated with a cephalosporin with an extended spectrum of gram-negative activity, such as ceftazidime (Fortaz) or cefepime (Maxipime). Carbapenem, such as imipenem (Primaxin) or meropenem (Merrem), can also be used for antibiotic-resistant gram-negative enteric and pseudomonas meningitis. Meropenem is associated with less risk of drug-induced seizures and may be a better choice for bacterial meningitis.

Patients with ventriculoatrial and ventriculoperitoneal shunt–associated meningitis and ventriculitis usually require removal of the shunt for cure, as well as the administration of antibiotics to clear the infection. Certain patients with infections caused by organisms of reduced virulence, such as coagulase-negative staphylococci, or those with exquisitely antibiotic-susceptible infections, can be treated with a trial of antibiotics alone.

TABLE 2 Antibiotic Recommendations for Bacterial Meningitis Acquired in the Community, by Age Group and Probable Pathogen

Age Group	Probable Pathogens	Empirical Therapy
Neonate < 1 mo	Group B streptococcus; Escherichia coli, or other gram-negative enteric rod; occasionally Listeria monocytogenes	Ampicillin plus cefotaxime (Claforan)
Infants 1–3 mo	H. influenzae, N. meningitidis, S. pneumoniae, Group B streptococci	Ceftriaxone (Rocephin) or cefotaxime (Claforan)
Children 3 mo–7 y and older children and adults 7–50 y	H. influenzae, S. pneumoniae, N. meningitidis	Ceftriaxone or cefotaxime plus vancomycin (Vancocin)
Older adults > 50 y	S. pneumoniae, N. meningitidis, and L. monocytogenes	Ceftriaxone plus ampicillin

TABLE 3 Antibiotic Recommendations for Presumed Bacterial Meningitis in Persons with Special Risks

Condition or Risk Factor	Common Pathogens	Antibiotic Recommendations
Impaired immunity (e.g., HIV, early complement deficiency, agammaglobulinemia)	Listeria monocytogenes, Streptococcus pneumoniae, Haemophilus influenzae	Ampicillin plus ceftriaxone (Rocephin) or cefotaxime (Claforan)
Closed head trauma with CSF leak	S. pneumoniae, H. influenzae	Ceftriaxone or cefotaxime plus vancomycin (Vancocin)
Asplenia	S. pneumoniae, H. influenzae	Ceftriaxone or cefotaxime plus vancomycin
Terminal complement deficiency	Neisseria meningitidis	Ceftriaxone or cefotaxime
Neurosurgical procedures	Staphylococcus aureus	Vancomycin plus ceftriaxone or cefotaxime
CSF shunt infections	Coagulase-negative staphylococci, gram-negative bacilli	
Elderly patients (> 65 y)	S. pneumoniae, Listeria monocytogenes	Ceftriaxone or cefotaxime plus vancomycin
Recurrent bacterial meningitis (see CSF leak)	Streptococcus pneumoniae	Ceftriaxone or cefotaxime plus vancomycin
Alcoholic patients	Streptococcus pneumoniae and gram-negative bacilli	Ceftriaxone or cefotaxime plus vancomycin

Abbreviation: CSF = cerebrospinal fluid.

Because of the extreme sensitivity of *Neisseria meningitidis* to antibiotics, uncomplicated meningitis may be treated with as little as 5 to 7 days of antibiotics. Pneumococcal meningitis may be treated with 10 to 14 days of antibiotics and haemophilus infections are treated successfully with 7 to 10 days of antibiotics. Gram-negative meningitis was treated in the past with 3 weeks of aminoglycosides, but current experience with newer extended-spectrum cephalosporins (ceftriaxone, cefotaxime, carbapenems) suggests that 2 weeks of therapy is often sufficient in neonates as well as in some elderly patients and postoperative infections.

All patients with bacterial meningitis should be monitored carefully throughout the treatment period. Infectious disease consultation is recommended for most infections of the central nervous system. Repeated lumbar punctures are not routinely recommended for patients with fully susceptible bacterial isolates or in those who show good response to therapy. Repeated sampling of the CSF with lumbar puncture or, when appropriate, shunt or ventricular reservoir puncture should be performed in those with known resistant bacterial isolates, in patients who have an inadequate response, in those patients who deteriorate on therapy, or in those for whom clinical response may correlate poorly with the microbiologic response (shunt infections, neonates, and elderly patients).

Adjunctive Therapy

Corticosteroids reduce the incidence of permanent neurologic sequelae in children with bacterial meningitis, particularly when caused by *Haemophilus influenza* type b. Data in support of steroids in either pneumococcal or meningococcal infections are less robust. Dexamethasone (Decadron[1]), 0.15 mg/kg every 6 hours for the first 2 to 4 days of treatment, was evaluated in children older than 2 months with bacterial meningitis. The first dose of dexamethasone should be given before, at the start, or within no later than 12 hours after beginning antibiotics.

Use of corticosteroids in adults is more controversial. Although doses of dexamethasone are recommended by some experts for adults with bacterial meningitis, its efficacy in adult meningitis has not been evaluated in a well-designed prospective trial. A recent study in adults found that corticosteroids significantly reduced the risk for unfavorable outcomes, particularly in patients with pneumococcal meningitis. There has been concern that the anti-inflammatory properties of dexamethasone may decrease the penetration of antibiotics, especially vancomycin, into the CSF. One study in children did not show this to be the case. Dexamethasone[1] should be administered in adults with proven or suspected pneumococcal meningitis, only if it can be given prior to the first dose of antibiotics in a dose of 10 mg every 6 hours for 4 days. In patients with meningitis caused by *Streptococcus pneumoniae* highly resistant to penicillin (minimum inhibitory concentration [MIC] >2.0 µg/mL) or cephalosporins (MIC >4.0 µg/mL), vancomycin should not be used as a single agent if corticosteroids are used. The addition of rifampin (Rifadin[1]) is often recommended in these situations.

CURRENT THERAPY

- Neonates < 2 mo
  - Group B streptococcal infection: cefotaxime (Claforan) or ampicillin
  - Gram-negative rods, other than *Pseudomonas*: cefotaxime
  - *Pseudomonas*: cefepime (Maxipime) or ceftazidime (Fortaz)
  - *Listeria*: Ampicillin + gentamicin (Garamycin)
- Children > 2 mo
  - Empirical for unknown etiology: cefotaxime or ceftriaxone (Rocephin)
  - *Streptococcus pneumoniae*: cefotaxime or ceftriaxone
  - *Haemophilus influenza*: cefotaxime or ceftriaxone
  - *Neisseria meningitidis*: ampicillin or cefotaxime
- Older children and adults
  - Empirical for unknown etiology: cefotaxime or ceftriaxone
  - *S. pneumoniae*: cefotaxime or ceftriaxone
  - *N. meningitidis*: ampicillin or cefotaxime
  - Gram negative, postoperative, or *Staphylococcus aureus* (see Tables 1–4)
  - Add vancomycin if at risk for infection with resistant pneumococcus

Chemoprophylaxis for Bacterial Meningitis

Prophylactic antibiotics are recommended in case of meningitis caused by *Neisseria meningitidis* and *Haemophilus influenzae* type b. Prophylaxis is provided to eliminate the carriage of organisms among contacts and prevent spread to hosts susceptible to invasive disease. In cases of meningococcal meningitis, prophylaxis is indicated only for those with household or close intimate contact with the

---

[1]Not FDA approved for this indication.

TABLE 4 Antibiotic Doses for Adults and Children for Treatment of Bacterial Meningitis

Antibiotic	Daily Adult Dose	Daily Pediatric Dose	Dose Interval
Amikacin (Amikin)	15 mg/kg	15–20 mg/kg	8 h
Ampicillin	12 g	200–400 mg/kg	4–6 h
Cefotaxime (Claforan)	12 g	200–300 mg/kg	4–6 h
Ceftriaxone (Rocephin)	4 g	100 mg/kg	12 h
Ceftazidime (Fortaz)	6 g	150–200 mg/kg	8 h
Cefepime (Maxipime)	6 g	100–150 mg/kg	8 h
Gentamicin (Garamycin)	5 mg/kg	7.5 mg/kg	8 h
Meropenem (Merrem)	6 g	120 mg/kg	8 h
Nafcillin (Unipen)	12 g	200 mg/kg	4–6 h
Penicillin G	24 million U	250,000 units/kg	4 h
Tobramycin (Nebcin)	5 mg/kg	6–7.5 mg/kg	8 h
Trimethoprim-sulfamethoxazole (Bactrim)	10–15 mg/kg	10–20 mg/kg	8 h
Vancomycin (Vancocin)	2 g	60 mg/kg	12 h

Adapted from Bradley JS, Nelson JD: 2002–2003 Nelson's Pocket Book of Pediatric Antimicrobial Therapy, 15th ed. Philadelphia and New York, Lippincott Williams & Wilkins, 2002.
Gilbert DN, Moellering RC, Sande MA: The Sanford Guide to Antimicrobial Therapy 2005. Hyde Park, Antimicrobial Therapy Inc., 2005.

index case. Administration of prophylaxis to large groups (e.g., college students, schoolchildren, or preschool classes) requires a special assessment and a recommendation of local or regional health departments. Chemoprophylaxis is not necessary for casual contacts or medical personnel unless there is a direct exposure to respiratory secretions. The recommended dose of rifampin (Rifadin) is 10 mg/kg (600 maximal, adults) twice a day for 2 days; ciprofloxacin (Cipro[1]), 500 mg as single dose, is also effective for adults. Third-generation cephalosporins used in treatment of the index case of meningitis are sufficient to eliminate carriage of the organism.

Chemoprophylaxis for *H. influenzae* type b is recommended for all household contacts of an index case if one of the contacts is an unvaccinated child younger than 4 years. If the index case is treated with ceftriaxone (Rocephin) or cefotaxime (Claforan), prophylaxis is not required, but if treated with ampicillin or chloramphenicol (Chloromycetin), prophylaxis is recommended to eliminate carriage. The recommended regimen for prophylaxis is rifampin,[1] 20 mg/kg (or 600 mg in adults) once a day for 4 days. With the near elimination of invasive infections caused by *Haemophilus influenzae* type b, with the use of routine immunization of children with conjugate haemophilus vaccines, *Haemophilus influenzae* types A, F, and rarely other serotypes have emerged, and the use of prophylaxis is not recommended in these situations because sufficient data are not available to support its efficacy, nor has spread within contacts been documented with any frequency.

Vaccines for Bacterial Meningitis

The universal recommendation for the use of protein-polysaccharide conjugate *Haemophilus influenzae* type b (HIB) vaccines in 1987 reduced the incidence of bacterial meningitis by this organism by greater than 97%. Three HIB vaccines (PedvaxHIB, ActHIB, HibTITER), licensed in the United States, are routinely given to children in dosage schedules employing three to four doses by 12 to 18 months of age (see www.cdc.gov).

A pneumococcal protein-polysaccharide conjugate vaccine (Prevnar) licensed in 2000 is routinely recommended for children and has markedly reduced the incidence of invasive infections with seven serotypes of pneumococci in children. This vaccine is also recommended for children at high risk of pneumococcal infections (e.g., HIV infection, asplenia, sickle cell disease, and others). A pneumococcal polysaccharide vaccine (Pneumovax 23) is recommended for adults older than 65 years or for those over 50 years with risk factors (e.g., alcoholism, diabetes or other metabolic or renal disease, chronic pulmonary or cardiac disease). Although clear evidence for prevention of bacterial meningitis is lacking, evidence supports its efficacy against invasive pneumococcal diseases, many of which are the preceding infections leading to bacteremia and meningitis.

Currently two vaccines remain available for prevention of meningococcal disease caused by four serotypes, A, C, Y, and W-135. The meningococcal polysaccharide vaccine (Menomune) is recommended for persons older than 2 years at high risk for severe meningococcal infections including adolescents and college students (particularly those residing in dormitories), military recruits, and those with complement deficiencies and asplenia. A quadrivalent protein-polysaccharide conjugate vaccines (Menactra) was licensed in 2005. This vaccine is recommended for routine immunization of all children 11 to 12 years of age and adolescents and college students at high risk as well as those more than 11 to 55 years of age with high-risk factors for meningococcal infection.

REFERENCES

Anderson EJ, Yogev LR: A rational approach to the management of ventricular shunt infections. Pediatric Infect Dis J 2005;24:557-558.
Andes DR, Craig WA: Pharmacokinetics and pharmacodynamics of antibiotics in meningitis. Infect Dis Clin North Am 1999;13(2):595-618.
De Gans J, van de Beek: Dexamethasone in adults with bacterial meningitis. N Engl J Med 2002;347:1549-1564.
Gray LD, Fedorko DP: Laboratory diagnosis of bacterial meningitis. Clin Microbiol Rev 1992;5:130-145.
Hussein AS, Shafran SD: Acute bacterial meningitis in adults: A 12-year review. Medicine (Baltimore) 2000;79:360-368.
Klinger G, Chin C-Y, Beyene J, et al: Predicting the outcome of neonatal bacterial meningitis. Pediatrics 2000;106:477-482.
Klein JO: Bacterial sepsis and meningitis. In Remington JS, Klein JO (eds): Infectious Diseases of the Fetus and Newborn Infant. 5th ed, New York and Saint Louis: WB Saunders, 2002, pp 943-998.
Odio CM, Faingezicht I, Paris M, et al: The beneficial effects of early dexamethasone administration in infants and children with bacterial meningitis. N Engl J Med 1991;324:1525-1531.
Ronan A, Hogg GG, Klug CL: Cerebrospinal fluid shunt infections in children. Pediatr Infect Dis J 1995;14:782-786.
Schuchat A, Robinson K, Wenger JD, et al: Bacterial meningitis in the United States in 1995. N Engl J Med 1997;337:970-976.
Unhanand M, Mustapha MM, McCracken GH, et al: Gram-negative enteric bacillary meningitis: A twenty-one year experience. J Pediatr 1993;122:15-17.
Van de Beek D, de Gans J, Spanjaard L, et al: Clinical features and prognostic factors in adults with bacterial meningitis. N Engl J Med 2004;351:1849-1858.

---

[1]Not FDA approved for this indication.

Infectious Mononucleosis

Method of
Leonard R. Krilov, MD

Infectious mononucleosis is a clinical illness characterized by fever (typically not higher than 39.5°C [103°F]), sore throat, tender cervical lymphadenopathy, fever, malaise, and anorexia; it occurs most commonly in adolescence and young adulthood. Initially described in the 19th century as glandular fever, the characteristic mononuclear response with atypical-appearing lymphocytes led to the name infectious mononucleosis.

Etiology

Epstein-Barr virus (EBV) was recognized as the primary cause of infectious mononucleosis in 1968. Other infectious agents such as cytomegalovirus (CMV), toxoplasma, or adenoviruses may cause a minority of cases of mononucleosis (or mononucleosis-like illness).

Epstein-Barr virus is an enveloped, double-stranded DNA virus of the Herpesviridae family. After primary EBV infection, as with other herpesviruses, the virus persists in a latent state throughout the patient's lifetime in a few B lymphocytes and is shed in saliva intermittently.

The virus has also been associated with African Burkitt's lymphoma, nasopharyngeal carcinoma, lymphoproliferative diseases after organ and bone marrow transplantation, and hairy leukoplakia and lymphocytic interstitial pneumonitis in HIV-infected patients. X-linked proliferative disease (Duncan syndrome) is a rare condition in which affected boys develop fulminant uncontrolled lymphoproliferation after acute infectious mononucleosis. Survivors develop severe chronic hypogammaglobulinemia, chronic EBV and enteroviral infections and B-cell lymphomas.

Epidemiology

Epstein-Barr virus infections occur at a younger age in lower socioeconomic groups; 70% to 90% of such children developing EBV antibodies by age 5 years compared to only 40% to 50% of those from higher socioeconomic groups. For unknown reasons primary infections occurring in adolescence and young adulthood are more likely to manifest as infectious mononucleosis than when initial infection occurs at a younger age. In younger children acute EBV infection is usually clinically inapparent or manifested by a nonspecific, uncomplicated upper respiratory tract infection or pharyngitis. Thus, infectious mononucleosis occurs most commonly among white high school and college students with an annual incidence of approximately 1 in 2500 among such individuals aged 15 to 25 years.

EBV transmission occurs through intimate sharing of saliva (thus, its description as the *kissing disease*) with an incubation period of 20 to 30 days (range 2 to 6 weeks). The efficiency of transmission is low, and outbreaks of disease are rare. Epstein-Barr virus' viral load in whole blood in the acute phase correlates with the severity of symptoms; but viral load in oral secretions is independent of symptoms. There is no seasonality or sex predilection to EBV infections.

CURRENT DIAGNOSIS

The clinical triad of fever, exudative pharyngitis, and lymphadenitis in association with atypical lymphocytosis and a positive heterophil response makes the diagnosis of infectious mononucleosis. Epstein-Barr virus serologies should be reserved for uncertain cases or to confirm the diagnosis in younger children who may not mount a heterophil response.

Post-transfusion development of symptoms of mononucleosis is most often associated with CMV infection.

Clinical Manifestations

The classic manifestations of infectious mononucleosis are fever, painful exudative pharyngitis, and lymphadenopathy. The enlarged nodes may be limited to the cervical regions (including posteriorly) or generalized. Splenomegaly and frequently hepatomegaly are the other hallmark findings of the illness. Elevated liver function tests are common in the acute phase of disease, but symptomatic jaundice is rare. Eyelid edema (Hoagland sign) has been reported in approximately 25% of cases. The acute symptoms typically resolve over 1 to 4 weeks, but lymphadenopathy and fatigue may last for 2 to 3 months.

Less common clinical manifestations include autoimmune hemolytic anemia (approximately 3%), severe neutropenia to less than 1000/mm^3 (approximately 3%), and neurologic involvement in up to 5% of cases. The reported neurologic manifestations of acute EBV infection include meningoencephalitis, Guillain-Barré syndrome, transverse myelitis, facial paralysis, optic neuritis, and metamorphopsia or Alice in Wonderland syndrome with altered perception of sizes, shapes, and spatial relationships.

Most cases of mononucleosis resolve uneventfully. Splenic rupture and the previously cited neurologic complications are the most frequent serious complications of mononucleosis with rare deaths reported.

Diagnosis

In the presence of the clinical features noted earlier, infectious mononucleosis is diagnosed by the presence of atypical lymphocytosis (>5% to 10% of all leukocytes) frequently in association with a decline in the number of granulocytes and platelets. Additionally, among school-age children and young adults, heterophil or Paul-Bunnell antibodies are detectable in 80% to 90% of cases beginning in the second week of illness and can be detected for up to 6 to 9 months after resolution of symptoms. These IgM antibodies react with horse, sheep, and beef erythrocytes but not guinea pig red cells. They are not EBV-specific and are present in only 50% or fewer of children younger than 4 years of age. Office-based commercial rapid slide kits for detecting heterophil response are 96% to 99% sensitive and give a result in 2 minutes.

Measurement of specific antibodies to EBV can be used to confirm the diagnosis. In the acute phase of illness, IgM and IgG antibodies

TABLE 1 Infectious Mononucleosis Serological Response Patterns (Typical Patterns)

	Heterophil Antibody	EBV VCA-IgM	EBV VCA-IgG	EBV EA	EBV EBNA
No Infection	−	−	−	−	−
Acute Infection	+	+	+/+	+/−	−
Past Infection	−	−	+	+/−	+

Abbreviations: EA = early antigen; EBNA = Epstein-Barr (virus) nuclear antigen; EBV = Epstein-Barr virus; VCA = viral capsid antigen.

CURRENT THERAPY

Rest and supportive care with limitation of physical activity during the first 1 to 4 weeks of illness are the mainstays of managing infectious mononucleosis. Corticosteroids are reserved for severe illness, especially with upper airway obstruction because of tonsillar hypertrophy.

to the viral capsid antigen (VCA) of EBV are detectable. The IgM response persists for approximately 4 months, whereas the IgG antibodies remain for life. Although the height of the VCA-IgG response decreases as the acute infection resolves, serial measurements of antibody titers are not clinically beneficial as a rule. Antibodies to the EBV nuclear antigen (EBNA) appear several weeks to months after a primary infection and are considered a marker for a past or convalescent infection, but 10% to 20% of individuals never develop detectable levels of EBNA antibodies. More than 80% of patients develop transient antibodies to the early antigen (EA) of the virus as the VCA-IgM clears and EBNA responses develop (Table 1).

Treatment

There is no effective antiviral therapy for EBV-associated infectious mononucleosis. Rest and supportive care are mainstays of therapy. Corticosteroids are frequently prescribed for severe cases, but critical evaluation of this modality is lacking. Indications include marked tonsillar hypertrophy with upper airway obstruction, neurologic manifestations, and hemolytic anemia. High-dose, short-term courses of steroids (dexamethasone [Decadron][1] [0.25 mg/kg every 6 hours]; methylprednisolone [Solu-Medrol][1] [1 mg/kg every 6 hours]; oral prednisone[1] [40 mg/day]) have been used with dramatic improvement typically noted over 24 to 72 hours.

[1]Not FDA approved for this indication.

REFERENCES

Ambinder RF, Lin L: Mononucleosis in the laboratory. J Infect Dis 2005;192:1503-1504.

Balfour HH Jr, Holman CJ, Hokanson KM, et al: A prospective clinical study of Epstein-Barr virus and host interactions during acute infectious mononucleosis. J Infect Dis 2005;192:1505-1512.

Barone SR, Krilov LR: Infectious mononucleosis and other Epstein-Barr virus infections. In Hoekelman RA (ed.): Primary Pediatric Care. (4th ed.). St. Louis: Mosby, 2001, pp 1573-1577.

Fafi-Kremer S, Morand P, Brion J-P, et al: Long-term shedding of infectious Epstein-Barr virus after infectious mononucleosis. J Infect Dis 2005;191:985-989.

Giffen BE, Xue S: Epstein-Barr virus infections and their association with human malignacies: Some key questions. Ann Med 1998;30:249-254.

Henle G, Henle W, Diehl V: Relation of Burkitt's tumor-associated herpestype virus to infectious mononucleosis. Proc Natl Acad Sci U S A 1968;59:94-101.

McGowan JE, Chesney PJ, Crossley KB, et al: Guidelines for the use of systemic glucococorticosteroids in the management of selected infections. Working group on steroid use, Antimicrobial Agents Committee, Infectious Diseases Society of America. J Infect Dis 1992;165:1-13.

Paul JR, Bunnell WW: Classics in infectious diseases. The presence of heterophile antibodies in infectious mononucleosis by John R. Paul and W. W. Bunnell. American Journal of the Medical Sciences, 1932. Rev Infect Dis 1982;4:1062-1068.

Sumaya CV, Ench Y: Epstein-Barr virus infectious mononucleosis in children. I. Clinical and general laboratory findings. Pediatrics 1985;75:1003-1010.

Sumaya CV, Ench Y: Epstein-Barr virus infectious mononucleosis in children. II. Heterophil antibody and viral-specific responses. Pediatrics 1985;75:1011-1019.

Chronic Fatigue Syndrome

Method of
James F. Jones, MD

Definition

Chronic fatigue syndrome (CFS) is the name applied to an illness of unknown origin that at face value resembles unresolved infections, depression, endocrinologic and metabolic disorders, sleep disorders, and many other conditions that include fatigue in their diagnostic criteria.

In the modern era, interest in this illness began with the question of a relationship with a chronic active Epstein-Barr virus infection. Subsequent studies did not support Epstein-Barr virus as the only cause of this syndrome, but several recent studies have found 10% of patients with acute infectious mononucleosis and other infectious diseases might have a similar illness or postinfection fatigue syndrome.

The lack of association with a specific infectious agent led to the generation in 1988 of a definition based on the presence of incapacitating fatigue and varying combinations of signs and symptoms. Any preexisting medical or psychiatric condition was exclusionary. Evaluation of this definition at a number of centers in the United States, Great Britain, and Australia led to the current definition published in 1994 (Box 1). The definition was altered so that preexisting medical conditions that were treated satisfactorily were allowed, as well as certain psychiatric and syndromic diagnoses. Additional changes in the definition included a decrease in the number of symptoms and removal of the signs; signs had been shown to be somewhat arbitrary, and patients could be identified in their absence. The greater number of symptoms in the 1988 version did not allow identification of a specific illness, and they increased the possibility that patients who had primary psychiatric illnesses (e.g., somatiform disorders) would be mislabeled with CFS. The 1994 definition still requires more than 6 months of fatigue, but it dropped the 50% level of activity present in the 1988 definition because the requirement was impossible to apply evenly across all patients.

The diagnostic criteria, including exclusion of other illnesses, are described in the Current Diagnosis box. The definition was originally designed as a research tool and included suggestions for unifying the measurement of fatigue and evaluation of the mental status of patients.

Epidemiology

The prevalence of the syndrome using the 1988 definition is approximately 13 per 100,000, whereas the 1994 definition identified approximately 300 per 100,000. Application of an empiric definition (see later) in a population recruited with unwellness, rather than fatigue, identified a higher prevalence of CFS (Reeves et al, 2007). An increase in CFS cases in an unwell population highlights the need to address illness in general and not just fatigue when considering this diagnosis. One demographic variable that has remained stable is the 3:1 ratio of women to men.

Diagnosis

Diagnosis of CFS begins with exclusion of other illness processes associated with fatigue and unwellness and subsequent suspicion of the syndrome after taking a history and performing a physical examination and screening laboratory tests (Box 2). It should not be assumed that a patient with fatigue as a presenting complaint has CFS. The history shows whether the illness began acutely or more

CURRENT DIAGNOSIS

- Identify duration of fatigue and its consequences.
- Identify primary symptoms.
- Exclude other illnesses/diseases.
- Reconsider the diagnosis on an ongoing basis.
- Chronic fatigue syndrome is a working diagnosis.

gradually and whether there are preexisting symptoms. History often provides insight into previously identified factors that influence patient perception of illness. Questioning about typical episodes provides information about cyclic events, possible triggers of symptoms, and possible exposures.

The interviewer gives the patients the opportunity to describe the history of the illness. The interviewer simply guides the patient and tries not to ask leading questions. This process not only gathers information but also serves as an ice breaker between the interviewer and the patient. It allows the interviewer to determine the mental status of the patient, the patient's concentration and memory capabilities, and what may be on the patient's agenda. It usually allows the examiner to determine the kind and scope of prior medical and alternative care evaluations the patients has received.

BOX 1 International Consensus Definition of Chronic Fatigue Syndrome

- Clinically evaluated, unexplained, persistent or relapsing chronic fatigue (lasting more than 6 months) that is of new or definite onset (has not been lifelong); is not the result of ongoing exertion; is not substantially alleviated by rest; and results in substantial reduction in previous levels of occupational, educational, social, or personal activities.
- Four or more of the following symptoms are concurrently present for more than 6 months:
  - Impaired memory or concentration
  - Multijoint pain
  - Muscle pain
  - New headaches
  - Postexertional malaise
  - Sore throat
  - Tender cervical or axillary lymph nodes
  - Unrefreshing sleep
- Exclusionary clinical diagnoses:
  - Any active medical condition that could explain the chronic fatigue
  - Any previously diagnosed medical condition whose resolution has not been documented beyond reasonable clinical doubt and whose continued activity can explain the chronic fatiguing illness
  - Psychotic major depression, bipolar affective disorder, schizophrenia, delusional disorders, dementias, anorexia nervosa, bulimia nervosa
  - Alcohol or other substance abuse within 2 years prior to the onset of the chronic fatigue and at any time afterward

Adapted from Fukuda K, Straus SE, Hickie I, et al: The chronic fatigue syndrome: A comprehensive approach to its definition and study. Ann Intern Med 1994;121:953-959.

The diagnosis of CFS should not be made on the first visit. Attempts should be made to determine the duration, the mode of onset, the magnitude, and the consequences of each complaint, although these are not included in the working definition. Only with such thorough questioning will an underlying process responsible for the illness be identified or suspected.

A more recent application of the definition uses three validated questionnaires: the Medical Outcomes Survey Short Form-36 (SF-36), the Multidimensional Fatigue Inventory (MFI), and the CDC Symptom Inventory. These questionnaires provide numeric scores that identify persons with CFS and provide a record of their level of impairment. The Symptom Inventory collects information about the presence, frequency, and intensity of 19 fatigue- and illness-related symptoms during the month preceding the interview; these include all eight CFS-defining symptoms (postexertional fatigue, unrefreshing sleep, problems remembering or concentrating, muscle aches and pains, joint pain, sore throat, tender lymph nodes and swollen glands, and headaches). Perceived frequency of each symptom is rated on a four-point scale (1 = a little of the time, 2 = some of the time, 3 = most of time, 4 = all of the time), and severity or intensity of symptoms is measured on a three-point scale (1 = mild, 2 = moderate, 3 = severe).

The case definition specifies that CFS causes substantial reduction in occupational, educational, social, or recreational activities. *Substantial reduction* is defined as scores lower than the 25th percentile on the SF-36 using the following four factors: physical function (≤ 70), or role physical (≤ 50), or social function (≤ 75), or role emotional (≤ 66.67) subscales of the SF-36, related to published norms of the U.S. population according to Ware and Sherbourne. We defined severe fatigue using the Multidimensional Fatigue Inventory as a score of 13 or higher on the general fatigue scale or 10 or higher on the reduced activity scales of the MFI (their respective medians). Finally, because the case definition specifies that characteristic symptoms accompany fatigue, subjects reporting at least 4 symptoms and scoring at least 25 on the Symptom Inventory Case Definition Subscale were considered to have substantial accompanying symptoms.

Routine laboratory evaluations are recommended to address contributory illnesses (see Box 2). Routine testing does not include specific antibody testing, tests of immune function per se, or single-photon emission computed tomography (SPECT) or magnetic resonance imaging (MRI) of the brain. Negative screening test results do not automatically exclude an alternative diagnosis. Specific testing, for example, for a sleep disorder or chronic sinusitis may be necessary. A mental status examination, either informally or by using a standard instrument when indicated, is equally important.

A working diagnosis of CFS may then be made if the evaluation fails to identify an underlying illness. This approach is warranted because the patient's underlying disease might declare itself in the future. Continued adherence to a diagnosis of CFS in the face of an evolving or readily identifiable medical or psychiatric illness is the

BOX 2 Screening Laboratory Tests

- Alanine aminotransferase
- Albumin
- Alkaline phosphatase
- C-reactive protein
- Complete blood count
- Creatinine
- Electrolytes
- Globulin
- Glucose
- Thyroid-stimulating hormone and free T_4
- Total protein
- Urinalysis

Abbreviation: T_4 = thyroxine.

single most detrimental outcome of a premature or prolonged diagnosis of CFS.

Additional laboratory or other diagnostic testing is based on the individual patient's complaints. The interview techniques listed earlier assist in this process. An additional valuable tool that will lead the interviewer to identify a specific illness or symptoms requiring intervention is simply to ask the patient to list the problems described in decreasing order of magnitude. Which problem causes the most difficulty? Or which problems interfere with the ability to carry out daily functions? Patients often use this exercise to list the consequences of their illness.

Therapy

Treatment regimens vary with the needs of the individual patient and how he or she perceives the illness. The goals of treatment depend on the person's specific symptoms and eventually the patient's identified needs within a framework of providing reentry into their premorbid condition. Complete return to normal might not be possible immediately, however, nor is this goal appropriate if it is too lofty. In fact, the desire for total immediate recovery can hamper clinical improvement. The patient's adaptation to this new, albeit temporary, state is often a more realistic short-term goal. Therapeutic modalities include education regarding the boundaries and limitations of the diagnosis, development of coping skills, institution of a graduated exercise program when possible, and use of medications to treat symptoms. If the patient is being seen in a multidisciplinary setting, these approaches may be combined into a specific program. If CFS is an infrequent diagnosis in a practice, identifying the problems that cause loss of function becomes critical.

EDUCATION

All physicians who make the diagnosis must provide information regarding the illness in general and the specific criteria that allowed recognition of the problem. Just as education regarding asthma and diabetes mellitus is a critical component of therapy for those diseases, education regarding the origin, specific components, and outcome of the syndrome is more critical in this situation.

The literature supports CFS as a condition that is not life threatening or progressive. Lay representations, which are readily available, are often incorrect in painting a uniformly dismal outcome. Physicians should counsel their patients that all illness symptoms should not be attributed to CFS, and patients should seek medical advice when new problems arise or old problems become more prominent. Patients should also be taught that persistent efforts to find a cure via experiences of their acquaintances or the newest information in magazines or on the Internet are not as productive as their participation in a specifically designed program as outlined here. Paramount in this process is their consideration of acceptance of their current, albeit temporary, status. Wanting their lives back and attempting to regain them with a pill are not effective approaches.

A major part of the education and treatment process is the interview process. Giving the patient the opportunity to describe the illness and its consequences in a nonjudgmental situation is critical to gaining the patient's confidence. A physician who makes the diagnosis of CFS literally establishes a contract for long-term care with the patient, and it must be based on mutual trust.

DEVELOPMENT OF COPING SKILLS

To recommend coping strategies, the provider must know the needs of the patient, another rationale for the patient-generated problem list. If the patient complains of problems with memory and concentration, simple advice regarding using lists and audiotaping activities or needs is logical. If they cannot perform on the job or their behavioral responses to these complaints aggravate the consequences, formal neuropsychological testing or therapy, or both, is required. Assistance with understanding losses is also very important. Depending on the magnitude of the consequences of their illness, patients can lose self-respect and the appreciation of their families, employees, and coworkers. They need to learn that as individuals they are not responsible for these losses but that they are responsible, at least in part, for their recovery. They need to go through a grieving process and then learn how to adapt to their current state. They need to learn to accept and desire incremental levels of progress. Formal psychological therapy may be required to achieve these goals.

The origin of the illness and the character of the fatigue dictate the approach in many cases. If the origin is with an apparent, usually unidentified, flu-like illness that does not resolve, or if the character of the fatigue simulates the malaise of such an illness, the patient needs to know that the symptoms are normal responses. The duration and consequences in the eyes of society and the individual patient are the factors that differentiate a normal resolution of an illness from a prolonged or chronic condition.

The patient also needs to know that resumption of normal activity is not the correct approach. Most patients have symptoms on a daily basis, but they also have days when the symptoms are more or less pronounced (bad and good days). A typical patient performs on the good days as if there were no illness. This action is then followed in 1 or 2 days by an exacerbation of symptoms. Learning to compartmentalize activities and to never exceed their personal limits are critical steps in coping with CFS.

On the other hand, total acceptance of such a program is not appropriate either. Usually, acute-onset patients notice that they can be more active without exacerbation of symptoms regardless of their therapeutic program. This observation usually heralds resolution of the illness. In some instances, the illness is resolving, but the patient perceives the outcome of increased physical activity (e.g., muscle aches and tiredness) as illness symptoms rather than simply the expected consequences of increased activity. The recurrence of the patient's whole syndrome following activity, however, suggests that resolution has not taken place.

EXERCISE

It seems contradictory to follow the discussion about listening to one's body and avoiding excessive activity with a section that recommends regular exercise. The studies on muscle function show that patients are tired after performing repetitive acts and that there appears to be no primary problem in muscle function. There may a problem in fitness or conditioning, however. Whether this result is a consequence of the illness or the inactivity that accompanies the syndrome is not known.

Lessons from the rehabilitation of patients with cardiac and pulmonary diseases teach us that anaerobic exercise to regain strength should precede exercises to improve aerobic fitness and overall conditioning. A program that includes active stretching followed by range-of-motion contractions and extensions that eventually includes resistance is usually an effective start. Five minutes per day is a typical starting point for a patient who has been totally inactive. The endpoint of each session should be preset by the clock or number of repetitions and should be reached before the patient becomes tired. This endpoint is based on the fact that either tiredness is a trigger for the production of biological changes that are a part of the host's attempt to limit activity or the perception that tiredness triggers illness behavior. At this stage in the understanding of the illness,

---

 CURRENT THERAPY

- Education regarding the advantages and disadvantages of CFS as a diagnosis
- Development of coping skills
- Cognitive behavior therapy
- Initiation of a graded exercise program
- Symptomatic medication

prevention of activation of either of these pathways and an increase in overall fitness are appropriate goals. This section may be summarized by the adage that no exercise is bad, some is good, and too much exercise is not helpful.

The previous sections on education, coping skills, and exercise provide the kinds of therapy that are offered in cognitive behavior therapy programs.

SYMPTOMATIC THERAPY

One usually associates symptomatic therapy with medication. Some interventions require alterations in patient habits or changes in biological processes that do not require medication per se.

Sleep Therapy

The primary example is treatment of sleep problems. A very large percentage of patients presenting for evaluation of fatigue, many of whom carry the diagnosis of CFS, have sleep disorders or disturbances. Some have problems with sleep hygiene. They may read or watch television for prolonged periods (longer than 15 minutes) before trying to go to sleep. This habit can actually allow arousal of the brain within several hours following sleep onset, thus leading to interrupted sleep. Caffeine ingestion after 6 PM and exercise within 4 hours of bedtime can impede getting to sleep.

Patients are often given medication for insomnia that is manifested by going to bed at 11 PM but not being able to get to sleep until 1 or 2 AM, with a waking time of 10 AM. A hypnotic might be prescribed that allows induction of sleep at an earlier time, but the patient might still not experience restorative sleep. One explanation for this series of events is that the patient has a phase-delay syndrome and needs to alter the sleep cycle with prescribed light therapy before improvement is expected. Appropriate use of hypnotics may be important in allowing initial normalization of sleep cycling, but these agents are not sufficient as the sole mode of therapy, nor should they be used for prolonged periods.

Daytime sleepiness is another common problem with multiple origins. Ill-advised symptomatic therapy includes self- or physician-generated use of stimulants. These drugs include caffeine, herbs that contain ephedrine such as Ma huang (Ephedra sinica), and antidepressants that actually serve as stimulants (serotonin and norepinephrine reuptake inhibitors [SNRIs]). These substances might allow short-term improvement in daytime function, but they block identification of the underlying nighttime or daytime origin of the sleep problem.

Pharmacologic Therapy

Premature treatment can prevent adequate diagnosis and treatment of readily remediated problems. However, symptomatic medications have a definite place in the therapy of CFS. Many CFS patients do not tolerate standard doses of any of the medications used for symptomatic relief.

Classes of drugs that might have beneficial effects for symptom relief include hypnotics of various types, antidepressants of several types if depression is evident, and non-narcotic analgesics. As used in the treatment of fibromyalgia, tricyclic antidepressants and SNRIs are used for symptomatic therapy in the absence of formal depression. Because these classes of medications are being used as adjuncts to the other modes of therapy, they are not always successful. They might need to be changed during the course of the illness.

Often patients come to the physician using a large number of medications. It might not be possible to determine by the history alone whether the patient's symptoms are not at least in part due to the medication regimen. Often the medications need to be tapered and stopped to sort out their influence on the manifesting complaints.

Popular remedies for CFS are discussed primarily to familiarize the practitioner with them and to support previous warnings regarding lack of efficacy. The primary problem with their use is that proof is lacking that such intervention has been uniformly beneficial. This statement is particularly true in cases of parenteral (injectable) repetitious therapy with any substance.

Alternative Therapies

The effectiveness of diet manipulations and ingestion of herbs, enzymes, amino acids, vitamins, minerals, or hormones, although usually safe, is equally unproven. These agents constitute a large component of the therapeutic armamentarium in use by patients with CFS. Herbs are particularly in vogue. Many of them have medicinal qualities and if taken in excessive amounts may be injurious. Because many of these substances are readily available, they are used by patients who are anxious for improvement in their illness. If the reader has such patients or is such a patient, one must make sure that the remedy in question is safe and that its use is affordable and does not hide illness parameters that require specific identification.

If patients are intent on taking these types of remedies, they should be advised to at least seek the advice of a responsible care provider who is knowledgeable in their use and adverse consequences. Alternative care in many forms is also in vogue and may be helpful if provided in a responsible fashion. Some patients with myalgias and other pain complaints find particular benefit from acupuncture and therapeutic massage.

Therapeutic Plan

Therapy for CFS patients continues to be directed at relieving symptoms and consequences of the syndrome. It is clear, however, that one approach or one medication is not satisfactory for all patients. Identifying the patient's most problematic symptoms and using a variety of modalities that address those problems in the treatment plan are the most effective ways of assisting the patient. Patients should be reminded not to expect total return to their premorbid state to occur immediately.

Because the use of medications remains arbitrary, failure of one regimen may be followed by successful relief using the more effective modes of therapy, such as cognitive behavior therapy and graduated exercise. Eventually the origins of symptom production will be understood and therapy can be directed with some authority. As it stands now, one must always be careful that whatever the treatment, it must not aggravate the illness.

REFERENCES

Bazelmans E, Prins JB, Lulofs R, et al; The Netherlands Fatigue Research Group Nijmegen. Cognitive behaviour group therapy for chronic fatigue syndrome: A non-randomised waiting list controlled study. Psychother Psychosom 2005;74(4):218-224.

Jones JF, Maloney EM, Boneva RS, et al: Complementary and alternative medical therapy utilization by people with chronic fatiguing illnesses in the United States. BMC Complement Altern Med 2007;7:12.

Jones JF, Nisenbaum R, Reeves WC: Medication use by persons with chronic fatigue syndrome: Results of a randomized telephone survey in Wichita, Kansas. Health Qual Life Outcomes 2003;1(1):74.

Moss-Morris R, Sharon C, Tobin R, Baldi JC: A randomized controlled graded exercise trial for chronic fatigue syndrome: Outcomes and mechanisms of change. J Health Psychol 2005;10(2):245-259.

Nater UM, Wagner D, Solomon L, et al: Coping styles in people with chronic fatigue syndrome identified from the general population of Wichita, KS. J Psychosom Res 2006;60(6):567-573.

Reeves WC, Jones JF, Maloney E, et al: Prevalence of chronic fatigue syndrome in metropolitan, urban, and rural Georgia. Popul Health Metr 2007;5:5.

Reeves WC, Wagner D, Nisenbaum R, et al: Chronic fatigue syndrome: A clinically empirical approach to its definition and study. BMC Med 2005;3(1):19.

Wagner D, Nisenbaum R, Heim C, et al: Psychometric properties of the CDC Symptom Inventory for assessment of Chronic Fatigue Syndrome. BioMed Central Popul Health Metr 2005;3:8.

Ware JE, Sherbourne CD: The MOS 36-item short form health survey (SF-36): Conceptual framework and item selection. Med Care 1992;30:473-483.

Whiting P, Bagnall AM, Sowden AJ, et al: Interventions for the treatment and management of chronic fatigue syndrome: A systematic review. JAMA 2001;286:1360-1368.

Mumps

Method of
Joel D. Klein, MD, FAAP

Mumps is a respiratory viral infection caused by mumps virus, an RNA virus in the family Paramyxoviridae. The virus is spread from human to human through direct contact with airborne droplets.

Epidemiology

Before the introduction of mumps vaccine, there were large yearly epidemics, usually occurring in the winter and early spring. Infection generally occurred among young children (younger than 15 years), with rare cases in young adults. With the introduction of the mumps vaccine in 1967, there was a dramatic decrease in the number of cases. However, in 1986 and 1987, there was a resurgence of mumps among teenagers and young adults, most of whom were born before routine immunization with the mumps vaccine.

Outbreaks were also seen among some children who had received mumps vaccine, because a single dose of the vaccine did not always confer immunity. In 1989, a second dose of mumps vaccine was recommended to address this issue. Mumps vaccine currently is usually administered as part of a combined vaccine such as measles-mumps-rubella (MMR) or most recently measles-mumps-rubella-varicella (MMRV) (Proquad).

Despite these changes, outbreaks of mumps occasionally occur, usually among college-aged persons. Recent examples include an epidemic in the United Kingdom in the winter of 2004 to 2005 and in the United States in 2006.

Clinical Manifestations

The incubation period of mumps is 14 to 25 days and involves nonspecific complaints of malaise, low-grade fever, and anorexia. The single most diagnostic physical finding in mumps is unilateral or bilateral parotitis, which occurs in up to 40% of cases. Mumps parotitis can occur early in the disease and may be associated with swelling and pain in other salivary glands. There often is erythema of the area and tenderness with palpation of the affected parotid. Patients at times also complain of earache and headache. Swelling over the parotid and related glands can occur rapidly and can result in distortion of the contours of the face, pushing the earlobe upward and outward. Edema can extend to the anterior chest wall as well. Examination of the oral cavity can reveal erythema of the orifice of Stensen's duct without purulent discharge. Parotitis generally resolves within 1 week.

The most commonly reported complications of mumps are aseptic meningitis and encephalitis, which can occur individually or together. Meningitis occurs in 10% to 15% of cases but probably is underreported. There is a typical viral-like pleocytosis in the cerebrospinal fluid (CSF), but the CSF glucose may be low. Encephalitis is rare and is seen in 1 or 2 per 100,000 cases.

TABLE 1 Complications of Mumps Infection

Mumps Complications	Incidence of Complications
Central nervous system	40%-50%
Orchitis and epididymitis	15%-30%
Oophoritis	7%
Pancreatitis	2%-5%
Deafness	1 in 20,000 reported cases
Myocarditis	Rare
Arthritis	Rare
Thyroiditis	Rare

Orchitis, either unilateral or bilateral, may be seen in as many as 50% of infected men. This complication can have a rapid onset and can be associated with increased fever, abdominal pain, nausea, and testicular swelling. This complication generally resolves within 1 week and can result in testicular atrophy but rarely infertility. Pancreatitis is sometimes seen, is usually mild, and may be associated with transient hyperglycemia. Table 1 lists the incidence of complications of mumps.

Diagnosis

Diagnosis of mumps is usually made by clinical examination and history. It should be considered in any patient with sudden onset of parotid swelling and fever. Mumps virus isolation may be attempted on fluids obtained by nasopharyngeal swab and urine. Virus may be excreted for 1 week before and 1 week after the onset of parotitis. When available, PCR may also be used to detect mumps virus in secretions.

Serum amylase determinations, although not specific, may be helpful in situations where mumps is suspected. Serology, which is readily available, may be diagnostic as well. Mumps IgM obtained during the acute infection is usually elevated and diagnostic. Acute and convalescent-paired sera can also be used to retrospectively confirm the diagnosis. Other commonly ordered laboratory tests, including complete blood count (CBC) are not particularly helpful. The CBC might show mild leukopenia with lymphocytosis.

Differential diagnosis of mumps parotitis includes many infections that are listed in Box 1.

Treatment

There is no specific therapy for mumps. Adequate analgesia is important, because many patients are quite uncomfortable. Because most patients are febrile, hydration also plays an important role. This is particularly critical because there may be difficulty swallowing and pain with mastication.

Children with mumps should be excluded from school for 9 days from onset of parotid swelling. Droplet precautions are recommended for patients with mumps admitted to the hospital for a period of 9 days from onset of parotid swelling.

CURRENT DIAGNOSIS

- Painful parotid swelling
- Edema of the face in the area of the parotid
- Elevation of serum amylase
- Headache and occasional meningismus
- Viral isolation or serology can confirm diagnosis

CURRENT THERAPY

- Analgesia for pain
- Warm or cold compresses
- Droplet isolation in the hospital
- Patient may return to school 9 days after the onset of parotid swelling

| BOX 1 | Differential Diagnosis of Mumps Parotitis |

- Parainfluenza virus infection
- Enterovirus infection
- Epstein-Barr virus
- Cytomegalovirus infection
- HIV
- Suppurative bacterial infection *(Staphylococcus aureus, Streptococcus pneumoniae)*
- Nontuberculous mycobacterial infection

Prevention

Mumps vaccine should be administered to children at age 12 to 15 months. A second dose should be given at age 4 to 6 years. Patients with HIV who are not severely immunocompromised may receive a combination mumps vaccine. Adults born in 1957 or later, in whom immunity is not known, should receive one dose of a mumps combination vaccine (MMR). Persons born before 1957 are usually considered immune, but they might benefit from immunization during a mumps community outbreak.

REFERENCES

American Academy of Pediatrics Committee on Infectious Diseases: Mumps. In Pickering LK (ed): Red Book: 2006 Report of the Committee on Infectious Diseases. 27th ed, Elk Grove Village, Ill: American Academy of Pediatrics, 2006, pp 464-468.
Cherry JD: Mumps Virus. In Feigin RD, Cherry JD, Demmler GJ, Kaplan SL (eds). Textbook of Pediatric Infectious Diseases. 5th ed. Philadelphia: WB Saunders, 2004 pp 2305-2314.
Gupta RK, Best J, MacMahon E: Mumps and the UK epidemic 2005. BMJ 2005;330:1132-1135.
Litman N, Baum SG: Mumps virus. In Mandell GL, Bennett JE, Dolin R (eds): Principles and Practice of Infectious Diseases. 6th ed. Philadelphia: Churchill Livingstone, 2005, pp 2003-2008.
Maldonado Y: Mumps. In Behrman RE (ed): Nelson Textbook of Pediatrics. 17th ed, Philadelphia: WB Saunders, 2004, pp 1035-1036.
McQuone SJ: Acute viral and bacterial infections of the salivary glands. Otolaryngol Clin North Am 1999;32(5):793-811.

Plague

Method of
Douglas A. Drevets, MD, DTM&H

Plague caused by *Yersinia pestis* is an ancient disease, and historical descriptions indicate that it probably caused Justinian's Plague (AD 541) that led into the first plague pandemic. The second plague pandemic, also known as the Black Death, began in Central Asia in 1347 and then spread to Europe, Asia, and Africa. It killed an estimated 50 million persons. The third and current plague pandemic began in China and then disseminated throughout the world by shipping routes in 1899–1900. *Y. pestis* is a gram-negative, nonmotile, facultatively anaerobic, non-spore-forming coccobacillus that is approximately 0.5 to 0.8 μm in diameter and 1 to 3 μm in length. Genomic sequencing shows that *Y. pestis* is a recently emerged clone of *Y. pseudotuberculosis*.

Epidemiology

Plague is a zoonosis that is usually spread between mammalian hosts by the bite of infected fleas. The most important enzootic reservoirs are urban and sylvatic rodents; however, domestic cats and dogs also are linked to human disease. Human plague occurs in North and South America, Asia, and Africa. An average of 2547 cases of human plague were reported yearly to the World Health Organization between 1988 and 1997, 76% of which were from Africa, with an overall case fatality rate of 7.1%. In North America, 82% of 295 indigenous cases were from Arizona, Colorado, and New Mexico. Bubonic plague is the most common form in humans, accounting for 97% of cases in a recent outbreak in Madagascar. Similarly, 84% of U.S. cases reported between 1947 and 1996 were the bubonic form, with septicemic and pneumonic plague accounting for 13% and 2%, respectively.

Modes of Transmission

Most human infections are transmitted from rodent to humans via the bite of an infected flea. Infection also can be acquired by contact with body fluids from infected animals, such as during field dressing of game or by inhalation of respiratory droplets from animals, particularly cats, or humans with pneumonic plague.

Bioterrorism Threat

Plague was used as an agent of biowarfare by the Japanese in World War II and was a focus of intensive research and development in the former Soviet Union during the Cold War. Primary pneumonic plague is the most likely form of exposure because of biowarfare or bioterrorism.

Pathogenesis and Clinical Syndromes

Transdermal inoculation of bacilli from the bite of an infected flea ultimately leads to infection of the regional lymph nodes in which massive replication of bacteria creates the bubo (derived from the Greek "bubon" or "groin"), a swollen, erythematous, and painful lymph node in the groin, axilla, or cervical region. Bacteremia and septicemia frequently develop and lead to secondary infection of other organs including lungs, spleen, and the central nervous system. Primary pneumonic plague is a rare natural occurrence and results from the inhalation of respiratory droplets containing *Y. pestis* bacilli from another case of pneumonic plague, usually in humans or in cats. Secondary pneumonic plague results from seeding of the lungs by blood-borne bacteria in the setting of either bubonic or septicemic plague. Septicemic plague also begins with a transdermal exposure but manifests as primary bacteremia/septicemia without the bubo. Less common manifestations include meningitis, pharyngitis, and gastroenteritis.

Bubonic plague is an acute febrile lymphadenitis that develops 2 to 8 days after inoculation. Inflamed lymph nodes are usually 1 to 6 cm and painful. Abrupt onset of fever is an almost universal finding and occurs simultaneously with, or up to 24 hours before, the appearance of the bubo. Headache, malaise, and chills are frequent, along with nausea, vomiting, and diarrhea. Most patients are tachycardic, hypotensive, and appear prostrate and lethargic with episodic restlessness. Leukocytosis with a left shift is typical. Complications include pneumonia, shock, disseminated intravascular coagulation, purpuric skin lesions, acral cyanosis, and gangrene. The differential diagnosis of bubonic plague includes tularemia and Group A β-hemolytic streptococcal adenitis with bacteremia.

The symptoms of septicemic plague are not distinct from those caused by other gram-negative bacteria, and they are very similar to those of bubonic plague except that abdominal pain is more common

CURRENT DIAGNOSIS

- Travel to a plague endemic area or contact with a case of animal or human plague.
- Abrupt onset of fever and prostration.
- Bubo in groin, axillae, or cervical areas.
- Gram-negative coccobacilli with bipolar staining identified in aspirate from bubo, on blood smear, or from blood-tinged sputum.

in septicemic plague. Septicemic plague must be differentiated from fulminate septicemia caused by other gram-negative bacteria. Primary pneumonic plague has an abrupt onset of fever and influenza-like symptoms 1 to 5 days after inhalation exposure. Symptoms include shortness of breath, cough, chest pain, and bloody sputum with rapid progression to fulminate pneumonia and respiratory failure. Patients with secondary pneumonic infection show respiratory symptoms in addition to those attributed to the bubo or sepsis. Radiographic findings include patchy bronchopneumonia, multilobar consolidations, cavitations, and alveolar hemorrhage and are not pathognomonic of *Y. pestis*. Plague pneumonia must be differentiated from severe influenza, inhalation anthrax, and overwhelming community-acquired pneumonia.

Diagnosis

Plague is diagnosed by demonstrating *Y. pestis* in blood or body fluids such as a lymph node aspirate, sputum, or cerebrospinal fluid. A tentative diagnosis of bubonic plague can be made rapidly with fluid aspirated from a bubo showing gram-negative coccobacilli with bipolar staining. Serology showing a fourfold rise in antibody titers to F1 antigen or a single titer of more than 1:128 is also diagnostic.

Treatment

The aminoglycosides gentamicin (Garamycin) and streptomycin, the fluoroquinolones ciprofloxacin (Cipro), levofloxacin (Levaquin), and ofloxacin (Floxin), and tetracyclines (i.e., doxycycline [Vibramycin]) are the first-, second-, and third-line classes of antibiotics, respectively. Typical minimal inhibitory concentrations for 90% (MIC_{90}) of tested strains for the fluoroquinolones are less than 0.03 to 0.25 μg/mL compared with less than 1.0 μg/mL and less than 1.0 μg/mL to 4.0 μg/mL for gentamicin and streptomycin, respectively, and less than 1.0 μg/mL for doxycycline. Streptomycin (15 mg/kg up to 1 g intermuscularly [IM] every 12 hours) and gentamicin (5 to 7 mg/kg/day intravenously [IV]/IM in one or two doses daily) are the drugs of choice for severe infection. Standard doses for the fluoroquinolones include ciprofloxacin, 400 mg IV/500 mg orally every 12 hours; levofloxacin, 500 mg IV/orally daily; and ofloxacin, 400 mg IV/orally every 12 hours. Doxycycline is administered at 100 mg IV/orally every 12 hours. Chloramphenicol (25 mg/kg IV/orally every 6 hours) can be used in select circumstances. Antibiotic therapy should be continued for a total of 10 days.

CURRENT THERAPY

- Prompt administration of gentamicin or ciprofloxacin.
- Aggressive supportive care.
- Respiratory isolation of hospitalized cases.
- Postexposure prophylaxis to close contacts.

Prevention and Control

Standard infection control procedures that should be used when caring for patients with suspected plague include a disposable surgical mask, latex gloves, devices to protect mucous membranes, and good hand washing. Hospitalized patients with known or suspected pneumonic plague should be placed in strict isolation for at least 48 hours after appropriate antibiotics are initiated. Postexposure prophylaxis should be given to individuals with close contact (defined as less than 2 meters) with an infectious case or who have had a potential respiratory exposure. The recommended adult antibiotics for prophylaxis are doxycycline or ciprofloxacin in the same doses used for treatment. Postexposure prophylaxis can be given orally and should be continued for 7 days following exposure. Currently, there is no licensed plague vaccine.

REFERENCES

Butler T: A clinical study of bubonic plague. Observations of the 1970 Vietnam epidemic with emphasis on coagulation studies, skin histology and electrocardiograms. Am J Med 1972;53:268-276.
Boulanger LL, Ettestad P, Fogarty JD, et al: Gentamicin and tetracyclines for the treatment of human plague: Review of 75 cases in New Mexico, 1985–1999. Clin Infect Dis 2004;38:663-669.
Cler DJ, Vernaleo JR, Lombardi LJ, et al: Plague pneumonia disease caused by *Yersinia pestis*. Semin Respir Infect 1997;12:12-23.
Gage KL, Dennis DT, Orloski KA, et al: Cases of cat-associated human plague in the Western US, 1977–1998. Clin Infect Dis 2000;30:893-900.
Hull HF, Montes JM, Mann JM: Septicemic plague in New Mexico. J Infect Dis 1987;155:113-118.
Inglesby TV, Dennis DT, Henderson DA, et al: Plague as a biological weapon: Medical and public health management. Working Group on Civilian Biodefense. JAMA 2000;283:2281-2290.
Perry RD, Fetherston JD: *Yersinia pestis*—etiologic agent of plague. Clin Microbiol Rev 1997;10:35-66.
Prentice MB, Rahalison L: Plague. Lancet 2007;369:1196-1207.
Ratsitorahina M, Chanteau S, Rahalison L, et al: Epidemiological and diagnostic aspects of the outbreak of pneumonic plague in Madagascar. Lancet 2000;355:111-113.
Wong JD, Barash JR, Sandfort RF, Janda JM: Susceptibilities of *Yersinia pestis* strains to 12 antimicrobial agents. Antimicrob Agents Chemother 2000;44:1995-1996.

Anthrax

Method of
Jon B. Woods, MD

Anthrax has been a significant disease for both humans and their livestock for millennia. It was the first disease to fulfill Koch's postulates in 1876, as well as the first bacterial disease for which an effective vaccine was developed, for livestock, in 1880. This gram-positive rod-shaped bacillus species differs from the more benign members of its genera in containing two additional plasmids, one encoding for an antiphagocytic poly-D-glutamic acid capsule and the other encoding for two toxins. Three distinct toxin components combine to form two toxins, edema toxin and lethal toxin; the common component, protective antigen (PA), forms a pore through eukaryotic cell walls that allows the other two toxin components, edema factor (EF) and lethal factor (LF), to enter affected host cells. EF is an adenylate cyclase affecting many cell types and is responsible for the edema associated with anthrax infections. LF is a zinc metalloprotease that seems to have its greatest affect on macrophages; within the cells it cleaves mitogen-activated protein kinase and disrupts the cellular response to infection.

Background

Anthrax is an enzootic, and occasionally epizootic, disease of grazing animals worldwide. The incredibly durable spores of this bacillus can persist in soil for decades. These spores, when inadvertently ingested by herbivores while grazing, can germinate and then replicate in a rapid progression to bacteremia and subsequent death of the animal. At the time of death these animals can have as many as 10^8 vegetative bacilli per milliliter of blood. Those bacilli, which are exposed to oxygen upon the animal's death, can sporulate and then reenter the soil to begin the cycle anew.

Human anthrax can take several forms, most commonly cutaneous, but also intestinal, oropharyngeal, and inhalational disease. Naturally occurring human anthrax disease has typically been the result of exposure to infected animals or contaminated animal products such as hair or wool, bone meal, hides, or meat. Less commonly, human cutaneous anthrax has resulted from the bites of flies that have recently fed on infected animals. Gastrointestinal and oropharyngeal anthrax can result from ingestion of the raw or inadequately cooked flesh of an animal infected with anthrax. Endemic inhalational anthrax, or woolsorter's disease, results from inhalation of anthrax spores aerosolized during the manipulation of contaminated animal products, especially hair or wool; this was an exceedingly rare form of disease even prior to the institution of more stringent control measures and closure of most of the U.S. textile mills processing foreign-acquired goat hair by the 1970s. More recently, inhalational anthrax and cutaneous cases have resulted from exposure to spores intentionally processed and disseminated as biologic weapons. The extreme environmental stability of the spores, their ease of production, and their infectivity via the aerosol route are some features that have made *Bacillus anthracis* a top candidate for both nations and terrorists seeking biologic weapons. An apparently accidental aerosol release of dried anthrax spores from a biologic weapons facility in the Soviet city of Sverdlovsk in 1979 resulted in as many as 68 deaths because of inhalational anthrax. More recently, anthrax spores intentionally sent through the U.S. postal system resulted in 11 cases of inhalational anthrax and perhaps as many as 11 cases of cutaneous anthrax.

Clinical Features

Cutaneous anthrax represents approximately 95% of naturally occurring human anthrax cases. It typically occurs 1 to 7 days after exposure to infected livestock or contaminated livestock products, but rarely it is transmitted to humans by the bites of flies that have recently fed on infected animals. The lesion begins as a painless or mildly pruritic papule at the site of spore inoculation, progressing into an expanding round ulcer by the following day. Over the following several days the ulcer dries to a dark, almost black eschar, which resolves over the ensuing 1 to 2 weeks. The lesion can be surrounded by significant local edema and may be accompanied by regional lymphadenopathy. Treated, cutaneous anthrax is rarely fatal, although without antibiotics, progression to bacteremia and ultimately death can occur in up to 10% to 20% of cases.

Both forms of gastrointestinal anthrax are acquired via ingestion of insufficiently cooked meat from infected animals. The infectious dose is unknown. Intestinal anthrax may be initially misdiagnosed as either gastroenteritis or acute abdomen, typically presenting 1 to 6 days following contaminated meat consumption with fever, nausea, vomiting, and focal abdominal pain. Without prompt initiation of antibiotic therapy, disease can progress to hematemesis, hematochezia or melena, massive serosanguineous or hemorrhagic ascites, and sepsis, with mortality rates greater than 50%. Oropharyngeal anthrax typically presents after a 1- to 6-day incubation period with severe pharyngitis and fever, followed by appearance of pharyngeal or tonsillar ulcers. Gray or tan pseudomembranes can form over the ulcers, which are often accompanied by significant cervical lymphadenopathy and unilateral neck edema. Mortality of oropharyngeal anthrax varies from 10% to 50%.

Inhalation of aerosolized anthrax spores into the pulmonary alveoli can result in inhalational anthrax. The lethal dose via inhalation for 50% of humans (LD_{50}) is thought to be between 8000 and 55,000 spores. The alveolar spores are ingested by macrophages and carried to regional lymphatics, where they can germinate and replicate, eventually leading to hemorrhagic mediastinitis. The incubation period is presumably dose dependent, and although typically 1 to 6 days was suspected in at least one human case to be 43 days. Early inhalational anthrax presents suddenly as a nonspecific syndrome consisting of fever, malaise, headache, fatigue, and drenching sweats. Other common symptoms include nausea, vomiting, confusion, a nonproductive cough, and mild chest discomfort. Upper respiratory symptoms are notably absent. Physical findings are nonspecific in the early phase of the disease, but tachycardia is common. Auscultatory lung exam is typically normal at this stage, but dullness to percussion can develop over time in the lower lung fields as hemorrhagic pleural effusions accumulate. These early findings generally persist for 2 to 5 days before progressing fulminantly to tachypnea, cyanosis, shock, and multiorgan system failure. These late findings typically herald impending death within 24 to 36 hours. Gastrointestinal hemorrhage and hemorrhagic meningitis are common at autopsy. Prognosis is poor in the absence of intensive supportive care and early initiation of appropriate antibiotic combinations. Mortality ranges from 45% to more than 85% historically.

Diagnosis

None of the forms of human anthrax disease can be diagnosed on the basis of clinical findings alone (Table 1). For example, diagnosis of cutaneous anthrax requires the presence of a compatible skin lesion accompanied by confirmatory laboratory studies; an exposure history, or a known risk may also be present. Both forms of gastrointestinal anthrax are typically accompanied by a history of ingestion of the meat of anthrax-infected animals. Early intestinal anthrax can be difficult to differentiate clinically from other causes of gastrointestinal illness to include acute gastroenteritis, dysentery, or even peritonitis. Later in the course of intestinal disease, surgical or autopsy findings may include ileal or cecal ulceration, and bowel edema and necrosis is associated with hemorrhagic mesenteric adenitis and serosanguineous to hemorrhagic ascites. Oropharyngeal anthrax can clinically resemble diphtheria, with pharyngeal lesions and an edematous so-called bull neck. Early inhalational anthrax is a nonspecific febrile syndrome that may be difficult to distinguish clinically from many other infectious diseases. However, the presence of mental status changes, profuse sweating, and absence of upper respiratory symptoms or pneumonia in inhalational anthrax may aid in differentiating it from influenza-like respiratory illnesses.

Gram stain and culture of skin lesions are ideally performed on the fluid of an unopened vesicle and are often positive in the cutaneous anthrax patient who has not received antibiotics. Tissue biopsy can be performed on lesions for immunohistochemical staining in culture-negative patients. Blood culture should be collected in any systemically ill patient suspected of having any form of anthrax disease. *B. anthracis* grows quickly in standard laboratory culture media. Paired acute and convalescent serologic studies may suggest infection in patents that have negative cultures, albeit these studies are not well validated. Stool culture can be positive in intestinal anthrax, although it is only variably so. Peritoneal fluid, pleural effusions, or cerebrospinal fluid (CSF) (when meningitis is present) can potentially demonstrate organisms on Gram stain and culture or may be positive via immunostaining or polymerase chain reaction (PCR) studies.

For patients with inhalation anthrax during the attacks of 2001, the complete blood count (CBC) revealed a mean white blood cell count of 9800/µL, with a predominance of neutrophils and a mildly elevated hematocrit. Mildly elevated serum sodium, aspartate transaminase (AST), and alanine aminotransferase (ALT) were common, as was hypoalbuminemia.

A widened mediastinum caused by adenitis, as well as pleural effusions, may be visible on chest radiograph in patients with inhalational anthrax. Negative chest radiograph in a patient suspected of inhalational anthrax should prompt a chest computerized tomography (CT) scan. In the 2001 attacks, either the chest radiograph or CT was

CURRENT DIAGNOSIS

Cutaneous/Oropharyngeal

- Painless or pruritic lesion beginning 1–7 d after exposure
    - Typical lesion progression from papule to ulcer to dark eschar (see text), often with significant edema

Plus

- Lesion gram stain, culture usually positive if patient has not received antibiotics
    - If negative, punch biopsy of lesion margin for IHC may still be positive
- Blood culture rarely positive in absence of systemic symptoms

Acute and convalescent serology or may give evidence of infection.

Gastrointestinal

- Gastrointestinal symptoms (variable) beginning 1–6 d after ingestion exposure.
    - Focal abdominal pain with hematochezia or melena common.
    - Nonspecific bowel wall edema, air–fluid levels, and ascites on radiographs.

Plus

- Stool culture (variably +).
- Blood culture (variably +).
- Acute and convalescent serology or blood sample for PCR may give evidence of infection.
- Ascites: often hemorrhagic.
    - Gram stain and culture, and IHC or PCR, if available, may be positive.

Surgical findings: hemorrhagic mesenteric adenitis, bowel edema, ileal and/or cecal ulcerations.

Inhalational

- Nonspecific febrile syndrome beginning abruptly 1–6 (but up to 43) d after aerosol exposure (see text).
    - Absence of upper respiratory findings, no pneumonia.
    - Widened mediastinum ± effusions on CXR or chest CT in *all* cases.

Plus

- Blood culture often positive if patient has not received antibiotics.
- Acute and convalescent serology or blood sample for PCR may give evidence of infection.
- Laboratory studies show hemoconcentration, mildly increased WBC with left shift, mildly increased AST and ALT, hypoalbuminemia.
- CSF (if meningitis) and pleural effusions are hemorrhagic.
- Gram stain and culture often positive.

If negative, IHC or PCR may be positive.

Abbreviations: AST = serum aspartate aminotransferase (level); ALT = serum alanine aminotransferase (level); CSF = cerebrospinal fluid; CXR = chest radiograph; CT = computed tomography study; IHC = immunohistochemical staining; PCR = polymerase chain reaction (study); WBC = white blood count.

---

abnormal in all cases of inhalational disease. Abdominal radiographs in intestinal anthrax may demonstrate any number of nonspecific findings, to include ascites, diffuse air–fluid levels, and bowel edema.

Treatment

Patient survival for all forms of severe anthrax disease hinges on prompt initiation of appropriate antibiotics. Initial empirical therapy for patients with inhalational anthrax, gastrointestinal anthrax, or cutaneous anthrax with systemic symptoms should include intravenous (IV) ciprofloxacin (Cipro IV) or doxycycline (Vibramycin IV) combined with one or two additional antibiotics effective against anthrax (Table 2). One suggested combination includes a quinolone (ciprofloxacin [Cipro IV]), clindamycin (Cleocin[1]), and rifampin (Rifadin[1]). Antibiotic choices should be adjusted to reflect the specific susceptibilities of the infecting strain. Rifampin (Rifadin[1]),

[1] Not FDA approved for this indication.

CURRENT THERAPY

Cutaneous Anthrax (without Systemic Symptoms)

- Oral antibiotics (see Table 2 for details)
    - Doxycycline (Vibramycin), or
    - Ciprofloxacin (Cipro[1])
- Consider nonsteroidal anti-inflammatory agents (NSAIDS) or corticosteroids for severe edema
- Infection control:
    - Contact precautions

Do not debride lesions

Inhalational, Gastrointestinal, or Cutaneous Disease with Systemic Symptoms

- Supportive care
    - May need assisted ventilation and/or vasopressors
    - Drain pleural effusions and large peritoneal fluid collections
- Combination IV antibiotics (see Table 2 for details)
    - Doxycycline (Vibramycin IV), or
    - Ciprofloxacin (Cipro IV[1])

Plus

- One or two additional antibiotics
- Consider corticosteroids for severe edema or meningitis
- Consider human anthrax immune globulin (investigational), if available
- Infection control:
    - Contact precautions (not transmitted by droplet or aerosol)

Avoid autopsy or invasive procedures prior to receipt of antibiotics.

---

[1] Not FDA approved for this indication.

TABLE 1 Empirical Antibiotic Therapy for Anthrax*

Cutaneous Anthrax (without Systemic Symptoms)	Inhalational, Gastrointestinal, or Cutaneous Disease with Systemic Symptoms
Ciprofloxacin (Cipro[1]) • 500 mg PO twice daily (adults) • 15 mg/kg (up to 500 mg/dose) PO twice daily (children) or Doxycycline (Vibramycin) • 100 mg PO twice daily (adults) • 2.2 mg/kg (up to 100 mg/dose) PO bid (children < 45 kg) or (if strain susceptible): Penicillin G procaine (Bicillin C-R) • 1,200,000 U IM q12h (adults) • 25,000 U/kg (maximum 1,200,000 U) q12h (children) or Penicillin V Potassium (Veetids) • 500 mg PO q6h (adults) or Amoxicillin (Amoxil[1]) • 500 mg PO q8h (adults and children > 40 kg) • 15 mg/kg q8h (children < 40 kg) According to CDC recommendations, amoxicillin prophylaxis is appropriate only after 14–21 d of fluoroquinolone or doxycycline and only for populations with relative contraindications to the other drugs (children pregnancy)	Ciprofloxacin (Cipro IV[1]) • 400 mg IV q12h (adult) • 15 mg/kg/dose (up to 400 mg/dose) q12h (children) or Doxycycline (Vibramycin IV) • 200 mg IV, then 100 mg IV q12h (adults) • 2.2 mg/kg (100 mg/dose maximum) q12h (children < 45 kg) or (if strain susceptible): Penicillin G (Pfizerpen) • 4 million U IV q4h (adults) • 50,000 U/kg (up to 4M U) IV q6h (children) plus One or two additional antibiotics with activity against anthrax. Clindamycin (Cleocin[1]) plus rifampin (Rifadin[1]) may be a good empiric choice, pending susceptibilities. Potential additional antibiotics include one or more of the following: clindamycin (Cleocin), rifampin (Rifadin), gentamicin[1] (generic), macrolides (erythromycin [generic], vancomycin (Vancocin[1]), imipenem (Pimaxin[1]), and chloramphenicol[1] (generic). Convert from IV to oral therapy when patient is stable, to complete at least 60 d of antibiotics. **Meningitis** Add Rifampin (Rifadin[1]) 20 mg/kg IV once daily or vancomycin (Vancocin[1]) 1 g IV q12h Oral dosing may be necessary for treatment of systemic disease in a mass casualty situation.

[1]Not FDA approved for this indication.
*Should be adjusted for susceptibilities.
Abbreviations: CDC = Centers for Disease Control and Prevention; IV = intravenous; PO = orally.
Adapted from Woods JB (ed): USAMRIID's Medical Management of Biological Warfare Casualties Handbook, 6th ed. 2005.

vancomycin (Vancocin[1]), or chloramphenicol[1] (generic) should be added if meningitis is suspected. IV antibiotics can be switched to oral treatment as the patent's clinical condition improves, to complete at least 60 days of total antibiotic therapy. Specific antidotes for anthrax toxins are in development, including human anthrax immune globulin, which may be available as an investigational therapy for severe anthrax disease through the Centers for Disease Control and Prevention (CDC).

Patients with systemic anthrax disease often require aggressive supportive therapy, including fluid resuscitation, blood products,

TABLE 2 Anthrax Aerosol Postexposure Prophylaxis*

Immunized[†]	Not Immunized and Vaccine Available	Not Immunized and Vaccine Not Available
Ciprofloxacin (Cipro) • 500 mg PO bid for adults • 10–15 mg/kg PO twice daily (up to 1 g/d) for children or Doxycycline (Vibramycin) • 100 mg PO bid for adults or children > 8 y and > 45 kg • 2.2 mg/kg PO bid (up to 200 mg/d) for children < 8 y		
If antibiotic susceptibilities allow, patients who cannot tolerate tetracyclines or quinolone antibiotics can be switched to amoxicillin (Amoxil[1]), 500 mg PO tid for adults and 80 mg/kg divided tid (≥ 1.5 g/d) in children.		
Continue antibiotics for *at least* 30 d.	Receive at least 3 doses of anthrax vaccine[1] (BioThrax) at 2-wk intervals, and then continue antibiotics for *at least* 1–2 wk after receipt of 3rd dose of vaccine.	Continue antibiotics for *at least* 60 d.

Patients should be closely observed after discontinuation of antibiotics.
If suspected clinical signs of anthrax disease occur, then resume empirical antibiotics.

[1]Not FDA approved for this indication.
*Unknown antibiotic susceptibilities.
[†]Immunized = completed 6 doses of anthrax vaccine and up to date on boosters, or minimum of 3 doses within past 6 mo. Those who have already received 3 doses within 6 mo of exposure should continue with their routine vaccine schedule.
Abbreviation: PO = orally.
Adapted from Woods JB (ed): USAMRIID's Medical Management of Biological Warfare Casualties Handbook, 6th ed. 2005.

vasopressor agents, and airway management. Patients may also benefit from drainage of large hemorrhagic pleural or peritoneal fluid accumulations. Although clinical data are lacking, severe edema or meningitis in anthrax disease may benefit from administration of corticosteroids.

Uncomplicated naturally acquired cutaneous anthrax should be treated empirically with 7 to 10 days of either oral ciprofloxacin (Cipro[1]) or doxycycline (Vibramycin). For cutaneous disease thought to have been acquired via exposure to an anthrax aerosol, at least 60 days of antibiotics is recommended.

A licensed anthrax vaccine (BioThrax) has been available in the United States to the armed forces, veterinarians, and textile and laboratory workers since 1970. It is derived from the sterile supernatant of a liquid culture of an attenuated (nonencapsulated) strain of B. anthracis and is administered subcutaneously in a six-shot primary series over 18 months followed by annual boosters. The vaccine is licensed only for preexposure prophylaxis of persons 18 to 65 years of age but is available investigationally for postexposure and pediatric use.

Individuals exposed to aerosolized anthrax spores should immediately receive postexposure prophylaxis consisting of both oral antibiotics and anthrax vaccine. Oral doxycycline (Vibramycin) or ciprofloxacin (Cipro) are the preferred empiric antibiotics for postexposure prophylaxis. Antibiotics should be continued for variable lengths of time depending on the patient's anthrax immune status and the suspected inhaled dose of anthrax (Table 2). Exposed individuals should also receive the anthrax vaccine[1] (BioThrax) to counter delayed incubation of residual alveolar anthrax after discontinuation of antibiotics.

---

[1]Not FDA approved for this indication.

REFERENCES

Beatty ME, Ashford DA, Griffin PM, et al: Gastrointestinal anthrax, a review of the literature. Arch Intern Med 2003;163:2527-2531.
Centers for Disease Control and Prevention: Notice to readers: Use of anthrax vaccine in response to terrorism: Supplemental recommendations of the Advisory Committee on Immunization Practices. MMWR 2002;51(45); 1024-1026.
Inglesby TV, O'Toole T, Henderson DA, et al: Anthrax as a biological weapon 2002: Updated Recommendations for Management. JAMA 2002;287(17): 2236-2252.
Jernigan JA, Stephens DS, Ashford DA, et al: Bioterrorism-related inhalational anthrax: The first 10 cases reported in the United States. Emerg Infect Dis 2001;7:933-944.
Kuehnert MJ, Doyle TJ, Hill HA, et al: Clinical features that discriminate inhalational anthrax from other acute respiratory illnesses. Clin Infect Dis 2003;36:328-336.
Turnbull PCB: Guidelines for the Surveillance and Control of Anthrax in Humans and Animals. 3rd ed. World Health Organization Report WHO/EMC/ZDI/98.6, 1998.
Woods JB (ed): USAMRIID's Medical Management of Biological Warfare Casualties Handbook, 6th ed. 2005.

Psittacosis

Method of
Julian Elliott, MB, BS, FRACP

Epidemiology

Psittacosis is the disease caused by infection with the bacterium *Chlamydophila psittaci*, formerly known as *Chlamydia psittaci*. It affects men more than women, and the main age group affected is adults older than 40 years. The main reservoir for psittacosis is birds, particularly psittacine birds (parrots, parakeets, budgerigars, and cockatoos), but other bird species and mammals can be infected. The most common form of acquisition is exposure to infected birds, by breathing in an aerosol of dried feces or from nose or eye secretions.

Risk factors for disease include contact with pet birds—especially a new, sick, or dead bird—and occupational exposure, for example work as a veterinarian, as a zoo keeper, or in a poultry-processing plant. Most cases are sporadic, but outbreaks have occurred associated with pet shops, aviaries, and poultry-processing plants and with mowing lawns in areas with large numbers of psittacine birds. Person-to-person transmission is rare. There is no evidence of infection acquired through ingestion of poultry products.

Clinical Features

The incubation period varies from 4 to 14 days or longer. The typical presentation of psittacosis is of an influenza-like illness with sudden onset of fever, chills, and prominent headache, but a more gradual onset is also seen. Rigors may be present. Cough is usually later in onset, dry, and not very marked. There may also be diarrhea, pharyngitis, altered mental state, or shortness of breath. Chest examination is usually abnormal, but the findings are often minimal and less prominent than symptoms or x-ray findings would suggest. Pleural effusions are rare.

Patients might present with a fever of unknown origin without obvious respiratory involvement, or the disease can be misdiagnosed as meningitis due to prominent headache, sometimes with photophobia. The degree of illness varies from asymptomatic to life threatening. Elderly persons and pregnant women are susceptible to more severe illness.

Other, less common findings include hemoptysis, proteinuria, hepatosplenomegaly, and encephalitis. Cardiac manifestations include relative bradycardia and rarely myocarditis, culture-negative endocarditis, and pericarditis. Erythema nodosum and other skin manifestations have also been described. *C. psittaci* has also been demonstrated by PCR to be present in a variable proportion of ocular adnexal MALT lymphomas with up to one half of cases responding to antibiotic treatment.

Diagnosis

Diagnosis depends on eliciting a history of recent bird contact from a patient with a compatible clinical syndrome, most commonly an influenza-like presentation, community-acquired pneumonia (CAP), or fever of unknown origin. The diagnosis should also be considered in a patient with CAP and prominent headache, splenomegaly, or failure to respond to β-lactam antibiotics. If the presentation is of an atypical CAP, the differential diagnosis includes infection with *Legionella* species, *Mycoplasma pneumoniae*, or *Chlamydophila pneumoniae*.

The white cell count is usually normal or slightly elevated, but there is often a left shift or toxic changes. Increases in the C-reactive protein (CRP) and erythrocyte sedimentation rate (ESR) are common. Mildly abnormal liver function tests, hyponatremia, and mild renal impairment are also common. The cerebrospinal fluid sometimes contains a few mononuclear cells but is otherwise normal. The chest x-ray usually shows more than predicted by the examination findings, but is nonspecific. The most common finding is lobar consolidation, but bilateral consolidation or interstitial opacities are also commonly seen.

Culture of *C. psittaci* is difficult and hazardous, so confirmation of diagnosis is more commonly performed using serology. The complement fixation (CF) test is widely used, but it cannot differentiate between *Chlamydophila* species. A fourfold rise in titer, using samples collected at least 14 days apart, or a single titer of 1:128 or higher, is

CURRENT DIAGNOSIS

- The key to successful management of psittacosis is considering it as a possible diagnosis and asking about bird contact.
- The commonest clinical scenarios are influenza-like illness, community-acquired pneumonia, or fever of unknown origin. The typical presentation is sudden onset of fever and chills, with prominent headache. The diagnosis should also be considered in a patient with community-acquired pneumonia and failure to respond to β-lactam antibiotics.
- Nonspecific findings on investigation include a normal or slightly elevated white blood cell count with a left shift or toxic changes, increase in C-reactive protein (CRP) or erythrocyte sedimentation rate (ESR), mildly abnormal liver function tests, hyponatremia, mild renal impairment, and a chest x-ray with more abnormalities than predicted by the examination findings.
- Diagnosis can be confirmed with serology using either the complement fixation test, which is widely used but unable to differentiate between *Chlamydia* species, or the microimmunofluorescent test, which is specific for individual *Chlamydia* species. Either a single high titer or a fourfold rise in titer using samples collected at least 14 days apart are interpreted as positive.

interpreted as a positive result. The antibody rise may be delayed or diminished by antibiotic treatment. A microimmunofluorescent (MIF) test is more specific for each *Chlamydophila* species, with a fourfold rise in titer or an IgM antibody titer of 1:16 interpreted as positive, but this test is not widely available. Polymerase chain reaction (PCR) assays have been developed, but they are not yet available for routine clinical use.

Management

When the diagnosis is suspected on clinical presentation and initial investigations, empiric therapy should be commenced. Tetracyclines are the drugs of choice, for example, doxycycline (Vibramycin) 100 mg bid for 10 to 14 days. This class usually leads to defervescence and improvement in symptoms within 24 to 48 hours, and subsequent mortality is less than 1%. Macrolides are usually recommended for pregnant women, children, and patients with intolerance of tetracyclines, but erythromycin (Erythrocin)[1] has been shown to fail in situations where a tetracycline was effective, and there are few clinical data on the efficacy of the other agents in this class. Some data suggest that quinolones may be effective, but further evidence is needed. Tetracycline hydrochloride[2] or doxycycline (4.4 mg/kg/d divided into two infusions) is given intravenously for critically ill patients.

Notification of health authorities is important for initiating public health investigations and interventions to reduce transmission and control of outbreaks.

[1]Not FDA approved for this indication.
[2]Not available in the United States.

REFERENCES

Centers for Disease Control and Prevention: Compendium of measures to control *Chlamydia psittaci* infection in humans (psittacosis) and pet birds (avian chlamydiosis), 2000. MMWR Morb Mortal Wkly Rep 2000;49(:RR08):1-17.
Crosse BA: Psittacosis: A clinical review. J Infect 1990;21:251-259.
Grayston JT, Thom DH: The chlamydial pneumonias. Curr Clin Top Infect Dis 1991;11:1-18.
Gregory DW, Schaffner W: Psittacosis. Semin Resp Infect 1997;12:7-11.
Hughes P, Chidley K, Cowie J: Neurological complications in psittacosis: A case report and literature review. Respir Med 1995;89:637-638.
Husain A, Roberts D, Pro B, et al: Meta-Analyses of the association between Chlamydia psittaci and ocular adnexal lymphoma and the response of ocular adnexal lymphoma and the response of ocular adnexal lymphoma to antibiotics. Cancer 2007;110:809-815.
Richards M: Psittacosis. UpToDate 2006 Available at http://www.uptodate.com/physicians/pulmonology_toclist.asp (accessed August 18, 2007; subscription required).
Williams J, Tallis G, Dalton C, et al: Community outbreak of psittacosis in a rural Australian town. Lancet 1998;351:1697-1699.
Yung AP, Grayson ML: Psittacosis: A review of 135 cases. Med J Aust 1988;148:228-233.

CURRENT THERAPY

- Empiric therapy should be commenced when the diagnosis is suspected on clinical presentation and initial investigations.
- Tetracyclines are the drugs of choice; for example, doxycycline (Vibramycin) 100 mg bid for 10 to 14 days.
- Macrolides are usually recommended for pregnant women, children, and people with intolerance of tetracyclines, but they are probably less effective.
- Defervescence and improvement in symptoms usually occur within 24 to 48 hours of initiating a tetracycline; subsequent mortality is less than 1%.
- Notification to health authorities facilitates public health investigation and interventions to reduce transmission and control outbreaks.

Q Fever

Method of
Didier Raoult, MD, PhD

Q fever is widespread zoonosis caused by *Coxiella burnetii*, a small, coccoid, strict intracellular gram-negative bacterium. It lives within the phagolysosome of its eukaryotic host cell at very low pH (4.5-4.8). It had previously been classified in the rickettsial family; however, recent phylogenic data based on study of the 16S rRNA gene sequence have shown that it belongs to *Legionellales* with the *Legionella* species and *Francisella tularensis*.

The bacterium has a spore-like life cycle, which explains its marked resistance to physicochemical agents. In cultures, *C. burnetii* exhibits a phase variation (from virulent phase I to avirulent phase II) caused by a spontaneous chromosome deletion. The avirulent form paradoxically generates high antibody levels in patients, but only patients with chronic infection have high antiphase I immunoglobulin G (IgG) and IgA antibody titers.

C. burnetii is a potent biological weapon. The reservoir of *C. burnetii* is wide, and nearly all tested mammals, birds, and ticks can be infected. Outbreaks have also been reported in association with the birth products of mammals (including ungulates and pets), raw milk, slaughterhouses, and farm work. Laboratory outbreaks have been reported. The disease is prevalent everywhere in the world but in

TABLE 1

Q Fever	Recommended Treatment	Alternative Treatment
Acute	Doxycycline (Vibramycin) 100 mg PO q8h × 14 d	Ofloxacin (Floxin)[1] 200 mg PO q8h × 14 d Cotrimoxazole (Bactrim)[1] 160/800 mg/PO q12h × 14 d
Chronic	Doxycycline 100 mg PO q12h *plus* hydroxychloroquine (Plaquenil)[1,2] 200 mg PO q8h × 18 to 36 mo	Doxycycline 100 mg PO q12h *plus* ofloxacin 200 mg PO q8h for 3 y to lifetime
Acute in a patient with a valvular lesion In pregnancy	Same as for chronic Q fever for 12 mo Cotrimoxazole (Bactrim)[1] 160/800 mg PO q12h until term	

[1] Not FDA approved for this indication.
[2] Hydroxychloroquine serum level should be 1 ± 0.2 μg/mL. Doxycycline serum level should be ≥ 4.5 μg/mL.

New Zealand, but because its clinical spectrum is wide and nonspecific, the observed incidence is directly related to physician interest in Q fever.

Clinical Features

Q fever is a reportable disease in the United States. In humans, infection is symptomatic in only 50% of patients. Most symptomatic patients experience a flu-like syndrome lasting 2 to 7 days and consisting of severe headaches and cough; 5% to 10% of infected patients may be sick enough to be investigated. They initially have high fever and one or several of pneumonia, hepatitis, meningoencephalitis, rash, myocarditis, and pericarditis. Routine laboratory investigation commonly shows mildly elevated transaminase levels and mild thrombocytopenia.

In special hosts such as immunocompromised patients (specifically those with lymphoma or splenectomy), *C. burnetii* can cause chronic infection. In pregnant women it can lead to recurrent miscarriage, low-birth-weight offspring, and prematurity.

In patients with valvular heart disease and those with arterial aneurysms or a vascular prosthesis, it can cause chronic endocarditis or vascular infection in patients in the two years following primary infection. The clinical picture is that of a chronic blood culture–negative endocarditis; the modified Duke criteria are of diagnostic value in such cases. It is spontaneously fatal in most cases.

Diagnosis

Because Q fever is pleomorphic, the diagnosis is based mainly on comprehensive serum testing in patients with an unexplained infectious syndrome. Liver biopsy may be of diagnostic value because the typical doughnut granuloma is quasispecific to Q fever. Valves obtained at surgery or autopsy can be used for culture, direct immunostaining, and polymerase chain reaction (PCR).

Three serologic techniques are used. Complement fixation lacks sensitivity, and one third of patients with acute Q fever do not exhibit complement-fixing antibodies within one month after onset of the disease. However, a fourfold increase in antibodies to phase II antigen indicates acute Q fever, and antibody levels against phase I that are higher than 1:200 indicate chronic Q fever. Indirect immunofluorescence assay is the reference method. A single titer of 1:200 for IgG antiphase II associated with a titer of 1:50 for IgM is diagnostic of acute infection. IgG antibody levels against phase I that are greater than 1:800 and IgA antibody levels greater than 1:50 are highly predictive of chronic infection. Enzyme-linked immunosorbent assay (ELISA) is useful for diagnosing acute infection in detecting IgM antiphase II.

PCR has recently been developed to detect *C. burnetii* DNA in the sera of patients with Q fever. Real-time PCR using multicopy gene *IS1111* is the more sensitive technique. It is positive in the sera of patients with acute Q fever before IgG antibodies to *C. burnetii* become apparent. It is also positive in patients with untreated chronic Q fever. Contamination of PCR can occur, and many unconfirmed results are reported in the literature.

Treatment

To be active against Q fever, an antibiotic compound has to enter the cell, be effective at an acidic pH (where *C. burnetii* multiplies), and have activity against *C. burnetii*. No antibiotic is bactericidal, but bactericidal activity can be achieved by the addition of hydroxychloroquine (Plaquenil) to doxycycline (Vibramycin).

For acute Q fever, the reference treatment is doxycycline 100 mg orally bid for 2 to 3 weeks. Other compounds have been reported to be effective, such as trimethoprim-sulfamethoxazole (TMP-SMX) (Bactrim),[1] Rifampin (Rifadin)[1] 300 mg bid, and ofloxacin (Floxin)[1] 200 mg bid. In the case of Q fever in pregnant women, one double-strength TMP-SMX[1] tablet (trimethoprim 160 mg, sulfamethoxazole 800 mg) twice daily until delivery prevents fetal death (Table 1).

Chronic endocarditis should be treated for three years, and antibody levels should be monitored. When IgG antiphase I is less than 800 and IgA is less than 50, treatment may be stopped before three years. Two protocols have been evaluated: doxycycline 200 mg daily combined with ofloxacin[1] 400 mg daily for four years to lifetime, and doxycycline combined with hydroxychloroquine[1] for 1.5 to 3 years in an amount to achieve a 1 ± 0.20 μg/mL plasma concentration. Doxycycline serum levels greater than 4.5 μg/mL of serum are associated with a more rapidly favorable outcome. This last regimen is apparently more efficacious in terms of relapse. However, regular ophthalmologic surveillance is critical to detect the accumulation of chloroquine in the retina. Both regimens expose the patient to a major risk of photosensitization.

The combination of doxycycline and hydroxychloroquine for one year has demonstrated efficacy in preventing endocarditis.

Prevention

Prevention depends on avoiding exposure, particularly by pregnant women and patients with valvulopathy. No vaccine is currently available outside Australia.

---

[1] Not FDA approved for this indication.

REFERENCES

Fenollar F, Fournier PE, Raoult D: Molecular detection of *Coxiella burnetii* in the sera of patients with Q fever endocarditis or vascular infection. J Clin Microbiol 2004;42(:11):4919-4924.

Klee SR, Tyczka J, Ellerbrok H, et al: Highly sensitive real-time PCR for specific detection and quantification of *Coxiella burnetii*. BMC Microbiol 2006;19:2.

Maurin M, Raoult D: Q fever. Clin Microbiol Rev 1999;12(4):518-553.

Raoult D, Marrie T, Mege J: Natural history and pathophysiology of Q fever. Lancet Infect Dis 2005;5(4):219-226.
Rolain JM, Raoult D: Molecular detection of *Coxiella burnetii* in blood and sera during Q fever. QJM 2005;98(8):615-617.
Rolain JM, Maurin M, Raoult D: Bacteriostatic and bactericidal activities of moxifloxacin against *Coxiella burnetii*. Antimicrob Agents Chemother 2001;45(1):301-302.

Rabies

Method of
Alan C. Jackson, MD, FRCPC

Rabies is an acute infection of the nervous system caused by rabies virus, which is a member of the family Rhabdoviridae in the genus *Lyssavirus*. Other lyssaviruses have only very rarely caused rabies in Europe, Africa, and Australia.

Pathogenesis

Rabies virus is usually transmitted by bites from rabid animals. Transmission has rarely occurred through an aerosol route (in a laboratory accident or bat cave containing millions of bats) or by transplantation of infected organs and tissues. The virus is in the saliva of the rabid animal and inoculated into subcutaneous tissues or muscles. During most of the long incubation period (lasting 20 to 90 days or longer), the virus is close to the site of inoculation. The virus binds to the nicotinic acetylcholine receptor at the postsynaptic neuromuscular junction and travels toward the central nervous system (CNS) in peripheral nerves by retrograde fast axonal transport. There is rapid dissemination throughout the CNS by fast axonal transport. Under natural conditions, degenerative neuronal changes are not prominent, and it is thought that the rabies virus induces neuronal dysfunction by mechanisms that are not well understood. In rabies vectors, the encephalitis is associated with behavioral changes that lead to transmission by biting. After the CNS infection is established, the virus spreads by autonomic and sensory nerves to multiple organs, including the salivary glands in which the virus is secreted in high titer.

Clinical Features

In North America, where the bat is the most common rabies vector, a history of an animal bite is usually absent, and there may be no known contact with animals. The incubation period is usually between 20 and 90 days, but it may occasionally last 1 or more years. Prodromal features are nonspecific and include malaise, headache, and fever, and patients may also have anxiety or agitation. Approximately half of patients may experience pain, paresthesias, or pruritus at the site of the wound, which has often healed; this may reflect involvement of local sensory ganglia. Approximately 80% of patients with rabies have encephalitic rabies; approximately 20% have paralytic rabies. In encephalitic rabies, there are characteristic periods of generalized arousal or hyperexcitability separated by lucid periods. Autonomic dysfunction occurs frequently and includes hypersalivation, gooseflesh, cardiac arrhythmias, and priapism. Hydrophobia is the most characteristic feature of rabies and occurs in 50% to 80% of patients; contractions of the diaphragm and other inspiratory muscles occur on swallowing. This may become a conditioned reflex, and even the sight or thought of water can precipitate the muscle contractions. Hydrophobia is thought to be caused by inhibition of inspiratory neurons near the nucleus ambiguus.

In paralytic rabies, prominent muscle weakness usually begins in the bitten extremity and progresses to quadriparesis; typically there is sphincter involvement. Patients have a longer clinical course than in encephalitic rabies. Paralytic rabies is frequently misdiagnosed as the Guillain-Barré syndrome. Coma subsequently develops in both clinical forms. With aggressive medical therapy, a variety of medical complications develop, and multiple organ failure is a frequent occurrence. Survival is very rare and has usually occurred in the context of incomplete postexposure rabies prophylaxis that included administration of some rabies vaccine.

Epidemiology

Worldwide more than 55,000 human deaths per year are attributed to rabies. The impact is particularly significant in terms of years of life lost because children are frequently the victims. Most human rabies cases occur through transmission from dogs in developing countries with endemic dog rabies, particularly in Asia and Africa. In the United States and Canada, the most common human cases are from insect-eating bats, and often, there is no known history of a bat bite or exposure to bats. A bat bite may not be recognized. The rabies virus variant responsible for most human cases is found in silver-haired bats and eastern pipistrelle bats. These are small bats not frequently in contact with humans. There are a variety of other rabies vectors in North American wildlife, including skunks, raccoons, and foxes, but these species are rarely responsible for transmission to humans. This is likely because of effective postexposure rabies prophylaxis.

Diagnosis

Most cases of rabies can be diagnosed clinically or the diagnosis strongly suspected, which is particularly important to initiate appropriate barrier nursing techniques and prevent exposures of many health care workers. Some cases may be candidates for an aggressive therapeutic approach. A serum neutralizing titer can be useful in a previously unimmunized individual, but a positive titer may not develop until the second week of clinical illness, and the result of the test may not be readily available. Detection of rabies virus antigen on a skin biopsy obtained from the nape of the neck using a fluorescent antibody technique is a useful diagnostic test. Detection of rabies virus ribonucleic acid (RNA) in saliva using reverse transcription polymerase chain reaction (RT-PCR) amplification is an important recent advance in rapid rabies diagnosis. Rabies virus antigen can be detected in brain tissue obtained by brain biopsy or postmortem.

 CURRENT DIAGNOSIS

- A history of animal bite or exposure is frequently absent in North America.
- Pain, paresthesias, and pruritus are early neurologic symptoms of rabies, probably reflecting infection in local sensory ganglia.
- Autonomic features are common.
- Hydrophobia is a highly specific feature of rabies.
- Paralytic features may be prominent, and the clinical presentation may resemble the Guillain-Barré syndrome.
- Saliva samples for reverse transcription polymerase chain reaction (RT-PCR) and a skin biopsy should be obtained for detection of rabies virus antigen.

Prevention

After recognition of a rabies exposure, rabies can be prevented with initiation of appropriate steps, including wound cleansing and active and passive immunization. After a human is bitten by a dog, cat, or ferret, the animal should be captured, confined, and observed for a period of at least 10 days. The animal should also be examined by a veterinarian prior to its release. If the animal is a stray, unwanted, shows signs, or develops signs of rabies during the observation period, the animal should be killed immediately, and its head should be transported under refrigeration for a laboratory examination. The brain should be examined via an antigen-detection method using the fluorescent antibody technique and viral isolation using cell culture or mouse inoculation.

The incubation period for animals other than dogs, cats, and ferrets is uncertain; these animals should be killed immediately after an exposure, and the head submitted for examination. If the result is negative, one may safely conclude that the animal's saliva did not contain rabies virus and, if immunization has been initiated, it should be discontinued. If an animal escapes after an exposure, it should be considered rabid unless information from public health officials indicates this is unlikely, and rabies prophylaxis should be initiated. The physical presence of a bat may warrant postexposure prophylaxis when a person (such as a small child or sleeping adult) is unable to reliably report contact that could have resulted in a bite.

Local wound care should be given as soon as possible after all exposures, even if immunization is delayed, pending the results of an observation period. All bite wounds and scratches should be washed thoroughly with soap and water. Devitalized tissues should be débrided.

Purified chick embryo cell culture vaccine (RabAvert), rabies vaccine absorbed (RVA), and human diploid cell vaccine (Imovax) are licensed rabies vaccines in the United States and Canada. Other vaccines grown in either primary cell lines (hamster or dog kidney) or continuous cell lines (Vero cells) are also satisfactory and available in other countries. A regimen of five 1-mL doses of rabies vaccine should be given intramuscularly (IM) in the deltoid area (anterolateral aspect of the thigh is also acceptable in children). Ideally, the first dose should be given as soon as possible after exposure, but failing that, it should be given regardless of the length of a delay. Four additional doses should be given on days 3, 7, 14, and 28. Pregnancy is not a contraindication for immunization. Live vaccines should not be given for 1 month after rabies immunization. Local and mild systemic reactions are common. Systemic allergic reactions are uncommon, and anaphylactic reactions may be treated with epinephrine and antihistamines. Corticosteroids may interfere with the development of active immunity. Immunosuppressive medications should not be administered during postexposure therapy unless they are essential. The risk of developing rabies should be carefully considered before deciding to discontinue vaccination because of an adverse reaction. A serum neutralizing antibody determination is necessary only after immunization of immunocompromised patients. Less expensive vaccines, derived from neural tissues, are still used in some developing countries; these vaccines are associated with serious neuroparalytic complications.

Human rabies immune globulin (Imogam or BayRab) should also be administered as passive immunization for protection before the development of immunity from the vaccine. It should be given at the same time as the first dose of vaccine and no later than 7 days after the first dose. Rabies vaccine and human rabies immune globulin should never be administered at the same site or in the same syringe. The recommended dose of human rabies immune globulin is 20 international units (IU)/kg; larger doses should not be given because they may suppress active immunity from the vaccine. After wounds are washed, they should be infiltrated with human rabies immune globulin (if anatomically feasible), and the remainder of the dose should be given IM in the gluteal area. If the exposure involves a mucous membrane, the entire dose should be administered IM. With multiple or large wounds, the human rabies immune globulin may need to be diluted for adequate infiltration of all of the wounds. Adverse effects of human rabies immune globulin include local pain and low-grade fever.

After an exposure, a previously immunized patient should receive two 1-mL doses of rabies vaccine on days 0 and 3, but the patient should not receive human rabies immune globulin.

Management of Human Rabies

Only six people have survived rabies, and five received rabies vaccine prior to the onset of their disease. The possibilities for an aggressive approach were recently reviewed (see Jackson et al., 2003). There was one survivor in Wisconsin in 2004 who did not receive rabies vaccine. It is now doubtful whether the therapy she received played a significant role in her favorable outcome because a similar approach has failed in many cases. Palliation is an alternative approach and may be appropriate for many patients who develop rabies.

REFERENCES

Centers for Disease Control and Prevention: Human rabies prevention—United States, 1999: Recommendations of the Advisory Committee on Immunization Practices (ACIP). MMWR 1999;48(No. RR-1):1-21.
Jackson AC: Human disease. In Jackson AC, Wunner WH (eds): Rabies. 2nd ed, London: Elsevier, Academic Press, 2007, pp 309-340.
Jackson AC: Rabies. Curr Treat Options Infect Dis 2003;5:35-40.
Jackson AC: Rabies: New insights into pathogenesis and treatment. Curr Opin Neurol 2006;19(3):267-270.
Jackson AC, Warrell MJ, Rupprecht CE, et al: Management of rabies in humans. Clin Infect Dis 2003;36:60-63.
Jackson AC, Wunner WH: Rabies. 2nd ed. London: Elsevier, Academic Press, 2007.
World Health Organization: WHO expert consultation on rabies: First report (First Report Edition). Geneva: WHO, 2005.

CURRENT THERAPY

- Details of an exposure determine whether postexposure rabies prophylaxis should be initiated.
- Wound cleansing is very important after a potential rabies exposure.
- Active immunization with a schedule of 5 doses of rabies vaccine at intervals is recommended.
- Passive immunization (if previously unimmunized) consists of human rabies immune globulin infiltrated into the wound and the remainder of the 20 IU/kg dosage given intramuscularly.

Rat-Bite Fever

Method of
Jean Dudler, MD

Rat-bite fever (RBF) is a systemic febrile disease caused by infection with *Streptobacillus moniliformis*. As its name implies, it is transmitted by rat bite. However, it can also be transmitted by simple contact with infected rats or even through ingestion of food contaminated with rat excreta. Diagnosis can be difficult, and a high degree of awareness is necessary to make a correct diagnosis. Recognition and early treatment are crucial, because case fatality can be higher than 10% in untreated cases.

Epidemiology

S. moniliformis is part of the normal respiratory flora of the rat. From 50% to 100% of healthy wild, laboratory, and pet rats harbor *S. moniliformis* in the nasopharynx. *S. moniliformis* is also excreted in the urine, and *Spirillum minus* has been demonstrated in conjunctival secretions and blood. Thus, rat-bite fever can be transmitted not only from a bite but also through scratches, handling of dead rats, and even handling of litter material.

Although the rat is the natural reservoir and major vector of the disease, *S. moniliformis* has also been found in other rodents such as mice, squirrels, and gerbils, as well as in other mammals such as weasels and in pets that prey on rodents, such as cats and dogs, which can also act as vectors of the disease.

The major risk factor is exposure to rats, either as an occupational hazard for persons such as laboratory workers, veterinarians, or pet shop employees, or for persons who have rats for pets or feed rats to snakes, especially children. Classically, homelessness and lower socioeconomic status were described as major factors, but most cases reported in the last few years have involved pet rats.

No precise data are available on the true incidence of rat-bite fever because it is not a reportable disease. It appears to be unusual in Western countries, a rarity that could reflect failed diagnosis or a spontaneous recovery in most cases, considering the high percentage of *S. moniliformis* carriage, the frequency of contacts between humans and rats in modern society, and the fairly high risk—estimated around 10%—of developing rat-bite fever after being bitten or scratched.

Clinical Presentation

Rat-bite fever is a systemic febrile disease. Classically, following a rat bite and a short incubation of 1 to 3 days (but up to 3 weeks), systemic dissemination of the organism is associated with an abrupt onset with intermittent relapsing fever, rigors, myalgias, arthralgias, headache, sore throat, malaise, and vomiting. These symptoms are followed within the first week by the development of a maculopapular rash in 75% of patients. The rash can be pustular, purpuric, or petechial, and it typically involves the extremities, in particular the palms and soles. The bite site typically heals promptly, with minimal inflammation and absent or minimal regional adenopathy.

Up to 50% of infected patients develop an asymmetric migrating polyarthritis, which appears to be exceedingly painful and affects large and middle-sized joints. Joint effusion appears more common in adults. Infection can occur in any tissues. Anemia, meningitis, bronchitis, pneumonia, endocarditis, myocarditis, pericarditis, brain abscess, and infarcts of the spleen and kidneys have been reported as complications of rat-bite fever.

Although most cases seem to resolve spontaneously within 2 weeks, persistence up to 2 years has been reported. The mortality rate in untreated cases is around 10% to 15%, and it rises to more than 50% in the rare cases with cardiac involvement.

Two closely related variants have been described. In Haverhill fever, the organism is transmitted by ingestion of contaminated food. It tends to occur in epidemics and also causes rashes and arthritis, but upper respiratory tract symptoms and vomiting appear more prominent. Sodoku is a rat-bite fever caused by *Spirillum minus*; it is common in Japan. The course is more subacute, arthritic symptoms are rare, and if the bite initially heals, it then ulcerates and is associated with regional lymphadenopathy and a distinctive rash.

Diagnosis

Diagnosis is difficult, with nonspecific clinical findings, broad differential diagnosis, and difficulties in identifying the responsible organism. Rat-bite fever should not be dismissed in the absence of bite history, because transmission can occur without a bite, and pet lovers

CURRENT DIAGNOSIS

- The examiner must maintain a high index of suspicion.
- Nonspecific initial symptoms are followed by a maculopapular rash and septic arthritis.
- Exposure to rats is the major risk factor. Transmission can occur with simple contact with infected animals or excreta.
- Notify microbiology laboratory of suspicion (slow growth, 5%-10% CO_2 microaerophilic conditions, 20% normal rabbit serum media supplementation, and avoidance of sodium polyanethol sulfonate).

or laboratory workers can minimize or forget the bite, especially in the absence of a local reaction.

No reliable serologic test is available, and the definitive diagnosis requires isolation of *S. moniliformis* from the wound, the blood, or the synovial fluid. The microbiology laboratory should be specifically notified of any clinical suspicion because of the hurdles in identification.

S. moniliformis is a highly pleomorphic, nonencapsulated, nonmotile gram-negative rod, which may stain positively on Gram stain. It is often dismissed as proteinaceous debris because of its numerous bulbous swellings with occasional clumping (*moniliformis* = "necklace-like"). It grows slowly and requires a microaerophilic environment with 5% to 10% CO_2 or anaerobic conditions and media supplementation with 20% normal rabbit serum. Cultures should be held for more than 5 days and should not be dismissed as contamination. *S. moniliformis* is also inhibited by sodium polyanethol sulfonate, a common adjunct in most commercial blood culture media. Identification using polymerase chain reaction amplification and gene sequencing has been used. It can be performed on samples from the patient or animal in question if available.

Differential Diagnosis

Differential diagnosis is broad and depends on the clinical presentation. Malaria, typhoid fever, and neoplastic disease can cause relapsing fevers, and the presence of a rash and polyarthritis might suggest viral and rickettsial diseases. An asymmetric oligoarthritis points more toward a bacterial etiology, in particular disseminated gonococcal and meningococcal diseases in the context of cutaneous lesions. Lyme disease or secondary syphilis occasionally have such a clinical presentation, but 25% to 50% of patients infected with *S. moniliformis* or *S. minus* have a false-positive VDRL (Venereal Disease Research Laboratory) test. Finally, when classic infectious symptoms such as fever or rash are missing, any causes of polyarthritis, from crystal-related arthropathies to rheumatoid arthritis, can be entertained.

Treatment

All established cases of rat-bite fever should be treated with antibiotics. Despite being potentially lethal, rat-bite fever is easily treatable by a simple course of penicillin. The Centers for Disease Control and Prevention recommends intravenous penicillin G 1.2 million units per day for 5 to 7 days followed by oral penicillin V (Pen Vee K)[1] or ampicillin (Omnipen)[1] 500 mg qid for an additional week. For allergic patients, or if an intravenous line cannot be established, oral tetracycline (Achromycin)[1] 500 mg qid or streptomycin[1] 7.5 mg/kg bid intramuscularly are alternatives. Numerous other antibiotics have been reported to be potentially useful, including clarithromycin

---

[1]Not FDA approved for this indication.

CURRENT THERAPY

Bite Site

- Clean and disinfect bite site.
- Local treatment does not prevent further dissemination.
- Administer tetanus toxoid (Td), if indicated.
- Do not give antirabies prophylaxis.

Established Cases

- Intravenous penicillin G (Bicillin) 1.2 million U/d for 5 to 7 d, followed by oral penicillin V[1] or ampicillin (Omnipen)[1] 500 mg qid for an additional wk (CDC recommendations).
- Oral tetracycline[1] 500 mg qid or streptomycin[1] 7.5 mg/kg bid IM are alternatives.
- Numerous other antibiotics are reported useful (macrolides, cephalosporins, quinolones)

Prophylaxis

- The role of prophylactic antibiotic is unknown. Some authors recommend oral penicillin V.[1]
- Encourage patients with an occupational risk to use protective gloves to handle animals or cages.

[1]Not FDA approved for this indication.

(Biaxin),[1] cephalosporins, and quinolones, but none has been subjected to any clinical trial.

Typically the bite site heals promptly. It should be cleaned and disinfected, even if local treatment does not appear to prevent further dissemination. Tetanus prophylaxis (Td) administration is indicated as required by the patient's immunization record, but antirabies prophylaxis is usually not required for rodent bite.

The role of prophylactic antibiotics is unknown, but some authors recommend the use of oral penicillin V.[1] Primary prevention by using protective gloves to handle animals or cages should be encouraged for patients with occupational risk.

[1]Not FDA approved for this indication.

REFERENCES

Abdulaziz H, Touchie C, Toye B, Karsh J: Haverhill fever with spine involvement. J Rheumatol 2006;33:1409-1410.
Albedwawi S, LeBlanc C, Show A, Slinger RW: A teenager with fever, rash and arthritis. CMAJ 2006;175:354.
Berger C, Altwegg M, Meyer A, Nadal D: Broad range polymerase chain reaction for diagnosis of rat-bite fever caused by *Streptobacillus moniliformis*. Pediatr Infect Dis J 2001;20:1181-1182.
Centers for Disease Control and Prevention: Fatal rat-bite fever—Florida and Washington, 2003. MMWR Morb Mortal Wkly Rep. 2005;53:1198-1202.
Holroyd KJ, Reiner AP, Dick JD: *Streptobacillus moniliformis* polyarthritis mimicking rheumatoid arthritis: An urban case of rat bite fever. Am J Med 1988;85:711-714.
Rupp ME: *Streptobacillus moniliformis* endocarditis: Case report and review. Clin Infect Dis 1992;14:769-772.
Schachter ME, Wilcox L, Rau N, et al: Rat-bite fever, Canada. Emerg Infect Dis 2006;12:1301-1302.
Stehle P, Dubuis O, So A, Dudler J: Rat bite fever without fever. Ann Rheum Dis 2003;62:894-896.
van Nood E, Peters SH: Rat-bite fever. Neth J Med 2005;63:319-321.
Washburn RG: *Streptobacillus moniliformis* (rat-bite fever). In Mandell GL, Bennett JE, Dolin R, eds. Mandell, Douglas, and Bennett's Principles and Practice of Infectious Diseases. 4th ed. Philadelphia: Churchill-Livingstone, 2000, pp 2422-2424.

Relapsing Fever

Method of
Diego Cadavid, MD

Relapsing fever is one of several diseases caused by spirochetes. Other human spirochetal diseases are syphilis, Lyme disease, and leptospirosis. Notable features of spirochetes are wavy and helical shapes, length-to-diameter ratios of as much as 100 to 1, and flagella that lie between the inner and outer cell membranes. The spirochetes that cause relapsing fever are in the genus *Borrelia*. Other *Borrelia* species cause Lyme disease, avian spirochetosis, and epidemic bovine abortion. Table 1 shows the main *Borrelia* species of relapsing fever, their vectors, and an estimate of their geographic ranges. In the United States relapsing fever was considered a disease endemic only in the West. However, the recent finding of relapsing fever–like *Borrelia* in ticks and dogs in the eastern United States suggests that the risk of relapsing fever may extend into the East.

Epidemiology

There are two forms of relapsing fever: epidemic transmitted to humans by the body louse *Pediculus humanus* (louse-borne relapsing fever, LBRF) and endemic transmitted to humans by soft-bodied ticks of the genus *Ornithodoros* (tick-borne relapsing fever, TBRF). In LBRF itching caused by skin infestation with lice leads to scratching, which may result in crushing of lice and release of infected hemolymph into areas of skin abrasion. Louse infestation is associated with cold weather and a lack of hygiene. Migrant workers and soldiers at war are particularly susceptible to this infection. Historically, massive outbreaks of LBRF occurred in Eurasia, Africa, and Latin America, but currently the disease is found only in Ethiopia and neighboring countries. However, immigrants can spread LBRF to other parts of the world.

The main risk factor for TBRF is exposure to endemic areas (Table 1). The risk of infection increases with outdoor activities in areas where rodents nest, like entering caves or sleeping in rustic cabins. *Ornithodoros* ticks are soft-bodied and feed for short periods of time (minutes), usually at night. They can live many years between blood meals and may transmit spirochetes to their offspring transovarially. Infection is produced by regurgitation of infected tick saliva into the skin wound during tick feeding. There are several natural vertebrate reservoirs for TBRF, but most common are rodents (deer mice, chipmunks, squirrels, and rats). In contrast, the body louse *Pediculus humanus* is a strict human parasite, living and multiplying in clothing.

Clinical Diagnosis

Relapsing fever should be suspected in any patient presenting with two or more episodes of high fever and constitutional symptoms spaced by periods of relative well-being. The index of suspicion increases if the patient has been exposed to endemic areas for TBRF or to countries where LBRF still occurs (Table 1). Whereas LBRF is usually associated with a single febrile relapse, TBRF usually has multiple relapses (up to 13). In LBRF the second episode of fever is typically milder than the first; in TBRF the multiple febrile periods are usually of equal severity. The febrile periods last from 1 to 3 days, and the intervals between fevers last from 3 to 10 days. During the febrile periods, numerous spirochetes are circulating in the blood. This is called spirochetemia and is sometimes unexpectedly detected during routine blood smear examinations. Between fevers, spirochetemia is not observed because the numbers are low. The fever pattern and recurrent spirochetemia are the consequences of antigenic variation of abundant outer membrane

CURRENT DIAGNOSIS

- There are two forms of relapsing fever: epidemic and endemic.
- Epidemic relapsing fever is transmitted from person to person by the body louse *Pediculus humanus*.
- Endemic relapsing fever is transmitted from rodent reservoirs to humans exposed to endemic areas by soft-bodied ticks of the genus *Ornithodoros*.
- The hallmark of relapsing fever is two or more febrile episodes separated by periods of relative well-being.
- The diagnosis is confirmed by visualization of the etiologic spirochetes in thin peripheral blood smears prepared at times of febrile peaks by phase-contrast or darkfield microscopy or light microscopy after Wright or Giemsa staining.

lipoproteins of relapsing fever *Borrelia* species that are the target for serotype-specific antibodies.

The mean latency between exposure to ticks in the endemic form or to lice in the epidemic form and onset of symptoms is 6 days (range, 3 to 18 days). Because *Ornithodoros* ticks feed briefly and painlessly at night, patients with TBRF may not be able to recall having been bitten by a tick. The clinical manifestations of TBRF and LBRF are similar, although some differences do exist. Table 2 lists the frequency of the most common manifestations of TBRF. The usual initial presentation is sudden onset of chills followed by high fever, tachycardia, severe headache, vomiting, myalgia and arthralgia, and often delirium. In the early stages, a reddish rash may be seen over the trunk, arms, or legs. The fever remains high for 3 to 5 days, and then it clears abruptly. After an asymptomatic period of 7 to 10 days, the fever and other constitutional symptoms can reappear suddenly. The febrile episodes gradually become less severe, and the person eventually recovers completely. As the disease progresses, fever, jaundice, hepatosplenomegaly, cardiac arrhythmias, and cardiac failure may occur, especially with LBRF. Jaundice is more common at times of relapses. Patients with LBRF are more likely to develop petechiae on the trunk, extremities, and mucous membranes; epistaxis; and blood-tinged sputum. Rupture of the spleen may rarely occur. Multiple neurologic complications can occur as a result of disseminated intravascular coagulation in LBRF and as a result of infection of the meninges and cranial and spinal nerve roots by spirochetes in TBRF. The most common neurologic complications of TBRF are aseptic meningitis and facial palsy. Relapsing fever in pregnant women can cause abortion, premature birth, and neonatal death. Sometimes patients can have nonfebrile relapses, consisting of periods of severe headache, backache, weakness, and other constitutional symptoms without fever that occur at the time of expected relapses. Delirium may persist for weeks after the fever resolves, and rarely symptoms may be protracted.

Relapsing fever may be confused with many diseases that are relapsing or cause high fevers. These include typhoid fever, yellow fever, dengue, African hemorrhagic fevers, African trypanosomiasis, brucellosis, malaria, leptospirosis, rat-bite fever, intermittent cholangitis, cat-scratch disease, echovirus 9 infection, among others. Relapsing fever *Borrelias* have antigens that are cross reactive with Lyme disease *Borrelias* and inasmuch as the endemic areas of relapsing fever and Lyme disease overlap to some extent, confusion between the two infections can be expected.

Laboratory Diagnosis

Although the pattern of recurring fever is the clue to diagnosing relapsing fever, confirmation of the diagnosis requires demonstration of spirochetes in peripheral blood taken during an episode of fever. The comparatively large number of spirochetes in the blood during relapsing fever provides the opportunity for the simplest method for laboratory diagnosis of the infection, light microscopy of Wright or Giemsa stained thin blood smears or darkfield or phase-contrast microscopy of a wet mount of plasma. The blood should be obtained during or just before peaks of body temperature. Between fever peaks, spirochetes often can be demonstrated by inoculation of blood or cerebrospinal fluid (CSF) into special culture medium (BSK-H with 6% rabbit serum available from Sigma) or experimental animals. Enrichment for spirochetes is achieved by using the platelet-rich fraction of plasma or the buffy coat of sedimented blood. In the United States the most common causes of relapsing fever are *Borrelia hermsii* and *Borrelia turicatae*; both grow in BSK-H medium and in young mice or rats. Whereas direct visual detection of organisms in the blood is the most common method for laboratory confirmation of relapsing fever, immunoassays for antibodies are the most common means of laboratory confirmation for Lyme disease. Although serologic assays have been developed for the agents of relapsing fever, these are not widely available and of dubious utility. The antigenic variation displayed by the relapsing fever species means there are hundreds of different "serotypes." If a different serotype or species is used for preparing the antigen, only antibodies to conserved antigens may be detected. For this reason, a standardized enzyme-linked immunosorbent assay (ELISA) with Lyme disease *Borrelia* as antigen may be the best available serologic assay for relapsing fever. ELISA for *Borrelia burgdorferi* antibodies is routinely done across the United States and Europe. If a positive result for IgM or IgG antibodies is obtained, the Western blot for antibodies to *B. burgdorferi* antigens would be expected to discriminate current or past Lyme disease from relapsing fever, as well as from syphilis, another cause of false-positive Lyme disease ELISA results. Other frequent laboratory abnormalities can occur in relapsing fever but are not diagnostic. These include elevated white blood cell count with increased neutrophils, thrombocytopenia, increased serum bilirubin, proteinuria, microhematuria, prolongation of the prothrombin time (PT) and partial thromboplastin time (PTT), and elevation of fibrin degradation products.

TABLE 1 Relapsing Fever *Borrelia* Species Pathogenic to Humans

Relapsing Fever	*Borrelia* Species	Arthropod Vector	Distribution of Disease
Endemic	B. hermsii	Ornithodoros hermsi	Western North America
	B. turicatae	O. turicata	Southwestern North America and northern Mexico
	B. venezuelensis	O. rudis	Central America and northern South America
	B. hispanica	O. marocanus	Iberian peninsula and northwestern Africa
	B. crocidurae	O. erraticus	North and East Africa, Middle East, southern Europe
	B. duttoni	O. moubata	Sub-Saharan Africa
	B. persica	O. tholozani	Middle East, Greece, Central Asia
	B. uzbekistan	O. pappilipes	Tajikistan, Uzbekistan
Epidemic	B. recurrentis	Pediculus humanus	Worldwide (recently only in East Africa including immigrants to Europe)

TABLE 2 Frequent Clinical Manifestations of Tick-Borne Relapsing Fever

Sign or Symptom	Frequency (%)
Headache	94
Myalgia	92
Chills	88
Nausea	76
Arthralgia	73
Vomiting	71
Abdominal pain	44
Confusion	38
Dry cough	27
Ocular pain	26
Diarrhea	25
Dizziness	25
Photophobia	25
Neck pain	24
Rash	18
Dysuria	13
Jaundice	10
Hepatomegaly	10
Splenomegaly	6

Treatment

Relapsing fever *Borrelias* are very sensitive to several antibiotics, and antimicrobial resistance is rare. Table 3 summarizes the treatment options for adults and children younger than 8 years. Children older than 8 years can be treated with the same antibiotics as adults, but the doses should be adjusted by weight. Before antibiotics are given, the possibility of causing the Jarisch-Herxheimer reaction should be considered (see later). The tetracycline antibiotics are most commonly used for treatment of LBRF and TBRF. The first antibiotic of choice in adults and children older than 8 years is doxycycline (Doryx). In general, shorter treatments are needed for LBRF than for TBRF. Single-dose therapy is usually recommended for LBRF. In contrast, in TBRF even multiple doses of tetracyclines for up to 10 days may fail to prevent relapses, and retreatment can be required.

CURRENT THERAPY

- The antibiotic of choice for treatment of relapsing fever is doxycycline (Doryx) except in children or pregnant women. In children < 8 y, erythromycin (E-Mycin)[1] or oral penicillin[1] is used instead of tetracycline (Table 3).
- Relapsing fever if severe or complicated with neuroborreliosis requires treatment with the intravenous antibiotics ceftriaxone (Rocephin) or penicillin G (Table 3).
- The louse-borne epidemic form is treated with a single dose, whereas the endemic tick-borne form is treated with multiple doses for at least 1 week (Table 3).
- Antibiotic treatment of relapsing fever results in the Jarisch-Herxheimer reaction in as many as 60% of cases, more often in the epidemic than in the endemic form. It is characterized by the sudden onset of tachycardia, hypotension, chills, rigors, diaphoresis, and high fever. To reduce the risk of the JHR, antibiotics should be started between but not at times of febrile peaks.

---

[1]Not FDA approved for this indication.

Alternative oral antibiotics to the tetracyclines are erythromycin (E-Mycin),[1] azithromycin (Zithromax),[1] amoxicillin (Amoxil),[1] penicillin,[1] and chloramphenicol (Chloromycetin).[1] However, oral chloramphenicol is no longer available in the United States. Erythromycin, azithromycin, and penicillin do not appear as effective as the tetracyclines; however, they are recommended for children younger than 8 years and for pregnant women. Amoxicillin is another alternative for young children with early Lyme disease; however, it is ineffective for human granulocytic ehrlichiosis, which sometimes occurs as a co-infection with Lyme disease.

Although treatment with antibiotics is usually given orally, they may need to be given intravenously if severe vomiting makes swallowing impractical. If there are symptoms and signs of meningitis or encephalitis without clinical and/or radiologic signs of increased intracranial pressure, the CSF should be examined to rule out central nervous system (CNS) infection. The finding of elevation of CSF cells and protein demands the use of parenteral antibiotics, such as penicillin G or ceftriaxone (Rocephin). Optimally, antibiotic treatment should be started during afebrile periods when the spirochetemia is low. Starting therapy near the peak of a febrile period may induce the Jarisch-Herxheimer reaction, in which high fever and a rise and subsequent fall in blood pressure, sometimes to dangerously low levels, may occur. Dehydration should be treated with fluids given intravenously. Severe headache can be treated with pain relievers such as codeine, and nausea or vomiting can be treated with prochlorperazine.

Jarisch-Herxheimer Reaction

Antibiotic treatment of relapsing fever causes the Jarisch-Herxheimer reaction (JHR) in as many as 60% of cases. The JHR is more common in LBRF than in TBRF. It is characterized by the sudden onset of tachycardia, hypotension, chills, rigors, diaphoresis, and high fever. Patients with the JHR have said that they felt as if they were going to die. The JHR is caused by the rapid killing of circulating spirochetes 1 to 4 hours after the first dose of antibiotic, which results in the release of large amounts of *Borrelia* lipoproteins in the circulation followed by massive release of tumor necrosis factor and other cytokines. If possible, patients with the JHR should be transferred to an intensive care unit for close monitoring and treatment. During several hours, the temperature declines and the patient feels better. Large amounts of intravenous fluids (0.9% sodium chloride solution) may be required to treat hypotension. Steroids and nonsteroidal anti-inflammatory agents have no effect on the frequency or severity of the JHR. One study found that pretreatment with anti-TNF-alpha monoclonal antibody (Humira)[1] suppressed the JHR after penicillin treatment for LBRF and reduced the associated increases in plasma cytokines. Death can occur as a result of the JHR secondary to cardiovascular collapse in up to 5% of patients with treated LBRF and much less frequently in TBRF.

Outcome

Complete recovery occurs in 95% or more of adequately treated patients. The prognosis for untreated cases or if treatment is delayed varies. Mortality as high as 40% is reported in untreated epidemics of LBRF. Relapsing fever also has a high mortality in neonates. Some neurologic sequelae can occur in patients with TBRF complicated with neuroborreliosis.

Prevention

Prevention of TBRF involves avoidance of rodent- and tick-infested dwellings such as animal burrows, caves, and abandoned cabins. Wearing clothing that protects skin from tick access (e.g., long

---

[1]Not FDA approved for this indication.

TABLE 3 Treatment Options for Tick-Borne Relapsing Fever*

Adults
Nonsevere forms

1. Doxycycline (Doryx oral), 100 mg PO bid for 1–2 wk[†]
2. Tetracycline (Sumycin), 500 mg PO qid for 1–2 wk
3. Erythromycin (Erythrocin),[1] 500 mg PO tid for 1–2 wk

Severe forms

1. Ceftriaxone (Rocephin),[1] 2 g IV qd for 1–2 wk
2. Penicillin G parenteral aqueous (Pfizerpen),[1] 4 million U IV q4h for 1–2 wk

Children (≤ 8 y)
Nonsevere forms

1. Erythromycin suspension oral (EryPed),[1] 30–50 mg/kg/d divided tid for 1–2 wk
2. Azithromycin oral suspension (Zithromax),[1] 20 mg/kg on the first day followed by 10 mg/kg/d for 4 more days
3. Penicillin V (Pen-Vee K),[1] 25–50 mg/kg/d divided qid for 1–2 wk
4. Amoxicillin (Amoxil),[1] 50 mg/kg/d divided tid for 1–2 wk

Severe forms

1. Ceftriaxone (Rocephin),[1] 75–100 mg/kg/d IV for 1–2 wk
2. Penicillin G parenteral aqueous (Pfizerpen),[1] 300,000 U/kg/d given IV in divided doses q4h for 1–2 wk

[1]Not FDA approved for this indication.
*The same oral agents are used for treatment of louse-borne (epidemic) relapsing fever but given as a single dose.
[†]In general, treatment for 1 wk is recommended in early/milder cases and for up to 2 wk for more severe cases.
Abbreviations: IV = intravenous; PO = orally.

---

pants and long-sleeved shirts) is also helpful. Repellents and acaricides provide additional protection. Diethyltoluamide (DEET) repels ticks when applied to clothing or skin, but it must be used with caution. It loses its effectiveness within 1 to several hours when applied to skin and must be reapplied; it is absorbed through the skin and may cause CNS toxicity if used excessively. Picaridin (KBR 3023), which has been used as an insect repellent for years in Europe and Australia, is now available in the United States in 7% solution as Cutter Advanced Repellent (Spectrum Brands). The U.S. Centers for Disease Control and Prevention (CDC) is recommending it as an alternative to DEET. Permethrin Insect Repellent, an acaricide, is more effective than DEET but should not be applied directly to skin. When applied to clothing, it provides good protection for 1 day or more. In LBRF, prevention can be achieved by promoting personal hygiene and by dusting undergarments and the inside of clothing with malathion[1,2] or lindane powder[2] when available. Widespread antibiotic use may be necessary to control epidemics of LBRF, using one or two doses of 100 mg doxycycline given within 1 week of exposure.

[1]Not FDA approved for this indication.
[2]Not available in the United States.

REFERENCES

Barbour AG, Hayes SF: Biology of *Borrelia* species. Microbiol Rev 1986;50:381-400.
Bryceson AD, Parry EH, Perine PL, et al: Louse-borne relapsing fever. Q J Med 1970;39:129-170.
Cadavid D, Barbour AG: Neuroborreliosis during relapsing fever: Review of the clinical manifestations, pathology, and treatment of infections in humans and experimental animals. Clin Infect Dis 1998;26:151-164.
Fekade D, Knox K, Hussein K, et al: Prevention of Jarisch-Herxheimer reactions by treatment with antibodies against tumor necrosis factor alpha. N Engl J Med 1996;335:311-315.
Kazragis RJ, Dever LL, Jorgensen JH, Barbour AG: In vivo activities of ceftriaxone and vancomycin against *Borrelia* spp. in the mouse brain and other sites. Antimicrob Agents Chemother 1996;40:2632-2636.
Melkert PW: Fatal Jarisch-Herxheimer reaction in a case of relapsing fever misdiagnosed as lobar pneumonia. Trop Geogr Med 1987;39:92-93.
Southern P, Sanford J: Relapsing fever. Medicine 1969;48:129-149.
Taft W, Pike J: Relapsing fever. Report of a sporadic outbreak including treatment with penicillin. JAMA 1945;129:1002-1005.

Lyme Disease

Method of
Arthur Weinstein, MD, FACP, FACR, and Shobha Wani, MD

Epidemiology

Lyme disease, or borreliosis, is a tick-transmitted infection caused by *Borrelia burgdorferi*. It is the most common insect-borne illness in the United States with more than 20,000 new cases reported annually. It occurs worldwide with hyperendemicity in temperate regions. In the United States, most cases originate from states in the Northeast, mid-Atlantic, upper Midwest, and Pacific coast regions. The life cycle of the Ixodes tick ensures that most cases of human borrelial infection occur from spring to fall. Three genospecies of *B. burgdorferi* account for human disease: *B. burgdorferi sensu stricto*, *B. garinii*, and *B. afzelii*. Although all three are found in Europe and the latter two in Asia, *B. burgdorferi sensu stricto* is the only cause of Lyme disease in the United States. Lyme disease occurs in all age groups with highest frequencies in young children and adults older than 30 years and is equally common in men and women. It often manifests clinically in stages, with exacerbations and remissions in each stage.

Clinical Features

EARLY LYME DISEASE

Localized skin infection and early disseminated infection occur within days to weeks after the bite of an infected tick. Erythema migrans (EM) rash, the hallmark of early Lyme disease, occurs in up to 70% to 80% of patients at the site of the tick bite. It usually is macular and asymptomatic but may burn or itch, and it is commonly found at the belt line, inguinal area, or in and around the axilla. It expands over days, often to a very large circumference and with central clearing, giving a bull's-eye appearance. Approximately 10% of patients have multiple skin lesions (disseminated EM), a sign of hematogenous spread of the borrelia. At this early stage, patients may have nonspecific flulike complaints, namely fever, fatigue, myalgia, arthralgia, and headache, resembling a viral syndrome. These symptoms occasionally occur without the rash. In untreated patients, EM resolves spontaneously within days to several weeks after onset, but treatment often accelerates its resolution.

Early disseminated disease occurs days to weeks after the tick bite and may occur without preceding localized EM. Certain subtypes of *B. burgdorferi* are associated with higher frequency of spirochetemia and dissemination to other organs. For instance, in Europe, EM is often an indolent, localized infection, whereas in the United States, it is associated with more intense inflammation and signs that suggest dissemination of the spirochete. The clinical manifestations of dissemination can be highly variable and may include disseminated EM rash and neurologic, cardiac, and musculoskeletal features either alone or in combination. Neurologic features (neuroborreliosis) are seen in approximately 10% of patients and include acute lymphocytic meningitis, cranial neuropathy, especially facial paresis, which may be bilateral, and radiculoneuritis. Neuroborreliosis is more common in Europe where neurotropic subspecies of borrelia (*B. garinii, B. afzelii*) are found. Meningitis usually resolves spontaneously, whereas treatment of other neurologic features can hasten recovery and prevent progression to the later stages of Lyme disease. Carditis, which includes varying degrees of atrioventricular block or mild myopericarditis, may develop in approximately 8% of untreated patients, but early treatment can prevent its occurrence. In more recent series, the incidence of Lyme carditis was reported as less than 1% in the United States. Rheumatic features at this stage consist of migratory, episodic joint, tendon, or bursal pains with or without objective signs of inflammation. Typically there is acute localized pain that lasts days to weeks, remits spontaneously, and then recurs in another region. Inflammatory polyarthritis is not a feature of early or late Lyme disease.

The diagnosis of early Lyme disease relies to a great degree on the clinical presentation. In an endemic area, with a history of possible tick exposure, the presence of a classical EM lesion is sufficient for the diagnosis. With very early infection and isolated EM, laboratory tests for antibodies to *B. burgdorferi* may be negative. Conversely, with disseminated early Lyme disease, antibody testing is frequently positive.

LATE LYME DISEASE

Late Lyme disease occurs months to years after initial infection (mean, 6 months) and may present de novo without prior features of early Lyme disease. Systemic symptoms are generally minimal or absent. Musculoskeletal complaints, the most common manifestation, are seen in 80% of untreated patients and include intermittent oligoarthritis (50%) and acute or subacute inflammatory arthritis that most often affects one or both knees. This arthritis may begin abruptly with knee pain and a large joint effusion. Synovial fluid is inflammatory with white counts ranging in the thousands or tens of thousands. Radiographs may be normal except for soft-tissue swelling and joint effusion but may also demonstrate osteopenia, bone cysts, and even mild cartilage loss with small erosions. Untreated, these attacks of arthritis generally last many months, recur for several years but eventually may remit. *B. burgdorferi* is not culturable from the synovial fluid of patients with Lyme arthritis, but borrelial DNA can be detected by polymerase chain reaction (PCR) in over 80% of untreated patients. The PCR test is generally negative after appropriate antibiotic therapy.

Neurologic features of late Lyme disease are seen more frequently in Europe because *B. garinii* is the most neurotropic subspecies. There are a wide range of neurologic abnormalities, especially encephalomyelitis and peripheral neuropathy. In the United States, Lyme encephalopathy or polyneuropathy is described with subtle disturbances of memory and concentration, spinal radicular pain, or distal paresthesias. Nerve conduction studies reveal axonal polyneuropathy. Pleocytosis of the cerebrospinal fluid (CSF) is unusual in late neurologic Lyme disease. High CSF protein may be seen, but borrelial organisms by culture or PCR are not commonly found. Important to the diagnosis of neuroborreliosis is the demonstration of increased intrathecal synthesis of borrelia-specific antibodies.

A chronic skin lesion, acrodermatitis chronica atrophicans, caused by *B. afzelii*, is seen most commonly in Europe.

Laboratory Testing in Lyme Disease

Lyme disease should not be diagnosed purely on serologic tests because false-positive tests are common. Instead, serologic tests

CURRENT DIAGNOSIS

- Erythema migrans is usually asymptomatic and expansile.
- Lyme disease can present with only flulike symptoms: fever, arthralgia, myalgia.
- Antibody testing for borrelial infection is often negative during early infection.
- A two-test strategy (serum ELISA, immunoblot) is recommended for diagnosis.
- IgM antibodies are commonly seen in early infection (4-8 wk) but may persist for many months.
- IgG antibodies are characteristic of late Lyme disease, especially Lyme arthritis.
- Intrathecal antibody synthesis is an important diagnostic marker for neuroborreliosis.
- Clinical symptoms combined with antibody status are of diagnostic importance.

Abbreviation: ELISA = enzyme-linked immunosorbent assay.

should be used to confirm the diagnosis in the appropriate clinical setting. Even a true positive test only confirms recent or past exposure to *B. burgdorferi*, but this must be evaluated in the context of the patient's past and current symptoms.

Despite these methodologic and diagnostic issues, measurement of antibodies to *B. burgdorferi* by enzyme-linked immunoassay (ELISA) is a useful screening test for early and late Lyme disease. This so-called Lyme test is positive in most cases of late Lyme disease and virtually always positive in late Lyme arthritis. It may be negative very early after infection or in those individuals who receive early antibiotic therapy. However, the high rate of false positivity has led to a two-test strategy whereby all sera that show positive or equivocal ELISA tests for borrelial antibodies are tested again by more specific Western (immuno) blotting. In patients with CNS disease, demonstration of intrathecal antibodies by ELISA in relatively higher concentration than serum antibodies is suggestive of neuroborreliosis.

Immunoblotting is usually performed for both IgM and IgG antibodies to borrelial proteins. Although this technique is not as automated or quantitative as ELISA, it is more specific because it identifies the borrelial antigens to which the antibodies are directed. There are recommendations for standardized testing and interpretation of Western blot results. IgM antibodies usually appear 2 to 4 weeks after EM, peak at 6 to 8 weeks, and decline thereafter, although IgM reactivity may occasionally persist for many years. An IgM blot is considered to be positive if two of three specified bands (23, 39, 41 kd) are present. The results of an IgM blot are best interpreted in the first weeks after symptom onset when the true positive rate exceeds the false-positive rate. A positive IgM blot found in a patient with long-standing symptoms should be interpreted with caution because it likely represents a false-positive result. IgG antibodies appear after 4 to 6 weeks, peak at 4 to 6 months, and then remain positive for many years, even decades. An IgG immunoblot is considered to be positive if 5 of 10 specified bands (18, 23, 28, 30, 39, 41, 45, 58, 66, 93 kd) are present. IgG seroconversion, with or without IgM seroconversion, can be taken as presumptive evidence of exposure to *B. burgdorferi* and in the proper clinical context supports the diagnosis of Lyme disease. However, a positive IgG immunoblot does not necessarily mean current or ongoing borreliosis. Conversely, a negative IgG immunoblot is presumptive evidence against the diagnosis of late Lyme disease. An ELISA assay for antibodies to a borrelial-specific surface protein (C6 peptide of VlsE) was demonstrated to be a sensitive and specific single test for the diagnosis of Lyme disease and is commercially available.

Culture of *B. burgdorferi* requires special medium and conditions and takes many weeks. Even so, in expert laboratories the organism can be recovered from the EM lesion in a high percentage of patients and from the blood in patients with disseminated early Lyme disease. Risk for spirochetemia starts the day the patient notices the rash and continues for 2 weeks.

B. burgdorferi is cultured only rarely from the CSF of patients with neuroborreliosis.

PCR to detect borrelial DNA is also positive with the same or higher frequency as culture from the skin, blood, and CSF. However, it is most useful in the synovial fluid of patients with suspected and untreated Lyme arthritis where it can be positive in more than 80% of patients despite universally negative cultures. PCR analysis of synovial tissue may be more likely to yield positive results than synovial fluid because *B. burgdorferi* associates with connective tissue. However, because virtually all cases of Lyme arthritis are strongly positive by ELISA and immunoblotting for IgG antibodies to *B. burgdorferi*, the diagnosis can usually be made with reasonable certainty using these tests alone.

Treatment

The goals of treatment of Lyme disease are to resolve the clinical symptoms by eradication of the organism and to prevent late stage disease with early therapy. Although most manifestations resolve spontaneously without treatment, clinical trials demonstrated that treatment with antibiotics hastens resolution and prevents late manifestations of Lyme borreliosis. In most of the trials, treatment of 3 weeks' duration was effective. Revised evidence-based guidelines for treatment have recently been published by the Infectious Diseases Society of America. Generally, early Lyme disease is treated with antimicrobials for 2 to 3 weeks, although studies showed that EM treatment with oral doxycycline for 10 days is as effective as treatment for 20 days. Effective oral medications include doxycycline (Vibramycin),[1] tetracycline, second-generation cephalosporins such as cefuroxime axetil (Ceftin), and amoxicillin (Amoxil).[1] Erythromycin (E-Mycin)[1] and azithromycin (Zithromax)[1] are somewhat less effective. Doxycycline and tetracycline should not be used in children younger than 8 years or in pregnant women. Oral therapy is sufficient for certain clinical features: EM, facial palsy without signs of meningitis, and first-degree heart block. Oral therapy with doxycycline (Vibramycin) is associated with fewer side effects and is much less expensive than the also employed intravenous (IV) therapy with ceftriaxone (Rocephin).[1] Although amoxicillin and doxycycline appear to be equally efficacious, doxycycline has the distinct advantage of also being effective in treating *Anaplasma phagocytophila* infection, which causes human granulocytic ehrlichiosis (HGE) and is also transmitted by the Ixodes tick. In general, patients with neurologic manifestations, either early or late, other than isolated facial palsy, are treated de novo with IV ceftriaxone (Rocephin)[1] for 3 to 4 weeks, although aqueous penicillin (Penicillin G)[1] is also effective. Carditis with heart block may resolve spontaneously, but patients with higher grades of heart block and with cardiomyopathy are generally treated with IV antibiotics. If the oral regimen fails, as may occur with 20% of patients, parenteral therapy with ceftriaxone or cefotaxime (Claforan)[1] is warranted. In patients with persistent symptoms, a second parenteral regimen is usually administered. There is no need to change the medication because *B. burgdorferi* does not show resistance to any of the antimicrobials recommended.

Oral and parenteral therapies are both used with success in treating Lyme arthritis with treatment duration of 3 to 4 weeks. Occasionally a second month of treatment is needed to eradicate the organism from the joint. Even with successful treatment, the arthritis may resolve quite slowly with synovitis persisting over several months (Table 1).

PERSISTENT (TREATMENT-RESISTANT) LYME ARTHRITIS

Approximately 10% of patients with Lyme arthritis in the United States are treatment resistant, with recurrent inflammatory effusions, usually in one knee, for months to several years despite appropriate antibiotic therapy. This antibiotic-resistant Lyme arthritis is thought to be related to an intra-articular autoimmune response in predisposed individuals. There is no evidence for persistent infection because borrelial DNA by PCR in synovial fluid or synovial tissue is not found in these individuals. A genetic predisposition is suggested by the increased frequency of HLA-DR4 and HLA-DRB1*0401, 0101, and related alleles, similar to that seen in rheumatoid arthritis. In this situation, treatment consists of nonsteroidal anti-inflammatory drugs, intraarticular steroid injections, and antirheumatic agents such as hydroxychloroquine (Plaquenil),[1] sulfasalazine (Azulfidine),[1] and even methotrexate (Rheumatrex).[1] In some cases, arthroscopic synovectomy proves effective. This arthritis usually remits after several years.

POST–LYME DISEASE SYNDROME

Although the long-term prognosis of treated Lyme disease is excellent, some patients develop arthralgia, myalgia, and fatigue, during or soon after infection, which persists despite adequate courses of antibiotics. Other features of this symptom complex include memory and concentration difficulties, neuropathic pains, headache, and unrefreshed sleep. This condition is often called post–Lyme disease syndrome, post-treatment chronic Lyme disease, or chronic Lyme disease. The actual frequency of this condition after Lyme disease is unclear but is likely no more than 5%. Some studies suggested that delay in initiating antibiotic treatment for borrelial infection is more likely to result in post–Lyme disease syndrome. In none of these studies did current serologic status correlate with persistent symptoms. Although these patients have significant somatic complaints and functional disability, they lack objective findings of an inflammatory condition. Although virtually all patients with this syndrome complain of problems with memory and concentration, demonstrable abnormalities on neurocognitive testing are not universally present. The pathogenesis of this chronic post-treatment symptomatic state and its relationship to Lyme disease are unclear. Patients may

---

[1]Not FDA approved for this indication.

CURRENT THERAPY

- Early antibiotic therapy hastens resolution of symptoms and prevents late complications.
- In adults, oral therapy with doxycycline (Vibramycin)[1] is preferred for most features of Lyme disease.
- Neuroborreliosis is usually treated with IV ceftriaxone.
- Duration of therapy is generally 2-4 wk.
- Lyme disease is cured after antibiotic treatment (one or two courses) in most patients.
- Some patients with Lyme arthritis develop persistent antibiotic-resistant synovitis, which may be autoimmune and is treated with antirheumatic drugs.
- Patients with chronic fatigue, arthralgia, and myalgia that begins, persists, or recurs after antibiotic treatment for Lyme disease generally have a post–Lyme disease syndrome and not ongoing infection.
- There is no scientific support for prolonged courses of oral or IV antibiotics for Lyme disease.

---

[1]Not FDA approved for this indication.
Abbreviation: IV = intravenous.

---

[1]Not FDA approved for this indication.

TABLE 1 Suggested Treatment of Lyme Disease

Clinical Features/ Indication	Antibiotic regimen	Adults	Children	Duration of Therapy
Early Infection (Local and Disseminated Disease)	Doxycycline (Vibramycin)[1]	100 mg bid	< 8 y: not recommended > 8 y: 1–2 mg/kg bid; maximum 100 mg	2–3 wk
	Tetracycline[1]	500 mg qid	Not for pregnant women	2–3 wk
	Amoxicillin[1]	500 mg tid	As above	2–3 wk
	Cefuroxime axetil (Ceftin)	500 mg bid	50 mg/kg/d in 3 divided doses	2–3 wk
	Azithromycin (Zithromax)[1]	500 mg daily	30 mg/kg/d in 2 divided doses	7–10 d
	Erythromycin[1]	500 mg qid	50 mg/kg/d	2–3 wk
Neuroborreliosis Failure to Respond to Oral Therapy	Ceftriaxone (Rocephin)[1] Cefotaxime (Claforan)[1]	2 g IV daily	75–100 mg/kg/d 90–180 mg/kg/d in 3–4 divided doses	2–4 wk 2–4 wk
	Penicillin G[1]	2 g IV tid		
		4–5 million U IV q4h	2–4 million U IV q4 h	2–4 wk
Carditis	Oral or IV regimen			2–3 wk
Late Lyme Arthritis	Oral or IV regimen			4 wk*
Pregnancy	Amoxicillin Penicillin G Ceftriaxone Cefotaxime			2–4 wk

*May give another course if poor response.
[1] Not FDA approved for this indication.
Abbreviation: IV = intravenous.

---

feel better during antibiotic therapy, but the effect is not durable and relapse is common when antibiotics are discontinued. The symptoms wax and wane, but the overall course is chronic. Controversy has raged as to whether chronic, relatively resistant borrelial infection plays a role and hence whether chronic antibiotic therapy is warranted. However, an important study on post–Lyme syndrome patients failed to document the presence of b. burgdorferi in the plasma or spinal fluid of these patients by culture or PCR. In addition, a controlled trial failed to show a response to a 3-month course of antibiotics (1 month of IV ceftriaxone [Rocephin][1] followed by 2 months of oral doxycycline[1]). This suggests that chronic infection is not the cause of post–Lyme disease syndrome, that the condition spontaneously waxes and wanes, and that prolonged antibiotic treatment does not result in long-term symptom remission.

Prevention

The best currently available method for preventing infection with B. burgdorferi and other tick-transmitted infections is to avoid tick infested areas through the summer. If exposure is unavoidable, use of protective clothing (shirt tucked into pants and pants tucked under socks) may interfere with attachment by ticks. Wearing light-colored clothing makes it easier to identify ticks. Daily inspection of the entire body to locate and remove ticks also decreases the transmission of infection. Attached ticks should promptly be removed with fine-toothed forceps, if possible. Tick and insect repellent applied to the skin and clothing provides additional protection. The most effective repellent is DEET (diethyltoluamide). Permethrin, a pesticide that kills ticks and mites when applied to clothing, decreases the risk of tick bite. Strategies to reduce the number of ticks may be somewhat effective in decreasing tick-borne illnesses, including the application of acaricides and landscaping to provide desiccating barriers. Although vaccination is available for dogs and a recombinant outer surface protein A (OspA)-based vaccine (LYMErix) is effective and relatively safe in humans, currently no marketed vaccine is available to prevent Lyme disease in humans.

---

[1] Not FDA approved for this indication.

AFTER TICK BITE

It is not recommended to treat all patients after a tick bite because several prospective studies demonstrated that the risk of drug-associated rash is as great as the risk of developing Lyme disease. Conversely, it may be reasonable to treat persons believed to be at higher risk for the development of borrelial infection prophylactically. Studies showed that transmission of B. burgdorferi from tick to host occurs with greater frequency when there has been tick attachment for more than 48 hours resulting in a blood-engorged tick. Because a controlled study demonstrated that a single 200-mg dose of doxycycline[1] effectively prevents Lyme disease when given within 72 hours of a tick bite, the threshold for treating patients after tick bites with this benign regimen is lower than in the past.

---

[1] Not FDA approved for this indication.

REFERENCES

Klempner MS, Hu LT, Evans J, et al: Two controlled trials of antibiotic treatment in patients with persistent symptoms and a history of Lyme disease. N Engl J Med 2001;345:85-92.

Nadelman RB, Nowakowski J, Fish D, et al: Prophylaxis with single dose doxycycline for the prevention of Lyme disease after an Ixodes scapularis tick bite. N. Engl J Med 2001;345:79-84.

Recommendations for test performance and interpretation from the Second National Conference on Serologic Diagnosis of Lyme Disease. MMWR 1995;44:590-591.

Steere AC: Lyme disease. N Engl J Med 2001;345:115-125.

Steere AC, Dhar A, Hernandez J, et al: Systemic symptoms without erythema migrans as the presenting picture of early Lyme disease. Am J Med 2003;114:58-62.

Steere AC, Sikand VK, et al: The presenting manifestations of Lyme disease and the outcomes of treatment. N Engl J Med 2003;348:2472-2474.

Treatment of Lyme disease. The Medical Letter 2005;47:41-43.

Tugwell P, Dennis DT, Weinstein A, et al: Clinical guideline 2: Laboratory evaluation in the diagnosis of Lyme disease. Ann Intern Med 1997;127:1109-1123.

Weinstein A, Britchkov M: Lyme arthritis and post-Lyme disease syndrome. Curr Opin Rheum 2002;14:383-387.

Wormser GP, Dattwyler RJ, Shapiro ED, et al: The clinical assessment, treatment, and prevention of Lyme disease, human granulocytic anaplasmosis, and babesiosis: Clinical practice guidelines by the Infectious Diseases Society of America. Clin Infect Dis 2006;43:1089-1134.

Wormser GP, Ramanathan R, Nowakowski J, et al: Duration of antibiotic therapy for early Lyme disease. A randomized, double-blind, placebo-controlled trial. Ann Intern Med 2003;138:697-704.

Rubella and Congenital Rubella Syndrome

Method of
Susan E. Reef, MD

Rubella, once thought to be a benign rash illness, gained public health significance when Norman Gregg in 1941 documented the association between rubella during pregnancy and congenital defects. The last pandemic occurred between 1962 and 1965. In the United States, this epidemic resulted in approximately 12.5 million rubella cases, 11,000 fetal deaths (including spontaneous and therapeutic abortions), and 20,000 infants born with congenital rubella syndrome (CRS).

Background and Epidemiology

Rubella virus is a member of the *Togaviridae* family and the genus *Rubivirus*. It is an enveloped RNA virus with a single antigenic type. Infection is limited to humans. Rubella is transmitted through person-to-person contact or droplets shed from the respiratory secretions of infected persons. The average incubation period is 14 days, with a range of 12 to 23 days. Persons with rubella are most infectious when the rash is erupting, but they can shed virus from 7 days before to 5 to 7 days after rash onset (i.e., the infectious period).

In the prevaccine era, rubella epidemics occurred approximately every 6 to 9 years in the United States. In 1969, live attenuated rubella vaccines were licensed in the United States, and the number of rubella cases decreased from 57,600 cases in 1969 to 223 cases in 1988. With the success of the rubella vaccination program, a goal was established to eliminate indigenous rubella transmission and congenital rubella syndrome (CRS) in the United States by 2000. In 2001 and 2002, fewer than 25 reported rubella cases occurred, and since 2003, 11 or fewer cases have been reported annually.

In October 2004, an independent expert panel was convened to assess progress toward elimination of rubella and CRS in the United States and concluded that rubella is no longer endemic in the United States. Since then, elimination of endemic rubella and CRS has been maintained in the United States. Even though rubella is no longer endemic in the United States, rubella continues to be endemic in many parts of the world. As a result, cases of rubella and CRS related to importation continue to be reported in the United States.

Clinical Features

The maculopapular erythematous rash of rubella usually starts on the face and neck and progresses downward. The rubella rash occurs in 50% to 80% of rubella-infected persons. The rash, which may be pruritic, usually lasts 1 to 3 days. The rash is fainter than measles rash and doesn't coalesce. However, rubella is sometimes misdiagnosed as measles or scarlet fever. Children usually develop few or no constitutional symptoms, but adults can experience a 1- to 5-day prodrome of low-grade fever, headache, malaise, mild coryza, and conjunctivitis. Postauricular, occipital, and posterior cervical lymphadenopathy is characteristic and typically precedes the rash by 5 to 10 days.

Diagnosis

Because many rash illnesses mimic rubella infection and 20% to 50% of rubella infections can be subclinical, laboratory testing is the only way to confirm the diagnosis. Acute rubella infection can be confirmed by the presence of serum rubella immunoglobulin M (IgM), a significant rise in IgG antibody titer in acute and convalescent serum specimens, positive rubella virus culture, or detection of the rubella virus by reverse transcriptase polymerase chain reaction (RT-PCR).

Serologic testing is the most common diagnostic methodology used. Because IgM antibodies might not be detectable before day five after rash onset, a repeat serum should be obtained for a negative rubella IgM in specimens taken before day five. False-positive serum rubella IgM tests have occurred in persons with parvovirus B19 infections, infectious mononucleosis, or a positive rheumatoid factor. To document a significant titer rise in IgG, paired specimens of acute and convalescent sera must be obtained, with the second serum collected about 14 to 21 days after the first specimen. Rubella virus can be isolated from nasal, blood, throat, urine, and cerebrospinal fluid specimens from patients with rubella and CRS. The most frequently positive results come from throat swabs. For viral cultures, the specimen should be obtained by day four after rash onset, which is the time for maximum viral shedding.

Laboratory confirmation of CRS can be obtained by demonstration of rubella-specific IgM antibodies in the infant's cord blood or sera, documentation of persistence of serum rubella IgG titer beyond the time expected from passive transfer of maternal IgG antibody (i.e., rubella titer that does not drop at the expected rate of a twofold dilution per month), isolation of rubella virus, or detection of rubella virus by RT-PCR.

Complications

Rubella disease is usually mild and results in very few complications. Transient arthralgia or arthritis occurs in up to 70% of women with rubella. Other complications include thrombocytopenic purpura (1 in 3000 rubella cases) and encephalitis (1 in 6000 rubella cases). However, intrauterine rubella infection, particularly during the first trimester, can result in serious consequences such as miscarriage, stillbirth, or the constellation of severe birth defects known as CRS.

 CURRENT DIAGNOSIS

- Even though the rubella virus no longer circulates endemically in the United States, rubella is endemic in many parts of the world.
- Rubella and congenital rubella syndrome cases continue to occur in the United States, however, due to importations.
- Diagnosis is based on clinical history and findings, epidemiologic history, and laboratory confirmation.
- Serologic testing is the most common method for diagnosis; viral isolation and reverse transcriptase polymerase chain reaction (RT-PCR) are also available.
- One dose of rubella-containing vaccine is recommended for full protection. Most infants and children receive two doses of rubella vaccine in the MMR (measles, mumps, and rubella) vaccine based on recommendations for measles.

CONGENITAL RUBELLA SYNDROME

For pregnant women infected with rubella during the first 11 weeks of gestation, 90% of the infants born will have CRS; the rate of CRS for infants born to women infected during the first 20 weeks of pregnancy is 20%. The most common congenital defects of CRS are eye defects (e.g., cataracts, congenital glaucoma, pigmentary retinopathy), cardiac defects (e.g., patent ductus arteriosus, peripheral pulmonic stenosis), and hearing impairment. Other clinical manifestations may include microcephaly, developmental delay, purpura, meningoencephalitis, hepatosplenomegaly, low birth weight, and radiolucent bone disease. The pregnant patient with rubella should be counseled about the risks of the congenital defects and her options. Infants with CRS can shed virus from body secretions for up to 1 year and are considered infectious. Persons in contact with these infants (e.g., health care workers, family members) should be immune to rubella either through vaccination or natural infection.

MANAGEMENT OF EXPOSURE DURING PREGNANCY

As part of routine prenatal care, all pregnant women should be tested for rubella immunity. Women who are IgG positive without recent history of exposure to rubella are considered immune. Reinfection with rubella occurs more often with vaccine-induced immunity than with natural disease; however, the risk of maternal reinfection is rare.

If a pregnant woman is suspected of being exposed to rubella, a blood specimen should be taken as soon as possible and tested for rubella IgG and IgM antibody. The specimen should be stored for possible retesting. A positive IgM regardless of the IgG result can indicate recent or acute infection or may be a false-positive IgM. Therefore, serology should be repeated in 7 to 10 days. Besides repeating the IgM and IgG, additional testing using special tests (e.g., avidity) may be warranted. If the IgM and IgG are negative with the first specimen, a second specimen should be taken 3 to 4 weeks after exposure and tested for IgM and IgG in parallel with the first specimen. Either a positive IgM in the second sera or IgG seroconversion indicates acute infection. As long as the pregnant woman is exposed to rubella, it is important to continue testing for IgG and IgM responses.

Treatment

There is no proven therapy for rubella. The best strategy is to ensure women are immune by vaccination before pregnancy. Health care providers who treat women of childbearing age should routinely determine rubella immunity and vaccinate those who are susceptible and not pregnant. Women found to be susceptible during pregnancy should be vaccinated immediately postpartum. There is no specific therapy for CRS; however, infants should be evaluated and provided early intervention by specialists who treat the identified CRS defects.

Rubella Vaccine

In 1969, three live attenuated rubella vaccines were licensed in the United States. In 1979, a new formulation of live attenuated rubella vaccine (RA 27/3 [Meruvax II]) replaced the other rubella vaccines in the United States, because the RA 27/3 vaccine was found to induce higher antibody titers and to produce an immune response more closely paralleling natural infection than did the other vaccines. Of the persons vaccinated in clinical trials, 95% had serologic evidence of rubella immunity after one dose. From longitudinal studies, rubella vaccine confers immunity for at least 15 years and probably for a lifetime.

A rubella virus–containing vaccine is recommended for persons 12 months old or older unless there is a medical contraindication such as severe immunodeficiency or pregnancy. In the United States, in 2001, the period of time to avoid getting pregnant following a rubella vaccination was shortened from 3 months to 28 days.

Rubella vaccine is available as monovalent formulation (Meruvax II) or in combination with measles and mumps (MMR) or measles, mumps, and varicella (MMRV [ProQuad]). With use of MMR for measles vaccination under the currently recommended two-dose schedule, most children and adolescents now receive two doses of rubella vaccine. The MMR vaccine is recommended at 12 to 15 months of age, with a second dose at 4 to 6 years of age. MMRV vaccine can be given to children aged 12 months to 12 years of age.

Documented evidence of rubella immunity is defined as serologic evidence (e.g., a positive serum rubella IgG), documented immunization with at least one dose of rubella-containing vaccine on or after the first birthday, or birth before 1957 (except women who could become pregnant). Clinical diagnosis of rubella is unreliable and should *not* be considered in assessing immune status.

REFERENCES

Centers for Disease Control and Prevention: Elimination of rubella and congenital rubella syndrome—United States, 1969-2004. MMWR Morb Mortal Wkly Rep 2005;54:279-282.
Centers for Disease Control and Prevention: Control and prevention of rubella: Evaluation and management of suspected outbreaks, rubella in pregnant women, and surveillance for congenital rubella syndrome. MMWR Recomm Rep 2001;50(RR-12):1-23Available at http://www.cdc.gov/mmwr/preview/mmwrhtml/rr5012a1.htm (accessed May 15, 2007).
Centers for Disease Control and Prevention: Revised ACIP recommendation for avoiding pregnancy after receiving a rubella-containing vaccine. MMWR Morb Mortal Wkly Rep 2001;50:1117.
Dayan GH, Reef SE, Orenstein WA: Rubella. In Burg FD, Ingelfinger JR, Polin RA, Gershon AA (eds): Current Pediatric Therapy, 18th ed. Philadelphia: WB Saunders, 2006, pp 803-807.
Miller E, Cradock-Watson JE, Pollock TM: Consequences of confirmed maternal rubella at successive stages of pregnancy. Lancet 1982;2:781-784.
Plotkin SA, Reef S: Rubella vaccine. In Plotkin SA, Orenstein WA (eds). Vaccines. 4th ed, Philadelphia: WB Saunders, 2004, pp 707-743.
Watson JC, Hadler SC, Dykewicz CA et al: Measles, mumps, and rubella—vaccine use and strategies for elimination of measles, rubella, and congenital rubella syndrome and control of mumps: Recommendations of the Advisory Committee on Immunization Practices (ACIP). MMWR Recomm Rep 1998;47:1-57.

CURRENT THERAPY

- There is no effective therapy for rubella.
- Vaccination provides excellent protection.
- Pregnant women with rubella should be counseled about the risk of congenital defects.
- Infants with congenital rubella syndrome should be evaluated and treated under the care of appropriate specialists.

Measles (Rubeola)

Method of
Claude P. Muller, MD, and
Jacques Kremer, PhD

Measles is an acute systemic disease associated with a maculopapular rash, fever, and respiratory symptoms caused by a single-stranded RNA virus of the family of Paramyxoviridae and the genus *Morbillivirus*.

Epidemiology

With a basic reproduction number of 15, measles virus is the most infectious pathogen. It is transmitted via aerosol to susceptibles (e.g., in kindergarten classes or doctors' offices), and humans are the only natural host. At least 95% of a population must be immune in order to prevent the virus from circulating.

Before the introduction of vaccination, epidemics occurred at regular intervals, and virtually all children had measles during early childhood. Measles induces high levels of antibodies and lifelong protection against the disease. Although vaccine-induced immunity is probably somewhat less robust than immunity after natural infection because of lower and waning antibodies, measles morbidity and mortality have dramatically declined since the introduction of a live-attenuated vaccine in 1963.

As of 2004, endemic circulation of the virus had been interrupted in the Western Hemisphere, as well as in several countries in Europe and the Western Pacific. The success in measles control has encouraged the World Health Organization (WHO) to introduce a timetable for measles elimination in most regions of the world.

In many developing countries, where 98% of global measles deaths occur, measles continues to be a serious condition. Although the 345,000 deaths estimated in 2005 represent a 60% reduction in global measles mortality compared with 1999, measles vaccines are still underused in developing countries.

Clinical Features

Eight to 14 days after infection, the patient develops characteristic prodromal symptoms including fever and cough, coryza, or conjunctivitis. A maculopapular rash appears 2 to 4 days later (typically on day 12 after exposure) behind the ears and the hairline, spreading from the head to the trunk and the extremities. One or 2 days before the onset of rash, Koplik's spots, the pathognomonic enanthema, appear on the buccal mucosa and fade again as the skin rash evolves.

Uneventful measles lasts about 7 to 10 days, and cough is usually the last symptom to disappear. Patients are infectious from 4 to 5 days before until 4 days after the onset of rash. The course of disease can be complicated by otitis media (3%-9%), bronchitis or bronchopneumonia (1%-6%), and gastrointestinal and neurologic involvement. Postinfectious encephalitis complicates about 1 in 1000 infections, and subacute sclerosing panencephalitis (SSPE) affects approximately 1 in 1,000,000 cases, usually 7 to 10 years after acute measles. Measles also causes immunosupression, facilitating secondary bacterial infections, which are responsible for most measles deaths, especially in developing countries.

Measles outbreaks have sometimes been observed in highly vaccinated populations. A mild, vaccine-modified form of measles, not necessarily covered by the clinical case definition, can occur in vaccinated persons with low-level immunity. In contrast, patients who contracted measles after vaccination with a formalin-inactivated measles vaccine, licensed in 1961 and withdrawn from the market in 1966, suffered from a severe illness referred to as *atypical measles*.

Diagnosis

The clinical case definition includes any person with fever (>38.3°C), maculopapular rash (≥3 d), and at least one of the symptoms of cough, coryza, or conjunctivitis. Laboratory confirmation is based on measles-specific IgM by enzyme-linked immunosorbent assay (ELISA), detected from onset of rash until weeks later. When IgM and IgG are negative early after onset of rash, repeat testing is warranted. The diagnosis can also be confirmed by an increase in measles-specific IgG between paired sera, detection of viral RNA by reverse-transcriptase polymerase chain reaction (RT-PCR), or virus isolation. Nasopharyngeal swabs, oral fluid, peripheral blood mononuclear cells (PBMCs), and the cellular fraction of urine are appropriate specimens for measles RT-PCR and virus isolation, as well as for genotyping of the virus in specialized laboratories. In most

CURRENT DIAGNOSIS

- Fever (>38.3°C) and maculopapular rash (≥3 d) in association with cough, conjunctivitis, or coryza or some combination of these (CDC clinical case definition)
- Pathognomonic Koplik's spots on the buccal mucosa
- Detection of measles-specific IgM or increase in measles-specific IgG in paired sera
- Detection of viral RNA by reverse transcriptase polymerase chain reaction (RT-PCR) in nasopharyngeal swabs, oral fluid, urine, peripheral blood mononuclear cells (PBMCs), (or dried blood spots) with or without virus isolation

countries, confirmed or even suspected cases must be reported to the national health authorities.

Treatment

There is no specific treatment for acute measles. Supportive therapy includes hydration, antipyretics, bedrest, and protection from light for patients with photophobia. Secondary bacterial infections are treated with antibiotics. Vitamin A supplementation[1] has been shown to improve the clinical outcome in malnourished patients and patients with vitamin A deficiency. Ribavirin (Virazole)[1] and isoprinosin,[2] combined with interferon-α (IFN-α), have been used with limited success in experimental treatments of SSPE.

Prevention

Measles virus has only one serotype, and current live-attenuated vaccines are effective against all of the 23 known genotypes. Vaccination induces long-lasting protection against the disease even after a single dose. Transplacentally acquired maternal antibodies and immaturity of the infant immune system interfere with seroconversion rates, which, after the first dose, range between 80% and 95% depending on the age of the vaccinee. Improper handling of the

---
[1]Not FDA approved for this indication.
[2]Not available in the United States.

CURRENT THERAPY

Treatment

- There is no specific therapy for treating acute measles.
- Patient care is limited to supportive therapy.
- Secondary bacterial infections are treated with antibiotics.
- Vitamin A supplementation[1] might improve the clinical outcome.

Supportive Therapy

- Hydration
- Antipyretics
- Rest
- Protection from light
- Vitamin A[1]
- Treatment for secondary bacterial infections

---
[1]Not FDA approved for this indication.

vaccine can be another reason for primary vaccine failures. Therefore, two-dose vaccination programs are necessary to achieve a population immunity greater than 95%, which is necessary to interrupt virus circulation.

Measles vaccination is recommended in virtually all countries, but immunization schedules depend on the specific epidemiologic situation of each country. Many industrialized countries use measles-mumps-rubella (MMR) combined vaccines, with a first dose given at 12 to 15 months of age and a second dose at 3 to 6 years of age to catch up children with primary or secondary vaccine failure after the first dose. In many developing countries with large birth cohorts and a higher measles incidence, monovalent measles vaccines (Attenuvax) are administered at 6 to 9 months of age to offset the higher risk of early exposure to wild-type virus and the earlier loss of maternal antibodies. A second dose should be provided as a routine revaccination during early childhood or in follow-up campaigns including broader age groups. Transient fever and rash are observed in 5% to 10% of patients vaccinated with live attenuated strains. Much publicized links to autism or other chronic diseases have never been confirmed by national or international scientific panels.

The vaccine is not recommended for children with primary or acquired severe immunodeficiency, except for children with asymptomatic HIV infection. The disease may be prevented in susceptible persons by hypergammaglobulin given within 6 days or by active immunization within 3 days after exposure. Passive immunization is also recommended in persons with some malignant diseases or deficits in cellular immunity.

REFERENCES

Bannister BA, Begg NT, Gillespie SH: Childhood Infections: Measles. Infectious Disease. Oxford: Blackwell Science, 1996, pp 256-260.
Campbell C, Levin S, Humphreys P, et al: Subacute sclerosing panencephalitis: Results of the Canadian Paediatric Surveillance Program and review of the literature. BMC Pediatr 2005;5:47.
Gershon AA: Measles virus. In Mandell GL, Bennett JE, Dolin R (eds): Principles and Practice of Infectious Diseases. New York: Churchill Livingstone, 1995, pp 1519-1525.
Griffin DE: Measles virus. In Knipe DM, Howley PM (eds): Fields Virology. Philadelphia: Lippincott Williams & Wilkins, 2001, pp 1401-1424.
World Health Organization: Progress in reducing global measles deaths: 1999-2004. Wkly Epidemiol Rec 2006;81(10):90-94.

Tetanus

Method of
Samuel S. Hsu, MD

Tetanus is a toxin-mediated infectious disease that is acquired from wounds and that results in muscular hyperexcitability and autonomic instability. It has a high mortality rate despite optimal treatment. It is best managed by prevention, which is accomplished with a highly effective low-cost vaccine. Victims are typically inadequately immunized.

Etiology

The causative agent of tetanus is *Clostridium tetani*, a spore-forming, gram-positive bacillus. The vegetative form is an obligate anaerobe, but the spores remain viable at ambient oxygen concentrations. The spores are ubiquitous in soil, are highly resistant to extremes in temperature and humidity, and can survive indefinitely. When spores enter wounds, they might not germinate immediately if tissue conditions are unfavorable. They can activate well after the wound has healed, which might account for cases of tetanus that have no identifiable source. When conditions are favorable, the spores germinate into mature bacilli, which release the toxin tetanospasmin.

Tetanospasmin is responsible for the clinical manifestations of tetanus. It enters peripheral nerves and travels via retrograde axonal transport to the central nervous system. Tetanospasmin then enters presynaptic neurons and disrupts the release of γ-amino butyric acid (GABA) and glycine, which are inhibitory neurotransmitters. This results in a disinhibition of end-organ neurons, such as motor neurons and those of the autonomic nervous system. Recovery depends on synthesis of new presynaptic components, a process that occurs over 2 to 3 weeks.

Epidemiology

Most cases occur in developing countries. In 2005, the World Health Organization (WHO) received reports of more than 15,000 cases, two thirds of which occurred in neonates. In contrast, tetanus is a disease of older adults in developed countries. According to the latest data from the Centers for Disease Control and Prevention (CDC), there are an average of 43 cases of tetanus per year in the United States, and the incidence is 0.16 per million population.

Even with optimal treatment, the mortality of tetanus is very high. The global fatality rate is estimated to be 30% to 50%. In the United States, the fatality rate ranges from 11% to 25%. Older adults have a higher mortality, 40% in those older than 60 years compared with 8% in those ages 20 to 59 years.

Lack of immunization is the greatest risk factor for contracting tetanus. The largest groups with the lowest rates of immunization in the United States are older adults and immigrants from Latin America. Serologic surveys show that although 95% of those 6 to 39 years old are adequately immunized, only 74% of those older than 60 years and 59% of those older than 70 years are adequately immunized. Only 75% of Latin American immigrants are adequately immunized. The result is a higher incidence of tetanus in these groups: 0.35 per million adults older than 60 years and 0.38 per million Latin Americans.

Clinical Features

An acute injury precedes most cases of tetanus, the most common being puncture wounds and lacerations. Nonacute etiologies include chronic wounds, IV drug use, and complications of diabetes. Cases have occurred without a clear etiology. The median time between an injury and onset of symptoms is 7 days, but there have been delayed presentations of up to 3 months. A more rapid onset correlates to a more severe clinical presentation.

There are four clinical forms of tetanus representing the extent and location of neurons involved: generalized, local, cephalic, and neonatal.

In the United States and other developed countries, generalized tetanus is the most common form. The initial symptom in 50% to 75% of cases is trismus ("lockjaw") secondary to masseter muscle spasm. Risus sardonicus, the "ironical smile of tetanus," can occur due to facial muscle contraction. Nuchal rigidity and dysphagia can also be initial complaints. As the disease spreads, generalized muscle spasms occur, either spontaneously or to minor stimuli such as touch or noise. Opisthotonos, a tonic contraction very similar to decorticate posturing, is classically described with tetanus. Severe spasms can result in bone fractures, tendon detachments, and rhabdomyolysis. Mental status is not affected, and spasms are experienced with severe pain.

In the acute phase, death results from acute respiratory failure due to diaphragmatic paralysis or laryngeal spasms. In severe cases, autonomic instability can occur, resulting most importantly in labile hypertension, tachycardia, and pyrexia. Hypotension and bradycardia can also occur. Arrhythmias and myocardial infarction are the most common fatal events. The exact mechanism of this syndrome is unclear but likely involves disinhibition of the sympathetic nervous system.

CURRENT DIAGNOSIS

- Tetanus is diagnosed on clinical grounds alone.
- Involuntary muscle spasms are the hallmark of tetanus.
- Generalized tetanus is the most common form. Characteristic features include trismus (lockjaw), risus sardonicus, and opisthotonos.
- Sensory function and mental status are preserved.
- Mimics of tetanus can be excluded by physical findings and select laboratory tests.

 CURRENT THERAPY

ACUTE TETANUS

- Human tetanus immune globulin (hTIG, BayTet) 500 IU IM neutralizes tetanus toxin.
- Metronidazole (Flagyl) eliminates reservoirs of *Clostridium tetani*.
- Wounds and abscess must be débrided and drained.
- Benzodiazepines are the drugs of choice to control muscle spasms. In severe cases, paralytics and mechanical ventilation may be required.
- Tetanus immunization must be initiated because surviving tetanus does not confer immunity.

PROPHYLAXIS IN ACUTE WOUNDS

- Administer tetanus toxoid (Td) if the last booster was more than 10 y ago in non–tetanus-prone or more than 5 y ago in tetanus-prone wounds.
- Administer hTIG 250 IU IM if the patient never completed a primary immunization series and has a tetanus-prone wound.
- Pregnancy is not a contraindication to appropriate use of Td or hTIG.

Local tetanus manifests as persistent muscle rigidity close to a site of injury. The rigidity can linger for weeks to months and often resolves without sequelae. Localized tetanus rarely progresses to generalized tetanus.

Cephalic tetanus is an uncommon variant of localized tetanus that involves the cranial nerves. Cephalic tetanus uniquely results in nerve palsies and muscle spasms. The seventh cranial nerve is most often involved, followed by the sixth, third, fourth, and 12th in decreasing order of frequency. With its predilection for the seventh cranial nerve, it commonly mimics Bell's palsy. Cephalic tetanus also manifests with trismus, but cranial nerve deficits precede the onset of trismus about 40% of the time. Head trauma and otitis media are commonly cited etiologies. About two thirds of cases progress to generalized tetanus.

Neonatal tetanus is generalized tetanus that occurs in newborns around the first week of life. Symptoms begin with nonspecific irritability and poor feeding, and they rapidly progress to generalized spasms. The portal of entry is the freshly cut umbilical cord. The risk of contracting neonatal tetanus is directly related to maternal immunization status, because passive transfer of maternal immunoglobulins is protective. Mortality is very high, 50% to 100%, due to the high load of toxin per body weight in neonates. In the United States, there were three reports of neonatal tetanus in the 1990s, all involving inadequately immunized mothers.

Diagnosis

The diagnosis of tetanus must be made on clinical grounds alone. There are no laboratory tests that can diagnose or exclude tetanus. Wound cultures rarely yield *C. tetani* and are not available quickly enough to aid diagnosis. Fortunately, the presentation of tetanus is so characteristic that a presumptive diagnosis can be made in most cases. When faced with a potential case of tetanus, it is useful to recall that sensory function and mental status remain normal.

The differential diagnosis is minimal. Most possibilities can be excluded by history, examination, and select laboratory tests. Exact mimics of tetanus occur with strychnine poisoning, which disables glycine release as tetanospasmin does, and hypocalcemia. These are easily excluded by laboratory tests. The differential for trismus includes peritonsillar/odontogenic abscesses and dystonic reactions. Cephalic tetanus without trismus can be easily mistaken for Bell's palsy, central nervous system tumor, or stroke. Neonatal tetanus initially manifests much like a host of other disorders. Once generalized spasms begin, the diagnosis is obvious.

Apte and Karnad describe a bedside test for tetanus in which a spatula is inserted into the pharynx. If the patient gags and tries to expel the spatula, the test is negative for tetanus; if the patient bites the spatula due to reflex masseter spasm, the test is positive for tetanus. The researchers reported 94% sensitivity and 100% specificity.

Treatment

Treatment involves neutralizing tetanospasmin, removing the source of the toxin, and providing supportive care for muscle spasms, respiration, and autonomic instability. Human tetanus immunoglobulin (hTIG, BayTet) 500 IU IM neutralizes circulating tetanospasmin. It cannot inactivate toxin already within neurons. Its half-life is 25 days; only a single dose is necessary. Doses of hTIG up to 10,000 IU have been used, but the lower dose is effective and has the advantage of requiring fewer injections to deliver. This feature is not insignificant, because hTIG is supplied in 250-IU doses, and injections are powerful stimuli for spasms. The adult and pediatric doses are the same. The burden of tetanospasmin, not the patient's size, determines the amount of hTIG needed.

To prevent ongoing production of toxin, antibiotics are needed to eliminate reservoirs of *C. tetani*. Metronidazole (Flagyl) in standard dose is the drug of choice. Penicillin, the historic drug of choice, does not penetrate devascularized wounds and abscesses well. Penicillin also has GABA-antagonist activity, which can potentiate the effects of tetanospasmin. In addition to antibiotics, obviously dirty wounds, abscesses, or devitalized tissue must be cleaned, drained, or excised to decrease the bacterial load.

Benzodiazepines are the drug of choice for muscle spasms because of their GABA-agonist and sedative properties. Daily doses of hundreds or thousands of milligrams have been used to control spasms. For severe cases, paralytics and mechanical ventilation may be needed. Vecuronium (Norcuron)[1] is an ideal agent for immediate and long-term control due to its minimal cardiovascular effects.

Treatment of autonomic instability has been problematic and is the subject of ongoing research. No therapeutic regimen has proved to be universally effective. α-Blockers,[1] β-blockers,[1] clonidine (Catapres),[1] and magnesium[1] have yielded variable success. Fentanyl (Sublimaze)[1] centrally decreases sympathetic outflow and has produced more consistent control of hypertension and tachycardia.

Supportive care includes placing the patient in a quiet, dark environment, minimizing patient manipulation, and treating for complications, most significantly rhabdomyolysis. Importantly, survivors must also receive a tetanus immunization series. The amount of tetanospasmin produced in clinical tetanus is small and partially sequestered in neurons; consequently, an immune response does not occur. Unimmunized survivors of tetanus have become victims a second time.

---

[1]Not FDA approved for this indication.

Prevention

Tetanus is preventable with proper use of tetanus toxoid and hTIG. Tetanus toxoid is an inactivated form of tetanospasmin. It is available as a single-antigen tetanus toxoid (TT) and combined with diphtheria and pertussis vaccine. The combination vaccines (e.g., Td for adults) are preferable because concurrent immunization is appropriate. The recommended primary immunization schedule is shown in Table 1. Adults should receive boosters every 10 years to maintain immunity.

Common adverse reactions to tetanus toxoid include erythema, swelling, and tenderness at the injection site. Nonspecific systemic effects such as fever, malaise, and anorexia can also occur. Reactions tend to occur more often and more severely if boosters are given more frequently than the recommended schedule. Patients who give a history of "allergy" to tetanus vaccine are most likely referring to a local or nonspecific systemic reaction. These are not contraindications to receiving tetanus toxoid. Other false contraindications include mild, acute illness; fever; and family history of an adverse reaction to vaccination. Anaphylactic reactions, neuropathies, and encephalopathies are rare and constitute the only true contraindications for giving toxoid. Patients who give a history of anaphylaxis should be referred for skin testing because they might no longer be reactive and can receive future vaccinations.

hTIG is derived from human plasma. It is available as 250-IU doses and is approved only for intramuscular use. Intradermal injection cause local irritation due to the concentration of the product and does not represent an allergy to hTIG. Because of this reaction, hTIG should not be infiltrated into the wound. Intravenous injection can cause hypotension. Adverse reactions to properly administered hTIG are rare and consist largely of discomfort at the injection site and slight temperature elevation.

In the setting of an acute injury, the CDC recommendations for tetanus prophylaxis depend on the wound characteristics and the patient's immunization history (Table 2). Many acute wounds can be considered not tetanus prone: recent wounds, linear wounds with sharp edges, well-vascularized wounds, and wounds not obviously contaminated or infected. All other wounds are considered tetanus prone, particularly those resulting from blunt trauma and bites and those that are grossly contaminated or infected.

If the patient has completed primary immunization, a booster is given if the last dose was longer than 5 years ago in a tetanus-prone wound or more than 10 years ago in a non–tetanus-prone wound. Patients with a contraindication to tetanus toxoid must be treated with hTIG alone.

If the patient has not completed primary immunization and the wound is tetanus prone, hTIG 250 IU IM is indicated. hTIG should be given at a site contralateral to the tetanus toxoid to prevent interaction between the two. A tetanus booster is also required, and the patient will need follow-up to complete primary immunization.

TABLE 1 Tetanus Primary Immunization

Age	Vaccine	No. of Doses	Schedule
<7 y	DTaP or DT	5	Doses 1-4 at 2, 4, 6, 15 mo Dose 5 between 4 and 6 y
>7 y	Td	3	First 2 doses more than 4 wk apart Dose 3 at 6 mo after dose 2

Abbreviations: DT = diphtheria and tetanus (adult); DTaP = diphtheria and tetanus toxoids and acellular pertussis; Td = diphtheria and tetanus (pediatric).
From Immunization Practices Advisory Committee: Diphtheria, tetanus, and pertussis: Recommendations for vaccine use and other preventive measures: Recommendations of the Immunization Practices Advisory Committee (ACIP). MMWR 1991;40(RR-10):1-28.

TABLE 2 Tetanus Prophylaxis in the Acute Wound

Wound Status	Primary Immunization Completed or Last Booster <5 y	>5 y	>10 y	Not Completed
Clean				
Td*	Yes	No	No	Yes
Tetanus-prone				
Td	Yes	No	Yes	Yes
TIG	Yes	No	No	No

*DTaP or DT for children younger than 7 years.
Abbreviations: DT = diphtheria and tetanus (adult); DTaP = diphtheria and tetanus toxoids and acellular pertussis; Td = diphtheria and tetanus (pediatric); TIG = tetanus immune globulin.
Adapted from Immunization Practices Advisory Committee: Diphtheria, tetanus, and pertussis: Recommendations for vaccine use and other preventive measures: Recommendations of the Immunization Practices Advisory Committee (ACIP). MMWR 1991;40(RR-10):1-28.

Due to an aging immune system, in elderly patients tetanus antibodies after vaccination do not form as quickly, do not have as high a peak, and do not persist as long as in younger persons. With low rates of baseline immunity, elderly patients who receive only a tetanus booster can not develop protective levels of antibodies quickly enough in the setting of an acute injury. More liberal use of hTIG in these patients, regardless of primary immunization, may be warranted to ensure protection against tetanus if the last booster was significantly longer than 10 years ago.

Td is safe in pregnancy. Generally, routine immunizations are avoided in the first trimester; however there is considerable evidence that Td is not teratogenic. In the setting of acute wounds, Td should not be withheld if indicated. hTIG is also safe in pregnancy. The main risk with donated biological products is infection, not teratogenesis. Other immune globulin products, such as Rh immune globulin (RhoGam), are commonly used during pregnancy without adverse effects.

REFERENCES

Ahmadsyah I, Salim A: Treatment of tetanus: An open study to compare the efficacy of procaine penicillin and metronidazole. Br J Med (Clin Res Ed) 1985;291:648-650.

American College of Obstetrics and Gynecology: Immunization during pregnancy. ACOG Committee Opinion No. 282. Obstet Gynecol 2003;101:207-212.

Apte NM, Karnad DR: Short report: The spatula test: A simple bedside test to diagnose tetanus. Am J Trop Med Hyg 1995;53(4):386-387.

Bleck TP, Brauner JS: Tetanus. In Scheld]WM, Whitely RJ, Durack DT (eds): Infections of the Central Nervous System. 2nd ed, Philadelphia: Lippincott-Raven, 1997, pp 629-653.

Centers for Disease Control: Prevention: Diphtheria, tetanus, and pertussis: Recommendations for vaccine use and other preventive measures: Recommendations of the Immunization Practices Advisory Committee (ACIP). MMWR 1991;40(RR-10):1-28.

Centers for Disease Control and Prevention: Tetanus surveillance—United States, 1998-2000. MMWR Surveill Summ 2003;52(SS-3):1-8.

Dietz V, Galazka A, Loon F, et al: Factors affecting the immunogenicity and potency of tetanus toxoid: Implications for the elimination of neonatal and non-neonatal tetanus as public health problems. Bull World Health Org 1997;75(1):81-93.

Sanford JP: Tetanus—forgotten but not gone. N Engl J Med 1995; 332(12):812-813.

Silveira CM, Caceres VM, Dutra MG, et al: Safety of tetanus toxoid in pregnant women: A hospital-based case-control study of congenital anomalies. Bull World Health Org 1995;73:605-608.

Talan D, Abrahamian F, Moran G, et al: Tetanus immunity and physician compliance with tetanus prophylaxis practices among emergency department patients presenting with wounds. Ann Emerg Med 2004; 43(3):305-314.

Pertussis

Method of
Michael E. Pichichero, MD

Pertussis, or whooping cough, is a highly contagious acute respiratory tract infection caused by *Bordetella pertussis*. It causes prolonged cough illness, without associated fever, characterized by paroxysms of coughing, inspiratory "whoops," and post-tussive vomiting in severe cases and persistent intermittent staccato cough episodes in teenagers and adults. The incidence of pertussis is rising in the United States despite record-high vaccination coverage. In 2004, more cases occurred in adolescents and in adults than children.

Microbiology and Pathophysiology

B. pertussis is a gram-negative coccobacillus that is difficult to grow with standard media. *B. pertussis* does not invade the human host; bacteremia does not occur. The systemic effects of illness are produced by the organism's toxins, especially pertussis toxin. *B. pertussis* attaches to the nasopharynx and tracheobronchial tree with adhesins such as fimbriae, filamentous hemagglutinin, and pertactin where it produces toxins such as pertussis toxin, adenylate cyclase toxin, and tracheal cytotoxin that paralyze the respiratory cilia, resulting in inflammation of the respiratory tract.

Epidemiology

B. pertussis is a human pathogen transmitted from person to person via aerosolized droplets. Pertussis is highly contagious, similar to varicella, infecting 80% to 90% of susceptible contacts. Persons with pertussis are most contagious in the 2 weeks before cough onset and during the first 2 weeks of cough, typically a time frame before medical care is sought or clinicians consider the possibility of the diagnosis.

In 2004, approximately 20,000 cases of pertussis were reported to the Centers for Disease Control and Prevention (CDC); because substantial underreporting is a recognized problem, current estimates of true pertussis incidence per year in the United States probably is in the range of 1 to 3 million cases. A new development is the recognition that pertussis is a disease of adolescents and adults as well as children. Several studies showed that among teenagers and adults who seek care for cough illness of more than 1 week duration, approximately 20% have pertussis.

Immunity

It has been known for decades that immunity to tetanus wanes over time and boosters are needed approximately every 10 years to sustain protective antibody levels. The phenomenon of waning immunity to pertussis is a newer observation and one of the explanations of the rising incidence of pertussis in the United States. Apparently boosters of pertussis vaccines are also needed, perhaps, like tetanus, approximately every 10 years. Two new adolescent/adult pertussis vaccine formulations that are combined with tetanus and diphtheria vaccines (Boostrix, Adacel) were licensed and recommended for universal use in 2005 to address this problem.

CURRENT DIAGNOSIS

- An illness marked by a staccato cough lasting >7 d in the absence of fever in an adolescent or adult may be pertussis.

Clinical Symptoms

Classic pertussis is a 30- to 90-day illness that presents in three stages: catarrhal, paroxysmal, and convalescent. The stages may be shorter in immunized children, adolescents, and adults. Pertussis is most severe when it occurs during the first 6 months of life.

In the catarrhal stage, nonspecific symptoms similar to the common cold predominate. The paroxysmal stage is characterized by a persistent cough, sometimes with bursts of numerous rapid coughs. A long inspiratory effort sometimes causes a high-pitched whoop. Typically, the patient is afebrile and, between coughing attacks, usually appears normal. The paroxysmal stage usually lasts 6 weeks. The cough gradually lessens over 2 to 3 weeks during the convalescent period. Milder paroxysms may recur with subsequent respiratory infections for many months following a pertussis infection. Infants may appear very ill and distressed during the paroxysmal stage and require close observation and supportive care. Older children, adolescents, and adults have a prolonged cough with paroxysms but no whoop.

Complications

Complications occur most commonly among young infants with pertussis. The most common complication is secondary bacterial pneumonia. Hypoxia or effects of pertussis toxin may contribute to neurologic complications including seizures and encephalopathy. In the United States, 90% of deaths occur in children younger than 6 months. Complications from pertussis in adolescents and adults are not uncommon (Table 1).

Diagnosis

A clinical diagnosis of pertussis is typically made based on the characteristic cough, although patients are often seen several times before the correct diagnosis is considered. absolute lymphocytosis (>10,000 lymphocytes/mm^3) may be seen during the late catarrhal and paroxysmal stages but is less common among adults and immunized children. Chest radiographs may show peribronchial consolidation, interstitial edema, or variable atelectasis. The presence of fever and consolidation with pertussis suggests a secondary bacterial pneumonia.

TABLE 1 Complications From Pertussis in Adolescents and Adults

Symptoms/Signs	Minnesota	Massachusetts	
		Adolescents	Adults
Paroxysmal cough	100%	85%	87%
Whooping	26%	30%	35%
Post-tussive emesis	56%	45%	41%
Apnea	—	19%	37%
Cyanosis	—	6%	9%
Hospitalization	0%	1.4%	3.5%

TABLE 2 Licensed Vaccines for the Prevention of Pertussis in Infants, Children, Adolescents, and Adults

Indicated Age Group	Sanofi Pasteur Tripedia infants/children[†]	GlaxoSmithKline Infanrix* infants/children[†]	Sanofi Pasteur Daptacel infants/children[†]	GlaxoSmithKline Boostrix adolescents[‡]	Sanofi Pasteur Adacel adults/adolescents[‡]
Antigens					
PT (μg)	23.4	25	10	8	2.5
FHA (μg)	23.4	25	5	8	5
PRN (μg)	—	8	3	2.5	3
FIM 2 + 3 (μg)	—	—	5	—	5
D (Lf)	6.7	25	15	2.5	2
T (Lf)	5	10	5	5	5

*PEDIARIX also contains these DTaP components.
[†]6 wk to <7 y.
[‡]Boostrix is indicated for 10–18 y; Adacel is indicated for 11–54 y.
Abbreviations: D = diphtheria toxoid; FHA = filamentous hemagglutinin; FIM 2 + 3 = fimbrial agglutinogen 2 and 3; PRN = pertactin; PT = pertussis toxoid; T = tetanus toxoid.

Isolation of *B. pertussis* from a culture of nasal secretions remains the gold standard for laboratory diagnosis. A nasopharyngeal specimen is obtained by inserting a small flexible Dacron or calcium alginate swab through the nose to the posterior nasopharynx (attempting to touch the adenoids) where it is held for a few seconds, perhaps inducing a cough. The specimen is transferred to *Bordetella*-specific transport media and subsequently plated on Regan-Lowe charcoal agar or Stainer-Scholte agar. Cultures are usually positive if obtained in the catarrhal or early paroxysmal stage of disease. Success in isolating *B. pertussis* diminishes if patients have received pertussis vaccine or recent antimicrobials or if specimens are obtained beyond the first 2 weeks of cough.

Polymerase chain reaction (PCR) is more sensitive among persons with mild or atypical symptoms and those who have received prior antimicrobial therapy. The CDC recommends using PCR as a presumptive assay in conjunction with culture. Direct fluorescent antibody (DFA) testing has a low sensitivity and variable specificity, requiring experienced laboratory personnel for consistent results. DFA testing should only be performed as a adjunct to culture or PCR. Serologic testing methods have recently emerged as a very valuable diagnostic tool. Single samples of 100 μL of blood can be used to measure pertussis antibodies that are compared to age-specific standards to confirm a clinical diagnosis. These methods are not widely available in hospitals or private laboratories, but state laboratories often can provide this testing.

Treatment

Infants and children with severe cough paroxysms associated with cyanosis or apnea require hospitalization and intensive care. Infants younger than 3 months should be admitted routinely for observation of their paroxysmal episodes, their need for supportive interventions, and their ability to feed appropriately. Continuous monitoring of heart rate, respiratory rate, and oxygen saturation is indicated.

All patients should receive antibiotics. Macrolides are the treatment of choice: erythromycin, clarithromycin (Biaxin),[1] azithromycin (Zithromax),[1] or telithromycin (Ketek).[1] Fluoroquinolones are also effective therapy for pertussis. Trimethoprim-sulfamethoxazole (Bactrim)[1] is an alternative choice although less effective.

Prevention

Pertussis is a preventable disease by vaccination. Vaccines are available and recommended for universal use in infants, children, adolescents, and selected adult populations (health care workers, adults caring for infants younger than 6 months, and those with chronic respiratory conditions, e.g., chronic obstructive pulmonary disease). Table 2 lists the vaccines licensed in the United States.

REFERENCES

Farizo KM, Cochi SL, Zell ER, et al: Epidemiological features of pertussis in the United States, 1980–1989. Clin Infect Dis 1992;14(3):708-719.
Lee LH, Pichichero ME. Costs of illness due to *Bordetella pertussis* in families. Arch Fam Med 2000;9(:10):989-996.
Pichichero ME, Rennels MB, Edwards KM, et al: Combined tetanus, diphtheria, and 5-component pertussis vaccine for use in adolescents and adults. JAMA 2005;293(24):3003-3011.
Purdy KW, Hay JW, Botteman MF, et al: Evaluation of strategies for use of acellular pertussis vaccine in adolescents and adults: A cost-benefit analysis. Clin Infect Dis 2004;39:20-28.
Skowronski DM, De Serres G, MacDonald D, et al: The changing age and seasonal profile of pertussis in Canada. J Infect Dis 2002;185(10):1448-1453. Epub 2002 Apr 22.
Strebel P, Nordin J, Edwards K, et al: Population-based incidence of pertussis among adolescents and adults, Minnesota, 1995–1996. J Infect Dis 2001;183(9):1353-1359. Epub 2001 Mar 30.
Yih WK, Lett SM, des Vignes FN, et al: The increasing incidence of pertussis in Massachusetts adolescents and adults. 1989–1998. J Infect Dis 2000;182(5):1409-1416. Epub 2000 Oct 09.

---

[1]Not FDA approved for this indication.

CURRENT THERAPY

- Early treatment of pertussis not only eliminates contagion, it also shortens the illness.
- Macrolides are the treatment of choice; azithromycin (Zithromax) is preferred for ease of dosing, tolerability, and short duration of treatment.

Office-Based Immunization Practices

Method of
Robert M. Jacobson, MD

Routine immunizations represent the cutting edge for consensus-driven, evidence-based practice guidelines in the care of children and adults. Perhaps no other office-based task is so universally accepted and practiced as well as evidenced as immunizations. We should be modeling the rest of our practices on the success that we have enjoyed with immunizations.

That is not to say that we are providing immunizations as well as we should; the practice of immunization is difficult, complex, and evolving. Other chapters deal with the specific diseases to which we direct our vaccines. Office practitioners must consider a variety of aspects that go beyond the understanding of the individual vaccine-preventable diseases. These include the adoption of a comprehensive immunization schedule, using a number of immunization-specific practices, and the understanding of common problems associated with immunization in the office.

The Adoption of a Comprehensive Immunization Schedule

In recent years, we have benefited from efforts made at the national level to harmonize and systematically update recommended schedules for routine immunizations (Tables 1 and 2). The Advisory Committee on Immunization Practices (ACIP), sponsored by the Centers for Disease Control and Prevention (CDC), works closely with the American Academy of Pediatrics (AAP) and the American Academy of Family Physicians (AAFP) to publish a single set of recommendations for routine immunizations for infants, children, and adolescents younger than 18 years. The Recommended Adult Immunization Schedule is similarly approved by the ACIP, the American College of Obstetricians and Gynecologists (ACOG), and the AAFP. These are published widely in a number of journals as well as on the internet. The harmonized schedules address the use of both individual vaccine components as well as all licensed combination vaccines. The vaccine schedules give ranges of target age ranges for immunization rather than prescribe individual ages. For example, the measles-mumps-rubella combination is to be given from 12 to 15 months of life rather than either 12 months or 15 months. Furthermore, the pediatric schedule includes catch-up schedules for children who did not receive immunizations at the recommended ages. The adult schedule includes common conditions with vaccine-specific recommendations (such as for pregnancy).

Each of the 50 states in the United States has specific immunization requirements for day care, school, and even college attendance. These vary state by state and in some states affect not only initial enrollment but also continued participation in schools. The Immunization Action Coalition collates and publishes online (www.immunize.org/laws/) an up-to-date listing of the state-specific state mandates on immunization and vaccine-preventable diseases as well as links to the individual state health departments.

For your office practice, you are encouraged to adopt a more specific schedule. For example, where the harmonized schedule might give you some latitude with what age to give the dose for the measles-mumps-rubella vaccine, it would be more appropriate for you and your colleagues to pick either 12 or 15 months. When all practitioners sharing an office adopt a uniform practice, they prevent parental and staff confusion and misunderstanding as well as mistakes in vaccine administration and patient scheduling.

Adoption of Immunization-Specific Practices

EDUCATION OF SELF AND STAFF

Immunization practices certainly have evolved over the last century, and much of the development has accelerated since the enactment of the National Childhood Vaccine Injury Act of 1986 (PL 99-660), which established the national Vaccine Injury Compensation Program (VICP), a no-fault alternative to the tort system for resolving vaccine injury claims. This legislation protects vaccine providers and manufacturers from frivolous lawsuits directed against routine childhood immunization.

Although in the 1980s it was routine for a child in the first year of life to receive three injections and three oral doses of polio, now the typical infant by 12 months of age may receive 24 separate injections against vaccine-preventable disease. Almost each year the routine childhood vaccine schedule is altered in a substantive way. Most recently, the newest routine vaccination schedule includes annual influenza vaccinations for children and adolescents through 18 years of age. Such changes require a practitioner's continuing education and practice advancement.

A number of electronic Web sites provide announcements and updates of vaccines in form delivered for health care practitioners; the CDC provides a Web site (www.cdc.gov/vaccines) with information resources for both parents and health care practitioners including sections on updates. In addition, the Immunization Action Coalition, a not-for-profit group dedicated to the dissemination of scientifically correct immunization information, also has a very useful Web site (www.immunize.org). The latter invites practitioners to sign up for routine mailings of updates on immunization practices. Similarly, providers can access the CDC's Morbidity and Mortality Weekly Report (MMWR) online. These provide updates and statements from ACIP. Furthermore, the AAP publishes on its Web site (www.aap.org) its policy statements and recommendation online for members and nonmembers alike.

Paper-based resources are more difficult to keep up to date, but important ones include the paper-based publication *MMWR* published by the CDC and the *Red Book* published by the AAP. The *Red Book* not only does an outstanding job with vaccine-related issues but also includes a host of information for a general practitioner on pediatric and adolescent infectious diseases. The CDC publishes the "Pink Book" both in paper and online. It is formally entitled *Epidemiology and Prevention of Vaccine Preventable Diseases*.

The CDC and the Medical University of South Carolina have sponsored the development of an electronic-based educational program called Teaching Immunization Delivery and Evaluation (TIDE). Its Web site is http://www2.edserv.musc.edu/tide, and the program is endorsed by the Ambulatory Pediatric Association and the Society of Adolescent Medicine. It is a flexible tool to teach immunization delivery, and it uses clinical scenarios that inspire problem solving. Self-contained modules are available that provide continued education credit.

ASSESSMENT OF INDIVIDUAL NEEDS

Each patient is unique, but the success of the routine immunization schedule depends on its universality. Precautions and contraindications exist, and the children and adults who most frequently attend health care providers' offices have relatively higher rates of chronic conditions than the general population. These conditions raise questions of contraindications and precautions. Therefore, individuals must be assessed for their individual needs. Even misperceptions of contraindications can lead to delays and require catch-up. Practitioners should be familiar with the routine schedules (Tables 1 and 2) as well as the general precautions of contraindications associated with each vaccine.

One of the most important resources available for the busy practitioner is a chart developed by the CDC organized by condition that specifies which vaccines are contraindicated by that condition. This chart is on the CDC Web site under the tab of Healthcare Professionals. It is entitled "Guide to Contraindications" (www.cdc.gov/vaccines/recs/vac-admin/contraindications.htm).

The CDC has developed survey tools that are available freely to download from its Web site (www.cdc.gov/vaccines). The practitioner can use this with the individual patient to assess vaccine needs. Assessment tools are available online for both adults and children.

PATIENT EDUCATION

Patient and parent education is incredibly important in applying immunizations. After all, we are giving a form of a biologic with known rates and associations with adverse events to large numbers of persons who are often well and without a medical need or condition. We should inform the patient, and, in the case of a child or adolescent not yet at the age of majority, the parent as best we can about the immunizations, the diseases for which we are vaccinating,

TABLE 1 Recommended Childhood and Adolescent Immunization Schedule

Recommended Immunization Schedule for Persons Aged 0–6 Years—UNITED STATES • 2008

For those who fall behind or start late, see the catch-up schedule

Vaccine ▼ Age ▶	Birth	1 month	2 months	4 months	6 months	12 months	15 months	18 months	19–23 months	2–3 years	4–6 years
Hepatitis B[1]	HepB	HepB		see footnote 1		HepB					
Rotavirus[2]			Rota	Rota	Rota						
Diphtheria, Tetanus, Pertussis[3]			DTaP	DTaP	DTaP	see footnote 3	DTaP				DTaP
Haemophilus influenzae type b[4]			Hib	Hib	Hib[4]	Hib					
Pneumococcal[5]			PCV	PCV	PCV	PCV				PPV	
Inactivated Poliovirus			IPV	IPV		IPV					IPV
Influenza[6]						Influenza (Yearly)					
Measles, Mumps, Rubella[7]						MMR					MMR
Varicella[8]						Varicella					Varicella
Hepatitis A[9]						HepA (2 doses)				HepA Series	
Meningococcal[10]											MCV4

Range of recommended ages

Certain high-risk groups

This schedule indicates the recommended ages for routine administration of currently licensed childhood vaccines, as of December 1, 2007, for children aged 0 through 6 years. Additional information is available at www.cdc.gov/vaccines/recs/schedules. Any dose not administered at the recommended age should be administered at any subsequent visit, when indicated and feasible. Additional vaccines may be licensed and recommended during the year. Licensed combination vaccines may be used whenever any components of the combination are indicated and other components of the vaccine are not contraindicated and if approved by the Food and Drug Administration for that dose of the series. Providers should consult the respective Advisory Committee on Immunization Practices statement for detailed recommendations, including for **high-risk conditions**: http://www.cdc.gov/vaccines/pubs/ACIP-list.htm. Clinically significant adverse events that follow immunization should be reported to the Vaccine Adverse Event Reporting System (VAERS). Guidance about how to obtain and complete a VAERS form is available at www.vaers.hhs.gov or by telephone, **800-822-7967**.

1. **Hepatitis B vaccine (HepB).** *(Minimum age: birth)*
   At birth:
   - Administer monovalent HepB to all newborns prior to hospital discharge.
   - If mother is hepatitis B surface antigen (HBsAg) positive, administer HepB and 0.5 mL of hepatitis B immune globulin (HBIG) within 12 hours of birth.
   - If mother's HBsAg status is unknown, administer HepB within 12 hours of birth. Determine the HBsAg status as soon as possible and if HBsAg positive, administer HBIG (no later than age 1 week).
   - If mother is HBsAg negative, the birth dose can be delayed, in rare cases, with a provider's order and a copy of the mother's negative HBsAg laboratory report in the infant's medical record.

   After the birth dose:
   - The HepB series should be completed with either monovalent HepB or a combination vaccine containing HepB. The second dose should be administered at age 1–2 months. The final dose should be administered no earlier than age 24 weeks. Infants born to HBsAg-positive mothers should be tested for HBsAg and antibody to HBsAg after completion of at least 3 doses of a licensed HepB series, at age 9–18 months (generally at the next well-child visit).

   4-month dose:
   - It is permissible to administer 4 doses of HepB when combination vaccines are administered after the birth dose. If monovalent HepB is used for doses after the birth dose, a dose at age 4 months is not needed.

2. **Rotavirus vaccine (Rota).** *(Minimum age: 6 weeks)*
   - Administer the first dose at age 6–12 weeks.
   - Do not start the series later than age 12 weeks.
   - Administer the final dose in the series by age 32 weeks. Do not administer any dose later than age 32 weeks.
   - Data on safety and efficacy outside of these age ranges are insufficient.

3. **Diphtheria and tetanus toxoids and acellular pertussis vaccine (DTaP).** *(Minimum age: 6 weeks)*
   - The fourth dose of DTaP may be administered as early as age 12 months, provided 6 months have elapsed since the third dose.
   - Administer the final dose in the series at age 4–6 years.

4. ***Haemophilus influenzae* type b conjugate vaccine (Hib).** *(Minimum age: 6 weeks)*
   - If PRP-OMP (PedvaxHIB® or ComVax® [Merck]) is administered at ages 2 and 4 months, a dose at age 6 months is not required.
   - TriHIBit® (DTaP/Hib) combination products should not be used for primary immunization but can be used as boosters following any Hib vaccine in children age 12 months or older.

5. **Pneumococcal vaccine.** *(Minimum age: 6 weeks for pneumococcal conjugate vaccine [PCV]; 2 years for pneumococcal polysaccharide vaccine [PPV])*
   - Administer one dose of PCV to all healthy children aged 24–59 months having any incomplete schedule.
   - Administer PPV to children aged 2 years and older with underlying medical conditions.

6. **Influenza vaccine.** *(Minimum age: 6 months for trivalent inactivated influenza vaccine [TIV]; 2 years for live, attenuated influenza vaccine [LAIV])*
   - Administer annually to children aged 6–59 months and to all eligible close contacts of children aged 0–59 months.
   - Administer annually to children 5 years of age and older with certain risk factors, to other persons (including household members) in close contact with persons in groups at higher risk, and to any child whose parents request vaccination.
   - For healthy persons (those who do not have underlying medical conditions that predispose them to influenza complications) ages 2–49 years, either LAIV or TIV may be used.
   - Children receiving TIV should receive 0.25 mL if age 6–35 months or 0.5 mL if age 3 years or older.
   - Administer 2 doses (separated by 4 weeks or longer) to children younger than 9 years who are receiving influenza vaccine for the first time or who were vaccinated for the first time last season but only received one dose.

7. **Measles, mumps, and rubella vaccine (MMR).** *(Minimum age: 12 months)*
   - Administer the second dose of MMR at age 4–6 years. MMR may be administered before age 4–6 years, provided 4 weeks or more have elapsed since the first dose.

8. **Varicella vaccine.** *(Minimum age: 12 months)*
   - Administer second dose at age 4–6 years; may be administered 3 months or more after first dose.
   - Do not repeat second dose if administered 28 days or more after first dose.

9. **Hepatitis A vaccine (HepA).** *(Minimum age: 12 months)*
   - Administer to all children aged 1 year (i.e., aged 12–23 months). Administer the 2 doses in the series at least 6 months apart.
   - Children not fully vaccinated by age 2 years can be vaccinated at subsequent visits.
   - HepA is recommended for certain other groups of children, including in areas where vaccination programs target older children.

10. **Meningococcal vaccine.** *(Minimum age: 2 years for meningococcal conjugate vaccine (MCV4) and for meningococcal polysaccharide vaccine (MPSV4))*
    - Administer MCV4 to children aged 2–10 years with terminal complement deficiencies or anatomic or functional asplenia and certain other high-risk groups. MPSV4 is also acceptable.
    - Administer MCV4 to persons who received MPSV4 3 or more years previously and remain at increased risk for meningococcal disease.

The Recommended Immunization Schedules for Persons Aged 0–18 Years are approved by the Advisory Committee on Immunization Practices (www.cdc.gov/vaccines/recs/acip), the American Academy of Pediatrics (http://www.aap.org), and the American Academy of Family Physicians (http://www.aafp.org).

DEPARTMENT OF HEALTH AND HUMAN SERVICES • CENTERS FOR DISEASE CONTROL AND PREVENTION • SAFER • HEATHIER • PEOPLE™

Continued

TABLE 1 Recommended Childhood and Adolescent Immunization Schedule—cont'd

Recommended Immunization Schedule for Persons Aged 7–18 Years—UNITED STATES • 2008
For those who fall behind or start late, see the green bars and the catch-up schedule

Vaccine ▼ Age ▶	7–10 years	11–12 years	13–18 years	
Diphtheria, Tetanus, Pertussis[1]	see footnote 1	Tdap	Tdap	Range of recommended ages
Human Papillomavirus[2]	see footnote 2	HPV (3 doses)	HPV Series	
Meningococcal[3]	MCV4	MCV4	MCV4	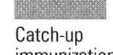 Catch-up immunization
Pneumococcal[4]	PPV			
Influenza[5]	Influenza (Yearly)			
Hepatitis A[6]	HepA Series			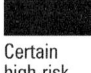 Certain high-risk groups
Hepatitis B[7]	HepB Series			
Inactivated Poliovirus[8]	IPV Series			
Measles, Mumps, Rubella[9]	MMR Series			
Varicella[10]	Varicella Series			

This schedule indicates the recommended ages for routine administration of currently licensed childhood vaccines, as of December 1, 2007, for children aged 7–18 years. Additional information is available at **www.cdc.gov/vaccines/recs/schedules**. Any dose not administered at the recommended age should be administered at any subsequent visit, when indicated and feasible. Additional vaccines may be licensed and recommended during the year. Licensed combination vaccines may be used whenever any components of the combination are indicated and other components of the vaccine are not contraindicated and if approved by the Food and Drug Administration for that dose of the series. Providers should consult the respective Advisory Committee on Immunization Practices statement for detailed recommendations, including for **high-risk conditions: http://www.cdc.gov/vaccines/pubs/ACIP-list.htm**. Clinically significant adverse events that follow immunization should be reported to the Vaccine Adverse Event Reporting System (VAERS). Guidance about how to obtain and complete a VAERS form is available at **www.vaers.hhs.gov** or by telephone, **800-822-7967**.

1. **Tetanus and diphtheria toxoids and acellular pertussis vaccine (Tdap).** *(Minimum age: 10 years for BOOSTRIX® and 11 years for ADACEL™)*
   - Administer at age 11–12 years for those who have completed the recommended childhood DTP/DTaP vaccination series and have not received a tetanus and diphtheria toxoids (Td) booster dose.
   - 13–18-year-olds who missed the 11–12 year Tdap or received Td only are encouraged to receive one dose of Tdap 5 years after the last Td/DTaP dose.

2. **Human papillomavirus vaccine (HPV).** *(Minimum age: 9 years)*
   - Administer the first dose of the HPV vaccine series to females at age 11–12 years.
   - Administer the second dose 2 months after the first dose and the third dose 6 months after the first dose.
   - Administer the HPV vaccine series to females at age 13–18 years if not previously vaccinated.

3. **Meningococcal vaccine.**
   - Administer MCV4 at age 11–12 years and at age 13–18 years if not previously vaccinated. MPSV4 is an acceptable alternative.
   - Administer MCV4 to previously unvaccinated college freshmen living in dormitories.
   - MCV4 is recommended for children aged 2–10 years with terminal complement deficiencies or anatomic or functional asplenia and certain other high-risk groups.
   - Persons who received MPSV4 3 or more years previously and remain at increased risk for meningococcal disease should be vaccinated with MCV4.

4. **Pneumococcal polysaccharide vaccine (PPV).**
   - Administer PPV to certain high-risk groups.

5. **Influenza vaccine.**
   - Administer annually to all close contacts of children aged 0–59 months.
   - Administer annually to persons with certain risk factors, health-care workers, and other persons (including household members) in close contact with persons in groups at higher risk.
   - Administer 2 doses (separated by 4 weeks or longer) to children younger than 9 years who are receiving influenza vaccine for the first time or who were vaccinated for the first time last season but only received one dose.
   - For healthy nonpregnant persons (those who do not have underlying medical conditions that predispose them to influenza complications) ages 2–49 years, either LAIV or TIV may be used.

6. **Hepatitis A vaccine (HepA).**
   - Administer the 2 doses in the series at least 6 months apart.
   - HepA is recommended for certain other groups of children, including in areas where vaccination programs target older children.

7. **Hepatitis B vaccine (HepB).**
   - Administer the 3-dose series to those who were not previously vaccinated.
   - A 2-dose series of Recombivax HB® is licensed for children aged 11–15 years.

8. **Inactivated poliovirus vaccine (IPV).**
   - For children who received an all-IPV or all-oral poliovirus (OPV) series, a fourth dose is not necessary if the third dose was administered at age 4 years or older.
   - If both OPV and IPV were administered as part of a series, a total of 4 doses should be administered, regardless of the child's current age.

9. **Measles, mumps, and rubella vaccine (MMR).**
   - If not previously vaccinated, administer 2 doses of MMR during any visit, with 4 or more weeks between the doses.

10. **Varicella vaccine.**
    - Administer 2 doses of varicella vaccine to persons younger than 13 years of age at least 3 months apart. Do not repeat the second dose if administered 28 or more days following the first dose.
    - Administer 2 doses of varicella vaccine to persons aged 13 years or older at least 4 weeks apart.

The Recommended Immunization Schedules for Persons Aged 0–18 Years are approved by the Advisory Committee on Immunization Practices (www.cdc.gov/vaccines/recs/acip), the American Academy of Pediatrics (http://www.aap.org), and the American Academy of Family Physicians (http://www.aafp.org).

DEPARTMENT OF HEALTH AND HUMAN SERVICES • CENTERS FOR DISEASE CONTROL AND PREVENTION
SAFER • HEALTHIER • PEOPLE™

TABLE 2 Recommended Catch-Up Immunization Schedule

Catch-up Immunization Schedule for Persons Aged 4 Months–18 Years Who Start Late or Who Are More Than 1 Month Behind
UNITED STATES • 2008

The table below provides catch-up schedules and minimum intervals between doses for children whose vaccinations have been delayed. A vaccine series does not need to be restarted, regardless of the time that has elapsed between doses. Use the section appropriate for the child's age.

CATCH-UP SCHEDULE FOR PERSONS AGED 4 MONTHS–6 YEARS

Vaccine	Minimum Age for Dose 1	Dose 1 to Dose 2	Dose 2 to Dose 3	Dose 3 to Dose 4	Dose 4 to Dose 5
Hepatitis B[1]	Birth	4 weeks	8 weeks (and 16 weeks after first dose)		
Rotavirus[2]	6 wks	4 weeks	4 weeks		
Diphtheria, Tetanus, Pertussis[3]	6 wks	4 weeks	4 weeks	6 months	6 months[3]
Haemophilus influenzae type b[4]	6 wks	4 weeks if first dose administered at younger than 12 months of age 8 weeks (as final dose) if first dose administered at age 12-14 months No further doses needed if first dose administered at 15 months of age or older	4 weeks[4] if current age is younger than 12 months 8 weeks (as final dose)[4] if current age is 12 months or older and second dose administered at younger than 15 months of age No further doses needed if previous dose administered at age 15 months or older	8 weeks (as final dose) This dose only necessary for children aged 12 months–5 years who received 3 doses before age 12 months	
Pneumococcal[5]	6 wks	4 weeks if first dose administered at younger than 12 months of age 8 weeks (as final dose) if first dose administered at age 12 months or older or current age 24–59 months No further doses needed for healthy children if first dose administered at age 24 months or older	4 weeks if current age is younger than 12 months 8 weeks (as final dose) if current age is 12 months or older No further doses needed for healthy children if previous dose administered at age 24 months or older	8 weeks (as final dose) This dose only necessary for children aged 12 months–5 years who received 3 doses before age 12 months	
Inactivated Poliovirus[6]	6 wks	4 weeks	4 weeks	4 weeks[6]	
Measles, Mumps, Rubella[7]	12 mos	4 weeks			
Varicella[8]	12 mos	3 months			
Hepatitis A[9]	12 mos	6 months			

CATCH-UP SCHEDULE FOR PERSONS AGED 7–18 YEARS

Vaccine	Minimum Age for Dose 1	Dose 1 to Dose 2	Dose 2 to Dose 3	Dose 3 to Dose 4	
Tetanus, Diphtheria/ Tetanus, Diphtheria, Pertussis[10]	7 yrs[10]	4 weeks	4 weeks if first dose administered at younger than 12 months of age 6 months if first dose administered at age 12 months or older	6 months if first dose administered at younger than 12 months of age	
Human Papillomavirus[11]	9 yrs	4 weeks	12 weeks (and 24 weeks after the first dose)		
Hepatitis A[9]	12 mos	6 months			
Hepatitis B[1]	Birth	4 weeks	8 weeks (and 16 weeks after first dose)		
Inactivated Poliovirus[6]	6 wks	4 weeks	4 weeks	4 weeks[6]	
Measles, Mumps, Rubella[7]	12 mos	4 weeks			
Varicella[8]	12 mos	4 weeks if first dose administered at age 13 years or older 3 months if first dose administered at younger than 13 years of age			

1. **Hepatitis B vaccine (HepB).**
   - Administer the 3-dose series to those who were not previously vaccinated.
   - A 2-dose series of Recombivax HB® is licensed for children aged 11–15 years.

2. **Rotavirus vaccine (Rota).**
   - Do not start the series later than age 12 weeks.
   - Administer the final dose in the series by age 32 weeks.
   - Do not administer a dose later than age 32 weeks.
   - Data on safety and efficacy outside of these age ranges are insufficient.

3. **Diphtheria and tetanus toxoids and acellular pertussis vaccine (DTaP).**
   - The fifth dose is not necessary if the fourth dose was administered at age 4 years or older.
   - DTaP is not indicated for persons aged 7 years or older.

4. *Haemophilus influenzae* **type b conjugate vaccine (Hib).**
   - Vaccine is not generally recommended for children aged 5 years or older.
   - If current age is younger than 12 months and the first 2 doses were PRP-OMP (PedvaxHIB® or ComVax® [Merck]), the third (and final) dose should be administered at age 12–15 months and at least 8 weeks after the second dose.
   - If first dose was administered at age 7–11 months, administer 2 doses separated by 4 weeks plus a booster at age 12–15 months.

5. **Pneumococcal conjugate vaccine (PCV).**
   - Administer one dose of PCV to all healthy children aged 24–59 months having any incomplete schedule.
   - For children with underlying medical conditions, administer 2 doses of PCV at least 8 weeks apart if previously received less than 3 doses, or 1 dose of PCV if previously received 3 doses.

6. **Inactivated poliovirus vaccine (IPV).**
   - For children who received an all-IPV or all-oral poliovirus (OPV) series, a fourth dose is not necessary if third dose was administered at age 4 years or older.
   - If both OPV and IPV were administered as part of a series, a total of 4 doses should be administered, regardless of the child's current age.
   - IPV is not routinely recommended for persons aged 18 years and older.

7. **Measles, mumps, and rubella vaccine (MMR).**
   - The second dose of MMR is recommended routinely at age 4–6 years but may be administered earlier if desired.
   - If not previously vaccinated, administer 2 doses of MMR during any visit with 4 or more weeks between the doses.

8. **Varicella vaccine.**
   - The second dose of varicella vaccine is recommended routinely at age 4–6 years but may be administered earlier if desired.
   - Do not repeat the second dose in persons younger than 13 years of age if administered 28 or more days after the first dose.

9. **Hepatitis A vaccine (HepA).**
   - HepA is recommended for certain groups of children, including in areas where vaccination programs target older children. See *MMWR* 2006;55(No. RR-7):1–23.

10. **Tetanus and diphtheria toxoids vaccine (Td) and tetanus and diphtheria toxoids and acellular pertussis vaccine (Tdap).**
    - Tdap should be substituted for a single dose of Td in the primary catch-up series or as a booster if age appropriate; use Td for other doses.
    - A 5-year interval from the last Td dose is encouraged when Tdap is used as a booster dose. A booster (fourth) dose is needed if any of the previous doses were administered at younger than 12 months of age. Refer to ACIP recommendations for further information. See *MMWR* 2006;55(No. RR-3).

11. **Human papillomavirus vaccine (HPV).**
    - Administer the HPV vaccine series to females at age 13–18 years if not previously vaccinated.

Information about reporting reactions after immunization is available online at http://www.vaers.hhs.gov or by telephone via the 24-hour national toll-free information line 800-822-7967. Suspected cases of vaccine-preventable diseases should be reported to the state or local health department. Additional information, including precautions and contraindications for immunization, is available from the National Center for Immunization and Respiratory Diseases at http://www.cdc.gov/vaccines or telephone, 800-CDC-INFO (800-232-4636).

DEPARTMENT OF HEALTH AND HUMAN SERVICES • CENTERS FOR DISEASE CONTROL AND PREVENTION • SAFER • HEALTHIER • PEOPLE

CURRENT DIAGNOSIS

- At each patient contact, practitioners should review the patient's immunization record for vaccines due and overdue.

the nature of the benefits from the vaccines, as well as the common adverse reactions and possible severe adverse reactions that might occur. The patients and parents should learn for whom the vaccines should be received as well as for whom the vaccines not be received and what they should do in case of an adverse event. This information is complex in depth and breadth, but the National Childhood Vaccine Injury Act of 1986 that created protection for vaccine providers and manufacturers at the same time created regulations with a uniform system of vaccine information statements to be provided. The National Immunization Program publishes brief vaccine-specific statements for all of the routine vaccines given to children and adults. These Vaccine Information Statements (VISs) are published in a highly readable format (www.cdc.gov/vaccines/pubs/vis) and are required by U.S. law to be provided to the parent and recipient before each dose of certain vaccines including those on a routine childhood vaccine schedule. VISs also exist for some of the more exotic vaccines, such as the Japanese encephalitis vaccine, the smallpox vaccine, the typhoid vaccines, the yellow fever vaccine, as well as for the rabies vaccines. The Immunization Action Coalition (www.immunize.org) has partnered with the CDC and has translated the VISs for each vaccine into more than 20 different languages. More detailed information for the vaccines can be obtained from the statements from the ACIP (www.cdc.gov/vaccines/recs/acip), the Food and Drug Administration–approved package inserts, and the AAP's *Red Book*.

PREVACCINATION PREPARATION

Not only should the parent and recipient of the vaccine be provided the VIS, but efforts should be taken to minimize the discomfort of the recipient. Information plays a large role. A study done at the Mayo Clinic demonstrated that informing the child prior to the visit actually decreased the amount of distress observed at the time of the visit. Furthermore, efforts at the time of the visit including distraction or relaxation techniques can prevent or reduce distress associated with the vaccine. Office staff should learn methods of successful communication, distraction, and relaxation techniques to facilitate routine immunizations.

For some of the vaccines, antipyretics such as acetaminophen (Tylenol) or ibuprofen (Advil) might be administered at the time of immunization and then at regular intervals specific to that drug for the following 24 hours to reduce the occurrence and the severity of fever as well as the local injection pain that might occur with immunization.

The *Red Book* Committee, the Committee on Infectious Diseases of the AAP, recommends that practitioners consider a variety of efforts to minimize the discomfort of immunization including specific injection techniques, the use of multiple vaccinators to immunize simultaneously rather than serially, as well as possibly local anesthetics and nonpharmacologic agents.

VACCINE DELIVERY

Some vaccines are given intramuscularly (IM) or subcutaneously (SC); still others, via the mouth or nose. IM vaccines should be

CURRENT THERAPY

- Providing routine immunizations requires an office to organize its educational activities, practice standards, communication methods, and documentation strategies.

given deep into a muscle mass. Practitioners should use the anterolateral thigh muscle injections for children younger than 18 months and then move to the deltoid muscle in children older than 18 months when the muscle mass of the deltoid is large enough. SC injections should be given in subcutaneous fat of the anterolateral thigh or triceps with a shorter needle inserted at an angle.

PREVENTION OF NEEDLE INJURY

For the safety of the patient, parent, and provider, efforts should be made to minimize the exposure to an accidental needle stick. Although the risk of accidental inoculation with the patient's blood is minimal in immunization, as with the use of sharps in any office, employees should examine the safety needles available and choose a safety needle appropriate for minimizing accidental needle sticks. The office should provide a child-proof sharps container that allows for rapid disposal of the needle with a minimal amount of effort. The container should be checked regularly for function and emptied frequently to avoid overfilling during the workday.

DOCUMENTATION AND RECORDS

All offices should adopt a standard of documentation of immunizations. The physician's or nurse's order for a vaccine should not be used in place of documentation that the vaccine was given. Documentation of the vaccine administered should include the species and the brand name given as well as the lot number. The patient record should also include the location, date, and time. Such a record would be made more useful if all the vaccine-antigens could be viewed at once with regard to series and dates. To best manage combinations currently available as well as future possibilities, the record should be organized by vaccine-antigen and not common vaccine combinations. This requires that a combination vaccine then appear in several antigen categories. Furthermore, the record would be enhanced by clarification when vaccines were not given because of precaution or contraindication as the basis. We have an ongoing problem with the adoption of chickenpox vaccine (Varivax). Those children who previously acquired chickenpox do not need the chickenpox vaccine, but we need to document the occurrence of that disease and its date to prevent overvaccination.

RECORD SHARING AND REGISTRIES

Vaccine registries at the community level or regional level dramatically reduce the miscommunication and the need for occurrence of both overimmunization as well as empowering physicians and nurses to feel better about taking advantage of missed opportunities in vaccinating children. Most parents whose children are undervaccinated report that their children are "up to date." Records that accurately reflect the child's full vaccine record would better equip the practitioner in best managing those patients.

VACCINE STORAGE

Storage requirements are much more complex than traditionally practiced. Offices must provide proper refrigeration as well as freezers for vaccines. Certain vaccines require refrigeration, other vaccines require freezing, and some vaccines are more heat labile or cold labile than others. Proper care and maintenance of refrigerator includes the purchase of appropriate dedicated equipment, the monitoring of the temperatures, the purchase of proper containers to be used on the shelves, and adequate space to allow for prevention of errors with storage. Furthermore, the staff must be trained and scheduled to provide oversight in the case of a power or equipment failure.

ASSESSMENT OF THE OVERALL PROCESS AND ITS OUTCOMES

Assessing an individual's immunization needs, providing the vaccines, and recording them properly in the individual's record is no longer adequate for the assessment of the overall process. Each office should make efforts to assess its overall practice. Each office must monitor the rates of on-time immunizations as well as up-to-date immunization and look for opportunities to improve these metrics. The effort of collecting this information has led to improvements in rates of on-time vaccination. Immunization practices are evolving and the maintenance of quality as well as the rapid adoption and improvement of practices require regular office meetings of staff. Physicians, nurses, and receptionists must be aware of new changes. Receptionists' misunderstanding of the vaccine needs frequently leads to missed opportunities to vaccinate. Misunderstanding between physicians and other clinicians can also lead to failed attempts. Regular office meetings should occur throughout the year to evaluate the vaccine schedule, the success of vaccinating the panel of patients, and considerations for practice improvements.

STANDING ORDERS

One of the most successful approaches in the office to make real efforts to improve immunization rates above and beyond that driven by the well child care schedule is to create standing orders that permit nursing staff to provide vaccines to patients without a doctor visit. This is particularly helpful with flu season and for acute care contacts with the patient. Such standing orders need to be written in such a way that they meet state law, facilitate nurse assessment of the patient's vaccine needs, as well as rule out any precautions or contraindications for the child's immunization. Materials exist online at the Immunization Action Coalition (www.immunize.org) that can help in writing such standing orders.

RECALL REMINDERS AND TRACKING

A second method for improving office vaccination rates are recall reminders and tracking. Providers should develop proactive approaches toward their patient panels to ensure compliance with the routine childhood schedule. Offices should contact patients when vaccines are due. Additional efforts should be made for those subjects who are behind in immunizations. Finally, offices should have systems to identify those children in families for whom the flu vaccine is indicated and make efforts every autumn to contact the families proactively and schedule immunization visits. The broadening of the flu vaccine indications has made this a major issue for office practices who care for either children or adults or both.

REPORTING ADVERSE EVENTS

The same laws that created the vaccine information statements and the protection for vaccine providers from frivolous lawsuits have also created the Vaccine Adverse Events Reporting System (VAERS). This system, set up by the federal government, collects information on adverse events believed to be related to immunization. These include certain ones required by regulation as well as those temporally associated with the immunizations that strike the provider or family as potentially significant. Vaccine manufacturers and providers are in fact required to report certain adverse events occurring after immunization whether or not they were caused by the immunization.

VAERS has actually led to the discontinuation of certain office-based immunization practices including the use of the tetravalent oral rhesus rotavirus vaccine (RotaShield). It has also helped to protect vaccines from unwarranted claims of harm. Although it has its weaknesses, statistical approaches have made it a powerful tool. Participation for providers of vaccines is required. All office staff, including receptionists, must understand the legal requirements of reporting.

VACCINES FOR CHILDREN

The U.S. government set up a program entitled Vaccines for Children (VFC) that enables providers to receive free-of-charge vaccines that can be given to patients with certain conditions including those who are younger than 18 years and are Medicaid eligible, uninsured, American Indian or Alaska Native, or whose health insurance benefit plan does not include vaccinations. Some recipients may be charged a vaccine provider fee, which is a limited amount. The federal government purchases vaccine for the VFC program and then distributes it to the state's health departments, which redistributes to the qualified providers. To learn how an office can participate, the VFC program can be contacted at the CDC through its web pages.

Common Problems

Offices that provide vaccines to their patients struggle with common problems in immunization practice. These include missed or delayed vaccinations, vaccine shortages, catch-up, change-ups, decisions not to vaccinate, true and false contraindications, multiple providers, and incomplete records. One cannot make these problems disappear, but one can prepare for them, prevent them from happening in many cases, and minimize the harm when they do occur.

MISSED OR DELAYED VACCINATIONS

Although daycare and school-based requirements have resulted in very high vaccine rates by school entry, on-time immunization is tragically low. Many children do not get their vaccines when due and are left at risk. Although this occurs more frequently among those with multiple providers and those who do not have health insurance, practitioners can change their office practices to reduce the problems in delayed immunizations. First of all, do not relegate routine immunization to the well child visit. Second, be assertive in obtaining the complete vaccine records from your patient's previous providers of health care. Third, create standing order policies to facilitate your office staff providing vaccines without a physician visit.

Furthermore, the practitioner should have charts available in the office explaining how to proceed with a child who has not received vaccines on time. Practitioners cannot be expected to memorize this information. It is complex, age dependent, and vaccine specific. The information must be available for ready reference. With the American Academies of Pediatrics and Family Practitioners, the ACIP has created catch-up schedules (www.cdc.gov/vaccines/recs/schedules). There are two catch-up schedules: one for children 4 months to 6 years of age and one for 7 to 18 years of age (Table 2).

LOCUS OF RESPONSIBILITY

Providers cannot expect their patients or their patients' parents, to take responsibility for timely vaccination. Patient-held immunization records have failed to improve vaccination rates. Office practitioners must also consider that even in a specialty practice their patients may be expecting them to monitor their immunization needs along with providing them the vaccines that they need. Providers, whether of specialty or primary care, must assess their individual patients and determine who is monitoring the patients' vaccination status and needs. Specialists must never assume that the patient is cognizant of the need or that a primary care provider is actively playing that role. All too often, patients relinquish their relationships with primary care providers once they begin an ongoing relationship with a specialist.

VACCINE SHORTAGES

Ongoing shortages do occur with vaccine supplies. Most famously are the shortages with the influenza vaccine, but we also have shortages with vaccines when there have been changes in use or recommendations such as the adoption of the adolescent diphtheria/tetanus (Td) at 11 years of age and the rapid acceptance of the pneumococcal conjugate vaccine (Prevar). Manufacturers struggle to produce adequate supplies knowing the expense of creating inadequate supplies actually leads to distrust and anger directed toward the manufacturer as well as difficulties in completing on-time immunizations. Manufacturing too much vaccine can lead to unusable stockpiles of expired vaccine product. Therefore manufacturers seek to reach a balance. Shortages are communicated best to office practices in the United States through the online Web site at the CDC where information is provided for the basis of shortages as well as explanations for what the practitioners should do during this time. In most situations the vaccine providers are expected to record those people who have not received the vaccine on time because of the shortage and are to be called back in a timely manner when vaccine supplies are available.

CATCH-UP

Catching children up on missed or delayed vaccinations is a major problem. This activity results not just because of shortages but because of parents' delays in immunization. The third and four child in a family often suffer delays in immunizations because of parents' issues with the organization and scheduling of appropriate on-time well child visits. Offices that rely on the well child visit schedules as the only basis for immunization have higher rates of vaccine delays and more problems with catch-up than those who use every opportunity of every visit to assess vaccine status of the child and to vaccinate on time. To make matters worse, the current schedule when on time can call for five injections at once. Imagine the child who has accumulated significant delays and now needs to be caught up. One of the major difficulties of catch-up is the problem of information. I previously mentioned the chart that all vaccine providers should have available to facilitate catching up immunizations (see Table 2).

CHANGE-UPS

Change-ups are also difficult because the new adoption of a vaccine can lead to some confusion for those who previously received an older moiety. For example, the recipients of the meningococcal polysaccharide vaccine (Menomune) are not due for the meningococcal conjugate vaccine (Menacta), but those who previously received the adolescent tetanus-diphtheria (Td) vaccine may certainly benefit from the new adolescent tetanus-diphtheria-reduced-dose-acellular pertussis vaccine (Tdap, Boostrix).

DECISIONS NOT TO VACCINATE

There are many reasons why patients may fail to be vaccinated. Common reasons include misunderstandings by the practitioner or parent of contraindications regarding vaccines. These are vaccine specific and complex in language in application. Many more people fail to get vaccines because of contraindications than those who truly have them. Other common reasons include parents' failure to attend to the well-visit schedule and the practitioners' failures to use other visits as the basis for immunization.

Some parents, however, actually consider immunization and choose to refuse. They are suspicious that the vaccines do not work, are not necessary or at least no longer necessary, are not safe, weaken the immune system, provide a poorer immunity than the actual diseases they target, that children receive too many vaccines, and that some vaccine lots are contaminated. Practitioners should be familiar with these concerns and their rebuttals. Two good sources for information on these include CDC (www.cdc.gov/vaccines) and the Immunization Action Coalition (www.immunize.org). The latter organization has actually collected stories of parents who chose not to vaccinate their children and then suffered the consequences of vaccine-preventable disease.

TRUE AND FALSE CONTRAINDICATIONS

Perhaps one of the most common problems with immunization delivery in the United States with regard to the failure of the provider stems from common misconceptions regarding the presence or absence of contraindication to immunization. Although some contraindications are vaccine specific, certain principles apply. First, family histories of adverse events are never contraindications to immunization. Second, household pregnancy or breast-feeding is never a contraindication to immunization. Third, the presence of an illness or injury by itself is not a contraindication. If the illness is moderate or severe, with or without a fever, then a vaccine's administration may be contraindicated. Although local and systemic adverse reactions do occur with vaccines, these are in general not contraindications to further doses.

It would be impossible for a practitioner to memorize contraindications. The CDC (www.cdc.gov/vaccines) has prepared a user-friendly online table that is indexed by disease and condition to guide the practitioner. This table should be available for ready use throughout the day.

MULTIPLE PROVIDERS AND INCOMPLETE RECORDS

Both under- and overimmunization occur much more frequently among patients who use more than one provider. Regional registries that allow practitioners to share their vaccine records greatly reduce both missed opportunities to vaccinate as well as the inadvertent administration of unnecessary doses. Practitioners should work with their local and state health departments to develop regional vaccine registries.

For all of the problems we face, for all of the intricacies of practices we must adopt, there is perhaps no one practice more important to the health of the community than the delivery of routine immunizations. Although it is worth the effort, it requires an ongoing commitment to continuing education, practice assessment, and evidence-based improvement of the office practice.

REFERENCES

American Academy of Family Physicians. "AAFP Immunization Resources." http://www.aafp.org/online/en/home/clinical/immunizationres.html. 2008. Accessed April 27, 2008. This web site provides links to specific AAFP recommendations for immunizations.

American Academy of Pediatrics. "AAP Policy." http://aappolicy.aappublications.org/. Accessed April 27, 2008. This web site provides links to the AAP policies including its online Red Book with its recommendations regarding vaccines and immunization.

Centers for Disease Control and Prevention. "ACIP Recommendations." http://www.cdc.gov/vaccines/pubs/ACIP-list.htm. This page last modified on April 3, 2008. Accessed April 27, 2008. This web site provides links to the ACIP recommendations, which are updated annually as new data dictate. All of the documents listed on this page are current, regardless of their publication dates.

Centers for Disease Control and Prevention. "2008 Child & Adolescent Immunization Schedules." http://www.cdc.gov/vaccines/recs/schedules/child-schedule.htm. This page last modified on March 17, 2008. Accessed April 27, 2008. This web site provides the harmonized schedule for children and adolescents with informative footnotes and additional charts for catch-up for children between the ages of 4 months and 18 years.

Centers for Disease Control and Prevention. "Adult Immunization Schedule." http://www.cdc.gov/vaccines/recs/schedules/adult-schedule.htm. This page last modified on January 28, 2008. Accessed April 27, 2008. This web site provides a harmonized schedule for anyone over 18 years old with informative footnotes.

Centers for Disease Control and Prevention. "Vaccine Information Statements." http://www.cdc.gov/vaccines/pubs/vis/default.htm. This page last modified on March 13, 2008. Accessed April 27, 2008. This web page lists links to all of the federally mandated Vaccine Information Statements that vaccine providers must use when informing parents of the recommended vaccines to be given to children.

Centers for Disease Control and Prevention. Vaccine Management: Recommendations for Storage and Handling Selected Biologicals. November 15, 2007. http://www.cdc.gov/vaccines/pubs/vac-mgt-book.htm. This page last modified on November 15, 2007. Last accessed April 27, 2008. This document provides vaccine-specific instructions on storage of vaccines.

Immunization Action Coalition. "State Mandates on Immunization and Vaccine-Preventable Diseases." http://www.immunize.org/laws/. Last updated April 27, 2007. Last access April 27, 2008. This web site provides specific state-by-state rules for school and day-care attendance.

Pickering LK, Baker CJ, Long SS, McMillan JA (eds): Red Book: 2006 Report of the Committee on Infectious Diseases. 27th ed, Elk Grove Village, IL: American Academy of Pediatrics, 2006.

Shefer A, Briss P, Rodewald L, et al: Improving immunization coverage rates: an evidence-based review of the literature. Epidemiologic Rev 1999;21(1):96-142. A systematic review of the published studies of interventions to improve vaccine uptake.

Travel Medicine

Method of
*Cynthia B. Snider, MD, MPH, and
William A. Petri, Jr., MD, PhD*

Travel medicine is an emerging subspecialty geared toward minimizing the risk of travel-related illness by educating travelers, providing immunization, and providing therapy, if needed, on their return. More than 50 million people from industrialized countries travel to the developing world annually, and 20% to 70% of travelers report some health problem associated with their recent travel. An estimated 4 million people seek medical care for their travel-related symptoms on an annual basis (Box 1).

Pretravel Counseling

In providing comprehensive medical advice to a patient about to embark on travel, it is important to know the preexisting medical conditions and assess the patient's risk of illness or injury. Pretravel counseling provides an excellent opportunity to review the need for vaccinations and provide general personal precautions. It is essential to obtain a detailed travel itinerary, type of travel, length of stay in each area, and expected activity. Because of the differences in local prevalence of infectious diseases, this information is necessary for determining appropriate chemoprophylaxis. Some activities, such as freshwater exposure, being exposed to wildlife, staying in a village while working for a nonprofit organization, or returning to visit family in rural settings can place travelers at added risk for contracting preventable diseases.

Travel-Related Infectious Illnesses

TRAVELER'S DIARRHEA

Traveler's diarrhea is defined as three or more watery stools in less than 24 hours. It is the most common illness to affect travelers. There is a 50% risk of having at least one attack of diarrhea in a 2-week trip.

BOX 1 Reducing the Number of Travel-Associated Illnesses

- Assess the patient's health at baseline prior to travel.
- Understand how the patient's preexisting medical condition can influence the options for chemoprophylaxis or immunizations for preventable diseases.
- Provide guidance and counseling in preparation for travel, including insect-bite and food and water precautions.
- Understand the spectrum of illness and the risk of acquiring certain infectious diseases in areas of travel by reviewing the patient's itinerary.
- Provide guidance regarding when to seek medical evaluation for post-travel illness.

Diarrhea affects 10% to 60% of travelers going to the developing world. In general, children are at greater risk for severe illness and are more susceptible to dehydration.

Pathogenesis

Traveler's diarrhea is usually contracted from contaminated food. Infection is often due to noninvasive enterotoxigenic *Escherichia coli* (ETEC), enteroaggregative *E. coli* (EAEC), or strains of *Campylobacter*, *Shigella*, or *Salmonella*. Viruses and parasites are less common causes but should still be considered in patients with chronic diarrhea. Viral threats include hepatitis A, hepatitis E, and Norwalk virus. Protozoa, including *Giardia intestinalis*, *Entomeba histolytica*, and *Cryptosporidium*, can also cause traveler's diarrhea. The cause of diarrhea is often unknown in 20% to 50% of cases.

Patients traveling to areas with poor hygiene should avoid consuming raw vegetables and fruits and unpasteurized dairy products. Pathogens can also be transmitted from contaminated tap water, ice, or improperly cooked foods (Box 2).

Treatment

Traveler's diarrhea is usually self-limited and lasts approximately 4 days. To minimize the morbidity associated with diarrhea, patients are encouraged to carry oral rehydration salts (CeraLyte) to be mixed with potable water to maintain electrolyte balance, particularly for children and the elderly (Table 1). Antibiotics should be reserved for moderate to severe disease. Up to 80% of patients are cured with a single dose of antibiotics. Drug treatment is summarized in Table 2.

For mild disease, bismuth subsalicylate (Pepto-Bismol) can reduce stool output and minimize the symptoms of diarrhea, nausea, and abdominal pain. Loperamide (Imodium), an over-the-counter synthetic opioid antimotility agent, can also be used. However,

BOX 2 Preventing Traveler's Diarrhea*

"Boil it, peel it, cook it, or forget it."
- Avoid vegetables or fruits that have not been peeled or cleaned.
- Avoid eating food from street vendors if it is not clear how the food is prepared or cooked.
- Eat food that is hot and cooked thoroughly. Avoid food that has been held at room temperature.
- Hot beverages such as tea and coffee, carbonated drinks, fruit juices, and bottled alcoholic beverages are safe to drink.
- Avoid ice unless is it made with bottled or boiled water.
- If safety of drinking water is questionable, drink bottled water.
- Boiling water for up to 1 minute is the most reliable method of treating possible contaminated water.
- Chemical treatment of water by either iodine or chloride is not effective against *Cryptosporidium* or *Giardia*.
- Filters may be used in some settings, such as hiking. Only the smaller microfilters with 0.1-0.3 μm pores can remove bacteria and protozoa; filters do not remove viruses. Filters with small pores can readily clog with large volumes of water, and they are often not effective for water with large sediment.
- Unpasteurized milk should be boiled before it is consumed.
- Ice cream that might have thawed and refrozen can be a potential source of foodborne illness. If the source is questionable, it should be avoided.

*Adapted from CDC information

TABLE 1 Composition of WHO Oral Rehydration Solution (ORS) for Diarrheal Illness			
Ingredient	Amount	Osmolality
Sodium chloride	2.6 g/L	75 mmol/L
Potassium chloride	1.5 g/L	20 mmol/L
Glucose	13.5 g/L	65 mmol/L
Trisodium citrate (or sodium bicarbonate)	2.9 g/L	10 mmol/L
Water	1 L	245 (Total)

loperamide should not be used in patients who have fever or bloody diarrhea. The side effect is constipation.

For moderate to severe diarrhea, as defined by persistent (>3 days) diarrhea or associated symptoms of fever or bloody stool, a short course of antibiotics is warranted. Self-treatment for 1 to 3 days with a fluoroquinolone such as ciprofloxacin (Cipro) is usually recommended.

Azithromycin (Zithromax)[1] is recommended for patients traveling to Southeast Asia, where there is a high prevalence of fluoroquinolone-resistant *Campylobacter*. Azithromycin can also be used for pregnant women, children, and patients who do not respond to a fluoroquinolone in 48 hours. Patients should see a physician if they do not respond to antibiotics or have bloody stools.

Another alternative is a nonabsorbed oral antibiotic, rifaximin, derived from rifampin. It is FDA approved for treating noninvasive forms of *E. coli* in travelers older than 12 years. Initial studies with travelers in Mexico showed efficacy similar to that of ciprofloxacin but with fewer side effects. It is still not known whether enteric organisms will develop resistance to rifaximin, as seen with rifampin.

Prophylaxis against traveler's diarrhea is not generally prescribed. Patients should be instructed to begin self-treatment if symptoms persist.

MALARIA

Malaria is a global public health problem. Forty percent of the world's population resides in endemic regions, and malaria causes 300 to 500 million infections each year. Despite taking a large human toll, malaria-related illness and death are largely preventable.

With the increase in international travel to malaria-endemic countries, a growing number of travelers are at risk for contracting this arthropod-borne illness. More than 500,000 travelers require chemoprophylaxis per year. In the United States, the Centers for Diseases Control and Prevention (CDC) reported 1324 malaria cases, including five fatalities, in 2004. In most of these cases, people were not taking the appropriate chemoprophylaxis regimen.

Epidemiology

In humans, malaria is an arthropod-borne illness transmitted by bites from infected female *Anopheles* mosquitos. It is caused by the parasite *Plasmodium*, with four species in particular: *Plasmodium falciparum*, *P. ovale*, *P. vivax*, and *P. malariae*. *P. falciparum* can cause rapid progressively severe illness with significant mortality.

The risk of acquiring malaria is influenced by geographic patterns. The predominant species of malaria transmitted in sub-Saharan Africa is *P. falciparum*, and there are higher malaria transmission rates in Africa than in other parts of the world. Due to decades of attempted disease eradication, drug-resistance patterns are seen throughout the world. Chloroquine-resistant *P. falciparum* (CRPF) is seen in sub-Saharan Africa and South America. A multi-drug resistant *P. falciparum* is now identified in border areas of Thailand with Cambodia and of Thailand with Myanmar.

Information about malaria risk in specific countries is tracked by various epidemiologic programs, including the CDC and World Health Organization (WHO). The most current information is on their Web sites (CDC travel information at http://www.cdc.gov/travel). The CDC has established a malaria hotline at 770-488-7788.

Chemoprophylaxis

Because there are no vaccines that completely guarantee protection against malaria, chemoprophylaxis and personal protection measures play a key role in malaria prevention (Table 3). Travelers should also be reminded that even if they have had malaria before, they can get it again, and so preventive measures are still necessary.

Atovaquone/proguanil (Malarone) is a fixed-combination antimalarial drug that is active on both blood and tissue schizonts. It can be used for both prophylaxis and treatment. Side effects include abdominal discomfort, nausea, vomiting, and headache. This medication is contraindicated in children who weigh less than 11 kg, pregnant women, mothers breast-feeding children who weigh less than 11 kg, patients with severe renal impairment, and patients with known allergies to either atovaquone or proguanil.

Doxycycline (Vibramycin) is effective against the erythrocytic stage of *Plasmodium* species but only minimally effective against liver schzonts, not enough to prevent relapse. It is effective for prophylaxis for chloroquine-resistant and mefloquine-resistant

---

[1]Not FDA approved for this indication.

TABLE 2 Self-Treatment for Traveler's Diarrhea		
Drug	Dosage	Comments
Antimotility Medications		
Bismuth subsalicylate (active ingredient in Pepto-Bismol)	1 oz liquid or 2 tablets q30min up to 8 doses Not to be used longer than 3 wk	Causes blackening of tongue, stool Not for those with renal insufficiency, anticoagulation therapy, or aspirin allergy Not for children with possible varicella or influenza because it can increase risk for Reye's syndrome
Loperamide (Imodium)	4 mg loading dose, then 2 mg after each loose stool, to a max 16 mg/d	Not for use in children <2 y Not to be used if patient has fever or bloody stools
Antibiotics		
Azithromycin (Zithromax)[1]	Adults: 1000 mg once or 500 mg qd for 3 d Children: 10 mg/kg/d	Preferred in children and in women who might be pregnant
Ciprofloxacin (Cipro)	500 mg bid for 1-3 d	Adjust dose for renal insufficiency Can interact with anticoagulation therapy
Levofloxacin (Levaquin)[1]	500 mg qd for 1-3 d	Adjust dose for renal insufficiency Can interact with anticoagulation therapy
Rifaximin (Xifaxan)	200 mg tid for 3 d	No need for renal or hepatic dosage adjustments

[1]Not FDA approved for this indication.
Abbreviation: max = maximum.

TABLE 3 Malaria Chemoprophylaxis

Medication	Adult Dosage	Pediatric Dosage
Areas of Chloroquine Resistance: Most of Africa, South America, except Paraguay, Argentina, Chile, Uruguay; parts of the Middle East, India, East Asia, and Southeast Asia		
Atovaquone-proguanil (Malarone)	250 mg/100 mg, take 1 tablet daily. Begin 1-2 d before entering the area and continue for 7 d after leaving	11-20 kg: 62.5 mg/25 mg, 1 pediatric tablet daily; 21-30 kg: 125 mg/50 mg, 2 pediatric tablets daily; 31-40 kg: 187.5 mg/75 mg, 3 pediatric tablets daily; >40 kg: 250 mg/100 mg dose, 1 adult tablet daily. All doses taken daily, as for adults. For >8 y old
Doxycycline (Vibramycin)	100 mg daily, take 1 tablet orally once daily. Begin 1-2 d before entering the area, and continue for 4 wk after leaving	2 mg/kg daily, (max dose, 100 mg/d)
Mefloquine HCl (Lariam)	228 mg base (250 mg salt) 1 tablet once per wk. Begin 1 wk before entering area and continue until 4 wk after leaving	<10 kg: 5 mg salt/kg weekly; 10-19 kg: one-quarter tablet; 20-30 kg: one-half tablet; 31-45 kg: three-quarters tablet; >45 kg, 1 tablet. All doses once/wk, as for adults. Can ask pharmacy to compound ingredients into 1 tablet if splitting medication is too difficult for the patient
Areas of Chloroquine Sensitivity: Haiti, the Dominican Republic, Central America west of the Panama Canal, and parts of the Middle East (resistance in Iran, Oman, Saudi Arabia, and Yemen)		
Chloroquine phosphate (Aralen)	300 mg base (500 mg salt) 1 tablet once per wk. Begin 1 wk before entering area and continue for 4 wk after leaving	5 mg base/kg body weight (8.3 mg salt/kg), up to adult dose, once/wk
Areas of Mefloquine Resistance: Parts of Southeast Asia, specifically borders between Thailand, Myanmar, and Cambodia		
Doxycycline	100 mg daily, take 1 tablet orally once daily. Begin 1-2 d before entering the area, and continue for 4 wk after leaving	2 mg/kg daily, (max dose, 100 mg/d)
Rare Circumstances: Alternative when other prophylactic agents are contraindicated or unavailable		
Primaquine	15 mg base daily, 2 tablets orally once daily. Begin 1-2 d before entering area and continue until 7 d after leaving	0.5 mg/kg daily, up to adult dose, as for adults

P. falciparum. Side effects include nausea, vomiting, abdominal discomfort, and photosensitivity. Patients should be cautioned to use sunscreen when taking doxycycline. Doxycycline can cause yeast infections in female patients and interferes with oral contraceptives. Doxycycline is contraindicated in pregnant women, children younger than 8 years, and patients with known allergies to tetracycline-related drugs.

Mefloquine (Lariam) is effective against the erythrocytic stages of *Plasmodium* species. It is commonly used for prophylaxis but does not prevent *P. vivax* or *P. ovale* relapses. Side effects include headache, nausea, dizziness, anxiety, sleep disturbances, vivid dreams, and visual hallucinations. The severe adverse effects include depression, seizure, and psychosis. Patients with active or recent history of depression, generalized anxiety disorder, schizophrenia, or psychosis should not take mefloquine. It should not be prescribed for those who have underlying seizure disorders or arrhythmias. Mefloquine prophylaxis in the second and third trimesters is not associated with adverse fetal or pregnancy outcome.

In instances where no other antimalarial drug is tolerated, primaquine may serve as an alternative primary prophylaxis. The use of primaquine for malaria chemoprophylaxis should be reviewed by infectious disease physicians or physicians certified in travel medicine. Primaquine can cause severe adverse effects, specifically a fatal hemolysis in those with glucose-6-phosphate dehydrogenase (G6PD) deficiency. Patients must be tested for G6PD deficiency, and normal G6PD levels must be documented before patients take this medication. The side effects include nausea, abdominal discomfort, and vomiting. Contraindications include G6PD deficiency, pregnancy, breast-feeding of children with unknown G6PD levels, and allergy to primaquine.

Personal Protective Measures

Personal protective measures (Box 3) also help minimize mosquito exposure. DEET (N,N-diethyl-m-tolulamide) is one of the most effective topical insect repellents that can be applied to exposed skin. It repels mosquitoes, fleas, ticks, chiggers, and some flies. Concentrations of 20% to 30% DEET protect for approximately 6 to 12 hours. Higher concentrations do not have higher efficacy rates but do last longer. DEET is not recommended for infants younger than 2 months, but it can be used on children and older infants. Side effects include skin sensitivity and decreased effectiveness of sunscreen. Higher concentrations of DEET are known for dissolving plastic-containing materials.

Permethrin 0.5% (Permanone) is an insecticide spray that can be used on clothing and mosquito nets, tents, and sleeping bags.

BOX 3 Personal Protective Measures to Prevent Insect Bites

- Malaria-transmitting mosquitoes are most active in the evening. Mosquitoes known to transmit dengue are active in the daytime.
- Sleep in screened areas, and use mosquito nets, preferably permethrin-impregnated nets.
- Wear clothing that covers arms and legs.
- Use insect repellent containing 20%-30% DEET.

Abbreviation: DEET = N,N-diethyl-m-toluamide.

> **BOX 4 Preventive Measures to Minimize Accident-Related Injury**
>
> - Wear shoes, long sleeves, and pants when engaging in off-road sports or riding on motorcycles.
> - Wear safety belts in motor vehicles.
> - Wear helmets when riding on motorcycles.
> - Minimize driving in the evening when there is poor visibility of road landmarks and increased incidence of drivers under the influence of alcohol.
> - Use safety flotation vests when engaging in water activities such as kayaking and rafting.

Pretreated clothing or sleeping bags retain its effects despite multiple launderings, up to 2 or more months.

Noninfectious Travel Risks

Travelers should be counseled to follow general safety precautions (Box 4). An estimated 5 million people were killed secondary to injuries in 2000. Ninety percent of these injury-related deaths are in middle- to lower-income countries. About 1.2 million fatalities are motor-vehicle related. A study assessing U.S. citizens traveling to Mexico showed 51% injury-related causes of death, 18% of which were motor vehicle related.[17]

Patients should consider purchasing supplemental health insurance policies that include 24-hour access to emergency evacuation and treatment.

TRAVEL KITS

Travelers should be encouraged to carry their medications with them in the original pharmacy bottles rather than packed in their luggage, in case the luggage is separated from the traveler. In addition, a list of the medications, including generic name, dosage, and reason for taking them, could be useful if the traveler needs to purchase more medication. If the patient uses syringes and needles for a health condition (e.g., diabetes), a medical letter detailing the necessity of these medical supplies can avert interrogation. A patient with a cardiac history should carry a copy of the latest electrocardiogram.

JET LAG

Jet lag is caused by the alteration in circadian rhythm caused by traveling through several time zones. It is more common in travelers going east to west across more than five time zones. Symptoms of jet lag include fatigue, malaise, headache, anorexia, insomnia, and difficulty with concentration. It is alleviated by acclimating to the destination's day and night schedule by not sleeping during daytime hours. Symptoms will dissipate once the biological clock adjusts to the destination time zone. Jet lag generally does not last more than a few days. Good sleep hygiene and hydration promote recovery from jet lag. The use of short-acting hypnotics is controversial. Some research suggests melatonin can reduce effects of jet lag; however, the safety of this remedy has not been scientifically established.

DEEP VENOUS THROMBOSIS

There are increasing reports of deep venous thrombosis and pulmonary embolism associated with airplane travel. A recent study reports a twofold increase in risk passengers traveling by plane, car, or train longer than 4 hours. The risk is highest in persons with factor V Leiden or body mass index greater than 30. Other risk factors include a prior history of deep venous thrombosis or pulmonary embolism, hypercoagulable states, and pregnancy. Travelers are encouraged to wear elastic stockings and to walk about the plane every 30 to 60 minutes.

MOTION SICKNESS

Motion sickness is often triggered by an inner ear imbalance. Motion sickness induces nausea, diaphoresis, anorexia, lethargy, and vomiting. Motion sickness is aggravated by up-and-down movement of the head and neck and by traveling in small aircraft or cars.

Many medications can remedy the symptoms of motion sickness. Children do best with antihistamines such as diphenhydramine (Benadryl), dimenhydrinate (Dramamine), or promethazine (Phenergan). The side effects of these antihistamines are largely sedation and drowsiness. They are most effective if taken before onset of motion sickness symptoms. Adults can also use these same antihistamine agents, or they may take meclizine (Bonine, Antivert) or scopolamine.

The scopolamine transdermal patch (Transderm-Scop) is effective for 72 hours. The side effects are chiefly anticholinergic, including dry mouth and mydriasis, but it is also known to cause hallucination and delirium in the elderly. The patch is contraindicated for children younger than 12 years and patients with glaucoma or urinary retention.

All of these medications should not be used concomitantly with alcoholic beverages, because alcohol can worsen effects on the sensorium.

HIGH-ALTITUDE SICKNESS

High-altitude sickness is seen not only in mountain climbers but also in patients traveling to high-altitude destinations. Some patients inquire about their risk of altitude-related illness. It is difficult to predict who will have symptoms, because some patients have mild symptoms at 4000 ft (1200 m). Risks are greatest with abrupt ascent above 9000 ft (2700 m). Minimizing morbidity associated with high-altitude sickness can be achieved through educating travelers to recognize symptoms and seek appropriate medical care.

High-altitude sickness includes the following syndromes: acute mountain sickness (AMS), high-altitude pulmonary edema (HAPE), and high-altitude cerebral edema (HAPE). Symptoms of AMS include headache, fatigue, anorexia, nausea, and vomiting. Symptoms of HAPE include dyspnea on exertion and productive cough, with progression to dyspnea at rest. Symptoms of HACE include altered mental status, severe lethargy, confusion, and truncal ataxia.

AMS can be prevented by acclimating to the specific altitude and not sleeping at a higher altitude if having symptoms of AMS. Drug prevention and treatment include acetazolamide (Diamox) 125 mg twice a day, starting 1 or 2 days before ascent and continuing for 2 or 3 days after reaching maximum altitude. Higher doses of acetazolamide are not proven to be more effective in treating AMS, but they do increase the medication's side effects. Prophylaxis is not routinely recommended.

HAPE and HACE must be urgently evaluated, and rapid descent is critical in managing these syndromes. Medications that can alleviate symptoms include acetazolamide, dexamethasone (Decadron), and nifedipine (Adalat).[1]

Immunizations

The traveler's recommended immunizations depend on their destination. Some countries require documentation of specific vaccinations, such as certain African countries requiring yellow fever vaccination or Saudi Arabia requiring meningococcal vaccination of travelers during the Hajj. Box 5 shows criteria for recommending immunizations. Table 4 describes the vaccines.

---
[1]Not FDA approved for this indication.

BOX 5 Vaccine Advice for Travelers

Vaccine advice should be based on the following factors:
- Prevalence of vaccine-preventable disease
- Risk behavior that can place the patient at risk for acquiring disease
- Potential side effects of the vaccine
- Previous vaccination records
- Underlying health problems that predispose the patient to adverse outcomes from the vaccine, such as immunocompromise, pregnancy, egg allergy

ROUTINE IMMUNIZATIONS

Travelers should be up to date with routine immunizations including measles, mumps, and rubella (MMR); tetanus, diphtheria, and pertussis (Tdap); varicella; *Haemophilus influenzae* type b and other influenza; polio; and hepatitis B. Adults should have had at least one polio booster (IPV) as an adult. Pneumococcal vaccination should be offered to travelers who are older than 65 years, those who are immunocompromised, patients with functional or anatomic asplenia, and those who have chronic illnesses such as diabetes, renal disease, or pulmonary disease. Refer to the CDC National Immunization Program (http://www.cdc.gov/Nip/) for guidelines.

TABLE 4 Travel Immunization Doses

Vaccine Name	Dosage	Comments
Hepatitis A Vaccines		
Havrix	Age 1–18 y: 720 EU IM (0.5 mL), 2nd dose at 0, 6-18 mo	Two doses provide lifelong immunity Vaqta may be substituted for the 2nd dose Giving the 2nd dose at a longer interval does not interfere with immune response
	Age $\geq$ 19 y: 1440 EU IM (1.0 mL), 2 doses at 0 and 6-12 mo	
Vaqta	Age 1-18 y: 25 U IM (0.5 mL), 2 doses at 0, 6-18 mo	Two doses provide lifelong immunity Havrix may be substituted for the 2nd dose Giving the 2nd dose at a longer interval does not interfere with immune response
	Age $\geq$ 19 y: 50 U IM (1.0 mL), 2 doses at 0, 6-12 mo	
Hepatitis B Vaccine		
Engerix-B	Age 0-19 y: 10 µg IM (0.5 mL), 3 doses given at 0, 1, 6 mo	No need to restart a series that has been interrupted Engerix-B and Recombivax-HB may be used interchangeably in the 3-dose schedule only the 3-dose schedule only
	Age $\geq$ 20 y: 20 µg IM (1.0 mL), 3 doses at 0, 1, 6 mo, or 4 doses at 0, 1, 2, 12 mo	
Recombivax-HB	Age 0-19 y: 5 µg, 3 doses at 0, 1, 6 mo	Engerix-B and Recombivax-HB may be used interchangeably in the 3-dose schedule only
	Age 11-15 y: 10 µg, 2 doses at 0, 4-6 mo Age $\geq$ 20 y: 10 µg, 3 doses at 0, 1, 6 mo	
Hepatitis A and B Vaccine		
Twinrix	Age $\geq$ 18 y: 720 EU or 20 µg IM (1.0 mL), 3 doses given at 0, 1, 6 mo	
Japanese Encephalitis		
JE Vax	Age 1-2 y: 0.5 mL SC $\geq$ 3 y 1.0 mL SC 3 doses given on d 0, 7, 30	High adverse reactions profile for JE vaccine, including generalized urticaria or angioedema, can occur within min or following vaccination. Most reactions occur in 48 h but can be as late as 17 d after vaccination. Vaccinated persons should be observed for 30 min after vaccination and warned about the possibility of delayed generalized urticaria, often in a generalized distribution or angioedema of the extremities, face, and oropharynx, especially of the lips. They should be advised to remain in areas where they have ready access to medical care and should not embark on international travel within 10 d after receiving a dose of JE vaccine Booster dose: 1 dose at 24 mo, but the full duration of protection is not known
Meningococcal Polysaccharide		
Menomune (quadrivalent A, C, Y, W-135)	Age $\geq$ 2 y: 50 µg SC (0.5 mL), 1 dose	May be given for short-term protection against group A to infants 3 mo Revaccination of a single 0.5-mL dose administered subcutaneously may be indicated for persons at high risk for infection, particularly children who were first vaccinated when they were < 4 y; such children should be considered for revaccination after 2 or 3 y if they remain at high risk Although the need for revaccination in older children and adults has not been determined, antibody levels decline rapidly over 2-3 y, and revaccination may be considered within 5 y

Continued

TABLE 4 Travel Immunization Doses—cont'd

Vaccine Name	Dosage	Comments
Meningococcal Polysaccharide Diptheria Toxoid Conjugate		
Menactra (quadrivalent A, C, Y, W-135)	Age 11-55 y: 4 µg of each antigen IM (0.5 mL)	The need for or timing of a booster dose has not been determined
Rabies		
Imovax (human diploid cell vaccine) HDCV, RVA (rabies vaccine adsorbed) RabAvert (purified chick embryo cell vaccine [PCEC])	All ages, 2.5 IU rabies antigen IM (1.0 mL), 3 doses given at 0, 7, and 21 or 28 d	The full course should be given with the same product. Travelers who are immunosuppressed should avoid travel to endemic areas and postpone vaccination. If this cannot be avoided, antibody titers should be checked after vaccination. If traveler has frequent exposure to rabies (spelunkers, veterinarians, rabies diagnostic laboratory workers, animal control workers in rabies-epizootic areas), check serologic testing for necessary booster doses
Typhoid		
Injectable (Typhim V)i	Age ≥ 2 y: 25 µg IM (0.5 mL)	Booster dose every 2 y if ongoing risk
Oral live attenuated (Vivotif Berna)	Age ≥ 6 y: 1 capsule every other d for 4 doses (on d 0, 2, 4, 6)	Booster dose: same as the initial four-capsule dose after 5 y. Do not take with antibiotics, which kill the attenuated Vivotif bacterium
Yellow Fever		
Attenuated virus vaccine (YF-VAX)	Age ≥ 9 mo: 1 injection 0.5 mL SC	African countries might require evidence of vaccination from all entering travelers, including if only in transit, and some might waive the requirements for travelers staying less than 2 wk who are coming from areas where there is no current evidence of significant risk of contracting yellow fever. The certificate becomes valid 10 d after vaccination with YF-VAX. Booster every 10 y if ongoing risk. Avoid in pregnant women, unless high-risk travel.

Note: Table is based on *Health Information for International Travel* 2005-2006, (http://www.cdc.gov/travel/yb/index.htm). manufacturer's full prescribing information should be consulted to confirm pediatric doses.

REQUIRED IMMUNIZATIONS

Meningitis

Meningococcal vaccine is a quadrivalent vaccine against *Neisseria meningitides*, serogroups A,C,Y, and W135. It does not protect against type B, which represents one third of meningitis cases in the United States. One form (Menactra) is conjugated to diphtheria toxoid. Side effects include headache, fatigue, and malaise, in addition to the pain, induration, and redness at the site of infection. These effects are reportedly more common than with Menomune, but they are similar to those with tetanus toxoid.

Saudi Arabia requires certification of immunization if traveling during the Hajj. It is also recommended for adults and children older than 2 years who are traveling to areas known as the *meningitis belt* in sub-Saharan Africa, from Senegal and Guinea eastward to Ethiopia. The vaccine should also be offered to persons who will have prolonged contact with people from this region or those living in refugee camps and to persons working in the health care settings in these regions.

Yellow Fever

Yellow fever vaccine (YF-Vax) is a single-dose live, attenuated virus preparation made from the 17D yellow fever virus strain, produced in chick embryo. Historically, it is reported to be one of the safest and most effective live virus vaccines. It should be administered at least 10 days before entering an endemic area, which includes sub-Saharan Africa and tropical South America. Various African countries require an international certification of vaccination or a physician's waiver letter for all entering travelers.

The vaccine can be administered concurrently with hepatitis A and B, typhoid fever, and meningococcal vaccines. Safety of the vaccine during pregnancy is not established, nor is it known if vaccine is excreted in human milk.

Adverse reactions include a vaccine virus–associated encephalitis, which occurs predominantly in infants and immunocompromised patients. Thus, the vaccine is not recommended for infants younger than 9 months, and it is contraindicated in infants younger than 6 months. Travelers with HIV/AIDS, leukemia, lymphoma, or other immunosuppressive disorders and travelers older than 65 years are at greater risk for systemic adverse effects. Risks and benefits of vaccination should be evaluated on a case-by-case basis. A rare risk of viscerotropic disease (estimated at 1 in 400,000 dose administered) is associated with the vaccine, which can result in fatal organ failure.

RECOMMENDED IMMUNIZATIONS

Hepatitis

Hepatitis A is the most common vaccine-preventable travel-related illness. Most hepatitis A cases are imported into the United States by travelers to Mexico and Central America. Hepatitis A virus vaccine (Havrix, Vagta) is now part of routine childhood immunization in the United States. It recommended to those traveling to countries other than the United States, Canada, Western Europe, Australia, New Zealand, Japan, and South Korea. It consists of two IM injections separated by 6 to 18 months. The initial dose should be given 2 to 4 weeks before departure. Antibodies reach protective levels in more than 95% of vaccinees after the first dose. The second dose confers more than 10 years of immunity. Two hepatitis A vaccines are available in the United States, and they can be used interchangeably.

Immunization is not recommended for children younger than 1 year. Children younger than 1 year and other travelers who cannot receive the vaccine should be given immune globulin (0.02 mL/kg IM if traveling for less than 3 months, or 0.06 mL/kg IM if traveling for longer than 3 months.

Hepatitis B virus vaccine (Engerix-B, Recombivax-HB) is a recombinant hepatitis B surface antigen vaccine composed of three doses taken at 0, 1, and 6 months. It is approved for all ages. It is recommended for travelers possibly engaging in voluntary medical care. It is also available as a combined vaccination with Hepatitis A (Twinrix).

Typhoid Fever

Typhoid vaccine is available in two formulations: as a live attenuated oral vaccine (Vivotif Berna) and as a purified capsular polysaccharide parenteral vaccine (Typhim Vi). This vaccine is recommended for those traveling to Central and South America, the Indian subcontinent, Africa, and Asia and to those traveling outside routine tourist destinations.

The parenteral formulation is a single IM injection given 2 weeks before departure for children older than 2 years and adults. It confers immunity for 2 to 3 years.

The oral formulation taken every other day for a total of 4 capsules, also administered 2 weeks before departure. It confers immunity for 5 years. The effectiveness of the oral vaccine is reduced if it is taken concomitantly with antibiotics. It is recommended for adults and children older than 6 years. Because the oral formulation is a live attenuated vaccine, it is not recommended for immunocompromised persons.

Rabies

Rabies is endemic in Africa, Asia, India, and Latin America. Preexposure immunization against rabies (Imovax, RVA, RabAvert) is recommended only for travelers with an occupational risk of exposure and for those planning to have animal exposure in endemic regions where immediate access to medical care might be limited.

After sustaining a skin-penetrating scratch or bite from a potentially rabid animal, the traveler should be seen by a physician for evaluation. Patients who have received preexposure prophylaxis should promptly receive two additional doses of vaccine on day 0 and day 3. Those who sustain exposure with no prior immunization require treatment with rabies immune globulin (Bayrab) and five doses over the course of 28 days of an approved vaccine.

Assessing Illness in the Return Traveler

Epidemiologic studies from the 1980s and 1990s estimated 50% of travelers report a health problem (based on 100,000 people traveling to developing countries for 1 month). About 8000 of these patients will seek care, and roughly 300 will be hospitalized for their illness.

The approach to assessing patients returning from international travel is to emphasize clinical manifestations and understand the importance of infectious diseases affecting these returned travelers. A few common infectious causes of illness to returning travelers are discussed here, but the list is by no means complete. Returning travelers should be seen by a physician with a specialty in travel medicine or infectious diseases to be evaluated for their symptoms.

A recent study using GeoSentinel surveillance data from 1998-2004 of 17,300 returned travelers from 230 countries found that two thirds of the diagnoses fell into four major syndromic categories of acute febrile illness, acute diarrhea, dermatologic disorders, and chronic diarrhea. Sixty-four percent presented within 1 month of travel. However, 10% had an indolent course and were not seen until 6 months after their return. Malaria was one of the three most frequent causes of systemic febrile illness and was disproportionately seen in persons traveling to sub-Saharan Africa and Southeast Asia. Acute diarrhea was seen more often in travelers returning from Southeast Asia. Acute diarrhea was predominantly bacterial diarrhea; however, travelers from other areas presented with parasite-induced diarrhea more often than bacterial diarrhea. More dermatologic problems were seen in those visiting Central and South America and the Caribbean (Figure 1).

FEVER

An estimated 3% of international travelers report new onset of fever. Undifferentiated fever can represent a large differential of diseases, including malaria, enteric fever, rickettsial infections, and meningitis. The potentially most dangerous causes of fever in returning travelers include malaria, typhoid, dengue, leptospirosis, and rickettsial

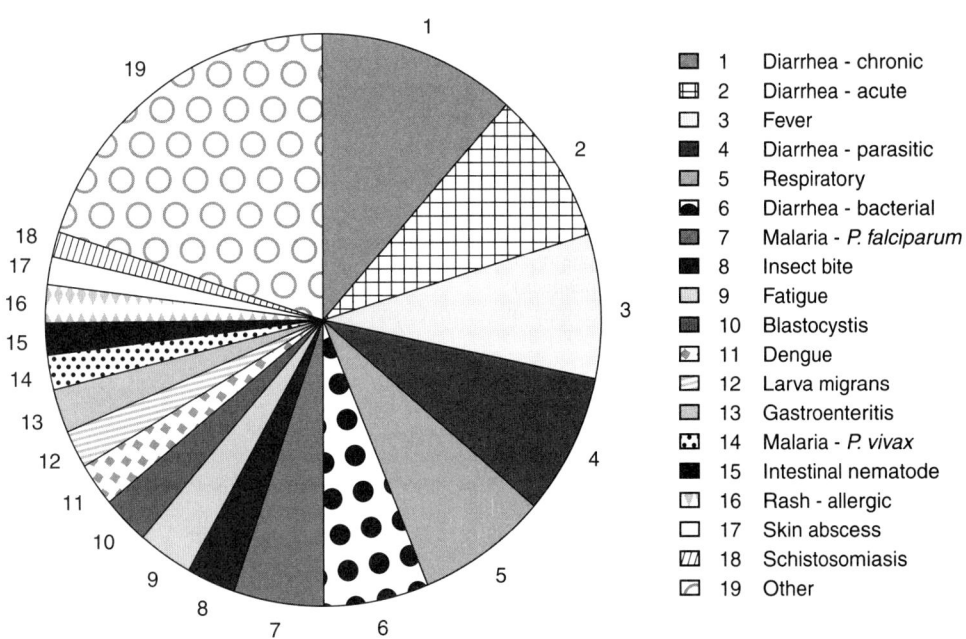

FIGURE 1. Illnesses occurring in travelers to the developing world.

diseases. Travel, incubation period, duration and pattern associated with symptoms, immunizations, and use of chemoprophylaxis for malaria should be carefully assessed.

Malaria

Malaria can pose a significant health risk to travelers due to the severity of illness in nonimmune patients. Ninety percent of travelers who contract malaria do not become ill until they return home. The estimated risk of a traveler acquiring malaria will differ depending on region of travel, the time and type of travel, and the intensity of transmission. In epidemiologic surveillance from 1985 through 2002, 11,896 cases of malaria among U.S. civilians were reported to the CDC. The majority, 6961 cases (59%), were acquired in sub-Saharan Africa in comparison with 2237 cases (19%) in Asia and 1672 cases (14%) in the Caribbean and Central and South America. During this period, 76 fatal malaria infections occurred among U.S. civilians; 71 (93%) were caused by *P. falciparum*, of which 52 (73%) were acquired in sub-Saharan Africa.

Studies suggest that the incubation times vary for different malaria species. *P. falciparum* malaria is typically evident within 4 weeks of the traveler's return. *P. ovale* and *P. vivax* malaria, however, can occur much later—as long as 2 to 12 months after the traveler's return. This is significant, because of those late-onset cases of malaria, 60% of the travelers were adherent to their chemoprophylaxis regimen.

Any person who has traveled to malaria-endemic regions and subsequently experiences a fever, chills, headache, nausea, vomiting, or influenza-like symptoms within 3 months of travel should seek immediate medical attention. This syndrome should be considered a medical emergency, and the traveler should report the travel history to the clinician. Thick and thin blood films should be collected as part of the investigations for malaria. The blood films should be repeated every 12 to 24 hours when the patient is symptomatic to catch different levels of blood parasites on stains. Delay in diagnosis and treatment of malaria infections results in serious and, perhaps, fatal outcomes.

Recommendations concerning diagnosis and treatment of malaria can be obtained through the CDC's malaria hotline and from http://www.cdc.gov/malaria/diagnosis_treatment/treatment.htm.

Dengue Fever

Dengue fever is one of most common causes of systemic febrile illness. It occurs in all regions of travel including sub-Saharan Africa and Central America. However, travelers from sub-Saharan Africa were noted to have more cases of fever caused by rickettsial and tickborne illness versus dengue fever.[8]

Dengue fever, also known as breakbone fever, is a flavivirus transmitted by day-biting mosquitoes, *Aedes aegypti*. There are four serotypes of dengue (DEN1 through DEN4) and no cross immunity among them. No vaccination is available, but repellents are an effective preventive measure.

Seasonal epidemics of dengue infections are common in tropical and subtropical regions. Dengue is endemic to the South Pacific, Asia, the Caribbean, the Americas, and Africa. It is responsible for 12,000 deaths per year. After a 4- to 7-day incubation period, dengue manifests with influenza-like symptoms, including high fevers, headache, myalgias, and arthralgias. Fifty percent of patients report signs of maculopapular rash 3 to 5 days after the onset of fever.

The disease is self-limited. Patients should be encouraged to rest, keep hydrated, and use acetaminophen for fevers. If the disease is a severe form, such as dengue shock syndrome or, rarer, dengue hemorrhagic fever, the patient will need intravenous fluid hydration and supportive care. This disease is diagnosed clinically and by comparison of acute and convalescent serum antibody titers. There is no specific treatment but only supportive care.

Typhoid Fever

Typhoid fever is caused by *Salmonella enterica typhi*, which produces an acute febrile illness. Typhoid fever is endemic to the Indian subcontinent, Asia, Africa, the Caribbean, and Central and South America. There are an estimated 22 million cases with 200,000 deaths worldwide. The CDC reports 400 cases per year in the United States, and 70% of these cases are associated with travel.

The vaccine does not provide 100% protection. Risks for typhoid fever are minimized by decreasing exposure to fecal-oral contaminated foods and using the "boil it, peel it, cook it, or forget it" strategy (see Box 2).

Typhoid can have an insidious onset, with ongoing fevers, malaise, abdominal discomfort, constipation, and, rarely, diarrhea. If typhoid fever is suspected in a returned traveler, serology assays should be ordered and the patient should be empirically treated with fluoroquinolones or a third-generation cephalosporin.

Rickettsia

Rickettsial infection is a tickborne illness transmitted by an arthropod vector. African tick typhus, Mediterranean tick typhus, and scrub typhus are a few of the rickettsial infections seen in returned travelers if they come into contact with environments that support these pathogens. Most patients with rickettsial infections recover with timely use of appropriate antibiotic therapy.

Clinical manifestations of rickettsial illnesses can start as a triad of nonspecific symptoms, fever, headache, and myalgias. Specific symptoms include regional lymphadenopathy, rash, and thrombocytopenia. A painless eschar is seen in scrub typhus.

Diagnosis of rickettsial disease is based on the clinical picture and epidemiologic history, isolation of the rickettsial agent by a positive polymerase chain reaction (PCR) test, immunohistologic detection of a microorganism, or by comparison of acute and convalescent serum titers. Patients should be promptly treated with antibiotic therapy and monitored for worsening condition.

DIARRHEA

Diarrhea in the acute setting is often caused by bacterial organism; however, diarrhea that is persistent and does not respond to antibiotics could be complicated by parasitic infections, antibiotic-resistant bacterial infections, and possibly a postinfectious irritable bowel syndrome. A recent study identified 60% of diarrhea in return travelers to be caused by parasites, except to cases coming from Southeast Asia. Patients with bacterial diarrhea often came from Southeast Asia with *Campylobacter* as one of the main causative organisms. The top causes for parasitic diarrhea include giardiasis and amebiasis. Sensitivities of diagnosis of *Giardia intestinalis*, *Cryptosporidium*, and *Entamoeba histolytica* have improved with use of reverse-transcriptase PCR testing. The key to managing return travelers with diarrhea is to properly investigate their history, especially their antibiotic use, and provide appropriate therapy while conducting investigatory testing to determine the cause of the diarrheal illness (Figure 2).

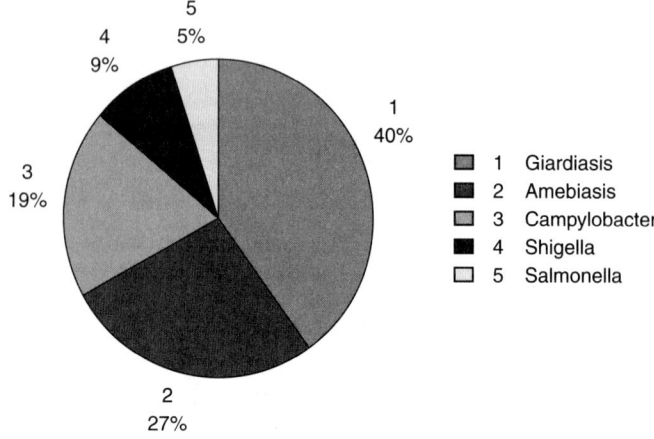

FIGURE 2. Distribution of causes of acute diarrhea in returned travelers.

BOX 6	Web Sites Giving Health Advice for Travelers

- American Society of Tropical Medicine and Hygiene: http://www.astmh.org/
- Centers for Diseases Control and Prevention, health information for international travel: http://www.cdc.gov/travel/index.htm
- Central Intelligence Agency, World Factbook: https://www.cia.gov/library/publications/the-world-factbook/index.html
- Health Canada, Current Travel Health Notices: https://www.cia.gov/library/publications/the-world-factbook/index.html
- International Society of Travel Medicine: http://www.istm.org/
- Travax, travel medicine subscription recommendations: http://www.shoreland.com/
- United States Department of Health, travel warnings: http://www.travel.state.gov/travel/travel_1744.html
- World Health Organization, international travel and health: http://www.who.int/ith/en/

DERMATOLOGIC CONDITIONS

Skin lesions and rashes represent up to 8% of illnesses of travelers seeking medical care after recent travel. The etiology of skin lesions can include insect bites, larval infestations, bacterial infections, or drug-related hypersensitivity. The diagnosis of the lesions will depend on identifying the location, their dermatologic pattern and other associated symptoms, and the patient's activity when first noticing the lesion.

Papules are often associated with insect bites, such as scabies. Subcutaneous painful nodules can be seen with myiasis, tungiasis, and furuncles. Myiasis is caused by invading larvae of the tumbu fly in Africa or the botfly in Latin America. Patients often report the sensation of movement under the lesion.

Cutaneous ulcers are often due to pyoderma secondarily infected with *Staphylococcus aureus* or group A streptococci. Painless ulcerative lesions with raised margins and isolated lymphadenopathy should suggest leishmania. Linear or serpiginous lesions, often found on the feet or buttocks, should bring to mind cutaneous larva migrans.

Summary

Clinicians who provide medical advice to travelers should be proficient in travel medicine and global epidemiology of infectious diseases. Travel medicine has become specialized, and thus the consultation with a specialist in travel or tropical medicine may be advantageous for travelers who live abroad for any length of time, who have multiple medical problems, who are immunocompromised, who are pregnant, or who are traveling with young children to developing countries. Patients presenting with illness and recent history of travel would also benefit from evaluation by such specialists, because travel medicine specialists have the expertise in seeing various infectious diseases in returning travelers and could expedite the appropriate diagnosis and treatment of the manifesting illness. A listing of travel clinics can be obtained through the American Society of Tropical Medicine and Hygiene. A list of helpful Web sites is given in Box 6.

REFERENCES

Advice for travelers. Treat Guidel Med Lett 2006;4(:45):25-34.
Cannegieter SC, Doggen CJ, Van Houwelingen HC, Rosendaal FR: Related venous thrombosis: Results from a large population-based case control study (MEGA study). PLoS Med 2006;3(8):e307.
Cetron MS, Marfin AA, Julian KG, et al: Yellow fever vaccine. Recommendations of the Advisory Committee on Immunization Practices (ACIP), 2002. MMWR Recomm Rep 2002;51(RR-17):1-10.
Dupont HL, Jiang ZD, Okhuysen PC, et al: Antibacterial chemoprophylaxis in the prevention of traveler's diarrhea: Evaluation of poorly absorbed oral rifaximin. Clin Infect Dis 2005;41:S571-S576.
Eliades MJ, Shah S, Nguyen-Dinh P, et al: Malaria surveillance—United States, 2003. MMWR Surveill Summ 2005;54(2):25-39.
Freedman DO, Weld LH, Kozarsky PE, et al: Spectrum of disease and relation to place of exposure among ill returned travelers. N Engl J Med 2006;354(2):119-130.
Guptill KS, Hargarten SW, Baker TD: American travel deaths in Mexico: Causes and prevention strategies. West J Med 1991;154(2):169-171.
Hill DR, Ericsson CD, Pearson RD, et al: The practice of travel medicine: Guidelines by the Infectious Diseases Society of America. Clin Infect Dis 2006;43(12):1499-1539.
McInnes RJ, Williamson LM, Morrison A: Unintentional injury during foreign travel: A review. J Travel Med 2002;9:297-307.
Peden M, Scurfield R, Sleet D, et al: World Report on Road Traffic Injury Prevention Geneva: World Health Organization, 2004.
Prevention of malaria. Med Lett Drugs Ther 2005;47(1223-1224):100-102.
Ryan ET, Kain KC: Health advice and immunizations for travelers. N Engl J Med 2000;342(23):1716-1725.
Ryan ET, Wilson ME, Kain KC: Illness after international travel. N Engl J Med 2002;347(7):505-516.
Schwartz E, Parise M, Kozarsky P, Cetron M: Delayed onset of malaria: Implications for chemoprophylaxis in travelers. N Engl J Med 2003;349(16):1510-1516.
Skarbinski J, James EM, Causer LM, et al: Malaria surveillance—United States, 2004. MMWR Surveill Summ 2006;55(SS-04):23-37.
Spira AM: Assessment of travelers who return home ill. Lancet 2003;361, 1459-1469.
Steffen R: Epidemiology of traveler's diarrhea. Clin Infect Dis 2005;41, S536-S540.
Steffen R, Lobel HO: Epidemiological basis for the practices of travel medicine. J Wilderness Med 1994;5:56-66.
Thielman NM, Guerrant RL: Clinical practice: Acute infectious diarrhea. N Engl J Med 2004;350:38-47.

Toxoplasmosis

Method of
Peter Mariuz, MD, and
Sumanth Rajagopal, MD

Toxoplasmosis, the disease caused by *Toxoplasma gondii*, is a worldwide zoonosis responsible for significant morbidity and mortality in both animals and humans. *T. gondii* is an obligate, intracellular protozoan, belonging to the subphylum Apicomplexa, subclass coccidian. With the advent of AIDS, cases of toxoplasma encephalitis (TE) began to occur in epidemic proportions. The availability of highly active antiretroviral therapy (HAART) and effective medications for prophylaxis against toxoplasmosis has significantly decreased the incidence and mortality of TE in the United States and Europe.

T. gondii exists in three morphologic forms: oocyst, tachyzoite, and tissue cyst.

Oocysts are formed after sexual gametogony, a process that occurs only in the gut of felines, the definitive hosts of *T. gondii*. Oocysts are excreted in large numbers in cat feces for up to 20 days. Sporulation of the oocyst, which requires 2 to 21 days to occur, results in the formation of two sporozoites per oocyst; these are infectious to humans, who, along with other warm-blooded animals, serve as intermediate hosts. The infectious sporozoites may remain viable in moist soil for up to 18 months, thus constituting a major environmental reservoir for *T. gondii*. The ingestion of food or water contaminated with oocysts is a common mode of acquisition of infection by humans. Boiling water for 5 minutes or exposing food to dry heat (>60°C) renders the oocyst noninfectious.

Ingestion of the sporozoites results in the formation of the rapidly dividing *tachyzoite* form. These invade the intestinal epithelial cells, spread to the mesenteric lymph nodes, and can disseminate to infect every kind of mammalian cell. The infected host cell is lysed; subsequently, contiguous cells are also infected and lysed. The presence of focal necrosis and tachyzoites surrounded by an acute inflammatory response is the hallmark of active infection. Tachyzoites are a source of infection in congenital toxoplasmosis and in infections acquired through blood transfusions and laboratory accidents.

An effective host immune response mediated by parasiticidal antibody, T lymphocytes, macrophages, interferon (IFN)-γ, and interleukin (IL)-12 significantly decreases the number of tachyzoites. This results in the development of *tissue cysts*, which contain *bradyzoites*. These are slowly replicating forms. Tissue cysts are especially common in the central nervous system (CNS); skeletal, smooth, and heart muscles; and eyes.

Toxoplasma infection can be acquired by ingesting tissue cysts contained in undercooked meat, particularly lamb, pork, bear, and deer; the risk of infection is lower with beef. After undercooked infected meat is ingested, bradyzoites enter the gut epithelium and transform into tachyzoites, which disseminate widely as described earlier. *T. gondii*–seronegative recipients of organ transplants can acquire the infection from tissue cysts in the transplanted organ (kidney and particularly heart transplants).

Infections in immunocompetent hosts are mostly benign and result in the development of an asymptomatic and latent infection with dormant tissue cysts. Evidence of latent infection can be detected serologically. Reactivation of infection can occur when a latently infected host becomes immunocompromised (particularly cell-mediated immunity).

In the United States, the prevalence of toxoplasmosis in adults as determined by serologic studies varies from 10% to 30%. The seroprevalence is much higher in France and Haiti and in countries in Africa and Latin America.

Diagnosis

A history of exposure to cats is of limited diagnostic value. Serology, demonstration of the organism (tachyzoites) in histologic specimens, polymerase chain reaction (PCR) testing for *T. gondii* DNA, and isolation of *T. gondii* from tissue cultures or intraperitoneal inoculation of mice may be used depending on the clinical context.

Serologic testing is the most commonly employed diagnostic method. With acute infection, immunoglobulin M (IgM) antibodies appear and persist for a few months, after which in most patients they are no longer detectable. Occasionally, IgM antibody remains detectable for months to years after acute infection. IgG antibodies are detectable within 1 to 2 weeks after acute infection; titers peak within 1 to 2 months and then decline but remain detectable for life. IgA and IgE antibodies can also be measured. Acute infection can be established if both IgG and IgM antibodies are simultaneously detected in serum. IgA antibodies may also be detected in sera of acutely infected adults and can persist for many months and sometimes for more than a year. Testing for IgA in this setting offers no further benefits; however, testing for IgA is important in diagnosing congenital toxoplasmosis. IgE antibodies are detected during acute infection and are most commonly used in conjunction with IgM and IgA serologies to diagnose congenital infection.

Because of variable methodologies and sensitivity and specificity of commercially available test kits, a combination of these tests, called a *toxoplasma serologic profile*, performed at a reference laboratory is often helpful in establishing a diagnosis of toxoplasmosis and distinguishing recently acquired from chronic infection. This is of utmost importance in the setting of possible acute maternal infection. The toxoplasma serology laboratory at the Palo Alto Medical Foundation (http://www.pamf.serology.org) is a well-known reference laboratory and offers all of the above-mentioned tests with expert interpretation of the results.

BOX 1 *Toxoplasma gondii* Infections Requiring Treatment

Infection in Immunocompetent Hosts
Congenital infection
Disseminated disease (e.g., encephalitis, pneumonitis, myocarditis, hepatitis)
Infections during pregnancy
Ocular disease
Unusually prolonged or severe adenopathy

Infection in Immunocompromised Hosts
AIDS
Chronic steroid use
Hematologic malignancies, particularly Hodgkin's disease
Transplantation

Other
Accidental infection of laboratory personnel
Transfusion-related infection

T. gondii DNA can be amplified by PCR from a variety of clinical specimens including amniotic fluid, cerebrospinal fluid (CSF), vitreous and aqueous fluids, bronchoalveolar lavage (BAL) fluid, fetal and placental tissues, and even blood in cases of disseminated toxoplasmosis. In general, the PCR-based tests are highly specific but can suffer from poor sensitivity. The reported sensitivities range from 64% to 81%. The sensitivity of the test on CSF in patients with TE is around 50% and only 30% on aqueous fluid. An early diagnosis of intrauterine infection can often be made by PCR amplification of toxoplasma DNA from amniotic fluid, which avoids the need for more invasive testing of the fetus. Although a negative PCR test does not necessarily rule out infection, a positive test can be a useful adjunct to serologic testing.

Immunoperoxidase staining of histologic sections demonstrating tachyzoites or multiple tissue cysts near an inflammatory necrotic lesion are diagnostic of an active infection. The presence of tissue cysts alone, seen often in cases of dormant or latent infection, do not indicate an active process.

Isolation of *T. gondii* by mouse inoculation or in tissue cultures represents an active infection.

Treatment

Most episodes of toxoplasmosis in immunocompetent hosts are asymptomatic and do not require therapy. There are, however, specific instances—based on the location of the infection, its severity, the mode of transmission (e.g., congenital disease), and the host's immune status—when treatment is necessary (Box 1).

Therapeutic regimens are based on data from in vitro and in vivo experimental animal models (mostly murine) and a few large, well-controlled clinical trials and the practice of physicians experienced in the treating toxoplasmosis (Tables 1 to 4). Drug therapy is primarily directed against tachyzoites; it does not eradicate tissue cysts. Treatment regimens usually include two drugs with activity against *T. gondii*.

Pyrimethamine (Daraprim), a folate antagonist, is the most active drug against *T. gondii* and is used whenever possible. Because pyrimethamine has significant bone marrow toxicity, folinic acid (leucovorin)[1] should be used in conjunction with it. Folic acid should not be used in place of folinic acid, because folic acid inhibits the activity of pyrimethamine.

---

[1]Not FDA approved for this indication.

TABLE 1 Overview of Drugs Currently Used to Treat Toxoplasmosis

Antimicrobial	Mode of Action	Metabolism	Recommended Dose — Immunocompromised	Recommended Dose — Immunocompetent	Adverse Effects
Clindamycin* (Cleocin)[1] oral and IV	Unknown; possibly inhibition of protein synthesis	Readily absorbed by gut; excellent tissue penetration	Acute: 600 mg q6h for 3-6 wk; Maintenance: same	300 mg q6h for 4 wk; repeat as needed	GI intolerance, rash, pseudomembranous colitis
Pyrimethamine (Daraprim) oral	Inhibits folic acid synthesis	Readily absorbed by gut; hepatic metabolism; lipid soluble	Acute: loading dose, 100-200 mg[3]; 50-75 mg daily for 3-6 wk, with oral folinic acid 10-20 mg/d; Maintenance: 25-50 mg/d, with oral folinic acid 10-20 mg/d	Loading dose, 2 mg/kg/d (max 100-200 mg)[3]; then 25-50 mg qd for 2-4 wk, with oral folinic acid 10-20 mg/d	Cytopenias, rash, GI intolerance
Sulfadiazine*	Inhibits folic acid synthesis; acts synergistically and sequentially with pyrimethamine	Readily absorbed by gut; penetrates blood–brain barrier; some hepatic metabolism	Acute: 4-6 g/d[3] for 3-6 wk; Maintenance: 2-4 g/d in 4 equally divided doses	100 mg/kg/d (max 4-8 g/d)[3] in 4 equally divided doses for 2-4 wk	GI intolerance, rash (Stevens-Johnson syndrome), cytopenias, nephrolithiasis, crystalluria, interstitial nephritis, encephalopathy

[1] Not FDA approved for this indication.
[3] Exceeds dosage recommended by the manufacturer.
*Most effective when used with pyrimethamine.
GI = gastrointestinal.

TABLE 2 Drugs Used to Treat Toxoplasmosis in Pregnant Women and for Congenital Toxoplasmosis

Antimicrobial	First Trimester	Second and Third Trimesters	Congenital	Adverse Effects
Pyrimethamine (Daraprim) oral	Not recommended: teratogenic	Loading dose: 100 mg/d for 2 d[3], then 50 mg/d with folinic acid 10 mg/d orally with sulfadiazine	Loading dose: 2 mg/kg for 2 d[3], then 1 mg/kg/d for 2-6 mo followed by this dose every Monday, Wednesday, Friday for 1 y, used in combination with folinic acid 10 mg three times weekly and sulfadiazine	Cytopenias, rash, GI intolerance
Spiramycin*[2] oral	1 g PO tid	1 g PO tid; If fetal infection is confirmed or suspected, pyrimethamine and sulfadiazine may be superior for treating fetus		Nausea, vomiting
Sulfadiazine	50-100 mg/kg/d in two equally divided doses; Has been used alone as an alternative to spiramycin	50-100 mg/kg/d in two equally divided doses with pyrimethamine	50-100 mg/kg/d in two equally divided doses for up to 1 y	GI intolerance, rash (Stevens-Johnson syndrome), cytopenias, nephrolithiasis, crystalluria, interstitial nephritis, encephalopathy

[2] Not available in the United States.
[3] Exceeds dosage recommended by the manufacturer.
*Spiramycin is available on request from the U.S. Food and Drug Administration, telephone 301-796-1600.
GI = gastrointestinal.
From Remington JS, McLeod R, Thulliez P, Desmonts G: Toxoplasmosis. In Remington JS, Klein JO, Wilson CB, Baker CJ (eds): Infectious Diseases of the Fetus and Newborn Infant, 6th ed. Philadelphia: WB Saunders, 2006, pp 1038-1039.

TABLE 3 Alternative Drugs Used to Treat Toxoplasmosis

Antimicrobial	Mode of Action	Metabolism	Recommended Dose	Adverse Effects
Atovaquone* (Mepron)[1] oral	Uncoupling electron biosynthesis; inhibition of de novo pyrimidine biosynthesis	Suspension has better bioavailability than old tablet formulation. Improved absorption if taken with food, particularly fatty foods	Acute: 1500 mg suspension bid for 3-6 wk. Maintenance: Same	Rash, elevated liver function tests
Azithromycin* (Zithromax)[1] oral	Unknown; possibly inhibition of protein synthesis	Readily absorbed by gut. High intracellular levels	Acute: 1250-1500 mg/d for 3-6 wk. Maintenance: Same	GI intolerance
Clarithromycin* (Biaxin)[1] oral	Unknown; possibly inhibition of protein synthesis	Readily absorbed by gut. High tissue levels	Acute: 1 g/d in two equally divided doses for 3-6 wk. Maintenance: Same	GI intolerance, hearing loss, elevated liver function tests

[1] Not FDA approved for this indication
*Most effective when used in combination with pyrimethamine
GI = gastrointestinal.

Sulfonamides, especially sulfadiazine, are synergistic with pyrimethamine, and these two drugs are often used together. Clindamycin (Cleocin)[1] is an alternative to sulfadiazine in patients who are sulfa intolerant. Pyrimethamine is teratogenic and should not be used before 16 weeks of gestation in pregnant women. For possible alternative regimens when combination pyrimethamine and sulfadiazine (or clindamycin) cannot be used, see Table 4.

TOXOPLASMOSIS IN IMMUNOCOMPETENT HOSTS

The majority of infections in immunocompetent hosts are asymptomatic and do not require therapy. Cervical lymphadenopathy, the most common manifestation, is self-limited and usually resolves within 1 to 3 weeks. Treatment in normal hosts should be considered only if systemic symptoms are severe or prolonged or in the rare event that there is visceral involvement (encephalitis, myocarditis, or pneumonitis). Acute infection as a result of laboratory accidents or transfusions may be severe and should be treated.

The treatment regimen of choice consists of a combination of pyrimethamine and sulfadiazine given for 2 to 4 weeks with folinic acid. Oral pyrimethamine is administered at a loading dose of 2 mg/kg/day[3], up to a maximum of 100 to 200 mg for 2 days, followed by 25 to 50 mg daily plus 10 mg folinic acid. Sulfadiazine, 100 mg/kg/day (maximum daily dose, 4-8 g)[3] in four divided doses, is given by mouth. In the event of pyrimethamine-induced hematologic toxicity (cytopenia), the dose of folinic acid may be increased to 20 mg/day.[3]

OCULAR TOXOPLASMOSIS

Toxoplasmosis is the most commonly identified etiologic agent of posterior uveitis worldwide. Involvement of the eye can be a result of either congenital or postnatally acquired infection. Outbreaks of ocular toxoplasmosis have been traced to water supplies contaminated with oocysts. When compared with postnatally acquired infection, congenital ocular infection is more likely to involve both eyes and the macular areas, resulting in visual impairment.

Clinical manifestations include blurred vision, scotomas, photophobia, pain, and excessive tearing. Vision loss can occur as a result of macular involvement. Symptoms can occur during the acute or chronic phase of infection. Typical finding on examination is an area of focal necrotizing chorioretinitis accompanied by an inflammatory reaction of the vitreous, leading to the classic headlight in fog appearance. Often there are adjacent scars from previous lesions. The active lesion may persist from 8 to 16 weeks, followed by scarring, with a disease-free interval or development of satellite lesions. Atypical manifestations such as large and bilateral lesions, endophthalmitis, and acute retinal necrosis are more common in immunodeficient and elderly persons. Optic nerve involvement is well described. Recurrence of disease, most commonly in the originally involved eye, occurs in both forms of infection. Signs of systemic involvement are uncommon except in patients with AIDS, in whom ocular toxoplasmosis can be a harbinger of CNS infection.

Diagnosis is based on the ophthalmic examination combined with serologic evidence of toxoplasmosis. PCR amplification of toxo-

[3] Exceeds dosage recommended by the manufacturer.

TABLE 4 Drugs Used for Primary Prophylaxis of Toxoplasmic Encephalitis in HIV-Positive Patients

Antimicrobial	Recommended Dose	Comments
Trimethoprim–sulfamethoxazole (Bactrim)[1] oral	1 double-strength tablet per d	
Dapsone[1] oral	100 mg twice weekly (with pyrimethamine)	Most effective when used in combination with pyrimethamine. Can cause hemolysis in persons with G6PD deficiency
Pyrimethamine (Daraprim) oral	25 mg/wk (with dapsone)	Most effective when used in combination with pyrimethamine. Can cause hemolysis in persons with G6PD deficiency

[1] Not FDA approved for this indication
G6PD = glucose-6-phosphate dehydrogenase.

plasma DNA from the aqueous fluid can help in select cases but lacks sensitivity.

Treatment is required in order to prevent relapse and the risk of progressive visual loss and other complications, such as glaucoma. The drugs of choice are oral pyrimethamine and sulfadiazine with folinic acid, in the same dosages as described in the previous section. For sulfa-allergic nonimmunocompromised patients, clindamycin,[1] 300 mg orally every 6 hours in combination with pyrimethamine and folinic acid has been used successfully; 600 mg every 6 hours is used for patients with AIDS. The usual duration of therapy is 4 to 6 weeks and is repeated as needed. Intraocular inflammation is thought to contribute to morbidity, so adjunctive therapy with systemic corticosteroids (prednisone 20-80 mg daily for a week and then tapered based on response) is indicated if the macula, optic nerve, or papillomacular bundle is involved. In particular cases, photocoagulation and vitrectomy may be necessary. Peripheral small lesions that are not immediately sight threatening might not require therapy, but they can be monitored because ocular toxoplasmosis can be self-limited in nonimmunosupressed patients. If relapses occur frequently or are severe, trimethoprim-sulfamethoxazole (TMP-SMX, Bactrim)[1] one double-strength tablet every 3 days may be of benefit.

TOXOPLASMOSIS IN IMMUNOCOMPROMISED HOSTS

Toxoplasmosis has a variety of clinical manifestations in immunosuppressed persons and is uniformly fatal if not treated. Patients with defective cell-mediated immunity are particularly at risk, including those receiving cytotoxic drugs or corticosteroids, patients with hematologic malignancies, and persons receiving bone marrow and solid organ transplantations. Persons infected with HIV, especially those with CD4$^+$ cell counts of $\leq 100/mm^3$ are at greatest risk for disease. TE is the most prevalent CNS disorder in persons with AIDS, both in the pre-HAART and the post-HAART eras (Box 2).

TE is the most common presentation of toxoplasmosis and manifests with hemiparesis, speech abnormalities, altered mental state, seizures, movement disorders, and cerebellar symptoms. Multiple ring-enhancing lesions, often involving the basal ganglia, are typical but not pathognomonic. The differential diagnosis includes primary CNS lymphoma, cryptococcomas, and tuberculomas. A definitive diagnosis requires a brain biopsy.

Therapy is generally initiated empirically, based on the clinical and neuroradiographic evidence in a patient with a CD4$^+$ cell count of less than 100/mm^3 and who is seropositive for anti–*T. gondii* IgG antibodies. Using these criteria, the predictive value according to one study was 80%. Seventy percent of patients with TE have a quantifiable clinical improvement by day 7 of therapy. Conversely, patients not responding to empiric therapy usually have evidence of progressive disease within the first 10 days. Ninety percent of patients show improvement on neuroradiographic studies within 6 weeks of starting therapy.

Less commonly encountered is a diffuse form of TE, which has a rapid onset of generalized neurologic decline, with normal neuroimaging studies leading to missed diagnosis.

Toxoplasma pneumonia and chorioretinitis have also been reported in patients with advanced AIDS.

In solid organ transplant and hematopoietic stem cell transplant recipients, toxoplasma infection manifests with fevers, pulmonary symptoms, CNS involvement, and graft dysfunction. A high index of suspicion is necessary to make a timely diagnosis and initiate therapy in this setting.

The combination of pyrimethamine (an initial loading dose of 100 mg/day for 2 days[3] followed by 50-75 mg/day) and sulfadiazine (4-6 g/day in four divided doses)[3] is the mainstay of treatment. Oral folinic acid 10 to 20 mg/day is added to preclude the hematologic toxicities associated with pyrimethamine. Acute therapy generally lasts 3 weeks; a longer course (up to 6 weeks or even longer) may be needed in severely ill patients and when a complete clinical or radiographic response has not been achieved. Clindamycin[1] 600 mg orally or intravenously every 6 hours in combination with pyrimethamine is an option in patients with significant sulfa allergy. Prophylactic anticonvulsants are not recommended. Corticosteroids should not be used routinely but are indicated if there is evidence of increased intracranial pressure. The use of corticosteroids can complicate the interpretation of the response to empiric therapy, because clinical and radiographic improvements may be related to a decrease in cerebral edema or the size of a steroid-sensitive CNS lymphoma.

In the rare instance when oral medications cannot be given, intravenous TMP-SMX[1] (10 mg/kg of the trimethoprim component every 12 hours) has been used. The currently available antimicrobials are active only against the tachyzoite form of *T. gondii*. Surviving tissue cysts can re-initiate TE if treatment is discontinued. Therefore, chronic suppressive therapy is used to decrease the rates of relapse. Pyrimethamine[1] 25 mg/day and sulfadiazine[1] 2 to 4 g/day orally in four equally divided doses, with 10 mg/day of oral folinic acid are recommended based on the low relapse rate associated with this combination (4.4 per 100 patient-years). In sulfa-allergic patients, clindamycin[1] is used; a daily dose of at least 2400 mg in four divided doses by mouth is recommended. Primary chemoprophylaxis is an attractive therapeutic option for patients known to be at risk for developing toxoplasmosis, such as HIV-infected patients seropositive for anti–*T. gondii* IgG antibodies and CD4$^+$ cell counts of less than 100/mm^3. Oral TMP-SMX[1] (one double-strength tablet per day) is effective. When used as single agents, dapsone[1] and pyrimethamine might not be effective. However, the combination of these drugs—pyrimethamine

---

> **BOX 2 Clinical Manifestations of Toxoplasmic Encephalitis in Patients with AIDS**
>
> **Focal Neurologic Deficits**
> Aphasia or impaired speech
> Ataxia
> Cerebellar tremor
> Cranial nerve palsies
> Diplopia
> Headache (severe localized)
> Hemiparesis
> Hemiplegia
> Hemisensory loss
> Movement disorders: Hemichorea, hemiballismus
> Parkinsonian symptoms
> Seizures
> Thalamic syndrome
> Visual field deficits
>
> **Generalized Cerebral Dysfunction**
> Coma
> Confusion
> Decreased attention
> Decreased recent memory
> Global cognitive impairment, e.g., AIDS dementia
> Lethargy
> Slowed motor responses
> Slowed verbal responses
>
> **Neuropsychiatric Abnormalities**
> Anxiety
> Dementia
> Personality changes
> Psychosis

---

[1]Not FDA approved for this indication.
[3]Exceeds dosage recommended by the manufacturer.

50 mg/week and dapsone 100 mg two times per week—has been used. In sulfa-allergic patients, desensitization is also an option.

In the past, lifelong suppressive therapy was recommended following TE. However, in patients receiving HAART, primary and secondary antitoxoplasma prophylaxis may be discontinued if the CD4$^+$ cell counts remain at 200/mm^3 for more than 3 months and 6 months, respectively.

TOXOPLASMOSIS IN PREGNANT WOMEN

Acute infection during pregnancy can result in transmission of infection to the fetus. Seroprevalence studies in the United States have shown that approximately 15% of girls and women between the ages of 15 and 44 years have IgG antibodies against *T. gondii*. Thus, the majority of women of reproductive age are susceptible to acute infection during pregnancy. The risk factors for seroconversion during pregnancy are not completely understood but include consuming raw or undercooked meat and oocyst-contaminated fruits and vegetables. As in the general population, most pregnant women who acquire infection remain asymptomatic. The most commonly recognized clinical manifestation is lymphadenopathy. The fetus is at risk for transplancental infection regardless of whether the mother is symptomatic or not.

Fetuses born to women infected with toxoplasma before conception are not at risk for congenital infection except in rare instances when the infection occurred within 3 months of conception or the mother is immunocompromised (e.g., AIDS) and has latent toxoplasma infection. The risk of transmitting infection to the fetus increases with the gestational age, from 9% for infections acquired in the first trimester to 27% in the second trimester and 59% in the third trimester. The severity of clinical manifestations in the newborn is inversely related to the timing of infection; first- and second-trimester infections are more symptomatic than infections in the third trimester.

Overall, transplacental transmission occurs in more than 50% of untreated and approximately 20% of treated women who are pregnant at the time of infection. Fetal infection can result in stillbirth, spontaneous abortion, or birth of a symptomatic or asymptomatic infant. Prenatal diagnosis is made by ultrasonography and PCR amplification of *T. gondii*–specific DNA from the amniotic fluid.

Pyrimethamine plus a sulfonamide or spiramycin[2] appears to decrease the incidence of congenital *T. gondii* infection when given to women who become infected during pregnancy. However, pyrimethamine is teratogenic and should not be used until after the first trimester. Because sulfonamides have been shown to be effective in acute toxoplasmosis in animal models, sulfadiazine can be used during the first trimester. However, most experience of maternal treatment to prevent transmission is with spiramycin (which can be obtained from the FDA, telephone 301-796-1600). Pregnant women acutely infected in the first trimester may be treated until term with 1 g orally every 8 hours. Treatment with spiramycin alone decreases the incidence of congenital infection by 60% but not the severity of established congenital toxoplasmosis. Maternal treatment with pyrimethamine plus sulfadiazine appears to attenuate the clinical manifestations in the fetus. If fetal infection is suspected after the first trimester, pyrimethamine, sulfadiazine, and folinic acid should be used to treat the mother.

CONGENITAL TOXOPLASMOSIS

Each year, there are 400 to 4000 cases of congenital toxoplasmosis in the United States. Congenital infection can manifest with varying degrees of severity, depending on the timing of maternal infection during pregnancy. Babies born to women infected in the first and second trimesters show evidence of severe disease, and those born to women infected in the last trimester are often asymptomatic at birth, although many develop chorioretinitis or developmental delays years later.

BOX 3 Clinical Manifestations of Toxoplasmosis in Newborns and Prominent Sequelae in Asymptomatic Newborns

Toxoplasmosis in Newborns
Neurologic
Cerebral calcification
Hydrocephalus
Microcephalus
Psychomotor retardation
Seizure disorders

Ophthalmic
Cataracts
Glaucoma
Micro-ophthalmia
Optic atrophy
Retinochoroiditis
Strabismus

Other
Hepatosplenomegaly
Lymphadenopathy
Myocarditis
Pneumonitis
Deafness
Diarrhea
Fever
Hypothermia
Jaundice
Rash
Vomiting

Prominent Sequelae in Asymptomatic Newborns
Blindness
Delayed psychomotor development
Hydrocephalus
Mental retardation
Retinochoroiditis
Seizures
Sensorineural hearing loss

The classic triad of chorioretinitis, hydrocephalus, and intracranial calcifications is neither common nor pathognomonic for toxoplasmosis. The clinical manifestations are nonspecific and include strabismus, epilepsy, mental retardation, hepatomegaly, anemia, jaundice, rash, thrombocytopenia, encephalitis, pneumonitis, diarrhea, and hypothermia. Infections due to cytomegalovirus, rubella, herpes simplex viruses, syphilis, and listeriosis can result in a similar presentation. One characteristic feature of congenital toxoplasmosis is a markedly increased CSF protein content.

Infants with clinically apparent disease at birth may have a combination of signs and symptoms (Box 3); 8% have severe impairment of the CNS or eyes. Seventy-five percent are asymptomatic. The incidence of untoward sequelae in the asymptomatic population has been studied prospectively and has been found to be greater than 85% (see Box 3). A serologic diagnosis is based on positive IgM and IgA antibody titers after the first week of life and the persistence of IgG antibodies. Maternally transferred antibodies usually decline over time and disappear in 6 to 12 months. Demonstration of IgA antibodies may be more sensitive than IgM antibodies in this setting. Ophthalmologic examinations, computed tomography scans of the brain (to demonstrate cerebral calcifications), and CSF evaluation should always be done. Direct demonstration of tachyzoites by mouse inoculation or tissue culture using placental tissue or other body fluids or PCR testing of these same specimens may be considered.

The National Collaborative Chicago-Based, Congenital Toxoplasmosis Study group treated 120 infants with congenital toxoplasmosis between 1981 and 2004 and have published their results.

---

[2] Not available in the United States.

The infants were treated with pyrimethamine and sulfadiazine. Treatment of children with moderate to severe neurologic disease at baseline resulted in normal neurologic or cognitive outcomes (or both) for more than 72% of patients. All children without substantial impairment at birth had normal cognitive, neurologic, and auditory outcomes after 1 year of therapy. These findings show the importance of diagnosis and treatment of congenital toxoplasmosis. Adjunctive corticosteroids (prednisolone 1 mg/kg/day in two divided doses) have been used when CSF protein is ≥1 g/dL and when chorioretinitis threatens vision.

Prevention

Primary infection can be prevented by consuming only meat that has been well cooked (>60° C or 140°F, and no longer pink inside) or that has been frozen (20°C for ≥ 24 hours) and thawed. Consistent handwashing after handling raw meat, vegetables, soil, and cats or their feces can decrease the chance of ingesting oocysts. Disposable gloves should be used when disposing of cat litter, and cat litter boxes should be emptied daily, before the oocysts can sporulate and become infectious. Cat owners should keep their cats indoors, if possible, and feed them commercial cat food or well-cooked table food only. Specifically, pregnant women and immunocompromised hosts (particularly HIV-positive persons) not previously infected with *T. gondii* (seronegative) should observe these prevention strategies. Serologic testing of pet cats plays no role in prevention because it does not show if oocysts are being excreted.

Cat-Scratch Disease

Method of
Michael J. Smith, MD, MSCE

Cat-scratch disease (CSD), regional lymphadenopathy following a cat scratch or bite, has been described since the 1950s. *Bartonella henselae*, a pleomorphic, facultative intracellular gram-negative bacillus, was not identified as the etiologic agent until 40 years later. As the laboratory detection of *B. henselae* has improved, it has become associated with an increasing number of clinical entities. These have traditionally been divided into typical CSD, the classic finding of unilateral regional lymphadenopathy following a cat scratch or bite, and atypical CSD, which includes all other presentations.

Epidemiology

As CSD is not a reportable disease, the true incidence remains unknown. However, there are an estimated 24,000 cases in the United States each year. Predominantly a disease of childhood and adolescence, CSD has the highest age-specific incidence rate occurring in children younger than 10 years of age. Although less frequent, CSD does occur in older individuals as well. A recent study found that 6% of patients with confirmed CSD were older than the age of 60 years.

Nearly 90% of patients with CSD have exposure to cats and approximately half recall a definitive scratch or bite. Early epidemiologic evidence suggested an increased risk of CSD in patients with kittens as compared to patients with adult cats. It was subsequently shown that kittens have a higher rate of *B. henselae* bacteremia than adult cats. In contrast, adult cats are more likely to have antibodies indicative of past infection. Most bacteremic cats are asymptomatic, so even a healthy-appearing animal can transmit disease.

The cat flea, *Ctenocephalides felis*, has been implicated in the transmission between cats. Consequently, CSD is more prevalent in warm and humid environments that support the growth of fleas with infection occurring primarily in the fall and winter months. To date, no evidence exists for human to human transmission.

Clinical Manifestations

Typical CSD is the most common form of CSD in immunocompetent patients. Initially, papules develop at the site of inoculation within the first week after a cat scratch or bite. This is followed by the gradual onset of unilateral regional lymphadenopathy over the next several weeks. Occasionally these lymph nodes may suppurate. The location of lymphadenopathy depends on the site of inoculation but most commonly occurs in the axillary, inguinal or cervical chains. In contrast to bacterial lymphadenitis, the lymph nodes are not inflamed. Patients are usually well-appearing and afebrile. Lymphadenopathy gradually resolves over several months without specific therapy.

The most common form of atypical CSD is Parinaud's oculoglandular syndrome (POGS), which occurs when bacteria are inoculated directly into the eye or eyelid. Small papules develop, almost always in the palpebral conjunctiva, in association with ipsilateral preauricular lymphadenopathy. There is also a painless, nonpurulent conjunctivitis. Similar to typical CSD, these symptoms resolve without antimicrobial therapy over several weeks.

Typical CSD and POGS share a similar pathophysiology; direct inoculation followed by a local immune response. In contrast, the other types of atypical CSD are due to systemic infection with *B. henselae*. These include hepatosplenic CSD, osteomyelitis, endocarditis, encephalitis, and neuroretinitis. *Bartonella* has also been implicated in the etiology of fever of unknown origin (FUO). One recent study revealed that 5% of all children with FUO of infectious etiology had antibodies against *B. henselae* indicative of current or recent infection.

In immunocompromised individuals, *B. henselae* can cause life-threatening invasive disease. Bacillary angiomatosis (BA), which is also caused by other *Bartonella* species, is caused by the angioproliferative effects of *Bartonella* and results in multiple vascular tumors in the skin and subcutaneous tissues. Bacillary peliosis (BP) is another form of vasoproliferative disease that leads to the development of blood-filled cysts in the reticuloendothelial element of the liver, spleen, and bone marrow of severely immunocompromised patients.

Diagnosis

A detailed history and physical examination are essential for the diagnosis of CSD. Any contact with cats or kittens, especially if bites or scratches occurred, should raise suspicion for CSD, regardless of the patient's age and clinical presentation.

Bartonella is a fastidious organism that takes several weeks to grow, making culture impractical. Therefore, serologic testing has become the mainstay of diagnosis. Indirect fluorescent antibody testing for IgM and IgG against *B. henselae* is performed by most commercial laboratories as well as the Center for Disease Control. A single

---

CURRENT DIAGNOSIS

- Suspect CSD in any patient with lymphadenopathy and a history of cat exposure, regardless of age.
- Serologic testing can confirm the diagnosis.
- If biopsy is performed, specimens should be sent for pathology as well as fungal, mycobacterial, and routine bacterial cultures.
- Granulomas with central necrosis are characteristic of CSD but are not specific. When available, PCR is highly specific for CSD.

Abbreviations: CSD = cat-scratch disease; PCR = polymerase chain reaction.

CURRENT THERAPY

Immunocompetent Patients

- Typical CSD only requires supportive treatment.
- No antibiotics are indicated.
- For atypical CSD there are no definitive treatment recommendations.
- Endocarditis requires surgery and antibiotic therapy, which should include at least 14 days of an aminoglycoside.

Immunocompromised Patients

- BA or BP treatment for at least 3 months with either
  - Erythromycin (E.E.S.)[1] 500 mg PO qid or
  - Doxycycline (Vibramycin) 100 mg PO bid.

---

[1]Not FDA approved for this indication.
Abbreviations: BA = bacillary angiomatosis; BP = bacillary peliosis; CSD = cat-scratch disease.

---

elevated titer or a fourfold or greater increase between acute and convalescent titers is diagnostic of CSD.

The combination of history, physical examination, and serologic testing may obviate the need for biopsy in cases of typical CSD. If a node is removed, the characteristic histopathologic finding is the formation of granulomas with microabscesses and central necrosis. Rarely, gram-negative bacilli may be identified using the Warthin-Starry silver stain. These are both non-specific findings, and any patient undergoing biopsy should have samples sent for cytology as well as fungal, mycobacterial, and standard bacterial culture and sensitivity to rule out other etiologies of lymphadenopathy. Polymerase chain reaction (PCR) testing of tissue is emerging as a highly specific diagnostic tool. Sensitivity of PCR testing varies with the specific DNA target used but is usually quite high. It is becoming increasingly available in commercial laboratories.

Treatment

Treatment of typical CSD is supportive and mainly consists of needle aspiration of suppurative lymph nodes when required. There is no evidence to suggest that treatment with antibiotics significantly alters the course of disease. In the only prospective, randomized, double blinded study of typical CSD, a 5-day course of azithromycin (Zithromax) or placebo was given to 29 patients with clinical CSD. Although the subjects who received azithromycin had a more rapid reduction in lymphadenopathy as measured by ultrasound at 30 days, the long-term outcomes were identical for both groups.

Evidence for the treatment of atypical CSD in immunocompetent patients is limited to case reports and retrospective reviews. Success has been reported using a range of oral antibiotics including trimethoprim-sulfamethoxazole[1] (Bactrim, Septra), rifampin (Rifadin),[1] azithromycin (Zithromax),[1] doxycycline (Vibramycin), and ciprofloxacin (Cipro[1]), as well as intravenous gentamicin (Garamycin).[1] Nevertheless, most cases of atypical CSD are thought to resolve without antibiotic therapy. A notable exception is endocarditis, which requires surgical replacement of the damaged valve in addition to antibiotic therapy. One retrospective review found that treatment of endocarditis with a regimen that included an aminoglycoside for at least 14 days was significantly associated with a higher rate of survival.

Immunocompromised patients with BA or BP warrant antimicrobial treatment. There have been no controlled studies to determine optimal therapy, but either erythromycin (E.E.S.)[1] or doxycycline

---

[1]Not FDA approved for this indication.

(Vibramycin) is effective. Most experts recommend a treatment course of at least 3 months to prevent relapse.

Prevention

Cat owners should avoid activities that may result in a cat scratch or bite, and should promptly wash any cat-inflicted wounds. Appropriate flea control will also reduce the likelihood of CSD. Because of the risk for invasive disease caused by *B. henselae*, immunocompromised individuals should be specifically warned of the risks of cat exposure. If possible, they should avoid purchasing or adopting kittens.

REFERENCES

American Academy of Pediatrics: Cat-scratch disease. In Pickering LK (ed): Red Book: 2003 Report of the Committee on Infectious Diseases. 26th ed, Elk Grove Village, IL: American Academy of Pediatrics, 2006, pp 232-234.
Bass JW, Freitas BC, Freitas AD, et al: Prospective randomized double blind placebo-controlled evaluation of azithromycin for treatment of cat-scratch disease. Pediatr Infect Dis J 1998;17:447-452.
Batts S, Demers DM: Spectrum and treatment of cat-scratch disease. Pediatr Infect Dis J 2004;23:1161-1162.
Ben-Ami R, Ephros M, Avidor B, et al: Cat-scratch disease in elderly patients. Clin Infect Dis 2005;41:969-974.
Hansmann Y, DeMartino S, Piemont Y, et al: Diagnosis of cat scratch disease with detection of *Bartonella henselae* PCR: A study of patients with lymph node enlargement. J Clin Microbiol 2005;43:3800-3806.
Jacobs RF, Schutze GE: *Bartonella henselae* as a cause of prolonged fever and fever of unknown origin in children. Clin Infect Dis 1998;26:80-84.
Massei F, Gori L, Machhia P, Maggiore G, et al: The extended spectrum of Bartonellosis in children. Infect Dis Clin North Am 2005;19:691-711.
Raoult D, Fournier PE, Vandenesch F, et al: Outcome and treatment of *Bartonella* endocarditis. Arch of Int Med 2003;163:226-230.
Rolain JM, Brouqui P, Koehler JE, et al: Recommendations for treatment of human infection caused by *Bartonella* species. Antimicrob Agents Chemother 2004;48:1921-1933.
Zangwill KM, Hamilton DH, Perkins BA, et al: Cat scratch disease in Connecticut: Epidemiology, risk factors, and evaluation of a new diagnostic test. N Engl J Med 1993;329:8-13.

Salmonellosis

Method of
Arvid E. Underman, MD, FACP, DTMH

Salmonellosis refers to a group of infections caused by members of the genus *Salmonella*. This genus is named after Salmon, a pathologist who first isolated the organism, later designated as *Salmonella choleraesuis*, from the intestine of pigs with diarrhea. *Salmonellae* are widely distributed throughout nature and are adapted to a myriad of warm and cold-blooded hosts. In humans there are four main clinical presentations:

1. Acute gastroenteritis
2. Bacteremia
3. Focal extraintestinal infection
4. Chronic carriage (Table 1)

Microbiology

Salmonellae are motile, Gram-stain negative, nonspore-forming bacilli that are differentiated from other *Enterobacteriaceae* by inability to ferment lactose and sucrose while producing acid, hydrogen sulfide, and gas (except *Salmonella typhi*). Members of the genus were

TABLE 1 Clinical Presentations of Salmonellosis
Acute gastroenteritis (90%–95% of cases)
Bacteremia (<5% of cases)
• Transient during acute gastroenteritis
• Enteric fever (nontyphoid)
• Persistent or recurrent (especially HIV)
Focal complications following bacteremia
• Bronchopneumonia, empyema, chest wall abscess
• Aortitis with mycotic aneurysm
• Prosthetic graft or valve infection
• Endocarditis, endarteritis
• Osteomyelitis (especially with sickle cell anemia)
• Septic arthritis
• Soft tissue abscess
• Hepatic or splenic abscess
• Meningitis or brain abscess
• Suppurative urogenital disease
Carriage (asymptomatic)
• Convalescent excretors (<2 mo)
• Convalescent carriers (2–12 mo)
• Chronic carriers (>12 mo)

TABLE 2 Predisposing Factors for Salmonellosis
Gastrointestinal
• Achlorhydria
• Gastric surgery
• Inflammatory bowel disease
Immune or structural compromise
• Age (<6 mo, >60 y)
• Lymphoma
• Splenectomy
• Cirrhosis with portal hypertension
• Diabetes mellitus
• Chronic uremia
• Hemolytic anemia (iron overload)
• Sickle cell (bone infarct, autosplenectomy)
• Systemic lupus
• Atheromata, aortic aneurysm
Infections
• HIV/AIDS (decreased T-cells)
• Malaria
• Bartonellosis
• Schistosomiasis
Drugs
• H_2-blockers, H^+ proton pump inhibitors
• Antibiotic administration
• Antimotility agents
• Chemotherapy
• Corticosteroids
• Transplant antirejection agents

more accurately classified into serotypes using the Kauffman-White schema that differentiated and grouped them serologically dependent on their lipopolysaccharide somatic (O) and flagellar (H) antigens.

More recently, DNA analysis has divided the genus into two species. Initially the first of the two species was named *Salmonella choleraesuis* and was divided into six subspecies, each of which was then divided into more than 2400 serotypes (serovars) by Kauffman-White methodology. The second species, *Salmonella Bongori*, is inconsequential. Serotypes were named historically from the host or the geographic locale of the first isolate, such as *Salmonella typhimurium* or *Salmonella dublin*. However, under the new DNA division, *choleraesuis* was both a species and a serotype. To avoid confusion the name *Salmonella enterica* has been widely adopted. The first of the six subspecies (Group I) is also named *enterica*. It contains the more than 1400 serotypes that occur in warm-blooded animals. Using nomenclature employed by the United States Centers for Disease Control and the World Health Organization (WHO), the species and subspecies name is understood; and the serotype is capitalized. Thus, the formal *S. enterica* subspecies *enterica* serotype *typhimurium* becomes simply *S. Typhimurium*, which except for the capital T is where we started!

Epidemiology

In the last 25 years, the incidence of nontyphoid salmonellosis has increased two- to threefold with approximately 1.5 million cases occurring annually in the United States. This is an underestimate because most cases are sporadic (endemic) and go unreported. Children younger than 5 years of age have the highest incidence of gastroenteritis and constitute the greatest number of cases.

Animals are the source of nontyphoid salmonella infection in humans. Infection occurs from food of animal origin such as meat, poultry, eggs, and dairy products. Contamination may occur during the production, slaughter, processing, or distribution of these products. Outbreaks have been associated with eggs, ice cream, and processed meats. Increasingly there have been outbreaks associated with raw vegetables (e.g., scallions) that are crosscontaminated during growth and distribution. Restaurant or home outbreaks occur in the context of improper preparation, cooking, and refrigeration. Most of the outbreaks can be attributed to centralized mass production and preparation of food along with globalization of the food trade. Novel sources of human salmonella include pet turtles, lizards, iguanas, African hedgehogs, rattlesnakes, and even marijuana contaminated by manure.

Emergence of antibiotic resistant species is a formidable problem. It is believed that resistance is driven worldwide by improper antibiotics use. However, in developed countries it is attributable to widespread use in animal feeds. Large numbers of transferable resistance plasmids have been described. Resistance rates of more than 50% to ampicillin, chloramphenicol (Chloromycetin), and trimethoprim-sulfamethoxazole (TMP-SMZ) (Bactrim) occur in parts of Asia, Africa, and Latin America. One strain of *S. Typhimurium* (DT104) is resistant to five antimicrobials; the three mentioned previously plus tetracycline and streptomycin. This organism has spread widely in livestock throughout the United States, Canada, United Kingdom, Europe, and the Middle East. Likewise, resistance to third-generation cephalosporins is increasing and is mediated by plasmids producing both regular and extended-spectrum beta-lactamases (ESBLs). Even more disturbing is fluoroquinolone resistance caused by mutated DNA gyrase, topoisomerase IV, or efflux pumps. The latter literally expel the quinolone from the bacterium before it can act on its target. Fluoroquinolone resistance is most pronounced in Southeast Asia, Europe, and the Middle East.

Pathogenesis

Human infection usually requires 10^6 organisms. Fewer organisms may cause disease in patients who have hypochlorhydria or achlorhydria, have impaired cellular immunity, are at the extremes of age, or are taking certain drugs (Table 2). *Salmonellae* predominately infect the terminal ileum and proximal colon through attachment. Initially host response is by neutrophils followed by lymphocytes and macrophages. Strains vary genetically in their virulence and invasiveness. The organisms can survive intracellularly, thus avoiding antibiotic agents that lack intracellular penetration. Bacteria that are not contained regionally in the gut or lymph nodes may enter the blood. There are many predisposing factors associated with this and subsequent focal complications (see Table 2).

Clinical Presentation

GASTOENTERITIS

Acute gastroenteritis is by far the most common clinical presentation of salmonellosis. It should be emphasized that there is considerable

CURRENT DIAGNOSIS

- More than 95% of nontyphoid Salmonellosis presents as uncomplicated acute gastroenteritis.
- The clinical presentation of different causes of gastroenteritis and diarrhea overlaps significantly.
- The physician should be familiar with groups of patients at risk for complicated Salmonellosis.
- Specific diagnosis requires culture of the stool or blood.
- Focal complications are always suspect in high-risk patients who are blood culture positive for nontyphoid *Salmonellae* (e.g., aortitis or mycotic aneurysm in patients older than age 60 years with atherosclerosis).

 CURRENT THERAPY

- Fluid and electrolyte replacement is of paramount importance.
- The physician should avoid routine empiric antibiotic in acute uncomplicated patients.
- The physician should avoid antimotility agents for diarrhea presenting with fever or with mucus and blood present.
- More than 95% of patients with nontyphoid salmonellosis *will get better* on their own.
- Fluoroquinolone antibiotics should be reserved for when they are truly indicated clinically.
- Increasing resistance mandates sensitivity testing (including tests for ESBL) to guide therapy of bacteremia and its complications.
- Do not prescribe *prophylactic* antibiotics to prevent diarrhea in travellers.
- Stress personal hygiene and prudent food choice with proper preparation.

Abbreviation: ESBL = extended spectrum beta lactamases.

overlap in its presentation with other infectious intestinal pathogens such as *Campylobacter* species. Given this, the incubation ranges from 6 to 96 hours but most commonly occurs between 12 and 48 hours. Initial symptoms include nausea and vomiting, followed by headaches, myalgias, malaise, chills, low-grade fever, abdominal cramps, and diarrhea. High temperatures (40°C [104°F]) should alert the clinician to invasive disease. Stools may be merely loose or profuse and watery. On direct examination, they may or may not contain polymorphonuclear leukocytes or occult blood. The presence of mucus or gross blood in the absence of hemorrhoids or fissures should alert the clinician to organisms causing dysentery such as *Shigella* species. The white count is most often normal or slightly elevated, with a left shift containing 10 to 15 bands. Low white counts with greater numbers of bands should alert the clinician to possible bacteremia or enteric fever. The diagnosis can be confirmed only by stool or blood culture. Serum serology examinations are not helpful. Most healthy adults have a self-limited, uncomplicated course, with resolution of symptoms without treatment within 48 to 72 hours.

Treatment

FLUID AND ELECTROLYTE REPLACEMENT

The sine qua non in the treatment of diarrhea is fluid and electrolyte replacement. In most cases increased oral intake of bland juices coupled with clear broth and temporary elimination of lactose-containing foods will suffice. Commercial electrolyte solutions (Pedialyte) may be useful. Although not readily available in the United States, rehydration salts are widely employed in many developing countries. WHO distributes packets containing its recommended formula of 90 mmol of sodium, 20 of potassium, 80 of chloride, 30 of bicarbonate, along with 111 mmol of glucose to dissolve in 1 L of sterile or boiled water. This mixture should be consumed at a rate sufficient to compensate for diarrheal losses while maintaining an adequate output of dilute appearing urine. Within 24 to 48 hours, the diet can be supplemented with bland, soft foods given in small, frequent feedings. If the patient has profuse vomiting or severe dehydration as determined by orthostatic changes in blood pressure, parenteral rehydration should be used. Frequently, this can be accomplished as an outpatient in an infusion room or with a home agency rather than through admission to hospital. When there is persistent emesis, profuse diarrhea, systemic toxicity, or abnormalities in serum electrolytes, parenteral rehydration in hospital is prudent.

ANTIMOTILITY AND ANTINAUSEA AGENTS

The use of agents such as atropine-diphenoxylate (Lomotil) or loperamide (Imodium) should be discouraged. Although they may result in symptomatic improvement in cramps and diarrhea, they can increase complications and even predispose to bacteremia. In general, if the patient has a fever and the diarrhea contains blood or mucus, their use should be eschewed. Most pediatricians feel they should never be used in children younger than 5 years of age. An alternative is bismuth subsalicylate (Pepto-Bismol). The adult dose is 1 ounce (2 tablespoons) or 2 tablets (262.5 mg) every 30 minutes for 8 hours. The pediatric dose is 1.1 mL/kg at 4-hour intervals for up to 5 days. Although nausea and vomiting are occasional presenting symptoms with enterocolitis, they rarely persist. Prochlorperazine (Compazine) or trimethobenzamide (Tigan) may be helpful. Both are available in oral, suppository, or parenteral form, even though injectable prochlorperazine (Compazine) has been in short supply. Suppositories usually stimulate further diarrhea. Vomiting may preclude oral administration. A singular muscular injection of prochlorperazine (Compazine) 5 to 10 mg, is often all that is needed. This may be repeated every 4 to 6 hours as needed. Promethazine hydrochloride (Phenergan) is more frequently used in children and may be used orally (0.5 mg/pound or 1 mg/kg every 6 hours) or intramuscularly in the same doses. A 5-HT$_3$ receptor antagonist such as ondansetron (Zofran)[1] is expensive and inefficacious.

ANTIBIOTICS

The routine empiric use of antibiotics, especially fluoroquinolones, for any and all cases of diarrhea is not only unjustifiable but should be decried. Certainly antibiotics are not needed in the treatment of uncomplicated *Salmonella* gastroenteritis in otherwise healthy children or adults. Studies have shown that they neither shorten the course nor improve symptoms. No doubt some of this usage is patient driven. However, overuse is contributing to the emergence of resistance, and may increase risk of symptomatic and bacteriologic relapse. Indeed antibiotic use may actually prolong the convalescent excretion or contribute to chronic carriage of the organism. Postponing antibiotic therapy until the return of a stool culture often provides the physician with a way to avert the frequent demand for antibiotic therapy. Often patients are better by the time results become available. Nevertheless, high-risk patients, as previously identified (see Table 2), should receive treatment to prevent potential complications from bacteremia. Additionally, if

---
[1]Not FDA approved for this indication.

patients are sick enough to require hospitalization, antibiotic therapy should be considered.

Appropriate antibiotic therapy should be guided by susceptibility testing. Initially, TMP-SMZ (cotrimoxazole, Bactrim, or Septra)[1] may be administered to the nonsulfonamide-sensitive patient. The dose is 5 to 8 mg/kg trimethoprim every 12 hours for children or 1 double-strength tablet (160 mg trimethoprim/800 mg sulfamethoxazole) every 12 hours for adults. Although widely used, trimethoprim-sulfamethoxazole has not yet received FDA approval. If the organism is susceptible, ampicillin, 50 mg/kg orally to 100 mg/kg/day intravenously, each in four divided doses for children, or 2 to 4 g/day in four divided doses for adults, may be administered. Amoxicillin (Amoxil)[1] in equivalent oral dosage may be substituted. The duration of therapy is generally 5 days.

Newer fluoroquinolone antibiotics, such as ciprofloxacin,[1] ofloxacin,[1] and norfloxacin,[1] are among the most effective agents with excellent oral bioavailability and intracellular concentration. They are contraindicated in prepubertal children and pregnant women. Adult doses are ciprofloxacin (Cipro), 500 mg twice daily; ofloxacin (Floxin), 400 mg twice daily; or norfloxacin (Noroxin), 400 mg twice daily. It must be emphasized that the trend in the United States to use these agents empirically for all suspected bacterial diarrhea should be vigorously resisted by the thoughtful clinician.

Bacteremia and Focal Infection

Bacteremia in acute uncomplicated *Salmonella* gastroenteritis is infrequent. Therefore, blood cultures are not routinely necessary except for patients who are in high-risk categories. Shaking chills or high fever (40°C [104°F]) should alert the clinician to possible bacteremia. Focal suppurative infection following bacteremia is also infrequent but may occur at any site. Thus, *Salmonella* has been associated with bronchopneumonia, soft tissue infection, aortic mycotic aneurysms, endocarditis, septic arthritis, splenic or hepatic abscesses, meningitis, and osteomyelitis. The clinician should suspect an endovascular mycotic aneurysm in all blood culture positive patients older than 50 years of age. *Salmonella* should always be suspected in individuals with sickle cell disease in whom bone and joint infection is the most frequent cause of extraintestinal infection. Meningitis occurs primarily in infants younger than 5 months of age. The diagnosis of a *Salmonella* bacteremia in HIV patients will almost always be accompanied by recurrent episodes.

Treatment

ANTIBIOTICS

Bacteremia and localized suppurative infection require antibiotic therapy. The choice of effective treatment is less predictable with the emergence of resistance. Therapy must be altered according to the results of susceptibility testing. Therefore the recovery of the organism is extremely important, and adequate cultures of blood or infected material must be obtained before initiation of therapy.

Parenteral ampicillin, 100 to 200 mg/kg/day divided into four doses, or TMP/SMZ,[1] 8 to 10 mg/kg of trimethoprim per day in three divided doses, may be used. In the case of resistance or allergy to the foregoing, third-generation cephalosporins such as cefotaxime (Claforan) or ceftriaxone (Rocephin) have reasonable activity, but intracellular concentrations are not optimal. Cefotaxime, 1 to 2 grams every 6 to 8 hours for adults, or 100 to 200 mg/kg/day in three or four divided doses for children, has been found effective in bacteremia, osteomyelitis, septic arthritis, and a variety of other focal *Salmonella* infections. The use of chloramphenicol (Chloromycetin) is not recommended but a preparation of it in oil (Typhomycine)[2] is in use in developing countries. Ciprofloxacin (Cipro)[1] 7.5 mg/kg intravenously twice daily is becoming a favored agent; not only is it effective but oral bioequivalence facilitates the change to 500 to 750 mg by mouth twice daily. If fluoroquinolone resistance is encountered, imipenem (Primaxin)[1] may be tried. Efficacy data for it or other agents such as azithromycin (Zithromax)[1] are scant.

SURGERY

Focal infection often requires surgery. Often this is as simple as the drainage of localized suppuration or lavage of a septic joint. However, in the case of infected aortic aneurysms, extensive resection and vascular reconstruction are required. Infected prosthetic grafts must be removed in nearly all cases with courses of antibiotics before and after surgery.

The duration of therapy for simple bacteremia is 10 to 14 days. Septic arthritis is usually treated 4 weeks whereas osteomyelitis and endovascular infections require 6 weeks. Oral fluoroquinolones such as ciprofloxacin (Cipro), 500 mg twice daily, may be helpful in treating osteomyelitis. TMP-SMZ (Bactrim)[1] can also be used in this manner. Both have adequate blood levels after oral administration. I have had to use continuous prophylaxis of either TMP-SMZ or ciprofloxacin in several HIV patients to prevent recurrent bacteremia. Because prophylactic TMP-SMZ is used chronically for *Pneumocystis*, it may be preferred.

Enteric Fever

The clinical picture of nontyphoid *Salmonella* enteric fever is indistinguishable from that of typhoid fever, which is discussed elsewhere in this publication. However, the following discussion also applies to enteric fever caused by nontyphoid *Salmonellae*.

TREATMENT

The adjunct and antibiotic therapy of nontyphoid enteric fever parallels that of the treatment of typhoid. Antibiotics should be adjusted and altered once the results of susceptibility testing are available. Acceptable regimens include ampicillin, amoxicillin,[1] and TMP-SMZ (Bactrim),[1] along with third-generation cephalosporins and fluoroquinolone antibiotics. My preference was cefotaxime (Claforan)[1] in the same doses as for bacteremic salmonellosis. The duration is 10 to 14 days. Relapse rates are low and is seen within 2 to 6 weeks. Relapse requires an equivalent course of therapy in both dose and duration. Currently, I prefer ciprofloxacin (Cipro)[1] intravenously 7.5 mg/kg every 12 hours continued until the patient is afebrile and clinically able to start it orally. Comparative studies are ongoing using both third-generation cephalosporins, such as ceftriaxone (Rocephin)[1] or cefixime (Suprax),[1] and oral fluoroquinolones in short-course therapy of typhoid as well as nontyphoid enteric fever. Although these show some promise, they are currently not the standard of practice in the United States. Nevertheless, a strong case can be made for oral fluoroquinolones use, with obvious cost saving. Otherwise healthy young adults may be treated orally as outpatients. This advantage, if for no other reason, should *prevent* the physician from prescribing quinolones for uncomplicated gastroenteritis or other self-limited diarrheas of bacterial origin.

Adjunctive measures are of importance, including attention to fluid and electrolyte balance and nutrition. As in typhoid the routine use of corticosteroids is controversial. Use in patients who are steroid dependent or believed to be hypoadrenal is indicated. In those who are delirious, obtunded, comatose, or in shock it may be warranted; but there are little supportive data. It has been my overall impression that nontyphoid enteric fever is somewhat milder than typhoid itself, and complications such as gastrointestinal bleeding or ileal perforation are exceedingly rare.

---

[1] Not FDA approved for this indication.
[2] Not available in the United States.

[1] Not FDA approved for this indication.

Carrier State

Asymptomatic excretion of organisms invariably occurs following clinical *Salmonella* gastroenteritis. It exceeds 8 weeks in 5% to 10% of patients. Chronic carriage, either in the stool or urine, is defined as excretion of the organism for more than 1 year. Its incidence is stated to be 1% in adults and 5% in children younger than 5 years of age. This is somewhat less than that seen with *S. typhi*. Convalescent excreters need only maintain strict personal hygiene to prevent transmission of the organism. Those involved in food preparation or in child and health care should be kept off work until three successive cultures are negative at intervals required by the public health department. It goes without saying that all positive cases of salmonellosis are reportable by law to local public health authorities.

Recently, oral quinolones have been used (ciprofloxacin [Cipro],[1] 500 to 750 mg twice daily for 5 to 14 days), to curtail institutional outbreaks, as in nursing homes or psychiatric facilities. Although this may be expeditious, eliminating or preventing the source of the outbreak in a prospective fashion is preferable. In the case of food handlers and health or child care workers, some feel that quinolone therapy eliminates the problem of convalescent excretion, hence individuals may return to work without delay. The data are debatable and the successive negative stool requirement will not be obviated.

The management of the chronic carriage of nontyphoidal salmonellosis is the same as that of *S. typhi*, which is discussed in detail elsewhere. A 4- to 6-week course of oral antibiotics may be tried when no evidence of gallbladder disease exists. However, if chronic cholecystitis and/or cholelithiasis are present, cholecystectomy is almost always necessary. Despite cholecystectomy, a certain number of individuals will continue to excrete organisms thought to be of hepatobiliary origin. Chronic carriage is seen, albeit rarely, in the United States with either *Schistosoma mansoni* or *Schistosoma haematobium*. When these parasites are treated, subsequent therapy of the *Salmonella* results in termination of the stool or urinary carrier state.

Prevention

Prevention of salmonellosis has both personal and public health dimensions. Food and leftovers should be rapidly refrigerated. I recommend separate plastic (not wood) cutting boards for meats and vegetables that are washed after each use. Spillage of raw animal juices should be immediately cleaned. All preparation surfaces should be washed and dried after each meal. Detergent rather than antibacterial cleaners should be used; bleach is beautiful.

Public health surveillance is essential with regular inspection of restaurants, food retailers, and industrial food processors. National efforts to coordinate and computerize surveillance systems such as FoodNet should be expanded and fully funded so as to guarantee our food supply. Preservation technologies including irradiation need study.

Finally, the practicing physician should take the time to reiterate to patients with HIV, malignancies or other immune compromised patients (see Table 2) how they can avoid food-borne pathogens.

REFERENCES

Brenner FW, Villar RG, Angulo FJ, et al: Salmonella nomenclature. J Clin Microbiol 2000;38:24652465.

Fierer J, Swancutt M: Non-typhoid *Salmonella*: A review. In Remington JS, Swartz MN (eds): Current Clinical Topics in Infectious Diseases 20. Boston: Blackwell Science, 2000, pp 134-157.

Herikstad H, Hayes P, Mokhtar M, et al: Emerging quinolone-resistant Salmonella in the United States. Emerg Infect Dis 1997;3:371-372.

Molbak K: Human health consequences of antimicrobial drug resistant *Salmonella* and other foodborne pathogens. Clin Infect Dis 2005;41:1613-1620.

Sirinivan S, Garner P: Antibiotics for treating Salmonella gut infections. Cochrane Database Sys Rev 2000;93:CD001167.

Su LH, Chiu CH, Chu CS, et al: Antimicrobial resistance in nontyphoid *Salmonella*: A global challenge. Clin Infect Dis 2004;39:546-551.

Voetsch AC, Van Gilder TJ, Angulo FJ, et al: FoodNet estimate of the burden of illness caused by nontyphoidal Salmonella infections in the United States. Clin Infect Dis 2004;38(Suppl 3):S127-134.

Typhoid Fever

Method of
Zulfiqar A. Bhutta, MB, BS, PhD

Despite vast advances in public health and hygiene in much of the developed world, typhoid fever remains endemic in many developing countries. Probably because of the ease of modern travel, cases are also reported in most developed countries.

Etiology

Typhoid fever is caused by *Salmonella typhi*, a gram-negative bacterium. A very similar but often less severe disease is caused by *Salmonella* serotype *paratyphi* A. The ratio of disease caused by *S. typhi* to that caused by *S. paratyphi* is approximately 10:1, although the proportion of *S. paratyphi* infections is increasing in some parts of the world. Although *S. typhi* shares many genes with *Escherichia coli* and at least 90% with *Salmonella typhimurium*, several unique gene clusters known as pathogenicity islands and others were acquired during evolution. One of the specific genes is for the polysaccharide capsule Vi. This is present in approximately 90% of all freshly isolated *S. typhi* organisms and has a protective effect against the bactericidal action of the serum of infected patients.

Epidemiology

Although accurate community-based figures are unavailable, an estimated 16 million cases occur annually, with more than 0.6 million deaths. The vast majority of cases occur in Asia. Given the paucity of microbiologic facilities in developing countries, these figures may largely represent the clinical syndrome. Regional incidence rates vary from 100 to 1000 cases per 100,000 population, and there may be differences in the spectrum of the disorder. Recent population-based studies from south Asia also indicate that, contrary to previous views, the disease may largely affect children younger than 5 years of age. In contrast, data from sub-Saharan Africa and HIV-endemic areas indicate that nontyphoidal *Salmonella* bacteremia far outstrips typhoid fever as a cause of community-acquired bacteremia.

In recent years, typhoid fever is notable for the emergence of drug resistance. Following sporadic outbreaks of chloramphenicol-resistant typhoid, many strains of *S. typhi* developed plasmid-mediated multidrug-resistance to all of the three primary antimicrobials (ampicillin [Chloromycetin], chloramphenicol, and trimethoprim-sulfamethoxazole [Septra]). More troubling, chromosomally acquired quinolone resistance in *S. typhi* was recently described in various parts of Asia and may be a consequence of widespread and indiscriminate use of these agents.

Pathogenesis

Typhoid fever occurs by the ingestion of the organism, and a variety of sources of fecal contamination are reported, including street vendor foods and contamination of water reservoirs. A larger infecting dose leads to a shorter incubation period and more severe infection. The organism crosses the intestinal mucosal barrier after attachment to the microvilli by an intricate mechanism involving membrane ruffling, actin rearrangement, and internalization in an intracellular vacuole. Once inside the intestinal cells, *S. typhi* find their way into the circulation and reside within the macrophages of the reticuloendothelial system. The clinical syndrome is produced by a release of proinflammatory cytokines (interleukin [IL]-6, IL-1β, and tumor necrosis factor [TNF]-α) from the infected cells. Some 1% to 5% of patients with acute typhoid infection may become chronic carriers of the infection in the gallbladder, depending on age, sex, and treatment regimen.

Clinical Features

Patients with typhoid fever usually present with high-grade fever and a wide variety of associated symptoms, such as abdominal pain, hepatosplenomegaly, diarrhea, and constipation. In the absence of localizing signs, the early stage of the disease may be difficult to differentiate from other endemic diseases including malaria and dengue fever. The classic stepladder rise of fever is relatively rare, but the presentation of typhoid fever may be tempered by coexisting morbidities and early administration of antibiotics. In malaria-endemic areas and in parts of the world where schistosomiasis is common, the presentation of typhoid may also be atypical.

Although data from South America and parts of Africa suggest typhoid may present as a mild illness in young children, this may vary in different parts of the world. Emerging evidence from south Asia indicates the presentation of typhoid may be more dramatic in children younger than 5 years of age, with comparatively higher rates of complications and hospitalization. Diarrhea, toxicity, and complications such as disseminated intravascular coagulopathy are also more common in infancy, with higher case fatality rates. Some of the other features of typhoid fever seen in adults, however, such as relative bradycardia, are rare, and rose spots may be visible only at an early stage of the illness in fair-skinned children.

It is also recognized that multidrug-resistant (MDR) typhoid is a more severe clinical illness with higher rates of toxicity, complications, and case fatality rates. This may be related to the increased virulence of MDR *S. typhi* as well as a higher number of circulating bacteria. These findings may have implications for treatment algorithms, especially in endemic areas with high rates of MDR typhoid.

Diagnosis

The mainstay of the diagnosis of typhoid fever is a positive culture from the blood or another anatomic site. But the sensitivity of blood cultures in diagnosing typhoid fever in many parts of the developing world is limited because widespread use of antibiotics may render bacteriologic confirmation difficult. Although bone marrow cultures may increase the likelihood of bacteriologic confirmation of typhoid, these are difficult to obtain and relatively invasive.

The serologic diagnosis of typhoid is also fraught with problems because results of a single Widal test may be positive in only 50% of cases in endemic areas, and serial tests may be required in cases presenting in the first week of illness. Newer serologic tests such as a dot enzyme-linked immunoabsorbent assay (ELISA) (TyphiDot) and the TUBEX tests are promising but require further evaluation in large-scale studies in community settings. In much of the developing world, the mainstay of diagnosis of typhoid remains clinical, and several diagnostic algorithms are being evaluated in endemic areas.

Therapy

An early diagnosis of typhoid fever and institution of appropriate treatment are essential. The vast majority of typhoid patients can be managed at home with oral antibiotics and close medical follow-up for complications or failure to respond to therapy. But

CURRENT DIAGNOSIS

- In the absence of localizing signs, the early stage of the disease may be difficult to differentiate from other endemic diseases such as malaria or dengue fever.
- The presentation and diagnosis of typhoid fever may be tempered by coexisting morbidities and early administration of antibiotics.
- The presentation of typhoid may be more dramatic in children younger than 5 years of age, with comparatively higher rates of complications and hospitalization.
- The sensitivity of blood cultures in diagnosing typhoid fever may be limited in many developing countries because of antibiotic prescribing.
- Multidrug-resistant (MDR) typhoid is a more severe clinical illness with higher rates of toxicity and complications. In particular, recent cases of quinolone-resistant typhoid may be more severe.

patients with persistent vomiting, severe diarrhea, and abdominal distention may require hospitalization and parenteral antibiotic therapy. These are the general principles of typhoid management:

- Adequate rest, hydration, and attention to correction of fluid-electrolyte imbalance
- Antipyretic therapy (acetaminophen, 120 to 750 mg orally every 4 to 6 hours[3]) as required
- Soft, easily digestible diet unless the patient has abdominal distention or ileus
- Antibiotic therapy (the right choice, dosage, and duration)
- Traditional therapy with either chloramphenicol (Chloromycetin) or amoxicillin,[1] associated with relapse rates of 5% to 15% and 4% to 8%, respectively; newer quinolones and third-generation cephalosporins associated with higher cure rates

Some authorities recommend treatment with second-line agents in all cases of typhoid. Others questioned this on the basis of adequate response to therapy among sensitive cases with first-line agents. Blanket administration of second-line agents such as fluoroquinolones and third-generation cephalosporins in all cases of suspected typhoid is expensive and may lead to the rapid development of further resistance. Table 1 gives the recommended therapy for typhoid fever based on a recent consensus document by the World Health Organization (2003).

---
[3]Exceeds dosage recommended by the manufacturer.
[1]Not FDA approved fot this indication.

CURRENT THERAPY

- The vast majority of typhoid patients can be managed at home with oral antibiotics and close medical follow-up for complications or failure to respond to therapy.
- Although newer quinolones are associated with better cure rates and clinical outcomes, there is insufficient evidence to recommend them as first-line agents in children.
- Recent emergence of quinolone resistance among *S. typhi* isolates requires treatment with alternatives such as third-generation cephalosporins and azithromycin.

TABLE 1 Treatment of Typhoid Fever Based on Diagnosis, Treatment, and Prevention

	Optimal Therapy			Alternative Effective Drugs		
Susceptibility	Antibiotic	Daily Dose (mg/kg)	Days	Antibiotic	Daily Dose (mg/kg)	Days
Uncomplicated Typhoid Fever						
Fully sensitive	Fluoroquinolone (e.g., ofloxacin [Floxin][1] or ciprofloxacin [Cipro])	15	5-7*	Chloramphenicol (Chloromycetin) Amoxicillin[1] TMP-SMX (Bactrim)[1]	50-75[3] 75-100[1] 8/40	14-21 14 14
Multidrug resistance	Fluoroquinolone or Cefixime (Suprax)[1]	15 15-20[3]	5-7 7-14	Azithromycin (Zithromax)[1] Cefixime	8-10[3] 15-20[3]	7 7-14
Quinolone resistance†	Azithromycin (Rocephin)[1] or Ceftriaxone (Rocephin)[1]	8-10[3] 75[3]	7 10-14	Cefixime[1]	20[3]	7-14
Severe Typhoid Fever						
Fully sensitive	Fluoroquinolone (e.g., ofloxacin)[1]	15	10-14	Chloramphenicol Ampicillin[1] TMP-SMX	100[3] 100[3] 8/40	14-21 14 14
Multidrug-resistant	Fluoroquinolone	15	10-14	Ceftriaxone[1] or Cefotaxime (Claforan)[1]	60[3] 80[3]	10-14
Quinolone-resistant	Ceftriaxone[1] or[1] cefotaxime	60[3] 80[3]	10-14	Fluoroquinolone	20[3]	14

[1] Not FDA approved for this indication.
[3] Exceeds dosage recommended by the manufacturer.
*Three-day courses are also effective and are particularly so in epidemic containment.
†The optimum treatment for quinolone-resistant typhoid fever is not determined. Azithromycin, the third-generation cephalosporins, or a 10- to 14-day course of high-dose fluoroquinolones is effective.
Abbreviation: TMX-SMZ = trimethoprim-sulfamethoxazole.
From World Health Organization (WHO)/Vaccines and Biologicals/03.07.

Preventive Strategies for Typhoid

Of the major risk factors for outbreaks of typhoid, contamination of water supplies with sewage is the most important. During outbreaks, therefore, a combination of central chlorination and domestic water purification is important. In endemic situations, consumption of street vendor foods, especially ice cream and cut-up fruit, is recognized as an important risk factor. The human-to-human spread by chronic carriers is also important, and attempts should be made to target food handlers and high-risk groups for *S. typhi* carriage screening.

The classic heat-inactivated whole cell vaccine is associated with an unacceptably high rate of side effects. Two newer vaccines that offer protection for school-age children and for adults are the Vi polysaccharide vaccine (Typhim Vi) and the orally administratable, attenuated Ty21a vaccine (Vivotif Berna). Both offer a protective efficacy of 70% to 80% for at least 3 to 5 years. In younger children, the experimental Vi-conjugate vaccine has a protective efficacy exceeding 90% and may offer protection in parts of the world where a large proportion of preschool children are at risk for the disease.

REFERENCES

Bhutta ZA: Impact of age and drug resistance on mortality in typhoid fever. Arch Dis Child 1996;75:214-217.
Chinh NT, Parry CM, Ly NT, et al: A randomized controlled comparison of azithromycin and ofloxacin for treatment of multidrug-resistant or nalidixic acid-resistant enteric fever. Antimicrob Agents Chemother 2000;44:1855-1859.
Communicable Disease Surveillance and Response Vaccines and Biologicals, World Health Organization: Treatment of Typhoid Fever. Background Document: The Diagnosis, Prevention and Treatment of Typhoid Fever, 2003, pp. 19-23. Available online at http://www.who.int/entity/vaccine_research/documents/en/typhoid_diagnosis.pdf
Crump JA, Luby SP, Mintz ED: The global burden of typhoid fever. Bull World Health Organ 2004;82:346-353.
Gasem MH, Keuter M, Dolmans WM, et al: Persistence of salmonellae in blood and bone marrow: Randomized controlled trial comparing ciprofloxacin and chloramphenicol treatments against enteric fever. Antimicrob Agents Chemother 2003;47:1727-1731.
Luby SP, Faizan MK, Fisher-Hoch SP, et al: Risk factors for typhoid fever in an endemic setting, Karachi, Pakistan. Epidemiol Infect 1998;120:129-138.
Parry CM, Hien TT, Dougan G, et al: Typhoid fever. N Engl J Med 2002;347:1770-1782.
Sinha A, Sazawal S, Kumar R, et al: Typhoid fever in children aged less than 5 years. Lancet 1999;354:734-737.
Thaver D, Zaidi AK, Critchley J, et al: Fluoroquinolones for treating typhoid and paratyphoid fever (enteric fever) (CD004530.pub2). Cochrane Database Syst Rev 2005;2.

Rickettsial and Ehrlichial Infections

Method of
Deverick J. Anderson, MD, and
Daniel J. Sexton, MD

Rickettsial Infections

ROCKY MOUNTAIN SPOTTED FEVER

Rocky Mountain spotted fever (RMSF) is the most lethal of several tickborne illnesses that occur in the United States. Between 20%

and 25% of infections are fatal if not treated appropriately. *Rickettsia rickettsii*, the obligate intracellular bacterium that causes RMSF, circulates in nature in a complex cycle between ticks and small rodents. Humans are only occasional and accidental hosts for this organism.

Epidemiology

RMSF is a highly seasonal disease that predominantly occurs in the spring and early summer months; cases occasionally occur in the autumn and even the winter in warmer climates. RMSF occurs with varying frequency in western Canada, much of the continental United States, Mexico, Central America, Brazil, and Colombia. The incidence of RMSF varies by geographic area and, although reporting of cases of RMSF is primarily through passive surveillance, the average reported annual incidence of RMSF is approximately 2.2 cases per 1 million persons.

Pathogenesis

In the United States, *R. rickettsii* is primarily transmitted by *Dermacentor variabilis* (the American dog tick) in the eastern United States and *Dermacentor andersoni* (the wood tick) in the western United States. Recently, *Rhipicephalus sanguineus* (the common brown dog tick) was recognized as the vector for RMSF in an outbreak in eastern Arizona; this finding is not surprising because this vector also transmits RMSF in Mexico and Central America. Although most infections occur after a tick bite, transmission rarely occurs from crushing or removing infected ticks from humans or animals. Indeed, infection can be experimentally induced with aerosols of infected tick tissues or by mucosal contact. Tick bites are painless and often go unnoticed. Thus, many patients with RMSF have no knowledge of a tick bite prior to the onset of their illness.

Clinical Features and Diagnosis

After inoculation from a tick bite, *R. rickettsii* proliferates and spreads throughout the body via the bloodstream and lymphatics, as well as by contiguous spread from cell to cell. *R. rickettsii* has a specific tropism for endothelial cells, resulting in widespread vasculitis, increased vascular permeability, edema, and activation of the humoral inflammatory and coagulation mechanisms. Organ dysfunction, hypovolemia, and shock can result from microvascular thrombosis and hemorrhage. Risk factors associated with increased severity and fatal outcomes include increasing age, male gender, diabetes mellitus, glucose-6-phosphate dehydrogenase (G6PD) deficiency, alcohol use, and delay in effective therapy for longer than 6 days after onset of symptoms.

The incubation period for RMSF ranges from 2 to 14 days. Most patients with RMSF develop a rash between the third and fifth days of illness. The typical rash of RMSF begins on the ankles and wrists and spreads both centrally and to the palms and soles. The skin rash often begins as a macular or maculopapular eruption and then usually becomes petechial. As many as 10% of patients do not, however, develop a rash *(spotless RMSF)*. Additionally, the rash can be difficult to recognize in patients with dark skin.

Other symptoms of RMSF are nonspecific and include fever, headache, myalgias, malaise, and anorexia. As the disease progresses and becomes more severe, symptoms such as cough, bleeding, nausea, vomiting, abdominal pain, edema (especially in children), delirium, and focal neurologic symptoms (including seizures) can occur. In the absence of the classic triad of tick bite, fever, and rash, patients with RMSF may be erroneously believed to have an array of other infections such as ehrlichiosis, infectious mononucleosis, viral hepatitis, viral meningitis, measles, influenza, toxic shock syndrome, meningococcemia, leptospirosis, or typhoid fever. Because of shared residence and shared risks for tick exposure, family clusters of infection occasionally occur. When such clusters do occur, assumed person-to-person transmission of a viral or bacterial pathogen may lead to misdiagnosis and delay in treatment. If ineffective antibiotics are prescribed empirically before a typical rash appears, patients with RMSF may be erroneously assumed to have a drug eruption. Such cases can end tragically if the rash is presumed to occur because of (ineffective) drug therapy rather than in spite of it.

Most patients with RMSF have normal white blood cell (WBC) counts. As the severity of illness progresses, thrombocytopenia almost always develops, and WBC counts can become quite low. Although fibrinogen concentrations may be low and fibrin split products can become elevated in patients with RMSF, disseminated intravascular coagulation is uncommon. Other common laboratory abnormalities in patients with RMSF include hyponatremia, elevated serum transaminases, hyperbilirubinemia, and elevated creatinine.

There is no timely diagnostic test for RMSF in the early phase of illness. Thus, it is imperative that therapy be based on individual clinical features and the epidemiologic setting. Patients who have symptoms suggesting RMSF and who present in the spring or summer in an endemic area usually require empiric therapy.

Treatment

The preferred therapy is doxycycline (Vibramycin) 100 mg orally or intravenously every 12 hours for adults and children who weigh more than 45 kg. For children younger than 8 years or for children older than 8 years but weighing less than 45 kg, the dose is 2.2 mg/kg divided into two doses (maximum dose 200 mg/day).[1] In severe cases, adjunctive therapy such as mechanical ventilation, oxygen therapy, or hemodialysis may be necessary and useful.

The optimal duration of therapy is unknown. Doxycycline can usually be discontinued 2 or 3 days after the patient becomes afebrile. Most clinicians treat patients with RMSF for 7 to 10 days, but this is probably longer than is necessary for cure in all but the most severe cases. Therapy can and should be discontinued within 4 or 5 days in children with RMSF who respond promptly to treatment because the risk of dental staining is minimal when short courses of doxycycline are given. In general, doxycycline use should be avoided in pregnant women. Instead, pregnant women should be given chloramphenicol (Chloromycetin) 500 mg intravenously or orally every 6 hours. Doxycycline may, however, be the preferred agent for treatment of RMSF in pregnant women at the end of pregnancy because chloramphenicol use in such situations can result in the gray baby syndrome, a potentially fatal drug reaction due to chloramphenicol's effect on bilirubin conjugation in term infants.

Although the diagnosis of RMSF can rarely be made in its acute phase by immunohistochemical staining of skin biopsy samples or by polymerase chain reaction, these diagnostic techniques are available only in a few large referral centers. In routine practice, the diagnosis of RMSF is usually proved long after symptoms and treatment have ceased. The mainstay of diagnosis is indirect fluorescent antibody testing, which is available through all state health laboratories. Antibodies typically appear 10 to 12 days after the onset of illness. The optimal time to obtain a convalescent antibody titer is 14 to 21 days after the onset of symptoms. The minimum diagnostic titer in most laboratories is 1:64.

Prevention

Prevention of many cases of RMSF is impossible because ticks are ubiquitous and many patients with RMSF are unaware of having had a tick bite. Persons with frequent exposure to tick-infested

---

CURRENT DIAGNOSIS

- There are no widely available tests to rapidly and accurately diagnose Rocky Mountain spotted fever (RMSF) in its early phases.
- If morulae are not found in patients with HME or HGA, the diagnosis cannot be established with certainty in the acute phases of these illnesses.

---

[1]Not FDA approved for this indication.

environments should frequently inspect their bodies and clothes for ticks. Early detection and removal of attached ticks can prevent disease transmission. Several hours of feeding are usually required for an infected tick to transmit *R. rickettsii*; thus, RMSF might not occur if infected ticks are removed during this preactivation period. Embedded ticks should be carefully removed by tweezers or by fingers shielded by a cloth, tissues, paper towels, or gloves. Prophylactic antimicrobial therapy is *not* recommended following tick exposure, because only a minuscule percentage of ticks in endemic areas are infected with *R. rickettsii*.

OTHER RICKETTSIAL INFECTIONS

Rickettsiae other than *R. rickettsii* can also cause human infection. For example, a single case of *Rickettsia parkeri* infection was reported in an otherwise healthy 40-year-old man from coastal Virginia in 2002. *R. parkeri* was first isolated from Gulf Coast ticks in the southern United States more than 60 years ago, but until this Virginia case was recognized, *R. parkeri* was not known to cause infections in humans. The patient presented with symptoms similar to those of RMSF and multiple eschars on his lower extremities. Erythematous papules, which then developed into eschars, preceded the other symptoms by 4 days. The patient failed to respond to other antibiotics but improved with doxycycline therapy. Subsequently, the authors of a serologic study of 15 patients with presumed RMSF reported that four of these 15 patients had higher titers for *R. parkeri* than for *R. rickettsii*, suggesting that infection with *R. parkeri* may be more common than previously realized and that some patients with presumed RMSF actually have *R. parkeri* infection.

Ehrlichial Infections

Ehrlichia and *Anaplasma* are obligate intracellular bacteria that grow within membrane-bound vacuoles in human and animal leukocytes. As yet, there is no clear understanding of the mechanism by which *Ehrlichia* produces disease in humans. Humans infected with *Ehrlichia* do not show tissue necrosis, abscess formation, or a severe inflammatory response. Ehrlichial and anaplasmal infections do not lead to vasculitis, thrombosis, or acute endothelial injury as seen in rickettsial infections. *Ehrlichia* replicates within phagosomes in infected leukocytes and produces intracellular colonies called *morulae*.

Ehrlichiosis typically leads to one of two types of illness in humans: human monocytotropic ehrlichiosis (HME) caused by *Ehrlichia chafeensis* or human granulocytic anaplasmosis (HGA) caused by *Anaplasma phagocytophilum*.

EPIDEMIOLOGY

Like other tickborne diseases, the actual incidence of ehrlichiosis is difficult to ascertain because reporting is based on a passive surveillance system that undoubtedly fails to detect or report many cases.

The best available evidence suggests that HME has an annual incidence of approximately 0.7 cases per 1 million persons and primarily occurs in the southeastern, south-central, and mid-Atlantic regions of the United States. *E. chafeensis* was first isolated from a soldier in Fort Chaffee, Arkansas, in 1990. Since then, cases of HME have been recognized in New England and the Pacific Northwest as well. First described in 1994, HGA has an annual incidence of approximately 1.6 cases per 1 million persons and has been described in the upper Midwest, California, and almost the entire Atlantic seaboard.

PATHOGENESIS

The principal vector of *E. chafeensis* is *Amblyomma americanum* (the Lone Star tick); the principal vector of *A. phagocytophilum* is *Ixodes scapularis* (the black-legged tick) in the eastern United States and *I. pacificus* (the western black-legged tick) in the western United States. As opposed to rickettsia, survival of ehrlichia requires horizontal transmission by ticks to and persistent infection in a wild vertebrate host (typically the white-tailed deer or white-footed mouse).

At least two other ehrlichial genogroups cause human disease. Infection of the neutrophils by *E. ewingii* causes mild disease that has mainly been diagnosed in immunocompromised patients in the Midwest. The ehrlichial-like *Neorickettsia sennetsu* group causes a mild mononucleosis-like illness that has never been reported outside East and Southeast Asia.

CLINICAL FEATURES AND DIAGNOSIS

Both HGE and HMA typically occur from May to September and have similar symptoms. After an incubation period of 7 to 14 days, patients most often present with fever, malaise, myalgias, headaches, and chills. An important minority of patients have nausea, vomiting, arthralgias, cough, or neurologic symptoms including altered mental status or stiff neck. Rash is uncommon in ehrlichiosis, though a faint rash occurs more commonly in patients with HGE than in those with HMA. When a rash is present as a prominent sign, coinfection with another rickettsial or other tickborne pathogen should be suspected. Rarely, patients with severe illness develop meningoencephalitis, septic shock, respiratory insufficiency, congestive heart failure, and acute renal failure.

Mortality rates of 3% for patients with HGE and 1% for patients with HMA have been reported, but these numbers may be inaccurate because many mild cases or cases that are empirically treated with doxycycline escape detection or definitive diagnosis. Immunocompromised patients may have severe illnesses and higher mortality rates.

The most common laboratory abnormalities seen in patients with ehrlichiosis are leukopenia and thrombocytopenia, but elevated serum transaminases, lactate dehydrogenase, and alkaline phosphatase levels also occur commonly. Cerebrospinal fluid abnormalities including pleocytosis are common and can mimic the changes seen in patients with viral or other forms of aseptic meningitis.

Distinguishing between RMSF and ehrlichiosis on the basis of clinical features may be impossible, although the presence of leukopenia and the absence of rash are more typical of ehrlichiosis. There are five methods to diagnose ehrlichiosis:

- Examination of peripheral blood or buffy coat for the presence of characteristic morulae in leukocytes
- Indirect fluorescent antibody (IFA) testing
- Polymerase chain reaction testing of tissues
- Immunochemical staining of erhlichial or anaplasmal antigens in tissue
- Synthesis of the history, clinical, laboratory, and epidemiologic features of individual cases

Culture of *Ehrlichia* is extremely difficult, and laboratories able to perform such cultures are few and often inaccessible to clinicians in daily practice. Although only a minority of patients with ehrlichiosis have morulae detectable in blood smears, a blood film should be examined in all patients with suspected infection; morulae are more commonly seen in patients with HGA than in those with HME.

Convalescent serologic antibody testing should be performed 2 to 3 weeks after onset of symptoms. The minimum diagnostic IFA titer is 1:64, and a fourfold-antibody rise is considered confirmatory of recent infection.

TREATMENT

As with rickettsial infection, doxycycline[1] is the treatment of choice for ehrlichiosis. Doxycycline can be administered either orally or intravenously at a dose of 100 mg twice per day. For children who weigh less than 45 kg or are younger than 8 years old, the recommended dose is 2.2 mg/kg each day in two divided doses.[1]

There have been no randomized trials of optimal therapy for either HME or HGA, but the consensus of most experienced clinicians is that therapy should be continued for approximately 7 days or for 3 days after defervescence. Defervescence typically occurs within 48 hours of initiation of therapy.

---

[1]Not FDA approved for this indication.

CURRENT THERAPY

- In most patients with Rocky Mountain spotted fever (RMSF), human monocytotropic ehrlichiosis (HME), or human granulocytic anaplasmosis (HGA), the cornerstone of management is empiric therapy based on clinical judgment and the epidemiologic setting.
- Doxycycline 100 mg PO or IV bid is the treatment of choice for patients with RMSF, HME, and HGA.
- For children who weigh <45 kg or who are younger than 8 y, the recommended dose of doxycycline is 2.2 mg/kg/d in two divided doses.[1]
- Most clinicians treat patients with RMSF for 7 to 10 d; treatment can usually be discontinued 2 to 3 d after the patient becomes afebrile.
- Treat ehrlichiosis for approximately 7 d or for 3 d after defervescence.
- Chloramphenicol (Chloromycetin) 500 mg IV every 6 h should be used to treat pregnant patients with RMSF and patients with adverse reactions to tetracyclines.
- Alternative therapies for HGE and HMA include chloramphenicol and rifampin (Rifadin),[1] although these should only be used to treat HGE or HMA in pregnant patients or in patients with adverse reaction to doxycycline. Doxycycline, however, may be necessary when life-threatening illness occurs in a pregnant patient.

[1]Not FDA approved for this indication.

All tetracyclines can cause dental staining, but this risk remains low if a short course is administered. Chloramphenicol[1] has also been used effectively, but, given the higher risk of hematologic toxicity, this medication should be reserved for pregnant patients or patients with adverse reaction to doxycycline. Additionally, some ehrlichia have been shown to be resistant to chloramphenicol in vitro. Thus, doxycycline may be necessary when life-threatening illness occurs in a pregnant patient. Rifampin (Rifadin)[1] has been used to successfully treat a few pregnant patients with HGA, but at present the efficacy of such therapy can only be considered an anecdotal observation; rifampin does not have an FDA approval for this indication.

[1]Not FDA approved for this indication.

REFERENCES

Bakken JS, Dumler JS: Human granulocytic ehrlichiosis. Clin Infect Dis 2000;31:554-560.
Chapman AS, Bakken JS, Folk SM, et al: Diagnosis and management of tickborne rickettsial diseases: Rocky Mountain spotted fever, ehrlichioses, and anaplasmosis—United States: A practical guide for physicians and other health-care and public health professionals. MMWR Recomm Rep 2006;55(RR-4):1-27.
Holman RC, Paddock CD, Curns AT, et al: Analysis of risk factors for fatal Rocky Mountain spotted fever: Evidence for superiority of tetracyclines for therapy. J Infect Dis. 2001;184:1437-1444.
Kaplan JE, Schonberger LB: The sensitivity of various serologic tests in the diagnosis of Rocky Mountain spotted fever. Am J Trop Med Hyg 1986;35:840-844.
Kirk JL, Sexton DJ, Fine DP, Muchmore HG: Rocky Mountain spotted fever: A clinical review based on 48 confirmed cases. Medicine (Baltimore) 1990;69:35-45.
Paddock CD, Holman RC, Krebs JW, Childs JE: Assessing the magnitude of fatal Rocky Mountain spotted fever in the United States: Comparison of two national data sources. Am J Trop Med Hyg 2002;67:349-354.
Parola P, Raoult D: Ticks and tickborne bacterial diseases in humans: An emerging infectious threat. Clin Infect Dis 2001;32:897-928.
Pretzman C, Daugherty N, Poetter K, Ralph D: The distribution and dynamics of *Rickettsia* in the tick population of Ohio. Ann N Y Acad Sci 1990;590:227-236.
Stone JH, Dierberg K, Aram G, Dumler JS: Human monocytic ehrlichiosis. JAMA 2004;292:2263-2270.

Smallpox

Method of
Isao Arita, MD

This chapter discusses the diagnosis and treatment of smallpox. However, in the unlikely event that a patient appears to have smallpox, it is essential to contact your local public health service office to obtain any updates, including vaccination, other methods of preventing further transmission, and protection for yourself and your personnel from the infection.

In 1980, the World Health Organization (WHO) declared that smallpox was eradiated throughout the world and would not return to the human community, and they recommended that smallpox vaccination be discontinued based on their assessment that risk of return of the disease is unlikely. Thus, all the nations in the world discontinued smallpox vaccination, and smallpox virus stocks in laboratories were destroyed except for those in two WHO collaborating centers in the United States and the Soviet Union. These stocks have been maintained to complete necessary research under strict biocontainment measures.

Since then, there has been no smallpox despite continuing global surveillance of the disease. Although the world has been apparently enjoying the benefit of successful smallpox eradication, the terrorist suicide attacks in New York City and Washington D.C. on September 11, 2001 completely altered the situation: Subsequent deliberate delivery of *Bacillus anthracis* from an unknown source alerted the U.S. and global community to the potential threat of bioterrorism, including smallpox as the bioweapon.

These circumstances urgently revived the necessity to remember the experience in smallpox eradication, which was once thought to be the technology of the past and which did not progress much in terms of prevention and treatment. Fortunately, such experience was described in detail and comprehensively by the experts who actually worked in the eradication program in WHO's 1988 publication "Smallpox and Its Eradication." In this section, special efforts are made to describe salient features of such experiences and knowledge for medical professionals at medical facilities, who may employ them in their emergency work for minimizing possible hazard, if smallpox infection occurs.

As in the past, there is no specific treatment for smallpox. In fact, this was one of the reasons international efforts were made to eradicate smallpox. Smallpox was greatly feared because of its 30% case-fatality rate and its ability to spread in any country and in any season. The second reason was that vaccination had been a very effective tool for prevention, but the complications, such as postvaccinal encephalitis, eczema vaccinatum, and progressive vaccinia, were relatively frequent and severe. For example, 10 to 50 persons per 1 million primary vaccinees suffered adverse effects in the United States. These complications prompted a strong consensus that the only way to eliminate such vaccine complications was to eradicate the disease, thereby making vaccination unnecessary.

Clinical Features

The clinical pictures of smallpox is distinct for diagnosis and surveillance. There is no subclinical infection of epidemiologic significance. If the national security office warns of a possible return of smallpox, the disease ought to be, without much difficulty, suspected by medical personnel, who are concerned about the risk.

Surveillance of deliberate release of smallpox virus will be done by the appropriate national security offices, which require full cooperation by medical professionals. In fact, such cooperation is indispensable. Experience has shown that medical facilities are a common contact point, where persons infected with such severe disease as smallpox will visit, seeking consultation and medical treatment.

Clinical Course

After the incubation period (usually 10-14 days, ranging rarely 7-19 days), prodromal symptoms begin with fever and malaise. The exanthem develops in a very regular stepwise fashion of macules, papules, vesicles, and pustules (Figure 1). The exanthem is quite characteristic, with uniform features at each step and typical distribution on the body. The lesions are distributed more on the face and extremities, the extensor side is more affected than the flexor side, and there are fewer lesions on the trunk. The appearance is so classic that medical personnel can suspect smallpox once they have seen the good pictures of smallpox exanthems.

Within one week, the skin lesions become pustules, which, in a few days, become confluent and reach maximum size. By the end of the second week, scabbing starts. The scabs fall from the skin, leaving depigmented spots in the affected skin (see Figure 1H). The scabs can persist for as long as 1 month. Within a few months, the depigmented areas become blackish pigmented spots. These are signs with which surveillance identified the presence of transmission retrospectively in the affected community in the recent past, if the surveillance missed the actual presence of smallpox. Finally, the pustules on the face become pockmark scars.

As for the severity of the disease, *Variola major* is the severest type, with a fatality rate of 30%. For smallpox terrorism, *V. major* is the likely strain. *V. minor* causes mild disease, with a fatality rate of a few percent. Intermediate-type disease has been found in some areas, including Africa. The clinical pictures of mild and intermediate smallpox are similar to those caused by *V. major*. Hence, *V. minor* disease should be treated just as *V. major* disease is in practice, when surveillance and control measures are to take place. Only laboratory study can verify the type of *V. virus*. Pregnancy appears to augment the severity of the disease.

History of smallpox vaccination modifies the course of the disease. Vaccinated patients who have smallpox have an accelerated clinical course and fewer skin lesions. This applies to persons vaccinated either before immunization programs ended, when smallpox had not yet been eradicated, or during special containment vaccination programs against the risk of infection. However, the percentage of unvaccinated persons among the global population is rapidly increasing. For clinical diagnosis, it is important to refer to the clinical characteristics, as described earlier.

Meanwhile, in emergency or unexpected circumstances, where the public health service has not yet been ready to organize personnel, persons who were vaccinated in the past may be requested (subject to their agreement to help), after a fresh vaccination, to participate in some emergency activities for surveillance or related activities.

Differential Diagnosis and Laboratory Studies

During the program of smallpox eradication (1967-1980), surveillance was based on the clinical diagnosis in endemic nations, and only during the last 3 years of the program was laboratory diagnosis practiced by WHO reference laboratories in the United States and the Soviet Union. However, in today's world, it is important to pay special attention to the differential diagnosis, both clinical and laboratory, because a diagnosis of smallpox will necessarily result in a

CURRENT DIAGNOSIS

- Smallpox was declared eradicated in 1980.
- Smallpox is one of the priority diseases requiring biodefense preparedness.
- Preliminary diagnosis of smallpox should be regarded as a national emergency.
- Smallpox has a characteristic progression of exanthems after prodromal symptoms: macules, papules, vesicles, and pustules. The entire rash is uniform at each stage. The rash lasts about 1 wk after the onset of fever. Check the type of rash on the patient against photos of the exanthems.
- If you suspect smallpox, report it to the local public health service office immediately to get instructions for further emergency action.
- Be prepared to collect specimens from the rash, based on established procedures, and to dispatch them to the designated laboratory.

national health emergency including control of traffic, social events, and economic affairs and psychological calamity.

The clinical differential diagnosis includes varicella and other diseases of rash and fever (Table 1). In varicella, the features of the exanthem are different from those of smallpox. The varicella exanthem is a mixture of different types of rash, and the lesions are more abundant on the trunk (Figure 2). For clinicians, it may be difficult to suspect smallpox for the first 2 to 3 days of smallpox rash, because the rash may be mistaken for varicella or some other skin eruption. However, by day 3 to 4, it should be apparent that the rash is smallpox. Human monkeypox is another possible diagnosis, because the type of rash and distribution on the skin are very similar to those of smallpox, but the lymphadenopathy (maxillar, inguinal, etc.) is distinctive in monkeypox (Figure 3).

In the differential diagnosis of smallpox, it is important to pay attention to the case history of the patient regarding whether the patient has had contact with a smallpox-like disease. In the case of a smallpox attack, there are two possible scenarios. In the first one, a case of deliberate release of smallpox virus through aerosol or contaminated materials, the case history does not arouse suspicion. The second scenario is a patient with secondary transmission from a primary smallpox patient. In this situation, the case history might show the contact with a smallpox-like disease within 17 days before the onset of rash.

The methods of laboratory diagnosis include electron microscopic test, rapid DNA test, virus isolation, and genetic sequence study. These should be operative services of a laboratory network of either a national reference laboratory or a contracted reference laboratory from another country. WHO should be in a position to assist in these laboratory networks.

The electron microscopic or rapid DNA test can be completed within a day, and virus isolation and genetic sequence tests can be completed in a few days in a designated laboratory in the network. Collection and dispatch of specimens (usually from skin lesions) should be according to the accepted protocol, namely, specimen placed in a leak-proof double container and packed according to the rules of the International Association of Transportation Regulators (IATR) (Figure 4).

The preparedness of the laboratory network is the first priority in any nation that wishes to handle smallpox bioterrorism surveillance properly.

Treatment

The patient with diagnosed smallpox must be safely transported and admitted to an isolated station or ward for treatment by

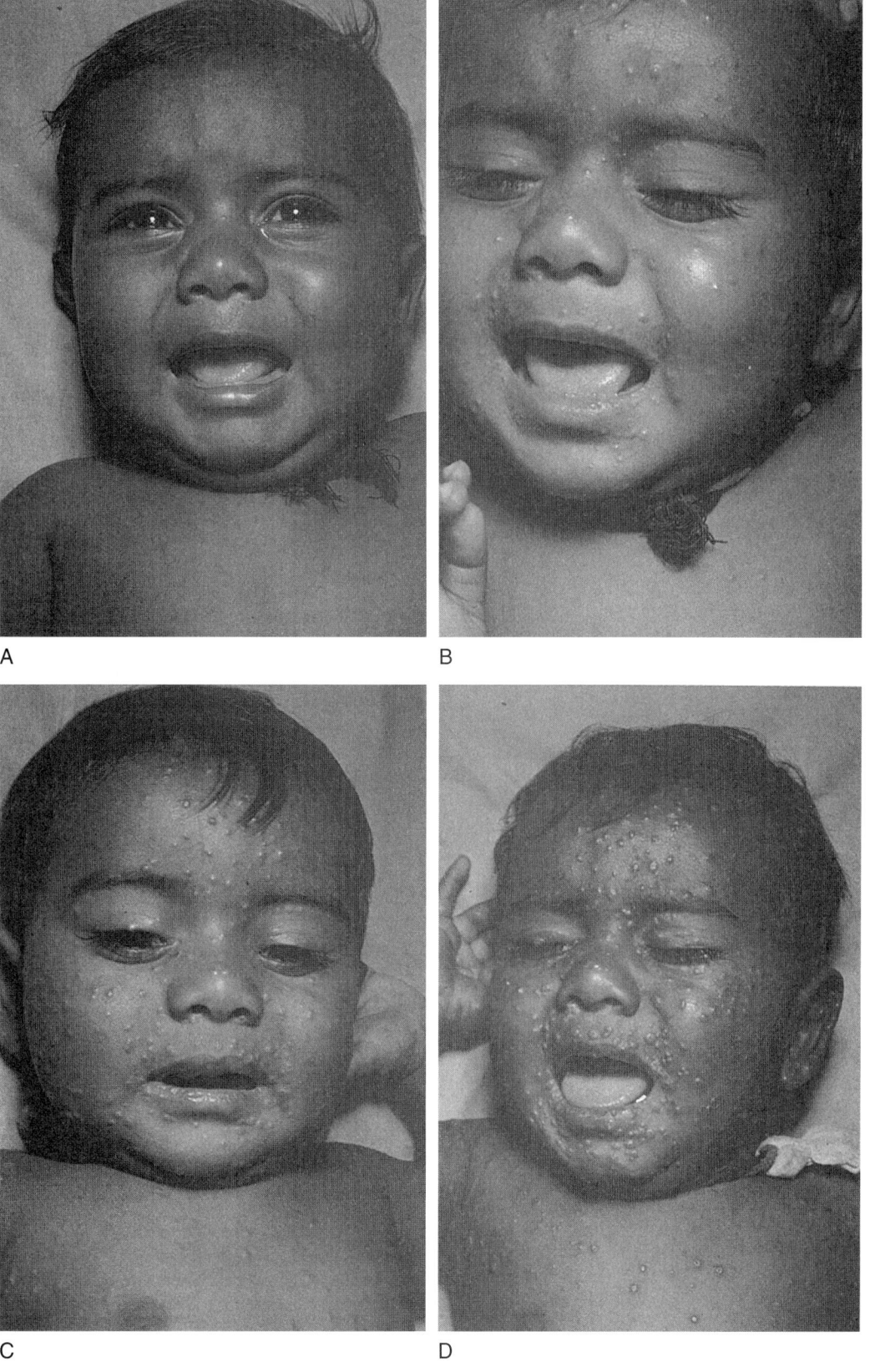

FIGURE 1. Lesions of smallpox. **A,** Day 1: The rash appears 1 day after the onset of fever. A few small papules are visible on the face and upper arms. An enanthem is usually present in the oropharynx at this time, but it cannot be seen in this photograph. **B,** Day 3: Additional lesions continue to appear, and some of the papules are becoming obviously vesicular. **C,** Day 4: All lesions have usually appeared by this time. Those that appeared earliest on the face and upper extremities are somewhat more mature than those that appeared later on other parts of the body, but on any specific area of the body all lesions are at approximately the same stage of development. Lesions are present on the palms. **D,** Day 5: Almost all the papules have now become vesicular or pustular, the true vesicular stage usually being very brief. Some of the lesions on the upper arms show early umbilication.

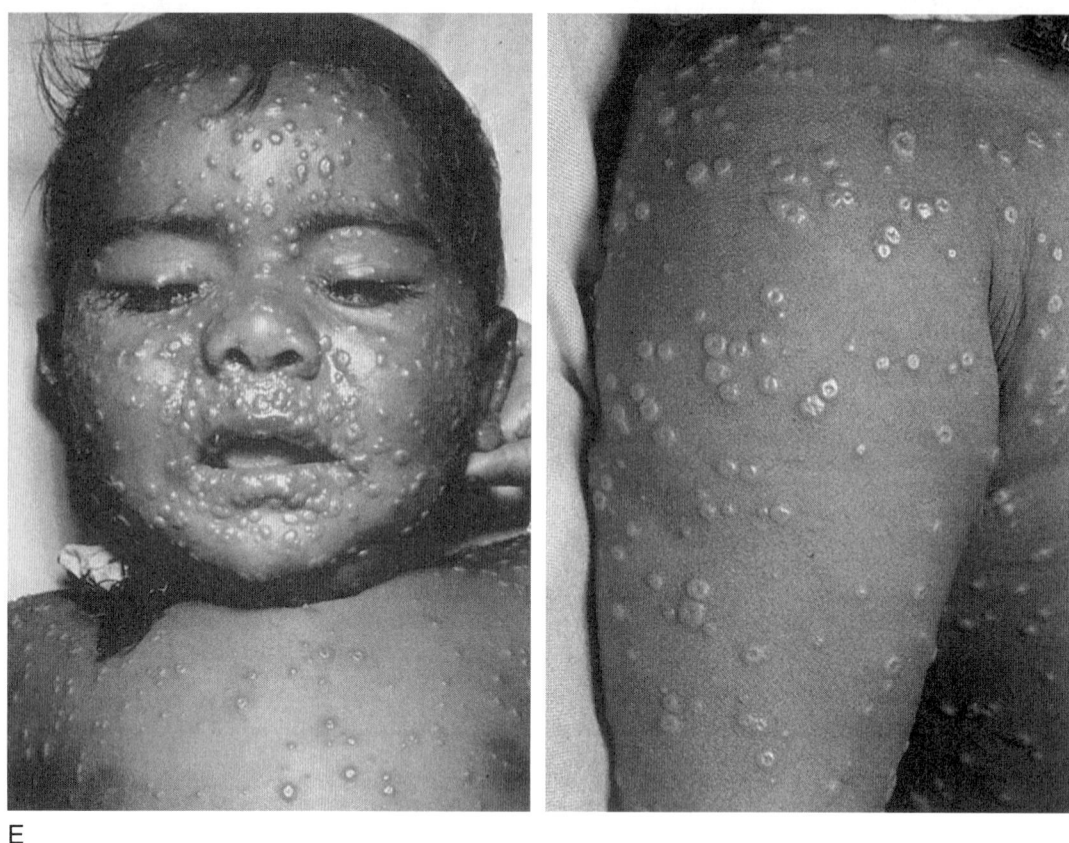

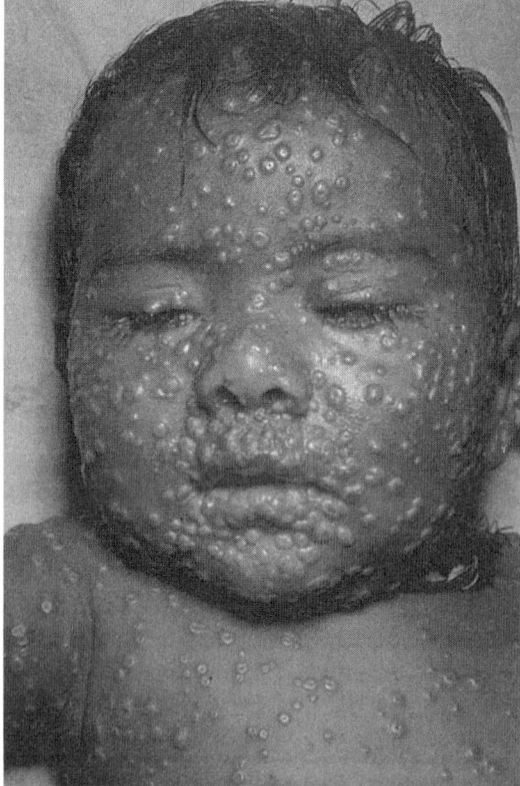

FIGURE 1, cont'd E, Day 6: All the vesicles have now become pustules, which feel round and hard to the touch ("shotty"), like a foreign body. **F,** Day 7: Many of the pustules are now umbilicated and all lesions now appear to be at the same stage of development.

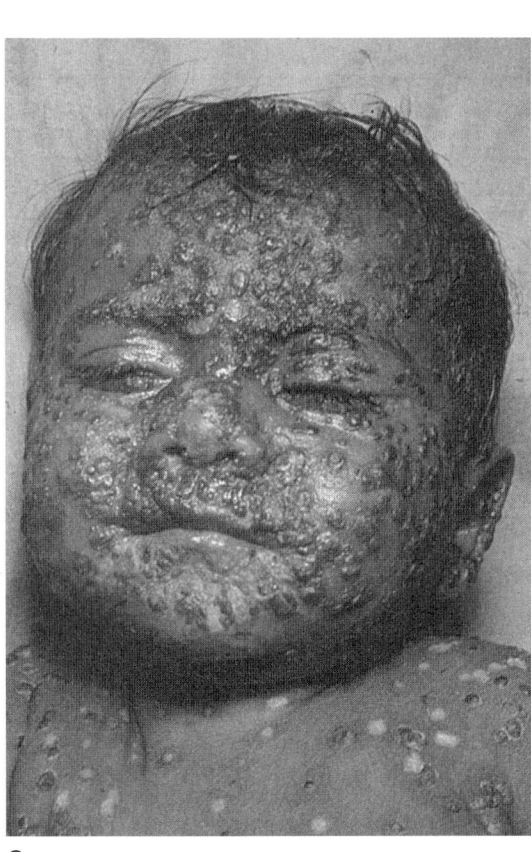
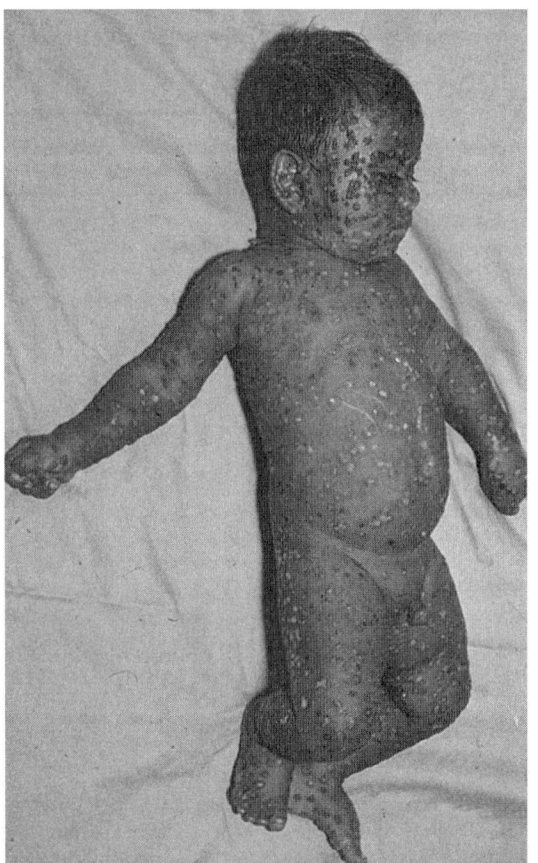
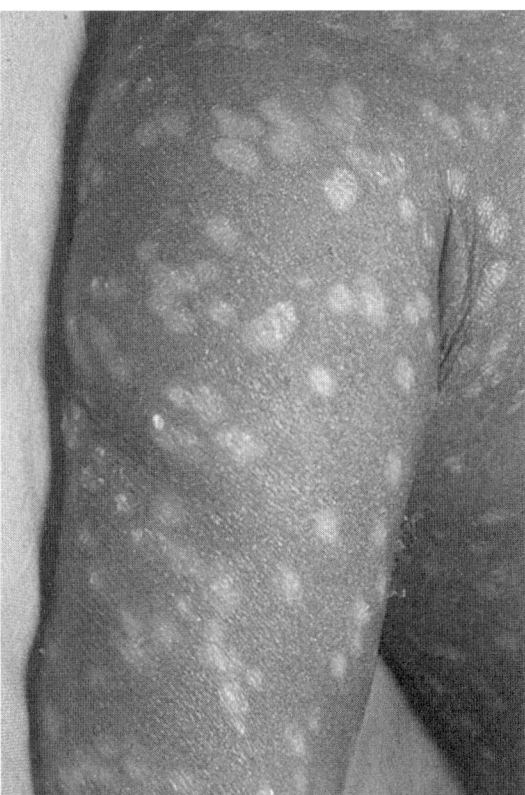

FIGURE 1, cont'd G, Day 13: The lesions are now scabbing, but the eyelids are more swollen than at earlier times. There is no evidence of secondary bacterial infection of the skin lesions. **H,** Day 20: The scabs have separated except on the palms and the soles, leaving depigmented areas.

TABLE 1 Alternative Diagnoses in Suspected but Unconfirmed Cases of Smallpox

Final Diagnosis	England and Wales, 1946-1948* (Variola major)	India, 1976[†] (Variola major)	Somalia, 1977-1979[‡] (Variola minor)
Chickenpox	41	53	20
Erythema multiforme	7	1	0
Allergic dermatitis	7	1	1
Drug rash	6	2	1
Syphilis	3	4	4
Impetigo	3	2	0
Scabies	1	1	0
Psoriasis	1	1	0
Vaccinia	5	0	1
Herpes	2	0	0
Measles	2	0	0
Rubella	1	0	0
Molluscum contagiosum	0	0	1
Septicemia	4	0	0
Skin diseases (various)	14	5	0
Other (including no diagnosis made)	0	30	1
Total	97	100	29

*Data from Conybeare ET: Cases in which smallpox was suspected but unconfirmed. Mon Bull Min Health Public Health Lab Serv 1950;9: 56-61.
[†]During posteradication surveillance in India. Data from Basu RN, Jezek Z, Ward NA: The eradication of smallpox from India. New Delhi: World Health Organization, 1979.
[‡]During posteradication surveillance in Somalia. Data from Jezek Z, Kriz B, Masar I, et al: [Liquidation of the last foci of variola in the world—Somalia (author's transl)] Cesk Epidemiol Mikrobiol Imunol 1981;30(2):113-124. Czech.
Source: World Health Organization.

trained hospital personnel. Patients with suspected smallpox should be also isolated and vaccinated. Patients with suspected smallpox *must not* be treated in the same isolation facilities with smallpox patients.

Currently, there is no effective therapeutic substance licensed for treating smallpox in humans. Before and after the smallpox eradication period (1967-1980), strenuous efforts were made to develop treatment for smallpox, but they have failed. As recently experienced in the United States, immunization of the population as preparedness for biodefense has also failed due to vaccine complications. Most nations, to date, are not in favor of conducting mass vaccination campaigns as preemptive measures. Thus, the research to produce a safer vaccine and the research on an antiviral drug are warranted and continued.

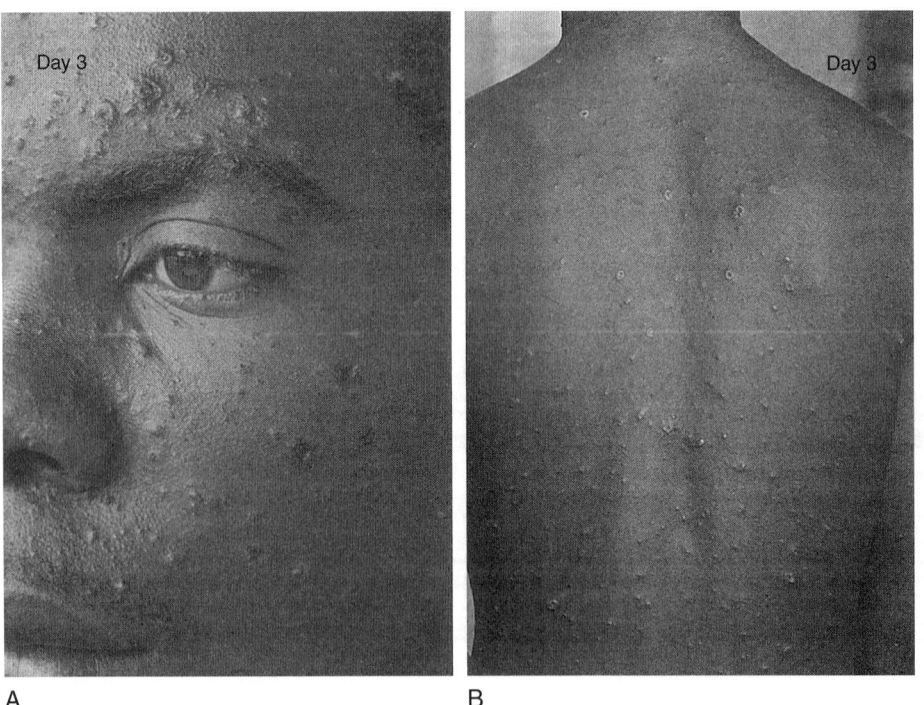

FIGURE 2. Chickenpox. **A** and **B,** On the third day of rash, pocks are at different stages of development (papules and vesicles). There are many lesions on the trunk (**B**) and few on the limbs. (Photographs from the World Health Organization.)

CURRENT THERAPY

- We have no specific antiviral drug or treatment of smallpox.
- Provide supportive care as symptoms suggest.
- Consult the local health service office for all the necessary pubic health measures, such as protection for yourself and your staff from infection, disinfection, isolation, vaccination, transport, and other relevant containment methods as required.

If smallpox reemerges, all patients should receive supportive care. Supportive care can include infection control, such as antibiotics to prevent secondary infection, and intensive rehydration therapy. Ventilator assistance may be needed. In special cases, such as the severe type of hemorrhagic smallpox, patients must also be treated for shock. Attention should be paid to likely renal failure and malnutrition. These medical practices are complicated by the precautions for protection and disinfection that are necessary to prevent smallpox virus contamination of the environment and population.

Experience has shown that smallpox vaccination during the incubation period, within 4 to 5 days after the exposure to the infection, can prevent the infection. However, in practice, any person in contact with a smallpox patient or suspected smallpox patient should be vaccinated as soon as possible. Vaccinia immune globulin intravenous (VIGIV) can reduce some complications of vaccination, but there has been no evidence that it is effective for treating smallpox.

Smallpox was once eradicated by the unified efforts of humankind. The strategy was through immunization as a preventive measure, not through curative treatment, which is not available even today, when bioterrorism by smallpox is threatening us. Research is needed to develop a further attenuated vaccine and antiviral drug as well, but use of the vaccine should still play a greater role, as was done in the eradication efforts a quarter century ago.

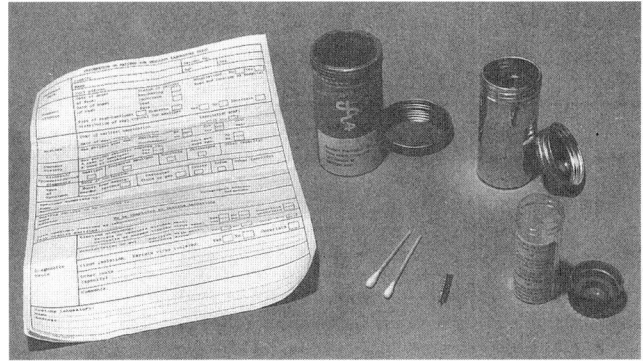

FIGURE 4. Container for smallpox specimen collection. Transportation of dangerous pathogens or specimens requires a special double container to ensure safety. (Photograph from the World Health Organization.)

This article was written in 2006, and because the technical progress will be very rapid, readers are requested to seek updated information that will be available from the World Health Organization (http://www.who.int/csr/disease/smallpox/en/) and the U.S. Centers for Disease Control and Prevention (http://www.bt.cdc.gov/agent/smallpox/index.asp) in 2008.

Acknowledgments

I am grateful to Dr. D. A. Henderson of Johns Hopkins University, who advised on the preparation of this article and to Ms. M. Nakane of the Agency for Cooperation in International Health (in Japan), who sorted out all important references during the preparation of this article.

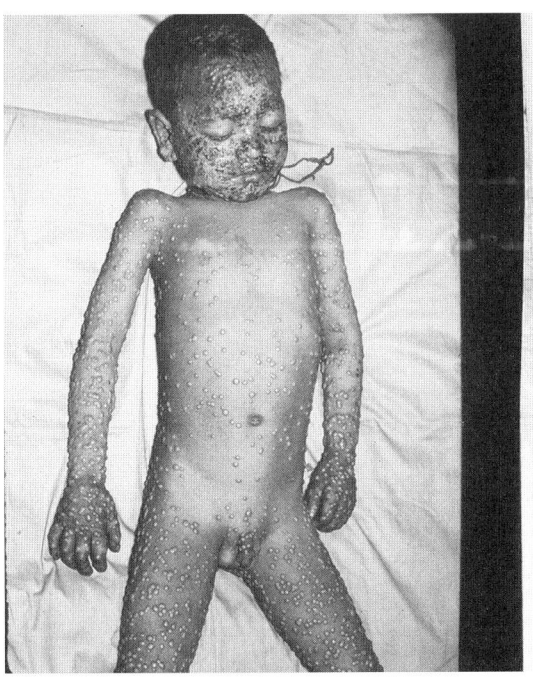

A

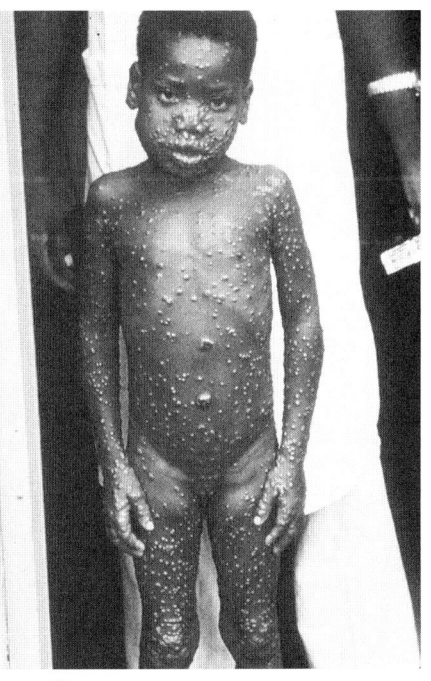

B

FIGURE 3. Similar exanthem in patients infected with smallpox virus (**A**) and monkeypox virus (**B**) on day 7 of exanthem. (Photographs from the World Health Organization.)

REFERENCES

Arita I: Smallpox vaccine and its stockpile in 2005. Lancet Infect Dis 2005;5(10):647-652.

Breman JG, Henderson DA: Diagnosis and management of smallpox. N Engl J Med 2002;346(17):1300-1308 Available from http://content.nejm.org/cgi/content/full/346/17/1300 (accessed May 30, 2007).

Centers for Disease Control and Prevention: Smallpox response plan and guidelines: Annex 1: Overview of smallpox, clinical presentations, and medical care of smallpox patients. Available from http://www.bt.cdc.gov/agent/smallpox/response-plan/files/annex-1-part1of3.pdf (accessed May 30, 2007).

Centers for Disease Control and Prevention: Smallpox response plan and guidelines: Annex 2: General Guidelines for Smallpox Vaccination Clinics. Available from http://www.bt.cdc.gov/agent/smallpox/response-plan/files/annex-2.pdf (accessed May 30, 2007).

Centers for Disease Control and Prevention: Smallpox response plan and guidelines: Annex 3: Guidelines for Large Scale Smallpox Vaccination Clinics: Logistical Considerations and Guidance for State and Local Planning for Emergency, Large-Scale, Voluntary Administration of Smallpox Vaccine in Response to a Smallpox Outbreak. Available from http://www.bt.cdc.gov/agent/smallpox/response-plan/files/annex-3.pdf (accessed May 30, 2007).

Centers for Disease Control and Prevention: Slides and notes: Smallpox disease and its clinical management. Available from http://www.bt.cdc.gov/agent/smallpox/training/overview/pdf/diseasemgmt.pdf (accessed May 30, 2007).

Centers for Disease Control and Prevention: Smallpox fact sheet: Reaction after smallpox vaccination. Available from http://www.bt.cdc.gov/agent/smallpox/vaccination/pdf/reactions-vacc-public.pdf (accessed May 30, 2007).

Fenner F, Henderson DA, Arita I, Jezek Z, Ladnyi ID: Smallpox and Its Eradication. Geneva, Switzerland: World Health Organization, 1988. PDF available at http://whqlibdoc.who.int/smallpox/9241561106.pdf (accessed May 15, 2007).

Institute of Medicine: Assessment of Future Scientific Needs for Live Variola Virus. Washington, DC: National Academies Press, 1999.

University of Pittsburgh Medical Center Center for Biosecurity: Smallpox FAQ, 2005. [on the Internet, cited October 2, 2006] Available from http://www.upmc-biosecurity.org/website/bioagents/smallpox/smallpox_faq_2005.html

SECTION 3

Diseases of the Head and Neck

Laser Vision Correction

Method of
Mitchell P. Weikert, MD, MS

The term *refractive error* describes any condition where light is poorly focused within the eye, resulting in blurred vision. This is the most common eye problem encountered in the United States and includes such conditions as nearsightedness, farsightedness, astigmatism, and age-related loss of near vision (presbyopia).

A wide variety of techniques are available for correcting refractive errors and restoring visual function. The most common methods employ corrective eyewear, such as eyeglasses and contact lenses. More than 150 million Americans are estimated to use corrective eyewear at a cost of approximately $15 billion per year. In addition to these noninvasive modalities, several surgical procedures can also be used to treat these conditions. These surgical techniques range from minimally invasive procedures, such as laser vision correction (LVC), to significantly invasive methods such as refractive lens exchange (RLE) or phakic intraocular lens implantation. LVC is considered minimally invasive because the treatment is extraocular and confined to the cornea. In RLE, the eye's natural lens is replaced with an artificial lens carefully chosen to correct the vision. Although phakic intraocular lens surgery also involves implanting an artificial lens, the natural lens is left in place, so the patient ends up with two lenses inside the eye. Because these techniques constitute intraocular surgery, they are considered more invasive and carry additional risks, such as intraocular infection and retinal detachment.

Whichever method is selected, the primary goal of every vision-correcting procedure should be to choose the technique that is most appropriate for each patient. The chosen method should not only correct the patient's visual deficit but also satisfy their goals for visual function. This chapter focuses on LVC, because it currently is the most popular surgical method for correcting vision. To set the groundwork for the discussion of LVC, we begin with some background information on ocular anatomy, refractive errors, and the clinical assessment of visual function.

Background

Although the human eye is a complex structure, from a conceptual standpoint, it can be thought to function much like a simple camera (Fig. 1). Light first enters through the cornea, a convex transparent window that performs approximately 66% to 75% of the focusing for the eye. After passing through the cornea, the light encounters the iris and pupil. The pupil is an aperture centered within the iris, a muscular diaphragm that controls the diameter of the pupil and thus the amount of light that continues into the eye. The crystalline lens sits behind the pupil and is suspended by a network of supporting cables called zonular fibers. These zonules insert into the ciliary body, a muscular ring that is a peripheral extension of the iris. The natural lens contains the remaining 25% to 33% of the eye's focusing ability. Although much less than that of the cornea, the lens's refractive power is adjustable and can be increased to move the focal point of the eye from distance to near, a process known as *accommodation*. Accommodation results from contraction of the ciliary muscle, which reduces the diameter of the ciliary ring, decreasing zonular tension on the crystalline lens, allowing the lens thickness and anterior curvature to increase, along with its refractive power. After being focused by the lens, light passes through the transparent vitreous humor until it reaches the retina that lines the inside of the back of the eye. The retina functions like the film in a camera, converting the focused image into an electrical signal that is transmitted to the brain via the optic nerve.

Refractive Errors

Refractive errors result when the cornea and lens inadequately focus incoming light, resulting in blurred images projected onto the retina. The unit of measure for refractive error is the diopter, which for a thin lens (in air) is defined as the reciprocal of the lens focal length. For example, a lens that focuses light over a distance of 0.5 m has a refractive power of +2.0 D. If the lens adds focusing power to the system and converges light, it is said to have positive power. Conversely, a lens has negative power if it decreases the system's focusing power and diverges light.

Most refractive errors refer to the patient's visual status when viewing objects in the distance. Emmetropia is the condition where the eye has essentially no refractive error and requires no correction for distance vision (Fig. 2A).

In myopic or nearsighted eyes, the focusing powers of the cornea and lens are too great for the axial length of the eye (see Fig. 2B). The resulting image comes into focus anterior to the retina and is out of focus by the time it reaches the back of the eye. As objects are brought closer to the observer, the focused image within the eye moves back toward the retina. Eventually, the object reaches a point near the observer where its image is correctly focused on the retina, which is why myopic eyes can see better at near, rather than distance. To correct a myopic eye, its refractive power must be decreased by using a lens with negative refractive power.

Hyperopes or farsighted persons are the opposite of myopes. The lens and cornea have inadequate focusing powers for the shorter axial length of the hyperopic eye (see Fig. 2C). The images from objects viewed at a distance are not yet in focus by the time they reach the retina. To see clearly, a hyperopic eye must accommodate to

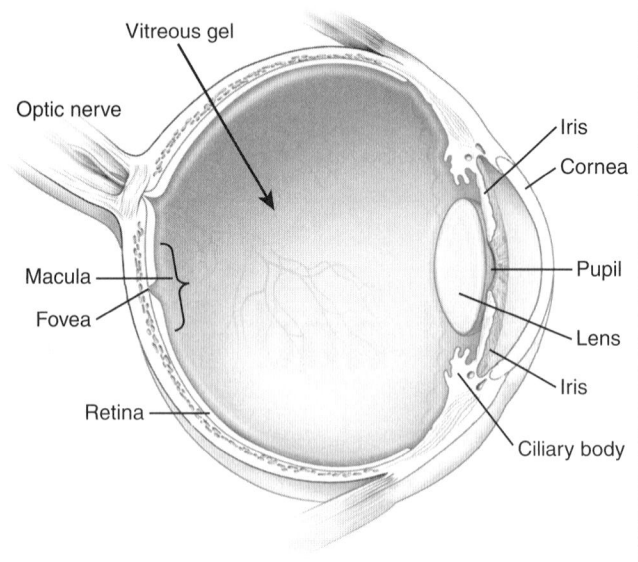

FIGURE 1. Cross-section of a human eye showing major anatomic features. Courtesy of the National Eye Institute, National Institutes of Health.

increase its lenticular power to bring distant objects into sharp focus. Because this requires contraction of the ciliary muscle, the farsighted eye is never at rest and must work even harder to see near objects clearly. Because of this, hyperopic refractive corrections must add focusing power to the eye.

In astigmatism, the eye has different refractive powers along different meridians; light entering in the vertical direction gets focused differently than light in the horizontal direction. Conceptually, it is easier to think of the astigmatic cornea or lens as shaped like a football rather than a basketball, with the meridian of steeper curvature having greater refractive power. The astigmatic eye requires different corrections along each of these meridians to produce a focused image on the retina.

Presbyopia describes the normal age-related loss of near vision. To see near objects clearly, young distance-corrected eyes must accommodate to increase their refractive power. However, this ability progressively declines with age, usually reaching clinical significance in the fifth decade. Several factors have been implicated in this process, including loss of lens elasticity, decreased zonular tension, and altered ciliary muscle function. Although there is currently no way to reverse this natural consequence of aging, several vision-correction options are available to improve near vision in presbyopic persons.

Assessment of Visual Function

The most common way to assess visual function is by measuring visual acuity. Visual acuity testing determines a patient's ability to read high-contrast symbols (usually black letters on a white background) of varying sizes at a standard testing distance. This reference distance approximates optical infinity and is typically 20 feet in the

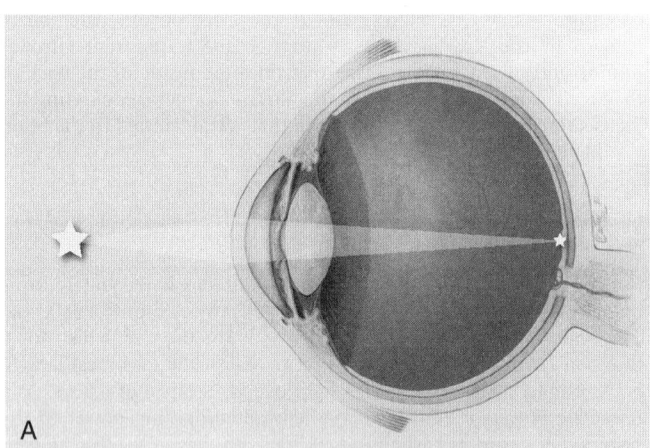
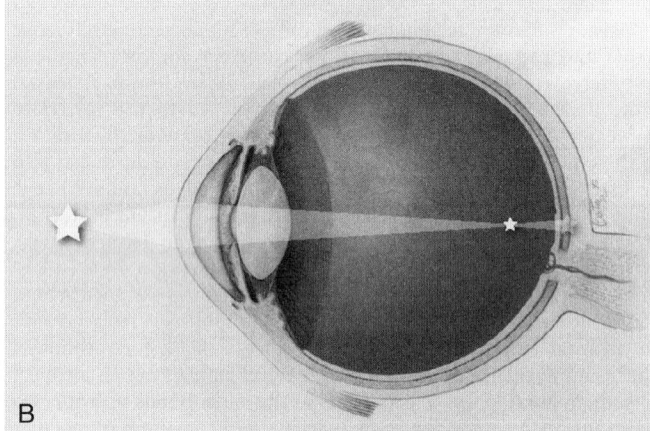
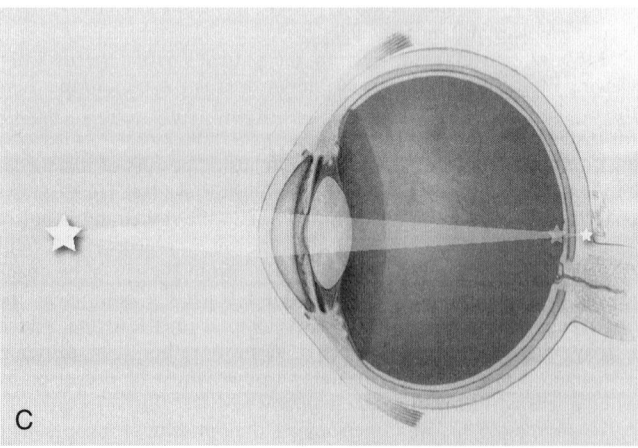

FIGURE 2. Refractive conditions of the eye. **A,** Emmetropia: Image focused on retina. **B,** Myopia: Image focused anterior to retina and out of focus at retina. **C,** Hyperopia: Image focused posterior to retina and out of focus at retina. Courtesy of the National Eye Institute, National Institutes of Health.

United States and 6 meters in Europe. A 20/20 letter on the standard eye chart devised by Snellen is approximately 3/8 inch tall at a distance of 20 feet (subtending a visual angle of 5 minutes of arc). Twenty-twenty vision is considered normal visual acuity.

Visual acuities less than 20/20 are represented by ratios whose denominator is greater than 20. For example, a visual acuity of 20/60 means that the smallest letter the eye can read is three times larger than a 20/20-size letter. A person is considered legally blind when both eyes have visual acuities of 20/200 or less. Although other aspects of visual function, such as contrast sensitivity, color perception, and peripheral vision, are often measured, visual acuity is by far the most commonly used method for rating visual performance.

Focusing or refractive errors can result in *uncorrected* visual acuities that fall below 20/20. However, in the absence of other disease, the conditions of myopia, hyperopia, astigmatism, and presbyopia can be corrected with restoration of normal visual function. Although noninvasive methods such as eyeglasses or contact lenses may be used, the remainder of this chapter is devoted to laser-based surgical methods for correcting refractive errors.

Laser Vision Correction

Laser in situ keratomileusis (LASIK) and photorefractive keratectomy (PRK) use an excimer laser to reshape the anterior surface of the cornea to correct the eye's refractive error. The excimer laser was developed in the 1970s and emits ultraviolet light at a wavelength of 193 nm. This particular wavelength has been found to accurately and efficiently ablate corneal tissue without causing thermal damage to the surrounding collagen. Each pulse of the laser removes approximately 0.25 µm, allowing precise contouring of the corneal surface. In myopia, the excimer laser treatment flattens the central cornea to decrease its focusing power. In hyperopia, laser pulses are applied to the periphery, indirectly steepening the central cornea and thereby increasing its refractive power. Astigmatism is corrected by combining central and peripheral treatments to differentially steepen the flattest corneal meridian and flatten the steepest meridian. The first excimer treatment on a seeing eye was performed in the late 1980s for the correction of myopia. Since that time, LASIK and PRK have been used to treat refractive errors in millions of patients.

LASER IN SITU KERATOMILEUSIS

In LASIK, a lamellar or partial-thickness corneal flap is first created in the cornea. The flap thickness typically varies from about 100 to 180 µm, as compared with a total corneal thickness that usually ranges from 500 to 600 µm. The LASIK flap is reflected at its hinge and the excimer laser ablation is applied to the underlying corneal stroma. Once the ablation is complete, the flap is returned to its original position. The most common way to create the LASIK flap is with a microkeratome, a device containing a motorized oscillating blade connected to a suction ring.

In recent years, flap creation has moved away from mechanical devices and toward the femtosecond laser (Fig. 3). The femtosecond laser uses ultrashort microscopic pulses of infrared light to define the lamellar flap. A spatula is then used to lyse any septa that remain between the laser spots, permitting reflection of the flap. The femtosecond laser can create flaps with greater predictability, and its nonmechanical nature eliminates the risk of certain serious complications, such as free, partial, or buttonhole flaps.

Recovery of vision usually takes a few days; some patients note gradual improvement over a few weeks. Postoperative medications usually include topical antibiotic and steroid eye drops for approximately 5 to 7 days.

PHOTOREFRACTIVE KERATECTOMY AND LASER-ASSISTED SUBEPITHELIAL KERATOMILEUSIS

PRK also uses the excimer laser to reshape the cornea, but this procedure requires no lamellar flap. In this method, the laser treatment is applied directly to the anterior stromal surface after the corneal epithelium is removed. Several techniques are available to remove the corneal epithelium. Mechanical débridement with a spatula or rotating brush is very common, as is devitalization with a 20% alcohol solution, followed by gentle débridement with a blunt spatula (Fig. 4). Newer techniques use an epikeratome (similar to a LASIK microkeratome) to separate a flap of epithelium at the level of the basement membrane. Each of these methods has certain advantages and disadvantages, but all do an effective job of preparing the corneal surface for laser ablation.

Once the laser treatment is complete, a soft contact lens is placed on the cornea. The corneal epithelium typically heals in 4 to 5 days, after which the contact lens is removed. Once the contact lens is removed, recovery of vision can take a few more weeks, although some patients experience improvement in vision that continues over several months. Antibiotic eye drops are used until the contact lens is removed, and steroid eye drops may be tapered over several months.

Laser-assisted subepithelial keratomileusis (LASEK) is a form of PRK. An epithelial flap is created with alcohol débridement or with an epikeratome. The epithelial flap is reflected and the laser treatment is performed, similar to LASIK. After the corneal ablation is completed, the epithelial flap is replaced and a contact lens is applied. Some surgeons believe that retention of the epithelium improves postoperative comfort, speeds epithelial healing, and decreases the risk of subepithelial haze following the procedure.

Recent Advances in Laser Refractive Surgery

The excimer laser treatments used in conventional LASIK and PRK are computed from the patient's manifest and cycloplegic refractions, that is, the measurement of the patient's eyeglass prescription before and after dilation, respectively. These treatments have been refined in the last few years using wavefront science. Wavefront technology measures the idiosyncratic focusing errors of the eye using an aberrometer. These individual focusing errors, or aberrations, can degrade the postoperative vision even if the patient's myopia, hyperopia, or astigmatism are virtually eliminated. By reducing postoperative aberrations, the probability of achieving uncorrected visual acuities of 20/20 or better significantly increases. The uncorrected visual acuity results for the U.S. Food and Drug Admnistration (FDA) clinical trials in wavefront-guided LASIK are presented in Table 1.

Successful laser refractive surgery depends on accurate calculation of the excimer ablation pattern and on precise placement of this treatment. Commercial lasers use several methods to optimize placement of the laser pattern. Fixation lights provide the patient with a visual target that aligns the center of the treatment with the line-of-sight. Trackers identify the edge of the pupil and monitor eye movement during the treatment. By tracking eye movement, the laser can continuously redirect the treatment to ensure alignment with the pupil center. Newer trackers can also identify landmarks on the iris to aid in accurately positioning the ablation pattern (Fig. 5). This technology is known as *iris registration* and helps to compensate for rotational misalignment and shifting of the pupil center under different lighting conditions. Although these automated techniques have made significant strides in improving treatment accuracy, there is still no substitute for a cooperative patient who steadily fixes on the target light during the laser ablation.

Screening Examinations

Laser vision correction is very successful, but it is still an elective procedure and might not be the best choice for every patient. A thorough screening examination is recommended to determine if a patient is a good candidate for LASIK or PRK. Essential elements of the screening visit include a thorough medical and ophthalmic history, combined with assessment of the Snellen visual acuity, manifest refraction, cycloplegic refraction, pupil sizes in dim and bright light, ocular surface condition, tear film quality, corneal thickness, corneal shape,

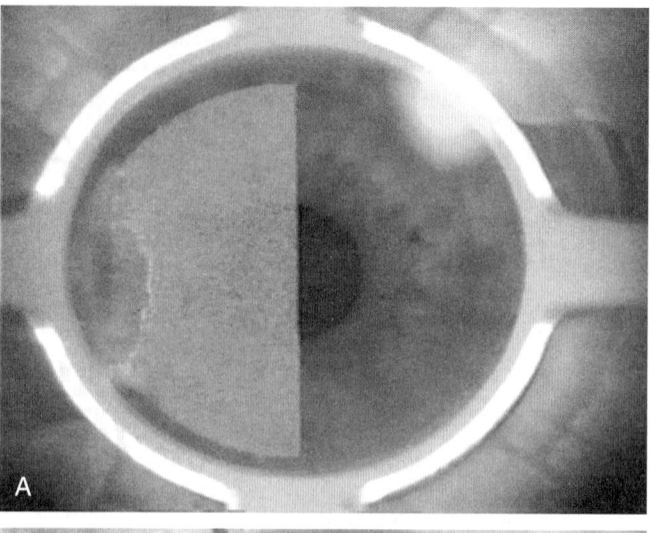
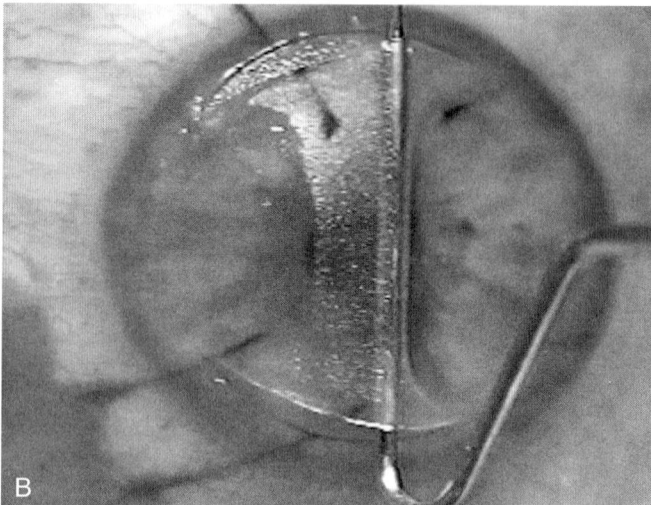
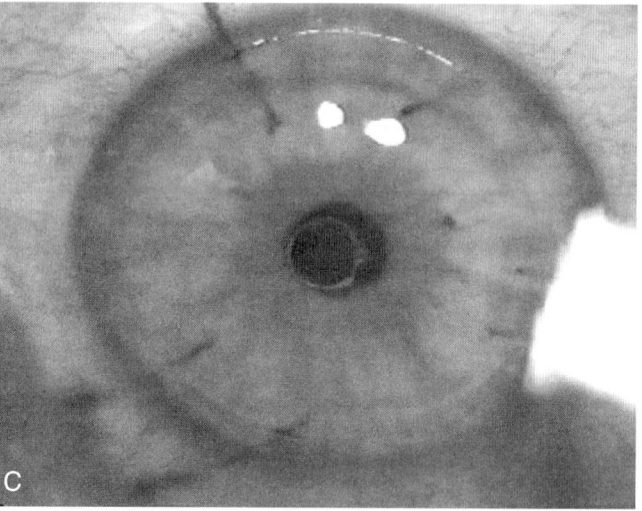

FIGURE 3. Laser in situ keratomileusis (LASIK) flap creation with the femtosecond laser. **A,** Laser treatment to bed of flap. **B,** Flap lift with spatula. **C,** Flap following replacement after laser ablation to correct myopia.

intraocular pressure, optic nerve health, and retinal status. If a patient cannot achieve a visual acuity of 20/20 with the best spectacle or contact lens correction in place, the vision is most likely not correctable with laser surgery either. If a vision-limiting condition has not been previously identified, the patient should receive a comprehensive examination to determine the etiology of the vision loss.

The manifest and cycloplegic (postdilation) refractions determine if the patient's correction falls within the approved treatment range of the laser. They are also valuable in setting patient expectations, because higher corrections may be associated with longer visual recovery and a slight reduction in the percentage of patients achieving uncorrected acuities of 20/20 or better.

The measurement of corneal thickness, also known as corneal pachymetry, can help direct the treatment choice toward LASIK or PRK. In LASIK, the laser treatment is applied under the lamellar flap and thus extends deeper into the cornea. Therefore, in eyes undergoing LASIK, the preoperative corneal pachymetry must be greater to ensure that the remaining, untouched cornea is thick enough to preserve its structural integrity. If the predicted thickness of the residual corneal bed falls below 250 to 300 μm, PRK may be the treatment of choice.

Certain corneal shapes can suggest a predisposition toward excessive weakening following laser vision correction. If corneal asymmetry is found (Fig. 6), the appropriate choice may be PRK or no surgery at all.

Finally, both PRK and LASIK damage corneal nerves. Although this denervation of the cornea is usually temporary, it can result in postoperative dryness, which may be greater in LASIK due to its greater treatment depth. If dryness is found in the screening examination, it should be managed before treatment, and PRK may be more appropriate.

Complications

Although laser refractive surgery is very safe, it is still surgery and is subject to complications, both during and after the procedure. Most intraoperative complications associated with LASIK involve the flap. The mechanical microkeratome and femtosecond laser both rely on a suction ring to hold the eye in place while the flap is being cut. Suction loss causes both devices to stop, which can result in partial flaps. Mechanical microkeratomes can produce erratic cuts in corneas that are excessively steep or flat, resulting in donut-shaped flaps with "buttonholes" or free flaps without hinges, respectively. The femtosecond laser eliminates the risk of buttonholes or free flaps, but it occasionally produces incomplete treatments that make the flap difficult to lift. In most cases, the excimer laser treatment can be completed at a later date with creation of a new flap. However, in certain instances, a case may require conversion to surface treatment with PRK.

Because laser-induced tissue cleavage creates gas bubbles, the femtosecond laser can produce temporary opacification of the cornea that can interfere with the laser's tracking mechanism. This opaque

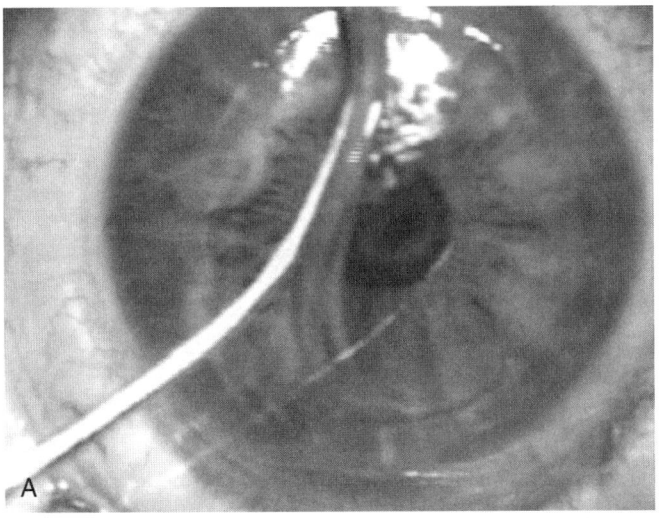
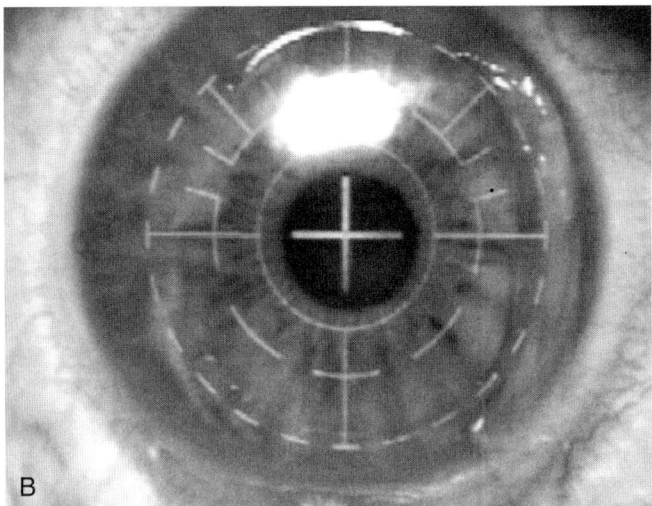
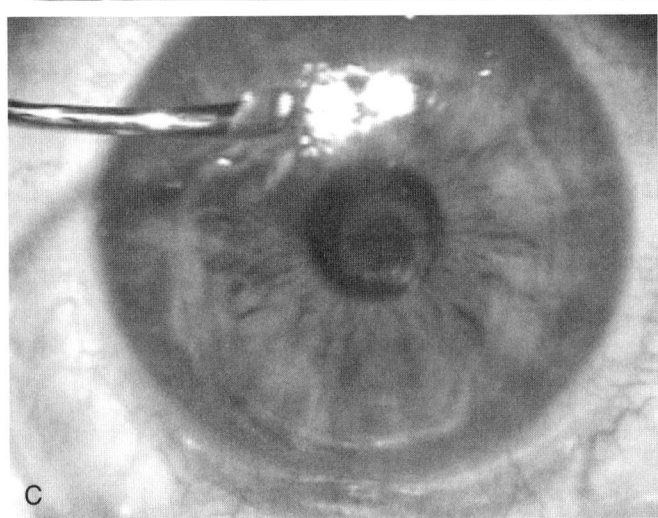

FIGURE 4. Corneal epithelial removal in laser-assisted subepithelial keratomileusis (LASEK). **A,** The epithelial flap is swept to the periphery of the cornea with a blunt spatula. **B,** The laser ablation is performed on the exposed corneal stroma. **C,** The epithelial flap is replaced following laser ablation.

bubble layer eventually clears, but it can prolong the procedure during this interval.

All modern excimer lasers use trackers to monitor the eye position during treatment, but they still require the patient to fix the gaze on a target during the laser ablation. Even with the best tracking mechanisms, fixation loss can result in decentration of the laser treatment, which can degrade the postoperative vision.

LASIK carries the postoperative risks of flap displacement or induction of flap striae. Flap displacement can occur spontaneously, and flap striae are usually associated with eye rubbing. Most of these cases require a flap lift and reposition. However, more severe or refractory cases can require further intervention, such as suturing.

On rare occasions, epithelial cells from the corneal surface can migrate underneath the LASIK flap and proliferate in the interface. Small peripheral nests of epithelial cells can be observed and can resolve without intervention. Large collections of cells can compromise vision or cause corneal necrosis and scarring, so they need to be removed. Epithelial ingrowth requires lifting of the flap and manual

TABLE 1 U.S. FDA Clinical Trial Results for Wavefront-Guided Lasik

		Uncorrected Vision Results (% Eyes)	
Refractive Category	Correction Range	≥ 20/20	≥ 20/40
Myopia	0 to −6.0 D	84%-93%	98%-99%
High myopia	−6.0 to −11.0 D	84%-93%	98%-100%
Hyperopia	0 to +3.0 D	56%-67%	93%-95%
Mixed astigmatism	Astigmatism up to 6 D	56%-87%	93%-99%

Note: Data are for four different laser platforms (AMO-VISX Star S4, Bausch & Lomb Zyoptix, Alcon LADARVision, Wavelight Allegretto). The percentage of eyes achieving uncorrected visual acuities ≥20/20 and 20/40 are listed. Although the clinical trials for wavefront-guided laser treatments were conducted for LASIK, most eye centers also use the same laser platforms to perform PRK as off-label procedures.
LASIK = laser in situ keratomileusis; PRK = photorefractive keratectomy.

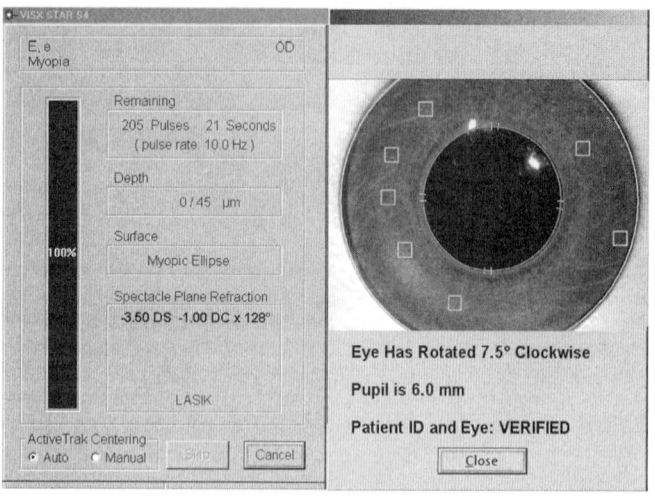

FIGURE 5. Display screen showing iris registration with identification of iris landmarks, ocular rotation, and the corneal limbus to allow proper alignment of the laser ablation pattern.

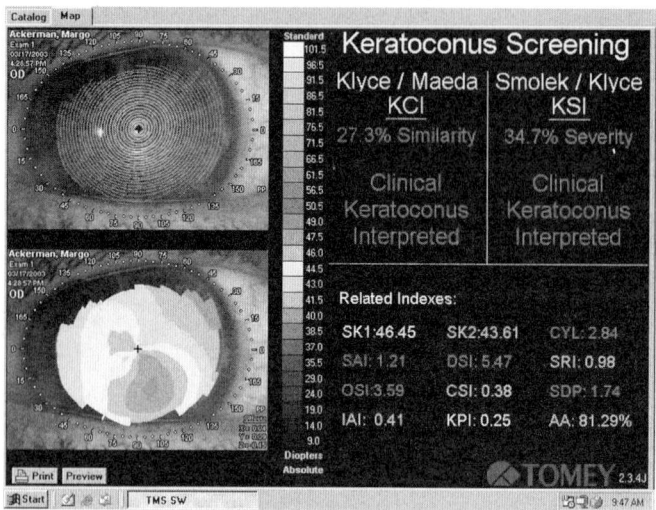

FIGURE 6. Abnormal corneal topography. The topographic map demonstrates steeper curvature in the inferior cornea *(red and orange areas)* as compared with the superior cornea *(yellow and green areas)*. This map is highly suspicious for keratoconus, a degenerative condition of the cornea. Laser treatment of this eye has a high risk for excessively weakening the cornea, with worsening of the keratoconus.

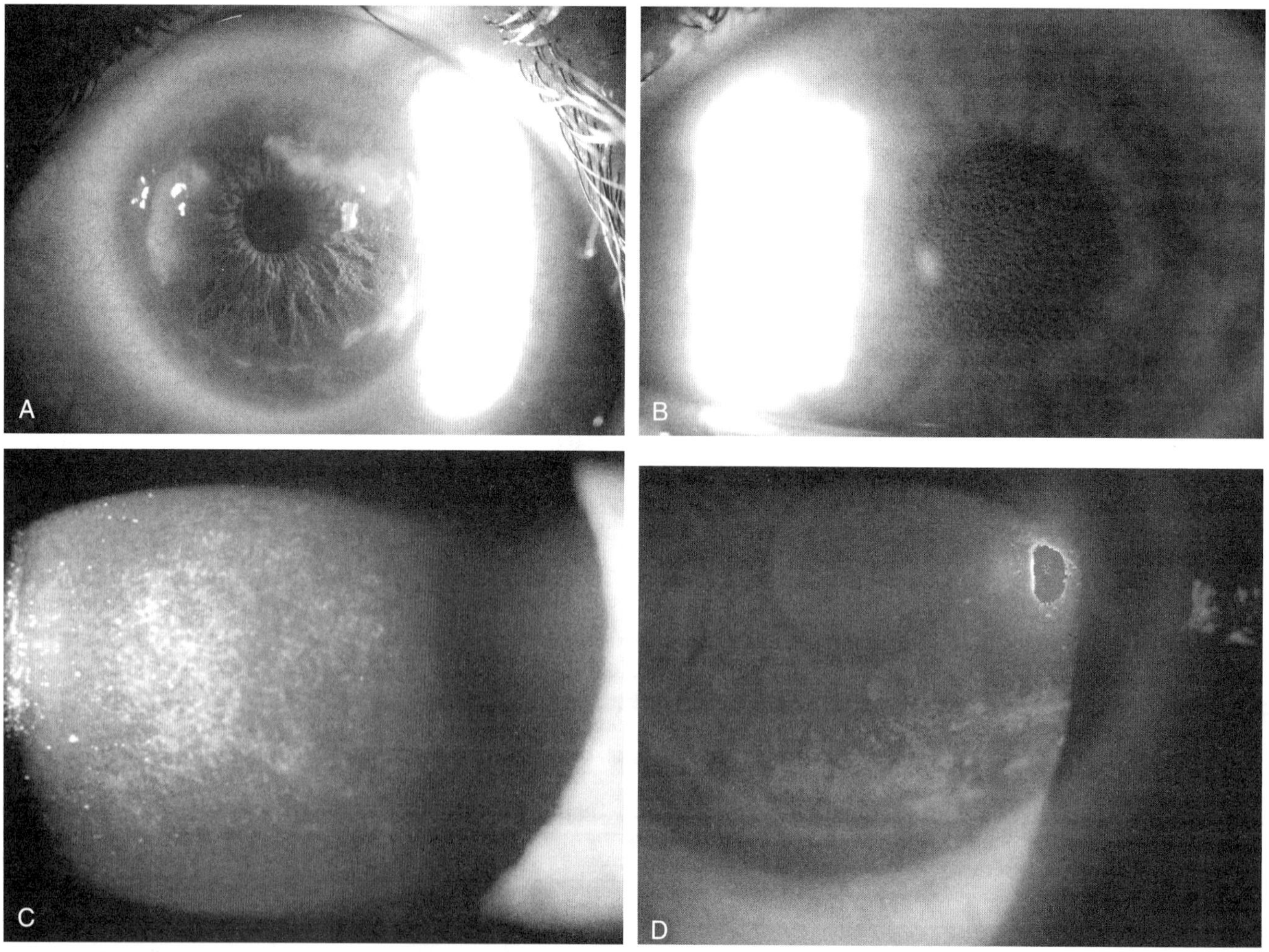

FIGURE 7. Potential complications of laser vision correction. **A,** Multifocal infiltrates following laser in situ keratomileusis (LASIK). This may be due to infection or sterile inflammation. **B,** Diffuse lamellar keratitis: Inflammation in the interface underneath a LASIK flap. **C,** Subepithelial corneal haze following photorefractive keratectomy (PRK). **D,** Post-LASIK dry eye with corneal epitheliopathy stained with fluorescein and illuminated via a cobalt-blue filter.

débridement of the cells. This treatment might need supplementation with alcohol or suturing, or both, to prevent recurrence.

Corneal weakening and subsequent distortion are other potential sequelae of laser vision correction. Certain preoperative corneal shapes suggest a predisposition toward weakening, especially those with steeper curvature in the inferior region as compared with the superior region (see Fig. 6). Preoperative corneal thicknesses less than 500 μm or post-LASIK residual stromal bed thicknesses less than 250 μm can also be associated with corneal weakening.

As with any surgery, LASIK and PRK are also associated with a risk of infection (Fig. 7A). The incidence varies, but published rates have been about 0.03%. Staphylococcal and streptococcal species are most common, but atypical organisms such as mycobacteria and fungi have also been reported. Management of post-LASIK corneal infections includes culturing, topical antibiotic eyedrops, flap interface irrigation, and, rarely, flap amputation or corneal transplant. Sterile inflammation can also occur in the flap interface and is known as *diffuse lamellar keratitis* (see Fig. 7B). Diffuse lamellar keratitis has been associated with bacterial endotoxin, cleaning solutions, corneal abrasions, and excessive femtosecond laser energy levels. Treatment primarily relies on topical steroid eyedrops, but it may also include oral steroids and flap-interface irrigation.

PRK does not carry the risk of flap complications, but it can be associated with subepithelial haze (see Fig. 7C). Fibroblastic transformation of keratinocytes can cause the deposition of disorganized collagen that decreases the smoothness and clarity of the post-PRK cornea. This development is usually associated with higher myopic corrections and may be reversed by increased application of topical steroid eyedrops. Short-duration intraoperative use of low-concentration topical mitomycin-C (Mutamycin)[1] (0.02%) appears to decrease the risk of haze formation.

Both PRK and LASIK damage corneal nerves, which appears to have a secondary effect on the ocular hydration status. Postoperative dry eye is greater in LASIK than PRK due to its greater depth of penetration into the cornea. The increased dryness appears to be temporary, and most patients return to baseline by 6 to 9 months, but a subset of patients experience chronic dry eyes following the procedure (see Fig. 7D). A careful preoperative assessment of dry eye risk factors is recommended, and those at risk may be steered toward PRK or toward no surgery at all.

Conclusions

Laser vision correction is currently the most popular surgical technique for correcting refractive errors, providing millions of patients with increased freedom from eyeglasses and contact lenses. Laser vision correction is safe and effective, but it is a surgical procedure and thus carries the risk for certain complications. A thorough preoperative interview and evaluation should be performed on each refractive surgery candidate to assess the patient's surgical risk and to identify the patient's goals and clarify expectations. Systematic application of these methods allows the refractive surgeon to choose the safest and most appropriate method for correcting the patient's refractive error, which sometimes is no surgery at all.

REFERENCES

Chang MA, Jain S, Azar DT: Infections following laser in situ keratomileusis: An integration of the published literature. Surv Ophthalmol 2004;49:269-280.

Friedman DS, Congdon N, Kempen J, Tielsch JM: Vision problems in the U.S. Prevent Blindness America, 2008 update to the 4th edition. Available at http://www.preventblindness.org/vpus/2008_update/VPUS_2008_update.pdf (accessed May 1, 2008).

Glasser A, Croft MA, Kaufman PL: Aging of the human crystalline lens and presbyopia. Int Ophthalmol Clin 2001;1(2):33-46.

Melki SA, Azar DT: LASIK complications: Etiology, management, and prevention. Surv Ophthalmol 2001;46:95-116.

McDonald MB, Kaufman HE, Frantz JM, et al: Excimer laser ablation in a human eye. Arch Ophthalmol 1989;107:641-642.

Sakimoto T, Rosenblatt MI, Azar DT: Laser eye surgery for refractive errors. Lancet 2006;367(9520):1432-1447.

Schallhorn SC, Amesbury EC, Tanzer DJ: Avoidance, recognition, and management of LASIK complications. Am J Ophthalmol 2006;141:733-739.

Trokel SL, Srinivasan R, Braren B: Excimer laser surgery of the cornea. Am J Ophthalmol 1983;96:710-715.

Conjunctivitis

Method of
Robert A. Copeland, Jr., MD

The conjunctiva is a unique mucous membrane that covers the inner surface of the eyelids and extends to the limbus on the surface of the globe. The major functions of the conjunctiva are to produce mucus for the tear film layer and to provide immune cells and antimicrobial agents to protect the ocular surface. The conjunctiva is divided into three anatomic areas: palpebral, forniceal (cul-de-sac), and bulbar. The conjunctiva is loosely attached to the eye and allows free movement. Similar to most mucous membranes, the conjunctiva has an epithelial layer and a deeper substantia propria.

Conjunctivitis is an inflammation of the conjunctiva that may have an infectious or noninfectious cause (Table 1). Noninfectious entities include allergic, immunologic, and toxic causes. Infectious agents include bacteria, viruses, and chlamydia.

Allergic Conjunctivitis

Ocular allergies encompass a variety of entities and are classically divided into five categories: seasonal allergic conjunctivitis, vernal keratoconjunctivitis, giant papillary conjunctivitis, atopic keratoconjunctivitis, and contact conjunctivitis. These varied diseases of the conjunctiva correlate with one or more of the four types of hypersensitive reactions described by Gell and Coomb. Allergic diseases affect approximately 10% of the general population, and most allergy sufferers have a family history. These patients develop symptoms and signs in childhood.

Seasonal allergic conjunctivitis is an acute process that is IgE mediated and triggered by airborne pollen, dander, mold, and house dust. This IgE mediation results in degranulation of conjunctiva, edema, erythema, and itching. Other, more severe forms of allergic conjunctivitis include vernal keratoconjunctivitis, which occurs in people with atopic dermatitis. Giant papillary conjunctivitis occurs in contact lens wearers who in most cases have lens surface deposits.

Seasonal allergic conjunctivitis is controlled by avoiding the offending allergen if possible. Initially, artificial tear supplements and a topical antihistamine and decongestant can be used to treat acute symptoms. The nonsteroidal antiinflammatory drug ketorolac (Acular) is effective in relieving itching. Cromolyn sodium 4% (Crolom) and lodoxamide (Alomide) are mast cell stabilizers and can be used prophylactically before exposure to offending allergens. A new classification of antihistamines and mast cell stabilizers, including ketotifen fumarate (Zaditor), levocabastine (Livostin),[8] olopatadine (Patanol), emedastine difumarate (Emadine), nedocromil sodium (Alocril), and azelastine (Optivar), is expected to play an increasing role in treating seasonal allergic conjunctivitis.

---

[1]Not FDA approved for this indication.

[8]Orphan drug in the United States.

TABLE 1 Differential Diagnosis of Conjunctivitis

Cause	Signs and Symptoms	Diagnostic Tests	Treatment	Differential Diagnosis
Bacterial	Lids stuck together in morning, visible discharge in tear film and/or caruncle, conjunctival injection, membrane or pseudomembranes	Gram stain, blood agar, chocolate agar, thioglycolate broth	Erythromycin, polymyxin B plus trimethoprim, bacitracin, aminoglycosides, fluoroquinolones	Allergic conjunctivitis, dry eye syndrome, viral conjunctivitis, chlamydial conjunctivitis, Parinaud's oculoglandular syndrome, sebaceous gland carcinoma, drug-induced allergic conjunctivitis, floppy lid syndrome
Chlamydial	Chronic unilateral or bilateral mucopurulent conjunctivitis	McCoy cell culture, ELISA, direct immunofluorescent monoclonal antibody stain	Tetracycline 250 mg PO qid for 3 wk Doxycycline 100 mg bid PO for 3 wk Erythromycin 500 mg PO qid[3]* for 3 wk	Bacterial conjunctivitis, viral conjunctivitis
Drug-induced allergic conjunctivitis	Ocular itching (moderate-severe), inferior conjunctiva vasodilation, lid edema (lower more than upper), ±dermatitis of the lower lid, relentless progression	Conjunctival scraping, acute eosinophils, chronic lymphocytes and mononuclear cells	Avoiding the offending agents, nonpreserved artificial tears and ointments, antihistamine and vasoconstrictor, cold compresses	Seasonal allergic conjunctivitis, bacterial conjunctivitis, bacterial conjunctivitis, superior limbic keratoconjunctivitis
Dry eye syndrome	Ocular burning, foreign body sensation, photophobia, blurred vision	Tear breakup test, fluorescein and rose Bengal stains, Schirmer's test, conjunctival impression cytology	Artificial tears, lubricants, ointments, restasis, punctal occlusion	Seasonal allergic conjunctivitis, drug-induced conjunctivitis, superior limbic keratoconjunctivitis
Gonococcal	Hyperpurulent conjunctivitis, beefy-red conjunctival injection	Gram stain, chocolate agar, Thayer-Martin media	Topical bacitracin or erythromycin; systemic antibiotics	Chlamydial conjunctivitis, viral conjunctivitis
Seasonal allergic conjunctivitis	Bilateral itching, conjunctival edema, injection, lid edema, tearing	Conjunctival scraping, eosinophils 20%-80%	Artificial tears, antihistamines, mast cell stabilizers, NSAIDs	Vernal keratoconjunctivitis, atopic keratoconjunctivitis, giant papillary conjunctivitis, contact conjunctivitis
Viral	Serous discharge starting unilaterally and then spreading bilaterally, itching, photophobia, conjunctival injection, membranes or pseudomembranes, preauricular and submandibular adenopathy	Viral cultures, immunofluorescent techniques	Cold compresses, dark glasses, vasoconstrictors, cycloplegia, antivirals	Allergic conjunctivitis, drug-induced allergic conjunctivitis, bacterial conjunctivitis

[3]Exceeds dosage recommended by the manufacturer
*Usually erythromycin is 250 mg qid or 500 mg bid.
ELISA = enzyme-linked immunosorbent assay; NSAID = nonsteroidal antiinflammatory drug.

The low-dose corticosteroid loteprednol etabonate (Alrex) has been used to relieve signs and symptoms of allergic conjunctivitis and in refractory cases. Because of the side effects of cataract formation and secondary glaucoma, however, this drug should be used with the supervision of an ophthalmologist.

Patients with vernal keratoconjunctivitis, atopic keratoconjunctivitis, and giant papillary conjunctivitis should usually be referred to an ophthalmologist for management.

Viral Conjunctivitis

Viral conjunctivitis can be caused by coxsackievirus, enterovirus, Epstein–Barr virus, herpes simplex virus (HSV), and herpes zoster virus (HZV). Most cases of conjunctivitis (pink eye) are caused by adenovirus. Two syndromes of external ocular adenovirus infection—epidemic keratoconjunctivitis and pharyngoconjunctival fever—have been described.

Epidemic keratoconjunctivitis has been reported to occur worldwide from 11 virus serotypes; 8, 11, and 19 are the most common causative strains. Patients present with watery discharge, redness, photophobia, mild foreign body sensation, and preauricular nodes. The peak intensity of the follicular conjunctivitis occurs 5 to 7 days after the onset of symptoms. The fellow eye is involved in at least 50% of cases. Adenovirus keratitis progresses through six stages characterized by an orderly sequence of superficial epithelial infiltrates. Often pharyngoconjunctival fever is indistinguishable from epidemic keratoconjunctivitis.

Diagnosis is usually based on clinical features, and only select cases are confirmed by rapid immunodetection of adenovirus antigens or viral cultures.

The treatment for adenovirus keratoconjunctivitis is mainly supportive. Cold compresses, artificial tears, topical decongestants, and prophylactic topical antibiotics may be given. The use of topical corticosteroids is controversial; corticosteroids should not be used without consultation with an ophthalmologist.

A primary ocular HSV infection typically manifests as a unilateral blepharokeratoconjunctivitis. If external vesicles of the skin are not present, this often is indistinguishable from epidemic keratoconjunctivitis. Primary ocular HSV is a self-limited condition, but topical and oral antiviral agents may be used for 1 week.

Bacterial Conjunctivitis

Bacterial conjunctivitis, which is uncommon, can be categorized into three subsets: acute, hyperacute, and chronic (Box 1). Bacterial conjunctivitis is the result of bacterial overgrowth with a secondary infiltrate of the conjunctival epithelium and sometimes the substantia propria as well. It is usually self-limited, but the severity depends on the inoculum size and the bacterial virulence factors.

ACUTE BACTERIAL CONJUNCTIVITIS

The most common form of bacterial conjunctivitis is the acute mucopurulent form. Cases can occur spontaneously or in epidemics. Common manifestations are modest mucopurulent discharge, diffuse conjunctival hyperemia, and, sometimes, preauricular nodes. In adults, acute mucopurulent conjunctivitis is usually caused by *Staphylococcus aureus*, *Streptococcus pneumoniae*, or *Streptococcus viridans*. In children, *Haemophilus influenzae*, *S. aureus*, and *S. pneumoniae* are the usual causes of acute mucopurulent conjunctivitis.

Topical antibiotic therapy should be based on Gram-stained morphology of conjunctivitis caused by gram-positive organisms. This condition can be treated with erythromycin or polymyxin B–bacitracin (Polysporin) ointment or polymyxin B–trimethoprim (Polytrim) solution. Cases caused by gram-negative coccobacilli should be treated with polymyxin B–trimethoprim. Topical aminoglycosides and fluoroquinolones should be reserved for cases refractory to initial therapy.

HYPERACUTE BACTERIAL CONJUNCTIVITIS

Hyperacute bacterial conjunctivitis manifests itself with an explosive onset of severe purulent conjunctivitis, severe chemosis, and massive exudation. If left untreated, it can progress to corneal infiltrates, melting, and perforation. The organism most commonly responsible is *Neisseria gonorrhoeae*. Cases of infection with *Neisseria meningitides* have been reported, however. Gram stain and cultures on Thayer-Martin medium should be performed. The treatment is with systemic and topical antibiotics.

CHRONIC BACTERIAL CONJUNCTIVITIS

A unilateral or bilateral conjunctivitis that lasts more than 3 to 4 weeks is considered chronic. *S. aureus* is the most common causative organism. A vigorous lid hygiene regimen and topical antibiotics are used initially. In refractory cases, conjunctival swabs for culture and sensitivity should be performed and the patient treated accordingly.

Adult Inclusion Conjunctivis

Adult inclusion conjunctivitis is a chronic follicular conjunctivitis associated with mucopurulent discharge and palpable preauricular adenopathy and is caused by *Chlamydia trachomatis* (serotypes D through K). The diagnosis is made by a direct fluorescent antibody assay, enzyme immunoassay, or a Giemsa stain of the conjunctiva. Treatment is with systemic tetracycline or erythromycin. Topical therapy is optional. The patient's sexual contacts should also be treated with systemic therapy.

Neonatal Conjunctivitis

Neonatal conjunctivitis, or ophthalmia neonatorum, is a distinct entity that occurs in the first 4 weeks of life. Because some of the infectious agents can lead to severe localized eye infection and possible serious systemic infection, precise identification and treatment are essential. Neonatal conjunctivitis is caused by a myriad of entities (Table 2).

Chemical conjunctivitis classically occurs in 90% of neonates from the instillation of silver nitrate drops used first by Crede in 1881 to protect against gonococcal infection. Although this form of conjunctivitis is 2.5 to 12 times more common when 1% silver nitrate is used, it has also been reported with topical erythromycin and tetracycline agents. The symptoms of a mild conjunctivitis and erythema and lid edema occur in the first 24 hours of life. Gram stain shows neutrophils with no organisms. This is a self-limited condition that resolves in 48 hours in most cases. In many countries, silver nitrate has been replaced by topical erythromycin or tetracycline ointment, both of which are effective against *Neisseria* and *Chlamydia* species.

Conjunctival cultures of vaginally delivered neonates reflect the flora of the vaginal canal, whereas the conjunctivae of neonates delivered by cesarean section within 3 hours of membrane rupture are culture negative. The conjunctival flora of the neonate is correlated with the method of delivery. The most common causes of neonatal bacterial conjunctivitis are *S. aureus*, *S. viridans*, *H. influenzae*, *S. pneumoniae*, *Branhamella catarrhalis*, *Enterococcus* species, *Escherichia coli*, and *Klebsiella* species. These bacterial species generally cause a mild, acute, mucopurulent conjunctivitis 3 to 5 days after birth. Serious complications are few except in the case of nosocomial infections caused by *Pseudomonas aeruginosa*, which can cause corneal complications and endophthalmitis. Systemically, there may be sepsis, which can lead to death. Gram stain and cultures are needed to make the diagnosis. Topical aminoglycosides are indicated for gram-negative organisms, and erythromycin or bacitracin ointment is recommended for gram-positive organisms and fortified antibiotics for *Pseudomonas aeruginosa*.

Neonatal conjunctivitis caused by *N. gonorrhoeae* has decreased significantly since the advent of prophylaxis. Gonococcal conjunctivitis in the neonate consists of excessive mucopurulent discharge, eyelid edema, and profound chemosis 24 to 48 hours after birth. This condition is a medical emergency. Therapy must be started immediately based on presumptive diagnosis from the Gram

---

BOX 1   Causes of Bacterial Conjunctivitis

Acute (hours to days)
Haemophilus influenzae biotype III
H. influenzae
Staphylococcus aureus
Streptococcus pneumoniae

Hyperacute (6 to 24 hours)
Neisseria gonorrhoeae
Neisseria meningitides

Chronic (days to weeks)
S. aureus
Moraxella lacunata
Enterobacteriaceae
Pseudomonas species

TABLE 2 Neonatal Conjunctivitis

Cause	Time of Onset	Microscopic Features of Conjunctival Smear	Culture	Treatment
Chemical (silver nitrate)	1-36 h	Neutrophils (Gram)	None	None
Neisseria gonorrhoeae	24-48 h	Bacteria, intracellular diplococci, neutrophils (Gram)	Chocolate agar, Thayer-Martin media	IM ceftriaxone (Rocephin) *or* IV/IM cefotaxime (Claforan) *plus* topical erythromycin
Bacteria *Staphylococcus* *Streptococcus* *Haemophilus*	3-5 d	Bacteria, neutrophils (Gram)	Blood agar, thioglycolate broth	Gram-positive: erythromycin ointment Gram-negative: tobramycin/gentamicin
Viruses	3-15 d	Lymphocytes, plasma cells, multinucleated giant cells (Gram); eosinophilic intranuclear inclusions in epithelial cells (Papanicolaou)	Viral culture	Topical trifluridine (Viroptic), systemic acyclovir (Zovirax)[1]
Chlamydial	5-14 d	Neutrophils, lymphocytes, plasma cells (Gram)	McCoy cell culture	Topical erythromycin and tetracycline ointment, systemic erythromycin

[1]Not FDA approved for this indication.

stain, which typically shows gram-negative intracellular diplococci. The neonate is hospitalized and the ophthalmologist is consulted. Recommended treatment consists of a single intramuscular dose of ceftriaxone (Rocephin) 25-50 mg/kg or IM or IV cefotaxime (Claforan) 100 mg/kg, (50 mg/kg in newborns) every 24 hours for 7 days. Either of these regimens should be combined with saline irrigation of the conjunctiva and application of topical erythromycin ointment.

The most common cause of neonatal conjunctivitis in the United States is C. *trachomatis* serotypes D through K. Infants whose mothers have untreated chlamydia infections have a 30% to 40% chance of developing conjunctivitis and a 10% to 20% chance of developing pneumonia. Neonatal chlamydial conjunctivitis differs clinically from the adult form of the infection: There is no follicular response in the newborn, newborns have greater amounts of mucopurulent discharge, and newborns have a greater percentage of Giemsa-stained intracytoplasmic inclusions. There is better response to topical medications in newborns. Gram and Giemsa stains of conjunctival scrapings are recommended with conjunctivitis to identify *C. trachomatis* and *N. gonorrhoeae* as well as other possible causative agents. Systemic erythromycin (Ery-Tab) 50 mg/kg orally divided into four doses a day for 14 days is recommended, even though inclusion conjunctivitis in the newborn usually responds to topical erythromycin.

Viral conjunctivitis is rare in neonates and is predominantly herpetic and seen in 40% to 50% of infants born to mothers with active genital infections. These infections are usually herpes type 2, but type 1 has been isolated. The onset of herpes keratoconjunctivitis is usually between 1 and 2 weeks postpartum, manifesting as serous discharge with moderate conjunctival infection. Herpes almost always manifests as a unilateral infection. This entity can be associated with central nervous system herpes or disseminated systemic disease. The diagnosis is confirmed by the characteristic vesicular skin lesions or a corneal dendrite, if present; otherwise a maternal history is helpful. To aid in the diagnosis, conjunctival smears and viral cultures can be implemented. The treatment for topical disease is trifluridine (Viroptic) 1 drop every 2 hours or vidarabine (Vira-A) ointment five times a day for 7 days. For systemic disease, treatment is oral acyclovir (Zovirax)[1] 30 mg/kg divided every 8 to 10 hours for 10 days.

---

[1]Not FDA approved for this indication.

Optic Neuritis

Method of
Anthony C. Arnold, MD

Diagnosis

Optic neuritis may be broadly classified as typical (the idiopathic demyelinative form most commonly associated with multiple sclerosis [MS]) and atypical (the form usually associated with infection or vasculitis). This chapter addresses only the typical form, which manifests as monocular central visual loss occurring over days, associated with pain on eye movement in the majority of cases. Examination reveals decreased visual acuity, color vision, and central visual field sensitivity in the presence of an afferent pupillary defect. The optic disc is normal in appearance initially in two thirds of cases, the other one third demonstrating optic disc edema at onset. In contrast, the atypical forms can develop visual loss at a different pace, lack associated pain, and demonstrate more severe optic disc edema with associated macular exudates, retinal hemorrhages, and possible uveitis.

Natural History

Typical demyelinative optic neuritis worsens over days to weeks, followed by spontaneous recovery. In the Optic Neuritis Treatment Trial (ONTT), acuity began to improve within 3 weeks in 79%. At 10 years, mean visual acuity for affected eyes (treated or untreated) was 20/16; visual acuity was better than 20/40 in 92%. Only 3% had 20/200 acuity or worse. Of those whose initial visual acuity fell in the range of counting fingers to no light perception, 76% had better than 20/40 at 10 years. About 35% of patients developed recurrence in either eye within 10 years.

Treatment

CORTICOSTEROID THERAPY

Current guidelines for using corticosteroids in treating optic neuritis are based on results of the ONTT.

CURRENT DIAGNOSIS

- Onset of central visual loss over days
- Pain with eye movement
- Decreased visual acuity and color vision
- Afferent pupillary defect
- Normal or edematous optic disc
- Central visual field depression

CURRENT THERAPY

- Consider methylprednisolone 1 g/day × 3 days to speed visual recovery.
- Standard dose (1 mg/kg/day) oral prednisone is contraindicated.
- Assess risk for multiple sclerosis using brain magnetic resonance imaging.
- Consider immunomodulating agents in patients with high risk for multiple sclerosis.

Intravenous methylprednisolone (Solu-Medrol) at a dose of 250 mg four times a day for 3 days, followed by 11 days of oral prednisone at 1 mg/kg/day resulted in increased rates of visual recovery during the first 2 weeks following visual loss. It did not, however, produce any significant long-term benefit for visual function at the 6-month or later follow-ups. Treatment for visual benefit is usually limited to patients who present within 8 to 10 days of onset of visual loss and who require more rapid visual recovery, for example, monocular patients, those with severe monocular or binocular visual loss, and those with occupational requirements, such as pilots. IVMP is typically administered now as a single outpatient dose of 1g IV daily for 3 days via heparin lock; authorities vary as to whether the oral tapering dose of prednisone at 1 mg/kg/day is required.

At 2-year follow-up in the ONTT, the intravenous treatment group showed a significantly decreased risk for the development of MS in patients with two or more white matter lesions on magnetic resonance imaging (MRI) (Fig. 1). The risk was 16% in the intravenous treatment group versus 36% in the placebo and the oral prednisone groups. This effect was not maintained, however, at 3 years (17% vs 21%) or after. Although the value of this therapy alone for reducing long-term MS risk is thus unclear, its use in conjunction with immunomodulation therapy for this purpose is more strongly supported (see later).

The use of oral prednisone alone at the standard dose (1 mg/kg/day) showed no visual benefit, either for speeding recovery or for long-term visual function. Moreover, its use was associated with a significantly higher rate of recurrence in the affected or fellow eye (44% in the oral group vs 29%-31% in the placebo or intravenous groups) at 10-year follow-up. Most authorities consider that the use of oral corticosteroids at this dose is contraindicated for typical optic neuritis. Some investigators, however, think that these effects were related to the relatively lower dose in the oral prednisone group of the ONTT, with resultant inadequate immune suppression, rather than the oral route of administration itself. The Quality Standards Committee of the American Academy of Neurology in 2000 supported the use of oral corticosteroids (prednisone or dexamethasone) at a higher dose, equivalent to the intravenous methylprednisolone dose used in the ONTT.

IMMUNOMODULATION THERAPY

At 10 years of follow-up in the ONTT, the overall risk for development of MS after an initial episode of optic neuritis was 38%. The MRI was the single most valuable predictor of risk (see Fig. 1); if T2-weighted MRI showed 0 typical (periventricular, > 3 mm in diameter) white matter demyelinating lesions at onset, the risk was 22%; if at least 1 such lesion was present, the risk increased to 56%. There was no significant additional increase in risk with more than one lesion.

The use of immunomodulation agents (interferon-β-1a [IFN-β-1a] [Avonex], IFN-β-1b [Betaseron], or glatiramer acetate [Copaxone]) has proved benefit for reducing morbidity in the relapsing–remitting form of MS. The CHAMPS (Controlled High-Risk Subjects Avonex Multiple Sclerosis Prevention Study) was an industry-sponsored clinical trial in North America to evaluate the effect of Avonex in lowering the rate of *developing* MS after a single demyelinating event. Of the 393 patients entered into this randomized, placebo-controlled trial, 192 (50%) had isolated optic neuritis as this initial event. All subjects had more than two MRI lesions, and all received intravenous methylpredisolone followed by oral corticosteroid therapy within 14 days of onset. They were then randomized to weekly intramuscular injections of either 30 μg IFN-β-1a or placebo. At the first interim analysis of study data, at 18-month follow-up, the study was terminated because a beneficial effect of therapy was indicated: Cumulative probability of MS development was 35% in the treated group versus 50% in the placebo group.

The Early Treatment of Multiple Sclerosis (ETOMS) studied the subcutaneous injectable form of IFN-β-1a (Rebif) in a similar manner in Europe; 98 of the 308 (32%) patients initially presented with optic neuritis. Results were similar, if less strongly supportive of a benefit for treatment: 34% of treated versus 45% of untreated patients developed MS.

The implications of these studies for optic neuritis therapy are significant. We recommend that all patients with optic neuritis undergo brain MRI to assess for MS risk and should be advised of this therapeutic option for reducing the risk of MS. If the MRI shows more than one lesion, IFN-β-1a should be strongly considered. Most authorities administer concomitant corticosteroids to patients treated with immunomodulation agents. If the MRI shows no lesions, the risk of MS development is much less and the benefit of immunomodulating agents unclear.

The use of immunomodulation agents for a single episode of optic neuritis remains controversial. The many issues involved include high cost of therapy, commitment to long-term weekly injections with side effects, and the possibility that therapy may be unnecessary (at least 44% of the high risk group will not develop MS at 10-year follow-up). Certain practitioners reserve therapy for those who, on repeat MRI at 3 to 6 months, show newly active lesions, suggesting ongoing demyelinative activity.

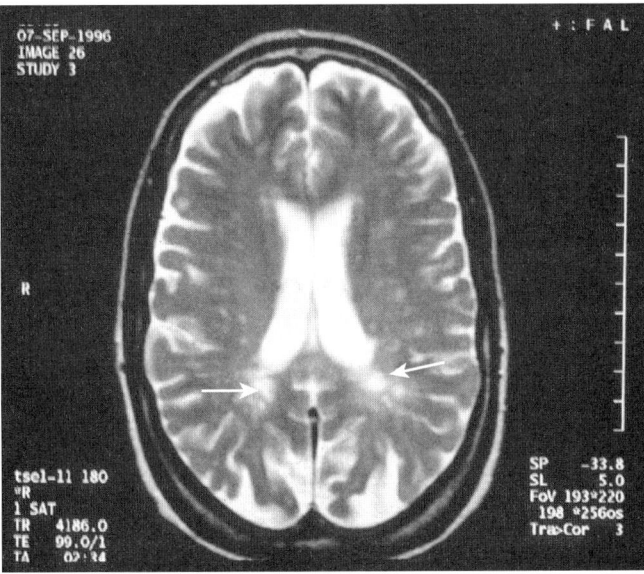

FIGURE 1. Axial T2-weighted magnetic resonance image demonstrating multiple white matter lesions consistent with demyelination *(arrows)*.

REFERENCES

Beck RW, Cleary PA, Anderson MM: and the Optic Neuritis Study Group: A randomized, controlled trial of corticosteroids in the treatment of acute optic neuritis. N Engl J Med 1992;326:581-588.

Beck RW, Cleary PA, Trobe JD, and the Optic Neuritis Study Group: The effect of corticosteroids for acute optic neuritis on the subsequent development of multiple sclerosis. N Engl J Med 1993;329:1764-1769.

Beck RW, and the Optic Neuritis Study Group: The Optic Neuritis Treatment Trial: Three year follow-up results. Arch Ophthalmol 1995;113:136-137.

CHAMPS Study Group: Interferon β-1a for optic neuritis patients at high risk for multiple sclerosis. Am J Ophthalmol 2001;132:463-471.

Comi G, Filipi M, Barkhof F, et al: Effect of early interferon treatment on conversion to definite multiple sclerosis: A randomized study. Lancet 2001;357:1576-1582.

Kaufman DI, Trobe JD, Eggenberger ER, et al: Practice parameter: The role of corticosteroids in the management of acute monosymptomatic optic neuritis. Report of the Quality Standards Subcommittee of the American Academy of Neurology. Neurology 2000;54:2039-2044.

Optic Neuritis Study Group: Visual function more than 10 years after optic neuritis. Experience of the Optic Neuritis Treatment Trial. Am J Ophthalmol 2004;137:77-83.

Optic Neuritis Study Group: High- and low-risk profiles for the development of multiple sclerosis within 10 years after optic neuritis. Arch Ophthalmol 2003;121:944-949.

Glaucoma

Method of
Misha F. Syed, MD, and Nicholas P. Bell, MD

Glaucoma is a group of disorders with various manifestations linked by a common optic neuropathy, resulting in characteristic, progressive optic nerve atrophy, and visual field loss. Glaucoma was once defined simply as intraocular pressure (IOP) greater than 21 mm Hg, but now this is recognized as only a risk factor. Elevated IOP dilates the optic cup, which subjects the ganglion cells to ischemic pressure forces. Peripheral visual field defects emerge in the areas subtended by the damaged retinal ganglion cells. Central vision loss is typically a late finding.

Glaucoma is classified by the anatomy of the anterior chamber angle, which may be *open* or *closed*. Gonioscopy, a detailed evaluation of the angle using a mirrored lens, is required to differentiate types of glaucoma. Childhood glaucoma may be primary or secondary to developmental ocular abnormalities. Patients who do not meet criteria for diagnosis within one of these groups are followed as glaucoma suspects.

Regardless of etiology, glaucoma is a leading cause of irreversible blindness. Of the 67 million people with glaucoma worldwide, 7 million are bilaterally blind. In the United States, more than 2.5 million people are diagnosed with glaucoma, and it is estimated that as many are undiagnosed. Glaucoma is the second leading cause of blindness in the United States; it is the most frequent cause among African Americans, in whom there is an earlier onset and more aggressive course. In 2000 the prevalence of blindness from glaucoma in the United States was greater than 1:130,000 people.

Types of Glaucoma

PRIMARY OPEN-ANGLE GLAUCOMA

The most common glaucoma is primary open-angle glaucoma (POAG). Increased resistance to outflow of the aqueous humor through the trabecular meshwork leads to gradual and painless

CURRENT DIAGNOSIS

- The most common form of glaucoma in the United States is POAG.
- Risk factors for POAG include increasing age, African American race, and a positive family history.
- Screening for POAG is recommended every 2 to 4 years after age 40 years and every 1 to 2 years after age 65 years.
- If risk factors for POAG are present, screening is recommended every 2 to 4 years after age 30 years and every 1 to 2 years after age 65 years.
- 95% of patients with POAG and 5% of normal patients may experience IOP elevation >15 mm Hg while taking steroids; therefore, patients with known glaucoma on long-term steroids (>1 month) need close follow-up with an ophthalmologist.
- Primary angle-closure glaucoma has an acute onset with pain, haloes, red eye, decreased vision, and nausea and/or vomiting. Emergent ophthalmologic referral is required.

Abbreviations: IOP = intraocular pressure; POAG = primary open-angle glaucoma.

elevation of IOP; hence, it is typically asymptomatic. It is bilateral but can be asymmetric. The existence of a subgroup of POAG patients without elevated IOP (normal-pressure glaucoma) suggests that other factors may be significant, such as insufficient vascular flow to the optic nerve head, accelerated programmed cell death (apoptosis), diurnal fluctuations of IOP, and autoimmunity.

Diseases such as diabetes mellitus, systemic hypertension, and vasospastic disorders have been associated with glaucoma but are not clearly linked to the disease. Increasing age is a risk factor, because 8% of the population older than 70 years old and only 0.1% of those younger than 40 years of age are affected. African American patients have a 5 to 15 times greater risk than white patients. Immediate family members of glaucoma patients have a 10- to 15-fold increased risk for developing glaucoma.

The prolonged asymptomatic phase of POAG can only be discovered by ocular evaluation. Complete eye examination is recommended every 2 to 4 years for patients older than 40 years of age and every 1 to 2 years for those older than 65 years. Patients with risk factors (age, race, family history) should be evaluated earlier and more frequently.

Screening in the primary care setting can include a family and medical history, vision (and possibly IOP) screening, and examination of the optic nerve head by direct ophthalmoscopy. Clinical findings may be subtle. Visual acuity is often normal, and decreased central vision secondary to glaucoma suggests advanced disease. Normal confrontation fields do not exclude glaucoma because this examination technique has a very low yield in identifying glaucomatous visual field loss. Formal visual field testing is preferred. Although not diagnostic, intraocular pressure greater than 21 mm Hg warrants thorough evaluation. Dilated fundus examination shows enlarged cupping of the optic nerve head and/or asymmetry between the optic nerves. Focal loss of neural rim tissue (notching) may occur, and flame hemorrhages may be seen at the disc margin, especially in actively progressing disease. If glaucoma is suspected, a patient should be referred for further ophthalmologic evaluation.

Patients with suggestive findings but no definitive glaucomatous damage are classified as glaucoma suspects. The Ocular Hypertension Treatment Study, a recent multicenter randomized, controlled clinical trial, conducted a long-term follow-up of glaucoma suspects with elevated IOP, normal optic nerve appearance, and no visual field defects. This study found that over 5 years, maintaining IOP 20%

below baseline reduced the rate of progression to POAG from 9.5% to 4.4%.

SECONDARY OPEN-ANGLE GLAUCOMA

Secondary open-angle glaucomas result from increased resistance to outflow through the trabecular meshwork because of a preexisting or underlying condition. Examples include pigmentary, pseudoexfoliative, traumatic, and steroid-induced glaucoma.

In pigment dispersion syndrome and pseudoexfoliation syndrome, deposition of iris pigment and fibrillar protein, respectively, in the trabecular meshwork may obstruct aqueous outflow and secondarily elevate IOP, leading to glaucoma. Blunt ocular trauma (often remote) is a common cause of unilateral glaucoma because of structural changes in the trabecular meshwork.

Chronic use of glucocorticosteroids can create resistance to trabecular outflow and IOP elevation, resulting in a glaucoma resembling POAG. Steroid-induced pressure elevation generally correlates with the dose and length of administration. Although most often seen with topical and periocular use, it can also result from systemic or inhaled administration. Steroid responses of greater than 15 mm Hg IOP elevation can develop in 95% of patients with POAG and in only 15% of patients without glaucoma. All patients with a known diagnosis of glaucoma should be evaluated by an ophthalmologist within 1 month of initiating a long-term steroid regimen for systemic diseases.

PRIMARY ANGLE-CLOSURE GLAUCOMA

Primary angle-closure glaucoma can have an acute, subacute, intermittent, or chronic presentation. Attacks of acute angle closure are ocular emergencies, because irreversible vision loss can occur within hours. Those at risk have an anatomic predisposition with narrow anterior chamber angles. If the pupillary margin of the iris contacts the lens for 360 degrees, which may occur in susceptible eyes when the iris is mid-dilated, flow of the aqueous humor from the posterior to the anterior chamber is blocked. The peripheral iris bows anteriorly and apposes the trabecular meshwork, obstructing outflow. The IOP may rise rapidly to greater than 60 mm Hg.

In Asian populations primary angle-closure glaucoma is more common than open-angle glaucoma. The risk increases with age, with most cases occurring during the sixth and seventh decades. Women have primary angle-closure glaucoma attacks 2 to 4 times as often as men. Environmental circumstances may trigger an acute attack of angle closure in predisposed eyes; these include movie theaters or dark rooms (physiologic mydriasis), sudden anxiety or pain (sympathetic stimulation causing pupil dilation), or medications causing mild mydriasis (anticholinergics and adrenergic stimulants such as sleep and cold medications).

The diagnosis of an acute angle-closure glaucoma attack requires gonioscopic evidence of a closed anterior chamber angle preventing aqueous flow into the trabecular meshwork. Patients may complain of ocular pain, brow ache, rainbow-colored halos around lights, and/ or blurred vision. They may experience intense nausea and vomiting, bradycardia, and sweating. Ocular exam reveals elevated IOP, conjunctival vascular injection, a cloudy cornea (if IOP rose acutely and recently), a shallow anterior chamber, a closed angle by gonioscopy, and a globe, which is firm to palpation.

SECONDARY ANGLE-CLOSURE GLAUCOMA

Scarring and adhesions between the peripheral iris and the anterior chamber angle may block outflow of aqueous. Diabetes mellitus may result in neovascularization of the retina, which can progress to neovascularization of the anterior segment including the iris and angle, blocking aqueous outflow and/or closing the angle. The resultant neovascular glaucoma can be devastating and refractory to treatment. Central retinal vein occlusion, a vascular accident closely linked to uncontrolled hypertension and diabetes, can also lead to retinal neovascularization and a similar process. Uveitis from systemic diseases such as sarcoidosis or autoimmune arthropathies can produce intraocular scarring and secondary angle closure if not controlled.

CURRENT THERAPY

- Although POAG is typically treated first medically, in select circumstances laser and incisional surgery may be appropriate first-line interventions.
- Glaucoma medications lower IOP by either decreasing production of aqueous humor or increasing its outflow.
- Topical β-blockers have been the traditional primary medical therapy for POAG, but prostaglandin analogues are now emerging as the first-line choice.
- Laser trabeculoplasty increases aqueous outflow through the trabecular meshwork.
- Incisional filtering surgery creates a new outflow drain, which bypasses the dysfunctional trabecular meshwork.
- Primary angle closure attacks require emergent treatment both medically and with laser iridotomy.
- Secondary angle closure glaucoma may be difficult to manage medically and often requires surgery.

Abbreviations: IOP = intraocular pressure; POAG = primary open-angle glaucoma.

Sulfonamide-based systemic medications can rarely cause swelling of the ciliary body, which anteriorly displaces the lens and iris. This can produce a secondary acute angle-closure glaucoma, which requires discontinuation of the medication and urgent lowering of the IOP. This phenomenon has also been reported with topiramate (Topamax).

CHILDHOOD GLAUCOMA

Congenital or childhood glaucoma develops from aqueous outflow obstruction because of abnormal anatomical development of the angle, ocular inflammation, or trauma. Primary congenital glaucoma often presents in infancy with the classic triad of photophobia, epiphora (tearing), and blepharospasm, but these signs are unnecessary for diagnosis. Buphthalmos (enlarged eye) may occur secondary to increased IOP if the glaucoma develops during the first 3 years of life. Juvenile glaucoma is similar in etiology to POAG and has been linked to several specific genetic loci. Enlargement of the cornea and sclera is not seen in this subtype.

Treatment

The Glaucoma Preferred Practice Pattern Committee of the American Academy of Ophthalmology suggests a target of 20% to 30% reduction of IOP from the untreated levels. Medical treatment is usually attempted first. Parameters that factor into selection of medications include efficacy in lowering IOP, systemic and localized side effect profiles, ease of compliance, and cost (Table 1). Noncompliance with treatment regimens may be responsible for 10% of visual loss in glaucoma; and in one study, approximately 60% of patients failed to use eyedrops as prescribed. If medications fail to control IOP, changes in optic nerve structure and visual field function may occur. Surgical treatment may become necessary to slow the progression of glaucomatous damage.

PROSTAGLANDIN ANALOGUES

This newest class of antiglaucoma agents has become a popular initial medical treatment because of the efficacy and lack of major systemic side effects. These medications reduce IOP by increasing aqueous humor outflow. Latanoprost (Xalatan), bimatoprost (Lumigan), and travoprost (Travatan) require only once daily dosing, whereas

TABLE 1

Topical Medications	Efficacy	Local Side Effects	Systemic Side Effects	Dosing	Cost
Prostaglandin analogues	+ + +	+ +	none to +	Once daily	+ + +
β-Blockers	+ + +	+	+ + +	bid	+ +*
α_2 Agonists	+ +	+ +	+ +	bid–tid	+ + +*
Carbonic anhydrase inhibitors	+ +	+ +	+ to + +	bid–tid	+ + +†

+ + + = high
+ + = moderate
+ = low
* = generic available
† = systemic form less costly

---

unoprostone (Rescula) is administered twice daily. Side effects include conjunctival hyperemia during the first several weeks of therapy, eyelash lengthening and thickening, occasional iris and periocular skin hyperpigmentation, and rarely, exacerbation of ocular inflammation.

BETA-ADRENERGIC ANTAGONISTS

Beta-adrenergic antagonists lower IOP by decreasing the production of aqueous humor. They are very effective at lowering IOP and include timolol (Timoptic, Betimol, Istalol), carteolol (Ocupress), metipranolol (OptiPranolol), and levobunolol (Betagan). Topical formulations may be absorbed into the bloodstream, and potential side effects are similar to systemic β-blockers, including exacerbation of chronic obstructive or reactive pulmonary disease, worsening of heart block or heart failure, bradycardia, systemic hypotension, mood effects/altered mental status, decreased libido, and masking of hypoglycemic symptoms in diabetic patients. Care should be taken in patients already taking systemic β-blockers, because additive side effects may develop. Betaxolol (Betoptic) is a selective β_1 antagonist, which may minimize the pulmonary side effects, but still must be used cautiously in patients suffering from asthma or COPD. Topical β-blockers are dosed once or twice daily, depending on the formulation of the eyedrop.

α_2 AGONISTS

α_2 Adrenergic agonists such as apraclonidine (Iopidine) and brimonidine (Alphagan) lower IOP by decreasing aqueous humor production. They are dosed 2 to 3 times daily. Major systemic side effects include somnolence and dry mouth. These medications should be used cautiously in infants and young children because of the risk of respiratory depression. α_2 Agonists are contraindicated in patients taking monoamine oxidase (MAO) inhibitors because of potential systemic hypertension. Ocular side effects include allergic follicular conjunctivitis, which may necessitate discontinuation.

CARBONIC ANHYDRASE INHIBITORS

Carbonic anhydrase inhibitors decrease production of aqueous humor. Systemic carbonic anhydrase inhibitors such as acetazolamide (Diamox) and methazolamide (Neptazane) have been used to treat glaucoma for decades, but up to 60% of patients are intolerant of the side effects. These include metallic taste alteration, loss of appetite, fatigue, confusion, nausea and vomiting, paresthesias, polyuria, urolithiasis, and hearing dysfunction or tinnitus. Rare side effects include Stevens-Johnson syndrome (in patients with sulfonamide allergies) and idiosyncratic aplastic anemia. Oral agents may also lower serum potassium levels, and patients on diuretics or digoxin should be monitored closely. Dorzolamide (Trusopt) and brinzolamide (Azopt) are topical preparations of carbonic anhydrase inhibitors dosed 2 to 3 times daily. Systemic side effects are minimized, but ocular stinging, localized allergic responses, and metallic taste alteration may occur. Systemic carbonic anhydrase inhibitors are more efficacious, but the improved tolerability of the topical agents has made them popular.

NONSPECIFIC SYMPATHOMIMETICS AND PARASYMPATHOMIMETICS

Nonspecific sympathomimetic and parasympathomimetic drugs have historically been used for the treatment of glaucoma, but with the newer agents available these are no longer commonly prescribed. The mechanism for both classes involves increasing aqueous humor outflow. The sympathomimetic agents include epinephrine (Epifrin) and dipivefrin (Propine). Potential adverse effects include systemic hypertension, headache, cardiac arrhythmias including premature ventricular contractions and tachycardia, and anorexia. Parasympathomimetic medications such as pilocarpine (Pilocar) can cause gastrointestinal cramping, diarrhea, vomiting, syncope, hypotension, increased sweating, and pupillary constriction.

ACUTE ANGLE CLOSURE

Acute angle closure patients require emergent ophthalmologic referral and treatment to prevent severe permanent sequelae. If this is not immediately possible, treatment should be initiated promptly with a topical β-blocker and a topical α_2 agonist every 30 minutes and a single dose of oral acetazolamide (Diamox) (250 mg × 2 tablets). Oral glycerin (Osmoglyn) or intravenous mannitol (Osmitrol) (1.0 to 1.5 g/kg) may be used if necessary. Pilocarpine should be used cautiously because it may worsen underlying inflammation. Once the attack has been broken medically, the corneal edema will clear and a laser peripheral iridotomy can be made to prevent future attacks. This opening in the peripheral iris allows aqueous flow to bypass any obstruction caused by pupillary block. Prophylactic iridotomy of the other eye is recommended if anatomically at risk. The management of *chronic* angle-closure glaucoma is generally similar to that for POAG.

LASER

Laser may also be used to treat open-angle glaucomas. Argon laser trabeculoplasty (ALT) or the newer selective laser trabeculoplasty (SLT) lowers IOP by facilitating aqueous outflow. For pigmentary, pseudoexfoliative, and select POAG patients, this may be an effective adjunct to medical therapy.

SURGERY

Surgical measures to control glaucoma include filtering procedures such as trabeculectomy or aqueous shunt placement, which increase aqueous outflow by creating alternative filtration pathways. After trabeculectomy, patients are warned of an increased lifetime risk for serious ocular infection and must report to an ophthalmologist immediately for any changes, including redness, pain, and/or decrease in vision. For poor surgical candidates with severely advanced disease, cyclodestructive procedures can be performed in the office to decrease aqueous production by ablating the ciliary body.

If glaucomatous damage has left an eye with no vision, the only reason to treat IOP is to control pain. In most cases, topical agents will suffice. If pain becomes frequent and severe, injections of retrobulbar absolute alcohol or even enucleation of the blind, painful eye may be offered.

REFERENCES

Allingham RR: Shields' Textbook of Glaucoma, 5th ed. Philadelphia, Lippincott Williams & Wilkins, 2005.
American Academy of Ophthalmology Online: Preferred practice patterns: Primary angle Closure glaucoma, primary open angle glaucoma, primary open angle glaucoma suspect 2003. Available at http://www.aao.org/
Kass MA, Heuer DK, Higginbotham EJ, et al: The ocular hypertension treatment study: A randomized trial determines that topical ocular hypotensive medication delays or prevents the onset of primary open-angle glaucoma, Arch Ophthalmol 2002;120:701-713.
Morrison JC, Pollack IP: Glaucoma: Science and Practice. New York, Thieme, 2003.
Tsai JC, Forbes M: Medical Management of Glaucoma, 2nd ed. West Islip, NY, Professional Communications, 2004.

Otitis Externa

Method of
Jeffrey T. Vrabec, MD

Otitis externa is defined as an acute infection originating in or limited to the external auditory canal. This common affliction may occur in any age group and may be caused by a variety of infectious agents.

Anatomy and Physiology

Functionally, the ear canal serves two purposes. It is important for sound localization and because of resonance effects it improves sound perception in the frequency range from 2500 to 4000 hertz (Hz). The ear canal is approximately 25 mm in length and has a diameter of approximately 7.5 mm. The medial half is an osseous channel formed by the merger of the tympanic bone with the mastoid posteriorly and the squamous portion of the temporal bone superiorly. The lateral half of the canal wall is cartilaginous with a thick squamous epithelium that contains sebaceous glands, sweat glands, and hair follicles. The medial skin covering the bony canal is quite thin, measuring only 0.2 mm in thickness. The medial skin lacks a subcutaneous layer and is in continuity with the outermost layer of the tympanic membrane.

The external canal receives its blood supply from the superficial temporal and posterior auricular branches of the external carotid artery. Venous drainage is to the external jugular vein. The external canal receives sensory innervation via multiple cranial nerves. The trigeminal nerve supplies sensation to the superior and anterior aspect of the canal, the facial nerve supplies the anterior inferior area, and the glossopharyngeal and vagus nerves innervate the inferior and posterior regions. Because of the diverse nerve supply, otalgia may often reflect referred pain from oral cavity, nasal, or pharyngeal sources.

Several anatomic features serve to protect the external canal and tympanic membrane (TM) from injury or infection. The gentle curvature of the canal and the narrowing at the bone–cartilage junction (the isthmus) reduce the probability of large objects penetrating the TM. The hair and cerumen also protect the canal, trapping airborne particles that enter the external meatus. Cerumen has the additional benefit of repelling water. The acidic composition of cerumen lowers the ambient pH of the external canal, making it less hospitable to infectious organisms. The phenomenon of epithelial migration is documented in the ear canal. Surface epithelium moves laterally from the umbo to the annulus of the TM and then laterally to the external meatus. Epithelial movement on the TM proceeds at a rate of 0.05 mm per day and is typically slower in the external canal. Lateral migration helps clear the medial canal of surface epithelium and attached debris. This migratory pattern is arrested in chronic infection of the external canal.

Diagnosis

Infections develop in the external canal when organisms breach the anatomic barriers. Trauma to the canal skin, excessive removal of the cerumen, and excessive moisture in the canal may all facilitate otitis externa. Presenting symptoms of an external ear infection include pain, itching, and hearing loss. Pain develops rapidly, is typically constant, and may be quite severe. Manipulation of the ear or jaw movement exacerbates the pain. Conductive hearing loss occurs because of accumulation of debris in the external canal and is exacerbated by concurrent edema. Persistent symptoms despite treatment are a matter of great concern and may indicate a developing osteitis. Cranial nerve deficits are ominous symptoms and indicate an advanced osteitis of the temporal bone.

Physical examination findings typically include erythema, edema, and drainage. Differences in examination findings can help distinguish bacterial from fungal infections. Bacterial infections usually produce marked edema of the canal skin, especially in the lateral cartilaginous canal. Drainage is usually scant and may have a mucoid or mucopurulent consistency and often has a foul odor. In contrast, fungal infections typically involve the medial canal skin and produce little edema. Drainage is thick and surface spore formation is evident. Focal granulation tissue develops in areas with invasive disease and TM perforations are occasionally present. Bloody drainage can be seen with either bacterial or fungal infections because of maceration of the canal skin or from granulation tissue formation.

Regional or systemic symptoms are uncommon in otitis externa. Periaural erythema, mild lymphadenopathy, and low-grade fever are possible. The presence of regional symptoms indicates a more virulent infection.

Treatment

The initial approach to outer ear infections involves aural toilet and avoidance of further trauma or moisture. Topical antibiotics are prescribed in accordance with the likely infectious organism. Many preparations have a rather broad spectrum of efficacy so routine culture of aural discharge is not performed. It is prudent to obtain culture and sensitivity data in recalcitrant cases. Analgesics are prescribed as necessary to control pain. Narcotics are occasionally required. Patients are instructed to avoid or minimize water exposure. With appropriate treatment, symptoms improve rapidly, and complete healing is seen in 2 weeks or less.

The most common organism identified in routine cases of external otitis is *Pseudomonas aeruginosa*. Staphylococcal species are the next most common. Topical fluoroquinolone or aminoglycoside antibiotics are the most appropriate choice for treatment. Preparations that include a steroid are recommended. Drops are instilled three times daily until resolution of the infection, usually 7 to 10 days. When severe edema of the canal skin is present, a wick is inserted into the canal to facilitate drug delivery. Persistent symptoms indicate inadequate treatment, although this may also be because of inappropriate antibiotic, inefficient drug delivery, noncompliance, or progressive infection.

Differential Diagnosis and Treatment

There are many other infectious disorders of the external canal, although each can usually be distinguished by characteristic

CURRENT DIAGNOSIS

Presenting symptoms include:

- Pain: develops rapidly, typically constant; exacerbated by movement of ear or jaw
- Itching
- Hearing loss: exacerbated by concurrent edema

Exam findings include:

- Erythema
- Edema
- Drainage: sometimes bloody
- Bacterial infections: often have edema of the canal skin with minimal drainage that has foul odor
- Fungal infections: involve the medial canal skin with slight edema, thick drainage, evident surface spore formation

CURRENT THERAPY

- Provide aural toilet and encourage avoidance of further trauma and water exposure.
- Obtain culture and sensitivity data in recalcitrant cases.
- Prescribe topical antibiotics that include a steroid and analgesics (for pain) as needed.

clinical findings. Malignancy may also mimic chronic infection. Biopsy is recommended for abnormal tissue that does not quickly resolve with treatment.

ACUTE INFECTIONS

Furuncles occur at the external meatus in the hair-bearing skin. Erythema and edema are localized, and skin a few millimeters away from the infection has a healthy appearance. Pain can be severe and is exacerbated by pressure or manipulation of the auricle. Furuncles are caused by staphylococcal infection. Spontaneous rupture of the lesion leads to resolution of the infection and pain. If fluctuance is present at presentation, the lesion is drained under local anesthesia. Topical antibiotics (bacitracin, neomycin, or mupirocin [Bactroban] ointment or solution) are a useful adjunct.

The physical findings in otomycosis were outlined earlier. The predominant organisms are *Aspergillus* and *Candida* with considerable variation in prevalence according to geographic region. Fungal infections produce more destruction of the canal skin but less edema. Granulation tissue and TM perforations are not uncommon, although most perforations heal spontaneously after eradication of the infection. Treatment requires meticulous cleaning of debris and topical antifungals. Clotrimazole (Lotrimin) solution is effective for *Candida* species, but eradication of *Aspergillus* species is most efficient with ketoconazole (Nizoral) cream applied directly to the affected skin.

Bullous external otitis is diagnosed based on the characteristic finding of hemorrhagic vesicles in the external canal. Spontaneous rupture of the lesions produces bloody otorrhea. The lesions are quite painful, and lancing the bullae to drain the fluid does not provide relief as is seen in bullous myringitis. Involvement of the medial canal skin is typical. The etiology of this infectious process is unclear. However, the disease responds to a broad spectrum of topical antibiotics. Topical or oral analgesics are a useful adjunctive treatment.

Herpes zoster oticus, or Ramsay Hunt syndrome, occurs because of reactivation of latent varicella zoster virus in the geniculate ganglion. Vesicles may develop in the sensory distribution of the facial nerve. The appearance of skin lesions is characteristic of zoster eruptions. Initially, the vesicles are erythematous with a straw-colored fluid. Spontaneous rupture results in a crusted ulcer that may take several weeks to heal. Facial paralysis, dysgeusia, dizziness, and sensorineural hearing loss are typical in herpes zoster oticus but extremely rare in other infectious diseases of the external ear canal. Treatment of the facial paralysis is the primary objective, necessitating systemic steroids and antivirals.

The skin lesions of the ear canal usually heal without incident, but secondary bacterial otitis externa is possible.

CHRONIC INFECTIOUS DISORDERS

Skull base osteitis occurs when disease extends from soft tissues of the canal into the temporal bone. Elderly patients, diabetics, and immunocompromised individuals are at increased risk of developing osteitis. The diagnosis is suspected when pain, discharge, fever, and/or granulation tissue persist despite treatment. Progressive involvement of the skull base may lead to cranial nerve palsies, vascular thrombosis, and intracranial infection. Laboratory testing reveals a markedly increased sedimentation rate. Technetium-99m bone scan displays increased uptake throughout the course of the disease and is useful for initial diagnosis. Computed tomography (CT) of the temporal bone displays bone erosion in advanced cases. Magnetic resonance imaging (MRI) is useful to detect soft-tissue and dural involvement. Biopsy of infected tissue or bone may be necessary to identify the responsible organism. Systemic antibiotics are selected according to culture and sensitivity data and should be continued until the sedimentation rate returns to normal. This may require months of treatment.

Osteoradionecrosis is a late complication of temporal bone irradiation. Contemporary stereotactic techniques should significantly reduce the incidence of this problem. The process is typically limited, and symptoms are much less severe than in skull base osteitis. Exposed necrotic bone with slight granulation and purulent drainage is seen on examination. Local débridement and topical antibiotics are usually sufficient to control the infection. Recurrence is common because the irradiated ear canal is highly susceptible to infection after exposure to water or minor trauma.

MISCELLANEOUS

With the exception of herpes zoster oticus, none of the entities just described typically involves the pinna. Inflammation of the external canal in conjunction with pinna involvement may signify dermatologic disease. Some common entities include eczema, neomycin allergy, relapsing polychondritis, and erysipelas.

REFERENCES

Clark WB, Brook I, Bianki D, Thompson DH: Microbiology of otitis externa. Otolaryngol Head Neck Surg 1997;116:23-25.
Hawke M, Wong J, Krajden S: Clinical and microbiological features of otitis externa. J Otolaryngol 1984;13:289-295.
Hurst WB: Outcome of 22 cases of perforated tympanic membrane caused by otomycosis. J Laryngol Otol 2001;115:879-880.
Litton WB: Epithelial migration over tympanic membrane and external canal. Arch Otolaryngol 1963;77:254-257.
Lucente FE: Fungal infections of the external ear. Otolaryngol Clin North Am 1993;26:995-1006.
Sreepada GS, Kwartler JA: Skull base osteomyelitis secondary to malignant otitis externa. Curr Opin Otolaryngol Head Neck Surg 2003;11: 316-323.
Sweeney CJ, Gilden DH: Ramsay Hunt syndrome. J Neurol Neurosurg Psychiatry 2001;71:149-154.

Otitis Media

Method of
J. Scott McMurray, MD

Ear infections, their complications and sequelae, comprise most patient-clinician interactions. Estimates suggest nearly $3 billion in direct and indirect cost for acute otitis media (AOM) and otitis media with effusion were spent in 1995 alone. In 2000 more than 16 million office visits were made for otitis media and 802 prescriptions per 1000 visits were written for a total of more than 13 million prescriptions. As common as the problem may be, it continues to be a source of confusion and controversy in terms of its diagnosis, treatment, and expectation for outcomes. Recently, there has been a renewed interest in determining the appropriate evaluation and management of these afflicted children, based on evidence-based medicine.

Along with new diagnostic protocols and realigned treatment strategies, there is a realization that children may fall into different at-risk groups and will therefore benefit from different treatment options. In his recent editorial in the International Journal of Pediatric Otolaryngology on a practical classification of otitis media subgroups, Richard Rosenfeld quoted Stanley Hoerr saying, "It is difficult to make the asymptomatic patient feel better." Yet, he added, much of the research on which we base our decisions to treat or not to treat children with otitis media has been formulated on those who would otherwise do well without treatment, the so-called innocent bystander. Children in the at-risk or suffering groups have been excluded from research trials for ethical reasons against withholding treatment. It is possible to group children into four subgroups with otitis media:

1. Innocent bystander
2. Susceptible child
3. At-risk child
4. Suffering child

These different subgroups imply different treatment limbs. The innocent bystander may do well without any therapy and may tolerate careful observation, whereas the suffering child with a similar disease process deserves rapid and intensive medical or surgical treatment or both.

The stratification of children into different subgroups may appear daunting at first glance but after closer reflection answers the problem of conflicting research data and perhaps uses more common sense (confirmed by clinical trials) in determining treatment. Otherwise developmentally and physically healthy children may be closely observed rather than treated medically or surgically for their acute ear infection or middle ear effusion (MEE). Other children who are at risk for developmental delays, physically challenged, or suffering from the effects or side effects of AOM or otitis media with effusion should be treated more aggressively with either the appropriate medical or surgical plan of care. Unfortunately, this increases the number of possible permutations when determining the appropriate treatment for the afflicted child. Fortunately, however, this new paradigm allows more freedom in determining the appropriate treatment option to be followed. Our challenge lies in honing our abilities to make a correct diagnosis and an accurate assessment of risk so that an appropriate treatment protocol with adequate follow-up can be implemented.

In 2004, the American Academy of Pediatrics, the American Academy of Family Practice, and the American Academy of Otolaryngology Head and Neck Surgery combined forces to create two separate clinical guidelines for AOM and otitis media with effusion. These guidelines serve as an excellent frame on which to build a knowledge base and understanding for the treatment of all children with AOM or otitis media with effusion. These references are invaluable and are recommended reading for all who treat children with ear pathology.

Definitions

Acute otitis media is defined as an abrupt onset of inflammation of the middle ear space. This contrasts with otitis media with effusion, which is fluid in the middle ear without signs and symptoms of inflammation. Otitis media with effusion is much more common than AOM but may be seen as a residual finding of a recently resolved infection. The distinction between the two and the ability of the clinician to distinguish between these disease entities is paramount to decision making and appropriate treatment.

The signs and symptoms of AOM are found in an abrupt onset of fluid in the middle ear with redness or distinct pain. Children suffering with AOM may or may not also exhibit systemic signs of infection, such as fever. Fever, pain, and irritability are seen in 90% of children with AOM, but it is also seen in 76% of children with upper aerodigestive tract viral illnesses as well. History alone may lead to an erroneous conclusions and unnecessary treatment. The distinction lies in the physical findings of MEE with inflammation. Fullness or bulging of the tympanic membrane, air fluid levels, opacification of the tympanic membrane, or bullous vesicles on the tympanic membrane are signs suggesting AOM when associated with acute inflammation. Visualization of the tympanic membrane and the use of pneumatic otoscopy should confirm the presence of a MEE and inflammation. Tympanometry can confirm suspicion of a MEE, but the clinician should work to be proficient with pneumatic otoscopy.

Otitis media with effusion alone may result from a resolved infection or from eustachian tube dysfunction alone. The physical findings are similar to those described but without the signs of acute inflammation. Although the tympanic membrane may be red in the otherwise healthy child crying at the displeasure of being examined, pain and an effusion are not generally associated with normal health.

Treatment Recommendations

Children with AOM should have adequate pain management. Acetaminophen, ibuprofen, and occasionally narcotics are useful in treating the pain of AOM. Rarely, myringotomy is required to relieve the discomfort of an acute ear infection.

If an acute bacterial infection in the middle ear is recognized, antibacterial therapy may be used in all age groups. If the diagnosis is uncertain, antibacterial therapy is recommended in the very young, younger than age 6 months. Antimicrobials may also be administered if one is uncertain of the diagnosis, if the illness is severe in those from 6 months to 2 years of age. If the child is older than age 2 years and the diagnosis is uncertain, observation and close follow-up is recommended.

If antibacterial treatment is instituted, amoxicillin at 80 to 90 mg/kg/day is used as a first line of therapy. If severe illness is encountered or if coverage for beta-lactamase–positive organisms such as *Haemophilus influenzae* or *Moraxella catarrhalis* is required,

---

 CURRENT THERAPY

- Adequate pain management is key in treating AOM.
- If a child has an acute bacterial otitis media, antibiotics are indicated.
- Amoxicillin at 80 to 90 mg/kg/day is the first therapy of choice in nonallergic children.
- Children older than age 2 years may be observed without antibiotic therapy if the diagnosis is uncertain.
- Children younger than age 2 years may be treated with antibiotics if the diagnosis is uncertain.

Abbreviation: AOM = acute otitis media.

CURRENT DIAGNOSIS

- The diagnosis of AOM requires acute signs of illness such as fever and pain along with signs of middle ear inflammation such as fluid and erythema.
- Associated symptoms of AOM include fever, pain, and irritability.
- Visualization of the tympanic membrane and pneumatic otoscopy are required to confirm the diagnosis of AOM.
- Fluid behind the tympanic membrane does not necessarily indicate an infection in the middle ear space.

Abbreviation: AOM = acute otitis media.

amoxicillin-clavulanate (Augmentin) is suggested (90 mg/kg/day of the amoxicillin component).

Children who are allergic to amoxicillin, but not with urticaria or anaphylaxis, may be given cefdinir (Omnicef), cefpodoxime (Vantin), or cefuroxime (Ceftin). Children with type-1 hypersensitivity to amoxicillin may be given azithromycin (Zithromax), clarithromycin (Biaxin), erythromycin-sulfisoxazole (Pediazole), or sulfamethoxazole-trimethoprim (Bactrim). In AOM where the organism is thought to be penicillin resistant *Streptococcus pneumoniae*, clindamycin is a reasonable choice.

Patients who fail to respond within 48 to 72 hours, whether in the observation or antibacterial therapy group, should be reassessed and treatment changed depending on the findings. Reduction of risk factors for AOM is encouraged for everyone. No recommendations were made regarding the efficacy of complementary and alternative medicine for the treatment of AOM.

Otitis media with effusion is common after resolution of acute otitis. Some children also present with asymptomatic otitis media with effusion as well. Treatment of children with persistent middle effusion depends on their at-risk grouping. Children at risk for speech, language, or other learning problems should be treated more promptly than other children not at risk. The at-risk groups include children with a permanent hearing loss independent of the otitis media, suspected or known speech and language delays, autism-spectrum disorder or other pervasive developmental disorder, syndromes or craniofacial disorders, blindness or uncorrectable visual impairment, cleft palate with or without associated syndrome, or developmental delay. The management of the child with otitis media with effusion in these at-risk groups should include hearing tests, speech and language assessment and therapy, hearing aids or other amplification devices for hearing loss independent of the otitis media, tympanostomy tube placement, and assessment of hearing after resolution of the otitis media with effusion to detect underlying hearing loss independent of the middle ear fluid.

Children who do not fall in the at-risk group may be watched for 3 months before intervention. If the MEE persists for longer than 3 months, audiometric assessment of hearing should be obtained. Intervention is then based on the presence of a hearing loss of generally greater than 20 decibels, suspicion of language development delay, or other impending complications related to the MEE. If the hearing loss is mild (21 to 39 decibels), strategies to optimize the listening and learning environment and/or surgical intervention should be suggested. If the hearing loss is greater than 40 decibels, surgical intervention to correct the MEE is indicated and most efficacious.

Initial surgical treatment of a problematic persistent MEE as described earlier is tympanostomy tube placement. Adenoidectomy is reserved for children who have other distinct indications, such as nasal airway obstruction or chronic adenitis, or in whom another set of pressure equalization tubes are necessary. Approximately 20% to 50% of children relapse after their tympanostomy tubes extrude and will require additional tubes. When adenoidectomy is performed with the second set of tubes, the rate of recidivism is decreased by 50%. This advantage is seen in children as young as age 2 years, with the greatest effect seen in children aged 3 years and older, regardless of adenoidal size. Children older than age 4 years may also benefit from adenoidectomy and myringotomy without tube placement. Myringotomy alone without tympanostomy tube insertion and/or tonsillectomy alone solely for the treatment of otitis media with effusion has not been found to be efficacious.

Conclusion

The key to successful management of a child with AOM or otitis media with effusion, as it is with any medical problem, is based on the clinician's ability to correctly diagnose and stratify at-risk groups. The new recommended clinical pathways developed by the AAP, AAFP, and AAO-HNS for AOM and otitis media with effusion may at first seem to increase complexity of treatment because it increases the number of pathways possible. Closer reflection, however, will reveal an easier paradigm. It is the clinician's responsibility to attain the skills and knowledge set to make the correct initial diagnosis and assessment of risk for the patient. The support from the evidence-based-medicine clinical pathways will then help in the decision making and treatment formulation.

REFERENCES

American Academy of Family Physicians, American Academy of Otolaryngology Head and Neck Surgery, American Academy of Pediatrics Subcommittee on Otitis Media with Effusion: Otitis media with effusion. Pediatrics 2004;113(5):1412-1429.
American Academy of Pediatrics Subcommittee on Acute Otitis Media: Diagnosis and management of acute otitis media. Pediatrics 2004; 113(5):1451-1465.
Bell LM: The new clinical practice guidelines for acute otitis media: An editorial. Ann Emerg Med 2005;45(5):514-516.
Bluestone CD: Epidemiology and pathogenesis of chronic suppurative otitis media: Implications for prevention and treatment. Int J Pediatr Otorhinolaryngol 1998;42(3):207-223.
Ohlms LA, Chen AY, Stewart MG, Franklin DJ: Establishing the etiology of childhood hearing loss. Otolaryngol Head Neck Surg 1999;120(2):159-163.
Paradise JL, Campbell TF, Dollaghan CA, et al: Developmental outcomes after early or delayed insertion of tympanostomy tubes. N Engl J Med 2005;353(6):576-586.
Rosenfeld RM: A practical classification of otitis media subgoups. Int J Pediatr Otorhinolaryngol 2005;69(8):1027-1029.
Rosenfeld RM, Culpepper L, Doyle KJ, et al: Clinical practice guideline: Otitis media with effusion. Otolaryngol Head Neck Surg 2004;130(5 Suppl): S95-S118.
Rosenfeld RM, Lous J, Bluestone CD, et al: Recent advances in otitis media. 8. Treatment. Ann Otol Rhinol Laryngol Suppl 2005;194:114-139.

Episodic Vertigo

Method of
Terry D. Fife, MD

Vertigo is the illusion of motion, particularly rotational motion or spinning. It generally implies localization to the vestibular pathways in the peripheral or central nervous system. One of the challenges of evaluating patients with dizziness is determining whether they have vertigo or some other form of dizziness that is not vestibular in origin. Table 1 outlines a general classification of dizziness; episodic vertigo is merely one type of episodic dizziness.

TABLE 1 Classification of Dizziness

Type	Symptom Description	Example
Disequilibrium without vertigo	Imbalance when standing or walking, unsteadiness, poor balance	Sensory ataxia, cerebellar ataxia, bilateral vestibular loss
Physiologic dizziness	Motion sickness, visual vertigo, nausea or queasiness, fatigue	Seasickness, carsickness, airsickness, visual vertigo*
Presyncope	Lightheadedness, near-faintness, fading-out feeling	Postural hypotension, neurally mediated hypotension, volume depletion
Psychiatric dizziness	Chronic floating or rocking, fatigue	Panic disorder, dizziness from anxiety, phobic vertigo
Vertigo	Spinning, tilting, toppling, free-falling sensation	Vestibular neuritis, Meniere's disease, BPPV, brainstem or cerebellar causes of vertigo, migrainous vertigo

*Visual vertigo is dizziness evoked by seeing objects in motion such as ceiling fans, moving traffic, moving scenery, and optokinetic stimulation from walking through grocery store aisles or from the movement of people in crowds.
BPPV = benign paroxysmal positional vertigo.

Episodic vertigo can be classified as being of *peripheral*, *central*, or *unknown* origin. Vertigo is of peripheral origin when there is dysfunction related primarily to the labyrinth or vestibulocochlear nerve. Central vertigo is caused by dysfunction of vestibular structures within the central nervous system, such as the vestibular nuclei or cerebellum. Vertigo of unknown origin includes conditions with vestibular symptoms but for which localization is unclear. Success in treating or managing dizziness is highly dependent on determining the cause of the disorder.

Vertigo of Peripheral Origin

Episodic vertigo is most often caused by peripheral vestibular conditions affecting the inner ear itself or the vestibulocochlear nerve. Some conditions, such as vestibular neuritis and labyrinthitis, probably simultaneously affect both the labyrinth and the nerve.

BENIGN PAROXYSMAL POSITIONAL VERTIGO

Benign paroxysmal positional vertigo (BPPV) is the most commonly seen cause of episodic vertigo in general practice, with a lifetime prevalence of 2.4%. BPPV is characterized by attacks of spinning evoked by certain movements such as lying back or getting out of bed, turning in bed, looking up, or straightening after bending over. The episodes of vertigo last 10 to 30 seconds and are not accompanied by any additional symptoms aside from nausea in some patients. The degrees of nausea, pallor, diaphoresis, and even diarrhea depend the patient's inherent tolerance to vertigo as well as on the severity of the BPPV. Patients prone to motion sickness can feel queasy and lightheaded for hours after the attack of vertigo, but most patients feel well between episodes of vertigo. If the patient reports spontaneous episodes or vertigo lasting more than 1 or 2 minutes or if episodes never occur in bed, then one should question the diagnosis of BPPV.

Diagnosis

The diagnosis of BPPV is confirmed by eliciting paroxysmal positional nystagmus on the Dix–Hallpike maneuver. The Dix–Hallpike maneuver is performed by rapidly moving the head from an upright to a head-hanging position with one ear 45 degrees to the side. In Figure 1, movement from position 1 to position 2 constitutes the Dix–Hallpike maneuver for the right side (right ear down). The Dix–Hallpike maneuver results in torsional upbeating nystagmus corresponding in duration to the patient's subjective vertigo and occurring only after Dix–Hallpike positioning on the affected side in those with typical BPPV affecting the posterior semicircular canal. A presumptive diagnosis can be made by history alone, but paroxysmal positional nystagmus confirms the diagnosis.

BPPV is a mechanical disorder of the inner ear caused by calcium carbonate crystals inappropriately located in the semicircular canal of the inner ear on one side and occasionally on both sides. The most commonly affected semicircular canal is the posterior canal; it accounts for approximately 90% of cases of BPPV. The calcium debris originates from the utricular otoconia, which can break off following trauma or viral infections or simply from degeneration. While the patient is supine, loose calcium debris from the utricle can become trapped in the semicircular canal, where it produces endolymph fluid movement during certain head movements, which stimulates the cupula and causes vertigo.

The features most useful in distinguishing typical BPPV of the posterior semicircular canal from central positional vertigo is the direction of the nystagmus, the tendency to fatigue (which lessens with each successive Dix–Hallpike maneuver), and the response to canalith repositioning. Factors such as latency and suppression of nystagmus by visual fixation are much less useful. Typical BPPV results in transient torsional nystagmus, with the top pole of the

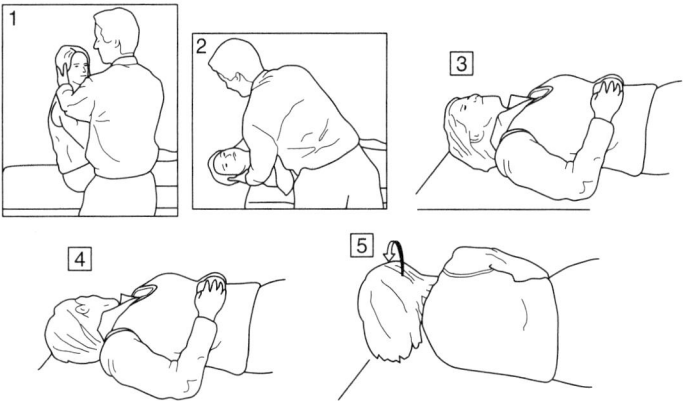

FIGURE 1. Canalith repositioning maneuver for right-sided benign paroxysmal positional vertigo. In position *1*, the patient is sitting up with the head turned 45 degrees toward the right. Position the patient rapidly to position *2* so the head is hanging back and still 45 degrees to the right. Hold this position for 30 seconds or until all nystagmus has stopped. Next, keeping the head back, turn the head through position *3* to position *4* so that the head is hanging back and 45 degrees to the left. Hold that position for 20 seconds. Next, turn the head down so the patient is almost facing the floor (position *5*) and hold in that position for 20 seconds. Finally, assist the patient to sit up, keeping the head toward the left shoulder until the patient is sitting upright. The whole maneuver can then be repeated until no further vertigo or nystagmus is evident in going from position 1 to position 2. (Modified from the Barrow Neurological Institute.)

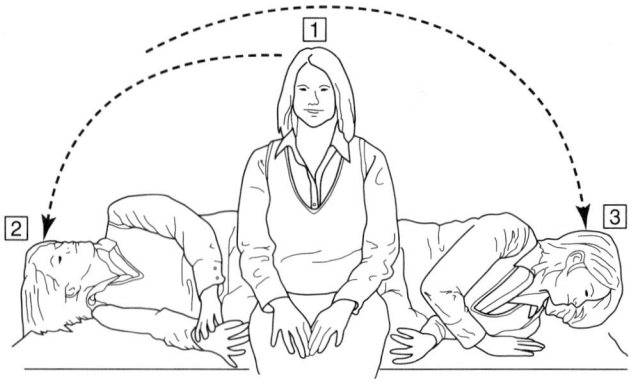

FIGURE 2. Liberatory maneuver or Semont maneuver for right-sided benign paroxysmal positional vertigo. In position *1*, turn the head 45 degrees toward the left (unaffected) side, then rapidly move the patient to the right side (position *2*). This will produce vertigo and nystagmus in active right benign paroxysmal positional vertigo. Hold the position for 1 minute, then rapidly move the patient from position *2* to position *3* and hold position *3* for 1 minute. During the whole maneuver, the head remains fixed 45 degrees toward the left (unaffected side). This maneuver moves debris from the right posterior canal to the utricle. (Modified from the Barrow Neurological Institute.)

eye beating with fast phases toward the ground and undermost ear. This torsional nystagmus is admixed with an upbeating component. Nystagmus straying from this pattern should raise suspicions for central positional nystagmus.

Treatment

Treatment of BPPV is illustrated in Figure 1, which depicts the canalith repositioning maneuver that is sometimes referred to as the Epley maneuver or particle repositioning maneuver. Figure 2 depicts the Liberatory maneuver or Semont maneuver, which is an effective alternative treatment method. Both maneuvers and variations of them are designed to clear calcium debris from the posterior semicircular canal by moving it back into the vestibule by the effects of gravity. This is possible because the calcium carbonate crystals sink in the endolymph. Once it is back in the vestibule it is generally absorbed or eliminated within a period of days in most patients through mechanisms yet to be determined. If properly done, the canalith repositioning maneuver eliminates BPPV immediately in more than 85% of patients. Similar success has been reported with the Semont maneuver.

Patients who do not respond to canalith repositioning have calcium particles that are immobile or that are attached to the cupula. BPPV that is disabling and refractory to all positioning treatments can be managed surgically, although this is rarely necessary.

BPPV is a mechanically produced disorder best managed by a mechanical remedy. Meclizine (Antivert) and other vestibular suppressants may be used to premedicate patients prone to motion sickness but are generally not useful for BPPV because the episodes are brief and because the therapeutic maneuvers are so immediate and effective.

ACUTE UNILATERAL LOSS
Etiology and Diagnosis

Sudden unilateral loss of inner ear balance (vestibular) function produces acute vertigo lasting days to weeks. The most common cause is viral or postinfectious vestibular neurolabyrinthitis. The term *vestibular neuritis* refers to the acute unilateral loss of vestibular function that spares hearing. *Labyrinthitis* refers to acute unilateral loss of both hearing and vestibular dysfunction due to viral infection. Other causes of acute vestibular loss include vestibular nerve sectioning and labyrithectomy, ischemia, trauma, or other infections. Herpes zoster oticus leads to blistering in the sensory distribution of the seventh cranial nerve, a small patch deep in the external ear canal or occasionally behind the ear. Otologic examination is usually painful and can reveal painful vesicles. When accompanied by ipsilateral Bell's palsy, the condition is referred to as Ramsay Hunt syndrome.

The time course of vestibular neuritis or labyrinthitis is about the same and usually evolves over a period of 30 minutes to several hours. Vertigo is present in all head positions but is aggravated by head motion and gradually abates in the ensuing days to weeks. The fast phases of the nystagmus beat away from the injured ear, increase during gaze in the direction of the fast phase, and diminish with gaze opposite the direction. This is referred to as *Alexander's law* and is characteristic of acute peripheral vestibular loss. The nystagmus of acute unilateral vestibular loss decreases daily so that spontaneous nystagmus is usually gone within a few days.

TABLE 2 Motion Sickness and Vestibular Suppressant Medications

Medication	Dosage	Sedation	Antiemetic Effect	Adverse Effects
Antihistamines				
Dimenhydrinate (Dramamine)	50 mg PO bid	+	+	Urinary retention, dry mouth
Meclizine (Antivert, Bonine)	12.5–50 mg PO tid or qid	++	+	Urinary retention, dry mouth
Promethazine (Phenergan)	12.5–50 mg PO or IM q4-6 h 50-mg suppository PR qid	++	++	Slightly lowered seizure threshold
Benzodiazepines				
Clonazepam[1] (Klonopin)	0.25–1 mg PO bid or tid	+++	+	Dose-dependent sedation
Diazepam[1] (Valium)	2–7.5 mg PO tid or qid	++	+	Dose-dependent sedation
Lorazepam[1] (Ativan)	0.5–2 mg bid or tid	++	+	Dose-dependent sedation
Others				
Metoclopramide[1] (Reglan)	10–20 mg PO q4-6 h 10–20 mg IV q 6 h	+	+++	Extrapyramidal effects
Ondansetron[1] (Zofran)	4–8 mg PO, SL, or IV q4-6 h	–	++++	
Prochlorperazine[1] (Compazine)	10–20 mg PO q4-6 h 10 mg IV q 6 h 25-mg suppository PR q 6 h	+	+++	Extrapyramidal effects
Scopalamine (Transderm Scop)	Patch 1 q 3 days	+	+	Urinary retention, dry mouth

[1]Not FDA approved for this indication

> **BOX 1 Home Habituation Exercises for Recovery from Vestibular Loss**
>
> **Thumb-Tracking Exercise**
> Turn the head quickly from side to side and then up and down while focusing on your thumb held out directly in front of you. As you move your head, move your thumb so that it is right in front of you and you can keep your focus on it. As you move your head, your focus should be fixed on your thumb. Repeat these exercises for 30 to 60 seconds at least five times daily. This exercise helps to improve your ability to focus on things while your head is moving from side to side.
>
> **Head Shaking**
> Practice slowly turning your head from side to side while seated and then later while standing with your feet shoulder width apart. Gradually increase the speed of head movements. The head turning can include side-to-side and up-and-down movements rapidly and repetitively with eyes open and in good lighting. Once you can do this standing still, try to walk (eyes open) forward while turning the head side to side, gradually increasing the speed of head turns. This helps you become more used to rapid movements of the head, which are often a source of momentary imbalance.
>
> **Walk While Turning Your Head**
> Walk down a hallway while turning your head side to side rapidly. Your head does not need to be turned far in each direction; it is more important to keep the head turning from side to side while you try to walk straight. This helps train your balance system to manage with less inner ear function.
>
> **Lie to Stand**
> Practice getting up from the lying down position to standing as quickly (but carefully) as possible. This may be done on a sofa or bed. Practice getting up toward the left and toward the right sides. Be careful not to fall. Get up quickly five times to each side; gradually try to increase the quickness but avoid falling. This helps improve the coordination of quick movements of the head and body.
>
> **Tightrope Exercise**
> Walk heel to toe as though walking a tightrope. This can be done in a corridor where there is something to hold on to if needed. Gradually try to achieve 10 steps (heel touching toe) without holding on or sidestepping. This trains the cerebellum in standing balance.
>
> **Standing Balance**
> Stand with feet together (touching) and try to maintain the position for 15 seconds. Once you accomplish that, try closing your eyes with someone nearby to keep you from falling. Try to eventually be able to stand with feet together and eyes closed for 8 seconds. This trains you to keep your balance using ankle sensation and inner ear signals. When you are able to do this for 8 seconds, then practice standing on one leg (with eyes open) or while standing on a foam pillow. Eventually try to stand for 10 seconds on a foam pillow with eyes closed and to stand on one leg for 12 seconds.
>
> **Pick-up Exercise**
> Rapidly bend over and straighten up five times. Do this exercise twice. Time yourself and try to gradually increase your speed. Eventually try adding an about face (180-degree turn) after each bend. Be especially careful if bending over tends to bother your back. This improves your balance with quick bending and turning movements.
>
> **Walk and Turn Test**
> Walk 10 steps down a corridor, then turn right, walk back to the starting point. Do this five times turning to the right, then five times turning toward the left. Time how long it takes you and try to improve your speed, being careful to avoid falling. This helps walking balance and balance with turns.

Treatment

Early in the course of acute unilateral vestibular loss, vestibular suppressants may be helpful in mitigating vertigo and nausea (Table 2). Within a few days, when nausea has subsided, vestibular suppressants should be used more sparingly or eliminated because these medications can delay or limit CNS adaptation to the acute vestibular loss. Initially patients should begin moving their head from side to side, extending the activity each day until they can undergo a full battery of vestibular exercises (Box 1). Eventually, through cerebellar adaptation, the brain can accommodate the unilateral vestibular loss and the patient makes a complete or nearly complete recovery. Studies in primates and humans indicate that vestibular exercises accelerate the recovery from a unilateral vestibular loss and improve overall balance function.

BILATERAL PERIPHERAL VESTIBULAR LOSS

Etiology and Diagnosis

Symmetrical bilateral loss of vestibular function does not usually manifest with a prominent complaints of vertigo. Patients more commonly report disequilibrium that is more prominent during head motion. Patients also might report bouncing of their vision during motion (oscillopsia) if their vestibular loss is severe and bilateral. This symptom occurs due to loss of the vestibulo-ocular reflex, a reflex that serves to stabilize gaze during head movement. Bilateral vestibular loss can often be detected in the bedside head thrust test. Quantitative vestibular testing by video- or electronystagmography or by rotational chair testing is confirmatory. The most well recognized cause of bilateral peripheral loss is aminoglycoside (especially gentamicin) ototoxicity. Other causes include idiopathic vestibular loss, bilateral sequential vestibular neuritis, bilateral Meniere's disease, luetic otitis, Lyme disease, ototoxicity from cisplatin or organic solvents, and trauma.

Treatment

There is no known therapy that restores vestibular function in humans. Treatment is therefore directed at retraining the patient to use visual, somatosensory, and other balance mechanisms that are still intact. Balance training includes exercises (see Box 1) that promote a retraining of balance so that joint position sensation and vision become the dominant senses used for balance maintenance. This requires a thorough neurologic examination to assess which components of balance are functional. The goal in such cases is to improve balance and reduce the risk of falling, although it is less helpful in reducing oscillopsia or the momentary sense of disequilibrium experienced during rapid head movements. Vestibular suppressants such as meclizine (Antivert) and diazepam (Valium) should be avoided in patients with bilateral vestibular loss because these medications suppress vestibular function further and may cause sedation. Hence, bilateral peripheral vestibular loss is one type of dizziness that may be aggravated by vestibular-suppressant medications.

OTOLITHIC VERTIGO

Spinning is often related to an asymmetry in the semicircular canal inputs. Tilting, flipping, pulling to one side, free falling, and translational sensations represent symptoms of otolithic dysfunction in the utricle or saccule. Otolithic vertigo can occur after motor vehicle accidents and trauma because the otolith structures are susceptible to acceleration–deceleration injury. The otolith organs normally detect gravity and translational movements. There is no well-established test of otolith function of the utricle, but vestibular evoked myogenic potentials (VEMPs) can detect the integrity of the saccular function on each side. Caloric or rotational vestibular testing assesses the horizontal semicircular canal function but can fail to detect vestibular dysfunctions that are predominantly otolithic in origin. When the central otolithic pathways are affected, skew diplopia can accompany the dizziness. Recovery may be incomplete with lesions of the central otolith pathways, but peripheral otolithic disorders often improve with rehabilitation and habituation exercises.

SUPERIOR CANAL DEHISCENCE SYNDROME

Superior canal dehiscence syndrome occurs when the bony covering of the superior semicircular canal in the temporal bone has dehisced or developed an abnormal opening. Studies indicate that 0.7% of temporal bone specimens show dehiscence of bony labyrinth of the temporal bone and another 1.3% are less than 0.1 mm thick. This is important because even the highest-resolution temporal bone scans cannot detect a bone thickness of 0.1 mm. Persons with a thin bone over the superior canal can subsequently develop superior canal dehiscence syndrome, perhaps from age-related erosion or barotrauma from straining.

Patients develop sound- or pressure-induced vertigo. This can result in unsteadiness, tilting, or nausea that increases during activities or when exposed to certain sounds or vibrations or air pressure changes.

Diagnosis

Examination might reveal increased sound sensitivity to bone conduction. The Weber tuning fork test can lateralize to the affected side, and bone conduction is greater than air conduction on Rinne testing.

Vestibular-evoked myogenic potential testing measures short latency relaxation potentials from sound-sensitive cells of the saccule that affect the ipsilateral sternocleidomastoid muscle. With superior canal dehiscence syndrome, decreased vestibular-evoked myogenic potential thresholds are present on the affected side.

High-resolution temporal bone CT radiographs confirm superior canal dehiscence. The images should be at 0.3 mm collimation taken directly in the coronal plane to allow one to see the bony roof of the superior canal.

Audiometry of superior canal dehiscence syndrome shows decreased bone conduction thresholds and an apparent conductive hearing loss that is most likely due to dissipation of sound due to the dehiscence.

Treatment

Treatment depends on severity. In mildly symptomatic cases, the patient may simply avoid aggravating factors and not have to undergo surgery. Superior canal resurfacing or canal plugging can be performed to eliminate the dehiscence in patients with more debilitating symptoms.

PERILYMPHATIC FISTULA

A perilymphatic fistula represents another type of abnormal opening of the labyrinth, often at the oval or round window, that allows transfer of pressure from the middle ear to the receptors of the inner ear. Patients experience momentary vertigo or illusions of movement with sneezing, coughing, lifting, or straining. A fistula test is performed by applying pressure to the external ear canal by insufflation to see if it can be transmitted across the middle ear to produce vertigo and nystagmus. The test is quite helpful when nystagmus is induced but it lacks sensitivity, being normal in some cases of confirmed fistula. Perilymphatic fistulas can occur following otologic surgery, trauma, or extreme straining. Perilymphatic fistulas that do not heal spontaneously generally require surgery.

ACOUSTIC NEUROMAS

Acoustic neuromas are benign schwannomas usually arising from the vestibular portion of the vestibulocochlear nerve. They gradually produce loss of vestibular and hearing function and usually manifest with a progressive unilateral hearing loss, perhaps with a history of intermittent disequilibrium or dizziness. Although a brainstem evoked potential may be helpful in detecting an acoustic neuroma, magnetic resonance imaging (MRI) with contrast is still the most sensitive method of detection. Not all acoustic neuromas require immediate treatment, particularly if they are small, are not affecting hearing, and do not appear to be growing quickly. Acoustic neuromas may be treated with surgical excision or by radiotherapy. The decision for treatment is based on the risks of treatment weighed against those of the untreated tumor.

OTHER CAUSES OF VERTIGO

Basilar meningitis is an inflammatory disorder, although it is generally taken to include neoplastic disorders that affect the structures in the posterior fossa near the prepontine cistern. Such disorders can include infectious meningitis and postinfectious inflammatory or carcinomatous meningitides. These conditions irritate or impair cranial nerves and subpial gray matter of the posterior fossa and can manifest with disequilibrium worsened by head turning. Cerebrospinal fluid is usually abnormal in basilar meningitis but is normal in some cases.

Neurovascular compression is a controversial diagnosis said to account for disabling positional vertigo by pulsating vessels abutting the vestibulocochlear nerve on one or both sides. This condition has vague diagnostic criteria and should be viewed with cautious skepticism before subjecting a patient to a craniotomy and microvascular decompressive surgery. Such patients should have a thorough neuro-otologic evaluation, particularly looking for refractory benign positional vertigo, uncompensated vestibular neuritis, and vestibular migraine, all of which could produce persisting vertigo worsened by positional changes.

Vertigo of Central Origin

VASCULAR CAUSES

Transient Ischemic Attacks

Transient ischemia of the brainstem or cerebellum can produce episodic vertigo or disequilibrium usually lasting 1 to 15 minutes. Although it is quite helpful when the patient concurrently experiences diplopia or dysarthria, ataxia, or clumsiness of the extremities, these findings may be absent in some cases. Vertebrobasilar transient ischemic attacks manifesting as isolated vertigo are usually related to vascular occlusion in the distal segments of the vertebral arteries between the posterior and anterior inferior cerebellar arteries. Many of the vital central and peripheral vestibular structures are supplied by this segment of vasculature including the labyrinth, which is supplied by a branch off the anterior inferior cerebellar artery.

Therapy for transient ischemic attacks suspected of causing episodic vertigo may include aspirin, 81 to 325 mg daily, dipyridamole (Persantin) with aspirin or clopidogrel bisulfate (Plavix) 75 mg daily, or systemic anticoagulation with heparin or warfarin (Coumadin). For select patients with concerning vertebrobasilar ischemic events despite maximal medical therapy, surgical stenting or focal angioplasty of the vertebral arteries may be considered.

Cerebral Infarction

Posterior Inferior Cerebellar Artery Syndrome

The posterior inferior cerebellar artery supplies the lateral medulla and the posterior and inferior sections of the cerebellum. An infarct to one or both of these structures can produce vertigo. Nystagmus is usually present if there is infarction of the lateral medulla. Diffusion MRI is the imaging procedure of choice.

If the infarct is less than 3 hours old, thrombolytic therapy with tissue plasminogen activator (Activase) 90 to 100 mg may be considered. Acute management of vertigo following a brainstem or cerebellar stroke includes minimizing movement and using vestibular suppressants such as promethazine (Phenergan) 12.5 to 50 mg three times a day or diazepam[1] 2 to 5 mg three times a day for the first 24 hours. As soon as the nausea subsides, these medications should be withdrawn and head movements resumed and rapidly increased to promote central nervous system adaptation. Balance training exercises under the guidance of a physical therapist is often helpful.

Anterior Inferior Cerebellar Artery Syndrome

The anterior inferior cerebellar artery supplies some crucial vestibular structures, including the flocculus and other anterior portions of the cerebellum important for ocular motor control, portions of the lateral pons and pontomedullary junction, and the inner ear itself. An infarct in the anterior inferior cerebellar artery can produce an isolated cerebellar stroke, a lateral pontine stroke, or both. When the lateral pons is affected, ipsilateral hearing loss and peripheral facial paresis can be seen. Treatment for this is similar to that for posterior inferior cerebellar artery syndrome.

NONVASCULAR CAUSES

Nonvascular causes of episodic vertigo can include space-occupying lesions, such as a tumor or abscess, that produce a gradual unsteadiness and imbalance, rather than discrete episodes of dizziness. Demyelinating or inflammatory disorders can also produce vertigo by affecting the root entry zone of the vestibular nerve or by affecting the CNS vestibular nuclei or connecting pathways to the cerebellum. Acute vertigo due to multiple sclerosis can improve with high-dose methylprednisolone (Solu-Medrol)[1] 1 g intravenously daily for 3 to 5 days.

Familial periodic ataxia is a rare dominantly inherited condition associated with *episodes* of vertigo and ataxia. It might respond to acetazolamide (Diamox)[1] 250 to 500 mg two or three times a day.

Rarely, epileptic vertigo manifests as episodic vertigo in isolation, although most vertigo associated with epilepsy occurs in patients with known epilepsy in or around the vestibular cortex. Treatment of epileptic vertigo is no different than that for other types of partial epilepsy.

Vertigo of Unknown Origin

VESTIBULAR MIGRAINE

Vestibular migraine can manifest with episodes of vertigo lasting minutes to hours at a time. In addition, some patients with a history of migraine experience chronic vertigo or severe motion sickness.

---

[1]Not FDA approved for this indication.

The mechanism for this is unclear but may be related to hypersensitivity of key brainstem nuclei including the superior salivatory nuclei and vestibular nuclei and the trigeminal nucleus caudalis. Migraine that manifests with predominantly vestibular manifestations is referred to as *vestibular migraine*.

Treatment includes symptomatic use of antivertiginous medications, as would be used in acute vertigo of any sort (see Table 2) when the vertigo episodes are consistently prolonged. When the episodes are frequent or interfere with daily functions, a migraine prophylactic medication such as verapamil (Verelan)[1] 180 to 360 mg daily, topiramate (Topamax) 50 to 100 mg at bedtime, imipramine (Tofranil)[1] 50 to 100 mg daily, propranolol (Inderal) 120 to 180 mg daily, venlafaxine (Effexor) 75 to 150 mg daily, or sodium valproate (Depakote) 125 mg twice daily may be useful.

POST-TRAUMATIC DIZZINESS

Post-traumatic dizziness, like postconcussive syndrome, in general is a difficult and perplexing problem. One of the challenges is disentangling vague, nonobjective symptoms, such as dizziness, pain, and headache from the potential secondary gain associated with litigation. However, there is a common story reported by many patients, including those who have no evident secondary gain. Constant rocking or floating dizziness is a common report, as is motion-related disequilibrium. Benign positional vertigo should always be excluded because it is fairly common in the aftermath of trauma. Migraine can sometimes be triggered by head injury and should be considered as well. Finally, partial vestibular loss or otolithic vertigo can occur after trauma, so vestibular habituation exercises may be helpful (see Box 1).

Psychiatric Dizziness

Dizziness associated with a psychiatric diagnoses is fairly common and is usually not the focus of treatment rendered by the treating psychiatrist, whose attention is usually directed at the behavioral and affective components of these disorders. Patients with panic syndrome often experience bouts of floating, rocking dizziness without nausea that are often not contemporaneous with panic attacks.

Medications that could be effective for this include imipramine 50-150 mg/d, or nortriptyline (Pamelor) 50 to 150 mg daily, venlafaxine 75 to 225 mg daily, or selective serotonin reuptake inhibitor medications such as paroxetine (Paxil) 20 to 60 mg daily or escitalopram (Lexapro) 10 to 40 mg daily. I generally avoid amitriptyline (Elavil) except in those with insomnia because it is quite sedating and can be difficult for patients to tolerate at higher doses. Alprazolam (Xanax) 0.25 mg tid is often helpful but is best used only intermittently rather than as the mainstay of daily management.

Other psychiatric conditions associated with dizziness include generalized anxiety, somatoform illnesses, and factitious disorder. Some phobias such as agoraphobia with or without panic attacks and acrophobia are associated with dizziness. These patients might respond to behavioral therapy or tricyclic amines such as imipramine 50 to 200 mg daily or clomipramine (Anafranil) 50 to 75 mg daily.

Physiologic Vertigo

Physiologic vertigo is dizziness that can be experienced by any person given the right environment or stimulation. Some patients develop excessive sensitivity to certain stimuli that can necessitate treatment.

MOTION SICKNESS

Motion sickness is usually described as a floating lightheadedness and drunken feeling, typically with significant nausea, with autonomic symptoms such as pallor, diaphoresis, and hypersalivation. Motion sickness develops with exposure to passive motion such as in a car (carsickness), airplane (airsickness), or on water (seasickness).

Etiology

The physiologic and molecular mechanisms for motion sickness are not known, though motion sickness has been attributed to poor reconciliation of conflicting visual and vestibular signals received. Certain exposures are more likely to evoke motion sickness than others: riding in the back seat of a car or bus travelling on a winding road while reading or being on a boat with large wave swells are strong stimuli. Driving the car rarely produces motion sickness, in part because of improved visualization in the front of the car and in part because of the predictability or anticipatory mechanism involved in controlling the car's direction. Motion sickness can occur in nearly anyone with normal vestibular function given sufficient exposure, but some people are more susceptible, possibly due to inherited factors.

Treatment

Prevention and avoidance are the first lines of defense. When travel or other activities are necessary, preemptive use of vestibular suppressants before motion exposure is more effective than using the same medications after the motion sickness has begun. Table 2 lists the medications most effective, including meclizine, dimenhydrinate, diazepam,[1] and promethazine. When these medications are too sedating, a morning dose of modafinil (Provigil)[1] 200 mg can be used to counteract their sedating effects. Hence, in patients with severe motion sickness, a regimen of diazepam[1] 4 mg, meclizine 25 mg, and, if needed to avert sedation, modafinil[1] may be taken 1 hour before exposure to motion. At the first hint of increasing motion sickness promethazine 25 to 50 mg may be added. Patients should be aware that this combination of medications can temporarily impair alertness.

Visual Vertigo

Visual vertigo is a motion sickness–like sensation brought on not by motion but by visual object motion or optokinetic stimulation. Many but not all patients also have a tendency for motion sickness. This symptom complex can be seen in some patients with acute vertigo, vestibular migraine, and some forms of psychiatric dizziness, or it can be a lifelong isolated trait.

Sometimes this can be severely disturbing to the extent that the patient cannot tolerate watching others in motion or visual commotion in general. Situations often reported as disturbing include grocery store aisles, crowded places such as malls or theaters, or watching moving ceiling fans, traffic, merry-go-rounds, or motion pictures. This syndrome should be distinguished from agoraphobia, although some patients with panic attacks have both.

If symptoms begin to intrude on daily activities, treatment is clonazepam (Klonopin)[1] 0.25 to 1 mg daily, imipramine[1] 75 mg daily, or duloxetine (Cymbalta)[1] 30 to 60 mg daily.

HYPERVENTILATION

Hyperventilation has been implied in some reports as the cause of vertigo in a large percentage of patients with dizziness. Because it is normal for patients to develop lightheadedness during hyperventilation, this is a physiologic form of lightheadedness. Some patients are pathologic hyperventilators and are not fully aware of it. Generally, however, if they are made aware of it they can manage their symptoms quite adequately. Many patients with hyperventilation have also had panic attacks or anxiety secondary to some other vestibular disturbance. Over-breathing is rarely a cause of chronic vertigo.

Ménière's Disease

Method of
*Ted A. Meyer, MD, PhD, and
Paul R. Lambert, MD*

Ménière's disease is a disorder of fluid balance of the endolymph of the peripheral auditory and vestibular systems. The inner ear contains an endolymph-filled membranous labyrinth housed inside the perilymph-filled bony labyrinth. The sensory receptor cells of the inner ear are contained in the membranous labyrinth. The composition of perilymph is very similar to cerebrospinal fluid (CSF) (high sodium, low potassium), whereas the composition of endolymph is like intracellular fluid (high potassium, low sodium). The uniqueness of endolymph lies in its high positive resting potential (+80 mV). Disturbances in the fluid dynamics of the endolymph appear to be involved in the hearing loss and peripheral vestibular disorders associated with Ménière's disease. The exact mechanism or mechanisms involved in Ménière's disease are not completely understood, but it appears that an overabundance of endolymph, either through overproduction and/or underabsorption, is the pathologic basis of the disease.

Clinical Presentation

The symptomatology of Ménière's disease was first described almost 150 years ago by the French physician for whom it is named, Prosper Ménière. Patients with Ménière's disease present with unilateral fluctuating sensorineural hearing loss, aural fullness, tinnitus, and spells of disabling vertigo that typically last between 20 minutes and 24 hours. Many patients with Ménière's disease have nonspecific dizziness and imbalance in between spells of vertigo as well. A small percentage of patients develop or present with drop attacks, or spells of Tumarkin. These attacks occur when a patient's vestibular system goes into a crisis and the patient loses extensor tone. Patients often describe an aura followed by a feeling that they are going to fall. Patients do not lose consciousness unless they hit their head. Patients with Ménière's disease may not present with all symptoms, and the severity and progression of hearing loss, tinnitus, and vertigo are variable. For the majority of patients, Ménière's disease occurs in a single ear; however, if patients are followed for a long enough time, the literature reports bilateral Ménière's disease in a wide percentage of patients. Patients with bilateral Ménière's disease whose hearing loss progresses to profound levels are excellent candidates for a cochlear implant.

Office Evaluation

The majority of patients with dizziness or vertigo present to their primary care physician (PCP) or to the emergency room. Many of these patients are given 25 mg of meclizine (Antivert) and are instructed to take it up to three times a day as needed. When the vertigo spells continue, they are often then referred to an otolaryngologist or otologist. Patients who are regularly taking meclizine as a prophylactic should stop the medication as quickly as possible.

When the patient with dizziness or vertigo presents to the clinic, the diagnosis of Ménière's disease can usually be obtained through the history and physical examination. The patient should give a history of disabling spells of vertigo, aural fullness or a "stuffy ear," fluctuating and progressive hearing loss, and tinnitus. The nature of the vertigo and the duration of the spells aids in the diagnosis. The vertigo is usually severe and can last between 20 minutes and 24 hours. Rarely does a Ménière's attack last longer than 24 hours. Longer attacks (days) are more consistent with vestibular neuritis. The attacks are not provoked by specific movements, such as the brief spell of benign paroxysmal positional vertigo (BPPV) that lasts seconds to a few minutes often after rolling over in bed. Aural fullness is variable, but when present it is often more pronounced during the attack.

CURRENT DIAGNOSIS

- Severe and often disabling vertigo lasting minutes to hours
- Fluctuating and progressive sensorineural hearing loss, often low-frequency
- Tinnitus: often low-pitched with roaring quality
- Aural fullness
- Complete neurologic evaluation
- Complete audiometric evaluation
- Consider further testing (MRI, FTA-ABS, tests for autoimmune disorders)

Abbreviations: FTA-ABS = fluorescent treponemal antibody absorption (test); MRI = magnetic resonance imaging.

CURRENT THERAPY

Medical
- Low sodium diet (<1500 mg/d)
- Smoking cessation
- Caffeine restriction
- Alcohol restriction
- Diuretic (hydrochlorothiazide, 25 mg, plus triamterene, 37.5 mg qd [Dyazide, Maxzide-25], may increase to bid)
- Vestibular suppressants for acute attacks

Surgical
- Hearing preservation:
  - Intratympanic gentamicin
  - Endolymphatic sac decompression/shunt
  - Vestibular nerve section (three approaches)
- Hearing ablative:
  - Labyrinthectomy

The sensorineural hearing loss associated with Ménière's disease is often a low-frequency loss that is fluctuant and progressive. The hearing loss is often worse during the attack; however, some patients are so vertiginous and nauseated during an attack that characteristics of their hearing loss or aural fullness are not appreciated. Tinnitus with Ménière's disease is variable, but many patients describe a low-pitched roaring sound, "like a refrigerator running."

A complete and thorough physical examination should be performed on all patients who present with dizziness or vertigo. The background and expertise of the PCP is different from that of the otologist, and the PCP should evaluate the patient for other causes of dizziness or lightheadedness. The physician should then perform a complete head and neck examination. Otoscopy is usually unremarkable unless the patient has a history of eustachian tube disease. Pneumatic otoscopy should be performed and should not be associated with any vertigo or nystagmus suggestive of a perilymphatic fistula. The cranial nerves and cerebellar function should be assessed. At a minimum, the patient should be evaluated for spontaneous and gaze-evoked nystagmus, and the Dix-Hallpike, Romberg, and Fukuda step tests should be performed. Tuning fork tests should be performed to determine the nature of the hearing loss. Assuming that hearing in the ear not in question is relatively normal, the sound from a tuning fork placed on the center of the head (Weber test) should lateralize to the normal ear. The Rinne test should confirm that hearing by air conduction is louder than bone-conduction hearing.

AUDIOMETRIC AND VESTIBULAR TESTING

Formal pure-tone and speech audiometry should be obtained on all patients with suspected Ménière's disease. Tympanometry and acoustic reflexes should be obtained as well. Patients usually present with a characteristic asymmetric low-frequency sensorineural loss that may recover to some degree between attacks. Patients with long-standing diagnoses of Ménière's disease rarely demonstrate normal and symmetric hearing. They often present with pure-tone thresholds in the 60-dB range, with diminished word recognition scores.

Vestibular testing is often performed on patients with Ménière's disease. Patients may have relatively normal responses to caloric irrigations in the affected ear; however with long-standing Ménière's disease, caloric responses are usually reduced. The patient should not have spontaneous, positional, or gaze-evoked nystagmus, and ocular motor testing should be unremarkable. Electrocochleography is rarely performed for patients with suspected Ménière's disease anymore.

LABORATORY AND RADIOLOGI TESTING

Some otologists believe that Ménière's disease is a clinical diagnosis and when they are confident in the diagnosis, they perform few other tests. With concerns about the exponential increase in the cost of health care, we as health care providers must have accurate data to justify this approach. Other clinicians feel that a battery of tests is warranted for patients who present with the clinical and audiologic manifestations of Ménière's disease, including a magnetic resonance imaging (MRI) scan to search for an acoustic neuroma or other retrocochlear pathology, fluorescent treponemal antibody absorption (FTA-ABS) test for syphilis, and the anti68-kD protein test for autoimmune inner ear disease. The clinician may take a prudent approach when ordering tests for patients with classic symptoms and signs of Ménière's disease and consider ordering more tests when the diagnosis is less clear.

Treatment

The therapeutic goal of treating patients with Ménière's disease is to prevent or minimize the disabling spells of vertigo. The mainstay of modern treatment for patients is management of dietary sodium intake and the use of a diuretic. Patients should be instructed to minimize the sodium in their diet. Patients should typically restrict their sodium intake to 1500 mg per day. Many patients consume 5 to 10 g of sodium per day, and a reduction to 1.5 g per day requires a major change in lifestyle. Patients are also asked to decrease their caffeine and alcohol input, and if they smoke, they are told to stop and given information on different options available for smoking cessation. If the patient is not allergic, and there are no medical contraindications, the diuretic of choice is a combination of 25 mg hydrochlorothiazide and 37.5 mg of triamterene (Dyazide, Maxzide-25). Although triamterene is a potassium-sparing diuretic, patients are still encouraged to eat foods containing potassium (bananas, oranges, potatoes) and watch for signs of hypokalemia.

Low-salt diet and diuretic therapy successfully control the spells of vertigo in the majority of patients with Ménière's disease. Before considering another treatment option when low-salt diet and diuretic therapy are not effective, patients should be counseled on maintaining an even more restrictive diet (1000 mg of sodium per day) and if not medically contraindicated, the diuretic can be increased from once to twice daily. For patients who continue to have spells of vertigo despite aggressive medical therapy, other treatment options should be discussed.

MENIETT

A mechanical device that delivers low-pressure bursts of air to the external auditory canal is now available and shows some promising early results. Patients who consider the Meniett (Xomed) device first undergo a myringotomy and placement of a tympanostomy tube. In an adult, this can often be performed under local anesthesia in the clinic. The Meniett is an expensive device, and many insurance providers do not cover it. However, Medicare currently reimburses for the device.

OTOTOXIC ANTIBIOTICS

Injecting gentamicin into the middle ear to create a partial chemical labyrinthectomy has become popular in recent years, and it is performed by many general otolaryngologists as well as otologists. The procedure is performed in the office under topical anesthesia. Most otologists use a low-dose titration method in hopes of damaging the vestibular system while causing as little hearing loss as possible. Patients often have vague dizziness or balance problems several days after the procedure, and they normally compensate for this partial chemical labyrinthectomy. Gentamicin is helpful in reducing or halting the disabling spells of vertigo in the majority of patients who undergo the procedure. The risk of profound hearing loss after a single gentamicin injection is low, but it can occur.

SURGERY

Three procedures are used for patients with Ménière's disease: endolymphatic sac decompression/shunting, vestibular nerve section, and labyrinthectomy. The procedure is chosen based on the patient's age, overall health, and hearing status. If the patient has good hearing, then an endolymphatic sac decompression/shunt is recommended as the primary surgical procedure. In this outpatient surgery, a mastoidectomy is completed, and the endolymphatic sac is identified. The bone covering the sac is removed to decompress the sac. The sac is opened, and a silastic stent is placed in the sac. The risks of major complications such as facial paralysis or hearing loss are minimized with this procedure. Approximately 65% to 75% of patients undergoing an endolymphatic sac procedure receive substantial benefit.

If the patient continues to have spells of vertigo, the endolymphatic sac decompression can be repeated, or if the hearing is still good, the patient may opt for a vestibular nerve section. The vestibular nerve may be sectioned by one of three approaches (middle fossa, retrosigmoid, or retrolabyrinthine) depending on the surgeon's training and expertise and the age and health status of the patient. These procedures are more involved and in general require an overnight stay in the intensive care unit. There is a slight risk of hearing loss with these procedures from disruption of the blood supply to the cochlea or from damage to the cochlear nerve. More than 90% of patients who undergo vestibular nerve section receive substantial benefit.

If a patient has poor hearing, then a labyrinthectomy is the procedure of choice. A labyrinthectomy is performed via a mastoidectomy. The three semicircular canals are removed and the vestibule is opened to remove the neuroepithelium of the utricle and saccule. Operative risks such as damage to the facial nerve and a CSF leak are low with this procedure. A somewhat less-complete labyrinthectomy can be performed through the external auditory canal. This procedure is typically reserved for an elderly patient. It can be performed while the patient is awake. After a labyrinthectomy, the patient loses all hearing in that ear. Patients undergoing a labyrinthectomy are often acutely vertiginous and many require overnight observation. Control of vertigo after a labyrinthectomy is excellent. Approximately 95% of patients are free from spells of vertigo following this procedure, and the vast majority of patients, even the elderly, recover from this total unilateral vestibular loss quite well.

In summary, Ménière's disease is often misdiagnosed, and despite a great deal of research, it remains poorly understood. Patients must receive proper treatment and be educated about simple methods that can be used to prevent their symptoms. When sodium restriction and diuretics do not control the severe disabling spells of vertigo, patients should be offered one of the treatment options described here.

REFERENCES

Gates GA, Green D: Intermittent pressure therapy of intractable Ménière's disease using the Meniett device: A preliminary report. Laryngoscope 2002;112:1489-1493.

Graham MD, Kemink JL: Transmastoid labyrinthectomy: Surgical management of vertigo in the nonserviceable hearing ear. A five-year experience. Am J Otol 1984;5:295-299.

Harner SG, Driscoll CL, Facer GW, et al: Long-term follow-up of transtympanic gentamicin for Ménière's syndrome. Otol Neurotol 2001;22:210-214.

Lustig LR, Yeagle J, Niparko JK, Minor LB: Cochlear implantation in patients with bilateral Ménière's syndrome. Otol Neurotol 2003;24:397-403.

Schessel DA, Minor LB, Nedzelski J: Ménière's disease and other peripheral disorders. In Cummings CW (ed): Cummings Otolaryngology Head and Neck Surgery, Philadelphia, Mosby, 2005, pp 3209-3253.

Welling DB, Pasha R, Roth LJ, Barin K: The effect of endolymphatic sac excision in Ménière disease. Am J Otol 1996;17:278-282.

Sinusitis

Method of
Richard R. Orlandi, MD

Classification and Etiologic Factors

Sinus inflammation is reported by more than 30 million adults in the United States and generates nearly 12 million office visits per year and at least $2.4 billion annually in direct medical costs. Loss of productivity likely has an even larger economic impact, with these patients reporting a quality-of-life impairment that is worse than patients with congestive heart failure.

The sinuses are air-filled chambers lined by respiratory epithelium that communicate with the nasal cavity through narrow openings or ostia. Mucus is produced by goblet cells within the respiratory mucosa and is propelled toward the ostia by the surface cilia. This mucociliary clearance is a self-cleaning mechanism for the nose and sinuses. Mucus and trapped particulate matter are transported into the nasopharynx and from there swallowed and eliminated via the gastrointestinal tract. The mucus blanket moves at approximately 8 mm per minute, resulting in a complete turnover every 10 minutes.

The anterior ethmoid and maxillary sinuses drain into a narrow trough within the middle meatus called the ethmoid infundibulum. This narrow system of drainage channels, called the ostiomeatal complex, can become easily blocked if the sinus and nasal mucosa swell because of inflammation, whatever the source. Mucociliary transport is then interrupted, trapping secretions and particulate matter, which can worsen the inflammation. This intensified inflammation can then spread to the frontal sinuses, as well as to the posterior ethmoid and sphenoid sinuses.

Inflammation within the nose has been traditionally referred to as *rhinitis*, whereas that in the paranasal sinuses has been called *sinusitis*. As understanding of the physiology and pathophysiology of the nose and sinuses has improved, it has become clear that the two conditions are interrelated and the term *rhinosinusitis* has been proposed. This disease has been categorized into a number of entities, including acute rhinosinusitis, where signs and symptoms last less than 4 weeks and chronic rhinosinusitis, where they are present for more than 12 weeks. Recurring acute rhinosinusitis, acute exacerbation of chronic rhinosinusitis, and subacute rhinosinusitis are also recognized subcategories.

Rhinosinusitis is an inflammatory condition with multiple etiologic factors. Anatomic variations, allergy, viruses, reflux, chronic bone inflammation (osteitis), fungi, and bacterial superantigens have all been postulated to play a role. Some of these factors, such as allergy or reflux, may create a background inflammation that makes patients more prone to an acute bacterial infection when another etiologic factor is introduced, such as a viral upper respiratory infection (URI). Other factors, such as biofilms, osteitis, fungi, or bacterial superantigens, may perpetuate inflammation in a positive feedback loop and lead to chronic sinus and nasal inflammation. Rarer underlying conditions, such as immunodeficiency, granulomatous diseases, cystic fibrosis, and immotile cilia syndromes, also may predispose patients to acute and chronic rhinosinusitis.

Rhinosinusitis may be a final common pathway of inflammation with multiple etiologies, a constellation of signs and symptoms comprising a syndrome rather than a disease. Acute rhinosinusitis is often a bacterial infection that follows the inflammation of a viral upper respiratory illness. Conversely, chronic rhinosinusitis appears to be a primarily inflammatory condition with acute bacterial exacerbations. Long-term treatment should therefore be anti-inflammatory with antibiotics reserved for acute flares.

Diagnosis

Diagnosing rhinosinusitis can be challenging. Headache syndromes, allergic and nonallergic rhinitis, nasal septal deviation, esophageal and laryngopharyngeal reflux, and temporomandibular joint disease all share signs and symptoms with rhinosinusitis. Multiple attempts to define one or two key diagnostic criteria have failed, and it appears that the diagnosis of rhinosinusitis rests, instead, on a constellation of signs or symptoms. Some more common ones include facial pain or pressure, a sense of nasal obstruction or congestion, altered sense of smell, discolored nasal discharge, and fever (in acute cases). Minor symptoms include headache, cough, halitosis, fatigue, dental pain, and ear pressure or pain. In children, irritability, fatigue, congestion, and nighttime cough may be the more prominent symptoms.

In differentiating viral upper respiratory infections from acute bacterial rhinosinusitis, the timing and severity of symptoms may be most important. Viral URIs are common in children and adults, and only 1 in 200 such infections progress to acute bacterial rhinosinusitis. When this does occur, symptoms of congestion, facial discomfort, and fever may persist longer than 10 days or worsen within 5 to 7 days of onset. Discolored discharge may be present from the start of the viral URI and does not necessarily correlate with bacterial infection, but rather is a sign of inflammation.

CURRENT DIAGNOSIS

- Acute rhinosinusitis lasts less than 4 weeks whereas chronic rhinosinusitis is primarily an inflammatory condition, lasting more than 12 weeks.
- Rhinosinusitis shares symptoms with headache syndromes, allergic and nonallergic rhinitis, nasal septal deviation, esophageal and laryngopharyngeal reflux, and temporomandibular joint disease, making diagnosis challenging.
- There are not one or two defining diagnostic characteristics for acute or chronic rhinosinusitis. Instead, the diagnosis is often made using the physician's overall impression.
- Discolored nasal discharge does not necessarily indicate a bacterial infection.
- Imaging cannot differentiate between viral and bacterial rhinosinusitis, making it less helpful in acute disease.
- Symptoms of a viral URI typically resolve within 5 to 7 days. Severe or worsening symptoms during this period, or failure of symptoms to resolve within 7 to 10 days, are more likely to represent an acute bacterial rhinosinusitis.

Because the symptoms of rhinosinusitis are nondescript, radiologic imaging may be called upon to make the diagnosis. Plain films of the sinuses have been all but supplanted by computed tomography (CT) because of the much greater information this modality affords. Nevertheless, the CT must be interpreted within the context of the patient's symptoms and prior treatment. Viral upper respiratory conditions generate inflammation within the nasal cavity as well as the sinuses, and CT during a URI will demonstrate changes consistent with "sinusitis." CT does not, therefore, play a prominent role in the diagnosis of acute rhinosinusitis, as it is unable to differentiate viral from bacterial disease. CT is more effective in diagnosing patients with chronic symptoms of rhinosinusitis, especially when performed after a trial of medical therapy and between acute exacerbations. Under these conditions, CT can determine the degree of inflammation and guide additional therapy. Unusual findings on CT mandate further evaluation, including unilateral disease, bone erosion, or sinus expansion. These findings may indicate neoplasia or an impending orbital or intracranial complication. In these cases, magnetic resonance imaging (MRI) may be helpful, but this modality is rarely indicated in uncomplicated rhinosinusitis because of its increased expense and lack of specificity.

Treatment Strategies

Whether the inflammation is acute or chronic, treatment is directed at diminishing the inflammation and re-establishing ostial patency and mucociliary clearance. Antibiotics form the mainstay for treatment of acute bacterial rhinosinusitis. Community-acquired acute bacterial rhinosinusitis is commonly caused by *Streptococcus pneumoniae* or *Haemophilus influenzae* in adults, with the addition of *Moraxella catarrhalis* in children. In acute exacerbations of chronic rhinosinusitis, *Staphylococcus aureus* and other staphylococcal species, as well as gram-negative enteric organisms, play a larger role.

Nearly 70% of patients with acute bacterial rhinosinusitis will improve without antibiotics, but that number goes up to 85% with appropriate antibiotics. The incidence of severe complications from acute rhinosinusitis is low and is not influenced by antibiotic use. Consequently, antibiotics should be prescribed for moderate to severe cases of acute bacterial rhinosinusitis or in immunocompromised individuals who may be more at risk for complications. Uncertain or mild cases of acute bacterial rhinosinusitis may be observed for spontaneous resolution, especially early in the course of disease.

Once the decision is made to prescribe antibiotics, the next complexity is which one to choose. Numerous studies and reviews still support the use of amoxicillin, either in standard or high doses (depending on local resistance patterns). Addition of clavulanate appears to improve the symptom resolution rate but is associated with increased gastrointestinal side effects. Second-line treatment for amoxicillin failures or allergic patients includes respiratory quinolone or macrolide antibiotics.

Adjunctive treatments to reduce inflammation and symptoms include mucolytics/expectorants, nasal saline spray, anticholinergics, and decongestants (both topical and systemic). Topical decongestant therapy should not be continued for more than 5 days because of its propensity to cause a rebound rhinitis medicamentosa. Antihistamines are also indicated in patients with an underlying allergic component. Despite their anti-inflammatory effect, nasal steroid sprays have not been shown to have a clear impact on acute disease.

Because chronic rhinosinusitis is primarily an inflammatory condition with periodic acute bacterial exacerbations, antibiotics play a much smaller role. Nasal corticosteroids instead form the mainstay of treatment for chronic rhinosinusitis. Treatment of underlying allergy, when present, typically also improves the patient's overall sinus and nasal inflammation. Leukotriene inhibitors, effective in treating asthma and allergic rhinitis, may play a role in patients with chronic rhinosinusitis, especially those with nasal polyps. Patients who are not sufficiently responsive to medical therapy often benefit from surgical intervention to widen the sinus drainage pathways, followed by continued medical management.

CURRENT THERAPY

- Treatment of rhinosinusitis is aimed toward decreasing mucosal inflammation and re-establishing patency and mucociliary clearance within the nose and sinuses.
- Acute rhinosinusitis is primarily an infectious condition. Approximately 70% of cases will resolve spontaneously. Antibiotics may be withheld for patients who have mild symptoms or a questionable diagnosis.
- Amoxicillin is the preferred first-line treatment for acute bacterial rhinosinusitis in an immunocompetent patient, with or without clavulanate. Respiratory quinolones or macrolides may be used for first-line treatment failures or for those that are allergic or more likely to suffer complications.
- Adjunctive treatments to reduce inflammation and symptoms in acute disease include mucolytics, nasal saline spray, anticholinergics, and decongestants.
- Chronic rhinosinusitis is primarily an inflammatory disease with secondary acute bacterial exacerbations. Consequently, therapy is principally anti-inflammatory with antibiotics reserved for periodic symptomatic flares.
- Nasal corticosteroids form the mainstay of treatment for chronic rhinosinusitis. Leukotriene inhibitors may play a role, especially in patients with associated asthma, allergic rhinitis, or nasal polyps.

Complications of Sinusitis

Complications of sinus disease are rare but potentially serious. The sinuses are separated from the orbit and intracranial cavity by thin bone perforated by venous and lymphatic channels, which can act as conduits for the spread of infection. Intracranial abscess, cerebritis, venous sinus thrombosis, or meningitis may complicate acute sinusitis, typically involving the frontal or sphenoid sinuses. Orbital cellulitis or abscess typically results from ethmoid or maxillary sinusitis and is more common in children. High fever, severe or worsening headache, meningeal signs, altered mental status, infraorbital hypesthesia, significant facial swelling, diplopia, ptosis, chemosis, proptosis, or pupillary or extraocular movement abnormalities should prompt a thorough evaluation, including dedicated imaging and more intensive therapy and observation.

Immunocompromised patients are at special risk for invasive fungal rhinosinusitis, a rare but lethal condition, where weakened host defenses allow tissue invasion and rapid spread of fungus. This disease has a predilection for neutropenic patients, poorly controlled diabetics (particularly during ketoacidosis), and patients undergoing hemodialysis. Early signs may be as subtle as a low-grade fever of unknown origin and can rapidly progress to orbital or cerebral symptoms as a result of extension of the disease to these areas. Therapy is directed toward swift reversal of the underlying immunocompromise, systemic antifungal therapy, and debridement of affected necrotic tissues, which can be disfiguring. Outcomes for this rare condition correlate with the ability to reverse the underlying immunocompromise.

Summary

Rhinosinusitis represents inflammation of the nose and paranasal sinuses and has many etiologies. The symptoms of rhinosinusitis overlap with many other conditions, making diagnosis somewhat difficult. Imaging may be helpful but must be interpreted in the context of the patient's symptoms. Acute bacterial rhinosinusitis typically follows a viral URI and is an infectious process while chronic rhinosinusitis is primarily an inflammatory process with infrequent bacterial exacerbations. Treatment is therefore primarily anti-infectious in acute disease and anti-inflammatory in chronic disease. As the etiologies and pathophysiology of acute and chronic rhinosinusitis are better defined, improved therapy will likely result.

REFERENCES

Benninger MS, Ferguson BJ, Hadley JA, et al: Adult chronic rhinosinusitis: definitions, diagnosis, epidemiology, and pathophysiology. Otolaryngol Head Neck Surg 2003;129(3 Suppl):S1-S32.

Lau J, Zucker D, Engels EA, et al: Diagnosis and Treatment of Acute Bacterial Rhinosinusitis. Evidence Report/Technology Assessment No. 9 (Contract 290-97-0019 to the New England Medical Center), Rockville, Md, Agency for Health Care Policy and Research, March 1999.

Orlandi RR, Kennedy DW: Surgical management of rhinosinusitis. Am J Med Sci 1998;316:29-38.

Sinus and Allergy Health Partnership: Antimicrobial treatment guidelines for acute bacterial rhinosinusitis. Otolaryngol Head Neck Surgery 2004; 130(1 Suppl):1-45.

Nonallergic Perennial Rhinitis

Method of
*Claus Bachert, MD, PhD, and
Nicholas Van Bruaene, MD*

Rhinitis is a very common disorder of the nose that is often trivialized although it is the cause of widespread morbidity, increased medical treatment costs, reduced work productivity, and lost school days.

Rhinitis strictly means "inflammation of the nasal mucosa," but it can practically be defined as a heterogeneous group of nasal diseases characterized by one or more of sneezing, nasal itching, rhinorrhea, and nasal congestion.

Rhinitis can be roughly divided into infectious, viral (common cold) or bacterial rhinitis, and noninfectious rhinitis. Recently, noninfectious rhinitis has generally been classified as either allergic or nonallergic, depending predominantly on whether or not an allergic etiology can be proven. However, mixed forms can occur.

Allergic rhinitis is the most common type of chronic rhinitis. Underlying pathomechanisms in allergic rhinitis have been comparably well understood, whereas for nonallergic rhinitis, such knowledge is scarce, and there are no specific diagnostic tests available. The term *nonallergic (noninfectious) rhinitis* is commonly applied to any nasal condition in which the symptoms are identical to those seen in allergic rhinitis but for which an allergic etiology has been excluded. Therefore, diagnosis of nonallergic perennial rhinitis is made on exclusion of an identifiable allergy (negative skin prick tests for allergy and a lack of symptoms following allergen exposure), structural abnormality (nasal endoscopy), sinus disease (sinus computed tomography [CT] scan), or other causes as discussed later.

Nonallergic rhinitis can broadly be classified as nonallergic occupational rhinitis, hormonal rhinitis, drug-induced rhinitis, other forms, and idiopathic rhinitis. The "other forms" include nonallergic rhinitis with eosinophilia syndrome (NARES), rhinitis due to physical and chemical factors, food-induced (nonallergic) rhinitis, emotion-induced rhinitis, and atrophic rhinitis. Idiopathic rhinitis is also referred to as vasomotor rhinitis or nonallergic, noninfectious perennial rhinitis (NANIPER).

Although it is difficult to readily diagnose nonallergic rhinitis, it has been suggested that in patients with perennial nonallergic rhinitis this condition persists for more than 3 months per year and produces two or more symptoms, including hypersecretion, blockage, sneezing, and postnasal drip.

Some studies are available on the prevalence of nonallergic rhinitis; however, these data show large variations ranging from around 20% to 50%. This is probably due to difficulties in definition and lack of specific diagnostic tests for nonallergic rhinitis.

Pathophysiology

Nasal hyperreactivity to various stimuli (e.g., odors, position, temperature, histamine) is a common feature of nonallergic rhinitis, allergic rhinitis, and postinfectious rhinitis and thus does not allow differentiation between allergic and nonallergic causes. Unlike for patients from defined subgroups of nonallergic rhinitis (particularly drug-induced, hormone-induced, and NARES) and patients with allergic rhinitis, the etiology and pathophysiology of nonallergic noninfectious rhinitis remain unknown.

The term *vasomotor rhinitis* has often been used as an equivalent to *rhinitis without clinical evidence for allergy or infection*. However, because allergic rhinitis also is characterized by a vasomotor dysfunction, it has been suggested that *idiopathic rhinitis* is probably a better term than vasomotor rhinitis.

Types of Nonallergic Rhinitis

NONALLERGIC OCCUPATIONAL RHINITIS

Occupational rhinitis (Box 1) arises in response to an airborne agent present in the workplace. These agents elicit predominantly sneezing, nasal discharge, and blockage and can act via both immunologic (IgE-mediated) and nonimmunologic mechanisms. The nonimmunologic triggers are often irritant or toxic low-molecular-weight compounds such as aldehydes, isocyanates, aircraft fuel and jet stream exhaust, solvents, ninhydrin, pharmaceutical compounds, or chlorine. They can also be physical, such as long-term exposure to cold or dry air.

HORMONAL RHINITIS

Hormonal rhinitis is known to occur during pregnancy in particular but also during the menstrual cycle, puberty, and in specific endocrine disorders such as acromegaly. Hormonal rhinitis can develop during pregnancy in otherwise healthy women. Neither asthma nor rhinitis is a risk factor for pregnancy rhinitis. Only 2% of patients with nonallergic rhinitis are afflicted with rhinitis due to hypothyroidism or acromegaly. Compared with pregnancy rhinitis, the evidence linking hypothyroidism with nasal pathology is sparse, and the reported increase in nasal secretion associated with thyroid disease is anecdotal.

BOX 1 Agents Causing Nonallergic Occupational Rhinitis

Toxic Low-Molecular-Weight Compounds
- Aircraft fuel and jet stream exhaust
- Aldehydes
- Isocyanates
- Nonallergenic microbial agents: endotoxin and β-1,3-glycan (compost workers)
- Solvents
- Vanadium pentoxide (boiler makers)

Physical
- Long-term exposure to cold, dry air or hot air

BOX 2 Medications Causing or Associated with Nonallergic Rhinitis

- Acetylsalicylic acid
- Angiotensin-converting enzyme (ACE) inhibitors
- Antihypertensives
- β-Blockers
- Immunosuppressive drugs: Cyclosporine (Neoral, Sandimmune)
- Methyldopa
- Nasal topical decongestants: Oxymetazoline (Afrin), naphazoline (Privine), xylometazoline (Otrivin)
- Nonsteroidal anti-inflammatory drugs (NSAIDs)
- Oral contraceptives
- Psychotropic agents: Chlorpromazine, thioridazine, chlordiazepoxide (Librium), amitriptyline (Elavil), perphenazine, alprazolam (Xanax)

DRUG-INDUCED RHINITIS

Several commonly employed medications can induce symptoms of rhinitis when they are administered either topically or systemically (Box 2). The symptoms may be either predictable, as would be the case for known side effects of particular drugs, or unpredictable, based on individual hypersensitivity to certain drugs, in particular aspirin, which commonly exacerbates rhinitis and asthma. However, intolerance to aspirin or nonsteroidal anti-inflammatory drugs (NSAIDs) predominantly produces rhinorrhea, which may be either isolated or part of a disease complex involving hyperplastic rhinosinusitis, nasal polyps, and asthma. In contrast, intolerance to angiotensin-converting enzyme (ACE) inhibitors, methyldopa, or oral contraceptives, which is less common than aspirin intolerance, leads to predominantly nasal blockage. Overuse of the topical nasal vasoconstrictors (xylometazoline and other α-adrenoceptor agonists) leads to nasal congestion by a mechanism involving a rebound effect hours after the last application. It can also lead to nasal hyperreactivity and hypertrophy of the nasal mucosa, a condition known as *rhinitis medicamentosa*.

OTHER FORMS OF RHINITIS

Nonallergic Rhinitis with Eosinophilia Syndrome

NARES was originally characterized on the basis of the presence of greater than 20% eosinophils in nasal smears of symptomatic patients with perennial sneezing attacks, a profuse watery rhinorrhea, nasal pruritus, incomplete nasal obstruction, and occasional loss of smell. In addition to these symptoms, a marked feature of the disease is the lack of evidence of allergy, as indicated by negative skin prick tests or absence of serum IgE antibodies to specific allergens.

Although the specific etiology of NARES is not clear, in view of the features shared by this syndrome and the triad of nasal polyposis, intrinsic asthma, and intolerance to aspirin, and because NARES patients frequently develop nasal polyps and asthma later on in life, it has been suggested that NARES may be an early expression of the triad.

The definition of NARES as a subgroup of nonallergic rhinitis is relevant for therapy because patients seem to respond well to nasal corticosteroids, in contrast to other subgroups of nonallergic rhinitis.

Rhinitis Due to Physical and Chemical Factors

Nasal symptoms similar to those of rhinitis can be induced by physical and chemical factors in persons with sensitized nasal mucous membranes. Cold, dry air has been shown to lead to a condition known as *skier's nose*, in which acetylcholine-induced rhinorrhea features prominently. Smoke, in particular cigarette smoke, is known for its direct irritating effect on the mucosa of both upper and lower airways. Eosinophil influx, increased IgE-positive cells, and increased interleukin-4 (IL-4) is found in nasal mucosa of smoking adults and passive smoking nonallergic children. Air pollutants derived from liquid petroleum fuels have also been shown to directly exacerbate symptoms of rhinitis in nonallergic persons. Although their effects have generally been extensively investigated and well documented in the lower airways of allergic persons, little information is available about the acute or chronic effects of air pollutants on the nasal mucosa.

Food-Induced Rhinitis

Certain foods and alcoholic beverages can induce nonallergic rhinitis; the underlying mechanisms are largely unknown. Hot and spicy foods, in particular, which contain capsaicin, lead to a watery rhinorrhea termed *gustatory rhinitis*, probably as a result of the capsaicin stimulating the sensory nerves to release neuropeptides and tachykinins. In contrast, alcoholic beverages are believed to induce symptoms as a result of vasodilation. Dyes, preservatives, and sulfites appear to play a role in a very few cases. Some foods may contain clinically relevant concentrations of histamine or other biogenic amines.

Emotionally Induced Rhinitis

Although not studied extensively, emotional factors such as stress and sexual arousal have been documented to affect the nose, likely as a result of autonomic stimulation. In patients suffering from postcoital rhinitis, anxiety appears to be a predominant feature, which leads to worsening of the disease.

Atrophic Rhinitis

Primary atrophic rhinitis is a progressive chronic nasal disease characterized by mucosal atrophy with resorption of the underlying bone of the conchae. It occurs predominantly in women. The atrophy leads to formation of thick crusts, which leave a distinct fetid odor in the nose (ozena). The nasal cavities are enlarged, but there is a sensation of nasal congestion. Although the precise etiology of this condition is not clear, it has been suggested that an infection with *Klebsiella ozaenae* and other bacteria might play a role. It is unknown whether primary atrophic rhinitis is purely an infectious entity or a combination of infectious, hereditary, dietary, and vascular disorders of the paranasal sinuses. However, primary atrophic rhinitis is distinct from secondary atrophic rhinitis, which develops directly as a result of granulomatous nasal infections, chronic sinusitis, excessive nasal surgery, trauma, or irradiation.

IDIOPATHIC RHINITIS

Once all previously mentioned causes are excluded, a significant percentage of nonallergic noninfectious rhinitis cases still remains. Syndromes of chronic rhinitis with an unknown etiology are categorized under the term *idiopathic rhinitis*.

Idiopathic rhinitis is a diagnosis of exclusion and is solely based on symptoms of nasal blockage, rhinorrhea, and sneezing, although the prevalence of sneezing, conjunctival symptoms, and pruritus is lower than that in allergic rhinitis. Although the subjects have traditionally been classified as either "runners" (those with predominantly rhinorrhea) or "blockers" (those with predominantly nasal congestion and blockage), many patients suffer from more than one type of these symptoms, therefore making it difficult to subdivide the patients into these groups.

Differential Diagnosis

Allergic rhinitis is the major disease to differentiate from nonallergic rhinitis. It is excluded by appropriate allergy tests. The possibility of a local IgE production within the nasal mucosa may account for some cases in which skin prick tests or IgE antibodies to common allergens are not yet indicative. Several other conditions are known to mimic

---

BOX 3 Differential Diagnosis

- Allergic rhinitis
- Benign and malignant tumors
- Cerebrospinal fluid leakage
- Ciliary defects
- Congenital and acquired abnormalities
  - Adenoid hypertrophy
  - Choanal atresia
  - Nasal septum deviation
  - Nasal turbinate hypertrophy
- Granulomas
- Nasal polyposis
- Sinusitis

---

symptoms of nonallergic noninfectious rhinitis and therefore have to be excluded by careful examination (Box 3).

Anatomic nasal abnormalities not only can cause obstruction but also can block the flow of nasal secretions and lead to rhinorrhea, postnasal drip, and nasal blockage. In children, unilateral congenital choanal atresia can lead to unilaterally reduced nasal airflow and secretions if not diagnosed early in life. Tumors are not very common in the nasal passages, but when established, they can grow rapidly and lead to unilateral nasal obstruction, bleeding, and pain in adults. Rhinorrhea and nasal congestion, in the absence of pruritus, are also characteristic features of nasal mastocytosis, an extremely rare condition in which eosinophils are absent and tests for IgE-mediated disease are negative.

In daily clinical practice, the diagnosis of nonallergic rhinitis and its subgroups is mainly based on a thorough case history. If the case history suggests clinically relevant noninfectious rhinitis, other possible diagnoses are excluded in a stepwise fashion:

1. Check possible stimuli, severity, and duration of disease
2. Check drug use (systemic and topical), exposure at the workplace, hormonal status (pregnancy, hypothyroidism, acromegaly), involvement of other organs (asthma, hormonal status)
3. Exclude other nasal disease (nasal rigid endoscopy)
4. Exclude allergy: skin prick test, serum IgE antibodies to the most common inhalant allergens, eventually nasal provocation testing
5. Exclude chronic rhinosinusitis (CT scan)
6. Perform nasal cytology (eosinophilia) and, if shown to be positive, consider performing an oral aspirin challenge

Management

First, an evaluation of the severity of the disease should be performed to confirm the need for therapy, in connection with counseling on how to avoid nonspecific stimuli. In case of drug-induced, food-induced, or occupational rhinitis, specific avoidance measures are employed as first-line therapy.

CURRENT DIAGNOSIS

- About one half of rhinitis patients suffer from nonallergic rhinitis or mixed forms.
- There are no clinically useful diagnostic tests for nonallergic rhinitis; it remains an exclusion diagnosis.
- A thorough case history is the best diagnostic tool available and should include drug intake, work exposure, and hormonal as well as emotional status to subdivide the symptoms into subgroups.

CURRENT THERAPY

- Whenever possible, the treatment should take into account the subgroups of nonallergic perennial rhinitis and lead to avoidance measures.
- In idiopathic rhinitis, although not efficacious in many cases, topical antihistamines and steroids are the two main classes of drugs for treatment. Topical steroids are to be preferred if an inflammatory pathogenesis is suggested.
- Intranasal capsaicin is still considered experimental.
- Surgery is an option in patients with persistent nasal obstruction and secretion not affected by medication.

BOX 4 Treatments for Nonallergic Rhinitis

Medications Used to Treat Nonallergic Rhinitis
- Azelastine (Astelin, Allergodil): 2 sprays each nostril qd-bid
- Fluticasone (Flonase, Flixonase AQ): 2 sprays each nostril qd or 1 spray each nostril bid
- Budesonide (Rhinocort AQ): 1 spray each nostril bid to 4 sprays each nostril qd
- Beclomethasone (Beconase AQ, Vancenase AQ): 1-2 sprays each nostril bid

Symptom-Specific Treatment
Nasal Secretion
- Ipratropium bromide (Atrovent 0.03%): 2 sprays each nostril bid-qid

Nasal Congestion
- Xylometazoline, oxymetazoline (Otrivine, Afrin, Nasivine): Dose varies; apply no longer than 1 wk

Experimental and Nonconventional Therapies
- Botulinum toxin (Botox)[1]
- Intranasal capsaicin[1]
- Silver nitrate[1]

Inferior Turbinate Surgery

[1] Not FDA approved for this indication.

CONVENTIONAL THERAPY

Several treatments (pharmaceutical, nonconventional, and surgical) have been employed for idiopathic nonallergic rhinitis (Box 4). In patients with nasal secretion as the predominant symptom, treatment with intranasal anticholinergics (ipratropium bromide [Atrovent]) has been shown to significantly reduce rhinorrhea, but it has little effect on the other rhinitis symptoms. A topical sympathomimetic provides instant relief of obstruction symptoms. However, it should be avoided or limited to 10 days in view of the risk of developing rhinitis medicamentosa. Systemic sympathomimetics, although commonly used in some countries, seem to have significant side effects when used long term.

In contrast to symptom-specific treatment, it is believed that topical steroids and antihistamines are the most appropriate first treatment options because the symptoms of nonallergic rhinitis are often variable and alternate from obstruction and congestion to secretion and rhinorrhea. Of these, fluticasone propionate (Flonase), budesonide (Rhinocort), beclomethasone (Beconase), and azelastine (Astelin) have been approved by the FDA for this indication.

Azelastine nasal spray has been found to be more effective than placebo for the control of rhinorrhea, postnasal drip, sneezing, and nasal congestion in most patients, although its effect on nasal congestion was marginal. Azelastine has a more rapid onset of action as compared with most other antihistamines and intranasal corticosteroids, and thus azelastine spray should be considered as primary therapy for patients who have symptoms of both allergic and nonallergic rhinitis.

Although the efficacy of intranasal steroids in patients with vasomotor rhinitis has been inconsistent, treatment with topical steroids has been mostly useful for treatment of more severe symptoms in patients in whom an inflammatory pathogenesis is a prominent feature of the disease, for example NARES.

NONCONVENTIONAL THERAPY

Recent evidence suggests that in patients who do not respond to treatment with nasal steroids or antihistamines, treatment with nonconventional therapies such as silver nitrate,[1] botulinum toxin (Botox),[1] and intranasal capsaicin[2] may be beneficial, because these treatments lead to significant reduction in nasal hyperreactivity, nasal airway resistance, and nasal symptom scores. Studies in patients suffering from NANIPER have demonstrated that intranasal capsaicin leads to a significant and long-term reduction in clinical visual analog scale scores compared with placebo. Treatment once daily for 5 weeks with intranasal capsaicin was also shown to significantly improve all symptoms and produce a larger vascular response throughout a 6-month follow-up period in patients suffering from severe chronic nonallergic rhinitis with nasal vasoconstrictor abuse. Recently, a double-blind randomized application regimen study showed that five treatments of capsaicin on a single day are at least as effective as five treatments of capsaicin in 2 weeks. However, there is no registered drug available for treatment containing capsaicin in whatever form.

SURGICAL THERAPY

In cases where nasal obstruction and secretion are resistant to medical treatment and the inferior turbinate is hyperplastic, surgical intervention to reduce the size of the turbinate by various procedures has been shown to be useful. Ethmoidal and vidian neurectomies have also been performed by excision, diathermy, and cryotherapy and have produced results with varying degrees and duration of success.

REFERENCES

Bousquet J, van Cauwenberge P, Khaltaev N, the ARIA Workshop Group: Allergic rhinitis and its impact on asthma—ARIA Workshop Report. J Allergy Clin Immunol 2001;108(5 suppl):S147-S333.

Dykewicz MS, Fineman S, Skoner DP, et al: Diagnosis and management of rhinitis: Complete guidelines of the Joint Task Force on Practice Parameter in Allergy, Asthma and Immunology. American Academy of Allergy, Asthma, and Immunology. Ann Allergy Asthma Immunol 1998;81(5 pt 2):478-518.

Fokkens WJ: Thoughts on the pathophysiology of nonallergic rhinitis. Curr Allergy Asthma Rep 2002;2:203-209.

Sanico A, Togias A: Noninfectious, nonallergic rhinitis (NINAR): Considerations on possible mechanisms. Am J Rhinol 1998;12:65-72.

van Cauwenberge PB, Wang D-Y, Ingels KJ, et al: Rhinitis: The spectrum of the disease. In Busse WW, Holgate ST, eds): Asthma and Rhinitis, 2nd ed. Oxford, Blackwell Science, 2000, pp 6-13.

---

[1] Not FDA approved for this indication.
[2] Not available in the United States.

Hoarseness and Laryngitis

Method of
Gayle Woodson, MD

Hoarseness is a broad term for an abnormality of the voice. It can be an alteration of sound or an increase in the amount of effort required to speak. Thus, it is a class of symptoms rather than a specific syndrome or disease. Laryngitis, the most common cause of acute hoarseness, is simply an inflammation of the larynx. Optimal management of acute laryngitis ranges from watchful waiting to pharmacologic therapy, but it always includes some degree of voice rest. If hoarseness becomes chronic, other diagnoses need to be considered.

Voice Production

In managing hoarseness, it is helpful to understand how vocal sound is produced. When the vocal folds are closed lightly, exhaled air causes the vocal folds to vibrate. If the closure is too loose, air escapes and the voice sounds breathy. If closure is too tight, the voice sounds strained. Vocal folds should be supple and without mass lesions. Even moderate swelling can markedly distort the voice. Friction between the two folds during vibration is diminished by the lubrication of mucus. Pitch is controlled by altering the length, tension, and thickness of the vocal folds, much like tuning a guitar string. The resulting sound is then filtered by the upper airway, and shaped into words by the lips, tongue, and palate (Box 1).

Laryngitis

ETIOLOGY

Infection

Acute inflammation of the larynx is most often the result of a respiratory infection. The vocal folds themselves can become swollen or stiff, but the most striking voice change is due to swelling of the posterior larynx, between the vocal folds, caused by the trauma of coughing.

A cough has three phases: deep inspiration, expiration against a tightly closed glottis, and then sudden opening of the glottis, with a sudden out rush of air. Frequent strong coughing causes repeated trauma to the mucosa of the posterior larynx, where closing pressure is maximal. Swelling increases the force required to close the larynx for phonation. This puts greater stress on posterior laryngeal tissue, leading to even more injury, and severity spirals upward. If swelling is sufficient to prevent closure, the voice becomes breathy or is lost completely.

The problem is compounded in the presence of nasal obstruction. Mouth breathing bypasses the normal humidifying influence of the nose, and the laryngeal mucus becomes thicker and sticky.

Vocal Abuse

Shouting or loud talking can cause significant edema or even bleeding into the vocal folds. Speaking in a noisy environment is also hard on the voice, because the speaker unconsciously increases volume. The effects of vocal abuse are often delayed until the morning after the big game or the cocktail party.

Reflux

Going to bed too soon after eating a large meal can result in acute laryngitis the following morning, particularly if the meal included alcoholic beverages. Vomiting can also expose the larynx to acid damage. The posterior larynx is the primary site of injury.

Other Causes

Other causes include allergies, smoke or chemical inhalation, tracheal intubation, and some systemic diseases. Some inhalant medications can cause significant laryngeal inflammation and even candidiasis.

Multifactorial Causes

More often than not, more than one mechanism is involved in laryngitis. For example, both upper respiratory infection and vocal abuse are more likely to cause acute loss of voice in a patient with chronic laryngopharyngeal reflux (LPR, discussed later). Treatment of hoarseness requires identification and treatment of all factors that are involved.

DIAGNOSIS

Duration of hoarseness is important in the diagnosis. If the problem has been present for less than 2 weeks, and onset was during an upper respiratory infection or after loud or abusive voice use, then the diagnosis of acute laryngitis can be presumed. A history of reflux problems in the past suggests that acid reflux may be a cause or contributing factor. Inhalers for pulmonary disease can cause laryngeal inflammation or predispose to laryngeal candidiasis.

Significant pain and dyspnea are red flags that the problem is not simple laryngitis, and requires urgent attention. Laryngitis per se is usually not painful. Significant pain may indicate tonsillitis, hemorrhage into the vocal folds, or the onset of a severe infection, such as epiglottitis or peritonsillar abscess. In adults and older children, laryngitis does not restrict the airway. Therefore, a complaint of dyspnea or stridor should prompt consideration of other diagnoses. Similarly, dysarthria, resonance changes, and associated dysphagia are signs that suggest a neurologic disorder.

Listening to the sound of the patient's voice is the first step in the physical examination. Laryngitis causes a tight, raspy voice or, not infrequently, no voice at all. On the other hand, laryngeal paralysis usually results in a breathy voice and often a weak cough. Nasal congestion can cause a hyponasal voice, with the inability to pronounce the voiced consonants *m* and *n*. Patients often perceive this voice change as hoarseness, but it does not reflect laryngeal inflammation. A "hot potato" voice is characteristic of airway swelling above the larynx, for example epiglottitis, peritonsillar abscess, or a large throat tumor.

 CURRENT DIAGNOSIS

- Acute laryngitis is hoarseness less than 2 weeks in duration. The patient might have reflux or upper respiratory infection, but no other associated symptoms and no history of steroid inhaler therapy. No laboratory investigation is indicated.
- Indications for emergent specialty referral of acute hoarseness include stridor, severe pain, and recent neck trauma.
- Chronic laryngitis requires a laryngeal examination and otolaryngology evaluation.

BOX 1 Requirements For Normal Phonation

Loosely approximated vocal folds
Adequate expiratory airflow and pressure
Supple, homogenous vocal fold mucosa
Appropriate mucus secretion
Control of vocal fold length and tension

Physical examination should include inspection of the nose, mouth, and oropharynx to seek signs of upper respiratory infection, sinusitis, or tonsillitis. The neck should be palpated for lymphadenopathy that could accompany a neck abscess or mononucleosis. Thyromegaly or nodules should be noted. Hypothyroidism occasionally manifests with hoarseness, and goiter and thyroid tumors can sometimes compress the recurrent laryngeal nerve, leading to weakness or paralysis. Examination of the larynx should confirm that the vocal folds move normally and that there are no lesions on the vocal folds. The posterior swelling of the larynx is sometimes quite impressive, preventing the vocal folds from closing completely during phonation. In the absence of the means to examine the larynx, patients who seem to have uncomplicated laryngitis can be managed expectantly, with referral for laryngeal examination if symptoms persist.

Laboratory studies and radiography are not required for the diagnosis of acute laryngitis.

TREATMENT

Treatment of acute laryngitis is symptomatic, supportive, and expectant. Voice use should be reduced in proportion to the severity of the hoarseness. For severe hoarseness, voice use should be drastically reduced. Absolute silence is not practical, but patients should be instructed to avoid talking whenever possible. If the voice is only moderately disturbed and does not decline with conversational use, then restrictions are milder.

Patients should refrain from shouting, talking on the telephone, or speaking over loud noises and should try to stop throat clearing. The urge to clear the throat can be diminished by the use of a mucolytic expectorant, guafenesin. This decreases mucus viscosity, so that it is less likely to cling to the larynx. A cough suppressant, such as dextromethorphan, can also be helpful; however a cough preparation that includes other drugs, such as an antihistamine or scopoloamine, can cause mucus to become thicker and stickier.

Nasal congestion may cause mouth breathing, which can dry out the throat. Topical or systemic decongestants to restore nasal breathing can be very helpful. In addition, systemic decongestants can effect laryngeal swelling, reducing the hoarseness and globus sensation.

If a bacterial infection such as tonsillitis or sinusitis is diagnosed, then appropriate antibiotic therapy should be instituted. Antibiotics are not indicated for laryngitis alone.

Steroids are not routinely recommended for the management of laryngitis, although they can produce prompt and often significant improvement in symptoms. The improvement is only temporary. Further, when the steroids improve symptoms, patients generally use their voices more, so that when the steroids wear off, the voice is worse, and healing is delayed. Steroids may be used with caution for the patient who has an urgent, short-term need to use the voice. This treatment should be for a one-time event, such as an important audition or speech, not a series of events over several days or weeks. Steroids should definitely not be used in an attempt to salvage the voice of a performer on a demanding tour. A laryngeal examination should be performed to confirm that the cause of the hoarseness is laryngeal edema, and to rule out hematoma or mucosal injury. The patient must be carefully counseled to strictly limit voice use while taking steroids. A single dose of 40 to 60 mg of prednisone should be taken by mouth, 1 to 2 hours before the performance, court case, or other major speaking event.

If gastroesophageal reflux is implicated, then acid suppression is indicated. First-line management would include the use of an H_2 blocker. If the patient is already taking such medication, or if first-line therapy fails, a proton pump inhibitor should be prescribed. Although once-a-day acid-suppressive therapy is adequate for gastroesophageal reflux disease, it is usually not sufficient to treat LPR, and so the medication should be taken twice a day, first thing in the morning and about an hour before the evening meal.

WHEN TO REFER ACUTE HOARSENESS

In the vast majority of cases, sudden onset of hoarseness is due to acute laryngitis that will resolve. Hoarseness is sometimes an urgent problem, however. Hoarseness after external neck trauma can represent a laryngeal fracture. This injury is potentially life threatening because sudden airway obstruction can occur, even hours after the injury. Physical signs include subcutaneous crepitus, hemoptysis, loss of the Adam's apple, and stridor. A patient with a suspected laryngeal fracture should be evaluated in an emergency department as soon as possible.

If the onset of hoarseness was during extreme vocal effort, or a strong Valsalva manuever, as in lifting a heavy object, then the problem may be hemorrhage into the vocal fold. Rebleeding could result in airway obstruction or permanent voice impairment. Strict reduction of vocal activity is required and sometimes surgical evacuation of the hematoma is necessary. If laryngeal hemorrhage is suspected, then the patient should be examined by an otolaryngologist as soon as possible.

Endotracheal intubation commonly results in some mild hoarseness, and further evaluation is not necessary for these patients unless hoarseness is severe or if there is significant pain. Urgent attention is required for patients with hoarseness who also have dyspnea or stridor.

Inhalant therapy for pulmonary disease can cause significant laryngeal inflammation and leukoplakia and can predispose to candidal infection. Patients who develop hoarseness while on inhalant therapy should have a laryngeal examination as soon as practical, even if they have been taking the same medication for months or years. In particular, the Advair disk has been frequently associated with severe laryngitis. If examination shows florid erythema and leukoplakia, then the inhalant medication should be stopped or changed and systemic antifungal treatment should be considered. This inflammation usually resolves dramatically within 3 to 4 weeks of discontinuing the inhaler.

Chronic Hoarseness

When hoarseness lasts more than 2 weeks and has not responded to appropriate medical management, the larynx should be evaluated by an otolaryngologist. This is particularly true for two groups of patients. In smokers, laryngeal cancer is a significant concern. In young children, chronic hoarseness may be due to laryngeal papilloma, which could progress to airway obstruction. A very breathy voice can indicate laryngeal paralysis. This requires prompt attention to identify the cause of the paralysis. The etiology of laryngeal paralysis is broad, and lung cancer is one of the leading causes.

PRESBYPHONIA

Chronic hoarseness in an older patient can represent presbyphonia (aging voice). Effects of aging in the voice include stiffness of the vocal folds and muscle atrophy, with weak closure of the larynx and thinning of the vocal folds. The voice becomes soft, weak, and often higher in pitch. Postmenopausal women, particularly smokers, often develop significant vocal fold edema, which results in a low-pitched, husky voice. Voice therapy and surgery can be helpful, but most patients are satisfied to accept the effects of aging if laryngeal examination rules out ominous pathology.

LARYNGOPHARYNGEAL REFLUX

The single most common diagnosis in patients with chronic hoarseness is LPR. It is estimated that up to 15% of all visits to the

CURRENT THERAPY

- Restricted voice use
- Hydration, expectorants
- Cough suppression
- Nasal decongestion
- Steroids only in selected cases

otolaryngology offices are manifestations of LPR. However, the role of acid reflux in laryngitis is controversial. Many clinical studies indicate that medical management of acid can reverse significant laryngeal pathology, but randomized, controlled trials do not consistently demonstrate improvement. The problem is likely due to a lack of a gold standard for the diagnosis of LPR.

It is not at all uncommon to have significant pathology in the larynx without inflammation of the esophagus. Patients seem to vary in the susceptibility of laryngeal and pharyngeal mucosa to acid irritation. Further, acid can pool in the hypopharynx after it has been rapidly cleared from the esophagus. Whatever the reason, esophagitis cannot be used as a marker for LPR. Further, pH criteria for LPR are not well established, and the results from a probe in the distal esophagus may be within normal limits. Pharyngeal acid exposure is the critical event for LPR. One episode of LPR can have sequelae that last for days, and so 24-hour monitoring may miss a significant event.

Characteristic findings on laryngeal examination have been described for LPR, including posterior and subglottic edema and erythema or ulceration. Not every patient with such findings responds to treatment. Thus the clinical diagnosis of LPR is based on laryngeal examination findings plus response to a therapeutic trial of acid suppression. Because prospective studies include LPR diagnosed by symptoms and laryngeal examination alone, the pool necessarily includes both responders and nonresponders. Definitive support for the role of acid suppression in treating chronic laryngitis requires an independent means of confirming the diagnosis of LPR, such as mucosal pepsin assay.

POSTNASAL DRIP

Postnasal drip is a common complaint from patients with chronic laryngitis, but the problem is rarely an overproduction of mucus, and chronic sinusitis is not often found in these patients. A normal person produces about a quart of nasal mucus each day. Normally this mucus is transported into the pharynx by ciliary action and is swallowed. In the presence of pharyngeal or laryngeal inflammation, mucus tends to cling to the larynx, and this can be observed on laryngeal examination. Also, the sensation of the laryngeal swelling is perceived as something in the throat and stimulates efforts to clear the throat. Throat clearing can dislodge some mucus, providing a temporary illusion of benefit. However, throat clearing is even more traumatic to the larynx than a cough.

OTHER CAUSES

Laryngeal edema can become self-perpetuating. It is not uncommon for an upper respiratory infection to result in acute laryngitis that never resolves, because of LPR, throat clearing, and maladaptive vocal habits.

Chronic hoarseness may be due to habitual or psychogenic voice misuse. Patients with habitual dysphonia can usually correct their behavior with voice therapy, but this requires having the patient take ownership of the problem. Those with psychogenic or factitious problems are more resistant to making changes during therapy. Psychiatric consultation is indicated for idiopathic chronic hoarseness that does not respond to voice therapy.

REFERENCES

Close LG, Woodson GE: Common upper airway disorders in the elderly and their management. Geriatrics 1989;44(1):67-68, 71-72.
Ford CN: Evaluation and management of laryngopharyngeal reflux. JAMA 2005;294:1534-1540.
Gallivan GJ, Gallivan KH, Gallivan HK: Inhaled corticosteroids: Hazardous effects on voice—an update. J Voice 2007;21:101-11.
Reveiz I, Cardona AF, Ospina EG: Antibiotics for acute laryngitis in adults. Cochrane Database Syst Rev 2007;(2):CD004783.
Roy N: Functional dysphonia. Curr Opin Otolaryngol Head Neck Surg 2003;11:144-148.

Streptococcal Pharyngitis

Method of
John Brusch, MD

The pharyngitis syndrome (sore throat) is characterized primarily by sore throat with associated fever and myalgias; occasionally with cough. It is responsible for 10% of outpatient visits and an estimated 50% of ambulatory care antibiotic usage. Of adult patients who receive treatment for a sore throat, 73% receive antibiotic treatment when at least 50% of these cases are of viral etiology. The increase in the overall resistance to antibiotics of the oral pharyngeal flora is due, in great part, to this overprescribing of antimicrobial agents. A variety of bacteria and viruses may produce this syndrome. Group A β-hemolytic streptococci (GABHS) is the most common bacterial cause of acute pharyngitis. The diagnosis of "strep throat" has long been a concern of the physician because of its suppurative and non-suppurative complications. There is such a great deal of overlap in their clinical presentations that the clinician must rely on the laboratory to diagnose GABHS from both other bacteria and viruses as the cause of the sore throat of his/her patient. The correct interpretation of the available diagnostic tests adds to the clinician's burden. For more than 50 years, the appropriate choice of antibiotic and duration of treatment of GABHS pharyngitis has been established. The real challenge of treating streptococcal pharyngitis lies not in the selection of treatment, but in deciding when to institute antibiotic therapy.

Microbiology

Most sore throats are viral in origin. GABHS is responsible for 10% of cases of adult pharyngitis. Its importance lies in the fact that its treatment can prevent the development of rheumatic fever and local complications. Gonorrheal pharyngitis primarily arises from oral sex, but may be a complication of disseminated gonorrhea. It is usually asymptomatic but may produce a typical sore throat. *Yersinia* pharyngitis, like that of groups C and G streptococci, is foodborne. In United States, *Corynebacterium diphtheriae* pharyngitis occurs primarily among the homeless often in outbreaks. It may not be associated with any systemic symptoms. *Arcanobacterium haemolyticum* is a true mimic of GABHS pharyngitis. This organism is more common in Scandinavia and in the United Kingdom than in other parts of the world. It produces a scarlatiniform rash involving the trunk and extremities (50% of cases) with a vesicular component. Occasionally a membranous exudate, resembling that of diphtheria, occurs. Anaerobic oral pharyngeal overgrowth can produce a severe sore throat (Plaut-Vincent or fusospirochetal angina). It is caused by an anaerobic, nonsporulating gram-negative rod. Infection with this organism classically results in an ulceration of the throat or tonsils that is covered by a grayish membrane. Widespread necrosis of surrounding tissue and sepsis may ensue. The presence of fusospirochetal angina may be a clue to a severe leukopenic state in the host. Cases of *Chlamydia pneumoniae* and *Mycoplasma pneumoniae* sore throat are usually seen with concurrent lung infection. The clinical courses may be quite prolonged. Unresponsiveness to the penicillins provides a useful clue to their presence. Many species of bacteria are commonly cultured from the upper airway. *Staphylococcus aureus*, *Streptococcus pneumoniae*, and *Haemophilus influenzae* are part of the normal pharyngeal flora, especially during the winter. They seldom cause pharyngitis. Their isolation from symptomatic individuals usually represents colonization.

Epstein-Barr virus (EBV) infections of the throat are marked by an exudate pharyngitis with palatal petechiae and a gelatinous uvula. In patients older than 30 years of age, only 25% of EBV pharyngitis presents with the classic picture of diffuse cervical adenopathy, diffuse adenopathy, lymphocytosis, and splenomegaly.

These patients often develop a diffuse scarlatiniform rash approximately 5 days into a course of ampicillin or other β-lactam antibiotics ("fifth-day rash"). The pharyngitis of *Cytomegalovirus* and herpesvirus type 6 may present in similar fashion to that of EBV without the fifth-day rash. Primary human immunodeficiency virus (HIV) infection may cause a sore throat that is characterized by a nonexudate pharyngitis fever, diffuse lymphadenopathy, and a maculopapular rash within 1 to 5 weeks of acquisition. Acute retroviral infection is truly a "cannot miss" diagnosis.

Epidemiology

GABHS pharyngitis primarily affects individuals 5 to 15 years of age. Up to 20% of these are carriers of GABHS. Infection is most commonly spread from human to human by large airborne droplets. The cold weather of winter and early spring produces the highest attack rates as a consequence of the indoor crowding that occurs during these seasons. Symptomatic patients, closeness of contact, and virulent strains are factors that promote spread of the disease. Transmission by both food and water is well documented.

During the acute phase of the illness, M-type streptococci are frequently isolated from the nares and oropharynx. Colonization of the upper airway with these strains can last for several months. Gradually, the streptococci lose their M proteins and with this loss their infectivity. Antibody to the M protein confers type-specific immunity to the host. The carrier state results from the ability of particular strains to penetrate the interior of respiratory epithelial cells. In this location, GABHS is protected from type-specific M protein antibody, from the suppressive effects of the host's oral flora, and from the actions of many types of antibiotics. In the developed world, both suppurative and nonsuppurative complications of GABHS pharyngitis have greatly lessened. This is a result of an overall improvement in living conditions (less crowding) and to the disappearance of M protein from many isolates of GABHS. This decreased pathogenicity has to be factored into any treatment strategy for "strep throat." However, the inner cities of the United States still provide conditions that are conducive to the development of poststreptococcal rheumatic fever.

Clinical Manifestations

Fever (>100.4°F [38°C]) and sore throat are invariably present in GABHS pharyngitis. The presence of rhinitis, laryngitis, diarrhea, conjunctivitis and bronchitis are inconsistent with this diagnosis and are more characteristic of a viral etiology. Examination reveals pharyngeal erythema or exudative pharyngitis, with or without palatal petechiae, that is associated with significant anterior cervical adenopathy. Untreated, 75% of patients defervesce within 3 days unless there is a local suppurative complication. This may include peritonsillar abscess, suppurative adenitis, and otitis media. Over a few more days, the individual's other signs and symptoms resolve. In the absence of antibiotic therapy, most patients carry streptococci for many months. With appropriate treatment, the carrier state is reduced to between 6% and 29% of patients.

Diagnosis

Although the diagnosis of GABHS pharyngitis cannot be based solely on clinical signs and symptoms, they have been quite useful in establishing the likelihood of streptococcal infection; especially in adults with an extremely low incidence of "strep throat." Determining the probability of GABHS pharyngitis is essential for establishing indications for diagnostic testing, as well as for interpreting the results of these tests. Several such scoring systems stratifying the importance of physical findings and symptoms have been developed. All are quite similar and include the presence of (a) fever higher than 99.9°F (37.7°C), (b) tonsillar exudate, and (c) anterior cervical

CURRENT DIAGNOSIS

Organism	% of Cases	Comments
Viral organisms	Total = 40%	Often associated with coryza, laryngitis, and diarrhea
Rhinovirus	20%	
Coronavirus	5%	
Herpes simplex	2%	
Retroviruses	?%	Present in 70% of cases of primary HIV infection
Primary Epstein-Barr	?%	Only 25% exhibit other manifestations of mononucleosis viral infection
Coxsackievirus	?%	Concurrent findings of herpangina and hand, foot, and mouth disease
Adenovirus	?%	Concurrent conjunctivitis
Bacterial organisms	Total = ?%	
GABHS	30%-50% in children; 10% in adults	1%-5% of adults are carriers of GABHS
Groups C, G streptococci	10%	Often foodborne
Nonstreptococcal bacteria	10%	
Neisseria gonorrhoeae	1%	May be the only manifestation of gonorrhea; associated with oral sex
Yersinia enterocolitica	?%	Often foodborne
Corynebacterium diphtheriae	?%	Seen in the homeless; often pharyngitis is the only manifestation
Arcanobacterium hemolyticum	0.4%	Causes a diffuse scarlatiniform rash; it is indistinguishable from GABHS pharyngitis

Abbreviations: GABHS, group A β-hemolytic streptococci.

adenopathy, and (d) absence of cough. The presence of all four makes the probability of GABHS 56%. When three conditions exist, the likelihood decreases to 32% and plummets to 15% and 6% when there are two and one positive indicators, respectively. If there are no positive indicators, the probability of a positive culture is less than 2.5%. At this level of risk, diagnostic testing is usually not required.

The throat culture remains the diagnostic gold standard. The throat should be swabbed under direct visualization in repeated sweeps extending from each tonsillar fossa and involving the posterior pharynx but avoiding any other area of the mouth. The swabs should be immediately cultured on sheep blood agar incubated in 10% CO_2. If there is no growth at 24 hours, the plate is re-incubated for another 24 hours. Sampling errors may cause false negatives in 9% to 12% of patients. Rarely, GABHS will not produce β hemolysis. False positives may be due to β hemolysis produced by non-GABHS organisms. The use of the bacitracin disk controls for this by inhibiting GABHS but not other types of β hemolytic flora. The specificity of the throat culture ranges from 95% to 99% with 88% to 91% sensitivity. When obtained in physicians' offices, the throat cultures are much less sensitive (<75%). The major disadvantage of the throat culture is the diagnostic delay. In adults, this may not be all that significant (see below).

Rapid antigen detection tests (RADTs) were developed to provide useful probability information at the time of the patient's visit. RADTs employ either enzyme or acid techniques to extract streptococcal antigen from the swabs, which is then measured by latex agglutination, coagglutination, or enzyme-linked immunosorbent assay (ELISA) techniques. Overall, the sensitivity of RADTs ranges from 77% to 95%. The higher range of values is associated with the newer optical immunoassay technique, which may approach the sensitivity of a well-performed throat culture. The specificity of the RADT is as high as that of the throat culture. Because of its low sensitivity, a negative RADT in any child or adolescent should be followed by a throat culture. In adults, this approach is not thought to be necessary because of the low incidence of GABHS pharyngitis and rheumatic fever in this population. However, when only an RADT is performed, the opportunity to detect a treatable non-GABHS cause of bacterial pharyngitis is lost.

Both throat culture and RADT are unable to distinguish streptococcal carriers from those whose symptoms are caused by GABHS and not by another organism. Of symptomatic adult patients with positive diagnostic tests, 30% to 50% are not infected with GABHS. Measurement of antibody titers against streptolysin O (ASL-O) or other streptococcal products is the most specific way to diagnose GABHS pharyngitis. Their levels require 2 to 4 weeks to peak and thus are not available to the clinician in a timely fashion.

TABLE 1 Reasons for Treating Streptococcal Pharyngitis

Item	Rationale
Preventing rheumatic fever	Rheumatic fever occurs in 2.1% of untreated patients and in 0.3% of treated patients
Preventing streptococcal glomerulonephritis	No evidence that treatment of streptococcal pharyngitis is effective
Preventing scarlet fever	Extremely rare in the antibiotic era
Reducing suppurative complications	They accounted for 13% of hospitalizations in the pre-antibiotic era; currently quite unusual
Reducing duration and severity of disease	Antibiotics have some mild effect when started early
Reducing spread of GABHS	Quite effective in preventing spread; patients become noncontagious after 24 hours of treatment

Abbreviation: GABHS, group A β-hemolytic streptococci.

TABLE 2 Management Strategies for GABHS Pharyngitis

Number of Positive Features	Action
1	No culture; no treatment
2	Culture; treat positive cultures
3	No culture or treatment
4	No culture or treatment

Abbreviation: GABHS, group A β-hemolytic streptococci.

Treatment

In the developed world, the reasons why we treat GABHS pharyngitis have markedly changed since the landmark studies that demonstrated such a significant drop in the incidence of poststreptococcal rheumatic fever. This is attributable to the change in epidemiology of the streptococcus (Table 1). In the early days of antimicrobial therapy, it was established that 10 days of treatment with oral penicillin or one intramuscular injection of penicillin G was effective in preventing rheumatic fever if begun within 5 to 9 days after the onset of clinical symptoms of GABHS pharyngitis. It was also demonstrated that for those patients in whom penicillin failed to eradicate GABHS, the risk of developing rheumatic fever was the same as that of an untreated patient. Table 2 presents the clinical indications for obtaining a throat culture/RADT and beginning antibiotic treatment. I prefer a culture over RADT as it is generally more sensitive and detects other possible pathogens. Its 1- to 2-day delay in receiving final results has little clinical significance. It was recently demonstrated that culture is the most effective and least expensive approach when the prevalence of GABHS pharyngitis is 10% or less. Empirical antibiotic treatment was found to be neither the most clinically useful nor cost-effective strategy for any degree of risk. This stepped approach holds true only for adults in the developed world who have no history of rheumatic fever, immunosuppression, or chronic pharyngitis. It is not applicable during an epidemic of GABHS/rheumatic fever. Eradication of the carrier state is not an indication for treatment unless the patient has a

CURRENT THERAPY

- Empirically treat all patients with 3 or more clinical predictors of GABHS pharyngitis.
- Optimal treatment still remains 10 days of oral penicillin or one injection of Bicillin.
- Avoid 3-day treatment regimens.
- Avoid trimethoprim-sulfamethoxazole and the tetracyclines (doxycycline). They have little effect on eradicating GABHS.
- Always keep in mind that culture of GABHS from an adult may represent a carrier state and that the pharyngitis is produced by another organism.
- Do not reculture at the end of clinically successful therapy unless the patient has an above-average risk for developing rheumatic fever.
- Always keep in mind the possibility of primary HIV infection as the cause of the pharyngitis.
- Do not culture family members unless there is an epidemic situation of or recurrence of proven GABHS pharyngitis in the family.

TABLE 3 Current Therapy

Drug	Dose	Duration of Therapy
Penicillin V (Pen-Vee K)	1000 mg bid,[3] 25 mg/kg bid*	10 d
Benzathine penicillin (Bicillin)	1.2 million U, 2500 U/kg*	1 dose
Cephalexin (Keflex)	500 mg bid, 25 mg/kg bid	10 d
Cefadroxil (Duricef)	1 g/d, 30 mg/kg/d*	5 d[†]
Cefuroxime (Ceftin)	250 mg bid, 10 mg/kg bid*	5 d[†]
Amoxicillin-clavulanate (Augmentin)[‡,1]	250 mg tid, 15 mg/kg tid*	10 d
Azithromycin (Zithromax)	500 mg first day, then 250 mg qd; 12 mg/kg qd	5 d[†]
Clarithromycin (Biaxin)	500 mg bid, 8 mg/kg bid*	10 d

*For children who weigh less than 40 kg (88 lb).
[†]Only azithromycin is approved by the Food and Drug Administration for less than 10 days of therapy.
[‡]Useful for recurrent GABHS pharyngitis or treatment of the carrier state if necessary.
[1]Not FDA approved for this indication.
[3]Exceeds dosage recommended by the manufacturer.
Abbreviation: GABHS, group A β-hemolytic streptococci.

TABLE 4 Reasons for Apparent Recurrent GABHS Pharyngitis

Cause	Solution
Not truly a GABHS pharyngitis (most likely to be of viral origin)	Document infection by ulture or RADT (see text)
Poor compliance (most frequent cause of recurrence)	Choose 5-day antibiotic regimen or intramuscular benzathine penicillin
Repeated exposure to GABHS, especially in families (ping-pong phenomenon)	Culture samples from all family members and treat culture-positive individuals
Decreased host immunity to GABHS because of initiation of antibiotic therapy within 48 hours of the onset of symptoms	Delay antibiotic treatment for 48 hours; this does not increase the risk for suppurative or nonsuppurative complications
Coexistence of β lactamase-producing bacteria (becoming a more common problem)	Use a β lactamase-resistant antibiotic (cephalosporin or amoxicillin-clavulanate)
Patient is carrier for GABHS and pharyngitis is caused by another organism, usually a virus	Confirm by positive culture or RADT in asymptomatic period; also obtain ASL-O titer for weeks after infection (should not show rise in the carrier state); generally no need to treat; if necessary to intervene, use a macrolide or amoxicillin-clavulanate
Deep-seated GABHS infection (i.e., tonsillar crypts)	Use intraleukocytic-active antibiotic such as a quinolone or a macrolide
Inadequate dose of penicillin	Increase dose or use better-absorbed form (amoxicillin)

Abbreviations: ASL-O, antistreptolysin O; GABHS, group A β-hemolytic streptococci; RADT, rapid antigen detection test.

---

history of rheumatic fever. It is unnecessary to do sensitivity testing of GABHS for any of the β-lactam antibiotics. GABHS remains quite sensitive to penicillin. The administration of oral penicillin for 10 days achieves almost 100% effectiveness in eradicating GABHS. In those who have been treated for 7 days or 5 days, the cure rate decreases to 89% and 50%, respectively.

In penicillin-allergic patients, erythromycin has traditionally been the alternative drug of choice. In the United States, 4% to 5% of isolates are resistant to erythromycin. Resistance to erythromycin is significantly higher in those countries where it is more commonly used as a first-line drug. The other macrolides hold no therapeutic advantage over erythromycin, but are much better tolerated, especially as regards the gastrointestinal tract. In my opinion, clindamycin (Cleocin) rarely should be used because of the significant risk of developing *Clostridium difficile* colitis. The most desirable treatment regimen remains 10 days of penicillin therapy. If compliance is in doubt, one dose of Bicillin is next best. The other β-lactams offer little advantage except for 5-day courses. There is some indication that they may have a somewhat higher clinical and bacteriologic success rate because of their resistance to breakdown by penicillinase-producing oral pharyngeal flora. They have as yet not stood the test of time. Three-day regimens should be avoided because of unacceptably high rates of failure and recurrence. More complete discussions of antibiotic therapy of GABHS pharyngitis are available in the referenced sources (Table 3).

Recurrence of GABHS has increased in the last 20 years from 9% of cases to greater than 30% currently. This has been paralleled by a slight decline in the bacteriologic and clinical success rates, currently 84% and 89%, respectively. Table 4 presents several possible reasons for these trends.

After a successful clinical result, there is no need to repeat the throat culture unless during an outbreak of rheumatic fever or in an individual who has already been stricken by the disease. In the antibiotic era, tonsillectomy for preventing relapse or recurrence is rarely necessary.

REFERENCES

Bisno AL: Acute pharyngitis, N Engl J Med 2001;344:205.
Bisno JL, Gerber MA, Gwaltney JM, et al: IDSA practice guidelines for the diagnosis and management of group A streptococcal pharyngitis. Clin Infect Dis 2002;35:113.
Gerber MA, Shulman ST: Rapid diagnosis of pharyngitis caused by group A streptococci. Clin Microbiol Rev 2004;17:571.
Komaroff AL: Pharyngitis coryza and related infections in adults. In Branch WT Jr, (ed): Office Practice of Medicine, Philadelphia, WB Saunders, 2003, p 153.
Stollerman GH: Global changes in group A streptococcal diseases and strategies for their prevention. Adv Intern Med 1982;27:373.

SECTION 4

The Respiratory System

Acute Respiratory Failure

Method of
Scott K. Epstein, MD

The respiratory system serves many complex physiologic functions, the most important of which is gas exchange. Using the interface between the alveolar space and capillaries, O_2 is taken up and CO_2 is eliminated. Acute respiratory failure, a life-threatening entity, is present when this system fails, over the course of minutes to hours, resulting in hypoxemia (type I) or hypercapnia (type II), or both. Most patients with acute respiratory failure present with dyspnea, although the correlation with disease severity is poor. Indeed, dyspnea might seem mild in those with baseline chronic respiratory failure, and it might be absent in those with an underlying neurologic process (e.g., drug overdose). Other symptoms and signs such as cough, chest pain, orthopnea, fever, tachypnea, rales, and wheezing are insensitive and nonspecific.

This chapter outlines the general pathophysiology and therapeutic approach to acute respiratory failure by using the examples of three common entities: acute lung injury (ALI), cardiogenic pulmonary edema (congestive heart failure [CHF]), and acute exacerbation of chronic obstructive pulmonary disease (COPD).

Definitions and Pathophysiology

ACUTE HYPOXIC RESPIRATORY FAILURE

Hypoxic respiratory failure is conventionally defined as an arterial oxygen tension (Pa_{O_2}) of less than 60 mm Hg. Because this definition ignores the inspired fraction of oxygen (Fi_{O_2}), some favor a Pa_{O_2}/Fi_{O_2} ratio of less than 300. To account for the arterial CO_2 tension (Pa_{CO_2}), others favor an alveolar–arterial (A–a) O_2 gradient greater than 250 mm Hg, using the equation

$$A - a\ O_2\ \text{gradient} = PA_{O_2} - Pa_{O_2}$$
$$= (713 \times Fi_{O_2}) - (PA_{O_2} + Pa_{CO_2}/0.8)$$

where 713 is the barometric pressure (760) minus the water vapor pressure. A normal A–a O_2 is less than 10 mm Hg, but this threshold value increases with age. The determination of Pa_{O_2} requires an invasive test, an arterial blood gas. Oxygenation can be continuously monitored noninvasively by pulse oximetry, which provides an estimate of arterial oxygen saturation (Sa_{O_2}). In general, an Sa_{O_2} of 0.90 corresponds to a Pa_{O_2} of 60 mm Hg, but the relation depends on temperature, pH, Pa_{CO_2}, and 2,3-diphosphoglycerate (2,3-DPG).

Accuracy is adversely affected by low perfusion states, dark skin pigmentation, nail polish, dyshemoglobins (e.g., carboxyhemoglobin, methemoglobin), intravascular dyes, motion, and ambient light.

Clinicians tend to focus on Pa_{O_2} and Sa_{O_2}, but the real parameter of interest is O_2 delivery (Do_2) to organs and tissues. Do_2 depends on cardiac output and O_2 carrying capacity of arterialized blood (Ca_{O_2}):

$$Do_2 = CO \times Ca_{O_2}$$

where

$$Ca_{O_2} = k\,(Hb \times Sa_{O_2}) + 0.003\,Pa_{O_2}$$

where k is a constant. Do_2 decreases when cardiac output or hemoglobin is reduced despite a normal Pa_{O_2} and Sa_{O_2}. The peripheral response to reduced Do_2 is an increased O_2 extraction ratio (O_2ER), allowing oxygen uptake ($\dot{V}o_2$), an indicator of metabolic demand, to remain constant. Cellular and organ dysfunction occurs when Do_2 and O_2ER are outstripped by metabolic demand. The balance between Do_2 and demand can be estimated by examining the mixed venous O_2 saturation (Mv_{O_2}) using the rearranged Fick equation:

$$Mv_{O_2} = Sa_{O_2} - (\dot{V}o_2/CO \times Hb)$$

When Mv_{O_2} falls below 65% to 75%, imbalance is present.

When cellular injury is present, extraction capabilities are limited and cellular hypoxia occurs despite "adequate" Do_2. Under these circumstances, the Mv_{O_2} can be paradoxically normal. These parameters can be determined using a pulmonary artery catheter. The data obtained may be useful in individual patients, but randomized, controlled trials show no benefit when the pulmonary artery catheter is used routinely to guide therapy.

The pathophysiologic mechanisms of type I respiratory failure are listed in Table 1. The most common mechanism is ventilation–perfusion ($\dot{V}/\dot{Q}$) mismatch, characterized by a widened A–ao_2 gradient, a dramatic increase in Pa_{O_2} in response to supplemental O_2, and a variable Pa_{CO_2}. When areas of low $\dot{V}/\dot{Q}$ predominate (e.g., reduced ventilation with normal perfusion), the Pa_{CO_2} may be low as the patient hyperventilates in an effort (only partially effective) to increase the Pa_{O_2}. When areas of high $\dot{V}/\dot{Q}$ predominate, much ventilation is wasted, and hypercapnia is also present. Areas of lung that are perfused but not ventilated characterize shunt. The resulting fall in Pa_{O_2} depends on the percentage of cardiac output circulating through the shunt and the O_2 content of that blood. Supplemental O_2 has minimal or small effect on Pa_{O_2} because the shunted blood is not exposed to the increased Fi_{O_2}. Therefore, treatment is aimed at decreasing shunt by improving ventilation to the effected area or reducing perfusion to that area. When shunt results from a unilateral process (e.g., pneumonia, atelectasis), placing the good lung down decreases shunt perfusion, and oxygenation improves.

TABLE 1 Pathophysiologic Mechanisms of Acute Hypoxic Respiratory Failure

Mechanism	A–ao$_2$ Gradient	Pa$_{CO_2}$	Response to 100% O$_2$	Cause
Diffusion abnormality	↑	↑, normal	↑↑	Severe interstitial lung disease
Hypoventilation	Normal	↑	↑↑↑	Narcotic overdose, obesity hypoventilation syndrome, respiratory muscle weakness
↓ Fi$_{O_2}$	Normal	Usually ↓	↑↑↑	High altitude, smoke inhalation
↓ Mv$_{O_2}$	↑	Usually ↓	↑	ALI, shock, CHF, PE
Shunt	↑	Usually ↓	None or ↑	ALI, CHF, atelectasis, PE
V̇/Q̇ mismatch	↑	↑, normal, ↓	↑↑↑	Acute exacerbation of COPD, asthma, PE

↑ = increased; ↓ = decreased; A–ao$_2$ = alveolar–arterial O$_2$; ALI = acute lung injury; CHF = cardiogenic pulmonary edema; COPD = chronic obstructive pulmonary disease; Fi$_{O_2}$ = fraction of inspired oxygen; Mv$_{O_2}$ = mixed venous oxygen saturation; Pa$_{CO_2}$ = partial pressure of arterial CO$_2$; PE = pulmonary embolism; V̇/Q̇ = ventilation–perfusion ratio.

ACUTE HYPERCAPNEIC RESPIRATORY FAILURE

Hypercapneic respiratory failure is defined as a Pa$_{CO_2}$ greater than 45 mm Hg. The equation used to determine Pa$_{CO_2}$ provides insight into the three basic mechanisms underlying hypercapnia:

$$Pa_{CO_2} = k\,(\dot{V}_{CO_2})/V_E(1 - V_D/V_T)$$

where k is a constant, V_E is total minute ventilation (respiratory rate times tidal volume) and V_D/V_T is the dead space. Therefore, hypercapnia can result from increased CO$_2$ production ($\dot{V}_{CO_2}$), increased physiologic dead space (V_D/V_T), and decreased minute ventilation (Box 1). Increased $\dot{V}_{CO_2}$ alone is usually insufficient to cause hypercapnia because the respiratory system responds by increasing minute ventilation to keep Pa$_{CO_2}$ normal (37-43 mm Hg). Conversely, with abnormalities of respiratory muscle function or respiratory drive or with increased dead space (and diminished reserve), the respiratory response to increased $\dot{V}_{CO_2}$ may be insufficient, and hypercapnia results.

Treatment

Treatment of acute hypoxemic and hypercapneic respiratory failure combines nonspecific (e.g., supplemental O$_2$, mechanical ventilation) and specific therapy (Boxes 2 and 3).

BOX 1 Pathophysiologic Mechanisms of Hypercapnia

Increased Carbon Dioxide Production (V̇$_{CO_2}$)
Fever
Overfeeding
Seizure
Sepsis
Thyrotoxicosis

Decreased Ventilation (V$_E$)
Depressed respiratory drive
Phrenic nerve injury
Respiratory muscle weakness

Increased Dead Space (V$_D$/V$_T$)
Acute exacerbation of chronic obstructive pulmonary disease
Interstitial lung disease
Pulmonary vascular disease

OXYGEN THERAPY

In the hospital, 100% O$_2$ is supplied from a wall source with a regulator determining flow rate in liters per minute. The final delivered oxygen concentration (Fi$_{O_2}$) depends on this flow rate and the amount of room air breathed by the patient. The O$_2$ flow rate is almost never sufficient to meet all of the patient's ventilatory demands, so varying amounts of room air are entrained to meet

---

BOX 2 Causes of and Treatments for Acute Hypoxemic Respiratory Failure

Acute Exacerbation of Chronic Obstructive Pulmonary Disease
Antibiotics
Bronchodilators
Systemic steroids

Acute Lung Injury or Acute Respiratory Distress Syndomre
Efforts to decrease lung water
Lung-protective mechanical ventilation

Congestive Heart Failure
Afterload reduction
Diuretics
Inotropes

Lobar Collapse or Atelectasis
Bronchoscopy
Pulmonary toilet (airway suctioning to improve clearance of secretions)

Pneumonia
Antibiotics
Chest physiotherapy

Pneumothorax
Tube thoracostomy to drain pleural air and facilitate lung re-expansion

Pulmonary Embolism
Anticoagulation
Thrombolytic therapy

Status Asthmaticus
Bronchodilators
Systemic steroids

BOX 3 Causes of and Treatments for Acute Hypercapnic Respiratory Failure

Acute Exacerbation of Chronic Obstructive Pulmonary Disease
Antibiotics
Bronchodilators
Systemic steroids

Acute Respiratory Muscle Weakness (e.g., myasthenic crisis)
Acetylcholinesterase therapy

Drug Overdose
Flumazenil (Romazicon)
Naloxone (Narcan)
Other antidotes

Guillain–Barré Syndrome
Immunoglobulin
Plasmapheresis

Spinal Cord Injury
Intravenous methylprednisolone

Status Asthmaticus
Bronchodilators
Systemic steroids

Toxin (e.g., botulinum toxin)
Antitoxin

---

of CO_2, and minute ventilation inadequate for the amount of CO_2 produced. Therefore, the goal in these patients is to achieve a PaO_2 of 55 to 60 mm Hg (SaO_2 88%-90%) with low-flow oxygen (~24%-28% O_2). If this (often delicate) balance between maintaining tissue oxygenation and avoiding significant respiratory acidosis cannot be achieved, short-term mechanical ventilation may be required. In most nonhypercapneic patients, high flow of oxygen (50%-100%) can be administered safely for 24 hours with a goal PaO_2 of between 65 and 80 mm Hg.

MECHANICAL VENTILATION

Mechanical ventilation can be delivered noninvasively through a tight-fitting face mask or invasively via an endotracheal tube. The goals of mechanical ventilation are to correct severe arterial blood gas abnormalities, provide respiratory support while specific therapy is used, and unload and rest the respiratory muscles. The ventilator should be set to optimize patient–ventilator interaction and avoid dynamic hyperinflation and intrinsic positive end-expiratory pressure (PEEPi). PEEPi can worsen gas exchange, predispose to barotrauma, and cause hypotension.

Noninvasive Ventilation

Noninvasive ventilation is most commonly applied as continuous positive airway pressure (CPAP), when airway pressure is kept constant throughout the respiratory cycle, or by bilevel positive airway pressure (BiPAP), when inspiratory pressure support actively assists each inspiration. Noninvasive ventilation offers numerous advantages over invasive ventilation, including increased comfort; maintenance of normal swallowing, speech, and cough; less need for sedation; and avoiding the trauma of intubation.

The effective application of noninvasive ventilation starts with carefully explaining the procedure to the patient, followed by selection of a proper-fitting face mask. The mask is placed close to the face to acclimate the patient to high inspiratory flow. The mask is then secured using straps (but not too tightly), and ventilator settings are adjusted to minimize leak and ensure comfort. The patient is reassessed frequently. Failure to improve within 2 to 4 hours (e.g., reduction in dyspnea, respiratory rate, accessory muscle use, and hypercapnia) signals noninvasive ventilation failure and need for intubation.

Noninvasive ventilation improves outcome (avoids intubation, decreases length of stay, improves survival) in a number of conditions (Table 3). Although randomized, controlled trials show dramatic benefit in AECOPD, other studies show no or uncertain benefit in

these needs. The final inspired oxygen concentration depends on the relative fraction of each gas, total minute ventilation, and the pattern of breathing (including the inspiratory to expiratory ratio). O_2 may be administered using nasal prongs, a facial mask, or high-flow devices designed to deliver higher FiO_2 (Table 2).

In hypercapneic patients (e.g., with acute exacerbation of COPD), high-flow O_2 can lead to worsening hypercapnia and acute respiratory acidosis. The mechanisms are multifactorial: worsening $\dot{V}/\dot{Q}$ matching (increased dead space), decreased intracellular binding

TABLE 2 Short-Term Oxygen Delivery Systems

Delivery System	O_2 Flow Rate (L/min)	FiO_2 Range	Comments
Basic Systems			
Nasal cannula (prongs)	1-6	0.22-0.40	Comfortable Facilitates communication and oral intake Humidification required at high flow rates
Simple masks	5-6	0.30-0.50	Mask acts as reservoir to increase FiO_2 High flow combats CO_2 rebreathing Less comfortable Must be removed to facilitate communication and oral intake Easily displaced with movement
Reservoir Masks			
Nonrebreathing	4-10	0.60-1.00	One-way valve between the mask and the reservoir bag Inspired O_2 from wall source and reservoir bag
Partial rebreathing	5-10	0.35-0.90	Lacks one-way valve
Venturi masks	4-10	0.24-0.40	Uses Bernoulli principle (fixed amount of entrained room air added to O_2) Maximum delivered FiO_2 can be controlled Often used in COPD to avoid excessive FiO_2 and risk for hypercapnia

COPD = chronic obstructive pulmonary disease; FiO_2 = fraction of inspired oxygen.

TABLE 3 Efficacy of Noninvasive Ventilation in Various Conditions

Condition	Quality of Evidence	Comment
AECOPD	Strong	↓Need for intubation ↑Survival
Acute cardiogenic pulmonary edema	Strong	↓Need for intubation ↑Survival
Hypoxemic respiratory in ICH with diffuse pulmonary infiltrates	Strong	↓Need for intubation ↑Survival
Facilitating weaning in select patients	Strong	↓Duration of intubation Most effective in AECOPD
High risk for extubation failure	Strong	↓Need for reintubation
Extubation failure in heterogeneous patient population	Moderate	Not effective, two RCTs
Routinely after extubation	Moderate	Not effective, single RCT
Extubation failure in acute exacerbation of COPD	Moderate	Single case-control study
Type I RF, diffuse infiltrates, not ICH	Moderate	↓Need for intubation
Asthma	No RCTs	Probably effective in ↓ need for intubation
Obesity hypoventilation	No RCTs	Probably effective in ↓ need for intubation
Postoperative respiratory failure	Small RCTs	Probably effective in ↓ need for reintubation
Do not intubate patients	Observational studies	Most effective with CHF, COPD
Pulmonary fibrosis	Observational studies	Not effective

AECOPD = acute exacerbation of chronic obstructive pulmonary disease; CHF = cardiogenic pulmonary edema; COPD = chronic obstructive pulmonary disease; FiO_2 = fraction of inspired oxygen; ICH = immunocompromised host; RCT = randomized, controlled trial; RF = respiratory failure.

BOX 4 Screening Criteria to Assess Readiness to Undergo a Trial of Spontaneous Breathing

Required Criteria
$PaO_2/FiO_2 \geq 150$ or $SaO_2 \geq 90\%$ or $FiO_2 \leq 40\%$ and (PEEP) ≤ 5 cm H_2O
Absence of hypotension

Additional Criteria (optional criteria)
Weaning parameters*
- Negative inspiratory force < −20- to −25 cm H_2O
- Respiratory rate (f) ≤ 35 breaths/min
- Spontaneous tidal volume (V_T) > 5mL/kg
- f/V_T < 105 breaths/L/min

Absence of significant anemia (e.g., Hb $\geq$ 8-10 mg/dL)
Absence of fever (e.g., core temperature $\leq 38.5°C$)
Adequate mental status: patient awake and alert or easily aroused

---
*Recent studies indicate that these parameters are often unnecessary in deciding whether to initiate trials of spontaneous breathing.
Hb = hemoglobin; PEEP = positive end-expiratory pressure

---

community acquired pneumonia, acute respiratory distress syndrome (ARDS), pulmonary fibrosis, and routinely after planned extubation. One mechanism for improved outcome is the reduction in infection (pneumonia, sepsis) seen with noninvasive ventilation compared with intubated patients. Noninvasive ventilation should not be used in the presence of respiratory arrest, shock, excessive secretions, inability to protect the airway, an agitated or uncooperative patient, and facial abnormalities that preclude proper application of the mask.

Invasive Ventilation

Invasive mechanical ventilation is delivered via an endotracheal tube. The set parameters include FiO_2 and positive end-expiratory pressure (PEEP). For volume-assist control, the clinician chooses respiratory rate and tidal volume. For pressure support, the clinician chooses the inspiratory pressure level above PEEP, and the patient determines respiratory rate. The resulting tidal volume depends on inspiratory pressure level and patient factors including respiratory muscle strength and respiratory system mechanics. Initially the ventilator is set to meet most of the patient's minute ventilation, allowing respiratory muscle rest. Such full support should not be prolonged because diaphragmatic dysfunction can result. Most patients require sedation, but excessive sedation levels are associated with worse outcomes. Therefore, strategies to minimize continuous intravenous sedation using a sedation protocol or once-daily interruption of sedation are recommended.

Invasive mechanical ventilation, especially when prolonged, is associated with numerous complications including ventilator-associated pneumonia, sinusitis, airway injury, thromboembolism, and gastrointestinal bleeding. Therefore, once significant clinical improvement occurs efforts should focus on rapidly removing the patient from the ventilator. This is achieved by daily screening for readiness (Box 4) followed by a 30- to 120-minute spontaneous breathing trial on minimal or no ventilator support. Patients tolerating the spontaneous breathing trial are extubated if they have a good cough, manageable respiratory secretions, and an adequate mental status to protect the airway. Approximately 25% of patients do not tolerate the spontaneous breathing trial; they should be returned to full ventilator support for 24 hours and undergo careful evaluation for reversible causes. The clinician should consider a more gradual approach to weaning these patients.

Specific Causes of Acute Respiratory Failure

ACUTE EXACERBATION OF CHRONIC OBSTRUCTIVE PULMONARY DISEASE

Patients with COPD can experience two or three exacerbations per year, especially if they are actively smoking, resulting in 500,000 hospitalizations every year in the United States. Hospital mortality ranges from 2% to 11%, rising to 25% for those requiring critical care.

Acute exacerbation of COPD is defined by increased sputum volume, purulence, and dyspnea. Physical examination is notable for tachypnea, use of accessory respiratory muscles, diminished breath sounds, prolonged expiratory phase with wheezing, thoracoabdominal paradox (inward inspiratory abdominal motion), and Hoover's sign (inward inspiratory motion of the lower rib cage). The latter two physical signs indicate the presence of dynamic hyperinflation and diaphragmatic dysfunction. Acute exacerbation of COPD is further characterized by hypoxemia (resulting from $\dot{V}/\dot{Q}$ mismatch) and hypercapnia. Patients with more severe underlying disease might demonstrate evidence of acute and chronic respiratory acidosis.

CURRENT DIAGNOSIS

- History and physical examination can give insight into the etiology of hypoxic and hypercapneic respiratory failure but may be insufficient to make a definitive diagnosis and guide therapy.
- An arterial blood gas is mandatory to define severity and whether hypoxic or hypercapneic (or both) respiratory failure is present.
- Additional diagnostic modalities, including chest radiograph, electrocardiogram, cardiac laboratory tests (troponin, brain natriuretic peptide), echocardiography, and selected use of a pulmonary artery catheter, can help identify a specific etiology.

Etiology and Diagnosis

Approximately 50% of acute exacerbations of COPD result from bacterial infection (e.g., *Pneumococcus* species, *Hemophilus influenzae*, *Moraxella catarrhalis*, and *Pseudomonas* species). The remainder result from viral infection and air pollution. In many cases a cause cannot be identified, although there is increasing appreciation that acute myocardial infarction and pulmonary embolism may be present in up to 25%. Pulmonary embolism may be suggested by a $Paco_2$ lower than baseline and the need for a higher than expected Fio_2 to maintain the Sao_2 at greater than 90%. Computed tomographic pulmonary arteriogram is recommended to make the diagnosis, because $\dot{V}/\dot{Q}$ scanning is nondiagnostic in nearly one half of COPD patients, and false-positive high-probability scans occur.

Treatment

Treatment for acute exacerbation of COPD is based on high-quality evidence consisting of numerous randomized, controlled trials and well-performed meta-analyses. Bronchodilator therapy is essential. Nebulized combination therapy (albuterol and ipratropium [DuoNeb]) is effective, but it is not demonstrably superior to single-agent therapy delivered via a metered-dose inhaler. Theophylline should generally be avoided because toxicity outweighs benefits.

Antibiotics improve outcome, especially in the presence of fever and increased sputum purulence and volume. Older agents, such as amoxicillin and tetracycline, appear as effective as newer agents.

Corticosteroids enhance β-agonist activity and counteract the inflammatory state seen in acute exacerbations of COPD. Oral prednisone at a dose of 30 to 40 mg is recommended. Intravenous therapy (methylprednisolone [SoluMedrol] 125 mg every 6 hours for 72 hours followed by oral prednisone) should be used in the critically ill patient or when response to oral therapy is suboptimal.

There is no role for mucolytic agents or chest physiotherapy.

Admission to the intensive care unit (ICU) is indicated for patients with hemodynamic instability, confusion, lethargy and coma, severe dyspnea unresponsive to emergency management, or severely abnormal gas exchange despite initial therapy (Pao_2 <40 mm Hg, $Paco_2$ >60 mm Hg, pH <7.25).

Randomized, controlled trials demonstrate that noninvasive ventilation decreases the risk for intubation and improves survival in acute exacerbations of COPD when there are severe dyspnea, hypoxemia, tachypnea, and significant respiratory acidosis ($Paco_2$ >45 mm Hg and pH <7.35). Patients who fail noninvasive ventilation or who are not candidates require intubation and mechanical ventilation.

A major risk is the development of dynamic hyperinflation (PEEPi), which can worsen gas exchange, predispose to barotrauma (e.g., pneumothorax), and cause hypotension. PEEPi is minimized by keeping delivered minute ventilation at 5 L/min or less; this is achieved by lowering tidal volume (e.g., 6 mL/kg ideal body weight) or respiratory rate (8-10 breaths/min), or by increasing inspiratory flow rate, allowing more time for expiration. PEEPi is suggested by an elevated plateau pressure or persistent expiratory flow at the time of the next ventilator breath. PEEPi can also increase work of breathing by increasing the patient's inspiratory effort to trigger the ventilator. When extrinsic PEEP is at or just below the PEEPi level, the patient triggers more easily and work of breathing is reduced.

The approach to weaning and extubation in acute exacerbations of COPD is similar to that for other conditions, although the risk of failing a spontaneous breathing trial is increased.

ACUTE LUNG INJURY AND ACUTE RESPIRATORY DISTRESS SYNDROME

ALI is the result of an acute process and is characterized by hypoxemia (Pao_2/Fio_2 < 300), bilateral diffuse alveolar infiltrates, and no evidence of cardiac etiology. When the Pao_2/Fio_2 is less than 200, the patient is said to have ARDS. ALI results from pulmonary and extrapulmonary etiologies. Pulmonary causes include pneumonia, gastric aspiration, near drowning, toxic gas inhalation, and lung contusion. Extrapulmonary causes include sepsis, pancreatitis, fat embolism, drug overdose, nonthoracic trauma, and massive transfusion. Conditions that can mimic the clinical findings of ALI include CHF, diffuse alveolar hemorrhage (DAH), acute cryptogenic organizing pneumonia (COP), and acute eosinophilic pneumonia (AEP). These latter three entities can be diagnosed by bronchoscopy (DAH, AEP) or by open lung biopsy (COP), all are treated with high doses of corticosteroids. Studies indicate that corticosteroids do not improve the outcome of ALI/ARDS.

Differentiating cardiogenic pulmonary edema from ALI can be challenging, especially because these conditions can coexist. Physical findings of jugular venous distention and a positive third heart sound, abnormal electrocardiogram (ECG), elevated brain natriuretic peptide (BNP), and positive cardiac enzymes (troponin) point to a cardiac etiology. A chest radiograph showing cardiomegaly, vascular redistribution, widened vascular pedicle, perihilar alveolar infiltrates and pleural effusions also suggest a cardiac cause. Bedside echocardiography can demonstrate reduced left ventricular function. A pulmonary artery catheter provides definitive evidence of an elevated pulmonary capillary wedge pressure and reduced cardiac output. That said, recent randomized, controlled trials demonstrate no

CURRENT THERAPY

- Treatment of acute respiratory failure often begins with nonspecific approaches such as oxygen and mechanical ventilation (noninvasive or invasive).
- The goal of mechanical ventilation is to improve gas exchange and rest the respiratory muscles while waiting for the beneficial effects of specific therapy aimed at the underlying cause (e.g., bronchodilators, antibiotics, and corticosteroids in acute exacerbations of chronic obstructive pulmonary disease [COPD]).
- Noninvasive ventilation avoids many complications associated with invasive ventilation and improves outcomes for patients with acute cardiogenic pulmonary edema and acute exacerbations of COPD.
- Invasive mechanical ventilation can be lifesaving but can cause clinical deterioration if not properly administered.
- Using low tidal volumes (6 mL/kg ideal body weight) can help avoid dangerous dynamic hyperinflation in acute exacerbations of COPD and further lung injury in acute lung injury (e.g., volutrauma, barotrauma).
- Once signs of improvement are evident, focus rapidly shifts to liberating the patient from the ventilator using spontaneous breathing trials to assess the need for ventilatory support followed by airway assessment to determine readiness for extubation.

improvement in survival with routine use of the pulmonary artery catheter in ALI.

ALI causes heterogeneous effects in the lung, resulting in poorly ventilated, atelectatic, dependent regions of lung. Traditional tidal volumes of 10 to 15 mL/kg can cause lung injury by creating significant shear stress by repeatedly opening these atelectatic areas (atelectrauma) and overdistending less affected areas (volutrauma, barotrauma). Indeed, experimental and clinical studies demonstrate that a lung-protective strategy, using a tidal volume of 6 mL/kg ideal body weight, improves survival in ALI. Using small tidal volumes often results in significant hypercapnia, which can have an independent protective effect (permissive hypercapnia). The application of PEEP recruits and opens atelectatic lung, thereby reducing harmful shear forces. The optimal level of PEEP remains uncertain: A recent multicenter study found no difference in mortality in patients randomized to high (~14 cm H_2O) or low (~8 cm H_2O) PEEP when all patients received a tidal volume of 6 mL/kg ideal body weight.

CARDIOGENIC PULMONARY EDEMA

CHF occurs in patients with cardiomyopathy or acutely when ischemia is present. Diagnosis is suggested by jugular venous distension, a third heart sound, diffuse rales, abnormal ECG, and a chest radiograph showing cardiomegaly, diffuse alveolar infiltrates, and bilateral pleural effusion. A markedly elevated BNP or pro-BNP further suggests a cardiac etiology.

Therapy consists of oxygen, nitrates, diuretics, afterload reduction, and anti-ischemic therapy if the history or ECG is suggestive. Mechanical ventilation produces positive intrathoracic pressure, which improves cardiac function by decreasing both left ventricular preload and afterload, reversing hypoxemia, and decreasing work of breathing. In hemodynamically stable patients without active ischemia, CPAP at levels of 8 to 12 cm H_2O should be used. A meta-analysis of 15 randomized, controlled trials showed that noninvasive ventilation decreased the need for intubation and improved survival. CPAP and BiPAP appear to be equivalent, although many prefer BiPAP when hypercapnia is present.

Because cardiogenic pulmonary edema is rapidly reversible, intubated patients can often be extubated within 24 hours. That said, the transition from positive pressure ventilation to negative ventilation (e.g., T-piece or extubation) can precipitate pulmonary edema.

REFERENCES

Acute Respiratory Distress Syndrome Network: Ventilation with lower tidal volumes as compared with traditional tidal volumes for acute lung injury and the acute respiratory distress syndrome. N Engl J Med 2000;342:1301-1308.
Bach PB, Brown C, Gelfand SE, et al: Management of acute exacerbations of chronic obstructive pulmonary disease: A summary and appraisal of published evidence. Ann Intern Med 2001;134:600-620.
Brower RG, Lanken PN, MacIntyre N, et al: Higher versus lower positive end-expiratory pressures in patients with the acute respiratory distress syndrome. N Engl J Med 2004;51:327-336.
Ely EW, Baker AM, Dunagan DP, et al: Effect on the duration of mechanical ventilation of identifying patients capable of breathing spontaneously. N Engl J Med 1996;335:1864-1869.
Epstein SK: Complications in ventilator supported patients. In Tobin M (ed): Principles and Practice of Mechanical Ventilation. New York: McGraw Hill, 2006, pp 877-902.
Kress JP, Pohlman AS, O'Connor MF, et al: Daily interruption of sedative infusions in critically ill patients undergoing mechanical ventilation. N Engl J Med 2000;342:1471-1477.
MacIntyre NR, Cook DJ, Ely EW Jr, et al: Evidence-based guidelines for weaning and discontinuing ventilatory support: A collective task force facilitated by the American College of Chest Physicians, the American Association for Respiratory Care, and the American College of Critical Care Medicine. Chest 2001;120:375S-395S.
Majid A, Hill NS: Noninvasive ventilation for acute respiratory failure. Curr Opin Crit Care 2005;11:77-81.
Masip J, Orque M, Sanchez B, et al: Noninvasive ventilation in acute cardiogenic pulmonary edema: Systematic review and meta-analysis. JAMA 2005;294:3124-3130.
Schumaker G, Epstein SK: Management of acute respiratory failure in acute exacerbations of COPD. Resp Care 2004;49:766-782.

Atelectasis

Method of
David R. Jones, MD, and
Matthew D. Taylor, MD

Atelectasis is defined as collapse of alveoli affecting segmental, lobar, or the entire lung, resulting in hypoventilation. In symptomatic patients, transient or persistent hypoxemia can ensue as a result of pulmonary shunting. The condition may be acute or chronic and might or might not result in symptoms. Acute atelectasis is most commonly encountered in the postoperative period. The incidence of atelectasis varies from 15% to 98% depending on the location and complexity of the surgical procedure (Table 1). Lobar atelectasis occurs in 8.5% of adult patients in the intensive care unit. Chronic atelectasis can be classified as rounded or folded atelectasis due to chronic pleural scarring.

Types of Atelectasis

OBSTRUCTIVE ATELECTASIS

Obstructive atelectasis is the most common form. It is caused by the reabsorption of alveolar gas in the setting of obstruction between the alveoli and the trachea. The etiology is commonly a foreign body, tumor, or mucus plug.

NONOBSTRUCTIVE ATELECTASIS

There are several subtypes of obstructive atelectasis. Passive atelectasis is a space-occupying process, such as a pneumothorax or pleural effusion, limiting approximation of parietal and visceral pleura. Compression atelectasis is a localized compression of the lung parenchyma as seen in lung adjacent to the chest wall, a pleural or intraparenchymal mass, loculated fluid collection, or bullae. Adhesive atelectasis is lung collapse due to surfactant deficiency resulting in pneumonia, hyaline membrane disease, or acute respiratory distress syndrome (ARDS). Cicatrization atelectasis involves severe parenchymal scarring associated with pulmonary fibrosis, chronic tuberculosis, fungal infection, or radiation fibrosis, resulting in lobar collapse. Rounded atelectasis is pleural scarring associated with asbestosis, tuberculosis, or parapneumonic effusions. It occurs in approximately 5 to 15 per 100,000 men older than 40 years.

Diagnosis

PRESENTATION

Signs and symptoms include tachypnea, dyspnea, hypoxia, diminished breath sounds, and dullness to percussion on physical examination. Tachypnea occurs as a result of compensation for low tidal

TABLE 1 Incidence of Atelectasis by Patient Population

Patient Population	Incidence (%)
All surgical patients	15-98
Abdominal surgery	20-30
Cardiac surgery	39-63
Thoracic surgery	5-15

CURRENT DIAGNOSIS

- Hypoxia
- Tachypnea
- Dyspnea
- Diminished breath sounds
- Radiologic signs of atelectasis

volumes and a need to maintain minute volumes. When a significant atelectatic proportion of lung parenchyma is present, hypoxia results due to inadequate oxygen exchange in the setting of unchanged alveolar blood flow.

DIAGNOSTIC STUDIES

The radiographic changes on chest x-ray are categorized as direct or indirect. Direct signs are displaced pulmonary vessels, air bronchograms, and displacement of the fissures. Indirect signs are pulmonary opacification; diaphragmatic elevation; hyperexpansion of unaffected lung; tracheal, heart, and mediastinal shift toward the atelectatic side; shift of the hilum toward the collapsed lobe or segment; and ipsilateral rib approximation. The most reliable sign of collapse is the displacement of interlobar fissures. Radiographic patterns of lower lobe collapse are similar on the right and left sides; upper lobe collapse is demonstrated by radiologic features that are different for the right and left lobes.

Treatment

Treatment is aimed at the cause of atelectasis. With regard to obstructive atelectasis, chest percussion or vibration and nasotracheal or bronchoscopic suctioning may be useful in clearing secretions or a mucus plug. Incentive spirometry, continuous or intermittent positive pressure ventilation, and early ambulation may be used to re-expand the lung. However, a meta-analysis of 35 trials evaluating the efficacy of respiratory physiotherapy following abdominal surgery found only four trials that had a significant decrease in pulmonary complications with the use of aggressive physiotherapy.

For nonobstructive atelectasis caused by a pneumothorax or pleural effusion, tube thoracostomy or thoracentesis may be indicated. Postoperative pain is another important cause of atelectasis following abdominal and thoracic surgery. In this patient population, epidural analgesia has been associated with a significant reduction in postoperative pulmonary complications.

CURRENT THERAPY

- Chest percussion and vibration therapy
- Nasotracheal suctioning
- Bronchoscopy
- Incentive spirometry
- Positive pressure ventilation
- Early ambulation
- Adequate postoperative pain control

REFERENCES

Ballantyne J, Carr DB, deFerranti S, et al: The comparative effects of postoperative analgesic therapies on pulmonary outcome: Cumulative meta-analyses of randomized, controlled trial. Anesth Analg 1998;86:598-612.
Goodman LR: Postoperative chest radiograph: I. Alterations after abdominal surgery. AJR Am J Roentgenol 1980;134: 533-541.
Groeben H: Epidural anesthesia and pulmonary function. J Anesth 2006; 20(4):290-299.
Hillerdal G: Rounded atelectasis: Clinical experience with 74 patients. Chest 1989;95(4):836-841.
Miller WT: Radiographic evaluation of the lungs and chest. In Shields TW(ed): General Thoracic Surgery, vol 1, 4th ed. Philadelphia: Williams & Wilkins, 1994, pp 145-148.
Pasquina P, Tramer MR, Granier JM, et al: Respiratory physiotherapy to prevent pulmonary complications after abdominal surgery: A systematic review. Chest 2006;130:1887-1899.
Verheij J, Van Lingen A, Raijmakers PG, et al: Pulmonary abnormalities after cardiac surgery are better explained by atelectasis than by increased permeability oedema. Acta Anaesthesiol Scand 2005;49:1302-1310.

Management of Chronic Obstructive Pulmonary Disease

Method of
Tamara Simpson, MD, Juan Armando Garcia, MD, Stephen G. Jenkinson, MD, and Jay Peters, MD

Chronic obstructive pulmonary disease (COPD) is characterized by airflow limitation that is not fully reversible. The airflow limitation is usually both progressive and associated with an abnormal inflammatory response of the lungs to noxious particles of gases. Under the direction of the National Heart, Lung, and Blood Institute (NHLBI) and the World Health Organization (WHO), collaborative guidelines on the diagnosis and management of chronic obstructive pulmonary disease (COPD) have been assembled by an expert panel: the Global Initiative for Chronic Obstructive Lung Disease (GOLD). These guidelines define the classifications of COPD on the basis of both severity and type of symptoms and explore all new information on the diagnosis and treatment of COPD. The GOLD initiative aims to improve prevention and management of COPD through a concerted worldwide effort of people involved in all facets of health care policy and to encourage a renewed research interest in this extremely prevalent disease.

To assure that recommendations for management of COPD are based on current scientific literature, the GOLD program established a science committee to update the sections of the report on recommendations for management of COPD each year. Although the update of these sections will occur each year and will be posted on the Web site (http://www.goldcopd.com), the full report will be updated and printed every 5 years. The latest update, including new modifications of management, was published in 2007.

Pathophysiology

The pathophysiology of COPD is somewhat different in various patients, and the terms *emphysema* or *chronic bronchitis* were used in the past. Both of these disorders cause airway obstruction. Emphysema is defined pathologically as abnormal permanent enlargement of airspaces distal to the terminal bronchioles, accompanied by destruction of their walls and without obvious fibrosis. This tissue destruction results in enlargement of proximal and distal airspaces and can ultimately form bullae in the lung parenchyma. These bullae result in loss of surface area for gas exchange in the involved lungs. There is also a genetically inherited form of emphysema which is caused by the α_1-antitrypsin (AAT) deficiency. This disorder accounts for less than 1% of COPD cases in the United States. AAT is a protease inhibitor produced by the liver that circulates into tissues. Active proteases are released into the lung by lung macrophages, which can contribute to the development of emphysema. When patients smoke cigarettes, they also recruit a neutrophil population into their lungs. These neutrophils release neutrophil elastase (another type of protease) and other toxic molecules, which can destroy alveolar walls and may also contribute to the production of emphysema. AAT offers protection from these effects, but the protection found in normal people is inadequate in patients with AAT deficiency. Patients who develop emphysema despite normal levels of AAT usually develop emphysema in the fifth or sixth decades of life, whereas patients with AAT deficiency can develop emphysema as early as the third or fourth decades of life, depending on the extent of their deficiency and smoking history.

All patients developing emphysema should be evaluated for AAT deficiency at least once, especially if they present with COPD before the age of 45-50. A normal serum level of AAT is greater than 11 mmol/L (>80 mg/dL). Patients with low levels of AAT should be evaluated by a pulmonologist and may be candidates for AAT replacement therapy.

Chronic bronchitis is defined clinically as the presence of chronic, productive cough for 3 months during each of 2 consecutive years, and for which other causes of chronic cough are excluded. The other most common causes of chronic cough include asthma, gastric reflux, or postnasal drip secondary to sinus disease. The pathologic findings of chronic bronchitis are enlargement of tracheobronchial mucus glands, variable amounts of airway smooth-muscle hyperplasia, inflammation, and bronchial wall thickening. Abnormalities of small airways may be present as well and are accompanied by fibrosis and the presence of a mononuclear inflammatory process. The forced expiratory volume at 1 second (FEV_1) of a COPD patient is inversely proportional to the number of inflammatory cells in the airways. Patients with chronic bronchitis also have increased mucus hypersecretion, goblet cell metaplasia, increased submucosal gland formation, and abnormal matrix deposition.

The use of the terms *emphysema* or *chronic bronchitis* is no longer specified in the GOLD definition of COPD. The inflammation seen in COPD is different from that seen in asthma, but some obstructive lung disease patients do have pathologic changes that can be seen in both diseases, so some overlap does occur.

Epidemiology and Risk Factors

In the United States COPD is presently the fourth leading cause of death and affects more than 21 million people. Death rates have risen more than 22% in the last decade and the disease is responsible for approximately 700,000 hospital stays each year. The disease is now more common in women than men because of increasing amounts of cigarette smoking in women and increased susceptibility. The primary risk factor associated with the development of COPD, cigarette smoking increases the death rate and disability caused by COPD and causes lung function to deteriorate over time much more rapidly than in a nonsmoker. Cigar and pipe smokers have greater COPD incidence than nonsmokers. Approximately 20% of smokers will develop COPD. The risk of development of COPD is increased in first-degree relatives of patients with COPD, which suggests the importance of genetic factors, but AAT deficiency is the only proved genetic risk factor in COPD. Exposures other than smoking that have been associated with COPD development include passive smoking, ambient air pollution, occupational dust and chemical exposure, and severe respiratory childhood infections.

Diagnosis

The diagnosis of COPD is suggested on the basis of symptoms, which may include those caused by the airway irritation (cough and sputum production) and those reflecting altered lung mechanics (dyspnea, wheezing, and occasionally chest pain). Individuals usually experience cough and sputum production years before the development of airflow limitation, while not all individuals with cough and sputum production go on to develop COPD.

Physical examination of individuals with COPD can reveal hyperinflation, wheezing, diminished breath sounds, hyperresonance, or prolonged expiration. Visual inspection during an examination can reveal signs of increased respiratory rate, increased anteroposterior (AP) chest diameter, hyperresonance to chest percussion, and impaired respiratory muscle function. Patients with COPD commonly have a respiration rate greater than 16 breaths per minute, and often this is proportional to disease severity; patients with COPD severe enough to exhibit hypercapnia (partial pressure of arterial carbon dioxide [$PaCO_2$] greater than 45 mm Hg) may have breathing rates of greater than 25 breaths per minute. Absence of wheezing does not exclude COPD. Patients with end-stage COPD may adopt body positions that help relieve dyspnea, such as leaning forward or expiring through pursed lips. Use of accessory muscles for respiration, such as the use of the abdominal rectus muscle on expiration, is a sign of advanced disease. Other signs of hyperinflation may include decreased diaphragm movement, tracheal tug, or pulsus paradoxus greater than 20 mm Hg.

Patients with advanced COPD may also have central cyanosis, peripheral edema, and signs of cor pulmonale associated with right heart failure. Other objective findings often include arterial blood gas changes demonstrating hypercapnia, severe hypoxemia, compensated respiratory acidosis with elevated carbon dioxide (CO_2), tension and a normal pH, and elevated serum bicarbonate level. Morning headaches in COPD patients may be indicative of hypercapnia.

The diagnosis of COPD is confirmed by spirometry. The standard pulmonary function test used to measure airway obstruction is the forced expiratory spirogram. This test assesses the rate of change in volume that occurs as a function of time. Pulmonary functions useful in the evaluation of patients presenting with symptoms of COPD include FEV_1, the forced vital capacity (FVC), and the ratio of FEV_1/FVC, which is also called the *timed vital capacity*. The FVC provides a measure of lung volume and the FEV_1 and FEV_1/FVC both provide a measure of obstruction. In most of these patients, other abnormal lung volumes that may exist include increases in both the total lung capacity (TLC) and the residual volume (RV). These increases in lung volumes are caused by hyperinflation of the lungs.

An FEV_1/FVC less than 70% of predicted confirms the presence of airflow obstruction. The FEV_1 serves as a marker of severity of the airflow obstruction. Other pulmonary function tests such as the flow volume loop or diffusing capacity for carbon monoxide (DL_{CO}) can help rule out other types of airway obstruction or help quantitate a patient's risk for surgery. Chest radiographs are only helpful for diagnosis in COPD if there are signs of bullous disease or severe hyperinflation or loss of vascular markings. Computed tomography (CT) scanning can show the location of bullous disease which can be helpful in narrowing the differential diagnosis of a patient with airway obstruction and also may be used to help determine if a patient is a candidate for lung reduction surgery.

COPD Classification

The GOLD committee presented a new classification of COPD. The management of COPD is largely symptom driven, and there is only an imperfect relationship between the degree of airflow limitation and the presence of symptoms. The staging therefore is aimed at practical implementation and should be only regarded as an educational tool, and a general indication of the approach to management. All FEV_1 values refer to postbronchodilator FEV_1.

This classification includes stages I to IV (Figure 1).

Stage I: Mild COPD—Characterized by mild airflow limitation (FEV_1/FVC <70% but FEV_1 >80% predicted) and usually, but not always, chronic cough and sputum production. At this stage, the individual may be unaware of abnormal lung function.

THERAPY AT EACH STAGE OF COPD

		I: Mild	II: Moderate	III: Severe	IV: Very severe
Characteristics		• $FEV_1/FVC < 70\%$ • $FEV_1 \geq 80\%$ • With or without symptoms	• $FEV_1/FVC < 70\%$ • $50\% \leq FEV_1 < 80\%$ • With or without symptoms	• $FEV_1/FVC < 70\%$ • $30\% \leq FEV_1 < 50\%$ • With or without symptoms	• $FEV_1/FVC < 70\%$ • $FEV_1 < 30\%$ or $FEV_1 < 50\%$ predicted plus chronic respiratory failure
		Avoidance of risk factor(s); influenza vaccination			
		*Add* short-acting bronchodilator when needed			
			Add regular treatment with one or more long-acting bronchodilators *Add* rehabilitation		
				Add inhaled glucocorticosteroid if repeated exacerbations	
					Add long-term oxygen if chronic respiratory failure. Consider surgical treatments

FIGURE 1. Therapy for different stages of COPD

Stage II: Moderate COPD—Characterized by worsening airflow limitation (<50% FEV_1 <80% predicted) and usually the progression of symptoms, with shortness of breath typically developing on exertion. This is the stage at which most patients typically first seek medical attention because of dyspnea or an exacerbation of their disease.

Stage III: Severe COPD—Characterized by further worsening of airflow limitation (<30% FEV_1 <50% predicted), increased shortness of breath, and repeated exacerbations which have an impact on the patient's quality of life.

Stage IV: Very Severe COPD—Characterized by severe airflow limitation (FEV_1 <30% predicted) or the presence of chronic respiratory failure. Patients may have very severe (Stage IV) COPD even if the FEV_1 is greater than 30% predicted, if respiratory failure is present. At this stage, quality of life is appreciably impaired and exacerbations may be life-threatening.

Management of Stable COPD

The general guidelines to management of COPD include the avoidance of risk factors to prevent disease progression and pharmacotherapy as needed to control symptoms. In addition, patient education including counseling about smoking cessation, instruction in physical exercise, and nutritional advice are necessary components of a comprehensive COPD management plan. The goals of management are to relieve symptoms, increase exercise tolerance, improve quality of life, prevent and treat complications, and decrease disease progression.

Smoking cessation is the single most effective (and cost-effective) intervention to reduce the risk of developing COPD and stop its progression. Comprehensive tobacco elimination policies and programs with clear and repeated nonsmoking messages should be delivered through every feasible system possible. Legislation to establish smoke-free schools, public facilities, and work environments should be encouraged by working with government officials, public health workers, and the public. Guidelines for smoking cessation were published by the U.S. Agency for Health Care Policy and Research (AHCPR) in 2000.

There are numerous effective pharmacotherapies for smoking cessation. Except in the presence of special circumstances, pharmacotherapy is recommended when counseling is insufficient. Nicotine replacement therapy in any form (nicotine gum, inhaler, nasal spray [Nicotrol NS], transdermal patch [Nicoderm], sublingual tablet [Nicorette Microtab],[2] or lozenge [Commit]) reliably increases long-term smoking abstinence rates. The antidepressants bupropion (Zyban) and the nicotinic receptor antagonist varenicline (Chantix), have been shown to significantly increase long-term quit rates. The antihypertensive drug clonidine (Catapres)[1] can also be used to help a patient quit smoking, but side effects should be carefully reviewed with each patient. Special consideration should be given before using pharmacotherapy in selected populations including patients smoking fewer than 10 cigarettes per day, pregnant patients, and adolescent smokers.

The overall approach to managing stable COPD should be characterized by a stepwise increase in treatment, depending on the severity of the disease. The management strategy is based on an individualized assessment of disease severity and response to various therapies. Disease severity is determined by the severity of symptoms and airflow limitation (using pulmonary function measurements) and other factors such as the frequency and severity of exacerbations, complications, respiratory failure, co-morbidities (cardiovascular disease and sleep-related disorders), and the general health status of the patient. Different types of pharmacologic agents treat patients with COPD (Box 1). Pharmacologic therapy is used to prevent and control symptoms, reduce the frequency and severity of exacerbations, improve health status, and improve exercise tolerance. Initial use should decrease airway obstruction and decrease dyspnea. None of the existing medications for COPD had been shown to alter the inevitable long-term decline in lung function that occurs with COPD; however, they can decrease morbidity and may also delay disability and mortality in some patients. Medications may also decrease the number of exacerbations of COPD occurring per year.

Bronchodilators are primary medications for symptomatic management of COPD. Bronchodilator drugs commonly used include anticholinergics (short and long acting), β_1 agonists (short and long acting), and long-acting methylxanthines. All of these medications have been shown to improve exercise capacity in COPD patients even if the FEV_1 is insignificantly changed. Inhaled drugs tend to have fewer side effects than oral drugs. Short-acting bronchodilators on an as-needed basis are recommended for mild (Stage I) COPD. The GOLD guidelines recommend the use of regular daily treatment with long-acting bronchodilators for moderate (Stage II) or severe (Stages III and IV) COPD and long-acting bronchodilators are preferred to short-acting drugs because of better compliance because of longer duration of action (Box 1). Regular use of a long-acting

---
[2] Not available in the United States.

> **BOX 1 Current Drugs Used to Manage Chronic Obstructive Pulmonary Disease**
>
> **SABAs**
> - Albuterol (multiple formulations)
>
> **LABAs**
> - Formoterol (Foradil)
> - Salmeterol (Serevent)
> - Short-acting anticholinergics
> - Ipratropium (Atrovent)
>
> **Long-acting anticholinergics**
> - Tiotropium (Spiriva)
> - Combination SABA + anticholinergic in 1 inhaler
> - Albuterol/ipratropium (Combivent)
>
> **Methylxanthines**
> - Theophylline (Theo-Dur)
>
> **Inhaled corticosteroids**
> - Beclomethasone (QVAR)
> - Budesonide (Pulmicort)
> - Fluticasone (Flovent)
> - Triamcinolone (Azmacort) and mometasone (Asmanex)
>
> **Combination LABA + ICS in 1 inhaler**
> - Formoterol/budesonide (Symbicort)
> - Salmeterol/fluticasone (Advair)
>
> **Systemic corticosteroids**
> - Prednisone
> - Methylprednisolone (Medrol)
>
> ---
>
> *Abbreviations:* LABAs = Long-acting β_2 agonists; SABAs = short-acting β_2 agonists.

anticholinergic (tiotropium [Spiriva]) or a long acting β_1-agonist (salmeterol [Serevent] or formoterol [Foradil]) improves health status. Theophylline (Theo-Dur) is effective in COPD, but because of its potential toxicity, inhaled bronchodilators are preferred when available. All studies that have shown efficacy of theophylline (Theo-Dur) in COPD were done with slow-release preparations (theophylline [Theo-Dur]). Each of the inhaled bronchodilators requires a delivery device which must be used correctly. Each type of device requires patient education and monitoring, and the GOLD guidelines recommend consideration of the delivery device as part of the selection process for drug treatment in a single patient. As symptoms of COPD worsen, several different types of COPD therapy are given simultaneously, and deletion of drug therapy is usually not possible. In general nebulized therapy for a stable patient is unnecessary unless it has been demonstrated to be more effective than conventional metered dose or dry powder inhaler dose therapy in that patient.

Combinations of bronchodilators with different mechanisms and durations of action tend to increase the degree of bronchodilation in COPD patients with increases in FEV_1, FEV_1/FVC, and peak expiratory flow (PEF). Changes in pulmonary function are indirectly additive with increasing the number of bronchodilators being administered, but combinations usually increase pulmonary function more than each agent alone. Short-acting β_2 agonists (SABAs) are quick-relief medications for use only when necessary rather than on a daily, regular schedule. The regular use of a SABA results in twice as much β_2 agonist use without any noted clinical benefits. Increasing use or daily use of a SABA for rescue indicates the need for additional therapy to achieve long-term control. Inhaled SABAs include albuterol (Proventil, Ventolin), bitolterol (Tornalate), pirbuterol (Maxair), and terbutaline (Brethaire). These medications are effective for 4 to 6 hours after use. Adverse effects of SABAs include palpitations, chest pain, tachycardia, tremor, unstable coronary artery disease or nervousness. Patients with coronary artery disease or cardiac dysrhythmias should also be monitored closely. Use caution in giving these medications to patients receiving monoamine oxidase inhibitors or tricyclic antidepressants. The short-acting anticholinergic agent, ipratropium bromide (Atrovent), causes bronchodilation by competitive inhibition of muscarinic receptors. This agent reverses cholinergically mediated bronchospasm and may decrease mucus-gland secretions. It is effective for 4 to 6 hours after use.

The most recent addition to the long-acting bronchodilators is tiotropium (Spiriva), a long-acting anticholinergic agent that lasts 24 hours, allowing for once-daily administration. Tiotropium (Spiriva) has shown in several recent studies with COPD patients to result in significant improvement in lung function compared with ipratropium (a short-acting anticholinergic) or salmeterol (Serevent, a long-acting β_2 agonist [LABA]). Inhaled LABAs are highly preferred than the extended-release oral formulation because of longer action and fewer side effects. Salmeterol (Serevent) and formoterol (Foradil) are both long-acting, inhaled β_2 agonists, and extended-release albuterol (Proventil Repetabs) are long-acting, β_2 agonists available as oral agents. The long-acting inhaled agents have a slower onset of action and longer duration of action, remaining active for more than 12 hours. The onset of action of formoterol (Foradil) is more rapid than salmeterol (Serevent), but it should not be used for rescue during episodes of acute shortness of breath. It remains a chronic bronchodilator therapy. Like the short-acting inhaled β_2 agonists, the long-acting agents produce bronchodilation by smooth muscle relaxation as a result of adenylate cyclase activation and increasing cyclic AMP in smooth muscle cells. Combining β_2 agonists and anticholinergics may increase the effects of these agents. Several studies have shown superior efficacy for either a SABA or LABA in combination with an anticholinergic.

Theophylline (Theo-Dur) inhibits phosphodiesterase action, which causes smooth muscle relaxation and leads to bronchodilation. It also increases central respiratory drive, diaphragm strength, promotes venous pooling in the legs, and may have some mild anti-inflammatory activity. Therapy with theophylline (Theo-Dur) should be individualized, taking into account such factors as drug interactions, current smoking, the patient's age, and the presence of congestive heart failure or liver disease. Serum theophylline (Theo-Dur) concentrations should be maintained at levels between 5 and 15 µg/mL. Dosage adjustment is based on the patient's clinical response, tolerance to the agent, and serum theophylline (Theo-Dur) levels. Some patients metabolize theophylline (Theo-Dur) very rapidly. Although theophylline (Theo-Dur) is not a preferred first line agent in the management of COPD, it may be a second-line agent in patients with severe COPD.

Inhaled corticosteroids (ICSs) are not recommended as single agents for chronic use in COPD management, which is quite different from the recommendations in asthma. They are recommended in combination therapy with other bronchodilators in severe COPD, and the only Food and Drug Administration (FDA)-approved combinations of ICS and a LABA are fluticasone plus salmeterol (Advair) or formoterol (Foradil) plus budesonide (Symbicort)[4] (see Box 1). Systemic steroids are clinically beneficial to patients hospitalized with COPD exacerbations and maximum effects of oral steroids after 3 days of intravenous (IV) steroids are achieved by 2 weeks of therapy. Longer use of oral steroids increases side effects without increasing pulmonary functions. Long-term treatment with oral glucocorticosteroids is not recommended in COPD. There is no evidence of a long-term benefit from this treatment. Moreover, a side effect of long-term treatment with systemic glucocorticosteroid is steroid myopathy, which contributes to muscle weakness, decreased functionality, and respiratory failure in patients with advanced COPD. Oral glucocorticosteroid use for long periods of time can also complicate control of diabetes and hypertension as well as causing bone demineralization.

Other pharmacologic treatments have been evaluated by the GOLD committee with some being beneficial. Use of influenza vaccines can reduce serious illness and death in COPD patients by approximately 50%. Use of the influenza vaccine has also been shown to reduce outpatient visits for influenza and reduces both

---

[4]Not yet approved for use in the United States.

hospital costs and death. Vaccines containing killed (Fluzone) or live, inactive viruses (FluMist)[1] are recommended and should be given once (in autumn) or twice[3] (in autumn and winter) each year. A pneumococcal vaccine containing 23 virulent serotypes (Pneumovax-23) has been used in an effort to decrease the number of cases of pneumococcal pneumonia in COPD patients but evidence supporting its effectiveness in COPD patients is lacking. An oral vaccine* using a strain of nontypeable *Haemophilus influenzae* has been shown to produce short-lived reduction in the number of exacerbations in some groups of COPD patients. The use of antibiotics, other than in treating infectious exacerbations of COPD or other bacterial infections such as pneumonia, is not recommended. Although a few patients with viscous sputum may benefit from mucolytics, the overall benefit is small. Therefore, the widespread use of these agents cannot be recommended.

Cough, although sometimes a troublesome symptom in COPD, has a significant protective role and the regular use of antitussives is contraindicated in stable COPD. The use of doxapram (Dopram), a nonspecific respiratory stimulant available as an intravenous formulation, is not recommended in stable COPD. Almitrine bismesylate (Duxil) also is not recommended for regular use in stable COPD patients. Narcotics are contraindicated in COPD because of their respiratory depressant effects and potential to worsen hypercapnia. Clinical studies suggest that morphine use to control dyspnea may have serious adverse effects, but it may provide benefits to a few select limited patients. Codeine and other narcotic analgesics should be avoided. Nonsteroidal anti-inflammatory agents (Nedocromil [Tilade]) and leukotriene modifiers have not been adequately tested in COPD patients and are not recommended for use. Alternative healing methods including herbal medicine, acupuncture, and homeopathy are not recommended for treatment in COPD.

Nonpharmacologic management of COPD patients includes pulmonary rehabilitation and long-term oxygen therapy. The principal goals of pulmonary rehabilitation are to improve quality of life, decrease symptoms, and increase physical participation in everyday activities. To accomplish these goals, pulmonary rehabilitation addresses a range of nonpulmonary problems, including exercise deconditioning, relative social isolation, altered mood states (especially depression), muscle wasting, and weight loss. COPD patients at all stages of disease benefit from exercise training programs and improve with respect to both exercise tolerance and symptoms of dyspnea and fatigue. These benefits can be sustained even after a single pulmonary rehabilitation program. Benefits have been reported from rehabilitation programs conducted in inpatient, outpatient, and home settings. Ideally, a comprehensive pulmonary rehabilitation program includes exercise training, nutrition counseling, and education. Baseline and outcome assessments of each participant in a pulmonary rehabilitation program should be made to quantify individual gains and target areas for improvement and include a detailed medical history and physical exam; measurement of spirometry before and after a bronchodilator drug; assessment of exercise capacity; measurement of the impact of breathlessness and/or health status; and assessment of inspiratory and expiratory muscle strength and lower limb strength (e.g., quadriceps) in patients who suffer from muscle wasting.

The long-term administration of oxygen (more than 15 hours per day) to COPD patients with chronic respiratory failure has been shown to increase survival. In studies done in Britain by the Medical Research Council Trial and in the United States in the Nocturnal Oxygen Therapy Trial, patients receiving continuous oxygen therapy had increased survival as compared with patients that did not receive oxygen or received oxygen only at night. Oxygen also has a beneficial impact on hemodynamics, hematologic characteristics, exercise capacity, lung mechanics, and mental state. Oxygen therapy also should be used if the patient has evidence of pulmonary hypertension, peripheral edema suggesting either right- or left-sided heart failure or evidence of polycythemia (hematocrit greater than 55%). Therapy can be given continuously, acutely to combat acute dyspnea, or intermittently during exercise. It is recommended to perform arterial blood gas measurement in patients with FEV_1 less than 40% predicted or with clinical findings suggestive of respiratory failure or cor pulmonale.

Management of Exacerbations

Patients with COPD will have usually two to three exacerbations of symptoms of their disease each year with some requiring hospitalization. The economic and social burden of COPD exacerbations is extremely high. The most common causes of an exacerbation are pulmonary infections (acute bacterial bronchitis) and air pollution. The exact cause of approximately one-third of severe exacerbations cannot be identified and may be related to reactive airway disease. Other conditions that may produce the symptoms of an acute exacerbation of COPD include pneumonia, myocardial ischemia, congestive heart failure, pneumothorax, formation of a pleural effusion, pulmonary embolism, cardiac arrhythmias, esophageal reflux, or noncompliance with medications. The clinical diagnosis of a COPD exacerbation is an increase in amount of sputum production, change in color of sputum, or increase in dyspnea. Exacerbations may also be accompanied by a number of nonspecific complaints such as malaise, insomnia, sleepiness, fatigue, anxiety, depression, confusion, or panic attacks. Patients with exacerbations of COPD may require hospital admission, and some patients will require ICU admission. There is a high incidence of *H. influenzae* infections in patients with a COPD exacerbation caused by infection. Other important bacterial causes include *Streptococcus pneumoniae*, *Moraxella catarrhalis*, and *Pseudomonas aeruginosum*. Hospital admission must be considered in COPD with an exacerbation if they have marked increase in symptoms, failure to respond to outpatient treatment, confusion, lethargy and coma, worsening oxygenation, or development of respiratory acidosis. Oxygen therapy is usually required in a hospitalized patient with an acute exacerbation of COPD; but this may lead to CO_2 retention and acidosis, which in turn could lead to either noninvasive mechanical ventilation, or mechanical ventilation depending on the cause of the exacerbation and the patient's wishes. Hospital mortality for patients with COPD admitted for an acute exacerbation is approximately 10%. Antibiotics, oral prednisone (40-60 mg/day for 5-10 days), and noninvasive positive pressure ventilation have been shown to reduce treatment failure, relapse, and length of hospital stay in patients hospitalized with acute exacerbation of COPD. Ventilator associated pneumonia is also an important risk in a COPD patient treated with invasive mechanical ventilation.

The primary objectives of mechanical ventilatory support in patients with acute exacerbations of severe COPD are to decrease mortality and morbidity and relieve symptoms. Ventilatory support can be given through an orotracheal or nasotracheal tube or tracheostomy connection, which is referred to as invasive (conventional) mechanical ventilation and is particularly suitable in severe acute exacerbations occurring in patients with end-stage disease. Ventilatory support can also be given through a noninvasive means using either negative or positive pressure devices. Fewer complications occur with noninvasive ventilation, but many patients presenting with severe exacerbations of COPD, including respiratory acidosis, may not be candidates for noninvasive ventilation. Noninvasive positive-pressure ventilation (NPPV) involves using a mechanical ventilator connected by tubing to an interface that allows airflow into the nose or the nose and mouth by using a mask or a mouthpiece. Head straps are used to secure the mask tightly to the patient. NPPV allows ventilation without the use of an endotracheal tube. Use of NPPV in acute respiratory failure has been studied in both uncontrolled and randomized controlled trials. The studies show consistently positive results with success rates of 80% to 85%. Taken together they provide evidence that NPPV increases pH, reduces $PaCO_2$, reduces the severity of breathlessness in the first 4 hours of treatment, and decreases the length of hospital stay. More importantly, mortality and intubation rates are reduced by this intervention. However, NPPV is not appropriate for all patients

---

*Investigational drug in the United States.
[1]Not FDA approved for this indication.
[3]Exceeds dosage recommended by the manufacturer.

and invasive mechanical ventilation may still be needed to maximize arterial blood gases values. NPPV can be delivered by different types of ventilators: volume-controlled, pressure-controlled, bilevel positive airway pressure, or continuous positive airway pressure. The use of NPPV together with long-term oxygen therapy has been shown to result in a significant improvement in daytime arterial blood gases, total sleep time, sleep efficiency, quality of life, and overnight $PaCO_2$.

Other treatments that can be useful in COPD patients who must be hospitalized include fluid administration as needed to keep the patient normovolemic; nutrition supplementation as needed with careful attention to the amount of carbohydrates given because excessive amounts can increase CO_2 production; and the use of low molecular weight heparin in immobilized patients with or without a history of thromboembolic disease. Manual or mechanical chest percussion and postural drainage may also be beneficial in patients producing greater than 25 mL sputum per day or those with lobar atelectasis.

Surgical Options

Surgical treatments of COPD include bullectomy, lung volume reduction surgery, and lung transplantation. In carefully selected patients, bullectomy can be effective in reducing dyspnea and improving lung function. A thoracic CT scan, arterial blood gases measurement and comprehensive respiratory function tests are essential before making a decision regarding a patient's suitability for resection of a bulla. Specific large bullae may be removed if they are compressing significant amounts of normal lung tissue.

Lung volume reduction surgery (LVRS) is another option for COPD patients and involves removing 20% to 30% of the upper lobes to improve airway mechanics and increase FEV_1. The National Emphysema Treatment Trial (NETT) study was a randomized controlled trial in 1218 patients with severe emphysema who received either LVRS or medical therapy. The results showed no overall survival benefit with LVRS compared with medical therapy, but improved exercise capacity and quality of life. The best outcome of this surgery was in patients with predominantly upper lobe emphysema and initial low exercise capacity. The surgery was prohibitive in patients with an FEV_1 of up to 20% and either a homogeneous distribution of emphysema or a concomitant diffusing capacity of lung for carbon monoxide (DL_{CO}) of up to 20%.

In appropriately selected patients with very advanced COPD, lung transplantation has been shown to improve quality of life and functional capacity. The average 5-year survival rate is approximately 50% when performed by highly skilled medical or surgical teams that specialize in lung transplantation. Appropriate criteria for lung transplantation referral include FEV_1 of up to 25% of predicted, $PaCO_2$ greater than 55 mm Hg, PaO_2 less than 50-60 mm Hg on room air, or the presence of secondary pulmonary hypertension.

Cystic Fibrosis

Method of
Robert Giusti, MD

Cystic fibrosis (CF), an autosomal recessive disease, is the most common lethal inherited disease in the white population. In this population the carrier rate is approximately 1 in 30, with an incidence of 1 in 3200 births. CF also occurs in African Americans (1 in 15,000), Hispanic Americans (1 in 8000) and Asian Americans (1 in 31,000), but diagnosis may be delayed because of a low index of suspicion in these ethnic groups. Lung disease is the primary cause of morbidity and mortality in CF. Progressive fibrosis and destruction of lung tissue from chronic cycles of infection and inflammation lead to respiratory failure. The median survival for CF patients is 36.5 years.

Pathophysiology

The defect that results in CF is an abnormal gene located on the long arm of chromosome 7 that codes for a protein known as the cystic fibrosis transmembrane regulator (CFTR). This protein becomes incorporated into the lipid bilayer of the epithelial surface of the cell and functions as a chloride channel. Defective cyclic adenosine monophosphate (cAMP)-regulated chloride secretion through a mutated CFTR protein results in dehydrated airway surface fluid, which impedes the normal ciliary function, resulting in chronic infection and atelectasis. In addition, CFTR also down-regulates an epithelial sodium channel (ENaC). When CFTR is defective, this down-regulation is diminished, resulting in increased sodium reabsorption and a further reduction in airway surface fluid. The *CFTR* gene is expressed in the biliary ducts, vas deferens, pancreatic ducts, sweat glands, and the mucous glands of the lung.

More than 1500 specific mutations have been discovered in the CF gene, and the functional consequences of these mutations at the cellular level have been classified into five types. Clinical features correlate with the amount of CFTR activity at the epithelial surface. As the amount of residual CFTR declines, more organ systems are involved. Classes I, II, and III mutations result from abnormal protein production, trafficking through the cell, and regulation at the apical cell surface. These mutations result in 1% CFTR activity and are associated with more severe disease, worse pulmonary function, and pancreatic insufficient (PI) phenotype. The ΔF508 mutation, the most common mutation affecting 70% of CF mutations in the U.S. population, results from the deletion of a phenylalanine at amino acid position 508. In the presence of two copies of this mutation, a patient manifests a PI phenotype.

In Classes IV and V mutations, CFTR is present on the apical surface but chloride channel conduction is defective, resulting in 5% residual CFTR activity and the pancreatic sufficient (PS) phenotype. In the PS phenotype, respiratory symptoms might not present until adulthood, and sufficient pancreatic function is maintained to prevent malabsorption. Because PS patients have residual pancreatic function, there is adequate pancreatic tissue to become inflamed, and these patients might present with recurrent pancreatitis. Residual CFTR function is also manifested in the sweat gland, with sweat tests in the borderline range (40-60 mEq/L). The presence of a class IV or V mutation with a Δ508 mutation results in a PS phenotype.

At the end of intron 8, a noncoding region of the *CFTR* gene, a stretch of 5, 7, or 9 thymidine residues is found, designated the 5T, 7T, or 9T allele. A lower number of thymidines results in less efficient splicing of CFTR transcripts and therefore a lower amount of functional CFTR protein. The 5T allele has been classified as a mutation causing mild disease with partial penetrance. The 5T polymorphism is found on about 21% of the *CFTR* genes derived from patients with congenital bilateral absence of the vas deferens (CBAVD). In CBAVD there is 10% CFTR activity, which is sufficient to have obstructive azoospermia as the only clinical manifestation (Box 1).

Clinical Presentation

GASTROINTESTINAL

About 15% of infants present with meconium ileus, obstruction of the distal ileum with thickened viscid meconium. Prenatal ultrasound might detect echogenic bowel, which suggests CF. Infants present shortly after birth with feeding intolerance and a distended abdomen that requires surgical intervention. Colostomies are placed to permit irrigation to dilate the underdeveloped microcolon, and resection of the terminal ileum is sometimes required. In utero perforation of the bowel can occur, manifesting with calcifications on abdominal x-ray.

The distal intestinal obstruction syndrome (DIOS) is an intestinal obstruction seen in older CF patients. It manifests with abdominal pain, constipation, and a palpable mass in the right lower quadrant consisting of viscous mucus and undigested fecal material that causes obstruction at the ileocecal valve. This can predispose to intussusception. The obstruction is treated by oral or nasogastric

> **BOX 1 Differentiating Between Criteria of CFTR Genotypes**
>
> **Pancreatic Insufficient**
>
> Class I, II, or III mutation
> 1% CFTR activity
> Absent or minimal chloride channel function
> Elevated sweat chloride > 60 mmol/L
> Classic early presentation (50% diagnosed by 6 months of age)
> Median survival is 36.5 years
> Patients require pancreatic enzymes
> Fecal pancreatic elastase-1 <100 µg/g
> Atrophic scarred pancreas
> Risk of diabetes mellitus increases with age
>
> **Pancreatic Sufficient**
>
> Class IV or V mutation
> 5% CFTR activity
> Some chloride channel function
> Borderline or mildly elevated sweat chloride (40-60 mmol/L)
> Atypical late presentation (sometimes in adulthood)
> Survival to 50 years is not uncommon
> No enzyme requirement
> Fecal pancreatic elastase-1 >100 µg/g
> Adequate functional pancreatic tissue to develop recurrent pancreatitis
> Lower risk of diabetes mellitus
>
> CFTR = cystic fibrosis transmembrane regulator (protein).

administration of polyethylene glycol and electrolytes (GoLYTELY),[1] an osmotic agent, which causes water to be retained in the intestine, inducing diarrhea. Rectal prolapse and the meconium plug syndrome, in which there is delayed passage of meconium in the newborn period, are additional reasons for referring a child for a sweat test.

Infants might also present with prolonged obstructive jaundice, which can progress to hepatic steatosis, complete biliary obstruction, and acholic stools. In the biliary tree, sludging of bile due to inadequate chloride and fluid transfer into the bile canaliculus can result in focal biliary cirrhosis and cholethiasis. Approximately 2% of patients progress to multilobular cirrhosis with portal hypertension, hypersplenism, and esophageal varices. Progression to liver failure and the need for transplantation is a possibility. Ursodeoxycholic acid (Actigall),[1] a cholorectic bile acid that increases the flow of bile, has been shown to lower hepatic enzymes and delay the progression of liver disease.

Chloride channel dysfunction in the pancreas results in thickened secretions within the pancreatic ducts and obstruction to the flow of pancreatic chyle. Approximately 85% of patients with CF develop exocrine pancreatic insufficiency. The inadequate production of pancreatic lipase and amylase results in fat and protein malabsorption, steatorrhea, failure to thrive, hypoalbuminemia, and edema. The buffering capacity of pancreatic chyle is diminished, resulting in decreased effectiveness of pancreatic enzyme replacement therapy, which is optimally effective at a neutral pH.

The 72-hour recording of dietary intake and stool collection for quantitative determination of fecal fat content is inconvenient and prone to collection errors in the nonresearch setting. The pancreatic enzyme elastase-1 is stable during intestinal transit and is not affected by porcine pancreatic replacement therapy. The measurement of fecal elastase-1 in stool has been found to be a less cumbersome and a sensitive assay to assess pancreatic function. This can be performed on a small specimen and does not require a timed collection.

Treatment with pancreatic enzyme replacement (pancrelipase [Creon, Pancrease] improves linear growth and weight gain. The recommended dose per meal is 1000 to 2500 U/kg/dose. A high-fat diet is recommended to increase caloric intake to 150 kcal/kg of body weight, which is necessary to ensure optimal growth. The report of the Cystic Fibrosis Foundation Patient Registry indicates that 14% of CF patients are below the 5th percentile for height and 22% are below the 10th percentile for weight. Becausee nutritional failure as measured by body mass index (BMI) has been shown to be a predictor of progressive pulmonary deterioration, aggressive use of nutritional supplementation and nighttime gastrostomy feeds are advocated to improve the quality of life and lung function. Supplementation of fat-soluble vitamins is necessary to prevent nutritional deficiency.

Because CF patients are living longer, progressive fibrosis of the pancreas results in an increased incidence of diabetes, which is seen in 15% of CF patients. Annual glucose tolerance testing has become the standard of care in adolescents and adults to diagnose glucose intolerance before the onset of diabetes, which has been found to result in deterioration of lung function. Respiratory infection and steroid therapy can result in hyperglycemia, leading to a need for insulin before the patient develops frank diabetes. Because there are reductions of both insulin and glucagon, ketoacidosis is rare.

Infants with CF lose a great deal of salt in their sweat and can develop hyponatremic dehydration, heat prostration, and hypochloremic alkalosis. Salt supplementation is the norm, especially during warm summer months.

PULMONARY

The lungs in CF are normal at birth. In young CF patients *Staphylococcus aureus* and *Haemophilus influenzae* are common early colonizers, but as patients age, *Pseudomonas aeruginosa* becomes the predominant organism and is present in the sputum of 80% of adults. *P. aeruginosa* undergoes a mucoid transformation, which interferes with the effectiveness of antibiotic therapy. Because the acquisition of *P. aeruginosa* has been correlated with a more rapid deterioration of lung function and decreased survival, aggressive antibiotic therapy is initiated when this organism is isolated to prevent chronic colonization of the airway.

Burkholderia cepacia, an organism that is intrinsically resistant to a broad range of antibiotics, has been associated with poorer lung function. Nine genetically distinct species, known as genomovars, make up the *B. cepacia* complex. *Burkholderia cenocepacia* and *Burkholderia multivorans* are most commonly isolated from CF patients. The transmission of these organisms and other multiply resistant gram-negative bacteria from person to person in CF clinics and summer camps has resulted in strict infection-control guidelines.

A chronic cough, recurrent chest infections, purulent sputum, digital clubbing, chronic sinusitis, and nasal polyps are common presenting symptoms in CF. The incidence of recurrent pneumothorax is increased in CF, and chemical pleurodesis or pleurectomy are often required. Massive hemoptysis and recurrent episodes of hemoptysis are often a result of collateral bronchial arteries that can require embolization. CF patients often have opacification of the sinuses and nasal polyposis (Box 2).

Diagnosis

Sweat testing remains the standard for making the diagnosis of CF. The elevation of the chloride results from CFTR chloride channel dysfunction in the sweat ducts, where reabsorption of chloride occurs. Pilocarpine is iontophoresized into the skin to stimulate sweating. A chloride level greater than 60 mEq/L is consistent with the diagnosis of CF, but the result must be interpreted in the context of the clinical picture. The borderline range for sweat chloride is 40 to 60 mEq/L. Additional testing is necessary to confirm the diagnosis when the sweat test is in the borderline range. False-positive sweat test

---
[1]Not FDA approved for this indication.

BOX 2 Clinical Presentation of Cystic Fibrosis

Gastrointesinal
Failure to thrive
Malabsorption
Meconium ileus
Meconium plug syndrome
Rectal prolapse
Recurrent pancreatitis
Steatorrhea

Pulmonary
Bronchiectasis
Chronic cough
Chronic sinusitis
Digital clubbing
Nasal polyps
Purulent bronchitis
Recurrent and persistent pneumonia

Other
Growth failure
Hyponatremia and dehydration
Male infertility

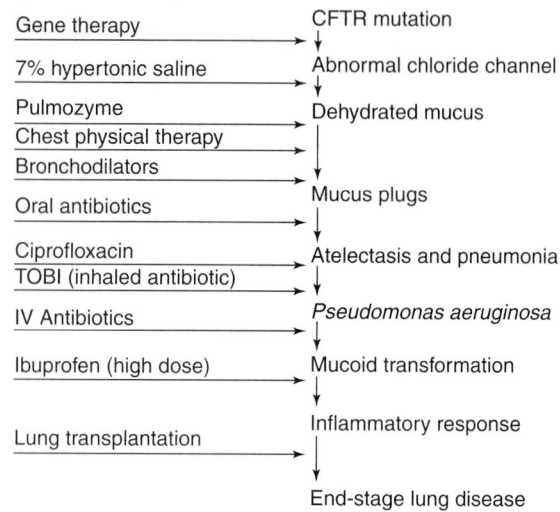

FIGURE 1. Therapeutic interventions for cystic fibrosis lung disease.

results can occur with malnutrition, Addison's disease, and ectodermal dysplasia, so it is essential to confirm the diagnosis with a confirmatory sweat test or a genetic analysis, or both. Sweat tests can be performed after 2 weeks of age or when an infant weighs about 8 lbs (3.6 kg), at which time a sufficient quantity of sweat can be collected to ensure a proper analysis.

Genetic analysis for mutations known to cause CF symptoms is an alternative diagnostic approach. The presence of two abnormal CFTR mutations known to cause CF disease predicts with a high degree of certainty that a patient has CF. Prenatal screening is recommended by the American College of Obstetrics and Gynecology for pregnant white women. When both parents are found to be carriers, amniocentesis and chorionic villous sampling can be used to assess the 25% chance of having an infant affected by CF.

The active transport of ions generates a transepithelial electrical potential difference (PD). Abnormalities of ion transport in respiratory in patients with CF are associated with a different pattern of PD compared with normal epithelium. This assay thus provides a direct view of the physiology at the ion channel level. Nasal PD measurements help to resolve diagnostic dilemmas in atypical patients.

Three features distinguish the nasal PD in a patient with CF. A high basal PD reflects enhanced sodium transport across a relatively chloride impermeable membrane. A larger inhibition of PD after nasal perfusion with the sodium channel inhibitor amilorlide reflects inhibition of accelerated sodium transport. Little or no change in PD in response to perfusion of the nasal epithelial surface with a chloride-free solution in conjunction with isoproterenol reflects an absence of CFTR-mediated chloride secretion.

Newborn screening for CF has been shown to improve nutritional and neurodevelopmental outcomes. Trypsinogen, a precursor of trypsin, is commonly elevated in the serum of newborns with CF because of in utero obstruction of pancreatic ducts. Infants with CF have elevated immunoreactive trypsinogen (IRT) levels for 2 to 3 weeks after birth. When the IRT is elevated in a blood specimen collected shortly after birth, then an analysis for the presence of CF mutations on the same blood specimen or a persistent elevation of IRT at 2 to 3 weeks of age in a repeat blood specimen are two different methods to determine which infants should be referred for sweat testing. Mutation analysis performed during newborn screening detects carriers of CF mutations, and genetic counseling for these families is warranted to permit informed decisions concerning future pregnancies.

Treatment

Therapeutic interventions are shown in Figure 1.

GENE THERAPY

The goal of gene therapy is to correct the basic defect by inserting a normal functioning gene into the ciliated cells in the submucous glands that express abnormal CFTR function. Initial attempts using the adenovirus as the vehicle for transporting the gene into the cells lining the airway appeared promising; however, the host immune response to the virus has limited the effectiveness of this approach. The ideal vector would efficiently deliver the gene to the appropriate target cell without causing toxicity or an inflammatory response. Although gene therapy offers the potential to correct the basic defect of CF, many technical barriers to effective gene therapy need to be addressed to permit this form of therapy to become an effective treatment.

HYDRATION OF AIRWAY SURFACE FLUID

Hypertonic saline, at a 7% concentration,[6] has been shown to increase the hydration of the airway surface fluid and reduce the frequency of pulmonary exacerbations. This recent addition to the therapeutic treatment regimen has been shown to facilitate the clearance of airway mucus, resulting in improved pulmonary function, and to decrease the frequency of pulmonary exacerbations. Hypertonic saline induces coughing and bronchospasm and is administered following bronchodilator therapy.

PHYSICAL THERAPY

Airway clearance can be performed using various techniques, including conventional percussion therapy, pneumatically inflated chest vest percussion device, oscillating positive pressure devices such as the Flutter or Acapella, autogenic drainage, and exercise. These techniques are recommended on a daily basis to help mobilize secretions and prevent the complications related to persistent accumulation of airway mucus.

BRONCHODILATORS

Airway hyperreactivity is present in 50% to 60% of CF patients. β-Agonists keep airways open and facilitate airway clearance by increasing ciliary beat frequency and smooth muscle relaxation. The spirometric response to β-agonists should be monitored because with worsening bronchiectasis and the development of floppy airways,

---

[6]May be compounded by pharmacists.

airflow may be impaired. Because anticholinergics alter viscosity of mucus and can have an adverse effect on gastrointestinal motility, this class of bronchodilator has not been recommended for routine use in CF by a consensus conference of the Cystic Fibrosis Foundation.

ANTIBIOTICS

Aggressive use of antibiotics for the chronic bacterial colonization of the airways in CF has resulted in improving longevity and quality of life. Prophylactic inhaled antibiotics have been effective in CF patients to decrease the bacterial burden in the CF airway. Alternate-month therapy with a 300-mg aerosol preparation of tobramycin (TOBI) improves lung function, delays the time to the onset of pulmonary exacerbation, and decreases the need for hospitalization. A preparation of aztreonam (Azactam) for inhalation,[1,6] which is administered by a very efficient portable nebulizer (eFlow), appears to be promising but has not yet been approved by the FDA.

Pulmonary exacerbations are characterized by an increased cough, copious purulent sputum, decreased appetite, weight loss, and decreased exercise tolerance. Quinolone antibiotics are effective for treating *P. aeruginosa* in an oral preparation, but the development of resistance to this class of drug is a limiting factor. Ciprofloxacin (Cipro) is not approved by the FDA for use in children, but there is considerable experience with this drug in children with CF. When oral and inhaled antibiotics are not effective, hospitalization for aggressive airway clearance and a 10- to 14-day course of IV antibiotics is indicated. A combination of two drugs (usually an aminoglycoside and a β-lactam semisynthetic penicillin or a cephalosporin) is selected based on susceptibility of the organism recovered by culture of sputum or a deep throat swab. In young children who are not able to produce sputum, bronchoscopy is employed to obtain a specimen for culture.

MUCOLYTIC THERAPY

DNase (Pulmozyme) is a nebulized mucolytic agent that cleaves neutrophil-derived DNA that contributes to the thick airway secretions that clog the CF airways. Daily inhalation therapy (2.5 mg) reduces sputum viscosity, facilitating airway clearance and resulting in a 5% improvement in lung function. This therapy has largely replaced treatment with *N*-acetylcysteine (Mucomyst),[1] which causes bronchial irritation.

ANTIINFLAMMATORY THERAPY

There has been growing awareness of the role of the host inflammatory response in the progression of CF lung disease. Chronic endobronchial colonization with bacteria results in the release of proinflammatory mediators interleukin (IL)-8 and nuclear factor (NF)-κB. These mediators recruit neutrophils into the airway; the neutrophils release elastase, protease, superoxide ions, and hydroxyl radicals, which damage lung tissue and contribute to the development of bronchiectasis.

Corticosteroids

Alternate day-systemic steroids were studied in a multicenter placebo-controlled study as a therapeutic intervention to decrease the inflammatory response in the CF airway. Significant risks of growth impairment, diabetes, and cataracts were found. Although inhaled steroids are commonly prescribed for CF patients, there is no double-blind study to demonstrate benefit of long-term therapy in CF patients who do not have a component of asthma.

Nonsteroidal Antiinflammatory Drugs

Oral administration of twice-daily high-dose ibuprofen[1] (20-30 mg/kg)[3] to achieve peak plasma concentration of 50 to 100 µg/mL interferes with neutrophil migration and inhibits the activation of NF-κB.

Konstan studied 85 CF patients and found that ibuprofen therapy results in less decline in lung function, fewer hospitalizations, and improved weight gain. This effect is most pronounced in patients who are younger than 13 years and have minimal lung disease. Although prolonged use of this therapy has been shown to have ongoing benefit, the risk of GI side effects has limited the implementation of this therapy by most CF patients.

Macrolide antibiotics (azithromycin [Zithromax])[1] are not considered effective in the treatment of infection with *P. aeruginosa*, but a number of clinical trials have demonstrated a modest improvement in lung function and a decrease in the frequency of infectious exacerbations and need for antibiotic therapy in CF patients chronically colonized with *P. aeruginosa*. The mechanisms of action are not well understood but are believed to be related to a number of antiinflammatory and immunomodulatory effects of this class of antibiotic. The expression of *P. aeruginosa* pathogenicity factors and neutrophil recruitment appear to be altered by chronic macrolide therapy.

Oxygen therapy to correct alveolar hypoxia is effective to prevent pulmonary hypertension in CF patients with severe lung disease. Pulmonary hypertension results from pulmonary vascular remodeling, which results in increased pulmonary vascular resistance. Cor pulmonale contributes to the morbidity of CF with right heart failure, progressive exercise intolerance, and risk of syncope.

LUNG TRANSPLANTATION

Approximately 150 patients receive bilateral cadaveric lung transplants per year. Evaluation at a lung transplant center is considered when progressive deterioration in lung function results in a forced expiratory volume in one second (FEV_1) less than 30% predicted. Survival rates in CF lung-transplant recipients are comparable with other groups of patients. The availability of donor organs continues to be a limiting factor, and the disparity between donor availability and a growing recipient pool has progressively lengthened the waiting time for organs and has increased the mortality for patients awaiting lung transplantation. Living-donor lobar transplantation, which involves removal of both diseased lungs from the recipient and the implantation of two lower lobes donated by two donors, is an alternative for CF patients awaiting lung transplantation.

REFERENCES

http://www.genet.sickkids.on.ca/cftr/app

Cystic Fibrosis Foundation: Cystic Fibrosis Foundation Patient Registry, 2005 Annual Data Report to the Center Directors. Bethesda Md: Cystic Fibrosis Foundation, 2006.

Solomon MP, Wilson DC, Corey M, et al: Glucose intolerance in children with cystic fibrosis. J Pediatr 2003;142:128-132.

Konstan MW, Byard PJ, Hoppel CL, Davis PB: Effect of high-dose ibuprofen in patients with cystic fibrosis. N Engl J Med 1995;332(13):848-854.

Sleep Apnea

Method of
Leon Rosenthal, MD

Obstructive sleep apnea (OSA) is a condition characterized by repetitive episodes of obstruction of the upper airway during sleep. The obstructions may be complete (apnea) or partial (hypopnea), and they result in fluctuations in blood oxygen saturation and disruption of sleep continuity.

By definition, apneic and hypopneic events last a minimum of 10 seconds. The apnea-hypopnea index (AHI) is defined as the total number of apneas and hypopneas during the time asleep divided by the number of hours of sleep. Respiratory effort—related arousal (RERA) is

---

[1]Not FDA approved for this indication.
[3]Exceeds dosage recommended by the manufacturer.
[6]May be compounded by pharmacists.

considered an additional type of sleep-related obstructive event. It presents a risk factor for the behavioral morbidity associated with OSA that is as great as those of obstructive apneas and hypopneas. RERAs also by definition last 10 seconds (or longer), reflect a sequence of breaths characterized by increasing respiratory effort, are not associated with oxygen fluctuations, and lead to an arousal from sleep.

In the adult population, the current classification of sleep disorders requires polysomnographic documentation of five or more obstructive respiratory events (obstructive apneas, hypopneas, or RERAs) per hour of sleep to diagnose OSA. To date, the diagnosis is established based on the sleep laboratory assessment using standard polysomnographic techniques. OSA should be suspected based on the clinical assessment, physical examination, and understanding of potential risk factors.

Epidemiology

The prevalence of OSA (defined as an apnea-hypopnea index of >5/hour) among adults between 30 and 60 years of age has been estimated at 9% for women and 24% for men. The prevalence of the OSA syndrome, which includes symptoms of excessive sleepiness, is estimated at 2% for women and 4% for men. Clearly, male gender represents an independent risk factor for OSA when compared with premenopausal women. The prevalence among women increases with menopause. In regard to ethnicity, African American, Pacific Islander, and Mexican American patients might be at increased risk for OSA.

Clinical Features

Snoring represents the most common feature of OSA and is usually reported by a bed partner. Many patients are prompted by their spouses to pursue consultation after many years of enduring the disruptive effects of snoring during sleep. The description of periods of snoring followed by periods of silence, which are terminated by breakthrough snoring make the diagnosis of OSA very likely. In many instances, the patients are described as experiencing stop-breathing episodes during their sleep.

Affected patients might not be aware of any difficulties during their sleep, but some report persistent nocturnal awakenings; some of the awakenings might be associated with a sensation of choking, smothering, or gasping. Nocturnal perspiration, nocturia, and symptoms of nocturnal gastroesophageal reflux are commonly associated with severe OSA. Patients might report awakening unrefreshed, with a dry mouth, and with a headache. Daytime symptoms are commonly encountered; the most frequent complaint is excessive sleepiness, which is a consequence of disrupted sleep.

Increased risk of motor vehicle accidents has been reported among OSA patients, and assessment of the patient's level of sleepiness in the context of their employment and their exposure to driving or operating machinery needs to be established during the clinical assessment. Associated features of excessive sleepiness may be manifested as fatigue, impaired memory and concentration, depression, and changes in personality. Among male patients, impotence due to low testosterone levels has been established in some severe cases of OSA.

Obesity is common in OSA, and a graded increase in OSA prevalence has been documented with increasing body mass index (BMI), neck circumference, and waist-to-hip ratio. However, a potential diagnosis of OSA should not be dismissed in a nonobese patient presenting with symptoms or having risk factors associated with a potential diagnosis of OSA. Physical findings such as a crowded oropharynx with evidence of a redundant soft palate, redundant soft tissue in the oropharyngeal examination, relative macroglossia, and tonsillar hypertrophy are often encountered among patients with OSA. A narrow oropharynx with a high arched palate and short intermolar distance has also been described among some patients with OSA. Retrognathia or micrognathia might also result in narrowing of the retroglossal area, which might increase the risk of OSA when sleeping in the supine position.

OSA has been shown to represent an independent risk factor for systemic arterial hypertension. Thus, difficult to control hypertension should raise the possibility of a diagnosis of OSA. Untreated OSA might also represent a risk factor for stroke; new-onset atrial fibrillation (in particular if triggered during sleep) should raise the clinical suspicion of OSA. Other medical conditions that appear to predispose to OSA include nasal obstruction, nasal septal deviation, hypothyroidism, acromegaly, and congestive heart failure.

Evidence of a potential link between OSA and insulin resistance (and diabetes mellitus) has been reported. Ongoing research is actively pursuing this pathophysiologic pathway, and the increased prevalence of the metabolic syndrome in the general population makes the clinical suspicion of OSA very relevant in these patients because both conditions share a number of clinical characteristics. In fact, it is conceivable that the increased cardiovascular risk conferred by OSA is, at least in part, mediated through the metabolic syndrome.

Screening and Testing

LABORATORY SLEEP TEST

The definitive diagnosis of OSA requires an in-laboratory attended sleep test (nocturnal polysomnography), which enables the characterization of multiple physiologic variables. Recording of a limited number of channels in the patient's home can be used for screening purposes (ambulatory oximetry or cardio-respiratory studies, which yield estimates of respiratory disturbance). Although in some cases ambulatory studies might render confirmation of the diagnosis, there is no consensus at present as to the ideal algorithm to be followed to allow the diagnosis of OSA without a sleep laboratory assessment. Ongoing research efforts will likely result in the diagnosis and treatment of some OSA populations without the need for in-laboratory testing.

The in-laboratory sleep test allows characterization of ventilation during sleep. Ventilation includes number of central and obstructive apneas, hypopneas, and RERAs and detailed information on oxygen saturation as well as the depiction of the potentially relevant positional effects on the frequency of respiratory events. Laboratory testing also includes a complete accounting of sleep variables, monitoring of cardiac rhythm, and assessment of possible restless legs syndrome (RLS) or periodic limb movements (PLMs) during sleep. This information enables the clinician to determine the severity of the condition and identifies potentially relevant comorbidities (RLS, PLMs, cardiac arrhythmias).

The split-night protocol during the laboratory assessment allows the clinician to derive the diagnosis of the condition during the first half of the night (ideally 4 hours of diagnostic testing with a minimum of 2 hours if an AHI >40 is confirmed). During the second half of the night, the clinician can titrate continuous positive airway pressure (CPAP), which requires a minimum of 3 hours of sleep. This protocol is a cost-effective use of laboratory resources that allows the clinician to identify therapeutic CPAP settings to help implement therapy at home, and in most instances there is no need for a second sleep study. This protocol is particularly well suited for patients with severe OSA. The possible implementation of CPAP titration should be discussed with the patient in advance, because the initial experience with CPAP is a major determinant of long-term use.

Several algorithms are available to make clinical predictions about the likelihood of a positive diagnosis of OSA. In general, an obese patient with a large neck size (≥ 17 in for male patients; ≥ 16.5 in for female patients) and symptoms of excessive sleepiness is likely to be a good candidate for split-night studies. In cases were a diagnostic polysomnography identified a diagnosis of OSA and CPAP is the therapy of choice, a second night in the laboratory for CPAP titration is indicated.

WHOM TO TEST AND THERAPEUTIC OPTIONS

Clinical signs and symptoms are not necessarily sensitive or specific enough to establish a definitive diagnosis of OSA. Therefore, sleep studies are required for patients who are symptomatic and for others who are asymptomatic but have clinical signs that suggest the diagnosis. Testing allows the examiner to define the severity of the condition, and the results (with adequate clinical correlation) should guide therapeutic intervention.

CURRENT DIAGNOSIS

Symptoms and Signs

- Excessive sleepiness
- Resuscitative snoring or loud snoring
- Witnessed stop-breathing episodes
- Nocturia

Risk Factors

- Obesity; large neck circumference (central obesity)
- Sex: men, postmenopausal women
- Age: 30 to 65 years
- Abnormal upper airway (e.g., nasal obstruction, large tongue, redundant soft tissue, large tonsils, retrognathia)
- Family history of obstructive sleep apnea

CURRENT THERAPY

- Continuous positive airway pressure (CPAP) represents the gold standard of therapy.
- Patient education, adequate CPAP settings, and a comfortable interface are critical to achieve a desirable level of treatment adherence.
- Integrated heated humidification minimizes nasal dryness and improves CPAP adherence.
- Clinical follow-up to assess tolerance to CPAP and resolution of symptoms is critical to achieve desired outcomes.
- Improved sleep schedule practices should be encouraged and comorbid conditions should be treated.
- Oral appliance therapy and surgical procedures represent alternative therapeutic options.

Epidemiologic data have helped define the index of severity. An AHI of 5 or higher has been shown to represent the minimum threshold value for increased risk of hypertension and an AHI greater than 30 has been associated with a substantial increase in the risk of hypertension. Thus, mild OSA is defined as an AHI of 5 to 15 per hour, moderate OSA is an AHI of 15 to 30 per hour, and severe OSH is an AHI greater than 30 per hour. In addition, a clinically derived index of severity of excessive sleepiness should be determined based on the presence of unwanted sleepiness or involuntary sleep episodes (mild if the episodes occur during activities that require little attention, moderate if the manifestations are associated with activities that require some attention, and severe if sleepiness is present in activities that require active attention).

Many patients are motivated to pursue treatment because of their desire to eliminate snoring, and others want relief of symptoms of excessive sleepiness. An increasing number of patients understand the potentially negative cardiovascular consequences of untreated OSA and expect therapy if the diagnosis is confirmed. Therapy is justified if the AHI is greater than 5 per hour, and it should not be delayed if the AHI is greater than 30 per hour.

Regardless of the severity of the condition, patients who are overweight should be encouraged to lose weight. In some patients with morbid obesity, bariatric surgery might be a means to enable effective weight loss and likely improvement of ventilation during sleep.

Patients should be counseled to avoid practices that can potentially worsen the severity of OSA. The use of CNS depressants before sleep (alcohol, sleep medications, pain medications) might worsen ventilation during sleep and should be discouraged. In some patients with positional OSA, avoiding the supine position during sleep might suffice in helping normalize ventilation during sleep. However, one needs to question how this can be done effectively over a long time. If upper airway pathology is identified (nasal septum deviation, enlarged tonsils, craniofacial abnormalities), surgical consultation should be pursued. If patients have symptoms of excessive sleepiness, they should be counseled to avoid driving or operating machinery, and the appropriate local laws should be followed regarding the need to notify the relevant administrative authorities.

Treatment

CPAP THERAPY

The proper positive airway pressure delivered by a flow generator through an interface of the patient's choice represents the gold standard in the therapy of OSA, because it is almost always successful in maintaining upper airway patency and oxygen saturation, and it improves sleep continuity and architecture. The main barrier to successful therapy is nonacceptance of the therapy or low therapeutic adherence. Treatment is effective as long as the patient uses the device for the entire night, every night. The use of integrated heated humidifiers has minimized issues of upper airway dryness and has helped improve adherence to therapy.

There are many manufacturers of CPAP devices and many interfaces that help maximize comfort with treatment. The clinician should be aware of the characteristics of the specific CPAP unit that is being prescribed to the patient and should monitor the level of comfort of the interface that the patient has selected. Expiratory pressure release (EPR) is available through a couple of CPAP manufacturers. EPR does not seem to compromise the effectiveness of CPAP therapy and improves the patient's sense of comfort with therapy, but it does not seem to systematically improve the level of adherence.

Autotitrating CPAP units are available, and their software has been greatly improved. They have been proved effective in improving ventilation during sleep, but no additional clinical benefits over standard CPAP therapy have been demonstrated.

Bilevel respiratory assist devices deliver alternating levels of positive airway pressure and might be considered as an alternative therapeutic option when standard CPAP is not tolerated or when oxygen saturation is not raised sufficiently with standard CPAP. In some cases of severe OSA (in particular among patients with underlying pulmonary conditions) supplemental oxygen can be used in conjunction with CPAP therapy.

ORAL APPLIANCE THERAPY

Prostheses worn in the mouth during sleep can help maintain a patent airway. In general, there are two types of appliances, mandibular advancement appliances and tongue-retaining devices. The mandibular advancement appliances are currently used more often and have been more widely studied. They require viable dentition for retention. They are fitted to the maxillary and mandibular dentition to enable the protrusion of the mandible and therefore increase oropharyngeal patency. The most common side effect is excessive salivation, but temporomandibular joint pain might limit the viability of this therapy. Chronic use of the appliance can result in a change of the dental occlusion and lead to discontinuation of therapy. A dentist with expertise in sleep medicine should ideally implement and monitor this type of treatment.

SURGICAL PROCEDURES

Patients with an identifiable anatomic upper airway (soft tissue) abnormality or craniofacial abnormality might benefit from surgery. There are a variety of soft-tissue procedures that might help stabilize the retropalatal region (the uvulopalatopharyngoplasty), and others are intended to stabilize the retrolingual airway (genioglossal advancement and hyoid myotomy). Office-based procedures have also become available, such as the injection snoreplasty and the pillar procedure, which are intended to stiffen the soft palate and thereby decrease snoring and respiratory events. A substantially more invasive procedure, the maxillomandibular advancement, has been shown very effective in a number of case series. However, it is not possible to predict which patients are likely to have a successful surgical outcome. As a result, many patients undergo a surgical procedure that fails to improve their condition and then require additional surgery or medical treatment of OSA. Surgical consultation with an otorhinolaryngologist or oral surgeon should be pursued for patients who might benefit from this therapeutic approach.

RESPONSE TO THERAPY

The patient's response to therapy needs to be monitored. In the case of CPAP therapy, monitoring of CPAP adherence is critical, because subjective reports are inaccurate. Resolution of excessive sleepiness is the desired outcome for patients who are symptomatic at baseline. If excessive sleepiness remains problematic despite documentation of desirable CPAP adherence, treatment with modafinil (Provigil) 100 to 400 mg in the morning might be considered.

Other potential conditions affecting sleep need to be monitored and, if needed, treated. Often, other conditions such as poor sleep hygiene, RLS, PLMs, or psychophysiologic insomnia interfere with adequate response to therapy.

For patients who undergo surgery, retesting is indicated. The interval at which retesting should be done depends on the type of surgery that was performed. Retesting 3 months following the surgical intervention is adequate in most cases.

REFERENCES

Dinges DF, Weaver TE: Effects of modafinil on sustained attention and quality of life in OSA patients with residual sleepiness while being treated with NCPAP. Sleep Med 2003;4:393-402.

Gay P, Weaver T, Loube D, et al: Evaluation of positive airway pressure treatment for sleep related breathing disorders in adults: A review by the positive airway pressure task force of the standards of practice committee of the American Academy of Sleep Medicine. Sleep 2006;29:381-401.

Lindberg E, Gislason T: Epidemiology of sleep-related obstructive breathing. Sleep Med Rev 2000;4:411-433.

Mulgrew AT, Fox N, Ayas NT, et al: Diagnosis and initial management of obstructive sleep apnea without polysomnography: A randomized validation study. Ann Intern Med 2007;146:157-166.

Rosenthal L, Bishop C, Guido P, et al: The sleep/wake habits of patients diagnosed as having obstructive sleep apnea. Chest 1997;111:1494-1499.

Rosenthal L, Gerhardstein R, Lumley A, et al: CPAP therapy in patients with mild OSA: Implementation and treatment outcome. Sleep Med 2000;3:215-220.

Sanders M, Givelber R: Overview of obstructive sleep apnea in adults. In Lee-Chiong TF (ed): Sleep: A Comprehensive Handbook, Hoboken, NJ: John Wiley and Sons, 2006, pp 231-240.

Senior B, Rosenthal L, Lumley A, Gerhardstein R, Day R: Efficacy of uvulopalatopharyngoplasty in unselected patients with mild obstructive sleep apnea. Otolaryngol Head Neck Surg 2000;123(3):179-182.

Sleep-related breathing disorders in adults: Recommendations for syndrome definition and measurement techniques in clinical research: The report of an American Academy of Sleep Medicine task force. Sleep 1999;22:667-689.

Lung Cancer

Method of
Gregory A. Otterson, MD

Epidemiology

Lung cancer is the leading cause of cancer death worldwide. In the United States, lung cancer represents about 13% of cancer diagnoses, but it causes a disproportionate 29% of cancer deaths. The American Cancer Society estimated that more than 160,000 patients died from lung cancer in 2007. These facts are all the more sobering when one recognizes that the vast majority of these cases are preventable in that 85% to 90% of lung cancers are directly attributable to smoking. The lung cancer epidemic in the United States directly mirrors the rise of smoking incidence in this country, albeit with a 20- to 30-year lag period.

Landmark epidemiologic studies in the 1950s demonstrated the link between cigarette smoking and lung cancer and led to the declaration by the U.S. Surgeon General in 1964 that smoking was a direct cause of lung and other cancers. Impressively, there has been a dramatic decrease in smoking incidence from the 1960s until the 1990s (from nearly 50% to 25% of Americans who smoke regularly). Unfortunately, this decrease has stabilized since the 1990s, and greater reductions in smoking incidence will require a concerted effort. Fortunately, the decrease in smoking has led to decreases in the incidence of and death rates from lung cancer in American men (again after a lag period of 30 years or longer).

Another sobering thought is that although there has been progress in decreasing smoking in developed countries, there has been a dramatic increase in smoking in less-developed countries, particularly in Asia. With history as a guide, one would surmise that the next wave of the lung cancer epidemic will occur in these countries.

Although smoking cigarettes (and cigars) is the greatest cause of lung cancer, approximately 10% to 15% of patients with lung cancer have never smoked. For an individual patient, the exact carcinogen is impossible to delineate, but it is thought that second-hand smoke, asbestos, radon, and other carcinogens cause the remainder of cases. Molecular evidence has recently suggested that although these cancers look pathologically similar, they likely represent a distinct disease with different treatment options and distinct prognoses.

Screening

Of the four major causes of cancer death in the United States (lung, colorectal, prostate, and breast), lung cancer is the only one without a widely used screening program. Although there is controversy about the proper timing and form of colorectal, prostate, or breast cancer screening, all public health and cancer-related advocacy groups recommend screening for these tumors. Why has no one recommended lung cancer screening?

In the 1970s, three influential screening trials in the United States suggested that screening of high-risk patients with chest radiography or sputum cytology was ineffective at decreasing lung cancer mortality. Little more was done until the 1990s. It was then recognized that there were serious concerns about the earlier studies, principally that they were underpowered to detect a realistic difference between screened and unscreened groups. Because of these concerns, the National Cancer Institute (NCI) launched a large-scale screening trial in the early 1990s called PLCO (for prostate, lung, colorectal, and ovarian), wherein 150,000 subjects at risk were randomized to screened and unscreened cohorts. The lung portion of the trial includes smokers or ex-smokers, and the screening tool is a posteroanterior chest x-ray performed annually for 5 years, compared with standard of care (chest x-ray for symptoms). Accrual is completed, and the primary outcome to be evaluated is lung cancer mortality rates in the screened and unscreened groups.

In 1999, a pivotal study from the Early Lung Cancer Action Project (ELCAP) hypothesized that annual low-dose computed tomography (CT) scans could detect early lung cancers and improve the survival of screened patients. This study has been updated and internationalized, with more than 31,000 subjects screened, and the answer is clear that spiral CT scans can detect more and earlier lung cancers than posteroanterior chest x-ray. In addition, most of the cancers detected by spiral CT are early stage, and the 5- and 10-year survival rates from these cancers appear excellent.

Despite this result, the American Cancer Society, the NCI, and other groups do not recommend spiral CT for smokers or ex-smokers. Why? A couple of issues remain unanswered. The survival from the single-arm studies of spiral CT screening appears excellent (patients with lung cancer diagnosed at an early stage are much more likely to survive 5 or 10 years than those with late stage, symptomatic cancer), it remains unclear if lung cancer mortality in the screened group will be superior to that in unscreened persons. Despite the apparently excellent results in the International ELCAP study, the study was uncontrolled, and concerns regarding lead time, length, and overdiagnosis bias remain.

The only way to successfully address these concerns is to perform a randomized trial comparing spiral CT screening with either no screening or annual chest x-ray. The NCI is performing such a study, the National Lung Screening Trial, with an endpoint of lung cancer mortality. Fifty thousand at-risk subjects have been enrolled, and early results are expected by 2010. Until then, most groups do not routinely recommend screening for asymptomatic smokers or ex-smokers.

Clinical Presentation

The clinical presentation of patients with lung cancer can be thought of in four categories related to local, regional, or metastatic disease or to paraneoplastic syndromes. The most common local symptoms are those related to the lungs: dyspnea, cough, hemoptysis, recurrent pneumonias, and chest pain. Unfortunately, these symptoms are often already present in patients with chronic obstructive pulmonary disease (COPD) and are often ignored until they cause significant morbidity. Regional symptoms are those related to critical structures close to the thoracic cavity: chest wall invasion, esophageal impingement (difficulty swallowing), and involvement of nerves such as the cervical plexus (Horner's syndrome), recurrent laryngeal nerve, brachial plexus, or phrenic nerve. Metastatic involvement can lead to a variety of symptoms depending on the organ involved. Although lung cancer can metastasize to any organ, common sites include bone, lung, liver, adrenal gland, and brain.

Paraneoplastic syndromes are distant effects of cancer not related to metastatic involvement. Paraneoplastic syndromes are mediated either immunologically or through hormone overproduction. Immunologic paraneoplastic syndromes seen in lung cancer include a variety of neurologic syndromes such as Eaton–Lambert syndrome (antibodies directed against the presynaptic motor neuron endplate), cerebellar ataxia, and sensory neuropathy. The neurologic syndromes are most commonly seen in small cell lung cancer and are presumably related to antigens recognized on the neuroendocrine tumor cells that cross-react with neural antigens. The endocrine abnormalities include the syndrome of inappropriate antidiuretic hormone secretion (SIADH) with hyponatremia, Cushing's syndrome from adrenocorticotropic hormone (ACTH) secretion, and hypercalcemia from parathyroid related peptide (PTHrp) secretion. All paraneoplastic syndromes tend to be more severe or more common in patients with more advanced disease. Although the endocrine syndromes tend to respond to therapy directed against the tumor, the neurologic syndromes do not.

Pathology

Lung cancer is divided into two categories, small cell lung cancer (SCLC) and non–small cell lung cancer (NSCLC).

SCLC represents about 15% of all lung cancers, behaves differently clinically, and appears distinct on hematoxylin and eosin (H&E) staining, with small to medium cells, high nuclear-to-cytoplasmic ratio, nuclear molding (i.e., conforming to the shape of the cell), and finely stippled nuclear chromatin (salt-and-pepper nucleus). SCLC is often defined as a poorly differentiated neuroendocrine carcinoma. The critical recognition is that SCLC is a poorly differentiated cancer and that other neuroendocrine cancers may be well differentiated (carcinoid tumors) or intermediately differentiated, with distinct treatment and prognostic issues.

NSCLC represents the majority of lung cancers. The most common varieties are adenocarcinomas (~40%), squamous carcinomas (~30%) and large cell carcinomas with or without neuroendocrine differentiation. The ratio of different histologic entities has subtly changed over the last half century, with a decreasing proportion of SCLC and squamous carcinomas and an increasing incidence of adenocarcinomas.

With the widespread incorporation of immunohistochemical staining as a routine test in clinical pathology laboratories, a number of common special stains have been developed to differentiate particular forms of lung cancer and to distinguish adenocarcinomas of the lung from adenocarcinomas derived from other organs. The most common stains performed include the cytokeratins (CKs), and particularly CK7 and CK20. Typically, CK7 is positive in lung cancer and CK20 is negative. In contrast, gastrointestinal tract cancers are typically CK20 positive and CK7 negative. An additional marker often positive in lung cancers is the thyroid transcription factor 1 (TTF1). The most commonly used neuroendocrine markers are chromogranin and synaptophysin. As suggested earlier, however, the diagnosis of a neuroendocrine cancer in the lung (positive chromogranin or synaptophysin staining) does not mean that the cancer is an SCLC. This determination is best made by the pathologist evaluating the H&E stain for the level of differentiation.

Newer technologies have allowed investigators to develop signatures of expressed genes that are specific for particular cancers. The most commonly used to date is expression profiling of RNA. In this technique, RNA from tumor can be labeled and the relative expression of nearly every gene in the body can be ascertained quickly and reproducibly such that the patterns derived from one sample can be compared with those from a different sample. For example, a number of laboratories have demonstrated that squamous carcinoma has an expression pattern that is distinct from that of adenocarcinoma. Similarly, adenocarcinoma derived from the lung has an expression pattern distinct from that of adenocarcinoma derived from other organs.

RNA expression patterns can have both prognostic and potentially predictive impact. To clarify the distinction, prognostic factors determine if someone is going to do well or poorly; in contrast, predictive factors, if present, suggest that a cancer will respond to a particular manipulation. A common prognostic factor is tumor differentiation, and the best-known predictive factor is estrogen-receptor expression in breast cancer, predicting responsiveness to hormonal manipulations. Molecular prognostic patterns and factors are now the basis of prospective clinical trials, intensifying therapy for those with a poorer prognosis. Similarly, molecular predictive patterns and factors form the basis of trials that assign therapy based on what one would predict to be useful therapy.

Currently available techniques are able to determine if a patient has a mutation within a number of therapeutically relevant genes, including the epidermal growth factor receptor (*EGFR*) and the *ras* oncogene. To perform this testing, however, a larger sample or biopsy is often necessary, and more than a fine-needle aspirate may be required. The therapeutic implications of this testing are discussed later.

Staging and Functional Evaluation

Appropriate treatment of lung cancer depends on proper staging as well as pathologic diagnosis. Because of the intricacies of staging and because treatment is based on stage, evaluation of patients with lung cancer should take place in a multimodality setting where medical oncologists, radiation oncologists, thoracic surgeons, and pulmonologists can all evaluate and discuss pertinent findings regarding a patient.

The staging system for SCLC is very simple and is defined by the ability of a radiation oncologist to incorporate all known areas of disease within a radiation port. If all known areas of disease can be confined within a radiation port, the disease is defined as *limited*; anything not limited is *extensive*. Typically, limited disease is confined to a single hemithorax, and extensive disease includes metastases (typically to bone, brain, liver, adrenal glands) or metastatic disease to pleura or pericardium leading to effusions in either organ.

In contrast to the simplicity of staging for SCLC, NSCLC staging is quite complex, but it can be simplified as local, regional, or

BOX 1 Tumor–Node–Metastasis Definitions

Primary Tumor

T0
No evidence of primary tumor

Tis
Carcinoma in situ

T1
Tumor ≤3 cm in greatest dimension

T2
Tumor 3-5 cm
Tumor involving the main bronchus
Tumor invading the visceral pleura
Tumor associated with atelectasis to the hilar region of less than the entire lung

T3
Tumor of any size invading chest wall, mediastinal pleura, or parietal pericardium
Tumor within 3 cm of the carina
Tumor associated with atelectasis of the entire lung

T4
Tumor of any size invading the mediastinum, great vessels, trachea, esophagus, vertebral body, or main carina
Satellite tumor nodules within the same lobe
Tumor associated with malignant pleural effusion

Node

N0
No regional lymph node involvement

N1
Involvement of ipsilateral bronchial, hilar, or intrapulmonary nodes

N2
Involvement of ipsilateral mediastinal and/or subcarinal nodes

N3
Involvement of contralateral mediastinal or hilar nodes
Involvement of scalene or supraclavicular nodes (either ipsilateral or contralateral)

Metastasis

M0
No distant metastases

M1
Distant metastases

---

metastatic disease. Modification of the staging system for NSCLC is expected in 2009. Box 1 includes the definitions of tumor, node, and metastasis determinations, and Table 1 shows the combination of these that lead to particular stages, with approximate 5-year survival data. In Table 1, note a distinction between dry and wet T4 (stage 3B) tumors. *Wet* refers to the presence of a malignant pleural effusion, which implies inability to deliver curative-intent radiation therapy.

Staging work-up starts with radiographic imaging. CT scanning of the chest (through the liver and adrenal glands), preferably with intravenous contrast, is performed to analyze the status of the tumor and the mediastinal lymph nodes and to get an assessment of other organs. Due to the incidence of brain metastases at presentation, imaging of the brain (MRI with contrast) is performed for all stages of SCLC and for stage 2 and higher NSCLC. In recent years, positron emission tomography (PET) scanning (particularly when fused with a CT scan) has become a de facto standard staging modality and has been shown to have improved sensitivity and specificity compared with CT scanning, particularly as applied to mediastinal lymphadenopathy. In SCLC, if PET has not been performed, then a bone scan is obtained. Further imaging depends on symptomatic complaints.

An important concept in staging is that radiographic imaging needs confirmation if it will change the stage, prognosis, and treatment strategy of a patient. For example, if a patient has a pleural effusion but no other sites of metastasis, it should not be assumed that the patient has an unresectable and incurable wet stage 3B cancer. It is incumbent on the physician to prove that the patient cannot be curatively treated. In this example, there may be other reasons for a pleural effusion including pneumonia, pulmonary embolus, or atelectasis. The most typical example that is faced by thoracic oncologists is the assessment of the mediastinal lymph nodes. Treatment and prognosis, as noted in Table 1, are dramatically influenced by the presence or absence of metastases to the ipsilateral or contralateral mediastinal lymph nodes. As with pleural effusions,

TABLE 1 Stage Groupings

Stage	Tumor Status	Node Status	Metastasis Status	Approximate 5-Year Survival
Stage 0	Tis	N0	M0	>90%
Stage 1A	T1	N0	M0	75%
Stage 1B	T2	N0	M0	60%
Stage 2A	T1	N1	M0	45%
Stage 2B	T2	N1	M0	~35%
	T3	N0	M0	~35%
Stage 3A	T1-T3	N2	M0	~25%
	T3	N1	M0	~25%
Stage 3B	Any T	N3	M0	~10%-15%
	T4 (dry)	Any N	M0	~10%-15%
	T4 (wet)	Any N	M0	<5%
Stage 4	Any T	Any N	M1	~1%

not all enlarged mediastinal nodes contain cancer, and not all PET-positive nodes are hypermetabolic due to cancer. For this reason, invasive staging is often called for when working up a patient with lung cancer.

Bronchoscopy is done in essentially all early-stage patients to evaluate the endobronchial anatomy and to evaluate for the presence of contralateral abnormalities. A number of techniques help to pathologically stage the mediastinal lymph nodes as well. These include blind transbronchial needle aspiration (TBNA) and ultrasonographically directed needle aspirations and biopsies. Certain mediastinal nodes are accessible through the esophagoscope and can be visualized and biopsied through endoscopic ultrasound (EUS); others are only visualized through the bronchoscope and can be biopsied through endobronchial ultrasonography (EBUS). Both of these techniques are quite valuable when they return positive results, but they are less helpful with a negative result.

Further work-up can intensify and lead to a mediastinoscopy or even a minithoracotomy or video-assisted thoracosopic surgery (VATS). Mediastinoscopy is a relatively minor surgical procedure performed under general anesthesia in which a small incision is made in the suprasternal notch, and a rigid endoscope is inserted into the retrosternal-prevascular space to allow visualization and direct biopsy of mediastinal lymph nodes. Unfortunately, not all lymph nodes are accessible through this, and at times, thoracotomy or VATS may be necessary for full staging.

Similarly, radiographic abnormalities in distant metastatic sites require biopsy confirmation. For example, adrenal metastases are a common and typical in both SCLC and NSCLC, but benign adrenal adenomas are also a common finding, and one should not assume that a patient has metastatic lung cancer on the basis of a small adrenal nodule.

If a patient is to be considered for surgery, then appropriate cardiovascular work-up is indicated because of the high incidence of cardiac disease in patients with lung cancer (given the common risk factor of smoking). For patients who are anticipated to receive treatment with surgery or radiation to the chest, pulmonary function testing with arterial blood gas is also indicated. Although there is no definite cutoff for pulmonary function testing results below which one dare not proceed with surgery, it is clear that patients with a predicted postoperative forced expiratory volume in 1 second (FEV_1) less than 800 mL have increased risk from surgery. Preoperatiive or postoperative pulmonary rehabilitation (or both) can often help the tenuous patient tolerate even major procedures.

A final clinical evaluation to be performed in all patients, regardless of their stage, is to assess functional status. It was recognized quite early in the history of oncology that patients who were doing well tended, stage for stage, to do better than those who were doing poorly. Although this might seem a obvious, it has been quite helpful for the physician to grade a patient's functional status. The most commonly used grading system is the five-point Eastern Cooperative Oncology Group (ECOG) performance status scale (Box 2). A physician's assessment of performance status might seem to be arbitrary and subjective, but performance status reliably and reproducibly helps to predict those who will do well or poorly and helps to predict toxicity from therapy.

Treatment

NON–SMALL CELL LUNG CANCER

Local Disease (Stages 1 and 2)

Localized disease is defined as not involving distant metastatic sites or mediastinum (lymph nodes or direct extension). In Table 1, this refers to stages 1 and 2, including those with intraparencymal tumors with no lymph node involvement (T1/T2 N0), tumors invading the chest wall (T3 N0), or those with intraparenchymal lymph node involvement (T1/T2 N1). Until recently, the treatment for fit patients (i.e., with adequate cardiopulmonary reserve) was surgical resection alone.

Studies performed in the surgical community demonstrated that anatomic (lobectomy and sometimes pneumonectomy) was superior to subanatomic (wedge) resection both in terms of local disease-free survival and overall survival. The Lung Cancer Study Group showed a 75% increase in risk of recurrence and a 50% increase in lung cancer death rate in those who had less surgery. Clearly, operative morbidity and mortality are associated with extent of resection such that pneumonectomy is associated with postoperative mortality as high as 5% or greater, and surgical mortality for lobectomy or wedge resection is close to 1% in appropriate patients.

Recent advances in minimally invasive surgical techniques have extended to thoracic surgery, and now many centers perform some of their lung cancer resections through a VATS approach. VATS appears to offer improved postoperative recovery time and less postoperative morbidity, and in experienced hands it is an appropriate oncologic surgical approach. No randomized data, however, demonstrate that VATS is equivalent or superior to open thoracotomy. It has been shown that overall outcome (hospital morbidity and mortality and overall survival) is linked with experience of the surgeon and the center where surgery is performed, and for this reason, elective oncologic thoracic surgical procedures should be performed at centers with experience.

Until recently, surgical resection alone was the standard for early stage NSCLC. In 1995, an influential meta-analysis was performed on 52 randomized clinical trials in NSCLC in all stages. Of these, 14 trials (involving 4357 patients) evaluated surgery with or without postoperative adjuvant chemotherapy. These results showed a detrimental effect of adding alkylating agents to surgery, but cisplatin-based therapy[1] tended to show a benefit, with an overall hazard ratio of 0.87 (13% reduction in the risk of death) and an absolute benefit of 5% at 5 years. Although not statistically significant, these results formed the basis of renewed enthusiasm in studying adjuvant therapy.

One of the assumptions in 1995 was that earlier studies failed to demonstrate definitive improvement because of overenthusiastic assumptions about the benefit of adding chemotherapy. Therefore, the International Adjuvant Lung Trial (IALT), launched at this time, was powered to demonstrate a benefit of approximately 5% in overall survival at 5 years. In 2004, the results were published in the *New England Journal of Medicine.* This study randomized more than

---

> **BOX 2 Eastern Cooperative Oncology Group (ECOG) Performance Status**
>
> **Grade 0**
> Fully active
> Able to carry on all predisease performance without restriction
>
> **Grade 1**
> Restricted in physically strenuous activity, but ambulatory
> Able to perform all activities of daily living
> Able to perform light or sedentary work
>
> **Grade 2**
> Ambulatory and capable of all self-care but not able to work
> Up and about >50% of waking hours
>
> **Grade 3**
> Capable of only limited self-care
> Confined to bed or chair for >50% of waking hours
>
> **Grade 4**
> Completely disabled
> Requires assistance for activities of daily living
> Confined to bed or chair

---

[1]Not FDA approved for this indication.

1800 patients following surgery for stages 1 to 3 NSCLC to either observation or chemotherapy; 36.5% of patients had stage 1 NSCLC, 24.2% had stage 2, and 39.3% had stage 3 disease. All chemotherapy included cisplatin; however, the choice of second agent was flexible, and four choices were allowed: vindesine (Eldisine),[2] vinblastine (Velban),[1] vinorelbine (Navelbine), or etoposide (VePesid).[1] More than 56% of patients were treated with etoposide, and 27% were treated with vinorelbine. At 5 years, there was a statistically significant improvement in overall survival (44.5% vs 40.4%; hazard ratio [HR], 0.86; $P < 0.03$) and disease-free survival. Toxicity was acceptable, although seven patients died from chemotherapy-related complications.

Since that time, two additional studies have been reported that demonstrate improvement with adjuvant cisplatin and vinorelbine. The National Cancer Institute of Canada reported in 2005 on 482 patients with stage 1B or 2 resected NSCLC who were randomized to receive postoperative cisplatin and vinorelbine for 16 weeks. Forty-five percent of patients had stage 1B disease and 55% had stage 2 disease. Increased fatigue, nausea, anorexia, vomiting, neuropathy, and constipation were associated with the chemotherapy (mostly mild). Overall and relapse-free survival rates were significantly improved in the chemotherapy arm (overall survival, 94 vs 73 months; HR, 0.69; $P = 0.04$). Five-year survival rates were 69% and 54%, respectively. Interestingly, a subgroup analysis showed that the benefit was restricted to patients with stage 2 disease. The ANITA study randomized 840 patients with stage 1B to 3A NSCLC to either observation or cisplatin and vinorelbine. Again, there was a demonstrable improvement in overall survival (median survival, 65.7 vs 43.7 months; HR, 0.8; $P = 0.017$), with an absolute benefit at 5 years of 8.7%.

One carboplatin-based adjuvant study has been reported. It showed, disappointingly, that paclitaxel (Taxol) and carboplatin (Paraplatin)[1] administered for 12 weeks following surgery for stage 1B NSCLC did not improve overall survival. In this Cancer and Leukemia Group B (CALGB) study, 344 patients with resected stage 1B NSCLC were randomized to chemotherapy or observation. Overall and disease-free survival rates were significantly improved at 3 years; however, further follow-up failed to maintain this benefit. A subset of patients with large tumors (>4 cm) appeared to have a benefit. Based on the results of this trial, most thoracic oncologists do not recommend carboplatin-based adjuvant therapy but might treat select patients with resected stage 1B disease.

The role of preoperative chemotherapy, although intriguing, has not been demonstrated to have any benefits and remains experimental in localized disease.

Patients with medically inoperable tumors (or patients who refuse surgery) are treated with radiation therapy alone. A typical course of curative-intent radiation therapy is administered daily (Monday to Friday) for 6 weeks or longer at doses of 6000 cGy or more (although studies increasing this dose have been performed). These patients potentially may be cured with radiation alone, but the 5-year survival is inferior to that seen with surgical resection. Whether this is because the patients are poorer candidates (i.e., unable to tolerate surgery) or because clinical and radiographic staging is inferior to pathologic-surgical staging or because radiation therapy is inadequate for local control is unknown.

Recent advances in imaging have led to the concept of using high-dose fractions (administration of 600 cGy or more instead of 180 to 200 cGy fractions) using multiple beams directed to a single focus as a potential strategy. Such stereotactic body radiotherapy offers the advantage of delivering a higher dose to the tumor while sparing normal structures. Whether it truly represents an advance in terms of patient survival has not yet been demonstrated. Complications associated with radiation therapy depend largely on how much normal structure is involved in the radiation port, but in the lung, potential toxicities include esophagitis, esophageal strictures, radiation pneumonitis, fatigue, skin reactions, and rarely, radiation-related tumors.

Locoregional Disease (Stages 3A and Dry 3B)

Stages 3A and 3B are most often considered together because they both involve typically regional lymph node metastatic disease, but stage 3A is often considered the cutoff for potentially resectable disease. However, not all patients with 3A NSCLC can undergo resection. As noted in Table 1, the most common presentation of stage 3A disease includes ipsilateral mediastinal (N2) lymph node involvement. Thoracic teams spend a great deal of time discussing the status of mediastinal lymph nodes. It may be helpful to think of three levels of involvement of mediastinal nodes:

- Incidental N2 involvement found at the time of surgical resection and mediastinal lymph node sampling or dissection
- Nonbulky but clinically evident N2 nodes seen on preoperative CT or PET imaging and pathologically documented by TBNA, EUS, EBUS, or mediastinoscopy
- Bulky mediastinal lymph nodes often involving multiple stations and visible on plain chest x-ray (unresectable N2 disease)

The prognosis and treatment of patients in these three categories are distinct.

Patients with incidental N2 involvement did not have suspected node involvement before surgery, and they are therefore treated with surgical resection followed by appropriate postoperative chemotherapy.

For patients with nonbulky, clinically evident N2 nodes, proceeding directly to surgery leaves inadequate results. Two small studies from the early 1990s randomized patients with pathologically confirmed stage 3A NSCLC to surgery alone or to preoperative cisplatin-based chemotherapy followed by surgery. Both studies were stopped prematurely because they demonstrated superiority of the preoperative therapy approach. Since then, this strategy has become the de facto standard approach for patients with clinically evident N2 disease. Unfortunately, the exact chemotherapy used or whether chemotherapy plus radiation would be superior to chemotherapy alone is not yet clear.

An intergroup study evaluating the role of surgery in this disease, not yet published, demonstrated superior 3-year disease-free survival but no difference in overall survival. In this study, all patients with pathologically documented stage 3A NSCLC received 4500 cGy radiation plus two cycles of cisplatin[1] plus etoposide[1] chemotherapy. Patients were randomized to either proceed to surgery at that time or to receive an additional 1500 cGy of radiation. The interpretation of the results has been quite varied, but one of the accepted facts is that surgical mortality was quite high, particularly if patients required a pneumonectomy; in patients requiring right-sided pneumonectomy, the operative mortality was approximately 24%. This has led some to argue that all clinically evident N2 disease (bulky or not) should be treated with chemotherapy plus radiation, whereas others argue that the best option is to restrict surgery to patients predicted to require a lobectomy. This remains an open question.

Patients with bulky N2 lymphadenopathy or those with dry 3B NSCLC are typically considered to have unresectable cancer. For many years, radiation therapy alone was the standard treatment, with a 5-year survival rate of approximately 7%. In 1990, the CALGB showed that 6 weeks of chemotherapy followed by radiation therapy doubled the 7-year survival rate from 6% to 13%. This result was subsequently confirmed in a Radiation Therapy Oncology Group (RTOG) study. Several years later, a European study demonstrated that cisplatin administered during radiation therapy (either daily or weekly) improved survival at 3 years to 16% (daily cisplatin) and 13% (weekly cisplatin) from 2% with radiation alone ($P = 0.009$). It was clear that radiation plus chemotherapy was superior to radiation alone for patients with locoregionally advanced (unresectable 3A and dry 3B) NSCLC.

The new question became whether sequential or concurrent therapy was superior. The first published study to resolve this question was in 1999 from Japan. In this study, 320 patients with unresectable stage 3 NSCLC were randomized to either sequential or concurrent cisplatin-based chemotherapy plus radiation to 5600 cGy. The results showed that response rate and survival were significantly improved

---

[1]Not FDA approved for this indication.
[1]Not FDA approved for this indication.

[1]Not FDA approved for this indication.

in the concurrent arm. In the concurrent arm, relative risk (RR) was 84%, compared with 66% in the sequential arm. Median survival was improved (16.5 vs 13.3 months). Two-year survival (34.6% vs 27.4%) and 5-year survival (15.8% vs. 8.9%) were significantly improved.

The relatively uncommon situation of a Pancoast or superior sulcus tumor is treated with preoperative chemotherapy plus radiation followed by surgical resection, if feasible.

Another strategy for concurrent chemoradiation is low-dose, weekly administration of carboplatin-based therapy. Although this is feasible and less toxic than cisplatin-based therapy, there are questions as to whether the cure rate of patients treated in such a fashion is equal to that seen with the more toxic alternatives. Randomized trial data do not exist comparing low-dose weekly carboplatin-based therapy with standard-dose cisplatin-based therapy.

The caveat for all of these studies is that toxicity is significantly increased in patients who receive combined modality therapy. Typical toxicity profiles include esophagitis, pneumonitis, myelosuppression, and fatigue. This points out that only patients with excellent performance status (ECOG 0 or 1) and minimal weight loss (<5%) should be considered candidates for this aggressive multimodality therapy.

Advanced and Metastatic Disease (Stages 3B Wet and 4)

Patients with malignant pleural or pericardial effusions and with distant metastatic disease have incurable disease. In this setting, the rationale for treatment is for palliation rather than with curative intent. This understanding is critical because the judicious initiation and discontinuation of therapy can positively affect the patient's quality of life, and the injudicious application of therapy to patients with poor performance status can worsen the patient's duration and quality of life.

In the 1995 meta-analysis, eleven trials comparing chemotherapy with best supportive care demonstrated significant improvement in patients treated with cisplatin-based chemotherapy but not in those treated with long-term alkylating-agent therapy. The hazard ratio was 0.73, correlating to a 27% reduction in the risk of death and an absolute 10% improvement in 1-year survival. Before this meta-analysis, there was significant pessimism about the benefit of therapy for NSCLC patients.

Since the early 1990s, sequential trials in patients with advanced disease have been conducted. Most have used cisplatin (and lately carboplatin) as the basis of treatment, and to this backbone they added additional agents. These studies have shown a steady increase in the response rate and in median and 1-year survival for patients so treated. All of these studies were performed in patients with good performance status (either ECOG 0-1 or, in some situations, 0-2). The novel agents that have been developed since the 1990s and successfully combined with either cisplatin or carboplatin include gemcitabine (Gemzar), paclitaxel, docetaxel (Taxotere), vinorelbine, irinotecan (Camptosar),[1] and pemetrexed (Alimta). A landmark study published in 2002 by ECOG compared three "modern" regimens of gemcitabine plus cisplatin, docetaxel plus cisplatin, and paclitaxel plus carboplatin against the ECOG reference arm of paclitaxel plus cisplatin. All four regimens were equally effective, leading to response rates of 15% to 20%, median survivals of about 8 to 9 months, and 1-year survivals of about 35%, but none proved superior to any of the others. Although distinct regimens offered different toxicity profiles, there was no significant difference in therapeutic outcome.

Subsequent to that study, a number of trials have been performed adding novel molecular-targeted agents onto the now-established NSCLC platinum-based doublet backbone. These trials included the addition of epidermal growth factor receptor (EGFR) antagonists, retinoid receptor–interacting agents, antisense molecules to oncogenes, and a product derived from shark cartilage (believed to have antiangiogenic properties). Unfortunately, all of these large randomized studies were negative. In one study of paclitaxel plus carboplatin with or without the EGFR tyrosine kinase inhibitor erlotinib (Tarceva), although the overall study was negative, analysis of a subset of never-smokers (approximately 15%) demonstrated a dramatic improvement for patients who received erlotinib (median survival improved from 10 to 22 months with the addition of erlotinib). Although this was an unplanned subgroup analysis, for reasons described later, this result generated some excitement.

In 2006, ECOG investigators published the results of a randomized trial comparing paclitaxel plus carboplatin with or without the addition of the anti-angiogenesis agent bevacizumab (Avastin). Bevacizumab is a humanized monoclonal antibody directed against the vascular endothelial growth factor (VEGF). Bevacizumab is the first in a new class of agents targeting angiogenesis in cancers. The hypothesis involved in angiogenesis is that in order for tumors to grow beyond a clinically insignificant size, they need to recruit nontumorigenic blood vessels. VEGF is one of a large group of growth factors (perhaps the most important one) involved in this process. Earlier studies demonstrated that bevacizumab could be added to paclitaxel plus carboplatin in the treatment of NSCLC, but significant toxicity was found. Specifically, of 66 patients treated with the combination, six had fatal or near-fatal hemoptysis. On further review, it was apparent that squamous histology was a major risk factor for this complication in that four of 13 patients with squamous histology had significant hemoptysis, whereas only two of 53 with adenocarcinoma or NSCLC (not otherwise specified) suffered this complication.

For this reason, the definitive phase III ECOG study excluded patients with squamous histology, patients with a history of hemoptysis, patients requiring anticoagulation, and patients with brain metastases. More than 800 patients were randomized, and the results were quite dramatic, showing improved response rate, median survival, and 1- and 2-year survival. Although there was increased toxicity (some hemoptysis, hypertension, and proteinuria and increased episodes of febrile neutropenia), the benefit was significant. Table 2 shows the improvements that have been seen since the 1980s, demonstrated through the sequential trials noted.

When discussing duration of chemotherapy, one needs to recall that this is an incurable malignancy and that chemotherapy causes acute and chronic toxicity. Two studies have addressed this question, looking at three versus six cycles of cisplatin-based therapy or four cycles versus eight cycles of paclitaxel plus carboplatin. In both studies, progression-free survival was improved with the longer duration, but overall survival was no better. For this reason, most thoracic oncologists would choose to treat for four to six cycles of chemotherapy as initial treatment, and then monitor the patient. In the bevacizumab trial, chemotherapy plus bevacizumab was administered for up to six cycles of three weekly treatments, and in patients with responding disease, bevacizumab alone was continued until progression.

Until 1999, there were no data supporting the use of second-line therapy. In that year, two studies demonstrated that fit patients (ECOG 0-2) had improvement in survival following treatment with docetaxel at 75 mg/m^2 every 3 weeks. Although the overall response rate was quite modest (7% to 8%), the survival benefit was apparently seen across the entire group. The assumption is that those who had stable disease (and improved symptom control) added to the overall

TABLE 2 Summary of Chemotherapy in Advanced Non–Small Cell Lung Cancer

Therapy	Response Rate	Median Survival	1-Year Survival
Best supportive care	NA	~4 mo	~10%
Cisplatin (Platinol AQ)[1]	10%–15%	~6 mo	~15%–20%
Platinum doublet	20%–25%	~8–10 mo	~35%
Platinum doublet plus bevacizumab (Avastin)	30%–35%	12 mo	50% (2-y survival ~15%)

[1]Not FDA approved for this indication.
NA = not applicable.

---

[1]Not FDA approved for this indication.

benefit seen by those who had bona fide responses. A subsequent randomized trial demonstrated that pemetrexed, a novel antimetabolite, had equivalent responses but improved toxicity when compared with docetaxel. Specifically, patients receiving pemetrexed had less neutropenia, fewer neutropenic fevers, and less alopecia.

The era of molecular targeted agents in NSCLC has dawned with the use of EGFR antagonist therapy, specifically the oral tyrosine kinase inhibitor erlotinib. The epidermal growth factor is commonly expressed on lung cancer cells and acts as a growth factor to increase the growth and proliferation of cells through a downstream signaling cascade. In vitro, inhibition of this cascade leads to diminished growth, and in some cells, it can lead to apoptosis and cellular death.

Phase I studies demonstrated that these agents were safe, with mild toxicity of acneiform rash and diarrhea. A phase III study of erlotinib compared with best supportive care as second-line therapy following failure of initial therapy in NSCLC demonstrated that erlotinib led to responses in about 8% of patients with stable disease in an additional 40% of patients, leading to improvement in overall survival. These results were quite similar to those seen with both docetaxel and pemetrexed. The best responses were seen in those who were never-smokers.

Subsequent data demonstrated that the tumors from approximately 10% to 13% of unselected patients bore mutations within the tyrosine kinase domain of EGFR. Patients who harbored these mutations were more likely to have never smoked, and the response rate in patients with the mutations was quite dramatic. Some studies in patients who carry these sensitizing mutations have demonstrated response rates of 75% lasting a year or longer.

Therefore, this novel molecular targeted agent has gained a firm foothold in the second- or third-line treatment of patients with NSCLC. In selected patients (e.g., clinically selected for never-smoking status or molecular selection with mutation analysis of the EGFR gene) it might show significant improvement without a great deal of toxicity in the first-line setting.

SMALL CELL LUNG CANCER

SCLC is a distinct clinical and pathologic entity. Clinically, it is characterized by a rapid growth rate and early metastatic spread. The staging for SCLC is quite simple. For patients with extensive disease, representing approximately two thirds of SCLC patients, treatment with chemotherapy alone is appropriate. Although chemotherapy is not curative, it does offer significant palliative relief. Since the early 1980s, the standard chemotherapy includes cisplatin (Platinol AQ)[1] and etoposide (VePesid). This gives response rates of 70% and improves overall survival from approximately 3 months with best supportive care to approximately 10 months.

Recently, Japanese investigators performed a phase III study in patients with extensive stage SCLC comparing etoposide and cisplatin with irinotecan (Camptosar)[1] and cisplatin. In their study, median survival was improved to nearly 13 months for patients treated with the irinotecan combination. Unfortunately, a study in the U.S. population using a slightly different irinotecan combination failed to demonstrate improvement. Therefore, at least in Western populations, etoposide and cisplatin remain the standard.

One of the reasons that etoposide and cisplatin has been such a successful combination is the relative ease of combining this with radiation therapy. In patients with limited disease (about one third of patients), potentially curative therapy can be delivered with chemotherapy combined with radiation therapy. Data show that radiation is best administered during chemotherapy (rather than sequentially), and twice-daily radiation offers superior survival compared with daily radiation when administered to 4500 cGy. Approximately 75% of patients treated in this way achieve complete response to treatment with chemotherapy plus radiation, and long-term survival is achieved in 20% to 25% of patients.

Following achievement of complete response, prophylactic radiation therapy to the brain has been demonstrated to lead to diminished recurrences in the brain and improved overall survival. Therefore, patients with both limited and extensive disease who achieve a complete (or even excellent partial) response can benefit from a short course of prophylactic cranial irradiation following the completion of therapy.

Follow-up

After patients complete therapy for NSCLC or SCLC, thoracic oncologists generally follow patients with clinical evaluations every 3 to 4 months and with CT scans of the chest every 6 to 12 months. In addition to evaluation for recurrent or progressive disease, another rationale for close radiographic imaging is the risk of second cancers. It has been estimated that those who have had one lung cancer have a 1% to 2% chance per year of a second lung or aerodigestive cancer.

REFERENCES

Furuse K, Fukuoka M, Kawahara M, et al: Phase III study of concurrent versus sequential thoracic radiotherapy in combination with mitomycin, vindesine, and cisplatin in unresectable stage III non–small-cell lung cancer. J Clin Oncol 1999;17:2692-2699.
Gould MK, Kuschner WG, Rydzak CE, et al: Test performance of positron emission tomography and computed tomography for mediastinal staging in patients with non–small-cell lung cancer, a meta-analysis. Ann Intern Med 2003;139:879-892.
Hecht SS: Tobacco smoke carcinogens and lung cancer. J Natl Cancer Inst 1999;91:1194-1210.
International Adjuvant Lung cancer Trial Collaborative Group: Cisplatin-based adjuvant chemotherapy in patients with completely resected non–small-cell lung cancer. N Engl J Med 2004;350:351-360.
Minna JD, Roth JA, Gazdar AF: Focus on lung cancer. Cancer Cell 2002;1:49-52.
Noda K, Nishiwaki Y, Kawahara M, et al: Irinotecan plus cisplatin compared with etoposide plus cisplatin for extensive small-cell lung cancer. N Engl J Med 2002;346:85-91.
Non–Small Cell Lung Cancer Collaborative Group: Chemotherapy in non–small cell lung cancer: A meta-analysis using updated data on individual patients from 52 randomised clinical trials. BMJ 1995;311:899-909.
Paez JG, Janne PA, Lee JC, et al: EGFR mutations in lung cancer: Correlation with clinical response to gefitinib therapy. Science 2004;304:1497-1500.
Patz EF, Goodman PC, Bepler G: Screening for lung cancer. N Engl J Med 2000;343:1627-1633.
Potti A, Mukherjee S, Petersen R, et al: A genomic strategy to refine prognosis in early-stage non–small-cell lung cancer. N Engl J Med 2006;355:570-580.
Sandler A, Gray R, Perry MC, et al: Paclitaxel–carboplatin alone or with bevacizumab for non–small-cell lung cancer. N Engl J Med 2006;355:2542-2550.
Shepherd FA, Pereira JR, Ciuleanu T, et al: Erlotinib in previously treated non–small-cell lung cancer. N Engl J Med 2005;353:123-132.

Coccidioidomycosis

Method of

Lynn L. Horvath, MD, and Duane R. Hospenthal, MD, PhD

Coccidioidomycosis (valley fever) is a fungal infection caused by *Coccidioides* species that produces mild to life-threatening disease. The disease was first described in an Argentinean soldier by Alejandro Posadas, when he was a medical student, in 1892. Initially, coccidioidomycosis was thought to be a rare, ultimately fatal disseminated infection. It is now known that most infections do not produce apparent disease, and those that do are generally self-limited pneumonias, often mistakenly diagnosed as influenza or community-acquired pneumonia.

Coccidioides species are dimorphic fungi that live in the soil as saprobic molds and in human disease produce unique thick-walled

---

[1]Not FDA approved for this indication.

spherical structures called *spherules,* which contain endospores. Infection occurs when the infectious particles, the arthroconidia, are inhaled. Previously believed to be a single species, two members of the genus are currently described, *C. immitis* and *C. posadasii.* Although this designation has little apparent clinical importance (and differentiating between the species is beyond the scope of most clinical laboratories), it is now known that *C. immitis* causes only disease originating from California and parts of Arizona.

Coccidioidomycosis is an endemic mycosis most commonly found in the southwestern United States and northern Mexico, with smaller areas of disease originating in Central and South America. The endemic niche appears to localize to areas with an arid climate and alkaline soils, the lower Sonoran life zone. Disease generally peaks in dry periods following rains, typically in the summer and fall. It has been estimated that about 150,000 infections occur each year, although many think the numbers are much higher. Filipinos and those of African descent (and perhaps other Asians and Native Americans), pregnant women, and immunocompromised persons are at the highest risk for severe or disseminated disease. Disease typically manifests 7 to 21 days after exposure, and infection appears to protect persons from subsequent repeat infections.

Clinical Manifestations

More than one half of infections are asymptomatic and were identified in past studies by skin testing of persons in the endemic areas. The majority of symptomatic infection is acute pulmonary disease, and chronic pulmonary and disseminated disease occurs only rarely (less than 1% of those infected).

ACUTE PNEUMONIA

Primary respiratory infection typically manifests with nonproductive cough, fever, pleuritic chest pain, malaise, headache, anorexia, myalgia, and often rash. Rash is usually diffuse, faint, and erythematous; however, some patients present with erythema multiforme or erythema nodosum. These latter two rashes tend to appear days to weeks after initial pulmonary symptoms and are more common in women. The triad of fever, arthralgias, and erythema nodosum is commonly referred to as *desert rheumatism.*

Acute respiratory coccidioidomycosis may be misdiagnosed as influenza or community-acquired pneumonia, but it typically produces longer duration of symptoms than those illnesses. Unlike typical bacterial pneumonias, acute coccidioidomycosis typically remits without therapy, although it may be followed by weeks to months of fatigue. Severe disease can manifest with protracted symptoms or even a sepsis syndrome. More severe infection (or infection requiring antifungal therapy) is typically defined as that occurring in persons older than 55 years; lasting longer than 2 months; impairing ability to go to work; and producing a weight loss of greater than 10%, night sweats longer than 3 weeks, infiltrates involving more than one half of one lung or both lungs, prominent or persistent hilar lymphadenopathy, or complement fixation antibody titers greater than 1:16.

PULMONARY NODULES AND CAVITIES

Following acute infection, pulmonary nodules or thin-walled cavities may be seen in about 5% to 10% of patients. Both of these presentations are often asymptomatic and found on follow-up or screening chest radiography. Most of these do not require specific therapy unless patients are symptomatic. Rupture of a cavity into the pleural space is a rare complication that typically requires both medical and surgical therapy.

CHRONIC PNEUMONIA

Chronic progressive fibrocavitary pneumonia can develop after primary infection. Most commonly seen in persons with diabetes and preexisting lung disease, this disease is typified by chronic infiltrates and cavitary lesions. This form of coccidioidomycosis can resemble tuberculosis and prove difficult to eradicate.

DISSEMINATED INFECTION

Extrapulmonary dissemination most commonly affects the skin, bones and joints, and meninges, although almost any organ can be involved. Occurring in 0.5% to 1% of those infected, disseminated infection has a much higher incidence (>15%) in the severely immunocompromised, including those with AIDS, lymphoma, and solid organ transplantation and in those receiving high-dose corticosteroids or tumor necrosis factor (TNF)-α–blocking agents.

Disseminated disease can manifest with localized or widespread involvement. Skin lesions are typically verrucous, but they may be maculopapular or ulcerative. Subcutaneous abscesses are also common. Bone and joint involvement can include any bone or joint, but the vertebrae are most commonly involved. Meningitis is the most feared form of coccidioidomycosis, because it is typically a fatal infection after a few months if left untreated; cure of this infection still eludes modern medicine. Meningitis manifests with chronic symptoms of headache, memory loss, lethargy, and confusion, and it can be complicated by hydrocephalus and vasculitis.

Diagnosis

The diagnosis of coccidioidomycosis must begin with awareness of the potential for this infection in the differential. Clinicians in the endemic areas typically include this disease and its many manifestations in their differential diagnosis. Those outside of the endemic areas must remember to obtain a travel history from every patient and to inquire about previous residence if reactivation is suspected in the immunosuppressed. Aside from endemic exposure, peripheral eosinophilia, and rarely eosinophils in cerebrospinal fluid (CSF), can indicate coccidioidomycosis. Diagnosis is typically made by direct observation or culture of *Coccidioides* or by serologic methods.

Direct examination and culture should be performed on sputum, lesion discharge, biopsy material, and CSF, based on presentation. The spherules and endospores of coccidioidomycosis can be seen with almost every stain (including hematoxylin and eosin [H&E] and Gram stain); typically Calcofluor white or KOH is used to examine sputum, aspirates, and CSF. The disease is confirmed on seeing the typical 10- to 80-μm thick-walled rounded structures (spherules) with 2- to 5-μm round endospores inside. Culture is performed by many laboratories; the diagnosis may be made by the identification of typical arthroconidia or using the commercially available DNA probe when indistinct, white, wooly colonies are recovered. *Coccidioides* grows well on most fungal and bacterial culture media, but the diagnostic yield of CSF is not very high. Although the disease is not communicable, the mold form growing in the laboratory (and producing arthroconidia) is highly infectious. Clinicians suspecting coccidioidomycosis should inform the clinical laboratory of their suspicion.

Nonculture diagnosis has included skin testing and serology; currently, a skin testing reagent is not available. Serologic testing may be done using several commercially available tests. Of these, complement fixation and immunodiffusion testing are most useful. Enzyme-linked immunoassay (EIA) (IgM) and latex-agglutination tests are highly

---

CURRENT DIAGNOSIS

- Coccidioidomycosis is a common cause of community-acquired pneumonia in endemic areas.
- Direct examinations of sputum, culture, and serologic testing are keys to making the diagnosis in respiratory disease.
- Disseminated infection should be suspected in those patients with complement fixation antibody titers >1:16.
- Peripheral eosinophilia or eosinophils in the cerebrospinal fluid should increase suspicion for coccidioidomycosis in the appropriate clinical setting.

sensitive and can be used for initial testing. Because of the potential for false-positive results with these tests, confirmation by complement fixation or immunodiffusion testing is suggested. In addition to their use in the diagnosis of coccidioidomycosis, serologic tests should be used to follow the care of patients with chronic or disseminated infections.

Radiology is often key to the diagnosis and management of coccidioidomycosis. Chest x-ray should be performed on all persons suspected to have disease. Chest computed tomography (CT) may be useful in chronic pulmonary disease and to follow asymptomatic nodules and cavities. With disseminated disease involving more than one site of infection, bone scanning may be useful in discovering the extent of disease and assisting in long-term follow-up. Plain x-rays of involved bones or joints and CT or magnetic resonance imaging (MRI) may be useful as well. Neuroradiologic studies may be normal in meningeal disease, but CT or MRI should be included in the diagnosis and management of this disease because hydrocephalus may be present initially and can develop subsequently. MRI can also reveal basilar leptomeningeal enhancement.

Treatment

ACUTE INFECTIONS

Untreated, most acute infections resolve spontaneously. Observation may be the treatment of choice for uncomplicated acute pulmonary disease in patients not at high risk for dissemination or severe disease. Some experts think all persons with infection should receive antifungal therapy (Table 1). Unfortunately, there are no randomized clinical trials to support treating or not treating in uncomplicated disease in low-risk patients.

CURRENT THERAPY

- Uncomplicated acute pneumonia in patients not at high risk for complications might not require antifungal therapy.
- Duration of antifungal therapy (when given) typically consists of months to years of oral azole (fluconazole[1] or itraconazole[1]) therapy: 3-6 months for acute pulmonary disease, 12 or more months for chronic pulmonary disease, years for disseminated disease, and life-long for meningitis.
- Amphotericin B (Fungizone) is now reserved for rapidly progressive disease, acute disease with respiratory failure, and treatment failure with azoles and for use in pregnancy (because of the teratogenicity of the azoles).
- Specialty consultation is warranted for disseminated disease.

[1]Not FDA approved for this indication.

Immunocompromised persons, those with preexisting lung disease or diabetes, and those at high risk for severe or disseminated disease should receive therapy. Pregnant patients and persons with severe disease should be treated with amphotericin B (Fungizone). Those with respiratory failure can be treated with amphotericin B or

TABLE 1 Treatment of Coccidioidomycosis

Disease	Primary Therapy	Alternative Therapy	Duration	Comments
Pulmonary Infection				
Acute				
Low-risk uncomplicated	Observation	Oral azole	3-6 mo	Typically, fluconazole (Diflucan)[1] or itraconazole (Sporanox)[1]
				Other azole alternatives include ketoconazole (Nizoral), posaconazole (Noxafil),[1] and voriconazole (Vfend)[1]
High-risk uncomplicated	Oral azole	Amphotericin B	3-6 mo	Patients may be switched to azole therapy on clinical improvement
				Azoles should not be used in pregnancy
Diffuse or severe	Amphotericin B	Oral azoles	≥12 mo	Patients may be switched to azole therapy on clinical improvement
				Azoles should not be used in pregnancy
				High-dose fluconazole[1] 800-1200 mg/day[3] is often used in severe disease, at least initially
Chronic				
All	Oral azole	Amphotericin B, surgical resection	≥12 mo	Patients may be switched to azole therapy on clinical improvement.
				Azoles should not be used in pregnancy.
Disseminated Infection				
Nonmeningeal	Oral azole	Amphotericin B	Years	Patients may be switched to azole therapy on clinical improvement
				Azoles should not be used in pregnancy
				High-dose fluconazole[1] 800-1200 mg/day[3] is often used in severe disease, at least initially
				Surgical resection may be used adjunctively
Meningeal	Oral fluconazole[1]	Itraconazole,[1] intrathecal amphotericin B[1]	Life-long	High-dose fluconazole[1] 800-1200 mg/day[3] is often used in severe disease, at least initially
				Consider early shunting if hydrocephalus is present and corticosteroids if vasculitis is present

[1]Not FDA approved for this indication.
[3]Exceeds dosage recommended by the manufacturer.

TABLE 2 Antifungal Agents Used in Coccidioidomycosis

Drug	Dosing
Fluconazole (Diflucan)[1]	400-1200 mg PO or IV qd[3]
Itraconazole (Sporanox)[1]	200 mg PO or IV bid or tid[3]
Ketoconazole (Nizoral)	200-400 mg PO qd
Posaconazole (Noxafil)[1]	400 mg PO qd
Voriconazole (Vfend)[1]	200 mg PO or IV bid
Amphotericin B (Fungizone)	0.5-1.5 mg/kg IV qd[3],*
Lipid formulations of amphotericin B (Ambisone,[1] Abelcet, Amphotec[1])	2-5 mg/kg IV qd

[1]Not FDA approved for this indication.
[3]Exceeds dosage recommended by the manufacturer.
*May be given on alternate days to decrease toxicity.

high-dose fluconazole (Diflucan).[1] All others may be treated with oral azole therapy (fluconazole [Diflucan][1] itraconazole [Sporanox][1] or ketoconazole [Nizoral]) (Table 2).

All infected persons, whether treated or not, should be followed up routinely (every 3-6 months) for at least 2 years to ensure that late complications, including dissemination, are not missed.

CHRONIC INFECTIONS

Treatment of chronic pulmonary disease and disseminated disease is generally given for years, sometimes for life. With the therapy options currently available, data do not support ever stopping therapy in those with meningitis.

Oral azole therapy is typically the treatment of choice for chronic infections (fluconazole,[1] itraconazole,[1] or ketoconazole). The two newest azole agents, posaconazole (Noxafil)[1] and voriconazole (Vfend),[1] are both highly active against *Coccidioides* in vitro. These agents may prove to be very useful in treating chronic infections in the future, but current clinical efficacy data are limited.

Amphotericin B can be used initially in severe infections and might have to be used in patients not responding to azole therapy. Intrathecal amphotericin B is still used by some experts initially in meningitis, and it may be used as a secondary regimen in persons failing azole therapy.

In meningeal disease, early shunting should be pursued if hydrocephalus is present, and corticosteroids should be considered if central nervous system vasculitis is suspected.

Follow-up of chronic or disseminated disease generally includes interval (typically every 3-6 months) history and physical examination and serologic and radiologic testing. In meningitis, this follow-up should also include CSF examination.

REFERENCES

Anstead GM, Corcoran G, Lewis J, et al: Refractory coccidioidomycosis treated with posaconazole. Clin Infect Dis 2005;40:1770-1776.
Anstead GM, Graybill JR: Coccidioidomycosis. Infect Dis Clin N Am 2006;20:621-643.
Catanzaro A, Cloud GA, Stevens DA, et al: Safety, tolerance, and efficacy of posaconzole in patients with nonmeningeal disseminated or chronic pulmonary coccidioidomycosis. Clin Infect Dis 2007;45:562-568.
Galgiani JN: *Coccidioides* species. In Mandell GL, Bennett JE, Dolin R, editors: Mandell, Douglas, and Bennett's Principles and Practice of Infectious Diseases, ed 6th, Philadelphia: Churchill Livingstone, 2005, pp 3040-3051.
Galgiani JN, Ampel NM, Blair JE, et al: Coccidioidomycosis [IDSA treatment guidelines]. Clin Infect Dis 2005;41:1217-1223.
Galgiani JN, Catanzaro A, Cloud GA, et al: Comparison of oral fluconazole and itraconazole for progressive, nonmeningeal coccidioidomycosis: A randomized, double-blind trial. Mycoses Study Group. Ann Intern Med 2000;133:676-686.
Galgiani JN, Catanzaro A, Cloud GA, et al: Fluconazole therapy for coccidioidal meningitis. Ann Intern Med 1993;119:28-35.
Johnson RH, Einstein HE: Coccidioidal meningitis. Clin Infect Dis 2006;42:103-107.
Prabhu RM, Bonnell M, Currier B, Orenstein R: Successful treatment of disseminated nonmeningeal coccidioidomycosis with voriconazole. Clin Infect Dis 2004;39:e74-e77.
Ramani R, Chaturvedi V: Antifungal susceptibility profiles of *Coccidioides immitis* and Coccidioides posadasii from endemic and non-endemic areas. Mycopathologia 2007;163:315-319.
Valdivia L, Mix D, Wright M, et al: Coccidioidomycosis as a common cause of community-acquired pneumonia. Emerg Infect Dis 2006;12:958-962.

[1]Not FDA approved for this indication.

Histoplasmosis

Method of
Linus H. Santo Tomas, MD, MS, and
Ralph M. Schapira, MD

Etiology and Epidemiology

The causative organism of histoplasmosis, *Histoplasma capsulatum*, is found worldwide, but thrives best in moist acidic soil with high organic content. In the United States, infection is highest in areas of the Ohio, Mississippi, and Missouri River valleys. Bat and avian droppings enhance soil characteristics that augment sporulation. Bats can also be infected, thereby transmitting the fungus in their droppings. *H. capsulatum* is a dimorphic fungus that exists in mycelial form in the environment. The infective spores are introduced to the lungs via inhalation and the organism is transformed to a yeast form in the mammalian host. Most infections are asymptomatic, but immunocompromised hosts and those exposed to large inoculums are more likely to develop progressive or severe disease.

Pathogenesis

Inhaled spores transform to the yeast form in the alveoli within hours to days. This leads to bronchopneumonia. The organism is ingested by macrophages and may be disseminated hematogenously to regional lymph nodes, liver, spleen, and other organs. Neutrophils, which can also phagocytose the organism and release antifungal proteins and granules, are thought to play an important role in limiting the initial phase of the infection. Yeasts may continue to multiply intracellularly within alveolar macrophages. Maturation of cell-mediated immunity is critical to effective control of the disease. The inflammatory response leads to the development of caseating lesions that heal, forming fibrotic lesions with granulomas. The dense fibrotic lesions frequently calcify. Yeast forms have been identified in these calcified lesions, and although attempts to culture the fungus from these lesions have been unsuccessful, the recrudescence of disease in immunocompromised individuals who are no longer in endemic areas suggests that some organisms may remain viable for years.

Clinical Manifestations

Most infections are asymptomatic, and in endemic areas it is not unusual for radiologic studies to show evidence of previous infection in the chest and abdomen, which most commonly appear as calcified granulomas in the lung parenchyma or spleen. The incubation period is from 3 to 21 days after exposure. The development of clinical disease is mainly dependent on the immune status of the host and the inoculum load. The more common presentations of the disease are discussed in the following section.

ACUTE PULMONARY HISTOPLASMOSIS

Localized Pulmonary Disease

Sixty percent of those who develop clinical disease present with acute pulmonary histoplasmosis. Initial symptoms are usually nonspecific and consist of fever, chills, fatigue, and cough. The chest radiograph may reveal mediastinal and hilar adenopathy accompanied by patchy pneumonic infiltrates, but may also be normal in some cases. Limited exposure in an immunocompetent host may manifest with a localized pneumonia that may be mistaken for a bacterial pneumonia. Most do not require antifungal treatment unless there is no improvement after a month.

Diffuse Pulmonary Involvement

More intense exposure, even in an immunocompetent host, can lead to diffuse pulmonary histoplasmosis. The typical chest radiograph may show bilateral reticulonodular or miliary-type infiltrates. Aside from fever, cough, chest pain, and chills, affected patients can have clinically significant hypoxemia that may require ventilatory support.

CHRONIC PULMONARY HISTOPLASMOSIS

In persons with underlying pulmonary disease, especially emphysema, the acute exposure can eventually lead to chronic pulmonary histoplasmosis that is characterized by fibrocavitary lesions on chest radiographs. Symptoms include cough, fatigue, fever, weight loss, and night sweats. Patients can also present with hemoptysis and progressive dyspnea. Chronic pulmonary histoplasmosis may mimic progressive mycobacterial disease, particularly tuberculosis.

GRANULOMATOUS MEDIASTINITIS

Occasionally, lymphadenopathy associated with histoplasmosis may be severe enough to cause compression of the airways, mediastinal vascular structures, and the esophagus. This can lead to cough, chest pain, hemoptysis, dysphagia, and signs of superior vena cava syndrome. Granulomatous mediastinitis has to be distinguished from fibrosing mediastinitis, a rare long-term sequelae of infection. Granulomatous mediastinitis can improve significantly with antifungal and corticosteroid treatment.

DISSEMINATED HISTOPLASMOSIS

Immunocompromised individuals, whether from extremes of age, debilitating comorbid disease, immunosuppressive medications, or immune deficiency syndromes, are at greater risk for disseminated disease. Symptoms may be nonspecific, and can include fever, chills, and weight loss. Physical examination may reveal pneumonitis, hepatosplenomegaly, and lymphadenopathy. Other manifestations depend on specific organs that may be involved. Five percent to 20% of cases may have central nervous system involvement.

OTHER MANIFESTATIONS

Less common manifestations of histoplasmosis include pericarditis, rheumatologic syndromes, broncholithiasis, and fibrosing mediastinitis. Pericarditis is thought to be caused by local immunologic response to release of inflammatory substances from adjacent necrotizing lymph nodes. Arthritis or arthralgia is usually polyarticular and symmetric, and is thought to be secondary to a systemic inflammatory response to the infection rather than actual joint invasion.

DIAGNOSIS

The nonspecific clinical manifestations of histoplasmosis can make diagnosis difficult, and maintaining a high clinical suspicion in the appropriate setting is important. It should be considered as a possible cause of nonresolving pneumonia and fever of unknown origin, especially in endemic areas. A high index of suspicion is also appropriate in immunocompromised hosts. A number of laboratory tests are available for confirmation of suspected disease, each with its own advantages and disadvantages. A combination of these laboratory tests may be needed to maximize the yield of diagnostic tests in less florid infections. Obtaining specimens from respiratory secretions, bronchoalveolar lavage, tissue biopsy, blood, and urine can also increase the overall yield.

CURRENT DIAGNOSIS

- Because clinical presentation is usually nonspecific, a high index of suspicion is needed to arrive at the diagnosis.
- Histoplasmosis should be considered in nonresolving pneumonia and fever of unknown etiology, especially in endemic areas and immunocompromised hosts.
- For rapid diagnosis, the urine *Histoplasma* polysaccharide antigen detection test has good sensitivity (89%) in disseminated histoplasmosis.
- A combination of tests using different specimen types may be needed to maximize the diagnostic yield and confirm the diagnosis.

FUNGAL STAINING

Rapid diagnosis of histoplasmosis can be made with identification of *H. capsulatum* with silver-methenamine stain of biologic specimens. The organism may also be identified by Wright stain of peripheral blood smears in individuals with severe disseminated disease. However, these have lower sensitivity compared to antigen detection and culture.

FUNGAL CULTURE

Blood and bone marrow culture can be positive in 85% to 90% of patients with disseminated and chronic pulmonary disease. The lysis-centrifugation method is best for blood cultures. Analyzing multiple specimens may improve yield. Bronchoalveolar lavage cultures should also be analyzed in patients with pulmonary involvement. The relatively long duration to obtain positive growth on culture limits its usefulness in an acute setting.

DETECTION OF SERUM ANTIBODIES

Serologic testing for antibodies to histoplasma antigen are positive in 80% to 90% of patients with diffuse pulmonary involvement and disseminated disease. Complement fixation and immunodiffusion assays are available. Precipitins to the M or H antigen may be detected but both have significant false positives as a consequence of cross-reactivity with other fungal infections. Other limitations of the test include false negatives early in the course of disease and reduced sensitivity in immunocompromised hosts.

POLYSACCHARIDE ANTIGEN DETECTION

The *Histoplasma* polysaccharide antigen can be detected by conventional radioimmunoassay (RIA) or enzyme immunoassay (EIA) in the urine of up to 92% of patients with disseminated disease and in 37% to 39% with self-limited disease. The same test can be used on serum and other body fluids, but the sensitivity may be lower. It is most useful when serologic tests are less likely to be positive, such as in the early phase of an infection or in immunocompromised hosts.

TABLE 1 Recommendations for Treatment of Histoplasmosis

Type of Histoplasmosis	Treatment Regimen
Acute Pulmonary Disease	
Mild to moderate, > 4 weeks	Itraconazole (Sporanox) 200 mg, once to twice daily for 6–12 weeks*
Severe	Amphotericin B (Fungizone) 0.7 mg/kg/d,[†] then itraconazole 200 mg once to twice daily for 12 weeks
	Consider corticosteroids (effectiveness not proven)
Chronic Pulmonary Disease	
Mild to moderate	Itraconazole 200 mg once to twice daily for 12–24 months
Severe	Amphotericin B 0.7 mg/kg/d,[†] then itraconazole 200 mg once to twice daily for 12–24 months
Granulomatous Mediastinitis	
Mild to moderate	Itraconazole 200 mg once to twice daily for 6–12 months
Severe	Amphotericin B 0.7 mg/kg/d,[†] then itraconazole 200 mg once to twice daily for 6–12 months
Disseminated Disease (without AIDS)	
Mild to moderate	Itraconazole 200 mg once to twice daily for 6–18 months
Severe	Amphotericin B 0.7 mg/kg/d,[†] then itraconazole 200 mg once to twice daily for 6–18 months[‡]
Disseminated Disease (with AIDS)	
Mild to moderate	Itraconazole 200 mg once to twice daily for life
Severe	Amphotericin B 0.7 mg/kg/d,[†] then itraconazole 200 mg once to twice daily for life
Meningitis	Amphotericin B 0.7 mg/kg/d[†] to total 35 mg/kg over 3–4 months, then fluconazole (Diflucan)[1] 800 mg daily[3] for 9–12 months

*Blood levels may be checked if poor absorption or increased metabolism is suspected.
[†]If amphotericin B is used exclusively, a total course dose of ≤35 mg/kg is recommended. Lipid preparation of amphotericin may be given at 3 mg/kg/d; recent studies in AIDS patients suggest better outcomes compared to deoxycholate amphotericin B (see text).
[‡]Continue treatment until *Histoplasma* urine and serum antigen concentrations <4 units.
[1]Not FDA approved for this indication.
[3]Exceeds dosage recommended by the manufacturer.

Antigen levels correlate with treatment response and recrudescence and can be used to guide treatment of disseminated histoplasmosis.

Treatment

Most patients who have histoplasmosis recover without treatment. The need for treatment is determined by the type of involvement, the severity and duration of the disease, and the immune status of the patient. Treatment is generally reserved for chronic pulmonary involvement, disseminated disease, or severe acute infections. Such infections most commonly occur in immunocompromised hosts or in those exposed to a large infectious inoculum. Table 1 summarizes the treatment recommendations.

In general, severe disease is initially treated with intravenous deoxycholate amphotericin B (Fungizone) at a dose of 0.7 mg/kg per day. The cumulative dose of amphotericin B depends on the clinical response, but for *Histoplasma* meningitis, completion of a 35-mg/kg course given over 3 to 4 months is recommended. The same cumulative dose of amphotericin B is recommended for other severe forms of histoplasmosis if the patient is unable to take oral medications. A shift from intravenous amphotericin to oral itraconazole (continuation phase) can be considered if there is clinical improvement (i.e., when the patient becomes afebrile, hemodynamically stable, or no longer requires ventilatory support) and is able to take oral medications. The duration of itraconazole (Sporanox) treatment also varies according to the type and severity of histoplasmosis (see Table 1). Monitoring of itraconazole blood levels should be considered if there is concern about absorption or use of medications that may reduce its bioavailability.

CURRENT THERAPY

- Treatment is indicated in severe acute (diffuse or localized) pulmonary disease, chronic pulmonary disease, granulomatous mediastinitis with obstructive or invasive symptoms, and disseminated infection.
- Mild to moderate acute pulmonary involvement that persists beyond 4 weeks also warrants treatment.
- Intravenous deoxycholate amphotericin B (Fungizone) is the drug of choice for initial treatment of severe disease. Although more expensive, liposomal amphotericin B (AmBisome)[1] may lead to better outcomes in AIDS patients with moderate to severe disease.
- Oral itraconazole (Sporanox) is the drug of choice for initial treatment of mild to moderate disease and in continuation phase therapy of severe disease that has improved after intravenous amphotericin treatment.
- Fluconazole (Diflucan),[1] which is less active than itraconazole against *H. capsulatum*, has special usefulness in continuation phase therapy of meningitis because of its good cerebrospinal fluid penetration.

[1]Not FDA approved for this indication.

The lipid formulations approved for use with invasive fungal infections include amphotericin lipid complex (Abelcet), amphotericin B colloidal dispersion (Amphotec), and liposomal amphotericin B (AmBisome), but only the latter has been studied with histoplasmosis. Recent studies involving AIDS patients suggest that liposomal amphotericin B may lead to better clinical outcomes, including earlier clearance of the fungal burden, as well as improved survival, when compared to deoxycholate amphotericin B and itraconazole for treatment of moderate to severe histoplasmosis. Thus, although liposomal amphotericin B[1] may be more costly, it should be considered as an alternative first-line drug for AIDS patients who have moderate to severe disease, especially for those who are at risk for, or who already have, renal insufficiency.

Among the oral agents itraconazole (Sporanox) has the greatest activity against *H. capsulatum*. Ketoconazole (Nizoral) is also active against *Histoplasma* but is less well tolerated than itraconazole. Although fluconazole (Diflucan)[1] is the least active against *Histoplasma*, it has special usefulness in meningitis because of its ability to reach 80% of the blood concentration in the cerebrospinal fluid. To reduce the relapse risk of meningitis, fluconazole 800 mg PO daily[3] is recommended for 9 to 12 months after the full course of intravenous amphotericin is completed. Itraconazole does not enter the cerebrospinal fluid.

Anti-inflammatory treatment, as an adjunct to antifungal therapy, may be considered in certain forms of histoplasmosis. The inflammatory response in diffuse pulmonary histoplasmosis is thought to add to the severity of respiratory dysfunction. In addition to antifungal treatment, a 2-week course of prednisone at 60 mg daily can be considered. Pericarditis may also respond to treatment with corticosteroids or nonsteroidal anti-inflammatory agents. For rheumatologic manifestations, nonsteroidal anti-inflammatory agents can be given for 2 to 12 weeks.

REFERENCES

Durkin MM, Connolly PA, Wheat LJ: Comparison of radioimmunoassay and enzyme-linked immunoassay methods for detection of *Histoplasma capsulatum* var. *capsulatum* antigen. J Clin Microbiol 1997;35(9):2252-2255.

Johnson PC, Wheat LJ, Cloud GA, et al: Safety and efficacy of liposomal amphotericin B compared with conventional amphotericin B for induction therapy of histoplasmosis in patients with AIDS. Ann Intern Med 2002;137(2):105-109.

Newman SL, Bucher C, Rhodes J, Bullock WE: Phagocytosis of *Histoplasma capsulatum* yeasts and microconidia by human cultured macrophages and alveolar macrophages. Cellular cytoskeleton requirement for attachment and ingestion. J Clin Invest 1990;85(1):223-230.

Newman SL, Gootee L, Gabay JE: Human neutrophil-mediated fungistasis against *Histoplasma capsulatum*. Localization of fungistatic activity to the azurophil granules. J Clin Invest 1993;92(2):624-631.

Sathapatayavongs B, Batteiger BE, Wheat J, et al: Clinical and laboratory features of disseminated histoplasmosis during two large urban outbreaks. Medicine (Baltimore) 1983;62(5):263-270.

Wheat J: Histoplasmosis. Experience during outbreaks in Indianapolis and review of the literature. Medicine (Baltimore) 1997;76(5):339-354.

Wheat J, Sarosi G, McKinsey D, et al: Practice guidelines for the management of patients with histoplasmosis. Infectious Diseases Society of America. Clin Infect Dis 2000;30(4):688-695.

Wheat LJ, Cloud G, Johnson PC, et al: Clearance of fungal burden during treatment of disseminated histoplasmosis with liposomal amphotericin B versus itraconazole. Antimicrob Agents Chemother 2001;45(8):2354-2357.

Wheat LJ, Connolly-Stringfield P, Kohler RB, et al: *Histoplasma capsulatum* polysaccharide antigen detection in diagnosis and management of disseminated histoplasmosis in patients with acquired immunodeficiency syndrome. Am J Med 1989;87(4):396-400.

Wheat LJ, Kauffman CA: Histoplasmosis. Infect Dis Clin North Am 2003;17(1):1-19vii.

Williams B, Fojtasek M, Connolly-Stringfield P, Wheat J: Diagnosis of histoplasmosis by antigen detection during an outbreak in Indianapolis, Ind. Arch Pathol Lab Med 1994;118(12):1205-1208.

---

[1]Not FDA approved for this indication.

Blastomycosis

Method of
*Robert Bradsher, MD, and
Anupama Menon, MD, MPH*

Epidemiology

Blastomycosis is caused by infection with the thermally dimorphic fungus *Blastomyces dermatitidis*. The organism grows as a yeast form at 98.6°F (37°C) and as a mycelial form at room temperature. In the environment, the fungus is thought to exist in warm, moist soil associated with decomposing vegetation and decaying wood. In North America, *B. dermatitidis* is endemic along the Mississippi and Ohio River basins, in the regions that surround the Great Lakes, and in a small area of New York and Canada along the St. Lawrence River. Hyperendemic areas with very high rates of blastomycosis have been reported within these endemic regions. Cases outside North America have been described most commonly in Africa, but there have been reports of blastomycosis on several continents.

Infection with *B. dermatitidis* usually occurs via inhalation of aerosolized conidia. Cutaneous inoculation has been reported after inadvertent exposure in the laboratory, at autopsy, and after dog bites. Person-to-person transmission has been described in rare cases of sexual and perinatal transmission. The median incubation period is approximately 30 to 45 days.

Clinical Manifestations

Approximately 50% of infected individuals may be asymptomatic. Pulmonary disease may be acute or chronic. Acute pulmonary blastomycosis presents similarly to bacterial pneumonia with abrupt onset of fever, chills, pleuritic chest pain, myalgias, arthralgias, and cough that is initially nonproductive but later becomes productive of purulent sputum. Chest radiography demonstrates lobar or segmental consolidation; pleural effusion and hilar adenopathy are unusual. Patients diagnosed with blastomycosis may develop progressive, chronic disease that may involve pulmonary and numerous extrapulmonary sites. Patients with chronic pulmonary blastomycosis present with productive cough, hemoptysis, weight loss, pleuritic chest pain, and low-grade fever. Alveolar or fibronodular infiltrates, mass lesions, nodular lesions, and cavitation are seen on chest radiography. Findings may mimic tuberculosis, other endemic mycoses, or bronchogenic carcinoma. Acute respiratory failure may be seen with miliary disease or diffuse pneumonitis and is associated with a very high mortality.

Hematogenous dissemination to almost any other organ may occur. Manifestations in the skin, bone, or genitourinary tract are the most common and may be seen after clearance of pulmonary manifestations. The skin is the most frequently encountered extrapulmonary site of infection. Lesions are usually characterized as verrucous or ulcerative; they may be mistaken for squamous cell carcinoma, atypical mycobacterial infection, pyoderma gangrenosum, or keratoacanthoma. After the skin, bone is the most frequent site of dissemination. Manifestations include osteolytic lesions with associated soft-tissue abscesses or chronic draining sinuses. Genitourinary disease occurs in some male cases, affecting the prostate and epididymis. Although central nervous system (CNS) infection is reported in only a small number of normal hosts, it is a relatively common complication in immunocompromised patients, in whom it may present as an abscess or meningitis. In a review of AIDS patients with blastomycosis, 40% had CNS involvement. Indeed, blastomycosis is more often disseminated and fulminant in patients with AIDS and other types of chronic immunosuppression; mortality rates of 30% to 40% have been reported in these groups.

CURRENT DIAGNOSIS

- Because colonization with *B. dermatitidis* does not occur, identification by culture or histology confirms infection.
- The gold standard for diagnosis is culture of the organism from clinical specimens, which may take up to 4 weeks.
- A presumptive diagnosis may be made by visualization of the typical yeast from clinical specimens in the appropriate setting

Diagnosis

The definitive diagnosis of blastomycosis is based on isolation of the organism from cultures of clinical specimens. Mycologic media usually demonstrate growth after an incubation period of 2 to 4 weeks. Conversion from the mycelial form to the yeast phase is required for confirmation.

Because isolation of the organism may take weeks, presumptive diagnosis of blastomycosis is established by identification of the characteristic yeast form in clinical specimens. With a compatible clinical picture, treatment should be initiated if round, broad-based budding yeasts with thick, doubly refractile cell walls are seen on a wet mount preparation with addition of 10% potassium hydroxide to digest mammalian cells. In histopathologic specimens, acute suppurative and granulomatous inflammation are found. Visualization in tissue is improved by the use of special stains, such as the Gomori methenamine silver and periodic acid-Schiff stains. Nucleic acid hybridization tests are now commercially available and significantly shorten identification time. Most serologic tests are neither adequately sensitive nor specific to be useful in diagnosing blastomycosis, although newer antigen assays may be more reliable. A recently developed assay detects *Blastomyces* antigen in urine, serum, and other body fluids, including cerebrospinal fluid. The test is most sensitive in urine samples, in which 70% to 80% are positive in disseminated blastomycosis, and almost 100% are positive in pulmonary disease. Antigen is detected in serum in approximately 50% of cases. Cross-reactivity can occur in patients with other endemic mycoses. The assay may be used to monitor response to therapy and to detect recurrence.

Treatment

Although spontaneous resolution of acute blastomycotic pneumonia has been reported in immunocompetent hosts, most patients with blastomycosis require treatment. Treatment is indicated in all immunocompromised individuals and in all patients with progressive pulmonary disease or extrapulmonary disease. Factors to consider when initiating therapy include the severity and extent of disease, the immune status of the patient, and the toxicities of the antifungal agents.

PULMONARY DISEASE

For mild to moderate lung disease, itraconazole (Sporanox) is the preferred oral agent because it is efficacious and well tolerated. The initial dose should be 200 to 400 mg daily. Treatment should continue for at least 6 months. Bioavailability of itraconazole capsules is enhanced with food, whereas the oral suspension should be taken while fasting. Attention should be given to the patient's concurrent medications because of the potential for drug–drug interactions. Intravenous itraconazole has not been studied in blastomycosis and has no major benefits to offer. Ketoconazole (Nizoral) at 400 to 800 mg daily is an alternative agent to itraconazole, but it is associated with significant adverse effects, serious drug interactions, and higher rates of relapse. Clinical experience with fluconazole

CURRENT THERAPY

- Itraconazole (Sporanox) is the agent used most commonly to treat blastomycosis. It is administered in an oral dose of 200 to 400 mg daily for 6–12 months, depending on the site of infection.
- For life-threatening pulmonary disease (acute respiratory distress syndrome [ARDS]) or severe disseminated disease, amphotericin B (Fungizone) is the drug of choice. After initial improvement, itraconazole may be substituted.
- For CNS blastomycosis, amphotericin is used because itraconazole does not adequately penetrate the CNS. Liposomal amphotericin is used when high doses are needed or adverse effects from amphotericin B are encountered.
- Fluconazole (Diflucan),[1] ketoconazole (Nizoral), and IV itraconazole have lesser roles in the treatment of blastomycosis. Voriconazole (Vfend)[1] has not been studied adequately, but it may hold promise for CNS disease.

[1]Not FDA approved for this indication.

(Diflucan)[1] indicates that this agent is as efficacious as ketoconazole at doses of 400 to 800 mg daily. In patients with life-threatening pulmonary disease, progression of disease while on an azole or inability to tolerate an azole, amphotericin B (Fungizone) remains the agent of choice. A dose of 0.7 to 1.0 mg/kg daily should be administered until a cumulative dose of 1.5 to 2.5 g is completed. Some patients may be switched to oral itraconazole at 200 to 400 mg daily after clinical stabilization with amphotericin B. Lipid formulations of amphotericin B have not been adequately studied, but have been used in patients unable to tolerate conventional amphotericin B.

NERVOUS SYSTEM DISEASE

CNS infection should be treated with amphotericin B at a dose of 0.7 to 1.0 mg/kg daily to complete a total dose of 2.0 to 2.5 g. Itraconazole and ketoconazole are not recommended because of inadequate CNS penetration; fluconazole at 800 mg daily may be considered if amphotericin B is not tolerated.

EXTRAPULMONARY DISEASE (WITHOUT CNS INVOLVEMENT)

For mild to moderate disease, itraconazole at 200 to 400 mg daily is recommended for a minimum of 6 months. Patients whose disease progresses on this agent should be switched to amphotericin B to complete at least 1.5 g. Bone disease should be treated for at least 1 year. For life-threatening disease, amphotericin B at 0.7 to 1.0 mg/kg daily should be administered for a total dose of 2.0 to 2.5 g. In immunocompromised individuals, many authorities recommend long-term suppressive therapy with itraconazole after a treatment course of amphotericin B. Pregnant women should be treated with amphotericin B because the azoles are teratogenic. Data on blastomycosis in children are sparse, but some authorities suggest initial amphotericin B because of a potential unfavorable response to azoles.

NEW ANTIFUNGAL AGENTS

Voriconazole (Vfend)[1] is active in vitro and in animal models of pulmonary blastomycosis; the in vitro activity against *B. dermatitidis*

[1]Not FDA approved for this indication.

is similar to itraconazole. Although clinical data in treating blastomycosis in humans are inadequate, voriconazole has good CNS penetration based on reports of successful treatment of CNS aspergillosis. Posaconazole (Noxafil),[1] which has recently been licensed in the United States, is also active in vitro and in animal models. Further data are needed before these agents may be recommended for use in blastomycosis. The echinocandin class of antifungal agents shows variable activity against *B. dermatitidis* and there are no clinical data to support their use.

REFERENCES

Bradsher RW: Clinical features of blastomycosis. Semin Respir Infect 1997;12:229-234.
Bradsher RW, Chapman SW, Pappas PG: Blastomycosis. Infect Dis Clin North Am 2003;17:21-40.
Chapman SW: Blastomyces dermatitidis. In Mandell GL, Bennett JE, Dolin R, (eds): Principles and Practice of Infectious Diseases, New York: Churchill Livingstone, 2005, pp. 3026-3040.
Chapman SW, Bradsher RW, Campbell GD, et al: Practice guidelines for the management of patients with blastomycosis. Clin Infect Dis 2000;30:679-683.
Chapman SW, Lin AC, Hendricks KA, et al: Endemic blastomycosis in Mississippi: Epidemiological and clinical studies. Semin Respir Infect 1997;12:219-228.
Lemos LB, Guo M, Baliga M: Blastomycosis: organ involvement and etiologic diagnosis. A review of 123 patients from Mississippi. Ann Diagn Pathol 2000;4:391-406.
Pappas PG: Blastomycosis in the immunocompromised patient. Semin Respir Infect 1997;12:243-251.
Schutze GE, Hickerson SL, Fortin EM, et al: Blastomycosis in children. Clin Infect Dis 1996;22:496-502.
Sugar AM, Liu X-P: Efficacy of voriconazole in treatment of murine pulmonary blastomycosis. Antimicrob Agents Chemother 2001;45:601-604.

[1]Not FDA approved for this indication.

Pleural Effusion and Empyema Thoracis

Method of
Craig E. Daniels, MD, and
Dennis A. Wigle, MD, PhD

The diagnosis and management of pleural effusion is a commonly encountered problem in clinical practice. Under normal conditions, pleural fluid continually enters and is cleared from the pleural space. The volume of pleural fluid is normally 0.1 to 0.2 mL/kg of body weight. Pleural effusions are associated with a variety of thoracic and systemic diseases and occur when fluid production is excessive or fluid clearance is disturbed. Symptoms related to pleural effusions depend on the size of the effusion as well as the underlying disease process causing fluid to accumulate. Large effusions are commonly associated with dyspnea and chest discomfort. Infections of the pleural space are usually associated with systemic symptoms and fever.

Etiology

In some situations, the cause of the pleural effusion may be apparent based on the clinical context and imaging studies. More commonly, however, multiple diagnostic possibilities exist that require further evaluation. The causes of pleural effusion are broad and are generally divided into transudative and exudative pleural effusions (Box 1).

BOX 1 Causes of Transudative and Exudative Pleural Effusions

Transudates
Cirrhosis
Congestive heart failure
Hypoalbuminemia
Peritoneal dialysis
Renal disease

Exudates
Asbestos pleural disease
Chylothorax
Connective tissue diseases and vasculitis
Drugs (e.g., methotrexate)
Hemothorax
Infection
Malignancy
Pancreatitis
Pleuropericarditis
Postcardiotomy injury syndrome
Pulmonary embolism
Trauma (including chest surgery)

Transudative effusions are protein poor and are most commonly caused by increased pulmonary capillary hydrostatic pressure (e.g., heart failure), but they can result from low oncotic pressure (e.g., hypoalbuminemia). Transdiaphragmatic movement of fluid (e.g., ascites) can also result in transudative pleural effusion.

Exudative effusions are caused by local inflammation, increased capillary permeability, or decreased lymphatic clearance. As a result, they contain higher levels of protein and cells. Many disease processes increase inflammation and permeability including infection, neoplasm, pulmonary infarction, and various local and systemic inflammatory conditions. Blockage of normal lymphatic pathways, as in metastatic cancer in mediastinal lymph nodes, can result in exudative effusion. Increased fibrin deposition from empyema can also result in impaired lymphatic clearance and cause exudative effusion. Rupture or blockage of the thoracic duct can also cause an exudative pleural effusion (chylothorax).

Evaluation

IMAGING

Patients should initially have an upright posteroanterior and lateral chest x-ray. On an upright chest x-ray, a pleural effusion of 200 to 500 mL will be apparent as blunting of the costophrenic sulcus. Lateral decubitus films can help distinguish loculated from free-flowing pleural effusion. Supine chest x-rays can show pleural effusion as increased haziness over the entire hemithorax and can be confused for parenchymal lung infiltrates. Computed tomography (CT) of the chest is most useful after large effusions have been drained or when planning treatment in empyema. Bronchoscopy is not typically helpful unless there is suspicion that pleural effusion is

---

 CURRENT DIAGNOSIS

- Begin with history and physical and chest x-ray.
- Is the effusion transudative or exudative? Is it infected?
- Computed tomography is most useful after effusion drainage.
- Video-assisted thoracoscopic surgery should be used for complex cases or cases of unknown etiology.

caused by atelectasis from a central airway lesion. Although it is less commonly used for diagnostic imaging, thoracic ultrasound can identify loculated effusions, pleural thickening, and masses, and can reduce complications when used before or during thoracentesis.

THORACENTESIS

If the cause of the pleural effusion is unclear based on clinical assessment, or if the patient has respiratory symptoms caused by effusion, thoracentesis should be performed with the goals of removing pleural fluid for symptom relief and analysis. Thoracentesis can be performed without image guidance at the bedside in a cooperative patient who has a moderate or large effusion. Thoracic ultrasound guidance should be used if it is easily available, if the effusion is small or loculated, or if the patient cannot be properly positioned. Contraindications to thoracentesis include insufficient patient cooperation and uncontrollable coagulopathy.

PLEURAL FLUID ANALYSIS

Analysis of pleural fluid to determine etiology should begin at the bedside at the time of thoracentesis. Fluid should always be examined for clarity, odor, cellularity, and presence of blood. Thickened or inflamed parietal pleura can be hard to penetrate, and drainage of fluid can elicit a pleural rub or pleuritic chest pain. Rapid fluid removal can cause re-expansion pulmonary edema.

Traditionally, Light's criteria have been employed in distinguishing transudative from exudative pleural effusions (Table 1). Light's criteria are highly sensitive for detection of exudates but less specific.

If a transudate is identified in a patient with a condition known to cause transudative effusion, further evaluation of the effusion is limited and therapy should be directed at the underlying cause. Exudative effusions should be evaluated until the etiology of the effusion is identified. As a general rule, diagnostic tests should be directed by the clinical and radiographic presentation, not from a preformed algorithm (Box 2). When there is a diagnostic possibility of malignancy, pleural fluid cytology should be ordered. Culture and pH are useful in the diagnosis and management of patients with suspected infection of the pleural space. In the appropriate setting, diagnosis of chylothorax can be made if the triglyceride concentration is greater than 110 mg/dL. The diagnosis of hemothorax can be confirmed by a ratio of pleural fluid to serum hematocrit of at least 0.5.

Despite a thorough initial evaluation, the etiology of 25% of pleural effusions remains uncertain. In these cases, it is important to reconsider cancer, tuberculosis, and pulmonary embolism as potential serious causes of exudative effusions of unknown etiology. Exudative pleural effusions of unknown etiology should be pursued with further evaluation or observed until resolution. Video-assisted thoracoscopic surgery (VATS) or medical thoracoscopy have largely replaced percutaneous closed pleural biopsy as the diagnostic procedures of preference in effusion of unknown etiology.

TABLE 1 Diagnostic Criteria for Exudative Pleural Effusion

Light's Criteria for Diagnosis of Exudate	Sensitivity	Specificity
Ratio of pleural-fluid protein level to serum protein level >0.5	86%	84%
Ratio of pleural-fluid LDH level to serum LDH level >0.6	90%	82%
Pleural-fluid LDH level greater than two thirds the upper limit of normal for serum LDH level	82%	89%

LDH = lactate dehydrogenase.

BOX 2 Disease-Specific Pleural Fluid Tests

Cancer: Cytology
Infection: Culture and pH
Pancreatitis: Amylase
Esophageal perforation: Salivary amylase
Lymphoma: Lymphocyte flow cytometry
Hemothorax: Spun hematocrit (>50% plasma hematocrit)
Chylothorax: Lipid analysis (triglyceride >110 mg/dL)
Eosinophilic pneumonia: Cell differential (% eosiniophils)
Tuberculosis: Adenosine deaminase

Treatment

Treatment of pleural effusion is usually directed at controlling the underlying disease that results in effusion. In specific cases, it is appropriate to direct therapeutic intervention to control the pleural effusion itself. Palliation of malignant pleural effusion can be performed with either pleurodesis or insertion of an indwelling long-term silicone-elastic catheter. Pleurodesis can be accomplished either via a bedside chest tube or VATS in suitable operative candidates. VATS may be preferable in malignant pleural effusion, because the patient's hospital stay is shorter and time to recurrence of effusion is also shorter when compared with tube thoracostomy pleurodesis. Talc (Sclerosol Intrapleural) is the most commonly used agent. Pleurodesis in patients with benign disease is less commonly performed. Failure and complication rates are high for attempted pleurodesis in hepatic hydrothorax due to ascites and in chylothorax. If trapped lung is diagnosed with demonstration of visceral pleural rind, thoracotomy with decortication is typically required to achieve lung re-expansion for benign disease. For malignant effusions with trapped lung, pleurodesis is rarely effective, and these patients benefit most from silicone-elastic tube insertion for chronic drainage.

Pleural Space Infection

Infection of the pleural space is most commonly a complication of bacterial pneumonia. Risk factors for development of pleural space infection include medical conditions such as diabetes, liver disease, alcoholism, or gastroesophageal reflux. Penetrating trauma and chest surgery are also associated with infection of the pleural space. Infected fluid or pus in the pleural space is termed *empyema*. Surgical and medical management depend on appropriate characterization of the phase of pleural space infection as defined by Light.

Parapneumonic effusions are caused by inflammatory cytokine-mediated increases in vascular permeability; these develop in 20% of patients with pneumonia. Parapneumonic effusion is characterized by free-flowing fluid that is an exudate, not pus, with negative Gram stain and culture. Because the fluid is not infected, drainage with thoracentesis coupled with appropriate antibiotic therapy are typically sufficient.

CURRENT THERAPY

- Drain symptomatic or effusions of unknown etiology by thoracentesis.
- Treat underlying cause of effusion.
- Undertake palliation of malignant effusions by pleurodesis or indwelling catheter.
- Perform early video-assisted thoracoscopic surgery for empyema not responding to drainage and antibiotics.

Complicated or fibropurulent effusions result from infection involving the pleural space. The inflammatory cascade results in fibrin sails that form progressive loculations. The fluid characteristics in the fibropurulent phase include a turbid or pus like appearance with positive bacterial studies and the demonstration of fluid pH lower than 7.2. Management at this stage requires complete evacuation of the infected fluid. Tube thoracostomy is recommended, and further imaging is often required to ensure adequate lung re-expansion and exclude persistent pockets of infected fluid. Some patients do not achieve effective drainage with tube thoracostomy and medical support alone. Although individual patients might have a favorable outcome with streptokinase (Streptase)[1] instillation, a recent large randomized, placebo-controlled clinical trial showed no difference in any favorable outcome for patients treated with streptokinase versus placebo. We recommend early identification and definitive surgical management by VATS in patients with complicated pleural effusions who do not respond to aggressive tube thoracostomy and medical therapy.

The final phase of pleural space infection is the organized or fibropurulent stage. It occurs when persistent undrained empyema causes cytokine-mediated fibroblast proliferation to form a thick inelastic pleural peel along both pleural surfaces. Characteristics include pleural thickening (CT and ultrasound), multiloculated pleural pockets, and failure of the lung to re-expand following tube thoracostomy and suction. These patients typically have a trapped lung at thoracoscopy and require an open thoracotomy for complete surgical decortication of parietal and visceral pleural surfaces.

REFERENCES

Ferrer JS, Muñoz XG, Orriols RM, et al: Evolution of idiopathic pleural effusion: A prospective, long-term follow-up study. Chest 1996;109(6):1508-1513.
Jones PW, Moyers JP, Rogers JT, et al: Ultrasound-guided thoracentesis: Is it a safer method? Chest 2003;123(2):418-423.
Light RW: Clinical practice: Pleural effusion. N Engl J Med 2002;346(25):1971-1977.
Light RW: Parapneumonic effusions and empyema. Proc Am Thorac Soc 2006;3(1):75-80.
Luh SP, Chen CY, Tzao CY: Malignant pleural effusion treatment outcomes: Pleurodesis via video-assisted thoracic surgery (VATS) versus tube thoracostomy. Thorac Cardiovasc Surg 2006;54(5):332-336.
Maskell NA, Davies CW, Nunn AJ, et al: U.K. Controlled trial of intrapleural streptokinase for pleural infection. N Engl J Med 2005;352(9):865-874.
Rahman NM, Chapman SJ, Davies RJ: Diagnosis and management of infectious pleural effusion. Treat Respir Med 2006;5(5):295-304.
Sahn SA: State of the art: The pleura. Am Rev Respir Dis 1988;138(1):184-234.

---

[1]Not FDA approved for this indication.

Primary Lung Abscess

Method of
Mark Krasna, MD, and Lei Yu, MD

Etiology

Primary lung abscesses generally arise from necrotizing pulmonary infections, including those occurring in immunocompromised patients or due to aspiration of either gastrointestinal contents or oropharyngeal secretions. Based on the duration of symptoms at presentation, lung abscesses may be further divided into acute (symptoms for 6 weeks or less before presentation) and chronic stages. The abscess formation may be single or multifocal depending on the etiology. Although lung abscesses can develop in any part of the lung, most abscesses tend to occur in the posterior segment of the right upper lobe and the superior segments of both lower lobes.

Lung abscess is usually caused by bacteria that normally live in the mouth or throat and that are inhaled into the lungs, resulting in an infection. Predisposing factors can contribute to compromising the body's normal defenses and making it susceptible to infection by invasive microorganisms. Depending on the cause, the predominating bacteria vary enormously.

Aspiration has long been considered the principal cause of primary lung abscesses. It is most likely to occur in patients who are unconscious or semiconscious due to anesthesia, seizures, alcohol and drug abuse, or stroke. Studies have shown that the abscess flora generally comprise a mixed spectrum of microbes, including microaerophilic and aerobic. About 65% of these infections are produced by anaerobes. When resulting from necrotizing pneumonia, the bacteria are predominantly gram-positive—such as α-hemolytic or β-hemolytic streptococci, *Staphylococcus aureus*, or *Streptococcus pneumoniae*—and gram-negative, including *Klebsiella pneumoniae* and *Haemophilus influenzae*.

Opportunistic organisms (e.g., *Salmonella*, *Legionella*, or *Nocardia* spp) predominate in the immunocompromised host. These opportunistic lung abscesses occur in patients at the extremes of age and in patients with multiple medical problems (e.g., substance abuse, diabetes, epilepsy, or poor dental hygiene). In children, the most vulnerable patients are those with weakened immune systems, malnutrition, or blunt injuries to the chest.

Clinical Features

The presenting symptoms of primary lung abscesses are similar to the clinical features of pneumonia: cough, fever, chills, chest pain, and even dyspnea. Sometimes symptoms are insidious, showing fatigue, malaise, weight loss, and chronicity. When abscesses have communication with the tracheobronchial tree, hemoptysis and production of copious foul-smelling sputum are characteristic. Hemoptysis can vary from blood-streaked sputum to life-threatening hemorrhage. Large quantities of foul sputum occasionally lead to contamination of the contralateral lung. Rupture into the pleural space can cause pyopneumothorax, which subsequently results in septic shock and respiratory failure.

Diagnosis

Bronchoscopy and percutaneous transthoracic tube drainage under computed tomography (CT) or ultrasound guidance are effective methods of diagnosis and providing guidance to the etiology of infection for suitable antibiotic treatment.

Based on the clinical presentation and a chest radiograph, the diagnosis of lung abscesses is not a difficult question. Posteroanterior and lateral chest films are likely to demonstrate lung abscess with air-fluid level, which can be confused with other diagnoses. Two important points are to rule out malignancy and to obtain an accurate bacteria culture. CT is helpful in distinguishing primary lung abscess from secondary lung abscess or other disorders that manifest with similar symptoms and for assessing the stage of the illness. Unlike cavitations secondary to tumor with thick, irregular walls, the CT scan usually shows features of primary lung abscess with

---

  CURRENT DIAGNOSIS

- Clinical presentation, chest radiograph, and computed tomography (CT) are useful for detecting lung abscesses.
- CT, various aspirates, and fiberoptic bronchoscopy can rule out malignancy and get an accurate bacteria culture.

the thin, smooth walls and response to antibiotic therapy. Infected cysts or bullae, which manifest with the same clinical picture as a lung abscess, show a smooth, thin-walled cavity with little surrounding inflammation. An interlobar fluid collection or empyema often has the presence of a lenticular shape, obtuse angle with the chest wall, and a split pleura.

Invasive diagnostic techniques, including transtracheal aspirates, transthoracic aspirates, and fiberoptic bronchoscopy, are often recommended to diagnose lung abscesses and obtain accurate and meaningful bacteriology. By these means, secretions obtained from the lower respiratory tract via either lavage or brush can be submitted for culture and sensitivity and for ruling out the possibility of lung cancer. These procedures should be performed before instituting antibiotic therapy in order to acquire dependable microbiological data, but not at the expense of unnecessary delay in treatment. Culture data should be correlated with the Gram stain result before narrowing antibiotic therapy.

Routine laboratory studies (e.g., complete blood count, electrolytes and glucose, renal and liver function tests, and assessment of oxygen saturation) and bacteriologic tests (including blood culture and sputum Gram stain and culture) identifying an etiologic agent should be performed on all patients, although the usefulness of blood and sputum cultures has been questioned. Patients with lung abscess usually have abnormally high white blood cell counts (leukocytosis), but this condition is not unique.

Treatment

Lung abscess is treated with a combination of antibiotic drugs, various drainage techniques, oxygen therapy, and surgery. About 85% to 90% of lung abscess patients can be treated successfully with antibiotics. Depending on accurate culture, prolonged effective and systemic antibiotic therapy is recommended. Therapy generally consists of 2 weeks of intravenous antibiotics and 4 to 8 weeks of oral antibiotics, such as high-dose penicillin, clindamycin (Cleocin), metronidazole (Flagyl) or a third-generation cephalosporin. Supportive therapy is also necessary. Supportive therapy includes nutritional support; postural drainage; inhalation of warm, humidified air; treatment of predisposing factors; and removal of underlying causes such as obstructing lesions, gastroesophageal reflux disease, and various dysphagia syndromes.

Bronchoscopy and percutaneous transthoracic tube drainage under CT or ultrasound guidance allow a means of treating refractory lung abscess, obviating possible surgery. CT-guided percutaneous tube drainage may be very helpful in patients who are too ill to tolerate thoracotomy and may be the treatment of choice for lung abscesses that are refractory to medical management. It is curative and obviates the unnecessary loss of functioning lung parenchyma. Adverse consequences, such as bronchoscopy-induced release of large amounts of purulent material into the contralateral lung, transthoracic drainage–related empyema, pneumothorax, or hemothorax, can occur and should be anticipated.

Surgical resection is required in less than 10% of cases of lung abscess. Candidates for a lobectomy or segmental pulmonary resection are those who do not respond to conservative management, who have underlying anatomic or physiologic comorbidities, who have larger and chronic abscesses, and who have significant hemoptysis. During surgery, a double-lumen endotracheal tube is used in all cases to protect the contralateral lung from contamination. The rate of major postoperative complications remains relatively high.

REFERENCES

Bartlett J: Anaerobic bacterial infections of the lung and pleural space. Clin Infect Dis 1993;16(suppl 4):S248-S255.
Chan PC, Huang LM, Wu PS, et al: Clinical management and outcome of childhood lung abscess: A 16-year experience. J Microbiol Immunol Infect 2005;38(3):183-188.
Hagan JL, Hardy JD: Lung abscess revisited. A survey of 184 cases. Ann Surg 1983;197(6):755-762.
Hammond JM, Potgieter PD, Hanslo D, et al: The etiology and antimicrobial susceptibility patterns of microorganisms in acute community-acquired lung abscess. Chest 1995;108:937-941.
Petrov D, Goranov E, Stanoev V, et al: Surgical treatment of chronic pulmonary abscesses—contemporary treatment. Khirurgiia (Sofiia) 2004;60(4-5):9-12.
Van Sonnenberg E, D'Agostino HB, Casola G, et al: Lung abscess: CT-guided drainage. Radiology 1991;178(2):347-351.
Wiedemann HP, Rice TW: Lung abscess and empyema. Semin Thorac Cardiovasc Surg 1995;7(2):119-128.
Weissberg D: Percutaneous drainage of lung abscess. J Thorac Cardiovasc Surg 1984;87(2):308-312.

Acute Bronchitis

Method of
Susan Davids, MD, MPH, and
Ralph M. Schapira, MD

Acute bronchitis is one of the most common diagnoses made by primary care physicians in the United States and accounts for nearly 10 million office visits per year. Acute bronchitis is a transient, self-limited inflammatory process of the upper respiratory tract, specifically the trachea and bronchi. Antibiotics are overprescribed to patients with acute bronchitis; this practice has raised significant concern related to the worldwide rise of antibiotic resistance, which is viewed as one of the world's most pressing public health problems.

Acute bronchitis manifests as an acute respiratory illness of less than 3 weeks' duration, with or without sputum production. Acute bronchitis is a clinical diagnosis and must be distinguished from other respiratory diseases, such as pneumonia, acute exacerbation of chronic bronchitis (episode of worsening of symptoms and expiratory airflow obstruction in patients with chronic obstructive pulmonary disease), and the onset of asthma. Most cases of acute bronchitis occur in the fall and winter. The etiology of acute bronchitis is infectious, and viruses appear to be the cause of most cases. Influenzas A and B are the most common viruses isolated, although a wide variety of infectious agents have been identified, such as adenovirus, coronavirus, parainfluenza virus, respiratory syncytial virus, coxsackievirus, *Mycoplasma pneumoniae*, *Bordetella pertussis*, and *Chlamydia pneumoniae*.

Diagnosis of acute bronchitis is based on findings of a prominent cough that may be accompanied by wheezing and sputum production. Most patients are otherwise healthy and without preexisting respiratory disease. Nonspecific constitutional symptoms may also be part of acute bronchitis. Appropriate management of acute bronchitis is essential because it is one of the most common illnesses that present to physicians in the outpatient setting. Antibiotics are often prescribed unnecessarily for acute bronchitis and other respiratory tract illnesses; these prescriptions may potentially lead to adverse

CURRENT THERAPY

- The primary treatment is intravenous antibiotics with certain supportive therapy.
- Predisposing factors must be eradicated.
- Bronchoscopy and various kinds of drainage can indicate the etiology of the infection and suitable antibiotic treatment, as well as supplying a way of treating refractory lung abscess.
- The role of surgery has decreased, but it is still necessary for certain lung abscesses.

CURRENT DIAGNOSIS

- Normal healthy adult with cough
- Predominance of cough
- Lasts 1 to 3 weeks
- With or without sputum
- Can be accompanied by other respiratory and constitutional symptoms
- Absence of abnormal vital signs and physical exam suggesting pneumonia, particularly
  - Heart rate >100 beats per minute
  - Respiratory rate >24 breaths per minute
  - Temperature >100.4°F (38°C)
  - Lung findings suggest a consolidation process

CURRENT THERAPY

- Antibiotics not routinely recommended
- If influenza is highly probable and patient is presenting within the first 48 hours, consider treatment with
  - Oseltamivir (Tamiflu) 75 mg PO bid with food for 5 days (influenza A/B)
  - Zanamivir (Relenza) 10 mg bid by inhalation for 5 days (influenza A/B)
  - *Amantadine (Symmetrel) 100 mg bid or 200 mg once daily for 5 days (influenza A)
  - *Rimantadine (Flumadine) 100 mg bid for 5 days (influenza A)
- In patients with evidence of bronchial hyperresponsiveness, consider treatment with
  - β_2-agonists for 1 to 2 weeks
  - Antitussives in those with cough for 2 to 3 weeks
  - Antipyretics and analgesics as needed
  - Smoking cessation
- Education: cough likely to last 3 weeks or more.

*Due to emergence of antiviral resistance, use of these agents has been discouraged by the CDC.

---

events (i.e., allergic reactions and gastrointestinal side effects) and bacterial resistance. Other medications, such as inhaled bronchodilators and antitussives, are often prescribed for acute bronchitis despite questionable evidence to support their routine use.

Pathophysiology of acute bronchitis involves an acute inflammatory response involving the mucosa of the trachea and bronchi, resulting in injury to the respiratory tract epithelium. Sputum production is increased and bronchoconstriction (potentially resulting in airflow obstruction and wheezing) can occur. Positron emission tomography (PET) of a patient with acute bronchitis confirms that the primary inflammatory changes occur in the trachea and bronchi and not the remainder of the lower respiratory track.

Diagnosis

Cough, phlegm (which may be purulent as both bacteria and viruses can cause purulent sputum), and wheezing help differentiate acute bronchitis from upper respiratory infections such as pharyngitis and sinusitis. Acute bronchitis must be differentiated from acute bacterial pneumonia. The absence of abnormalities in vital signs (heart rate >100 bpm, respiratory rate >24 breath/min, oral temperature >100.4°F [38°C] and physical examination of the chest) supports the diagnosis of acute bronchitis and makes the need for chest radiography unnecessary in most cases. The treatment and outcome of acute bronchitis and pneumonia are very different; a chest radiograph should always be obtained if there is uncertainty about the diagnosis. Chest radiography will demonstrate no lung infiltrates in a patient with acute bronchitis. In contrast, lung infiltrates are present in pneumonia. Pertussis or whooping cough should be considered in adults with cough in the setting of what appears to be an upper respiratory infection, even in those previously immunized. Typically, the cough of pertussis, unlike acute bronchitis, lasts for longer than 3 weeks. Other respiratory diseases, such as previously undiagnosed asthma, can also mimic acute bronchitis, although several features differentiate asthma from acute bronchitis (see Section 12). Rapid testing to diagnose influenza viruses A and B (the most common causes of acute bronchitis) as a cause of acute bronchitis should be considered given the availability of effective treatment if initiated in the first 48 hours.

Treatment

ANTIBIOTICS, INHALED BRONCHODILATORS, AND ANTITUSSIVES

Existing evidence does not support the routine use of antibiotics for uncomplicated cases of acute bronchitis. Although most cases of acute bronchitis are caused by viral infections, upwards of 60% of patients are prescribed antibiotic therapy, which is contributing to the rise of bacterial resistance to commonly used antibiotics.

Meta-analyses examining the effectiveness of antibiotic therapy in patients without underlying lung disease suggest no consistent effect of antibiotics on the severity or duration of acute bronchitis. A recent study evaluated children and patients with colored sputum and found that they also did not benefit from antibiotics. This study also found that compared to other populations, the elderly were less likely to benefit from antibiotics. Smokers with acute bronchitis are even more likely to be prescribed antibiotics. Their response to antibiotics was either equal to or worse than that of nonsmokers.

One possible reason for overuse of antibiotics is the concern by physicians about patient satisfaction. Studies show that patients presenting to the doctor expecting antibiotics were more likely to be prescribed antibiotics; studies also suggest that satisfaction is more related to appropriate patient education than to receiving antibiotics. Patient education should include information regarding the duration of symptoms associated with acute bronchitis. It was found that patients presented on average after 9 days of cough and that the cough persisted for an additional 12 days after the physician visit. This information can impart a realistic expectation of illness duration to the patient.

If influenza is highly suspected and the patient presents within 48 hours of the onset of symptoms, rapid diagnostic testing and treatment should be considered. Both amantadine (Symmetrel) and rimantadine (Flumadine) are effective for influenza A, and neuraminidase inhibitors, inhaled zanamivir (Relenza), and oral oseltamivir (Tamiflu) are effective for influenzas A and B. If these medications are initiated within the first 48 hours of symptoms (and ideally within 30 hours), the duration of illness can be shortened.

The evidence supporting the use of inhaled bronchodilators for the treatment of the symptoms has been variable. Two small trials reported a shorter duration of cough with the use of inhaled β-agonists; another study reported benefit in those with evidence of bronchial hyperresponsiveness. Current recommendations support the use of β-agonists only in patients with evidence of bronchial hyperresponsiveness (wheezing or spirometry demonstrating a forced expiration volume in 1 second [FEV_1] <80% of predicted).

Antitussive agents have not been shown to improve the acute or early cough but did show some improvements in cough lasting longer than 3 weeks. The current recommendations are to use antitussives, namely dextromethorphan (Benylin) or codeine, in patients with cough of 2 to 3 weeks' duration.

Acute uncomplicated bronchitis is most often a viral illness in which antibiotics are not routinely indicated. Patients presenting with an acute respiratory illness, who are younger than 65 years old without existing pulmonary disease or other significant comorbid illness, should have a thorough physical examination, including vital signs. If the vital signs are normal and physical examination of the chest is clear, pneumonia can most likely be ruled out. In patients who present within 48 hours of onset of symptoms, influenza should be considered as effective therapy is available for acute bronchitis caused by influenzas A or B. Otherwise, the evidence for treatment with antibiotics does not support their routine use. Bronchodilators should be considered in those with evidence of bronchial hyperresponsiveness; cough suppressants should be considered in those with 2 to 3 weeks of cough. Patient education is an integral part of the treatment, and patients should receive information that provides realistic expectations regarding the duration of cough.

REFERENCES

Aagaard E, Gonzales R: Management of acute bronchitis in healthy adults. Infect Dis Clin North Am 2004;18:919-937.

Ebell MH: Antibiotic prescribing for cough and symptoms of respiratory tract infection. JAMA 2005;294(3):3062-3064.

Fahey T, Smucny J, Becker L, Glazier R: Antibiotics for acute bronchitis. Cochrane Database Syst Rev 2004;(4):CD000245.

Gonzales R, Sande M: Uncomplicated acute bronchitis. Ann Intern Med 2000;133:981-991.

Kicska G, Zhuang H, Alavi A: Acute bronchitis imaged with F-18 FDG positron emission tomography. Clin Nucl Med 2003;28(6):511-512.

Little R, Rumsby K, Kelly J, et al: Information leaflet and antibiotic prescribing strategies for acute lower respiratory tract infection. JAMA 2005;293(24):3029-3035.

Linder JA, Sim I: Antibiotic treatment of acute bronchitis in smokers. J Gen Intern Med 2002;17:230-234.

Martinez FJ: Acute bronchitis: State of the art diagnosis and therapy. Compr Ther 2004;30(1):55-59.

Smucny J, Flynn C, Becker L, Glazier R: Beta$_2$-agonists for acute bronchitis. Cochrane Database Syst Rev 2004;1):CD001726.

Bacterial Pneumonia

Method of
Edward Septimus, MD

Pneumonia occurs in about 3 to 4 million patients per year in the United States with approximately 1 million patients requiring hospitalization. The symptoms of pneumonia include cough, shortness of breath, sputum production, and chest pain. Physical examination includes fever in most, with crackles and bronchial breath sounds on auscultation in about 80% of cases. Pneumonia is classified by where it was acquired: community-acquired pneumonia (CAP) and health care–acquired pneumonia (HAP, sometimes called *hospital-acquired pneumonia*). This chapter focuses on adult patients with CAP or HAP.

Community-Acquired Pneumonia

CAP remains a leading cause of death in the United States. One study estimated that more than 900,000 cases of CAP occur in persons older than 65 years each year. The emergence of drug-resistant *Streptococcus pneumoniae* (DRSP) and less common pathogens including methicillin-resistant *Staphylococcus aureus* (MRSA) is well documented. Pneumonia in long-term care institutions usually resembles HAP and is discussed later.

DIAGNOSTIC TESTING

Symptoms plus an infiltrate by chest radiograph or other imaging studies are required for the diagnosis. Clinical features and physical findings may be absent in the elderly. All patients should be screened by pulse oximetry. Arterial blood gases should be reserved for patients with suspected CO_2 retention. Routine diagnostic studies to determine the etiology for outpatients with CAP are optional. For patients requiring admission, diagnostic studies to determine the etiology of CAP should be attempted. Increased mortality is more common with inappropriate initial empiric therapy. De-escalation of antimicrobial therapy based on pathogen-specific treatment has been shown to decrease adverse drug effects and selection of antimicrobial resistance.

Blood cultures and sputum for Gram stain and culture (in patients with a productive cough) should be obtained in most patients who are admitted to the hospital. Pretreatment blood cultures have a 5% to 14% yield in patients hospitalized with CAP. The most common positive blood culture to be considered a pathogen is *S. pneumoniae*. In some series, false-positive blood cultures (contaminants) exceed positive blood culture with true pathogens. A false-positive blood culture can lead to extra days in the hospital and unnecessary use of antibiotics, especially vancomycin (Vancocin). The highest yield has been demonstrated with severe CAP (Box 1). Pretreatment Gram stain and culture should be performed only if a good quality specimen can be obtained. A Gram stain can direct initial empiric therapy, especially with less common pathogens such as *S. aureus* or gram-negative bacteria.

Patients with pleural effusions greater than 5 cm on a lateral upright chest radiograph or greater than 1 cm on a lateral decubitus film should undergo a thoracentesis for Gram stain and culture. Urinary antigen tests are available for *S. pneumoniae* and *Legionella pneumophila*. These tests are rapid and specific in adults. For pneumococcal pneumonia, studies in adults show a sensitivity of 50% to 80% and a specificity of greater than 90%. False-positives are seen in children colonized with *S. pneumoniae*; therefore, this test is not recommended in children. For *L. pneumophila*, the urinary antigen can only detect *L. pneumophila* serogroup 1, which accounts for 80% to 90% of legionnaires' disease cases in the United States. The urinary antigen has a sensitivity of 70% to 90% and a specificity of greater than 95%. A new polymerase chain reaction (PCR) test can

---

BOX 1 Criteria for Severe Community-Acquired Pneumonia

Minor Criteria

Confusion or disorientation
Hypotension requiring fluid resuscitation
Hypothermia (<36°C)
Leukopenia (WBC <4000 cell/mm^3)
Multilobar infiltrates
Pao$_2$/Fio$_2$ ≤ 250
Respiratory rate ≥ 30
Thrombocytopenia (platelet count <100,000 cells/mm^3)
Uremia (BUN ≥20 mg/dL)

Major Criteria

Invasive mechanical ventilation
Septic shock requiring vasopressors

BUN = blood urea nitrogen; Fio$_2$ = fraction of inspired oxygen; Pao$_2$ = partial pressure of arterial oxygen; WBC = white blood cell count.
Adapted from Mandell LA, Wunderink RG, Anzueto, et al: Infectious Diseases Society of America/American Thoracic Society Consensus Guidelines on the Management of Community-Acquired Pneumonia in Adults. Clin Infect Dis 2007;44:S27-S72.

detect all serotypes of *L. pneumophila* in sputum; however, clinical experience is currently limited.

The diagnosis of atypical pneumonia such as *Chlamydophila pneumoniae*, *Mycoplasma pneumoniae*, and *Legionella* species other than *L. pneumophila* rely on acute and convalescent serologies. In general, management on a single acute serology is unreliable; therefore, serologies are often retrospective and usually do not affect initial antimicrobial therapy.

ADMISSION CRITERIA

The initial decision of the treatment of CAP often revolves around severity of illness and if the patient requires hospitalization. Two severity-of-illness scores are commonly used, CURB-65 and the pneumonia severity index (PSI). CURB-65 stands for *c*onfusion, *u*remia (blood urea nitrogen >20 mg/dL), *r*espiratory rate greater than 30 breaths/minute, systolic *b*lood pressure less than 90 mm Hg, and age older than 64 years. The PSI score is based primarily on history of underlying diseases and age that increase the risk of mortality, whereas CURB-65 does not rely on underlying diseases.

With CURB-65, mortality was higher when three (14.5%), four (40%), or five (57%) factors were present. Patients with a score of 0 or 1 can be treated on an outpatient basis, patients with a score of 2 can be admitted to the floor, and patients with scores higher than 3 often require admission to the intensive care unit (ICU). PSI uses 20 different variables and places patients into five risk groups (Table 1). Risk classes I and II patients can be treated as outpatients, risk class III patients can be treated on a short hospitalization or observational unit, and risk classes IV and V patients should be treated as inpatients.

ETIOLOGY

CAP may be caused by a number of pathogens, but only a few account for the majority of cases. Box 2 lists the more common pathogens divided by site of care and severity. According to most studies, an etiology is established in only about 40% of patients with CAP. In confirmed cases, *S. pneumoniae* is the most common bacterial pathogen identified. Atypical pathogens are the most common in mild to moderate CAP; *S. aureus*, gram-negative bacilli, and *L. pneumophila* are more common in severe CAP. Nontypable *Haemophilus influenzae* can be seen in patients with underlying chronic lung disease. *S. aureus* is often associated with preceding influenza. Gram-negative bacilli, including *Pseudomonas aeruginosa*, can be seen in patients who are taking steroids or chemotherapy, who have previously used antibiotics, are alcoholics, or who have underlying pulmonary disease.

TREATMENT

Antimicrobial therapy remains the mainstay of treatment. Until better diagnostic tests are available, initial treatment remains largely empiric. Box 3 reviews the most recent recommended empiric antibiotics. Anaerobic coverage should be considered with a history of loss of consciousness in patients with gingival or esophageal disease. Antibiotics should be modified based on local epidemiology and susceptibilities.

Current levels of penicillin and cephalosporin resistance to *S. pneumoniae* do not usually result in failure when appropriate doses are administered. However, recent studies indicate that resistance to macrolides and older fluoroquinolones (levofloxacin [Levaquin] and ciprofloxacin [Cipro]) have resulted in clinical failures in patients with CAP caused by *S. pneumoniae*. Pneumonia caused by community-acquired MRSA may be increasing, especially associated with influenza. Many of these cases are genotypically and phenotypically different from hospital-acquired MRSA. Community-acquired MRSA isolates are less antibiotic resistant and often contain the gene for Panton-Valentine leukocidin (PVL), a toxin associated with necrotizing pneumonia. Anecdotal and in vitro studies suggest clindamycin (Cleocin) (if susceptible) or linezolid (Zyvox) can affect toxin production and improve outcome. More studies are needed to determine the most effective treatment for CAP caused by community-acquired MRSA. Several studies have reported that combination therapy with the combination of a macrolide and a β-lactam for bacteremic pneumococcal pneumonia is associated with lower

---

BOX 2 Community-Acquired Pneumonia Pathogens by Site

Outpatient Setting
Chlamydophlia pneumoniae
Haemophilus influenzae
Mycoplasma pneumoniae
Respiratory viruses: adenovirus, influenza, parainfluenza, respiratory syncytial virus
Streptococcus pneumoniae

Inpatient outside Intensive Care Unit
Aspiration
Chlamydophlia pneumoniae
Haemophilus influenzae
Legionella species
Mycoplasma pneumoniae
Respiratory viruses
Streptococcus pneumoniae

Inpatient in Intensive Care Unit
Gram-negative bacilli
Haemophilus influenzae
Legionella species
Staphylococcus aureus
Streptococcus pneumoniae

Adapted from File TM: Community-acquired pneumonia. Lancet 2003;362:1991-2001.

TABLE 1 Pneumonia Severity Index

Risk Factors	Points
Demographic factors	
Age for men	Age (yr)
Age for women	Age (yr) −10
Nursing home resident	+10
Coexisting illnesses	
Active neoplastic disease	+30
Chronic liver disease	+20
CHF	+10
Cerebrovascular disease	+10
Chronic renal disease	+10
Physical examination	
Altered mental status	+20
Respiratory rate ≥30	+20
Blood pressure <90 mm Hg	+20
Temperature <35°C or ≥40°C	+15
Pulse ≥125	+10
Laboratory and radiographic findings	
Arterial pH <7.35	+30
BUN ≥30 mg/dL	+20
Sodium <130 mmo/L	+20
Glucose ≥250 mg/dL	+10
Hematocrit <30%	+10
Pao$_2$ <60 mm Hg	+10
Pleural effusion	+10

Risk classes: I = 0; II = 70 (low risk); III = 71-90 (low risk); IV = 91-130 (moderate risk); V >130 (high risk).
BUN = blood urea nitrogen; CHF = congestive heart failure; Pao$_2$ = partial pressure of arterial oxygen.
Adapted from Fine MJ, Auble TE, Yealy DM, et al: A predictive rule to identify low-risk patients with community-acquired pneumonia. N Engl J Med 1997;336:243-250.

> **BOX 3 Empiric Antimicrobial Choice for Community-Acquired Pneumonia**
>
> **Outpatient Treatment**
> Healthy patient, no prior antibiotics within the previous 3 months
> - Macrolide (azithromycin [Zithromax], clarithromycin [Biaxin], or erythromycin) *or*
> - Doxycycline (Vibramycin) (weak recommendation)
>
> Patient with comorbidity (e.g., chronic heart, lung, liver, or renal disease; malignancies; alcoholism; asplenia; diabetes mellitus; immunosuppression) or use of antibiotics in previous 3 months
> - Respiratory fluoroquinolone (moxifloxacin [Avelox], gemifloxacin [Factive], or levofloxacin [Levaquin] (750 mg) *or*
> - β-Lactam (high-dose amoxicillin or amoxicillin-clavulanate [Augmentin]); alternatives are ceftriaxone (Rocephin), cefpodoxime (Vantin), or cefuroxime (Ceftin) plus a macrolide
>
> In regions with a high rate (>25%) of infection with high-level (MIC ≥16 µg/mL) macrolide-resistant *Streptococcus pneumoniae*
> - Use a fluoroquinolone or a β-lactam plus either a macrolide or doxycycline
>
> **Inpatients Not in Intensive Care**
> - Fluroquinolone alone *or*
> - β-Lactam (e.g., ceftriaxone, cefotaxime [Claforan], ampicillin, ertapenem [Invanz]) plus a macrolide
>
> **Intensive Care Unit Patients**
> - β-Lactam (e.g., ceftriaxone, cefotaxime, or ampicillin-sulbactam [Unasyn]) *plus* either azithromycin or a fluoroquinolone
>
> For *Pseudomonas* infection
>   - Antipneumococcal, antipseudomonal β-lactam (piperacillin-tazobactam [Zosyn], cefepime [Maxipime], imipenem [Primaxin], or meropenem [Merrem]) plus either ciprofloxacin (Cipro) or levofloxacin (750 mg) *or*
>   - Antipneumococcal, antipseudomonal β-lactam *plus* an aminoglycoside and azithromycin
>
> **Community-Acquired MRSA**
> - Add vancomycin (Vancocin) or linezolid (Zyvox)
>
> ---
> MIC = minimum inhibitory concentration;
> MRSA = methicillin-resistant *Streptococcus aureus*.
> Adapted from Mandell LA, Wunderink RG, Anzueto, et al: Infectious Diseases Society of America/American Thoracic Society Consensus Guidelines on the Management of Community-Acquired Pneumonia in Adults. Clin Infect Dis 2007;44:S27-S72.

mortality compared with a single effective drug. A possible explanation might relate to the fact that macrolides have immunomodulatory effects, including cytokine production.

Time to first antibiotic dose for CAP has been studied in two retrospective studies in Medicare patients. These studies demonstrated lower mortality in patients who received timely antimicrobial treatment. The first study showed that if the first dose was given within 8 hours of arrival, mortality was reduced. The second study demonstrated that a 4-hour interval was associated with better outcomes. Treatment should be given for a minimum of 5 days; the patient should be afebrile for 48 to 72 hours and clinically stable. Longer treatment may be needed for CAP caused by *S. aureus*, *L. pneumophila*, or *P. aeruginosa* and in patients with evidence of associated endocarditis, septic arthritis, or meningitis.

PREVENTION

Patients older than 50 years, others at risk for influenza complications, household contacts of high-risk patients, and health care workers with direct patient contact should receive a yearly influenza vaccine. Several reviews have demonstrated that influenza vaccination not only prevents pneumonia but also decreases hospitalizations, decreases cerebrovascular events, and decreases deaths from all causes.

Pneumococcal polysaccharide vaccine (Pneumovax 23) is recommended for all persons older than 65 years and persons with certain underlying illnesses (e.g., functional and anatomic asplenia, cardiopulmonary disease, diabetes). Studies have documented moderate effectiveness for preventing invasive pneumococcal disease (bacteremia and meningitis). The overall efficacy in patients older than 65 years is reported to be between 44% and 75%.

Vaccination status should be determined in all patients admitted to the hospital. Vaccination should be offered year-round for pneumococcal vaccine and during the fall and winter months for influenza vaccine.

Health Care–Acquired Pneumonia

HAP is defined as a pneumonia that occurred more than 48 hours after admission and that was not incubating at the time of admission. Ventilator-associated pneumonia (VAP) is defined as pneumonia that develops 48 to 72 hours after intubation. Health care–associated pneumonia (HCAP) is a new category; HCAP occurs in a patient who attended a hospital or hemodialysis clinic, who was hospitalized in an acute-care hospital for more than 2 days within the prior 90 days, or who resided in a long-term care facility or nursing home. The remaining comments are directed at HAP and VAP.

HAP is the second or third most common health care–associated infection in the United States and is associated with significant morbidity and mortality, resulting in increased length of stay and costs. HAP accounts for about 25% of all ICU infections. VAP occurs in 9% to 27% of intubated patients, and the mortality is double that of similar patients without VAP. The risk of VAP is highest in the first 1 to 2 weeks. Some investigators consider time of onset an important factor in terms of outcomes and pathogens. Early-onset HAP and VAP are pneumonia occurring within 4 to 7 days of hospitalization. Early-onset HAP and VAP usually carry a better prognosis and are more likely to be caused by more sensitive pathogens. Late-onset HAP and VAP are more likely to be caused by multidrug-resistant organisms (MDRO) with a higher mortality.

Aspiration of oropharyngeal secretions or leakage of bacteria around the endotracheal tube is the primary source of bacteria causing HAP or VAP. The stomach and sinuses, blood, and contaminated aerosols are much less common sources. Contaminated biofilm in the endotracheal tube, with subsequent embolization into the lower airway, may be an important factor in the pathogenesis of VAP.

DIAGNOSIS

Unfortunately, there is no universally accepted gold standard for the diagnosis of HAP or VAP. The diagnosis is suspected if a patient has a new or progressive infiltrate along with new-onset fever, purulent sputum (>25 neutrophils per low-power field), leukocytosis, and decreased oxygenation.

Unfortunately, the clinical parameters are overly sensitive; therefore, other diagnostic tests are desirable. For a start, blood and lower respiratory secretions should be collected for culture in all patients with suspected HAP or VAP. A thoracentesis should be performed if a large pleural effusion is present. The microbiological approach favors quantitation or semiquantitation of lower respiratory secretions. The diagnostic threshold used to differentiate colonization versus true infection varies by specimen collection. The proposed diagnostic threshold for endotracheal aspirate is greater than 10^5

colony-forming units (CFU)/mL; for bronchoalveolar lavage, greater than 10^4 CFU/mL; and for protected-specimen brush, greater than 10^3 CFU/mL. A major reservation to this approach is the possibility of false-negative results, which can result if a patient has been started on an antimicrobial agent before the specimens are collected.

TREATMENT

For patients with suspected HAP or VAP, appropriate broad-spectrum antimicrobial therapy should be ordered to cover anticipated pathogens. Consider a Gram stain to guide initial therapy. Whenever possible, select antimicrobial therapy based on local microbiology and epidemiology. Use combination therapy in patients whenever an MDRO is suspected until culture results are available. Risk factors include prolonged hospitalization (>5-7 days), admission from another health care facility, and recent antibiotic therapy. Table 2 summarizes suggested empiric therapy. De-escalation of therapy is strongly recommended when culture results become available. Discontinue antimicrobial therapy if results of cultures and other clinical parameters do not confirm pneumonia. Based on recent studies, a shorter duration of therapy (7-8 days) is now recommended in patients with uncomplicated HAP or VAP who received initial appropriate therapy and have had a good clinical response. *P. aeruginosa*, *Acinetobacter* species, and MRSA can require longer durations of therapy.

TABLE 2 Initial Empiric Therapy for Suspected Health Care–Acquired Pneumonia or Ventilator-Associated Pneumonia

Suspected Pathogen	Recommended Therapy
Patients with No Known Risk Factors for MDRO and Early Onset	
Streptococcus pneumoniae	One of the following:
Haemophilus influenzae	Ceftriaxone (Rocephin) or
Methicillin-sensitive *Streptococcus aureus*	Fluoroquinolone (levofloxacin [Levaquin], moxifloxacin [Avelox], or ciprofloxacin [Cipro])
Antibiotic-sensitive enteric gram-negative *Escherichia coli*	or Ertapenem (Invanz)
Klebsiella pneumoniae	or
Enterobacter species	Piperacillin-tazobactam (Zosyn)
Proteus species	
Serratia marcescens	
Patients with Risk Factors for MDRO or Late Onset	
Pathogens listed above and MDRO	Antipseudomonal cephalosporin (e.g., cefepime [Maxipime] or ceftazidime [Fortaz])
Pseudomonas aeruginosa	or
K. pneumoniae (ESBL)*	Antipseudomonal carbepenem (e.g., imipenem [Primaxin] or meropenem [Merrem])
Acinetobacter species	or
MRSA	Piperacillin-tazobactam (Zosyn)
Legionella species†	**plus** Aminoglycoside
	or
	Antipseudomonal fluoroquinolone (e.g., ciprofloxacin [Cipro] or levofloxacin [Levaquin])
	plus Vancomycin (Vancocin) or linezolid (Zyvox)

*If an ESBL strain, a carbepenem is preferred.
†If *Legionella* suspected, the combination regimen should include either a macrolide (e.g., azithromycin) or a fluoroquinolone.
ESBL = extended-spectrum β-lactamase; MDRO = multidrug-resistant organisms; MRSA = methicillin-resistant *Staphylococcus aureus*.
Modified from American Thoracic Society; Infectious Diseases Society of America: Guidelines for the management of adults with hospital-acquired, ventilator-associated, and healthcare-associated pneumonia. Am J Respir Crit Care Med 171:388-416, 2005.

PREVENTION

The incidence of HAP and VAP can be reduced by following certain proved measures. An effective infection control program, which includes education, hand-washing compliance, surveillance of ICU infections, and isolation of patients with MDRO to reduce cross-infection should be followed. Noninvasive ventilation should be used whenever possible. If intubation is required, the orotracheal route is preferred to reduce health care–associated infections due to sinusitis and VAP. Consider continuous aspiration of subglottic secretions, if available. Follow a protocol for using sedation with daily interruptions. Perform daily assessment for extubation. For patients on a ventilator, keep the head of the bed at 30 to 45 degrees to prevent aspiration (except when contraindicated). Use agents such as oral chlorhexidine (Peridex) to reduce oropharyngeal colonization. In diabetic patients, use intensive insulin therapy to maintain glucose levels below 110 mg/dL.

REFERENCES

American Thoracic Society; Infectious Diseases Society of America: Guidelines for the management of adults with hospital-acquired, ventilator-associated, and healthcare-associated pneumonia. Am J Respir Crit Care Med 2005;171:388-416.
Chastre J, Wolff M, Fagon JY, et al: Comparison of 8 vs 15 days of antibiotic therapy for ventilator-associated pneumonia in adults: A randomized trial. JAMA 2003;290:2588-2598.
Fagon JY, Chastre J, Wolff M, et al: Invasive and noninvasive strategies for management of suspected ventilator-associated pneumonia: A randomized trial. Ann Intern Med 2000;132:621-630.
File TM: Community-acquired pneumonia. Lancet 2003;362:1991-2001.
Fine MJ, Auble TE, Yealy DM, et al: A predictive rule to identify low-risk patients with community-acquired pneumonia. N Engl J Med 1997; 336:243-250.
Houck PM, Bratzler DW, Nsa W, et al: Timing of antibiotic administration and outcomes for Medicare patients hospitalized with community-acquired pneumonia. Arch Intern Med 2004;164:637-644.
Lim WS, van der Eerden MM, Laing R, et al: Defining community acquired pneumonia severity on presentation to hospital: An international derivation and validation study. Thorax 2003;58:377-382.
Mandell LA, Wunderink RG, Anzueto, et al: Infectious Diseases Society of America/American Thoracic Society Consensus Guidelines on the Management of Community-Acquired Pneumonia in Adults. Clin Infect Dis 2007;44:S27-S72.
Metersky ML, Ma A, Houck PM, Bratzler DW: Antibiotics for bacteremic pneumonia: Improved outcomes with macrolides but not fluoroquinolones. Chest 2007;131:466-473.
Richards MJ, Edwards JR, Culver DH, Gaynes RP: Nosocomial infections in medical ICUs in the United States: National Nosocomial Infections Surveillance System. Crit Care Med 1999;27:887-892.
van den Berghe G, Wilmer A, Hermans G, et al: Intensive insulin therapy in the medical ICU. N Engl J Med 2006;354:449-461.

Viral Respiratory Infections

Method of
Robert C. Welliver, Sr., MD

Viral infections of the respiratory tract are among the most common infections in humans, and they account for significant morbidity at all ages. Infants and young children can sustain six to eight such infections annually, and adults have an average of nearly two such infections per year.

Rhinoviruses are the most commonly identified etiologic agents and cause illness year-round. Other common causative agents during winter months include influenza viruses and respiratory syncytial virus, and enteroviruses predominate in summer months. The parainfluenza viruses also commonly cause respiratory infection, particularly in autumn (type 1) and late spring or summer (type 3). Coronaviruses, metapneumoviruses, adenoviruses, and other agents are identified less often.

Although each of these agents can cause a common cold, some viral infections are associated with characteristic patterns of respiratory disease. Most of these viruses can also exacerbate asthma, cystic fibrosis, and chronic obstructive pulmonary disease (COPD).

Common Colds

Colds are the most common of the viral respiratory illnesses. Pharyngitis is usually the earliest sign of a cold, beginning a few days after infection has taken place. Nasal congestion and clear or slightly cloudy rhinorrhea usually follow within 24 to 48 hours. Cough occurs in approximately 30% to 40% of those infected, and fluid can accumulate in middle ear or sinus cavities that have become blocked as a result of mucosal swelling. Ear and sinus cavity infections occur when this fluid is trapped for a week or more. Treatment with antibiotics is ineffective before this time, and they are ineffective especially in the absence of other clinical signs of ear and sinus infections.

Colds are a frequent cause of missed school and work, and even of mild morbidity, but they are rarely serious in otherwise healthy persons. The most appropriate approach to treatment therefore entails rest, with adequate nutrition and hydration. Agents that inhibit the activity of cyclooxygenase probably represent the most effective form of pharmacologic intervention. These compounds include acetaminophen (Tylenol) and the nonsteroidal anti-inflammatory agents (NSAIDs) such as ibuprofen (Motrin). They are effective in reducing fever and, perhaps more importantly in most colds, reducing malaise, headache, and pharyngitis.

Nasal congestion and some rhinorrhea during colds are related to dilation of blood vessels in the nose and sinuses. Vasoconstrictors have therefore been used extensively to attempt to reverse these symptoms. Oral decongestants such as pseudoephedrine (Sudafed) have minimal effect on nasal congestion, and can result in systemic hypertension, anxiety, and difficulty sleeping. The propensity for these compounds to cause cardiac arrhythmias in the very young child has led to recommendations against their use in the first year or two of life. Nasal sprays containing vasoconstricting agents such as oxymetazoline (Afrin) can result in mild temporary relief of nasal obstruction. However, the use of these compounds for more than 3 or 4 days can result in rebound vasodilation and paradoxically increased rhinorrhea.

Numerous investigations have evaluated the role of antihistamines in colds. The release of histamine itself is not associated with fever, cough, or malaise, so effects on these symptoms would not be expected. Furthermore, nasal congestion and discharge may be more related to the release of kinins, and not histamine. Indeed, the administration of antihistamines in adults and, particularly, in children has not demonstrated strikingly positive results. As many as 40% of subjects treated with placebo report beneficial effects. Side effects of histamine use, primarily sedation and dry mouth, are commonly encountered.

Cough can be one of the most irritating symptoms during colds. Cough during colds is principally caused by secretions entering the airway (postnasal drip) and not by inflammation of the airway itself. Therefore, it is not surprising that cough suppressants, especially codeine, have little effect on cough induced by colds. Antihistamines have also been found to be ineffective in relief of cough during colds.

Influenza-Like Illness

The influenza syndrome is defined as the abrupt onset of fever, headache, and striking degrees of malaise and prostration, often with intense myalgia. Respiratory symptoms can occur concurrently, but they might not be prominent features. The principal cause is, of course, influenza virus, although infection with many other viruses can cause similar (although not as intense) symptoms. The illness is generally self-limited, and most symptoms resolve over 4 or 5 days. Lassitude can persist for up to 2 weeks.

CURRENT DIAGNOSIS

- Rapid diagnostic kits are available for many common respiratory viruses. These tests are used increasingly to establish that antibiotic therapy is not necessary in many patients with febrile respiratory illnesses or with lower respiratory tract infections.
- The presence of wheezing on physical examination virtually excludes bacterial infection from consideration in subjects with lower respiratory disease.

Influenza virus infection and influenza-like illness are best treated symptomatically, relying on rest, adequate intake of fluids and calories, and appropriate analgesic therapy. Compounds referred to as *M2 inhibitors* such as amantadine (Symmetrel) and rimantadine (Flumadine) have been approved for therapy. Positive outcomes from therapy with these agents are observed only when therapy is instituted within 48 hours after the onset of symptoms, and benefits are not striking. In recent years, resistance to M2 inhibitors has been commonly observed among circulating epidemic strains of influenza virus.

More recently, inhibitors of the activity of influenza viral neuraminidase have been used in treatment and prevention of influenza virus infection in adults and children. The first such compound released, zanamivir (Relenza,) was administered by inhalation but was unpopular because of its irritating effects on the airway. An oral compound, oseltamivir (TamiFlu), has been used to prevent and to treat influenza virus infection. As with M2 inhibitors, it is believed that treatment should be started within the first 48 hours of symptoms and that prophylaxis should be instituted within 48 hours of exposure. Treatment with oseltamivir shortens the duration of subsequent illness by only about 24 hours. Treatment can prevent some of the complications of influenza infection, including pneumonia. The drug may be more effective as a therapeutic agent, because it may be up to 90% effective in preventing culture-positive symptomatic influenza illness. The recommended dose for adults is 75 mg orally every 12 hours for 5 days. In children, the appropriate dose based on body weight is 30 mg twice daily for children weighing less than 15 kg, 45 mg twice daily for children weighing 15 to 23 kg, 60 mg twice daily for children weighing 23 to 40 kg, and 75 mg twice daily for children weighing more than 40 kg. The principal side effect is nausea, which can be reduced by taking the drug with food.

Croup

Croup is defined by the occurrence of hoarseness or laryngitis, a deep, brassy or barking cough, and inspiratory stridor. Airway obstruction in croup is caused by constriction in the subglottic area, often noted on radiographs by a steeple-shaped narrowing of the air column in

CURRENT THERAPY

- The management of most viral respiratory infections consists of rest, adequate caloric and fluid intake, and management of fever and malaise.
- Corticosteroids are essential in the management of croup.
- Specific antiviral therapy is available only for influenza virus infection, and beneficial effects have been more readily achieved in prevention rather than treatment.

this region. Affected children are usually afebrile and nontoxic in appearance.

Parainfluenza virus type 1 is the primary cause of croup, although infection with many different viruses can produce this illness, and influenza virus can cause a particularly severe form of croup. Bacterial secondary infection occurs uncommonly, but it can result in fever and severe obstruction of the airway. Administration of dexamethasone (Decadron)[1] at 0.6 mg/kg either orally or intramuscularly markedly reduces the rate of hospitalization, admission to the intensive care unit, and intubation for croup.

Bronchiolitis

Bronchiolitis represents the most common cause for hospitalization of infants in developed countries. Infants present with a history of several days of upper respiratory symptoms, followed by the rapid onset of wheezing and labored breathing. Respiratory syncytial virus (RSV) is the most common cause and is the agent found in the most severe cases that result in respiratory failure. Contrasting with asthma, obstruction of the airway in bronchiolitis is a result of plugging of bronchioles with detached epithelium and inflammatory cells. Mucus plugging and constriction of smooth muscle are not prominent. Also in contrast with asthma is the absence of a sustained response to bronchodilators and corticosteroids among infants with bronchiolitis.

Therapy of bronchiolitis primarily consists of administration of supplemental oxygen and replacement of fluid deficits as needed. Ribavirin (Virazole)[1] is a compound with antiviral activity against RSV, but controlled studies have not demonstrated meaningful differences in outcomes between treated and untreated subjects. The compound is quite expensive and must be delivered via a special aerosol generator.

Palivizumab (Synagis), a preparation consisting of a monoclonal antibody against the fusion protein of RSV, has proved to be effective in reducing the rate of hospitalization for RSV infection by approximately 50% when given to high-risk infants. Infants who may be considered candidates for therapy include those with chronic lung disease, those born prematurely, and those with hemodynamically significant congenital heart disease. Doses of palivizumab (15 mg/kg) are given on a monthly basis throughout the local RSV season, usually November through March.

REFERENCES

Akerlund A, Klint T, Olen L, Runderantz H: Nasal decongestant effect of oxymetazoline in the common cold: An objective dose-response study in 106 patients. J Laryngol Otol 1989;103:743-746.
Buckingham SC, Jafri HS, Bush AN, et al: A randomized, double-blind, placebo-controlled trial of dexamethasone in severe respiratory syncytial virus (RSV) infection: Effects on RSV quantity and clinical outcome. J Infect Dis 2002;185:1222-1228.
Curley FJ, Irwin RS, Pratter MR, et al: Cough and the common cold. Am J Respir Crit Care Med 1988;138:305-311.
Flores G, Horwitz RI: Efficacy of β2-agonists in bronchiolitis: A reappraisal and meta-analysis. Pediatrics 1997;100:233-239.
Johnson DW, Jacobson S, Edney PC, et al: A comparison of nebulized budesonide, intramuscular dexamethasone, and placebo for moderately severe croup. N Engl J Med 1998;339:498-503.
Muether PS, Gwaltney JM Jr: Variant effect of first- and second-generation antihistamines as clues to their mechanism of action on the sneeze reflex in the common cold. Clin Infect Dis 1001;33:1483-1488.
Randolph AG, Wang EL: Ribavirin for respiratory syncytial virus lower respiratory tract infection. Arch Pediatr Adolesc Med 1996;150:942-947.
Tavorner D, Danz C, Economos D: The effects of oral pseudoephedrine on nasal patency in the common cold: A double-blind single-dose placebo-controlled trial. Clin Otolaryngol 1999;24:47-51.
Treanor JJ, Hayden FG, Vrooman PS, et al: Efficacy and safety of the oral neuraminidase inhibitor oseltamivir in treating acute influenza: A randomized controlled trial. US Oral Neuraminnidase Study Group. JAMA 2000;283:1016-1024.
Van Voris LP, Betts RF, Hayden FG, et al: Successful treatment of naturally occurring influenza A/USSR/77 H1N1. JAMA 1981;245:1128-1131.

---

[1]Not FDA approved for this indication.

Viral and Mycoplasmal Pneumonias

Method of
Burke A. Cunha, MD

Influenza pneumonia is the most important cause of viral pneumonia in adults. Influenza A is the predominant type of influenza found in adults, and influenza B is more common in children. Influenza A has the potential for severe disease, occurs seasonally, and is the predominant type involved in influenza pandemics. *Mycoplasma pneumoniae* community-acquired pneumonia (CAP) was first recognized decades ago as distinctive from bacterial and viral pneumonias. It was originally described by Eaton as "Eaton agent" pneumonia caused by a pleuropneumonia-like organism (PPLO), later shown to be caused by *M. pneumoniae*. *M. pneumoniae* is a common cause of pneumonia in all age groups, but the peak incidence of *M. pneumoniae* CAP is in young adults. *M. pneumoniae* CAP is a common cause of ambulatory CAP.

The term *atypical pneumonia* was first applied to viral pneumonias because the clinical laboratory and radiologic findings were different from those caused by typical bacterial pulmonary pathogens. In influenza pneumonia, the clinical findings are confined to the trachea, bronchi, lung parenchyma, and central nervous system. *M. pneumoniae* CAP is a systemic infection with a pulmonary component. Over the years, atypical pneumonia has come to refer to pneumonia caused by systemic nonviral/nonbacterial pathogen agents that have a pulmonary component. Viral pneumonias are no longer considered atypical pneumonias. Atypical pneumonias may be divided into nonzoonotic and zoonotic atypical CAPs. Nonzoonotic CAPs are most commonly caused by *M. pneumoniae, Chlamydia pneumoniae,* or *Legionella* species; whereas the three most common zoonotic atypical pneumonias are caused by *Chlamydia psittaci* (psittacosis), *Francisella tularensis* (tularemia), or *Coxiella burnetii* (Q fever). All of the atypical pneumonias are distinct clinical entities that may be differentiated on the basis of their characteristic pattern of extrapulmonary organ involvement. Although some viruses may occasionally have extrapulmonary manifestations (i.e., influenza, adenovirus with viral pneumonias), the primary clinical features are confined to the lungs. *M. pneumoniae* is a critical cause of nonzoonotic atypical CAP, particularly in the ambulatory setting. *M. pneumoniae* CAP may be severe in patients with impaired host defenses or those with severe, preexisting cardiopulmonary disease.

Viral Influenza Pneumonia

Viral influenza pneumonia affects children and adults. Influenza B is the primary type, causing mild influenza in children and adults. Influenza A is primarily an infection of adults that may be mild to severe. Influenza A has the potential for pandemic spread.

Influenza occurs during the winter months, usually peaking in February. Influenza is spread by aerosolized droplet infection from person to person and via fomites. Viral influenza A is classified into subtypes based on neuramidase (N) [YG1] and hemagglutinin (H) surface proteins. An important characteristic of influenza A virus is antigenic drift, which refers to a change in surface protein shift in the neuramidase or hemagglutinin receptors. With influenza A, these surface receptor proteins are important in cellular adherence of the influenza virus and the spread of influenza from respiratory epithelial cells. The vaccine for the flu season most often includes the influenza hemagglutinin and neuramidase types seen at the end of the preceding year's season. Prevention of attachment and spread of the virus is helpful to controlling the spread of influenza; vaccine protection conferred by specific antibody response to influenza A is highly protective (approximately 80% in noncompromised hosts).

During the years when influenza B has been important, vaccines for the subsequent year contain an influenza B component.

TABLE 1 Adult Anti-Influenza Antivirals

Antiviral	Treatment Dose	Prophylactic Dose
Mild Influenza A/B		
Zanamivir (Relenza)[†]	2 inhalations (5 mg per inhalation) q12h × 5d	No FDA indication
Severe Influenza A		
Amantadine (Symmetrel)[†]	200 mg (PO) q24h Persons age 65: 100 mg	200 mg (PO) q24h Persons age 65: 100 mg
	or	
Rimantadine (Flumadine)	100 mg (PO) q12h Persons with hepatic/renal failure (CrCl <10 mL/min) or elderly 100 mg (PO) q24h	100 mg (PO) q12h Persons with hepatic/renal failure (CrCl <10 mL/min) or elderly 100 mg (PO) q24h
	plus	
Oseltamivir[1] (Tamiflu)[†]	75 mg (PO) q12d × 5d*	75 mg (PO) q24h × 7d

[1]Not FDA approved for this indication.
*For avian influenza, 150 mg (PO) q12h may be more effective.
[†]Some avian influenza strains may be resistant.

The prophylactic effects of amantadine (Symmetrel) and rimantadine (Flumadine) are based on preventing viral adherence, thus preventing entry and infection of respiratory epithelial cells. Neuramidase inhibitors have anti-influenza activity.

Clinical manifestations of influenza A in adults varies considerably from mild to fatal infection. Mild infection is usually manifested as an acute febrile illness characterized by headache and myalgias with dry unproductive cough, rhinorrhea, and tracheobronchitis. Mild viral influenza may be a result of influenza A or B and usually resolves in a few days without complications in normal hosts who have good cardiopulmonary function.

Severe viral influenza A occurs in normal healthy adults and may be fatal. The onset of severe influenza A is sudden, and the patient often recalls the exact hour of onset. The patient is febrile with early/extreme prostration rendering the patient bedridden. Fever rapidly rises and may be accompanied by chills. Neck soreness, severe headache, and myalgias are typical. Sore throat, eye pain, conjunctival injection, and hemoptysis are frequently present. Chest pain worsened by deep inspiration is not truly pleuritic but rather reflects influenza A myositis of the intracostal muscles. Shortness of breath is related to the degree of hypoxemia. Severe influenza A causes an oxygen diffusion defect as manifested by an increased A-a gradient (>35). Profound hypoxemia may be accompanied by cyanosis. Hypotension caused by hypoxemia and vascular collapse may follow. The course of severe viral influenza A is fulminant and of short duration.

Physical findings are few in viral influenza (i.e., conjunctival suffusion). Auscultation reveals absolutely quiet lungs because the infectious process is interstitial and not alveolar. Routine blood tests are usually unremarkable except for leukopenia/lymphopenia and, less commonly, thrombocytopenia. Few atypical lymphocytes may be noted, and low titers of cold agglutinins may be present. Cold agglutinins (if present) have low titers less than or equal to 1:16. In severe cases, a pale bluelike hue of the skin may be noted, and there may be bleeding from diffuse intravascular coagulation (DIC) from multiple orifices preterminally. The chest radiograph in uncomplicated viral influenza A is unremarkable or may have minimal perihilar bilateral increased prominence of interstitial markings. In severe influenza A pneumonia, the chest radiograph shows bilateral symmetrical perihilar infiltrates without pleural effusions.

Patients may die from severe influenza A without superimposed bacterial pneumonia. Most deaths during the 1918 pandemic were young military recruits who died of influenza A pneumonia without bacterial superinfection. Viral influenza may be complicated by bacterial pneumonia. Bacterial pneumonias complicating viral influenza may occur concurrently at presentation or may present 1 to 2 weeks after the presentation of viral influenza. Viral influenza A presenting concurrently with a bacterial pneumonia is usually caused by *Staphylococcus aureus*. In contrast to uncomplicated viral influenza, bacterial superinfection is manifested by an increase in fever, shaking chills, leukocytosis, purulent sputum, localized rales on auscultation, bacteremia, and focal/segmental infiltrates on chest radiograph. Alternately, patients with viral influenza A may develop a secondary bacterial infection (same manifestations as noted previously) 1 to 2 weeks later. Secondary bacterial pneumonia is less severe than with concurrent *S. aureus* and is usually caused by *Streptococcus pneumoniae* or *Haemophilus influenzae*.

ANTI-INFLUENZA THERAPY

Therapy of viral influenza is directed at inhibiting viral replication and preventing further infection of respiratory epithelial cells. The neuramidase inhibitors zanamivir (Relenza) and oseltamivir (Tamiflu) have anti-influenza A and B activity. Neuramidase inhibitors decrease the severity and duration of influenza symptoms by 1 to 2 days. Amantadine (Symmetrel) and rimantadine (Flumadine) are useful prophylactically and therapeutically in influenza. Amantadine and rimantadine have anti-influenza A activity, but no influenza B activity. Amantadine and rimantadine inhibit early M2 protein-dependent replication and prevent adherence of the influenza virus to respiratory epithelial cells, thus preventing progression of infection and minimizing further cell to cell spread. Amantadine and rimantadine also affect peripheral airway dilatation and oxygenation is improved, which is of critical importance because patients with severe influenza A uncomplicated by bacterial superinfection die of severe hypoxemia. Mild influenza A/B may be treated with neuramidase inhibitors. Mild cases of influenza A should be treated at the onset of the illness. For severe influenza A, amantadine or rimantadine in combination[1] with neuramidase inhibitors provide optimal anti-influenza therapy (Table 1). For avian influenza (H_5N_1), these antiviral drugs may be ineffective.

---

[1]Not FDA approved for this indication.

Mycoplasma pneumoniae Pneumonia

M. pneumoniae is a common cause of ambulatory CAP. It affects all age groups, and in normal hosts with intact cardiopulmonary function, *Mycoplasma* CAP is usually a mild, self-limiting infection. However, *M. pneumoniae* derives its importance from difficulty in diagnosis, the necessity for non–β-lactam therapy, and because of its effect on peripheral airways.

Mycoplasma CAP is one of the nonzoonotic causes of CAP (the others being *Legionella* and *Chlamydia pneumoniae*). *M. pneumoniae* is an atypical pneumonia that is a systemic infectious disease with a pulmonary component. It may be distinguished from other atypical pneumonias by its characteristic pattern of extrapulmonary organ involvement. *M. pneumoniae* CAP most closely resembles *C. pneumoniae* CAP clinically, but is very different from Legionnaires' disease in terms of its epidemiology, age distribution, pattern of extrapulmonary organ involvement, and severity.

Clinically, *M. pneumoniae* presents as a subacute febrile illness. Temperatures rarely exceed 102°F (38.9°C). Rigors are not a feature of *M. pneumoniae* CAP, but patients may complain of chilly sensations. Mild headache and/or myalgias are not uncommon. The most common presenting symptom in *Mycoplasma* CAP is the prolonged, nonproductive dry cough. Patients with *Mycoplasma* CAP often complain of or have mild nonexudative pharyngitis. Rhinorrhea and conjunctivitis are not features of *M. pneumoniae* CAP. Watery diarrhea is commonly present in *Mycoplasma* CAP, but abdominal pain is not a clinical finding. Other extrapulmonary manifestations are uncommon or rare (e.g., meningoencephalitis, pericarditis, hemolytic anemia, glomerular nephritis, Guillain-Barré syndrome, erythema multiforme). *M. pneumoniae* has a distinctive pattern of extrapulmonary organ involvement that does not include cardiac involvement (relative bradycardia) or hepatic involvement, including normal serum glutamate-oxaloacetate transaminase (SGOT) or serum glutamate-pyruvate transaminase (SGPT). The distinguishing laboratory feature of *M. pneumoniae* CAP is elevated cold agglutinin titers. Although a variety of infectious and noninfectious diseases are associated with cold agglutinin elevations, they are usually of low titer (i.e., <1:16). There are no pulmonary infections presenting as CAP that are associated with high elevations of cold agglutinin titers (i.e., ≥1:64). Although elevated cold agglutinins occur early in up to 75% of patients with *M. pneumoniae* CAP, they are still diagnostically important when present. In a patient with CAP and a cold agglutinin titer greater than or equal to 1:64, the diagnosis of *M. pneumoniae* CAP is very likely.

M. pneumoniae may be differentiated from the typical bacterial pneumonias because of the presence of extrapulmonary findings, including nonexudative pharyngitis, loose stools or watery diarrhea, erythema multiforme, and high cold agglutinin. Patients with typical bacterial CAP usually have a more acute onset of presentation, a productive cough, and temperatures that may exceed 102°F (38.9°C),

CURRENT DIAGNOSIS

Viral Influenza
- Mild influenza A or B presents acutely with headache, fever, sore throat, plus/minus rhinorrhea.
- Severe influenza A presents with an acute onset (patients often able to name the hour the influenza began) and rapidly become bed bound.
- Headache, myalgias, and prostration are severe.
- Auscultation of the lungs is quiet, disproportionate to the degree of respiratory distress. Influenza is an interstitial process and not alveolar, which explains the absence of rales.
- With severe influenza, patients rapidly become hypoxemic. Hypoxemia is accompanied by an AA gradient (>35), which suggests an interstitial oxygen diffusing defect typical of severe viral influenza pneumonia.
- Severe tracheobronchitis is common and is manifested by hemoptysis.
- Leukopenia/lymphopenia is typical; thrombocytopenia may occur. Low titer elevations of cold agglutinins are not infrequent (≥1:16).
- Patients may have chest pain exacerbated by breathing mimicking pleuritic chest pain. This is the result of direct intracostal muscle involvement with the influenza virus, which results in myositis and pain on inspiration.
- The chest radiograph in early viral influenza, in mild to moderate cases, is normal or near normal, with minimal, if any, increase in perihilar interstitial markings. The chest radiograph in fulminant cases shows symmetrical bilateral patchy infiltrates without pleural effusion in 24 to 48 hours.
- Severe viral influenza A is accompanied by severe hypoxemia or cyanosis, which may be followed by a fatal outcome.
- Influenza pneumonia may present alone without bacterial superinfection. Bacterial infection may accompany or follow.
- Purulent sputum with viral influenza indicates concurrent bacterial pneumonia usually caused by *S. aureus*. Bacterial pneumonia following influenza (after 1 to 2 weeks), is suggested by leukocytosis, focal or segmental pulmonary infiltrates, and purulent sputum; the pathogens are not *S. aureus*, but most commonly are *S. pneumoniae* or *H. influenzae*.
- A laboratory diagnosis may be made by DFA staining of respiratory secretions, viral influenza titers, or viral cultures.

Mycoplasma pneumoniae
- In a patient with CAP and a dry nonproductive cough, without severe headache or myalgias, the most likely diagnosis is *M. pneumoniae*. *M. pneumoniae* CAP is commonly accompanied by nonexudative pharyngitis and/or loose stools or watery diarrhea.
- The temperature is usually less than 102°F (38.9°C) and is not accompanied by frank rigors or pleuritic chest pain.
- Relative bradycardia and elevations in the serum transaminases are not features of *M. pneumoniae* CAP.
- Respiratory viruses are often associated with mild elevations of cold agglutinins (≤1:16) but *M. pneumoniae* is the only pathogen causing CAP associated with highly elevated cold agglutinin titers (≥1:64). Elevated cold agglutinin titers occur in up to 75% of patients with *M. pneumoniae*, and occur early and transiently.
- In a patient with CAP, elevated cold agglutinin titers (>1:8) effectively rule out the typical pathogens, as well as *Legionella* species and *C. pneumoniae*.
- Elevated *M. pneumoniae* ELISA IgG titers indicate past exposure/infection and not current infection or co-infection with another pathogen.
- In the absence of an antecedent respiratory tract infection (e.g., nonexudative pharyngitis, otitis, etc., in the preceding 3 months), the presence of an increased *M. pneumoniae* ELISA IgM titer is diagnostic of acute infection.

CURRENT THERAPY

Viral Influenza
- The aim of therapy is to inhibit the influenza virus and prevent its attachment/spread to uninfected respiratory epithelial cells.
- The neuramidase inhibitors shorten the course of influenza by 1 to 2 days and have antiviral activity. These agents are active against both influenza A and B.
    - Amantadine (Symmetrel) or rimantadine (Flumadine) do not have antiviral properties but are important in prevention/therapy.
    - Amantadine and rimantadine prevent the adherence of influenza virus to uninfected upper respiratory epithelial cells, thereby limiting the extent of the infection.
    - Amantadine and rimantadine also have an important therapeutic effect in influenza A by increasing distal airway dilation and increasing oxygen action; their effect on peripheral airways is important in severe influenza A. Amantadine and rimantadine are not active against influenza B.
    - Amantadine and rimantadine should be given for the duration of viral influenza. Used prophylactically, amantadine and rimantadine should be given before, during, and following an outbreak of influenza A.

Mycoplasma pneumoniae
- The agents active against *M. pneumoniae* are macrolides, tetracyclines, quinolones, and ketolides. β-Lactam antibiotics are not active against *M. pneumoniae* because the organisms do not contain a bacterial cell wall.
- Goals of therapy of *M. pneumoniae* CAP are to eradicate the infection, decrease the shedding of *Mycoplasma* in respiratory secretions posttherapy, and to prevent posttreatment asthma.
- Therapy is equally efficacious with macrolides, doxycycline (Vibramycin), respiratory quinolones, or telithromycin (Ketek) intravenously, orally, or in combination for 1 to 2 weeks.
- The mode of administration is determined by the severity of the CAP and the setting. Outpatients are usually treated orally. Patients hospitalized with severe CAP are initially treated intravenously and then changed to an oral agent.
- Resistance to *M. pneumoniae* with antimicrobials has not been described and is not a clinical consideration.

often accompanied by chills. Patients with typical pneumonia often have pleuritic chest pain, which is not a feature of *M. pneumoniae* CAP. Among the atypical pneumonias, the zoonotic pneumonias (i.e., tularemia, psittacosis, Q fever) may be eliminated from consideration if there is a recent zoonotic contact history with the appropriate vector.

C. pneumoniae resembles closely *M. pneumoniae* CAP. *C. pneumoniae* may be distinguished by the absence of cold agglutinins and the presence of hoarseness, which is a feature of *C. pneumoniae* but not *M. pneumoniae* CAP. Loose stools or watery diarrhea are not usual features of *C. pneumoniae* CAP. The most common clinical problem is differentiating *Legionella* from *Mycoplasma* CAP; this may be done by appreciating the differences in the pattern of extrapulmonary organ involvement with each of these pathogens. *Legionella* may be clinically differentiated from *Mycoplasma* by acuteness of onset or severity, the presence of relative bradycardia, temperatures greater than 102°F (38.9°C), and the presence of abdominal pain.

From a laboratory standpoint, highly elevated cold agglutinin titers argue strongly against the diagnosis of *Legionella* and point to *M. pneumoniae*. Nonspecific laboratory tests in a patient with CAP that suggest *Legionella* and argue against *M. pneumoniae* include otherwise unexplained hypophosphatemia, hyponatremia, microscopic hematuria, and increased creatinine. *Legionella* does not affect the upper respiratory tract as does *Mycoplasma* (e.g., nonexudative pharyngitis). Ear findings are not a feature of Legionnaires' disease but are common in *M. pneumoniae* CAP. The finding most likely to cause confusion between *M. pneumoniae* and *Legionella pneumophila* is the presence of loose stools or watery diarrhea, which is found in both.

M. pneumoniae may be cultured from the throat in viral culture media, but the diagnosis is usually made serologically. An elevated enzyme-linked immunosorbent assay (ELISA) or enzyme immunoassay (EIA) IgM titer suggests acute or recent infection, but an elevated IgG titer indicates past exposure but not acute infection. Elevated IgG titers regardless of degree of elevation are not diagnostic of current infection with *M. pneumoniae* and only indicate previous antigenic exposure. *M. pneumoniae* ELISA IgM levels may take up to 3 months to decrease. Therefore, clinicians should take into account recent antecedent respiratory illness in order to properly interpret elevated IgM titers, including patients with nonexudative pharyngitis within 3 months prior to the presentation of CAP. The combination of an increased *M. pneumoniae* IgM titer and highly elevated cold agglutinin titers is virtually diagnostic of acute infection. Cold agglutinin titers are elevated transiently early and rapidly fall; the simultaneously elevated cold agglutinins and IgM titers of *M. pneumoniae* indicate active or current infection. In patients with CAP caused by another organism (e.g., *S. pneumoniae*), the presence of elevated *Mycoplasma* IgG titers does not indicate co-infection but only preexisting serologic exposure to *M. pneumoniae*.

THERAPY

M. pneumoniae has a predilection for the respiratory epithelial cells and resides literally on their surface. Mycoplasmas have no definite cell wall like the typical pathogens causing CAP. Their position on the surface of the respiratory epithelium and their absence of a cell wall necessitates the therapeutic approach, which includes non–β-lactam antibiotics with the capacity to penetrate into the *Mycoplasma* organisms. Traditionally, macrolides and tetracyclines have been used successfully to treat *M. pneumoniae*. Both CAP tetracyclines and macrolides are effective against *Mycoplasma* because they interfere with intracellular protein synthesis at the ribosomal level. Tetracyclines penetrate intracellularly better than macrolides, with the exception of penetration into the alveolar macrophage, which is relevant in *Legionella*, but not *M. pneumoniae*, infections. Macrolides and tetracyclines are both active against *Mycoplasma*; the relative lack of penetration by macrolides into respiratory epithelial cells accounts for differences in therapeutic response. Patients treated with macrolides or tetracyclines defervesce rapidly over 24 to 48 hours. Clinical deferevescence manifests by an increased feeling of well-being and a decrease in fever. The dry cough persists during and after therapy regardless of the anti-*Mycoplasma* antimicrobial used.

There are important differences in the shedding rates of *Mycoplasma* from respiratory epithelial cells posttherapy when using tetracyclines instead of macrolides. Tetracycline therapy is associated with a more rapid decrease in shedding. Tetracyclines with better ability to penetrate intracellularly, such as doxycycline (Vibramycin), are the most rapid at decreasing *Mycoplasma* shedding, which is an important public health consideration. Mycoplasmas are transmitted by aerosolized droplet infection. Because patients with *Mycoplasma* have a prolonged cough, organisms not eliminated from respiratory epithelial cells may be aerosolized during coughing for weeks following the acute infection, spreading the infection to susceptible individuals via aerosolized droplets. The aim of therapy is to rapidly treat the patient's pneumonia and extrapulmonary sites of involvement. The secondary goal is to rapidly decrease shedding and aerosolization to prevent the spread of *Mycoplasma*

TABLE 2 Antibiotics Effective Against *M. pneumoniae*

Antibiotic	Dose (Adult)
Mild/Moderate CAP	
Erythromycin	500 mg (base, estolate, stearate) (PO) q6h
Erythromycin lactobionate	1 g (IV) q6h
Clarithromycin (Biaxin)	500 mg (PO) q12h
Azithromycin (Zithromax)	500 mg (IV) q24h × 2 doses, followed by 500 mg (PO) q24h
Gemifloxacin (Factive)	320 mg (PO) q24h
Telithromycin (Ketek)	800 mg (PO) q24h
Doxycycline	100 mg (IV/PO) q12h
Severe CAP	
Doxycycline	100 mg (IV/PO) q12h
Levofloxacin (Levaquin)	500 mg (IV/PO) q24h, or 750 mg IV/PO q24h (may allow for shorter duration of therapy)
Gatifloxacin (Tequin)	400 mg (IV/PO) q24h
Moxifloxacin (Avelox)	400 mg (IV/PO) q24h

to other individuals. An additional therapeutic goal is to decrease the incidence of post-*Mycoplasma* asthma seen in some patients. *M. pneumoniae* CAP may exacerbate preexisting asthma, but may also cause permanent post-CAP asthma in some individuals.

Until recently, doxycycline was the most active antimicrobial to use against *M. pneumoniae*. Currently, the "respiratory quinolones," levofloxacin (Levaquin), gatifloxacin (Tequin), moxifloxacin (Avelox), and gemifloxacin (Factive), are all highly active anti-*M. pneumoniae* antimicrobials. Telithromycin (Ketek), a ketolide antibiotic, also has a high degree of anti-*M. pneumoniae* activity. The respiratory quinolones and telithromycin all penetrate cells efficiently and interfere with intracellular enzymes or protein synthesis of intracellular organisms. Respiratory quinolones and telithromycin are highly effective anti-*Mycoplasma* agents and rapidly decrease shedding of *M. pneumoniae* in respiratory secretions.

Therapy for *M. pneumoniae* is ordinarily 1 to 2 weeks. Patients who have impaired cardiopulmonary disease or compromised host may require 2 full weeks of therapy. In patients with borderline cardiopulmonary function, *M. pneumoniae* as with other relatively low virulence pathogens may present as severe CAP. Antimicrobial therapy for typical or atypical CAP should be directed against the presumed pathogen and not based on co-morbidities. Normal healthy hosts are treated with the same antimicrobial as patients hospitalized with severe CAP. Patients hospitalized with compromised cardiopulmonary function severe *Mycoplasma* CAP are most often initially treated intravenously with doxycycline (Vibramycin), a macrolide, or a respiratory quinolone. Most patients with *M. pneumoniae* CAP present in the ambulatory setting, which permits therapy with oral doxycycline, macrolide, a respiratory quinolone, or telithromycin (Ketek) (Table 2).

REFERENCES

Ali NJ, Sillis M, Andrews BE, et al: The clinical spectrum and diagnosis of *Mycoplasma pneumoniae* infection. Q J Med 1986;58:241-251.
Cunha BA: Influenza and its complications. Emerg Med 2000;2:56-67.
Cunha BA: Hepatic involvement in *Mycoplasma pneumoniae* community-acquired pneumonia. J Clin Microbiol 2003;3:385-386.
Cunha BA: Influenza: Historical aspects of epidemics and pandemics. Infect Dis Clin North Am 2004;18:141-155.
Cunha BA: The atypical pneumonia: Clinical diagnosis and importance. Clin Microbiol Infect 2006;12:12-24.
Cunha BA: Pneumonia Essentials, Royal Oak, MI: Physicians' Press, 2007.
Cunha BA: Urosepsis in the Critical Care Unit. In: Cunha BA (ed): Infectious Diseases in Critical Care Medicine, 2nd ed. New York, NY, Informa Healthcare USA, Inc., pp 527-534.
Cunha BA: Antibiotic Essentials, 6th ed., Royal Oak, MI, Physicians' Press, pp 79-85.
Debré R, Couvreur J: Influenza: Clinical features. In Debré R, Celers J, eds:Clinical Virology: The Evaluation and Management of Human Viral Infections, Philadelphia: WB Saunders, 1970, pp 507-515.
File TM, Tan JS: *Mycoplasma pneumoniae* pneumonia. In TJMarrie, editor: Community-Acquired Pneumonia, New York: Kluwer Academic/Plenum Publishers, 2001, pp 487-500.
Hammerschlag MR: *Mycoplasma pneumoniae* infections. Curr Opin Infect Dis 2001;14:181-186.
Hurt AC, Selleck P, Komadina N, et al: Susceptibility of highly pathogenic A(H5N1) avian influenza viruses to the neuraminidase inhibitors and adamantanes. Antiviral Res 2007;73:228-231.
Louria DB, Blumenfield HL, Ellis JT: Studies on influenza in the pandemic of 1957-1958. II. Pulmonary complications of influenza. J Clin Invest 1959;38:213-265.
Marrie TJ: Empiric treatment of ambulatory community-acquired pneumonia: Always include treatment for atypical agents. Infect Dis Clin North Am 2004;18:829-841.
Murray HW, Masur H, Senterfit LS, Roberts RB: The protean manifestations of *Mycoplasma pneumoniae* infection in adults. Am J Med 1975;58:229-242.
Nisar N, Guleria R, Kumar S, et al: Mycoplasma pneumoniae and its role in asthma. Postgrad Med J 2007;83:100-104.
Schmidt AC: Antiviral therapy for influenza: A clinical and economic comparative review. Drugs 2004;6:2031-2046.
Waites KB, Talkington DF: *Mycoplasma pneumoniae* and its role as a human pathogen. Clin Microbiol Rev 2004;17:697-728.

Legionellosis

Method of
Julio A. Ramirez, MD

In the summer of 1976, an outbreak of approximately 182 cases of pneumonia occurred in persons attending the American Legion convention in Philadelphia. One year later, Dr. McDade reported the identification of *Legionella pneumophila*, the bacterium responsible for the infection. Today, the family of Legionellaceae is composed of more than 40 species, with some species having different serogroups. *L pneumophila* causes approximately 85% of all *Legionella* infections. *L. pneumophila* serogroup 1 is the single most common member of the family causing clinical infections.

Epidemiology

Legionella is an intracellular organism that lives in natural water. In the aquatic environment, the bacteria live and multiply within freshwater amebae. The number of *Legionella* organisms in the water can increase significantly with appropriate local conditions such as warm temperature, lack of biocides, stagnant water, and presence of amebae and other nutrients. These special conditions can be present in artificial water systems such as cooling towers, whirlpools, decorative fountains, and respiratory therapy devices.

The susceptible host acquires the bacteria from water containing the organism. Infection can be acquired by inhaling aerosols containing *Legionella* organisms or by microaspiration of water contaminated with *Legionella*. The hospitalized patient with *Legionella* pneumonia does not require respiratory isolation because legionellosis is not transmitted from person to person.

Clinical Features

Once *Legionella* organisms reach the respiratory tract, based on the interactions of the organism with the host immune system, the patient can have four possible clinical outcomes: asymptomatic infection, Pontiac fever, legionnaires' disease, or extrapulmonary disease involving the liver, heart, brain, or other organs. Pontiac fever is a nonpneumonic form of disease characterized by fever, headaches, myalgias, and malaise. The patient has an influenza-like illness, with resolution of disease in a few days without specific antimicrobial therapy. Patients with legionnaires' disease present with community-acquired pneumonia associated with high fever, gastrointestinal complaints such as diarrhea, and central nervous system complaints such as headaches or mental status changes. Hospital-acquired pneumonia can occur if *Legionella* is present in the hospital water supply.

Diagnosis

The currently available laboratory tests for diagnosis of *Legionella* infections include the direct fluorescent antibody stain (DFA), culture, antigen detection in the urine, antibody detection in serum by indirect fluorescent antibody testing (IFA), and DNA amplification using the polymerase chain reaction (PCR). The DFA stain can detect all *L. pneumophila* serogroups, but a large number of bacteria need to be present in sputum for a positive result. *Legionella* can be cultured from respiratory specimens on selective media composed of buffered charcoal–yeast extract agar. The urinary antigen detection has a specificity greater than 95%; the disadvantage is that the test detects only the antigen of *L. pneumophila* serogroup 1. Clinical specimens that have been used to detect *Legionella* by PCR include throat swabs, sputum, tracheal suction, bronchoalveolar lavage fluid, pleural fluid, and lung tissue.

Treatment

In the pulmonary parenchyma, *Legionella* can infect and multiply inside alveolar macrophages, alveolar epithelial cells, and capillary endothelial cells. The poor clinical outcome with β-lactam antibiotics is due to their lack of penetration into cells. Antibiotics with good intracellular penetration that can be used as monotherapy for *Legionella* infections include macrolides, ketolides, tetracyclines, and quinolones (Table 1). Rifampin (Rifadin)[1] is not used as monotherapy because resistance can rapidly emerge when it is used alone.

Therapy of the patient with severe disease is initiated with intravenous antibiotics. Once the patient reaches clinical stability, the intravenous therapy can be switched to oral therapy. Doses for the most common antibiotics for intravenous and oral therapy are depicted in Table 1. In the nonimmunocompromised patient, the recommended duration of therapy is 7 to 10 days. In immunocompromised patients, because they are at risk for relapsing infection, the recommended duration of therapy is 14 to 21 days.

Several antibiotics have demonstrated clinical efficacy in legionnaires' disease. Data with several in vitro and animal studies comparing different anti-*Legionella* antibiotics indicate that erythromycin (Ery-Tab) is a weak anti-*Legionella* agent. If erythromycin is selected for therapy, it is important to add rifampin to the regimen to increase intracellular killing. From the family of macrolides, azithromycin (Zithromax)[1] is the most active. The best bactericidal activity in the laboratory is achieved with quinolones. Retrospective observational studies indicate that patients treated with levofloxacin (Levaquin) have a shorter time to reach clinical stability and shorter duration of hospital stay. These antibiotics are considered primary anti-*Legionella* agents.

In clinical practice, I treat immunocompromised patients who have severe legionnaires' disease with a combination of an intravenous quinolone plus an intravenous macrolide (e.g., levofloxacin plus azithromycin). This regimen is based only on the theoretical consideration that synergistic killing may be obtained using a quinolone to alter DNA synthesis and a macrolide to alter protein synthesis.

TABLE 1 Antibiotic Therapy for *Legionella* Infections

Antibiotic	Oral Dose	Intravenous Dose
Ketolides		
Telithromycin (Ketek)[1]	800 mg qd	—
Macrolides		
Azithromycin (Zithromax)[1]	500 mg qd	500 mg qd
Clarithromycin (Biaxin)[1]	500 mg bid	—
Erythromycin (Ery-Tab)	500 mg q6h	1 g q6h
Quinolones		
Ciprofloxacin (Cipro)[1]	750 mg bid	400 mg bid
Levofloxacin (Levaquin)	750 mg qd	750 mg qd
Moxifloxacin (Avelox)[1]	400 mg qd	400 mg qd
Rifamycins		
Rifampin (Rifadin)[1]	300 mg bid	300 mg bid
Tetracyclines		
Doxycycline (Vibramycin)[1]	100 mg bid	100 mg bid

[1]Not FDA approved for this indication.

Pulmonary Embolism

Method of
Victor J. Test, MD, FCCP

There are estimated to be at least 600,000 episodes of pulmonary embolism (PE) in the United States annually, resulting in between 100,000 and 200,000 deaths. The overwhelming majority of deaths occur when the disease is not suspected or is misdiagnosed. Once the diagnosis is made and effective treatment is initiated, the risk of death diminishes dramatically. The patient who presents with shock has a dramatically higher risk of death from pulmonary embolism.

Pulmonary embolism is closely liked to deep venous thrombosis (DVT). Classically, proximal lower extremity venous thrombosis has been reported to be the source of 90% of emboli, but upper extremity thrombosis and catheter-associated thrombosis are often associated with PE as well. The possibility of thromboembolic disease should be considered in patients who present with chest pain, dyspnea, hemoptysis, syncope, or palpitations. The clinical signs of PE are often quite subtle and can include tachycardia, tachypnea, pleural effusion, jugular venous distention, fever, tricuspid regurgitation, and an increased pulmonic heart tone. Lower extremity findings such as asymmetric edema, leg and calf tenderness, erythema, venous cords, and Homan's signs can indicate a lower extremity DVT.

Diagnosis

CLINICAL RISK

The diagnosis of PE and DVT depends on suspicion of the disease. A number of methods can determine the probability that a patient will have a PE. The traditional risk factors have included age greater than 40 years, previous DVT/PE, surgery requiring anesthesia for more than 30 minutes, prolonged immobilization, stroke, heart

---

[1]Not FDA approved for this indication.

TABLE 1 Studies that Exclude the Diagnosis of Embolism

Test	Clinical Probability Low	Intermediate	High
Computed tomography	Normal	Normal	—
Contrast angiography	Normal	Normal	Normal
ELISA D-dimer	Negative	Negative	—
V̇/Q̇ Scan	Normal or low	Normal	Normal

Abbreviations: ELISA = enzyme-linked immunosorbent assay; Q̇ = perfusion; V̇ = ventilation.

TABLE 2 Studies that Confirm the Diagnosis of Embolism

Test	Clinical Probability Low	Intermediate	High
Computed tomography	Positive	Positive	Positive
Contrast angiography	Positive	Positive	Positive
Duplex ultrasound	Positive	Positive	Positive
V̇/Q̇ Scan	—	High	High

Abbreviations: Q̇ = perfusion; V̇ = ventilation.

failure, malignancy (adenocarcinoma and pancreatic carcinoma), fractures of the long bones or pelvis, spinal cord injury, obesity, smoking, pregnancy, estrogen therapy, inflammatory bowel disease, and genetic or acquired thrombophilia. Renal failure, the nephrotic syndrome, central venous catheterization, chronic obstructive pulmonary disease (COPD), and long-distance travel have been identified as risk factors.

CLINICAL DIAGNOSIS

Traditional tests include arterial blood gas, electrocardiogram, and chest x-ray. Unfortunately, these tests are neither specific nor sensitive. Over the past decade, a bewildering array of diagnostic studies, used alone or in combination, have been evaluated as a means of excluding or confirming the diagnosis of embolism. Patients can be stratified into high-risk, moderate-risk, or low-risk categories by empiric assessment or by using structured clinical prediction rules such as those devised by Wells, which use a point system based on historical factors such as malignancy, hemoptysis, previous DVT/PE, immobilization, recent surgery, tachycardia, clinical evidence of DVT, and absence of an equally likely alternative diagnosis. Clinical prediction rules seem to be less influenced by experience and allow a more standardized approach to the diagnostic process.

Table 1 shows studies that can exclude the diagnosis of embolism at different levels of clinical probability. Table 2 shows studies that can confirm the diagnosis of embolism at different levels of clinical probability.

Often I use a combination of tests to help me rule out the diagnosis of pulmonary embolism. The enzyme-linked immunosorbent assay (ELISA) D-dimer is most useful in ruling out the diagnosis in outpatients at low risk or who have a low pretest probability of pulmonary embolism. In patients who are low risk based on the scoring systems, the incidence of pulmonary embolism at 3 months in the setting of a negative highly sensitive D-dimer assay is extremely low.

CURRENT DIAGNOSIS

- The diagnosis of pulmonary embolism is guided by suspicion for the disease.
- Interpretation of the diagnostic testing should be guided by the clinical probability for the presence of pulmonary embolism.
- Multiple diagnostic tests and evaluations may be required for assessment of pulmonary embolic disease.
- In the absence of a contraindication to anticoagulant therapy, therapy should be begun while awaiting confirmatory testing in patients at intermediate or high risk.

The sensitivities of the different assays result in a wide variability of sensitivities. In general, intermediate-risk and high-risk patients should receive diagnostic imaging.

As documented in the PIOPED 1 study, a normal ventilation-perfusion (V̇/Q̇) scan virtually rules out a pulmonary embolism. A high-probability scan in someone with a moderate or high risk of pulmonary embolism strongly suggests a pulmonary embolism. Unfortunately, the underlying chest x-rays strongly affect the effectiveness of this test. It is still quite useful but is less available because computed tomography (CT) scanning is now the preferred choice in many centers.

The advent of the multislice, multidetector CT scanner has had a substantial impact on the diagnosis of pulmonary embolism. The technology associated with CT scanning has been evolving, whereas the technology associated with (V̇/Q̇) scanning has been more or less static. The PIOPED 2 study compared CT angiogram (CTA) with CT angiography with venography (CTA/CTV). The sensitivity of CTA was 83% and the specificity was 96% for PE. The sensitivity of CTA/CTV was 90% and the specificity was 95%. It is clear from this study that clinicians must still use the concept of pretest probability in assessing for PE. Unfortunately, most centers do not use this technology, and I am often forced to use duplex ultrasonography to augment the negative CT to rule out a significant pulmonary embolism.

The CT angiogram also has the benefit of evaluating for lymphadenopathy and for parenchymal lung disease. The crucial disadvantages are the need to obtain a high-quality and well-timed bolus of contrast to obtain an optimal scan as well as the use of intravenous contrast. CTA typically uses more contrast than standard pulmonary angiography. Pulmonary angiography is the standard imaging procedure but in general has fallen out of use in most centers due to its perceived risk and the increased use of CT scanning. Duplex ultrasonography of the venous system may be used to rule out proximal deep venous thrombosis of the lower extremity.

A radiographic or anatomically massive pulmonary embolism does not always cause hemodynamic instability.

Transthoracic echocardiogram is often used to assess chest pain. In acute pulmonary embolism, the echocardiogram is useful to stratify hemodynamically stable patients to determine which patient is at risk for a poor outcome. The findings of right ventricular dilatation and pulmonary hypertension are poor markers for increased mortality. The echocardiogram may show evidence of right ventricular strain or overload. In addition, the echocardiogram is often used to identify patients at risk for developing hemodynamic decompensation.

Therapy

Therapy for DVT/PE should be initiated empirically when there is a significant clinical suspicion for the disease and if the risk of systemic anticoagulation is low, because PE is associated with significant mortality. Tests to confirm or exclude pulmonary embolism should be arranged as soon as possible. Supplemental therapies such as oxygen should be employed as indicated by the clinical situation.

CURRENT THERAPY

- If the clinical suspicion is high and there are no contraindications, therapy should begin while confirmatory testing is being arranged
- For hemodynamically stable patients, therapy with dose-adjusted unfractionated heparin or low-molecular-weight heparin is indicated in the absence of complications.
  - Unfractionated heparin: 80 IU/kg ideal body weight bolus; 18 IU/kg/h infusion with monitoring of the aPTT every 4-6 h. Adjust to an aPTT 1.5-3 times control.
  - Low-molecular-weight heparin: Enoxaparin (Lovenox)[1] 1 mg/kg SC twice a d or tinzaparin (Innohep)[1] 175 anti-Xa IU/kg SC once daily
- Warfarin therapy (5 mg/d) should be started on d 1 of therapy with heparin in the absence of contraindications.

[1]Not FDA approved for this indication.

UNFRACTIONATED HEPARIN

Unfractionated heparin (UFH) has been the mainstay of therapy for DVT/PE since the 1970s. Heparin acts by accelerating the activity of antithrombin III. Heparin does not directly dissolve the thrombus, but it prevents the formation of new thrombi. Heparin can be administered subcutaneously or by intermittent intravenous bolus, but is usually given as a constant intravenous infusion to ensure that an adequate therapeutic level has been achieved.

Unfractionated heparin requires monitoring of the activated partial thromboplastin time (aPTT). The typical goal for the aPTT is 1.5 to 3.0 times the control value, which corresponds to a plasma heparin level from 0.3 to 0.7 IU/mL anti-Xa activity. In certain circumstances, such as the presence of a lupus anticoagulant, anti-Xa levels might have to be monitored.

It is crucial to achieve a therapeutic level of anticoagulation within 12 to 24 hours of starting therapy or the morbidity and mortality will increase. The therapy should begin with a heparin bolus of 80 U/kg followed by a continuous infusion of 18 U/kg/hour. The aPTT should be monitored every 6 hours and adjusted according to a weight-based nomogram until a therapeutic range has been reached; aPTT can then be monitored daily.

The chief complications of unfractionated heparin are bleeding and heparin-induced thrombocytopenia. It is necessary to monitor the platelet count every other day in patients treated with heparin.

LOW-MOLECULAR-WEIGHT HEPARIN

Low-molecular-weight heparins (LMWHs) are single-molecular-weight heparin molecules that act on factor Xa. They have the advantage of being more predictable in their dose effect. For most patients, the LMWH preparations do not require monitoring of their effect for short-term therapy. Monitoring of the anti-Xa levels should be undertaken with long-term therapy, in obese patients (>150 kg), in very small patients (<40 kg), and in pregnant patients. LMWH has a prolonged half-life in patients with renal insufficiency (creatinine clearance <30 mL/min) and are relatively contraindicated in these patients. There also may be a lower risk of heparin-induced thrombocytopenia, but the platelet count should still be monitored. Enoxaparin (Lovenox) and tinzaparin (Innohep) are currently approved by the FDA for the management of acute deep venous thrombosis with or without pulmonary embolism.

WARFARIN

Warfarin (Coumadin) is the only vitamin K antagonist available in the United States and is used for the subacute and long-term management of DVT/PE. It prevents the formation of the vitamin K–dependent clotting factors (factors II, V, VII, and IX). It also decreases the levels of protein S and protein C, which are antithrombotic proteins. It can induce hypercoagulability by depleting proteins C and S levels if it is initiated without heparin or LMWH.

Warfarin therapy should begin on the day that anticoagulation is begun with heparin or LMWH unless there is a contraindication to therapy with warfarin. Warfarin is contraindicated in patients who have a known reaction to warfarin, who have a high risk of bleeding, or who are pregnant. In addition, warfarin interacts with many foods and pharmaceutical agents.

The protime (PT) as reflected by the international normalized ratio (INR) should be monitored daily with initiation of therapy. The goal therapeutic INR for most patients is 2.0 to 3.0. The patient should take unfractionated heparin or LMWH for a minimum of 5 days and the INR should be greater than 2.0 for two consecutive days before the unfractionated heparin or LMWH is discontinued.

ALTERNATIVE AGENTS FOR INITIAL MANAGEMENT

In the setting of a contraindication to the use of heparin, several agents can be used for the initial management of acute DVT/PE. Fondaparinux (Arixtra) is a pentasaccharide that has an anti–factor Xa effect. It has been shown to be effective in the treatment of DVT/PE. It is administered subcutaneously and is cleared renally. It has been demonstrated to be useful in the treatment of DVT/PE. Fondaparinux is now FDA approved for the treatment of DVT and PE, but it is not FDA approved for acute management. Liver enzymes must be monitored. Argatroban (Novastan) and hirudin (lepirudin [Refludan])[1] have been used to manage DVT/PE in the setting of heparin-associated thrombocytopenia.

LONG-TERM MANAGEMENT

The determination of the duration of therapy for DVT/PE is based on the balance between the risk of bleeding and the risk of recurrence. Patients who have an identifiable reversible risk factor, such as surgery, should receive treatment for 3 months. Patients with an initial episode of idiopathic DVT/PE are at higher risk for recurrence than patients with an identifiable risk factor and should be treated for 6 to 12 months. The exact duration should be determined based on the patient's risk of bleeding. For patients with identifiable risk factors, the duration of treatment is often at least 1 year or longer. In patients with malignancy, long-term therapy with LMWH may be preferable to therapy with warfarin. These patients should be treated for life or until the malignancy is resolved.

ALTERNATIVE MODES OF THERAPY FOR ACUTE PULMONARY EMBOLISM

Venocaval Interruption and Inferior Vena Cava Filter Placement

Interruption of the inferior vena cava (IVC) was originally accomplished via surgical ligation of the vena cava or surgical placement of a filter to prevent pulmonary embolism. The IVC filter is now placed percutaneously to prevent recurrence of pulmonary embolism in selected groups. These groups include patients with contraindications to systemic anticoagulation, patients who are undergoing surgical intervention for acute pulmonary embolism, patients with chronic thromboembolic pulmonary hypertension, and possibly patients with limited cardiopulmonary reserve. The IVC filter has been shown to decrease the risk of recurrent pulmonary embolism after placement, but it is associated with an increased risk of venous thrombosis without a survival benefit.

[1]Not FDA approved for this indication.

Thrombolytic Therapy

Thrombolytic agents actively destroy a clot by activating plasminogen. Three agents are FDA approved for acute management of massive PE. These agents are urokinase (Abbokinase), streptokinase (Streptase), and tissue plasminogen activator (TPA; Activase). They have been associated with a significant risk of severe bleeding, including intracranial hemorrhage, and should be used cautiously. They are typically used in patients who are hemodynamically unstable or have suffered sudden death from PE.

Patients with evidence of right ventricular dysfunction by echocardiogram or with substantial elevations of troponin or brain natriuretic peptide (BNP) levels at the time of admission have been demonstrated to be at risk of hemodynamic deterioration. Patients with right ventricular thrombi are at increased risk for hemodynamic decompensation and can benefit from the use of thrombolytic agents. Routine use of thrombolytic agents in this group of patients, which represents approximately 50% of patients with symptomatic emboli, remains controversial.

The use of thrombolytic drugs has been demonstrated to show improvement in right ventricular function by echocardiogram and improvement in lung V/Q scans at 1 to 3 days. At 7 days after therapy, there is no difference in the degree of pulmonary perfusion abnormalities in patients treated with thrombolytics versus those treated with heparin. Thrombolytic agents are contraindicated in patients with intracranial pathology, recent neurosurgery, recent operations, and active bleeding.

HEMODYNAMIC MANAGEMENT OF HYPOTENSION ASSOCIATED WITH MASSIVE PULMONARY EMBOLISM

Shock is a marker for increased mortality in patients with massive pulmonary embolus. In one study, the mortality rate increased to 31% when the patient presented with shock. Pulmonary embolus should be suspected in patients who ahve cardiac arrest with pulseless electrical activity or who have shock associated with hypoxemia. It is important to maintain an adequate systemic arterial pressure to prevent right ventricular infarction. Intravenous fluids should be used cautiously to prevent overdistention of the overloaded right ventricle. The blood pressure is typically supported with dopamine (Intropin), norepinephrine (Levophed), or phenylephrine (Neo-Synephrine). Inotropic agents such as dobutamine (Dobutrex) can improve cardiac output but can also increase myocardial oxygen consumption and hypotension, so they should be used cautiously.

INTERVENTIONS FOR MANAGEMENT OF PULMONARY EMBOLISM

The indications for surgical embolectomy include massive pulmonary embolism, persistent shock, and failure of or contraindications to thrombolytic therapy. The morbidity and mortality of surgical intervention in the setting of hemodynamic collapse are significant, and surgery should be performed by experienced teams with readily available cardiopulmonary bypass. Catheter-based embolectomy[1] is available in some centers and is an alternative for some patients.

REFERENCES

Buller HR, Agnelli G, Hull RD, et al: Antithrombotic therapy for venous thromboembolic disease: The Seventh ACCP Conference on Antithrombotic and Thrombolytic Therapy. Chest 2004;126:401S-428S.
Dalen JE, Alpert JS: Natural history of pulmonary embolism. Prog Cardiovasc Dis 1975;17:257-270.
Elliot CG, Goldhaber SZ, Visani L, De Rosa M: Chest radiographs in acute pulmonary embolism. Chest 2000;118:33-38.
Kearon C, Ginsberg JS, Douketis J, et al: An evaluation of D-dimer in the diagnosis of pulmonary embolism: A randomized controlled trial. Ann Intern Med 2006;144:812-821.
PIOPED Investigators: Value of the ventilation-perfusion lung scan in acute pulmonary embolism. JAMA 1990;263(20):2753-2759.
PIOPED Investigators: Tissue plasminogen activator for the treatment of acute pulmonary embolism: A collaborative study by the PIOPED Investigators. Chest 1990;97:528-533.
PIOPED II Investigators: Multidectector computed tomography for acute pulmonary embolism. N Engl J Med 2006;354:2317-2327.
Pulido T, Aranda A, Zevallos MA, et al: Pulmonary embolism as a cause of death in patients with heart disease: An autopsy study. Chest 2006;129:1282-1287.
Ryu JH, Olson EJ, Pellikka PA: Clinical recognition of pulmonary embolism: Problem of unrecognized and asymptomatic cases. Mayo Clin Proc 1998;73:873-879.
Sors II, Pacouret G, Azarian, et al: Hemodynamic effects of bolus vs. 2 hours infusion of alteplase in acute massive pulmonary embolism: A randomized controlled trial. Chest 1994;106:712-717.
Stein PD, Terrin ML, Hales CA, et al: Clinical, laboratory roentgenographic, and electrocardiographic findings in patients with acute pulmonary embolism and no preexisting cardiac or pulmonary disease. Chest 1991;100:598-603.
Urokinase Pulmonary Embolism Trial: Phase 1 results: A COOPERATIVE Study. JAMA 1970;214:2163-2172.
Wells PS, Anderson DR, Rodger M, et al: Derivation of a simple clinical model to categorize the patients' probability of pulmonary embolism: Increasing the model's utility with the SimpliRED D-dimer. Thromb Haemost 2000;83(3):416-420.
Wicki J, Perneger T, Junod A, et al: Assessing clinical probability of the pulmonary embolism in the emergency ward: A simple score. Arch Intern Med 2001;161:92-97.
Wood KE: Major pulmonary embolism: Review of a pathophysiologic approach to the golden hour of hemodynamically significant pulmonary embolism. Chest 2002;121:877-905.

Sarcoidosis

Method of
Marc A. Judson, MD

Sarcoidosis is a multisystem granulomatous disease of unknown cause. The lung is most commonly affected, but any organ may be involved. The clinical presentation of sarcoidosis is variable for two main reasons. First, the manifestations of pulmonary sarcoidosis are variable and can range from an asymptomatic state to significant pulmonary dysfunction. Second, extrapulmonary manifestations of sarcoidosis are common and can cause the prominent symptoms of the disease. This variability in disease presentation often makes the diagnosis of sarcoidosis problematic.

Epidemiology

Sarcoidosis occurs worldwide and affects all races and ages. Although the disease shows a predilection for the third decade of life, a smaller second peak in diagnosis occurs in women older than 50 years. There is a slightly higher disease rate in women at younger ages as well. The highest prevalence of sarcoidosis is found in whites in Scandinavia and in persons of African descent in the United States. In the United States, the lifetime risk of sarcoidosis is 0.85% in whites and 2.4% in African Americans, with an age-adjusted incidence rate of 10.9 per 100,000 persons for the white population and 35.5 per 100,000 persons for African Americans. The relative risk for having sarcoidosis increases significantly if a family member has it as well. In the United States, nearly 20% of African Americans with sarcoidosis have an affected first-degree relative, compared with 5% in whites.

---

[1]Not FDA approved for this indication.

The clinical presentation and severity of sarcoidosis vary among racial and ethnic groups. The disease tends to be more severe in African Americans, whereas whites are more likely to be asymptomatic at presentation. Extrathoracic manifestations are more common in certain populations, such as ocular and cardiac sarcoidosis in Japanese populations, chronic uveitis in African Americans, and erythema nodosum in Europeans. There is increasing evidence that genetic polymorphisms affect the risks and manifestations of the disease. This is consistent with the current theory that sarcoidosis does not have a single cause but is the result of an abnormal host (granulomatous) response to one of many potential antigens in a genetically susceptible person.

Immunopathogenesis

The exact immunopathogenesis of sarcoidosis is unknown, but it is thought to be similar to that of other granulomatous diseases. That is, antigen-presenting cells (APCs), usually either macrophages or dendritic cells, process and present an antigen via a human leukocyte antibody (HLA) class II molecule to T lymphocytes and their receptors. These T lymphocytes are usually of the CD4 T-helper 1 (Th1) class. The antigen involved in this reaction is unknown, and there may be many antigens that are each associated with a specific HLA class II molecule and T-cell receptor. This could explain the inability to determine one specific cause of sarcoidosis and the varied phenotypic expressions of the disease.

The interaction of APCs and T lymphocytes activates the APCs to produce tumor necrosis factor α (TNF-α), and other cytokines. A proliferation of CD4 Th1 lymphocytes also ensues that results in the secretion of interferon-γ (INF-γ), interleukin (IL)-2, IL-12, and other cytokines. These cytokines activate and recruit monocytes and macrophages and transform them into giant cells, which are important building blocks of the granuloma.

The typical sarcoidosis lesion is a noncaseating (non-necrotic) granuloma. The sarcoid granuloma consists of a compact core of macrophage-derived epithelioid and multinucleated giant cells surrounded by a perimeter of monocytes, lymphocytes, and fibroblasts. Granulomas can resolve spontaneously or with therapy; however, they can also persist and lead to peripheral hyalinization and fibrosis. The development of such fibrosis can cause permanent organ damage and in large part determines the prognosis.

Clinical Features and Clinical Course

PULMONARY SARCOIDOSIS

Between 30% and 60% of patients with pulmonary sarcoidosis are asymptomatic, and the disease is detected incidentally on chest x-ray. Some patients present with nonspecific pulmonary symptoms, such as dyspnea, cough, wheezing, and chest pain. Respiratory failure from sarcoidosis is extremely rare at presentation. Unlike many other interstitial lung diseases, crackles are rarely heard on chest auscultation. Abnormalities on the chest radiograph occur in more than 90% of patients with pulmonary sarcoidosis. Bilateral hilar adenopathy occurs in 50% to 85% at disease presentation, and 25% to 50% have parenchymal infiltrates. Sarcoid granulomas have a predilection for the bronchovascular bundles, subpleural locations, intralobular septa, and the airways.

A radiographic staging system was developed several decades ago (Table 1). Groups of patients with higher radiographic stages have more severe pulmonary dysfunction, lower remission rates, and greater mortality. However, there is significant overlap between these groups, and predictions concerning individual patients based on stage are highly inaccurate.

Advanced pulmonary stage IV sarcoidosis displays destruction of the lung architecture, with upward traction of the hila, lung distortion, upper-lobe volume loss, fibrocystic disease, honeycombed cysts, and decreased lung volumes. Aspergillomas can develop in these large

TABLE 1 Chest Radiograph Stages of Sarcoidosis

Stage	Lymph Node Enlargement	Parenchymal Disease
1	Yes	No
2	Yes	Nonfibrotic
3	No	Nonfibrotic
4	No or yes	Fibrotic

Adapted from Judson MA, Baughman RP: Sarcoidosis. In Baughman RP, du Bois RM, Lynch JP, Wells AU (eds): Diffuse Lung Disease: A Practical Approach. London: Arnold, 2004, pp 109-129.

cystic lesions and may be associated with life-threatening hemoptysis. Bronchiectasis from airway distortion also can occur and is an additional potential cause of hemoptysis.

The majority of patients with pulmonary sarcoidosis have a vital capacity of greater than 70% of predicted at diagnosis. Pulmonary function and the chest radiographic findings are often discordant. In pulmonary sarcoidosis patients with a normal lung parenchyma (stage 1), the vital capacity, diffusing capacity, partial pressure of arterial oxygen (PaO_2) at rest, PaO_2 with exercise, and lung compliance are abnormal in 20% to 40% of cases. Patients with abnormal lung parenchyma have abnormal pulmonary function tests 50% to 70% of the time. Patients with stage IV fibrocystic sarcoidosis tend to have the most severe pulmonary dysfunction.

Sarcoidosis is an interstitial lung disease with a restrictive ventilatory defect often found on spirometry. It is underappreciated, however, that endobronchial involvement is common in sarcoidosis, and therefore airflow obstruction may be the major abnormality found on pulmonary function testing. Wheezing may be the prominent presenting symptom of sarcoidosis, and many cases of sarcoidosis are misdiagnosed as asthma in many patients. Airflow obstruction is also common in chronic pulmonary sarcoidosis, where it is caused by airway distortion from fibrosis. The cause of dyspnea in pulmonary sarcoidosis is multifactorial. It may be the result of abnormalities of gas exchange or lung mechanics, weakness of the respiratory muscles, obesity from corticosteroid therapy, pulmonary hypertension, or sarcoidosis involvement of the heart.

Only 3% to 5% of patients die of sarcoidosis. In the United States, 75% of these deaths are the result of pulmonary involvement. Death from pulmonary involvement is rarely acute but normally is an insidious process that develops over 5 to 25 years with the development of progressive pulmonary fibrosis. Several studies have suggested that pulmonary hypertension is a major risk factor for death from pulmonary sarcoidosis. Patients with aspergillomas and stage IV fibrocystic sarcoidosis are also at risk for death from episodes of life-threatening hemoptysis. Other organs that result in fatalities from sarcoidosis are the heart and the central nervous system. In Japan, death from sarcoidosis is more commonly caused by cardiac than pulmonary involvement.

EXTRAPULMONARY SARCOIDOSIS

Sarcoidosis is a multisystem disease that can affect any organ in the body. The extrapulmonary manifestations of sarcoidosis can predominate in many patients. Extrapulmonary disease can affect the prognosis and treatment options for sarcoidosis.

The eyes and skin are the most common extrapulmonary organs involved with sarcoidosis. Ocular manifestations occur in 25% to 50% of patients; anterior uveitis is the most common manifestation. Symptoms of anterior uveitis include red eyes, painful eyes, and photophobia. However, in one third of patients with anterior uveitis from sarcoidosis, the eye is quiet and without symptoms. In addition, an intermediate or posterior uveitis can cause vision problems or be asymptomatic. For this reason, all patients with sarcoidosis should undergo an eye examination by an ophthalmologist. Other ocular manifestations of sarcoidosis include conjunctivitis, keratoconjunctivitis sicca (dry eyes), scleritis, and optic neuritis.

Skin lesions in sarcoidosis can be classified into two categories: specific lesions that demonstrate noncaseating granulomas on biopsy and nonspecific lesions that do not. The specific skin lesions are often papular and have a predilection for areas of previous scars and tattoos. Lupus pernio is a type of specific skin lesion causing disfiguring lesions on the face, often with erythema and significant induration. These lesions have a predilection for the nose, cheeks, medial and lateral sides of the eyes, and lateral sides of the mouth. Lupus pernio lesions are relatively recalcitrant to therapy and often respond only partially to corticosteroids. The most common nonspecific skin lesion is erythema nodosum, which is often seen with an acute sarcoidosis presentation of fever, arthritis (especially in the ankles), pulmonary symptoms, and bilateral hilaradenopathy on chest radiograph. This syndrome is known as *Löfgren's syndrome* and tends to have a good long-term prognosis.

Cardiac and neurologic sarcoidosis can be life threatening and is therefore important to recognize. Cardiac involvement is detected clinically in 5% of sarcoidosis patients during life but in 25% at autopsy. Cardiac sarcoidosis can cause left ventricular dysfunction and cardiac arrhythmias, possibly resulting in sudden death. All patients with sarcoidosis are recommended to have a 12-lead electrocardiogram; an abnormal result should prompt further evaluation. The diagnosis of cardiac sarcoidosis is problematic, because the disease is patchy and diagnosed less than 25% of the time by endomyocardial biopsy because of sampling error. Often the diagnosis is made noninvasively, if a typical clinical presentation is coupled with detection of abnormalities on echocardiography, gallium scanning, thallium scanning, cardiac magnetic resonance imaging (MRI), or positron emission tomography (PET).

Clinically apparent neurosarcoidosis occurs in less than 10% of sarcoidosis patients. Palsy of the seventh cranial nerve is the most common manifestation of neurosarcoidosis, and it often predates the diagnosis of the disease. Sarcoidosis can affect any part of the peripheral nervous system and central nervous system and can cause a cranial nerve palsy, mononeuropathy or polyneuropathy, aseptic meningitis, seizures, mass lesions in the brain and spinal cord, and encephalopathy.

Sarcoidosis causes clinically apparent peripheral lymphadenopathy in more than 10% of patients. Splenic involvement may be present in up to 50% of patients, but it is usually asymptomatic and rarely causes hypersplenism.

Bone involvement is occasional, usually occurring as small cysts or cortical defects found in the small bones of the hands and feet. An acute sarcoid arthritis often is present at disease onset and has a good prognosis. This is commonly found in the ankles of patients who present with Löfgren's syndrome. Chronic sarcoid arthritis is rare. It is usually a nondestructive arthropathy of the shoulders, wrists, knees, ankles, and small joints of the hands and feet.

Sarcoidosis of the sinuses is underappreciated. It can occur in the nasopharynx, hypopharynx, larynx, or any of the sinuses and is known as *sarcoidosis of the upper respiratory tract*. Sarcoidosis of the upper respiratory tract is often relatively recalcitrant to therapy.

Histologic evidence of hepatic sarcoidosis is present in 50% to 80% of sarcoidosis patients, although most are asymptomatic and have normal liver function tests. Hepatomegaly, abdominal pain, and pruritus are the most common symptoms associated with hepatic sarcoidosis but are present only in 15% to 25% of patients with hepatic involvement. Elevation of the serum alkaline phosphatase is the most common liver function test abnormality.

Hypercalcemia or hypercalciuria leading to nephrolithiasis and renal dysfunction can occur with sarcoidosis. These phenomena are the result of the enzyme 1α-hydroxylase in activated macrophages that convert 25-hydroxyvitamin D to 1,25-dihydroxyvitamin D, the active form of the vitamin. This results in increased gut absorption and increased renal excretion of calcium that can cause nephrolithiasis.

Sarcoidosis rarely involves the thyroid, renal parenchyma, and GI tract.

Patients can have constitutional symptoms such as fever, night sweats, weight loss, malaise, and fatigue at presentation.

BOX 1 Factors Associated with a Poor Prognosis in Sarcoidosis

African American race
Extrathoracic disease
Stage II-III versus stage I on chest x-ray
Age >40 years
Splenic involvement
Lupus pernio
Disease duration >2 years
Forced vital capacity <1.5 L
Stage IV chest x-ray or aspergilloma

Data from Judson MA, Baughman RP: Sarcoidosis. In Baughman RP, du Bois RM, Lynch JP, Wells AU (eds): Diffuse Lung Disease: A Practical Approach. London: Arnold, 2004, pp 109-129.

These symptoms occasionally are associated with hepatic sarcoid involvement but together may be a sign of the systemic nature of the disease, presumably from cytokine release, rather than specific organ involvement. Patients who present with Löfgren's syndrome or with asymptomatic bilateral hilar adenopathy on chest radiograph have a good prognosis. African Americans tend to have a worse prognosis than whites, with lower forced vital capacity and more new organ involvement within 2 years of diagnosis. Box 1 lists risk factors associated with a poor prognosis.

Diagnosis and Initial Workup

The diagnosis of sarcoidosis requires a compatible clinical picture, histologic demonstration of noncaseating granulomas, and exclusion of other diseases capable of producing a similar histologic and clinical picture. Mycobacterial and fungal diseases always must be considered as alternative diagnoses. Therefore, stains and cultures of tissue specimens for mycobacteria and fungi always should be obtained when the diagnosis of sarcoidosis is considered. Because sarcoidosis is a diagnosis of exclusion (granulomatous inflammation of unknown cause), bear a healthy degree of skepticism in the diagnosis and follow the patient closely for additional clues supporting an alternative diagnosis.

Sarcoidosis is a systemic disease, so the signs or symptoms of extrathoracic disease such as uveitis, skin lesions, or an elevated serum alkaline phosphatase should be sought. The diagnosis in a patient with granulomas on lung biopsy who has interstitial infiltrates without adenopathy on radiographic studies is suspect. In this situation, granulomatous infections and bioaerosol exposure causing hypersensitivity pneumonitis should be strongly considered. Because of the varied clinical presentation of sarcoidosis, there is no single diagnostic algorithm.

It is prudent to select a biopsy site associated with less morbidity, such as the skin if a lesion is present. Transbronchial lung biopsy has a diagnostic yield of 40% to more than 90% in pulmonary sarcoidosis. It is recommended that at least four lung biopsy specimens be collected to maximize the diagnostic yield. Endobronchial biopsy has a 40% to 60% sensitivity and adds to the yield of transbronchial biopsy.

Bronchoalveolar lavage (BAL) with examination of lymphocyte populations has been used in the evaluation of possible pulmonary sarcoidosis. In sarcoidosis, there is an increased number of BAL lymphocytes, and these are predominantly CD4+. It has been proposed that an increase in BAL lymphocytes and a BAL CD4/CD8 ratio greater than 3.5 make the diagnosis of sarcoidosis highly likely.

Although serum angiotensin-converting enzyme (ACE) often is elevated in active sarcoidosis, the specificity and sensitivity of this test are inadequate for it to be used diagnostically. Serum ACE may be used as supportive evidence for the diagnosis, and it also may be used in some instances to follow disease activity.

CURRENT DIAGNOSIS

- The diagnosis of sarcoidosis is one of exclusion.
- Tissue biopsy, confirming noncaseating granulomatous inflammation, is required in most cases.
- Efforts should be made to search for the least invasive biopsy site.

CURRENT THERAPY

- Many cases of sarcoidosis do not require treatment.
- All patients should be evaluated for possible pulmonary, eye, and cardiac disease.
- When therapy is indicated, corticosteroids are most commonly used.
- Topical corticosteroids should be given whenever possible.

Gallium-67 (^{67}Ga) scanning is cumbersome because it takes several days to complete and is infrequently used as a diagnostic test. However, bilateral hilar uptake and right paratracheal uptake (lambda sign) coupled with lacrimal and parotid uptake (panda sign) with ^{67}Ga strongly suggest a diagnosis of sarcoidosis.

Ideally, the diagnosis of sarcoidosis requires demonstration of noncaseating granulomas in at least one organ. However, certain clinical presentations are so specific for the diagnosis of sarcoidosis that the diagnosis may be accepted without tissue biopsy. Extreme caution must be used in these situations to ensure that there is no clinical information that would suggest an alternative diagnosis that should prompt a tissue biopsy. Clinical or laboratory findings that strongly support the diagnosis of sarcoidosis without a tissue biopsy are listed in Box 2.

Treatment

Therapy is not mandated for sarcoidosis because the disease can remit spontaneously. Therapy is indicated for potentially dangerous disease that includes neurosarcoidosis, cardiac sarcoidosis, hypercalcemia that does not respond to dietary measures, ocular sarcoidosis that does not respond to topical (eyedrop) therapy, and other life- or organ-threatening disease. Therapy also should be considered when the disease is progressive. Relative indications for therapy include arthritis that fails to respond to nonsteroidal antiinflammatory drugs (NSAIDs); a systemic inflammatory response syndrome of fever, night sweats, fatigue, and arthralgias; and symptomatic hepatic disease. In general, treatment is discouraged for asymptomatic elevations of serum liver function tests, specific levels of ACE, or asymptomatic uptake on ^{67}Ga scan (with the possible exceptions of the heart or brain).

The decision to treat sarcoidosis can be problematic, because the disease has a variable prognosis that must be weighed against the potential side effects of therapy. It is often most prudent to monitor patients without therapy if they are asymptomatic or have only mild organ dysfunction. For pulmonary sarcoidosis, asymptomatic patients and those with mild disease that might spontaneously remit usually are not treated. For patients with clinical findings that predict spontaneous remission (e.g., erythema nodosum), the benefits of treatment often are offset by the toxicity of therapy. Often these patients can be managed with palliative therapy such as NSAIDs for arthralgias and fever and bronchodilators and inhaled corticosteroids for wheezing and cough.

It is recommended that patients with mild to moderate pulmonary sarcoidosis be observed for 2 to 6 months, if possible. Patients who improve will have avoided the toxicity of corticosteroids, and patients who deteriorate over this period should be considered for treatment. Patients with pulmonary dysfunction who neither improve nor deteriorate during the observation period may be given a corticosteroid trial, or they may be observed further. Patients with severe pulmonary dysfunction or pulmonary symptoms causing significant impairment should be treated.

Corticosteroids often are used to treat sarcoidosis, but the dose, duration of therapy, and method by which one can assess effectiveness have not been standardized. Topical corticosteroid therapy should be used whenever possible in an attempt to minimize systemic complications. This would include corticosteroid eye drops for anterior sarcoid uveitis and corticosteroid creams and injections for localized skin lesions. Pulmonary sarcoidosis usually is treated initially with 20 to 40 mg/day of prednisone or its equivalent. Higher doses may be required for neurosarcoidosis and cardiac sarcoidosis. The patient usually is evaluated within 2 to 12 weeks for a response. Patients failing to respond to therapy within 3 months are unlikely to respond to a more protracted course of therapy or a higher dose. Among the responders, the corticosteroid dose is tapered to 5 to 10 mg/day of a prednisone equivalent or an every-other-day regimen. Treatment is usually continued for 12 months.

The relapse rate after corticosteroid therapy is withdrawn may be as high as 70%, and therefore patients need to be followed closely as the corticosteroid dose is tapered and discontinued. In some patients, there may be recurrent relapses requiring long-term, low-dose therapy. On occasion, the chronic prednisone dose needed to prevent relapse is less than 5 mg/day. Patients who relapse after corticosteroids have been withdrawn should be re-treated with corticosteroids. Alternative agents, such as corticosteroid-sparing agents, to control the disease in a patient on a chronic low dose of prednisone should be considered. On occasion, alternative agents may completely replace corticosteroid therapy. In general, corticosteroid-sparing agents should not be considered unless the patient requires more than 7.5 mg/day of prednisone to control the disease.

Methotrexate (Rheumatrex)[1] and hydroxychloroquine (Plaquenil)[1] are the most-studied alternative sarcoidosis medications. They are usually used as corticosteroid-sparing agents but at times can be used as replacement therapy. Methotrexate is most useful for pulmonary, skin, joint, and eye sarcoidosis. Hydroxychloroquine is often used for sarcoidosis of the skin, joints, and nerves and for hypercalcemia from sarcoidosis. Azathioprine (Imuran)[1] may be useful for sarcoid uveitis, but usually it is added to corticosteroid plus methotrexate in this instance. Monocycline (Minocin)[1] and doxycycline (Vibramycin)[1] may be useful for skin sarcoidosis. Cyclophosphamide (Cytoxan)[1] is used occasionally and seems to have a potential role in neurosarcoidosis. Recently anti–TNF-α therapies have shown promise in the treatment of sarcoidosis. Such agents include pentoxifylline (Trental),[1] thalidomide (Thalomid),[1] and monoclonal antibodies against TNF-α, such as infliximab (Remicade).[1]

REFERENCES

Baughman RP, Teirstein AS, Judson MA, et al: Clinical characteristics of patients in a case control study of sarcoidosis. Am J Respir Crit Care Med 2001;164:1885-1889.

Gibson GJ, Prescott RJ, Muers MF, et al: British Thoracic Society Sarcoidosis study: Effects of long term corticosteroid treatment. Thorax 1996;51:238-247.

---

[1]Not FDA approved for this indication.

BOX 2 Clinical or Laboratory Findings that Strongly Support a Diagnosis of Sarcoidosis without a Tissue Biopsy

Löfgren's syndrome
Heerfordt's syndrome (uveoparotid fever)
Asymptomatic bilateral hilar adenopathy on chest x-ray
^{67}Ga scan showing a lambda sign and a panda sign

Hunninghake GW, Costabel U, Ando M, et al: ATS/ERS/WASOG statement on sarcoidosis. Am J Respir Crit Care Med 1999;160:736-755.

Hunninghake GW, Gilbert S, Pueringer R, et al: Outcome of treatment for sarcoidosis. Am J Respir Crit Care Med 1994;149:893-898.

Judson MA: An approach to the treatment of pulmonary sarcoidosis with corticosteroids. Chest 1999;111:623-631.

Judson MA, Baughman RP: Sarcoidosis. In Baughman RP, du Bois RM, Lynch JP, Wells AU (eds): Diffuse Lung Disease: A Practical Approach. London: Arnold, 2004, pp 109-129.

Judson MA, Baughman RP, Teirstein AS, et al: Defining organ involvement in sarcoidosis: The ACCESS proposed instrument. Sarcoidosis Vasc Diffuse Lung Dis 1999;16:75-86.

Lower EE, Baughman RP: Prolonged use of methotrexate in refractory sarcoidosis. Arch Intern Med 1995;155:846-851.

Lynch JP, Kazerooni EA, Gay SE: Pulmonary sarcoidosis. Clin Chest Med 1997;755-785.

Newman LS, Rose CS, Maier LA: Sarcoidosis. N Engl J Med 1997;1224-1234.

Sharma OR: Pulmonary sarcoidosis and corticosteroids. Am Rev Respir Dis 1993;147:1598-1600.

Pneumoconiosis

Method of
*Richard D. deShazo, MD, and
David N. Weissman, MD*

Pneumoconiosis

The pneumoconioses are a group of interstitial fibrotic lung diseases predominantly associated with occupational exposures. They are caused by inhalation of particulate matter in the respirable size range (0.3-5 µm mean aerodynamic diameter), especially mineral or metallic dusts (Table 1). These agents interact with pulmonary target cells, including alveolar macrophages and alveolar epithelial cells, to activate a cascade of inflammatory mediators including growth factors. Although exposure to these dusts can induce other types of respiratory disease as well, the final common pathway is alveolar epithelial cell damage and interstitial fibrosis. This chapter focuses on silicosis and asbestosis, two common forms of pneumoconiosis.

Asbestosis

Asbestos is composed of strong, heat-resistant fibers of hydrated magnesium silicate classified morphologically as serpentine (chrysotile) or amphibole (crocidolite [riebeckite asbestos]), amosite [cummingtonite-grunerite asbestos], anthophyllite asbestos, actinolite asbestos, and tremolite asbestos. In addition, certain asbestiform fibers (winchite, richterite, erionite) can cause adverse health effects identical to those of asbestos. Fiber dimensions and persistence in tissues are key determinants of toxicity. There is a dose–response effect between the quantity of asbestos inhaled and the severity of fibrotic lung disease. Asbestos is also a carcinogen, and increasing exposure is associated with increased risk, particularly for lung cancer and mesothelioma.

Although asbestos is no longer mined in the United States, importation of asbestos-containing products continues. Exposures also continue to occur, especially in construction and renovation (due to reservoirs of asbestos that are still present in many older buildings), the heating trades (where asbestos is often encountered), and with exposure to older or imported asbestos-containing automotive friction products such as brake linings and clutch facings. Workers exposed to asbestos can carry it home on their clothing, resulting in exposure of family members. Living near natural amphibole deposits in California has been implicated as a risk factor for mesothelioma.

The Occupational Safety and Health Administration (OSHA) permissible exposure limit (PEL) for asbestos is 0.1 fiber per cc air. This limit was affected in part by the limits of the analytical methodology used in exposure assessment. Exposure to the PEL every day over a 45-year working lifetime has been estimated to be associated with an increased risk of cancer (lung, mesothelioma, and gastrointestinal) of 336 cases per 100,000 exposed persons and an increased risk of asbestosis of 250 cases per 100,000 exposed persons.

Asbestosis causes symptoms of dyspnea and cough. Latency between initial exposure and disease onset is related to exposure intensity. In the United States, this period is generally about two decades. The disease can lead to chronic respiratory failure. Effects of smoking add to the severity of the disease and can cause obstructive findings in addition to the expected decreased lung volume and diffusion capacity associated with fibrotic lung diseases. Bibasilar rubs and inspiratory crackles on auscultation, finger clubbing, and diffuse, bilateral, small, irregular parenchymal opacities and linear streaking at the lung bases on chest x-ray are characteristic.

The International Labour Organization (ILO) has established a system for classification (grading) of radiographs for the presence of radiographic abnormalities in lung parenchyma and pleura that are associated with pneumoconiosis, as well as their severity. The ILO classification system is widely used in epidemiology, surveillance, administrative, and legal settings. The small opacity profusion grades of 0/1 and 1/0 are often considered as defining the boundary between normal and abnormal lung parenchyma.

High-resolution computed tomography (CT) is the most sensitive imaging method for suspected asbestosis. It detects a range of parenchymal abnormalities related to the fibrotic process, such as ground glass and honeycombing, and pleural abnormalities, such as pleural plaques and diffuse pleural thickening. The presence of pleural plaques on radiography (particularly bilateral calcified pleural plaques); uncoated asbestos fibers or fibers coated with an iron-rich proteinaceous material (asbestos bodies) in sputum, bronchoalveolar lavage, or lung biopsy; and the slower progression of symptoms help differentiate asbestosis from idiopathic pulmonary fibrosis.

TABLE 1 Representative Pneumoconioses

Source	Clinical Features	Occupation	Dust
Crystalline silica	Silicosis, increased susceptibility to TB, airways obstruction, lung cancer	Mining, stone cutting, pottery, foundry work	Free crystalline silica (SiO2)
Asbestiform fibers	Asbestosis, bronchogenic carcinoma, mesothelioma, various forms of benign pleural disease	Insulation, shipbuilding, construction, some mining (e.g., vermiculite mining in Libby, Mont)	Various asbestiform fibers
Coal	Coal workers' pneumoconiosis, COPD	Coal mining	Coal mine dust
Hard metal	Hard metal lung disease (cobalt lung), asthma	Machinists, metal workers	Hard metal, composed primarily of tungsten carbide and cobalt

COPD = chronic obstructive pulmonary disease; TB = tuberculosis.

CURRENT DIAGNOSIS

- History of inhalation of mineral or metal dust
- Respiratory symptoms such as cough and dyspnea
- Spirometry and lung volumes show restriction in advanced disease
- Interstitial lung disease can usually be demonstrated by chest imaging. Biopsy is usually unnecessary
- No other likely cause of interstitial lung disease is present

CRITERIA FOR DIAGNOSIS

Diagnosis is supported by radiographic chest imaging or lung biopsy findings of interstitial lung disease compatible with asbestos; documentation of exposure to asbestos by history, the presence of pleural plaques (bilateral pleural plaques are essentially pathognomonic for asbestos exposure), or the presence of asbestos bodies or an excessive burden of uncoated asbestos fibers in lung biopsy tissue or possibly via bronchoalveolar lavage or sputum; and no other likely explanation for the diffuse fibrotic lung disease.

ASBESTOS-RELATED BENIGN PLEURAL DISEASE

Pleural plaques are characteristic forms of localized parietal pleural thickening that are usually bilateral and asymmetrical, involve the lower lung fields or the diaphragm, and spare the costophrenic angles and apices. Pleural plaques are a marker for exposure to asbestos and are often associated with other asbestos-related conditions. Pleural plaques result in minimal reductions in forced vital capacity and do not degenerate into malignant lesions.

In contrast, *diffuse visceral pleural thickening* can result in adhesions between the visceral and parietal pleura with major decreases in forced vital capacity, respiratory insufficiency, and the requirement for decortication.

Benign pleural effusions can occur in the first decade after asbestos exposure and contain erythrocytes and a mixed inflammatory cell infiltrate of lymphocytes, neutrophils, and eosinophils. The thickened visceral pleura and adjacent atelectatic lung tissue can result in a pleural-based area of *rounded atelectasis*, simulating a lung mass on chest radiography. CT can reveal the comet sign, a pleural band connecting the apparent mass to an area of thickened pleura.

LUNG CANCER AND MALIGNANT MESOTHELIOMA

Exposure to all forms of asbestos increases the risk of lung cancer. The peak risk occurs at about 30 to 35 years after the onset of exposure. Tobacco smoking increases this risk in a multiplicative fashion, increasing the sixfold risk associated with asbestos exposure alone to a relative risk of about 60-fold. In contrast, smoking does not further increase the asbestos-associated risk for *malignant mesothelioma*. Asbestos-associated malignant mesothelioma can also affect the peritoneum (and sometimes the pericardium), but when it affects the pleura, this disease manifests with dyspnea, chest pain, and bloody pleural effusion (most often unilateral). A latency period of 30 years or longer after initial exposure is common. Special immunochemical stains and electron microscopy of pleural fluid or pleural biopsies may be necessary to differentiate mesothelioma from adenocarcinoma. There is no evidence of benefit from surveillance for lung cancer in asbestos-exposed populations.

TREATMENT

Treatment of asbestosis is symptomatic and similar to that for other patients with chronic lung disease (Box 1). Lung transplantation should be considered in the setting of end-stage lung disease.

BOX 1 Recommendations for Managing Patients with Silicosis or Asbestos-Related Lung Disease

Patients
Stop further exposure to silica or asbestos.
Stop smoking, avoid exposure to tobacco products.

Physicians
Provide early treatment of respiratory infections with antibiotics.
Give pneumococcal and influenza vaccinations.
Maintain a high index of suspicion and provide early evaluation of symptoms for lung, laryngeal, and gastrointestinal cancers and mesothelioma in asbestos-exposed patients.
Maintain a high index of suspicion for pulmonary infection with *Mycobacterium tuberculosis*, nontuberculous mycobacteria, and fungi in silica-exposed patients.
Screen silica-exposed patients for latent tuberculosis infection with tuberculin skin test. Treat latent infections with isoniazid (9 mo) or rifampin (4 mo).
Provide empiric treatment with short- and long-acting inhaled bronchodilators and inhaled corticosteroids when they are found to provide symptomatic relief.
Give supplemental oxygen therapy if pulmonary hypertension is present or to prevent pulmonary hypertension if O_2 saturation is less than 85% at rest, with exercise, or with sleep.
Consider lung transplantation in the setting of end-stage lung disease.

Treatment of benign pleural disease is also symptomatic; as already noted, decortication is sometimes required for managing diffuse visceral pleural thickening. Depending on extent of disease, mesothelioma may be treated with surgery, radiation, chemotherapy, or some combination of these. In general, prognosis is poor. Mesothelioma-associated malignant pleural effusion can require palliation through procedures such as pleurodesis, pleurectomy, and decortication. Asbestos-associated lung cancer is managed in the same fashion as lung cancer occurring without a history of exposure to asbestos.

Silicosis

Silicosis is a fibrosing interstitial lung disease resulting from the inhalation of crystalline silicon dioxide (silica) in dust of respirable size. The commonest form of crystalline silica is quartz, which is the main component of sand and is present in most rocks. Noncrystalline (amorphous) silica, like that in diatomaceous earth or glass, does not cause silicosis. However, heating amorphous silica, as occurs in foundries when molten metal is poured into clay castings, can convert amorphous silica into cristobalite, a hazardous form of crystalline silica. Mining, stone cutting, sandblasting, and foundry work are all examples of trades associated with exposure to respirable dust containing crystalline silica. The International Agency for Research on Cancer (IARC) has designated crystalline silica from occupational sources as a Group 1 human lung carcinogen.

The current OSHA PEL for respirable dusts containing crystalline silica is defined according to specified formulas, including one that is most commonly used:

$$(10 \text{ mg/m}^3)/(\% \text{ SiO}_2 \text{ content} + 2)$$

According to this formula, if a respirable dust contains 100% crystalline silica, the PEL for that dust approximates 0.1 mg/m^3.

A number of studies have suggested that this PEL is not fully protective for exposures over an entire working lifetime. The National

Institute for Occupational Safety and Health (NIOSH) recommended exposure limit (REL) for respirable crystalline silica should be lower than the PEL, at 0.05 mg/m^3. Reporting of silicosis cases to public health authorities is required in some states.

RADIOGRAPHIC PATTERNS OF SILICOSIS

Three main radiographic patterns of silicosis have been described. Two are nodular interstitial patterns and one is an alveolar-filling pattern. The *simple* pattern is associated with nodules that are smaller than 10 mm and that are predominantly rounded and in the upper lung zones. *Progressive massive fibrosis* (PMF) is found in more advanced interstitial disease. It is associated with multiple coalescent larger nodules, upper lobe fibrosis, upward retraction of the hila, and compensatory hyperinflation of the lower lobes. The large upper-zone opacities can cavitate, sometimes in the setting of superimposed mycobacterial infection. Hilar adenopathy can occur, sometimes with an egg-shell pattern of hilar node calcification. A third radiographic pattern is an alveolar-filling process. Overwhelming silica exposure over a short period can cause a pathologic response called *silicoproteinosis*, in which alveoli become flooded with proteinaceous fluid. The condition resembles idiopathic pulmonary alveolar proteinosis. The radiographic alveolar filling pattern favors the lower lung zones and is not associated with the changes of simple silicosis or PMF.

SILICOSIS SYNDROMES

Three syndromes of silicosis can be defined based on clinical course and radiographic pattern. *Chronic silicosis* develops slowly, usually 10 to 30 years after first exposure. It most often has the simple radiographic pattern, but it can be associated with PMF.

Accelerated silicosis develops more rapidly, within 10 years after first exposure. It is associated with higher intensity exposures and can be associated with either the simple or PMF radiographic patterns. Accelerated silicosis is differentiated from chronic silicosis by its more rapid course. Patients with accelerated courses are at greater risk for developing PMF. The clinical presentations of chronic and accelerated silicosis are variable but include cough, dyspnea, and a variety of chest findings ranging from a normal chest examination to crackles, rhonchi, or wheezing. PMF is associated with more severe symptoms and respiratory impairment. Findings compatible with both restrictive and obstructive lung disease (decreased forced vital capacity [FVC], forced expiratory volume at 1 sec [FEV$_1$], FEV$_1$/FVC, diffusion capacity) can occur, potentially leading to cor pulmonale and respiratory failure.

Acute silicosis is associated with very intense exposures to silica, leading to symptoms within a few weeks to a few years after exposure. Intense exposure results in lung injury caused by flooding of alveoli with proteinaceous material, or silicoproteinosis. As already noted, the radiographic appearance is that of an alveolar-filling pattern favoring the lower lung zones. Patients present weeks to a few years after exposure with cough, weight loss, fatigue, and occasional pleuritic chest pain, crackles on auscultation, and progression to respiratory failure often complicated by mycobacterial infection.

CRITERIA FOR DIAGNOSIS

The diagnosis of silicosis is predicated on a history of exposure to respirable crystalline silica, typical chest x-ray findings, and the lack of a more likely diagnosis. There is no consensus on the use of high-resolution CT, and lung biopsy is seldom required for diagnosis.

TREATMENT

Treatment is symptomatic and similar to that for other patients with chronic lung disease (see Box 1). Experimental therapies such as oral corticosteroid therapy and whole-lung lavage have been reported, but clinical benefit is unclear. Lung transplantation should be considered for patients with end-stage lung disease.

All forms of silicosis, as well as substantial exposure to crystalline silica in the absence of silicosis, are associated with an increased risk of pulmonary tuberculosis and fungal infections. Patients should be evaluated for latent tuberculosis infection by skin testing with tuberculin purified protein derivative. A positive tuberculin skin test in a patient with a history of substantial silica exposure of at least 10 mm of induration should be considered evidence of tuberculosis infection, regardless of previous immunization with bacille Calmette-Guérin. If the tuberculin skin test is positive, an evaluation for active tuberculosis should be performed and active disease treated. If active tuberculosis is not present, treat for latent infection. For adults, isoniazid (Nydrazid) 5 mg/kg (300 mg maximum) daily or 15 mg/kg (900 mg maximum) twice weekly for 9 months; or rifampin (Rifadin) 10 mg/kg (600 mg maximum) daily for 4 months are effective regimens. Pediatric doses are isoniazid (Nydrazid) 10-20 mg/kg (300 mg maximum) daily or 20-40 mg/kg (900 mg maximum) twice weekly for 9 months; or rifampin (Rifadin) 10-20 mg/kg (600 mg maximum) daily for 4 months. Directly observed therapy must be used with twice-weekly dosing. Pneumococcal vaccine polyvalent (Pneumovax 23, 0.5 mL intramuscularly every 10 years[3]) and yearly influenza immunization should be provided.

Disclaimer

The findings and conclusions in this report are those of the authors and do not necessarily represent the views of the National Institute for Occupational Safety and Health or the Centers for Disease Control and Prevention.

REFERENCES

American Thoracic Society: Targeted tuberculin testing and treatment of latent tuberculosis infection. MMWR Recomm Rep 2000;49(RR-6):1-54.
Department of Labor, Mine Safety and Health Administration: 30 CFR Parts 56, 57, and 71. Asbestos exposure limit; proposed rule. Fed Reg 2005;70:43950-43989.
Miller A: Radiographic readings for asbestosis: Misuse of science—validation of the ILO classification. Am J Ind Med 2007;50:63-67.
Rimal B, Greenberg AK, Rom WN: Basic pathogenic mechanisms of silicosis: Current understanding. Curr Opin Pulm Med 2005;11:169-173.
Ross MH, Murray J: Occupational respiratory disease in mining. Occup Med 2004;54:304-310.
Weissman DN, Banks DE: Silicosis. In King TEJr, Schwarz MI (ed): Interstitial Lung Disease, 4th ed, Hamilton, Ontario: B.C. Decker, 2003, pp 387-402.
World Health Organization: Concise international chemical assessment document 24. Crystalline silica quartz, Stuttgart: Wissenschaftliche Verlags GmbH, 2000.

---

[3]Exceeds dosage recommended by the manufacturer.

Hypersensitivity Pneumonitis

Method of
Yvon Cormier, MD and Yves Lacasse, MD

Hypersensitivity pneumonitis is a respiratory disease caused by a hyperimmune response to a variety of inhaled antigens. These antigens include animal proteins, bacterial or fungal particles, and nonorganic compounds that act as haptens with human albumin. The clinical manifestations vary from an acute form characterized by fever, shortness of breath, and chest tightness that start 3 to 8 hours from exposure to a more insidious presentation where the patient develops progressive shortness of breath with cough and weight loss.

Physical examination is unremarkable, with inspiratory crackles, sometimes fever, and in some chronic cases digital clubbing. Early in the disease the physiologic abnormalities are restrictive, with a marked

BOX 1	Predictors of Hypersensitivity Pneumonitis

Exposure to a known antigen
Serum antibodies to that antigen
Weight loss
Inspiratory crackles
Recurrent symptoms
Symptoms occurring 4 to 8 hours after exposure

Data from Lalancette P, Carrier G, Ferland S, et al: Long-term outcome and predictive value of bronchoalveolar lavage fibrosing factors in farmer's lung. Am Rev Respir Dis 1993;148:216-221.

BOX 2	Treatment of Hypersensitivity Pneumonitis

Prevention
Primary: education in high-risk environments
Secondary: avoidance of contact in subjects with the disease

Pharmaceutical
Oral corticosteroids
Short course, high dose (prednisone 50 mg/day)
Maintenance low dose (prednisone 20 mg/day)

---

reduction in lung-diffusion capacity. In acute cases or after a lengthy subacute presentation, hypoxemia is usually present. Lung functions can revert to normal when the disease is diagnosed early and prevented from progressing. If, however, the disease is allowed to continue for repeated bouts of acute reactions or for a prolonged period, irreversible lung damage can occur. The long-term outcome can be either lung fibrosis with restrictive lung functions or emphysema with associated irreversible airflow obstruction and hyperinflation.

Diagnosis

There are no robust diagnostic criteria for hypersensitivity pneumonitis. Previously published criteria were based on expert opinions and on the characteristics of the disease. These criteria were not validated. The Hypersensitivity Pneumonitis Study Group has published a simple predictive rule for the diagnosis or exclusion of hypersensitivity pneumonitis. These simple criteria are given in Box 1. This predictive rule can be sufficient to rule in or out hypersensitivity pneumonitis in typical settings, but additional investigative procedures are often required.

Additional procedures include bronchoalveolar lavage; the absence of a typical high-intensity lymphocytic alveolitis rules out active hypersensitivity pneumonitis. Chest radiographs, especially high-resolution computed tomography (HRCT), can be very useful. Typically one sees patchy alveolitis and ground-glass infiltrations on the HRCT. Chest radiographs are normal in up to 20% of cases. Lung biopsy is sometimes required in difficult cases to confirm the diagnosis or rule out other diseases.

Coleman and Colby's diagnostic triad of hypersensitivity pneumonitis includes cellular infiltrates of lymphocytes and plasma cells of varying density along airways; interstitial infiltrates of lymphocytes and plasma cells varying from mild to very dense; and single, non-necrotizing, randomly scattered granulomata in the parenchyma, with some in bronchiolar and alveolar walls, but without mural vascular involvement. Eosinophils are scant or absent.

Treatment

The treatment of hypersensitivity pneumonitis is based on contact avoidance when possible. In high-risk environments (such as farming activities), education can prevent respiratory problems. Complete elimination of antigenic exposure is often difficult. This is especially obvious when the antigen is in the work place (e.g., dairy farmer) or where pigeons are part of the living environment. Even when the responsible source can be eliminated and cleaning measures are applied, a significant amount of antigen can persist for months. Wearing a protective respirator can be effective, but these are uncomfortable and cumbersome and must always be worn when the patient is in contact with the offending environment. It is likely that if all contact is eliminated, the disease will stop progressing and that some or total recovery will occur. The amount of recovery depends on the extent of irreversible damage present (alveolar wall destruction or interstitial fibrosis) when the contact is elimi-nated (Box 2).

Systemic corticosteroids are the only drugs currently recognized for treating hypersensitivity pneumonitis. Oral steroids attenuate the clinical symptoms and are as effective as contact avoidance in the early outcome of hypersensitivity pneumonitis. The long-term outcome is probably not altered by corticosteroid use. An empiric recommendation is to give high-dose steroids (e.g., prednisone 50 mg/day) in acute severe cases. In this setting, the steroids can usually be withdrawn within a few days, as soon as the acute manifestations have waned. One could also consider giving oral steroids at lower doses (20 mg/day) over a longer period of time as a maintenance treatment (for a month or two) when contact cannot be avoided (e.g., a dairy farmer). Appropriate treatment of the potential side effects of long-term corticosteroids must also be considered when this approach is used.

REFERENCES

Coleman A, Colby TV: Histologic diagnosis of extrinsic allergic alveolitis. Am J Surg Pathol 1988;2:514-518.

Cormier Y, Israel-Assayag E, Desmeules M, Lesur O: Effect of contact avoidance or treatment with oral prednisolone on bronchoalveolar lavage surfactant protein A levels in subjects with farmer's lung. Thorax 1996;51:1210-1215.

Hodgson MJ, Parkinson DK, Karpf M: Chest X-rays in hypersensitivity pneumonitis: A meta-analysis of secular trends. Am J Ind Med 1989; 16:45-53.

Kokkarinen JI, Tukiainen HO, Terho EO: Effect of corticosteroid treatment on the recovery of pulmonary function in farmer's lung. Am Rev Respir Dis 1992;145:3-5.

Lacasse Y, Selman M, Costabel U, et al: Clinical prediction rule for the diagnosis of active hypersensitivity pneumonitis (HP): The HP study. Am J Respir Crit Care Med 2003;168:952-958.

Lalancette P, Carrier G, Ferland S, et al: Long-term outcome and predictive value of bronchoalveolar lavage fibrosing factors in farmer's lung. Am Rev Respir Dis 1993;148:216-221.

Monkare S, Haahtela T: Farmer's lung—a 5-year follow-up of eighty-six patients. Clin Allergy 1987;17:143-151.

Perez-Padilla R, Salas J, Chapela R, et al: Mortality in Mexican patients with chronic pigeon breeder's lung compared to those with usual interstitial pneumonitis. Am Rev Respir Dis 1993;148:49-53.

Richerson HB, Bernstein IL, Fink JN, et al: Guidelines for the clinical evaluation of hypersensitivity pneumonitis. J Allergy Clin Immunol 1989;84: 839-844.

Schuyler M: The diagnosis of hypersensitivity pneumonitis. Chest 1997; 111:534-536.

Silver SF, Muller NL, Miller RR, Lefcoe MS: Hypersensitivity pneumonitis: Evaluation with CT. Radiology 1989;173:441-445.

Terho EO: Diagnostic criteria for farmer's lung disease. Am J Ind Med 1986;10:329.

Tuberculosis and Other Mycobacterial Diseases

Method of
*Surendra Kumar Sharma, MD, PhD, and
Alladi Mohan, MD*

Declared a global emergency in 1993 by the World health Organization (WHO), tuberculosis (TB) continues to be a major public health problem throughout the world despite relentless global efforts directed at containing the scourge. The HIV infection and AIDS pandemic in the context of increased demographic pressure and poorly run control programs with low case finding and cure rates have been implicated as the cause of the global resurgence of TB.

Epidemiology

It has been estimated that 2 billion people are infected with *Mycobacterium tuberculosis* globally. In 2006, there were an estimated 9.2 million new TB cases (8% HIV-seropositive); there were 1.5 million deaths in HIV-seronegative people, and 0.2 million deaths among people co-infected with HIV. TB kills more women than all causes of maternal mortality combined.

The WHO Asian region (South-East Asia and Western Pacific regions) accounts for 55% of global cases, and Africa accounts for 31%. Current estimates reveal that India, China, Indonesia, South Africa, and Kenya rank first to fifth in terms of incident cases. As a result of HIV/AIDS, incidence rates of TB in certain countries have gone up by more than 6% per year, crippling the already overburdened health care resources. In 2007, a total of 13,293 TB cases were reported in the United States; the TB rate declined 4.2% from 2006 to 4.4 cases per 100,000 population. The TB rate in foreign-born persons in the United States was 9.7 times that of native-born persons. Despite a decreasing trend observed since 1993 (7.3% per year between 1993 and 2000 to 3.8% between 2000 and 2007), TB still remains a serious public health problem among certain patient populations.

Natural History

As the natural history of pulmonary TB is understood today, 70% of persons exposed do not get infected and only 30% develop infection. Among those infected, only about 10% develop progressive primary TB, in most cases within 2 years. The infection gets contained in the remaining 90% of the infected subjects, a condition termed *latent TB infection* (LTBI).

The unique ability of *M. tuberculosis* to persist for long periods unrecognized by the human immune system by as yet poorly understood mechanisms results in LTBI. Persons with LTBI are noninfectious and remain symptom free. Immunocompetent patients with LTBI have a 10% lifetime risk of developing reactivation of infection, resulting in postprimary TB; 50% of reactivations occur during the first 2 years of primary infection. In comparison, in HIV-infected persons with LTBI, the risk of reactivation is about 10% per year. Therefore, early diagnosis of persons with LTBI and institution of treatment can be rewarding, especially in industrialized nations, where prevalence of the active disease is low, because patients with LTBI act as reservoirs to contribute to the pool of active disease. On the other hand, in developing nations, the problem of LTBI might not be an important issue because of high prevalence of the active disease.

Multidrug-resistant tuberculosis (MDR-TB), caused by *M. tuberculosis* that is resistant to both isoniazid (INH, Nydrazid) *and* rifampin (Rifadin) with or without resistance to other drugs, is a phenomenon that is threatening to destabilize global TB control. According to the 2008 report of the World Health Organization (WHO) and the International Union Against Tuberculosis and Lung Disease (IUATLD) Global Project on Antituberculosis Drug-resistance Surveillance estimates, the prevalence of MDR-TB among new cases ranged from 0% to 22.3%. The proportion, however, is considerably higher in patients who have previously received antituberculosis treatment (ranging from 0% to 62.5%). Incomplete and inadequate treatment are the most important factors leading to development of MDR-TB, suggesting that it is often a human-made tragedy. MDR-TB is a worldwide problem, being present in virtually all countries that were surveyed.

Extensively drug-resistant tuberculosis (XDR-TB), caused by isolates resistant to at least rifampicin and isoniazid (which is the definition of MDR-TB), in addition to any fluoroquinolone, and to at least one of the three following injectable drugs used in antituberculosis treatment; namely, capreomycin, kanamycin, and amikacin has recently been documented from many parts of the world and appears to be a threat to global TB control.

Diagnosis

LATENT INFECTION

The tuberculin skin test (TST) has been the most widely employed tool to detect LTBI. Published evidence suggests that treatment of LTBI results in considerable reduction of active disease. This has prompted the evolution of programs for targeted skin testing and latent tuberculosis treatment in countries such as the United States. In this approach, emphasis is on targeted tuberculin testing among persons at high risk for recent LTBI or with clinical conditions that increase the risk of progression of LTBI to active TB. Infected persons considered to be at high risk for developing active TB are offered treatment of LTBI irrespective of age.

The Mantoux method has been the preferred skin test for detecting LTBI caused by *M. tuberculosis*. It is administered by injecting 0.1 mL of 5 tuberculin units (TU) of purified protein derivative (PPD) intradermally into the volar or dorsal surface of the forearm.

 CURRENT DIAGNOSIS

- It is important to distinguish infection with *M. tuberculosis* from active TB disease.
- Diagnosing latent TB infection by targeted tuberculin skin testing and use of interferon-γ–based assays can facilitate institution of treatment for this condition.
- Patients with active TB disease present with constitutional symptoms such as fever, malaise, anorexia, weight loss, night sweats, and fatigue. They might also present with symptoms related to the organ system(s) involved. The symptoms classically evolve over 4 to 6 weeks.
- Atypical presentation is common in immunosuppressed persons, such as those with late HIV-infection, miliary TB, or occult extrapulmonary TB, resulting in a delay in the diagnosis.
- In patients suspected to have active TB disease, appropriate specimens must be collected for microscopic examination and mycobacterial culture and sensitivity testing, molecular diagnosis, and histopathologic examination.
- Diagnosis is established when clinical and radiologic findings are supported by microbiological, molecular, or histologic evidence of TB.

Abbreviation: TB = tuberculosis.

The test is read 48 to 72 hours after administration, and the transverse diameter of induration is recorded in millimeters. Based on the patient scenario, three cut-off levels have been recommended for defining a positive tuberculin reaction: larger than 5 mm (for subjects who are at highest risk for developing TB disease), larger than 10 mm (for subjects with an increased probability of recent infection or with other clinical conditions that increase the risk of TB), and larger than 15 mm of induration (or subjects with no risk factors for TB) (Box 1).

For patients with a negative TST reaction who are subject to repeat TST testing, an increase in reaction size of greater than 10 mm within a period of 2 years should be considered a skin-test conversion suggesting recent infection with *M. tuberculosis*. TST is not contraindicated for persons who have been vaccinated with bacille Calmette-Guérin (BCG), and a positive reaction to tuberculin in BCG-vaccinated persons indicates infection with *M. tuberculosis* when the person tested is at increased risk for recent infection or has medical conditions that increase the risk of disease.

Use of TST for detecting LTBI is hampered by poor specificity in BCG-vaccinated populations and by its low sensitivity in immunosuppressed persons, who are at highest risk for progression. Furthermore, good quality tuberculin in various strengths is seldom available in many parts of the world. Recently, blood tests based on detection of interferon-γ (IFN-γ) released by T lymphocytes in response to *M. tuberculosis*–specific antigens have become available, and these tests seem to offer an improvement over the TST. Compared with the TST, the IFN-γ–based assays that use *M. tuberculosis*–specific region of difference 1 (RD1) antigens such as early secretory antigenic target 6 (ESAT6) and culture filtrate protein 10 (CFP10) might have advantages over the TST. The IFN-γ assays are available in enzyme-linked immunosorbent assay (ELISA) (e.g., QuantiFERON-TB and the enhanced QuantiFERON-TB Gold assay) and enzyme-linked immunospot (ELISPOT) (e.g., T SPOT-TB assay) formats. The QuantiFERON-TB Gold assay is available in two formats, a 24-well culture plate format (approved by the FDA) and a newer, simplified in-tube format.[1,2] T SPOT-TB is marketed for use in Europe and is likely to receive FDA approval in the future. Recently, QuantiFERON-TB Gold assay received final approval from the FDA as an aid for diagnosing *M. tuberculosis* infection. These tests are more specific than TST in the BCG-vaccinated population, do not require patient's return visit, give results by the next day, and do not have boosting with repeated testing. However, like the TST, IFN-γ assays cannot reliably differentiate active TB disease from LTBI. The performance of QuantiFERON-TB Gold assay is being evaluated in the United States in certain populations targeted by TB control programs for detecting LTBI.

A chest radiograph (posteroanterior view for adults, with appropriate shielding if the subject is pregnant; posteroanterior and lateral views for children) is indicated for all patients being considered for treatment of LTBI to exclude active pulmonary TB. If the subject does not present with symptoms of active TB disease and the chest radiograph is normal, sputum smear examination for acid-fast bacilli (AFB) is not considered necessary, and the patient should be considered for treatment of LTBI.

ACTIVE DISEASE

In immunocompetent persons with TB disease, pulmonary involvement occurs in 80% of patients, 15% have isolated extrapulmonary TB, and 5% can have pulmonary and extrapulmonary involvement. In contrast, in immunosuppressed persons such as those with late HIV infection, pulmonary involvement occurs in 30% of patients, 20% have isolated extrapulmonary TB, and 50% can have pulmonary and extrapulmonary involvement.

Patients with active TB disease present with constitutional symptoms such as fever, malaise, anorexia, weight loss, night sweats, and fatigue. They also present with symptoms related to the organ system(s) involved. For example, those with pulmonary TB complain of cough, sputum, and hemoptysis. The symptoms classically evolve over 4 to 6 weeks. However, atypical presentation is common in immunosuppressed patients such as those with late HIV infection, miliary TB, or occult extrapulmonary TB. This results in a delay in the diagnosis and treatment.

Treatment

PRETREATMENT EVALUATION

In many countries, the WHO guidelines that target resource-poor nations that have a high burden of TB are followed in national programs for control of TB. For operational, logistic, and economic reasons, these guidelines differ from those advocated by the guidelines of the American Thoracic Society, Centers for Disease Control and Prevention, and the Infectious Diseases Society of America (ATS/CDC/IDSA guidelines), which are followed in the United States.

In patients suspected to have active TB disease, the ATS/CDC/IDSA guidelines state that appropriate specimens must be collected for microscopic examination and mycobacterial culture and

---

BOX 1 Cut-off Levels for Defining a Positive Tuberculin Reaction

Reaction >5 mm of induration
- HIV-positive patients
- Recent contacts of patients with TB
- Patients with fibrotic changes on chest radiograph consistent with past TB
- Organ transplant recipients and other immunosuppressed patients (receiving ≥15 mg/day of prednisone for ≥1 month*)
- Patients receiving tumor necrosis factor-α inhibitors such as infliximab (Remicade), etanercept (Enbrel), adalimumab (Humira)

Reaction >10 mm of Induration
- Recent immigrants from high-prevalence countries
- Injection drug users
- Residents and employees[†] of prisons and jails, nursing homes and other long-term facilities for the elderly, hospitals and other health care facilities, residential facilities for patients with AIDS, and homeless shelters
- Personnel working in a mycobacteriology laboratory
- Persons with silicosis, diabetes mellitus, chronic renal failure, certain hematologic disorders, some malignancies (e.g., carcinomas of the head or neck and lung), weight loss of >10% of ideal body weight, gastrectomy, and jejunoileal bypass patients who are at a high risk for developing TB
- Children younger than 4 years or infants, children, and adolescents exposed to adults at high risk

Reaction >15 mm of Induration
- Any person with no risk factors for TB

Abbreviation: TB = tuberculosis.
*In patients treated with corticosteroids, risk of TB increases with increasing dosage and duration.
[†]For persons who are otherwise at low risk and are tested at the start of employment, a reaction of >15 mm induration is considered positive.

---

[1]Not FDA approved for this indication.
[2]Not available in the United States.

CURRENT THERAPY

- Treatment of TB has been considered the most cost-effective health intervention ever conceived. Antituberculosis treatment aims to kill the tubercle bacilli rapidly, prevent the emergence of drug resistance, and eliminate persistent bacilli from the host's tissues to prevent relapse.
- To accomplish these goals, several antituberculosis drugs must be taken together for a sufficiently long time.
- The decision to initiate antituberculosis treatment should be based on clinical, radiographic, microbiological, and histopathologic information.
- When the patient is seriously ill with a life-threatening condition (such as miliary disease, meningitis) that is believed to be possibly due to TB, treatment using one of the recommended regimens should be initiated promptly, often before AFB smear results are known and usually before mycobacterial culture results have been obtained.
- DOTS is considered an effective way to control TB. Efficiently run TB-control programs based on a policy of DOTS are essential for preventing the emergence of MDR-TB.
- Treatment of patients coinfected with HIV and TB is essentially similar to the treatment of TB in HIV-negative patients. Differences include potential for drug interactions between the rifamycins and antiretroviral agents and immune reconstitution inflammatory syndrome (IRIS) (paradoxical reactions). Efavirenz-based HAART is the preferred regimen for use along with rifampin-based antituberculosis treatment. Co-administration of PI-based HAART and rifampin should be avoided and rifabutin should be used instead of rifampin. In patients co-infected with HIV and TB, CPT reduces case fatality rates.
- Management of MDR-TB is a challenge that should be undertaken by experienced clinicians at centers equipped with reliable laboratory services for mycobacterial cultures and in vitro sensitivity testing because it requires prolonged use of costly second-line drugs with a significant potential for toxicity. Treatment of MDR-TB with DOTS-Plus strategy will prevent the emergence of XDR-TB.

Abbreviations: CPT = cotrimoxazole preventive treatment; DOTS = directly observed therapy, short course; HAART = highly active antiretroviral therapy; HIV = human immunodeficiency virus; MDR = multidrug resistant; TB = tuberculosis.

sensitivity testing. In patients with suspected pulmonary TB, three sputum specimens must be obtained. If the patient is unable to produce adequate sputum, induction of sputum using hypertonic saline and bronchoscopy may be performed under appropriate infection-control measures. All patients with TB should have counseling and testing for HIV infection. A CD4+ T-lymphocyte count should be obtained for HIV-seropositive patients. These guidelines also suggest serologic testing for hepatitis B and C viruses (in patients with risk factors); baseline measurement of serum aminotransferases, bilirubin, alkaline phosphates, creatinine, and platelet count; and testing of visual acuity and red-green color discrimination if ethambutol (Myambutol) will be used.

PRINCIPLES OF TREATMENT

Treatment of TB has been considered the most cost-effective health intervention ever conceived. Antituberculosis treatment aims to kill the tubercle bacilli rapidly, prevent the emergence of drug resistance, and eliminate persistent bacilli from the host's tissues to prevent relapse. To accomplish these goals, several antituberculosis drugs must be taken together for a sufficiently long period. WHO recommends the directly observed treatment short-course (DOTS) approach as the only way to control TB globally, and DOTS is the key principle on which many of the TB control programs are run globally. The WHO categorization of patients with TB and the appropriate treatment regimens for each category that is followed in many of the national TB control programs is shown in Table 1. Drugs currently used for treating TB, preparations available currently, the recommend dosage schedule, and regimens described in the ATS/CDC/IDSA guidelines for patients with drug-susceptible TB are listed in Tables 2, 3, and 4 and Box 2.

In the ATS/CDC/IDSA guidelines, the decision to initiate antituberculosis treatment should be based on any clinical, radiographic, microbiological, and histopathologic information that is available. In situations where the patient is seriously ill with a life-threatening condition (such as miliary disease, meningitis) that might be due to TB, treatment using one of the recommended regimens should be initiated promptly, often before AFB smear results are known and usually before mycobacterial culture results have been obtained. A positive smear for AFB provides strong inferential evidence for the diagnosis of TB. However, if clinical suspicion of active TB is high, TST is positive, the initial AFB smears are negative, and no other diagnosis is established, empiric treatment with the appropriate standard treatment regimen should be initiated. If the diagnosis is confirmed by isolation of *M. tuberculosis* or a positive nucleic acid amplification test, there is a clinical or radiographic response within 2 months of initiation of therapy, and no other diagnosis has been established, treatment may be continued to complete a standard course of therapy. If the patient is smear negative, *M. tuberculosis* cannot be isolated, and there is no clinical and radiologic improvement at the end of 2 months, antituberculosis treatment may have to be stopped and an alternative diagnosis must be considered.

In patients with drug-susceptible TB, antituberculosis treatment has two phases: the initial intensive phase, which consists of 2 months of treatment, and the maintenance (continuation) phase, which is usually 4 months. In some patients with potential for relapse, such as those with cavitary disease, and in patients with extrapulmonary disease, the maintenance phase might have to be extended by 3 more months beyond the scheduled 4 months. In TB meningitis, the continuation phase is administered for 10 months. The ATS/CDC/IDSA guidelines advocate the use of corticosteroids in patients with central nervous system TB (including meningitis) and TB pericarditis.

MONITORING DURING TREATMENT

The patient must be closely monitored clinically, radiographically, and microbiologically at least monthly during the period of treatment to assess the response to treatment and identify possible adverse drug reactions. As per the ATS/CDC/IDSA guidelines, during treatment of patients with pulmonary TB, a sputum specimen for AFB smear and culture should be obtained at monthly intervals until two consecutive specimens are negative on culture. For patients who had positive AFB smears at the time of diagnosis, follow-up smears may be obtained at more frequent intervals until two consecutive specimens are negative. Drug susceptibility tests should be repeated on isolates from patients who have positive cultures after 3 months of treatment. Patients who have positive cultures after 4 months of treatment should be considered to have failed treatment and should be managed accordingly. For patients with extrapulmonary TB, the frequency and kind of evaluation will depend on the site involved and the ease with which specimens can be obtained.

In drug-naïve pulmonary TB, patients with positive cultures at diagnosis, a repeat chest radiograph at the completion of 2 months of treatment and at the completion of treatment is desirable but is not essential. In patients with negative initial cultures, a chest radiograph is necessary after 2 months of treatment, and a radiograph at the completion of treatment is desirable.

TABLE 1 World Health Organization Standard Regimens for Treating Tuberculosis

	TB Treatment Regimens*	
TB Patients	**Initial Phase**	**Continuation Phase**
Diagnostic Category I		
New sputum smear–positive PTB	2 $H_3R_3Z_3E_3$	4 H_3R_3
New smear–negative PTB[†] with extensive parenchymal involvement	2 HRZE	4 HR
Severe concomitant HIV disease or severe forms of EPTB[‡§]	2 HRZS	4 HR
Diagnostic Category II		
Sputum smear–positive relapse	2 $S_3H_3R_3Z_3E_3$	5 $H_3R_3E_3$
Sputum smear–positive treatment failure	1 $H_3R_3Z_3E_3$	5 HRE
Sputum smear–positive after treatment interruption	2 HRZES/1HRZE	
Diagnostic Category III		
Sputum smear–negative PTB and EPTB, not severe[¶]	2 $H_3R_3Z_3$	4 H_3R_3
	2 HRZE	4 HR
	2 HRZS	4 HR
Diagnostic Category IV		
Chronic and MDR-TB cases	Specially designed standardized and individualized regimens will be required	

*Either daily or three times per week. The number before the letters refers to the number of months of treatment. The subscript number after the letter refers to the number of doses per week.
[†]New sputum smear–negative PTB includes all forms of PTB other than primary complex.
[‡]Severe forms of EPTB include TBM, disseminated/miliary TB, TB pericarditis, TB peritonitis and intestinal TB, bilateral or extensive pleurisy, spinal TB with or without neurologic complications, genitourinary tract TB, and bone and joint TB.
[§]In patients with TBM on Category I treatment, the four drugs used during the intensive phase should be HRZS (instead of HRZE). Continuation phase of treatment in TBM and spinal TB with neurologic complications should be given for 6-7 months, extending the total duration of treatment to 8-9 months.
[¶]Not severe EPTB includes lymph node TB and unilateral small pleural effusion.
Abbreviations: E = ethambutol (Myambutol); EPTB = extrapulmonary tuberculosis; H = isoniazid (INH); PTB = pulmonary tuberculosis; R = rifampin (Rifadin); S = streptomycin; TB = tuberculosis.; TBM = tuberculosis meningitis; Z = pyrazinamide.
Adapted from World Health Organization: Treatment of Tuberculosis: Guidelines for National Programmes. 3rd ed. Geneva: World Health Organization, 2003.

TABLE 2 Drugs Used to Treat Tuberculosis

Drug	Preparations
First-Line Drugs	
Isoniazid (INH, Nydrazid)	Tab: 50 mg,[2] 100 mg, 300 mg
	Elixir: 50 mg/5 mL
	Aqueous sol'n for IM or IV injection: 100 mg/mL
Ethambutol (Myambutol)	Tab: 100 mg, 400 mg, 800 mg,[2] 1000 mg[2]
Pyrazinamide	Tab: 500 mg (scored), 750 mg,[2] 1000 mg[2]
Rifabutin (Mycobutin)[1]	Cap: 150 mg
Rifampin (Rifadin)	Cap: 150 mg, 300 mg, 450 mg,[2] 600 mg[2] (powder may be suspended for PO dosing)
	Aqueous sol'n for IV injection[2]
	Powder for injection: 600 mg
Rifapentine (Priftin)	Tab: 150 mg (film coated)
Second-Line Drugs	
Amikacin[1] (Amikin)	Aqueous sol'n for IM or IV injection: 0.5-g and 1-g vials
p-Aminosalicylic acid (PAS) (Paser)	Granules: 4-g packets (can be mixed with food)
	Tab: 0.5 g, 1 g (film coated)[2]
	Sol'n for IV injection[2]
Capreomycin (Capastat)	Aqueous sol'n[2] for IM or IV injection
	Powder: 1-g vials for IM or IV injection
Cycloserine (Seromycin)	Cap: 250 mg
Ethionamide (Trecator-SC)	Tab: 250 mg
Gatifloxacin (Tequin)[1]	Tab: 200 mg, 400 mg
	Aqueous sol'n for IV injection: 200 mg/20 mL
Kanamycin[1] (Kantrex)	Aqueous sol'n for IM or IV injection: 0.5-g and 1-g vials
Levofloxacin (Levaquin)[1]	Tab: 250 mg, 500 mg, 750 mg
	Aqueous sol'n for IV injection: 0.5-g, 0.75-g vials
Moxifloxacin (Avelox)[1]	Tab: 400 mg
	Aqueous sol'n for IM or IV injection: 400 mg/250 mL
Streptomycin	Aqueous sol'n for IM or IV injection: 0.5-g and 1-g vials[2]
	Powder: 1-g vials for injection

[1]Not FDA approved for this indication.
[2]Not available in the United States.
Abbreviations: cap = capsule; sol'n = solution; tab = tablet.

TABLE 3 Dosage Schedule of First-Line Drugs Used in the Treatment of Tuberculosis

Drug*	Daily	2 Days/Week	3 Days/Week	Important Adverse Effects
Ethambutol (Myambutol)[†]				Ocular toxicity, retrobulbar neuritis
Adults 40-55 kg[‡]	14.5-20.0 mg/kg (800 mg)	36.4-50.0 mg/kg (2000 mg)	21.8-30.0 mg/kg (1200 mg)	
Adults 56-75 kg[‡]	16.0-21.4 mg/kg (1200 mg)	37.3-50.0 mg/kg (2800 mg)	26.7-35.7 mg/kg (2000 mg)	
Adults 76-90 kg[‡]	17.8-21.1 mg/kg (1600 mg)[§]	44.4-52.6 mg/kg (4000 mg)[§]	26.7-31.6 mg/kg (2400 mg)[§]	
Children	15-20 mg/kg (1000 mg)	50 mg/kg (2500 mg)	NA	
Isoniazid (INH)				Hepatotoxicity, CNS effects, lupus-like syndrome, hypersensitivity reactions
Adults	5 mg/kg (300 mg)	15 mg/kg (900 mg)	15 mg/kg (900 mg)[¶]	
Children	10-15 mg/kg (300 mg)[¶]	20-30 mg/kg (900 mg)	NA	
Pyrazinamide				Hepatotoxicity, hyperuricemia, arthralgias, GI tract upset
Adults 40-55 kg[‡]	18.2-25.0 mg/kg (1000 mg)	36.4-50.0 mg/kg (2000 mg)	27.3-37.5 mg/kg (1500 mg)	
Adults 56-75 kg[‡]	20.0-26.8 mg/kg (1500 mg)	40.0-53.6 mg/kg (3000 mg)	33.3-44.6 mg/kg (2500 mg)	
Adults 76-90 kg[‡]	22.2-26.3 mg/kg (2000 mg)[§]	44.4-52.6 mg/kg (4000 mg)[§]	33.3-39.5 mg/kg (3000 mg)[§]	
Children	15-30 mg/kg (2000 mg)	50 mg/kg (2000 mg)	NA	
Rifabutin (Mycobutin)[1]				Hepatotoxicity, cutaneous reactions; GI reactions, flu-like syndrome, orange discoloration of body fluids, drug interactions, uveitis
Adults	5 mg/kg (300 mg)	5 mg/kg (300 mg)	5 mg/kg (300 mg)	
Children	NA	NA	NA	
Rifampin (Rifadin)				Hepatotoxicity, cutaneous reactions; GI reactions, flu-like syndrome, orange discoloration of body fluids, drug interactions, uveitis
Adults	10 mg/kg (600 mg)	10 mg/kg (600 mg)	10 mg/kg (600 mg)	
Children	10-20 mg/kg (600 mg)	NA	10-20 mg/kg (600 mg)	

[1]Not FDA approved for this indication.
*Maximum dosages are given in parentheses.
[†]Ethambutol can be used safely in older children, but it should be used with caution in children younger than 5 years, in whom visual acuity cannot be monitored. In younger children, ethambutol may be used at 15 mg/kg/d if there is suspected or proven resistance to isoniazid or rifampin.
[‡]Based on estimated lean body weight. Children weighing more than 40 kg should receive adult doses.
[§]Maximum dose regardless of weight.
[¶]The WHO recommends 10 mg/kg as the dose of isoniazid for adults for the thrice-weekly regimen. The WHO recommends 5 mg/kg as the dose of isoniazid for children for the daily regimen.
Adapted from Blumberg HM, Burman WJ, Chaisson RE, et al: American Thoracic Society, Centers for Disease Control and Prevention, and the Infectious Diseases Society: Treatment of tuberculosis. Am J Respir Crit Care Med 2003;167:603-662; and World Health Organization: Treatment of Tuberculosis: Guidelines for National Programmes, 3rd ed. Geneva: World Health Organization; 2003.
Abbreviations: CNS = central nervous system; GI = gastrointestinal; max = maximum; NA = no recommendation.

In patients with baseline laboratory abnormalities, liver and renal functions and platelet count might have to be repeated during the course of treatment to ensure that they are not deteriorating. Patients receiving ethambutol according to the standard dosage schedule should be questioned regarding vision symptoms during the monthly visits. If ethambutol is used in a higher dosage or if it is used for more than 2 months, monthly visual acuity and color vision checking must also be done.

Treatment is considered to be completed if the total number of doses are taken in the stipulated duration of treatment. Management of a patient who has interrupted treatment is beyond the scope of this chapter, and the reader is referred to the ATS/CDC/IDSA guidelines for details.

SPECIAL SITUATIONS
Latent Infection

Various regimens available for treating LTBI are listed in Table 5. Completion of treatment for LTBI is based not only on the duration of treatment alone but also on the total number of doses administered. For example, the 9-month regimen of daily isoniazid should consist of 270 doses, at minimum, administered within 12 months, allowing for minor interruptions in therapy.

Antituberculosis drug induced liver injury (DILI) is an important concern when isoniazid, pyrazinamide, and rifampin are being used. As per the official ATS statement on hepatotoxicity of

TABLE 4 Treatment Regimens for Patients with Drug-Susceptible Tuberculosis

	Intensive Phase		Maintenance Phase	
Regimen	Interval and Doses* (Minimum Duration)	Regimen	Interval and Doses*[†] (Minimum Duration)	Range of Total Doses (Minimum Duration)
Regimen 1 RHZE	7 d/wk for 56 doses (8 wk) or 5 d/wk for 40 doses (8 wk)[‡]	RH	7 d/wk for 126 doses (18 wk) or 5 d/wk for 90 doses (18 wk)[‡]	130-182 (26 wk)
		RH	Twice weekly for 36 doses (18 wk)[§]	76-92 (26 wk)
		RpH	Once weekly for 18 doses (18 wk)[¶]	58-74 (26 wk)
Regimen 2 RHZE	7 d/wk for 14 doses (2 wk), then twice weekly for 12 doses (6 wk) or 5 d/wk for 10 doses (2 wk),[‡] then twice weekly for 12 doses (6 wk)	RH	Twice weekly for 36 doses (18 wk)[§]	62-58 (26 wk)
		RpH	Once weekly for 18 doses (18 wk)[¶]	44-40 (26 wk)
Regimen 3 RHZE	Three times weekly for 24 doses (8 wk)	RH	Three times weekly for 54 doses (18 wk)	78 (26 wk)
Regimen 4 RHE	7 d/wk for 56 doses (8 wk) or 5 d/wk for 40 doses (8 wk)[‡]	RH	7 d/wk for 217 doses (31 wk) or 5 d/wk for 155 doses (31 wk)[‡]	273-195 (39 wk)
		RH	Twice weekly for 62 doses (31 wk)	118-102 (39 wk)

*When DOT is used, drugs may be given 5 d/wk and the necessary number of doses adjusted accordingly. Although there are no studies that compare 5 with 7 daily doses, extensive experience indicates this would be an effective practice.
[†]Patients with cavitation on initial chest radiograph and positive cultures at completion of 2 months of therapy should receive a 7-month maintenance phase. The 7-month maintenance phase is 31 weeks, either 217 doses (daily) or 62 doses (twice weekly).
[‡]5 d/wk administration is always given by DOT.
[§]Not recommended for HIV-infected patients with CD4+ T lymphocyte count <100/µL.
[¶]Should be used only in HIV-negative patients who have negative sputum smears at the time of completion of 2 months of therapy and who do not have cavitation on the initial chest radiograph. For patients who are started on this regimen and who have a positive culture in the 2-month specimen, treatment should be extended by an extra 3 months.
Abbreviations: DOT = directly observed therapy; E = ethambutol; H = isoniazid; R = rifampin; Rp = rifapentine; Z = pyrazinamide.
Adapted from Blumberg HM, Burman WJ, Chaisson RE, et al: American Thoracic Society, Centers for Disease Control and Prevention, and the Infectious Diseases Society: Treatment of tuberculosis. Am J Respir Crit Care Med 2003;167:603-662

BOX 2 Fixed-Dose Combination Preparations

These preparations are not available in the United States but are listed by the World Health Organization. Quality assurance is essential for ensuring adequate bioavailability while using fixed-dose combinations.

Daily Regimens

- Isoniazid + rifampin: 75 mg +150 mg tab, 150 mg +300 mg tab, 30 mg + 60 mg tab, or pack of granules for pediatric use
- Isoniazid + ethambutol: 150 mg + 400 mg tab
- Isoniazid + rifampin + pyrazinamide: 75 mg + 150 mg + 400 mg tab, 30 mg + 60 mg + 150 mg tab, or pack of granules for pediatric use
- Isoniazid + rifampin + pyrazinamide + ethambutol: 75 mg + 150 mg + 400 mg + 275 mg tab

Thrice-Weekly Regimens

- Isoniazid + rifampin: 150 mg +150 mg tab, 60 mg + 60 mg tab, or pack of granules for pediatric use
- Isoniazid + rifampin + pyrazinamide: 150 mg + 150 mg + 500 mg tab

Abbreviation: tab = tablet.

---

antituberculosis drugs, baseline laboratory testing is not routinely indicated for all patients at the start of treatment for LTBI. However, liver function testing should be performed in persons with a history of liver disease, persons who consume alcohol regularly, HIV-positive individuals, pregnant women and those in the immediate postpartum period (up to 3 months), among others. All patients receiving treatment should be monitored clinically; laboratory monitoring is indicated for patients whose baseline liver function tests are abnormal and for persons at risk for hepatic disease.

Laboratory monitoring should be used to evaluate possible adverse drug reactions that occur during the course of treatment. Isoniazid taken for nine months is the preferred regimen for the treatment of LTBI. Rifampin is an option for those who cannot tolerate isoniazid, but potential drug interactions must be considered. Revised guidelines recommended that the rifampicin and pyrazinamide regimen is no longer generally recommended for the treatment of LTBI.

Coinfection with HIV

Treatment of patients coinfected with HIV and TB is essentially similar to the treatment of TB in HIV-negative persons but with important differences. These include potential for drug interactions between rifamycins and antiretroviral agents and the immune reconstitution inflammatory syndrome (IRIS) (paradoxical reactions), which may be interpreted as clinical deterioration, treatment failure, or drug-resistant TB, among others. A low baseline CD4+ count, a higher baseline viral load at initiation of highly active antiretroviral

TABLE 5 Recommended Treatment Regimens for Latent Tuberculosis

Drug Regimen	Dosage Children	Dosage Adults	Comments
Isoniazid daily for 9 mo	10-20 mg/kg (max 300 mg)	5 mg/kg (max 300 mg)	In HIV-infected patients, isoniazid may be administered concurrently with NRTIs or NNRTIs
Isoniazid twice-weekly for 9 mo	20-40 mg/kg (max 900 mg)	15 mg/kg (max 900 mg)	DOT must be used with twice-weekly dosing
Isoniazid daily for 6 mo	10-20 mg/kg (max 300 mg)	5 mg/kg (max 300 mg)	Not indicated for HIV-infected persons, those with fibrotic lesions on chest radiographs, or children
Isoniazid, twice-weekly for 6 mo	20-40 mg/kg (max 900 mg)	15 mg/kg (max 900 mg)	DOT must be used with twice-weekly dosing
Rifampin (Rifadin) daily for 4 mo	10-20 mg/kg (max 600 mg)	10 mg/kg (max 600 mg)	For persons who are contacts of patients with isoniazid-resistant, rifampin-susceptible TB who cannot tolerate pyrazinamide

Abbreviations: DOT = directly observed therapy; HIV = human immunodeficiency virus; max = maximum; NRTIs = nucleoside reverse transcriptase inhibitors; NNRTIs = non-nucleoside reverse transcriptase inhibitors; TB = tuberculosis.
Data from American Thoracic Society and the Centers for Disease Control and Prevention: Targeted tuberculin testing and treatment of latent tuberculosis infection. Am J Respir Crit Care Med 2000;161(4 Pt 2):S221-S247; and Centers for Disease Control and Prevention (CDC); American Thoracic Society: Update: Adverse event data and revised American Thoracic Society/CDC recommendations against the use of rifampin and pyrazinamide for treatment of latent tuberculosis infection—United States, 2003. MMWR Morb Mortal Weekly Rep 2003;52:735-739.

therapy (HAART) and a rapid reduction in viral load and a greater increase in CD4+ cell count in response to HAART and a shorter interval between antituberculosis treatment and HAART are risk factors for the development of IRIS.

In HIV-coinfected patients, once-weekly isoniazid-rifapentine (Priftin) should not be used in the continuation phase, and twice weekly isoniazid-rifampin or rifabutin (Mycobutin)[1] should not be used for patients with CD4+ T-lymphocyte counts less than 100/µL because these regimens can result in acquired rifamycin resistance. The optimal time of initiation of antiretroviral treatment in HIV-TB coinfected patients is not known. The ATS/IDSA/CDC guidelines advocate delaying the initiation of HAART until the intensive phase of antituberculosis treatment is completed, if possible. Treatment of HIV-TB coinfected patients must be undertaken by clinicians experienced in this area, and the timing of initiation of HAART should be carefully individualized, weighing the risk of progression of disease and development of IRIS, drug-drug interactions, and the benefits from treatment.

Relapse, Treatment Failure, and Drug-Resistant Tuberculosis

A patient who becomes and remains culture-negative while receiving antituberculosis treatment but, at some point after completion of therapy, either becomes culture-positive again or experiences clinical or radiographic deterioration consistent with active tuberculosis is said to have developed *relapse*. Both drug-susceptible and drug-resistant strains can result in relapse. *Treatment failure* is defined as continued or recurrently positive cultures in a patient receiving appropriate antituberculosis treatment. Vigorous microbiological evaluation must be undertaken in patients who present with relapse or treatment failure so that true relapse and drug-resistant TB are identified.

Efficiently run TB control programs based on a policy of DOTS are essential for preventing the emergence of MDR-TB. The management of MDR-TB is a challenge that should be undertaken by experienced clinicians at periodically accredited centers equipped with reliable laboratory services for mycobacterial cultures and in vitro sensitivity testing because it requires the prolonged use of costly second-line drugs with a significant potential for toxicity. Already several countries, with the help of the WHO's Green Light Committee, are rolling out DOTS-Plus, WHO's supplemental strategy to treat MDR-TB, for use in areas with a high prevalence of MDR-TB. The DOTS-Plus strategy is expected to help in the prevention of the emergence of XDR-TB. The judicious use of drugs; supervised standardized treatment; focused clinical, radiologic, and bacteriologic follow-up; and surgery at the appropriate juncture are key factors in the successful management of these patients.

Nontuberculous Mycobacterial Disease

The term *nontuberculous mycobacteria* (NTM) is applied to mycobacteria other than *M. tuberculosis* complex that are ubiquitously found in the environment. NTM can cause transient infection, colonize the airways, or contaminate clinical specimens. Pulmonary disease due to NTM usually occurs in patients with structural lung disease such as old healed TB lesions, cystic fibrosis, pneumoconiosis, chronic obstructive pulmonary disease, and bronchiectasis. Classification of NTM recovered from humans is shown in Box 3.

CLINICAL PRESENTATION AND DIAGNOSTIC CRITERIA

NTM can cause localized pulmonary disease; lymphadenitis; skin, soft tissue, and skeletal infection; infection of bursae, joints, tendon sheaths, and bones; or disseminated disease that may be found in patients with and without AIDS. Recently, an NTM pulmonary syndrome (previously termed *hot tub lung*) with a presentation similar to hypersensitivity lung disease has also been recognized. The diagnosis of NTM infection is suspected based on the clinical presentation and radiographic abnormalities, and it is confirmed by microbiological characterization. The staining and culture methods, species identification, and susceptibility testing for NTM are beyond the scope of this chapter, and the reader is referred to the ATS 2007 guidelines for details.

TREATMENT

Treatment of NTM disease requires prolonged administration of multiple drugs. At the time of initial presentation, NTM disease can closely mimic TB, and antituberculosis treatment is often initiated in many of these patients. Thus, by the time the

---
[1]Not FDA approved for this indication.

BOX 3 Classification of Nontuberculous *Mycobacterium* Species Recovered from Humans

Common Etiologic Species

Pulmonary disease
- M. abscessus
- M. avium complex
- M. kansasii
- M. malmoense
- M. xenopi

Lymphadenitis
- M. avium complex
- M. malmoense
- M. scrofulaceum

Disseminated disease
- M. avium complex
- M. chelonae
- M. haemophilum
- M. kansasii

Skin, Soft Tissue, and Bone Disease
- M. abscessus
- M. chelonae
- M. fortuitum
- M. marinum
- M. ulcerans

Unusual Etiologic Species

Pulmonary disease
- M. asiaticum
- M. celatum
- M. chelonae
- M. fortuitum
- M. haemophilum
- M. scrofulaceum
- M. shimoidei
- M. simiae
- M. smegmatis
- M. szulgai

Lymph adenitis
- M. abscessus
- M. chelonae
- M. fortuitum
- M. genavense
- M. haemophilum
- M. kansasii
- M. szulgai

Disseminated disease
- M. abscessus
- M. celatum
- M. conspicuum
- M. fortuitum
- M. genavense
- M. kansasii
- M. immunogenum
- M. malmoense
- M. marinum
- M. mucogenicum
- M. scrofulaceum
- M. simiae
- M. szulgai
- M. xenopi

Skin, Soft Tissue, and Bone Disease
- M. avium complex
- M. haemophilum
- M. immunogenum
- M. kansasii
- M. malmoense
- M. nonchromogenicum
- M. smegmatis
- M. szulgai
- M. terrae complex

Adapted from the American Thoracic Society. Diagnosis, treatment, and prevention of nontuberculous mycobacterial diseases. Am J Respir Crit Care Med 2007;175:367-416.

---

microbiological confirmation is obtained, many patients would have completed the intensive phase of standard antituberculosis treatment. Once laboratory confirmation is obtained, the treatment must be modified to include specific regimens. Direct observation of treatment might not be required in NTM disease because there is no person-to-person transmission and NTM disease does not constitute a public health hazard. Unlike TB, in vitro susceptibilities for many of the NTM do not correlate well with clinical response to any of the antituberculosis drugs. Empiric therapy for NTM lung disease is not recommended.

Adult patients with *M. kansasii* pulmonary disease can be treated with a daily three-drug regimen containing isoniazid[1] (300 mg), rifampin[1] (600 mg), and ethambutol[1] (15 mg/kg) for 18 months. A minimum of 1 year of culture negativity must be ensured. In HIV-positive patients who take protease inhibitors, clarithromycin (Biaxin)[1] or rifabutin[1] should be substituted for rifampin.

HIV-negative adult patients with *M. avium intracellulare complex* (MAC) pulmonary disease (nodular/bronchiectatic disease), can be treated with a thrice-weekly regimen containing clarithromycin (1000 mg) or azithromycin (500-600 mg), rifampin (600 mg), and ethambutol (25 mg/kg). Patients with fibrocavitary or severe nodular/bronchiectatic MAC disease should be treated with a daily regimen containing clarithromycin (500-1000 mg) or azithromycin (250-300 mg), rifampin (10 mg/kg, maximum 600 mg), ethambutol (15 mg/kg), and intermittent streptomycin or amikacin for the initial 2 to 3 months. The ATS guidelines (2007) suggest that patients tolerate amikacin or streptomycin at 25 mg/kg three times weekly during the initial 3 months of therapy. For patients 50 years or older who require treatment for more than 6 months, some experts recommend administration of streptomycin/amikacin at a dosage of 8 to 10 mg/kg two to three times weekly (maximum dose of 500 mg for patients 50 years or older). Patients should receive treatment until they remain culture negative for 12 months. Adult HIV-negative patients with disseminated MAC disease should receive daily clarithromycin (500-1000 mg) or azithromycin (250-300 mg), ethambutol (15 mg/kg /day) and rifabutin (150-300 mg) or rifampin (450-600 mg). In HIV-positive patients with disseminated MAC disease, daily clarithromycin (500 mg twice a day) or azithromycin (500 mg, daily), ethambutol (15 mg/kg, daily), with or without rifabutin (300-450 mg, daily) may have to be used. When ART is also being administered, drug interactions with rifamycins should be kept in mind. Therapy is continued as long as the cultures remain positive, and discontinuation of treatment can only be considered if the culture remains negative for 12 months; often patients may receive treatment lifelong.

Surgical excision still remains the primary treatment for NTM cervical lymphadenitis, with cure rates of about 95%. In patients with extensive disease or a poor response to surgery, a clarithromycin-containing regimen[1] may be tried. Nonpulmonary disease caused by *M. fortuitum*, *M. abscessus*, or *M. chelonae* responds to amikacin (Amikin)[1] and clarithromycin,[1] and therapy should be based on in vitro susceptibility tests.

In adult patients with AIDS and a CD4+ T-lymphocyte count of less than 50 cells/μL, especially with a previous history of an opportunistic infection, the preferred prophylactic drug regimen for prevention of disseminated MAC disease consists of azithromycin (1200 mg once weekly). Alternatively, clarithromycin (500 mg twice daily), or rifabutin (300 mg daily) can be used. Rifabutin dosage may need to be modified based on drug-drug interactions. Preventive therapy may be stopped if the CD4+ T-lymphocyte count is more than 100 cells/μL for more than 3 months.

REFERENCES

American Thoracic Society: Diagnostic standards and classification of tuberculosis in adults and children. This statement was endorsed by the Council of the Infectious Diseases Society of America. (IDSA), September 1999. Am J Respir Crit Care Med 2000;161:1376-1395.

American Thoracic Society: Diagnosis, treatment, and prevention of nontuberculous mycobacterial diseases. Am J Respir Crit Care Med 2007; 175:367-416.

American Thoracic Society and the Centers for Disease Control and Prevention: Targeted tuberculin testing and treatment of latent tuberculosis infection. This statement was endorsed by the Council of the Infectious Diseases Society of America. (IDSA), September 1999. Am J Respir Crit Care Med 2000;161(4 Pt 2):S221-S247.

American Thoracic Society, Centers for Disease Control and Prevention, Infectious Diseases Society of America: Controlling tuberculosis in the United States. Am J Respir Crit Care Med 2005;172:1169-1227.

Blumberg HM, Burman WJ, Chaisson RE, et alAmerican Thoracic Society, Centers for Disease Control and Prevention, the Infectious Diseases

---

[1]Not FDA approved for this indication.

Society: Treatment of tuberculosis. Am J Respir Crit Care Med 2003;167:603-662.

Centers for Disease Control and Prevention (CDC): American Thoracic Society. Update: adverse event data and revised American Thoracic Society/CDC recommendations against the use of rifampin and pyrazinamide for treatment of latent tuberculosis infection—United States, 2003. MMWR Morb Mortal Wkly Rep 2003;52:735-739.

Centers for Disease Control and Prevention (CDC): Guidelines for the investigation of contacts of persons with infectious tuberculosis: Recommendations from the National Tuberculosis Controllers Association and CDC. MMWR Morb Mortal Wkly Rep 2005;54:1-47.

Centers for Disease Control and Prevention (CDC): Trends in tuberculosis—United States, 2007. MMWR Morb Mortal Wkly Rep 2008;57:281-285.

Dye C: Global epidemiology of tuberculosis. Lancet 2006;367:938-940.

Gopi A, Madhavan SM, Sharma SK, Sahn SA: Diagnosis and treatment of tuberculous pleural effusion in 2006. Chest 2007;131:880-889.

Sharma SK, Liu JJ: Progress of DOTS in global tuberculosis control. Lancet 2006;367:951-952.

Sharma SK, Mohan A: Multidrug-resistant tuberculosis: A menace that threatens to destabilize tuberculosis control. Chest 2006;130:261-272.

The WHO/1UATLD Global Project on Anti-tuberculosis Drug Resistance Surveillance 1999-2002. Antituberculosis drug resistance in the world. Report No.4. Geneva: World Health Organization; 2008. WHO/HTM/TB/2008.394.

World Health Organization: Treatment of tuberculosis: Guidelines for National Programmes, 3rd ed, Geneva: World Health Organization; 2003. WHO/CDS/TB/2003.313.

SECTION 5

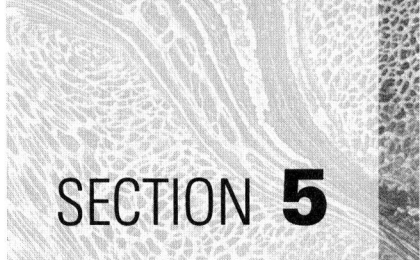

The Cardiovascular System

Acquired Diseases of the Aorta

Method of
Gorav Ailawadi, MD, and Irving L. Kron, MD

Aortic pathology occurs along the entire length of the aorta. Traditional open surgical treatment of these disorders has been, in part, replaced by less invasive endovascular therapy. A role for medical therapy has also been defined for specific diseases of the aorta. This article covers acquired diseases including aortic aneurysm, aortic occlusive disease, and aortic dissection, as well as traumatic aortic injury.

Aortic Aneurysm

An *aneurysm* is a dilation of a blood vessel of at least 50% over baseline, and *ectasia* is arterial dilation of less than 50% over baseline. The normal diameters of the ascending, descending, and abdominal aorta vary from person to person but are roughly 2.8 cm, 2.5 cm, and 2 cm, respectively. Aneurysms most commonly affect the infrarenal abdominal aorta (AAA).

Whether aneurysms are atherosclerotic in nature is a subject of great debate. Although many risk factors for aneurysmal and occlusive disease are similar, the pathophysiology of the two diseases appears different. At a molecular level, aneurysms are characterized by inflammatory cell infiltration, release of matrix-degrading enzymes, and destruction of the aortic wall media. Specifically, matrix metalloproteinases (MMPs)-1, -2, -3, -9, -12, and -13 are known to be up-regulated in aortic aneurysm walls. The inciting event for this process is unclear, although an immune-regulated phenomenon has been suggested.

Thoracic aortic aneurysms include both ascending aortic aneurysms and descending thoracic aortic aneurysms (DTAAs). The etiology for thoracic aneurysms includes cystic medial necrosis, familial diseases (see later), Takayasu's arteritis, and previous aortic dissection.

Inflammatory aneurysms are nonbacterial, sterile aneurysms with an intense periaortic inflammatory infiltrate and are associated with retroperitoneal fibrosis. *Mycotic aneurysms* are bacterial (not fungal) infiltration of the vessel wall, most commonly by *Staphylococcus aureus*, *Salmonella* species, and *Streptococcus* species, resulting in subacute aneurysmal dilation.

INCIDENCE AND NATURAL HISTORY

The incidence of aortic aneurysms is as high as 100 per 100,000 person-years, and aortic aneurysms are the tenth leading cause of death in elderly men in the United States. Nine percent of men older than 65 years have an AAA, and 15% of men older than 75 years have an AAA. Aneurysms typically grow at a rate of approximately 10% or 2 to 4 mm per year. Risk factors for aneurysms include smoking history (fivefold risk), male gender (fourfold risk), family history (20% have a first-degree relative affected), chronic obstructive pulmonary disease (COPD), age older than 60 years, hypertension, and hyperlipidemia. Notably, black race, female gender, and diabetes are negatively associated with AAA.

The risk of rupture depends on the size of the aneurysm and the patient's gender. Randomized trials in small aneurysms (<5.0 cm) have demonstrated no advantage to early surgical repair and a 1% yearly rate of rupture. Estimates for annual AAA rupture risk are stratified by diameter: Those 5 to 6 cm have a 6% rupture risk, those 6 to 7 cm have a 20% rupture risk, those 7 to 8 cm have a 30% rupture risk, and those larger than 8 cm have a greater than 40% rupture risk. Early repair may be warranted in women, who have a higher risk of rupture at a given aortic diameter compared to men.

Ascending aortic aneurysms greater than 5.5 cm have a 5% annual risk of dissection. DTAAs greater than 6 cm have an annual rupture risk of 8%.

DIAGNOSIS

Most aneurysms are asymptomatic and are found incidentally. Abdominal ultrasound screening for AAA is inexpensive and reproducible, and echocardiography can identify thoracic aortic aneurysms. Conventional angiography to diagnose aortic aneurysms is no longer routinely used because the best evaluation for aortic aneurysms is computed tomography (CT) angiography. Magnetic resonance angiography can be used in patients unable to tolerate intravenous (IV) dye. In patients with ascending aortic aneurysms, echocardiography should be performed to evaluate for aortic valve pathology.

Symptomatic thoracic aortic aneurysms and AAAs with chest, abdominal, or back pain warrant urgent or emergent surgical evaluation. Ruptured aneurysms manifest with acute onset of pain and patients often present in hypovolemic shock.

TREATMENT

Medical Therapy

To date, there is no proven medical treatment to prevent aneurysm expansion or to induce aneurysm regression. Blood pressure control with β-blockers did not slow the growth of aneurysm progression in a randomized trial. This intent-to-treat analysis was limited by a 40% dropout rate due to side effects of the medication. Doxycycline,[1] an antibiotic with known MMP inhibitory effects, has not demonstrated any effect on aneurysm growth in small trials despite lowering plasma MMP-9. Statins have been shown in nonrandomized

---
[1]Not FDA approved for this indication.

trials to reduce AAA growth by 50%, which may be due to their MMP inhibitory effects. Thus, medical therapy in patients with aortic aneurysms includes blood pressure control and a statin.

Surgical Therapy

Surgical treatment is warranted when the risk of rupture is greater than the morbidity and mortality of surgical repair. The surgical approach is determined by the location and extent of the aneurysm.

Ascending and Arch Aneurysms

Mortality rates for elective ascending aortic aneurysm and AAA are 2% to 5% and increase to 6% to 15% with the repair of aortic arch aneurysms because of the necessity of circulatory arrest and reimplantation of arch vessels. The approach for repair of these aneurysms is through a sternotomy with the use of cardiopulmonary bypass. Typically, ascending aortic aneurysms 5.5 cm are referred for repair in low- to moderate-risk patients. In the setting of concomitant cardiac surgery or bicuspid aortic valve, the ascending aorta is replaced when it is 5.0 cm. In Marfan syndrome patients, due to a high risk of dissection, the ascending aorta and root should be replaced when the aneurysm is 4.5 cm. Repair or replacement of the aortic valve depends on the presence and severity of aortic stenosis or insufficiency.

Descending and Thoracoabdominal Aneurysms

Repair of DTAA and thoracoabdominal aneurysms carries a risk of mortality of 5% to 15% and risk of paraplegia of 3% to 20% depending on the anatomy. In adequate-risk patients, repair is recommended when the aneurysm is 6 cm. DTAA can often be performed through an endovascular repair, but thoracoabdominal aneurysms are difficult to perform with an endovascular approach due to the involvement of visceral vessels. Open repair is performed through a left thoracotomy, often with the assistance of partial bypass and lumbar CSF drainage to decrease the risk of paraplegia. Whether reimplantation of intercostal vessels minimizes the risk of paraplegia is controversial.

Infrarenal Abdominal Aorta Aneurysms

Mortality for open repair of AAA is 2% to 5%. Less than 50% of operative repair of AAA is performed open at our institution. Open repair is most commonly performed through a vertical or transverse laparotomy, although retroperitoneal approaches have excellent results as well.

Endovascular Repair

Endovascular repair is gradually becoming more common than open repair of AAA and DTAA. Considerations to determine if a patient is a candidate for endovascular repair include adequacy of nondiseased proximal and distal landing zones for the stent graft; size, tortuosity, and disease of the iliac vessels; and renal function. Manufacturer-derived guidelines for proximal and distal landing zones for DTAA are 2 cm and 1.5 cm for AAA, although many referral centers performing these procedures have challenged these guidelines. Lifetime follow-up is necessary, because up to 20% develop an endoleak, or leak around or through the graft into the aneurysm sac. Midterm results for endovascular repair have demonstrated less morbidity and mortality for AAA and DTAA compared to open repair. Long-term results are currently being evaluated.

Screening

Clinical examination alone can miss the diagnosis of AAA. Ultrasound screening programs have not been performed routinely in the United States. Studies indicate that ultrasound screening in men older than 50 years can reduce the AAA rupture rate by 50%. Cost-analysis studies support ultrasound screening in men older than 50 years who have a history of smoking.

Familial Diseases: Marfan and Ehlers–Danlos Syndromes

Marfan syndrome is an autosomal dominant defect of the fibrillin gene resulting in abnormal elastic fibers with a predisposition to aneurysmal dilation and dissection. Ehlers–Danlos type IV is an autosomal dominant disorder of type III collagen synthesis that can lead to aneurysmal dilation and rupture.

Aortic Occlusive Disease

Atherosclerosis can affect the thoracic or the abdominal aorta. Abdominal disease often occurs in concert with iliac disease. The spectrum can span from mild atheromatous disease to complete occlusion of these large vessels. Symptoms include embolic disease from mobile plaques, limb or thigh claudication, rest pain, or tissue loss of the lower extremities. Occasionally, symptoms include impotence, diminished femoral pulses, and buttock claudication (Leriche's syndrome). Treatment depends on the severity of symptoms.

INCIDENCE AND NATURAL HISTORY

Peripheral vascular disease affects 8 million Americans and is a sign of decreased life expectancy. Risk factors include smoking, diabetes, hypertension, atherosclerosis, coronary artery disease, hyperhomocysteinemia, and African American ethnicity. The natural history is not determined by the severity and length of the stenosis but by patient factors including continued tobacco use, diabetes, and renal failure.

DIAGNOSIS

History and physical examination are often sufficient to make the diagnosis. Claudication is defined as reproducible pain with exertion relieved by rest, typically occurring in the calf, thigh, or buttock. Embolic disease manifests as infarcts affecting toes bilaterally, termed *blue-toe syndrome*. Examination demonstrates diminished femoral pulses. Ankle–brachial index and pulse volume recording (PVR) can confirm clinical suspicion. Once the diagnosis is suggested, characterization of disease extent can be determined by CT angiography, magnetic resonance (MR) angiography, or conventional angiography.

Thoracic aortic plaques are found secondary to embolic disease or as incidental findings. These are at risk for embolization during cardiac and aortic surgery and are best diagnosed by transesophageal echocardiography (TEE) or CT angiography.

TREATMENT

Treatment choice is determined by the severity of symptoms. Mild to moderate claudication should initially be treated with medical therapy. Smoking cessation should be reinforced no matter the severity of the disease. Severe claudication, rest pain, and tissue loss warrant intervention.

Medical Therapy

Control of diabetes, hypertension, and hyperlipidemia, in addition to smoking cessation, can slow the progression of disease. Patients should take aspirin. Exercise programs can help recruit collateral vessels and improve symptoms, although they do not change objective criteria of the ankle–brachial index. Cilostazol (Pletal) in some studies has documented symptomatic benefit in patients with claudication.

Endovascular Therapy

Minimally invasive techniques including balloon angioplasty and stenting have become the preferred treatment for isolated or bilateral iliac occlusive disease. Extensive aortic or aortoiliac disease is treated surgically.

CURRENT DIAGNOSIS

Abdominal Aortic Aneurysms and Descending Thoracic Aortic Aneurysms

- Men with a smoking history and older than 60 years are at greatest risk.
- Aneurysms are usually asymptomatic and found incidentally.
- Ultrasound can be used to screen.
- Gold standard diagnostic test is computed tomographic (CT) angiography.

Ascending Aortic Aneurysm

- Men and women are affected equally.
- Aneurysm is associated with aortic valve pathology and familial disorders, such as Marfan syndrome.
- Conventional or CT aortography is diagnostic.
- Echocardiography should be performed to evaluate for aortic valve pathology.

Aortoiliac Occlusive Disease

- Diagnosis is made by history and examination.
- Ankle–brachial index or pulse volume recording confirms the diagnosis.
- Conventional or CT arteriography or magnetic resonance angiography can identify location and extent of disease.

Acute Aortic Dissection

- Diagnosis is often delayed; this is the great imitator.
- CT angiography is gold standard and identifies malperfused branches.
- Transesophageal echocardiography is diagnostic and is preferred in an unstable patient.

Traumatic Aortic Injury

- High index of suspicion is based on mechanism of injury.
- Chest x-ray may be suggestive.
- CT angiography is the gold standard.

Surgical Therapy

Approaches to improve blood flow to the lower extremities include aortobifemoral bypass, thoracobifemoral bypass, or axillobifemoral bypass. Mortality with aortobifemoral bypass is 5%. At 10 years, patency for aortobifemoral and thoracobifemoral bypass is 85% to 90%, and patency of an axillofemoral bypass is 60% due to the longer length and smaller caliber of the conduit. As a consequence, axillofemoral bypass is reserved for high-risk patients unable to tolerate the other approaches.

Aortic Dissection

An aortic dissection occurs when an intimal tear results in blood propagating into the media of the aortic wall. Dissections are classified by location. *Stanford A dissections* (62.5%) always involve the ascending aorta and can involve the descending aorta. *Stanford B dissections* (37.5%) involve the descending aorta and can include the aortic arch but *not* the ascending aorta. An alternative classification is the DeBakey classification: *DeBakey type I* occurs in the ascending and descending aorta, *DeBakey type II* occurs in the ascending aorta only, and *DeBakey type III* occurs in the descending aorta only. Aortic dissection develops in 30% of patients with Marfan syndrome. The most common and important risk factor is preoperative hypertension. Subacute dissections are those present longer than 2 weeks, and chronic dissections have been present longer than 2 months. These less acute dissections do not have the same risk of early mortality as acute dissections. *Intramural hematoma* is a focal intimal tear that can lead to aortic dissection in 15% of cases.

INCIDENCE AND NATURAL HISTORY

The incidence of aortic dissection is estimated to be 3 per 100,000 patient-years. The natural history of dissections varies based on location. The mortality rate for Stanford A dissections is estimated to be 25% at 24 hours, 50% at 48 hours, and 90% at 1 month.

DIAGNOSIS

Sudden onset of severe, migrating chest or back pain is classic for an aortic dissection and is present in up to 80% of patients. Chest x-ray shows a widened mediastinum in 50%, but the definitive diagnostic test is a CT scan, which has a sensitivity and specificity of greater than 99%. If CT scan is unavailable or the patient is unstable, TEE provides greater than 97% specificity and sensitivity when performed by an experienced operator. Physical examination should evaluate for an aortic valve murmur, quality of pulses in the carotids and extremities, presence of abdominal pain indicating visceral ischemia, and neurologic deficits indicating propagation of the dissection into the cerebrovascular system.

TREATMENT

Stanford Type A Dissection

Initial management is blood pressure control. Urgent surgical intervention is warranted because these aortic catastrophes can lead to acute aortic insufficiency, propagation of the dissection into the coronary arteries, pericardial tamponade, or frank rupture. Operative intervention requires cardiopulmonary bypass and replacement of the ascending aorta. Occasionally, coronary artery bypass or aortic valve replacement is necessary. The remaining descending aorta, if involved, will need to be followed long term.

Stanford Type B Dissection

The initial management involves control of blood pressure with a systolic goal of less than 100 mm Hg. β-Blockers are the preferred agent because they decrease the pulsatility (dp/dt; change in pressure per change in time) of blood the aorta receives. An arterial line for continuous blood pressure monitoring and serial examination is recommended. Visceral or extremity ischemia (20% of type B dissection) warrants urgent intervention. If available, angiographic guided fenestration of the dissection flap should be performed. A less desirable alternative is operative intervention. The mortality is 10% for medically managed type B dissection and more than 30% for surgically treated type B dissection. Patients must be followed for life because up to 30% require surgical intervention for recurrent pain, visceral ischemia, or aneurysmal dilation of the dissected aorta.

Traumatic Aortic Injury

Traumatic aortic injury occurs due to sheer stress on the mobile aorta distal to the fixed ligamentum arteriosum with rapid decelerating injuries, most commonly during motor vehicle crashes. With a high mortality, the risk of early repair must be weighed against associated injuries and should be patient specific. Cardiovascular surgery consultation should be obtained early even in patients with significant concomitant injuries.

INCIDENCE AND NATURAL HISTORY

Traumatic aortic injury occurs most often in young men. Eighty percent of patients with traumatic aortic injury die before reaching the hospital. Of the remaining 20%, 50% die within the first 24 hours and 25% die over the subsequent 2 weeks without treatment. In these

CURRENT THERAPY

Abdominal Aortic Aneurysm
- No medical treatments can prevent growth of the aneurysm.
- Repair is considered when the aneurysm is larger than 5.0-5.5 cm.
- Endovascular repair is being performed more commonly with good results.

Thoracic Aortic Aneurysm
- Repair of ascending aortic aneurysm is considered when it is larger than 5.5 cm or when it is larger than 5.0 cm with concomitant cardiac disease or a bicuspid aortic valve.
- Ascending aortic aneurysm is repaired in Marfan syndrome patients when it is greater than 4.5 cm.
- Repair is considered when the aneurysm is larger than 6 cm.
- Select repair is being done endovascularly with good results.

Aortoiliac Occlusive Disease
- Medical treatment includes smoking cessation, glycemic control, statin therapy, and exercise program.
- Severely symptomatic patients can undergo stenting for isolated lesions.
- Low-risk patients can undergo aortobifemoral bypass; axillofemoral bypass is reserved for high-risk patients.

Acute Aortic Dissection
- Stanford A dissections are treated with emergent intervention, usually sparing the aortic valve.
- Stanford B dissections are treated medically, but 30% develop aneurysms late.

Traumatic Aortic Injury
- Must have a high index of suspicion based on mechanism of injury.
- Careful medical observation can be performed with severe concomitant injuries.
- Endovascular repair is being performed more commonly with good results.

patients, the transected aorta is kept intact by the overlying adventitia and mediastinal pleura.

DIAGNOSIS

A conscious patient can present with chest or back pain, hoarseness, dyspnea, dysphagia, or paralysis and signs of trauma to the chest. Commonly, these patients are unconscious, and diagnosis is based on imaging. Chest x-ray can demonstrate a constellation of findings including a widened mediastinum, rib fractures, and a left pleural effusion. CT angiography has replaced conventional arteriography as the gold standard at many institutions. TEE, although operator dependent, can be useful in the unstable patient.

TREATMENT

Medical Therapy

Initial treatment includes blood pressure control as in aortic dissection primarily using β-blockers and afterload reduction if necessary. This is important to allow the treatment of other life-threatening traumatic injuries and proceed with diagnostic evaluation. Many centers are reporting experience with delayed repair after treatment of other injuries with careful hemodynamic monitoring.

Surgical Therapy

Surgical therapy for traumatic aortic injury is evolving. Traditional open repair involves a left thoracotomy in the fourth interspace, clamping the aorta proximal and distal to the injury and replacing the aorta. Use of left heart bypass and spinal cord drainage can decrease the risk of paraplegia and renal failure. Mortality of 30% often depends on concomitant injuries.

Endovascular repair is becoming more common for traumatic aortic injury. Current limitations include endograft sizes designed for aneurysmal aortas, small-caliber iliac vessels in these previously healthy young patients, less-than-ideal proximal landing zone, and poor long-term follow-up. Nonetheless, endovascular repair may be the preferred treatment in patients with significant traumatic injuries.

REFERENCES

Ailawadi G, Eliason JL, Upchurch GR: Current concepts in the pathogenesis of abdominal aortic aneurysm. J Vasc Surg 2003;38:584-588.

Anderson PL, Arons RR, Moskowitz AJ, et al: A statewide experience with endovascular abdominal aortic aneurysm repair: Rapid diffusion with excellent early results. J Vasc Surg 2004;39:10-19.

Baxter BT, Pearce WH, Waltke EA, et al: Prolonged administration of doxycycline in patients with small asymptomatic abdominal aortic aneurysms: Report of a prospective (Phase II) multicenter study. J Vasc Surg 2002;36:1-12.

Birkmeyer JD, Upchurch GR Jr: Evidence-based screening and management of abdominal aortic aneurysm. Ann Intern Med 2007;146:749-750.

Brown SL, Busuttil RW, Baker JD, et al: Bacteriologic and surgical determinants of survival in patients with mycotic aneurysms. J Vasc Surg 1984;1:541-547.

Cao P, Verzini F, Parlani G, et al: Clinical effect of abdominal aortic aneurysm endografting: 7-year concurrent comparison with open repair. J Vasc Surg 2004;40:841-848.

Castañer E, Andreu M, Gallardo X, et al: CT in nontraumatic acute thoracic aortic disease: Typical and atypical features and complications. Radiographics 2003;23:S93-S110.

Cosford PA, Leng GC: Screening for abdominal aortic aneurysm. Cochrane Database Syst Rev 2007;(2):CD002945.

Evangelista A, Avegliano G, Elorz C, et al: Transesophageal echocardiography in the diagnosis of acute aortic syndrome. J Card Surg 2002;17:95-106.

Evangelista A, Mukherjee D, Mehta RH, et al; International Registry of Aortic Dissection (IRAD) Investigators: Acute intramural hematoma of the aorta: A mystery in evolution. Circulation 2005;111:1063-1070.

Etz CD, Halstead JC, Spielvogel D, et al: Thoracic and thoracoabdominal aneurysm repair: Is reimplantation of spinal cord arteries a waste of time? Ann Thorac Surg 2006;82:1670-1677.

Golledge J, Muller J, Daugherty A, Norman P: Abdominal aortic aneurysm: Pathogenesis and implications for management. Arterioscler Thromb Vasc Biol 2006;26:2605-2613.

Golledge J, Powell JT: Medical management of abdominal aortic aneurysm. Eur J Vasc Endovasc Surg 2007;34(3):267-273.

Hagan PG, Nienababer CA, Isselbacher EM, et al: The International Registry of Acute Aortic Dissection (IRAD): New insights into an old disease. JAMA 2000;283:897-903.

Hertzer NR, Bena JF, Karafa MT: A personal experience with direct reconstruction and extra-anatomic bypass for aortoiliofemoral occlusive disease. J Vasc Surg 2007;45:527-535.

Hirsch AT, Criqui MH, Treat-Jacobson D, et al: Peripheral arterial disease detection, awareness, and treatment in primary care. JAMA 2001;286:1317-1324.

Johnston KW, Rutherford RB, Tilson MD, et al: Suggested standard for reporting on arterial aneurysms. Subcommittee on Reporting Standards for Arterial Aneurysms, Ad Hoc Committee on Reporting Standards, Society for Vascular Surgery and North American Chapter, International Society for Cardiovascular Surgery. J Vasc Surg 1991;13:452-458.

Kazui T, Yamashita K, Washiyama N, et al: Aortic arch replacement using selective cerebral perfusion. Ann Thorac Surg 2007;83(2):S796-S798.

Lederle FA: A summary of the contributions of the VA cooperative studies on abdominal aortic aneurysms. Ann N Y Acad Sci 2006;1085:29-38.

Lederle FA, Johnson GR, Wilson SE, et al: Prevalence and associations of abdominal aortic aneurysm detected through screening. Aneurysm Detection and Management (ADAM) Veterans Affairs Cooperative Study Group. Ann Intern Med 1997;126:441-449.

Lettinga-van de Poll T, Schurink GW, De Haan MW, et al: Endovascular treatment of traumatic rupture of the thoracic aorta. Br J Surg 2007;94:525-533.

Mészáros I, Mórocz J, Szlávi J, et al: Epidemiology and clinicopathology of aortic dissection. Chest 2000;117:1271-1278.

Powell JT, Brown LC, Forbes JF, et al: Final 12-year follow-up of surgery versus surveillance in the UK Small Aneurysm Trial. Br J Surg 2007;94:702-708.

Propanolol Aneurysm Trial Investigators: Propranolol for small abdominal aortic aneurysms: Results of a randomized trial. J Vasc Surg 2002;35:72-79.

Reed AB, Thompson JK, Crafton CJ, et al: Timing of endovascular repair of blunt traumatic thoracic aortic transections. J Vasc Surg 2006;43:684-688.

Roberts WC, Honig HS: The spectrum of cardiovascular disease in the Marfan syndrome: A clinico-morphologic study of 18 necropsy patients and comparison to 151 previously reported necropsy patients. Am Heart J 1982;104:115-135.

Selvin E, Erlinger TP: Prevalence of and risk factors for peripheral arterial disease in the United States: Results from the National Health and Nutrition Examination Survey, 1999-2000. Circulation 2004;110:738-743.

Singh K, Bonaa KH, Jacobsen BK, et al: Prevalence of and risk factors for abdominal aortic aneurysms in a population-based study: The Tromso Study. Am J Epidemiol 2001p154:236-244.

Sukhija R, Aronow WS, Sandhu R, et al: Mortality and size of abdominal aortic aneurysm at long-term follow-up of patients not treated surgically and treated with and without statins. Am J Cardiol 2006;97:279-280.

Thomas SM, Beard JD, Ireland M, et al: Results from the prospective registry of endovascular treatment of abdominal aortic aneurysms (RETA): Mid term results to five years. Eur J Vasc Endovasc Surg 2005;29:563-570.

Tsai TT, Evangelista A, Nienaber CA, et al: Long-term survival in patients presenting with type A acute aortic dissection: insights from the International Registry of Acute Aortic Dissection (IRAD). Circulation 2006;114(1 suppl):I350-I356.

Tsai TT, Fattori R, Trimarchi S, et al: International Registry of Acute Aortic Dissection: Long-term survival in patients presenting with type B acute aortic dissection: Insights from the International Registry of Acute Aortic Dissection. Circulation 2006;114:2226-2231.

Wilmink AB, Hubbard CS, Day NE, et al: The incidence of small abdominal aortic aneurysms and the change in normal infrarenal aortic diameter: Implications for screening. Eur J Vasc Endovasc Surg 2001;21:165-170.

Angina Pectoris

Method of
John F. Moran, MD

The diagnosis and management of chest pain remain an important challenge. Although there can be a long differential diagnosis of chest pain to be considered, the diagnosis of angina pectoris is especially important. According to the American Heart Association statistics, chronic stable coronary artery disease is the leading cause of mortality in the United States, accounting for one in five deaths. More than 1.2 million Americans had a myocardial infarction in 2001 out of a total of 13.2 million with coronary disease. Of these 1.2 million patients, 700,000 had a new attack and 500,000 had a recurrent attack.

Clinical Features

GENERAL FEATURES

Angina pectoris is associated with myocardial ischemia and left ventricular dysfunction but not necessarily myocardial necrosis. Angina pectoris is usually provoked by exercise and relieved by rest. Patients give a variety of descriptions of their chest discomfort: strangling, suffocating, chest pressure, chest tightness, or heaviness. Often the patient suffering from effort angina can predict the amount of physical exercise that causes his or her angina and might be a candidate for preventive therapy. The chest discomfort can be characterized in terms of its frequency, duration, and intensity as well as precipitating factors and the time of day that it occurs. The anginal threshold can be influenced by emotional stress, exposure to cold weather, superfluous meals, and cigarette smoking. Angina can last from 10 to 15 minutes and rarely longer. If the chest discomfort lasts for 15 to 30 minutes or more, myocardial necrosis should be suspected. The discomfort can radiate up the left arm along the ulnar aspect, occasionally to the right arm, and occasionally to both arms. Radiation of the discomfort can occur up into the neck and the jaw, shoulders, and back.

Angina pectoris equivalents can consist of exertional dyspnea probably related to diastolic dysfunction or changes in left ventricular compliance that occurs with ischemia. In elderly patients fatigue can be an angina equivalent related to poor cardiac output, when the left ventricle becomes ischemic. Atypical angina has some of these characteristics.

Angina can be classified as stable when its characteristics are unchanged for 60 days. Stable angina pectoris responds to sublingual nitroglycerin (Nitrostat) or rest. Unstable angina pectoris consists of the chest discomfort syndrome, occurring more frequently, lasting longer, and manifesting with lesser degrees of exertion. Unstable angina can occur at rest and at night.

ANGINA IN WOMEN

There are gender differences reported in the language and the history of angina. Atypical chest pain is more common in female patients. Female patients describe more throat, neck, or jaw discomfort for angina, and the chest discomfort is more likely to occur at rest, during sleep, or with periods of mental stress. Women can have neck and shoulder discomfort. Fatigue, shortness of breath, and nausea with vomiting are often present.

In a recent Finnish study, female patients who use nitrates had increased coronary mortality risks similar in magnitude to those observed in men. This seemed to be true up into the ninth decade of life in their study.

Diagnostic cardiac catheterization is listed as the sixth most commonly performed health care procedure in more than 500,000 women, and total charges exceeded $4 billion. In the Women's Ischemic Syndrome Evaluation (WISE) studies, the data suggest that symptom-driven care is costly even for women with nonobstructive coronary artery disease. They suggested that health conditions may be detected earlier in women because of more frequent use of physician's services.

Five-year rates of hospitalization for women with chest pain and nonobstructive coronary artery disease increased for women with one-vessel to three-vessel coronary artery disease. Similarly, 5-year cardiovascular death or myocardial infarction (MI) rates ranged from 4% to 38% for women with nonobstructive to three-vessel coronary artery disease.

MANAGEMENT

Because the angina chest pain syndrome is believed to be caused by an imbalance of oxygen supply and demand to the myocardium, management of angina is directed toward increasing the oxygen supply or decreasing oxygen demands. Increasing coronary blood flow with percutaneous interventions or coronary artery bypass graft (CABG) surgery increases oxygen supply to the heart, whereas medication decreases oxygen demand. In any event, the goals of management of angina pectoris include increasing the quantity and quality of life. The American College of Cardiology and the American Heart Association issue periodic updates in guidelines for the management of stable angina pectoris.

Diagnosis

Box 1 lists the differential diagnosis of chest pain. The diagnosis of angina pectoris presumes a mismatch between myocardial oxygen consumption and oxygen delivery to the myocardium. Angina occurs when there is an area of myocardial ischemia caused by

> **BOX 1 Differential Diagnosis of Chest Pain**
>
> - Acute aortic dissection
> - Acute myocardial infarction
> - Acute pericarditis
> - Angina pectoris
> - Biliary colic
> - Costochondritis
> - Esophageal motility disorders, reflux
> - Idiopathic hypertrophic aortic stenosis
> - Musculoskeletal disorders
> - Pulmonary embolism
> - Severe aortic stenosis
> - Severe pulmonary hypertension

inadequate coronary perfusion and thus insufficient oxygen supply to match oxygen demand. Angina pectoris is a predictable and reproducible anterior chest discomfort after physical activity, or emotional stress. The patient must stop all activities when the chest discomfort occurs. This discomfort is usually relieved within a few minutes of taking nitroglycerin or stopping the activity.

HISTORY

A successful interview with a potential angina patient requires a consideration of the prevalence of coronary artery disease in that patient. The interpretation of the chest pain is based on a prior probability of disease in that patient, which includes a review of the patient's lifestyle. A likely candidate for coronary artery disease is a man who is older than 60 years and has a history of cigarette smoking. Precipitating factors such as anemia or hyperthyroidism should be considered. The differential diagnosis listed in Box 1 is a short list of disorders that can cause chest discomfort, and these can often be differentiated in the history and physical examination.

TESTING

Electrocardiogram

After the history and physical examination are completed, a 12-lead electrocardiogram (ECG) is often made. However, it is normal in more than 50% of patients with angina.

Stress Testing

The next consideration is often the exercise ECG or some noninvasive stress test. This allows an evaluation of ST segment changes. The Duke treadmill score takes ST segment depression, the duration of exercise, and the development of chest discomfort into consideration to increase the sensitivity of the test. The Duke treadmill score allows the patient to be stratified according to the score. A score of 5 or higher carries an annual mortality rate of 0.25%; a high-risk Duke score is −10 or more and carries a 5% annual mortality risk.

The exercise ECG can also be combined with echocardiography or myocardial perfusion scans such as technetium Tc-99m tetrofosmin (Myoview) or thallium. Some patients are unable to walk on the treadmill, and pharmacologic stress testing is available with adenosine (Adenoscan), dipyridamole (Persantine), or dobutamine.[1] Nuclear myocardial perfusion with thallium, myoview, or echocardiography can also be combined with pharmacologic stress.

Electron beam computed tomography (CT) is a technique that identifies calcification of the coronaries, suggesting atherosclerotic disease. The volume of atherosclerotic plaque can also be estimated. Asymptomatic thoracic or abdominal aortic calcifications can also help identify the patient with atherosclerosis and possible coronary artery disease.

A more recent development in diagnostic techniques for coronary artery disease is the 16-detector multislice CT. Studies comparing the multislice CT with coronary angiography have shown positive and negative predictive values of as high at 87% and 99%, respectively. Patients must be able to hold their breath for 20 seconds and have a heart rate less than 70 bpm. β-Blockade usually allows this heart rate. The coronary arteries cannot be assessed well if there is motion artifact, and severe calcification can obscure the coronary lumen. The estimated radiation dose for multislice CT scanning of the coronary arteries can be as high as 13.0 to 16.3 mSv compared with conventional coronary angiography, which has a radiation dose of 3 to 5 mSv.

The specificity of multislice CT scanning can be improved if the test is followed by a dobutamine stress echocardiogram. Cost effectiveness for the diagnosis becomes a factor here. The treadmill and the Duke treadmill scores with or without a myocardial scan might suffice to confirm the diagnosis of angina pectoris and stratify the patient's risk for future cardiac events. ST segment depression alone on the exercise ECG had a sensitivity of 68% and a specificity of 77% in a meta-analysis of 24,074 patients.

In addition to helping to confirm a diagnosis of angina, the ability to walk on the treadmill can stratify patients into a functional class as described by the Canadian Cardiovascular Society (CCS) functional classification. The CCS class I allows patients activity up to 7 metabolic equivalents of exercise (METs). This would be the equivalent of performing 6 minutes of exercise on the Bruce Protocol exercise ECG. CCS class II is any activity of up to 5 METs of exercise. This is the equivalent of completing 3 minutes on the Bruce Protocol test. CCS class III allows any activity up to 2 METs of exercise. This means the patient would not complete the first 3 minutes of the Bruce Protocol exercise test. CCS class IV implies the patient can do less than 2 METs of work; 1 MET is the metabolic equivalent of rest. Clearly, patients with CCS classes II, III, and IV are limited by angina pectoris. Moreover, ST segment depression of 1 mm in the first stage of the Bruce Protocol exercise test or 2 mm of ST depression in the second stage of exercise strongly suggest serious coronary artery disease.

In addition to marked ST segment depression and a high-risk Duke treadmill score, other noninvasive tests suggesting high-risk angina include severe left ventricular dysfunction in exercise with an ejection fraction of less than 35%, large perfusion defects on nuclear scanning that are stress induced, and multiple perfusion defects of moderate size with left ventricular dilation or increased pulmonary uptake. Echocardiographic wall motion abnormalities following dobutamine stress that involve more than two segments indicate high risk. In contrast, low-risk noninvasive test results include a low-risk Duke treadmill score, normal wall motion on echocardiography, or a limited resting wall abnormality and a small myocardial perfusion defect on nuclear scanning or a totally normal scan. Intermediate-risk patients fall somewhere between these two.

Treatment

STRATEGY FOR MANAGING STABLE ANGINA PECTORIS

Box 2 lists the reasonable strategy for managing patients with angina pectoris. Coronary risk factor reduction fits well with the aggressive management of angina pectoris patients. After precipitating factors for angina are ruled out, lifestyle modifications that include weight control, an exercise program, smoking cessation, and control of diabetes (if it is present) are necessary. Management of hypertension should include a goal that brings blood pressure down in the range of 130/80 mm Hg or lower.

Blood Pressure

Framingham Heart Study data have indicated the effect of high-normal blood pressure on the risk of cardiovascular disease. The researchers defined high-normal blood pressure as blood

---

[1] Not FDA approved for this indication.

> **BOX 2 Strategy for Managing Stable Angina Pectoris**
>
> - Identify precipitating factors such as anemia, hyperthyroidism, valvular heart disease (e.g., aortic stenosis, tachyarrhythmias, hypertension).
> - Start sublingual nitroglycerin, β-blockers, and aspirin and consider ACE inhibitors.
> - Start risk factor modification, statin medication to the ATP III goal of cholesterol <200 mg and LDL cholesterol <100.
> - Add a calcium channel blocker if the angina is more frequent than two or three times a week, and consider prophylactic sublingual nitroglycerin before activities.
> - Count the use of sublingual nitroglycerin to monitor the success of treatment.
> - Use of nitroglycerin patch or ointment at bedtime for nocturnal angina.
> - Consider coronary angiography if angina pectoris symptoms are refractory or if the exercise electrocardiogram is abnormal, especially with poor work capacity.
>
> *Abbreviations:* ACE = angiotensin-converting enzyme; ATP III = Adult Treatment Panel III; LDL = low-density lipoprotein

pressures ranging from 130/85 to 139/89 mm Hg. An optimal blood pressure was less than 120 mm Hg systolic and less than 80 mm Hg diastolic. The high-normal blood pressure was associated with a risk factor adjusted hazard ratio of 2.5 for women and 1.6 for men. These were not significantly different, but the accrued event rates per 1000 patient-years for persons younger than 65 years were 4.7 for women and 9.2 for men. The numbers needed to treat (NNT) for patients older than 65 years were estimated to be 24 to 71 men and 34 to 102 women to prevent any cardiovascular events in the 5 years of follow-up.

Although the HOPE (Heart Outcomes Prevention Evaluation) Trial results seem to fit well with this management of blood pressure, overall results of randomized studies of angiotensin-converting enzyme (ACE) inhibitors in patients with coronary artery disease and normal left ventricular function are conflicting. In the HOPE trial, ramipril (Altace) 10 mg/day orally was compared with placebo in 9297 high-risk men and women of at least age 55 years with a history of coronary artery disease, stroke, peripheral vascular disease, or diabetes. In the ramipril group, 14% of the patients died of combined endpoints of MI or stroke; 18% of the patients in the placebo group succumbed to these. In the HOPE trial, blood pressure at entry was 139/79 mm Hg. Both the ramipril and the placebo groups had systolic blood pressures that were in the 130s. The difference in the HOPE Trial endpoint was highly significant. Fewer patients in the ramipril group under-went revascularization, and there were reductions in the new diagnosis of diabetes and in the complications of diabetes in patients who had it.

A recent meta-analysis of seven trials of ACE inhibitors that included a total of 33,960 patients followed for a mean of 4.4 years suggested decreased overall mortality, cardiovascular mortality, MI, and stroke. Of the seven trials studied, five trials enrolled patients with documented coronary artery disease. One trial enrolled patients with coronary disease or patients with diabetes who were 55 years or older, and 80% of that population had documented coronary artery disease. The last trial enrolled patients who had coronary disease, intermittent claudication, or transient ischemic attack. Five different ACE inhibitors were tested, and two of the trials used higher doses than those usually necessary for antihypertensive therapy.

All-cause mortality was lower in the treatment arms compared with the placebo arms in all of the trials except one, and the reduction was significant in HOPE. The cardiovascular mortality was consistently reduced by ACE inhibitors across all trials except CAMELOT (Comparison of Amlodipine versus Enalapril to Limit Occurrences of Thrombosis). The meta-analysis showed a 14% reduction in mortality. In the HOPE Trial, a highly significant 19% reduction was seen in the meta-analysis. In addition, significant reductions in the acute MI were found in both HOPE and EUROPA (European Trial on Reduction of Cardiac Events with Perindopril in Stable Coronary Artery Disease) Trials. There seemed to be no effect on the MI rate in the PEACE (Prevention of Events with ACE Inhibition) Trial, and nonsignificant reductions were observed in the other trials. Overall, there was an 18% reduction in MI with ACE inhibitor therapy. Stroke was less frequent in patients receiving ACE inhibitors in all trials except Part II of the Prevention of Atherosclerosis with Ramipril Trial-2. Overall, there was a 23% relative reduction in the occurrence of stroke in these trials.

In the summary article from the American College of Cardiology/American Heart Association 2002 Guidelines, the use of ACE inhibitors with coronary artery disease or other vascular disease without diabetes or left ventricular dysfunction was a class IIA recommendation. However, the use of ACE inhibitors in all patients with coronary artery disease who have diabetes or left ventricular systolic dysfunction was a class I recommendation.

Weight and Diet

In addition to blood pressure, other coronary risk factors are important, as is body weight. The ideal body mass index (BMI) goal is 18.5 to 24.9 kg/m^2. The Lyon Diet Heart Study suggested an increase in survival for patients on the Mediterranean diet, with a reduction of all-cause as well as cardiovascular mortality. MIs were reduced in the treatment group. The Nurses' Health Study follow-up enrolled some 121,700 female registered nurses, and the Health Professionals follow-up recruited 51,529 male health professionals. These studies found that consumption of fruits and vegetables, particularly green leafy vegetables and vitamin C–rich fruits and vegetables, appeared to have a protective effect against coronary heart disease.

Cholesterol

In addition to diet, lowering the total cholesterol and the LDL cholesterol reduces total mortality by 22% to 30%, coronary events by 24% to 37%, and CABG surgery and angioplasty by 22% to 37%. A recent prospective meta-analysis of 90,056 participants in 14 randomized trials of statins by the Cholesterol Treatment Trialists' (CTT) Collaborators have confirmed these data. In addition, data were available on first strokes after randomization in this meta-analysis. Overall, there was a significant 17% proportional reduction in the incidence of first stroke of any type in the statin group versus control group. In strokes not attributed to hemorrhage and presumed to be ischemic, the overall reduction in stroke reflected a highly significant 19% reduction. The CCT calculations revealed that a reduction in LDL cholesterol of 39 mg/dL (1 mmol/L) sustained for 5 years could produce a reduction in major vascular events of about 23%. This was more than the 21% reductions observed in the weighted analysis. Moreover, a reduction of the LDL cholesterol by 78 mg/dL (2 mmol/L) might be expected to reduce the risk of vascular disease by as much as 40%. In the case of stroke, cohort studies showed no associations between serum cholesterol levels and stroke. However, there is no question that the randomized trials showed that statins reduced the incidence of stroke by about 30%.

Several trials have demonstrated that high-dose aggressive LDL cholesterol lowering therapy can increase benefit to patients. The PROVE-IT (Pravastatin or Atorvastatin Evaluation and Infection Therapy) trial and the MIRACL (Myocardial Ischemia Reduction with Acute Cholesterol Lowering) trial used acute coronary syndrome patients and high-dose (80 mg) atorvastatin (Lipitor). PROVE-IT compared atorvastatin with pravastatin (Pravachol) 40 mg. The IDEAL (Incremental Decrease in Endpoints Through Aggressive Lipid Lowering) study compared 80 mg of atorvastatin with 20 mg of simvastatin (Zocor). Phase Z of the A to Z Trial compared 20 mg of simvastatin with 80 mg of simvastatin. The REVERSAL (Reversing Atherosclerosis with Aggressive Lipid Lowering) trial compared 80 mg of atorvastatin with 40 mg of pravastatin. The TACTICS TIMI 22 trial compared 80 mg of atorvastatin with 40 mg of pravastatin. The ASTEROID (A Study to Evaluate the Effect of Rosuvastatin on Intravascular Ultrasound-Derived Coronary Atheroma Burden) trial used rosuvastatin (Crestor) 40 mg per day.

These trials compared a variety of patients who had hypercholesterolemia. There seemed to be good data to suggest that some patients would be better off with an LDL cholesterol in the range of 75 mg/dL. There clearly was no adverse effect on safety in these trials although there was improved clinical benefit. The meta-analysis data of 90,056 participants lowering the LDL cholesterol by 39 mg/dL with 5 years of statin therapy failed to show any increased risk of any specific nonvascular cause of death or any specific type of cancer. In that meta-analysis of 14 trials, 39,884 patients allocated to a statin, nine patients developed rhabdomyolysis compared with six patients in 39,817 patients allocated to control. The 5-year risk was not significant, with an absolute incidence of 0.01%. High-risk patients would particularly benefit from lowered LDL cholesterol. These patients include those with MI, CABG surgery, or any percutaneous intervention.

The pertinent findings from the Adult Treatment Panel III are presented in Table 1. The goal of an LDL cholesterol of less than 100 mg/dL for coronary artery disease patients might well be reduced with further review by the National Cholesterol Education Program (NCEP). That panel defined diabetes as the equivalent of coronary heart disease even though there may be no symptoms or signs of coronary artery disease in diabetic patients.

Metabolic Syndrome

The metabolic syndrome requires intensive lifestyle changes as a baseline. The NCEP defined the waist circumference for abdominal obesity for men as greater than 40 inches and for women as greater than 35 inches. They also advocated a higher high-density lipoprotein to 40 mg/dL for men and 50 mg/dL for women. The blood pressure should be in the range of 130/85 mm Hg, and a fasting glucose should be less than 110 mg/dL.

The sub-study of the Treating to New Targets (TNT) trial that compared 80 mg of atorvastatin with 10 mg of atorvastatin in 5584 patients with the metabolic syndrome suggested statistically significant benefit with the 80-mg dose. At 3 months, the LDL cholesterol was reduced to 72.6 mg/dL with the 80-mg dose versus 99.3 mg/dL with the low dose of atorvastatin.

For most statin medications the evening dose has a greater effect, probably because of a short biological half-life, and because peak cholesterol synthesis occurs at night. Atorvastatin and rosuvastatin have longer half-lives and do not have this problem. All statin medications lower LDL cholesterol but at different doses. For example, rosuvastatin 5 mg/day, atorvastatin 10 mg/day, and lovastatin (Mevacor) or simvastatin 40 mg/day reduce LDL cholesterol by 35% or approximately 72 mg/dL. Fluvastatin (Lescol) and pravastatin produce smaller reductions even at the higher doses tested. All statins can reach NCEP goals in certain patients.

Anticoagulants

The antiplatelet aspirin is recommended if not contraindicated. Doses of 75 to 325 mg/day are the usual. The dose of 75 mg/day in the Swedish Angina Pectoris Aspirin Trial (SAPAT) resulted in a 34% reduction in the outcome of MI and sudden death, with a 32% drop in secondary vascular events.

If patients cannot tolerate aspirin or it is contraindicated, clopidogrel (Plavix) 75 mg a day or warfarin (Coumadin) can be used. Clopidogrel was studied in the CAPRIE (Clopidogrel versus Aspirin in Patients at Risk of Ischemic Events) trial; more than 19,000 patients were recruited who had a recent ischemic stroke, MI, or peripheral arterial disease. Clopidogrel and aspirin were compared with aspirin alone. There was a relative risk reduction of 8.7% for the combination of clopidogrel and aspirin against aspirin alone. The greatest benefit and risk reduction were in the peripheral arterial disease patients.

Clopidogrel and ticlopidine (Ticlid) are theinopyridine derivatives. Clopidogrel is favored because of the side effects associated with ticlopidine. Both drugs inhibit platelet aggregation induced by adenosine diphosphate (ADP). In the absence of contraindications, aspirin 75 to 325 mg/day is recommended for routine use in patients with chronic ischemic heart disease.

Combination drug therapy can also help patients reach ATP III goals. Simvastatin and long-acting niacin (Slow-Niacin) reduced major clinical events 90% as compared with a placebo. Statins themselves can significantly lower LDL cholesterol from all pretreatment levels. The absolute reductions were greater in patients with higher pretreatment levels of cholesterol.

PHARMACOLOGIC THERAPY

Anti-Anginal Drug Therapy

Nitrates in the treatment of angina pectoris have been a time-honored treatment and are still an important part of therapy. The nitrates seem to work primarily in the venous circulation and reduce preload to the left ventricle. Nitrate preparations are available in sublingual tablets, nitroglycerin spray bottles, ointments, and transdermal nitroglycerin patches. Nitroglycerin ointment or the nitroglycerin patch can be placed at bedtime to prevent nocturnal angina and allow some prevention of angina pectoris in the early morning hours before the patient first awakens.

Isosorbide dinitrate (Isordil) is an anti-anginal agent but has relatively low bioavailability after oral administration. The active metabolite of isosorbide dinitrate is isosorbide mononitrate (Imdur). This is completely bioavailable with oral administration because it does not undergo first-pass hepatic metabolism. Either of these preparations requires a 12-hour nitrate-free interval to avoid nitroglycerin tolerance.

The mechanism of nitroglycerin tolerance is not well understood. Currently the best evidence seems to suggest that there is an impairment of nitrate bioconversion as the mechanism of tolerance induction. Several agents have been suggested to limit or reverse the development of nitrate tolerance, although the evidence is not consistent.

ACE inhibitors have not been associated with amelioration of nitrate efficacy, despite their effects on reversing endothelial dysfunction. Folic acid seems to improve endothelial dysfunction in many situations and can potentiate hemodynamic responses to

TABLE 1 Cholesterol Treatment Cutpoints and Targets for Therapy

Risk Category	10-Year Risk*	Cholesterol Goals (mg/dL) LDL	Non-HDL
CAD and CAD equivalent†	>20%	<100	<130
Multiple risk factors (2+)‡	10%-20%	<130	<160
0-1 risk factors	<10%	<160	<190

*Based on projections from the Framingham Heart Study for 10-year risk of having a CAD event.
†Diabetes is considered a CAD equivalent, even if the patient has no CAD symptoms.
‡Identifies patients with metabolic syndrome for extensive lifestyle changes.
Abbreviations: CAD = coronary artery disease; HDL = high-density lipoprotein; LDL = low-density lipoprotein
Data from the National Cholesterol Education Program Adult Treatment Panel III (ATP III).

nitrates. At present, the only management for nitroglycerin tolerance is to allow a nitrate-free interval of at least 12 hours.

A combination of nitrates and sildenafil (Viagra) can cause a prolonged and potentially life-threatening drop in blood pressure. Sildenafil therapy is contraindicated in patients who use nitrates.

β-Adrenergic Antagonists

β-Blockers, or β-adrenergic receptor blocking agents, are an important part of the therapy for angina pectoris and are often started early in the management of these patients. They can be antihypertensive and antiarrhythmic. Information suggests these medications prolong survival and prevent reinfarction in patients who have had an MI. These agents have different pharmacology, some being selective of β_1-receptor block and others being nonselective β-blocking drugs (Table 2). For example, nadolol, pindolol, sotalol, and timolol, all block both β_1- and β_2-receptors. β-Blockers with less effect on β_2-receptors and more effect on β_1-receptors are acebutolol, atenolol, metoprolol, and esmolol.

The β_1-receptors are primarily found in the heart, and stimulation of these receptors leads to increased atrial ventricular nodal conduction, an increase in heart rate, an increase in contractility, and an increase in norepinephrine release. In contrast, stimulation of β_2-receptors causes bronchodilation and vasodilation. Cardioselectivity of β_1-blocking drugs disappears as the dose of these drugs increased.

Doses of β-blockers required to control angina might reach a point where they do cause some degree of bronchoconstriction in sensitive patients. Labetolol and carvedilol have α-blocking capabilities as well as β_1-blocking capability. Acebutolol and pindolol have some intrinsic sympathomimetic activity. This means they can produce low-grade β-stimulation when sympathetic activity is low, for instance, at rest. For these reasons they might not be as effective in reducing heart rate or the magnitude of ST segment depression in patients with angina.

The gastrointestinal tract does not as readily absorb the β-blockers propanolol, metoprolol, and pindolol. Because of the gastrointestinal absorption, intravenous doses of metoprolol or propanolol can result in much higher concentrations in the bloodstream than oral dosing. Therefore, lower doses of these medications given intravenously will produce an adequate effect (see Table 2).

Barring contraindications, indefinite use of β-blockers in patients with angina pectoris is recommended. Abrupt cessation in patients with angina should be avoided because of the possibility of exacerbation of the angina pectoris.

Calcium Channel Antagonists

Calcium channel blockers can be considered third-choice agents in the treatment of stable angina pectoris. These medications block the entry of calcium into smooth muscle cells as well as myocytes. Calcium channel antagonists reduce smooth muscle tension in the peripheral vascular bed, producing arterial vasodilation and thereby reducing arterial blood pressure and afterload. They also reduce myocardial contractility. Altogether, they reduce myocardial oxygen consumption. Diltiazem and verapamil reduce the heart rate. Dihydropyridine calcium channel blockers such as nifedipine and amlodipine are among the most potent calcium blocking agents.

Short-acting calcium channel blockers are to be avoided. Only long-acting calcium channel blockers are recommended. Although β-blockers are recommended as first-line treatment for angina pectoris, calcium channel blockers can be used and are equally effective in angina pectoris if β-blockers are not tolerated.

Diltiazem and verapamil depress contractility more than the dihydropyridines, which is a disadvantage. Adverse effects of calcium channel blockers include ankle edema, palpitations, flushing, headaches, and hypotension. These agents can be combined with a β-blocker, especially a long-acting dihydropyridine such as amlodipine or nifedipine XL. These decrease ischemic events and increase exercise time.

Long-acting metoprolol 200 mg/day or nifedipine XL 40 mg/day were more effective when used together than either drug when used separately. The combination showed a greater increase in exercise tolerance over monotherapy with either drug. To avoid complications, the β-blocker should be started first, then the calcium channel blocker should be added for angina control. Dosing is also important. A therapeutic dose of metoprolol is 50 mg twice daily with the goal of bringing the resting heart rate into the 50s. Calcium channel blockers are also effective in the treatment of vasospastic angina.

Even when dosing of these medications is appropriate, most patients with angina pectoris benefit from three agents: nitrates, β-blockers, and calcium channel blockers. Despite these efforts at therapy, many angina patients still fail therapy and continue to have disabling angina classified as class III or IV limitations. The goal of therapy is not only symptomatic relief but also prolonged survival. Probably more than 50% of patients with stable angina will have coronary angiography in an attempt to relieve symptoms. Data show that left main coronary artery disease, triple vessel disease, and double vessel disease involving a proximal left anterior descending coronary artery all benefit from revascularization with prolonged survival. Patients with high-risk noninvasive testing are candidates for angiography (Box 3).

The Asymptomatic Cardiac Ischemia Pilot (ACIP) study randomized patients into three treatment strategies if they were candidates for revascularization. These strategies were angina-guided therapy, angina plus ischemic medications, and revascularization by angioplasty or CABG surgery.

Titrated doses of atenolol with long-acting nifedipine or sustained-release diltiazem and the addition of sustained-release isosorbide dinitrate were used. Mortality rates in the 2-year follow-up in the guided therapy were 6.6% for ischemic-guided therapy, 4.4% for angina plus ischemic medications, and 1.1% for the revascularization strategy. This suggests that revascularization can improve the 2-year prognosis of patients who have objective evidence of ischemia, even if their angina is well controlled on aggressive medical management.

TABLE 2 Commonly Used Medications in Angina Pectoris

Drug	Form	Dose
Nitrates		
Isosorbide dinitrate(Isordil)	Tab	20-40 mg PO bid
Isosorbide mononitrate (Imdur)	Tab	30-120 mg PO qd
Nitroglycerin (Nitrostat)	Sublingual tab	0.4 mg PO prn
Nitroglycerin (Nitrolingual)	Spray	0.4 mg prn
Nitroglycerin (Nitrol)	Ointment	½-1 inch qid
Nitroglycerin (Nitroglyn)	Cap slow release	2.5 to 13 mg PO bid or tid
β-Blockers		
Atenolol (Tenormin)	Tab	50-200 mg PO qd
	Soln	5 mg IV q15 min
Carvedilol (Coreg)	Tab	12.5-50 PO mg bid
Esmolol (Brevibloc)	Soln	50-300 µg/kg/min continuous infusion
Labetalol (Normodyne, Trandate)	Tab	200-600 mg PO bid or tid
Metoprolol (Lopressor)	Tab	50-200 mg PO bid
	Soln	5 mg q15 min
Propranolol (Inderal)	Cap, tab	20-80 mg PO bid
Calcium Channel Blockers		
Amlodipine (Norvasc)	Tab	5-10 mg qd
Diltiazem (Cardizem CD)	Tab slow release	120-480 mg qd
Nifedipine (Procardia XL)	Tab slow release	30-90 mg qd
Verapamil (Calan SR)	Caplet slow release	120-480 mg qd

Abbreviations: cap = capsule; soln = IV solution; tab = tablet.

Future Therapies

Because chronic angina can impair quality of life and is associated with decreased life expectancy affecting 6.4 million Americans, newer therapies are being developed. These current therapies reduce demand-induced myocardial ischemic symptoms but often they are not sufficient. Newer drugs under evaluation include ivabradine[1], omapatrilat[2], fasudil[2], and nicorandil.[1]

Ranolazine (Ranexa) has recently been approved. Ranolazine is an active piperazine derivative with a short half-life of 1.4 to 1.9 hours. Only the prolonged or sustained-release ranolazine is available for patients who still have limiting angina despite triple therapy. Ranolazine should always be used in combination with other medications: amlodipine, β-blockers, or nitrates. It should not be used as an alternative to β-blocker therapy. The therapeutic dose range is 500 to 1000 mg twice a day. This dosage range is generally well tolerated, but constipation, nausea, and dizziness are the most common adverse effects reported.

Ranolazine is extensively metabolized through the CYP3A4 pathway. The medication is contraindicated in patients with hepatic impairment or those with QTc prolongation or who are taking medications known to prolong the QT interval. It is also contraindicated if the patient is taking drugs that are moderately potent CYP3A inhibitors. A baseline ECG to evaluate the QT interval should be performed. At present, ranolazine is only recommended for patients who have failed angina control with triple therapy.

Other Forms of Angina

REFRACTORY ANGINA PECTORIS

Despite optimal medical management, angiography with angioplasty, and CABG surgery, many patients still have severe limiting angina. These patents are survivors. There are estimates that as many as 100,000 patients with refractory angina are alive in the United States. For these patients with no options there are methods that will palliate the angina pectoris. The treatment might not affect the basic disease process, but it will decrease the angina pain and increase the patient's quality of life. The prognosis for survival in these patients appears to be low, estimated at a 5% annual mortality.

The OPTIMIST (Options in Myocardial Syndrome Therapies) trial suggested patients with refractory angina have low long-term mortality; during their 3.5-year follow-up period, 11.8% of their patients died. They treated some of their patients with enhanced external counterpulsation (EECP), transmyocardial laser revascularization, and neurostimulation. The international EECP ($n = 978$ patients) patient registry demonstrated an improvement of at least one angina class in 81% of the patients with class III or IV refractory anginas. Transmyocardial laser revascularization has been shown to reduce cardiac pain, although the information that it affects myocardial ischemia is lacking. Neurostimulation in the form of transcutaneous electrical nerve stimulation (TENS) or spinal cord stimulation has been found useful in relieving pain. Symptom relief with neurostimulation has been found effective in managing patients with refractory angina pectoris.

A recent paper evaluated the prognosis of post-MI patients who had preinfarction stable angina pectoris versus those who did not. Patients who had stable angina pectoris before they developed an MI had less remodeling of the left ventricular volumes. This could improve survival without necessarily improving chest pain.

UNSTABLE ANGINA PECTORIS

Unstable angina has a changing pattern. The pain or discomfort comes more frequently, lasts longer (perhaps >20 minutes), comes with lesser degrees of exertion, occurs at rest, or occurs at night, and requires additional sublingual nitroglycerin for control. Unstable angina suggests the disruption of a vulnerable atherosclerotic plaque and partial or total closure of a coronary artery as opposed to a fixed athero-sclerotic obstruction.

Unstable angina is part of the acute coronary syndrome, which accounts for nearly 1.7 million patients who are hospitalized after presenting to the emergency department in the United States every year. Risk stratification of these patients is performed on the basis of the 12-lead ECG as well as biochemical markers. The acute coronary syndrome also includes ST segment elevation MI and non–ST segment elevation MI or the non–Q wave MI. A rapid evaluation of these patients with acute coronary syndrome is critical. Unstable angina is the part of the acute coronary syndrome where no biochemical marker is elevated. There is no sign of myocardial necrosis.

Much new material on the acute coronary syndrome has been published in the last few years. The data focus on the best treatment for these patients as well as the diagnosis, prognosis, and risk stratification. Biochemical markers such as troponin, creatinine kinase, creatinine kinase MB, B-naturetic peptide, C-reactive protein (CRP), and myoglobin are used. Myoglobin and troponin markers are measured at the onset of the chest pain and at 6 hours and again at 12 hours after admission to the hospital.

Clinical Findings

Box 3 lists the findings of high-risk patients. They can have accelerating chest pain as well as left ventricular dysfunction or pulmonary edema. New-onset mitral regurgitation, ventricular gallops, hypotension, the extremes of heart rate, and age older than 75 years are all abnormalities found in a high-risk patient. These are usually associated with acute MI and ST segment changes or new-onset bundle branch block. Cardiac enzymes are elevated in these cases. Low-risk chest pain patients have a new-onset or progressive angina and at least a moderate or perhaps a high likelihood of coronary artery disease based on their history. The ECG may be normal in these patients, and biochemical markers may also be normal.

Treatment

The problem in the acute coronary syndrome is an abnormal physiology in the vessel wall, that is, plaque, platelets, and thrombus. Therefore, antithrombotic therapy is very important. All patients receive an aspirin, which blocks the thromboxane A_2 within 15 to 30 minutes of the oral dose. Clopidogrel is also indicated as an adenosine-mediated platelet blocker, particularly if the patient has an aspirin allergy. Unfractionated heparin is used. Data now suggest a preference for low-molecular-weight heparin. Enoxaparin might have an advantage over unfractionated heparin for patients who have the acute coronary syndrome (ESSENCE).

The results of the CURE (Clopidogrel in Unstable angina to prevent Recurrent Events) trial make clopidogrel a class I indication for the treatment of patients with unstable angina even in patients in whom an early coronary intervention is not considered. The treatment might be continued for 9 months. If a coronary intervention is performed, clopidogrel should be started at 300 mg and continued for at least 3 months at a dose

---

BOX 3 Findings in High-Risk Patients

- Hemodynamic instability
- High-risk noninvasive stress testing with depressed ejection fraction, extensive wall motion abnormalities
- Recent revascularization with coronary intervention or coronary bypass graft surgery
- Recurrent ischemia at rest or low levels of activity with medical management
- Recurrent ischemia with heart failure, ventricular gallop, extremes of heart rate, or mitral regurgitation
- Sustained ventricular tachycardia

---

[1] Not available in the United States.
[2] Investigational drug in the United States.

TABLE 3 Antithrombotic Drugs

Drug(s)	Dosing
Abciximab (Reopro) with unfractionated heparin and aspirin	0.25 mg/kg IV bolus followed by an infusion of 0.125 µg/kg/min for 12-24 h up to 10 µg/min
Eptifibatide (Integrilin) with unfractionated heparin and aspirin	180 µg/kg followed by an infusion of 2 µg/kg/min up to 72 h for intervention Max infusion dose 15 mg/h
Tirofiban (Aggrastat) with unfractionated heparin and aspirin	0.4 µg/kg/min for 30 min 0.1 µg/kg/min infusion for 48 h up to 108 hours (PRISM-PLUS)
Enoxaparin (Lovenox)	1 mg/kg SC q 12 h
Clopidrogrel (Plavix)	300 mg initially followed by 75 mg/d

Abbreviations: max = maximum; PRISM-PLUS = Platelet Receptor Inhibition in Ischemic Syndrome Management in Patients Limited by Unstable Signs and Symptoms.

of 75 mg/day. There are trials suggesting that an initial dose of 600 mg clopidogrel can shorten the onset of action.

There are rare cases of thrombotic thrombocytopenic purpura from the use of clopidogrel. These are manifested by thrombocytopenia and microangiopathic hemolytic anemia sometimes associated with neurologic or renal dysfunction. These patients must discontinue clopidogrel and in some instances undergo plasma exchange. Postmyocardial infarction patients who cannot tolerate aspirin or clopidogrel can be given warfarin and titrated to an international normalized ratio (INR) of 2.0 to 3.0. All of these medications have a tendency to increase bleeding, particularly in female and elderly patients. Studies have shown that the risk of bleeding in these patients doubles. However, the risk-to-benefit ratio still favors treatment with these agents.

A platelet glycoprotein (GP) IIb/IIIa inhibitor is also indicated. The GPIIb/IIIa receptors on a platelet number between 60,000 and 80,000 and are regarded as the final common pathway for binding fibrinogen. Table 3 lists the three current drugs that are available: abciximab (Reopro), epitifibatide (Integralin), and tirofiban (Aggrastat). All three of these GPIIb/IIIa receptor blockers have been studied with the simultaneous use of unfractionated heparin and aspirin treatments. Most of the trials of these agents have involved coronary interventions and have shown significant benefits.

A meta-analysis of seven contemporary randomized trials in more than 8000 patients has been reported. Potent antiplatelet therapy and coronary angioplasty with stent placement decreased mortality by 25% at a mean of 2 years of follow-up when compared with a more conservative approach. These data showed that to save one life, 62 patients needed to be treated with invasive therapy. Early invasive therapy also decreased nonfatal infarction by 17% and recurrent unstable angina requiring hospitalization by 31%.

A patient who has thrombocytopenia of less than 100,000 platelets should not be treated with GPIIb/IIIa inhibitors. Tirofiban needs renal adjustment because it is cleared by the kidney. Ideally, abciximab should be administered 10 to 60 minutes before percutaneous intervention. If there is no intervention, abciximab is not indicated. Tirofiban and eptifibatide are useful in patients with continuing ischemia where no percutaneous intervention in planned. These two medications can also be used in patients with continuing ischemia or other high-risk features in whom a percutaneous intervention is planned.

There are other antithrombin agents, such as lepirudin (Refludin), argatroban (Novostan), and the low-molecular-weight heparin dalteparin (Fragmin). Thrombolytic therapy in the presence of unstable angina is of no benefit to these patients, in contrast to the benefits seen with an acute MI.

Biomarkers

Much research has been done in the field of biomarkers, and currently several biomarkers are under study. Most experience is with creatinine kinase, creatinine kinase MB, troponin I or T, and myoglobin, but others are under study. Currently available biomarkers include CRP and brain-natriuretic peptide (BNP). BNP has been found to be elevated in patients with congestive heart failure. However, in addition, transient myocardial ischemia can result in an elevation of BNP. This suggests that BNP is linked to ischemic injury in addition to left ventricular dysfunction.

An exercise study using the Bruce protocol evaluated transient myocardial ischemia in 112 patients. If patients had no inducible ischemia, BNP levels were low at baseline (43 pg/mL) and unchanged during and after exercise. If patients developed inducible ischemia by electrocardiographic and technetium Tc-99m tetrofosmin scans, BNP levels rose from a median of 62 to 92 and returned to baseline at 4 hours after exercise. In patients with severe ischemia and median BNP levels (101 pg/mL) at baseline, BNP levels increased to 123 pg/mL and were still elevated at 4 hours after exercise. In that study, patients with no ischemia (43 pg/mL), mild to moderate ischemia (60 pg/mL), and severe ischemia (101 pg/mL) were statistically different. The differences were increased with exercise stress.

Currently, an important inflammatory biomarker is CRP. CRP can identify inflammation, and inflammation predicts the prognosis with acute coronary syndrome. It is also possible that CRP is a marker for atherosclerosis and not necessarily atherothrombosis. One study of 2554 patients with angina but not MI found that CRP significantly correlated with the extent of coronary vascular disease. A high CRP and severe coronary artery disease indicated the highest risk in the 5-year follow-up. There was still a high predictive risk for MI or death in the follow-up regardless of the extent of coronary artery disease if the CRP was elevated. There was a 10-fold difference in the lowest level and the highest level of CRP (2.5% versus 25%). It is likely that more research will result in a panel of biochemical markers that will be useful in stratifying the patients with the acute coronary syndrome in the emergency department.

Summary

Most patients in the high-risk and intermediate-risk acute coronary syndrome groups receive coronary angiography for the full assessment because of the survival benefit of revascularization. Patients in the low-risk group of unstable angina with no biochemical markers or ECG changes may be considered for a stress test. The abnormal stress tests with echocardiographic or nuclear scans direct further aggressive therapy (see Box 3). Studies in these patients show that an early invasive strategy reduces the incidence of major cardiac events. The data for high-risk acute MI and non–Q-wave MI suggest angiography should be part of the early plan. The data for unstable angina with no biochemical marker elevation are less clear at present.

All patients who present with stable angina or unstable angina should receive aggressive medical management and coronary risk factor reduction. Medication should include β-blockers, lipid-lowering medications, antiplatelet medications, aspirin, and nitrates. Because some studies show a relatively low rate of use of these medications, the American Heart Association has mounted a nationwide effort entitled "Get With the Guidelines." The relative risk reductions for each of the class 1–indicated medications in the study trials vary from 15% to 20% for aspirin, β-blockers, ACE inhibitors, statins, and clopidogrel. It is now clear that the goal of prolonging survival and enhancing the quality of life can only be met by a polypharmacy approach often associated with coronary angiography and revascularization.

REFERENCES

Baigent C, Keech A, Kearney PM, et al: Cholesterol Treatment Trialists' (CTT) Collaborators: Efficacy and safety of cholesterol-lowering treatment: Perspective meta-analysis of data from 90,056 participants in 14 randomised trials of statins. Lancet 2005;366:1267-1278.

Bavry AA, Kumbhani DJ, Rassi AN, et al: Benefit of early invasive therapy in acute coronary syndromes: A meta-analysis of contemporary randomized clinical trials. J Am Coll Cardiol 2006;48:1319-1325.

Chaitman BR: Ranolazine for the treatment of chronic angina and potential use in other cardiovascular conditions. Circulation 2006;113:2462-2472.

Cohen M, Demers C, Gurfinkel EP, et al: A comparison of low-molecular-weight heparin with unfractionated heparin for unstable coronary artery disease: Efficacy and Safety of Subcutaneous Enoxaparin in Non-Q-Wave Coronary Events Study Group. N Engl J Med 1997;337:447-452.

Danchin N, Cucherat M, Thuillez C, et al: Angiotensin converting enzyme inhibitors in patients with coronary artery disease and absence of heart failure or left ventricular systolic dysfunction: An overview of long-term randomized control trials. Arch Intern Med 2006;166:787-796.

DeJongste M, Tio RA, Foreman RD: Chronic therapeutically refractory angina pectoris. Heart 2004;90:225-230.

Hemingway H, McCallum A, Shipley M, et al: Incidence and prognostic implications of stable angina pectoris among women and men. JAMA 2006;295:1404-1411.

Law MR, Wald NJ, Rudnicka AR: Quantifying the effect of statins on low density lipoprotein cholesterol, ischemic heart disease, and stroke: Systemic review and meta-analysis. BMJ 2003;326:1423.

Nelson GI, Silke B, Ahuja RC, et al: The effect of left ventricular performance of nifedipine and metroprolol singly and together in exercise-induced angina pectoris. Eur Heart J 1984;5:67-79.

Third Report of the National Cholesterol Education Program (NCEP) Expert Panel on Detection, Evaluation, and Treatment of High Blood Cholesterol in Adults (Adult Treatment Panel III) final report. Circulation 2002;106:3143.

Cardiac Arrest: Sudden Cardiac Death

Method of
Robert W. Rho, MD

Sudden cardiac arrest is the cause of death in up to 250,000 people per year in the United States. This accounts for more than 50% of all cardiovascular deaths. Sudden cardiac arrest is responsible for more deaths in the United States than stroke, breast cancer, and lung cancer combined. Approximately 1 sudden cardiac arrest occurs every 1.5 minutes in the United States. Unfortunately, 80% of cardiac arrests occur outside of the hospital and resuscitation is only attempted in approximately two thirds of these patients. Even in most urban communities, where an organized emergency medical system (EMS) is available, the survival rate of patients who suffer an out-of-hospital cardiac arrest is less than 10%. Approximately 10% to 40% of these patients have severe neurologic impairment at the time of discharge. This chapter provides a contemporary overview of the epidemiology, mechanism, diagnosis, and treatment of cardiac arrest.

Definitions

- Cardiac arrest: A primary cardiac disorder that results in sudden loss of cardiac output and a resultant loss of end-organ perfusion resulting in death unless the primary cardiac disorder is corrected.
- Sudden death: Death that occurs unexpectedly within a short interval of time from the onset of symptoms. (Definition varies in the literature from 1 hour to 24 hours from the onset of symptoms.)
- Aborted sudden cardiac death: An intervention or spontaneous event that reverses a life-threatening but modifiable cardiac process (malignant arrhythmia, pump failure, or ischemia) that would have otherwise resulted in sudden death.

Epidemiology

Approximately 250,000–400,000 patients suffer a cardiac arrest annually in the United States. The incidence of cardiac arrest in the United States is estimated to be approximately 1.5 to 2.0 per 1000 subject-years.

The incidence of cardiac arrest based on a retrospective review of death certificates in Multnomah County, Oregon, was 1.5 per 1000 subject-years. The incidence of cardiac arrest reported in a population based case-control study in Seattle was 1.9 per 1000 subject-years. The incidence varies across clinical subsets known to be at greater risk of cardiac arrest. In the Seattle study, the incidence in patients with prior myocardial infarction was 13.7 per 1000 subject-years and in those with a history of heart failure was 21.9 per 1000 subject-years.

Prognosis

Patients who suffer an out-of-hospital cardiac arrest have a poor prognosis. Survival depends on the availability and quality of bystander cardiopulmonary resuscitation (CPR), early defibrillation, and the availability of EMS. In many densely populated urban communities (such as Chicago and New York City), survival to hospital discharge is less than 5%. In smaller urban communities with well-coordinated EMS systems, survival can approach 15% to 20% (Rochester, Minnesota, and Seattle, Washington). The initial rhythm when a defibrillator is available for monitoring has significant prognostic implications. Among patients who have ventricular fibrillation (VF) as their initial rhythm, 10% to 40% survive to hospital discharge. In contrast, patients who are found to be in asystole or pulseless electrical activity (PEA) have a grim prognosis, and less than 5% survive to hospital discharge.

Etiology

Cardiac arrhythmias account for the vast majority of all causes of cardiac arrests. The remaining minority of patients have cardiac arrest due to nonarrhythmic mechanisms such as left ventricular pump failure and cardiac tamponade.

The majority of patients suffering a cardiac arrest have coronary artery disease (CAD), but other conditions that predispose to cardiac arrest include hypertrophic cardiomyopathy, dilated cardiomyopathy, arrhythmogenic right ventricular cardiomyopathy, myocarditis, drug toxicities (antiarrhythmic agents, cocaine, amphetamines), congenital heart disease (especially tetralogy of Fallot and transposition of the great vessels [after a Mustard or Senning procedure]), ion-channel disorders such as long QT syndrome, Brugada syndrome, and short QT syndrome (Table 1).

Patients with abnormalities in myocardial substrate are predisposed to ventricular tachycardia because of a reentry mechanism. Most patients who suffer a cardiac arrest develop a rapid monomorphic ventricular tachycardia that degenerates to ventricular fibrillation and then ultimately (after 8 to 10 minutes) to asystole (Figure 1).

Management of Cardiac Arrest

The International Liaison Committee on Resuscitation (ILCOR) published its most recent recommendations for management of patients of cardiac arrest in November 2005. The recommendations from 2000 were updated based on an up-to-date review of resuscitation science between 2000 and 2005. Figure 2 shows the ILCOR universal cardiac arrest algorithm.

The initial rhythm encountered by EMS in patients suffering a cardiac arrest are ventricular fibrillation, pulseless ventricular tachycardia (VT), asystole, and PEA. Most patients who suffer an out-of-hospital cardiac arrest are found to be in ventricular fibrillation, but asystole or PEA has been found to be the initial rhythm in increasing frequency in the more recent literature.

Acute Management of Cardiac Arrest

Survival from a cardiac arrest depends critically on what the American Heart Association describes as the "chain of survival." The chain of

TABLE 1 Causes of Cardiac Arrest

1. **Coronary Artery Disease**
   a. Atherosclerotic coronary artery disease
   b. Nonatherosclerotic coronary artery disease
      - Anomalous coronary origin
      - Acute coronary spasm
      - Coronary vasculitis (Kawasaki's disease, connective tissue disease)
      - Aortic dissection
      - Embolic coronary obstruction

2. **Structural Heart Disease**
   a. Ischemic cardiomyopathy
   b. Idiopathic dilated cardiomyopathy
   c. Hypertrophic cardiomyopathy
   d. Arrhythmogenic right ventricular cardiomyopathy
   e. Myocarditis
   f. Prior myocardial infarction
   g. Heart failure exacerbation

3. **Ion Channel Abnormality**
   a. Brugada syndrome
   b. Congenital or acquired long QT syndrome
   c. Short QT syndrome
   d. Idiopathic ventricular fibrillation

4. **Drug Toxicity**
   a. Cocaine
   b. Amphetamines
   c. Antiarrhythmic agents
   d. Digoxin toxicity
   e. Drug-induced long QT syndrome

5. **Metabolic Abnormalities**
   a. Severe hypokalemia or hyperkalemia
   b. Severe hypomagnesemia
   c. Severe acidosis

survival includes early recognition and initiation of bystander CPR, activation of the EMS system, early defibrillation (which may include automated external defibrillators), and advanced cardiac life support. Because a bystander may provide three of the four links to the chain of survival, community awareness and education in basic life support is a key element in increasing the likelihood of survival of cardiac arrest victims.

RECOGNITION

The initial management of patients experiencing cardiac arrest should be focused on the patient's ABCs: airway, breathing, and circulation. Delay in the recognition that a patient is experiencing cardiac arrest can waste critical minutes in initiating CPR and providing timely defibrillation. Rescuers should suspect cardiac arrest in any individual who is not moving, not breathing, and unresponsive. Involuntary gasps for air should not be confused for spontaneous respiration because agonal breathing patterns can be present in the early phases of 40% of all cardiac arrests and should not delay initiation of CPR.

ACTIVATION OF THE EMS SYSTEM

As soon as a patient is recognized to be experiencing a cardiac arrest, the EMS system should be activated. In most communities the system can be activated by calling the universal emergency number 911. The interval of time from onset of the cardiac arrest to arrival of EMS is critical. The shorter this interval of time, the more likely the patient will survive without neurologic injury. Survival is improved in those communities that have a well-organized and well-trained EMS system. Response times can be shortened when other professionals (e.g., firefighters or police officers) trained in CPR and equipped with a defibrillator are employed as first responders.

AIRWAY

The airway should be opened using a head-tilt, chin-lift technique. If a foreign object is visible, a finger sweep of the oropharynx may be performed. Endotracheal intubation is the optimal means to establish control of the airway. Care must be taken to rule out esophageal intubation once the tube is inserted. While performing intubation, interruption of CPR must be minimized. Other invasive airway adjuncts have been developed and have proven field success. These include the Combitube and the laryngeal mask airway (LMA).

BREATHING (VENTILATION)

Ventilation can be achieved by mouth-to-mouth or bag-valve-mask. Each breath should be given a 1-second inspiratory time to achieve a chest rise. A tidal volume of approximately 500 mL to 750 mL should be delivered with a ventilatory rate of 8 to 10 breaths per minute. When an advanced airway is in place (endotracheal tube or LMA), the rescuer should provide ventilation without interruption in CPR.

CIRCULATION

The quality of CPR and minimizing interruption of CPR received significant emphasis in the 2005 ILCOR guidelines. Even with optimal chest compressions, the maximum cardiac output achieved is only a third of normal. Chest compressions should be performed with the patient on the floor or with a backboard placed under the patient. The rescuer should place the dominant hand on the lower half of the sternum with the nondominant hand placed over the lower hand. The rescuer should use the weight of his or her torso to compress the chest by 1.5 to 2 cm. After each compression, adequate decompression should be allowed while maintaining a compression-decompression rate of 100 compressions per minute. The ratio of time for decompression should be at least 50% of the total compression-decompression cycle. Several studies have demonstrated that chest compression rate, depth, and decompression are inadequate even among trained professionals. Inadequate chest compressions may not provide satisfactory hemodynamic support and result in worse survival and neurologic outcome. The quality of CPR (compression, decompression, rate, and depth)should be monitored by all rescuers involved in the resuscitative effort. During prolonged resuscitation, a fatigued rescuer performing CPR should be replaced by a fresh rescuer.

DEFIBRILLATION

The most critical intervention in patients who have cardiac arrest during ventricular fibrillation or pulseless VT is immediate initiation of chest compressions by a bystander and early defibrillation. In patients with VF, every 1-minute delay in defibrillation reduces the chance of survival by approximately 8% to 10%. The priority of defibrillation and CPR is time dependent. Several studies have demonstrated that when myocardial energy supplies are depleted from prolonged ischemia, coronary perfusion must be achieved before defibrillation. In a study conducted in Seattle, patients who received 90 seconds of CPR before defibrillation had significantly better survival to hospital discharge compared to patients who received defibrillation first. This finding was only significant among patients who had EMS response times of greater than 4 minutes. In patients with EMS response intervals of less than 4 minutes, there was no difference in survival between the two groups. In a prospective randomized study from Oslo, Norway, 3 minutes of CPR before defibrillation was compared with defibrillation first. In this study, return of spontaneous circulation (ROSC) was observed more frequently in patients who received CPR first compared to defibrillation first (58% vs. 38%; $p < 0.04$) if the EMS response time was more than 5 minutes. There was no difference between the two groups when EMS response time was less than 5 minutes. Survival to hospital discharge was significantly improved in this study in patients who had CPR before

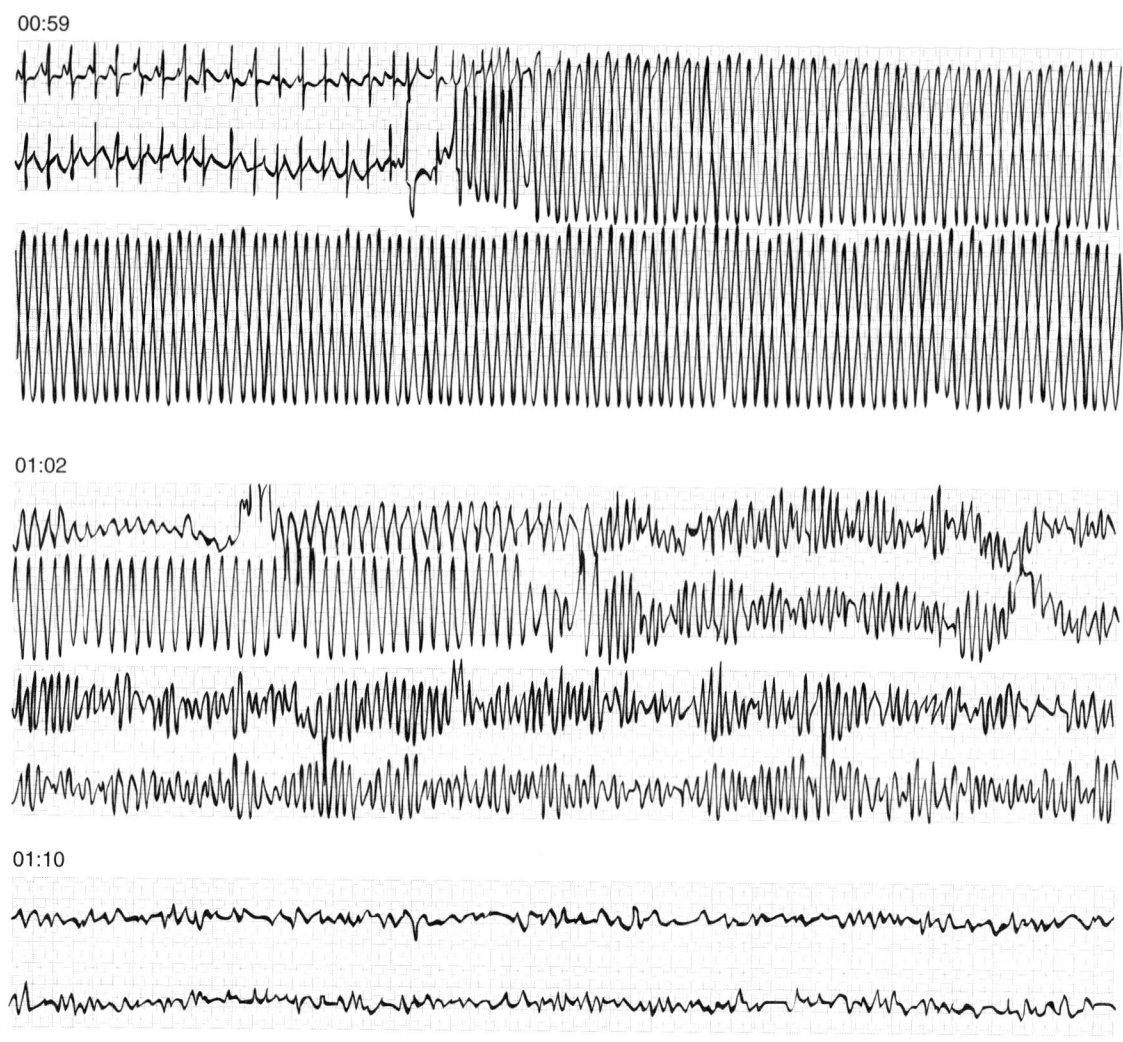

FIGURE 1. A Holter tracing of sudden death starting with monomorphic ventricular tachycardia and degenerating into ventricular fibrillation. (From Aziz S, McMahon RF, Garratt CJ: Images in cardiovascular medicine. Sudden cardiac death in arrhythmogenic right ventricular dysplasia. Circulation 2000;101:825-827. Reprinted with permission.)

defibrillation when EMS response times were more than 5 minutes (22% CPR first vs. 4% defibrillation first; $p = 0.006$). No difference in survival to hospitalization was observed in patients who had EMS response times of less than 5 minutes. These studies demonstrated that CPR prior to defibrillation improved survival in patients who had prolonged VF arrests and did not seem to worsen survival (by delaying defibrillation) in patients who had shorter periods of VF arrest. Based on these data and others, the 2005 ILCOR recommends CPR preceding defibrillation in patients who have an unwitnessed out-of-hospital VF arrest. Furthermore, ILCOR recommends that one shock should be given rather than three successive shocks. This is based on the fact that, in patients who are likely to be successfully defibrillated, the first shock success is very high and a significant interruption in CPR may occur when three successive shocks are delivered because of the time needed to charge the defibrillator, deliver the shock, and check a pulse three times.

When a defibrillator becomes available, the rescuer should continue CPR while the defibrillator is charging. The rescuer should give one shock and continue CPR for five cycles before checking for a pulse. The initial shock energy should be 200 J for a biphasic defibrillator and 360 J for a monophasic defibrillator.

AUTOMATED EXTERNAL DEFIBRILLATORS

The automated external defibrillator (AED) is a portable device with a battery, capacitor, and a processor that provides an accurate analysis of the cardiac rhythm and an algorithm that instructs the operator if a shock is indicated. The arrhythmia analysis algorithm in the AED has the capacity to interpret complicated cardiac rhythms and to recommend appropriate therapy with a high degree of accuracy. Several studies have demonstrated that AED arrhythmia detection for VF has a 100% sensitivity and specificity. The operation of the AED is simple and involves four steps:

1. Turn on the AED.
2. Connect the pads to the patient.
3. Wait for the AED to analyze cardiac rhythm.
4. Press the shock button (if shock is advised by the AED).

The AED uses voice and text prompts to guide the user through these steps. Because of ease of use, the AED can be safely and reliably operated by a nonmedically trained person.

Since the majority of cardiac arrests occur out of the hospital, the efficacy of AEDs has been tested in a number of conditions. In a 2-year study of AEDs used in a major airline, an AED was used in 200 patients. Of the 15 patients with VF, 6 patients (40%) were successfully defibrillated and survived to hospital discharge. The sensitivity and specificity of VF detection by the AED was 100%.

The efficacy of AEDs was also tested in casinos. This is a unique setting where a large population of patients are monitored by closed-circuit surveillance cameras. In this study, 56 of 105 (53%) patients who suffered a cardiac arrest because of ventricular fibrillation were successfully defibrillated and survived to hospital discharge. The mean time to first shock from the AED in this study was 4.4 minutes, and the mean time for arrival of paramedics was

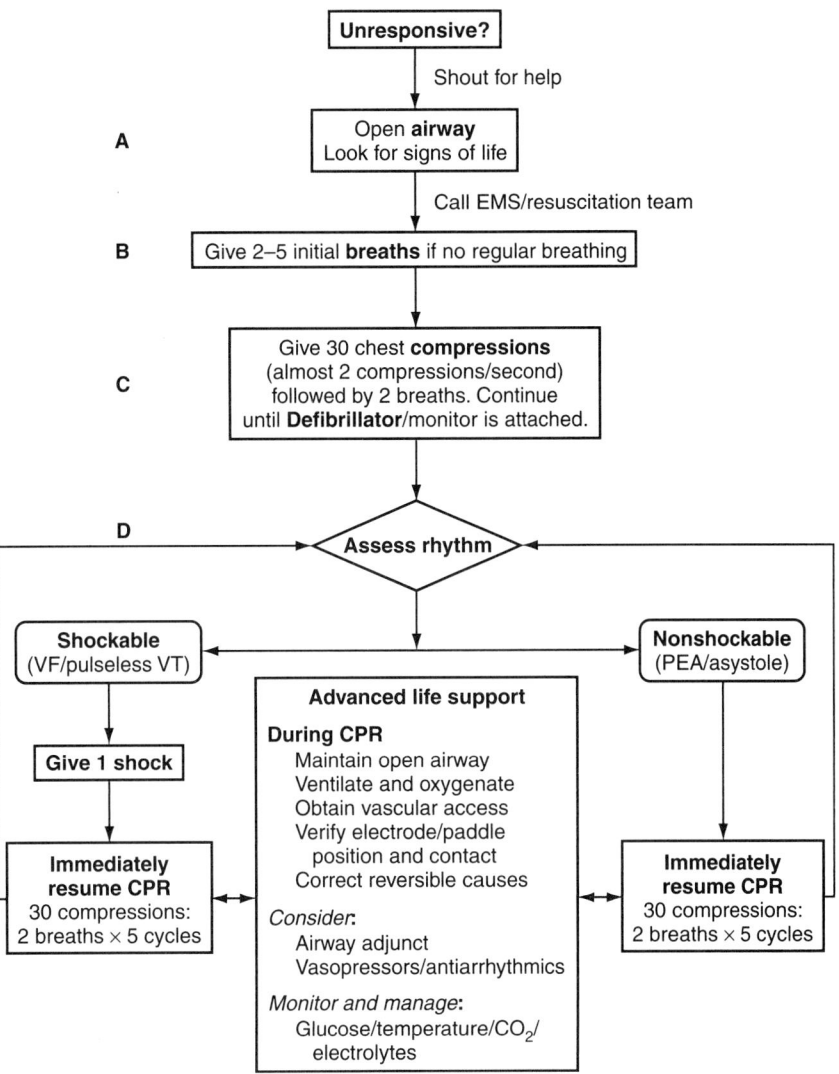

FIGURE 2. 2005 ILCOR universal cardiac arrest algorithm. CPR = cardiovascular resuscitation; PEA = pulseless electrical activity; VF = ventricular fibrillation; VT = ventricular tachycardia. (From Circulation 2005;112:1-11. Reprinted with permission.)

9.8 minutes. In another study of public access defibrillation (PAD) conducted in Seattle; 475 AEDs were placed in a variety of public settings, and more than 4000 persons were trained in CPR and AED operation. A total of 50 cases of cardiac arrest were treated by PAD before EMS arrival, representing 1.33% of all EMS-treated cardiac arrests in the county. Of the 50 patients treated by PAD, 25 (50%) patients survived to hospital discharge.

CARDIAC ARREST FROM PULSELESS ELECTRICAL ACTIVITY

PEA is defined by the presence of a heart rhythm that does not generate a pulse. Patients who are found in PEA generally have a poor prognosis but may be successfully resuscitated if a correctable cause is identified and treated promptly. Some correctable causes of PEA include:

1. Hypovolemia
2. Exsanguination
3. Tension pneumothorax
4. Acute pulmonary embolism
5. Cardiac tamponade from a pericardial effusion
6. Hypothermia
7. Hyperkalemia
8. Metabolic acidosis (preexisting)

Patients suspected to be hypovolemic from obvious bleeding should be resuscitated with volume expanders (normal saline, lactated Ringer's) and transfused as soon as blood is available. O negative blood (universal donor) may be transfused in patients in extremis. A tension pneumothorax results from a tear in the pleura that serves as a one-way valve, allowing air to enter but not leave the pleural space. This results in significant increase in pleural pressure and intrathoracic pressures. It should be suspected in patients with absence of breath sounds and a deviated trachea toward the contralateral lung. A large-bore needle may be inserted at the midclavicular line over the second rib to decompress the affected lung rapidly, followed by insertion of a chest tube. In selective cases an acute pulmonary embolism may be successfully treated with thrombolytic medication. Cardiac tamponade should be treated with a pericardiocentesis. Hypothermia may be treated with rewarming. Hyperkalemia should be treated with intravenous (IV) calcium, insulin and glucose, or sodium bicarbonate. Rapid assessment of these secondary causes and immediate treatment may be life saving in some patients who present with reversible causes of PEA.

CARDIAC ARREST CAUSED BY ASYSTOLE

Asystole is usually a terminal rhythm in cardiac arrest victims who have had a prolonged episode of hypoxia and ischemic injury.

External pacing has demonstrated no improvement in survival in patients who present in the field with asystole. Hyperkalemia is a reversible cause of asystole. Patients who present with asystole because of hyperkalemia may be successfully resuscitated with early bystander CPR and rapid treatment of hyperkalemia.

Pharmacologic Treatment in Cardiac Arrest

The primary goals in the successful resuscitation of a patient with cardiac arrest is to restore a rhythm that results in adequate perfusion of the two most vulnerable organs to hypoxemia, the heart and the brain, and maintain adequate perfusion to the heart and brain to prevent irreversible injury during the arrest until a rhythm and adequate hemodynamics are restored. To date, no randomized clinical trials have demonstrated an improvement in survival to hospital discharge among patients who have suffered a cardiac arrest attributable to any drugs currently used in advanced cardiac life support.

Drugs Used to Restore Rhythm

No randomized human studies have demonstrated that the use of antiarrhythmic agents in cardiac arrest improves survival to hospital discharge. Despite the lack of evidence supporting the role of antiarrhythmic agents, these agents are used routinely in shock refractory ventricular arrhythmias.

AMIODARONE

A randomized, double-blind, placebo-controlled study of IV amiodarone (Cordarone) in out-of-hospital cardiac arrest demonstrated an improvement in survival to hospitalization in patients treated with IV amiodarone versus placebo (44% vs. 34%; $p = 0.03$). This study demonstrated no difference in survival to hospital discharge (13.4% vs. 13.2%) but was not powered to evaluate this endpoint. Furthermore, there was no difference among survivors in the ability to resume independent living activities (55% vs. 50%). In another randomized, controlled study of amiodarone versus lidocaine in out-of-hospital cardiac arrest, amiodarone was superior to lidocaine in survival to hospitalization (22.8% vs. 12%; $p = 0.009$), but there was no difference in survival to hospital discharge.

LIDOCAINE

No randomized, placebo-controlled studies of lidocaine have been performed in out-of-hospital cardiac arrest. In one study with historical controls, lidocaine was associated with an improvement in return of spontaneous circulation and survival to hospitalization but not in survival to discharge. However, other studies have demonstrated no benefit in survival with lidocaine.

Drugs Used to Support Blood Pressure

Despite the standard use of vasopressors in cardiac arrest, there is a lack of clinical evidence demonstrating improved survival with these interventions.

EPINEPHRINE

Epinephrine is a mixed adrenergic agonist and acts on α-1, α-2, β-1 and β-2 adrenergic receptors. It is the α actions of epinephrine that provide the most benefit during resuscitation. Through its α actions, epinephrine increases coronary perfusion pressure and maintains peripheral vascular tone. The beta-adrenergic effects of epinephrine may be detrimental in patients during cardiac arrest. Stimulation of β-1 receptors results in an increase in myocardial oxygen consumption and decreases subendocardial perfusion.

There are no randomized trials of standard dose epinephrine versus placebo in cardiac arrest. Herlitz et al. compared 417 patients with out-of-hospital VF who received epinephrine (1 mg every 3 to 5 minutes) with 786 patients (historical control) who did not receive epinephrine. Although more patients had return of spontaneous circulation and survived to hospitalization when treated with epinephrine, there was no significant difference in survival to hospital discharge.

Evidence on high-dose epinephrine (5 to 15 mg) in cardiac arrest did not show a benefit in survival in out-of-hospital arrest. Although high-dose epinephrine is associated with a higher rate of return of spontaneous circulation, there is no difference in survival to discharge. These patients who survive to hospitalization are likely to have significant neurologic injury. Most of these patients do not survive to hospital discharge.

Despite the lack of clinical data demonstrating an improvement in survival with epinephrine in cardiac arrest, the ILCOR recommends the continued use of epinephrine at standard dose (1 mg every 3 to 5 minutes) on a routine basis for cardiac arrest. High-dose epinephrine is not recommended.

VASOPRESSIN

Vasopressin (Pitressin) is an endogenous vasopressor that causes selective vasoconstriction of resistance vessels. Although vasopressin appears to have pharmacologic properties well suited for cardiac arrest (increases vascular tone without β-adrenergic stimulation), clinical trials comparing vasopressin to epinephrine showed no difference in outcomes. However, in a study of vasopressin versus epinephrine in 1186 patients with cardiac arrest because of VF, PEA, or asystole, vasopressin was superior to epinephrine with the endpoint of survival to discharge in the subset of patients who had asystole (4.7% vs. 1.5%; $p = 0.04$). This study, like others, demonstrated no difference in survival to hospital discharge in the subset of patients who presented with VF or PEA.

The ILCOR concluded that "There is insufficient evidence to support or refute the use of vasopressin as an alternative to, or in combination with, epinephrine in any cardiac arrest rhythm." For the management of cardiac arrest because of VF refractory to defibrillation, asystole, or PEA, a dose of epinephrine (1 mg) IV may be repeated every 3 to 5 minutes. Vasopressin may substitute for the first or second dose of epinephrine. In patients who present with asystole, vasopressin may be preferred over epinephrine. Drugs should be administered without interruption of CPR.

Alternative Routes for Drug Administration

IV access cannot always be established during a resuscitation attempt. CPR and defibrillation should not be delayed to establish IV access. As an alternative to IV access, resuscitative drugs may be given via the endotracheal tube. Drugs that are absorbed via the trachea can be remembered by the mnemonic *navel*: *n*aloxone, *a*tropine, *v*asopressin, *e*pinephrine, and *l*idocaine. When drugs are administered via the endotracheal tube, two to three times the usual IV dose should be given to achieve the same serum levels.

Management and Evaluation of Survivors of Cardiac Arrest

The management of survivors of cardiac arrest begins with a continuous effort to identify the cause of the cardiac arrest at the onset of the resuscitation. After return of spontaneous rhythm and circulation, the patient should be monitored in an intensive care setting. During the initial period of hospitalization, the patient is vulnerable to cardiac arrhythmias and hemodynamic and respiratory instability. Patients are also prone to ongoing ischemic neurologic injury. Other issues encountered in the postarrest period include acute renal failure, shock liver, ischemic bowel, sepsis, and acute respiratory distress syndrome. The patients may require antiarrhythmic agents, inotropic support, and ventilatory support during the early period after a cardiac arrest. Frequent monitoring of arterial blood gas and electrolytes should be performed, and abnormalities should be corrected. Recent studies showed an improvement in neurologic outcomes in patients treated with hypothermia (32° to 34°C [90° to 93°F]) for 12 to 24 hours post-resuscitation. The ILCOR recommends therapeutic hypothermia in all patients who are unconscious for a period of 12 to 24 hours after a cardiac arrest.

The physician should begin a detailed history and physical examination. Family members should be contacted to see whether the patient had an advance directive. A myocardial infarction should be ruled out with an electrocardiogram (EKG) and serial cardiac enzymes, and a thorough review of available medical records including a complete review of current medications should be performed. Minimum initial workup should include a chest radiograph and laboratory evaluation (electrolytes, arterial blood gas, liver and renal function tests, and toxicology screening). An echocardiogram should be performed to assess the presence or absence of structural heart disease. Because the majority of all cardiac arrests occur in patients with significant coronary artery disease, coronary angiography should be performed in most patients who have suffered a cardiac arrest.

HISTORY

It is often difficult to obtain any history from the patient. If the patient is awake, he or she may have significant neurologic impairment and retrograde amnesia of events preceding the arrest. History taken from witnesses to the cardiac arrest and family members and friends close to the victim may be valuable. Important information gained from the history would include any recent medications, heart failure symptoms preceding the arrest, angina preceding the arrest, illicit drug use, and a family history of sudden death.

12-LEAD ELECTROCARDIOGRAM

A 12-lead EKG may demonstrate signs of myocardial ischemia or injury. Other findings on the 12-lead EKG include the presence of epsilon waves suggesting arrhythmogenic right ventricular cardiomyopathy; incomplete right bundle branch block with ST-segment elevations in the right precordial leads (suggestive of Brugada syndrome); a prolonged or abnormally short (<300 ms) QT segment, which may suggest long QT syndrome or short QT syndrome, respectively; ventricular pre-excitation because of a bypass tract; and severe conduction system disease (bifascicular block or evidence of heart block). The 12-lead EKG should be screened carefully for these abnormalities.

LABORATORY EVALUATION

Laboratory evaluation should include electrolytes, arterial blood gas, liver and renal function tests, serial cardiac enzymes, complete blood count, and a toxicology screen. The causal role of the abnormalities detected should be interpreted carefully. Hypokalemia may occur because of intracellular shifting of potassium secondary to endogenous catecholamines or epinephrine given during the cardiac arrest. Elevations in myocardial band enzymes of creatine phosphokinase (MB CK) and troponins indicate myocardial infarction; however, mild elevations in cardiac enzymes may result from prolonged CPR and defibrillation and may not be indicative of a primary myocardial infarction.

Other laboratory findings may be helpful in screening for end organ damage. Significant elevations in transaminases and elevated protime may be evidence of ischemic liver injury. Bloody stools and persistent lactic acidosis should increase the suspicion for ischemic bowel. Acute renal failure is commonly seen after an arrest.

ECHOCARDIOGRAM

An echocardiogram is essential in the workup of patients who have survived a cardiac arrest. The echocardiogram may detect evidence of hypertrophic cardiomyopathy, left ventricular dysfunction, regional wall motion abnormalities, abnormalities in the RV that might be suggestive of arrhythmogenic right ventricular cardiomyopathy, significant valvular disease, and other structural cardiac abnormalities. The presence of left ventricular dysfunction early postarrest may be because of "stunning" (caused by ischemia and defibrillation) and may not be representative of the patient's true left ventricular function.

CARDIAC CATHETERIZATION

Coronary angiography should be performed in most patients who have suffered a cardiac arrest to rule out significant epicardial coronary artery disease or congenital coronary anomalies.

ELECTROPHYSIOLOGIC STUDY

Currently, the electrophysiologic study in cardiac arrest victims has a limited role. However, an electrophysiologic study may be useful in a select group of patients: those with ventricular preexcitation (Wolff-Parkinson-White [WPW] pattern) on the EKG because the electrophysiologic study will allow characterization of the antero-grade conduction properties of the bypass tract and may offer a curative strategy; patients with suspected bundle branch reentry ventricular tachycardia, which occurs in patients with dilated cardiomyopathy; and provocative drug testing for concealed long QT syndrome (epinephrine), Brugada syndrome (sodium channel blocker), or significant His-Purkinje disease. The electrophysiologic study is not routinely indicated in patients who have suffered a cardiac arrest.

Neurologic Assessment

Patients who are unconscious after cardiac arrest require an assessment of the degree of irreversible global neurologic injury. Patients should be assessed while normothermic and after all sedation is withheld. Assessment of neurologic status in a comatose patient includes apnea testing and assessment of brainstem reflexes. Absence of reflexes and abnormal apnea testing is associated with a grim prognosis. Additional neurologic testing with excellent predictive accuracy includes a median nerve somatosensory evoked potential (SSEP) and an electroencephalogram (EEG). An abnormal SSEP assessed at 72 hours postresuscitation predicts a poor outcome with 100% specificity. An EEG may also be a useful prognostic tool.

Patients who are conscious may still suffer from varying degrees of amnesia, short term memory loss, and from motor or sensory deficits. They may require physical therapy, occupational therapy, speech therapy, and rehabilitation.

ROLE OF IMPLANTABLE CARDIAC DEFIBRILLATORS

Currently, most patients who are survivors of a ventricular fibrillation or ventricular tachycardia—related cardiac arrest are treated with an implantable cardiac defibrillator (ICD) even if there is an identifiable reversible cause. A randomized controlled study of amiodarone versus implantable cardiac defibrillator among cardiac arrest survivors (Antiarrhythmics Versus Implantable Defibrillators [AVID]) demonstrated a survival advantage in patients treated with an ICD. A subset analysis revealed that survival benefit was observed only in patients with ejection fraction (EF) less than 35%. Patients with EF more than 35% had no difference in survival whether treated with an ICD or amiodarone. Patients in AVID with reversible or correctable causes were excluded from and followed in a registry. The mortality among the 278 patients followed in the registry at 3 years was found to be higher than in patients who did not have transient or reversible causes. Contemporary practice is that most patients who have suffered a VT/VF cardiac arrest are treated with an ICD regardless of whether their arrest was because of a transient or reversible cause and regardless of their EF. An important exception are patients with preserved left ventricular function who had a VT/VF arrest within 72 hours of an acute transmural myocardial infarction. These patients have a low recurrence rate of cardiac arrest if they have no evidence of residual ischemia and preserved left ventricular function. Amiodarone is a reasonable option for patients with preserved EF with contraindications for an ICD.

Some situations where an ICD may not be appropriate are patients who have a cardiac arrest less than 72 hours after a transmural myocardial infarction, patients who do not wish to have an ICD, patients who had a cardiac arrest because of rapidly conducting atrial fibrillation via a bypass tract (WPW) that was treated successfully with a radiofrequency ablation procedure, and patients of advanced age and significant co-morbidities (the risks and benefits of ICD implantation should be carefully considered in such patients).

Cardiac arrest is a major public health concern killing hundreds of thousands of people annually in the United States. The cornerstone of treatment of patients suffering a cardiac arrest is early recognition, early activation of EMS, early bystander CPR, early defibrillation, and advanced cardiac life support. Despite our best efforts, the prognosis of cardiac arrest victims remains poor. Recent advances in the science of resuscitation have provided grounds to make some significant changes to the guidelines for resuscitation of cardiac arrest. Communities with a well-established EMS system, public access defibrillation programs, and citizens who are well educated in basic life support have the highest rates of survival for cardiac arrest victims.

REFERENCES

Antiarrhythmics versus implantable defibrillators (AVID) investigators: A comparison of antiarrhythmic-drug therapy with implantable defibrillators in patients resuscitated from near-fatal ventricular arrhythmias. N Engl J Med 1997;337:1576–1583.
Cobb LA, Fahrenbruch CE, Walsh TR, et al: Influence of cardiopulmonary resuscitation prior to defibrillation in patients with out-of-hospital ventricular fibrillation. JAMA 1999;281:1182–1188.
Connolly SJ, Hallstrom AP, Cappato R, et al: Meta-analysis of the implantable cardioverter defibrillator secondary prevention trials. Eur Heart J 2000;21:2071–2078.
Cully CL, Rea TD, Murray JA, et al: Public access defibrillation in out-of-hospital cardiac arrest. Circulation 2004;109:1859–1863.
Dorian P, Cass D, Schwartz B, et al: Amiodarone as compared with lidocaine for shock-resistant ventricular fibrillation. N Engl J Med 2002;346:884–890.
2005 International consensus on cardiopulmonary resuscitation (CPR) and emergency cardiovascular care (ECC) science with treatment recommendations. Circulation 2005;112:1–11.
Kudenchuk PJ, Cobb LA, Copass MK, et al: Amiodarone for resuscitation after out-of-hospital cardiac arrest due to ventricular fibrillation. N Engl J Med 1999;341:871–878.
Page RL, Joglar JA, Kowal RC, et al: Use of automated external defibrillators by a US airline, N Engl J Med 2000;343:1210–1216.
Pepe PE, Fowler RL, Roppolo LP, et al: Clinical review: Reappraising the concept of immediate defibrillatory attempts for out-of-hospital ventricular fibrillation. Crit Care 2004;8:41–45.
Rea TD, Eisenberg MS, Sinibaldi G, et al: Incidence of EMS-treated out-of-hospital cardiac arrest in the United States. Resuscitation 2004;63:17–24.
Wyse DG, Friedman PL, Brodsky MA, et al: Life threatening ventricular arrhythmias due to transient or correctable causes: high risk for death in follow-up. J Am Col Cardiol 2001;38:1718–1724.
Zhong J, Dorian P: Epinephrine and vasopressin during cardiopulmonary resuscitation. Resuscitation 2005;66:263–269.

Atrial Fibrillation

Method of
Anne B. Curtis, MD

Atrial fibrillation (AF) is the most common arrhythmia seen in clinical practice, and it accounts for about one third of hospitalizations for cardiac arrhythmias. The prevalence of AF is 0.4% to 1.0% in the general population, but it increases to about 8% in those older than 80 years. More than 2.3 million people in the United States are estimated to have AF.

Classification

Paroxysmal AF is AF that begins and terminates spontaneously. *Persistent* AF is AF that lasts longer than 7 days or requires intervention, either pharmacologic treatment or electrical cardioversion, to restore sinus rhythm. AF is *permanent* when the arrhythmia has failed to respond to cardioversion or when attempts to restore sinus rhythm have been abandoned.

Presentation

Patients may or may not have symptoms with AF. If they do, they may complain of palpitations, shortness of breath, exercise intolerance, chest discomfort, or fatigue. Many patients have symptomatic as well as asymptomatic episodes of AF, as demonstrated from arrhythmia logs in permanent pacemakers.

AF increases the risk of stroke and impairs quality of life. It is often found in patients with valvular heart disease, particularly mitral valve disease, and is found in many patients with heart failure from any etiology.

Clinical Evaluation

The most common finding on physical examination in a patient with AF is an irregular pulse. The S1 can vary in intensity, an S3 may be

 CURRENT DIAGNOSIS

Minimum Evaluation

- Detailed history and physical examination
- 12-lead electrocardiogram
- Transthoracic echocardiogram
- Laboratory tests including thyroid function tests

Additional Tests

- 24-hour Holter monitor or event monitor (to establish diagnosis or to assess rate or rhythm control)
- Exercise testing (to assess adequacy of rate control, reproduce exercise-induced atrial fibrillation, or exclude ischemia)
- Transesophageal echocardiogram (to evaluate for thrombus in the left atrial appendage before cardioversion)

present if there is coexisting heart failure, and an S4 is absent. The A wave is absent in the jugular venous pulse.

When a patient presents with AF, initial evaluation beyond a history and physical examination should include an electrocardiogram and a transthoracic echocardiogram and routine blood chemistries including thyroid function tests. The electrocardiogram (ECG) shows an absence of P waves and irregular R-R intervals. An echocardiogram is useful to evaluate the patient for valvular heart disease, assess left ventricular function, and measure left atrial size. Event monitors may be used to confirm the diagnosis of AF in patients with unexplained palpitations. Holter monitors and exercise stress tests may be useful in assessing the adequacy of rate control in patients with persistent or permanent AF. For a first episode of AF, reversible causes such as pericarditis, pulmonary embolism, or hyperthyroidism, among others, should be considered.

Treatment

When the diagnosis of AF has been established, several decisions must be made regarding patient management. First, the patient should be evaluated for the risk of thromboembolism, and anticoagulation should be initiated as appropriate. Second, a decision must be made about the need for treatment. If treatment is needed, a decision is needed as to whether rate control or rhythm control should be the initial management strategy.

ANTICOAGULATION

The most useful scheme for stratification of patients for risk of thromboembolism is the CHADS$_2$ score (Table 1). In this approach, one point each is assigned for the presence of congestive heart failure, hypertension, age (>75 years), and diabetes mellitus, and two points are assigned for a history of stroke or transient ischemic attack. Patients with no risk factors for thromboembolism do not need anticoagulation with warfarin (Coumadin). They may be managed with aspirin 81 to 325 mg daily. Patients with a CHADS score greater than or equal to 2 and patients with rheumatic mitral stenosis should be managed with adjusted-dose warfarin to achieve an international normalized ratio (INR) of 2 to 3. For patients with a CHADS score of 1, anticoagulation with either aspirin or warfarin is reasonable. Patients with AF and no risk factors do not need anticoagulation.

The decision whether and how to anticoagulate should be made on the basis of an assessment of risk factors and not on the type of AF, because there is no evidence that the risk of thromboembolism is different in patients with paroxysmal versus permanent AF. Patients with atrial flutter, although they appear to have a somewhat lower risk of thromboembolism compared with patients with AF, should still receive anticoagulation based on the considerations outlined earlier.

A recent study showed that bleeding risks in elderly patients given warfarin may be higher than previously appreciated, creating some challenges in managing these patients. Elderly patients who are given warfarin should be followed very closely after the drug is initiated because the risk of hemorrhage is highest in the initial months of treatment.

RATE VERSUS RHYTHM CONTROL

When AF is diagnosed, a decision must be made about the management approach. A patient with a first episode of AF that terminates spontaneously or after cardioversion might need no specific therapy aside from consideration of anticoagulation. For patients with recurrent AF, the management approach should be determined based on the patient's symptoms and underlying heart disease. There have been several randomized trials of rate versus rhythm-control strategies for the management of AF. The two largest, the Atrial Fibrillation Follow-up Investigation of Rhythm Management (AFFIRM) and the Rate Control vs. Electrical Cardioversion (RACE) trials, found no significant difference in morbidity or mortality with either strategy. Generally speaking, patients with minimal symptoms or long-standing AF are best managed with a rate-control strategy, and highly symptomatic patients benefit most from a rhythm-control approach.

Rate Control

Rate control often must be initiated first in any patient presenting with AF, regardless of whether the ultimate goal is rhythm control or rate control, in order to control symptoms from an elevated heart rate. Particularly in elderly patients with minimal to no symptoms from AF, rate control may be the preferred long-term strategy. The goal for heart rate control should be 60 to 80 bpm at rest and 90 to 115 bpm with moderate exercise.

For acute management of the ventricular response in AF, either intravenous β-blockers or non–dihydropyridine calcium channel blockers (diltiazem [Cardizem] or verapamil) may be used. The same drugs may be used orally for long-term control of heart rate in patients with persistent or permanent AF (Box 1). Digoxin (Lanoxin) is not the best choice as a sole agent for controlling the ventricular response in patients with paroxysmal AF. However, it is useful for controlling resting heart rate in sedentary patients or patients with heart failure. In addition, digoxin may be added to other atrioventricular (AV) nodal blockers if heart rate control is not adequate with single agents. Although amiodarone can slow the heart rate in patients with AF, it is not advisable to use this drug for the long term solely for the purpose of rate control because of the side effects potentially associated with its use.

Rhythm Control

The approach to rhythm control in AF depends heavily on the patient's symptoms, the frequency of recurrences, and any underlying

TABLE 1 The CHADS$_2$ Score for Assessing Risk of Thromboembolism in Patients with Nonvalvular Atrial Fibrillation

Risk Criterion	Score
Cardiac failure	1
Hypertension	1
Age >75 years	1
Diabetes mellitus	1
Stroke or prior transient ischemic attack	2

CURRENT THERAPY

Stroke Prevention
- Aspirin
- Warfarin (Coumadin)

Rate Control
- β-Blockers
- Non-dihydropyridine calcium channel blockers: Diltiazem, verapamil
- Digoxin (Lanoxin)
- AV junction ablation and permanent pacemaker

Rhythm Control
- Cardioversion: Electrical and pharmacologic
- Antiarrhythmic drugs
- Atrial fibrillation ablation
- Surgical maze procedure

BOX 1 Long-Term Treatment Options

Stroke Prevention
Aspirin 325 mg/d
Warfarin (Coumadin) (dosed for target INR of 2-3)

Rate Control
Pharmacologic
β-Blockers
- Atenolol (Tenormin) (PO)
- Esmolol (Brevibloc) (IV)
- Metoprolol (Lopressor) (PO or IV; IV drip available)

Calcium channel blockers
- Diltiazem (Cardizem) (PO or IV; IV drip available)
- Digoxin (Lanoxin) (PO or IV)
- Verapamil (Calan) (PO or IV)

Nonpharmacologic
AV junction ablation and pacemaker

Rhythm Control
Antiarrhythmic Drugs*
Amiodarone (Cordarone) 100-400 mg/d
Propafenone (Rythmol) 150-300 mg tid (450-900 mg daily)
Propafenone (Rythmol SR) 225-425 mg bid (450-850 mg daily)
Flecainide (Tambocor) 50-150 mg bid (100-300 mg daily)
Sotalol (Betapace) 80-160 mg bid (160-320 mg daily)
Dofetilide (Tikosyn) 125-500 μg bid (250-1000 μg daily)

Nonpharmacologic Treatment
Catheter ablation
Surgical maze procedure

---

*Quinidine, procainamide, and disopyramide (Norpace) are rarely used anymore for long-term treatment unless patients are intolerant of amiodarone.
AV = atrioventricular; INR = international normalized ratio.

---

structural heart disease (Table 2). For patients with an initial episode of AF or rare recurrences of AF, particularly those that terminate spontaneously, no specific therapy to control rhythm may be indicated. For patients who have occasional episodes of symptomatic AF in the setting of a structurally normal heart or only mild left ventricular hypertrophy, an excellent option is the pill-in-the-pocket approach. A patient may take either flecainide (Tambocor) 300 mg or propafenone (Rythmol) 600 mg[3] orally as a single dose. It may be best to give either of these drugs in a monitored setting the first time they are administered, in case there are side effects such as marked sinus arrest on termination of AF.

For management of recurrent AF, the presence of underlying heart disease dictates to a large extent the choice of antiarrhythmic drug therapy. Patients with normal hearts or at most mild left ventricular hypertrophy may be treated with flecainide or propafenone orally. Propafenone has β-blocking properties, so it may be used as a sole agent. It is particularly attractive in its sustained-release preparation, in which it is dosed twice daily. Because flecainide has no AV nodal blocking properties, it is usually given in conjunction with either a β-blocker or a calcium channel blocker. Both drugs are usually well tolerated, with minimal extracardiac side effects, and neither prolongs the QT interval. An alternative antiarrhythmic drug in this setting is sotalol (Betapace), which has β-blocking properties as well and can prolong the QT interval. Sotalol is particularly attractive as an initial choice of antiarrhythmic drug therapy in patients with coronary artery disease and preserved ventricular function, both because of its β-blocking properties and because flecainide and propafenone are not recommended in patients with established ischemic heart disease.

When these drugs are ineffective or not tolerated, either amiodarone (Cordarone) or dofetilide (Tikosyn) can be used. However, catheter ablation is now considered an acceptable alternative management approach in such patients when initial antiarrhythmic drug therapy fails to control symptoms.

For patients with heart failure, amiodarone and dofetilide are the drugs of choice for rhythm control. The latter requires in-hospital initiation because of the slight risk of QT prolongation and torsades de pointes. Patients with significant left ventricular hypertrophy should also be treated with amiodarone for rhythm control.

CATHETER ABLATION

One of the most important changes in the 2006 Guidelines for the Management of Patients with Atrial Fibrillation was the elevation of catheter ablation from its status as a last-resort therapeutic approach after failure of all antiarrhythmic drugs (including amiodarone) to a coequal option with amiodarone. The reasons for the change include the increasing success rate with catheter ablation and the better understanding and standardization of the procedure itself.

In the course of management of a patient with AF, when one would recommend catheter ablation depends on the type of AF, the presence and severity of underlying heart disease, and the comorbidities of the patient. An ideal candidate is a patient younger than 60 years with paroxysmal AF and a structurally normal heart. In such cases, pulmonary vein isolation alone is often sufficient to cure AF, with success rates approaching 85% to 90% if one includes patients who require second procedures.

Patients with persistent or permanent AF usually require more than just pulmonary vein isolation, with additional ablation lines in both atria and ablation of complex fractionated electrograms as well, depending on the approach in the particular electrophysiology laboratory. Success rates for these patients for an initial procedure are much lower than for patients with paroxysmal AF, often around 33% even in experienced laboratories.

At present, catheter ablation for AF is not recommended solely for the purpose of allowing discontinuation of anticoagulation with warfarin. Long-term studies have not yet been done to show that this approach is safe, and the procedure itself has a number of potentially serious complications associated with it.

Surgical maze procedures have success rates similar to those for catheter-based procedures for AF. Because surgery is more invasive, surgical procedures for management of AF are most often performed

---

TABLE 2 Guidelines for Choosing Antiarrhythmic Drugs

Underlying Disorder	First Line	Second Line
No structural heart disease	Flecainide (Tambocor) Propafenone (Rythmol) Sotalol (Betapace)	Amiodarone (Cordarone) Dofetilide (Tikosyn)
Left ventricular dysfunction	Amiodarone Dofetilide	
Coronary artery disease	Sotalol	Amiodarone Dofetilide
Hypertension with left ventricular hypertrophy <1.4 cm	Flecainide Propafenone	Amiodarone Dofetilide Sotalol
Hypertension with left ventricular hypertrophy >1.4 cm	Amiodarone	

---

[3]Exceeds dosage recommended by the manufacturer.

TABLE 3 Advantages and Disadvantages of Different Approaches to Cardioversion

Method	Advantages	Disadvantages
Electrical (direct current; 200-J biphasic shocks)	Rapid conversion to sinus rhythm	Need for general anesthesia Early recurrence
Ibutilide, 1 mg IV; may repeat one time	No need for general anesthesia	Requires ECG monitoring for at least 4 hours after administration
Flecainide 300 mg PO or propafenone 600 mg PO[3]	No need for general anesthesia Outpatient use (consider observation of response in-hospital for first use)	Effect may be delayed for several hours
Amiodarone IV	No need for general anesthesia Prevention of early recurrence Ideal in postoperative setting	Delayed onset of action

[3]Exceeds dosage recommended by the manufacturer.
ECG = electrocardiogram.

in conjunction with cardiac surgery for another reason, such as mitral valve repair for mitral regurgitation.

PACING

In patients who have the tachy–brady syndrome manifested as sinus bradycardia alternating with AF, permanent pacemakers are often considered for managing the bradycardia, and antiarrhythmic drugs and AV nodal blockers are used to manage the tachycardia. Given the success of radiofrequency ablation for cure of paroxysmal AF in patients without significant structural heart disease, ablation should be considered as an initial approach instead of a pacemaker if medical therapy fails, particularly in younger patients.

A number of pacing algorithms have been investigated for preventing AF in order to suppress bradycardia or pauses that can promote the development of AF. None of these approaches has been demonstrated to have a significant impact on AF burden, and so pacemaker therapy cannot be recommended solely for that purpose.

Ablation of the AV node with permanent pacing has fallen out of favor to a large extent, particularly for paroxysmal AF, where curative ablation is preferred. AV node ablation might still be a viable option in patients with existing pacemakers and uncontrollable heart rates from AF, especially when there are significant comorbidities that make a prolonged catheter ablation procedure unattractive.

CARDIOVERSION

Patients who present with AF that does not convert spontaneously may be candidates for cardioversion. If the onset of AF can confidently be determined to have been within 48 hours of presentation, and if anticoagulation with heparin is instituted promptly, one may proceed with cardioversion immediately. If patients are hemodynamically unstable or experiencing acute ischemia from elevated rates in AF, cardioversion should also be performed without delay.

There are several options for cardioversion (Table 3). Electrical cardioversion requires general anesthesia. It should be performed with patches placed in an anterior–posterior configuration, and 200-J biphasic shocks are recommended initially to maximize the chances of conversion to sinus rhythm with a minimal number of shocks. Ibutilide (Corvert) can be used intravenously if the patient has a normal QT interval. Monitoring of the patient must be continued for at least 4 hours after conversion to sinus rhythm, because there is a risk of torsades de pointes if significant QT prolongation occurs. Oral flecainide or propafenone can be administered if the patient has minimal heart disease. These drugs do not prolong the QT interval, so they pose no risk of torsades de pointes. An additional advantage of these drugs is that the patient can be observed in a monitored situation as sinus rhythm is restored. If there are no untoward side effects, such as marked sinus arrest on termination of AF, patients can be given a prescription for either drug to use in the future for recurrent AF according to the pill-in-the-pocket approach. Finally, intravenous amiodarone is another option for chemical cardioversion. Conversion to sinus rhythm may be delayed, but this is a good option for patients in intensive care settings who need ongoing suppression of AF after cardioversion.

If the duration of AF cannot be determined, or if it is known to be longer than 48 hours without adequate anticoagulation, there are two options. A transesophageal echocardiogram can be performed to rule out the presence of thrombus in the left atrium. A transthoracic echocardiogram is inadequate for this purpose. If no clot is seen, cardioversion may be performed, with the patient subsequently anticoagulated with warfarin for a minimum of 4 weeks afterward. Alternatively, the patient may be anticoagulated with warfarin for at least 3 weeks with documented therapeutic INRs before cardioversion, without a transesophageal echocardiogram, followed again by a minimum of 4 weeks of anticoagulation.

POSTOPERATIVE ATRIAL FIBRILLATION

AF commonly occurs postoperatively, especially after cardiothoracic surgery. Both sotalol and amiodarone have been shown to reduce the incidence of AF when used prophylactically. β-Blockers have also been shown to be effective in preventing AF in the postoperative setting. Amiodarone is usually used when AF occurs postoperatively and requires treatment, because it can be given intravenously and has a high efficacy rate.

REFERENCES

Alboni P, Botto GL, Baldi N, et al: Outpatient treatment of recent-onset atrial fibrillation with the "pill-in-the-pocket" approach. N Engl J Med 2004;351:2384-2391.

Atrial Fibrillation Follow-up Investigation of Rhythm Management (AFFIRM) Investigators: A comparison of rate control and rhythm control in patients with atrial fibrillation. N Engl J Med 2002;347:1825-1833.

Calkins H, Brugada J, Packer DL, et al. HRS/EHRA/ECAS Expert Consensus Statement on catheter and surgical ablation of atrial fibrillation: recommendations for personnel, policy, procedures and follow-up. A report of the Heart Rhythm Society (HRS) Task Force on catheter and surgical ablation of atrial fibrillation. Heart Rhythm 2007;4:816-861.

Fuster V, Ryden LE, Cannom DS, et al: ACC/AHA/ESC 2006 Guidelines for the Management of Patients with Atrial Fibrillation—Executive Summary. Circulation 2006;114:700-752.

Hylek EM, Evans-Molina C, Shea C, et al: Major hemorrhage and tolerability of warfarin in the first year of therapy among elderly patients with atrial fibrillation. Circulation 2007;115:2689-2696.

Van Gelder IC, Hagens VE, Bosker HA, et al: A comparison of rate control and rhythm control in patients with recurrent persistent atrial fibrillation. N Engl J Med 2002;347:1834-1840.

Van Walraven WC, Hart RG, Wells GA, et al: A clinical prediction rule to identify patients with atrial fibrillation and a low risk for stroke while taking aspirin. Arch Intern Med 2003;163:936-943.

Premature Beats

Method of
*Prakash C. Deedwania, MD, and
Enrique V. Carbajal, MD*

Premature beats are the most common form of cardiac arrhythmia encountered in clinical practice. Premature beats are one of the most common causes of irregular pulse and palpitations. In many instances, premature beats are not associated with any symptoms. They result from electrical depolarization of myocardium that occurs earlier than the sinus impulse. Premature beats have been referred to by a variety of names, including premature contractions, premature complexes, ectopic beats, and early depolarizations. Although no single term is ideal, most electrophysiologists refer to them as premature complexes because although the term *ectopic beat* denotes the abnormal site of origin of the depolarization, it does not necessarily require the beat to be premature, and, in some cases, ectopic rhythm indeed occurs as an escape phenomenon.

Although premature beats generally occur in patients with organic heart disease, they frequently can be seen in the absence of any structural heart disease, especially in elderly patients. Premature beats can be triggered by, or increase in frequency with, myocardial ischemia and heart failure. Premature beats can be provoked by, or occur in association with, a variety of systemic abnormalities, including electrolyte disturbances, acid-base imbalance, toxins from recreational drug and/or alcohol abuse, metabolic perturbations, systemic illnesses such as thyroid disorders, pulmonary disease, infections, and febrile illnesses, and any condition associated with increased catecholamine levels.

Most premature beats occur as a result of enhanced automaticity, but other electrophysiologic mechanisms, including reentry and triggered activity, might play a role. Based on the corresponding site of origin, premature electrical depolarizations are called *premature atrial complexes* (PACs), *premature junctional complexes* (PJCs), and *premature ventricular complexes* (PVCs). Morphologic features and timing of the premature beat on electrocardiographic (ECG) recording(s) help determine the site of origin and the nature of premature complexes. Premature beats can occur in a repetitive fashion as *bigeminy* (after every other normal beat), *trigeminy* (after each sequence of two normal beats), or *quadrigeminy* (after each sequence of three normal beats). They also can occur as two or three successive premature beats, defined as *couplets* and *triplets*, respectively. In this article, the primary focus is on single premature beats.

Premature Atrial Complexes

PACs are the most common form of atrial arrhythmias that can originate at any site in the atria. The exact morphology of the atrial activation (P wave) varies depending on the site of origin of the PAC. Careful and systematic examination of the ECG features of PACs usually can distinguish them from PVCs.

ELECTROCARDIOGRAPHIC FEATURES

The cardinal features of PACs include their prematurity with reference to sinus beats, abnormal P wave morphology, and, in most cases, QRS morphology that is similar to that of sinus beats. The P wave morphology of the PAC generally differs from the sinus P wave unless the premature complex originates in the high right atrial area adjacent to the sinus node, in which case distinguishing PACs from sinus arrhythmia may be difficult. Although sinus arrhythmias are generally phasic in nature, being influenced by the respiratory cycle, this feature would be helpful in differentiating from high right atrial PACs only when the PACs are frequent and repetitive. When the PAC occurs quite early in the diastolic phase, the P wave

CURRENT DIAGNOSIS

- Premature beats are identified by their occurrence at times considerably shorter than the regular sinus rhythm cycles.
- The origin of the premature beats is determined by the presence or absence of P waves, morphology of the P wave (when present), QRS configuration, and the presence or absence of a compensatory period.
- The presence of frequent PVCs (≥ 10 per hour) during the postdischarge evaluation of survivors of acute MI predicts increased risk of arrhythmic death and overall cardiac mortality.

may not be obvious on surface ECG because it is often hidden in the preceding T wave and would be evident only by watching carefully for the notched or peaked T wave.

If the PAC is too premature, it might fail to conduct to the ventricles if the atrioventricular (AV) node is refractory owing to conduction of the preceding sinus impulse. Such nonconducted PACs are called *blocked PACs*, and they are important because they can be confused with instances of AV block. Such erroneous interpretation can be avoided by simply remembering a common rule of thumb that requires normal successive P-P intervals for all sinus beats, including the interval for a blocked P wave, before considering the diagnosis of AV block. Although most PACs have a normal or prolonged PR interval, the relationship of the PAC to the subsequent QRS complex depends on the site of origin of the PAC and the prematurity index. For example, a PAC originating in the lower atrial area near the AV node generally has a shorter PR interval, whereas a PAC that is quite premature and originates in the upper left atrial area might have a longer than usual PR interval. In general, the PR interval of a PAC is inversely related to its prematurity.

Because most PACs are able to depolarize the sinus node, they usually can reset the sinus automaticity; therefore, the subsequent pause following most PACs is generally less than compensatory because the sinus node fires earlier than expected. In this case, measurement of the P-P interval between the sinus P wave preceding the PAC and the P wave following the PAC is generally less than twice the basic sinus cycle length. This is in contrast to the full compensatory pause often observed in conjunction with PVCs. In some cases, the PAC collides with the sinus impulse in the perinodal tissue and thus fails to reset the sinus node, thereby resulting in a full compensatory pause.

In general, electrical depolarization below the AV node is normal with PAC and results in an unchanged (baseline) QRS complex. Aberrant conduction, however, may be encountered when the PAC reaches the infranodal tissue during the period when it is still partially refractory. Most frequently, the aberrant conduction usually occurs when a short coupled PAC follows a long pause in patients with sinus bradycardia (long-short cycle). This usually results in a right bundle-branch block pattern and is commonly referred to as the *Ashman phenomenon*.

CLINICAL FEATURES

Although PACs can occur in normal individuals of all ages, they are quite infrequent except in the elderly. Their frequency increases with age; as many as 50% to 70% of the elderly may have occasional PACs. Some elderly individuals without organic heart disease have frequent PACs and occasionally atrial bigeminy or two to three PACs in a row. Whether the increased frequency of PACs in these individuals is secondary to senile amyloidosis, myocardial fibrosis, or diastolic dysfunction secondary to aging-related changes in the heart is not known. PACs are extremely common in patients with heart disease and in patients with acute as well as chronic respiratory failure.

The frequency of PACs can increase markedly during periods of acute febrile illness, shock states, and metabolic disorders, especially in patients with hyperthyroidism and conditions associated with increased catecholamine levels. Use of excessive caffeine, alcohol, tobacco, and recreational drugs can increase the frequency of PACs. In patients with acute myocardial infarction (MI), frequent PACs usually are precursors of atrial fibrillation and occur in association with ventricular failure. In general, the presence of frequent PACs in the setting of acute MI is an indicator of poor prognosis.

In general, PACs are benign except when they are a marker of an underlying cardiopulmonary disorder(s). The major clinical importance of PACs is related to the increased risk of atrial tachyarrhythmias in patients with an established history of such arrhythmias as well as in the elderly who are generally at high risk for atrial fibrillation. As indicated earlier, in rare instances the blocked PACs may be confused with episodes of AV nodal block; however, careful examination of the ECG features described previously easily establishes the correct diagnosis and avoids unnecessary pacemaker implantation.

TREATMENT

The correction of an underlying structural cardiopulmonary disorder and other precipitating factors (e.g., electrolyte or metabolic abnormalities) usually is all the treatment that is needed. No specific treatment is generally required in most patients because PACs usually are benign except in patients with a history of recurrent atrial tachyarrhythmias, for example, atrial flutter/fibrillation. In such patients, specific treatment may be indicated and could include a β-blocker or a heart rate-modulating calcium channel blocking agent such as verapamil (Calan) or diltiazem (Cardizem). Recent studies have shown that verapamil is quite effective in patients with frequent PACs and multifocal atrial tachycardia in the setting of acute or chronic ventilatory insufficiency. In patients who are at risk for recurrent atrial fibrillation, treatment with a specific antiarrhythmic agent, such as propafenone (Rythmol) or flecainide (Tambocor), may be beneficial; however, these drugs should be used only when the patient has a history of recurrent atrial flutter/fibrillation because of the increased risk of proarrhythmia, especially in the presence of organic heart disease such as recurrent ischemia or heart failure.

Premature Junctional Complexes

PJCs are rarely seen in normal individuals and are infrequently encountered even in patients with organic heart disease. When present, PJCs can occur due to abnormal automaticity or reentry phenomenon. Although digitalis toxicity is cited as a common etiologic factor, PJCs also can occur in the setting of MI, myocarditis, and electrolyte/metabolic disturbances.

ELECTROCARDIOGRAPHIC FEATURES

The ECG characteristics of PJCs are distinct from those of PACs in that the P wave usually is inverted in the inferior leads (II, III, and aVF) because of retrograde conduction to the atria from the ectopic foci in the junctional area. The second feature of PJCs is that the PR interval almost always is shorter than the normal PR interval because of the proximity of ectopic foci to the AV node and bundle of His. In most cases, the P wave might not even be visible on surface ECGs because it lies hidden within the QRS complex. Rarely, the P wave precedes the QRS complex when the ectopic impulse traverses the atria before traveling down to depolarize the ventricle. In general, the infranodal conduction of PJCs is normal, and thus the QRS morphology of the conducted PJCs is similar to that noted during sinus rhythm. When the PJC is closely coupled to the preceding sinus beat, aberrant conduction might occur if the impulse traverses down the bundle branch during the relative refractory period (most frequently manifesting as a right bundle-branch block pattern). Because in many instances no obvious P wave accompanies a PJC, aberrantly conducted PJCs may be hard to differentiate from PVCs.

In some instances when PJCs occur during the period when the AV node as well as the infranodal conduction systems both are refractory, the PJC may encounter both retrograde and antegrade blocks for impulse propagation. In such situations, no P wave or QRS complex is related tothe PJC. Although the ectopic impulse would be invisible on a surface ECG, it would penetrate a portion of the conduction system and thus make it partially or completely refractory to conduction of the subsequent sinus impulse. This would be manifested as a sudden prolongation of subsequent PR interval in case of partial refractoriness or as an episode of "pseudo AV nodal block" due to the blocked sinus beat if the infranodal tissue were unable to conduct the sinus impulse. Thus, even though some PJCs might not have any surface ECG complexes, their presence can be suspected based on their influence on the conduction of the following sinus beat owing to the electrophysiologic phenomenon described as "concealed conduction."

CLINICAL FEATURES

PJCs usually are not seen in normal persons and are rarely encountered in cardiac patients except in the setting of digitalis intoxication and infrequently in the setting of MI or myocarditis. In patients with digitalis toxicity, PJCs may lead to junctional tachycardia, occasionally resulting in palpitation, but are rarely associated with hemodynamic compromise. Because in some cases concealed conduction of PJCs might result in periods of varying degrees of pseudo AV blocks, it is clinically important to recognize their presence in order to prevent undue concern and avoid inappropriate pacemaker implantation.

Premature Ventricular Complexes

PVCs are the most common form of arrhythmia and can be encountered frequently in both healthy individuals as well as in patients with a variety of cardiac disorders. PVCs are often triggered by electrolyte abnormalities, acid-base imbalance, metabolic perturbations, hypoxia, and ischemia.

ELECTROCARDIOGRAPHIC FEATURES

PVCs occur as a result of premature depolarization of the ventricles due to ectopic foci in the ventricular myocardium or Purkinje fibers. In general, PVCs result in wide QRS complexes with the T wave axis usually opposite to that of the QRS. In the vast majority of cases,

CURRENT THERAPY

- In general, premature beats in patients without evidence of organic heart disease do not require any specific antiarrhythmic therapy because generally there is no significant increased risk of life-threatening arrhythmia.
- Correction of any underlying structural cardiopulmonary disorder and other precipitating factors (e.g., electrolyte or metabolic abnormalities).
- Suppression of PVCs using currently available antiarrhythmic drugs (except for amiodarone) is notadvisable for most patients primarily because of the increased risk of proarrhythmic effects of these drugs.
- In the occasional patient who is disabled by annoying symptoms due to PVCs, a trial of β-blocker therapy should be considered and often is effective in many patients.

PVCs do not conduct retrogradely and thus do not result in a distinct P wave. The sinus beats may, however, continue uninterrupted and thus manifest as an instance of AV dissociation in conjunction with PVCs. For the same reason, because PVCs usually do not conduct retrogradely and depolarize the atrium and the sinus node, there usually is a full compensatory pause in contrast to the partial compensatory pause generally seen with PACs. In patients with slow sinus rates, however, interpolated PVCs might occur. If the ectopic foci for PVCs are located high in the His-Purkinje system, the resulting premature complexes may have a narrow QRS morphology quite similar to that seen during sinus rhythm. Additionally, if the PVCs occur rather late, in close proximity to the sinus impulse, there may also be a narrow complex QRS because of fusion between the normal depolarization due to sinus impulse and the abnormal activation sequence from the ectopic foci. In the instance of fusion beats, a normal P wave precedes the QRS. The PR interval is shorter, and the QRS morphology may be only partially altered. In some cases, this might give the appearance of an intermittent bundle-branch block or preexcitation (Wolff-Parkinson-White syndrome) pattern.

Based on the morphologic features of PVCs, they have been classified as *uniform* or *multiform;* they also have been referred to as *unifocal* or *multifocal*. Also recommended is classification of PVCs based on their coupling interval with the preceding sinus beat. PVCs with a short coupling interval near or on the previous T wave have been described as showing R-on-T phenomenon; alternatively PVCs may have long coupling intervals. Based on the underlying electrophysiologic mechanism responsible for PVCs, the coupling interval may be *fixed*, as in reentrant beats, or *variable*, as seen with ventricular parasystole. PVCs may have a repetitive pattern, for example, bigeminy or trigeminy, or they may occur in pairs. It is now believed that repetitive PVCs, such as couplets and triplets, are prognostically more important than just the frequency of isolated PVCs.

CLINICAL FEATURES

PVCs can be recorded frequently in normal individuals, and, similar to PACs, their frequency increases with age. In patients without organic heart disease or without prior evidence of sustained ventricular tachyarrhythmias, the mere presence of frequent PVCs is not considered prognostically important. However, individual exceptions do exist, and the clinician is advised to evaluate each given patient accordingly. In patients with organic heart disease, PVCs are the most common form of arrhythmia and carry significant prognostic importance, especially in survivors of acute MI and patients with recurrent ischemia and advanced heart failure. It has been well established during the past 2 decades that frequent PVCs occurring during the acute phase of MI are associated with an increased risk of sustained ventricular arrhythmias in the initial 48 hours, but they do not predict long-term outcome or risk of arrhythmic events. More recently, it has been shown in patients receiving thrombolytic therapy that PVCs, particularly episodes of nonsustained ventricular tachycardia, increase in frequency but are generally short-lived and represent a sign of myocardial reperfusion. However, the presence of frequent PVCs during the postdischarge evaluation of survivors of MI is indicative of a poor prognosis.

Although as many as 80% to 90% of patients with chronic heart failure have frequent PVCs, the results of several recent studies have shown that only the presence of nonsustained ventricular tachycardia (defined as three or more PVCs in a row) at a rate greater than 100 bpm is strongly predictive of an increased risk of sudden cardiac death in these patients. This is in clear contrast to the findings of several large clinical trials, which showed that more than 10 PVCs per hour in post-MI patients are predictive of a poor prognosis and an increased risk of arrhythmic death.

Overall, the association between PVCs and an increased risk of ventricular tachyarrhythmias and sudden cardiac death appears to be related not only to the frequency and complexity of PVCs but also to the severity of underlying structural heart disease. For example, a patient with mitral valve prolapse and frequent PVCs would be at relatively lower risk for arrhythmic events compared to a patient with advanced heart failure who has repetitive PVCs and episodes of nonsustained ventricular tachycardia. Proper evaluation of the risk of PVCs has become more crucial than ever because most currently available antiarrhythmic drugs have the potential for causing serious adverse reactions, including proarrhythmias, in patients with advanced cardiac disorders.

TREATMENT

In general, PVCs in patients without evidence of organic heart disease do not require any specific antiarrhythmic therapy because generally there is no significantly increased risk of life-threatening arrhythmia. However, when PVCs are associated with disabling palpitations, reassurance and treatment with β-blockers (atenolol [Tenormin], metoprolol [Toprol-XL]) may help in relieving symptoms. In patients with systemic illness or other provoking factors (e.g., electrolyte abnormalities or acid-base imbalance), immediate correction of the underlying abnormality usually is associated with beneficial effects.

Because of the associated poor prognosis with PVCs in the setting of acute MI, common practice in the past consisted of routine administration of intravenous lidocaine (Xylocaine) in an effort to suppress PVCs during the initial phase of acute MI. However, because recent data suggest that the routine use of lidocaine is not necessary and often can be harmful, lidocaine should be avoided because of the risk of serious adverse reactions, especially central nervous system side effects such as seizures in the elderly. With the ready availability of cardiac monitoring, it now is possible to accurately identify a harbinger of ventricular tachyarrhythmias early in the coronary care unit, so prophylactic use of lidocaine is generally not recommended. Furthermore, results from several studies and their meta-analyses have demonstrated that routine use of prophylactic lidocaine during the acute or healing phase of MI does not alter the overall mortality in patients with acute MI.

In contrast, it is well established that the presence of frequent PVCs (≥ 10 per hour) during the postdischarge evaluation of survivors of acute MI predicts an increased risk of arrhythmic death and overall cardiac mortality. Numerous trials have been conducted with a variety of different antiarrhythmic drugs. Many of the studies demonstrated that suppression of PVCs with most currently available antiarrhythmic drugs is not beneficial in reducing the increased risk associated with PVCs. The Cardiac Arrhythmia Suppression Trials (CAST I and II) clearly demonstrated that, compared to placebo, treatmentwith class Ic antiarrhythmic drugs (which primarily work by slowing conduction) was associated with an increased risk of arrhythmic death despite adequate suppression of PVCs. The findings from CAST I and II, as well as several other clinical trials, indicate that although frequent PVCs may be a marker for an adverse event, suppression of PVCs with type I antiarrhythmic agents does not favorably influence the associated increased riskof death. Results from the Canadian Amiodarone Myocardial Infarction Arrhythmia Trial (CAMIAT) and the European Myocardial Infarct Amiodarone Trial (EMIAT) suggest that in patients with frequent PVCs in the post-MI setting, use of amiodarone (Cordarone), a complex drug with predominantly class III antiarrhythmic properties, in combination with β-blockers is associated with improved outcome. However, because of the associated drug toxicity with long-term amiodarone use, it is generally considered suitable only for the high-risk cohort (although many patients with low left ventricular ejection fraction now undergo implantation of an automatic internal cardiac defibrillator).

In general, suppression of PVCs using currently available antiarrhythmic drugs (except for amiodarone) is not advisable for most patients, primarily because of the increased risk of proarrhythmic effects of these drugs. In the occasional patient who is disabled by annoying symptoms due to PVCs, an initial trial of β-blocker therapy should be considered and is effective in many patients. Correction of the provoking factors and appropriate management of any underlying heart disease often are beneficial in managing patients with frequent PVCs.

REFERENCES

Barrett PA, Peter CT, Swan HJ, et al: The frequency and prognostic significance of electrocardiographic abnormalities in clinically normal individuals. Prog Cardiovasc Dis 1981;23:299.

Boutitie F, Boissel J-P, Connolly SJ, et al, EMIAT and CAMIAT Investigators: Amiodarone interaction with β-blockers: Analysis of the merged EMIAT (European Myocardial Infarct Amiodarone Trial) and CAMIAT (Canadian Amiodarone Myocardial Infarction Trial) databases. Circulation 1999;99:2268.

Brodsky M, Wu D, Denes P, et al: Arrhythmias documented by 24 hour continuous electrocardiographic monitoring in 50 male medical students without apparent heart disease. Am J Cardiol 1977;39:390.

Cairns JA, Connolly SJ, Roberts R, et al: Randomised trial of outcome after myocardial infarction in patients with frequent or repetitive ventricular premature depolarisations: CAMIAT. Lancet 1997;349:675.

Echt DS, Liebson PR, Mitchell B, et al: Mortality and morbidity in patients receiving encainide, flecainide, or placebo. N Engl J Med 1991;324:781.

Fleg J, Kennedy H: Cardiac arrhythmias in a healthy elderly population. Chest 1982;81:302.

Julian DG, Camm AJ, Frangin G, et al: Randomised trial of effect of amiodarone on mortality in patients with left-ventricular dysfunction after recent myocardial infarction: EMIAT. Lancet 1997;349:667.

Morganroth J: Premature ventricular complexes. Diagnosis and indications for therapy. JAMA 1984;252:673.

Romhilt D, Chaffin C, Choi S, et al: Arrhythmias on ambulatory electrocardiographic monitoring in women without apparent heart disease. Am J Cardiol 1984;54:582.

Rosen KM, Rahimtoola SH, Gunnar RM: Pseudo A-V block secondary to premature nonpropagated His bundle depolarizations: Documentation by His bundle electrocardiography. Circulation 1970;42:367.

Ruskin JN: Ventricular extrasystoles in healthy subjects. N Engl J Med 1985;312:238.

Simpson RJ Jr, Cascio WE, Schreiner PJ, et al: Prevalence of premature ventricular contractions in a population of African American and white men and women: The Atherosclerosis Risk in Communities (ARIC) study. Am Heart J 2002;143:535.

Heart Block

Method of
Kelley P. Anderson, MD

Heart block is at once a syndrome, a set of electrocardiographic (ECG) patterns, and a mechanism of serious signs and symptoms including sudden death and syncope. Interest has accelerated since conventional pacemaker therapy, once considered to be a straightforward, definitive treatment, has been associated with serious consequences in many patients. The development of new forms of pacing has magnified the complexity of pacemaker therapy selection and many aspects remain controversial. This has underscored the importance of recognizing preventable and reversible causes of heart block to reduce the need for permanent pacing and to eliminate unnecessary implantation.

The details of risk stratification of heart block, assessment of the benefits and risks of the therapeutic options, and patient education and guidance are largely in the domain of heart rhythm specialists. However, heart block may be encountered unexpectedly in any patient during any clinical encounter. Furthermore, some patients can require evaluation in the absence of known cardiac disease because of increased risk of conduction disorders in themselves, family members, or future children. A basic understanding of heart block may be useful in order to initiate emergency treatment when necessary and to recognize patients who might benefit from further evaluation or specialist referral.

Mechanisms

The function of the cardiac conduction system is to initiate and coordinate cardiac contractions in order to circulate blood according to physiologic needs. Electrical activation is initiated by pacemaker cells of the sinus node regulated by the autonomic nervous system. Unlike conduction in common electrical circuits in which electrons flow along a conductor according to the voltage gradient, electrical activity in cardiac cells propagates from segment to segment of the cell membrane in cardiac myocytes (myocardial cells) and in specialized cardiac conduction cells. Energy-requiring ion pumps maintain an electrochemical gradient across the insulating cell membrane. Electrical activity opens voltage-sensitive ion channels, causing regenerative electrical activity as ions shift along their electrochemical gradient.

Electrical activity in a single cell excites several adjacent cells via gap junctions. This cascade effect makes it possible for a single cell impulse to spread rapidly throughout the myocardium so that myocytes are excited in the shortest possible time to enhance contraction synchrony, and it provides a vital safety mechanism in that each myocardial cell can be activated by many electrical paths. In addition, specialized conduction cells exhibit automaticity. Although normally latent, because normal activation inhibits spontaneous discharge, when the normal impulse is blocked, discharges from these subsidiary pacemakers provide vital heart rate support.

Block of electrical activation can occur due to failure of any step in the process, such as lack of energy, electrolyte imbalance, inflammatory disruption of the membrane, block of ion channels by drugs, or loss of gap junctions with infiltration of fibrous tissue (Box 1). Because of the extensive redundancy and interconnectedness of system elements and because of the capacity to compensate for injury by electrical and anatomic remodeling, extensive damage can occur before signs or symptoms of heart block. Regions of the heart where there are fewer alternative paths for electrical activation, such as proximal portions of the His–Purkinje system, where all conducting fibers are confined to a relatively small area, are more vulnerable to complete block. Subclinical preexisting injury might explain why subsidiary pacemakers often fail to provide adequate rate support when heart block occurs.

If the patient survives the initial insult, there is a possibility for recovery due to remodeling. However, remodeling can be maladaptive and result in an adverse long-term outcome by further conduction system damage, by left ventricular dysfunction, and perhaps by increasing the propensity for bradycardia-induced ventricular tachyarrhythmias (VTAs). The mechanisms of bradycardia-induced VTA are not known, but bradyarrhythmias precipitate torsades de pointes, a specific form of VTA, in the presence of drugs that block potassium channels, electrolyte disturbances, certain genetic abnormalities of ion channel function, heart failure, and myocardial hypertrophy. A comprehensive list of drugs that can account for bradyarrhythmia-related ventricular arrhythmias is available at www.torsades.org.

Etiology

Although there are many potential causes of heart block, the pathophysiology is not known for the vast majority of cases because there are no tests that allow detailed structural or functional examination in patients. By the time of death, morphologic examination can reveal only nonspecific changes such as fibrosis. Instead, most etiologies are inferred by history of recent or past exposures (e.g., trauma or radiation), concomitant disorders (e.g., muscular dystrophy, amyloidosis), abnormal test results (Lyme disease), or family history (Lenègre's disease) (Box 2). Because most etiologies cannot be verified, the clinician must remain open to alternative explanations and accept the likelihood of multiple contributors.

Some patients, usually young, otherwise healthy persons, present with prolonged asystole due to heart block but have no other

> **BOX 1 Some Mechanisms of Conduction Disturbances**
>
> Calcium channel blockade
> - Diltiazem
> - Verapamil
>
> Cell death
> - Ablation
> - Apoptosis
> - Inflammatory necrosis
> - Ischemic necrosis
> - Surgical trauma
>
> Cell dysfunction
> - Barotrauma
> - Inflammation
> - Thermal injury
>
> Congenital structural defects
> - Endocardial cushion defects
>
> Energy depletion
> - Cyanide
> - Ischemia
>
> Gap junction disturbances
> - Edema
> - Fibrosis
> - Genetic defects
> - Inflammation
>
> Genetic defects
> - *NKX2.5* mutation
> - *SCN5A* mutation
>
> Prolonged refractory period
> - Drugs
> - Ischemia
> - Vagal activity
>
> Sarcolemmal ion gradient disturbances
> - Hyperkalemia
> - Hypokalemia
>
> Sodium channel dysfunction
> - *SCN5A* mutations
> - Sodium channel blocking drugs such as lidocaine, procainamide, flecainide, amiodarone, and imipramine

> **BOX 2 Etiologies of Heart Block**
>
> **Often Permanent or Progressive**
>
> Alcohol septal ablation (acute, delayed)
> Cardiomyopathies (hypertrophic, idiopathic, mitochondrial)
> Catheter ablation (atrioventricular nodal reentry, accessory atrioventricular connections)
> Congenital heart block (neonatal lupus)
> Congenital heart disease (endocardial cushion defects)
> Genetic disorders (sodium channel mutations, Lenègre's disease)
> Hypertension
> Idiopathic fibrosis and calcification (previously Lev's disease, Lenègre's disease)
> Infectious disorders (destructive, e.g., endocarditis)
> Infiltrative disorders (amyloidosis)
> Myocardial infarction
> Neuromyopathic disorders (myotonic dystrophy, Erb's dystrophy, peroneal muscular atrophy)
> Noninfectious inflammatory disorders (HLA-B27–associated disorder, sarcoidosis)
> Tumors (mesothelioma)
> Valvular heart disease
>
> **Often Transient or Reversible**
>
> Blunt trauma (baseball)
> Cardiac surgery (valve replacement)
> Cardiac transplant rejection
> Central nervous system
> Drugs (antiarrhythmics, digoxin, edrophonium [Tensilon])
> Electrolyte disturbances (hyperkalemia)
> Increased vagal activity
> Infectious disorders—nondestructive (Eyme diseas)
> Metabolic disturbances (hypothermia, hypothyroidism)
> Myocardial ischemia
> Myocarditis (Chagas' disease, giant cell myocarditis)
> Rheumatic fever

detectable abnormalities and have excellent outcomes in the absence of intervention beyond counseling. This suggests that autonomic influences alone can cause severe heart block and suppression of subsidiary pacemakers. It is not known if such responses result from an abnormality or an exaggerated normal reflex. However, the identification of such patients is important because most can be managed without pacemakers.

Other patients who should be identified are those with conditions that place them, their relatives, or their unborn children at risk for heart block. This includes patients and family members with genetic disorders associated with heart block. It also includes women with anti-Ro/SSA and/or anti-La/SSB antibodies whose children are at increased risk for congenital heart block, a rare, but devastating disorder. Members of this group can benefit from counseling and anticipatory evaluation and treatment of offspring.

Signs and Symptoms

Most of the symptoms experienced by patients with heart block are common and nonspecific, such as syncope, lightheadedness, fatigue, and dyspnea. Because other arrhythmias and other cardiac and noncardiac disturbances may be responsible for the same symptoms, it is important to document the cause. Proof, which requires documentation of rhythm and the abnormal hemodynamics responsible for the symptoms, is almost never accomplished. Sometimes a cardiac rhythm disturbance can be related to a clinical event, such as several seconds of asystole due to atrioventricular (AV) block and syncope. More commonly, a patient complaining of fatigue or lightheadedness is bradycardic due to high-grade AV block. Asymptomatic complete AV block is also not uncommon. A favorable response to pacemaker implantation is inconclusive due to a powerful placebo effect. Rarely, first-degree AV block results in significant symptoms (e.g., fatigue, palpitations, chest fullness) due to atrial contraction against a partially closed mitral valve. In such cases it is often possible to identify a recent change in PR interval.

ELECTROCARDIOGRAPHIC PATTERNS

Cardiac conduction disturbances are classified by the pattern of ECG complexes. A normal 12-lead ECG lessens the probability of significant fixed conduction disturbances, but it does not eliminate the possibility of transient third-degree block due to reversible functional effects such as intense vagal activity or ischemia. A normal ECG rhythm during symptoms is very helpful for excluding heart block as the mechanism.

PR prolongation and intraatrial delay rarely require immediate action but can have adverse hemodynamic consequences and occasionally cause symptoms due to suboptimal coordination between atrial and ventricular contraction. Significant disease of the His bundle may be electrocardiographically silent, but more often, concomitant distal disease is evident in the form of fascicular or bundle branch block or a nonspecific intraventricular conduction delay. In a patient with syncope, the presence of bifascicular block raises the possibility of transient third-degree block as the mechanism and of progression to permanent complete block.

Most patients with conduction disorders are not symptomatic and do not progress to complete block. However, the combination of right bundle branch block (RBBB) and left posterior fascicle block has a greater tendency to progress to complete block than the more common RBBB and left anterior fascicle block. Nevertheless, conduction disturbances of the His–Purkinje system should not be assumed to be responsible for syncope or cardiac arrest because they are relatively common in patients with cardiovascular disorders that cause syncope or cardiac arrest due to other mechanisms. Conduction disturbances can cause dyssynchronous contraction and result in adverse remodeling. In addition, they can mask or mimic the ECG signs of myocardial infarction.

Alternating bundle branch block is a changing ECG pattern in which both RBBB and left bundle branch block are observed or when the bifascicular block pattern switches between the anterior and posterior fascicle involvement. This pattern is considered a harbinger of complete block with or without symptoms and warrants continuous monitoring and evaluation for permanent pacemaker implantation.

The challenge in second-degree and transient third-degree AV block is distinguishing between block in the AV node, which is rarely permanent, and infranodal block, which often progresses to permanent third-degree block. ECG clues that block is in the AV node include normal QRS duration (<100 ms), type I (Wenckebach) pattern, PR prolongation before blocked impulses and PR shortening after pauses, occurrence during enhanced vagal activity (e.g., sleep), narrow QRS escape complexes, and no factors favoring infranodal block. ECG clues for infranodal block include prolonged QRS duration (120 ms), type II pattern, and escape QRS complexes broader than intrinsic complexes. Whereas type II second-degree AV block is almost always due to block in the His–Purkinje system, other second-degree AV block ECG patterns have poor sensitivity and specificity for the site of the block.

Unsustained polymorphic ventricular tachycardia is an ominous sign in any context and can result from a variety of cardiac, metabolic, and autonomic abnormalities. However, in the presence of heart block it suggests that heart rate support may be necessary to prevent sustained VTA. QT prolongation and post-pause U-wave accentuation should be sought as other harbingers of bradycardia-related VTA.

The importance and value of ECG documentation of heart block to the patient's management and well-being cannot be overemphasized. ECGs are subject to artifact and may be misleading when standards for acquisition and analysis are not followed. Multiple tracings of suspicious events should be obtained in multiple leads when possible. A 12-lead simultaneous rhythm recording mode is available on most modern ECG machines and should be used when continuous recordings are obtained to document arrhythmias.

METHODS USED IN THE ASSESSMENT OF HEART BLOCK

Clinicians encounter heart block in three general contexts. For the patient with documented heart block, the clinician selects therapy based, in part, on whether or not the arrhythmia is permanent or likely to recur. There are no tests that provide information about the pathologic state of the AV conduction system; therefore, these outcomes must be inferred from the ECG and past experience. Additional testing including invasive tests such as electrophysiologic studies, coronary angiography, and myocardial biopsy, as well as a large number of specific laboratory tests are occasionally helpful but usually do not provide information about the choice of therapy for heart block.

Another common context is the patient with symptoms for whom the objective is to verify or exclude heart block as the mechanism by correlating the cardiac rhythm with symptoms. Real-time monitoring, such as inpatient telemetry, is used for patients who might require immediate access to drugs or pacing devices to prevent or terminate asystole or bradycardia-dependent VTA. Holter monitoring is useful for patients who have more than one event in a 24-hour window and for capturing asymptomatic rhythm events. External loop recorders are carried for a month or longer and are very helpful to associate rhythm abnormalities with symptoms and to rule out a rhythm disorder as the cause of symptoms. Patients with infrequent events may be candidates for implantable loop recorders that monitor for longer than 1 year.

 CURRENT DIAGNOSIS

- Assess risk for heart block in the absence of symptoms or evidence of asystole
- Review ECG pattern, family history, maternal antibodies, cardiac interventions, and surgery
- Evaluate documented heart block with asystole or bradycardia
- Classify bradyarrhythmia: Transient, recurrent, progressive, permanent
- Grade signs and symptoms: none, mild, severe
- Evaluate signs or symptoms of possible transient heart block with no documentation
- Establish temporal pattern: Single, recurrent, rare, often, recent onset, long-standing
- Grade signs and symptoms: none, mild, severe
- Document rhythm during symptoms: Telemetry monitoring, Holter monitor, external loop recorder, implantable recorder

Electrophysiologic studies allow precise measurements of AV node and His–Purkinje system function and can provide definitive information regarding the site of block if the conduction disturbance occurs during the study. Additional tests have been developed that stress the AV conduction system, including rapid atrial and ventricular pacing, administration of antiarrhythmic drugs such as procainamide and disopyramide, combinations of drugs, and pacing maneuvers. The provocation of heart block is assumed to indicate a propensity for spontaneous AV block. Unfortunately, the sensitivity is low and a negative test does not imply a low risk of future episodes. Electrophysiologic studies have the additional advantage of providing immediate test results, as well as providing the results of programmed stimulation for provocation of supraventricular and ventricular tachyarrhythmias.

The third important context for clinicians is patients who might be at high risk for adverse consequences of heart block but are asymptomatic. Addressing this is a challenge for the future because few methods are currently available. Possible applications include screening for mutations and polymorphisms that predispose to heart block, measurements of mechanical dyssynchrony to identify patients prone to develop adverse cardiac remodeling due to conduction disorders or right ventricular pacing, and methods capable of assessing electrophysiologic and metabolic function of conducting tissue in vivo.

Treatment

Selecting the correct therapeutic approach balances the risks and benefits of therapy against the risks of heart block for both immediate and long-term management. Pharmacologic agents are useful for emergency, temporary, and standby heart support in select circumstances. The standby mode is accomplished by a prepared infusion at the bedside. To avoid excessive doses at the time of sudden heart block, the optimal dose can be established in advance by test doses starting at low infusion rates.

PHARMACOLOGIC TREATMENT

Atropine 0.5 to 3.0 mg[3] or 0.04 mg/kg IV is useful for treatment or pretreatment of patients who develop heart block at the level of the

---

[3] Exceeds dosage recommended by the manufacturer.

CURRENT THERAPY

Methods of Heart Rate Support

- Immediate: Intravenous catecholamines, transcutaneous pacing
- Short-term: Transvenous temporary pacing
- Long-term: Permanent pacemakers

Pacemaker Configuration

- Number of leads: 1,2,3,4
- Lead locations: Right atrial appendage, Bachmann's bundle, right ventricular apex, outflow tract, left ventricle, coronary sinus
- Programming to minimize ventricular pacing (manufacturer dependent)

AV node in the context of elevated vagal tone, such as in association with nausea or endotracheal tube suction. Atropine should be avoided in patients with infranodal AV block because prolonged asystole sometimes occurs due to more frequent His–Purkinje system depolarization from increased sinus rate. Vagal activity inhibits sympathetic activity, and therefore reduction of vagal tone by atropine disinhibits sympathetic activity and can account for the unpredictable effects of atropine on heart rate. Elevations in heart rate after atropine can persist for hours and cannot be readily reversed.

Aminophylline 2.5 to 6.3 mg/kg IV is reported to reverse heart block resistant to atropine and epinephrine by antagonizing adenosine. Stimulation of β-adrenergic receptors increases sinus and subsidiary pacemaker rates, AV node and His–Purkinje system conduction velocities, and myocardial contractility. The effective refractory period shortens in most tissue, but this effect varies with dose and specific tissue type.

Dobutamine 2.5 to 40 μg/kg/minute is a useful β-receptor agonist because it increases cardiac output and lowers filling pressures without excessive rise or fall of blood pressure.

Isoproterenol (Isuprel) in a 0.02 to 0.06 mg IV bolus or 0.5 to 10.0^3 μg/min IV infusion, stimulates $β_1$- and $β_2$-adrenergic receptors and enhances vasodilation more than the other catecholamines. This can result in unwanted hypotension in some circumstances, but it is also less likely to cause a reflex increase in vagal tone than other drugs.

Epinephrine in 1 mg IV boluses for cardiac arrest, 0.2 to 1 mg subcutaneously, or 0.5-5 μg/min IV stimulates both α- and β-adrenergic receptors. It is recommended for asystolic cardiac arrest in part because it increases myocardial and cerebral flow. However, the increase of systemic vascular resistance may be detrimental by augmenting metabolic acidosis and decreasing cardiac performance in patients with poor left ventricular function. The suggested dose ranges are broad because the response, such as improved AV conduction, to β-adrenergic stimulants varies widely and may be affected by β-adrenergic receptor down-regulation in patients with chronic elevations in sympathetic activity, such as patients with long-standing heart failure.

Any of these agents can precipitate tachyarrhythmias by direct electrophysiologic effects mediated by adrenergic receptors and indirect effects such as myocardial ischemia, and they can worsen hemodynamic status. The adverse effects of catecholamines are time dependent and cumulative. Ischemia and receptor-mediated electrophysiologic effects occur immediately after administration, and changes in gene expression of ion channels begin as early as several hours. Long-term changes such as myocardial hypertrophy, apoptosis, and fibrosis usually begin to occur within 24 hours but can progress over much longer periods. This suggests that the duration and dose of catecholamine infusions should be minimized.

PACING

Temporary pacing includes transcutaneous, transvenous, transthoracic, transesophogeal, and transgastric approaches. Transcutaneous pacing provides noninvasive heart rate support as well as immediate access to countershock, but it is often painful, so most patients require sedation, and capture is not achieved in some patients. For these reasons, its principal uses are for short-term pacing during cardiopulmonary resuscitation and for standby pacing in patients at risk for bradyarrhythmias. If the risk of bradycardia is high, ventricular capture should be verified in advance. Capture is often difficult to ascertain because transcutaneous stimuli cause large deflections on the ECG, and pectoral muscle stimulation can be confused with a pulse. Capture should be verified by careful ECG analysis at sub- and suprathreshold stimulus amplitudes and confirmed by appropriately timed femoral artery pulses, Korotkoff sounds, or arterial pressure waveforms.

Transvenous insertion of an electrode catheter is the method of choice for most patients who require temporary pacing. This approach is reliable and safe when performed by competent staff with strict aseptic technique, fluoroscopic guidance, and appropriate catheters. Complications include inadequate pacing or sensing thresholds, vascular complications, pneumothorax, myocardial perforation, infection, and dislodgment. Small studies suggest that long-term (>5 days) temporary pacing can be accomplished with active-fixation permanent pacemaker leads attached to an external pulse generator.[1] Tunneling the lead can enhance stability and reduce the risk of infection.

Permanent pacemakers are highly effective, safe, and cost-effective and have few contraindications. Although the complications are rarely life threatening, they should be carefully considered and acknowledged. Septicemia or endocarditis has been reported in 0.5% of patients. In patients with pacemaker-related endocarditis, the in-hospital mortality rate is reported to be greater than 7%, with a 20-month mortality greater than 25%. The rate of significant complications has been reported to be 3.5%. About 10% of pacemakers become infected or develop some other type of failure that can require extraction. In one series, the rate of major complications associated with extraction was 1.4%. There is a long-term continuous risk of infection, thrombosis, and erosion. Conventional pacing, that is, from the right ventricular apex, is now known to be detrimental and can cause adverse ventricular remodeling, atrial fibrillation, heart failure, and premature death.

In young persons there is a periodic need to replace generators and leads, which limits venous access sites, and unused leads accumulate or must be extracted. Perhaps of greater consequence is the constant inconvenience of lifelong follow-up, electromagnetic interference, and false alarms from electronic surveillance devices as well as exclusion from important procedures, such as magnetic resonance imaging of the thorax.

Although it has been shown that patients with reduced left ventricular function are at greater risk for adverse effects, it is not known how to identify other patients at risk. Many strategies for reducing the adverse effects of conventional pacing have been proposed and many have been studied, but there is no consensus about which method should be used in the many settings that are encountered. Therefore, the decision for pacemaker implantation also includes selection of lead configuration, lead locations, and pacing mode. Because some configurations change the short- and long-term risks of implantation, patient guidance and education are more complex as well.

Approach to the Patient

The object of the evaluation and management for heart block is to prevent adverse effects by heart rate support in patients with poorly tolerated bradycardia; monitoring and standby heart rate support in stable patients at high risk for asystole or severe bradycardia; identifying and treating reversible causes of heart block; identifying patients at high risk for sudden death, syncope, or recurrent symptoms; and selecting and implanting the appropriate rate support device as soon as safety permits.

Advanced cardiac life-support guidelines apply to the patient who is unresponsive or severely compromised by heart block.

---

[1]Not FDA approved for this indication.

However, heart block is rarely the primary problem. Therefore, evaluation and treatment of other disorders should continue while efforts to increase heart rate are under way.

The initial evaluation should include a thorough history and physical examination, review of current and previous ECGs and rhythm strips, and laboratory tests to determine if heart block is present or if there is a significant risk of heart block occurring in the future and, if so, a differential diagnosis of possible etiologies. The patient should then be stratified for the appropriate level of care: the unstable patient who requires on-going evaluation and treatment in an intensive care setting, the stable patient at high risk for asystole or complications who needs temporary transvenous pacing or other invasive procedures, the patient at moderate risk who requires continuous monitoring and standby noninvasive heart rate support measures, the patient at low risk who requires rapid but not immediate access to heart-rate support measures that hospital monitoring provides, and the patient at low risk who can be evaluated and managed as an outpatient.

Patients who present after resuscitated cardiac arrest or syncope or with ECG abnormalities that indicate conduction system abnormalities usually belong in one of the first four categories. The fifth category usually includes patients with mild symptoms and no suggestive ECG abnormalities and patients whose risk is estimated to be low after in-patient monitoring or previous evaluation. The most common presentation is the patient who has symptoms that could be due to heart block as well as other arrhythmic or nonarrhythmic causes. In such patients, ECG confirmation of the relationship between heart block and symptoms should be obtained.

Determining the need for long-term heart rate support, as well as other issues that can affect selection of implantable devices (e.g., risk for VTAs), should be accomplished as soon as possible because the risks of complications and anxiety associated with temporary heart rate support measures increase over time. Medical societies have developed guidelines for implantable rhythm management devices (http://www.cardiosource/guidelines/index.asp). The reasons for the selected therapy, including the rationale for any deviation from established guidelines, should be documented and provided to the patient. This will reduce future confusion or misunderstanding about the original rationale for implantation that can affect management of patients with device complications and those with a compelling need for device upgrade or explanation.

Patients with acute coronary syndromes require special consideration. The incidence of heart block in patients with myocardial infarction based on creatine phosphokinase as the marker of necrosis is approximately 10%. Although the incidence is probably lower using more sensitive markers such as troponin, heart block is still likely to be associated with increased in-hospital mortality due to larger infarct size. Bradycardia reduces myocardial oxygen consumption. Therefore, overcorrection of heart rate must be avoided, and ischemia should be relieved by increasing perfusion as soon as possible.

Studies in the prethrombolytic era did not demonstrate a benefit in mortality with prophylactic temporary transvenous pacing, and complications were common. The risks of transvenous insertion may be higher in patients requiring administration of thrombolytics and other anticoagulants. Catheter-based revascularization methods should be given strong consideration because of established effectiveness, because thrombolytic drugs might be avoided, and because transvenous temporary pacing, if needed, is readily and safely accomplished during the procedure. Suggestions for standby temporary pacing (Box 3) should take into consideration the risks of transvenous pacing based on local circumstances (e.g., experience, fluoroscopic guidance, insertion site, use of anticoagulants).

Most conduction disturbances associated with myocardial ischemia or infarction resolve quickly but can persist for days or weeks. The need for permanent pacemaker implantation as a consequence of myocardial infarction is rare, and prophylactic pacemaker implantation in high-risk subsets has not been shown to reduce mortality. Guidelines for temporary and permanent pacing in acute myocardial infarction have been published (http://www.escardio.org/guidelines-surveys/esc-guidelines/pages/cardiac-pacing-and-cardiac-resynchronisation-therapy.aspx).

BOX 3 Suggestions for Temporary Pacing in Acute Myocardial Infarction

Transvenous Pacing

Asystole or poorly tolerated bradycardia unresponsive to atropine or aminophylline
Persistent third-degree AV block
Alternating RBBB and LBBB, or RBBB and alternating LAFB and LPFB
Bifascicular block (new)
Second-degree AV block (any type) and QRS $\geq$110 ms
Any indication listed for standby transcutaneous pacing at time of cardiac catheterization if performed

Standby Transcutaneous Pacing

Any indication listed for transvenous pacing until the transvenous pacing system is inserted
Transient asystole or poorly tolerated bradycardia
Bifascicular block (uncertain time of onset or old)
Second-degree AV block (any type) and QRS <110 ms
New first-degree AV block

AV = atrioventricular; LAFB= left anterior fascicle block; LPFB = left posterior fascicle block; LBBB = left bundle branch block; RBBB = right bundle branch block.

Conclusions

Heart block remains a challenge because the cellular mechanisms responsible are poorly understood, prediction of symptomatic heart block (who and when) is unreliable, treatments that restore normal conduction do not exist for most conditions, and pacemaker therapy can have significant long-term adverse consequences. Fortunately, ongoing clinical trials will provide guidance in pacemaker configurations and programming that will minimize adverse effects. Recent achievements in molecular biology suggest we are on the threshold of advances that will elucidate mechanisms and produce treatments that will relegate artificial pacemakers to museum pieces.

Acknowledgments

The author thanks the Marshfield Clinic Research Foundation for its support through the assistance of Linda Weis and Alice Stargardt in the preparation of this chapter.

REFERENCES

Barold SS, Hayes DL: Second-degree atrioventricular block: A reappraisal. Mayo Clin Proc 2001;76:44-57.

Carlson MD, Wilkoff BL, Maisel WH, et al: Recommendations from the Heart Rhythm Society Task Force on Device Performance Policies and Guidelines Endorsed by the American College of Cardiology Foundation (ACCF) and the American Heart Association (AHA) and the International Coalition of Pacing and Electrophysiology Organizations (COPE). Heart Rhythm 2006;3:1250-1273.

Elizari MV, Acunzo RS, Ferreiro M: Hemiblocks revisited. Circulation 2007;115:1154-1163.

Pierpont ME, Basson CT, Benson DW Jr, et al: Genetic basis for congenital heart defects: Current knowledge: A scientific statement from the American Heart Association Congenital Cardiac Defects Committee, Council on Cardiovascular Disease in the Young: Endorsed by the American Academy of Pediatrics. Circulation 2007;115:3015-3038.

Zipes DP, Camm AJ, Borggrefe M, et al: ACC/AHA/ESC 2006 guidelines for management of patients with ventricular arrhythmias and the prevention of sudden cardiac death: A report of the American College of

Cardiology/American Heart Association Task Force and the European Society of Cardiology Committee for Practice Guidelines (writing committee to develop Guidelines for Management of Patients with Ventricular Arrhythmias and the Prevention of Sudden Cardiac Death): Developed in collaboration with the European Heart Rhythm Association and the Heart Rhythm Society. Circulation 2006;114:e385-e484.

Tachycardias

Method of
Sei Iwai, MD, and Bruce B. Lerman, MD

The term *tachycardia* translates literally into "fast" (tachy-) "heart" (cardia). Cardiac arrhythmias that result in electrical activation more than 100 times per minute fall under the category of tachycardia.

Mechanisms of Tachyarrhythmias

Tachycardias are initiated or sustained by one of three general mechanisms: reentry, abnormal automaticity, or triggered activity.

Reentry is the most common mechanism of arrhythmogenesis. Reentry typically requires a region of relatively slow conduction in order to become sustained. This creates an excitable gap, preventing the leading edge of a wavefront from colliding with its back end (Fig. 1). Reentry can occur in the setting of an abnormal electrical pathway or connection (e.g., accessory atrioventricular [AV] pathway or dual AV nodal pathway physiology). Alternatively, a barrier to conduction, either anatomic (e.g., tricuspid or mitral valve, venae cavae), or functional (e.g., crista terminalis—due to anisotropic conduction), can provide a setting favorable for reentry. Finally, abnormal impulse propagation, such as through diseased cardiac tissue, can cause sufficient slowing of conduction, allowing recovery of neighboring cells, initiating reentry.

Rhythmic pacemaker activity can occur in various types of cardiac cells. However, there is a normal hierarchy in the frequency of the initiated action potentials from these sites; the sinoatrial node is the dominant pacemaker. Automaticity in the distal conduction system (or myocardium) can compete with that in the sinoatrial node on the basis of enhanced normal or *abnormal automaticity*.

Under certain pathologic conditions, a decrease in the resting membrane potential can occur, resulting in spontaneous phase-4 depolarization in cardiac cells. Abnormal automaticity is defined as spontaneous impulse initiation in cells that are not fully polarized. Perturbations in the ionic balance (state of depolarization), which result in abnormal automaticity, may be due to disturbances in various ion channel currents. For example, during the subacute phase of a myocardial infarction, automatic arrhythmias can arise from the infarct border zones.

Triggered activity has become an increasingly appreciated cause of cardiac arrhythmias. In cardiac cells, oscillations of membrane potential that occur during repolarization or after the action potential are referred to as *afterdepolarizations*. They are divided into two subtypes: early and delayed afterdepolarizations, depending on when they occur relative to the cardiac action potential. When an afterdepolarization achieves sufficient amplitude to reach a threshold potential, a new action potential, or triggered response, is evoked. If this process repeats itself, sustained triggered arrhythmias can develop.

An early afterdepolarization can appear during the plateau (phase 2) or repolarization phase (phase 3) of the action potential (Fig. 2). A prolongation of repolarization by a reduction in outward currents, an increase in inward currents, or a combination of the two is required for the manifestation of early afterdepolarization–induced ectopic activity. Bradycardia or pauses, which prolong repolarization, can potentiate early afterdepolarizations.

Delayed afterdepolarizations are oscillations in membrane potential that occur after repolarization, during phase 4 of the action potential (see Fig. 2). In contrast to automatic rhythms that originate *de novo* during spontaneous diastolic depolarization, delayed afterdepolarizations depend on the preceding action potential and do not occur in the absence of a previous action potential.

During the plateau phase of the normal action potential, calcium enters the cell. The increase in intracellular calcium triggers release of calcium from the sarcoplasmic reticulum. This further elevates intracellular calcium and initiates contraction. Relaxation occurs through sequestration of calcium by the sarcoplasmic reticulum. Delayed afterdepolarizations arise when the cytosol becomes overloaded with calcium and triggers a transient inward current, I_{Ti}. I_{Ti} is generated by the sodium–calcium exchanger (I_{NaCa}). Delayed afterdepolarizations can originate from myocardial cells, Purkinje fibers, and even mitral valve and coronary sinus tissue.

Tachyarrhythmias can be broadly classified as either supraventricular, which arise from the atria or AV junction, or ventricular, which arise from the ventricles.

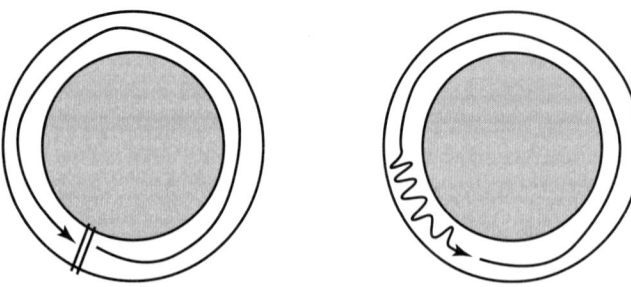

FIGURE 1. Diagrams demonstrate the effect of slow conduction in promoting reentrant circuits. *Gray area* represents an obstacle (e.g., scar). *Left*, In this example, normal conduction velocity around the scar results in termination of the wavefront *(circular line with arrow)*, as the head *(arrow)* of the wavefront meets the tail during refractoriness *(double line)*. *Right*, Due to an area of slow conduction, the head of the wavefront meets the tail after it has recovered *(circular line with arrow)* and can perpetuate reentry.

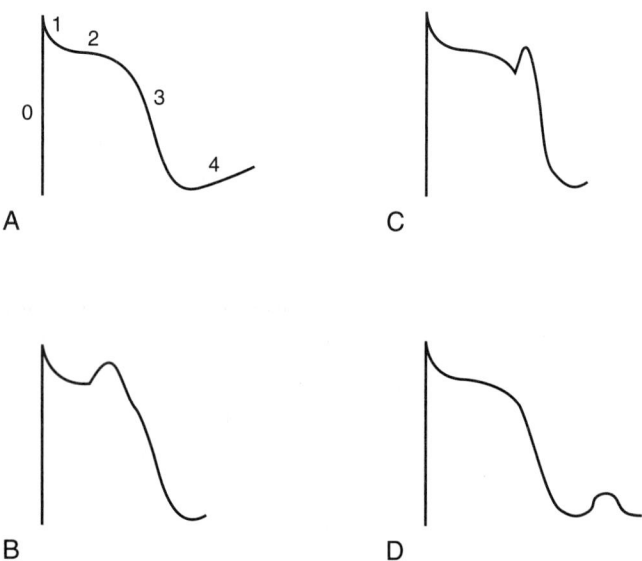

FIGURE 2. A, Normal action potential of myocardial tissue and the corresponding phases (0-4). **B,** Early afterdepolarization during phase 2. **C,** Early afterdepolarization during phase 3. **D,** Delayed afterdepolarization occurring during phase 4.

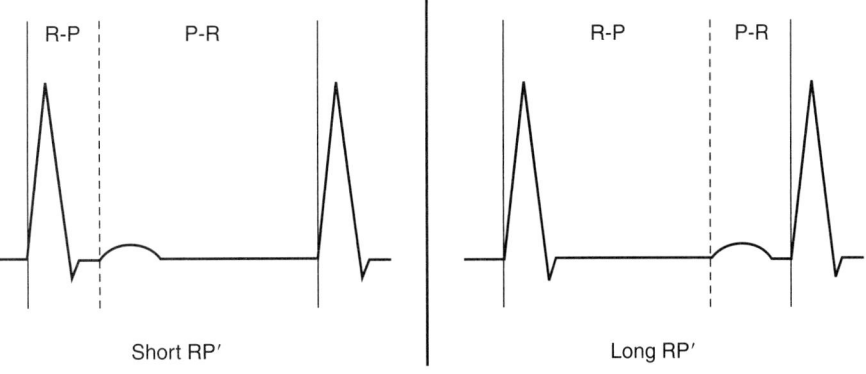

FIGURE 3. Schematic demonstrating the relation of the P wave with respect to the R-R interval. *Left*, Short RP′ tachycardia, with P wave occurring shortly after the preceding QRS complex; thus the R-P interval is short (compared with the P-R interval). *Right*, The P wave occurs just before the following QRS complex (long RP′ tachycardia).

Supraventricular Tachyarrhythmias

ATRIOVENTRICULAR NODAL REENTRY

Excluding atrial fibrillation (discussed in the chapter on atrial fibrillation), the most common supraventricular arrhythmia is AV node reentrant tachycardia (AVNRT). AVNRT accounts for more than 50% of the supraventricular tachycardias (SVTs) with a 1:1 atrial-to-ventricular activation pattern. The initiation of AVNRT depends on the presence of dual AV nodal pathway physiology. A fast pathway, located in the anterior portion of the septum, typically has a relatively longer refractory period. A slow AV nodal pathway, usually located in the posterior aspect of the septum, has a shorter refractory period.

The anatomy of the AV node is quite complex and incompletely understood. It appears that the reentry circuit of AVNRT also contains transitional cells in between the atrial portions of the fast and slow pathways. During the typical form of AVNRT, anterograde conduction occurs over the slow pathway, and retrograde conduction is via the fast pathway. Therefore, activation of the atria and ventricles occurs almost simultaneously. As a result, this tachycardia can be described as a short RP′ tachycardia, based on the relation between the R and P waves; that is, the R-P interval is less than the P-R interval (Fig. 3). Thus, in typical AVNRT, the P wave occurs during the QRS complex, or it occurs shortly afterward, in which case it can appear as a pseudo-R′ (Fig. 4). Less common forms of AVNRT include fast–slow (i.e., anterograde conduction down the fast pathway and retrograde conduction via the slow pathway) and slow–slow variants (in which there are two different slow pathways). The former results in a long RP′ tachycardia, and the latter results in an RP′ interval approximately equal to the PR interval. The relation between P wave and QRS complex on an electrocardiogram (ECG) can help in forming a differential diagnosis for the SVT (Box 1).

Initiation of AVNRT is usually due to an atrial or ventricular premature complex that blocks in one pathway but conducts via the other with enough delay to allow recovery and activation of the initially refractory pathway in the retrograde direction. First-line therapy for acute termination of AVNRT is adenosine (Adenocard) (typically 6 or 12 mg IV). Other options include intravenous β-blockers or calcium channel blockers such as metoprolol (Lopressor)[1] 5 mg IV or diltiazem (Cardizem) 20 mg IV. Therapeutic options for long-term therapy include oral β-blockers or calcium channel blockers and radiofrequency catheter ablation.

ATRIOVENTRICULAR RECIPROCATING TACHYCARDIA

The presence of an accessory pathway between the atria and ventricles can result in a reentrant tachycardia called *atrioventricular reciprocating tachycardia* (AVRT). The most common location (>50%) for an accessory pathway is the left free wall. Orthodromic reciprocating tachycardia (ORT) results when anterograde conduction occurs over the AV node, with retrograde conduction occurring over the accessory pathway. Conversely, antidromic reciprocating tachycardia (ART) describes reentry in the opposite direction (Fig. 5). Anterograde conduction evident on ECG during sinus rhythm is a Wolff-Parkinson-White (WPW) pattern.

[1]Not FDA approved for this indication.

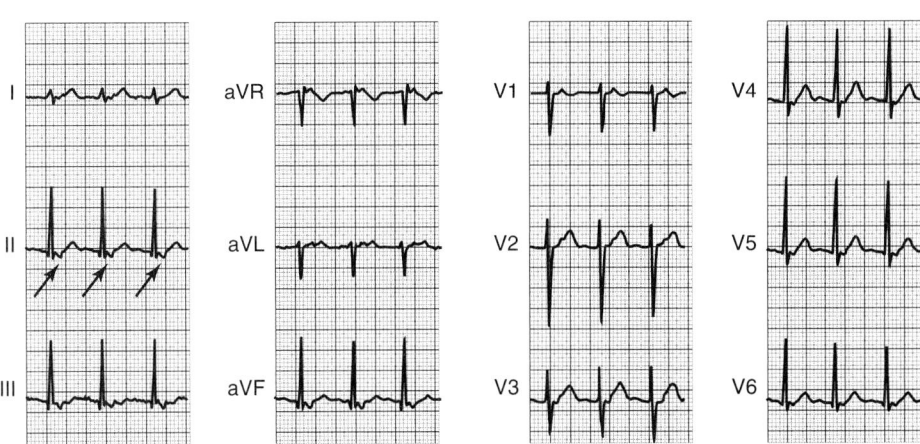

FIGURE 4. A 12-lead electrocardiogram of a short RP′ tachycardia, consistent with typical atrioventricular nodal reentrant tachycardia. *Arrows* identify the retrograde P waves.

BOX 1 Differential Diagnosis of Narrow Complex Supraventricular Tachycardia with 1:1 Atrioventricular Conduction

Short RP' Tachycardias
Typical atrioventricular (AV) nodal reentry
Orthodromic reciprocating tachycardia
Atrial tachycardia with first-degree AV delay
Junctional tachycardia

Long RP' Tachycardias
Atypical AV node reentry
Atrial tachycardia
Sinus tachycardia
Permanent form of junctional reciprocating tachycardia

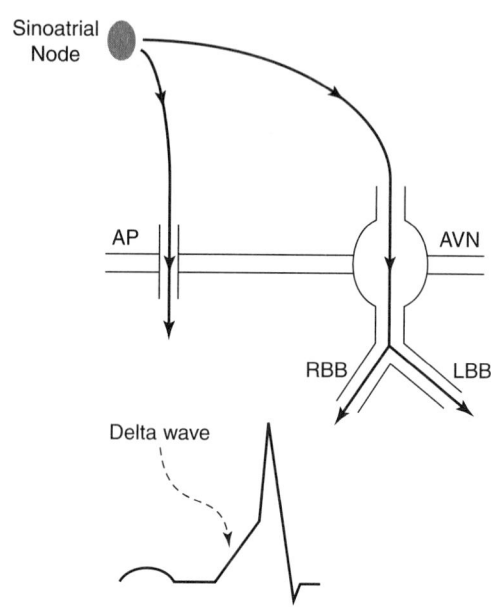

FIGURE 6. The delta wave is a result of fusion of ventricular activation via the atrioventricular node (AVN) and conduction via the accessory pathway (AP). Due to the normal slowing of conduction down the AVN (to the right and left bundle branches [RBB and LBB, respectively], and subsequently the ventricles), a portion of the ventricles is preexcited via the AP, manifesting as a slurred upstroke (curved dashed arrow) of the initial portion of the QRS complex (the delta wave).

The combination of a WPW pattern and a history of tachycardia is WPW syndrome. Ventricular preexcitation is present, as manifested by a delta wave on the ECG. A delta wave is formed by AV conduction via the accessory pathway, which occurs without the delay seen during conduction via the AV node and His–Purkinje system (Fig. 6). Thus, the PR interval is shortened. The magnitude of PR interval shortening is related to the proximity of the accessory pathway to the sinus node. Right-sided accessory pathways therefore usually result in shorter PR intervals than left-sided accessory pathways. The accessory pathway can often be concealed; that is, the pathway is capable of retrograde conduction only. In this case, no delta wave is present.

ORT results in a short RP' tachycardia, owing to relatively rapid conduction over the accessory pathway. However, the RP' interval is typically longer than that seen in typical AVNRT. This is because the reentry circuit in ORT results in serial, or sequential, activation of the ventricles and the atria, whereas it occurs in parallel in AVNRT. RP' intervals in AVNRT are rarely greater than 70 ms, and they are rarely less than this in ORT.

ART manifests as a wide complex tachycardia rhythm, with QRS morphology dependent on the location of the accessory pathway. ART is an uncommon arrhythmia. In fact, in patients with WPW syndrome, atrial fibrillation is more common, occurring in up to 40% of patients. The combination of an accessory pathway and atrial fibrillation can result in very rapid activation of the ventricles (via the accessory pathway), with bizarre QRS complexes. Atrial fibrillation with WPW syndrome can lead to syncope or even ventricular fibrillation due to the rapid ventricular stimulation.

Rarely, ORT can result due to reentry using a long, slowly conducting serpentine pathway, with decremental (similar to the AV node) conduction. These tachycardias can be incessant and are termed *permanent form of junctional reciprocating tachycardia*. Permanent form of junctional reciprocating tachycardia often results in a tachycardia-mediated cardiomyopathy, due to its incessant nature.

Similar to AVNRT, both ORT and ART are usually initiated by an atrial or ventricular premature complex. First-line therapy for acute termination of AVRT is adenosine (typically 6 or 12 mg IV). ART, however, can be difficult to differentiate from ventricular tachycardia, due to its wide QRS complex. Other options include intravenous β-blockers or calcium channel blockers, as well as intravenous procainamide (Pronestyl), amiodarone (Cordarone), or ibutilide (Corvert). Therapeutic options for long-term therapy include oral β-blockers or calcium channel blockers, class I or III antiarrhythmic agents, as well as catheter ablation. Recently, the availability of cryoablation energy has increased the safety of ablation of accessory pathways in close proximity to the AV node.

Lastly, in patients with dual-chamber permanent pacemakers only, a specific form of iatrogenic AV reciprocating tachycardia can occur, called *pacemaker-mediated tachycardia*. Typically in this case, a ventricular premature complex conducts retrogradely up to the atria, with enough delay to result in atrial activation after the end of the postventricular atrial refractory period. This atrial activation is sensed by the pacemaker and tracked, resulting in a ventricular paced beat. The paced beat then conducts up to the atria, perpetuating the tachycardia. Pacemaker-mediated tachycardia can be avoided by extending the postventricular atrial refractory period, or, if intrinsic AV conduction is present, switching from a tracking mode (DDD) to a nontracking mode (DDI).

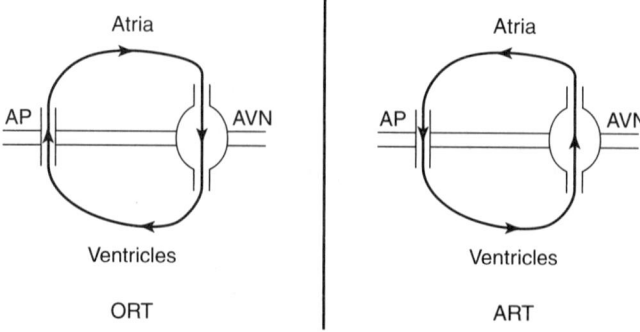

FIGURE 5. Demonstration of activation pattern in orthodromic reciprocating tachycardia (ORT) and antidromic reciprocating tachycardia (ART). ORT involves anterograde conduction down the atrioventricular node (AVN), with retrograde conduction back to the atria via the accessory pathway (AP). ART is due to conduction in the opposite direction and results in a wide (preexcited) QRS complex due to ventricular activation originating at the site of the AP.

ATRIAL TACHYCARDIA

Atrial tachycardias (ATs) can be broadly subdivided into those that are focal (i.e., arising from a discrete region) and those that are macroreentrant (i.e., reentry occurs around obstacles, either anatomic or functional).

Focal ATs appear to arise preferentially from certain anatomic areas. The most common regions include the tricuspid and mitral valve annuli, crista terminalis, pulmonary vein ostia, and atrial appendages. Although it is difficult to conclusively determine the mechanism of these arrhythmias, triggered activity appears to be the underlying mechanism for most ATs, with microreentry and abnormal automaticity responsible for a smaller fraction.

Macroreentrant AT, as the term implies, involves a reentry circuit that revolves around a relatively large area. As stated above, boundaries that stabilize this form of AT can include anatomic structures (valves, venae cavae, pulmonary veins) as well as functional obstacles (crista terminalis, diseased atrial myocardium). The classic example of macroreentrant AT is typical atrial flutter. The reentry circuit for this arrhythmia revolves around the tricuspid valve (outer, or anterior boundary) with the venae cavae, coronary sinus, fossa ovalis, and crista terminalis helping to form the inner (or posterior) boundary. Macroreentrant ATs can also occur due to the presence of surgical scars (e.g., from prior valve surgery). These are often termed *lesional tachycardias*. In addition, incomplete ablation lesion sets, with gaps within linear lesion sets, can result in an area of slow conduction. This can lead to a larger excitable gap, a favorable condition for the occurrence of macroreentry.

Management of ATs can involve either (ventricular) rate control or attempt at conversion of the arrhythmia to sinus rhythm. Rate control can be attempted with β-blockers or calcium channel blockers, either intravenously (acute management) or orally (chronic). Conversion of a focal AT to sinus rhythm can often be achieved with adenosine (6-12 mg IV), which can terminate ATs resulting from cyclic AMP–mediated triggered activity. In addition, adenosine can transiently suppress (typically for <20 sec) focal ATs that result from abnormal automaticity. Other therapeutic options for these ATs include β-blockers or calcium channel blockers. For ATs that are insensitive to adenosine, class I or III antiarrhythmic agents can be considered. Long-term therapy includes oral forms of the effective agents used in acute management (except for adenosine). In addition, catheter ablation is effective, especially when used in conjunction with a three-dimensional mapping system to help localize the arrhythmia focus or circuit.

Sinus tachycardia has not been included in this discussion, because this arrhythmia is usually secondary to another condition, such as fever, pain, hypotension, hyperthyroidism, or anemia.

Ventricular Tachyarrhythmias

In this section, we highlight the more common and the more important forms of ventricular tachycardia (VT). VTs can be either monomorphic or polymorphic. The term monomorphic signifies that the QRS complex has a consistent morphology from beat to beat. This implies that either the site of origin of each ventricular depolarization is the same, or that the reentrant circuit is uniform for each beat of the tachycardia. Ventricular fibrillation (VF), characterized by chaotic electrical ventricular activity, is discussed in the chapter on cardiac arrest.

OUTFLOW TRACT VENTRICULAR TACHYCARDIA

The most common form of idiopathic VT in North America is outflow tract tachycardia. Although this form of VT was first appreciated in the right ventricular (RV) outflow tract and occurs more commonly (∼80% of the time) from this region, origin from the left ventricular outflow tract region is also possible. Less commonly, these arrhythmias can arise from other sites, including the mitral annulus and the RV inflow tract, as well as epicardial sites. These tachycardias are focal in origin, are monomorphic, and most commonly have a left bundle branch block (LBBB) and inferior axis morphology (due to its RV outflow tract origin). Patients with this form of arrhythmia can present with frequent premature ventricular complexes (at rest), with salvos of nonsustained VT, or with sustained VT (usually exertional). This arrhythmia appears to be highly dependent on autonomic tone.

The underlying mechanism of outflow tract VT is delayed afterdepolarizations due to cyclic AMP-mediated triggered activity. β-Adrenergic receptor stimulation increases cyclic AMP, ultimately increasing intracellular calcium via stimulation of L-type calcium current (I_{CaL}) and subsequent calcium-induced calcium release and activation of a transient inward current (I_{ti}). This form of VT is uniquely sensitive to adenosine. Adenosine binds to a G-protein–coupled (A_1-adenosine) receptor and exerts its antiarrhythmic effect on ventricular myocytes via antagonism of β-adrenergic receptor activity. Other pharmacologic options for acute termination of outflow tract VT include intravenous β-blockers and intravenous verapamil (Calan). Long-term therapy includes administration of oral β-blockers or verapamil. Catheter ablation is extremely effective in curing outflow tract tachycardia.

INTRAFASCICULAR VENTRICULAR TACHYCARDIA

After outflow tract tachycardias, intrafascicular VT is the next most common form of monomorphic VT arising in the absence of structural heart disease. This form of VT is usually diagnosed in the second through fourth decades of life and has a male predominance. The distinguishing characteristics of intrafascicular VT include inducibility with rapid atrial pacing, right bundle branch block (RBBB) morphology with relatively narrow QRS complex (≤140 ms), and sensitivity to verapamil. Although there has been some debate regarding the exact mechanism of intrafascicular VT, it appears that it is due to a small reentrant circuit involving a portion of one of the fascicles of the left bundle branch (more commonly the posterior fascicle), as well as peri-Purkinje fibers. As a result, this tachycardia most commonly manifests with a RBBB and left superior axis morphology on ECG. However, RBBB and right inferior axis VT can also be observed when the circuit involves the left anterior fascicle. This form of VT is initiated due to conduction block down the fascicle, with conduction down the peri-Purkinje circuit. Retrograde conduction occurs up the adjacent fascicle.

Regarding acute management of intrafascicular VT, intravenous verapamil is effective in terminating the arrhythmia. The efficacy of oral verapamil in chronic therapy for intrafascicular VT is less clear, however. Catheter ablation has emerged as a viable alternative. Current strategies include targeting the earliest retrograde Purkinje potentials in the region of the reentrant circuit.

ARRHYTHMOGENIC RIGHT VENTRICULAR DYSPLASIA OR CARDIOMYOPATHY

It is extremely important to differentiate RV outflow tract VT from VT due to arrhythmogenic right ventricular dysplasia/cardiomyopathy (ARVD/C). Similar to RV outflow tract VT, ARVD/C can manifest with monomorphic VT of LBBB, inferior axis morphology.

ARVD/C is a condition involving progressive infiltration of the right ventricle with fibrosis and fat. The entity appears to have a male predominance, and diagnosis is usually made in the second through fourth decades of life, although this can be quite variable. Because there is no gold standard to diagnose ARVD/C, identifying patients can sometimes be difficult. Currently, diagnosis is made using Task Force criteria, published in 1994, which includes morphologic, functional, ECG, and histologic characteristics of the right ventricle, along with family history. Cardiac magnetic resonance imaging of the RV can demonstrate thinning of the walls and fibrofatty replacement, although this might not be evident early on in the disease. Modified, less stringent, criteria have been proposed for use in screening relatives of patients with ARVD/C to improve sensitivity.

Classically, the fibrofatty infiltration in ARVD/C has been described to involve predominantly the RV apex, diaphragmatic, and infundibular regions, the *triangle of dysplasia*. However, this can progress to involve other parts of the RV as well as the left ventricle. This fibrofatty infiltration predisposes the patient to VT due to reentry.

Several theories have been hypothesized regarding the etiology of ARVD/C. However, recent reports of mutations in plakoglobin, plakophilin, desmoplakin, and desmocollin genes have been reported in families with ARVD/C, pointing to a disorder of the desmosome as the underlying etiology of the disease process.

ARVD patients can present with ventricular arrhythmias as well as progressive RV failure. Due to the catecholamine dependence of VT in patients with ARVD/C, management includes avoidance of extreme physical activity and administration of β-blockers for low-risk patients. Those with a history of ventricular arrhythmias, unexplained syncope, sudden death, or family history of sudden death should consider receiving an implantable cardioverter-defibrillator (ICD) and possibly arrhythmia suppression with antiarrhythmic agents. ICD implantation can be technically difficult because of the thinning of the RV commonly seen in these patients. In some cases, palliative catheter ablation of VT can be performed. If either intractable ventricular tachycardia or end-stage right (or, less commonly, left) ventricular failure occurs, cardiac transplantation may be the only viable option.

LONG QT SYNDROME AND TORSADE DE POINTES

The clinical entity of long QT syndrome (LQTS) is heterogeneous with respect to phenotype and genotype. However, as the name suggests, there is a common ECG manifestation, a prolonged corrected QT interval (>440 ms in men, >460 ms in women), which is associated with an increased risk of syncope and sudden death. The estimated prevalence of LQTS is approximately 1:5000.

LQTS is considered a channelopathy. Hundreds of mutations have been reported in eight distinct ion channel genes, as well as in a structural protein (Ankyrin B) and a caveolin protein that helps form invaginations in the plasma membrane (Table 1). LQTS demonstrates both autosomal dominant (more common) and recessive patterns of inheritance. In addition to the congenital form of LQTS, an acquired form can also occur. In this form, after administration of certain medications, QT prolongation occurs due to electrolyte abnormalities or due to marked bradycardia. Most patients with acquired LQTS also have an underlying genetic predisposition to QT prolongation.

The most commonly affected gene, *KCNQ1* (LQT1) on chromosome 11, encodes the α-subunit of the slowly activating delayed rectifier potassium channel (I_{Ks}), leading to a loss of function. The next most commonly affected gene, *KCNH2* (or *HERG*; [LQT2]) is located on chromosome 7, resulting in loss of function of the rapidly activating delayed rectifier potassium channel, I_{Kr}. These two gene loci account for approximately 95% of cases of LQTS. LQT3 is due to mutations in a sodium channel (*SCN5A*; chromosome 3), leading to a gain of function of the channel. Abnormalities in this gene account for 3% to 5% of cases of LQTS.

Increased dispersion of repolarization within the ventricular myocardium serves as the substrate for torsade de pointes (TdP), a form of polymorphic VT that has a characteristic appearance of twisting around an isoelectric point. TdP is initiated by an early afterdepolarization (enabled by the prolonged QT interval). The maintenance of TdP is due to reentry facilitated by the dispersion of repolarization between the different layers and regions of the ventricular myocardium. TdP can either terminate spontaneously or can degenerate into VF, causing sudden death.

The circumstances in which TdP is initiated can provide clues regarding the underlying gene involved. Emotional or physical stress or exertion is a common trigger of TdP in LQT1 patients. LQT2 patients can also experience arrhythmias during stress, but sudden auditory stimuli (e.g., alarm clock) are often the culprits. In contrast, LQT3 patients often have TdP during rest or sleep. The ECG can also help differentiate between the genotypes. LQT1 patients often have a prominent, broad-based T wave, and LQT2 manifests with low-amplitude notched T waves. LQT3 patients typically have a long ST segment with a fairly normal T wave. Recently, clinical screening for many of the LQTS mutations has become available.

All patients with suspected LQT1, as well as those with LQT2, should be treated with β-adrenergic antagonists. In addition, these patients should refrain from competitive sports. Higher-risk patients (those with syncope, aborted sudden death, or marked QT prolongation) should consider implantation of an ICD. Family members of those with LQTS should also be screened by careful history an a 12-lead ECG.

CATECHOLAMINERGIC POLYMORPHIC VENTRICULAR TACHYCARDIA

Catecholaminergic polymorphic VT (CPVT) was first described by Reid in 1975 and by Coumel in 1978. Three distinct features were noted: a structurally normal heart, onset of arrhythmia during adrenergic activation, and a typical pattern of bidirectional VT with normal resting ECG. These patients have been found to have polymorphic VT as well. The degree and complexity of ectopy are correlated with increase in physical or emotional stress, and ectopy occurs with heart rates greater than 110 to 120 bpm. Patients usually present early in childhood (mean age 7-9 years; although CPVT is diagnosed in some during their adult years) with syncope or sudden death.

CPVT has a familial distribution, with both autosomal dominant and recessive patterns. Mutations in the gene encoding the cardiac ryanodine receptor *(RyR2)* have been reported, and they occur in an autosomal dominant fashion. *RyR2* mutations account for approximately 50% of patients with CPVT. The autosomal recessive form of CPVT results from mutations in the calsequestrin gene *(CASQ2)*, which encodes a protein involved in controlling calcium release from the sarcoplasmic reticulum. CPVT occurs because of uncontrolled calcium release from the sarcoplasmic reticulum, leading to VT due to delayed afterdepolarization—dependent triggered activity. CPVT typically arises from the left and right ventricular outflow tracts or the RV apex. Interestingly, CPVT patients often have supraventricular arrhythmias, including isolated atrial ectopy, and nonsustained atrial fibrillation.

β-Blocker therapy should be administered to all patients with CPVT, including silent carriers of *RyR2* mutations. ICD implantation should be considered for all CPVT patients with aborted sudden death and for those with syncope or VT despite therapy with β-blockers.

Brugada Syndrome

In 1992, the Brugadas described eight patients with aborted sudden death and a distinct ECG pattern. This ECG pattern included RBBB and coved ST segment elevation in leads V1 through V3 (with inverted T wave) in the absence of structural heart disease (Fig. 7). This ECG pattern can be intermittent; the findings can be unmasked by the administration of sodium channel blockers such as procainamide (Pronestyl), flecainide (Tambocor), or ajmaline.[2]

---

[2]Not available in the United States.

TABLE 1 Long QT Syndrome: Mutations

Gene	Locus	Ion Channel or Protein
LQT1	11p15	I_{Ks}
LQT2	7q35	I_{Kr}
LQT3	3p21	I_{Na}
LQT4	4q25	Ankyrin B
LQT5	21q22	I_{Ks}
LQT6	21q22	I_{Kr}
LQT7	17q23	I_{K1}
LQT8	9q8A	I_{Ca-L}
LQT9	3p25	I_{Na} or caveolin-3
LQT10	11q23.3	I_{Na}

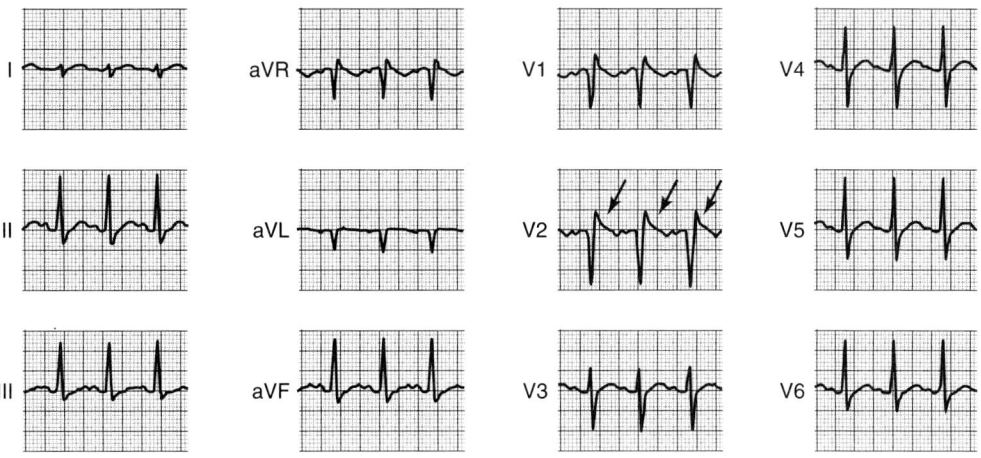

FIGURE 7. 12-lead electrocardiogram in a patient with Brugada syndrome. Note the J-point elevation and coved ST segments in the right precordial leads, most prominent in lead V₂ *(arrows)*.

Although mutations in *SCN5A*, the gene encoding the α-subunit of the sodium channel, have been reported in patients with Brugada syndrome, the majority of patients do not have a mutation in this gene. In contrast to mutations causing LQTS, SCN5A mutations causing Brugada syndrome lead to a *loss* of function. Other mutations reported to cause Brugada syndrome include those involving the glycerol-3-phosphate dehydrogenase 1-like gene *(GPD1L)* on chromosome 3, which leads to a reduction in sodium current, as well as two other genes encoding the α1-(CACNA1C) and β-(CACNB2b) subunits of the L-type calcium channel.

The underlying abnormality, loss of function of the sodium channel, leaves the transient outward potassium current (I_{to}) unopposed during phase 1 of the action potential. This results in a loss of the normal spike and dome and truncation of the action potential (Fig. 8). The RV subepicardial region is most severely affected, likely due to a higher concentration of I_{to} in this region. As a result, this leads to heterogeneity of repolarization between the epi- and endocardial layers and polymorphic VT/VF due to phase 2 reentry.

There have been isolated case reports of the use of intravenous isoproterenol (Isuprel)[1] in improving the ST segment elevation as well as in preventing VF episodes in patients with Brugada syndrome. The data are limited, however. Recently, oral quinidine has been reported to be efficacious in reducing VT and VF in these patients. Quinidine, although a sodium channel blocker, also blocks I_{to}, which reduces the effect on the action potential of the loss of sodium channel function. Symptomatic patients should be treated with implantation of an ICD.

Much more controversial is the management of the asymptomatic patient with Brugada pattern. The inducibility of ventricular arrhythmias during electrophysiologic testing has met with conflicting results regarding its prognostic usefulness. A spontaneous Brugada pattern on ECG and family history of sudden death from VF, have also been proposed as adverse prognostic risk factors. ICD implantation can be considered on an individual basis in those thought to be at high risk for sudden death.

VENTRICULAR ARRHYTHMIAS IN ISCHEMIC HEART DISEASE

Patients who have had a prior myocardial infarction (MI) are at increased risk for sudden cardiac death due to ventricular arrhythmias. Approximately 2% to 5% of patients develop sustained monomorphic VT during the chronic (healed) phase of an MI. Areas of infarction (scar) provide anatomic obstacles for perpetuation of reentry. Also, the peri-infarct border zone, as well as surviving myocardial cells within the scar, provides the substrate for slow conduction. These areas of slow conduction provide the optimal milieu for sustaining reentrant circuits.

Patients with sustained, hemodynamically significant VT and coronary artery disease should be managed with ICD implantation. ICDs have been shown, in numerous randomized multicenter studies, to reduce overall mortality in patients undergoing implantation for both primary and secondary prevention of sudden death. In those with frequent episodes of VT, suppressive therapy with antiarrhythmic agents can be considered. However, antiarrhythmic therapy is often ineffective, and it has not been shown to reduce overall mortality. Use of class IC antiarrhythmic agents (e.g., flecainide) is contraindicated in MI patients due to increased mortality. Alternatively, catheter ablation

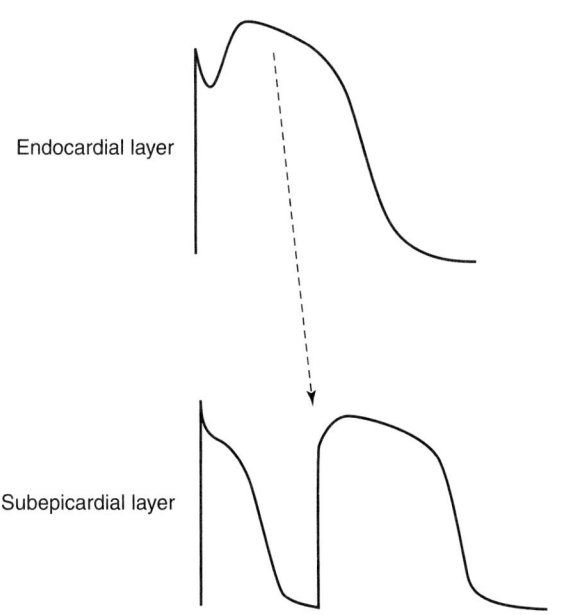

FIGURE 8. Typical action potentials in the endocardial *(top)* and subepicardial *(bottom)* layers of the right ventricle in a patient with Brugada syndrome. Note the loss of the spike-and-dome appearance (all-or-none phenomenon) in the subepicardial layer from loss of sodium channel function. This results in heterogeneity of repolarization (i.e., epicardium is fully repolarized when the endocardium is depolarized), which can lead to phase 2 reentry. In this example, propagation proceeds from phase 2 of the endocardial layer to the epicardial layer *(dashed arrow)*, which has already fully repolarized.

---

[1]Not FDA approved for this indication.

can be effective in decreasing the frequency of VT by disruption of the reentrant circuits.

REFERENCES

Ackerman MJ, Clapham DE: Normal cardiac electrophysiology. In Chien K (ed): Molecular Basis of Cardiovascular Disease. Philadelphia: WB Saunders, 1999, pp 281-301.
Antzelevitch CA: Brugada syndrome. PACE 2006;29:1130-1159.
Brugada P, Brugada J: Right bundle branch block, persistent ST segment elevation and sudden cardiac death: A distinct clinical and electrocardiographic syndrome. J Am Coll Cardiol 1992;20:1391-1396.
Hulot J-S, Jouven X, Empana J-P, et al: Natural history and risk stratification of arrhythmogenic right ventricular dysplasia/cardiomyopathy. Circulation. 2004;110:1879-1884.
Iwai S, Markowitz SM, Stein KM, et al: Response to adenosine differentiates focal from macroreentrant atrial tachycardia: Validation using three-dimensional electroanatomic mapping. Circulation 2002;106:2793-2799.
Jalife J, Delmar M, Davidenko J, et al: Basic Cardiac Electrophysiology For The Clinician. Armonk, NY: Futura, 1999.
Kim RJ, Iwai S, Markowitz SM, et al: Clinical and electrophysiologic spectrum of idiopathic ventricular outflow tract arrhythmias. J Am Coll Cardiol 2007;49:2035-2043.
Lerman BB, Stein KM, Markowitz SM: Adenosine-sensitive ventricular tachycardia: A conceptual approach. J Cardiovasc Electrophysiol. 1996;7:559-569.
Markowitz SM, Nemirovsky D, Stein KM, et al: Adenosine-insensitive focal atrial tachycardia: Evidence for de novo microreentry in the human atrium. J Am Coll Cardiol 2007;49:1324-1333.
McKenna WJ, Thiene G, Nava A, et al: Diagnosis of arrhythmogenic right ventricular dysplasia/cardiomyopathy. Br Heart J 1994;71:215-218.
Napolitano C, Priori SG: Diagnosis and treatment of catecholaminergic polymorphic ventricular tachycardia. Heart Rhythm 2007;4:675-678.
Zipes DP, Camm AJ, Borggrefe M, et al: ACC/AHA/ESC 2006 guidelines for management of patients with ventricular arrhythmias and the prevention of sudden cardiac death. Circulation 2006;114:e385-e484.

Congenital Heart Disease

Method of
Robb L. Romp, MD, and Yung R. Lau, MD

Congenital heart disease is the most common type of severe congenital malformation, with a prevalence of approximately 8 per 1000 live births. Proper evaluation of patients for congenital heart disease includes reviewing the past medical history, performing a systematic physical examination, and using selective ancillary testing.

The etiology of most congenital heart disease is unknown, but numerous high-risk populations have been identified. Fetal exposure to maternal diabetes, rubella, or teratogens such as ethanol and retinoic acid leads to an increased incidence of cardiac malformation. Certain chromosomal abnormalities, including Down syndrome (trisomy 21), DiGeorge's syndrome (22q11 deletion), and Turner's syndrome (XO) are associated with specific cardiac lesions. Some forms of congenital heart disease carry increased risk for familial transmission.

Cardiac Evaluation

The physical examination begins with gross inspection for dysmorphic features suggesting syndromes related to congenital heart disease. Next, a thorough review of vital signs including growth parameters, four extremity blood pressures, and oxygen saturation should be conducted. Normal arterial saturations should be greater than 93% in newborns. In the presence of desaturation, a hyperoxia challenge (measuring partial oxygen pressure of blood while breathing 100% oxygen) can be helpful. Infants with pulmonary disease can typically achieve a partial oxygen pressure in excess of 150 mm Hg, whereas infants with intracardiac right-to-left shunting cannot. Respiratory symptoms, including tachypnea and hyperpnea, are frequent findings in cardiac malformations that cause increased pulmonary blood flow. Hepatomegaly is also common in cardiac malformations with important pulmonary overcirculation. The extremities should be evaluated for evidence of impaired perfusion, clubbing, or edema. Abnormal pulses and brachiofemoral pulse delay are markers for certain types of congenital heart disease.

Evaluation of the heart itself includes observing and palpating the location and size of the cardiac impulse on the precordium. Auscultation of cardiac sounds should focus sequentially on the first and second heart sounds and then on murmurs. The first heart sound is typically single in pediatric patients. The second heart sound varies with respiration, with splitting that widens during inspiration and narrows to a single sound during expiration.

Murmurs are described based on intensity from I (quietest) to VI (loudest), and a palpable thrill is present in murmurs of grades IV to VI. The timing and amplitude of murmurs help to identify the cause of the sound. Systolic ejection murmurs have an onset after the first heart sound and a crescendo-decrescendo quality that terminates before the second heart sound. When such murmurs are soft and vibratory and vary with patient position, they are generally benign or innocent. Harsher and louder ejection murmurs are more likely to represent obstructed blood flow, such as valve stenosis.

Holosystolic murmurs have an onset coincident with the first heart sound. These murmurs are caused most commonly by ventricular septal defects but are also associated with mitral or tricuspid valve insufficiency. Continuous murmurs extend from systole

CURRENT DIAGNOSIS

- History and physical examination, including growth parameters, blood pressures, respiratory rate, pulse oximetry, work of breathing, hepatomegaly, and peripheral pulses
- Cardiac examination, including description of murmur and heart sounds
- Ancillary testing, including chest radiograph and electrocardiogram
- Consultation with pediatric cardiologist for:
- Abnormal examination suggesting congenital heart disease
- High-risk populations (trisomy 21)

CURRENT THERAPY

- Endocarditis prophylaxis is recommended for:
  - Unrepaired cyanotic CHD
  - Recently repaired CHD (<6 months from surgical or catheterization repair)
  - Repaired CHD with residual defects near prosthetic material
- Catheterization and surgical techniques have improved outcomes for complex congenital heart disease
- Exercise restrictions exist for certain congenital heart disease
- All congenital heart disease patients should have long-term follow-up for complications of disease

Abbreviations: ASD = atrial septal defect; PDA = patent ductus arteriosus; VSD = ventricular septal defect.

through the second heart sound into diastole and represent flow from the systemic arterial circulation into the pulmonary or venous circulation. Diastolic murmurs are isolated in diastole and can be caused by aortic or pulmonary valve insufficiency. Diastolic rumbles can also be caused by excess flow across the tricuspid or mitral valve due to intracardiac left-to-right shunting. The location of the murmur and direction of radiation are helpful in determining the cause of the sound.

Ancillary testing plays an important role in diagnosing congenital heart disease. Chest radiography can help identify the presence of cardiac enlargement and the prominence of the pulmonary vascularity. These findings help determine whether a heart defect is causing increased, normal, or decreased pulmonary blood flow. The electrocardiogram (ECG) can identify conduction abnormalities that are associated with certain congenital malformations. In experienced hands, echocardiography is the primary tool for diagnosis of congenital heart disease. Most malformations of the heart can be delineated completely by transthoracic echocardiography, and fetal echocardiography can be used to diagnose many cardiac abnormalities prenatally. Although cardiac catheterization has, in the past, played a role in defining congenital heart disease, most catheterizations are now performed for interventional purposes, such as closing septal defects, dilating stenotic valves, or stenting open narrowed vessels. Cardiac computed tomography (CT) and magnetic resonance imaging (MRI) are becoming increasingly important noninvasive diagnostic tools for extracardiac vascular abnormalities and patients in whom only limited transthoracic echocardiographic images can be obtained.

Using an evaluation including only the physical examination, oxygen saturation, and chest x-ray, it should be possible to identify patients with significant congenital heart disease and in turn the urgency of an evaluation by a pediatric cardiologist. This same basic evaluation permits patients to be readily categorized based on the presence or absence of cyanosis and the amount of pulmonary blood flow. Acyanotic lesions include those with increased pulmonary blood flow and those with normal pulmonary blood flow but obstruction of flow from the heart. Cyanotic lesions include those with increased or decreased pulmonary blood flow.

Acyanotic Lesions with Increased Pulmonary Blood Flow

Acyanotic cardiac defects with increased pulmonary blood flow make up the largest category of congenital heart disease and include ventricular septal defect, atrial septal defect, atrioventricular canal defect, and patent ductus arteriosus. Such defects permit left-to-right shunting, the magnitude of which depends on the size of the defect and the relative resistances of the pulmonary and systemic vascular beds. As the pulmonary vascular resistance falls within the first weeks of life, the quantity of shunting increases substantially. This leads to the typical findings of cardiomegaly and increased pulmonary vascularity on the chest radiograph. Symptoms are related to the magnitude of additional pulmonary flow.

VENTRICULAR SEPTAL DEFECT

A ventricular septal defect (VSD), an opening in the ventricular septum, is the most common cardiac malformation. It is present as an isolated lesion in one quarter and as a component of a cardiac malformation in one half of all patients with congenital heart disease. The hemodynamic importance and natural history of a VSD are related to its location and size. A VSD located in the muscular septum, remote from the valves, is the most common type and fortunately the most likely to undergo spontaneous closure. Defects of the perimembranous septum can also decrease in size over time, but perimembranous defects are more likely to be associated with other abnormalities and to require surgical closure. Defects of the inlet and outlet portions of the ventricular septum are relatively rare. Large defects (approaching the size of the aortic annulus) are almost certain to cause symptoms from pulmonary overcirculation and to require surgical closure. Moderate-sized defects (about one half the size of the aortic annulus) can cause sufficient symptoms to require medical management but often spontaneously decrease in size to the point where they no longer require surgical or medical intervention. Small defects (less than one half the aortic annulus) are unlikely to cause symptoms or require intervention.

Most often, a newborn with a VSD has no murmur immediately after birth, due to the relatively high pulmonary vascular resistance, which prevents significant left-to-right shunting. As the pulmonary resistance falls in the first few weeks of life, shunting increases. In small and moderate VSDs, a concomitant decrease in right ventricular pressure occurs and a characteristic harsh holosystolic murmur is heard. In a large VSD, there is little restriction of flow, and no holosystolic murmur is present. Patients with pulmonary overcirculation caused by important left-to-right shunts typically develop symptoms in the first weeks to months of life. Tachypnea is often the first sign, followed by poor feeding, diaphoresis, and eventual failure to thrive. The chest x-ray shows increased cardiac size and pulmonary vascular markings in proportion to the size of the shunt. In rare circumstances, a large VSD can lead to persistent elevation of the pulmonary resistance. Though such patients have no murmur and few symptoms, they are at risk for developing pulmonary vascular obstructive disease.

Management of ventricular septal defects depends on the patient's symptoms and the magnitude of shunting permitted by the defect. Symptomatic patients are usually treated with a combination of diuretics, digoxin (Lanoxin), and afterload reduction. Patients who are refractory to medical management and those with large nonrestrictive defects should undergo surgical closure during infancy to prevent the development of irreversible pulmonary vascular obstructive disease. Surgical closure might also be indicated in asymptomatic children with significant shunting that persists, due to long-term risk of pulmonary vascular obstructive disease. Surgical closure is currently the standard of care for defects requiring closure, but trials are under way for catheter-delivered devices that will play an increasingly important role in VSD closure in the future.

ATRIAL SEPTAL DEFECT

An atrial septal defect (ASD) is an opening in the atrial septum that permits important left-to-right shunting. The magnitude of the shunt depends on the size of the defect and the relative compliance of the ventricles. Despite the increased pulmonary blood flow permitted by a large ASD, such a defect generally does not cause pulmonary hypertension or symptoms during childhood. The increased right ventricular output and flow across the pulmonary valve cause the systolic ejection murmur and widely split second heart sound, which does not narrow during expiration.

If the magnitude of the shunt is substantial, ASD closure should be performed during childhood to avoid the long-term risks of pulmonary vascular disease and atrial arrhythmias. With the exception of large ASDs and some defects located eccentrically within the atrial septum that require surgical closure, most ASDs are now closed using a catheter-delivery system in which a device is positioned within the defect to prevent shunting. Medical therapy is rarely necessary.

ATRIOVENTRICULAR CANAL DEFECT

Atrioventricular (AV) canal defects are malformations caused by incomplete fusion of the endocardial cushions during embryonic development. These cushions normally fuse to form the tricuspid and mitral valves as well as the adjacent portions of the atrial and ventricular septum. Endocardial cushion defects include a spectrum of abnormalities ranging from an isolated defect in the atrial septum, known as a primum ASD, to a common AV canal defect in which there is a single AV valve in association with a large ASD and VSD. A common AV canal defect permits substantial left-to-right shunting at both the atrial and ventricular levels, which leads to early symptoms from both excess pulmonary blood flow and pulmonary hypertension. Patients typically develop early symptoms of congestive heart failure in the first months of life.

Physical findings include tachypnea and hepatomegaly. The cardiac examination reveals a hyperdynamic precordium and a systolic ejection murmur from increased flow across the pulmonary valve. A holosystolic murmur is likely caused by AV valve insufficiency, which is commonly present, rather than VSD shunting. The chest x-ray shows cardiomegaly and increased pulmonary vascularity. The EGC characteristically reveals left axis deviation.

AV canal defects require surgical repair. Although such patients can benefit from medical treatment with diuretics, digoxin, and afterload reduction, the onset of heart failure symptoms is generally the point at which surgery is considered. Surgical techniques vary and include use of one or two patches (depending on the size of the septal defects) and division of the common AV valve into two separate components.

PATENT DUCTUS ARTERIOSUS

The patent ductus arteriosus (PDA) is a normal prenatal vessel connecting the pulmonary artery and the aorta that permits the output of the right ventricle to bypass the fetal lungs. The PDA typically constricts and closes within the first days of postnatal life. Persistent PDA is present in one in 1250 live births, with an increasing prevalence in premature infants (as common as 80% for infants with a birth weight of less than 750 g). The presence of a PDA permits left-to-right shunting that is related to the size of the PDA and the relative resistance of the pulmonary and systemic vascular beds. Significant shunting leads to volume overload of the left heart and pulmonary vascular bed that manifest clinically as tachycardia, tachypnea, and widened pulse pressures. A large ductus in a patient with low pulmonary vascular resistance causes a continuous murmur. Often the diastolic component of the murmur is diminished in newborns who might have elevated pulmonary resistance, making clinical diagnosis more challenging.

In the infant, the need for closure of a PDA depends on the clinical significance of the shunt. As a general rule, a PDA that causes symptoms or results in dilation of the left heart should be closed. In an older child, closure of a PDA is advisable if a classic murmur is present in order to eliminate the lifetime risk of endocarditis.

Several options are available to close a PDA. Preterm infants often respond to medical management with prostaglandin inhibitors such as indomethacin (Indocin) or ibuprofen (Motrin). If medical therapy is unsuccessful or contraindicated, surgical ligation of the ductus is performed. In older children, interventional catheterization techniques using several available devices are widely used to occlude the ductus.

Acyanotic Lesions With Obstruction

Obstruction of blood flow from the heart can be caused by aortic stenosis, pulmonary stenosis, or coarctation of the aorta. These lesions are not associated with cyanosis, except in cases of critically severe obstruction in neonates.

COARCTATION OF THE AORTA

Coarctation, which has a prevalence of 1 in 3000 live births, is a narrowing of the aortic arch between the origin of the left subclavian artery and the insertion of the ductus arteriosus—ligamentum. Coarctation can manifest in two ways: neonatal critical coarctation and non-neonatal coarctation. Critical coarctation manifests as shock caused by impaired systemic cardiac output when the ductus arteriosus closes spontaneously in the neonatal period. Less severe forms of coarctation cause hypertension in the proximal aorta (best measured in the right arm) and both delayed and diminished pulses in the femoral arteries.

Coarctation should be excluded as the etiology of hypertension in any pediatric patient. The heart sounds are normal unless there is an associated anomaly, such as a bicuspid aortic valve. A continuous murmur may be heard over the back. Chest x-ray findings can include the "3 sign" caused by indentation of the aorta at the point of coarctation and rib notching due to engorged intercostal arteries carrying collateral flow.

Treatment of coarctation depends on the age at presentation. Critical coarctation is initially treated medically with prostaglandin E_1 (Alprostadil) to maintain ductal patency. Surgical repair, involving resection of the coarctation site and elongated anastomosis of the proximal and descending ends of the aorta, is the most widely used therapy in infants. After repair, infants can develop re-coarctation from anastomotic scarring, which responds well to balloon angioplasty in the catheterization laboratory. Older children and adults may be candidates for catheterization interventions including balloon angioplasty or stenting of native coarctation as an initial intervention (Figure 1).

AORTIC STENOSIS

The incidence of aortic stenosis is as great as 1 in 2600 live births. Obstruction most commonly occurs at the level of the valve itself, due to dysplasia or fusion of the valve leaflets, but it can also involve the region below or above the valve. Critical aortic stenosis manifests as shock in the neonatal period, when systemic cardiac output is compromised. Severe aortic stenosis can manifest with exertional chest pain, syncope, or even sudden death. Mild to moderate aortic stenosis is generally asymptomatic.

Cardiac examination reveals an ejection click and a systolic ejection murmur that radiates to the carotids and increases in intensity in relation to severity of stenosis. With moderate to severe stenosis, a thrill may also be palpated in the suprasternal notch. The ECG is normal with mild stenosis but shows evidence of left ventricular hypertrophy and strain with increasingly severe aortic stenosis. Dilation of the ascending aorta may be apparent on chest x-ray.

Aortic stenosis has a tendency to progress over time and therefore requires close follow-up. With higher degrees of severity, exercise restrictions are recommended. For moderate and severe aortic stenosis, balloon valvuloplasty performed in the catheterization laboratory is recommended to reduce the obstruction. Though generally effective in reducing the stenosis, valvuloplasty can cause aortic insufficiency. Surgery is reserved for patients who have aortic stenosis associated with important insufficiency or stenosis caused by a severely dysplastic valve not responsive to balloon dilation.

PULMONARY STENOSIS

Pulmonary stenosis is a common form of congenital heart disease, with an incidence of 1 in 1250 live births. As in aortic stenosis, the valve leaflets are thickened and they separate incompletely from one another. Critical pulmonary stenosis can result in impaired pulmonary blood flow and cyanosis in newborns (due to right-to-left shunting through the patent foramen ovale), but less severe forms of pulmonary stenosis are generally asymptomatic. An ejection click and systolic ejection murmur are present, with the intensity and duration of the murmur proportional to the severity of stenosis. ECG findings may include right ventricular hypertrophy or strain. Echocardiography can accurately grade the severity of stenosis. Balloon valvuloplasty is the treatment of choice for moderate and severe valvular pulmonary stenosis and provides excellent long-term relief of obstruction.

Cyanotic Lesions with Decreased Pulmonary Blood Flow

Cyanotic lesions with decreased pulmonary vascularity are caused by obstructed pulmonary blood flow and right-to-left shunting within the heart. The most common lesions are tetralogy of Fallot and tricuspid atresia. Affected patients have varying degrees of cyanosis. The absence of pulmonary overcirculation prevents the development of tachypnea seen in patients with congestive heart failure.

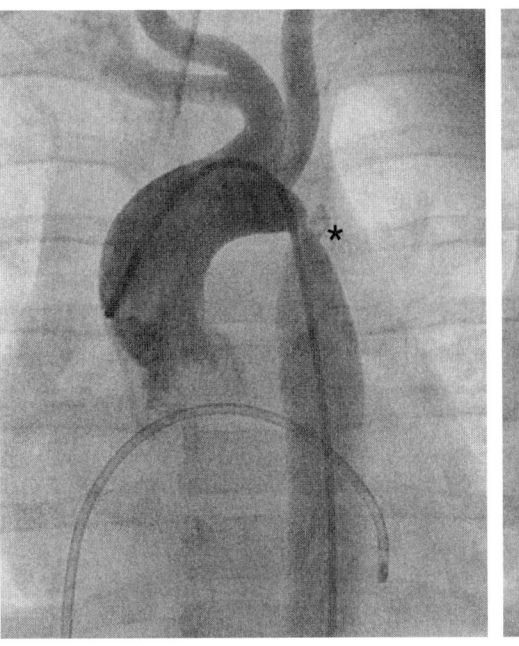 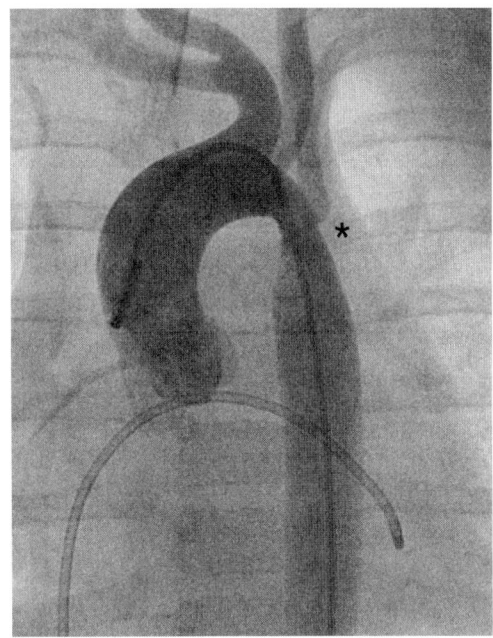

FIGURE 1. Angiography demonstrating aortic coarctation. **A,** There is moderate to severe coarctation with reduced blood flow into the left subclavian artery (*). **B,** Following balloon angioplasty, the obstruction is reduced and filling of the subclavian artery is normalized.

TETRALOGY OF FALLOT

Tetralogy of Fallot is the most common form of cyanotic congenital heart disease, with an incidence of about 1 in 3000 live births. Malalignment of the perimembranous ventricular septum leads to the tetralogy, which consists of pulmonary outflow tract obstruction, large ventricular septal defect with aortic override, and right ventricular hypertrophy. The severity of pulmonary outflow tract obstruction dictates the degree of cyanosis, ranging from pulmonary atresia with severe cyanosis to more mild pulmonary stenosis with normal saturations. Hypercyanotic spells are precipitated by spasm of the subpulmonary infundibular muscle, which causes acute worsening of pulmonary outflow tract obstruction and potentially life-threatening cyanosis. Squatting is a maneuver used by older unrepaired patients to increase the systemic vascular resistance and overcome the pulmonary obstruction causing a hypercyanotic spell.

The examination is notable for cyanosis in the case of more severe obstruction of the pulmonary outflow tract. A harsh systolic ejection murmur is present in the pulmonary region. The chest x-ray shows decreased pulmonary vascularity with an absent pulmonary segment and upturned apex of the cardiac silhouette, which gives the classic boot-shaped heart.

Tetralogy does not typically require medical management, and in fact, diuretics and positive inotropes can increase the likelihood of hypercyanotic spells. Hypercyanotic spells are a medical emergency and must be treated aggressively (Box 1). Patients with pulmonary atresia are ductal dependent and require prostaglandin therapy to maintain ductal patency. These patients commonly undergo surgical placement of a modified Blalock-Taussig shunt between the subclavian artery and the pulmonary artery to secure pulmonary blood flow during infancy. Repair of the intracardiac abnormalities can be undertaken as early as the neonatal period, but it is often delayed until later in infancy in the patient with only mild cyanosis.

Surgical repair involves patch closure of the VSD with enlargement of the pulmonary outflow tract by resection of subpulmonary muscle bundles and enlargement of the pulmonary valve with a transannular patch. Lifelong endocarditis prophylaxis is recommended, but most patients require no other long-term medical management. Although the functional outcomes are excellent during childhood, right ventricular dilation and dysfunction are common long-term complications that can require surgical placement of a competent pulmonary valve.

TRICUSPID ATRESIA

Tricuspid atresia is a rare cardiac malformation with an incidence of 1 in 17,500 live births. In this condition, the tricuspid valve is platelike and does not permit flow from the right atrium to the right ventricle. Instead, the systemic venous return shunts right to left across an atrial septal defect, mixing with the pulmonary venous return in the left atrium. Blood flow to the lungs is either through a VSD to a hypoplastic right ventricle and thereby to the pulmonary artery or is ductal dependent from the aorta to the pulmonary arteries by way of a PDA.

Patients are severely cyanotic from the time of birth but can have relatively quiet hearts without pathologic murmurs. The ECG is helpful in making the diagnosis due to the presence of left axis deviation. The chest x-ray shows diminished pulmonary vascularity and relatively small heart size, similar to tetralogy of Fallot.

BOX 1 Management of Hypercyanotic "Tet" Spells

Noninvasive Treatments

Patient in calm environment (mother's lap)
Supplemental oxygen
Swaddled knee-chest position to increase systemic afterload

Invasive Treatments

- Morphine or ketamine (Ketalar)
- Volume expansion (packed red blood cells if anemic)
- Phenylephrine (Neo-Synephrine) to increase systemic afterload
- Esmolol (Brevibloc) to relax the infundibular spasm
- Anesthetize and paralyze
- Surgical repair or palliation

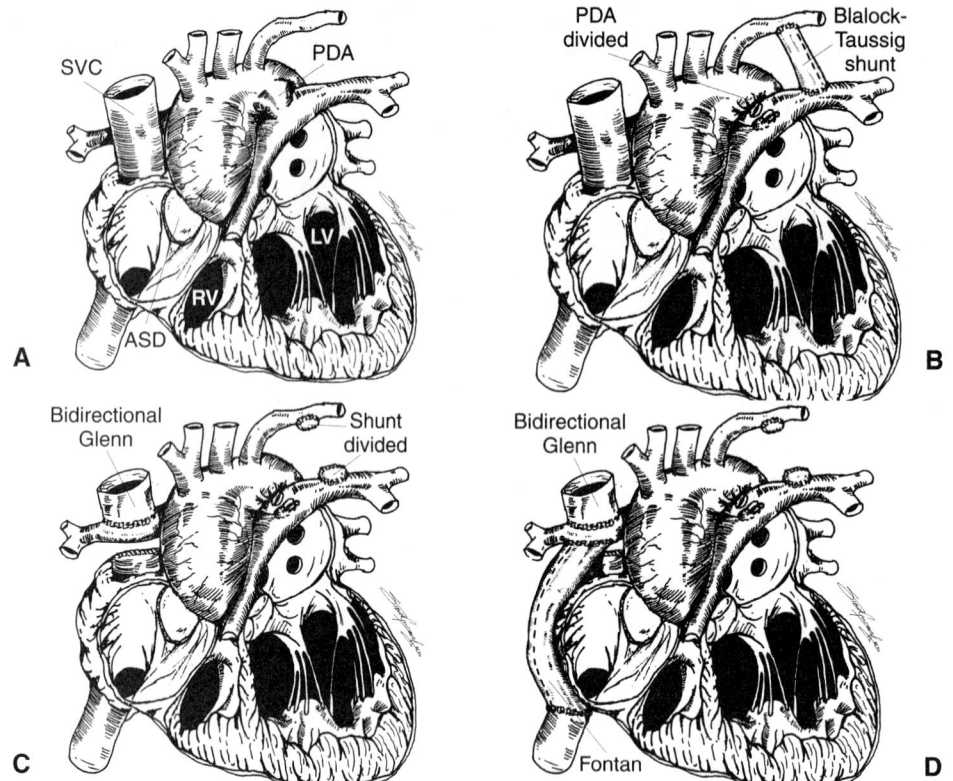

FIGURE 2. Illustrations of tricuspid atresia and surgical palliations. **A,** Pulmonary blood flow originates from the patent ductus arteriosus (PDA). **B,** A modified Blalock-Taussig shunt replaces the PDA as the source of pulmonary blood flow. **C,** Pulmonary blood flow is through the bidirectional Glenn connection of the superior vena cava (SVC) to the right pulmonary artery. **D,** Following the modified Fontan connection of the inferior vena cava to the right pulmonary artery, the systemic venous return bypasses the heart, entirely separating the deoxygenated blood from the oxygenated blood. *Abbreviation:* ASD = atrial septal defect.

Treatment of tricuspid atresia depends on the degree of flow through the hypoplastic right ventricle. Ductal-dependent patients require prostaglandin to maintain ductal patency until placement of a modified Blalock-Taussig shunt in the neonatal period. All patients eventually undergo cavopulmonary anastomosis by means of a modified Glenn operation (superior vena caval anastomosis to pulmonary artery) during infancy and a modified Fontan operation (inferior vena caval anastomosis to pulmonary artery) during early childhood (Figure 2). The cavopulmonary anastomoses permit the systemic venous return to bypass the heart and flow passively through the lungs, allowing the functional single ventricle to be used as the systemic ventricle. The modified Glenn and modified Fontan operations are used as a common final pathway in most cardiac malformations resulting in a functional single ventricle.

Cyanotic Lesions with Increased Pulmonary Blood Flow

Cyanosis with increased pulmonary blood flow suggests the presence of an admixture lesion that has both right-to-left and left-to-right shunting. Patients in this category have both cyanosis and early development of tachypnea due to pulmonary overcirculation. The most common lesions include transposition of the great arteries, truncus arteriosus, total anomalous pulmonary venous connection, and hypoplastic left heart syndrome.

TRANSPOSITION OF THE GREAT ARTERIES

Transposition of the great arteries (TGA) has a prevalence of 1 in 4000 live births. In TGA, the aorta arises from the right ventricle and the pulmonary artery arises from the left ventricle. This arrangement of parallel systemic and pulmonary circulations causes severe cyanosis. Mixing between the systemic and pulmonary circulations depends on the presence of an ASD, which permits shunting of the oxygenated pulmonary venous return to the right heart, where it is pumped to the systemic circulation. Cardiac examination reveals a single second heart sound without pathologic murmurs. The chest x-ray shows cardiomegaly with a narrow superior mediastinum related to the parallel orientation of the great arteries.

Treatment of TGA involves prompt recognition and institution of prostaglandin infusion to maintain ductal patency. If an adequate ASD is not present, a balloon atrial septostomy is performed urgently to enhance mixing of systemic and pulmonary circulations. Repair is done in the first week of life by means of an arterial switch operation, which involves transection and relocation of the great arteries so they arise from the correct ventricle.

TRUNCUS ARTERIOSUS

Truncus arteriosus is a rare cardiac malformation with a prevalence of about 1 in 25,000 live births. A single great artery is situated above a large VSD, receiving the outputs of both the right and left ventricles. This ascending truncal artery supplies the coronary, pulmonary, and systemic circulations. There is severe pulmonary overcirculation with relatively mild cyanosis but early development of tachypnea and respiratory distress related to severe congestive heart failure. A continuous murmur of flow into the pulmonary arteries is present and there is often a diastolic murmur and ejection click caused by an insufficient and dysplastic truncal valve. The chest x-ray shows cardiomegaly and prominent pulmonary vascular markings.

Medical management with diuretics and digoxin can alleviate symptoms, but definitive treatment involves early surgical repair within days to weeks of diagnosis. The VSD is closed in such a way as to direct blood from the left ventricle to the truncal valve (which serves as the new aortic valve), and a conduit is placed between the right ventricle and the detached pulmonary arteries. Repeat catheterizations and surgical replacement of obstructed conduits are inevitable during childhood.

TOTAL ANOMALOUS PULMONARY VENOUS CONNECTION

Total anomalous pulmonary venous connection (TAPVC) is a rare form of congenital heart disease, with a prevalence of 1 in 17,500 live births. The pulmonary veins drain to a confluence that connects anomalously to either the innominate vein, the coronary sinus, or below the diaphragm to the inferior vena cava. In all types, the pulmonary venous return mixes with the systemic venous return in the right atrium. The systemic cardiac output is dependent on right-to-left shunting through an ASD. Pulmonary blood flow is increased and the level of cyanosis is generally mild. A systolic ejection murmur is present over the pulmonary valve. The chest x-ray shows cardiomegaly and vascular engorgement. Subdiaphragmatic forms of TAPVC can have obstruction of the anomalous pulmonary venous connection, which can cause respiratory distress and severe cyanosis within hours of birth. Surgical repair is performed in the neonatal period and involves ASD closure and anastomosis of the pulmonary venous confluence to the left atrium.

HYPOPLASTIC LEFT HEART

Hypoplastic left heart (HLH) is relatively rare, with a prevalence of 1 3500 live births. There is hypoplasia of the mitral valve, left ventricle, aortic valve, and ascending aorta to a degree that the left heart is not able to support the systemic circulation. The pulmonary venous return shunts left to right across an ASD to mix with the systemic venous return in the right atrium, and the systemic circulation is dependent on right-to-left shunting across the PDA.

Patients are cyanotic and develop severe pulmonary overcirculation as newborns. Presentation often involves circulatory collapse when the PDA closes, causing impaired systemic perfusion. The examination is notable for cyanosis and a single second heart sound but no important murmurs. The chest x-ray shows cardiomegaly and increased pulmonary vascularity.

Treatment involves early recognition and institution of prostaglandin infusion to maintain ductal patency. Surgical palliation in the first week of life involves the Norwood stage 1 procedure, which has mortality rates approaching 10% at many larger medical centers. Patients require future surgeries during infancy and childhood, including the Glenn and Fontan cavopulmonary anastomoses, which permit passive systemic venous return to the lungs and establish the single right ventricle as the systemic pump. Although such patients have a diminished exercise tolerance and risk of right ventricular failure long term, they can have a reasonable quality of life through childhood.

REFERENCES

Allen, HD, Gutgesell, HP, Clark, EB, Driscoll, DK (eds): Moss and Adams' Heart Disease in Infants, Children, and Adolescents, 6th ed. Philadelphia: Lippincott Williams & Wilkins, 2001.
Garson, A, Bricker, JT, Fisher, DJ, Neish, SR (eds): The Science and Practice of Pediatric Cardiology, 2nd ed. Baltimore: Williams & Wilkins, 1998.
Johnson, WH, Moller, JH: Pediatric Cardiology. Philadelphia: Lippincott Williams & Wilkins, 2001.
Keane, JF, Lock, JE, Fyler, DC (eds): Nadas' Pediatric Cardiology, 2nd ed. Philadelphia: Saunders, 2006.
Maron, BJ, Zipes, DP: 36th Bethesda conference: Eligibility recommendations for competitive athletes with cardiovascular abnormalities. J Am Coll Cardiol 2005;45(8):1312-1375.
Nichols, DG, Ungerleider, RM, Spevak, PJ, et al (eds): Critical Heart Disease in Infants and Children, 2nd ed. Philadelphia: Mosby, 2006.
Rudolph, AM: Congenital Diseases of the Heart: Clinical Physiological Considerations, 2nd ed. Armonk, NY: Futura, 2001.

Hypertrophic Cardiomyopathy

Method of
Ali J. Marian, MD

Definition

Hypertrophic cardiomyopathy (HCM) is a primary disease of the myocardium characterized by unexplained cardiac hypertrophy, a hyperdynamic left ventricle with a small cavity, and often dynamic outflow tract obstruction. The pathologic features of HCM include myocyte hypertrophy, disarray, and interstitial fibrosis. Myocyte disarray is considered the pathologic hallmark of HCM.

The current clinical diagnosis of HCM is neither specific nor highly sensitive. For example, the presence of systemic hypertension, per convention, excludes the diagnosis of HCM, despite the possibility of concomitant HCM in hypertensive individuals. "Unexplained cardiac hypertrophy" also can occur in storage diseases, mitochondrial disorders, and triplet repeat syndromes. The presence of a hyperdynamic left ventricle, outflow tract obstruction, and asymmetric hypertrophy favors the diagnosis of true HCM. In contrast, depressed global cardiac systolic function, conduction defects, neurologic abnormalities, and skeletal myopathy favor the possibility of a phenocopy.

Prevalence

The prevalence of HCM, defined as a wall thickness of 15 mm or greater on echocardiogram in the absence of a secondary cause, is estimated to be 1:500 in individuals 23 to 35 years old. However, the disease probably is more common, as expression of cardiac hypertrophy is age dependent. Many young individuals with the disease-causing mutation may exhibit mild hypertrophy or express cardiac hypertrophy late in life.

Clinical Manifestations

Clinical manifestations of HCM are variable, ranging from an asymptomatic course to that of severe heart failure and sudden cardiac death (SCD). The majority of patients with HCM are asymptomatic or minimally symptomatic. The most common symptoms are dyspnea, chest pain, palpitations, and lightheadedness. Syncope is an infrequent symptom that often indicates serious cardiac arrhythmias. Atrial fibrillation and nonsustained ventricular tachycardia are the most common cardiac arrhythmias in patients with HCM.

HCM is the most common cause of SCD and often is the first manifestation of the disease in young competitive athletes, accounting for almost half of cases. A history of SCD, syncope, a strong family history of SCD, serious ventricular arrhythmias including frequent episodes of nonsustained ventricular tachycardia, severe cardiac hypertrophy, exertional hypotension, and genetic factors are considered risk factors for SCD. None of the risk factors alone is a reliable predictor; hence, the global risk, which is derived from a combination of multiple risk factors, should be assessed. The overall

---

CURRENT DIAGNOSIS

- Cardiac hypertrophy in the absence of known etiology, usually asymmetric with predominant involvement of the interventricular septum.
- Hyperdynamic left ventricle with a small cavity size
- Outflow tract obstruction

estimated annual mortality rate of patients with HCM is about 1% in the adult population.

Molecular Genetics

HCM is a genetic disease with an autosomal dominant mode of inheritance. A family history of HCM can be elicited in approximately half to two thirds of cases. The seminal report by Seidman and colleagues in 1999 of the R403Q mutation in the β-myosin heavy chain (β-MyHC) led to elucidation of the molecular genetic basis of HCM. To date, more than 400 causal mutations in more than a dozen different genes, all encoding the sarcomeric proteins, have been identified. Accordingly, HCM is considered a disease of mutant sarcomeric proteins (excluding HCM phenocopy). Mutations in *MYH7* and *MYBPC3*, which encode β-MyHC and myosin-binding protein-C (MyBP-C), respectively, are the most common, each accounting for approximately 30% of HCM cases. Mutations in *TNNT2* and *TNNI3*, which encode cardiac troponin T and cardiac troponin I, respectively, each accounts for 3% to 5% of HCM cases. The vast majority of causal mutations are missense and private mutations; hence, the frequency of each specific mutation is low.

There is considerable variability in the phenotypic expression of HCM, even among patients with similar or identical causal mutations. Multiple mutations are often associated with more severe phenotypes but are present in only a small fraction of cases. The genetic background of individuals, defined by the presence of single nucleotide polymorphisms, is considered an important determinant of phenotypic variability of HCM. In addition, environmental factors, such as isometric exercises, are expected to affect phenotypic expression of HCM.

 CURRENT THERAPY

Asymptomatic

- Periodic follow-up for symptoms and risk factors assessment for SCD
- ICD implantation in patients at high risk for SCD

Symptomatic

- ICD implantation in patients at high risk for SCD
- Medical therapy with β-blockers and calcium channel blockers
- Surgical myectomy, transcoronary septal ablation, and dual-chamber pacing in patients refractory to medical therapy, septal thickness >15 mm, and outflow tract obstruction >50 mm Hg
- Atrial fibrillation
  1. Acute: Cardioversion
  2. Chronic: β-Blockers and amiodarone (Cordarone), anticoagulation, and radiofrequency ablation if refractory to medical therapy
- Syncope
  1. β-Blockers and clonidine in patients with inappropriate vasodilatory response
  2. ICD and antiarrhythmic drugs in patients with ventricular arrhythmias
  3. Antiarrhythmic drugs in patients with supraventricular arrhythmias and radiofrequency ablation for refractory cases
  4. Myectomy or transcoronary septal ablation in patients with severe outflow tract obstruction

---

Abbreviations: ICD = internal cardioverter-defibrillator; SCD = sudden cardiac death.

GENETIC SCREENING

There is considerable interest in genetic testing for the diagnosis and prognostication of HCM patients. Currently, the primary utility of genetic testing is in families in which the causal mutation is already known, which makes possible the accurate diagnosis of mutation carriers from noncarriers. In families in which the causal mutation is unknown, initial genetic linkage mapping could help to identify the putative candidate gene, followed by mutation screening. Genetic testing in isolated cases of HCM is complicated by the need for extensive genetic screening of a large number of genes and a 30% to 40% chance of not finding the causal mutation. However, advances in rapid and high-throughput screening techniques are expected to change the current approach. The significance of genetic testing in clinical prognostication and identification of individuals at risk for SCD remains to be established. In general, information on the causal genes as well as the modifier genes and the environmental factors will be necessary for accurate prognostication and genetic counseling of HCM patients.

Pathogenesis

Elucidation of the molecular genetic basis of HCM has provided significant clues to its pathogenesis. The evolution of phenotype can be categorized into three sets: the initial functional phenotype, the intermediary molecular phenotype, and the final morphologic phenotype. The collective results of a large number of in vitro and in vivo mechanistic studies indicate that the initial defects are diverse and encompass reduced ATPase activity of the myofibrils, impaired actomyosin cross-bridging, and enhanced Ca^{2+} sensitivity of myofibrils. The intermediary molecular phenotype occurs in response to the functional phenotype and is largely unknown but is expected to include expression and activation of intracellular signaling molecules. The morphologic and histologic phenotypes are the consequence of the intermediary molecular phenotype and, hence, are considered secondary and potentially reversible.

Treatment

The goals in the management of patients with HCM are fourfold: to determine the risk of SCD, to reduce the risk of SCD, to alleviate symptoms, and to provide genetic counseling to patients and family members.

MANAGEMENT ACCORDING TO THE RISK OF SUDDEN CARDIAC DEATH

There is no close correlation between the risk of SCD and the presence of symptoms. Overall, the majority of patients with HCM are at low risk for SCD and are asymptomatic or minimally symptomatic. These individuals require periodic evaluation to determine risk of SCD and to assess symptoms. Accordingly, history, physical examination, electrocardiography, Holter monitoring, and two-dimensional and Doppler echocardiography are performed at least annually. Asymptomatic individuals at high risk for SCD should undergo internal cardioverter-defibrillator (ICD) implantation. Otherwise, no pharmacologic or nonpharmacologic intervention is necessary in asymptomatic patients who are at low risk for SCD.

MANAGEMENT OF SYMPTOMATIC PATIENTS

Therapeutic options in symptomatic patients include pharmacologic therapy, surgical myectomy, and transcatheter septal ablation; the latter two are options for those with significant outflow tract obstruction. Symptomatic patients at high risk for SCD should undergo ICD implantation in addition to medical therapy. Medical treatment of symptomatic patients is largely empiric and limited to β-blockers, verapamil hydrochloride[1] (Calan and Verelan), disopyramide[1]

---

[1]Not FDA approved for this indication.

(Norpace), low-dose diuretics, and amiodarone[1] (Cordarone and Pacerone[1]). The goals are to improve diastolic function, reduce outflow tract obstruction, and prevent cardiac arrhythmias. β-Blockers such as atenolol (Tenormin[1]) and metoprolol (Lopressor and Toprol XL[1]) are the first line of therapy and are generally well tolerated. β-Blockers with intrinsic sympathetic activity are avoided. β-Blockers are also the preferred choice in patients with sympathetic-driven symptoms, such as exercise-induced dyspnea, outflow tract obstruction, and chest pain. The most common side effect of β-blocker therapy is easy fatigability. Other side effects include excess bradycardia, hypotension, and bronchospasm.

Verapamil and, to lesser extent, diltiazem (Cardizem, Cartia XT, Dilacor, Tiazac[1]) are the most commonly used calcium channel blockers in patients with HCM. They are commonly used in conjunction with β-blockers. Symptomatic relief with calcium channel blockers presumably is achieved through improving left ventricular relaxation and reducing left ventricular filling pressure. Calcium channel blockers impart a negative inotropic effect, which could contribute to reduction of outflow tract obstruction. Nonetheless, the use of verapamil is primarily restricted to patients without an outflow tract obstruction because of concern about the vasodilatory effect inducing hypotension, syncope, and rarely death. The most common side effect of verapamil is constipation. Nifedipine (Adalat and Procardia) is avoided because of its potent vasodilatory effect.

Disopyramide is commonly reserved for patients who do not respond to β-blockers and/or calcium channel blockers, because of the relatively higher rate of anticholinergic side effects with disopyramide. The beneficial effect of disopyramide is mediated through its negative inotropic effect, which results in a significant reduction in left ventricular outflow tract gradient and symptomatic improvement. Diuretics are used judiciously to relieve dyspnea while avoiding intravascular volume depletion. Rapid changes in intravascular volume should be avoided because of enhanced susceptibility to hypotension. Mineralocorticoid receptor blockers may be preferable because of their antihypertrophic and antifibrotic effects in addition to their diuretic effects. Angiotensin-converting enzyme inhibitors and angiotensin-II receptor blockers are not conventionally used. However, experimental data favor their use because of their antihypertrophic and antifibrotic effects.

In a small fraction of patients, HCM evolves into advanced heart failure with systolic dysfunction and a congestive state. These patients are treated, as are those with other forms of systolic heart failure, with β-blockers, angiotensin-converting enzyme inhibitors, angiotensin-II receptor blockers, digoxin, and diuretics.

MANAGEMENT OF CARDIAC ARRHYTHMIAS

Patients with palpitations should undergo 12-lead electrocardiography, Holter monitoring, and electrophysiologic studies, if needed, to delineate the etiology and to provide appropriate therapy. Chronic or intermittent atrial fibrillation occurs in approximately 20% of patients. Atrial fibrillation with a fast ventricular rate is not well tolerated and often results in severe dyspnea and hypotension, particularly in those with severe cardiac hypertrophy or left ventricular outflow tract obstruction. Electrical cardioversion is indicated in such patients. Electrical or chemical cardioversion is also warranted in patients with new-onset atrial fibrillation (<48 hours in duration) if they are at low risk for intracardiac thrombus. Otherwise, transesophageal echocardiography should be performed to exclude intracardiac thrombi prior to cardioversion. Patients with chronic or intermittent atrial fibrillation require chronic anticoagulation. Medical treatment of atrial fibrillation includes use of β-blockers, verapamil, diltiazem, and amiodarone. Amiodarone is the most effective, but its long-term use is associated with considerable toxicity; therefore, only low-dose amiodarone (up to 200 mg daily) is recommended. Experience with other antiarrhythmic agents, such as flecainide (Tambocor), for treatment of arrhythmias in patients with HCM is limited. Radiofrequency ablation is reserved for patients refractory to medical therapy.

Patients with frequent nonsustained ventricular tachycardia or sustained ventricular tachycardia should undergo ICD implantation because they are considered at high risk for SCD. In addition, medical treatment with antiarrhythmic drugs such as amiodarone or β-blockers is recommended. Patients with rare episodes of nonsustained ventricular tachycardia should undergo further evaluation to assess the risk of SCD and then treated according to the risk of SCD.

MANAGEMENT OF SYNCOPE

Recurrent syncope is a serious event in patients with HCM because it often heralds SCD. The most common causes of syncope are malignant ventricular or supraventricular arrhythmias, exercise-induced hypotension, severe outflow tract obstruction, and neurally mediated syncope (vasodepressor syncope). Evaluation of patients with syncope includes Holter monitoring, exercise test, tilt-table testing, and, if needed, electrophysiologic studies. Patients with repetitive bursts of nonsustained ventricular tachycardia and those with sustained ventricular tachycardia are candidates for ICD implantation. Ventricular arrhythmia is the main cause of SCD in individuals with HCM. Implantation of an ICD as a preventive measure reduces the risk of SCD.

Patients with syncope due to supraventricular arrhythmias are treated with antiarrhythmic drugs, and those refractory to medical therapy are treated with radiofrequency ablation. Surgical myectomy and transcoronary septal ablation are considered in patients with syncope due to severe outflow tract obstruction. Treatment of patients with syncope due to an inappropriate peripheral vascular response to exercise includes propranolol (Inderal[1]), clonidine (Catapres[1]), and sometimes paroxetine (Paxil[1]).

MANAGEMENT OF OUTFLOW TRACT OBSTRUCTION

Left ventricular outflow tract obstruction is a dynamic phenotype that is associated with symptoms of heart failure, but its contribution to the risk of SCD is not well established. Most patients with outflow tract obstruction respond well to medical therapy and remain asymptomatic or mildly symptomatic. Treatment with β-blockers alone may suffice. A subset of patients who exhibit significant resting or exercise-induced outflow tract obstruction (>50 mm Hg) remain in New York Heart Association functional class III and IV despite optimal medical therapy. These patients are candidates for percutaneous transcoronary septal ablation or surgical myectomy. The prerequisite for invasive interventions is an interventricular septal thickness of 15 mm and greater. Otherwise, invasive procedures are not warranted because of a potentially excessive risk-to-benefit ratio. Instead, treatment should focus on diastolic dysfunction.

No prospective randomized studies have compared clinical outcomes after surgical myectomy and percutaneous transcoronary septal ablation. Several observational studies suggest the two interventions are equally effective in reducing the left ventricular outflow tract gradient and alleviating symptoms. However, neither is a curative intervention, and additional treatment usually is necessary.

A. **Surgical Myectomy (Myomectomy):** Surgical myectomy involves resection of a small portion of the interventricular septum, commonly at the base, through a transaortic approach (Morrow procedure). It reduces outflow tract obstruction and results in significant improvement of heart failure symptoms. It is best reserved for symptomatic patients with significant outflow tract obstruction at rest who are refractory to pharmacologic therapy. It is the procedure of choice in patients with concomitant valvular disease and/or coronary artery disease. The recurrence rate of outflow tract obstruction is low, and a second intervention is seldom required. The overall mortality rate of surgical myectomy in experienced centers is 1% to 5%, but the rate is higher among the elderly and those with concomitant cardiac surgeries. Surgical myectomy is associated with excellent short-term and long-term symptomatic relief and survival, and it has a favorable impact on the risk of SCD.

---

[1]Not FDA approved for this indication.

B. *Transcoronary Septal Ablation:* The procedure is performed through percutaneous coronary catheterization and injection of 1 to 3 mL of pure ethanol into the main septal perforators of the left anterior descending artery. Accordingly, focal myocardial necrosis, emulating surgical myectomy, is induced. It reduces the outflow tract gradient significantly and improves symptoms. It is indicated in symptomatic patients who are refractory to medical therapy, have an interventricular septal thickness of 15 mm and greater, and have a significant resting left ventricular outflow tract gradient. In those with significant exertional dyspnea, a provoked exercise-induced gradient can be used as a surrogate phenotype for septal ablation.

Overall, the procedure is well tolerated and has relatively low perioperative morbidity and mortality. The most common complication is the development of advanced atrioventricular (AV) conduction defect requiring permanent pacemaker placement in 15% to 20% of patients. There is a small risk of ventricular arrhythmias arising from the localized myocardial necrosis. Progressive left ventricular remodeling occurs predominantly within the first 6 months. Short-term and intermediary follow-up data show favorable outcome that is largely comparable, but probably not equal, to that of surgical myectomy.

C. *Dual-Chamber Pacing:* Dual-chamber pacing is designed to reduce outflow tract obstruction by inducing dyssynchronized left ventricular contraction. Thus, optimal timing of the AV interval is considered essential. Randomized clinical studies show no significant direct benefit to pacing strategy but rather a considerable placebo effect and no discernible improvement in exercise tolerance. Accordingly, dual-chamber pacing is reserved for occasional symptomatic patients who are refractory to medical therapy and are not candidates for either surgical or transcatheter septal ablation.

Experimental Pharmacologic Agents

Recent experimental studies have suggested the potential utility of β-hydroxy-β-methylglutaryl-coenzyme A (HMG-CoA) reductase inhibitors (statins), angiotensin-II receptor blockers, aldosterone blockers, and antioxidants in the prevention, attenuation, and reversal of cardiac phenotype in patients with HCM. Clinical studies testing the potential utility of these agents for treatment of patients with HCM are ongoing.

REFERENCES

Cannan CR, Reeder GS, Bailey KR, et al: Natural history of hypertrophic cardiomyopathy. A population-based study, 1976 through 1990. Circulation 1995;92:2488-2495.

Geisterfer-Lowrance AA, Kass S, Tanigawa G, et al: A molecular basis for familial hypertrophic cardiomyopathy: a beta cardiac myosin heavy chain gene missense mutation. Cell 1990;62:999-1006.

Hess OM, Sigwart U: New treatment strategies for hypertrophic obstructive cardiomyopathy: Alcohol ablation of the septum: the new gold standard? J Am Coll Cardiol 2004;44:2054-2055.

Marian AJ: Pathogenesis of diverse clinical and pathological phenotypes in hypertrophic cardiomyopathy. Lancet 2000;355:58-60.

Marian AJ: Recent advances in genetics and treatment of hypertrophic cardiomyopathy. Future Cardiol 2005;1:341-353.

Maron BJ, Gardin JM, Flack JM, et al: Prevalence of hypertrophic cardiomyopathy in a general population of young adults. Echocardiographic analysis of 4111 subjects in the CARDIA Study. Coronary Artery Risk Development in (Young) Adults. Circulation 1995;92:785-789.

Maron BJ, Shen WK, Link MS, et al: Efficacy of implantable cardioverter-defibrillators for the prevention of sudden death in patients with hypertrophic cardiomyopathy. N Engl J Med 2000;342:365-373.

Maron BJ, Shirani J, Poliac LC, et al: Sudden death in young competitive athletes. Clinical, demographic, and pathological profiles. JAMA 1996;276:199-204.

Ommen SR, Maron BJ, Olivotto I, et al: Long-term effects of surgical septal myectomy on survival in patients with obstructive hypertrophic cardiomyopathy. J Am Coll Cardiol 2005;46:470-476.

Woo A, Williams WG, Choi R, et al: Clinical and echocardiographic determinants of long-term survival after surgical myectomy in obstructive hypertrophic cardiomyopathy. Circulation 2005;111:2033-2041.

Mitral Valve Prolapse: The Floppy Mitral Valve, Mitral Valve Prolapse, and Mitral Valvular Regurgitation

Method of
Charles F. Wooley, MD, and
Harisios Boudoulas, MD, PhD*

The floppy mitral valve (FMV) is the central theme in the mitral valve prolapse (MVP) narrative. It has taken 6 decades to reconcile the observations by the pathologists who described the FMV morphology in the 1940s with the role of the FMV in clinical mitral valvular regurgitation (MVR). When the early cardiac surgeons encountered floppy, myxomatous mitral valves at open heart surgery, they described prolapse (MVP) of the FMV into the left atrium and used the FMV terminology for descriptive purposes, a term also used by the early cardiac pathologists. The clinicians initially described, and later recorded, apical systolic clicks and late systolic murmurs, but with a few exceptions they tended to regard these auscultatory findings as extracardiac in origin. When left ventricular angiography became feasible, the pathologic, surgical, and auscultatory phenomena were reconciled and came into clear focus. The nonejection systolic clicks were clearly related to prolapse (MVP) of an FMV into the left atrium, and the mid to late apical systolic murmurs represented a unique form of MVR. At this stage of clinical understanding, the auscultatory, angiographic, surgical, and pathologic correlates were quite distinct.

When the M-mode echocardiogram came into clinical usage, the result was a mixed blessing for diagnostic accuracy in patients with the FMV–MVP–MVR triad. Clinical auscultatory findings were ignored, and the nonspecific echocardiographic criteria produced a prolonged period of diagnostic confusion, elements of which persist to the present. This era was characterized by the separation of MVP from FMV, and the result was grossly exaggerated estimates of the incidence and prevalence of MVP. Gradually, however, with the use of the evolving technologic advances in multidimensional echo-Doppler transthoracic and esophageal techniques, close attention to in vivo mitral valve anatomy, and rigorous clinical conference, reason was restored to the diagnostic process. Revised imaging diagnostic criteria once again were based on fundamental FMV morphology, the mechanisms of MVP, and precise identification and quantification of MVR.

These developmental observations are highly significant because no other valvular lesion has a lineage similar to that of FMV. Thus, recognition and definition of an FMV as a discrete pathologic entity producing mitral valvular dysfunction was the key step to our current understanding (Figure 1). Essential steps in comprehending the clinical significance of the FMV–MVP–MVR triad was the recognition that the mitral valve dysfunction associated with FMV resulted in prolapse of the mitral valve into the left atrium (MVP) and that FMV/MVP resulted in a specific form of mitral valvular regurgitation (MVR).

Pathologic Observations

Early cardiac pathologists also called attention to the long natural history of patients with FMVs. In 1944 Bailey and Hickam pointed out the discrete nature of FMV and emphasized that this type of valve was a nonrheumatic entity. They noted fibrosis of the mitral valve without rheumatic stenosis, increased valve thickness with

---

*Deceased.

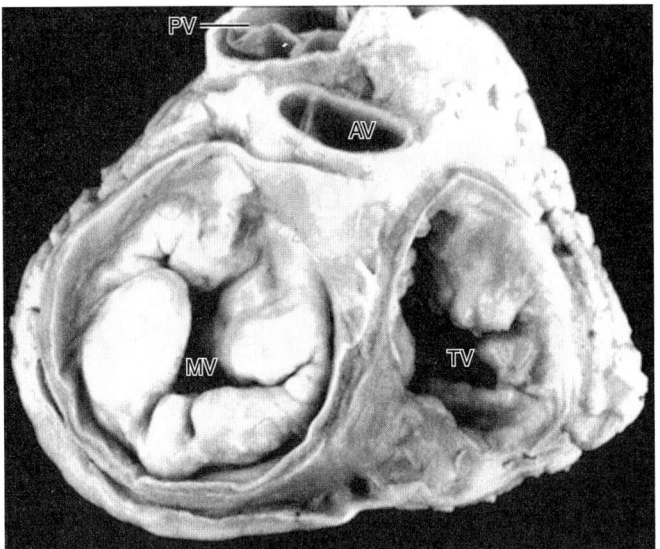

FIGURE 1. Floppy mitral valve. *Abbreviations:* AV = aortic valve; MV = mitral valve; PV = pulmonic valve; TV = tricuspid valve. Photograph courtesy of Dr. William D. Edwards, Mayo Clinic.

histologic evidence of dense acellular connective tissue thickening and basophilic areas of degeneration. The long natural history of the disorder, the susceptibility to infectious endocarditis, and the late onset of rapidly progressive congestive heart failure were important clinical correlates. Subsequent studies of FMV incidence, pathobiology, and complications by Davies and other cardiac pathologists provided clinicians with a new chapter in valvular heart disease. Thus, the natural history of patients with FMVs was reasonably well defined early on; however, the translation of these early observations into the clinical realm took much longer than generally appreciated.

Surgical Observations

Open heart surgery allowed cardiac surgeons to visualize the mitral valve in the beating heart. In 1965, Read and colleagues used the term *floppy valve syndrome* to describe patients with significant mitral and aortic valvular regurgitation due to myxomatous transformation of the mitral and aortic valves. Valvular regurgitation was related to "valve prolapse" because of loss of valve integrity from structural fatigue, ruptured chordae, or interference with valvular coaptation. Their report was marked by descriptive language—floppy valve for myxomatous changes in valve tissue; dynamic terminology—valve prolapse as a mechanism for valvular regurgitation; and the recognition of connective tissue disorders as the etiology for valvular disease. Subsequently, cardiac surgeons developed FMV reconstructive procedures from careful analysis of FMV morphology and dynamics.

Clinical Observations

During the 1960s, the clinicians' approach to FMV and MVR, in particular by Barlow, Criley, and their coworkers, resulted from auscultatory–phonocardiographic, hemodynamic, and angiographic studies of patients with apical systolic clicks and apical mid and late systolic murmurs. Apical systolic clicks were shown to be of intracardiac origin, distinct from aortic and pulmonary ejection clicks, and were classified as nonejection clicks; apical mid and late systolic murmurs were related to a unique anatomic type of MVR associated with FMV prolapse into the left atrium (i.e., MVP); and bulging of the mitral leaflets was identified as the angiographic counterpart of the balloon deformity seen at necropsy by Bailey and Hickam in 1944.

MVP postural auscultatory phenomena (i.e., postural exercise hemodynamic abnormalities and changes in timing and intensity of the systolic click–apical systolic murmur) were explained in hemodynamic terms as changes in the timing and extent of MVP, and the time of onset and duration of MVR were related to postural changes in left ventricular volume and contractility (Figure 2). Thus, by the 1970s and 1980s, clinical auscultatory observations, postural auscultatory dynamics, and angiographic definition of FMV characteristics with established pathologic correlates provided a reasonable clinical diagnostic profile for the FMV–MVP–MVR triad.

A number of events transpired that obscured this relatively simple diagnostic profile. Clinical phonocardiography virtually disappeared as remuneration for phonocardiograms was halted and production of phonocardiographic equipment ceased. This was followed by an auscultatory "silent spring" phenomenon, when physicians in training were not exposed to the self-critique that phonocardiography imposed on the discipline of auscultation.

Sensitivity and specificity diagnostic criteria suffered, as studies that relied on unproven M-mode echocardiographic criteria proliferated, FMV was uncoupled from MVP, and estimates of MVP incidence and prevalence reached epidemic proportions. Patients or individuals with small, hyperdynamic left ventricles were placed into

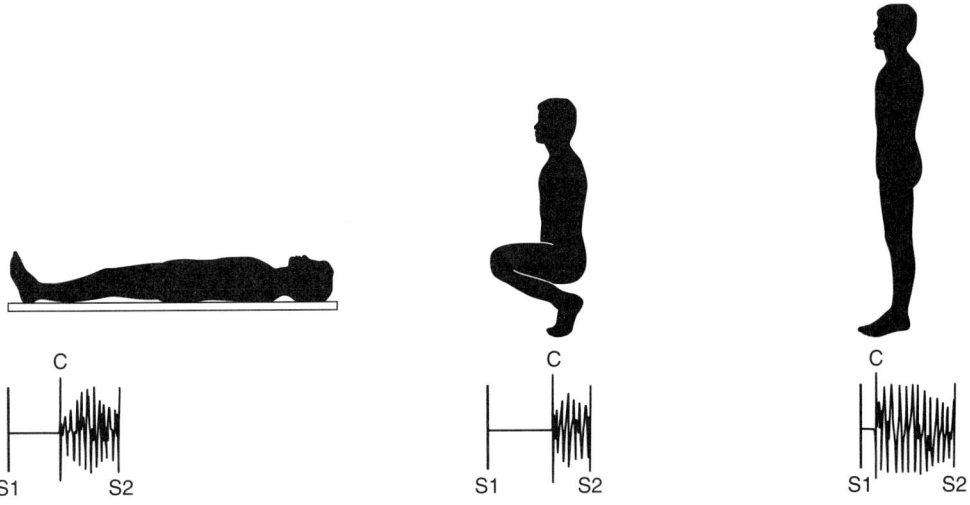

FIGURE 2. Floppy mitral valve–mitral valve prolapse–mitral valvular regurgitation: Postural auscultatory complex. *Abbreviations:* C = systolic click; S_1 = first heart sound; S_2 = second heart sound.

the same category as patients with the FMV–MVP–MVR triad. When the M-mode echocardiographic prolapse comet swept across psychiatry, individuals with anxiety and panic syndromes were engulfed, and the epidemic became pandemic.

Historical Perspective

Why introduce the historical perspective? First, recalling the ways in which MVR, FMV, and MVP diagnostic criteria evolved during the past 50 years helps us understand that these clinical entities were moving targets, constantly being defined and redefined by pathologists, surgeons, auscultors, imagers, and epidemiologists, and hence the multitude of names for the clinical entities and the variability of diagnostic criteria. Second, when the FMV–MVP–MVR clinical auscultatory–phonocardiographic–angiographic profile was separated from the prolapse imaging diagnosis that ignored FMV morphology and focused on a 1- to 2-mm disputed zone, cardiologists wandered into areas fraught with difficulties. As the MVP pendulum moved away from the exaggerated incidence/prevalence figures of the past 2 decades, it is apparent that the FMV occupies the high ground and is the central issue in the FMV–MVP–MVR triad (see Figure 1).

Heritable Disorders of Connective Tissue

FMV may be an inherited lesion, either as an isolated event or as part of the recognized or incompletely defined heritable disorders of connective tissue. FMV–MVP inheritance and phenotypic features have been well described. FMV has gradually become recognized as a common cardiac lesion in the Marfan syndrome. Although FMV–MVP may be genetically determined, clinical manifestations do not usually become evident before childhood. Although children and adolescents with FMV–MVP may have the same symptoms as adults, the frequency of symptoms appears to be less in children. At present, the family history remains the cornerstone in clinical genetic analysis, as FMV genetic diagnostic testing has not entered clinical practice.

DIAGNOSTIC CONSIDERATIONS

FMV is a common mitral valve abnormality with a broad spectrum of structural and functional changes. Although the pathobiology of FMV has been, and continues to be, re-examined in contemporary terms, we are still dealing with gross structural and morphologic characteristics at the clinical level. Distinguishing between a normal mitral valve with its minor variants and an FMV mitral valve with an intrinsic structural derangement remains a central issue. Thus, it is important to emphasize the necessity for clinical coherence in the FMV–MVP–MVR dialogue.

Tic-tac-toe has its origins in the ancient "three in a row" category of games of strategy. Diagnostic tic-tac-toe avoids the pitfalls of a diagnosis based on a single phenomenon and places emphasis on a multidimensional approach to FMV–MVP–MVR diagnostics similar to our diagnostic approach to any complex cardiac disorder or disease (Figure 3).

We are more comfortable with the FMV–MVP–MVR diagnosis when (1) the clinical auscultatory phenomena are precisely described, preferably recorded, and dynamic auscultation has been performed; (2) the clinical auscultatory phenomena are matched with an imaging procedure that captures and quantitates FMV morphology and function; and (3) the imaging procedure demonstrates MVP and the presence, absence, or quantification of MVR.

Postural auscultation, electrocardiogram, and echocardiogram with Doppler, assessment of orthostasis, dynamic exercise testing, ambulatory electrocardiographic or blood pressure monitoring, and dynamic interventional imaging or hemodynamic studies may be required, depending on the patient's symptoms or the specific clinical situation.

FLOPPY MITRAL VALVE—MITRAL VALVE PROLAPSE—MITRAL VALVULAR REGURGITATION: CLASSIFICATION

The classification of cardiovascular diseases is in constant evolution, and our textbooks and literature do not always reflect the dynamics of this process. At present, we classify patients with the FMV–MVP–MVR triad into two general categories (Table 1). The first category places emphasis on the FMV anatomy and pathobiology and includes patients whose symptoms, physical findings, laboratory abnormalities, and clinical course are directly related to the progressive mitral valve dysfunction and complications associated with the FMV–MVP–MVR triad. The second category includes FMV–MVP patients whose symptoms cannot be explained on the basis of the valvular abnormality alone but result from the occurrence, or coexistence, of various forms of neuroendocrine or autonomic nervous system dysfunction. We refer to this group as patients with the FMV–MVP syndrome.

We have found this to be a clinically useful classification, but one that should be subject to revision or modification as we better understand the pathogenesis and mechanisms of symptoms in patients with the FMV–MVP–MVR triad.

FLOPPY MITRAL VALVE—MITRAL VALVE PROLAPSE—MITRAL VALVULAR REGURGITATION: COMPLICATIONS AND NATURAL HISTORY

Profiles of the natural history of the FMV–MVP–MVR triad have been limited by variations in diagnostic criteria, the nature of the populations studied, and the duration of clinical follow-up.

The FMV–MVP association has well-defined clinical auscultatory correlates; however, the sensitivity and specificity of these clinical

---

MEDICAL HISTORY, PHYSICAL EXAMINATION, LABORATORY

Diagnostic tic-tac-toe

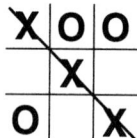

Multidimensional approach to FMV, MVP, MVR diagnosis

FIGURE 3. Diagnostic tic-tac-toe. Emphasis is placed on a multidimensional approach to the diagnosis. *Abbreviations:* FMV = floppy mitral valve; MVP = mitral valve prolapse; MVR = mitral valvular regurgitation.

 CURRENT DIAGNOSIS

- Clinical coherence should exist among the medical history, the physical examination, and the imaging procedure.
- Because the floppy mitral valve–mitral valve prolapse–mitral valvular regurgitation triad is accompanied by dynamic clinical phenomena, dynamic examination procedures may be indicated in individual situations.
- A family pedigree is a vital part of the clinical evaluation.

TABLE 1 Classification of Floppy Mitral Valve–Mitral Valve Prolapse–Mitral Valvular Regurgitation (FMV-MVP-MVR)

FMV-MVP-MVR
Common mitral valve abnormality with a spectrum of structural and functional changes, mild to severe

The Basis for
Systolic click; mid-late systolic murmur
Mild or progressive mitral valve dysfunction
Progressive mitral regurgitation, atrial fibrillation, congestive heart failure
Infectious endocarditis
Embolic phenomena
Characterized by long natural history
May be heritable or associated with heritable disorders of connective tissue
Conduction system involvement possibly leading to arrhythmias and conduction defects

FMV-MVP-MVR Syndrome
Patients with mitral valve prolapse
Symptom complex; chest pain, palpitations, arrhythmias, fatigue, exercise intolerance, dyspnea, postural phenomena, syncope-presyncope, neuropsychiatric symptoms
Neuroendocrine or autonomic dysfunction (high catecholamine levels, catecholamine regulation abnormality, hyperresponse to adrenergic stimulation, parasympathetic abnormality, baroreflex modulation abnormality, renin-aldosterone regulation abnormality, decreased intravascular volume, decreased ventricular diastolic volume in the upright posture, atrial natriuretic factor secretion abnormality) may provide explanation for symptoms
Mitral valve prolapse—a possible marker for autonomic dysfunction

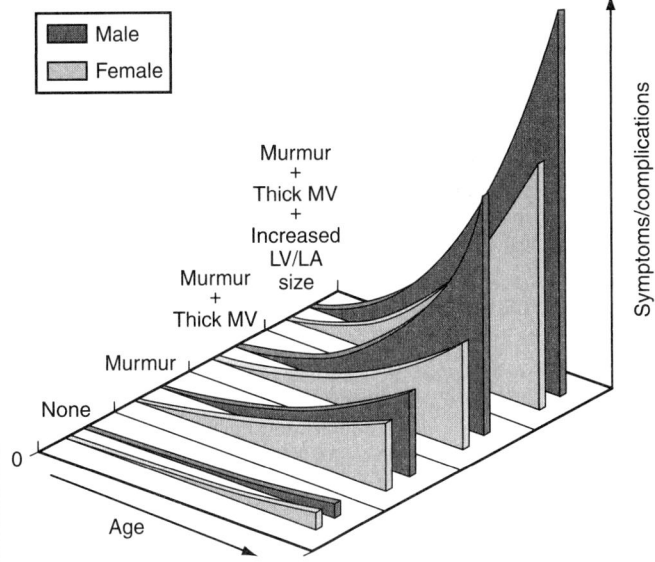

FIGURE 4. Floppy mitral valve–mitral valve prolapse–mitral valvular regurgitation: High-risk patient. Symptoms and complications plotted against age. *Abbreviations:* LA = left atrium; LV = left ventricle; MV = mitral valve.

phenomena have not been determined with contemporary objective methods. Similarly, the FMV–MVP association has specific imaging correlates, yet these are being constantly redefined as echo-Doppler, magnetic resonance imaging, and angiographic technologies improve and diagnostic criteria are reassessed.

The FMV–MVP association may lead to progressive mitral valvular dysfunction and severe MVR over time; however, the individual patient's natural history may not fully develop for 7 to 8 decades. Hence, studies or evaluations at one point in time have limitations (Figure 4).

Valve surface phenomena occur in patients with FMVs. A FMV is particularly vulnerable to infection and may be a site for infective endocarditis. The pathogenesis is poorly understood, and we currently mask our lack of understanding by using incident-related antibiotic prophylaxis prior to dental, gastrointestinal, and genitourinary procedures. Although guidelines have been evolving, simply stated, infectious endocarditis prophylaxis is indicated for patients with FMVs. Thromboemboli are additional valve surface complications of FMV; however, this is an area that is not well defined.

Chordal rupture, progressive MVR, left atrial and left ventricular failures, and atrial and ventricular arrhythmias occur in varying combinations and permutations, usually as late complications in certain patients with FMV. FMVs have been documented as being one of the leading causes of MVR requiring mitral valve surgery. Sudden cardiac death has been reported in a small subset of patients with FMV.

Therapeutic Implications

Each of the FMV–MVP–MVR complications has implications involving prevention, recognition, and treatment. Individual patient evaluation and management are fundamental considerations, as is the necessity of regular, long-term clinical follow-up.

Individuals with progressive mitral valvular dysfunction require initial and periodic assessment of their hemodynamic status. Individuals with the MVP syndrome as defined earlier whose symptoms may be related to autonomic dysfunction, neuroendocrine abnormalities, volume depletion, or vasoconstriction require investigation and therapeutic approaches aimed at these pathogenetic mechanisms. Both groups require careful explanations of their individual situation, the rationale for regular follow-up, and infective endocarditis prophylaxis.

High-risk Patients

Individuals with FMV–MVP and thick, redundant mitral valve leaflets are at high risk for developing complications; those older than 50 years with arterial hypertension are at particularly high risk (see Figure 4). A mitral systolic murmur also is a risk factor for complications. Left atrial and left ventricular enlargement and dysfunction in patients with FMV–MVP–MVR have been used as predictors for the need for mitral valve surgery. When two or more of

CURRENT THERAPY

- Guidelines for surgical intervention in patients with floppy mitral valve–mitral valve prolapse–mitral valvular regurgitation should include the feasibility of floppy mitral valve repair, surgical competence, low operative mortality and morbidity, and long-term clinical results.
- Careful explanation of the clinical findings and the nature of mitral valve prolapse will help reassure the anxious patient with the mitral valve prolapse syndrome.
- As is always the case, individual patient evaluation and diagnostic certainty precede rational therapy.

these abnormalities coexist, the possibility of complications increases. In contrast, the absence of all three of these features identifies patients at low risk (see Figure 4). These individuals, whether or not they are symptomatic, may require more sophisticated imaging studies, exercise testing, or hemodynamic and angiographic assessment. Individuals with a history of atrial or ventricular arrhythmias should be evaluated with contemporary electrophysiologic monitoring or testing. Patients who have a history of syncope, lightheadedness, or unexplained collapse or who are postresuscitation require further diagnostic testing.

SURGICAL CONSIDERATIONS

Decisions regarding surgical intervention (mitral valve repair or replacement) in symptomatic FMV patients have been based on the impact of MVR on left atrial and left ventricular functions expressed in both hemodynamic terms and echocardiographic measurements. Improvements in FMV repair techniques and intraoperative imaging coupled with better echo-Doppler methods of quantitating MVR severity prompted recommendations for earlier intervention extending into the asymptomatic state. This is another moving target in the FMV–MVP–MVR lineage that requires careful assessment and analysis by thoughtful clinicians.

Patients with MVP syndrome are sensitive to volume depletion and increased adrenergic activity. Thus, prophylaxis for volume depletion before, during, or immediately after physical exercise may be particularly beneficial to patients with low intravascular volume. Removing catecholamine and cyclic adenosine monophosphate stimulation by abstaining from caffeine, tobacco, alcohol, and prescription or over-the-counter drugs containing epinephrine may help. Low doses of β-blocking drugs administered for a short time during stressful periods or in a single dose may be beneficial. Exercise programs are frequently beneficial in patients with the MVP syndrome.

Summing up, the concept of a triad, a group of three closely related things, as expressed in the floppy mitral valve–mitral valve prolapse–mitral valvular regurgitation triad, emphasizes the central role of the FMV in the MVP–MVR lineage. A recent in-depth review of the subject by Hayek, Gring, and Griffin contains clinical wisdom for clinicians involved in the diagnosis, care, and management of patients with the FMV–MVP–MVR triad.

REFERENCES

Bailey OT, Hickam JB: Rupture of mitral chordae tendineae. Am Heart J 1944;28:578-600.
Barlow JB, Pocock WA, Marchand P, et al: The significance of late systolic murmurs. Am Heart J 1963;66:443-452.
Bashore TM, Grines CL, Utlak D, et al: Postural exercise abnormalities in symptomatic patients with mitral valve prolapse. J Am Coll Cardiol 1988;3:499-507.
Boudoulas H, Wooley CF: Mitral Valve: Floppy Mitral Valve, Mitral Valve Prolapse, Mitral Valvular Regurgitation. Armonk, NY, Futura, 2000.
Carpentier A: Cardiac valve surgery: The "French correction." J Thorac Cardiovasc Surg 1983;3:323-337.
Criley JM, Lewis KB, Humphries JO, et al: Prolapse of the mitral valve: Clinical and cineangiographic findings. Br Heart J 1966;28:488-496.
Davies MJ, Moore BP, Braimbridge MV: The floppy mitral valve. Study of incidence, pathology, and complications in surgical, necropsy and forensic material. Br Heart J 1978;40:468-481.
Enriquez-Sarano M, Avierinos JF, Messika-Zeitoun D, et al: Quantitative determinants of the outcome of asymptomatic mitral regurgitation. N Engl J Med 2005;352:875-883.
Fontana ME, Wooley CF, Leighton RF, Lewis RP: Postural changes in left ventricular and mitral valvular dynamics in the systolic click-late systolic murmur syndrome. Circulation 1975;1:165-173.
Glesby MJ, Pyeritz RE: Association of mitral valve prolapse and systemic abnormalities of connective tissue. JAMA 1989;262:523-528.
Hayek E, Gring CN, Griffin BP: Mitral valve prolapse. Lancet 2005;365:507-518.
Otto CM, Salerno CT: Timing of surgery in asymptomatic mitral regurgitation. N Engl J Med 2005;352:928-929.
Read RC, Thal AP, Wendt VE: Symptomatic valvular myxomatous transformation (the floppy valve syndrome). A possible forme fruste of the Marfan syndrome. Circulation 1965;32:897-910.

Heart Failure

Method of
Marc A. Silver, MD

Heart failure is an epidemic in the United States. Every day, clinicians face the task of caring for more patients with heart failure in all its forms. Heart failure is the primary reason for hospitalization of Americans older than 65 years, and although 6 million Americans are estimated to have symptomatic heart failure, that number is expected to double over the next 7 years. Many millions more have asymptomatic left ventricular dysfunction or existing medical conditions that make it quite likely heart failure will develop and they will die.

It is truly in the hands of primary care physicians, who care for most heart failure patients, as well as those with common precursors of heart failure, to understand heart failure and its natural history better and thereby make an impact on this challenging epidemic. With this concept in mind, heart failure is discussed here from the perspective of understanding its natural history or stages, as well as a chronic disease process amenable to strategic planning.

Definitions

All clinicians define heart failure differently. Some choose to think about heart failure only when the patient has advanced disease characterized by significant volume overload and exercise limitation. Others consider heart failure to be present only when the left ventricle is dilated. Although broad by intent, *heart failure* is usually defined as a complex clinical syndrome that affects cardiac function (its ability to fill and/or eject blood) and is often preceded by and certainly accompanied by systemic neurohormonal abnormalities that participate in and perpetuate the dysfunction of the heart as well as other target organs, including the vasculature and muscles.

Although a wide range of signs and symptoms may accompany the heart failure syndrome of whatever cause, once symptomatic, patients usually have evidence of dyspnea, fatigue, and sodium and water retention manifested as congestion in the lungs, legs, and gut. It is useful, however, to think about heart failure not only as a symptomatic disease but also as a disease whose development begins decades before the patient crosses the threshold of clinical symptoms.

Classification and Stages of Heart Failure

Although many clinicians bristle at the concept of prescribed sets of recommendations or guidelines applied to a diverse disease process such as heart failure, these guidelines are frequently a place where available evidence is evaluated in a critical way and balanced with consensus to provide a distillation of what might work when caring for a patient with a disease process.

One of the well-accepted standard guidelines for heart failure recently was revised. Within the 2001 Revision of the American College of Cardiology/American Heart Association Guidelines for the Evaluation and Management of Chronic Heart Failure for the Adult (executive summary and full text available online at http://www.acc.org/clinical/guidelines/failure/hf_index.htm), aside from detailed information on the testing and therapies currently supported by evidence, appears a new classification for heart failure (Table 1). The classification most clinicians are familiar with is that of the New York Heart Association (NYHA) (Box 1). The NYHA classification is generally applied to patients who at some point become symptomatic. Although they may revert to a

TABLE 1 Common Heart Failure Drugs and Their Therapeutic Targets

Drug	Dose	Comment
Loop diuretics (expressed as furosemide [Lasix] equivalent units)	40-100 mg once or twice daily	Many factors affect the doses required, such as patient compliance with dietary restrictions, fluid intake, and associated titration of other medication, including ACE inhibitors and β-blockers.
ACE inhibitors (expressed as enalapril [Vasotec] equivalent units)	10-20 mg twice daily	Higher doses seem to have an impact on hospitalization rates. Be aware of adverse events that will limit use, including hyperkalemia. To allow adequate titration of β-blockers, reduced doses may be used.
β-Blockers (expressed as carvedilol [Coreg] equivalent units)	25-50 mg twice daily	Dependent on body size. Although data suggest clinical improvement and decreased mortality with smaller doses, the target remains full dose.
Digoxin	0.125-0.25 mg daily	Adjustment needed for renal function. Routine measurement of serum levels is not required unless done to confirm toxicity.

Abbreviation: ACE = angiotensin-converting enzyme.

symptom-free status (NYHA functional class I), it is still implied the patient has overt heart failure. Even though the NYHA classification is of great value and carries prognostic value, it also tends to allow us to think of a patient with mild or moderate symptoms (i.e., NYHA functional class II to III) as having a mild or moderate disease, but indeed, patients in this category have a markedly shortened life span and by definition less than optimal functional status.

The new classification (Box 2), in contrast, identifies four stages of heart failure based on the spectrum of common clinical syndromes from which they have evolved. By so doing, it is hoped the clinician recognizes the patient's increased risk for the clinical syndrome and then acts aggressively to reduce the risk and/or intervene earlier just as one would with a patient at risk for cancer.

The classification addresses four stages. Unlike the NYHA classification, in which a patient may easily pass back and forth through several functional classes over a period of days to weeks, as the patient passes through each stage of the new classification, there is no longer any hope of reverting to an earlier stage, which should act as an impetus to capture the patient at the earliest stage and prevent progression to the next stage by using the proper diagnostics and therapeutics.

Stage A refers to patients who by virtue of having other common clinical conditions are at increased risk of heart failure ultimately developing. These conditions include hypertension, diabetes mellitus, and coronary artery disease. Similarly, patients with a family history of heart failure have an increased risk. The heart failure syndrome clearly does not develop in all these patients, but acknowledging their at-risk status gives the clinician and the patient fair warning of the potential risk of development of heart failure and may serve as an early warning detection system for the insidious progression to more advanced heart failure. Progression to the next stage is preventable, and disease progression is usually measured in years or decades.

Stage B refers to patients in whom structural and even functional abnormalities in heart function are already developed, but because of enormous cardiac reserve, the signs or symptoms that usually bring these patients to medical attention are not yet developed. This stage has also been referred to as "asymptomatic left ventricular dysfunction." Progression to the next stage may be slowed and again may be measured in years.

Stage C represents most of what is called heart failure today: specifically, a patient who has structural and functional disease but who has now progressed and used up enough cardiac reserve actually to have signs and symptoms of the disease. By looking at heart failure in this perspective, it becomes clear that any symptomatic heart failure indeed represents a serious condition that the clinician must diagnose and treat accordingly. In this stage of the disease, clinicians can intervene to improve symptoms and quality of life, as well as improve, but not completely abolish, the increased mortality. Progression to the next stage is quite variable but is usually measured in months to years.

Stage D represents very advanced disease in which even standard measures cannot overcome its severity and advanced measures need to be undertaken. During this stage, despite best efforts, patients usually have increased use of resources, decreased quality of life, and progressive limitation. Although many advanced resources are applied during this stage, including heart transplantation and ventricular restraint and assist devices, generally these patients ultimately die of either progressive heart failure or sudden cardiac death.

Steps for Appropriate Heart Failure Management

Physicians often take a reflex approach to initiating drug therapy in a patient with symptomatic heart failure. For example, a patient who is volume overloaded might be treated with diuretics as monotherapy while overlooking the need not only to treat the current symptoms but also plan a strategy to limit progression of disease. Thus a useful approach in planning patient care involves two broad steps. The first is assessing the information needed to create a management plan, and the second is understanding the therapeutic targets in heart failure treatment.

An assessment of what is known or yet needed to be known to best make the diagnosis and treat a patient with heart failure is a very useful step. This assessment generally involves an understanding of the etiology of the heart failure, the current stage or functional class, and so forth. Even after a detailed history and physical examination and collection of some diagnostic data, however, a gap can remain

---

BOX 1 New York Heart Association Functional Classification of Heart Failure*

I. Symptoms occur only at a level that would cause normal individuals to become symptomatic.
II. Symptoms occur with ordinary exertion or moderate levels of activity.
III. Symptoms occur with less than ordinary degrees of activity.
IV. Symptoms occur even at rest.

*This classification scheme is generally applied to patients once they are or have been symptomatic with heart failure (stages C and D). Note: In general, the classification implies the patient's worst level of functioning related to a heart failure symptom (e.g., fatigue, dyspnea, exercise intolerance).

> **BOX 2 Stages of Heart Failure**
>
> **Stage A**
> - Patients who are at increased risk for heart failure because of associated medical conditions (e.g., hypertension, coronary artery disease, or diabetes mellitus).
> - Heart structure and function: Not yet affected.
> - Potential therapies: Treatment of hypertension, smoking cessation, and weight loss; ACE inhibitors in appropriate patients.
>
> **Stage B**
> - Patients who have abnormal heart structure and/or function but who have not manifested signs or symptoms.
> - Heart structure and function: Abnormal.
> - Potential therapies: Same as for stage A, plus ACE inhibitors and β-blockers in all appropriate patients.
>
> **Stage C**
> - Patients with symptomatic heart failure. These patients indeed have advanced heart failure. Note that signs and symptoms develop as late phenomena after significant perturbation of many homeostatic mechanisms and the consumption of large cardiac reserves.
> - Heart structure and function: Abnormal.
> - Potential therapies: Same as for stages A and B, plus ACE inhibitors, β-blockers, and digoxin and diuretics in most patients; also, coronary revascularization and repair of mitral regurgitation in select patients.
>
> **Stage D**
> - Patients with extremely advanced heart failure.
> - Heart structure and function: Extremely abnormal.
> - Potential therapies: Same as for stages A, B, and C, plus consideration of advanced therapies including investigational therapies, consideration for left ventricular assist devices, heart transplantation for appropriate patients, as well as end-of-life counseling and hospice.
>
> *Abbreviation:* ACE = angiotensin-converting enzyme.

in the information needed to complete the therapeutic plan. Generally, the clinician can group the areas that need to be completed into three main categories: diagnostics, therapeutics, and prognostics. In fact, these three areas are useful to consider each time a patient is seen in the office or hospital. Even though treatment is often initiated without complete information in each of these areas, not asking what other information is needed often leads to an incomplete understanding of the disease syndrome, as well as suboptimal therapy.

Diagnostics refers to any additional information that allows a better understanding of the etiology, status, degree of limitation, and signs and symptoms of a patient. For example, an echocardiogram allows assessment of the nature and degree of left ventricular function and may lead to consideration of myocardial ischemia (wall motion abnormalities) or valvular disease (valvular regurgitation or stenosis) as a therapeutic target. Often in this category are tests that might reveal an easily addressable cause of the heart failure and even a form of heart failure that is potentially reversible (such as hyperthyroidism).

Therapeutics refers to the design of the treatment strategy based on what is currently known about the patient and that patient's disease. It is also useful to write down a therapeutic plan, including the one or two next steps that might be taken should the patient's signs or symptoms not abate with the current regimen. For example, the clinician might begin with using angiotensin-converting enzyme (ACE) inhibitors but indicate that if the patient is found to have underlying coronary artery disease, the addition of long-acting nitrates should be considered.

Prognostics refers to focusing in on what is known about the patient's heart failure in terms of predicting what might be the path of progression in the near future. Although imperfect, many pieces of information are closely linked to survival and disease progression, including functional status, exercise tolerance, and left ventricular ejection fraction. In considering any additional prognostics, the clinician should always ask what might be done differently given the result. Over the years we have become more willing to intervene earlier with therapeutics, which can alter progression of the disease, and therefore we depend less on a bad set of prognostic markers to make these decisions. Nevertheless, awareness of a low peak oxygen consumption, a low right ventricular ejection fraction, or a markedly elevated neurohormonal marker often serves to alert the physician and the patient and family to review the current therapeutic plan and broaden considerations to include the next level of care and treatment, which might consist of investigational therapies and evaluation for heart transplantation. The role of measurement of B-type natriuretic peptide in this regard is of some interest and may prove to be a prognostic marker against which to target our therapies.

TREATMENT TARGETS

In designing the drug treatment plan, the following treatment targets for patients with heart failure should be considered: improved survival, improved symptoms, slowing and/or reversal of disease progression, improved functional status and quality of life, avoidance of troublesome adverse events, and decreased use of resources, including hospitalization. With the recognition that not all these targets are concordant or attainable, the drug regimen reflects these targets and our understanding of the ability of drugs to address them.

In general, patients with symptomatic heart failure are managed with a core group of four drug classes, including diuretics, an ACE inhibitor, a β-blocker, and, usually, digoxin. The former and the latter are generally applied to relieve symptoms or to improve functional status or exercise tolerance, whereas the middle two are also administered with the specific intention of altering disease progression, reversing the structural and/or functional abnormalities of the heart and other target organs, and improving medium- and long-term survival.

Increasing evidence supports the initiation of ACE inhibitors and β-blocker jointly when caring for a symptomatic patient. Diuretics often need to be adjusted up or down, depending on a patient's level of compensation, as well as where they are in terms of other (β-blocker) titration. Target doses for most of the commonly used drugs come from clinical trials suggesting their benefit (ACE inhibitors) or from tradition, as well as from attempts to balance drug efficacy with drug safety (digoxin and diuretics). Target doses are listed in Table 1. Excellent details and practical considerations of implementing and titrating heart failure drugs can be found in recent guidelines (http://www.acc.org/clinical/guidelines/failure/hf_index.htm).

NONPHARMACOLOGIC MEASURES

An enormous armamentarium outside routine drug therapy is available to clinicians caring for patients with heart failure. In general, most nonpharmacologic measures should be used in a simultaneous fashion with the initiation and titration of drug therapy. Although most of these therapies either have not or will not undergo rigorous clinical investigation, they nonetheless remain therapeutic cornerstones of complete heart failure care. Dramatic functional improvement can often be observed with more careful attention to nonpharmacologic therapies. Of particular interest is an understanding that sleep-disordered breathing (including obstructive and central forms of sleep apnea) may be present in nearly 40% of heart failure patients. Increasing evidence suggests therapy that includes continuous positive airway pressure may alter symptoms, disease progression, and even survival (Box 3).

BOX 3 Nonpharmacologic Therapies for Patients with Heart Failure

Definitely Helps Reduce Symptoms or Improve Functional Status
- Salt restriction (target: 2.3 g of salt per day)
- Exercise
- Stress reduction
- Screening for depression
- Smoking cessation
- Weight loss
- Treatment of documented sleep-disordered breathing

May Be of Use in Selected Patients
- Fluid restriction
- Avoidance of alcohol

As far as dietary advice, generally admonitions for avoidance of excessive sodium intake and fluid are given along with specific information on lowering dietary saturated fat. Emerging information is that the patient with heart failure suffers a significant energy imbalance, however, and may well benefit from nutritional assessment, including measurement of nitrogen balance.

Use of Disease Management and Other Resources

Perhaps one of the greatest tools at hand for clinicians caring for patients with heart failure, as well as for their families, is providing a thorough understanding of the heart failure syndrome and how self-empowered actions may have a significant impact on how they feel, what they can do, and how long they might live. Studies have repeatedly demonstrated the benefits of a structured disease management program in reducing symptoms, improving functional status, and, in particular, reducing heart failure hospitalizations. The clinician frequently can best serve the patient by fostering and supporting a heart failure disease management program. Although not present in all communities yet, the resources required (a physician and/or a nurse champion) are often accessible.

CURRENT DIAGNOSIS

- Determine the etiology. It is critical to determine the underlying cause of a patient's heart failure; common clinical conditions including hypertension, diabetes mellitus, and coronary artery disease increase the risk of developing heart failure.
- Assess a patient's stage and functional class (see text). These are good guides to help recognize disease severity and guide treatment. Symptoms include evidence of dyspnea, fatigue, and sodium and water retention as congestion in the lungs, legs, and gut; these are usually late symptoms.
- Assess the volume status on every patient at every visit. Inability to assess volume carefully often leads to errors in therapeutics.
- Use additional tests and biomarkers such as peak oxygen consumption, ventricular ejection fraction, and elevated neurohormonal markers (B-type natriuretic peptide), which may provide early clues to disease severity.

CURRENT THERAPY

Targets
- Improved survival
- Improved symptoms
- Slowing and/or reversal of disease progression
- Improved functional status, quality of life
- Avoidance of adverse events
- Decreased use of resources including hospitalization

Care for Patients With Heart Failure
- Treatment of hypertension
- Smoking cessation
- Dietary counseling
- Exercise
- Weight loss
- Treatment of sleep-disordered breathing
- Angiotensin-converting enzyme (ACE) inhibitors (at target doses)
- β-Blockers (at target doses)
- Digoxin and diuretics
- Coronary revascularization
- Repair of mitral regurgitation
- Investigational therapies
- End-of-life counseling and hospice

Abundant educational patient-oriented books and materials are available to support these programs.

Disease management programs are often part of a larger specialized heart failure center. Within these structures are advanced strategies, including investigational therapies. It is incumbent on clinicians to be aware of these local and regional resources and refer patients when appropriate. Even with advanced disease, these centers can often offer improved outcomes and strategies not available to all clinicians.

Another area within the disease management spectrum is the home care programs that exist in most communities. These services frequently provide a link between intensive hospital-based care and infrequent, less intensive office-based care. In addition, for many patients with advanced disease, home care meets the constraints of patients and families.

For patients with advanced disease, physicians often begin discussions surrounding end-of-life issues too late. Patients who have advanced disease requiring frequent hospitalization and treatment generally are aware of their likelihood of death and, in fact, they value regaining some control of their lives through discussion of end-of-life planning and preferences. For some, hospice care is the choice made, whereas for others, referral to specialized centers and participation in emerging therapies through clinical trials might be the correct choice. Understanding comes only with an open and frank discussion with each patient and family.

Emerging and Emerged New Therapeutic Areas

Because of the intense interest in heart failure, a variety of important additional therapies are undergoing clinical investigation. These therapies include new application of biventricular pacemakers, aggressive mitral valve repair for patients with ongoing mitral valve regurgitation, and the use of left ventricular assist devices as bridges to heart recovery, as well as destination or permanent therapies. Moreover, several new cardiac restraint devices are being applied with some success. Within years, genomic therapies will broaden, as will areas of vascular and myogenic regeneration. Again, although most clinicians are not aware of all these newly emerging therapies, they can offer their patients referrals to specialized centers where suitable therapies can be sought.

REFERENCES

Gattis WA, O'Connor CM, Gallup DS, et al: Predischarge initiation of carvedilol in patients hospitalized for decompensated heart failure: Results of the Initiation Management Predischarge: Process for Assessment of Carvedilol Therapy in Heart Failure (IMPACT_HF) trial. J Am Coll Cardiol 2004;43:1534-1541.

Hunt SA, Baker DW, Chin MH, et al: ACC/AHA guidelines for the evaluation and management of heart failure in the adult: A report of the American College of Cardiology/American Heart Association Task Force on Practice Guidelines (Committee to Revise the 1995 Guidelines for the Evaluation and Management of Heart Failure), 2001. American College of Cardiology Web site. Available online at http://www.acc.org/clinical/guidelines/failure/hf_index.htm

Konstam MA: Systolic and diastolic dysfunction in heart failure? Time for a new paradigm. J Card Fail 2003;9:1-3.

Pitt B, Remme W, Zannad F, et al: Eplerenone, a selective aldosterone blocker in patients with left ventricular dysfunction after myocardial infarction. N Engl J Med 2003;348:1309-1321.

Poole-Wilson PA, Swedberg K, Cleland JG, et al: Comparison of carvedilol and metoprolol on clinical outcomes in patients with chronic heart failure in the Carvedilol or Metoprolol European Trial (COMET): Randomized controlled trial. Lancet 2003;362:7-13.

Redfield MM: Heart failure—an epidemic of uncertain proportions. N Engl J Med 2002;347:1442-1444.

Infective Endocarditis

Method of
Navin M. Amin, MD

Epidemiologic Changes

Infective endocarditis denotes microbial infection of the cardiac valves and, less frequently, infection of the mural endocardium or of septal defects. At present, infective endocarditis accounts for 1 case per 1000 hospital admissions. The age of patients with endocarditis has increased. In the preantibiotic era, the average age of patients with endocarditis was 32 to 39 years old; currently more than half the cases occur in patients older than 60 years of age. Men are affected twice as often as women; the ratio increases to 5:1 in men older than 60 years of age.

Three major epidemiologic changes are observed in endocarditis:

1. The pattern of infective organisms has changed. Early in the antibiotic era, group A *Streptococci* (β hemolyticus), *Pneumococci*, *Gonococci*, and *Meningococci* were the predominant pathogens. *Streptococcus viridans*, *Staphylococcus aureus* (methicillin-sensitive [MSSA] or methicillin resistant [MRSA]), coagulase—negative *Staphylococcus epidermidis* or *lugdunensis*—and gram-negative organisms are more common today.
2. Certain signs and symptoms, once characteristic of endocarditis, are seen in less than 5% of cases today: peripheral lesions involving skin, nails, and eyes—petechiae, subungual hemorrhage, Janeway lesions, Osler nodes, or Roth's spots.
3. Surgical procedures can be both a cause and a cure of endocarditis. Prosthetic valves inserted to improve mechanically malfunctioning valves can predispose recipients to endocarditis. But surgery can be lifesaving in patients with refractory congestive heart failure (CHF) or resistant infections.

Forms of Endocarditis

Endocarditis is classified as acute or subacute on the basis of its clinical course. The acute form, which evolves over days to weeks, is diagnosed within 2 weeks. Invasive organisms such as *Staphylococcus aureus, Staphylococcus epidermidis, Streptococcus pneumoniae*, group A streptococci, *Neisseria gonorrhoeae, Haemophilus influenzae, Salmonella*, other Enterobacteriaceae, Serratia, and *Pseudomonas aeruginosa* are usually the cause. Clinically acute endocarditis is associated with high fever, systemic toxicity, and leukocytosis with rapid destruction of the valves. It carries high morbidity and mortality.

Subacute endocarditis has a duration of more than 6 weeks and an indolent course. The most common agents are streptococcal species, with *Streptococcus viridans* the most predominant: *Enterococcus*, HACEK (*Haemophilus, Actinobacillus, Cardiobacterium, Eikenella, Kingella*) organisms, fungi, and *Coxiella burnetii*. Clinically subacute endocarditis is associated with prolonged low-grade fever (fever of unknown origin [FUO]), night sweats, weight loss, and vague symptoms such as generalized weakness, lethargy, and myalgia.

Infective endocarditis can also be grouped into three categories:

1. *Native valve endocarditis* usually develops when there is structural damage to the heart valve. Rheumatic/syphilitic valvular disease is responsible in 20% to 40% of the cases. The mitral valve is involved in 85%, and the aortic valve is affected in 50% of the cases. In patients older than age 60 years, 30% of cases occur with degenerative cardiac lesions such as calcified mitral valve annulus and calcified nodular lesions secondary to atherosclerosis or postmyocardial infarction thrombus. Twenty percent of cases with mitral valve prolapse (with thickened leaflets or significant mitral regurgitation) and obstructive cardiomyopathy can predispose to endocarditis. In 6% to 25% of cases, congenital heart disease is a risk factor as is evident in ventricular septal defect (VSD), patent ductus arteriosus (PDA), tetralogy of Fallot, or coarctation of the aorta. It can also occur with a stenotic or regurgitant valve such as bicuspid aortic valve and pulmonary stenosis. Endocarditis is rare in patients with atrial septal defect (secundum type) because of the low-pressure gradient between the atria. Finally is a group of patients without any structural defect who are susceptible to endocarditis. Tricuspid valve endocarditis can develop in intravenous drug abusers and immunocompromised patients (with chronic renal failure, severe burns, chronic active hepatitis, collagen vascular disease, or neoplasm involving the pancreas, lung, or stomach).
2. *Prosthetic valve endocarditis* (PVE) at present constitutes 20% of all cases of endocarditis. It occurs in 2% to 4% of patients with a prosthetic valve. It can be early or late. Early PVE occurs within 60 days of the valve replacement, and predominant organisms are *Staphylococcus epidermidis* and *S. aureus* (MSSA or MRSA). In the case of late-onset endocarditis, which occurs after 2 months, *Streptococcus viridans* is the main offending pathogen.
3. *Nosocomial endocarditis* commonly affects patients older than age 60 years and seriously ill hospitalized patients. These individuals are subjected to invasive procedures such as insertion of central venous pressure, monitoring lines, hyperalimentation catheters, or intracardiac pacemaker wires that represent nidus of infection. Box 1 summarizes the factors predisposing to endocarditis.

Microbiology

Any microorganism can cause endocarditis (Table 1). Certain pathogens have increased ability to adhere to valvular leaflets, thereby

> **BOX 1   Factors Predisposing to Endocarditis**
>
> **Native Valve Endocarditis**
> - Structural Damage
>   Rheumatic valvular disease
>   Syphilitic valvular disease
>   Degenerative
>   Calcified mitral/aortic valve
>   Calcified post-MI thrombus
>   Mitral valve prolapse
>   IHSS
>   Congenital heart disease
>   Regurgitant or stenotic valve, bicuspid aortic valve, PS, Ebstein's anomaly, Marfan's syndrome
>   High-pressure shunt, VSD, PDA, coarctation of the aorta, tetralogy of Fallot
> - No Structural Damage
>   Catheter Induced
>   IVDA
>   Immunocompromised
>
> **Prosthetic Valve Endocarditis**
> - Early (<2 mo)
>   *Staphylococcus epidermidis*
>   *Staphylococcus aureus*
> - Late (>2 mo)
>   *Staphylococcus viridans*
>
> **Nosocomial Endocarditis**
> - Invasive procedures
>
> ---
>
> *Abbreviations*: IHSS = idiopathic hypertrophic subaortic stenosis; IVDA = intravenous drug abuse; MI = myocardial infarction; PDA = patent ductus arteriosus; PS = pulmonary stenosis; VSD = ventricular septal defect.
> Adapted with permission from Amin NM: Infective endocarditis. Consultant 1994;34(3):319-343.

establishing infection. Approximately 70% of the cases are caused by streptococci and staphylococci.

Staphylococci (MSSA or MRSA) are encountered predominantly in intravenous drug abuse (IVDA), in early PVE, in an immunocompromised host, and in nosocomial endocarditis. *S. viridans* is more commonly seen in native valve endocarditis and in late PVE. Gram-negative bacilli commonly cause right-sided endocarditis as in IVDA and in patients with intravascular catheters.

Approximately 10% of patients with endocarditis have a negative blood culture after 48 to 72 hours of incubation. Factors that produce culture-negative endocarditis are (1) antibiotic therapy before cultures are obtained; (2) a low level of bacteremia (common with right-sided and mural endocarditis); (3) infection with fastidious or nutritionally deficient bacteria that require prolonged cultures (2 to 3 weeks) or additional supplements (e.g., pyridoxine) for growth; this group includes HACEK organisms, *Brucella*, and nutritionally deficient streptococci; (4) nonbacterial infectious agents such as fungi, viruses, spirochetes, *Rickettsia*, *Chlamydia*, or parasites; and (5) noninfectious causes: left atrial myxoma, Libman-Sacks endocarditis, systemic lupus erythematosus, Löffler's hypereosinophilic endocarditis, carcinoid syndromes, and marantic endocarditis associated with malignancies of the pancreas, stomach, or lung.

Clinical Manifestations

The clinical manifestations of infective endocarditis are extremely diverse and can mimic pulmonary, neurologic, renal, or bone and joint disease. The classic manifestations of fever, heart murmur, splenomegaly, and petechiae of the skin and the mucous membranes help establish the diagnosis.

The onset may be abrupt or insidious. The early manifestations may be vague flulike symptoms that occur within 3 weeks after an invasive procedure. The patient may complain of malaise, fatigue, weakness, myalgia, arthralgia, low-grade fever, night sweats, or weight loss. Anorexia is almost universal. When the onset is acute, as in intravenous (IV) drug abuse, PVE, or nosocomial endocarditis, there may be evidence of severe infection heralded by high fever (90% to 95%), shaking chills and rigors, or, more ominous, symptoms of frank heart failure or embolic phenomena.

In patients older than age 60 years, diagnosis is often delayed because 5% may not have fever or are admitted with diagnosis of cerebral vascular accident (CVA), pneumonia, occult neoplasm, degenerative joint disease, or osteomyelitis. Infective endocarditis should always be considered in patients older than age 60 years who have fever and associated unexplained CHF, CVA, renal failure, weight loss, anemia, new-onset murmur, or confusional state.

In 85% of the cases, cardiac manifestations include a heart murmur. In right-sided endocarditis and mural infection, murmur is absent. A new or changing murmur (usually of aortic regurgitation) occurs in 5% to 10% of patients and is a very helpful diagnostic sign. Persistent or progressive CHF is indicative of a serious complication that carries a high mortality rate.

Peripheral cutaneous manifestations take a variety of forms: skin pallor caused by secondary anemia; petechiae found in 20% to 40% of cases concentrated on the conjunctiva, palate, buccal mucosa, and distal extremities; clubbing of nails in 10% to 20% if infection is long-standing; splinter hemorrhages as linear red-to-brown streaks in the middle of the nail bed of fingers and toes; Osler nodes (5% to 20% cases), which are small painful, tender, purplish subcutaneous nodules in the pads of fingers and toes; and Janeway lesions, which are small macular, painless, erythematous or hemorrhagic plaques on the palms or soles.

Ocular manifestations include Roth's spots, which occur in 5% of the patients and appear as oval or boat-shaped white or pale retinal lesions surrounded by hemorrhage and located near the optic disk. In a few cases there may be presence of cotton-wool exudates, petechiae, or flame-shaped hemorrhages.

Embolization can occur in 15% to 35% of cases. A cerebral emboli may produce hemiplegia, monoplegia, aphasia, or unilateral blindness. Mesenteric emboli can result in acute abdominal pain, ileus, or melena. Splenic emboli may cause left upper quadrant pain that radiates to the left shoulder of the chest with a small pleural effusion or splenic frictional rub. Flank pain with hematuria indicates a renal infarction. Peripheral arterial emboli may produce pain or gangrene. Large arterial occlusions are frequently seen with fungal endocarditis. Very rarely, emboli to coronary arteries cause acute myocardial infarction, myocardial abscess, or mycotic aneurysm.

Neurologic complications (30% to 40%) include CVA from embolization, mycotic aneurysm causing cerebral of subdural hemorrhage and seizure, and brain abscess or toxic encephalopathy with confusion and nonspecific obtundation.

Renal manifestations are accompanied by microscopic or frank hematuria secondary to renal infarct, diffuse membranoproliferative glomerulonephritis, focal embolic glomerulonephritis, or renal abscess.

Splenomegaly occurs in 25% to 45% of the patients and is more common in subacute than in acute endocarditis.

Diagnosis

Infective endocarditis may mimic any systemic disorder. For this reason and because of its high morbidity and mortality, the diagnosis should be kept in mind whenever a high-risk patient has an unexplained fever, constitutional symptoms, or multiple systemic involvement with a changing or new heart murmur. A high index

TABLE 1 Microbiology of Infective Endocarditis

Type of Infection	Specific Associated Risk Factors
Bacterial	
Gram Positive	
Streptococci (40%-60%)	
S. viridans, S. pneumoniae, S. bovis, S. pyogenes, S. sanguis	NVE, late-onset PVE
Enterococci (Group D) (5%-20%)	
S. faecalis, S. faecium, S. durans	Gastrointestinal malignancies
Staphylococci (17%-40%)	IVDA, early PVE
S. aureus (MRSA), S. epidermidis (MRSE), S. lugdunensis	
Diphtheroids	
Listeria	IVDA, early PVE
Gram Negative	
Cultured easily	
Pseudomonas aeruginosa, Serratia marcescens, Salmonella, Proteus mirabilis, Shigella, Providencia, Enterobacter, Neisseria gonorrhoeae, Escherichia coli	IVDA, immunocompromised, nosocomial endocarditis
Difficult to culture	
(HACEK) (1%-10%)	
Haemophilus, Actinobacillus, Cardiobacterium, Eikenella, Kingella	
(not HACEK)	
Brucella, Legionella	
Nonbacterial	
Fungi (2%-4%)	
Candida, Aspergillus, Histoplasma, Coccidioides, Blastomyces	IVDA, PVE, cardiac surgery, IV catheters, immunosuppressed
Viruses	
Coxsackie B, adenovirus	
Spirochetes	
Borrelia burgdorferi	Tick bite
Spirillum minus	Rat bite
Rickettsiae	
Coxiella burnetii	Infected livestock or unpasteurized milk
Chlamydia	
C. psittaci	Infected birds
Parasites	
Trypanosoma cruzi (Chagas' disease)	Kissing bug bite

Abbreviations: IVDA, intravenous drug abuse; MRSA, methicillin-resistant staphylococcus aureus; MRSE, methicillin-resistant staphylococcus epidermidis; NVE, native valve endocarditis; PVE, prosthetic valve endocarditis.
Modified from Amin NM: Infective endocarditis. Consultant 1994;34(3):319-343.

---

of suspicion for endocarditis in certain clinical situations is very helpful:

- Intravenous drug abusers with high fever
- Patients older than age 60 years with nonspecific vague symptoms with a calcified mitral valve annulus
- Unknown source of embolization
- Certain virulent infections caused by organisms such as *Staphylococcus* or *Enterococcus*

A thorough history, complete examination, and laboratory tests should establish the correct diagnosis. Box 2 outlines the various laboratory abnormalities in infective endocarditis.

A baseline electrocardiogram (ECG) is helpful to detect chamber enlargement or possible conduction defect that may indicate underlying valvular or congenital anomalies. Later development of first-degree atrioventricular (AV) block, new bundle branch block, or new ectopic beats may indicate a myocardial abscess, especially in aortic valve endocarditis.

Echocardiography (transesophageal [TEE], M mode, two-dimensional, or Doppler) can confirm the diagnosis, detect complications, and help assess the prognosis. The echocardiogram can detect vegetations larger than 2 to 3 mm on mitral or aortic valves. Sensitivity in detecting vegetations is approximately 87% to 90% with TEE, 30% to 75% with M-mode, 40% to 50% with two-dimensional, and 50% with Doppler echocardiography. False-positive results are seen with old healed vegetations, myxomatous valvular degeneration, arterial myxoma, or a thrombus.

Echocardiogram can detect complications such as torn or perforated valves, ruptured chordae tendineae, myocardial abscess, or pericardial effusion that may require surgical intervention. Large-sized vegetations in the left side of the heart or in the aortic valve, or myocardial abscess, suggest a relatively poor prognosis, and surgery may be indicated.

Serial blood cultures are required to establish the diagnosis by isolating the offending bacterium or fungus. A minimum of three blood samples should be drawn 30 to 60 minutes apart before initiating empiric antibiotic therapy. If the patient has taken antibiotics in the preceding 2 weeks, two or three additional sets of blood cultures should be taken. Cultures of arterial blood offer no additional advantage over venous blood. Ninety percent of the blood cultures become positive within 7 days of incubation. Negative blood cultures are likely seen in patients who have received prior antibiotics or who have endocarditis caused by fastidious gram-negative (HACEK) bacilli, fungi, or nutritionally deficient streptococci. The microbiology laboratory should be alerted to the suspected endocarditis, and a report for prolonged incubation for 2 weeks included.

In fungal endocarditis, in which there is embolization of large arteries, a culture of the removed embolus can establish the diagnosis. Serologic studies can be helpful in fungal infection

> **BOX 2 Laboratory Abnormalities in Endocarditis**
>
> Hematologic
>   Leukocytosis
>   Anemia of chronic disorder
>   Thrombocytopenia (10% SBE)
>   Elevated ESR
>   Urine analysis
>   Hematuria, microscopic
>   Proteinuria
> Cardiac abnormality
>   ECG: chamber enlargement, conduction defect
> Chest x-ray
>   Cardiomegaly
>   Evidence of congestive heart failure
>   Nodular infiltrate (staphylococcal endocarditis)
> Diagnostic gold standards
>   Echocardiography (transesophageal preferred)
>   Three sets of blood (embolus) cultures
> Immunologic abnormalities
>   Rheumatoid factor (disappears after treatment)
>   Hypergammaglobulinemia
>   Cryoglobulinemia
>   Circulating immune complexes
>   Low complement levels
>
> *Abbreviations*: ECG = electrocardiogram; ESR = erythrocyte sedimentation rate; SBE = subacute bacterial endocarditis.

(histoplasmosis or coccidioidomycosis) or when rickettsial (Q fever) *Legionella* or *Chlamydia* infections are suspected.

Treatment of Infective Endocarditis

The main goal is eradicating the infecting pathogens as quickly as possible to reduce the risks of morbidity and mortality. This can be achieved with antibiotic therapy, surgical intervention, or both.

ANTIBIOTIC THERAPY

In using antibiotics to treat infective endocarditis, the following guidelines are helpful:

- Parental antibiotics are used to sustain bactericidal activity.
- Bactericidal antimicrobials are used for complete eradication of the pathogens. Synergistic bactericidal activity is achieved with combination therapy such as ampicillin and aminoglycosides in treatment of enterococcal endocarditis.
- The drug regimen and appropriate duration of course, 2 to 6 weeks, must be tailored to prevent relapse.
- The bactericidal activity of the antibiotic is monitored by determining the minimum inhibitory concentration (MIC) and the minimum bactericidal concentration (MBC) against the infecting organisms.
- Antibiotic therapy is initiated as quickly as possible. When endocarditis is severe and/or complicated, empiric treatment should be instituted immediately with antibiotics effective against *S. aureus* and enterococci. A combination of vancomycin (Vancocin) and gentamicin (Garamycin) is recommended. Once a specific organism is identified, appropriate bactericidal antibiotics should be used.

Most streptococci other than enterococci are exquisitely sensitive to penicillin. If MIC is less than 0.2 μg per mL, high-dose penicillin alone or in combination with either gentamicin (Garamycin) or streptomycin or ceftriaxone (Rocephin) can be used for 4 weeks. If the MIC is below 0.1 μg per mL, treatment should be for 2 weeks. If MIC is greater than 0.2 μg per mL or the MBC to MIC ratio exceeds 10:1, as it occurs in 15% to 20% of cases with *S. viridans* infection, higher dose of penicillin with aminoglycoside should be used. In penicillin-allergic patients, vancomycin is the best alternative with or without aminoglycoside (Table 2).

In enterococcal endocarditis, ampicillin is recommended in combination with an aminoglycoside. Gentamicin is preferred because 40% of the isolates are resistant to streptomycin. In penicillin-allergic patients, vancomycin with an aminoglycoside is the best choice.

In *S. aureus* infection, semisynthetic penicillin or first-generation cephalosporins are the agents of first choice. Addition of gentamicin or rifampin (Rifadin)[1] during the first few days rapidly reduces bacteremia. Vancomycin is recommended for patients allergic to penicillin or if the organism is methicillin resistant (MRSA). Addition of rifampin, although controversial, is recommended in patients demonstrating poor bactericidal activity during therapy with beta-lactams or vancomycin and for patients with suppurative complication, such as a valve ring abscess.

Endocarditis with *S. epidermidis*, which commonly develops on prosthetic valves, is ideally treated with vancomycin and rifampin.[1] An aminoglycoside may be added for 2 weeks.

Gram-negative infections causing high mortality are best treated with broad-spectrum penicillin or, preferably, a third-generation cephalosporin with an aminoglycoside. In most of these patients, valve replacement is necessary.

SURGICAL INTERVENTIONS

Approximately 25% of patients with severe or complicated endocarditis undergo surgery. The chief indications for surgery are refractory moderate or severe CHF; perivalvular invasion or myocardial abscess as evident by persistent fever despite antibiotics or electrocardiographic changes of conduction defects; systemic or arterial embolization; fungal endocarditis; PVE of early onset; large bulky vegetations that increase risk of CHF; persistent infection (particularly with gram-negative bacilli) that does not respond to 7 to 10 days of antibiotic therapy; and staphylococcal endocarditis in IV drug abusers that does not respond to antimicrobials.

PREVENTION OF BACTERIAL ENDOCARDITIS

Transient bacteremia that develops after a variety of manipulations or surgical procedures in patients with structural heart defects causes endocarditis. Prophylactic antibiotics in this situation can be highly effective when given before the procedure. Administration of these agents only once is required 30 minutes to 2 hours before the procedure (Table 3).

In choosing prophylactic therapy, the following questions (Table 4) are useful:

- Is the patient at increased risk for endocarditis with underlying structural defect?
- Is there a high risk the procedure will produce bacteremia with organisms that cause endocarditis, such as *S. viridans* infection with oral cavity procedures or enterococcal with gastrointestinal or genitourinary procedures?

Antibiotic prophylaxis is recommended for patients with VSD, PDA, pulmonary or aortic stenosis, tetralogy of Fallot, or coarctation of the aorta. Such therapy is needed for patients with rheumatic or syphilitic valvular defects, prosthetic valves, calcified valves, obstructive cardiomyopathy, or mitral valve prolapse with either regurgitant murmur or with thickened mitral valve leaflets.

Endocarditis prophylaxis is not advised for patients with isolated secundum atrial septal defect or those who have undergone surgical repair for VSD or PDA and have no residual defect beyond 6 months. The same is true for those who have coronary artery bypass graft, previous rheumatic fever, or Kawasaki disease without any valve dysfunction. Prophylaxis is not recommended for those who have mitral valve prolapse (MVP) without mitral regurgitation (MR) and for persons with a cardiac pacemaker or implanted defibrillator (Table 5).

---

[1]Not FDA approved for this indication.

Procedures for which antibiotic prophylaxis is needed are those in which transient bacteremia develops when mucosal surfaces colonized with microorganisms are traumatized. For example, bacteremia may occur following dental manipulation in 80% of cases or in 20% of patients after urethral instrumentation. Prophylactic antimicrobials are recommended for high-risk patients who are scheduled to have certain dental, oropharyngeal, gastrointestinal, or genitourinary manipulations.

Standard antibiotic prophylaxis for patients undergoing oral, dental, or upper respiratory tract manipulations include oral amoxicillin. Clindamycin (Cleocin),[1] cefadroxil (Duricef),[1] cephalexin (Keflex),[1] or azithromycin (Zithromax)[1] or clarithromycin (Biaxin)[1] should be given to those who cannot tolerate or are allergic to penicillin.

[1]Not FDA approved for this indication.

CURRENT DIAGNOSIS

- High index of suspicion
- Febrile patient (temperature >38°C [100.4°F]) with
  Valvular or congenital heart defects
  Intravenous drug abuse
  Prosthetic or vascular access
  New onset or changing cardiac murmur
  Unknown source of embolization
- Positive blood cultures on at least two different specimens.
- Presence of vegetation detected on echocardiography (transesophageal [TEE] preferred)

TABLE 2 Antibiotic Regimens for Bacterial Endocarditis

Infecting Organism	Antibiotic	Dosage, Route, and Frequency	Duration in Weeks
Penicillin susceptible *Streptococcus viridans*, and *S. bovis* (MIC <0.2 µg/dL)	*Preferred Regimen* Penicillin G	12-16 million U/d IV in 6 divided doses	4
	or Penicillin G PLUS	12-16 million U/d IV in 6 divided doses	4
	Gentamicin	1 mg/kg IM or IV q8h	2
	or Penicillin G PLUS Gentamicin	Dosages same as above regimen	2
	or Ceftriaxone	2 g IV or IM q24h	4
	Alternative Regimen Vancomycin	0.5 g IV q6h	4
Relative penicillin-resistant streptococci (MIC >0.2 µg/dL)	*Preferred Regimen* Penicillin G PLUS	20-30 million U/d IV in 6 divided doses	4
	Gentamicin	1 mg/kg IV or IM q8h	4
	Alternative Regimen Vancomycin	0.5 g IV q6h	4
Staphylococcus epidermidis (MRSE)	*Native Valve* Vancomycin	0.5 g IV q6h	4
	Prosthetic Valve Vancomycin PLUS	0.5 g IV q6h	4-6
	Gentamicin	1 mg/kg IV or IM q8h	2
	or Rifampin	300 mg PO/IV q12h	2
Enterococcus (*S. faecalis, S. faecium, S. durans*)	*Preferred Regimen* Penicillin G PLUS	20-30 million U/d IV in 6 divided doses	4-6
	Gentamicin	1 mg/kg IM or IV q8h	4-6
	or Ampicillin PLUS	2 g IV q4h	4-6
	Gentamicin	1 mg/kg IM or IV q8h	4-6
	Alternative Regimen Vancomycin PLUS	0.5 g IV q6h	4-6
	Gentamicin	1 mg/kg IM or IV q8h	4-6
Staphylococcus aureus (methicillin sensitive)	*Preferred Regimen* Nafcillin or Oxacillin	2 g IV q4h	4-6
	or Oxacillin PLUS	2 g IV q4h	4-6
	Gentamicin OR/PLUS	1 mg/kg IM or IV q8h	2
	Rifampin	300 mg PO/IV q12h	2
	Alternative Regimen Cefazolin	2 g IV q6h	4-6
	or Vancomycin	0.5 g IV q6h	4-6

TABLE 2 Antibiotic Regimens for Bacterial Endocarditis—cont'd

S. aureus (methicillin resistant [MRSA])	Daptomycin	6 mg/kg IV once a day	6
	Vancomycin PLUS	0.5 g IV q6h	4-6
	Gentamicin OR/PLUS	1 mg/kg IM or IV q8h	2
	Rifampin[1]	300 mg PO/IV q12h	2
HACEK group (Haemophilus, Actinobacillus, Cardiobacterium, Eikenella, Kingella)	Ampicillin or	2 g IV q6h	4
	Ampicillin PLUS	2 g IV q6h	4
	Gentamicin or	1 mg/kg IM or IV q8h	4
	Ceftriaxone	2 g IV q24h	4
Culture negative	Vancomycin PLUS	0.5 g IV q8h	6
	Gentamicin	1 mg/kg IM or IV q8h	6

Abbreviations: MIC = minimum inhibitory concentration
[1]Not FDA approved for this indication
Modified from Amin NM: Infective Endocarditis. Consultant 1994;34(3):319-343.

Parenteral ampicillin is recommended for patients who cannot take oral antibiotics and for those at high risk for infective endocarditis, such as patients with a prosthetic valve, previous endocarditis, or surgical systemic pulmonary shunts. Clindamycin[1] or cefazolin (Ancef) can be used as an alternative. Patients undergoing gastrointestinal or genitourinary instrumentation should be given vancomycin.

As recommended by the American Heart Association, all prophylactic antibiotics should be used only once before the procedure. There is no need for additional antibiotic administration except in high-risk patients who are undergoing gastrointestinal or genitourinary manipulation and who are given an ampicillin and gentamicin combination.

[1]Not FDA approved for this indication.

TABLE 3 Preprocedural Antibiotic Prophylaxis for At-Risk Patients

Type of Procedure and Situation	Antibiotic	Dosage, Route, and Frequency
Dental, oral respiratory tract, and esophageal procedures		
Standard prophylaxis	Amoxicillin	2 g PO 1 h before procedure
Patient unable to take oral medication	Ampicillin	2 g IM/IV within 30 min before procedure
Patient allergic to penicillin	Clindamycin (Cleocin*) or	600 mg PO 1 h before procedure
	cefadroxil (Duricef*) or	2 g PO 1 h before procedure
	cephalexin (Keflex*) or azithromycin (Zithromax*) or	2 g PO 1 h before procedure 500 mg PO 1 h before procedure
	clarithromycin (Biaxin*)	500 mg PO 1 h before procedure
Patient allergic to penicillin and unable to take oral medication	Clindamycin (Cleocin*) or	600 g IV within 30 min of starting procedure
	cefazolin (Ancef) or	1 g IV within 30 min of starting procedure
	vancomycin (Vancocin)	1 g IV over 1-2 h within 60 min of starting procedure
Genitourinary/gastrointestinal procedures		
Moderate-risk patient	Amoxicillin or	2 g PO 1 h before procedure
	ampicillin	2 g IM/IV within 30 min of starting procedure
Moderate-risk penicillin-allergic patient	Vancomycin	1 g IV over 1-2 h infusion completed within 30-60 min of starting procedure
High-risk patient	Ampicillin PLUS	2 g IM/IV given within 30 min of starting procedure
	gentamicin 6 h later	1.5 mg/kg IV given within 30 min of starting procedure
	Ampicillin or	1 g IM or IV
	amoxicillin	1 g PO
High-risk penicillin-allergic patient	Vancomycin PLUS	1 g IV over 1-2 h
	gentamicin	1.5 mg/kg IV given within 30 min of starting procedure

*Not FDA approved for this indication
Modified from Dajani AS, Taubert KA, Wilson W, et al: Prevention of bacterial endocarditis: Recommendation by the American Heart Association. JAMA 1997;277(22):1794-1801.

TABLE 4 Indications for Endocardial Prophylaxis

Cardiac Conditions

High-risk category
Prosthetic valve
Previous endocarditis
Complex cyanotic disease
   Tetralogy of Fallot, single ventricle
Surgically conducted systemic-pulmonary shunt

Moderate-risk category
Congenital heart disease: VSD, PDA, AS, PS
Acquired valvular dysfunction
   Rheumatic/syphilitic
Hypertrophic cardiomyopathy

MVP with MR or thickened leaflets

Procedures

Dental
Dental extraction
Periodontal procedures: surgery, scaling, root planing
Dental implant replacement
Subgingival placement of antibiotic fibers
Intraligamentary local anesthetic injection
Cleaning of teeth or implants

Respiratory
Tonsillectomy/adenoidectomy
Rigid bronchoscopy

Gastrointestinal
Sclerotherapy
Esophageal stricture dilation
ERCP with biliary obstruction
Biliary tract surgery
Surgery involving intestinal mucosa

Genitourinary
Prostatic surgery
Cystoscopy
Urethral dilation
Septic abortion

Abbreviations: AS = aortic stenosis; ERCP = endoscopic retrograde cholangiopancreatography; MVP = mitral valve prolapse; MR = mitral regurgitation; PDA = patent ductus arteriosus; PS = pulmonary stenosis; VSD = ventricular septal defect.
Modified from Dajani AS, Taubert KA, Wilson W, et al: Prevention of bacterial endocarditis: Recommendations by the American Heart Association. JAMA 1997;277(22):1794-1801.

TABLE 5 Endocardial Prophylaxis Not Recommended

Cardiac Conditions

Isolated secundum ASD
Surgical repair of ASD, VSD, PDA (without residue > 6 mo)
Previous CABG surgery
MVP without valvular dysfunction
Functional murmur
Kawasaki disease without valvular dysfunction
Previous rheumatic fever without valve dysfunction
Cardiac pacemaker and implanted defibrillators
Cardiac catheterization, balloon angioplasty
Coronary stent placement

Procedures

Dental
Restorative dentistry
Local anesthetic injections
Intracanal treatment
Postoperative suture removal
Oral impression/radiograph
Fluoride treatment
Shedding of primary teeth

Respiratory
Endotracheal intubation
Fiberoptic bronchoscopy
Tympanostomy tube insertion

Gastrointestinal
TEE*
Endoscopy with/without biopsy*

Genitourinary
Vaginal delivery/hysterectomy*
Cesarean section
Urethral catheterization
Uterine dilation and curettage
Insertion/removal of IUD
Circumcision

*Prophylaxis optional for high-risk category.
Abbreviations: ASD = atrial septal defect; CABG = coronary artery bypass graft; IUD = intrauterine device; MVP = mitral valve prolapse; PDA = patent ductus arteriosus; TEE = transesophageal echocardiogram; VSD = ventricular septal defect.
Modified from Dajani AS, Taubert KA, Wilson W, et al: Prevention of bacterial endocarditis: Recommendations by the American Heart Association. JAMA 1997;277(22):1794-1801.

CURRENT THERAPY

- Empiric antibiotics should be started immediately with vancomycin and gentamicin.
- Specific therapy should be started once the pathogen is identified:
  Use combination therapy for synergetic activity.
  Monitor MIC/MBC level whenever possible.
  Administer therapy for 2 to 6 weeks.
- Surgical interventions should be undertaken for severe, refractory, and complicated endocarditis.
- Prophylactic antibiotics are recommended in patients with structural heart defects undergoing surgical procedures or manipulations that can cause transient bacteremia, as recommended by the American Heart Association.
- Administration of antibiotic is usually once and 30 minutes to 1 to 2 hours before the procedure.

Abbreviations: MBC = minimum bactericidal concentration; MIC = minimum inhibitory concentration.

REFERENCES

Amin NM: Infective endocarditis. Consultant 1994;34(3):319-343.
Bansal RC: Infective endocarditis. Med Clin North Am 1995;79:1205-1220.
Bayer AS, Bolger AF, Taubert KA, et al: Diagnosis and management of infective endocarditis and its complications. Circulation 1998;98:2936-2948.
Bayer AS, Ward JI, Ginzton LE, Shapiro SM: Evaluation of new clinical criteria for diagnosis of infective endocarditis. Am J Med 1994;96:211-219.
Cunha BA, Gill MV, Lazar JM: Acute infective endocarditis. Infect Dis Clin North Am 1996;10(4):811-834.
Dajanai AS, Taubert KA, Wilson W, et al: Prevention of bacterial endocarditis. Recommendations by American Heart Association. JAMA 1997;277:1794-1801.
Giessel BE, Koenig CJ, Blake RL: Management of bacterial endocarditis. Am Fam Physician 2000;61:1725-1732.
Karchner AW: Infections on prosthetic valves and intravascular infections. In Mandell GL, Bennett JE, Dolin R (eds): Mandell, Douglas and Bennett's Principles and Practice of Infectious Diseases, 5th ed. Philadelphia: Churchill Livingstone, 2000, pp 903-917.
Li JS, Sexton DJ, Mick N, et al: Proposed modification to Duke criteria for diagnosis of infective endocarditis. Clin Infect Dis 2000;30:633-638.
Mylonakis E, Calderwood SB: Infective endocarditis in adults. N Engl J Med 2001;345(18):1318-1330.

Hypertension

Method of
L. Michael Prisant, MD

Physiologic Variability of Blood Pressure

Like temperature and heart rate, blood pressure is a continuous physiologic variable. Blood pressure progressively increases from birth. The 90th percentile blood pressure for boys in the United States is 87/68 mm Hg at birth and 136/84 mm Hg by 18 years. With aging, progressive fragmentation of elastin occurs in the aorta and other large blood vessels and results in loss of the dampening or buffering function of the aorta. Thus, the recoil or pump function of the aorta diminishes. When the aorta is less elastic, systolic blood pressure is amplified because more blood is delivered to the periphery during systole. The reflected waves from the periphery return to the aortic root before the end of systole and augment systolic blood pressure. Diastolic blood pressure drops because there is less residual stroke volume to be delivered to the periphery during diastole. Thus, the hallmark of the loss of the recoil function of the aorta is a widened pulse pressure, which is the difference between systolic and diastolic blood pressures.

Differences in physiology according to the time of the day, time of the month, or season of the year encompass the discipline of chronobiology. There are daily and seasonal variations in blood pressure. During summer months, blood pressure is lower, and winter months it is higher. With the daily activation of the sympathetic nervous system prior to awakening, blood pressure and heart rate increase (Figure 1). These changes in blood pressure parallel the morning activation in catecholamines, renin, and angiotensin.

The peak blood pressure is between 6 AM and noon. Associated with the morning surge in blood pressure, there is a disproportionately higher rate of myocardial infarction, stroke, aortic dissection, and sudden cardiac death in the morning than other times of the day.

Activity and sleep influence the level of blood pressure throughout the day. Between midnight and 6 AM, blood pressure is generally lowest. The systolic blood pressure normally increases with pain, stress, or dynamic exercise.

Normally, blood pressure declines 10% to 20% from the daytime activity period to the sleep period. Patients with less than a 10% reduction in daytime blood pressure are referred to as *nondippers* and have more target organ damage.

Definitions

Blood pressure is a continuous physiologic variable associated with vascular disease (Figure 2). Diastolic blood pressure confers risk, but systolic blood pressure is a more potent risk factor. Furthermore, as pulse pressure widens, so does the risk. Although our cutpoint for a normal and an abnormal blood pressure is arbitrary, definitions for a treatment threshold are based on outcome trials.

The current classification of blood pressure is shown in Table 1. For adults aged 18 years and older, a blood pressure less than 120/80 mm Hg is normal, and 140/90 mm Hg or higher is hypertension. A diagnosis of hypertension is based on the average of two or more properly measured blood pressure readings on each of two or more office visits. The higher systolic or diastolic blood pressure from the four or more measurements determines the classification. The stage of hypertension at the initial visit indicates the time frame for follow-up assessment and subsequently the magnitude of therapy required.

Prehypertension is a category that identifies persons at high risk for developing hypertension and alerts patients and clinicians to intervene and prevent or delay disease from developing. The prevalence of prehypertension for adults 18 years or older was 29.6% in the 2003-2004 National Health and Nutrition Examination Survey (NHANES). In the Trial of Preventing Hypertension (TROPHY) Study ($N = 772$), despite nonpharmacologic treatment, 40% of prehypertensive study participants developed hypertension after 2 years and 63% after 4 years. Patients with prehypertension often have the concomitant risk factors of hypercholesterolemia, hypertriglyceridemia, low HDL cholesterol, glucose intolerance, increased waist circumference, and obesity. Furthermore, prehypertension has a higher risk of cardiovascular disease than normal blood pressure.

PREVALENCE

In the United States among persons 20 years or older, 69.7 million have prehypertension (Figure 3). In 1999 and 2000, there were at least 65.2 million adults with hypertension, a 30% increase from 1988 to 1994, and this condition affects more than 30% of the population. It is the

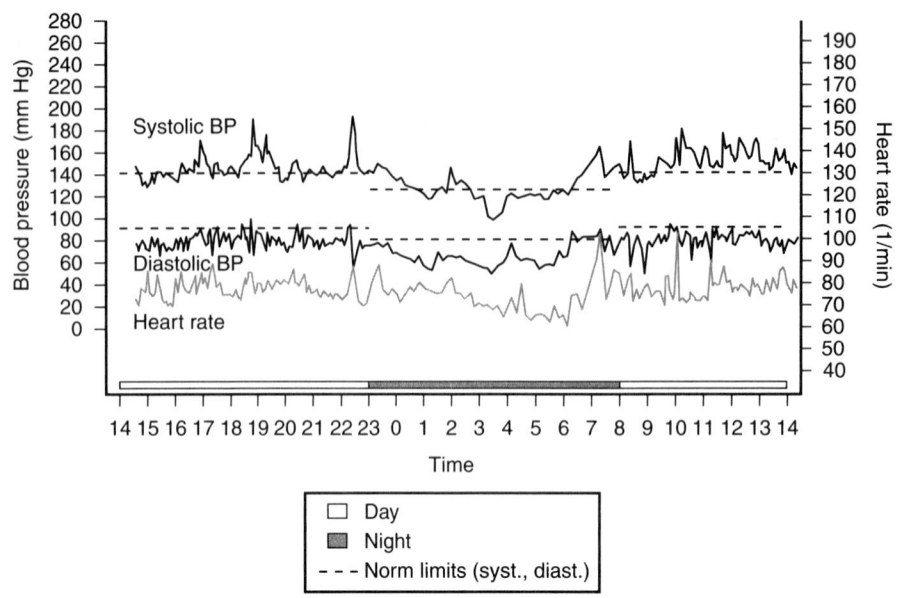

FIGURE 1. Ambulatory blood pressure recording. *Abbreviations*: diast = diastole; syst = systole.

most common medical reason for an office visit. The prevalence of hypertension (Figure 4) is slightly higher among women than men, significantly higher among non-Hispanic blacks compared with whites or Latin Americans, and increases with age. As the population becomes more obese, it is likely that hypertension, diabetes mellitus, cardiovascular disease, and end-stage renal disease will escalate.

VASCULAR RISKS OF HYPERTENSION

Hypertension promotes alteration or rupture of arteries or arterioles in the brain, eyes, heart, and kidneys (hypertensive events) and progressive atherosclerosis involving the aorta or carotid, coronary, iliofemoral, and renal arteries (atherosclerotic events).

The cardiovascular sequelae of hypertension include angina, unstable angina, myocardial infarction, atrial fibrillation, sudden death, left ventricular hypertrophy, and congestive heart failure (both systolic and diastolic). Left ventricular hypertrophy is not only a target organ response to increased afterload, but is also the most potent cardiovascular risk factor. When left ventricular hypertrophy is present, it is associated with a higher prevalence of coronary heart disease, cardiovascular death (including sudden cardiac death), stroke, heart failure, and atrial fibrillation. Even without obstructive coronary disease, left ventricular hypertrophy impedes perfusion of blood from the epicardial to the endocardial surface, promoting angina, myocardial infarction, ventricular ectopy, myocardial fibrosis, and heart failure (Figure 5). Seventy-five percent of all patients with heart failure have antecedent hypertension. Chronic heart failure can occur early in the natural history of the disease due to diastolic filling abnormalities with normal systolic function without a dilated ventricle, or it can occur late due to reduced systolic function with a dilated ventricle. Patients with diastolic or preserved ejection fraction heart failure have a mortality rate similar to that of asymptomatic patients with a reduced ejection fraction. Chronic heart failure is the only cardiovascular disease increasing in incidence and prevalence.

The cerebrovascular consequences of hypertension include stroke, cerebral edema, and dementia. Acute intracerebral hemorrhage is usually due to rupture of a small, penetrating intraparenchymal artery. Ischemic strokes result from obstruction of arterial flow by local atherothrombosis, embolization, or small vessel occlusion. Uncontrolled hypertension is more likely to rupture a berry aneurysm, causing a subarachnoid hemorrhage. Hypertensive encephalopathy results from the consequence of increased blood pressure (accelerated or malignant hypertension) exceeding the confines of cerebral autoregulation. Cerebral edema, microinfarcts, petechial hemorrhages, and fibrinoid necrosis of the arterioles are present. Manifestations of hypertensive encephalopathy include headaches, nausea, vomiting, visual disturbances, seizures, impaired consciousness, and reversible focal neurologic symptoms and signs.

Hypertension is only second to diabetes mellitus as a cause of chronic kidney disease. Hypertensive nephropathy is the consequence of alteration in small arteries and arterioles producing hyaline arteriosclerosis with chronic hypertension and myointimal hyperplasia and fibrinoid necrosis with accelerated or malignant hypertension. Preglomerular arteriolar destruction, glomerular collapse, tubular atrophy, and interstitial fibrosis occur in a progressive fashion. Nephrosclerosis reduces renal blood flow, resulting in early increases of uric acid and progressive excretory failure, characterized by a rising blood urea nitrogen and creatinine. Microalbuminuria (30-300 mg/d) is an incipient manifestation of hypertensive renal disease and a cardiovascular risk factor. Atherosclerotic renal artery stenosis independently causes renal ischemia, excessive renin secretion, and further elevation in blood pressure.

Examination of the retinal vessels provides a window to examine the vascular effects of hypertension. The ocular manifestations of

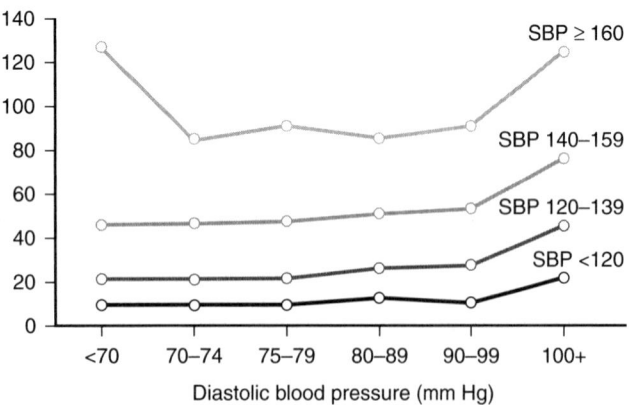

FIGURE 2. Age-adjusted coronary heart disease death rates per 10,000 person-years among 316,099 men by level of blood pressure. *Abbreviation*: SBP = systolic blood pressure. Derived from Neaton JD, Wentworth D: Serum cholesterol, blood pressure, cigarette smoking, and death from coronary heart disease. Overall findings and differences by age for 316,099 white men. Multiple Risk Factor Intervention Trial Research Group. Arch Intern Med 1992;152:56-64.

TABLE 1 Classification of Blood Pressure for Adults

Classification*	Systolic BP (mm Hg)		Diastolic BP (mm Hg)	Follow-up Recommended[†]
Normal	<120	and	<80	Recheck within 2 y
Prehypertension	120-139	or	80-89	Recheck within 1 y
Stage 1 hypertension	140-159	or	90-99	Recheck within 2 mo
Stage 2 hypertension	≥160	or	≥100	Evaluate or refer to source of care within 1 mo[‡]

*The classification is based on the average of *two or more* properly measured, seated, blood pressure readings on each of *two or more* office visits. The *higher* systolic or diastolic blood pressure from the *four or more* measurements determines the classification.
[†]Based on initial average blood pressure measurements.
[‡]For patients with higher blood pressures (e.g., >180/110 mm Hg), evaluate and treat immediately or within 1 week depending on clinical situation and complications.
Modified from Chobanian AV, Bakris GL, Black HR, et al: Seventh report of the Joint National Committee on Prevention, Detection, Evaluation, and Treatment of High Blood Pressure. Hypertension 2003;42:1206-1252.

hypertension include retinopathy, optic neuropathy, choroidopathy with retinal detachment, and central or branch retinal vein occlusion. The normal arteriole-to-venule ratio is 2:3. Arteriolar narrowing occurs early in hypertension. Retinal arterioles normally have a yellow-white appearance, but as arteriosclerosis develops, the appearance becomes reddish-brown (copper wiring) and then white (silver wiring). Arterioles and venules share a common adventitial sheath. Arteriosclerosis compresses the venules, causing arteriovenous nicking, a predictor for mortality and stroke. The interruption of venous flow where a retinal artery crosses a vein can result in central or branch retinal vein occlusion. Uncontrolled severe hypertension causes flame-shaped retinal hemorrhages, cotton-wool spots (retinal infarcts), and blurring of the optic disk margin (papilledema). Retinal hard exudates can indicate prior accelerated or malignant hypertension. They are yellow-white lipid deposits with sharp borders. A macular star, a hard exudate, radiates out from the fovea and is the consequence of retinal edema.

Large artery involvement from hypertension causes dilation or dissection of the thoracic aorta. Hypertension is present in 69% of ascending aortic dissections and 77% of descending aortic dissections. The definition of an abdominal aortic aneurysm is a segment of aorta that exceeds 3 cm in diameter, or the ratio of the abnormal to normal segment of aortic diameter is 1.5 or greater. Hypertension may be an important factor in the pathogenesis and growth of abdominal aneurysms.

Hypertension, diabetes, and cigarette smoking are associated with lower extremity peripheral arterial disease. Hypertension increased the risk of intermittent claudication 2.5-fold in men and 4-fold in women in the Framingham Heart Study. The risk was proportional to the magnitude of high blood pressure. One should remember that lower extremity peripheral arterial disease predicts a high prevalence of coronary disease.

MEASUREMENT OF BLOOD PRESSURE

Health care providers need to be trained to perform blood pressure measurements correctly to avoid inaccurate labeling (and insurance premium hikes), psychological trauma, and inappropriate medication use. At least two or three measurements at 1-minute intervals should be performed at every visit. My preference is three measurements; the first of these three blood pressure measurements is used to locate the systolic and diastolic blood pressures, and the average of the last two is used for decision making. Initial blood pressure measurements should include measurement in the contralateral arm. A mercury manometer should be used to measure blood pressure because it is the gold standard and the most accurate. If an aneroid or electronic sphygmomanometer is used, it must be calibrated against a mercury manometer every 3 to 6 months using a Y-connection to determine if there is more than 4 mm Hg difference between devices over a range of blood pressures (40-260 mm Hg) for assessment of the accuracy of the nonmercury equipment. White-coat effect can be limited by teaching, monitoring, and retraining office personnel to perform blood pressure measurements according to the standards of the American Heart Association.

The patient should be seated in a quiet room in a chair with the back and arm supported and the legs uncrossed. There should be no talking during the measurements. Abstinence from tobacco use or caffeine ingestion within 30 minutes of the initial measurements of blood pressure is necessary. Subsequent readings are performed after a 5- to 15-minute period of rest. Cuff application is on an uncovered and supported arm at heart level. The length of the cuff bladder should encircle 80% of the arm circumference, and the width of the cuff bladder should be 40% of the arm circumference. Placing a small cuff on obese patients is a common cause of pseudohypertension. *Pseudohypertension* refers to falsely elevated blood pressure that is an artifact of measurement.

Radial artery palpation is used to estimate the systolic blood pressure once the cuff is applied snugly and evenly over the brachial artery. The cuff should be distended about 20 to 30 mm Hg above the palpable systolic blood pressure. Radial artery palpation prevents underestimating systolic blood pressure or overestimating diastolic blood pressure, which is associated with the silent period (auscultatory gap) between the systolic and diastolic blood pressures, and prevents the pain of excess cuff inflation pressure that elevates systolic blood pressure. Osler's sign is a palpable pulseless radial artery present after the cuff is inflated above the systolic blood pressure. This sign, a clue for pseudohypertension from atherosclerosis, is not discriminatory.

The bell of the stethoscope is used to auscultate low-intensity Korotkoff sounds over the brachial artery, and then the cuff is slowly deflated with each heart beat, or 2 to 3 mm Hg per second. The systolic blood pressure is the first faint tapping sound of two

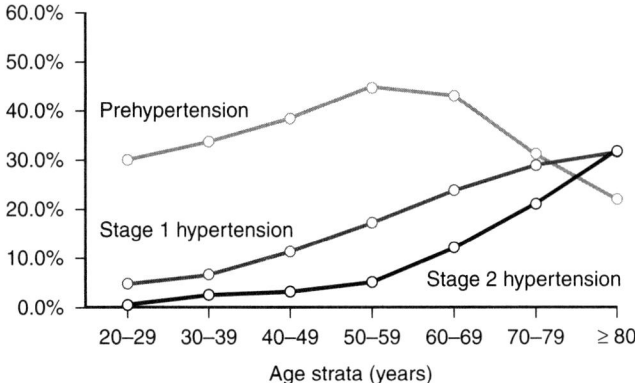

FIGURE 3. Prevalence of prehypertension and stages 1 and 2 hypertension by age strata. Derived from Qureshi AI, Suri MF, Kirmani JF, Divani AA: Prevalence and trends of prehypertension and hypertension in United States: National Health and Nutrition Examination Surveys 1976 to 2000. Med Sci Monit 2005;11(9):CR403-CR409.

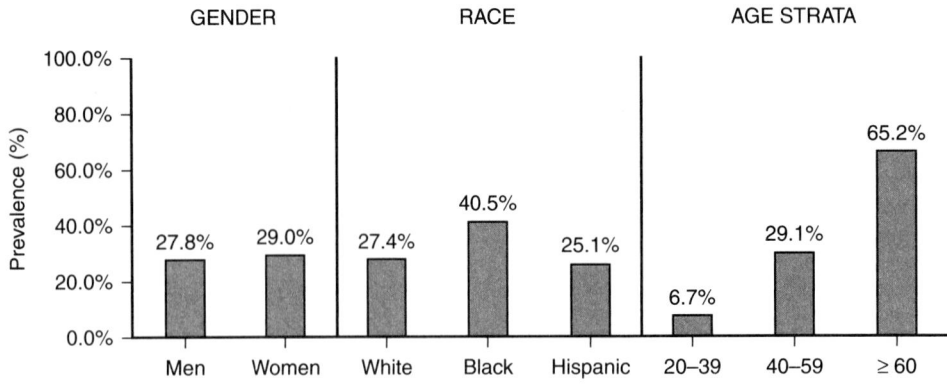

FIGURE 4. Prevalence of hypertension by race, gender, and age strata in the united states, 1999-2002. Derived from Centers for Disease control and Prevention: Racial/ethnic disparities in prevalence, treatment, and control of hypertension—United States, 1999-2002. MMWR Morb Mortal Wkly Rep. 2005;54(1):7-9.

successive beats after cuff deflation, and the diastolic blood pressure is the point at which Korotkoff sounds completely cease. If the diastolic blood pressure approaches zero, then the diastolic blood pressure is reported as the period marked by an abrupt muffling sound quality. All values are reported to the nearest 2 mm Hg. If more than 20% of the measurements end in zero, then a zero-digit preference is documented and retraining is necessary.

Blood pressure can decline over subsequent visits even without active drug therapy. This has been referred to as the *placebo effect*. It highlights the importance of not making a diagnosis of hypertension at a single office visit (see Table 1).

Home blood pressure monitoring may be useful for the care of patients. *White coat hypertension* (also called *office hypertension*) refers to elevated blood pressure that occurs in the medical environment. Home blood pressure monitoring is advocated to assess this condition in hypertensive patients who do not have target organ involvement. However, research documents that patients with this diagnosis have target organ involvement that is intermediate between true normotensive and true hypertensive patients. Furthermore, many patients with white coat hypertension develop true hypertension. Another application is masked hypertension, defined as normal office blood pressure and elevated home or ambulatory blood pressure. More research is required, but these patients appear to have increased cardiovascular risk. However, the best argument for the use of home blood pressure measurements is the involvement of patients with their disease.

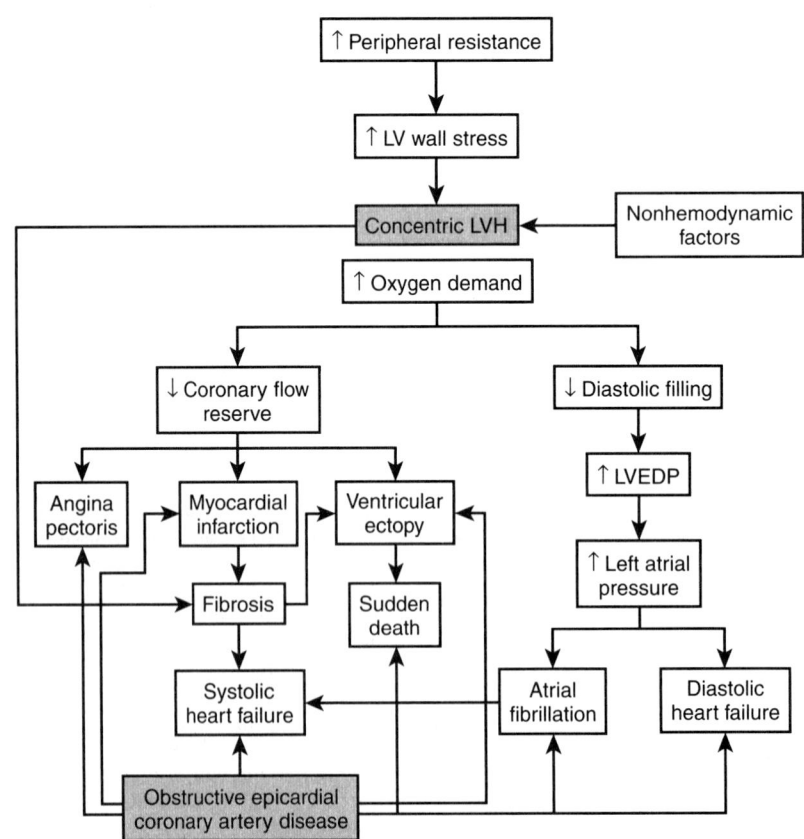

FIGURE 5. Hypertensive heart disease. *Abbreviations* LF = left ventricle; LVEDP = left ventricular diastolic filling pressure; LVH = left ventricular hypertrophy. Reproduced with permission from Prisant LM: Hypertensive heart disease. J Clin Hypertens (Greenwich) 2005;7:231-238. Copyright 2005 by Le Jacq, Ltd.

Many home devices (e.g., wrist devices) are not accurate for decision-making. An objective source of information at http://www.dableducational.com/sphygmomanometers.html helps to guide physician recommendations. The patient should be told to take two seated measurements twice daily after resting for 5 minutes. Values consistently less than 130/80 mm Hg are normal.

Ambulatory blood pressure monitoring provides information on the average 24-hour blood pressure, diurnal variation of blood pressure, and the variability of blood pressure. It is the only means for recording sleep blood pressure. Daytime and sleep blood pressures that exceed 135/85 mm Hg and 120/75 mm Hg, respectively, are abnormal. Medicare currently reimburses ambulatory blood pressure for the diagnosis of white coat hypertension in patients who have three office measurements exceeding 140/90 mm Hg, two out-of-office measurements less than 140/90 mm Hg, and no evidence of target organ damage. However, individual test repeatability is limited.

OTHER DEFINITIONS

Labile hypertension refers to episodically normal and abnormal blood pressures, but *borderline hypertension* is a preferable term because there is no more or less blood pressure variability in normotensive versus sustained hypertensive patients. Secondary hypertension is hypertension of a known cause (e.g., renovascular disease, hyperthyroidism, pheochromocytoma, primary renal disease). In the absence of a secondary cause, the diagnosis of essential hypertension (also called *idiopathic* or *primary hypertension*) is established by default. Isolated systolic hypertension is defined as a systolic blood pressure of 140 mm Hg or greater and a diastolic blood pressure of less than 90 mm Hg.

The presence of resistant, accelerated, or malignant hypertension should provoke suspicion of secondary hypertension. *Resistant hypertension* defines hypertension greater than 160/100 mm Hg despite rational, maximal three-drug therapy in an adherent patient. *Refractory hypertension* refers to a blood pressure greater than 140/90 mm Hg (or greater than 160/90 mm Hg in patients older than 60 years) in patients without secondary hypertension who are treated with maximal doses of two appropriate drugs that are given adequate time to be effective. *Accelerated hypertension* is severe hypertension associated with ongoing target organ damage (e.g., heart failure, kidney failure, unstable angina) and flame-shaped hemorrhages and cotton-wool spots. *Malignant hypertension* requires the presence of papilledema.

Pathogenesis

There is no single mechanism that explains the genesis of essential hypertension, unlike the mechanisms for secondary hypertension. Essential hypertension is viewed as a polygenic trait with various subsets of genes that are additive. In contrast to first-degree relatives of normotensive patients, first-degree relatives of hypertensive patients are more likely to develop hypertension. African Americans tend to have an earlier onset and more severe hypertension than whites. Excess body weight, psychosocial stress, sodium and potassium ingestion, alcohol consumption, and physical activity modify the level of blood pressure in an individual patient.

Other factors are also important. The impact of the sympathetic nervous system on blood pressure is appreciated in patients who have a cervical spinal cord injury and chronically low blood pressure. The distal portion of the spinal cord retains function, and activation of spinal cord reflexes working independently can result in paroxysmal hypertension or autonomic dysreflexia. Increased sympathetic nervous system activity is present in younger and older persons with essential hypertension. The role of the heart in elevating systolic blood pressure is suggested in high cardiac output states associated with low systemic vascular resistance, such as hyperthyroidism, anemia, and aortic insufficiency. The importance of the kidney is supported by normalization of blood pressure after transplantation of a kidney from a normotensive patient into a patient with renal failure due to hypertension.

EVALUATION

The goals for the initial evaluation (Box 1) are to document that the patient has a sustained elevation in blood pressure, to identify the presence of hypertensive and atherosclerotic target organ involvement, to screen for other cardiovascular risk factors (diabetes mellitus, dyslipidemia, tobacco use, physical inactivity, obesity, family history), to identify factors (e.g., gout, asthma) that might modify treatment, and to diagnose correctable causes of secondary hypertension. Box 1 lists the components of the physical examination and their implications. Initial tests prior to treatment are a fasting glucose, hematocrit, serum potassium, calcium, creatinine, complete lipid profile, urinalysis, and electrocardiogram. Box 2 lists the components of the laboratory studies and their implications. Additional studies may be needed based on the history, physical examination, and results of the laboratory studies.

Therapy

NONPHARMACOLOGIC THERAPY

Lifestyle modification is recommended for all patients with prehypertension and hypertension. Weight reduction, sodium restriction, alcohol restriction, and increased physical activity lower blood pressure, but recidivism is common. The DASH (Dietary Approaches to Stop Hypertension) diet lowered systolic blood pressure 8 to 14 mm Hg in a feeding trial.

PHARMACOLOGIC THERAPY

There is a proliferation of antihypertensive medications that target different mechanisms. Although the number of pharmacologic agents may seem bewildering, selecting drugs within a class that have outcome data simplifies selection (see Box 2). Dosing frequency, side effects, cost, and many other factors influence adherence to treatment. Low-dose, fixed-dose combination therapy reduces dose-dependent side effects and maximizes attainment of blood pressure control.

The blood pressure goal for hypertensive patients with diabetes mellitus and chronic kidney disease is less than 130/80 mm Hg. With protein excretion greater than 1 g/day, a goal of less than 125/75 mm Hg is often advocated. The American Heart Association now recommends a target blood pressure of less than 130/80 mm Hg in patients with ischemic heart disease and less than 120/80 mm Hg with left ventricular dysfunction. The target blood pressure for the remaining patients is less than 140/90 mm Hg. To achieve blood pressure control, most patients require more than one drug.

Factors in Drug Selection

Characteristics to consider when selecting an antihypertensive drug include mode of action, route of elimination, and potential drug interactions. Assuming a drug within a drug class has a class effect in protecting or reducing target organ damage is an error, especially among hypertensive patients who have compelling indications for specific drug classes (Table 2). Age, race, comorbid conditions, and renal function influence initial drug selection. For instance, β-blockers, angiotensin-converting enzyme (ACE) inhibitors, and angiotensin receptor blockers (ARBs) are less effective as initial therapy in African American patients than in whites. Older patients respond better to diuretics and calcium channel blockers (CCBs) than to ACE inhibitors. A diminished glomerular filtration rate requires reduction of the drug dose or avoidance of the drug. The highest priority for drug selection is based on comorbid illness to prevent target organ damage.

A conservation-of-medication approach can be used to treat more than one disease with a single drug and lessen pharmaceutical costs. For instance, a nonselective β-blocker could be used to treat both hypertension and migraine headaches or essential tremor. Another example is treating a patient who has heart failure, diabetes, and hypertension with an ACE inhibitor and a diuretic.

BOX 1 Physical Examination

Blood Pressure Measurement
Isolated Increased Systolic Blood Pressure
- Anemia
- Aortic regurgitation
- Arteriovenous fistula
- Atherosclerosis
- Hyperthyroidism

Inequality of Pressure Between Arms
- Coarctation of the aorta
- Cervical rib
- Dissection of the aorta
- Subclavian atherosclerosis
- Subclavian steal syndrome
- Supravalvular aortic stenosis
- Variability of measurements

Orthostatic Changes
- Autonomic failure
- Diabetes mellitus
- Hypovolemia
- Pheochromocytoma

General Appearance
Angioneurotic Edema
- ACE inhibitor therapy

Café-au-lait Spots, Neurofibromatosis
- Pheochromocytoma
- Renal artery stenosis

Central Obesity, Acne, Moon Face, Hirsutism, Thin Skin, Striae, Bruises, Wasted Limbs, Buffalo Hump
- Cushing's syndrome

Coarse Hair, Thick Lips and Tongue, Puffy Eyelids, Myxedema
- Hypothyroidism

Exogenous Obesity
- Sleep apnea
- Diabetes mellitus
- Pseudohypertension

Exophthalmos, Lid Retraction, Tremulousness, Goiter
- Hyperthyroidism

Gynecomastia
- Adrenal hyperplasia or tumor
- Anabolic steroids
- Calcium channel blockers
- Chronic renal failure
- Cyclosporine (Sandimmune)
- Hyperthyroidism
- Methyldopa (Aldomet)
- Reserpine
- Spironolactone (Aldactone)

Marfanoid Features, Mucosal Neuromas
- Pheochromocytoma

Periorbital Edema, Pallor
- Renal disease

Plethora, Conjunctival Suffusion
- Polycythemia

Prognathism; Enlarged Tongue, Nose, Hands, and Feet
- Acromegaly

Webbing of the Neck, Broad Chest, Wide-Spaced Nipples, Low Posterior Hairline, Short Stature
- Coarctation of the aorta
- Turner's syndrome

Fundus
Arteriole-to-Venule Ratio < 2:3
- Advanced age
- Hypertensive retinopathy

Arteriovenous Nicking
- Hypertensive retinopathy

Copper or Silver Wire Reflex
- Advanced age
- Hypertensive arteriosclerosis

Cotton-Wool Spots
- Anemia
- Accelerated hypertension
- Diabetic retinopathy
- Hyperviscosity
- Vasculitis

Flame-Shaped Retinal Hemorrhages
- Accelerated hypertension

Papilledema
- Hypertensive encephalopathy
- Intracranial hypertension
- Malignant hypertension

Neck
Carotid Bruits
- Atherosclerosis of carotid artery

Jugular Venous Distention
- Right-sided heart failure

Thyroid Enlargement
- Hyperthyroidism
- Hypothyroidism

Lungs
Rales
- Heart failure

Wheezes
- Asthma
- β-Blocker therapy
- Chronic lung disease
- Heart failure

Heart
Tachycardia
- Anemia
- Heart failure
- Hyperthyroidism
- Pheochromocytoma

Atrial fibrillation
- Hyperthyroidism
- Ischemic heart disease
- Left atrial enlargement

BOX 1 Physical Examination—cont'd

Palpable Pulses of Intercostal Arteries of Posterior Thorax
- Coarctation of the aorta

Sustained, Enlarged (>3 cm) Apical Impulse
- Left ventricular hypertrophy

Apical Impulse Outside Midclavicular Line
- Left ventricular dilation
- Left ventricular hypertrophy

Tambour S₂
- Aortic root dilatation

S₃ Gallop
- Anemia
- Arteriovenous fistula
- Cardiomyopathy
- Heart failure
- Hyperthyroidism
- Regurgitant valvular disease

S₄ Gallop
- Anemia
- Arteriovenous fistula
- Cardiomyopathy
- Coronary artery disease
- Hyperthyroidism
- Left ventricular hypertrophy

Basal Systolic Murmur
- Aortic stenosis
- Benign murmur
- Coarctation of aorta
- Hypertension

Basal Diastolic Murmur
- Aortic insufficiency
- Dissecting aorta

Pericardial Rub
- Uremic pericarditis

Abdomen and Genitalia
Palpable Kidneys
- Polycystic kidney disease

Mass with Expansile Pulsation
- Abdominal aneurysm

Suprapubic Mass
- Distended urinary bladder

Systolic or Systolic-Diastolic Bruit
- Arteriovenous malformation
- Mesenteric artery stenosis
- Renal artery stenosis

Small Testes or Clitoromegaly
- Anabolic steroid use

Extremities
Decreased Femoral Pulses
- Aortofemoral atherosclerosis
- Coarctation of the aorta

Femoral Bruits
- Aortofemoral atherosclerosis

Radial-Femoral Delay
- Aortofemoral atherosclerosis
- Coarctation of the aorta

Peripheral Edema
- Calcium antagonist therapy
- Chronic renal failure
- Direct vasodilator therapy
- Nephrotic syndrome
- Right-sided heart failure

Abbreviation ACE=angiotensin-converting enzyme.
Modified from Prisant LM: Hypertension. In Conn RB, Borer WZ, Snyder JW (eds): Current Diagnosis 9. Philadelphia: WB Saunders, 1997, pp 349-359.

Most patients require more than one drug to achieve their target blood pressure. The current recommendation is to use two drugs from the outset with stage II hypertension. This approach does require caution to avoid hypotension, especially in elderly patients. African Americans, patients with systolic hypertension, hypertensive diabetic patients, and patients with chronic kidney disease need the most drugs.

Dosing Strategies and Drug Efficacy

Stage I hypertensive or frail, elderly patients are treated initially with a low initial dose. Assessment of efficacy is in 4 to 6 weeks. At that follow-up visit, the patient is questioned about drug-specific side effects. If the medication is tolerated, but the blood pressure is not at goal, then the drug should be titrated or a second drug added. Titrated monotherapy for any drug class is unlikely to achieve a placebo-corrected control rate greater than 50%.

As the dose of a drug is doubled, there is a decrement of additional blood pressure lowering when compared with the previous dose, and drug-induced adverse effects increase. However, not all side effects are dose-dependent. For example, ACE inhibitors have the dose-independent side effects of cough and angioneurotic edema. The balance of blood pressure lowering and unacceptable adverse drug reactions is about two titrations.

Because adherence to therapy decreases if drugs are dosed frequently throughout the day, drugs should be selected that are dosed once or twice daily. Fixed-dose combinations also improve adherence and provide financial advantages for patients. Synchronizing the dosing of antihypertensive medications with other medications can improve overall adherence.

Drugs that combine different pharmacologic mechanisms increase the likelihood of reaching the target blood pressure. Not all antihypertensive drugs are additive to one another. Diuretics tend to augment the blood pressure–lowering effect of most antihypertensive agents.

Drug Classes

Hypertension may be treated with diuretics, β-blockers, CCBs, ACE inhibitors, ARBs, α₂-stimulants, α₁-blockers, peripheral sympatholytics, and direct vasodilators. The oral direct renin inhibitor aliskiren, the first of a new class of drugs, was recently released. Endothelin antagonists,

BOX 2 Laboratory Assessment of Hypertension

Hypokalemia
- Cushing's syndrome
- Diuretic use
- Primary hyperaldosteronism

Hypercalcemia
- Hyperparathyroidism
- Thiazide diuretics

Hyperglycemia
- Acromegaly
- β-Blockers
- Corticosteroids
- Cushing's syndrome
- Diabetes mellitus
- Diuretics
- Pheochromocytoma

Hypercholesterolemia
- Anabolic steroids
- Hypercortisolism
- Hyperparathyroidism
- Hypothyroidism
- Nephrotic syndrome
- Primary lipid disorder
- Progestational agents

Increased serum creatinine
- Acromegaly
- ACE inhibitor or ARB use
- Avoid renally excreted drugs
- Primary renal disease
- Renovascular hypertension

Hyperkalemia
- ACE inhibitor or ARB use
- Chronic renal failure
- NSAIDs
- Potassium chloride supplement
- Potassium-sparing diuretics
- Salt substitutes
- Type IV renal tubular acidosis

Hyperuricemia
- Chronic renal failure
- Diuretics
- Early sign of renal disease
- Gout
- Hyperparathyroidism
- Hypothyroidism
- Polycystic kidney disease
- Polycythemia
- Toxemia of pregnancy

Hypertriglyceridemia
- β-Blocker use
- Chronic renal failure
- Diabetes mellitus
- Diuretic use
- Estrogen use
- Ethanol abuse
- Liver disease
- Obesity

Abnormal liver function
- Avoid hepatically metabolized drugs
- Ethanol abuse
- Hypertriglyceridemia

Abbreviations ACE = angiotensin-converting enzyme; ARB = angiotensin receptor blocker; NSAID = nonsteroidal anti-inflammatory drug.
Modified from Prisant LM: Hypertension. In Conn RB, Borer WZ, Snyder JW (eds): Current Diagnosis 9. Philadelphia: WB Saunders, 1997, pp 349-359.

---

selective I1-imidazoline receptor agonists, and vasopeptidase inhibitors may be added to our treatment armamentarium in the future.

α₂-Stimulants, sympatholytics, and direct vasodilators are not used initially for the treatment of hypertension. α₂-Stimulants include clonidine (Catapres), methyldopa (Aldomet), guanabenz (Wytensin), and guanfacine (Tenex); peripheral sympatholytics include reserpine; and direct vasodilators include hydralazine (Apresoline) and minoxidil (Loniten). α1-Blockers (prazosin [Minipress], terazosin [Hytrin], and doxazosin [Cardura]) have fallen out of favor as initial therapy for hypertension but have been safely used for many years. Peripheral sympatholytics are not used often, although low-dose reserpine (0.05-0.1 mg daily) with a diuretic is effective for patients who have limited resources.

Diuretics

There are thiazide or thiazide-like, loop, and potassium-sparing diuretics. Thiazide (e.g., hydrochlorothiazide [Esidrix]) and thiazide-like diuretics (e.g., chlorthalidone [Hygroton], indapamide [Lozol], and metolazone [Zaroxolyn]) increase sodium excretion by inhibiting the

---

TABLE 2 Drug Choices for Compelling Indications

Indication	Aldosterone Antagonist	ACE Inhibitor	ARB	β-Blocker	CCB	Diuretic
Chronic kidney disease		×	×			
Diabetes mellitus		×	×	×	×	×
Heart failure	×	×	×	×		×
High coronary disease risk		×	×	×	×	×
Prior myocardial infarction	×	×	×	×		
Recurrent stroke		×	×			×

Abbreviations: ACE = angiotensin-converting enzyme; ARB = angiotensin receptor blocker; CCB = calcium channel blocker.
Modified from Chobanian AV, Bakris GL, Black HR, et al; and the National Blood Pressure Education Program: The Seventh Report of the Joint National Committee on Prevention, Detection, Evaluation, and Treatment of High Blood Pressure. JAMA 2003;289:2073-2082.

sodium-chloride pump in the early segment of the distal convoluted tubule and reduce plasma volume initially. This results in increased plasma renin activity and aldosterone, which facilitates potassium loss. Systemic vascular resistance progressively declines and plasma volume approaches pretreatment levels.

Thiazide or thiazide-like diuretics reduce strokes, heart failure, and total cardiovascular mortality. Diuretics are proven in isolated systolic hypertension and diastolic hypertension trials. Diuretics are especially effective for obese patients, African Americans, the elderly, diabetic patients, patients with systolic heart failure, and patients with excess sodium intake. Thiazides decrease osteoporosis.

Thiazide diuretics enhance the efficacy of other drug classes and are required as a triple component with direct vasodilators. Nonsteroidal anti-inflammatory drugs (NSAIDs) attenuate the antihypertensive effect of diuretics. The side effects of thiazide diuretics include volume depletion, hyponatremia, hypokalemic alkalosis, hypomagnesemia, hypercalcemia, hyperuricemia, gout, sexual dysfunction, and occasionally sulfonamide-related skin eruptions. Glucose intolerance and diabetes mellitus with diuretics are due to hypokalemia. Thiazides must be avoided in patients with severe recurrent gout, hyponatremia, and volume depletion.

Loop diuretics—furosemide (Lasix), bumetanide (Bumex), torsemide (Demadex), and ethacrynic acid (Edecrin)—act at the thick ascending loop of Henle to prevent chloride and sodium reabsorption. They have a rapid onset of action compared with thiazide diuretics. The longest-acting loop diuretic is torsemide. Loop diuretics should not be used for hypertensive patients who have normal renal function. They are required in patients whose serum creatinine exceeds 2.5 mg/dL. For patients who have a true sulfur allergy, ethacrynic acid is the only nonsulfonamide diuretic available. However, permanent ototoxicity occurs at high doses.

The potassium-sparing diuretics—amiloride (Midamor), triamterene (Dyrenium), spironolactone (Aldactone), and eplerenone (Inspra)—are often used in combination with hydrochlorothiazide. They decrease magnesium and potassium excretion. Amiloride and triamterene block the epithelial sodium transport channel, and, unlike aldosterone blockers, they do not lower blood pressure much. Spironolactone is a potent nonselective aldosterone blocker, acting also on androgen and progesterone receptors, and eplerenone is a selective aldosterone blocker. Spironolactone reduces mortality in advanced heart failure, and eplerenone decreases mortality in postinfarction patients with left ventricular dysfunction. Both drugs are effective for resistant hypertension. Hyperkalemia can occur in patients with chronic kidney disease and type IV renal tubular acidosis. Concomitant treatment with potassium supplements, over-the-counter salt substitutes, ACE inhibitors, ARBs, and NSAIDs requires careful monitoring. Spironolactone causes sexual dysfunction, gynecomastia, mastodynia, and menorrhagia at higher doses.

β-Blockers

β-blockers are a heterogeneous class of drugs. Their antihypertensive mechanism of action is unclear because most β-blockers increase peripheral vascular resistance acutely. However, they inhibit renin release, decrease angiotensin II and aldosterone, and reduce heart rate, cardiac output, and blood pressure. Labetalol and carvedilol also block the α_1-receptor and cause vasodilation. Acebutolol, carteolol, pindolol, and penbutolol possess intrinsic sympathomimetic activity, a characteristic that causes vasodilation and stimulates the β-receptor if resting sympathetic activity is low. Nebivolol uniquely has nitric oxide–mediated vasodilating properties. Cardioselective β_1-blockers—acebutolol, atenolol, betaxolol, bisoprolol, metoprolol tartrate, metoprolol succinate, and nebivolol—cause less bronchospasm and claudication in low doses. Atenolol, nadolol, betaxolol, and carteolol are hydrophilic β-blockers that are renally eliminated. Intravenous β-blockers include atenolol, esmolol, metoprolol tartrate, and labetalol.

Although β-blockers have fallen into disfavor as initial therapy for uncomplicated hypertension, the combination of β-blockers and diuretics reduced total mortality in elderly hypertensive patients. The most important mandatory indications are for myocardial infarction and heart failure patients. Timolol, metoprolol tartrate, propranolol, acebutolol, and carvedilol reduced postinfarction mortality. Bisoprolol, carvedilol, and metoprolol succinate (but not metoprolol tartrate) decrease total mortality in chronic heart failure. In addition, atenolol and bisoprolol diminish cardiovascular events in the perioperative period.

Hypertensive younger patients who are anxious or who have hyperkinetic heart syndrome benefit from β-blocker treatment. Nonselective β-blockers, such as propranolol, are useful in the treatment of essential tremor and migraine headaches because they block the β_2-receptor. β-Blockers diminish the ventricular response rate of atrial fibrillation and other supraventricular tachycardias. β-Blockers reduce blood pressure less in African Americans compared with whites unless the β-blocker is combined with a diuretic. Cardioselective β_1-blockers are preferred for bronchospastic pulmonary disease, peripheral vascular disease, and diabetes mellitus, although no β-blocker is selective at large doses. Nonselective β-blockers should not be used with insulin-requiring diabetes mellitus because hypoglycemic symptoms are masked and a hypertensive response to hypoglycemia ensues.

β-blockers are not additive to ACE inhibitors, ARBs, and α_2-stimulants to further reduce blood pressure. The use of α_2-stimulants and β-blockers together increases blood pressure, and abrupt withdrawal of either drug results in a markedly elevated blood pressure from unopposed α-receptor–induced vasoconstriction. Verapamil or diltiazem with a β-blocker can cause heart failure, extreme bradycardia, and advanced heart block.

Fatigue, weight gain, depression, erectile dysfunction, claudication, and lipid abnormalities are reported as adverse drug reactions to β-blockers. Care must be taken to taper β-blockers over a 14-day period in patients with coronary artery disease.

Angiotensin-Converting Enzyme Inhibitors

ACE inhibitors inhibit the angiotensin-converting enzyme, blocking the conversion of angiotensin I to angiotensin II and bradykinin breakdown. However, there are other pathways by which angiotensin II is generated, which cause angiotensin II levels to drift toward baseline levels. Other blood pressure lowering effects of ACE inhibitors involve bradykinin, prostacyclin (prostaglandin I_2 [PGI_2]), nitric oxide, aldosterone, endothelin, the sympathetic nervous system, and venodilation.

Several characteristics differentiate ACE inhibitors: the zinc-binding ligand (carboxyl, phosphoryl, sulfhydryl), which permits attachment of the ACE inhibitor to the angiotensin-converting enzyme; whether or not the drug is a prodrug; tissue ACE inhibition; and lipophilicity. Captopril has a sulfhydryl zinc-binding ligand that can cause a skin rash and taste disturbances, and fosinopril uses a phosphoryl group. Prodrugs remain inactive until converted by the liver, which improves absorption. Captopril and lisinopril are not prodrugs. The prodrug characteristic is not used to select a drug unless the patient has severe hepatic dysfunction. Tissue ACE inhibition and lipophilicity are not proven to be therapeutically important.

Trandolapril, ramipril, perindopril, and lisinopril are the longest-acting ACE inhibitors. Captopril is dosed 2 to 3 times per day. Because most ACE inhibitors require renal excretion, the dose is reduced with chronic kidney disease. However, fosinopril and trandolapril use hepatic and renal excretion. Food reduces the absorption of captopril and moexipril. Enalaprilat is an intravenous formulation.

Enalapril is the only ACE inhibitor proven to reduce the total mortality in chronic heart failure. Captopril, lisinopril, ramipril, and trandolapril reduce cardiovascular mortality in patients having left ventricular dysfunction after a myocardial infarction. Ramipril is proven to prevent myocardial infarction, stroke, and cardiovascular death in patients with vascular disease. Benazepril, captopril, and ramipril reduce progression of renal insufficiency.

ACE inhibitors are necessary treatment for heart failure, postinfarction left ventricular dysfunction, recurrent stroke, diabetes mellitus, and chronic kidney disease, and they are required in patients with a high risk of cardiovascular events (see Table 2). Like β-blockers, ACE inhibitors are less effective in African Americans compared with whites unless they are combined with a diuretic. In the African

American Study of Kidney Disease (AASK), which researched hypertensive renal insufficiency, ramipril was superior to amlodipine or metoprolol in slowing the rate of glomerular filtration rate decline. ACE inhibitors are also used for scleroderma renal crisis. They also reduce the rate of development of diabetes.

ACE inhibitors are additive with diuretics or CCBs, but not with β-blockers or ARBs. NSAIDs attenuate the blood-pressure–lowering effect of ACE inhibitors.

Hypotension occurs if ACE inhibitors are given to patients who have high renin levels or volume depletion or who are taking diuretics. ACE inhibitors rarely cause cholestatic jaundice and pancreatitis. Side effects of ACE inhibitors are an intractable cough, hyperkalemia, deteriorating creatinine, and angioneurotic edema. ACE inhibitors cause reversible renal insufficiency with bilateral renal artery stenosis, renal artery stenosis in a solitary kidney, or renal artery compression from a polycystic kidney.

Creatinine rises with chronic disease, heart failure, volume depletion, sepsis, and the use of NSAIDs, cyclosporine, and tacrolimus. When the creatinine increase is greater than 30%, the ACE inhibitor should be stopped and the cause determined. NSAIDs, potassium-sparing diuretics, potassium supplements, chronic kidney disease, and type IV renal tubular acidosis elevate potassium in patients treated with an ACE inhibitor. Cough is reported in 10% of patients. Angioneurotic edema can be life threatening if the larynx is involved. The face is most often affected, but edema also can involve the hands, feet, genitalia, and bowel. Angioneurotic edema affects 0.72% of African American versus 0.31% of non African American patients. ACE inhibitors are contraindicated during pregnancy.

Angiotensin Receptor Blockers

ARBs attach to the type I angiotensin II (AT1) receptor and cause plasma renin, angiotensin I, and angiotensin II to increase. Blockade of the AT1 receptor can stimulate the AT2 receptor to increase nitric oxide production and dilate arterioles.

The ARBs are not as heterogenous as ACE inhibitors and β-blockers. Telmisartan has the longest terminal half-life. Losartan, which is uricosuric, has an active E3174 metabolite that lowers blood pressure. Candesartan cilexetil and olmesartan medoxomil are pro-drugs. Food reduces the absorption of valsartan.

ARBs do not reduce blood pressure as much in African American patients as in white patients unless they are combined with a diuretic. Outcomes document a benefit for diabetic nephropathy (losartan and irbesartan), strokes (losartan, candesartan, and eprosartan), heart failure (candesartan and valsartan), postmyocardial infarction with left ventricular dysfunction (valsartan), and left ventricular hypertrophy (losartan). Telmisartan is as effective as enalapril for renoprotection in type 2 diabetes mellitus. Hypertensive diabetic patients with left ventricular hypertrophy had a reduction in total mortality with losartan compared with atenolol. ARBs reduce the rate of development of diabetes. A large outcomes trial comparing ramipril, telmisartan, or the combination in high-risk patients reported no difference in cardiovascular events among the treatment groups.

ARBs are additive to diuretics and CCBs; however, there are fewer data on the combination with other antihypertensive agents. The combination of valsartan or candesartan added to an ACE reduces cardiovascular death and heart failure hospitalizations.

The side effects of ARBs are similar to placebo. Angioedema is quite rare. Like ACE inhibitors, ARBs are contraindicated in pregnancy, and increases in serum creatinine and potassium can occur.

Calcium Channel Blockers

The three classes of CCBs are dihydropyridine (nifedipine and others), benzothiazepine (diltiazem), and phenylalkylamine (verapamil). They block the calcium flux into cells, causing vasodilation. They also cause acute and repetitive natriuresis, inhibit aldosterone, and interfere with α_2-stimulated angiotensin II vasoconstriction. The nondihydropyridine CCBs reduce myocardial contractility and alter sinoatrial and atrioventricular conduction. Dihydropyridines have a dose-dependent negative inotropic effect, but this is counterbalanced by systemic vasodilation.

All CCBs have a short duration of action, except amlodipine, and require drug delivery systems to prolong their duration of action. Three CCBs (Covera HS, Verelan PM, Cardizem LA) are chronotherapeutic formulations that are dosed at 10:00 PM and achieve a peak concentration in the early morning hours when most cardiovascular events occur. Intravenous nicardipine is used for hypertensive emergencies without myocardial ischemia. Diltiazem and verapamil can be given intravenously.

CCBs reduce blood pressure in white and African American patients. CCBs are less susceptible to blood pressure attenuation from excessive sodium ingestion and NSAIDs than are other antihypertensive drugs. Nitrendipine decreased strokes in elderly patients with isolated systolic hypertension. The combination of amlodipine and perindopril decreased total mortality when compared with a diuretic and atenolol in an open label, blinded endpoint study.

CCBs are contraindicated in patients with systolic heart failure, acute myocardial infarction, or unstable angina. It is used for cocaine-induced vasospasm (not first-line therapy) and cyclosporine-induced hypertension. Amlodipine offered no protection against hypertensive nephrosclerosis in African American patients or diabetic nephropathy when compared with ARBs or ACE inhibitors. Amlodipine, diltiazem, nicardipine, nifedipine, and verapamil have an indication for stable angina. Diltiazem and verapamil are approved for atrial fibrillation, atrial flutter, and paroxysmal supraventricular tachycardia.

Most drugs are additive to CCBs. The combination of amlodipine and the α_1-blocker doxazosin appears to be synergistic. The use of a dihydropyridine and nondihydropyridine CCB is also additive.

Constipation is a dose-dependent side effect of verapamil. Diltiazem can cause sinus bradycardia, peripheral edema, headache, dizziness, asthenia, fatigue, and rash. Dose-dependent peripheral edema with dihydropyridines is not a result of salt and water retention. It is caused by precapillary arterial vasodilation and relative venular constriction and is ameliorated by an ACE inhibitor or ARB. Gingival overgrowth and esophageal reflux occur with CCBs.

α_1-Blockers

Norepinephrine interacts with the postsynaptic α_1-receptors on vascular smooth muscle cells to cause vasoconstriction. Selective α_1-blockers (prazosin, terazosin, and doxazosin) cause venous and arterial dilation. Although tachycardia is unexpected, sodium and water retention can occur. This class of drugs is no longer considered for initial therapy because the Antihypertensive and Lipid-lowering Treatment to Prevent Heart Attack Trial (ALLHAT) observed more heart failure and strokes with doxazosin than with chlorthalidone.

The α_1-blockers are additive to most drugs except α_2-stimulants. They improve urinary flow with prostatism by lessening urinary sphincter constriction. They reduce LDL cholesterol and triglycerides, increase HDL cholesterol, improve insulin sensitivity, and are unlikely to cause erectile dysfunction.

Volume depletion can produce first-dose hypotension or syncope; thus, slow titration is necessary. If the drug is stopped, retitration is required. Stress urinary incontinence, asthenia, nasal congestion, and priapism are known adverse drug reactions.

Central α_2-Stimulants

Methyldopa, clonidine, guanabenz, and guanfacine reduce sympathetic outflow from the nucleus tractus solitarii and rostral ventrolateral medulla and decrease norepinephrine and renin. However, high doses paradoxically raise blood pressure by stimulating peripheral α_2-receptors.

This drug class is not recommended as initial therapy for hypertension due to sodium and water retention. These drugs are effective for most patient groups, but they are poorly tolerated. They are ineffective in patients with spinal cord transection. Guanfacine is the longest-acting oral drug. The transdermal clonidine preparation is effective for 7 days, but it requires 3 days initially to achieve adequate blood levels. Methyldopa is safely used for pregnancy-induced hypertension. α_2-Stimulants are additive to diuretics, but they are not additive to α_1-blockers or β-blockers.

Common adverse drug reactions are sedation, erectile dysfunction, dry mouth, dental caries, and periodontal disease. A discontinuation syndrome, characterized by very high blood pressure, tachycardia, tremulousness, and anxiety, is precipitated within 24 to 36 hours after stopping the medication and is magnified with concomitant β-blocker therapy. Bradycardia occurs when used with rate-lowering medications or sick sinus syndrome. Skin irritation or an allergic skin reaction is seen with the transdermal preparation. Hepatotoxicity, Coombs' positive hemolytic anemia, and galactorrhea occur with methyldopa.

Direct Vasodilators

Hydralazine and minoxidil dilate resistance and capacitance vessels; increase renin, norepinephrine, cardiac output; and cause salt and water retention. Minoxidil is the most potent oral antihypertensive drug and the longest-acting direct vasodilator.

Direct vasodilators are used for refractory hypertension. A diuretic and a heart rate–lowering drug is given as a part of a triple drug regimen. Hydralazine is used safely during pregnancy. The combination of hydralazine and nitrates (BiDil) reduced mortality and heart failure hospitalizations in African Americans with chronic systolic dysfunction.

Hydralazine is inactivated in the liver by acetylation, which has a genetically determined rate. Toxicity is more likely to occur with slow acetylators. The dose is limited to 200 mg/day to avoid a lupus-like reaction, which is characterized by arthralgias, weight loss, splenomegaly, and pleural and pericardial effusions. Minoxidil causes fluid retention, hypertrichosis, and pericardial effusion.

Other Conditions

RESISTANT HYPERTENSION

There are a number of reasons why patients fail to achieve blood pressure control with appropriate doses of three antihypertensive drugs. Improper blood pressure measurement from a noncalibrated, inaccurate sphygmomanometer or wrong cuff size is common. Volume overload due to excess sodium intake, excretory failure, and inadequate or improper diuretic dosing are important considerations. Using medications that are not complementary is a common reason for resistant hypertension. Concomitant medications that interfere with antihypertensive drugs or raise blood pressure are listed in Box 3. Consumption of more than 30 grams of ethanol daily raises blood pressure and increases the risk of a stroke. Exogenous obesity and insulin resistance are patient factors associated with resistant hypertension.

Clues to nonadherence are suggested by evasive answers to direct questions about medications, failure to keep appointments, complaints about costs or side effects, and lack of knowledge about medications and their dosing. A simple way to evaluate nonadherence is to bring the patient to the clinic in the morning, observe the patient swallowing the medications, and measure the blood pressure hourly for 5 hours. Assessment of secondary hypertension or noninvasive hemodynamic measurements may be undertaken if the cause of resistant hypertension is not apparent.

SECONDARY HYPERTENSION

Age, history, physical examination (see Box 2), severity of hypertension, or initial laboratory studies (see Box 3) provide clues to secondary causes of hypertension. Resistant hypertension, well-controlled blood pressure that increases without explanation, and abrupt-onset hypertension are additional signs.

Chronic kidney disease and renovascular hypertension are the most common etiologies. An abnormal serum creatinine, estimated glomerular filtration rate, or urinary sediment point to renal parenchymal disease. A renal ultrasound may be helpful for further evaluation. Acute or chronic bladder outlet obstruction also elevates blood pressure. In the absence of a family history, onset of hypertension before age 30 years may be from renovascular hypertension due to fibromuscular dysplasia. After age 55 years, atherosclerotic renovascular hypertension should be suspected, especially in tobacco users and with carotid and femoral bruits. Other findings suggestive of renovascular hypertension include an abdominal bruit that has a diastolic component, accelerated hypertension, recurrent flash pulmonary edema, renal failure of uncertain etiology, and acute renal failure precipitated by an ACE inhibitor or an ARB. A renal arteriogram defines the anatomy of the renal arteries, but it does not say if the anatomic obstruction is causing renovascular hypertension. Captopril renography, duplex Doppler sonography, and magnetic resonance imaging (MRI) are used to screen patients, but they are not always accurate.

There are a number of endocrine causes of hypertension. Hypothyroidism is the most common and causes diastolic hypertension. Hyperthyroidism raises systolic blood pressure. Hyperparathyroidism elevates calcium and parathyroid hormone levels and causes osteopenia

---

BOX 3 Drug Causes of Increased Blood Pressure

- Anabolic steroids
- Anesthetics: Ketamine, desflurane (Suprane)
- Bromocriptine (Parlodel)
- Buspirone (BuSpar)
- Carbamazepine (Tegretol)
- Clonidine (Catapres), β-blocker combination
- Clozapine (Clozaril)
- Cocaine and cocaine withdrawal
- Cortisone and other steroids (both corticosteroids and mineralocorticoids), ACTH
- Cyclosporine (Sandimmune) and tacrolimus (Prograf)
- Ergotamine and ergot-containing herbal preparations
- Erythropoietin
- Estrogens (usually birth control pills with high estrogenic activity)
- Licorice
- Ma huang, "herbal ecstasy," and other ephedrine analogues
- Methylphenidate (Ritalin, Concerta, and others)
- Metoclopramide (Reglan)
- NSAIDs (including cyclooxygenase-2 inhibitors)
- Phencyclidine
- Phenylpropanolamine and analogues
- St. John's wort
- Sibutramine (Meridia)
- Tyramine-containing foods (with monoamine oxidase inhibitors)
- Venlafaxine (Effexor)

Abbreviation: NSAID = nonsteroidal anti-inflammatory drug.

CURRENT DIAGNOSIS

- Perform two or three blood measurements on two or more visits to diagnose hypertension.
- Assess the patient with a targeted history, physical examination, and laboratory tests.
- Recognize hypertensive and atherosclerotic target organ involvement.
- Screen for other cardiovascular risk factors.
- Identify comorbid conditions that alter treatment.
- Discover correctable secondary causes of hypertension.

CURRENT THERAPY

- Choose initial antihypertensive medication based on age, race, target organ damage, and coexisting illnesses.
- Question patients about adverse drug reactions before initiating therapy and during follow-up visits.
- Titrate the initial drug choice once or twice at 4- to 6-week intervals (2007 American Heart Association recommendation).
- Use additional complementary medications to reach blood pressure treatment goals.
- Target a blood pressure of 130/80 mm Hg for diabetes mellitus, ischemic heart disease, and chronic kidney disease, and 140/90 mm Hg for all other patients.
- Investigate over-the-counter, herbal, and prescribed (including ophthalmic) medications for possible pharmacokinetic and pharmacodynamic interactions with antihypertensive drugs.

and nephrolithiasis. Cushing's syndrome is tested with a dexamethasone suppression test. Increased urinary potassium with low serum potassium suggests hyperaldosteronism. Measuring an elevated 24-hour aldosterone level in a salt-loaded patient and finding suppressed renin levels under conditions of ambulation and sodium depletion locates the defect to the adrenal gland. Paroxysms of hypertension with headache, palpitations, pallor, and perspiration occur in patients with a pheochromocytoma. Orthostatic changes in blood pressure are present. Unless the patient is treated with an α-blocker and is sodium repleted, β-blockers must be avoided because they further elevate blood pressure. Plasma-free metanephrines and fractionated urinary metanephrines are the most sensitive tests. Inaccurate results may be due to comorbid conditions or concomitant medications. MRI can help locate the tumor. ^{131}I-metaiodobenzylguanidine concentrates in up to 85% of tumors.

Diminished and delayed pulses in the right femoral artery compared with the right brachial artery, the presence of a systolic murmur over the anterior chest, bruits over the back, and visible notching of the posterior ribs on a chest x-ray are important clues of aortic coarctation. If the obstruction occurs before the left subclavian artery, systolic blood pressure is higher in the right arm than the left arm, and there is a decreased or absent left brachial pulse. A transesophageal echocardiogram can be used to confirm the diagnosis.

HYPERTENSIVE EMERGENCIES

A hypertensive emergency is defined as a blood pressure greater than 180/120 mm Hg and the presence of ongoing vascular damage. Cardiac causes include unstable angina pectoris, acute myocardial infarction, aortic dissection, and acute pulmonary edema. Cerebrovascular causes are hypertensive encephalopathy, ischemic stroke, intracerebral hemorrhage, and subarachnoid hemorrhage. Eclampsia is another cause.

These patients are admitted to an intensive care unit for continuous monitoring of blood pressure, volume status, urinary output, electrocardiogram, and mental status. Intravenous medication should be titrated to reduce mean arterial pressure 15% to 25%. An attempt to normalize blood pressure can cause coronary, cerebral, and renal ischemia. However, for aortic dissection patients, systolic blood pressure is lowered to 100 mm Hg with sodium nitroprusside after the heart rate is reduced with β-blockers, unless myocardial or cerebral ischemia limits the goal. The treatment of blood pressure with ischemic strokes is very controversial among neurologists.

Intravenous nitroglycerin is needed for coronary ischemia. Nitroprusside is an ideal agent for most hypertensive emergencies because it is titratable and hypotension resolves within 2 minutes of stopping the infusion. It is given at 0.3 μg/kg/min with the head of the bed elevated. If dosed at < 2 μg/kg/min, cyanide toxicity is unlikely. Fenoldopam, a dopamine-1 receptor agonist, is advocated when renal insufficiency prevents the use of nitroprusside. Esmolol is helpful for aortic dissections and perioperative hypertension. Intravenous hydralazine and magnesium sulfate are given for eclampsia.

Asymptomatic patients with very high blood pressure and no evidence of ongoing vascular damage do not require immediate normalization of blood pressure. Drug therapy is initiated, and the patient is scheduled for an evaluation in 1 week.

REFERENCES

Calhoun DA, Zaman MA, Nishizaka MK: Resistant hypertension. Curr Hypertens Rep 2002;4:221-228.
Chobanian AV, Bakris GL, Black HR, et al: Seventh report of the Joint National Committee on Prevention, Detection, Evaluation, and Treatment of High Blood Pressure. Hypertension 2003;42:1206-1252.
Pickering TG, Hall JE, Appel LJ, et al: Recommendations for blood pressure measurement in humans and experimental animals: Part 1: Blood pressure measurement in humans: A statement for professionals from the Subcommittee of Professional and Public Education of the American Heart Association Council on High Blood Pressure Research. Hypertension 2005;45:142-161.
Prisant LM (ed): Hypertension in the Elderly. Totowa, NJ: Humana Press, 2005.
Prisant LM: Hypertensive heart disease. J Clin Hypertens (Greenwich) 2005;7:231-238.
Prisant LM: Pharmacology of antihypertensive drugs. In MR Weir (ed): Hypertension. Philadelphia: American College of Physicians, 2005, pp 85-114.
Prisant LM: Nutritional treatment of blood pressure: Major nonpharmacologic trials of prevention or treatment of hypertension. In Berdanier CD (ed): CRC Handbook of Nutrition and Food. Boca Raton, FL: CRC Press, 2002, pp 999-1010.
Taler SJ, Textor SC, Augustine JE: Resistant hypertension: Comparing hemodynamic management to specialist care. Hypertension 2002;39:982-988.

Acute Myocardial Infarction

Method of

Guy S. Reeder, MD, and Abhiram Prasad, MD

The diagnosis of myocardial infarction (MI) is confirmed by a typical rise and fall in biochemical markers of myocardial necrosis with at least one of the following: ischemic symptoms, changes on the electrocardiogram (ECG) of ischemia (ST elevation or depression), development of pathologic Q waves, or percutaneous coronary intervention (PCI).

Incidence

More than 1 million patients suffer an MI every year in the United States. Despite a 50% decline in cardiovascular death due to advances in diagnosis and management related to MI since the 1970s, MI remains a fatal event in one out of three patients.

Pathophysiology

MI results from reduction in myocardial perfusion sufficient to cause cell necrosis. Atherosclerotic plaque rupture or erosion allows the thrombogenic lipid core to be exposed with complete or partial thrombotic occlusion. Epicardial occlusion may also be accompanied by downstream microvascular constriction. Coronary spasm is an uncommon cause of MI, and spontaneous coronary artery dissection, coronary embolus, and hypercoagulable states are among the rare causes.

Clinical Presentation

Patients with MI usually present with central pressure-like chest discomfort that can radiate to the arms, neck, or back. This is often associated with nausea, diaphoresis, and dyspnea. At least 20% of MIs are clinically unrecognized due to atypical presentation without chest pain, especially in elderly, diabetic, or postoperative patients. Symptoms include back pain, epigastric pain, syncope, dyspnea, or confusion. The differential diagnosis of acute MI includes aortic dissection, acute pulmonary embolus, perimyocarditis, musculoskeletal pain, esophagitis, peptic ulcer disease, cholecystitis, biliary colic, and pancreatitis.

Physical examination is often normal. Some patients have signs of left ventricular (LV) dysfunction including tachycardia, pulmonary rales, and third heart sound. Infarction or ischemia leading to papillary muscle dysfunction or rupture can lead to a murmur of mitral regurgitation. Patients with right ventricular (RV) infarction might have an elevated jugular venous pressure and a positive Kussmaul sign, and those with severe LV dysfunction present with cardiogenic shock. An estimation of prognosis at presentation is possible using the Killip classification or the TIMI (Thombolysis in Myocardial Infarction [trial] risk scores (Table 1).

Evaluation of Suspected Acute Myocardial Infarction

The initial evaluation of a patient with suspected MI should include a focused history, physical examination, ECG, blood sample for cardiac biomarkers, and chest radiograph. The patient's rhythm should be continuously monitored and intravenous access should be established.

ELECTROCARDIOGRAM

A 12-lead ECG should be performed within 10 minutes of arrival into an emergency department. In addition, posterior leads (V7-V9) and leads V3R and V4R should be used in patients with suspected posterior and RV infarctions, respectively. The ECG findings differentiate patients with ST elevation MI (STEMI) and ST depression MI (NSTEMI) (Fig. 1). Patients with STEMI require immediate reperfusion therapy, but those with NSTEMI do not unless there is ongoing ischemic pain or hemodynamic instability.

The ECG diagnosis of MI is difficult in the presence of left bundle branch block (LBBB). However, the presence of ST segment elevation of greater than 1 mm concordant with a QRS complex, ST segment depression greater than 1 mm in leads V1 to V3, or ST segment elevation greater than 5 mm discordant with a QRS complex supports the diagnosis.

SERUM MARKERS

Serum biomarkers of myocardial necrosis include troponins, MB isoforms of creatine kinase (CK-MB), creatine kinase (CK), and myoglobin. Measurement of troponin has replaced other biomarkers due to higher sensitivity, specificity, and prognostic value. Measurements of troponin I or T should be performed at presentation and 6 to 9 hours after the onset of symptoms. If troponin levels are elevated, confirmation with CK-MB may be performed to determine acuteness, because troponin can remain elevated for 10 to 15 days after MI. Likewise, CK-MB is useful for detecting reinfarction during a period of persistent troponin elevations from the initial event. Troponin and CK-MB may be elevated following cardiac surgery, myopericarditis, PCI, tachyarrhythmias, and cardioversion. Troponins may be elevated following pulmonary embolus and decompensated congestive heart failure. All cardiac markers may be initially negative early in acute MI; treatment must never be withheld based on negative initial biomarkers.

Treatment

ST ELEVATION MYOCARDIAL INFARCTION

Initial Approach

These goals should be achieved expeditiously and simultaneously (see Fig. 1): relief of pain, initiation of reperfusion and ancillary therapy, and assessment and treatment of hemodynamic abnormalities. Pain relief is best achieved with oxygen (2 L nasal cannula), nitroglycerin, and morphine sulfate. Patients with ST segment elevation or new LBBB with symptoms for 12 hours or less are candidates for reperfusion therapy.

Reperfusion Therapy

The diagnosis of STEMI mandates immediate reperfusion. PCI is preferred, but it is not promptly available in many areas. Fibrinolytic therapy is widely available, but it is slightly less effective in randomized trials and carries a higher risk of hemorrhagic stroke. The decision regarding which therapy to employ should be made on the basis of a written institution-specific protocol that considers symptom duration, availability of PCI locally, time to transfer to a PCI facility, and fibrinolytic contraindications (Fig. 2). In general, patients presenting within 3 hours of symptom onset derive a large benefit from fibrinolytics; if transfer time to a PCI facility results in a door-to-balloon time of longer than 90 minutes, fibrinolysis is preferred. Guidelines for door-to-needle (30 min) and door-to-balloon (90 min) times recommended by the American College of Cardiology and American Heart Association (ACC/AHA) are one of a number of quality indicators for acute MI care.

Fibrinolytic Therapy

Fibrinolytic therapy should be administered within 30 minutes of arrival to the emergency department. The greatest benefit is seen when this is performed within the first 4 hours of onset of pain resulting in an absolute 3% reduction in mortality, but it is associated with a small (0.4%) increase in stroke rate. There is a 2% absolute reduction in mortality rate for every hour saved in administration of therapy, and no benefit is seen after 12 hours of symptom duration. A benefit is observed in all age groups, including those with prior MI and diabetes, as well as in patients presenting with hypotension and tachycardia. Age older than 75 years, Killip class higher than II, resting tachycardia, hypotension, anterior MI location, and time to reperfusion longer than 4 hours are useful predictors of early mortality, ranging from 0.8% with none of these factors to more

TABLE 1 Killip Class and Hospital Mortality

Killip Class	Clinical Classification	Mortality (%)
I	No heart failure	6
II	Mild heart failure, rales, S₃, congestion on chest radiograph	17
III	Pulmonary edema	38
IV	Cardiogenic shock	81

Data from Killip T 3rd, Kimball JT: Treatment of myocardial infarction in a coronary care unit. A two year experience with 250 patients. Am J Cardiol 1967;20(4):457-464.

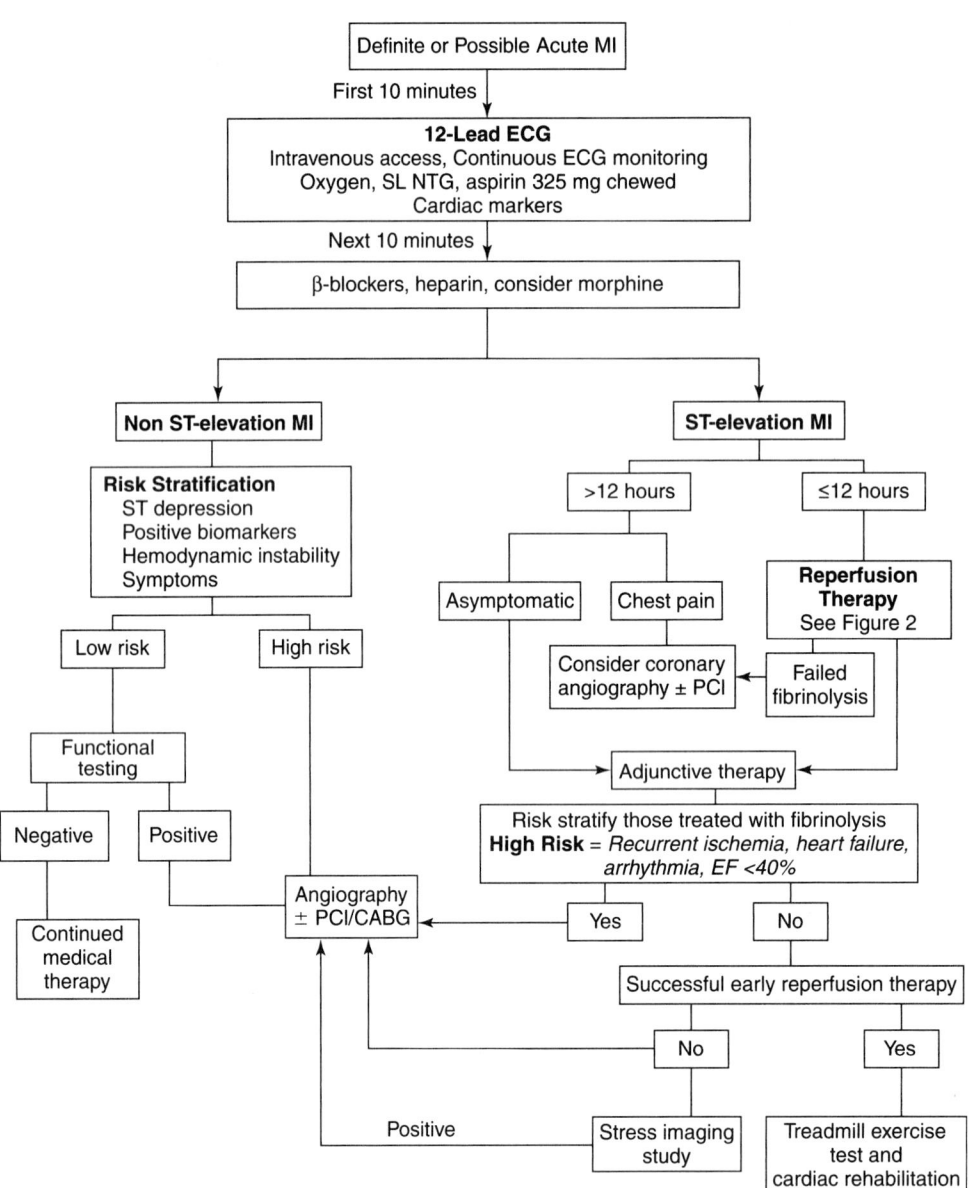

FIGURE 1. Definite or possible acute myocardial infarction (MI). CABG = coronary artery bypass graft; ECG = electrocardiogram; EF = ejection fraction; PCI = percutaneous coronary intervention; SL NTG = sublingual nitroglycerin.

than 36% for all (Table 2). Box 1 lists indications and contraindications for fibrinolysis.

Table 3 lists the currently available fibrinolytic agents. These differ primarily with respect to plasma half-life; the longest-acting agent, tenecteplase, requires a single bolus injection. Intravenous heparin must be administered concurrently to reduce the risk of late reocclusion of infarct-related artery.

Primary Percutaneous Coronary Intervention

Although fibrinolytic therapy is easy to administer and widely available, it provides early reperfusion in only 80% of patients and is often not administered due to perceived or actual contraindications in a significant number of patients. In contrast, primary PCI has only rare contraindications and leads to higher reperfusion (approximately 90%). Randomized trials performed in high-volume academic centers comparing fibrinolytic therapy with PCI for acute MI have demonstrated approximately 30% reduction in mortality and reinfarction rates and a significant reduction in cerebrovascular accidents with PCI. Stent deployment during acute MI leads to similar early outcome compared with balloon angioplasty, but it reduces restenosis rates and target vessel revascularization.

Primary PCI should be performed within 60 to 90 minutes of arrival to the hospital by an interventional cardiologist who performs at least 75 procedures a year in a center that has a volume of at least 200 procedures a year and has cardiac surgery capabilities. PCI should also be considered in specific patient populations listed in Box 2. Transfer from one hospital to another for primary PCI should only be considered if it can be achieved within 60 to 90 minutes (total door-to-balloon time); otherwise, fibrinolytic therapy should be administered without delay.

Adjunct Therapy for STEMI

Agents proved to reduce mortality in patients with STEMI include aspirin, β-blockers, statins, and angiotensin-converting enzyme (ACE) inhibitors (Table 4).

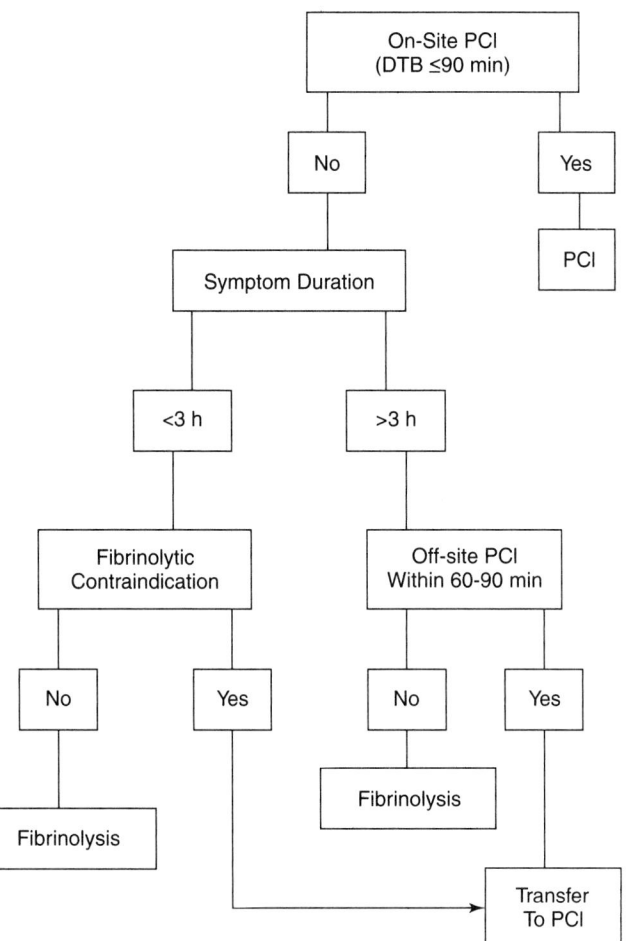

FIGURE 2. Selection of reperfusion therapy. DTB = door-to-balloon time; PCI = percutaneous coronary intervention.

BOX 1 Indications and Contraindications for Fibrinolytic Therapy in Acute Myocardial Infarction

Indications

ST segment elevation ≥1 mV in ≥2 contiguous limb leads or ≥2 mV in contiguous precordial leads
New left bundle branch block
Posterior MI: ST segment depression >2 mV in leads V1 and V2 with either imaging evidence of posterior LV wall motion abnormality or ST segment elevation of 1 mV in the posterior leads V7-V9

Contraindications

Absolute

Active bleeding
Prior intracranial hemorrhage; other strokes or neurologic events within 1 year; intracranial neoplasm
Recent major surgery (<6 wk) or major trauma (<2 wk)
Recent vascular puncture in a noncompressible site (<2 wk)
Suspected aortic dissection

Relative

Active peptic ulcer disease or recent gastrointestinal bleeding (<4 wk)
Severe uncontrolled hypertension on presentation (BP >180/110 mm Hg) or chronic severe hypertension
Cardiopulmonary resuscitation >10 min
Prior nonhemorrhagic stroke
Pregnancy
Bleeding diathesis or INR >2

BP = blood pressure; INR = international normalized ratio.

Aspirin

Unless there is history of allergic reaction, aspirin 325 mg should be administered immediately on the patient's arrival to the emergency room and continued indefinitely at a dose of at least 81 mg/day. Chewed aspirin has the most rapid onset of action due to absorption from the buccal mucosa, with inhibition of platelets within minutes. Clopidogrel (Plavix) may be administered to patients with an aspirin allergy.

Clopidogrel

is a thienopyridine which blocks the platelet ADP receptor, resulting in reduced platelet aggregation. A loading dose of 300 to 600[3] mg is typically administered at the time of PCI. Some data suggest a benefit of 75 to 300 mg administered with thrombolytic therapy; the lower dose might reduce the bleeding risk in patients older than 75 years. Maintenance dose is 75 mg/day; duration of therapy in PCI with stenting is defined by type of stent. Duration of therapy when administered with fibrinolytics is not well established.

Unfractionated Heparin

Unfractionated heparin has been shown to decrease reocclusion following fibrinolytic therapy, and it should be administered at the time of fibrinolytic infusion. A bolus of 60 U/kg (maximum 4000 units) of unfractionated heparin followed by an infusion of 7-12 U/kg/h may be used to initiate therapy. The activated partial thromboplastin time (aPTT) should be checked at 4 to 6 hours after initiation of heparin and then every 6 to 8 hours. The aPTT should be maintained between 50 and 70 seconds, and therapy should be continued for approximately 48 hours. Heparin may be continued for a longer duration in patients with atrial fibrillation or large anterior MI who are at risk for embolic events. Long-term anticoagulation with warfarin may be indicated in patients with LV thrombus, atrial fibrillation, or an

TABLE 2 TIMI Risk Score for ST-Elevation Myocardial Infarction

Risk Factor	Points	Risk Score	30-Day Mortality (%)
Age ≥75 y	3	0	0.8
Age 65-74 y	2	1	1.6
Diabetes or hypertension	1	2	2.2
Systolic BP <100 mm Hg	3	3	4.4
Heart rate >100/min	2	4	7.3
Killip class II-IV	2	5	12.4
Anterior MI or LBBB	1	6	16.1
Weight <67 kg	1	7	23.4
Time to treatment >4 h	1	8	26.8
		>8	35.9

BP = blood pressure; TIMI = Thombolysis in Myocardial Infarction (trial).
Data from Morrow DA, Antman EM, Charlesworth A, et al: TIMI risk score for ST-elevation myocardial infarction: A convenient, bedside, clinical score for risk assessment at presentation: An intravenous nPA for treatment of infarcting myocardium early II trial substudy. Circulation 2000;102:2031-2037.

---

[3]Exceeds dosage recommended by the manufacturer.

TABLE 3 Comparison of Fibrinolytics

Characteristic	Alteplase (Activase) (tPA)	Reteplase (Retavase) (rPA)	Tenecteplase (TNKase)
Dose	15-mg bolus, then 0.75 mg/kg over 30 min (max 50 mg), then 0.5 mg/kg over 60 min (max 35 mg)	10 + 10 MU double bolus 30 min apart	0.5 mg/kg single bolus (max 50 mg)
Plasma half-life	4-6 min	18 min	20 min
Fibrin specificity	++	+	+++
Plasminogen activation	Direct	Direct	Direct
Antigenicity	No	No	No

max = maximum; MU = megaunit; rPA = recombinant plasminogen activator; tPA = tissue plasminogen activator.

ejection fraction (EF) less than 30% following MI with a target international normalized ratio (INR) of 2 to 3.

Low-Molecular-Weight Heparin

Low-molecular-weight heparins (LMWHs) are produced by fragmentation of unfractionated heparin. These agents have advantages over unfractionated heparin, including a more predictable dose response, greater bioavailability, no need for laboratory monitoring, and a lower rate of thrombocytopenia. LMWH possess greater anti-Xa activity relative to anti-IIa (antithrombin) activity. This may be of potential benefit, because factor Xa generation occurs several steps earlier in the coagulation cascade.

Enoxaparin (Lovenox) is the most widely studied LMWH in STEMI and acute coronary syndromes. Trials of enoxaparin in conjunction with fibrinolysis have shown benefit in terms of preventing reinfarction, no significant mortality advantage, and somewhat increased risk of bleeding. LMWH should be avoided in men with creatinine higher than 2.5 or women with creatinine higher than 2.0.

Glycoprotein IIb/IIIa Antagonists

Platelet glycoprotein IIb/IIIa receptor inhibitors block the final common pathway in platelet aggregation. Currently available drugs include the chimeric monoclonal antibody abciximab (Reopro) and the nonantibody agents tirofiban (Aggrastat) and eptifibatide (Integrilin). Several studies have investigated the role of glycoprotein IIb/IIIa antagonists in STEMI and demonstrated a reduction in the composite endpoints of death, MI, and target vessel revascularization in patients treated with primary PCI. This benefit is due to higher TIMI-3 flow rate in the infarct-related artery, both before and after the coronary intervention procedure. Initial studies investigating the use of glycoprotein IIb/IIIa receptor antagonists with fibrinolytic agents suggested higher TIMI-3 flow rates, but phase III trials have failed to show a superiority of combined therapy over fibrinolytic therapy alone. Thus, intravenous glycoprotein IIb/IIIa inhibitors are indicated in patients being reperfused with PCI, but no indication exists for their combination with fibrinolytic therapy.

β-Adrenergic Antagonist Drugs

Early intravenous β-blocker therapy—metoprolol (Lopressor) 5 mg IV × 3 q5 min, followed by oral administration—is indicated in all patients without contraindications. In patients with borderline LV function, a test dose of intravenous esmolol can be given to assess tolerance to β-blockade. Patients with relative contraindications, such as chronic obstructive pulmonary disease or insulin-dependent diabetes, appear to derive benefit from treatment. Major contraindications to β-blockade include moderate to severe asthma, second- or third-degree atrioventricular block, severe bradycardia, hypotension, and pulmonary edema. β-Blockade should be withheld in these settings.

Angiotensin-Converting Enzyme Inhibitors

ACE activity is markedly increased at the edge of the infarct, and clinical trials have confirmed that ACE inhibitors reduce deleterious LV remodeling. The optimal selection of patients for ACE-inhibitor therapy remains controversial, but the most cost-effective approach is to selectively treat high-risk patients (those with impaired LV function or an anterior MI). However, demonstration of asymptomatic LV dysfunction requires bedside imaging studies, and selection of patients by infarct location alone might not result in early identification of all patients with significant LV dysfunction. Thus, unless the infarct is known to be small, it may be most reasonable to consider initial administration of ACE inhibitors in a nonselective fashion (i.e., in all patients with an acute MI) and then withdraw therapy later based on the absence of high-risk features. Exclusion criteria include allergy to ACE inhibitors, hypotension (systolic blood pressure [BP] <90 mm Hg), shock, history of bilateral renal artery stenosis, and prior worsening of renal function with ACE inhibitors.

ACE inhibitors have a class effect and should be administered orally, initially at low doses, with careful monitoring of the BP. Treatment should be continued indefinitely in patients with symptomatic heart failure or asymptomatic LV dysfunction (LVEF <45%), hemodynamically significant mitral regurgitation, or hypertension. Angiotensin receptor blockers (ARBs) may be used in patients intolerant of ACE inhibitors.

HMG CoA Reductase Inhibitors

Low-density lipoprotein (LDL) cholesterol plays a critical role in the pathogenesis of atherosclerosis. Lipid lowering with HMG CoA (3-hydroxy-3-methyl-glutaryl coenzyme A) reductase inhibitors (statins) are effective in secondary prevention by reducing mortality, recurrent infarction, ischemia, and heart failure. Preliminary studies indicate that treatment with statins can also lead to modest reductions in recurrent ischemia and infarction during acute coronary syndromes. Thus, a lipid profile should be assessed within 24 hours of the MI (before the inflammatory response from the MI leads to a

---

BOX 2 Indications for Percutaneous Coronary Intervention in Acute Myocardial Infarction

Failed fibrinolysis (rescue PCI)
Contraindication to fibrinolytics
Shock or markers of increased mortality such as TIMI risk score ≥5 or Killips classes III-IV
Nondiagnostic ECG changes with ongoing pain or hemodynamic instability
As a preferred strategy when available promptly

ECG = electrocardiogram; PCI = percutaneous coronary intervention; TIMI = Thrombolysis in Myocardial Infarction (trial).

TABLE 4 Adjunctive Therapies that Reduce Mortality in Patients with Myocardial Infarction

Drug	Indication	Suggested Drugs and Initial Dose	NNT
Aspirin	All	160-325 mg/day	42 patients for 1 mo
β-Blocker	All except patients with moderate or severe asthma, cardiogenic shock, pulmonary edema or ≥second-degree AV block	Metoprolol (Lopressor) 5 mg IV × 3 (at 5-min intervals), and then 50 mg PO bid or Esmolol (Brevibloc) bolus 500 µg/kg and infuse at 50 µg/kg/min	38 patients for 2 y
HMG CoA reductase inhibitors	All	Simvastatin (Zocor) or atorvastatin (Lipitor) 40-80 mg/day	30 patients for 5 y
ACE Inhibitors	Anterior MI, EF <40%, diabetes May consider using in all CAD patients	Captopril (Capoten) 6.25 mg PO tid, increasing at 6h-8h intervals to a maximum of 50 mg tid or Lisinopril (Prinivil, Zestril) 2.5-10 mg PO qd Maintain systolic BP >90 mm Hg	20 patients for 3.5 y

ACE, angiotensin-converting enzyme; AV = atrioventricular; BP= blood pressure; CAD = coronary artery disease; EF = ejection fraction; HMG CoA = 3-hydroxy-3-methyl-glutaryl coenzyme A; MI = myocardial infarction; NNT = number needed to treat to save one life.

temporary reduction in lipids) or 6 to 8 weeks later. Either way, improved outcomes have been demonstrated by early intensive statin therapy started in the hospital, with a target LDL cholesterol of 60 to 85 mg/dL.

Nitrates

Potential benefits of nitrate therapy include increased perfusion of ischemic zones, decrease in oxygen consumption, improved diastolic function, and enhanced collateral flow. The infusion of intravenous nitroglycerin should be initiated at 5 to 10 µg/min and gradually increased. The goal should be a 10% reduction in systolic BP in normotensive patients and approximately a 30% reduction in systolic pressure in hypertensive patients. Nitrates should be used with caution in patients with RV infarction or dehydration (who are preload dependent) to avoid excessive hypotension. Long-acting oral nitrates may be indicated with significant residual ischemia or heart failure. A nitrate-free interval of 8 to 12 hours must be provided to prevent nitrate tolerance.

Calcium Channel Blockers

Calcium channel blockers have vasodilative, antianginal, and antihypertensive actions. Calcium channel blockers do not reduce mortality in patients with MI and are not recommended for routine therapy or secondary prevention. In patients in whom β-adrenergic antagonists are contraindicated, verapamil or diltiazem may be appropriate as an alternative.

Antiarrhythmic Therapy

Potentially fatal ventricular arrhythmia occurs most commonly in the first 48 hours after an MI, and numerous trials have investigated the effects of antiarrhythmic agents on mortality and the incidence of ventricular fibrillation. Prophylactic therapy with antiarrhythmic drugs has been shown to be ineffective. Lidocaine may be used for 24 to 48 hours to treat ventricular tachycardia and following resuscitation for ventricular fibrillation. Amiodarone (Cordarone) is safe to use in the setting of MI and is the drug of choice for treating symptomatic ventricular arrhythmia.

Implantable Cardioverter-Defibrillator

ICD implantation reduces the occurrence of sudden death in certain high-risk patients such as those with late (>24 hours after the onset of symptoms) sustained ventricular tachycardia and ventricular fibrillation and in patients with EF persistently less than 30% to 35%. An ICD may also be beneficial in patients with late nonsustained ventricular tachycardia who have an EF of less than 40% and ventricular tachycardia induced during an electrophysiology study. ICD implantation should be considered if the patient is judged to be at continuous high risk for ventricular arrhythmia after revascularization for significant spontaneous or inducible ischemia.

NON–ST ELEVATION MYOCARDIAL INFARCTION

Incompletely occluding coronary thrombus, or extensive collateral arterial supply (or both) is the underlying pathology of NSTEMI. More common than STEMI, especially in the elderly, the presentation is identical except for the absence of ST elevation.

Initial Therapy

Management differs from STEMI in that urgent reperfusion therapy is not indicated; the administration of fibrinolytics may be harmful. Instead, the focus of initial therapy is intensive medical stabilization with antiplatelet and antithrombotic agents to prevent clot propagation, nitrates and β-blockers for anti-ischemic effects, statins for cholesterol lowering, and other agents to control pain and hemodynamic compromise. For patients with continued pain or hemodynamic deterioration, immediate angiography and PCI are indicated. All other patients should undergo risk stratification (see Fig. 1). The TIMI risk score for unstable angina and NSTEMI (Table 5) allows separation of low risk from intermediate and high risks. Low-risk patients are suitable for functional testing,

TABLE 5 TIMI Risk Score for Unstable Angina and Non–ST-Elevation Myocardial Infarction

Risk Factor	Points	Risk Score	14-Day D, MI, Revascularization
Age ≥65	1	1	4.7
Three risk factors	1	2	8.3
Stenosis ≥50%	1	3	13.2
ST deviation	1	4	19.9
Angina × 2/24 h	1	5	26.2
ASA use	1	6	
Elevated biomarkers	1	7	40.9

ASA = aspirin; MI = myocardial infarction.

TABLE 6 Complications Associated with Acute Myocardial Infarction

Complications	Clinical Features	Treatment
Ischemic		
Postinfarction angina	Recurrent chest pain after resolution of symptoms	Medical therapy or revascularization
Infarct extension	Recurrent chest pain and biomarker elevation	Urgent angiography and revascularization
Mitral regurgitation	Murmur, heart failure	Treat ischemia, ACE inhibitors
		Consider revascularization with or without mitral valve repair
Mechanical		
LV dysfunction (see Killip classification)	Dyspnea, hypoxia, elevated jugular venous pressure, third heart sound, rales	Diuretics, vasodilators
		Consider revascularization
		Treat associated mechanical complications
Cardiogenic shock	See text	Inotropes and IABP
		Urgent revascularization
Papillary muscle rupture	New mitral regurgitation, pulmonary edema, or shock 2-7 days after MI	IABP
		Emergency mitral valve replacement or repair
Myocardial rupture (lateral wall most often involved)	More common in women, elderly, non-reperfused patients, and inferior MI	Emergency surgery
	3-5 days post MI	
	Recurrent chest pain, pericarditis, vomiting, agitation, bradycardia	
Ventricular septal defect	Equally prevalent with anterior or inferior MI	IABP
	New pansystolic murmur, heart failure, shock	Urgent surgery
Electrical		
Second-degree AV block Mobitz type I	Asymptomatic, syncope More common after inferior MI	Observe Avoid AV node–blocking drugs
Second-degree AV block Mobitz type II	Asymptomatic presyncope/syncope Presyncope/syncope	Observe if asymptomatic and temporary pacing with symptoms after inferior MI
Third-degree AV block		Temporary ± permanent pacing after anterior MI
Atrial fibrillation/flutter	Asymptomatic, palpitations, heart failure	IV heparin for thromboembolic risk
		DC cardioversion for ischemia or hemodynamic compromise
		β-Blockers and digoxin for rate control in asymptomatic patients
		Sotalol or amiodarone for recurrent episodes
Ventricular premature complexes	Asymptomatic, palpitations	No antiarrhythmics indicated
		β-Blockers
		Correct electrolytes
Ventricular tachycardia Ventricular fibrillation	Hemodynamic collapse, syncope, palpitations, sudden cardiac death Sudden cardiac death	CPR and DC cardioversion for hemodynamic collapse; otherwise, IV lidocaine or amiodarone
		Treat associated ischemia and heart failure
		Correct electrolytes
		Consider revascularization
		If >24 hours after MI, consider EPS and ICD
Torsades de pointes	Hemodynamic collapse, sudden cardiac death	CPR and DC cardioversion
		Correct hypokalemia or hypomagnesemia
		Consider temporary pacing for bradycardia or IV phenytoin

ACE = angiotensin-converting enzyme; AV = atrioventricular; CPR = cardiopulmonary resuscitation; DC = direct current; EPS = electrophysiologic study; IABP = intraaortic balloon counterpulsation; ICD = implantable cardioverter-defibrillator; LV = left ventricular; MI = myocardial infarction.

whereas all others undergo elective catheterization plus PCI in 4 to 48 hours.

Adjunct Therapy

In addition to aspirin, clopidogrel is beneficial in NSTEMI. The benefit must be weighed against the bleeding risk if coronary bypass surgery is performed within 5 days of drug administration. We elect to not administer clopidogrel until establishment of coronary anatomy and decision regarding need for bypass surgery. Once started, the drug has shown benefit for 9 to 12 months.

Several large studies have investigated the role of glycoprotein IIb/IIIa antagonists in patients with unstable angina or NSTEMI. Overall, the studies using tirofiban and eptifibatide have demonstrated a small but significant risk reduction in composite endpoints, with the greatest benefit in patients with diabetes, patients with troponin elevations, and patients undergoing PCI. In contrast, the GUSTO-IV ACS (Global Utilization of Strategies To open Occluded coronary arteries trial IV in Acute Coronary Syndromes) trial did not demonstrate any benefit of abciximab in the treatment of NSTEMI. Thus, these studies lead us to recommend that glycoprotein IIb/IIIa receptor antagonists should not be routinely used in all patients with NSTEMI, but they should be considered for high-risk patients requiring PCI, especially those with diabetes, resting ST depression, or elevated troponin.

Enoxaparin has shown modest outcome benefits over unfractionated heparin in patients with NSTEMI. This benefit may be counterbalanced by the inability to measure drug effect if PCI is performed. In our center, where PCI is readily available, we prefer unfractionated heparin.

Bivalirudin (Angiomax) is a direct thrombin inhibitor that compares favorably with unfractionated heparin plus glycoprotein IIb/IIIa inhibition in patients with acute coronary syndromes undergoing PCI. It is also commonly used in the catheterization laboratory for patients with a history of heparin-induced thrombocytopenia. We reserve its use for the latter case.

Fondaparinux (Arixtra) is a synthetic pentasaccharide that binds to antithrombin and compares favorably with enoxaparin in patients with NSTEMI.

The use of β-blockers and statins is similar to that in STEMI. The role of ACE inhibitors is less well defined for all patients, but they are selectively useful for treatment of hypertension and in those with LVEF less than 45%.

Meta-analyses of trials of early elective catheterization and PCI versus initial medical therapy have shown lower rates of mortality, recurrent MI, and rehospitalization for recurrent unstable angina after an early invasive approach. Benefits are predominantly limited to higher-risk patients, especially those older than 65 years and those who have resting ST depression or elevated biomarkers.

SPECIAL SITUATIONS

Cardiogenic Shock

Cardiogenic shock occurs in approximately 7% of patients with MI and has a mortality rate of approximately 80%. It is characterized by systemic hypotension (systolic BP <80 mm Hg), reduced cardiac index (<2.2 L/min/m^2), and elevated pulmonary artery wedge pressure (>16 mm Hg). Initial stabilization should be attempted with inotropes such as dopamine, dobutamine, or epinephrine together with intraaortic balloon counterpulsation. Intraaortic balloon counterpulsation reduces cardiac afterload, improves coronary artery perfusion, and increases systolic BP. However, these interventions do not reduce mortality. Early angiography and revascularization with either PCI or surgery have a significant effect in reducing mortality and should be considered in patients with cardiogenic shock.

Right Ventricular Infarction

RV infarction occurs in approximately 40% of patients with acute inferior MI; however, hemodynamically significant RV dysfunction is less common. Patients usually present with an elevated jugular venous pressure without hemodynamic compromise. Some patients present with hypotension, particularly after the administration of vasodilators such as nitrates. On physical examination, patients might have an elevated jugular venous pressure, Kussmaul sign, clear lungs, and a right-sided gallop. The diagnosis is strengthened by demonstrating the presence of at least 1 mm of ST segment elevation in leads V1, V3R, or V4R or RV dysfunction by echocardiography. The treatment is supportive, with intravenous fluids and inotropic support with dopamine or dobutamine if needed. These interventions may be tailored using guidance from hemodynamic data obtained from a pulmonary artery catheter. Patients with RV infarction are more likely to have complications with bradycardia or atrioventricular block that can require temporary atrial and ventricular pacing. Most patients improve spontaneously after 48 to 72 hours. Patients with shock might benefit from early revascularization with PCI to the right coronary artery.

Mechanical Complications of Acute Myocardial Infarction

Successful reperfusion therapy leads to lower complication rates. Table 6 lists the major ischemic, mechanical, and electrical complications of acute MI and their management.

Cardiac Rehabilitation and Secondary Prevention

Cardiac rehabilitation should be initiated before discharge from the hospital, with the goals of improving quality of life, facilitating return to normal activities, encouraging regular exercise, and promoting secondary prevention. Secondary prevention is aimed at smoking cessation and at aggressive dietary and pharmacologic treatment for hyperlipidemia, hypertension, and diabetes mellitus. Patients with uncomplicated MI may drive a car after 1 to 2 weeks and return to work at 2 to 4 weeks, whereas those with complicated MI require longer cardiac rehabilitation.

Summary

Early recognition and prompt treatment are essential for management of MI. Atypical and painless presentation must always be considered. Urgent reperfusion with fibrinolytic or primary PCI is lifesaving in STEMI, and in-hospital revascularization is beneficial in high-risk NSTEMI and unstable coronary syndromes. Agents that reduce mortality, including aspirin, β-blockers, ACE inhibitors, and lipid-lowering drugs, should always be employed in the absence of contraindications. Most patients benefit from lifestyle changes and risk factor modification in a continuing outpatient setting.

REFERENCES

Alpert JS, Thygesen K, Antman E, et al: Myocardial infarction redefined—a consensus document of the Joint European Society of Cardiology/American College of Cardiology Committee for the redefinition of myocardial infarction. J Am Coll Cardiol 2000;36:959-969.

Anderson JL, Adams CD, Antman EM, et al. ACC/AHA 2007 guidelines for the management of patients with unstable angina/non-ST-elevation myocardial infarction. J Am Coll Cardiol 2007;50:e1-e157.

Antman EM, Anbe DT, Armstrong PW, et al: ACC/AHA guidelines for the management of patients with ST-elevation myocardial infarction: A report of the American College of Cardiology/American Heart Association Task Force on Practice Guidelines (Committee to Revise the 1999 Guidelines for the Management of Patients With Acute Myocardial Infarction). J Am Coll Cardiol. 2004;44(3):E1-E211.

Antman EM, Cohen M, Bernink PJ, et al: The TIMI risk score for unstable angina/non-ST elevation MI: A method for prognostication and therapeutic decision making. JAMA 2000;284:835-842.

Cannon CP, Hand MH, Bahr R, et al: Critical pathways for management of patients with acute coronary syndromes: An assessment by the National Heart Attack Alert Program. Am Heart J 2002;143:777-789.

Krumholz HM, Anderson JL, Brooks NH, et al: ACC/AHA clinical performance measures for adults with ST-elevation and non–ST-elevation myocardial infarction: A report of the ACC/AHA task force on performance measures (ST-Elevation and Non-ST-Elevation Myocardial Infarction Performance Measures Writing Committee). J Am Coll Cardiol 2006;47:236-265.

Mehta SR, Cannon CP, Fox KA, et al: Routine vs selective invasive strategies in patients with acute coronary syndromes: A collaborative meta-analysis of randomized trials. JAMA 2005;293:2908-2917.

Smith SC Jr, Allen J, Blair SN, et al: AHA/ACC guidelines for secondary prevention for patients with coronary and other atherosclerotic vascular disease: 2006 update endorsed by the National Heart, Lung, and Blood Institute. J Am Coll Cardiol 2006;47:2130-2139.

Smith SC Jr, Feldman TE, Hirshfeld JW Jr, et al: ACC/AHA/SCAI 2005 guideline update for percutaneous coronary intervention: A report of the American College of Cardiology/American Heart Association Task Force on Practice Guidelines (ACC/AHA/SCAI Writing Committee to Update the 2001 Guidelines for Percutaneous Coronary Intervention). Circulation 2006;113(7):e166-e286.

Weaver WD, Cerqueira M, Hallstrom AP, et al: Prehospital-initiated vs hospital-initiated thrombolytic therapy. The Myocardial Infarction Triage and Intervention Trial. JAMA 1993;270:1211-1216.

Acute Pericarditis

Method of
José G. Díez, MD

The pericardium is a fibroelastic sac made up of visceral and parietal layers separated by a (potential) space, the pericardial cavity. In healthy persons, the pericardial cavity contains 25 to 50 mL of an ultrafiltrate of plasma secreted by the visceral pericardium.

The pericardium provides mechanical protection for the heart and lubrication to reduce friction between the heart and surrounding structures. It also has a significant hemodynamic impact on the atria and contributes to the diastolic coupling between the two ventricles (the distention of one ventricle alters the filling of the other).

Acute pericarditis is usually self-limited unless it is caused by malignancy or other systemic disease. Its clinical presentation can vary, but usually it manifests in one of four ways: acute fibrinous pericarditis, pericardial effusion without major hemodynamic compromise, cardiac tamponade, or constrictive pericarditis.

The pericardium may be involved in a large number of systemic disorders or may be diseased as an isolated process. The principal manifestations of pericardial disease are pericarditis and pericardial effusion. The most prominent symptom is pleuropericardial chest pain, which is generated by the parietal layer, because the visceral layer is devoid of pain fibers.

Etiology

OVERVIEW

The causes of acute pericarditis are numerous (Box 1). The major causes include viral infection (including HIV), purulent bacterial pericarditis, tuberculosis, mediastinal radiation, recent or remote myocardial infarction (MI), cardiac surgery (recent or remote), chest trauma, cardiac diagnostic or interventional procedures (stents, occluding devices), drugs and toxins, metabolic disorders, malignancy (breast, lung, Hodgkin's disease), collagen vascular diseases, or idiopathic causes.

Pericardial disease may also be a feature of other disorders, including inflammatory bowel disease and meningitis. Work-up and evaluation of systemic disorders are beyond the scope of this chapter. Additional studies are appropriate if the history and initial evaluation suggest a specific cause.

In patients with acute pericarditis in whom no cause is identified (idiopathic pericarditis), the etiology is usually presumed to be viral or autoimmune. Autoimmune factors may be particularly important in patients with recurrent acute pericarditis.

The yield of the standard diagnostic evaluation for identification of the etiology in patients with acute pericarditis is relatively low. We discuss here the infectious etiology.

INFECTION

Any infectious organism (virus, bacterium [e.g., *Rickettsia* or *Chlamydia* spp], spirochete, fungus, parasite) can infect the pericardium. Bacteria and fungi can cause a purulent inflammatory exudate. Infectious pericarditis can result in chronic constriction.

Viral

The most common viral infections causing pericarditis include Coxsackieviruses A and B, echovirus, adenovirus, and HIV. Because the same viruses that are responsible for acute pericarditis can also cause myocarditis, it is not uncommon to find some degree of myocardial involvement in patients who have acute pericarditis. This combination is referred to as *myopericarditis*.

BOX 1 Causes of Pericarditis

Autoimmune
Behçet's disease
Giant cell arteritis
Inflammatory bowel disease (Crohn's, ulcerative colitis)
Mixed connective tissue disease
Polyarteritis nodosa
Rheumatic diseases (lupus, rheumatoid arthritis)
Sarcoidosis
Scleroderma
Vasculitis
Wegener's granulomatosis
Whipple's disease

Idiopathic (Nonspecific, Probably Viral)

Infectious Causes
Bacteria
• Gram-positive and gram-negative organisms
• *Mycobacterium tuberculosis*
Fungi (most common in immunocompromised patients)
• *Blastomyces dermatitidis*
• *Candida* species
• *Echinococcus granulosus*
• *Histoplasma capsulatum*
Viruses
• Coxsackieviruses A and B
• Hepatitis viruses
• Human immunodeficiency virus
• Influenza viruses
• Measles virus
• Mumps virus
• Varicella virus

Noninfectious Causes
Acute myocardial infarction
Aortic dissection
Chest trauma
Iatrogenic
• Cardiopulmonary resuscitation
• Catheter and pacemaker perforations
• Following thoracic surgery
Malignancy
• Breast cancer
• Hodgkin's disease
• Leukemia
• Lung cancer
• Lymphoma
• Paraneoplastic syndromes
Radiation therapy (usually for breast or lung cancer)
Renal failure

Medications
Anticoagulants
Cromolyn sodium (Intal)
Dantrolene (Dantrium)
Doxorubicin (Adriamycin)
Hydralazine (Apresoline)
Isoniazid
Methysergide (Sansert)
Penicillin
Phenylbutazone (Butazolidine)
Phenytoin (Dilantin)
Procainamide (Pronestyl)
Thrombolytics

Metabolic
Hypothyroidism
Ovarian hyperstimulation syndrome
Uremia

Bacterial

The most common bacterial genera causing pericarditis are *Staphylococcus*, *Pneumococcus*, *Streptococcus* (rheumatic pancarditis), and *Haemophilus*.

Mycobacterium tuberculosis is also a common bacterial cause. Tuberculosis deserves particular attention because it is responsible for approximately 70% of cases of large pericardial effusion and most cases of constrictive pericarditis in developing countries, but it has also affected the HIV-infected population. In industrialized countries, tuberculosis accounts for only 4% of cases of pericardial effusion. Tuberculous pericarditis is a dangerous disease with a mortality rate of 17% to 40%; constriction occurs in a similar fraction of cases after tuberculous pericardial effusion. A *definite* diagnosis of tuberculous pericarditis is based on the demonstration of tubercle bacilli in pericardial fluid or on a histologic section of the pericardium; *probable* tuberculous pericarditis is based on the proof of tuberculosis elsewhere in a patient with otherwise unexplained pericarditis, a lymphocytic pericardial exudate with elevated adenosine deaminase levels, or appropriate response to a trial of antituberculosis chemotherapy.

Treatment consists of four-drug therapy (isoniazid, rifampin (Rifadin), pyrazinamide, and ethambutol (Myambutol)) for 2 months followed by two drugs (isoniazid and rifampin) for 4 months regardless of HIV status. It is uncertain whether adjunctive corticosteroids are effective in reducing mortality or progression to constriction. Surgical resection of the pericardium remains the appropriate treatment for constrictive pericarditis. The timing of surgical intervention is controversial, but many experts recommend a trial of medical therapy for noncalcific pericardial constriction, and pericardiectomy is indicated for patients with calcific constrictive pericarditis or with persistent signs of constriction after a 6- to 8-week trial of antituberculosis treatment in patients with noncalcific constrictive pericarditis.

Fungal

Histoplasma is the most common genus causing fungal pericarditis in patients with an intact immune system. In immunocompromised patients, pathogens include *Aspergillus*, *Candida*, and *Coccidioides* species.

Diagnostic Criteria and Clinical Presentation

The major clinical manifestations of acute pericarditis include chest pain, pericardial friction rub, electrocardiographic (ECG) changes (widespread ST elevation or PR depression), and pericardial effusion. At least two of these features are usually considered necessary to make the diagnosis. Absence of pericardial effusion does not exclude pericarditis. The presence of an elevated C-reactive protein level also supports the diagnosis.

CHEST PAIN

The chest pain of acute pericarditis is sudden in onset and occurs over the anterior chest. It is usually pleuritic, sharp, and exacerbated by inspiration. It can also manifest as pressure-like pain, which is difficult to distinguish from that of myocardial ischemia. The differential diagnosis of pericarditic chest pain includes myocardial ischemia, pulmonary embolism, gastroesophageal reflux disease, and musculoskeletal pain.

PERICARDIAL FRICTION RUB

A pericardial friction rub is highly specific for acute pericarditis. Pericardial rubs may be easier to hear in patients without a pericardial effusion. Pericardial friction rubs are generated by friction of the two inflamed layers of the pericardium. Three phases have been described corresponding to atrial systole, ventricular systole, and the rapid filling phase of early ventricular diastole.

Some rubs are present only during one (one component) or two phases (two components) of the cardiac cycle. By breath holding it is possible to distinguish a pericardial rub from a pleural friction rub.

ELECTROCARDIOGRAM

The ECG is often the most helpful test in patients with suspected acute pericarditis. The electrocardiographic changes in acute pericarditis signify inflammation of the epicardium, because the parietal pericardium itself is electrically inert. The electrocardiogram in acute pericarditis evolves through four stages. Stage 1 (first hours to days) is characterized by diffuse ST elevation (typically concave up) with reciprocal ST depression in leads aVR and V1. There is also an atrial current of injury, reflected by elevation of the PR segment in lead aVR and depression of the PR segment in other limb leads and in the left chest leads, primarily V5 and V6. Thus, the PR and ST segments typically change in opposite directions. Stage 2 is characterized by normalization of the ST and PR segments. Stage 3 is characterized by the development of diffuse T wave inversions, generally after the ST segments have become isoelectric. In stage 4, the ECG may be normal or the T wave inversions may persist indefinitely (chronic pericarditis).

The typical ECG evolution can be noted in up to 60% of patients. Treatment can accelerate or alter ECG progression. Modern advances have reduced the number of infectious cases and restricted the ECG stage sequence. The electrocardiographic changes should be distinguished from acute MI (in which case they are more localized and associated with reciprocal ST segment changes) and from early repolarization (a variant in as many as 30% of young adults).

Arrhythmias are uncommon in acute pericarditis. The presence of atrial or ventricular arrhythmias suggests concomitant myocarditis.

PERICARDIAL EFFUSION

Pericardial effusion is typically diagnosed by echocardiography. Pericardial fluid and tissue can be tested with tumor markers, fluorescence-activated cell sorting, polymerase chain reaction, and immunohistochemistry.

In cases of hemorrhagic pericardial effusion, malignancy and tuberculosis need to be considered, but viral pericarditis can also cause hemorrhagic effusion. Other causes include percutaneous interventional procedures, postpericardiotomy syndrome, MI (free wall rupture), uremia, aortic dissection, and trauma.

ECHOCARDIOGRAM

Echocardiogram is an essential part of the evaluation, due to the possibility of an associated pericardial effusion and tamponade. In tamponade, the clinical signs include pulsus paradoxus, an inspiratory fall in arterial pressure of at least 10 mm Hg. The echocardiogram commonly shows diastolic chamber collapses of the right atrium, right ventricle, or both, occasionally the left atrium, and rarely the left ventricle. Right atrium and right ventricle collapses are sensitive and become more specific if they last for at least a third of the cardiac cycle.

CHEST X-RAY

Chest x-ray is typically normal in patients with acute pericarditis. A large pericardial effusion can explain an enlarged cardiac silhouette with clear lung fields. A large cardiac silhouette on x-ray requires chronic and slow fluid accumulation.

BIOMARKERS

Acute pericarditis can cause modest elevations in the MB fraction of creatine kinase (CK-MB) and serum cardiac troponin I (cTnI). This elevation is related to the extent of myocardial involvement. Due to the sensitivity of troponins, mild increases in cTnI often occur in

> **BOX 2 Indications for Hospitalization of Patients with Acute Pericarditis**
>
> Anticoagulation therapy
> Echocardiographic findings of a large pericardial effusion (>20 mm)
> Echocardiographic findings of hemodynamically significant effusion
> Findings of cardiac tamponade (hypotension and neck vein distention or echocardiographic signs, e.g., chamber collapse, respiratory variability in inflow)
> Immunocompromised system
> Myopericarditis
> Temperature >100.4°F (38°C)
> Trauma
> Troponin I elevation

the absence of elevations in CK-MB. Other signs of inflammation are common, including elevated white blood cell count, erythrocyte sedimentation rate, and serum C-reactive protein concentration.

ADDITIONAL TESTS

Additional tests include tuberculin skin test, antinuclear antibody titer, HIV serology, and blood cultures if the patient is febrile. Viral studies are not obtained routinely, because the yield is low and management is not altered. Additional studies are appropriate if the history and initial evaluation suggest a specific cause, such as malignancy.

DETERMINATION OF RISK AND NEED FOR HOSPITALIZATION

Patients with high-risk features are at increased risk for short-term complications. These features of high risk include subacute symptoms (e.g., developing over several days or weeks), fever (>38°C [100.4°F]) and leukocytosis, clinical or echocardiographic evidence of cardiac tamponade, a large pericardial effusion (an echo-free space >20 mm), immunosuppression, oral anticoagulant therapy, trauma, and failure to respond within 7 days to nonsteroidal antiinflammatory drug (NSAID) therapy (Box 2).

Treatment

VIRAL OR IDIOPATHIC PERICARDITIS

In patients with an identified cause other than viral or idiopathic disease, specific therapy appropriate to the underlying disorder is indicated. In the treatment of idiopathic or viral pericarditis, the goals of therapy are the relief of pain and resolution of inflammation and pericardial effusion.

Aspirin or Other Nonsteroidal Antiinflammatory Drugs

Primary therapy has been aspirin 2 to 4 g/day. An alternative protocol consists of aspirin 800 mg every 6 to 8 hours, followed by gradual tapering of 800 mg every week for a treatment period of 3 to 4 weeks.

In pericarditis associated with an acute MI, aspirin is preferred. Aspirin may also be the first choice in patients who require concomitant antiplatelet therapy for other reasons. In observational series of low-risk patients, almost 90% responded to aspirin alone within 7 days, and most of the nonresponders had an autoimmune disease or tuberculosis. Aspirin resistance has been associated with significant increases in the rates of recurrent pericarditis and constrictive pericarditis.

Ibuprofen (Motrin, Advil) has the advantage of relatively few adverse effects and the potential advantage of increasing coronary flow. Ibuprofen 300 to 800 mg every six to eight hours can be continued for days or weeks (2-4 weeks). NSAID dose tapering may be prescribed in an attempt to reduce the subsequent recurrence rate. Ketorolac, a parenteral NSAID, is also effective. In contrast, indomethacin (Indocin)[1] usually controls pain but has a poor adverse effect profile and reduces coronary flow.

Both aspirin and NSAID regimens require gastrointestinal protection, using either proton pump inhibitors or antihistamine H_2 blockers.

Failure to respond to aspirin or NSAID therapy within 1 week (defined as persistence of fever, pericarditic chest pain, a new pericardial effusion, or worsening of general illness) suggests that a cause other than idiopathic or viral pericarditis is present.

Colchicine

Initial observational studies suggested that colchicine[1] might prevent recurrence of acute idiopathic or viral pericarditis.

The effect of colchicine in the primary management of acute pericarditis was directly evaluated in the prospective, randomized, open label COPE (COlchicine for acute PEricarditis) trial of 120 patients with a first episode of acute pericarditis (84% idiopathic; mean age, 57 years). The patients were assigned to aspirin 800 mg every 6 or 8 hours for 7 to 10 days with gradual tapering (e.g., 800 mg/week) over 3 to 4 weeks, either alone or in combination with colchicine 1 to 2 mg on the first day, followed by 0.5 once or twice daily for 3 months. The lower colchicine dose (1 mg initial dose followed by 0.5 mg once daily) was given to patients who weighed less than 70 kg or who did not tolerate the higher dose. Corticosteroids were given only for contraindications to or intolerance of aspirin, which were present in 19 patients (16%).

The following findings were noted: The primary endpoint, the recurrence rate, was significantly lower in the colchicine group (10.7 vs 32.3% with aspirin alone at 18 months). Colchicine significantly reduced the secondary endpoint, the rate of persistent symptoms at 72 hours (11.7 vs 36.7%). Colchicine was discontinued because of diarrhea in five patients (8.3%), two of whom had recurrent pericarditis after cessation of therapy.

The findings in COPE, including the relative lack of toxicity, provide a stronger evidence base for the use of colchicine[1] in acute pericarditis. Based on the totality of the evidence, colchicine is an optional additional treatment in patients with a first episode of acute idiopathic or viral pericarditis, using the regimen in the COPE trial (0.5-1 mg twice on the first day, followed by 0.5 once or twice daily for 3 months).

The 2004 European Society of Cardiology guidelines supported the use of colchicine[1] 0.5-1 mg/day, alone or in combination with NSAIDs, to treat acute pericarditis. On the basis of COPE and of the CORE (COlchicine for REcurrent pericarditis) trial of patients with recurrent pericarditis, colchicine appears to be effective in both first episodes and recurrent disease.

Corticosteroids

Corticosteroids should be considered only if the patient is clearly refractory to NSAIDs and colchicine. The use of corticosteroid therapy early in the course of the disease has been associated with recurrent episodes of pericarditis. The confounding issue with corticosteroid therapy is that it may be more likely to be used in patients with disease resistant to initial therapy, which would be a predictor of recurrence independent of prior administration of corticosteroids. Corticosteroids may be useful in refractory acute pericarditis. In the COPE trial of colchicine therapy, corticosteroids were given only when aspirin was contraindicated or not tolerated. On multivariate analysis, corticosteroid use was a significant predictor of recurrence (odds ratio, 4.30). The same effect has been reported for patients with the first recurrence or multiple recurrences and might result from promotion of viral replication.

---

[1]Not FDA approved for this indication.

CURRENT DIAGNOSIS

- The typical clinical manifestations of acute pericarditis are chest pain (usually pleuritic), a pericardial friction rub, and widespread ST segment elevation on the electrocardiogram or PR depression. At least two of these features, with or without a pericardial effusion, should usually be present for the diagnosis.
- Acute pericarditis has a wide spectrum of etiologies.
- Iatrogenic pericarditis occurs following surgery and invasive medical procedures (percutaneous coronary interventions, structural and electrophysiology).
- Echocardiography is recommended for patients with suspected pericardial disease in order to evaluate effusion, constriction, or effusive-constrictive process.
- In patients with acute pericarditis in whom no cause is identified (idiopathic pericarditis), the etiology is usually presumed to be viral. A complex and exhaustive testing strategy is typically not justified by the limited implications for clinical management. An exception to this recommendation is the absence of a prompt and adequate response to standard treatment.
- In multivariable analysis, specific clinical features included female gender, fever >38°C, subacute course, large effusion or tamponade, and aspirin or NSAID failure. These features were useful for identifying a higher risk of complications and need for hospitalization.

The 2004 European Society of Cardiology guidelines recommended that systemic steroid therapy be restricted to patients with acute pericarditis due to connective tissue disease, immune-mediated pericarditis, or uremic pericarditis

When corticosteroid therapy is necessary, initiate therapy at a high dose (prednisone 1 mg/kg daily) and taper slowly over 2 to 4 weeks after C-reactive protein normalizes. Tapering can be done in decrements of 2.5 to 5 mg at intervals of 1 to 4 weeks. Aspirin or another NSAID is introduced toward the end of tapering. A very slow taper becomes critical in recurrent pericarditis.

Combination Therapy

Because of the demonstrated effectiveness of colchicine[1] (as monotherapy or combined therapy), the best combination may be ibuprofen 800 mg every 8 hours and colchicine 0.6 mg twice daily. Colchicine also tends to prevent recurrent pericarditis. Combined therapy could be continued for 7 to 14 days followed by tapering for another 1 or 2 weeks because of the possibility of early recurrence. An oral corticosteroid should only be used if it is also indicated for an underlying disease or if the patient's syndrome is severe and resistant to NSAIDs. It appears that the early use of corticosteroids in most forms of pericarditis actually contributes to recurrent pericarditis. Physical activity could exacerbate accompanying superficial myocarditis.

Pericardiocentesis

In patients with a pericardial effusion, pericardiocentesis or surgical drainage (with pericardial biopsy) can serve both diagnostic and therapeutic purposes. In patients with acute pericarditis, decisions are based on the presence of a moderate to large effusion and on clinical significance (e.g., causing hemodynamic compromise). Pericardiocentesis is generally performed for moderate to severe tamponade; purulent, tuberculous, or neoplastic pericarditis is suspected or if there is a persistent symptomatic pericardial effusion.

---

[1]Not FDA approved for this indication.

Prognosis

Generally, acute pericarditis is benign and self-limited. Occasionally, acute pericarditis is complicated by tamponade, constriction, or recurrence. Nearly 24% of patients with acute pericarditis have recurrence. Most of these patients have a single recurrence within the first weeks after the initial episode, and a minority have repeated episodes for months or years. The first episode of viral pericarditis is usually the most severe, and recurrences are less severe and might manifest only with chest pain.

BACTERIAL PERICARDITIS

Bacterial pericarditis occurs by direct infection during trauma, thoracic surgery, or catheter drainage; by spread from an intrathoracic, myocardial, or subdiaphragmatic focus; and by hematogenous dissemination. The frequent causes are *Staphylococcus* and *Streptococcus* species (rheumatic pancarditis), *Haemophilus* species, and *M. tuberculosis*. In AIDS pericarditis, the incidence of bacterial infection is much higher than in the general population, with a high percentage of *Mycobacterium avium-intracellulare* infection.

Purulent pericarditis is the most serious manifestation of bacterial pericarditis, characterized by gross pus in the pericardium or microscopically purulent effusion. It is an acute, fulminant illness with fever in virtually all patients. Chest pain is uncommon. Purulent pericarditis is always fatal if untreated. The mortality rate in treated patients is 40%, and death is mostly due to cardiac tamponade, systemic toxicity, cardiac decompensation, and constriction.

Tuberculous infection can manifest as acute pericarditis, cardiac tamponade, silent (often large) relapsing pericardial effusion, effusive-constrictive pericarditis, toxic symptoms with persistent fever, and acute, subacute, or chronic constriction. The mortality rate in untreated patients approaches 85%. Urgent pericardial drainage, combined with intravenous antibacterial therapy (e.g., vancomycin [Vancocin] 1 g twice daily, ceftriaxone [Rocephin][1] 1-2 g twice daily, or ciprofloxacin [Cipro][1] 400 mg/day) is mandatory in purulent pericarditis. Irrigation with urokinase (Abbokinase) or streptokinase[1], using large catheters, can liquefy the purulent exudate, but open surgical drainage is preferable. The initial treatment of tuberculous pericarditis should include isoniazid 300 mg/day, rifampin 600 mg/day, pyrazinamide 15 to 30 mg/kg/day, and ethambutol 15 to 25 mg/kg/day. Prednisone 1 to 2 mg/kg/day is given for 5 to 7 days and progressively reduced to discontinuation in 6 to 8 weeks. Drug-sensitivity testing is essential. Pericardiectomy is reserved for recurrent effusions or continued elevation of central venous pressure after 4 to 6 weeks of antituberculous and corticosteroid therapy.

RECURRENT PERICARDITIS

Recurrent pericarditis is a syndrome in which pericarditis recurs after the agent inciting the original acute attack has disappeared or has ceased to be active. The exact recurrence rate after initial attacks of idiopathic pericarditis is unknown, but it may be as high as 15% to 30% in patients not treated with colchicine. Some patients, however, have more persistent pericarditis in which symptoms can only be controlled with steroid therapy.

Recurrent pericarditis usually manifests with a pericardial effusion. Immune mechanisms appear to be of primary importance in most cases. Lack of response to aspirin or other NSAIDs, corticosteroid therapy, and inappropriate pericardiotomy or creation of a window are risk factors for recurrent disease.

Therapy for recurrent pericarditis can be a prolonged and frustrating. Due to the need to maintain compliance, effective communication with the patient is important. It is important to explain to the patient the nature of the disease, the likely course, and the treatment alternatives. The patient should be informed about the symptoms of cardiac tamponade and constrictive pericarditis.

---

[1]Not FDA approved for this indication.

CURRENT THERAPY

- Pericardiocentesis is indicated in cardiac tamponade (clinical and/or echocardiographic) and suspected purulent pericarditis.
- The nonsteroidal antiinflammatory drugs (NSAIDs), with the addition of colchicine,[1] have been rapidly effective in most appropriately diagnosed cases.
- Colchicine[1] should be considered as an adjunct to NSAID therapy in patients with acute viral or idiopathic pericarditis.
- Corticosteroids are restricted to patients with pericarditis caused by connective tissue disease, autoreactive (immune-mediated) pericarditis, and uremic pericarditis and to patients with idiopathic or viral pericarditis that is refractory to treatment with NSAIDs and colchicine.[1] Initiate at high initial dosing (e.g., 1 mg/kg/day of prednisone) with slow tapering.

[1]Not FDA approved for this indication.

The possibility of pericardiectomy and the complications of immunosuppression should be discussed.

The vast majority of patients respond to prednisone, initially given in a high dose, which is maintained for a short period and subsequently tapered.

Nonsteroidal Antiinflammatory Drugs

The 2004 European Society of Cardiology guidelines support the use of NSAIDs with an agent such as ibuprofen 800 mg four times daily. If the patient responds well to the initial regimen, the dose of ibuprofen is reduced to 600 mg four times daily at 2 weeks and to 400 mg four times daily at 4 weeks. Treatment is discontinued after 3 months. Gastrointestinal protection should be provided during therapy.

Colchicine[1]

The use of colchicine with or without NSAIDs can reduce or eliminate the need for corticosteroids in patients with recurrent pericarditis. The best available data come from the CORE study, which evaluated the safety and efficacy of colchicine therapy as adjuncts to conventional therapy for the first episode of recurrent pericarditis. Eighty-four consecutive patients with a first episode of recurrent pericarditis were randomly assigned to receive conventional treatment with aspirin alone or conventional treatment plus colchicine (1.0-2.0 mg the first day and then 0.5-1.0 mg/day for 6 months). When aspirin was contraindicated, prednisone (1.0-1.5 mg/kg daily) was given for 1 month and then was gradually tapered. The primary end point was the recurrence rate.

During a mean follow-up of 20 months, treatment with colchicine significantly decreased the recurrence rate (actuarial rates at 18 months were 24.0% vs 50.6%; $P = 0.02$; number needed to treat, 4.0; 95% confidence [CI] interval, 2.5-7.1) and symptom persistence at 72 hours (10% vs 31%; $P = 0.03$). In multivariate analysis, previous corticosteroid use was an independent risk factor for further recurrences (odds ratio, 2.89; 95% CI, 1.10-8.26; $P = 0.04$). No serious adverse effects were observed. The authors conclude that colchicine therapy led to a clinically important and statistically significant benefit over conventional treatment, decreasing the recurrence rate in patients with a first episode of recurrent pericarditis.

Given the results of the CORE trial, aspirin or other NSAID plus colchicine[1] are recommended for initial therapy of recurrent pericarditis due to idiopathic or viral causes.

[1]Not FDA approved for this indication.

Corticosteroids

Failure of NSAIDs and colchicine indicates the need to use prednisone. The starting dose is 1 mg/kg; this dose should be maintained for 1 month, even if the patient shows no clinical evidence of pericarditis. In the small number of patients who do not respond adequately, azathioprine (Imuran)[1] (75-100 mg/day) has been used. Methotrexate (Trexall)[1] has also been evaluated.

A recent nonrandomized observation suggests that in cases of recurrent pericarditis, lower doses of prednisone (0.2 to 0.5 mg/kg per day), maintained for 4 weeks and then slowly tapered, are superior to higher doses. Doses of 1 mg/kg per day for recurrent pericarditis were associated with more side effects, recurrences, and hospitalizations. Based on the accumulated evidence, unless the use of corticosteroids is deemed inevitable, the superior strategy seems to be the use of a NSAID and colchicine.

Intrapericardial Therapy

A method to minimize systemic steroid-induced side effects while maintaining efficacy is intrapericardial steroid therapy to achieve high local concentration. Pericardiocentesis with antibiotic prophylaxis was followed by the intrapericardial administration of triamcinolone (Kenalog) 300 to 600 mg/m^2 given in 100 mL of isotonic saline at body temperature as a single injection and then removed at 24 hours; maintenance therapy consisted of colchicine[1] 0.5 mg three times daily for 6 months.

The 2004 European Society of Cardiology guidelines gave a class IIa recommendation (weight of evidence or opinion is in favor of usefulness or efficacy) to the use of intrapericardial steroid therapy. Technical considerations might limit the usefulness of this approach, and more research is required. If the patient has a large or moderate-sized pericardial effusion, intrapericardial therapy is straightforward. If the patient has a small or no pericardial effusion, pericardioscopy technique is needed for this form of treatment.

REFERENCES

Imazio M, Bobbio M, Cecchi E, et al: Colchicine in addition to conventional therapy for acute pericarditis: Results of the COlchicine for acute PEricarditis (COPE) trial. Circulation 2005;112:2012-2016.

Imazio M, Brucato A, Cumetti D, et al: Corticosteroids for recurrent pericarditis. High versus low doses: A nonrandomized observation. Circulation 2008;118:667-671.

Imazio M, Cecchi E, Demichelis B, et al: Indicators of poor prognosis of acute pericarditis. Circulation 2007;115(21):2739-2744.

Imazio M, Demichelis B, Parrini I, et al: Management, risk factors, and outcomes in recurrent pericarditis. Am J Cardiol 2005;96:736-739.

Lange RA, Hillis LD: Clinical practice. Acute pericarditis. N Engl J Med 2004;351:2195-2202.

Maisch B, Ristic AD: The classification of pericardial disease in the age of modern medicine. Curr Cardiol Rep 2002;4:13-21.

Maisch B, Seferovic PM, Ristic AD, et al: Guidelines on the diagnosis and management of pericardial diseases executive summary; The task force on the diagnosis and management of pericardial diseases of the European Society of Cardiology. Eur Heart J 2004;25:587-610.

Mayosi BM, Burgess LJ, Doubell AF: Tuberculous pericarditis. Circulation 6 2005;112(23):3608-3616.

Pankuweit S, Ristic AD, Seferovic PM, Maisch B: Bacterial pericarditis: Diagnosis and management. Am J Cardiovasc Drugs 2005;5(2):103-112.

Spodick DH: Acute pericarditis: Current concepts and practice. JAMA 2003;289:1150-1153.

Troughton RW, Asher CR, Klein AL: Pericarditis. Lancet 2004;363:717-727.

Spodick DH: Pericardial diseases. In Braunwald E, Zipes DP, Libby P (eds): Heart Disease. 6th ed. Philadelphia: WB Saunders, 2001, pp 823-866.

Syed FF, Mayosi BM: A modern approach to tuberculous pericarditis. Prog Cardiovasc Dis 2007;50(3):218-236.

[1]Not FDA approved for this indication.

Peripheral Arterial Disease

Method of
Jeffrey L. Ballard, MD

Peripheral arterial disease (PAD) is a prevalent atherosclerotic disease process that affects millions of Americans and is associated with significant morbidity and loss of life. Until symptoms arise or a critical problem is serendipitously discovered via imaging for another disease process, most patients and even physicians are not aware of this silent syndrome. The consequences of undiagnosed and untreated PAD include nonfatal but debilitating thromboembolic ischemic events, decreased quality of life, and increased mortality risk. Despite these potentially devastating outcomes, PAD has not yet emerged as a major focus of public health awareness efforts. In the absence of a national PAD education and detection program, increased diagnostic efforts in primary care offices and community-based programs may be able to identify a sizable number of at-risk patients with modifiable atherosclerotic risk factors or threatening arterial lesions. This is particularly important because clinical examination findings are not independently sufficient to include or exclude the diagnosis of PAD with certainty.

Selective screening for PAD based on specific risk factors results in the highest yield of significant atherosclerotic findings. For instance, in community-based stroke screening programs, occult carotid artery stenosis is often diagnosed among patients who are older than 60 years and have a personal history of hypertension, heart disease, or cigarette smoking or a family history of stroke. Screening for PAD has been shown to be cost-effective and compares favorably with screening programs for other disorders in adults. Establishing a diagnosis of PAD based on focused risk factors and clinical findings is important because of prognostic and therapeutic implications. Even nonselective screening programs can identify a sizable number of at-risk patients with modifiable atherosclerotic risk factors or threatening arterial lesions.

Short of screening every adult patient for PAD, recognition of the signs and symptoms of the more common PAD processes by the primary care physician facilitates the formulation of a precise differential diagnosis. This PAD recognition combined with focused diagnostic testing are important tools because PAD can manifest acutely or as a smoldering chronic disease process. Definitive care is then accomplished by prompt referral to a vascular or endovascular surgeon, who is best equipped to offer a complete battery of treatment options and to optimize patient outcomes. This article focuses on three common manifestations of PAD: chronic lower extremity ischemia, carotid occlusive disease, and aneurysm of the abdominal aorta.

Chronic Limb Ischemia

Symptomatic disease caused by atherosclerosis primarily occurs in the coronary arteries, the arteries of the lower extremities, and the extracranial carotid arteries. Of the three arterial sites, lower extremity ischemia is probably the most underdiagnosed and least aggressively managed. The two primary operative indications for infrainguinal bypass are disabling claudication and chronic limb ischemia (CLI).

Patients with claudication who are unable to perform their primary occupation, who are unable to comfortably carry out activities of daily living, or whose lifestyles are significantly limited are potential candidates for infrainguinal revascularization after a conservative trial of risk factor modification and a daily exercise program with or without available medical therapy. The primary reason for intervention in patients with claudication is to improve lifestyle, because the risk of clinical deterioration (20%) or major limb amputation (5%) over a 3- to 5-year period is quite low. In most vascular practices with large infrainguinal bypass experience, patients with

CURRENT DIAGNOSIS

- In addition to a detailed history, complete evaluation of the patient with peripheral arterial disease requires palpation of extremity pulses; auscultation of the neck, chest, and abdomen for bruits, murmurs, and rubs; and palpation of the abdomen, groin, and popliteal fossa for aneurysm.
- Arterial and venous duplex ultrasound and other noninvasive testing modalities performed in an accredited vascular laboratory are the primary tools to be used for diagnosis of and screening for peripheral arterial disease.

claudication account for a small percentage (<20%) of patients undergoing revascularization; the remaining bypasses are performed in patients with CLI.

Patients with CLI generally require prompt intervention and pose a complex medical and surgical problem, because there is a high anticipated amputation rate without lower extremity arterial reconstruction. Such patients usually have rest pain and nonhealing ulceration or gangrene. In addition, CLI patients have a high prevalence of coronary artery disease (CAD) and, as a result, significantly reduced 5-year survival. Furthermore, CLI patients tend to be older and have a greater number of associated comorbidities. Cardiac intervention in such patients has higher reported morbidity and mortality rates than in the general population of patients with isolated CAD targeted for intervention.

Therefore, all CLI patients should be assumed to have significant CAD. Perioperative blood pressure control, antianginal regimens, and treatment for CHF should be optimized, and based on level I data, perioperative β-blockade should be employed if there are no contraindications. Postponement of infrainguinal bypass to allow focused and expeditious cardiac evaluation is reasonable in the presence of frequent or unstable angina, recent myocardial infarction, poorly controlled CHF, or symptomatic cardiac dysrhythmias. Invasive coronary intervention should only be pursued if patient and anatomic characteristics are favorable, if the benefit-to-risk ratio is high, and if intervention can be performed without prolonged delay. In the

CURRENT THERAPY

- Smoking cessation, medical management of vascular risk factors, and lifestyle modification including a supervised exercise program are paramount for the conservative management of peripheral arterial disease.
- Aggressive treatment of chronic limb ischemia prevents limb loss in most patients, and a more aggressive posture than previously considered is warranted for patients with claudication to prevent the ravages of the metabolic syndrome.
- Carotid endarterectomy is a durable and safe procedure that is appropriate for asymptomatic carotid stenosis greater than 70% and symptomatic carotid stenosis greater than 50%. Carotid stenting performed in centers of excellence may be a viable alternative in select patients.
- Open abdominal aortic aneurysm repair via a left flank retroperitoneal approach is the current benchmark. Stent-graft repair is appropriate for older patients with suitable arterial anatomy who are willing to undergo lifelong postoperative endograft surveillance.

absence of such cardiac instability, CLI patients are best treated with meticulous perioperative medical care and expeditious lower extremity revascularization.

Nearly all patients in whom infrainguinal bypass is indicated have suitable target vessels if diagnostic angiography is properly performed. Only a small number of patients, usually following multiple failed previous reconstructions, do not have an identifiable target artery. Very few patients are truly unsuitable for reconstruction from an anatomic standpoint due to the lack of a suitable outflow target vessel. Infrainguinal bypass for CLI taxes surgeon ingenuity and requires thoughtful consideration of numerous alternatives and potential complications both in the preoperative evaluation and during the conduct of the surgical arterial reconstruction.

Surgical outcomes such as graft patency and limb salvage are important endpoints; however, numerous investigators have recognized that functional outcomes are at least of equal importance. The ideal functional outcome, as defined by the expectations of a patent graft, healed wound, no need for reoperation, independent living status, and continued ambulation is actually extremely difficult to achieve in patients with CLI. Only a small fraction of treated patients (<20%) meet these basic criteria for success. Preoperative independence and ambulation are the two best predictors of postoperative independence and continued ambulation. These findings emphasize the severity of underlying comorbidities in CLI patients and the difficulties encountered in obtaining functional limb salvage.

Further studies using such functional or patient-relative outcomes are needed to put the role of infrainguinal bypass in perspective, particularly to allow comparison with evolving less-invasive techniques such as subintimal angioplasty and atherectomy or even primary amputation in select high-risk subsets of patients with CLI. Although it is generally agreed that nearly all patients with CLI are best treated with surgical revascularization, it is clear that both economic and functional outcomes mandate consideration of alternative therapies, at least in certain subsets of patients with CLI, such as those living in nursing facilities or who are minimally ambulatory.

All PAD patients require treatment to maintain or improve function, reduce or eliminate ischemic symptoms, and prevent disease progression. Modification of risk factors such as smoking, hypertension, dyslipidemia, and diabetes is crucial. In addition, patients with non–limb-threatening ischemia benefit from a supervised exercise program, available medical therapy as needed, and selective use of revascularization for those who are truly disabled by claudication symptoms. Patients who present with rest pain, foot gangrene, or nonhealing ulceration have CLI and require prompt revascularization to avoid major limb amputation.

Progressive evolution in patient evaluation, selection, and conduct of infrainguinal bypass procedures has resulted in a more successful approach to distal arterial reconstructions, especially for patients with CLI. Graft patency and limb salvage rates have demonstrated parallel improvements; however, there remains a need for detailed clinical studies that examine the cost effectiveness of infrainguinal bypass procedures as well as patient quality of life outcomes in order to ensure their appropriate use and to permit meaningful comparison with evolving less-invasive endovascular therapies.

Carotid Occlusive Disease

The natural sequela of an untreated critical atherosclerotic lesion of the carotid artery is associated with significant morbidity and mortality. A stroke can have a devastating impact on the life of its victim and family as well as on the economic resources of our already taxed health care system. In appropriately selected patients, carotid artery repair has a positive effect on the occurrence of stroke, and now it is widely recognized that this therapy has greater impact on morbidity and mortality compared with medical management alone.

Several population studies have demonstrated an alarming progression of stroke risk with advancing age. In the age group 55 to 64 years, the cerebral infarction rate is roughly 277 per 100,000 population per year. However, this figure escalates to 1786 per 100,000 per year in persons older than 75 years. In addition, men have a 1.5 times greater risk of stroke than women in all age groups. In the United States, there are approximately 160 new strokes per 100,000 population per year. Symptoms are usually the result of debris embolization from plaque rupture or platelet or thrombus aggregate embolization from an ulcer or severely stenotic lesion.

Episodes of transient cerebral ischemia (TIA) can herald subsequent stroke or other neurologic disability. In this regard, it is extremely important to distinguish focal neurologic events from global symptoms, such as dizziness or vertigo. This is because the ultimate stroke risk is greater following a true TIA than for the latter. Carotid-based TIAs clearly indicate instability of the plaque lesion, and the stroke risk is highest in the first year after diagnosis. Asymptomatic lesions can also lead to stroke. Prospective natural history data demonstrate an annual stroke incidence of approximately 4% ipsilateral to an asymptomatic stenosis greater than 50%. However, the stroke risk increases significantly when the carotid lesion progresses to greater than 70% stenosis.

The overwhelming majority (~90%) of lesions that affect the extracranial cerebrovascular system are the result of progressive atherosclerosis. This disease process characteristically occurs at the carotid bifurcation and more specifically at the proximal portion of the internal carotid artery. Duplex ultrasound is the imaging modality of choice for cerebrovascular occlusive disease. The test is noninvasive and has a high diagnostic accuracy if performed in an accredited vascular laboratory. In the acute setting, head computed tomography (CT), magnetic resonance imaging (MRI), or magnetic resonance angiography (MRA) is useful to differentiate between hemorrhagic and ischemic stroke. MRI can also provide images of the extracranial and intracranial arterial anatomy, but the degree of stenosis tends to be over-read by the modality. CT angiography is evolving as a useful diagnostic tool, but the gold standard still remains duplex ultrasound. Carotid angiography, infrequently used as a diagnostic tool, can be used to delineate difficult anatomy that could not be successfully imaged with ultrasound and to plan for potential angioplasty and stenting of appropriately chosen carotid artery lesions.

The purpose of carotid artery treatment is to eliminate recurrent neurologic symptoms or to prevent stroke. Carotid endarterectomy has been the mainstay of treatment since 1950. However, recent clinical trials have also confirmed the safety and efficacy of carotid artery stenting. In general, symptomatic patients with greater than 50% stenosis and asymptomatic patients with greater than 70% stenosis should be considered candidates for intervention. Appropriate selection of treatment modality is then based on patient risk factors, arterial anatomy, and plaque morphology. In experienced hands, results of either carotid endarterectomy or stenting are superb, with a low incidence of procedure-related complications.

Abdominal Aortic Aneurysm

PAD is usually thought of in terms of arterial stenosis and ischemia; however, the same atherosclerotic process can lead to abnormal weakness or swelling in the wall of the abdominal aorta or any other intracranial or peripheral artery. Dilation of the coronary arteries is rare (1%-2% of all aneurysms) and may be congenital, atherosclerotic, or associated with Kawasaki's disease. AAA is defined as abdominal aorta increased by more than 1.5 times its normal diameter at the level of the renal arteries. Arterial aneurysms are associated with very few signs or symptoms. In fact, most AAAs are first discovered during the work-up for another problem such as low back pain, kidney dysfunction, or vague abdominal pain. Therefore, screening for AAA can be truly lifesaving.

The Deficit Reduction Act of 2005 contains the Screening Abdominal Aortic Aneurysms Very Efficiently (SAAAVE) Act, a provision that included aortic aneurysm screening as a Medicare benefit. As of January 1, 2007, SAAAVE provides for a one-time AAA screening, at the Welcome to Medicare physical, for men with a family history of AAA and for those who currently smoke or who have ever smoked. The National Aneurysm Alliance, under the direction of the Society for Vascular Surgery, is lobbying to extend this Medicare benefit to women with appropriate risk factors.

Aneurysm rupture affects at least 15,000 people every year in the United States, making it the 13th leading cause of death. This sobering statistic is the primary reason vascular surgeons focus on early detection and treatment of this silent killer. Timely AAA diagnosis and treatment are paramount, because the mortality rate after AAA rupture exceeds 50% even if the broken blood vessel is promptly repaired with a graft in the standard open surgical fashion. Regarding endovascular repair, the results of single-center and multicenter trials have been published, with mortality rates that range from 10.8% to 35.0%. These results do demonstrate that endovascular repair of ruptured AAA is technically possible. However, these procedures were all specialized centers of excellence in AAA repair, and patients who were selected for this type of repair had favorable arterial anatomy and presented in a relatively hemodynamically stable condition.

Cigarette smoking, high blood pressure, and pulmonary disease are the primary risk factors associated with aortic aneurysms. Additional factors include family history, elevated cholesterol, high triglyceride levels, and a few rare connective tissue diseases such as Marfan and Ehlers–Danlos syndromes. Diagnosis can be made by clinical examination in fit patients. However, most aneurysms are diagnosed with ultrasound or abdominal CT. The risk of AAA rupture increases with advancing age as well as with aneurysm size. Most vascular surgeons agree that an aneurysm larger than 5 cm in an otherwise healthy person is an indication for surgical repair to prevent the risk of rupture. Treatment may also be recommended for smaller aneurysms in certain patients. These include but are not limited to patients with high blood pressure, pulmonary disease, or a positive family history of AAA and persons who live far away from major medical centers.

Traditional open treatment of an abdominal aortic aneurysm involves replacement of the diseased blood vessel with graft material. Modern AAA repair by trained vascular surgeons has evolved from a chest-to-pelvis incision with multiple ICU and in-hospital days to a relatively small left- or right-flank incision and a much quicker recovery. In our vascular practice, the average ICU stay is 1 day and the average hospital stay is 3 to 4 days. Most patients tolerate this type of open surgery very well and experience few, if any, complications. Death after elective aneurysm repair is exceedingly unusual in centers of excellence and in the hands of a vascular surgeon who performs a large number of these procedures on a yearly basis. Long-term problems are also uncommon, and the risk of rupture is essentially reduced to zero. Life quality is well maintained by the overwhelming majority of patients who have timely treatment.

Although open AAA repair is the gold standard, many patients desire a less invasive treatment option. Endovascular repair of AAA is now mainstream and within the armamentarium of the trained vascular surgeon. This endovascular procedure begins with two-incisions over each artery in the groin instead of a left-flank incision. In some cases, the entire procedure can be accomplished with percutaneous vessel access. Then using x-ray imaging and endovascular techniques, a stent graft (endograft) is guided through the femoral artery into the infrarenal abdominal aneurysm. The stent graft is then deployed inside the aneurysm using balloon angioplasty techniques and appropriately positioned to fully exclude the aneurysm sac. Because the endograft is secured to the healthy artery above and below the aneurysm, blood flow and arterial pressure are essentially diverted away from the aneurysm through the endograft by bridging the aneurysm sac.

Advantages of this treatment option include no ICU stay, a slightly shorter hospital stay, and in most cases, a remarkably quick overall recovery. However, this procedure is not recommended for every patient with an aneurysm. Rigorous long-term radiographic follow-up is mandatory to ensure that the device remains stable without failure, fracture, or migration and that the aneurysm sac remains stable or decreases in size. In some cases, secondary procedures are required to ensure that the aneurysm sac remains out of circulation or that the stent graft limbs remain patent. Nevertheless, midterm data are encouraging regarding this evolving technology, and the morbidity of this procedure compared with an open surgical procedure is certainly reduced. This decrease in surgical morbidity is most evident after endovascular repair of thoracic aneurysms and hybrid open and endovascular repair of thoracoabdominal aortic aneurysms. In any case, AAA repair via open surgery or by endovascular means is highly successful in preventing untimely death from rupture.

REFERENCES

Aronow WS: Management of peripheral arterial disease of the lower extremities in elderly patients. J Gerontol A Biol Sci Med Sci 2004;59:172-177.

Ballard JL (ed): Aortic Surgery. Georgetown, Tex: Landes Bioscience, 2000.

Mohler ER: Peripheral arterial disease: Identification and implications. Arch Intern Med 2003;163:2306-2314.

Moore WS: Fundamental considerations in cerebrovascular disease. In Rutherford RB (ed): Vascular Surgery, 6th ed. Philadelphia: WB Saunders, 2005, pp 1879-1896.

Norgren L, Hiatt WR, Dormandy JA, et al: TASC II Working Group: Inter-Society Consensus for the Management of Peripheral Arterial Disease (TASC II). J Vasc Surg 2007;45(Suppl S):S5-S67.

Venous Thrombosis

Method of
Paul L. F. Giangrande, MD

Air Travel And Thrombosis

The subject of air travel and thrombosis has been the subject of much debate in both the lay and medical press in recent years, although a possible link has been recognized for many years, and the very first report concerned a physician who traveled from Boston to Venezuela in 1946. However, venous thromboembolism is not exclusively associated with air travel, and it has also been documented following long car, bus, and train journeys.

A case-control study of 160 consecutive patients with deep venous thrombosis (DVT) showed that 39 of 160 (24.5%) had recently completed a journey by car, train, or plane of longer than 4 hours; nine of these patients had traveled by air. When the patients with DVT were compared with the control group, a history of recent travel was reported four times more often in the subjects with venous thromboembolism (odds ratio [OR] = 4). This correlation has been confirmed by a recent and much larger case-control study, the Multiple Environment and Genetic Assessment (MEGA) study, from the Netherlands, which confirmed that travel by car, bus, train, or plane is associated with an increased risk of venous thrombosis. Thrombosis associated with flight is also by no means restricted to those in the relatively confined conditions of economy class, and thus the alternative term of "travelers' thrombosis" has been suggested.

It is possible to derive some general conclusions from published cases of venous thromboembolism associated with travel. Thromboembolism is rarely observed after flights of less than 5 hours, and typically, the flights are 12 hours or longer. The risk rises with age, and persons older than 50 years are more at risk, whereas those younger than 40 years are less vulnerable. Symptoms of thromboembolism do not usually develop during or immediately after the flight but tend to appear within 3 days of arrival, when the patient may present far away from the airport, and thus the causal link might not be immediately apparent. Symptoms of thrombosis or pulmonary embolism have been reported up to 2 weeks after a long flight. Pulmonary embolism may also be the first manifestation, without any symptoms in the lower limbs. Although most case reports and studies involve DVT in the lower limbs, there are also reports of cerebral venous thrombosis and arterial thrombosis associated with long flights.

The consequences of venous thromboembolism are not insignificant. Quite apart from the pain and discomfort, which can ruin a holiday or business trip, pulmonary embolism is estimated to develop in approximately 10% of cases. The mortality associated with pulmonary embolism rises with increasing age, but it is in the range of 2% to 15% of cases. The inconvenience and side effects of warfarin treatment should also not be overlooked.

Approximately 60% of patients develop postphlebitis syndrome (persistent swelling and discomfort of the leg, often associated with ulceration) within 2 years despite appropriate anticoagulant therapy. A history of thrombosis precludes future prescription of hormone replacement therapy (HRT) or oral contraceptive pills (OCPs) for women, and it can make it difficult to secure travel insurance in the future because of the increased risk of recurrence.

Epidemiology

The precise incidence of thromboembolism in relation to air travel is uncertain, though it has been estimated that at least 5% of all cases of DVT may be linked to air travel. A study based on 56 confirmed cases of pulmonary embolism among 135.3 million passengers passing through one airport in the period between 1993 and 2000 clearly demonstrated an association between duration of travel and risk of pulmonary was significantly higher (1.5 cases per million) for passengers traveling more than 5000 km when compared with a risk of only 0.01 cases per million among passengers traveling less than 5000 km.

Cases of pulmonary embolism clearly only represent the tip of the iceberg of cases of DVT. A recent observational study from New Zealand, based on the study of 878 passengers who traveled extensively (at least 10 hours; mean, 39 hours) reported an incidence of venous thromboembolism of 1%, including four cases of pulmonary embolism and five of DVT. However, the incidence of latent, asymptomatic thrombosis is likely to be even higher. A prospective study of long-haul air passengers older than 50 years reported that 12 of 116 passengers (10%) were found by duplex scanning to have asymptomatic DVT confined to the calf.

Etiology

The etiology of venous thrombosis is usually multifactorial, with a combination of both constitutional and environmental factors responsible for causing a thrombosis in a patient at a given time. The three underlying causes of thrombosis are classically defined as Virchow's triad: stasis, hypercoagulability of the blood, and vessel wall disease.

Stasis in the venous circulation of the lower limbs is undoubtedly the major factor in promoting the development of venous thromboembolism associated with travel. The potential danger of confinement in cramped conditions has been recognized for some years. An increase in the incidence of fatal pulmonary embolism was reported during the Blitz in London during the Second World War. Simpson recognized that the primary cause was mechanical impairment of venous circulation due to squatting for a prolonged period in air raid shelters, and he recommended that bunks should be installed. The term *economy class syndrome* was coined to describe the phenomenon, and this also emphasizes the role of impaired venous circulation due to prolonged immobility in a cramped position. Ingestion of alcohol also encourages immobility during a flight, and the use of strong sedative medication may also be associated with an increased risk of venous thrombosis.

A number of other risk factors are now also recognized, primarily through clinical experience in the setting of surgery, which predispose to venous thromboembolism. These are listed in Box 1.

BOX 1 Risk Factors for Venous Thromboembolism

- Age greater than 40 years (but especially the elderly)
- Previous thrombotic episode (especially pulmonary embolism)
- Documented thrombophilic abnormality (e.g., antithrombin deficiency)
- Other hematologic disorders (polycythemia and thrombocythemia)
- Pregnancy and puerperium
- Malignancy
- Congestive heart failure or recent myocardial infarction
- Recent surgery (especially lower limb)
- Chronic venous insufficiency
- Estrogen therapy (e.g., OCP, HRT)
- Obesity
- Prolonged recent immobility (e.g., after recent stroke)
- Dehydration (diarrhea)

Abbreviations: HRT = hormone-replacement therapy; OCP = oral contraceptive pill.

The effect of age was highlighted in a recent study from Australia, which concluded that the annual risk of venous thromboembolism is increased by 12% if one long-haul flight is undertaken annually. However, the incidence of thromboembolism was less than 1 per 100,000 arriving passengers younger than 40 years, but it rose steadily to exceed 14 per 100,000 in those aged 75 years or older.

A hematologic abnormality might predispose a person to development of venous thromboembolism. Such disorders include the relatively rare congenital (inherited) deficiencies of natural anticoagulants, such as antithrombin, protein C, or protein S. A recent study demonstrated that an inherited thrombophilic defect or use of an OCP increased the risk of thrombosis associated with air travel 16-fold and 14-fold, respectively. The MEGA study has also demonstrated that positivity for the factor V Leiden thrombophilic mutation, body mass index greater than 30, height greater than 1.9 or less than 1.6 meters, and use of OCPs are strong susceptibility factors. In one small uncontrolled, retrospective study of patients with flight-related DVT, 6 of 20 (30%) subjects had a thrombophilic defect (factor V Leiden in 5). Four subjects had a history of a previous episode of thrombosis, and other potential risk factors were identified in 10 subjects (including malignancy, leg in plaster cast, use of OCP or HRT). Five of the 20 patients had a negative thrombophilia screen and no other identifiable risk factor.

The value of screening passengers for thrombophilic defects before long-haul flights has been raised. It is generally accepted that routine screening of passengers or screening of pilots as part of their medical screening is not justified or cost-effective. Such screening is not, of course, routinely offered in other circumstances associated with an increased risk of thrombosis (e.g., before starting an OCP, pregnancy, before orthopedic surgery), and no case has yet been established for air travel to be treated differently from current practice for thrombophilia screening in other fields.

Some evidence now suggests that exposure to the mild hypobaric hypoxia encountered in pressurized aircraft might also result in activation of the coagulation and thus encourage thrombosis. Aircraft typically fly at altitudes of between 35,000 and 40,000 feet to avoid turbulence and drag, thus benefiting fuel consumption. The cabin air is derived from the outside atmospheric air, which is drawn in and compressed. The maximum pressure in the cabin at cruising altitude is influenced by the allowable differential pressure across the wall of the cabin. This varies with aircraft design, but the lowest pressure permitted by the regulatory authorities for civil aircraft is equivalent to atmospheric pressure at an altitude of 8000 feet. Although the percentage of oxygen in the cabin remains unchanged at around

21%, the partial pressure of oxygen is reduced to around 74% of the sea level value. The very cold air at this altitude (typically around −50°C) contains only negligible water vapor, and the humidity in the cabin is thus typically very low.

Markers of activation of coagulation were transiently elevated in an uncontrolled study of 20 healthy male volunteers who were exposed to a hypobaric environment designed to simulate the conditions of an airplane cabin. The plasma levels of prothrombin fragments 1 and 2, thrombin-antithrombin (TAT) complex, and activated coagulation factor VII increased significantly, although the D-dimer level remained unchanged. Treatment with heparin inhibited the development of this apparent activation of the coagulation cascade. Another study of eight subjects who ascended rapidly to high altitudes by helicopter in Nepal documented increases in the levels of prothrombin fragments 1 and 2 and PAI-1 (plasminogen activator inhibitor, a key inhibitor of fibrinolysis). Activation of coagulation associated with flight, reflected by an increase in plasma levels of TAT complex, was also demonstrated in a crossover study in which 71 healthy volunteers were studied in the setting of an 8-hour flight, with the same volunteers monitored in two controlled-exposure situations.

Contrary to the widespread belief that passengers on long-haul flights can develop dehydration through increased insensible loss of water across the skin and mucous surfaces, it has been calculated that the maximum possible increase in insensible loss of water over an 8-hour period in such conditions is only around 100 mL. Although systemic dehydration is not a significant factor in healthy persons, the low humidity in an aircraft cabin can certainly lead to dryness of the mucous membranes and a sensation of thirst. Excessive consumption of alcohol or gastrointestinal infections associated with vomiting and diarrhea can also exacerbate dehydration.

Prevention

A number of general measures may be taken to minimize the risk of thrombosis associated with long flights. Perhaps the most important step is to consider at the outset whether the passenger is actually fit to fly in the first place. For example, it is probably wise to defer long-haul travel after recent major orthopedic surgery. Passengers should be encouraged to carry out leg exercises from time to time while seated (e.g., flexion, extension, and rotation of the ankles help to promote circulation in the lower limbs). However, many airlines discourage unnecessary walking about in the cabin because there is always the possibility of encountering unexpected air turbulence. Hand luggage stowed under seats also restricts movement. Passengers should take advantage of refueling stops on long-haul flights to get off the plane and walk around for awhile. Adequate hydration should be ensured during the flight. It is not necessary to abstain from alcohol, but excessive consumption should be avoided because it promotes diuresis and discourages mobility. Similarly, sedatives are best avoided. Although estrogen-containing OCPs and HRT are recognized risk factors for venous thrombosis, I do not advocate interrupting such hormonal medication for the period of travel.

A recent review of 10 randomized studies for the Cochrane database has confirmed the value of compression hosiery (flight socks). In the very first study performed, 231 passengers were recruited before long-haul flights and randomized into two groups. Of those who did not wear compression hosiery, 12 of 116 (10%) were found after the flight to have asymptomatic calf DVT with duplex ultrasonography, but none of the 115 who wore compression hosiery was affected. In the LONFLIT-4 study of 372 passengers considered to be at medium to high risk of thromboembolism, none of the 179 subjects wearing compression hosiery developed DVT, but six of 179 (3.35%) controls developed asymptomatic DVT (four DVT, two superficial) ($P < 0.002$). In the subsequent LONFLIT-5 study of 224 high-risk passengers who went on an even longer flight, DVT was observed in six of 102 (5.8%) control subjects and only one of 103 (0.97%) subjects wearing compression hosiery ($P < 0.0025$). Quite apart from reducing the risk of thrombosis, compression hosiery helps to prevent edema of the legs and feet, which can itself cause discomfort after a long flight.

Flight socks have the advantage of being readily available without prescription and are washable and thus reusable. They apply graduated pressure to the leg that is maximal at the ankle, thus encouraging venous return. The usual full-length stockings used in hospitals for prophylaxis of thromboembolism in patients undergoing surgery are not suitable for use in flight because they provide a lower pressure at the ankle (UK Class I standard: 14-17 mm Hg) because they are designed for recumbent patients. It is also important that the patient is provided with the correct type and size of compression stocking; unfortunately, there is no internationally agreed standard with regard to the degree of compression. The stockings also need to be worn correctly, taking care to ensure that there is no constriction in the popliteal area. Stockings are contraindicated in cases of peripheral vascular disease because the additional compression could provoke ischemia.

Aspirin[1] has been advocated by some in the general prophylaxis of thrombosis associated with travel, but any beneficial effect is weak in absolute terms. Aspirin is certainly very effective in preventing arterial thrombosis, because platelets play a major role in thrombosis in the arterial circulation. Arterial thrombi are rich in platelets on histologic examination, whereas thrombi in the venous circulation consist primarily of red cells enmeshed in fibrin strands but contain few platelets. It has been estimated that if the rate of travel-related DVT is 20 per 100,000 travelers, then 17,000 people would need to be treated with aspirin to prevent just one episode of DVT. Furthermore, there is a significant FDA potential for adverse reactions: 13% of subjects taking aspirin in a study to evaluate its potential in preventing venous thrombosis associated with air travel reported gastrointestinal symptoms such as dyspepsia. Heparin may be considered in the relatively few passengers considered to be at particularly high risk for thrombosis (e.g., history of more than one thrombotic episode and an identified thrombophilic abnormality), although many such subjects are already likely to be on long-term oral anticoagulation anyway.

Unfortunately, there are no consensus guidelines yet and it is clear that there is still a wide difference in practice. This was emphasized by the results of a survey of more than 2000 delegates attending an international conference on thrombosis in Australia, which noted that 80% had taken precautions to prevent travel-related thrombosis. Just 17% wore compression hosiery and 21% relied on aspirin either alone or in combination with other measures.

Summary

It is now generally accepted that there is an association between long-distance air travel as well as other forms of long-distance travel and venous thromboembolism. The risk is largely confined to those with recognized additional risk factors for venous thromboembolism. Leg exercises while seated help to reduce the risk of DVT. There is also clear evidence from prospective and randomized clinical trials to support the use of compression hosiery as a preventive measure. By contrast, there is no firm evidence to support the indiscriminate use of aspirin as a routine prophylactic measure.

REFERENCES

Ashkan K, Nasim A, Dennis MJ, Sayers RD: Acute arterial thrombosis after a long-haul flight. J R Soc Med 1998;91:324.

Belcaro G, Cesarone MR, Shah SS, et al: Prevention of edema, flight microangiopathy and venous thrombosis in long flights with elastic stockings. A randomized trial: The LONFLIT 4 Concorde Edema-SSL Study. Angiology 2002;53:635-645.

Belcaro G, Cesarone MR, Nicolaides AN, et al: Prevention of venous thrombosis with elastic stockings during long-haul flights: The LONFLIT 5 JAP study. Clin Appl Thromb Hemost 2003;9:197-201.

Bendz B, Rostrup M, Sevre K, et al: Association between hypobaric hypoxia and activation of coagulation in human beings. Lancet 2000;356:1657-1658.

---

[1]Not FDA approved for this indication.

Bendz B, Sevre K, Andersen TO, Sandset PM: Low molecular weight heparin prevents activation of coagulation in a hypobaric environment. Blood Coagul Fibrinolysis 2001;12:371-374.

Cannegieter SC, Doggen CJ, van Houwelingen HC, Rosendaal FR: Travel-related venous thrombosis: Results from a large population-based case control study (MEGA study). PLoS Med 2006;3:e307.

Cesarone MR, Belcaro G, Nicolaides AN, et al: Venous thrombosis from air travel: The LONFLIT 3 study—prevention with aspirin vs. low molecular weight heparin (LMWH) in high risk subjects: A randomized trial. Angiology 2002;53:1-6.

Clarke M, Hopewell S, Juszczak E, et al: Compression stockings for preventing deep vein thrombosis in airline passengers. Cochrane Database Syst Rev 2006;(2):CD004002.

Collins REC, Field S, Castleden WM: Thrombosis of leg arteries after prolonged travel. BMJ 1979;2:1478.

Cruickshank JM, Gorlin R, Jennett B: Air travel and thrombotic episodes: The economy class syndrome. Lancet 1988;2:497-498.

Giangrande PLF: Air travel and thrombosis. Br J Haematol 2002;117:509-512.

Hagg S, Spigset O: Antipsychotic-induced venous thromboembolism: A review of the evidence. CNS Drugs 2002;16:765-776.

Homans J: Thrombosis of the deep leg veins due to prolonged sitting. N Engl J Med 1954;250:148-149.

Hughes RJ, Hopkins RJ, Hill S, et al: Frequency of venous thromboembolism in low to moderate risk long distance air travellers: The New Zealand Air Traveller's Thrombosis (NZATT) Study. Lancet 2003;362:2039-2044.

Kelman CW, Kortt MA, Becker NG, et al: Deep vein thrombosis and air travel: Record linkage study. BMJ 2003;327:1072-1075.

Kuipers S, Cannegieter SC, Middeldorp S, et al: Use of preventive measures for air travel–related venous thrombosis in professionals who attend medical conferences. J Thromb Haemost 2006;4:2373-2376.

Lapostolle F, Surget V, Borron SW, et al: Severe pulmonary embolism associated with air travel. N Engl J Med 2001;345:779-783.

Loke YK, Derry S: Air travel and venous thrombosis: How much help might aspirin be? Med Gen Med 2002;4:4 Available at http://www.medscape.com/viewarticle/441153 (accessed June 1, 2007).

Martinelli I, Taioli E, Battaglioli T, et al: Risk of venous thromboembolism after air travel: Interaction with thrombophilia and oral contraceptives. Arch Intern Med 2006;163:2674-2676.

Mannucci PM, Gringeri A, Peyvandi F, et al: Short-term exposure to high altitude causes coagulation activation and inhibits fibrinolysis. Thromb Haemost 2002;87:342-343.

Nicholson AN: Dehydration and long haul flights. Travel Med Int 1998;16:177-181.

Pfausler B, Vollert H, Bosch S, Schmutzhard E: Cerebral venous thrombosis: A new diagnosis in travel medicine. J Travel Med 1996;3:165-167.

Rege KP, Bevan DH, Chitolie A, Shannon MS: Risk factors and thrombosis after airline flight. Thromb Haemost 1999;81:995-996.

Rosendaal FR: Venous thrombosis: A multicausal disease. Lancet 1999;353:1167-1173.

Schreijer AJM, Cannegieter SC, Meijers JCM, et al: Activation of coagulation system during air travel: A crossover study. Lancet 2006;367:832-838.

Scurr JH, Machin SJ, Bailey-King S, et al: Frequency and prevention of symptomless deep-vein thrombosis in long-haul flights: A randomized trial. Lancet 2001;357:1485-1489.

Simpson K: Shelter deaths from pulmonary embolism. Lancet 1940;11:744.

Teenen RP, MacKay AJ: Peripheral arterial thrombosis related to commercial airline flights: Another manifestation of the economy class syndrome. Br J Clin Prac 1992;46:165-166.

Thomassen R, Vandenbroucke JP, Rosendaal FR: Antipsychotic drugs and venous thrombosis. Br J Psychiatry 2001;179:63-66.

Zornberg GL, Jick H: Antipsychotic drug use and risk of first-time idiopathic venous thromboembolism: A case-control study. Lancet 2000;356:1219-1223.

SECTION 6

The Blood and Spleen

Aplastic Anemia

Method of
Eva C. Guinan, MD

The survival of patients with aplastic anemia has improved dramatically in the past several decades. Improved testing for underlying acquired and congenital genetic defects has served to better segregate patients with idiopathic aplastic anemia from those with the very different prognoses associated with an inherited bone marrow failure syndrome (IBMFS) and myelodysplasia (MDS). For patients in the idiopathic (or acquired) aplastic anemia group, advances in transfusion medicine and other supportive care have also certainly contributed. Refinements in both major arms of treatment, immunosuppressive therapy (IST), and allogeneic hematopoietic stem cell transplantation (HSCT), have also contributed to current outcomes (Fig. 1). Although IST survival curves have been stable in the last decade, survival after HSCT regardless of donor source has continued to improve. Greater understanding of pathophysiology and long-term treatment outcomes are having the largest impact on triage of therapy and standards of practice.

Definition

There is no pathognomonic diagnostic test for aplastic anemia. Accordingly, aplastic anemia continues to be diagnosed by a combination of inclusion and exclusion criteria. The definition established by the International Agranulocytosis and Aplastic Anaemia Study states that patients must have bone marrow hypocellularity with two or more of the following: hemoglobin of less than 10 g/dL, platelet count of less than 50×10^9/L, and neutrophil count of less than 1.5×10^9/L. Most commonly, patients said to have aplastic anemia in fact have severe aplastic anemia, which is defined by the absolute neutrophil count (ANC) as shown in Box 1. Severity grading has become part of the diagnostic algorithm and is increasingly used as a predictor of outcome.

Differential Diagnosis

Because many conditions can fulfill these inclusion criteria, care must be taken to consider infectious, metabolic, and toxic exposures that could result in transient pancytopenia. Specific considerations are listed in many current reviews. These diagnoses are wide ranging and include hypoplastic presentations of lymphoma, leukemia, and MDS; anorexia; and transient severe bone marrow suppression due to drug exposure or, albeit rarely, a spectrum of acute viral illnesses.

Patients should be carefully evaluated for other conditions that can require an alternative management approach. A small fraction of pancytopenic and hypocellular patients have clonal cytogenetic abnormalities despite well-reviewed histology that appears to be free of any evidence of dysplasia or infiltrative disease. Accordingly, best practice should include both fluorescent in situ hybridization (FISH) and routine cytogenetics, because the yield for the latter analysis may be inadequate given the hypocellularity of the bone marrow compartment.

Although the prognostic relevance of clonal cytogenetics remains somewhat debatable, evidence of clonality at diagnosis should certainly provoke consideration of MDS as an alternative diagnosis and mandate an aggressive plan of follow-up and determination of HSCT donor status. Clonality also potentially alters immediate treatment depending on the clinical setting and most current literature. Among infectious problems, perhaps the most important consideration from a diagnostic and management perspective is HIV. However, viruses rarely cause a true aplastic picture, and their diagnosis, at present, does not have much therapeutic importance. Aplastic anemia can occur or recur during pregnancy and can resolve with either delivery or termination.

The most important alternative diagnoses are the IBMFSs (Table 1), which should be considered in virtually all patients and certainly in all pediatric patients. Such a diagnosis has important implications for medical management of the extended family, for genetic counseling, for the choice of therapy, for prognosis of the patient, and, in the setting of HSCT, for donor evaluation. A meticulous patient and family history and physical examination should be performed, although uninformative results do not eliminate the possibility of an IBMFS. Genetic testing is now widely available for some IBMFSs; however, it is clear that these syndromes are polygenic, and the relevant genetic defects have not all been defined. Therefore, testing might not be diagnostic. As additional mutations are described and as the natural history and phenotype of various mutations and polymorphisms become better elucidated, this information should be of increasing value.

In addition to IBMFS, an evaluation for paroxysmal nocturnal hemoglobinuria (PNH) should be undertaken. A clonal populations of cells deficient in glycosylphosphatidylinositol (GPI)-linked proteins that characterize PNH can be found in 20% to 40% of adults with aplastic anemia without a concurrent history of clotting or hemolysis. A similar percentage of children has been found to have such cells in their bone marrow. The presence of such cells does not imply a diagnosis of classic PNH, although some patients with apparent aplastic anemia do develop classic PNH. Ongoing clinical investigation into the relation of aplastic anemia and PNH might yield further information that will assist in therapeutic decision making.

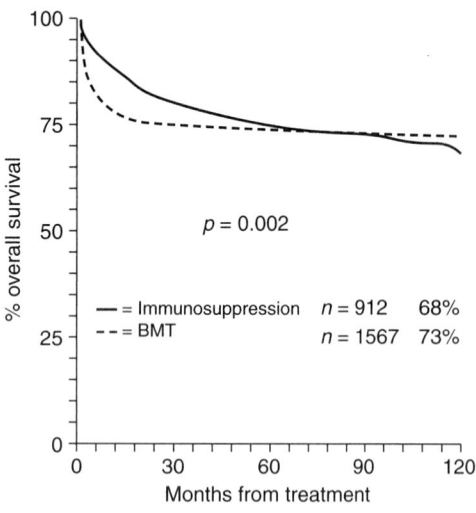

FIGURE 1. The actuarial survival of 2479 patients with acquired severe aplastic anemia. Group A received immunosuppressive therapy (IST) *(solid line)* as first-line therapy and Group B underwent hematopoietic stem cell transplant (BMT) *(dashed line)*. Ten-year survival was 73% with BMT and 68% with IST ($P < 0.002$). Data from Locasciulli A, Oneto R, Bacigalupo A, et al: Outcome of patients with acquired aplastic anemia given first-line bone marrow transplantation or immunosuppressive treatment in the last decade: A report from the European Group for Blood and Marrow Transplantation (EBMT). Haematologica 2007;92:11-18.

Supportive Care

The goals of supportive care in aplastic anemia are alleviating symptoms of anemia and addressing the risks of hemorrhage and infection that result from pancytopenia. Appropriate precautions for minimizing alloimmunization should be taken, such as use of leukodepletion techniques and conservative transfusion goals.

Preemptive counseling can play as important a role as symptom management. There are few evidence-based guidelines for activities of daily living, such as the quality of diet, extent of exercise, and travel restrictions. The best standard is frequent, open communication between physician and patient. Some practical issues, however, are common. For example, the menstrual status of female patients should be ascertained immediately on diagnosis. Because severe menorrhagia can occur in the setting of protracted thrombocytopenia, use of hormonal therapy to suppress menstruation

---

BOX 1   Severity Classification of Aplastic Anemia

Severe
Bone marrow cellularity <25%
and
Two peripheral blood findings:
- Absolute neutrophil count $<0.5 \times 10^9$/L
- Platelet count $<20 \times 10^9$/L
- Reticulocyte count $<20 \times 10^9$/L

Very Severe
Same criteria as for severe
and
Peripheral blood absolute neutrophil count $<0.2 \times 10^9$/L

Nonsevere (Moderate)
Hypocellullar bone marrow
and
Peripheral blood cytopenias not meeting criteria for severe aplastic anemia

---

 CURRENT DIAGNOSIS

- Patient must all meet hematologic criteria.
- Assess severity.
- Adequate cytogenetic analysis is essential.
- Consider diagnoses with treatment implications:
  - Causes of transient pancytopenia.
  - Evaluate for inherited bone marrow failure syndromes, paroxysmal nocturnal hemoglobinuria, myelodysplasia syndrome.
  - Evaluate for malignancy (leukemia, lymphoma), HIV.

---

should be addressed with patients and with families of younger patients. Particular regard should be paid to anticipation of menarche in pubertal girls.

With regard to infectious risks, standards widely vary by practitioner and institution. Although the largest single cause of death in patients undergoing either HSCT or IST is infection, there is no current standard for infection prophylaxis in aplastic anemia. Clinical trials to define the best possible approaches to this issue, including the role of novel broad-spectrum anti-infectives and their schedule of use, would be very important. At the least, a detailed history taken in the context of exposure and lifestyle issues should be used to develop a plan for fever and infection prophylaxis with which the patient can be compliant.

Benefit from the use of hematopoietic growth factors to support the ANC, or indeed any lineage, has been unclear in patients with idiopathic aplastic anemia. Some concern has been raised about the association of long-term use of granulocyte colony-stimulating factor (G-CSF) (Neupogen)[1] by patients, particularly children, with aplastic anemia and subsequent development of MDS and acute myelogenous leukemia (AML), although this remains uncertain.

Monitoring of iron status should be routine for patients with ongoing red cell transfusion needs. Chelation should be initiated according to accepted guidelines to minimize complications of iron overload.

Treatment

Observation is not a successful treatment option for patients with severe aplastic anemia; older, retrospective data demonstrate a 1-year mortality with supportive care alone of more than 80%, although clearly more effective current transfusion and support strategies would improve on this outcome. Nonetheless, a recent large report from the European Group for Blood and Marrow Transplantation demonstrates that decreased time from diagnosis to treatment, whether IST or HSCT, is a highly significant predictor of survival. A triage of therapy is shown in Figure 2.

IMMUNOSUPPRESSIVE THERAPY

It is generally held that a significant percentage of aplastic anemia has an immune pathogenesis. A variety of data on immune effector cell function and repertoire, cell surface phenotype, and cytokine production support this belief. In practice, this hypothesis is also supported by the observation that IST with cyclosporine (Neoral)[1] (CSA), antithymocyte globulin (Atgam) (ATG), and corticosteroids results in response in roughly 75% of patients.

Age and response are related, and younger patients generally have a higher likelihood of response. It has also been reported that children with IST and very severe aplastic anemia do better than their age peers with severe aplastic anemia and that children (<16 years) with very severe aplastic anemia have better survival rates than

---

[1]Not FDA approved for this indication.

TABLE 1 Inherited Bone Marrow Failure Syndromes Commonly Associated with Pancytopenia*

Syndrome	Common Hematologic Findings	Diagnostic Tests Available[†]
Amegakaryocytic thrombocytopenia	Thrombocytopenia with absent or hypolobulated megakaryocytes Macrocytosis Progressive pancytopenia with marrow hypoplasia	Gene mutation analysis
Dyskeratosis congenita	Macrocytosis Thrombocytopenia Progressive pancytopenia with marrow hypoplasia	Gene mutation analysis Telomere length (may be shortened)
Fanconi's anemia	Macrocytosis Single, bilineage or trilineage cytopenia Progressive pancytopenia with marrow hypoplasia	Abnormal chromosomal breakage or sister-chromatid exchange in the presence of DNA cross-linkers Cell cycle progression in the presence of DNA cross-linkers Gene mutation analysis
Shwachman–Diamond syndrome	Neutropenia Progressive pancytopenia with marrow hypoplasia	Radiologic bony abnormalities Serum trypsinogen and isoamylase levels (may be decreased) Gene mutation analysis

*Diamond–Blackfan anemia, as well as less common disorders such as Pearson's, Seckel's, and Noonan's syndromes; cartilage–hair hypoplasia; and reticular dysgenesis, can progress to marrow failure meeting the definition of aplastic anemia.
[†]Clinically approved mutation testing is becoming increasingly available, but not all genetic defects have been defined for any of these disorders.

similarly affected adults. Age does not affect the relative survival rate of patients with less severe aplastic anemia.

Randomized studies have demonstrated better response when IST agents are used in combination. In addition to their general immunomodulatory capacity, the immunologic effects of IST may be specific, because direct lympholytic and bone marrow stimulatory activities have been described. The addition of further immunosuppressive medications, such as mycophenolate, to this regimen has thus far not improved outcomes.

IST responses can be of varying degree and duration and can take 3 to 6 months to become evident. Often, responding patients continue to manifest some evidence of bone marrow failure, with mild degrees of cytopenia or residual macrocytosis commonly observed. Slow taper of CSA in IST responders is advisable, generally over longer than 6 months, and a significant fraction of patients demonstrate prolonged dependence on CSA for persistent hematologic improvement. A second course of IST in patients who failed a first course can produce response in 35% to 50% of patients. Complete or

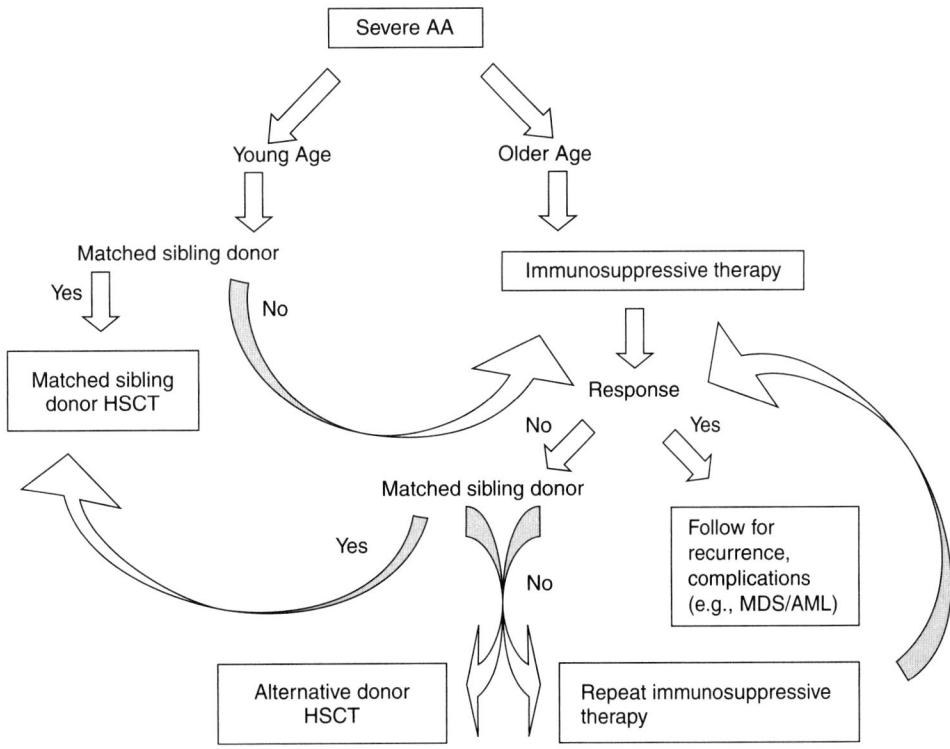

FIGURE 2. Triage of aplastic anemia (AA) therapies. The age limit suggested by young/old is variable from report to report, but generally sits in the 30 to 40-year-old range. AML = acute myelogenous leukemia; HSCT = hematopoietic stem cell transplant; MDS = myelodysplasia.

CURRENT THERAPY

- Minimize interval between diagnosis and initiation of treatment.
- Determine if an MSD is available.
- If the patient is young and has an MSD, proceed to HSCT with non-TBI regimen.
- If has no MSD or is older, proceed to IST with CSA/ATG/steroid.
- For treatment failure, reconsider IST versus HSCT options.

ATG = antithymocyte globulin; CSA = cyclosporine; HSCT = hematopoietic stem cell transplantation; IST = immunosuppressive therapy; MSD = matched sibling donor; TBI = total body irradiation.

partial loss of response occurs in an appreciable number of patients, approximately one third, and can become manifest years after cessation of IST or immediately on CSA taper. Re-treatment with the same or a similar regimen is often successful.

HEMATOPOIETIC STEM CELL TRANSPLANTATION

HSCT is the only truly curative therapy for aplastic anemia and produces stable survival rates in the range of 60% to 80%, depending on donor type and other HSCT variables (Fig. 3). In young patients with matched sibling donors (MSDs), a short interval from diagnosis to HSCT, and little prior therapy, survival rates up to 97% have been recently reported. Conversely, prior IST or excessive transfusion (or both) are associated with worse outcome. Thus, the general recommendation is for young patients with MSDs to proceed to HSCT as soon as the diagnosis is confirmed. The age cutoff for this decision varies somewhat, but the recommendation certainly holds for patients younger than 30 years and is often implemented for those younger than 40 years.

HSCT for aplastic anemia from MSD can be successfully achieved with radiation-free preparative regimens, of which the most standard and widely used is cyclophosphamide (Cytoxan)[1] (CY) and ATG conditioning. CSA and short-course methotrexate (Trexall)[1] (MTX) provide highly effective graft-versus-host disease (GVHD) prophylaxis in this setting. In a group of adults and children undergoing MSD allogeneic HSCT, this classic CY/ATG/CSA/MTX regimen produced a 96% rate of sustained engraftment, 3% rate of severe acute GVHD, 26% rate of chronic GVHD, and overall survival of 88% at median follow-up of 9 years. A recent study suggests that ATG may not be as essential to this outcome as previously thought. All stem cell sources, including sibling umbilical cord blood, have been used successfully, although use of peripheral blood stem cells appears to result in an unacceptably high rate of chronic GHVD and is not currently advised.

The dearth of alternative therapies for those who fail to respond to IST, coupled with the success of MSD HSCT, have encouraged the use of alternative-donor HSCT for aplastic anemia. Originally, the use of somewhat more aggressive regimens than those necessary with MSD engendered more regimen-related toxicity, and patients coming to alternative-donor HSCT were often late in their clinical course with significant aplastic anemia–associated morbidity. Outcomes were somewhat disappointing. Results have improved significantly over the past decade, and even more so over the past 5 years (see Fig. 3B). Moving HSCT treatment earlier in therapeutic triage, coupled with improvements in histocompatibility typing, better supportive care, and the successful implementation of reduced-intensity regimens and alternative immunosuppressive strategies have produced highly encouraging results, with an overall survival in excess of 70% in some reports. However, the best results are seen when patients are younger, and outcomes in those older than 40 years remain less satisfactory.

[1]Not FDA approved for this indication.

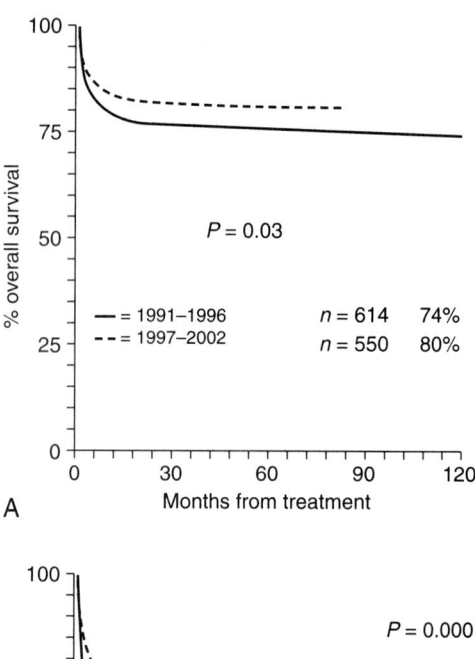

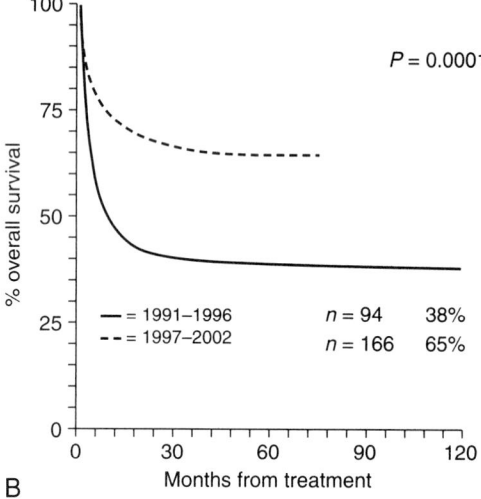

FIGURE 3. The actuarial survival of patients undergoing hematopoietic stem cell transplantation (HSCT) from matched sibling donors (**A**) or alternative donors (**B**) by time periods. Results improved for both donor groups in the later time period (matched sibling donors 74% vs 80%, $P = 0.03$) and alternative donors (38% vs 65%, $P = 0.0001$). Data from Locasciulli A, Oneto R, Bacigalupo A, et al: Outcome of patients with acquired aplastic anemia given first line bone marrow transplantation or immunosuppressive treatment in the last decade: A report from the European Group for Blood and Marrow Transplantation (EBMT). Haematologica 2007; 92:11-18.

Long-Term Complications of Treatment

All aplastic anemia treatments can be associated with significant morbidity, be it the iron-overload of chronic transfusion or the more protean problems of IST or HSCT. These include, in both cases, significant regimen-related end-organ toxicity. The development of clonal cytogenetic abnormalities after IST is well described and occurs in patients of all ages, regardless of treatment response, and over a broad time frame. The rate of progression to frank AML is not predictable, although progression is most common in those with monosomy 7 or complex cytogenetic abnormalities. Patients with aplastic anemia who undergo HSCT generally experience fewer toxicities than does the overall HSCT population, in part due to the reduced intensity of aplastic anemia regimens. Growth and fertility may be well preserved, but persistent infectious complications, pulmonary insufficiency, dermatologic pathology, avascular necrosis, and other bone and joint issues, as well as hypothyroidism or other endocrine disturbances, can occur, as can secondary malignancies. Some of these conditions reflect the sequelae of chronic GVHD itself, and others reflect the toxicity of drugs used to manage GVHD. The toll of GVHD is real; decreased quality of life and overall survival are observed in the nearly one half of aplastic anemia patients experiencing chronic GVHD.

Conclusions

Improvements in diagnosis, supportive care, IST, and HSCT have led to significant improvements in survival for patients with severe aplastic anemia. However, there are still controversies over the optimal choice of therapy for individual patients, and any given choice can lead to a number of serious regimen-related toxicities. Further insights into the pathophysiology of bone marrow failure, increased diagnostic accuracy for IBMFS, greater appreciation of the risk and epidemiology of late complications, and steady progress in therapeutics will hopefully combine to yield increasingly well-targeted and more-successful treatment.

Acknowledgments

Eva C. Guinan is a recipient of a Specified Established Researcher Award from the Aplastic Anemia & MDS International Foundation.

REFERENCES

Ades L, Mary JY, Robin M, et al: Long-term outcome after bone marrow transplantation for severe aplastic anemia. Blood 2004;103:2490-2497.
Alter BP: Bone marrow failure: A child is not just a small adult (but an adult can have a childhood disease). Hematology (Am Soc Hematol Educ Program) 2005:96-103.
Frickhofen N, Heimpel H, Kaltwasser JP, Schrezenmeier H: Antithymocyte globulin with or without cyclosporin A: 11-year follow-up of a randomized trial comparing treatments of aplastic anemia. Blood 2003;101:1236-1242.
Fuhrer M, Burdach S, Ebell W, et al: Relapse and clonal disease in children with aplastic anemia (AA) after immunosuppressive therapy (IST): The SAA 94 experience. German/Austrian Pediatric Aplastic Anemia Working Group. Klin Padiatr 1998;210:173-179.
Kojima S, Horibe K, Inaba J, et al: Long-term outcome of acquired aplastic anaemia in children: Comparison between immunosuppressive therapy and bone marrow transplantation. Br J Haematol 2000;111:321-328.
Kurre P, Johnson FL, Deeg HJ: Diagnosis and treatment of children with aplastic anemia. Pediatr Blood Cancer 2005;45:770-780.
Locasciulli A, Oneto R, Bacigalupo A, et al: Outcome of patients with acquired aplastic anemia given first line bone marrow transplantation or immunosuppressive treatment in the last decade: A report from the European Group for Blood and Marrow Transplantation (EBMT). Haematologica 2007;92:11-18.
Maciejewski JP, Risitano A, Sloand EM, et al: Distinct clinical outcomes for cytogenetic abnormalities evolving from aplastic anemia. Blood 2002; 99:3129-3135.
Marsh JCW, Ball SE, Darbyshire P, et al: Guidelines for the diagnosis and management of acquired aplastic anaemia. Br J Haematol 2003;123:782-801.
Parker C, Omine M, Richards S, et al: Diagnosis and management of paroxysmal nocturnal hemoglobinuria. Blood 2005;106:3699-3709.
Schrezenmeier H, Passweg JR, Marsh JC, et al: Worse outcome and more chronic GVHD with peripheral blood progenitor cells than bone marrow in HLA-matched sibling donor transplants for young patients with severe acquired aplastic anemia: A report from the European Group for Blood and Marrow Transplantation and the Center for International Blood and Marrow Transplant Research. Blood 2007; 110(4):1397-1400.
Socie G, Gluckman E: Cure from severe aplastic anemia in vivo and late effects. Acta Haematologica 2000;103:49-54.
Socie G, Mary JY, Schrezenmeier H, et al: Granulocyte-stimulating factor and severe aplastic anemia: a survey by the European Group for Blood and Marrow Transplantation (EBMT). Blood 2007;109:2794-2796.
Young NS: Paroxysmal nocturnal hemoglobinuria: Current issues in pathophysiology and treatment. Curr Hematol Rep 2005;4:103-109.
Young NS, Calado RT, Scheinberg P: Current concepts in the pathophysiology and treatment of aplastic anemia. Blood 2006;108:2509-2519.

Iron Deficiency

Method of
James C. Barton, MD

Iron deficiency is common worldwide. In developed countries, iron requirements of reproductive-age women (menstruation, pregnancy, lactation) and the increased iron requirements for growth in infants and children often exceed dietary iron availability and absorption. Pathologic blood loss in men and postmenopausal women, especially that from the gastrointestinal tract, is also a common cause of iron deficiency. In less well-developed areas, diets poor in absorbable iron, vegetarianism, intestinal parasitism, chronic diarrhea, and multiparity are common causes of iron deficiency.

Successful treatment of iron deficiency depends on identification and management of its cause(s) and administration of a regimen that takes into account the cause and severity of iron deficiency, comorbid disorders, and concomitant medications.

Normal Iron Metabolism

Body iron quantities are regulated by controlled absorption that responds to the rate of erythropoiesis and other body demands. Quantities of total body iron in healthy adults are approximately 4.0 g in men and 3.5 g in women. Hemoglobin in men contains about 2.0 g Fe and in women about 1.5 g Fe. Storage sites in men contain about 1.0 g and in women about 0.3 g. The remaining iron, approximately 6% of total body quantities, is incorporated in myoglobin, heme-containing enzymes, transferrin, and other compounds.

Dietary iron typically consists of heme derived from animal products, nonheme ionic iron in vegetable foods, and inorganic iron added to fortify certain foodstuffs. Iron compounds must be soluble for absorption to occur. Heme iron is readily soluble. Absorption of nonheme iron is facilitated by gastric acid, ascorbic acid (vitamin C), and certain amino acids and sugars that maintain iron solubility at acid values of pH. Other substances commonly present in food, such as tannate in tea and phytates in vegetables, inhibit iron absorption.

Iron is absorbed only from the small intestine, especially the duodenum. Transport of nonheme iron across the microvilli of absorptive enterocytes requires its reduction to a soluble ferrous form and binding to DCT1 (divalent cation transporter), quantities of which are increased in iron deficiency. Heme enters enterocytes via a surface receptor and is cleaved thereafter to release iron. Other iron uptake mechanisms also exist in enterocytes. Transport of iron to transferrin in the blood is modulated by ferroportin (an iron export protein), HFE (hemochromatosis) protein, and transferrin receptor at the basolateral surfaces of enterocytes. On average, 5% to 10% of food iron is absorbed daily.

Iron is highly conserved due to phagocytosis and digestion of senescent erythrocytes by macrophages in the spleen, marrow, and liver and by iron storage in ferritin molecules (or degraded ferritin aggregates known as *hemosiderin*). Hepcidin, a liver-derived polypeptide that is a potent regulator of iron absorption and transport, controls the release of conserved iron into the circulation from macrophages via ferroportin. Iron is delivered by transferrin to erythrocytes and other cells via their surface transferrin receptors. Unavoidable iron losses of about 1.0 mg daily occur due to exfoliation of skin and gastrointestinal tract cells, perspiration, and minor trauma. In menstruating women, additional average daily iron losses average 0.5 to 1.0 mg. Average net iron losses with normal term pregnancies are 700 mg. If insufficient quantities of iron are presented to the gastrointestinal tract in a form acceptable for absorption, or if iron absorptive mechanisms are not intact, iron depletion, iron-deficient erythropoiesis, and iron-deficiency anemia develop sequentially in accordance with the rate of net iron loss.

Causes of Iron Deficiency

Some infants and adolescents ingest insufficient dietary iron to meet physiologic demands of rapid growth. Many women of childbearing age develop iron deficiency due to the high iron requirements of menstruation, pregnancy, and lactation. Many otherwise healthy regular blood donors and highly trained athletes develop iron deficiency.

Pathologic blood loss from gastrointestinal tract lesions of diverse etiologies is a common cause. These include erosion or ulceration of the esophagus, stomach, or duodenum, malignant neoplasms (particularly those of the colon, esophagus, or stomach), microangiopathy (inherited or acquired), inflammatory disorders (especially Crohn's disease), diverticula, and polyps. Chronic intestinal blood loss due to hookworms is common in tropical regions. Some patients who receive warfarin (Coumadin) or aspirin therapy have chronic gastrointestinal blood loss without demonstrable anatomic lesions. Nonbleeding gastrointestinal causes in patients with few or no gastrointestinal symptoms include atrophic gastritis, celiac disease, and *Helicobacter pylori* gastritis.

Less commonly, there is urinary tract blood loss from lesions within the kidneys, ureters, or bladder or due to conditions that cause hemoglobinuria (e.g., defective heart valve prostheses, paroxysmal nocturnal hemoglobinuria). Chronic blood loss from the respiratory tract is sometimes caused by recurrent epistaxis or hemoptysis (e.g., idiopathic pulmonary hemosiderosis, lung fluke infestation).

Blood loss during major chest operations or with hip or knee replacement can induce iron deficiency that is unapparent until weeks or months later. Patients on chronic hemodialysis develop iron deficiency due to blood retained in dialysis apparatus, hemolysis, and laboratory testing. Antitransferrin antibodies or mutations of the ceruloplasmin gene have been reported as rare causes.

Signs and Symptoms of Iron Deficiency

Many persons develop weakness, ease of fatigue, or dyspnea with exertion, often before anemia develops. Infants or children can present with retarded motor and intellectual skills.

Pica, the compulsive ingestion of (often) non-nutritive substances, is a distinctive consequence that occurs in approximately one half of persons with iron deficiency, especially women. Ice eating (pagophagia) is the most common form of pica; some patients prefer dirt or clay, salt, sand, paper, cold fruit or lettuce, laundry starch, or other substances.

Some patients report evidence of bleeding. In adults with severe, chronic iron deficiency, sore mouth or tongue, nail and hair changes, dysphagia, paresthesias, and loss of memory and normal affect sometimes occur. Others present with restless legs.

Iron deficiency is diagnosed in a high percentage of children and adults coincidentally when routine physical and laboratory evaluations are performed. The most common physical sign of iron deficiency is pallor, although some patients have angular stomatitis, glossitis, koilonychia, or cricoid or esophageal web.

Laboratory Abnormalities

Laboratory abnormalities associated with iron deficiency and other forms of anemia in the differential diagnosis are displayed in Table 1. Because iron deficiency is more common in women, many laboratories report lower reference limits for iron measures in women than men. Nonetheless, astute clinicians recognize that serum iron measures characteristic of iron deficiency are equally applicable to men and women. Persons with serum ferritin less than 50 ng/mL often have iron depletion or deficiency by bone marrow examination criteria, regardless of the laboratory's lower reference limit for serum ferritin. Other causes of abnormal serum iron measures or anemia occur in some patients with iron deficiency (see Table 1).

TABLE 1 Laboratory Assessment of Iron Deficiency*

Laboratory Measurement	Diagnostic Result
Depletion of Iron Stores	
Serum ferritin concentration	<50 ng/mL
Serum total iron-binding capacity	Increased
Stainable marrow iron	Absent
Iron-Deficient Erythropoiesis	
Serum transferrin saturation	<15%
Mean corpuscular volume	<80 fL
RDW	Increased
Free erythrocyte protoporphyrin concentration	Increased
Reticulocyte index	Low
Serum transferrin receptor concentration	Increased
Iron-Deficiency Anemia	
Hemoglobin concentration	Men: <13.0 g/dL
	Women: <12.0 g/dL

*Consult laboratory-specific reference ranges. The differential diagnosis often includes anemia of chronic disease or inflammation, renal insufficiency, or malignancy, in which total iron-binding capacity is usually decreased, serum ferritin concentration is normal or increased, and RDW is normal. These forms of anemia can also occur concomitantly with iron deficiency. In some patients, the differential diagnosis also includes thalassemia minor, hemoglobinopathy E or Lepore hemoglobinopathy, various forms of sideroblastic anemia, anemia of chronic liver disease, anemia of chronic hemolysis, hypoplastic and aplastic anemias, myeloproliferative and myelodysplastic disorders, congenital dyserythropoietic anemias, anemia of myxedema, and megaloblastic anemia.
Abbreviation: RDW = red blood cell distribution width.

Principles of Iron Replacement Therapy

Treatment should be undertaken after the diagnosis is established and potential benefits and adverse effects of therapy options have been considered (Table 2). Therapy must be individualized and monitored regularly. Many patients can be treated with oral iron preparations. Hematinic combinations should not be used in lieu of an adequate pretreatment evaluation. There is no indication for administering iron therapy except to treat iron deficiency.

Intravenous iron therapy should be reserved for noncompliant patients, those unable to take oral iron, patients who absorb iron poorly, patients who have not had a satisfactory therapeutic response to oral iron replacement, and patients in whom recurrent bleeding causes iron loss in excess of what can be replaced at an acceptable rate with oral therapy. For chronic hemodialysis patients, intravenous iron administration is the only suitable route of replacement. However, intravenous therapy does not induce a more rapid erythropoietic response than is possible with oral replacement. Intravenous iron therapy should be given only by physicians experienced in such treatment who are prepared to treat hypotension or other hypersensitivity symptoms that sometimes occur. I do not recommend single intravenous iron doses greater than 500 mg (see Table 2).

Increasing the quantity of food iron is important in children with iron deficiency, many of whom have other nutritional deficits. Infants and some children need iron supplements; these should be prescribed by experienced pediatricians. In adults, dietary maneuvers as treatment are often ineffective. Multivitamins that contain "daily" amounts of iron (usually 10-20 mg Fe as inorganic iron salts) are usually inadequate for replacement therapy, and there is no basis for advising patients to take these preparations routinely unless they are premenopausal women, vigorous athletes, chronic blood donors, or

TABLE 2 Adverse Effects of Iron Replacement Therapy*

Adverse Effect	Form of Iron Therapy	Relative Frequency	Susceptible Patients
Black discoloration of stools	Iron salts,[†] carbonyl iron[†]	Very common	Children, adults
Epigastric pain, nausea, constipation, abdominal cramps, metallic taste	Iron salts[†] (more likely, especially with ascorbic acid), carbonyl iron[†] (less likely), intravenous iron[‡] (unlikely)	Common	Children, adults
Acute iron poisoning	Iron salts[†]	Common in children; rare in adults	Children: accidental ingestion Adults: accidental ingestion, suicide attempt
Arthralgias, myalgias, bone aches, low-grade fever	Intravenous iron[‡] (likely with doses >500 mg Fe), oral iron (less likely)[†]	Uncommon	Children, adults
Decreased absorption of other medications	Iron salts, carbonyl iron[†]	Uncommon	Children, adults
Flushing, hypotension	Intravenous iron[‡]	Uncommon with proper administration	Children, adults
Skin discoloration due to extravasation	Intravenous iron[‡]	Very uncommon with proper administration	Children, adults
Tooth discoloration (temporary)	Liquid oral iron elixir[§]	Very uncommon with proper administration	Children
Severe hypersensitivity, anaphylaxis	Intravenous iron[‡]	Very uncommon with proper administration	Children, adults
Increased susceptibility to infections with *Vibrio vulnificus* and other *Vibrio* species	Intravenous iron (dose-related)[‡]	Probably uncommon	Hemodialysis patients who consume raw shellfish or are exposed to water from warm seas
Iron overload	Intravenous iron (more likely),[‡] oral iron (less likely)[†]	Rare	Adults

*I do not recommend single intravenous iron doses >500 mg due to risk of post-treatment myalgias, arthralgias, and low-grade fever. I do not recommend intramuscular iron therapy due to risk of severe allergy or anaphylaxis; pain, discoloration, and atrophy of subcutaneous tissues at injection sites; therapy failure due to limitations of iron doses; and rare occurrence of sarcomas at injection sites. Avoid intravenous iron therapy in pregnant women unless the benefit outweighs the potential risk to the fetus. Intravenous iron therapy for children should be undertaken only by pediatricians experienced in such management.
[†]Feosol Ferrous Sulfate Tablets, 65 mg Fe/tablet; Niferex Film Coated Tablets, 50 mg Fe/tablet; Feosol Carbonyl Iron Tablets, 45 mg Fe; ICAR Pediatric Chewables, 15 mg Fe/tablet; ICAR Pediatric Suspension, 15 mg Fe/1.25 mL.
[‡]InFeD, 50 mg Fe/mL; Dexferrum, 50 mg Fe/mL; Venofer, 20 mg Fe/mL; Ferrlecit, 12.5 mg Fe/mL.
[§]Niferex Elixir, 100 mg Fe/5 mL.

vegetarians with uncomplicated iron depletion. Erythrocyte transfusion is indicated to elevate the circulating red blood cell mass in persons with iron-deficiency anemia who have vigorous bleeding or cardiac or respiratory compromise.

ORAL IRON THERAPY

Carbonyl Iron

Carbonyl iron consists of microspheres of pure iron precipitated from the gas iron pentacarbonyl; it is widely used for food iron fortification. This is the oral therapy of choice for most persons, because it causes less gastrointestinal toxicity than iron salts and is equally effective in correcting iron deficiency. Increasing the dosage gradually over a few weeks until the target dose is reached can improve tolerance in some patients.

The usual adult dosage is 45 mg three times daily (Feosol Carbonyl Iron tablets, 45 mg Fe/tablet), preferably taken on an empty stomach. Doses for adolescents (to be divided into three or four equal portions) are higher: For adolescent boys younger than 18 years, the dose is 90 to 135 mg daily, and for menstruating adolescent girls 12 to 18 years, the dose is 45 to 135 mg daily. In preadolescent school-age children, administer up to 6 mg/kg/day (ICAR Pediatric Chewables, 15 mg Fe/tablet); in infants and young children, administer 3 mg/kg/day (ICAR Pediatric Suspension, 15 mg Fe/1.25 mL).

In patients with anemia, the hemoglobin concentration usually increases about 1.0 g/dL weekly. Continue treatment until anemia is corrected and serum ferritin concentration is higher than 50 ng/mL; microcytosis, if present, typically resolves several months after iron stores are replete. In patients who have gastrointestinal symptoms, administer iron with meals or reduce dosing frequency, but expect delayed correction of iron deficiency. Completion of therapy in patients without continuing blood loss typically requires several months.

Iron Salts

Iron salts are suitable for many children and adults. The most commonly used preparation is ferrous sulfate (Feosol Ferrous Sulfate Tablets, 65 mg Fe/tablet; many generic brands); a polysaccharide-iron complex is also popular (Niferex Film Coated Tablets, 50 mg Fe/tablet).

CURRENT DIAGNOSIS

- Weakness, fatigue, pica, and pallor are common.
- Transferrin saturation is usually <15% (decreased serum iron level, normal or elevated total iron-binding capacity).
- Serum transferrin receptor concentration is elevated in most cases.
- Serum ferritin level is typically <20 ng/mL.
- Serum ferritin level is normal or elevated in patients who also have anemia of chronic disease, active liver disease, renal insufficiency, or malignancy.
- Reticulocytopenia and normal or low erythrocyte count are typical.
- Anemia with or without microcytosis is a late development.

CURRENT THERAPY

- Identify and correct causes of inadequate nutrition and blood loss.
- Individualize therapy and monitor outcomes regularly.
- Many patients can be treated with oral preparations; noncompliance is the most common cause of treatment failure.
- Oral therapy often fails in patients who take antacids, H_2 blockers, proton pump antagonists, or calcium supplements.
- Use intravenous therapy for noncompliance or inadequate response to oral iron, severe iron deficiency, recurrent blood loss, malabsorption, or hemodialysis.
- Many patients with nondialysis chronic renal disease, chronic inflammation, or malignancy and all hemodialysis patients require erythropoietin (Epogen, Procrit, Aranesp) therapy to maximize response to iron replacement.

In adults, the dose is one tablet three times daily, preferably on an empty stomach. In older children, the dose is 5 mg/kg of iron daily as tablets or elixir (administered by an adult).

Rate of response of anemia, monitoring of hemoglobin and ferritin concentrations, and dose adjustments for adverse gastrointestinal symptoms attributed to treatment are similar to those for carbonyl iron therapy. Ferrous gluconate, ferrous fumarate, polysaccharide-iron complex, and enteric-coated iron preparations can be used similarly. However, they might contain less iron per tablet than ferrous sulfate or be less absorbable, and thus induce therapeutic responses less rapidly. Most are more expensive.

INTRAVENOUS IRON THERAPY

Iron Dextran

Iron dextran preparations (InFeD or Dexferrum, 50 mg Fe/mL) are indicated for treatment of iron deficiency in persons with normal renal function who fail to respond to or do not tolerate oral iron supplementation. Iron dextran is safe and effective when administered properly (see Table 2). Each infusion in adults should consist of 500 mg Fe in 250 to 500 mL of normal saline. I recommend premedication with intravenous dexamethasone (Deltasone) (10 mg) plus either diphenhydramine (Benadryl) (25 mg), cimetidine (Tagamet) (400 mg), or famotidine (Pepcid) (20 mg) and giving a test dose of 25 mg Fe or approximately 5 mL over 10 to 15 minutes in a freely flowing intravenous line. If there is no immediate adverse effect, the remaining dose should be infused over 2 to 3 hours. Infusions are repeated every 2 to 3 weeks until anemia is corrected and iron stores are replete, as described for oral iron preparations. Many patients who require intravenous iron dextran for initial management have recurrent bleeding and thus require periodic maintenance infusions.

Iron Sucrose

Iron sucrose (Venofer, 20 mg Fe/mL) is indicated for treatment of iron deficiency in patients undergoing chronic hemodialysis who also receive erythropoietin therapy (epoetin alfa, epoetin beta, or darbepoetin). In previously untreated patients, a test dose should be administered before the first infusion as described for iron dextran. Doses of 200 to 300 mg[1] Fe administered intravenously over 2 hours during hemodialysis are safe and effective. In anemic patients with non–dialysis-dependent chronic kidney disease, oral and intravenous iron therapies yield similar hemoglobin responses, but intravenous iron is more effective in increasing iron stores. Goals of therapy include maintenance of serum transferrin saturation at least 30%, serum ferritin concentration at least 300 ng/mL, and hemoglobin greater than 11.0 g/dL. Most hemodialysis patients require ongoing or recurrent therapy.

Iron Gluconate

This product (Ferrlicit, 12.5 mg Fe/mL) is also indicated for treating iron deficiency in patients undergoing chronic hemodialysis who are receiving erythropoietin therapy. A test dose should be administered before the first infusion, as described for iron dextran. Typical treatments consist of 125 mg of Fe administered intravenously at each hemodialysis treatment. Adequacy of therapy is monitored in the same manner as for iron sucrose therapy.

FAILURE OF IRON REPLACEMENT THERAPY

The most common cause of unsuccessful therapy with oral iron supplements is poor compliance due to adverse gastrointestinal effects. Another common cause is unrecognized or uncorrectable chronic or recurrent blood loss associated with angiodysplasia of the gastrointestinal tract or chronic anticoagulant therapy. Some commonly prescribed drugs markedly decrease iron absorption, including antacids, H_2 blockers, proton pump antagonists, calcium supplements, and tetracycline. Gastrectomy, duodenectomy, achlorhydria, celiac disease, and gastric or intestinal bypass are often associated with iron malabsorption. Patients suspected to have suboptimal iron absorption unrelated to medications should be evaluated for additional causes of anemia. Many patients who have inadequate responses to oral iron therapy require intravenous iron replacement. In persons with chronic disease or renal insufficiency and in those receiving anticancer chemotherapy, erythropoietin therapy is often necessary to induce a satisfactory erythropoietic response.

REFERENCES

Annibale B, Capurso G, Chistolini A, et al: Gastrointestinal causes of refractory iron deficiency anemia in patients without gastrointestinal symptoms. Am J Med 2001;111:439-445.

Barton JC, Barton EH, Bertoli LF, et al: Intravenous iron dextran therapy in patients with iron deficiency and normal renal function who failed to respond to or did not tolerate oral iron supplementation. Am J Med 2000;109:27-32.

Cook JD, Flowers CH, Skikne BS: The quantitative assessment of body iron. Blood 2003;101:3359-3364.

Ferguson BJ, Skikne BS, Simpson KM, et al: Serum transferrin receptor distinguishes the anemia of chronic disease from iron deficiency anemia. J Lab Clin Med 1992;119:385-390.

Hershko C, Bar-Or D, Gaziel Y, et al: Diagnosis of iron deficiency anemia in a rural population of children: Relative usefulness of serum ferritin, red cell protoporphyrin, red cell indices, and transferrin saturation determinations. Am J Clin Nutr 1981;34:1600-1610.

Hershko C, Hoffbrand AV, Keret D, et al: Role of autoimmune gastritis, *Helicobacter pylori* and celiac disease in refractory or unexplained iron deficiency anemia. Haematologica 2005;90:585-595.

Ioannou GN, Rockey DC, Bryson CL, et al: Iron deficiency and gastrointestinal malignancy: A population-based cohort study. Am J Med 2002; 113:276-280.

Lozoff B, Beard J, Connor J, et al: Long-lasting neural and behavioral effects of iron deficiency in infancy. Nutr Rev 2006;64:S34-S43.

Van Wyck DB, Roppolo M, Martinez CO, et al: A randomized, controlled trial comparing IV iron sucrose to oral iron in anemic patients with nondialysis-dependent CKD. Kidney Int 2005;68:2846-2856.

Yates JM, Logan EC, Stewart RM: Iron deficiency anaemia in general practice: Clinical outcomes over three years and factors influencing diagnostic investigations. Postgrad Med J 2004;80:405-410.

---

[1]Not FDA approved for this indication.

Autoimmune Hemolytic Anemia

Method of
Stephen R. Larsen, MB BS

Autoimmune hemolytic anemias are characterized by the combination of decreased red blood cell survival and the presence of autoantibodies directed against red blood cell antigens. Patients with these disorders have symptoms and signs of anemia; however, the patterns of presentation vary according to the specific type. These disorders are classified according to the in vivo and in vitro characteristics of the causative antibody (Table 1). This classification reflects our understanding of the underlying pathogenesis and divides these disorders into warm autoimmune hemolytic anemia and the two cold autoantibody syndromes: cold agglutinin syndrome and paroxysmal cold hemoglobinuria. Each of these is discussed in turn. Drug-induced autoimmune hemolytic anemia is treated separately.

Warm Autoimmune Hemolytic Anemia

Warm autoimmune hemolytic anemia accounts for 60% to 70% of all patients with autoimmune hemolytic anemia. Approximately one half of cases are idiopathic or primary and the remainder are secondary to various disorders including lymphoproliferative disorders, connective tissue disorders, immunodeficient states, solid tumors, or infectious diseases. The peak incidence of warm autoimmune hemolytic anemia is between the ages of 40 and 70 years, with a mean of approximately 49 years.

DIAGNOSIS

Warm autoimmune hemolytic anemia is diagnosed on the basis of laboratory findings consistent with shortened red cell survival and serologic evidence of autoantibodies directed against red cell antigens, optimally reactive at 37°C. The peripheral blood film shows anisocytosis, polychromasia (suggesting elevated reticulocytes), and spherocytes. When the hemolytic process has been extensive and rapid, nucleated red blood cells can appear. Reticulocytosis is confirmed with direct testing and indicates increased erythropoiesis as part of bone marrow compensation. Other laboratory evidence of hemolysis, but not specific to warm autoimmune hemolytic anemia, includes an elevated bilirubin (unconjugated), increased serum lactate dehydrogenase, and decreased haptoglobins.

The direct antiglobulin test is used to determine the presence of red cell surface antibodies. It is used to identify the presence of immunoglobulin G (IgG) or complement, or both, which can give a clue to the underlying cause (see Box 1). The antibody is usually classified as a panagglutinin because it causes agglutination of all of the red blood cells in the panel used to characterize the reactivity of anti–red cell antibodies. In approximately 2% to 4% of cases of warm autoimmune hemolytic anemia, the direct antiglobulin test is negative. This is due to low levels of IgG bound to the red cell, to an IgG autoantibody of low affinity, or to an autoantibody that is IgA.

TREATMENT

The natural course of autoimmune hemolytic anemia varies with age, such that in children it is often self-limited, occurring after a viral infection and resolving over 2 to 3 months. In adults, however, it is often chronic and can manifest for many years, requiring a protracted course of treatment. The treatment of warm autoimmune hemolytic anemia is summarized in the Current Therapy box and can be divided into direct therapy, which reduces the pathogenic antibodies or their effectiveness, and supportive care. Usually these two management principles are undertaken simultaneously. The various options to reduce antibodies include immunosuppressive therapies, and there is often a degree of balancing such that there is control of anemia while minimizing the risk of infection due to immunosuppression.

Direct Treatment

Corticosteroids (e.g., prednisone at a starting dose of 1 mg/kg) are usually used as the first therapy for warm autoimmune hemolytic anemia. This approach can result in improvement in the hemoglobin within several days and achieves a remission in approximately 60% to 70% of patients. On evidence of efficacy, the dose of corticosteroid is tapered gradually, with the aim of finding the lowest dose that will maintain adequate control of hemolysis. In adults, this tapering should be more gradual than in children, because evidence of an insufficient dose will not be apparent for 3 to 4 weeks. If remission is not achieved in 2 to 3 weeks, or if at any time during the tapering process the remission is not maintained, other measures are warranted as described later.

The production of antibodies is also reduced by the use of other immunosuppressive agents or cytotoxic drugs. Azathioprine (Imuran)[1] can be given in a dose of 100 to 150 mg/day and is tolerated quite well. It can affect liver function tests and cause a mild degree of bone marrow suppression. As well as in the context of steroid-refractory disease, it can also be used as a steroid-sparing agent in patients who require moderate long-term doses of corticosteroids. Cyclophosphamide (Cytoxan)[1] is a cytotoxic drug that can be administered orally (e.g., 100 mg daily) or intravenously (e.g., 500-700 mg monthly) and can be more effective than azathioprine; however, it is does have more side effects including bone marrow suppression, bladder irritation, hair loss, and potential gonadal suppression.

Rituximab (Rituxan)[1] is a genetically engineered monoclonal anti-CD20 antibody being used in an increasing number of patients with malignant and nonmalignant disorders. Rituximab targets B-cell precursors and mature B-cells and is used successfully in a number of autoimmune disorders, especially idiopathic thrombocytopenic purpura (ITP), as well as warm autoimmune hemolytic anemia. Rituximab is usually given at a dose of 375 mg/m^2 weekly for 4 weeks. Worldwide experience with rituximab in the treatment of these patients is steadily increasing. In one report, 11 patients

---
[1]Not FDA approved for this indication.

TABLE 1 Classification and Serology of Autoimmune Hemolytic Anemia

Classification	Warm Autoimmune Hemolytic Anemia	Cold Agglutinin Syndrome	Paroxysmal Cold Hemoglobinuria
Direct antiglobulin test	IgG or IgG and C3	C3 only	C3
Immunoglobulin class	IgG	IgM	IgG
Specificity	Rh	I, i	IgG
Serum	IgG agglutinating red cells at the anti–human globulin phase	IgM agglutinating antibody reacting at 30°C	IgG biphasic hemolysin (Donath–Landsteiner antibody)

CURRENT THERAPY

Warm Autoimmune Hemolytic Anemia

- Initial treatment consists of corticosteroids (e.g., prednisone 1 mg/kg).
- For poorly responsive or resistant disease: splenectomy, cyclophosphamide (Cytoxan),[1] cyclosporin (Neoral),[1] rituximab (Rituxan),[1] azathioprine (Imuran),[1] intravenous immunoglobulin,[1] danazol.[1]
- Supportive care consists of red cell transfusion.

Cold Agglutinin Disease

- Avoidance of the cold
- Alkylating agent: chlorambucil (Leukeran) 0.1-0.2 mg/kg/day or cyclophosphamide (Cytoxan)[1] 1.5-2.0 mg/kg/day
- Corticosteroids (not usually effective except in cases of polyclonal cold agglutinin syndrome such as in infections with *Mycoplasma pneumoniae*)
- Rituximab (Rituxan)[1]
- Plasmapheresis
- Blood transfusion, if indicated, using blood warmer

[1]Not FDA approved for this indication.

---

refractory to steroids or immunosuppressive drugs received rituximab, and all achieved remission after a mean follow-up of 604 days. Eight patients remained in complete remission and three in partial remission.

Splenectomy can now be performed safely using a laparoscopic technique and results in improvement of anemia in 60% to 70% of patients within 2 weeks. Of those who obtain remission, about 50% require low doses of corticosteroids to maintain hemoglobin levels.

Other reagents that can be used in refractory cases include intravenous immunoglobulin (IVIg) and danazol.[1] Reports of the effectiveness of IVIg in warm autoimmune hemolytic anemia are varying. High doses may be necessary (e.g., 1 g/kg[3] daily for 5 days), only about 40% of patients respond, and often the effect is transient, necessitating repeat courses. Danazol is an attenuated androgen that has shown some efficacy in ITP. There are anecdotal reports of successful responses with the use of this agent in warm autoimmune hemolytic anemia.

Supportive Care: Transfusion Support

Red cell transfusion plays an important role in managing warm autoimmune hemolytic anemia. If a patient has mild to moderate anemia and is not symptomatic, transfusion might not be necessary, especially because the therapies just described result in an improvement in the hemoglobin over several days. However, with more significant anemia, and especially if the patient is symptomatic, a blood transfusion is appropriate.

The autoantibodies present in the serum of patients with warm autoimmune hemolytic anemia usually react against antigens present on the red cells of almost all patients in the donor population. The result of this is the inability to find fully compatible blood during the compatibility-testing process. Of greatest importance is detecting coexisting alloantibodies, which can develop if the patient has had previous pregnancies or received blood transfusions in the past. The exclusion of clinically significant alloantibodies requires time-consuming adsorption techniques. In the case of the need for an urgent blood transfusion, completion of these studies might not be possible.

[1]Not FDA approved for this indication.
[3]Exceeds dosage recommended by the manufacturer.

If the patient has not received a transfusion in the last 3 months, determination of the red cell phenotype is invaluable. The erythrocyte phenotype can guide which alloantibodies are possible and allow the transfusion of phenotype-matched red cells, which should be safe for transfusion. A close liaison between the hematologist and blood bank personnel is crucial to establish the urgency of blood transfusion, minimize delays in providing blood, and prevent misunderstandings relating to the compatibility of donor units.

Cold Agglutinin Syndrome

DIAGNOSIS

Cold agglutinin syndrome represents about 15% to 25% of cases of autoimmune hemolytic anemia and can be acute or chronic. It is usually seen either in response to an infection (such as that caused by *Mycoplasma pneumoniae* or Epstein–Barr virus) or in lymphoproliferative disorders. Patients often present with symptoms and signs of a progressive anemia rather than an acute hemolytic process that can occur in warm autoimmune hemolytic anemia. The patient might also complain of Raynaud's phenomenon or of acrocyanosis of the fingers, ears, or nose tip that resolves on warming. Symptoms are often exacerbated in the colder season and only occasionally can be associated with an acute hemolytic crisis with frank hemoglobinuria.

In cold agglutinin syndrome, the red blood cells are sensitized with IgM antibody and can activate complement. The specificity of the IgM antibody is most often directed against the I antigen (reacts best against untreated adult red cells), although it can be directed against the i antigen in patients with infectious mononucleosis (reacts best against fetal or cord cells). Rarely, IgG cold-reacting antibodies are seen, either alone or in combination with IgM cold-reacting antibodies.

In general, the cold autoantibodies that cause clinical cold agglutinin syndrome have a high titer (1 in 1000) and can be higher than 1 in 10,000 in many patients. The observation of cold agglutination in the laboratory is not sufficient to make a diagnosis of cold agglutinin disease. Also, the antibody titer does not correlate well with the degree of hemolysis in vivo. More important is the thermal amplitude, which is the highest temperature at which the antibody causes agglutination. In most patients with clinically significant hemolysis, the thermal amplitude is usually greater than 30°C.

TREATMENT

The treatment of cold agglutinin syndrome is summarized in the Current Therapy box. Avoiding the cold is the most important aspect of the management of this disorder. Staying indoors in a heated environment and wearing appropriate warm clothes can prevent acute hemolytic crises. This requires ongoing vigilance and can be difficult for some patients. When possible, it is recommended to move to a warmer climate, at least during the colder months.

Cytotoxic agents can be given with a view to reducing antibody production in patients who have significant anemia despite attempts to avoid the cold. The most commonly used agents are the alkylating agents chlorambucil (Leukeran)[1] (0.1-0.2mg/kg/day) or cyclophosphamide (1.5-2.0mg/kg/day). Unlike in warm autoimmune hemolytic anemia, corticosteroids are usually not effective in patients with cold agglutinin syndrome. There are a couple of exceptions to this: some patients with a polyclonal cold agglutinin, such as those with *Mycoplasma* pneumonia, and the rare patient with IgG cold-reacting antibodies. Similarly, splenectomy is not usually effective, presumably because the liver is the dominant site of sequestration of red cells sensitized with C3. Experience with rituximab is growing. In 27 patients with primary cold agglutinin disease, rituximab achieved an overall response of 54%. The median time to response and duration of response were 1.5 and 11 months, respectively.

[1]Not FDA approved for this indication.

Plasmapheresis can be used to physically remove the IgM antibody from the plasma. Because the IgM antibody is confined to the intravascular space, this treatment is effective but short lived because the half-life for replacement of the protein is only 5 days. There are two clinical situations when plasmapheresis may play a role. Firstly, it can be used to reduce severe hemolysis at initial presentation when the syndrome is due to an infection and the thermal amplitude is high. Secondly, it can be used to prepare a patient for surgery when performed 1 to 2 days prior. Patients undertaking hypothermic surgical procedures represent a special group in whom precautions such as plasmapheresis can be important (for example, patients undergoing cardiopulmonary bypass surgery).

Transfusion may be necessary in patients with severe symptomatic anemia and, as in warm autoimmune hemolytic anemia, transfusion represents a challenge. Cross-match testing is often difficult to perform because all red blood cells are reactive. Warm washing of red blood cells may be necessary to remove the IgM autoantibody to facilitate accurate determination of the ABO group. If ABO typing remains uncertain, group O red cells can be administered. It is generally recommended that a blood warmer be used for the transfusion.

Paroxysmal Cold Hemoglobinuria

DIAGNOSIS

Paroxysmal cold hemoglobinuria was recognized as a distinct entity in 1872. The causative antibody was first described by Donath and Landsteiner in 1904; Landsteiner received the 1930 Nobel Prize in medicine for the discovery of the ABO blood groups. The Donath–Landsteiner antibody is an IgG directed against the P blood group antigen and identified using a bithermal assay. Two aliquots of the patient's red blood cells are collected; one is incubated for 60 minutes at 37°C, and the other is incubated for 30 minutes at 3°C and then 30 minutes at 37°C. After centrifugation, the blood is inspected for evidence of hemoglobin. Complement-mediated hemolysis in the control tube is not seen because the anti-P antibodies do not bind the red blood cell surface, and complement is not fixed. Incubation at 3°C allows the binding of polyclonal anti-P antibody and complement fixation.

Patients are usually children and can present in a dramatic fashion with hemoglobinuria, jaundice, pallor, and fever. Often there is a history of a recent viral infection, and exposure to cold is not necessarily elicited. The anemia can be severe and the blood film can be dramatic, showing typical morphologic features of immune hemolysis.

TREATMENT

Most cases of paroxysmal cold hemoglobinuria are self-limited and require only supportive care during the acute illness. The patient must be kept warm, and often blood transfusion is not necessary. If anemia is severe, blood transfusion may be necessary. The Donath–Landsteiner antibody does not react above 4°C and therefore does not interfere with routine compatibility testing. Corticosteroids may be used but their usefulness has not been ascertained. The transfusion of P phenotype red cells has been suggested, but donors are uncommon and blood would be difficult to obtain under urgent circumstances. The issue of whether blood warmers are required is also not clear, but using them can reassure the clinician in an urgent situation.

Drug-Induced Autoimmune Hemolytic Anemia

Drug-induced hemolytic anemia accounts for a significant percentage of cases of acquired autoimmune hemolytic anemia. Some drugs are associated with nonimmune hemolysis; the typical example of this is some antimalarial drugs in patients with glucose-6-phosphate dehydrogenase (G6PD) deficiency who develop hemolysis due to excess oxidative stress.

Three mechanisms have been proposed to explain the development of autoantibodies caused by medications. In the autoantibody theory, an antibody is produced with serologic similarities to a warm autoimmune hemolytic anemia. Methyldopa is the drug classically associated with this mechanism. In the hapten (or drug-adsorption) theory, an antibody is formed against the drug, which acts as a hapten and binds to the surface of red cells. Penicillin is the drug most commonly associated with this mechanism, and the hemolysis is usually extravascular. Hemolysis occurs because the antigen–antibody reaction occurs at the surface of the red cell. In the immune-complex theory, free circulating drug stimulates the production of drug-specific antibody, which binds to the drug and binds to red cells. Hemolysis can be rapid and is usually intravascular. Quinidine is the prototypic drug that causes hemolysis via this mechanism. A list of drugs and their respective mechanisms are summarized in Box 1. Because some patients have features consistent with more than one of these mechanisms, a unifying theory has been proposed. In this theory, antibody is directed against red cells depending on the specific interaction between the drug and the red cell. Therefore, the antibody is directed against predominantly the red cell, predominantly the drug, or a portion of both.

Serologic tests can be used to help determine the mechanism. When autoantibodies are formed, the serology is the same as that in idiopathic warm autoimmune hemolytic anemia. This antibody can show specificity for Rh blood group antigens and can persist even after the patient stops taking the drug. For the hapten mechanism, the antibody is usually a warm-reactive IgG antibody. With immune-complex formation, the antibody may be IgG, IgM or both. The direct antiglobulin is usually positive, with evidence of complement coating the red cells.

The treatment consists of immediately ceasing the implicated drug and providing supportive care. There are no supportive data to recommend the use of corticosteroids, although they are often administered. The prognosis is excellent, with the expectation of a full recovery.

BOX 1 Causes of Drug-Induced Hemolytic Anemia

Autoantibody Mechanism
Cephalosporins
L-Dopa
Ibuprofen (Motrin)
α-Methyldopa
Procainamide (Pronestyl)

Hapten Mechanism
Cephalosporins
Penicillins
Tetracycline
Tolbutamide (Orinase)

Immune Complex Mechanism
Amphotericin B
Cephalosporins
Chlorpropamide (Diabinese)
Diclofenac (Arthrotec)
Doxepin (Sinequan)
Quinidine
Quinine
Probenecid
Rifampicin (Rifadin)

REFERENCES

Arndt PA, Garratty G: The changing spectrum of drug-induced immune hemolytic anemia. Semin Hematol 2005;42:137-144.
Berentsen S, Beiske K, Tjonnfjord GE: Primary chronic cold agglutinin disease: An update on pathogenesis, clinical features and therapy. Hematology 2007;12:361-370.
Brodsky RA: New insights into paroxysmal nocturnal hemoglobinuria. Hematology Am Soc Hematol Educ Program 2006;24-28, 516.
D'Arena G, Califano C, Annunziata M, et al: Rituximab for warm-type idiopathic autoimmune hemolytic anemia: A retrospective study of 11 adult patients. Eur J Haematol 2007;79:53-58.
Gertz MA: Management of cold haemolytic syndrome. Br J Haematol 2007; 138:422-429.
Ness PM: How do I encourage clinicians to transfuse mismatched blood to patients with autoimmune hemolytic anemia in urgent situations? Transfusion 2006;46:1859-1862.
Petz LD: A physician's guide to transfusion in autoimmune haemolytic anaemia. Br J Haematol 2004;124:712-716.
Schollkopf C, Kjeldsen L, Bjerrum OW, et al: Rituximab in chronic cold agglutinin disease: A prospective study of 20 patients. Leuk Lymphoma 2006;47:253-260.

Nonimmune Hemolytic Anemia

Method of
Stella T. Chou, MD, and
Mitchell J. Weiss, MD, PhD

The hemolytic anemias (HAs) are a heterogeneous group of disorders characterized by accelerated erythrocyte destruction. Intrinsic causes of hemolysis are usually inherited and include abnormalities in the erythrocyte membrane, metabolic defects, and altered hemoglobin structure. Extrinsic causes include erythrocyte-directed antibodies, trauma, infections, and toxins. Within these categories, there are virtually hundreds of specific etiologies. Here we address the most common and clinically significant disorders, focusing mainly on the congenital HAs.

Diagnosis

Anemia with reticulocytosis, hyperbilirubinemia, and an elevated lactate dehydrogenase (LDH) level strongly suggests hemolysis. The family history is often helpful for diagnosis. In particular, the clinician should inquire about ethnic background and family members with anemia, splenectomy, early gallstones/cholecystectomy, or significant neonatal jaundice. Several forms of HA confer protection against *Plasmodium falciparum* malaria. Accordingly, these disorders are relatively common in malaria endemic regions such as Africa, the Mediterranean basin, and Asia because of positive selective genetic pressure. Assessment of erythrocyte indexes and morphology are critical and frequently reveal distinct diagnostic clues (Table 1). Together, these initial data usually point to a specific diagnosis that can be confirmed by directed specialized testing that includes more detailed examination of erythrocytes and DNA analysis.

In addition, patients with primary hemolytic disorders may present during an aplastic episode, most typically from Parvovirus B19 infection. In this case, erythrocyte production stops temporarily resulting in reticulocytopenia and declining hemoglobin.

CURRENT DIAGNOSIS

- Anemia, reticulocytosis and hyperbilirubinemia suggest hemolytic anemia (HA).
- Reticulocytopenia in the context of chronic HA suggests a Parvovirus-induced aplastic crisis.
- Erythrocyte-intrinsic etiologies for HA are usually inherited abnormalities affecting the erythrocyte membrane, enzymes, or hemoglobin structure.
- Congenital HA can present with severe neonatal jaundice.
- Extrinsic causes for HA include antierythrocyte antibodies, trauma, infection, and toxins.
- History, physical examination, and examination of erythrocyte morphology combined with more specialized testing usually provides a specific diagnosis.
- Paroxysmal nocturnal hemoglobinuria is a clonal somatically acquired hematopoietic disorder characterized by intravascular hemolysis, thromboses, and sometimes cytopenias. Diagnosis is made by flow cytometry demonstrating a population of cells that lack glycosyl phosphatidylinositol (GPI)-anchored membrane proteins.

Management

Folate replacement is recommended for most patients with moderate to severe congenital hemolytic anemia. Iron from hemolyzed erythrocytes is usually reabsorbed, and supplementation is not necessary. Formation of gallstones is a common complication of HA, and therefore periodic screening abdominal ultrasounds are warranted. Concomitant Gilbert's syndrome, caused by a variant in the uridine diphosphoglucuronate glucuronosyltransferase 1A (UGT1A) gene promoter, increases the propensity for gallstones. Neonatal jaundice is common in many of the inherited disorders and may necessitate exchange transfusion for severe hyperbilirubinemia. Parvovirus B19–induced aplastic crisis is a life-threatening complication of congenital HA that frequently requires blood transfusion. Therefore, it is essential that patients with known hemolytic disorders be counseled to seek medical attention if they experience symptoms of viral illness, increased pallor, and lethargy.

CURRENT THERAPY

- Many forms of congenital severe HA are ameliorated by splenectomy.
- Long-term risks of splenectomy include susceptibility to sepsis from encapsulated organisms and possibly increased risk of thrombosis.
- Splenectomized patients should be immunized against *Streptococcus pneumoniae*, *Haemophilus influenzae* type B, and *Neisseria meningitidis*. Daily penicillin prophylaxis is recommended for children.
- Splenectomized patients presenting with fever should receive appropriate parenteral antibiotics until a negative blood culture is documented.
- Aplastic crisis and hyperhemolytic episodes associated with HA are managed with erythrocyte transfusion.
- Folate (folic acid) replacement, 1 mg/d, is recommended for moderate to severe HA.

TABLE 1 Causes of Nonimmune Hemolytic Anemia

Type of Defect	Disease Mechanism	Example	Erythrocyte Morphology
Intrinsic erythrocyte defect	Membranopathy	Hereditary spherocytosis Hereditary elliptocytosis Hereditary stomatocytosis Hereditary xerocytosis Hereditary pyropoikilocytosis Paroxysmal nocturnal hemoglobinuria	Spherocytes Elliptocytes Stomatocytes Target cells, echinocytes Micropoikilocytes, microspherocytes, fragmented erythrocytes Macrocytosis
	Enzymopathy	G6PD deficiency Pyruvate kinase deficiency	Heinz bodies, bite cells, blister cells, anisocytosis, poikilocytosis Echinocytes
	Hemoglobinopathy	Sickle cell disease Thalassemia Unstable hemoglobinopathies	Sickle cells Microcytosis, target cells Heinz bodies
Extrinsic erythrocyte defect	Trauma	Heart valve hemolysis (macrovascular) DIC/TTP/HUS (microvascular)	Schistocytes Schistocytes
	Thermal injury	Severe burns	Schistocytes
	Chemicals	Arsenic, lead, copper, and chlorates	Varied
	Toxins	Bee and wasp stings, spider bites, and snake venom	Schistocytes
	Infections	Malaria, *Babesia*, *Bartonella*, clostridia, streptococci, staphylococci, enterococcus, salmonella, mycoplasma, EBV, CMV, HSV, rubeola, influenza A	Intraerythrocytic parasites Schistocytes with bacterial infections

Abbreviations: CMV = cytomegalovirus; DIC = disseminated intravascular coagulation; EBV = Epstein-Barr virus; HSV = herpes simplex virus; HUS = hemolytic uremic syndrome; TTP = thrombotic thrombocytopenic purpura.

Splenectomy is an effective treatment for many forms of severe congenital HA. The most significant problem from splenectomy is increased risk of life-threatening infections from encapsulated organisms. Prior to splenectomy, patients should be vaccinated against *Streptococcus pneumoniae*, *Haemophilus influenzae* type B, and *Neisseria meningitidis*. Daily penicillin prophylaxis is recommended postsplenectomy, particularly for children. Splenectomized patients presenting with fever should be managed promptly with physical examination, blood culture, and appropriate parenteral antibiotics.

Congenital Hemolytic Anemias

ERYTHROCYTE MEMBRANE ABNORMALITIES

The erythrocyte membrane must be flexible and strong enough to withstand multiple passages through small capillary beds. A specialized membrane composed of a lipid bilayer, integral membrane proteins, and an underlying skeletal network formed by numerous proteins supports these requirements. Erythrocyte membrane proteins include alpha and beta spectrin, ankyrin, protein 4.1, and actin. Inherited mutations in these proteins disrupts the integrity of the membrane to cause HA.

Hereditary Spherocytosis

Hereditary spherocytosis is the most common cause of nonimmune HA in populations from Northern Europe and North America, with a prevalence of approximately 1 in 2000.

Pathophysiology

Hereditary spherocytosis is caused by varying degrees of spectrin loss, usually from deficient or dysfunctional ankyrin, band 3 and/or protein 4.2, or, less frequently, a primary spectrin defect. Disruption of the membrane skeleton destabilizes the lipid bilayer causing splenic removal of microvesicles and subsequent spherocyte formation. The molecular basis of hereditary spherocytosis is heterogeneous. Approximately two thirds of cases are autosomal dominant, with the remaining one third being autosomal recessive or arising from new mutations.

Clinical Manifestations and Diagnosis

The severity of hereditary spherocytosis varies from asymptomatic to severe and typically correlates with the degree of spectrin deficiency. Most diagnoses of hereditary spherocytosis are made in childhood, from a positive family history or a clinical presentation of anemia, jaundice, and splenomegaly. New patients occasionally present with a Parvovirus-induced aplastic crisis. In these clinical contexts, an elevated mean corpuscular hemoglobin concentration (MCHC) strongly indicates hereditary spherocytosis. This value reflects a decreased surface-to-volume ratio caused by splenic removal of the erythrocyte membrane. In addition, the red cell distribution width (RDW) reflecting size variation, is elevated. The blood smear demonstrates spherocytes (erythrocytes lacking central pallor). A positive incubated osmotic fragility test, which demonstrates increased susceptibility to hypotonic lysis, supports the diagnosis. However, it is important to note that osmotic fragility is normal in 10% to 20% of hereditary spherocytosis cases. Moreover, other disorders, most notably immune HAs, are also characterized by spherocytes with increased osmotic fragility. A positive direct antiglobulin test (Coombs test) usually distinguishes immune HA from hereditary spherocytosis.

Patients with mild hereditary spherocytosis may have normal or near normal hemoglobin levels, mild reticulocytosis and hyperbilirubinemia, and typically have an uncomplicated course. More severely affected patients experience additional complications including severe neonatal hyperbilirubinemia and hyperhemolytic episodes later in life. The latter are frequently precipitated by viral illness and are characterized by worsening anemia, signs of accelerated hemolysis, and often, splenic enlargement. Rare complications of severe hereditary spherocytosis include leg ulcers, gout, and extramedullary hematopoiesis.

Management

Aplastic and hyperhemolytic episodes are supported with erythrocyte transfusions. Although splenectomy improves the anemia and reduces the risk of gallstones by removing the site of erythrocyte destruction, splenectomy should be reserved for patients with severe hemolysis, recurrent life-threatening hyperhemolytic episodes, or growth failure. Most clinicians prefer to treat as needed with transfusions until after 5 years of age when the postsplenectomy infection risk declines. In less severely affected patients, the threshold for recommending splenectomy varies among clinicians. In most centers, splenectomy is performed laparoscopically with very low morbidity and rapid recovery times. Moreover, improved vaccines, particularly pneumococcal, reduce the risk for postsplenectomy sepsis. However, some data indicate that splenectomy increases the long-term risk for venous and arterial thromboses, cardiovascular disease, and pulmonary hypertension. Accessory spleens are relatively common and should be searched for at the time of surgery.

Hereditary Elliptocytosis and Pyropoikilocytosis

The hereditary elliptocytoses are a heterogeneous group of inherited HAs with oval-shaped erythrocytes. Hereditary elliptocytosis is relatively common in African, Mediterranean, and Asian populations. Hereditary pyropoikilocytosis is a more rare and severe form of HA with erythrocyte fragmentation in which one parent usually has hereditary elliptocytosis.

Pathophysiology

Most forms of hereditary elliptocytoses are inherited in an autosomal dominant fashion and are relatively mild. The underlying molecular defects are usually mutations in genes encoding alpha or beta spectrin, band 3, or protein 4.1. These mutations all destabilize the latticework of spectrin organization underlying the plasma membrane to induce an oval or elliptical shape. Assorted hereditary elliptocytoses mutations that qualitatively alter membrane proteins produce subtle variations in cell shape that distinguish different clinical subtypes, which are categorized according to erythrocyte morphology. In hereditary pyropoikilocytosis, the patient usually inherits a common hereditary elliptocytosis mutation from one parent and a milder subclinical defect in spectrin synthesis from the other parent.

Clinical Manifestations and Diagnosis

Hereditary elliptocytosis is classified into three subtypes according to morphology: common hereditary elliptocytosis, the most prevalent form, which is characterized by biconcave elliptocytes; spherocytic hereditary elliptocytosis, a phenotype between hereditary spherocytosis and hereditary elliptocytosis; and Southeast Asian ovalocytosis, characterized by oval erythrocytes. Most patients are asymptomatic and diagnosed incidentally with minimal or mild compensated hemolysis. The peripheral smear demonstrates more than 30% elliptocytes. Patients who are homozygous or compound heterozygous have more severe HA. The peripheral blood smear also has budding erythrocytes, fragments, and other poikilocytes. Hereditary pyropoikilocytosis, at the extreme end of this spectrum, causes bizarre fragmented erythrocytes with microspherocytosis and micropoikilocytosis. The mean corpuscular volume is very low (25 to 75 fL), the osmotic fragility is abnormal, and erythrocytes characteristically demonstrate thermal instability. Hereditary pyropoikilocytosis typically presents in newborns or infants with jaundice and anemia.

Management

Most hereditary elliptocytoses patients have a mild course and do not require treatment. In cases of severe hemolysis because of homozygous or compound heterozygous hereditary elliptocytosis or hereditary pyropoikilocytosis, splenectomy is indicated.

Hereditary Stomatocytosis and Xerocytosis

Hereditary stomatocytosis and xerocytosis are rare inherited causes of hemolytic anemia associated with abnormal erythrocyte cation permeability and volume (increased in stomatocytosis and decreased in xerocytosis). Both disorders are autosomal dominant. Hereditary stomatocytosis patients have erythrocytes with a mouth-shaped (stoma) area of central pallor, whereas hereditary xerocytosis patients demonstrate target cells and echinocytes. The clinical courses of these diseases are highly variable, ranging from asymptomatic to moderate hemolysis and subsequent anemia. Most patients do not require treatment. Importantly, splenectomy is contraindicated in hereditary stomatocytosis because of an increased incidence of life-threatening thrombosis.

ERYTHROCYTE METABOLISM ABNORMALITIES

Erythrocytes rely on two major biochemical pathways: glycolysis for energy to maintain metabolic needs and the hexose-monophosphate shunt for antioxidant pathways. More than 20 enzymes are involved in these two pathways, and defects in each one are associated with various forms of HA. The two most common enzymopathies are deficiencies in glucose-6-phosphate dehydrogenase (G6PD) and pyruvate kinase (PK).

Glucose-6-Phosphate Dehydrogenase Deficiency

G6PD deficiency is the most common erythrocyte metabolism disorder, affecting as much as 3% of the world's population.

Pathophysiology

G6PD is the first enzyme in the hexose-monophosphate pathway, which is required to maintain a high level of reduced glutathione, an important antioxidant. G6PD-deficient erythrocytes undergo increased hemoglobin oxidation leading to hemolysis. G6PD deficiency is an X-linked recessive disorder. More than 300 G6PD genetic variants affect enzyme activity to different extents that determine the severity of HA. Type A$^-$ is a genetic variant seen in 10% to 15% of African American males and is associated with mild to moderate G6PD deficiency. Variants causing more severe HA are more prevalent in Mediterranean and Asian populations.

Clinical Manifestations and Diagnosis

G6PD deficiency is an X-linked disorder; therefore, hemizygous males and homozygous females are typically affected. Many G6PD variants are associated with neonatal jaundice. Severe forms of G6PD deficiency can cause chronic ongoing HA, but most commonly, affected individuals are asymptomatic in between hemolytic episodes. However, anemia develops rapidly following a precipitating event related to oxidative stress that induces acute intravascular hemolysis with the severity determined by the G6PD variant and the offending agent. Drugs are the most common inciting event in Africans with the A$^-$ variant (Table 2). Other precipitating events include mothball (naphthalene) exposure and infections. In some Mediterranean and Asian variants, ingestion of fava beans can cause acute life-threatening hemolysis. Symptoms can include fever, abdominal pain, nausea, diarrhea, and impressive hemoglobinuria, frequently described as Coca-Cola colored. The spleen is often enlarged and tender. Anemia ranges from mild to life-threatening and is normocytic and normochromic. Morphologic abnormalities include anisocytosis, poikilocytosis, "bite cells" (erythrocytes that are partially destroyed in the spleen), and "blister cells" (a thin strip of membrane overlying a bleb of clear cytoplasm). A methyl violet stain to detect Heinz bodies, indicative of denatured hemoglobin, is typically positive. Immediately after an acute hemolytic event, G6PD levels can be deceptively normal because of an elevated reticulocyte count, which can express significant enzymatic activity in some variants. Therefore, G6PD levels should be tested weeks to months later to obtain a true baseline level.

TABLE 2 Drugs Capable of Precipitating Hemolysis in G6PD Deficiency

Analgesics and Antipyretics	Acetanilid*
	Acetylsalicylic acid (aspirin)
Antibacterials	Chloramphenicol
	Furazolidone (Furoxone)*
	Nalidixic acid (NeGram)*
	Nitrofurantoin (Furadantin)*
	Sulfonamides*
	Trimethoprim-sulfamethoxazole (Bactrim)
Antimalarials	Pamaquine*
	Pentaquine*
	Primaquine*
	Quinacrine
Miscellaneous	Dimercaptosuccinic acid (Succimer)
	Methylene blue*
	Phenazopyridine (Pyridium)*
	Urate oxidase*
	Vitamin K

*These drugs have an increased tendency to cause clinically significant hemolysis. Most patients with mild G6PD deficiency alleles tolerate drugs that are not marked by the asterisk. For a more comprehensive list of drug–G6PD interactions, see reading by Beutler.
Abbreviation: G6PD = glucose-6-phosphate dehydrogenase.

Management

Treatment of the A⁻ variant of G6PD deficiency is mostly preventive by avoiding oxidant stresses. When acute hemolytic episodes result in symptomatic anemia, erythrocyte transfusions are indicated. Rarely, acute renal failure develops secondary to severe intravascular hemolysis. This is managed by vigorous hydration, alkalinization, electrolyte monitoring, and occasionally hemodialysis.

Pyruvate Kinase Deficiency

Pyruvate kinase (PK) deficiency, which is most commonly seen in Northern European populations, accounts for more than 80% of the HAs due to glycolytic disorders.

Pathophysiology

PK deficiency is genetically heterogeneous, with many different mutations impairing enzyme activity to different extents. Pyruvate kinase deficiency causes decreased production of ATP, impairing erythrocyte survival. Inheritance is usually autosomal recessive; simple heterozygotes with 50% enzyme activity are unaffected.

Clinical Manifestations and Diagnosis

PK deficiency is extremely heterogeneous, ranging from life-threatening HA to asymptomatic compensated hemolysis. Erythrocyte morphology may be normal or show echinocytes (small dense crenated erythrocytes). Quantitation of erythrocyte enzyme activity is usually diagnostic.

Management

General supportive care for chronic hemolysis and supportive erythrocyte transfusions when needed are the mainstays of therapy. Patients with severe hemolysis may benefit from splenectomy, although the response is variable and unpredictable.

HEMOGLOBINOPATHIES

HA can be caused by mutations that alter the α- or β-like globin proteins that contribute to hemoglobin structure. Quantitative defects that impair globin gene expression comprise the thalassemia syndromes, discussed in the article on thalassemia. Qualitative defects are usually caused by missense mutations that alter hemoglobin structure and stability. The most important examples are the sickle syndromes, discussed in the article on sickle cell disease. Numerous other missense mutations that destabilize hemoglobin also cause HA. In these cases, hemoglobin precipitates may be detected by a Heinz body stain. Unstable hemoglobins can also be detected by hemoglobin electrophoresis or increased precipitation upon exposure to heat or isopropanol. If any of these tests are positive in the context of hemolysis, direct globin gene sequencing can provide a definitive diagnosis.

Acquired Nonimmune Hemolytic Anemias

PAROXYSMAL NOCTURNAL HEMOGLOBINURIA

Paroxysmal nocturnal hemoglobinuria (PNH) is a rare acquired disease with chronic HA, thrombosis, and often pancytopenia. The hemolytic anemia results from increased erythrocyte sensitivity to complement-mediated hemolysis.

Pathophysiology

PNH is an acquired clonal disorder caused by a somatically acquired inactivating mutation in the X-linked phosphatidylinositol glycan, class A (PIGA) gene, which encodes an enzyme involved in the synthesis of glycosyl phosphatidylinositol (GPI) anchor proteins. All blood cells derived from the abnormal clone lack surface proteins that require the GPI anchor. Hemolysis occurs from the deficiency of specific GPI-linked surface proteins that inhibit complement activation. The hypercoagulable state seen in PNH is most likely related to complement-mediated platelet activation and elevated levels of ADP from lysed erythrocytes, leading to platelet aggregation. For unknown reasons, PNH commonly progresses to aplastic anemia.

Clinical Manifestations and Diagnosis

PNH can present as a primary hemolytic syndrome with chronic intravascular HA, a thrombotic event, or with pancytopenia. Few patients exhibit the classic nocturnal hemoglobinuria, reporting red or brownish urine in the morning. In most patients hemoglobinuria occurs irregularly and is often precipitated by infection or stress. Iron deficiency can occur from urinary loss. Associated thromboses may be venous or arterial and can involve extremities, the hepatic vein (Budd-Chiari syndrome), other intraabdominal veins, and cerebral veins. Hence, PNH can present as severe abdominal pain or headaches. The majority of patients have defective hematopoiesis, ranging from a macrocytic anemia to severe aplastic anemia and pancytopenia. Rarely, PNH can also evolve into a myelodysplastic syndrome or acute leukemia. The median survival for patients diagnosed with PNH is 10 to 15 years.

Laboratory findings include anemia, variable reticulocytosis, leukopenia, and thrombocytopenia. The bone marrow examination typically reveals erythroid hyperplasia or, in the case of associated aplastic anemia, hypocellularity. Urine hemosiderin is typical. Laboratory diagnosis of PNH previously relied on assays that demonstrated abnormal erythrocyte sensitivity to complement (Ham test, sucrose hemolysis test). The current standard is flow cytometry demonstrating the absence of hematopoietic GPI-linked proteins, typically CD55 and CD59, on some or all circulating cells.

Management

Oral iron supplementation is recommended to replace the urinary losses associated with intravascular hemolysis. Corticosteroids can sometimes improve the hemolysis in the first 24 to 72 hours of a hemolytic episode. A recent phase 3 trial showed that eculizumab, a monoclonal antibody that inhibits activation of the terminal complement complex, is effective for the hemolytic anemia of PNH. Eculizamab was recently FDA-approved and is entering clinical practice. Anticoagulation is indicated for documented thromboses, and thrombolytic therapy can be effective for patients with hepatic vein thrombosis or massive thrombotic events. Short-term prophylactic therapy should be used in the setting of surgery or prolonged immobilization, even if there is no history of thrombosis. HLA-identical bone marrow transplantation is indicated for bone marrow failure associated with PNH. Alternatively, immunosuppressive therapy with antithymocyte globulin and cyclosporine is used for patients without a suitable bone marrow donor.

Hemolytic Anemia Caused by Erythrocyte Fragmentation

Erythrocyte fragmentation can occur in the macrovascular or microvascular circulations. Shear stress produces fragmented erythrocytes (schistocytes). Macroangiopathic hemolysis can occur with prosthetic surfaces, large thromboses, and aged or damaged heart valves, but it is usually mild. Microangiopathic causes of hemolysis include disseminated intravascular coagulation, thrombotic thrombocytopenic purpura, and hemolytic uremic syndrome, which are discussed in their respective articles.

Hemolytic Anemia Caused by Chemical and Physical Agents

Arsenic, lead, copper, and chlorates can cause hemolysis through numerous mechanisms. Most notably, hemolytic anemia may be the presenting feature of the copper toxicity of Wilson's disease. Animal toxins associated with intravascular hemolysis include bee and wasp stings, brown recluse spider bites, and snake venom. Severe burns can also cause fragmentation hemolysis from the thermal injury.

Hemolytic Anemia Caused by Infection

Infections cause hemolysis by direct invasion of the erythrocyte, toxin production, or by immune-mediated mechanisms. Malaria is the most common infectious cause of hemolytic anemia worldwide. *Plasmodium falciparum* invades erythrocytes and is associated with severe hemolysis and hemoglobinuria (blackwater fever). Other parasitic infections associated with hemolysis are *Babesia microti* and *Bartonella bacilliformis*. Bacterial organisms that cause hemolysis via erythrocyte membrane injury and toxins include clostridia, streptococci, staphylococci, enterococcus, and salmonella. Immune hemolysis is associated with *Mycoplasma pneumoniae*, Epstein-Barr virus, cytomegalovirus, herpes simplex, rubeola, and influenza A (see topic in Section 2). Hemolysis improves once the underlying infection resolves.

REFERENCES

Beutler E: Glucose-6-phosphate dehydrogenase deficiency and other red cell enzyme abnormalities. in Beutler E, et al. (eds): Williams Hematology. New York, McGraw-Hill, 2001, pp 527-545.

Bolton-Maggs PH, Stevens RF, Dodd NJ, et al: Guidelines for the diagnosis and management of hereditary spherocytosis. Br J Haematol 2004; 126(4):455-474.

Gallagher P, Lux S: Disorders of the erythrocyte membrane, in Nathan D, et al, (eds): Nathan and Oski's Hematology of Infancy and Childhood. Philadelphia, WB Saunders, 2003, pp 560-684.

Hillmen P, Young NS, Schubert J, et al: The complement inhibitor eculizumab in paroxysmal nocturnal hemoglobinuria. N Engl J Med 2006;355(12): 1233-1243.

Parker C, Omine M, Richards S, et al: Diagnosis and management of paroxysmal nocturnal hemoglobinuria. Blood 2005;106(12):3699-3709.

Tse WT, Lux SE: Red blood cell membrane disorders. Br J Haematol 1999;104(1):2-13.

Zanella A, Fermo E, Bianchi P, Valentini G: Red cell pyruvate kinase deficiency: Molecular and clinical aspects. Br J Haematol 2005;130(1):11-25.

Pernicious Anemia and Other Megaloblastic Anemias

Method of
Eugene P. Frenkel, MD

Historically, pernicious anemia was the prevalent prototypic megaloblastic anemia. At present, its diagnostic incidence, when appropriately defined, has been overshadowed by many other pathophysiologic mechanisms that produce similar hematologic and neurologic changes.

The term *megaloblastic anemia* identifies peripheral blood findings of red cell macrocytosis (mean corpuscular volume [MCV] >96 fL) associated with macro-ovalocytes and anisocytosis. Because macrocytosis can be seen in many clinical circumstances in the absence of a megaloblastic state (Box 1), the true diagnosis defines defective erythroid maturation in the bone marrow, wherein the red cell precursors have enlarged reticulated nuclear chromatin characteristic of defective DNA synthesis with normal permissive RNA synthesis,

---

BOX 1 Etiologic and Pathophysiologic Mechanisms for Macrocytosis and Megaloblastosis

Nonmegaloblastic Macrocytosis*

These are nonprogressive over time, usually associated with a normal RDW, and banal macrocytes (nonovalocytic macrocytes seen in true megaloblastic states)
- Aplastic anemia
- Chronic alcohol use
- Chronic liver disease
- Myelodysplastic syndromes
- Postsplenectomy states

Megaloblastic Anemia
- Deficiency or defects in vitamin B_{12} (cobalamin) metabolism
  - Inadequate diet: Strict vegan patients
  - Inadequate absorption: Lack of intrinsic factor
- Classic pernicious anemia
- Aging stomach
- Intrinsic factor inhibition
- Small intestinal disease/resection
- Abnormal utilization (e.g., nitrous oxide anesthesia, etc.)
- Deficiency or defects in folate metabolism
  - Inadequate intake
  - Altered absorption
  - Abnormal utilization—especially chemotherapeutic drugs, anticonvulsants, alcoholism
  - Increased excretion, renal dialysis

---

*Mean corpuscular volume is usually 96 to 100 μm^3.

resulting in a large cytoplasmic mass. Because the defective DNA synthesis is not exclusive to the red cells, giant metamyelocytes reflect the defect in white cells, and macro-megakaryocytes also occur. Indeed, defective DNA synthesis is seen not only in the bone marrow but also in all proliferating cells (e.g., buccal mucosa, gastrointestinal tract, etc.)

Etiology

Almost one century after Addison's (1855) annotation of an unusual anemia, termed *pernicious anemia*, Minot and Murphy (1926) showed that the anemia could be "abolished" by (almost) raw liver, and in 1929 Dr. William Castle described an "intrinsic factor" in the stomach, which was required for liver extract to correct the anemia. Then in 1938, Lucy Wills and Barbara Evans described a nutritional anemia in pregnant women that failed to respond to liver extract, thereby posing the conundrum that a second form of megaloblastic anemia existed. Important resolution of this dilemma came when Pfiffner and Stokstad found a relevant growth factor in yeast and green plants, which they named folic acid. In 1948, Karl Folkers identified and crystallized vitamin B_{12}, which was subsequently shown to require intrinsic factor for facilitated absorption in the terminal ileum. Absorption was defined in the upper small intestine. Subsequently, the finding of circulating autoantibodies to intrinsic factor in patients with (genetic) pernicious anemia appeared to complete the pathogenesis and clinical picture related to these two moieties.

Almost immediately this simplistic clinical construct began to unravel. As shown in Box 1, vitamin B_{12} (cobalamin) absorption was related to the increasing incidence of megaloblastic anemia with age. The concept of the aging stomach changed the clinical expression of megaloblastic anemia. As we age (after 50 years), the release of vitamin B_{12} from food proteins declines due to reduced pepsin activity at a low pH. The known decrease in gastric acidity with aging may be the most important factor of such decreased extraction of vitamin B_{12} from food, but it is clearly not the only factor. However, such patients have normal absorption of crystalline vitamin B_{12}, so that treatment with nonfood vitamin B_{12} results in a physiologic response.

Clearly a very common addition to the effects with aging is the new ubiquitous use of proton pump inhibitors for the treatment of gastric reflux and heartburn. These agents reduce secretion of intrinsic factor as well as pepsin and gastric acid, and they are now recognized as an important factor in decreased vitamin B_{12} absorption.

Clinical Features

A very important aspect of vitamin B_{12} deficiency is that in addition to the anemia, neurologic deficits are a significant part of the clinical expression. Neurologic deficits are being seen with remarkable frequency, and in the past two decades they are actually the common presenting complaint, often occurring in the *absence* of anemia. These include posterolateral spinal column dysmyelinization with resultant peripheral paresthesias, loss of vibratory and positional sense, decreased deep tendon reflexes, and even ataxia. In addition, classic peripheral neuropathy or even cerebral dysfunction with depression, irritability, and memory loss can occur. Because these signs and symptoms are often present in the absence of anemia, the clinician needs special vigilance to evaluate the neurologic findings and relate them to vitamin B_{12} deficiency. The explanation for the dichotomy of progressive neurologic deficits in the absence of anemia appears to be the increased availability of folate in fortified food, because folate can replace vitamin B_{12} in blood cell production but not in neural function.

Another correlative clinical event has been the recognition of severe and rapid progressive neurologic lesions in patients undergoing nitrous oxide exposure. This has been seen after its use in open heart surgery and even when used for 2 to 3 hours for oral surgery. We now know that nitrous oxide interferes with the two known enzymatic pathways in vitamin B_{12} metabolism. As noted earlier, the methylcobalamin methyltransferase biochemical pathway can be bypassed by folate. However, functional inactivation and interference of the second pathway (methylmalonyl coenzyme–mutase reaction) occur. This alteration cannot be bypassed by folate and has been demonstrated to result in nerve dysmyelinization.

The changing pattern of the causes of megaloblastic anemia is also related to folate metabolism. The FDA-mandated addition of folate to whole grain products beginning in 1998 has remarkably changed the occurrence of folate deficiency in the United States and the development of megaloblastic anemia. It, of course, may be the basis for the prominent increase in the neurologic presentation in vitamin B_{12} deficiency. A very important observation relative to folate metabolism is the clear requirement for supplemental folate during pregnancy. The most important reason is that folate is critical for normal neural tube formation in the first weeks of pregnancy.

CURRENT DIAGNOSIS

- Pernicious anemia is the result of autoantibody loss of gastric intrinsic factor, resulting in failure of facilitated absorption of vitamin B_{12} in the terminal ileum.
- Megaloblastic anemia is almost entirely related to deficiency or defective (altered) utilization of vitamin B_{12} or folate.
- Megaloblastic anemia in association with neurologic deficit is due to vitamin B_{12}.
- Determination of serum methylmalonic acid and homocysteine are the best, most sensitive, and most specific tests for the etiologic basis of megaloblastic anemia and demonstrate presence of the metabolic defect.
- Repletement of vitamin B_{12} or folate is best defined by identifying the pathophysiologic mechanism for the defect.
- With age, the effective extraction of vitamin B_{12} from food declines, with resultant vitamin B_{12} deficiency.
- Folate supplementation is very important in the first trimester of pregnancy to protect from neural tube abnormalities in the fetus.

Diagnosis

LABORATORY DIAGNOSIS OF VITAMIN B_{12} AND FOLATE METABOLIC DEFICIENCIES

Diagnostic value of a low serum vitamin B_{12} value in patients with megaloblastic anemia is well confirmed. However, evaluation of patients with little or no hematologic abnormalities, but with a variety of neurologic or psychiatric changes, particularly in the older age group, has defined a significantly decreased sensitivity and specificity for the serum vitamin B_{12} assay.

Characterization of the only two metabolic pathways for vitamin B_{12} metabolism had long ago provided assays of the intermediates of the two functional coenzymes: methylcobalamin active in the homocysteine-to-methonine pathway and adenosylcobalamine in the salvage pathway. Vitamin B_{12} deficiency results in an increase in serum methylmalonic acid and serum (or plasma) total homocysteine. Normally, serum methylmalonic acid (MMA) is undetectable (commonly defined as <0.4 mmol/L). An increase in serum and urine MMA has been shown to be highly sensitive and specific for the diagnosis of vitamin B_{12} deficiency. It is now clearly the gold standard in the clinical evaluation of suspected vitamin B_{12} deficiency because it defines true tissue depletion. As would be expected, homocysteine is also increased with tissue vitamin B_{12} deficiency.

The laboratory diagnosis of folate deficiency has been even more difficult than that of vitamin B_{12}. The serum folate assay has been commonly used. Unfortunately, it is remarkably affected by a short period of dietary deprivation or recent alcohol ingestion, and slight hemolysis will increase the serum value. Red cell folate levels have been considered a more stable site to measure. Because the red cell life span is 120 days, the red cell folate measurement is a mean of the events over a prolonged period. Unfortunately, it is difficult to perform and is insensitive to issues relating to alcohol ingestion and pregnancy.

By contrast, measurements of homocysteine levels are very sensitive and serve as an excellent assessment of folate deficiency, when the serum MMA is *normal*. The assay of MMA and homocysteine provides approximately a 99% sensitivity and specificity for the diagnosis of vitamin B_{12}– or folate-deficient states and are truly the tests of choice.

PHYSIOLOGIC ISSUES RELATIVE TO VITAMIN B_{12} AND FOLATE

The average American diet contains 5 to 30 μg of vitamin B_{12}, and the absorption has been considered to be 1 to 2 μg/day, with a projected daily requirement of 0.5 to 1.0 μg/day. Issues related to the efficiency of the enterohepatic circulation make these numbers far from precise, because it has been projected that 1 to 10 μg of cobalamins are recycled daily.

The folate content of the mean American diet is about 280 μg for men and 210 μg for women. Although previous estimates of daily requirements had been 400 μg/day, recent daily recommendations have been 200 μg/day for men and 180 μg/day for women. Tissue stores of folate are limited and levels begin to decline within 2 weeks of deprivation. Indeed, acute clinical deprivation is a recognized event in intensive care units. Studies of this rapid deprivation suggest that our daily needs are closer to 400 μg per day and that the mean tissue storage content is approximately 5000 μg.

Treatment

GENERAL PRINCIPLES OF THERAPY

The first and most critical therapeutic concern is the clinical stability of the patient who presents with severe anemia or rapidly progressive neurologic deficit, especially where an impending or pseudo spinal cord transection appears to be developing. However, because megaloblastic anemias usually develop slowly, compensatory cardiopulmonary responses are often associated with only modest symptoms, even when patients present with hemoglobin levels less than 3 or 4 g/dL. Often the impulse is to quickly treat with multiple hematinics

CURRENT THERAPY

- The decision for therapy depends on the determination of the etiology (vitamin B_{12} or folate) and the definition of the pathophysiologic mechanism for the deficiency or altered metabolism.
- The cardiopulmonary status of the patient with anemia determines the therapeutic initiation, because hematologic repair will take 7 to 14 days regardless of the hematinic used. Cautious red cell transfusions should be used to stabilize the cardiopulmonary issues.
- Parenteral vitamin B_{12} is the therapy of choice in classic pernicious anemia.
- Oral vitamin B_{12} (at pharmacologic doses) is very effective in the management of patients with the aging stomach.
- Folate supplementation is essential during the first trimester of pregnancy to protect neural tube development.

while awaiting diagnostic data from the laboratory. The appropriate approach is to recognize that even with specific diagnosis and therapy, the red cell values will not improve for at least 7 to 14 days. The red cell needs must be judged solely on the cardiopulmonary and cerebral functional status of the patient, and if required, cautious transfusion is the urgent treatment of choice. Commonly, only a single unit of packed red cells is needed. Transfusion(s) should be given slowly (over 3 to 4 hours), because rapid volume shifts can precipitate functional problems related to the precarious hemodynamic status of these patients.

Less commonly, the neurologic deterioration (such as with the nitrous oxide effect) of the patient encourages urgency of therapy. Such rapid progression virtually defines the etiology to be due to vitamin B_{12}. Although rare, if progression appears rapid, serum should be collected and treatment with parenteral vitamin B_{12} instituted immediately.

The second important principle is the requirement for a specific etiologic diagnosis, because the pathophysiologic mechanism that produced the defect must be defined to determine reversibility of the cause and the duration of therapy (e.g., short term, lifetime). Thus, (genetic) pernicious anemia will demand a lifetime of vitamin B_{12} replacement therapy, whereas vitamin B_{12} deficiency due to jejunal diverticula can be approached with short-term vitamin B_{12} therapy, antibiotics, and the consideration of surgical repair. Similarly, the aged stomach syndrome can easily be managed with oral vitamin B_{12} supplements.

The third issue relates to an understanding of the rate and pattern of repair of the clinical abnormalities. When the anemia fails to respond in the expected time frame, the question of an incorrect diagnosis or an unrecognized associated lesion must be considered. For instance, iron deficiency is often unrecognized when it is associated with megaloblastosis; it will, however, result in a suboptimal therapeutic response. This can be particularly noteworthy in vitamin B_{12} deficiency, when patients with pernicious anemia have an increased risk of gastric cancer, and the finding of iron deficiency can provide the clue to its diagnostic pursuit.

Fourth, the serial follow-up of patients after therapeutic restitution requires an understanding of the natural history of the underlying disease status. Patients can only be educated about the need for therapy and follow-up when the physician understands the cause and mechanism. This is important, because the ease with which repair can be achieved sometimes belies the significance of the problem. For instance, pernicious anemia patients have an increased incidence of gastric cancer and have the potential to develop endocrinopathies (especially hypothyroidism and hypoadrenalism) secondary to autoantibodies. Thus, they will need a lifetime of therapy and serial clinical evaluation.

Finally, the concept of a therapeutic trial in patients with megaloblastic states does not eliminate the need for a specific diagnosis and determination of the pathophysiologic mechanism. Certainly, an elevated MMA or homocysteine S can be used as a parameter for a trial of therapy; correction of the defect should similarly correct the metabolic abnormality in 10 to 14 days. This allows affirmation of the diagnosis and confirms the presence of tissue deficiency.

TREATMENT OF VITAMIN B_{12} (COBALAMIN) DEFICIENCY

Normal tissue vitamin B_{12} stores (primarily in liver and bone marrow) range between 7 and 15 mg. Clinically significant deficiency is expressed when tissue stores are reduced to 30% to 50% of normal. The goal of therapy is to replete tissue stores. However, with each dose of vitamin B_{12}, the percentage of the given dose retained by tissues declines. In essence, fractional urinary excretion of an administered dose increases as the stores are progressively repleted. Therefore, significantly more must be administered than one would calculate from the amount known to exist in total body tissues. The fractional retention is better when temporal gaps (daily or every few days) are left between doses. These physiologic issues help explain the many repletement schedules found in literature, and further allow the clinician to adopt a sequence most appropriate to the patient and the related clinical issues.

Because most of the mechanisms of vitamin B_{12} deficiency relate to decreased absorption, the initial therapy should begin with cyanocobalamin or hydroxycobalamin 1 mg (1000 μm) given subcutaneously or intramuscularly. This is rapidly absorbed from either site, with peak serum levels in approximately 1 hour after injection. Following this initial dose, approximately 65% will be retained. Intravenous injection produces a much greater urinary loss and should not be used. A simple repletement schedule from that point is 1 mg given daily or every other day during the first 2 weeks and then weekly for the next month, by which time normal peripheral hematologic values are expected.

Thereafter, the pathophysiologic mechanism of the deficiency will determine the approach to future therapy. For patients in whom gastric intrinsic factor secretion is defective (pernicious anemia), vitamin B_{12} must be given for life. Monthly or bimonthly injections of 1 mg provide simple, inexpensive, and effective therapy that requires no special monitoring. In patients with neurologic deficits, more frequent administration (weekly) of vitamin B_{12} has been used in the first 6 months, a time when neurologic repair is at the maximum. It must be emphasized that such an increased frequency is empiric, with no defined supportive data. Similarly, shortening the interval between injections, often requested by elderly patients who express having an improved sense of well-being with the treatment, is not based on specific evidence.

The elderly most often have vitamin B_{12} deficiency due to ineffective liberation of vitamin B_{12} bound to protein in food. In these patients the absorption of crystalline vitamin B_{12} is normal. In such circumstances, as well as in the strict vegan (no dietary animal products) patient, oral vitamin B_{12} can be used. Oral 1 mg (1000 μg) tablets are inexpensive and available for such use and should be given daily. We have successfully treated patients with the aged stomach with oral vitamin B_{12} alone, without initial parenteral repair.

Increased daily vitamin B_{12} requirements occur in pregnancy and lactation, thyrotoxicosis, and liver or renal disease, especially where protein loss is extensive. Because tissue concentrations of vitamin B_{12} are in the milligram range and daily requirements are in the microgram range, the normal stores are adequate for 1 to 3 years in the absence of supplementation. Deficiency is therefore uncommonly associated with such an increased need, except in the pregnant vegan patient.

Side effects from vitamin B_{12} therapy are extremely rare. Patients with the very rare early Leber's disease (hereditary optic nerve atrophy) have been reported in the past to have increased atrophy with institution of high-dose therapy. Rarely, pruritus and skin rash have occurred, and more rarely anaphylactic shock has been reported.

Short-term sequelae of repletement therapy in megaloblastic states can occur regardless of the etiology of the deficiency. These include hypokalemia and hyperuricemia, especially in the first 48 to 72 hours of institution of therapy. Therefore, potassium supplementation is wise when therapy is started.

TREATMENT OF FOLATE DEFICIENCY

Normal tissue stores of folate are approximately 5000 μg (5 mg) with a projected daily requirement of 200 to 400 μg. These limited stores result in folate deficiency more quickly with dietary deprivation than in vitamin B_{12} deficiency. Because most clinical circumstances of folate deficiency are due to inadequate intake or drug interference, oral repletement is the usual mode, giving 1 mg (or 5 mg[3]) folic acid pills, a commonly available form, per day. In general, 1 mg/day provides a significant excess and allows rapid repletement of tissue stores. In known malabsorption syndromes, the 5 mg[3] daily folic acid oral dose is preferable. Tissue stores can be repleted easily in a few weeks with daily oral therapy, and therefore the duration of therapy is determined on the persistence of the cause.

---

[3]Exceeds dosage recommended by the manufacturer.

Folate prophylaxis is very important through pregnancy, where at least 600 μg of folate per day is desirable. However, because of its critical need in neurologic development, doses in the range of 4 mg/day are recommended to prevent neural tube defects. This should begin 4 weeks before the pregnancy and continue at least through the first 3 months of gestation. High doses of folate (>500 μg/day) have allegedly reduced zinc absorption; thus, mineral supplementation during pregnancy may be appropriate. Another circumstance that merits folate prophylaxis is in patients on longstanding anticonvulsant therapy, because folate deficiency has been associated with an increased seizure frequency.

It again merits emphasis that empiric folate therapy in a patient with megaloblastic anemia will repair the anemia, but if the correct diagnosis is vitamin B_{12} deficiency, a fulminant neurologic deficit can ensue.

REFERENCES

Carmel R: Cobalamin, the stomach, and aging. Am J Clin Nutr 1997; 66:750-759.
Herbert VD, Colman N: Folic acid and vitamin B_{12}. In Shils ME, Young VR (eds): Modern Nutrition in Health and Disease, 7th ed. Philadelphia: Lea & Febiger, 1988, pp 388-416.
Lindenbaum J, Healton EB, Savage DG, et al: Neuropsychiatric disorders caused by cobalamin deficiency in the absence of anemia or macrocytosis. N Engl J Med 1988;318:1720-1728.
Stabler SP, Allen RH, Savage DG, et al: Clinical spectrum and diagnosis of cobalamin deficiency. Blood 1990;76:871-881.

Thalassemia

Method of
Ashutosh Lal, MD, and Sylvia T. Singer, MD

The thalassemias, inherited disorders of hemoglobin synthesis, result from a defective synthesis of one of the two globin chains that constitute hemoglobin, α or β. It is the most common single-gene disease worldwide. The highest incidence of thalassemia is among ethnic groups in the regions of the malaria belt around the equator, because heterozygous inheritance reflects an advantage against *Plasmodium falciparum* malaria. Therefore, 95% of affected births occur in Asia, India, and the Mediterranean region. Due to recent trends in population migration, however, thalassemia is found throughout the world.

Most forms are inherited in a Mendelian recessive fashion from asymptomatic gene-carrying parents, who have one chance in four of having an affected child. Clinically, there is wide variation, ranging from a very mild disease to a severe anemia requiring transfusions for survival.

Prenatal diagnosis, improved supportive care, and cure with bone marrow transplantation characterize the current preventive and therapeutic approach for the more severe cases of thalassemia major. Moreover, advances in the care of these transfusion-dependent patients has resulted in decreased morbidity and prolonged life expectancy. In particular, major progress has occurred over the last several years in developing methods for improved chelation, reducing iron toxicity, and applying noninvasive techniques for measuring the extent of tissue iron. Some of these newer diagnostic tools or treatment combinations are not readily available in many thalassemia centers. Determining optimal care of the disease complications and continued monitoring for patients who live in underserved areas far from larger thalassemia clinics is a continuing challenge in many countries.

Pathophysiology and Diagnosis

Thalassemia is caused by defective or absent synthesis of either of the two chains, α or β, of the adult hemoglobin tetramer as a result of a gene deletion or mutation. Classification is according to the particular globin chain that is ineffectively produced. The most important types are α and β thalassemias; more than 200 mutations leading to β thalassemia and about 60 mutations or deletions leading to α thalassemia have been described so far.

Decreased or absent globin chain synthesis results in a diminished amount of normal functional hemoglobin, increased hemolysis causing anemia, and an imbalance between the two globin types as the unaffected chain is continuously produced. The unpaired globin chain alters red cell (RBC) cellular and membrane properties, leading to early destruction of cells in the bone marrow or ineffective erythropoiesis. Ineffective erythropoiesis is mainly a feature of β thalassemia, as the relative excess unstable α chains precipitate and disintegrate, causing oxidative damage to the RBC membrane. The excess of β chains in α thalassemia results in more stable globin chain aggregates and less intramedullary cell death. Therefore, there is a difference in disease symptoms and severity between α and β thalassemias. Beyond the actual globin gene mutations, other globin chain factors and genetic modifiers are involved in altering the phenotype. Predicting with certainty a phenotype from the genotype is not always possible.

Most β mutations result from point mutations that affect transcription, translation, or RNA stability. If only a single β globin gene is affected, the result is β thalassemia minor, a mild microcytic anemia and erythrocytosis sometimes mistaken to be iron-deficiency anemia. In homozygous or compound heterozygous states, there is absence (β^0 thalassemia) of normal β globin chain production, in most cases resulting in a transfusion-dependent phenotype referred to as *thalassemia major* or *Cooley's anemia*. If there is only reduction of normal β globin chain synthesis (β^+ thalassemia), the phenotype is generally that of a milder disease, *thalassemia intermedia*. Other hemoglobinopathies involve genes for structural hemoglobin variants, such as hemoglobins S, C, and E, which are often inherited from one parent along with a gene for thalassemia from another parent. Important examples are hemoglobin E-β thalassemia and S-β thalassemia, the latter having clinical manifestations of sickle-cell disease.

The majority of α thalassemia mutations are gene deletions, and phenotypic expression depends on the number of available α genes. Normal persons inherit two α globin genes from each parent, resulting in an αα/αα genotype. A homozygous state with deletion of four α globin genes (−−/−−), results in hydrops fetalis, a severe, usually fatal disease in utero or shortly after birth. Hemoglobin H disease is characterized by three α globin gene deletions (α−/−−), resulting in a moderately severe anemia. The remaining unpaired β-globin chains form tetramers, named hemoglobin H. Hydrops fetalis and hemoglobin H disease are generally found in Southeast Asian persons because both require *cis* α gene deletion, known as (−−SEA), which is endemic to that area. α thalassemia trait is expressed by two α gene deletions, *trans* deletion (α−/α−) or *cis* deletion (αα/−−), causing mild microcytic hypochromic anemia. Silent carriers have one gene deletion and three intact α globin genes (αα/α−) and are clinically and hematologically undetectable. One important nondeletion α mutation, Constant Spring (CS), results in an elongated α chain due to a mutation in the stop codon of the α gene, and if inherited in conjunction with two other deleted α genes, it results in a more severe phenotype than hemoglobin H disease, occasionally requiring transfusions.

Carrier State and Diagnosis

Diagnosis of a carrier for thalassemia is very important for female and male patients of reproductive age. Awareness and alertness of providers, especially those caring for women of ethnic groups at high risk for thalassemia, can result in prevention of the birth of an affected child. Prevention requires laboratory work for a patient with a positive family history or a suspicious complete blood count (CBC) and informing the family of their risk for having an affected child with a hemoglobin disorder. Once a couple at risk for having a child with thalassemia has been identified, genetic counseling and education regarding prenatal testing should be offered.

In the CBC, a hypochromic microcytic anemia without a decrease in RBC count or an increase in RBC distribution width (RDW) makes thalassemia trait a likely diagnosis. Ruling out concomitant iron deficiency by performing iron studies is often helpful. Quantification of HbA2 and HbF, commonly elevated in β thalassemia, can be followed by DNA methods to define the mutation or the deletion present, in particular for the purpose of genetic counseling. For unknown mutations, the amplified globin gene DNA is sometimes sequenced. Newborn screening, currently implemented in all states in the United States, detects new cases, which are then referred for further laboratory evaluation and clinical follow-up. Prenatal testing is accomplished by fetal DNA polymerase chain reaction (PCR) methods or by direct fetal hemoglobin testing. The relation between genotype and phenotype enables a prediction of the likely prognosis for a particular genotype, although it is difficult to predict with certainty.

Clinical Manifestations

The clinical forms of β thalassemia are classified based on their severity into thalassemia major (TM) and thalassemia intermedia (TI). The important clinical forms of α thalassemia include HbH disease and HbH-CS; the latter, a more severe form, is considered a type of TI.

Even within these categories, in particular TI and E-β thalassemia, there is a remarkable variability from a mild anemia to complete transfusion dependency for survival. With the advances in treatment of TM in developed countries, clinical problems have shifted to consequences of transfusion therapy, particularly iron overload, its diagnosis, and treatment. In less developed countries, the full spectrum of undertreated TM can be seen in addition to some of the transfusion-related side effects.

 CURRENT DIAGNOSIS

Thalassemia Trait
- Microcytic anemia (<75 fL), increased RBC count (>5×10^6/mm^3)
- Hb electrophoresis: Elevated HbA2 ($\alpha_2\delta_2$) and possibly elevated HbF ($\alpha_2\gamma_2$)

β Thalassemia Major
- Microcytic hypochromic anemia (usually <5 g/dL), target cells, increased reticulocytes and nucleated RBCs
- Hb electrophoresis: Mostly absence of HbA ($\alpha_2\beta_2$), β^0 thalassemia
- DNA analysis: Mutations in both β globin genes

β Thalassemia Intermedia
- Milder microcytic hypochromic anemia (6-9 g/dL)
- Hb electrophoresis: Decreased HbA ($\alpha_2\beta_2$), β^+ thalassemia; or decreased HbA with HbE, E-β^0 thalassemia
- DNA analysis: Varies; mutations in one or both β globin genes (β^+/β^0)

α Thalassemia
- Microcytic anemia, inclusion bodies
- Hb electrophoresis: Hb Barts (γ^4) in cord blood, HbH (β^4) in fresh blood
- DNA analysis: Specific deletions

Hb = hemoglobin; RBC = red blood cell.

β THALASSEMIA MAJOR

Patients with β-thalassemia major usually develop severe anemia (hemoglobin <5 g/dL) within the first 6 to 12 months of life. Transfusion therapy is usually initiated to turn off the marrow and halt continuous marrow expansion. Lifelong supportive care is indicated, unless a curative procedure with bone marrow transplantation is performed. If regular transfusion therapy is not initiated, a clinical picture of severe untreated β thalassemia, typical Cooley's anemia, will develop: profound anemia, splenomegaly, progressive bone changes, and masses of extramedullary hematopoiesis due to marrow expansion. For transfused patients, the consequences of iron toxicity to the heart, liver, and endocrine system, as well as the side effects of the particular iron chelation agent in use, determine the spectrum of clinical issues, as discussed further in this chapter.

THALASSEMIA INTERMEDIA

β Thalassemia intermedia, an intermediate-severity thalassemia, has a remarkable clinical variability and can be better classified as two syndromes: mild TI and moderately severe TI. The symptoms start beyond infancy, usually during the second year of life, and include mild to moderate anemia (Hb 6-9 g/dL). The genetic basis is variable, and the resultant extent of anemia and erythropoietic activity determines the clinical findings and severity. Those with a milder anemia (Hb >8 g/dL) will usually grow and develop well, whereas those with more severe disease (Hb 6-8 g/dL) have more remarkable splenomegaly, delayed growth, bone abnormalities, and an occasional need for transfusions with infections or fever. Some require regular blood transfusions and chelation to promote growth and development during childhood and early adolescence. However, in both milder and more severe TI, not infrequently symptoms of progressive anemia, heart failure, pulmonary hypertension, hypersplenism, and bone expansion will evolve during the second and third decades of life, necessitating initiation of regular transfusion therapy, essentially categorizing the patient as having thalassemia major.

Because TI patients do not require regular medical intervention, as TM patients do, they often do not receive adequate monitoring and screening of their symptoms, which at times are preventable or diagnosed in late stages. It is important to keep monitoring these patients every 3 to 6 months for early detection and intervention of complications (Table 1). Common clinical complications are

TABLE 1 Supportive Care and Monitoring for Patients with Thalassemia Major

Complication	Evaluation	Frequency	Comments, Desired Values
Transfusions			
Alloimmunization	Antibody screen	Monthly	Baseline extended RBC phenotype
Increased iron loading	Transfused packed RBC volume, chelation	6-12 mo	<200 mL/kg/y
Insufficient transfusions	Pretransfusion hemoglobin	3-4 wk	9-10 g/dL
Transfusion-transmitted infections	Hepatitis B and C serology, HIV	Yearly	More often if unexplained ↑ liver enzymes
Iron Overload			
Systemic	Ferritin	3 mo	500-1000 ng/mL
Liver			
Fibrosis, inflammation	Liver biopsy or SQUID or MRI R2	Yearly	3-7 mg/g dry weight
Hepatocellular injury	Bilirubin, transaminases, alkaline phosphatase	3 mo	
Heart			
Cardiac iron overload	MRI T2	Yearly	>20 msec
Pulmonary hypertension	Echocardiogram	Yearly	Pulmonary artery pressure <25 mm Hg
Ventricular dysfunction Arrhythmias	Echocardiogram or MRI, Holter monitoring, ECG	Yearly	Shortening fraction >32%, LVEF >56%
Endocrine			
Adrenal insufficiency	Cortisol stimulation tests	Yearly or every 2 y	
Delayed puberty	FSH, LH, testosterone, estradiol, DHEAS	Yearly	Bone age if concern for delayed puberty
Diabetes mellitus	Oral glucose tolerance test	Yearly	
Growth failure	Height	3 mo	Consistent growth on same percentile
	Sitting height, bone age	Yearly	
	GH, IGF-1, IGF-BP3	Yearly	
Hypothyroidism	T3, T4, TSH	Yearly	
Hypoparathyroidism	Calcium, phosphate, parathormone	Yearly	
Osteopenia or osteoporosis	Bone mineral density	Yearly or every 2 y	Stable or improved z score on bone scan, normal vitamin D and Ca levels
Nutrition			
Insufficient weight gain	Weight	Monthly	
Trace elements deficiency	Daily vitamin	Yearly	
Vitamin deficiency	supplements to include: Zn, Cu, Se, vitamin E, vitamin C, 25-OH vitamin D	Yearly	

DHEAS = dehydroepiandrosterone sulfate; ECG = electrocardiogram; FSH = follicle-stimulating hormone; GH = growth hormone; IGF-1 = insulin-like growth factor 1; IGF-BP3 = Insulin-like growth factor 2 mRNA binding protein 3; LH = luteinizing hormone; LVEF = left ventricular ejection fraction; MRI = magnetic resonance imaging; RBC = red blood cell; SQUID = superconducting quantum interface device; T3 = triiodothyronine; T4 = thyroxine; TSH = thyroid-stimulating hormone.

progressive splenomegaly, gallstone formation, reduced bone mass and higher incidence of consequential fractures, and chronic joint and bone pain. The increased erythropoiesis also results in increased intestinal iron absorption, which tends to accumulate mostly in the liver and is less likely to cause the cardiac and endocrine problems seen in TM patents with iron overload from transfusions. Hypercoagulability causing increased risk of thrombosis and pulmonary hypertension are complications more often seen in TI patients, and they can cause significant morbidity. As patients' symptoms worsen, therapeutic choices include initiation of transfusions, splenectomy, and medications aimed at fetal hemoglobin augmentation (mostly hydroxyurea [Hydrea]) which, if successful, can ameliorate the anemia and severity of the disease.

E-β thalassemia, the most common type of β thalassemia in Southeast Asia, manifests as a thalassemia intermedia phenotype in 50% to 60% of cases. Others have a more severe phenotype and require early transfusion treatment. Confusion can occur in newborn screening between the clinically mild HbEE and the more severe E-β⁰ thalassemia because the electrophoresis shows absence of HbA and similar HbE and HbF levels. In such cases, parental testing or DNA studies are occasionally required.

α THALASSEMIA

Hemoglobin H disease, a three-α gene deletion, is common in persons of East Asian descent and causes a chronic moderately severe hemolytic anemia. Patients can develop splenomegaly or cholelithiasis, and they can require transfusions during episodes of oxidative stress induced by infections, fever, or certain medications. Hemoglobin H Constant Spring, the coinheritance of a nondeletional α gene variant, manifests with more severe hemolytic anemia and hypersplenism, requiring more frequent transfusions. Patients are followed periodically, in 3- to 6-month intervals, for monitoring of spleen size, hemoglobin level, and growth pattern. Special attention is required during febrile episodes, when the hemoglobin can drop precipitously. The main treatment measures are supplementation with daily folic acid and family education on the potential hemolytic risks involved with high fevers and the use of certain medications. A partial list includes sulfa, antimalaria agents, aspirin, and naphthalene.

Treatment

APPROACH TO THE NEW PATIENT

The diagnosis of a severe thalassemia syndrome is a time of great stress for the entire family due to the implications for a lifelong need for monitoring and complex therapy. A referral to a comprehensive thalassemia care center is appropriate at this time and is highly encouraged. Understanding the complexity of the thalassemia syndromes and treatment options requires care by a team including a hematology expert, subspecialists, and thalassemia support services familiar with the disease and its treatment options. It is important to obtain genotypic diagnosis and provide genetic counseling and information on the likelihood of transfusion dependence. It is also important to emphasize that when thalassemia is adequately managed, it is not a life-threatening diagnosis. Most families are interested in learning about cure and stem cell transplantation, and they should be provided with the information and assured that these options will be explored once a stable treatment plan has been achieved. The discussion about iron overload and chelation should be brief in the initial stages.

MEDICAL THERAPY

Blood Transfusion Therapy

The decision to start regular transfusions is clear when the hemoglobin level is well below 6 g/dL in the absence of an infectious illness. A genotype consistent with a phenotype of severe thalassemia can support this decision. Occasionally, a child might have started receiving regular transfusions due to a transient drop of hemoglobin because of concomitant infection or fever before a full evaluation.

CURRENT THERAPY

Clinical Findings in Thalassemia Intermedia
- Children: Delayed growth, bone changes, frequent illness
- Adolescents and young adults: Delayed growth, delayed pubertal development, low bone mass, splenomegaly and hypersplenism, gallstones.
- Young adults and adults: Low bone mass, osteoporosis, fractures, iron overload, pulmonary hypertension, thrombotic events, extramedullary masses

Annual Monitoring in Thalassemia Intermedia
- First decade: Linear growth and development, photos for facial bone changes, head circumference
- Second decade and adulthood: Right heart pressure on echocardiogram, liver iron, bone density, spinal imaging for nerve compression by masses

Treatment in Thalassemia Intermedia
- Low-iron diet, multivitamin without iron
- Ca 1200-1500 mg/day and vitamin D 400 IU/day
- Warfarin 2 mg/day or aspirin 81 mg/day for splenectomized patients
- Oral chelator for patients with high liver iron
- Regular transfusions when symptoms worsen

Regular transfusions should be commenced if the hemoglobin level is less than 6 to 7 g/dL on two occasions at 2-week intervals. For patients with a higher hemoglobin level (>7 g/dL), the decision is made mostly on a clinical basis considering growth impairment, marked skeletal changes, or extramedullary hematopoiesis. The aim of transfusion therapy is to permit normal growth and activity level, prevent skeletal changes associated with marrow hyperplasia, reduce splenomegaly, and decrease absorption of dietary iron.

Before starting regular transfusions during this long term-therapy, an extended RBC antigen phenotype should be obtained to reduce the future probability of developing alloantibodies. If a child has already started transfusions, the RBC antigen genotype can be determined by DNA testing and, at a minimum, should include the C, E, and Kell alleles. Antibodies to hepatitis B, hepatitis C, and HIV are determined at baseline and then annually (or more often if an unexplained increase in liver function tests occurs). The liver function and serum ferritin level should be checked at baseline and every 3 months.

Packed RBCs, prestorage leukodepleted, is the preferred choice of transfusion for preventing viral transmitted diseases and transfusion reactions. If a febrile or allergic reaction occurs, it might respond to acetaminophen and diphenhydramine (Benadryl) before the transfusion, but persistence of allergic reaction can require administration of washed units to remove the excess plasma. Patients should be assessed for hemolytic reaction if any adverse event is noted during transfusion. The development of new alloantibodies requires extended matching of RBC phenotype, but it can complicate transfusion therapy and might require use of frozen packed RBC units of rare compatible blood types.

The target pretransfusion hemoglobin level is 9 to 10 g/dL and a post-transfusion hemoglobin not to exceed 14 g/dL; this is usually obtained by transfusions given every 3 to 4 weeks. If cardiac insufficiency is present, a higher pretransfusion hemoglobin (10-12 g/dL) is aimed for, with smaller-volume transfusions given every 1 to 2 weeks. The transfusion rate is about 5 mL/kg/hour, or at a slower rate in first-time anemic patients. At each transfusion, the patient's weight, pretransfusion hemoglobin, and the volume of transfusion should be recorded. These values are reviewed periodically (every 6 months) aiming for an annual blood transfusion requirement of 200 mL/kg/ year or less.

The very best practices for blood transfusion must be employed, because lifelong transfusions lead to cumulative increase in the risk of adverse reactions in patients with thalassemia, making future transfusion administration very complex.

Splenectomy

The use of splenectomy in thalassemia has declined in recent years. This is due to the less common occurrence of hypersplenism in patients who are now receiving adequate transfusions from early childhood. In addition, the short- and long-term risks have been of increasing concern, in particular, the association of absence of spleen with thrombosis and pulmonary hypertension.

Occasionally splenectomy is indicated, mostly in TI patients who have not received transfusions or who have received intermittent transfusions; these patients inevitably develop splenomegaly over time. Splenectomy can increase their hemoglobin by 1 to 2 g/dL and allow discontinuation of occasional transfusions. However, if high cardiac output and increased pulmonary artery pressure are present, they are not ameliorated by this procedure. Either laparoscopic or open procedure may be used to remove the spleen.

Patients must receive adequate immunization against *Streptococcus pneumoniae*, *Haemophilus influenzae* type B, and *Neisseria meningitides* before surgery. Splenectomy should be avoided in children younger than 5 years owing to a greater risk of overwhelming postsplenectomy sepsis.

After splenectomy, patients should receive oral penicillin prophylaxis (250 mg twice daily) and are instructed to seek urgent medical attention for fever. Postsplenectomy thrombocytosis is common, and low-dose aspirin should be given during this time.

It is now well recognized that removal of the spleen adds to the risk of a hypercoagulable state and venous thromboembolism, especially in TI patients. In addition, in conjunction with other vascular and hemolysis-induced risk factors, the likelihood of developing pulmonary hypertension increases as splenectomized patients get older. Patients should have annual echocardiographic measurement of pulmonary artery pressure and should be referred to a cardiologist familiar with the monitoring and treatment of this serious complication.

Hematopoietic Stem-Cell Transplantation

Stem cell transplantation is currently the only available cure for thalassemia, with increasing success (>90% engraftment and survival rates), even in older patients (14-18 years old). Matched unrelated transplants are now achieving results similar to those of related transplants with the use of extended haplotypes and improved preparatory regimens.

It is important to obtain HLA type of siblings of an affected child and inform the family of their option and success rates of transplantation, ideally provided by transplant experts. An additional method that families often inquire about is preimplantation genetic diagnosis, which enables in vitro PCR detection of thalassemia mutation within blastomeres (after conventional in vitro fertilization), so that unaffected blastomeres are then implanted. This technology can include HLA typing for a possible unaffected HLA match and has been increasingly used by families with an affected child.

Fetal Hemoglobin Augmentation

Several clinical trials have used agents aimed at increasing fetal hemoglobin concentration via γ globin induction. The success rate has been variable and a significant sustained response has been obtained only in a few patients, usually with specific hemoglobinopathies or a higher baseline fetal hemoglobin. For TI patients without severe complications, and especially in the absence of a large spleen, a trial of treatment with hydroxyurea (15-20 mg/kg/day) for 6 months or longer can show whether an increase in total hemoglobin can be achieved. Monitoring of the WBC monthly or more often is indicated due to hydroxyurea's myelosuppressive potential. Similarly, the use of erythropoietin and butyrate compounds can be considered. A very promising agent for fetal hemoglobin augmentation, decitabine,[5] is currently being assessed in clinical trials.

MANAGING IRON OVERLOAD

Assessment of Iron Overload

Transfusion therapy inevitably results in iron accumulation, because there is no physiologic mechanism that can remove the excess iron involved with transfusions. Iron-induced tissue damage and organ dysfunction are the causes of most of the morbidity and mortality in thalassemia. The deleterious effect is caused by the measurable tissue iron stores and by the non–transferrin-bound iron, a very toxic form of iron. An accurate assessment of body iron overload is essential to assess the risk for organ damage and guide iron chelation therapy. Recent advances in magnetic resonance imaging (MRI) technology have resulted in better assessment of cardiac and liver iron, a major benefit in understanding the selective iron-induced organ damage and subsequent chelation needs. Now that oral iron chelators are available, new approaches can tailor the chelation therapy, with single or combination therapy according to the specific iron-loaded organ.

The most readily available measure of body iron stores is serum ferritin. Serial measurement of serum ferritin is a valuable marker so long as the limitations are recognized. Ferritin level is elevated with infection, inflammation, and hepatitis, and it is reduced with deficiency of vitamin C; all these occur commonly in thalassemia. Levels greater than 3000 ng/mL no longer have a linear relation with body iron stores. Patients with TI have lower ferritin levels for the same degree of liver iron concentration compared with patients receiving transfusions. Levels greater than 2500 ng/mL increase the risk of cardiac disease, but the relative risk of death progressively decreases at lower ferritin levels. Hence, when used to guide chelation therapy, chelation should be started in patients receiving transfusions when the levels approach 1000 ng/mL, with a target level of 500 to 1000 ng/mL.

Because approximately 85% of the body's iron is stored in the liver, methods to measure iron concentration have been a major focus for research. Liver biopsy provides a direct measure of tissue iron loading, and biopsy provides the benefit of the histologic assessment of liver parenchyma. The latter is indicated in patients with severe iron overload or concomitant hepatitis C disease who are at an increased risk for progressive fibrosis and cirrhosis of the liver. Values greater than 15 mg/g dry weight increase the risk of cardiac disease, and the target liver iron concentration should be 4 to 7 mg/g dry weight. Noninvasive assessment of liver iron concentration correlates very well with biopsy and is now used more often where available. The superconducting quantum interface device (SQUID) has shown good correlation with liver iron concentration, but it is available in only few locations around the world. MRI R2 technique is expected to be used by more centers in the future because MRI is more readily available.

Liver iron concentration might not always represent cardiac iron, nor can it always predict the risk of cardiac disease in thalassemia major, although in patients who have a lifelong pattern of adequate chelation, a good correlation exists. Still, a direct assessment of heart iron is desirable and can be accomplished by MRI using T2* technique. T2* values less than 20 ms indicate elevated cardiac iron, and values less than 10 ms indicate increased risk of cardiac dysfunction. Further validation with long-term cardiac function studies and effect of chelation therapy are needed. Accurate assessment of endocrine iron deposition is still not available.

Chelation Regimens

Adequate chelation and continuous medical and psychosocial support to assure optimal compliance are imperative in treating patients receiving transfusions. Iron chelation is a rapidly evolving field owing to the recent introduction of two oral iron chelators into clinical practice.

---

[5]Investigational drug in the United States.

Three chelating agents are available: Deferoxamine (DFO, Desferal) has been used for more than 30 years and still has a major role in chelation therapy for thalassemia. Administered parenterally in an average dose of 30 to 40 mg/kg over 8 to 10 hours for 5 days a week, this method of delivering deferoxamine has caused reduced adherence to treatment in many patients.

Two oral chelators are also available. Deferiprone[1,2] (DFP), not yet approved in the United States but in use in many countries, can penetrate cell membranes better than deferoxamine and therefore is probably more effective in removing myocardial iron. It has several serious potential side effects that need to be carefully watched for (Table 2). Deferasirox (DFS, Exjade), the other iron chelator currently approved for use in thalassemia in the United States, is well absorbed from the gastrointestinal tract and has a long half-life. The starting dose is 20 mg/kg/day, and the dose can be increased to 30 mg/kg/day if negative iron balance is not achieved. Preliminary data also suggest an advantage in removing cardiac iron. Studies on the combined use of deferiprone and deferoxamine suggest an advantage compared with each agent alone. Preliminary studies on combination deferoxamine and deferasirox are under way.

In the United States, deferasirox is becoming the drug of choice for many patients who either start with this agent or switch to it from deferoxamine. However, more long-term trials on its effectiveness are still required. For those who are unable to tolerate this drug, mostly due to gastrointestinal side effects or abnormal renal or hepatic function tests as the dose is escalated, deferoxamine is still prescribed. Deferoxamine is also used in severe iron overload, particularly in the presence of cardiac dysfunction. Continuous intravenous or subcutaneous infusion of deferoxamine[2] at a dose of 50 mg/kg/24 hours or higher is required for prolonged periods, occasionally best administered via a central line catheter.

An additional measure to decrease iron load includes avoiding iron-rich or iron-enriched (e.g., cereals, multivitamins with iron) foods. Drinking black tea with meals can reduce iron absorption from the diet, due to the inhibitory effect of tannic acid in tea leaves.

A more experimental approach is the addition of antioxidants to reduce the oxidative damage induced by thalassemia and iron overload.

Periodic assessment of diet composition, calories, and blood levels of vitamins E, C, and D and chelatable trace elements (selenium, copper, zinc) should be performed, and modifications or supplements provided.

MANAGING DISEASE AND IRON-INDUCED COMPLICATIONS

In less optimally controlled TM or TI, ineffective erythropoiesis results in bone expansion, hepatosplenomegaly, and extramedullary masses. Iron overload, mostly transfusion-induced, results in cardiac, hepatic, and endocrine damage.

Cardiac Disease

Cardiac disease continues to be the most common cause of death in patients with thalassemia major with reduced compliance with chelation treatment. Starting in the second decade, or earlier if indicated, regular monitoring of cardiac function and, where available, of cardiac iron deposition (by MRI using the T2* technique) is extremely important. Patients with significant cardiac iron deposition or decrease in cardiac function should have a reevaluation of chelation therapy and transfusional iron loading and should increase their chelation regimen. Patients with cardiac dysfunction should also maintain a higher pretransfusion hemoglobin level (10-12 g/dL) by more frequent, smaller volume transfusions.

Patients usually present with a rapid change in left ventricular dysfunction, which quickly progresses to congestive heart failure. They can present with arrhythmia and occasionally with acute myocarditis followed by congestive heart failure. Aggressive chelation (continuous deferoxamine infusion at 50 mg/kg/24 hours) is critical. The combination of deferoxamine with deferiprone, owing to the latter's greater efficacy in mobilizing cardiac iron, may be more effective. In addition, angiotensin-converting enzyme inhibitors, diuretics, antiarrhythmic drugs, and inotropic agents are often indicated. Parallel exploration of options for cardiac transplantation should be done in severe cases, a procedure that has been successful in some thalassemia patients with end-stage heart disease.

Liver Disease

Monitoring liver damage and infectious hepatitis is indicated in all patients receiving transfusions. In addition, liver iron concentration is an important measure of total body iron load. Progressive iron deposition can result in hepatomegaly and hepatocellular injury manifesting as elevated transaminases. This can progress to fibrosis and cirrhosis, and the process is accelerated if the patient also acquires viral hepatitis. Pigmentary gallstones can occur in the second or third decade, mostly in TI patients or in older TM patients. Transfusion-transmitted hepatitis C is still prevalent in less developed countries. It can be successfully treated in some cases with a combination of interferon and ribavarin (Rebetol).

Endocrinopathies and Bone Disease

Endocrinopathies can be prevented or minimized with meticulous chelation but are generally not reversible once apparent. Regular monitoring of growth in children is important because intervention with adjustment of transfusion and chelation regimens as well as growth hormone treatment can be very helpful if these treatments are not delayed. In early childhood, impaired growth can result from inadequacy of transfusions as well as from the use of deferoxamine, especially in higher doses, which can suppress linear growth, mostly of the spine. Growth velocity should be monitored every 6 months. In older children, growth failure arises from deficiency of growth hormone, which should be evaluated by measuring hormone levels. Failure of pubertal growth spurt is a common manifestation of hypogonadotropic hypogonadism.

Skeletal changes are common among TM and TI patients due to erythroid hyperplasia and marrow expansion if transfusions are not adequate. A majority of patients develop low bone mass and eventually osteoporosis in the second and third decades. Their management requires sex hormone replacement, supplementation of calcium and vitamin D, and, occasionally, specific treatment to decrease the bone resorption rate. Patients should have annual monitoring of the bone mineral density after the first decade.

The incidence of delayed sexual development is decreasing. Still, the anterior pituitary is extremely sensitive to iron overload and, once hypogonadotropic hypogonadism is established, it cannot be reversed with chelation therapy. Additionally, impaired sexual maturation affects the growth velocity and bone mineral acquisition. Thus, monitoring the levels of sex hormone and obtaining bone age films as well as a full endocrine evaluation are important. Often, sex hormone replacement therapy is indicated, occasionally preceded with growth hormone treatment, in those with delayed bone age in order to maximize the child's potential height.

Glucose intolerance is important to monitor, because diabetes mellitus develops among patients with iron overload. Although diabetes is initially responsive to oral hypoglycemic agents, most patients become insulin dependent. Less commonly, abnormalities in thyroid, parathyroid, and adrenal function can occur and should be monitored periodically. Replacement therapy is required in the occasional patient.

PSYCHOSOCIAL SUPPORT

It is important to support the family during the initial difficult period of diagnosis of an affected child and provide them with information and resources about thalassemia. As children grow older, each life stage poses separate challenges to providing the complex medical care

---
[1] Not FDA approved for this indication.
[2] Not available in the United States.

TABLE 2 Iron-Chelating Agents in Clinical Use

Drug	Half-Life	Route	Average Dose (Range)	Frequency	Iron Excretion	Side Effects	Monitoring	Intervention
Deferoxamine (Desferal)	20 min	SC, IV	35 mg/kg/d (30-50 mg/kg/d)	8-24 h infusion	Urine, stool	Hearing, vision, growth, local skin reactions, pulmonary	Every 6-12 mo: ophthalmology, audiometry Linear growth	Hold, restart at lower dose for audiology abnormalities Discontinue if retinal changes ↓ vision Lower dose, prolong infusion time for ↓ growth
Deferiprone[2] (Ferriprox, Kelfer)	2-3 h	PO	75 mg/kg/d	Three times daily	Urine	Agranulocytosis, neutropenia, gastric upset, arthritis	Weekly CBC	Hold for total neutrophil <1500/mcL Lower dose when restarted
Deferasirox (Exjade)	8-16 h	PO	25 mg/kg/d (20-30 mg/kg/d)	Once daily	Stool	Skin rash, abdominal pain, diarrhea, ↑ creatinine, proteinuria, ↑ transaminases	Monthly creatinine, urine protein, liver enzymes	Hold if persistent ↑ in creatinine Hold for transaminase >5 times normal

[2]Not available in the United States.
CBC = complete blood count.

needed for an optimal outcome. Adolescence is a particularly vulnerable period when compliance with chelation therapy can be greatly compromised. Thalassemia patients now live into adulthood, and they face problems of occupation, insurance and financial challenges, problems with relationships, and desire for a family. They are often compromised due to multisystem iron-induced complications. Thalassemia programs should be able to provide multidisciplinary support to improve patients' quality of life and outcome.

REFERENCES

Aessopos A, Kati M, Farmakis D: Heart disease in thalassemia intermedia: A review of the underlying pathophysiology. Haematologica 2007; 92(5):658-665.
Borgna-Pignatti C: Modern treatment of thalassaemia intermedia. Br J Haematol 2007;138(3):291-304.
Borgna-Pignatti C, Cappellini MD, De Stefano P, et al: Survival and complications in thalassemia. Ann N Y Acad Sci 2005;1054:40-47.
Chui DH, Fucharoen S, Chan V: Hemoglobin H disease: Not necessarily a benign disorder. Blood 2003;101:791-800.
Cohen AR: New advances in iron chelation therapy. Hematology Am Soc Hematol Educ Program 2006;42-47.
Lucarelli G, Andreani M, Angelucci E: The cure of thalassemia by bone marrow transplantation. Blood Rev 2002;16:81-85.
Old JM: Screening and genetic diagnosis of haemoglobin disorders. Blood Rev 2003;17:43-53.
Porter JB: Practical management of iron overload. Br J Haematol 2001;115: 239-252.
Rund D, Rachmilewitz E: Beta-thalassemia. N Engl J Med 2005;353:1135-1146.
Vichinsky EP: Changing patterns of thalassemia worldwide. Ann N Y Acad Sci 2005;1054:18-24.
Weatherall DJ, Clegg JB: The Thalassemia Syndromes, Oxford, Blackwell Science, 2001.

Sickle Cell Disease

Method of
*Lewis L. Hsu, MD, PhD, and
Griffin P. Rodgers, MD**

Fluid Therapy

Renal tubular insufficiency occurs early in childhood in sickle cell disease (SCD), and inability to concentrate urine causes very high susceptibility to dehydration. Dehydration greatly increases sickling of erythrocytes. When a person with SCD cannot take fluids orally (such as before general anesthesia), administer intravenous fluids. In periods of high risk for dehydration, such as the second day after tonsillectomy, a prudent clinician will not shut off IV fluids "to promote thirst." Dehydration also occurs easily in hot weather or dry environments such as airline travel, so that people with SCD should carry their own water. Hydration is fundamental to management of vasoocclusive pain and splenic sequestration. An exception to this principle of liberal hydration is during acute chest syndrome: Parenteral fluid supplements

---

*Adapted from Hsu LL, Rodgers G: Sickle cell disease and other hemoglobinopathies. In Young NS, Gerson SL, High K (eds): Clinical Hematology. Philadelphia: Elsevier, 2006, pp 259-280.

BOX 1 Common Subtypes and Rankings of Disease Severity

Very Mild
SS HPFH
S δβ thalassemia

Milder
Sβ⁺ thalassemia
SC
SE

Similar to SS
Sβ⁰ thalassemia
SD^{Punjab}
SC^{Harlem}

More Severe than SS
SO^{Arab}

HPFH = hereditary persistence of fetal hemoglobin.

---

should be moderate (maintenance replacement), to avoid adding pulmonary edema to the region of pneumonitis.

Sickle cell anemia is a severe hemoglobinopathy with multisystem complications and is the most common of the hemoglobinopathies worldwide. A single nucleotide substitution in codon 6 of the β globin gene causes the abnormal sickled hemoglobin, HbS. The underlying pathophysiologic mechanism common to all genotypes of sickle cell disease involves the intracellular polymerization of deoxy-HbS. Homozygous HbS is termed *sickle cell anemia* or *sickle cell disease SS* and is the most common type of sickle cell disease, with an incidence of approximately 1 in 360 African Americans and 1 in 1200 Latin Americans in Florida. Coinheriting other abnormal hemoglobins with HbS can produce compound heterozygote types of sickle cell disease (Box 1), even when one parent does not have the sickle trait (an important point during genetic counseling). Incidence of HbC is high in many of the populations with HbS, so that typically one third of the people followed at U.S. sickle cell centers have the sickle cell disease SC. Mutations of the α globin genes can also be coinherited, and α-thalassemia has mixed effects in modulating HbSS: decreased hemolytic anemia, fewer strokes and leg ulcers, but higher risk of osteonecrosis and splenic sequestration.

Clinical Features

HEMATOLOGY

Each hemoglobin genotype of SCD has a *likely* range of hematologic values and risks of complications. These are generally most severe in HbSS or HbS β⁰-thalassemia, less severe for HbSC and HbS β⁺-thalassemia, and modified by inheritance of other traits such as α-thalassemia and hereditary persistence of fetal hemoglobin (HPFH). However, each individual patient appears to have his or her own baseline anemia or steady-state hemolysis, which can change gradually over the patient's lifetime. These baseline blood counts are crucial (Box 2) for proper evaluation of acute SCD complications. Therefore, empowering SCD patients to know their own blood counts is a major goal of quality medical care. Acute anemia exacerbation (especially dips 2 g/dL below the baseline anemia) should trigger a search for a new acute complication, such as aplastic crisis, splenic sequestration, accelerated hemolysis, or acute chest syndrome (Table 1).

Leukocytosis is common in SCD (baseline can be 10,000 to 30,000/mm³), which can confuse an evaluation for infection. From this baseline, however, neutrophil counts change acutely as in normal hosts. Severe leukocytosis is also associated epidemiologically with more severe morbidity and mortality. Thrombocytosis is also common.

> **BOX 2 Key Medical History for Sickle Cell Disease and Disease-Specific Review of Systems**
>
> **Sickle Cell Disease Type and Baseline Key Data**
> Sickle cell type
> Baseline hemoglobin
> Reticulocyte fraction
> White blood cell count
> Pulse oximetry
> Spleen size
>
> **Potentially Life-Threatening Problems**
> Allergies
> Red blood cell alloantibodies
> Transfusion reaction
>
> **Sickle Cell Complications (Disease-Specific Review of Systems)**
> Frequent pain
> Recurrent acute chest syndrome
> Sepsis
> Splenic sequestration
> Stroke
> Abnormal transcranial Doppler or brain magnetic resonance imaging
> Priapism
> Leg ulcer
> Avascular necrosis
> Renal insufficiency
> Pulmonary hypertension
> Iron overload
>
> **Past Surgical History**
> Cholecystectomy
> Splenectomy
> Central venous line
> Subcutaneous port
> Hip coring or hip prosthesis
> Tonsillectomy
>
> **Other Problems**
> Asthma
> Chronic hypoxia
> Obstructive sleep apnea
> Psychological, psychiatric, family, social
>
> **Medical Home**
> Health care provider
> Recent and future appointments
>
> **Chronic Transfusion**
> Latest transfusion
> Next transfusion
> Percent HbS
>
> **Immunizations**
> *Streptococcus pneumoniae* conjugate and polysaccharide vaccine
> Hepatitis B vaccine
>
> **Other Long-Term Issues**
> Plans for surgery
> Immunizations or hormone injections due
>
> **Individualized Pain Management Plan**
> Effective medication and nonpharmacologic measures for pain management in the hospital, clinic, emergency department and home.

During acute complications such as splenic sequestration, acute chest syndrome, and sepsis, platelet counts can acutely fall into the thrombocytopenic range. Sickle cell disease and thalassemia share a prothrombotic tendency, so that plasma markers of activated coagulation (D-dimers, prothrombin fragment 1.2 [F1.2], and thrombin–antithrombin [TAT] complex) are often encountered at baseline.

Vasoocclusive pain

The hallmark of sickle cell disease is also its most distressing feature: episodic severe painful vasoocclusion. Triggers for vasoocclusive pain include dehydration, cold temperature or skin cooling, exhaustion or lactic acidosis, infection, weather, emotional stress (including major academic examinations), and menstruation. These triggers appear to be linked to the pathophysiology of increased HbS polymerization, vasoconstriction, and increased endothelial activation. Vasoocclusion often has no objective signs, either on physical examination or laboratory tests. Recognizing one of the characteristic patterns of pain can be the principal clue to diagnosing sickle cell vasoocclusion (Box 3) and spares the patient from unnecessary medical testing. For example, symmetrical bilateral painful hands is probably vasoocclusive dactylitis, but unilateral metacarpal pain may be osteomyelitis. Pain assessment should include a quantitative intensity rating, anatomic location(s), descriptive terms for the pain, time course, aggravating and mitigating factors, and patient self-report about whether this pain feels like previous episodes. Vasoocclusive pain often varies throughout the day and can migrate to different anatomic locations.

Infection

Infection dominates sickle cell disease in natural history studies, but comprehensive care and acute interventions have greatly decreased the mortality and morbidity from infectious disease. Research continues on the mechanisms of immunocompromise in sickle cell disease, but the list of mechanisms includes opsonic defect, functional asplenia, complement activation, altered lymphocyte function, impaired antibody response, impaired phagocytosis, and abnormal cytokine production.

Sepsis

Until the 1970s, people with SCD in the United States usually died in childhood of bacterial sepsis, and the childhood fatality rate is still high in the developing world where immunizations and prophylactic

---

 CURRENT DIAGNOSIS

- In the United States, sickle cell disease is most commonly diagnosed by newborn screening. The public health goal is to confirm the diagnosis of sickle cell disease and start prophylactic antibiotics by 4 to 6 weeks of age to prevent deaths from *Streptococcus pneumoniae* sepsis.
- Diagnosis missed at newborn screening (e.g., new immigrants, errors in the screening program) depends on the alert clinician.
- Anemia, anisocytosis, and reticulocytosis can be detected by automated blood count.
- Sickle deformation is readily seen on the blood smear, and hemoglobin electrophoresis confirms the diagnosis (exceptional compound heterozygotes with unusual hemoglobins can be confusing).
- Infants can present with dactylitis or the life-threatening complications of splenic sequestration or sepsis.
- Later in life, adults may be diagnosed when chronic complications such as gallstones or infarcted vertebral bodies on radiograph.

TABLE 1 Evaluating A Falling Hematocrit in Sickle Cell Disease

Reticulocyte Fraction	Associated Features	Diagnosis
High	Enlarged spleen or liver, pulmonary infiltrate, decreased platelet count	Splenic sequestration, hepatic sequestration, or acute chest syndrome
Baseline	Hemoglobinuria (Coca-Cola urine), autoantibodies, alloantibodies	Accelerated hemolysis, transfusion reaction
0	Parvovirus B19 exposure, Epstein–Barr virus exposure, excessive oxygen supplementation	Aplastic crisis

antibiotics are not available. Sepsis mortality due to *Streptococcus pneumoniae* was 100- to 400-fold greater in children with SCD than in the general childhood population in historical studies. Sepsis in SCD historically also included other encapsulated bacteria (*Haemophilus influenzae, Neisseria meningitides*). *Yersinia* sepsis is a particular problem for patients with iron overload, because this family of bacteria has an unusually high requirement for iron.

Pneumonia

Acute chest syndrome is defined as a new infiltrate on chest x-ray in a person with SCD, combined with fever, cough, or chest pain. Acute chest syndrome (ACS) often results in rapid deterioration, with a mortality rate as high as 6%. ACS can have multiple etiologies, but respiratory infection is involved in most episodes of ACS in children. Organisms identified in ACS include typical community-acquired bacterial pneumonia, atypical bacteria such as *Chlamydia pneumoniae* and *Mycoplasma hominis,* and respiratory viruses.

Osteomyelitis and Septic Arthritis

The devitalized ischemic bones in sickle cell disease are more susceptible to bacterial infections of bones and joints than in normal hosts. *Staphylococcus aureus, Salmonella,* and other enteric bacteria are common etiologies for osteomyelitis. However, diagnosing these infections can be extremely challenging because the signs, symptoms, and imaging results of osteomyelitis and septic arthritis overlap with those of sickle cell vasoocclusion.

Parvovirus

One of the ordinary respiratory viruses, parvovirus B19, causes a transient erythroblastopenia (reticulocyte counts are typically zero for 7 to 10 days) that can become aplastic crisis in persons with SCD and other hemolytic anemias. This sudden cessation of erythrocyte production while chronic hemolytic destruction continues can lead to fatal anemia, stroke, or heart failure. In some patients, parvovirus B19 triggers a spectrum of other sickle cell complications (ACS, stroke) and thrombocytopenia, neutropenia, or hemophagocytic syndrome.

BOX 3 Patterns of Pain in Differential Diagnosis

Avascular necrosis of femoral head: Recurrent vasoocclusive pain, sciatica
Biliary colic: Constipation
Dactylitis: Osteomyelitis, trauma
Hepatic sequestration: Hepatitis, ascending cholangitis
Menstrual trigger: Unexplained recurrent pain
Mesenteric vasoocclusion: Acute surgical abdomen, constipation
Priapism: Normal erection, urinary tract infection
Rib infarct: Pulmonary embolism
Skull infarct: Hemorrhagic stroke, skull abscess
Vasoocclusion with joint effusion: Septic arthritis, fracture

---

RESPIRATORY

Acute chest syndrome is a leading cause of death in sickle cell disease. The most common trigger for ACS in adults is marrow fat embolism and the most common trigger in children is respiratory infection, but multiple etiologies often contribute to ACS: vasoocclusive pain of the chest wall, atelectasis from a splinting respiratory pattern and hypoventilation, and rib infarctions. These problems all lead to hypoxemia and increased sickling, which can then worsen the vasoocclusive contribution to ACS and further compromise respiratory function in a positive feedback loop. ACS can worsen rapidly to include acute respiratory distress syndrome or multi-organ failure syndrome, or both. Other sickle cell complications can accompany ACS, including neurologic complications, splenic or hepatic sequestration, and priapism.

Chronic hypoxemia occurs in a significant fraction of patients with SCD. Abnormally low pulse oximetry in SCD can be caused by complex artifacts in some cases, but true chronic hypoxemia can be determined by arterial blood gas analysis, and this can be a useful part of the patient's record. Obstructive sleep apnea due to adenoidal hypertrophy appears to be more common in children with sickle cell disease than in the general population, but it can be relieved surgically. For unknown reasons, the prevalence of hyperreactive airways is high in sickle cell disease, and pulmonary function testing generally reveals a mixture of restrictive and obstructive dysfunction. Coordinating and optimizing pulmonary and hematologic management can significantly decrease the rate of hospitalizations in children with asthma and SCD.

Pulmonary hypertension has gained recognition as a major concern in sickle cell disease, affecting one third of adults with sickle cell disease SS, with onset in adolescence or earlier. Pulmonary hypertension can be detected by Doppler echocardiogram measurement of a tricuspid regurgitant jet velocity (TRJV) greater than 2.5 m/sec performed when the patient is at steady-state baseline. Although this level of TRJV might be considered trivially mild in patients without hemoglobinopathy, TRJV greater than 2.5 m/sec in patients with SCD is associated with a 10-fold increased rate of mortality in 18 months. The etiology of pulmonary hypertension may be tonic vasoconstriction from low nitric oxide bioavailability due to high hemolysis. Microemboli might also be involved, with significant plexogenic vascular remodeling in the later stages of pulmonary hypertension in autopsy series.

CENTRAL NERVOUS SYSTEM

Cerebrovascular complications are prominent manifestations of SCD vasculopathy, ranging from fatal hemorrhagic stroke to subtle neuropsychological damage, and commonly seen as ischemic changes in children with SCD-SS and SCD-Sβ^0-thalassemia. Arteries around the circle of Willis are susceptible to focal segments of stenosis with intimal hyperplasia and disrupted elastic lamina. Atherosclerosis is rare in sickle cell cerebrovasculopathy. These stenoses can be detected by magnetic resonance angiography (MRA, with data acquisition adjustments to suppress artifacts of turbulent flow). Infarcts can manifest as major sensory, motor, or cognitive deficits. Infarcts can also be completely silent and detected only by imaging. Small infarcts in the deep white matter are associated with abnormalities of smaller arteries, called *small-vessel disease,* which are not detectable by MRA.

Ischemic stroke can occur in association with other sickle cell complications: as a watershed bilateral infarct distribution with transient acute anemia such as splenic sequestration or aplastic crisis or as focal infarcts due to emboli from marrow fat embolism or priapism.

Regular screening of children for high risk of stroke using transcranial Doppler ultrasound is part of the standard comprehensive care of SCD types SS and S-β^0-thalassemia. A large fraction of ischemic strokes in children with SCD can be prevented by using transcranial Doppler screening to identify a high-risk group and then treating this group with a blood-transfusion program. Without treatment, children with cerebrovascular stenosis are likely to progress to recurrent stroke and the moyamoya pattern of vasculopathy.

Hemorrhagic stroke is more common in adults with SCD than in children, and it is often rapidly fatal. The patient typically complains of "the worst headache of my life," and remarks that the pain is different from sickle cell vasoocclusive pain. The etiology is often an aneurysm, associated with a weakened medial layer of the arterial wall. Multiple aneurysms may be present, and further bleeds may be prevented by vascular clip. Bleeding can also occur from moyamoya collateral vessels.

RENAL

Sickle cells cause renal tubular damage from very early in childhood, causing isosthenuria. As a result, the urine specific gravity is not a reliable sign of hydration status in patients with SCD. Renal tubular damage also leads to nocturia or enuresis, because the urine produced all night is fairly dilute, and the bladder is filled with the larger volume of urine produced by the kidneys during the night. Hematuria is common in SCD, attributable to papillary necrosis from red blood cell (RBC) sickling in the renal medulla.

Proliferative glomerulopathy and microalbuminuria can also begin early in life. By young adulthood, some patients have frank albuminuria and the nephrotic syndrome. Approximately 4% of patients with HbSS and one half as many with HbSC progress to end-stage renal disease requiring hemodialysis.

OTHER COMPLICATIONS

Several other organ systems can suffer complications of sickle cell disease. Proliferative retinopathy can be silent until catastrophic complications like hyphema or retinal detachment occur; a screening ophthalmologic examination can permit early intervention to prevent such problems. Cholelithiasis with pigment stones is present in over one half of adults, but there is a controversy about when to perform elective cholecystectomy on asymptomatic gallstones. Impaired growth and delayed puberty are common, and have been linked to elevated energy expenditure and micronutrient and endocrine abnormalities, but patients usually reach normal adult height eventually.

Leg Ulcers

Leg ulcers occur in patients with SS and S β^0-thalassemia in the United States with an incidence of 2 to 6 per 100 patient-years, but they are more common in patients living in the tropics. Ulcers typically involve the skin overlying the medial malleoli after trauma, insect bites, or dry skin. Ulcers can be extremely painful and slow to heal, causing functional disability for months to years. Infectious complications can include cellulitis, lymphadenitis, or osteomyelitis. Skin edema can herald recurrence of a leg ulcer. It is controversial whether hydroxyurea therapy worsens leg ulcers.

Bone Infarcts and Osteonecrosis of Femoral and Humeral Heads

Vertebral bone infarcts lead to a characteristic radiographic sign of SCD: the H-shaped vertebral body. Vertebral distortion can lead to nerve compression syndromes. Rib infarcts are significant contributors to ACS pathophysiology.

Osteonecrosis or avascular necrosis causes pain in the hip or shoulder with weight bearing or motion and often aches at night. Avascular necrosis is more common in HbSC and HbS-β^+-thalassemia. X-rays reveal degeneration of the head of the femur or humerus in advanced cases. MRI is useful in early diagnosis. Bone scan shows decreased uptake early in the course of avascular necrosis, then increased uptake later in the course.

Priapism

Priapism is a prolonged, painful penile erection that probably arises from dysregulated nitric oxide and increased vasoconstrictor tone. Priapism affects more than 30% of male SCD patients at some stage, from early school age to adulthood. Priapism occurs in two patterns: stuttering episodes of 2 to 4 hours, which might precede a major episode, and severe ischemic events that last more than 4 hours and can cause fibrosis and impotence.

Splenic Sequestration

The spleen usually infarcts and involutes, so that normal splenic filtration function is lost in the first years of life in SCD-SS but much later in SCD-SC. Sometimes, however, the spleen enlarges and sequesters a significant fraction of RBCs and platelets, transiently removing them from circulation. Acute splenic sequestration can suddenly drop the hemoglobin level by 2 g/dL, typically accompanied by thrombocytopenia and painful splenomegaly. Simply palpating the acutely enlarged spleen provides the diagnosis of acute splenic sequestration. The patient's activity level decreases as the anemia exacerbates. Additional splenic sequestration can worsen to life-threatening hypovolemic shock and profound anemia exacerbation.

Acute splenic sequestration can resolve spontaneously with intravenous hydration or with blood transfusion. Recurrent acute splenic sequestration can enlarge the spleen again within hours, a pattern called *yo-yo spleen*. Alternatively, the spleen can enlarge gradually over weeks or months without pain, leading to persistently palpable splenomegaly, mild anemia, and thrombocytopenia. This chronic splenomegaly can fluctuate for years and then can spontaneously resolve.

Treatment

COMPREHENSIVE APPROACH TO CARE

Comprehensive care is important in SCD: treating chronic problems, individualizing pain management, screening and preventive care (Table 2 and Box 4). Multidisciplinary comprehensive care is less costly than episode acute care, improves patient satisfaction, and can even be implemented in developing countries. Family education is crucial to significant lifesaving home care (see Table 2) (prophylactic antibiotics for children and spleen palpation), and it can also lay the foundation for home pain management and coping skills. When a patient must receive care at different institutions, key points of the medical history can be given to families as a "health passport" or "travel letter" to promote medical communication and continuity of care (see Box 2).

VASOOCCLUSIVE PAIN

Sickle cell vasoocclusive pain is the leading reason for patients to seek medical care. Vasoocclusion often targets certain sites (Table 3 and Box 5). Patterns often recur in a given patient, and deviations from a previous pattern can be subtle but important in distinguishing vasoocclusive pain from other complications. For example, painful limping could be due to acute vasoocclusion or avascular necrosis of the hip, but painless limp may be due to stroke.

Pain Management Principles

Pain management in SCD is challenging and sometimes frustrating because the vasoocclusive pain can be episodic, unpredictable, and

TABLE 2 Comprehensive Care and Family and Patient Education

Care	Newborn	Infant and Toddler	School Age	Adolescent	Adult
Screening	Confirm SCD type	Establish baseline CBC and reticulocytes, pulse oximetry	TCD, hip exam, dental, pulse oximetry, consider gallstones, ECG	Proteinuria, retinopathy, dental care, echocardiogram, pulse oximetry	Proteinuria, retinopathy, ECG, dental care, pulse oximetry
Immunizations	Routine, including conjugated pneumococcal	Routine, including influenza and conjugated pneumococcal	Routine, including influenza, polysaccharide pneumococcal	Routine, including influenza	Routine, including influenza
Education	Fever, spleen palpation, prophylactic antibiotics, dactylitis, sickle pathophysiology	Pain prevention and management, stroke symptoms	Pain prevention and management, priapism, academic and career choices	Academic and career choices, HbS genetics and reproduction, personal responsibility, pain management, dependence vs independence, transition to adult health care program	Career and family choices, health insurance, HbS genetics and reproduction, pain management
Prevention	Penicillin prophylaxis	Penicillin prophylaxis, RBC phenotype	Penicillin prophylaxis becomes optional	Healthy habits and hydration	Healthy habits and hydration

CBC = complete blood count; ECG = echocardiogram; Hb = hemoglobin; RBC = red blood cell; SCD = sickle cell disease; TCD = transcranial Doppler.

variable, and it might have no objective signs. However, the basic principles of pain management still apply: quantify the pain, give analgesic combinations to match the intensity of therapy to the intensity of pain, check frequently for response to interventions and adjust therapy. Use the WHO staircase of analgesics strategy (Fig. 1) to add analgesics in a rational sequence. Inflammation plays a large role in SCD, making nonsteroidal antiinflammatory agents (NSAIDs) a rational first choice for pharmacologic intervention. For a patient coming to the emergency department because his or her home pain management was not sufficient, a strong NSAID such as ketorolac can be combined with a parenteral opioid. Maximal analgesia is achieved by combining an NSAID with escalating doses of opioids, plus sometimes other classes of analgesics; however, there have been few clinical trials to determine whether any one combination is superior for vasoocclusive pain. Patient-controlled analgesia (PCA) pumps permit great flexibility of parenteral opioid administration and can be used safely by children as young as 6 years old. Some centers use PCA subcutaneous opioid infusion in patients with poor venous access.

During a hospitalization for sickle cell pain, complications to avoid are acute chest syndrome, constipation, and loss of venous access. Several strategies are available to minimize the adverse effects of parenteral opioids: agonist–antagonist agents such as nalbuphine (Nubain), continuous infusion of a very low dose of antagonist such as naloxone (Narcan), or pharmacologic combinations to manage specific adverse effects (antiemetics for nausea, antihistamine for pruritus, laxatives and stool softeners for constipation, and stimulants for sedation). Incentive spirometry to reduce atelectasis in patients with sickle cell pain in the chest wall has been proved to reduce acute chest syndrome by a factor of 9, and therefore incentive spirometry is part of the standard of care for hospitalized patients with sickle cell pain. Adjunct corticosteroids can provide some benefit for vasoocclusive pain, perhaps with a short steroid taper to avoid rebound pain.

Nonpharmacologic pain management adjuncts can be very important, increasing comfort with little or no adverse effects: warm compresses, cushioned mattress pads, recreational therapy and music for distraction, massage, hydrotherapy, hypnosis, relaxation imagery, and transcutaneous electrical nerve stimulators. Sickle cell centers in Cuba report that laser acupuncture is helpful for pain management.

Improving Hospital Pain Management

Individualized pain management plans can list those combinations that have been effective for the patient (see Table 3), and the patient and continuity doctors can update the list periodically. Vasoocclusive pain intensity and duration of hospitalization can vary widely between and within individual patients. A small subset of patients can have very frequent hospitalizations, and focusing individualized case management on these complex patients may reap a greater economic and clinical impact than broad guidelines for the majority of SCD patients to shorten their already-short hospital stays. Psychosocial staff are vital to the multidisciplinary case management approach. When resources permit sickle cell pain management in a day hospital or a dedicated urgent-care center, 8 hours of parenteral analgesic treatment can provide enough pain relief to allow 80% of patients to avoid admission to the hospital.

BOX 4 FARMS

The mnemonic FARMS summarizes major points of self-care for sickle cell disease at every age.

F: Fluids, folic acid.
A: Air. Oxygenation is important to prevent sickling. Avoid smoking. Treat asthma, sleep apnea, and other respiratory diseases.
R: Rest, relaxation. Rest breaks when exercising or working can prevent lactic acidosis, which promotes sickling. Relaxation exercises can help with pain management.
M: Medications, medical care. Know your medications: their names, doses, desired effects and side effects. Communicate with your health care team and try to maintain a medical home to avoid fragmenting care among several medical facilities.
S: Situations, support. Avoid situations that can trigger pain or other problems: dehydration, exhaustion, extremes of temperature, infection, high stress. Seek support from family, friends, and the community.

TABLE 3 Preventing and Managing Vasoocclusive Pain

Degree	Opioid	NSAID	Adjunct Medications	Nonpharmacologic
Prevention			Influenza prophylaxis: Penicillin VK (Veetids) PO bid *or* Pen G (Bicillin) IM monthly *or* erythromycin PO bid Folic acid Consider hydroxyurea (Droxia)	Maintain good hydration Avoid extremes of temperature Avoid exhaustion and lactic acidosis Reduce stress and epinephrine Avoid hypoxia (treat asthma, sleep apnea)
Mild		Acetaminophen (Tylenol) Ibuprofen (Motrin, Advil) Naproxen (Naprosyn)		
Moderate	Codeine with acetaminophen Oxycodone with acetaminophen	Ketorolac	Laxative ± stool softener Antihistamine	
Severe	Nalbuphine (Nubain) Morphine Hydromorphone (Dilaudid) Oxycodone (OxyContin) Fentanyl (Actiq)	Ketorolac	Low-dose naloxone (Narcan) Antiemetic Antihistamine Laxative ± stool softener	

Home Pain Management

The vast majority of vasoocclusive pain is managed at home. Typically, pain management starts with rest, fluids, and warmth, then adding an NSAID such as ibuprofen (Motrin, Advil), acetaminophen (Tylenol), or naproxyn (Naprosyn). More intense pain may be managed by adding oral opioid combinations such as acetaminophen and codeine or acetaminophen and oxycodone. Prescribing stronger oral opioids for home use might permit patients to avoid some hospitalizations, but other patients find that severe vasoocclusive pain can only be managed with parenteral opioids. Families can prevent some vasoocclusive pain by avoiding triggers of HbS polymerization (see Table 3). Menstruation is a trigger for sickle vasoocclusive pain in some patients, and hormonal regulation to suspend the menses may be offered as a pain-management strategy. Recognizing such pain patterns is important for individualized case management, but many pain episodes have no identifiable trigger. More complete discussion of sickle cell pain management and current analgesic considerations are available in the references.

INFECTION

Sepsis

For patients with SCD and fever, the standard of care is prompt medical evaluation, blood culture, and empiric antibiotics targeting *S. pneumoniae*. Vaccines have successfully reduced sepsis from the bacteria covered by the conjugated vaccines against *S. pneumoniae* and *H. influenzae* type B and the 23-valent polysaccharide vaccine against *S. pneumoniae*. However, vaccinated SCD patients still suffer more cases of *S. pneumoniae* sepsis than the normal population, sometimes with bacteria not covered by the vaccines, and *S. pneumoniae* is becoming increasingly resistant to antibiotics.

Another special consideration arises in patients with SCD and iron overload, due to bacterial avidity for iron. Iron chelators should be withheld temporarily in febrile patients, especially those with abdominal pain, diarrhea and vomiting, or fever and sore throat. The clinician should strongly consider *Yersinia* in an iron-overloaded patient with sepsis and gastrointestinal symptoms.

Acute Chest Syndrome

Because acute chest syndrome often has an infectious etiology, part of the management for acute chest syndrome is empiric antibiotic coverage for both respiratory bacteria and atypical bacteria (e.g., ceftriaxone [Rocephin] or ampicillin-sulbactam [Unasyn], plus a macrolide antibiotic). Antiviral agents are generally not warranted for respiratory infections in sickle cell patients.

Osteomyelitis

When osteomyelitis is suspected on clinical grounds, sickle cell patients should not be overtreated with antibiotics for osteomyelitis unless infection is proven by bacterial culture, because bone infarction is estimated to be 50 times more likely than osteomyelitis. Note that the erythrocyte sedimentation rate is subject to artifacts from the sickle erythrocytes, and the C-reactive protein may be elevated by vasoocclusive ischemic tissue damage, thus diminishing their value as markers for diagnosing and following osteomyelitis. In patients with culture-proved bone or joint infection, surgical curettage and drainage should be followed by 2 to 6 weeks of antibiotics. Initial empiric antibiotics should cover *Salmonella* and *Staphylococcus* species and then should be adjusted for specific susceptibilities once an organism is isolated. Most patients can be cured with this therapy but, unfortunately, recurrences and refractory infection can occur.

BOX 5   Mnemonic for Sickle Cell Pain Management: BACK PAIN

Believe the patient
Assess pain
Combine therapy (staircase concept)
Kinetics of medications guide dosing intervals
Primum non nocere
Acute chest syndrome and other complications
Individualize but provide consistency
You are **N**ot alone — involve the patient and team

CURRENT THERAPY

- Sickle cell disease (SCD) is more than hemolytic anemia and vasoocclusive pain, and the clinician must be alert for complications in nearly every organ system. Multidisciplinary care and a medical home are optimal.
- Diagnosis by newborn screening permits early enrollment in preventive and comprehensive care.
- Much of sickle cell care is based on evidence from randomized clinical trials: transcranial Doppler ultrasound screening for stroke risk, pneumococcal vaccination (Pneumovax) and prophylactic antibiotics, incentive spirometry, extended matching of red blood cell antigens for blood transfusion.
- A patient's baseline hemoglobin level and reticulocytosis are critically important for management, especially for aplastic crisis and splenic sequestration.
- *Streptococcus pneumoniae* is particularly lethal in persons with SCD, so rapid evaluation of the febrile patient and empiric parenteral antibiotics is the current standard of care.
- Acute chest syndrome is potentially fatal, and so an SCD patient with a new radiographic infiltrate and chest symptoms merits close observation.
- Begin acute vasoocclusive pain management with swift assessment and standardized treatment. Subsequent treatment often requires individualized combinations of opioids, nonsteroidal antiinflammatory agents, and nonpharmacologic and pharmacologic adjuncts.
- Extending the transfusion cross-matching to C, E, and Kell antigens can decrease the risk of alloimmunization.
- Environmental triggers for vasoocclusive pain can be mitigated by family and patient education.
- Reduce the risk of leg ulcers by avoiding venipuncture and other trauma to the ankles and avoiding prolonged standing.
- Hydroxyurea (Droxia) can reduce the severity of sickle cell disease, but not all patients respond.
- Sickle cell disease can be cured by hematopoietic stem cell transplantation from an HLA-matched related donor, including sibling umbilical cord–placental blood.

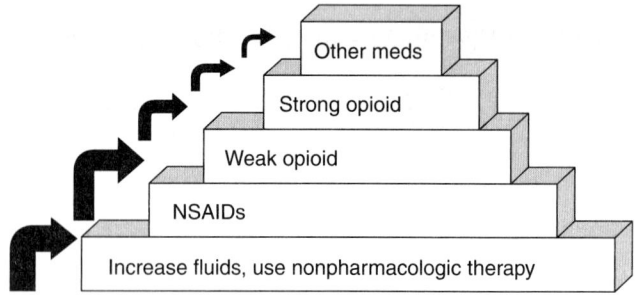

FIGURE 1. Staircase concept for management of vasoocclusive pain. Titrate analgesia upward by adding analgesics of different modalities. Nonpharmacologic measures and increased fluids are fundamental. NSAID = nonsteroidal antiinflammatory drug. (Adapted from Cancer Pain Relief and Palliative Care: Report of a WHO Expert Committee. Geneva, World Health Organization, 1990, p 7-21.)

Parvovirus B19

Parvovirus B19 infection usually suppresses erythrocyte production for 7 to 10 days, causing a falling hematocrit and reticulocytopenia. This period of aplastic crisis might be managed by supportive care without transfusion in patients with milder hemolytic anemia and no complications. Deciding whether to give a blood transfusion depends on the severity of anemia (compared with the patient's baseline) and cardiopulmonary compromise, not a specific hematocrit. Additional considerations may include severe RBC alloimmunization or religious objection to transfusion. The patient suspected of parvovirus should be isolated from immunocompromised or pregnant persons, at least until reticulocyte counts begin to rise.

Other Infections

Annual influenza immunization is recommended for persons with sickle cell disease, because influenza can cause acute chest syndrome.

Persons with SCD are quite susceptible to malaria, even though sickle trait confers improved survival with malaria. Malaria treatment should include prompt antimalarials plus fluid supplements to prevent dehydration and splenic sequestration.

The theoretical risk of subacute bacterial endocarditis in SCD patients with hyperdynamic and dilated hearts has led some clinicians to advocate routine antibiotic prophylaxis for dental care of SCD patients. However, the 2007 American Heart Association guidelines indicate that such conditions of turbulent flow no longer require prophylaxis against endocarditis.

RESPIRATORY

Due to the potential for rapid deterioration, patients with ACS should have prompt treatment and initial observation in the hospital. The multiple etiologies of ACS should be addressed by empiric therapy that comprises empiric antibiotics, including a macrolide to cover atypical bacteria, bronchodilators, analgesics, supplemental oxygen, and measures to reduce atelectasis (incentive spirometry, continuous positive airway pressure, or intermittent positive airway pressure). RBC transfusion can produce prompt clinical improvement and should be considered when the patient has hemoglobin dropping by more than 1 g/dL from baseline and pulse oximetry falling below 93% (being cautious not to overtransfuse into hyperviscosity or volume overload). Be moderate with parenteral fluid supplements to avoid adding pulmonary edema to the region of pneumonitis. If the patient requires high supplemental oxygen despite RBC transfusion, consider a double-volume exchange transfusion to reduce the fraction of sickle RBCs below 30%.

Bronchoscopy can provide useful diagnostic information for a patient with worsening ACS, and in rare cases, bronchoscopy has cured ACS by removing bronchial casts from the airway (plastic bronchitis). Severe ACS has many features of acute respiratory distress syndrome and appears to benefit from the same therapies if there is respiratory failure: careful mechanical ventilation, extracorporeal membrane oxygenation, inhaled nitric oxide, and high-frequency ventilation. People with recurrent ACS often have reactive airways disease and benefit from pulmonology consultation.

Pulmonary hypertension in sickle cell disease might respond to antisickling therapy in addition to specific therapy for pulmonary arterial hypertension. Patients can benefit from referral to a pulmonary hypertension center offering clinical trials for this high-risk condition.

Obstructive sleep apnea can be relieved by tonsillectomy or adenoidectomy (or both), with careful perioperative management to avoid sickle cell complications in this moderate-risk surgery.

NEUROLOGIC

The neurologic complications of SCD were reduced dramatically after a landmark clinical trial established a new standard of care: screening children with transcranial Doppler ultrasound to detect those at high risk for stroke, and then protecting them from primary stroke by a long-term program of blood transfusion to maintain the sickle RBC fraction below 30%. After implementing this strategy, California's rate of first stroke in SCD children decreased from 0.88 per 100 person-years to 0.17 per 100 person-years.

In acute stroke, many centers use exchange transfusion to rapidly maintain sickle erythrocytes below 30% to limit the ischemic damage. Acute anticoagulation has not been studied in this setting. Neurology consultation and neurocognitive evaluation can guide a plan for vigorous rehabilitation therapy, and many neurologic deficits in children are reversible.

After a stroke, a chronic transfusion program to maintain sickle erythrocytes below 30% for at least 3 years reduces the risk of recurrent stroke by as much as 90%. Hydroxyurea appears to confer partial protection against recurrent stroke in children with contraindications to chronic transfusion; a clinical trial is in progress. Hematopoietic stem cell transplantation prevents stroke recurrence and appears to halt cerebrovascular stenosis, and the family should have HLA typing to identify possible related donors.

Intracranial hemorrhage can arise from two features of cerebrovascular disease: aneurysms (which may be in unusual locations) and moyamoya vasculopathy. Patients can present dramatically with severe headache, vomiting, and coma for a subarachnoid hemorrhage. The presentation can have more subtle neurologic deficits for intraparenchymal bleeding. Acute neurologic symptoms should be evaluated with emergent noncontrast head computed tomography (CT) to determine whether neurosurgical intervention is needed. Guidelines for intracranial hemorrhage should be followed, and preoperative transfusion plans may need to be pragmatically modified for the individual circumstances.

If the patient's hemoglobin is less than 10 g/dL, an RBC transfusion should improve cerebral oxygenation, but excessive transfusion to hemoglobin greater than 12 g/dL risks hampering oxygen delivery through hyperviscosity and hypertension. Many clinicians proceed to erythrocytapheresis or manual exchange transfusion to reduce HbS fraction to below 30% to optimize blood flow and oxygenation for the weeks of critical care and recovery ahead. Most clinicians recommend chronic transfusion for a child with severe vasculopathy or unrepaired aneurysm.

RENAL

Enuresis

Desmopressin (DDAVP) and anticholinergics have only modest benefit in children with SCD and enuresis, presumably because the damaged renal tubules have a blunted pharmacologic response. Behavioral training can be effective if applied for at least 3 weeks: reduce fluid intake for a couple of hours before bedtime, urinate just before going to bed, set an alarm and nightlight to wake up and go to the bathroom during the night, and have the child participate in laundering any wet sheets the next day.

Hematuria

An SCD patient with hematuria should be assessed for possible malignancy, infection, and other causes, leaving SCD renal papillary necrosis as the diagnosis of exclusion. The treatment of hematuria in SCD involves bedrest and maintenance of a high urinary flow documented by monitoring of intake and output. If blood loss is significant, iron replacement or blood transfusion, or both, may be indicated.

Glomerulopathy

Microalbuminuria and frank proteinuria are markers of deterioration of glomerular function. Coordinated nephrology and hematology management of patients with renal insufficiency can include angiotensin-converting enzyme inhibitors and hydroxyurea (Droxia), erythropoietin supplementation, and managing the higher risk of thrombotic complications. Renal transplants for people with SCD can be similar to renal transplantation for other end-stage renal disease and might have lower mortality than dialysis.

LEG ULCERS

Leg ulcer treatment requires a consistent, systematic approach to maximize patient compliance over several months: elevation of the legs, meticulous débridement, zinc supplements, antibiotics, and analgesics for chronic pain (see the National Heart, Lung, and Blood Institute guidelines at www.SCInfo.org). Leg ulcers commonly recur. Prevention must be stressed, especially avoiding venipuncture of the lower extremities and avoiding occupations that involve prolonged standing.

BONE INFARCTS AND AVASCULAR NECROSIS

The pain of bone infarcts, sickle arthritis, or other joint complications can persist for weeks, with a waxing and waning course. Physical therapy and NSAIDs are preferable to persistent administration of narcotics, and patients can learn to differentiate the treatment of this chronic pain from treatment of acute pain episodes. During periods of exacerbation of pain in avascular necrosis of the femoral head, for example, non–weight bearing improves the acute problem and can slow progression. Options to reduce the disability caused by avascular necrosis are emerging: early physical therapy, core decompression of the femoral head, and prosthetic hips with improved materials.

PRIAPISM

SCD priapism resulted in impotence in nearly one half of historical cases, but current guidelines for swift intervention aim to reduce this long-term sequela as well as acute suffering. Home therapy may be sufficient to relieve an episode of stuttering priapism: oral fluids, analgesics, urination, moderate exercise, or bathing or showering. Patients with stuttering priapism can be evaluated for priapism prophylaxis using several months of pseudoephedrine (Sudafed),[1] terbutaline (Brethine),[1] or low-dose hydroxyurea (Droxia). Preliminary reports suggest that sildenafil may also be effective prophylaxis for stuttering priapism.

Priapism that fails to resolve within 2 to 4 hours is considered an acute ischemic emergency requiring prompt aspiration of the corpora cavernosa by a urologist, who may also consider intracavernous injection of sympathomimetic drugs and creation of vascular shunts. Intravenous hydration and analgesics are used as in other vasoocclusive pain. The use of exchange transfusion for priapism has become controversial, but it permits further management options that might otherwise trigger vasoocclusion, such as cooling the penis.

Other Therapeutic Issues

PREGNANCY AND CONTRACEPTION

Pregnancy is not contraindicated in women with SCD, but there are increased risks of pregnancy-induced hypertension, vasoocclusive pain, urinary tract infections, hypercoagulability, renal and pulmonary complications, and perinatal mortality. Ideally, managing the pregnancy starts with preconception planning and genetic counseling, gathering a multidisciplinary team with expertise in sickle cell hematology, obstetrics, nutrition, and primary care. Hyperemesis in early pregnancy should be managed early with antiemetics, because dehydration can cause sickle vasoocclusion. Prophylactic transfusions are reserved for women with additional obstetric or hematologic high-risk features. Postpartum care must include screening for SCD in the infant and counseling on plans for future pregnancies.

There is no evidence of increased thrombotic events with modern low-estrogen oral contraceptive formulations in women with SCD. Factors to weigh when choosing contraception include the adverse

---

[1]Not FDA approved for this indication.

health effects of pregnancy in SCD and the potential for hormonal therapy to reduce vasoocclusive pain. Men and women on hydroxyurea therapy should use contraceptive methods, because hydroxyurea is well known to be teratogenic in animal models. However, if there is a conception while the patient is taking hydroxyurea, counselors should mention that no birth defects occurred in 14 reported cases of hydroxyurea in human pregnancies.

SURGERY AND PERIOPERATIVE CARE

Coordinated attention to the unique needs of SCD by the anesthesiology, surgery, and hematology teams can significantly reduce the risk of perioperative complications. Older age, regional anesthesia, tonsillectomy, and abdominal surgery are associated with greater risk of SCD-related complications. Sickle cell patients can tolerate major procedures (e.g., neurosurgery, organ transplantation) with preoperative exchange transfusion, perioperative hydration, and close attention to oxygenation and warmth. For procedures with moderate risk of vasoocclusion, the standard of care is to administer a preoperative RBC transfusion to a hemoglobin level of approximately 10 g/dL instead of exchange transfusion and to administer postoperative respiratory therapy with incentive spirometry. With meticulous supportive care, SCD patients with religious objections to blood transfusion have tolerated low- to moderate-risk surgery without transfusion, sometimes with careful doses of erythropoietin to raise blood counts preoperatively.

BLOOD TRANSFUSION

Transfusion of normal red blood cells has two broad indications in patients with SCD: to improve the oxygen-carrying capacity and to dilute sickled RBCs and prevent extensive sickling in situations of acidosis, hypoxia, or stasis. However, each blood transfusion carries risks (Table 4).

Acute Indications for Transfusion

In various scenarios of acute complications, experts disagree on the indications for transfusion and generally do not fix a standard hemoglobin level that triggers transfusion for all SCD patients. Key considerations are the patient's baseline hemoglobin level and reticulocyte fraction compared with the current levels, the physiologic reserve of cardiorespiratory function, and the likelihood of triggering more sickling with severe acidosis and hypoxemia. Typically, transfusions are given for acute complications like aplastic crisis, splenic sequestration, or acute chest syndrome when the patient's hemoglobin level has fallen by 2 g/dL and symptoms of anemia or hypoxemia emerge.

The typical transfusion goal is to raise the hemoglobin to 10 g/dL, taking care to avoid excessive transfusion to hemoglobin greater than 12 g/dL, where oxygen delivery can be hampered by hyperviscosity and hypertension. Typically, exchange transfusion should be considered when a patient is so physiologically compromised as to require management in an intensive care unit. Exchange transfusion can simultaneously raise the hemoglobin to 10 g/dL and dilute the sickle RBCs to 30%.

Alloimmunization to RBC antigens affects a high percentage of patients with SCD. Extended RBC phenotyping should be done as part of comprehensive care so that whenever possible, RBC units can be matched to the recipient not only for ABO antigens but also C, E, and Kell antigens to decrease the risk of alloantibody formation. Blood banks serving large populations of sickle cell patients often keep a supply of a few RBC units for urgent use that are negative for C, E, and Kell antigens. Hyperhemolysis in an SCD patient receiving transfusions can be life threatening but very difficult to evaluate, because transfusion reaction symptoms overlap with SCD symptoms. Alloimmunized patients who receive transfusions at different medical institutions should be advised to wear medical alert bracelets or to have the blood banks share information about alloantibody history, because routine cross-matching might not detect all alloantibodies.

Chronic Transfusion Programs

Regularly scheduled blood transfusion every 3 or 4 weeks can maintain the sickled RBC fraction at 30%, and this level of dilution of sickled RBCs effectively reduces the risk of stroke and other sickle cell complications. Less intense transfusion programs can prevent recurrence of splenic sequestration or acute chest syndrome. Chronic transfusions should use extended RBC phenotyping and matching of at least antigens C, E, and Kell, to reduce risks of alloimmunization. Complications of chronic transfusion programs include poor venous access, transfusion-transmitted infection, and iron overload. Exchange transfusion, generally by automated erythrocytapheresis, can reduce or eliminate iron overload in a chronic transfusion program. However, erythrocytapheresis has disadvantages: increased exposure to blood donors, need for large-bore venous access, and need for a pheresis team.

Iron overload becomes a concern after about 20 lifetime RBC transfusions. Iron is removed from the body by the chelation medications deferoxamine (Desferal) or deferasirox (Exjade). Patient compliance with deferoxamine is usually poor because it is administered as an overnight subcutaneous infusion. The newer chelator, deferasirox, is administered as an oral solution. Monitoring iron overload and the side effects of the chelators is best coordinated with hematologist and hepatologist consultants.

TABLE 4 Three Major Antisickling Therapies

Therapy	Indications	Contraindications	Advantages	Disadvantages
Bone marrow or cord blood stem cell transplantation	Ischemic CVA Recurrent ACS Frequent pain Avascular necrosis	No matched donor	Curative Prevents further cerebrovascular disease	Risk of procedure-related death, infection, organ failure, GVHD Risk of chronic GVHD
Chronic transfusion	Ischemic CVA Recurrent ACS Splenic sequestration Severe anemia due to renal failure	Multiple RBC alloantibodies Poor venous access	Reduces severity of sickle cell complications Prevents stroke in children	Requires good venous access RBC alloimmunization Iron overload except when using erythrocytapheresis Not curative
Hydroxyurea	Recurrent ACS Frequent pain	Pregnancy	Reduces severity of sickle cell complications Improves longevity Increases Hb Promotes weight gain	Requires monitoring myelosuppression Not curative

ACS = acute chest syndrome; CVA = cerebrovascular accident; GVHD = graft-versus-host disease; Hb = hemoglobin; RBC = red blood cell.

Hydroxyurea

Hydroxyurea (Droxia), an S-phase cytotoxic drug that raises HbF, is FDA approved as antisickling therapy for adults with severe sickle cell disease complications (see Table 4). HbF modulates the severity of SCD by reducing the concentration of HbS, inhibiting polymerization of HbS, and possibly conferring other beneficial effects on the RBCs. Hydroxyurea daily treatment can reduce the frequency of vaso-occlusive pain, acute chest syndrome, hospitalizations, transfusions, and priapism. Hydroxyurea improves longevity and is cost effective. However, some patients do not respond to hydroxyurea. Results of hydroxyurea clinical trials with adolescents and children are similar to those in adults, and an infant study is in progress. Hydroxyurea therapy requires close monitoring for excessive myelosuppression and individualized adjustment of dosage, as well as precautions due to theoretical risks of teratogenicity and leukemia.

TRANSPLANTATION

Curative therapy for sickle cell disease and other hemoglobinopathies is available through hematopoietic stem cell transplantation (HSCT). More than 200 children with severe complications of SCD have had HSCT using HLA-matched related donors through SCD-specific protocols in international consortia of transplant centers. HSCT for children under these conditions is now accepted as a standard care option, with mortality 5% or less, few transplant-related complications, and elimination of sickle-related complications in the majority of patients (see Table 4). In contrast, adults had high mortality rates with HSCT under the same conditions, attributable to age-related impaired organ function, and so new approaches such as reduced-intensity preparative regimens are still in clinical trials for adults with SCD. The major barrier to curing more people through transplantation is the lack of HLA-identical related donors, and additional clinical trials are under way to offer HCT using alternative donors.

REFERENCES

Ballas SK: Sickle Cell Pain. Progress in pain research and management, vol. 11. Seattle: IASP Press, 1998.
Benjamin LJ, Dampier CD, Jacox AK, et al: Guideline For the Management of Acute and Chronic Pain in Sickle Cell Disease. APS Clinical Practice Guidelines Series no. 1. Glenview, Ill: American Pain Society, 1999.
Castro O, Brambilla DJ, Thorington B, et al: The acute chest syndrome in sickle cell disease: Incidence and risk factors. The Cooperative Study of Sickle Cell Disease. Blood 1994;84(2):643-649.
Davies EG, Riddington C, Lottenberg R, Dower N: Pneumococcal vaccines for sickle cell disease. Cochrane Database Syst Rev 2004;(1):CD003885.
Gladwin MT, Sachdev V, Jison ML, et al: Pulmonary hypertension as a risk factor for death in patients with sickle cell disease. N Engl J Med 2004;350(9):886-895.
Information Center for Sickle Cell and Thalassemic Disorders. Available at http://sickle.bwh.harvard.edu/ (accessed May 26, 2008).
Krishnamurti L: Hematopoietic cell transplantation for sickle cell disease: State of the art. Expert Opin Biol Ther 2007;7(2):161-172.
Lane PA, Buchanan GR, Hutter JJ, Austin RF, et al: Sickle cell disease in children and adolescents: Diagnosis, guidelines for comprehensive care, and care paths and protocols for management of acute and chronic complications. Available at http://www.scinfo.org/protchildindex.htm (accessed May 26, 2008).
National Heart, Lung, and Blood Institute: The Management of Sickle Cell Disease. NIH Publication No. 02-2117, 4th ed, June 2002. Available at http://www.nhlbi.nih.gov/health/prof/blood/sickle/sc_mngt.pdf (accessed May 26, 2008).
Sickle Cell Disease [entire issue]. Hematol Oncol Clin North Am 2005; 9(5):771-987.
Sickle Cell Disease Association of America: Home page. Available at http://www.sicklecelldisease.org/ (accessed May 26, 2008).
Sickle Cell Information Center: Home page. Available at http://www.SCInfo.org (accessed May 26, 2008).
Steinberg MH: Pathophysiologically based drug treatment of sickle cell disease. Trends Pharmacol Sci 2006;27(4):204-210.
Stuart MJ, Nagel RL: Sickle-cell disease. Lancet 2004;364(9442):1343-1360.
Vichinsky EP, Neumayr LD, Earles AN, et al: Causes and outcomes of the acute chest syndrome in sickle cell disease. National Acute Chest Syndrome Study Group. N Engl J Med 2000;342(25):1855-1865.

Neutropenia

Method of
Peter E. Newburger, MD

Neutropenia is defined as a below-normal number of peripheral blood neutrophils, as determined by calculation of the absolute neutrophil count (ANC). The ANC equals the total white blood cell count multiplied by the fraction of neutrophils (including both segmented and band forms) on the differential count. The clinical significance of neutropenia depends on the level of depression of the ANC, as indicated in Table 1. Severe neutropenia, with ANC less than 200, is also termed *agranulocytosis*. The normal range for the ANC extends down to 1000/mm^3 in persons of African origin.

Fever in the setting of ANC less than 500 is a medical emergency that compels immediate evaluation and antibiotic treatment.

Clinical Presentation

Neutropenia can cause few or no clinical symptoms per se, so the clinical presentation usually derives from secondary infections or mucositis. Patients may be asymptomatic, but they usually present with fever, with or without localizing signs of infection. Gingivitis or ulcerative stomatitis, often with thrush, occurs commonly; periodic stomatitis occurring every 21 days is a hallmark of cyclic neutropenia.

Neutropenic patients can develop infection in virtually any organ system. The most common forms are cellulitis; pneumonia and lung abscess; enteritis, which can progress rapidly to peritonitis; perirectal abscess; lymphadenitis; and sepsis. Bacteremia or fungemia is particularly likely in patients with indwelling central venous catheters, mucositis, or additional defects in host defense. With agranulocytosis, local inflammation may be attenuated or absent, and clinical signs may be limited to fever, which occurs even in the complete absence of granulocytes. Common pathogens include *Staphylococcus aureus* and enteric gram-negative bacilli. Fungi and opportunistic or multiple-antibiotic-resistant bacteria generally enter the clinical spectrum only after prolonged neutropenia and broad-spectrum antibiotic therapy, but they need to be considered even at initial presentation. Isolated neutropenia does not impair host defense against viral infection.

Evaluation

Box 1 presents the differential diagnosis of neutropenia. In an acutely ill patient, the initial evaluation for infection needs to be completed rapidly (within hours at the most) and should include assessment of potential sites and causes of infection, but with minimal manipulation of the anus and rectum, where minor trauma could induce a perirectal abscess. The diagnostic approach requires a step-by-step evaluation of a differential diagnosis based on the history, the severity and duration of neutropenia, the leukocyte and bone marrow morphology, the associated hematologic or congenital abnormalities, and tests for specific disorders.

Acquired neutropenia often accompanies viral infection and requires only monitoring of blood counts until recovery. Depletion of bone marrow reserves can reduce the ANC in bacterial sepsis in the newborn or in overwhelming bacteremia, as with meningococcus. Drug-induced neutropenia can be associated with a large number of agents including, but by no means limited to, antibiotics, anticonvulsants, antiinflammatories, antithyroid drugs, diuretics, and phenothiazines. Antineutrophil antibodies may be detected by flow cytometry or agglutination assays, but false-negative and borderline-positive results can obscure the diagnosis of immune neutropenia. Careful review of the peripheral blood smear can reveal blasts or nucleated erythrocytes (suggesting bone marrow involvement by malignancy), large granular lymphocytosis, or specific neutrophil

TABLE 1 Clinical Significance of Absolute Neutrophil Counts

ANC (neutrophils/mm^3)	Clinical Significance	Treatment
>1500	Normal	None
1000-1500	Not clinically significant	None
500-1000	Very slight predisposition to infection	Outpatient antibiotic treatment for febrile illness
200-500	Significant predisposition to infection	G–CSF if symptomatic Inpatient IV antibiotics for febrile illness
<200 (agranulocytosis)	Very high risk of infection, decreased local signs of inflammation	G–CSF if responsive Aggressive IV antibiotics for febrile illness

ANC = absolute neutrophil count; G-CSF = granulocyte colony-stimulating factor.

BOX 1 Differential Diagnosis of Neutropenia

Acquired
Antibody-mediated (aminopyrine, other drugs)
Bacterial or fungal sepsis with exhaustion of bone marrow storage pool
Bone marrow aplasia, dysplasia, or replacement
Drug-induced
Hypersplenism
Immune-mediated (alloimmune and autoimmune)
Impaired production (chemotherapy, phenothiazines, other drugs)
Nutritional (folate, vitamin B$_{12}$)
Viral bone marrow suppression

Congenital
Disorders of granulocytopoiesis
Cyclic neutropenia
Familial benign neutropenia
Fanconi's anemia
Reticular dysgenesis
Severe congenital neutropenia (including Kostmann's disease)

Disorders of Ribosomal Function
Dyskeratosis congenita
Shwachman–Diamond syndrome

Disorders of Vesicular Transport
Chédiak–Higashi syndrome
Cohen's syndrome
Griscelli's syndrome, type II
Hermansky–Pudlak syndrome, type II

Neutropenia Associated with Immunologic Abnormalities
Common variable immunodeficiency
Hyper-IgM syndrome
IgA deficiency
Myelokathexis and WHIM syndrome
X-linked hyper-IgM syndrome
X-linked agammaglobunemia

Disorders of Metabolism
Barth's syndrome
Glycogen storage disease type 1b
Organic acidurias
Pearson's syndrome
Pseudoneutropenia

Ig = immunoglobulin; WHIM = warts, hypogammaglobulinemia, infection, and myelokathexis.

---

morphology associated with a congenital disorder, such as the giant granules of Chédiak–Higashi syndrome.

Serial blood counts, two to three times weekly over 6 to 9 weeks, are necessary to make the diagnosis of cyclic neutropenia and to document the period of cycles and depths of nadirs. In some of the less severe forms of congenital neutropenia, such as familial benign neutropenia, adequate bone marrow reserves of mature granulocytes can be demonstrated by steroid stimulation of neutrophil release into the peripheral blood, evaluated by white blood cell and differential counts before and 6 hours after prednisone 1 to 2 mg/kg.

Bone marrow examination, including cytogenetics, is indicated in cases of severe neutropenia or when other bone marrow lineages are abnormal. Bone marrow neutrophil morphology can be diagnostic for myelokathexis or Chédiak–Higashi syndrome; in the latter, characteristic granules may be difficult to detect in peripheral blood but plainly evident in bone marrow.

Several of the syndromes listed in the table include unique phenotypic features that aid in the diagnosis; pediatric hematology texts or the Online Mendelian Inheritance in Man website provide detailed descriptions. Quantitative measurement of immunoglobulins G, A, and M can not only contribute to the diagnosis of neutropenia associated with immunologic abnormalities but can also indicate a need for more aggressive management if the humoral arm of host defense is also impaired.

In infants with hypoglycemia or neurologic abnormalities, blood and urine testing may reveal a metabolic disorder such as glycogen storage disease type 1b, Barth's syndrome, hyperglycinemia, tyrosinemia, or an organic acidemia.

Treatment

SUPPORTIVE CARE

Fever or other signs of infection require immediate, aggressive antibiotic therapy in the neutropenic patient with an ANC less than 500. Antibiotics tailored to the susceptibility of identified organisms provide ideal treatment for infections with positive cultures. However, the initial treatment of most febrile illnesses and the entire therapy of many with negative cultures rely on an empiric choice of antibiotics.

Empiric therapy can consist of a single broad-spectrum antibiotic (such as a third-generation cephalosporin) or a combination of broad-spectrum antibiotics such as an aminoglycoside (e.g., gentamycin, tobramycin) plus either a third-generation cephalosporin (e.g., ceftazidime [Fortaz]) or a semisynthetic penicillin with anti-*Pseudomonas* activity (e.g. piperacillin, ticarcillin [Ticar]). Patients with indwelling central venous catheters might require substitution of an agent with better gram-positive coverage (e.g., nafcillin or vancomycin) for the aminoglycoside.

Each institution needs to base its empiric antibiotic selection on the identity and antibiotic susceptibilities of microorganisms in the community or hospital (depending on the likely site of acquisition of

CURRENT DIAGNOSIS

- The clinical significance of neutropenia depends on the level of depression of the ANC.
- Fever in the setting of ANC <500 is a medical emergency that compels immediate evaluation and antibiotic treatment.
- Patients may be asymptomatic, but they usually present with fever, with or without localizing signs of infection, which may be attenuated or absent.
- Common complications include gingivitis, ulcerative stomatitis, cellulitis, pneumonia, lung abscess, enteritis, peritonitis, perirectal abscess, lymphadenitis, and sepsis.
- Common pathogens include *Staphylococcus aureus* and enteric gram-negative bacilli. Infections with fungi and other opportunistic organisms can appear in the setting of prolonged neutropenia and antibiotic therapy.
- The diagnostic approach requires a step-by-step evaluation of a differential diagnosis based on the history, severity, and duration of neutropenia; leukocyte and bone marrow morphology; associated hematologic or congenital abnormalities; and tests for specific disorders.
- Bone marrow examination, including cytogenetics, is indicated in cases of severe neutropenia or when other bone marrow lineages are abnormal.

ANC = absolute neutrophil count.

CURRENT THERAPY

- Fever or other signs of infection require immediate, aggressive antibiotic therapy in the neutropenic patient with ANC < 500.
- Antibiotics tailored to the susceptibility of identified organisms provide ideal therapy, but empiric antibiotics are usually necessary for the initial treatment of febrile neutropenia.
- Treatment of febrile neutropenia accompanied by abdominal pain should include antibiotic coverage of intestinal anaerobes, including *Clostridium* species.
- Prophylactic antibiotics can be useful in uncorrected chronic neutropenia.
- Granulocyte colony-stimulating factor (filgrastim; Neupogen) is the most important highly specific drug for the treatment of congenital and some forms of acquired neutropenia.
- Granulocyte transfusion is indicated only for patients with agranulocytosis complicated by persistent life-threatening bacterial or fungal infection.

ANC = absolute neutrophil count.

infection), and the final choices should be made in consultation with the local microbiology or infectious disease division.

Fever persisting for longer than 5 days generally indicates the need for modification of antibiotic coverage, generally including addition of empiric antifungal therapy such as caspofungin (Cancidas), voriconazole (Vfend), or other triazole agent. Treatment of febrile neutropenia accompanied by abdominal pain should include antibiotics (e.g., piperacillin–tazobactam [Zosyn] or clindamycin) for intestinal anaerobes, including *Clostridium* species.

For hospitalized patients, hand washing needs to be strictly enforced. More aggressive reverse precautions do little to prevent the majority of infections, which derive from the patient's own skin, mucosa, and gastrointestinal flora. Careful oral, perianal, and skin hygiene can help reduce the prevalence of infection in patients with acute or chronic neutropenia.

Prophylactic antibiotics can be useful in uncorrected chronic neutropenia, particularly for the prevention of *Staphylococcus* colonization and infection. Cephalosporins or trimethoprim-sulfamethoxazole (TMP-SMX, Bactrim) are appropriate for this indication. TMP-SMX, a widely used combination, provides broad-spectrum coverage with very little toxicity, but it can itself cause neutropenia.

SPECIFIC THERAPY

Granulocyte colony-stimulating factor (G-CSF), marketed as filgrastim (Neupogen), is the most important highly specific drug for the treatment of neutropenia. FDA-approved indications for G-CSF include neutropenia associated with cancer chemotherapy and severe congenital neutropenia. The pegylated long-acting form of the drug (pegfilgrastim, Neulasta) is a single-dose formulation that can be administered once in each chemotherapy cycle.

Treatment with G-CSF can correct the ANC to the normal range in most patients with severe congenital neutropenia or cyclic neutropenia. Successful correction of the peripheral blood count also prevents stomatitis and other infection-related symptoms and risks.

At the initiation of therapy, or if the ANC rises far above normal, expansion of myelopoiesis may cause bone pain or splenomegaly. The major long-term risk in these patients is a conversion to myelodysplasia or leukemia. Most reported cases of myelodysplasia or secondary myeloid leukemia in severe congenital neutropenia patients, both treated and untreated, have been associated with an acquired deletion or abnormality of chromosome 7. Therefore, bone marrow cytogenetics need to be examined before initiating G-CSF and yearly during its chronic administration. Sensitivity to G-CSF varies considerably in severe congenital neutropenia, so dosage needs to be titrated for each patient, usually starting at 5 µg/kg/day. Patients with cyclic neutropenia generally respond to lower doses of G-CSF (usual starting dose 1-2 µg/kg/day) and have a much lower risk of myelodysplasia or leukemia.

The use of G-CSF for acquired neutropenia is more controversial. Although it hastens recovery in drug-induced neutropenia, discontinuation of the offending drug is usually sufficient. An empiric trial of G-CSF in other acquired forms of chronic neutropenia may be warranted for symptomatic patients. Patients with autoimmune or idiopathic neutropenia often respond to low doses of G-CSF and can experience considerable bone pain at the standard dosage used for postchemotherapy myelosuppression; they should be started at doses of 0.5-1 µg/kg/day.

Granulocyte transfusions, although rarely indicated, provide additional therapeutic support for newborns with sepsis and bone marrow neutrophil depletion as well as for older children or adults with agranulocytosis complicated by life-threatening bacterial or fungal infections that persist after adequate trials of appropriate antibiotic therapy.

Patients with systemic rheumatologic disorders, including Felty's syndrome, can benefit from therapy with glucocorticosteroids (e.g., prednisone), but there is rarely any indication to use steroids in other forms of neutropenia. Administration of steroids to a patient with neutropenia can do more harm than good, particularly if there is little or no response.

REFERENCES

Bal AM, Gould IM: Empirical antimicrobial treatment for chemotherapy-induced febrile neutropenia. Int J Antimicrob Agents 2007;29:501-509.
Berliner N, Horwitz M, Loughran TP Jr: Congenital and acquired neutropenia. Hematology Am Soc Hematol Educ Program 2004:63-79.

Bhatt V, Saleem A: Drug-induced neutropenia—pathophysiology, clinical features, and management. Ann Clin Lab Sci 2004;34:131-137.
Boxer LA, Newburger PE: A molecular classification of congenital neutropenia syndromes. Pediatr Blood Cancer 2007;49(5):609-614.
Dale DC, Cottle TE, Fier CJ, et al: Severe chronic neutropenia: Treatment and follow-up of patients in the Severe Chronic Neutropenia International Registry. Am J Hematol 2003;72:82-93.
Online Mendelian Inheritance in Man. Available at http://www.ncbi.nlm.nih.gov/sites/entrez?db=omim (accessed May 23, 2008).
Rosenberg PS, Alter BP, Bolyard AA, et al, for the Severe Chronic Neutropenia International Registry: The incidence of leukemia and mortality from sepsis in patients with severe congenital neutropenia receiving long-term G-CSF therapy. Blood 2006;107:4628-4635.
Severe Chronic Neutropenia Registry. Available at http://depts.washington.edu/registry/(acessed May 23, 2008).
Walsh TJ, Teppler H, Donowitz GR, et al: Caspofungin versus liposomal amphotericin B for empirical antifungal therapy in patients with persistent fever and neutropenia. N Engl J Med 2004;351:1391-1402.

Hemolytic Disease of the Fetus and Newborn

Method of
Douglas S. Richards, MD

Since the 1960s there has been a marked reduction in the number of fetuses and neonates dying from alloimmune hemolytic anemia. This is primarily because the administration of Rh immune globulin (RhoGAM) to RhD-negative pregnant women has been very effective in preventing sensitization. This article emphasizes measures that ensure adequate prophylaxis and discusses the intensive management that is required for the few women who become sensitized.

The RhD Antigen

In the 1940s the Rh antigen was discovered in Rhesus monkeys, and it was determined that antibodies against this antigen were responsible for most cases of hemolytic disease of the human newborn. Two genes located on the first chromosome determine the Rh type. The *RhD* gene determines the presence or absence of the D antigen, and the *RhCE* gene determines whether the C, c, E, or e antigens will be expressed.

ALLOIMMUNIZATION

Alloimmunization can occur when fetal cells bearing an antigen foreign to the mother enter the maternal circulation. As little as 0.1 mL of RhD-positive blood is sufficient to cause sensitization in an RhD-negative woman. The risk of fetomaternal hemorrhage is low in the first and second trimesters but increases in the third trimester, and at delivery up to 50% of women have sufficient fetomaternal hemorrhage to be at risk for sensitization. Pathologic processes such as abortion and ectopic pregnancy and invasive procedures such as amniocentesis and chorionic villus sampling are associated with an increased risk of fetomaternal hemorrhage and maternal sensitization.

For alloimmunization to occur, the mother must be negative and the fetus must be positive for a particular antigen. The incidence of the RhD negative state varies by ethic origin. Fifteen percent of whites of European ancestry are RhD negative, and 8% of African Americans and Latin Americans from Mexico and Central America are RhD negative. The rate is even lower (<1%) for Native Americans, and persons of Chinese and Japanese ancestries.

CURRENT DIAGNOSIS

- An antibody screen should be performed in all pregnant women at the time of registration.
- Anti-RhD titers >4 indicate sensitization and require careful follow-up. Titers <16 should be repeated monthly. Titers >16 or the birth of a previous affected child should prompt referral to a maternal–fetal medicine specialist for appropriate fetal surveillance.
- For sensitized women with significant anti-RhD titers, measurement of the middle cerebral artery peak velocity has replaced amniocentesis for ΔOD 450 measurement as the best way to diagnose severe fetal anemia.
- Amniocentesis with determination of the fetal RhD type by polymerase chain reaction techniques allows discontinuation of surveillance when the fetus is found to be RhD negative.
- With sensitization for many of the minor antigens, the father's antigen status should be determined. This is particularly true for the Kell antigen, because only 9% of the population is positive for this antigen. Surveillance can be discontinued when the father is negative for the antigen against which the mother is sensitized.

PREVENTION OF ALLOIMMUNIZATION

The principle of antibody-mediated immune suppression was first applied to the Rh problem in the 1960s. Postpartum Rh immune globulin administration in Rh-negative pregnant women results in a 10-fold reduction in sensitization rates compared with untreated controls. Consequently, the administration of Rh immune globulin to RhD-negative women after the delivery of RhD positive infants is the standard of care. Administration of Rh immune globulin to RhD-negative women at 28 weeks to prevent third-trimester sensitization is also cost-effective. Although sensitization can rarely occur before 28 weeks, early administration of Rh immune globulin is only indicated when there are complications or procedures that can allow a fetomaternal hemorrhage.

Treatment

MANAGEMENT OF PREGNANT WOMEN NOT KNOWN TO BE SENSITIZED

A blood type and antibody screen should be performed at the first prenatal visit on all pregnant women. Because of the possibility of laboratory and clerical errors, repeat typing is indicated even if the woman has previously been typed. The antibody screen is performed on all women, even those who are RhD positive, to allow detection of antibodies against other red cell antigens. Patients who are found to be weak RhD positive (previously termed D^u-positive) are not at risk for RhD-alloimmunization and do not require Rh immune globulin.

RhD-negative women with an initial negative antibody screen should have the screen repeated at 28 weeks' gestation. If the antibody screen is still negative, Rh immune globulin, 300 μg, should be given. If anti-RhD antibodies are detected at the time of the repeat screen, the patient is already sensitized, and Rh immune globulin will be of no benefit. Rh immune globulin administration is not harmful in this setting, so it is permissible to administer it before the results of the antibody screen are available.

Because more than 85% of partners of RhD-negative women are RhD positive, and because paternity is not always certain, it is usually best to assume the possibility of an RhD-positive fetus. If a woman

CURRENT THERAPY

- All nonsensitized RhD-negative women should have Rh immune globulin (RhoGAM) administered at 28 weeks' gestation.
- Those whose babies are RhD positive should have Rh immune globulin administered within 72 hours of delivery. A rosette test should be performed to determine whether more than one vial of immune globulin is needed.
- Rh immune globulin should be given to RhD-negative women who experience induced abortion, spontaneous abortion, vaginal bleeding in pregnancy, ectopic pregnancy, abdominal trauma in pregnancy, or external cephalic version attempt or who undergo chorionic villus sampling or amniocentesis. If Rh immune globulin is given before 28 weeks, the dose should be repeated within 12 weeks.
- When a fetus is found to be severely anemic, direct transfusion of packed red cells into the umbilical vein under ultrasound guidance can usually allow safe delay of delivery until after 34 weeks' gestation.
- Fetuses who receive intrauterine transfusions rarely require exchange transfusions after birth.

declines to receive antepartum Rh immune globulin because she believes the baby's father has RhD-negative blood, I have her sign the following statement in her chart. "I understand that if the father of my baby has RhD-positive blood I should receive Rh immune globulin. Knowing this, I decline to receive Rh immune globulin." Rh immune globulin is also indicated for women who experience induced abortion, spontaneous abortion, vaginal bleeding in pregnancy, ectopic pregnancy, abdominal trauma in pregnancy, or external cephalic version attempt or who undergo chorionic villus sampling or amniocentesis. If there is an indication for Rh immune globulin before 28 weeks, it is generally accepted that repeat doses should be given at least every 12 weeks.

Based on the initial studies with male volunteers, it is recommended that Rh immune globulin be administered within 72 hours of the time of suspected fetomaternal hemorrhage. However, it has never been shown that Rh immune globulin is ineffective if the interval is longer. Therefore, even if there is a delay of greater than 72 hours, Rh immune globulin should be given.

POSTPARTUM Rh IMMUNE GLOBULIN

Delivery represents the time of greatest risk for fetomaternal hemorrhage. At birth, the antibody screen should be repeated, and the neonatal blood type should be determined. If the baby is RhD positive or weak RhD positive, Rh immune globulin should be given. If the mother received antepartum Rh immune globulin at 28 weeks, low levels of residual passive antibodies are not uncommon. This does not represent sensitization, and Rh immune globulin should be given. If the last dose of antepartum Rh immune globulin was given within 3 weeks of delivery, and there was no large fetomaternal hemorrhage, Rh immune globulin does not need to be repeated.

A standard 300-µg vial of Rh immune globulin is sufficient to cover a fetomaternal bleed of 15 mL of red blood cells (30 mL of whole blood). To avoid sensitization in the 1% of women in whom there is a larger bleed, a screening test for the presence of RhD-positive cells in the maternal circulation is recommended. If the commercially available rosette test (Fetalscreen) is positive, the Kleihauer–Betke test is performed to quantify the fetomaternal hemorrhage. One 300-µg vial should be given to the mother for every 15 mL of fetal red blood cells that have entered the maternal circulation. Because the calculated fetomaternal hemorrhage from the Kleihauer–Betke test is not precise, it is best to be liberal in calculating the Rh immune globulin dose.

MANAGEMENT OF RhD SENSITIZED WOMEN

Antibody Titers

An initial positive antibody screen with a titer of 4 or greater indicates that the patient is sensitized. A titer of 2 may be due to laboratory error, so the screen should be repeated. If the initial titer is less than 16, and there is no history of a previously affected infant, titers should be repeated monthly. When antibody titers are 16 or greater, the fetus should be considered at risk for significant hemolytic disease, and subsequent titers are not helpful. When there has been a prior affected infant, the current fetus is considered to be at risk, and serial titers are not done.

When a woman has significant sensitization, the next step is to determine the father's RhD antigen status and CcEe genotype. If paternity is assured and the father is RhD negative, the fetus is not at risk. If the father is RhD positive, the chance that he is heterozygous can be calculated from his race, his CcEc genotype, and the number of RhD-positive infants he has previously fathered (see the table in Moise 2002).

Amniocentesis

Determination of the fetal RhD antigen status can be determined by polymerase chain reaction (PCR) methods from an amniotic fluid sample. For women with a previously significantly affected baby in whom early intensive surveillance will be required, amniocentesis to determine fetal genotype is usually done at 15 to 16 weeks. If the fetus is found to be RhD negative, no further surveillance is needed. To avoid the small risk of amniocentesis, some sensitized women with lower risk prefer to be followed with noninvasive fetal surveillance as described later. However, amniocentesis is usually indicated to plan the timing of delivery.

Amniocentesis with spectrophotometric analysis of the amniotic fluid is the traditional method of determining the degree of hemolysis in an at-risk fetus. The deviation of optical density reading from the expected value at 450 nm (the $\Delta OD\ 450$ reading) reflects the amount of bilirubin in the amniotic fluid and is directly related to the severity of hemolysis.

The $\Delta OD\ 450$ value is plotted on a semilogarithmic graph that has the weeks of gestation on the horizontal axis and the $\Delta OD\ 450$ on the logarithmic vertical axis. Based on Liley's pioneering work in the 1960s, with subsequent modifications by Queenan, the graph is divided into three zones that describe the degree of fetal risk. Zone I, the lowest zone, indicates mild or no hemolytic disease, and zone III, the upper zone, indicates severe hemolytic disease. Without intrauterine transfusion or delivery, there is a high probability of fetal hydrops and death for fetuses in this zone.

Middle Cerebral Artery Peak Velocity

In recent years, measurement of the middle cerebral artery peak velocity (MCA-PV) in the fetus using Doppler ultrasound has supplanted amniocentesis as the preferred method of fetal surveillance in RhD-sensitized pregnancies. The flow velocity in the middle cerebral artery is increased in severely anemic fetuses as a result of decreased blood viscosity and increased cardiac output. The MCA-PV can be readily and reproducibly measured by a well-trained sonographer. Precise attention to technique is essential for an accurate reading. With an axial view of the fetal head, The MCA is visualized with color Doppler, and the Doppler gate is placed close to its origin at the internal carotid artery, with the angle of insonation as close as possible to 0 degrees. It is important that the fetus is quiescent and apneic.

Not only does MCA-PV measurement avoid the risks of amniocentesis (e.g., rupture of membranes, infection, and worsening fetal sensitization by causing a fetal-to-maternal hemorrhage), it has been proved to be more accurate for predicting severe fetal anemia, especially in the second trimester. The sensitivity of this test is 88%, and an abnormal test (>1.5 multiples of the median for the gestational age) has an 85% predictive value for moderate or severe anemia.

In sensitized patients without a previously affected infant, testing is usually started at 22 to 24 weeks of gestation. Surveillance is begun at 18 weeks if there was a prior fetus with significant hemolysis. The test is usually repeated every 1 to 2 weeks, depending on prior pregnancy outcomes and whether values are approaching the abnormal range.

Fetal Blood Sampling and Intravascular Transfusions

When the MCA-PV is abnormally elevated, ultrasound-guided puncture of the umbilical cord for direct determination of fetal hematocrit is indicated. Intrauterine fetal blood transfusions are begun when the hematocrit falls to less than 30%. Historically, fetal blood transfusions were given into the peritoneal cavity, from which about 50% of the transfused red cells are absorbed. Most practitioners now give the transfusion directly into the umbilical vein.

Intravascular transfusion can be performed as early as 22 weeks' gestation. If the procedure is done at a time when the fetus is potentially viable, intramuscular betamethasone (Celestone; 12 mg IM q24h for 2 doses) is given to the mother in case a transfusion-related complication leads to delivery. An ultrasound estimate of the fetal weight is obtained to aid in the calculation of the required transfusion volume. The blood bank is asked to prepare irradiated, leukocyte-poor, cytomegalovirus-negative, type O-negative blood with a hematocrit of 80% to 85%, cross-matched against the mother.

We perform the procedure in an operating room, observing full sterile technique. Before we begin, we give an intravenous dose of cefazolin (Kefzol 1 g IV) for antimicrobial prophylaxis. Under ultrasound guidance, a 20- or 22-gauge needle is advanced into the umbilical vein at the point that the cord inserts into the placenta. A transplacental approach is often easier with an anterior placenta, but this is avoided because of a greater chance of a fetomaternal hemorrhage, which could augment the mother's immune response.

Once intravascular access is obtained, an aliquot of fetal blood is aspirated for initial determination of hematocrit. The amount of blood to be transfused is calculated, based on the initial fetal hematocrit, the estimated fetal blood volume, the desired final hematocrit, and the hematocrit of the transfused blood. Vecuronium bromide (Norcuron) 0.3 mg/kg is injected directly into the umbilical vein to paralyze the fetus. Once the desired volume is transfused, a fetal blood sample is drawn to check the final hematocrit and to calculate the percentage of circulating red cells that are native fetal cells (the Kleihauer–Betke test).

The fetal hematocrit falls rapidly after the first transfusion, because ongoing hemolysis of the remaining RhD-positive cells occurs and because fetal hematopoiesis slows dramatically. For this reason, the second transfusion is scheduled 2 weeks after the first. After the second transfusion, the majority of cells in the fetal circulation are RhD negative, so the rate of fall of the hematocrit is governed by the natural senescence of the donor cells. A good general rule is to expect a 1-point drop in the hematocrit per day. Subsequent transfusions are given when the calculated hematocrit falls below 25%. Intervals of 3 to 4 weeks are often possible.

Timing of Delivery

Controversy exists about whether to give a transfusion to a fetus who is due for a final transfusion between 32 and 34 weeks' gestation. Because the chance of extrauterine survival is excellent, one could argue that the risks of prematurity are less at this gestational age than a repeated intrauterine transfusion. I make this determination based on the lecithin-to-sphingomyelin (L/S) ratio, the expected difficulty of performing the transfusion, and the desires of the patient. An intrauterine transfusion would almost never be done after 34 to 35 weeks, so a fetus who reaches this gestational age would be delivered 3 weeks after the last transfusion.

For fetuses in sensitized pregnancies who have not required a transfusion, amniocentesis is performed at 35 weeks' gestation. If not already done, the fetal RhD type is determined. If the fetus is RhD negative, no further special care is needed. The ΔOD 450 value is determined to confirm that the MCA-PV has not been falsely reassuring. Fetal lung-maturity tests are obtained (the FLM test and/or L/S ratio). If the lungs are mature and the ΔOD 450 value or MCA-PV is borderline high, delivery is indicated. If the lungs are mature, delivery at 37 weeks is appropriate even with reassuring testing, because ongoing hemolysis in the last part of pregnancy can lead to hyperbilirubinemia in the baby.

While awaiting the proper time to deliver, the clinician should assess fetal well-being with nonstress testing and daily fetal movement counting. Nonstress tests should be performed at least weekly starting at 34 weeks in all RhD-sensitized women with an RhD-positive baby. The testing can be started earlier and performed more frequently if fetal transfusions have been required.

Neonatal Care

The three greatest problems facing the neonate from an alloimmunized pregnancy are prematurity, hyperbilirubinemia, and anemia. When the management scheme outlined previously is followed, serious problems from prematurity are uncommon, because almost all fetuses can successfully receive transfusions in utero until near term. When there have been two or more intrauterine transfusions, neonatal hyperbilirubinemia is not a serious problem. Most of the circulating red cells are RhD-negative donor cells, and significant hemolysis has long since ceased. Hyperbilirubinemia can usually be managed with phototherapy, and it is uncommon for exchange transfusions to be required.

Hematopoiesis is severely depressed in neonates who have received transfusions in utero. For this reason, these babies should be followed carefully, with weekly hematocrit and reticulocyte counts until normal erythropoetic function returns. It is expected that the postnatal hematocrit will gradually fall, but in order to not further depress hematopoiesis, blood transfusions are given only to symptomatic neonates. In recent years, administration of erythropoietin (Epogen) has proved useful in stimulating neonatal reticulocytosis.

Immunomodulation Therapy

In some cases of RhD sensitization, the disease process is so severe that fetal hydrops and death occur at a gestational age that is earlier than intrauterine transfusion is feasible. Trials including women such as these have shown a benefit of immunomodulation therapy. Treatment has consisted of plasmapheresis three times during the 10th week of gestation, then, after the final plasmapheresis, intravenous immunoglobulin is given weekly until 20 weeks of gestation. In a trial in which this approach was used, all fetuses still required intrauterine transfusions, but the maternal antibody titer was significantly reduced, and all babies survived.

Hemolytic Disease of the Fetus and Newborn From non-RhD Antibodies

Historically, less than 2% of cases of hemolytic disease of the newborn were caused by antigens other than the RhD antigen. With the successful elimination of most cases of RhD sensitization, the so-called minor antigens have assumed a relatively greater importance. Sensitization to these other antigens usually results from a blood transfusion before the current pregnancy. Antibodies against the Lewis, I, and P antigens are not associated with hemolytic disease, because they are of the IgM type and do not cross the placenta. The two most common potentially serious antibody types are anti-Kell, occurring in 10% of sensitized pregnancies requiring intrauterine transfusion, and anti-c, occurring in 3.5%. There are numerous other IgG antibodies that have rarely been reported to cause severe hemolytic disease in the fetus.

Anti-c sensitization is very similar to RhD disease in its propensity to cause hemolytic disease, and affected patients should be followed in the same manner as described earlier. RhC, RhE, and Rhe antibodies are often found in low titers in patients with RhD sensitizationm and these antibodies can contribute to fetal hemolysis. When found alone, they rarely cause sufficient hemolysis to require intrauterine treatment.

The Kell antigen system contains many specific antigens. The most concerning of these is the K1 antigen. This antibody not only causes significant hemolysis but also suppresses fetal hematopoiesis. For this reason, fetal surveillance should be started at a lower antibody titer (8), and MCA-PV testing is clearly superior to ΔOD 450 testing of amniotic fluid. This is because the latter test measures bilirubin products from hemolyis and cannot assess the component of fetal anemia that results from impaired red cell production.

REFERENCES

Mari G, Deter RL, Carpenter RL, et al: Noninvasive diagnosis by Doppler ultrasonography of fetal anemia due to maternal red-cell alloimmunization. N Engl J Med 2000;342:9-14.

Moise KJ Jr: Management of rhesus alloimmunization in pregnancy. Obstet Gynecol 2002;100:600-611.

Oepkes D, Seaward PG, Vandenbussche FP, et al: Dopper ultrasonography versus amniocentesis to predict fetal anemia. N Engl J Med 2006; 355:156-164.

Ruma MS, Moise KJ Jr, Kim E, et al: Combined plasmapheresis and intravenous immune globulin for the treatment of severe maternal red cell alloimmunization. Am J Obstet Gynecol 2007;196:138.e1-138.e6.

Van Kamp IL, Klumper FJ, Oepkes D, et al: Complications of intrauterine intravascular transfusion for fetal anemia due to maternal red-cell alloimmunization. Am J Obstet Gynecol 2005;192:171-177.

Hemophilia and Related Bleeding Disorders

Method of
Meera Chitlur, MD, and Roshni Kulkarni, MD

Hemophilia A and Hemophilia B

Hemophilia is an X-linked congenital bleeding disorder caused by a deficiency of factor VIII (hemophilia A) or factor IX (hemophilia B). Hemophilia A is the most common severe bleeding disorder and affects 1 in 5000 males in the United States; hemophilia B occurs in 1 in 30,000 males.

PATHOPHYSIOLOGY

The factor VIII gene is one of the largest genes and spans 186 kb of genomic DNA at Xq28. Inversion mutations account for 40% of severe hemophilia A, and deletions, point mutations, and insertions account for the remainder.

Hepatic and reticuloendothelial cells are presumed sites of factor VIII synthesis. Factor VIII is synthesized as a single chain polypeptide with three A domains (A1, A2, and A3), a large central B domain, and two C domains (Fig. 1). The binding sites for von Willebrand's factor (vWF), thrombin, and factor Xa are on the C2 domain, and factor IXa binding sites are on the A2 and A3 domains. The B domain can be deleted without any consequences. vWF protects factor VIII from proteolytic degradation in the plasma and concentrates it at the site of injury.

The factor IX gene is 34kb long and located at Xq26. It is a vitamin K–dependent serine protease composed of 415 amino acids. It is synthesized in the liver and its plasma concentration is about 50 times that of factor VIII. Gene deletions and point mutations result in hemophilia B.

ROLE OF FACTORS VIII AND IX IN COAGULATION

Factor VIII circulates bound to vWF. It is a cofactor for factor IX and is essential for factor X activation. In the classic coagulation cascade, activation of the intrinsic or extrinsic pathway of coagulation results in sufficient thrombin generation. However, this does not explain bleeding in hemophilia, because the extrinsic pathway is intact. This led to the revised cell-based model of coagulation.

The revised pathway incorporates all coagulation factors into a single pathway initiated by FVII and tissue factor. The contact factors (XI, XII, kallikrein, and high-molecular-weight kininogen) are not essential but serve as a backup. Following injury, encrypted tissue factor is exposed and forms a complex with factor VIIa. The tissue factor–factor VIIa complex activates factor IX to IXa (which moves to the platelet surface) and factor X to Xa. This generates small amounts of thrombin that activates platelets, converts platelet factor V to Va and factor XI to XIa, and releases factor VIII from vWF and activates it. The factor XIa activates plasma factor IX to IXa on the platelet surface, which together with factor VIIIa forms the tenase complex (factor VIIIa/IXa) that converts large amounts of factor X to Xa. Factor Xa forms a prothrombinase complex with FVa and converts large amounts of prothrombin to thrombin, called *thrombin burst*. This results in the conversion of sufficient fibrinogen to fibrin to form a stable clot. (An interactive animation on cell-based coagulation is available at http://www.hemostasiscme.org/Activities/CellBasedCoagulation/content/).

In hemophilia, lack of factor VIII or IX produces a profound abnormality. Factor Xa generated by FVIIa and tissue factor is insufficient because it is soon inhibited by tissue factor pathway inhibitor (negative feedback), and factors VIII and IX, which are required for amplifying the production of Xa are absent. The primary platelet plug formation and initiation phases of coagulation are normal. Any clot that is formed (from the initiation phase) is friable and porous.

CLINICAL FEATURES

The diagnosis of hemophilia is often made following a bleeding episode or because of a family history; 30% of cases, however, have no family history. Based on the plasma levels of factor VIII or IX (normal levels are 50%-150%) that correlate with severity and predict bleeding risk, hemophilia is classified as mild (>5%), moderate (1%-5%) and severe (<1%) (Table 1). Approximately 65% of persons with hemophilia have severe disease, 15% have moderate disease, and 20% have mild disease. Most severe disease manifests by 4 years of age; moderate or mild disease is diagnosed later and often following bleeding secondary to trauma or surgery.

Hemophilia can be diagnosed in the first trimester, using chorionic villus sampling and gene analysis. In the second trimester, fetal blood sampling can be performed. Prenatal diagnosis to determine fetal gender can aid in the management of pregnancy and delivery.

The hallmark of severe hemophilia is hemarthrosis, or bleeding into the joint, that can occur spontaneously or with minimal trauma. Although the immediate effects of a joint bleed are excruciating pain, swelling, warmth, and muscle spasm, the long-term effects of recurrent hemarthrosis include hemophilic arthropathy, which is characterized by synovial thickening, chronic inflammation, and repeated hemorrhages resulting in a target joint. Knees, elbows, ankles, hips,

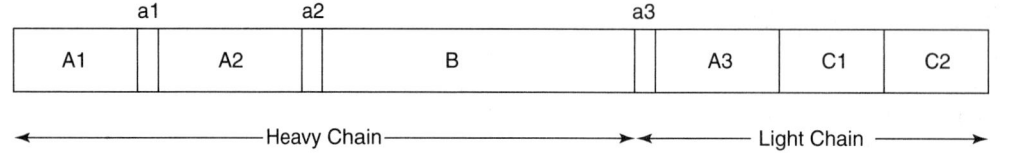

FIGURE 1. Factor VIII protein structure.

and shoulders are commonly affected. Disuse atrophy of surrounding muscles leads to further joint instability. Limitation of joint range of motion due to hemarthrosis often correlates positively with older age, nonwhite race, and increased body mass index, and it affects quality of life.

Muscle hematomas, another characteristic site of bleeding, can lead to compartment syndrome, with eventual fibrosis and peripheral nerve damage. Iliopsoas bleeds manifest with pain and flexion deformity. Gastrointestinal bleeding and hematuria occur less often.

Central nervous system (CNS) hemorrhage is a rare but serious complication with a 10% recurrence rate and is the leading cause of mortality in hemophiliacs. Although most newborns with severe hemophilia experience an uneventful course following vaginal delivery, vacuum extraction is associated with an increased CNS bleeding risk. The incidence of intracranial hemorrhage in newborns with hemophilia is 1% to 4%.

DIAGNOSIS

Hemophilia A and B are clinically indistinguishable, and specific factor assays are the only way to differentiate and confirm the diagnosis. Both should be differentiated from von Willebrand's disease (vWD). The prothrombin time (PT), platelet function analyzer (PFA-100), and fibrinogen are normal. (PFA, a platelet-function screening test, is replacing bleeding time, because the bleeding time has low sensitivity and specificity and is operator dependent.) The activated partial thromboplastin time (aPTT) is prolonged when the factor levels are below 30%. Table 2 shows the characteristics and differences between the hemophilias and vWD. Female carriers are usually asymptomatic except for those with extreme lyonization resulting in low factor VIII or IX levels. Factor VIII levels increase throughout pregnancy and drop to prepregnancy levels following delivery, but factor IX levels remain constant throughout pregnancy.

TREATMENT

The treatment for hemophilia consists of replacement therapy with intravenous factor VIII or factor IX concentrates produced by purification of donor plasma (plasma derived) or in cell culture bioreactors (recombinant). Careful screening of donors combined with heat treatment and viral inactivation methods have made plasma-derived products safer. Plasma-derived and recombinant products appear to have equivalent clinical efficacy. Recombinant factor concentrates

 CURRENT DIAGNOSIS

- The hemophilias and von Willebrand's disease (vWD) account for 80% to 85% of inherited bleeding disorders. Hemophilia A and B are X-linked, whereas vWD and rare bleeding disorders (RBDs) are autosomal disorders.
- The diagnosis of hemophilia and other inherited bleeding disorders should be confirmed by specific assays, because screening tests such as prothrombin time (PT) and activated partial thromboplastin time (aPTT) may be normal. Plasma levels of deficient factor determine clinical severity and management.
- Hemarthrosis is the most common and debilitating complication, and central nervous system bleeding is the most common cause of mortality in hemophilia. Mucosal bleeding and menorrhagia are the most common manifestations of vWD. Bleeding manifestations of RBDs are mild, although homozygotes can present with severe disease.
- Newborns have normal levels of factor VIII; therefore, the diagnosis of hemophilia A can be established at birth. Vacuum delivery should be avoided to prevent head bleeds.
- Women and adolescents with menorrhagia and no underlying pathology should be investigated for a bleeding disorder.

are recommended, but if they are not available, plasma-derived concentrates can be used. Cryoprecipitate is no longer recommended because of concerns regarding pathogen safety.

Treatment administered only during bleeding symptoms is known as *episodic therapy*, and periodic administration of factor concentrates to prevent bleeding is known as *prophylactic therapy*. Response to treatment is more effective when it is administered early. Although prophylaxis prevents the development of joint disease, the high cost of factor replacement coupled with the need for venous access makes it expensive and difficult.

The goal of treatment is to raise factor levels to approximately 30% or more for minor bleeds (hematomas or joint bleeds) and

TABLE 1 Hemophilia Severity and Clinical Manifestations

Characteristics	Severe (50%-70%)	Moderate (10%)	Mild 30%-40%
Factor VIII or IX activity (normal 50%-150%)	<1%	1%-5%	>5%
Age of diagnosis	At birth to 2 y	Childhood or adolescence	Adolescence or adult
Bleeding patterns	2-4/mo	4-6/y	Rare
Clinical manifestations	Hemarthroses, muscle, central nervous system, gastrointestinal bleeding, hematuria	Bleeding into joints or muscle following minor trauma, surgical procedure, dental bleeding Rarely spontaneous	Surgical procedures (including dental) and major trauma

TABLE 2 Hemophilias and von Willebrand's Disease: Key Characteristics and Differences

Characteristic	Hemophilia A	Hemophilia B	von Willebrand's Disease
Incidence	1:5000	1:30,000	1%-3% of U.S. population
Abnormality	Factor VIII deficiency	Factor IX deficiency	vWF (qualitative and quantitative defect)
Inheritance	X-linked, affects males Gene at the tip of X-chromosome	X-linked, affects males Gene at the tip of X-chromosome	Autosomal dominant (gene: chromosome 12) Some are recessive or compound heterozygotes
Production site	Unknown. liver endothelium	Liver (vitamin K dependent)	Megakaryocytes and endothelial cells
Function	Cofactor; forms tenase complex with factor IX and activates factor X, leading to thrombin burst that results in conversion of large amounts of fibrinogen to fibrin	Serine protease (inactive form: zymogen) Activated by factor XI or VIIa; forms a tenase complex with factor VIII and activates factor X	Platelet adhesion to site of injury or damaged endothelium Protects factor VIII from proteolysis
Classification (normal levels 50%-150%)	Mild (>5%) Moderate (1-5%) Severe (<1%)	Mild (>5%) Moderate (1-5%) Severe (<1%)	Type 1 Type 2 (2A, 2B, 2M, 2N) Type 3
Clinical presentation	Positive family history (30% new mutation) Hemarthroses, hematomas, hematuria, intracranial hemorrhage, gastrointestinal hemorrhage, etc.	Positive family history (30% new mutation) Milder disease, although identical hemorrhage sites as hemophilia A	Positive family history Mucocutaneous bleeding (epistaxis, menorrhagia, postdental bleeding) Type 3 can manifest as hemophilia A.
PFA, bleeding time	Normal	Normal	May be prolonged
PT	Normal	Normal	Normal
aPTT	Prolonged	Prolonged	Prolonged or normal
Factor VIII assay	Decreased or absent	Normal	Decreased or normal (absent type 3)
Factor IX assay	Normal	Decreased or absent	Normal
vWF antigen	Normal	Normal	Decreased or absent (type 3)
vWF:RCo	Normal	Normal	Decreased or abnormal
vWF multimers	Normal	Normal	Abnormal in types 1, 2A, 2B; absent in type 3
Specific treatment	Recombinant factor VIII (preferred) Pathogen-safe plasma-derived concentrates DDAVP for mild cases	Recombinant factor IX Pathogen-safe plasma-derived concentrates DDAVP ineffective	DDAVP (intranasal or intravenous) vWF concentrates (pathogen-safe plasma derived)
Inhibitor patients	Immune tolerance, recombinant factor VIIa, APCC	Immune tolerance, recombinant factor VIIa	Inhibitors are rare
Adjunct therapy	Antifibrinolytics	Antifibrinolytics	Oral contraceptives, antifibrinolytics

APCC = activated prothrombin complex concentrates; aPTT = activated partial thromboplastin time; DDAVP = desmopressin; PFA = platelet function analyzer; PT = prothrombin time; RCo = ristocetin cofactor; vWF = von Willebrand's factor.

100% for major bleeds (CNS or surgery). Giving 1 U/kg of factor concentrate raises plasma factor VIII levels by 2% and factor IX levels by 1.5% (except with the recombinant factor IX product, where it increases by 0.8%). The half-life of factor VIII is approximately 8 to 12 hours and that of factor IX is up to 24 hours. Factor concentrates can also be given by continuous infusion (3-4 U/kg/hour). The bolus dose varies from 25 to 50 U/kg depending on the severity, site, and type of bleeding and is dosed to the closest vial because of the cost of the products. Table 3 lists the dosing schedule for various types of bleeds.

For short-term therapy (before dental procedures and minor bleeding episodes) in mild hemophilia A and vWD, the synthetic vasopressin analogue desmopressin acetate (DDAVP [Stimate]) is useful. It increases plasma concentrations of coagulation factor VIII and vWF three- to fivefold by releasing the endothelial stores. A DDAVP trial to determine response is helpful in selecting patients who might benefit from such therapy. For hemostatic purposes, intravenous (0.3 µg/kg in 50 mL of normal saline infused over 15-30 min) or intranasal dose (150 µg) can be used. The intranasal dose is 15 times larger than that recommended for diabetes insipidus. A multidose intranasal spray formulation (Stimate nasal spray) delivers 150 µg per spray. The recommended dosage is one spray for patients who weigh less than 50 kg and two sprays (one in each nostril) for those who weigh more than 50 kg. Desmopressin is ineffective in hemophilia B. Aspirin and aspirin-containing compounds should be avoided in persons with bleeding disorders because they interfere with platelet function and can exacerbate bleeding.

CURRENT THERAPY

- Early and effective treatment and prophylaxis can prevent repeated hemarthrosis and joint destruction in persons with hemophilia. Patients should be tested annually for the presence of inhibitors.
- Wherever available and indicated, recombinant factor concentrates are preferred over plasma-derived products due to potential risk of pathogen transmission. Cryoprecipitate is not recommended. For mild and moderate hemophilia A and von Willebrand's disease, the use of desmopressin coupled with antifibrinolytics can obviate the use of concentrates. Continued vigilance should be implemented for new and emerging blood-borne pathogens.
- All patients with inherited bleeding disorders should be immunized against hepatitis A and B and followed in close collaboration with the local hemophilia treatment center (http://www2a.cdc.gov/ncbddd/htcweb/index.asp). The National Hemophilia Foundation's (www.hemophilia.org) Medical and Scientific Advisory Committee (MASAC) guidelines for updated recommendations and product choice should be followed.

TABLE 3 Treatment of Bleeding Episodes and Desired Plasma Levels in Hemophilias A and B

Type of bleeding	Desired Factor Level (%)	Factor VIII Dose (U/kg)	Factor IX Dose (U/kg)	Duration of Treatment (Days)	Comments (Dose Factor to the Closest Vial)
Persistent or profuse epistaxis Oral mucosal bleeding (including tongue and mouth lacerations)	20-30	10-15	20-30	1-2	Local pressure, antifibrinolytics, fibrin glue for local control, nosebleed QR for epistaxis Sedation in small children with tongue laceration
Dental procedures	30-50	15-25	30-50	1 h before procedure	Antifibrinolytics for 7-10 d
Acute hemarthrosis, intramuscular hematomas	30-60	15-50	30-60	1-3	Use lower doses if treated early. Non–weight bearing on affected joint.
Physical therapy	30-50	15-25	30-50	Treat before PT	Consider synovectomy (surgical, radioisotope or chemical) for target joints.
Life-threatening bleeding such as intracranial hemorrhage, major surgery, and trauma	80-100	40-50	80-100	10-14 d	Bolus dose followed by continuous infusion (3-4 U/kg/h); may switch to bolus before discharge
Gastrointestinal bleeding	30-50	15-25	30-50	2-3	May use oral antifibrinolytics
Persistent painless gross hematuria	30-50	15-25	30-50	1-2	Increase PO or IV fluids with low-dose antifibrinolytics

PT = physical therapy.

Antifibrinolytics such as ε-aminocaproic acid (Amicar) and tranexamic acid (Cyklokapron) are used as adjunct therapies and in mild hemophilia and can obviate the need for factor concentrates. The recommended dosage for ε-aminocaproic acid is 75 to 100 mg/kg/dose IV or orally every 4 to 6 hours (maximum 30 g/24 hours). The recommended dosage for tranexamic acid is 10 mg/kg/dose IV or 25 mg/kg body weight orally, three times daily.

For prophylaxis, factor VIII 25 to 40 U/kg administered every other day or factor IX 25 to 40 U/kg twice weekly (because of the longer half-life of factor IX) is aimed at preventing joint disease. Prophylaxis may begin at 1 to 2 years of age and is continued lifelong. Self-infusion before any planned strenuous activity is recommended. Because of the complications of central venous catheters (infections, thrombosis, and mechanical), use of a peripheral vein is encouraged.

COMPLICATIONS OF TREATMENT

One of the most serious complications of hemophilia treatment is the development of inhibitors or neutralizing antibodies (immunoglobulin [Ig]G) that inhibit the function of substituted factor VIII and factor IX. Approximately 5% to 10% of all hemophiliacs and up to 30% of patients with severe hemophilia A develop inhibitors. The incidence of inhibitors in hemophilia B is lower (1%-3%). Most factor VIII inhibitors arise after a median exposure of 9 to 12 days in patients with severe hemophilia A. They can be transient or permanent and should be suspected if a patient fails to respond to an appropriate dose of clotting factor concentrate. Inhibitors can exacerbate bleeding episodes and hemophilic arthropathy.

Inhibitor levels, measured using Bethesda units (BU), are classified as high titer (>5 BU) or low titer (<5 BU). In patients with low titer, inhibitors higher than normal doses of factor VIII or IX may be used to treat bleeding. For those with high-titer inhibitors, agents that bypass factor VIII or factor IX are used. These include recombinant activated factor VII and, in the case of hemophilia A, activated prothrombin complex concentrates (APCC) or recombinant porcine factor VIII (currently in prelicensure clinical trials). Immune tolerance induction, a long-term approach designed to eradicate inhibitors, is effective in 70% to 85% of patients with severe hemophilia A; the most important predictor of success of immune tolerance induction is an inhibitor titer of less than 10 BU at the start of immune tolerance induction.

Although inhibitors are rare in hemophilia B, they can result in anaphylaxis with exposure to factor IX–containing products. Immune-tolerance regimens are associated with the nephrotic syndrome and are successful in eradicating the inhibitor only in 40% of cases.

Another important complication of treatment is the transmission of bloodborne pathogens such as hepatitis B and C viruses and HIV. In the 1970s, lyophilized plasma factor concentrates of low purity resulted in the transmission of HIV, causing the deaths of many hemophiliacs. Currently, donor screening for pathogens coupled with viral attenuation by heat or solvent detergent technology make these products pathogen safe. However, nonenveloped virus (parvovirus and hepatitis A) and prions can resist inactivation and can be potentially transmitted.

Patients with bleeding disorders should be encouraged to attend the comprehensive hemophilia treatment centers, where they are educated, trained to self-infuse and calculate dosage, maintain treatment logs, and call for serious bleeding episodes. Hemovigilance at the hemophilia treatment centers is maintained through participation in the Centers for Disease Control and Prevention's (CDC) Universal Data Collection project. The mortality rate among patients who receive care at hemophilia treatment centers is lower than among those who do not: 28.1% versus 38.3%, respectively.

Routine vaccination against hepatitis A and B is recommended. Gene therapy offers promise of a cure but has not yet become reality. Two gene-therapy trials for hemophilia B have shown subtherapeutic or transient expression of factor IX.

Von Willebrand's Disease

von Willebrand's disease (vWD) is an inherited (autosomal dominant) bleeding disorder caused by deficiency or dysfunction of von Willebrand Factor (vWF), a plasma protein that mediates platelet adhesion at the site of vascular injury and prevents degradation of factor VIII. A defect in vWF results in bleeding by impairing platelet adhesion or by decreasing factor VIII.

vWF is synthesized in endothelial cells and undergoes dimerization and multimerization, forming low-, intermediate-, and high-molecular-weight (HMW) multimers. The HMW multimers are most effective in promoting platelet aggregation and adhesion. Circulating HMW multimers are cleaved by the protease ADAMTS13, which is deficient in patients with thrombotic thrombocytopenic purpura.

vWD is the most common bleeding disorder, affecting 1% or more of the population. It occurs worldwide and affects all races. vWD is classified into three major categories: partial quantitative deficiency (type 1), qualitative deficiency (type 2), and total deficiency (type 3). There are several different variants of type 2 vWD: 2A, 2B, 2N, and 2M based on the phenotype. About 75% of patients have type 1 vWD.

CLINICAL PRESENTATION

Mucous membrane–type bleeding (e.g., menorrhagia, epistaxis) and excessive bruising are characteristic clinical features in vWD. Bleeding manifestations vary considerably, and in some cases, the diagnosis is not suspected until excessive bleeding occurs with a surgical procedure or trauma. Although excessive menstrual bleeding may be the initial manifestation, it takes 16 years for a diagnosis of bleeding disorder. It is for this reason that the American College of Obstetrics and Gynecology recommended screening for hemostatic disorders in all adolescents and women presenting with menorrhagia and no pathology and before hysterectomy for menorrhagia. In infants or small children with type 3 (severe) vWD, excessive bruising and even joint bleeding (due to very low levels of factor VIII) can mimic hemophilia A.

DIAGNOSIS

Laboratory evaluation for vWD requires several assays to quantitate vWF and characterize its structure and function. Many variables affect vWF assay results, including the patient's ABO blood type. Persons of blood group AB have 60% to 70% higher vWF levels than those of blood group O. Thus, some laboratories interpret vWF levels referenced to specific normal ranges for blood types.

Clinical conditions and disorders with elevated vWF levels include pregnancy (third trimester), collagen vascular disorders, following surgery, in liver disease, and in disseminated intravascular coagulation. Low levels are seen in hypothyroidism and days 1 to 4 of the menstrual cycle.

Symptoms are modified by medications like aspirin or nonsteroidal antiinflammatory drugs (NSAIDs), which can exacerbate the bleeding; oral contraceptives can decrease the bleeding in women with vWD by increasing vWF levels. vWF levels in African American women are 15% higher than in white women. Clinical symptoms and family history are important for establishing the diagnosis of vWD, and a single test is sometimes not sufficient to rule out the diagnosis.

Initial work-up should include a complete blood count, aPTT, PT, fibrinogen level, or thrombin time. These tests do not rule out vWD but help to rule out thrombocytopenia or factor deficiency as the cause for bleeding. The closure times on the PFA-100, which has replaced the bleeding time as a screening test in some centers, may be prolonged. The aPTT in vWD is only abnormal when factor VIII is sufficiently reduced.

Specific tests for vWD include ristocetin cofactor assay, a factor VIII activity, and vWF antigen (vWF Ag) assay. The Ristocetin cofactor activity measures induced binding of vWF to platelet glycoprotein Ib and is the best functional assay of vWF activity. Multimer analysis is done by agarose gel electrophoresis using anti-vWF polyclonal antibody and is available at reference laboratories.

In type I vWD, the vWF is subnormal in amount, with normal multimer structure. Those with types 2A and 2B vWD lack the HMW multimers. In type 2B, the vWF has a heightened affinity for platelets, often resulting in some degree of thrombocytopenia from platelet aggregation. A useful laboratory test for type 2B is the low-dose ristocetin-induced platelet aggregation (RIPA) assay.

In type 3 (severe) vWD, the affected person has inherited a gene for type I vWD from each parent, resulting in very low levels (3%) of vWF (and low factor VIII, because there is no vWF to protect factor VIII from proteolytic degradation). Less commonly, a person with type 3 is doubly heterozygous. Table 4 provides a quick overview of the laboratory findings in the different variants of vWD.

TREATMENT

In type 1 vWD (with subnormal levels of normally functioning vWF), the treatment of choice is DDAVP, which causes a rapid release of vWF from storage sites. It can be given intravenously or by the intranasal route. The recommended dose for IV use is 0.3 µg/kg, given in saline over 10 minutes. Most persons with type 1 vWD have a two- to four-fold increase in plasma levels of vWF within 15 to 30 minutes following infusion. The IV route is often used for surgical coverage or for a severe bleeding episode requiring hospitalization. When necessary, repeat doses may be given at 12- to 24-hour intervals. Tachyphylaxis is less commonly seen in vWD patients than in hemophilia patients. It is important to monitor free water intake following DDAVP administration because it can cause hyponatremia and seizures.

The concentrated form of desmopressin for intranasal use (Stimate nasal spray) may be used. The recommended dosage is one 150-µg spray for patients who weigh less than 50 kg and two sprays (one in each nostril) for those who weigh more than 50 kg. Some young women with menorrhagia have benefited from its use at the onset of menses, with a second dose after 24 hours. Others have used it approximately 45 minutes before invasive dentistry, with good results.

In the type 2 variants (vWF produced is abnormal), desmopressin can cause an increase in abnormal vWF. Although some persons with type 2A might respond, desmopressin is seldom useful in type 2 and might even be contraindicated (as in type 2B, where it can exacerbate the thrombocytopenia).

In type 3 vWD, desmopressin is ineffective because there is no vWF to be released from storage sites. For type 3 patients and in persons with type 1 vWD who do not respond adequately to desmopressin, an intermediate-purity plasma-derived concentrate rich in the hemostatically effective HMW multimers of vWF (such as

TABLE 4 Clinical Variants of von Willebrand's Disease

Type	Factor VIII	vWF Ag	Ristocetin Cofactor	RIPA	Multimer
1	↓	↓	↓	↓ or normal	Normal
2A	↓ or normal	↓↓	↓	↓↓	Large and intermediate multimers absent
2B	↓ or normal	↓↓	↓ or normal	↓ to low dose	Large multimers absent
2M	Variably ↓	Variably ↓	↓	Variably ↓	Normal
2N	↓↓	Normal	Normal	Normal	Normal
3	↓↓↓↓	↓↓↓↓	↓↓↓↓	None	Absent
Platelet type	↓ or normal	↓ or normal	↓	↓ to low dose	Large multimers absent

Ag = antigen; RIPA = ristocetin-induced platelet aggregation; vWF = von Willebrand's factor.

TABLE 5 Rare Bleeding Disorders: Inheritance, Clinical Features, and Treatment

Factor	Prevalence	Type	Inheritance	Manifestation and Diagnosis	Treatment	Hemostatic Levels	Half-life
Factor I	1:1,000,000	Afibrinogenemia Dysfibrinogenemia Hypofibrinogenemia	AR AD AD	Mild bleeding CNS, umbilical, joint bleeding Recurrent miscarriage PT, aPTT, TT prolonged Low FI levels Paradoxical thrombosis	FFP 15-20 mL/kg Cryoprecipitate 1 bag/5-10 kg Plasma-derived concentrate[2]* Treatment q3-5d	50 mg-1g/dL	2-5 d
Factor II	1:2,000,000	Type I: hypoprothrombinemia Type II: dysprothrombinemia	AR AR	Hematomas, hemarthroses, menorrhagia CNS, umbilical, postpartum hemorrhage PT abnormal	FFP, PCC 20-30 U/kg for prophylaxis or treatment	20%-30%	3-4 d
Factor V	1:1,000,000	Parahemophilia, labile factor, proaccelerin, Owren's disease	AR	Mucosal bleeding, postpartum hemorrhage, CNS bleeding Platelet factor V deficiency more reflective of bleeding potential Prolonged PT, aPTT Normal TT	FFP Platelet transfusions Antiplatelet antibodies can develop with repeated platelet transfusions	15%-20%	36 h
Factor VII	1:500,000	Proconvertin or stable factor	AR	Menorrhagia; mucosal, muscle, intracranial bleeds (15%-60%); hemarthrosis Prolonged PT Normal aPTT, TT, FI, liver functions	Recombinant factor VIIa, 15-30 μg/kg q2h for major bleeds FFP, PCC 20-30 U/kg for prophylaxis or treatment Plasma-derived factor VII concentrates[2]*	15%-20%	4-6 h
Factor X	1:1,000,000		AR	Menorrhagia; umbilical, joint, mucosal, muscle, intracranial bleeding Prolonged PT, aPTT	FFP, PCCs 20-30 U/kg	15%-20%	24-48 h
Factor XI (common in Ashkenazi Jews)	1:1,000,000		AR	Post-traumatic bleeding, menorrhagia Prolonged aPTT Normal PT	Hemoeleven,[2]* FFP 15-20 mL/kg Inhibitors can occur	15%-20%	
Factor XIII	1:2,000,000		Ar	Intracranial, joint, umbilical bleeding Delayed wound healing Recurrent miscarriages PT, APTT normal ↓FXIII assay	Fibrogammin p[2†] 10-20 U/kg FFP 15-20mL/kg Cryoprecipitate 1 bag/5-10 kg q3-4wk	2%-5%	11-14 d
Combined factor V and VIII	1:2,000,000			Mucosal bleeding Prolonged PT, aPTT (disproportionately)	Factor VIII concentrates and FFP	15%-20%	
Vitamin K–dependent multiple deficiencies	1:2,000,000			Umbilical stump, intracranial, postsurgical bleeding Skeletal abnormalities Hearing loss	Oral vitamin K, FFP, PCC	15%-20%	

[2]Not available in the United States.
*Available in Europe.
†Compassionate use in the United States.
AD = autosomal dominant; aPTT = activated partial thromboplastin time; AR = autosomal recessive; CNS = central nervous system; FFP = fresh frozen plasma; FI = fibrinogen; PCC = prothrombin complex concentrate; PT = prothrombin time; TT = thrombin time.

Humate P) should be used to treat moderately severe or severe bleeding episodes and for before surgery.

As in hemophilia, antifibrinolytics are an effective adjunctive treatment for invasive dental procedures or other bleeding in the oropharyngeal cavity. These may be effective even when used alone in some vWD women with menorrhagia. For epistaxis, Nosebleed QR, a hydrophilic powder, can help.

SPECIAL SITUATIONS

Pregnancy

vWF (and factor VIII) levels increase during the third trimester of pregnancy, and women with type 1 vWD have a decrease in bruising or other bleeding symptoms. However, those with type 2 vWD (abnormal vWF) and type 3 (no vWF) have no change in the bleeding tendency. Even in type 1 vWD, vWF levels fall following delivery, so treatment (with IV desmopressin or Humate P) may be needed.

Acquired von Willebrand's Disease

Acquired vWD occurs in persons who do not have a lifelong bleeding disorder. Conditions associated with acquired vWD include underlying autoimmune disease (lymphoproliferative disorders, myeloproliferative disorders, or plasma cell dyscrasias), valvular and congenital heart disease, Wilms' tumor, chronic renal failure, and hypothyroidism. The mechanism of acquired vWD is unknown. Medications such as valproic acid can also cause vWD. Removal of the underlying condition often corrects the vWF. Desmopressin, Humate P, recombinant factor VIIa, or plasma exchange may be tried, if necessary, to treat bleeding.

Rare Bleeding Disorders

The rare bleeding disorders account for 3% to 5% of inherited coagulation deficiencies, other than factor VIII, factor IX, or vWF deficiencies. They are autosomal recessive and affect both sexes. The prevalence of rare bleeding disorders ranges from 1:500,000 to 1:2 million. Bleeding manifestations are restricted to persons who are homozygotes or compound heterozygotes. Rare bleeding disorders are common in countries such as Iran, where consanguineous marriages are customary. Ashkenazi Jews are particularly affected by factor XI deficiency. Deficiency of factor XII is a risk factor for thrombosis, but not for bleeding. Most cases of rare bleeding disorders are identified by abnormal screening tests coupled with specific factor assays.

Factor concentrates (recombinant or plasma derived) are available for some of the deficiencies (mostly in Europe, but not in the United States). Fibrogammin P, a plasma-derived virally purified factor XIII concentrate, is not yet licensed in the United States but is available under an Investigational New Drug (IND) protocol of the Food and Drug Administration through Dr. Diane Nugent, Children's Hospital of Orange County, 500 S. Main St., Orange County, Calif 92868. The advantages of concentrates are pathogen safety and small volume. The use of antifibrinolytics and fibrin glue as adjunct therapy for bleeding manifestations is encouraged. Table 5 lists the inheritance, frequency, manifestations, and treatments of the rare bleeding disorders.

REFERENCES

Arnold WD, Hilgartner MW: Hemophilic arthropathy. Current concepts of pathogenesis and management. J Bone Joint Surg Am 1977;59(3):287-305.
Bolton-Maggs PH, Pasi KJ: Haemophilias A and B. Lancet 2003; 361(9371):1801-1809.
Gill JC, Wilson AD, Endres-Brooks J, Montgomery RR: Loss of the largest von Willebrand factor multimers from the plasma of patients with congenital cardiac defects. Blood 1986;67(3):758-761.
Hoffman M, Monroe DM 3rd: A cell-based model of hemostasis. Thromb Haemost 2001;85(6):958-965.
Miller CH, Dilley AB, Drews C, et al: Changes in von Willebrand factor and factor VIII levels during the menstrual cycle. Thromb Haemost 2002; 87(6):1082-1083.
Miller CH, Dilley A, Richardson L, et al: Population differences in von Willebrand factor levels affect the diagnosis of von Willebrand disease in African-American women. Am J Hematol 2001;67(2):125-129.
Mulder K, Llinas A. The target joint. Haemophilia 2004;10(Suppl 4):152-156.
National Hemophilia Foundation Medical and Scientific Advisory Council (MASAC): MASAC recommendations concerning the treatment of hemophilia and other bleeding disorders (Revised October 2006). Available at http://www.hemophilia.org/NHFWeb/MainPgs/MainNHF.aspx?menuid= 57&contentid=693 (accessed May 21, 2008).
Pierce GF, Lillicrap D, Pipe SW, Vandendriessche T: Gene therapy, bioengineered clotting factors and novel technologies for hemophilia treatment. J Thromb Haemost 2007;5(5):901-906.
Soucie JM, Nuss R, Evatt B, et al: Mortality among males with hemophilia: Relations with source of medical care. The Hemophilia Surveillance System Project Investigators. Blood 2000;96(2):437-442.
Veldman A, Hoffman M, Ehrenforth S: New insights into the coagulation system and implications for new therapeutic options with recombinant factor VIIa. Curr Med Chem 2003;10(10):797-811.
Warrier I, Ewenstein BM, Koerper MA, et al: Factor IX inhibitors and anaphylaxis in hemophilia B. J Pediatr Hematol Oncol 1997;19(1):23-27.

Platelet-Mediated Bleeding Disorders

Method of
Suman Sood, MD, and
Charles S. Abrams, MD

Quantitative and qualitative platelet defects are commonly encountered in clinical practice and can result in bleeding diatheses.

Elements of Platelet Function

The vascular endothelium separates platelets from adhesive substrates in the subendothelial connective tissue. Platelet-mediated hemostasis is initiated by adherence to exposed collagen, fibronectin, and laminin following a breach to the vessel wall. Intracellular signaling cascades lead to secretion of platelet granules, synthesis, and release of thromboxane A_2, and a conformational change in platelet surface glycoprotein IIb/IIIa (GPIIb/IIIa) that enables it to bind soluble fibrinogen or von Willebrand's factor (vWF). Release of thromboxane A_2 and agonists within the secretion granules, such as adenosine diphosphate (ADP) and serotonin, activate neighboring platelets to perpetuate the process.

Fibrinogen binding to GPIIb/IIIa cross-links the platelets into a hemostatic plug, resulting in platelet aggregation and accumulation at the site of injury. Other signaling pathways initiated by agonists such as thrombin, thromboxane A_2, and collagen help promote the process of aggregation. Activated platelet plasma membrane interacts with circulating coagulation factors and provides a surface for assembly and generation of active factor X and thrombin. Secondary hemostasis occurs when the platelet plug is stabilized further by a thrombin-mediated fibrin mesh. The arrest of bleeding in a superficial wound almost exclusively results from the primary hemostatic plug.

Platelet-mediated bleeding disorders are characterized by a prolonged bleeding time, mucocutaneous bleeding, petechiae, and purpura. In contrast, deficiencies in secondary hemostasis result in delayed deep bleeding, such as bleeding into muscles and joints.

Quantitative Bleeding Disorders

Adequate numbers of platelets are required to achieve primary hemostasis. Thrombocytopenia can result from decreased platelet production by bone marrow megakaryocytes, accelerated platelet removal, or platelet sequestration in an enlarged spleen. The clinical context is essential because there is no easy test to differentiate among these possibilities. Most commonly, thrombocytopenia is caused by accelerated platelet removal.

Hemorrhage following trauma or surgery generally does not occur if the platelet count is more than 50,000/µL. In an otherwise hemostatically normal patient, significant spontaneous bleeding usually does not occur with a platelet count greater than 5000 to 10,000/µL. However, there is no absolute threshold for spontaneous bleeding due to thrombocytopenia, and spontaneous bleeding can occur at higher counts when fever, sepsis, severe anemia, and other hemostatic defects are present or when platelet function is impaired by medication. Notably, a prolonged cutaneous bleeding time does not accurately predict clinical bleeding.

THROMBOCYTOPENIA DUE TO DECREASED PLATELET PRODUCTION

Decreased platelet production occurs in primary diseases of the bone marrow such as acute leukemia and aplastic anemia; myelophthisic processes in which marrow is replaced by metastatic carcinoma, fibrosis, or multiple myeloma; following chemotherapy or radiation therapy; with ethanol toxicity; and during infections with viruses such as HIV, cytomegalovirus (CMV), Epstein-Barr virus (EBV), and varicella. Thrombocytopenia also occurs when megakaryocyte proliferation is impaired by myelodysplasia.

Overt bleeding in these disorders, when clearly a result of thrombocytopenia, is treated by platelet transfusion. Prophylactic platelet transfusion, however, is an area of controversy and is complicated by the short life span of platelets (10 days), the 5-day shelf life of stored platelets, and platelet immunogenicity. In patients undergoing treatment for acute leukemia, outcome is unchanged when platelet counts of 5,000 to 10,000/µL are used as the threshold for prophylactic transfusion. Single-donor apheresis platelets or platelet donors who are HLA identical to the recipient should be considered to prevent alloimmunization. The multicenter Platelet Dose trial in patients with malignancy is currently accruing and should help clarify these issues.

THROMBOCYTOPENIA DUE TO INCREASED PLATELET DESTRUCTION

Nonimmune and immune processes can lead to a shortened platelet life span. Nonimmune causes include sepsis, disseminated intravascular coagulation (DIC), thrombotic thrombocytopenic purpura/hemolytic uremic syndrome (TTP/HUS), preeclampsia and eclampsia, cardiopulmonary bypass, and giant cavernous hemangiomas. The thrombocytopenia resolves with treatment of the underlying disorder, and platelet transfusion is rarely necessary. In TTP/HUS, thrombocytopenia is associated with thrombosis rather than bleeding, and controversial reports exist of clinical deterioration following platelet transfusion.

Immune-mediated platelet destruction can occur due to medication, alloimmune sensitization, or autoimmunity. Medications should always be considered a possible cause of thrombocytopenia. The potential list is long, but drugs with strong evidence of antibody-mediated platelet destruction include quinine (Qualaquin), quinidine, sulfonamides, and gold salts. Besides stopping the offending medication, emergent treatment for severe thrombocytopenia with bleeding includes platelet transfusion, and corticosteroids with or without intravenous immunoglobulin (IVIg).

Heparin-induced thrombocytopenia (HIT) is a special case of drug-induced thrombocytopenia associated with arterial and venous thrombosis rather than bleeding. HIT occurs in 2% to 5% of patients given unfractionated heparin by any route for 5 to 10 days. Antibodies develop to a heparin–platelet factor 4 (PF4) complex. HIT must always be considered when thrombocytopenia is detected in a hospitalized patient. If a patient has HIT, all heparin administration should be stopped, and alternative anticoagulation such as the direct thrombin inhibitors recombinant hirudin and argatroban should be instituted, at least until the platelet count normalizes. Warfarin (Coumadin) should not be used in acute HIT because of its delayed therapeutic effect and association with a syndrome of venous limb gangrene. Platelet transfusions in this disease are controversial, because some reports suggest that they can precipitate thrombotic complications.

Alloimmune thrombocytopenia due to sensitization to alloantigens such as Pl^{A1} can result from transfusion (post-transfusion purpura, PTP) or maternal sensitization during pregnancy (neonatal alloimmune thrombocytopenia, NAIT). PTP causes profound thrombocytopenia 7 to 10 days after transfusion and can be treated with IVIg or plasma exchange. NAIT can cause severe thrombocytopenia and bleeding in neonates and is treated with platelet transfusion, corticosteroids, and IVIg.

Autoimmune thrombocytopenia, also known as idiopathic thrombocytopenic purpura (ITP), is caused by circulating antiplatelet autoantibodies. An ITP-like picture can also occur in autoimmune diseases such as systemic lupus erythematosus, in patients with low-grade lymphoproliferative disorders such as chronic lymphocytic leukemia, and in patients with HIV infections. ITP can occur at any age in both sexes and manifests with either mucocutaneous bleeding or unexplained asymptomatic thrombocytopenia. The complete blood count (CBC) is otherwise normal, splenomegaly is absent, and peripheral blood smears are only remarkable for a decreased number of platelets, some of which may be larger than normal. Bone marrow examination is usually not necessary in the absence of other findings suggesting myelodysplasia, but it typically shows normal or increased numbers of megakaryocytes.

 CURRENT DIAGNOSIS

- Platelet-mediated bleeding disorders are characterized by a prolonged bleeding time, mucocutaneous bleeding, petechiae, and purpura.
- Thrombocytopenia can result from decreased platelet production, accelerated platelet removal, or platelet sequestration in an enlarged spleen.
- In an otherwise hemostatically normal patient, significant spontaneous bleeding generally does not occur until the platelet count declines to <5000-10,000/µL. A prolonged bleeding time does not predict clinical bleeding.
- Medications are common causes of quantitative and qualitative platelet defects.
- Heparin-induced thrombocytopenia must always be considered when thrombocytopenia is detected in a hospitalized patient.
- Idiopathic thrombocytopenic purpura manifests as otherwise unexplained spontaneous mucocutaneous bleeding or asymptomatic thrombocytopenia and is a diagnosis of exclusion.
- Although many medications impair platelet function in vitro, only a few, including aspirin, ticlopidine (Ticlid), clopidogrel (Plavix), and the glycoprotein IIb/IIIa antagonists induce clinically significant bleeding.
- While hereditary disorders of platelet adhesion and aggregation are rare, hereditary disorders of platelet secretion are not uncommon causes of easy bruising, menorrhagia, and excessive postoperative and postpartum blood loss. Platelet aggregation studies are helpful for diagnosis.

Management of ITP is guided by symptoms and platelet count. Asymptomatic patients with platelet counts greater than 30,000/μL can be followed without treatment. With bleeding or a platelet count less than 30,000/μL, treatment with prednisone is initiated. Refractory patients may require splenectomy (60%-75% remission rate), other immunosuppressive medications, or new thrombopoiesis-stimulating agents. Emergent presentation with severe thrombocytopenia (<5000/μL) or internal bleeding should be treated with high doses of pulse corticosteroids or IVIg, or both. Platelet transfusion may be given concurrently with the IVIg for critical bleeding. Anti-D immune globulin may be substituted for IVIg in Rh$^+$ patients who have not undergone splenectomy; however, occasional patients develop severe autoimmune hemolysis.

THROMBOCYTOPENIA DUE TO HYPERSPLENISM

Approximately 30% of the circulating platelet mass is normally present in the spleen. Additional platelets may be sequestered when the spleen enlarges due to portal hypertension or infiltrative diseases. Platelet counts in patients with hypersplenism generally are not lower than 40,000 to 50,000/μL. Consequently, bleeding due to thrombocytopenia from hypersplenism alone is unusual.

Qualitative Platelet Disorders

ACQUIRED QUALITATIVE PLATELET DISORDERS

Acquired disorders of platelet function are relatively common but are usually asymptomatic or mild. Nonetheless, they can be of substantial clinical importance when engrafted on another hemostatic abnormality. They are subclassified as resulting from drugs, hematologic diseases, and systemic disorders. Drugs are the most common cause of dysfunction, most notably aspirin, which irreversibly inactivates the enzyme cyclooxygenase-1 (COX-1), thus inducing a permanent blockade in platelet prostaglandin synthesis and consequently thromboxane A_2 synthesis. Although the antihemostatic effect is minimal in normal persons, it may be quite prominent in a patient with an underlying bleeding disorder. Nonsteroidal anti-inflammatory drugs (NSAIDs) reversibly inhibit platelet prostaglandin synthesis and generally have little effect on hemostasis. Other medications that interfere significantly with platelet function include clopidogrel (Plavix), ticlopidine (Ticlid), and GPIIb/IIIa receptor antagonists. Numerous other drugs have been implicated in platelet dysfunction in case reports, but the evidence for most of these medications is less well established.

Bone marrow processes that can produce intrinsically abnormal platelets include myeloproliferative disorders, leukemias, myelodysplastic syndromes, and dysproteinemias such as multiple myeloma and Waldenström's macroglobulinemia, in which abnormal plasma proteins impair platelet function. In addition, acquired forms of von Willebrand's disease, a rare disorder that can arise secondary to critical aortic stenosis, multiple myeloma, or other clonal lymphoproliferative disorders, can lead to a bleeding diathesis.

Renal failure is the most prominent systemic disorder associated with abnormal platelet function. The hemostatic defect is generally mild and corrects rapidly with the initiation of dialysis. Intravenous desmopressin (DDAVP), a vasopressin analogue that causes release of von Willebrand factor (vWF) from tissue stores, is helpful in uremia, shortening bleeding time in 50% to 75% of patients. Dosing may be repeated, although tachyphylaxis can occur. Maintaining the hemoglobin greater than 10 g/dL can optimize the efficiency of platelets by enhancing the interactions between platelets and the blood vessel wall. DIC can also lead to impaired platelet function. Thrombocytopenia is a consistent feature of cardiopulmonary bypass surgery, typically secondary to hemodilution, platelet membrane activation from interaction with the bypass circuit, and fragmentation from hypothermia. It generally resolves spontaneously within several days after bypass, but platelet transfusions may be helpful if bleeding persists.

CURRENT THERAPY

- In the absence of bleeding, platelet counts of 5000-10,000/μL are used as the threshold for prophylactic transfusion. Single-donor apheresis platelets should be considered to prevent alloimmunization.
- For hemorrhaging patients or for patients scheduled to undergo delicate operations such as neurosurgery, maintaining the platelet count greater than 75,000 to 100,000/μL is recommended.
- When heparin-induced thrombocytopenia is a possibility, all heparin administration must be stopped and alternative anticoagulation instituted, at least until the platelet count returns to normal.
- Because bleeding in patients with ITP is usually minimal to absent until platelet counts decline to <30,000/μL, asymptomatic patients with platelet counts >30,000 can be followed without treatment.
- Treatment for ITP is initiated with prednisone (1 mg/kg); patients who fail to enter clinical remission are candidates for splenectomy or treatment with immunosuppressive agents including rituximab[1] (Rituxan) and azathioprine[1] (Imuran).
- High doses of corticosteroids (methylprednisolone [Solu-Medrol], 1 g/d for 3 d) or IVIg (1 g/kg/d for 2 d) are indicated for emergency treatment of ITP. Platelet transfusion given concurrently with IVIg can be effective for critical bleeding. Anti-D immune globulin (WinRho) may be used instead of IVIg in Rh$^+$ patients, although this treatment can induce clinically significant hemolysis.
- The platelet dysfunction of uremia is usually corrected by dialysis. Maintaining the hemoglobin above 10 g/dL helps minimize bleeding by increasing interactions between platelets and the blood vessel wall. Intravenous desmopressin (DDAVP) given at a dose of 0.3 μg/kg IV over 15 to 30 minutes shortens the bleeding time in most patients with uremia for approximately 4 hours.
- When necessary, treatment of hereditary disorders of platelet adhesion and aggregation usually requires platelet transfusion.

[1]Not FDA approved for this indication.
Abbreviations: ITP = idiopathic thrombocytopenic purpura; IVIg = intravenous immunoglobulin.

HEREDITARY QUALITATIVE PLATELET DISORDERS

Bernard-Soulier syndrome (BSS) and Glanzmann's thrombasthenia (GT) are rare autosomal recessive disorders of the platelet membrane glycoproteins GPIb/IX and GPIIb/IIIa, respectively. They manifest with mucocutaneous bleeding in infancy or childhood. Patients with BSS are also thrombocytopenic and have very large platelets that do not agglutinate when exposed to ristocetin. Platelet counts and morphology are normal in GT, but the platelets cannot aggregate in response to ADP or thrombin. Reliable treatment of bleeding in both conditions requires platelet transfusion.

Hereditary disorders of platelet secretion are not uncommon causes of mucocutaneous bleeding and can be due to alpha granule deficiency (gray platelet syndrome), the more common dense granule deficiency (δ storage pool disease [δSPD]), or to aspirin-like defects resulting from abnormalities of the platelet secretory mechanism. δSPD may be associated with albinism (Hermansky-Pudlack and Chédiak-Higashi syndromes) or occur in otherwise normal persons.

Patients with δSPD have normal platelet counts with prolonged bleeding times and abnormal platelet aggregation studies with a diagnostic increased adenosine triphosphate-to-adenosine diphosphate (ATP/ADP) ratio due to the absence of platelet dense granule ADP. Although bleeding in patients with secretion disorders can be controlled by platelet transfusion, DDAVP sometimes shortens the bleeding times and improves hemostasis.

REFERENCES

Aster RH, Bougie DW: Drug-induced immune thrombocytopenia. N Engl J Med 2007;357:580-587.

Bennett JS: Novel platelet inhibitors. Ann Rev Med 2001;52:161-184.

Bolton-Maggs PHB, Chalmers EA, Collins PW, et al: A review of inherited platelet disorders with guidelines for their management on behalf of the UKHCDO. Br J Haematol 2006;135:603-633.

Cines DB, Blanchette VS: Immune thrombocytopenic purpura. N Engl J Med 2002;346:995-1008.

Hedges SJ, Dehoney SB, Hooper JS, et al: Evidence-based treatment recommendations for uremic bleeding. Nat Clin Pract Nephrol 2007;3:138-153.

Lind SE: The bleeding time does not predict surgical bleeding. Blood 1991;77:2547-2552.

Mannucci PM: Drug therapy: Treatment of von Willebrand's disease. N Engl J Med 2004;351:683-694.

Nurden AT: Qualitative disorders of platelets and megakaryocytes. J Thromb Hemostasis 2006;3:1773-1782.

Stanworth SJ, Hyde C, Brunskill S, et al: Platelet transfusion prophylaxis for patients with hematological malignancies: Where to now?. Br J Haematol 2005;131:588-595.

Warkentin TE: Heparin-induced thrombocytopenia: Pathogenesis and management. Br J Haematol 2003;121:535-555.

Disseminated Intravascular Coagulation

Method of
John J. Byrnes, MD

The hemostatic system is in a balanced and highly regulated matrix of coagulant and anticoagulant activities that keep the blood fluid and maintain hemostasis. Disseminated intravascular coagulation (DIC) is a clinicopathologic syndrome of excessive procoagulant imbalance and dysregulation that occur secondary to a variety of disorders. Generally, a primary disorder causes tissue injury and the release of excessive tissue factor or other endogenous or exogenous procoagulant material into the circulation. Endotoxins or exotoxins, venoms, or proteases from granulocytic or pancreatic cells and other products from cancerous tissues can activate the coagulant cascade.

Thrombin is generated by combined activation of the extrinsic and intrinsic pathways in excess of the normal counter-regulatory capacities such as antithrombin III, activated protein C, and tissue factor pathway inhibitor. Excessive intravascular thrombin produces soluble fibrin, which deposits as microthrombi in the smaller vessels of the circulation. Fibrinogen and factors II, V, VIII, and XIII are consumed; platelets are trapped in the fibrin mesh. In addition, exposure of platelets to thrombin causes them to aggregate, which contributes to clot formation and thrombocytopenia. Thrombin in lesser concentrations causes secretion of platelet granules, which leads to a functional deficit of platelets remaining in the circulation.

Fibrinolysis begins as plasminogen is activated to plasmin in response to intravascular fibrin deposition. Plasmin also degrades fibrinogen and factors V, VIII, and XIII, which causes even more severe depletion of coagulation factors. Degradation products of fibrinogen and fibrin inhibit fibrin polymerization and platelet–platelet interaction, further compromising hemostasis; a severely hypocoagulable state can result. Conversely, a hypercoagulable state can ensue because of activated procoagulant factors in the circulation and the depletion of anticoagulant factors such as antithrombins and protein C and protein S and tissue factor pathway inhibitor along with the up-regulation of fibrinolytic inhibitors such as plasminogen activator inhibitor.

The clinical presentation of DIC may be either acute and fulminant or less severe and chronic, depending in large part on the initiating process. Thrombotic or hemorrhagic clinical manifestations can predominate in a given patient, or both manifestations can occur simultaneously. In general, hemorrhagic problems more often complicate acute DIC, whereas chronic DIC is more commonly associated with thrombotic disorders. In acute DIC, the precipitating disorder is generally readily evident and often catastrophic; common etiologies are given in Box 1. Chronic DIC is more subtle and may be manifest long before or after the underlying disorder is evident.

Hemorrhagic manifestations seen with DIC can reflect associated trauma or breaches in skin or mucosal integrity that may be relatively minor. Organ systems that are often involved are the skin, gastrointestinal tract, lungs, and brain. Continued bleeding or rebleeding from sites of minor trauma such as venipunctures is typically seen.

Thrombotic manifestations of DIC can result from widespread microthrombus formation, leading to impaired perfusion of multiple organs. Fulminant DIC can lead to occlusion of the terminal arterioles in the skin and thus to necrosis of the digits, nose, and ears and occasionally to diffuse skin infarction (purpura fulminans). Renal dysfunction may be extreme and can result in complete renal failure. Involvement of cerebral microvessels often produces nonfocal dysfunction or seizures. Occlusions in the pulmonary microcirculation can manifest as the respiratory distress syndrome.

BOX 1 Etiologies of Intravascular Coagulation

Disseminated

Hypotension shock of any etiology
Immunologic disorders
- Anaphylaxis
- Hemolytic transfusion reaction

Infections
- Gram-negative sepsis
- Meningococcemia
- Postsplenectomy sepsis
- Rocky Mountain spotted fever

Injuries
- Brain trauma
- Burns
- Extensive tissue damage
- Snakebite

Malignant disorders
- Mucin-producing adenocarcinomas, especially prostatic and gastric
- Promyelocytic leukemia

Metabolic disorders
- Acidosis
- Hyperthermia

Obstetric complications
- Abruptio placentae
- Amniotic fluid embolism
- Retained dead fetus
- Saline-induced abortions

Localized

Vascular malformations
- Aortic aneurysm
- Giant hemangioma

Diagnosis

The laboratory picture of DIC may be obvious or subtle. In acute DIC, the platelet count is low; 50% of the time it is less than 50,000/µL. The prothrombin time and partial thromboplastin time are prolonged, and the fibrinogen level is below normal. Fibrinogen levels may be normal if the patient initially had elevated levels because of pregnancy or a response to infection. Fibrin (and fibrinogen) degradation products are a hallmark of the disorder; cross-linked fibrin degradation products, D-dimers, indicate fibrin clot lysis. Impaired microvascular blood flow by fibrin strands leads to fragmentation of red blood cells, microangiopathic hemolysis, especially in severe acute DIC. Close monitoring of the parameters of fibrinogen consumption and fibrinolysis and the trend from day to day are the best indicators of the patient's response to treatment. The thrombocytopenia is multifactorial and often protracted, slowly reflecting clinical improvement.

In chronic DIC, fibrin degradation products are present, but the prothrombin time and partial thromboplastin time might or might not be prolonged; the partial thromboplastin time can actually be shorter than normal because of activated factors and depletion of antithrombin. Liver failure can complicate the diagnosis of DIC, because clotting factor deficiency often occurs, together with thrombocytopenia and impaired clearance of fibrin-degradation products, leading to elevated levels.

Syndromes sharing common findings with DIC must be excluded because many have specific and effective treatments. These include thrombotic thrombocytopenic purpura, the hemolytic uremic syndrome, the heparin-induced thrombocytopenia and thrombosis syndrome, and the catastrophic antiphospholipid syndrome. Sometimes these syndromes are difficult to distinguish from DIC and sometimes they are complicated by DIC.

Treatment

Successful resolution of DIC is contingent on successful management of the underlying initiating process. Supportive measures to maintain adequate blood pressure, hemoglobin concentration, oxygenation, and acid–base and electrolyte balances to minimize organ damage consequent to the impaired microvascular perfusion are critical. Therapeutic interventions aimed at the coagulation disorder must be considered in the full clinical context, and the risks of therapy must, as usual, be weighed against the potential benefit. If there is only laboratory evidence of DIC but no significant hemorrhage or thrombosis, measures other than addressing the underlying process are not required. If bleeding is the predominant problem, factor replacement with fresh frozen plasma 2 to 4 U/day or greater and as hemodynamically tolerated, cryoprecipitate, and platelet transfusion are used to replenish diminished levels. A platelet count of at least 50,000/µL should be strived for if there is significant bleeding. Cryoprecipitate is given to maintain a fibrinogen level higher than 100 mg/dL.

When thrombotic complications resulting in severe organ hypoperfusion occur, anticoagulation with heparin may be considered. In adults, a loading dose of heparin 5000 U followed by the continuous intravenous infusion of 1000 U/hour is usually given to start. Adjustment of the dose of heparin is determined by the clinical and laboratory response. Improvement in organ perfusion and a rising fibrinogen level and platelet count with diminished signs of intravascular hemolysis point to a satisfactory response. The evidence for heparin effectiveness is limited to small and uncontrolled series. A specific contraindication to the use of heparin is head trauma or intracerebral hemorrhage.

Acute promyelocytic leukemia (AML-M3) often manifests with DIC and requires specific management. AML-M3 is associated with the release of granule contents from the hypergranulated promyelocytes into the circulation, thus activating the coagulation cascade. Cytolysis caused by treatment of the leukemia releases even more granule contents into the circulation, causing acceleration of DIC. AML-M3 is a very treatable and often curable form of acute leukemia, which responds to all-*trans*-retinoic acid and arsenic-based treatment regimens. However the primary cause of failure is due to DIC at presentation often associated with intracerebral hemorrhage. To minimize this risk of this complication, all-*trans*-retinoic acid must be started promptly and DIC parameters must be monitored closely during remission induction, with blood product support given as needed.

In most obstetric patients, management of acute DIC consists of removing the products of conception and supportive care. Transfusions are used to replace clotting factor in patients with significant bleeding. The role of heparin remains controversial; the effectiveness of heparin in controlling bleeding manifestations when there was an unavoidable delay in the resolution of the underlying cause has been reported.

Certain disease states are associated with the consumption of platelet and clotting factors at localized anatomic sites. These states include aortic aneurysm, large hemanginomas (Kasabach–Merritt syndrome), and certain renal disorders, including hyperacute allograft rejection. The laboratory values are often compatible with DIC. The risk of not recognizing the limited nature of the disorder is that inappropriate therapy may be given for a presumed disseminated state. If surgery for an aortic aneurysm is to be done, hemostasis is best obtained first. Most patients with chronic DIC of this nature respond to treatment with heparin and factor replacement.

Chronic low-grade DIC associated with venous thromboses, such as Trousseau's syndrome, requires treatment with adjusted full-dose heparin, a loading dose of 5000 to 10,000 U, followed by continuous intravenous infusion of 1000 to 2000 U/hour. After resolution of the venous thrombosis, prophylactic-dose heparin should be given to prevent recurrence; warfarin (Coumadin) is not as effective in this setting. (Comparable doses of low-molecular-weight heparin may also be used).

Based on the pathophysiologic concepts and encouraging preclinical studies, the protease inhibitors and concentrates of antithrombin III, activated protein C, and tissue factor pathway inhibitor have been used to treat DIC. However, thus far, only recombinant activated protein C has shown a significant reduction in DIC mortality when used early in patients with sepsis. The product is contraindicated in patients with bleeding tendencies or a platelet count of less than 30×10^6/L.

Recombinant activated factor VII has been used with some success in patients who are bleeding and with coagulopathy due to massive severe trauma.

REFERENCES

Abraham E, Reinhart K, Demeyer I: Efficacy and safety of Tifacogin (recombinant tissue pathway factor inhibitor) in severe sepsis: A randomized controlled trial. JAMA 2003;290:238-247.

Franchini M, Lippi G, Manzato F: Recent acquisitions in the pathophysiology, diagnosis and treatment of disseminated intravascular coagulation. Thromb J 2006;4.

Levi M, de Jonge, van der Poll T: New treatment strategies for disseminated intravascular coagulation based on current understanding of the pathophysiology. Ann Med 2004;36(1):41-49.

Sallah S, Hussain A, Nguyen NP: Recombinant activated factor VII in patients with cancer and hemorrhagic disseminated intravascular coagulation. Blood Coagul Fibrinolysis 2004;15:577-582.

Tallman MS, Abutalib SA, Altman JK: The double hazard of thrombophilia and bleeding in acute promyelocytic leukemia. Semin Thromb Hemost 2007;33(4):330-338.

Vincent JL, Bernard GR, Beale R, et al: Drotrecogin alfa (activated) treatment in severe sepsis from global open-label trial ENHANCE: Further evidence for survival and safety and implications for early treatment. Crit Care Med 2005;33:2266-2277.

Zeeleder S, Hack CE, Wuillemin WA: Disseminated intravascular coagulation in sepsis. Chest 2005;128:2864-2875.

Thrombotic Thrombocytopenic Purpura

Method of
Joseph E. Kiss, MD

Thrombotic thrombocytopenic purpura (TTP) is a life-threatening thrombotic disorder in which unrestrained platelet deposition occurs in the microcirculation of many organs including the brain, kidneys, heart, and abdominal viscera. Thrombocytopenia develops as platelets are progressively consumed. The term *microangiopathic hemolytic anemia* refers to the fragmentation of red blood cells (schistocytes) during their passage through partially occluded arterioles and capillaries. Therapeutic plasma exchange, the mainstay of therapy, has markedly improved mortality from more than 90% in the past to 10% to 20% currently. A high index of suspicion for the diagnosis is necessary, because delays in recognizing the disorder can increase treatment failure and death. Because plasma exchange is very effective, it is appropriate to consider TTP as a provisional diagnosis and initiate therapy when thrombocytopenia and microangiopathic hemolytic anemia are present without another apparent etiology.

Classification

A wide variety of disorders can be associated with TTP or can develop TTP-like manifestations. The primary causes and major secondary forms are outlined in Box 1. This classification is based on clinical and laboratory similarities. There is ongoing controversy as to whether certain secondary causes should be considered in this classification and whether they should be treated using plasma exchange. For example, a TTP-like syndrome can occur in the setting of hematopoietic stem cell transplantation, but the efficacy of plasma exchange has been questioned. Experienced clinical judgment may be necessary to decide on the appropriate diagnosis and the best course of therapy.

Pathogenesis

Remarkable progress has been made over the last few years in understanding the pathogenesis of TTP. Defects in ADAMTS13, a key enzyme that normally clips large, sticky multimers of von Willebrand's factor into smaller subunits, have been found in patients with congenital TTP and in patients with idiopathic TTP. Without the enzyme, long strings of ultra-large von Willebrand's factor (ULVWF) remain anchored to the surface of endothelial cells, binding platelets and forming occlusive microthrombi throughout many organs, especially the brain and kidneys. A second hit, presumably endothelial cell injury following the stress of infection, surgery, or pregnancy, triggers an acute episode in the setting of ADAMTS13 deficiency.

Dysfunctional enzyme is found in all cases of congenital TTP. Severe ADAMTS13 deficiency (defined as <10% normal) due to an immunoglobulin G (IgG) autoantibody to ADAMTS13 is reported in 30% to 100% of cases of idiopathic TTP. Typical TTP patients have also been described who do not have ADAMTS13 deficiency, suggesting that alternative mechanisms that are not yet known also lead to TTP.

Clinical Presentation

Idiopathic TTP often occurs in young healthy persons. The peak age group is between 20 and 40 years; women are affected twice as often as men. African Americans are disproportionately affected. The classic diagnostic pentad, consisting of thrombocytopenia, microangiopathic anemia, fever, neurologic abnormalities, and renal failure occurs in only a minority of cases, perhaps because with increased clinical awareness the diagnosis is being considered earlier in the course of the disease. Patients might have vague symptoms at first, such as malaise, weakness, and headache several days before developing worrisome

---

BOX 1 Clinical Classification and Distinguishing Features of Thrombotic Thrombocytopenic Purpura

Primary Disease

Congenital
Due to mutations in ADAMTS13 gene
Very rare

Idiopathic
Due to IgG autoantibody that binds to ADAMTS13
Diagnosed by exclusion of secondary causes
Most common form

Secondary Disease

Human Immunodeficiency Virus
High response rate reported to plasma infusion and anti-retroviral therapy

Collagen Vascular Diseases
Treated in the same way as idiopathic TTP using plasma exchange, immunosuppressants

Drug-Induced Immunologic Disease
Quinine is the most common cause—anti-platelet antibodies associated—ADAMTS13 auto-antibody associated
Ticlopidine (Ticlid) ± clopidogrel (Plavix) is also associated
Treatment is by withdrawing offending drug and performing plasma exchange
Rapid recovery is typical

Drug-Induced, Dose-Dependent Toxicity
Associated with cancer chemotherapeutic agents including mitomycin C (Mutamycin) and gemcitabine (Gemzar)
Can develop slowly, sometimes after drug is discontinued
Can also be seen with immunosuppressive agents including cyclosporin (Neoral) and tacrolimus (Prograf)
Treated by stopping drug
Uncertain benefit of plasma exchange

Pregnancy and Postpartum
May be due to a IgG inhibitor of ADAMTS13
Must be distinguished from HELLP syndrome (HELLP usually occurs during the third trimester of pregnancy or immediately postpartum in association with severe preeclampsia)

Hematopoietic Stem Cell Transplant–Associated Disease
A TTP-like syndrome that may be caused by infection or graft-versus-host disease
Doubtful benefit of plasma exchange

Note: If laboratory studies are to be drawn to evaluate a secondary cause (e.g., SLE), it is important to obtain these before instituting plasma exchange therapy to avoid a dilution effect.
HELLP = hemolysis with elevated liver enzymes and low platelets; HUS = hemolytic uremic syndrome; IgG = immunoglobulin G; SLE = systemic lupus erythematosus; TTP = thrombotic thrombocytic purpura.

neurologic complaints including visual disturbances, paresthesias, focal motor weakness, and aphasia (i.e., transient ischemic attacks) or more generalized manifestations such as confusion, seizures, stupor, and coma. The neurologic abnormalities in conjunction with thrombocytopenia and anemia form a common triad that should lead to high diagnostic suspicion. Fever occurs in about 50% at the time of presentation.

Renal injury is associated with rising creatinine and proteinuria and is typically mild in TTP. Cases in which renal failure predominates are termed *hemolytic uremic syndrome* (HUS). Diarrhea (usually but not always bloody) should prompt consideration of enterotoxin-associated epidemic HUS. Because of frequent clinical overlap with both neurologic and renal manifestations, however, it may be difficult to distinguish between TTP and HUS in adults.

Gastrointestinal complaints are also common. Abdominal pain, nausea, vomiting, and diarrhea can reflect the presence of visceral ischemia or pancreatitis. These symptoms along with mental status changes, elevated bilirubin, and thrombocytopenia may be mistaken for liver disease, further delaying diagnosis. Chest pain and arrhythmias due to small vessel myocardial involvement have been reported up to 18% of patients in some series. These protean clinical manifestations of TTP reflect its multisystemic pathophysiology.

Diagnosis

The hallmark of microangiopathic hemolytic anemia is the presence of fragmented red blood cells on the blood smear. A number of disorders are known to cause microangiopathic hemolysis and thrombocytopenia, which can mimic the clinical and laboratory features of TTP. These include severe hypertension (persisting blood pressure >200/100 with or without papilledema), prosthetic cardiac devices (e.g., left ventricular assist devices, intra-aortic balloon pump), HELLP syndrome (hemolysis with elevated liver enzymes and low platelets) with severe preeclampsia, and vasculitis. Disseminated intravascular coagulation (DIC) may be seen in association with sepsis or a low-grade form associated with carcinoma. In contrast to DIC, the fibrinogen level in TTP is normal and fibrin degradation products are also normal or minimally increased. The direct antiglobulin test is used to exclude immune hemolysis, which can occur concomitantly with thrombocytopenia (Evan's syndrome).

Although measurement of ADAMTS13 is becoming more widely available in clinical laboratories, the usefulness of this test still needs to be validated as a diagnostic and management tool. A number of technical issues affect the analytical sensitivity and specificity of the various assays in use. A normal level should not be used to exclude the diagnosis. Severe deficiency of ADAMTS13 has been proposed as a specific test for TTP, but it has also been noted in severe sepsis, disseminated intravascular coagulation, and metastatic malignancy. If these entities can be confidently excluded, a severe deficiency of ADAMTS13 reported by an experienced laboratory strongly supports the diagnosis of TTP.

CURRENT DIAGNOSIS

Recommended Diagnostic Tests for Initial Evaluation

- Complete blood count with differential white blood cell, platelet, and reticulocyte count
- Review of peripheral blood smear
- Coagulation studies including fibrinogen and fibrin degradation products
- Lactate dehydrogenase (LDH)
- Blood urea nitrogen, creatinine, electrolytes
- Liver function tests, including direct and indirect bilirubin
- Direct antiglobulin test
- Urinalysis

Treatment

Plasma exchange is the only therapy that has been shown to be effective in a randomized, controlled clinical trial. It is believed to work by replacing ADAMTS13 and by removing inhibitory antibodies to the enzyme. It also appears to be effective in patients who are not deficient in ADAMTS13, so other mechanisms may be involved.

If there is a delay in instituting plasma exchange, 15-30 mL/kg plasma should be infused, with attention to avoiding volume overload. Cardiac monitoring in the initial stages of management is advisable in light of the relatively high frequency of cardiac involvement. In the absence of serious bleeding, platelet transfusions are contraindicated because of the potential deposition in platelet microthrombi and the risk of serious clinical sequelae (e.g., transient ischemic attack, myocardial infarction). The role of adjuvant therapy, such as corticosteroids, antiplatelet drugs, and other immunosuppressives, is not firmly established in the routine management of TTP.

Between 1 and 1.5 plasma volumes are exchanged daily, using fresh frozen plasma or alternative products that have been shown to contain ADAMTS13 (e.g., plasma frozen within 24 hours, cryoprecipitate-reduced plasma, thawed plasma). Plasma exchanges are continued daily while assessing the clinical and laboratory responses (Fig. 1). The platelet count is the single most useful laboratory parameter to follow. Lactate dehydrogenase (LDH), an indicator of tissue ischemia and hemolysis, typically lags behind changes in platelet levels. The therapeutic goal is to induce remission, consisting of a normal platelet count and near-normal LDH (<1.5 times normal levels).

Plasma exchange is generally continued on a daily schedule for 1 to 2 days after remission is achieved. It is not unusual for the disease activity to quickly reappear, leading some to taper the plasma exchanges over a short period (e.g., every other day three times, then every 3 days twice, then stop). A study comparing different institutional tapering practices found no differences in exacerbation rates. A total of 10 to 20 procedures may be needed to achieve a durable response.

Although plasma exchange is considered a safe procedure, serious complications including catheter-related sepsis, venous thrombosis, and death have been reported. Patients should be observed closely for 30 days following cessation of plasma exchange. This is a critical time for exacerbation of the disease, occurring in about 20% of patients. In those who do not respond or who respond slowly, the plasma volume may be increased and immunosuppressive therapy may be considered (e.g., prednisone 1 mg/kg/day). Continuation of the daily plasma-exchange regimen (i.e., patience on the part of the treater) is probably the single most important therapeutic strategy.

Patients who remain refractory or who are plasma exchange–dependent over several weeks are considered for additional immunosuppressive therapy. Use of the anti-CD20 monoclonal antibody rituximab (Rituxan)[1] has shown very good results leading to disease remission in the majority of patients with refractory disease who were treated with it. Relapses occur in 30% to 40% of patients with idiopathic TTP, months to years later, reflecting the relapsing and remitting autoimmune nature of this disorder.

Prognosis

Due to increased recognition and earlier treatment of TTP, most patients achieve remission and go on to complete recovery. More than one half of the deaths occur early, within 48 hours of admission to the hospital. A recent clinical analysis found that age older than 40 years, hemoglobin less than 9 g/dL, and temperature higher than 38.5°C at presentation were associated with increased mortality. Outcome cannot be predicted from the severity of thrombocytopenia or LDH level. The ADAMTS13 level also appears to have prognostic value: Patients who have severe deficiency have more autoimmune manifestations, lower platelet count, less renal insufficiency, and a higher risk of relapse. Unfortunately, TTP in association with

---

[1]Not FDA approved for this indication.

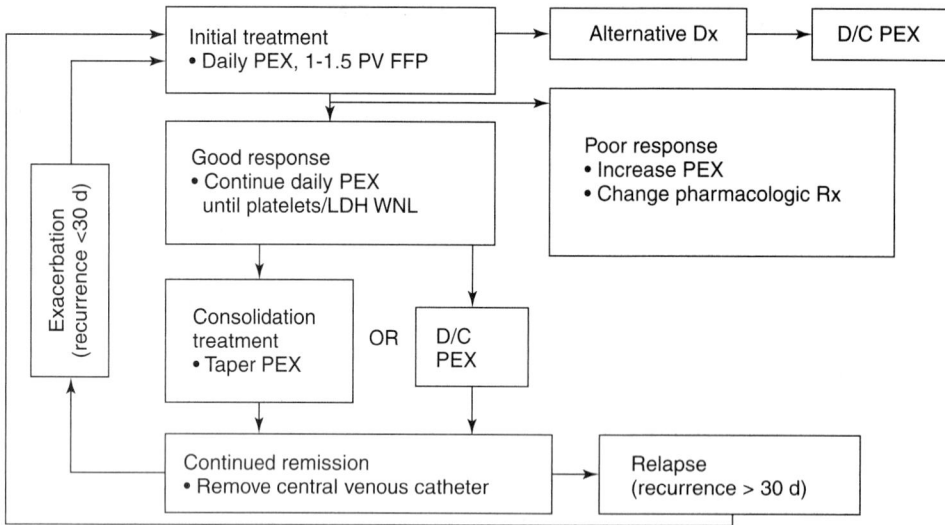

FIGURE 1. Management of patients with thrombotic thrombocytopenic purpura. D/C = discontinue; Dx = diagnosis; FFP = fresh frozen plasma; LDH = lactate dehydrogenase; PEX = plasma exchange; PV = plasma volume; Rx = prescription; WNL = within normal limits. (Adapted from George JN: How I treat patients with thrombotic thrombocytopenic purpura–hemolytic uremic syndrome. Blood 2000;96:4:1223-1229.)

transplantation and malignancy is often resistant to therapy, and novel approaches are needed.

REFERENCES

Allford S, Hunt B, Rose P, et al: Guidelines on the diagnosis and management of the thrombotic microangiopathic haemolytic anaemias. Br J Haematol 2003;120:556-573.

Bandarenko N, and members of the US TTP Apheresis Study Group; United States Thrombotic Thrombocytopenic Purpura apheresis study group (US TTP ASG): Multicenter survey and retrospective analysis of current efficacy of therapeutic plasma exchange. J Clin Apheresis 1998;13:133-141.

Fakhouri F, Vernant JP, Veyradier A, et al: Efficiency of curative and prophylactic treatment with rituximab in ADAMTS13-deficient thrombotic thrombocytopenic purpura: A study of 11 cases. Blood 2005;106:1932-1937.

George JN: How I treat patients with thrombotic thrombocytopenic purpura–hemolytic uremic syndrome. Blood 2000;96:4:1223-1229.

Howard MA, Williams LA, Terrell DR: complications of plasma exchange in patients treated for clinically suspected thrombotic thrombocytopenic purpur–hemolytic uremic syndrome. III. An additional study of 54 consecutive patients. Transfusion 2006;46:154-156.

Moake JL: Thrombotic microangiopathies. NEJM 2002;347:8:589-600.

Qu L, Kiss JE: Thrombotic microangiopathy in transplantation and malignancy. Semin Thromb Hemost 2005;31:691-699.

Vesely SK, George JN, Lammle B, et al: ADAMTS13 activity in thrombotic thrombocytopenic purpura–hemolytic uremic syndrome: Relation to presenting features and clinical outcomes in a prospective cohort of 142 patients. Blood 2003;102(1):60-68.

Hemochromatosis

Method of
Bruce R. Bacon, MD

In 1996, the *HFE* gene was identified on the short arm of chromosome 6, allowing genetic testing for the two major mutations (C282Y, H63D) that are responsible for *HFE*-linked hereditary hemochromatosis (HH). Several prospective population surveys have now shown that the incidence of the C282Y homozygous state is approximately 1:200 to 1:250 in white persons of Northern European descent. Several additional genes and proteins involved in regulating iron homeostasis have been identified, providing a better understanding of cellular iron uptake and release. *HFE*-linked HH is a common autosomal recessive disorder of iron metabolism, and if it is diagnosed early and treated appropriately, all patients can have a normal lifespan.

Clinical Features

In the past, HH was recognized by a constellation of symptoms and physical findings that are related to significant iron loading in the liver, pancreas, heart, skin, and pituitary (see Current Diagnosis box). More recently, many HH patients have been identified because of screening laboratory data obtained as part of a routine health physical, identification of *HFE* mutations as part of family screening, and prospective population-screening studies. Most patients identified in these ways are asymptomatic, and phlebotomy treatment may be started before the patient develops any significant manifestations of the disease.

Large population studies using *HFE* genotyping have shown differing results. Some have observed that the incidence of symptoms in C282Y homozygotes is not substantially different from that of a matched control population and that cirrhosis is infrequent in C282Y homozygotes in the absence of concomitant alcohol use. Conversely, more recent studies have shown an increase in fatigue, arthritis symptoms, and a history of liver disease, particularly when serum ferritin levels are greater than 1000 ng/mL. These differences in results relate to differences in study design. The latter is probably more representative.

Characteristic iron studies that occur in patients with typical HH are an elevation in transferrin saturation (serum iron divided by transferrin or total iron-binding capacity, times 100) of more than 45% and an elevation in serum ferritin level. In the absence of any other underlying disease states, serum ferritin levels reflect tissue iron stores. However, ferritin can be influenced by numerous other conditions such as inflammatory diseases, other chronic liver diseases, or malignancies, and thus an elevated serum ferritin in these disorders does not necessarily reflect increased iron stores. Conversely, some persons who are homozygous for the C282Y mutation do not have evidence of phenotypic expression (either an elevated ferritin or an elevated transferrin saturation). The reasons for this lack of phenotypic expression are not yet known but probably relate to the existence of modifying genes.

CURRENT DIAGNOSIS

Symptoms
- None
- Fatigue
- Arthropathy
- Liver disease

Findings
- None
- Hepatomegaly
- Second and third metacarpophalangeal joint arthritis

Laboratory Testing
- * C282Y/C282Y or C282Y/H63D
- * Elevated transferrin saturation >45%
- * Elevated ferritin

CURRENT THERAPY

- Perform phlebotomy of 500 mL (1 unit) of whole blood weekly
- Check transferrin saturation and ferritin levels at 2- to 3-month intervals to monitor response
- Once iron stores are depleted (ferritin <50 ng/mL; transferrin saturation <50%), proceed to maintenance phlebotomy of 1 unit of whole blood every 2 to 3 months. The goal is to keep transferrin saturation <50%; if successful, the ferritin level will remain <50 ng/mL.

Alcohol and chronic hepatitis C are potentiating factors in the development of hepatic fibrosis in HH patients. For example, C282Y homozygotes who drink more than 60 g of alcohol per day have a ninefold increase in the prevalence of cirrhosis.

Diagnosis

The inclusion of iron studies during routine clinical visits coupled with the availability of *HFE* genotyping for family and population studies has facilitated the detection of HH. It has also led to identification of C282Y homozygotes who do not have phenotypic expression. In the past, liver biopsy provided important information to determine whether or not a patient had HH; liver biopsy is no longer considered essential for the diagnosis of HH. Nonetheless, it still provides an important assessment of liver fibrosis and it can give the clinician a qualitative assessment of iron loading that can be useful in determining the amount of phlebotomy that may be required to eliminate excess iron stores. Liver biopsy is generally restricted to HH patients with suspected significant fibrosis or cirrhosis. Several studies have examined criteria for liver biopsy in the era of genetic diagnosis, concluding that biopsy is unnecessary with normal liver enzymes, with a serum ferritin of less than 1000 ng/mL, and without hepatomegaly on physical examination. Thus, it is currently recommended that liver biopsy be performed in C282Y homozygotes if liver enzymes are abnormal or if serum ferritin is higher than 1000 ng/mL.

Although liver biopsies are being performed less often to confirm a diagnosis of HH, it is still important to understand the findings that are apparent on biopsies. Using the Perls' Prussian blue stain for storage iron, iron is found in a periportal to pericentral gradient, and the highest amount is found in periportal hepatocytes. Iron is typically in hepatocytes rather than in sinusoidal lining cells (Kupffer cells). The fibrosis that occurs in HH is portal based, and in the absence of complicating factors, cirrhosis is uncommon at hepatic iron concentrations of less than 16,000 μg/g dry weight. Whenever liver biopsy is done in a patient with suspected HH, it is reasonable to measure the hepatic iron concentration to determine the relative degree of iron loading.

Treatment

Once the diagnosis of HH is confirmed by genetic testing, and there is an elevated ferritin or transferrin saturation (or both), the therapeutic approach is relatively simple, cheap, and effective. Weekly therapeutic phlebotomy should be initiated with the goal of removing 250 mg of iron with each phlebotomy (each unit of blood contains 200 to 250 mg of iron, depending on the hemoglobin concentration). The goal should be to continue weekly phlebotomy until the patient's serum ferritin level is less than 50 ng/mL and the transferrin saturation is less than 50%. In the patient with uncomplicated disease, each unit of blood removed results in a decrease in the serum ferritin level by about 30 ng/mL. This can be used as a rough guideline to predict phlebotomy requirements to deplete excess iron stores.

The goal of treatment is not to make patients iron deficient or anemic but rather to deplete excess iron stores and to achieve serum iron levels in the low-normal range. Once initial therapeutic phlebotomy has been accomplished, maintenance phlebotomy should be performed, with one unit of blood being removed every 2 to 4 months with subsequent assessment of iron status by measuring serum ferritin and transferrin saturation. Most patients require maintenance phlebotomy, but some patients do not reaccumulate excess iron.

Family Screening

Once a proband has been identified and treated, it must be remembered that this is a familial disorder and all first-degree relatives should be offered the opportunity to be screened for HH. Generally, this is done by measuring fasting transferrin saturation and ferritin as well as genetic testing in all first-degree relatives. If elevated iron levels are found, or if any relatives are C282Y homozygotes or compound heterozygotes (C282Y/H63D), then therapeutic phlebotomy may be initiated using the guidelines mentioned earlier. For evaluation of children of a proband, it is appropriate to first perform *HFE* mutation analysis in the other parent. This can obviate the need to do blood testing in the child. For example, if the proband is a C282Y homozygote and the other parent does not carry either the C282Y or H63D mutation, then it is known that the children will be obligate C282Y heterozygotes and will not be at any increased risk for iron loading. This avoids labeling the child with a genetic diagnosis that could have consequences in terms of genetic discrimination for insurance or a job.

Population Screening

After the original discovery of *HFE*, it was suggested that population screening using genetic testing might be ideal for *HFE*-related HH. This was because the disorder is known to be common, there is a long latent phase before the disease manifests, treatment is simple and effective, and tests of phenotypic markers are available and reliable. However, it has become apparent that not all C282Y homozygotes have phenotypic expression, and this then raises questions about the advisability of large-scale population screening. A summary of the results of some studies that have used *HFE* genotyping for population screening (excluding studies of blood donors), indicates that about 25% to 60% of C282Y homozygotes have a normal serum ferritin concentration and thus are not iron loaded.

Phenotypic testing based on serum iron studies has traditionally been the standard for detecting iron overload. An elevated transferrin saturation has usually been considered the main test for detecting iron overload given its excellent sensitivity, acceptable specificity, relatively low cost, and widespread availability. Methodologic issues need to be taken into consideration, and some investigators have suggested using the unbound iron-binding capacity (UIBC) as a screening tool given its reproducibility, low cost, and high sensitivity and specificity. The serum ferritin level is often elevated in iron overload, and its sensitivity is quite high. Unfortunately, it has a low specificity and it is best used in conjunction with transferrin saturation. Population screening for HH using a combination of phenotypic testing followed by focused *HFE* genotyping may be feasible. However, the cost-effectiveness of screening remains a key factor when considering public health recommendations, and population screening for HH requires further evaluation.

Summary

HH should be distinguished from the other syndromes of iron overload such as secondary iron overload and transfusional iron overload. Many patients with *HFE*-related HH have abnormal serum iron values before they develop any significant symptoms or clinical findings, and liver biopsy is less important in evaluating these patients. Treatment by phlebotomy is safe and effective and prevents the sequelae of iron overload. It must be recognized that hepatic iron can play a contributory role in the pathogenesis of porphyria cutanea tarda (PCT), nonalcoholic steatohepatitis (NASH), and chronic hepatitis C. *HFE* genotyping for the C282Y and H63D mutations has strengthened our ability to diagnose HH accurately and it is very useful in family studies. It is now clear that a substantial fraction of C282Y homozygotes do not have evidence of phenotypic expression, thereby suggesting the existence of genetic modifiers.

Our understanding of the normal physiology of iron absorption and homeostasis is growing and the ability to decipher the contribution of interindividual genetic differences in this process will be enhanced in the future.

REFERENCES

Adams PC, Reboussin DM, Barton JC, et al: Hemochromatosis and iron-overload screening in a racially diverse population. N Engl J Med 2005; 352:1769-1778.

Beutler E, Felitti VJ, Koziol JA, et al: Penetrance of 845G→A (C282Y) HFE hereditary haemochromatosis mutation in the USA. Lancet 2002;359: 211-218.

Harrison SA, Bacon BR: Hereditary hemochromatosis: Update for 2003. J Hepatol 2003;38:S14-S23.

Iron and the Liver [entire issue]. Semin Liver Dis 2005;25(4):381-472.

Pietrangelo A: Hereditary hemochromatosis: A new look at an old disease. N Engl J Med 2004;350:2383-2397.

Hodgkin's Lymphoma

Method of
Ralph M. Meyer, MD, and
David C. Hodgson, MD, MPH

Current estimates of the incidence and mortality of Hodgkin's lymphoma in the United States come from American Cancer Society statistics, which predicts approximately 7800 diagnoses and 1800 deaths in 2006. This mortality-to-incidence rate ratio of 0.19 reflects the high potential for cure of this disease and emphasizes that long-term issues of survivorship are important for these patients, but it also demonstrates that curative potential is not achieved in an important fraction of patients. Historically, understandings of the biology and management of Hodgkin's lymphoma have played pivotal roles in developing broader understandings of cancer; this continues to be the case. In this article, we describe these principles and review current management strategies.

Histologic Classification

The diagnosis of Hodgkin's lymphoma requires an adequate tissue biopsy and expert interpretation. The histologic classification of Hodgkin's lymphoma, and lymphomas in general, exemplifies how new understandings of biology, including advances in molecular oncology, require that categorization schema be continuously updated to accommodate new discoveries. Since the initial description of this lymphoma by Thomas Hodgkin in 1832 and the reporting of the hallmark features of the Reed–Sternberg cell in 1902, the classification of Hodgkin's disease has undergone sequential updating. Landmark schemata include those described by Jackson and Parker in 1943 and Lukes and Butler in 1966. This latter classification system was modified at the 1966 Rye Conference and included four separate entities: lymphocyte predominant, nodular sclerosing, mixed cellularity, and lymphocyte deplete. It is this classification system that has been used in the vast majority of clinical trials that have determined current treatments.

The most current classification schema was determined as part of the Revised European American Lymphoma (REAL) classification of 1994 and was updated in the World Heath Organization classification described in 1997 (Fig. 1). Major changes include recognition of nodular lymphocyte predominant disease as a distinct clinical entity that is separate from the other forms of Hodgkin's lymphoma, which are now grouped under the umbrella term of classic Hodgkin's lymphoma. Within classic Hodgkin's lymphoma are four entities: lymphocyte rich, nodular sclerosing, mixed cellularity, and lymphocyte deplete. As we describe later, the new clinical ramifications of incorporating recent biological findings into the WHO classification system are that an entity that is associated with a different clinical course and might require a different form of therapy has been defined (i.e., nodular lymphocyte predominant disease), and criteria that separate Hodgkin's from non-Hodgkin's lymphomas have been made more explicit. It is crucial that evaluation of biopsy material be performed by an expert pathologist, with necessary ancillary studies such as immunohistochemistry, flow cytometry, and molecular studies completed as appropriate to ensure that the Hodgkin's and non-Hodgkin's lymphomas have been distinguished and that subtypes of lymphoma have been properly characterized.

Staging and Risk Categorization

As with histologic classifications, the variables that determine the extent of disease and prognosis of patients with Hodgkin's lymphoma have evolved to account for new biological understandings and the relevance of these variables within the context of current therapies. Beginning with the initial observations of Peters in 1950, risk categorization of patients with Hodgkin's lymphoma has historically emphasized the anatomic spread of the disease. Subsequently, the Ann Arbor Staging Classification was devised in 1971; this was modified at the Cotswold meeting in 1989. The Cotswold criteria continue to be applied to newly diagnosed cases (Table 1).

Current management strategies for patients with classic Hodgkin's lymphoma involve collapsing the Ann Arbor and Cotswold classifications into two or three categories. These categories include at least limited-stage and advanced-stage disease. In North America, cooperative group clinical trials have defined limited-stage disease as clinical stage I to IIA and an absence of bulky disease. Bulky disease is defined as a mass that is at least 10 cm in diameter or that measures more than one third of the maximum transthoracic diameter on a standard posteroanterior chest radiograph. Other factors that have been considered of potential prognostic importance, such as erythrocyte sedimentation rate (ESR) and histologic subtype within classic

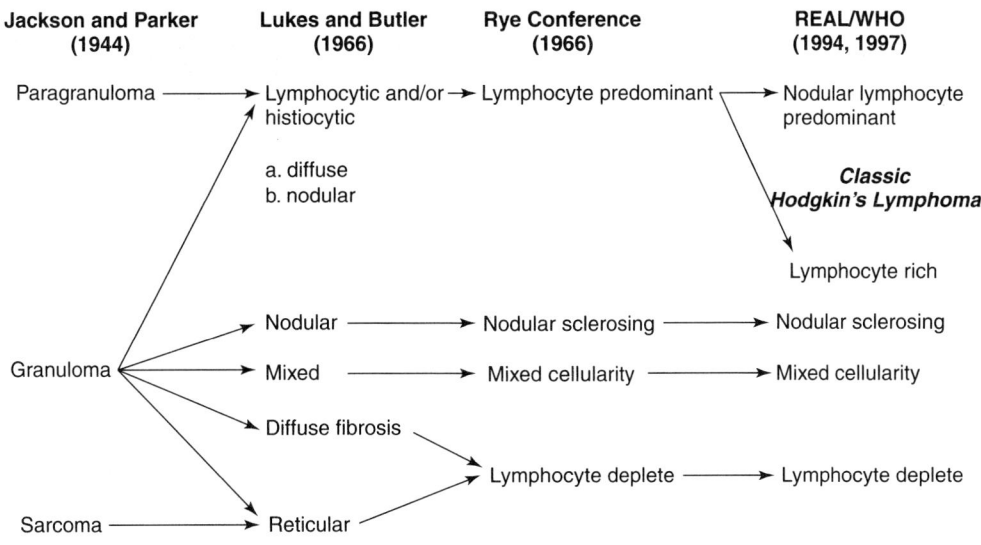

FIGURE 1. Histologic classifications of Hodgkin's lymphoma. REAL = Revised European American Lymphoma; WHO = World Health Organization.

Hodgkin's lymphoma, are no longer deemed to be important in defining therapy, because the prognostic properties of these factors have been obviated by current therapies. Patients with stages IIB, III, IV, and bulky disease associated with any stage are considered to have advanced-stage disease. Within this article, these definitions of limited and advanced-stage disease will be used to describe treatment practices. For the purposes of determining prognosis, and for designing clinical trials, patients with advanced-stage disease may be further assessed through use of the International Prognostic Index (IPI), which includes anatomic stage as a variable, but also includes six other parameters that have been shown to be prognostic through evaluation of large databases (Table 2).

Cooperative group practices in Europe use schemata that have considerable overlap with those used in North America. Patients who in North America would be classified in Europe as having limited-stage disease may be classified as having *favorable early-stage* disease. A separate category of *intermediate-stage* or *unfavorable early-stage* disease is used to include patients with stage I, IIA, or IIB disease and presence of one or more predefined risk factors, such as the presence of bulky disease, elevation of the ESR, or an increased number of nodal sites of disease. *Advanced stage* includes those with stage III or IV disease. Despite these minor variations, these classification systems result in similar stage-related treatment practices in both geographic regions.

Clinical Presentation and Initial Investigations

Patients with Hodgkin's lymphoma are typically young, with the peak incidence of disease occurring in those in late adolescence to their early 40s. The median age observed in most clinical trials is approximately 35 years. Although a bimodal age distribution has been historically described, with a second age peak occurring in elderly patients, recent revisions of lymphoma histologic classification have resulted in changing the diagnosis in many older patients from Hodgkin's disease to non-Hodgkin's lymphoma.

The presentation of patients with Hodgkin's lymphoma typically falls into two major categories: those who present with painless lymphadenopathy and those who present with other symptoms. Usually those with painless adenopathy present with supradiaphragmatic disease, with an enlarged lymph node in the neck or axilla. The lymph nodes are typically described as firm, hard, or rubbery as opposed to the softer or fleshy nodes in patients with lymphadenopathy that is reactive to an inflammatory condition. Nodes that are anatomically asymmetrical (unilateral) and that are present in the posterior

TABLE 1 Ann Arbor Staging System Including Cotswold Modifications

Stage	Disease Involvement
I	Single lymph node region (I) or one extralymphatic site (I$_E$)
II	Two or more lymph node regions, on the same side of the diaphragm (II) or local extralymphatic extension plus one or more lymph node regions on the same side of the diaphragm (II$_E$).
III	Lymph node regions on both sides of the diaphragm (III), which may be accompanied by local extralymphatic extension (III$_E$)
IV	Diffuse involvement of one or more extralymphatic organs or sites
A	No B symptoms
B	Presence of at least one of unexplained weight loss >10% baseline during 6 mo before staging, recurrent unexplained fever >38°C, recurrent night sweats
X	Bulky tumor: either a single mass exceeding 10 cm in largest diameter or a mediastinal mass exceeding one third of the maximum transverse transthoracic diameter measured on a standard posteroanterior chest radiograph

TABLE 2 The International Prognostic Index*

Variable	Risk Level
Serum albumin	<40 g/L
Hemoglobin	<105 g/L
Sex	Male
Stage	Stage IV
Age	≥45 y
White cell count	≥15 × 10^9/L
Lymphocyte count	<0.6 × 10^9/L or <8% of total while cell count

*The number of factors present is totaled.

CURRENT DIAGNOSIS

- The most common age of patients is late adolescence to the early 40s.
- Many patients present with painless adenopathy that is often in the neck or axilla and is asymmetrical.
- Due to the frequency of mediastinal lymph node involvement, a chest radiograph can be helpful in evaluating patients with persistent symptoms for which an etiology has not been discovered.
- The diagnosis requires an adequate biopsy with expert review to confirm the diagnosis, distinguish Hodgkin's lymphoma from non-Hodgkin's lymphoma, and determine the histologic subtype of the disease.

BOX 1 Baseline Investigations for Patients with Hodgkin's Lymphoma

History
Fever
Night sweats
Weight loss

Physical Examination
Hepatosplenomegaly
Lymphadenopathy
Pleural effusion

Laboratory
Complete blood count and white cell differential
Serum bilirubin and liver enzymes
Serum creatinine and calcium
Total protein and albumin

Imaging
Bone marrow: Aspirate and biopsy (can be omitted with limited–stage disease and a normal complete blood count)
Chest radiograph
Computed tomography scanning of the chest, abdomen, and pelvis

Biopsy
Lymph node biopsy with specialized review (see text)

Other
Positron emission tomographic (PET) scanning (see text)
Specialized imaging according to symptoms and signs

---

triangle of the neck, as opposed to the internal jugular chain, are more suspicious for lymphoma, as opposed to a reactive condition. Only 5% of Hodgkin's lymphoma patients present with disease that is confined to the subdiaphragmatic regions; typically these patients present with adenopathy in the inguinal or femoral region and disproportionately may have the nodular lymphocyte–predominant histologic subtype. Symptoms can relate to local disease or be constitutional. Patients with mediastinal disease may present with chest fullness and cough. Constitutional symptoms often include fatigue, lethargy or the prognostic B symptoms of fevers, night sweats, or weight loss. Unusual, but potentially distinct, symptoms can include intractable pruritus or pain in a region affected by adenopathy associated with alcohol intake.

Evaluation of patients with suspected Hodgkin's lymphoma includes a thorough history and physical examination with particular attention to the presence of the above-described symptoms and of lymphadenopathy, hepatosplenomegaly, or a pleural effusion on physical examination. In patients with chest symptoms, a chest x-ray can be extremely valuable. The definitive diagnosis requires an adequate tissue biopsy; although cytologic evaluations of material obtained from a fine-needle aspirate might suggest a diagnosis of Hodgkin's lymphoma, at present, this technology is not consistently reliable to ensure a correct diagnosis. Material for histologic evaluation obtained from an adequate large-bore core biopsy might, in select circumstances, be sufficient for diagnosis, but in general, an excisional biopsy should be expected to achieve a definitive diagnosis.

Once a diagnosis of Hodgkin's lymphoma is confirmed, patients require systematic evaluation to assess prognostic features that will influence therapy and determine whether complications of the disease are present. Standard investigations are listed in Box 1. At present, the role of ^{18}F-fluorodeoxyglucose positron emission tomography (FDG-PET scanning) is under evaluation. Potential roles might include pretreatment disease staging, evaluation during therapy for purposes of prognosis or prediction of benefit with specific therapy, and determination of remission status at the completion of therapy. Currently, the utility of PET scanning is least well defined as a pretreatment staging tool and cannot yet be considered a standard test for this purpose.

Treatment

Treatment of patients with Hodgkin's lymphoma can be subdivided into categories that are determined by the histologic subtype and the stage of disease with the added potential that risk factors, such as those identified in the Hodgkin's lymphoma IPI, might further influence treatment options. Principles of management include careful balancing of the desire to maximally control the underlying disease, while minimizing the risks of long-term treatment-related toxicities (also referred to as late effects). Late effects include increased risks of developing acute leukemia, which is associated with use of chemotherapy regimens that include alkylating agents or epipodophyllotoxins, and second cancers and cardiovascular events, which are associated with radiation therapy. In addition, chemotherapy regimens that include alkylating agents are associated with dose-dependent risks of gonadal failure and infertility.

LIMITED-STAGE CLASSIC HODGKIN'S LYMPHOMA

The management of patients with limited-stage Hodgkin's lymphoma has changed dramatically over the past 15 to 20 years. As recently as 1990, standard management included a staging laparotomy with splenectomy followed by treatment with subtotal nodal radiation. With this treatment, other prognostic factors were identified and used to refine therapy; these included ESR, number of disease sites, and histologic subtype (e.g., nodular sclerosing vs mixed cellularity). These practices have been improved on by advances in diagnostic imaging and through the availability of more-efficacious and less-toxic systemic chemotherapy. Further improvements should be expected as other technologies, such as PET scanning, become validated.

Based on current data, patients and physicians have two main options for the treatment of limited-stage Hodgkin's lymphoma. These options are associated with specific trade-offs.

The first option is treatment with combined modality therapy that includes two cycles of doxorubicin (Adriamycin), bleomycin (Bleoxane), vinblastine (Velban) and dacarbazine (DTIC-Dome) (ABVD), and radiation therapy to the involved field. The advantage of this approach is that long-term disease control is maximized with initial therapy; this is expected in approximately 95% of patients. The disadvantage relates to use of radiation therapy and the associated risks of late effects such as second cancers and, with mediastinal radiation, cardiovascular events. Advances in radiation technology,

CURRENT THERAPY

Limited Stage Classic Hodgkin's Lymphoma

- Option 1: Combined modality therapy consisting of two cycles of ABVD and involved-field radiation therapy. The advantage is long-term disease control with initial therapy in more than 90% of patients.
- Option 2: Treatment with ABVD (4-6 cycles). The advantage is that, although long-term disease control with initial therapy is about 7% less than with combined modality therapy, the risks of late effects of radiation therapy are avoided

Advanced Stage Classic Hodgkin's Lymphoma

- Option 1: Treatment with ABVD (6-8 cycles). The advantage is that long-term disease control with initial therapy in at least 65% of patients. Gonadal function and fertility are preserved.
- Option 2: Treatment with escalated BEACOPP. The advantage is that long-term disease control with initial therapy is approximately 10% better than that associated with ABVD, but treatment is associated with more toxicity, including high rates of infertility (see text).

Refractory or Recurrent Classic Hodgkin's Lymphoma

- Usual initial treatment is with high-dose chemotherapy and autologous stem cell transplantation.
- Subsequent treatments require individualized approaches.

Nodular Lymphocyte–Predominant Hodgkin's Lymphoma

- The most common option is involved-field radiation therapy.
- Numerous new options, including use of rituximab and observation have been described.
- Advanced-stage disease is treated the same as classic Hodgkin's lymphoma.

such as conformal treatment, use of PET scanning for planning, and limiting the treatment field to the affected nodes as opposed to nodal regions, significantly reduces the radiation dose to normal tissues compared with radiation treatments given in the 1970s to the 1990s. Further data are required before we can confidently conclude that important long-term risks do not remain.

The second option is therapy with four to six cycles of ABVD alone. The advantage of this approach is avoidance of radiation therapy and the associated risks of late effects, with the disadvantage being a decrement in long-term disease control with initial therapy that is estimated to be about 7% (i.e., to approximately 88%). To date, no differences in long-term overall survival have been detected between these options. Ongoing randomized trials that assign use of radiation according to patients' early response to chemotherapy might clarify which patients can be treated with chemotherapy alone without increasing the risk of relapse. In the meantime, balancing these options requires careful discussions with patients about their preferences.

ADVANCED-STAGE CLASSIC HODGKIN'S LYMPHOMA

The management of patients with advanced-stage disease has also evolved over the past 15 to 20 years. In 1990, standard therapy would have included six to eight cycles of nitrogen mustard, vincristine (Oncovin), prednisone, and procarbazine (Matulane) in combination with ABVD (± dacarbazine) (MOPP-ABVD or MOPP-ABV). Recent randomized, controlled trials have demonstrated that these regimens and ABVD all provide long-term disease control in approximately 65% of patients. However, there is less short-term toxicity with ABVD, and importantly, this regimen avoids the long-term risks of infertility and leukemogenesis associated with nitrogen mustard and procarbazine. Treatment with ABVD is therefore considered a standard.

An alternative strategy is to intensify therapy with use of the bleomycin, etoposide (Vepesid),[1] doxorubicin (Adriamycin), cyclophosphamide (Cytoxan), vincristine (Oncovin), prednisone, and procarbazine (BEACOPP) regimen. Use of this regimen, particularly in its escalated-dose form, has been associated with superior disease control and an improvement in overall survival that is in the range of 8% to 10% at 5 years (i.e., 91% with escalated BEACOPP versus 83% with ABVD). In comparison with ABVD, the magnitude of disease-control benefits associated with the BEACOPP regimens may be greatest in patients who have more than three IPI risk factors. However, the BEACOPP regimens are associated with more severe toxicities, including more severe myelosuppression and risks of infection during the treatment period, and a greater risk of acute leukemia and myelodysplasia as a late effect. Furthermore, risks of infertility are markedly increased: Preliminary reports suggest that escalated BEACOPP is associated with gonadal failure in 85% to 90% of all men and women who are older than 30 years and in 50% of female patients younger than 30 years.

Another strategy uses weekly chemotherapy that is administered over a shorter time course than ABVD. The prototype of this therapy is the Stanford V regimen. Although this treatment has shown promising results in a phase II trial, in three randomized, controlled trials testing this concept, outcomes were inferior in comparison with ABVD or an equivalent regimen. A large North American Intergroup study has completed accrual to a randomized comparison of Stanford V and ABVD. Until the results of this trial are known, use of regimens based on this concept should be limited to clinical trials testing.

The role of combining radiation therapy with chemotherapy has been studied in a number of randomized trials and an individual patient-data meta-analysis. A summary of these results shows that no differences in overall survival are detected, and particularly in patients with stage III or IV disease who are treated with ABVD or BEACOPP, there are also no differences in disease control. At present, there continues to be a role for combined modality therapy for patients with stage I or II disease who are considered to have advanced-stage disease because of the presence of a bulky mediastinal mass. The need for all of these patients to receive radiation therapy will require reevaluation as the utility of PET scanning is better understood.

Therefore, as with limited-stage disease, practitioners and patients are faced with a decision involving trade-offs as the treatment associated with the best long-term disease control is also associated with the greatest long-term risk. At an individual patient level, the risks of infertility associated with BEACOPP should be regarded as likely. Provided patients are aware of these trade-offs, treatment with either escalated BEACOPP or ABVD is a reasonable option.

RELAPSED OR REFRACTORY DISEASE

Unfortunately, an important number of patients have disease that is refractory to initial therapy or that is associated with subsequent recurrence. The vast majority of these patients present with advanced-stage disease and receive a full course of chemotherapy with ABVD. Based on the results of two randomized trials that have shown significant improvements in progression-free or event-free survival, treatment with high-dose chemotherapy and autologous stem cell transplantation is considered standard. Autologous transplantation is particularly recommended for patients with primary refractory disease and disease that recurs within 1 year of completing initial therapy; it is also a reasonable option for most other patients

---

[1]Not FDA approved for this indication.

who experience disease recurrence after a longer disease-free interval. Patients with recurrent disease that includes a site of bulky disease, such as the mediastinum, should also receive radiation therapy to that site following confirmed stem cell engraftment.

Treatment options for recurrent Hodgkin's lymphoma in patients who initially present with limited-stage disease are poorly characterized due to the uncommon occurrence of this event. The choice of therapy is strongly influenced by specifics of the pattern of disease recurrence. Options for patients with recurrent disease after receiving combined modality therapy include receiving a full course of a standard regimen (e.g., ABVD) or, more commonly, stem cell transplantation. For patients whose disease recurs after receiving ABVD alone, and particularly when this recurrence is confined to the initial sites of disease, the option of treatment with combined-modality therapy that includes involved-field radiation is preferred over stem cell transplantation.

The treatment of patients with recurrent disease after stem cell transplantation has been poorly evaluated; there are no randomized, controlled trials. Management must be individualized and should account for the demographic features of the patient, the temporal profile, burden and symptoms associated with the disease, and natures of the previous therapies. A common option includes single-agent vinblastine for purposes of palliation, but additional options can include radiation therapy, including wide-field radiation, use of other standard-dose chemotherapy regimens, and for select patients, observation. For very select patients, the option of allogeneic stem cell transplantation, including with reduced-intensity conditioning regimens, has been described.

NODULAR LYMPHOCYTE–PREDOMINANT HODGKIN'S LYMPHOMA

There are now robust data indicating that nodular lymphocyte–predominant Hodgkin's lymphoma is a distinct biological entity and is associated with a clinical course that differs from classic Hodgkin's lymphoma. Most patients present with limited-stage disease and have an indolent clinical course; extensive mediastinal involvement is rare. An important biological feature is expression by the malignant cell of the CD20 antigen, which raises the opportunity for potential treatment with immunotherapy using the monoclonal antibody rituximab.

The uncommon incidence of this disease means that the clinical trials that inform current practices generally consist of case series, many of which are retrospective, and small subset analyses from larger randomized trials that evaluate patients with all histologic subtypes. From these data, a commonly preferred therapy is with involved-field radiation therapy as a single modality. An alternative option is combined-modality therapy as given for patients with limited-stage classic Hodgkin's lymphoma, but the curative potential of this option is uncertain. Small case series have evaluated observation alone or rituximab treatment, but sufficient data do not yet exist to permit recommending these as standard therapies. Patients with advanced-stage disease should receive the same therapy as patients with classic Hodgkin's lymphoma.

SPECIAL CIRCUMSTANCES

Special circumstances can arise that require modification of these treatment strategies. For each of these circumstances, the data on which current recommendations are based are limited and largely consist of case reports, case series, and generalizations from other diseases or biological principles.

A first circumstance is managing older patients with Hodgkin's lymphoma. As with the therapy of older patients with non-Hodgkin's lymphoma, the treatment plan must initially account for the presence of any comorbidities or specific patient preferences related to individual values. When no additional factors are identified, treatment that incorporates the principles for managing younger patients should be followed. For these patients, the BEACOPP regimens are associated with excessive toxicity and should not be used. For patients with cardiac compromise who cannot receive doxorubicin, treatment with chlorambucil, vinblastine, prednisone, and procarbazine (ChlVPP) may be considered.

A second circumstance is management of female patients in whom Hodgkin's lymphoma is diagnosed during pregnancy. Diagnostic staging of these patients should include replacement of computed tomography with ultrasound examination. Provided that the disease is sufficiently indolent, many patients can be carefully observed until the postnatal period and then complete standard staging tests and therapy. For patients who must receive therapy before delivery, a common option is treatment with single-agent vinblastine, which is not teratogenic, followed by postnatal therapy with a full course of standard chemotherapy. In very select circumstances, patients who have rapidly progressing disease after their first trimester of pregnancy may, after thorough consideration and discussion of options, be treated with ABVD.

A third special circumstance is management of the HIV patient who develops Hodgkin's lymphoma. These patients might not be as profoundly immunosuppressed as HIV patients who develop non-Hodgkin's lymphoma, but unfortunately risks of infection associated with standard chemotherapy are increased. These patients should receive optimal antiretroviral therapy and ideally treatment that is otherwise considered standard for their stage of disease. Due to insufficient data, therapy with BEACOPP is not recommended and these patients should receive ABVD.

Issues of Survivorship

Studies of survivors have shown that delayed morbidity and excess mortality not directly attributable to Hodgkin's lymphoma is an important problem. For patients whose disease was diagnosed in the 1960s to 1980s, deaths from other causes exceeded deaths due to Hodgkin's lymphoma after 15 years of follow-up. A major cause of other deaths is the occurrence of a second cancer. A man whose disease was diagnosed at age 30 and who was treated with historical approaches, the 30-year cumulative incidence of developing a solid-tumor cancer is approximately 15% to 20%, which is 10% higher than expected in the gender- and age-matched general population. Comparable values for a 30-year-old woman include a 30-year cumulative incidence of a subsequent solid cancer of 25%, which is 15% higher than expected. The incremental risk of solid cancers among younger female patients is even more pronounced, largely due to the excess risk of breast cancer related to radiation therapy to the mediastinum.

A second major cause of late morbidity and mortality is cardiovascular diseases. These may be related to doxorubicin, which produces free radicals that are directly toxic to the myocardium, and mediastinal radiation to a field that includes the heart. The cumulative incidence of significant cardiac morbidity 10 years after treatment is approximately 2% to 6% and increases to 15% to 20% by 20 years. This represents a 1.5- to 3-fold increased relative risk and is largely related to the radiation therapy. Technical interventions that reduce the dose of radiation to the heart reduce this risk.

The persistence of symptoms associated with nonfatal complications is also common. Even following modern therapy, many survivors experience persistent fatigue; its cause is uncertain. Although persistent anemia and hypothyroidism are known late effects of treatment, these do not usually provide the reason for fatigue.

Specifically focused follow-up of survivors can reduce the morbidity of late treatment effects. Among patients who receive neck or mediastinal radiation, thyroid function should be evaluated at least annually to detect preclinical hypothyroidism. Female patients treated with mediastinal radiation should undergo annual breast cancer screening beginning 8 years after this treatment or beginning at age 25 years. Due to the suboptimal performance of mammography in women with dense breast tissue, which includes most young women, this screening should include magnetic resonance imaging (MRI) for women younger than 30 years. For women ages 30 to 50 years, mammography can be initiated and the adequacy of mammographic images can guide decisions regarding the appropriate screening modality.

For those with good mammographic images (i.e., predominantly fatty breast tissue) mammography alone is recommended, whereas those with dense breast tissue should be screened with MRI plus mammography. Mammographic screening alone is recommended for women older than 50 years.

Recommendations for colorectal cancer screening for patients who have received abdominal radiation therapy are less clear. Some recommendations include initiation of colorectal cancer screening 15 years after treatment, or by age 35 years, whichever comes later. The evidence supporting this recommendation is indirect and there are no data to indicate whether colonoscopy or fecal occult blood testing is superior.

Most cardiac morbidity occurs in survivors who have conventional cardiac risk factors. Consequently, blood pressure and serum lipids should be monitored and, if elevated, treated aggressively. Similarly, strong efforts should be made to help survivors quit smoking, because the smoking-related risks of heart disease and lung cancer appear to be even greater than among the general population. Young survivors who experience progressive fatigue or chest pain require cardiac evaluation; these symptoms should not be attributed to noncardiac causes until heart disease has been excluded. Preliminary data suggest that screening stress echocardiography can detect clinically important valvular or coronary artery disease among long-term survivors who received mediastinal radiation to doses greater than 35 Gy; future studies are required to clarify the value of routine screening of all asymptomatic patients. Female survivors who become pregnant, however, should undergo cardiac evaluation because of the significant cardiac stress associated with pregnancy and childbirth.

Persistent fatigue among survivors can be a challenging management problem. Depression or dysthymia, hypothyroidism, impaired cardiac function, and anemia should be considered as potential causes. Regular exercise can significantly reduce fatigue and in severe cases, referral to a mental health professional should be considered for cognitive behavior therapy or short-term pharmacotherapy.

Given the nature of these and other survivorship issues, standard oncology clinics might not be well suited to deal with the types of issues that patients who have been otherwise successfully treated for Hodgkin's lymphoma. Specialized clinics for survivors, which focus on these late-effect issues as opposed to the less likely potentials of disease recurrence, are now more common and may be a preferred way to provide this health care.

REFERENCES

Connors JM: State-of-the-art therapeutics: Hodgkin's lymphoma. J Clin Oncol 2005;23(26):6400-6408.

Diehl V, Franklin J, Pfreundschuh M, et al: Standard and increased-dose BEACOPP chemotherapy compared with COPP–ABVD for advanced Hodgkin's disease. N Engl J Med 2003;348(24):2386-2395.

Duggan DB, Petroni GR, Johnson JL, et al: Randomized comparison of ABVD and MOPP/ABV hybrid for the treatment of advanced Hodgkin's disease: Report of an Intergroup trial. J Clin Oncol 2003;21(4):607-614.

Gospodarowicz MK, Meyer RM: The management of patients with limited-stage classical Hodgkin lymphoma. Hematology 2006;2006(1):253-258.

Harris NL, Jaffe ES, Diebold J, et al: World Health Organization classification of neoplastic diseases of the hematopoietic and lymphoid tissues: Report of the Clinical Advisory Committee Meeting, Airlie House, Virginia, November 1997. J Clin Oncol 1999;17(12):3835-3849.

Harris NL, Jaffe ES, Stein H, et al: A revised European–American classification of lymphoid neoplasms: A proposal from the International Lymphoma Study Group. Blood 1994;84(5):1361-1392.

Hasenclever D, Diehl V, Armitage JO, et al: A prognostic score for advanced Hodgkin's disease. N Engl J Med 1998;339(21):1506-1514.

Hodgson DC, Gilbert ES, Dores GM, et al: Long-term solid cancer risk among 5-year survivors of Hodgkin's lymphoma. J Clin Oncol 2007;25(12):1489-1497.

Lister TA, Crowther D, Sutcliffe SB, et al: Report of a committee convened to discuss the evaluation and staging of patients with Hodgkin's disease: Cotswolds meeting. J Clin Oncol 1989;7(11):1630-1636.

Meyer RM, Gospodarowicz MK, Connors JM, et al: Randomized comparison of ABVD chemotherapy with a strategy that includes radiation therapy in patients with limited-stage Hodgkin's lymphoma: National Cancer Institute of Canada Clinical Trials Group and the Eastern Cooperative Oncology Group. J Clin Oncol 2005;23(21):4634-4642.

Nogova L, Rudiger T, Engert A: Biology, clinical course and management of nodular lymphocyte–predominant Hodgkin lymphoma. Hematology 2006;2006(1):266-272.

Ralleigh G, Given-Wilson R: Breast cancer risk and possible screening strategies for young women following supradiaphragmatic radiation for Hodgkin's disease. Clinical Radiology 2004;59:647-650.

Hodgkin's Disease: Radiation Therapy

Method of
Pelayo C. Besa, MD

Hodgkin's disease is a malignancy of lymph nodes with a predictable pattern of spread. Advances in treatment have made Hodgkin's disease a highly curable cancer with a long-term survival rate of more than 90%. Cure rate, defined as 10-year freedom from relapse, for early-stage disease is in the range of 80% to 90%; for intermediate-stage disease, 70% to 80%; and for advanced disease, 30% to 50%.

Radiation therapy plays a major role in the management of Hodgkin's disease. Treatment planning and patient selection are based on thorough clinical staging and review of the pathology. Most patients afflicted with Hodgkin's disease are less than 30 years old and will be cured; therefore, they will be at risk of late toxicity from treatment. Ideal therapy should provide the highest cure rate with minimal long-term toxicity. With this goal, treatment programs have gradually adjusted therapy to the different clinical settings.

Adequate radiation therapy requires pretreatment simulation and therapy with a linear accelerator with a minimal photon beam energy of 6 MV through parallel opposed fields that deliver a tumoricidal dose in a fractionated fashion. Treatment reproducibility is verified periodically with portal films. After completion of therapy, the patient is observed regularly to detect early relapse and evaluate treatment-related toxicity.

Patient Evaluation and Staging

To determine the best treatment approach, the patient needs to undergo disease staging. A complete medical history is obtained with special attention to the tumor history, presence of B symptoms (unexplained fever, drenching night sweats, and unexplained weight loss), and general performance status. The physical examination should be thorough, with special attention to all nodal areas, Waldeyer's ring, liver, and spleen. When a single nodal site is involved, the low neck or supraclavicular area is involved in 60% of the cases, the mediastinum in 15%, axillae in 10%, and the inguinal-femoral regions in 10%. The disease progresses with involvement of contiguous nodal regions. Upper abdominal nodes are considered contiguous to the supraclavicular nodes through the thoracic duct. A biopsy must be performed, preferably with sampling from the most clinically suspicious node.

The hematologic assessment should include complete blood cell and platelet counts, erythrocyte sedimentation rate, and screen chemistries, including lactate dehydrogenase and thyroid function studies. An elevated erythrocyte sedimentation rate is associated with high risk of subclinical disease in the abdomen. An abnormal blood cell count and an elevated lactic dehydrogenase level suggest bone marrow involvement. Thyroid function testing must be done as a

CURRENT DIAGNOSIS

History	Tumor history
	B symptoms (unexplained fever, drenching night sweats, unexplained weight loss)
Physical	All nodal areas
	Waldeyer's ring
	Liver/spleen
Laboratory tests	Complete CBC
	Erythrocyte sedimentation rate
	LDH
	Screen chemistries
Radiologic studies	CT chest/abdomen/pelvis
	PET-CT
Pathology	Lymph node or extranodal site
	Bone marrow

Abbreviations: CBC = complete blood count; CT = computed tomography; LDH = lactate dehydrogenase; PET-CT = positron emission tomography fused with computed tomography.

follow-up study because of a substantial risk of late dysfunction caused by radiation therapy.

Routine imaging studies include chest radiographs and computed tomography (CT) of the chest, abdomen, and pelvis. Magnetic resonance imaging (MRI) is used occasionally to better delineate hilar adenopathy and chest wall and pericardial extension and, in the abdomen, to distinguish unfilled bowel and vessels from adenopathy. Positron emission tomography fused with computed tomography (PET-CT) scans are most useful for distinguishing active disease in enlarged lymph nodes. Treatment response is evaluated with repeated PET-CT.

Bone marrow biopsies are performed in all patients except those with early stage (stage I or II) disease and no B symptoms. The overall frequency of bone marrow involvement in Hodgkin's disease is only 5%. Hodgkin's disease is staged according to the Ann Arbor staging classification system (Table 1). Figure 1 shows the lymphoid regions used in this system. Note that the infraclavicular, cervical occipital, and preauricular areas are a single region.

TABLE 1 Ann Arbor Staging Classification System

Stage I
Involvement of single lymph node region (I) or localized involvement of an extralymphatic organ or site (IE)

Stage II
Involvement of two or more lymph node regions on the same side of the diaphragm (II) or localized involvement of an extra lymphatic organ or site and one or more nodal regions on the same side of the diaphragm (IIE)

Stage III
Involvement of lymph node regions on both sides of the diaphragm (III), which may be accompanied by localized involvement of an extralymphatic organ or site (IIIE)

Stage IV
Diffuse involvement of one or more extralymphatic organs with or without associated lymph node involvement

Systemic Symptoms
A: Absence of systemic symptoms defined as B.
B: Unexplained fever with temperatures above 38 C (100 F), unexplained weight loss >10%, body weight, or drenching night sweats

Radiation Treatment Technique

Treatment planning starts by reviewing the staging evaluation and pathology report. Clinical and radiologic studies are used to outline the extent of disease. The treatment fields include the known disease areas and adjacent nodal regions. Treatment volume varies according to the treatment plan. The *treatment volumes* are defined as involved field, extended field, and subtotal nodal irradiation. *Involved field irradiation* includes the entire nodal area in which nodes with Hodgkin's disease are noted; for example, if a low neck node is involved, the entire neck and supraclavicular areas are treated. *Extended field irradiation* treats the entire nodal region. *Subtotal nodal irradiation* includes all the regions at risk: the supradiaphragmatic area including neck, supraclavicular, infraclavicular, axillary, mediastinal, and hilar nodes, and the infradiaphragmatic area, including para-aortic nodes, spleen, pelvic, and inguinal-femoral nodes. The nodal areas not included are mesenteric, presacral, popliteal, brachial, and epitrochlear nodes because they are only rarely involved with Hodgkin's disease. These regions are treated in three areas: the mantle for the supradiaphragmatic region, the abdomen, and the pelvis, including inguinal and femoral nodes (Figure 2). The junction between the fields must be placed away from the tumor to prevent underdosing, and normal tissue tolerance must be considered to avoid organ toxicity.

After the treatment plan is determined, the radiation field is simulated and marked on the patient. The simulator is a diagnostic radiography unit that reproduces the geometry of the therapy machine and takes verification films of the treatment fields. CT simulation is used to better outline the treatment areas and protect the normal tissue. CT cuts are used to outline the areas at risk, treatment volume, and the organs. Digital reconstructed images from CT simulation match the verification films from the simulator. To optimize reproducibility of the daily setup, patient immobilization devices are used; for example, a face mask of low-temperature thermal plastic (polycarbolactone) or vacuum body mold can be used for the mantle. Treatment fields include lymphoid regions, and to encompass all these areas, large and irregular fields are necessary.

The treatment volume generated with the CT simulation is used to outline the field to be treated and to design the blocks for the areas to be protected from irradiation. Divergent blocks are constructed from the drawings on the digital reconstructed images using either a low-melting-point alloy such as Lipowitz metal (Cerrobend) or a multileaf collimator, a machine device that shapes the beam with small movable leaves. Typically, the dose is prescribed to be delivered along the central axis at the midplane. The dose is higher for thin areas where diameters are small. To calculate the dose in the different areas, the three-dimensional reconstruction from the CT simulation is used and a dose distribution is obtained. Partial transmission blocks or shrinking field technique are used to compensate for the difference in the diameters and to make the dose homogeneous throughout the treatment field. Better dose distributions are obtained with intensity modulated radiation therapy, using an electronic compensator, which modifies the beam moving the multileaf collimator to block the areas when they reach the prescribed dose.

Patients are treated on a linear accelerator at a 100-cm source-to-surface distance, usually using 6-MV photons for the upper torso and 18-MV photons for the abdomen and pelvis. The patient is seen on the treatment table by the radiation oncologist to verify the proper location of the fields. Machine portal films for verification are taken at the beginning of treatment and weekly thereafter. The dose delivered to the visible tumor areas is 39.6 Gy in 22 fractions over 4.5 weeks. The nodal areas treated prophylactically receive 30.6 Gy in 17 fractions over 3.5 weeks. In general, the treatment field is arranged with parallel opposed fields, using even-weighted beams, and all fields are treated daily. When two fields are matched (e.g., mantle and abdomen), special gap calculations are used to avoid overlap. If the adjacent fields overlie the spinal cord, CT simulation is used to computer-generated isodose calculations to determine the dose at the cord.

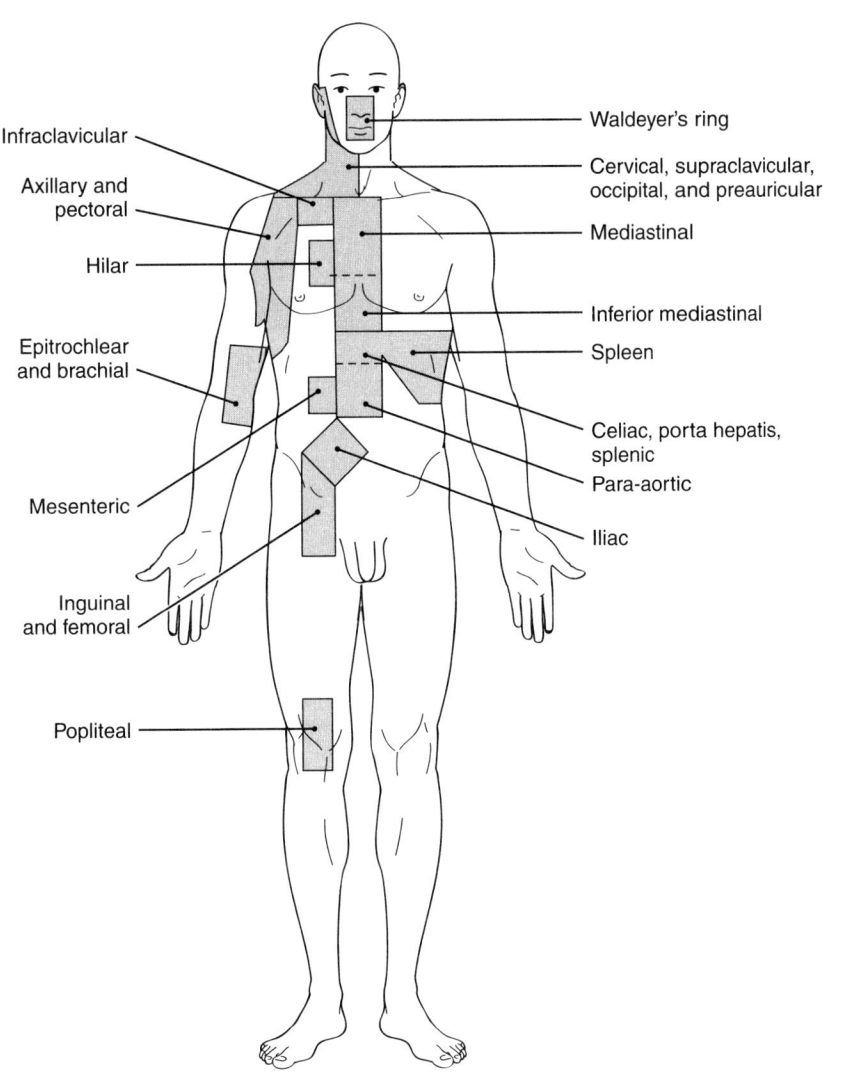

FIGURE 1. Lymphoid regions for Ann Arbor staging of Hodgkin's disease.

Mantle Field Irradiation

Radiation to the mantle field treats the supradiaphragmatic nodal regions. The mantle field extends from the mastoid and base of the mandible to the diaphragm and encompasses the submental, occipital, cervical, supraclavicular, infraclavicular, axillary, mediastinal, and hilar nodes. The patient is treated using parallel opposed anteroposterior fields, with individually contoured lung and heart blocks. Usually, the cervical spine is blocked posteriorly, the larynx anteriorly, and both humeral heads anteriorly and posteriorly. The mantle is treated with equally loaded beams to a dose of 30.6 Gy in 17 fractions. At this point, treatment is stopped for the areas of prophylactic irradiation and continues only for the areas of gross involvement to a dose of 39.6 Gy. Obese patients have a wide mediastinum when they lie on their back and can be treated sitting in a specially designed chair to decrease the amount of normal lung treated.

Subdiaphragmatic Irradiation

Subdiaphragmatic nodal areas are usually divided into two treatment fields: the abdomen, which includes the para-aortic nodes and spleen, with or without the pelvis, which includes the common and external iliac nodes and the inguinal-femoral regions. If the pelvic field is treated concurrently with the para-aortic field, the term *inverted Y* is used.

The field encompassing the para-aortic and spleen areas extends from the diaphragm to the bottom of the fourth lumbar vertebra; field edges are matched with those of the mantle with an appropriate skin gap; to encompass the para-aortic nodes, the field is drawn to the width of the transverse processes of the lumbar vertebral bodies, provided that the abdominal CT scan does not show nodes in a more lateral position. Radiation is delivered using parallel opposed anteroposterior fields with equally loaded beams that deliver a dose of 30.6 Gy in 17 fractions. An additional 9-Gy boost in five fractions is given to areas with tumor involvement. Individually contoured blocks are made to protect the kidneys and bowel. Often, it is not necessary to treat the pelvic lymph nodes and the radiation treatment stops at the level of the fourth lumbar vertebra. If needed, pelvic treatment is given through parallel opposed anteroposterior fields with 6-MV photons from the front (because the inguinal-femoral nodes are superficial) and 18-MV photons from the back. The pelvic field matches the abdomen field at the level of the fourth lumbar vertebra and extends to encompass the femoral lymph nodes. The nodal areas must be evaluated on the CT scan.

Careful blocking is used to spare the bone marrow as much as possible and, in young women, the ovaries. The ovaries are transposed medially and placed as low as possible behind the uterus to avoid radiation-induced amenorrhea and sterility. The ovaries are

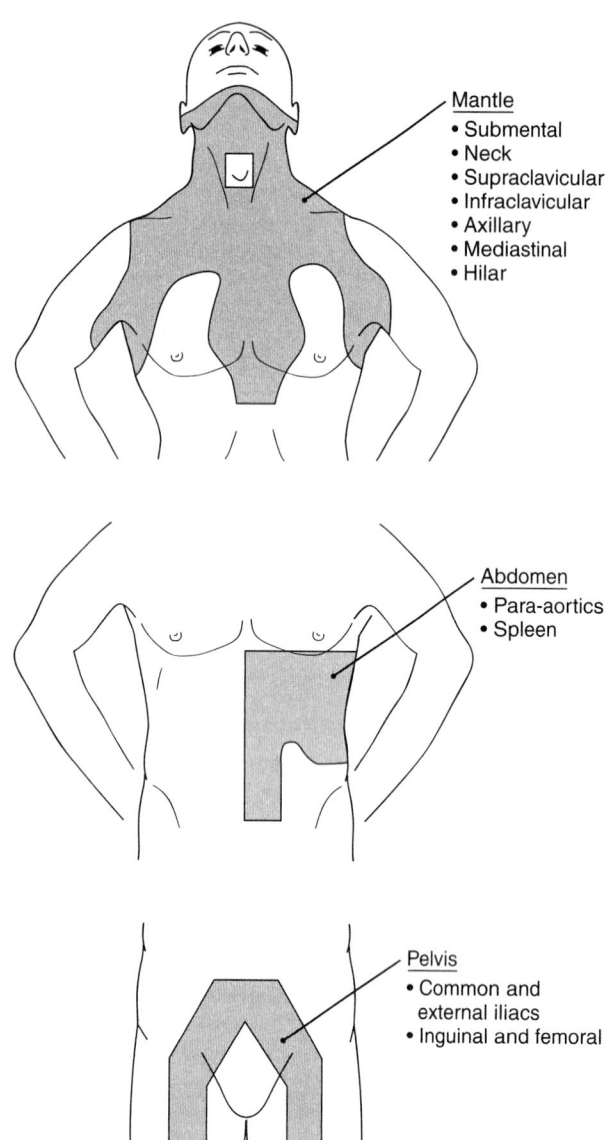

FIGURE 2. Radiation therapy extended fields: supradiaphragmatic: mantle; infradiaphragmatic: abdomen and pelvis.

marked with radiopaque clips to aid in the placement of a double-thickness block. At a distance of 2 cm from the edge of the block, the ovaries receive approximately 8% of the pelvic dose.

Combined Modality Therapy

Many patients with intermediate or advanced Hodgkin's disease benefit from combined chemotherapy and radiation therapy. To reduce the toxicity from the combined modality approach, treatment must be tailored to the extent of disease and the risk of normal tissue injury. Special attention must be paid to the chemotherapy drugs, the number of cycles, the total dose, the time frequency between cycles or intensity, the radiation fields, the volume of tissue irradiated, and doses. Both the medical oncologist and the radiation oncologist must work together from the beginning to tailor the treatment plan.

Most patients with Hodgkin's disease treated with combined modality receive initially four or six cycles of a combination of doxorubicin (Adriamycin), bleomycin (Blenoxane), vinblastine (Velban), and dacarbazine (DTIC), the ABVD regimen, followed by radiation therapy to the involved areas. For patients with advanced Hodgkin's disease (stage IIIB or IV) or mediastinal masses larger than 15 cm, six cycles of chemotherapy are given, followed by radiation therapy to the involved sites.

PET-CT is used to evaluate the treatment response to chemotherapy. The test is done before chemotherapy begins and, if positive, repeated before radiation is delivered. Patients who become negative have a lower relapse rate.

Treatment Recommendations and Results

SUPRADIAPHRAGMATIC FAVORABLE STAGES I AND IIA

Upper torso presentation in patients younger than 40 years, with three or fewer sites of involvement, no large mediastinal mass, no B symptoms, and erythrocyte sedimentation rate less than 50 mm/hour should be treated with radiation therapy alone. Radiation is given to the mantle field and the para-aortic and spleen areas (Figure 2). Patients with mediastinal disease are excluded because they benefit from induction chemotherapy, which reduces the mediastinal mass and decreases radiation to normal lung. Freedom from relapse for this group of patients is 80% to 90% (Table 2).

Patients with stage IA nodular lymphocyte predominant Hodgkin's disease are a special subgroup who tend to have disease localized and have a late relapse pattern similar to low-grade nodular lymphomas. These patients must be treated to the involved field (Figure 3).

SUPRADIAPHRAGMATIC UNFAVORABLE STAGES I THROUGH IIA AND IIB

This group includes all patients with stages I and II disease who do not meet the so-called favorable criteria. These patients have an increased risk of abdominal involvement, approaching 30% according to the laparotomy data. Treatment is with combined modality therapy. Chemotherapy (four or six cycles of ABVD) is given first, followed by radiation therapy to the involved fields. The radiotherapy dose varies according to the chemotherapy response: For complete response 30 Gy is used, and for partial response, 40 Gy. Patients in this group, treated with chemotherapy followed by radiation therapy, have a disease-free survival between 80% and 90% and a survival rate of 90% at 6 years (Table 2).

STAGES I AND II WITH MEDIASTINAL INVOLVEMENT

Mediastinal involvement in very common in Hodgkin's disease and presents a special challenge to the radiation oncologist because toxicity to the lungs and heart must be avoided. The extent of mediastinal tumor involvement is determined by measuring the maximum single horizontal width of the mediastinum on a standing

 CURRENT THERAPY

Disease Extension	Treatment
Favorable I–IIA	XRT
Unfavorable I–IIB and favorable III	ABVD + IF-XRT
Advanced III–IV	ABVD or ABVD + IF-XRT
Relapse or refractory	High-dose chemotherapy + IF-XRT

Abbreviations: ABVD = doxorubicin/bleomycin/vinblastine/dacarbazine; IF = Involved field. XRT = radiotherapy.

TABLE 2 Treatment Results for Hodgkin's Disease

Series	Stage	Treatment	Survival % (y)	Freedom from Relapse % (y)
EORTC	I—IIA Favorable	XRT	96 (6)	81 (6)
EORTC	I—II Unfavorable	MOPP/ABV-XRT	89 (6)	94 (6)
JCRT	I—II large mediastinal mass	MOPP-XRT	88 (10)	89 (10)
MDACC	III (except III$_3$)	MOPP-XRT	87 (10)	83 (10)
EORTC	IIIB—IV	MOPP/ABV	85 (5)	85 (5)

Abbreviations: ABV = doxorubicin, bleomycin, vinblastine; EORTC = European Organization for Research and Treatment of Cancer; JCRT = Joint Center for Radiation Therapy; MDACC = MD Anderson Cancer Center; MOPP = mechlorethamine, vincristine, procarbazine, prednisone; XRT = radiotherapy.

posteroanterior chest radiograph. Three categories are defined as follows: Tumors less than 7.5 cm are small, those larger than 7.5 cm to less than 15 cm are large or bulky, and those larger than 15 cm are massive.

Patients with mediastinal involvement mass are treated with combined modality therapy. Chemotherapy is administered first to decrease the size of the mediastinal tumor. Patients receive six cycles of combination chemotherapy followed by radiation therapy to the involved field. Bleomycin is stopped after the fourth cycle if mediastinal irradiation is planned. Patients in this group, treated with combination chemotherapy followed by radiation therapy, have a disease-free survival of 80% and an 89% survival rate at 10 years (see Table 2).

STAGES I AND II: SUBDIAPHRAGMATIC INVOLVEMENT

Fewer than 10% of patients with stage I or II Hodgkin's disease present with disease limited to the subdiaphragmatic areas. CT of the abdomen and pelvis is used to evaluate nodal and spleen involvement, and treatment is adjusted to the extent of tumor involvement.

For stage IA inguinal presentation, radiation is delivered to the involved field. More advanced cases receive combined modality therapy. Radiation therapy fields include the para-aortic nodes, the spleen, the common and external iliac nodes, and the inguinal-femoral regions. Treatment results for these patients are similar to those with supradiaphragmatic presentations.

FAVORABLE STAGE III

Nodal involvement in patients with stage III disease varies greatly. This heterogeneous group of patients is divided into subgroups according to extent of abdominal disease. Stage III$_1$ includes patients with disease limited to the upper abdomen (involving the celiac region, splenic hilum, and spleen). When the disease extends to the para-aortic region, it is classified as stage III$_2$; and if the pelvis or inguinal region is involved, the classification is stage III$_3$. With the exception of patients presenting with stage III$_3$ disease or IIIB, all patients with stage III receive six cycles of combination chemotherapy (ABVD), followed by radiation therapy to the involved areas (Figure 3). The relapse-free rate for this group is 85% with a cause-specific survival of 80% at 10 years.

ADVANCED STAGES III AND IV

The majority of patients with stage III$_3$ and many with stage IV receive combined modality therapy. Radiotherapy can be omitted for the patients that achieve a complete response to chemotherapy. Only approximately 35% of patients with advanced-stage disease treated with chemotherapy alone are alive and well at 10 years. Patterns of failure after chemotherapy show that recurrence overwhelmingly occurs in previously involved areas. Patients with stage III$_3$ ant IV Hodgkin's disease are treated initially with six cycles of combination chemotherapy (ABVD), followed by irradiation to the involved sites. With combined modality therapy, relapse-free survival of 85% and overall survival of 85% at 5 years is reported (see Table 2).

For relapsed or refractory Hodgkin's disease, involved field radiotherapy is used after high-dose chemotherapy and autologous bone marrow transplantation, with better local control and probable

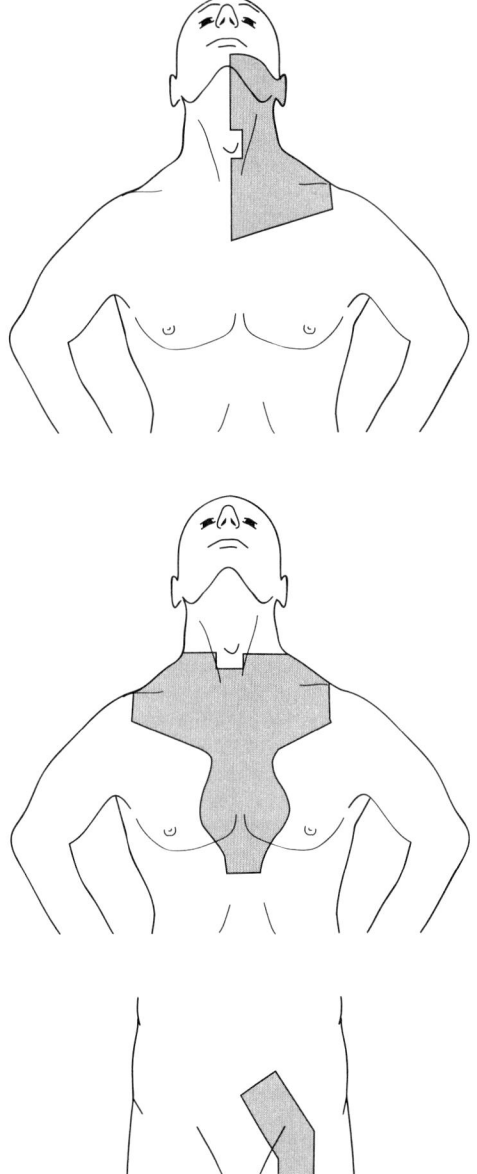

FIGURE 3. Radiation therapy involved field examples: neck, mediastinum, and inguinal-femoral.

improved survival. The disease-free survival at 3 years is 66% and the survival is 57%.

Complications

Complications are classified as acute or late. Acute complications occur during or shortly after the course of radiation therapy; they are treated symptomatically and resolve quickly after the completion of treatment. Acute complications include mild skin reactions and hair loss in the irradiated areas, dysphasia, dry cough, nausea, and diarrhea. These complications are treated symptomatically with skin ointments, analgesics, cough suppressants, and antinausea and antidiarrheal agents.

Late complications occur after treatment is complete, months or years later, and tend to be permanent. Late complications include pneumonitis, pericarditis, hypothyroidism, dental caries, and second malignancies. These reported toxicities observed in long-term survivors are clearly associated with treatment techniques that are different from the ones used today; therefore, in the future a decrease in these toxicities is expected.

Radiation pneumonitis occurs infrequently, and its risk is proportional to the volume of lung irradiated, the total dose, and the fraction size. The patient typically presents 6 to 12 weeks after the completion of the radiation therapy with dry cough, shortness of breath, pleuritic chest pain, and fever. The chest radiograph reveals interstitial infiltrates. Severe cases require treatment with high doses of corticosteroids for 4 to 6 weeks, with gradual tapering to avoid recurrence of symptoms.

Pericarditis is rare, occurring 6 to 12 months after treatment and usually after irradiation of the entire heart. Pericarditis presents as an acute episode of chest pain, fatigue, fever, and friction rubs or sometimes with decreased heart sounds because of pericardial effusion. Patients with mild pericarditis are managed with nonsteroidal anti-inflammatory agents, and for severe cases corticosteroids are used. Constrictive pericarditis and pericardial tamponade are rare complications that require surgical correction.

Subclinical hypothyroidism develops in a third of patients treated with mantle field irradiation. Patients are asymptomatic, and the physician is alerted by the elevation in the thyroid-stimulating hormone seen on the routine yearly blood measurement. Thyroid hormone replacement is necessary to avoid development of symptomatic hypothyroidism with weight gain, lethargy, temperature intolerance, irritability, and changes in skin and hair.

Xerostomia (mouth dryness) develops during irradiation of the mantle field that treats a portion of the salivary glands. There is minimal risk of clinically significant xerostomia, but partial decrease in saliva produces a favorable environment for dental caries. This complication can be prevented with pretreatment dental evaluation, careful dental care, and the daily use of fluoride.

Serious abdominal complications are extremely rare. An occasional gastric ulcer may occur. Bowel obstruction is related to prior laparotomy. In men, pelvic irradiation with adequate testicular shielding produces only temporary azoospermia. In women, ovariopexy is needed before pelvic irradiation to preserve fertility. The ovaries are meticulously shielded, but even this may not preserve ovarian function, especially in women older than 30 years.

The improved survival of patients with Hodgkin's disease is associated with an increase in the frequency of second malignancies. Leukemias are associated with the use of alkylating agents, and solid tumors are associated with radiation therapy. The most common cancers seen are breast cancer that occurs at a younger age, lung cancer in smokers, thyroid cancer, and non-Hodgkin's lymphoma. Shrink in the irradiation volume, with the use of involved fields, and the decrease in the total dose delivered should reduce the incidence of solid tumors in the future. Workup for early detection of cancer must be included in the yearly follow-up, and recommendations to avoid smoking given to all patients.

REFERENCES

Berthe MP, Aleman MD, John MM, et al: Involved-field radiotherapy for advanced Hodgkin's lymphoma. N Engl J Med 2003;348:24.

Eich H, Mueller R, Engert A, et al: Comparison of 30 Gy versus 20 Gy involved field radiotherapy after two versus four cycles ABVD in early stage Hodgkin's lymphoma: Interim analysis of the German Hodgkin Study Group Trial HD10. Int J Radiat Oncol Biol Phys 2005;63(S1):S1-S2. Proceedings of the 47th Annual ASTRO meeting.

Hughes-Davies L, Tarbell NJ, Coleman CN, et al: Stage IA-IIB Hodgkin's disease: Management and outcome of extensive thoracic involvement. Int J Radiat Oncol Biol Phys 1997;39(2):361-369.

Noordijk EM, Carde P, Dupouy N, et al: Combined-modality therapy for clinical stage I or II Hodgkin's lymphoma: Long-term results of the European Organisation for Research and Treatment of Cancer H7 randomized controlled trails. J Clin Oncol 2006;24(19):3128-3135.

Poen JC, Hoppe RT, Horning SJ: High-dose therapy and autologous bone marrow transplantation for relapsed/refractory Hodgkin's disease: The impact of involved field radiotherapy on patterns of failure and survival. Int J Radiat Oncol Biol Phys 1996;36(1):3-12.

Acute Leukemias in Adults

Method of
Jonathan E. Kolitz, MD

The acute leukemias are clonal hematopoietic neoplasms that cause death by usurping the bone marrow's ability to produce normal blood elements. The replacement of marrow by primitive progenitor cells (blasts) leads to infection from neutropenia, bleeding from thrombocytopenia and coagulopathies, and anemia. The two major subtypes of acute leukemia are acute lymphoblastic leukemia (ALL) and acute myeloid leukemia (AML). ALL is the predominant acute leukemia of childhood, and the incidence of AML increases with age.

AML may be associated with antecedent hematologic disorders such as the myeloproliferative disorders and the myelodysplastic syndrome (MDS). Such cases of AML, along with those associated with prior exposure to chemotherapy or radiation, are associated with especially poor outcomes.

Diagnosis

Once acute leukemia is suspected, diagnostic measures must be rapidly undertaken (Table 1). Readily available in most centers are tools that can categorize the acute leukemia in preparation for specific therapy. In addition to morphology, flow cytometry can rapidly establish a diagnosis of acute leukemia by applying combinations of monoclonal antibody stains directed at antigens known as *cluster designation (CD) groups*. A panel of 10 or more antigens is generally studied to properly assign lineage. Acute leukemia with minimal expression of lineage-specific antigens may be difficult to categorize. In addition, an occasional leukemia expresses antigens common to more than one lineage (biphenotypic leukemia) or even manifests as two distinct clonal processes. Most often, the combination of morphologic review and the application of the tests outlined in Table 1 satisfactorily establish a diagnosis.

Cytogenetics has become an essential tool both for categorizing leukemias and for establishing prognosis and detecting minimal residual disease (MRD), the remnant of leukemia that is almost invariably subclinically present when a patient is clinically in complete remission (CR). The eradication of MRD is a principal goal of leukemia therapy.

CURRENT DIAGNOSIS

- Leukocytosis and increased blasts or leukopenia (aleukemic leukemia)
- Anemia and/or thrombocytopenia
- Adenopathy, organomegaly, bone pain more common in ALL
- Central nervous system and/or testicular involvement more common in ALL
- High LDH, tumor lysis syndrome more common in L3 All (Burkitt's leukemia).
- Coagulopathy typical in APL.
- Bone marrow aspirate and biopsy must include routine Wright-Giemsa stain, complete immunophenotype using flow cytometry and immunohistochemistry, and cytogenetics for appropriate diagnostic categorization and for prognostic purposes.

Abbreviations: ALL = acute lymphoblastic leukemia; AML = Acute myeloid leukemia; LDH = lactate dehydrogenase; APL = acute promyelocytic leukemia.

Classification

The categorization of acute leukemia has shifted from the original French-American-British (FAB) classification system, which was based on morphology, to the World Health Organization (WHO) classification scheme (Box 1). The WHO system recognizes the original FAB categories but specifies wherever possible subtypes that have distinct clinical and cytogenetic features. It is hoped that as the molecular understanding of acute leukemia evolves, subsets will be shifted from the original FAB to an expanded WHO classification.

Prognostic Factors

The prognosis of patients with acute leukemia depends on multiple variables. Outcomes of patients with acute leukemia are strongly influenced by the cytogenetic abnormalities present at diagnosis. Important prognostic factors are outlined in Box 2. Listed in Box 2 are several recently identified gene mutations that have been associated with distinct outcomes in the 50% or so of patients with AML who have a normal karyotype, a group regarded as a whole to have an intermediate prognosis.

Treatment

ACUTE MYELOID LEUKEMIA

The therapy of acute leukemia is divided into sequential components. For both AML and ALL, induction therapy involves a period of intensive antileukemic therapy generally given in an inpatient hospital setting. Typically, a central venous catheter is placed to ensure the venous access needed for the chemotherapy and vigorous antibiotic and blood product support required during the period of severe myelosuppression.

Induction

The backbone of induction chemotherapy for AML consists of a combination of 3 days of an anthracycline given by short IV bolus with a 7-day continuous IV (CIV) infusion of cytarabine (Ara-C, Cytosar-U) 100-200 mg/m^2/day (3- and 7-day regimens). Anthracyclines include daunorubicin (cerubidine) given at doses between 45 and 90 mg/m^2, idarubicin (Idamycin) 12 mg/m^2, and mitoxantrone (Novantrone) 12 mg/m^2, each given daily for 3 days. There are no conclusive data showing that the choice of anthracycline is fundamentally important. Randomized trials have not compared pharmacologically and pharmacodynamically equivalent doses of these agents. An ongoing randomized trial will help clarify if daunorubicin 45 mg/m^2 given daily for 3 days differs from twice that dose given in the same manner, both combined with infusional cytarabine, in untreated patients with AML.[3]

Increasing the cytarabine infusional dose from 100 mg/m^2 to twice that dose has not improved outcomes. Neither has extending the 7-day cytarabine infusion to 10 days. Escalating the dose of cytarabine to 3000 mg/m^2 (High-Dose Ara-C, or HiDAC) has not increased the incidence of CR when given during induction. Typical schedules of high-dose cytarabine entail once- or twice-daily administration for 5 or 6 days. A phase III trial suggested that even in the absence of improvements in CR, high-dose cytarabine given during induction improved relapse-free survival. Similar data exist for the use of etoposide[1] (VePesid) during induction, an important third class (epidophyllotoxins) of drugs active against acute leukemia, when given at a dose of 75 mg/m^2 IV daily for 7 days. High-dose cytarabine or etoposide has been used by clinicians during induction but is not considered standard of care at this time, particularly in the elderly.

Typically, in patients undergoing induction, a bone marrow aspirate and biopsy is done 14 days after starting therapy. Residual leukemia is then treated with a second course of therapy using an abbreviated schedule of the original induction. Therapy may be

---

[3]Exceeds dosage recommended by the manufacturer.
[1]Not FDA approved for this indication.

TABLE 1 Diagnostic Tests in Acute Leukemia

Test	Comment
Complete blood count and differential	
DIC screen	Especially in APL, monocytic leukemias
Chemistry profile, including uric acid, phosphorus, LDH	
HLA typing	Irrespective of transplantation intent, to identify compatible platelets units if needed
Bone marrow aspirate	Dry tap can occur in extensively infiltrated (packed) marrow or in the presence of fibrosis
Bone marrow biopsy	Permits determination of cellularity, immunophenotyping
Immunohistochemistry	Chemical stains for lineage, monoclonal antibody stains for specific antigens on paraffin sections from biopsy
Flow cytometry	Stain blasts with monoclonal antibodies directed at lineage-specific antigens
FISH	Rapidly diagnoses suspected subtypes of acute leukemia, especially APL
Cytogenetics	Analyzes metaphases for numeric and structural changes in banded chromosomes
PCR	Sensitive technique to measure minimal residual disease. Sensitivity is 1 in 10^4 to 10^6 leukemic cells.

Abbreviations: APL = acute promyelocytic leukemia; DIC = disseminated intravascular coagulation; FISH = fluorescence-in-situ-hybridization; HLA = human leukocyte antigen; LDH = lactate dehydrogenase; PCR = polymerase chain reaction.

> **BOX 1** World Health Organization Classification of the Acute Leukemias
>
> **Acute Myeloid Leukemias**
> - With recurrent genetic abnormalities
>   - AML with t(8;21) (AML-1-ETO)
>   - AML with abnormal marrow eosinophils
>   - AML with inv(16)(p13q22) or t(16;16)(p13q22) (*CBFβ-MYH11*) [FAB M4Eo]
>   - Acute promyelocytic leukemia: AML with t(15;17)(q22q12) (*PML-RARα*) [FAB M3]
>   - AML with MLL (11q23) abnormalities
> - With multilineage dysplasia
> - With or without antecedent myelodysplastic or myeloproliferative disorder
> - Therapy-related
>   - Alkylating agent related
>   - Topoisomerase II inhibitor related
>   - Other types
> - Not otherwise categorized
>   - AML, minimally differentiated [FAB M0]
>   - AML without maturation [FAB M1]
>   - AML with maturation [FAB M2]
>   - Acute myelomonocytic leukemia [FAB M4]
>   - Acute monoblastic and monocytic leukemias [FAB M5]
>   - Acute erythroid leukemia [FAB M6]
>   - Acute megakaryoblastic leukemia [FAB M7]
>   - Acute basophilic leukemia
>   - Acute panmyelosis with myelofibrosis
>   - Myeloid sarcoma
>
> **Acute Leukemias of Ambiguous Lineage**
> - Undifferentiated acute leukemia
> - Bilineal acute leukemia
> - Biphenotypic acute leukemia
>
> **Acute Lymphoblastic Leukemia/Lymphoblastic Lymphoma**
> - Precursor B ALL
> - Precursor T ALL
>
> *Note*: FAB classifications are given in square brackets following some classifications.
> *Abbreviations*: ALL = acute lymphoblastic leukemia; AML = acute myeloid leukemia; ETO = ETO (eight twenty-one) gene; FAB = French-American-British classification system; MLL = mixed lineage leukemia.

> **BOX 2** Prognostic Factors in Acute Leukemia
>
> **Favorable**
> *Acute Myeloid Leukemia*
> - Age <60 years
> - t(15;17), t(8;21), inv(16), t(16;16), t(8;21)
> - De novo disease
> - Nucleophosmin gene mutation*
> - CCAAT/enhancer binding protein mutation*
>
> *Acute Lymphoblastic Leukemia*
> - Age 2-10 years
> - Hyperdiploidy
> - Early blast clearance with chemotherapy
> - Mature B cell (Burkitt's leukemia) or T cell phenotype
> - WBC <30,000/µL
> - t(12;21)
>
> **Unfavorable**
> *Acute Myeloid Leukemia*
> - Age >70 years
> - Chromosome 7 abnormalities, complex karyotypes, t(6;9); inv(3); t(3;3)
> - Multidrug resistance gene expression
> - WBC >100,000/µL
> - Fms-like tyrosine kinase (flt3) mutation
> - Brain and leukemia cytoplasmic (BAALC) gene mutation*
> - ETS-related gene (ERG) mutation*
> - Antecedent MDS or myeloproliferative disorder
> - Therapy-related AML
>
> *Acute Lymphoblastic Leukemia*
> - Age <2 or >10 years
> - t(9;22); t(4;11); −7; +8
> - Pro-B (very early B lineage) phenotype
> - Hypodiploidy
> - WBC >30,000/µlL
> - Time to CR >4-5 weeks
> - MLL gene mutation
>
> *Among the approximately 50% of patients with AML and normal cytogenetics
> *Abbreviations*: AML = acute myeloid leukemia; CR = complete remission; MDS = myelodysplastic syndrome; MLL = mixed lineage leukemia; WBC = white blood cell.

changed and intensified at that time in select younger patients with minimal evidence of an antileukemic effect, often including high-dose cytarabine.

About 60% to 80% of younger patients with previously untreated, de novo AML achieve CR, most with one course of induction therapy. Therapy-related mortality is between 5% and 10%, with deaths occurring most often as a result of sepsis or hemorrhage, with or without the accompaniment of resistant leukemia.

Consolidation

Once CR is attained, it is essential for the younger patient to move on to intensive treatments aimed at eradicating MRD. By the time a morphologic CR is attained, the total body leukemic cell burden may have fallen only 3 logs (from 10^{12} to 10^{9} cells), so substantial further treatment is needed. Patients with very poor risk karyotypes (complex cytogenetics, chromosome 7 or 3 abnormalities, t(6;9), among others) may be best served by allogeneic transplantation (myeloablative chemotherapy followed by infusion of stem cells from an immunologically matched donor) if a suitable human leukocyte antigen (HLA)-matched donor can be identified.

For most patients, intensive, repeated cycles of chemotherapy are given, usually with high-dose cytarabine alone or a high-dose cytarabine–containing combination. Older patients in CR often receive one or two courses of consolidation using the less-intensive combination of 2 days of an anthracycline and 5 days of infusional cytarabine (2 and 5 regimen). Repeated courses of high-dose cytarabine are especially benefit patients with the favorable cytogenetics of t(8;21), inv(16), and t(16;16), with a cure fraction of more than 50%.

Stem-Cell Transplantation

For the bulk of the patients (about 50%) with normal cytogenetics, the choice is between several courses of high-dose cytarabine or a similar variant, or an allogeneic or autologous stem-cell transplant (ASCT). ASCT involves collecting stem cells from a patient in CR, which are then infused back to the patient after myeloablative chemotherapy is given.

CURRENT THERAPY

- AML in patients younger than 60 years and favorable cytogenetics
  - Anthracycline/cytarabine induction
  - High-dose cytarabine consolidation × 3-4 cycles
- AML under age 60, unfavorable cytogenetics, including normal
  - Anthracycline/cytarabine induction followed by either high-dose cytarabine consolidation or stem cell transplantation
- Acute promyelocytic leukemia
  - Anthracycline with or without cytarabine plus all-*trans*-retinoic acid induction
  - Anthracycline consolidation × 2 cycles generally with all-*trans*-retinoic acid
  - Maintenance therapy with all-*trans*-retinoic acid, with or without PO 6-mercaptopurine and methotrexate (role being determined)
  - High-dose cytarabine, mylotarg, and arsenic trioxide in untreated patients being studied
- AML in patients older than 60 years
  - Options as in patients younger than 60 years in select patients
  - Investigational therapies.
- ALL
  - Five-drug induction regimen (see text)
  - Consolidation therapy with high-dose cytarabine and methotrexate, l-asparaginase, 6-mercaptopurine, cyclophosphamide
  - Maintenance therapy with vincristine, steroids, PO 6-mercaptopurine, and methotrexate for 18 months
  - CNS prophylaxis with systemic and intrathecal therapies
  - Cranial radiotherapy is an option but is potentially toxic
- L3 ALL (Burkitt's leukemia)
  - Short-course intensive high-dose cytarabine, methotrexate therapy plus anthracycline, vincristine, cyclophosphamide; intensive systemic and intrathecal CNS prophylactic therapy
  - No maintenance
  - Rituximab[1] (Rituxan) may be effective
- Myeloid growth factors more effective in reducing periods of neutropenia and infectious risk in ALL than in AML.

[1]Not FDA approved for this indication.

Prognostic factors are being increasingly described in normal-karyotype AML, but it is premature to make treatment recommendations based on these early data. Several trials have compared intensive chemotherapy with ASCT, and although trends favoring relapse-free survival in patients undergoing ASCT have been seen, only one phase III trial has demonstrated that patients benefited from ASCT given late in their clinical course. The Cancer and Leukemia Group B has shown that ASCT yields results similar to those achieved with four courses of high-dose cytarabine followed by maintenance therapy in patients with normal cytogenetics. It has been suggested that ASCT may be associated with less morbidity than multiple courses of high-dose chemotherapy.

The advantage presented by ASCT, that of administering myeloablative doses of chemotherapy, might be negated by failure to eradicate residual leukemia in the infused stem cells. Attempts to improve outcomes have included intensifying the chemotherapy given prior to stem cell collection (in vivo purging) as well as ex vivo purging of stem cell collections with high doses of cytotoxic agents or monoclonal antibodies (or both). The use of peripheral stem cells reduces the time to hematopoietic engraftment. Whether overall treatment outcomes will improve with the increased use of peripheral blood rather than marrow as a source of stem cells remains to be seen.

Allogeneic transplants are limited to the 30% to 35% or so of eligible patients who have a donor. Although the risk of infusing leukemic cells is eliminated in allogeneic transplants, greater risks exist related to the immunologic effect of infused donor T cells against host tissues (graft-versus-host disease, GVHD). The other important consequence is the development of a direct antileukemic effect called *graft-versus-leukemia* (GVL). In younger patients, especially those younger than 30 years, GVHD tends to be manageable, and outcomes in AML patients receiving transplants in first CR can be excellent. The risk of GVHD and associated complications greatly increases with age. The high-dose chemotherapy, given with or without total body irradiation, can cause unacceptable toxicities in older patients.

An attempt to counter this problem has been the ongoing exploration of reduced-intensity transplants, in which low doses of immunosuppressive agents such as fludarabine[1] (Fludara), antithymocyte globulin (Atgam, others), alemtuzumab[1] (CamPath), melphalan[1] (Alkeran), or busulfan[1] (Myleran PO or Busulfex IV) are used to suppress host defenses sufficiently to permit engraftment of donor stem cells. This can lead to a curative GVL effect in some patients. The relative safety of the preparative regimen can be negated, however, by the development of severe GVHD. Methodologies to enhance the GVL effect while limiting the sequelae of GVHD are being actively studied. Select patients older than 60 years, and even older than 70 years, have been treated using this approach.

Maintenance

Unlike in ALL, there is no evidence that lower doses of chemotherapy given for prolonged periods after induction and consolidation (maintenance therapy) improve survival, although time to relapse may be favorably affected. Overall, about 30% of patients with AML younger than 60 years with other than favorable cytogenetics are cured.

Older Patients

Older patients present a special challenge. Patients older than 60 years, and especially older than 70 years, are more likely to harbor resistant forms of AML associated with poor-risk cytogenetic features and multidrug-resistance phenotypes. Comorbid conditions limit tolerance for severely myelotoxic therapies. Nonetheless, a good performance status predicts a more favorable outcome, even in older patients. The patient's physiologic state must be factored in with other established predictors of outcome in deciding whether or with what to treat older patients with AML.

Several randomized trials suggest that treatment of older patients who have AML can lead to better outcomes with respect to survival than purely supportive or palliative approaches. Ideally, investigational therapies should be evaluated in this high-risk patient population. Select older patients can benefit from intensive therapies used in younger patients, such as the 7- and 3-day regimens described earlier. Depending on performance status and other prognostic factors, the probability of a patient older than 60 years entering CR using conventional induction treatment is 30% to 50%, with therapy-related mortality of 20% to 40%. Only about 10% are long survivors.

For many patients, investigational agents, attenuated doses of conventional induction regimens, or alternative therapies that have been most often used in high-risk MDS may be considered. A non–anthracycline-containing combination of the topoisomerase

[1]Not FDA approved for this indication.

I inhibitor topotecan[1] (Hycamptin, 1.5 mg/m^2/day by CIV) and cytarabine 2 g/m^2, each given daily for 5 days, has moderate activity in older patients with AML, as does the non–cytarabine-containing combination of mitoxantrone (Novantrone) 10 mg/m^2 and etoposide[1] (Toposar) 100 mg/m^2 each given daily IV for 5 days.

Fludarabine[1] 25 to 30 mg/m^2 IV daily for 4 days has been combined with high-dose cytarabine and filgrastim (Neupogen) in the non–anthracycline-containing FLAG (fludarabine, cytarabine, granulocyte colony-stimulating factor [G-CSF]) regimen.

Hypomethylating agents that induce the expression of silenced genes such as 5-azacytidine[1] (Vidaza, 75 mg/m^2 SC daily for 7 days every 4 weeks) or* decitabine[1] (Dacogen), using various doses and schedules, may have activity in select older patients with AML, as may low doses of cytarabine (10 mg/m^2 SC bid for 14-21 days every 28 days). Low-dose cytarabine has also been recently combined with arsenic trioxide[8] (Trisenox) in an investigational regimen for elderly patients with AML.

Clofarabine (Clolar) is a newly developed nucleoside analogue that might have activity in older patients with AML. The optimal dose and schedule remain under study.

The anti-CD33 monoclonal antibody–calicheamycin construct gemtuzumab ozogamycin (Mylotarg) can induce CR in a small fraction (about 20%) of older patients with untreated AML. The approved dose and schedule when used as a single agent is 9 mg/m^2 IV on days 1 and 15. Various combinations of this antibody with chemotherapy are being investigated.

The orally available farnesyl transferase inhibitor tipifarnib (Zarnestra)[1] has proven disappointing when used as a single agent.

Investigational Therapy

Relapsed and refractory disease and AML in the elderly demand the use of investigational therapies. High-dose cytarabine can occasionally induce response in a patient resistant to a conventional anthracycline-cytarabine regimen. For almost all suitable patients, a CR achieved after an initial induction failure or a second CR must be rapidly consolidated with a transplant-based strategy.

Investigational approaches have involved novel agents with inhibitory properties directed against proliferative, differentiation, immunomodulatory, angiogenic, and drug-resistance pathways. Efforts to improve outcomes by inhibiting P-glycoprotein, a transmembrane drug efflux pump that confers multidrug resistance, have had limited success. A partial list of novel agents, most of which are being studied in AML but some of which may be active in ALL, is presented in Table 2. Ongoing efforts are assessing the use of these agents alone and in combination with chemotherapy.

Filgrastim[1] (and sargramostin (Leukine) are myeloid growth factors that have been studied in AML to hasten myeloid recovery as well as to stimulate proliferation of leukemic cells in order to increase their susceptibility to cell cycle–active cytotoxic agents such as cytarabine. Benefits have been, at best, marginal, with some indication that periods of neutropenia and hospital stays are reduced but without clear evidence that survival is increased. Studies looking at cell cycle activation effects have been conflicting but mostly negative.

ACUTE PROMYELOCYTIC LEUKEMIA

Acute promyelocytic leukemia (APL) represents a paradigm for a malignancy that is yielding to targeted strategies that are not principally dependent on cytotoxic agents. Representing only about 5% to 10% of adult AML, 70% to 80% of patients with newly diagnosed disease can now expect to be cured.

All-*trans*-retinoic acid (ATRA, tretinoin, Vesanoid) induces terminal differentiation and apoptosis in APL cells. It can induce CR in most patients with APL given alone at a dose of 45 mg/m^2 PO daily in 2 divided doses for 30 to 45 days, but it cannot eradicate

---

[1]Not FDA approved for this indication.
*Approved for MDS, not acute leukemia.
[8]Orphan drug in the United States.

TABLE 2 Investigational Therapies of Acute Leukemia

Drug	Mechanism of Action
Bevacizumab (Avastin)[1]	VEGF inhibitor
SU5416 (Semaxanib)[5]	VEGF-R, c-kit, and flt-3 inhibitor
SU11248 (Sugen)[5]	VEGF-R, c-kit, and flt-3 inhibitor
Tipifarnib (Zarnestra)[5]	Farnesyl transferase inhibitor
Lonafarnib (SCH66336)[5]	Farnesyl transferase inhibitor
Valproic acid (Depakote)[1]	Histone deacetylase inhibitor
SAHA[1]	Histone deacetylase inhibitor
PKC412[5]	flt-3 inhibitor
MLN518[5]	flt-3 inhibitor
CEP701[5]	flt-3 inhibitor
Decitabine[1]	DNA methyltransferase inhibitor
Imatinib (Gleevec)[1]	bcr-abl inhibitor: Ph$^+$ ALL, AML
Dasatinib (BMS-354825)*	bcr-abl, src inhibitor, Ph$^+$ ALL, AML
Oblimersen (Genasense)[5]	bcl-2 mRNA inhibitor (antisense therapy)
Interleukin-2 (Proleukin)[1]	T and NK cell stimulant
PR-1[5]	Vaccine for AML
Hum-195-Bismuth 213[5]	Radiolabeled monoclonal antibody for AML
Alemtuzumab (CamPath)[1]	Monoclonal antibody for ALL
VNP40101M (Cloretazine)[5]	Alkylating agent
Troxacitabine (Troxatyl)[5]	Purine nucleoside analogue
Zosuquidar[5]	Inhibitor of multidrug resistance
Cyclosporin A (Sandimmune)[1]	Inhibitor of multidrug resistance

[1]Not FDA approved for this indication.
[5]Investigational drug in the United States.
*Approved for ALL in 2006. http://www.fda.gov/cder/foi/label/2006/022072lbl.pdf
Abbreviations: ALL = acute lymphoblastic leukemia; AML = acute myeloid leukemia; NK = natural killer cells; Ph = Philadelphia chromosome; SAHA = suberoylanilide hydroxamic acid; VEGF = vascular endothelial growth factor; VEGF-R = vascular endothelial growth factor receptor.
Definitions: bcr-abl = gene product of the Ph (Philadelphia) chromosome translocation t(9;22); c-kit = transmembrane tyrosine kinase (CD117); DNA methyltransferase = inhibition promotes gene transcription; farnesyl transferase = enzyme in ras pathway; flt-3 = fms-like transmembrane tyrosine kinase; histone deacetylase = inhibition promotes histone disassembly and gene transcription; multidrug resistance = major mediator of resistance to anthracyclines, vinca alkaloids, and epipodophyllotoxins is a transmembrane drug efflux pump, p-glycoprotein, or mdr-1.

---

the disease by itself. The combination of anthracycline-based chemotherapy and ATRA induces CR and polymerase chain reaction (PCR, a highly sensitive assay for MRD, see Table 1) negativity in 70% to 80% of patients. A non–anthracycline-containing combination using arsenic trioxide (Trisenox, 0.15 mg/kg IV over 2 hours daily until CR and then repeated for 4 to 6 cycles) with or without ATRA induces similar outcomes, although long-term follow-up is shorter than with chemotherapy-containing regimens.

APL is sensitive to anthracyclines, so consolidation courses consisting, for example, of two courses of daunorubicin 50 mg/m^2 IV daily for 3 days, usually given in combination with ATRA, induces a high cure fraction. The results of a phase III North American Intergroup trial in which untreated patients were randomized to receive or not receive two courses of arsenic trioxide in addition to anthracycline-based chemotherapy have shown results favoring the arsenic arm.

Patients with APL who present with high WBC counts (>10,000/μL) have adverse outcomes, and attempts have been made to improve their prognosis using strategies that include gemtuzumab ozogamicin (Mylotarg) (APL strongly expresses CD33) or treatment with high-dose cytarabine.

Maintenance therapy with ATRA for a year, with or without the oral chemotherapy agents methotrexate (Rheumatrex, others) 20 mg/m^2 orally once per week and 6-mercaptopurine (Purinethol) 60 mg/m^2 orally daily, has been used to prevent relapse in APL. It may be that patients who are molecularly negative by PCR after completing induction and consolidation do not need maintenance. This question is posed in a planned phase III trial.

ATRA needs to be given intermittently because it can induce its own metabolism. Patients treated with ATRA or arsenic trioxide can develop a differentiation syndrome marked by fever, dyspnea, weight gain, pulmonary infiltrates, pleural effusions, and even death. This can result, in part, from interactions between maturing leukemic promyelocytes and the pulmonary vascular endothelium as well as cytokine release. Most patients respond to interruptions in drug therapy and brief courses of dexamethasone 10 mg IV twice daily.

APL generally manifests with a low WBC count and evidence of coagulopathy, including severe hypofibrinogenemia. ATRA helps to reverse the coagulopathy, but it is critical to maintain the fibrinogen greater than 100 mg/dL and the platelet count higher than the traditional 10,000 to 20,000/μL. Nonrandomized clinical experience suggests that keeping the platelet count higher than 50,000/μL in APL is important until laboratory evidence of disseminated intravascular coagulation (DIC) reverses. There are no convincing data to support the use of low-dose heparin or antifibrinolytic agents in APL.

Relapsed APL is generally approached with an attempt at reinduction using regimens similar to those that were initially effective. ASCT has been an active salvage therapy in APL in second CR, although an allogeneic transplant could be considered in suitable high-risk patients.

ACUTE LYMPHOBLASTIC LEUKEMIA

Approximately 30% to 40% of adults with ALL are cured. CR rates are high, approaching 90% in patients younger than 60 years, but relapse rates are substantially higher than in childhood ALL. One important reason for this disparity is that the Ph chromosome is far more common in adults than in children (30%-40% vs. 5%). Also, the favorable t(12;21) is overrepresented in childhood ALL. Furthermore, children with ALL have been treated more intensively than adults, using higher doses of cytotoxic agents with shorter treatment-free intervals and more aggressive use of prophylactic therapy aimed at preventing central nervous system (CNS) relapse.

The backbone of induction therapy for ALL consists of weekly doses of vincristine 2 mg IV weekly for 4 weeks combined with prednisone 60 mg/m^2 PO daily for 21 days or dexamethasone 6 mg/m^2 orally daily for 14 to 21 days. Response rates have increased as additional drugs have been added to the induction framework, so that a typical induction regimen for adult ALL often includes cyclophosphamide (600-1200 mg/m^2 IV once on day 1 or 300 mg/m^2 IV bid for 3 days in a regimen called HyperCVAD), daunorubicin (45-80 mg/m^2 IV daily on days 1 to 3 and L-asparaginase (Elspar, 6000 U/m^2) SC or IM biweekly for 6 doses. PEG-asparaginase (Oncaspar) 2500 IU/m^2 IM or IV given twice during induction 2 weeks apart has also been used. A two-drug induction regimen using a high-dose anthracycline (e.g., mitoxantrone 60-80 mg/m^2 IV[3] given once) with high-dose cytarabine has been studied, which is then followed in patients achieving CR by more traditional anti-ALL regimens. Childhood regimens have intensified further the use of L-asparaginase.

Achieving CR by 4 to 5 weeks after starting induction is prognostically important. For the majority of patients in CR, repeated cycles of multiple agents with both antileukemia effects and the capacity for crossing the blood-brain barrier are given. This is because the CNS is a major sanctuary site in ALL. Efforts are directed early in therapy to identify or eradicate occult disease in the CSF. High doses of methotrexate (1000 to 3500 mg/m^2 IV) are given, followed by rescue with folinic acid (leucovorin) 25 to 50 mg PO every 6 hours until serum methotrexate levels drop to less than .05 M. High-dose cytarabine (3000 mg/m^2 IV daily for 2-3 days) is also an active anti-ALL agent that, along with methotrexate, penetrates well into the CSF. Repeated courses using these agents, with or without cyclophosphamide, L-asparaginase, and 6-mercaptopurine, are given over a period of about 6 months, after which about 18 months of lower-dose maintenance therapy is given, usually using monthly courses of vincristine (2 mg IV day 1), and oral pulses of prednisone (60 mg/m^2) or dexamethasone (6 mg/m^2) on days 1 to 5, daily doses of oral 6-mercaptopurine (60 mg/m^2), and weekly doses of oral methotrexate (20 mg/m^2). Variants of these regimens are described in the references.

The incidence of CNS disease has been reduced to 5% to 10% using prophylactic therapies as discussed earlier, along with repeated intrathecal instillations of methotrexate (6 mg/m^2/dose) and cytarabine (30 mg/m^2/dose), alone or in combination, via the lumbar route or intraventricularly using an Omaya reservoir. Commonly, 6 to 12 prophylactic treatments are given during induction and consolidation. Prophylactic cranial irradiation (up to 2400 cGy) has also been used. Because radiotherapy can induce cognitive defects, especially when combined with high-dose antimetabolite-based treatments, attempts are being made to clarify whether or not systemic and intrathecal treatments can suffice to prevent CNS disease, without cranial radiotherapy. In the setting of established CNS disease, most practitioners favor using whole-brain radiotherapy in addition to vigorous intrathecal treatments.

Drug resistance in the significant minority of patients with Ph$^+$ ALL is being countered using targeted therapies that inhibit the specific product of the fusion gene that occurs in that disease (bcr-abl). Imatinib[1] (Gleevec) 600 to 800 mg orally daily induces transient remissions in a significant minority of patients with Ph$^+$ ALL. Other inhibitors include nilotinib (Tasigna)[1], a more potent bcr-abl inhibitor, and dasatinib (Sprycel) which inhibits additional oncogenic pathways besides bcr-abl. Ongoing trials are clarifying the efficacy of cytotoxic therapies in combination with imatinib.[1] It is still critical to identify donors for allogeneic transplantation in patients with Ph$^+$ ALL entering into CR. ASCT is also being studied in Ph$^+$ ALL in conjunction with imatinib[1] and chemotherapy.

T-lineage ALL has been believed to have an inferior outcome to B-lineage ALL, but current intensive adult regimens have yielded outcomes in T-cell disease that are at least as good as those seen in the other ALL subtypes.

Mature B lineage ALL (Burkitt's leukemia or L3 ALL) is a highly proliferative form of acute leukemia, which demands distinct treatment that concentrates on the use of antimetabolites (high-dose methotrexate and high-dose cytarabine as described earlier for consolidation therapy of ALL) early in therapy along with an anthracycline, vincristine, cyclophosphamide, and corticosteroids. The risk of CNS disease is especially high in Burkitt's leukemia, and vigorous prophylactic CNS therapy is needed. Unlike typical ALL regimens, short-term (3 months or less) cyclic therapy without maintenance therapy is curative. Somewhat more prolonged regimens using similar drugs and most recently including the anti-CD20 monoclonal antibody rituximab[1] (375 mg/m^2 given every 3 weeks) have also been studied. Older patients might better tolerate such less dose-intense regimens. More than 80% of younger adults and perhaps 40% to 50% of older adults are cured. For both typical B lineage ALL and Burkitt's leukemia, judicious use of filgrastim (5 μg/kg/day SC) given daily after chemotherapy cycles will hasten myeloid recovery and reduce infectious risk.

Future directions in treating ALL include improving prognostic factor analysis, studying the more intensive childhood regimens in younger adults (younger than 30 years), continuing to refine CNS prophylactic measures, and evaluating new agents. Alemtuzumab[1] is being studied in the MRD setting in patients with ALL. Clofarabine is active in relapsed ALL and will be studied in earlier patients. Except for very poor risk patients, the role of early allogenic transplant in ALL remains undefined. Nelarabine (Arranon) is a newly approved purine nucleoside analogue. At a dose of 1500 mg/m^2 IV on days 1, 3, and 5 every 21 days, it is active in relapsed and refractory T-ALL. It is hoped that outcomes in both forms of acute leukemia will improve with the intelligent use of new agents in the context of carefully designed and conducted clinical trials.

---

[3]Exceeds dosage recommended by the manufacturer.

[1]Not FDA approved for this indication.

REFERENCES

Kolitz JE: Acute myeloid leukemia and the myelodysplastic syndromes. In AEChang, PAGanz, DFHayes, et al, editors: Oncology: An Evidence-Based Approach. New York, Springer, 2006, pp 1151-1172.

Odenike OM, Michaelis LC, Stock W: Acute lymphoblastic leukemia. In Chang AE, Ganz PA, Hayes DF et al, (eds): Oncology: An Evidence-Based Approach. New York, Springer, 2006, pp 1173-1201.

Pui CH, Evans WE: Treatment of acute lymphoblastic leukemia. N Engl J Med 2006;354:166-178.

Sanz MA, Tallman MS, Lo-Coco F: Tricks of the trade for the appropriate management of newly diagnosed acute promyelocytic leukemia. Blood 2005;105:3019-3025.

Tallman MS, Gilliland DG, Rowe JM: Drug therapy of acute myeloid leukemia. Blood 2005;106:1154-1163.

Acute Leukemia in Children

Method of
Patrick Brown, MD, and
Stephen P. Hunger, MD

The word "leukemia" is derived from the Greek roots *leukos* (white) and *haima* (blood). Leukemia, cancer of the blood-forming cells, is characterized by a marked proliferation of abnormal leukocytes in the bone marrow and blood that may be associated with widespread infiltration in extramedullary sites including the central nervous system (CNS), testes, thymus, liver, spleen, and lymph nodes.

Classification

The first level of classification of leukemia is *acute* versus *chronic*. Acute leukemia is characterized by the predominance of very immature white blood cell precursors, or blasts, and is an aggressive, rapidly fatal disease if left untreated. Chronic leukemia is characterized by proliferation of relatively mature white blood cells and is typically an indolent disease.

The second level of classification is *lymphoid* versus *myeloid*, depending on whether the leukemic cells display characteristics of lymphocyte precursors or myelocyte (granulocyte, erythrocyte, monocyte, or megakaryocyte) precursors. Acute lymphoblastic leukemia (ALL) and acute myeloid leukemia (AML) account for the overwhelming majority of pediatric leukemias. Chronic leukemias are uncommon in pediatrics.

ALL and AML are further subclassified by morphology and expression of cell surface antigens using flow cytometry. For ALL, classification is largely based on cell surface and cytoplasmic marker expression (Table 1). AML cases are classified by characteristic chromosomal abnormalities (if present) or by light microscopic morphology in cases where these specific chromosomal changes are absent (Box 1).

BOX 1 Classification of Childhood Acute Myeloid Leukemia (World Health Organization Criteria)

Acute Myeloid Leukemia with Recurrent Genetic Abnormalities

Acute myeloid leukemia with t(8;21)(q22;q22), *(AML1/ETO)*
Acute myeloid leukemia with abnormal bone marrow eosinophils and inv(16)(p13q22) or t(16;16)(p13;q22), *(CBFβ/MYH11)*
Acute promyelocytic leukemia with t(15;17)(q22;q12), *(PML/RARα)*, and variants
Acute myeloid leukemia with 11q23 *(MLL)* abnormalities

Acute Myeloid Leukemia, Not Otherwise Categorized

Acute myeloid leukemia, minimally differentiated (FAB M0)
Acute myeloid leukemia without maturation (FAB M1)
Acute myeloid leukemia with maturation (FAB M2)
Acute myelomonocytic leukemia (FAB M4)
Acute monoblastic/acute monocytic leukemia (FAB M5)
Acute erythroid leukemia (FAB M6)
Acute megakaryoblastic leukemia (FAB M7)

FAB = French–American–British classification.

Epidemiology

The incidence of childhood cancer is 14 cases per 100,000 children younger than 16 years of age per year, which translates into approximately 11,000 new cases per year in the United States. Leukemia accounts for approximately 30% of childhood cancers, making it the most common form of childhood cancer. The distribution of the major forms of leukemia is vastly different in children than in adults (Fig. 1). In general, children are far more likely to have acute leukemia, and ALL is much more common than AML. In adults, most cases of leukemia are chronic, and AML is much more common than ALL.

The incidence of the various forms of leukemia varies by age in both children and adults (Fig. 2). This is especially true for childhood ALL, for which there is a marked incidence peak in the 2- to 4-year-old age group. This ALL age peak is primarily found in children living in industrialized nations, leading to speculation that a common environmental exposure, coupled with age-related immunologic susceptibility, is at least partially responsible for many cases of ALL.

TABLE 1 Classification of Childhood Acute Lymphoblastic Leukemia

ALL Subtype	CD19	CD10	cIg	sIg	%	Comment
Pre-pre B	+	−	−	−	5	Mostly infants, poor prognosis, frequent *MLL* 11q23 rearrangements
Early pre-B	+	+	−	−	63	Common ALL, young children, good prognosis
Pre-B	+	+	+	−	16	Older children, good prognosis with intense therapy
B-cell	+	+	+	+	4	Burkitt's leukemia, *MYC/Ig* fusion genes, good prognosis with lymphoma-type therapy
T-cell	−	−	−	−	12	Adolescents, anterior mediastinal mass, CNS involvement, good prognosis with intense therapy

ALL = acute myeloid leukemia; cIg = cytoplasmic immunoglobulin; sIg = surface immunoglobulin; CNS, central nervous system.

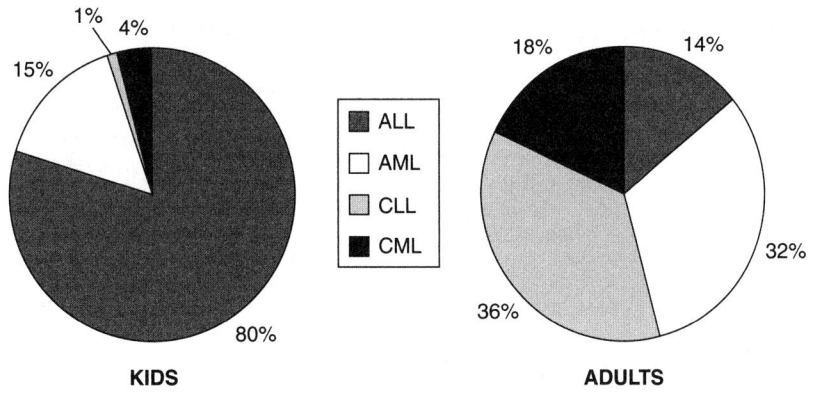

FIGURE 1. Relative incidence of four major leukemia subtypes in children and adults. ALL = acute lymphoblastic leukemia; AML = Acute myeloid leukemia; CLL = chronic lymphoblastic leukemia; CML = chronic myeloid leukemia.

Except for a small peak in infants, the incidence of AML is fairly constant in childhood but rises quickly in later adulthood.

Prognosis

One of the most dramatic success stories in modern medicine is the improvement in survival of children with ALL over the past four decades. Leukemia was once a uniformly fatal diagnosis, with less than a 5% to 10% cure rate until the mid to late 1960s. Today, approximately 85% of children with ALL are cured. The improved prognosis is built on pioneering observations on the efficacy of multiagent systemic therapy and the importance of presymptomatic CNS treatment in the late 1960s and early 1970s. Further successive, incremental improvements in outcome have been achieved due to clinical trials conducted by large single centers and national and international cooperative groups that have successfully enrolled a high percentage of eligible children.

Similar approaches have unfortunately not been quite so successful in improving the prognosis of children with AML. Although approximately one half of children with AML are cured today, this has been accomplished by intensifying therapy to the point that the toxic death rate in the early phases of therapy is about 10%. Current research in AML is therefore focusing on developing novel molecularly targeted agents that hold the promise of improving efficacy and limiting toxicity.

Etiology

The question, "What is the cause of leukemia?" can be considered on a few different levels. First, what is wrong with *this child* that caused the child to develop leukemia? Second, what is wrong with *the leukemia cell* that causes it to behave so badly? Third, what is wrong with *the leukemia cell's genes* that cause the cell to behave that way?

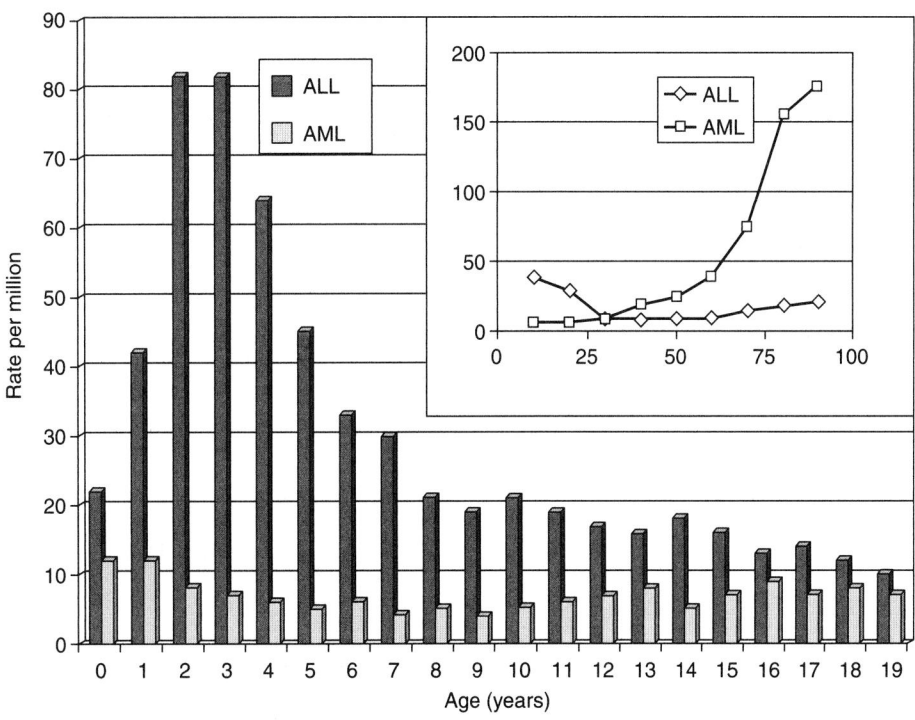

FIGURE 2. Age-specific incidence of acute lymphoblastic leukemia (ALL) and acute myeloid leukemia (ALL) in children and in adults *(inset).*

TABLE 2 Summary of Known Constitutional and Heritable Childhood Leukemia Predispositions

Disorder	Inheritance	Malignancy Type	Comments
Ataxia–telangiectasia	AR	ALL, NHL	*ATM* gene mutations lead to defective DNA repair
Bloom's syndrome	AR	AML, ALL	Chromosomal instability, sister chromatid exchanges
Down syndrome	Sporadic	AML, ALL	See text
Li–Fraumeni syndrome	AD	AML, ALL, many others	*p53* mutations; leukemias less common than solid tumors
Fanconi's anemia	AR	AML	Chromosomal instability, increased sensitivity to DNA damage
Kostmann's syndrome	AR	AML	G-CSF receptor mutations lead to agranulocytosis
Neurofibromatosis type 1	AD	AML, JMML, MPNST	*NF1* gene mutations lead to enhanced *RAS* signaling

AD, autosomal dominant; ALL = acute lymphoblastic leukemia; AML = acute myeloid leukemia; AR, autosomal recessive; G-CSF = granulocyte colony-stimulating factor; JMML, juvenile myelomonocytic leukemia; MPNST, malignant peripheral nerve sheath tumor; NHL, non-Hodgkin's lymphoma.

PREDISPOSITIONS

The answer to the first question is unknown in the vast majority of cases. Attempts to correlate various genetic features or environmental or infectious exposures with risk of childhood leukemia have been largely uninformative. It is presumed that children are particularly susceptible to ALL because of the marked expansion and genetic rearrangement of lymphocytes that occurs during early childhood as the result of exposure to a multitude of immunogenic antigens for the first time. The proliferation required to meet the constant demand for granulocytes, erythrocytes, and platelets is likely a setup for the development of AML in children.

Although a number of constitutional and single-gene disorders are known to confer an increased risk of childhood leukemia (Table 2), in total, these are involved in only a very small minority of cases. The most common of these is Down syndrome. Children with Down syndrome have a 10- to 20-fold increased risk of leukemia, with an approximately equal incidence of ALL and AML. The peak age at onset of leukemia for children with Down syndrome is earlier than for other children. Approximately 30% of Down syndrome children with AML have the megakaryoblastic form (M7 AML), a subtype that is extremely rare in children without Down syndrome. In the newborn period, Down syndrome patients can present with transient myeloproliferative disease, a disorder distinguishable from congenital AML primarily by its spontaneous resolution within 3 months. Children with Down syndrome tend to present with biologically favorable subtypes of leukemia, but they also suffer increased toxicity from therapy. On balance, the prognosis of leukemia in Down syndrome patients is similar to that in other children.

The only environmental exposures that are known to predispose to leukemia are ionizing radiation (such as was seen with atomic bomb survivors) and prior exposure to certain chemotherapy drugs (cyclophosphamide [Cytoxan], etoposide [Vepesid]). There is good evidence that in utero exposure to maternal diagnostic radiation also increases the risk of childhood cancer (including leukemia), particularly if the exposure is in the first trimester. Other environmental or infectious exposures remain unproved as risk factors for childhood leukemia, including electromagnetic fields from power lines.

CELLULAR PATHOGENESIS

Three major characteristics of leukemia cells distinguish them from normal hematopoietic cells. They proliferate rapidly, they do not differentiate, and they have defects in apoptosis. This results in a growth advantage for leukemia cells, leading to progressive replacement of the normal bone marrow with a massive clonal population of poorly differentiated leukemic blasts. Another characteristic of leukemia cells is their tendency to spread throughout the body and infiltrate organs other than the bone marrow. This is discussed in more detail in the section on clinical presentation.

MOLECULAR PATHOGENESIS

As is true of most human cancers, development of leukemia is a multihit process. The initiating or permissive mutation (first hit) in childhood ALL often occurs in utero or early infancy, which is the peak of lymphocyte expansion and recombinase activity.

The initiating events are typically chromosomal rearrangements that activate expression of cellular proto-oncogenes by fusing them to transcriptionally active immunoglobulin or T-cell receptor genes or by joining two genes from different chromosomes to create a new fusion gene that encodes a chimeric protein with unique functional properties. The most common of these sentinel chromosomal rearrangements are translocations (exchanges of genetic material between chromosomes), which can serve as a unique marker of the malignant clone. Retrospective studies of blood obtained at birth and preserved on filter paper used for diagnosis of genetic disorders (Guthrie cards) of children who developed leukemia in early childhood have shown that leukemia-associated fusion genes were present at birth in a large percentage of children, including some who did not develop leukemia for one or more years.

In ALL, the promotional mutation (second hit) likely occurs during the proliferative stress generated by immune responses to exogenous antigens. Because these are maximal in the 2- to 4-year-old age group, this is thought to explain the age peak of childhood ALL during these years. The lack of such a peak in AML suggests that the promotional mutations can occur at any time or are not triggered by immune stimulation. Examples of specific genetic hits known to be associated with the development of childhood leukemia are summarized in Table 3.

TABLE 3 Summary of Common Leukemogenic Genetic Events

Acute Lymphoblastic Leukemia	Acute Myeloid Leukemia
Chimeric Transcription Factors	
t(12;21): *TEL-AML1* fusion	t(8;21): *AML1-ETO* fusion
t(1;19): *E2A-PBX1* fusion	t(15;17): *PML-RAR* α fusion
t(4;11), et al: *MLL* fusions	t(9;11), et al: *MLL* fusions
t(8;14), t(8;22), t(2;8): *Ig-MYC* fusions	inv(16): MYH11-CBFB
T-cell receptor fusions	
Mutationally Activated Oncogenes	
t(9;22): *BCR-ABL* fusion	*FLT3* mutation
PTPN11 mutation	*RAS* mutation
FLT3 mutation	*KIT* mutation
Altered *Rb/p53* Tumor-Suppressor Network	
p16INK4a/p14ARF deletion or silencing	Nucleophosmin mutations
p21CIP1 silencing	*p53* mutations
HDM2 overexpression	*HDM2* overexpression

Clinical Presentation

Most symptoms and signs of childhood leukemia are the result of the propensity of leukemia cells to replace the bone marrow and infiltrate multiple other organs throughout the body. It is estimated that approximately 10^9 (1 trillion) leukemia cells are present in the child's body at diagnosis.

The replacement of normal bone marrow is responsible for the characteristic abnormal blood counts, which in most cases include the triad of neutropenia, anemia, and thrombocytopenia. Depending on the number of circulating leukemic blasts in the peripheral blood, the total white blood cell count may be low, normal, or high. The neutropenia is often profound (absolute neutrophil count <500/μL), and is associated with an increased risk of serious infection. Blood cultures and broad-spectrum intravenous antibiotic coverage are indicated in any patient with newly diagnosed leukemia and fever. Anemia is often manifested by fatigue, lethargy, headache, pallor, and, in extreme cases, congestive heart failure that may be precipitated by vigorous transfusion or intravenous hydration. Thrombocytopenia often leads to bruising and petechiae; however, clinically significant hemorrhage is uncommon in industrialized countries. Platelet transfusion is indicated for bleeding or for very low platelet counts (<10,000-20,000/μL).

Infiltration of organs other than the bone marrow with leukemia cells is responsible for additional presenting clinical features. Box 2 summarizes the organ systems most often involved in leukemia and the typical clinical manifestations.

BOX 2   Summary of Clinical Manifestations of Childhood Leukemia*

Bone Marrow
Pancytopenia, bone pain

Reticuloendothelial System
Lymphadenopathy
Hepatosplenomegaly

Thymus
Anterior mediastinal mass (T-cell leukemia)

Bones
Bone pain is common
Fractures and chloromas are rare

Gums
Gingival hypertrophy (M4 and M5 AML)

Skin
Leukemia cutis and chloromas (M2, M4, and M5 AML, infant ALL)

Central Nervous System
Meningitis
Cranial nerve palsies
Rarely intracranial epidural or orbital chloromas (M4 and M5 AML, T-cell ALL)

Kidneys
Often infiltrated or enlarged
Rarely acute renal failure (except in tumor lysis syndrome)

Genitourinary
Testicular enlargement (T-cell ALL)

*See Box 1 for descriptions of classifications.
ALL = acute lymphoblastic leukemia; AML = acute myeloid leukemia.

Medical Emergencies in Childhood Leukemia

Newly diagnosed leukemia in a child is a medical emergency. There are several potentially life-threatening complications that may be present at diagnosis or can develop within a short time after diagnosis. The need to diagnose and treat potential infection in patients who are febrile and neutropenic was discussed earlier.

Tumor lysis syndrome (TLS) is a complication resulting from the rapid lysis of large numbers of tumor cells, releasing intracellular contents. Although TLS is seen most often after initial treatment with chemotherapy, it can also be present before therapy is initiated due to spontaneous lysis. Risk factors include high white blood cell (WBC) count, lymphadenopathy, hepatosplenomegaly, high mitotic index, and a diagnosis of ALL (especially Burkitt's leukemia or lymphoma and T-cell ALL). TLS is characterized by the triad of hyperuricemia (from breakdown of purines by xanthine oxidase), hyperkalemia, and hyperphosphatemia (with secondary hypocalcemia). Renal insufficiency can develop due to the nephrotoxic effects of precipitated urate crystals in the renal tubules; in severe cases, dialysis may be necessary.

Management consists of aggressive hydration to reduce tubular uric acid concentration and alkalinization of urine to promote solubility of urate crystals. The xanthine oxidase inhibitor allopurinol (Zyloprim) is routinely used during the first 3 to 7 days of leukemia treatment to decrease uric acid production. Rasburicase (Elitek) (recombinant urate oxidase) is a new agent used in severe cases of TLS to almost instantaneously convert uric acid to the more soluble allantoin. Frequent electrolyte monitoring with standard management of abnormal levels is essential.

Hyperleukocytosis becomes a potential clinical problem when the WBC count rises above 100,000/μL. Markedly elevated WBCs lead to increased blood viscosity that can produce sludging of blood in the brain, lungs, kidneys, and other organs, causing clinical features such as depressed level of consciousness, stroke, intracranial hemorrhage, respiratory distress, hypoxia, diffuse pulmonary infiltrates, and renal insufficiency. The risk of hyperviscosity is higher with AML than ALL, because myeloblasts are generally larger and stickier than lymphoblasts (likely due to increased expression of integrins and other mediators of cell–cell adherence on the surface of myeloblasts). Management consists of treating the leukemia as soon as possible and performing exchange transfusion or leukopheresis in cases where symptoms are prominent.

Life-threatening bleeding is another potential complication of leukemia. Although all patients with thrombocytopenia are at risk, patients with concomitant coagulopathy due to disseminated intravascular coagulation (DIC) are at particularly high risk. The leukemia subtype most commonly complicated by DIC and serious bleeding is acute promyelocytic leukemia (APL). This association results from the release of thromboplastin from the cytoplasmic granules in promyelocytic blasts. Aggressive blood product support and early treatment with the differentiation-inducing agent all-*trans* retinoic acid (ATRA) has been shown to decrease the risk of bleeding in APL. Despite these measures, up to 10% of patients die of bleeding complications during the initial weeks of therapy, and additional patients suffer lasting morbidity from retinal hemorrhages and nonfatal central nervous system hemorrhages.

Tracheal compression and superior vena cava syndrome can result from large anterior mediastinal masses, which are commonly present in T-cell ALL but are rare in other forms of leukemia. Patients can present with respiratory distress, cough, orthopnea, headaches, syncope, dizziness, facial swelling, or plethora. A chest x-ray should be performed to assess the mediastinum in any patient suspected to have ALL. If the mediastinum is enlarged, a CT is indicated to assess airway patency. This evaluation must precede any attempts at sedation for diagnostic procedures, because even light sedation can precipitate acute airway collapse. Diagnostic material should be obtained by the least invasive method possible before treatment. If necessary, emergent airway compromise can be treated with radiation or steroids, or both.

Differential Diagnosis

Although leukemia should be considered in cases of isolated neutropenia, anemia, or thrombocytopenia, the vast majority of leukemia patients present with depressions in more than one cell line. In suspected cases of immune thrombocytopenic purpura (ITP), for example, a careful review of the peripheral blood smear should be performed to rule out the presence of circulating leukemic blasts. Routine bone marrow aspiration is not necessary for children with ITP, but it should be performed in patients with atypical features, such as concomitant anemia or neutropenia, hepatosplenomegaly, bone pain, or significant weight loss. Treatment of ITP with corticosteroids should only be instituted after evaluation by an experienced hematologist.

Pancytopenia can be caused by diseases other than leukemia. Some viral infections have a propensity to suppress bone marrow function and cause low peripheral blood cell counts, including Epstein–Barr virus (EBV), herpes simplex virus (HSV), influenza, hepatitis viruses, and HIV. Infectious mononucleosis from EBV infection can be particularly difficult to differentiate from leukemia, because patients often have hepatosplenomegaly and circulating atypical lymphocytes (which can appear very similar to leukemic blasts). Pancytopenia on the basis of bone marrow failure (from acquired aplastic anemia or rare inherited bone marrow failure syndromes) can be distinguished from leukemia by bone marrow biopsy for assessment of overall marrow cellularity. Certain solid tumors have a tendency to metastasize to the bone marrow and cause cytopenias, including neuroblastoma, rhabdomyosarcoma, and retinoblastoma, but it is rare for pancytopenia to be the primary presenting feature in these cases.

Joint pain, fever, hepatosplenomegaly, and pallor are common presenting features in both systemic-onset juvenile rheumatoid arthritis (JRA) and leukemia. A bone marrow aspirate should be performed to rule out leukemia before treatment with steroids in suspected cases of systemic-onset JRA.

Risk Stratification

In the last several years, treatment decisions for children with newly diagnosed acute leukemia have been based on the concept of risk stratification. Using factors identified during clinical trials to predict a high or low risk of relapse, patients are separated into risk groups before the start of treatment or at the end of the first month of induction therapy. The treatment plan is then tailored to the degree of risk. The desired result is that patients with relatively low-risk disease can be treated with less toxic therapy without compromising cure rates, and patients with high-risk disease receive more-intensive, potentially toxic therapy. The risk groups are currently defined based on several criteria and differ for ALL and AML. Different centers and cooperative groups typically employ different risk-stratification strategies.

In ALL, the initial risk assessment is based on two simple clinical parameters that are available immediately at the time of diagnosis (the National Cancer Institute [NCI] or Rome criteria): WBC count (>50,000/µL is high risk), and age (<1 year or >9 years is high risk). Further refinement of risk assignment is often based on a combination of leukemia phenotype (B- vs T-lineage), the presence of certain sentinel cytogenetic lesions, and how quickly the patient's leukemia responds to the first few weeks of therapy (rapid clearance of leukemia cells from the blood or marrow is associated with a lower risk of relapse).

Low-risk cytogenetic features include hyperdiploidy (≥50 chromosomes in the leukemia cells) or trisomies of specific chromosomes and the presence of a t(12;21) that results in *TEL/AML1* fusion.

High-risk cytogenetic features include hypodiploidy (<44 chromosomes in the leukemia cells) and the presence of either an 11q23 (*MLL* gene) rearrangement or a t(9;22), or Philadelphia chromosome, that creates a *BCR/ABL* fusion gene.

Early response has historically been measured by the response to a prednisone prophase that includes a single dose of intrathecal methotrexate and 7 days of prednisone, or by the percentage of blast cells remaining in the bone marrow after 7 to 14 days of multiagent therapy. Over the past 10 to 15 years, measures of tumor burden remaining in the marrow at the end of induction therapy (minimal residual disease) have been shown to be highly predictive of outcome and have been integrated into risk-stratification schemata of all of the major leukemia cooperative groups.

In AML, risk stratification is based largely on cytogenetics. Low-risk features include a t(8;21), which results in the *AML1/ETO* fusion, and either inv(16) or a t(16;16), both of which create the *CBFβ/MYH11* fusion. High-risk features include monosomy 7 and abnormalities in the long arm of chromosome 5. In addition to these cytogenetic abnormalities, failure to achieve remission with induction chemotherapy is another high-risk feature in AML. All other cytogenetic abnormalities, as well as normal cytogenetics (which are seen in approximately 60% of cases), are considered intermediate risk. More recently, a specific type of genetic mutation in the tyrosine kinase gene *FLT3* has been identified as another high-risk feature. This type of *FLT3* mutation (called an internal tandem duplication [ITD]) occurs in 10% to 15% of childhood AML.

Treatment

There are significant differences in the specific treatments for ALL and AML, so they will be discussed separately. Table 4 summarizes the most salient features of the treatment for each.

ACUTE LYMPHOBLASTIC LEUKEMIA

Treatment for ALL generally occurs in four phases: remission induction, CNS preventive therapy, consolidation, and maintenance. Remission induction in ALL typically lasts 4 to 6 weeks and includes three to five systemic agents. Common to almost all regimens are a corticosteroid (either prednisone [Deltasone] or dexamethasone [Decadron]), vincristine [Vincasar], and L-asparaginase [Elspar], which compose the three-drug induction. An anthracycline, typically doxorubicin (Adriamycin), is also included in many regimens (four-drug induction), with other agents such as cyclophosphamide (Cytoxan) or etoposide (VePesid) used in a small minority of centers. More than 98% of children enter remission by the end of 4 weeks of induction therapy, and the mortality rate from toxicity during induction therapy is generally less than 2% to 3% in industrialized countries.

The concept that the CNS could be a sanctuary site for leukemia emerged in the mid 1960s when the introduction of multiagent systemic chemotherapy led to high remission rates, but a majority of patients relapsed within 6 to 12 months, with many of these recurrences being limited to the CNS. Routine introduction of presymptomatic CNS radiation in the late 1960s and early 1970s led to substantial increases in cure rates to approximately 50%. Modern CNS preventive therapy includes periodic administration of intrathecal chemotherapy (usually methotrexate) starting at the time of the first diagnostic lumbar puncture. Systemic agents with improved CNS penetration (dexamethasone rather than prednisone, higher doses of intravenous methotrexate) might also play an important role in CNS control. Cranial irradiation is currently reserved for patients at the highest risk for CNS relapse (e.g., those with high diagnostic WBC count or leukemic blasts in CSF at diagnosis). Over time, CNS radiation has been given to fewer and fewer ALL patients; some groups believe that it can be eliminated for all patients. With these modern strategies, the risk of isolated CNS relapse is less than 5%.

Following the induction of remission, patients receive additional chemotherapy designed to consolidate the remission. The intensity and duration of the consolidation phase are risk based, and

TABLE 4 Summary of Treatment for Childhood Leukemia

Characteristics	Acute Lymphoblastic Leukemia	Acute Myeloid Leukemia
Remission Induction		
Chemotherapy	4 wk with prednisone or dexamethasone, vincristine, L-asparaginase, doxorubicin (not all cases)	Two courses (6-8 wk) with cytarabine (Ara-C), doxorubicin, others (e.g., etoposide, thioguanine)
Toxic death rate	Low (<3%)	High (>10%)
Remission rate	>98%	75%-85%
CNS Preventive Therapy		
Intrathecal chemotherapy	Methotrexate	Cytarabine
Cranial irradiation	For high risk (blasts in CSF at diagnosis and/or high WBC count)	None
Consolidation		
Chemotherapy	Combinations of various drugs (not cross-resistant) Intensity/duration based on risk stratification	Based on cytogenetic risk group Low risk: 2-3 additional courses Intermediate risk: BMT for patients with HLA-matched related donors High risk: BMT for patients with any suitable donor (including unrelated)
Maintenance		
Chemotherapy	Low-dose oral (6-mercaptopurine and methotrexate) Total duration of therapy 2-3 y	No maintenance therapy (does not improve survival)

BMT = bone marrow transplant; CNS = central nervous system; CSF = cerebrospinal fluid; HLA = human leukocyte antigen; WBC = white blood cell.

alternating cycles of non–cross-resistant chemotherapy drugs are typically used. These consolidation or intensification phases typically last about 6 months and often include a reinduction phase similar to the first month of treatment.

It has been clearly demonstrated that the risk of relapse in ALL can be reduced with an extended phase of continuous low-dose chemotherapy (maintenance) that lasts until 2 to 3 years from the time of diagnosis. Oral 6-mercaptopurine (Purinethol) and methotrexate are used universally, with variable administration of intrathecal chemotherapy. Some centers or groups also employ periodic doses of vincristine and 5- to 7-day pulses of prednisone or dexamethasone. The optimal frequency of intrathecal chemotherapy treatments and vincristine and steroid pulses is uncertain and might depend on the intensity of therapy delivered during the induction and consolidation phases.

ACUTE MYELOID LEUKEMIA

Remission induction in AML typically consists of two courses of very intensive chemotherapy with cytarabine (Tarabine) and doxorubicin, often combined with thioguanine (Tabloid) or etoposide. Remission rates are 75% to 85%, with about one half of the failures due to resistant leukemia and the others to mortality from toxicity (usually infection).

Similar to ALL, CNS preventive therapy in AML begins at diagnosis with intrathecal chemotherapy (usually cytarabine) and continues with additional periodic intrathecal treatments during consolidation. High-dose cytarabine, which is a key component of most AML treatment regimens, also contributes to CNS treatment. Cranial radiation is not typically administered by most groups to children with AML, except for treatment of chloromas (solid masses of leukemia cells) that do not resolve with chemotherapy.

Consolidation in AML is risk dependent. For intermediate-risk patients, most groups have reported the best results using allogeneic bone marrow transplant (BMT) with a histocompatible (i.e., human leukocyte antigen (HLA)-identical or matched) sibling donor. However, only about 25% to 30% of children with AML with have a matched sibling donor. For the remaining intermediate-risk patients, consolidation consists of two to three additional chemotherapy courses that are slightly less intense and usually consist of cytarabine combined with drugs not used in induction such as mitoxantrone (Novantrone) and L-asparaginase. High-risk patients can be identified who have a less than 20% to 25% chance of cure with intensive chemotherapy. Most groups consider these patients to be candidates for BMT. If a matched sibling is unavailable, then alternative donor sources (e.g., matched unrelated bone marrow or umbilical cord blood) are usually offered. For low-risk patients, for whom the cure rate with chemotherapy alone approaches 70%, BMT is usually not offered in first remission, even for patients with a matched sibling donor. In addition, relapses in low-risk patients, unlike relapses in intermediate-risk or high-risk patients, can often be successfully treated with BMT in second remission, justifying reserving BMT for use as a salvage therapy for low-risk patients. Unlike ALL, most groups have found no benefit to extended maintenance therapy in children with AML.

Relapse

The most common site of relapsed leukemia is the bone marrow (with or without concomitant CNS involvement). Less common are isolated extramedullary relapses (CNS or testicular relapse in ALL, chloromas in AML). For both ALL and AML, a critical determinant of outcome following relapse is the time from diagnosis to relapse.

ALL patients who relapse within 18 months of initial diagnosis have a dismal outcome, with only about one half able to attain a second remission and less than 10% overall cure rate; the outcome is marginally better for those who relapse between 18 and 36 months after diagnosis. ALL patients with such early relapses are typically treated with 3 to 4 months of intensive therapy in an attempt to achieve a second remission and attain further cytoreduction, followed by BMT using a matched sibling or unrelated donor. In contrast, children with ALL who relapse more than 3 years after initial diagnosis have an approximately 95% chance of entering a second remission, and 40% to 45% can be cured with intensive chemotherapy; these patients are generally considered to be candidates for matched sibling, but not unrelated donor, BMT in second remission.

Overall, relapsed AML has a dismal outcome (long-term survival approximately 20%), and the approach is to attempt to reinduce remission and then proceed to BMT or investigational treatments. Even in this setting, there is clearly an improved outcome for

TABLE 5 Summary of Late Effects of Leukemia Treatment

Late Effect	Treatment-Related Risk Factors	Diagnostic Approach
Bone	Avascular necrosis, osteonecrosis	X-ray and/or MRI of major joints for persistent pain
Cardiac dysfunction	Anthracyclines: cardiomyopathy (risk related to cumulative dose, higher risk in AML)	ECG or echocardiogram every 3 y (cardiomyopathy can occur decades after treatment)
Cataracts	CNS RT	Yearly eye exam
CNS and psychosocial	CNS RT, IT chemotherapy: learning problems, neurocognitive dysfunction	Yearly educational assessment, neurocognitive testing
Dental abnormalities	CNS RT	Dental exam at age 5
Endocrine and reproductive	CNS RT: pituitary dysfunction Alkylators: primary gonadal failure	Yearly growth curves, TSH, LH, FSH LH, FSH, estradiol or testosterone, semen analysis
Hepatic dysfunction	Methotrexate, 6-mercaptopurine, 6-thioguanine: late hepatic fibrosis	Yearly LFTs
Secondary neoplasms	CNS RT: brain tumors Alkylators or epipodophyllotoxins: secondary AML	MRI for symptoms Yearly CBC

ALL = acute lymphoblastic leukemia; AML = acute myeloid leukemia; CNS = central nervous system; ECG = electrocardiogram; FSH = follicle stimulating hormone; IT = intrathecal; LFT = liver function test; LH = leutenizing hormone; MRI = magnetic resonance imaging; RT = radiation therapy; TSH = thyroid stimulating hormone.

---

patients who relapse after a prolonged initial remission (>12 months from the end of remission-induction therapy) compared with patients who have refractory disease or who relapse after a shorter period of remission.

New treatment strategies are urgently needed for patients with relapsed ALL and AML, because the current regimens produce poor results and are associated with a great deal of toxicity. The major clinical trial groups are testing novel and targeted therapies in these patient populations.

Late Effects

Approximately 70% of children with leukemia are cured of their disease. As the numbers of long-term survivors of childhood leukemia has grown, there has been increasing interest in assessing the late effects of leukemic therapy. In childhood ALL, with cure rates of 85%, a major effort is being made in ongoing clinical trials to reduce the intensity of therapy for lower-risk patients, with the hope of reducing late effects of therapy without compromising high cure rates. The most common late effects of leukemia therapy, with the known treatment-related risk factors and recommended diagnostic approach for each, are summarized in Table 5. Many pediatric oncology centers have developed late-effects programs to conduct surveillance for the development of these problems and provide follow-up care to patients who develop late complications of therapy.

REFERENCES

Brown P, Small D: FLT3 inhibitors: A paradigm for the development of targeted therapeutics for paediatric cancer. Eur J Cance 2004;40:707-721.

Gaynon PS, Qu RP, Chappell RJ, et al: Survival after relapse in childhood acute lymphoblastic leukemia: Impact of site and time to first relapse—the Children's Cancer Group Experience. Cancer 1998;82:1387-1395.

Gibson BE, Wheatley K, Hann IM, et al: Treatment strategy and long-term results in paediatric patients treated in consecutive UK AML trials. Leukemia 2005;19:2130-2138.

Greaves MF, Wiemels J: Origins of chromosome translocations in childhood leukaemia. Nat Rev Cancer 2003;3:639-649.

Hitzler JK, Zipursky A: Origins of leukaemia in children with Down syndrome. Nat Rev Cancer 2005;5:11-20.

Meshinchi S, Alonzo TA, Stirewalt DL, et al: Clinical implications of FLT3 mutations in pediatric AML. Blood 2006;108:3654-3661.

Moghrabi A, Levy DE, Asselin B, et al: Results of the Dana–Farber Cancer Institute ALL Consortium Protocol 95-01 for children with acute lymphoblastic leukemia. Blood 2007;109:896-904.

Mrozek K, Heinonen K, Bloomfield CD: Clinical importance of cytogenetics in acute myeloid leukaemia. Best Pract Res Clin Haematol 2001;14:19-47.

Pinkel D, Simone J, Hustu HO, Aur RJ: Nine years' experience with "total therapy" of childhood acute lymphocytic leukemia. Pediatrics 1972;50:246-251.

Pui CH, Cheng C, Leung W, et al: Extended follow-up of long-term survivors of childhood acute lymphoblastic leukemia. N Engl J Med 2003;349:640-649.

Pui CH, Evans WE: Treatment of acute lymphoblastic leukemia. N Engl J Med 2006;354:166-178.

Pui CH, Mahmoud HH, Rivera GK, et al: Early intensification of intrathecal chemotherapy virtually eliminates central nervous system relapse in children with acute lymphoblastic leukemia. Blood 1998;92:411-415.

Pui CH, Sandlund JT, Pei D, et al: Improved outcome for children with acute lymphoblastic leukemia: Results of Total Therapy Study XIIIB at St Jude Children's Research Hospital. Blood 2004;104:2690-2696.

Ries LAG, Melbert D, Krapcho M, et al: SEER Cancer Statistics Review, 1975-2004. Bethesda, Md: National Cancer Institute, 2007.

Schrappe M, Reiter A, Zimmermann M, et al: Long-term results of four consecutive trials in childhood ALL performed by the ALL-BFM study group from 1981 to 1995. Berlin–Frankfurt–Munster. Leukemia. 2000;14:2205-2222.

Stahnke K, Boos J, Bender-Gotze C, et al: Duration of first remission predicts remission rates and long-term survival in children with relapsed acute myelogenous leukemia. Leukemia 1998;12:1534-1538.

Wakeford R, Little MP: Risk coefficients for childhood cancer after intrauterine irradiation: A review. Int J Radiat Biol 2003;79:293-309.

Woods WG, Kobrinsky N, Buckley JD, et al: Timed-sequential induction therapy improves postremission outcome in acute myeloid leukemia: A report from the Children's Cancer Group. Blood 1996;87:4979-4989.

Woods WG, Neudorf S, Gold S, et al: A comparison of allogeneic bone marrow transplantation, autologous bone marrow transplantation, and aggressive chemotherapy in children with acute myeloid leukemia in remission. Blood 2001;97:56-62.

Chronic Leukemias

Method of
Jorge E. Cortes, MD, Hagop M. Kantarjian, MD, and William Wierda, MD, PhD

Chronic Myeloid Leukemia

CLINICAL FEATURES AND DIAGNOSIS

Chronic myelogenous leukemia (CML) is a clonal myeloproliferative disorder characterized by leukocytosis and the presence of immature white blood cells (WBCs) in the peripheral blood with all maturation stages present. Bone marrow examination reveals a hypercellular

CURRENT DIAGNOSIS

Chronic Myeloid Leukemia

- Initial Evaluation
  - History: Visual disturbances, neurologic symptoms, abdominal pain, weight loss, or fever
  - Physical examination: Degree of splenomegaly, signs of leukostasis (visual abnormalities, priapism, focal neurologic deficits), chloromas
  - Peripheral blood: CBC with differential, blood chemistry analysis, molecular ratio (BCR-ABL/ABL ratio by real-time PCR), FISH
  - Bone marrow: Morphology, cytogenetics, BCR-ABL/ABL ratio
  - The diagnosis of CML is established by the presence of the Philadelphia chromosome and/or the BCR-ABL rearrangement
  - Bone marrow aspiration for morphology is necessary for adequate stage classification
- Follow-up
  - CBC: Every 1-2 weeks until counts stabilize (usually 2-3 mo), then every 6-12 weeks
  - Cytogenetic: Every 3-6 months until CCyR, then every 12 months. After major molecular response, less frequent depending on clinical, hematologic, and molecular findings
  - FISH: Can be used to monitor cytogenetic response until down to 5% to 10% Ph$^+$
  - PCR: Every 3-6 months

Chronic Lymphocytic Leukemia

- Initial Diagnosis
  - Absolute lymphocytosis (>5000 lymphocytes/μL)
  - Well-differentiated, monotonous-appearing lymphocytes
  - <55% blood prolymphocytes
  - Flow cytometry on blood: monoclonal light chain, CD19$^+$, CD23$^+$, CD5$^+$
  - Evaluation of prognostic factors
  - β$_2$ Microglobulin
  - FISH for 17p del, 11q del, +12, 13q del (sole)
  - IgV$_H$ mutation status
  - ZAP70 expression
  - CD38 expression

CBC = complete blood count; CCyR = complete cytogenetic response; CML = chronic myeloid leukemia; FISH = fluorescent in situ hybridization; Ph = Philadelphia chromosome; PCR = polymerase chain reaction.

---

marrow with myeloid hyperplasia. The hallmark of the disease is the presence of the Philadelphia (Ph) chromosome, which represents a balanced translocation between the long arms of chromosomes 9 and 22: t(9;22)(q34;q11.2). This juxtaposes the *c-abl* gene located in chromosome 9q34 with the *bcr* gene located in chromosome 22q11.2. The chimeric *BCR-ABL* gene translates into a protein (p210$^{Bcr/Abl}$) that is a tyrosine kinase with increased kinase activity that promotes cellular proliferation and suppresses apoptosis. This kinase activity is critical to the development of CML.

The manifesting features of CML have changed over time. In the past, most patients presented with fatigue, fever, or other features of leukostasis (e.g., headache, priapism) and splenomegaly (e.g., right upper quadrant pain). Now, approximately 70% of patients are asymptomatic and diagnosis is based on a routine blood examination.

NATURAL HISTORY

CML usually runs a biphasic or triphasic course, with an initial chronic phase that, unless adequately treated, eventually transforms into a blastic phase resembling an acute leukemia. An intermediate or accelerated phase precedes the blastic phase in 60% to 80% of patients. Although no definition of these stages is universally accepted, some of the most commonly used criteria are presented in Table 1. Historically, the median survival of patients in chronic, accelerated, and blastic phases was 4 to 5 years, 6 to 18 months, and 2 to 6 months, respectively. Modern therapy with tyrosine kinase inhibitors has significantly improved the outcome, with 95% survival at 5 years for patients in the chronic phase.

Clinical features at diagnosis help segregate patients into different prognostic categories. The most commonly used prognostic system is the Sokal score. In this system, the hazard ratio for death is calculated from baseline characteristics using the following formula:

$$\lambda^i(+)/\lambda_o(t) = \text{Exp } 0.0116 \text{ (age} - 43.4) + 0.0345 \text{ (spleen} - 7.51)$$
$$+ 0.188 \, [(\text{platelets}/700)^2 - 0.563] + 0.0887 \text{ (blasts} - 2.10)$$

Three prognostic groups are identified with hazard ratios of less than 0.8, 0.8 to 1.2, and greater than 1.2, and historical median survivals of 2.5, 3.5, and 4.5 years, respectively.

INITIAL EVALUATION AND TREATMENT OBJECTIVES

The diagnosis of CML requires the documentation of the Philadelphia chromosome or its corresponding gene rearrangement, BCR-ABL. In 90% to 95% of patients this is found in a karyotype analysis; in all others it can be identified by polymerase chain reaction (PCR). To properly diagnose and stage CML, all patients need a bone marrow aspiration at the time of diagnosis. In addition, the BCR-ABL/ABL ratio should be determined in peripheral blood or bone marrow. Although PCR results obtained from both sources correlate well with each other, it is not recommended to use them interchangeably. Thus, it is better to measure BCR-ABL transcripts in peripheral blood because it is easier to monitor more frequently during therapy.

Conventional chemotherapy with hydroxyurea (Hydrea) or busulfan (Myleran) was used for many years to control the WBC count and splenomegaly (i.e., hematologic response). However, a hematologic response alone does not change the natural history of the disease. With the introduction of interferon (IFN)-α, cytogenetic responses (disappearance of the Philadelphia chromosome) were for the first time achieved in up to 50% to 60% of patients. The response criteria used for patients with CML are detailed in Box 1. Complete cytogenetic response (CCyR) is associated with an improved survival probability of 78% at 10 years compared with 25% to 40% for those with lesser responses. The goal of therapy therefore became to eliminate the malignant clone represented by the Philadelphia chromosome (cytogenetic response). In addition, approximately 30% of patients with CCyR after IFN-α had undetectable disease by PCR; none of them has relapsed after a median follow-up of 10 years and are therefore probably cured. With imatinib, most patients can achieve a CCyR, and the achieving molecular response is more likely and might further improve the long-term outcome. Thus, proper monitoring is required during therapy to ensure adequate response and optimize the long-term outcome. An approach to the work-up and management of patients with newly diagnosed CML is summarized in the Current Diagnosis box.

Treatment

The first line of therapy for patients with CML is imatinib 400 mg daily. Patients should be monitored closely with cytogenetics and PCR to ensure that treatment goals are met at specific times. If this is the case, treatment should be continued indefinitely, avoiding unnecessary dose reductions or treatment interruptions. Patients who fail imatinib should be offered therapy with a second-generation

TABLE 1 Criteria for Accelerated Phase

Feature	MDACC	IBMTR	WHO
Blasts	15%-29%	10%-29%	10%-19%[†]
Blasts + promyelocytes	30%	20%	NA
Basophils	20%	20%*	20%
Platelets	<100	Unresponsive increase or persistent decrease	<100 $\cdot$ 10^9/L, or >1000 $\cdot$ 10^9/L unresponsive to treatment
Cytogenetics	CE	CE	CE not at the time of diagnosis
WBC	NA	Difficult to control, or doubling in <5 d	NA
Anemia	NA	Unresponsive	NA
Splenomegaly	NA	Increasing	NA
Other	NA	Chloromas, myelofibrosis	Megakaryocyte proliferation, fibrosis

*Basophils plus eosinophils.
CE = clonal evolution; IBMTR = International Bone Marrow Transplant Registry; MDACC = MD Anderson Cancer Center; NA = not applicable; WBC = white blood cell count; WHO = World Health Organization.

tyrosine kinase inhibitor (dasatinib, nilotinib). Stem cell transplantation (SCT) should be considered for patients who have failed imatinib, and in many instances it is considered as third option if a second-generation tyrosine kinase inhibitor has also failed. There is no significant cross-resistance between these agents, so patients who fail imatinib and one second-generation tyrosine kinase inhibitor sometimes respond to a different second-generation inhibitor.

Patients in accelerated-phase CML might still respond well to imatinib. Although responses can be observed in patients in blast phase, these are usually transient, and SCT should be considered after returning to chronic phase.

IMATINIB MESYLATE

Imatinib (Gleevec) is an orally administered tyrosine kinase inhibitor. By inhibiting *BCR-ABL*, it blocks proliferation and induces apoptosis of *BCR-ABL*–expressing cells. Imatinib has become the standard therapy for CML due to its remarkable activity and mild toxicity profile.

The efficacy of imatinib in chronic-phase CML was established in a randomized study in patients with CML in chronic phase compared with the combination of IFN-α (Intron A) and cytarabine (Tarabine). After 5 years of follow-up, the projected CCyR rate with imatinib was 87%, with most responses occurring by 12 months of therapy.

BOX 1 Response Criteria in Chronic Myelogenous Leukemia

Hematologic Remission

Complete: Normalization of peripheral counts and differential, and disappearance of all signs and symptoms of CML including splenomegaly

Cytogenetic Remission (Major Cytogenic Response)*

Complete: 0% Ph$^+$ metaphases
Partial: 1% to 34% Ph$^+$ metaphases
Minor: 35% to 95% Ph$^+$ metaphases
None: >95% Ph$^+$ metaphases

Molecular Remission[†]

Complete: Undetectable *BCR-ABL* transcripts
Major: ≥3-log reduction in *BCR-ABL/ABL* from standardized baseline or a ratio of <0.1% on a proposed international scale

*Cytogenetic response is based on a routine karyotype analyzing at least 20 metaphases.
[†]Molecular response is based on real-time polymerase chain reaction.
CML = Chronic myelogenous leukemia.

Responses are durable, with an event-free survival of 83% at 6 years of follow-up and overall survival of 95%. This compares favorably with the 50% 5-year survival with prior therapies.

Earlier responses are associated with improved outcome. Patients with CCyR or PCyR at 12 months from start of therapy have a 93% to 97% probability of being alive and free from transformation to accelerated or blast phase, compared to 81% for those without CCyR or PCyR. Among patients who achieved a CCyR by 12 months of therapy, 100% of those with a major molecular response (MMR) (*BCR-ABL/ABL* <0.1% on an international harmonized scale, or ≥3-log reduction from a standardized baseline) were alive and free from transformation at 5 years, compared to 95% for those with CCyR but not MMR.

The standard dose of imatinib is 400 mg daily. Among patients who fail imatinib therapy, increasing their dose from 400 mg to 800 mg daily induces a major cytogenetic response in 40% to 50%. Some studies have suggested that initiating therapy with 800 mg daily on diagnosis may be associated with improved outcome. These observations are being confirmed in randomized trials.

Management of Toxicity

Imatinib is overall well tolerated. Although some adverse events occur in 30% to 40% of patients, these are usually mild and manageable. The most commonly encountered side effects and suggestions for management are included in Box 2. Grade 3 or 4 toxicity that is related to imatinib requires treatment interruption. When toxicity resolves to grade 1, treatment should be resumed, usually at a reduced dose, but doses less than 300 mg daily are not recommended. Less than 5% of patients are intolerant to imatinib and require change of therapy.

Myelosuppression is a more common adverse event. Dose interruptions are not recommended unless the patient develops grade-3 neutropenia or thrombocytopenia (neutrophils <10^9/L, platelets <50 × 10^9/L). Treatment is restarted when counts recover above these thresholds. If recovery occurs within 2 weeks, treatment is resumed at the same dose. If recovery takes longer than 2 weeks, the dose can be reduced (e.g., from 600 mg to 400 mg, or from 400 mg to 300 mg). Most commonly, myelosuppression occurs within the first 2 to 3 months of therapy, is self-limited, and does not lead to clinical consequences. No interruptions or dose adjustments are usually recommended for anemia.

Monitoring Patients

Adequate monitoring is needed to optimize treatment outcome. The primary goal of therapy is to achieve CCyR. In addition, achieving an MMR can improve the probability of a durable remission and transformation-free survival. However, although achieving a molecular response is an important objective, failure to achieve MMR or increasing transcript levels should not by itself be considered therapy failure. A description of the techniques and proposed guidelines for monitoring patients is presented earlier and in the Current Diagnosis box.

CURRENT THERAPY

Chronic Myeloid Leukemia
- Therapy Initiation
  - Initiate imatinib (Gleevec) 400 mg/day as soon as the diagnosis is confirmed
  - Educate patients and family members about objectives of therapy, adequate monitoring, importance of dose, and potential adverse events
- Therapeutic Monitoring
  - Weekly CBC and blood chemistry weekly until counts are stable, then every 4-6 weeks.
  - Monitor for adverse events; identify adverse events early and manage them properly
  - Cytogenetic analysis and bone marrow aspirate every 3-6 months until CCyR, then every 12 months
  - PCR every 3 months in peripheral blood; frequency may be decreased to every 6 months after stable major molecular response is achieved
- Dose Modifications
  - Interrupt imatinib for grades 3-4 nonhematologic toxicities, then resume with dose reduction (i.e., from 800 mg to 600 mg, from 600 mg to 400 mg, from 400 mg to 300 mg).
  - Reduce dose schedule by 25% for grade 2 persistent chronic toxicities.
  - Interrupt imatinib for grades 3-4 hematologic toxicities (i.e., ANC $<10^9$/L, platelets $<50 \times 10^9$/L). Resume therapy once counts recover above these levels. If recovery is within 2 weeks, restart at same dose. Reduce as per nonhematologic toxicity if recovery takes >2 weeks.
- Suboptimal Response
  - Assess compliance and measure imatinib plasma levels
  - Optimize therapy; consider dose increase (i.e, from 300 mg to 600 mg or from 400 mg to 800 mg)
- Failure to Imatinib
  - Assess for mutations of the Abl kinase domain
  - Change therapy to dasatinib (Sprycel) 100 mg daily (70 mg bid for patients in accelerated or blast phase) or nilotinib (Tasigna) 400 mg bid

Chronic Lymphocytic Leukemia
- Initial Evaluation
  - History: Fatigue, weight loss, fever, bleeding, recurrent infections, new adenopathy or change in previously noted adenopathy, prior blood work
  - Physical examination: Extent of lymphadenopathy, degree of splenomegaly and hepatomegaly, signs of infection or anemia
  - Laboratory: CBC with differential, blood chemistry analysis, tests for β_2-microglobulin and LDH levels, immunophenotyping, and HLA typing.
  - Prognostic factors: FISH for 17p del, 11q del, +12, and 13q del; IgV$_H$ gene mutation status; ZAP70 expression; CD38 expression
  - Bone marrow (optional): Morphology, immunophenotyping, metaphase karyotpying
- Initial Management:
  - Determine need for therapy (symptoms, stage, lymphocyte doubling time).
  - If WBC count $>2 \times 10^{11}$/L, consider admission, hydration, allopurinol (Zyloprim) therapy, and leukapheresis followed by chemotherapy.
  - Treat patients with autoimmune disorders with corticosteroids.
- Subsequent Management:
  - Patients are encouraged to participate in clinical trials.
  - Patients requiring therapy and but who are ineligible for investigational therapy can receive fludarabine-based therapy. A combination of fludarabine plus cyclophosphamide ± rituximab is preferable for younger patients.
  - Patients who have failed fludarabine-based therapy should be offered alemtuzumab.
  - Allogeneic stem cell transplant might be considered for patients who have failed fludarabine-based regimens.

BMT = bone marrow transplantation; CBC = complete blood count; CCyR = complete cytogenetic response; CML = chronic myeloid leukemia; FISH = fluorescent in situ hybridization; HLA = human leukocyte antigen; IgV$_H$ = Ig heavy chain variable gene; Ph = Philadelphia chromosome; LDH = lactate dehydrogenase; PCR = polymerase chain reaction; WBC = white blood cell.

Imatinib Failure

Despite the favorable results achieved with imatinib, approximately 10% to 15% of patients lose their response after 5 years. Several mechanisms of resistance have been described, including amplification or overexpression of *BCR-ABL* or its protein product, point mutations of the Abl kinase domain, a defective transporter (OCT-1) of imatinib into the cell, overexpression of the multidrug-resistance (MDR) phenotype, and overexpression of Src-related kinases. Among them, mutations in the Abl kinase domain is the most commonly identified, occurring in 40% to 60% of patients who develop resistance to imatinib. More than 50 different mutations have been described. Although some mutations retain relative sensitivity to imatinib, others, particularly T315I, are nearly completely insensitive.

Imatinib failure can be defined based on the response achieved and the time to achieve such response. The current definitions of failure are presented in Table 2. Patients who meet these criteria have a significantly worse outcome, with a median survival of only 5 years in chronic phase and much shorter in the advanced stages.

In addition, some patients have a suboptimal response to therapy. These patients have an outcome that is not quite as poor as that of patients with failure, but they do not have the same favorable outcome as those with what would be considered to be an optimal response.

Second-Line Therapy

A second generation of tyrosine kinase inhibitors has been developed to treat patients who develop resistance or intolerance to imatinib. Two agents have been already approved and others are being investigated.

Dasatinib (Sprycel) is a dual inhibitor of Abl and Src-related kinases. It is approximately 300 times more potent than imatinib against Abl and inhibits most mutated variants, except T315I. Studies with dasatinib in patients who have failed imatinib have demonstrated significant efficacy. In the chronic phase, nearly 50% of patients have achieved a complete cytogenetic response, with approximately 90% of patients alive and free from progression after 12 months.

BOX 2 Recommended Management of the Most Common Adverse Events Associated with Imatinib

Nausea and Vomiting
Take with food, fluids
Antiemetics

Diarrhea
Loperamide (Imodium)
Diphenoxylate atropine (Lomotil)

Peripheral Edema
Diuretics

Periorbital Edema
Steroid-containing cream

Rash
Avoid sun exposure
Topical steroids
Systemic steroids
(Early intervention is important)

Muscle Cramps
Tonic water or quinine
Electrolyte replacement as needed
Calcium gluconate

Arthralgia, Bone Pain
Nonsteroidal antiinflamatory agents

Elevated Transaminases (uncommon)
Hold therapy and monitor closely
Dose reduction upon resolution

Myelosuppression

Anemia
Treatment interruption and dose reduction are usually not indicated
Erythropoietin (Procrit) or darbopoetin (Aranesp)

Neutropenia
Hold therapy if grade ≥3 (i.e., ANC <1×10^9/L)
Consider G-CSF (Neupogen) if recurrent or persistent neutropenia or with sepsis

Thrombocytopenia
Hold therapy if grade ≥3 (platelets <50 ×10^9/L)
Consider IL-11 10 µg/kg 3-7 days/week

ANC = absolute neutrophil count; G-CSF = granulocyte colony-stimulating factor; IL = interleukin.

TABLE 2 Definitions of Failure and Suboptimal Response to Imatinib According to the European Leukemianet

Time (mo)	Failure	Suboptimal
3	No HR	No CHR
6	No CHR	35% Ph$^+$
	100% Ph$^+$	
12	35% Ph$^+$	5% Ph$^+$
18	5% Ph$^+$	No MMR (<3-log ↓ BCR-ABL/ABL)
Any	Loss of CHR	CE
	Loss of CCgR	Loss of MMR
	Mutation	Mutation

CCgR = complete cytogenetic response; CE = clonal evolution; CHR = complete hematologic remission; HR = hematologic remission; MMR = major molecular response; Ph+ = Philadelphia chromosome positive.

disease have suggested that a once-daily dose (100 mg in chronic phase, 140 mg in accelerated phase) may be better tolerated, with decreased incidence of myelosuppression (in chronic phase) and other nonhematologic adverse events such as pleural effusions and gastrointestinal hemorrhage. The approved dose for chronic phase is now 100 mg once daily.

Nilotinib (Tasigna) is a more selective Abl tyrosine kinase inhibitor structurally similar to imatinib. Nilotinib is approximately 30 times more potent than imatinib against Abl, including most of the known mutants, but not more potent against other kinases. Phase II studies with nilotinib after imatinib failure have demonstrated significant activity among patients with resistance or intolerance to imatinib with CCyR in more than 40% of patients. Despite the similar biochemical structure, there is minimal cross-intolerance between imatinib and nilotinib. The standard dose of nilotinib is 400 mg twice daily. Myelosuppression grade 3 or 4 occurs in approximately 30% of patients. Other adverse events include elevation of lipase or bilirubin and hypophosphatemia. All of these are usually transient and asymptomatic.

ALLOGENEIC BONE MARROW TRANSPLANTATION

Allogeneic bone marrow transplantation (BMT) is an established strategy for patients with CML. The best results are reported for young patients (≤30 years) receiving transplants early in chronic phase with a disease-free survival of approximately 70% to 80%. The overall disease-free survival is 40% to 60%, with a 10% to 20% leukemic relapse rate. Allogeneic BMT may be associated with serious morbidity and an early mortality rate of 20% to 30%. Major complications include graft-versus-host disease (GVHD), interstitial pneumonitis, serious viral and fungal infections, organ damage from the conditioning regimen, and bleeding. Improvements in supportive and conditioning regimens (e.g., intravenous busulfan) have decreased the treatment-related mortality but have not affected relapse rates. Today SCT is rarely recommended as first-line therapy in CML and is mostly reserved for second- or third-line therapy.

Chronic Lymphocytic Leukemia

INCIDENCE AND RISK FACTORS

Chronic lymphocytic leukemia (CLL) is the most common type of adult leukemia in the United States and Western Europe. It is most common in persons of European or Russian descent. CLL is a disease of older persons; the median age at diagnosis is 72 years. It is more

Dasatinib is overall well tolerated. Grade 3 neutropenia or thrombocytopenia occurs in approximately 50% of patients. This is usually transient and can be managed with temporary treatment interruptions and, occasionally, dose reductions. Among nonhematologic adverse events, fatigue, headache, diarrhea, dyspnea, and rash are the most common and are usually mild and manageable. Pleural effusions occur in 25% to 35% of patients in the chronic phase, usually grade 1 or 2, and more often in advanced stages. This is best managed with temporary treatment interruptions, diuretics, and occasionally corticosteroids.

Initially, dasatinib was used at a dose of 70 mg twice daily. However, randomized trials in both chronic and advanced-stage

TABLE 3 Differential Diagnosis of CLL

Disease	Immunophenotype sIg	CD5	CD23	CD10	CD103	Chromosome Abnormality	Morphology
CLL	Weak	++	++	-	-	Varied	Small, well-differentiated
B-PLL	Strong	/+	/+	-	-	Varied	Large, open chromatin, nucleoli
HCL	Strong	-	-	-	++	None	Villous cytoplasmic projections
SLVL	Strong	/+	/+	/+	-	Varied	Short cytoplasmic projections
FL	Strong	-;	-	++	-	t(14;18)	Follicular LN architecture
MCL	Strong	++	-	-	-	t(11;14)	Small, irregular nuclei

+ = present; - = not present; B-PLL = B-cell prolymphocytic leukemia; CLL = chronic lymphocytic leukemia; FL = follicular lymphoma; HCL = hairy cell leukemia; LN = lymph node; MCL = mantle cell lymphoma; sIg = surface immunoglobulin; SLVL = splenic lymphoma with villous lymphocytes.

common in men than women. In contrast to other leukemias, there are no definite environmental exposures associated with this disease. Approximately 10% of cases have a familial association, suggesting a genetic predisposition for some individuals.

DIAGNOSIS

CLL is diagnosed based on finding an absolute blood lymphocytosis consisting of well-differentiated cells with monoclonal immunoglobulin (Ig) light chain expression and expressing CD19, CD5, CD23, and CD20. Chronic lymphoproliferative diseases can be differentiated by morphology, immunophenotype, and cytogenetics. The malignant lymphocytes accumulate in blood and other lymphoid tissues including bone marrow, lymph nodes, spleen, and liver. The differential diagnosis is shown in Table 3.

CLINICAL STAGING AND PROGNOSTIC FACTORS

The original Rai classification characterized CLL into five stages (Table 4). This system was simplified to low-risk (0), intermediate-risk (I and II), and high-risk (III and IV) disease. The Binet system categorizes CLL into three stages: A, B, and C (see Table 4). Both Rai and Binet stages are prognostic for survival, with earlier stages having superior survival.

CLL cells are not rapidly proliferating, making it difficult to generate metaphase chromosome preparations of these cells. Fluorescence in situ hybridization (FISH) is a way to probe interphase cells for specific chromosome abnormalities. Chromosome abnormalities can be identified in leukemia cells of more than 80% of patients with CLL by FISH analysis. A hierarchical categorization was developed in which patients are grouped according to their most unfavorable FISH abnormality in the following order: 17p deletion, 11q deletion, trisomy 12, no abnormality, and 13q deletion (sole).

There are at least four distinct prognostic groups associated with specific chromosome abnormalities. The two noted unfavorable groups are those with the 17p deletion or 11q deletion, with estimated median survivals of 32 and 79 months, respectively. The del(17p) and del(11q) abnormalities are associated with loss of *P53* and *ATM* genes, respectively. Patients with a 13q deletion as a sole abnormality had the best outcome, with an estimated median survival of 133 months.

Normal germinal center B cells can undergo somatic hypermutation, a mechanism to increase the affinity of their antibody for the stimulating antigen. These mutations occur in the Ig heavy chain variable gene (IgV$_H$), predominantly the CDR3 region. The clonal expressed IgV$_H$ gene can be sequenced, and this sequence compared with the expected germline sequence to determine if the leukemia clone has undergone somatic hypermutation. Homology of 98% or greater to germline indicates an unmutated IgV$_H$ gene, and less than 98% homology indicates a mutated IgV$_H$ gene. The mutation status has prognostic importance, particularly for patients with early-stage CLL. IgV$_H$ mutation status is likely static and does not change over time. In retrospective analyses of select patient populations, survival was shorter for patients with an unmutated IgV$_H$ gene compared with those with a mutated IgV$_H$ gene. Surrogate markers for IgV$_H$ mutation status have been sought, owing to the technical complexity of sequencing the IgV$_H$ gene. As a result, expression of ZAP-70 or CD38 were correlated with having an unmutated IgV$_H$ gene and with shorter survival in retrospective studies. Prospective evaluation of all these biomarkers is needed.

TREATMENT

The National Cancer Institute Working Group proposed formal recommendations or criteria in 1996 for initiating therapy for patients with CLL. These indications include bone marrow failure

TABLE 4 Staging of Chronic Lymphocytic Leukemia

Rai Stage	Modified Rai Stage	Description	Binet Stage	Description	Approximate Median Survival (y)
0	Low risk	Lymphocytosis only	A	Two or fewer lymphoid-bearing areas	>10
1	Intermediate risk	Lymphocytosis and lymphadenopathy	B	Three or more lymphoid-bearing areas	8
2		Lymphocytosis and splenomegaly ± lymphadenopathy	—	—	>6
3	High risk	Lymphocytosis and anemia (hemoglobin, <11 g/dL)	C	Anemia (hemoglobin, <10 g/dL) or thrombocytopenia (platelets 10^8/dL)	2
4		Lymphocytosis and thrombocytopenia (platelets <10^8/dL)	—	—	<2

(anemia and thrombocytopenia), symptomatic disease, or rapidly progressing disease. Prognostic factor results are not used as indicators to initiate treatment. For patients with these indications, it is also important to exclude other confounding factors such as infection, immune thrombocytopenic purpura, or hemolytic anemia.

Historically, the approach to treatment was palliation, based on the observations that no treatment was shown to prolong survival and that no standard-dose chemotherapy or regimen results in cure. This approach focuses on improving symptoms and maintains that treatment should be nontoxic and reduce bulk of disease but does not need to result in complete remission. Historical therapy was often initiated with oral chlorambucil, with or without corticosteroids. Patients who progressed on this therapy were then treated with a combination such as cyclophosphamide (Cytoxan), vincristine (Vincasar),[1] and prednisone (Prelone) (CVP), and when this regimen failed, patients would then be treated with cyclophosphamide, doxorubicin (Adriamycin), vincristine, and prednisone (CHOP). Although this paradigm was widely followed, most patients who became refractory to chlorambucil failed to respond to these subsequent treatments.

Clinical research has been aimed at developing new treatments that prolong survival and potentially cure patients with CLL. A response-driven approach is used, based on the observation that patients who achieve complete remission live longer than those who achieve partial remission or those who fail treatment. In general, clinical trials aim to increase the complete remission rate and demonstrate prolonged remission duration with the expectation that this will result in improved survival. New drugs and combinations have dramatically expanded treatment options and are significantly improving response rates for patients with CLL.

The superiority of purine analogues compared with alkylating agents was confirmed by at least three large randomized trials. The large Intergroup trial demonstrated superior complete remission rate for patients treated with fludarabine (Fludara) (Table 5). In addition, response duration was longer for patients treated with fludarabine. Despite greater activity, no overall survival advantage was demonstrated for treatment with fludarabine.

Cyclophosphamide induces DNA interstrand cross-links as the mechanism of inducing cell death. Leukemia cells, to some extent, can recover from this damage by DNA excision repair. Excision repair is inhibited by fludarabine, thus giving a rationale for combining fludarabine with cyclophosphamide (FC). A similar rationale applies to cladribine (Leustatin)[1] combined with cyclophosphamide. Recently, results from three large randomized trials have demonstrated that patients who received FC had higher complete and overall response rates and longer progression-free survival than those treated with fludarabine alone. None of the trials showed overall survival difference between patient groups (see Table 5).

Alemtuzumab (Campath), the monoclonal antibody (mAb) against CD52, was approved for treatment of fludarabine-refractory patients with CLL. Refractoriness was defined by failure to achieve at least partial remission with the last fludarabine-based regimen or relapse within 6 months of response. In the pivotal trial of alemtuzumab, one third of patients responded (most with partial remission), and the estimated median overall survival was 16 months with alemtuzumab treatment. Higher response rates were seen in a phase II single-arm trial of alemtuzumab for previously treated, but not refractory, patients. Some of these patients were free of minimal residual disease, which correlated with longer overall survival.

[1]Not FDA approved for this indication.

TABLE 5 Randomized Trials of Chemotherapy as Initial Treatment For Chronic Lymphocytic Leukemia

Agent*	No. Pts	% CR	% OR	RD	Survival
Intergroup Study					
F: 20 mg/m² IV d 1-5 plus CHL: 20 mg/m² PO d 1 or	123	20	61	NR	55 mo OS
F: 25 mg/m² IV d 1-5 or	170	20	63	25 mo (TTP)	66 mo OS
CHL: 40 mg/m² PO d 1	181	4	37	14 mo (TTP)	56 mo OS
GCLLSG Study					
F: 30 mg/m² IV d 1-3 plus CYT: 250 mg/m² IV d 1-3 or	164	24	95	48 mo (PFS)	80% at 3 y
F: 25 mg/m² IV d 1-5	164	7	83	20 mo (PFS)	81% at 3 y
ECOG Study					
F: 20 mg/m² IV d 1-5 plus CYT: 600 mg/m² IV d 1 or	137	23	74	32 mo (PFS)	79% at 2 y
F: 25 mg/m² IV d 1-5	132	6	60	19 mo (PFS)	80% at 2 y
UK LRF Study					
F: 25 mg/m² IV d 1-3 plus CYT: 250 mg/m² IV d 1-3 or	182	38	95	43 mo (PFS)	54% at 5 y
F: 25 mg/m² IV d 1-5 or	181	15	80	23 mo (PFS)	52% at 5 y
CHL-10 mg/m² PO d 1-7	366	7	72	20 mo (PFS)	59% at 5 y
PALG Study					
CDA: 0.12 mg/kg IV d 1-5 or	166	21	77	24 mo (PFS)	50 mo OS
CDA: 0.12 mg/kg IV d 1-3 plus CYT: 650 mg/m² IV d 1 or	162	29	83	22 mo (PFS)	NR
CDA: 0.12 mg/kg IV d 1-3 plus CYT: 650 mg/m² IV d 1 plus MIT: 10 mg/m² IV d 1	151	36	80	24 mo (PFS)	NR

[1]Not FDA approved for this indication.
*All courses are 28 days

CDA = cladribine (Leustatin)[1]; CHL = chlorambucil (Leukeran); CR = complete remission; CYT = cyclophosphamide (Cytoxan); ECOG = Eastern Cooperative Oncology Group; F = fludarabine (Fludara); GCLLSG = German CLL Study Group; MIT = mitoxantrone (Novantrone)[1]; NR = not reached; OR = overall response; OS = median overall survival; PALG = Polish Adult Leukemia Group; PFS = median progression-free survival; Pts = patients; RD = median remission duration; TTP = median time-to-progression; UK LRF = United Kingdom Leukaemia Research Fund.

TABLE 6 Chemoimmunotherapy for Patients with Chronic Lymphocytic Leukemia

Treatment	Prior Treatment	No. Evaluable	% CR	% OR
FluCam Regimen (4-wk course)	Yes	36	30	83
F: 30 mg/m^2 d 1-3, courses 1-6				
A: 30 mg d 1-3, courses 1-6				
MD Anderson Cancer Center Regimen (4-wk course)	No	224	70	95
F: 25 mg/m^2 IV d 2-4, course 1; d 1-3, courses 2-6	Yes	177	25	73
C: 250 mg/m^2 IV d 2-4, course 1; d 1-3, courses 2-6				
R: 375-500 mg/m^2 IV d 1, courses 1-6				
CALGB 9712 Study, Randomized				
Concurrent (4-wk course)	No	51	47	90
F: 25 mg/m^2 IV d 1-5, courses 1-6				
R: 375 mg/m^2 IV d 1 and 4, course 1; d1, courses 2-6				
2 months' observation, then				
R: 375 mg/m^2 IV weekly × 4				
Sequential (4-wk course)	No	53	28	77
F: 25 mg/m^2 IV d 1-5, courses 1-6				
2 months observation, then				
R: 375 mg/m^2 IV weekly × 4				
Mayo Clinic and Ohio State University Study (3-wk course)	No	64	41	91
P: 2 mg/m^2 IV d 1, courses 1-6				
C: 600 mg/m^2 IV d 1, courses 1-6				
R: 375 mg/m^2 IV d 1, courses 2-6				
Memorial Sloan Kettering Study (3-wk course)	Yes	32	25	75
P: 4 mg/m^2 IV d 1, courses 1-6				
C: 600 mg/m^2 IV d 1, courses 1-6				
R: 375 mg/m^2 IV d 1, courses 2-6				

A = alemtuzumab (Campath); C = cyclophosphamide (Cytoxan); CALGB = Cancer and Leukemia Group B; CR = complete remission; F = fludarabine (Fludara); FluCam = fludarabine phosphate and alemtuzumab; OR = overall response; P = pentostatin (Nipent); R = rituximab (Rituxan).

The highest response rate for single-agent alemtuzumab was reported in previously untreated patients.

Rituximab (Rituxan), the mAb against CD20, has very limited activity at 375 mg/m^2/week for 4 weeks in patients with CLL. The pivotal trial for rituximab demonstrated an overall response rate of 12% in previously treated patients with IWF (International Working Formulation) A non-Hodgkin's lymphoma, the CLL/SLL equivalent. Dose-intense or dose-dense single-agent rituximab markedly improves response rate over the standard dose and schedule and is well tolerated. Rituximab has been evaluated in a dose-intense regimen of up to 2.25 g/m^2 weekly for 4 weeks and in a dose-dense regimen of 375 mg/m^2 thrice weekly for 4 weeks. These phase II studies showed improved activity compared with that seen with standard-dose single-agent rituximab in the pivotal trial.

Purine analogue-based chemotherapy has been combined with mAbs, referred to as chemoimmunotheapy, for treatment of chemotherapy-naïve, relapsed, and refractory patients with CLL (Table 6). The phase II randomized CALGB 9712 (Cancer and Leukemia Group B) trial compared concurrent with sequential fludarabine and rituximab and demonstrated a higher complete remission rate with concurrent treatment, indicating potentiation of activity with the combination. Significant activity has been seen with front-line and salvage phase II single-arm trials with chemoimmunotherapy regimens, and randomized phase III controlled clinical trials are ongoing. Overall, management of patients with CLL has changed significantly with the development of new therapeutic agents and combinations.

REFERENCES

Apperley JF: Part I: Mechanisms of resistance to imatinib in chronic myeloid leukaemia. Lancet Oncol 2007;8:1018-1029.

Baccarani M, Saglio G, Goldman J, et al: Evolving concepts in the management of chronic myeloid leukemia: Recommendations from an expert panel on behalf of the European LeukemiaNet. Blood 2006;108:1809-1820.

Cheson BD, Bennett JM, Grever M, et al: National Cancer Institute–sponsored Working Group guidelines for chronic lymphocytic leukemia: Revised guidelines for diagnosis and treatment. Blood 1996;87:4990-4997.

Crespo M, Bosch F, Villamor N, et al: ZAP-70 expression as a surrogate for immunoglobulin-variable-region mutations in chronic lymphocytic leukemia. N Engl J Med 2003;348:1764-1775.

Damle RN, Wasil T, Fais F, et al: Ig V gene mutation status and CD38 expression as novel prognostic indicators in chronic lymphocytic leukemia. Blood 1999;94:1840-1847.

Dohner H, Stilgenbauer S, Dohner K, et al: Chromosome aberrations in B-cell chronic lymphocytic leukemia: Reassessment based on molecular cytogenetic analysis. J Mol Med 1999;77:266-281.

Druker BJ, Guilhot F, O'Brien SG, et al: Five-year follow-up of patients receiving imatinib for chronic myeloid leukemia. N Engl J Med 2006;355:2408-2417.

Hochhaus A, Kantarjian HM, Baccarani M, et al: Dasatinib induces notable hematologic and cytogenetic responses in chronic-phase chronic myeloid leukemia after failure of imatinib therapy. Blood 2007;109:2303-2309.

Kantarjian HM, Giles F, Gattermann N, et al: Nilotinib (formerly AMN107), a highly selective Bcr-Abl tyrosine kinase inhibitor, is effective in patients with Philadelphia chromosome–positive chronic myelogenous leukemia in chronic phase following imatinib resistance and intolerance. Blood 2007;110(10):3540-3546.

Kantarjian H, Schiffer C, Jones D, Cortes J: Monitoring the response and course of chronic myeloid leukemia in the modern era of BCR-ABL tyrosine kinase inhibitors: Practical advice on the use and interpretation of monitoring methods. Blood 2008;111:1774-1780.

Keating MJ, O'Brien S, Albitar M, et al: Early results of a chemoimmunotherapy regimen of fludarabine, cyclophosphamide, and rituximab as initial therapy for chronic lymphocytic leukemia. J Clin Oncol 2005;23:4079-4088.

Rai KR, Peterson BL, Appelbaum FR, et al: Fludarabine compared with chlorambucil as primary therapy for chronic lymphocytic leukemia. N Engl J Med 2000;343:1750-1757.

Non-Hodgkin's Lymphoma

Method of
Lawrence Rice, MD, and Uday Popat, MD

Rather than representing a single disease, non-Hodgkin's lymphomas (NHLs) comprise a diverse spectrum of disorders, varying from the most rapidly growing cancer known to the most indolent of neoplasms having no impact on well-being and requiring no treatment. Together these clonal lymphocyte proliferations comprise 5% of all cancers, ranking fifth in incidence, yet their importance is far greater than their frequency. Reasons for this include that lymphomas have critically accelerated scientific understanding of neoplasia, displaying the roles of oncogenic viruses, specific genetic alterations, and the interplay of tumor with host immune factors. Lymphomas are the most common cancers in adolescents and young adults. Regarding therapy, breakthroughs in lymphomas are being applied to curing cancers more generally. The efficacy of the earliest chemotherapy drugs were established in lymphomas; the principles of combination chemotherapy and of curative radiotherapy were gleaned.

Epidemiology and Genetics

Indolent NHLs are disorders of older individuals (rare younger than age 40 years). Although large B-cell lymphomas are also most common after age 65 years, the incidence curve is much flatter such that they also represent the most common cancer in adolescents and young adults. Other lymphomas have distinctive epidemiologic patterns, such as T-cell lymphoblastic lymphoma occurring mainly in adolescent and young adult men and primary mediastinal large B-cell lymphoma in young women. Burkitt's lymphoma presents as jaw tumors in children in third-world countries related to Epstein-Barr virus (EBV) infection, but presents as abdominal masses or leukemia in young adults in developed Western countries. Hepatitis C increases the risk for several lymphomas, particularly primary splenic marginal zone B-cell lymphoma. Many lymphomas increase with HIV infection, but Burkitt's lymphoma and large B-cell lymphomas with CNS primaries are particularly common. Mucosa-associated lymphoid tissue lymphoma (MALToma) of the stomach is associated with *Helicobacter pylori*.

Lymphomas often display distinctive acquired cytogenetic abnormalities. The abnormal gene products provide clues to pathogenesis and targets for therapy. Examples include Burkitt's lymphoma where translocations involve the c-myc oncogene on chromosome 8 and immunoglobulin heavy- or light-chain genes. Follicular lymphomas have a characteristic t(14;18) affecting BCL-2 gene regulation of cellular apoptosis. In many lymphomas cytogenetic patterns provide prognostic information (e.g., small lymphocytic lymphoma) or can help establish the proper diagnosis, such as (11;14) with cyclin D overexpression in mantle cell lymphoma.

Classification of Lymphomas and Leukemias

Differentiating lymphomas from lymphoid leukemias is arbitrary and semantic, based on whether a clonal neoplasm presents mainly in lymph nodes and tissues versus prominent peripheral blood involvement. Thus, B-cell chronic lymphocytic leukemia and small lymphocytic lymphoma represent different clinical presentations of the same malignant disorder; disease behavior and treatment principles are identical. Similarly, B-cell (L3 type) acute lymphoblastic leukemia and Burkitt's lymphoma are the same disorder, as are T-cell acute lymphoblastic leukemia and lymphoblastic lymphoma.

A major advance in understanding and managing NHLs emerged 40 years ago with the Rappaport classification system. Morphologic parameters such as whether malignant cells were large or small and whether they showed a nodular (follicular) growth pattern separated disorders into clinically useful categories predicting disease behavior and responsiveness to therapies. Proliferating alternative classification schemes since have daunted students and clinicians, becoming an object for satires. Nevertheless, modern classification goes beyond morphology, bringing to bear advances in molecular biology, flow cytometry, and cytogenetics to establish homogeneous disease entities that behave more predictably. Optimizing a patient's treatment requires familiarity with up-to-date classification (Table 1).

TABLE 1 Proposed World Health Organization Classification Scheme for Non-Hodgkin's Lymphoma

B-Cell Neoplasms
Precursor B-cell neoplasm
Precursor B-lymphoblastic leukemia/lymphoma

Mature B-cell neoplasms
B-cell chronic lymphocytic leukemia/small lymphocytic lymphoma
B-cell prolymphocytic leukemia
Lymphoplasmacytic lymphoma
Splenic marginal zone B-cell lymphoma (± villous lymphocytes)
Hairy cell leukemia
Plasma cell myeloma/plasmacytoma
Extranodal marginal zone B-cell lymphoma of the MALT type
Nodal marginal zone B-cell lymphoma (± monocytoid B cells)
Follicular lymphoma
Mantle cell lymphoma
Diffuse large-B-cell lymphoma
    Mediastinal large-B-cell lymphoma
    Primary effusion lymphoma
Burkitt lymphoma

T-Cell and NK Cell Neoplasms
Precursor T-cell neoplasm
Precursor T-lymphoblastic lymphoma/leukemia

Mature T-cell neoplasms
T-cell prolymphocytic leukemia
T-cell granular lymphocytic leukemia
Aggressive NK cell leukemia
Adult T-cell lymphoma/leukemia (HTLV-1-positive)
Extranodal NK/T-cell lymphoma, nasal type
Enteropathy-type T-cell lymphoma
Hepatosplenic γδ T-cell lymphoma
Subcutaneous panniculitis-like T-cell lymphoma
Mycosis fungoides/Sézary syndrome
Anaplastic large-cell lymphoma, T/null cell, primary cutaneous type
Anaplastic large-cell lymphoma, T/null cell, primary systemic type
Peripheral T-cell lymphoma, not otherwise characterized
Angioimmunoblastic T-cell lymphoma

Abbreviations: HTLV-1 = human T-cell leukemia virus 1; MALT = mucosa-associated lymphoid tissue; NK = natural killer.

Evaluation, Staging, and Prognosis

A thorough history specifically addresses whether the *B symptoms* of fevers, night sweats, and weight loss are present. Physical exam pays extra attention to palpating lymph nodes and abdominal viscera. All patients require a complete blood count (CBC) with differential, blood chemistries including tests of renal function, hepatic function, calcium and lactate dehydrogenase (LD), and chest radiograph. Essential staging procedures are computed tomography (CT) scans (chest, abdomen, pelvis) and bone marrow. Bone marrow biopsy must be obtained but bilateral biopsies are not routinely indicated. Nonroutine tests for certain patients and certain disease subtypes

CURRENT DIAGNOSIS

- Precise histologic diagnosis is mandatory.
- Currently, this requires assessment of cell surface markers (e.g., by flow cytometry) and increasingly of cytogenetic and molecular markers.
- Clinical staging requires history of systemic symptoms (weight loss, fever, sweats) and careful palpation of lymph node areas, spleen, and liver.
- Evaluation requires CBC, hepatic and renal function and LD.
- Routine staging is completed by CT scans of nodal areas and bone marrow biopsy.
- Other modalities (lumbar puncture; PET scan) are for select cases or investigational.
- An international prognostic index (age, stage, number of extranodal sites, performance status, serum LD) is clinically useful.

Abbreviations: CBC = complete blood count; CT = computed tomography; LD = lactate dehydrogenase; PET = positron emission tomography.

CURRENT THERAPY

- Low-grade (indolent) lymphomas are usually advanced (stage III or IV) and asymptomatic—these can be followed without therapy (*watch and wait*).
- Most common indications for therapy of low-grade lymphomas are emergence of systemic systems, progressive cytopenias, or histologic transformation.
- Most effective therapies for low-grade lymphomas are alkylating agents (cyclophosphamide), nucleoside analogues (fludarabine), monoclonal antibodies (rituximab), or combinations of these.
- Corticosteroids, anthracyclines and analogues, and alkaloids are also effective.
- Large B-cell lymphomas (intermediate to high grade) require moderately aggressive chemotherapy and are potentially curable.
- The regimen of choice for large B-cell lymphomas is CHOP-R.
- High-grade lymphomas (lymphoblastic, Burkitt's) are tissue variants of acute lymphoid leukemias and should be treated with ALL-type regimens.

Abbreviations: ALL = acute lymphoblastic leukemia; CHOP-R = cyclophosphamide, hydroxydaunomycin (doxorubicin), Oncovin (vincristine), prednisone, and rituximab.

include lumbar puncture and gallium scanning. Positron emission tomography appears promising, and its role is being investigated. The Ann Arbor staging system remains standard: Stage I is involvement of one lymph node region (or IE single extranodal site); stage II, multiple lymph node regions on the same side of the diaphragm; stage III, lymph nodes on both sides of the diaphragm; and stage IV, extralymphatic spread such as to bone marrow, liver or pleura. A follows the stage if B symptoms are absent.

The most important factors guiding treatment and prognosis are histology and stage. Age and co-morbidities must be considered. An international prognostic index developed for large-cell lymphomas can, with some modification, also be applied to other lymphomas. Scores are generated from five parameters:

1. Age
2. Stage
3. Number of extranodal sites
4. Performance status
5. Serum LD

Another modality applicable to prognostic stratification with diffuse large-cell lymphoma is microarray gene expression profiling, able to separate good risk "germinal center like large-cell lymphoma" from poor risk "activated B-cell lymphoma."

Treatment of Some Specific Disease Entities

INDOLENT LYMPHOMAS

The common indolent lymphomas are small lymphocytic lymphoma and grade 1 follicular lymphoma, representing more than one third of NHLs. The great majority (85% to 90%) present with stage III or IV disease; in fact 90% to 100% of small lymphocytic lymphomas and 40% to 90% of follicular lymphomas have bone marrow involvement, marking them stage IV. Patients with apparent localized presentations are candidates for radiotherapy with curative intent (recognizing that two thirds will eventually relapse). Adjuvant chemotherapy is under study for such patients.

Stage III and IV patients cannot be cured with standard therapies, yet median survival for asymptomatic subgroups exceeds 10 years. So, a *watch and wait* approach with no initial therapy is appropriate for most patients, given that the disease is often asymptomatic, indolent in behavior, incurable, and associated with prolonged survival. (One cannot deliver palliative therapy to individuals who are asymptomatic.) Initially untreated patients average 4 years or more before disease progression mandates treatment, with no decrement in survival attributable to treatment delay. Twenty percent of patients with follicular lymphoma, and a greater number with small lymphocytic lymphoma may never require treatment even after more than 10 years of follow-up.

Factors that mandate treatment at presentation or during follow-up are mainly related to emerging cytopenias (e.g., significant anemia) or systemic symptoms. Young age and psychoemotional factors can be reasons for early therapy, but most patients readily accept no initial treatment when the rationale is fully explained. A major problem impacting survival is transformation to more histologically aggressive lymphomas (Richter-like syndrome); this may occur at 5% per year regardless of treatment.

When treatment is warranted, additions to our armamentarium have increased choices, making decisions less clear-cut. Single oral alkylating agents such as cyclophosphamide (Cytoxan) and chlorambucil (Leukeran) were mainstays and remain reasonable choices for many. Response rates are approximately 50%, few complete, but clinical problems may be dramatically reversed for years. These agents are inexpensive, convenient, and most patients experience no side-effects. Potential toxicities are myelosuppression, leukemogenesis emerging after few years (in approximately 1%), and bladder toxicity with cyclophosphamide. Cyclophosphamide (often intravenous) is the backbone of the traditional CVP regimen, with vincristine (Oncovin) and prednisone. Adding doxorubicin (Adriamycin)—the CHOP (cyclophosphamide, hydroxydaunomycin [doxorubicin], Oncovin [vincristine], and prednisone) regimen—adds toxicity without survival benefit in indolent lymphomas. Nucleoside analogues, particularly fludarabine, are active in these disorders. Response rates may exceed those of alkylating agents at the costs of toxicities and inconvenience (several days monthly of intravenous therapy). Beyond myelosuppression, long-lasting immunosuppression creates significant risks for serious opportunistic infection. Newer combinations such as FC (fludarabine, cyclophosphamide) and FND (fludarabine, mitoxantrone [Novantrone], dexamethasone) reduce the fludarabine dose, reducing toxicities. Spectacular remission rates have been observed with these regimens, making them attractive choices both for initial and salvage therapy.

The promise of monoclonal antibody therapy is realized in these disorders. Rituximab (Rituxan), an anti-CD20 monoclonal antibody, can be administered singly or in combination with any chemotherapy regimen, either initially or for salvage. It has rapidly become the world's largest selling antineoplastic agent, even though the only cancers for which it is used are B-cell lymphoproliferative disorders. It is remarkably nontoxic, with fever, chills, and manageable hypotension occurring mainly during the first infusion; infectious risks are low. Understandably, regimens such as FC-R and FND-R are becoming popular. Molecular remissions emerge with these regimens, fueling hopes that curative goals may become realistic. Other monoclonal antibodies for indolent lymphomas are more toxic and used for salvage therapy. These include anti-CD52 alemtuzumab (Campath) for small lymphocytic lymphoma, associated with high opportunistic infection risks, and anti-CD20 antibodies conjugated to radioisotopes. Recurrent or refractory disease is treated with approaches discussed earlier, but rate and duration of response shortens with each subsequent relapse. To re-emphasize, observation without treatment is reasonable for asymptomatic relapse; more harm has resulted from overly aggressive treatment than the reverse. Patients transforming to large-cell lymphoma have a worse prognosis than de novo large-cell lymphoma, but some respond to combination chemotherapy with or without stem cell transplants. Transplants, both autologous and allogeneic, have benefited selected patients, but utility is limited by the age of patients, the anticipation of long survival, and the frequency of bone marrow involvement, which could contaminate autografts. Grade 1 and 2 follicular lymphomas are considered indolent, but grade 3 (follicular large cell) should be treated as diffuse large-cell lymphoma (in the following text), because it progresses more rapidly and because long-lasting remissions can be achieved.

DIFFUSE LARGE B-CELL LYMPHOMA

This most common lymphoma subtype comprises another one third of cases. Unlike indolent lymphomas, these are clinically aggressive with survival of few months untreated. Alkylating agents or monoclonal antibodies used alone are ineffective. Contrasting with indolent lymphomas, there is a reasonable possibility of cure with appropriate chemotherapy. Localized presentations (Stage I or II) occur in less than 30% of large-cell cases. Nonbulky localized disease is treated with three cycles of CHOP or CHOP-R (cyclophosphamide, hydroxydaunomycin [doxorubicin], Oncovin [vincristine], prednisone, and rituximab) followed by involved-field radiotherapy. A good majority of such patients are cured, as demonstrated in a randomized trial showing progression-free survival of 76% with chemoradiation compared to 67% with eight cycles of CHOP. Patients with stage III or IV disease are given six to eight cycles of CHOP or CHOP-R. Complete response to CHOP will occur in two thirds, and one third will be cured. More intensive regimens like MACOP-B (methotrexate, doxorubicin, cyclophosphamide, Oncovin, prednisone, and bleomycin), ProMACE-CytaBOM (prednisone, methotrexate [with leucovorin rescue], Adriamycin, cyclophosphamide, etoposide, cytarabine, bleomycin, Oncovin, dexamethasone), or m-BACOD (methotrexate, bleomycin, Adriamycin, cyclophosphamide, Oncovin dexamethasone) are more toxic, more difficult to administer, and no more efficacious than CHOP. The addition of rituximab improves the progression-free survival to 54% compared with 30% in patients receiving CHOP without rituximab. Hence, CHOP-R is the standard of care in patients with advanced CD20 positive diffuse large B-cell lymphomas. A baseline echocardiogram is performed because of the potential cardiotoxicity of doxorubicin. Restaging procedures are usually done after four treatment courses. Two additional courses are delivered after remission is confirmed. Prophylactic intrathecal chemotherapy should be strongly considered with involvement of the testis, ovary, breast, sinuses, bone marrow, more than one extranodal site, or a high LD. Recurrent or refractory disease carries a poor prognosis. Cure is still reasonably possible in candidates for autologous stem cell transplantation (those relatively young without serious co-morbidities). It is crucial that they have *chemotherapy-sensitive* relapse; that is, the disease is not progressing during therapy. Common salvage regimens include ICE (ifosfamide, carboplatin, etoposide), ESHAP (etoposide, Solu-Medrol, high-dose ara-C, Platinol), and DHAP (dexamethasone, high-dose ara-C, Platinol), using ifosfamide, platinums, etoposide, cytosine arabinoside, and corticosteroids. Two thirds of patients respond, but longer outlook remains bleak unless stem cell transplant ensues (event-free survival improved from 12% to 46% in a randomized study). Patients refractory to salvage therapy may be candidates for investigational agents, allogeneic transplantation or palliative care.

Peripheral T-cell lymphoma and anaplastic large-cell lymphoma are treated similarly to diffuse large B-cell lymphoma.

LYMPHOBLASTIC AND BURKITT'S LYMPHOMAS

These represent variant presentations of T-cell and B-cell acute lymphoblastic leukemia, respectively, and they are treated with acute lymphoblastic leukemia (ALL) protocols, which employ vincristine, anthracyclines, cyclophosphamide, cytosine arabinoside, and methotrexate (e.g., Hyper-CVAD [cyclophosphamide, vincristine, Adriamycin, dexamethasone, methotrexate, cytarabine]). Prophylactic CNS therapy is mandatory. Care must be taken to avoid the tumor lysis syndrome (especially with Burkitt's lymphoma) by vigorous hydration, alkalinization of urine, allopurinol, and close monitoring. Approximately one third of patients with these disorders can be cured by chemotherapy (higher in some patient subsets).

LYMPHOMAS RELATED TO INFECTIOUS AGENTS

HIV predisposes to many lymphomas but particularly to Burkitt's lymphoma and primary CNS large-cell lymphoma. The addition of antiretroviral therapy to chemotherapy improves results. Hepatitis C also predisposes to several lymphomas, particularly primary splenic marginal zone lymphoma. Interferon therapy is highly efficacious for this lymphoma when associated with hepatitis C. (The toxicities of interferon relative to any benefit mitigate against its use in other lymphomas.) With MALToma of the stomach related to *Helicobacter pylori* infection, eradication of the organism with antibiotics results in *spontaneous* regression of the neoplasm in patients with superficial, node-negative, low-grade disease; but others often require chemotherapy or radiotherapy.

LYMPHOMAS RELATED TO IMMUNE SUPPRESSION OR DEFICIENCY

It has been known for decades that lymphomas complicate primary immunodeficiency disorders. Lymphomas with AIDS are addressed above. Post-transplant lymphoproliferative disorder is usually (but not always) a monoclonal proliferation of B-cells expressing large amounts of EBV DNA. Incidence varies from 1% in renal transplant recipients to 2% to 5% in more heavily immunosuppressed organ transplant recipients. The main therapeutic maneuver is to stop or substantially decrease immunosuppressive therapies. This leads to lymphoma resolution in half. Rituximab may be added, but antivirals have not proven beneficial. The prognosis is poor for patients who progress despite these actions, but some respond well to combination chemotherapy. Immunosuppressive drugs also relate to lymphomas apart from transplantation. Withdrawal of methotrexate from rheumatoid arthritis patients can produce *spontaneous* lymphoma regression.

Other Treatment Modalities

SURGICAL THERAPY

This has been advocated for isolated extranodal lymphomas, such as stomach or bowel, but its role should be relegated to obtaining biopsy material for diagnosis. Even here, it may be supplanted by needle biopsy with ancillary flow cytometry, histochemistry, and cytogenetics, sometimes allowing definitive diagnosis. (Nonsurgical therapies of gastrointestinal lymphomas do entail a small risk of bowel perforation.)

STEM CELL (BONE MARROW) TRANSPLANT

Autologous stem cell transplants, now usually collected from peripheral blood by cytapheresis, have been favored for lymphomas. This is the preferred therapy (after cytoreduction) for patients with *chemotherapy-sensitive* relapse where cure remains the goal. *Up-front* use as a form of consolidation intensification for high-risk patients is under investigation. Continuing investigations address the necessity for and means to accomplish purging of tumor cells from autografts. Allogeneic transplants, seeking the advantage of *graft versus tumor* effects, afford a chance of cure for selected patients but with increased risks of toxicity. Toxicities are being reduced by less intensive conditioning regimens.

FUTURE THERAPIES

Tumor vaccines are in clinical trials and new monoclonal antibodies loom. Molecular advances bring forth agents such as BCL-2 antisense oligonucleotides, currently in clinical trials.

REFERENCES

A predictive model for aggressive non-Hodgkin's lymphoma. The international Non-Hodgkin's Lymphoma Prognostic Factors Project. N Engl J Med 1993;329:987-994.
Ardeshna KM, Smith P, Norton A, et al: Long-term effect of a watch and wait policy versus immediate systemic treatment for asymptomatic advanced-stage non-Hodgkin lymphoma: A randomised controlled trial. Lancet 2003;362:516-522.
Coiffier B, Lepage E, Briere J, et al: CHOP chemotherapy plus rituximab compared with CHOP alone in elderly patients with diffuse large-B-cell lymphoma. N Engl J Med 2002;346:235-242.
Fisher R, Gaynor E, Dahlberg S, et al: Comparison of a standard regimen (CHOP) with three intensive chemotherapy regimens for advanced non-Hodgkin's lymphoma. N Engl J Med 1993;328:1002-1006.
Horning SJ, Rosenberg SA: The natural history of initially untreated low-grade non-Hodgkin's lymphoma. N Engl J Med 1984;311:1471-1475.
MacManus M, Hoppe RT: Is radiotherapy curative for stage I and II low-grade follicular lymphoma? Results of a long-term follow-up study of patients treated at Stanford University. J Clin Oncol 1996;14:1282-1290.
Marcus R, Imrie K, Belch A, et al: CVP chemotherapy plus rituximab compared with CVP as first-line treatment for advanced follicular lymphoma. Blood 2005;105:1417-1423.
Miller T, Dahlberg S, Cassady J, et al: Chemotherapy alone compared with chemotherapy plus radiotherapy for localized intermediate- and high-grade non-Hodgkin's lymphoma. N Engl J Med 1998;339:21-26.
Philip T, Guglielmi C, Hagenbeek A, et al: Autologous bone marrow transplantation as compared with salvage chemotherapy in relapses of chemotherapy-sensitive non-Hodgkin's lymphoma. N Engl J Med 1995;333:1540-1545.

Multiple Myeloma

Method of
*Rodger E. Tiedemann, MB, ChB, PhD, and
A. Keith Stewart, MB, ChB*

Multiple myeloma is a malignancy of clonal plasma cells that proliferate and accumulate in the bone marrow. The neoplastic plasma cells typically produce a monoclonal immunoglobulin (or M protein) that can be detected in blood or urine. In the United States, myeloma accounts for 15% of hematologic malignancies and for nearly 2% of all deaths due to cancer. The incidence is 4 in 100,000 per year, although African Americans have an incidence twice that of whites. The median age at diagnosis is 65 to 70 years.

Multiple myeloma is often but not always preceded by a premalignant phase known as *monoclonal gammopathy of undetermined significance* (MGUS). MGUS is found in up to 3% of patients older than 50 years, and studies with 30-year follow-ups indicate that approximately 1% of MGUS patients per year progress to myeloma.

Myeloma remains incurable and is associated with a median survival of only 3 to 4 years, although its clinical course can be extremely variable, ranging from indolent disease that progresses only over the space of a decade to aggressive disease causing death within months.

Diagnosis

CLINICAL FEATURES

Bone pain, recurrent infection and symptoms of anemia, renal impairment, or hypercalcemia should raise suspicion of a diagnosis of myeloma. These clinical features can result directly from the mass effect of plasma cells lesions (plasmacytoma) or can arise indirectly from the M-protein or cytokines secreted by plasma cells. Common nonspecific laboratory findings such as an elevated erythrocyte sedimentation rate, normocytic anemia, rouleaux formation, and hypergammaglobulinemia should also prompt consideration of a diagnosis of myeloma, among other possibilities.

INVESTIGATIONS

Laboratory

Patients suspected of having myeloma require careful investigation (Box 1). Most patients (98%) with myeloma have an M protein detectable either by serum or urine protein electrophoresis. Serum electrophoresis alone shows a monoclonal band in 80% of cases. The components of the monoclonal immunoglobulin are identified by immunoelectrophoresis and immunofixation. Sixty percent of myeloma patients have a monoclonal immunoglobulin (Ig)G paraprotein, and 20% have a monoclonal IgA. Isolated monoclonal light chain

---

 CURRENT DIAGNOSIS

Multiple Myeloma

- Monoclonal protein in the serum or urine* *and*
- Bone marrow (clonal) plasmacytosis or soft tissue plasmacytoma *and*
- Evidence of related end-organ damage or tissue injury[†]

Smoldering Myeloma

- Serum monoclonal protein ≥3.0 g/dL *and/or*
- Bone marrow (clonal) plasma cells ≥10% *and*
- *No* related organ or tissue impairment[†]

Monoclonal Gammopathy of Undetermined Significance

- Serum monoclonal protein <3.0 g/dL *and*
- Bone marrow plasma cells <10% *and*
- *No* related organ or tissue impairment[†] *and*
- *No* evidence of other B cell proliferative disorder or amyloidosis

*A monoclonal protein is not detected in approximately 1% of MM patients.
[†]Myeloma-related end-organ damage can consist of hypercalcemia (>2.75 mmol/L or >0.25 mmol/L above normal limits), renal impairment (serum creatinine>173 mmol/L or >1.96 mg/dL), anemia (hemoglobin <10 g/dL or >2 g/dL below normal limits), or bone lesions (lytic lesions or osteopenia with compression fracture), abbreviated to the acronym CRAB. Based on the International Working Group criteria for multiple myeloma (MM), smoldering myeloma (SMM), and monoclonal gammopathy of undetermined significance (MGUS).

BOX 1 Investigations in Multiple Myeloma

- Serum protein electrophoresis
- 24-Hour urine collection for total and Bence Jones protein quantitation
- Immunoelectrophoresis or immunofixation of serum and urine
- CBC with differential and reticulocyte count
- Serum creatinine, calcium, uric acid, electrolytes, lactic acid dehydrogenase, alkaline phosphatase
- Bone marrow aspirate and biopsy
- Cytogenetics and/or FISH [e.g., for del(13) and t(4;14)] recommended
- Skeletal survey
- β_2-microglobulin, C-reactive protein, plasma cell labeling index if available
- If indicated: Biopsy of soft tissue masses
- If hyperviscosity is suspected: Serum viscosity
- If indicated: Cryoglobulins, MRI or CT of affected areas, biopsy for amyloidosis

Abbreviations: CBC = complete blood count; CT = computed tomography; MRI = magnetic resonance imaging; FISH = fluorescence in situ hybridization.

without identifiable heavy chain is detected in another 15% of myeloma patients (commonly known as *light-chain myeloma* or *Bence Jones myeloma*). Monoclonal IgD and biclonal gammopathies are rarer; each accounts for 1% to 2% of myeloma cases. In 1% of cases, malignant plasma cells synthesize but do not secrete immunoglobulin, and an M protein cannot be detected (nonsecretory myeloma).

Bone marrow aspiration and biopsy are essential in the diagnostic process and typically show increased numbers of plasma cells (>10%). Aspiration and biopsy might also reveal abnormal plasma cell morphology or amyloid deposition in the marrow space or within blood vessel walls.

Radiology

Plain x-rays of the axial skeleton and long bones are used to survey for skeletal evidence of myeloma and to assess for impending pathologic fracture. Magnetic resonance imaging (MRI) (using T1/T2 settings plus STIR [short T1 inversion recovery] sequences) can also be used and is particularly sensitive in detecting less overt patchy plasma cell involvement of the bone marrow. MRI may be especially useful when plain x-ray films are negative but the index of suspicion for myeloma remains high. In patients with confirmed multiple myeloma, the size and number of lesions on MRI correlate with prognosis. Computed tomography (CT) is less sensitive than MRI but is useful in defining lesions when cord compression is suspected and urgent treatment may be required. Because myeloma lesions are *osteolytic*, a nuclear bone scan, which best detects *osteoblastic* lesions, is not generally useful.

DIAGNOSTIC CRITERIA

Various minimal criteria for the diagnosis of myeloma have been published, most recently those of the International Myeloma Working Group (see the Current Diagnosis box), which has sought to provide standardization.

The presence or absence of myeloma-related end-organ damage and the levels of monoclonal protein and bone marrow involvement by clonal plasmacytosis are keys to distinguishing symptomatic multiple myeloma (MM) from smoldering myeloma (SMM) and MGUS. Myeloma-related end-organ damage can consist of hyper*c*alcemia, *r*enal impairment, *a*nemia, or *b*one lesions (CRAB). Other less common criteria for end-organ damage due to myeloma include symptomatic hyperviscosity or recurrent bacterial infections (≥ 2 in 12 months).

In most MM patients, plasma cells account for more than 10% of nucleated marrow cells; however, rare symptomatic MM patients can present with plasma cells less than 10%, and a lower limit is not specified in the Working Group criteria. Approximately 1% of patients with symptomatic multiple myeloma do not have a detectable monoclonal protein when highly sensitive techniques are employed.

MGUS may be difficult to distinguish from SMM or early stage MM. Features that help to support a diagnosis of myeloma include depression of the normal immunoglobulin levels and high paraprotein concentration (>30 g/L in serum or >1 g/24 h in urine). Although MGUS and SMM do not usually require immediate therapy, it is nevertheless important to distinguish between the two because the prognoses differ.

Primary or immunoglobulin light chain (AL) amyloidosis is a plasma cell neoplasm related to myeloma that secretes an abnormal immunoglobulin that deposits in tissues in a β-pleated sheet conformation. Notably, 20% of AL amyloid patients have overt myeloma, whereas among myeloma patients nearly 15% develop primary amyloidosis. Amyloidosis should be suspected in myeloma patients who develop progressive neuropathy, cardiac dysfunction with hypotension, enlarged tongue, swollen joints, hepatomegaly, or nephrotic syndrome. A needle biopsy of the involved tissue is the most reliable method to yield a diagnosis, but if involved tissue is inaccessible, blind abdominal fat pad needle aspiration may be helpful. Samples are assessed by Congo red staining for birefringence.

Staging and Prognosis

Several staging systems are in existence. The Salmon/Durie system, developed in 1975, remains widely used and integrates the results of CBC, serum creatinine, calcium, serum and urine M protein levels, and radiology to correlate approximate tumor mass with survival. More recently, the new International Staging System (ISS) has been derived and validated by the International Myeloma Working Group from a cohort of 11,000 patients with newly diagnosed untreated myeloma. The ISS (Table 1) uses a simple combination of serum β_2 microglobulin and serum albumin to provide a reproducible and powerful three-stage classification that stratifies patients to groups with median overall survivals of 62, 44, or 29 months.

TABLE 1 International Staging System for Myeloma

Stage	Criteria	Median Survival*
1	Serum β_2 microglobulin <3.5 mg/dL and serum albumin $\geq$3.5 g/dL	62 months
2	Serum β_2 microglobulin < 3.5 mg/dL and serum albumin <3.5 g/dL	44 months
	or	
	Serum β_2 microglobulin 3.5-5.5 mg/dL (irrespective of serum albumin)	
3	Serum β_2 microglobulin >5.5 mg/dL	29 months

*Times reflect median overall survival by International Staging System stage.

More sophisticated prognostic tests including tumor cytogenetics and fluorescence-in-situ-hybridization (FISH) are now increasingly recognized as powerful determinants of outcome, and in the near future molecular stratification of tumors may be used to guide therapy. Aberrations such as deletion of chromosome 13, deletion of 17p, or translocation between chromosomes 4 and 14, t(4;14), causing overexpression of fibroblast growth factor receptor 3 *(FGFR3)* and *MMSET* genes, have been associated with significantly poorer survival compared with the absence of any informative abnormality or with t(11;14) translocation or hyperdiploidy.

Therapy

OVERVIEW

Although there are many treatment options for patients with multiple myeloma, at present there is no cure. The disease may remain indolent for many years in some patients, particularly in those with smoldering myeloma or in those with low-level M protein (<30 g/L) and absent bone lesions. There is no evidence that early treatment prolongs survival. Therefore, therapy is generally reserved for patients with symptoms. The decision to begin therapy is based on the patient's symptoms and physical status and results of laboratory and radiographic investigations. Those with smoldering myeloma are not usually treated except within clinical trials. Treatment should be initiated in patients with impending complications (such as renal insufficiency or impending pathologic fracture) even if the patient is not yet symptomatic.

CURRENT THERAPY

Transplant Candidate (Often ≥65-70 Years)

- Induction therapy:
  - High-dose dexamethasone (HDD), often used in combination with vincristine and doxorubicin (VAD) or with thalidomide (thal/dex). Follow with collection of stem cells
  - High-dose melphalan (HDM) and autologous hematopoietic stem cell transplantation (SCT)
- For relapse or induction failure consider:
  - Thal/dex
  - Lenalidomide (Revlimid)/dexamethasone (rev/dex)
  - Bortezomib (Velcade)/dexamethasone (velcade/dex)
  - Cyclophosphamide/prednisone
- Repeat autologous SCT if first remission is longer than 18-24 months

Not a Transplant Candidate (Often >65-70 Years)

- Melphalan/prednisone (MP) ± thalidomide (MPT)
- For relapse or induction failure consider:
  - MPT or thal/dex, if no prior thalidomide
  - Rev/dex
  - Velcade/dex
  - Cyclophosphamide/prednisone

Select Patients

- Bisphosphonates, particularly for previous or present bone disease: Zoledronic acid (Zometa) 4 mg IV or pamidronate (Aredia) 60-90 mg IV, repeated every 4-6 weeks
- Erythropoietin for Hb <10 g/dL (caution: should not be used together with thalidomide or lenalidomide due to increased venous thrombosis)

Because multiple myeloma is a systemic disorder from the onset, the primary treatment modality is chemotherapy (Box 2). For eligible patients, the physician should consider a treatment strategy that includes high-dose melphalan combined with autologous peripheral blood stem cell transplantation (ASCT). Four randomized trials comparing high-dose therapy (HDT) plus ASCT with conventional chemotherapy have each shown a survival advantage for HDT, on the order of 5 to 13 months (depending on the alternative treatment strategy provided). These randomized trials were all conducted in patients younger than 65 to 70 years; however, occasional patients

BOX 2 Chemotherapy Regimens for Multiple Myeloma

High-Dose Dexamethasone (HDD)
- Dexamethasone (Decadron) 40 mg PO on days 1-4, 9-12, 17-20
- Repeat every 4 weeks

Thal/Dex
- Thalidomide 100-200 mg PO qd, plus HDD
- Prophylactic anticoagulation required (aspirin 325 mg PO qd or full-dose anticoagulation)

Rev/Dex
- Lenalidomide (Revlimid) 25 mg PO on days 1-21, plus HDD
- Repeat every 4 weeks
- Anticoagulation required

VAD
- Vincristine 0.4 mg IV on days 1-4
- Doxorubicin (Adriamycin) 9 mg/m^2/day IV on days 1-4
- HDD days 1-4, 9-12, 17-20 all cycles
- Repeat every 4 weeks (typically × 4) (short-infusional regimen)

High-Dose Melphalan (HDM)
- Melphalan (Alkeran) 200 mg/m^2 IV,[3] followed by SCT

Velcade/Dex
- Bortezomib (Velcade) 1.3 mg/m^2 IV on days 1, 4, 8, and 11, plus HDD
- Repeat every 3 weeks (e.g., × 8)

MP
- Melphalan (Alkeran) 9 mg/m^2 PO on days 1-4
- Prednisone 100 mg PO on days 1-4
- Repeat both every 4-6 weeks

MPT
- Melphalan (Alkeran) 9 mg/m^2 PO on days 1-4
- Prednisone 100 mg/m^2 PO on days 1-7
- Thalidomide 100 mg PO qd, continuous
- Repeat melphalan and prednisone every 4-6 weeks × 12 cycles
- Requires prophylactic anticoagulation

Cyclophosphamide
- Cyclophosphamide (Cytoxan) 300 mg/m^2 weekly PO or IV
- Often given together with prednisone 100 mg PO on alternate days

[3]Exceeds dosage recommended by the manufacturer.
Abbreviation: SCT = stem cell transplantation.
Note: Dose reductions may be necessary for side effects, advanced age, frailty, cytopenias, or impaired renal or liver function.

older than 70 years might also be candidates for HDT and ASCT on the basis of superior physiologic status.

HIGH-DOSE THERAPY WITH AUTOLOGOUS STEM CELL TRANSPLANTATION

In patients in whom ASCT is planned, induction therapy is used to control the presenting disease before stem cell harvest. Care must be taken to avoid the use of agents excessively toxic to hematopoietic stem cells (e.g., melphalan). Historically, common induction regimens have included high-dose dexamethasone alone or combined with vincristine and doxorubicin (VAD). VAD is generally given as vincristine 0.4 mg/day IV plus doxorubicin 9 mg/m^2/day IV on days 1 to 4, and dexamethasone 40 mg orally on days 1 to 4, 9 to 12, and 17 to 20. This is usually repeated every 28 days for four cycles. VAD induces partial remission (PR) in approximately 50% to 70% of patients and complete remission (CR) in 5% to 10% of patients. Dexamethasone alone is only mildly less effective and is useful as initial treatment in patients with severe cytopenia, with renal failure, or requiring extensive radiotherapy.

An alternative oral induction regimen consists of thalidomide (Thalomid) 200 mg daily plus dexamethasone (thal/dex). The dexamethasone is given 40 mg/day on days 1 to 4, 9 to 12, and 17 to 20 on odd cycles and days 1 to 4 on even cycles. Thal/dex produces response rates comparable with VAD and superior to dexamethasone alone. Adverse effects include an increased rate of venous thrombosis (15%), which necessitates prophylactic anticoagulation; neuropathy; somnolence; and constipation.

Use of thalidomide within the induction regimen can limit the efficacy of thalidomide-based regimens at relapse. No overall survival advantage is conferred by using this agent upfront instead of as a de novo agent at relapse. In one large study, approximately 50% of 668 myeloma patients were randomly assigned to receive daily thalidomide starting alongside standard HDT plus ASCT therapy. Incorporation of thalidomide into HDT had no effect on overall survival (OS). Use of thalidomide alongside HDT did result in increased event-free survival (EFS). However, this was balanced by substantially shortened survival following relapse and by higher rates of severe peripheral neuropathy and deep venous thrombosis (DVT).

Combination therapies using newer agents such as bortezomib (Velcade) or lenalidomide (Revlimid) are being investigated as induction regimens. These offer the promise of deeper remissions in greater numbers of patients than current induction treatments. However, their benefit on OS following HDT and ASCT remains to be determined.

Following recovery from induction treatment, peripheral blood stem cells are collected from the patient via a cell separator (apheresis) and are frozen until their reinfusion after high-dose chemotherapy. Stem cell mobilization typically requires pretreatment with cyclophosphamide and granulocyte colony-stimulating factor (G-CSF). High-dose melphalan[2] (Alkeran), 200 mg/m^2, is the most common HDT used and in patients younger than 65 years is associated with an upfront mortality rate of approximately 1%.

Unfortunately, many patients continue to have evidence of myeloma after ASCT and all patients eventually relapse. The median time to progression in myeloma patients treated with HDT and ASCT is 18 to 24 months. Pre-relapse maintenance therapy following HDT using various agents (e.g., interferon-α [IFN-α], steroids, thalidomide, or combination chemotherapy) is being tested in several clinical trials; however, evidence of significant benefit in OS is currently lacking.

Tandem sequential ASCTs have been reported to improve OS compared with single ASCT. This benefit was not seen within the first 2 years of follow-up; however, it was subsequently observed up to 7 years after ASCT. The benefits of early tandem transplantation are unlikely to be universal; advantages appear to accrue primarily in patients who fail to achieve satisfactory remission following their first ASCT procedure.

There is no clear standard of treatment following relapse after HDT. Treatment with standard alkylating agents or newer agents, repeat HDT plus ASCT, entry into a clinical trial, or allogeneic transplantation can each be considered.

ALLOGENEIC TRANSPLANTATION

An allogeneic transplant uses stem cells obtained from an HLA-matched donor, usually a sibling, to repopulate the bone marrow following chemotherapy. Allogeneic transplantation can theoretically provide an immunologic graft-versus-myeloma effect that can lead to significant reductions in tumor mass and prolonged remission. However, this potential benefit is balanced by high rates of transplant-related mortality (TRM) and a risk of troublesome graft-versus-host disease (GVHD). Less than 10% of myeloma patients are eligible for intensive myeloablative allogeneic protocols because 90% are aged 50 years or older, and only one third have an HLA-compatible donor. Nonmyeloablative (mini) allogeneic transplantation may be achievable in greater numbers of patients and offers a lower risk of early TRM. However, this approach is again associated with significant risk of GVHD (45% acute GVHD, 55% chronic GVHD reported), and we believe it should be considered primarily in the setting of well-planned clinical trials.

STANDARD ALKYLATING AGENT THERAPY

For elderly patients or those who do not want, or cannot tolerate, aggressive therapy, various oral chemotherapy regimens may be used. Oral melphalan plus prednisone (MP), given as melphalan 9 mg/m^2 plus prednisone 100 mg daily for 4 days at 4- to 6-week intervals, is the gold standard in this setting and induces objective responses in 50% to 60% of patients and a median OS of 2 to 3 years. Because melphalan absorption is reduced by food, it should be given in the morning on an empty stomach. Dose reduction should be considered in the elderly and for renal insufficiency. Melphalan doses are titrated to induce mild midcycle cytopenia. A mild neutropenic nadir (1.0-1.5 × 10^9/L) or thrombocytopenia (<100 × 10^9/L) is often targeted to ensure maximal efficacy. Severe cytopenia should be avoided by delaying treatment in weekly increments if significant cytopenias persist at follow-up and by reducing subsequent melphalan dosing in 2-to 4-mg/day decrements. MP is generally continued until maximal reduction in the M protein has occurred plus 2 to 4 months (plateau), or for approximately 1 year. At this point, treatment is stopped because cumulative melphalan exposure can result in late development of myelodysplastic syndrome or leukemia. Objective responses can occur slowly, and unless rapidly progressive disease occurs, treatment should not be abandoned until at least three cycles of treatment can be assessed.

Addition of thalidomide to MP (MPT) has recently been shown to improve the results of MP therapy. MPT is given as melphalan 4 mg/m^2 for 7 days, prednisone 40 mg/m^2 for 7 days, and thalidomide 100 mg daily continuously, repeated every 4 weeks for six cycles. Use of MPT in patients older than 65 years resulted in an increased response rate (76%) compared with MP (48%), more complete responses or near-complete responses (28 vs. 7%), and longer EFS (33 vs. 14 months). These gains were balanced, however, by increased toxicity (grade 3-4 toxicity: 49% vs. 25%) and by the need for concurrent anticoagulation (e.g., enoxaparin [Lovenox] 40 mg SC daily). In patients who tolerated six cycles of MPT, there was a trend to survival advantage at 3 years compared with patients treated with similar doses of MP (80 vs. 64%; hazard ratio [HR], 0.68; $P = 0.19$), even when MP patients were permitted to cross over and receive thalidomide following disease progression.

Cyclophosphamide (Cytoxan) can be used as an alternative to melphalan in select patients with a weekly dose of 400 to 500 mg orally or intravenously. Cyclophosphamide is less likely to suppress thrombopoiesis and has less myelosuppressive potentiation in renal failure. It is often administered in conjunction with prednisone 100 mg orally on alternate days.

Multidrug regimens using combinations of vincristine, anthracyclines, melphalan, BCNU [1,3 bis(2-chloroethyl)-1-nitrosourea],

---

[2]Not available in the United States.

cyclophosphamide and corticosteroids can provide a faster onset of action than MP and may be useful in patients with high tumor loads or acute complications. Significantly, however, a large meta-analysis of more than 6000 patients indicates that conventional multiagent chemotherapy regimens do not improve overall survival beyond that achieved with standard MP, even in poor-risk patients.

REFRACTORY MYELOMA AND NOVEL AGENTS

All patients with multiple myeloma who initially respond to treatment subsequently relapse. If relapse occurs more than 6 months after treatment response, a repeat trial of the previous treatment should be considered. Similarly, for patients who have experienced lasting remission (several years) after HDT, repeat HDT and ASCT may be useful. Myeloma patients often continue to show useful responses to prior therapies, although the quality and duration of response generally diminish with repeated exposure.

Patients who become refractory to alkylating agents typically respond poorly to ensuing chemotherapy and traditionally have had a poor prognosis. Dexamethasone often continues to be useful in relapsed patients. Unfortunately, complications of corticosteroids such as depression or agitation, infection, diabetes, hypertension, osteoporosis, and osteonecrosis can limit long-term use.

Importantly, thalidomide has been found to induce response rates of 30% to 35% in patients with relapsed or refractory myeloma when used as a single agent, with a median progression-free survival of 5 months. A greater response rate of approximately 55% is seen when thalidomide is used in combination with corticosteroids, with an improved median time to progression of 12 months and median OS of 27 months, providing a statistically significant advantage over conventional salvage chemotherapy in relapse. Most studies using thalidomide have used a dose of at least 200 mg daily; however, lower doses of 50 to 100 mg daily might also be effective. Adverse effects of thalidomide, which can influence the maximum obtainable dose, include sedation, constipation, and peripheral neuropathy. Rash, venous thrombosis, and the risk of birth defects are also problematic.

Lenalidomide (Revlimid, CC-5013), a derivative of thalidomide with greater potency and less toxicity, has shown promising activity in relapsed or refractory and untreated myeloma. In preliminary studies, lenalidomide 25mg daily on days 1 to 21, repeated every 4 weeks, plus dexamethasone (rev/dex), caused objective responses in 91% of patients with newly diagnosed myeloma, including CR in 6%, and very good PR in 32%. In relapsed patients, rev/dex has been shown to be superior to dexamethasone alone in a multicenter randomized trial of more than 350 patients with progressive myeloma, achieving an overall response rate of 58% (versus 22% for dexamethasone alone) and a median time to progression of 13.1 months (versus 5.1 months for dexamethasone). Other trials have demonstrated lenalidomide efficacy in patients refractory or intolerant to thalidomide. Head-to-head randomized comparisons with thalidomide are awaited at the time of writing.

Bortezomib (Velcade, PS-341), a first-in-class proteosome inhibitor, is an FDA-approved novel antimyeloma agent. When given intravenously at a dose of 1.3 mg/m^2 on days 1, 4, 8, and 11 on a 21-day schedule for eight cycles, followed by a lower intensity 35-day maintenance schedule, bortezomib resulted in objective responses in 46% of relapsed patients, including CR or near CR in 13%. Notably, the APEX (Assessment of Proteasome Inhibition for Extending Remissions) trial has shown bortezomib to be superior to single-agent dexamethasone as a salvage therapy for relapsed patients, 99% of whom have been exposed to prior corticosteroid therapy. Bortezomib provided an OS at 1 year of 80%, versus 66% for dexamethasone ($P = 0.003$), and median time to disease progression of 6.2 months, compared with 3.5 months for dexamethasone. In patients who do not respond to bortezomib alone, cotreatment with dexamethasone can result in additional partial or minimal responses in 15% to 20%. Notable toxicities of bortezomib include fatigue, gastrointestinal disturbance, painful peripheral neuropathy, and thrombocytopenia.

A multitude of clinical trials evaluating thalidomide, lenalidomide, or bortezomib, in combination with conventional therapies or with each other, are now accruing patients worldwide. These might result in rapid changes in the approach to myeloma treatment in coming years.

SUPPORTIVE THERAPY

Renal Failure

Approximately 20% of patients with myeloma have significant renal dysfunction, with serum creatinine >2.0 mg/dL at diagnosis. Common causes include cast nephropathy, dehydration, hypercalcemia, infection, use of nephrotoxic drugs, or amyloid deposition. Cast nephropathy involves deposition of amorphous nonfibrillary material (monoclonal immunoglobulin, usually light chain—thus *light chain deposition disease* or *myeloma kidney*) in the distal tubules and differs from renal amyloidosis in its distribution, absence of β-pleated sheet structure, and absence of Congo red staining. Additionally, the nephrotic syndrome is rare in myeloma kidney and should raise a suspicion of amyloidosis.

Adequate hydration and prompt chemotherapy are pivotal to management and can reverse mild dysfunction in 50% of patients. Allopurinol (Zyloprim) 300 mg daily (or less, according to creatinine clearance) is useful for controlling or preventing secondary hyperuricemia. Nonsteroidal anti-inflammatory drugs (NSAIDs) and nephrotoxic antibiotics should generally be stopped or avoided in the presence of renal impairment. Severe renal failure can require hemodialysis support in order to administer chemotherapy. In addition, plasmapheresis to reduce the plasma M protein can help limit acute renal damage and perhaps reduce the risk of long-term dialysis. However, randomized trials are lacking.

Hypercalcemia

Aggressive hydration with isotonic saline (150-200 mL/h) and steroid therapy (prednisone 100 mg/day) generally leads to rapid resolution of hypercalcemia. Treatment directed at the myeloma should then be instituted. Intravenous bisphosphonates such as pamidronate (Aredia) 60 to 90 mg or zoledronic acid (Zometa) 4 mg, are also commonly employed after resolution of coexisting renal dysfunction and can provide additional bone protection.

Anemia

Most patients with myeloma develop anemia, whose etiology is often multifactorial. Where anemia is caused primarily by marrow infiltration, specific antimyeloma therapy (with or without transfusion) may be beneficial. Recombinant erythropoietin (Eprex)[2] may be helpful in severe anemia (Hb ≤80 g/L), even in the absence of renal failure, because myeloma patients often have decreased levels or impaired response to endogenous erythropoietin. Doses of 150 U/kg three times weekly have led to hematologic responses in up to 70% of patients. Lower doses may be effective in patients with renal failure.

Skeletal Lesions

Bone lesions causing pain or impending pathologic fracture should be treated early. Skeletal imaging should be performed and repeated at regular intervals if pain develops. Internal fixation of impending long bone fractures (usually indicated when >50% cortical erosion is present) can prevent the significant pain and immobility associated with fracture. Advanced bone lesions that threaten fracture or are painful and unresponsive to systemic chemotherapy are best managed with localized radiation (20-30 Gy). Adequate analgesia is vital and often requires narcotics. Vertebroplasty or kyphoplasty can help decrease pain caused by compression fractures of the spine.

All myeloma patients with active bone disease, including those with significant osteopenia, should be treated with intravenous bisphosphonates unless contraindications exist. Pamidronate 90 mg

---

[2]Not available in the United States.

over 2 hours or zoledronic acid 4 mg over 15 minutes IV every 4 weeks show equal efficacy. Common side effects include flulike symptoms such as fatigue, anorexia, nausea, and bone pain; these can last 3 to 5 days but generally diminish with repeated exposure. More problematic is the recently reported association between prolonged bisphosphonate therapy and osteonecrosis of the mandible. Most cases have been reported in patients also receiving chemotherapy and corticosteroids who had undergone a dental procedure such as tooth extraction. A dental examination with preventive intervention should be considered before bisphosphonate therapy, and invasive dental procedures should, if possible, be avoided in patients receiving bisphosphonate treatment. Because hypocalcemia, renal impairment, and proteinuria can occur in patients receiving bisphosphonates, regular monitoring of serum calcium, electrolytes, creatinine, and urine protein is recommended.

Hyperviscosity Syndrome

Impaired vision, cognitive changes, mucosal bleeding, and congestive heart failure can occur as a consequence of increased serum protein concentration. Symptoms generally do not occur with serum viscosities less than 4.0 Cp (viscosity of water = 1 Cp, normal serum viscosity is 1.4-1.8 Cp), although the relationship between clinical signs and measured viscosity is imprecise. Hyperviscosity is most commonly seen in disorders associated with elevated IgM and is more common in IgA myeloma than in IgG myeloma. Plasmapheresis is used to acutely reduce the level of M protein, and myeloma chemotherapy should be instituted to decrease paraprotein production.

Spinal Cord Compression

Compression of the spinal cord or nerve roots can result from expansion of an extradural soft tissue plasmacytoma or from vertebral collapse and is a medical emergency. Lower back or radicular pain is a typical manifesting symptom. Leg weakness, urinary retention, incontinence, or obstipation can indicate impending cord damage. Urgent MRI or CT scanning is indicated to identify the extent of compression. To prevent permanent paraplegia, high-dose steroids (dexamethasone 16-96 mg/day) should be started immediately to reduce cord edema, and local irradiation (25-30 Gy) should be administered.

REFERENCES

Attal M, Harousseau JL, Facon T, et al: Single versus double autologous stem-cell transplantation for multiple myeloma. N Engl J Med 2003;349: 2495-2502.
Barlogie B, Tricot G, Anaissie E, et al: Thalidomide and hematopoietic-cell transplantation for multiple myeloma. N Engl J Med 2006;354:1021-1030.
Dimopoulos MA, Zervas K, Kouvatseas G, et al: Thalidomide and dexamethasone combination for refractory multiple myeloma. Ann Oncol 2001;12: 991-995.
Durie BG, Kyle RA, Belch A, et al: Myeloma management guidelines: A consensus report from the Scientific Advisors of the International Myeloma Foundation. Hematol J 2003;4:379-398.
Fonseca R, Blood E, Rue M, et al: Clinical and biologic implications of recurrent genomic aberrations in myeloma. Blood 2003;101:4569-4575.
Greipp PR, San Miguel J, Durie BG, et al: International staging system for multiple myeloma. J Clin Oncol 2005;23:3412-3420.
Harousseau JL, Attal, M: The role of stem cell transplantation in multiple myeloma. Blood Rev 2002;16:245-253.
International Myeloma Working Group: Criteria for the classification of monoclonal gammopathies, multiple myeloma and related disorders. Br J Haematol 2003;121:749-757.
Kyle RA, Therneau TM, Rajkumar SV, et al: A long-term study of prognosis in monoclonal gammopathy of undetermined significance. N Engl J Med 2002;346:564-569.
Palumbo A, Bringhen S, Caravita T, et al: Oral melphalan and prednisone chemotherapy plus thalidomide compared with melphalan and prednisone alone in elderly patients with multiple myeloma: Randomised controlled trial. Lancet 2006;367:825-831.
Rajkumar SV, Hayman SR, Lacy MQ, et al: Combination therapy with lenalidomide plus dexamethasone (rev/dex) for newly diagnosed myeloma. Blood 2005;106:4050-4053.
Reece DE: An update of the management of multiple myeloma: The changing landscape. Hematology (Am Soc Hematol Educ Program) 2005;353-359.
Richardson PG, Sonneveld P, Schuster MW, et al: Bortezomib or high-dose dexamethasone for relapsed multiple myeloma. N Engl J Med 2005;352: 2487-2498.

Polycythemia Vera

Method of
Michael Kroll, MD, and Jennifer Wright, MD

Polycythemia vera (PV) is a clonal disorder of myeloid progenitors resulting in erythrocytosis and varying degrees of thrombocytosis and leukocytosis. The erythrocytosis persists in spite of low levels of erythropoietin.

A mutation in the Janus kinase 2 *(JAK2)* gene is observed in most cases of PV. This mutation results in a substitution of phenylalanine for valine at amino acid residue 617 (V617F). This substitution in a critical binding partner of the cytoplasmic domain of the erythropoietin receptor leads to proliferation signals in the absence of erythropoietin binding. The presence of the mutation assists in diagnosis by distinguishing PV from secondary causes of erythrocytosis and it provides a potential target for new therapies.

Clinical Presentation

Patients with PV are usually identified by abnormal blood counts obtained for unrelated reasons, although some visit a physician with complaints related to arterial or venous thrombosis. The median age at diagnosis is 60 years. Male and female patients are equally affected.

As many as 40% of PV patients suffer some form of thrombosis. The first thrombotic event might occur prior to the diagnosis of PV. In a large retrospective review by the Italian Polycythemia Study Group of 1213 PV patients evaluated over 20 years, 20% received the diagnosis at the time of their first thrombosis and 14% reported a history of thrombosis, mainly within the 2 years preceding a diagnosis of PV. Arterial thromboses, such as ischemic stroke and myocardial infarction, outnumber venous thrombosis by two to one. Sites of venous thrombosis may be unusual, such as hepatic vein thrombosis (Budd-Chiari syndrome), and the presence of an unusual venous thrombosis should prompt an evaluation for PV. PV patients older than 60 years or with a prior thrombosis are at increased risk for PV-associated thromboses.

Bleeding is also a problem. It is most likely to occur with extreme thrombocytosis (platelet counts >1,000,000-1,500,000/μL). GI bleeding, often associated with aspirin use, can occur with lower platelet counts and is sometimes the chief complaint leading to a diagnosis of PV. Bleeding might bring the hematocrit to within normal limits, thereby confusing the clinical picture. One should think of the possibility of PV when normal red cell counts are maintained in the face of iron deficiency.

Other symptoms that could prompt medical attention are erythromelalgia (painful inflammation in the distal extremities), pruritis (especially after a hot bath or shower), and discomfort or early satiety from splenomegaly.

Natural History

The median survival for PV patients is 15 to 20 years, although it is considerably shorter in patients whose PV is undiagnosed or untreated. Even with appropriate treatment, however, PV carries with it a slight increase in mortality as compared with age-, sex-, and comorbid condition–matched controls. Decreased survival is due mainly to thrombosis.

There is a higher incidence of acute leukemia among PV patients, particularly when they have been treated with an alkylating agent or radioactive phosphorous (^{32}P). The development of myelofibrosis also complicates the clinical course of PV, perhaps more often in patients with uncontrolled thrombocytosis. Overall, about 4% of all PV patients suffer at some time from a hematologic transformation, with myelofibrosis occurring in about 2.5% and an acute myeloid leukemia occurring in about 1.5%.

Diagnosis

The initial goal in the evaluation of a patient with a persistently elevated hematocrit is to determine whether the erythrocytosis is absolute or relative. This goal is accomplished by measuring an elevated red cell mass accompanied by a normal plasma volume. Relative (or apparent) erythrocytosis, which is defined as a normal red cell mass with a low plasma volume, includes a heterogeneous group of benign and reversible conditions, such as diuretic use or smoker's polycythemia. With long-term follow-up, nearly one third of those with apparent erythrocytosis have normalization of the hematocrit following routine interventions, such as changing medications or quitting smoking.

Levels of hemoglobin or hematocrit are sometimes used as surrogates for red cell mass measurements, but one must be aware of their limitations. PV patients often have normal hemoglobin concentrations. For example, in one study only 35% of men and 63% of women with PV had elevated hemoglobin (defined as >18.5 g/dL for men and >16.5 g/dL for women). This is the reason for using several additional diagnostic elements when making the diagnosis of PV. These diagnostic elements are broadly described as the clinicopathologic features that are associated with erythrocytosis in PV patients (rule-in criteria) and those that are associated with secondary erythrocytosis (rule-out criteria).

A medical history should identify most causes of secondary erythrocytosis. A history of cyanotic congenital heart disease, chronic lung disease, kidney transplantation, or medications such as androgens or exogenous erythropoietin excludes PV as the cause of erythrocytosis. Smoking elevates hematocrit not only by inducing lung injury and hypoxemia but also by increasing carboxyhemoglobin concentrations and decreasing plasma volume. One must also be aware of rare inherited polycythemias, and a lifetime personal or family history of erythrocytosis should prompt an evaluation for high oxygen affinity hemoglobin or some other syndrome of hereditary erythrocytosis.

Hypoxemia-induced erythrocytosis is evaluated by measuring arterial oxygen saturation. Oxygen saturation is unaffected by carboxyhemoglobin, however, and normal O_2 saturation does not eliminate a diagnosis of smoker's polycythemia. Patients with obstructive sleep apnea can have normal saturations during the day and yet suffer a secondary erythrocytosis because of nighttime hypoxemia. Renal cell carcinoma and benign renal disease (such as hydronephrosis and polycystic kidneys) can stimulate erythropoietin production and cause erythrocytosis. Nonrenal neoplasms, such as hepatocellular carcinoma and uterine leiomyoma, also lead to pathologic elevations of serum erythropoietin levels directing elevated red cell counts. Elevated levels of erythropoietin rule out PV and point to a diagnosis of secondary erythrocytosis.

A low serum erythropoietin level is consistent with a diagnosis of PV. Normal levels are not helpful because they are seen in PV, secondary erythrocytoses, and apparent erythrocytoses. Other laboratory abnormalities observed in PV include elevated serum vitamin B_{12} and leukocyte alkaline phosphatase. Iron deficiency may be present because iron is being consumed by the hyperproliferative erythron or because of GI bleeding or therapeutic phlebotomy. Neutrophilia and thrombocytosis often occur and are useful diagnostic adjuncts. The bone marrow typically shows trilineage hyperplasia, varying amounts of reticulin, and absent or low iron, and it is the best test for excluding a diagnosis of myelofibrosis. Erythroid colonies can be cultured from PV blood or bone marrow without adding erythropoietin, and erythropoietin-independent erythroid colony formation is sometimes used as a diagnostic test.

An activating mutation has been identified in the JAK2 protein that associates with the cytoplasmic tail of the erythropoietin receptor. This mutation—V617F—is found in patients with all myeloproliferative disorders, but it is most commonly associated with PV. The mutation leads to continual activation of genes usually signaled when erythropoietin binds to its receptor. These genes drive erythropoiesis totally independent of the influence of erythropoietin. The JAK2 mutation has been identified in 65% to 97% of patients with PV. Detection of the JAK2 V617F mutation requires only a simple polymerase chain reaction–based test. A positive test is a major criterion for making the diagnosis of PV.

 CURRENT DIAGNOSIS

Diagnosis requires both absolute criteria plus one major criterion or two minor criteria.

Absolute Criteria

- Elevated red cell mass
  - >25% predicted *or*
  - Hb >18.5 or Hct >60 in male patients *or*
  - Hb >16.5 or Hct >56 in female patients
- No secondary erythrocytosis
  - No elevation of erythropoietin
  - Normal arterial oxygen saturation
  - Carboxyhemoglobin levels normal

Major Criteria

- Splenomegaly on examination
- JAK2 V617F mutation or other evidence of clonality (excluding *bcr/abl*)

Minor Criteria

- Thrombocytosis
- Leukocytosis
- Low serum erythropoietin
- Spontaneous erythroid colony growth

Adapted from Campbell PJ, Green AR? Management of polycythemia vera and essential thrombocythemia. Hematol Am Soc Hematol Educ Program 2005;201-208; McMullin MF, Bareford D, Campbell P, et al: Guidelines for the diagnosis, investigation and management of polycythaemia/erythrocytosis. Br J Haem 2005;130:174-195; and Michiels JJ, De Raeve H, Berneman Z, et al: The 2001 World Health Organization and updated European clinical and pathological criteria for the diagnosis, classification, and staging of the Philadelphia chromosome-negative chronic myeloproliferative disorders. Semin Thromb Hemost 2006;32(4)?307-340.

Treatment

Morbidity and mortality associated with PV are reduced by lowering the risk of thrombosis and by controlling bleeding and other symptoms.

THROMBOSIS

The hematocrit (Hct) correlates with the risk of thrombosis, and higher rates of thrombosis are seen at Hct levels greater than 0.45. The cornerstone of treatment is to maintain the Hct below this level using phlebotomy. Moderate iron deficiency should emerge,

CURRENT THERAPY

Hematocrit <45%

- Phlebotomy
- Cytoreduction with hydroxyurea (Hydrea)[1] beginning at 500 mg PO daily
  - Intolerance to phlebotomy
  - Thrombocytosis develops
  - Symptomatic splenomegaly

Platelets <450,000/μL

- Cytoreduction with hydroxyurea[1]
  - Age ≥60
  - Prior thrombosis
- Anagrelide (Agrylin) beginning at 0.5 mg PO bid if the patient is hydroxyurea intolerant
- Interferon-α-2 (Roferon, Intron A)[1]
  - During pregnancy
- Prevent thrombosis
  - Daily baby (81 mg) aspirin
- Control reversible cardiovascular risks
  - Smoking
  - Diabetes
  - Hyperlipidemia
  - Hypertension
  - Obesity
- Control bleeding
  - Plateletpheresis for extremely high platelet counts (≥1,000,000/μL)
  - Stop aspirin

[1]Not FDA approved for this indication.

---

if it is not present initially, but it does not pose any threat. Patients should be cautioned against taking iron supplements. If iron is required, the hemoglobin (Hb) or Hct should be monitored closely.

Some patients cannot tolerate phlebotomy, and therefore chemotherapy is required to control the Hct. Hydroxyurea (Hydrea)[1] is effective at reducing both the hematocrit and the platelet count. Adverse effects include pancytopenia, leg ulcers, and gastrointestinal complaints. Although there has been concern about a potential increased risk of leukemia associated with hydroxyurea, this risk has not been demonstrated conclusively. Other agents such as busulfan (Myleran)[1] or ^{32}P, however, are clearly associated with a significant risk of leukemic transformation. These agents are very rarely used today, although oral busulfan, because it can be given intermittently, is sometimes employed for patients who are unable to comply with daily hydroxyurea dosing. Interferon-α-2 (Roferon or Intron A)[1] is also effective at controlling the Hct, carries no increased risk of leukemia, and is the recommended treatment for pregnant PV patients who cannot tolerate phlebotomy. Flulike symptoms and fatigue are common side effects of interferon-α-2.

Platelets contribute to thrombotic risk. The European Collaboration on Low-Dose Aspirin in Polycythemia Vera trial demonstrated in a prospective, randomized fashion that daily low-dose aspirin effectively reduces the risk of thrombosis without significantly increasing the risk of major bleeding episodes. Therefore, unless there is a clear contraindication, low-dose aspirin should be included in the treatment of all PV patients, including pregnant women. Reduction of the platelet count to normal also reduces the risk of thrombosis. Hydroxyurea[1] is used to reduce the platelet count when thrombocytosis develops, especially if other risk factors for thrombosis are present. Anagrelide (Agrylin) selectively reduces the platelet count and is an FDA-approved alternative to hydroxyurea.

Other known risk factors for cardiovascular disease, such as smoking, dyslipidemia, hypertension, diabetes, and obesity, should be identified and treated.

BLEEDING

Extremely high platelet counts, high doses of aspirin, or a history of gastrointestinal bleeding increases the risk of hemorrhagic events. Bleeding is typically mucocutaneous and from the gastrointestinal tract. Management of bleeding depends on the clinical severity of the event. It is usually first managed by stopping aspirin. If the platelet counts are extremely high (>1,000,000-1,500,000/μL), plateletpheresis is used to control bleeding. It works by rapidly reducing the platelet count and thereby reversing a hemostatic defect resulting from platelets absorbing plasma von Willebrand's factor (causing an acquired von Willebrand's syndrome).

OTHER SYMPTOMS

Erythromelalgia often resolves with aspirin therapy. Higher (antiinflammatory) doses of aspirin may be required initially, but reduction of the dose to 81 mg/day is usually possible after symptoms are controlled. Pruritis usually improves when the Hct is controlled, but H$_2$-blockers or selective serotonin reuptake inhibitors[1] can help those with more severe or intractable itching. Symptoms of splenomegaly are improved by hydroxyurea.[1]

REFERENCES

Campbell PJ, Green AR: Management of polycythemia vera and essential thrombocythemia. Hematol Am Soc Hematol Educ Program 2005; 201-208. Available at http://asheducationbook.hematologylibrary.org/cgi/content/full/2005/1/201 (accessed May 27, 2007).

Coretlazzo S, Finazzi G: Hydroxyurea for patients with essential thrombocythemia and a high risk of thrombosis. N Engl J Med 1995;332:1132-1136.

Gruppo Italiano Studio Policitemia: Polycythemia vera: The natural history of 1213 patients followed for 20 years. Ann Intern Med 1995;123:656-664.

James C, Ugo V, Le Couedic JP, et al: A unique clonal JAK2 mutation leading to constitutive signaling causes polycythaemia vera. Nature 2005;434:1144-1148.

Johansson PL, Safai-Kutti S, Kutti J: An elevated venous hemoglobin concentration cannot be used as a surrogate marker for absolute erythrocytosis: A study of patients with polycythaemia vera and apparent polycythaemia. Br J Haem 2005;129:701-705.

Kralovics R, Passamonti F, Buser AS, et al: A gain-of-function mutation of JAK2 in myeloproliferative disorders. N Engl J Med 2005;352:1779-1790.

Landolfi R, Marchioli R, Kutti J, et al: Efficacy and safety of low-dose aspirin in polycythemia vera. N Engl J Med 2004;350:114-124.

Marchioli R, Finazzi G: Vascular and neoplastic risk in a large cohort of patients with polycythemia vera. J Clin Oncol 2005;23:2224-2232.

McMullin MF, Bareford D, Campbell P, et al: Guidelines for the diagnosis, investigation and management of polycythaemia/erythrocytosis. Br J Haem 2005;130:174-195.

Michiels JJ, De Raeve H, Berneman Z, et al: The 2001 World Health Organization and updated European clinical and pathological criteria for the diagnosis, classification, and staging of the Philadelphia chromosome-negative chronic myeloproliferative disorders. Semin Thromb Hemost 2006;32(4):307-340.

Pearson TC, Wetherley-Mein G: Vascular occlusive episodes and venous haematocrit in primary proliferative polycythaemia. Lancet 1978;2:1219-1222.

Schafer AI: Molecular basis of the diagnosis and treatment if polycythemia vera and essential thrombocythemia. Blood 2006;107:4214-4222.

Spivak JL: Polycythemia vera: Myths, mechanisms, and management. Blood 2002;100:4272-4290.

---

[1]Not FDA approved for this indication.

Porphyria

Method of
Herbert L. Bonkovsky, MD, and
Manish Thapar, MD

The porphyrias are metabolic disorders caused primarily by inherited defects in heme synthesis (Table 1). They manifest clinically in two major ways: with neurovisceral symptoms and signs (including abdominal pain, constipation, and weakness) and with cutaneous symptoms and signs. In hereditary coproporphyria and variegate porphyria, patients can present with both kinds of symptoms; in the other forms of porphyria, patients have one or the other kind of clinical presentation.

Classification

In considering therapy for the porphyrias, it is useful to classify them into two major categories: acute or inducible porphyrias and chronic cutaneous porphyrias (see Table 1). Regardless of the specific form of acute porphyria or associated enzymatic defect, all of the acute porphyrias produce similar neurovisceral manifestations and should be managed in a similar manner. Management of cutaneous porphyria, although more specific to the particular type, also involves application of some general principles.

Diagnosis

A complete discussion of the diagnosis of porphyria is beyond the scope of this article. However, a correct and definitive diagnosis at the outset is of paramount importance. Box 1 and Table 2 give the recommended approach to diagnosis. Because of the complicated and unfamiliar tests often required for diagnosis, it is recommended that physicians without special training in the porphyrias discuss

---

BOX 1 Key to Diagnosis: Screening Tests for Porphyrias

Urinary PBG (porphobilinogen) is substantially elevated in all patients with acute attacks of AIP, HCP, and VP and often during latent periods as well, a finding that occurs in no other medical condition. Urinary PBG offers both sensitivity and specificity in diagnosing the acute porphyrias. PBG is not increased in ADP; diagnosis of this rare condition requires measurement of ALA.

If serum or urine ALA and/or PBG are increased, second-line testing is done to determine the precise disorder of porphyrin metabolism, although treatment (which is the same regardless of the type of acute porphyria) should not be delayed pending these results.

A simple test of considerable value for diagnosis and differential diagnosis of the cutaneous porphyrias is the plasma porphyrin fluorescence pattern. In this test, the fluorescence emission spectrum of diluted plasma is measured. The exciting wavelength is the Soret band (400-410 nm). Uroporphyrin and coproporphyrin, which accumulate in PCT and HCP, have a peak at 618 nm, and protoporphyrin, which accumulates in PP, has a peak at 636 nm. A protein-porphyrin complex unique to VP has a peak at 626 nm. The latter is nearly always present in postpubertal VP patients, and it is the simplest and most reliable method for making a presumptive diagnosis of VP.

Abbreviations: AIP = acute intermittent porphyria; ALA = 5-aminolevulinic acid; CEP = congenital erythopoietic porphyria; EPP = erythopoietic protoporphyria; HEP = hepatoerythopoietic porphyria, HCP = hereditary corproporphyria; PBG = porphobilinogen; PCT = porphyria cutanea tarda; VP = variegate porphyria

---

TABLE 1 Classification and Major Features of Human Porphyrias

Disease	Primary Enzymatic Defect	Autosomal Inheritance	Neurovisceral Symptoms	Photosensitivity Dermatosis
Acute or Inducible Porphyrias				
ALA-D deficiency porphyria	ALA dehydratase	Recessive	+	−
Acute intermittent porphyria	PBG deaminase	Dominant	+	−
Hereditary coproporphyria	Coproporphyrinogen oxidase	Dominant	+	+
Variegate porphyria	Protoporphyrinogen oxidase	Dominant	+	+
Chronic Cutaneous Porphyrias				
Congenital erythropoietic	Uroporphyrinogen III (co)-synthase	Recessive	−	+ +
Hepatoerythopoietic porphyria	Uroporphyrinogen decarboxylase	Recessive	±	+
Porphyria cutanea tarda	Uroporphyrinogen decarboxylase	Dominant (acquired variant exists)	−	+
Protoporphyria	Ferrochelatase	Recessive	− *	+

Abbreviations: ALA = 5-aminolevulinic acid, the first intermediate in the heme biosynthetic pathway; ALA-D = ALA dehydratase; PBG = porphobilinogen, the second intermediate in the heme biosynthetic pathway.
*A neurovisceral syndrome reminiscent of those observed in the acute porphyrias has been described in a few patients with protoporphyria and hepatic failure around the time of orthotopic liver transplantation.

TABLE 2 Further Testing to Confirm the Diagnosis of Acute Porphyrias

Type of Porphyria	RBC PBGB Deaminase	Urinary Porphyrins	Fecal Porphyrins	Plasma Porphyrins	Peak of Porphyrin Emission Fluorescence (nm)
Acute intermittent (AIP)	Low: <50%	Markedly increased (uroporphyrins)	Normal or slightly Increased	Normal or slightly increased	618
Variegate porphyria (VP)	Normal	Markedly increased (coproporphyrins)	Markedly increased (copro- and protoporphyrin)	Markedly increased	626
Hereditary coproporphyria (HCP)	Normal	Markedly increased (coproporphyrins)	Markedly increased (coproporphyrins)	Mostly normal	618
ALA dehydratase porphyria	Normal	Increased (5-aminolevulinic acid and coproporphyrin)	Normal or slightly increased	Increased	618

Abbreviations: PBG = porphobilinogen; RBC = red blood cell.

possible patients with, or refer patients to, physicians who have such expertise. See http://www.porphyriafoundation.com/index.html or call 713-266-9617 for an updated listing. Resources with descriptions on how to diagnose or exclude porphyrias are listed in the references.

CURRENT DIAGNOSIS

Suspected Acute Porphyria

- In suspected acute porphyria, the screening test of choice is random spot urine for qualitative or quantitative porphobilinogen and creatinine. Urinary porphobilinogen is markedly (>10× ULN) increased.
- Mild to moderate increases of urinary porphyrins, with normal urinary ALA and PBG are *not* diagnostic of porphyria but more likely due to secondary porphyrinurias.
- The most useful test for diagnosis of variegate porphyria is the emission fluorescence of plasma excited by the Soret band (excitation wavelength ∼ 400 nm). Peak emission at 626 nm is pathognomic of variegate porphyria.

Suspected Cutaneous Porphyria

- Typical skin lesions of CEP, PCT, or HEP are vesicles and bullae on the hands and face.
- Typical skin lesions of EPP are solar urticaria, acute burning and itching.
- The single most useful screening test is plasma porphyrin and fluorescence emission pattern.
- In clinically manifest cutaneous porphyria, plasma porphyrins are increased and the fluorescence emission pattern is helpful in the differential diagnosis (with excitation light of ∼400 nm, peak emission wavelengths are ∼618 nm in CEP, HEP, PCT, HCP; 626 nm in VP; and 634 nm in EPP).
- In EPP, urinary porphyrins and porphyrin precursors are completely normal.

Abbreviations: ALA = 5-aminolevulinic acid; CEP = congenital erythopoietic prophyria; EPP = erythopoietic protoporphyria; HCP = hereditary coproporphyria; HEP = hepatoerythopoietic porphyria, PBG = prophobilinogen; PCT = porphyria cutanea tarda; ULN = upper limit of normal; VP = variegate porphyria

Treatment

ACUTE HEPATIC PORPHYRIAS

Management of Acute Attacks

The cardinal symptom of acute porphyria is severe colicky abdominal pain. Nausea, vomiting, constipation, and pain or paresthesias in the extremities are present in about one half of patients. Tachycardia and dark urine are the most common signs. The pathogenesis of acute porphyric attacks involves a deficiency of hepatic heme and induction of hepatic 5-aminolevulinic acid (ALA) synthase by stressors, with resultant overproduction of ALA, which is neurotoxic.

General measures should include parenteral hydration and pain control with meperidine (Demerol) 50 to 150 mg or morphine 3 to 10 mg. Addition of a phenothiazine (e.g., chlorpromazine [Thorazine], 25 to 50 mg) enhances the analgesic and sedative effects of the narcotic. Propranolol (Inderal) may be given for control of severe tachycardia or arterial hypertension. The dose should be titrated carefully because of the risk of serious bradycardia and hypotension from propranolol. Frequent checks (every 6 hours) of neuromuscular function, looking for developing weakness of crucial muscles such as the diaphragm, by measuring the vital capacity are recommended.

Specific treatment is directed at correcting the deficiency of hepatic heme and decreasing activity of ALA synthase. The treatment of choice of an acute attack requiring hospital admission is intravenous heme.

Heme is administered intravenously at a dose of 3 to 4 mg/kg/day for 4 days; it is taken up primarily by the liver and replenishes the depleted heme pool. Heme should be started early for most attacks. At this time in the United States, only one FDA-approved form of heme is available: heme hydroxide or hematin (Panhematin, Ovation Pharmaceuticals, Deerfield, IL; www.ovationpharma.com). Each vial of hematin contains 313 mg of heme, supplied as a lyophilized powder that also contains sodium carbonate. The manufacturer recommends dissolving the powder in sterile water. In this form, the resultant hematin solution is unstable and must be administered within 1 hour of preparation. It is also irritating to veins, often producing thrombophlebitis, and causes a mild coagulopathy due to adverse effects on clotting factors and platelets.

It is now recommended that lyophilized hematin be reconstituted with human albumin (1:1 molar complex), which increases its stability and decreases unwanted side effects. To prepare such a solution, add 132 mL of 25% human serum albumin (33 g) to a vial containing lyophilized hematin and mix gently. Heme given in this form has biochemical and clinical effects on porphyria that appear equivalent to those of freshly prepared aqueous solutions of hematin and are superior to those of aged aqueous solutions of hematin. Hematin can

CURRENT THERAPY

Acute Porphyria

- Remove inciting factors: Alcohol, drugs, toxins and chemicals (see Box 2)
- Nutritional supplementation: ≥300 g glucose/day may be given enterally if tolerated
- Intravenous heme: 3-5 mg/kg/d for 3-5 days
- Frequent checks of neurologic status: Especially watch for development of paresis of muscles of respiration
- Monitor for hypokalemia, hypomagnesemia, or hyponatremia and treat vigorously, if found
- Parenteral meperidine (Demerol) 50-150 mg or morphine 3-10 mg q4-6h for pain
- Chlorpromazine (Thorazine) 25-50 mg q4-6h for nausea and agitation
- Propranolol (Inderal) 10-40 mg q6h for tachycardia and hypertension
- Magnesium sulfate, gabapentin (Neurontin), and/or vigabatrin (Sabril)[2] for seizures
- All cases should undergo hepatocellular carcinoma screening every 6 months even in the absence of cirrhosis.
- All first-degree family members should be screened for porphyria

Cutaneous Porphyria

- General measures: Protect skin from light and trauma; treat secondary skin infections
- Congenital erythropoietic porphyria: Oral activated charcoal; hypertransfusion to suppress erythropoiesis; heme infusion; splenectomy for hemolysis; glucocorticoid trial for anemia; bone marrow transplantation (gene therapy in the future)
- Hepatoerythropoietic porphyria: Uncertain; probably the same as for congenital erythropoietic porphyria (phlebotomy and antimalarials are not effective)
- Porphyria cutanea tarda: Stop ethanol, estrogen, or other precipitating chemicals; iron depletion by phlebotomy; treat chronic hepatitis C, if present; chloroquine (Aralen)[1] or hydroxychloroquine (Plaquenil)[3]; urinary alkalinization
- Protoporphyria: β-Carotene; adequate iron; oral charcoal; cholecystectomy for gallstones; plasmapheresis; intravenous heme; hypertransfusion; liver transplantation; (gene therapy in the future)

[1]Not FDA approved in this indication.
[2]Not available in the United States.

be delivered within a few hours to anywhere in the United States by calling the 24/7 Ovation hotline at 1-888-514-5204.

In some other countries, another effective form of heme is available: heme arginate (Normosang).[2] This preparation consists of heme complexed to arginine and is supplied as a solution that usually is also diluted in approximately 5% human serum albumin just before administration. Usual doses are as for Panhematin.

Another way to decrease ALA synthase is to administer glucose or other readily metabolized carbohydrates, taking advantage of the phenomenon of carbohydrate repression of the enzyme, the so-called glucose effect. This may be used for mild attacks or when awaiting IV hematin. At least 300 g of glucose per day is given, enterally if tolerated or as a 10% infusion. Some patients have elevations of antidiuretic hormone (ADH) and can rapidly develop profound symptomatic hyponatremia and hypomagnesemia, especially when dextrose in water is given intravenously. As a rule, it is best to give dextrose in half-normal saline. Serum electrolytes including magnesium should be checked every 12 hours for the first few days. Hypokalemia or hypomagnesemia should be corrected promptly.

Many drugs and chemicals are known to exacerbate acute porphyrias, and many others are theoretically risky because they induce hepatic cytochrome P-450, deplete hepatic regulatory heme, and induce ALA synthase, especially in animals with a partial block in heme synthesis (Box 2). Among dangerous drugs, the worst offenders are barbiturates, ethanol excess, hydantoins, and sulfonamides. These drugs are absolutely contraindicated in patients with acute porphyric attacks; others, listed in the first two sections of Box 2, should be avoided if possible. The last section of Box 2 lists drugs believed to be safe; however, a wise practice is to use as few systemically absorbed drugs as possible.

Therapy of Seizures in Patients with Acute Porphyria

Treatment of seizures in porphyric patients has been particularly problematic because most of the commonly used anticonvulsants also induce cytochrome P-450 and can precipitate or worsen acute attacks (see Box 2). Seizures in acute attacks can also occur due to hyponatremia or hypomagnesemia. Seizures in patients with acute porphyria have been treated with bromides, which are effective and do not exacerbate porphyria, but they have a narrow therapeutic window. High doses of magnesium sulfate (3 g loading dose; then 1 g/h in 0.15 M NaCl, with or without 5% dextrose) have been of benefit. A suggested therapeutic range for serum magnesium level is 4 to 8 mEq/L. Clonazepam (Klonopin) has helped some patients, but in large doses it has made others worse. High doses of clonazepam must be considered a potential hazard, because it induces cytochrome P-450 and ALA synthase in cultured hepatocytes (see Box 2).

The safety of newer anticonvulsant medications has been studied in cultured liver cells. Phenobarbital, felbamate (Felbatol), lamotrigine (Lamictal), or tiagabine (Gabitril), but not gabapentin (Neurontin) or vigabatrin (Sabril),[2] increased levels of porphyrins and the mRNA of ALA synthase, the first and rate-controlling enzyme of porphyrin synthesis. Vigabatrin[2] or gabapentin is therefore recommended in patients with acute porphyria and seizures. Administration of gabapentin should be individualized; the usual dose range for adults is 900 to 1800 mg/day, given in three divided doses.

Management of Frequent Recurrent Attacks

Some unfortunate women suffer attacks of acute porphyria nearly every month during the luteal phase of their menstrual cycles. Some are helped by oral contraceptives, which are believed to act by interrupting their endogenous cyclic production of sex hormones. However, such therapy is a double-edged sword, because exogenous estrogens and progestogens can induce ALA synthase (see Box 2). Minimal effective doses should be used, and patients should be followed closely, particularly in the first few months. Regular infusions of heme have also been of benefit but require frequent IV access. Also, chronic heme therapy can lead to iron overload, because heme is about 8% iron by weight.

For most women with cyclic attacks of acute porphyria, the treatment of choice is a luteinizing hormone-releasing hormone (LHRH) analogue. Leuprolide (Lupron)[1] has been used most often. The usual daily dose is 1 mg (0.2 mL), subcutaneously, although higher doses are occasionally required. LHRH analogues can produce initial worsening of porphyric symptoms due to partial agonist effects, followed by improvement due to chronic antagonist effects.

[2]Not available in the United States.
[1]Not FDA approved in this indication.

BOX 2 Some Drugs and Chemicals in Acute Hepatic Porphyrias

Reported to Exacerbate Disease

Aminoglutethimide (Cytadren)
Antipyrine
Aminopyrine
Barbiturates
Barbamazepine
Carbamazepine (Tegretol)
Carisoprodol (Soma)
Chloramphenicol (Chloromycetin)
Clindamycin (Cleocin)
Danazol (Danocrine)
Dihydralazine
Diclofenac (Voltaren)
Erythromycin
Estrogens
Ethanol excess
Fosphenytoin (Cerebyx)
Griseofulvin (Grifulvin)
Hydralazine
Hydantoins
Hydroxyzine (Vistaril)
Indinavir (Crixivan)
Ketoconazole (Nizoral)
Ketamine (Ketalar)
Lidocaine
Lynestrenol
Medroxyprogesterone (Provera)
Methyldopa (Aldomet)
Metoclopramide (Reglan)
Norethisterone (Micronor, Aygestin)
Nitrofurantoin (Microdantin)
Oral contraceptives
Orphenadrine (Norflex)
Phenylbutazone
Phenytoin (Dilantin)
Primidone (Mysoline)
Progestogens
Pyrazinamide
Rifampicin (Rifadin)
Sulfonamides
Spironolactone (Aldactone)
Tamoxifen (Nolvadex)
Testosterone
Theophylline and its derivatives
Trimethoprim
Valproic acid (Depakote)

Theoretically Risky

Amlodipine (Norvasc)
Amiodarone (Cordarone)
Amitriptyline (Elavil)
Azathioprine (Imuran)
Amphetamines
Atorvastatin (Lipitor)
Bosentan (Tracleer)
Buspirone (Buspar)
Clonidine (Catapres)
Clonazepam (Klonopin) (large doses)
Ceftriaxone (Rocephin)
Cervistatin (Baycol)
Cetirizine (Zyrtec)
Diazepam(Valium)
Diltiazem (Cardizem)
Diphenhydramine (Benadryl)
Econazole (Spectazole)
Ethosuximide (Zarontin)
Felodipine (Plendil)
Fluconazole (Diflucan)
Fluvastatin (Lescol)
Glibenclamide (Diabeta)
Glipizide (Glucotrol)
Guaifenesin (Robitussin)
Heavy metals
Halothane
Hyoscyamine (Levsin)
Imipramine (Tofranil)
Isoniazid
Itraconazole (Sporanox)
Lansoprazole (Prevacid)
Lamotrigine (Lamictal)
Lamivudine (Epivir)
Metronidazole (Flagyl)
Montelukast (Singulair)
Nortriptyline (Pamelor)
Nifedipine (Adalat)
Oxytetracycline
Oxcarbazepine (Trileptal)
Pioglitazone (Actos)
Probenecid
Quinine (Qualaquin)
Rabeprazole (Aciphex)
Rosiglitazone (Avandia)
Sulfonylureas
Simvastatin (Zocor)
Telithromycin (Ketek)
Tetracycline
Topiramate (Topamax)
Tramadol (Ultram)
Verapamil (Calan)
Voriconazole (VFEND)
All agents known to induce cytochrome P-450 or to increase hepatic heme turnover

Believed to be Safe

Acetaminophen (Tylenol)
Allopurinol (Zyloprim)
Aspirin
Atropine
Azithromycin (Zithromax)
Bisacodyl (Dulcolax)
Bromides
Cimetidine (Tagamet)
Chlorpromazine
Cephalexin (Keflex)
Ciprofloxacin (Cipro)
Candesartan (Atacand)
Captopril (Capoten)
Dopamine
Digoxin (Lanoxin)
Enalapril (Vasotec)
Ezetimibe (Zetia)
Furosemide (Lasix)
Fondaparinux (Arixtra)
Gabapentin (Neurontin)
Glucocorticoids
Gemfibrozil (Lopid)
Heparin
Hydrochlorothiazide (Microzide)
Ibuprofen (Motrin, Advil)
Insulin
Iron
Irbesartan (Avapro)
Labetalol (Trandate)
Lisinopril (Prinivil, Zestril)
Lithium (Lithobid)
Meperidine (Demerol)
Morphine
Nicotinic Acid (Niaspan)
Nystatin (Mycostatin)
Naproxen (Naprosyn)
Ofloxacin (Floxin)
Ondansetron (Zofran)
Penicillin and its derivatives
Phenylephrine
Phenylpropanolamine
Propranolol (Inderal)
Quinapril (Accupril)
Ramipril (Altace)
Streptomycin
Tetanus toxoid
Thiamine (vitamin B_1)
Tobramycin (Tobrex)
Valsartan (Diovan)
Vancomycin (Vancocin)
Vitamins A, B, C, D, and E
Vigabatrin (Sabril)[2]

[2]Not available in the United States.
Refer to http://www.porphyriafoundation.com/ and http://www.porphyria-europe.com/ for more detailed lists.

Therapy with LHRH analogues is usually continued for at least 1 year and sometimes longer. The use of bisphosphonates to minimize development of osteoporosis is advised when prolonged therapy with LHRH analogues is undertaken.

Prevention of Attacks

Patients should be counseled not to use ethanol and avoid drugs not known to be safe (see Box 2). The use of herbal remedies and alternative therapies is also to be discouraged because many such preparations are likely to contain porphyrogenic compounds. Patients should also avoid very-low-calorie diets or prolonged periods of fasting and should receive prompt and vigorous management of intercurrent illnesses or other stressors. Pregnancy does not usually cause acute porphyria to worsen, and termination of pregnancy is not usually indicated on medical grounds, even if both mother and fetus have acute porphyria.

A small fraction of patients with frequent attacks require chronic infusions of heme. In some, the heme needs to be given weekly or even twice weekly. These patients need to be watched for the development of iron overload and can require iron-reduction therapy by therapeutic phlebotomies if serum ferritin exceeds 1000 ng/mL.

Relatives at risk should be evaluated thoroughly and all probands and relatives found to be carriers should be educated and encouraged to wear medical alert bracelets and to carry medical alert cards.

In a rare patient with recalcitrant and unremitting disease, consideration may be given to orthotopic liver transplantation. Liver transplantation has been described in case reports as resulting in biochemical and clinical remission.

Studies have shown a 60- to 70-fold increased prevalence of hepatocellular carcinoma in patients with hepatic porphyrias even in the absence of cirrhosis or steatohepatitis. This lends credence to periodic screening for hepatocellular cancer in this patient population.

CHRONIC CUTANEOUS PORPHYRIAS

Porphyrin accumulations in the skin, red cells, and hepatocytes are responsible for the pathophysiologic changes of the chronic porphyrias. The general principles of therapy of chronic cutaneous porphyrias are to decrease the overproduction and increase the excretion of porphyrins as much as possible. Protection of the skin from light (opaque sunscreens and/or clothing) and physical trauma should also be recommended. Oral activated charcoal or cholestyramine (Questran) can improve symptoms by absorbing porphyrins and hastening their excretion in the urine. In several diseases, the chronic blistering and ulcerating skin lesions are prone to secondary infection, which requires prompt treatment to minimize further damage.

Congenital Erythropoietic Porphyria

Congenital erythropoietic porphyria (CEP; Günther's disease) is a rare autosomal recessive disorder that manifests in infancy with red urine, erythrodontia, anemia, and a severe blistering dermatosis. The marked overproduction of uroporphyrin I characteristic of CEP arises from erythroid precursors. Elevated levels of porphyrins have been improved by large oral doses of activated charcoal (30-60 g every 6 hours), by hypertransfusion, and by infusions of heme. Unfortunately, long-term therapy with any of these is difficult, and chronic transfusions exacerbate iron overload, which is often a preexisting problem related to ineffective erythropoiesis and increased iron absorption. Some patients with hemolysis have responded to splenectomy, and glucocorticoids have also been reported to improve anemia. Because of the rarity and phenotypic heterogeneity of CEP, a consensus regarding therapy has not emerged. A few patients have been cured by bone marrow transplantation. In the future, gene replacement therapy will deserve serious consideration for treatment of severely affected patients.

Hepatoerythropoietic Porphyria

Hepatoerythropoietic porphyria (HEP) is even rarer than CEP, which it resembles clinically. HEP is due to homozygous or compound heterozygous defects, leading to severe deficiency of uroporphyrinogen decarboxylase. Infants present with severe skin fragility and extensive vesicle and bulla formation, leading to scarring and mutilation of sun-exposed skin. They also present with hypertrichosis, erythrodontia, anemia, and hepatosplenomegaly.

The general and specific measures outlined earlier for therapy of CEP are rational in HEP as well, although none has been shown clearly effective in HEP. HEP shows no response to therapeutic phlebotomy, unlike porphyria cutanea tarda, even though both share a defect in uroporphyrinogen decarboxylase.

Porphyria Cutanea Tarda (PCT)

Porphyria cutanea tarda (PCT) is the most common type of porphyria. It is characterized by an inherited or acquired defect in activity of hepatic uroporphyrinogen decarboxylase. In the common inherited form(s) of PCT, there is a 50% decrease in activity of the decarboxylase, usually identifiable in nonliver tissues as well as in the liver. A defect in the decarboxylase is not sufficient to produce clinical manifestations; other factors, such as iron overload, chronic hepatitis C, ethanol abuse, estrogens, and porphyrogenic toxins, are important pathogenic elements. The typical patient is a middle-aged man with a vesiculobullous eruption on the dorsa of the hands. Patients usually abuse ethanol and have evidence of modest iron overload and liver injury. In some parts of the world, including the United States, most patients with PCT also have chronic hepatitis C.

Patients with mild PCT often respond simply to the general measures and removal of the precipitating agent such as estrogen, ethanol, or halo-aromatic chemical exposure. For those with more severe disease, the treatment of choice is phlebotomy for depletion of hepatic iron stores. The initial treatment regimen should be removal of a pint of blood each week, continued until the patient has developed a mild degree of anemia with decreased serum ferritin, transferrin saturation, and erythrocytic mean corpuscular volume (MCV). Although most patients with PCT have moderate iron overload (~3-4 g), phlebotomy therapy is effective even when hepatic iron stores are not increased.

Unfortunately, the response to iron removal or other therapy of PCT is slow, and evidence of improvement in the skin might not appear for months. It is important to let patients know this and to encourage them to persist in therapy, for it will eventually succeed. Patients should not take medicinal iron and are encouraged to decrease their intake of red meats, which contain relatively large amounts of heme iron, a form of iron particularly well absorbed.

Recent results from our center and others showed that most patients with active PCT also have chronic hepatitis C infection and one or both of the mutations of the *HFE* gene associated with HLA-linked hereditary hemochromatosis. All patients with PCT should be screened for hepatitis C infection and for *HFE* gene mutations (C282Y and H63D).

Chloroquine (Aralen)[1] and hydroxychloroquine (Plaquenil)[1] form water-soluble complexes with uroporphyrin, increasing porphyrin removal from tissue stores and excretion in the urine. However, in previously untreated PCT, the doses of these drugs usually used for other disorders can cause acute hepatic injury with fever, jaundice, and right upper quadrant pain. This is due to excessively rapid mobilization of porphyrin from the liver. For this reason, such drugs should be started slowly at low doses (125 mg 2-3 times per week) with gradual increase to 500 mg/day. Monitoring for possible retinal damage is advisable whenever chronic chloroquine or hydroxychloroquine therapy is used.

PCT can occur in association with end-stage renal disease. Because the chloroquine-porphyrin complex is poorly dialyzable, chloroquine is ineffective. Because of anemia, phlebotomy is relatively contraindicated in such patients. However, administration of recombinant human erythropoietin (Epogen, Procrit) stimulates iron mobilization for red cell production sufficient to support therapeutic phlebotomyies.

Protoporphyria

Also called erythropoietic protoporphyria (EPP), protoporphyria (PP) is a disorder with highly variable clinical expression. Infants and children develop intense burning pain of sun-exposed skin following brief exposure in the spring and summer. A few hours later, erythema, edema, and itching become prominent. Vesicles only develop with prolonged exposure. With chronic and repeated exposure, involved skin can become leathery and hyperkeratotic. This is especially prominent in a malar butterfly distribution on the face and over the knuckles of the hands. Diagnosis of PP requires demonstration of increased amounts of protoporphyrin, without increased coproporphyrin, in the stool, red cells, or both. It is the only form of clinically manifested porphyria in which urinary heme precursors are normal. A common complication of PP is development of pigment gallstones, which contain a high content of protoporphyrin.

---

[1]Not FDA approved in this indication.

A rare, but serious, complication is development of severe liver disease, due to precipitation of protoporphyrin in hepatocytes and biliary radicles. Such disease can progress and produce liver failure with all its usual complications.

In addition to the usual general measures, PP is treated with β-carotene (Solatene). The usual adult dose is 120 to 180 mg/day. The recommended therapeutic serum β-carotene level is 600 to 800 μg/dL. Drugs or chemicals that can increase protoporphyrin production or decrease its utilization should be avoided. Griseofulvin (Grifulvin) is the most obvious example, because it can cause a protoporphyric condition in mice. Any drug or toxin (e.g., excess alcohol) that produces cholestasis is a risk, because protoporphyrin must be excreted through the bile. Patients should be immunized against hepatitis A and B unless they clearly are immune. Avoidance of iron deficiency is important, because iron deficiency can exacerbate overproduction of protoporphyrin. Oral cholestyramine and activated charcoal have been suggested as treatments to prevent the enterohepatic circulation of protoporphyrin, which appears to be substantial. Patients with symptomatic gallstones are best treated by cholecystectomy, as long as they do not have severe liver disease or other contraindications to surgery.

Patients with evidence of liver disease require regular and frequent monitoring, because decompensation can occur quickly. Those with abnormal liver chemistries or very high red cell (>1500 μg/dL) or plasma (>150 μg/dL) protoporphyrin concentrations should undergo liver biopsy. Patients with liver injury must avoid ethanol or other hepatotoxins that can act synergistically to accelerate liver damage. Liver transplantation is an option for those with advanced liver disease, although it does not correct the biochemical abnormality because ferrochelatase deficiency in the bone marrow persists.

Unfortunately, some patients with PP who have undergone liver transplantation have redeveloped pigmentary fibrosis quite rapidly. Thus, transplantation of bone marrow before, during, or after liver transplantation is considered. In the future, gene therapy (the normal ferrochelatase gene targeted to the bone marrow stem cells) will be a major advance. Transient improvements in PP have been achieved by plasmapheresis followed by intravenous heme infusions. The dose of heme used has been 3 to 5 mg/kg/day. Such therapy is recommended, particularly as a way to stabilize hepatic function while transplantation is awaited or to decrease plasma protoporphyrin concentrations just prior to transplantation. Without such therapy, several patients have suffered severe neuromuscular complications, requiring prolonged and expensive convalescence.

REFERENCES

Anderson KE, Bishop DF, Desnick RJ, Sassa S: Disorders of heme biosynthesis. In Scriver CR, Beaudet AL, Sly WS, Valle D, (eds):The Metabolic and Molecular Bases of Inherited Disease, 8th ed. New York, McGraw-Hill, 2001, pp 2991-3042.

Anderson KE, Bloomer JR, Bonkovsky HL, et al: Recommendations for the diagnosis and treatment of the acute porphyrias. Ann Intern Med 2005;142:439-450.

Anderson KE, Bonkovsky HL, Bloomer JR, Shedlofsky SI: Reconstitution of hematin for intravenous infusion. Ann Intern Med 2006;144:537-538.

Bonkovsky HL, Barnard GF: Diagnosis of porphyric syndromes: A practical approach in the era of molecular biology. Semin Liver Dis 1998;18:57-65.

Bonkovsky HL, Barnard GF: The hepatic porphyrias. In Brandt L (ed): Clinical Practice of Gastroenterology. Philadelphia: Current Medicine, 1998, pp 947-960.

Bonkovsky HL, Healey JF, Lourie AN, Gerron GG: Intravenous heme-albumin in acute intermittent porphyria: Evidence for repletion of hepatic hemoproteins and regulatory heme pools. Am J Gastroenterol 1991;86:1050-1056.

Bonkovsky HL, Poh-Fitzpatrick M, Pimstone N, et al: Porphyria cutanea tarda, hepatitis C, and HFE gene mutations in North America. Hepatology 1998;27:1661-1669.

Chemmanur AT, Bonkovsky HL: Hepatic porphyrias: Diagnosis and management. Clin Liver Dis 2004;8:807-838.

McGuire BM, Bonkovsky HL, Carithers RL Jr, et al: Liver transplantation for erythropoietic protoporphyria liver disease. Liver Transpl 2005;11:1590-1596.

Therapeutic Use of Blood Components

Method of
Peter A. Millward, MD, and
Mark E. Brecher, MD

The transfusion of blood was the first successful transplantation of living tissue in humans. Today, transfusion is so commonplace that it is rarely thought of as a transplant. In 2001, for allogeneic transfusions within the United States alone, it is estimated that 13,898,000 units of whole blood or red blood cells, 2,614,000 units of whole blood—derived platelets, 1,264,000 units of apheresis platelets, and 3,926,000 units of plasma were administered. For red blood cell—containing products alone, this equates to 1 unit transfused every 2.3 seconds. A basic understanding of indications for blood component therapy is essential to optimally treat patients.

Red Blood Cells

Red blood cells are collected via whole blood donation or automated erythrocytapheresis. Both collection techniques employ a sterile closed system for blood collection. The blood is collected into plastic blood bags containing a sufficient formulation of anticoagulant and preservative solution.

The components of the anticoagulant solution determine the maximum shelf life (ranging from 21 to 35 days) of collected blood and blood components. The solution can contain citrate (trisodium citrate and citric acid), dextrose, phosphate (monobasic sodium phosphate), and adenine. Citrate is for anticoagulation, dextrose and adenine are for metabolic energy, and phosphate is for buffering pH.

Shelf life of red cells may be extended to 42 days with the addition of an preservative-additive solution, such as Adsol (AS-1), Nutricel (AS-3), or Optisol (AS-5). This additive solution must be added within 72 hours from primary collection. Additive solution contains dextrose, adenine, and sodium chloride and contains either monobasic sodium phosphate or mannitol.

Even with anticoagulant and preservative-additive solutions, biochemical changes, called storage lesions, develop with stored red blood cells. These biochemical changes are decreased pH, adenosine triphosphate (ATP), and 2,3-diphosphoglycerate (DPG) and increased plasma potassium and plasma hemoglobin (Hb). Even in massively transfused patients, storage lesions do not routinely cause significant clinical consequences when transfused.

The standard collection volume for a whole blood donation is 450 mL ± 45 mL. Because whole blood is rarely indicated, centrifugation is used to separate a whole-blood donation into various components, which maximizes this limited resource. One red blood cell (RBC) unit, also known as *packed RBCs*, is made by removing a significant portion of plasma from a whole-blood donation. Using apheresis technique, one or two RBC units can be specifically collected with each donation. With either technique, an RBC unit volume is approximately 300 mL. Based on the preservative-additive solution used, an RBC unit averages a hematocrit of 60% to 80%.

After initial processing of whole blood, an RBC unit is composed of RBCs, white blood cells (WBCs), platelets, and plasma. An erythrocytapheresis RBC unit is composed of RBCs with decreased platelets and plasma and are *leukocyte reduced* ($<5 \times 10^6$ leukocytes per component) due to intraprocedural leukocyte filtration.

RBC units can be further modified for specific needs of the patient to leukoreduced RBCs, washed RBCs, irradiated RBCs, and frozen deglycerolized RBCs.

LEUKOREDUCED RED BLOOD CELLS

In the United States, a leukoreduced RBC unit must have less than 5 million leukocytes per unit. This decrease in leukocytes is achieved using a leukocyte filter that extracts leukocytes based on their relative larger size and propensity to adhere to certain fiber types. Current leukoreduction filters remove between 3 and 5 log of leukocytes in an RBC unit. Leukocyte filtration can occur during or immediately after collection (prestorage leukocyte reduction) or at the time of transfusion (poststorage leukocyte reduction).

Common indications for leukoreduced RBCs are multiple febrile, nonhemolytic transfusion reactions (FNHTR), prevention of HLA alloimmunization, and reduction of cytomegalovirus (CMV) transmission.

An FNHTR is defined by a greater than 1°C (2°F) temperature rise occurring up to 2 hours after transfusion and unexplained by the patient's underlying medical condition; it may be accompanied by chills, rigors, nausea, vomiting, malaise, and headache. Two mechanisms of FNHTR with RBC transfusion have been proposed: recipient anti-HLA or antigranulocyte antibodies react with donor leukocytes and induce cytokine release, or donor leukocytes form an antigen-antibody complex resulting in recipient monocytes to release cytokines. Both mechanisms depend on the presence of donor leukocytes, and therefore leukoreduction effectively decreases the incidence of FNHTR associated with red blood cell transfusions.

The formation of HLA antibodies (also known as HLA alloimmunization) can lead to platelet transfusion refractoriness, which is especially problematic for patients requiring substantial platelet transfusion support (e.g., hematology-oncology patients). All potential candidates for bone marrow (BMT) or solid organ transplantation should receive leukoreduced RBCs to minimize the formation of HLA antibodies.

Transfusion-transmitted CMV (TT-CMV) infections in high-risk populations, such as CMV-negative neonates, AIDS patients, and BMT candidates or patients, are associated with considerable mortality and morbidity. CMV is latent in leukocytes, specifically in the monocyte-macrophage lineage. Based on Bowden and colleagues' findings in 1995, leukoreduced RBCs offer a CMV-safe blood product that is an equivalent alternative to providing blood from a CMV-seronegative donor. These findings and other confirming studies led to numerous institutions using leukoreduced RBCs as their sole method for providing CMV-safe blood products and abandoning a CMV-seronegative inventory. Recently, Nicholas and colleagues questioned the equivalence of leukoreduced blood products versus CMV-seronegative blood products and called for further investigation.

WASHED RED BLOOD CELLS

The objective of washing RBCs is to effectively remove 99% of antibodies, plasma proteins, and electrolytes contained within the RBC component. The washing process involves repetitive steps of infusion of normal (0.9%) saline and centrifugation, with final resuspension of washed RBCs in normal saline. Because this process is an open system and the anticoagulant-preservative solution is removed, washed red cells must be transfused within 24 hours. This process can be automated or achieved with a manual technique, leading to up to 20% red cell loss. Approximately 20% to 90% of the platelets and 90% of the leukocytes are removed during this procedure. This decrease in leukocytes is not effective enough to render the component leukoreduced ($<5 \times 10^6$ leukocytes per unit).

Common indications for washed RBCs are recurrent severe allergic reactions not controlled with antihistamines and immunoglobulin A (IgA) deficiency. Washed RBCs also reduce the potassium load of the product. IgA-deficient patients can develop anti-IgA antibodies that react to donor IgA in plasma and lead to anaphylaxis. Potassium accumulates in the plasma during storage of the RBC unit or following irradiation.

IRRADIATED RED BLOOD CELLS

The goal of irradiation is to prevent proliferation of transfused immunocompetent T lymphocytes. This goal is accomplished by using cesium-137 or cobalt-60 as a radiation source, which administers a dose of 2500 cGy (25 Gy or 2500 rad) to the central portion of the RBC unit and a minimum of 1500 cGy to all other areas of the component. Due to decreased survival and viability of the RBCs and increased potassium leakage, irradiated RBCs expire on their original assigned outdate or 28 days after irradiation, whichever occurs first.

The only indication for the irradiated RBCs is to prevent transfusion-associated graft-versus-host disease (TA-GVHD). TA-GVHD is a rare, fatal complication (mortality >90%) caused by the engraftment and proliferation of donor T lymphocytes in the transfused recipient. Irradiated RBCs are indicated for patients receiving hematopoietic stem cell or bone marrow transplantation, patients with congenital immunodeficiency syndromes, intrauterine transfusions, neonates, HLA-matched platelet transfusions, patients with Hodgkin's disease, and patients with chronic lymphocytic leukemia treated with purine analogues (e.g., fludarabine [Fludara]).

Patients receiving transfusions from first-degree relatives require irradiation because of the increased risk of TA-GVHD due to HLA similarity of donor and recipient.

FROZEN RED BLOOD CELLS

The purpose of frozen RBCs is to store units with rare blood types and autologous units for extended periods of time (routinely up to 10 years, but storage may be extended for certain circumstances). Before freezing the RBCs, glycerol, a cryoprotective agent, is added to the system, which allows freezing of the red cells without damage. Based on the concentration of glycerol used (~20% or ~40%), the storage temperatures vary. Most commonly in the United States, 40% glycerol is used, and therefore the frozen RBCs are stored at −65°C.

Frozen RBCs must be deglycerolized before transfusion. Washing the product in saline solutions of progressively decreasing osmolarity achieves glycerol removal. During the process, 99.9% of the plasma along with the vast majority of WBCs and platelets are removed. Depending on the technique used to deglycerolize the RBCs, once deglycerolized, these units have a 24-hour (open system) or 14-day (closed system) shelf life.

Frozen RBCs are indicated for heavily alloimmunized patients (e.g., multiple clinically significant RBC antigens) who require rare phenotypic RBCs for compatible transfusions.

Due to the multiple washing steps in the deglycerolized procedure, these units can be considered equivalent to a washed RBC unit.

INDICATIONS FOR RED BLOOD CELL TRANSFUSION

The purpose of RBC transfusions is to provide oxygen-carrying capacity and to maintain tissue oxygenation when the intravascular volume and cardiac function are adequate for perfusion. In a 70-kg recipient, 1 unit of transfused RBCs should increase the hemoglobin by 1 g/dL and the hematocrit by 3%. To obtain the same expected response in a pediatric patient, the RBC transfusion dose should be 15 mL/kg. RBC transfusions should only be used when time or underlying pathophysiology precludes other management (e.g., iron, erythropoietin, folic acid [folate]).

Criteria for administering RBC transfusions include:

- Hb <8 g/dL in an otherwise healthy patient
- Hb <11 g/dL in cases of increased risk of ischemia (e.g., pulmonary disease, coronary artery disease, cerebral vascular disease)
- Acute blood loss >15% of total blood volume (e.g., 750 mL in 70-kg man) or with evidence of inadequate oxygen delivery (e.g., electrocardiographic signs of cardiac ischemia, tachycardia, cyanosis)
- Symptomatic anemia in a normovolemic patient (e.g., tachycardia, mental status changes, electrocardiographic signs of cardiac ischemia, angina, shortness of breath, lightheadedness or dizziness with mild exertion)
- Regular predetermined therapeutic program for severe hypoplastic or aplastic anemia or for bone marrow suppression for hemoglobinopathies

The post-transfusion hemoglobin should not exceed 11.5 g/dL (12.5 g/dL in cases of increased risk of organ or tissue ischemia). Attempts to increase wound healing or merely to take advantage of available predonated autologous blood without a valid medical indication are not acceptable uses for RBC transfusions.

Platelets

Platelets are often a limited resource because of their relatively short shelf life and the inability to stockpile this product through freezing techniques. Temperature, pH, and gas exchange are critical issues for platelet viability and function, and they all determine the storage shelf life. Platelets remain viable for up to 7 days after collection, but the current 5-day shelf life has been instituted because of increased rates of clinically significant bacterial contamination on days 6 and 7. At a temperature lower than 20°C, platelets can be damaged and become nonfunctional. Platelets must be maintained at room temperature (20°–24°C) with gentle agitation in gas-permeable bags. Gas-permeable bags are required for platelet storage to ensure proper oxygenation and facilitate removal of carbon dioxide buildup. Constant gentle agitation is required to facilitate this gas exchange.

At present, two methods to obtain platelets are employed in the United States. First, platelets may be prepared from whole blood donations via centrifugation separation. These platelets are commonly referred to as *platelet concentrates, random donor platelets,* or *whole blood–derived platelets*. One platelet concentrate can be manufactured from a single whole blood donation. This platelet concentrate should have 5.5×10^{10} platelets per unit in 40 to 70 mL of plasma. One platelet concentrate should increase the platelet count by 7 to 10×10^9/L in a 70-kg recipient. Therefore, general platelet-concentrate dosing consists of a pool of 4 to 6 platelet concentrates, also known as a *four-pack* or *six-pack*, respectively. Second, platelets may be prepared using apheresis technology. These products are called *apheresis platelets, single-donor platelets,* or *platelet pheresis.*

Due to current apheresis technology, most apheresis platelets are leukoreduced at the time of collection. Apheresis platelets should have 3.0×10^{11} platelets per unit in 300 to 500 mL of plasma. One apheresis unit should increase the platelet count by 40 to 60×10^9/L in a 70-kg recipient.

One apheresis platelet product has an equivalent dose of a six-pack of platelet concentrates. In the United States, the use of apheresis platelets has been increasing annually. In 2004, it was estimated that 77% of all therapeutic doses of platelets transfused were apheresis platelets.

Once a platelet component is collected, it may be further modified in the same manner as RBCs: leukoreduced, washed, or irradiated.

LEUKOREDUCED PLATELETS

As with leukoreduced RBCs, common indications for leukoreduced platelets are multiple FNHTRs, prevention of human leukocyte antigen (HLA) alloimmunization, and reduction of CMV transmission. The proposed mechanisms by which leukoreduction prevents these conditions are discussed in the leukoreduced RBCs section. These mechanisms are the same with one exception. FNHTRs with RBCs are associated with an active release of cytokines induced by leukocyte-antibody interaction. The mechanism of FNHTR with platelets differs and is due to passively transfused cytokines. At room temperature, residual donor leukocytes release cytokines that accumulate during storage. Therefore, prestorage leukocyte reduction is the only effective way to prevent FNHTR with platelet transfusions because the leukocytes are removed before releasing their cytokines.

It has been determined that cytokine accumulation does not occur if a blood product is refrigerated, which explains why both prestorage and poststorage RBC leukoreductions prevent FNHTRs.

WASHED PLATELETS

As with RBCs, the goal of washing platelets is to effectively remove 99% of antibodies, plasma proteins, and electrolytes contained within the component. The process involves washing platelets with normal saline or saline buffered with ACD-A (acid citrate dextrose) or citrate. This process can be achieved via automated or manual technique, leading to approximately 33% platelet loss. Once a platelet component is washed, it must be transfused within 4 hours because it is now an open system with removed anticoagulant-preservative solution at room temperature. This differs from washed RBCs that have a 24-hour shelf life after washing.

The two most common indications for washed platelets are recurrent severe allergic or anaphylactic reactions and IgA-deficiency in patients with IgA antibodies.

IRRADIATED PLATELETS

As with RBCs, the objective of irradiating platelets is to prevent immunocompetent T lymphocytes from proliferating and leading to TA-GVHD in the transfused recipient. The current dose (2500 cGy to the central portion of the unit and 1500 cGy to other portions of the unit) inactivates the T lymphocytes within the product and achieves this goal without significantly altering platelet function during their maximum shelf life.

Indications for irradiated platelets are the same as for irradiated RBCs: hematopoietic stem cell or BMT patients, congenital immunodeficiency syndrome patients, intrauterine transfusions, neonates, HLA-matched platelet transfusions, Hodgkin's disease patients, and chronic lymphocytic leukemia patients treated with purine analogues (e.g., fludarabine).

Patients receiving transfusions from first-degree relatives require irradiation because of the increased risk of TA-GVHD due to HLA similarity of donor and recipient.

INDICATIONS FOR PLATELET TRANSFUSION

Criteria for instituting a platelet transfusion include:

- Platelet count $<10 \times 10^9$/L for prophylaxis in a stable, nonfebrile patient
- Platelet count $<20 \times 10^9$/L for prophylaxis with fever or instability
- Platelet count $<50 \times 10^9$/L in a patient with documented hemorrhage or rapidly decreasing platelet count or planned invasive or surgical procedure
- Diffuse microvascular bleeding in a patient with disseminated intravascular coagulation or following a massive blood loss (>1 blood volume) with a platelet count not yet available
- Bleeding in a patient with platelet dysfunction

It is unacceptable to empirically transfuse platelets for a massively transfused patient not exhibiting a clinical coagulopathy or for extrinsic platelet dysfunction (e.g., renal failure, hyperproteinemia, or von Willebrand's disease). Platelet transfusion is contraindicated in thrombotic thrombocytopenic purpura (TTP), hemolytic-uremic syndrome (HUS), or idiopathic thrombocytopenic purpura (ITP) unless the patient is experiencing life-threatening bleeding or coagulopathy.

PLATELET REFRACTORINESS

Both nonimmune and immune causes lead to poor platelet increment following transfusion. To accurately assess response to platelet transfusion, a post-transfusion platelet count should be obtained 10 to 60 minutes after the transfusion is complete. If the patient does not respond appropriately, platelet refractoriness must be considered.

Platelet refractoriness is defined as failure to achieve an appropriate post-transfusion response on more than one occasion. A post-transfusion corrected count increment (CCI) can be calculated to more accurately assess refractoriness. The CCI is calculated as follows:

$$CCI = \frac{(\text{post} - \text{transfusion count} - \text{pretransfusion count}) \times \text{body surface area}}{\text{platelets tranfused} \times 10^{11}}$$

where platelet counts are in microliters and body surface area is in square meters. A CCI less than 5000 (using a 10- to 60-minute post-transfusion platelet count) on two separate occasions is consistent with platelet refractoriness.

The most common causes for poor platelet increments are nonimmune causes, including splenomegaly, bleeding, fever, sepsis, and disseminated intravascular coagulation (DIC). If refractoriness is determined to be nonimmune in etiology, management often consists of increasing the dose or frequency (or both) of transfused platelets. HLA alloimmunization is the primary cause of immune-mediated platelet refractoriness. Other immune-mediated causes for poor platelet increment are anti–platelet-specific antibodies, drug-induced antibodies, and immune or idiopathic thrombocytopenia purpura (ITP). If HLA alloimmunization is the cause, three common treatment options can be employed:

- Give platelets that are platelet crossmatch compatible with recipient plasma
- Provide HLA antigen-negative platelets (for the identified HLA antibodies)
- Give HLA matched (class I: HLA A and HLA B) platelets

Plasma

FROZEN PLASMA

Platelet-poor plasma is obtained by centrifugation and separation of a whole-blood donation or direct collection with apheresis technique. If this plasma is frozen at −18°C within 8 hours of original collection, the product contains adequate levels of all labile (factor V and factor VIII) and nonlabile coagulation factors and is called *fresh frozen plasma* (FFP). If this plasma is frozen at −18°C for more than 8 hours but within 24 hours from original collection, the product contains adequate levels of all nonlabile and decreased levels of labile coagulation factors and is called *plasma frozen within 24 hours*. Both types of plasma units have a volume of approximately 220 mL, and both can be stored for 12 months at −18°C.

These products are indicated for the correction of multiple or specific coagulation factor deficiencies or for the empiric treatment of TTP or HUS. The usual starting dose is 5 to 15 mL/kg (2 to 4 units in a 70-kg recipient).

INDICATIONS FOR PLASMA TRANSFUSION

Criteria for implementing a plasma infusion include:

- Treatment or prophylaxis of multiple or specific coagulation factor deficiencies (PT and/or PTT >1.5 times the mean normal value)
- Congenital coagulation factor deficiencies (antithrombin III; factors II, V, VII, IX, X, and XI; plasminogen; antiplasmin)
- Acquired coagulation factor deficiencies related to warfarin (Coumadin) therapy, vitamin K deficiency, liver disease, massive transfusion (>1 blood volume in 24 h), and disseminated intravascular coagulation
- Patients with a suspected coagulation deficiency (PT/PTT pending) who are bleeding, or at risk of bleeding, from an invasive procedure

Unacceptable criteria are empiric use during massive transfusion in which the patient does not exhibit clinical coagulopathy, nutritional supplementation, or volume replacement. There is little evidence to support prophylactic plasma infusion in patients with mild prolongation of the prothrombin time (<1.5 times the mean normal value).

CRYOPRECIPITATE

Cryoprecipitate is a cold insoluble fraction of FFP that precipitates when FFP is thawed at 4°C. A unit of cryoprecipitate contains approximately 10 mL, which can be stored for 12 months at −18°C. Each unit contains approximately 80 to 100 U of factor VIII and 250 mg of fibrinogen, along with factor XIII, von Willebrand's factor, and fibronectin.

The usual starting dose is one unit per 7 to 10 kg, and therefore multiple units must be pooled for a therapeutic dose. Once pooled, cryoprecipitate must be transfused within 4 hours. In a 70-kg man, 14 units would be expected to raise the fibrinogen 100 mg/dL. Cryoprecipitate (2-4 units) may also be applied topically, with an equal volume of bovine thrombin, taking advantage of its adhesive, hemostatic, and sealant properties.

Appropriate indications for cryoprecipitate include:

- A bleeding patient with congenital or acquired hypofibrinogenemia, dysfibrinogenemia, or afibrinogenmia (fibrinogen <150 mg/dL)
- Treatment or prevention of bleeding associated with certain known or suspected clotting factor deficiencies (factor VIII, von Willebrand's, factor XIII, or factor I)
- Treatment of surface oozing and maintenance of tissues in tight apposition to each other or sealing of leaking spaces (fibrin glue)

Rather than cryoprecipitate, factor concentrates are mostly used to treat hemophilia A and type I von Willebrand's disease. Desmopressin acetate (DDAVP) may be used as an alternative treatment for these patients and for patients with certain platelet dysfunctional disorders.

Granulocytes

Using apheresis techniques, granulocytes contain approximately 20 to 30×10^9 granulocytes per collection, 200 to 400 mL of donor plasma, 10 to 30 mL of donor RBCs, and some donor platelets. Like platelets, this product is stored at room temperature but without agitation. Granulocytes have a 24-hour shelf life, but they should be transfused as soon as possible because of rapid decline of function and viability of the leukocytes.

There are several special considerations for this product. Granulocytes must be ABO compatible with the recipient because of significant RBC contamination. This is an Rh-specific product for female patients of childbearing age. CMV-negative donors must be used for CMV-negative recipients because the product cannot be leukoreduced. It is an HLA-matched product for alloimmunized patients. Granulocytes should be irradiated to prevent TA-GVHD.

Granulocyte infusions are indicated for adult neutropenic patients (granulocyte count <500/μL) who have fever for 24 to 48 hours due to bacterial or fungal sepsis that is unresponsive to appropriate antibiotic or antifungal treatment. In infants, granulocyte therapy should be considered in bacterial septicemic patients with a granulocyte count less than 3000/μL. Daily granulocyte transfusion should be continued until infection resolves or the granulocyte count remains greater than 500/μL for 48 hours.

REFERENCES

Bowden RA, Slichter SJ, Sayers M, et al: A comparison of filtered leukocyte-reduced and cytomegalovirus (CMV) seronegative blood products for the prevention of transfusion-associated CMV infection after marrow transplant. Blood 1995;86:3598-3603.

Brecher ME (ed): Technical Manual, 15th ed. Bethesda, MD: American Association of Blood Banks, 2005.

British Committee for Standards in Haematology, Blood Transfusion Task Force: Guidelines for the use of platelet transfusions. Br J Haematol 2003;122:10-23.

Development Task Force of the College of American Pathologists: Practice parameters for the use of fresh frozen plasma, cryoprecipitate and platelets. JAMA 1994;271:777.

Goodnough LT, Brecher ME, Kanter MH, AuBuchon JP: Transfusion medicine. First of two parts—blood transfusion. N Engl J Med 1999;340:438-447.

Goodnough LT, Brecher ME, Kanter MH, AuBuchon JP: Transfusion medicine. Second of two parts—blood conservation. N Engl J Med 1999;340:525-533.

Menitove JE, McElligott MC, Aster RH: Febrile transfusion reaction: What blood component should be given next? Vox Sang 1978;5:101-106.

Nichols WG, Price TH, Corey L, Boeckh M: Transfusion-transmitted cytomegalovirus infection after receipt of leukoreduced blood products. Blood 2003;101:4195-4200.

Strauss R: Neutrophil (granulocyte) transfusions in the new millennium. Transfusion 1998;38:710-712.

The Trial to Reduce Alloimmunization to Platelets Study Group: Leukocyte reduction and ultraviolet B irradiation of platelets to prevent alloimmunization and refractoriness to platelet transfusions. N Engl J Med 1997;337:1861-1869.

Wandt H, Frank M, Ehninger G, et al: Safety and cost effectiveness of a 10 × 10⁹/L trigger for prophylactic platelet transfusions compared with the traditional 20 × 10⁹/L trigger: A prospective comparative trial in 105 patients with acute myeloid leukemia. Blood 1998;91:3601-3606.

Adverse Effects of Blood Transfusion

Method of
Chelsea A. Sheppard, MD, and
Christopher D. Hillyer, MD

Although blood transfusion is a beneficial and not uncommonly lifesaving therapy, it carries inherent risks or adverse effects. These adverse effects are commonly classified either as *transfusion reactions* (Table 1), which occur immediately or shortly following the transfusion event, or as *transfusion-related complications*, which can occur up to many years following transfusion. These latter complications are commonly divided into *infectious* (Table 2) and *noninfectious* (Table 3) categories. Indeed, 0.5% to 3% of all transfusions result in an adverse event; however, the majority of these are minor reactions with no long-term sequelae.

Herein we describe a large number of adverse events so that the physician can determine if his or her patient has had an adverse effect from a transfusion, assign a diagnosis, and consider if an intervention is needed. For a complete discussion of all of the adverse events related to transfusion, as well as more detailed references, the reader is referred to *Blood Banking and Transfusion Medicine* (see References).

Transfusion Reactions

When a patient experiences an immediate reaction to a transfusion, the most important question to answer is whether hemolysis is occurring. Thus, transfusion medicine specialists usually classify transfusion reactions as either *hemolytic* or *nonhemolytic*.

Hemolytic reactions are caused by recipient antibodies targeted against donor red cell antigens and the resultant response, which attempts to destroy or clear those foreign cells. These antibodies may be naturally occurring (e.g., a recipient with group A blood has antibodies to B-group red cells) or they can occur after exposure to foreign blood from past transfusion, pregnancy, or transplantation. This process is termed *alloimmunization*.

Nonhemolytic reactions occur via a variety of mechanisms usually involving recipient response to donor leukocytes or their byproducts, including inflammatory cytokines.

HEMOLYTIC TRANSFUSION REACTIONS

Acute Hemolytic Transfusion Reaction

Clinical Description

Arguably, the most devastating transfusion reaction is an acute hemolytic reaction caused by the mistransfusion of ABO incompatible blood. *Mistransfusion* is defined as failure to give the right blood product to the right person at the right time and for the right reason. The severity of the reaction is dose dependent; however, infusion of even a small amount of incompatible blood can cause intravascular hemolysis, resulting in a range of signs and symptoms including pain at the infusion site, back, or flank; fever; chills or rigors; hemoglobinuria or hemoglobinemia; chest pain; circulatory collapse or shock; vasoconstriction with resultant end organ ischemia; and activation of the coagulation system, resulting in microangiopathic thrombosis.

The annual incidence of ABO-mismatched transfusion according to observed errors in the New York State database and the FDA

TABLE 1 Transfusion Reactions

Type	Frequency	Common Signs and Symptoms	Laboratory Diagnosis	Therapy
Hemolytic				
AHTR	Rare	Pain at the infusion site, back, or flanks Fever, chills, rigors Hemoglobinuria or hemoglobinemia Chest pain Circulatory collapse and shock Vasoconstriction resultant end organ ischemia Activation of the coagulation system, resulting in microangiopathic thrombosis	Schistocytes on peripheral smear Indirect bilirubinemia and jaundice Decreased haptoglobin Elevated LDH and reticulocyte count	Stop the transfusion Maintain IV fluids (1 L NS over 1-2 h) to maintain urine flow >1 mL/kg/h Diuresis with furosemide or mannitol Support cardiovascular and respiratory function with vasopressors Intubate if necessary
Bacterial contamination	Rare	Fever, chills, rigors Hypotension Intravascular hemolysis	Positive blood cultures Similar organism found in product and recipient	Antibiotics Treat shock if appropriate
DHTR	Rare	Intra- or extravascular hemolysis	Same as AHTR, with spherocytes on peripheral smear if hemolysis is predominantly extravascular	Monitor renal function; forced diuresis or dialysis may be required to support renal function if extravascular hemolysis is severe Transfuse with antigen-negative blood if anemia is symptomatic

TABLE 1 Transfusion Reactions—cont'd

Nonhemolytic

Allergic	Common	Itching, urticaria, generalized flushing or rash, angioedema Wheezing, cough	No abnormal laboratory tests	Diphenhydramine 25-50 mg PO or IV May premedicate for future transfusions if recurrent
Anaphylactic	Rare	Shortness of breath, vasomotor instability, bronchospasm	No abnormal laboratory tests	Epinephrine 1:1000 0.3 mL IM Secure airway
FNHTR	Common	Fever, chills, rigors Absence of hemolysis	No abnormal laboratory tests R/o hemolysis	Acetaminophen 650 mg PO if not contraindicated May premedicate for future transfusions if recurrent
TA-GVHD	Rare	Fever, mucositis, dermatitis, hepatitis, enterocolitis, pancytopenia	Low blood counts, low reticulocyte count, elevated liver enzymes, elevated inflammatory markers	Treatment is usually ineffective High dose steroids, OKT3, cyclosporine A, and anti-thymocyte globulin may be helpful Irradiate blood for high-risk patients to prevent TA-GVHD
TRALI	Rare	Noncardiogenic pulmonary edema with dyspnea, acute hypoxemia, hypotension, occasionally fever Bilateral infiltrates on CXR Signs of congestive heart failure (increased jugular venous pressure and/or a third heart sound) absent Normal pulmonary capillary wedge pressure.	HLA/HNA antibody or antigen cognates between recipient and donor can support diagnosis	Respiratory support High-dose steroids Avoid diuretics in hypotensive patients

Abbreviations: AHTR = acute hemolytic transfusion reaction; CXR = chest x-ray; DHTR = delayed hemolytic transfusion reaction; FNHTR = febrile nonhemolytic transfusion reaction; HLA = human leukocyte antigen; HNA = human neutrophil antigen; LDH = lactate dehydrogenase; NS = normal saline; OKT3 = muromonab CD3; r/o = rule out; TA-GVHD = transfusion-associated graft-versus-host disease; TRALI = transfusion-related acute lung injury.

---

database of transfusion-associated fatalities has been reported at between 1 in 12,000 and 1 in 19,000 transfused units. The fatality rate ranges from 1 in 800,000 to 1 in 2,000,000 transfused units. However, these numbers do not take into account the large number of near misses, which have been reported to be as common as 1 in 3000 to 4000 units transfused per year.

TABLE 2 Infectious Complications of Transfusion

Type	Risk of Transfusion Transmitted Infection from Screened Units
Viruses	
CMV	Leukoreduction has made transfusion transmission rare (~1% remaining risk)
EBV	Rare
HAV	Rare
HBV	~1:200,000
HCV*	~1:2 million
HHV	
HIV*	~1:2 million to 4 million
HTLV	<1:3 million
WNV*	Rare
Parasitic Infections	
Babesia spp.	Rare
Plasmodium spp.	1:4 million
Trypanosoma cruzi	Rare
Prions	
CJD, BSE	Rare

*Risk after nucleic acid testing was implemented.
Abbreviations: BSE = bovine spongiform encephalopathy; CJD = Creutzfeldt-Jakob disease; CMV = cytomegalovirus; EBV = Epstein-Barr virus; HAV = hepatitis A virus; HBV = hepatitis B virus; HCV = hepatitis C virus; HHV = human herpesvirus; HTLV = human T-cell lymphotropic virus; WNV = West Nile virus.

Diagnosis

The first signs of an acute hemolytic transfusion reaction (AHTR) are usually fever and pain. However, a decrease in blood pressure, tachycardia, and hemoglobinuria may be the only signs in an anesthetized patient.

Laboratory studies can help confirm a diagnosis of intravascular hemolysis. Red cell abnormalities including schistocytes on peripheral smear, increased indirect bilirubin and jaundice, and decreased haptoglobin are signs of increased red cell destruction. Elevated lactate dehydrogenase (LDH) and reticulocyte count indicate increased red cell turnover. It is important to maintain adequate renal function; therefore, it is necessary to monitor blood urea nitrogen (BUN), creatinine, and urine output.

Occasionally, patients with severe intravascular hemolysis can develop disseminated intravascular coagulation (DIC). Serial measurements including prothrombin time (PT), activated partial thromboplastin time (aPTT), D-dimer, fibrinogen, antithrombin, and platelet count can be used to evaluate for the presence of an ongoing consumptive process. After the transfusion is stopped, the unit itself and a post-transfusion sample should be immediately sent to the blood bank for further analysis. The blood bank will perform a clerical check for correct patient identification, look for the presence of visible hemolysis in the post-transfusion plasma, and compare direct Coombs' test results from the pre- and post-transfusion samples for evidence of in vivo antibody adsorption on the red cells.

Treatment and Prevention

If an acute hemolytic transfusion reaction is suspected, the transfusion should be stopped immediately. Intravenous fluids should be given to maintain an adequate blood pressure and to aid the kidneys in expelling circulating hemoglobin. Some experts recommend furosemide (Lasix) or mannitol (Osmitrol) to induce diuresis; however, this has not been studied in a randomized fashion. A patient who develops signs of shock should be treated accordingly. Vasopressors

TABLE 3 Noninfectious Complications of Transfusion

Type	Frequency	Common Signs and Symptoms	Laboratory Diagnosis	Therapy
Massive Transfusion Reactions				
Coagulopathy	Common in massive transfusion	Hemorrhage usually described as mucosal bleeding or oozing from suture lines	Prolonged PT, PTT Fibrinogen <100 mg/dL Rapidly decreasing platelet count and antithrombin level	Replace clotting factors with FFP In massive transfusion, RBC/FFP ratio should be 1:1-2 If fibrinogen <100 mg/dL transfuse 1 cryoprecipitate pool and recheck fibrinogen Transfuse platelets if count <50,000/L
Citrate toxicity	Rare	Muscle cramping, shortness of breath secondary to bronchospasm, tetanic contractions, distal extremity numbness, tingling sensations, seizures	Decreased ionized calcium Monitor for hypomagnesemia	Calcium gluconate 2 g/250 mL NS Replete magnesium if indicated
Hyperkalemia	Rare	Generalized fatigue, weakness, paresthesias, paralysis, palpitations ECG changes: peaked T waves, shortened QT interval, ST segment depression	Elevated serum potassium Monitor for evidence of metabolic alkalosis Monitor for ECG changes	Replete with oral or IV potassium preparations if indicated
Iron overload	Rare	Iron deposition with end-organ damage in heart, liver, lungs, pituitary, thyroid, adrenals, exocrine pancreas	Elevated iron, ferritin (~10-20 g in patients with SCD are typical), and transferrin saturation	Phlebotomy or iron chelators if indicated
Transfusion-Related Immunomodulation				
Platelet refractoriness (HLA)	Occasional in highly sensitized patients	FNHTR No response or inadequate response to platelet transfusion	Corrected count increment (see text), flow cytomtery, or ELISA screen for anti-HLA antibodies or platelet-specific antibodies	Consider appropriateness of HLA-matched or crossmatched platelets, contact transfusion medicine specialist
Post-transfusion purpura (HPA)	Rare	Severe thrombocytopenia 5-10 d after transfusion Bruising and petechiae Can result in severe hemorrhage	Flow cytomtery or ELISA screen for anti–platelet-specific antibodies Must r/o other causes of thrombocytopenia, including HIT and DIC	Self-limited IVIg Efficacy of antigen-negative platelets is controversial
Other				
Volume overload	Common	Cardiogenic pulmonary edema with dyspnea, acute hypoxemia, hypertension Bilateral infiltrates on CXR Signs of congestive heart failure, increased jugular venous pressure, and/or absent third heart sound Elevated pulmonary capillary wedge pressure.	BNP can help distinguish volume overload from TRALI	Diuresis If transfusion is required, slow the rate

Abbreviations: BNP = brain natriuretic peptide; CXR = chest x-ray; DIC = disseminated intravascular coagulation; ECG = electorcardiogram; ELISA = enzyme-linked immunosorbent assay; FNHTR = febrile nonhemolytic transfusion reaction; FFP = fresh frozen plasma; HIT = heparin-induced thrombocytopenia; HLA = human leukocyte antigen; HPA = human platelet antigen; IVIg = intravenous immunoglobulin; NS = normal saline; PT = prothrombin time; PTT = partial thromboplastin time; RBC = red blood cells; r/o = rule out; SCD = sickle cell disease; TRALI = transfusion-related acute lung injury.

and mechanical ventilation may be required in cases of circulatory collapse and respiratory failure.

Most cases of mistransfusion are the result of human error. More than one half of these errors occur from misidentification of the patient at the bedside. Approximately one third of these errors occur in the blood bank as a result of either a clerical misprint or the misidentification of a specimen. Despite strict transfusion procedures and protocols, the use of hospital identification wrist bands, and multiple redundant check systems, mistransfusions still occur at an alarming rate. Therefore, systems including the use of bar codes, barrier technology (Blood-Loc), and radiofrequency identification (RFID) systems are under investigation.

Delayed Hemolytic Transfusion Reaction

Clinical Description

Red blood cell antibodies acquired through exposure to foreign antigen can cause a delayed hemolytic transfusion reaction (DHTR). These patients can develop signs and symptoms of intra- or extravascular hemolysis approximately 2 weeks after transfusion due to the formation of a de novo alloantibody. Alternatively, symptoms appearing 3 to 4 days after transfusion support previous exposure to the antigen and a robust amnestic response on reexposure to antigen-positive blood.

Diagnosis

Patients with a history of a recent transfusion and signs and symptoms of hemolysis should be evaluated for a possible DHTR. Laboratory studies for intra- and extravascular hemolysis are described earlier. However, in delayed hemolytic transfusion reactions, extravascular hemolysis is more common; thus, spherocytes rather than schistocytes may be the predominant abnormal morphologic red cell type on peripheral smear.

Alloantibodies are usually detected during the antibody screen carried in blood banks as a "type and screen." If the screen is positive, the specificity of the antibody is determined. For patients with multiple antibodies, this can significantly lengthen the time it takes for the pretransfusion work-up. If the patient has not recently received a transfusion, antibody titers may be too low to be detected at the time of screening. However, if the patient is rechallenged with the antigen, an amnestic antibody response can cause destruction of the transfused cells. Intravascular and extravascular hemolysis can be severe and life threatening.

Treatment and Prevention

Treatment of intra- and extravascular hemolysis is discussed under acute hemolytic transfusion reactions.

The inherent immunogenicity of the antigen, antigen concentration per erythrocyte, transfused cell dosage, and individual patient factors determine the rate of alloimmunization. Patients with sickle cell disease are at greater risk, and immunosuppressed patients may be at less risk. Highly immunogenic antigens such as Kell, Duffy, and Kidd are generally associated with more severe reactions. These antigens are also commonly implicated in hemolytic disease of the newborn because these antibodies can cross the placenta.

Antibody screening is required before transfusion in any patient who has received a transfusion or been pregnant in the last 30 days; thus, it is important to take a thorough transfusion history. Additionally, hospitalized patients receiving transfusions should be rescreened every 3 days because antibodies that are initially too low in titer to be detected might be identified later.

Bacterial Contamination of Blood Products

Clinical Description

Bacterial contamination at the time of collection usually occurs through one of three mechanisms: asymptomatic donor bacteremia, introduction of skin flora to the unit, or manufacturing processes and manipulation of the unit. Initially, the amount of bacteria present is low; however, during storage the bacteria can proliferate to levels of 10^6/mL or greater. This amount of bacteria transfused over a short time can result in a spectrum of clinical signs and symptoms including bacteremia, fever, chills, hypotension, nausea, vomiting, diarrhea, and oliguria, which can progress to sepsis and ultimately multisystem organ failure and death.

Pathophysiology

The most common bacteria identified in 70% to 80% of contaminated platelets are gram-positive skin flora introduced to the unit during collection; however, 40% to 80% of fatalities are due to endotoxin-producing gram-negative organisms. The severity of the reaction depends on the species of bacteria present, the inoculum, the rate of bacterial propagation, and patient factors including underlying disease, including leukocyte count, the status of the immune system, and use of concomitant antibiotics in the recipient.

Diagnosis

Blood cultures should be obtained both from the recipient (cultures should not be drawn from the same line used for the transfusion) and from the blood product in question. Confirmation requires that the same organism be cultured from both sites. False negatives can occur in patients taking antibiotics. False-positive cultures are common due to improper collection of the sample.

Additional laboratory tests can help evaluate for end-organ damage including tests of renal and liver function. Endotoxin-induced DIC is a common complication; therefore, serial measurements of the PT, APTT, D-dimer, fibrinogen, antithrombin, and platelet count may be useful in evaluating for the presence of an ongoing consumptive process.

Treatment and Prevention

Sepsis caused by transfusion of a bacterially contaminated unit can be fatal. Antibiotics should be given empirically as soon as symptoms appear. The patient can develop septic shock and should be treated accordingly.

Bacterial contamination is the third most common cause of transfusion-associated fatality reported to the FDA. Improved phlebotomy practices (strict arm preparation standards and diversion of the first 10 mL containing the skin plug), donor questioning for recent illnesses or travel to endemic areas, better materials used in product collection and storage, and implementation of platelet culturing have helped reduce the incidence of fatality as a result of bacterial contamination of blood products. Red cell units and plasma, which are stored refrigerated or frozen, are less often implicated in bacteria-related transfusion reactions. However, platelets, which are stored at room temperature in a large volume of plasma and in a bag that allows oxygen diffusion, are most commonly implicated.

Prior to 2004 and the implementation of American Association of Blood Banks (AABB) Standard 5.1.5.1, which charged blood banks with the responsibility of limiting and detecting bacterial contamination, the infectious risk of receiving a contaminated unit was estimated at 1 in 2000 to 1 in 3000 platelet units per year. Risk of death was 1 in 60,000 to 1 in 85,000 units transfused. Since implementation of the AABB standard, many of the nation's blood collection systems have begun culturing platelet units using automated systems, which detect CO_2 generation or O_2 consumption by bacteria for 24 hours prior to hospital distribution. Despite a marked reduction in the number of cases of transfusion-transmitted bacterial infections, rare fatal consequences have been reported.

Pathogen reduction technology aims at eradicating pathogens without harming the blood cells or generating toxic chemical agents. Several methods under investigation include a number of photodynamic processes that use psoralen-based chemicals, phenothiazine dyes (methylene blue [urolene blue]), or riboflavin (vitamin B_2) followed by ultraviolet light to inactivate bacteria and viruses by degrading nucleic acids. Other methods include solvent-detergent treatment and treatment with FRALEs (frangible anchor linker effectors). The appeal of pathogen reduction is that it is proactive and may be able to prevent new and emerging infections. Nonetheless, serious regulatory hurdles remain before these methods are approved for use in the United States.

NONHEMOLYTIC TRANSFUSION REACTIONS

Transfusion-Related Acute Lung Injury

Clinical Description

Transfusion-related acute lung injury (TRALI) has now become the most common cause of transfusion-associated death *reported* to the FDA, with an incidence that ranges widely from 1 case per 432 whole blood units transfused to 1 case per 557,000 red blood cell units transfused. Because it was not until 2004 that standardized criteria were widely accepted for defining and diagnosing TRALI, these previous figures might not reflect current incidence, and thus most authorities agree that the true incidence of TRALI is unknown. Nonetheless, it is becoming increasingly clear that platelets and FFP are the most commonly implicated blood products due to the large plasma volume of these products and the likelihood of alloantibodies being passively transferred (see later).

TRALI is a clinical syndrome characterized by noncardiogenic pulmonary edema with dyspnea, acute hypoxemia, hypotension, and occasionally fever. Bilateral infiltrates in a white-out pattern are commonly described on chest x-ray. Signs of congestive heart failure (increased jugular venous pressure and/or a third heart sound) are usually absent. The pulmonary capillary wedge pressure is typically normal. Symptoms usually appear 1 to 6 hours after transfusion and resolve in 96 hours.

Diagnosis

Until recently, accepted criteria allowing standardized diagnosis of TRALI were lacking, thus complicating the ability to make accurate diagnoses and hindering attempts at determining true incidence rates. In April 2004, a consensus conference convened in Toronto, Ontario, and attempted to further adapt and improve previously proposed definitions of TRALI. The consensus panel recommended criteria for *TRALI* and *possible TRALI*.

TRALI was defined as a new occurrence of acute-onset acute lung injury (ALI) with hypoxemia and bilateral infiltrates on chest x-ray, but no evidence of left atrial hypertension. The ALI cannot have been preexisting, but it must emerge during or within 6 hours of the end the transfusion and have no temporal relation to an alternative ALI risk factor. *Possible TRALI* included cases in which there was a temporal association with an alternative ALI risk factor.

These proposed definitions continue to suffer the limitations inherent in the American-European Consensus Conference definition of ALI (including the subjectivity of certain findings, including chest x-ray and volume status and the influence of PEEP on measurements of the PaO_2/FiO_2 ratio). Brain natriuretic protein (BNP) might help to distinguish cardiogenic from noncardiogenic pulmonary edema.

Pathophysiology

The events and mechanisms that cause TRALI are incompletely understood. They have been described as antibody-mediated and non–antibody-mediated. Antibody-mediated mechanisms implicate alloantibodies directed toward human leukocyte antigen (HLA) or human neutrophil antigen (HNA) on leukocytes or lung tissue, which lead to granulocyte activation and pulmonary injury. In approximately 90% of TRALI cases where antibodies are identified, the antibodies are of donor origin and react with recipient leukocyte epitopes. Multiparous women and recipients of previous transfusions are more likely to be alloimmunized. Many investigators have suggested that a number of hits may be required to cause a full-blown case of TRALI.

The two-hit model of TRALI may be antibody- or non–antibody-mediated. In this model, the first hit is usually described as an underlying illness that primes recipient pulmonary endothelial cells and leukocytes. *Priming* refers to the development of a heightened stage of (cellular) activation. The second hit is delivered by the transfusion, which contains factors (either antibodies or biological response modifiers [BRMs], such as cytokines or certain lipids) capable of inducing complete activation of the presequestered primed neutrophils in the recipient's lungs. This results in the release of cytotoxic compounds in the pulmonary vasculature, leading to endothelial damage, capillary leak, and noncardiogenic pulmonary edema, namely, TRALI.

Treatment and Prevention

Treatment is primarily respiratory support until the injury resolves (usually in 24-96 hours); however, high-dose intravenous steroids may be beneficial. Approximately 20% of patients with TRALI require 1 week or more to fully recover. Death is estimated to occur in 6% to 23% of cases; survivors have no permanent sequelae.

Without a simple laboratory test to prospectively eliminate high-risk blood products, recommended strategies to prevent TRALI are currently based on deferral of donors implicated in TRALI cases. The United Kingdom has preemptively deferred all women from donating plasma. In the United States, the use of male-only plasma is under consideration, as is the testing of all plasma and platelet units for anti-HLA or anti-HNA antibodies.

Febrile Nonhemolytic Transfusion Reaction

Clinical Description

Febrile nonhemolytic transfusion reaction (FNHTR) is defined as an increase in the recipient's temperature of at least 1°C or 2°F during transfusion in the absence of another cause of fever. Some patients develop chills or rigors. FNHTRs are very common, occurring in 0.1% to 0.5% of all leukodepleted transfusions occurring per year in the United States. The incidence is significantly higher in nonleukoreduced blood products. Additionally, transfusion reactions such as FNHTRs and allergic reactions are believed to be underreported in patients with frequent febrile episodes due to underlying diseases such as cancer and sepsis. Other causes for transfusion-associated fever, including hemolysis or bacterial contamination, must be excluded before a diagnosis of FNHTR can be made.

Pathophysiology

FNHTRS are attributed to white blood cells (WBCs) in blood products that synthesize and release proinflammatory cytokines during storage. Preformed recipient antibodies that target donor WBCs can also lead to cytokine release after transfusion.

Treatment and Prevention

Antipyretics are often used to treat these reactions. Patients prone to FNHTRs can require premedication with antipyretics. Many transfusion medicine services have implemented universal leukoreduction protocols to prevent FNHTRs.

Allergic Reactions

Clinical Description

Allergic transfusion reactions are very common. Allergic reactions are variably severe and result in a spectrum of clinical signs and symptoms. Uncomplicated or simple reactions manifest as itching, urticaria, generalized flushing or rash, or local swelling, also known as *angioedema*. However, recipients can also develop anaphylactoid reactions in which wheezing, cough, shortness of breath, vasomotor instability, and bronchospasm are typically observed. IgA-deficient patients with circulating anti-IgA antibodies can develop life-threatening anaphylaxis and cardiovascular collapse requiring emergent therapy. Most reactions are afebrile. The incidence of uncomplicated allergic reactions is 1% to 3%; however, anaphylactic reactions are very rare (0.002%-0.005% of all transfusions).

Pathophysiology

Simple allergic reactions occur when donor plasma proteins are targeted by preformed IgE antibodies on recipient mast cells, leading to histamine release. More severe reactions have been attributed to antibodies against IgA, C4 determinants, or other nonbiological elements (ethylene oxide used for sterilization of tubing sets). The presence of anti-IgA antibodies in IgA-deficient patients cannot predict the occurrence of allergic reactions.

Treatment and Prevention

Most simple allergic reactions can be treated with antihistamines or anticholinergic medications (e.g., diphenhydramine). Patients with more severe reactions can require IV steroids or epinephrine. Patients with respiratory failure require supportive therapy. In patients with recurrent allergic reactions, prophylactic antihistamine therapy administered 30 minutes before transfusion may be helpful. In patients with simple allergic reactions involving only the skin, the transfusion may be restarted 15 to 30 minutes after the administration of antihistamines; however, transfusions should never be restarted in patients with more severe reactions.

Transfusion-Associated Graft-Versus-Host Disease

Clinical Description

Transfusion-associated graft-versus-host disease (TA-GVHD) is a rare but uniformly fatal complication of blood transfusions in severely immunosuppressed patients in which donor lymphocytes escape immune clearance in the recipient and engraft. Following clonal expansion, these cells cause immune destruction of host tissues including the skin, gastrointestinal (GI) tract, liver, and bone marrow. These patients develop fever, mucositis, dermatitis (starting as a blistering rash on the palms, soles, and face, which then can generalize), hepatitis, enterocolitis with large volumes of secretory diarrhea, and pancytopenia, 1 to 2 weeks after transfusion. Infections are the most common cause of death, which generally occurs within 3 to 4 weeks of the transfusion.

The degree of immunosuppression and the dose of T lymphocytes are factors in determining an individual patient's risk of developing TA-GVHD. Patients with hematologic malignancy, patients with congenital immunodeficiency, premature infants weighing less than 1200 g, bone marrow transplant recipients, and patients receiving fludarabine (Fludara) (see Box 1 for a complete list) are susceptible. Patients with HIV, healthy newborns, and patients who are neutropenic due to sepsis are generally considered to be at low risk. There is a minimally increased risk associated with solid tumor transplants (especially heart and liver) or solid tumor malignancies. There have been reports of TA-GVHD associated with neuroblastomas, rhabdomyosarcomas, bladder tumors, and small cell lung cancer. It is possible that more immunosuppressive and myeloablative chemotherapy protocols are responsible for these cases.

The degree of HLA similarity between the donor and recipient is also an important determinant of a patient's risk of developing TA-GVHD. These patients may be immunocompetent heterozygotes of an HLA haplotype for which the donor is homozygous. Therefore, patients receiving transfusions from first-degree relatives or populations in which there is a great deal of HLA homology (including some Asian populations) might also require irradiated blood products.

Treatment and Prevention

The mortality rate of TA-GVHD approximates 100%. Currently, there is no effective treatment; however, high-dose steroids, muromonab-CD3 (OKT-3), cyclosporine A (Neoral, Sandimmune) and antithy-mocyte globulin (Atgam, Thymoglobin) have been used with few successes.

Prevention of TA-GVHD via irradiation of blood products in at-risk populations is absolutely required. A minimum dose of 25 Gy delivered to the midline of the container (with a minimum of 15 Gy to the distal parts of the bag) cross-links the DNA of T cells, thereby preventing replication and potential engraftment and expansion.

Transfusion-Related Complications

INFECTIOUS COMPLICATIONS

Viral Transmission

Clinical Description

A large number of viruses, including HIV-1 and HIV-2; hepatitis A, B, and C (HAV, HBV, HCV); human T-lymphotrophic viruses (HTLV) 1 and 2; cytomegalovirus (CMV); and West Nile virus can be transmitted via transfusion. These viruses, with the exception of CMV, are acquired from cellular and noncellular blood and blood products including plasma-derived clotting factors, intravenous immunoglobulin (IVIg), and anti-D immunoglobulin. CMV remains latent in monocytes and is essentially therefore transmitted only in cellular products. Other viruses that are potentially transmitted via transfusion are HAV, transfusion-transmitted virus (TTV), Epstein-Barr virus (EBV), human herpesvirus 8 (HHV 8), and parvovirus B19.

Hepatitis

Hepatitis viruses (especially B and C) are readily transfusion transmissible. About 70% of patients infected with HCV develop chronic infections resulting in chronic active hepatitis, cirrhosis, or hepatocellular carcinoma (HCC). A smaller but significant fraction of patients infected with HBV develop chronic disease proceeding to cirrhosis. Hepatitis viruses A and E are rarely transmitted through blood transfusion. Hepatitis G, TTV, and SEN viruses emerged as candidates for non–A to E type post-transfusion hepatitis, but no clear association has been demonstrated.

Human Immunodeficiency Virus

The annual risk of transfusion-transmitted HIV with the addition of nucleic acid testing is reported to be less than 1 in 2,000,000 units in the United States (1:4,000,000 in Canada). However, despite the implementation of this very sensitive testing, cases of transfusion-transmitted HIV have been reported. The average survival after diagnosis for adults and children with transfusion-transmitted HIV is approximately 5.6 months and 13.7 months, respectively.

BOX 1   Risk Factors for the Development of TA-GVHD

Significantly Increased Risk
- Bone marrow transplantation
  - Allogeneic and autologous
  - HLA-matched platelet transfusions
  - Hodgkin's disease
  - Intrauterine transfusions
  - Patients treated with purine analogue drugs
  - Transfusions from blood relatives
- Congenital immunodeficiency syndromes

Minimally Increased Risk
- Acute leukemia
- Exchange transfusions
- Non-Hodgkin's lymphoma
- Preterm infants (<1200 g)
- Solid organ transplant recipients
- Solid tumors treated with intensive chemotherapy or radiotherapy

Perceived but No Reported Increased Risk
- Healthy newborns
- Patients with AIDS

Abbreviations: HLA = human leukocyte antigen; TA-GVHD = transfusion-associated graft-versus-host disease. Modified from Schroeder ML: Transfusion-associated graft-versus-host disease. Br J Haematol 2002;117:275-287.

West Nile Virus and Other Flaviviruses

In 2002, there was an emergence of West Nile virus in the United States, and several cases of transfusion-transmitted disease were identified. Infected elderly and immunocompromised patients developed a severe flulike illness rarely resulting in death. Other flaviviruses including dengue are transfusion transmissible and could threaten the blood supply if an epidemic were to emerge in the United States.

Parvovirus B19

Parvovirus B19 has been transmitted through plasma-derived products including clotting factors. Immunocompromised patients can develop erythema infectiosum, arthralgias, and aplastic crises with chronic anemia after infection with parvovirus B19.

Cytomegalovirus

Transfusion transmission of CMV to immunocompetent patients usually causes an asymptomatic infection or rarely an infectious mononucleosis. However, in seronegative immunocompromised patients, transfusion transmission can lead to lethal CMV disease. Seronegative immunocompromised patients include premature low-birth-weight infants (<1500 g) born to seronegative mothers and seronegative recipients of autologous or seronegative allogeneic bone marrow or peripheral blood stem cell transplantation.

Following primary infection, CMV remains latent and can reactivate, with subsequent production of progeny virus in macrophages. Transfusion-transmitted CMV can be mitigated through the transfusion of leukoreduced or seronegative blood. The rate of infectivity with either leukoreduced or seronegative blood is approximately the same (1%). Box 2 lists the indications for which many hospital blood banks dispense CMV seronegative blood or leukoreduced blood.

Parasitic and Emerging Infections

Clinical Description

Trypanosoma cruzi, *Plasmodium* spp., and *Babesia* spp. can be transmitted by blood transfusion. *T. cruzi* can cause fatal cardiac and GI disease (Chagas' disease). Malaria, the disease caused by *Plasmodium*, can cause fatal intravascular hemolysis and DIC. Human babesiosis generally causes a mild flulike syndrome, but it can be lethal in the elderly and in immunocompromised patients. At the time of this writing, no agent is tested for in the United States, but it appears likely that tests for *T. cruzi* will commence by early 2007.

TRYPANOSOMA CRUZI

There have been fewer than 10 cases of transfusion-transmitted *T. cruzi* reported in the United States and Canada since 1990.

BOX 2 Indications for CMV Seronegative or Leukoreduced Blood

- Intrauterine transfusions
- Premature low-birth-weight infants (<1500 g) born to SN mothers
- SN recipients of autologous bone marrow or peripheral blood stem cell transplantation
- SN recipients of seronegative allogeneic bone marrow or peripheral blood stem cell transplantation
- SN recipients of solid organ transplants from SN donors

Abbreviations: CMV = cytomegalovirus; SN = seronegative.

Many of these patients were immunocompromised as a result of hematologic malignancy, AIDS, or bone marrow transplantation. Some of these recipients received platelets only, others received multiple blood products. A majority of the patients developed Chagas' disease. At least one case was fatal. Others did respond to nitrofurtimox[2] (Nifurtimox), interferon-γ[1] (Actimmune), and benznidazole,[1] followed by itraconazole[1] (Sporanox) and fluconazole[1] (Diflucan). In endemic areas, transfusion transmission of Chagas' disease is more common. No screening is currently done for these parasites in blood donors. In the United States, 1 in 25,000 donors are estimated to be seropositive, and as many as one half of these donors are actively parasitemic.

PLASMODIUM SPECIES AND BABESIA SPECIES

Annually, approximately two cases of transfusion-transmitted *Plasmodium* infections are reported in the United States. Donors who have traveled to malaria-endemic countries are deferred from donation for a period of 1 year. Red cell exchange may be helpful in patients with high parasitemia loads and intravascular hemolysis; however, this is controversial.

There have been more than 50 cases of transfusion-transmitted *Babesia* infections in the world. Currently, there are no licensed tests for screening the blood supply. Human babesiosis is treated with antibiotics.

PRIONS

The agent of variant Creutzfeldt-Jakob disease (vCJD), a novel human prion disease that results in a rare and fatal human neurodegenerative condition, can be transmitted via blood transfusion. Although this agent has no nucleic acids, the transmission results in the conversion of normal prion protein to the abnormal β-sheet amyloid responsible for the clinical disease.

Since 2003, it has been established that prion infection could be transmitted via blood transfusion in animals. Additionally, in 2003 the first case of probable transfusion-transmitted vCJD was reported. The recipient received a transfusion in 1996 from a donor now known to have been incubating vCJD. The recipient died in 1996 from complications of vCJD.

In 2006, the National CJD Surveillance Unit (NCJDSU) and the UK Blood Services (UKBS) released the Transfusion Medicine Epidemiology Review (TMER), a look-back investigation that confirmed three separate incidents of probable transfusion transmission of vCJD infection. Two of these patients died less than 7 years after infection. At this time, sporadic CJD and familial CJD have still not been shown conclusively to be transfusion transmitted.

To date there is no known treatment for transmissible spongiform encephalopathy. The AABB Standard 5.4.1A Requirements for Allogeneic Donor Qualification states that donors with a risk of vCJD as defined by the FDA Guidance for Industry (January 2002) should be indefinitely deferred from giving blood. Currently those donors include anyone who has traveled to or resided in the United Kingdom for a cumulative period of 3 or more months between 1980 and the end of 1996, those with a history of 5 or more years of cumulative residence or travel in France since 1980, and current and former U.S. military personnel, civilian military personnel, and their dependents who were stationed at European bases for 6 months or more between 1980 and 1996.

NONINFECTIOUS COMPLICATIONS

Transfusion-Related Immunomodulation

Clinical Description

Transfusion-related immunomodulation (TRIM) describes the immunosuppression that occurs after transfusion. TRIM was first

---

[2]Not available in the United States.
[1]Not FDA approved for this indication.

recognized in the 1960s and 1970s in renal allograft recipients who had less rejection and improved graft survival after receiving blood transfusions from their donors. Since then, TRIM has been implicated in the development of postoperative infections, the recurrence of resected malignancies (especially colorectal cancer), spontaneous abortions, and inflammatory bowel disease. TRIM has been suggested to cause reactivation of latent viruses such as CMV.

Pathophysiology

Most authorities agree that TRIM exists, although the mechanisms and magnitude are unclear. However, it is believed that donor WBCs, BRMs, and soluble HLA antigens that have accumulated during storage exert an effect on cell-mediated immunity. TRIM appears to be dose dependent, and thus conservative transfusion triggers might decrease the incidence.

Treatment and Prevention

There is no known treatment for TRIM. Leukoreduction and washing might reduce the incidence of TRIM.

Alloimmunization

Alloimmunization is the development of an antibody to a foreign donor antigen after exposure through blood transfusion, pregnancy, or transplantation. These antibodies, if directed against RBC antigens, can cause DHTRs and AHTRs. Anti-HLA antibodies can cause FNHTRs and platelet refractoriness. These patients may be difficult to match for bone marrow or solid organ transplants. Thrombocytopenia can result in patients who develop platelet-specific antigens either in utero (neonatal alloimmune thrombocytopenia) or after transfusion (post-transfusion purpura).

Refractoriness to Platelet Transfusions

Patients who become refractory to platelet transfusion can do so by several different mechanisms including immune-mediated and non–immune-mediated mechanisms. Immune-mediated refractoriness occurs in highly sensitized patients with anti-HLA or anti–platelet-specific antibodies to donor-specific antigens. Alternatively, patients with sepsis, DIC, fever, splenomegaly, or portal hypertension and persons taking certain drugs can also appear refractory to platelet transfusion due to the sequestration or accelerated clearance of the transfused platelets.

Diagnosis

The expected corrected count index (CCI) can help distinguish between immune-mediated and non–immune-mediated platelet refractoriness. The CCI is calculated 15 minutes to 1 hour after transfusion using the following equation:

$$CCI = \frac{(Post - transfusion\ platelet\ count - Pretransfusion\ platelet\ count) \times Body\ surface\ area}{Number\ of\ platelets\ tranfused \times 10^{11}}$$

A CCI less than 5000 after two sequential platelet transfusions suggests immune-mediated platelet refractoriness. These patients should be screened for anti-HLA and anti–platelet-specific antibodies if other causes of non–immune-mediated refractoriness have been excluded.

Pathophysiology

HLA antibodies are not routinely tested for in most clinical laboratories and blood banks. Additionally, because platelets are not crossmatched prior to transfusion, the only clue to a significant HLA antibody may be FNHTR or the lack of response to a platelet transfusion. Patients who develop multiple HLA antibodies can become refractory to platelet transfusion. Rarely, patients develop platelet-specific antibodies, causing platelet refractoriness.

Treatment and Prevention

Treatment depends on the etiology of platelet refractoriness. Patients with non–immune-mediated refractoriness (including those with splenic sequestration, sepsis, or DIC) require treatment of the underlying disease. If an immune-mediated mechanism is more likely, HLA-matched or crossmatched platelets can be supplied on request. Leukoreduction can potentially reduce HLA-alloimmunization.

Post-transfusion Purpura

Post-transfusion purpura (PTP) is a rare disorder caused by alloantibodies to platelet-specific glycoprotein, most commonly human platelet antigen (HPA)-1a, resulting in destruction of both transfused platelets and the patient's own platelets, leading to severe thrombocytopenia and risk of life-threatening hemorrhage. Thrombocytopenia can last 1 to 2 weeks after transfusion. IVIg is the first-line treatment. The use of washed antigen-negative platelets is controversial.

Volume Overload

Clinical Description

The development of cardiogenic pulmonary edema and other signs of congestive heart failure after transfusion suggest volume overload. The annual reported incidence in the United States of volume overload secondary to transfusion is greatly variable, anywhere from 1 in 100 to 1 in 15,000 units, and largely depends on patient population. The elderly and newborn, as well as patients with cardiac disease, renal insufficiency, and anemia with expanded plasma volumes, are at greater risk for developing volume overload, especially with massive transfusions.

Diagnosis

Diagnosis depends on establishing a cardiac etiology for the resulting dyspnea and pulmonary edema. Elevated central venous pressures or pulmonary wedge pressures, chest x-ray consistent with pulmonary edema, and response to diuretics are used to confirm the suspected diagnosis. It is important to rule out TRALI and other etiologies of acute respiratory distress syndrome (ARDS). BNP may be a useful adjuvant marker in establishing a diagnosis of volume overload secondary to transfusion.

Treatment and Prevention

Some patients respond simply to slowing the rate of the transfusion. Others require diuretics and supportive therapy.

Massive Transfusion Coagulopathy

Clinical Description

Massive transfusion is usually defined as transfusion of 10 or more units of RBCs in less than 24 hours. Massive transfusion usually occurs in the setting of trauma and can be complicated by coagulopathy secondary to dilution of clotting factors and platelets, hypothermia, and hypofibrinogenemia. Patients often receive crystalloid fluids and numerous uncrossmatched group O packed red cells in transit to the hospital or in the emergency department to correct hypovolemia before receiving plasma (which requires at least 30 minutes' thawing time) or platelets. This results in dilution of platelets, clotting proteins, and fibrinogen. Additionally, as the patient's blood pressure is normalized, bleeding becomes brisker resulting in further losses of platelets and clotting factors.

Treatment and Prevention

Ideally, patients with massive bleeding are transfused with whole blood, thereby minimizing the complications of dilution. Additionally, current guidelines are based on whole-blood transfusion and wash-out equations, simple mathematical models that calculate exponential decay of blood components during bleeding, assuming that the blood volume of the patient is stable and the replacement rates are constant and equal. Blood volumes and bleeding rates are usually quite variable, and replacement tends to lag behind blood loss; therefore, these guidelines and equations tend to underestimate needs. Computer modeling has demonstrated that patients with penetrating traumas have generally lost 2500 mL (or one half the average blood volume) by the time they arrive in the emergency department, 3200 mL (or two thirds the average blood volume) by the start of surgery, and 11,000 mL (or more than two blood volumes) at the end of surgery. PT will be prolonged (>1.5 times normal) after a loss of less than one blood volume. Fibrinogen is next, dropping below 0.8 g/L, in a little over one blood volume. Platelets stay above $50,000 \times 10^9$/L until after losses of more than two blood volumes.

Various massive transfusion protocols have been reviewed extensively in the literature. Early plasma replacement at higher plasma–to–red cells ratios (~1:1) is gaining popularity in this clinical setting despite the fear that some patients may be overtransfused. However, there are few studies comparing conservative with liberal plasma and platelet transfusion with regard to outcome.

Hypothermia due to massive transfusion of refrigerated and recently thawed products contributes to the coagulopathy associated with massive transfusion. For this reason, many products are transfused through blood warmers. The use of cryoprecipitate for fibrinogen replacement is often necessary and more efficient than use of plasma.

OTHER ADVERSE EVENTS

Less frequent adverse events of transfusion include hypocalcemia due to large infusions of citrate anticoagulant, hyperkalemia due to RBC leakage during storage, mechanical hemolysis, and iron overload. These events are rare and typically affect infants receiving large amounts of old blood or patients receiving chronic transfusions; thus they are outside of the scope of this article. However, it is important to be aware of their existence and to monitor patients accordingly for signs of their development.

REFERENCES

Allain JP, Bianco C, Blajchman MA, et al: Protecting the blood supply from emerging pathogens: The role of pathogen inactivation. Transfus Med Rev 2005;19(2):110-126.

Blumberg N: Deleterious clinical effects of transfusion immunomodulation proven beyond a reasonable doubt. Transfusion 2005;45(suppl):33S-39S.

Blumberg N, Heal JM, Gettings KEJ: WBC reduction of RBC transfusions is associated with decreased incidence of RBC alloimmunization. Transfusion 2003;43:945-952.

Dodd RY, Notari IV, Stramer SL: Current prevalence and incidence of infectious disease markers and estimated window-period risk in the American Red Cross blood donor population. Transfusion 2002;42(8):975-979.

Goldman M, Webert KE, Arnold DM, et al; TRALI Consensus Panel: Proceedings of a consensus conference: Towards an understanding of TRALI. Transfus Med Rev 2005;19(1):2-31.

Hillyer CD, Silberstein LE, Ness PM, et al (eds): Blood Banking and Transfusion Medicine, 2nd ed. Philadelphia. Churchill Livingstone, 2007.

Hirschberg A, Dugas M, Banez EI, et al: Minimizing dilutional coagulopathy in exsanguinating hemorrhage: A computer simulation. J Trauma 2003;54:454-463.

Kleinman S, Caulfield T, Chan P, et al: Toward an understanding of transfusion-related acute lung injury: Statement of a consensus panel. Transfusion 2004;44(12):1774-1789.

Lee D: Perception of blood transfusion risk. Transfus Med Rev 2006;20(2):141-148.

Linden JV, Wagner K, Voytovich AE, Sheehan J: Transfusion errors in New York State: An analysis of 10 years' experience. Transfusion 2000;40:1207-1213.

Luban NC: Transfusion safety: Where are we today? Ann N Y Acad Sci 2005;1054:325-341.

Schroeder ML. Transfusion-associated graft-versus-host disease. Br J Haematol 2002;117:275-287.

Sheppard CA, Roback JD, Hillyer CD: Transfusion-transmitted cytomegalovirus infection: Consideration toward an optimal plan for its mitigation. Blood Ther Med 2005;5(1):6-14.

Zhou L, Giacherio D, Cooling L, Davenport RD: Use of B-natriuretic peptide as a diagnostic marker in the differential diagnosis of transfusion-associated circulatory overload. Transfusion 2005;45:1056-1063.

Zou S, Dodd RY, Stramer SL, Strong DM, for the Tissue Safety Group: Probability of Viremia with HBV, HCV, HIV and HTLV among tissue donors in the United States. N Engl J Med 2004;351(8):751-759.

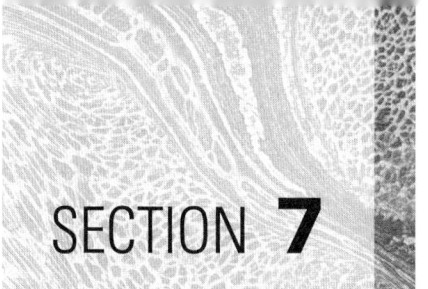

SECTION 7

The Digestive System

Cholelithiasis and Cholecystitis

Method of
Grant R. Caddy, MD

Cholelithiasis

Gallstones affect 10% to 12% of people in Western populations, and the prevalence increases with age. The majority of patients with gallstones (approximately 80%) remain asymptomatic. The risk of complications, mainly that of acute cholecystitis, occurs in around 2% of patients with symptomatic gallstones.

Gallstones can be classified depending on their composition. The commonest stones are cholesterol or cholesterol-predominant stones (mixed stones), which make up around 80% to 85% of all gallstones. Mixed stones can be multiple, of varying sizes, and faceted. Most are radiolucent but 10% are radiopaque. Pure cholesterol stones are commonly solitary but may be multiple and are radiolucent. Pigment stones are less common in Western populations and are associated with hemolytic disorders such as hemolytic anemias, malaria and cirrhosis.

Risk factors for cholesterol-predominant stone formation are shown in Box 1. Female patients have a 2 to 8 times greater risk of developing gallstones than male patients. This increased risk appears to decline following menopause. High intake of carbohydrate, high glycemic load, and high glycemic index foods increases the risk of symptomatic gallstone disease by approximately 1.5 times. Other risk factors include a high body mass index (BMI), rapid weight loss (> 1.5 kg/week), and history of dieting or gastric bypass surgery. In a 10-year follow-up study, patients who were overweight (defined as BMI > 25) were approximately twice as likely to develop gallstones compared with controls. It has also been documented that following antiobesity surgery, 20% to 35% of patients develop gallstones in the postoperative period.

Complications of symptomatic gallstones are shown in Box 2.

Acute Cholecystitis

Acute cholecystitis is suspected when patients present with pain localized to the right upper quadrant (RUQ), pain aggravated by palpation in the RUQ (with or without a positive Murphy's sign), and an inflammatory response (e.g., fever and elevation in white blood cell count, C-reactive protein, and/or erythrocyte sedimentation rate). The exact mechanism of acute cholecystitis is uncertain, but blockage of the cystic duct in addition to irritation to the gallbladder mucosa result in further recruitment of inflammatory mediators such as prostaglandins (PG) I_2 and E_2. Secondary infection develops in approximately 20% of patients, usually with *Escherichia coli*, *Klebsiella* species, or *Streptococcus faecalis*. Mild elevations in bilirubin, aspartate aminotransferase (AST), alkaline phosphatase (ALP), and γ-glutamyl transpeptidase (GGT) are not uncommon (in up to one third of patients), but high levels often indicate concomitant choledocholithiasis, cholangitis, or Mirizzi's syndrome (see later).

DIAGNOSIS

First-line radiologic investigation should be a transabdominal ultrasound (TUS), which has a high specificity for cholecystitis (> 98%).

BOX 1 Risk Factors for Developing Gallstones

- Age > 50 years (relative risk, 2.5; $P < .001$)
- Bile salt loss (e.g., terminal ileal disease)
- Diabetes mellitus
- Female gender
- First-degree relative with symptomatic gallstone disease
- Gallbladder dysmotility and stasis
- Genetic factors
- High intake of carbohydrates and high glycemic load
- Hyperlipidemia
- Overweight and obesity
- Positive family history of previous cholecystectomy in a first-degree family member
- Pregnancy
- Starvation
- Total parenteral nutrition

BOX 2 Complications of Gallstones

- Acalculous cholecystitis
- Acute cholecystitis
- Biliary colic
- Cholecystoenteric fistulas
- Choledocholithiasis ± ascending cholangitis
- Chronic cholecystitis
- Gallstone ileus
- Gallstone pancreatitis
- Gangrenous gallbladder and gallbladder perforation
- Mirizzi's syndrome

CURRENT DIAGNOSIS

- The majority of patients with gallstones (approximately 80%) remain asymptomatic. The risk of complications, mainly acute cholecystitis, occurs in around 2% of patients with symptomatic gallstones.
- Mild elevations in bilirubin, AST, ALP, and GGT occur in approximately one third of patients but high levels often indicate concomitant choledocholithiasis or cholangitis.
- TUS has a high specificity for cholecystitis (> 98%). A HIDA scan has a sensitivity of > 95% and a specificity of 90%.
- Approximately 10% to 18% of patients undergoing cholecystectomy have coexisting bile duct stones.
- In choledocholithiasis, TUS is particularly sensitive if there is biliary dilatation (sensitivity is 96%) but is less sensitive in detecting stones within the duct (sensitivity is 63%).
- EUS, MRCP, and ERCP are equivalent in accuracy rates for detecting choledocholithiasis, but because of the complication rate of ERCP, this procedure should be reserved for patients with a high probability of choledocholithiasis.

Abbreviations: ALP = alkaline phosphatase; AST = aspartate aminotransferase; ERCP = endoscopic retrograde cholangiopancreatography; EUS = endoscopic ultrasound; GGT = γ-glutamyl transpeptidase; HIDA = hepatobiliary iminodiacetic acid; MRCP = magnetic resonance cholangiopancreatography; TUS = transabdominal ultrasound.

In addition to identifying gallstones, gallbladder thickening (> 4-5 mm), edema, adjacent pericolic fluid, and tenderness with the transducer strongly suggest cholecystitis. Hepatobiliary iminodiacetic acid (HIDA) scan should be reserved for second-line investigation if the diagnosis remains in doubt. If the cystic duct is patent, HIDA will be taken up by the gallbladder and will be evident on scanning the abdomen after 1 hour. A positive test fails to detect any localization of HIDA within the gallbladder due to obstruction of the cystic duct. The test has a sensitivity of greater than 95% but a specificity of 90%.

TREATMENT

Patients should receive supportive care as first-line treatment with intravenous hydration and analgesia. There is evidence that nonsteroidal anti-inflammatory drugs (NSAIDs) have additional benefits other than their analgesic properties, due to their antagonist effect on prostaglandins, which are central to the inflammation of cholecystitis. NSAIDs reduce intraluminal pressure in the gallbladder, which is increased in acute cholecystitis. In addition, NSAIDs have been shown to reduce the rate of progression of biliary colic to acute cholecystitis. Due to the risk of secondary infection, antibiotics such as cephalosporin (Zinacef) and metronidazole (Flagyl) are generally recommended, but in uncomplicated cholecystitis, the routine use of antibiotics does not appear to reduce the risk of gallbladder empyema.

Laparoscopic cholecystectomy remains the most common surgical treatment for acute cholecystitis and is considered the treatment of choice for most patients. The advantages of laparoscopic cholecystectomy over open cholecystectomy are well documented and include reduced mortality, reduced postoperative pain, better cosmetic result, and a reduction in hospital stay. Studies investigating the optimal timing of laparoscopic cholecystectomy following acute cholecystitis suggest that early cholecystectomy (within 72 hours) compared with delayed cholecystectomy results in a reduction in hospital stay and readmission rate but no overall differences in operation time, conversion rate, or complication rates. Patient symptom scores (diarrhea, indigestion, and abdominal pain) at 4 weeks are significantly better in patients undergoing early cholecystectomy versus supportive treatment followed by delayed cholecystectomy.

There is evidence supporting mini-laparotomy cholecystectomy (usually defined as open cholecystectomy through an incision of 4 to 7 cm) with similar overall results to laparoscopic cholecystectomy. In one prospective study, laparoscopic cholecystectomy took a longer time to perform but produced a slightly shorter postoperative hospital stay and a smoother postoperative course than mini-laparotomy. The choice of which operation to perform is often determined by the experience of individual surgical centers.

COMPLICATIONS

Emphysematous Cholecystitis

Acute emphysematous cholecystitis is characterized by the presence of gas within the wall or lumen of the gallbladder caused by the gas-forming organisms (e.g., *Clostridium welchii* or *E.coli*). Symptoms can be identical to those of acute cholecystitis. In contrast to acute cholecystitis, emphysematous cholecystitis occurs more commonly in elderly and diabetic patients. Its importance lies in the increased rates of early gangrene and perforation of the gallbladder. Treatment is with empiric antibiotic therapy and early cholecystectomy.

Gangrenous Cholecystitis

Gangrenous cholecystitis occurs in 2% to 20% of patients admitted with acute cholecystitis. The risk factors for gangrenous cholecystitis is increased in male patients older than 50 years; in patients with diabetes, history of cardiovascular disease, or white blood cell count greater than 15,000/mm^3; and in those who delay seeking medical treatment. The risk of gallbladder perforation and mortality is increased with gangrenous cholecystitis. Treatment is with empiric antibiotic therapy and early cholecystectomy.

Gallbladder Perforation

Gallbladder perforation can occur following gangrenous cholecystitis. It is estimated to occur in 3% to 10% of patients with acute cholecystitis. Like gangrenous cholecystitis, patients with gallbladder perforations have similar characteristics including older age and cardiovascular disease. In addition, perforations were associated with more postoperative complications that required more ICU admissions and longer hospital stays. Perforations may be localized, resulting in a pericholecystic abscess, or, less commonly, free perforations may occur into the peritoneum. Diagnosis is often difficult preoperatively.

Acalculous Cholecystitis

Acalculous cholecystitis occurs in 5% to 10% of cases of cholecystitis. It is often associated with critically ill patients, severe trauma, burns, and cardiovascular surgery but is also associated with patients who have diabetes, cardiovascular disease, or AIDS and in patients on total parenteral nutrition or opiates. Without treatment, the mortality rate is 30% to 50%.

Characteristic features on TUS are thickened gallbladder wall, absence of gallstones, gallbladder distension, Murphy's sign induced by probe, and emphysematous cholecystitis with or without perforation. Treatment is initially with supportive therapy with antibiotics and urgent referral for laparoscopic cholecystectomy. In patients with high operative risk, percutaneous cholecystostomy (insertion of a drain into the gallbladder) under radiologic guidance is an alternative treatment.

Other complications of cholelithiasis include gallstone ileus, cholecystoenteric fistulas, and Mirizzi's syndrome (obstruction of the bile duct secondary to extrinsic compression from an impacted stone in the cystic duct)

Acute Cholecystitis in Pregnancy

Overall acute cholecystitis in pregnancy is relatively uncommon. The optimal treatment remains controversial. Conservative management of a pregnant patient results in resolution of symptoms in approximately 90% of patients. However, up to 60% of patients have recurrent symptoms (readmission with acute cholecystitis, biliary colic, and premature delivery). Due to concerns of fetal loss, a conservative approach is often adopted. However, studies have supported the role of laparoscopic cholecystectomy as a safe procedure in pregnant patients with acute cholecystitis, resulting in decreased hospital stay, reduced rate of labor induction, and reduced preterm deliveries.

Chronic Cholecystitis

Chronic cholecystitis refers to recurrent episodes of gallbladder inflammation usually due to stones. These episodes may be asymptomatic but they can also result in recurrent episodes of pain. However, there does not appear to be any correlation of symptoms and degree of fibrosis and thickening of the gallbladder wall. Patients with symptomatic gallstones with recurrent biliary colic should be referred for laparoscopic cholecystectomy.

Biliary Sludge

Biliary sludge is usually diagnosed on ultrasonography. Its appearance on ultrasonography is of layered echoes in the dependent portion of the gallbladder, with no associated acoustic shadows. It is often made up of cholesterol crystals and calcium salts.

Precipitating factors include total parenteral nutrition, rapid weight loss, pregnancy, prolonged fasting, bone marrow and solid organ transplants, and drugs such as octreotide (Sandostatin) and ceftriaxone (Rocephin). In one study, 50% of patients presenting with symptomatic biliary sludge had complete resolution of gallbladder sludge on repeat imaging. In the remaining group, in 50% the sludge remained but patients were asymptomatic and in 50% further symptoms developed.

The management of biliary sludge should be managed similar to gallbladder stones. Asymptomatic sludge should be managed conservatively. Symptomatic patients should be considered for laparoscopic cholecystectomy.

Choledocholithiasis

PRESENTATION

Approximately 10% to 18% of patients undergoing cholecystectomy have coexisting bile duct stones. The symptoms of choledocholithiasis are varied and include biliary colic, jaundice, cholangitis, and pancreatitis. Conversely, a portion of patients with choledocholithiasis are asymptomatic, with a prevalence estimated to be up to 12%. In patients who present with symptoms of retained bile duct stones, the risk of subsequent symptoms is up to 50%, and the risk of complications is up to 25% if the stones are left untreated.

Patients with choledocholithiasis often present with biliary colic—pain that is often located in the RUQ and lasting between 30 minutes and several hours. There is often associated nausea and vomiting. If there is partial or complete obstruction of the common bile duct, then patients develop jaundice with associated pale stools and dark urine. Infection often occurs, resulting in a cholangitis. Approximately three fourths of patients with cholangitis have Charcot's triad of jaundice, fever, and pain. However, in 10% of patients pain may be the only feature of cholangitis. Due to bacterial translocation from the bile duct to the bloodstream, 20% of patients with cholangitis have a bacteremia, usually with gram-negative organisms.

Smaller bile duct stones (up to 8 mm) are more likely to pass spontaneously through the ampulla into the duodenum. However, it is the passage of smaller stones through the ampulla that is more likely to result in gallstone pancreatitis compared with larger stones. For example, one study found that patients who presented with gallstone pancreatitis had a mean stone diameter of 4 mm compared with patients presenting with obstructive jaundice, who had a mean stone diameter of 9 mm.

DIFFERENTIAL DIAGNOSIS

The differential of choledocholithiasis will depend on the clinical presentation. Differentials are shown in Box 3.

DIAGNOSIS

Patients presenting with symptomatic choledocholithiasis often have elevations in serum GGT and ALP (increased in 94% and 91% of cases, respectively). Bilirubin levels may be increased depending on if obstruction of the bile duct has occurred.

TUS is the commonest method of imaging the gallbladder and biliary tree in choledocholithiasis. TUS is particularly sensitive if there is biliary dilation (sensitivity up to 96%). It is less sensitive in detecting stones within the duct (sensitivity up to 63%) but has high specificity (specificity 95%). Therefore, a negative TUS does not rule out suspected choledocholithiasis.

Other radiologic investigations include computed tomography (CT), endoscopic ultrasound (EUS), magnetic resonance cholangiopancreatography (MRCP), and endoscopic retrograde cholangiopancreatography (ERCP). A National Institutes of Health (NIH) consensus statement found that EUS, MRCP, and ERCP were equivalent in accuracy rates. However, due to the risks of ERCP (pancreatitis, bleeding, perforation, infection), ERCP is recommended in patients with a high probability of choledocholithiasis. In patients with an intermediate probability, other imaging modalities, such as MRCP or EUS, should be considered.

TREATMENT

Generally, patients with symptomatic choledocholithiasis should be offered treatment because of the high risk of recurrent symptoms and complications if stones are left in situ as already discussed. In some special circumstances, adopting a conservative approach may be appropriate such as severe end-stage dementia or severe comorbid factors that make removal hazardous.

The two main methods of bile duct stone removal are at ERCP or, in patients with an intact gallbladder, laparoscopic cholecystectomy and bile duct exploration (LC+BDE). Current practice in choosing between the two methods depends on center preference and local

---

CURRENT THERAPY

- Patients with symptomatic gallstones should undergo laparoscopic cholecystectomy if there is no contraindication.
- For acute cholecystitis, first-line treatment is supportive care with intravenous hydration, analgesia (NSAIDs), and antibiotics. If there are no contraindications, patients should undergo laparoscopic cholecystectomy within 72 hours.
- Percutaneous cholecystostomy is an alternative option in patients with acalculous cholecystitis who are too unwell to undergo cholecystectomy.
- Treatment options for patients with choledocholithiasis include ERCP and stone removal followed by laparoscopic cholecystectomy or, in patients with an intact gallbladder, cholecystectomy and bile duct exploration. Overall, there are no differences in morbidity and mortality between the two procedures.
- There is a limited role for other techniques such as extracorporeal shockwave lithotripsy and endoscopic laser lithotripsy or oral dissolution therapy.

Abbreviation: ERCP = endoscopic retrograde cholangio-pancreatography.

> **BOX 3 Differential Diagnosis of Choledocholithiasis by Presentation**
>
> **Jaundice with or without Pain**
> - Alcoholic liver disease
> - Benign stricture
> - Bile duct injuries
> - Drug induced
> - Malignant stricture
> - Parasitic infection of the biliary tree
> - Primary biliary cirrhosis
> - Sclerosing cholangitis
> - Viral hepatitis
>
> **Biliary Colic**
> - Acute pancreatitis
> - Cholecystitis
> - Duodenitis
> - Esophageal spasm
> - Inferior myocardial infarction
> - Peptic ulcer disease
> - Sphincter of Oddi dysfunction
>
> **Pancreatitis**
> - Appendicitis
> - Biliary colic
> - Dissecting aneurysm
> - Diverticulitis
> - Ectopic pregnancy
> - Hematoma of abdominal muscles
> - Inferior myocardial infarction
> - Mesenteric infarction
> - Perforated gastric or duodenal ulcer
>
> **Cholestatic Liver Function Tests**
> - Alcoholic liver disease
> - Ampullary carcinoma
> - Biliary strictures
> - Drugs
> - Granulomatous hepatitis
> - Malignant infiltration of the liver
> - Nonalcoholic fatty liver disease (NAFLD)
> - Primary biliary cirrhosis
> - Sclerosing cholangitis

expertise in laparoscopic bile duct exploration. A recent Cochrane Database of systematic review comparing LC+BDE and ERCP found that both methods were equally effective, with no significant difference in morbidity and mortality. However, shorter hospital stay was achieved in patients undergoing LC+BDE.

There is a limited role for other techniques, such as extracorporeal shockwave lithotripsy and endoscopic laser lithotripsy, and these techniques should be reserved for bile duct stones that cannot be removed at ERCP or LC+CBE due to technical or safety reasons.

REFERENCES

Al-Waili N, Saloom KY: The analgesic effect of intravenous tenoxicam in symptomatic treatment of biliary colic: A comparison with hyoscine N-butylbromide. Eur J Med Res 1998;3(10):475-479.

Field AE, Coakley EH, Must A, et al: Impact of overweight on the risk of developing common chronic diseases during a 10-year period. Arch Intern Med 2001;161(13):1581-1586.

Johansson M, Thune A, Blomqvist A, et al: Impact of choice of therapeutic strategy for acute cholecystitis on patient's health-related quality of life. Results of a randomized, controlled clinical trial. Dig Surg 2004; 21(5-6):359-362.

Lau H, Lo CY, Patil NG, Yuen WK: Early versus delayed-interval laparoscopic cholecystectomy for acute cholecystitis: A meta-analysis. Surg Endosc 2006;20(1):82-87.

Lu EJ, Curet MJ, El-Sayed YY, Kirkwood KS: Medical versus surgical management of biliary tract disease in pregnancy. Am J Surg. 2004;188(6):755-759.

Martin DJ, Vernon DR, Toouli J: Surgical versus endoscopic treatment of bile duct stones. Cochrane Database Syst Rev 2006;(2):CD003327.

Miller K, Hell E, Lang B, Lengauer E: Gallstone formation prophylaxis after gastric restrictive procedures for weight loss: A randomized double-blind placebo-controlled trial. Ann Surg 2003;238(5):697-702.

NIH state-of-the-science statement on endoscopic retrograde cholangiopancreatography (ERCP) for diagnosis and therapy. NIH Consens State Sci Statements. 2002;19(1):1-26.

Papi C, Catarci M, D'Ambrosio L, et al: Timing of cholecystectomy for acute calculous cholecystitis: A meta-analysis. Am J Gastroenterol. 2004; 99(1):147-155.

Ros A, Gustafsson L, Krook H, et al: Laparoscopic cholecystectomy versus mini-laparotomy cholecystectomy: A prospective, randomized, single-blind study. Ann Surg 2001;234(6):741-749.

Thornell E, Nilsson B, Jansson R, Svanvik J: Effect of short-term indomethacin treatment on the clinical course of acute obstructive cholecystitis. Eur J Surg 1991;157(2):127-130.

Tsai CJ, Leitzmann MF, Willett WC, Giovannucci EL: Dietary carbohydrates and glycaemic load and the incidence of symptomatic gall stone disease in men. Gut 2005;54(6):823-828.

Cirrhosis

Method of
Richard K. Sterling, MD, MSc, Wissam E. Mattar, MD, and Paul Y. Kwo, MD

Cirrhosis is defined as the development of fibrosis of the liver with the formation of regenerative nodules. Typically it follows a chronic injury to hepatocytes that activate the perisinusoidal stellate cells by cytokines, which transforms them into myofibroblasts capable of proliferating and depositing collagen type 1. Progressively the normal liver histology is replaced by the fibrotic, distorted architecture. It is the resultant impairment in the synthetic, metabolic, and hemodynamic functions of the liver that defines cirrhosis clinically.

Common Clinical Manifestations

In addition to the particular expression of every etiology, most cirrhotic patients have little or no clinical features in the early stages, and many are already being followed up for abnormal liver panels before the development of cirrhosis. Patients may present with fatigue, weakness, nausea, abdominal discomfort, loss of appetite with weight loss, and pruritus. On physical examination, there may be jaundice, skin hematomas, spider angiomas, palmar erythema, gynecomastia, testicular atrophy, and caput medusae. The spleen and the liver could be palpable with tenderness in the right upper quadrant. Attention should also be given to the so-called seven hand signs of cirrhosis: palmar erythema, Dupuytren's contracture, telangiectasias, thenar wasting, leukonychia or Terry's nails, clubbing, and asterixis. As liver function decompensates, the more specific clinical manifestations of complications appear. Ascites, spontaneous bacterial peritonitis (SBP), hepatic encephalopathy (HE), esophageal varices, hepatorenal syndrome (HRS), hepatopulmonary syndrome (HPS), portopulmonary hypertension, and hepatocellular carcinoma (HCC), as well as other less apparent complications such as hematologic disturbances and hepatic osteodystrophy, are problems to address in the decompensated stage (Table 1).

TABLE 1 Key Current Diagnoses

Ascites	Shifting dullness on physical exam, abdominal ultrasound, diagnostic paracentesis
SBP	Ascitic fluid: PMN cells count above 250/mm^3, positive gram stain, positive cultures
Esophageal/ gastric varices	EGD
HE	Neuropsychiatric abnormalities; rule out other etiologies, search for precipitating factors
HRS I	Decrease of >50% in creatinine clearance or doubling of serum creatinine in less than 2 wk; rule out other etiologies of ARF
HRS II	Progressive renal failure, refractory ascites
Hepatopulmonary syndrome	Hypoxia, intrapulmonary vascular dilations, contrast-enhanced echocardiography or technetium-labeled macroaggregated albumin scanning
Portopulmonary hypertension	Pulmonary hypertension without secondary etiologies other than portal hypertension
Hepatocellular carcinoma	Lesion >2 cm with arterial enhancement or AFP >400 µg/mL, FNA in other suspicious lesions

Abbreviations: AFP = alpha-fetoprotein; ARF = acute renal failure; EGD = esophagogastroduodenoscopy; FNA = fine-needle aspiration; HE = hepatic encephalopathy; HRS = hepatorenal syndrome; PMN = polymorphonuclear neutrophil (leukocyte).

Common Laboratory and Imaging Findings

Frequently, tests confirm the clinical suspicion of cirrhosis in the presence of the characteristic physical findings of advanced liver disease. Laboratory studies could help establish the etiologic diagnosis and screen or confirm complications. In general, alanine aminotransferase (ALT) and aspartate aminotransferase (AST) are elevated but can be in the normal range. In the absence of chronic alcohol use, cirrhosis may be indicated by a higher AST than ALT. Bilirubin often increases only in advanced stages. High alkaline phosphatase pinpoints to a cholestatic component. Albumin trends to lower levels and the prothrombin time (PT) or international normalized ratio (INR) increases with the severity of the synthetic disturbance. Cytopenias, especially thrombocytopenia, are common. A low platelet count is often the only initial laboratory finding. Several non-invasive indices have been developed.

Imaging studies such as abdominal ultrasound (US), computed tomography (CT) scan, and magnetic resonance imaging (MRI) can suggest the diagnosis by revealing abnormalities in size, shape, and contour of the liver. However, they are not perfect, and liver biopsy remains the gold standard. Liver imaging can be helpful for the evaluation of portal hypertension and biliary tree abnormalities and to look for complications of advanced liver disease such as ascites, vascular thrombosis, and HCC.

Diagnosis

Obtaining adequate tissue from the liver confirms the diagnosis of cirrhosis. Biopsies could be obtained percutaneously except in the presence of a prolonged PT more than 3 seconds, thrombocytopenia of less than 60,000 to 80,000, or the presence of ascites. In these instances, an open biopsy or a transjugular approach can be used.

CURRENT DIAGNOSIS

- Symptoms: fatigue, weakness, nausea, abdominal discomfort, loss of appetite with weight loss, pruritus
- Physical exam (general): jaundice, skin hematomas, spider angiomas, palmar erythema, gynecomastia, testicular atrophy, caput medusae, Dupuytren's contracture, thenar wasting, leukonychia or Terry's nails, clubbing, splenomegaly
- Physical exam (in decompensation): ascites, hepatic encephalopathy (asterixis)
- Complications: spontaneous bacterial peritonitis, esophageal/gastric varices, portal hypertensive gastropathy, hepatorenal syndrome, hepatopulmonary syndrome, portopulmonary hypertension, hepatocellular carcinoma

Severity of Cirrhosis

Multiple scores have been created to categorize the severity of disease. The Child-Pugh score is the most widely used (Table 2). It incorporates three laboratory values (PT, bilirubin, and albumin) and two clinical features (ascites and encephalopathy). Class A patients have an 85% 2-year survival, compared with 60% and 35% for classes B and C, respectively. The MELD (Model for End-stage Liver Disease) score has now supplanted the Child-Pugh classification for listing the patient for liver transplantation (Table 2) and is calculated by a formula that includes bilirubin, creatinine, and the INR instead of PT.

Causes

The etiologies that could lead to cirrhosis are very diverse and can be categorized into toxins and drugs, viruses, autoimmune diseases, biliary disease, metabolic, vascular and idiopathic (Table 3).

TABLE 2 Classification of Cirrhosis

	Child-Pugh Points		
	1	2	3
Bilirubin (mg/dL)	<2.0	2.1–3.0	>3.0
Prothrombin time (seconds prolonged)	<4	4–6	>6
Albumin (g/L)	>3.5	2.8–3.5	<2.8
Ascites	None	Mild–moderate	Severe
Encephalopathy	None	Mild–moderate	Severe

Child's class A: 5–6, Child's class B: 7–9, Child's class C: 10–15.

MELD Score	3-mo Mortality
<10	2%–8%
10–19	6%–29%
20–29	50%–76%
30–39	62%–83%
≥40	100%

Abbreviations: INR = international normalized ratio; MELD = Model for End-stage Liver Disease. MELD Score = 11.2 ln (INR) + 3.78 ln (bilirubin) + 9.57 ln (creatinine) + 6.43

TABLE 3 Common Causes of Cirrhosis

Etiology	Diagnostic Test
Alcohol	History, AST-to-ALT ratio > 2, liver biopsy
Viral hepatitis B	Surface antigen, E antigen, HBV DNA
Viral hepatitis C	HCV antibody, HCV RNA, HCV genotype
Autoimmune hepatitis	ANA, ASMA, A-LKM
Primary biliary cirrhosis	AMA
Primary sclerosing cholangitis	P-ANCA, ERCP, MRCP
Alpha 1 antitrypsin deficiency	A_1AT level, phenotype
Wilson's disease	Ceruloplasmin, serum Cu, Kayser-Fleischer rings
NASH	Liver biopsy, history of metabolic syndrome
Budd-Chiari syndrome	Duplex of the hepatic vein
Cryptogenic	Diagnosis of exclusion

Abbreviations: A-LKM = antich-liver/kidney microsome; ALT = alanine aminotransferase; AMA = antimitochondrial antibody; ANA = antinuclear antibody; ASMA = antismooth muscle antibody; AST = aspartate aminotransferase; Cu = copper; ERCP = endoscopic retrograde cholangiopancreatography; HBV = hepatitis B virus; HCV = hepatitis C virus; MRCP = magnetic retrograde cholangiopancreatography; NASH = nonalcoholic steatohepatitis; P-ANCA = perinuclear antineutrophil cytoplasmic antibody.

Treatment

There are limited treatments to reverse advanced fibrosis, but controlling the etiology preferably before end-stage disease ensues is highly recommended. Treatment of the complications of cirrhosis could be lifesaving or palliative.

Treatment of the Etiologies

CHRONIC VIRAL HEPATITIS

More information can be obtained from the article on viral hepatitis in this volume.

ALCOHOL

Alcohol abuse could lead to a spectrum of liver disease states that range from asymptomatic fatty liver to cirrhosis. The average total intake to develop cirrhosis is 80 g of ethanol per day for 20 years. Lesser doses in women, chronic viral hepatitis, and hemochromatosis could lead to higher risks of developing cirrhosis.

History, physical examination, and laboratory features can be specific for alcoholic hepatitis. An AST value more than two times the level of the ALT (related both to the deficiency in pyridoxal-6-phosphate and the direct mitochondrial toxicity of alcohol) suggests alcohol as the culprit of liver injury. If this ratio is less than 2, alcohol is unlikely to be the cause of liver injury. Aminotransferases usually do not exceed 500 UI/L. If they do, other coexisting etiologies, such as acetaminophen or acute viral hepatitis, should be excluded. Elevations in gamma glutamyl transferase (GGT) and carbohydrate-deficient transferase (CDT) could also suggest alcohol as the etiology of hepatitis. Thrombocytopenia and anemia with macrocytosis are classical findings but not specific. In acute alcoholic hepatitis (AH), alkaline phosphatase and GGT are typically and persistently elevated. Approximately 10% of the cases of AH are atypical or unclear, and in these a liver biopsy is required. A rapid bedside screening by looking for encephalopathy and ascites could evaluate the severity of alcohol-induced liver injury. If one or both are present, then calculating the MELD score and the discriminant function

CURRENT THERAPY

Procedure/Reason

- Upper endoscopy: Screen for varices.
  - If moderate or large, primary prophylaxis with non-selective β-blocker to prevent bleeding.
  - If none, then repeat q2y.
- Liver imaging (ultrasound or CT): screen/surveillance for hepatocellular carcinoma.
  - Repeat q6–12 mo.
- Alpha fetoprotein: Screen/surveillance for hepatocellular carcinoma.
- Repeat q3–6 mo.
- Diagnostic paracentesis: Send fluid for WBC, differential, albumin, and total protein.
  - Exclude SBP (PMN < 250).
  - Calculate SAAG.
- Hepatitis A and B serology: Vaccinate if negative.
- Diet: Low sodium:
  - 2 g/d if ascites.
  - 3–5 g if no ascites.
  - Avoid protein restriction unless uncontrolled encephalopathy.
- Medications: Avoid NSAIDs.
- Avoid aminoglycosides.
- Liver transplant referral/evaluation: if hepatic decompensation, variceal bleeding, or hepatocellular carcinoma.

Abbreviations: NSAIDs = nonsteroidal anti-inflammatory drugs; PMN = polymorphonuclear neutrophil (leukocyte); SAAG = serum ascites-albumin gradient; SBP = spontaneous bacterial peritonitis; WBC = white blood cell count.

(DF), 4.6 × (PT patient − PT control) + bilirubin in mg/dL, help assess the mortality risk and the subsequent management plan. A DF value greater than 32 predicts a 50% mortality in 1 month in those with acute alcoholic hepatitis.

The best treatment for alcoholic liver disease is total abstinence. Progression of disease and accelerated mortality are likely in patients who continue to drink. It should be emphasized that nutritional needs are to be addressed (protein 1 to 1.5 g/kg/day with caloric needs being 1.2 to 1.4 × resting energy expenditure divided as 50% from carbohydrate and 30% from fat mainly unsaturated). If dietary intake is insufficient, supplements are indicated. A nighttime snack is encouraged. The administration of 50 to 100 mg/day of thiamine along with intravenous (IV) glucose, 100 mg/day of pyridoxine (vitamin B_6), and 1 mg/day of folic acid is often required. Supplementation with phosphorus, magnesium, and potassium are necessary if serum levels are low. Colchicine[1] has no benefits and should not be prescribed. Pentoxifylline (Trental),[1] at a dose of 400 mg every 8 hours for 4 weeks, showed significant survival benefit equivalent to those reported with corticosteroids. Infliximab (Remicade)[1] with corticosteroids increased mortality from infectious complications in one study and should not be administered in acute alcoholic hepatitis.

In acute AH with a DF of 32 or with hepatic encephalopathy, it is recommended to administer 40 mg of prednisone or 32 mg of methylprednisolone for 28 days, which can increase survival. A MELD score of 21 is suggested as a cutoff for beginning treatment with steroids. Predictors of the response to corticosteroids are decreasing

---

[1]Not FDA approved for this indication.

DF, MELD score, and creatinine and bilirubin levels after 1 week of treatment. If these improvements are not seen, continued steroids are of little benefit. Liver transplantation is the best treatment for advanced alcoholic liver disease. Alcohol abstinence for 6 months is routinely required before transplantation in alcoholics. This time frame can be changed on an individual basis.

AUTOIMMUNE HEPATITIS

The exclusion of replicating hepatitis virus infection together with female sex, hypergammaglobulinemia, and response to immunosuppressive treatment are the hallmarks of an accurate diagnosis of autoimmune hepatitis (AIH). A score based mainly on gender, liver chemistries, immunoglobulins titers, histology, absence of viral hepatitis, and alcohol abuse was created to predict the chance of diagnosing AIH. Liver biopsy, which is helpful for diagnosis, management, and prognosis, shows characteristically an increase in plasma cells with interface hepatitis.

AIH can be divided into two categories. In type 1, antibodies to nuclei (ANA) and/or to smooth muscle (SMA) are present. In type 2, anti–liver/kidney microsome-1 (ALKM-1) antibodies are most common. Untreated disease has a mortality rate of 50% at 5 years. Two fundamental goals are distinguished: induction of remission and maintenance of remission. Treatment is guided by the American Association for the Study of Liver Diseases (AASLD) guidelines, which recommend treating active disease and observing closely milder forms; severe disease is considered when aminotransferases are 10 times the normal limit, or five times the normal limit with gammaglobulins that are twice the normal, or if on histology central necrosis or bridging fibrosis is present. Some authors recommend treatment of any symptomatic patient.

The AASLD recommends treatment by corticosteroids alone or in combination with azathioprine (Imuran)[1] for its steroid-sparing effects in patients who are susceptible to the side effects of steroids. For initial induction, adults who are on prednisone alone should be on 60 mg/day and then the dose tapered by 10 mg/week to a dose of 15 to 20 mg/day by 6 months. Prednisone at 20 to 30 mg/day is sufficient if given with azathioprine[1] at a dose of 50 mg/day. Prednisone can be reduced to 15 mg/day in 5-mg decrements every 2 weeks. Once the liver panel is normalized, azathioprine[1] at 50 to 75 mg/day and prednisone at 10 to 20 mg/day are continued, and then prednisone can be decreased to 10 mg/day by 2.5 mg every 3 months. Remission is defined by a decrease by half of the aminotransferase levels and normalization of the bilirubin and the gammaglobulin levels with improvement of the histologic features. In addition to the blood work including immunoglobulins, a liver biopsy, although not required to stop therapy, is essential to confirm complete remission and is helpful in the decision process. Most patients require both drugs for a year, at which time prednisone could be tapered. Ninety percent are responders to this regimen. However, recurrence rates after stopping treatment are as high as 90% and are inversely correlated with the pathology findings. It is for this reason that many patients remain on long-term azathioprine[1] at a dose of 0.5 mg/kg/day. In those who cannot tolerate azathioprine,[1] mycophenolate mofetil[1] has been used successfully.

PRIMARY BILIARY CIRRHOSIS

Primary biliary cirrhosis (PBC) is an autoimmune disease affecting middle-aged women. PBC results in progressive granulomatous destruction of the bile ducts. Manifestations classic of the disease are fatigue, pruritus, osteoporosis, hypercholesterolemia and skin xanthomas, sicca syndrome, vitamin deficiencies, and recurrent urinary tract infections. Most patients with PBC when discovered have no symptoms, and it is often suspected when alkaline phosphatase is elevated. Bilirubin stays in the normal range until late in the progression and is strongly correlated with prognosis. The AMA (antimitochondrial antibody) is positive in 95% of the cases. SMA and ANA can be positive in a third of the patients with PBC. Diagnosis is made by the constellation of cholestatic picture, exclusion of extrahepatic disease, positivity for AMA, and a compatible liver biopsy with granulomatous nonsuppurative cholangitis.

The first-line treatment is ursodeoxycholic acid (UDCA). It is a safe drug that lowers toxic bile acid levels and has a protective effect on the membranes of the liver cells. It is administered at a dose of 13 to 15 mg/kg/day. Cholestatic enzymes can fall to normal or near normal levels, and UDCA can delay disease progression and increase survival. It is a second-line agent for unresponsive pruritus. Although immunosuppressive therapy with methotrexate[1] at 0.25 mg/kg/week and colchicine[1] at 0.6 mg twice daily needs more verification, some authors use it in advanced stages of PBC. Their association with UDCA was additive in some reports.

Pruritus is difficult to manage; in mild cases, skin hydration (emollients and warm baths) with hydroxyzine (Atarax), 25 mg, or cyproheptadine (Periactin), 4 mg every 8 hours, can be sufficient. The first-line therapies for moderate to severe pruritus are cholestyramine (Questran) and colestipol (Colestid). Cholestyramine is taken apart from any other medication. The dose is 4 g before breakfast and dinner, with extra doses to be taken before lunch or bedtime. Second-line therapies for severe pruritus include rifampin (Rifadin),[1] at 300 to 600 mg/day twice daily, phenobarbital,[1] at 120 mg/day, opioid antagonists like naltrexone (ReVia)[1] 10 to 50 mg/day which can lead to significant decrease in the perception of pruritus. In patients who fail to respond, methotrexate,[1] colchicine,[1] sertraline (Zoloft)[1] at 75 mg/day, paroxetine (Paxil)[1] at 20 mg/day, or phototherapy (UVB) could be tried. Because plasmapheresis is inconvenient it is only used when none of the treatments just cited work because it will only give temporary relief. Liver transplantation is the only definitive treatment for severe pruritus.

Hypothyroidism and sicca syndrome associated with PBC should be addressed. Because of chronic cholestasis, fat-soluble vitamin deficiencies (A, D, and K) may occur in PBC. For osteoporosis, the only proven treatment is liver transplant, but vitamin D at 50,000 U/week can prevent osteopenia and is indicated with calcium at 1 to 1.5 g/day if osteopenia is documented. If levels of 25-hydroxy vitamin D are low, supplementation at a dose of 20 μg/day is ideal. Hormone replacement therapy (HRT) is recommended in postmenopausal women. Calcitonin (Miacalcin) or alendronate (Fosamax) are considered if osteoporosis is documented. If vitamin A, which correlates to retinol-binding protein and albumin and inversely to bilirubin, is low, then 15,000 UI/day should be used; otherwise 5000 UI/day is considered as the maintenance regimen. Vitamin E at a regular dose of 400 IU/day can be supplemented. Vitamin K at 5 to 10 mg/day is only supplemented if the patient has bleeding tendencies that are obvious, which only is present if the patient is on cholestyramine or has advanced liver disease. If the patient has a steatorrhea of more than 40 g/day, then restriction of fat is indicated, with replacement by medium chain fatty acids up to a dose of 60 mL/day (medium-chain triglycerides [MCT] oil, 1 tablespoon three to four times a day).

PRIMARY SCLEROSING CHOLANGITIS (PSC)

PSC is an uncommon disease characterized by progressive diffuse inflammation of the intra- and extrahepatic bile ducts. An estimated 70% to 90% of the patients are men older than 20 years. These ducts are intermittently strictured and dilated. Up to 90% of the cases have ulcerative colitis, less commonly Crohn's disease. PSC harbors a 15% lifetime risk for developing cholangiocarcinoma. No screening for cholangiocarcinoma in patients with PSC has proven beneficial.

Suggestive symptoms of PSC include right upper quadrant pain, fatigue, pruritus, and jaundice; 25% are asymptomatic. Typically liver tests demonstrate a cholestatic pattern with transaminases less than 300 IU/L. Perinuclear antineutrophil cytoplasmic antibodies (P-ANCA) are associated with 70% of PSC and of inflammatory bowel disease and can be helpful in the diagnosis in difficult cases.

---

[1]Not FDA approved for this indication.

Endoscopic retrograde cholangiopancreatography (ERCP) and magnetic resonance cholangiopancreatography (MRCP) confirm the diagnosis by showing the intra- and/or extrahepatic bile strictures, beading, and dilations and ruling out secondary causes of stenosis. Liver biopsy supports the diagnosis and determines the severity of the disease but is unnecessary to make the diagnosis. Typical findings include ductopenic and periductal fibrosis.

Treatment is limited and there are no approved therapies for PSC. Ursodiol (UDCA) at standard doses (12 to 15 mg/kg/day) is not effective and unlike in PBC, UDCA did not show survival improvement in this condition. In the presence of a dominant stricture anywhere in the biliary tree, cytologic brushing should be performed to rule out cholangiocarcinoma. Endoscopic or radiologic dilation or stent placement should be attempted while knowing that the risk of restenosis is 30% to 50% with the same failure rate for reintervention; no survival benefit is shown, but jaundice, pruritus, and liver tests improve significantly. It is recommended to administer antibiotics 1 hour before any hepatobiliary procedure for cholangitis prophylaxis. The treatment of choice for advanced PSC is liver transplantation with 70% to 80% survival at 5 years. Treatment of pruritus, osteoporosis, steatorrhea, and fat-soluble vitamin deficiencies are the same as those for PBC. No test is recommended for cholangiocarcinoma screening; in suspicious cases, percutaneous guided-needle biopsy is the procedure of choice.

NONALCOHOLIC STEATOHEPATITIS

The majority of cryptogenic cirrhosis is caused by nonalcoholic steatohepatitis (NASH), which presents almost identically as alcoholic hepatitis, with the exception that the patient drinks less than 40 g of alcohol per week. NASH is correlated to obesity and central obesity, insulin resistance, type II diabetes, hyperlipidemia; it is now called the metabolic syndrome. Drugs like corticosteroids, estrogens, tamoxifen, and amiodarone are also associated with NASH. Total parenteral nutrition, rapid weight loss, and starvation can induce NASH. It is often suspected in patients with constantly enlarged liver, unexplained increased levels of aminotransferases, and the presence of a fatty liver on imaging studies. NASH is diagnosed on liver biopsy when steatosis and inflammation are present and after the exclusion of alcoholic, viral, metabolic, and autoimmune hepatitis by their respective laboratory tests. It is now recognized that NASH can progress to cirrhosis in a fourth of the cases. Diabetes, high body mass index (BMI), and fibrosis on diagnosis are predictors of progression. Usually ALT and AST levels are elevated, and unlike in alcoholic liver disease, ALT is the same or greater than AST.

The first-line treatment of NASH is always related to the underlying cause if present. Essentially lowering insulin resistance, which is universal in NASH, targets all components of the metabolic syndrome. Diabetes should be controlled. Weight reduction and exercise are correlated with improvement in liver enzymes. Rapid weight loss, especially after bypass surgeries, is ill advised in those with fibrosis/cirrhosis because it may precipitate liver failure by necroinflammation, portal fibrosis, and bile stasis. Although there is no proven medical therapy for NASH, some small studies encourage the use of insulin-sensitizing agents and antioxidants, either alone or in combination. However, until results from ongoing clinical trials are available, these agents cannot be recommended.

HEMOCHROMATOSIS

Hemochromatosis (HC) is defined as an excessive deposition of iron in major organs such as the liver, kidneys, heart, endocrine glands (pancreas and pituitary), and joints. The main etiology, hereditary HC, results from a genetic mutation on the short arm of chromosome 6. Most patients with clinical HC are homozygous for C282Y, whereas those with only H63D mutations are not at increased risk of liver disease. Most patients are in their 40s or 50s, and cirrhosis develops in more than 60% of the cases. Screening is recommended in persons who are symptomatic (e.g., liver disease, skin pigmentation, diabetes), who are first-degree relatives of patients with hemochromatosis, or who have abnormal iron studies. Fasting iron saturation (total iron-binding capacity [TIBC]) and ferritin levels are the first tests to be done; then genotyping is required if the iron studies are suggestive (TIBC more than 45%) or if the patient is a first-degree relative of a C282Y homozygous patient. In patients who are homozygous and older than 40 years, have signs of liver disease, or have ferritin levels above 1000 µg/mL, a biopsy is recommended to exclude cirrhosis. A patient with a serum ferritin less than 1000 µg/mL without hepatomegaly and a normal AST is unlikely to have cirrhosis. Conversely, patients with a ferritin greater than 1000 µg/mL, a platelet count less than 200,000, and an elevated AST have a high probability of cirrhosis. Biopsy rules out secondary causes of iron overload (like alcohol or HCV) and assesses the fibrotic changes, which determine the prognosis.

An effective treatment of HC is serial phlebotomies. It is recommended to withdraw 1 U of blood, which contains 200 to 250 mg of iron every week and, if not tolerated, one phlebotomy every 2 to 4 weeks until the patient adapts to blood withdrawal. Once iron stores return to normal, reflected by a serum ferritin level of less than 50 µg/mL and a transferrin saturation of less than 50%, maintenance phlebotomy every 2 to 6 months is done. Hemoglobin should be monitored to avoid anemia. Levels of approximately 10 to 12 g/dL are acceptable.

HC patients must be regularly screened for hepatocellular carcinoma. Most foods are not restricted, except for iron and vitamin C supplements. Vitamin C increases iron absorption and can induce arrhythmias, but fruits and vegetables should not be limited. Daily alcohol consumption is ill advised because it will increase iron absorption, but occasional drinking is permitted in those without advanced liver disease. Liver transplantation is the definitive therapy, but cardiac involvement should be carefully evaluated. Even in acceptable candidates, survival following liver transplantation is reduced compared to most other indications.

WILSON'S DISEASE

Wilson's disease (WD), an autosomal recessive disorder, is the inability to excrete copper into bile properly and to incorporate it into ceruloplasmin (CP), leading first to inappropriate copper accumulation in the liver and later in the eyes, kidneys, and central nervous system. Liver abnormalities in WD are particular for their association with psychiatric and neurologic symptoms like dystonia, tremor, unsteady gait, slurred speech, and drooling because of the involvement of the basal ganglia. Recurrent or chronic low-grade hemolysis can be a presenting manifestation in approximately 10% of the patients.

Diagnosis of WD is confirmed when Kayser-Fleischer (KF) rings are present along with a CP level of less than 20 mg/dL. A ceruloplasmin level under 5 mg/dL or a basal 24-hour urinary copper excretion of more than 100 µg is a strong evidence of WD. If KF rings are absent or CP levels are normal, a liver biopsy should be done. Abnormal liver tests with a 24-hour urinary copper excretion of more than 40 µg with a decreased ceruloplasmin level are also an indication for liver biopsy. On quantitative copper measurement, levels greater than 250 µg/g of dry liver weight are indicative of WD. Neurologic evaluation and MR imaging are recommended prior to treatment in all patients. Screening of first-degree relatives by clinical and biologic means is indicated.

The chelating agents D-penicillamine (Cuprimine) or trientine (Syprine) are initially given at 250 to 500 mg per day, then increased to 1 to 1.5 g a day in four divided doses. Improvement appears 2 to 12 months later, and monitoring is obtained by the 24-hour urinary copper excretion, which should stay above 200 µg. Nonceruloplasmin-bound copper concentration and aminotransferases should normalize with successful treatment. The maintenance regimen is approximately 750 to 1000 mg per day. Supplementation with 25 to 50 mg of pyridoxine is required with D-penicillamine, and iron should not be administered with trientine. Many severe hypersensitivity reactions could limit their use; thus blood counts, liver function tests, creatinine, and urinalysis should be obtained regularly. Zinc gluconate, which eliminates copper from the gut, is given at

50 mg three times a day. It is the first choice for maintenance therapy and can be used in presymptomatic patients. Urinary copper excretion is required for monitoring and should be less than 75 µg in 24 hours. Maintenance therapy is lifelong. Liver and shellfish are the only banned food for patients on initiation of treatment; during maintenance therapy once a week ingestion of these foods is acceptable.

ALPHA$_1$-ANTITRYPSIN DEFICIENCY

Liver damage is caused by the accumulation of the mutant A$_1$AT in the hepatocytes. An estimated 10% to 15% of individuals with the homozygous form PiZZ (protease inhibitor phenotype ZZ) eventually develop cirrhosis with older age, Male gender and obesity are the only known predisposing factors. Most patients with liver damage are children. After excluding the most common causes of cirrhosis, diagnosis is done by phenotyping the A$_1$AT protein and not by measurement of the total A$_1$AT protein in the serum. Patients with chronic disease should be screened for hepatocellular carcinoma. An effective treatment is liver transplantation with a 5-year survival rate of 80%. Hepatocyte transplantation holds promise in this disease.

Treatment of Complications

Many patients with cirrhosis have no serious outward complications from the disease that are clinically evident. These patients are described as having compensated cirrhosis (Child's class A). For the remaining patients, several classic complications may occur, and this is described as the decompensated state. The onset of the decompensated state may herald a clinical decline with reduced survival compared to the compensated state. The major complications include ascites, bleeding from esophagogastric varices, and hepatic encephalopathy. Other common and serious complications include SBP, hepatorenal syndrome, and hepatocellular carcinoma (Table 4).

ASCITES

Ascites is the most common complication of cirrhosis. In 50% of those with compensated cirrhosis, ascites will develop within 10 years (30% in 5 years). The onset of ascites is associated with a poor prognosis, with ascites associated with a 50% mortality rate at 1 to 2 years, compared to a 10% mortality rate at 1 year in those with compensated cirrhosis. In diuretic responsive ascites, there is a 50% 2-year survival rate, but in those with diuretic-resistant ascites, there is increased mortality with a 50% 6-month survival and a 25% 1-year survival.

Portal hypertension is a prerequisite for the formation of ascites. In response to portal hypertension, there is vasodilation of the arterioles of the splanchnic bed that is mediated by nitric oxide. In response to this vasodilation with decreased effective arterial blood volume, and as a compensatory mechanism, there is activation of the renin-angiotensin system. This leads to significant sodium retention, which, when coupled with an increase in hydrostatic pressure in the portal system and a decrease in oncotic pressure caused by hypoalbuminemia, leads to accumulation of ascitic fluid in the abdomen with ascitic fluid primarily weeping off the surface of the liver into the peritoneal cavity. The formation of ascites secondary to cirrhosis is one of the considerations for liver transplantation.

Clinical examination is unreliable in detecting small amounts of ascites (less than 2 L), especially in obese patients. Therefore US is the ideal test to detect small amounts of peritoneal fluid (as low as 100 mL) and can also be used to determine patency or thrombosis of the hepatic and portal vasculature. A paracentesis should be performed for newly diagnosed ascites and the fluid examined for total protein, cell count, cultures (inoculated at the bedside), and albumin. The serum ascites-albumin gradient (SAAG), determined by subtracting the ascitic fluid albumin from the serum albumin determined at the same time, confirms the presence of portal hypertension as having a role in the development of ascites with more than 97% accuracy if the gradient is greater than 1.1 g/dL. If the total protein in the ascitic fluid is less than 1.1 g/dL, this suggests the patient is at high risk for spontaneous bacterial peritonitis, and prophylaxis should be considered. A polymorphonuclear neutrophil (leukocyte) (PMN) count of greater than 250/mm^3 is essential for diagnosing SBP. Paracentesis carries a small risk of bowel perforation and abdominal wall hematoma (less than 1 in 1000 patients).

Ascites may be graded in severity and treatment can be tailored based on this grade. In 15% of the patients who have mild ascites, sodium restriction to 3 to 5 g/day may be sufficient if they have the ability to excrete this sodium load. For those patients with higher-grade ascites, sodium restriction to 2 g/day is recommended, as well as the initiation of diuretics. Oral spironolactone (Aldactone) is effective in 20% to 50% when used alone; additive effect is obtained when used with furosemide (Lasix). Initial doses are 100 mg and 40 mg daily, respectively, and are given once in the morning. Painful gynecomastia may result from spironolactone, and if this occurs, amiloride (Midamor), 5 to 20 mg/day, or triamterene (Dyrenium), 50 to 100 mg/day, may be substituted. Amiloride is less effective than spironolactone in reducing ascites. The dosage of furosemide and spironolactone can be increased in case of resistance every 3 to 5 days up to a maximum of 160 mg/day for furosemide and 400 mg for spironolactone or 40 mg for amiloride. Tense ascites should be treated first with therapeutic paracentesis followed by administration of diuretics and salt restriction.

A key indicator of response to diuretics is a random spot urine test to see if the ratio of sodium to potassium concentration is greater than 1. If so, then it is 90% certain that the patient is excreting a satisfactory amount of sodium (minimum 78 mmol/day). Urine sodium of less than 10 mEq/day is considered a diuretic-resistant state. A 24-hour urinary sodium more than 78 mmol is the best indicator of adequate natriuresis. The ideal weight loss should be 0.5 kg/day in patients without edema, and 1 kg/day in those with lower extremity edema. If it is observed that there is no weight loss, but patients have a good sodium clearance, then the compliance with

TABLE 4 Key Current Treatments

Ascites and peripheral edema	Sodium restriction, spironolactone and furosemide, therapeutic paracentesis with and without albumin infusion, TIPSS, OLT
SBP	Cefotaxime, ceftriaxone, ofloxacin, albumin infusion, discontinue diuretics
SBP prophylaxis	TMP-SMX, norfloxacin, ciprofloxacin
Hepatic encephalopathy	Treat precipitating etiologies, lactulose or Lactinol, metronidazole, rifaximin, or vancomycin, low-protein diet
Bleeding from esophageal/gastric varices	Hemodynamic stabilization, balloon tamponade, vasopressin, octreotide, nitroglycerin, band ligation, sclerotherapy, TIPSS
Esophageal/gastric varices prophylaxis	Propranolol or nadolol, nitrates, sclerotherapy, band ligation, TIPSS, OLT
HRS I	Treat precipitating etiologies, OLT, antibiotics, albumin, midodrine, octreotide, terlipressin, TIPSS
HRS II	Serial paracentesis, diuretics, TIPSS, OLT
Portopulmonary hypertension	Calcium channel blockers, bosentan, isoproterenol
Hepatopulmonary syndrome	OLT
Hepatocellular carcinoma	Surgical resection, OLT, chemoembolization, radiofrequency, irradiation

Abbreviations: HRS = hepatorenal syndrome; OLT = orthotopic liver transplantation; SBP = spontaneous bacterial peritonitis; TIPPS = transjugular intrahepatic portosystemic shunt; TMP-SMX = trimethoprim-sulfamethoxazole.

sodium restriction must be considered and reviewed with the patient. Inpatient treatment is indicated with significant encephalopathy, bacterial infections, or gastrointestinal (GI) hemorrhage. If patients do not have these complications and are steadily losing weight, they may be followed as outpatients. Fluid restriction to 1.5 L/day or less may be required with development of severe (sodium less than 125 mmol/L) or symptomatic hyponatremia.

In 10% of cases of ascites, patients do not respond to diuretic therapy, reaccumulate fluid rapidly after paracentesis, or have a contraindication to the use of diuretics (encephalopathy, hyponatremia with the fluid restriction, or a creatinine more than 2 mg/dL). Then two other methods are available: serial paracentesis and transjugular intrahepatic portosystemic stent shunt (TIPSS) placement. Large-volume paracentesis is highly effective and should be followed by diuretics, which lengthen the period of reaccumulation of fluid, and should always be accompanied by cell counts to rule out SBP. Circulatory disturbance and hepatorenal syndrome are potential complications that could be prevented by the infusion of 5 to 10 g of albumin for every liter of ascites drained when removing volumes larger than 5 L.

TIPSS is a radiologically placed shunt that relieves portal hypertension by shunting blood between the portal vein and the hepatic vein. TIPSS is effective in approximately 66% of patients with refractory ascites and has the same survival benefit as serial paracentesis with a decrease in the incidence of HRS. TIPSS is recommended when it becomes necessary to draw fluid more than two times in a month or when it is impractical. The major complication of TIPSS is hepatic encephalopathy (up to 60%); thus it should be recommended with caution in those with Child-Pugh class C or in those with a MELD greater than 19. Other requirements for the successful placement of TIPSS is relatively preserved cardiac function without significant elevation of right-sided heart pressures, patency of the portal vein, and the absence of severe hepatic encephalopathy. Liver transplantation is the definitive treatment for refractory ascites and may be considered for all appropriate candidates. Another treatment for patients ineligible for transplant, TIPSS, and serial paracentesis are peritoneovenous shunts, although infection and long-term patency with these remain a problem.

SPONTANEOUS BACTERIAL PERITONITIS

SBP is the spontaneous proliferation of bacteria in the ascitic fluid in the absence of intra-abdominal source of infection. Hospitalized patients with decompensated cirrhosis have a 10% to 30% chance of having SBP. Once it occurs there is a 20% mortality rate per treated episode (90% if untreated), and SBP recurs in approximately 70% of patients at 1 year. In patients with cirrhosis and ascites, with sudden onset of fever, encephalopathy of unclear etiology, abdominal pain, renal failure, acidosis, or peripheral leukocytosis, there should be high clinical suspicion for SBP, and they should receive immediate antibiotic therapy before the data from the paracentesis and cultures are available. Cirrhotic patients with SBP may also remain clinically silent. All patients with an ascitic fluid with PMN counts above 250/mm^3 must receive empirical antibiotic therapy and be tested in their ascitic fluid for total protein, lactate dehydrogenase (LDH), glucose, and Gram stain to differentiate it from secondary peritonitis. Culture-negative neutrocytic ascites are treated as SBP. Blood and urine cultures should be done, and ascitic fluid cultures should always be in blood culture bottles at the patient's bedside. Aerobic gram-negative organisms account for 70% of the cases, with *Escherichia coli* and *Klebsiella* species predominating. Gram-positive cocci are present in 30% of the cases, with streptococci dominating. Anaerobic organisms are rare, and when isolated they should raise the suspicion of secondary peritonitis from a perforated viscus.

The treatments of choice for SBP are the third-generation cephalosporins cefotaxime (Claforan), at a dose of 2 g IV every 8 hours, and ceftriaxone (Rocephin), at 1 g every 12 hours for 5 days. Aminoglycosides should not be used because of increased nephrotoxicity. For atypical presentations a paracentesis should be considered after 48 hours and a PMN count performed again. In SBP, the PMN count should be 50% of its previous level, whereas in other sources of peritonitis, the PMN count may be higher or unchanged. Alternatively, the patient may take oral ofloxacin (Floxin) if the patient has no vomiting, shock, or hemorrhage, has a creatinine of less than 3 mg/dL and no or mild encephalopathy. Albumin infusion at a rate of 1.5 g/kg of body weight within 6 hours after starting antibiotic treatment and readministered on the third day of treatment at 1 g/kg decreases mortality after an episode of SBP. All diuretics should be stopped during infection.

The incidence of recurrent SBP may be reduced by administration of prophylactic antibiotics. Norfloxacin (Noroxin),[1] at 400 mg/day, or trimethoprim-sulfamethoxazole (TMX) (Bactrim), at one double-strength tablet daily for 5 days a week, are indicated for prophylaxis in patients who already had an episode of SBP and those who have ascitic protein levels less than 1 g/dL on diagnostic paracentesis. Norfloxacin prophylaxis has reduced SBP occurrence by 60% and is highly cost effective. Ciprofloxacin (Cipro), at a dose of 750 mg once weekly, is also efficacious. For patients admitted to the hospital for cirrhosis and GI hemorrhage, norfloxacin,[1] at 400 mg twice a day, ofloxacin, 400 mg/day or TMX, one tablet twice a day for 7 days, decreases infection rates and prolongs survival.

ESOPHAGEAL VARICES

Patients with cirrhosis should be screened for varices when first diagnosed and then every 3 years until found. Refer to the article on esophageal varices in this volume for more information.

ENCEPHALOPATHY

HE is characterized by neuropsychiatric abnormalities that are primarily caused by nitrogenous products, endogenous ligands for benzodiazepines, and other unknown toxins released by bacteria from the colon that are incompletely metabolized by the cirrhotic liver or bypass the liver because of portal hypertension and portosystemic shunting. HE can develop in 28% of cirrhotic patients within 10 years of the diagnosis of cirrhosis and portal hypertension. Older age and severity of cirrhosis are the only known factors to predict the risk of developing HE. HE has five stages for its severity: Stage 0 is normal or only features abnormal results on psychometric tests, referred to as minimal HE, and stage 4 represents the most severe form with deep coma (Table 5).

Precipitating causes of HE include infection (usually urinary tract, pneumonia, or SBP), renal insufficiency, GI bleed, hypokalemia, excess protein in the diet, use of sedatives such as benzodiazepines and other tranquilizers and sedatives, constipation or noncompliance with lactulose, portal vein thrombosis, further hepatic parenchymal damage, hepatocellular carcinoma, and recent TIPSS placement. When assessing a mental status change in a patient with cirrhosis, other causes of motor and mental disturbance other than hepatic encephalopathy should be investigated. CT of the head must be obtained if there is any neurologic sign concerning an intracranial lesion.

Most cases of HE are preventable, and recognition of the precipitating causes just described will help prevent this complication. Lactulose (Cephulac), at 30 to 60 g/day, titrated to achieve a goal of three to four soft bowel movements a day with a pH less than 6, is effective in 90% of the patients. Lactinol is slightly better tolerated. Excessive use leading to diarrhea is to be avoided because it can lead to prerenal azotemia and other electrolyte imbalances. In patients who have profound HE and are unable to take medications orally, Lactinol and lactulose can be administered via a nasogastric tube or as enemas at a dose of 300 mL in 700 mL of tap water two to three times a day with a response in 4 to 6 hours. Opiate analgesics, calcium, and iron supplements can all exacerbate HE and should be avoided. Also oral nonabsorbable antibiotics such as metronidazole (Flagyl),[1] at 250 mg three times a day, rifaximin (Xifaxan),[1] at 400 mg two to three times a day, and vancomycin (Vancocin),[1] at 2 g/day, can help alleviate HE in the remaining 10% of cases resistant to disaccharides.

---

[1]Not FDA approved for this indication.

TABLE 5 Grades and Clinical Manifestations of Hepatic Encephalopathy

Encephalopathy Grade	Level of Consciousness	Mental Status	Neurologic Signs	EEG Abnormalities
0	Normal	Normal	None	None
Subclinical	Normal	Normal	Psychometric tests may be abnormal	None
1	Day-night reversal, restlessness	Forgetful, mild confusion, Irritable	Tremor, apraxia, impaired handwriting	Triphasic waves (5 cycles/s)
2	Lethargy	Disorientation to time, inappropriate behavior	Asterixis, ataxia, dysarthria	Triphasic waves (5 cycles/s)
3	Somnolent, confused	Disorientation to time, inappropriate behavior	Asterixis, hyperreflexia, Babinski signs	Triphasic waves (5 cycles/s)
4	Coma	None	Decerebration	Delta activity

Abbreviation: EEG = electroencephalogram.

Because of renal toxicity, neomycin should be avoided. In severe HE, oral intake should be held. In milder forms, protein intake should be titrated by increasing the protein intake by 10 g/day over 3 to 5 days starting from 20 g/day to a maximum dose of 80 g/day depending on individual tolerances. Avoidance of negative nitrogen balance is crucial. An infusion of dextrose helps decrease protein catabolism. For chronic HE, lactulose and moderate protein restriction to 0.8 g/kg/day are recommended.

HEPATORENAL SYNDROME

Approximately 40% of patients with cirrhosis and ascites will develop HRS within 5 years. This complication occurs when there is avid continuous sodium retention with dilutional hyponatremia and activation of the renin-angiotensin system, in the setting of ineffective arterial blood flow because of splanchnic vasodilation. Initially, renal perfusion is maintained because of renal vasodilatation that is mediated by prostaglandins. With progressive disease, renal vasoconstriction occurs in response to arterial vasodilation, leading to reduction of renal blood flow and the glomerular filtration rates with subsequent hepatorenal syndrome. A common precipitant of HRS is the use of nonsteroidal anti-inflammatory drugs (NSAIDs). Patients with ascites should scrupulously avoid other nephrotoxic agents such as aminoglycosides. Other precipitants are aggressive use of diuretics with volume depletion, large-volume paracentesis without albumin infusion, SBP, and sepsis. In the diagnosis of HRS, several key criteria are almost always present (Table 6).

There are two clinical types of hepatorenal syndrome, type I and type II. In type I there is a decrease of more than 50% in creatinine clearance to less than 20 mL/minute or a doubling of the creatinine level to more than 2.5 mg/dL in 2 weeks. The prognosis for type I HRS is dismal, with 80% mortality within 2 weeks after diagnosis. Type II is a more progressive form and can evolve into type I. In type II the renal deterioration does not fulfill the criteria for type I and it presents in the form of refractory ascites. Survival is 50% in type II after 6 months.

TABLE 6 Diagnostic Criteria for Hepatorenal Syndrome as Proposed by the International Ascites Club

1. Serum creatinine >1.5 mg/dL indicating low glomerular filtration rate
2. Exclusion of shock, volume depletion, bacterial infection, nephrotoxic drugs
3. Failure to improve with discontinuing diuretics, volume expansion with 1.5 L normal saline
4. No evidence of proteinuria, obstruction, parenchymal renal disease

Clinical management of these patients includes an investigation for a precipitating cause, including infection such as SBP, bacteremia, or catheter-related bacteremia, and appropriate cultures should be sent. Broad-spectrum antibiotics should be started irrespective of proof of infection.

The most successful treatment for HRS is liver transplantation, with survival rates greater than 80% over 1 year. The next most effective treatment for type I HRS is albumin infusion (20 to 40 g/day for 20 days) with concomitant arterial vasoconstrictors. Midodrine (ProAmatine), titrated to 7.5 to 15 mg three times a day for 20 days, to achieve an increase in mean arterial blood pressure of 15 mm Hg in combination with octreotide (Sandostatin),[1] at a dose of 100 to 300 μg subcutaneously three times a day, improves renal function in selected patients with type 1 HRS in small uncontrolled trials. Similarly, terlipressin,[2] a synthetic analogue of vasopressin, infused at 0.5 to 2 mg over 4 to 6 hours for 15 days, increases the glomerular filtration rate (GFR) in up to 75% of the patients. TIPS can improve creatinine clearance and survival in well-selected patients with MELD scores less than 18. It is reasonable in patients not eligible for or awaiting liver transplantation. TIPSS in combination with midodrine, octreotide,[1] and albumin may have some benefit in HRS patients. Type II HRS is treated as refractory ascites in an outpatient setting.

HEPATOPULMONARY SYNDROME

HPS is defined in patients with cirrhosis as the increase in the alveolar-arterial gradient on room air and the documentation of intrapulmonary vascular dilations, which cause right to left shunting corrected partially by oxygen at 100%. It is associated with spider angiomata and presents as platypnea and orthodeoxia. Diagnosis is confirmed by contrast-enhanced echocardiography or technetium-labeled macroaggregated albumin scanning. The only treatment in highly selected populations is liver transplantation.

PORTOPULMONARY HYPERTENSION

Portopulmonary hypertension (PPHTN) is characterized by a mean pulmonary artery pressure measured by cardiac catheterization above 25 mm Hg on rest with a pulmonary capillary wedge pressure less than 15 mm Hg, a pulmonary vascular resistance (PVR) greater than 120 dynes/second/cm-5, and the presence of portal hypertension without any other secondary cause of pulmonary hypertension. Clinical manifestations are similar to those with primary PHTN. Treatment with calcium channel blockers is indicated if the patient has more than 20% reduction in mPAP during the trial with vasodilators on cardiac catheterization. Bosentan (Tracleer), at 62.5 mg per day for 4 weeks, increased thereafter to 125 mg daily, improves

---
[1]Not FDA approved for this indication.
[2]Not available in the United States.

symptoms and exercise capacity. Preoperatively, Epoprostenol (Flolan) is given at 10 to 28 μg/kg/mm^3 for a few months to decrease the mPAP to levels acceptable for liver transplantation. Liver transplantation may reverse minor or moderate degrees of pulmonary hypertension but is contraindicated in patients with pulmonary hypertension above 40 to 45 mm Hg because of high postoperative mortality related to cardiac failure.

HEPATOCELLULAR CARCINOMA

Patients with cirrhosis, regardless of etiology, have an increased risk for the development of HCC. An estimated 10% to 15% of patients with cirrhosis develop HCC after 10 years of diagnosis with a median survival of 6 to 20 months. Selected patients who successfully undergo orthotopic liver transplantation (OLT) for HCC have survival rates equal to those without HCC.

Screening for HCC is best accomplished by measuring serum alpha fetoprotein (AFP) and abdominal US every 6 months. Because of a sensitivity ranging between 20% and 65% (depending on the cutoff value), AFP is not proven to improve the outcome in cirrhotics from HCC. The positive predictive value for AFP levels above 20 or for a suspicious lesion on ultrasound is low; therefore imaging with triple-phase helical CT, MRI, or magnetic resonance angiography is indicated if any one of these two situations is present. These imaging modalities can reliably diagnose HCC if tumors are greater than 2 cm and there is an arterial enhancing lesion seen on two of the imaging tests just cited or seen on one test with an AFP level above 400 μg/mL. In these cases a biopsy is not required. Suspicious lesions between 1 and 2 cm should be biopsied by fine-needle aspiration (FNA), which does not worsen the outcome from tumor seeding along the needle tack, and tumors less than 1 cm should be monitored by repeat scanning every 3 months until they grow above 1 cm. Des-gamma-carboxy prothrombin (DCP) and lectin reactive AFP (AFP-L3)-to-AFP ratio are tumor markers that are measured alone or in combination with AFP and can increase the sensitivity and specificity of HCC screening.

Treatment of HCC is approached in an algorithmic fashion with surgery the ultimate goal because it is the only curative treatment. A tumor is resectable when it is confined to the liver and shows no vascular invasion and no portal hypertension. Size alone should not influence the decision. General performance of the patient, tumor stage, and assessment of liver function determine if the procedure is practical (Child's class A) or not (Child's class B/C). Prior to resection, a search for metastatic disease should be undertaken. Ninety percent of cirrhotic patients with HCC have decompensation of their cirrhosis, which contraindicates surgical resection. With earlier detection of HCC there is greater likelihood of successful outcomes with transplantation. To be a candidate for liver transplantation, the patient must have no vascular invasion, no metastatic disease, no lymphatic spread, and no more than three suspected lesions in the liver. If there are multiple lesions in the liver, all must be less than 3 cm in diameter; if only one lesion is present, it must be less than 5 cm in diameter. A major drawback of liver transplantation is long waiting times for cadaveric donor matching.

Other alternative therapies include chemoembolization, ethanol or acetic acid injection into the tumor, radiofrequency ablation, and irradiation with intra-arterial yttrium-tagged microspheres. All patients should be considered candidates for some kind of intervention. These therapies should be considered palliative, although survival for radiofrequency ablation and percutaneous ethanol injection may approach survival in surgical resection for tumors less than 3 cm. Any approach can be considered in nonresectable tumors depending on the team preferences and/or local expertise. Chemotherapy is only indicated in the context of a clinical trial.

Prevention of the development of HCC is also possible: Hepatitis B vaccine has decreased the incidence of HCC by a third in highly infected areas. Also in clinical trials for the treatment of chronic hepatitis C with interferon-based therapies, studies have suggested that patients with compensated liver cirrhosis, whether or not they have a sustained response, may have reduction of their risk of HCC.

Other Considerations

VACCINATION

Hepatitis A and B vaccines should be given to all patients with chronic liver disease who are found to be nonimmune to these viruses. Pneumonia and SBP because of streptococcal pneumonia are very common in cirrhotic patients; thus all patients in this population should receive a single dose of the polyvalent pneumococcal vaccine. An annual injection of the influenza vaccine protects against influenza.

LIVER TRANSPLANTATION

Liver transplantation (LT) is the definitive treatment for a variety of irreversible problems associated with chronic liver disease. Patients with Child's class B, and those with complications from cirrhosis such as refractory ascites, variceal bleeding, and any other condition that is irreversible and progressive should be referred early for liver transplantation evaluation. HRS type 1 and HPS should expedite the referral for transplantation. The MELD score was developed to replace the Child-Pugh score as a disease severity score. A score of more than 10 is an indication for referral to a transplantation center. The MELD score (for calculation, visit www.unos.org/resources/MeldPeldCalculator.asp?index=98) is designed to improve the organ allocation system, so that available organs are directed to patients based on the severity of their liver disease rather than on the total time on the waiting list. Contraindications for liver transplantation depend on the local approach, but universal contraindications are high perioperative risk (e.g., severe cardiac failure), uncontrolled malignancies within the previous 5 years, and active alcohol or drug abuse. LT offers an overall 5-year survival rate of greater than 60% to 70%.

REFERENCES

Boyer TD, Haskal ZJ: The role of transjugular intrahepatic portosystemic shunt in the management of portal hypertension. Hepatology 2005;41:386-400.

Cardenas A, Gines P: Management of complications of cirrhosis in patients awaiting liver transplantation. J Hepatology 2005;42:S124-S133.

Czaja AJ, Freese DK: Diagnosis and treatment of autoimmune hepatitis. Hepatology 2002;36:479-497.

D'Amico G, Luca A, Morabito A, et al: Uncovered transjugular intrahepatic portosystemic shunt for refractory ascites: A meta-analysis. Gastroenterology 2005;129:1282-1293.

Levitsky J, Mailliard ME: Diagnosis and therapy of alcoholic liver disease. Semin Liver Dis 2004;24:233-247.

Moore KP, Wong F, Gines P, et al: The management of ascites in cirrhosis: Report on the consensus conference of the International Ascites Club. Hepatology 2003;38:258-266.

Murray KF, Carithers RL Jr: AASLD Practice Guidelines: Evaluation of the patient for liver transplantation. Hepatology 2005;41:1407-1432.

Runyon BA: Management of adult patients with ascites due to cirrhosis. Hepatology 2004;39:841-856.

Sanyal AJ: AGA technical review on nonalcoholic fatty liver disease. Gastroenterology 2002;123:1705-1725.

Tavill AS: Diagnosis and management of hemochromatosis. Hepatology 2001;33:1321-1328.

Bleeding Esophageal Varices

Method of
Vijay H. Shah, MD, and Patrick S. Kamath, MD

The three major and potentially fatal complications of portal hypertension are gastrointestinal (GI) bleeding from gastroesophageal varices, ascites, and hepatic encephalopathy. Of these, hemorrhage from varices is the most dramatic presentation. The prognosis of patients with variceal bleeding has improved over the past decade, with the risk of mortality at 1 week being approximately 5% to 8% and at 6 weeks approximately 20%.

Variceal Bleeding: Scope of the Problem

Upper GI endoscopy is currently the gold standard used to detect varices. Although computed tomography, ultrasound, and magnetic resonance imaging can detect consequences of portal hypertension and varices, they are currently not accurate enough to detect all large varices. Similarly, platelet counts, splenomegaly, or hypoalbuminemia are unreliable as markers to target patients at risk for large varices. Endoscopic ultrasound is still considered an investigational tool in the diagnosis of portal hypertension.

There are numerous causes of portal hypertension. In the Western world, the most common cause of portal hypertension is cirrhosis but worldwide, schistosomiasis could be the most common cause of portal hypertension. Portal venous thrombosis and idiopathic portal hypertension are more common in the Far East.

Esophageal varices are present in about 40% of patients with cirrhosis. However, in patients with cirrhotic ascites, varices are detected in about 60% of patients. The prevalence of large varices in patients with cirrhosis is approximately 20%, and these patients have a 30% risk of bleeding from varices within 2 years. Because of the high risk of mortality from bleeding varices, it is recommended that all patients with cirrhosis be screened for varices with upper GI endoscopy so that prophylactic therapy can be initiated. If no varices are noted on the initial endoscopy, then a repeat endoscopy should be performed in 2 to 3 years. If small varices are noted at the initial endoscopy, then a repeat endoscopy should be performed in 1 to 2 years.

In the presence of variceal bleeding, spontaneous control is seen in about one half of patients. Hypovolemia that occurs as a result of hypotension and splanchnic vasoconstriction results in a decrease in portal pressure, which might result in control of bleeding. Excessive transfusions, therefore, might result in an increased risk of bleeding.

In patients in whom bleeding has been controlled, rebleeding occurs in about one third of patients within the first 6 weeks, and approximately 40% of these episodes occur within the first 5 days. The risk of rebleeding and risk of mortality are related to the degree of liver dysfunction.

Because of the high risk of morbidity and mortality with a variceal bleed, significant effort needs to be made to prevent initial bleeding (primary prophylaxis), control the acute variceal bleed, and prevent rebleeding from varices (secondary prophylaxis).

 CURRENT DIAGNOSIS

- Upper gastrointestinal endoscopy is the gold standard for diagnosis of varices.
- Large esophageal varices that are at risk of bleeding are present in approximately 20% of all patients with cirrhosis.
- Ultrasonography, computed tomography, and magnetic resonance imaging may be less accurate than endoscopy in detecting varices.
- Measurement of portal pressure is the most accurate method of determining which patients are at risk for variceal bleeding.
- Bleeding esophageal varices should be suspected in all patients with gastrointestinal bleeding and jaundice, ascites, and other stigmata of liver disease.

Treatment

Portal hypertension results from an increase in resistance to portal blood flow, along with an increase in portal blood flow. Therefore, treatment of portal hypertension is aimed either at reducing portal blood flow with pharmacologic agents like β-blockers or vasopressin and its analogues or by decreasing intrahepatic resistance. At this time, there are no effective drugs that decrease intrahepatic resistance. The major method of reducing intrahepatic resistance is by creating a surgical portosystemic shunt or a radiologic portosystemic shunt (transjugular intrahepatic portosystemic shunt, TIPS). Bleeding from the varices can be controlled directly by endoscopic methods.

PREVENTION OF FIRST BLEED (PRIMARY PROPHYLAXIS)

Currently, pharmacologic treatment of all cirrhosis patients with the goal of preventing the development of esophageal varices is not recommended. In the absence of such contraindications as significant comorbidity, all patients with large varices—varices larger than 5 mm in diameter on endoscopy—should receive prophylaxis against variceal bleeding. Patients with smaller varices but with more advanced liver disease (Child–Pugh class C) may also receive prophylactic treatment.

The two current modalities used to prevent variceal bleeding are nonselective β-blockers and endoscopic variceal ligation. It is important to use nonselective β-blockers rather than selective β-blockers. β_1-blockade decreases cardiac output, whereas β_2-blockade prevents splanchnic vasodilation, allowing unrestricted action of α_1-adrenergic receptors, which causes a reduction in portal blood flow. Therefore, a combination of the decreased cardiac output and decreased portal flow decreases portal pressure. The two nonselective β-blockers that are used most commonly are nadolol (Corgard)[1] and propranolol (Inderal).[1] The advantage of nadolol over propranolol is that the excretion is predominantly in the kidneys (rather than by the liver), and it is not very lipid soluble, which decreases central side effects such as depression. The use of nitrates or drugs such as spironolactone (Aldactone)[1] alone or in combination with β-blockers is not recommended for primary prophylaxis.

When β-blockers are used, the dose should be titrated such that the resting heart rate decreases by about 25%, or to about 55 to 60 bpm, provided the systolic blood pressure remains greater than 90 mm Hg. Long-acting preparations of propranolol[1] are preferred and may be started in a dose of 60 mg daily. If nadolol[1] is used, the initial dose is 20 mg once daily. The medications are best administered in the evening. The dose of propranolol or nadolol is gradually increased every 3 to 5 days until the target reduction in heart rate is reached. It is possible to increase the dose even further if patients continue to tolerate treatment. The typical dose of long-acting propranolol or nadolol required to reach target heart rates ranges between 40 and 160 mg daily.

In patients on pharmacologic therapy, there is no need for follow-up endoscopy. In general, if only patients with large varices are selected for prophylactic treatment, approximately six patients require treatment to prevent one variceal bleed. However, approximately 22 patients need to be treated to prevent one death. If patients tolerate the medications and have no further bleeding, then the medication is continued indefinitely.

Prophylactic endoscopic injection sclerotherapy is no longer recommended as primary prophylaxis against variceal hemorrhage in view of the significant complications. Endoscopic variceal ligation is the preferred modality and is as effective as β-blockers. Endoscopic variceal ligation is carried out at 2- to 4-week intervals until the varices are obliterated.

Because of ease of use and probable lower costs, pharmacologic therapy with β-blockers is considered the first-line treatment for preventing variceal bleeding. In patients who have contraindications

---

[1]Not FDA approved for this indication.

CURRENT THERAPY

- Upper endoscopy is recommended to screen for esophageal varices in all patients with cirrhosis who are candidates for prophylactic therapy. If no varices are seen at initial endoscopy, a repeat endoscopy is recommended in 2 to 3 years. If small varices are noted at initial endoscopy, a repeat endoscopy is recommended in 1 to 2 years.
- Patients with large varices and patients with Child–Pugh class C cirrhosis and small varices may be considered for primary prophylactic therapy.
- Either nonselective β-blockers or endoscopic variceal ligation may be used to prevent esophageal variceal bleeding, although β-blockers are preferred (primary prophylaxis).
- Endoscopic therapy combined with vasoactive drugs and antibiotics form the mainstay of treatment of bleeding esophageal varices.
- Patients with acute bleeding require prompt resuscitation. The target for red cell transfusion is a hematocrit of 24%.
- When bleeding cannot be controlled in spite of two sessions of endoscopic therapy, placement of a transjugular intrahepatic portosystemic shunt (TIPS) is recommended.
- Secondary prophylaxis is best carried out with a combination of β-blockers and endoscopic variceal ligation.
- TIPS is carried out when patients continue to bleed in spite of the use of both variceal ligation and β-blockers as secondary prophylaxis.

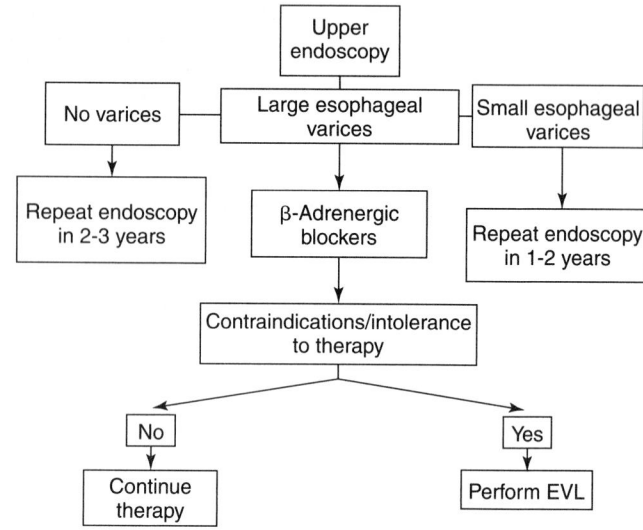

FIGURE 1. Algorithm for primary prophylaxis of esophageal variceal hemorrhage. EVL, endoscopic variceal ligation

to β-blockers, who are intolerant to β-blockers, or in whom β-blockers are not effective in preventing variceal bleeding, then endoscopic therapy is recommended.

An algorithm on how to approach primary prophylaxis is given in Figure 1.

CONTROL OF ACUTE ESOPHAGEAL VARICEAL BLEEDING

It cannot be overemphasized that controlling acute variceal bleeding is a team effort because of the high risk of morbidity and mortality in these patients. Variceal bleeding is ideally carried out by a team of hepatologists, endoscopists, intensive care physicians, radiologists, and hepatobiliary surgeons.

The goals of treatment are to resuscitate the patient, control the acute bleeding episode, prevent complications, and prevent rebleeding. It is recommended that the patient have two large-bore intravenous lines placed immediately on arrival to the emergency department. Red blood cells should be transfused as required to provide a hematocrit of no greater than 24% (hemoglobin of 8 g/dL). Until red blood cells are available for transfusion, normal saline may be used for resuscitation. If there is active bleeding, endotracheal intubation is mandatory.

All patients with cirrhosis and GI bleeding, even in the absence of ascites, should receive prophylactic antibiotics with norfloxacin (Noroxin) 400 mg twice daily for 7 days. If patients have ascites, then a diagnostic paracentesis needs to be carried out before initiating therapy with norfloxacin. This is because some of these patients might have spontaneous bacterial peritonitis, which is better treated with cefotaxime (Claforan) 2 g every 12 hours for 5 days rather than oral norfloxacin. If oral ingestion of antibiotics is not possible, then intravenous antibiotics such as ciprofloxacin (Cipro) or levofloxacin (Levaquin) should be used. The recent reduction in mortality with variceal bleeding is believed to be related to the use of antibiotics.

Pharmacologic therapy should be started as early as possible. Terlipressin[8] is the only vasoactive drug that has been associated with improved survival, but this drug is not currently available in the United States. Octreotide (Sandostatin)[1] is the agent most commonly used in the United States, although the efficacy in such situations is still debatable. It is generally recommended that pharmacologic treatment be continued for up to 5 days to prevent early rebleeding. Octreotide is generally infused intravenously in a dose of 50 μg/hour following a bolus of 50 μg. Side effects with octreotide are few, but hyperglycemia and abdominal discomfort can occur. The most serious side effects are cardiac dysrhythmias, including sinus bradycardia.

Once the vasoactive drug has been infused for about 30 minutes, the patient is hemodynamically stable, and endotracheal intubation has been carried out if the patient has active bleeding, upper endoscopy may be carried out. At upper endoscopy, the actively bleeding varix is ligated. Other large varices can also be ligated at the same session. Following endoscopic ligation, most experts use proton pump inhibitors to prevent the development of variceal ligation ulcers, although there are insufficient data to support this recommendation.

In about 10% of patients, bleeding cannot be controlled in spite of all these measures. Failure to control bleeding is defined usually by the requirement of greater than four units of red blood cells to maintain the hematocrit at about 24%. In such patients, a repeat endoscopy may be carried out within 24 hours. However, if in spite of two endoscopic sessions within a 24-hour period bleeding has not been controlled, then a TIPS may be carried out by an interventional radiologist. Unfortunately, mortality in this group is high.

The algorithm for control of acute variceal bleeding is given in Figure 2.

PREVENTION OF VARICEAL REBLEEDING (SECONDARY PROPHYLAXIS)

Initiation of secondary prophylaxis is important, because up to 80% of all patients who have a variceal bleed will rebleed within 2 years without such measures. Patients with a Child–Pugh score of 7 should be referred for evaluation for liver transplantation.

---

[1]Not FDA approved for this indication.
[8]Orphan drug in the United States.

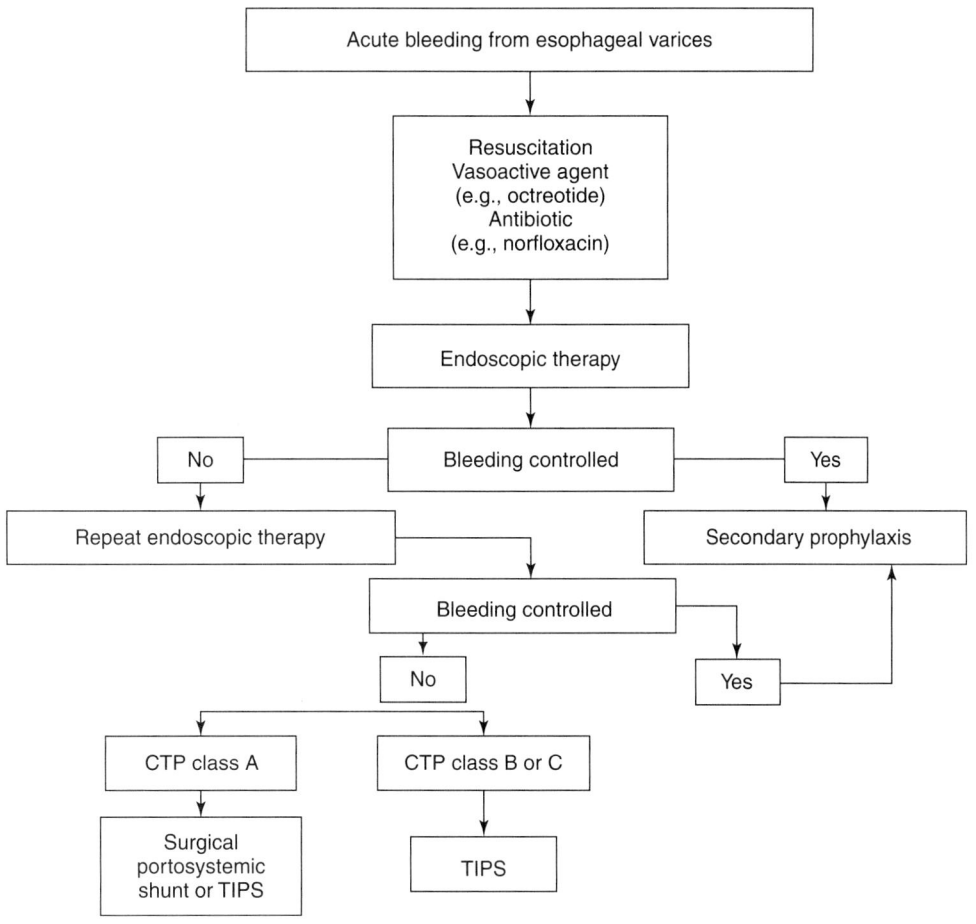

FIGURE 2. Algorithm for managing bleeding esophageal varices. CTP = Child–Turcotte–Pugh, TIPS = Transjugular intrahepatic portosystemic shunt.

Variceal bleeding can be prevented by using pharmacologic agents, endoscopic therapy, TIPS, or surgical portosystemic shunts.

Usually, a combination of endoscopic therapy (endoscopic variceal ligation and nonselective β-blockers) is initiated to prevent variceal bleeding. The combination is superior to either modality alone. However, endoscopic therapy alone may be used in patients with contraindications or intolerance to β-blockers. The ideal interval between sessions of endoscopic variceal ligation is not clear, but it usually ranges between 2 and 4 weeks. Nonselective β-blockers alone may be used in patients who find it difficult to return frequently for endoscopic treatment. Whereas isosorbide mononitrate (Imdur),[1] when added to β-blockers, can make pharmacologic treatment more effective, it is unusual for most patients to tolerate nitrates after they have been adequately β-blocked.

If patients have variceal rebleeding in spite of receiving a combination of endoscopic and pharmacologic treatments (β-blockers and endoscopic variceal ligation), then a portosystemic shunt is considered. A TIPS is the shunt most widely used because of limited availability of surgical expertise and lower procedure related morbidity. A surgical shunt is recommended only in patients who have good liver function as determined by Child–Pugh class A.

The algorithm for secondary prophylaxis is given in Figure 3.

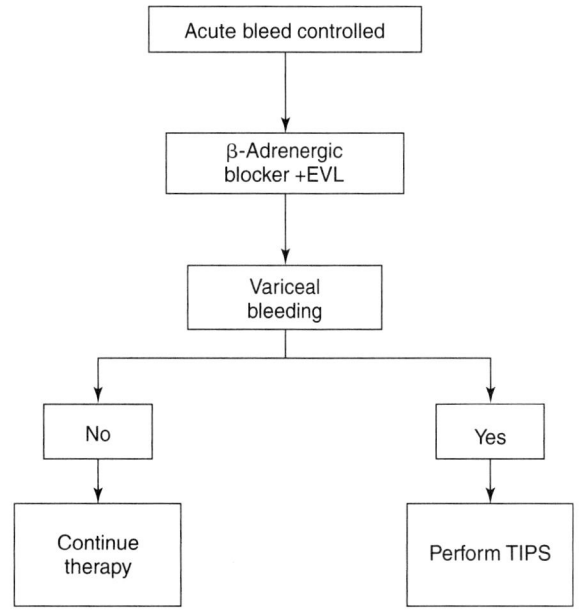

FIGURE 3. Algorithm for preventing recurrent bleeding from esophageal varices (secondary prophylaxis). EVL = endoscopic variceal ligation; TIPS = transjugular intrahepatic portosystemic shunt.

---

[1]Not FDA approved for this indication.

REFERENCES

D'Amico G, Garcia-Pagan JC, Luca A, Bosch J: Hepatic vein pressure gradient reduction and prevention of variceal bleeding in cirrhosis: A systematic review. Gastroenterology 2006;131(5):1611-1624.

Garcia-Pagan JC, Bosch J: Endoscopic band ligation in the treatment of portal hypertension. Nat Clin Pract Gastroenterol Hepatol 2005;2(11):526-535.

Garcia-Tsao G: Portal hypertension. Curr Opin Gastroenterol 2006; 22(3): 254-262.

Henderson JM: Surgery versus transjugular intrahepatic portal systemic shunt in the treatment of severe variceal bleeding. Clin Liver Dis 2006; 10(3):599-612.

Kamath PS, Shah V: Does nadolol improve the efficacy of endoscopic variceal ligation in the treatment of variceal bleeding? Nat Clin Pract Gastroenterol Hepatol 2005;2(6):254-255.

Longacre AV, Garcia-Tsao G: A commonsense approach to esophageal varices. Clin Liver Dis 2006;10(3):613-625.

Shah VH, Kamath PS: Portal hypertension and gastrointestinal bleeding. In Feldman M, Friedman LS, Brandt LJ (eds): Sleisenger & Fordtran's Gastrointestinal and Liver Disease: Pathophysiology, Diagnosis, Management, 8th ed. Vol 2. Philadelphia: Saunders, 2006, pp 1899-1934.

Zaman A: Portal hypertension-related bleeding: Management of difficult cases. Clin Liver Dis 2006;10(2):353-370.

Zaman A, Chalasani N: Bleeding caused by portal hypertension. Gastroenterol Clin North Am 2005;34(4):623-642.

Dysphagia and Esophageal Obstruction

Method of
Philip O. Katz, MD, and Girish Anand, MD

Dysphagia refers to a subjective sensation of the delayed passage of food from the mouth through the esophagus to the stomach. It derives its origin from Greek *dys* meaning "difficulty" and *phagia* meaning "eat."

Dysphagia has been reported in about 2% of healthy adults older than 65 years. The incidence increases to 12% to 13% in the hospitalized elderly. Dysphagia has been reported in about 50% to 60% of patients in nursing homes and other chronic care facilities.

There may be associated pain with swallowing (odynophagia) if there is coexistent inflammation. Most patients describe dysphagia as a feeling of food getting "stuck" or "not going down right." The history plays an important role in understanding the anatomic location and the severity of the symptoms. Key questions like the exact location where the food is getting stuck, associated regurgitation, types of foods causing dysphagia, and presence of weight loss or heartburn are crucial in assessing the symptom of dysphagia.

Pathophysiology

In the swallowing process, the oropharyngeal and esophageal phases transport solid or liquid boluses rapidly from the mouth to the stomach. *Primary peristalsis* is the classic coordinated motor pattern of the esophagus, combined with almost simultaneous upper and lower esophageal sphincter relaxation initiated by the act of swallowing. The food bolus is transferred by a progressive pharyngeal contraction through the relaxed upper esophageal sphincter (UES) into the esophagus. The UES closure is followed by a progressive circular contraction beginning in the upper esophagus and proceeding distally along the esophageal body to propel the bolus through the relaxed lower esophageal sphincter (LES), which subsequently closes with a prolonged contraction.

Secondary peristalsis is a progressive contraction in the esophageal body occurring in response to its distention by stimulation of sensory receptors in the esophageal body. It usually begins at or above a level corresponding to the location of the stimulus and is limited to the esophagus. A local intramural mechanism can at times take over as a reserve mechanism to produce peristalsis in the smooth muscle segment of the esophagus. This has been called *tertiary peristalsis.*

Any problem with either the strength or coordination of the musculature causes difficulty with movement of food, leading to obstruction. Similarly, any narrowing in the path of transit causes obstruction and distention of the lumen, leading to the sensation of dysphagia. The motility abnormalities might not be constant, thus giving intermittent dysphagia. The extent of luminal obstruction guides the diagnosis. Partial obstruction might initially give only solid food dysphagia related to large food boluses (e.g., steak). When the extent of obstruction progresses to near total occlusion, the symptoms involve both solid and liquid dysphagia. The extent of associated inflammation (esophagitis) determines whether or not odynophagia is an associated symptom.

Diagnosis

A careful history helps to localize the site of abnormality, and this forms the basis of further work-up. The evaluation of dysphagia begins with a complete history. A problem initiating a swallow and associated coughing or choking indicates a more proximal or oropharyngeal cause for the symptoms. Pure solid food dysphagia suggests a structural lesion, stricture, ring, or malignancy. A problem initially with solids progressing later to liquids suggests a benign or malignant stricture.

Rapidly progressive dysphagia is concerning for malignancy. The presence of other medical problems such as stroke or scleroderma might point to a systemic cause of the symptoms. A careful history of medications is important, because many drugs have been implicated in pill esophagitis and can cause dysphagia as well as odynophagia. The history can also differentiate dysphagia from globus sensation (feeling of a lump in the throat), which has a different evaluation from dysphagia.

Dysphagia for all practical purposes can be classified into oropharyngeal and esophageal dysphagia.

OROPHARYNGEAL DYSPHAGIA

Difficulty in transferring a food bolus from the hypopharyngeal area to the esophageal body across the upper esophageal sphincter gives rise to the suspicion of oropharyngeal or transfer dysphagia. Several clues in the patient's history help to establish the cause.

The onset of symptoms in oropharyngeal dysphagia is almost immediate. The patient describes the feeling of choking or coughing on initiation of swallowing and frequently points to the cervical region as the site of dysphagia. Patients might describe regurgitation of food, aspiration, or halitosis, which can point to a structural abnormality such as a Zenker's diverticulum.

CURRENT DIAGNOSIS

- Differentiate between oropharyngeal and esophageal dysphagia.
- Pure solid food dysphagia implies a mechanical (obstructive) cause.
- Mixed solid and liquid dysphagia suggests functional (motility) abnormality.
- Eosinophilic esophagitis should be considered in young men with solid dysphagia.
- Barium swallow (with solid bolus) and endoscopy are complementary.
- Esophageal function testing (manometry) should be performed for nonobstructive dysphagia.

Patients might have to resort to certain physical maneuvers, such as extending their arms and neck and using their fingers to move the bolus. There may be associated speech abnormalities such as hoarseness, nasal quality, or dysarthria, which points to a neuromuscular cause for the oropharyngeal dysphagia. The various causes of oropharyngeal dysphagia are listed in Box 1.

In patients with oropharyngeal dysphagia, the oral cavity, head, and neck should be carefully examined. Special attention should be paid to the neurologic examination, especially the nerves involved in the act of swallowing, namely cranial nerves V, VII, IX, X, XI, and XII. Clues in the physical examination might suggest polymyositis or dermatomyositis as the cause of symptoms.

Video fluoroscopy (barium swallow) is a good first test that permits visualization of the swallowing mechanism. It can identify aspiration, pooling, and abnormal motor activities. This examination concentrates on the cervical esophageal region. A barium swallow can delineate the anatomic anomalies and also can show the remainder of the esophagus. The study starts with liquid barium, progressing to a solid phase. Different consistencies of food are used to assess the oropharynx, UES, and proximal esophagus.

A structural abnormality found on the barium examination generally requires an endoscopy for confirmation or treatment. Endoscopy is not the first test to use to evaluate oropharyngeal dysphagia, because the chances of missing an abnormality in the upper part of esophagus are higher than in the distal esophagus.

A nasopharyngeal laryngoscopy performed by the otolaryngologist provides detailed information of the hypopharynx, larynx, and oropharynx. It also allows a clear visualization of the vocal cords, valleculae, and the pyriform sinuses to assess any pooling of secretions.

Patients with oropharyngeal dysphagia who have an unrevealing barium study or endoscopy might need an esophageal manometry study with careful attention to the UES. Incoordination between UES opening and pharyngeal contractions can cause relaxation (opening) or shortening opening may be associated with dysphagia as well.

Zenker's diverticulum is an outpouching of the mucosa through an area of muscular weakness between the transverse fibers of the cricopharyngeus and the oblique fibers of the lower inferior constrictor. These generally occur in older adults and can show symptoms of pulmonary aspirations, gurgling, or regurgitation. Rarely, they become large enough to manifest as a mass and even cause esophageal obstruction.

ESOPHAGEAL DYSPHAGIA

Esophageal dysphagia occurs either from mechanical or motility causes. The abnormality lies within the body of the esophagus or the lower esophageal sphincter. Patients often complain of symptoms localizing to the upper epigastric region or lower sternum although the association is less significant than in oropharyngeal dysphagia. The type of food producing symptoms and its temporal progression help to identify the cause of symptoms. Dysphagia progressing from solids to liquids usually indicates a mechanical cause, and dysphagia to both solids and liquids from the outset favors a motility disorder. Symptoms of associated heartburn, weight loss, anemia, and regurgitation further narrow the differential diagnosis. Other medical conditions such as radiation therapy and medication use may be associated with dysphagia, as may infectious esophagitis. Both are often associated with odynophagia as well. Opportunistic infections—especially in the setting of HIV disease and AIDS—such as candida, cytomegalovirus, and herpes virus, are the most common and can be managed adequately with medical therapy.

The various causes of esophageal dysphagia are listed in Box 2.

The most common initial diagnostic approach to esophageal dysphagia is to perform endoscopy. In addition to the diagnostic value, endoscopy affords an opportunity to obtain tissue samples and do

---

BOX 1 Causes of Oropharyngeal Dysphagia

Structural (Mechanical)
- Carcinoma
- Cervical and proximal esophageal webs
- Cricopharyngeal bar
- Osteophytes and other skeletal abnormalities
- Prior surgery or radiation therapy

Neuromuscular
- Amyotrophic lateral sclerosis
- Brainstem tumors
- Dermatomyositis, polymyositis
- Head trauma
- Idiopathic upper esophageal sphincter dysfunction
- Multiple sclerosis
- Myasthenia gravis
- Myotonic dystrophy
- Paraneoplastic syndromes
- Parkinson's disease
- Postpolio syndrome
- Sarcoidosis
- Stroke

Infection
- Botulism
- Diphtheria
- Lyme disease
- Syphilis

BOX 2 Causes of Esophageal Dysphagia

Structural (Mechanical)
Intrinsic
- Benign tumors
- Carcinoma: Adenocarcinoma and squamous cell cancer
- Diverticula
- Eosinophilic esophagitis
- Esophageal rings and webs: Schatzki's ring
- Foreign body
- Infections: Herpes, CMV, EBV, MAI, *Candida*, *Pneumocystis*
- Peptic strictures
- Pill esophagitis
- Radiation strictures or esophagitis

Extrinsic
- Cervical osteophytes
- Mediastinal masses
- Vascular compression: Dysphagia lusoria

Motility (Neuromuscular)
- Achalasia
- Diffuse esophageal spasm (DES)
- Hypertensive lower esophageal sphincter
- Ineffective esophageal motility disorder
- Nutcracker esophagus
- Secondary causes like scleroderma, Sjögren's syndrome, Chagas' disease

Functional
- Functional dysphagia

Abbreviations: CMV = cytomegalovirus; EBV = Epstein-Barr virus; MAI = *Mycobacterium avium-intracellulare*.

therapeutic intervention. A barium swallow with a solid bolus challenge is a reasonable alternative, especially with patients in whom oropharyngeal causes are a possibility or when the history suggests a complex stricture or achalasia. An endoscopy is required if a structural abnormality is discovered on the barium study.

STRUCTURAL CAUSES

Patients reporting only solid food dysphagia typically have a mechanical cause for their symptoms. This can progress to both solid and liquid dysphagia in cases of a high-grade obstruction. These patients tend to develop food impaction and might regurgitate. Benign causes for these symptoms include an esophageal web or a distal esophageal ring. The rings, also called Schatzki's rings, are smooth, thin mucosal structures at the gastroesophageal junction covered by squamous mucosa above and columnar epithelium below. Muscular rings, on the other hand, are characterized by hypertrophic esophageal musculature and are generally located about 2 cm above the gastroesophageal junction. Nonprogressive, episodic dysphagia is a characteristic of esophageal rings. Dysphagia becomes prominent when the diameter is smaller than 13 mm. Rings can manifest with acute dysphagia associated with impaction of a piece of meat, often referred to as "steakhouse syndrome." Esophageal webs, often asymptomatic, have been associated with iron deficiency anemia (Plummer-Vinson syndrome).

Peptic strictures occur in 8% to 10% of patients with symptomatic gastroesophageal reflux disease (GERD). Peptic strictures are associated with a long duration of reflux symptoms, male sex, and older age. Symptoms of dysphagia occur when the luminal diameter narrows to 13 mm or less.

Radiation-related strictures or esophagitis are seen in persons undergoing radiotherapy for thoracic or head or neck tumors. In the acute setting esophagitis is the predominant finding and can progress to fibrosis and strictures in the chronic phase.

Malignancy is the primary concern in patients with rapidly progressive solid food dysphagia associated with weight loss and anorexia. The staging of esophageal cancer involves CT scanning of the chest and abdomen and endoscopic ultrasonography (EUS). EUS provides the most accurate estimate of disease stage and assists with management decisions. The 5-year survival rate for patients with advanced esophageal cancer continues to be less than 5%.

Eosinophilic esophagitis is seen more often as a cause of dysphagia, particularly in young adults. Extensive diffuse eosinophilic infiltration (>20 per high power field), particularly in the proximal esophagus, is seen. The disease can manifest for the first time as a food impaction requiring emergency endoscopic therapy. Feline esophagus, concentric mucosal rings, or ringed esophagus is the classic endoscopic description of eosinophilic esophagitis.

Pill-induced esophagitis has been shown to occur with a variety of medications including bisphosphonates, doxycycline, potassium chloride, quinidine, nonsteroidal anti-inflammatory drugs (NSAIDs), aspirin, and iron preparations.

Vascular anomalies such as double aortic arch or aberrant right subclavian artery can cause dysphagia.

MOTILITY CAUSES

Patients reporting both solid and liquid dysphagia are more likely to have a motility disorder. Achalasia is a disease in which there is a loss of peristalsis in the distal esophagus and a failure of LES relaxation. These patients complain of chest pain, regurgitation, heartburn, and weight loss in addition to dysphagia. A barium swallow is the primary screening test when achalasia is suspected and manometry is confirmatory. The characteristic features on manometry include elevated resting LES pressure, incomplete LES relaxation, and aperistalsis.

Spastic motility disorders also manifest with dysphagia and often associated chest pain. The group of spastic motility disorders includes distal esophageal spasm, nutcracker esophagus, and hypertensive LES. The clinical relevance of these abnormalities identified during esophageal manometry is debated, and their management can be challenging.

Treatment

OROPHARYNGEAL DYSPHAGIA

Surgical and endoscopic therapeutic options are available, and these should be based on the patient's age and surgical risk. Surgery has been the mainstay of symptomatic Zenker's diverticulum. These involve cricopharyngeal myotomy with or without diverticulectomy or diverticulopexy. The efficacy of myotomy has been observed to be in excess of 80%. More recently, endoscopic techniques involving coagulation or cutting of the bridge, especially the cricopharyngeal muscle, between the esophagus and the diverticulum have been used. This approach is especially good for patients who are poor surgical risks and is now being used widely by experts in this technique.

Botulinum toxin injection might be an alternative to cricopharyngeal myotomy, although results are variable. Injection is usually performed under electromyographic guidance and has been shown to relieve dysphagia in small trials.

The presence of other structural abnormalities such as proximal strictures, can require endoscopic measures such as dilatation. A neoplasm requires appropriate intervention with surgical resection, chemotherapy, or radiation therapy.

If the oropharyngeal dysphagia is believed to be from nonstructural causes, swallowing rehabilitation may be the best option available. Swallowing rehabilitation is carried out by trained speech and language therapists, who teach patients maneuvers to overcome the risks of aspiration and improve dysphagia. These can involve proper positioning of the head and neck during swallowing, oral motor exercises, and deliberate multiple swallows. Certain diet modifications can improve swallowing and prevent aspirations.

The risk of malnutrition or recurrent aspiration can require placement of gastrostomy tubes for managing long-term nutritional needs.

ESOPHAGEAL DYSPHAGIA

The treatment of peptic strictures can involve dilatation, biopsies to rule out malignancy, and medical therapy for reflux. Proton pump inhibitor therapy has been shown to reduce the development of these strictures and the need for future dilatation.

Radiation-related strictures or esophagitis may be difficult to treat and require frequent esophageal dilatation.

The treatment of esophageal cancer depends on the stage of the cancer at the time of diagnosis. The various options available include surgery, chemotherapy, radiation therapy, palliative intraluminal stenting, and, more recently, photodynamic therapy.

Eosinophilic esophagitis is treated with topical steroid therapy with fluticasone[1] (Flovent), oral methylprednisolone, or montelukast in addition to dietary restrictions. These treatments have been studied in small series and have been shown to be beneficial. Dilatation may be helpful but must be done with care.

Treatment of pill-induced esophagitis involves stopping the offending agent and dilatation of strictures as needed.

Treatment modalities for achalasia include pneumatic dilatation of the LES, laparoscopic myotomy, botulinum toxin injection, and

---

[1]Not FDA approved for this indication.

CURRENT THERAPY

- Treat the underlying disorder (e.g., GERD).
- Dilatation and antireflux therapy manage most peptic strictures.
- Multimodality therapy should be considered for malignant dysphagia.
- Achalasia can be effectively treated with pneumatic dilatation or surgery.
- Swallowing rehabilitation is helpful for oropharyngeal dysphagia following stroke.

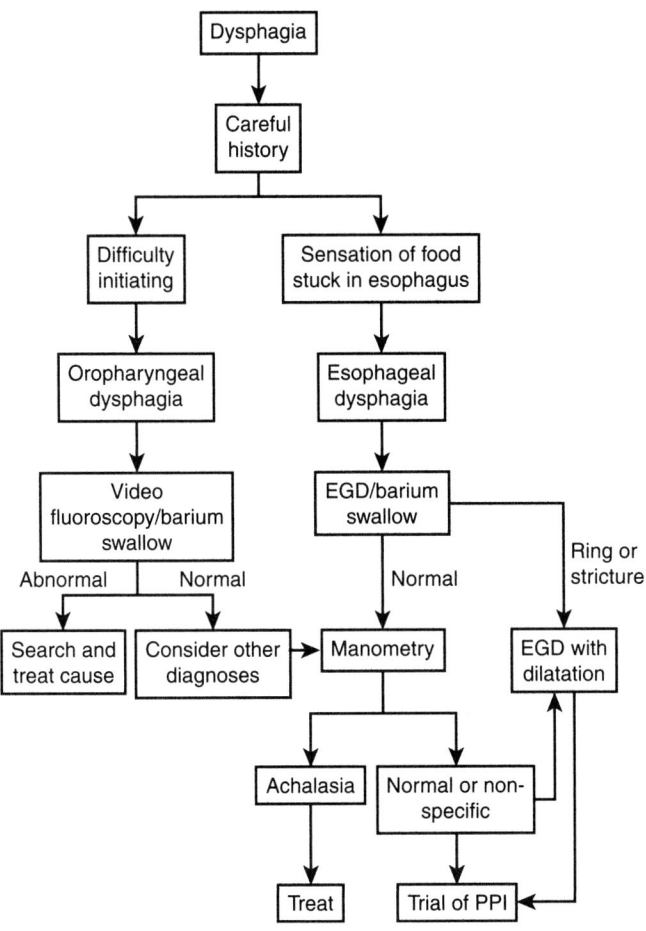

FIGURE 1. Diagnostic algorithm for patients with dysphagia. *Abbreviations:* EGD = esophagogastroduodenoscopy; PPI = proton pump inhibitor.

medical therapy with nitrates and calcium channel blockers. Medical therapy should be considered only for people who are not candidates for other modalities. Good to excellent relief of dysphagia can be achieved in patients with achalasia whether treated with pneumatic dilatation or myotomy. Many patients require multiple approaches and should be managed by experts in the field. Minimally invasive (laparoscopic or thoracoscopic) myotomy is gaining popularity, and in some centers it has become the procedure of choice.

Proposed treatments for distal esophageal spasm, nutcracker esophagus, and hypertensive LES include proton pump inhibitors, nitrates, calcium channel blockers, phosphodiesterase inhibitors, and tricyclic antidepressants or selective serotonin reuptake inhibitors.[1] Botulinum toxin[1] application and endoscopic dilatation have been tried in small series with varying results.

Summary

This review outlines the various causes and management of dysphagia. A careful history and examination with use of certain diagnostic tests help in establishing the reason for the symptom of dysphagia. Most of the conditions can be managed by medical therapy, endoscopic therapy, or surgery. A possible approach is outlined in Figure 1.

REFERENCES

Cook IJ, Kahrilas PJ: AGA technical review on management of oropharyngeal dysphagia. Gastroenterology 1999;116(2):455-479.

---

[1]Not FDA approved for this indication.

Katz PO, Gilbert J, Castell DO: Pneumatic dilatation is effective long-term treatment for achalasia. Dig Dis Sci 1998;43(9):1973-1977.
Khazanchi A, Katz PO: Strategies for treating severe refractory dysphagia. Gastrointest Endosc Clin N Am 2001;11(2):371-386. viii.
Spechler SJ: American Gastroenterological Association medical position statement on treatment of patients with dysphagia caused by benign disorders of the distal esophagus. Gastroenterology 1999;117(1):229-233.
Trate DM, Parkman HP, Fisher RS: Dysphagia: Evaluation, diagnosis and treatment. Prim Care 1996;(3):417-432.
Tutuian R, Castell DO: Esophageal motility disorders (distal esophageal spasm, nutcracker esophagus, and hypertensive lower esophageal sphincter): Modern management. Curr Treat Options Gastroenterol 2006;9(4):283-294.
Yan BM, Shaffer EA: Eosinophilic esophagitis: A newly established cause of dysphagia. World J Gastroenterol. 2006;12(15):2328-2334.

Diverticula of the Alimentary Tract

Method of
Pinckney J. Maxwell IV, MD, and
Charles W. Chappuis, MD

A diverticulum is a pouch or sac branching out from a hollow or fluid-filled organ or structure. Diverticula can occur throughout all levels of the gastrointestinal (GI) tract from the esophagus, stomach, and duodenum to the small intestine and colon. True diverticula contain all layers of the bowel wall including mucosa, submucosa, and muscular wall. False diverticula, also known as pseudodiverticula, are herniations of mucosa and submucosa through the muscular wall of the bowel, often at the site of a penetrating blood vessel. True diverticula are generally congenital structures, and false diverticula are generally structures acquired from pulsion forces, traction forces, or abnormalities of the muscular wall. Complications associated with diverticula of the alimentary tract include pain, bleeding, and perforation.

Zencker's Diverticula

A Zencker, or pharyngoesophageal, diverticulum occurs in the distal hypopharynx within the fibers of the inferior pharyngeal constrictor between the cricopharyngeus muscle and the oblique fibers of the posterior pharyngeal constrictor muscle, an area also known as Killian's triangle. This is the most common type of esophageal diverticulum, generally occurring in patients older than 60 years. Men are affected twice as commonly as women. Pulsion forces create this diverticulum, resulting from transient incomplete relaxation of the upper esophageal sphincter (UES), causing mucosa and submucosa to herniate.

CLINICAL FEATURES

Zencker's diverticula are generally asymptomatic initially, but they can develop symptoms including intermittent cough, excessive salivation, halitosis, dysphagia, and regurgitation of undigested food. Aspiration, often nocturnal, can lead to recurrent pneumonia. Large diverticula can cause more significant symptoms, including esophageal or respiratory obstruction and retrosternal chest pain.

DIAGNOSIS

These diverticula are often only discovered during routine plain film radiologic evaluations, revealing an air-fluid level. The diagnosis is usually confirmed by barium esophagogram, revealing the lesion most often on the left posteriorly. Endoscopy may be indicated to rule out ulceration or a malignancy.

CURRENT DIAGNOSIS

Colonic Diverticula
- Most commonly asymptomatic; diagnosis by endoscopy
- Abdominal pain, nausea, fever; diagnosis by air-contrast barium enema
- Hemorrhage, obstruction, fistulas; diagnosis by CT scan with oral or rectal contrast

Duodenal Diverticula
- Most commonly asymptomatic; diagnosis by upper GI contrast studies
- Cholangitis, pancreatitis; diagnosis by ERCP

Gastric Diverticula
- Most commonly asymptomatic; diagnosis by upper GI contrast studies
- Mild epigastric pain; diagnosis by endoscopy

Jejunoileal Diverticula
- Most commonly asymptomatic; diagnosis by upper GI contrast studies
- Chronic vague abdominal pain; diagnosis by laparotomy
- Low-grade obstruction, hemorrhage

Meckel's Diverticula
- Often asymptomatic; diagnosis by Meckel's nuclear scan
- Ulceration, hemorrhage; diagnosis by laparotomy
- Obstruction, incarceration; diagnosis by angiography, enteroclysis

Midesophageal or Epiphrenic
- Often asymptomatic; diagnosis by barium esophagogram
- Dysphagia, chest pain, heartburn; diagnosis by esophageal manometry
- Regurgitation, anorexia, weight loss; diagnosis by endoscopy

Zencker's Diverticula
- Asymptomatic initially; diagnosis by plain film x-rays
- Cough, salivation, halitosis, regurgitation; diagnosis by barium esophagogram
- Dysphagia, chest pain, aspiration pneumonia; diagnosis by endoscopy
- Esophageal or respiratory obstruction

CT = computed tomography; ERCP = endoscopic retrograde cholangiopancreatography; GI = gastrointestinal;

TREATMENT

Therapy is indicated for symptomatic patients and is directed primarily toward correcting the underlying motility disorder. The most common approach in dealing with this problem is the combination of a cervical esophagomyotomy in conjunction with resection of the diverticulum.

The procedure is usually performed through an oblique left neck incision that parallels the sternocleidomastoid muscle. It is recommended that a 40- to 50-F bougie be inserted in the esophagus before resecting the diverticulum to prevent narrowing the esophagus. The myotomy is performed from the base of the diverticulum, extending 7 to 10 cm proximally and distally. Small diverticula often blend into the exposed mucosa following the esophagomyotomy. Excision of larger pouches is best done with the surgical stapler. Another, less morbid, approach is a diverticulopexy, suspending the distal free end of the diverticulum proximally to prevent matter from becoming trapped.

Myotomy and diverticulectomy yield excellent results, with few recurrences. Recurrence rates are significantly higher if a myotomy is not performed.

Midesophageal and Epiphrenic Diverticula

CLINICAL FEATURES

Midesophageal diverticula are true diverticula found in the middle third of the esophagus, most often within 4 to 5 cm of the carina, and epiphrenic diverticula appear in the distal third of the esophagus, most often within 10 cm of the gastroesophageal junction. Midesophageal diverticula have been historically associated with traction forces, resulting from inflammatory changes from mediastinal lymphadenopathy, fibrosis, tuberculosis, or histoplasmosis. However, as with epiphrenic diverticula, midesophageal diverticula are more commonly the result of pulsion forces of motility disorders, such as achalasia or diffuse esophageal spasm.

These diverticula are often asymptomatic. However, symptoms are usually those common to an underlying motility disorder, including dysphagia, regurgitation or emesis, belching, epigastric or substernal chest pain, heartburn, anorexia, and weight loss. Although complications are unusual, they can include spontaneous rupture, aspiration, tracheobronchial fistula, hemorrhage, and carcinoma.

DIAGNOSIS

The best diagnostic test is a barium esophagogram; however, manometry is generally indicated to rule out an esophageal motility disorder. Midesophageal diverticula are often wide-mouthed, singular, and smaller than 5 cm. Epiphrenic diverticula are multiple in 19% of cases. Both are more common on the right side. Generally, endoscopy is also performed preoperatively.

TREATMENT

Therapy is indicated for symptomatic disease. A left thoracotomy is performed to provide access for a diverticulectomy and a long extramucosal esophagomyotomy. If an antireflux procedure is indicated following myotomy, a partial fundoplication (Belsey type) should be performed rather than a full 360-degree Nissen fundoplication. Although diverticulectomy and esophagomyotomy are associated with a 9% operative mortality, they also have good long-term results.

Gastric Diverticula

CLINICAL FEATURES

Gastric diverticula are exceedingly rare and are most commonly asymptomatic. These diverticula can be either true or false and generally occur between the ages of 20 and 60 years. Symptoms can include mild epigastric pain, and infrequent complications include hemorrhage, diverticulitis, and perforation.

DIAGNOSIS

Most gastric diverticula are discovered on upper GI contrast studies. They are most often located in the cardiac portion of the stomach and are small, 1 to 3 cm.

TREATMENT

Therapy is not indicated for asymptomatic diverticula and is reserved for complicated or symptomatic diverticula. Diverticulectomy is the treatment of choice, which can require partial gastric resection depending on the size and location of the diverticulum.

Duodenal Diverticula

Diverticula of the duodenum are relatively common, with some autopsy series reporting the incidence as high as 15% to 20%. This is the second most common site of GI diverticula after the colon. They are the most common acquired diverticula of the small bowel and are usually false. They are rare in patients younger than 40 years and are twice as common in women as in men.

DIAGNOSIS

Most duodenal diverticula are found incidentally on upper GI contrast studies or endoscopic retrograde cholangiopancreatography (ERCP) studies, located in the second portion of the duodenum near the ampulla of Vater. The common bile duct and pancreatic duct occasionally open into the diverticulum itself. The vast majority are asymptomatic, but complications include obstruction of the biliary or pancreatic ducts, with associated cholangitis or pancreatitis, perforation, or hemorrhage.

TREATMENT

Diverticulectomy is reserved for complicated disease and can require extensive dissection and reconstruction if located in the head of the pancreas or associated with the ampulla of Vater. Great care should be taken to preserve the integrity of the biliary and pancreatic ductal systems.

Jejunoileal Diverticula

CLINICAL FEATURES

Jejunoileal diverticula are false diverticula and are much less common than duodenal diverticula, occurring in approximately 1% of autopsy series. Most occur in the jejunum, are multiple, and are found in patients older than 60 years. These diverticula are usually the result of a motor disorder of the smooth muscle or myenteric plexus, which causes uncoordinated contractions of the small bowel. As with other upper GI diverticula, jejunoileal diverticula are asymptomatic in the vast majority of patients. Symptoms, when present, include chronic vague abdominal pain, malabsorption, and low-grade obstruction or hemorrhage. Complications include hemorrhage, diverticulitis, or perforation.

DIAGNOSIS

These diverticula are usually located on the mesenteric border or in the mesentery of the proximal jejunum. They are found incidentally on upper GI with small bowel follow through contrast studies or at the time of laparotomy for other reasons.

TREATMENT

Therapy is reserved for symptomatic or complicated disease. Resection is performed with primary end-to-end anastomosis. Patients who present with malabsorption secondary to bacterial overgrowth in a diverticulum can initially be treated with antibiotics followed by resection of the diverticulum.

Meckel's Diverticula

A Meckel's diverticulum is a true diverticulum that occurs on the antimesenteric border of the ileum approximately 45 to 60 cm from the ileocecal valve. It is present in 2% of the population equally

CURRENT THERAPY

- Most gastrointestinal diverticula are asymptomatic and require no treatment; however, symptomatic or complicated diverticular disease usually requires intervention, most often in the form of surgical resection.
- Colonic diverticulitis: Bowel rest, intravenous fluids and antibiotics
- Complicated colonic: Partial to subtotal colectomy
- Duodenal: Diverticulectomy, with potential extensive reconstruction
- Gastric: Diverticulectomy, with potential partial gastrectomy
- Jejunoileal: Segmental small bowel resection
- Meckel's: Diverticulectomy, with potential segmental bowel resection
- Midesophageal or epiphrenic: Diverticulectomy and myotomy, only partial fundoplication
- Zencker's: Diverticulectomy and cervical myotomy, or diverticulopexy

among male and female patients. It results from the failure of obliteration of the vitelline or omphalomesenteric duct, the structure connecting the yolk sac to the midgut in the embryo.

CLINICAL FEATURES

Although the size and shape of the diverticulum can vary greatly, it is usually wide-mouthed, between 3 and 5 cm in length, and about 2 cm in diameter. It can be lined with ileal mucosa, but heterotopic mucosa is also found. The most common lining is gastric mucosa, present in approximately one half of all Meckel's diverticula. Pancreatic mucosa is present in 5%, and colonic mucosa is present in even fewer cases.

DIAGNOSIS

The vast majority of these diverticula are asymptomatic; however, gastric mucosa, when present produces acid and can lead to ulceration in the diverticula or in adjacent tissue. Hemorrhage is the most common manifesting symptom, especially in patients younger than 2 years. Other complications include intestinal obstruction, intussusception, volvulus around a fibrous persistent band from the diverticulum to the umbilicus, incarceration in an inguinal hernia (Littre's hernia), diverticulitis, or a neoplastic process. Diverticulitis is a more common presentation in adults and is clinically indistinguishable from acute appendicitis. A search for a Meckel's diverticulum should be undertaken when an exploration is negative for appendicitis.

Diagnosis of a Meckel's diverticulum can be more difficult than with other GI diverticular diseases. Plain film x-rays, upper GI contrast studies, ultrasounds, and computed tomography (CT) rarely establish the diagnosis. The most sensitive and specific modality is a ^{99m}Tc-pertechnetate scan (Meckel's scan), especially in pediatric patients who have a higher incidence of gastric mucosa in the diverticulum. Angiography in an acute hemorrhage or enteroclysis, the introduction of barium directly into the small bowel through a nasogastric tube positioned beyond the ligament of Treitz, are often useful diagnostic adjuncts.

TREATMENT

Surgical resection is the treatment for symptomatic Meckel's diverticulum. Resection of the adjacent segment of ileum is often indicated when peptic ulceration is present. There is no clinical evidence to support resection of asymptomatic Meckel's diverticula discovered either at laparotomy or by contrast study.

Colonic Diverticula

Colonic diverticulosis occurs equally between the sexes and in less than 10% of the population between 30 and 40 years of age, 20% to 35% between 50 and 60 years, more than 40% older than 70 years, and more than 66% older than 90 years. With advancing age, there are increases in both the size and number of diverticula.

ETIOLOGY AND PATHOGENESIS

Most colonic diverticula are false diverticula, acquired as a result of pulsion forces of the circular muscle layer. High intraluminal pressures result from segmental and circular muscular contraction, forcing the mucosa and submucosa to herniate, generally at the points of entrance of the arteriae rectae of the colon wall. They form only between the mesenteric taenia and the two lateral taenia. Eighty percent to 95% of diverticula are limited to the sigmoid colon. Cecal or right-sided diverticula are usually true diverticula, containing all layers of the colon wall; they are thought to be congenital. It is generally agreed that a lack of dietary fiber contributes significantly to the development of diverticulosis by decreasing the bulk of stool, requiring greater muscular contraction and higher intraluminal pressures.

Although a large percentage of the population develops diverticula at some point in their lives, more than 80% of these remain asymptomatic. Symptoms develop as a result of complications of diverticular disease, including inflammation (diverticulitis) and perforation, hemorrhage, obstruction from stricturing, and fistulas.

CLINICAL FEATURES

Diverticulitis typically manifests with left lower quadrant abdominal pain, low-grade fever, leukocytosis, nausea with occasional vomiting, and mild to moderate abdominal distention. Occasionally, one can appreciate a palpable mass in the left lower quadrant on physical examination. Perforation of a single diverticulum is thought to be the initial event that results in a peridiverticulitis. The perforation may be contained within the mesocolon or might freely perforate into the peritoneal cavity, resulting in peritonitis. Abscesses can develop into the mesentery, as localized fluid collections, or as uncontained collections throughout the abdomen. Fistulas can result from the inflammatory process to adjacent organs such as the small bowel, bladder, vagina, or even the skin in delayed cases. Hemorrhage can result in acute lower GI bleeding, and repeated episodes of diverticulitis can lead to stricturing, causing symptoms of obstruction.

DIAGNOSIS

The diagnosis is usually established via endoscopy or contrast enema studies. CT scanning can also be used with oral and rectal luminal contrast. Hemorrhage can require nuclear medicine scanning or angiography.

TREATMENT

Mild attacks of diverticulitis can be treated with bowel rest, intravenous fluids, and parenteral antibiotics. Some cases may be amenable to management on an outpatient basis with a clear liquid diet and a 10-day course of oral antibiotics with broad-spectrum coverage to include anaerobes and gram-negative rods. Most patients requiring hospitalization show improvement in 3 to 5 days. Patients with more severe cases of diverticulitis or with associated complications can require a more prolonged hospitalization.

CT often demonstrates the extent and complications of diverticulitis and should be obtained early in patients with suspected complications of diverticular disease. Diverticulitis complicated by the development of an abscess can require drainage, either by CT-guided percutaneous drainage or by laparotomy with resection.

Patients with recurrent attacks of diverticulitis may undergo elective primary resection of the involved segment of colon, although this is somewhat controversial. Surgery is also indicated in cases of peritonitis secondary to perforated diverticulitis. The involved segment of perforated colon is resected, sometimes requiring the formation of a temporary colostomy.

Colovesicular fistulas, the most common type of spontaneous internal fistula, occur in 2% to 4% of patients with diverticulitis. Patients can present with recurrent urinary tract infections or even pneumaturia or fecaluria in more advanced cases. Female patients are more protected from this complication secondary to the interposition of the uterus between the colon and bladder. Colovesicular fistulas can usually be treated with primary resection of the involved segment of bowel and fistula tract with primary anastomosis. Obvious defects in the bladder wall are sutured with layered absorbable suture in conjunction with urethral catheter drainage. If neoplasm is suspected as a cause of the fistula, a segment of bladder including the fistula should be resected en bloc with the colon.

Gastrointestinal hemorrhage should be managed by resuscitation initially to replace hypovolemia and achieve hemodynamic stability. Blood losses are replaced as needed. Diagnosis then depends on cessation of bleeding. Hemorrhage stops spontaneously without intervention in more than 80% of cases; however, recurrent bleeding occurs in nearly one quarter of these patients. Attempts should be made to identify the source of hemorrhage, and this can be aided with colonoscopy, nuclear medicine scanning, and angiography. In cases of persistent or recurrent bleeding in which the site of bleeding has been identified, a segmental colectomy may be performed. Persistent hemorrhage and inability to localize the site of bleeding can necessitate subtotal colectomy.

REFERENCES

Afridi SA, Fichtenbaum CJ, Taubin H: Review of duodenal diverticulum. Am J Gastroenterol 2002;97(3):935-938.
Akhrass R, Yaffe MB, Fischer C, et al: Small bowel diverticulosis: Perceptions and reality. J Am Coll Surg 1997;184:383-388.
Allen MS: Treatment of epiphrenic diverticula. Semin Thoracic Cardiovasc Surg 1999;11(4):358-362.
Benacci JC, Deschamps C, Trastek VF, et al: Epiphrenic diverticulum: Results of surgical treatment. Ann Thorac Surg 1993;55:1109-1113.
Longo WE, Vernava AM: Clinical implications of jejunoileal diverticular disease. Dis Colon Rectum 1992;35(4):381-388.
Martin JP, Connor PD, Charles K: Meckel's diverticulum. Am Fam Physician 2000;61(4):1037-1042.
Rice TW, Baker ME: Midthoracic esophageal diverticula. Semin Thoracic Cardiovasc Surg 1999;11(4):352-357.
Simpson J, Scholefield JH, Spiller RC: Pathogenesis of colonic diverticula. Br J Surg 2002;89(5):546-554.
Stollman NH, Raskin JB: Diverticular disease of the colon. J Clin Gastroenterol 1999;29(3):241-252.

Inflammatory Bowel Disease

Method of
*Mark A. Peppercorn, MD, and
Alan C. Moss, MD*

Inflammatory bowel disease (IBD) describes the spectrum of chronic intestinal inflammation from Crohn's disease to ulcerative colitis. This condition is currently thought to occur as a consequence of a persistent and inappropriate immunologic response to gut luminal antigens. The absence of enteric parasites in developed societies and defects in mucosal innate defenses are recent additions to the many

CURRENT DIAGNOSIS

- Diagnosis should only be based on a combination of clinical, radiologic, endoscopic, and histologic features.
- Exclude tuberculosis, *Yersinia* infection, and NSAID use in suspected Crohn's disease.
- Exclude *Clostridium difficile, Campylobacter, Shigella,* and *Salmonella* infection, NSAID use, and ischemic colitis in suspected ulcerative colitis.
- Distinction between Crohn's disease and ulcerative colitis has implications for surgical interventions and prognosis.
- Nocturnal diarrhea, bloody diarrhea, weight loss, and low energy levels suggest severe disease.
- CBC, ESR, CRP, and albumin levels are useful in distinguishing disease exacerbations from functional symptoms.

Abbreviations: CBC = complete blood count; CRP = C-reactive protein; ESR = erythrocyte sedimentation rate; NSAID = nonsteroidal anti-inflammatory drug.

hypotheses on the pathogenesis. Irrespective of the cause, Crohn's disease (CD) and ulcerative colitis (UC) respond to a similar range of anti-inflammatory and immunomodulator therapy in inducing and maintaining remission.

Both CD and UC are characterized by mucosal ulceration, which is patchy in CD but continuous in UC. In CD the focal areas (skip lesions) of transmural inflammation and ulceration can penetrate the gut wall, leading to fistulous tracts. In 80% of patients the terminal ileum is involved, and half of these have both ileal and colonic disease. These patients typically present with crampy abdominal pain, diarrhea, and evidence of weight loss or fevers. Up to a third of patients develop perianal disease, characterized by fistulas or abscesses during their life span. Patients may also present with mouth ulcers, gastric ulceration, or skin manifestations such as erythema nodosum. These clinical patterns are dynamic, with more than 60% of patients having a change in clinical behavior over 10 years. For small intestinal disease, computed tomography (CT) with contrast is the investigation of choice, with a sensitivity of 95% in most studies. A small bowel series has advantages over CT in early disease and fistula and sinus tract delineation; magnetic resonance imaging (MRI) is superior in perianal disease. Assessment of colonic disease and tissue diagnosis is best performed with full colonoscopy and terminal ileum intubation; this allows staging of the condition and exclusion of other causes of terminal ileum inflammation such as tuberculosis (TB) or *Yersinia* infection. There are no diagnostic blood tests for CD per se, although erythrocyte sedimentation rate (ESR), C-reactive protein (CRP), and complete blood count (CBC) are useful markers of disease activity. CRP elevation is positively associated with clinical and endoscopic activity and severe histologic disease. Anti-*Saccharomyces cerevisiae* antibodies (ASCA) are positive in 40% to 70% of patients with CD, with a reported specificity of 95%; this may be useful in patients where the clinical pattern of colitis is nondiagnostic. In patients with a family history of CD, polymorphisms in the NOD2 gene confer an increased risk of ileal disease and fibrostenotic disease. These mutations can be found in up to 30% of patients with CD, depending on ethnic group. However, 3% of the population may also harbor such mutations, limiting their role at the diagnostic level.

UC, in contrast, is characterized by continuous inflammation proximally from the rectum; two thirds of patients have disease limited to distal to the splenic flexure at presentation, and the rest have more extensive disease. The geography of the disease is usually described in terms of its extent: proctitis (rectum), distal colitis (rectum to descending), left-sided colitis (to splenic flexure), extensive colitis (beyond splenic flexure), and pancolitis (to cecum). UC usually causes bloody diarrhea, urgency, and lower abdominal pain, progressing to fecal incontinence and nocturnal symptoms in severe disease. Up to 30% of patients progress from distal to pancolitis over 10 years. Colonoscopy remains the investigation of choice in mapping disease geography and confirming tissue diagnosis. Similar to CD, inflammatory markers such as ESR and CRP are useful to confirm clinical disease activity and predict those likely to require surgery. Antineutrophil cytoplasmic antibodies (P-ANCA) can be detected in 50% to 70% of patients with UC but in only 5% to 10% of patients with CD. These patients tend to have more aggressive disease, leading to early surgery. The main diagnoses to exclude are infective colitides, such as infection with *Clostridium difficile, Campylobacter, Shigella,* or *Salmonella.* Ischemic colitis and nonsteroidal anti-inflammatory drug (NSAID)-induced colitis can also mimic UC.

The natural history of IBD is of frequent flares of the condition in response to unknown triggers. In CD, for example, 75% of patients have a chronic intermittent course, 15% have chronically active disease, and 10% remain in remission. The management of active disease can be divided into pharmacologic therapy, surgery, and nonpharmacologic interventions. Agents are usually described in terms of obtaining remission during flare-ups and maintaining remission in the medium to long term. We describe each of these in detail and then specifically in relation to disease subtypes.

Pharmacologic Therapy

AMINOSALICYLATES

Sulfasalazine (Azulfidine), the original aminosalicylate compound, consists of sulfapyridine (an antibiotic) and 5-aminosalicylic acid (5-ASA) (an anti-inflammatory) bound with an azo bond. After ingestion, sulfasalazine reaches the colon practically unabsorbed, where the enzymatic action of colonic bacteria cleaves the azo bond to release the active 5-ASA from sulfapyridine. Because the sulfapyridine moiety is the cause of most of the adverse effects of sulfasalazine, most modern aminosalicylates contain 5-ASA alone or combined with an inert carrier via the azo bond. For the purposes of this discussion, we refer to the nonsulfa aminosalicylates, such as mesalamine (Asacol), balsalazide (Colazal), and olsalazine (Dipentum), as "5-ASA." The exact mechanism of action of aminosalicylates is unclear, but they appear to orchestrate a broad range of anti-inflammatory properties within the intestinal mucosa. At a molecular level they inhibit arachidonic acid metabolism and are free-radical scavengers, two pathways through which local inflammation and necrosis occurs in the intestine. They inhibit activation of peripheral and intestinal lymphocytes and their release of

CURRENT THERAPY

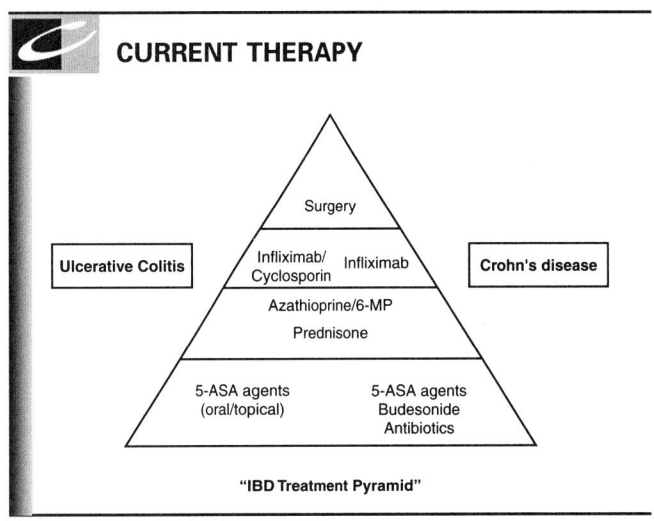

"IBD Treatment Pyramid"

immunoglobulin and proinflammatory cytokines. The therapeutic effects of these alterations are dose dependent and can take up to 14 days to reach their peak clinical response. Doses of more than 2 g/day of 5-ASA are required to obtain benefit in inducing remission, occurring in 40% to 80% of patients after 4 to 8 weeks of treatment in UC. In the longer term, sulfasalazine and the 5-ASA preparations maintain remission in 60% to 80% of these patients.

A number of oral 5-ASA are preparations available. Asacol and Salofalk (in Canada) contain mesalamine coated with a pH-sensitive acrylic polymer that dissolves above pH of 6/7, typically releasing mesalamine in the terminal ileum and colon. Recently Multi-Matrix (MMX) mesalamine (Lialda) was introduced. After dissolution of the coating at a pH>7, the contents form a viscous gel for colonic distribution. This theoretically allows once a day dosing. Pentasa contains mesalamine microspheres that release 5-ASA throughout the gastrointestinal (GI) tract as these microspheres become hydrated and diffuse out of the capsule; this potentially makes it suitable for treatment of proximal small bowel disease. Olsalazine (Dipentum) contains two 5-ASA molecules joined by an azo bond that is cleaved by colonic bacteria. Balsalazide (Colazal) consists of 5-ASA bound by an azo bond to an inactive molecule, which also requires bacterial digestion to release the active 5-ASA molecules. In addition to oral therapy, topical preparations in the form of suppositories, foam, and enemas are widely used in treating distal disease. Mesalamine enemas (Rowasa) reach up to the proximal sigmoid, foam extends to the midsigmoid, whereas mesalamine suppositories (Canasa) reach the first 10 to 12 cm of the rectosigmoid region only. Patients with proctitis often find the foam preparations less irritating and easier to retain than enemas. The side-effect profile of topical therapy is superior to oral 5-ASAs in patients with distal disease. Recent data have demonstrated efficacy of topical 5-ASAs even in patients with pancolitis when used in conjunction with oral therapy.

Adverse effects from the aminosalicylate compounds are uncommon, but a number of potentially severe effects can occur. The majority of side effects occur more commonly in patients treated with sulfasalazine. The most common adverse events reported are headache, fever, and rash in up to 10% of patients. These are generally dose dependent and can be ameliorated by reducing the dose. In some patients (1% to 2%), 5-ASA can ironically cause an intolerance syndrome marked by severe diarrhea and abdominal pain; this should be considered in any patients whose symptoms worsen with therapy. Rare hypersensitivity side effects of sulfasalazine and 5-ASA include pancreatitis, nephritis, pneumonitis, pericarditis, and hepatitis. Agranulocytosis is a severe but rare side effect of sulfasalazine, which typically occurs within the first 8 weeks of therapy; it usually responds to discontinuation of sulfasalazine within 2 weeks. Infertility may also occur because of sulfasalazine in male patients by causing a reversible reduction in sperm function and number. This effect is dose dependent and can be avoided by using nonsulfa-containing 5-ASAs in these patients.

CORTICOSTEROIDS

Corticosteroids have long been used, and continue to be used, in the acute management of flares of IBD. Their exact mechanism of action is unclear, although they are a potent inhibitor of cytokine release by inducing inactivation of NFkB. This leads to a reduction in lymphocyte recruitment to inflamed areas, reduced vascular permeability, and inhibition of cytokine-mediated tissue necrosis. Although oral corticosteroids are absorbed rapidly, their biologic anti-inflammatory effects take 4 to 9 hours to take effect, regardless of mode of delivery. There appears to be no difference in the benefits of oral steroids when compared to parenteral steroids in rates of remission in IBD.

Methylprednisolone (Solu-Medrol) or hydrocortisone (Solu-Cortef) can be given parenterally in patients with severe disease or in those unable to tolerate oral intake. They are given either as bolus or continuous infusion, although no evidence indicates that either is more efficacious in obtaining remission. Intramuscular methylprednisolone induces response faster than oral prednisolone in the outpatient setting in patients with moderately active colitis. Prednisone is the most commonly used oral corticosteroid in IBD, usually at doses of 30 to 60 mg as a starting dose. The dose-response effect occurs at doses of 20 to 60 mg/day, with side effects occurring at doses greater than 40 mg. It is absorbed within 30 minutes and undergoes first-pass metabolism in the liver to produce the active drug prednisolone. In both UC and CD, steroids induce a response in approximately 80% of patients, and approximately half of these obtain remission.

These corticosteroids have little mineralocorticoid or androgenic effects, but the main risk is of suppression of the hypothalamic-pituitary-adrenal axis and Cushing's syndrome. Chronic steroid use for less than 3 weeks does not appear to suppress the hypothalamic-pituitary axis, significantly, regardless of dose. Patients receiving steroid therapy for IBD for longer than this period should have any future reduction in steroid dose undertaken slowly (e.g., 5 mg weekly) to prevent hypoadrenalism. The main other side effect of concern is osteoporosis because up to 25% of patients with IBD have osteoporosis on bone density scans. Corticosteroid use is a major risk factor for vertebral fractures in these patients. Adequate calcium (1200 mg/day) and vitamin D (800 IU/day) are essential for patients receiving chronic steroids in IBD.

Such adverse effects with conventional synthetic steroids may be reduced with use of newer steroids such as budesonide (Entocort EC) and beclomethasone. Budesonide capsules are designed to release the active drug in the distal small bowel, where there is rapid mucosal uptake. Because of extensive hepatic metabolism, less than 10% becomes systemically available, thus reducing side effects. Beclomethasone also has high mucosal absorption with minimal systemic bioavailability.

AZATHIOPRINE/6-MERCAPTOPURINE

Azathioprine (Imuran, Azasan)[1] is a prodrug that is converted into 6-mercaptopurine[1] (6-MP, [Purinethol]) by glutathione in red blood cells. The 6-MP product is subsequently metabolized to both 6-methylmercaptopurine (6-MMP) by the TPMT enzyme, and to 6-thioguanine (6-TG) by a series of enzymatic alterations. The incorporation of 6-TG into activated lymphocytes results in activation of apoptotic pathways and inhibition of cytokine release, thus inhibiting the role of lymphocytes in IBD. These therapeutic effects take approximately 8 to 12 weeks to manifest in clinical response, which reflects the chronic inflammatory role of activated lymphocytes in IBD. Both azathioprine[1] and 6-MP (Purinethol)[1] are used in inducing and maintaining remission in both CD and UC, with efficacy rates of 60% to 70%. Azathioprine is equivalent to 6-MP in efficacy because 88% of azathioprine is metabolized to 6-MP. In practice, 6-MP is usually underdosed, whereas azathioprine is overdosed by clinicians. Full dose is 1.5 to 2.5 mg/kg for azathioprine and 1.5 mg/kg for 6-MP, although most gastroenterologists begin at a lower dose and titrate upward if no adverse effects are noted.

Side effects occur in up to 25% of patients on azathioprine[1]/6-MP,[1] but these are usually mild. Nausea and vomiting is common soon after initiation of azathioprine therapy, but in most cases this subsides or requires a trial of 6-MP instead. Bone marrow suppression and pancreatitis are two more serious adverse effects seen in patients with IBD. Leukopenia is usually dose dependent and should be prevented by monitoring CBC. We check the CBC weekly for 1 month, then every 2 weeks for 1 month, then every 3 months. Pancreatitis occurs more commonly in patients with CD and appears to be idiosyncratic. Hepatitis in the form of elevated aspartate transaminase/alanine transaminase (AST/ALT) may also occur, but this usually responds to dose reduction. There is a theoretical increased risk of infections and neoplasia in patients on immunomodulators such as azathioprine/6-MP. Meta-analysis of cohort studies reported an increased risk of lymphoma in patients with IBD treated with azathioprine/6-MP, but risk-benefit models suggest the benefits of such therapy still outweigh this risk.

In recent years it was recognized that an individual's level of the TPMT enzyme influences the amount of the active 6-TG metabolite they produce during azathioprine[1]/6-MP therapy.[1] Patients with low

---

[1]Not FDA approved for this indication.

TPMT levels because of genetic polymorphisms, approximately 1 in 300 of population, produce higher levels of 6-TG and are at higher risk of leukopenia. In theory, the measurement of TPMT levels prior to commencement of therapy might identify individuals at high risk of toxicity. However, integration of TPMT testing in patients with IBD has produced mixed results in preventing toxicity; prospective data have only shown a correlation between TPMT levels and early leukopenia in patients with IBD.

METHOTREXATE

Methotrexate (MTX)[1] is a folate analogue that prevents conversion of folic acid to folinic acid, its active intracellular metabolite. This action leads to accumulation of adenosine, a potent anti-inflammatory that inhibits the production of a number of cytokines from neutrophils, macrophages, and lymphocytes. MTX also causes inhibition of proliferation and induction of apoptosis in activated T-lymphocytes. Similar to azathioprine, this effect takes up to 12 weeks to manifest clinically, and is therefore often used in patients who are steroid dependent or have failed azathioprine[1]/6-MP therapy.[1] MTX given intramuscularly shows results in 40% to 65% of patients in inducing and maintaining remission in CD. Trials using oral MTX failed to show a benefit over placebo, possibly because of variable absorption.

The main adverse effects of MTX are hepatotoxicity, myelosuppression, pneumonitis, infertility, and teratogenicity. Myelosuppression is uncommon in those receiving MTX for more than 1 year, but they should be screened for by checking the CBC every 1 to 3 months. The hepatic toxicity of MTX is well documented in other conditions where it is used at high doses, such as psoriasis. Series of IBD patients taking MTX show low prevalence of liver fibrosis with accumulated dosage greater than 2.5 g. Patients who receive MTX should have CBC and liver function tests (LFTs) frequently and further investigation if serial abnormalities appear. Folic acid supplementation is recommended in all patients who receive MTX, at least 4 hours after MTX administration.

ANTICYTOKINE THERAPY

Anticytokine therapy refers to the development of antibody therapy targeted against specific cytokines that play a role in the pathogenesis of CD, including TNF, IL-12, IL-6, and IL-8. Only anti-TNF is accepted so far into mainstream therapy based on clinical trials. Infliximab (Remicade) is a chimeric antibody (75% human, 25% mouse) against the TNF-α molecule, which leads to induction of apoptosis in activated lymphocytes. It also appears to reduce the number of inflammatory cells at the site of mucosal inflammation, possibly by inhibiting leukocyte migration. Infliximab induces and maintains remission in patients with luminal and fistulizing CD and recently induced remission in active UC. It is given as an intravenous (IV) infusion over 2 hours at 0, 2, and 6 weeks, and 8 weeks thereafter to maintain remission. In patients with CD, approximately 60% of patients respond within 2 weeks, and 30% to 50% of responders maintain response for up to 1 year. Patients who do not smoke, are also taking immunomodulators, and have nonstricturing disease achieve the best response to this therapy in CD. Recent trials in ulcerative colitis reported response rates of 70% in patients with pancolitis refractory to steroids and immunomodulators.

Adverse effects to infliximab primarily relate to immunologic reactions to the TNF antibody, which is mouse derived. Up to 60% of patients receiving infliximab develop anti-infliximab antibodies, which may cause infusion reactions and flulike illness after subsequent therapy. Thankfully these are usually mild and can be prevented by using prednisone and antihistamines prior to infusions. In the longer term up to 50% of patients may require a higher dose or shorter interval between doses to overcome loss of efficacy. More serious side effects such as reactivation of TB, cardiac events in patients with congestive cardiac failure, demyelination, and lymphoma are reported.

Reactivation of latent TB occurs with an incidence of 0.46 per 1000 patient-years; therefore all patients should undergo a purified protein derivative (PPD) test and chest radiograph prior to commencement of therapy. The use of infliximab in patients with intra-abdominal collections and strictures is relatively contraindicated. A rare hepatosplenic T-cell lymphoma has been reported in young patients who had received both azathioprine or 6MP with infliximab.

In the area of TNF inhibition, similar response and remission rates, and potential adverse events, have been reported with the humanized anti-TNF antibody adalimumab (Humira), and the humanized pegylated anti-TNF fragment certolizumab (Cimzia). Both agents are now FDA-approved for moderate to severe CD. The advantage of these agents over infliximab is that they are administered subcutaneously and appear to induce fewer antibodies.

CYCLOSPORINE

Cyclosporine (Neoral)[1] inhibits cytokine production primarily in activated T-helper cells by binding to calcineurin and inhibiting proinflammatory transcription factors. Its role in UC is mainly in steroid-refractory patients (no response to 72 hours of high-dose steroids) with severe colitis. It has a response rate of 80% when administered as an IV infusion for a mean of 7 days in clinical trials. However, up to 60% of responders relapse within 6 months, and by 7 years approximately 60% will have required a colectomy. The relapse rate may be reduced by immunomodulator therapy. Tacrolimus (Prograf),[1] which acts via similar pathways, shows a similar response, up to 80% in severe colitis in small studies. Cyclosporine has a number of side effects, including renal impairment, hyperkalemia, tremor, hypertension, and hirsutism. Patients with low magnesium or cholesterol are at risk of seizures. In addition there is a risk of *Pneumocystis* pneumonia, aspergillus, and cytomegalovirus (CMV) infection because of immunosuppression. Data from Europe reported mortality rates as high as 3% in patients receiving cyclosporine, although this would not be the U.S. experience.

ANTIBIOTICS/PROBIOTICS

Because the intestinal microflora plays a role in the pathogenesis of intestinal inflammation, manipulating the composition of this environment would be expected to ameliorate the disease process in IBD. Recent advances in the understanding of IBD suggest an impaired mucosal bacterial sensing, leading to invasion by the microflora and sustained immune response. It appears certain bacteria may be phenotype specific in the inflammatory response they elicit.

In UC, oral vancomycin (Vancocin), tobramycin (Nebcin), ciprofloxacin (Cipro), and rifaximin (Xifaxan) all improve response rates in the short term in patients with moderate to severe disease activity. IV metronidazole and tobramycin also show better response rates than placebo. These responses are not maintained in the longer term in clinical trials, however, and in the majority of trials patients were also on steroids. In practice, antibiotics are often administered to patients with severe disease requiring hospitalization as an adjunct to immunosuppressive therapy. The role of the novel nonabsorbed antibiotic rifaximin remains to be determined in active colitis and pouchitis.

The results in CD are more impressive with antibiotic therapy. Metronidazole (Flagyl) has intracellular activity against anaerobes and parasites primarily. In clinical trials it reduced colonic disease activity compared to sulfasalazine and placebo. Metronidazole is most successful in treating perianal disease, with demonstrated complete healing of chronic fistulas and symptom improvement. Finally, in patients who have undergone resection for CD, metronidazole taken for 12 weeks reduces the recurrence of endoscopic lesions at 3 months and clinical recurrence for up to 1 year. The chronicity of therapy requires close monitoring for peripheral neuropathy, the most serious adverse effect. This is unlikely to occur at daily doses less than 1 g. Patients who develop paresthesia should initially

---
[1] Not FDA approved for this indication.

have dose reduction, followed by cessation if symptoms persist. Ciprofloxacin also produces clinical response, with 72% of patients with CD achieving complete or partial remission in recent trials. The combination of metronidazole and ciprofloxacin produces results similar to both steroids and mesalamine in patients with active disease and is a commonly used alternative to steroids. Ciprofloxacin also provides synergistic results when administered with infliximab for CD fistulas. Many gastroenterologists use antibiotic therapy in colonic and perianal CD as adjunctive therapy or as an alternative to steroids. Broad-spectrum antibiotics are also the mainstay of therapy for patients with CD who present with localized peritonitis because of a microperforation or bacterial overgrowth secondary to chronic strictures.

At the opposite end of the bacterial spectrum, probiotics have more recently been used to treat IBD. Probiotics are viable bacteria that induce beneficial therapeutic effects in intestinal mucosa. The rationale is that laboratory studies suggest that a balance between beneficial and aggressive commensal enteric microflora determines mucosal immune response in genetically susceptible individuals. Patients with IBD tend to have higher concentrations of adherent and invasive strains of bacteria such as *Bacteroides*, *Enterococci*, and *Escherichia coli*. The most studied probiotics in controlled trials to date are *Saccharomyces boulardii*, *E. coli Nissle 1917*, *Lactobacillus GG*, and a combination of eight species (*VSL#3*). In CD these randomized controlled trials produced mixed results, with some benefit demonstrated in small trials in maintenance of medically induced remission but no benefit in preventing postoperative recurrence. In ulcerative colitis, *E. coli Nissle 1917* was equal to mesalamine, and *Bifidobacteria*-fermented milk superior to placebo, in maintaining medically induced remission. No randomized controlled trials have been published in obtaining remission in patients with active disease, although a combination of bacteria showed benefit in a recent open trial. The most impressive results to date emerged in treatment of patients with pouchitis, inflammation in the ileo-anal pouch that is constructed after colectomy in patients with ulcerative colitis. *VSL#3*, a combination of eight bacterial species, is superior to placebo in preventing the development of pouchitis after pouch closure and maintaining remission after a treated episode of pouchitis. Thus, at present, the evidence suggests a definite role for probiotics as an alternative to standard therapy in prevention of pouchitis and maintenance of remission in ulcerative colitis. A number of topics in our understanding of probiotics remain to be elucidated, such as their exact anti-inflammatory mechanisms, and which probiotic strains are best suited to which conditions. A more rigorous comparison of different strains to each other and standard therapy is required. An additional approach is to stimulate the growth of an individual's commensal bacteria through dietary substances, such as oligosaccharides, inulin, and psyllium. These so-called prebiotics may tip the balance of enteric growth in favor of *Lactobacilli*, which alter luminal pH and impair invasion of disease-associated species. Some evidence indicates a potential role for this strategy in mild to moderate UC.

EXPERIMENTAL THERAPIES

As with many chronic conditions, IBD treatment still lacks a therapy that can induce high remission rates that are sustained in the long term without significant side effects. In particular, ileal CD and pancolitis that do not respond to standard therapy can prove problematic for clinicians. A high placebo response rate in CD trials (up to 50%) can make it difficult to judge the benefits of novel therapies. In response, molecular approaches targeted against specific inflammatory mediators are used with mixed effects in IBD. These include IL-11 (Oprelvekin [Neumega]),[1] thalidomide,[1] anti-IL12,[*] growth hormone,[1] and bone marrow transplantation. Antibodies against integrins (MLNO2, natalizumab [Tysabri]), which promote translocation of lymphocytes into inflamed mucosa, improve response and remission rates in active IBD. Natalizumab has recently been FDA approved for moderate to severe Crohn's disease in patients who have failed an anti-TNF agent. However, the development of JC virus-related progressive multifocal leukoencephalopathy (PML) in a number of patients treated with natalizumab has raised concerns about anti-integrin therapy at present. MLNO2, which inhibits integrins specific to the gut, may avoid this rare complication. Two alternative approaches include removal of leukocytes using apheresis columns or administration of granulocyte colony-stimulating factor in patients with CD. Although many of these agents demonstrated efficacy in small trials, they are not used routinely in practice or are not licensed for treatment of IBD.

NUTRITIONAL SUPPORT

Patients with IBD tend to have a high prevalence of protein-calorie malnutrition; up to 80% in some series. This tends to develop gradually in patients with small bowel CD but more rapidly in patients with UC during severe attacks. In addition to general malnutrition, specific deficits in calcium, vitamin D, vitamin B_{12}, folate, iron, zinc, and selenium are common in patients with IBD. Calcium/vitamin D depletion, in conjunction with steroid use and chronic inflammation, can lead to osteopenia in 40% to 50% of patients and to osteoporosis in up to 25%. This is associated with a 40% greater relative risk of fractures in these patients. Folate deficiency has an epidemiologic association with colorectal cancer, and supplementation may have a protective effect against dysplasia in ulcerative colitis. Zinc deficiency impairs mucosal healing, especially fistula closure, whereas selenium depletion can lead to cardiomyopathy.

Nutrition in IBD can be divided into general supportive nutrition and nutrition as primary therapy. All patients should be encouraged to maintain a balanced healthy diet without restrictions. Patients with strictures should adhere to a low-residue diet, and patients with overlap irritable bowel syndrome should avoid high-fiber foods. Calcium (1200 mg/day) and vitamin D (800 IU/day) should be taken by all patients if dietary calcium is inadequate. Folate deficiency should be sought and corrected if found. These approaches are yet to be validated in controlled trials. There is a high prevalence of lactose intolerance (40%) in patients with CD, and this should be considered and excluded if diarrhea persists despite minimal inflammatory activity. In patients with malnutrition, enteral nutrition is the preferred option as general nutritional support in most cases. Total parenteral nutrition (TPN) is associated with higher costs, greater length of stay, and more complications than enteral nutrition and should be restricted on a short term to patients with bowel obstruction or perforation, toxic megacolon, preoperatively, or for postoperative fistulas. Rarely home TPN may be required in the longer term for short-bowel syndrome after multiple resections.

Enteral nutrition as primary therapy in CD has been examined in a number of trials since the early 1980s. Systematic review of these trials concluded that enteral nutrition is superior to placebo but inferior to steroids in inducing remission in active Crohn's ileitis. Elemental diets do not appear to differ from nonelemental diets in this regard. The main problem with enteral nutrition is that it can take up to 4 weeks to demonstrate an effect, which can be difficult to comply with for these patients. Additionally, factors such as palatability, motivation, and resources can limit its use in adults. However, it remains a viable option to avoid or reduce steroids in patients with intestinal CD. There are no data to support use of enteral nutrition in ulcerative colitis, but it may be required in patients with severe colitis to supplement calorific intake.

Surgery

In the era of biologic therapy for IBD, surgery still remains an important therapeutic option for patients. In patients with UC, toxic megacolon, fulminant colitis, steroid-refractory disease, high-grade dysplasia, and cancer are all indications for colectomy. Where possible, panproctocolectomy and ileal pouch–anal anastomosis (IPAA) is the procedure of choice. This has a technical success rate of up to 95%, with the advantage of removing the diseased organ and thus cancer

---
[*]Investigational drug in the United States.
[1]Not FDA approved for this indication.

risk. Most patients defecate from six to eight times per day after IPAA because of the lack of colonic reservoir. Postoperative impotence in men and dyspareunia in women occurs in less than 5% of patients. In addition there is a 15% risk per year of pouchitis in the long term, which can be problematic in some patients. Hospitalized patients with severe pancolitis who do not respond to IV steroids within 72 hours should either be referred for surgery or started on cyclosporin (Neoral)[1] or infliximab (Remicade) based on current evidence. It is worthwhile for all patients with refractory UC to meet an experienced colorectal surgeon and ostomy nurse during the course of the illness to prepare them psychologically for possible surgery.

For patients with CD, indications for surgery include strictures, inflammatory collections or abscesses, fistulas, perforation, and neoplasia. Up to 70% of patients require surgery during their lifetime. Those patients who smoke or have NOD2 mutations are more likely to require surgery during the course of their disease because they are more associated with penetrating and/or stricturing disease. Local surgical therapy, such as strictureplasty, seton placement, and limited resection, are preferred in CD because of the high rate of postoperative recurrence; approximately 50% at 5 years. Immunomodulators, such as 6-MP, and 5-ASA appear to reduce this risk and should be offered to all patients postoperatively. In those who have terminal ileum resection, bile salt diarrhea is common postoperatively and can be treated with cholestyramine. Vitamin B_{12} deficiency may occur and should be prevented with regular B_{12} injections or intranasal therapy.

Alternative Therapy

It is recognized that approximately half of all patients with IBD try nonconventional therapies during the course of their illness. The majority of these have not been assessed in randomized controlled trials or even reported in the medical literature. However, there are a number of alternative treatments we recommend to patients with mild to moderate disease who do not wish to advance to immunomodulators or biologic therapy. These are not evidence based but rather experience and anecdote based.

Aloe vera[1] has established healing properties, particularly in skin disorders. A single randomized clinical trial (RCT) in patients with mild to moderate ulcerative colitis reported that oral aloe vera gel for 4 weeks produced a significant clinical and histologic response in a small trial of 44 patients. The dose used was 100 mL of aloe vera gel taken orally per day.

Short-chain fatty acid (SCFA)[1] enemas administered daily show some promise in subsets of patients with proctitis, including those with diversion and radiation proctitis. SCFAs are an important component of mucosal nutrition, hence the rationale for their use. RCTs in ulcerative colitis reported mixed results, but they remain an option in proctitis and distal colitis that is refractory to conventional therapy.

Finally, dietary manipulation, in the form of the "Specific Carbohydrate Diet,"[1] has been used by a number of our patients. This involves minimizing the dietary intake of carbohydrates to monosaccharides, in an attempt to reduce the carbohydrates available for pathogenic gut bacteria. It is a restrictive diet that requires motivation. The efficacy of this dietary manipulation has not been reported in RCTs.

Management Strategies: Ulcerative Colitis

Management of UC depends on the disease geography and severity, based on prior endoscopy and symptoms. The Simple Colitis Activity Index can be used to assess disease severity in the office without laboratory results (Walmsley, 1998).

MILD TO MODERATE DISEASE

Aminosalicylates are the agents of choice for inducing remission in patients with mild to moderate UC. Patients with proctitis obtain the best response with topical therapy such as mesalamine suppositories (Canasa), 1 g once a day, whereas distal disease requires enemas (Rowasa), 4 g per day. Topical therapy is associated with a more rapid clinical response than oral 5-ASAs alone and a greater efficacy than topical steroids. Up to 80% of patients should be in remission by 6 weeks. We advise patients to insert the enema at bedtime to increase its retention. In the event of poor response or difficulty with the rectal route, oral 5-ASAs should be used. In addition, the combination of oral and topical 5-ASA agents produces better clinical results than either alone. Because the topical therapy can take up to 2 weeks to produce a clinical response, topical steroids (Cortifoam) may be used concomitantly for this period in patients who are particularly symptomatic.

In patients with left-sided extensive pancolitis, oral sulfasalazine (Azulfidine), at 2 to 4 g/day, and 5-ASA agents, at 2 to 4.8 g/day[3] should be prescribed because lower doses are not effective in inducing remission. Doses of 5-ASAs up to 4.8 g are usually well tolerated and produce clinical response in 60% of patients by 3 weeks and up to 80% in remission by 8 weeks. The dose used is probably more important than the 5-ASA agent used because there has been little comparison between the agents. Sulfasalazine has similar response rates but at a higher risk of adverse events than the other aminosalicylates, and it should be avoided in men considering fatherhood. It is significantly less expensive than the other 5-ASA agents, however, and thus more cost effective given its low absolute risk of side effects. Once remission is achieved, the same 5-ASA dose should be continued to maintain remission. As many as 90% of patients remain in remission at 1 year. Other than steroids, little evidence supports other therapies in mild to moderate disease; antibiotics, probiotics, or aloe gel may be tried in patients who cannot tolerate 5-ASAs.

SEVERE DISEASE

Approximately 9% of patients present with severely active disease, requiring supplementary therapy to 5-ASAs. It is worth excluding surreptitious NSAID use, concomitant infection by stool culture, and 5-ASA intolerance, prior to proceeding to more potent agents. In particular, *Clostridium difficile* infection in those recently hospitalized or on antibiotics, and CMV infection in those receiving steroids can cause severe colitis.

The mainstay of induction of remission in severe disease is an oral steroid. Prednisone at a dose of 40 to 60 mg/day is highly effective in inducing remission in patients with moderate to severe disease. Approximately 80% of patients respond, and 54% are in remission at 1 month. No studies have compared the efficacy of oral to IV administration. Hydrocortisone (Solu-Cortef), at 100 mg IV every 6 hours, or methylprednisolone (Solu-Medrol), 40 mg/day IV, can be used in the few patients who do not respond or have difficulty with oral absorption. Hyperglycemia occurs commonly and should be monitored for, especially in those receiving IV steroids. In those patients who respond to steroids, the aim should be to begin a steroid taper after approximately 2 weeks of high-dose therapy. The dose should be reduced by 5 mg weekly until either the steroids are withdrawn or the patient develops recurrence of symptoms. If patients are not already on 5-ASAs, they should be started during the steroid taper as maintenance therapy. If patients cannot be withdrawn from steroid therapy because of recurrence of symptoms (steroid dependent), azathioprine (Imuran, Azasan),[1] at a dose of 1.5 to 2.5 mg/kg, or 6-MP (Purinethol),[1] at a dose of 1.5 mg/kg, should be started as maintenance therapy. As discussed previously, it may take 12 weeks for full effect, and patients should have their AST, ALT, and CBC checked regularly for adverse effects. The strategy here is to remove the steroids gradually as the therapeutic effect of azathioprine/6-MP

---

[1]Not FDA approved for this indication.

[3]Exceeds dosage recommended by the manufacturer.
[1]Not FDA approved for this indication.

manifests. Once in remission, treatment should continue indefinitely because patients who later have their maintenance drugs stopped have a higher rate of relapse. These agents can be used for induction of remission also, but the long time to clinical effect is usually too long when patients have severe disease.

In those cases with severe colitis where steroids do not induce a clinical response, the options then are cyclosporine (Neoral),[1]b infliximab (Remicade), or surgery at present. Steroids are usually given for 72 hours to determine their response before proceeding to these options, although surgery is indicated sooner for toxic megacolon, fulminant colitis, or hemorrhage. One study demonstrated that those patients with a bowel frequency of more than eight times per day or a CRP greater than 45 have an 85% chance of colectomy after 3 days of medical therapy. Cyclosporine,[1] at a dose of 2 to 4 mg/kg/day by infusion, produces a response in up to 80% of patients after 8 days of therapy. Recent data suggest the response from 2 mg/kg is similar to 4 mg/kg with less adverse events. Renal function, blood pressure, magnesium levels, cholesterol, and cyclosporine levels should be monitored during treatment. Magnesium less than 0.5 mg/dL or a cholesterol level less than 120 mg/dL increases the risk of seizures. Opportunistic infections such as *Pneumocystis* pneumonia (PCP) and *Aspergillus* should be considered if patients develop respiratory symptoms. We routinely prescribe prophylaxis against PCP with sulfamethoxazole/trimethoprim (Bactrim) because deaths from this infection are reported in patients receiving cyclosporine for ulcerative colitis. Patients usually respond within 4 days of treatment; in this case they can be switched to oral cyclosporine[1] at a dose of 5 to 7 mg/kg/day, with maintenance of serum trough levels between 150 and 250 µg/mL.

The other medical option is infliximab (Remicade) at a dose of 5 mg/kg by IV infusion. In patients with severe ulcerative colitis who are hospitalized, this halves the risk of colectomy at 90 days. For patients with moderate to severe UC, infliximab produces response in 65% and puts approximately 30% of patients into remission at 30 weeks if given at 0, 2, 6 weeks, and at 8 weeks thereafter. The precautions and side effects are similar to its use in CD. All patients should have a PPD and chest radiograph (CXR) prior to instigation of therapy, and infusion reactions can be prevented with prednisone or IV hydrocortisone. No comparison between cyclosporine and infliximab has been made in these patients to date. If these medical options do not improve individual cases, surgery will be required.

Management Strategy: Crohn's Disease

At any one time, approximately 50% of patients with CD will be in remission or have mild disease that is responsive to therapy. Of the rest, 40% will be postsurgery and 10% will have severe or treatment-refractory disease.

MILD TO MODERATE DISEASE

In patients with ileocolonic disease, there are three initial treatment options: antibiotics, 5-ASAs, or budesonide (Entocort EC). Evidence from clinical trials and clinical experience differs as to which agent to use, but all three show moderate efficacy in this setting. There is significant controversy among IBD experts about which agent should be used as first-line therapy. We generally use mesalamine (Asacol, Pentasa, Salofalk) first for ileal disease, followed by ciprofloxacin (Cipro) or metronidazole (Flagyl) in nonresponders. For ileocolonic disease we use sulfasalazine (Azulfidine) as first-line therapy, followed by the other 5-ASAs. Other experts in the field start with budesonide (Entocort EC), whereas we reserve this for nonresponders to initial therapy.

Metronidazole, at doses of 500 mg three times daily, and ciprofloxacin, at 500 mg twice daily, produce a moderate clinical response in patients with ileal and colonic disease and more marked improvements in those with perianal disease. Therapy should continue for at least 3 months to maximize the therapeutic benefit, and the development of paresthesia should warrant dose reduction or discon-tinuation of metronidazole. Patients on ciprofloxacin should be warned about the risk of tendon rupture. In the event of a partial response to one agent, the combination of metronidazole and ciprofloxacin is often used prior to proceeding to steroids. Antibiotic resistance does not seem to be a problem in our practice, despite prolonged therapy.

Budesonide (Entocort EC), at 3 mg three times daily, is as effective as prednisone and superior to mesalamine with fewer side effects in ileitis and ileocolonic disease. Patients who respond may be continued at a maintenance dose of 6 mg/day because this reduces relapse rates. For colonic disease, 5-ASAs are first-line therapy in CD. Mesalamine at 4 g/day or sulfasalazine (Azulfidine) at 3 g/day produces a clinical response in 50% to 60% of patients. This response takes up to 2 weeks to develop and requires adequate doses of 5-ASA. The role of 5-ASAs in maintaining remission once achieved is controversial, although probably worthwhile if patients have responded. Regardless of which agent is used to induce remission, if therapy cannot be tapered without worsening of symptoms, immunomodulator therapy should be initiated. Azathioprine (Imuran[1]), 6-MP (Purinethol[1]), and methotrexate[1] should be started in this setting.

SEVERE DISEASE

The selection of more aggressive therapy for CD should be individualized for each patient because this area is rapidly evolving. As in UC, oral steroids are highly effective first-line therapy for severe CD. Approximately 60% to 80% of cases respond to prednisone, 40 to 60 mg/day, and this should be tapered once the clinical status stabilizes. In this setting, azathioprine,[1] 1.5 to 2.5 mg/kg, or 6-MP,[1] 1.5 mg/kg, may be started during the steroid taper period or withheld until further episodes. Patients treated with immunomodulator maintenance therapy have a reduced risk of relapse in the medium term.

If patients do not respond to steroids, or they are concerned about their adverse effects, the next options are infliximab or methotrexate. Infliximab should be administered at a dose of 5 mg/kg at 0, 2 and 6 weeks initially. Patients usually notice a response within 1 to 2 weeks in the 60% of patients who respond. The development of infusion-related reactions can be prevented on subsequent doses by slowing the rate of infusion or administering prednisone, 50 mg twice daily, on the day before administration, or hydrocortisone, 200 mg IV, prior to the infusion. In those who respond to infliximab, repeated infusions every 8 weeks maintain approximately 30% to 40% in remission in the medium term. If this response wanes with time, either increase the dose to 10 mg/kg or shorten the duration between infusions. It is debatable whether the addition of azathioprine[1] or 6-MP[1] to infliximab produces major benefits in clinical efficacy, but it may increase the risk of adverse effects of immunosuppression. The addition of adalimumab (Humira) and certolizumab (Cimzia) provides alternatives to infliximab, or options for those who fail infliximab therapy. In addition, netalizumab (Tysabri) is also an option for patients who failed anti-TNF agents.

An alternative to infliximab in steroid-refractory disease is methotrexate.[1] Induction of remission with 25 mg IM weekly, followed by 15 mg IM weekly, induced remission in approximately 40% of patients treated and maintained 65% in remission in clinical trials at 1 year. All patients should have their AST/ALT and CBC monitored and take folic acid supplementation. This therapy is teratogenic so should be discussed prior to its use in women of child-bearing age or women intending to conceive.

Strictures that do not respond to medical therapy require surgical intervention because some of these will be "cold" stenotic strictures without mucosa inflammation. Draining fistulas are primarily treated with antibiotics as above or infliximab with azathioprine[1]/6-MP[1] in more resistant cases. Deep perianal fistulas can be treated with seton placement and superficial ones with fistulotomy.

---

[1]Not FDA approved for this indication.

Pregnancy

Pregnancy often raises questions about both pregnancy and disease outcomes and about drug therapy for women with IBD. There is a small increased risk of low birth weight and premature delivery in women with IBD, especially those with CD. The risk of a child of an affected parent developing UC is 2% to 5% and developing CD is 5% to 10% over their lifetime. Patients in remission at the time of conception are no more likely to develop a relapse than at other times of life, although if this occurs it is most often in the first trimester. Many cases of relapse in disease activity are actually because of discontinuation of maintenance therapy once the pregnancy is confirmed. In general, patients in remission with IBD have better pregnancy outcomes than those with active disease; therefore continuation of suitable maintenance medications is important in this setting. Apart from methotrexate, most drugs used for management of IBD can safely be used during pregnancy. This includes 5-ASAs, steroids, azathioprine,[1] 6-MP,[1] cyclosporine,[1] infliximab, and metronidazole (after the first trimester). As with all drugs, the benefits need to be weighed against potential adverse effects that are unknown. Drugs that should be avoided if possible during breast-feeding include olsalazine (Dipentum), azathioprine1/6-MP,[1] methotrexate,[1] cyclosporine,[1] and infliximab[1] if possible. Apart from the 5-ASA agents and steroids, there is little experience documented in breast-feeding with these drugs; women in this situation should consult with their pediatrician.

Colon Cancer Surveillance

The risk of colorectal cancer (CRC) is increased in patients who have colitis for greater than 8 years; the excess risk is 19.2 for those with pancolitis and 2.8 for those with left-sided disease. At 20 years since onset of diagnosis, patients have an 8% risk of cancer. In particular, patients with primary sclerosing cholangitis and UC have a 31% risk of CRC at 20 years.

Surveillance for CRC should begin at 8 years after diagnosis for patients with disease beyond the descending colon and continue every 2 years. In patients with distal colitis and Crohn's colitis, the ideal surveillance intervals are more difficult to determine because the risk may not be similar to more extensive colitis. Our personal practice is to perform surveillance on all those with UC above the rectum or extensive colonic CD after 8 years of disease. Because of the higher risk of CRC, all patients with primary sclerosing cholangitis should have surveillance regardless of their duration of UC or CD. Those patients in whom dysplasia or adenomas are detected require more intensive surveillance or consideration of colectomy. The finding of high-grade dysplasia or dysplasia-associated lesion or mass (DALM) is an indication for colectomy. However, when low-grade dysplasia is found, the risk of neoplasia progression is controversial, varying between 5% and 50%. We most often recommend colectomy for patients with long-standing colitis and low-grade dysplasia.

In those at high risk of CRC (e.g., family history of CRC, long disease history, primary sclerosing cholangitis [PSC], extensive colitis), chemoprophylaxis should be advised. 5-ASA at doses of 1.5 to 2 g/day in some case-control studies reduced CRC risk by at least 50%. Folic acid supplements, calcium, and NSAIDs such as aspirin reduce the risk of CRC in the general population. It is not known whether a combination of these produces an additive benefit, and they have not specifically been studied in IBD.

REFERENCES

Aberra FN, Lichtenstein GR: Review article: Monitoring of immunomodulators in inflammatory bowel disease. Aliment Pharmacol Ther 2005;21:307-319.

Banerjee S, Peppercorn MA: Inflammatory bowel disease. Medical therapy of specific clinical presentations. Gastroenterol Clin North Am 2002;31:185-202.

Campieri M: New steroids and new salicylates in inflammatory bowel disease: A critical appraisal. Gut 2002;50(Suppl 3):III43-III46.

Farrell RJ, Peppercorn MA: Ulcerative colitis. Lancet 2002;359:331-340.

Ferrero S, Ragni N: Inflammatory bowel disease: Management issues during pregnancy. Arch Gynecol Obstet 2004;270:79-85.

Hanauer SB, Korelitz BI, Rutgeerts P: Postoperative maintenance of Crohn's disease remission with 6-mercaptopurine, mesalamine, or placebo: A 2-year trial. Gastroenterology 2004;127:723-729.

Jain SK, Peppercorn MA: Inflammatory bowel disease and colon cancer: A review. Dig Dis 1997;15:243-252.

Loftus EV Jr, Schoenfeld P, Sandborn WJ: The epidemiology and natural history of Crohn's disease in population-based patient cohorts from North America: A systematic review. Aliment Pharmacol Ther 2002;16:51-60.

Rutgeerts P, Van AG, Vermeire S: Optimizing anti-TNF treatment in inflammatory bowel disease. Gastroenterology 2004;126:1593-1610.

Thukral C, Travassos WJ, Peppercorn MA: The role of antibiotics in inflammatory bowel disease. Curr Treat Options Gastroenterol 2005;8:223-228.

Velayos FS, Terdiman JP, Walsh JM: Effect of 5-aminosalicylate use on colorectal cancer and dysplasia risk: A systematic review and metaanalysis of observational studies. Am J Gastroenterol 2005;100:1345-1353.

Walmsley RS, Ayres RC, Pounder RE, Allan RN: A simple clinical colitis activity index. Gut 1998;43:29-32.

Irritable Bowel Syndrome

Method of
Michael D. Crowell, PhD, John K. DiBaise, MD, and Lucinda A. Harris, MD

Irritable bowel syndrome (IBS), the most common of the functional gastrointestinal (GI) disorders, is characterized by chronic episodic abdominal pain or discomfort associated with altered bowel function. The alteration in bowel function can include constipation, diarrhea, or both. IBS is defined by symptoms because there are no known structural, mechanical, or biochemical abnormalities.

The most recent diagnostic criteria proposed by the Rome III international working group on functional GI disorders are presented in Box 1. Although these diagnostic criteria can be used clinically, they have most commonly been used in the setting of patient-oriented research studies in an attempt to select a more homogeneous study population. The Rome III criteria proposed to classify patients, based on stool characteristics, as having IBS with constipation (IBS-C), IBS with diarrhea (IBS-D), IBS mixed type (IBS-M), or IBS unsubtyped (IBS-U) (Box 2).

Because perceptions of diarrhea and constipation differ substantially among patients and clinicians, determination of stool consistency using a scale such as the Bristol stool form scale (Fig. 1) is advocated by the criteria as a more reliable method of classifying IBS patients' bowel function. Subclassification of these patients has been important because treatments have traditionally targeted the predominant symptoms in IBS.

Epidemiology

In North America, IBS has been reported in up to 20% of the population. However, IBS is not just a Western disease, and similar prevalence rates have been demonstrated throughout the world. IBS usually manifests in early adulthood, has an approximate 2:1 female predominance, and has been reported in a primary care setting. The prevalence of IBS among whites, African Americans, and Latin Americans appears to be very similar.

Although most IBS patients do not seek medical attention, health care visits related to IBS still represent a substantial portion of visits to primary care providers and gastroenterologists, accounting for approximately 12% of primary care clinic visits and up to 28% of gastroenterology visits in the United States. IBS sufferers experience a threefold increase in absences from work and undergo more frequent medical testing and abdominal surgery than do patients without IBS. As a consequence, considerable costs, both direct and indirect, are associated with IBS.

> **BOX 1 Diagnosis of Irritable Bowel Syndrome: The Rome III Diagnostic Criteria***
>
> Recurrent abdominal pain or discomfort[†] at least 3 days per month in the last 3 months associated with two or all of the following:
> - Improvement with defecation
> - Onset associated with a change in frequency of stool
> - Onset associated with a change in form (appearance) of stool
>
> Other symptoms that are not essential but support the diagnosis of IBS:
> - Abnormal stool frequency (more than three bowel movements a day or less than three bowel movements per week)
> - Abnormal stool form (lumpy/hard or loose/watery stool)
> - Abnormal stool passage (straining, urgency, or feeling of incomplete bowel movement)
> - Passage of mucus
> - Bloating or feeling of abdominal distention
>
> *Criteria fulfilled for the last 3 months with symptom onset at least 6 months prior to diagnosis.
> [†]"Discomfort" means an uncomfortable sensation not described as pain.

A variety of non-GI somatic complaints such as chronic fatigue, myalgia, sleep disturbance, headache, dysuria, and sexual dysfunction often coexist in IBS patients. Consequently, IBS is commonly associated with comorbid conditions such as fibromyalgia, chronic fatigue syndrome, interstitial cystitis, migraine headaches, and other pain syndromes. Anxiety and depression occur more commonly in IBS patients, particularly as the severity of symptoms worsens. As a result of the GI and non-GI symptoms and psychological comorbidity, a number of studies have demonstrated impaired quality of life in patients with IBS. A history of abuse, sexual, physical, or both, has been associated with severe symptoms of IBS and is more commonly seen in patients referred to tertiary IBS clinics.

> **BOX 2 Subtypes of Irritable Bowel Syndrome by Predominant Stool Pattern**
>
> **IBS-C**
> IBS with constipation: Hard or lumpy stools ≥ 25% and loose (mushy) or watery stools < 25% of bowel movements, in the absence of antidiarrheals or laxatives
>
> **IBS-D**
> IBS with diarrhea: Loose (mushy) or watery stools ≥ 25% and hard or lumpy stools < 25% of bowel movements, in the absence of antidiarrheals or laxatives
>
> **IBS-M**
> Mixed IBS: Hard or lumpy stools ≥ 25% and loose (mushy) or watery stools ≥ 25% of bowel movements, in the absence of antidiarrheals or laxatives
>
> **IBS-U**
> Unsubtyped IBS: Insufficient abnormality of stool consistency to meet criteria for IBS-C, IBS-D, or IBS-M
>
> IBS = irritable towel syndrome.

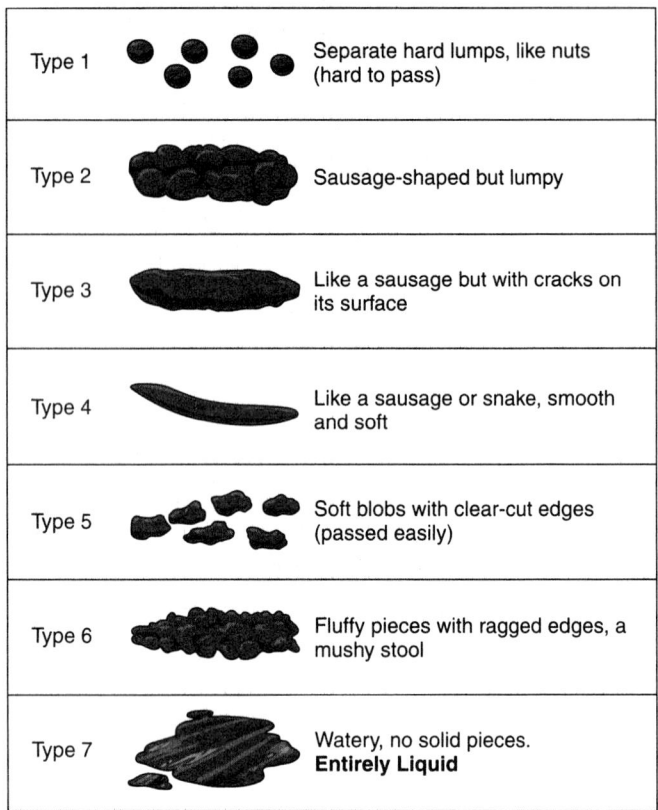

FIGURE 1. Perceptions of diarrhea and constipation differ substantially among patients and clinicians. A scale such as the Bristol stool form scale can help determine stool consistency.

The overall prognosis of IBS is good. No studies have demonstrated significant morbidity or mortality over the long term in IBS patients. In contrast, although symptoms can improve over time, they rarely resolve completely in patients with IBS, and overlap with other functional GI disorders (e.g., functional dyspepsia) is common.

Pathogenesis

Although progress has been made in understanding its pathophysiology, the cause(s) of IBS remain(s) unclear and continue to evolve. Important mechanisms responsible for IBS symptoms that have been described include abnormalities of GI sensation (e.g., visceral hypersensitivity), altered motor function, and dysregulation of brain–gut interactions including the autonomic nervous system and the hypothalamic–pituitary–adrenal axis. However, none of these abnormalities is present in all IBS patients, and it is likely that multiple factors play a role in generating symptoms in individual patients. A number of factors have been implicated in the development of the physiologic alterations noted earlier and include genetic predisposition, environment, stress, food intolerances, psychological conditions, low-grade intestinal mucosal inflammation, and GI infection or dysbiosis.

Recent advances in the development of pharmacologic therapies for IBS have resulted in a better understanding of the role that serotonin and other neurohumoral mechanisms play in modulating intestinal function. These findings have led to increased research into the role of specific hormones and receptors that might prove effective for treating IBS including neurokinins, corticotrophin releasing factors, opioids, and epithelial chloride channel activators.

BOX 3 Alarm Symptoms in Irritable Bowel Syndrome*

Anemia
Positive fecal occult blood tests
Hematochezia
Weight loss of ≥10 lb
Family history of colon cancer or inflammatory bowel disease
Recurring fever
Chronic severe diarrhea

*Might not represent a complete list of symptoms.

Diagnosis

IBS should no longer be considered a diagnosis of exclusion. A symptom-based diagnostic approach (e.g., Rome criteria) together with a thorough history and physical examination to assess for alarm symptoms (Box 3) and selected tests to exclude organic disease are effective and rarely result in missed IBS diagnoses. In the absence of alarm symptoms, the Rome criteria have been shown to be reasonably sensitive and specific for the diagnosis of IBS. The presence of alarm symptoms, however, should prompt further investigation. Other conditions to consider in the differential diagnosis of IBS include inflammatory bowel diseases, malabsorptive processes (e.g., celiac disease, small intestinal bacterial overgrowth), intestinal infections, food intolerances (e.g., lactose, fructose, fat), neoplasms, intestinal obstruction, eosinophilic gastroenteritis, and endometriosis, to name just a few.

CURRENT DIAGNOSIS

- Take a symptom-based diagnostic approach rather than assuming that IBS is a diagnosis of exclusion.
- Use Rome III criteria to diagnose IBS (see Box 1) and define stool consistency (see Box 2).
- Rule out alarm symptoms (see Box 3).

IBS = irritable bowel syndrome.

The American College of Gastroenterology (ACG) Functional Gastrointestinal Disorder Task Force issued a position statement on the diagnosis of IBS. It recommended that the diagnostic work-up of patients with IBS be limited in patients younger than 50 years and without the presence of alarm symptoms. For those aged 50 years or older, it was recommended that standard screening guidelines for colorectal cancer be followed. In patients with IBS-D, serologic testing for celiac disease was suggested as reasonable given a higher likelihood of celiac disease in IBS-D patients compared with the general population. The routine use of endoscopic procedures, radiologic imaging, stool studies, complete blood count, erythrocyte sedimentation rate, and thyroid function testing was not recommended. The current recommendations for the diagnosis of IBS do not support extensive testing in patients who meet the symptom-based criteria for IBS and do not present with alarm features. A symptom-based diagnostic algorithm for IBS is presented in Figure 2.

Treatment

Once a confident diagnosis of IBS has been made, it is essential to provide a basic level of education to the patient about the syndrome

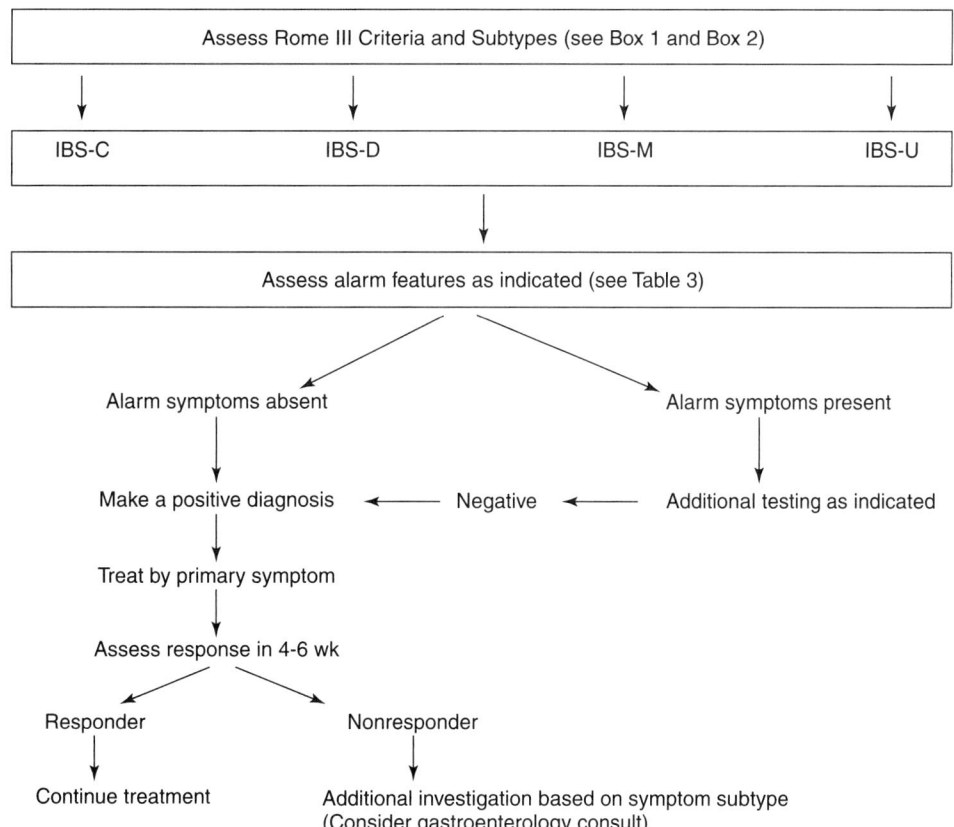

FIGURE 2. A symptom-based diagnostic algorithm for irritable bowel syndrome (IBS). IBS-C = IBS with constipation; IBS-D = IBS with diarrhea; IBS-M = IBS mixed type; IBS-U = IBS unsubtyped.

CURRENT THERAPY

- Reassurance and education are the basis of an effective doctor–patient relationship.
- Set realistic goals and expectations of therapy.
- Direct therapy to symptoms and severity with a goal toward global improvement.
- Treat comorbid psychiatric diagnoses.

and the treatments used. Careful reassurance regarding the diagnosis and prognosis and establishing an effective patient–physician relationship with realistic goals and expectations and regular clinic follow-up are critical to the successful management of the IBS patient, particularly those with more severe symptoms. Treatments may include self-care and lifestyle management and physician-directed options. These options include dietary changes, over-the-counter medications, prescription medications, and behavioral interventions; however, the evidence of benefit from these options varies widely.

The pharmacologic management of IBS has traditionally focused on specific symptoms such as diarrhea, constipation, and pain. The ACG Task Force recently reported the evidence relating to the therapeutic effectiveness of currently available IBS treatments based on the quality of trial evidence (Grade A, B, or C). Although traditional IBS interventions such as antispasmodic agents, bulking agents, loperamide (Imodium), and antidepressants[1] might improve individual symptoms such as constipation, diarrhea, and pain, they found very limited data supporting their usefulness in terms of improving the multiple symptoms of IBS (Table 1). In addition, the benefit of these agents is particularly inadequate as the severity of symptoms worsens. These agents also can have adverse effects such as bloating, gas, and abdominal discomfort that can further exacerbate IBS symptoms. Indeed, recent evidence suggests that although these therapies are commonly used to treat IBS, the vast majority of IBS patients are not satisfied with these treatments.

A variety of behavioral interventions have been evaluated in the treatment of IBS including relaxation therapy to relieve stress, biofeedback regulation of bowel habits, hypnotherapy directed at intestinal muscle contraction, cognitive behavior therapy, and psychotherapy. Behavioral treatments have been shown to be more effective than placebo at relieving individual symptoms of IBS; however, few quality randomized, controlled trials have been completed in this area. As a result, behavioral therapies received a Grade B recommendation based on available evidence from the ACG Task Force.

Despite the focus of traditional therapies on relief of individual symptoms, the Rome working groups, the American Gastroenterological Association and the ACG have all agreed that the most important measures of efficacy in IBS should be relief of multiple IBS symptoms and improvement in overall well-being. Recent pathophysiologic insights have led to the development of agents that improve multiple symptoms.

Serotonin is an important mediator of multiple GI functions including intestinal motility, sensation, and secretion. Serotonin receptor subtype agonists and antagonists have, to date, demonstrated the greatest benefit and thus the strongest recommendations based on the findings of several randomized, placebo-controlled trials. Primary serotonin receptor subtypes studied have included $5\text{-}HT_3$, $5\text{-}HT_{1A}$, $5\text{-}HT_4$, and $5\text{-}HT_{2B}$. Serotoninergic drugs that affect mixed receptor sites are also under investigation, but none is currently approved for treating IBS. Both SSRIs and newer antidepressant agents that block the reuptake of both serotonin and norepinephrine (SNRIs) are an emerging area of interest. Some of the SSRIs have been shown in small trials to improve abdominal pain, bloating, and impact of IBS symptoms on daily life independent of any effect on anxiety or depression. Larger, more rigorous trials are thought to be indicated.

Recent evidence suggests that SNRIs can reduce colonic sensation and alter colonic tone. Tegaserod (Zelnorm; Novartis), a $5HT_4$ receptor partial agonist, has been shown to be more effective than placebo at relieving global IBS symptoms in female IBS patients with constipation and received a Grade A recommendation from the ACG Task Force. Alosetron (Lotronex), a $5HT_3$ receptor antagonist, has also been demonstrated to be more effective than placebo at relieving global IBS symptoms in female IBS patients with diarrhea and received a Grade A recommendation. However, marketing of both of these compounds was halted in the United States because of

---

[1]Not FDA approved for this indication.

TABLE 1 American College Of Gastroenterology Task Force Ratings Of Traditional Therapies in Irritable Bowel Syndrome

Therapy	Drug/Treatment	Grade	Comments
Antispasmodic agents	Hyoscyamine (Levsin) Dicyclomine (Bentyl)	B	Only one of three studies meeting the required standards showed a statistically significant benefit on global IBS symptoms At high doses, antispasmodics can produce atropine-like side-effects
Bulking agents	Wheat bran, corn fiber, calcium polycarbophil, psyllium (Metamucil) Ispaghula husk	B	Zero of 13 trials had adequate methodology Evidence of benefit from ispaghula husk was slight, if any The conclusion: fiber is appropriate for treatment of constipation but may not be recommended for treatment of IBS
Antidepressants	TCAs:[1] Nortriptyline (Pamelor), desipramine (Norpramin), amitriptyline (Elavil), doxepin (Sinequan) SSRIs:[1] Fluoxetine (Prozac), paroxetine (Paxil)	B	TCAs are not more effective than placebo at relieving global IBS symptoms, but they do improve abdominal pain The effectiveness of SSRIs in IBS has not yet been fully documented
Antidiarrheal agents	Loperamide (Imodium, lomotil[1])	B	Loperimide: Three acceptable trials in IBS patients with diarrhea Diphenoxylate: Stool frequency and stool consistency were improved, but bloating and abdominal pain were unaffected
Behavioral therapy	Relaxation therapy, biofeedback, hypnotherapy, cognitive therapy, and psychotherapy	B	In 11/16 studies IBS symptoms were significantly improved, compared with control groups; five showed no significant improvements

[1]Not FDA approved for this indication.
IBS = irritable bowel syndrome; SSRI = selective serotonin reuptake inhibitor; TCA = tricyclic antidepressant.

concerns about serious adverse events in some patients. The FDA has now permitted restricted marketing of alosetron for treating "women with severe, diarrhea-predominant IBS who have failed to respond to conventional IBS therapy." A number of investigational compounds with different mechanisms of action targeted at a variety of receptor sites are currently being evaluated.

Considerable interest has developed regarding the potential role of intestinal infection (e.g., postinfectious IBS) and the intestinal microflora (e.g., small intestinal bacterial overgrowth) in the pathogenesis of IBS and modulation of the gut flora as a possible treatment. Encouraging results have been demonstrated in controlled studies using antibiotics and probiotics in patients with IBS; however, these studies are limited by differences in study design, outcome measures, antibiotics used, and probiotic strains, doses, and delivery, making a definitive statement regarding their clinical usefulness impossible at this time.

Conclusion

Irritable bowel syndrome, the prototypic functional GI disorder, is a common chronic disorder that is associated with considerable disability and cost. Although progress has been made in understanding its pathophysiology, the causes of IBS remain unclear and continue to evolve. A symptom-based diagnostic approach with selected tests to exclude organic disease is effective and rarely results in missed diagnoses. Although treatment remains largely aimed at individual symptoms, recent pathophysiologic insights have led to the development of agents that can improve multiple symptoms. It is only with a clearer understanding of the pathophysiologic disturbances involved that more effective treatments will be developed.

REFERENCES

American College of Gastroenterology Functional Gastrointestinal Disorders Task Force: Evidence-based position statement on the management of irritable bowel syndrome in North America. Am J Gastroenterol 2002;97(11 Suppl):S1-S5.

Brandt LJ, Bjorkman D, Fennerty MB, et al: Systematic review on the management of irritable bowel syndrome in North America. Am J Gastroenterol 2002;97:S7-S26.

Camilleri M, Talley NJ: Pathophysiology as a basis for understanding symptom complexes and therapeutic targets. Neurogastroenterol Motil 2004;16(2):135-142.

Cash BD, Schoenfeld PS, Chey WD: The utility of diagnostic tests in irritable bowel syndrome patients: A systematic review. Am J Gastroenterol 2002;97:2812-2819.

Crowell MD: The role of serotonin in the pathophysiology of irritable bowel syndrome. Am J Manag Care 2001;7(Suppl):S252-S260.

Drossman DA, Camilleri M, Mayer EA, Whitehead WE: AGA technical review on irritable bowel syndrome. Gastroenterology 2002;123:2108-2131.

Longstreth GF, Thompson WG, Chey WD, et al: Functional bowel disorders. Gastroenterology 2006;130:1480-1491.

Ownevs DM, Nelson DK, Talley NJ: The irritable bowel syndrome: Long-term prognosis and the physician–patient interaction. Ann Intern Med 1995;122:107-112.

Vanner SJ, Depew WT, Paterson WG, et al: Predictive value of the Rome criteria for diagnosing the irritable bowel syndrome. Am J Gastroenterol 1999;94:2803-2807.

Hemorrhoids, Anal Fissure, and Anorectal Abscess and Fistula

Method of
Neil H. Hyman, MD

Anal canal diseases such as hemorrhoids, anal fissures, anorectal abscesses, and fistulas are very common. Although these conditions seldom cause life-threatening complications, they are a major cause of patient discomfort, morbidity, and diminished quality of life. Because most anorectal disorders are diagnosed and treated in the outpatient setting, physicians receive little exposure to them during their medical training. Further, relatively little attention is given to anorectal disease in most medical and surgical textbooks. Therefore, misperceptions and misdiagnoses are extremely common, leading to considerable unnecessary suffering.

The vast majority of the time, the diagnosis is readily made based on the patient's symptoms. An accurate history is the key to appropriate diagnosis and successful management.

History

Patients most often ascribe any perianal symptom to a "hemorrhoid" problem. When using this term, the patient might mean that there is a palpable perianal lesion, anal itching, pain, rectal bleeding, or abnormal discharge, to name a few common anorectal symptoms. However, the correct diagnosis and treatment often are unrelated to hemorrhoidal disease.

Two of the most common complaints are pain and bleeding (Table 1). Pain that occurs with defecation, often associated with bright red blood on the toilet tissue, is typical for an anal fissure. Constant pain of acute onset is most often caused by a thrombosed external hemorrhoid or a perianal abscess. Anal outlet bleeding is characterized by bright red blood that appears on the toilet tissue or perhaps drips into the toilet water. This type of bleeding associated with pain on defecation strongly suggests an anal fissure. Painless bleeding of this type is typical for internal hemorrhoids.

Physical Examination

An accurate patient history is usually sufficient to make the diagnosis. The physical examination is usually confirmatory, especially when a patient is having pain and only a brief physical examination is possible. The practitioner needs to know what he or she is looking for.

Hemorrhoids

The anal cushions consist of redundant rectal mucosa, arterioles, venules, and arteriovenous malformations that are supported by elastic connective tissue and smooth muscle fibers. These can be found in all patients, classically in the right anterior, right posterior, and left lateral position. In this light, hemorrhoids really are normal anatomic structures. When there is weakening of the supportive tissue and these cushions prolapse, or there is erosion into the submucosal vascular plexus and there is bleeding, one uses the term *hemorrhoids*.

Internal hemorrhoids occur above the dentate line, where there is typically columnar or transitional epithelium. Common symptoms include prolapse or bleeding. Internal hemorrhoids are typically classified on the basis of the degree of prolapse (Table 2).

The external hemorrhoidal plexuses lie below the dentate line and are prone to thrombosis. Perianal skin tags are often called external hemorrhoids. Numerous symptoms are often ascribed to these skin tags because they are readily apparent to the patient. Most often,

TABLE 1 Differential Diagnosis of Anal Lesions

Lesion	Pain	Bleeding
Anal fissure	With defecation	Yes
Internal hemorrhoids	Usually not	Yes
Thrombosed external hemorrhoid	Constant	Only if ulcerated
Perianal abscess	Constant	Mixed with pus

TABLE 2 Classification of Internal Hemorrhoids

Grade	Physical Findings
I	Prominent hemorrhoidal vessels, no prolapse
II	Prolapse with Valsalva and spontaneous reduction
III	Prolapse with Valsalva, requires manual reduction
IV	Chronically prolapsed, manual reduction ineffective

these skin tags are an incidental finding and not the cause of the patient's symptoms.

EVALUATION

A targeted history and physical examination is the most important determinant of the need for further evaluation and treatment. Painless bleeding is a common symptom from internal hemorrhoids. Physical examination should typically include visual inspection of the anal canal, a digital rectal examination, and often anoscopy. Generally speaking, patients older than 50 years, those with a family history of colorectal neoplasm, and those with more worrisome symptoms (e.g., blood mixed in with the stool, change in stool caliber, abdominal pain) typically require full colonic evaluation with colonoscopy. Most other patients require at most a flexible sigmoidoscopy to evaluate their bleeding. Colonoscopy does not cure bleeding hemorrhoids!

External hemorrhoids or skin tags are usually an innocent finding. However, external hemorrhoids can cause pain owing to acute thrombosis or can present anal hygiene problems when stool collects on them, making cleansing difficult. Although anal itching is often ascribed to the skin tags, the tags are usually the result of irritation and scratching rather than the cause.

TREATMENT

Dietary management consisting of adequate fluid and fiber supplementation is the primary treatment for most patients with hemorrhoids. Patients should also be instructed to avoid excessive straining during defecation.

Patients with significant prolapse (typically grade 3 or 4) require a more aggressive treatment modality. The vast majority can be treated with office-based procedures such as hemorrhoid banding. The aim of these treatments is to decrease vascularity, diminish hemorrhoidal volume, and increase fixation of the fibrovascular cushion to the rectal wall. Rubber band ligation has been associated with a 65% to 85% success rate but often requires repeating. Surgical hemorrhoidectomy should be reserved for patients whose hemorrhoids are refractory to less-invasive procedures, patients who are unable to tolerate office-based procedures, and patients with large combined internal and external hemorrhoids.

Thrombosed external hemorrhoids may be treated conservatively with sitz baths, avoidance of constipation, and analgesics. However, if the pain is increasing or excessive, or conservative management fails, then excision is warranted. Thrombosed external hemorrhoids should be excised, and simple enucleation of the clot is generally inadequate. The most painful aspect of the treatment is the injection of local anesthesia; excising the hemorrhoid does not increase the morbidity. Simple enucleation of the clot often leads to repeat thrombosis within the next 24 to 48 hours. Large skin tags that create significant hygiene problems can also be readily excised on an outpatient basis with local anesthesia.

Anal Fissures

An anal fissure is a crack or tear in the richly innervated squamous lining of the anal canal between the anal verge and the dentate line. The classic symptoms are ripping or tearing with defecation, which is associated with blood on the toilet tissue. Patients often feel like they are passing glass or sharp objects in their stool and have a sensation that the anal canal is too small to allow passage of the stool. Anal fissures can be agonizingly painful. They are commonly associated with extremes of bowel function such as excessively hard and large stools or frequent diarrhea, which abrades the anoderm.

EVALUATION

The diagnosis is typically readily made on the basis of the characteristic history. An effort should be made to identify the cause of the patient's fissure (e.g., constipation or diarrhea) and manage it appropriately. Because fissures are so often painful, physical examination is necessarily limited. Simply spreading the buttocks to observe the anal canal is often very uncomfortable. Most fissures occur in the posterior midline, and this is where attention should initially be directed. Chronic anal fissures are often associated with secondary findings such as an external skin tag and a hypertrophied anal papilla. It is the sentinel anal tag that explains why patients with a fissure most often think they have a hemorrhoid. The true culprit, an anal fissure, is usually lurking at the cephalad aspect of the anal tag. Digital examination is often impossible owing to the pain and sphincter spasm.

Most anal fissures are associated with very high pressures in the anal canal. In fact, the pressures can exceed those of systemic blood pressure, impairing perfusion to the fissure and preventing healing. Most fissures are elliptic and located in the midline. Fissures with an atypical appearance, those not associated with sphincter hypertonia, or those in a lateral position suggest an alternative pathogenesis such as Crohn's disease or a sexually transmitted disease.

TREATMENT

Acute anal fissures typically respond to conservative measures. This includes fluid and fiber supplementation, sitz baths, and possibly stool softeners if the patient has hard stools. Adjunctive measures such as topical anesthetics may be used for patient comfort.

Topical nitrates[1] have been associated with pain relief and a marginal improvement in fissure healing rates. However, the principal side effect has been headaches, which are dose related. Topical calcium channel blockers such as nifedipine (Adalat, Procardia)[1] appear to be at least equally efficacious and are associated with fewer side effects. Botulinum toxin (Botox)[1] injections have been used for anal fissures that fail to respond to these conservative measures; however, even if the injections are effective, recurrence rates over time appear to be high.

Patients with symptoms that are refractory to conservative measures should be considered for surgery. The treatment of choice is usually a lateral internal sphincterotomy; this corrects the markedly elevated anal canal pressures that are associated with an anal fissure and leads to healing in well over of 90% of cases. The very low morbidity and almost immediate pain relief make this procedure among the most effective of any surgical intervention. However, surgical sphincterotomy is associated with a small risk of minor fecal incontinence.

Anorectal Abscess And Fistula

Most perianal abscesses arise from cryptoglandular obstruction. Specifically, the duct of an anal gland becomes occluded, with subsequent bacterial overgrowth and retrograde infection. Fortunately, at least one half of anorectal abscesses resolve after adequate drainage. However, many patients develop a persistent epithelialized tract from the infected gland inside the anal canal to the external drainage site (anal fistula).

---

[1]Not FDA approved for this indication.

EVALUATION

Patients with an anorectal abscess typically present with acute pain. Often there are systemic signs of infection such as malaise and fever.

There are relatively few causes of acute anorectal pain. Pain that occurs with defecation is typically caused by an anal fissure. Thrombosed external hemorrhoids are also readily apparent on physical examination. Most patients with an anorectal abscess present with an obvious red, tender, fluctuant mass. However, more deep-seated abscesses can manifest in a far more subtle manner.

Physical examination typically consists of only visual inspection. If the abscess is identified, no further evaluation is really required at that time. Patients with pain who do not have a discernible abnormality should undergo a careful digital examination; in some patients, this examination requires a formal anesthetic. Imaging studies such as computed tomography (CT) or magnetic resonance imaging (MRI) are only required in select ambiguous circumstances.

In the chronic phase, patients typically present with an external opening on the perianal skin that drains purulent material. Quite often, the patient describes a cycle of perianal pain followed by drainage and relief of symptoms. This sequence repeats itself over and over again. Alternatively, the patient might seem to be abscess prone; specifically, the patient presents every few months with an acute abscess requiring drainage. All of these clinical scenarios suggest an anal fistula.

TREATMENT

A perianal abscess should be adequately drained. Lack of fluctuance is not an appropriate reason to delay timely drainage. Perianal erythema typically indicates that the abscess will be found deeper in the anal canal or ischiorectal fossa. Outside of unusual circumstances or specific immunocompromised states, perianal cellulitis does not occur.

Most abscesses are readily localized and easily drained in the outpatient setting under local anesthesia. Packing the abscess cavity is typically painful and usually unnecessary. Rather, a cruciate incision should be made that is adequate to facilitate complete drainage of the abscess cavity. An inadequate incision often leads to recurrent abscess formation.

Patients with diffuse erythema, in whom precise localization is not possible, commonly require drainage under anesthesia. Similarly, patients who appear toxic or are immunocompromised might need drainage in the operating room to ensure there are no loculations.

Antibiotics are an unnecessary addition to routine incision and drainage of uncomplicated perianal abscesses. Similarly, a culture is not required in most cases. The addition of antibiotics does not improve healing times or reduce recurrences. However, in patients with immunosuppression, diabetes, prosthetic devices, or excessive cellulitis, adjunctive antibiotic therapy should be considered.

An anal fistula denotes the chronic phase of anorectal sepsis and is the natural history in up to 50% of perianal abscesses. A fistula is believed to arise from persistent sepsis or the development of an epithelialized tract. Anal fistulas are characterized based on their location relative to the sphincter muscles. Fortunately, most anal fistulas involve a relatively small amount of muscle and can be readily treated by fistulotomy, or unroofing of the anal fistula tract. However, complex fistulas can be among the most difficult and frustrating problems for patient and colorectal surgeon alike. Generally speaking, patients with deep tracts involving considerable portions of this sphincter muscle or patients with preexisting fecal incontinence require an alternative approach. These might include injection of fibrin glue, endoanal advancement flap repair of the internal opening, or perhaps placement of a biological plug. These techniques appear to have a substantially lower success rate than fistulotomy.

REFERENCES

Boyum J, Hyman N: Fissure-in-ano. Semin Colon Rectal Surg 2003;14:107-110.
Cataldo P, Ellis N, Gregorcyk S, Hyman N, et al: Practice parameter for the management of hemorrhoids. Dis Colon Rectum 2005;48:189-194.
Hyman NH: Anorectal abscess and fistula. Prim Care 1999;26:69-80.
Hyman N: Incontinence after lateral internal sphincterotomy: A prospective study and quality of life assessment. Dis Colon Rectum 2004;47:35-38.
Keighley MR, Buchmann P, Minervium S, et al: Prospective trials of minor surgical procedures and high fibre diet for haemorrhoids. BMJ 1997;2:967-969.
Orsay C, Rakinic J, Perry B, et al: Practice parameter for the management of anal fissures. Dis Colon Rectum 2004;47:2003-2007.
Nelson R: Operative procedures for fissure in ano. Cochrane Database Syst Rev 2005;2):CD002199.
Richard CS, Gregoire R, Plewes EA, et al: Internal sphincterotomy is superior to topical nitroglycerin in the treatment of chronic anal fissure: Results of a randomized, controlled trial by the Canadian Colorectal Surgical Trials Group. Dis Colon Rectum 2000;43:1048-1057.
Whiteford M, Kilkenny J, Hyman N, et al: Practice parameter for the treatment of perianal abscess and fistula-in-ano. Dis Colon Rectum 2005;48:1337-1342.

Gastritis and Peptic Ulcer Disease

Method of
*Sripathi R. Kethu, MD, and
Steven F. Moss, MD*

Gastritis is by definition a histopathologic diagnosis, and peptic ulcer disease (PUD) is an endoscopic or radiologic diagnosis. Neither of these conditions has a specific symptom complex to help the clinician arrive at a diagnosis. Instead, physicians encounter patients with symptoms of dyspepsia that might or might not be secondary to gastritis or PUD. Thus, for the primary care provider, the discussion of gastritis and PUD must be prefaced by first considering the approach to the patient with dyspeptic symptoms.

Dyspepsia

Dyspepsia refers to pain or discomfort centered in the upper abdomen, which may be intermittent or continuous and might or might not be related to meals. The symptoms may be described by several other terms, including *bloating, fullness, belching,* and *nausea* or simply as *indigestion*.

The prevalence of uninvestigated dyspepsia in the general population is not well documented. However, up to 25% of people in the community each year report chronic or recurrent pain or discomfort in the upper abdomen, and approximately 2% to 5% of family practice consultations are for dyspepsia.

ETIOLOGY AND DIFFERENTIAL DIAGNOSIS

Dyspepsia can result from an identifiable cause such as peptic ulcer disease, malignancy, gastroesophageal reflux, or the use of specific medications. Other rare causes include pancreatic-biliary disease, gastroparesis, celiac disease, lactose intolerance, and parasitic diseases such as giardiasis. Patients who have no definite structural or biochemical explanation for their symptoms are considered to have functional dyspepsia (nonulcer dyspepsia). There is a subset of patients in whom dyspepsia might coexist with a microbiological or structural abnormality such as *Helicobacter pylori* gastritis or duodenitis or with gallstones, but a causal relation between these abnormalities and dyspepsia may be unclear.

The patient's age is one of the most important factors in tailoring the management of patients with dyspepsia because of the very low probability of stomach cancer in younger patients (typically this cut-off is arbitrarily fixed at 55 years). Thus, if a patient older than 55 years presents with new-onset upper abdominal complaints, or patients younger than this age develop alarm symptoms (anemia, anorexia, weight loss >10% of body weight, early satiety, dysphagia, or gastrointestinal (GI) bleeding either overt or occult), prompt endoscopic evaluation is required to detect the cause before administering empiric therapy.

In a primary care setting, the patient's history is crucial in elucidating the cause of dyspepsia. Peptic ulcer disease is an important consideration in the differential diagnosis of dyspepsia, accounting for up to 15% of cases. Although it is impossible to distinguish gastric and duodenal ulcers by symptoms alone, the pain of gastric and duodenal ulcers is typically epigastric, episodic, and often worse at night. Symptoms are often temporarily relieved with food or antacids in duodenal ulcer; in contrast, food can precipitate gastric ulcer pain. Associated symptoms such as anorexia, nausea, or vomiting can point toward the diagnosis of gastric ulcer or pyloric stenosis. Patients with gastric malignancy, which accounts for less than 2% of all cases of dyspepsia, can also present with similar symptoms.

Gastroesophageal reflux disease (GERD) may be the underlying disorder in 10% to 15% of patients with dyspepsia. Other typical symptoms in GERD include heartburn or a retrosternal burning pain or a feeling of regurgitation of food or acid. However, about 20% of patients with GERD present with epigastric pain alone, thereby creating a diagnostic problem. If medications are responsible for dyspepsia, generally a temporal relationship can be established between the medication intake and the onset of dyspeptic symptoms. Nonsteroidal anti-inflammatory drugs (NSAIDs) are the most common offending agents; other medications that cause dyspepsia are corticosteroids, iron preparations, digitalis, potassium supplements, bisphosphonates, niacin, and antibiotics, particularly erythromycin and ampicillin.

Functional, or nonulcer, dyspepsia accounts for up to 60% of all cases of dyspepsia. Functional dyspepsia and PUD share many symptoms, thus making the distinction by history alone impossible. By definition, the cause of functional dyspepsia is obscure; the putative pathophysiologic abnormalities that have been proposed to cause or to be associated with functional dyspepsia are gastric acid hypersecretion, H. pylori infection, gastroduodenal dysmotility, visceral hyperalgesia, and psychological distress including physical or sexual abuse. Although functional dyspepsia is a benign condition, it is the hardest to treat given the uncertain interplay between numerous pathogenic mechanisms.

EVALUATION

Currently the best test in the evaluation of dyspepsia is upper endoscopy. Barium meal radiographs are less sensitive and specific.

In a younger patient (age < 55 years), in the absence of alarm symptoms, and after excluding other causes such as GERD and NSAID use by history, an H. pylori test and treat strategy, followed by proton pump inhibitor (PPI) treatment if the patient remains symptomatic or is not infected by H. pylori, is the management strategy of choice. The justification for this approach is that among patients with uninvestigated dyspepsia who are H. pylori positive, a substantial number have peptic ulcers, and a few without ulcers can improve symptomatically following eradication of H. pylori. Whether this strategy is suitable for affluent populations in the United States who have a very low prevalence of H. pylori is debatable because it can result in the diagnosis of almost as many false-positive H. pylori infections and lead to inappropriate eradication therapy. Furthermore, the cost benefits of the test and treat approach over one with early invasive testing remains unproven in practice. In other populations, noninvasive testing for H. pylori either by stool antigen test or urea breath test is reasonable. These tests are relatively less expensive compared with either upper endoscopy or indefinite empiric acid-suppressive therapy and are more accurate than serology.

If symptoms persist after H. pylori eradication therapy, or if empiric acid-suppressive therapy in H. pylori–negative patients fails, upper endoscopy should be undertaken. Ultrasonography is not recommended as a routine next step unless the history or biochemical tests suggest pancreatic-biliary disease. In patients with diabetes or a history suggesting autonomic neuropathy, a gastric emptying scan (scintigraphy) may be considered to document gastroparesis. Even though functional dyspepsia should be considered a diagnosis of exclusion, clinicians should use their judgment on a case-by-case basis to limit the use of numerous invasive and expensive investigations whenever possible.

MANAGEMENT

Once the cause of dyspepsia is established, management involves treating the underlying cause. The most challenging task is managing patients with functional dyspepsia. H. pylori eradication therapy for patients who do not have an ulcer can result in symptomatic improvement in a small minority, approximately in 15% of patients, at best, over placebo. However, most patients remain symptomatic after eradication therapy, thus requiring other therapies.

Reassurance and explanation are important first steps in management. Proving that the symptoms do not represent a malignancy may be sufficient. Patients should be educated to avoid any obvious offending agents, such as coffee, alcohol, smoking, NSAIDs, and spicy and fatty foods; this helps relieve symptoms in some patients. Precipitant psychosocial factors including anxiety and depression should also be explored and treated appropriately. Pharmacologic therapy is not always required, and if required, it should be individualized. No single drug has been clearly shown to be beneficial over the long term, and the results of pharmacologic therapy are disappointing overall.

First-line therapies usually involve a therapeutic trial of either antisecretory agents such as H_2-receptor antagonists (H_2-RAs) or PPIs. A prokinetic agent such as metoclopramide (Reglan) 10 mg 1 hour after meals and at bedtime for 4 to 6 weeks may be useful as an alternative therapy. A drug holiday during therapy can help determine if the medication is still needed. The benefits of individual drugs should be weighed against the side-effect profile and cost. Metoclopramide, for example, is associated with neuropsychiatric complications and therefore cannot be recommended for the long term. Antidepressants such as amitriptyline (Elavil)[1] 150 mg at bedtime or antispasmodics such as dicyclomine (Bentyl)[1] 20 to 40 mg every 6 hours, can be tried as a next step, but the results are marginal at best. Alternative therapies such as acupuncture, cognitive behavior therapy, and hypnotherapy have been anecdotally reported to be beneficial.

Gastritis

Exposure of the gastric mucosa to various insults can lead to epithelial damage and regeneration with minimal or no inflammation (gastropathy), or the epithelial damage may be associated with significant inflammation (gastritis). For an endoscopist, gastritis usually means petechiae or erosions of the gastric mucosa. These endoscopic findings might not have a good correlation with the presence of inflammatory cells on biopsy. Strictly speaking, gastritis is a histopathologic diagnosis associated with the presence of inflammatory cells. Gastritis and gastropathy can be categorized according to the histologic features and the etiology (Box 1).

ACUTE EROSIVE AND HEMORRHAGIC GASTROPATHY

The most common causes of acute erosive and hemorrhagic gastropathy include NSAIDs, alcohol, and stress due to critical illness. Clinically, the patient might present with nonspecific complaints such as epigastric pain, nausea, or vomiting and occasionally with upper bleeding alone. Upper endoscopy usually reveals erythema or erosions. Histologically, there is usually no or minimal inflammation, hence the term *gastropathy* instead of *gastritis*. Stress gastritis, most likely due to chronic gastric ischemia, can lead to gastric ulceration, usually multiple small ulcers involving the proximal part of the stomach.

---

[1]Not FDA approved for this indication.

> **BOX 1 Classification of Gastritis**
>
> - Acute erosive and hemorrhagic gastropathy
> - Chronic gastritis
>   - *Helicobacter pylori* gastritis (may be atrophic or nonatrophic)
>   - Pernicious anemia–associated atrophic gastritis (type A gastritis or autoimmune gastritis)
> - Others
>   - Eosinophilic gastritis
>   - Infectious (Cytomegalovirus, Herpes virus)
>   - Granulomatous gastritis (Crohn's disease)
>   - Portal gastropathy

Management of symptomatic gastropathy caused by NSAIDs or alcohol involves minimizing or avoiding the offending agents or taking the NSAIDs with food. A short course of H_2-RAs or PPIs is recommended if the patient has persistent symptoms despite conservative measures. Long-term acid-suppression therapy with PPIs may be necessary for patients believed to be at high risk for bleeding but in whom chronic NSAID use is necessary. The development of cyclooxygenase-2 (COX-2) selective NSAIDs has diminished but not eliminated clinically important gastroduodenal bleeding, and the benefit of these agents should be weighed against their reported risk of cardiovascular complications.

Endoscopy is recommended only for patients with risk factors for developing an ulcer (see the section on peptic ulcer disease). Many critically ill hospitalized patients develop superficial erosions ("stress gastritis) from chronic gastric ischemia, but this rarely leads to clinically significant gastric bleeding. Two risk factors that are associated with a high risk of clinically significant bleeding are mechanical ventilation and a coagulopathy. In the absence of these two risk factors, the risk of significant bleeding is less than 0.1%. Preventing stress gastritis and ulcers with the use of acid-suppression medications is strongly recommended in all critically ill patients, particularly if they have the previously mentioned risk factors. The superiority of oral or intravenous PPIs over H_2-RAs in this setting has not been definitely established.

CHRONIC *HELICOBACTER PYLORI* GASTRITIS

H. pylori is a gram-negative spiral bacterium acquired in childhood that colonizes the gastric mucosa and usually causes an antral-predominant gastritis. In the developed world, infection is more prevalent in the elderly, the poor, and immigrants from high-incidence regions such as Asia, Africa, and Central and South America.

Inflammation associated with chronic *H. pylori* colonization may be confined to the superficial mucosa or can extend deeper into the gastric glands, leading in some cases to gastric atrophy (atrophic gastritis) and intestinal metaplasia of the gastric epithelium. The majority of all gastric and duodenal ulcers are caused by *H. pylori*; approximately 10% of all patients with chronic gastritis due to *H. pylori* eventually develop peptic ulcer disease.

A more uncommon consequence of *H. pylori* infection is adenocarcinoma of the stomach, typically developing after many decades of infection and after histologic progression from atrophic gastritis through intestinal metaplasia and dysplasia. *H. pylori* infection is associated with a threefold to sixfold increased risk of distal gastric cancer, leading to its designation by the World Health Organization as a carcinogen. It is also a major risk factor for the relatively rare mucosa-associated lymphoid tissue (MALT) gastric B-cell lymphoma. (See the section on peptic ulcer disease for detailed discussion of diagnosis and management of *H. pylori*.)

Factors believed to be important determinants of individual clinical outcome following *H. pylori* infection include host genetics, nutritional and general health status, and specific *H. pylori* virulence genes.

PERNICIOUS ANEMIA–ASSOCIATED ATROPHIC GASTRITIS

Pernicious anemia–associated atrophic gastritis (type A gastritis or autoimmune gastritis) is an autoimmune disorder characterized by antiparietal cell antibodies leading to parietal cell destruction. The disease is more common in women and in persons of northern European descent. Parietal cell destruction in the gastric fundus leads to achlorhydria, and the impaired intrinsic factor production results in vitamin B_{12} malabsorption. Generally, patients are asymptomatic until extreme vitamin B_{12} deficiency causes anemia leading to neurologic syndromes. Patients are at increased risk for developing carcinoid tumors (secondary to prolonged hypergastrinemia) and adenocarcinoma of the stomach. Treatment involves vitamin B_{12} supplementation even if the serum vitamin B_{12} level is not low. The usefulness of periodic endoscopic screening to detect carcinoma or carcinoid tumors is controversial in this condition.

Peptic Ulcer Disease

Peptic ulcer disease is a generic term used to indicate a mucosal defect in the stomach or duodenum. As opposed to an erosion, which is a superficial lesion, an ulcer has a perceivable depth extending through the submucosa. PUD is believed to occur when factors aggressive to the gastric mucosa dominate (such as *H. pylori* infection or gastric acid hypersecretion) or when mucosal defense mechanisms are impaired (by NSAIDs, for example), or both.

The lifetime risk of PUD in the United States is approximately 10%, with a male-to-female ratio of 1.3:1 for a duodenal ulcer and 1:1 for a gastric ulcer. Duodenal ulcer occurs more commonly between ages 25 and 55 years, whereas gastric ulcer affects a slightly older population (ages 40-70 years). NSAID use or *H. pylori* infection increases the peptic ulcer risk by about 20-fold. Cigarette smoking not only increases the ulcer risk (by twofold), but also retards ulcer healing and increases the risk of bleeding. Despite popular beliefs, alcohol and dietary factors have no established relation with the cause of ulcers or their healing. Psychological stress can play some role in idiopathic ulcers.

ETIOLOGY

Depending on their etiology, ulcers can be classified in four groups: *H. pylori*–associated ulcers, NSAID-induced ulcers, idiopathic (non-*H. pylori*, non-NSAID) ulcers, and Zollinger-Ellison syndrome (discussed later). Other less-common causes include ulcers secondary to drugs other than NSAIDs (e.g., potassium chloride, bisphosphonates), stress ulcers due to a critical illness, ulcers of Crohn's disease, and infectious causes (*Cytomegalovirus* ulcers in HIV patients, *Herpes simplex*).

Helicobacter pylori–Associated Ulcers

H. pylori infection is responsible for the majority of peptic ulcers. *H. pylori* is believed to be transmitted from person to person, probably via the fecal–oral route. The prevalence of *H. pylori* is between 20% and 50% in the Western world, including the United States. However, *H. pylori* is much more prevalent in developing nations, affecting as many as 90% of the population. In the United States, the prevalence is higher in the elderly, probably reflecting the poor sanitary conditions that existed in the early part of the century, and is more common in those of African American or Latin American ethnicity. *H. pylori* is also more prevalent in persons of low socioeconomic status, possibly related to crowded childhood living conditions.

Initial studies reported that *H. pylori* was present in about 90% of patients with duodenal ulcers and 60% of patients with gastric ulcer. More recent estimates show slightly lower prevalence of *H. pylori* in both duodenal ulcer and gastric ulcer, probably reflecting the relative increase in NSAID-associated ulcers. Approximately 10% of all persons infected with *H. pylori* develop PUD over their lifetime.

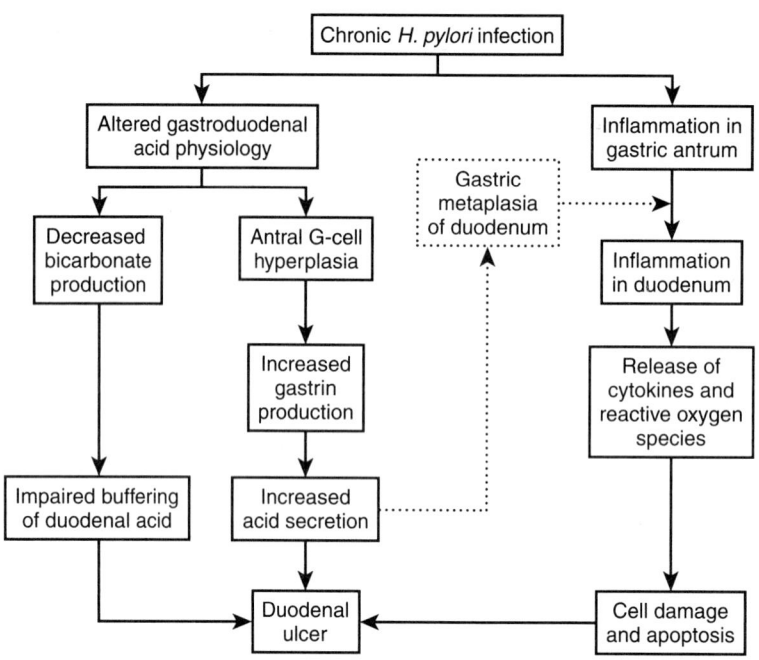

FIGURE 1. Proposed pathogenic mechanisms leading to *Helicobacter pylori*–induced duodenal ulcer.

The exact pathophysiologic mechanism(s) by which *H. pylori* causes either duodenal or gastric ulcer and why only a minority of infected persons develop clinically overt disease is not known. Generally, duodenal ulcer is a disease of acid hypersecretion and gastric ulcer is associated with states of low acid secretion. *H. pylori* can potentially cause both of these secretory abnormalities. Gastric acid hypersecretion in duodenal ulcer occurs secondary to increased gastrin release by a healthy acid-secreting gastric body mucosa (Figure 1). In contrast, when *H. pylori*–associated gastritis affects the proximal stomach too, this results in loss of gastric glands (atrophic gastritis) and hypochlorhydria with impaired mucosal defense, leading to gastric ulceration and even gastric cancer.

NSAID-Induced Ulcers

NSAIDs are among the most prescribed medications in the United States. The incidence of ulcers in chronic NSAID users is approximately 15% to 20%. The risk of NSAID-induced ulcers increases dramatically with the presence of specific risk factors (particularly with age >60 years and a prior history of peptic ulcer) and also with high doses of NSAIDs and concurrent use of either anticoagulants or high-dose corticosteroids. NSAIDs cause gastric ulcers much more commonly than duodenal ulcers. Up to 40% of these persons remain asymptomatic, and patients commonly present with complications.

The most important mechanism by which NSAIDs cause ulcers is by indirectly decreasing prostaglandin production via the inhibition of COX-1. Prostaglandins are important in maintaining mucosal integrity by producing mucus, stimulating bicarbonate production, decreasing acid production, and maintaining mucosal blood flow. The analgesic and anti-inflammatory effects of NSAIDs result from the inhibition of the COX-2 isoenzyme. Nonselective NSAIDs cause inhibition of both COX-2 and COX-1, resulting in considerable GI toxicity. The more recently developed selective COX-2 inhibitors, such as celecoxib (Celebrex), as the name implies, inhibit COX-2 to a much greater extent than COX-1, leading to their better GI safety profile. However, recent reports of cardiovascular complications attributed to COX-2 inhibitors have severely restricted their use.

Idiopathic Ulcers

In a specific subgroup of patients who develop ulcers, all the known etiologic factors are excluded. This subgroup should not be confused with patients who have unexplained ulcers, 60% of whom have a history of surreptitious NSAID use. The true incidence of idiopathic ulcers is hard to assess in various studies as a result of false-negative *H. pylori* tests or surreptitious use of NSAIDs, and the exact pathogenic mechanism that causes these idiopathic ulcers remains unknown. Various abnormalities including genetic predisposition, defective mucosal defense mechanisms, and increased acid production have all been postulated.

CLINICAL FEATURES

Clinical signs and symptoms are unreliable and are not specific enough to make a diagnosis of a peptic ulcer. Upper abdominal pain (dyspepsia) is present in more than 80% of patients; however, only 15% of patients with dyspepsia have PUD. Pain is typically epigastric, described as burning and nonradiating. Food or antacids can relieve duodenal ulcer pain. Nausea or anorexia can occur with gastric ulcers. Nocturnal symptoms awaken patients in two thirds of duodenal ulcer and one third of gastric ulcer cases. Symptoms usually wax and wane over a period of months. The physical examination is usually normal in PUD patients. Epigastric tenderness may be present on palpation, but it is an unreliable sign with a positive predictive value of less than 50%. Stool tests for occult blood may be positive in one third of patients.

DIAGNOSTIC WORK-UP

Routine laboratory studies are not helpful in establishing a diagnosis of PUD. Upper endoscopy is the gold standard in making a diagnosis of peptic ulcer. Endoscopy has the advantage of taking biopsies for the presence of *H. pylori* infection and, in the case of gastric ulcer, to rule out malignancy. However, endoscopy is more expensive and invasive. In the absence of alarm symptoms, double-contrast barium radiography may be a suitable second choice. If barium radiography shows an ulcer (gastric or duodenal), *H. pylori* must be tested noninvasively. Treatment can be instituted with

CURRENT DIAGNOSIS

- In the majority of cases of dyspepsia, no structural abnormality can be identified after investigation.
- Patients with dyspepsia who are older than 55 years or who have alarm symptoms (anemia, anorexia, weight loss, early satiety, dysphagia, or gastrointestinal bleeding) should undergo upper endoscopy.
- *Helicobacter pylori* infection and NSAIDs are the two most common causes of peptic ulcer disease.
- Endoscopic biopsy, urea breath test, and stool antigen testing are the most accurate ways to diagnose active *H. pylori* infection.
- Zollinger-Ellison syndrome should be suspected if there are multiple duodenal ulcers, ulcers that are refractory to treatment, or peptic ulcers associated with diarrhea.

TABLE 1 Diagnostic Tests for *H. pylori*

Diagnostic Test	Sensitivity (%)	Specificity (%)
Noninvasive Tests		
Serum ELISA test for antibody	85	80
Urea breath test (^{14}C or ^{13}C)	95-100	91-98
Stool antigen test	91-98	94-99
Invasive (Endoscopy-Based) Tests		
Rapid urease test	93-97	95-100
Histology	>95	98-99
Culture	70-80	100

Abbreviation: ELISA = enzyme-linked immunosorbent assay.

acid-suppression therapy with or without antibiotics depending on the presence of *H. pylori*. Gastric pH and fasting gastrin levels should be obtained only if there is clinical suspicion for gastrinoma (see the section on Zollinger-Ellison syndrome). For gastric ulcers, it is advisable to repeat the endoscopy after 6 to 8 weeks of therapy to confirm the healing of the ulcer and re-biopsy if it is not healed, because 5% of gastric ulcers can be malignant.

Many tests are available for *H. pylori*. Testing for *H. pylori* can be made by either noninvasive or invasive methods (Table 1). An appropriate test should be chosen depending on the clinical situation. For example, testing for serologic antibodies against *H. pylori* may be appropriate for the initial testing for *H. pylori* though it is not as accurate as breath or stool tests. Also, serology is not useful to check for eradication after therapy, because it will not distinguish current active infection from prior infection that was treated (antibody levels fall slowly and unpredictably). Office-based qualitative antibody tests are cheaper compared with enzyme-linked immunosorbent assay (ELISA) test done in the laboratory but not as accurate, and they have been superseded by stool antigen and breath testing. Patients with alarm symptoms and all patients older than 55 years who have dyspeptic symptoms should undergo endoscopy, at which time *H. pylori* testing can be done by biopsy if an ulcer is found.

Confirmation of the eradication of *H. pylori* should be considered after treating this infection in ulcer patients, by either the stool antigen test or the urea breath test, depending on the local resources. Confirmation of eradication by gastric biopsy is only recommended if endoscopy is performed for another reason, for example, to confirm healing of a gastric ulcer.

DIFFERENTIAL DIAGNOSIS

Functional dyspepsia is a major differential diagnostic consideration in all patients with upper abdominal pain (see the section on functional dyspepsia). Other diseases that mimic the symptoms of PUD include cancers of the upper gastrointestinal tract, biliary colic, and mesenteric ischemia.

TREATMENT

Different classes of drugs are available to treat PUD (Table 2). Antacids heal the ulcers and are cheap but are relatively ineffective, are slow to produce healing, and have many side effects. Both PPIs and H_2-RAs block acid secretion, but PPIs inhibit more than 90% of the 24-acid output compared with 65% with H_2-RAs; hence, PPIs heal the ulcer and relieve symptoms faster. Ulcer-healing rates of

TABLE 2 Treatment Options for Peptic Ulcers*

Pharmacologic Agent	Active Ulcer (Gastric or Duodenal)[†]	Prevention of NSAID-Induced Ulcer Recurrence
Antisecretory Agents		
H_2-Receptor Antagonists		
Cimetidine (Tagamet)	400 mg bid or 800 mg qhs	Double the dose indicated for active ulcer[1]
Famotidine (Pepcid)	20 mg bid or 40 mg qhs	
Nizatidine (Axid)	150 mg bid or 300 mg qhs	
Ranitidine (Zantac)	150 mg bid or 300 mg qhs	
Proton Pump Inhibitors		
Esomeprazole (Nexium)	40 mg qd	40 mg qd[1]
Lansoprazole (Prevacid)	30 mg qd	30 mg qd
Omeprazole (Prilosec)	20 mg qd	20 mg qd[1]
Pantoprazole (Protonix)	40 mg qd	40 mg qd[1]
Rabeprazole (Aciphex)	20 mg qd	20 mg qd[1]
Mucosal Protectants		
Misoprostol (Cytotec)	200 μg qid	200 μg qid or 400 μg bid
Sucralfate (Carafate)	1 gm qid	Not effective

[1]Not FDA approved for this indication.
*All patients should be tested for *H. pylori* and treated if positive.
[†]Duration of treatment for duodenal ulcer is 4 weeks with proton pump inhibitor (PPI) and 6 weeks with H_2-receptor antagonist. Duration of treatment for gastric ulcer is 8 weeks with either PPI or H_2-receptor antagonist.

TABLE 3 Select FDA-Approved *Helicobacter pylori* Eradication Regimens

Drug Combination	Dosing Schedule
PPI* (omeprazole 20 mg or lansoprazole 30 mg) + amoxicillin 1 g + clarithromycin 500 mg	Each bid for 10-14 d
Esomeprazole* 40 mg qd + amoxicillin 1 g bid + clarithromycin 500 mg bid	For 10 d
PPI* (omeprazole 20 mg or lansoprazole 30 mg) + amoxicillin 1 g + metronidazole 500 mg	Each bid for 10-14 d
Rabeprazole* 20 mg + amoxicillin 1 g + clarithromycin 500 mg	Each bid for 7 d
Bismuth subsalicylate 525 mg + metronidazole 250 mg + tetracycline 500 mg[†]	Each qid for 2 wk plus H$_2$-RA for 4 wk

*Although not yet approved, pantoprazole (Protonix) can be substituted.
[†]In patients with penicillin allergy, this regimen can be used. Alternatively, PPI + clarithromycin + metronidazole can be used.
Abbreviations: FDA = U.S. Food and Drug Administration; PPI = proton pump inhibitor.

sucralfate (Carafate) are similar to those for H$_2$-RAs. The mechanism of action of sucralfate is unknown; it probably coats the ulcer base, thereby promoting ulcer healing, and might have other effects too. The frequent dosing schedule and large tablet size of sucralfate is not conducive to good compliance. Misoprostol (Cytotec) is a prostaglandin analogue approved for preventing NSAID-induced ulcers. Compliance with misoprostol treatment is also a problem, particularly at high doses, owing to its GI side effects of abdominal cramping and diarrhea.

H. pylori eradication is recommended in all ulcer patients who are *H. pylori* positive, but *H. pylori* infection should not be assumed without a documented positive test. *H. pylori* eradication heals ulcers and reduces the ulcer recurrence dramatically, to less than 20% after 2 years. Select *H. pylori* eradication regimens are summarized in Table 3. Confirmation of eradication is mandatory for complicated ulcer associated with bleeding, perforation, or obstruction and is recommended in all ulcer patients receiving *H. pylori* therapy. Treatment of idiopathic ulcers is difficult and often requires indefinite maintenance antisecretory therapy, particularly for a complicated ulcer.

PREVENTION

Ulcers can recur either with continued use of NSAIDs or with *H. pylori* infection that persists after the initial antibiotic course. The incidence of antibiotic resistance to *H. pylori* is rising all over the world. In the United States, approximately 40% of *H. pylori* strains are now resistant to metronidazole (Flagyl), and 10% to 12% are resistant to clarithromycin (Biaxin), which decreases the cure rates by as much as 50% and 37%, respectively. If the patient has persistent symptoms after therapy, eradication failure should be strongly suspected and noninvasive testing for *H. pylori* should be performed. If the initial diagnosis of the ulcer was made by radiography, endoscopy is the next reasonable test. Drugs that are clearly shown to be superior to placebo in preventing NSAID-induced ulcers are PPIs and misoprostol (Cytotec). Double the standard doses of H$_2$-RAs used for active ulcers are significantly better than placebo in preventing NSAID-induced gastroduodenal ulcers (see Table 2). PPIs are generally preferred over H$_2$-RAs given the simplicity of the dosing schedule and comparable cost. Elderly patients who require long-term NSAID therapy should receive *H. pylori* eradication therapy if they are infected with this bacterium.

COMPLICATIONS

Hemorrhage

Gastrointestinal bleeding is the most common complication of PUD. Approximately 10% to 20% of ulcer patients develop significant GI bleeding, with overall mortality of up to 10%. Patients generally present with either melena or hematemesis. Endoscopy is indicated for diagnosis, risk stratification, and therapy in all patients with significant bleeding. High-dose oral or intravenous PPIs should be instituted before endoscopy if upper bleeding is suspected. All *H. pylori*–positive patients must have confirmation of eradication after therapy.

Perforation

Perforations occur in approximately 5% to 7% of ulcer patients. The incidence has not changed in spite of decreasing prevalence of *H. pylori*, because the use of NSAIDs continues to increase. The decision whether to manage operatively or nonoperatively should be made on a case-by-case basis.

Obstruction

Duodenal bulb or pyloric channel ulcers cause scarring and gastric outlet obstruction in approximately 2% of patients with PUD. Patients then present with early satiety, vomiting, and weight loss. Management involves *H. pylori* eradication and acid suppression along with endoscopic dilatation. Surgery is reserved for patients who do not respond to endoscopic therapy.

Zollinger-Ellison Syndrome

Less than 1% of PUD is caused by Zollinger-Ellison syndrome (ZES). This syndrome results from a gastrin-producing neuroendocrine tumor (gastrinoma), two thirds of which are malignant. PUD is caused by increased acid production from very high serum gastrin levels. Most gastrinomas arise in the gastrinoma triangle, bounded by the porta hepatis, neck of the pancreas, and third portion of the

CURRENT TREATMENT

- In patients with dyspepsia who are younger than 55 years, a *Helicobacter pylori* test-and-treat strategy, followed by PPI treatment (if the patient remains symptomatic or is not infected by *H. pylori*) is the management strategy of choice.
- Long-term acid-suppression therapy with PPIs may be necessary for patients believed to be at high risk for bleeding but in whom chronic NSAID use is necessary.
- PPIs inhibit more than 90% of the 24-acid output compared with 65% with H$_2$-RAs; hence PPIs heal peptic ulcers and relieve symptoms faster.
- Elderly patients who require long-term NSAID therapy should receive *H. pylori* eradication therapy if they are infected with this bacterium.
- Triple therapy (PPI plus amoxicillin and clarithromycin) is the most widely used treatment strategy for *H. pylori* in the United States.

Abbreviations: H$_2$-RA = H$_2$-receptor antagonist; NSAID = nonsteroidal anti-inflammatory drug; PPI = proton pump inhibitor.

duodenum. The pancreas and the duodenum are the two organs most commonly involved. Approximately one quarter of gastrinomas are part of the multiple endocrine neoplasia type 1 (MEN-1) syndrome, which is associated with parathyroid hyperplasia, pituitary tumors, and pancreatic endocrine tumors.

Gastrinomas commonly manifest between ages 30 and 50 years and have a male-to-female ratio of 2:1. The clinical features include peptic ulcers (90%), diarrhea (60%), and GERD (20%), all of which are due to gastric acid hypersecretion. The majority of ulcers occur in the duodenum. ZES should be suspected if the ulcers are multiple, in unusual locations, refractory to treatment, or associated with diarrhea.

Diagnosis is made by measuring fasting gastrin levels and gastric pH. If the gastrin levels are elevated to more than 1000 pg/mL in the right clinical setting, the diagnosis of ZES is established. Hypochlorhydria secondary to gastric atrophy from *H. pylori* or autoimmune gastritis, or due to acid suppression therapy by H$_2$-RAs and PPIs, can increase gastrin levels. Therefore, gastrin levels should be measured after H$_2$-RAs are held for 24 hours and PPIs for 1 week.

The gastric pH should be measured to distinguish ZES from hypochlorhydria. Gastric pH is less than 2 in ZES, whereas in achlorhydria secondary to gastric atrophy, gastric pH is greater than 2.

Provocative tests, such as the secretin test, can also be used to diagnose gastrinoma. Intravenous administration of secretin can decrease or slightly increase gastrin levels in normal patients and in patients with antral G-cell hyperplasia. In cases of gastrinoma, gastrin levels are significantly increased (>200 pg/mL) from the basal levels.

Tumor localization should be investigated by somatostatin receptor scintigraphy (Octreoscan), computed tomography, magnetic resonance imaging, and endoscopic ultrasound.

Treatment involves medical therapy with a high-dose PPI titrated against symptoms, gastric pH, and endoscopic findings. Surgical resection of isolated hepatic metastasis will decrease symptoms and prolongs survival.

REFERENCES

Chan FK, Graham DY: Review article: Prevention of non-steroidal anti-inflammatory drug gastrointestinal complications: Review and recommendations based on risk assessment. Aliment Pharmacol Ther 2004;19(10):1051-1061.

Chan FK, Leung WK: Peptic-ulcer disease. Lancet 2002;360(9337):933-941.

Stollman N, Metz DC: Pathophysiology and prophylaxis of stress ulcer in intensive care unit patients. J Crit Care 2005;20(1):35-45.

Suerbaum S, Michetti P: *Helicobacter pylori* infection. N Engl J Med 2002;347(15):1175-1186.

Talley NJ: American Gastroenterological Association: American Gastroenterological Association medical position statement: Evaluation of dyspepsia. Gastroenterology 2005;129(5):1753-1755.

Talley NJ: Vakil N, Practice Parameters Committee of the American College of Gastroenterology: Guidelines for the management of dyspepsia. Am J Gastroenterol. 2005;100(10):2324-2337.

Acute and Chronic Hepatitis

Method of
*Mamta K. Jain, MD, MPH, and
Daniel M. Brailita, MD*

Viral hepatitis is the most common cause of acute and chronic liver disease worldwide. Given the increasing number of new diagnoses and the risk of chronic liver disease, cirrhosis, and hepatocellular carcinoma, viral hepatitis is a serious health care problem. This article focuses on the epidemiology, diagnosis, prevention, and, in some cases, therapies that are available.

Several viruses are considered hepatotropic because viremia is associated with elevation of serum aminotransferases. However, *viral hepatitis* refers to infections caused by hepatitis viruses A through E. Hepatitis A (HAV) and E (HEV) viruses have a fecal-oral transmission route and do not produce chronic infection; hepatitis B (HBV), C (HCV), and D (HDV) viruses have a parenteral transmission route and can lead to chronic liver disease, hepatocellular carcinoma, and cirrhosis.

Other viral infections, which can involve the liver as one manifestation of a systemic infection, include HIV, Epstein–Barr virus (EBV), cytomegalovirus (CMV), herpes simplex virus (HSV), and varicella-zoster virus (VZV). These viruses can cause acute hepatitis, which can be fatal, especially in immunocompromised patients. Only hepatitis A, B, C, D, and E viral infections (characteristics are outlined in Table 1) are discussed in this article.

Acute Hepatitis Versus Chronic Hepatitis

ACUTE HEPATITIS

Acute hepatitis can be either symptomatic or asymptomatic. Generally, asymptomatic disease occurs in younger children. Symptomatic clinical disease is often seen in adolescents and adults. In the prodromal phase, a person can experience flulike illness with malaise, fever, anorexia, nausea, vomiting, and mild abdominal pain. During the icteric phase, jaundice appears, often accompanied by dark-brown urine and acholic or clay-colored stools. However, these signs may be seen in some persons without jaundice. Less frequent symptoms include arthralgias, rash, diarrhea, and lymphadenopathy.

Typical laboratory tests show high elevations of liver enzymes including alanine aminotransferase (ALT) and aspartate aminotransferase (AST) (often in the 1000 IU/mL range), an increase in bilirubin, and sometimes an increase in alkaline phosphatase. Fulminant hepatic failure, a rare complication, can be seen, with prolongation of prothrombin time (PT), coagulopathy, encephalopathy, and jaundice.

Patients with fulminant hepatic failure, because of the high mortality rate, should be managed in specialized centers with access to liver transplantation and close monitoring of coagulopathy, volume status, and neurologic status.

CHRONIC HEPATITIS

HBV and HCV can cause acute infection, either symptomatic or asymptomatic, and can progress to chronic liver disease. Most patients with chronic viral hepatitis are asymptomatic or complain of mild fatigue only; progression to cirrhosis, hepatocellular carcinoma, and end-stage liver disease is possible. The clinical examination can be normal or stigmata of chronic liver disease may be observed, such as spider angiomas, palmar erythema, testicular atrophy, and gynecomastia. The laboratory tests might show mild to moderate transaminitis in the chronic phase. The degree of ALT and AST elevation might not reflect the severity of liver fibrosis. Often, patients with cirrhosis have normal ALT and AST levels. The degree of fibrosis in chronic liver disease is based on histologic findings on liver biopsy.

Cirrhotic patients can develop portal hypertension leading to an enlarged spleen, variceal bleeding, ascites, and encephalopathy. Other clinical parameters that indicate progressive liver disease include: decrease in serum albumin and platelet count, rise of serum bilirubin, and prolongation of PT. In these patients, transplantation may be necessary. Cirrhotic patients are also at increased risk for developing hepatocellular cancer (HCC) and should be screened by alpha fetoprotein (AFP) and abdominal ultrasound every 6 months. In addition, these patients are at risk for fulminant hepatitis due to other viruses and should be vaccinated for vaccine-preventable

TABLE 1 Characteristics of Hepatitis A through E

Virus	HAV	HBV	HCV	HDV	HEV
Family	Picornaviridae	Hepadnaviridae	Flaviviridae	Deltavirus (no separate family)	Hepeviridae
Size	27 nm	42 nm	50-55 nm	36 nm	32 nm
Nucleic acid	ssRNA	dsDNA	ssRNA	ssRNA	ssRNA
Transmission	Fecal-oral	Vertical, percutaneous, sexual	Blood products, percutaneous, sexual	Mainly percutaneous	Fecal-oral
Incubation	15-45 d	1-6 mo	7 wk	3-20 wk	15-60 d
Chronic infection?	No	Yes	Yes	Yes	No
Vaccine available?	Yes	Yes	No	No	Experimental

Abbreviations: HAV = hepatitis A virus; HBV = hepatitis B virus; HCV = hepatitis C virus; HDV = hepatitis D virus; HEV = hepatitis E virus; ss = single-stranded; ds = double-stranded.

infections. For example, patients with HCV-related cirrhosis should be vaccinated for HAV and HBV. Vaccination schedules are shown in Table 2.

Hepatitis A

EPIDEMIOLOGY

HAV is the leading cause of acute viral hepatitis worldwide and is a reportable disease in the United States, but significant shifts in HAV epidemiology have been seen since the introduction of licensed vaccines from 1995 to 1999. In 2004, an estimated 56,000 new infections occurred in the United States, which represents a historically low rate; to compare, more than 356,000 infections occurred in 1995. Higher prevalence of HAV is seen in children in less developed countries where sanitation is poor and infection occurs at an early age.

The virus is transmitted mainly by the fecal–oral route via contaminated food or water. In industrialized countries, like the United States, sporadic cases are more common and the prevalence of acute HAV is higher in adults. Populations at risk include children in daycare centers, close contacts of viremic patients, persons with substandard hygiene habits, or eating undercooked food, travelers in endemic areas, and men who have sex with men (MSM). Waterborne outbreaks are rare in developed countries but can be seen in less developed countries.

CLINICAL FEATURES

Infection with HAV does not lead to chronic liver disease. Acute infection is asymptomatic in most children, especially children younger than 2 years, but it is symptomatic in children older than 5 years. Symptomatic illness occurs after an incubation of 15 to 45 days. The viral prodrome before the onset of jaundice (see acute hepatitis) typically lasts 2 to 7 days. Hepatomegaly is possible. Typically, significant improvement occurs by the end of the third week, with normalization of ALT and AST, fading jaundice, and resolution of hepatomegaly.

The clinical patterns include asymptomatic infection without jaundice, symptomatic infection with jaundice but with a limited 8-week course, cholestatic infection with jaundice with usually a longer course, relapsing infection with two or more episodes over a 6- to 10-week period, and, rarely, fulminant hepatic failure. Complete recovery is achieved in most persons by 6 months. The prognosis is excellent, with no progression to chronic disease. Mortality, occurring in less than 0.4%, is more common in the extremes of age (infants and the elderly, especially those with diabetes).

DIAGNOSIS

Acute HAV infection is diagnosed by detecting anti-HAV immunoglobulin M (IgM) (see Table 3) in the acute serum sample, which

TABLE 2 Vaccination Schedules for Hepatitis Vaccines Licensed in the United States

Vaccine	Type	Dose	Schedule
Hepatitis A Virus			
Havrix (GlaxoSmithKline)	Inactivated HAV	12 mo-18 y: 0.5 mL (720 EL.U) > 18 y: 1 mL (1440 EL.U)	0 and 6-12 mo
Vaqta (Merck)	Inactivated HAV	12 mo-18 y: 0.5 mL (25 U) > 18 y: 1 mL (50 U)	0 and 6-18 mo
Hepatitis A and B Viruses			
Twinrix (GlaxoSmithKline)	Inactivated HAV and recombinant HBV	> 18 y: 1 mL	0, 1, and 6 mo
Hepatitis B Virus			
Recombivax-HB (Merck)	Recombinant HBV	0-19 y: 0.5 mL (5 µg)	Infants: birth, 1-4, and 6-18 mo Older children: 0, 1-2, and 4 mo
		> 20 y: 1 mL (10 µg)	0, 1, and 6 mo
Engerix-B (GlaxoSmithKline)	Recombinant HBV	0-19 y: 0.5 mL (10 µg)	Infants: birth, 1-4, and 6-18 mo Older children: 0, 1-2, and 4 mo
		> 20 y: 1 mL (20 µg) Dialysis patients: double adult dose	0, 1, and 6 mo 0, 1, 2, and 6 mo.
Comvax (Merck)	Recombinant HBV, HiB	Approved for 6 wk-4y of age: 1 dose	2, 4, and 12-15 mo
Pediarix (GlaxoSmithKline)	Recombinant HBV, DTaP, IPV	Approved for 6 wk-6y of age.: 1 dose	2, 4, and 6 mo

Abbreviations: DTaP = diphtheria, tetanus toxoids, and acellular pertussis vaccine; EL.U = enzyme-linked immunosorbent assay units of HAV antigen; HiB = *Haemophilus influenzae* group B vaccine; IPV = inactivated polio vaccine; U = units of HAV antigen.

CURRENT DIAGNOSIS

- Acute hepatitis is self-limited and does not cause progressive liver disease.
- Chronic hepatitis can lead to cirrhosis and end-stage liver disease.
- Hepatitis A is a vaccine-preventable disease, but sporadic outbreaks still occur.
- Travelers to less developed countries should be vaccinated for hepatitis A.
- Hepatitis B can cause both acute and chronic liver disease. In most cases, infection resolves through natural immune clearance. For patients with chronic infection, several therapies exist.
- Hepatitis B is a vaccine-preventable disease.
- Hepatitis C is a leading cause of chronic liver disease.
- Combination therapies for hepatitis C with pegylated interferon and ribavirin are available but are only effective in 50% of patients.
- Hepatitis E is a self-limited disease seen mostly in less developed countries. Travelers should drink bottled or boiled water in endemic countries to avoid infection.
- Mortality is high in pregnant women who acquire hepatitis E.
- Hepatocellular cancer is a complication of chronic liver disease and should be screened for regularly.

appears before the onset of clinical symptoms and persists for 3 to 6 months. Anti-HAV IgG appears after IgM and persists for years, indicating immunity. Although different variants of HAV have been identified, only one serotype is responsible for cross-reactivity to all variants. HAV antigen is detectable in the stool 1 to 2 weeks before the onset of symptoms, disappears before jaundice, and reappears during relapses. ALT and AST are typically very high and recover in 3 weeks. Bilirubin peaks at 12 to 30 mg/dL and starts declining in 2 to 3 weeks. The patient is no longer infectious 1 week after the onset of jaundice.

TREATMENT AND PREVENTION

The treatment of HAV is supportive. Hygiene is important in prevention of infection.

Persons with documented HAV immunity (previous infection) do not need passive or active prophylaxis. Active prophylaxis, obtained by HAV vaccines, offers prolonged immunity. Prevaccination testing of children is not indicated due to low incidence of infection in the United States, but it may be cost-effective in select adult populations. Currently in the United States three licensed vaccines are available: Havrix, Vaqta, and the combination HAV/HBV vaccine Twinrix. The vaccines are highly effective if used appropriately. Immunity occurs in 1 month.

TABLE 3 Serologic Parameters for Hepatitis A Virus

Type	Anti-HAV IgM	Anti-HAV IgG
Acute	+	−
Exposed	±	+
Immunized	±	+

Abbreviations: anti-HAV = antibodies to hepatitis A; HAV = hepatitis A virus; Ig = immunoglobulin.

HAV vaccine should be given to all children ages 1 to 18 years, travelers to endemic areas, MSM, recreational drug users, those with chronic liver disease, persons with clotting factor disorders, and persons at risk for occupational exposure. During outbreaks, unvaccinated children should receive both active and passive prophylaxis.

Passive prophylaxis, obtained by administration of pooled immunoglobulins (Ig), offers limited protection, but it is important during HAV outbreaks in daycare centers and among food handlers, household contacts of patients with acute HAV, and persons traveling to HAV-endemic areas within 4 weeks from the first dose of HAV vaccine. A 0.02 mL/kg Ig dose is 80% to 90% effective as postexposure prophylaxis if given within 2 weeks, but it also attenuates the clinical disease if given after 2 weeks. A 0.06 mL/kg Ig dose given before travel confers immunity for 3 to 5 months. (See Table 2 for the vaccination schedules.)

Hepatitis B

EPIDEMIOLOGY

Worldwide, the number of HBV infections exceeds 350 million. In the United States, an estimated 1.25 million people are chronically infected. The number of acute infections in the United States has decreased from 260,000 per year in the 1980s to 60,000 per year in 2004. The decline is largely due to the routine use of HBV vaccine.

In areas of high prevalence, such as Southeast Asia, China, and Africa, the most common route of transmission is vertically from mother to child and horizontally among children. However, in the United States and other Western countries, which are considered low-prevalence areas, horizontal spread among adults is the most common, especially through sexual contact or through injection drug use. The virus is transmitted by passage of infectious bodily fluids through percutaneous routes or disrupted mucosal membranes. HBV is 100 times more infectious than HIV and approximately 8 to 10 times more infectious than HCV.

Routine testing for HBV should be offered to persons with multiple sexual partners, MSM, parenteral drug users, household contacts of infected persons, children born to infected mothers or to immigrants from highly endemic areas, hemodialysis patients, pregnant women, HIV-positive persons, and health care and public safety workers.

CLINICAL FEATURES

Acute HBV infection occurs after an incubation period of 30 to 180 days. The age and immune status of the exposed person are correlated with the outcome of the acute infection, but why some patients ultimately clear the viral infection is not known. Acute HBV is subclinical in 90% of young children but 30% to 80% of adults have anicteric or icteric forms (see the discussion of acute hepatitis). Resolution of jaundice generally occurs within 1 to 3 months. Eighty percent of acute HBV resolves with disappearance of hepatitis B surface antigen (HBsAg) by 12 to 24 weeks. As in HAV, less than 1% of the cases progress to fulminant hepatic failure, which generally occurs within 4 weeks of onset of symptoms.

Chronic hepatitis following acute infection develops in 90% of infants born to hepatitis B e antigen (HBeAg)-positive mothers, 30% of children infected at 1 to 5 years of age, and 6% of those infected after 5 years of age. Immunosuppressed persons are more likely to develop chronic infection. From 15% to 25% of the chronically infected patients die from complications of HBV including cirrhosis and HCC.

Extrahepatic manifestations are common in both acute and chronic HBV infection. Arthritis-dermatitis is manifested with fever, arthralgia, rash, and edema. Polyarteritis nodosa (PAN), a systemic necrotizing vasculitis, is a serious complication of HBV infection. Glomerulonephritis occurs with several different glomerular lesions and can manifest with the nephrotic syndrome. Essential mixed cryoglobulinemia is not seen as commonly as in HCV and is often asymptomatic.

TABLE 4 Serologic Parameters for Hepatitis B Virus

Type	HBsAg	Anti-HBs	HBeAg	Anti-HBe	Anti-HBc	HBV DNA
Acute	±	−	+	−	IgM	+
Immune clearance (recovered)	−	+	−	+	IgG	−*
Chronic	+	−	±	±	IgG	+
Vaccination	−	+	−	−	−	−

*May have detectable HBV DNA by more sensitive assays.
Abbreviations: anti-HBc = antibodies to hepatitis B core antigen; anti-HBe = antibodies to hepatitis B e antigen; anti-HBs = antibodies to hepatitis B surface; HBeAg = hepatitis B e antigen; HBsAg = hepatitis B surface antigen; HBV = hepatitis B virus.

DIAGNOSIS

The diagnosis of acute HBV infection (Table 4) is made by the presence of HBsAg and antibodies to hepatitis B core antigen (anti-HBcAg). During the replicative phase of the infection, HBV DNA and HBeAg, a marker of viral replication, are also positive. HBsAg appears first, before the onset of symptoms, and disappears 3 to 6 months after the infection in persons who recover without chronic infection. Hepatitis B surface antibodies (anti-HBs) are protective and appear after the clearance of HBsAg. Anti-HBs also appear after successful vaccination. The persistence of HBsAg longer than 6 months usually indicates chronic infection; however, clearance after 6 to 12 months is possible. There is a serologic window between the disappearance of HBsAg and the appearance of HBsAb when the diagnosis of acute infection is only possible by detection of anti-HBcAg IgM. Anti-HBcAg is detectable throughout the course of disease (IgM is replaced by IgG in chronic infection), but it does not give protection and its presence means natural infection.

HBeAg seroconversion, referring to loss of HBeAg and development of antibodies to HBeAg (anti-HBe), can occur through immune clearance during acute infection or through antiviral therapies in chronic infection. However, mutations in the precore and basal core promoter regions of HBV can give rise to HBeAg mutants in which patients are HBeAg-negative, but produce HBV DNA and can develop progressive liver disease.

Inactive carriers are persons who have evidence of HBV DNA by highly sensitive polymerase chain reaction (PCR) methods and also have normal serum aminotransferases. Long-term follow-ups of these persons suggest that they do not develop progressive liver disease. Liver function tests may need to be monitored every 6 to 12 months. Active carriers have evidence of HBV DNA by non-PCR methods and elevated or intermittently elevated serum aminotransferases.

TREATMENT

Treatment goals include HBeAg seroconversion, significant decrease in HBV DNA or viral suppression, normalization of aminotransferases, and improvement of fibrosis on liver biopsy. Patients with more than 10^4 copies/mL of HBV DNA and abnormal liver function tests may need to be considered for therapy, especially if they are cirrhotic (see Table 5 for guidelines). A specialist should evaluate those who do not meet the guidelines outlined in Table 5 but have detectable HBV DNA levels to determine risk of disease progression.

Older therapies such as interferon-α-2b (IFN-α-2b) (Intron A) given three times weekly for 4 months have been replaced with the newer pegylated IFN-α-2a (Pegasys) once-weekly

TABLE 5 Current Therapies for Chronic Hepatitis B and C Viruses

Virus and Type	Treatment Decision Factors	Treatment Strategy	Therapy Options
HBV, HBeAg-positive*	HBV DNA > 20,000 copies/mL, elevated ALT†	Treat until HBV DNA is undetectable and HBeAg seroconversion plus 6 additional mo	Lamivudine (Epivir) 100 mg PO qd Adefovir (Hepsera) 10 mg PO qd Entecavir (Baraclude) 0.5 mg PO qd for naive, 1 mg PO qd for experienced Telbivudine (Tyzeka) 600 mg PO qd IFN-α-2b (Intron A) 10 million units SC 3 ×/wk for 16 wk PEG-IFN-α-2a (Pegasys) 180 µg SC weekly for 48 wk
HBV, liver cirrhosis	Decompensated	Combination therapy with lamivudine or entecavir *plus* adefovir; place on transplant list	Adefovir *plus* entecavir or lamivudine (dose as for HBeAg-positive) Interferon therapy is contraindicated
	Compensated	If HBV DNA > 2000 copies, treat long term with adefovir or entecavir	Adefovir or entecavir (dose as for HBeAg-positive)
HCV, genotype 1	If no contraindications	Treatment for 48 wk Discontinue if no virologic response at 12 wk	PEG-IFN-α-2a (Pegasys) 180 µg SC weekly *or* PEG-IFN-α-2b (PEG-Intron) 1.5 µg/kg SC weekly *plus* Ribavirin (Rebetol, Ribasphere, Copegus) 1200 mg (> 75 kg) or 1000 mg (< 75 kg) in 2 divided doses
HCV, genotype 2 and 3	If no contraindications	Treatment for 24 wk	PEG-IFN (dose as for genotype 1) *plus* Ribavirin 800 mg PO qd in 2 divided doses

*HBeAg-negative, threshold for treatment > 2000 copies/mL.
†Normal ALT may need to have liver biopsy to determine if treatment is necessary
Abbreviations: HBV = hepatitis B; HBeAg = hepatitis B e antigen; HCV = hepatitis C; IFN = interferon; PEG = pegylated.

treatment given for 12 months (see Table 5), in which one third of patients who are HBeAg-positive at baseline obtain HBeAg loss. Interferon is more effective in patients with high ALT and low HBV DNA.

Lamivudine (Epivir), adefovir (Hepsera), entecavir (Baraclude), and telbivudine (Tyzeka) are oral agents directed against viral replication. They have few adverse effects in comparison with interferon-based therapies (see discussion of HCV for side effects) but HBeAg loss rates are not as high as with interferon therapies. Lamivudine is also safe for use in decompensated liver disease. For lamivudine, response rates in HBeAg-positive patients have been 16% to 18% in loss of antigen and 49% to 56% in histologic improvement; higher ALT predicted better response. In HBeAg-negative patients, good response rates were offset by the greater than 90% relapse rate after 1 year. Over time, lamivudine resistance (70% with 5 years of therapy) can develop, making lamivudine ineffective.

Adefovir can be used either initially in treatment-naive persons or as second-line treatment for those with lamivudine resistance. Long-term therapy with adefovir has revealed development of resistance in 3% with 2 years of therapy and 30% with 5 years of therapy. The relapse rate is high if medication is stopped.

Entecavir can suppress HBV replication significantly and is active for both lamivudine- and adefovir-resistant mutations. Entecavir is administered at two doses depending on whether the drug is being used in a naive or treatment-experienced patient. Telbivudine has been used for the treatment of chronic HBV, however, resistance can develop in 10% of patients after one year of treatment.

Several other agents including tenofovir (Viread)[1] and emtricitabine (Emtriva)[1] (used in HIV infection) also have activity against HBV.

PREVENTION

Vaccination against HBV with newer DNA recombinant vaccines has changed the epidemiology of the disease and significantly decreased the number of new infections. The currently available HBV vaccines are Engerix-B and Recombivax HB (see Table 2 for vaccine schedule and dose). Combination vaccines effective against both HAV and HBV are available (see the discussion of hepatitis A).

Due to the high risk of vertical transmission, all infants born to HBsAg-positive mothers should receive a first dose of HBV vaccine and passive prophylaxis with hepatitis B immune globulin (HBIg) 0.5 mL IM, in a separate site from the vaccine, in the first 12 hours after delivery. Vaccination of all other stable infants before hospital discharge is now recommended. All children and adolescents are currently included in a catch-up vaccination program.

Vaccination is also recommended for health care workers, persons with chronic liver disease, and all persons considered at risk (i.e., persons recommended to be screened for HBV). Generally, a postvaccine HBsAb titer of greater than 10 IU/mL is considered protective, but postvaccination testing is necessary only for health care workers. Boosting is indicated for hemodialysis patients. The vaccine is more than 95% efficacious in immunocompetent patients.

Hepatitis C

EPIDEMIOLOGY

Worldwide, an estimated 3% of persons have HCV antibodies and more than 170 million people are chronically infected. No available HCV vaccine exists. In the United States, as well as most developed countries, the number of new infections has decreased significantly due to screening of blood products. However, the number of new diagnoses continues to rise, with an estimated burden of 3.2 million chronic infections in the United States; most of these persons were infected through intravenous drug use or receipt of blood products decades ago. Transmission from mother to child is also possible. In 1992, a commercial assay became available for HCV testing and has been used to test blood products since then. Other routes of transmission include tattoos, especially if occurring during incarceration, and intranasal cocaine use. Sexual transmission is rare among heterosexual couples. The Centers for Disease Control and Prevention (CDC) does not recommend changes in sexual practices in monogamous couples. However, risk of sexual transmission might be increased in persons with multiple sexual partners or MSM.

The CDC and the American Association for the Study of Liver Diseases (AASLD) recommend HCV testing for parenteral drug users, hemophiliacs, and other persons receiving blood products or organ transplants before 1992, HIV-positive persons, hemodialysis patients, health care workers with occupational exposure to HCV-positive blood, children born to infected mothers, partners of HCV-positive patients, and persons with unexplained liver function test abnormalities. HCV-positive persons should be counseled about how to avoid transmitting the disease to others.

CLINICAL FEATURES

There are six major genotypes of HCV, and they have a geographic distribution. In the United States, 60% to 70% of persons are infected with genotype 1, whereas genotypes 2 and 3 are more common in Europe. In Egypt, the predominant genotype is 4. The importance of genotype lies in its predictive value for treatment response to combination therapy with PEG-IFN and ribavirin.

Following an incubation period averaging 7 weeks, acute hepatitis C usually is asymptomatic; it manifests as a flulike illness or rarely as a mild icteric disease. Following acute infection, 50% to 85% of the patients develop chronic infection. Of these, 70% progress to chronic liver disease. Overall, 1% to 5% of infected persons die of HCV-related complications.

Progression to HCC occurs in the setting of cirrhosis, and all HCV-infected cirrhotic patients should be screened for HCC regularly. Extrahepatic manifestations are rare during acute infection but common in chronic infection. Well-described extrahepatic manifestations are essential mixed cryoglobulinemias, membranoproliferative glomerulopathy, leukocytoclastic vasculitis, immune arthropathies, and porphyria cutanea tarda. There may be an increased incidence of non-Hodgkin's lymphoma in HCV-infected patients.

DIAGNOSIS

The diagnosis (Table 6) is based on detection of antibodies against HCV (anti-HCV). HCV antibodies are not protective and only serve as a marker of infection. The third-generation enzyme immunoassay (EIA) has 97% sensitivity in detecting total antibodies and can be confirmed by direct detection using HCV RNA. If the HCV RNA is negative, a recombinant immunoblot assay (RIBA) can be performed; if RIBA is negative, EIA is a false positive. If the EIA and RIBA are positive but HCV RNA is repeatedly negative, prior infection and natural immune clearance have occurred, which can be seen in 15% to 50% of acute infections, and no further testing is required.

TABLE 6 Serologic Parameters for Hepatitis C Virus

HCV	Anti-HCV	HCV RNA
Acute	+	+
Chronic	+	+
Past Infection	+	−

Abbreviations: anti-HCV = antibodies to hepatitis C; HCV = hepatitis C.

---

[1]Not FDA approved for this indication.

The quantitative HCV RNA assays have lower sensitivity than the qualitative assays. A quantitative assay is obtained to confirm infection (presence of virus) and determine the level of viremia; however, the actual RNA level is only important as a prognostic factor for treatment response. It does not correlate with severity of liver disease. A genotypes should also be ordered because it affects the treatment duration and predicts therapeutic response.

Qualitative HCV RNA assays are available with limits of detection of 50 UI/mL. The only FDA-approved quantitative test is Bayer's Versant HCV RNA 3.0, with limits of detection of 615,000 to 7,700,000 copies/mL, but other quantitative assays are available. The same quantitative test should be used to monitor treatment response.

TREATMENT

The goal of treatment is eradication of infection and prevention of complications from chronic HCV infection such as end-stage liver disease. Sustained virologic response (SVR) is defined as an undetectable HCV RNA by qualitative assays (< 50 IU/mL) 6 months after completion of HCV treatment. Follow-up studies in patients who have achieved an SVR were unable to detect reemergence of HCV RNA up to 5 years after therapy. Currently, the treatment of choice is combination therapy with pegylated interferon (Pegasys or PEG-Intron) and ribavirin (Rebetol, Ribasphere, or Copegus). Pegylated interferon, a synthetic compound with weekly subcutaneous dosing, is used in combination with oral ribavirin (see Table 5 for treatment options).

Patients with genotype 1 and high HCV viral loads achieved a SVR of 41% with pegylated interferon–ribavirin combination therapy, and the SVR in genotype 1 patients with low viral loads was 56%; genotypes 2 and 3 achieved higher rates, of 74% and 81%, respectively. Race appears to affect treatment response in genotype 1 African Americans, who respond less often (< 20%) compared with whites (~50%). HIV-infected persons with genotype 1 also respond less often (~30%).

Treatment can be considered in patients who do not have uncontrolled depression, thyroid disease, diabetes, or heart disease; transplant recipients; pregnant or lactating women; patients with autoimmune diseases; and patients with malignancies. Side effects of pegylated interferon include flulike symptoms, thrombocytopenia, leukopenia, anemia, depression, thyroid dysfunction, fatigue, and alopecia. Ribavirin, a teratogen, is contraindicated in renal failure and often causes anemia and a rash. Determining candidates for therapy is an individualized decision based on HCV genotype, degree of fibrosis, HCV RNA level, and other comorbid illnesses. For genotype 1 patients, treatment should be given for 48 weeks; treatment should be discontinued if there is no evidence of response by week 12. For genotypes 2 and 3 patients, treatment should be given for 24 weeks. Retreatment is not indicated in patients who have failed the combination therapy using pegylated interferon.

Treatments targeting the HCV genome transcriptions and translation, currently under evaluation, may be a new therapeutic option for genotype 1 patients in the near future.

Hepatitis D

HDV is a defective virus only found in HBV-infected persons. It consists of an RNA genome and a hepatitis delta antigen (HDAg); the viral envelope is composed of HBsAg. HDV depends on HBV to acquire the HBsAg needed for viral envelope assembly and transport into the hepatocyte, which is the only target cell. The HDV genome can replicate independently, and nonencapsulated particles circulate in the blood of the infected persons, but because they lack HBsAg, these forms are not pathogenic.

EPIDEMIOLOGY AND CLINICAL FEATURES

The distribution of HDV is variable but is estimated to infect 5% of those with chronic HBV. The prevalence rate is highest in South America and the Mediterranean basin. Prevalence rates in northern Europe and North America are low, and the population at risk seems to be confined to injection drug users. There are two forms of acquisition: coinfection (simultaneously with HBV) and superinfection (in previously HBV-infected persons). In coinfection, seen primarily in injection drug users, HDV is usually self-limited because acute HBV infection generally resolves, but chronic HDV infection can develop in 5% of patients who are coinfected. A biphasic elevation in liver enzymes may be seen in coinfection because of delay in HDV replication, but it is not seen in acute HBV infection alone. Coinfected persons may be at increased risk for fulminant HBV. HDV superinfection occurs in the setting of chronic liver disease and should be suspected in any HBsAg-positive patient with an acute flare of hepatitis or decompensation of preexisting liver disease. HDV superinfection develops into chronic HDV infection in 70% of patients characterized by persistent HDV viremia.

DIAGNOSIS AND TREATMENT

The most useful test for diagnosis is the HDV IgM or total anti-HDV (both IgM and IgG) (Table 7). In chronic HDV infection, anti-HDV IgM can persist for some time and is a marker of serious liver disease. Anti-HDV IgG develops over time and can persist, but detection of anti-HDV IgG does not indicate chronic disease and may be seen in patients who have recovered. HDV RNA testing is available mainly for treatment follow-up.

The only treatment option available for chronic infection is interferon therapy. High doses are needed for up to 48 weeks. Nucleoside therapy is not effective for HDV infection. The success rate is controversial but the relapse rate is low. Vaccination against HBV is the most effective prevention.

Hepatitis E

EPIDEMIOLOGY

HEV causes an acute, icteric, self-limited hepatitis. HEV is endemic in Southeast and Central Asia, North Africa, and, most recently, Iraq. Epidemic outbreaks of HEV occur, affecting hundreds to thousands of persons. Attack rates are lower in children (0.2%-10%) but higher in adults (3%-30%). A high mortality rate is seen in pregnant women (5%-25%) who acquire HEV. Transmission is through the fecal-oral route and is associated with contaminated water. Recurrent epidemics are seen in countries where sanitation is poor. Person-to-person transmission is unlikely in epidemics. Sporadic HEV in endemic areas accounts for up to 50% to 70% of acute hepatitis but less than 1% in nonendemic areas.

CLINICAL FEATURES

The incubation period is 15 to 60 days. HEV can be detected in the stool approximately 1 week before clinical disease appears and up to 2 weeks after onset of clinical symptoms. The prodromal phase typically lasts 1 to 4 days, followed by an icteric phase and clinical signs and symptoms typical of any viral hepatitis.

TABLE 7 Serologic Parameters for Hepatitis D Virus

HDV	HBsAg	Anti-HBc	Anti-HDV	HDV Ag
Coinfection	+	IgM	IgM	+
Superinfection	+	IgG	IgM	+
Chronic Infection	+	IgG	IgM/IgG	+

Abbreviations: anti-HDV = antibodies to hepatitis D; HDV = hepatitis D; HDV Ag = hepatitis D antigen.

TABLE 8 Serologic Parameters for Hepatitis E Virus

HEV	Anti-HEV
Acute	IgM
Recovered	IgG

Abbreviations: anti-HEV = antibodies to hepatitis E; HEV = hepatitis E.

DIAGNOSIS, TREATMENT, AND PREVENTION

Diagnosis is made by detection of anti-HEV IgM (Table 8) that can be detected at onset of illness; it is unclear if HEV antibodies confer immunity. Treatment is supportive. Because no vaccine is available, travelers to endemic areas should drink boiled or bottled water.

Hepatocellular Carcinoma Screening

Both HBV and HCV are associated with hepatocellular carcinoma, with higher incidence in cirrhotic patients. By contrast, HDV appears to lower the chance of HBV-infected patients to develop HCC. AASLD guidelines recommend screening with a AFP and liver ultrasound every 6 months in all HBV carriers at risk for HCC, such as adults older than 45 years, cirrhotic patients, and patients with a family history of HCC. Computed tomography or magnetic resonance imaging studies are more sensitive but more expensive methods of screening for HCC. Routine screening of HBV carriers from endemic areas without other known risk factors may be performed although there is no proven benefit. Based on current clinical data, all HCV-positive cirrhotic patients should be screened because the HCC incidence is 2% to 8% per year in this group.

HIV Coinfection

Patients coinfected with HIV and hepatitis B or C are difficult to manage. The treatment options should be carefully weighed and an experienced physician should help manage them. Several drugs are active against both HIV and HBV, and their value in treating coinfections is under evaluation. All chronic hepatitis patients should be tested for HIV because of shared transmission routes.

REFERENCES

Chang T, Gish R, De Man RA, et al: A comparison of entecavir and lamivudine for HBeAg-positive chronic hepatitis B. N Engl J Med 2006;354:1001-1010.
Dienstag JL, Schiff ER, Wright TL, et al: Lamivudine as the initial treatment for chronic hepatitis B virus in the United States. N Engl J Med 1999;341:1256-1263.
Emerson SU, Purcell RH: Running like water: The Omnipresence of hepatitis E. N Engl J Med 2004;351:2367-2368.
Erhard A, Gerlich W, Starke C, et al: Treatment of chronic hepatitis delta with pegylated interferon alfa-2b. Liver Int 2006;26(7):805-810.
Fiore AE., Wasley A, Bell BP: Prevention of hepatitis A through active or passive immunization. Recommendations of the Advisory Committee on Immunization Practices (ACIP). MMWR Recomm Rep 2006; 55(RR-07):1-23.
Fried MW, Shiffman ML, Reddy KR, et al: Peginterferon-alfa 2a plus ribavirin for chronic hepatitis C virus infection. N Engl J Med 2002;347(13):975-982.
Hadziyannis SJ, Sette H, Morgan TR, et al: Peginterferon alfa 2a (40 kilodaltons) and ribavirin combination therapy in chronic hepatitis C: Randomized study of the effect of treatment duration and ribavirin dose. Ann Intern Med 2004;140:346-355.
Keeffe EB, Dieterich DT, Han SH, et al: A treatment algorithm for the management of chronic hepatitis B virus infection in the United States: An update. Clin Gastroenterol Hepatol 2006;4(8):936-962.
Lok A, McMahon B: Chronic hepatitis B: Update of recommendations. AASLD Guideline. Hepatology 2004;39:857-861.
Manns MP, McHutchinson JG, Gordon SC, et al: Peginterferon alfa-2b plus ribavirin compared with interferon alfa-2b plus ribavirin for initial treatment of chronic hepatitis C: A randomized trial. Lancet 2001;358:958-965.
Marcellin P, Chang TT, Lim SG, et al: Adefovir dipivoxil for the treatment of hepatitis B e antigen–positive chronic hepatitis B. N Engl J Med 2003; 348:808-816.
Strader BD, Wright T, Thomas DL, et al: Diagnosis, management, and treatment of hepatitis C. AASLD Practice Guideline. Hepatology 2004;39(4):1147-1171.

Malabsorption

Method of
Lawrence R. Schiller, MD

Every day the average human being consumes 2000-3000 kcal of food, much of it in the form of polymers or other complex molecules that must be digested and absorbed by the gut. The processes of digestion and absorption are complex and are readily disturbed by pathologic processes. More than 200 conditions have been described that can adversely affect nutrient absorption.

Strictly speaking, *maldigestion* refers to impaired hydrolysis of nutrients, usually due to lack of luminal factors, such as bile acids and pancreatic enzymes, and *malabsorption* refers to impaired mucosal transport. For clinical purposes, "malabsorption" is used to describe both processes.

Malabsorption can be generalized (panmalabsorption) or limited to a specific category of nutrients. Generalized malabsorption is usually due to maldigestion or to extensive mucosal dysfunction. Specific malabsorption occurs when a single transporter is disabled.

The causes of malabsorption can be divided into three categories: impaired luminal hydrolysis, impaired mucosal function (mucosal hydrolysis, uptake, packaging, and excretion), and impaired removal of nutrients from the mucosa (Box 1).

Diagnosis

SYMPTOMS AND SIGNS

Most patients with panmalabsorption have changes in their stools (Box 2). Steatorrhea (excess fat in stools) is characterized by pale color, bulkiness, greasiness, and a tendency to float (probably because of incorporated gas). Occasionally patients with malabsorption present with watery stools due to the osmotic effects of unabsorbed carbohydrates and short-chain fatty acids.

Abdominal distention and excess flatus also commonly occur due to fermentation of unabsorbed carbohydrate by colonic bacteria. This can occur not only with panmalabsorption but also with specific malabsorption of carbohydrate (e.g., lactase deficiency).

Weight loss is typical with severe panmalabsorption, but it might not be very prominent with lesser degrees of malabsorption due to compensatory hyperphagia. Weight loss is most prominent early in the course of the illness, but body weight usually stabilizes as calorie absorption and body weight come into balance again. This is in contrast to illnesses like cancer or tuberculosis that produce continuing weight loss. If a patient with malabsorption has continuing weight loss, inflammatory bowel disease or lymphoma should be considered.

Abdominal pain is usually not present with malabsorption, although some cramping may be associated with diarrhea. Severe pain should bring chronic pancreatitis, Zollinger-Ellison syndrome, lymphoma, Crohn's disease, or mesenteric ischemia to mind.

Constitutional symptoms of fatigue and weakness commonly occur, even early in the course. In contrast, appetite is impaired only late in the course of most malabsorption states. Edema is uncommon until late in the course unless protein-losing enteropathy is present.

CURRENT DIAGNOSIS

- Recognize the presence of generalized malabsorption by the combination of typical symptoms: diarrhea, greasy stools, flatulence, weight loss, fatigue, edema.
- Recognize the presence of specific malabsorption by associated symptoms and those symptoms particular to deficiency states of the malabsorbed substance: flatus, diarrhea, anemia, dermatitis, glossitis, neuropathy, paresthesias, tetany, ecchymosis.
- Documentation of generalized malabsorption is best done by stool analysis demonstrating steatorrhea and acid stools (reflecting carbohydrate malabsorption). Diagnosis depends on visualization of the small bowel by endoscopy or radiography and small bowel biopsy. Additional tests may be needed.
- Documentation of specific malabsorption is best done by demonstrating low blood levels of the malabsorbed substance or by tests designed to measure absorption of that substance. Diagnosis depends on studies designed to identify the likely diagnosis for a given situation.

BOX 1 Causes of Malabsorption or Maldigestion

- Impaired luminal hydrolysis or solublization
  - Bile acid deficiency
  - Impaired mucosal hydrolysis, uptake, or packaging
  - Pancreatic exocrine insufficiency
  - Postgastrectomy syndrome
  - Rapid intestinal transit
  - Small bowel bacterial overgrowth
  - Zollinger-Ellison syndrome
- Brush border or metabolic disorders
  - Abetalipoproteinemia
  - Glucose-galactose malabsorption
  - Lactase deficiency
  - Sucrase-isomaltase deficiency
- Mucosal diseases
  - Amyloidosis
  - Chronic mesenteric ischemia
  - Crohn's disease
  - Celiac sprue
  - Collagenous sprue
  - Eosinophilic gastroenteritis
  - Immunoproliferative small intestinal disease (IPSID)
  - Lymphoma
  - Nongranulomatous ulcerative jejunoileitis
  - Radiation enteritis
  - Systemic mastocytosis
- Infectious diseases
  - AIDS enteropathy
  - *Mycobacterium avium-intracellulare*
  - Parasitic diseases
  - Small bowel bacterial overgrowth
  - Tropical sprue
  - Whipple's disease
- After intestinal resection
- Chronic mesenteric ischemia
- Impaired removal of nutrients
  - Lymphangiectasia

BOX 2 Symptoms and Signs of Malabsorption or Maldigestion

- Changes in stool characteristics
  - Floating stools
  - Pale, bulky, greasy stools
  - Watery diarrhea
- Increased colonic gas production
  - Abdominal distention
  - Borborygmi
- Vitamin and mineral deficiencies
  - Anemia
  - Cheilosis
  - Glossitis
  - Dermatitis
  - Neuropathy
  - Night blindness
  - Osteomalacia
  - Paresthesia
  - Tetany
- Ecchymosis
- Fatigue, weakness
- Edema
- Weight loss, muscle wasting

Vitamin and mineral deficiencies can lead to several symptoms or signs. Glossitis and cheilosis are common in patients with water-soluble vitamin deficiencies. Florid beriberi, pellagra, and scurvy are not commonly seen unless malabsorption has been particularly severe or long-lasting. Fat-soluble vitamin deficiencies also are unlikely to develop except when malabsorption has been long-standing because of substantial body stores.

Miscellaneous findings occasionally seen in patients with malabsorption can provide clues to the diagnosis. Aphthous ulcers in the mouth may be seen with celiac disease, Behçet's syndrome, or Crohn's disease. Hyperpigmentation is seen in Whipple's disease, and dermatitis herpetiformis (pruritic, blistering skin lesions) is seen in celiac disease. Scleroderma can manifest with tight skin, digital ulceration, nail changes, and Raynaud's phenomenon. Chronic sinusitis, bronchitis, and recurrent pneumonia suggest cystic fibrosis or IgA deficiency. Several systemic diseases can be associated with malabsorption syndrome (Box 3).

TESTS

Routine Laboratory Tests

Routine laboratory tests (Box 4) commonly are abnormal in patients with established malabsorption syndrome. Anemia is common but

BOX 3 Systemic Diseases Associated with Malabsorption or Maldigestion

Endocrine Diseases
- Addison's disease
- Diabetes mellitus
- Hypoparathyroidism
- Hyperthyroidism, hypothyroidism

Collagen-Vascular and Miscellaneous Diseases
- AIDS
- Amyloidosis
- Scleroderma
- Vasculitis (systemic lupus erythematosus, polyarteritis nodosa)

BOX 4 Laboratory Tests for Evaluation of Malabsorption or Maldigestion

Routine Blood Tests
- Complete blood count
- Hemoglobin/hematocrit
- Platelet count
- WBC differential count

Biochemistry Tests
- Blood urea nitrogen
- Potassium
- Prothrombin time
- Serum albumin
- Serum calcium
- Serum creatinine

Blood Levels of Potentially Malabsorbed Substances
- Serum iron, vitamin B_{12}, folate, 25-OH vitamin D, carotene

Fat absorption
- Qualitative fecal fat
- Quantitative fecal fat

Protein Absorption and Protein-Losing Enteropathy
- α_1-Antitrypsin clearance
- Fecal nitrogen excretion

Carbohydrate Absorption
- Osmotic gap in stool water
- Quantitative excretion (anthrone)
- Stool pH < 5.5
- Stool reducing substances
- D-Xylose absorption test
- Oral glucose, sucrose, and lactose tolerance tests
- Breath hydrogen tests

Vitamin B_{12} Absorption
- Schilling test with intrinsic factor

Bile Acid Malabsorption
- ^{14}C-glycocholic acid breath test
- Fecal bile acid excretion
- Radiolabeled bile acid excretion
- ^{75}SeHCAT retention

Small Bowel Bacterial Overgrowth
- ^{14}C-glycocholic acid breath test
- ^{14}C-xylose breath test
- Glucose breath hydrogen test
- Quantitative culture of jejunal aspirate

Exocrine Pancreatic Insufficiency
- Dual-labeled Schilling test
- Secretin/CCK test
- Stool chymotrypsin concentration

Serologic Testing for Celiac Disease
- Anti-tissue transglutaminase antibody (IgA)
- Anti-endomysial antibody (IgA)

Abbreviations: CCK = cholecystokinin; SLE = systemic lupus erythematosus; ^{75}SeHCAT = selenium-75-labeled taurohomocholic acid.

CURRENT THERAPY

- Once a diagnosis is reached, therapy can be directed toward that specific problem:
    - Gluten-free diet for celiac disease
    - Antibiotics for bacterial overgrowth
    - Lactose-free diet for lactase deficiency

not universal. Iron deficiency anemia may be the only finding in some patients with celiac disease. Microcytic anemia may be present in Whipple's disease (due to occult blood loss) and in lymphomas manifesting with malabsorption. Macrocytic anemia due to folate or vitamin B_{12} deficiency can occur in short bowel syndrome, small bowel bacterial overgrowth, or ileal disease. Lymphopenia may be present in patients with AIDS or lymphangiectasia.

Electrolyte abnormalities may be due to a combination of poor intake and excess loss in stool. Renal function usually is well maintained in malabsorption syndrome, but blood urea nitrogen may be low due to poor protein absorption, and serum creatinine concentration may be low due to depletion of muscle mass. Serum calcium levels may be low due to malabsorption, vitamin D deficiency, or intraluminal complexing of calcium by fatty acids. Hypomagnesemia can produce hypocalcemia or hypokalemia that is resistant to intravenous repletion. Serum phosphorus, cholesterol, and triglyceride levels may be reduced due to poor intake or malabsorption. Liver tests may be abnormal due to fatty liver. Serum protein and albumin levels are well preserved in patients with malabsorption unless protein-losing enteropathy or an acute illness is present.

Prothrombin time is normal unless vitamin K malabsorption (typically associated with steatorrhea), anticoagulant therapy, antibiotic therapy, or colectomy is present.

Assays are available for several potentially malabsorbed substances, including iron, vitamin B_{12}, folate, 25-hydroxyvitamin D, and β-carotene. Malabsorption tends to lower blood levels, but substantial body stores of many of these can mitigate the reduction in concentration that otherwise might occur. Thus, the sensitivity and specificity of these assays for malabsorption are poor.

Tests for Malabsorption

Fat Malabsorption

The simplest test for fat malabsorption is a qualitative microscopic examination of stool using a fat-soluble stain, such as Sudan III. The finding of more than 5 stained droplets per high power field is abnormal and correlates well with quantitative measurement of fecal fat excretion. The test is subject to false-positive results with some drugs and food additives, such as mineral oil, orlistat, and olestra.

A more precise estimate of fat absorption is obtained by a quantitative analysis of a timed stool collection (48 or 72 hours). During the collection, a diary of dietary intake should be maintained so that fat excretion can be assessed as a percentage of intake. Normal fat excretion is < 7% of intake when stool weight is normal, but it can be twice as high due to voluminous diarrhea without indicating defective mucosal transport of fat. Thus, fat excretion must be judged against stool weight. Stool fat concentration (grams of fat per 100 grams of stool) also is of value. Pancreatic exocrine insufficiency is associated with high fecal fat concentration (> 10 g/100 g stool) because unlike hydrolyzed fat, unhydrolyzed fat does not stimulate colonic water and electrolyte secretion that would dilute fecal fat concentration.

Protein Malabsorption

Fecal nitrogen excretion can be employed as a marker of protein malabsorption, but is not often used in clinical medicine because it adds little to the evaluation. If protein-losing enteropathy is suspected, an α_1-antitrypsin clearance study can be done. In this study, *fecal* excretion of α_1-antitrypsin, a serum protein that is relatively resistant to hydrolysis by luminal enzymes, is divided by *serum* concentration of α_1-antitrypsin, and the volume of serum leaked into the lumen can be calculated. Values of more than 180 mL/day are associated with hypoalbuminemia.

Carbohydrate Malabsorption

Carbohydrate malabsorption is difficult to measure directly because fermentation of malabsorbed carbohydrate by colonic bacteria reduces the amount of intact carbohydrate that can be recovered in stool. Indirect estimates of carbohydrate malabsorption can be made by examining fecal pH (<5.5 with carbohydrate malabsorption) or fecal osmotic gap (>100 mOsm/kg with osmotic diarrhea). Oral carbohydrate tolerance tests may be used to evaluate absorption of sugars, such as lactose or fructose. Following an oral load of a given sugar, blood glucose levels are monitored; failure of blood glucose to increase suggests malabsorption.

Another test for carbohydrate malabsorption is the D-xylose absorption test. In this test, a 25-gram dose of D-xylose is given orally; blood xylose levels are measured 1 and 3 hours later, and urinary excretion of xylose is measured for 5 hours. Failure of blood xylose to rise above 20 mg/dL at 1 hour or above 22.5 mg/dL at 3 hours or failure of urinary excretion to exceed 5 g in 5 hours suggests malabsorption. In addition, because xylose does not require pancreatic enzymes or bile acids for absorption, an abnormal D-xylose test suggests a mucosal problem as the cause for malabsorption. The results of this test can be misleading if the patient is dehydrated or has ascites, if renal function is compromised, or if bacterial overgrowth is present in the upper small bowel.

Breath hydrogen testing is another method to assess carbohydrate absorption. If substrates such as lactose or sucrose are not absorbed in the small intestine, they pass into the colon, where bacterial fermentation produces hydrogen gas. The hydrogen is absorbed into the bloodstream and then is exhaled. The concentration of hydrogen in exhaled breath can be measured easily; a rise of more than 10 to 20 ppm after ingestion of a specific substrate is consistent with malabsorption. False-positive results can be seen in patients with small bowel bacterial overgrowth, and false-negative results can be seen in patients who lack hydrogen-producing flora or who have been on antibiotics recently.

Vitamin B$_{12}$ Malabsorption

The Schilling test can be used to measure vitamin B$_{12}$ absorption. For purposes of a malabsorption evaluation, part II of the Schilling test (measurement of radiolabeled B$_{12}$ absorption *with* intrinsic factor) is all that is needed. Recovery of less than 9% of the radiolabel in the urine is abnormal and suggests ileal dysfunction. The test may be falsely positive in patients with pancreatic exocrine insufficiency, small bowel bacterial overgrowth, or renal failure.

Bile Acid Malabsorption

Tests for bile acid malabsorption are not widely available in the United States. Direct measurement of bile acid excretion has been used mainly in research studies. Retention of a radioactive taurocholic acid analogue (SeHCAT, selenium-75-labeled taurohomocholic acid) is used in Europe to assess bile acid malabsorption. A breath test using ^{14}C-glycocholic acid has been used for evaluating small bowel bacterial overgrowth, but it may have application for assessing bile acid malabsorption as well.

Small Bowel Bacterial Overgrowth

The gold standard method used to test for small bowel bacterial overgrowth in the upper intestine is quantitative culture of jejunal fluid. The sample can be obtained during endoscopy and sent to the laboratory with instructions to quantitate the aerobic and anaerobic flora. Finding more than 10^5 bacteria per mL confirms bacterial overgrowth. Breath tests using glucose, ^{14}C-xylose, and lactulose also have been described for this purpose.

Pancreatic Exocrine Insufficiency

Tests for pancreatic exocrine insufficiency are not commonly used. The gold standard test is a secretin test. This study requires duodenal intubation, injection of secretin, and measurement of bicarbonate output. A tubeless test, the bentiromide test, had average clinical utility; it is no longer available in the United States. Measurement of fecal chymotrypsin or elastase activity is only moderately useful in predicting the presence of exocrine pancreatic insufficiency. For most situations, a therapeutic trial using a high dose of pancreatic enzymes with monitoring of the effect on steatorrhea is the best that can be done.

Evaluation of Suspected Malabsorption

When malabsorption is suspected because of the history, physical findings, and setting, the physician must decide if the malabsorption involves a specific nutrient or represents a generalized process (Figure 1). If the malabsorption seems to be specific, a diet and symptom diary, breath tests using the presumptively malabsorbed substrate, and stool pH to identify acid stools seen with carbohydrate malabsorption are reasonable diagnostic maneuvers.

Suspected generalized malabsorption requires a more intense evaluation. Steatorrhea should be confirmed with either a qualitative fecal fat test (e.g., Sudan stain) or a quantitative stool collection for measurement of fat excretion. If steatorrhea is confirmed, the small bowel should be visualized with either capsule endoscopy or radiography (small bowel follow-through examination or computed tomography) and biopsied from above by enteroscopy and from below by colonoscopy. During enteroscopy, an aspirate of small bowel contents can be obtained for quantitative culture to look for small bowel bacterial overgrowth. An alternative method to detect small bowel bacterial overgrowth is breath testing (see earlier). Stool samples also should be examined with microscopy or immunoassay for the presence of parasites that may be associated with malabsorption.

This sequence of evaluation often leads to a specific diagnosis. When it does not, empiric trials of pancreatic enzyme replacement

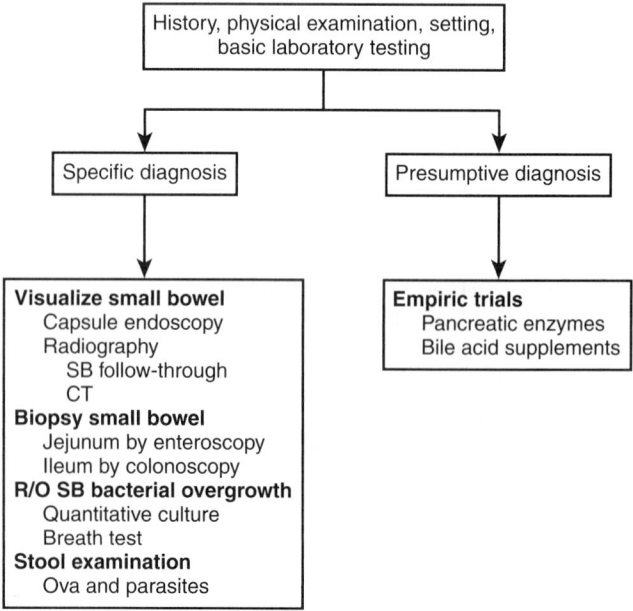

FIGURE 1. Flow chart for evaluation of malabsorption or maldigestion. *Abbreviations:* CT = computed tomography; R/O = rule out; SB = small bowel.

or bile acid supplementation can lead to a presumptive diagnosis of pancreatic exocrine insufficiency or bile acid deficiency. Hard endpoints (e.g., quantitative fat excretion) should be used to assess the effectiveness of these empiric trials.

Specific Disorders Associated with Malabsorption

MALABSORPTION OF SPECIFIC NUTRIENTS

Disaccharidase Deficiency

Ingested disaccharides such as lactose and sucrose and starch-digestion products such as maltotriose and α-limit dextrins must be hydrolyzed by brush border enzymes into monosaccharides for absorption by the mucosa. If these brush border enzymes are not active or if the brush border is damaged, malabsorption of the specific carbohydrate substrate results. This can result in gaseousness or osmotic diarrhea when those substrates are ingested. This rarely occurs on a congenital basis, but it commonly occurs as an acquired disorder.

Lactase deficiency is the most common acquired disaccharidase deficiency. Infant mammals all rely on lactose as the carbohydrate source in milk, but lactase activity is shut off after weaning in most species. Most human populations lose lactase activity during adolescence as a normal part of maturation. Members of the northern European gene pool might maintain lactase activity into adult life, but lactase activity declines gradually in many. At some point the amount of lactose ingested might exceed the ability of the remaining enzyme to hydrolyze it, resulting in lactose malabsorption and symptoms. This also can occur with acute conditions such as gastroenteritis that can disturb the mucosa and temporarily reduce lactase activity. Patients might not recognize lactose ingestion as a cause of their problem because they have not had difficulty tolerating lactose in the past. Restriction of lactose in the diet (or use of products that have predigested lactose) mitigates symptoms. Use of exogenous lactase as a tablet may only be partially effective because of incomplete hydrolysis of ingested lactose.

Transport Defects at the Brush Border

Glucose-galactose malabsorption is a rare congenital disorder resulting from an inactive hexose transporter in the brush border. Hydrolysis of lactose is intact, but transport across the apical membrane of the enterocyte fails to occur. Fructose absorption, which is mediated by a different carrier, is unaffected.

In all human beings the ability to absorb fructose is limited by the availability of carriers in the brush border and may be overwhelmed when excess fructose is ingested. This can occur relatively easily nowadays, because high-fructose corn syrup is used frequently as a sweetener in commercial products such as soda pop. Limiting the amount of fructose ingested will reduce symptoms.

Abetalipoproteinemia is a rare condition that prevents absorption of long-chain fatty acids due to failure to form chylomicrons. Use of medium-chain triglycerides that do not require transport in chylomicrons can bypass this defect.

Pernicious anemia develops when failure to secrete intrinsic factor in the stomach prevents vitamin B_{12} absorption by the ileal mucosa. Parenteral replacement with cyanocobalamin by injection (Cyanoject) or nasal spray (Nascobal) is necessary.

GENERALIZED MALABSORPTION

Celiac Disease

Celiac disease (also known as celiac sprue) is a disorder in which the mucosa of the small bowel is damaged due to activation of the mucosal immune system by ingestion of gluten, a protein component found in wheat, barley, and rye. People who have HLA-DQ2 or DQ8 are susceptible to this condition because these specific antigen-presenting proteins produce particularly strong reactions by interacting with a unique peptide digestion product of gluten. Tissue transglutaminase, an enzyme produced in the mucosa, is an important cofactor in pathogenesis by amplifying the immunogenicity of gluten peptide fragments and is the target of autoantibodies that are characteristic of this disease. The condition produces generalized malabsorption by destroying the villi of the small intestine, reducing the surface area available for absorption.

In addition to malabsorption syndrome with diarrhea and weight loss, celiac disease can produce a host of nonspecific symptoms, including abdominal pain, fatigue, muscle and joint pains, and headaches and seemingly unrelated problems such as iron deficiency anemia, abnormal liver tests, and osteoporosis. These protean manifestations mean that celiac disease must be considered in the differential diagnosis of many conditions. The clinical course is quite variable, with symptoms coming and going. Symptoms can develop during childhood and produce growth retardation or first become manifest in adulthood.

Testing for celiac disease has been simplified by the development of an assay for anti–tissue transglutaminase antibodies. This test largely supplants measurement of antigluten antibodies, although these remain of some use in evaluating adherence to a gluten-free diet. IgA antibodies are the most useful for diagnosis, but IgA deficiency is common enough that an IgA level should be measured concomitantly.

Although serologic tests have high sensitivity and specificity, the implications of adhering to a gluten-free diet are so extreme that the diagnosis of celiac disease should be confirmed whenever possible by small bowel mucosal biopsy, now obtained routinely by endoscopy. An empiric trial of a gluten-free diet may be difficult to interpret because many persons with gastrointestinal symptoms improve with dietary carbohydrate restriction. Wheat starch is particularly hard to digest (due to gluten coating wheat starch granules), and ordinarily 20% of wheat starch are not absorbed by the small bowel and enter the colon.

Treatment of celiac disease at present involves strict lifetime exclusion of gluten from the diet. This is a difficult regimen that excludes most processed foods. Assistance of a dietitian is most helpful. The prognosis with effective treatment is very good. Symptoms should respond to the diet within weeks; failure to do so should prompt an examination of compliance with the diet or reconsideration of the diagnosis. Failure to respond may be seen when lymphoma or adenocarcinoma complicate the course of celiac disease or in cases of "refractory sprue" or "collagenous sprue" which can have a different autoimmune basis from classic celiac disease and which might respond to immunosuppressive drugs such as corticosteroids or azathioprine (Imuran)[1]. Persistent diarrhea may be observed in patients with celiac disease who have concomitant microscopic colitis, another condition that is linked to HLA-DQ2 and HLA-DQ8.

Inflammatory Diseases

Diseases that produce extensive mucosal damage by inflammation cause generalized malabsorption by reduction of mucosal surface area, by promotion of small bowel bacterial overgrowth, by ileal dysfunction, or by development of enteroenteral or enterocolic fistulas. Examples include jejunoileitis due to Crohn's disease, nongranulomatous ulcerative jejunoileitis, radiation enteritis, and chronic mesenteric ischemia. With Crohn's disease, previous resection can add to the problem (see later). Therapy aimed at the underlying process can improve absorption; in some cases (e.g., radiation enteritis) no effective therapy is available for the underlying problem, and symptomatic management is all that is possible. This includes use of antidiarrheal drugs to prolong contact time between luminal contents and the small bowel mucosa, ingestion of a reduced fat diet to reduce steatorrhea, and use of vitamin and mineral supplements to prevent deficiency states.

Infiltrative Disorders

Several conditions involve infiltration of the intestinal mucosa with cells or extracellular matrix that impede absorption or modify mucosal function by secretion of cytokines and other regulatory

---

[1]Not FDA approved for this indication.

substances. These include eosinophilic gastroenteritis, systemic mastocytosis, immunoproliferative small intestinal disease (IPSID), lymphoma, and amyloidosis. These conditions are diagnosed by mucosal biopsy, but special stains might have to be employed to identify the infiltrating cells or matrix accurately.

Treatment of the underlying processes can improve absorption, but it is not uniformly effective. For eosinophilic gastroenteritis, a hypoallergenic (elimination) diet and corticosteroids may be useful. Mild systemic mastocytosis is treated with the mast cell-stabilizer sodium chromoglycate, H_1- and H_2-receptor antagonists, and low-dose aspirin. More advanced disease might respond to interferon or cytotoxic chemotherapy. IPSID initially is treated with antibiotics because small bowel bacterial overgrowth may be a causative factor. Once malignant change has occurred, it is treated like lymphoma with cytotoxic chemotherapy. Amyloidosis affecting the gut is not amenable to therapy and is usually fatal.

Infectious Diseases

Small Bowel Bacterial Overgrowth

Small bowel bacterial overgrowth in the jejunum can produce generalized malabsorption. It can occur whenever the mechanisms that reduce overgrowth are compromised. These situations include achlorhydria or hypochlorhydria, motility disorders of the small intestine (e.g., diabetes mellitus or scleroderma), and anatomic alterations (e.g., diverticulosis, gastrocolic fistula, or blind loops postoperatively). Fat malabsorption is attributed to bacterial deconjugation of bile acid. Bacterial toxins or free fatty acids can produce patchy mucosal damage, leading to less efficient carbohydrate and protein absorption. Bacteria also can compete with the mucosa for uptake of certain nutrients such as vitamin B_{12}.

Diagnosis of small bowel bacterial overgrowth can be difficult (see earlier). Treatment consists of antibiotic therapy unless a surgically correctable anatomic defect is discovered. Tetracycline is no longer uniformly effective; amoxicillin–clavulinic acid (Augmentin), cephalosporins, ciprofloxacin (Cipro), metronidazole (Flagyl), and rifaximin (Xifaxan) may be employed. Therapy should be given for 1 to 2 weeks initially and then discontinued. It should be restarted when symptoms recur. If this occurs quickly, longer treatment periods should be considered. Continuous antibiotic therapy is needed rarely.

Tropical Sprue

Tropical sprue is a progressive, chronic malabsorptive condition occurring in both the indigenous population and in visitors residing in certain tropical countries for extended periods. The prevalence of tropical sprue seems to be decreasing for uncertain reasons. The disease starts as an acute diarrheal disease that becomes a persistent diarrhea associated with substantial weight loss and typically megaloblastic anemia. Villi become shortened and thickened (partial villous atrophy), but the flat mucosa of celiac disease is not usually present. Enterocytes have disrupted brush borders and can have megaloblastic changes; the submucosa has a chronic inflammatory infiltrate. Intestinal biopsy is required for diagnosis.

Currently, tropical sprue is believed to represent a form of bacterial overgrowth with organisms that secrete enterotoxins. Most patients have evidence of excessive gram-negative bacterial colonization of the jejunum. The declining prevalence of tropical sprue may be due to improved nutrition, better sanitation, or prompt treatment of acute diarrhea with antibiotics. Treatment consists of pharmacologic doses of folic acid (folate) (5 mg daily[3]), injection of cyanocobalamin (if deficient), and antibiotic therapy for 1 to 6 months. Tetracycline 250 mg four times a day or sulfonamide is the treatment of choice. Newer antibiotics have not been tested extensively in this condition. Improvement should be noted after a few weeks. The prognosis with treatment is excellent; without treatment, tropical sprue can be fatal. Recurrence can occur.

Whipple's Disease

Whipple's disease is a rare chronic bacterial infection with multisystem involvement. The small bowel typically is heavily infiltrated with foamy macrophages containing periodic acid–Schiff (PAS)-positive material, distorting the villi. Small bowel biopsy with special stains or electron microscopy or a specific polymerase chain reaction (PCR) is diagnostic. Foamy macrophages and bacteria can be found outside the intestine in lymph nodes, spleen, liver, central nervous system, heart, and synovium. Accordingly, symptoms are protean. The bacterium has been identified as *Tropheryma whippelii*, a relative of *Acinetobacter*. It does not appear to be very contagious, and no direct person-to-person transmission has been demonstrated. Presumably differences in host resistance allow proliferation within macrophages without clearance of the bacteria.

Whipple's disease occurs mainly in older white men, but women and all ethnic groups are susceptible. Patients can present with malabsorption syndrome or with symptoms related to the extraintestinal disease (arthritis, fever, dementia, headache, or muscle weakness). Gross or occult gastrointestinal bleeding can occur. Protein-losing enteropathy may be present.

Treatment with any of several antibiotics (penicillin, erythromycin, ampicillin, tetracycline, chloramphenicol, or trimethoprim-sulfamethoxazole (TMP-SMX) produces excellent symptomatic responses within days to weeks, but it should be continued for months to years. Even with protracted courses, relapses are common.

Other Infections

Mycobacterium avium–intracellulare is another chronic bacterial infection that can cause malabsorption, particularly in patients with AIDS. Mucosal biopsy with special stains to distinguish it from Whipple's disease is essential. Antibiotic therapy can reduce the intensity of infection; clearance depends on immunologic reconstitution with antiretroviral therapy. Clarithromycin (Biaxin) and ethambutol (Myambutol) are recommended as initial therapy.

Parasitic diseases can produce malabsorption by competing for nutrients and causing mechanical occlusion of the absorptive surface and epithelial damage. Protozoa that may be associated with malabsorption include *Giardia lamblia*, *Isospora belli*, *Cryptosporidium*, and *Enterocytozoon bieneusi*. Tapeworms associated with malabsorption include *Taenia saginata* (beef tapeworm), *Hymenolepis nana* (dwarf tapeworm), and *Diphyllobothrium latum* (fish tapeworm).

Giardia lamblia is a cosmopolitan parasite acquired from contaminated water or from another person by fecal-oral transmission. Cysts are relatively hardy, and ingestion of as few as 10 cysts is sufficient to establish infection. Patients with dysgammaglobulinemia (especially IgA deficiency) are likely to become infected. Diagnosis depends on finding the organism (cysts or trophozoites) in stool by microscopy (sensitivity ~50% for a single specimen), or detection of giardia antigens by immunologic testing of stool (sensitivity >90%), or discovery of the organism on small bowel biopsy.

Therapy consists of a single dose of tinidazole (Tindamax) (2 g), metronidazole (Flagyl)[1] (250 mg three times a day for a week), nitazoxanide (Alinia) (500 mg twice a day for three days), or quinacrine[2] (100 mg three times a day for a week).

Isospora belli and *Cryptosporidium* spp. are coccidia, protozoa that disrupt the epithelium by intracellular invasion (*Isospora*) or by attaching to the brush border, destroying microvilli (*Crptosporidium*). Stool examination or small bowel biopsy can identify the organism. *Cryptosporidium* antigen can be discovered by immunoassay on stool with excellent sensitivity. *Isospora* can be treated with TMP-SMX[1] or furazolidone.[2] *Cryptosporidium* can be treated by nitazoxanide.

Microsporidia are intracellular organisms now believed to be most closely related to fungi and are implicated in diarrhea and malabsorption in patients with AIDS and other immunodeficiency states. Small bowel biopsy can show partial villous atrophy, and electron

---

[3]Exceeds dosage recommended by the manufacturer.

[1]Not FDA approved for this indication.
[2]Not available in the United States.

microscopy displays characteristic changes. Stool examination occasionally is helpful. No treatment is of proven value.

Tapeworms compete with their hosts for nutrients in the lumen. *Diphyllobothrium latum* can produce vitamin B_{12} deficiency. The others can result in more extensive nutritional deficiencies. Diagnosis is based on stool examination, and treatment depends on the particular organism identified.

Luminal Problems Causing Malabsorption

Pancreatic Exocrine Insufficiency

Pancreatic exocrine insufficiency is the most common luminal problem that results in maldigestion. Patients develop symptoms of malabsorption when pancreatic enzyme secretion is reduced by >90%. There are several clinical features that distinguish pancreatic exocrine insufficiency from mucosal disorders, such as celiac disease. When fat is not digested, it is transported through the gastrointestinal tract as intact triglyceride, which can appear as oil in the stool. In contrast, if fat is digested but not absorbed, it is in the form of fatty acids that can produce secretory diarrhea in the colon, resulting in more voluminous, even watery stools. This has two important ramifications: Fecal fat concentration is lower with mucosal disease (typically < 9% by weight), and hypocalcemia due to formation of soaps (calcium plus 2 fatty acids) is seen with mucosal disease but not with pancreatic exocrine insufficiency. In addition, patients with mucosal disease tend to have more problems with water-soluble vitamin deficiencies than those with pancreatic exocrine insufficiency. In some patients with pancreatic exocrine insufficiency, carbohydrate malabsorption can produce substantial bloating, flatulence, and watery diarrhea.

Tests to document pancreatic exocrine insufficiency are not widely available or are nonspecific (see earlier), and so diagnosis usually hinges on a consistent history, demonstration of anatomic problems in the pancreas (calcification or abnormal ducts), and documentation of a response of steatorrhea to empiric treatment with a large dose of exogenous enzymes.

Bile Acid Deficiency

Bile acid deficiency is a less common cause of maldigestion, and malabsorption in this setting is limited to fat and fat-soluble vitamins. The usual setting is a patient with an extensive ileal resection (see later), but this also occurs in certain cholestatic conditions in which bile acid secretion by the liver is markedly compromised, such as advanced primary biliary cirrhosis, or complete extrahepatic biliary obstruction. As with pancreatic exocrine insufficiency, stools tend to have high fat concentrations (>9% by weight) when bile acid secretion is limited by hepatic or biliary disorders.

Zollinger-Ellison Syndrome

Zollinger-Ellison syndrome produces several abnormalities that can affect absorption. High rates of gastric acid secretion produce persistently low pH in the duodenum, which precipitates bile acid and inactivates pancreatic enzymes. In addition, excess acid can damage the absorptive cells directly.

Postoperative Malabsorption

Substantial malabsorption can result from gastric surgeries. Weight loss can result from inadequate intake due to early satiety or symptoms of dumping syndrome. Malabsorption can result from impaired mechanical disruption of food, mismatching of chyme delivery and enzyme secretion, rapid transit, or small bowel bacterial overgrowth due to loss of the gastric acid barrier. In addition, gastric surgery sometimes brings out latent celiac disease.

Short intestinal resections are well tolerated, but more extensive resections produce diarrhea and malabsorption of variable severity. When these symptoms are associated with weight loss or dehydrating diarrhea, short bowel syndrome is said to exist. In general, nutrient absorptive needs can be met if at least 100 cm of jejunum are preserved, but fluid absorption will be insufficient and diarrhea may be profuse.

The process of intestinal adaptation permits improved absorption with time; it depends on exposure of the absorptive surface to nutrients. Absorption of specific substances, such as bile acids or vitamin B_{12}, is reduced permanently by resection of the terminal ileum.

Malabsorption in short bowel syndrome is not due solely to loss of absorptive surface area. Gastric acid hypersecretion, bile acid deficiency, rapid transit (due to loss of the ileal brake), and bacterial overgrowth may be present. These conditions are amenable to treatment and therapy with antisecretory drugs, exogenous bile acids, opiate antidiarrheals, or antibiotics can produce substantial improvement. Injection of growth hormone in combination with glutamine and a special diet has been approved as treatment for short bowel syndrome; it can reduce the volume of parenteral fluid or nutrients required. Results with small bowel transplantation are improving with the use of better immunosuppressive regimens, and it remains the only cure for select patients with postresection malabsorption.

Attention to nutrition is vital in any patient with malabsorption. If adequate nutrition cannot be maintained by oral intake, nutritional therapy is needed. Because of impaired bowel function, success with enteral nutrition may be impossible; parenteral nutrition may be needed. It is important to distinguish between the need for supplemental fluid and electrolytes and the need for nutrients; total parenteral nutrition is not a good choice for patients who only require fluids and electrolytes.

REFERENCES

Bai JC, Mazure RM, Vazquez H, et al: Whipple's disease. Clin Gastroenterol Hepatol 2004;2:849-860.
Culliford AN, Green PH: Refractory sprue. Curr Gastroenterol Rep 2003;5:373-378.
Green PH, Jabri B: Celiac disease. Annu Rev Med 2006;57:207-221.
Gupta V, Toskes PP: Diagnosis and management of chronic pancreatitis. Postgrad Med J 2005;81:491-497.
Horslen SP: Optimal management of the post-intestinal transplant patient. Gastroenterology 2006;130(2 suppl 1):S132-S137.
Jeejeebhoy KN: Management of short bowel syndrome: Avoidance of total parenteral nutrition. Gastroenterology 2006;130(2 suppl 1):S60-S66.
Nath SK: Tropical sprue. Curr Gastroenterol Rep 2005;7:343-349.
O'Keefe SJ, Buchman AL, Fishbein TM, et al: Short bowel syndrome and intestinal failure: Consensus definitions and review. Clin Gastroenterol Hepatol 2006;4:6-10.
Petroniene R, Dubcenco E, Baker JP, et al: Given capsule endoscopy in celiac disease. Gastrointest Endosc Clin N Am 2004;14:115-127.
Schiller LR: Nutrition management of chronic diarrhea and malabsorption. Nutr Clin Pract 2006;21:34-39.
Simren M, Stotzer PO: Use and abuse of hydrogen breath tests. Gut 2006;55:297-303.
Singh VV, Toskes PP: Small bowel bacterial overgrowth: Presentation, diagnosis, and treatment. Curr Gastroenterol Rep 2003;5:365-372.
Swallow DM: Genetics of lactase persistence and lactose intolerance. Annu Rev Genet 2003;37:197-219.

Acute and Chronic Pancreatitis

Method of
Carmen C. Solorzano, MD, and
Richard A. Prinz, MD

Acute Pancreatitis

Acute pancreatitis is an inflammatory process of the pancreas, with variable involvement of adjacent regional tissues or remote organ systems. The clinical manifestations of acute pancreatitis are heterogeneous but usually are of rapid onset. Most patients have epigastric pain, which can range from very mild to severe with associated hemodynamic instability. Early diagnosis and staging are necessary to provide appropriate treatment.

INCIDENCE AND ETIOLOGY

The incidence of acute pancreatitis has been reported to be as high as 38 per 100,000 population per year and appears to be increasing. Around 15% to 20% of patients will develop severe life-threatening complications requiring prolonged intensive care support at considerable cost.

Gallstones and alcohol abuse are the leading causes of acute pancreatitis in the United States, accounting for up to 80% of cases. Acute alcoholic pancreatitis may occur after binge drinking, but in most cases the patient has a minimum 5- to 7-year history of regular, heavy ethanol ingestion. Controversy exists as to whether alcohol alone, without prior gland injury, can cause the condition, as only a minority of alcoholics ever develop acute pancreatitis, implying multifactorial causation. A gallstone in the common bile duct (choledocholithiasis) may incite acute pancreatitis as it passes through the sphincter of Oddi en route to the duodenum. It does so, at least in principle, by transiently obstructing pancreatic duct flow and perhaps also by promoting reflux of bile into the pancreatic duct. As with alcoholic acute pancreatitis, the exact mechanisms remain uncertain. Perhaps 10% of attacks remain "idiopathic" in spite of thorough investigation. Other infrequent causes of acute pancreatitis are listed in Table 1.

PATHOGENESIS

Although the etiologic factor is known in 85% of patients with acute pancreatitis, the pathologic basis for the condition is incompletely understood. Most patients have a mild form of acute pancreatitis, which is associated with minimal organ dysfunction and an uneventful recovery. These patients respond to appropriate fluid administration, with rapid normalization of physical signs and laboratory values. The predominant pathologic finding in mild acute pancreatitis is interstitial edema with occasional parenchymal necrosis. On the other hand, 10% to 15% of patients have severe acute pancreatitis, which is associated with organ failure and/or local complications, such as acute fluid collections, necrosis, abscess, and pseudocyst formation.

In most experimental models of acute pancreatitis, secretion of digestive enzymes from the acinar cell is disturbed. Inappropriate activation of the proteolytic enzyme trypsin outside the gastrointestinal tract leads to inflammation and autodigestion. Tissue destruction results in an influx of leukocytes and macrophages, which, together with the pancreas itself, elaborate numerous inflammatory mediators leading to systemic inflammatory response syndrome. This is thought to be the first step in the development of pancreatitis. Trypsinogen is activated through hydrolysis of an N-terminal peptide called *trypsinogen-activating peptide*. Several natural mechanisms prevent pancreatic autodigestion by activated trypsin. These include: production of serine protease inhibitor Kazal type 1 (SPINK1), also known as *pancreatic secretory trypsin inhibitor* (PSTI), which reversibly inhibits activated trypsin; trypsin-activated trypsin-like enzymes that degrade trypsinogen; and bicarbonate-rich secretions, which are dependent on the normal production of the cystic fibrosis transmembrane conductance receptor (CFTR). SPINK1 mutations have been identified in familial pancreatitis and in children with idiopathic chronic pancreatitis. Because SPINK1 mutations are more common than is pancreatitis, they are thought to be modifiers or promoters rather than the cause of the disease.

The cationic trypsinogen gene that causes hereditary pancreatitis was discovered in 1996. Its mutation leads to a conformational change in the structure of the trypsinogen–SPINK1 complex and may lead to an impaired SPINK1-mediated defense mechanism against activated trypsin. Hereditary pancreatitis is an autosomal dominant condition with clinical and pathologic manifestations identical to those of sporadic pancreatitis. It has an 80% penetrance and is manifested by recurrent episodes of acute pancreatitis, progression to chronic pancreatitis, and development of pancreatic cancer. Many of these mutations have also been noted in patients with idiopathic pancreatitis.

DIAGNOSIS

The predominant symptom of acute pancreatitis is severe, constant epigastric pain. The onset is rapid, although not as sudden as that of perforated duodenal ulcer. The pain frequently radiates through to the back and may be partially diminished by sitting and leaning forward, or by lying curled in a fetal position. The signs of Cullen and Grey-Turner, periumbilical and flank bruising, respectively, are rare. Nausea and vomiting are frequent. These symptoms cause most patients to seek medical attention within 6 to 12 hours of the onset of pancreatitis, although delay is often seen among inebriated patients. Patients appear acutely ill, and they are usually tachycardic. Hypotension denotes a severe attack. The abdomen is quiet, tender, and full to palpation in the epigastrium.

The simplest laboratory test that suggests the diagnosis of acute pancreatitis is an elevated serum amylase level. Acute acinar cell injury causes a rapid rise in serum amylase level. Normal kidneys efficiently clear amylase, so typically the serum amylase level returns toward normal by the third or fourth day of the attack. A number of acute abdominal surgical emergencies cause hyperamylasemia, such as perforated duodenal ulcer, but rarely to the level of elevation seen

TABLE 1 Causes of Acute Pancreatitis

Biliary tract disease (gallstones and microlithiasis)
Alcohol abuse
Drug reaction
Pancreatic or ampullary tumors
Ampullary stenosis
Congenital anomalies of the pancreatic or biliary anatomy
Hypertriglyceridemia
Hypercalcemia
Trauma (external or iatrogenic)
Infection (mumps...)
Bites (scorpion, spiders, Gila monster)
Tropical pancreatitis
Idiopathic

 CURRENT DIAGNOSIS

Acute Pancreatitis

CLINICAL MANIFESTATIONS

- Severe constant epigastric pain
- Pain radiates to the back
- Nausea and vomiting
- Mild pancreatitis responds to supportive treatment with no organ failure

RADIOLOGIC AND LABORATORY TESTS

- Flat and upright plain abdominal film to rule out small-bowel obstruction, perforated ulcer
- Serum amylase and lipase levels
- Ultrasound of the abdomen, with attention to the right upper quadrant (gallbladder, bile ducts, pancreas)
- Contrast-enhanced computed tomography

EVALUATE SEVERITY OF PANCREATITIS

- Ranson criteria
- Acute Physiology and Chronic Health Evaluation (APACHE) II
- Degree of pancreatic necrosis on contrast-enhanced computed tomography

with acute pancreatitis. The severity of pancreatitis does not correlate with the degree of amylase elevation. Patients with acute biliary pancreatitis tend to have very high amylase levels, even during a mild attack, presumably because the pancreas was completely normal at the outset. A lesser elevation of serum amylase is usually observed in acute alcoholic pancreatitis, especially during a second or subsequent attack. Serum lipase concentration rises within 4 to 8 hours and returns to normal after 8 to 14 days, making it a useful method for patients presenting late. Lipase elevation may be more sensitive than amylase elevation in patients with alcoholic pancreatitis and is more specific as a marker of acute pancreatitis than is elevated amylase.

Plain abdominal radiographs are useful mainly to exclude other conditions, such as perforated peptic ulcer and mechanical small-bowel obstruction. Ultrasound of the abdomen may disclose edema of the pancreatic parenchyma. However, this finding is often obscured by overlying bowel gas, which acts as an acoustic barrier. Ultrasound is most useful for diagnosing gallbladder stones. It can also accurately calibrate the common bile duct diameter, suggesting choledocholithiasis if distended. A contrast-enhanced abdominal computed tomography (CT) scan (although often unnecessary) more reliably diagnoses acute pancreatitis. The severity of the attack and its outcome can be graded and correlated to the CT appearance of the pancreas and parapancreatic tissues (see next section).

QUANTIFICATION OF SEVERITY

Between 70% and 80% of all attacks of acute pancreatitis are mild, resulting in little short- or long-term morbidity and virtually no mortality. The remainder are severe attacks, involving a variable fraction of pancreatic necrosis, extensive short- and long-term morbidity, and a mortality rate between 10% and 30%. Predicting severe pancreatitis soon after hospital admission allows early triage to intensive care for supportive treatment. To this end, several systems of severity measurement have been developed and correlated with outcome. Of these systems, the best known is the scoring system devised by Ranson and associates (Table 2). They identified 11 "criteria," five of which were determined on admission and six others at 48 hours after admission, which correlated with ultimate risk of morbidity and mortality. Patients exhibiting two or fewer of the prognostic criteria are likely to survive a relatively mild attack, those with three to six criteria have progressively more severe disease and a greater probability of death, and those with seven or more criteria will almost certainly not survive. The Ranson prognostic score has the advantages of strong clinical correlation and a simple, universally available data set. Its disadvantages are that it requires 48 hours to complete, and it is not useful after 48 hours. It was originally developed to grade acute alcoholic pancreatitis. The Acute Physiology and Chronic Health Evaluation (APACHE) II evaluates 12 prognostic variables that cover all organ systems. Scores greater than 13 in acute pancreatitis have been associated with poor prognosis. An advantage of APACHE II is that it can be used at any time during the hospital course. The Balthazar Score predicts severity of acute pancreatitis based on CT appearance of the pancreas, including presence or absence of pancreatic necrosis. According to these criteria, if 30% of the pancreas is nonperfused, the chances are high that the patient will progress to complicated acute pancreatitis. The Atlanta Classification defines severe acute pancreatitis using standard clinical manifestations, three or more Ranson criteria or an APACHE II score of eight or more, evidence of organ failure, and intrapancreatic pathologic findings such as necrosis (Table 3).

MANAGEMENT OF MILD ACUTE PANCREATITIS

Although recovery without specific treatment is the rule, all patients are watched closely in a hospital setting because rapid deterioration is not always predictable. Management consists of nothing by mouth, hydration with intravenous crystalloid solution, and analgesia as needed. Prophylaxis against deep venous thrombosis with low-dose subcutaneous heparin and/or sequential calf compression should be routine. Alcoholic patients must be assessed for risk of alcohol withdrawal syndromes. Laboratory tests on admission should include either an arterial blood gas measurement or oxygen saturation measured by pulse oximetry. Oral intake of liquids is resumed when the abdomen is soft and nontender, which usually correlates with a normalized serum amylase level. If the liquids do not exacerbate the attack, the diet can be advanced as tolerated. A right upper quadrant ultrasound is performed in all patients, even alcoholic patients, because they too may harbor gallstones. Nasogastric suction is indicated if ileus and vomiting are present because of the risk of aspiration. Likewise, gastric antisecretory agents are given only if there is concern about peptic ulcer or stress gastritis.

MANAGEMENT OF SEVERE ACUTE PANCREATITIS

Severe acute pancreatitis is usually evident on initial clinical assessment; if not, the grave situation declares itself within the subsequent 24 to 48 hours. Early mortality from severe acute pancreatitis results from cardiovascular and/or respiratory failure. Thus, patients are managed in an intensive care unit, with urinary, central venous pressure, and arterial catheters, cardiac and pulse oximetry monitoring,

TABLE 2 Ranson Criteria of Severity of Acute Pancreatitis*

On Admission	At 48 Hours
1. Age > 55 years 2. White blood cell count > 16,000 cells/mm^3 3. Serum glucose > 200 mg/dL 4. Serum lactate dehydrogenase > 350 IU/L 5. Aspartate transaminase > 250 U/dL	6. Hematocrit fall > 10%[†] 7. Serum calcium < 8 mg/dL 8. Base deficit > 4 mEq/L 9. Blood urea nitrogen increase > 5 mg/dL[†] 10. Arterial PO$_2$ < 60 mm Hg 11. Fluid sequestration > 6L[‡]

*Criteria are modified slightly for gallstone pancreatitis.
[†]Compared to admission values.
[‡]Fluid volume infused minus urine and nasogastric tube output.

TABLE 3 Atlanta Symposium Clinically Based Classification System for Acute Pancreatitis*

Mild Acute Pancreatitis (75%)
Clinical manifestations (abdominal tenderness, vomiting, hypoactive bowel sounds)
Lacks features of severe pancreatitis
Patients respond appropriately to fluid administration
Minimal organ dysfunction
Contrast enhancement of pancreatic parenchyma is usually normal
Intrapancreatic pathology: Interstitial edema rarely necrosis

Severe Acute Pancreatitis (25%)
Clinical manifestations (abdominal tenderness, vomiting, hypoactive bowel sounds)
Ranson ≥3, Acute Physiology and Chronic Health Evaluation (APACHE) II ≥ 8
Organ failure
Intrapancreatic pathology: Necrosis, less commonly interstitial edema

Pancreatic Necrosis
Nonenhanced parenchyma on contrast-enhanced computed tomography > 3 cm or involving > 30% of the gland
Pathology: Macroscopic focal or diffuse areas of devitalized pancreatic tissue and peripancreatic fat necrosis

*Adapted from Arch Surg 1993;128:586-990.

and close observation. Profound and ongoing intravascular volume loss results from fluid sequestration within the retroperitoneum as well as a diffuse capillary leak, which causes generalized edema. Intravascular volume is maintained by crystalloid infusion, titrated to maintain adequate tissue perfusion. Inotropic cardiac support is used as needed once intravascular volume repletion is achieved. Packed red blood cells are transfused as needed to maintain adequate oxygen-carrying capacity. Respiratory function frequently worsens precipitously in the first 24 hours, requiring endotracheal intubation and ventilatory support. Analgesia and sedation are liberally administered, as is stress ulcer prophylaxis.

At present, no pharmacologic therapy dependably ameliorates the severity of the pancreatitis or decreases the risk of systemic complications. Neither octreotide (Sandostatin),[1] a somatostatin analogue that inhibits pancreatic exocrine secretion, nor various protease inhibitors have improved mortality. Newer therapies targeting mediators of the pancreatic and systemic inflammatory response could in theory improve outcome, especially if administered very early in the attack. One such agent, a platelet-activating factor antagonist called *lexipafant*, showed promise in initial laboratory investigations but did not prove beneficial in clinical trials. Because retroperitoneal and peritoneal exudates contain activated digestive enzymes and a host of other vasoactive and inflammatory mediators, peritoneal dialysis might logically improve the condition of patients with severe acute pancreatitis. Indeed, several trials report amelioration of the cardiovascular collapse associated with a severe attack, although overall hospital mortality due mainly to late infectious sequela was not altered. Finally, operation has almost no role early in the course of severe acute pancreatitis (first 14 days), except to rule out another suspected cause of the acute abdomen or to resect gangrenous bowel, which has developed as a complication of the severe pancreatitis.

NECROSIS AND INFECTION

The presence of pancreatic necrosis can be detected by dynamic CT scanning or by serum markers, if available. The probability of complications and of death correlates with the amount of pancreas that is necrotic. When 20% or less of the gland undergoes necrosis, secondary pancreatic infection is rare, and survival is expected. If 50% or more of the gland is necrotic, secondary infection becomes very probable, and mortality is as high as 50%. Secondary infection of necrotic pancreatic and peripancreatic tissues is relatively common and is the principal cause of mortality from severe acute pancreatitis. Infecting organisms are usually enteric gram-negative bacilli, but infection with gram-positive organisms and fungi is now recognized as well. A trend toward reduced pancreatic infection (as well as other systemic infection) has been shown following the prolonged use of newer antibiotics, which effectively penetrate pancreatic tissue. However, infections that develop in patients treated with prophylactic antibiotics tend to involve resistant organisms. One standard prophylactic antibiotic regimen gaining acceptance uses imipenem-cilastatin (Primaxin) started soon after admission and continued for at least 2 weeks. These patients have many intravenous and invasive monitoring catheters, which are potential portals for entry of gram-positive organisms that can secondarily infect the pancreas. Rigid adherence to appropriate infection control measures is required to minimize this risk.

Infected pancreatic necrosis is the most dreaded and lethal complication of severe acute pancreatitis. The condition becomes apparent most frequently during the third and fourth weeks of hospitalization and is marked by fever, increasing pain, tenderness, and fullness in the upper abdomen. The patient usually appears septic. Contrastenhanced CT may reveal extraluminal retroperitoneal gas, which is a radiographic hallmark of infected necrosis. Percutaneous image-guided fine-needle aspiration of the pancreas, with immediate gram stain and culture of the aspirate, can reveal the presence of organisms, which is diagnostic of infected necrosis. Infected pancreatic necrosis is almost always fatal without aggressive débridement and drainage of the retroperitoneum. The standard for wide débridement is an open laparotomy, although laparoscopic, endoscopic, and percutaneous techniques are being described and developed. Surgical strategy ranges from débridement with closed suction and irrigation of the retroperitoneum to multiple planned operative débridements every 2 to 3 days until all necrotic material is removed. All approaches are time and labor intensive, but they offer the only chance for survival of the majority of patients.

Sterile pancreatic necrosis is associated with severe acute pancreatitis but, unlike infected pancreatic necrosis, is usually managed without the need for urgent operation. Acute peripancreatic fluid collections frequently arise. They may include reactive serous effusions but likely represent secondary or even main pancreatic ductal disruption, with resultant leak of pancreatic juice into the lesser peritoneal sac or other anatomic spaces surrounding the pancreas. These acute collections often resorb spontaneously, requiring no specific treatment. If infection of the fluid is suspected or if pain and tenderness are increasing, the collections may be percutaneously aspirated or even drained. In some centers, endoscopically placed transpapillary drains are inserted into the pancreatic duct, occasionally through the disruption into the fluid collection, to accomplish drainage. Finally, if such collections do not spontaneously disappear and do not require early drainage, they may evolve into a pancreatic pseudocyst.

A few patients with sterile pancreatic necrosis fail to improve in spite of optimal, protracted conservative care. These patients deserve operative exploration and pancreatic débridement on the grounds of failed nonoperative treatment, coupled perhaps with the suspicion that a smoldering, occult infection has eluded discovery. The operation is delayed as long as is practical, to allow areas undergoing necrosis to demarcate and liquefy. This makes the débridement technically easier. The pancreas and adjacent tissues are débrided and drained, provision for enteric feeding is established, and the abdomen is closed with the expectation that the need for reoperation will be likely.

BILIARY (GALLSTONE) PANCREATITIS

Gallstone pancreatitis is caused by transient obstruction of the pancreatic duct at the ampulla of Vater. The offending gallstone need not be large; "biliary sludge" and even biliary "microlithiasis" appear to be capable of provoking acute pancreatitis. As a rule, patients with gallstone pancreatitis have multiple small gallstones within the gallbladder, a comparatively wide cystic duct (promoting passage into the common bile duct), and a distinct "common channel" of the bile and pancreatic ducts.

Nonalcoholic patients with acute pancreatitis very likely have biliary lithiasis as the underlying cause. The presence of gallstones within the gallbladder virtually makes the diagnosis. A distended common bile duct seen by ultrasound further suggests the recent passage of a stone. Serum bilirubin and/or alkaline phosphatase levels may be mildly elevated, but often both are normal. If the

---

[1]Not FDA approved for this indication.

CURRENT THERAPY

Acute Pancreatitis

MILD ACUTE PANCREATITIS

- Supportive therapy: Intravenous fluids, pain control, diet as tolerated
- If gallstones: Cholecystectomy and cholangiogram during same hospitalization or shortly thereafter

SEVERE ACUTE PANCREATITIS

- Admission to intensive care unit
- Supportive therapy: Intravenous fluids, pain control, antibiotics, enteral or parenteral nutrition
- Surgical treatment of infected pancreatic necrosis
- Surgical or endoscopic treatment of pseudocyst

ultrasound fails to reveal gallbladder stones or sludge and other rare causes are excluded, an endoscopic ultrasound may identify sludge or microlithiasis in a stable patient. Endoscopic ultrasound can also complement the pancreatic anatomic findings on CT. If endoscopic ultrasound is not available or is inconclusive, the next diagnostic step includes endoscopic retrograde cholangiopancreatography (ERCP). A sample of bile can be obtained to examine for microscopic crystals (this can be achieved by duodenal drainage as well), and small stones or anatomic anomalies may be identified.

Gallstone pancreatitis is usually mild, resolving clinically within 2 to 4 days. Serum bilirubin and alkaline phosphatase levels are typically normal or return to normal within this period, suggesting a low probability of persistent stone(s) within the common bile duct. Cholecystectomy eliminates the source of further stones and thus prevents recurrent pancreatitis; it should be performed during the same hospitalization or shortly thereafter. An intraoperative cholangiogram is performed, unless it has been undertaken preoperatively. If pancreatitis resolves but liver function tests suggest a persistent stone in the bile duct, then preoperative ERCP with papillotomy and stone extraction is appropriate, followed by prompt cholecystectomy.

If the intraoperative cholangiogram shows choledocholithiasis, a laparoscopic or open common bile duct exploration or a postoperative ERCP with papillotomy with stone removal can be performed, depending on the available expertise. Severe gallstone pancreatitis is managed like severe pancreatitis of any cause. Usually, the inciting stone has passed, leaving the bile and pancreatic ducts unobstructed; therefore, routine, early ERCP is not warranted. However, if a stone is persistently obstructing the ampulla of Vater, if the patient has jaundice, or if the patient has signs of cholangitis, urgent ERCP and stone extraction may be necessary.

Chronic Pancreatitis

Chronic pancreatitis (CP) is an irreversible, progressive inflammatory disease of the pancreas characterized by pain, fibrosis, and progressive loss of exocrine and/or endocrine function. The early course of this disease may often manifest as repeated attacks of acute pancreatitis. It occurs in men more frequently than in women. Excessive alcohol consumption is usually the cause in developed countries.

INCIDENCE

In several Western industrialized countries, the estimated prevalence of CP is approximately 10 to 15 per 100,000 population, with an annual incidence of 3.5 to 4 per 100,000 population. These rates may actually underestimate the problem because the diagnosis of CP is not based on advanced diagnostic tools such as ERCP and CT scan. In a recent report from Japan using CT and ERCP, the incidence of CP is 12 per 100,000 and prevalence is 45 per 100,000 population, which are much higher than in Western countries. In southern India, the prevalence of CP has been estimated to be 125 per 100,000 with the majority being calcific pancreatitis. The cause of this tropical pancreatitis is thought to be dietary. According to estimates of the Commission on Professional and Hospital Activities, CP ranks as the 27th most common digestive disease in the United States, with a threefold higher prevalence in the black male population.

The majority of care for CP is directed toward ameliorating pain, but a substantial amount of resources is also spent on treating complications. More than half of CP patients will develop pancreatic diabetes; one third of these patients will be insulin dependent, and nearly 50% will eventually require surgical intervention for pain or other complications. Optimal care of the patient with CP relies on supportive medical management of endocrine and exocrine insufficiency and of pain. Surgical intervention is generally reserved for intractable pain and specific complications such as pseudocyst and biliary or intestinal obstruction. As many as half of all patients will die within 20 years of their diagnosis of CP, a rate much higher than their age-matched population.

TABLE 4 Causes of Chronic Pancreatitis

Alcohol
Obstruction
    Pancreas divisum
    Congenital strictures
    Acquired strictures
    Acute pancreatitis
    Trauma
    Endoscopic retrograde cholangiopancreatography
    Neoplasm
        Pancreatic
        Periampullary
Toxic Substances
    Tropical pancreatitis
    Hypercalcemia
    Hyperlipidemia
Genetic
Autoimmune
Idiopathic

ETIOLOGY AND PATHOGENESIS

CP appears to be a multifactorial process involving both a genetic predisposition and environmental factors (see Table 4). Alcohol use is by far the number one cause of CP in the Western world, accounting for an estimated 70% of the cases in the United States and Europe. About 10% of chronic alcoholics will develop CP, roughly the same percentage of alcoholics who develop hepatic cirrhosis. Average age at diagnosis of alcoholic pancreatitis is 35 to 45 years with an 11- to 18-year history of 150 to 175 g of alcohol ingestion daily.

Ingested alcohol results in direct damage to the acinar cell with increased concentration of protein secretion, decreased production of bicarbonate, and decreased fluid volume as demonstrated in experimental models and in patients with alcoholic pancreatitis. This combination appears to result in protein and calcium precipitation within the pancreatic duct system, subsequent ductal obstruction, activation of pancreatic enzymes, and autodigestion of the gland. Over time, a fibrotic response results in permanent ductal abnormalities, calcification, and stone formation.

Dietary factors, such as high-fat and high-protein intake and trace mineral insufficiency, seem to be epidemiologically associated with CP. Another theory suggests the presence of an acinar cell product, lithostatin or pancreatic stone protein, that prevents calcium precipitation. Decreased concentrations of lithostatin and decreased levels of lithostatin messenger RNA have been found in the pancreatic juice and acini of patients with chronic calcific pancreatitis, suggesting a genetic component of risk for developing the disease. Alcohol-induced derangement of lipid metabolism has also been postulated as inducing the periacinar fibrosis and changes associated with alcoholic pancreatitis. The range of experimentally identified abnormalities supports the multifactorial nature of the disease.

Another form of CP, tropical pancreatitis, may be caused by protein malnutrition and cyanogens found in cassava root. The clinical and histologic features of tropical pancreatitis are nearly identical to those of alcoholic CP. Obstructive pancreatitis results from both congenital and acquired ductal obstruction, as in pancreas divisum, congenital and acquired strictures, and neoplasia. Unlike alcoholic pancreatitis, the obstructed pancreas shows uniform inflammatory changes with preserved ductal epithelium and rare protein plugs. The hypothesis that high intraductal pressure results in pancreatitis has been proposed based partly on the demonstration of high intraductal pressures in these patients.

Additional causes of CP include hypercalcemia, hyperlipidemia, autoimmune diseases, and genetic alterations, as seen in hereditary and idiopathic pancreatitis (see section on acute pancreatitis). The mechanism by which pancreatitis develops in these situations is unclear.

CURRENT DIAGNOSIS

Chronic Pancreatitis

CLINICAL MANIFESTATIONS

- Persistent midepigastric pain exacerbated by eating or alcohol consumption
- One or more present: Malnutrition, steatorrhea, glucose intolerance

RADIOLOGIC AND LABORATORY TESTS

- Computed tomography scan of the pancreas may show calcifications, pancreatic duct dilation, and/or pseudocyst formation
- Endoscopic retrograde cholangiopancreatography is the gold standard diagnostic test but is used only when computed tomography is not sufficient to make the diagnosis or clarify anatomy
- Amylase and lipase levels are not useful
- Functional pancreatic studies are cumbersome and rarely required

DIAGNOSIS

Patients with CP typically present with persistent midepigastric pain, often with a thoracolumbar component. The pain may be exacerbated by eating and by alcohol consumption. Nausea, vomiting, and hemodynamic instability are less frequent than with acute pancreatitis. Examination often reveals upper abdominal fullness and tenderness with frequent associated signs of malnutrition and occasionally jaundice. The classic triad of CP—pancreatic calcification, diabetes mellitus, and steatorrhea—occurs in fewer than 25% of cases, although two thirds of patients will have an abnormal glucose tolerance test at the time of presentation. Because of the difficulty of obtaining pancreatic tissue for histologic analysis, CP is usually diagnosed by pancreatic imaging with or without tests of exocrine function. Radiologic evidence of pancreatic calcification is pathognomonic and is present in only 30% to 50% of patients.

Pain is present in 75% of patients. Initially the pain is characterized by recurrent attacks but tends to become persistent with variable periods of remission. Occasionally it will "burn out" over time. The etiology of pain is uncertain. Table 5 lists some of the proposed factors. The most recent theory suggests hypoxia and damage to local sensory nerves with exposure to inflammatory irritants such as histamine, prostaglandins, and pancreatic enzymes.

Laboratory values are of limited value in evaluating CP. Pancreatic enzyme levels (amylase, lipase) may be elevated in acute exacerbations but are not a good measure of chronic disease, pancreatic function, or pancreatic reserve, nor do they correlate with symptoms. Functional studies are cumbersome and are rarely required to diagnose CP. However, stimulated pancreatic secretions collected from the duodenum (amylase, lipase, trypsin, chymotrypsin, and bicarbonate), urine tests (nitroblue tetrazolium–*para*-aminobenzoic acid [NBT-PABA] test, and pancreolauryl test), or serum studies (P-isoamylase and trypsin), provide reliable estimates of pancreatic functional reserve and can be useful in evaluating treatment strategies. Serum liver enzyme levels and leukocyte counts may provide important information regarding complications of the disease.

Imaging

Plain abdominal radiographs reveal pancreatic calcification in less than 50% of patients and are otherwise nonspecific in CP. Transabdominal ultrasound can determine the size and consistency of the gland, characteristics of the biliary tree, and the presence of complications. A skilled ultrasonographer may achieve 70% sensitivity in diagnosing the disease.

CT approaches 90% sensitivity and greater than 90% specificity in diagnosing CP and should be considered in all suspected patients to classify their disease and determine the presence of complications and surgically correctable lesions. CT scan is the best radiologic modality for detecting calcifications, pancreatic ductal dilation, and pseudocysts and may be the only imaging study necessary in most cases.

ERCP remains the gold standard for diagnosis and staging of CP, with a sensitivity up to 95% and specificity greater than 90%. The small but finite incidence of serious complications related to ERCP should limit its use to those patients who require anatomic definition not provided by other imaging studies and in patients suspected of ampullary or ductal obstruction amenable to ERCP treatment.

Magnetic resonance imaging (MRI), magnetic resonance cholangiopancreatography (MRCP), and CT cholangiopancreatography/angiography are rapidly evolving and can replace diagnostic ERCP in most situations. This technology provides definition of soft tissues and ductal anatomy but remains institutional and operator dependent. Likewise, endoscopic ultrasound is becoming more available and may play a role in the early diagnosis of CP.

MEDICAL TREATMENT

Medical treatment of CP consists primarily of supportive care. Pain relief, metabolic and nutritional support, as well as pancreatic endocrine and exocrine support, are the mainstays of medical therapy. Pain control is difficult, often requiring opiate analgesics. Abstinence from alcohol must be the initial goal, as alcohol consumption predicts recurrent pain even after surgical intervention. Oral pancreatic enzyme supplementation and octreotide[1] may provide modest pain relief, probably due to reduced pancreatic secretion. Because opiate addiction increases in proportion to duration of disease, nonsteroidal anti-inflammatory drugs should be prescribed early and chronically. Opiates should be reserved for exacerbations and intractable pain. Some authorities recommend surgical intervention prior to the chronic administration of opiates.

Malnutrition is common due to fear of pain after eating, as well as poor dietary habits and nutritional problems, in the alcoholic population. Attention should be directed at providing a low-fat diet with adequate protein and calories and vitamin supplementation. Parenteral or jejunal feedings may be required in certain situations, such as preoperative preparation and episodes of acute exacerbation.

Pancreatic exocrine insufficiency necessary to produce protein malabsorption does not occur until 90% of acinar mass has been lost. However, steatorrhea, or fat malabsorption, is a common and often troublesome problem in patents with CP. In addition to lipase from the pancreas, digestion of lipids depends on salivary and gastric hydrolysis, alkalinization in the duodenum, and adequate bile acid concentrations, all of which may be diminished in alcoholics. Pancreatic exocrine enzyme replacement is indicated to ameliorate steatorrhea. Present enzyme preparations include enteric-coated and encapsulated forms to aid delivery of active enzymes and decrease the volume of administration. Gastric acid suppression may also be necessary to provide an adequate pH environment for enzyme activity.

Endocrine insufficiency in CP is primarily manifested as pancreatic diabetes. Its treatment is similar to that for other forms of diabetes in that it may be controlled by diet, oral hypoglycemic agents, or insulin.

TABLE 5 Proposed Factors Producing Pain in Chronic Pancreatitis

Ductal hypertension
Autodigestion
Parenchymal ischemia
Perineural inflammation

---

[1]Not FDA approved for this indication.

TABLE 6 Indications for Surgery in Chronic Pancreatitis

Pain refractory to medical management
Inability to exclude pancreatic malignancy
Complications
Pseudocyst
Biliary obstruction
Duodenal obstruction
Splenic vein thrombosis
Pancreatic fistula
Colonic obstruction
Pancreatic ascites
Pancreatic abscess

SURGICAL TREATMENT

The first line of therapy in CP should be noninjurious; surgical intervention should be reserved for intractable disease. Additional indications for surgical intervention are listed in Table 6. The choice of operation depends on the anatomic findings in each patient (Table 7). Pancreatic and biliary duct anatomy should be carefully evaluated preoperatively. Improvements in perioperative preparation and care have enabled routine performance of surgical procedures on the pancreas, with very low mortality and morbidity. Contemporary series of operations for CP demonstrate mortality rates less than 3% and complication rates less than 30%, comparable to the rates of other major intra-abdominal operations.

In a minority of patients, stenosis or stricture of the ampulla of Vater can be treated with simple sphincterotomy or sphincteroplasty. Initial results with this technique revealed improvement in pain, but the results were short lived and correlated with alcohol abstinence. Although these procedures have been successful in limiting recurrent acute bouts of pancreatitis in pancreas divisum, no benefit has been realized for patients with CP. This experience suggests that sphincterotomy and pancreatic duct stenting will have little effect on the long-term management of CP from other etiologies.

The pancreatic duct in CP usually is either dilated diffusely or in a beaded ("chain-of-lakes") pattern. A dilated pancreatic duct is best treated with internal drainage of the pancreatic duct into a Roux-en-Y limb of jejunum. Historically, 8 mm was considered the lower limit of dilation amenable to internal drainage, but the procedure has proved tenable and successful in relieving pain in patients with duct dilation of greater than 5 mm. The Partington-Rochelle modification of the Puestow operation (lateral pancreaticojejunostomy) has resulted in good to excellent relief of pain in 70% to 80% of patients. Concomitant procedures to address complications such as pseudocyst and biliary obstruction can be incorporated into the jejunal limb. There is no evidence that surgery improves pancreatic function, as was hoped by the pioneers of ductal drainage procedures.

The Frey procedure is based on the concept that the head of the pancreas and uncinate process may not be completely drained by longitudinal pancreaticojejunostomy. This procedure entails a "coring out" or local resection of the head of the gland combined with lateral pancreaticojejunostomy. Results have been promising; only 13% of patients have reported no pain relief. Another proposed mechanism for the success of this operation is the reversal of ischemia or ductal hypertension that irritates sensory nerves in the head of the gland.

When the pancreatic duct is not dilated, decompressing procedures are not feasible. However, patients may obtain relief of pain with pancreatic resection. Debate continues on the merits and complications of partial (40%–80%) distal pancreatectomy, subtotal (95%) distal pancreatectomy (Child's procedure), pancreaticoduodenectomy (Whipple's procedure), and total pancreatectomy. Duodenum-preserving pancreatic head resection (Beger's procedure) performed in the 10% to 30% of CP patients with an inflammatory mass in the head of the gland has shown excellent pain relief, comparable to that of a Whipple procedure. Pancreatic insufficiency resulting from resection procedures is generally proportional to the extent of resection, with severe exocrine insufficiency and a particularly brittle and difficult to control form of pancreatic diabetes at the extreme. Attempts at autologous pancreatic islet cell transplantation at the time of pancreas resection were initially promising, but enthusiasm for the technique has waned because of less than satisfactory long-term results.

Several approaches to nerve ablation have been proposed based on the theory that the pain of CP is related to inflammatory involvement of the splanchnic nerves. Extraperitoneal, intraperitoneal, thoracic, and thoracoscopic splanchnicectomy as well as complete denervation procedures have been attempted to treat the pain of CP. Results have been unpredictable, often unconfirmed, and with limited follow-up. Neurotomy may be considered in patients who have not obtained relief of pain after surgical drainage or resection procedures.

PANCREATIC PSEUDOCYST

Pancreatic pseudocysts are walled-off collections of fluid and debris resulting from disruption of the pancreatic duct and are most commonly associated with acute and chronic pancreatitis. Pseudocysts will develop in up to 10% of patients after an episode of acute alcoholic pancreatitis. They may also occur after trauma or in association with a neoplasm. The wall is vascularized inflammatory tissue without an epithelial lining and may contain pancreatic parenchyma. Pseudocysts may occur in any region of the gland and are multiple in 10% to 15% of patients. Fluid collections occurring within 3 weeks of an acute episode of pancreatitis are considered acute fluid collections, and 30% to 40% of these collections will resolve spontaneously.

The most common presentation is abdominal pain, present in 90% of patients. Physical examination often reveals a tender abdominal fullness or mass. Nonspecific complaints of nausea, vomiting, early satiety, and weight loss are common. More dramatic presentations may result from free intraperitoneal rupture, intracystic hemorrhage or infection, gastric variceal bleeding resulting from splenic or portal vein thrombosis, or intraperitoneal hemorrhage from adjacent pseudoaneurysm rupture. Laboratory findings are nonspecific, although persistent amylase elevation is common. Imaging with CT is preferable, but ultrasound is nearly as sensitive and can be recommended for follow-up to determine interval changes in size.

Sampling of a postpancreatitis fluid collection is rarely indicated. However, if there has not been a preceding episode of pancreatitis, fluid cytology and chemistry can help differentiate a pseudocyst from a more likely mucinous or serous cystic neoplasm.

The natural history of asymptomatic pseudocysts reveals that nearly half remain stable, decrease in size, or completely resolve at 1-year follow-up, irrespective of size. However, pseudocysts larger

TABLE 7 Selection of Operation for Chronic Pancreatitis

Disease limited to tail of gland	Distal pancreatectomy
Obstruction in head of gland	
Dilated pancreatic duct	LR-LPJ
Nondilated pancreatic duct	Whipple, DPPHR
No obstruction in head of gland	
Dilated pancreatic duct	LPJ
Nondilated pancreatic duct	Distal resection (40%–95%), total pancreatectomy
Unable to tolerate major operation	Neurolysis?
Failure of primary drainage/resection	Additional drainage/resection, neurolysis
Inability to rule out malignancy	Resection

Abbreviations: DPPHR = duodenal preserving pancreatic head resection; LR-LPJ = local resection–longitudinal pancreaticojejunostomy.

than 6 cm are more likely to require operation during follow-up. Pseudocysts present for more than 12 weeks almost never resolve spontaneously and have a high rate of complications. Therefore, current management of pancreatic pseudocysts takes into account the presence or absence of symptoms, the age and size of the pseudocyst, and the presence or absence of complications. Postpancreatitis fluid collections that are asymptomatic in a stable patient can be followed with monthly imaging to evaluate resolution, stability, and enlargement. Failure to resolve and evidence of enlargement are indications for intervention. If, on the other hand, the pseudocyst is symptomatic, early intervention should be considered. Generally, a period of 6 weeks is desired prior to surgical intervention to assure adequate maturation of the cyst wall.

The preferred operative management of a pseudocyst is internal drainage into the gastrointestinal tract. This can be accomplished by anastomosis of the opened cyst wall to the stomach (cystogastrostomy), duodenum (cystoduodenostomy), or a Roux-en-Y limb of jejunum (cystojejunostomy), depending on the location of the pseudocyst. Multiple pseudocysts can be addressed simultaneously by connecting the pseudocysts and draining them as one, separately draining each cyst into a Roux-en-Y jejunal limb, or a combination of the internal drainage procedures. A lateral pancreaticojejunostomy should be added when the pancreatic duct is dilated. The cyst wall should be biopsied on all occasions, as cystic neoplasms of the pancreas can mimic a pseudocyst. Infected pseudocysts are generally treated as pancreatic abscesses.

Simple aspiration of pseudocysts will fail to resolve the fluid collection in as many as 80% of patients. Prolonged catheter drainage has demonstrated better resolution rates but may take months of drain maintenance. New endoscopic techniques that place an endoprosthesis through the intestinal lumen into the pseudocyst and that bridge the pancreatic duct disruption with a pancreatic duct stent are currently being analyzed.

ENDOSCOPIC THERAPY

Endoscopic approaches to ductal decompression have been attempted in CP. These include endoscopic clearance of the main pancreatic duct with pancreatic sphincterotomy and basketing of stones for removal, extracorporeal shock wave lithotripsy, transpapillary drainage of pseudocysts, and dilation and stenting of ductal strictures. Various endoscopic series have reported success rates of 50% to 70% for clearing the pancreatic duct and 60% to 80% for long-term pain relief. The risk of complications is approximately 10%. The early results of endoscopic therapy are comparable with those of surgery, but all endoscopic reports have been case series, some with little long-term follow-up. Randomized controlled studies using adequate and constant methods for evaluating and reporting results and comparing endoscopic, medical, and surgical treatment modalities are now required.

REFERENCES

Balthazar EJ, Robinson DL, Megibow AJ, Ranson JH: Acute pancreatitis: Value of CT in establishing prognosis. Radiology 1990;174:331-336.
Baron TH, Morgan DE: Acute necrotizing pancreatis. N Engl J Med 1999;340:1412-1417.
Bradley EL 3rd: A clinically based classification system for acute pancreatitis. Summary of the International Symposium on Acute Pancreatitis, Atlanta, Ga, September 11 through 13, 1992. Arch Surg 1993;128:586-590.
Howare J, Idezuki Y, Ihse I, Prinz RA: Surgical Diseases of the Pancreas, 3rd ed, Baltimore: Williams & Wilkins, 1998.
Mitchell RM, Byrne MF, Baillie J: Pancreatitis. Lancet 2003;361:1447-1455.
Tandon RK, Sato N, Garg PK; Consensus Study Group: Chronic pancreatitis: Asia-Pacific consensus report. J Gastroenterol Hepatol 2002;17:508-518.
Triester SL, Kowdley KV: Prognostic factors in acute pancreatitis. J Clin Gastroenterol 2002;34:167-176.
Uhl W, Warshaw A, Imrie C, et al, International Association of Pancreatology: IAP guidelines for the surgical management of acute pancreatitis. Pancreatology 2002;2:565-573.
Working Party of the British Society of Gastroenterology: Association of Surgeons of Great Britain and Ireland: Pancreatic Society of Great Britain and Ireland: Association of Upper GI Surgeons of Great Britain and Ireland: UK guidelines for the management of acute pancreatitis. Gut 2005;54(Suppl. 3):iii1-iii9.

Gastroesophageal Reflux Disease

Method of
Kenneth R. DeVault, MD

Gastroesophageal reflux disease (GERD) is defined as symptoms or mucosa damage resulting from the reflux of gastric content into the esophagus. GERD is one of the most common disorders in the western world, affecting up to 20% of the U.S. population on at least a weekly basis.

The classic symptoms of GERD are heartburn and regurgitation, but there have been other symptoms and diseases associated with this condition including noncardiac chest pain, chronic cough, asthma, sleep disturbances, and many others. Mucosa damage can vary from none, to mild esophagitis, to more severe esophagitis and, less commonly, Barrett's esophagus and esophageal carcinoma. The goal of therapy is to control both the symptoms and mucosal damage.

GERD is commonly a chronic condition, requiring chronic, often lifelong treatment. GERD is also a very costly condition. For example, in the United States it has been estimated to cost up to $10 billion annually, $6 billion of which are drug costs. In addition, there are substantial indirect costs of decreased work productivity and significant GERD-related impairments in the quality of life.

Diagnosis

There is no gold-standard test to confirm the diagnosis, and most experts believe a trial of medication to be the best diagnostic and therapeutic approach to most patients with symptoms suggesting GERD. This approach has resulted in the exponential growth in

CURRENT THERAPY

Chronic Pancreatitis

MEDICAL TREATMENT

- Abstinence from alcohol
- Pain control, preferably with nonopioid analgesics, pancreatic enzymes, octreotide
- Nutritional support: Low-fat foods, adequate protein and vitamins
- Management of diabetes
- Management of exocrine insufficiency with pancreatic enzymes

MEDICAL TREATMENT

- Indications: Pain refractory to medical management, inability to exclude malignancy, biliary or enteral obstruction, pseudocyst, pancreatic ascites, pancreatic fistula
- Dilated pancreatic duct: Internal drainage procedure
- Nondilated pancreatic duct: Resection
- Pseudocyst: Internal surgical drainage or endoscopic techniques

CURRENT DIAGNOSIS

- Empiric therapy (usually with a proton pump inhibitor) is indicated in most GERD patients.
- Endoscopy is indicated in patients with warning symptoms and in some patients with chronic disease to screen for Barrett's esophagus.
- Barium testing is generally not helpful in GERD.
- Ambulatory reflux testing is indicated in patients who do not respond to empiric therapy and in whom GERD is still a concern and to confirm the disease before endoscopic or surgical therapy.

GERD = gastroesophageal reflux disease.

CURRENT THERAPY

- Lifestyle modifications can help some patients, but most patients require additional therapy for symptom control.
- Acid suppression remains the mainstay of GERD therapy in the majority of patients.
- Proton pump inhibitors provide outstanding acid suppression given once daily.
- There are no currently available promotility agents with an acceptable efficacy and side effect profile to make them viable agents for most GERD patients.
- Surgical therapy, performed by an experienced surgeon, is a maintenance option for the patient with well-documented GERD.
- Research is ongoing into less invasive endoscopic therapies for GERD, but most of the currently available methods should remain in investigational environments.

GERD = gastroesophageal reflux disease.

GERD-related prescriptions. Testing is only mandated when patients have symptoms suggesting a complication of their disease or when the empiric trial of therapy is not successful.

THERAPEUTIC TRIALS AS DIAGNOSTIC TOOLS

Correctly making the diagnosis of GERD is an essential element of the management strategy. A careful history may be the most important aspect in establishing the diagnosis. For patients with heartburn or regurgitation, response to high-dose proton pump inhibitors (PPIs) has a sensitivity of 75% and specificity of 55% when compared with ambulatory pH testing. Although using response to acid suppression is not a perfect strategy to diagnose GERD, it is cost-effective and has become the preferred initial approach to patients with GERD-related symptoms. That having been said, although most experts would continue to use empiric acid suppression when an untested patient responds, they would also require confirmatory testing (usually with ambulatory reflux testing) before a more invasive endoscopic or surgical approach.

TESTING

Endoscopy is indicated mainly in two situations; when the warning symptoms (dysphagia, odynophagia, weight loss, signs of gastrointestinal [GI] blood loss) are present and in patients thought to be at risk for Barrett's esophagus. The former patients should be easily identified with a carefully obtained history, but whom to screen for Barrett's esophagus is more problematic. Current guidelines suggest screening patients who are at least 40 to 50 years old and who have had a history of symptoms for at least 5 to 10 years. Other groups that can benefit from endoscopy include those who develop new symptoms at an older age and those with severe symptoms that do not respond to medical therapy.

Barium studies do not provide accurate data for evaluating GERD and should not be routinely used except in patients with dysphagia and in some select patients before endoscopic or surgical therapy. Several methods have been developed to test for reflux from the stomach to the esophagus. Traditionally, these have consisted of a nasal tube with an electrode that measures pH and therefore can detect only acid reflux. Recently both a tubeless pH monitoring device and impedance-based devices (to look for nonacid reflux) have been developed. Ambulatory reflux tests are most useful in patients with GERD symptoms that have not responded to empiric therapy and to confirm GERD in patients under evaluation for endoscopic or surgical therapy.

Treatment

LIFESTYLE CHANGES

Educating the patient about factors that can precipitate reflux remains reasonable. Numerous studies have indicated that elevating the head of the bed, decreasing fat intake, quitting smoking, and avoiding recumbency for 3 hours postprandially all decrease distal esophageal acid exposure, although data reflecting the true efficacy of these maneuvers in patients is almost completely lacking. Certain foods (chocolate, alcohol, peppermint, coffee, and perhaps onions and garlic) have been noted to lower pressure in the lower esophageal sphincter (LES), although randomized trials are not available to test the efficacy of these maneuvers. Many clinicians assume the 20% to 30% placebo response rate seen in most randomized trials is due to lifestyle changes, but this has not been rigorously tested. The potential negative effect of lifestyle changes on a patient's quality of life has also not been examined.

PHARMACOLOGIC TREATMENT

Acid Suppression

Acid suppression is the mainstay of GERD therapy. This has evolved quickly over the past few decades. The H_2 receptor antagonists (H_2RAs) were introduced in the 1980s and, for the first time, provided a specific pharmacologic approach to control acid secretion. Eventually, four of these agents were marketed in the United States (cimetidine [Tagamet], ranitidine [Zantac], famotidine [Pepcid], and nizatidine [Axid]). H_2RAs are relatively effective in treating heartburn symptoms with a rapid onset of action. Although H_2RAs offer an improvement over placebo for healing of mild esophagitis, they have limited usefulness, regardless of dose, in healing more-severe esophagitis. Patients who continue to have heartburn after 6 weeks of treatment with H_2RAs are unlikely to respond to prolonged courses or increased dosages. These agents have various approved doses and there are small differences in side effects, but overall, their efficacy is quite similar (Table 1).

In 1989, the first PPI (omeprazole [Prilosec]) was developed. This was followed by the introduction of three additional agents (lansoprazole [Prevacid], pantoprazole [Protonix], and rabeprazole [Aciphex]) that, similar to the H_2RAs, were minimally different from the original agent. PPIs are the most potent gastric acid suppressants, and their efficacy is superior to that of other antisecretory agents such as H_2RAs, because PPIs suppress not only basal nighttime secretion but also daytime food-stimulated gastric acid secretion. This is important because pathologic esophageal reflux occurs mostly during the day (following meals). A review of 33 randomized trials including more than 3000 patients showed that symptomatic relief can be expected in 27% of patients treated with placebo, 60% treated with H_2RAs, and 83% treated with PPIs. Of patients with

TABLE 1 Acid Suppressants

Generic (Brand)	Usual Dose
Proton Pump Inhibitor	
Esomeprazole (Nexium)	20-40 mg once daily
Lansoprazole (Prevacid)	30 mg once daily
Omeprazole* (Prilosec, Zegerid†)	20-40 mg once daily
Pantoprazole (Protonix)	40 mg once daily
Rabeprazole (Aciphex)	20 mg once daily
H$_2$ Receptor Antagonists	
Cimetidine* (Tagamet)	300-400 mg twice daily
Famotidine* (Pepcid, Pepcid Complete†)	20-40 mg twice daily
Nizatidine* (Axid)	150 mg twice daily
Ranitidine* (Zantac)	150 mg twice daily

*Over the counter and generics available.
†Combination of agent with antacid

esophagitis, 24% treated with placebo, 50% treated with H$_2$RAs, and 78% treated with a PPI had mucosal healing.

The optimal benefit of PPIs is achieved with appropriate timing of dosages. The best timing for maximum serum concentration is when the largest number of proton pumps are active. Meals stimulate proton pumps, so having a high serum concentration of these drugs at the time of a meal results in the most effective acid suppression. Therefore, these drugs should be given before meals with enough time for systemic absorption, which is typically 15 to 60 minutes. It has been suggested that patients on once-daily PPIs take the dose before breakfast. However, a recent study has shown that nighttime acid is better controlled if the PPI is taken before the evening meal.

PPI therapy does have some limitations. Once-daily therapy suppresses gastric acid for 11.2 to 15.3 hours during a 24-hour day. Even a powerful PPI given twice daily still leaves the stomach with a pH of less than 4.0 at least 20% of the time, with most of this acidity occurring at night. PPI therapy also has a delayed onset of action that achieves optimal acid suppression after 3 to 5 days from initiation of treatment.

An optically pure preparation of omeprazole was tested and approved as a different agent (esomeprazole [Nexium]). Esomeprazole has shown some increased efficacy when compared with omeprazole, lansoprazole, and pantoprazole in certain subsets of patients, although huge studies were required in order to achieve statistical significance. Omeprazole has also been combined with an antacid in a new formulation that might have some advantages over the parent compound, including the ability to be taken without meals and perhaps a more rapid onset of action.

Antacids and Antirefluxants

Antacids are better than placebo in achieving relief of heartburn. In certain circumstances, antacids may be preferred to other acid-suppressing medications. They are inexpensive and have a very rapid onset. Alginate-based formulations have been available since the 1970s and have been marketed under a variety of brand names, the most common of which is Gaviscon. Alginates act by a unique mechanism in which the alginate precipitates in the presence of gastric acid, forming a gel. The gel then traps carbon dioxide, creating foam that floats on the surface of gastric contents like a raft on water. It is thought that this raft preferentially moves into the esophagus ahead of acidic gastric contents during episodes of reflux and might work as a physical barrier to reduce reflux episodes.

Prokinetic (Motility) Therapy

Prokinetic drugs are appealing in the treatment of GERD because they can increase gastric emptying, improve peristalsis, and increase LES pressure. Unfortunately, these agents are typically not effective as monotherapy, and their side effect profiles often limit their use.

The prokinetic drugs that have been used in GERD include bethanechol (Urecholine),[1] metoclopramide (Reglan), cisapride (Propulsid),[2] domperidone (Motilium),[2] baclofen (Lioresal),[1] and tegaserod (Zelnorm).[1,5] Bethanechol[1] and metoclopramide have poor efficacy and common sideeffects and are not recommended for routine use in GERD. Cisapride[2] has been associated with fatal cardiac arrhythmias and significant cardiotoxicity, especially when taken together with protease inhibitors, macrolide antibiotics, and imidazoles, and has been withdrawn from regular availability in the United States. Baclofen[1] is a γ-amino butyric acid (GABA) receptor agonist. It appears to suppress transient LES relaxation and therefore reduces the number of reflux episodes and the amount of esophageal acid exposure with a single dose (40 mg). Unfortunately, baclofen has a limiting side effect profile (e.g., nausea, vomiting, somnolence, seizures, death on withdrawal).

There is much ongoing research attempting to design a compound with the efficacy of baclofen, yet without the side effects. Tegaserod[1,5] is a 5-HT$_4$ receptor agonist with promotility effects. It has been shown to reduce esophageal acid exposure, but it does not appear to be effective as monotherapy in the treatment of GERD symptoms. Originally, it was not associated with as many side effects as the other prokinetic agents, but because of reports of an increase in cardiovascular events with the medication, it has been withdrawn from the U.S. market.

Step Therapy

A great deal of discussion over the years has involved the concept of step therapy in GERD. Step-up therapy starts with a less expensive, perhaps less-effective agent and then progressively increases the intensity of therapy until symptoms are controlled. Step-down therapy starts with the most-effective, perhaps more-expensive therapy to control symptoms, then therapy is decreased until symptoms return, and medication is stepped back up slightly to the weakest therapy that keeps symptoms controlled.

Because there are no real differences in safety profile between the available agents, these concepts were mainly driven by cost, with antacids being less expensive than H$_2$RAs, which likewise are less expensive than PPIs. Lately, these cost differentials have narrowed, which has strengthened PPI therapy as the best initial and long-term therapy for GERD. With the exception of the rare patient who is allergic or does not respond to a PPI, H$_2$RAs or prokinetic therapies are now used less commonly and the concept of step therapy has become mostly obsolete.

On-Demand Therapy

Intermittent therapy with an H$_2$RA or PPI is most likely to be successful in patients without esophagitis and with mild to moderate heartburn. There is very little evidence to support any one approach for on-demand therapy. H$_2$RAs taken as needed provide acceptable control in patients with mild, intermittent symptoms. Slightly better outcomes were achieved in an open trial of 68 patients with mild or nonulcerative GERD who were given ranitidine (150 mg effervescent tablets) on demand. PPIs do not seem to be a good choice for on-demand therapy because their onset of action does not maximize for a few days. However, there are data and experience to suggest this approach may be beneficial in some patients. A more reasonable use of PPIs is on an intermittent basis, where rather taking one pill, the patient takes a few-day course when the symptoms are more bothersome. This approach has not been approved as an indication in the United States (with the exception of the label for over-the-counter Prilosec), but it is an accepted approach in Europe.

---

[1] Not FDA approved for this indication.
[2] Not available in the United States.
[5] Investigational drug in the United States.

Long-Term (Maintenance) Therapy

Although GERD symptoms and mucosal damage can be brought under control in the majority of patients, that control is usually lost when the medications are discontinued. Many patients with GERD require long-term, possibly lifelong, therapy; therefore, maintenance therapy to keep symptoms comfortably under control and prevent complications is a major concern. This varies in each patient and might require only antacids and lifestyle modifications in up to 20% of patients.

Patients whose disease has required PPIs for control often have symptomatic relapses and failure of healing of esophagitis on standard-dose or even higher-dose H_2RAs or prokinetic therapy. A full dose of H_2RA given once daily, although effective for peptic ulcer disease, is not appropriate for GERD. There does not appear to be a safety advantage with using a lower PPI dose for maintenance, but the indications for some PPIs do suggest a lower maintenance dose (e.g., esomeprazole 20 mg/day and lansoprazole 15 mg/day). Ultimately, whatever dose of medication is needed to control symptoms is the dose that should be used and may include full or even increased-dose PPIs in many patients.

There are clear data that full-dose PPIs lengthen the interval between symptomatic relapses in patients with esophageal strictures requiring dilation. There are no similar data regarding the prevention or prevention of progression of Barrett's esophagus. It does not appear that Barrett's esophagus will regress with either medical or surgical therapy. There have been reports of occasional islands of squamous epithelium appearing with chronic PPI therapy, but the significance of this is not known. One retrospective study suggests less dysplasia in patients with Barrett's esophagus who take PPIs, but this needs confirmation in a large, properly designed trial.

Because many patients are treated with PPIs on a long-term basis, safety is a prominent concern. Effective gastric acid suppression produces varying degrees of hypergastrinemia, although there are no significant, documented adverse effects of elevated gastrin in PPI-treated patients. Several retrospective studies have suggested small but significant increases in community-acquired pneumonia, *Clostridium difficile* infection and hip fractures in patients on PPIs (particularly higher-than-indicated doses). Atrophic gastritis in chronic omeprazole users is common, but it seems to occur predominantly in patients who are infected with *Helicobacter pylori*. No patients have developed PPI-induced gastric dysplasia or cancer. Patients on long-term omeprazole can develop vitamin B_{12} malabsorption and should have their vitamin B_{12} levels periodically assessed. Drugs that require acid for absorption and that are potentially altered with PPI therapy include ketoconazole (Nizoral), iron salts, and digoxin (Lanoxin). When PPI therapy is initiated, the international normalized ratio and prothrombin time may be altered in patients on warfarin (Coumadin).

ENDOSCOPIC AND SURGICAL APPROACHES

The vast majority of GERD patients have mucosal disease, and symptoms are controlled with medical therapy. There is a small subset of patients with symptoms that either are or appear to be refractory to medical therapy. Of these symptoms, regurgitation seems the most reasonable, because current therapy addresses the acid content of the refluxate but probably allows continued reflux of neutralized material in some patients. A trial that randomized 310 patients between surgery and PPIs found surgery to be slightly superior to omeprazole 20 mg/day at the end of 7 years, but if doses up to 40 to 60 mg/day of omeprazole were used, the two treatments were almost equal.

Proper selection and preoperative evaluation of patients are very important. In a study of 100 patients, the best predictors of a good outcome were age younger than 50 years and typical reflux symptoms that had completely resolved on medical therapy. It is also clear that these typical reflux symptoms are more likely to resolve after surgery than the other atypical and supraesophageal symptoms. If typical reflux esophagitis is not present endoscopically, ambulatory pH testing should be performed to confirm the disease.

One study found significantly lower cost and shorter lengths of hospital stay with the laparoscopic approach, although patient satisfaction was similar between the open and laparoscopic groups. The only adverse affect of switching from an open to laparoscopic approach appears to be an increase in dysphagia in those treated laparoscopically. The decreased postoperative morbidity involved in this approach should not change the indications or evaluations for surgery, but it does make this option more attractive for some patients whose alternative would be long-term medical therapy. However, postoperative symptoms are common and include dysphagia, difficulty with belching, increased flatulence, and diarrhea.

A great deal of excitement had been generated by the introduction of techniques designed to control reflux endoscopically, although some of that excitement has waned. There are three broad categories of endoscopic therapy: radiofrequency application to the LES area, techniques designed to decrease reflux using endoscopic sewing devices, and techniques using an injection into the LES region.

Radiofrequency application (Stretta, Curon Medical) is designed to increase the reflux barrier of the LES by creating a scar or perhaps changing the neurologic function of the sphincter. Endoscopic sewing techniques have also been developed in an attempt to replicate the fundoplication from an intragastric approach. Most recently, early data from the full-thickness plication device (NDO Surgical) have been reported. Finally, injection of a nonresorbable polymer (Enteryx, Boston Scientific) has been reported, although complications have resulted in a market withdrawal for this technique. All of these techniques seem to produce an improvement in reflux symptoms, although significant changes in LES pressure have not been documented and less than 35% of patients have been demonstrated to have normalization of intraesophageal acid exposure (measured with ambulatory pH testing).

When the results of the available studies (both published manuscripts and abstracts) are critically examined, many issues remain unresolved, including long-term durability and safety, efficacy of these procedures performed outside of clinical trials, and efficacy in atypical presentations of GERD, among others. Systematic reviews of the radiofrequency, endoscopic sewing, and injection techniques were unable to identify any clear indications for these techniques, but they did support their use in clinical trials and outside of clinical trials in certain well-informed patients who have documented GERD that is responsive to PPI therapy.

REFERENCES

American Gastroenterological Association: Medical position statement: Guidelines on the use of esophageal pH recording. Gastroenterology 1996;110(6):1981.

DeVault KR, Castell DO: Updated guidelines for the diagnosis and treatment of gastroesophageal reflux disease. Am J Gastroenterol 2005;100(1):190-200.

El-Serag HB, Aguirre TV, Davis S, et al: Proton pump inhibitors are associated with reduced incidence of dysplasia in Barrett's esophagus. Am J Gastroenterol 2004;99:1877-1883.

Jackson PG, Cleiber MA, Askari R, Evans SRT: Predictors of outcome in 100 consecutive laparoscopic antireflux procedures. Am J Surg 2001;181:231-235.

Johnsson F, Weywadt L, Solhaug JH, et al: One-week omeprazole treatment in the diagnosis of gastro-oesophageal reflux disease. Scand J Gastroenterol 1998;33:15-20.

Lundell L, Miettinen P, Myrvold HE Nordic GORD Study Group: Seven-year follow-up of a randomized clinical trial comparing proton-pump inhibition with surgical therapy for reflux oesophagitis. British J Surg 2007;94:198-203.

Miner P, Katz Po, et al: Gastric acid control with esomeprazole, lansoprazole, omeprazole, pantoprazole and rabeprazole: A five-way crossover trial. Am J Gastroenterol 2003;98:2616-2620.

Pasricha PJ: Desperately seeking serotonin. A commentary on the withdrawal of tegaserod and the state of drug development for functional motility disorders. Gastroenterology 2007;132:2287-2290.

Sampliner RE Practice Parameters Committee of the American College of Gastroenterology: Updated guidelines for the diagnosis, surveillance, and therapy of Barrett's esophagus. Am J Gastroenterol 2002;97:1888-1895.

Scarpignato C, Pelosini I, Di Mario F: Acid suppression therapy: Where do we go from here? Dig Dis 2006;24:11-46.

Triadafilopoulos G: Endotherapy and surgery for GERD. J Clin Gastroenterol 2007;41:S87-S96.

Tumors of the Stomach

Method of
Scott A. Hundahl, MD

Gastric Adenocarcinoma

Thanks to happy accident rather than specific planning, over the past 80 years, gastric adenocarcinoma has changed from the most-common solid organ malignancy in the United States to a relatively uncommon disease. Worldwide, however, it remains a scourge second only to lung cancer.

CLASSIFICATION AND EPIDEMIOLOGY

Several classification schemes exist. Two are commonly used. Borrmann's morphologic classification relies on gross characteristics of the tumor. The histologic classification of Lauren, first described by Jarvi and Lauren in 1951, divides gastric adenocarcinomas into intestinal (gland-forming) and diffuse (discohesive) types, based on their microscopic appearance. Several other classification schemes have been proposed, including Broder's classification of differentiation, the WHO (World Health Organization) classification, the Nagayo–Komagome classification, the Ming classification, and the Goseki classification, but none eclipses the Lauren classification.

Epidemiologically, three patterns of disease can be discerned, with *Helicobacter pylori* infection playing an important role in the first two patterns: intestinal-type tumors arising from the lesser curve and distal stomach, related to *H. pylori*–associated atrophic gastritis and intestinal metaplasia; diffuse-type tumors involving the body of the stomach, often associated with intense *H. pylori*–associated inflammation but not associated with significant intestinal metaplasia; and intestinal-type tumors of the gastroesophageal junction.

In high-incidence regions of the world, such as Japan and Korea, up to two thirds of gastric adenocarcinomas are of the first type and are strongly associated with chronic multifocal atrophic gastritis and intestinal metaplasia from chronic *H. pylori* infection. The process usually begins at the antrum–corpus junction along the lesser curvature and predisposes to cancers of the intestinal type occurring in the sixth or seventh decades of life. The second type of gastric adenocarcinoma, also associated with *H. pylori*, afflicts younger persons in the fourth and fifth decades of life. The last type, seen in lower-incidence regions of the world such as the United States, is associated with chronic gastroesophageal reflux and Barrett's esophagitis.

Epidemiologists and public health experts estimate that more than 40% of gastric adenocarcinomas worldwide can be attributed to chronic *H. pylori* infection. Strains containing the *cagA* gene appear more dangerous. The infection usually starts by the second or third decade, and unless it is successfully treated, it gives rise to chronic inflammation, atrophic gastritis, and eventually intestinal metaplasia, which is a premalignant histologic condition. Dietary factors such as high salt and high nitrates can accentuate this progression as well as the march to cancer. As the condition progresses, acid-producing oxyntic mucosa is progressively wiped out, gastric pH increases, and bacterial overgrowth with non–*H. pylori* bacteria is facilitated. The original *H. pylori*, which requires an acid environment to thrive, often disappears at this point.

Once intestinal metaplasia is established, dietary factors become particularly important in mitigating the risk of cancer development. Protective factors include intake of vitamin C, fresh fruits and vegetables, and antioxidants. The association of *H. pylori* infection with the development of intestinal metaplasia suggests that early detection and elimination of this infection might prevent gastric cancer. Unfortunately, in high-incidence areas, reinfection from contaminated water supply and other sources is common, thus undermining the strategy. Also, in prevention trials to date, benefit appears restricted to the subgroups without preexisting intestinal metaplasia.

RISK FACTORS

Risk factors other than *H. pylori* infection include low socioeconomic status, smoking, a diet deficient in fresh fruits and vegetables or high in salt-preserved high-nitrate foods, previous gastric ulcer, ionizing radiation, family history, and previous gastric resection. Blood group A is associated with higher risk of developing a diffuse-type tumor. Predisposing genetic conditions include the Lynch's syndrome (hereditary nonpolyposis colorectal cancer [HNPCC], a condition with microsatellite instability due to deficient DNA repair enzymes), as well as dominantly inherited germline mutations in the E-cadherin gene.

DIAGNOSIS

In Western populations, by the time gastric cancer causes symptoms, the disease is often relatively advanced. In a large National Cancer Data Base survey of U.S. patients, presenting ascribable symptoms included weight loss (62%), abdominal or epigastric pain (52%), nausea (34%), anorexia (32%), early satiety (32%), dysphagia (26%), and melena (18%).

Mass screening combining upper GI series, endoscopy, and serum pepsinogen I/II ratio have proved beneficial in high-incidence areas such as Japan, but they cannot be justified in the United States, where incidence is low. However, for defined risk groups, such as those with established atrophic gastritis and established intestinal metaplasia, strong family history, and those with HNPCC syndrome, surveillance screening should definitely be considered. For those with hereditary E-cadherin mutations associated with gastric cancer, prophylactic total gastrectomy is recommended.

In the United States, diagnosis is usually made by upper endoscopy. One should be aware that diffuse-type cancers manifesting as linitis plastica are often associated with minimal visible mucosal changes, and deep biopsies are often required for establishing the diagnosis. Furthermore, small, early gastric cancers (defined by the Japanese as in situ and T-1 cancers, with or without node involvement) can be associated with particularly subtle mucosal changes, presenting a challenge for even the most experienced endoscopist. Chromoendoscopy and other sophisticated mucosal imaging techniques have been used to identify such changes but are not yet standard.

Extent-of-disease studies for gastric adenocarcinoma include endoscopic ultrasound (good for estimating depth of tumor and visualizing immediately adjacent nodes), and helical CT scanning, which is good for evaluating extraluminal extent of disease, intraabdominal or mediastinal extension or spread, and liver or lung

---

 CURRENT DIAGNOSIS

- Intestinal metaplasia, which predisposes to cancer, results from chronic *Helicobacter pylori* infection.
- In the United States, screening studies are reserved for those with definite risk factors.
- Pretreatment staging drives subsequent treatment and involves endoscopy, endoscopic ultrasound, helical computed tomography, and often laparoscopy or mini-laparotomy.
- Mucosal abnormalities can be largely absent in early gastrointestinal stromal tumors, small carcinoids, and even diffuse-type linitis plastica. Deep endoscopic biopsies are required.

CURRENT THERAPY

Adenocarcinoma

- To ensure complete surgical resection, resection should be customized (e.g. gross margin, use of endoscopic mucosal resection for certain mucosal tumors).
- Survival is highest with low Maruyama Index surgery.
- Adjuvant therapy options include preoperative chemotherapy (± postoperative treatment), or postoperative chemoradiation

Gastrointestinal Stromal Tumors

- Node dissection is not indicated.

Gastric Lymphoma

- For aggressive diffuse-type lymphomas, chemotherapy with or without radiation therapy is now the mainstay of treatment. Surgery is reserved for complications such as acute perforation.
- Superficial mucosa-associated lymphoid tissue tumors can sometimes be treated by simply eliminating *Helicobacter pylori* infection. It comes back if reinfection occurs, however.

metastases. Because even high-resolution CT scanning can miss small peritoneal implants, extraregional nodal spread, and small liver metastases, staging laparoscopy or minilaparotomy are valuable adjuncts and should be considered mandatory if any preoperative chemotherapy is considered.

STAGING

Although a long-established, much-modified Japanese staging system, the General Rules, finds widespread use in many areas of the world, the AJCC/UICC (American Joint Committee on Cancer/International Union Against Cancer) TNM (tumor, nodes, metastases) system is by far the dominant staging system used. T stage is defined a bit differently than that for colorectal cancer: Muscularis propria penetration short of serosal penetration is still considered T2 disease, a serosal breach is required for T3 disease, and a T4 designation requires direct involvement of adjacent structures. Optimally, accurate nodal designation requires that more than 15 nodes be examined by the pathologist. N1 disease means metastases in 1 to 6 regional nodes, N2 disease means metastases in 7 to 15 regional nodes, and N3 disease means metastases in more than 15 nodes. Any N3 disease, any node-positive T4 disease, any M1 distant metastatic disease, and any involved extra-regional M1 nodes translate in the staging matrix to stage IV disease. The reader is referred to the AJCC staging manual referenced at the end of this chapter.

TREATMENT

Curative treatment of gastric cancer involves, as main therapy, complete negative-margin surgical resection of disease. For select tumors, such resection sometimes follows up-front chemotherapy. For localized in situ and select T1 tumors, endoscopic mucosal resection and minimally invasive techniques have been successfully employed. Unfortunately, most tumors in the United States are discovered at a stage where formal open surgery is required.

To secure a histologically negative mural margin of resection, a gross margin of 2 cm is usually adequate for exophytic, noninfiltrating tumors, and a margin of at least 5 to 6 cm of grossly normal tissue is recommended for ulcerated or infiltrating tumors or diffuse histology. Closest mural margins are generally checked by frozen section at the time of surgery to confirm adequacy of resection. Total gastrectomy is not indicated as a routine procedure, except in diffuse-type tumors involving most of the stomach (linitis plastica), but it is warranted whenever required for a negative-margin resection.

Routine splenectomy in the treatment of gastric cancer, as well as routine distal pancreatectomy (performed in the past to clear splenic nodes), should be avoided unless definitely required for complete resection of visible or palpable disease.

The optimal extent of lymph node dissection in this disease has generated—and continues to generate—international controversy. Although several prospective randomized trials to date in non-Asian populations—none perfect—fail to demonstrate that routine extensive lymphadenectomy increases survival, it has also been shown that insufficient lymphadenectomy definitely compromises survival. A prospective randomized single-institution trial in Taipei has documented survival benefit associated with radical lymph node dissection. The adequacy of lymphadenectomy for a given case can be quantified using the Maruyama Index of Unresected Disease. In both a large U.S. adjuvant chemoradiation trial and in a blinded reanalysis of a large Dutch surgical trial, low Maruyama Index score correlates with survival. Moreover, a dose–response effect is seen for the extent of surgical clearance of node groups at risk. Using the Maruyama computer program to predict the extent of nodal spread for a given cancer case before surgery is one way to facilitate a low Maruyama Index operation.

Sentinel node biopsy, an established technique in the treatment of other cancers, has largely failed to win support in cancer of the stomach owing to the organ's lymphatic complexity and relatively high reported false-negative rates.

A large North American prospective randomized trial of postoperative adjuvant 5-fluorouracil–based chemoradiation in completely resected gastric cancer revealed a significant increase in disease-free and overall survival with this treatment. The postoperative nature of this trial thwarted implementation of surgical guidelines, and the extent of node dissection for most patients in the trial was suboptimal. Practitioners in some countries, such as Japan, dismiss the necessity of adjuvant postoperative adjuvant chemoradiation with the (unproved but reasonable) argument that this is only a salvage technique for inadequate surgery. A separate Korean chemoradiation series has shown benefit even for radically treated cases, however. For patients with good postoperative performance status, good organ function, and adequate nutrition, postoperative adjuvant chemoradiation therapy remains the standard in North America.

A recent U.K. study of preoperative plus postoperative ECF (epirubicin [Ellence],[1] *cis*-platinum, and continuous-infusion 5-fluorouracil [Adrucil]) chemotherapy versus surgery alone has shown encouraging results for ECF, with a significant improvement in survival. Previous preoperative chemotherapy trials, using other regimens, have been negative, however. Preoperative ECF chemotherapy is now recommended by some, and this is especially the case for localized advanced tumors considered borderline resectable.

In Korea, a positive trial of adjuvant perioperative intraperitoneal chemotherapy has been reported. Considerable morbidity and mortality are associated with this adjuvant treatment, however, and it is unlikely it will be implemented without refinement and successful independent duplication of results.

For localized disease deemed not resectable to negative margins, both chemotherapy and chemoradiation have been used to convert such tumors to potentially resectable status. With successful negative-margin resection, some of these patients indeed survive free of disease long term. When localized unresected disease is documented to exist, administering chemoradiation with 5-fluorouracil as a radiation sensitizer can also result in some degree of 5-year survival (per reports, >10%).

Gastrointestinal Stromal Tumors

Gastrointestinal stromal tumors (GISTs) manifest as submucosal spindle cell tumors in the sarcoma family. In contrast to

---

[1]Not FDA approved for this indication.

leiomyosarcomas and other spindle cell sarcomas, they express the antigen CD117 and most (>80%) tumors have activating mutations of *c-KIT*. Formerly considered rare, approximately 5000 of these tumors per year are now diagnosed in the United States. Owing to pattern of growth in the gastric wall, deep to the mucosa, early symptoms are unusual and these tumors often grow to massive size before mucosal ulceration and hemorrhage (or other major symptoms) finally develop. GISTs are classified as sarcomas. Even low-risk GISTs (< 5 cm and < 1 mitosis per 10 high power fields) can metastasize, and no GIST can be considered truly benign.

Treatment of localized primary GISTs consists of complete surgical resection, and a 2-cm margin of grossly normal tissue usually accomplishes this. Specific lymph node dissection is not indicated for this histology. Surgical series indicate that approximately 50% of primary gastric tumors metastasize and recur within 5 years. For patients with widespread metastases, generally located in the peritoneal cavity or the liver, first-line therapy is now a well-tolerated oral agent, imatinib mesylate (Gleevec or STI-571) at an initial dose of 400 mg daily, which generates partial responses in more than 50% of cases and stable disease in an additional 25% of cases. Side effects are minimal, and 1-year survival in treated patients is approximately 85%. On the basis of a completed American College of Surgeons Oncology Group (ACOSOG) trial, patients who have all disease completely resected should receive postoperative adjuvant therapy for 1 year.

For tumors resistant to imatinib, SU11248, sunitinib malate (Sutent), is now used as effective second-line therapy. Additional targeted biological agents are under active investigation.

Carcinoid Tumors

Carcinoid tumors of the stomach are similar in behavior to small bowel carcinoids. When small (<1 cm), and unassociated with invasion of the muscularis propria, local excision to negative margins is generally deemed sufficient. For such tumors, endoscopic resection has an established role. However, even small tumors can metastasize to lymph nodes. Wider gastrectomy with lymph node dissection is generally recommended for gastric tumors larger than 1 cm. Many of these tumors are associated with serum hypergastrinemia; those without this finding tend to be more aggressive. When metastatic to the liver or other organs, surgical cytoreduction (or other means of tumor ablation) can offer considerable palliation to those with carcinoid syndrome, and this should always be considered. Octreotide therapy is now a palliative mainstay in all patients with carcinoid syndrome.

Gastric Lymphomas

Gastric lymphomas encompass most of the lymphoma subtypes, but low-grade, mucosa-associated B-cell lymphomas (B-cell MALT lymphomas) deserve special mention because they are strongly associated with *H. pylori* infection. Indeed, localized cases can be controlled simply by treating the *H. pylori* infection. In such cases, molecular studies indicate persistence of the offending lymphoid clone in about one half of cases. However, and, particularly if *H. pylori* infection recurs, the lymphoma in such cases returns.

Aggressive high-grade diffuse-type B-cell gastric lymphomas, stage IE and IIE, once treated with multimodal therapy, are now treated with chemotherapy alone as the primary treatment, with or without radiotherapy. Surgical intervention is now reserved for emergencies, such as perforation.

For further information on this and other gastrointestinal lymphomas, please see the chapter on lymphoma.

REFERENCES

Cunningham D, Allum WH, Stenning SP, et al: Perioperative chemotherapy versus surgery alone for resectable gastroesophageal cancer. N Engl J Med 2006;355(1):11-20.

Ferrucci PF, Zucca E: Primary gastric lymphoma pathogenesis and treatment: What has changed over the past 10 years? Br J Haematol 2007;136(4):521-538.

Hundahl SA, Macdonald JS, Benedetti J, et al: Surgical treatment variation in a prospective, randomized trial of chemoradiotherapy in gastric cancer: The effect of undertreatment. Ann Surg Oncol 2002;9(3):278-286.

Hundahl SA, Peeters KC, Kranenbarg EK, et al: Improved regional control and survival with "low Maruyama Index" surgery in gastric cancer: Autopsy findings from the Dutch D1-D2 Trial. Gastric Cancer 2007;10(2):84-86.

Macdonald JS, Smalley SR, Benedetti J, et al: Chemoradiotherapy after surgery compared with surgery alone for adenocarcinoma of the stomach or gastroesophageal junction. N Engl J Med 2001;345(10):725-730.

Modlin IM, Kidd M, Latich I, et al: Current status of gastrointestinal carcinoids. Gastroenterology 2005;128(6):1717-1751.

Siehl J, Thiel E. C-kit, GIST, and imatinib. Recent Results Cancer Res 2007;176:145-151.

Tumors of the Colon and Rectum

Method of
Daniel Albo, MD, PhD

Epidemiology

Colorectal cancer is the second leading cause of cancer-related death in the United States and the third most common malignancy in men and women. In 2005, there were approximately 145,000 new cases (104,500 colon and 40,340 rectal) diagnosed and an estimated 54,290 deaths (10% of all cancer deaths in the United States) due to the disease. The overall incidence is identical in men and women, with the risk beginning at age 40 years and increasing with age. The incidence is also higher in the industrialized nations.

Etiology and Risk Factors

The causes of colon and rectal cancer are unknown, but risk appears associated with genetic factors. Those with a personal or family history of colorectal cancer or polyps are at a higher risk for developing colorectal cancer. The two most common forms of hereditary colorectal cancer are familial adenomatous polyposis (FAP) and hereditary nonpolyposis colorectal cancer (HNPCC). By the age of 40 years, the risk of developing colon cancer for people with untreated FAP is 100%. Colorectal cancer is diagnosed in approximately 50% of patients with HNPCC by the age of 80 years. HNPCC patients can also develop endometrial, breast, ovarian, and gastric carcinomas.

Dietary factors also influence the development of colorectal cancer. Diets high in unsaturated fats and low in fiber have been strongly implicated. Inflammatory bowel disease can also increase the risk of colorectal cancer. Patients with ulcerative colitis have a 5 to 10 times higher risk of developing colorectal cancer. Similarly, Crohn's disease predisposes to colorectal cancer, although the relative risk is slightly lower.

Screening

Colorectal cancers arise from adenomatous polyps. The National Polyp Study showed that colonoscopic removal of adenomatous polyps significantly reduces the risk of developing colorectal cancer. The natural history of polyps supports an aggressive approach to their treatment. Adenomatous polyps coexist with colorectal cancer in 60% of patients and are associated with an increased incidence of synchronous and metachronous colorectal cancers. Features of adenomatous polyps that are particularly worrisome include villous type (40% are malignant), large size (46% of adenomatous polyps >2 cm are malignant), and the presence of dysplasia (35% are malignant).

The value of routine screening for colorectal cancer of asymptomatic populations has been established. The goals of screening are detection of early colorectal cancers and prevention of colorectal cancer by finding and removing adenomatous polyps. In 2003, the U.S. Multisociety Task Force on colorectal cancer met to update the original 1997 consensus guidelines for colorectal cancer screening and surveillance and made recommendations regarding screening (Box 1).

Staging

The American Joint Committee on Cancer (AJCC) and the International Union Against Cancer (IUAC) recommend the TNM classification system for colorectal cancer (Table 1 and Box 2). Treatment decisions should be made based on the TNM classification rather than the older Dukes' or the modified Astler–Coller classifications.

Clinical Presentation

Most people with colorectal cancer experience no symptoms until the disease is at a late stage. This is the reason that screening tests, such as a colonoscopy, are so important. When present, signs and symptoms of colorectal cancer are nonspecific and can include diarrhea, constipation, and narrow-caliber stools; blood in the stool; unexplained anemia; abdominal discomfort, pain, or tenderness; intestinal obstruction; unexplained weight loss; constant tiredness; tenesmus; and iron-deficiency anemia.

BOX 1 2003 U.S. Multisociety Task Force on Colorectal Cancer Screening Recommendations

Average risk, asymptomatic, age 50 years or older
- FOBT once a year (colonoscopy or DCBE/flexible sigmoidoscopy if positive)
  and
- Colonoscopy every 10 years
  or
- Flexible sigmoidoscopy every 5 years (consider colonoscopy if positive)
  or
- DCBE every 5 years (consider colonoscopy if positive)

First-degree relative with CRC or adenomatous polyps at age 60 years or older, or two second-degree relatives affected with CRC: Same as for average risk but starting at age 40 years

Two or more first-degree relatives with CRC or single first-degree relative with CRC or adenomatous polyps or adenomatous polyps diagnosed when younger than 60 years: Colonoscopy every 5 years beginning at age 40 or 10 years younger than the earliest diagnosis in the family

One second-degree or any third-degree relative with CRC: Same as for average risk

Gene carrier or at risk for FAP: Annual flexible sigmoidoscopy beginning at age 10-12 years

Gene carrier or at risk for HNPCC: Colonoscopy every 1-2 years beginning at age 20-25 years or 10 years younger than the earliest case in the family

CRC = colorectal cancer; DCBE = double-contrast barium enema. FAP = familial adenomatous polyposis; HNPCC = hereditary nonpolyposis colorectal cancer.

TABLE 1 TNM Staging Systems

TNM Staging	Primary Tumor	Lymph Node Status	Metastases
Stage 0	Tis	N0	M0
Stage 1	T1	N0	M0
	T2	N0	M0
Stage 2	T3	N0	M0
	T4	N0	M0
Stage 3A	Any T	N1	M0
Stage 3B	Any T	N2 or N3	M0
Stage 4	Any T	Any N	M1

Diagnosis and Work-up

The diagnosis of colorectal cancer should be confirmed by colonoscopy and biopsy. The entire colon and rectum are evaluated to avoid missing synchronous tumors. Metastatic work-up includes computed tomography (CT) or magnetic resonance imaging (MRI) of the abdomen and pelvis (Fig. 1) (to evaluate for potential local invasion of adjacent organs, liver metastases, or carcinomatosis) and a carcinoembryonic antigen (CEA) blood test. CEA levels are not accurate for screening (low sensitivity and specificity) but are useful for both prognostic and follow-up purposes in colorectal cancer.

Rectal cancer patients also require an endoluminal rectal ultrasound (EUS) (see Fig. 1). EUS is up to 95% accurate for evaluating the T stage and 74% accurate for detecting nodal metastases. Accurate staging can help select candidates for sphincter preservation or neoadjuvant therapy.

Positron emission tomography (PET) and now PET-CT, although not useful for primary colorectal cancer, can be a useful imaging modality in recurrent colorectal cancer. It is also useful to assess response to neoadjuvant therapies and to detect occult metastases in patients with postoperative elevations in CEA levels that are not detectable on CT scan.

BOX 2 TNM Definitions

Tumor

Tis: Carcinoma in situ
T1: Tumor invades submucosa
T2: Tumor invades muscularis propria
T3: Tumor invades through muscularis propria into the sub serosa or into nonperitoneal pericolic or perirectal tissues
T4: Tumor perforates the visceral peritoneum or directly invades other organs or structures

Node

N0: No regional lymph node metastasis
N1: Metastases in one to three pericolic or perirectal lymph nodes
N2: Metastases in four or more pericolic or perirectal lymph nodes
N3: Metastases in any lymph node along the course of a named vascular trunk

Metastasis

M0: No distant metastasis
M1: Distant metastasis

CURRENT DIAGNOSIS

- Cancer is usually asymptomatic early.
- Men or postmenopausal women with unexplained iron-deficiency anemia should be evaluated for colorectal cancer.
- Symptoms are usually vague, nonspecific, and late.
- There are no available reliable tumor markers for screening or diagnosis.
- Colorectal cancer arises from premalignant polyps.
- Screening colonoscopy is paramount for detecting polyps or early cancer.

 CURRENT THERAPY

- Margin-negative anatomic surgical resection with en-bloc resection of nodal basin
- Total mesorectal excision for distal rectal cancer
- Adjuvant chemotherapy for stage III colon cancer and stages II and III rectal cancer
- Neoadjuvant chemoradiation for locally advanced rectal cancer
- Anatomic metastasectomy for resectable liver-only metastases (consider adjuvant or neoadjuvant chemotherapy, or both)
- Palliative chemotherapy for unresectable metastases

Treatment

Colorectal cancer patients requires multidisciplinary treatment, including surgery, chemotherapy, radiation therapy, and, increasingly, biological cancer therapies. Surgery is the only potentially curative therapy for colorectal cancer. Chemotherapy, radiation therapy, and biological cancer therapies have roles in the adjuvant (after surgery), neoadjuvant (before surgery), and palliative settings.

SURGERY

Principles of surgical therapy for colorectal cancer include mobilization of colon and rectum following embryologic (avascular) planes, use of sharp dissection techniques, anatomic resections including intact vascular and lymphatic basins (Table 2), and reconstruction of intestinal continuity when feasible.

Patients with rectal cancer deserve special consideration. The rectum lies in a confined space. It is surrounded by autonomic nerve structures of critical functional importance; if these nerve structures are violated, severe autonomic dysfunction will occur (e.g. urinary retention, impotence, incontinence). It is also in very close proximity to vascular structures (hypogastric vein, presacral venous plexus) that if injured can produce life-threatening hemorrhage. As a result, the technical expertise of the surgeon is the single most important prognostic factor of oncologic and functional outcomes in rectal cancer. Prospective randomized trials have shown a 60% reduction in local recurrence rates, a 40% reduction in rectal cancer–specific death

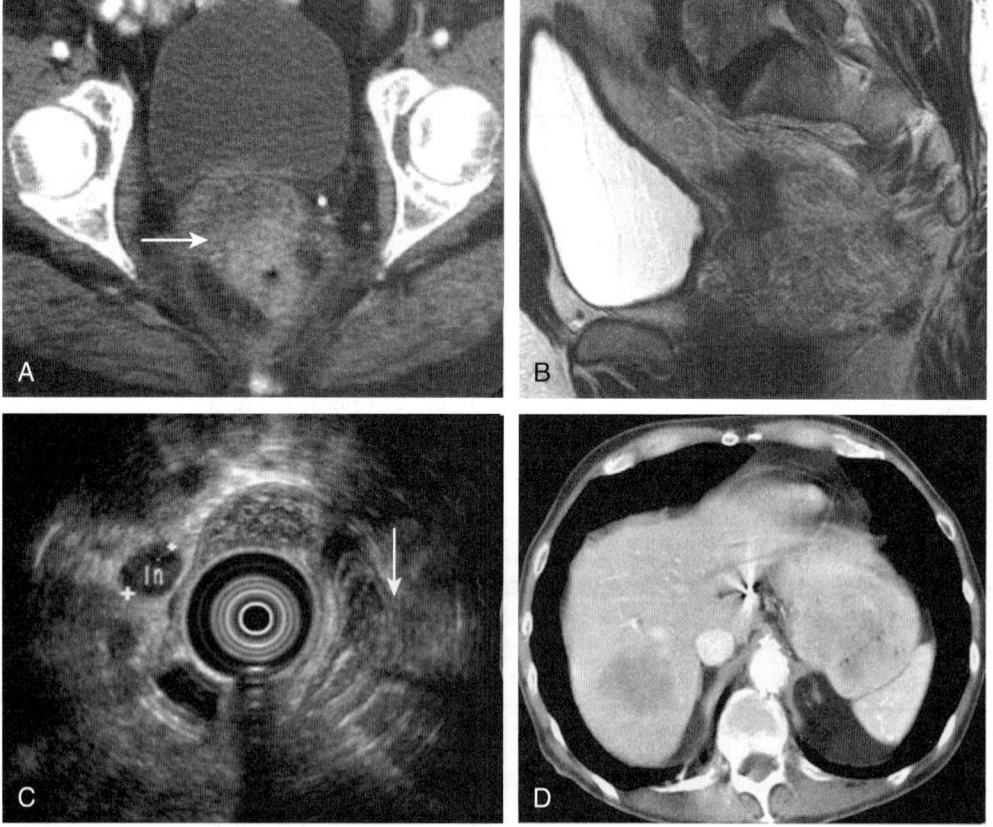

FIGURE 1. Imaging in colorectal cancer cancer. **A,** Computed tomography (CT) scan of a rectal cancer with direct extension into the seminal vesicles *(arrow)*. **B,** Magnetic resonance image of the pelvis (sagittal view) showing a locally advanced rectal cancer occupying the entire pelvis with posterior extension into the sacrum *(arrow)*. **C,** Endoluminal rectal ultrasound of a T4 N1 rectal cancer with invasion into the prostate *(arrow)* and lymphadenopathy in the mesorectum *(ln)*. **D,** CT scan (liver protocol) showing a colorectal cancer metastasis in the posterior sector of the right lobe of the liver.

TABLE 2 Surgical Therapy For Colorectal Cancer

Tumor Location	Operation
Ascending colon	Right hemicolectomy
Hepatic flexure	Extended right hemicolectomy
Transverse colon	Transverse colectomy
Splenic flexure	Extended left hemicolectomy
Descending colon	Left hemicolectomy
Sigmoid colon	Sigmoid colectomy
Upper or mid rectum	Low anterior resection
Distal rectum	Proctectomy with total mesorectal excision and coloanal anastomosis *or* abdominoperineal resection *or* transanal excision

rates, and better functional outcomes when rectal cancer surgery is performed by specialty-trained surgeons in high-volume centers.

It is paramount to obtain negative distal and radial margins during colorectal cancer operations. Although traditionally a distal margin of 5 cm has been advocated, more recently it has been established that distal margins of 2 cm (and even subcentimeter margins) are safe. From a practical standpoint, this means that even very distal rectal tumors are potential candidates for sphincter-preserving radical resections. Of more importance is the radial margin. Positive radial margins are associated with three times higher local recurrence and metastasis rates and lower survivals.

Another important consideration is the extent of mesorectal excision in rectal cancer patients. For tumors in the upper rectum, a mesorectal excision of 5 cm distal to the tumor site is adequate. For tumors within 5 cm of the anal verge, a total proctectomy with total mesorectal excision is indicated (Fig. 2). Total mesorectal excision combined with low colorectal or coloanal anastomosis obviates the need, in many patients, for abdominoperineal resections and the associated permanent stoma. The risk of anastomotic dehiscence with these sphincter-preserving procedures, however, is considerable (>15%), often requiring temporary proximal diversion. In these patients, the creation of a colonic pouch improves functional outcomes.

Transanal excision of rectal tumors is an alternative way of achieving sphincter preservation. Although this technique is feasible in a small subset of patients, it increases recurrence rates and, for patients with T2 or greater tumors, decreases survival rates. To qualify for transanal excision, rectal tumors must be T1 (or some selected T2) exophitic lesions, less than 4 cm in diameter, and less than 10 cm from the anal verge. They must have cell-differentiated histology, no lymphatic or vascular invasion, and no lymph node involvement. Potential exceptions include patients unfit for major surgery or patients with extensive metastases.

The Clinical Outcomes of Surgical Therapy (COST) Study multicenter prospective randomized trial recently compared laparoscopic-assisted colectomy with open colectomy. Recurrence rates and 3-year overall survival rates were similar in both groups. Potential advantages of laparoscopic-assisted colectomy included minimal decreases in hospital stay (5 days for laparoscopic-assisted colectomy vs 6 days for open colectomy) and a modest decrease in the use of analgesics. Disadvantages of laparoscopic-assisted colectomy included a 21% conversion rate from laparoscopic-assisted colectomy to open procedure, longer operating times, and higher costs. The quality-of-life component of this trial showed minimal short-term quality-of-life benefits with laparoscopic-assisted colectomy.

ADJUVANT AND NEOADJUVANT THERAPIES

In 1997, the American Society of Clinical Oncology, based on data from several randomized clinical trials, stated that 5-fluorouracil(5-FU)—based chemotherapy improves survivals and should be considered for postoperative treatment of patients with stage III colon cancer. After the approval of irinotecan (Camptosar) and oxaliplatin (Eloxatin) for the treatment of patients with advanced colorectal cancer, these drugs are now being tested in patients with local or recurrent disease. A preliminary analysis of the MOSAIC (Multicenter International Study of Oxaliplatin/5FU-LV in the Adjuvant Treatment of Colon Cancer) study in patients with resected stage III colon cancer has demonstrated a significant improvement in disease-free survival at 3 years in favor of an oxaliplatin-containing regimen compared with 5-FU (Adrucil) and leucovorin alone.

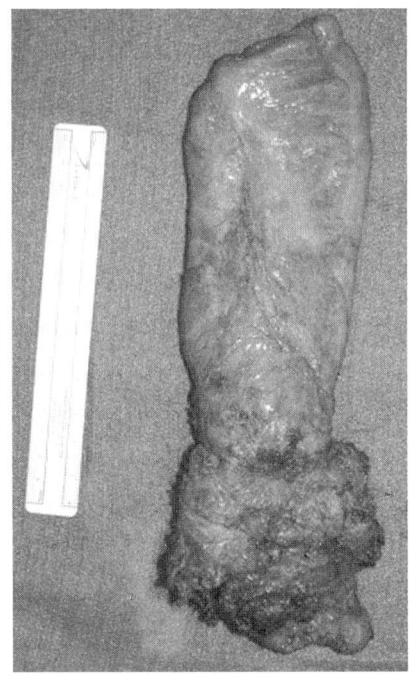 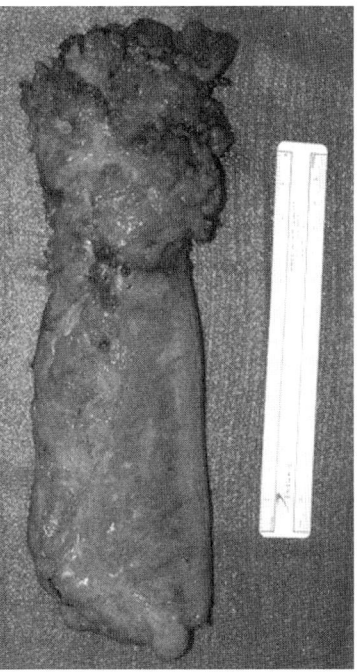

FIGURE 2. Total mesorectal excision for distal rectal cancer. Note the shiny surface on the specimen indicating that the entire intact mesorectum was excised en bloc with the tumor in this total proctectomy specimen. *Left*, anterior; *right*, posterior.

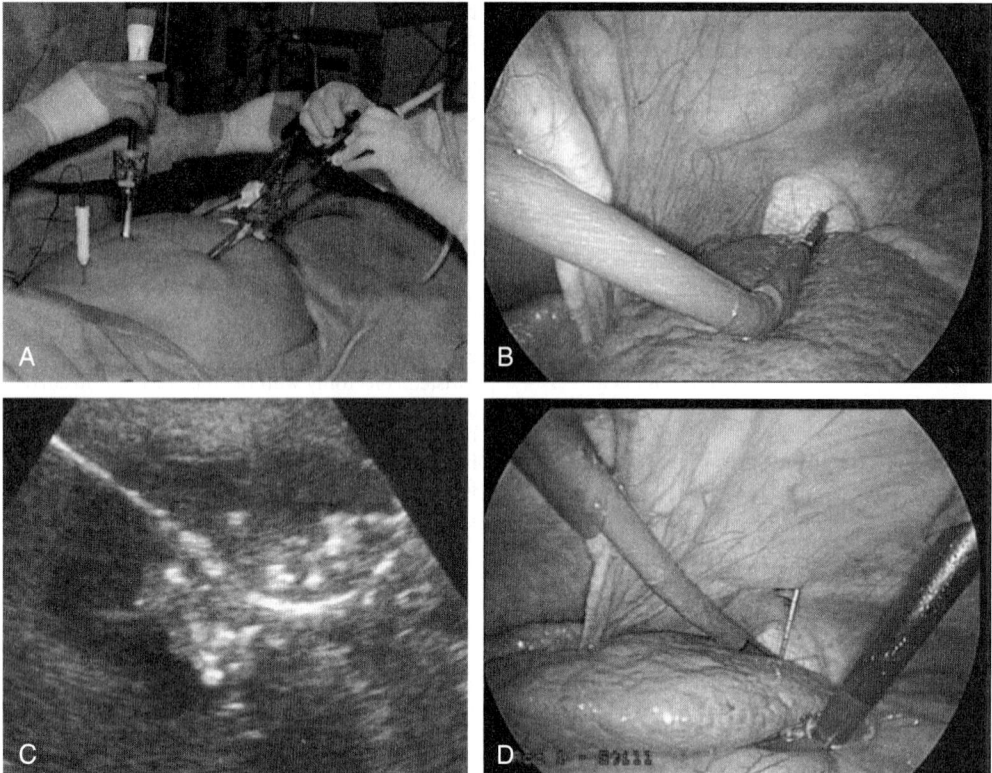

FIGURE 3. Minimally invasive treatment for colorectal cancer liver metastases: Laparoscopic radiofrequency ablation (RFA). **A,** Port placement. **B,** Laparoscopic intraoperative ultrasound (IOUS) probe. **C,** IOUS on ongoing RFA of a liver metastasis. Note the RFA array deployed into the tumor (dark area) with ongoing tumor ablation (white areas). **D,** Intraoperative ultrasound guided radiofrequency ablation of liver metastases.

Treatment of patients with recurrent colon cancer depends on the location and extent of disease. For patients with liver-only or lung-only metastatic disease, surgical resection is the only potentially curative treatment (≤30%-40% 5-year survival rates). Patients with liver-only metastases who are not candidates for resection can be considered for ablative therapies such as radiofrequency ablation. Radiofrequency ablation can be performed laparoscopically with excellent results and minimal morbidity (Fig. 3). Patients with unresectable disease are treated with systemic chemotherapy.

Irinotecan or oxaliplatin, or both, combined with 5-FU–leucovorin have demonstrated improved survival in patients with advanced or metastatic disease compared with 5-FU–leucovorin alone. In addition, novel biological cancer therapies such as vascular endothelial growth factor (VEGF) and epidermal growth factor receptor (EGFR) inhibitors are used with increasing frequency, showing marked improvements in survival in patients with unresectable metastatic disease. These agents are being investigated in patients with resectable disease as well.

Based on analysis of several randomized prospective clinical trials, the National Cancer Institute concluded at a consensus development conference in 1990 that postoperative combined-modality treatment is recommended for patients with stage II and stage III rectal carcinoma. 5FU-based chemotherapy improves survival, and radiation therapy decreases locoregional treatment failures in patients with resectable rectal cancer. Patients with locally advanced disease (T3 or N$^+$) benefit from neoadjuvant chemoradiation, with a significant improvement in disease-free survival and sphincter-preservation rates reported in recent clinical trials.

Surveillance

The objective of surveillance for colorectal cancer is to detect early, potentially resectable recurrences or metastases as well as metachronous colorectal cancer primaries. Approximately 80% of colorectal cancer recurrences occur within 2 years of resection, and the majority of additional recurrences occur within 5 years. The most common site of distant metastases is the liver. There is considerable variation among practitioners in regard to the ideal surveillance for colorectal cancer patients. Table 3 summarizes the recommended colorectal cancer surveillance guidelines by the American Society of Clinical Oncology (ASCO).

TABLE 3 Recommended Colorectal Cancer Surveillance Guidelines By the American Society of Clinical Oncology

Test	Guideline
Carcinoembryonic antigen	Every 3 mo for stages II and III disease for at least 3 y if the patient is a potential candidate for surgery or chemotherapy of metastatic disease
History and physical examination	Every 3 to 6 mo for the first 3 y and annually thereafter
Liver function tests	Against routine use
Fecal occult blood test	Against routine use
Computed tomography	Against routine use
Chest x-ray	Against routine use
Colonoscopy	Every 3 to 5 y to detect new cancers and polyps
Pelvic imaging	Against routine use
Complete blood cell counts	Against routine use

REFERENCES

Anthony T: Colorectal cancer. Surg Oncol Clin North Am 2006;15(1):175-193.
Chang GJ, Feig BF: Cancer of the colon, rectum, and anus. In Feig BW, Berger DH, Fuhrman GM (ed): The M.D. Anderson Surgical Oncology Handbook, 4th ed. Philadelphia: Lippincott Williams & Wilkins, 2006, pp 261-319.
Desch CE, Benson AB III, Smith TJ, et al: Recommended colorectal cancer surveillance guidelines by the American Society of Clinical Oncology. J Clin Oncol 1999;17(4):1312.
Guillem JG, Chessin DB, Cohen AM, et al: Long-term oncologic outcome following preoperative combined modality therapy and total mesorectal excision of locally advanced rectal cancer. Ann Surg 2005;241(5):829-836.
Meyerhardt JA, Mayer RJ: Systemic therapy for colorectal cancer. N Engl J Med 2005;352(5):476-487.
Meyerhardt JA, Tepper JE, Niedzwiecki D, et al: Impact of hospital procedure volume on surgical operation and long-term outcomes in high-risk curatively resected rectal cancer: Findings from the Intergroup 0114 Study. J Clin Oncol 2004;22(1):166-174.
Nelson H, Petrelli N, Carlin A, et al: Guidelines 2000 for colon and rectal cancer surgery. J Natl Cancer Inst 2001;93(8):583-596.
Winawer S, Fletcher S, Rex D, et al: American Gastroenterological Association: Colorectal cancer screening and surveillance: Clinical guidelines and rationale—update based on new evidence. Gastroenterology 2003;124:544-560.

Intestinal Parasites

Method of
Nathan Thielman, MD, MPH, and
Elizabeth Reddy, MD

Intestinal parasites are a diverse group of pathogens with local and global significance. Immigration, international adoption, travel, and the frequency of HIV, AIDS, and other immune-compromising conditions (e.g., malignancy, organ transplantation) have all contributed to a need for ongoing or increased awareness of parasitic infections in the United States. Persons who reside in chronic care facilities, children in daycare, and persons whose sexual practices increase the likelihood of fecal–oral contact are also at risk for acquiring intestinal parasitic infection.

Globally, intestinal parasites are responsible for an enormous burden of disease. Although these pathogens are rarely fatal, ongoing exposure to intestinal parasites among persons in endemic areas exacerbates malnutrition, carries multiple morbidities, and causes stunting of growth and development in children, all of which have far-reaching consequences.

Patients who present with diarrheal illness (especially prolonged or travel-associated), unexplained eosinophilia, or expulsion of worms should be evaluated for intestinal parasites. In such cases, a careful history should focus on the patient's country of origin, detailed travel and recreational activities, dietary habits and new or unusual food exposures, occupation, sexual history, sick contacts, and risks for or known immunodeficiency. Some specialists advocate obtaining a complete blood count with differential to assess eosinophil count in all international adoptees and immigrants from areas where parasitic infections are common. If eosinophilia is present, antibody testing for schistosomiasis and strongyloidiasis—two chronic parasitic infections with potentially serious consequences—should be performed, and appropriate therapy should be administered if infection is discovered. For key features of common intestinal parasitic infections, see the Current Diagnosis box.

Diagnosis of intestinal parasites has improved recently with the advent of quick, simple, and accurate stool antigen tests for some major pathogens, such as *Entamoeba, Giardia* and *Cryptosporidium* species. However, the fecal examination for ova and parasites is still the mainstay of diagnosis in many cases. Whenever possible, stool specimens should be sent to a laboratory with clinical expertise in parasitology, where wet preparation, concentration, or staining can identify most pathogens. Evaluation of fresh specimens and repeated examinations improve diagnostic sensitivity. Key diagnostic points are summarized in the Current Diagnosis box.

This review focuses on basic understanding, recognition, diagnosis and treatment of common intestinal parasites in the United States and throughout the world. Within each section, parasites are listed in order of relative clinical significance.

Protozoa: Amoebae, Flagellates, Ciliates

ENTAMOEBA HISTOLYTICA

Entamoeba histolytica, the cause of amoebic dysentery and amebic liver abscess, is a worldwide pathogen of major clinical significance. Approximately 10% of the world's population and up to 60% of children in highly endemic areas show serologic evidence of infection, and *E. histolytica* is estimated to cause 100,000 deaths per year globally. In the United States, infection is almost exclusively found among returned travelers, immigrants from endemic areas (especially Mexico and Central and South America), men who have sex with men (MSM), and institutionalized persons. *E. histolytica* exists in only two forms, the hardy cyst characterized by four nuclei, and the trophozoite, which has a single nucleus and survives poorly outside the human body. It is important to note that *Entamoeba dispar* and *Entamoeba moshkovskii*, which are morphologically identical to *E. histolytica* in stool microscopy, are now known to be non-pathogenic species. Other *Entamoeba*, including *Entamoeba hartmanni, Entamoeba coli, Entamoeba polecki* and others can be individually identified on microscopy but are of uncertain pathogenicity and thought to be benign.

E. histolytica infection is acquired by ingestion of cysts in contaminated water or food or by fecal–oral contact, as can occur in chronic care facilities or with anal–oral sexual practices. Acquisition of the parasite can result in asymptomatic infection (most common), diarrheal illness, or extraintestinal infection, the latter most commonly manifest as amebic liver abscess. An appropriately robust layer of colonic mucin may be protective against symptomatic infection, whereas attachment to intestinal epithelium results in penetration of the organism into the submucosal layer, where extensive tissue destruction can take place in the form of apoptosis and lysis of cells, hence the name "histolytica."

Symptoms of classic amebic dysentery begin insidiously 1 to 2 weeks after infection. Diarrhea is almost universal and typically consists of numerous small-volume stools that can contain mucous or frank blood, or both. Stools are almost always heme positive if not grossly bloody. Abdominal pain and tenesmus are common; fever is present in approximately 30% of cases. Some persons have a chronic course characterized by weight loss, intermittent loose stools, and abdominal pain. Rare presentations of amebic dysentery include amebomas, which can mimic malignancy, and perianal ulcerations or fistulae. Severe disease can occur in the form of fulminant colitis or toxic megacolon; the latter almost universally requires colectomy. Young age, pregnancy, and corticosteroid use predispose to severe infection. Although persons with HIV infection or AIDS can develop invasive disease, *E. histolytica* does not appear to be a common opportunistic infection, and infection is curable in this population.

Amebic liver abscess is the most common extraintestinal complication of *E. histolytica*; cerebral and ocular amebiasis have also been reported. Amebic liver abscess affects children of both sexes equally, but it is up to nine times more common in men, indicating that hormonal milieu likely plays a role. Amebic liver abscess almost always manifests within 3 to 5 months of initial infection, but it can surface years later. Illness is characterized by fever and abdominal tenderness that worsen over several days to weeks. Weight loss, jaundice, and cough from diaphragmatic irritation can also occur. Symptoms of dysentery usually are not present, and diarrhea is reported in less than one third of cases. Laboratory abnormalities include leukocytosis, transaminitis, elevated alkaline phosphatase, and elevated sedimentation rate. Chest radiograph often demonstrates elevation of the right hemidiaphragm, and pleural effusion may be present. Rupture of the abscess can occur into the abdomen or pleuropulmonary space, manifesting as acute abdmen or empyema.

Diagnosis of intraintestinal *E. histolytica* infection has classically relied on stool microscopy, and this remains the only available method in much of the world. At least three stool specimens should be examined to improve sensitivity. Cysts visualized in stool might or might not indicate active infection and cannot be distinguished from *E. dispar* and *E. moshkovskii*. Presence of trophozoites with ingested red blood cells on stool preparation is diagnostic of dysentery secondary to *E. histolytica*, as are mobile amebae if seen within freshly examined biopsy material.

Diagnosis of *E. histolytica* infection has improved greatly with the advent of antigen tests, now available as enzyme-linked immunosorbent assays (ELISAs) and immunoflorescent probes. The Techlab ELISA antigen test is highly sensitive and specific and can be used on a freshly passed stool specimen, serum, or hepatic abscess material. It becomes positive with onset of symptomatic disease and resolves on treatment of infection. Other available antigen tests appear to function well but have not been as rigorously studied. Aspirate of liver abscess material may be necessary to distinguish from pyogenic liver abscess; a negative stool examination for *E. histolytica* does not preclude amebic liver abscess. In a patient at high risk for amebic liver abscess (e.g., young male immigrants), a trial of antimicrobial therapy can help in diagnosis because infection typically responds rapidly.

 CURRENT DIAGNOSIS

Signs and Symptoms

- Watery diarrhea: Most protozoal infections, e.g., *Giardia, Blastocystis, Dientamoeba, Cryptosporidium, Cyclospora, Isospora, Microsporidia*
- Dysentery: Most commonly *Entamoeba histolytica*; less commonly, *Balantidium coli, Trichuris trichuria* (whipworm)
- Eosinophilia: Throughout chronic infection, *Strongyloides*, schistosomiasis, *Isospora*; usually only in early infection, *Ascaris*, hookworm, whipworm
- Prolonged or severe diarrhea in HIV infection sporeforming protozoal infections: *Cryptosporidium, Cyclospora, Isospora, Microsporidia*
- Visible worms passed in stool: *Ascaris*, Taeniasis, *Diphyllobothrium*

Diagnosis of Parasitic Infections

- Stool antigen assay: *Entamoeba histolytica, Giardia, Cryptosporidium*
- Serology:* *Strongyloides*, schistosomiasis
- Stool for ova and parasites: All intestinal parasites. Sensitivity increased with repeat exams if necessary. Concentration, preservation, and staining improve diagnosis of certain pathogens.

Note: Key features of intestinal parasitic infection may overlap with other conditions, including non-parasitic infections, and extra-intestinal parasites

*Optimal method of diagnosis in returned travelers and immigrants from endemic to nonendemic areas. Does not distinguish between active and resolved infections.

All patients who have confirmed *E. histolytica* infection and reside in nonendemic areas should be treated regardless of whether they are symptomatic, because invasive disease can develop in the future. Asymptomatic cyst passers may be treated with an intralumnal agent alone, such as paromomycin (Humatin) or iodoquinol (Yodoxin). In the United States, the most readily available effective treatment for patients with amebic colitis or liver abscess is metronidazole (Flagyl). It can be given intravenously for patients unable to tolerate oral medications. Experts recommend that a course of therapy with an intraluminal agent be given following the completed course of the systemic agent for all cases of invasive *E. histolytica*. See Table 1 for medications and doses.

GIARDIASIS

Giardia lamblia, also known as *Giardia intestinalis* or *Giardia duodenalis*, is the most commonly identified diarrheal parasitic infection in the United States, with an estimated 100,000 to 2.5 million cases per year. It is globally distributed and found in fresh water throughout mountainous regions of the United States and Canada. The organism is a flagellated aerotolerant anaerobe that exists in a cyst and trophozoite form. Cysts can survive for several weeks in cold water. Contaminated food and water are the most common sources of infection, but the organism can also be passed by person-to-person contact. In the United States, giardiasis is primarily diagnosed among international travelers, persons with recreational water exposure, institutionalized persons and children in day care, and persons with anal–oral sexual practices.

Illness can result from ingestion of as few as 10 to 25 cysts, which transform into trophozoites in the small intestine and attach to and damage the small bowel wall. Symptomatic disease begins insidiously over approximately 2 weeks in 25% to 50% of persons who ingest *Giardia* cysts. Others become asymptomatic cyst passers (5%-15%) or have no signs of infection (35%-50%). Hallmarks of infection are watery diarrhea, bloating, gas, abdominal pain, and weight loss; less commonly, patients have nausea, vomiting, or low-grade fever. Steatorrhea and malabsorption, particularly secondary to *Giardia*-induced lactase deficiency, can be observed. Chronic *Giardia* infection should be considered in the differential diagnosis for a long-standing diarrheal illness, especially if there is history of exposure to possibly contaminated water. Patients with common variable immune deficiency, X-linked agammglobulinemia, and IgA deficiency syndromes are at risk for fulminant and sometimes incurable disease, suggesting a significant role for humoral immunity in control of infection. Persons with HIV infection or AIDS have symptoms similar to those in patients without HIV and typically can be cured of infection with standard therapy.

Diagnosis of giardiasis is made by examination of fresh or preserved stool or by stool antigen assays. In the case of fecal examination, trophozoites may be directly visualized in fresh liquid stool; semiformed and preserved stool should be stained before examination. Currently, there are immunochromographic, direct fluorescence antibody, and ELISA tests for diagnosis of *Giardia*, including the ImmunoCard STAT! Cryptosporidium/Giardia Rapid Assay (Meridian Bioscience, Cincinnati, Ohio), which tests for both pathogens simultaneously. Although it is rarely necessary, the diagnosis can sometimes be made on duodenal biopsy.

For details of treatment options, see Table 1. Metronidazole is the most commonly prescribed treatment in the United States and should be given for a 10-day course. Tinidazole (Tindamax), recently approved in the United States, appears to have excellent efficacy and improved tolerability over metronidazole. Nitazoxanide (Alinia) has also been shown to eradicate infection well and can be used as an alternative or in patients who fail a first course of treatment. Patients who fail first-line therapy might have a persistent source of infection (contaminated water source, close contact with an infected person), immune deficiency predisposing to difficult eradication, or persistence of cysts. Once possible sources of reinfection have been investigated and eliminated, relapsed infections should either be re-treated with a longer course of therapy (21-28 days) or

TABLE 1 Pharmacologic Treatment of Major Protozoan Infections

Clinical Situation	Drug	Adult Dose	Pediatric Dose	Comments
Amebiasis *Entamoeba histolytica*				
Asymptomatic	Recommended: Paromomycin (Humatin) or	25-35 mg/kg/d in 3 doses × 7 d	25-35 mg/kg/d in 3 doses × 7 d	
	Iodoquinol (Yodoxin)	650 mg tid × 20 d	30-40 mg/kg/d (max 2g) in 3 doses × 20 d	
	Alternative: Diloxanide furoate (Furamide)[2,*]	500 mg tid × 10 d	20 mg/kg/d in 3 doses × 10 d	
Mild to moderate intestinal disease	Recommended: Metronidazole (Flagyl) or	500-750 mg tid × 7-10 d	35-50 mg/kg/d in 3 doses × 7-10 d	Treatment should be followed by a course of iodoquinol or paromomycin in the dosage used to treat asymptomatic amebiasis
	Tinidazole (Tindamax)	2 g once daily × 3 d	50 mg/kg once daily (max 2 g) × 3 d	
Severe intestinal or extraintestinal disease*	Metronidazole or	750 mg tid × 7-10 d	35-50 mg/kg/d in 3 doses × 7-10 d	
	Tinidazole	2 g once daily × 5 d	50 mg/kg once daily (max 2 g) × 5 d	A nitroimidazole similar to metronidazole, tinidazole is FDA approved and appears to be as effective and better tolerated than metronidazole. It should be taken with food to minimize GI adverse effects. For children and patients unable to take tablets, a pharmacist may crush the tablets and mix them with cherry syrup. The syrup suspension is good for 7 d at room temperature and must be shaken before use. Ornidazole, a similar drug, is also used outside the United States.
Balantidiasis *Balantidium coli*				
Symptomatic and asymptomatic disease	Recommended: Tetracycline[1,†]	500 mg qid × 10 d	40 mg/kg/d (max 2 g) in 4 doses × 10 d[5]	Contraindicated in pregnant and breastfeeding women and children <8 y
	Alternatives: Metronidazole[1] or	750 mg PO tid × 5 d	35-50 mg/kg/d in 3 doses × 5 d	
	Iodoquinol[1]	650 mg tid × 20d	40 mg/kg/d in 3 doses × 20 d	
Blastocystis hominis Symptomatic disease only				Organism's pathogenicity is uncertain.[‡]
Cryptosporidiosis *Cryptosporidium parvum*				
Immune competent	Nitazoxanide	500 mg bid × 3 d	1-3 y: 100 mg bid × 3 d 4-11 y: 200 mg bid × 3 d	FDA approved as a pediatric oral suspension for treating Cryptosporidium in immunocompetent children <12 y and for *Giardia*. It might also be effective for mild to moderate amebiasis. Nitazoxanide is available in 500-mg tabs and an oral suspension; it should be taken with food.
HIV-infected	No optimal therapy available[§]			All HIV-infected patients with cryptosporidiosis should receive HAART whenever possible. Limited data suggest nitazoxanide might have some benefit in patients with CD4 counts >50. Recent meta-analysis showed no efficacy over placebo for any antiparasitic therapy for cryptosporidiosis.

[1] Not FDA approved for this indication.
[2] Not available in the United States.
[5] Investigational drug in the United States.
*The drug is not available commercially, but as a service it can be compounded by Panorama Compounding Pharmacy, 6744 Balboa Blvd., Van Nuys, CA 91406 (800-247-9767) or Medical Center Pharmacy, New Haven, CT (203-688-6816).
[†] An approved drug, but considered investigational for this condition by the FDA.
[‡] Clinical significance of these organisms is controversial; metronidazole 750 mg tid × 10 d, iodoquinol 650 mg tid × 20 d, or TMP-SMX[11] double-strength tab bid × 7 d are effective. Metronidazole resistance may be common. Nitazoxanide is effective in children.

TABLE 1 Pharmacologic Treatment of Major Protozoan Infections—cont'd

Clinical Situation	Drug	Adult Dose	Pediatric Dose	Comments
Cyclosporiasis Cyclospora cayetanensis	Recommended: TMP-SMX (Bactrim, Septra)[1]	160 mg TMP, 800 mg SMX (1 DS tab) bid × 7-10 d	5 mg/kg TMP, 25 mg/kg SMX bid × 7-10 d	In immunocompetent patients, usually a self-limited illness. Immunosuppressed patients might need higher doses, longer duration (TMP-SMX qid × 10 d, followed by bid × 3 wk) and long-term maintenance. For isosporiasis in sulfonamide-sensitive patients, pyrimethamine, 50-75 mg qd in divided doses (*plus* leucovorin 10-25 mg/d) is effective.
	Alternative: Ciprofloxacin[1]	500 mg bid × 7-10 d		Quinolones currently not approved for use in children <18 y
Dientamoebiasis Dientamoeba fragilis Symptomatic disease only	Iodoquinol[1] *or*	650 mg tid × 20 d	30-40 mg/kg/d (max 2g) in 3 doses × 20 d	
	Paromomycin[1] *or*	25-35 mg/kg/d in 3 doses × 7 d	25-35 mg/kg/d in 3 doses × 7 d	
	Tetracycline[1] *or*	500 mg qid × 7-10 d	40 mg/kg/d (max 2g) in 4 doses × 10 d[5]	
	Metronidazole	500-750 mg tid × 10 d	20-40 mg/kg/d in 3 doses × 10 d	
Giardiasis Giardia lamblia All symptomatic disease and asymptomatic carriage in nonendemic areas	Recommended: Metronidazole[1] *or*	250 mg tid × 5 d	15 mg/kg/d in 3 doses × 5 d	
	Nitazoxanide[†] *or*	500 mg bid × 3 d	1-3 y: 100 mg bid × 3 d 4-11 y: 200 mg bid × 3 d	
	Tinidazole	2g once	50 mg/kg (max 2g) once	Treatment should be followed by a course of iodoquinol or paromomycin in the dosage used to treat asymptomatic amebiasis. Albendazole, 400 mg daily × 5 d alone or in combination with metronidazole may also be effective. Combination treatment with standard doses of metronidazole and quinacrine for 3 wk is effective for a small number of refractory infections. In one study, nitazoxanide was used successfully in high doses to treat a case of *Giardia* resistant to metronidazole and albendazole.
	Alternatives: Quinacrine[1,2] *or*	100 mg tid × 5 d	2 mg/kg/d (max 300 mg/d) tid × 5 d	
	Furazolidone (Furoxone) *or*	100 mg qid × 7-10 d	6 mg/kg/d in 4 doses × 10 d	
	Paromomycin[1] *or*	25-35 mg/kg/d in 3 doses × 7 d	25-35 mg/kg/d in 3 doses × 7 d	Nonabsorbed luminal agent; may be useful for treating giardiasis in pregnancy
	Albendazole (Albenza)[1]	400 mg daily × 5 d		
Isosporiasis Isospora belli[‡]	Recommended: TMP-SMX[1]	160 mg TMP, 800 mg SMX bid × 7-10 d	5 mg/kg TMP, 25 mg/kg SMX bid × 7-10 d	
	Alternatives: Ciprofloxacin[1]	500 mg bid × 7-10 d		
Microsporidiosis *Enterocytozoon bineusi* Diarrheal or disseminated disease	Fumagillin[2]	60 mg/d PO × 14 d		Oral fumagillin (Sanofi Recherche, Gentilly, France) is effective in treating *E. bieneusi* but is associated with thrombocytopenia. HAART can lead to microbiological and clinical response in HIV-infected patients with microsporidial diarrhea. Octreotide (Sandostatin) has provided symptomatic relief in some patients with large-volume diarrhea.
Encephalocytozoon intestinalis Diarrheal or disseminated disease	Albendazole	400 mg bid × 21 d		

DS = double strength; GI = gastrointestinal; HAART = highly active antiretroviral therapy; max = maximum; tab = tablet; TMP-SMX = trimethoprim-sulfamethoxazole.
Adapted from Drugs for parasitic infections. Med Lett Drug Ther, August 2004

treated with a different agent. Patients who fail more than one course of therapy should undergo immunologic work-up.

Prevention of *Giardia* infection, as with other parasitic infections, involves primarily close attention to personal hygiene, hand washing, and avoidance of ingestion of fresh unfiltered water. Boiling water or use of a 0.2- to 1-μm water filter offer optimal protection against *Giardia* and other parasitic pathogens, although such filters still might not protect against *Cryptosporidium*.

BLASTOCYSTIS HOMINIS

Blastocystis hominis is a protozoan with worldwide distribution found most commonly in tropical regions; it is present in humans and several other animals. In temperate regions, *B. hominis* is detected at a high rate among men who have sex with men. *B. hominis* was long thought to cause only asymptomatic colonization, but there is some evidence to suggest a role in human disease, although this remains controversial. Ongoing molecular analysis might elucidate subtypes of *B. hominis* with varying degrees of pathogenicity in humans.

B. hominis has four forms: vacuolated, ameba-like, granular, and cyst, the latter of which is likely to be the infectious form. It appears to be transmitted via the fecal–oral route, possibly from waterborne sources.

As suggested previously, the majority of infections appear to be entirely asymptomatic, and number of organisms does not appear to accurately predict severity of illness. Symptoms consist mainly of watery diarrhea, bloating, and abdominal cramps. There are typically no pathologic findings on colonoscopy and there are no reports of invasive disease. Infection is diagnosed by stool microscopy with use of a trichrome or hematoxylin-stained preserved specimen. The organism is susceptible in vitro to numerous antimicrobials. Bactrim[1] or metronidazole is the treatment of choice; details are listed in Table 1.

DIENTAMOEBA FRAGILIS

Dientamoeba fragilis was originally classified as an amoeba, but it is more closely related to the flagellates such as *Trichomonas vaginalis*. It is distributed worldwide, including in Western nations, and has only recently been recognized as a clinically significant pathogen, possibly because it is difficult to visualize without specific staining techniques. Illness has commonly been found in travelers and MSM, but it can affect anyone.

The parasite exists only in the trophozoite form. Despite its genetic relationship to the flagellates, *D. fragilis* does not have a flagellum and is immotile. Trophozoites range in size from 4 to 20 μm and are binucleate. Patients in the United States who have *D. fragilis* were found in some studies to harbor other intestinal parasites as well, such as *E. vermicularis* and *B. hominis*, and in general *D. fragilis* is more prevalent in areas of the world with limited public sanitation. These features support a fecal–oral mode of transmission for *D. fragilis*.

Most patients are asymptomatic; however, numerous case reports and small series describe patients with no other organisms identified to cause their symptoms who improve significantly after treatment and documented clearance of *D. fragilis* from their stool. Illness is typically subacute to chronic, characterized by abdominal pain, watery diarrhea, anorexia, fatigue, and malaise. Diagnosis can be difficult, because the parasite is fastidious. If *D. fragilis* is suspected, stool should be preserved with polyvinyl alcohol and quickly stained with iron–hematoxylin and trichrome. Polymerase chain reaction (PCR) has been used for diagnosis as well, but it is not readily available for use in most clinical settings.

For full treatment information, see Table 1. Iodoquinol (Yodoxin) and metronidazole have both been used successfully to treat *D. fragilis*.

BALANTIDIUM COLI

Balantidium coli is the largest protozoan that infects humans, and the only ciliate. Balantidiasis is a relatively rare cause of illness and is found primarily in rural agrarian communities in Southeast Asia, Central and South America, and Papua New Guinea. *B. coli* is highly associated with animal farming, in particular, pigs; humans are incidental hosts. The parasite is transmitted by direct contact with animals or on ingestion of water or food contaminated by animal excrement. Persons with malnutrition or immune deficiency are particularly susceptible to infection.

B. coli invades the intestinal mucosa from the terminal ileum to the rectum. About one half of infections are asymptomatic; the other one half result in a subacute or chronic diarrheal illness with abdominal cramping, nausea, vomiting, weight loss, and occasional low-grade fever. Fewer than 5% of patients present with severe or even fulminant dysentery, and rare cases of colonic penetration with peritonitis, mesenteric lymphadenitis, or hepatic infection have been reported.

Diagnosis is made by visualization of trophozoites in fresh stool specimens or preserved and permanently stained samples. The trophozoite is large and ciliated; cysts are difficult to distinguish. It displays a distinct spiraling motility that can be seen under low power. On stained sample, visualization of *B. coli*'s characteristic macronucleus and spiral micronucleus can help confirm the diagnosis. All patients should be treated regardless of symptoms. Tetracycline (Sumycin) is the therapy of choice; the infection also responds to metronidazole[1]; see Table 1 for dosing information.

Spore-Forming Protozoa and Microsporidia

CRYPTOSPORIDIOSIS

Cryptosporidium is a pathogen with worldwide distribution that is endemic to the United States. Humans are most commonly infected by the recently reclassified *Cryptosporidium hominis*, but *Cryptosporidium parvum*, primarily a bovine pathogen, also causes human disease. *Cryptosporidium* has caused multiple waterborne outbreaks in the United States and can be acquired secondary to recreational water exposure (e.g., swimming pools, water parks). The best-known outbreak occurred secondary to heavy rains that brought farm runoff into the drinking water supply in Wisconsin in 1984. It resulted in 430,000 documented cases of cryptosporidiosis and contributed to the deaths of dozens of persons with advanced HIV infection or malignancy.

Cryptosporidium is a coccidian, part of a group of spore-forming protozoa with a complex life cycle and a structure that allows mechanical penetration into host cells. *Cryptosporidium* can mature and reproduce entirely within human hosts, thereby enabling infection to occur both from environmental sources and by direct person-to-person contact. Its oocysts, the source of infection on ingestion, are markedly hardy; they can withstand heavy chlorination, survive for months in cold water, and are small enough to occasionally evade even the smallest available water filtration systems.

All persons are susceptible to infection, which usually is self-limited. Fulminant or chronic infection, or both, can be seen among patients with immune compromise secondary to HIV infection or AIDS (especially those with CD4 < 50), in patients with malignancy, and in malnourished children. As few as 100 oocysts can cause infection, which results when the parasite penetrates small bowel epithelium and replicates just beneath its surface. Villous flattening and small bowel wall edema are seen on pathologic examination from infected persons.

Asymptomatic infections occur but are relatively rare. Symptoms begin within several days to 1 week of ingestion of oocysts. The hallmark of infection is explosive watery diarrhea, which can be so

---

[1]Not FDA approved for this indication.

voluminous as to resemble cholera and can cause significant dehydration and electrolyte imbalance. Abdominal discomfort, nausea, vomiting, fever, malaise, and myalgia can also be present, and weight loss is common. Illness lasts 1 to 2 weeks, but a substantial percentage of patients report a relapse of symptoms after initial improvement. The biliary tract can be involved, particularly in patients with HIV infection, and infection at other distant sites, such as the lungs, has rarely been reported.

Diagnosis of *Cryptosporidium* has improved dramatically in recent years with the advent of antigen tests, which are highly sensitive and specific and can be used on a single sample of fresh stool. The ImmunoCard STAT! Cryptosporidium/Giardia Rapid Assay is useful because it can detect both pathogens. When such tests are not available, stools submitted for examination should be fixed in formalin and stained for trophozoites or cysts; multiple stool specimens improves the diagnostic sensitivity. Luminal fluid or biopsy specimens obtained during endoscopy can also reveal the organism.

Infection with *Cryptosporidium* is typically a self-limited illness in otherwise healthy persons, but symptoms can be improved and the course shortened with the antiparasitic nitazoxanide. *Cryptosporidium* remains an extremely challenging and potentially devastating infection in immunocompromised patients, especially those with HIV and a low CD4 count (counts < 200 increase risk of severe illness, and counts < 50 markedly increase risk). Although anticryptosporidial therapies in this population have shown very limited efficacy, restoration of immune function with HAART often effects cure. Limited data suggest a trial of nitazoxanide may be reasonable in this circumstance as well. Appropriate supportive measures are also crucial in all patients with *Cryptosporidium*, including fluid and electrolyte replacement; avoiding lactose products is likely to be beneficial during the first 2 weeks after infection as the brush border regenerates. Appropriate treatment doses for nitazoxanide are listed in Table 1.

Prevention of *Cryptosporidium* infection requires a highly developed public water purification system including flocculation, sedimentation, and filtration. Use of 0.2- to 1-μm personal water filters for campers and hikers greatly reduces but does not eliminate risk of infection, whereas boiling water before drinking kills oocysts. Close attention to hygiene and avoidance of fecal–oral contact is the mainstay of prevention in the settings of institutional and community outbreaks.

CYCLOSPORA SPECIES

Cyclospora cayetanensis is a coccidian with structure similar to that of *Cryptosporidium*. Unlike *Cryptosporidium*, *C. cayetanensis* requires a period of development outside the human body, thereby eliminating the possibility of close person-to-person contact as a means of acquiring the infection. *C. cayetanensis* is distributed worldwide, most commonly in the tropics and subtropics where infection tends to exhibit seasonality. It has also been associated with food (e.g., raspberries) and waterborne outbreaks in temperate regions, including the United States, and in recent years it has become increasingly recognized as a cause of infectious diarrhea in returned travelers.

All persons are susceptible to infection, but those with HIV are at risk for more severe and prolonged disease, as seen with cryptosporidiosis and isosporiasis. Symptomatic disease appears to be most common in adults who do not have previous exposure to *Cyclospora*, such as travelers or persons who have relocated to endemic areas. Illness begins about a week after ingestion of sporulated oocysts and is characterized by watery diarrhea, abdominal cramping, bloating, anorexia, and weight loss. Low-grade fever can occur; marked fatigue is common and can last weeks or even months, and untreated infections can relapse after apparent resolution. Biliary involvement can occur in patients with HIV coinfection, as with cryptosporidiosis. Cyclosporiasis, similar to infection with other coccidians, causes damage to the small bowel epithelium, with resultant crypt flattening, edema, and inflammatory infiltrate. Lactose deficiency can remain for months following initial infection.

Diagnosis is made by stool examination. As with diagnosis of other parasitic infections, multiple stool specimens improve sensitivity. In the case of *Cyclospora*, concentration of the stool specimen also increases yield. If cyclosporiasis is suspected, specific testing should be requested, because the organism exhibits unique properties. Organisms are about two times the size of *Cryptosporidium* and can be seen with Kinyoun acid-fast stain. They also autofluoresce and can be visualized under ultraviolet microscopy. Currently there is no stool antigen assay, but PCR testing has been used in experimental and limited clinical settings to assist in diagnosis.

Cyclosporiasis is best treated with trimethoprim-sulfamethoxazole (Bactrim)[1]; ciprofloxacin[1] may be effective for patients who have a sulfa allergy. Patients with HIV infection can require longer courses of treatment or chronic suppressive therapy; appropriate antiretroviral therapy is also important in the treatment of severe or relapsing infections. See Table 1 for details.

ISOSPORA SPECIES

Isospora belli is a large coccidian native to tropical areas. Similar to *Cyclospora*, it requires a period of maturation outside the human body and therefore cannot be spread directly from person to person. It appears to cause largely asymptomatic or mild infection in tropical areas to which it is endemic; the exception is among patients coinfected with HIV and particularly those with AIDS, in which it is a very common cause of chronic diarrhea in the Caribbean and Central America. Currently in wealthy countries it is found primarily in travelers returning from endemic areas.

Illness is typically mild and self-limited, consisting primarily of watery diarrhea. However, some immunocompetent persons can develop a chronic spruelike syndrome with malabsorption, and those with HIV infection or AIDS often have severe and prolonged diarrhea. *Isospora* can invade to the lamina propria and can cause eosinophilia, which is different from other coccidian infections.

Diagnosis is made by observation of cysts in stool. As with *Cyclospora*, they can be visualized with acid-fast stains or ultraviolet microscopy. Stool may also contain Charcot–Leiden crystals. Infection in immunocompetent hosts responds well to antimicrobials; persons coinfected with HIV can require longer courses of therapy or chronic suppression, and appropriate antiretroviral therapy may be helpful as well. Trimethoprim-sulfamethoxazole[1] is the treatment of choice. Ciprofloxacin (Cipro)[1] or pyrimethamine (Daraprim)[1] may be used in cases of sulfa allergy. Doses are listed Table 1.

MICROSPORIDIOSIS

Microsporidia are eukaryotic organisms that have been recently reclassified as fungi based on molecular genotyping. They are distributed globally, and more than 100 genera have been identified, seven of which contain species known to be pathogenic in humans: *Encephalitozoon*, *Enterocytozoon*, *Trachipleistophora*, *Pleistophora*, *Nosema*, *Vittaforma*, and *Microsporidium*. These pathogens cause a wide variety of systemic and focal illness throughout the world.

Many immunocompetent patients in wealthy nations exhibit positive serology for certain types of microsporidial infections without a history of disease or travel. Microsporidia are most commonly associated with systemic infection in immunosuppressed persons, particularly those with HIV and a CD4 count of less than 100 or patients with organ transplants. Mode of transmission is not entirely clear, but the pathogen likely is spread both from water sources and possibly from close household contact.

Encephalitozoon intestinalis and *Enterocytozoon bieneusi* are responsible for intestinal microsporidial infections. *E. bieneusi* has been associated with self-limited diarrheal illness; *E. intestinalis* is commonly found in stool specimens throughout the developing world, but its pathogenicity is often not certain. Symptomatic infections, most often in patients coinfected with HIV, typically include a

---

[1]Not FDA approved for this indication.

gradual onset of watery diarrhea, which may be worse in the morning and after oral intake. Significant volume and electrolyte depletion can occur, as well as fatigue, anorexia, weight loss, and malabsorption. *E. intestinalis* can disseminate and cause acute abdomen with peritonitis, cholangitis, nephritis, and keratoconjunctivitis, and *E. bieneusi* infection can result in cholangitis and nephritis as well as rhinitis, bronchitis, and wheezing. Other microsporidia are implicated in a wide variety of illness both in previously healthy and immunosuppressed hosts and include several ocular pathogens.

Diagnosis of microsporidiosis is attained by visualization of spores in stool or in tissue specimens. As suggested by their name, microsporidial spores are much smaller than those produced by spore-forming protozoal infections; most are approximately 1 μm in length and can easily be confused with bacteria or debris on slides. Special staining techniques have been described, but electron microscopy is required for species identification. See Table 1 for details of treatment. Albendazole (Albenza)[1] is the treatment of choice for *Encephalocytozoon intestinalis*.

Treatment of *Enterocytozoon bieneusi* is more challenging. Although some response to albendazole has been reported, oral fumagillin[2] may have more efficacy. Unfortunately, it is not currently commercially available in the United States. Use of appropriate antiretroviral therapy is perhaps the most important treatment for patients with HIV infection or AIDS and chronic microsporidial infections.

Helminths

NEMATODES

Nematodes (roundworms) are cylindrical nonsegmented organisms that are found throughout the world both as free-living species and as human and animal pathogens. Nematodes are the most common type of human parasitic infestation, found in approximately one quarter of the world's population; often susceptible hosts carry multiple different pathogenic nematodes. There are at least 60 species that have been shown to infect humans and 10 times that many that cause disease in other animals, but a few pathogens account for the bulk of human infections, in particular *Ascaris*, hookworm, and whipworm. These three organisms all require a period of maturation outside the human body—typically in warm, moist soil—underscoring the fact that repeated contact with fecally contaminated soil or food and water is necessary to sustain the cycle of infestation. *Strongyloides* and *Enterobius* are unique in that they can both complete their life cycle on or within human hosts and therefore can cause chronic infection and be transmitted directly by close person-to-person contact where there is the possibility of fecal–oral contamination.

Ascaris

Ascaris lumbricoides, the most common human helminthic infection, is estimated to affect 20% to 25% of the world's population. Up to 80% of community members are infected in heavily endemic areas, namely in Africa, Asia, and Central and South America. Cases of *Ascaris* infestation are also seen in rural areas in the southeastern United States. *A. lumbricoides* are white to pinkish worms that range from 10 to 40 cm in length; the infectious eggs are oval white bodies with an adherent mucopolysaccharide capsule that clings to multiple surfaces and aids in transmissibility of the parasite. Eggs are also remarkably durable, capable of surviving up to 6 years in moist soil and able to weather brief droughts and periods of freezing.

Fecal contamination of water, food, and environmental surfaces such as doorknobs and countertops provide the means of transmission for *Ascaris*, and recurrent infection occurs as long as living conditions that predispose people to infection remain unchanged. Lack of adequate public sanitation, use of human feces as fertilizer (night soil), and frequent contact with soil or shared contaminated surfaces among close household members are risk factors for infection. Persons who move to environments with improved sanitation typically lose their infection within 2 years as all the adult worms die. Eggs excreted by an infected person must mature outside the human body for approximately 2 weeks. On ingestion by a susceptible host, mature eggs hatch in the small intestine and release larvae, which penetrate the intestinal wall and travel through the venous circulation to the lungs, where they are coughed up and swallowed. They then undergo maturation into adult worms in the intestine and produce eggs by 2 to 3 months after initial infection, which are excreted in the feces and mature outside the body to continue the cycle.

Most persons with *Ascaris* infection are asymptomatic. Approximately 15% of people have morbidity as a result of infection, which is associated with young age, large burden of worms, coinfection with other intestinal parasites, and genetic predisposition. In children, infection contributes to malabsorption of protein, fat, and vitamins A and C, and treatment of heavily infected children can improve their nutritional status. *Ascaris* infection can also cause intestinal, pancreatic, or biliary obstruction as a result of worm mass or worm migration. Despite the low incidence of obstructive complications per infected person, the *Ascaris*-related acute abdomen is a significant problem on a global level given the enormous number of people infected. Some patients with intestinal *Ascaris* infection report vague abdominal complaints, such as abdominal discomfort, nausea, vomiting or diarrhea, but these are relatively rare. Pulmonary migration of a large quantity of worms can produce Loeffler's syndrome, or eosinophilic pneumonitis.

Diagnosis is easily attained with standard saline stool preparation, and large numbers of eggs are typically seen. Larvae or worms can also sometimes be seen in sputum or stool samples. In cases of intestinal obstruction, worms may be visualized on upper gastrointestinal series, computed tomography, and even ultrasound. Eosinophilia with *Ascaris* infection is found only during the larval migratory phase, but not at all times. Chronic eosinophilia in an at-risk person suggests another parasitic infection, often *Strongyloides*.

All persons documented to carry *Ascaris* who have migrated to nonendemic areas should be treated to prevent complications in the future; in endemic areas, adults need only be treated if they are symptomatic. Children have been shown to benefit from intermittent anthelminthic therapy in heavily affected areas of the world.

For patients with intestinal obstruction, bowel rest and intravenous hydration are usually sufficient to relieve the obstruction, at which time anthelminthic therapy can be administered. In such cases, gastroenterology consultation should be obtained. In rare cases, surgical intervention is required. Treatment of pulmonary infection is controversial; however, most experts recommend steroid therapy for severe infections followed 2 to 3 weeks later (at the time full-grown worms will have migrated to the intestine) by administration of anthelminthic therapy.

The benzimadazoles (mebendazole [Vermox], albendazole,[1] levamisole,[2] and pyrantel [Pin-X]) all exhibit excellent activity against *Ascaris*. Doses and other options are listed in Table 2. Although albendazole and mebendazole carry a pregnancy class B label, they have been used in pregnant women, adolescent girls, and women of reproductive age without demonstrable effects on fetuses; most experts recommend holding treatment until the second trimester whenever possible.

Sanitary conditions that allow for proper management of human feces are crucial in control and prevention of *Ascaris* infection; boiling water kills the eggs.

Whipworm (Trichuriasis)

Trichuris trichuria has become recognized in recent years as a worldwide pathogen with a scope similar to that of *Ascaris*. Sanitary conditions that predispose to ingestion of food and water contaminated with human feces place people at risk for infection; in many

---

[1]Not FDA approved for this indication.
[2]Not available in the United States.

TABLE 2 Pharmacologic Treatment of Nematode, Trematode, and Cestode Infections

Clinical Situation	Drug	Adult Dose	Pediatric Dose	Comments
Anisakiasis *Anisaka* spp. or *Pseudoterranova decipiens*	No recommended medical therapy. Surgical or endoscopic removal of worm	—	—	Successful treatment of a patient with Anisakiasis with albendazole has been reported
Ascariasis *Ascaris lumbricoides*	Albendazole (Albenza)[1,†] or Mebendazole* (Vermox) or Ivermectin[1] (Stromectol)	400 mg once 100 mg bid × 3 d 150-200 μg/kg once	??? 100 mg bid × 3 d 150-200 μg/kg once	In heavy infection, therapy may be given for 3 d
Enterobiasis (Pinworm) *Enterobius vermicularis*	Pyrantel pamoate or	11 mg/kg base (max 1g) once; repeat in 2 wk	11 mg/kg base (max 1g) once; repeat in 2 wk	Because all family members are usually infected, treatment of the entire household is recommended.
	Mebendazole* or	100 mg once, repeat in 2 wk	100 mg once, repeat in 2 wk	
	Albendazole[1,]*	400 mg once, repeat in 2 wk	400 mg once, repeat in 2 wk	
Hookworm *Ancylostoma duodenale, Necator americanus*	Albendazole* or Mebendazole or Pyrantel pamoate*	400 mg once 100 mg bid × 3 d or 500 mg once 11 mg/kg (max 1g) × 3 d	400 mg once 100 mg bid × 3 d or 500 mg once 11 mg/kg (max 1g) × 3 d	
Schistosomiasis *Schistosoma haematobium, Schistosoma mansoni*	Praziquantel or	40 mg/kg/d in 2 doses × 1 d	40 mg/kg/d in 2 doses × 1 d	
S. mansoni only	Oxamniquine[2]	15 mg/kg once	20 mg/kg/d in 2 doses × 1d	Effective in some patients in whom praziquantel is less effective Contraindicated in pregnancy
Schistosoma japonicum, Schistosoma mekongi	Praziquantel	60 mg/kg/d in 3 doses × 1 d	60 mg/kg/d in 3 doses × 1 d	
Strongyloidiasis	Recommended: Ivermectin	200 μg/kg/d × 2 d or × 1 d with repeat dose in 2 wk	200 μg/kg/d × 2 d or × 1 d with repeat dose in 2 wk	In immunocompromised patients or in patients with disseminated disease, it may be necessary to prolong or repeat therapy or use other agents Veterinary parenteral and enema formulations of ivermectin are used in severely ill patients unable to take oral medications
	Alternatives: Albendazole* or	400 mg bid × 7 d	400 mg bid × 7 d	
	Thiabendazole (Minetezol)	50 mg/kg/d (max 3g/d) in 2 doses × 2 d	50 mg/kg/d (max 3g/d) in 2 doses × 2 d	This is the recommended dose, but it might need to be reduced secondary to side effects
Tapeworm *Taenia solium* (intestinal disease), *Taenia sanguinata, Diphyllobothrium latum*	Praziquantel[1,]* (Biltricide) or Niclosamide[2] (Yomesan)	5-10 mg/kg once 2 g once	5-10 mg/kg once 50 mg/kg once	Available in the United States only from the manufacturer
Trichuriasis (Whipworm) *Trichuris trichuria*	Recommended: Mebendazole Alternatives: Albendazole[1,]* or Ivermectin[1,]*	100 mg bid × 3 d or 500 mg once 400 mg daily × 3 d 200 μg/kg daily × 3 d	100 mg bid × 3 d or 500 mg once 400 mg daily × 3 d 200 μg/kg daily × 3 d	

[1] Not FDA approved for this indication.
[2] Not available in the United States.
*The drug is not available commercially, but as a service it can be compounded by Panorama Compounding Pharmacy, 6744 Balboa Blvd., Van Nuys, CA 91406 (800-247-9767) or Medical Center Pharmacy, New Haven, CT (203-688-6816).
†An approved drug, but considered investigational for this condition by the FDA.
max = maximum.
Adapted from Drugs for parasitic infections. Med Lett Drug Ther, August 2004.

communities infection is hyperendemic, with almost universal carriage of the pathogen.

The adult organism is a small worm about 4 cm in length with a unique whip-like structure that allows its thin tail to become embedded in colonic crypts. Whipworm eggs have a characteristic barrel shape with mucous plugs at either end. Infection is acquired by ingesting *Trichuris* eggs that have undergone embryonation in the soil for 2 to 4 weeks after excretion from a previous host. Larvae emerge from eggs in the intestine and migrate into crypts, where they begin to mature. Egg production begins approximately 3 months later.

Most persons with whipworm carry few worms (approximately 20) and are asymptomatic. As with many other intestinal parasites, children are at greater risk for symptomatic infection, which can cause failure to thrive, anemia, clubbing, inflammatory colitis, and rectal prolapse. Adults with a high worm burden can also experience inflammatory colitis characterized by frequent—often bloody—diarrhea and tenesmus. Infection has been shown to result in production of tumor necrosis factor (TNF)-α by lamina propria cells in the colon, which can contribute to poor appetite and wasting that can be seen with significant infection.

Diagnosis is made by standard stool microscopy without a need to concentrate stool, because large numbers of eggs are excreted. Worms can also be seen on colonoscopy, or they can be visualized grossly in cases of rectal prolapse. Eosinophilia may be seen.

Treatment of symptomatic infections can be accomplished with mebendazole, albendazole,[1] or ivermectin (Stromectal)[1]; see Table 2 for details.

Hookworm (*Necator americanus* and *Ancylostoma duodenale*)

Like other helminthic infections, hookworm affects a substantial portion of the world's population, particularly in rural subtropical and tropical communities where human feces is used as a component of fertilizer. Infection results primarily from parasite penetration into the skin; therefore persons with an agrarian lifestyle and significant soil contact are at greatest risk.

Two species are responsible for the majority of human hookworm: *Necator americanus* and *Ancylostoma duodenale*. *Ancylostoma braziliense*, a canine intestinal pathogen, causes cutaneous larval migrans in humans because the pathogen cannot penetrate the human dermis. Of the two common forms of human hookworm, *N. americanus* is smaller and a less aggressive pathogen with a longer life span than *A. duodenale*. Both parasites are found in warm climates throughout the world; *A. doudenale* exists in smaller pockets, whereas *N. americanus* is widely distributed throughout impoverished rural areas of the tropics in the Americas, Asia, and Africa.

Hookworms are small helminths, between 0.5 and 1 cm in length. Infection results from larval penetration of the skin on contact with contaminated soil. An intensely pruritic, erythematous, papulovesicular rash called *ground itch* can develop at the site of entry. Parasites then enter the venous or lymphatic circulation and travel to the lungs, at which point an urticarial rash with cough can develop. The larvae are swallowed and migrate to the small intestine, where they attach to the bowel wall with teeth or biting plates and take a continuous blood meal by sucking with strong esophageal muscles. As the hookworms lodge in the small intestine, peripheral eosinophilia peaks, and gastrointestinal discomfort with or without diarrhea can result. Large oral ingestion of *A. duodenale* can cause Wakana syndrome, characterized by cough, shortness of breath, nausea, vomiting, and eosinophilia. The most important clinical manifestation of hookworm infection is iron-deficiency anemia, which can be mild or severe and may be accompanied by malabsorption of protein in hosts with heavy burden of disease. Infants and pregnant women can become extremely ill or even die as a result of the anemia.

Hookworm may be difficult to diagnose because light infections often do not produce enough eggs to be readily seen on stool examination; stool should therefore be concentrated if infection is suspected. Eggs do not appear in stool until approximately 2 months after infection, so patients with pulmonary complaints will not yet have a positive stool examination.

Hookworm infection can be eradicated with benzimidazole anthelminthics; see Table 2 for details. Prevention of hookworm infection, as with other parasites, lies in improved sanitary conditions; wearing shoes is especially important because the majority of infections are acquired through the skin. Mass anthelminthic treatment campaigns have shown some efficacy in reducing disease in children; however, reinfection and concern for development of resistance continue to present significant challenges. Candidate vaccines are currently under investigation.

Strongyloides

Strongyloides stercoralis is a global pathogen that is estimated to affect as many as 100 million people, mostly in tropical regions of the world. In recent years, it has become more commonly recognized in the United States among immigrants as a cause of chronic eosinophilia as well as symptomatic infection.

Strongyloides infection results when filariform larvae dwelling in fecally contaminated soil penetrate the skin or mucous membranes of a susceptible host. Larvae move to the lungs and subsequently to the trachea, where they are coughed up and swallowed. Females, about 2 cm in length, lodge in the lamina propria of the duodenum and proximal jejunum where they begin to oviposit. Rhabtidiform larvae emerge from these eggs and either repenetrate the intestinal wall or are passed into the feces, at which point they can begin a free-living cycle and reproduce sexually, or can molt directly into an infectious form ready to enter a subsequent susceptible host.

Persons infected with *Strongyloides* are typically asymptomatic. Those who have symptoms might report abdominal discomfort, diarrhea alternating with constipation, or rarely blood-tinged stool. Severe intestinal infections can occur and are manifest by chronic watery or mucousy diarrhea. In such cases, colonoscopy reveals excessive bowel wall thickening and copious secretions, or edema (catarrhal enteritis or edematous enteritis). Parasite migration through the dermis can manifest as serpiginous, erythematous, and pruritic patches along the buttocks, perineum, and thighs, known as *larvae currens*.

Strongyloides appear to attain a balanced state in their host, with similar numbers of adult worms throughout the many years of infection. During periods of host immunocompromise, in particular in patients taking corticosteroids, *Strongyloides* can enter into a state of rapid autoinfection and rampant reproduction called *hyperinfection syndrome*, which results in devastating illness. Persons with HIV infection do not seem to be at particular risk for symptomatic disease or hyperinfection, but hyperinfection has been linked to HTLV-1 infection. *Strongyloides* has also caused hyperinfection in organ-transplant patients whose donor had been infected asymptomatically with the parasite. Although it has long been thought that steroid-induced immune compromise was the major trigger for hyperinfection, growing evidence suggests that steroids themselves may be the culprit by directly inducing the accelerated life cycle in the parasite.

The hyperinfection syndrome is characterized by systemic illness with fever, cough, hypoxia, patchy or diffuse pulmonary infiltrates with alveolar microhemorrhages, and dermatitis; it can include myocarditis, hepatitis, splenic abscess, meningitis and cerebral abscess, and endocrine organ involvement. Larvae migrating out of the intestines can drag bacteria with them, resulting in gram-negative or polymicrobial sepsis. The prognosis of *Strongyloides* hyperinfection syndrome is grave even with highly effective anthelminthic treatment given the diffuse nature of this disease. However, earlier recognition and intensive supportive care can result in cure.

Diagnosis of uncomplicated *Strongyloides* infection in endemic areas can be challenging because few larvae are passed in stool, and numerous examinations may be necessary to detect them. ELISA is available and is highly sensitive, but it does not distinguish between active and past infections. It is, however, the test of choice for persons who have migrated to nonendemic areas, and all persons in this setting should be treated. Ivermectin is the treatment of choice; see

---

[1] Not FDA approved for this indication.

Table 2 for dosing. During the first days of treatment, patients can experience intense dermal pruritis as parasites die. Eosinophilia and positive ELISA can persist for months even after effective therapy.

Enterobius vermicularis

Human pinworm infection, caused by the thread-like nematode *Enterobius vermicularis*, is found throughout the world and continues to be diagnosed commonly in the United States, especially in children. Its persistence is likely related to the fact that pinworm does not require a period of maturation outside the human body, and autoinfection or transmission by very close contact sustains the parasite within communities. *E. vermicularis* is at maximum 1 cm long with a tapered tail, and dwells in the cecum, appendix, and adjacent colon. At night, female worms travel to the anus and lay small (25-50 μm), double-walled oval eggs in the perianal skin. Within 6 hours, the eggs embryonate within their capsule and are infectious. In scratching the perianal area and subsequently bringing his or her hand to the mouth, the host ingests the embryos, which then hatch in the bowel about 2 months later and continue the cycle of infection. Embryonated eggs can also attach to bedclothes, thereby placing other household members with close contact at risk for infection. In family groups, infection is associated with close living quarters, poor hand washing, and infrequent washing of clothes and sheets. It can also be prevalent in among institutionalized persons.

Infection is often asymptomatic, but it can cause perianal itching, which helps to facilitate persistent infection by encouraging frequent touching of the perianal area. Rarely, worms migrate into ectopic foci and produce painful genitourinary tract disease with granulomatous inflammation; pinworm infection rarely results in pain that mimics acute appendicitis.

Pinworm infestation is best diagnosed by the classic Scotch tape test, which involves placing and immediately removing a piece sticky tape firmly across the perianal area early in the morning when the eggs have been deposited. The tape can then be brought into a physician's office or laboratory, where it is placed sticky-side down for microscopic examination to detect the eggs. Three specimens should be examined if necessary to improve the sensitivity. It is also sometimes possible to see the worms directly on the perianal region, although they are so small that they may easily be mistaken for residual bits of toilet paper. *E.vermicularis* is susceptible to standard anthelminthic therapies as listed in Table 2. All household contacts should be empirically treated with the same regimen to avoid reintroducing infection from family members who may be asymptomatically carrying the parasite. Careful laundering of all bedclothes is recommended as well.

Anisakiasis

Anisakiasis is a descriptive term for human infection with parasites of two distinct genuses: *Anisakis* and *Pseudoterranova*. Humans are incidental hosts for these roundworms that inhabit multiple species of fish and other marine animals (tuna, mackerel, hake, cod, sardines, and cephalopods) as intermediate hosts, and marine mammals such as whales, seals, sea lions, and walruses as final hosts. Humans acquire the parasite in its larval stage by eating raw fish (e.g., sushi, ceviche), and therefore the condition predominates in cultures where uncooked fish is consumed. Cases are most commonly reported from Japan but are seen throughout the world in other coastal nations and among restaurateurs.

On consumption of fish with anisakid larvae embedded in its musculature, humans can experience immediate symptoms in the form of itching or burning in the throat, which can provoke coughing that expels the parasite. If the parasite is swallowed, the larva attempts to embed in the gastric musculature at the pylorus. This can produce acute, short-lived epigastric abdominal pain and possibly immediate vomiting, at which point the parasite might again be ejected. If the larva does manage to penetrate gastric tissue, it dies because it is incapable of further tissue invasion in humans. An intense inflammatory response to the dead pathogen can then result, with gastric pain, nausea, and occasionally diarrhea with blood or mucus if a gastric ulcerative lesion has resulted.

Rare cases have been reported in which the larva penetrates the peritoneum, causing focal peritonitis and abscess formation. *Pseudoterranova* appears to cause milder symptoms and less tissue invasion, and the worm might simply be vomited several days after initial ingestion and presented to a physician, often by an alarmed patient. Because the vast majority of infections are caused by a single organism, vomiting of the parasite results in a definitive cure and patients can be reassured. Diagnosis in patients with ongoing symptoms related to an embedded parasite is ultimately endoscopic. Effective cure results on endoscopic or surgical removal of the worm.

TREMATODES

Schistosomiasis

Schistosomes are freshwater pathogens with areas of endeminicity in Africa, South America, Southeast Asia, and parts of the Middle East. These small trematodes cause varied, often chronic infections that can carry significant morbidity, although some species cannot invade beyond the dermis in humans and result strictly in cercarial dermatitis or swimmer's itch. There are five species of schistosomes known to cause disease in humans: *Schistosoma haematobium*, found through much of Africa and parts of the Middle East; *Schistosoma mansoni*, also native to Africa and the Middle East as well as Latin America; *Schistosoma japonicum*, present in China, Southeast Asia, and the Philippines; *Schistosoma mekongi*, found only in the Mekong River basin in Southeast Asia; and *Schistosoma intercalatum*, endemic only in West Africa.

All persons who come in contact with schistosomes are at risk for infection, even after only very brief exposure to fecally contaminated freshwater in which the intermediate hosts of the pathogen (snails) reside. Frequency and degree of infection tend to be highest in children in endemic areas and then levels off in the early teenage years, likely secondary to level of environmental exposure and possibly to host immunity. *S. mansoni* causes disease in the genitourinary system; the others cause intestinal, hepatic, and sometimes pulmonary diseases.

Infection is acquired rapidly on contact with freshwater (including brief swims or by repeated splashing, as can occur during river rafting), when free-living fork-tailed schistosomal larvae penetrate human skin and lose their tail. These schistomorulae can cause intense itching and a papulovesicular, pruritic rash at the site of penetration, swimmer's itch. Invasive schistomorulae then enter the venous bloodstream and ultimately lodge in gut mesenteric and portal venules, where maturation occurs, and male and female forms join and mate for life. Females begin to oviposit, and the resultant inflammatory response to the eggs can cause either acute illness or chronic fibrosis and granulomatous inflammation of the tissues in which they reside.

Acute illness, called *Katayama's fever*, is more common among hosts who have not been previously exposed to the organism and can be quite severe, even fatal. Katayama's fever begins 4 to 8 weeks after exposure to the schistosomes, with fever, cough, abdominal pain, hepatomegaly, and lymphadenopathy. Eggs might not yet be present in the stool at the time of diagnosis. Chronic schistosomiasis is a slowly progressive illness. *S. haematobium* infection is manifest by gross or microscopic hematuria, urinary symptoms, and chronic bacterial urinary tract infections; ultimately ureteral fibrosis, hydronephrosis, and granulomatous genital lesions also can ensue. In infection with other invasive schistosomes, chronic illness can manifest as abdominal pain and diarrhea, which is often bloody, with associated iron-deficiency anemia. Hepatomegaly is often the first clinical finding in chronic intestinal schistosomiasis. Over many years, hepatic congestion and fibrosis can result in liver failure, and the pulmonary vasculature can be involved as well, which causes pulmonary hypertension and cor pulmonale.

Diagnosis of schistosomiasis is by observation of eggs in stool (intestinal disease), urine (urinary tract disease), or biopsy specimens, or by serum antibody testing. Concentration of stool may be necessary to detect the pathogen. The eggs of the three most common species of schistosomes can be readily identified microscopically: *S. haematobium* has an inferior spine, *S. mansoni* an inferolateral spine, and *S. japonicum* lacks a spine. Eosinophilia is a hallmark of chronic infection and is a common cause of asymptomatic eosinophilia among immigrants from schistoendemic regions of the world. Serology is highly sensitive and specific but cannot distinguish acute, chronic, or cleared infection; it is very useful when attempting to diagnose infection in returned travelers.

All patients with schistosomiasis should be treated, and those with chronic manifestations might experience significant regression of even late-stage organ-specific disease. Treatment of choice is with praziquantel; see Table 2 for details.

Prevention of schistosomiasis involves improving access to treated water and exploration of avenues to eliminate the intermediate snail hosts. Host immunity does appear to occur, and efforts are under way to better understand and induce such immunity in the form of a vaccine.

CESTODES

Taeniasis

Human tapeworm infection has long been implicated in North American oral folklore as a cause of insatiable appetite and excessive weight loss. In reality, despite their impressive size of up to 12 meters, tapeworm infection tends to be minimally symptomatic.

Taenia solium, pork tapeworm, and *Taenia sanguinata*, beef tapeworm, are the two most common flatworm infections of humans worldwide and occur in any setting in which raw or undercooked meat is served and cattle and pigs have access to feed contaminated with human feces. *T. sanguinata* is still found in areas of North America and Europe, as well as in Central and South America and Africa; *T. solium* is common throughout Mexico, Central and South America, Africa, China, and the Indian subcontinent. Although humans are the definitive hosts for both parasites, *T. solium* is best known for its pathogenicity in the form of cysticercosis. Cysticercosis is not an intestinal parasitic infection.

Domesticated animals acquire infection on ingestion of eggs excreted by humans; the eggs mature in their musculature and develop a scolex. When humans consume infected meat, the scolex attaches in the small intestine, and the adult tapeworm develops over approximately 2 months. Adult tapeworms are made up of hundreds to thousands of gravid proglottids and can live for up to 25 years. Symptoms tend to be mild or absent but can include nausea, abdominal pain, loose stools, anal pruritus, and occasionally weakness or increased appetite, especially in children. Serious illness rarely results when a tapeworm becomes lodged in the biliary or pancreatic ducts or is coughed up and aspirated. Some patients come to medical attention when the worm is noted emerging from the anus or on extrusion of proglottids in the stool.

Diagnosis of taeniasis can be made on visualizing the round eggs in stool; however, the species cannot be determined unless a segment of the worm is examined. Serum antibody and antigen tests, as well as stool PCR, have been developed for diagnosis but are not widely used in clinical practice. Eosinophilia and elevated IgE levels may be present. Single dose praziquantel[1] (see Table 2) is curative in almost all cases, but infectious eggs can still be released in the feces for a time; ingestion of these could result in the subsequent development if cysticercosis, so patients should be counseled to avoid fecal–oral contact.

---

[1]Not FDA approved for this indication.

Proper cooking of meat is the mainstay of prevention; disposal of human waste away from animals would also be effective in interrupting the life cycle.

Diphyllobothriasis

Diphyllobothrium latum is the longest parasite known to infect humans (10 to 12 m). It is found in freshwater lakes in areas of the Americas, Northern Europe, Africa, China, and Japan and has a complex life cycle involving two intermediate hosts: crustaceans and small fish. Humans and other fish-eating mammals are the definitive hosts and acquire the infection on ingestion of raw fish or roe.

The organism attaches within the small intestine, and hosts are usually asymptomatic. Infected persons might complain of increased appetite, nausea, or abdominal discomfort. Many present after passage of portions of the tapeworm in stool, as with taeniasis; in others, diagnosis is on stool examination done for other purposes or during screening colonoscopy. As with other worms, the parasite occasionally migrates into biliary ducts or causes intestinal obstruction. Attachment of the parasite higher in the intestine can result in decreased levels of vitamin B_{12}. Rarely, pernicious anemia develops as a result (tapeworm anemia).

Diagnosis is made either by seeing eggs in unconcentrated stool or by encountering the adult worm. Eosinophilia is present in a minority of cases. Treatment with praziquantel[1] is curative; see Table 2. Vitamin B_{12} supplementation is necessary in cases of severe or symptomatic deficiency, but it will not recur once the tapeworm is eliminated. Prevention involves not ingesting undercooked fish.

REFERENCES

Abubakar I, Aliyu SH, Hunter PR, Usman NK: Prevention and treatment of cryptosporidiosis in immunocompromised patients. Cochrane Database Syst Rev 2007;(1):CD004932.

Bethony J, Brooker S, Albonico M, et al: Soil-transmitted helminth infections: Ascariasis, trichuriasis, and hookworm. Lancet 2006;367(9521):1521-1532.

Boggild A, Yohanna S, Keystone J, Kain K: Prospective analysis of parasitic infections in Canadian travelers and immigrants. J Travel Med 2006; 13:138-144, 2006.

Boulware DR, Stauffer WM, Hendel-Paterson RR, et al: Maltreatment of Strongyloides infection: Case series and worldwide physicians-in-training survey. Am J Med 2007;120:545. e1-545.e8.

Concha R, Harrington W Jr, Rogers AI: Intestinal strongyloidiasis: Recognition, management, and determinants of outcome. J Clin Gastroenterol 2005;39(3):203-211.

Drugs for parasitic infections, The Medical Letter [serial online]. 2004, 46. Available at: www.medicalletter.org. Accessed June 17, 2007.

Goodgame RW: Understanding intestinal spore-forming protozoa: Cryptosporidia, microsporidia, isospora, and cyclospora. Ann Intern Med 1996;124(4):429-441.

Guerrant R, Walker D, Weller P, editors: Tropical Infectious Diseases: Principles, Pathogens, and Practice, Philadelphia: Churchill Livingstone, 1999.

Huang DB, White AC: An updated review on Cryptosporidium and Giardia. Gastroenterol Clin North Am 2006;35:291-314.

Mandell G, Bennett J, Dolin R, editors: Mandell, Douglas and Bennett's Principles and Practice of Infectious Diseases, ed 5th, Philadelphia: Churchill Livingstone, 2005.

Pardo J, Carranza C, Muro A, et al: Helminth-related eosinophilia in African immigrants, Gran Canaria. Emerg Infect Dis 2006;12(10):1587-1589.

Stark D, Beebe N, Marriott D, et al: Dientamoebiasis: Clinical importance and recent advances. Trends Parasitol 2006;22(2):92-96.

---

[1]Not FDA approved for this indication.

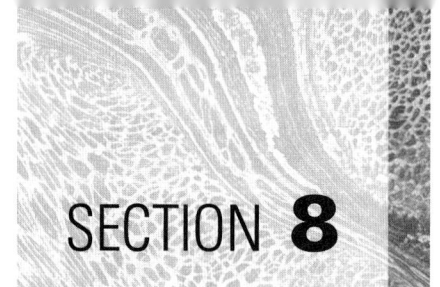

SECTION 8

Metabolic Disorders

Diabetes Mellitus in Adults

Method of
Anthony L. McCall, MD, PhD, and
J. Terry Saunders, PhD

Epidemiology

The Centers for Disease Control and Prevention (CDC) estimated that in 2007 the prevalence of diabetes in the United States was 23.6 million. Diabetes is diagnosed in 17.9 million persons and undiagnosed in 5.7 million. Type 2 diabetes mellitus (T2DM) is 90% to 95% of prevalent diabetes, and type 1 diabetes (T1DM) is about 5% to 10%. There are fewer persons with secondary or monogenic forms of diabetes, called *maturity-onset diabetes of the young* (MODY). About 57 million people in the United States are believed to have prediabetes.

The focus of this article is T2DM because it is the most prevalent form and is increasing rapidly in the United States and worldwide. A few comments are made on adult T1DM. This chapter emphasizes both lifestyle and pharmacologic treatments.

Diagnosis and Classification of Diabetes and Prediabetes

DIAGNOSIS

Most diabetes is diagnosed by random or fasting glucose (Table 1). Symptoms should be present if random glucose criteria are used, but surprisingly, many people with diabetes are relatively asymptomatic. In the elderly, cognitive changes can occur and atypical symptoms such as prostatism can appear. The American Diabetes Association (ADA) screening recommendations suggest screening every 3 years starting at age 45 for the general population, but they suggest earlier and more frequent screening in those with high risk. Recently, a case has been made for using elevated A1c as an adjunct combined with glucose measurement or as a sole criterion when >7% for screening and diagnosis of diabetes.

Patients from diabetes-prone ethnic groups (e.g., Latin Americans, African Americans, Native Americans) or with a strong family history, polycystic ovary syndrome (PCOS), or gestational diabetes should have early and frequent screenings. High-risk persons include those with prediabetes (impaired glucose tolerance, impaired fasting glucose) or who meet the National Cholesterol Education Program (NCEP) criteria for the metabolic syndrome or its individual components (dyslipidemia, hypertension, central obesity, prediabetes). The metabolic syndrome as defined by the NCEP is criticized as flawed, but such critique does not reduce the importance of fully documenting and treating cardiometabolic risk components in those with or at risk for T2DM in a targeted manner (see Box 1). The metabolic syndrome concept is useful to teach patients and clinicians about these risks and the response of the overweight and sedentary to a healthier lifestyle.

CLASSIFICATION

The classification of diabetes into its two most prominent types (T1DM and T2DM) seems straightforward in theory but in practice is increasingly confusing as more Americans become overweight. Although T1DM patients are traditionally lean, many now are overweight and some have metabolic syndrome characteristics. About 80% to 90% of persons with T2DM are overweight or have metabolic syndrome characteristics, but some are leaner and more active and do not have the metabolic syndrome. C-peptide measurements are not very helpful for those who are difficult to classify, but measuring three antibodies—including IA-2 (islet cell antigen 512), anti-GAD$_{65}$ (glutamic acid decarboxylase), and anti-insulin antibodies in high titers—can clarify a diagnosis of latent autoimmune diabetes. Younger age at onset, lean body habitus, severe loss of glycemic control with or without ketonemia, and weight loss all suggest insulin deficiency but might not be definitive.

Pathophysiology

The primary causes of most adult diabetes are insulin resistance and lack of compensatory insulin secretion. Insulin resistance is typically longstanding and begins at a young age because of heredity combined with environmental causes (sedentary lifestyle and calorie overconsumption with resultant overweight). Insulin secretory defects usually start about 10 years before diagnosis, and no therapy is proven so far to prevent progressive loss of insulin secretion. A few patients develop diabetes associated with malnutrition, but this is much less common. Longstanding insulin resistance is associated with dyslipidemia, central obesity, hypertension, and hyperglycemia. This long prodrome accounts for the common coexistence of cardiovascular disease and diabetes.

CARDIOVASCULAR RISK MANAGEMENT

Cardiovascular risk management in diabetes starts with lifestyle counseling and education. It is paramount that patients understand the intimate and direct links among diabetes, glycemic control, and cardiovascular

TABLE 1 Diagnosis and Classification of Diabetes and Prediabetes

Diagnosis	Glucose Test	Diagnostic Level	Comments
Diabetes	Random	≥200 mg/dL	Plus classic symptoms*
Diabetes	Fasting	≥126 mg/dL	8-hour fast; need confirmation
Diabetes	Postglucose load (75 g in nonpregnant adults)	≥200 mg/dL at 2 h	Need confirmation
Prediabetes IFG	Fasting	≥100 mg/dL	Decreased insulin secretion
Prediabetes IGT	Postglucose load (75 g)	140-199 mg/dL at 2 h	Increased insulin resistance

*Polyuria, polydipsia, unexplained weight loss.
Abbreviations: IFG = impaired fasting glucose; IGT = impaired glucose tolerance

---

disease. Drug interventions are ultimately needed for glycemia, lipid risks, and blood pressure in most patients. Women have higher relative risk and similar overall risk as men and are often undertreated. Specific recommended targets of therapy for diabetes in glycemia, blood pressure, dyslipidemia, and lifestyle are shown in Box 1.

DOCUMENTING AND FOLLOWING COMPLICATIONS

Patients should have a thorough examination and evaluation for complications at the time of diabetes diagnosis. About one half of patients with newly diagnosed T2DM have established chronic complications, indicating delayed recognition of this disorder.

Neuropathy and circulatory signs and symptoms on foot examination should be assessed. Risk of ulcer and amputation can be gauged by 10-g Semmes-Weinstein monofilaments that test for severe neuropathy and attendant risk of ulceration. Retina examinations should be done by skilled eye professionals likely to pick up significant eye disease. High-risk patients (poor glycemic control, established retinopathy, especially if preproliferative or worse) should be referred promptly to an eye specialist. Pregnancy counseling should be given to all women of childbearing age with diabetes. Microalbumin-to-creatinine ratio in the urine should be assessed and kidney function (serum creatinine and blood urea nitrogen [BUN]) should be tracked yearly.

Home glucose monitoring should be taught to patients so they understand the effects of food, stress, and exercise on glycemic patterns. Diabetes education should be arranged for all patients, preferably by a diabetes educator. Diabetes is unique in being a self-managed condition where patient knowledge and skills are critical to avoiding complications.

BOX 1 Summary of Goals for Treatment

Lifestyle
Medical Nutrition Therapy (individualized)
- Appropriate calories
- Low saturated and *trans* fats
- Moderate, consistent carbohydrates (whole grains, vegetables, fruits)
- Healthy fats and proteins (decreased saturated and trans fats, increased monosaturated fat; reduced consumption of animal protein)

Activity
- Consistent, regular activity tailored to complications and safety (ECG or stress test may be needed before starting an exercise program)

Glycemia
- Best possible without frequent or severe hypoglycemia
- HbA1c <7% minimally; 6% or less if possible

Self-Monitored Blood Glucose
- Preprandial 90-130 mg/dL; <110 ideally
- Postprandial (1 to 2 h) <180 minimal; <140 ideally

Lipids
- LDL <100 mg/dL; optional <70 mg/dL (ACS, clinical ASCVD)
- Non-HDL <130 mg/dL; optional <100 mg/dL
- HDL >40 mg/dL (men); >50 mg/dL (women)
- Triglycerides <150 mg/dL

Blood Pressure
- Systolic <130 mm Hg
- Diastolic <80 mm Hg

Abbreviations: ACS = acute coronary syndrome, ASCVD = atherosclerotic cardiovascular disease (also multiple severe risk factors that are difficult to control); HDL = high-density lipoprotein; LDL = low-density lipoprotein.

CURRENT DIAGNOSIS

- Screening for diabetes should be done in high-risk populations, especially:
  - Those with prediabetes or the metabolic syndrome.
  - High-risk ethnic groups (e.g., Native American, Latino American, African American).
  - Gestational diabetes.
  - Patients might present with atypical symptoms.
  - Most diabetes is type 2 in adults, but type 1 does occur in adults, and delayed diagnosis is common.
- Cardiovascular risk should be aggressively screened for and treated.
- Complications should be documented and tracked.
  - Check fasting lipids.
- Check renal function and albuminuria yearly.
  - Have a low threshold for stress testing, with imaging for all patients.
  - Refer for yearly eye examinations.
  - Check feet for sensation, deformity, and circulation at regular visits.
- All patients should receive an educational assessment and training in self-management and self-monitoring of blood glucose.
- Take a diet history; this is especially important for patients on insulin.
- Get a baseline HbA1c and repeat 2 to 4 times per year (twice yearly if at glycemic goal).

Treatment

BEHAVIORAL SELF-MANAGEMENT

Self-management of behavioral factors, including eating, physical activity, and psychological stress, is essential to good diabetes self-care. Ideally, professional support for behavioral self-management should be a coordinated, multidisciplinary effort involving expertise appropriate to a given patient from the areas of nutrition, nursing, exercise training, and behavioral counseling. The provider should develop a referral network of available multidisciplinary resources and make regular use of any appropriate community-based resources (e.g., weight loss programs, fitness programs, diabetes support groups). Unfortunately, multidisciplinary resources are often in short supply or difficult to pay for. Therefore, it is essential that the provider develop basic skills and techniques for working with patients on behavior change.

Behavior change is slow and is inherently a multisession activity. Quick, one-shot interventions seldom change longstanding patterns of behavior. Initial sessions should be scheduled closely together (1-2 weeks), then further apart as the patient gains momentum and confidence. If multiple one-on-one sessions are impossible, other options such as group meetings, telephone support, or e-mail messaging should be considered.

Behavior change interventions should be highly individualized and specific. General advice about diet and exercise does not address the life experience or problems of a given patient and is often perceived as insensitive or unhelpful. Arriving at individualized objectives for behavior change can be accomplished using a simple three-step process composed of initial assessment, setting behavioral objectives, and follow-up and reassessment.

Initial Assessment

Initial assessment includes identifying salient features of social and family history that can affect efforts to change behavior. A nutrition assessment should be performed, including an appraisal of usual food intake, the patient's perception of problem eating behavior, and weight history. A physical activity assessment should also be conducted, focusing on past and current physical activity, preferences, perceived barriers, and general attitudes. Readiness to make changes in behavior should be assessed by asking how important a patient thinks it is to change a given area of behavior and how confident she or he is that she or he can succeed in making changes (on a 1 to 10 scale). Discussion of specific objectives for behavioral change should occur in areas where the patient indicates a definite readiness to begin. Other areas of change should be discussed, but not forced or driven by the provider. Finally, ask patients about current levels and sources of stress. Because depression is common with diabetes, patients should be screened for possible depression.

Behavioral Objectives

Setting behavioral objectives is initiated and facilitated by the provider, but the patient is responsible for selecting his or her own behavioral objectives. Resist the temptation to take over responsibility for this function. Objectives should be FIRM: *f*ew (1-3 at a time is plenty), *i*ndividualized to the patient's specific behavioral challenges, *r*ealistic (beware of trying to make big strides quickly), and *m*easurable. For measurement, the patient should be given a tracking form (such as the example in Figure 1) to use in recording daily progress on each objective. Note that although the patient might have long-term goals in the areas of weight loss, calorie intake, or general fitness, specific behavioral objectives such as eating a bowl of cereal for breakfast or walking one-half hour on five mornings each week are the means to achieving those outcomes. The primary focus of provider-patient discussions of progress should be on behavioral objectives, not outcomes.

Follow-up and Reassessment

Follow-up and reassessment occur during each return visit, following a period of patient efforts to carry out mutually agreed on behavioral objectives. Reassessment focuses on the behavioral records kept by patients as well as on their verbal reports of difficulties and successes. Praise and encouragement are the order of the day. Efforts to initiate behavior change are highly responsive to external positive reinforcement, and the patient will need maximum external reinforcement until new behavior becomes self-sustaining. After review and discussion of patient records, new behavioral objectives or incremental changes in existing objectives are selected by mutual agreement, with the patient taking the lead.

A modest weight loss of 5% to 10% has a positive impact on cardiovascular risk factors and progression of diabetes. Reassure patients that medical goals for weight loss are achievable and worth the effort.

When discussing changes in eating with patients, distinguish dieting from gradual behavioral changes that result in a lasting pattern of healthy eating. Diets are impermanent and run the risk of large weight losses followed by even larger weight gains. Gradual behavioral changes offer the possibility of permanent lifestyle changes.

Prohibiting or demonizing foods is counterproductive. It leads patients to think of food in moral extremes (e.g., "sugar is bad for my diabetes") rather than along a continuum of nutritional benefit and blood glucose control. Food prohibition also casts the provider as withholding and overly controlling. These traps can be avoided by exploring very small changes that are not perceived as significant losses.

Patients may be extremely confused about the role of carbohydrates in weight loss and weight maintenance because of popular myths about sugar and the controversy surrounding low-carbohydrate diets. Low-carbohydrate diets (<130 g/day) are not recommended as an approach to weight loss. Carbohydrates should be included as an

---

 CURRENT THERAPY

- Diabetes requires nutrition and behavioral self-management counseling as well as drug therapy.
- Repeatedly encourage healthy eating and an active lifestyle.
- Prediabetes diagnosis represents an opportunity for behavioral and drug interventions.
- Metformin (Glucophage) is usually the first drug therapy.
- Don't expect one drug to do the job for very poorly controlled glycemia.
- Dual defects (insulin resistance and secretion) should be addressed in most patients.
- Very insulin resistant patients might need a dual insulin resistance strategy.
- Therapy goals for both HbA1c and self-monitored blood glucose can be achieved in most patients.
- Cardiovascular risk reduction therapy is a very high priority.
- When patients have not met goals on dual oral agent therapy, basal insulin is often the most appropriate choice, particularly when patients are not near glycemic goals.
- For oral agent therapy, add don't switch unless side effects require it.
- When adding basal insulin, continue oral agent therapies.
- Threatening patients with insulin therapy is counter productive.
- Follow the 3F rule: Fix the fasting glucose first, especially in patients with poor glycemic control.
- Prompt recognition of the need for meal insulin is critical to achieve glycemic goals.
- Balance meal and basal insulin.

My Behavioral Goals

To take better care of my diabetes and improve my health, I will:
(Write your behavioral goal in the blank spaces below and track your daily progress in the boxes on the tracking form. Make notes about your successes and challenges.)

Walk for 30 minutes, 5 days per week

Circle the day you will start and mark your progress every day with a check or number.

Monday	Tuesday	Wednesday	Thursday	Friday	Saturday	Sunday
		(20)	10	25	30	25
0	30					

Date	My Successes
11/30	Finally did 30 minutes on Saturday!
	My Challenges

FIGURE 1. Example of a behavioral goals tracking form.

important part of a healthy diet for people with diabetes. Recommendations for achieving consistent, appropriate carbohydrate intake at meals are based on controlling postprandial blood glucose (<180 mg/dL 1 to 2 hours after beginning a meal). Carbohydrate counting and blood glucose pattern management are complicated and time consuming to teach. Referral to a dietitian for medical nutrition therapy (MNT) or nutrition education through an ADA-recognized diabetes patient education program is recommended.

The best place to begin setting behavioral objectives for nutrition and exercise is where the patient is currently. Obtaining a 3-day food record (2 work days and one nonwork day) and a baseline for activity (we generally use a week of daily steps measured with a pedometer) provide a solid baseline for setting objectives.

An irregular pattern of eating often underlies unhealthy food choices. For example, staying up late encourages late-night snacking, which in turn can suppress interest in eating breakfast. Eating tends to be deferred to the afternoon or evening, perpetuating the cycle.

A modest reduction in caloric consumption of around 250 to 500 kcal/day and moderate physical activity on the order of at least 150 minutes a week are the recommended approaches to weight loss. Reducing calories through decreased food consumption is more effective for weight loss than increasing energy expenditure through physical activity. Box 2 contains a checklist of healthy eating behaviors that can be used to stimulate patients' thinking about places they might like to make changes. Physical activity plays an important role in weight maintenance, but higher levels of activity (200 min/week) may be required to prevent long-term weight regain. Box 3 lists ways that patients can become more active. It is worth repeating that the point of these and other suggestions is not to direct patients but to expand their thinking about what might work for them.

Stress reduction is important in controlling blood glucose, but it can also play a role by helping patients achieve a mental focus on their behavior-management efforts. We encourage patients to sit calmly for a period of 5 to 10 minutes each day, focusing on slow deep breathing and muscle relaxation. Activities such as yoga or tai chi also reduce stress and support awareness of body and mind. Box 4 contains suggestions for coping behaviors that may be useful to patients in dealing with stress.

PHARMACOLOGIC THERAPY

Overview

Eventually, most patients with T2DM require drug treatment, often with multiple agents (combination therapy). Progressive insulin secretory loss probably is the primary explanation for the need to advance treatment. A resultant general rule with all therapies is *add, don't switch.* Table 2 lists major types of pharmacotherapeutic interventions with their usual hemoglobin (Hb) A1c lowering, balance of preprandial versus postprandial effects, and some comments on their actions and side effects. Table 3 lists classes of drugs, commonly used agents, and typical doses.

Recently the ADA and European Association for the Study of Diabetes (EASD) have issued a joint consensus algorithm on controlling hyperglycemia in T2DM. In our practice, we similarly initiate behavioral self-management along with medication, typically metformin unless there are contraindications or intolerance. Commonly, ineffective early attempts by physicians to change behavior (e.g., giving general advice) lead to abandonment of this therapy. A second oral medication may be initiated if patients cannot achieve glycemic goals. Commonly, we favor insulin secretagogues especially glimepiride (Amaryl) or extended-release glipizide (Glucotrol XL) for their relatively low risk of hypoglycemia, convenient once-daily dosing, and low expense. An alternative treatment strategy for heavier, more insulin-resistant patients is use of a thiazolidinedione, effectively a dual insulin-resistance strategy (see thiazolidinediones).

BOX 2 Checklist of Healthy Eating Behaviors

☑ **Eat meals and snacks at set times to promote health.**
Examples:
- I will eat breakfast within 1 hour of getting up.
- I will not skip meals.
- Other: ....
  ....

☑ **Eat healthy carbohydrates.**
Examples:
- I will avoid regular soft drinks and choose water or diet soft drinks instead.
- I will eat 5-7 servings of fruits and vegetables every day.
- I will choose whole-grain breads and cereals.
- Other: ....
  ....

☑ **Decrease serving sizes.**
Examples:
- I will keep a record of the food I eat and drink.
- I will know what counts as a serving size.
- When I am eating out, I will share or split an entrée and eat a salad.
- Other: ....
  ....

☑ **Eat less fat and choose healthy fats.**
Examples:
- I will bake, broil, roast, grill, or boil instead of fry food.
- I will have a meatless meal at least once a week.
- I will choose fried or high-fat foods no more than once a week.
- I will drink fat-free or low-fat milk.
- I will use healthy oils (olive oil, canola oil) and buy tub margarine.
- Other: ....
  ....

☑ **Make other healthy choices.**
Examples:
- I will drink plenty of fluids (at least 8 glasses of water or low-calorie fluid per day).
- I will limit how much alcohol I drink. (Women should drink no more than 1 alcoholic drink per day. Men should drink no more than 2 alcoholic drinks per day.)
- Other: ....
  ....

Unpublished source: Virginia Center for Diabetes Professional Education, University of Virginia; Virginia Diabetes Council.

More reliably effective is the use of basal insulin treatment as a second agent to achieve control. Insulin initiation should be preceded by an open discussion of the patient's attitudes, beliefs, and possible fears regarding insulin. Insulin therapy should never be used as a threat or possible negative consequence for failure to carry out behavioral management. Many patients associate insulin with serious diabetes complications and mortality. A positive attitude about the value of insulin therapy and a reassuring, educational approach can help to reduce initial fears enough to begin. Self-demonstration of injection technique using saline is also useful in overcoming fear of injections. Improvement in blood glucose control with insulin generally makes patients feel better, which further reinforces its perceived value. Use of insulin pens may increase acceptance of insulin treatment, patient convenience, and dosing accuracy.

Oral Agents

Secretagogues

These drugs enhance insulin secretion. There are first- and second-generation oral sulfonylureas; the latter are most commonly used. They are inexpensive, are moderately effective, and often can be dosed once daily. First-generation agents such as tolbutamide, chlorpropamide (Diabenese), and tolazamide (Tolinase) are less often used than the second-generation agents glyburide (Diabeta, Glynase), glipizide (Glucotrol), and glimepiride (Amaryl).

The dose-response characteristics of sulfonylureas suggest that one half the approved maximum dose achieves maximum HbA1c lowering, typically 1 to 1.5 percentage points. If the patient is not at goal with half-maximum doses, it is more effective to add a second agent

---

BOX 3 Checklist for Physical Activity

☑ **Do something that you enjoy.**
Examples:
- I will take the stairs.
- I will park my car farther away and walk.
- I will walk.
- I will swim or do water exercises.
- I will ride a bike.
- I will use an exercise video.
- I will do yoga.
- Other: ....
  ....

☑ **How often?**
Examples:
❑ Every day
❑ 3x/week
❑ 5x/week
❑ ....

☑ **How long?**
Examples:
❑ 10 minutes
❑ 15 minutes
❑ 20 minutes
❑ 30 minutes
❑ 60 minutes
❑ __ minutes

☑ **Limit inactivity.**
Examples:
- I will watch no more than 1 hour of television per day.
- I will spend no more than 2 hour(s) per day on the computer.
- Other: ....
  ....

Unpublished source: Virginia Center for Diabetes Professional Education, University of Virginia; Virginia Diabetes Council.

BOX 4 Checklist of Coping Behaviors

Examples:
- Talk about how you feel to people you trust.
- Decide one small way to change your mood or old habit, and do it.
- Write down 10 good things about your life and think about and appreciate them.
- Organize your day with a To Do list.
- Learn how to relax through yoga, meditation, biofeedback, tai chi, deep breathing, or visual imagery.
- Take 30 minutes each day to relax through music, yoga, bath, writing, etc.
- Take time to have fun every day by exploring a new interest, watching a funny movie, going shopping, playing with a pet, etc.
- Get in touch with your spiritual side to help you feel better about yourself.
- Keep a stress diary to see what triggers your stress and discover better ways to react.
- Exercise every day to help you focus your energy on a more positive path.
- Keep your sleep cycle as regular as possible.
- Develop a favorite hobby.
- Other: ....
  ....

Unpublished source: Virginia Center for Diabetes Professional Education, University of Virginia; Virginia Diabetes Council.

than raise the dose. Common side effects include hypoglycemia, weight gain of about 2 kg, and, more rarely, hematologic or skin reactions.

Rapid secretagogues, the glinides (repaglinide [Prandin] and nateglinide [Starlix]), are more expensive and should be considered for patients who are sulfonylurea allergic, extremely erratic in eating, or at high risk for hypoglycemia.

TABLE 3 Dosing Used for Various Agents

Agent	Dose
Thiazolidinediones	
Pioglitazone (Actos)	15, 30, 45 mg
Rosiglitazone (Avandia)	2, 4, 8 mg
α-Glucosidase inhibitors	
Acarbose (Precose)	25, 50, 100 mg ac
Miglitol (Glycet)	25, 50 mg ac
Biguanides	
Metformin (Glucophage) IR	500, 850, 1000 mg
Metformin SR	500, 750 mg
Glinides	
Nateglinide (Starlix)	60-120 mg ac
Repaglinide (Prandin)	0.5-4 mg ac
Sulfonylureas (Second Generation)	
Glimepiride (Amaryl)	1-4 mg
Glipizide (Glucotrol) IR	2.5-20 mg
Glipizide SR	2.5-10 mg
Glyburide (Glynase)	1.25-10; 1.5-6 mg
Incretins	
Exenatide (Byetta)	5, 10 μg
Sitagliptin (Januvia)	25, 50, 100 mg*
Vildagliptin (Galvus)[4]	50, 100 mg
Amylin Agonists	
Pramlintide (Symlin)	15, 30, 60, 90, 120 μg
Insulin	
Aspart (Novolog)	No dose limit
Detemir (Levemir)	No dose limit
Glargine (Lantus)	No dose limit
Glulisine (Apidra)	No dose limit
Inhaled powder insulin (Exubera)	No dose limit
Lispro (Humalog)	No dose limit
NPH	No dose limit
Regular	No dose limit

[4] Not yet approved for use in the United States.
Abbreviations: ac = before meals; IR = immediate release; NPH = neutral protamine Hagedorn; SR = sustained release.
*Based on renal function.

TABLE 2 Overview and Characteristics of Therapy Interventions

Drug Type	HbA1c Lowering (Percentage Points)	Effect on Glycemia Levels — Preprandial	Postprandial	Actions	Side Effects
SUs and non-SU rapid secretagogues**	1.5-2*	++	+	Direct and indirect secretagogue	Hypoglycemia, weight gain
Biguanides	1.5-2*	+++	0	↓ hepatic glucose output	GI, lactic acidosis, weight neutral
Thiazolidinediones	0.7-1.5	+++	0	↓muscle insulin sensitivity	Edema, CHF, fractures
Incretin agonists	0.9-1.1	+	++	Strong GLP-1 effects ↑ insulin ↓glucagon	Nausea, vomiting, weight loss
DPP-4 inhibitors	0.6-0.8	+	++	Moderate GLP-1 effects ↑ insulin ↓ glucagon	Weight neutral
Basal insulin	1.5-2.5	+++*	0*	↓ hepatic glucose output, ↑ muscle glucose disposal	Hypoglycemia, weight gain
Meal insulin	1.0-2.0	0-+*	++*	↓ hepatic glucose output, ↑ muscle glucose disposal	Hypoglycemia, weight gain
Pramlintide	0.5-0.7	0-+	++	↑ insulin ↓ glucagon	Nausea, vomiting

Abbreviations: CHF = congestive heart failure; DPP = dipeptidyl peptidase; GI = gastrointestinal; GLP = glucagon-like peptide; Hb = hemoglobin; PFT = pulmonary function test; SU = sulfonylurea.
*Older drugs may be less effective in well-controlled patients.
**Rapid secretagogues have more postprandial effects and less preprandial effects.

Biguanides

Metformin is the only available agent in this class. It is useful in both obese and normal weight T2DM patients. HbA1c lowering is typically about 1.5 percentage points in monotherapy or in combination therapy. Maximum efficacy is achieved with 2000 mg daily. The sustained-release preparation will last 24 hours if given with the evening meal.

Metformin's hypoglycemic mechanism is primarily by reduction of liver glucose production. It is cleared by the kidney, and the risk of lactic acidosis, a rare side effect with 50% mortality, may be increased in renal dysfunction. Serum creatinine should be less than 1.4 mg/dL in women and less than 1.5 mg/dL in men, and glomerular filtration rate (GFR) should be assessed in patients 80 years and older. It is also an increased lactic acidosis risk in patients with drug-treated congestive heart failure (CHF) or respiratory insufficiency. Intravascular contrast administration should prompt holding the drug for 24 to 48 hours until renal function is assured to be adequate. GI side effects are common initially and are dose dependent but wane; they can require gradual titration. Sustained-release preparations have fewer GI side effects. Weight gain is less with this drug than with many others for diabetes. The United Kingdom Prospective Diabetes Study (UKPDS) found that risk of MI and death was reduced, making it a first choice for pharmacotherapy in most patients.

Thiazolidinediones

Two drugs of the thiazolidinedione (TZD) class are available, rosiglitazone (Avandia) and pioglitazone (Actos). Both have similar glycemic-lowering effects and side effects. These drugs work by increasing the sensitivity of muscle tissue and fat to insulin action, probably through action of adipokines like adiponectin and muscle effects on adenosine monophosphate–activated protein kinase (AMPK), a fuel sensor enzyme. HbA1c lowering varies considerably, dependent on whether patients are very insulin resistant (central adiposity, often hypertriglyceridemia) and whether there is adequate endogenous insulin secretion (short diabetes duration or secretagogues) or insulin is given.

Diabetes may be prevented with rosiglitazone, and this is being tested for pioglitazone. Both TZDs can precipitate edema, weight gain due to obesity, and occasionally congestive heart failure even absent a prior heart failure history. It is thus wise to track weight in all patients and limit it to 5 or 6 pounds. The risk of heart failure is increased when TZDs are combined with insulin. Both TZDs have beneficial effects on some lipid parameters, but pioglitazone appears more effective in reducing hypertriglyceridemia. Recent analyses suggest, but do not prove, increased coronary ischemic events with rosiglitazone. Pioglitazone studies suggest reduced ischemic risk (stroke or myocardial infarction). Both medicines may increase heart failure, and new studies suggest more self-reported fractures in women, which will need further study.

Incretins

Incretins are gut hormones that enhance food-induced insulin secretion. Incretin drugs either are receptor agonists (e.g., exenatide) for glucagon-like peptide-1 (GLP-1), perhaps the most important incretin, or they enhance endogenous levels for both GLP-1 and gastrointestinal insulinotropic polypeptide (GIP).

Exenatide (Byetta) is the only available GLP-1 receptor agonist. Its actions increase meal insulin, decrease meal hyperglucagonemia, decrease rate of stomach emptying, and suppress appetite, which may cause a moderate weight loss. It works rapidly on injection. It has substantial GI side effects including nausea, vomiting, and diarrhea in a large minority of patients. Despite this, many patients favor it, probably because the side effects generally wane within weeks and there can be substantial weight loss in some very overweight patients. Typically, exenatide is given in doses of 5 μg twice daily at meals, advancing after a month to 10 μg twice daily. Patients might report that nausea is more tolerable if they have a little food in their stomach at the time of dosing. Pancreatitis may rarely occur (case reports).

Because incretin drugs all have a glucose-dependent insulin secretion and glucagon suppression, there is little tendency for hypoglycemia used alone or when they are combined with metformin and TZDs in comparison with sulfonylureas. HbA1c lowering with exenatide has been 0.9 to 1.1 percentage points.

Dipeptidyl Peptidase-4 Inhibitors

Dipeptidyl peptidase-4 (DPP-4) is the peptidase that normally rapidly degrades the incretins GLP-1 and GIP to inactive proteolytic products. Inhibitors of DPP-4 have been shown to enhance GLP-1 and GIP levels to high physiologic levels and thereby reduce HbA1c concentrations, typically about 0.6 to 0.8 percentage points. At this writing, one of two drugs, sitagliptin (Januvia), has been approved and appears to be effective in doses of 100 mg once daily. This drug is excreted by the kidney largely unchanged and therefore should be given in lower doses (50 mg once daily) for those with moderate renal insufficiency (GFR 30-50 mL/min) and further reduced (25 mg) for those with severe renal dysfunction (GFR <30 mL/min).

Because DPP-4 inhibitors are oral, they may be preferred to the injectable exenatide. The side effects for these drugs are relatively minor and cause little nausea, vomiting, or diarrhea. They also do not cause significant weight loss but, like metformin, appear to be weight neutral. Recently, rare but serious allergic reactions such as angioedema and Stevens-Johnson syndrome have been reported in a few patients.

Amylin Agonists

Insulin is cosecreted with another beta cell hormone called amylin. The effects of amylin appear to be to help lower glycemia, reduce excess glucagon levels, curb appetite, and possibly reduce the rate of gastric emptying. A synthetic analogue of amylin, pramlintide (Symlin), is available as an injectable agent for treating both T1DM and T2DM as an adjunct to insulin. It lowers HbA1c about 0.5 to 0.7 percentage points. It also appears to have some weight loss effect, typically around 1 to 2 kg. Its action primarily controls glucose postprandially. Nausea and vomiting can occur in patients with either T2DM or T1DM but are worse in T1DM patients who require low doses at first (15 μg or less with meals) and slower titration. Those with T2DM usually start with 60 μg and can usually advance to 90 to 120 μg at meals.

Insulin

Barriers to Insulin Use

Insulin deficiency underlies the genesis of both T1DM and T2DM. Progression of therapy to use of insulin typically with oral agents in T2DM also seems predicated on progressive loss of insulin secretion. Nonetheless, it is often started too late, and patients often are in very poor control when this is done. Reluctance by patients and physicians alike might underlie this. Physicians should understand that exogenous insulin in T2DM is needed, does not negatively alter life quality, and is more likely to achieve therapeutic targets. Moreover, exogenous insulin does not worsen insulin resistance, does not cause excess cardiovascular disease, and has a low frequency of severe hypoglycemia, especially when used relatively early in the disease. Table 4 lists common insulin preparations and some notes about kinetics and timing.

Starting Insulin: Use of Basal Insulin in Type 2 Diabetes

How should insulin be started? Practitioners should use temporary insulin for patients whose glycemia is initially poorly controlled or when patients temporarily have worse control due to illness or medications, such as glucocorticoids. It is unwise to use insulin as a threat because it creates a sense of personal failure and dread of insulin use. When therapy progresses but there is failure to achieve glycemic goals after one or two oral medications, use of basal insulin is often the best

TABLE 4 Insulin Preparations

Insulin Type	Onset (h)	Peak (h)	Duration (h)	Comments
Basal Insulin				
NPH (Humulin N, Novolin N)	0.5	4-10	18	Kinetics is dose dependent; Peak effects exert meal action; Dose at breakfast, bedtime, supper*
Glargine[†] (Lantus)	2-4	none	24*	Up to 1/3 of C-peptide-negative T1DM need bid administration; Dose can be given at any time of day if consistent
Detemir[†] (Levemir)		Less peak activity than NPH		Kinetics is dose dependent; Dose at breakfast, bedtime, supper*
Meal Insulin				
Regular (Humulin R, Novolin R)	15-30	2-3	5-8	Give 1/2 hour before meals
Lispro (Humalog)	0.1-0.2	1.5-2.0	4	Dose at mealtime or immediately after
Aspart (Novolog)	0.1-0.2	1.5-2.0	4	Dose at mealtime or immediately after
Glulisine (Apidra)	0.1-0.2	1.5-2.0	4	Dose at mealtime or immediately after
Mixed Preparations				
NPH/regular (Humulin, Novolin)	70/30 dual kinetics based on components			Dosing 1/2 hour before meals; Should not be dosed at bedtime
Lispro/NPLispro (Humalog Mix75/25)	25/75 dual kinetics			Dosing at mealtime; should not be dosed at bedtime
Lispro/NPLispro Humalog Mix 50/50	50/50 dual kinetics			Dosing at mealtime; should not be dosed at bedtime
Aspart/NPAspart (NovoLog Mix 70/30)	30/70 dual kinetics			Dosing at mealtime; should not be dosed at bedtime

*Bedtime dosing may be preferred for some patients, especially those on low doses.
[†]Should not be mixed with other insulins or used in the same syringe that other insulin has been in.
Abbreviations: NPH = neutral protamine Hagedorn.

---

way to achieve euglycemia, especially if patients are much more than 1 percentage point from HbA1c goal (< 7%).

The Treat-to-Target Trial offers a good example of how to initiate insulin therapy. In this study, as often in our practice, patients start with a basal insulin either with NPH insulin or insulin glargine (Lantus). Insulin detemir (Levemir) represents another new option to be used similarly. Insulin is instituted as 10 U once daily, commonly in the evening near bedtime, followed by weekly increases between 2 and 8 units depending on proximity to glucose goals, focusing on the fasting glucose.

This strategy is sometimes called the *fix the fasting first* rule. Average doses in that study were around 45 to 50 units for patients whose BMI was about 31 kg/m². An alternative initial dosing might be 0.2 U/kg body weight, but whatever the starting dose, a forced titration guided by patient self-monitoring with clear communication of target fasting glucose (90-130 mg/dL), size of increment (or decrement in case of hypoglycemia; usually 10%-20% of dose), and frequency of change (every 3-7 days) is necessary to get most patients to overall glycemic (HbA1c) goal. This strategy is referred to as *pattern management*. The intent is to use monitoring to adjust the insulin dose likely to affect the fasting glucose for basal insulin therapy. NPH and detemir usually can be used once daily, typically at bedtime. Patients using glargine may choose any time of the day as long as it is reasonably consistent, usually within an hour. Occasionally, twice-daily NPH or detemir is used.

At some point, basal insulin therapy alone may be insufficient for glycemic control for T2DM patients. Usually this is a consideration in patients whose HbA1c values are over 9% to 9.5% or where the fasting goal is met but HbA1c or daytime glycemia remains elevated. The need for meal insulin is particularly likely to occur with larger meals, such as supper. Diagnostically, what is important is to have patients check either both before and after large meals or, if they are unwilling to check frequently, simply check about 2 to 3 hours after meals. Self-monitored glucose values that exceed even minimum postprandial glycemic guidelines (<180 mg/dL) indicate the need for meal insulin. A common mistake made in practice is to treat fasting hyperglycemia only with increases in basal insulin, when in some patients, the cause is overeating or lack of meal insulin the previous evening. This can be discerned by observing the pattern of glycemia, with lows often between meals or overnight and highs occurring after meals or at bedtime.

FIXED-RATIO COMBINED INSULINS

A commonly employed strategy is to use fixed-ratio combination short-acting (either regular or rapid analogue) insulin combined with intermediate insulin (NPH or neutral protamine modified rapid analogue that mimics NPH timing). Examples of these preparations include 70/30 NPH and regular insulin, 75/25 neutral protamine lispro and lispro insulin (Humalog), and 70/30 neutral protamine aspart and aspart insulin (Novolog). These have the advantage of being able to achieve control very conveniently in T2DM patients who have quite poor control (HbA1c of 9.5% or more) with a simple twice-daily injection regimen. They also offer the advantage of greater dosing accuracy, especially when used with insulin pens. Important to the success of these formulations is consistent eating and carbohydrate intake with meals. Unfortunately, when such consistency is not advised or followed, patterns of glycemia can be erratic and hypoglycemia can be significantly increased due to both components of the combination. Patients who skip meals are poor candidates for such treatments and should either switch to individual dosing of an insulin mixture or, even safer, use a basal bolus insulin regimen.

Colesevelam hydrochloride (WelChol) in doses of 3.8 g/day altogether or in divided doses has been shown to reduce hyperglycemia when compared with placebo in patients with type 2 diabetes mellitus. A1c reductions range from 0.4% to 0.8% in comparison with placebo when used alone, with patients on metformin alone or in combination with other oral agents, with sulfonylureas, on sulfonylureas and other oral agents and when used with insulin and other oral agents. Although this drug has already been approved for hyperlipidemia, it is now FDA approved also for type 2 diabetes. It has the potential, however, to increase triglycerides, and thus baseline fasting lipid values should be obtained and tracked, especially in hypertriglyceridemic patients. There is little reason to justify its use alone or with thiazolidinediones but may be appropriate for some patients with type 2 diabetes not at goal on other therapies.

ADULTS WITH TYPE 1 DM

A significant minority of patients with a diagnosis of T2DM actually have a late onset of T1DM and typical autoimmunity (IA-2 antibodies, GAD-65 antibodies, and insulin antibodies). The diagnosis should certainly be suspected in patients who rapidly fail combination oral agent therapy. Nonobese body habitus, marked weight loss, extremely elevated glucose values, or a family or personal history of autoimmune disease (e.g., Hashimoto's or Graves' thyroid problems) should lead to diagnostic evaluation for such signs of autoimmunity.

T1DM patients need combined mealtime and basal insulin therapy. Although it is tempting to do so in a convenient fashion with combined preparations such as those with analogue fixed ratios, it usually is far preferable to use a better basal insulin, such as glargine or detemir combined with a rapid-acting analogue (separately injected) before meals. Sometimes an insulin pump is the best way for patients who have frequent hypoglycemia or marked variability to achieve good glycemic control safely. T1DM patients should preferably be seen by an endocrine specialist or other practitioner with extensive experience in T1DM management. Ready access to diabetes educators is an important key to success with both T1DM and T2DM.

ADULTS WITH TYPE 2 DM

Many T2DM patients eventually need mealtime insulin. For those on insulin alone, incretin mimetics[1] can be successfully used for mealtime control, because they effectively lower prandial hyperglycemia. If using exenatide, then additional injections will be required at the two major meals of the day. If using an incretin-enhancer drug such as sitagliptin, injections are not required. There are no published data yet to provide guidelines for this strategy, but we have occasionally used this approach with exenatide in patients who need to lose weight, who gain considerable weight with meal insulin, or who experience poor control despite attempts to regulate meal glycemia with short-acting insulins.

REFERENCES

American Diabetes Association: Diagnosis and classification of diabetes mellitus. Diabetes Care 2006;29(Suppl. 1):S43-S48.

Diabetes Prevention Program Research Group: The Diabetes Prevention Program (DPP): Description of lifestyle intervention. Diabetes Care 2002;25:2165-2171.

Grundy SM, Cleeman JI, Daniels SR, et al: Diagnosis and management of the metabolic syndrome. An American Heart Association/National Heart, Lung, and Blood Institute Scientific Statement. Executive summary. Circulation 2005;112:2735-2752.

Kahn R, Buse J, Ferrannini E, Stern M: The metabolic syndrome: Time for a critical appraisal. Joint statement from the American Diabetes Association and the European Association for the Study of Diabetes. Diabetes Care 2005;8:2289-2304.

Knowler WC, Barrett-Connor E, Fowler SE, et al: Reduction in the incidence of type 2 diabetes with lifestyle intervention or metformin. N Engl J Med 2002;346:393-403.

Monnier L, Lapinski H, Colette C: Contributions of fasting and postprandial plasma glucose increments to the overall diurnal hyperglycemia of type 2 diabetic patients: Variations with increasing levels of HbA1c. Diabetes Care 2003;26:881-885.

Nathan DM, Buse JB, Davidson MB, et al: Management of hyperglycemia in type 2 diabetes: A consensus algorithm for the initiation and adjustment of therapy. A consensus statement from the American Diabetes Association and the European Association for the Study of Diabetes. Diabetes Care 2006;29:1963-1972.

Nesto RW, Bell D, Bonow RO, et al: Thiazolidinedione use, fluid retention, and congestive heart failure. A consensus statement from the American Heart Association and American Diabetes Association. Diabetes Care 2004;27:256-263.

Pihoker C, Gilliam LK, Hampe CS, Lernmark A: Autoantibodies in diabetes. Diabetes 2005;54:S52-S61.

Riddle MC, Rosenstock J, Gerich J: The treat-to-target trial: Randomized addition of glargine or human NPH insulin to oral therapy of type 2 diabetic patients. Diabetes Care 2003;26:3080-3086.

Saudek CD, Herman WH, Sacks DB, et al: A new look at screening and diagnosis of diabetes mellitus. J Clin Endocrinol Metab 2008;May 6, epub ahead of print.

Diabetes Mellitus in Children and Adolescents

Method of
Lori M. B. Laffel, MD, MPH, and
Jamie R. S. Wood, MD

Diabetes mellitus is a group of metabolic disorders that have hyperglycemia as a common feature caused by inadequate insulin secretion, insulin action, or both. Chronic hyperglycemia and its numerous downstream effects lead to micro- and macrovascular complications involving the eyes, kidneys, nerves, and blood vessels. Childhood and adolescent years are periods of rapid physical growth and psychosocial change, and these two factors make the care of children and adolescents with diabetes both challenging and rewarding. The health care professional must balance the important goals of optimal glycemic control and normal growth and development along with the risks of hypoglycemia and the challenges of expected glycemic excursions during childhood. Multidisciplinary care is the hallmark of successful diabetes management for the child and adolescent with diabetes and for family members.

The American Diabetes Association (ADA) classifies diabetes mellitus into four main types: type 1 diabetes (T1D), type 2 diabetes (T2D), other specific types, and gestational diabetes mellitus (Table 1). T1D is caused by insulin deficiency, which results from the autoimmune destruction of the pancreatic β cells. There are multiple genetic loci in the major histocompatibility region of chromosome 6 that predispose (DR 3/4, DQ 0201/0302, DR 4/4, and DQ 0300/0302) or protect against (DQB1∗0602, DQA1∗0102) the development of T1D. T2D is caused by the combination of insulin resistance and relative insulin deficiency.

Genetic forms of diabetes include maturity-onset diabetes in the young (MODY), mitochondrial diabetes, and certain syndromes of insulin resistance. MODY is characterized by young age of onset, autosomal dominant inheritance, the lack of association with obesity,

---

[1]Not FDA approved for this indication.

TABLE 1 Classification of Diabetes Mellitus*

Type 1 diabetes
Type 2 diabetes
Other specific types:
- Genetic defects of β-cell function
  - MODY 1: chromosome 20, HNF-4α
  - MODY 2: chromosome 7, glucokinase
  - MODY 3: chromosome 12, HNF-1α
  - MODY 4: chromosome 13, IPF-1
  - MODY 5: chromosome 17, HNF-1β
  - MODY 6: chromosome 2, NeuroD1
  - Mitochondrial diabetes
- Genetic defects in insulin action
  - Leprechaunism
  - Rabson-Mendenhall syndrome
- Diseases of the exocrine pancreas
  - Pancreatitis
  - Cystic fibrosis
  - Pancreatectomy
- Endocrinopathies
  - Acromegaly
  - Cushing's syndrome
  - Glucagonoma
  - Pheochromocytoma
- Drug or chemical induced
  - Glucocorticoids
- Infections
  - Congenital rubella
  - Cytomegalovirus
- Other genetic syndromes associated with diabetes
  - Down's syndrome
  - Klinefelter's syndrome
  - Turner's syndrome
Gestational diabetes mellitus (GDM)

*Table is not all inconclusive and gives examples of each subtype of diabetes mellitus. For complete list, see American Diabetes Association: Diagnosis and classification of diabetes mellitus. Diabetes Care 2005;28 (Suppl 1):S37-S42.
Abbreviations: MODY = maturity-onset diabetes in the young.

CURRENT DIAGNOSIS

ADA Recommendations for the Diagnosis of Diabetes

- Symptoms (polyuria, polydipsia, unexplained weight loss) and a casual plasma glucose (any time of day without regard to time since last meal) ≥200 mg/dL (11.1 mmol/L) or
- Fasting (no caloric intake for at least 8 h) plasma glucose ≥126 mg/dL (7.0 mmol/L) or
- 2-hour plasma glucose ≥200 mg/dL (11.1 mmol/L) during an oral glucose tolerance test (glucose load of 75 g anhydrous glucose dissolved in water or 1.75 g/kg body weight if weight <43 kg).

Note: Criteria 2 and 3 should be confirmed on a second day if child/adolescent is asymptomatic. The OGTT is not recommended for routine clinical use and should be reserved for the asymptomatic child with incidental glucosuria/hyperglycemia or in the child with suspected diabetes but normal fasting plasma glucose.
Adapted from American Diabetes Association: Care of children and adolescents with type 1 diabetes. Diabetes Care 2005;28(1):186-212.

---

and a variable phenotype. The most common disease of the exocrine pancreas that causes diabetes in children and adolescents is cystic fibrosis. Glucocorticoids used in the treatment of systemic illnesses are also commonly associated with hyperglycemia and diabetes. Certain genetic syndromes, such as Down syndrome, Klinefelter's syndrome, and Turner's syndrome, increase the risk for diabetes.

Diagnosis

The diagnosis of T1D in children and adolescents is typically straightforward. The classic symptoms of polyuria, polydipsia, polyphagia, and weight loss over a several-week period are common. A thorough history and physical exam may reveal perineal candidiasis or thrush. Such symptoms may be followed by nausea, abdominal pain, vomiting, lethargy, and Kussmaul respirations if diabetic ketoacidosis (DKA) and lactic acidosis develop. The presentation of T2D in children and adolescents can be more subtle and sometimes even clinically silent. However, approximately a third of adolescents with T2D have ketosis and a quarter have ketoacidosis at presentation.

The Current Diagnosis box outlines the diagnosis of diabetes mellitus. In the asymptomatic child or adolescent, diabetes is diagnosed when a fasting plasma glucose is 126 mg/dL or more, a 2-hour plasma glucose during an oral glucose tolerance test (OGTT) is 200 mg/dL or more, or a random plasma glucose is 200 mg/dL or more with confirmation on a second day. The symptomatic child or adolescent with a random plasma glucose of 200 mg/dL or more does not need repeat testing to confirm the diagnosis. Measurement of islet cell autoantibodies consistent with T1D (GAD, insulin, IA2) at diagnosis may help distinguish between type 1 and T2D. Care must be taken to avoid delay in the diagnosis and initiation of treatment because of the risk of rapid metabolic deterioration with insulin deficiency.

Initial Management

The goals of initial management of the child or adolescent newly diagnosed with diabetes mellitus are to correct fluid and electrolyte imbalances, reverse hepatic gluconeogenesis and ketogenesis by halting lipolysis with insulin replacement, and begin the process of diabetes education. The location of this initial management depends on the severity of the clinical presentation, the age of the patient, the psychosocial assessment of the child or adolescent and caregiver, and the diabetes-related resources available in the family's geographic location (availability of an outpatient education program).

Diabetic Ketoacidosis

Approximately 30% of children with newly diagnosed T1D present with diabetic ketoacidosis (DKA). Children who are younger (less than 4 years), without a first-degree relative with T1D, and from a family of lower socioeconomic status are at higher risk of DKA at onset of T1D. The majority of DKA episodes occur in patients with established diabetes, not in those newly diagnosed. Children or adolescents with established T1D are at higher risk for DKA if they are in poor metabolic control, have had a previous episode of DKA, are peripubertal/adolescent girls, have a psychiatric disorder, or are from a disadvantaged background.

Management of DKA in children and adolescents is based on the same principles used in adults and therefore is covered in a separate chapter in this book. The development of cerebral edema, however, warrants discussion because this complication is seen primarily in children and is associated with both high morbidity and mortality. Risk factors for the development of cerebral edema include lower initial partial pressure of carbon dioxide, higher initial serum urea nitrogen concentrations, treatment with bicarbonate, and an attenuated rise in measured serum sodium concentrations during therapy. In addition, children who are younger (less than 5 years), have new-onset T1D, and longer duration of symptoms may also be at an increased risk. A high index of suspicion is needed with mannitol (Osmitrol) at the bedside to allow for timely intervention.

Initiation of Insulin Replacement Therapy

Subcutaneous insulin is initiated in the patient who does not present in DKA or following intravenous insulin therapy in the child with resolved DKA who is tolerating oral intake (pH of ≥ 7.3, $tCO_2 \geq 18$, anion gap 12 ± 2 mEq/L). The starting dose of insulin replacement therapy depends on the age, weight, and pubertal status of the patient, as well as the presence or absence of DKA. For the prepubertal child without DKA, the starting dose is usually 0.25 to 0.5 U/kg/day. For the prepubertal child with resolved DKA, the usual starting dose is 0.5 to 0.75 U/kg/day. For the pubertal child without DKA, the starting dose is 0.5 to 0.75 U/kg/day and for the pubertal child with resolved DKA, 0.75 to 1 U/kg/day. This total daily dose (TDD) of insulin is typically divided into either two or three injections per day, with the latter the preference toward implementation of intensive therapy (Figure 1). The twice-daily regimen may be selected for the younger (less than 4 years) child or if the psychosocial assessment determines that fewer injections per day would be beneficial. The use of an insulin pump at diagnosis remains within the research realm currently.

When the patient is metabolically stable, the focus turns to the psychosocial assessment of the child or adolescent and caregiver(s) and the initiation of diabetes education. A licensed social worker or other mental health professional evaluates each family and screens for circumstances that might complicate diabetes management: family composition, alternative caregiver(s), financial concerns, lack of health insurance, psychiatric or medical illness in a family member, or severe emotional distress of caregiver secondary to the diabetes diagnosis.

Diabetes education is provided by a certified diabetes nurse educator (DNE) and focuses on the set of essential skills needed to keep a child or adolescent with diabetes safe at home and school. These survival skills include techniques of blood glucose monitoring, urine or blood ketone measurement, drawing up and administration of subcutaneous insulin and glucagon, recognition and treatment of hypoglycemia and hyperglycemia, basics of sick day management, and indications for and methods of contacting the child's diabetes team. In addition to the survival skills, the child or adolescent and family should meet with a registered dietician who will assist them in developing an individualized meal plan and introduce the family to the concept of carbohydrate counting or exchanges. Once the child or adolescent (if developmentally appropriate) and caregiver(s) demonstrate the knowledge and skills needed, they are discharged with the expectation of daily phone contact with a member of their diabetes team to further titrate insulin doses and answer questions. When available and clinically indicated, a visiting nurse may assist with ongoing home-based education and support in the short term.

Outpatient Diabetes Care

The management of children and adolescents with diabetes requires a multidisciplinary team approach. Members of this team include either a pediatric endocrinologist or pediatrician with training in diabetes, a pediatric DNE, a dietician, and a mental health professional (social worker and psychologist). Members of this team need to be easily accessible to the family in times of illness or metabolic crisis. Another member of the child/adolescent's team is a pediatrician or family doctor who will continue to provide routine well child care including anticipatory guidance, immunizations, and general medical care.

In the first few months of outpatient diabetes care, patients are seen frequently by members of the diabetes team to assess the family's adaptation to the new diagnosis, reinforce skills and knowledge learned during the first few days, and expand on the skills and knowledge needed for intensive diabetes management. Patients are subsequently seen at a minimum frequency of every 3 months, alternating between their DNE and their pediatric endocrinologist. Visits with the dietician are recommended yearly or more frequently if circumstances warrant (e.g., young child or toddler, desired weight loss, initiating pump therapy, etc.).

Diabetes Education

Diabetes education is an ongoing process with continuous need for review of previously learned material and introduction of new concepts as the family develops a more sophisticated understanding of intensive diabetes management. The educator should evaluate the patient and his or her caregiver's knowledge and skills regularly. In addition, age-appropriate issues need to be discussed as the patient matures (e.g., driving guidelines, issues related to alcohol and smoking, etc.). Diabetes education needs to be tailored to each family taking into account their educational level and cultural practices. The educator must be sensitive to the age and developmental stage of the child or adolescent, and shift his or her educational efforts from the caregiver(s) to the adolescent when it is developmentally appropriate. Continued parental involvement and supervision of the adolescent with diabetes is crucial to good metabolic control.

The health care provider should complete a focused interval history at each visit that includes recent illnesses, visits to the emergency department, hospitalizations, medications prescribed other than insulin, types of insulin and current doses, daily routine including meal plan and activity level, self-care behaviors and identifying who performs them, episodes of hypoglycemia and their precipitants, school performance, emotional health, and a review of systems focusing on symptoms of hyperglycemia (polyuria, polydipsia, polyphagia, weight loss, candidal infections) and the possible development

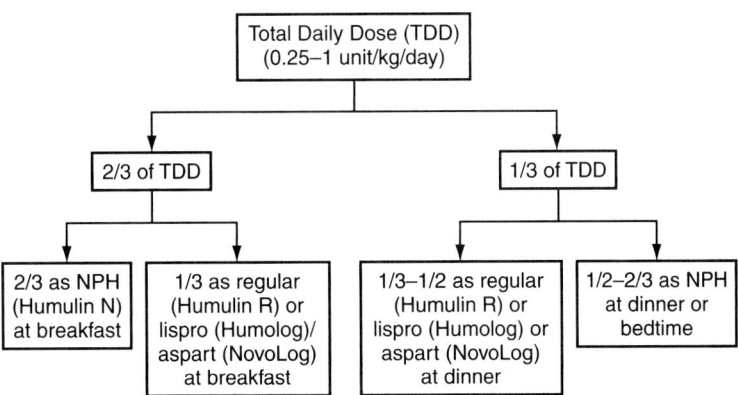

FIGURE 1. Initiation of Insulin Replacement Therapy. Two thirds of the total daily dose (TDD) is given at breakfast and further divided into NPH (two thirds) and short/rapid-acting insulin (one third). The remaining one third is either given in one injection at dinner (in a twice-daily regimen) or divided between dinner and bedtime (in a thrice-daily regimen), and should also be divided into NPH (two thirds) and short/rapid-acting insulin (one third). Short/rapid-acting insulin can be regular (Humulin R), lispro (Humalog), or aspart (NovoLog).

of other autoimmune disorders. If appropriate, a history of tobacco, alcohol, recreational drugs, and sexual activity should be elicited. A focused physical examination that includes measurement of blood pressure and heart rate, weight, height, body mass index (BMI), and examination of the thyroid gland, sites of blood glucose monitoring, and insulin injections should be completed at each visit. A more thorough physical examination including Tanner staging should be performed once per year or more frequently if indicated.

The hemoglobin A1C, the fraction of hemoglobin that has glucose attached to it, is a measure of the average level of blood glucose over the preceding 2 to 3 months. It should be measured every 3 months and serves as an objective measure of blood glucose control. A discrepancy between the hemoglobin A1C and the average blood glucose levels from self-monitoring records suggests that the patient needs to monitor at different times of day, may benefit from a review of blood glucose monitoring technique and equipment, or there may be fabrication of results. Obtaining computer downloaded data helps eliminate the latter possibility.

Goals of Therapy

The Diabetes Control and Complications Trial (DCCT) demonstrated that the incidence of microvascular complications was reduced with improved blood glucose control (hemoglobin A1C approximately 7%). The reduction in complications, however, was accompanied by an increased risk of severe hypoglycemia. Because young children are more vulnerable to hypoglycemia (reduced catecholamine response to hypoglycemia, decreased ability to communicate symptoms of hypoglycemia, and risk for neuropsychologic impairment from hypoglycemia), the ADA has developed age-specific glycemic targets (Table 2).

Insulin Therapy

The ideal insulin replacement therapy would be one that mirrors the basal and prandial insulin secretion in individuals without diabetes. Numerous insulin preparations are available that vary in time to onset, peak, and duration of action (Table 3). No single regimen is superior to another; thus individualization of the insulin regimen to the child or adolescent and family remains a major determinant. Important factors for consideration include blood glucose monitoring frequency, number of daily injections the family can perform, the need for flexibility in meal planning, and the unique family schedule. Regimens range in intensity from twice-a-day injections with a set dose of premixed insulin to intensive diabetes management with multiple injections per day of two or more types of insulin or use of an insulin pump (continuous subcutaneous insulin infusion [CSII]).

TABLE 2 Blood Glucose and A1C Goals for Type 1 Diabetes by Age Group

Age Group	Plasma Blood Glucose Range (mg/dL) Before Meals	Bedtime/ Overnight	A1C
<6 y	100–180	110–200	7.5%–8.5%
6–12 y	90–180	100–180	<8%
13–19 y	90–130	90–150	<7.5%

Goals should be individualized; lower goals may be reasonable and achievable without hypoglycemia.
Goals should be higher in patients with frequent hypoglycemia or hypoglycemia unawareness.
Adapted from American Diabetes Association: Care of children and adolescents with type 1 diabetes. Diabetes Care 2005;28(1):186-212.

CURRENT THERAPY

Examples of Insulin Regimens

Injections bid:
- Insulin mixtures (70/30, 75/25) given at breakfast and dinner
- NPH and rapid- or short-acting insulin given at breakfast and dinner

Injections tid:
- NPH and rapid- or short-acting insulin given at breakfast, rapid- or short-acting insulin given at dinner, and NPH given at bedtime
- NPH and rapid- or short-acting insulin given at breakfast, rapid- or short-acting insulin given at dinner, and NPH or glargine (Lantus) given at bedtime

Injections qid:
- NPH and rapid-acting insulin given at breakfast, rapid-acting insulin given at lunch and dinner, and rapid-acting insulin and NPH given at bedtime
- NPH and rapid-acting insulin given at breakfast and lunch, rapid-acting insulin given at dinner, and NPH given at bedtime
- Rapid-acting insulin given at breakfast, lunch, and dinner, and glargine (Lantus) given at breakfast, dinner, or bedtime

Continuous subcutaneous insulin infusion (CSII)
- Rapid-acting insulin given for basal requirements and as bolus at every meal/snack and periodically to correct hyperglycemia (no more frequent than q2-3h)

The typical regimen that children or adolescents begin at diagnosis was described previously (Figure 1). Some centers initiate a basal-bolus regimen in which insulin is replaced in a manner that attempts to mimic physiologic insulin release. Basal-bolus regimens include the insulin pump and glargine (Lantus) given once a day with rapid-acting insulin (lispro [Humalog] or aspart [NovoLog]) before each meal/snack and as needed for correction of hyperglycemia. The school-age child who hopes to avoid an injection at lunch often benefits from a regimen of glargine (Lantus) at dinner or bedtime, along with NPH (Humulin N) and a rapid-acting insulin at breakfast, plus a rapid-acting insulin at dinner. The peak of the NPH covers carbohydrate intake at lunch. The use of basal insulin analogue glargine (Lantus) in the evening is associated with less nocturnal hypoglycemia.

Patients on a basal-bolus regimen determine their insulin doses based on an insulin-to-carbohydrate ratio and a correction factor or sensitivity index (CF or SI). The insulin-to-carbohydrate ratio is the number of grams of carbohydrate covered by 1 U of insulin (roughly 450 divided by TDD) for each meal and snack. The CF/SI is the expected decrement in glucose following 1 U of rapid-acting insulin (roughly 1650 divided by TDD). The CF/SI is applied no more than every 2 to 3 hours to lower an elevated blood glucose toward the target range to avoid so-called stacking of insulin action and subsequent hypoglycemia. For patients on a combination of intermediate-acting insulin (NPH) and rapid- or short-acting insulin, meals typically contain a certain amount of carbohydrates (e.g., 60 g or 4 carbohydrate exchanges) and require consistency in timing to avoid hypoglycemia.

The CSII, otherwise known as insulin pump therapy, comes the closest to mimicking the basal and prandial insulin secretion of an individual without diabetes. The insulin pump is steadily becoming a commonly used method to replace insulin, especially in the pediatric population. There are many advantages to the insulin pump including the elimination of multiple daily injections, increased flexibility in meal planning,

TABLE 3 Insulin Analogues

Insulin Preparation	Onset of Action	Peak Action	Effective Duration
Rapid Acting			
Insulin lispro	5–15 min	30–90 min	2–4 h
Insulin aspart	5–10 min	60–180 min	3–5 h
Insulin glulisine*	5–15 min	30–90 min	3–5 h
Short Acting			
Regular (soluble insulin)	30–60 min	2–3 h	3–6 h
Intermediate Acting			
Lente (insulin zinc preparation)[†]	3–4 h	4–12 h	12–18 h
NPH (isophane insulin)	2–4 h	4–10 h	10–16 h
Long Acting			
Ultralente (extended insulin zinc preparation)[†]	4–6 h	8–20 h	20–24 h
Insulin glargine	1.1 h	None	24 h
Insulin detemir*	2–3 h	6–14 h	16–24 h
Insulin mixtures			
70/30 human mix[‡] (70% NPH, 30% regular)	30–60 min	dual	10–16 h
70/30 aspart analogue mix (70% intermediate, 30% aspart)[‡]	5–15 min	dual	10–16 h
75/25 lispro analog mix[‡] (75% intermediate, 25% lispro)	5–15 min	dual	10–16 h
50/50 human mix (50% NPH, 50% regular)	30–60 min	dual	10–16 h

*FDA approved for adult use only.
In many countries, including the United States, insulin preparations contain 100 U/mL and are referred to as U-100 insulin. Highly concentrated U-500 short-acting insulin is available and used primarily in adults with severe insulin resistance.
[†]Recently discontinued by manufacturer (Lilly); estimated to be available until end of 2005.
[‡]Typically used in fixed doses in twice-a-day insulin regimens.
Profiles for each insulin preparation are reasonable estimates only, based on data from adult study participants. There is variation between individuals, and time of onset, peak, and duration are also affected by size of dose, site and depth of injection, dilution, exercise, and temperature.

ease of decreasing insulin for physical activity, fewer hypoglycemic events, and the ability to deliver very small amounts of insulin. The disadvantages are more frequent blood glucose monitoring, always being tethered to the pump, and increased risk for the development of DKA. Because only rapid-acting insulin (lispro [Humalog] or aspart [NovoLog]) is used in the insulin pump, discontinuation of insulin delivery can result in ketone production within hours. Increased vigilance, therefore, is necessary to ensure proper functioning of the insulin pump with frequent blood glucose monitoring and checking for ketones if hyperglycemia develops.

Self-Monitoring

One of the main goals of diabetes education is to teach and empower the patient and family in the self-management of diabetes. Self-management of diabetes includes measuring blood glucose and blood/urine ketone levels, recording the results along with amount of carbohydrate intake and amount of insulin administered, and the ability to make insulin dosing decisions based on the interpretation of these records. Monitoring blood glucose four or more times daily is recommended in children with T1D. Additional monitoring may be necessary postprandially, overnight, or during periods of increased physical activity to help optimize control and prevent severe hypoglycemia. Preschool or early school-age children may require more frequent monitoring because of their inability to recognize symptoms or to communicate during episodes of hypoglycemia. In addition, children and adolescents using the insulin pump typically check their blood sugar six or more times per day. Ketone measurements should be done whenever the blood glucose is greater than 250 to 300 mg/dL and/or if the patient is ill, especially with nausea, vomiting, or abdominal pain. Ketones can be measured either in the urine (acetoacetate and acetone) or blood (β-hydroxybutyric acid). Measurement of blood ketones is now available on a home meter and is the preferred method in the current era stressing blood glucose monitoring. The key to successful intensive diabetes management is frequent blood glucose monitoring, good record keeping, and communication of these results with the diabetes team at frequent intervals so that timely modifications can be made to the insulin regimen and/or meal plan.

Medical Nutrition Therapy

The meal plan remains an important component of management aimed at good glycemic control, although it is often the most difficult aspect of intensive diabetes management for families. A dietician trained in pediatric nutrition and diabetes should meet with the family at the time of T1D diagnosis and periodically thereafter. The dietician should help develop a meal plan that is individualized to the patient's daily schedule, food preferences, cultural influences, and physical activity. The meal plan is more likely to be successful if it is designed to fit into the family's already established schedule and preferences. The patient and family should also be instructed on carbohydrate counting so that either carbohydrate exchanges or insulin-to-carbohydrate ratios can be used. Like the child without diabetes, the total number of recommended calories follows the child's growth requirements along with consideration of the need for weight gain or loss. Growth velocity, weight gain, and BMI should be monitored at every visit to ensure that the meal plan is sufficient to meet the energy requirements of the patient. Unexpected weight loss or poor weight gain should prompt consideration of suboptimal metabolic control, as well as eating disorders, thyroid dysfunction, or gastrointestinal disease.

The ADA does not have pediatric specific guidelines for medical nutrition therapy, but the recommendations for adults can be extrapolated to children. The ADA recommends that carbohydrates provide 45% to 65% of total calories, with protein and fat contributing 15% and 30%, respectively. The patient and family should be educated to avoid foods high in cholesterol, saturated fat, and concentrated sweets and select foods high in complex carbohydrate and dietary fiber.

All children and adolescents are recommended to have three meals per day. If they receive intermediate-acting insulin preparations, they should also receive three snacks per day (morning, afternoon, and bedtime) to match anticipated peaks of insulin action. If the child or adolescent is on a basal-bolus regimen, snacks are optional and require insulin coverage based on insulin-to-carbohydrate ratios.

Exercise

Exercise, or periods of sustained physical activity, can be beneficial to the patient by contributing to a sense of well-being, helping achieve the recommended BMI, improving glycemic control (exercise enhances insulin sensitivity), improving the lipid panel (increasing HDL), and lowering blood pressure and improving cardiovascular fitness. All children and adolescents, especially those with diabetes, should be encouraged to participate in routine physical activity.

The child or adolescent with diabetes needs to take precautions to avoid hypoglycemia during periods of increased physical activity. The patient and family need to check blood glucose before the initiation of activity, every hour during sustained activity, and at the completion of physical activity. For the first several days of increased activity, the child should also check his or her blood sugar frequently during the 12-hour postexercise period because there is often a delayed drop in the blood glucose following exercise (i.e., the lag effect). Some children require additional carbohydrate before, during, and after activity; lower insulin doses on the days of increased physical activity; or both. It is suggested that the child take 5 to 15 g of carbohydrates, depending on age and exercise intensity, before exercise if the blood sugar is below target, and repeat the 5 to 15 g of carbohydrate for every 30 minutes of sustained activity. Rapid-acting carbohydrate should be readily available, and coaches and trainers should be aware of the diagnosis of diabetes and trained in the treatment of hypoglycemia.

Psychosocial Support

The mental health professional is an important member of the diabetes team. A thorough family assessment generally accompanies the diabetes diagnosis with appropriate referrals for additional services as needed. Thereafter, children or adolescents should be referred back to a mental health professional if social, emotional, or economic barriers to the achievement of good glycemic control are identified. Family conflict, especially conflict over diabetes care, can be associated with deterioration in glycemic control. Encouragement of ongoing family teamwork in the management of childhood diabetes promotes successful outcomes with respect to glycemic control, reducing diabetes-specific conflict, and preventing acute complications and emergency assessments.

Sick Day Management

The goals for the management of children and adolescents during sick days are never omit insulin, prevent dehydration and hypoglycemia, monitor blood glucose frequently (every 2 to 4 hours), monitor for ketosis, provide supplemental rapid- or short-acting insulin doses (5% to 20% of TDD) depending on degree of hyperglycemia and ketosis, treat underlying illness, and have frequent contact with the diabetes team. The majority of DKA among children or adolescents with established diabetes is caused by insulin omission or errors in administration of insulin. Inadequate insulin therapy in the context of an intercurrent illness accounts for the remaining small percentage. Although it is more common for children to require more insulin during illnesses, some children require a reduction of the basal and/or rapid-acting insulin dose if he or she is unable to eat and the blood glucose is less than 200 mg/dL.

Families need to be educated about symptoms that warrant immediate medical attention, including signs of dehydration (dry mouth, sunken eyes, cracked lips, weight loss, dry skin), persistent vomiting for more than 2 to 4 hours, persistence of blood glucose levels greater than 300 mg/dL or ketones for more than 12 hours, or symptoms of DKA (nausea, abdominal pain, chest pain, vomiting, ketotic breath, hyperventilation, or altered consciousness). It is helpful for the diabetes team to review sick day management annually with the family (can accompany flu immunization) to avoid metabolic decompensation during intercurrent illness.

Hypoglycemia

Fear of hypoglycemia can be a common occurrence in the management of childhood diabetes, especially among caregivers, and can be a barrier to optimal glycemic control. Recognition and treatment of hypoglycemia are important topics for diabetes education. Families are trained to treat hypoglycemia with 10 to 15 g of rapid-acting carbohydrate, recheck blood glucose in 15 minutes, repeat treatment with 10 to 15 g if blood sugar remains below target, and follow with a protein-containing snack if a meal will not follow within 1 to 2 hours. This technique avoids the natural tendency to overtreat low blood glucose levels. Caregivers should also receive glucagon training (20 to 30 µg/kg; maximum 1 mg) for severe hypoglycemia and low-dose glucagon (1 U on an insulin syringe for every year of life up to 15 years) for impending hypoglycemia, for example, in the context of a gastrointestinal illness or inadvertent insulin administration (lispro given instead of NPH). A member of the diabetes team should assess frequency, treatment, awareness, and circumstances of hypoglycemia at each visit.

Screening for Diabetes-Related Complications

Patients, families, and caregivers worry about the risk of diabetes-related complications, and therefore the diabetes team must educate families and screen for complications with sensitivity and optimism, emphasizing prevention of complications and the maintenance of health. Screening for nephropathy, hypertension, dyslipidemia, and retinopathy are indicated.

Microalbuminuria (MA) is the first sign of diabetic nephropathy, and patients who develop persistent MA are at increased risk of progression to macroalbuminuria. Poor glycemic control, smoking, and a family history of essential hypertension are risk factors for the development of MA and nephropathy. Identification of persistent MA provides an opportunity for intervention and prevention of progressive renal disease through improvements in glycemic control and/or therapy with angiotensin-converting enzyme (ACE) inhibitors. There are currently no pediatric data on the use of angiotensin receptor blockers (ARBs). Table 4 outlines definitions, screening recommendations, and treatment.

Hypertension is an important predictor of the progression of diabetic nephropathy to end-stage renal disease. Hypertension in children and adolescents may go unrecognized because providers are not familiar with the gender-, age-, and height-specific definitions. Blood pressure should be measured every 3 months with standardized technique, using the proper size cuff. If elevated blood pressures are detected and confirmed, the first step is to exclude causes not related to diabetes. Table 4 outlines the definitions, screening recommendations, and treatment.

Dyslipidemia and diabetes are established risk factors for cardiovascular disease, and recent research suggests that a significant proportion of adolescents with diabetes already have evidence of atherosclerosis. Low-density lipoprotein (LDL) cholesterol is most closely associated with cardiovascular disease, and therefore, the ADA has developed guidelines for LDL cholesterol. Screening may be delayed until puberty if family history is negative for cardiovascular disease. A lipid profile should be performed on prepubertal children with diabetes who are older than 2 years if there is a positive family history of cardiovascular disease or if the family history is unknown. If the LDL cholesterol is less than 100 mg/dL, screening

TABLE 4 Screening for Diabetes-Related Complications

Complication	How to Screen	Definition	When to Screen	Therapy
Microalbuminuria	Spot urine sample timed overnight or 24-h collection	Spot urine albumin/creatinine ratio 30–299 µg/g or AER 20–199 µg/min from timed collection	Annual screening begins at 10 y or after ≥5 y duration of diabetes	Optimize glucose control, smoking cessation, normalize BP
Persistent microalbuminuria		2/3 of urine samples meet above criteria		Above, plus addition of ACE inhibitor
High-normal BP	Manual BP measurement with standard technique	Systolic or diastolic BP within the 90th–95th percentile for age, gender, and height	At every clinic visit	Dietary intervention, weight control, and exercise; if target BP not reached within 3–6 mo, then initiate pharmacologic therapy
Hypertension		Systolic or diastolic BP above the 95th percentile for age, gender, and height, or >130/80 on ≥3 occasions (whichever is lower)		Above, plus pharmacologic therapy titrated to achieve target BP

Note: Urine collection should not be performed following vigorous exercise, during an acute infection, during a female patient's menstrual cycle, or following an episode of severe hypoglycemia. Once angiotensin-converting enzyme (ACE) inhibitor is started, microalbumin excretion should be monitored q3–6 mo.
Target BP is <130/80 or <90th percentile for age, gender, and height. Initial drug treatment is ACE inhibition.
Abbreviations: AER = albumin excretion rate; BP = blood pressure.

---

can be repeated every 5 years. The mainstay of therapy for dyslipidemia is dietary management (saturated fat less than 7% of calories and less than 200 mg/day of cholesterol). Children with levels between 130 and 159 mg/dL should be started on medication if diet and lifestyle modification are unsuccessful after 6 months or if the child has additional risk factors for cardiovascular disease, such as obesity or hypertension. Pharmacotherapy is recommended if the LDL cholesterol is more than 160 mg/dL. The LDL goal for children with diabetes is less than 100 mg/dL.

Diabetic retinopathy is a feared complication because it is the leading cause of vision loss. According to the ADA, the first ophthalmologic exam should be requested when the child is 10 years or older and has had diabetes for more than 3 to 5 years. Examinations with an eye care professional with expertise in diabetic retinopathy should occur early.

Screening for Other Autoimmune Diseases

Children and adolescents with T1D are at an increased risk for other autoimmune diseases and should be screened accordingly. Approximately 15% of patients with T1D also have autoimmune thyroid disease. All children and adolescents should be screened for autoimmune thyroid disease at the time of diabetes diagnosis once metabolic control is established. TSH measurement is a useful initial screen, with and without measuring the presence of thyroid autoantibodies. Screening should be repeated yearly or if there is any clinical suspicion of thyroid disease (abnormal growth rate, symptoms of hypo- or hyperthyroidism, goiter on examination, erratic blood glucose control).

Another commonly associated disorder is celiac disease. Nearly 6% of patients with T1D have elevated levels of circulating autoantibodies to tissue transglutaminase. Celiac disease can cause diarrhea, weight loss or failure to gain weight, abdominal pain, fatigue, and unexplained hypoglycemia or erratic blood glucose secondary to malabsorption. Patients with T1D should be screened with circulating IgA autoantibody to tissue transglutaminase. A quantitative serum IgA level should be drawn at the same time to rule out IgA deficiency as a cause for falsely low IgA tissue transglutaminase levels. Positive antibodies should be confirmed with a second measurement, and if positive, a referral should be made to a gastroenterologist for small bowel biopsy. If the diagnosis is confirmed, celiac disease is treated with a gluten-free diet with recommendations and support from a registered dietician with pediatric expertise in diabetes and celiac management.

TABLE 5 Risk Factors and Screening for Type 2 Diabetes in Children

Criteria	Age of Initiation	Frequency	Method
Overweight (BMI >85th percentile for age and gender), weight for height >85th percentile, or weight >120% of ideal for height Plus 2 of the following risk factors: Family history of T2D in 1st- or 2nd-degree relative Race/ethnicity (American Indian, African American, Hispanic, Asian/Pacific Islander) Signs of or conditions associated with insulin resistance (acanthosis nigricans, PCOS, HTN, dyslipidemia)	10 y or at pubertal onset if puberty occurs at a younger age	q2y	Fasting plasma glucose

Note: Clinical judgment should be used to test for diabetes in high-risk patients who do not meet these criteria.
Abbreviations: BMI = body mass index; T2D = type 2 diabetes; HTN = hypertension; PCOS = polycystic ovarian syndrome.
Adapted from American Diabetes Association: Type 2 diabetes in children. Diabetes Care 2000;23(3):381-389.

TABLE 6 Medications to Treat Type 2 Diabetes

Class	Mechanism of Action	Adverse Effects
Biguanides (metformin)*	Decrease hepatic glucose production Increase peripheral glucose disposal	Gastrointestinal upset Lactic acidosis
Sulfonylureas (glimepiride, glyburide, glipizide)	Insulin secretagogues	Hypoglycemia Weight gain
Meglitinides (repaglinide, nateglinide)	Insulin secretagogues	Hypoglycemia Weight gain
α-Glucosidase inhibitors (acarbose)	Decrease gut carbohydrate absorption	Gastrointestinal upset
Thiazolidinediones (rosiglitazone and pioglitazone)	Decrease hepatic glucose production Increase peripheral glucose disposal	Weight gain Edema Increased liver enzymes Anemia

*Metformin (Glucophage) is the only medication with FDA approval for use in children.

Type 2 Diabetes Mellitus in Youth

With the increasing prevalence of childhood obesity during the last two decades, there is an increased occurrence of T2D in youth. Based on National Health and Nutrition Examination survey data, the prevalence of overweight children (defined as a body mass index greater than the 95th percentile for children and youth) increased from 5% in the 1970s to more than 15% by 1999. The epidemic of obesity follows the increased consumption of fast foods, increased consumption of soft drinks, increased sedentary behavior with more television watching, and decreased physical activity. Mirroring this epidemic of childhood obesity is the occurrence of T2D in children and adolescents. Before 1990, T2D in youth was a rare occurrence. By 2000, between 8% and 45% of all newly diagnosed cases of childhood diabetes were caused by T2D. T2D occurs most commonly in those with a family history of T2D; individuals from certain racial and ethnic minority groups including Native Americans, Hispanics, African Americans, and Asian and Pacific Islanders; those with obesity falling above the 85th percentile for BMI based on age and gender; and in association with markers of insulin resistance (Table 5). Markers of insulin resistance include the occurrence of acanthosis nigricans and polycystic ovarian syndrome (PCOS). In addition, other well-known risk factors include hypertension and hyperlipidemia.

As noted earlier, the diagnosis of T2D is based on fasting plasma glucose (FPG), 2-hour glucose value during an OGTT, or a casual glucose level. Because T2D often goes without symptoms, individuals who are overweight, have a positive family history of T2D, come from one of the high-risk racial and ethnic minority groups, and/or have markers of insulin resistance warrant screening for T2D. Screening can be performed with a FPG or OGTT when clinical concerns are high and the FPG is normal.

Currently one oral medication is approved for the treatment of T2D in youth. This medication is metformin (Glucophage), which is also available in a liquid formulation. The maximum recommended daily dose of metformin (Glucophage) in youth is 2000 mg/day divided as 1000 mg twice daily. Often patients with T2D present in ketoacidosis and require initial insulin therapy. The goal of management of the child with T2D is initial stabilization often with insulin therapy, metformin (Glucophage) directed at managing the insulin resistance, and education. Once glucose levels are stabilized, insulin dosage may be lowered along with continued treatment with metformin (Glucophage) and approaches to lifestyle management. Lifestyle management involves a healthy diet, increasing exercise, and decreasing sedentary behaviors.

Other medications used to treat T2D include second-generation sulfonylureas, meglitinides, thiazolidinediones, and α-glucosidase inhibitors, none of which is currently approved for use in pediatric patients. There is ongoing studies to assess the efficacy and safety of these medications (Table 6).

REFERENCES

American Diabetes Association: Diagnosis and classification of diabetes mellitus. Diabetes Care 2005;28(Suppl 1):S37-S42.
American Diabetes Association: Type 2 diabetes in children. Diabetes Care 2000;23(3):381-389.
Barroso I: Genetics of type 2 diabetes. Diabet Med 2005;22:517-535.
Dunger DB, Sperling MA, Acerini CL, et al: ESPE/LWPES consensus statement on diabetic ketoacidosis in children and adolescents. Arch Dis Child 2004;89:188-194.
Fox LA, Buckloh LM, Smith SD, et al: A randomized controlled trial of insulin pump therapy in young children with type 1 diabetes. Diabetes Care 2005;28:1277-1281.
Glaser N, Barnett P, McCaslin I, et al: The Pediatric Emergency Medicine Collaborative Research Committee of the American Academy of Pediatrics. N Engl J Med 2001;344(4):264-269.
Goodwin G, Volkening LK, Laffel LM: Younger age at onset of type 1 diabetes in concordant sibling pairs is associated with increased risk for autoimmune thyroid disease. Diabetes Care 2006;29(6):1397-1398.
Hannon TS, Rao G, Arslanian SA: Childhood obesity and type 2 diabetes mellitus. Pediatrics 2005;116(2):473-480.
Hirsch IB: Insulin analogues. N Engl J Med 2005;352:174-183.
Laffel LM, Vangsness L, Connell A, et al: Impact of ambulatory, family-focused teamwork intervention on glycemic control in youth with type 1 diabetes. J Pediatr 2003;142(4):409-416.
Rosenbloom AL: Cerebral edema in diabetic ketoacidosis and other acute devastating complications: Recent observations. Pediatr Diabetes 2005;6:41-49.
Silverstein J, Klingensmith G, Copeland K, et al: American Diabetes Association: Care of children and adolescents with type 1 diabetes. Diabetes Care 2005;28(1):186-212.
Wysocki T, Harris MA, Mauras N, et al: Absence of adverse effects of severe hypoglycemia on cognitive function in school-aged children with diabetes over 18 months. Diabetes Care 2003;26(4):1100-1105.

Diabetic Ketoacidosis

Method of
Isaiah D. Wexler, MD, PhD

Diabetic ketoacidosis (DKA) and the hyperglycemic hyperosmolar state (HHS) are two acute life-threatening complications associated with diabetes mellitus (DM). The mortality for DKA is declining, but it remains high for HHS. The morbidity and mortality are also higher at the extremes of age, possibly because of the delay in diagnosis or because of the presence of comorbid conditions, especially among the elderly.

Classically, DKA was considered a complication of type 1 DM (T1DM) and HHS of type 2 DM (T2DM). However, there is significant overlap, and children and adults with T2DM can present with DKA (especially among the nonwhite population), and HHS can occur in those with T1DM. Both DKA and HHS may be the presenting manifestation of new-onset diabetes.

Diagnosis

The diagnosis of DKA and HHS is laboratory based, but there are clinical manifestations that suggest the diagnosis. For both HHS and DKA, there are signs of dehydration and hypovolemia. However, as the dehydration in these entities is hypertonic; signs such as significant tachycardia and low blood pressure may only be prominent in advanced DKA and HHS. In DKA, there is a fruity or acetone smell to the breath, emesis, and abdominal pain, and when the pH is especially low (<7.1), the breathing pattern may be aberrant (Kussmaul breathing). Mental status changes can occur in both DKA and HHS, and patients may be frankly obtunded and even comatose. In HHS, the changes in sensorium may be gradual, and the index of suspicion for HHS should be high, especially in elderly or moribund patients with unexplained changes in mental status.

The diagnostic criteria for DKA and HHS are based on blood pH, serum bicarbonate, and the presence of significant ketosis as manifested by high levels of serum or urine ketones. The presence of acidosis defined as an arterial blood pH less than 7.3 and or serum bicarbonate less than 15 mmol, or both, in children and adults distinguish DKA from HHS. When the bicarbonate is in the range of 15 to 18 mmol, other criteria including the degree of ketonemia and ketonuria assist in the diagnosis of DKA. Serum bicarbonate is often a more accurate indication because the arterial pH is also affected by the ventilatory rate. For a diagnosis of HHS, the blood glucose must be greater than 600 mg/dL and the effective serum osmolality greater than 320 mOsm/L (which can be calculated by the formula 2 × serum Na [mEq/L] + serum glucose [mg/dL]/18). In HHS, the fluid and electrolytes losses are often more severe than in DKA. The presence of ketones in the urine does not negate the diagnosis of HHS.

Treatment

PRECIPITATING CAUSES

Key elements in the treatment of DKA and HHS are the identification of precipitating causes and stabilization of the patient. The pathophysiologic basis of hyperglycemic crisis is insulinopenia and elevation of counter-regulatory stress hormones including catecholamines, cortisol, and growth hormone. Among patients with an established diagnosis of DM, infection (even mild) and noncompliance with the medical regimen are the leading causes of DKA and HHS. As the use of insulin pumps is increasing, pump malfunction or misuse has also become a more common cause of DKA. A source of infection should be sought in any patient presenting with DKA.

Abdominal pain, which is often attributed to ketosis, may be a manifestation of acute appendicitis or pelvic inflammatory disease. Conversely, the diagnosis of DKA may be delayed because abdominal pain is attributed to an acute abdominal process.

Other factors associated with DKA and HHS include cardiovascular disease and the use of medications such as corticosteroids, thiazides, and sympathomimetic agents. DKA and HHS have also been associated with the use of atypical (second-generation) antipsychotic agents. Cocaine use has been found to precipitate DKA.

HHS can often occur in obtunded or intellectually limited persons whose fluid intake is restricted. Fluid restriction can precipitate dehydration and decreased renal function, leading to both hyperglycemia and hyperosmolarity.

Identification and treatment of the precipitating cause of DKA and HHS are extremely important because it is often difficult to stabilize the patient if the precipitant is not dealt with appropriately.

MANAGEMENT

The management of DKA and HHS is based on repairing the fluid deficit and correcting the metabolic derangements. The mainstay of DKA management is fluid replacement and insulin administration. Other supporting interventions include providing potassium and, when clinically indicated, phosphate and bicarbonate. Most patients respond well to treatment if it is instituted in a timely fashion. Pitfalls associated with the treatment of hyperglycemic crises include excessive fluids; inappropriate administration of insulin, bicarbonate, or potassium; and iatrogenically induced hypoglycemia.

In recent years, the American Diabetic Association, the Lawson Wilkins Pediatric Endocrine Society, and the European Society for Pediatric Endocrinology have developed consensus evidence-based protocols for treating DKA and HHS. These protocols are summarized in Tables 1 to 3. The basis for these protocols is discussed below.

Fluids

Patients with DKA and HHS often have a fluid deficit of 100 to 200 mL/kg of body weight. Patients with hyperglycemic crises can present with severe hypovolemic shock, and if signs of shock are present, patients should be given resuscitation fluids, usually with a 0.9% sodium chloride solution (normal saline). Normal saline is continued until the hemodynamic status is stabilized. Subsequently, 0.45% NaCl is substituted for normal saline to prevent sodium overload, especially in older patients who might have compromised cardiac function.

The rate of fluid administration is designed to correct the fluid deficits over 48 hours. In children, this means providing fluid at a rate that approximates 1.5 times the daily fluid maintenance requirement. For adults, the rate of fluid administration should be based on the hemodynamic and hydration status of the patient as determined by vital signs, the physical examination, urine output, and repeated measurements of renal function.

In patients with diminished cardiac or renal function, the rate of fluid administration might have to be modified, and in these situations, hemodynamic monitoring is appropriate. Caution needs to be exercised in terms of the amount of fluid administered, especially during the early hours of treatment, because excessive fluid administration has been associated with cerebral edema in children and adolescents, and it can cause fluid overload states or rapid osmotic shifts.

Insulin

Administration of insulin corrects hyperglycemia and the metabolic acidosis and ketosis of DKA. Many different modes of insulin administration have been used. Most authorities prefer providing insulin as an intravenous drip because this mode of delivery is easily regulated; there is a more-rapid attainment of pharmacologic levels of insulin in the blood. Intravenous administration of insulin is not associated with problems of absorption that can occur with insulin that is administered intramuscularly or subcutaneously, especially in states of dehydration and poor perfusion. Regular insulin has been the insulin of choice for treating hyperglycemic crises, but recent studies indicate that short-acting insulin analogues administered subcutaneously may be equally effective in the treatment of DKA in children and adults.

Optimally, the rate of decline for serum glucose levels should be between 50 and 75 mg/dL/hour so as to avoid rapid osmotic shifts. In some cases, serum glucose might not fall appropriately. This may be due to mistakes in preparing the insulin drip or failure to prime the tubing of the intravenous administration setup. Alternatively, the patient might have severe insulin resistance, excessive hepatic glucose production related to stress, or compromised renal function. In these

TABLE 1 Management of Diabetic Ketoacidosis and Hyperglycemic Hyperosmolar State in Children and Adolescents

Treatment	Precautions
Fluids	
Initial Treatment	
NS, 10-20 mL/kg during the first h	Amount of fluid administered depends on hydration status
	For a patient in shock, continue NS, 20 mL/kg/h until vital signs are stable
Subsequent Treatment	
Continue intravenous NS, 10 mL/kg/h for 1 h, then correct estimated fluid deficit over 48 h with 0.45% NaCl (usually at a rate equal to 1.5-2 times the daily maintenance requirement)	Overhydration must be avoided
	Do not exceed 3.5 L/m^2/24 h
	Use NS if patient has hyponatremia
Dextrose and Insulin	
Dextrose	
Add dextrose (5%) to 0.45% NaCl when serum glucose declines to ≤250 mg/dL	Maintain serum glucose at 150-250 mg/dL
	Might need to increase dextrose concentration to 10% if serum glucose is less than target levels
Insulin	
Intravenous regular insulin drip at a rate of 0.1 U/kg/h	If continuous intravenous insulin administration is not feasible, an alternative is to give SC or IM rapid-acting insulin or short-acting analogues at a dose of 0.1 U/kg/h after an initial insulin bolus of 0.3 U/kg
When pH is >7.25 and HCO$_3$ >15 mEq/L, lower insulin infusion to 0.05 U/kg/h until SC insulin therapy is begun	
Electrolytes	
Potassium	
Starting K$^+$ concentration in intravenous fluids 40 mEq/L	If serum K$^+$ <2.5 mEq/L, hold insulin drip, and administer KCl, 1 mEq/kg over 1 h; continue until serum K$^+$ ≥2.5 mEq/L
Maintain K$^+$ concentration at 3.5-5 mEq/L	
If necessary, adjust K$^+$ concentrations in infusate to 20-40 mEq/L	If serum K$^+$ >5 mEq/L, do not add KCl
	Some authorities recommend using both the chloride and phosphate salts of K$^+$ at a ratio of 2:1
Bicarbonate	
Only consider administering HCO$_3$ if pH <7.0	Do not administer HCO$_3$ if pH ≥7.0
HCO$_3$ 75 mEq should be added to a liter bag containing 0.45% NS and given at a rate that does not exceed 2 mEq/kg/h of HCO$_3$	
Monitoring	
Monitor vital signs and perform frequent neurologic examinations, including fundoscopic evaluation	Monitor blood gases, serum glucose, and serum electrolytes more frequently if pH <7.0 or is not rising appropriately, serum glucose is <150 mg/dL or declining at a rapid rate, and/or serum K$^+$ is <3.5 mEq/L or >5 mEq/L
Initially obtain blood gases, serum electrolytes including BUN and creatinine, glucose, and urinary ketones	
ECG monitoring in severe DKA	
Monitor fluid input, urine output, blood gases, electrolytes, and serum glucose every 2-4 h until stable	Check neurologic signs for evidence of cerebral edema (e.g., headache, drowsiness)

BUN = blood urea nitrogen; DKA = diabetic ktoacidosis; ECG = electrocardiogram; NS = normal saline.

situations, the insulin drip can be increased stepwise until the desired rate of serum glucose reduction is achieved. Too rapid a decline in the level of serum glucose may be the result of excessive fluid administration.

Dextrose

A major challenge in the treatment of hyperglycemic crises is the prevention of treatment-induced hypoglycemia, which can lead to changes in the level of consciousness due to reduced glucose delivery to the brain. When serum glucose levels reach target levels as listed in the tables, dextrose as a 5% solution is added to the intravenous fluids. Sometimes, especially in children, 5% dextrose is not adequate to maintain serum glucose in the target range, and it may be necessary to increase the concentration of dextrose in the administered intravenous fluids. A common mistake made in managing DKA is to lower the rate of insulin administration as a means of regulating the serum glucose. The fallacy of this approach is that the reduction in insulin administration slows the correction of acidosis and ketosis.

Potassium

During DKA and its treatment, there are significant shifts in total body and serum potassium. Before treatment, there is significant depletion of total body potassium associated with polyuria, but at the same time, the acidosis associated with DKA causes cellular extrusion of potassium into the blood, leading to an increase in serum potassium. During treatment of DKA, both insulin administration and correction of the acidosis drive potassium back into cells, thereby lowering serum potassium. Because changes in serum potassium may be difficult to predict, it is important to monitor serum potassium at the time of admission and frequently during treatment. Potassium should not be administered when the serum potassium is too high, and potassium replacement should be given simultaneously with insulin if serum potassium is low or even in the normal range (see Tables 1 and 2 for specific guidelines). Electrocardiogram monitoring is useful for early detection of potentially symptomatic hyperkalemia or hypokalemia.

TABLE 2 Management of Diabetic Ketoacidosis in Adults

Treatment	Precautions
Fluids	
Initial Treatment	
NS, 1 L/h for 1 h or until hemodynamically stable	Hemodynamic monitoring if evidence of cardiogenic or severe hypovolemic shock
	Rate of fluid administration may have to be modified in patients with cardiac compromise
Subsequent Treatment	
Patients with high or normal serum Na$^+$ should receive 0.45% NaCl at a rate of 250-500 mL/h depending on hydration status	Use NS in place of 0.45 NaCl if patient has hyponatremia
Continue fluid therapy until patient's hydration status is stabilized and the patient can take oral feeds	
Dextrose and Insulin	
Dextrose	
Add dextrose (5%) to 0.45% NaCl when serum glucose declines to $\leq$200 mg/dL	Maintain serum glucose at 150-200 mg/dL by adjusting the rate of fluid infusion (150-250 mL/h) and insulin administration (0.05-0.1 U/kg/h)
Insulin	
Intravenous regular insulin drip is initially administered as a bolus of 0.1 U/kg and then continued at a rate of 0.1 U/kg/h	An alternative is to give SC rapid-acting insulin short-acting analogues with an initial bolus of 0.2 U/kg
Monitor serum glucose hourly and if rate of glucose decline is <50-75 mg/dL, double rate of insulin infusion every h until the glucose falls at a rate of 50-75 mg/dL/h	Subsequently, the patient is given SC or IM regular or short-acting analogue insulin at a rate of 0.1 U/kg every hour
Continue insulin and glucose intravenous treatment until metabolic stability is achieved (glucose <200 mg/dL, pH >7.30, and HCO$_3$ >18 mEq/L) and the patient can begin SC insulin treatments	Monitor serum glucose hourly and if rate of glucose decline is <50-75 mg/dL, double the dose of the hourly insulin injection
Electrolytes	
Potassium	
K$^+$ concentration in intravenous fluids is 20-30 mEq/L	If serum K$^+$ is <3.3 mEq/L, hold insulin and administer KCl, 20-30 mEq/h; continue until serum K$^+$ is $\geq$3.3 mEq/L
Maintain serum K$^+$ concentration at 4-5 mEq/L	If serum K$^+$ is >5.3 mEq/L, do not add K$^+$
	Some authorities recommend giving both the chloride and phosphate salts of K$^+$ at a ratio of 2:1.
Bicarbonate	
Only consider administering HCO$_3$ if blood pH is $\leq$7.0	Do not administer HCO$_3$ if pH is >7.0
If pH is <6.9, give NaHCO$_3$ 100 mmol diluted in 400 mL of H$_2$O at a rate of 200 mL/h. For pH 6.9-7.0, administer NaHCO$_3$ 50 mmol in 200 mL of H$_2$O at a rate of 100 mL/h	
Continue administering HCO$_3$ until pH is >7.0	
Monitoring	
Monitor vital signs and perform frequent neurologic examinations, including fundoscopic evaluation	Monitor blood gases, serum glucose, and serum electrolytes more frequently if the pH is <7.0 or is not rising appropriately, serum glucose is <150 mg/dL or the rate is not falling appropriately, and/or serum K$^+$ is $\leq$3.3 or $\geq$5.3 mEq/L
Initially obtain blood gases, serum electrolytes, including BUN and creatinine, glucose, urinary ketones, and an ECG	
Monitor fluid input, urine output, blood gases, serum electrolytes, and serum glucose every 2-4 h until stable	Check hemodynamic, respiratory, and neurologic status for signs of overhydration

BUN = blood urea nitrogen; ECG = electrocardiogram; NS = normal saline.

Phosphate

Similar to serum potassium, there is a significant depletion in cellular phosphate as a result of hyperglycemic crises, and serum phosphate declines during treatment. Phosphate is an important molecule for energy metabolism, and severe hypophosphatemia is associated with muscle weakness, diminished cardiac contractility, and respiratory insufficiency. Reduced 2,3-diphosphoglycerate concentrations resulting from hypophosphatemia can impair tissue oxygenation. Repletion of phosphate remains a theoretical benefit because no clinical trials have conclusively shown a benefit to phosphate administration for treating hyperglycemic crises. However, it seems prudent to administer phosphate as a potassium salt (as detailed in the tables) to patients in whom the impact of hypophosphatemia may be significant, such as those with cardiac or pulmonary disease. If phosphate is administered, serum calcium should be monitored.

Bicarbonate

Significant controversy surrounds the use of bicarbonate in DKA. There is little evidence supporting a beneficial effect of bicarbonate administration in terms of improved outcomes, and there is some evidence from both clinical studies and animal models that the treatment of acidosis with bicarbonate might even be deleterious. Current recommendations are to not administer bicarbonate if the pH is 7.0 because insulin administration is sufficient to correct the acidosis. For cases in which the pH is

TABLE 3 Management of Hyperglycemic Hyperosmolar State in Adults

Treatment	Precautions
Fluids	
Initial Treatment	
NS, 1 L/h for 1 h or until hemodynamically stable	Hemodynamic monitoring if evidence of cardiogenic or severe hypovolemic shock
	Rate of fluid administration might have to be modified in patients with cardiac compromise
Subsequent Treatment	
Patients with high or normal serum Na+ should receive 0.45% NaCl at a rate of 250-500 mL/h depending on the hydration status	Use NS in place of 0.45 NaCl if patient has hyponatremia
Continue fluid therapy until patient's hydration status is stabilized, the serum osmolality is ≤315 mOsm/L, and the patient's mental status has returned to baseline	
Dextrose and Insulin	
Dextrose	
Add dextrose (5%) to 0.45% NaCl when serum glucose declines to ≤ 200-250 mg/dL	Maintain serum glucose at 150-200 mg/dL by adjusting the rate of fluid infusion (150-250 mL/h) and insulin administration (0.05-0.1 U/kg/h)
Insulin	
Intravenous regular insulin drip is initially administered as a bolus of 0.1 U/kg and then continued at a rate of 0.1 U/kg/h	Monitor serum glucose frequently to avoid hypoglycemia. Clinical signs of hypoglycemia may be unapparent due to obtunded state and underlying neurologic disease
Monitor serum glucose hourly, and if rate of glucose decline is <50 mg/dL, double rate of insulin infusion every h until the serum glucose falls at a rate of 50-75 mg/dL/h	
When serum glucose falls under 300 mg/dL, reduce insulin infusion to 0.05-0.1 U/kg/h to maintain the serum glucose at 250-300 mg/dL	
Continue insulin and glucose IV treatment until serum glucose is stabilized at 250-300 mg/dL and the patient can begin SC insulin therapy	
Electrolytes	
K+ concentration in intravenous fluids is 20-30 mEq/L	If serum K+ is <3.3 mEq/L, hold insulin and administer KCl 20-30 mEq/h; continue until serum K+ is >3.3 mEq/L
Maintain serum K+ concentration at 4-5 mEq/L	If serum K+ is >5 mEq/L, do not add K+
	Some authorities recommend giving both the chloride and phosphate salts of K+ at a ratio of 2:1
Monitoring	
Initially obtain arterial blood gas, CBC, serum electrolytes including BUN and creatinine, glucose, urinalysis, and an ECG	Monitor more frequently if serum glucose is <250 mg/dL or the rate is not falling appropriately and/or serum K+ is ≤3.3 or ≥5.3 mEq/L
Obtain serum or calculated osmolality	Check hemodynamic, respiratory, and neurologic status for signs of overhydration
Monitor electrolytes, serum glucose, serum osmolality, fluid input, and urine output every 2-4 h until stable	

BUN = blood urea nitrogen; CBC = complete blood count; ECG = electrocardiogram.

less than 7.0, recommendations are less clear. If bicarbonate is to be administered, it should be done slowly, and by the methods listed in Tables 1 and 2.

MONITORING

The treatment of DKA and HHS is based on physiology, and with appropriate treatment, most patients will respond. Difficulties in the management of DKA and HHS usually result from too-aggressive treatment with fluids, electrolytes, insulin, or bicarbonate. To prevent such problems, it is very important to monitor the clinical and biochemical status of the patient. Clinically, the neurologic status of patients must be monitored closely. The sudden development of lethargy, obtundation, or headache can herald cerebral edema in pediatric patients. Respiratory difficulties, signs of congestive heart failure, or mental status changes can indicate fluid overload or rapid osmotic shifts. Biochemically, it is important to monitor response to treatment in terms of correcting the acidosis and lowering serum glucose. Patients are also at risk for electrolyte abnormalities and hypoglycemia, and frequent measurement of serum glucose and electrolytes, including phosphate, should be performed. Because the management of DKA and HHS is fairly complicated, it is imperative that there be a bedside flowchart in which vital signs, central nervous system status, fluid input, type of fluid, urine output, and laboratory values are recorded as a function of time.

Complications

Many of the complications of DKA, including hypoglycemia and hypokalemia, have been addressed.

A significant complication, most prevalent among the pediatric population, is cerebral edema. Cerebral edema developing during the course of treatment of DKA is a major cause of morbidity and mortality in children with DKA. The causes of cerebral edema are unclear, but studies suggest that it may be due to excessive fluid administration, especially during the early course of treatment, severity of the initial presentation, rapid osmotic shifts, or administration of bicarbonate. In cases in which cerebral edema is suspected (e.g., headache, lethargy, confusion), the rate of fluid administration should be decreased immediately and the patient should be carefully monitored. If there are clinical signs of cerebral edema (e.g., posturing, changes in papillary reflexes, Cushing's triad), mannitol (Osmitrol) should be administered at a dose of 0.25 to 1.0 g/kg over 20 minutes. Alternatively, hypertonic saline (3%) can be given at a dose of 5 to 10 mL over 30 minutes. The decision to intubate and hyperventilate patients with cerebral edema should be based on the clinical situation and in consultation with medical intensivists.

Adults should be monitored for pulmonary edema, cerebral edema, vascular accidents related to thrombotic conditions, hyperviscosity, and disseminated intravascular coagulation.

Summary

DKA and HHS, in most cases, remain preventable. Compliance with treatment, frequent monitoring, and close contact with a physician or diabetes health professionals during times of illness can reduce the frequency of DKA and HHS. Early consultation with a diabetologist is warranted at the beginning of an intercurrent illness and can often prevent development of DKA or HHS at the earliest stages. Patient education regarding the appropriate use of insulin, sick day management, early signs of DKA and HHS, drug interactions, and the dangers of certain recreational drugs will continue to have a major role in reducing the incidence of recurrent DKA or HHS.

REFERENCES

Dunger DB, Sperling MA, Acerini CL, et al: ESPE/LWPES consensus statement on diabetic ketoacidosis in children and adolescents. Arch Dis Child 2004;89:188-194.

Kitabchi AE, Nyenwe EA: Hyperglycemic crises in diabetes mellitus: Diabetic ketoacidosis and hyperglycemic hypersosmolar state. Endocrinol Metab Clin N Am 2006;35:725-751.

Kitabchi AE, Umpierrez GE, Murphy MB, Kreisberg RA: Hyperglycemic crises in adult patients with diabetes: A consensus statement from the American Diabetes Association. Diabetes Care 2006;29:2739-2748.

Wolfsdorf J, Craig ME, Daneman D, et al: Diabetic ketoacidosis. ISPAD clinical practice consensus guidelines 2006-2007. Pediatric Diabetes 2007;8:28-43.

Hyponatremia

Method of
Gregory Proctor, MD, and Moshe Levi, MD

Hyponatremia is defined as plasma sodium (Na$^+$) concentration of less than 135 mEq/L. It is a common finding in the hospitalized patient, with an estimated inpatient incidence of 10% to 15%.

Hyponatremia arises when water intake exceeds the kidney's ability to excrete free water. Normal renal excretion of electrolyte free water requires that three processes be intact. First, glomerular filtration must occur with delivery of ultrafiltrate to the tubular lumen. Second, solute removal must occur in the thick ascending limb and distal tubule, where tubular fluid can be diluted. Third, circulating levels of antidiuretic hormone (ADH) must be appropriately low, minimizing tubular aquaporin channel expression and water reabsorption. When all three processes are intact, minimally dilute urine of 50 to 60 mOsm/kg is excreted. Therefore, a patient who excretes a normal dietary solute intake of 600 to 900 mOsm/day can excrete a maximum urine volume of 10 to 18 L/day. Most cases of hyponatremia are due to a renal impairment in water excretion arising from high circulating levels of ADH. The remainder of cases result from water intake in excess of renal water excretory capacity limited by renal solute abundance or glomerular filtration rate (GFR).

BOX 1 Causes and Classification of Hyponatremia

High Plasma Osmolality
- Hyperglycemia
- Hypertonic mannitol

Normal Plasma Osmolality (Pseudohyponatremia)
- Hyperlipidemia
- Hyperparaproteinemia

Low Plasma Osmolality
High Circulating ADH
- Cirrhosis
- Drugs
- ECV depletion
- Glucocorticoid deficiency
- Heart failure
- Hypothyroidism
- Pregnancy
- Severe hypoalbuminemia
- SIADH
- True volume depletion

Low Circulating ADH
- Acute or chronic renal failure
- Low solute intake (beer potomania)
- Primary polydipsia

Abbreviations: ADH = antidiuretic hormone (vasopressin); CKD = chronic kidney disease; ECV = effective circulating volume depletion; SIADH = secretion of inappropriate antidiuretic hormone.

Approach to Hyponatremia

Preliminary evaluation of hyponatremia should begin with measurement of the serum osmolality and classification into hypo-osmolar, normo-osmolar, or hyperosmolar hyponatremia (Box 1).

Hyperosmolar hyponatremia is most commonly caused by severe hyperglycemia as seen in diabetic ketoacidosis (DKA) or uncontrolled type 2 diabetes mellitus. It may also be seen during hypertonic infusion of mannitol (Osmitrol) used to treat intracranial hypertension. High serum concentrations of glucose resulting from insulinopenic states in types 1 and 2 diabetes mellitus cause water movement out of the intracellular space into the extracellular space, leading to dilution of the serum sodium (S_{Na}). For every 100 mg/dL increase in serum glucose, the serum sodium decreases by approximately 1.6 mEq/L. Treatment of hyperglycemia with insulin rapidly moves glucose into cells followed by water movement in the same direction, resulting in correction of the hyponatremia.

Normo-osmolar hyponatremia, also known as pseudohyponatremia, occurs when a component of the solid phase of plasma is increased, as seen in severe hypertriglyceridemia or paraproteinemia. Normo-osmolar hyponatremia is a laboratory artifact resulting in falsely low serum sodium. It occurs when flame photometry methods are used to measure sodium concentration in whole plasma and does not occur when serum is analyzed with direct potentiometry, which measures actual serum sodium concentration.

Hypo-osmolar hyponatremia is by far the most common form of hyponatremia and is the focus of the remainder of this chapter.

HYPO-OSMOLAR HYPONATREMIA: ASSESSMENT OF VOLUME STATUS

Following measurement of serum osmolality and exclusion of pseudohyponatremia and hyperosmolar hypernatremia, the next step in

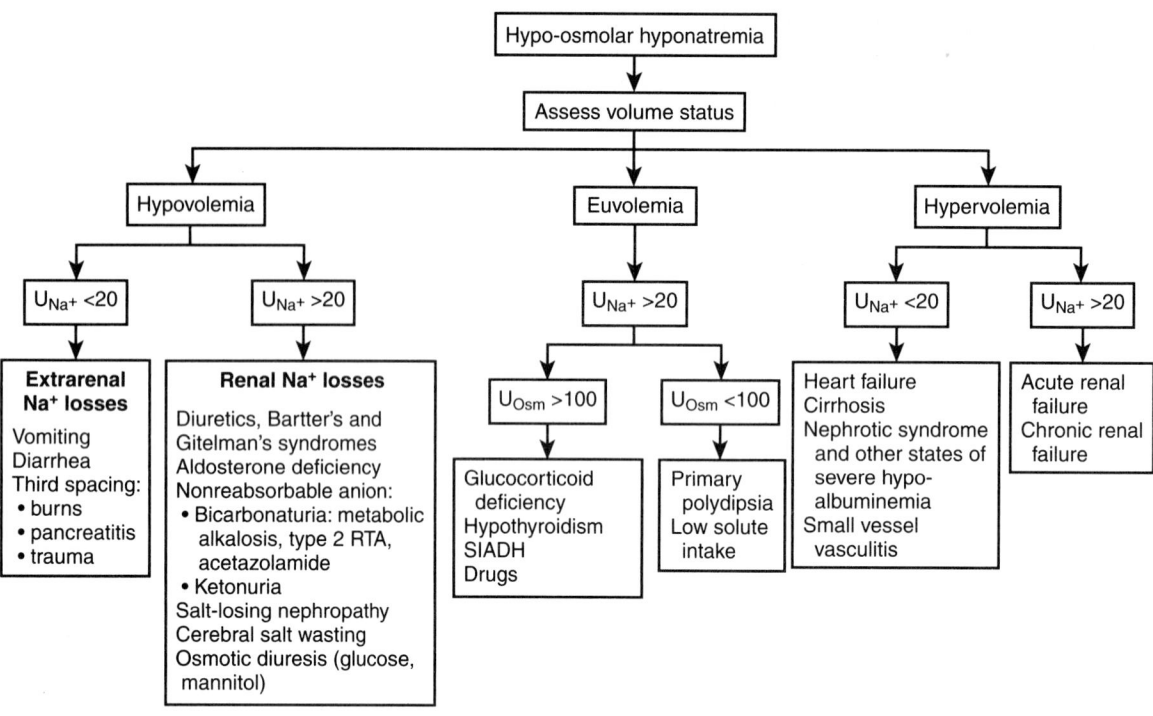

FIGURE 1. Diagnostic approach to hypo-osmolar hyponatremia. *Abbreviations:* RTA, renal tubular acidosis; SIADH, syndrome of inappropriate antidiuretic hormone secretion; U_{Na^+}, urinary sodium concentration (mEq/L); U_{Osm}, urine osmolality (mOsm/kg water).

evaluating hyponatremia is assessing the patient's volume status (Figure 1). A careful physical examination should be performed to determine the patient's effective circulating volume (ECV) and net total body sodium. This allows classification of the patient into one of three categories: hypovolemic hyponatremia (with a deficit in total body sodium), hypervolemic hyponatremia (with excess total body sodium), or euvolemic hyponatremia (with near-normal total body sodium).

Patients with *hypovolemic hyponatremia* have a deficit in total body sodium causing low ECV and nonosmotic release of antidiuretic hormone (ADH). High circulating ADH levels stimulate excessive renal water reabsorption and subsequent development of hyponatremia. Physical examination typically shows flat neck veins, absence of edema, dry mucous membranes and axillae, orthostatic hypotension, and tachycardia. When volume losses are nonrenal (due to hemorrhage, diarrhea, dermal losses, or third spacing of fluids as in pancreatitis or peritonitis), the spot urine sodium concentration (U_{Na^+}) is low, typically less than 20 mEq/L (see Figure 1). When volume losses are due in part to renal sodium wasting, the U_{Na^+} is greater than 20 mEq/L. Such renal sodium wasting may be seen in the presence of active diuretics, mineralocorticoid deficiency, osmotic diuresis, salt-losing nephropathy, bicarbonaturia (most commonly from vomiting), and ketonuria.

Hypervolemic hyponatremic patients have excess total body sodium manifested by edema. These patients have low ECV secondary to heart failure, cirrhosis, or severe hypoalbuminemia (as may be seen in the nephrotic syndrome). Low ECV stimulates nonosmotic release of vasopressin, renal water reabsorption, and subsequent hyponatremia. Spot urinary sodium is very low (often <10 mEq/L) due to avid renal sodium retention. Physical examination demonstrates any combination of peripheral edema, ascites, pulmonary congestion, and jugular venous distention. Hypervolemic hyponatremia may also be seen in acute or chronic renal failure where appropriate renal excretion of sodium and water is greatly decreased. In such situations, hyponatremia is dilutional, occurring as a result of water intake in excess of sodium intake. It is a common finding in patients with end-stage renal disease (ESRD) who cannot excrete large dietary water intake. The U_{Na^+} may be greater than 20 mEq/L in these cases because of either appropriate sodium excretion in the setting of high ECV or sodium wasting from frank tubular dysfunction.

Euvolemic hyponatremia is commonly seen in hospitalized patients. These patients have normal ECV and manifest no signs of edema or hypovolemia. They are in sodium balance and therefore have spot urinary sodium concentrations that reflect excretion of dietary intake (U_{Na^+} >20 mEq/L). Causes of euvolemic hyponatremia are hypothyroidism, glucocorticoid deficiency, acute emotional stress or psychosis, certain drugs, secretion of inappropriate ADH (SIADH), primary polydipsia, or very low solute intake. Circulating ADH levels are high in all these disorders except for primary polydipsia and low solute intake. High ADH levels are reflected by less than maximally concentrated urine (U_{Osm} >100 mOsm/kg). ADH levels are appropriately low in primary polydipsia and low solute intake as reflected by U_{Osm} less than 100 mOsm/kg. Drugs associated with euvolemic hyponatremia are believed to act largely by stimulating release of ADH from the posterior pituitary gland (Box 2) but can act to potentiate the effect of ADH on the distal tubule. SIADH may be caused by a wide variety of central nervous

---

BOX 2   Medications Associated with Euvolemic Hyponatremia

- Amitriptyline (Elavil)
- Antidepressants (especially SSRIs)
- Carbamazepine (Tegretol)
- Chlorpropamide (Diabinese)
- Clofibrate (Atromid-S)[2]
- Cyclophosphamide (Cytoxan)
- DDAVP (Desmopressin)
- Haloperidol (Haldol), thioridazine, thiothixene (Navane)
- Nonsteroidal anti-inflammatory drugs
- Oxytocin (Pitocin)
- Vincristine (Vincasar)

[2]Not available in the United States.
Abbreviation: SSRI = selective serotonin reuptake inhibitor.

CURRENT DIAGNOSIS

- Determine if hyponatremia is hypo-osmolar, normo-osmolar or hyperosmolar.
- If a hypo-osmolar state exists, perform a careful physical examination to establish the patient's volume status (presence of edema, jugular venous distention, ascites, orthostatic hypotension, dry mucous membranes).
- Then measure the urine sodium and osmolality to further narrow the differential diagnosis.

system (CNS) and pulmonary disorders as well as carcinomas of the lung, pancreas, and duodenum (Box 3).

SYMPTOMS

Symptoms of acute hyponatremia occur directly as a result of water movement into the brain and the development of cerebral edema. Early symptoms are anorexia and nausea and may occur even with mild reductions in serum sodium concentration. As hyponatremia worsens, depressed sensorium, seizures, coma, and death from cerebral herniation may occur. These symptoms cam occur even with mild reductions in serum sodium in young patients and constitute a medical emergency.

CEREBRAL ADAPTATION TO HYPONATREMIA

Cerebral adaptation to hypotonicity involves early movement of water (within 1-3 hours) out of cells into the CSF, followed by shunting into the systemic circulation. Next, brain cells adapt by losing cellular potassium, organic solutes, and then other organic osmolytes such as phosphocreatine, myoinositol, and amino acids. This adaptation requires 48 to 72 hours and is very effective in reducing brain swelling. Thus, when hyponatremia occurs slowly, allowing time for adaptation to occur, patients can present with few or no symptoms. When hyponatremia develops acutely, in less than 48 hours, adaptation has not had time to occur and patients are at high risk for developing cerebral edema and intracranial hypertension. Whereas patients with acute hyponatremia are particularly at risk for cerebral edema, those with chronic, asymptomatic hyponatremia (in whom cerebral adaptation has occurred) are at risk for osmotic demyelination syndrome if correction occurs too rapidly.

Treatment

Treatment of hyponatremia is dictated by presence or absence of symptoms and acute versus chronic development (Figure 2). Hyponatremia that develops in less than 48 hours is considered acute. If the time course is greater than 48 hours *or if the time-course is unknown*, then hyponatremia is considered chronic.

ACUTE HYPONATREMIA

Acute symptomatic hyponatremia should be treated promptly because of the high morbidity associated with acute cerebral edema. Serum Na$^+$ should be raised by 2 mEq/L/hour until symptoms resolve by infusing hypertonic saline (3% NaCl) at 1 to 2[3] mL/kg/hour. The rate of correction should aim for approximately 2 mEq/L/hour. Full correction is probably safe but is not necessary. In the setting of antidiuresis, where spot urinary sodium (U_{Na}) and potassium (U_K) concentrations sum to greater than 150 mEq/L ($U_{Na} + U_K > 150$ mEq/L), administration of furosemide (Lasix) with hypertonic saline ensures electrolyte-free water excretion and correction of hyponatremia.

CHRONIC HYOPNATREMIA

Chronic symptomatic hyponatremia must be handled with care. Promptly increase the serum Na$^+$ concentration by 10% (or by approximately 10 mEq/L). After completing this initial rapid correction, further correction should not exceed a rate of 1.0 to 1.5 mEq/L/hour or 12 mEq/L/24 hours.

Chronic asymptomatic hyponatremia is treated conservatively, because these patients are at risk for osmotic demyelination syndrome if correction is too rapid. No immediate intervention is needed. The underlying cause of hyponatremia should be carefully sought. If hypothyroidism or cortisol deficiency is present, then hormone replacement is indicated followed by close observation of the serum sodium. Likewise, if the cause is congestive heart failure, gentle diuresis and a trial of inotropes can improve myocardial function and ECV leading to improvement in hyponatremia. If the cause is hypovolemic hyponatremia, careful restoration of ECV by administration of 0.9% saline with careful observation of serum sodium is indicated. In general, if the underlying cause of hyponatremia cannot be identified or corrected (as in end-stage liver or heart disease, severe nephrotic syndrome, and some forms of SIADH) several approaches are available.

Fluid Restriction

Fluid restriction is usually successful if the patient is compliant. The degree of fluid restriction can be estimated by two methods. Division of the daily osmolar load by the minimal urine osmolality approximates the maximal urine volume and hence the daily fluid allowance. The daily osmolar load in a North American diet is estimated at approximately 10 mOsm per kilogram of body weight, and the minimal urine osmolality is obtained directly by measurement of the patient's urine osmolality. Therefore, fluid restriction (liters) is less than the daily osmolar load (mOsm/day)/U_{Osm} (mOsm/L). The second method employs simultaneous measurement of spot urinary sodium, potassium, and serum sodium concentrations and a calculation of:

$$\text{Urine osmolality} = \frac{(U_{Na} + U_K)}{S_{Na}}$$

BOX 3 Causes of SIADH

- Acute emotional stress, psychosis, or physical pain
- Pulmonary disease
  - Pulmonary abscess
  - Tuberculosis
  - Viral, bacterial, or fungal pneumonia
- CNS disease
  - Brain abscess
  - Brain trauma
  - Encephalitis
  - Guillain-Barré syndrome
  - Intraparenchymal, subarachnoid, or subdural hemorrhage
  - Ischemic CVA
  - Meningitis
- Carcinomas
  - Duodenum
  - Lung
  - Pancreas

Abbreviations: CNS, central nervous system; CVA, cerebral vascular accident; SIADH = secretion of inappropriate antidiuretic hormone.

---

[3]Exceeds dosage recommended by the manufacturer.

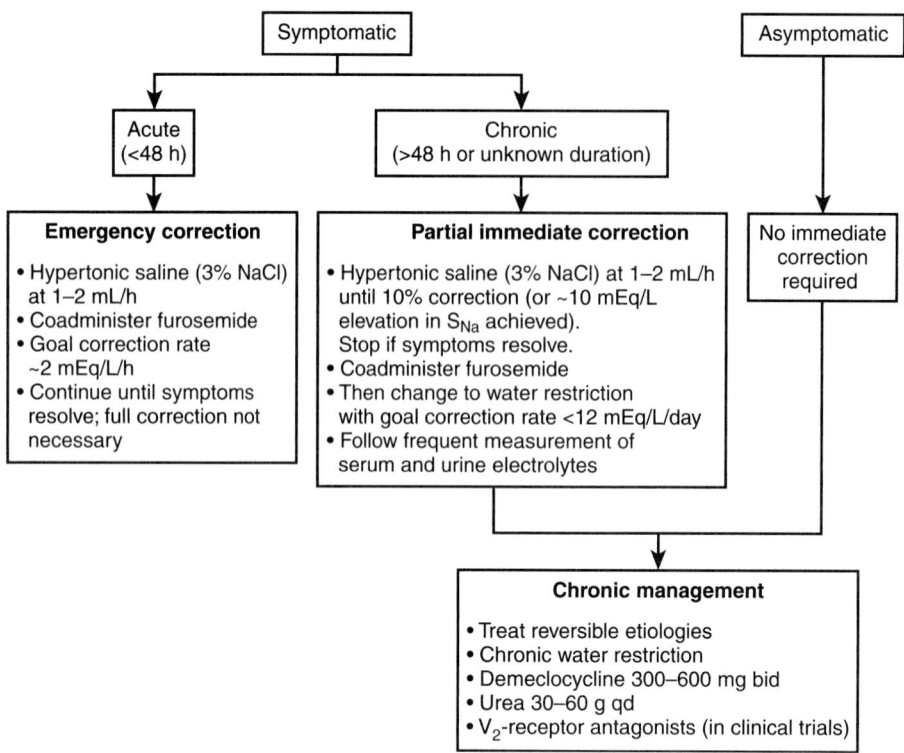

FIGURE 2. Treatment algorithm for severe euvolemic hyponatremia: serum sodium (S_{Na}) <125 mEq/L.

If the value is <0.5, then fluid is restricted to a maximum of 1 L/day. If the value is 0.5 to 1.0, fluid is restricted to a maximum of 500 mL/day. If the value is greater than 1.0, then fluid restriction alone might not be sufficient to raise the serum sodium concentration.

CURRENT THERAPY

- Symptomatic acute hyponatremia (<48 h duration) warrants immediate correction with hypertonic saline (3% NaCl) infused at 1-2³ mL/kg/h with coadministration of furosemide (Lasix) until symptoms resolve.
- Symptomatic chronic hyponatremia (>48 h duration) warrants immediate partial correction of approximately 10% of the sodium deficit (~10 mEq/L elevation in S_{Na^+}) using hypertonic saline (3% NaCl) infused at 1-2³ mL/kg/h coadministered with furosemide, followed by slower correction not faster than 1-1.5 mEq/L/h or 12 mEq/L/day.
- Asymptomatic hyponatremia requires no immediate intervention and may be treated with correction of the underlying etiology (e.g., discontinuation of drugs that cause hyponatremia, hormone replacement in hypothyroidism or cortisol deficiency, 0.9% saline in hypovolemic hyponatremia, diuresis, inotropes and water restriction for heart failure, water restriction for SIADH and cirrhosis.

³Exceeds dosage recommended by the manufacturer.
Abbreviations: S_{Na^+} = serum sodium, SIADH = secretion of inappropriate antidiuretic hormone.

Pharmacologic Therapy

Pharmacologic agents include demeclocycline, urea, daily sodium chloride tablets plus low-dose furosemide, and V_2-receptor antagonists, which inhibit vasopressin-mediated water reabsorption. One IV formulation, conivaptan (Vaprisol), has been approved for treatment of euvolemic hyponatremia, and several oral V_2 antagonists are undergoing clinical trials for approval by the U.S Food and Drug Administration. V_2-receptor antagonists will likely become the first-line treatment for euvolemic and hypervolemic hypernatremia.

Until broad clinical experience with V_2 antagonists is obtained, demeclocycline (Declomycin),[1] a drug that inhibits renal tubular responsiveness to ADH, leading to increased water excretion, is currently the agent of choice. Onset is 3 to 6 days. Demeclocycline is prescribed in doses of 300 to 900 mg/day with unrestricted water intake. Furosemide 40 mg/day in combination with 2 to 3 grams of sodium chloride tablets will force increased urine volume and allow a patient to consume more water. Finally, prescription of urea (Ureaphil)[1] 30 to 60 g/day increases urinary solute, and hence water excretion is limited by unpalatable taste and gastrointestinal symptoms.

[1]Not FDA approved for this indication.

REFERENCES

Berl T, Schrier RW: The patient with hyponatremia or hypernatremia. In Schrier RW, (ed): Manual of Nephrology, 6th ed, Philadelphia: Lippincott Williams & Wilkins, 2005, pp 21-36.
Kumar S, Berl T: Sodium. Lancet 1998;352:220-228.
Thurman J, Halterman R, Berl T: Therapy of dysnatremic disorders. In Brady N, Wilcox C, (eds): Therapy of Nephrology and Hypertension, Philadelphia: WB Saunders, 2003, pp 335-348.

Hyperuricemia and Gout

Method of
Beth K. Rubinstein, MD, and Christopher M. Wise, MD

Gout is a common cause of inflammatory arthritis typically affecting middle-aged men. However, women and men older than 65 years are affected equally. Gout classically evolves through various stages, starting with a period of asymptomatic hyperuricemia and progressing to a period during which episodes of acute intermittent gouty arthritis occur. Over many years, attacks become more frequent and prolonged, and chronic tophaceous gout develops.

Asymptomatic hyperuricemia is associated with an increased risk of gout. The annual incidence increases from 0.1% to 5% with rising serum urate levels (<7 mg/dL to >9 mg/dL). The cumulative incidence of gouty arthritis reaches 22% in 5 years with serum uric acid levels greater than 9 mg/dL. Risk factors for hyperuricemia and gout include elevated serum creatinine, obesity, insulin resistance, elevated blood pressure, diuretic use, alcohol consumption, and higher meat and seafood intake. Higher intake of dairy products might decrease the risk. Hyperuricemia and gout are now considered elements of the metabolic syndrome, and gout may be an independent risk factor for myocardial infarction.

Diagnosis

Acute gouty arthritis, a mono- or oligoarthritis escalating over a 6- to 12-hour period with pain, swelling, and erythema, is usually easily recognized, but the presence of fever, chills, or leukocytosis broaden the differential diagnosis to include infection and pseudogout. A definitive diagnosis of gout can be accomplished by arthrocentesis of a symptomatic joint and identification of monosodium urate crystals in the joint fluid. Aspiration of an asymptomatic joint can reveal crystals even between attacks.

In many patients, a gradual transition from acute intermittent gout to chronic tophaceous gout occurs over the next 10 to 20 years. Tophi and erosions form due to the deposition of urate crystals in the subcutaneous tissue and articular cartilage, respectively. Eventually, joint destruction and deformity occur, which can mimic rheumatoid arthritis.

Treatment

ACUTE GOUT

Acute gouty arthritis tends to resolve spontaneously, but attacks can be quite painful and disabling, necessitating early therapeutic intervention. Nonsteroidal antiinflammatory drugs (NSAIDs), colchicine, and intraarticular or systemic corticosteroids are used most often to terminate an acute gout attack. NSAIDs have a relatively rapid onset of effect and low toxicity profile in the acute setting but their use may be limited by the potential for gastric ulceration and gastritis, acute or chronic renal failure, fluid retention, exacerbation of congestive heart failure, interference with antihypertensive therapy, and alteration of mentation in the elderly. Indomethacin (Indocin) has been the most widely used NSAID, but other agents in the same class are comparable in efficacy and may be better tolerated.

Colchicine begins to relieve symptoms of acute gout within 12 to 24 hours. It is often administered in oral dosages of 0.6 to 1.2 mg initially, followed by 0.6 mg every 2 hours until improvement, but most patients experience gastrointestinal symptoms with these dosages. More serious toxicities, including bone marrow suppression, renal and hepatic injury, central nervous system (CNS) dysfunction, or neuromyopathy can occur if an inappropriately high cumulative dose is given acutely, in the elderly, or in patients with renal or hepatic insufficiency. Low doses of colchicine (0.6 mg bid) may be effective in milder attacks and are less toxic. Intravenous colchicine has been used in the past for treating acute attacks, but it is currently not widely available and is seldom used given its potential to reach toxic levels if not used judiciously.

Corticosteroids have become more widely used to treat acute gout, particularly in patients with contraindications to NSAIDs and colchicine. Intraarticular steroid injection can be done after arthrocentesis and usually provides rapid relief of pain in patients with monoarticular attacks. Systemic corticosteroids (intramuscular or oral) are very useful in patients with polyarticular involvement. Oral prednisone can be given as a taper starting at doses of 40 to 60 mg daily, with gradual decreases in the dose over a period of 7 to 14 days to prevent rebound flares in the first several days after therapy. A single intramuscular injection of triamcinolone (Kenalog) (40-60 mg) has been shown to be comparable to NSAIDs in efficacy and may be preferable in patients who have difficulty taking oral medications.

INTERCRITICAL GOUT

After the initial attack of gout resolves, management should be aimed at preventing further attacks, assessing the baseline serum urate level (with or without urinary urate excretion), and determining the need for long-term urate-lowering therapy. There is a general correlation between the serum urate levels and frequency of subsequent attacks, although serum urate levels can vary and may be falsely low in the setting of an acute attack. Measurements of serum urate levels during asymptomatic periods, therefore, can provide a more accurate assessment of chronic hyperuricemia.

Patients are at increased risk for a recurrent attack of gout for several weeks after an initial attack, although 40% of patients might not have another attack within the next year. During this intercritical period, prophylaxis with small doses of NSAIDs or colchicine (0.6 mg once or twice daily) should be used for most patients and will prevent recurrences in about 85% of patients if used for 6 to 12 months after the last attack.

INDICATIONS FOR URATE-LOWERING THERAPY

Not all patients with hyperuricemia need to be treated with urate-lowering therapy. Some patients with gout never have another attack and will not develop renal stones or renal damage. However, most patients have microscopic evidence of synovial urate deposition (microtophi) at the time of the first attack. Indications for urate-lowering therapy are listed in Box 1. Patients should only be started on urate-lowering therapy if they are willing to comply with a long-term regimen and accept the cost and potential risks of such therapy.

CHRONIC HYPERURICEMIA

Urate levels can be lowered by agents that either decrease production or increase renal excretion of urate. Most patients with gout are underexcretors of urate; therefore, drugs that increase urate excretion can be used to lower serum levels. However, these agents promote urate nephrolithiasis and should only be considered for patients who have normal renal function (glomerular filtration rate >50-60 mL/min), have no history of nephrolithiasis, have a 24-hour urate excretion of less than 700 mg/day, and are willing to drink at least 2 L of fluid daily and maintain good urine flow. Probenecid (1-2 g/day) is the most commonly used agent in this class, although sulfinpyrazone (Anturane) (up to 400-800 mg/day) may also be used. Gastrointestinal side effects and rash can occur.

Allopurinol (Zyloprim), an inhibitor of xanthine oxidase, reduces serum urate levels in nearly all compliant patients and eventually prevents further attacks and promotes resorption of tophi. The dose of allopurinol should be titrated up as frequently as every 2 to 3 weeks to achieve a serum urate level of less than 6 mg/dL. Allopurinol is well tolerated except for occasional skin rashes, which are seen in about 2% of patients, and gastrointestinal symptoms. Other rare but serious reactions include bone marrow suppression, alopecia, and the allopurinol hypersensitivity syndrome. This syndrome, which has a

BOX 1 General Indications for Hypouricemic Therapy

Tophaceous gout
Destructive arthropathy attributable to gout
Marked overproduction of urate (>1000 mg urate excretion daily)
History of nephrolithiasis (urate or other)
Chronic urate nephropathy (due to deposition of monosodium urate crystals in the renal medulla and pyramids)
Gout with renal insufficiency
Frequent attacks of acute gout (>2/year)
Patients *without* documented gout should be treated or considered for treatment:
Acute uric acid nephropathy (acute renal failure seen in tumor lysis syndrome from chemotherapy or rapidly proliferating lymphomas/leukemias)
Asymptomatic hyperuricemia with marked (>1000 mg/day) hyperuricosuria or serum urate level >10 mg/dL
Hyperuricemia associated with heritable disorders of purine metabolism leading to urate overproduction (hypoxanthine-guanine phosphoribosyltransferase [HGPRT] deficiency, Phosphoriboxyl-pyrophosphate synthetase polypeptide [PRPP] synthetase superactivity)

TABLE 1 Adult Maintenance Dosages of Allopurinol and Colchicine Based on Creatinine Clearance

Creatinine Clearance (mL/min)	Maintenance Dose of Allopurinol (mg)	Maintenance Dose of Colchicine (mg)
≧100	300-600 qd	0.6 bid-tid
80	250 qd	0.6 bid
60	200 qd	0.6 bid
40	150 qd	0.6 qd
20	100 qd	0.6 q2-3d
10	100 qod	Contraindicated
<10	50-100 q3d	Contraindicated

mortality rate of up to 25%, is manifested by rash, fever, eosinophilia, hepatic injury, and renal failure. Allopurinol should be discontinued in any patient who experiences an unexplained rash or fever and should be restarted only if the rash is mild. Allopurinol hypersensitivity can be overcome through desensitization protocols if needed.

Urate-lowering therapy should generally not be initiated during an acute gout attack, but it may be started 2 to 3 weeks after an acute attack has resolved. In addition, urate-lowering therapy should not be stopped in the setting of an acute flare, even if the serum urate level appears to be at goal. Prophylactic agents, such as NSAIDs and low-dose colchicine, may be started a few weeks before, and given concomitantly with, urate-lowering therapy to prevent attacks during initiation of such therapy, and it should be continued until the serum urate level is less than 6 mg/dL and the patient has been free of attacks for at least 6 months. Chronic colchicine use can be associated with neuromyopathy and bone marrow suppression in patients with renal or hepatic insufficiency. Maintenance doses of both allopurinol and colchicine should be adjusted according to renal function (Table 1).

Other agents that appear to have modest urate-lowering effects include fenofibrate (Tricor),[1] losartan (Cozaar),[1] amlodipine (Norvasc),[1] and vitamin C[1] (500 mg daily). Dietary adjustments such as decreasing the intake of purine-rich foods (organ meats, shellfish, anchovies) and alcohol, especially beer and distilled spirits, should be part of a urate-lowering regimen, and medications known to decrease urate excretion (cyclosporine [Neoral], nicotinic acid [Niaspan], furosemide [Lasix], thiazide diuretics, ethambutol [Myambutol], pyrazinamide, and aspirin) should also be switched or dose-adjusted if possible.

ELDERLY PATIENTS

Gout is the most common inflammatory arthritis affecting the elderly, but it may be difficult to recognize in this population. The incidence of gout increases in postmenopausal women when the level of estrogen, which has uricosuric effects, decreases. Women can also get gouty arthritis in atypical joints such as the distal interphalangeal (DIP) joints of the hands. The treatment of gout in the elderly is the same as that in younger patients; however, the doses of medications used should be decreased to avoid potential toxic effects. Joint aspiration and corticosteroids may be safer alternatives for some patients. Analgesics can also be used alone when other agents are contraindicated because acute attacks are usually self-limited.

RESISTANT GOUT

Most patients treated for acute gouty arthritis respond to initial therapy with NSAIDs or colchicine; however, an occasional patient responds poorly. In this circumstance, one should consider an alternative diagnosis, such as infectious arthritis, and perform arthrocentesis and culture of the synovial fluid. In the absence of an infection, a corticosteroid (systemic or intraarticular) can be added to achieve a therapeutic response. In a patient with polyarticular involvement who has had inadequate response to an intramuscular corticosteroid, it is not unreasonable to repeat injection 2 to 3 days later. When giving oral corticosteroids for acute gout, one should ensure that the length of therapy is sufficient to prevent rebound attacks.

Patients receiving urate-lowering therapy who continue to have frequent attacks are usually found to have persistently elevated serum urate levels (>6 mg/dL). Medication noncompliance can explain the lack of efficacy of urate-lowering agents; however, urate levels also remain elevated in compliant patients if the dose of the urate-lowering medication is not adjusted to achieve goal urate levels.

CRITICALLY ILL PATIENTS

Acute gouty arthritis often occurs in hospitalized or critically ill patients due to fluctuations in the urate levels related to trauma, surgery, or serious infections. This usually occurs in patients with established gout, but initial gout attacks are also seen in this setting. Treatment of gout is often difficult in these patients due to

CURRENT DIAGNOSIS

- Definitive diagnosis of gout depends on the finding of intracellular monosodium urate crystals in synovial fluid or from tophaceous deposits.
- Even in acute settings where gout is the most likely diagnosis, alternative diagnoses such as infection and pseudogout should be considered.
- Chronic polyarticular gout can mimic rheumatoid arthritis.
- Most patients with gout have elevated serum urate levels at some point during their clinical course, but hyperuricemia alone is not diagnostic of gout.

---
[1]Not FDA approved for this indication.

CURRENT THERAPY

- The goals of gout treatment include termination of the acute attack, prevention of further attacks, identification and management of associated conditions and risk factors, and consideration of long-term urate-lowering therapy.
- NSAIDs, colchicine, and corticosteroids remain the mainstay of treatment of acute gouty arthritis.
- A serum uric acid level of 6 mg/dL is the initial target when using urate-lowering therapy.
- Urate-lowering medications should not be stopped (or started) during an acute gout flare.
- Prophylactic agents such as colchicine or NSAIDs should be administered when initiating urate-lowering therapy for a period of 3 to 12 months.
- Lifestyle changes, dietary adjustments, and medication alterations may be useful in preventing acute gout and its progression to chronic tophaceous gout.

NSAID = nonsteroidal antiinflammatory drug.

hemodynamic instability, renal or hepatic dysfunction, or altered oral intake status. Intraarticular corticosteroid injections may be the safest treatment if a single joint or small number of joints are involved and provide an opportunity to aspirate the joint fluid to exclude infection, which can coexist with gout. If multiple joints are involved and oral medication is contraindicated, then intramuscular corticosteroids may be preferable. Urate-lowering therapy should not be initiated in a hospitalized or critically ill patient.

TRANSPLANT PATIENTS

Organ transplant patients have typically been more susceptible to the development of gout within a few years of the transplant due to the interference of urate excretion by certain immunosuppressive medications, but use of these agents (cyclosporine) is less common in recent years and can, in turn, decrease the incidence of gout in this patient population. In addition, allopurinol interferes with the metabolism of other immunosuppressive medications (azathioprine [Imuran] and 6-mercaptopurine [Purinethol]), necessitating a decrease in the dose of these medications or a switch to another medication such as mycophenolate mofetil (Cellcept).

POTENTIAL NEW AND ALTERNATIVE THERAPIES

No new urate-lowering agents have become available since 1964; however, there are agents that have been studied and may have potential efficacy. Febuxostat,[5] a nonpurine selective xanthine oxidase inhibitor, has been shown to lower urate levels at least as effectively as allopurinol, and it might have an advantage over allopurinol in patients with renal insufficiency or in those who have had hypersensitivity reactions to allopurinol. Recombinant uricase (rasburicase [Elitek]), which is primarily used in malignancy-associated hyperuricemia, has been shown to rapidly lower serum urate levels and resorb tophi when given intravenously, but it has a short half-life and may be associated with allergic reactions and anaphylaxis. Subcutaneous and intravenous forms of polyethylene glycol–modified uricase[5] have been studied and found to greatly reduce serum urate levels in patients with severe or refractory gout, but acute gout flares occurred commonly.

[5]Investigational drug in the United States.

REFERENCES

Becker MA, Schumacher HR Jr, Wortmann RL: Febuxostat compared with allopurinol in patients with hyperuricemia and gout. N Engl J Med 2005;353:2450-2461.
Campion EW, Glynn RJ, DeLabry LO: Asymptomatic hyperuricemia: risks and consequences in the Normative Aging Study. Am J Med 1987;82:421-426.
Choi HK, Atkinson K, Karlson EW, Curhan G: Obesity, weight change, hypertension, diuretic use, and risk of gout in men: The health professionals follow-up study. Arch Intern Med 2005;165:742-748.
Choi HK, Liu S, Curhan G: Intake of purine-rich foods, protein, and dairy products and relationship to serum levels of uric acid: The Third National Health and Nutritional Examination Survey. Arthritis Rheum 2005;52:283-289.
Hoskison KT, Wortmann RL: Management of gout in older adults: Barriers to optimal control. Drugs Aging 2007;24:21-36.
Keith MP, Gilliland WR: Updates in the management of gout. Am J Med 2007;120:221-224.
Krishnan E, Baker JF, Furst DE, Schumacher HR: Gout and the risk of acute myocardial infarction. Arthritis Rheum 2006;54:2688-2696.
Lee SJ, Terkeltaub RA, Kavanaugh A: Recent developments in diet and gout. Curr Opin Rheumatol 2006;18:193-198.
Pascual E, Sivera F: Therapeutic advances in gout. Curr Opin Rheumatol 2007;19:122-127.
Sundy JS, Ganson NJ, Kelly SJ, et al: Pharmacokinetics and pharmacodynamics of intravenous PEGylated recombinant mammalian urate oxidase in patients with refractory gout. Arthritis Rheum 2007;6:1021-1028.
Vogt B: Urate oxidase (rasburicase) for treatment of severe tophaceous gout. Nephrol Dial Transplant 2005;20:431-433.

Management of Patients with Dyslipoproteinemias (Cholesterol and Triglyceride Disorders)

Method of
Michael A. Crouch, MD, MSPH

Dyslipoproteinemias are abnormal levels of low-density lipoprotein (LDL), very-low-density lipoprotein (VLDL), high-density lipoprotein (HDL), or intermediate-density lipoprotein (IDL). *Dyslipidemia* refers to numerous lipid disorders with primary genetic, secondary metabolic, lifestyle, and iatrogenic contributing factors. *Hyperlipidemia* refers to elevated low-density lipoprotein (LDL) cholesterol or triglyceride (TG) levels (or both). Familial combined (mixed) hyperlipidemia is elevated LDL cholesterol and TGs. LDL cholesterol is one of the main risk factors for coronary artery disease (CAD). Cholesterol and triglycerides cutpoints are shown in Table 1.

Epidemiology

The prevalence of hypercholesterolemia increases with age, peaking around age 60 years. About 50% of adults have borderline or elevated LDL cholesterol (>130 mg/dL or 3.35 mmol/L). Five percent to 10% of adults have low HDL cholesterol (<40 mg/dL or 1.0 mmol/L). Elevated TGs are seen in 20% to 25% of adults.

Pathogenesis

Primary lipid disorders are familial, expressing both genetic factors and learned behavior. Secondary causes of dyslipidemia include

TABLE 1 Lipid Categories from the National Cholesterol Education Program

Lipid	Level mg/dL	mmol/L
Low-Density Lipoprotein Cholesterol		
High	≥160 mg	≥4.2
Borderline high	130-159	3.4-4.1
Above optimal	100-129	2.6-3.3
Desirable	<100	<2.6
Optimal	<70	<1.8
High-Density Lipoprotein Cholesterol		
Desirable	≥50	≥1.3
Borderline	40-49	1.0-1.2
Low	<40	<1.0
Triglycerides (Fasting)		
Elevated	≥200	>1.7
Borderline	150-199	1.3-1.7
Normal	<150	<1.3

BOX 1 Other Risk Factors for Coronary Artery Disease

Factors Cited by the National Cholesterol Education Program
Male gender
Cigarette smoking
Diabetes mellitus
Hypertension
Low HDL cholesterol
Obesity
Personal history of atherosclerotic disease
Family history of lipid disorder
Family history of atherosclerotic disease (especially men <55 years and women <65 years)

Other Factors (Not Specifically Cited by the National Cholesterol Education Program)
Apolipoprotein B elevation
C-reactive protein elevation
Coronary-prone (Type A) behavior or personality
Lipoprotein(a) elevation
Low apolipoprotein A-I level
Lp-PLA2 elevation
Menopause
Old age (risk rises with increasing age)
Proinflammatory high-density lipoprotein
Small, dense low-density lipoprotein particles

diabetes mellitus, hypothyroidism, pregnancy, the nephrotic syndrome, obstructive jaundice, chronic renal failure, dysgammaglobulinemia, anorexia nervosa, porphyria, and glycogen storage disease. Familial heterozygous and homozygous hypercholesterolemias display mendelian dominant inheritance, but most cases of hypercholesterolemia are polygenic.

Excessive dietary intake of saturated fat raises LDL and total cholesterol more than does excessive cholesterol intake. Triglycerides are elevated by genetic predisposition and by sedentary lifestyle, overweight, and excessive intake of alcohol, sugars, and rapidly digested starches. Stress and coronary-prone (Type A) behavior can markedly elevate LDL cholesterol in susceptible persons.

HDL particles facilitate LDL metabolism, carrying LDL back to the liver from peripheral tissues. Patients with low HDL cholesterol and elevated TGs tend to have smaller, more dense LDL particles that are more atherogenic. Physical inactivity or being overweight decreases HDL_2 cholesterol. Alcohol in moderation raises HDL_3 cholesterol.

Several medications can cause or worsen lipid problems. β-Blockers can lower HDL cholesterol and raise LDL cholesterol. Oral contraceptives with strongly androgenic progestins lower HDL cholesterol, raise TGs, and can raise LDL cholesterol. High-dose steroids, disulfiram (Antabuse), and isotretinoin (Retin-A) raise TGs.

Natural History

Lipid problems are asymptomatic for decades. In childhood and adolescence, fatty streaks form on the lining of susceptible arteries and later develop into atheromas. Atherosclerotic progression, plaque rupture, and thrombus formation can eventually block crucial arteries, causing ischemic symptoms or tissue infarction. The clinical course of lipid problems depends on the type and severity of lipid disorder and on the presence of other risk factors (Box 1).

The physical examination findings of arcus senilis, xanthelasma, tendon xanthomas, and eruptive xanthomas are uncommon signs of lipid problems. Angina pectoris, intermittent claudication, and erectile dysfunction can warn of advanced atherosclerosis. Myocardial infarction, cerebrovascular accident (stroke), or sudden death is often the first overt sign of a lipid problem. Severe TG elevation (>1000 mg/dL or 11 mmol/L) can cause acute pancreatitis, requiring urgent intravenous heparin.

Screening

Screening is recommended by the National Cholesterol Education Program (NCEP) every 3 to 5 years for adults younger than 70 years. Adults with LDL cholesterol levels lower than 130 mg/dL (3.35 mmol/L) and HDL levels higher than 50 mg/dL (1.3 mmol/L) need not be rescreened this often unless they experience major changes in weight, diet, or physical activity. Children and adolescents with a family history of severe dyslipidemia or early atherosclerotic disease also should be screened.

A random or fasting lipid profile (with total, LDL, and HDL cholesterol and TGs) should be obtained initially. The more-convenient random lipid profile increases compliance with screening, and it gives useful information about the extent of postprandial hyperlipemia. Blood lipids change acutely in response to food intake. The TG level is lowest in the fasting state, rises by an average of 50 mg/dL postprandially, and peaks 3 to 6 hours after a meal. As the TG level rises, total and LDL cholesterol each fall by an average of 5 to 15 mg/dL. Thus, total and LDL cholesterol tend to be higher when fasting. HDL cholesterol varies little between the fasting and postprandial states, averaging 45 mg/dL (1.16 mmol/L) for men and 55 mg/dL (1.42 mmol/L) for women. Blood lipids can fluctuate within minutes, days, or weeks in response to illness, emotional stress, or malnutrition.

Diagnosis

If a screening lipid profile shows borderline or elevated LDL cholesterol, low HDL cholesterol, or high TGs (cutpoints in Table 1), a second lipid profile should be obtained (fasting) before starting treatment. Thyroid, renal, and liver function tests should be ordered to rule out secondary causes of dyslipidemia.

Prognosis categorization identifies patients at highest risk. The higher the LDL cholesterol level, the higher the risk for coronary heart disease (CHD) and stroke. Patients with markedly elevated LDL cholesterol levels (>190 mg/dL, or 4.9 mmol/L) are at increased risk even if they have HDL cholesterol levels at or above average. Lipid ratios (total to HDL cholesterol or LDL:HDL cholesterol) predict outcome only marginally better than absolute HDL and LDL cholesterol values. At highest risk are patients with other major risk factors (listed in Box 2). Patients with high fasting TG levels are at increased risk, especially obese women with diabetes mellitus. Low

| BOX 2 | Drugs that Interact with Statins |

Amiodarone (Cordarone)
Amlodipine (Norvasc)
Cimetidine (Tagamet)
Clarithromycin (Biaxin)
Clindamycin (Cleocin)
Cyclosporine (Neoral)
Diltiazem (Cardizem, Cartia, Dilacor, Diltia, Tiazac)
Erythromycin (EES, E-Mycin, EryC, PCE, Ery-Tab)
Femfibrate (Tricor)
Gemfibrozil (Lopid)
Indinavir (Crixivan)
Itraconazole (Sporanox)
Nelfinavir (Viracept)
Niacin (nicotinic acid; Slo-Niacin, Niacor, Niaspan, Nico-400, NIA delay, Endur-Acin)
Ritonavir (Norvir)
Saquinavir (Invirase)
Tacrolimus (Prograf)
Verapamil (Calan, Covera, Isoptin, Verelan)

TABLE 2 LDL Cholesterol Levels for Initiating Drug Therapy

Risk Category	10-Year Estimated Risk for CHD	LDL Level for Considering Drug Therapy
CHD or CHD risk equivalent (diabetes, stroke)	>20%	Regardless of LDL level*
2+ risk factors	10%-20%	≥130 mg/dL (3.35 mmol/L)
	<10%	>160 mg/dL (4.2 mmol/L)
0-1 risk factors (not diabetes)	Usually <10%	>190 mg/dL (4.9 mmol/L) (160-189 mg/dL or 4.2-4.9 mmol/L: drug optional)

*Statins stabilize existing atherosclerotic plaque and reduce the risk of lesion rupture and thrombosis.
CHD = coronary heart disease; LDL = low-density lipoprotein.

HDL cholesterol is the best single lipid predictor of adverse outcome. Patients with low HDL cholesterol levels are at some increased risk even if their LDL cholesterol levels are not notably elevated. Above-average or high HDL cholesterol levels (>60 mg/dL or 1.55 mmol/L) however, do not guarantee immunity from CAD. A proinflammatory form of HDL is present in the blood of some with high HDL levels; this form of HDL greatly increases the risk for atherosclerosis.

C-reactive protein (CRP) can be helpful to refine a patient's estimated risk and adjust the aggressiveness of lipid treatment, especially in those with a strong family history of CAD or stroke. About 25% of patients have high-CHD-risk levels of CRP in the moderately elevated range of 3.0 to 10.0 mg/L. A CRP level of greater than 10.0 mg/L usually indicates acute or chronic illness. It is unknown how often CRP should be retested. Because it is not known whether lowering CRP with aspirin or a statin improves clinical outcomes, the cost of CRP testing is not reimbursed by most health insurance plans.

Homocysteine elevation is a weak risk predictor for myocardial infarction and stroke. Intervention study results have shown no benefit from lowering homocysteine with folate, pyridoxine, and vitamin B_{12}; thus, homocysteine testing is not recommended.

Apolipoprotein levels predict outcome somewhat more accurately than does LDL or HDL cholesterol, but their clinical usefulness is unproved. Elevation of lipoprotein(a), a modified LDL moiety similar to plasminogen, independently predicts a bad prognosis. A new test, PLAC, measures the enzyme lipoprotein-associated phospholipase A2 (Lp-PLA2), which, when elevated, is associated with a twofold-increased CAD risk.

CURRENT DIAGNOSIS

- Low-density-lipoprotein (LDL) cholesterol elevation is a crucial risk factor for coronary artery disease.
- One half of all myocardial infarctions occur in those with LDL cholesterol levels in the suboptimal (100-129 mg/dL) or borderline (130-159 mg/dL) ranges; most of these patients have multiple other risk factors.
- Recommendations for screening, diagnosis, and treatment are detailed in the National Cholesterol Education Program Adult Treatment Panel III guidelines (2001); ATP IV guidelines are scheduled to be issued in 2009.

Treatment

Treatment recommendations and goals should be established based on the patient's clinical status, other risk factors (Box 1), and estimated 10-year risk for CHD (Table 2). The estimated 10-year risk for CHD is a key step in evaluating candidacy for medication treatment for patients not known to have CHD, diabetes, or other CHD-equivalent. Ten-year CHD risk can be estimated manually using the NCEP risk-calculator sheet or by using any reliable Internet risk calculator or downloading a risk-calculator program.

The treatment goals are to lower LDL cholesterol to less than 70 mg/dL (2.60 mmol/L) in patients with clinical CAD or CAD

CURRENT THERAPY

- Lowering intake of dietary saturated fat, trans fat, and cholesterol is the cornerstone for treating hyperlipidemias to reduce risk of coronary heart disease.
- Other useful dietary measures include regular intake of fiber, fish or fish oil (omega-3 fatty acids), nuts, soy protein, and plant sterols or stanols.
- Many patients with elevated low-density-lipoprotein (LDL) cholesterol require medication in addition to diet modification to achieve primary prevention treatment target goals for LDL cholesterol (<100 mg/dL).
- Suggested modifications of the National Cholesterol Education Program guidelines (2004) advocate a more aggressive LDL cholesterol target goal of less than 70 mg/dL for secondary prevention in patients with coronary heart disease (CHD) or CHD-equivalent.
- Statin therapy is the treatment of choice for most cases of hyperlipidemia.
- Patient-perceived statin intolerance and fear of potential side effects greatly undermine acceptance of and long-term adherence to statin therapy.
- Ongoing monitoring of patient adherence and repetitive interactive patient education are needed to maximize the likelihood of long-term continuation of statin therapy.

TABLE 3 LDL Cholesterol Medication Treatment Goals

	Treatment Goal for LDL Cholesterol	
10-Year Risk	2 or More CAD Risk Factors (mg/dL [mmol/L])	<2 CAD Risk Factors (mg/dL [mmol/L])
Known CAD or Diabetes		
Any	<70 (<1.8)	<70 (<1.8)
No known CAD or Diabetes		
>20%	<100 (<2.6)	<100 (<2.6)
10%-20%	<130 (<3.35)	<160 (<4.2)
<10%	<160 (<4.2)	<190 (<4.9)

CAD, coronary artery disease; LDL, low-density lipoprotein.

BOX 3 Key Dietary Changes for Lowering Cholesterol

Eat less beef and pork (especially fatty cuts).
Eat cold-water fish twice a week (salmon, tuna, herring, mackerel). Fish with high mercury content (e.g., swordfish) should be limited to once a month.
Eat more chicken and turkey (white skinless meat).
Eat 40-50 g of soy protein a day (tofu, soy burger, soy dog, soy milk).
Drink nonfat, ½%, or 1% fat milk. Eat minimal amounts of other whole-milk dairy products (cheese, butter, ice cream, sour cream).
Use polyunsaturated oil products (safflower, corn, soybean) or monounsaturated oil products (olive) for margarine and cooking oil.
Minimize intake of commercial fried fast foods (high in trans fats).
Eat oat bran as cereal or muffins, three to six servings per day.
Eat nuts (walnuts, pecans, almonds, peanuts, cashews), 1 oz a day.
Eat fish oil high in omega-3 fatty acids. Fish oils reduce blood triglycerides but can elevate LDL cholesterol. If regular fish intake is impractical, three capsules a day of fish oil provides the 1 g/day of EPA plus DHA recommended for prevention. To lower triglycerides, the recommended dose of fish oil is 2 to 4 g/day.
Use products enhanced with plant stanols or sterols (e.g., Benecol, Take Control).

---

equivalent or with an estimated 10-year CHD risk greater than 20%. CAD equivalents are diabetes, peripheral artery disease, abdominal aortic aneurysm, or symptomatic carotid artery disease, including transient ischemic attack and stroke. Treatment goals for other levels of risk are shown in Table 3. For all hyperlipidemic patients, the TG goal is to lower fasting TG to less than 150 mg/dL (1.3 mmol/L).

HYGIENIC MANAGEMENT OPTIONS

Hygienic approaches can sometimes improve lipid levels effectively. Encourage lifestyle changes in anyone with LDL cholesterol greater than 130 mg/dL or HDL cholesterol less than 40 mg/dL (1.0 mmol/L). Those with HDL cholesterol levels in the borderline 40- to 49-mg/dL (1.03-1.16 mmol/L) range also should be urged to exercise regularly. Diet modification is often feasible in the short term, but for many it is difficult to sustain over the long term. Depending on baseline diet, eating less saturated fat and cholesterol often lowers total blood cholesterol by 10% to 20%. Key dietary changes are listed in Box 3.

Regular vigorous exercise, at least 30 minutes at a time, three or more times a week, raises HDL cholesterol by 5 to 15 mg/dL, lowers TGs and VLDL cholesterol, and sometimes lowers LDL cholesterol. Walking daily for several miles has smaller favorable effects on lipids. Weight loss lowers TG and VLDL cholesterol and raises HDL cholesterol by 5 to 10 mg/dL, but it lowers LDL cholesterol only transiently during weight reduction.

MEDICATION

For most patients with diabetes, coronary or carotid artery disease, or a 10-year estimated CHD risk greater than 20%, statin medication is recommended, regardless of LDL cholesterol level. Beside lowering LDL cholesterol and triglycerides, statins stabilize existing atherosclerotic plaque and reduce the risk of lesion rupture and thrombosis. The 2001 NCEP Adult Treatment Panel III recommends medical treatment if LDL cholesterol remains greater than 190 mg/dL (4.9 mmol/L) despite hygienic management, regardless of the patient's clinical status and other CAD risk factors. The guidelines for drug therapy with other combinations of risk factors and LDL cholesterol levels are shown in Table 2.

Psyllium

Over-the-counter drugs are preferred by some patients for medical lipid treatment because they cost less and seem less intimidating. Psyllium hydrophilic mucilloid[1] (Metamucil, others) lowers LDL cholesterol 5 to 10%; it can be used to treat mildly elevated LDL cholesterol (130-159 mg/dL), especially in elderly patients. It promotes bowel regularity and causes flatulence but causes no serious adverse effects.

Niacin

Niacin (Niaspan) is a logical choice for treating healthy patients with moderately elevated LDL cholesterol, low HDL cholesterol, or high TGs. Niacin can reduce risk for myocardial infarction and CAD death. At 1 to 3 g/day, it lowers LDL cholesterol 15% to 20%, variably lowers elevated TGs, and raises HDL cholesterol by 5 to 15 mg/dL. Begin with a low dose of 100 to 200 mg of regular release form or 250 to 500 mg of sustained release; gradually increase to a maximum of 2 to 3 g/day, based on patient tolerance. Most patients experience some flushing and itching when taking sustained-release niacin; side effects can be reduced by taking 325 mg of aspirin daily before the first dose. Although usually safe, niacin can worsen hyperglycemia, exacerbate gout, precipitate serious arrhythmias in patients with heart disease, and cause severe liver toxicity. Niacin is also available in expensive prescription form (Niaspan), which might have less risk for hepatotoxicity.

Statins

Prescription drugs for modifying lipids are much more effective for lowering LDL cholesterol. Statins (HMG-CoA reductase inhibitors) are the best choice for most patients with moderately or severely elevated LDL cholesterol and for most high-risk patients. Statins lower LDL cholesterol by 30% to 60%, more than any other medication. In controlled trials, statins reduced heart attack, stroke, CHD death, and total mortality by 25% to 40%.

Cost-effectiveness analyses of statin therapy have shown relatively favorable cost-to-benefit ratios, even before the emergence of less-expensive generic statins such as lovastatin, pravastatin, and simvastatin greatly improved statins' cost-effectiveness. The cost-effectiveness of

---

[1] Not FDA approved for this indication

treatment may be improved by prescribing twice the intended dose and having patients take one-half tablet doses. Statins are usually well tolerated, and serious adverse effects are uncommon. The most-often reported side effects of statins are muscle aches, headache, flatulence, constipation, dyspepsia, insomnia, and mild harmless elevation of hepatic transaminases. Rare side effects of statin therapy include pruritus, rashes, myopathy, rhabdomyolysis, acute renal failure, and memory loss.

Statin use is relatively contraindicated in patients with active hepatic disease (e.g., viral hepatitis) or significantly elevated serum transaminases (more than three times normal upper limit). Statin use appears to be safe and beneficial in patients with mildly elevated alanine aminotransferase (ALT) due to fatty liver disease; over time, statin therapy usually normalizes ALT in such persons. Because significant asymptomatic elevation of ALT) occurs in 1% to 2% and mildly elevated ALT (less than three times normal) occurs in about 5% to 10% of treated patients, it is prudent to obtain a baseline ALT and to recheck it 6 to 12 weeks after initiating treatment or after increasing a statin dose. It is unnecessary to monitor aspartate transaminase (AST) or other liver enzymes. No cases of serious or life-threatening liver toxicity have thus far been attributed to statin therapy.

Myalgias or muscle weakness occur in about 10% of patients, usually resolving within a few weeks after stopping the statin. Taking coenzyme Q-10 (100 mg twice a day)[7] with a statin appears to prevent muscle symptoms in some patients. Myopathy occurs rarely; it sometimes causes rhabdomyolysis, with or without acute renal failure. Muscle toxicity occurs more often when statins are used along with niacin, gemfibrozil (Lopid), fenofibrate (Tricor), and other drugs (Box 2); these medications should be avoided if possible when taking a statin, or the statin dose should be adjusted downward while these drugs are being taken. Because they are metabolized differently, pravastatin, rosuvastatin (Crestor), and fluvastatin (Lescol) are least likely to cause drug interactions. Grapefruit juice interferes with the metabolism of simvastatin, atorvastatin (Lipitor), and lovastatin, raising their blood level and increasing the risk of adverse effects. Because the grapefruit juice effect lasts about 24 hours, it should be avoided or minimized when taking simvastatin, atorvastatin, or lovastatin. Renal failure is a risk factor for muscle side effects only with pravastatin.

Concurrent intake of the antioxidant vitamin E does not appear to be advisable because it interfered with the beneficial effects of statin therapy in the Heart Protection Study.

Once started, statin therapy should be continued indefinitely, barring unacceptable side effects or allergic reactions. Perceived side effects from one statin can often be avoided by switching to a different statin. Because they are hydrophilic, pravastatin or fluvastatin are least likely to cause side effects.

Because of potential teratogenicity, statins should not be used in women of childbearing age unless contraception effectiveness is maximized and potential benefit appears to exceed risk. Statins are not approved by the FDA for use in children younger than 14 years except for atorvastatin for homozygous familial hypercholesterolemia.

The average effect of each statin on LDL cholesterol is shown in Table 4. Until generic atorvastatin becomes available, generic simvastatin may be the most cost-effective statin.

Pravastatin, the only statin with prominent renal excretion (about 50% renal), should be used cautiously, if at all, in patients with renal insufficiency or renal failure. Proteinuria occasionally occurs with rosuvastatin (usually at the 40-mg dose), so periodic spot microalbumin-to-creatine ratio testing is advisable. Caduet (atorvastatin-amlodipine), is a logical choice for patients with hyperlipidemia and hypertension.

Ezetimibe

Nonstatin prescription lipid medicines have a place at times. Numerous patients do not accept or tolerate statin therapy. Ezetemibe (Zetia), lowers cholesterol by interfering with the

---

[7] Available as a dietary supplement.

TABLE 4 Lipid Medication Preparations and LDL-Lowering Efficacy

Medication	Average LDL-Lowering Effect (%)
Statins	
Atorvastatin (Lipitor)	38-55
Atorvastatin-amlodipine (Caduet)	38-55
Fluvastatin (Lescol)	23-33
Lovastatin (generic, Mevacor, Altocor)	25-35
Pravastatin (generic, Pravachol)	25-35
Pravastatin-aspirin (Pravigard)	25-35
Rosuvastatin (Crestor)	40-65
Simvastatin (generic, Zocor)	35-50
Simvastatin-ezetemibe (Vytorin)	40-65
Resins and Other GI-Active Meds	
Cholestyramine (generic, Questran, Questran Lite)	15-20
Colestipol (Colestid)	15-20
Colesevelam (Welchol)	15-20
Ezetemibe (Zetia)	15-20
Fibrates	
Fenofibrate (generic, Tricor)	5-15
Gemfibrozil (generic, Lopid)	5-15

GI = gastrointestinal; LDL = low-density lipoprotein.

absorption of cholesterol in the gut, but it is not a resin. Used alone, ezetimibe lowers LDL cholesterol and triglycerides only 15% to 20%. Vytorin (simvastatin-ezetemide), low dose (10 mg of each) lowers LDL cholesterol as much or more than the maximum dose of any statin by itself. Large ongoing outcome studies will compare Vytorin's efficacy for reducing risk for heart attack and stroke with the efficacy of a statin alone. However, preliminary results from the relatively small ENHANCE (Ezetimibe and Simvastatin in Hypercholesterolemia Enhances Atherosclerosis Regression) study showed no advantage of Vytorin over simvastatin alone, based on serial ultrasound measurements of carotid artery plaque in 720 high-risk patients, despite Vytorin's greater reduction of LDL cholesterol.

Resins

Resin medications—cholestyramine (Questran), colestipol (Colestid), and colesevelam (Welchol)—lower cholesterol and triglycerides by binding bile acids in the gut. Cholestyramine is appropriate for the patient with moderate LDL cholesterol elevation who can tolerate its inconvenient form; 2 scoops, or packs two to three times a day, lowers LDL cholesterol by 15% to 20%. Because the maximum dose of six scoops or packs a day causes severe constipation, it is poorly tolerated. Colestipol is very similar to cholestyramine, with no advantages. Another resin, colesevelam comes as a large pill.

Fibrates

Fibrates (gemfibrozil and fenofibrate) change the hepatic metabolism of lipoproteins. Gemfibrozil (Lopid) is a logical choice for the patient with low HDL cholesterol and elevated TGs who has not tolerated or responded well to niacin. It is well tolerated. Gemfibrozil 600 mg twice a day lowers LDL cholesterol by 5% to 15%, markedly lowers TGs, and raises HDL cholesterol by 5 to 15 mg/dL. Gemfibrozil lowered CAD morbidity and mortality by 40% in patients with elevated LDL cholesterol or TGs (or both) and HDL cholesterol less than 45 mg/dL. Fenofibrate (Tricor) is similar to gemfibrozil, with comparable efficacy and long-term safety. Use of a fibrate in combination with a statin increases the absolute risk for rhabdomyolysis and acute renal failure over that of statin monotherapy.

MANAGEMENT STRATEGIES

Long-term adherence to lipid-altering medications is poor. Many patients are reluctant to take preventive medications for asymptomatic conditions. Some patients prefer taking "natural" supplements and express general distrust of the long-term safety of prescription medications. Fear of potential adverse effects from chronic statin therapy appears to be a major deterrent to adherence.

Patient education and discussions with family members are needed to foster a thorough understanding of the importance of a lifelong commitment to hygienic and medical management of lipid problems. Explanations of important concepts need to be expressed in lay terms, accompanied by memory devices to help people remember them. Many good educational materials are available from the American Heart Association, the NCEP, and commercial sources.

Family-oriented care entails screening as many family members as possible and educating nuclear and extended families who have a member with an identified lipid problem. It is particularly important to work with the persons who buy and prepare the family's food, so that they thoroughly understand how to select and prepare heart-healthy foods.

Systematic follow-up at regular intervals is essential for effective long-term management of lipid problems. Initial visits every 1 to 3 months are advisable to monitor progress and sustain motivation. The interval can be gradually lengthened to every 6 to 12 months for dietary and medication management when treatment goals have been reached. A manual or computerized flowchart in the medical record documenting blood lipid results, dietary and exercise modifications, and medication regimens facilitates management.

SPECIAL POPULATIONS

Elderly patients are at a greatly increased risk for myocardial infarction or sudden death. Treating dyslipidemia in patients aged 65 to 85 years decreases the risk of first and recurrent coronary events about 30%. The use of benign inexpensive medications such as psyllium seems prudent. Because outcome studies show similar benefits and no increase in adverse effects for elderly patients, the expense and small risk of statin therapy seem justified for those wishing to preserve their current quality of life as long as possible.

Children and adolescents with dyslipidemias should receive ongoing family-oriented education about diet, exercise, and weight control. Extremely low-fat diets should be avoided in children younger than 6 years because of the risk of essential fatty acid malnutrition, which has deleterious effects on nervous system development. No information is available on the cost-effectiveness and long-term safety of lipid-altering medication treatment in children and adolescents. Children and adolescents with severe dyslipidemias should be treated with lipid-altering medications only with caution and preferably with written parental and minor informed consent.

Secondary prevention focuses on identifying and treating persons who already have atherosclerosis. Many times these patients' lipid problems are ignored or discounted, based on the faulty logic of "it is too late now to prevent atherosclerosis complications." Persons with atherosclerosis have clearly demonstrated their high vulnerability to death from CAD. They are the most likely to benefit from treatment to prevent further atheroma progression and rupture and to regress existing atheromas. The lowering of LDL cholesterol has clearly demonstrated substantial benefit in secondary prevention trials. Long-term adherence is improved when statin therapy is started before hospital discharge for patients admitted with acute myocardial infarction or unstable angina.

ADJUNCTIVE AND OVERALL MANAGEMENT

Other valuable measures for curtailing atherosclerosis or minimizing its damage in patients with lipid disorders include smoking cessation, good control of hypertension and diabetes, and daily aspirin (81 or 325 mg, enteric coated). Some studies indicate that getting a flu shot annually might lower the risk for CAD events. For maximum preventive benefit, these adjunctive measures should be combined with hygienic and lipid medication treatment that is as intensive as individual patients are able to sustain in the long term.

REFERENCES

Ballantyne CM: Current and future aims of lipid-lowering therapy: Changing paradigms and lessons from the Heart Protection Study on standards of efficacy and safety. Am J Cardiol 2003;21(4B):92-9K.

Grundy SM, Cleeman JI, Merz NB, et al: Implications of recent clinical trials for the National Cholesterol Education Program Adult Treatment Panel III guidelines. Circulation 2004;110:227-239.

Heart Protection Study Collaborative Group: MRC/BHF heart protection study of cholesterol lowering with simvastatin in 20,536 high risk individuals: A randomised placebo-controlled trial. Lancet 2002;360:7-22.

Hu FB, Willett WC: Optimal diets for prevention of coronary heart disease. JAMA 2002;288:2569-2578.

Kris-Etherton PM, Harris WS, Appel LJAmerican Heart Association Nutrition Committee: Fish consumption, fish oil, omega-3 fatty acids and cardiovascular disease. Circulation 2002;106:2747-2757.

Expert Panel on Detection, Evaluation, and Treatment of High Blood Cholesterol in Adults: Summary of the third report of the National Cholesterol Education Program (NCEP) Expert Panel on Detection, Evaluation, and Treatment of High Blood Cholesterol in Adults (Adult Treatment Panel III). JAMA 2001;285:2486-2497.

Obesity

Method of
Christopher D. Still, DO, and
Gordon L. Jensen, MD, PhD

Obesity is a heterogeneous disease that has reached epidemic proportions in the United States. For most individuals, it is chronic, relapsing, and multifactorial in origin. It encompasses genetic, environmental, socioeconomic, psychological, and behavioral factors. According to the National Health and Nutrition Examination Survey (NHANES), the prevalence of obesity in the United States has increased from approximately 25% to 33% over a single decade, and obesity now affects nearly 26 million men and 32 million women. Unfortunately, obesity does not spare children or adolescents. NHANES data indicate that approximately 30% of children are overweight (more than 10 million).

The magnitude of obesity differs widely among gender and ethnic groups. There is a marked increase in the prevalence of obesity among females of African American and Mexican American ethnic groups. Some studies estimate nearly 70% of this population is overweight.

Health care providers can no longer view obesity as simply a cosmetic issue caused by a lack of willpower. They need to have an appreciation of its complexity and the related multiple co-morbid medical problems. This chapter discusses the epidemiology, definitions, and assessment of obesity with an emphasis on its clinical consequences and the current techniques in evaluating and treating the obese patient.

Definition and Assessment

The definition of obesity has always been quite ambiguous. The once widely used determination of so-called ideal body weight based on standard height/weight tables such as the Metropolitan Life Insurance Table has fallen out of favor. Experts now recommend the routine use of the body mass index (BMI). The BMI is defined as the ratio of body weight in kilograms to the height in meters squared (kg/m^2). The BMI correlates with body fat and morbidity and mortality (Figure 1).

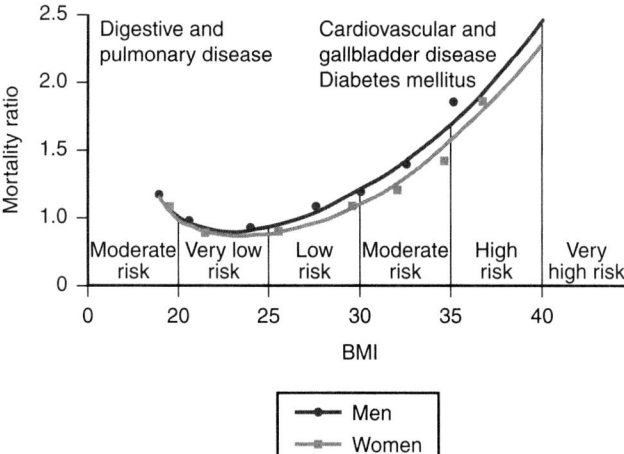

FIGURE 1. Correlation between mortality risk and increasing body mass index (BMI). As BMI increases to higher than 25, the risk for mortality from all causes increases. (Adapted with permission from Gray DS: Diagnosis and prevalence of obesity. Med Clin North Am 1989;73:1.)

The BMI differentiates between overweight and obesity. Moreover, as the BMI increases, so does the risk of mortality. A so-called desirable weight individual has a BMI between 20 and 24.9 kg/m². The National Heart, Blood and Lung Institute defines overweight as a body mass index between 25 and 29.9 kg/m². Obesity, therefore, is defined as a BMI more than 30. Patients with a BMI more than 27 with a co-morbid medical problem, such as diabetes mellitus, hypercholesterolemia, hypertension, or sleep apnea, are also at a higher risk of overall mortality and, therefore, more aggressive treatment options may be warranted (Table 1).

In addition to the BMI, waist circumference is another useful tool in assessing the overweight individual. A waist circumference is measured at the smallest area between the xiphoid process and the iliac crest. A waist circumference more than 35 inches in women and more than 39 inches in men reflects an android or visceral fat distribution. This visceral fat upper body distribution puts one at greater risk for developing co-morbid medical problems such as diabetes, heart disease, lipid dyscrasias, insulin resistance, and possibly cancer. In contrast, the gynoid or lower body weight obesity of the hips and buttocks is mainly subcutaneous adipose tissue that is cardioprotective and not associated with adverse sequelae.

Etiology and Pathophysiology of Obesity

Several etiologic factors classify obesity. Neuroendocrine disorder and single gene deletion syndromes include Cushing's, polycystic ovarian, gonadal failure, Prader-Willi, Cowen's, Carpenter's, and Bardet-Biedl.

Commonly prescribed medications may also promote weight gain. These include, but are not limited to, classes of drugs such as antidiabetics, antipsychotics, antidepressants, antiepileptics, steroids, hormones and adrenergic agonists (Table 2). It is always important to take a thorough medication history to ensure that no medications, either prescription or over the counter, are taken that promote weight gain.

CURRENT DIAGNOSIS

- Height, weight, and body mass index
- Waist circumference
- Exclusion of co morbid medical problems such as diabetes, obstructive sleep apnea, and hypercholesterolemia

TABLE 1 Clinical Use of the Body Mass Index (BMI)

BMI = ratio of weight in kilograms or weight in pounds to (height in meters)² or (height in inches)²
Obesity is defined as BMI >30. If risk factors such as heart disease, hypertension, or elevated serum cholesterol levels are present, more aggressive intervention may be warranted for a BMI >27.

Medical Consequences of Obesity

Obesity and its multiple medical co-morbidities are associated with a profound increase in morbidity and premature mortality. With increasing BMI there is an increased prevalence of metabolic syndrome/insulin resistance, diabetes mellitus, hypertension, coronary artery disease, lipid and cholesterol dyscrasias, gallbladder disease, respiratory compromise, degenerative joint disease, infertility, and some cancers. The major complications associated with obesity are addressed next.

INSULIN RESISTANCE/METABOLIC SYNDROME

The fundamental pathophysiologic defect that often leads to non–insulin-dependent diabetes mellitus (NIDDM) is insulin resistance. It is estimated that 25% of the population is insulin resistant, which is especially prevalent in individuals with the android type of weight distribution. Hyperinsulinemia results from compensatory pancreatic cell hypersecretion and therefore serves as a biologic and laboratory marker of insulin resistance. After prolonged hypersecretion, the insulin secretory capacity of the β cells diminishes, possibly because of the accumulation of amyloid deposits in the islet cells and eventually decompensation of insulin resistant to overt hyperglycemia. In addition, undetermined genetic factors and acquired factors such as aging, sedentary lifestyle, and obesity all contribute to insulin resistance.

Clinically, this syndrome can be associated with abdominal obesity (android adiposity), hypertension, hypertriglyceridemia, high-density lipoprotein/low-density lipoprotein (HDL/LDL) cholesterol abnormalities, hyperuricemia, fluid retention, polycystic ovarian

TABLE 2 Prescription Medications That May Promote Weight Gain

Class of Medication	Examples
Antidiabetics	Insulin, thioglitazones, sulfonylureas
Antipsychotics	Risperidone (Risperdal), clozapine (Clozaril), olanzapine (Zyprexa)
Antidepressants	Amitriptyline (Elavil), imipramine (Tofranil), doxepin (Sinequan), lithium desipramine (Norpramin), trazodone (Desyrel), tranylcypromine (Parnate)
Antiepileptics	Valproate (Depakote), carbamazepine (Tegretol)
Steroids	Glucocorticoids
Antihistamines	Astemizole[2]

[2]Not available in the United States.

syndrome, hypofibrinolysis, acanthosis nigracans, and skin tags. Studies revealed that treatment options in this patient population favor complex carbohydrate modification, reduced fat intake, regular exercise, and possibly the use of medications, such as metformin, that increase insulin sensitivity.

DIABETES MELLITUS

Undoubtedly, the increasing prevalence of obesity is associated with the growing prevalence of NIDDM in the United States. Some 70% to 80% of patients with NIDDM are overweight. NHANES data clearly reveal a strong correlation between the relative risk of development of NIDDM and increasing body mass index beyond 27 kg/m^2. Moreover, there exists a 10-fold increase in the prevalence of obesity in individuals with a BMI more than 40 kg/m^2. Additional individual risk factors for the development of diabetes mellitus, regardless of gender, include increasing age, family history of NIDDM, and central adipose distribution. What must be emphasized, however, is that even a modest weight loss (5% to 10% of presenting weight) can have tremendous benefit on glycemic control as well as curtailing the development and progression of the multiple co-morbidities associated with diabetes mellitus.

HYPERTENSION

Hypertension is a common, chronic disease affecting millions of individuals worldwide. A strong correlation exists between hypertension and obesity, with obesity associated with approximately 30% to 50% of the hypertension in the United States. In addition to a reduction in blood pressure, left ventricular mass, which is often associated with long-standing hypertension, has been shown to be reduced with a modest weight loss (5% to 10% of presenting weight). Moreover, a modest weight loss often leads to reduction or elimination of the need for hypertensive pharmacotherapy.

CORONARY HEART DISEASE

Until recently, obesity was considered only a minor contributor to coronary artery disease (CAD). However, in response to the emerging body of scientific, medical, and behavioral data about the link between excess adiposity and CAD, the American Heart Association reclassified obesity as a major, modifiable risk factor for CAD. In addition to obesity alone, studies suggest when other co-morbidities are present (such as hypertension, elevated LDL cholesterol, diabetes mellitus, and elevated serum triglycerides), obese individuals are at even greater risk for the development of CAD, and more aggressive treatment options may be warranted.

LIPID DYSCRASIAS

Blood lipid abnormalities are common in the obese individual. Obese individuals who possess the upper body, android, visceral adiposity often have lower HDL cholesterol leading to an increased risk of the development of CAD. On the contrary, individuals who possess the lower body, gynoid, more subcutaneous adiposity are predisposed to an elevated HDL cholesterol concentration that is cardioprotective. Overweight and obese individuals routinely have normal or slightly elevated total or LDL cholesterol levels. Therefore, individuals with a random total cholesterol level greater than 200 mg/dL warrant a fasting lipid profile.

Unlike cholesterol, obesity predisposes individuals to higher triglyceride levels compared to normal weight individuals. Although hypertriglyceridemia alone and its association with increased morbidity and mortality have been controversial, increased portal free fatty acid availability and hyperinsulinemia increase the synthesis of very low density lipoprotein (VLDL), which is a risk factor for CAD. Pharmacologic intervention is often required when obese individuals exhibit Frederickson class IV or V hyperlipidemia.

PULMONARY ABNORMALITIES

Severe respiratory insufficiency, commonly known as pickwickian syndrome, may develop in patients with morbid obesity. Obstructive sleep apnea syndrome and obesity hypoventilation syndrome are two primary breathing disorders of the pickwickian syndrome. With obstructive sleep apnea, the tongue obstructs the glottis during sleep impeding air entry to the trachea. In moderately and morbidly obese individuals, obstructive sleep apnea is very common and often misdiagnosed. Symptoms of obstructive sleep apnea include snoring, apneic episodes, excessive daytime somnolence, memory loss, irritability, fatigue, and erectile dysfunction. Nocturnal hypoxemia, a consequence of sleep apnea, may contribute to arrhythmias, pulmonary hypertension, and right-sided heart failure. The most important and first-line intervention should be weight reduction. Moderate weight loss as a result of modified caloric intake improves oxygenation and sleep apnea in obese subjects. The most likely mechanism of improvement after a modest weight loss results from an increase in airway size or from changes in ventilatory drive, which increases upper airway muscle activity.

Treatment Options

Successful comprehensive weight management programs combine the use of nutritionally balanced, mildly hypocaloric diet regimens, modest regular activity, behavior modification techniques and, when indicated, pharmacotherapy. High rates of recidivism are seen in programs not proportionally balanced or requiring drastic dietary modification.

INITIAL EVALUATION

Individuals should undergo a comprehensive history and physical examination before initiating any diet and exercise program. Secondary causes of obesity such as Cushing's syndrome, hypothyroidism, and diabetes mellitus should be considered in the initial evaluation. In addition, contraindications to weight reduction such as pregnancy, lactation, unstable mental illness, and medical conditions such as unstable angina or uncontrolled blood pressure should all be evaluated prior to initiation. Eating disorders such as anorexia and bulimia must also be considered. The physical examination should include both the BMI and waist circumference. These are critical to stratify patients to predict and guide various treatment options (Figure 2).

Initial blood chemistry studies including complete blood cell count, liver function studies, fasting lipid profile, determination of thyroid-stimulating hormone concentration, fasting glucose level, and renal panel should be considered as well as an electrocardiogram in appropriate individuals.

BMI category	Health risk based on BMI
<25	Minimal–low
25–<27	Low–moderate
27–<30	Moderate–low
30–<35	High–very high
35–<40	Very high–extremely high
>40	Extremely high

Health risk	Treatment options
Minimal and low	Healthful eating Increased physical activity Life style changes
Moderate	All of the above plus caloric restriction
High + very high	All of the above plus pharmacotherapy
Extremely high	All of the above plus surgical considerations

FIGURE 2. Determination of health risk based on body mass index (BMI) and various treatment options. (Adapted from the National Institute of Health: Practical Guide to the Identification, Evaluation, and Treatment of Overweight and Obesity in Adults, 1998.)

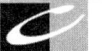

CURRENT THERAPY

- Diet, exercise, and behavior modification
- Pharmacotherapy
- Bariatric surgery

DIET

Once any secondary causes of obesity (hypothyroidism, Cushing's syndrome, etc.) are ruled out, determination of what diet regimen to best fit the overweight or obese individual is critical. The implementation of drastic, unrealistic dietary limitations makes long-term compliance difficult.

Popularized in the 1970s, very low calorie diets (VLCDs) were widely used to promote initial rapid weight loss. VLCDs are drastically limited in energy, usually between 600 and 800 calories per day, resulting in significant but usually short-term results.

VLCDs can be beneficial in the instance where rapid weight loss is needed for a specific procedure to be performed (i.e., cardiac catheterization) or life-threatening obstructive sleep apnea where rapid weight loss can significantly reduce the frequency and duration of apneic episodes. Individuals on VLCDs should be closely monitored, and additional supplementation of at least 1500 mL of water, multiple vitamins, calcium, magnesium, and potassium are usually required. VLCDs should be used as an initial step to a less drastic conventional balance deficit meal plan.

Contraindications to VLCDs include recent myocardial infarction, unstable angina, malignant arrhythmias, type I diabetes mellitus, and pregnancy. Medications such as insulin, sulfonylurea hypoglycemics, and antihypertensives must be carefully monitored and often tapered as weight loss ensues.

Popular commercial liquid diet preparations usually contain approximately 10 to 15 g of protein, 30 to 45 g of carbohydrate, and 2 to 3 g of fat. The vastly protein-rich supplements contribute to caloric energy levels and usually range between 180 and 250 calories per serving. Rates of recidivism remain quite high with most commercial diet preparations. This is mostly because of the failure of liquid diets to provide an opportunity for the patient to alter fundamental eating and lifestyle behaviors needed for sustained weight loss.

Over the last several years, low-carbohydrate ketogenic diets such as the Atkins diet have been popular in the lay press. Although initially one may see increased satiety and rapid weight loss because of fluid loss, long-term studies on cardiovascular risk reduction and sustained weight loss over other diet options are ongoing.

What is probably most beneficial for the majority of overweight and obese individuals is a less drastic hypocaloric and balanced meal plan. These typically provide 1200 to 1800 calories per day, 20% to 30% of calories from fat, 50% to 55% from carbohydrates, and 15% to 20% from protein. These conventional diets should result in losses of approximately 1 to 2 lbs per week or 4 to 8 lbs per month. These less drastic meal plans allow individuals to make lifestyle changes, ideally long term.

To recommend a caloric concentration adequately, one must determine the caloric requirement to maintain a patient's weight upon presentation. This is crucial so unrealistic goals are not placed on individuals, setting them up for failure. For instance, in most instances it is unrealistic for a 275-lb man to adhere to 1200 calories per day. As a general rule, a 500-calorie per day deficit promotes a weight loss of 1 lb per week. A moderate degree of restriction is better tolerated, and long-term compliance should be superior to more restrictive caloric plans.

In addition to calories consumed by eating, it is also important to discern how many calories individuals are drinking. Individuals can drink thousands of calories per day and not equate them to "total calories consumed per day." Maintaining blood volume by drinking at least 64 oz of water per day and limiting or avoiding liquids with calories (i.e., regular sodas, juices, alcoholic beverages) has proven beneficial.

BEHAVIOR MODIFICATION

Behavior modification must be an integral part of any diet plan to promote the best chance of success. Several controlled trials have validated the effectiveness of behavioral techniques. However, in a busy primary care office this can be time consuming. A concise and comprehensive manual that provides specific monthly goals for the practitioner to review with patients is the Learn Program for Weight Control from the American Health Publishing Company in Dallas, Texas. This provides excellent behavior modification lessons for the patient to work through between office visits.

EXERCISE

In reviewing national weight loss registries in patients who have lost a significant amount of weight and kept it off for greater than 1 year, regular exercise is the most common denominator for weight maintenance. Unfortunately, exercise is the most difficult component of a comprehensive weight management program, partly because of unrealistic expectations placed on obese individuals. Many experts agree that 30 minutes a day, 5 days a week, of aerobic activity is the minimum exercise prescription required for weight loss and maintenance. However, it is unrealistic to expect an obese individual to sustain himself or herself, at least initially, for 30 minutes and therefore, compliance drops precipitously.

A more reasonable starting point is an occurrence type of activity program several times per day. For instance, 3 to 5 minutes of aerobic activity five to six times a day is much better tolerated by a patient, and long-term compliance is greatly enhanced. The use of a pedometer can objectively measure one's number of steps, and goals of 8000 to 10,000 steps per day should be recommended. Also, common everyday activities such as walking up stairs rather than taking the elevator or escalator, parking farther away from an entrance, or not using the television remote control add up to small but meaningful periods of increased activity, thereby increasing energy expenditure. Increased exercise, however, increases muscle mass, which weighs more than adipose tissue. Once a patient progresses to 30 minutes of occurrence exercise, 5 days per week, studies have determined a greater than 50% chance of achieving weight maintenance.

PHARMACOTHERAPY

During the 1990s, there were great ups and downs in the development of pharmacotherapy for the treatment of obesity. What must be emphasized, however, is that if pharmacotherapy is considered, it must be used as an adjunct to diet, behavior modification, and exercise to attain the best results for patients.

One of the oldest medications that is still available and used is phentermine (Ionamin). Phentermine is adrenergic medication that mildly increases norepinephrine release. This medication was popularized in the early 1990s when Weintraub studied the efficacy of phentermine used in combination with fenfluramine[1,2] or the so-called fen-phen combination. Phentermine, used alone, is not associated with cardiac valvular defects and remains available for use as a single agent for short-term use (3 months). It is available as phentermine HCl and phentermine resin. The resinate, when compared to HCl, is absorbed more slowly and blood levels reach a lower, later, and flatter peak, which is likely to result in more consistent and sustained blood levels. Potential side effects of phentermine include dry mouth, palpitations, tachycardia, hypertension, insomnia, or overstimulation.

Early in 1998, the Food and Drug Administration (FDA) approved the use of sibutramine (Meridia) for the treatment of obesity. Sibutramine is a beta-phenylethylamine that acts as a reuptake inhibitor for both norepinephrine and serotonin. Unlike fenfluramine and dexfenfluramine, sibutramine does not possess any

---

[1] Not FDA approved for this indication.
[2] Not available in the United States.

releasing ability of serotonin. It is the potent releasing ability of dexfenfluramine and fenfluramine that has been suggested to be the cause of the valvular heart disease and pulmonary hypertension associated with these medications. To date, there have been no reports of any valvulopathies or primary pulmonary hypertension with the use of sibutramine.

Most common side effects associated with sibutramine include dry mouth, insomnia, and constipation. In addition, tachycardia and hypertension (mean blood pressure increase of 2 to 3 mm Hg and increase in pulse rate by four to five beats per minute) are reported. Therefore, pulse and blood pressure should be monitored when initiating sibutramine. Efficacy studies using sibutramine revealed an approximate 8% weight loss at the end of 12 months when used in combination with diet. Contraindications to sibutramine include use with any monoamine oxidative inhibitors or selective serotonin reuptake inhibitors or in patients with severe renal or hepatic impairment. In addition, it is contraindicated for patients with a history of CAD, congestive heart failure, arrhythmias, stroke, glaucoma, or uncontrolled hypertension.

In May 1999, the FDA approved another medication for the treatment of obesity, orlistat (Xenical). Orlistat tetrahydrolipstatin is a selective inhibitor of pancreatic lipase and thus is a novel approach to weight loss medications. Orlistat is the first nonsystemically acting medication that acts locally in the gastrointestinal tract to block gastric and pancreatic lipase and results in decreased fat absorption. Orlistat inhibits lipases for approximately 90 minutes after ingestion. Approximately a third of digested fat is excreted in the stool by patients taking orlistat. Recently, orlistat has been approved, at the 60-mg dose, for over-the-counter use under the name Alli.

Certain adverse events can be predicted from the mode of action of orlistat including steatorrhea, oily spotting, flatulence with discharge, and fecal urgency. Fat-soluble vitamins A, D, E, and K as well as beta carotene may be modestly decreased in individuals taking orlistat; therefore, multivitamin supplementation is recommended daily. Efficacy studies after 2 years revealed an approximate 9% weight loss when used in combination with a mildly hypocaloric meal plan.

The use of pharmacotherapy as an adjunct to diet, exercise, and behavior modification is indicated for individuals with a BMI more than 30 kg/m^2 or more than 27 kg/m^2 with a co-morbid medical problem relating to their obesity such as diabetes, hypercholesterolemia, or hypertension. Pharmacotherapy alone is neither indicated nor recommended. Table 3 summarizes commonly prescribed medications for the treatment of obesity.

BARIATRIC SURGERY

Bariatric surgery for the treatment of obesity, despite impressive outcomes, should be considered for patients suffering from morbid obesity. The surgical candidates who can benefit the most include patients who have failed medical management and who have a BMI more than 40 kg/m^2 or have a BMI 35 kg/m^2 and also suffer from diabetes, hypertension, obstructive sleep apnea, cardiovascular disease, gastroesophageal reflux disease, degenerative joint disease, or steatohepatitis (fatty liver). Amelioration of those common medical problems should be the prominent reason for considering bariatric surgery.

Contraindications to bariatric surgery include untreated major depression/psychosis, certain personality disorders, active alcohol or drug abuse, and noncompliance with preoperative medical, nutritional, and psychological management. Age greater than 65 years is no longer an absolute contraindication to bariatric surgery, but the risk may outweigh the benefits for patients older than 70 years.

Bariatric surgery for children and adolescents remains highly controversial. However, surgery on patients between 12 and 18 years of age who have significant medical problems relating to their obesity (diabetes mellitus, obstructive sleep apnea, reactive airway disease, steatohepatitis, and metabolic syndrome) has resolved their co-morbidities.

PREOPERATIVE EVALUATION

A comprehensive team approach is supported and recommended by most physicians and insurance carriers. An ideal program would encompass a minimum of four components: medical, nutritional, psychological, and surgical. This multidisciplinary team is involved in evaluating the patient before surgery and in the education and treatment after surgery. This team ensures optimal medical, nutritional, and psychological care and ensures good insight into the lifelong lifestyle changes after bariatric surgery.

SURGICAL ASSESSMENT

Once the patient completes the preoperative medical, nutritional, and psychological evaluation and has achieved adequate metabolic control of any medical problems, he or she can be referred to the bariatric surgeon. The surgeon evaluates the patient's motivation and expectations, discusses the risks and benefits of the different surgical interventions, and chooses the most appropriate surgery for each individual patient.

Most Common Surgical Options

RESTRICTIVE PROCEDURES: GASTRIC BANDING AND THE ADJUSTABLE LAPAROSCOPIC BAND

Gastric banding has been popular in Europe, but until the 1980s did not receive much attention in the United States. Initial stapling procedures (Figure 3A) were complicated by staple-line ruptures. This has given rise to the more commonly performed verticalbanded gastroplasty (VBG) (Figure 3A). The VBG separates the stomach, forming a small pouch that joins the rest of the stomach through a small channel. This channel is banded, so to speak, with a ring of nonexpandable material that prevents the opening from enlarging. This procedure is relatively easy to perform and involves no bypass of the intestines. The VBG is not routinely performed any longer and has since been replaced by the laparoscopic adjustable band (Figure 3B).

The adjustable laparoscopic band is also a purely restrictive and relatively noninvasive procedure that requires no malabsorption. These restricted procedures are generally best suited for patients who eat large quantities of protein and carbohydrates because

---

TABLE 3 Commonly Prescribed Medications for the Treatment of Obesity

Generic Name	Phentermine	Sibutramine	Orlistat
Trade Name	Ionamin Fastin Adipex-P	Meridia	Xenical
Mechanism of Action	Adrenergic agonist	Norepinephrine and serotonin inhibitor	Lipase inhibitor
Dose	15–30 mg 37.5 mg	5–15 mg	120 mg
Side Effects	CNS CV	CNS CV	GI

Abbreviations: CNS = central nervous system; CV = cardiovascular; GI = gastrointestinal.

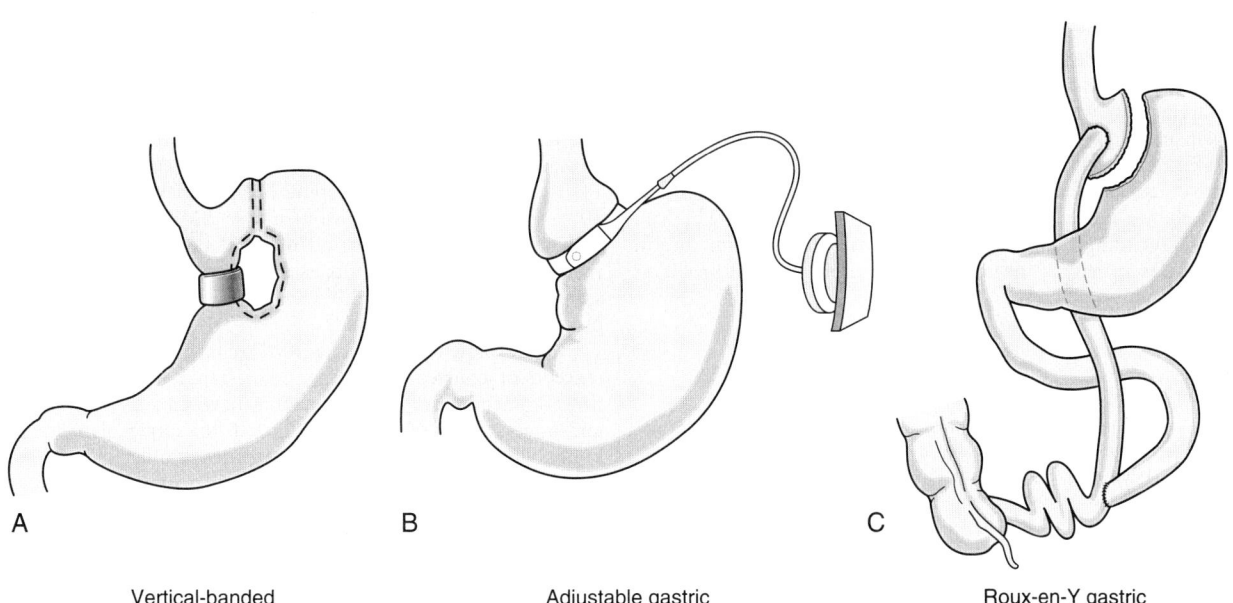

FIGURE 3. Techniques commonly used for the surgical treatment of obesity: vertical-banded gastroplasty (**A**), adjustable laparoscopic band (**B**), Roux-en-Y gastric bypass (**C**).

surgery prevents entry of a large quantity of food. Weight loss may be less adequate in patients who consume high-calorie soft foods and liquids (such as cakes, milkshakes, and ice cream) because these can rapidly pass through the banded channel. Expected weight loss with the adjustable lap band approximates 40% to 60% of excess body weight in properly selected individuals. However, with patients that consume soft foods and liquid calories, long-term weight loss (3 to 5 years postoperatively) may be somewhat variable.

COMBINED RESTRICTIVE AND MALABSORPTIVE PROCEDURES: ROUX-EN-Y GASTROPLASTY

The Roux-en-Y gastroplasty combines stomach restriction with a bypass procedure and modest malabsorption of a vast majority of the stomach and the first part of the small intestine called the duodenum. This procedure prevents entry of large amounts of food at one time while bypassing the duodenum, where calories are normally absorbed (Figure 3C).

In most instances, the malabsorptive procedures are more effective than VBG and the adjustable lap band for causing and maintaining weight loss. The expected weight loss for the malabsorptive procedures are approximately 70% to 80% of a patient's excess body weight 3 years following surgery and continued maintenance 50% to 60% of excess body weight after 10 years depending on which procedure. Most importantly, co-morbid medical problems relating to obesity such as diabetes, high cholesterol, obstructive sleep apnea, fatty liver, and high blood pressure diminish or resolve after malabsorptive bariatric surgery.

All of the bariatric procedures just discussed are relatively safe, with an overall mortality of less than 2% when performed by an experienced surgeon who has performed at least 75 surgeries.

Pregnancy should be avoided for at least 12 to 18 months after undergoing malabsorptive bariatric surgery. With changes in absorption of iron/vitamins, vitamin B_{12}/folate, and protein along with rapid weight loss, women are at higher risk for spinal cord defects and other pregnancy complications. As with other medications during this period, adequate blood levels of oral birth control pills cannot be assured, and additional measures of birth control using barrier methods, patches, or injections are necessary.

Benefits of Modest Weight Loss

What is often overlooked in the obese individual with multiple co-morbid medical problems is the benefit of a modest weight loss. As health care providers, of primary importance is managing, not curing, the co-morbid medical problems of obese patients (e.g., blood sugar control, reducing cholesterol, etc.). Modest (10% to 15%) weight loss is documented in several studies to produce significant benefit in glucose control, blood pressure, and lipid management. A goal of metabolic fitness, as defined as the absence of biochemical risk factors associated with obesity, such as elevated fasting concentration of cholesterol, triglycerides, glucose, or elevated blood pressure, should be sought. Although in many instances achieving metabolic fitness still leaves patients obese by many practitioners' standards, there is tangible benefit in health risk reduction, increase in quality of life, and improved physical function.

Future Treatment Options for Obesity

Over the last decade, great advancements have been made in the treatment of obesity. This is related in part to a better understanding of appetite regulation on the neural-hormonal level, discovery of various human obesity genes, molecular targets for obesity treatment as well as various signals that regulate food intake and energy homeostasis. Characterization of obesity-associated gene products has revealed new biochemical pathways and molecular targets for potential pharmacologic intervention that will likely lead to new treatments into the millennium.

Although great strides have been made in the discovery of various hormones, genes, and gene products to develop the ideal antiobesity agent, it is likely that pharmacologic treatments will require combination therapy likely tailored to phenotype and genotype; each requiring a distinct mechanism of action. Optimism remains high for a magic bullet for the cure of obesity; however, one cannot lose sight of the fact that diet, exercise, and behavior modification will remain the cornerstone for any potential future pharmacotherapy.

In conclusion, obesity in the United States has reached epidemic proportions, leading to a significant health crisis. Health care providers can no longer view obesity as a social issue but rather they must acknowledge it as a chronic medical condition, like diabetes, requiring long-term treatment. A realistic goal set at the outset to achieve metabolic fitness via a comprehensive weight management program consisting of prudent dietary changes, behavior modification, and regular aerobic exercise, with or without the adjunctive use of pharmacotherapy and/or surgery, will provide the best chance for modest weight loss and maintenance. This will be most rewarding, not only for patients, but also for health care providers managing the multiple co-morbid medical problems relating to obesity.

REFERENCES

Apovain C: The medical management of obesity and the role of pharmacotherapy: An update. Nutr Clin Pract 2000;15:5-12.

Brownell KD, Wadden TA. The Learn Program for Weight Control. Dallas, Tex, American Health Publishing Company.

Buchwald H, Avidor Y, Braunwald E, et al: Bariatric surgery: A systematic review and meta-analysis. JAMA 2004;292(14):1724-1737.

Kushner RF: Roadmaps for Clinical Practice: Case Studies in Disease Prevention and Health Promotion—Assessment and Management of Adult Obesity: A Primer for Physicians, Chicago: American Medical Association, 2003.

National Institutes of Health, National Heart, Lung and Blood Institute: North American Association for the Study of Obesity: The Practical Guide to the Identification, Evaluation, and Treatment of Overweight and Obesity in Adults, Bethesda, Md: National Institutes of Health, 2000.

National Task Force on the Prevention and Treatment of Obesity: Overweight, obesity and health risk. Arch Intern Med 2000;160:898-904.

NIH Consensus Development Conference Panel: Gastrointestinal surgery for severe obesity. Ann Intern Med 1991;115:956-961.

Still C: Geisinger Frequently Asked Questions: Weight Management in Adults: Decker Publishing Company, Hamilton, Ontarió, Canada.

Osteoporosis

Method of
Bart L. Clarke, MD, and Sundeep Khosla, MD

Osteoporosis is defined by the World Health Organization (WHO) as a systemic skeletal disease characterized by compromised bone strength predisposing to increased risk of fracture, where bone strength reflects the integration of bone density and bone quality. Bone quality reflects bone architecture, bone turnover, bone microfracture accumulation, and bone mineralization.

Etiology

Osteoporosis results from changes in the bone remodeling process that occur during the skeletal life cycle. Postmenopausal osteoporosis generally results from high-turnover bone loss due to estrogen deficiency in the early menopause, in which osteoblasts fail to completely fill in resorption pits formed by osteoclasts, resulting in minor deficits with each bone remodeling cycle. Over time, this results in significant bone loss. Osteoblast precursors and osteoblasts synthesize and secrete receptor activator of nuclear factor (NF)-kB ligand (RANKL), which stimulates receptor activator of NF-kB (RANK) on osteoclast precursors to differentiate and begin resorbing bone. Osteoblast precursors and osteoblasts also synthesize and secrete osteoprotegerin, which serves as a decoy receptor for RANKL. The balance between RANKL and osteoprotegerin in the local bone environment determines osteoclast activity.

A variety of changes occur in bone mineral density (BMD) measured by dual energy X-ray absorptiometry (DXA) with age in women. Girls experience a rapid increase in BMD starting shortly before puberty. This increase continues until the late teenage years, at which time the rate of increase slows down, until peak BMD is achieved in the late 20s to mid-30s. After about age 35 years, women lose 0.5% to 1.0% of their lumbar spine BMD each year until menopause. Beginning shortly before menopause, women lose as much as 1% to 3% of their lumbar spine BMD each year for the next 5 to 10 years. Postmenopausal women lose BMD less rapidly at other skeletal sites. After this period of rapid bone loss during the early menopause, late postmenopausal women continue to lose lumbar spine BMD at 0.5% to 1.0% each year indefinitely and BMD at other skeletal sites less rapidly.

Men experience the same BMD changes with age as women (except, of course, for the period of rapid bone loss around the time of menopause). Men generally have greater peak areal BMD and bone strength than women due to the larger diameter of their bones, which is a major reason that bones in older men fracture less frequently than older women. Men with osteoporosis often have abnormal gonadal sex steroid levels.

Recent studies using peripheral quantitative computed tomography (CT) scanning, which can distinguish between cortical and trabecular bone loss, show that women and men begin to lose trabecular bone beginning in their 20s, whereas cortical bone loss doesn't start until the mid-50s. With normal aging, women lose greater amounts of trabecular bone than men, whereas men have greater trabecular thinning than women.

Epidemiology

About 44 million persons in the United States are estimated to be affected by low bone mass, based on the 2000 U.S. Census and projections from the third U.S. National Health and Nutritional Examination Survey (NHANES III). Roughly two thirds of these patients meet current WHO criteria for low bone density and one third for osteoporosis. Eighty percent of those with low bone mass are women, but about 20% are men.

RISK FACTORS

A variety of risk factors for osteoporosis are recognized. Female gender, postmenopausal status, nulliparity, late onset of menarche, and early menopause from any cause increase risk of bone loss. Women of northern European or Asian background are at higher risk for osteoporosis, as are those with a positive family history for osteoporosis or fracture, regardless of ethnicity. It is estimated that genetic inheritance explains about 60% to 70% of the variance in BMD within populations.

Environmental and dietary factors play key roles in a patient's risk for osteoporosis. Low calcium or vitamin D intake, alcohol abuse, cigarette smoking, and high-protein, high-caffeine, or high-sodium diets all increase risk of bone loss. U.S. National Health and Nutrition Examination Survey III data show that total daily elemental calcium intake in the United States averages 500 to 600 mg for women from age 20 to 90 years and 600 to 700 mg for men in the same age range. Certain medications, such as glucocorticoids, anticonvulsants, or excess thyroid hormone replacement, may cause bone loss. Lack of regular physical exercise, defined as 30 minutes of weight-bearing exercise each day at least 5 days each week, and a slender body frame, with an average adult weight of less than 127 lb, increase the risk of developing osteoporosis.

Risk factors for osteoporotic fracture include a positive family history of osteoporotic fracture, previous personal history of osteoporotic fracture, propensity to fall, and use of medications predisposing to falls (e.g., sedatives, hypnotics, antihypertensives, narcotics).

Patients with significant bone loss are often completely asymptomatic until they experience a fracture. Patients with clinical fractures are easily identified, but the significance of their fractures may be overlooked, because both patients and physicians might believe that fractures that have occurred are a normal part of the aging process. Osteoporotic fractures by definition occur with minimal trauma, often with falls from standing height or less.

FRACTURES

The average 50-year-old white woman in the United States has a 40% remaining lifetime risk of clinically recognized fracture, with the risk of vertebral, hip, and wrist fractures about equal (16% for each). The estimated remaining lifetime fracture risk increases to more than 50% if asymptomatic vertebral compression fractures are included in this estimate. The average 50-year-old white man has a 4.6% remaining lifetime risk of clinically recognized fracture.

Each year, an estimated 1.5 million fractures occur due to osteoporosis in the United States. Fracture rates are highest in whites and Asians and lower in Latin Americans, Native Americans, and African Americans. The economic cost of these fractures was estimated to be between $12 billion and $18 billion per year in 2002, with 63% of the total cost due to hospital services and 28% due to long-term rehabilitation and nursing home care.

In the United States, more than 250,000 hip fractures result from osteoporosis, with an estimated 20% excess mortality within the first year after fracture and significant functional loss for those who survive. The overall prevalence of hip fracture exceeds 15% by age 80 years and 25% by age 90 years. By age 90 years, 31% of women and 17% of men have had a hip fracture. Hip fractures account for 63% of the total direct costs of osteoporosis. More than 500,000 vertebral fractures occur annually, with resultant loss of height and chronic back pain. It is estimated that more than 25% of women older than 65 years have a vertebral fracture and that as many as 40% of these are asymptomatic. More than 200,000 distal forearm fractures and more than 300,000 other limb fractures occur annually. Limb fractures double every 5 to 8 years after the fifth decade in women, but they do not occur frequently in men until after the seventh decade.

Diagnosis

CLINICAL AND LABORATORY DIAGNOSIS

Men or postmenopausal women found to have significant bone loss, with or without fractures, should undergo physical examination and laboratory evaluation to assess for secondary causes of bone loss. Serum total calcium, phosphorus, alkaline phosphatase, creatinine, aspartate aminotransferase (AST), sensitive thyroid-stimulating hormone (TSH), erythrocyte sedimentation rate (ESR), serum protein electrophoresis, and appropriate x-rays (e.g., spine films), should be obtained to rule out the majority of the recognized secondary causes of osteoporosis, if not checked within the 6 months preceding evaluation. Serum parathyroid hormone, 25-hydroxyvitamin D, urine protein electrophoresis, and serum or urine protein immunoelectrophoresis should be assessed when appropriate. Twenty-four-hour urine calcium and creatinine are helpful to establish that patients are taking and absorbing adequate calcium and to make sure they do not have idiopathic hypercalciuria. The most common secondary causes of bone loss found in postmenopausal women are vitamin D insufficiency or deficiency, hyperparathyroidism, hyperthyroidism in women taking l-thyroxine replacement therapy, and hypercalciuria.

BONE MINERAL DENSITY

Low bone density remains the single most accurate predictor of increased fracture risk. For every 1.0 standard deviation decrease in BMD below the mean for young adults of the same sex and ethnicity, fracture risk roughly doubles at the spine and hip.

BMD should be checked, preferably by DXA, in all patients with a history of osteoporotic fractures or suspected low bone density to quantify the severity of bone loss. All women older than 65 years should undergo bone density testing if it was not done earlier. Postmenopausal women younger than 65 who have risk factors for osteoporosis should be considered for bone density testing. All men older than 70 years should undergo bone density testing if it was not done earlier. BMD testing by any technique may be done to confirm the presence and severity of bone loss, but DXA is required to assess bone loss over time and to monitor effects of therapy. Medicare-approved indications for BMD testing include osteoporotic fractures of the hip, spine, wrist, or other bones; x-ray evidence of vertebral deformity or fracture suggesting osteoporosis; postmenopausal estrogen-deficient women at clinical risk for osteoporosis; monitoring osteoporosis therapy with an FDA-approved drug; primary hyperparathyroidism; and glucocorticoid therapy equivalent to or greater than prednisone 7.5 mg/day for more than 3 months or if the expected duration of therapy is more than 3 months.

The BMD T-score, representing the number of standard deviations above or below the young adult mean for persons of the same sex and ethnicity, is currently used to diagnose osteoporosis and low bone density in men or women older than 50 years. The International Society for Clinical Densitometry advises using the Z-score, representing the number of standard deviation above or below the age-matched mean for persons of the same sex and ethnicity, to diagnose low bone density in men or women younger than 50. The WHO currently defines low bone density in postmenopausal women or older men as a BMD T-score of −1.5 to −2.5 and osteoporosis as a BMD T-score of less than −2.5. The International Society for Clinical Densitometry defines low bone density as a Z-score of less than −2.0 in men or in women less than 50. A WHO Working Group recently released a country-specific FRAX fracture prediction tool to predict an individual's 10-year absolute risk of hip fracture and major osteoporotic fracture for men and women from ages 40 to 90, based on a combination of femoral neck BMD and weighted risk factors including age, gender, height, weight, personal history of fracture, parental history of fracture, current smoking habits, oral glucocorticoids, rheumatoid arthritis, secondary causes of osteoporosis, and alcohol intake.

Biochemical markers of bone turnover are not a substitute for bone density as a means of diagnosing osteoporosis. Several markers of bone resorption have been described, including urine amino- or carboxy-telopeptide of type I collagen (NTx or CTx) and urinary pyridinoline and deoxypyridinoline. Several markers of formation have also been described, including serum bone-specific alkaline phosphatase, osteocalcin, and procollagen type I extension peptides (e.g., procollagen type I intact N-terminal propeptide [PINP]). Bone markers are currently used to monitor the response to treatment with anticatabolic agents and might predict the response to treatment with these drugs better than bone density changes.

Differential Diagnosis

The differential diagnosis for low bone density and osteoporosis is shown in Box 1.

CURRENT DIAGNOSIS

- Serum calcium
- Serum phosphorus
- Serum bone alkaline phosphatase
- Serum creatinine
- Serum AST
- Serum TSH
- Serum 25-hydroxyvitamin D
- Serum PTH
- 24-Hour urine calcium, creatinine, and sodium
- 24-Hour urine NTx or CTx

Abbreviations: AST = aspartate aminotransferase; CTx = Carboxyterminal cross-linking telopeptide of bone collagen; NTx = aminoterminal cross-linking telopeptide of bone collagen; PTH = parathyroid hormone; TSH = thyroid-stimulating hormone.

BOX 1 Differential Diagnosis of Low Bone Density or Osteoporosis

- Celiac disease or other malabsorptive disorders
- Chronic liver disease
- Chronic kidney disease
- Endogenous or exogenous glucocorticoid excess
- Hypercalciuria
- Hyperparathyroidism
- Hyperthyroidism
- Hypogonadism of any cause
- Multiple myeloma
- Osteomalacia
- Prolonged heparin therapy
- Prolonged immobilization
- Systemic mastocytosis
- Type 1 diabetes mellitus
- Vitamin D insufficiency or deficiency

Treatment

Treatment of osteoporosis begins with maximizing acquisition of bone mass during growth and development and preventing bone loss after peak bone mass is achieved. All patients should be encouraged to make healthy lifestyle choices in childhood, adolescence, and their young adult years that are likely to maximize their peak BMD in their late 20s to mid-30s and to follow practices later in life known to minimize bone loss. Patients with known bone loss should decrease their subsequent likelihood of fracture by minimizing their fall risk and avoiding high-risk activities likely to cause fracture. Modifiable risk factors should be adzdressed to assist in preserving bone density.

EXERCISE

Patients with bone loss should perform weight-bearing exercise for a minimum of 3 hours each week to help preserve or increase their BMD and reduce their fall risk. Moderate or higher impact activities, or weight lifting, can help preserve BMD in younger persons.

CALCIUM

Calcium supplementation can help prevent bone loss, cause mild increases in BMD in some women, and prevent hip fracture in postmenopausal women compliant and persistent with treatment. Women with low BMD or osteoporosis should optimize their total daily elemental calcium intake to 1000 mg until age 50, and then increase this to 1500 mg after age 50. Men should optimize their total daily elemental calcium intake to 1000 mg until age 50, and then increase this to 1500 mg after age 50. The 1997 U.S. National Academy of Sciences dietary reference intakes were established to preserve bone health in healthy adults without osteoporosis or bone loss, and they call for healthy adults to take 1000 mg elemental calcium daily until age 50, and to increase this to 1200 mg/day at age 50 and older. Healthy men younger than 50 years should take 1000 mg elemental calcium per day, and healthy men older than 50 years should take 1200 mg/day. The Women's Health Initiative (WHI) study showed that calcium 1000 mg/day and vitamin D 400 IU/day does not prevent fractures in noncompliant patients, but it does prevent hip fractures in those who comply with recommendations.

VITAMIN D

Vitamin D supplementation might prevent loss of BMD or cause mild increases in BMD. Vitamin D stimulates intestinal absorption of calcium and phosphorus. Although adequate sunlight exposure can maintain a normal vitamin D level of serum 25-hydroxyvitamin D of >30 ng/mL in some persons, vitamin D 400 IU/day, in the form of one multivitamin or vitamin D tablet daily, is typically recommended for postmenopausal women and men older than 50 years. Some patients may need as much as 3,000 IU of vitamin D/day to achieve this goal. Patients taking prednisone at more than 10 mg/day should take vitamin D 800 IU/day. Recent meta-analyses of vitamin D clinical trials show that vitamin D can prevent falls and fractures at doses of 700 to 800 IU/day.

ANTICATABOLIC AGENTS

Bisphosphonates are currently the most potent oral antiresorptive agents available to prevent or treat osteoporosis. Approved oral bisphosphonates include alendronate (Fosamax), risedronate (Actonel), and ibandronate (Boniva). Approved intravenous bisphosphonates include ibandronate and zoledronic acid. Bisphosphonates block bone resorption by inhibiting osteoclast activity by several mechanisms, with long-term incorporation into bone. Less than 1% of a dose of an oral bisphosphonate is normally absorbed via the intestine. Oral alendronate and risedronate are proven to decrease bone turnover and reduce vertebral and hip fractures by 50% to 60% in postmenopausal women, whereas oral ibandronate reduces vertebral fractures by 50% to 60%, but it has not yet been proved to reduce nonvertebral, including hip, fractures. Intravenous ibandronate has been shown to prevent bone loss but not fractures. Alendronate 35 or 70 mg once a week is approved for prevention or treatment, respectively, of postmenopausal osteoporosis. Alendronate is also approved for treatment of glucocorticoid-induced osteoporosis and male osteoporosis. Oral risedronate 35 mg once a week, 75 mg once daily for two days each month, and 150 mg once a month are approved for the prevention and treatment of corticosteroid-induced osteoporosis and male osteoporosis. Oral ibandronate 150 mg once a month and intravenous ibandronate 3 mg over 15 minutes every three months are approved for the prevention and treatment of postmenopausal osteoporosis. Intravenous zoledronic acid 5 mg over 15 minutes once a year is approved for the prevention and treatment of postmenopausal osteoporosis.

The first head-to-head comparison trial of oral bisphosphonates showed alendronate to be more effective than risedronate at increasing BMD over 24 months, with no difference in side effects. Fracture numbers were too small to assess in this trial. Patients who stop alendronate after several years of therapy lose bone beginning about 6 months after stopping the drug, but the rate of bone loss is slower than in subjects who had never taken alendronate, and fracture risk does not increase during the first 2 years off the drug. Alendronate appears to be safe when taken for up to 10 years of continuous therapy and risedronate for up to 7 years of continuous therapy.

CURRENT THERAPY

Nonpharmacologic Therapies
- Adequate calcium intake
- Adequate exercise
- Adequate protein intake
- Adequate vitamin D intake
- Low sodium intake

Pharmacologic Therapies
- Alendronate (Fosamax)
- Calcitonin nasal spray (Miacalcin)
- Hormone therapy
- Ibandronate (Boniva)
- Raloxifene (Evista)
- Risedronate (Actonel)
- Teriparatide (Forteo)
- Zoledronic acid (Reclast)

Patients with hypocalcemia, hypersensitivity to medication, or esophageal irritation or strictures should avoid oral bisphosphonates. Patients with renal insufficiency should not take alendronate if their creatinine clearance is less than 35 mL/min and should not take risedronate, ibandronate, or zoledronic acid if their creatinine clearance is less than 30 mL/min. Patients with malignancy treated with high doses of intravenous bisphosphonates appear to have a significant risk of developing osteonecrosis of the jaw (ONJ), particularly following dental procedures, but the risk of ONJ appears to be extremely low with the oral bisphosphonates at doses used to treat osteoporosis.

Raloxifene (Evista) is the first marketed selective estrogen receptor modulator (SERM), and is approved for prevention or treatment of osteoporosis at 60 mg/day. Raloxifene has been shown to decrease vertebral fractures, but not hip fractures. Raloxifene interacts with estrogen receptor (ER)-α and ER-β similar to estrogen, but it causes a different ligand-receptor conformational change that results in tissue-specific effects. Raloxifene is contraindicated in patients with a history of deep venous thrombosis or pulmonary embolus due to increased clotting risk, and it can worsen vasomotor symptoms. Raloxifene has been shown to reduce the risk of breast cancer, but it does not increase or decrease the risk of cardiovascular disease.

Salmon calcitonin nasal spray (Miacalcin) is approved for treatment of osteoporosis at 200 IU in alternating nostrils each day. Salmon calcitonin nasal spray prevents bone loss and vertebral fractures but not nonvertebral fractures, and it can decrease postvertebral fracture pain. The main side effect of nasal spray salmon calcitonin is rhinitis in 12% of treated patients.

The role of hormone therapy remains controversial. The WHI clinical trial showed that estrogen alone, or combination estrogen and progesterone, decreased bone turnover, bone loss, and fractures as expected, but that heart attack, stroke, venous thromboembolism, and invasive breast cancer occurred more frequently. Hormone therapy is currently approved for prevention, but not treatment, of osteoporosis. The FDA advises using hormone therapy in postmenopausal women in doses as low as possible, for as short a time as possible, before stopping therapy. The WHI study showed benefit of hormone therapy in preventing hot flashes, but not in preventing age-related memory loss or improving quality of life.

ANABOLIC AGENTS

Recombinant human parathyroid hormone analogues are potent bone anabolic agents. Teriparatide (Forteo) is the first anabolic agent approved for treating women who have severe postmenopausal osteoporosis and high risk of fracture and for treating men who have primary or hypogonadal osteoporosis and high risk of fracture. Teriparatide is given as 20 μg subcutaneously injected once a day for up to 2 years of therapy. Teriparatide might increase bone density more potently than oral bisphosphonates, and it reduces vertebral fractures by 65% and nonvertebral fractures by 53%. Teriparatide used in combination with alendronate in previously untreated postmenopausal women with osteoporosis is less effective than teriparatide alone, but raloxifene in combination with teriparatide does not appear to impair teriparatide effects on bone. Teriparatide used in combination with alendronate in postmenopausal women previously treated with alendronate is more effective than teriparatide alone. However, it is clear that following 2 years of teriparatide therapy, treatment with an anticatabolic agent, such as a bisphosphonate, is necessary in order to maintain gains in BMD.

Side effects of teriparatide include lightheadedness, dizziness, nausea, or pain at the injection site. Risk of postinjection hypercalcemia is not sufficient to warrant routine monitoring of serum calcium. Teriparatide is contraindicated in patients with a history of osteogenic sarcoma, Paget's disease of bone, unexplained hypercalcemia, history of skeletal radiation exposure, or age less than 18 years. Other anabolic parathyroid hormone analogues are under development.

FRACTURES

Patients with hip or wrist fractures often require surgical treatment, whereas patients with vertebral fractures usually require pain medication and supportive therapy. Vertebroplasty or kyphoplasty can help with pain relief in patients with significant pain due to vertebral fracture. Patients with vertebral fractures and kyphosis can benefit from a lumbar or other support brace. Patients with fractures should be evaluated for secondary causes of bone loss to increase the likelihood that therapy will be effective when it is given. Medications used to treat osteoporosis after fracture are identical to those used to treat or prevent osteoporosis before fracture. The occurrence of a fracture on therapy does not necessarily mean patients have failed therapy, because patients on therapy still have a 20% to 65% chance of fracturing, depending on the therapy selected.

REFERENCES

Cranney A, Guyatt G, Griffith L, et al: Meta-analyses of therapies for postmenopausal osteoporosis. IX: Summary of meta-analyses of therapies for postmenopausal osteoporosis. Endocr Rev 2002;23:570-578.
Epstein S: The roles of bone mineral density, bone turnover, and other properties in reducing fracture risk during antiresorptive therapy. Mayo Clin Proc 2005;80:379-388.
Hodsman AB, Bauer DC, Dempster DW, et al: Parathyroid hormone and teriparatide for the treatment of osteoporosis: A review of the evidence and suggested guidelines for its use. Endocr Rev 2005;26:688-703.
Khosla S, Melton LJ III: Clinical practice. Osteopenia. N Engl J Med 2007;356:2293-2300.
Khosla S, Melton LJ 3rd, Robb RA, et al: Relationship of volumetric BMD and structural parameters at different skeletal sites to sex steroid levels in men. J Bone Miner Res 2005;20:730-740.
Khosla S, Riggs BL: Pathophysiology of age-related bone loss and osteoporosis. Endocrinol Metab Clin North America 2005;34:1015-1030, xi.
Khosla S, Riggs BL, Robb RA, et al: Relationship of volumetric bone density and structural parameters at different skeletal sites to sex steroid levels in women. J Clin Endocrinol Metab 2005;90(9):5096-5103.
Mauck KF, Clarke BL: Diagnosis, screening, prevention, and treatment of osteoporosis. Mayo Clin Proc 2006;81:662-672.
National Osteoporosis Foundation: America's Bone Health: The State of Osteoporosis and Low Bone Mass in Our Nation, Washington, DC: National Osteoporosis Foundation, 2002.
NIH Consensus Development Panel on Osteoporosis Prevention, Diagnosis, and Therapy. Jama 2001;285:785-795.
Raisz LG: Pathogenesis of osteoporosis: Concepts, conflicts, and prospects. J Clin Invest 2005;115:3318-3325.
Riggs BL, Hartmann LC: Selective estrogen-receptor modulators—mechanisms of action and application to clinical practice. N Engl J Med 2003;348: 618-629.
Riggs BL, Melton JL III, Robb RA, et al: Population-based study of age and sex differences in bone volumetric density, size, geometry, and structure at different skeletal sites. J Bone Miner Res 2004;19:1945-1954.
Sambrook P, Cooper C: Osteoporosis. Lancet 2006;367:2010-2018.
Seeman E, Delmas PD: Bone quality—the material and structural basis of bone strength and fragility. N Engl J Med 2006;354:2250-2261.
Tanaka S, Nakamura K, Takahasi N, Suda T: Role of RANKL in physiological and pathological bone resorption and therapeutics targeting the RANKL-RANK signaling system. Immunol Rev 2005;208:30-49.

Paget's Disease of Bone

Method of
Paul D. Miller, MD

Diagnosis

Paget's disease is characterized by excessively high bone turnover in the involved skeletal site(s). Although the bone may appear "osteosclerotic" on radiographic evaluation, the bone strength is actually compromised and may easily fracture. Paget's disease may present with pain in the involved skeleton, or it may be asymptomatic and suspected when a patient is discovered to have either an elevated total serum alkaline phosphatase level or an unexplained elevated bone resorption marker (e.g., urine or serum collagen cross-link of type I collagen: N- or C-telopeptide). If a physician discovers an unexplained elevated total alkaline phosphatase level, then the source of this elevated enzyme must be differentiated as either hepatic or bone (assuming the patient is not pregnant because the placenta also produces alkaline phosphatase). If the alkaline phosphatase originates from bone, differential diagnosis of the possible causes of an elevated bone-specific alkaline phosphatase (BSAP) level is as follows:

1. Paget's disease
2. Metastatic cancer in bone
3. Recent large bone fracture
4. Osteomalacia
5. Hyperthyroidism
6. Hyperparathyroidism
7. Medication induced (antiseizure drugs, parathyroid hormone used for treatment of osteoporosis)
8. Immobilization/space travel
9. Vitamin D deficiency without osteomalacia

Many of these potential causes of an elevated BSAP level can be differentiated clinically and by laboratory testing. In patients who still have an elevated BSAP level of undeterminable etiology, a total body bone scan is required to locate any "hot spots" that could suggest Paget's disease. I always simultaneously order a routine radiograph of any hot spots seen on a radioisotope bone scan because Paget's disease is a radiographic, not a bone scan, diagnosis. The one radiographic finding that can be confused with Paget's disease is metastatic prostatic carcinoma. However, metastatic prostatic cancer is associated with an elevated prostate-specific antigen level and other clinical findings of prostatic abnormalities. Given any radiographic finding that one has difficulty distinguishing between Paget's disease and prostatic cancer, a magnetic resonance image is more distinctly abnormal in metastatic cancer to bone, or, if necessary, a bone biopsy is definitive.

Painful Paget's disease requires treatment. Bisphosphonates are the treatment of choice because of their exceptional efficacy and safety when used appropriately in Paget's disease. Bisphosphonates may have the potential of "curing" Paget's disease or, at least, putting the disease into very prolonged and sustained biochemical and clinical remission.

Asymptomatic Paget's disease should also be treated. Although the proportion of patients with asymptomatic Paget's disease who progress to become symptomatic is not known, progression does occur in many patients, and who might or who might not progress cannot be predicted from the initial assessment. Because progression can lead to bony deformities, fractures, hearing loss, neurologic complications (spinal cord compression, nerve entrapment), high-output congestive heart failure, and osteogenic sarcoma, asymptomatic patients merit strong consideration for treatment. To reiterate, because the bisphosphonates are very safe, especially when required only intermittently in Paget's patients, and can be administered either by the oral or intravenous route, they should not be withheld in asymptomatic Paget's patients.

CURRENT DIAGNOSIS

- No known cause.
- Diagnosed by radiography, not by bone scan or magnetic resonance imaging.
- Often asymptomatic.
- May be active with normal biochemical markers of bone turnover: collagen cross-links or bone-specific alkaline phosphatase.

A few patients with Paget's disease may have normal BSAP but elevated bone resorption (NTX/CTX) markers. In my opinion, this combination of disassociated bone formation versus bone resorption markers may be seen in two circumstances: very early Paget's disease—classic or type 1 Paget's disease, and type 2 Paget's disease, in which the BSAP level never becomes elevated despite sustained elevation of the bone resorption markers.

Paget's disease is a disease of the osteoclasts, the cells that induce bone resorption. In pagetic bone biopsies, these osteoclasts are larger, have many more nuclei, and are increased in number compared to osteoclasts seen in normal patients or in patients with osteoporosis. The initial pathophysiologic process in Paget's disease is excessive bone resorption. Thus, the first radiologic defect seen is an osteolytic lesion (a "black" hole) in bone. Hence, early in the pagetic process, an increase in bone resorption markers is seen before the bone formation markers increase. Owing to the normal coupling process between the bone cell lines (increasing or decreasing bone resorption is followed by a directional increase or a decrease in bone formation), bone formation will, in time, also increase, and the BSAP level will ultimately rise. As the BSAP level rises, the osteolytic lesion begins to develop sclerosis and fill in with the white-appearing honeycombed pagetic features. This is the classic sequence in most pagetic patients.

Type 2 Paget's disease looks just like type 1 on radiography: the initial osteolytic lesion is present. The difference between the two forms of Paget's disease is that the osteolytic lesion persists: the bone resorption markers remain elevated without a rise in BSAP or filling in of the osteolytic lesion. There is something different about this very uncommon form of Paget's disease that both I and my colleagues, who see many Paget's patients, have observed in clinical practice. The normal coupling between bone cell lines seems to be absent. It is possible that these patients started out with a low BSAP level, and that it did increase but never above the upper limits of the normal reference range. It may also be true that type 2 Paget's disease is a different disease from a pathophysiologic point of view than type 1 Paget's disease. It is important, however, to stress that even if the BSAP level never becomes elevated, the high NTX/CTX ratio confers enough evidence of high bone turnover of a sufficient magnitude to warrant treatment because these persistent osteolytic pagetic lesions are highly prone to fracture. Multiple myeloma is another clinical condition characterized by high bone resorption and elevated bone resorption markers without an increase in either bone formation or in the bone formation markers BSAP. Despite the presence of many osteolytic lesions in patients with advanced multiple myeloma, the BSAP level never becomes elevated. Hence, myeloma represents another situation in which there is uncoupling between bone resorption and bone formation, as may be seen in type 2 Paget's disease.

Do the two different forms of Paget's disease respond differently to treatment? Probably not, although the proportion of patients with type 2 Paget's disease is small and insufficient for a head-to-head study with type 1 disease to determine any differences in treatment response.

Treatment

The Food and Drug Administration (FDA)–approved therapies for treatment of Paget's disease are calcitonin and bisphosphonates. Off-label use of gallium nitrate (Ganite)[1] or pliamycin[2] is available for the very rare recalcitrant patient. I have not needed to use either gallium nitrate or pliamycin for more than 20 years because of the exceptional response rate to bisphosphonates. In addition, the response rate seems far greater with bisphosphonates than with calcitonin, which for Paget's disease must be given parenterally and has a high nausea side-effect profile.

Injectable calcitonin has been used for more than 25 years as therapy for Paget's disease and may be considered an option in

---
[1]Not FDA approved for this indication.
[2]Not available in the United States.

CURRENT THERAPY

- Bisphosphonates are the treatment of choice.
- Bisphosphonates should be used in asymptomatic patients who have elevated bone turnover markers.
- May be mono-ostotic (single bone involvement) or polyostotic (more than one bone involved). Once the patient is diagnosed with either mono-ostotic or polyostotic Paget's disease, those bones will be the only ones ever involved. Paget's disease does not spread from one bone to another.
- Recent data suggest that the greater the magnitude of normalization of the total or bone-specific alkaline phosphatase level achieved with treatment, the longer the duration of remission.
- Prevalence is highly variable throughout the world: estimated to be 2% of the white population of North America, declining in northern England, and very rare in China. However, the accuracy of prevalence data must be interpreted in the context that many asymptomatic patients are radiographed, and population radiographic studies that assessed prevalence radiographed only specific skeletal sites, so some involved areas could have been missed.

patients who might not be able to tolerate or to be given a bisphosphonate. Subcutaneous administration of 100 IU/day[3] often leads to an average 50% reduction in bone turnover markers 3 to 6 months after therapy. The nasal spray formulation of calcitonin (Miacalcin) is not FDA approved for Paget's disease.

The bisphosphonates available for treatment of Paget's disease are: etidronate (Didronel), alendronate (Fosamax), risedronate (Actonel, oral formulations), and pamidronate (Aredia). Zolendronic acid[4] is currently under review by the FDA for registration for Paget's disease.

The bisphosphonates alendronate and risedronate have the most robust data showing an exceptional positive effect in the treatment of Paget's disease. Alendronate (Fosamax) at a dose of 40 mg/day for 6 months or risedronate (Actonel) at a dose of 30 mg/day for 2 months can rapidly normalize the NTX/CTX ratio or BSAP level in the majority of patients. No head-to-head clinical trials have compared the efficacy of these two bisphosphonates in Paget's disease, although a head-to-head study did compare etidronate to risedronate in active Paget's disease. Risedronate was clearly more effective in reducing the BSAP level and inducing a longer remission than was etidronate. Selection between the two aminobisphosphonates (alendronate and risedronate) probably is based on physician preference, tolerability, and costs. With either bisphosphonate, bone turnover marker should be measured at the end of the treatment period. If the BSAP level has not normalized, either a second course of the oral bisphosphonate or a change to an intravenous bisphosphonate should be considered. As previously stated, normalization of the BSAP level is the goal of treatment, and the lower the BSAP level, the greater the probability of a longer duration of remission.

Recently, clinical trial data on the efficacy of intravenous zoledronic acid[4] in the treatment of Paget's disease were published. The study showed that 5 mg of intravenous zolendronic acid given over 15 minutes induced a more rapid therapeutic response along with a larger proportion of patients who responded with normalization of BSAP level than was seen with risedronate. In addition, in the 6-month posttreatment follow-up, a greater proportion of patients who received zolendronic acid were still in remission than those who had received risedronate. This finding is consistent with the observations suggesting that the duration of remission is related to the magnitude of suppression of BSAP.

Zolendronic acid[4] has also been shown to have a greater effect on alkaline phosphatase than pamidronate, the other available intravenous nitrogen-containing bisphosphonate.

Hence, with highly effective oral and intravenous bisphosphonates available for treatment of Paget's disease, the clinician must choose which one to use. In my practice, all Paget's disease patients who have pain receive an intravenous bisphosphonate because the pain reduction or elimination is very fast. On the other hand, for asymptomatic Paget's patients, I often use an oral bisphosphonate, saving the intravenous formulations for recalcitrant patients or for patients with relapses. This approach may change as the data evolve, confirming that the duration of remission is prolonged with greater suppression of BSAP. Certainly, costs may become a consideration in the choice, as will upper gastrointestinal conditions that could make an oral bisphosphonate risky. On the other hand, in the zolendronic acid versus risedronate clinical trial, more patients receiving zolendronic acid experienced the acute-phase reaction (fever, muscle pain), which was transient and without sequelae. Nevertheless, intravenous formulations may not be preferred in some patients.

Resistance to bisphosphonates may develop in Paget's disease. After repeated doses of a particular bisphosphonate, some patients stop responding to that particular bisphosphonate but do respond to a different bisphosphonate. The reason for resistance development is unknown because it has not been described in patients treated with bisphosphonates for osteoporosis. Another unexplained phenomenon in Paget's patients who develop resistance to a particular bisphosphonate is that often they again become responsive to the bisphosphonate to which they had become unresponsive after a period of not receiving that specific bisphosphonate.

Finally, there are a few instances in the treatment of Paget's disease in which the clinician must use extra diligence. One is the patient with a painful osteolytic lesion in the proximal femur. Bisphosphonate administration will often relieve the pain promptly, which may encourage the patient to increase activity and weight bearing, and then the hip may fracture. In these circumstances, the patient should be cautioned about this potential and provided with a cane to support the leg until the osteolytic lesion fills in (several months). Another area of caution is the patient who does not respond to any treatment, who relapses quickly and has a rapidly progressive radiographic pagetic change, or develops more pain, swelling, and redness over the pagetic bone. Osteogenic sarcoma could be a distinct possibility, and the lesion may require biopsy. Finally, a third area of caution is the patient in whom neurologic impairment may be related to pagetic bone encroachment, spinal cord compression with long-tract signs, spinal stenosis, or basilar skull invagination with neural compromise. Close consultation with a neurosurgeon is needed to help decide on a possible surgical intervention through a highly vascular pagetic bone. Administration of intravenous bisphosphonate 1 to 2 days before surgery might mitigate bleeding because bisphosphonates reduce blood flow in highly vascular areas for a period of time.

Paget's disease is manageable and may be put into very long-term remission by normalization of the biochemical markers of bone turnover. Asymptomatic patients with high bone turnover should be treated to prevent potential long-term complications. Treatment in these patients is very reasonable given the evidence that the newer aminobisphosphonates are highly effective and very safe when used appropriately.

---

[4]Not yet approved for use in the United States.

REFERENCES

Altman RD, Bloch DA, Hochberg MC, Murphy WA: Prevalence of pelvic Paget's disease of bone in the United States. J Bone Miner Res 2000; 15:461-465.

---

[3]Exceeds dosage recommended by the manufacturer.
[4]Not yet approved for use in the United States.

Miller PD, Brown JP, Siris ES, et al: A randomized, double-blind comparison of risedronate and etidronate in the treatment of Paget's disease of bone. Am J Med 1999;106:513-520.

Reid IR, Miller PD, Lyles K, et al: Comparison of a single infusion of zolendronic acid with risedronate for Paget's disease. N Engl J Med 2005;353:22-32.

Reid IR, Nicholson GC, Weinstein RS, et al: Biochemical and radiologic improvement in Paget's disease of bone treated with alendronate: A randomized, placebo-controlled trial. Am J Med 1996;101:341-348.

Parenteral Nutrition in Adults

Method of
*Elaine B. Trujillo, MS, RD, and
Malcolm K. Robinson, MD*

Since the inception of parenteral nutrition (PN) in the 1960s, the science of PN has matured in a number of ways. The initial excitement of being able to feed basic nutrients, vitamins, and trace elements intravenously has been tempered by the realization that indiscriminant use of PN can be harmful. Although PN can still be lifesaving, it is imperative that it be used judiciously and only as long as necessary. This chapter discusses the current use of PN in adult patients.

Indications and Contraindications

Enteral nutrition is the preferred method of nutrition support, primarily because it is associated with fewer infectious and metabolic complications. However, total PN (TPN), which is the provision of all nutrient requirements intravenously, may be indicated when feeding through the gastrointestinal (GI) tract is not possible. PN may be appropriately initiated in those who cannot receive enteral nourishment and are malnourished or at risk for developing malnourishment. Malnourishment can be defined as unintentional loss of more than 10% of usual body weight or greater than 7 to 10 days of inadequate nutrient intake. The body stores of well-nourished persons are generally sufficient to provide the essential nutrients, resist infection, promote wound healing, and support other necessary physiologic functions for this time period. In patients who are anticipated not to be able to receive adequate enteral nutrition for longer than 10 days, it is not necessary to wait 10 days before initiating PN. This may include patients with short-bowel syndrome and others who are expected to have prolonged GI dysfunction.

According to the American Society of Parenteral and Enteral Nutrition guidelines, enteral nutrition is contraindicated in conditions such as diffuse peritonitis, intestinal obstruction, early stages of short-bowel syndrome, intractable vomiting, paralytic ileus, severe GI bleeding and severe diarrhea and malabsorption syndromes. Other relative contraindications to enteral nutrition include pancreatitis and enterocutaneous fistulae, although depending on the clinical circumstances, enteral nutrition may be indicated. PN and enteral nutrition may be provided concomitantly, although in patients who are critically ill, PN should not be started until all strategies to maximize enteral feeding (such as the use of postpyloric feeding tubes and motility agents) have been attempted. PN support is unlikely to benefit a patient who will be able to take enteral nutrition within 4 or 5 days after the onset of illness or who has a relatively minor injury (Fig. 1).

There are four key steps to consider before initiating PN, including assessing nutritional status, determining energy needs, evaluating GI function, and estimating the length of time a patient will require PN (Box 1).

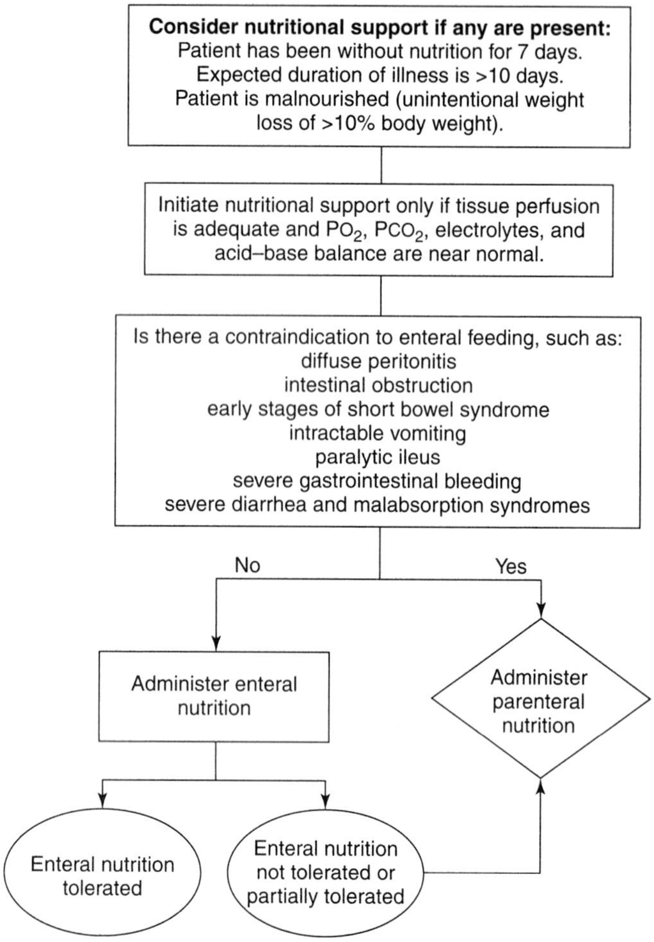

FIGURE 1. Determining route of feeding.

BOX 1 Decision-Making Steps When Initiating Parenteral Nutrition

Assess the patient's nutritional status. Nutrition support (PN and/or EN) should not be initiated in well-nourished patients unless they have received a suboptimal diet for more than 7 days.

Determine if the patient has extreme energy needs (hypermetabolism) that warrant the early use of nutrition support (PN and/or EN) within 7 days of injury or illness. These are typically critically ill patients who have suffered severe burns or trauma.

Evaluate the function of the GI tract; if it is intact and can be used safely, PN should be avoided. PN support is indicated until enteral access is established and the patient can meet nutrient needs via tube feedings.

Estimate how long the patient will require PN support. If GI function is expected to return within 5 days, there is no known benefit of initiating PN.

EN = enteral nutrition; GI = gastrointestinal; PN = parenteral nutrition.

Assessment of Nutritional Status

Nutrient depletion is associated with increased morbidity and mortality, and the prevalence of malnutrition in hospitalized patients is approximately 50%. Therefore, it is imperative to identify patients who have or are at risk for developing protein-energy malnutrition or specific nutrient deficiencies. A patient's risk of developing malnutrition-related medical complications needs to be quantified, and it is necessary to monitor the adequacy of nutritional therapy.

Nutrition assessment begins with a thorough history and physical examination in conjunction with select laboratory tests aimed at detecting specific nutrient deficiencies in patients who are at high risk for future abnormalities. The nutrition assessment should establish whether the patient will need maintenance therapy or nutrition repletion and should assess the status of the patient's GI tract, especially if nutrition support will be required.

A thorough history includes an assessment of recent weight changes, dietary habits, GI symptoms, and changes in exercise tolerance or physical abilities that would indicate functional capacity deficiencies. The physical examination includes inspecting for a loss of subcutaneous fat and muscle wasting, which indicate a loss of body energy and protein stores; edema and ascites, which can also indicate altered energy demands or decreased energy intake; and signs of vitamin and mineral deficits such as dermatitis, glossitis, cheilosis, neuromuscular irritability, and coarse, easily pluckable hair.

Several laboratory measurements have been used as nutritional biomarkers to aid the nutritional assessment. The serum proteins prealbumin, transferrin, and retinol binding protein have a rapid turnover rate and short half-lives and therefore may be used as indicators of recent nutritional intake. However, these proteins are affected by the metabolic responses to stress and illness, as well as other conditions, including iron status (transferrin) and renal status (retinol binding protein, prealbumin). This can limit their usefulness during acute illness states.

Prealbumin is least affected by fluctuations in hydrations status and by liver and renal function compared with other plasma proteins. However, prealbumin levels drop in acute inflammatory conditions during which the liver switches to acute phase protein production and decreases prealbumin synthesis. A rise in C-reactive protein, a protein synthesized by the liver as part of the acute-phase response, indicates inflammatory states. Thus, C-reactive protein when measured along with prealbumin, can help differentiate a low prealbumin due to nutritional inadequacy versus low prealbumin due to an acute-phase response.

The serum albumin concentration has traditionally been used as an indicator of nutritional status. Although it is a good preoperative predictor of outcome for patients undergoing surgery, it is affected by too many variables in the acute care setting to make it a reliable marker of nutritional status under such conditions or in the immediate postoperative period.

A simple and practical index of malnutrition is the degree of weight loss. Unintentional weight loss of greater than 10% within the previous 6 months indicates protein-energy malnutrition and is a good prognosticator of clinical outcome. Weight can also be compared with an ideal or desirable weight, or an index of body weight relative to height. The body mass index (BMI) is the best known such index and can be used to detect both undernutrition and overnutrition: BMI equals weight in kilograms divided by height in meters squared. This index is independent of height, and the same standards apply to both men and women. A BMI of 18.5 to 25 is considered normal, 25 to 29.9 is considered overweight, and greater than 30 is considered obese. Patients with a normal or high BMI can still have nutrient deficiencies and therefore can be malnourished if they have recently lost a significant amount of weight. In addition, a BMI of 18 kg/m^2 or less in an adult indicates moderate malnutrition and a BMI less than 15 kg/m^2 is associated with increased morbidity.

Another practical tool for evaluating nutritional status is the subjective global assessment (SGA) that encompasses historical, symptomatic, and physical parameters. The SGA technique determines if nutrient assimilation has been restricted because of decreased food intake, maldigestion, or malabsorption; if any effects of malnutrition on organ function and body composition have occurred; and if the patient's disease process influences nutrient requirements. The findings of the history and physical examination are subjectively weighted to rank patients as being well-nourished, moderately malnourished, or severely malnourished and are used to predict their risk for medical complications (Box 2).

BOX 2 Subjective Global Assessment

Select the appropriate category with a checkmark, or enter a numerical value where indicated by #.

History
1. Weight change
   Overall loss in past 6 months: amount = # ___ kg; %loss = # ___.
   Change in past 2 weeks: ___ increase, ___ no change, ___ decrease.
2. Dietary intake change (relative to normal)
   ___ No change
   ___ Change ___ duration = # ___ weeks.
   ___ Type: ___ suboptimal solid diet, ___ full liquid diet, ___ hypocaloric liquids, ___ starvation.
3. Gastrointestinal symptoms (that persisted for >2 weeks)
   ___ None, ___ nausea, ___ vomiting, ___ diarrhea, ___ anorexia.
4. Functional capacity
   ___ No dysfunction (e.g., full capacity),
   ___ Dysfunction ___ duration = # ___ weeks.
   ___ Type: ___ working suboptimally, ___ ambulatory, ___ bedridden.
5. Disease and its relation to nutritional requirements
   Primary diagnosis (specify) _____.
   Metabolic demand (stress): ___ no stress, ___ low stress, ___ moderate stress, ___ high stress.

Physical (for each trait specify: 0 = normal, 1+ = mild, 2+ = moderate, 3+ = severe)
___ Loss of subcutaneous fat (triceps, chest)
___ Muscle wasting (quadriceps, deltoids)
___ Ankle edema
___ Sacral edema
___ Ascites

SGA Rating (select one)
___ A = Well nourished
___ B = Moderately (or suspected of being) malnourished
___ C = Severely malnourished

Reprinted with permission from Detsky AS, McLaughlin JR, Baker JP, et al: What is subjective global assessment of nutritional status? JPEN 1987;11:8-13.

Estimating Nutritional Requirements

Historically, TPN often provided nutrients in excess of actual requirements. This was based on the assumption that patients requiring nutritional intervention were severely depleted and required aggressive repletion, hence the misnomer "hyperalimentation." Overfeeding is associated with increased carbon dioxide production and difficulty weaning from a ventilator as well as metabolic complications, such as hyperglycemia, which can lead to increased infection, morbidity, and mortality. Thus, nutritional support should be titrated to match actual metabolic requirements.

ENERGY REQUIREMENTS

There are four components of daily energy requirement. The first component is the basal metabolic rate (BMR), which is the amount of energy expended under complete rest, shortly after awakening and in a fasting state (12-14 hours). BMR varies with age, sex, and body size, correlates roughly with body surface area, and is proportional to lean tissue mass. This relationship holds true even among persons of different ages and sexes. Resting metabolic rate or resting energy expenditure (REE) represents the amount of energy expended 2 hours after a meal under conditions of rest and thermal neutrality. However, although it is often used synonymously with BMR, the REE is typically 10% higher.

The second component of daily energy expenditure is the thermic effect of exercise or the energy used in physical activity. The contribution of this component increases markedly during intense muscular work, and admission to a hospital generally results in a marked decrease in physical activity. Hospital activity in ambulatory patients accounts for a 20% to 30% increase in BMR. Critically ill patients who are on a ventilator generally have low activity levels (BMR increases by only 5% to 10%) because the ventilator performs the work of breathing, and they are not ambulatory.

The third component of energy expenditure is dietary thermogenesis, the increase in BMR that follows food intake. The digestion and metabolism of exogenous nutrients, whether delivered to the gut or vein, result in an increase in metabolic rate. The magnitude of the thermic effect of food varies depending on the amount and composition of the diet and accounts for approximately 10% of daily energy expenditure.

Finally, acute illness adds an additional stress factor to the daily energy expenditure and correlates with disease severity. For example, a patient's metabolic rate increases by 10% to 30% after a major fracture, from 20% to 60% with severe infection, and from 40% to 110% with a severe third-degree burn. In addition, fever accelerates chemical reactions and the BMR rises approximately 10% for each degree Celsius increase in temperature. Alternatively, cooling of febrile patients produces a reduction in BMR of approximately 10% per degree Celsius.

The first step of estimating calorie requirements is to estimate the BMR. This is usually accomplished using one of several predictive equations. The most commonly used method is based on the predictive equations reported by Harris and Benedict in 1909. The Harris–Benedict equations are as follows:

$$\text{BMR (men)} = 66.47 + 13.75(W) + 5.0(H) - 6.76(A)$$

$$\text{BMR (women)} = 655.1 + 9.56(W) + 1.85(H) - 4.68(A)$$

where W is weight in kg, H is height in cm, and A is age in years.

After the BMR is calculated, it is adjusted for the level of stress induced by injury or the disease process (Fig. 2) and activity level. Activity factors for hospitalized patients are 1.0 to 1.1 for intubated patients, 1.2 for patients confined to bed, and 1.3 for patients out of bed. Therefore, the patient's energy requirements (total energy expenditure [TEE]) are finally calculated:

$$\text{TEE} = \text{BMR} \times \text{Activity factor} \times \text{Stress factor}$$

The thermic effect of feeding is generally not included in the calculation of energy requirements for hospitalized patients.

Alternatively, some clinicians estimate energy requirements based on actual body weight. Thus, 20 to 25 calories (kcal)/kg is administered to the critically ill intubated patient and 30 kcal/kg is given to nonventilated patients in whom excessive intake is not a major concern.

Predicting energy expenditure in obese patients can be difficult, because using predictive formulas with current body weight can lead to high TEE and potentially to overfeeding. A factor of 18 to 21 kcal/kg has been validated in obese patients, and the Harris–Benedict equation using the average of actual and ideal weight and a stress factor of 1.3 accurately predicts REE in acutely ill obese patients with a BMI of 30 to 50 kg/m^2.

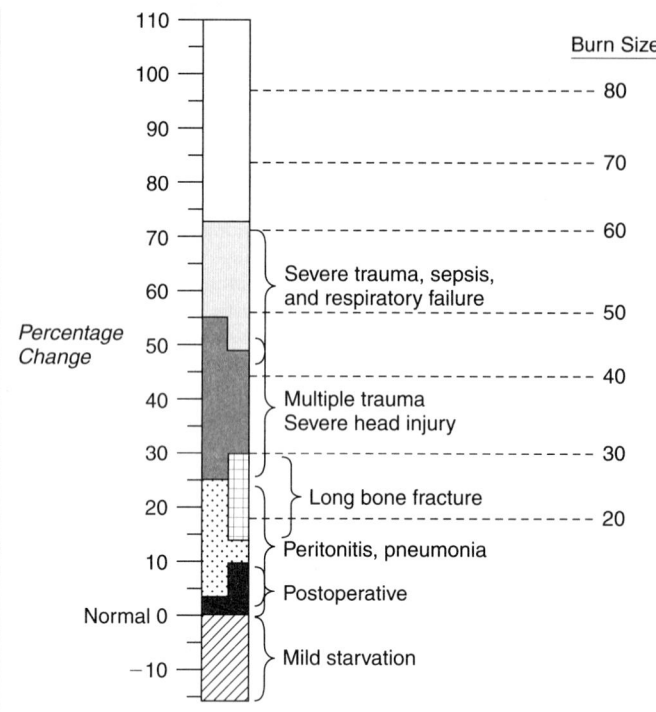

FIGURE 2. Percentage change in metabolic rate due to injury. (Adapted from Wilmore DW: The Metabolic Management of the Critically Ill, New York: Plenum Medical Books, 1977.)

Indirect calorimetry is a more precise, clinically practical and individualized method to determine energy expenditure, particularly in patients in whom estimating requirements through predictive equations are difficult, such as those who continue to lose weight despite what appears to be an adequate caloric intake, who are critically ill, or who have rapidly changing energy needs.

Indirect calorimetry measures changes in oxygen consumption and carbon dioxide production to calculate the REE. Including a stress factor to account for injury is not necessary with indirect calorimetry because the measured energy expenditure accounts for the effects of disease state, stress, and trauma. However, the measurement occurs at rest, and therefore an activity factor of 1.0 to 1.3, depending on whether the patient is intubated, bedridden, or ambulatory, must be applied.

NUTRIENT REQUIREMENTS

The recommended daily protein allowance for most healthy persons who are not hospitalized is 0.8 g/kg or about 60 to 70 g of protein each day. The stressed, critically ill patient generally needs a higher dose of protein in the range of 1.0 to 1.5 g/kg/day. For most patients, providing protein beyond 1.5 g/kg/day is not beneficial. In fact, providing excess protein does not enhance uptake and can lead to increased ureagenesis, which can cause renal injury in some patients.

The calorie-to-nitrogen ratio for most PN solutions typically is around 150:1, with an acceptable range of 100:1 to 180:1. Nitrogen content is used as a marker for protein, and hence the two terms are used interchangeably. Usually, 6.25 g of protein is equal to 1.0 g of nitrogen. The conversion factor is slightly higher (6.4) for PN solutions, such as those with higher concentrations of crystalline amino acids.

Vitamin and mineral requirements are altered in certain disease states due to increased losses, greater use or both. Guidelines for parenteral vitamin and trace elements, developed by the Nutrition Advisory Group of the American Medical Association, were approved by the U.S. Food and Drug Administration (FDA) in 1979 and amended in 2000 (Table 1).

TABLE 1 Recommended Daily Doses of Parenteral Vitamins and Trace Elements

Micronutrient	Parenteral Dose
Vitamins	
Vitamin A	3300 IU
Vitamin D	200 IU
Vitamin E	10 IU
Vitamin K	150 µg
Ascorbic acid (Vitamin C)	200 µg
Folic acid	600 µg
Niacin	40 mg
Riboflavin (Vitamin B_2)	3.6 mg
Thiamine (Vitamin B_1)	6 mg
Pyridoxine (Vitamin B_6)	6 mg
Cyanocobalamin (Vitamin B_{12})	5 µg
Pantothenic acid	15 mg
Biotin	60 µg
Trace Elements	
Zinc	2.5-5 mg
Copper	0.3-0.5 mg
Chromium	10-15 µg
Manganese	60-100 µg
Selenium	20-60 µg

Data from American Medical Association, Department of Foods and Nutrition: Multivitamin preparations for parenteral use. A statement by the Nutrition Advisory Group, JPEN J Parenter Enteral Nutr 1979;3:258-262; Food and Drug Administration: Parenteral multivitamin products: Drugs for human use: Drug efficacy study implementation: Amendment, Federal Register 2000;65(77):21200-21201.

TABLE 2 Central Versus Peripheral Parenteral Nutrition

Property	Central Nutrition	Peripheral Nutrition
Daily calories	2000-3000	1000-1500
Protein	Variable	56-87 g
Volume of fluid required	1000-3000 mL	2000-3500 mL
Duration of therapy	≥ 7 d	5-7 d
Route of administration	Dedicated central venous catheter	Peripheral vein or multi-use central catheter
Substrate profile	55%-60% carbohydrate 15%-20% protein 25% fat	30% carbohydrate 20% protein 50% fat
Osmolarity	~2000 mOsm/L	~600-900 mOsm/L

Composition of Central and Peripheral Venous Solutions

Central venous access is required for providing TPN because of the hypertonicity of the formulas infused (1900 mOsm/kg). The infusion of a hypertonic solution into a peripheral vein, known as *peripheral parenteral nutrition* (PPN), can result in thrombophlebitis and venous sclerosis unless the PN is drastically diluted to lower the tonicity. To minimize the hypertonicity of PPN solutions, dextrose is limited to 5% to 10% and amino acids are limited to 2.5% to 3.5%. Lipids are isotonic and therefore provide a significant portion of the caloric substrate of PPN formulas.

Central venous solutions, which are prepared by the hospital's pharmacy, typically combine carbohydrate in the form of dextrose, protein as crystalline amino acids, and lipids from polyunsaturated long-chain triglycerides such as soybean oil or a safflower/soybean oil mixture. Vitamins, electrolytes, and trace elements are added to the formulation as needed. Typical substrate profiles of carbohydrate, protein, and lipids in central PN are shown in Table 2. A usual PN prescription administers 1 to 2 L of a solution each day. Administration of 500 mL of a 20% fat emulsion 1 day each week is sufficient to prevent essential fatty acid deficiency. Alternatively, if additional calories from lipids are needed on a daily basis, they can be administered as a separate infusion or most commonly as part of the mixture of dextrose and amino acids, a technique known as *triple mix* or *three-in-one*.

Including intravenous fat emulsion into a parenteral admixture changes the conventional nutritional solution into an emulsion. Various electrolytes and micronutrients can adversely influence emulsion stability, and therefore their concentration in three-in-one solutions is limited to prevent cracking of the TPN solution, in which microscopic or macroscopic precipitates are formed. The higher the cation valence, the greater the destabilizing influence to the emulsifier. Therefore, trivalent cations such as ferric ion (iron dextran) are more disruptive than divalent cations such as calcium or magnesium ions, which are more disruptive than monovalent cations such as sodium or potassium. No concentration of iron dextran is safe in triple-mix formulations. In-line filtration is necessary for all PN solutions, including triple-mix solutions because it is impossible to visually detect precipitates until they are grossly incompatible and unsafe for infusion.

Once the basic solution is created, electrolytes are added as needed (Table 3). Sodium or potassium salts are given as chloride or acetate depending on the patient's requirements. Normally, equal amounts of chloride and acetate are provided. However, if chloride losses from the body are increased, such as can occur in patients who have nasogastric tubes, then most of the salts should be given as chloride. Similarly, more acetate should be given to patients when additional base is required because acetate generates bicarbonate when it is metabolized. Sodium bicarbonate is incompatible with PN solutions and so cannot be added to the mixture. Phosphate may be given as the sodium or potassium salt. Lipid emulsions contain an additional 15 mmol/L of phosphate.

Commercially available preparations of fat-soluble and water-soluble vitamins, minerals, and trace elements are added to the nutrient mix unless they are contraindicated. Adequate thiamine is essential for patients receiving PN and can be provided separately. Vitamin K is not a component of any of the vitamin mixtures formulated for adults. Maintenance requirements can be satisfied by adding 10 mg of vitamin K weekly in the PN solution for patients who are not receiving anticoagulants such as warfarin (Coumadin).

Trace element preparations that include zinc, copper, manganese, and chromium are added to the PN solution in amounts consistent with the American Medical Association guidelines (Table 1). Manganese accumulation can be toxic, and overexposure can lead to progressive neurodegenerative damage. Manganese is usually supplied in the PN solution at a daily dose of 0.5 mg as part of a multiple trace element additive. Because manganese is primarily eliminated via biliary excretion, patients with biliary obstruction or cholestasis can accumulate potentially toxic levels of manganese. Hence, manganese should be removed from the PN of patients with hyperbilirubinemia. Higher doses, 10 to 15 mg/day, of zinc are provided to patients with excessive GI losses.

Iron is not a part of commercial additive preparations because it is incompatible with triple mix solutions and can cause anaphylactic reactions when it is given intravenously. Patients who need this trace element should receive it orally or by injection. Iron is not given to patients who are critically ill because hyperferremia can increase bacterial virulence, alter polymorphonuclear cell function, and increase host susceptibility to infection.

PPN is less commonly used than central PN or TPN and can be disadvantageous. Because of the low concentration of dextrose, greater volumes (≥ 2 L/day) are required to provide sufficient calories, which might not be feasible in fluid-restricted patients. PPN generally does not approximate a patient's energy needs, because PPN provides only 1000 to 1500 kcal/day and a large percentage of the calories (50%)

TABLE 3 Electrolyte Concentrations in Parenteral Nutrition

Electrolyte	Recommended Central PN Doses	Recommended Peripheral PN Doses	Usual Range of Doses
Potassium (mEq/L)	30	30	0-120 (CVL)
			0-80 (PV)
Sodium (mEq/L)	30	30	0-150
Phosphate (mmol/L)	15	5	0-20
Magnesium (mEq/L)	5	5	0-16
Calcium (mEq/L) (as gluconate)	4.7	4.7	0-10
Chloride (mEq/L)	50	50	0-150
Acetate (mEq/L)	40	40	0-100

CVL = central venous line; PN = parenteral nutrition; PV = peripheral vein.

are derived from fat. High-fat infusions are undesirable because they are associated with impaired reticuloendothelial system function and are potentially immunosuppressive. There is no evidence that IV lipids improve outcomes or significantly decrease nitrogen losses. Generally, PPN should be avoided unless it is combined with enteral feeding in patients who can not tolerate full enteral feeding, patients who cannot get a central venous catheter, or patients with low body weights in whom PPN can meet at least two thirds of estimated needs.

Administration and Venous Access

Typically, central PN solutions are administered into the superior vena cava. Access to this vein can be achieved by cannulation of the subclavian or internal jugular veins. Peripherally inserted central venous catheters (PICC) (typically inserted via an antecubital vein and advanced into the superior vena cava) are the most commonly used central venous access devices for providing PN. PICC placement offers the advantage of central venous access while avoiding the risks associated with accessing the subclavian or jugular veins, such as hemothorax, pneomothorax, and arterial injury.

Tunneled catheters or catheters with indwelling ports should be considered for patients who will need prolonged central venous nutrition (e.g., >6 weeks). Patients who will be using their catheters solely for daily central PN and who require home IV feeding may be best served by a tunneled catheter rather than an indwelling port. Tunneled catheters may be more easily manipulated and cared for, which can minimize the risk of infection.

Inserting a dedicated line for infusing hypertonic solutions requires strict aseptic technique or maximal barrier protection: Hat, mask, gown, and gloves must be worn. The position of the catheter tip in the superior vena cava is confirmed by chest x-ray before any concentrated solutions are administered. Once the position of the tip has been confirmed, the line should be used exclusively for administering the hypertonic nutrient solution based on the Centers for Disease Control and Prevention (CDC) guidelines.

Multiple-lumen central venous catheters are most commonly used. Although at least one lumen is dedicated to the infusion of the PN solutions, the other(s) may be used for monitoring, blood drawing, or medication. The rate of catheter sepsis associated with multiple-port catheters may be the same as or slightly greater than the rate associated with the use of single-port catheters. However, multiple-port PICCs are used to infuse PN solutions for a shorter time, which can minimize their inherent risk. Multiple-port catheters should be carefully maintained, including dressing changes, maintaining the dedicated lumen, careful handling of the other lumens, and removing the catheter as soon as it is no longer needed.

Infusion and Patient Monitoring

It is advisable to start with 1 L of central PN and increase the volume as needed, depending on the patient's metabolic stability. Blood sugar levels should be closely monitored and maintained at 80 to 110 mg/dL, tissue perfusion should be adequate, and Po_2, Pco_2, electrolytes (especially potassium, phosphate, and magnesium) and acid-base balance should be near normal before starting or advancing to the goal solution. The solutions should be administered using a volumetric pump set at a constant rate. It is important not to modify the infusion rate during any given day to try to compensate for excess or inadequate administration of the PN solution, such as when the PN solution arrives later than expected. A cyclic schedule (10-16 h/day) for patients requiring long-term PN can be initiated once the patient is metabolically stable. In situations when the central PN solution must be suddenly discontinued, a 10% dextrose solution may be given at the same infusion rate as was used for the PN unless the patient is severely hyperglycemic. PN solutions may be administered at one half the infusion rate to patients who are undergoing surgical procedures because circulating glucose and electrolyte levels are easier to control.

In addition to hyperglycemia, metabolic complications include hyper- and hypophosphatemia, hyper- and hypokalemia, hyper- and hypomagnesemia, and hyper- and hypocalcemia. Thus, it is important to monitor the patient's serum electrolytes closely, especially when initiating TPN. Once the patient has stabilized on the individual nutritional prescription, serum chemistries should be obtained at least twice weekly to measure chloride, CO_2, potassium, sodium, blood urea nitrogen, creatinine, calcium, and phosphate levels and once weekly for a full profile that includes liver function, magnesium, and triglyceride levels.

Patients with Special Needs

GLUCOSE INTOLERANCE

Hyperglycemia is the most common metabolic complication related to PN, and glucose regulation may be especially difficult in patients who have diabetes mellitus or who develop insulin resistance in response to severe stress or infection. Control of blood glucose levels is important for all patients who receive PN because uncontrolled hyperglycemia may be associated with complications such as fluid and electrolyte disturbances and increased infection risk due to impairment of host defenses, including decreased polymorphonuclear leukocyte mobilization, chemotaxis, and phagocytic activity. Evidence suggests that maintaining tight blood glucose concentrations between 80 and 110 mg/dL decreases morbidity and mortality in critically ill surgical patients. Intensive insulin therapy minimizes derangements in normal host defense mechanisms and modulates release of inflammatory mediators.

TABLE 4 Management of Hyperglycemia in Critically Ill Patients Receiving Parenteral Nutrition

Blood Glucose	Treatment
Before Parenteral Nutrition or Insulin Infusion	
>220 mg/dL	Start insulin infusion at 2-4 U/h
110-220 mg/dL	Start insulin infusion at 1-2 U/h
<110 mg/dL	Do not start insulin infusion
	Check BG every 4 h
During Insulin Infusion	
Above Normal Range	
>140 mg/dL	Increase insulin infusion by 1-2 U/h
	Monitor BG every 1-2 h until in normal range
110-140 mg/dL	Increase insulin infusion by 0.5-1 U/h
	Monitor BG every 1-2 h until in normal range
Normal Range	
80-110 mg/dL	No change
	Monitor BG every 4 h
Below Normal Range	
60-80 mg/dL	Reduce insulin dosage
	Monitor BG every 4 h
	Recheck BG within 1 h
40-60 mg/dL	Stop insulin, ensure adequate baseline glucose intake
	Recheck BG within 1 h
<40 mg/dL	Stop insulin, ensure adequate baseline glucose intake, give 10 g IV glucose bolus
	Recheck BG within 1 h
Steeply Falling	
Any	Reduce insulin dosage by one half
	Monitor BG every h

BG = blood glucose.
Adapted from Butler SO, Btaiche IF, Alaniz C: Relationship between hyperglycemia and infection in critically ill patients. Pharmacotherapy 22005;5(7):963-976.

Patients with difficult glycemic control may best be managed by continuous insulin infusion, which is safe, effective, and more timely than subcutaneous insulin therapy. Hypoglycemia that occurs during this type of infusion generally is short lived and more easily corrected than hypoglycemia resulting from subcutaneous insulin administration. A separate IV insulin infusion can be used rather than adding incremental doses of insulin to the PN bag every 24 hours in patients in whom glycemic control is difficult. Many intensive care units (ICUs) have an insulin drip infusion protocol in which there are frequent checks of serum glucose and adjustments of the insulin infusion drip (e.g. every 1-2 hours) to maintain tight control of glucose levels. The conventional approach of using sliding scale insulin to cover high blood glucose levels may be unsafe and ineffective, and repetitive doses of subcutaneous insulin in the edematous patient can have a cumulative effect leading to prolonged hypoglycemia. In addition, adjusting insulin in the TPN bag every 24 hours might not achieve the desired rapid correction of hyperglycemia deemed appropriate based on the literature, which indicates worse outcomes for those with poor glucose control. See Table 4 for guidelines for managing hyperglycemia in critically ill patients receiving PN.

Abrupt discontinuation of PN can lead to hypoglycemia and should be avoided. Instead, it is recommended to decrease the PN infusion rate by one half before discontinuation to prevent rebound hypoglycemia.

PANCREATITIS

Most cases of pancreatitis are mild, and nutritional support is not needed. However, 10% to 20% of patients with pancreatitis develop severe disease that results in a hypermetabolic, hyperdynamic, systemic inflammatory response syndrome that creates a highly catabolic stress state. Although the usual care of pancreatitis had been gut rest, with or without PN, an evidence-based review found a trend toward reductions in the adverse outcomes of acute pancreatitis after administration of enteral nutrition. Hence, if feasible, enteral nutrition should be used in patients with pancreatitis because it is associated with a significant reduction in infectious morbidity and hospital length of stay compared with PN.

Initiation of PN should be delayed in patients with acute pancreatitis who cannot tolerate enteral nutrition even though they might eventually require PN. providing PN within 24 hours of admission has been shown to worsen outcome, and providing PN after resuscitation and abatement of the acute inflammatory process appears to improve outcome compared with standard therapy. Consequently, if enteral nutrition is not feasible, the initiation of PN should be delayed for at least 5 days after admission to the hospital, when the peak period of inflammation has abated.

ACUTE RENAL FAILURE

Acute renal failure (ARF) is associated with severe nutritional deficits. Most patients with ARF are catabolic and have energy requirements of 50% to 100% greater than resting requirements, likely the result of other coexisting conditions such as sepsis, trauma, and burns. Calories are provided to patients with ARF in sufficient quantities to minimize protein degradation, generally in the range of 25 to 35 kcal/kg/day. Lipid emulsions can be used as a source of concentrated energy in patients who are on fluid restriction.

Protein loss is accelerated and protein synthesis is impaired in patients with ARF. Loss of amino acids in the dialysate and renal replacement therapies add to the protein deficit and increase individual protein needs. Approximately 10 to 12 g of amino acids are lost with each dialysis therapy, depending on the type of dialyzer membrane, blood flow rate, and dialyzer reuse procedure, and approximately 10 to 16 g/day of amino acids are lost through continuous renal replacement therapies (CRRT). The provision of protein 1.0 to 1.4 g/kg/day and 1.5 to 2.5 g/kg/day is recommended for ARF patients receiving hemodialysis and CRRT, respectively.

Protein is provided with a standard solution containing both essential and nonessential amino acids. Traditionally, formulas designed for renal failure contained predominantly essential amino acids. These formulas often were insufficient in calories and protein for metabolic needs and further compromised the patient's nutritional status. They also increase the risk for hyperammonemia and metabolic encephalopathy when used for longer than 2 to 3 weeks. The current recommendations are to provide adequate protein while treating the patient aggressively with dialysis to prevent the accumulation of nitrogenous waste products.

Fluid and electrolyte balance are often impaired in patients with ARF. The amount of fluid from the PN might need to be adjusted daily, depending on the phase of ARF, whether the patient is receiving dialysis, and whether dialysis is continuous or intermittent. Serum potassium and phosphate levels typically rise in patients with ARF until dialysis is initiated, at which time levels might drop, especially with the provision of PN. Potassium, phosphate, and magnesium levels need close monitoring and adjusting to correct imbalances. Acetate salts of potassium or sodium can be administered to help correct a metabolic acidosis.

Standard doses of the water-soluble vitamins and additional folic acid (1 mg/day total) and pyridoxine (vitamin B_6) (10 mg/day) might need to be added to the solution for patients who are being dialyzed because these vitamins are lost from the body in the dialysate bath. The dose of vitamin C might need to be restricted to 100 mg/day to prevent oxalate deposits. The supplementation of fat-soluble vitamins is usually not required, especially in patients who also are eating, because excretion of fat-soluble vitamins is reduced in renal failure. For example, serum vitamin A levels may be elevated in ARF due to enhanced hepatic release of retinol and retinol-binding protein, decreased renal catabolism, and decreased degradation of vitamin A transport protein by the kidneys. Vitamin D levels may be decreased because of impaired activation of 1,25-dihydroxycholecalciferol in the kidneys. In anuric patients, trace elements may be withheld from the PN solution; however, for prolonged PN, trace elements and fat-soluble vitamins should be monitored and replaced accordingly.

Patients with chronic renal failure (CRF) also have nutritional deficits due to anorexia, amino acid losses into the dialysate, concurrent illness, metabolic acidosis, and endocrine disorders. However, unlike those suffering from ARF, patients with CRF have normal energy requirements. Protein intake generally is restricted in predialysis patients to 0.5 to 0.6 g/kg/day but required in higher amounts in patients on dialysis, depending on the type of dialysis (1.2 g/kg/day for hemodialysis; 1.2 to 1.5 g/kg/day for peritoneal dialysis). Predialysis patients who become acutely ill should be given protein 1.2 to 1.5 g/kg/day even if this precipitates the need for dialysis. Starvation from insufficient calories or protein in the patient with renal dysfunction increases the risk of nutritionally related complications and should be avoided in the severely ill patient regardless of the potential need for dialysis.

Intradialytic PN is the provision of IV amino acids, carbohydrates, and fat directly into the venous drip chamber of the hemodialysis unit during treatment. It is a method of providing additional calories and protein in malnourished chronic hemodialysis patients. It is associated with significant increases in body weight and serum albumin in patients with chronic renal failure. However, intradialytic PN is expensive and the benefits have not been fully elucidated. A typical solution contains about 1100 kcal and 50 g of protein, which is provided three times per week with dialysis. For example, intradialytic PN provides a patient with energy and protein requirements of 2500 kcal and 70 g of protein/day, respectively, only 20% of the weekly calorie and 30% of the weekly protein needs. Thus, intradialytic PN is reserved for patients with CRF who cannot ingest sufficient nutrients by mouth and who are not candidates for nutritional support via enteral nutrition on PN due to GI intolerance or venous access problems or for other reasons. Appropriate use of intradialytic PN should be limited to a very small fraction of people who are on dialysis.

HEPATIC DYSFUNCTION AND LIVER FAILURE

Hepatic dysfunction is associated with a variety of abnormalities including metabolic abnormalities, malabsorption, maldigestion, anorexia, and early satiety due to ascites. Dietary restrictions also can contribute to malnutrition.

Protein intake in patients with stable chronic liver disease depends on the patient's nutritional status and protein tolerance. Nutritionally depleted patients can require as much protein as 1.5 g/kg estimated dry weight. In a minority of patients who have protein-sensitive hepatic encephalopathy, protein intake might need to be decreased to 0.5 to 0.7 g/kg/day and gradually increased to 1.0 to 1.5 g/kg/day, as tolerated. These patients have deranged plasma amino acid profiles, with increased concentrations of aromatic amino acids (phenylalanine, tyrosine, and tryptophan) and methionine and decreased branched-chain amino acids (valine, leucine, and isoleucine). Randomized, controlled trials that provided parenteral or enteral formulas enriched with branched-chain amino acids have been inconsistent and have had results including no benefit, improved morbidity, no change in mortality, and improvement in encephalopathy. These specialty products should be reserved for patients with disabling encephalopathy who do not tolerate standard proteins and have not responded to other therapies, such as lactulose or neomycin administration.

Energy requirements are difficult to predict in patients with liver failure. Whereas most patients have a normal metabolic rate, up to one third may be hypermetabolic. Although providing 25 to 30 kcal/kg/day is a guideline for providing energy needs, basing requirements on indirect calorimetry is often recommended.

Fluid restriction due to ascites and edema often necessitates increasing the dextrose concentration in the PN so as to maintain sufficient calories in a restricted volume. Sodium is reduced in the formula because liver-failure patients excrete nearly sodium-free urine. Vitamin and mineral deficiencies often occur as a result of suboptimal nutrient intake, decreased absorption, decreased storage, and in some cases alcohol use, which decreases thiamine (vitamin B_1) and folate absorption. Copper and manganese may be contraindicated because a major route of excretion for these substances is the biliary system. Zinc deficiency is common in cirrhotic patients, and supplementation of this mineral may be necessary, especially if there are excessive GI losses.

ACUTE RESPIRATORY DISTRESS SYNDROME

Patients with protein-calorie malnutrition have an increased incidence of pneumonia, respiratory failure, and acute respiratory distress syndrome (ARDS). Nutritional support is indicated in patients with ARDS, and underfeeding and overfeeding can be detrimental to pulmonary function.

Overfeeding calories, and particularly glucose, can lead to increased minute ventilation, increased dead space, and increased carbon dioxide production and ultimately to difficulty weaning from a ventilator. Hypercapnia from increased carbon dioxide production is the result of glucose combustion causing more carbon dioxide production and excess calories triggering lipogenesis. A healthy person increases ventilation in response to increased calories and thus avoids hypercapnia. However, patients with compromised ventilatory status might not be able to compensate with increased ventilation and can develop respiratory distress, acute respiratory failure, and difficulty weaning from mechanical ventilation. Thus, the use of indirect calorimetry measurements to determine respiratory quotient and energy expenditure is imperative in patients with ARDS.

OTHER CONDITIONS AND NUTRITIONAL TREATMENTS

The catabolic response to major surgery, trauma, burn, and sepsis is characterized by a net breakdown of body protein stores to provide substrates for gluconeogenesis and acute-phase protein synthesis. Adequate nutrition can attenuate whole-body catabolism but rarely, if ever, prevents or reverses the loss of lean body mass during the acute phase of injury. Several strategies to prevent the loss of lean body mass have been investigated, including growth hormone, growth factors, and conditionally essential amino acids, such as glutamine.

Growth hormone is a potent anabolic agent, and administration to humans increases the rate of wound healing, decreases rates of wound infection, and decreases the catabolism and muscle wasting of critical illness. However, a large European trial found increased morbidity and mortality in patients with prolonged critical illness who received high doses of growth hormone. Thus, the use of growth hormone in patients who are in the acute phase of critical illness is not recommended.

Alternative anabolic agents, such as oxandrolone (Oxandrin) and testosterone[1] are being pursued to induce positive nitrogen balance and enhance wound healing in critically ill patients. These anabolic steroid hormones increase protein synthesis and can reduce the rate of protein breakdown. In a study of patients with alcoholic hepatitis, administration of oxandrolone was associated with lower mortality compared with patients receiving placebo. The patients receiving oxandrolone had improvements in the severity of their liver injury and the degree of malnutrition. Several studies have demonstrated a benefit of oxandrolone use in the burn patient population. Other anabolic steroid hormones, such as methandieone and nandrolone decanoate, have been shown to increase protein anabolism and nitrogen balance in hospitalized patients.

Growth factors should be reserved for patients with major burns and documented impaired healing, patients who have large wounds or enterocutaneous fistulae and who have impaired healing, and patients with muscle wasting and weakness associated with AIDS, other failure to thrive conditions, and in general, patients who have not responded to aggressive nutritional support but whose underlying disease processes are controlled. Growth factors have not

---

[1] Not FDA approved for this indication.

been shown to decrease length of time on a respiratory in ICU patients. In fact, such factors can increase ventilator time and worsen outcome.

Glutamine-supplemented PN solutions administered to trauma or stressed patients can improve overall nitrogen balance, enhance muscle protein synthesis, improve intestinal nutrient absorption, decrease gut permeability, improve immune function, and decrease hospital stays and costs in some patient populations. A review of 14 randomized trials in surgical and critically ill patients found that glutamine supplementation was associated with reduced mortality, lower rates of infectious complications, and a decreased hospital stay. The greatest benefit was in patients receiving high-dose (>0.29 g/kg/day) parenteral glutamine.

Patients with intestinal dysfunction requiring PN, such as those with short bowel syndrome, mucosal damage following chemotherapy, irradiation, or critical illness might benefit from glutamine-containing PN. Glutamine-containing PN might also be beneficial in patients with immunodeficiency syndromes, including AIDS, immune-system dysfunction associated with critical illness, and bone marrow transplantation; patients with severe catabolic illness, such as major burns; patients with multiple trauma; and patients with other diseases associated with a prolonged ICU stay. Glutamine-supplemented solutions should not yet be considered routine care and should not be used in patients with significant renal insufficiency or in patients with significant hepatic failure.

Common Complications and Management

CATHETER SEPSIS

Central venous catheter–related bloodstream infection ranges from 3% to 20% in hospitalized patients and is the most common complication of central venous catheters. The migration of microorganisms along the external surface of the catheter is likely the most common cause, followed by intraluminal contamination from manipulation of the catheter hub or IV connectors. The most common organisms associated with catheter-related bloodstream infections include *Staphylococcus epidermidis*, *Staphylococcus aureus*, *Enterococcus* spp, *Candida albicans*, and *Enterobacter* spp as well as resistant strains such as methicillin-resistant *S. aureus* and vancomycin-resistant enterococci. Primary catheter sepsis occurs when there are signs and symptoms of infection and the indwelling catheter is the only anatomic focus of infection. Secondary catheter infections are

TABLE 5 Possible Etiologies and Treatment of Common Complications of Central Parenteral Nutrition

Problem	Possible Etiology	Treatment
Glucose		
Hyperglycemia, glycosuria, hyperosmolar nonketotic dehydration, or coma	Excessive dose or rate of infusion, inadequate insulin production, steroid administration, infection	Decrease the amount of glucose given, increase insulin, administer a portion of calories as fat
Diabetic ketoacidosis	Inadequate endogenous insulin production and/or inadequate insulin therapy	Give insulin Decrease glucose intake
Rebound hypoglycemia	Persistent endogenous insulin production by islet cells after long-term high-carbohydrate infusion	Give 5%-10% glucose before parenteral infusion is discontinued
Hypercarbia	Carbohydrate load exceeds the ability to increase minute ventilation and excrete excess CO_2	Limit glucose dose to 5 mg/kg/min Give greater percentage of total caloric needs as fat (up to 30%-40%)
Fat		
Hypertriglyceridemia	Rapid infusion Decreased clearance	Decrease rate of PN infusion Allow clearance (~12 h) before testing blood
Essential fatty acid deficiency	Inadequate essential fatty acid administration	Administer essential fatty acids in doses of 4%-7% of total calories
Amino Acids		
Hyperchloremia metabolic acidosis	Excessive chloride content of amino acid solutions	Administer Na^+ and K^+ as acetate salts
Prerenal azotemia	Excessive amino acids with inadequate caloric supplementation	Reduce amino acids Increase the amount of glucose calories
Miscellaneous		
Hypophosphatemia	Inadequate phosphorus administration with redistribution into tissues	Give 15 mmol phosphate/1000 IV kcal Evaluate antacid and Ca^{2+} administration
Hypomagnesemia	Inadequate administration relative to increased losses (diarrhea, diuresis, medications)	Administer Mg^{2+} (15-20 mEq/1000 kcal)
Hypermagnesemia	Excessive administration; renal failure	Decrease Mg^{2+} supplementation
Hypokalemia	Inadequate K^+ intake relative to increased needs for anabolism; diuresis	Increase K^+ supplementation
Hyperkalemia	Excessive K^+ administration, especially in metabolic acidosis; renal decompensation	Reduce or stop exogenous K^+ If ECG changes are present, treat with calcium gluconate, insulin, diuretics, and or Kayexalate
Hypocalcemia	Inadequate Ca^{2+} administration; reciprocal response to phosphorus repletion without simultaneous calcium infusion	Increase Ca^{2+} dose
Hypercalcemia	Excessive Ca^{2+} administration; excessive vitamin D administration	Decrease Ca^{2+} and/or vitamin D administration
Elevated liver transaminases or serum alkaline phosphatase and bilirubin	Enzyme induction secondary to amino acid imbalances or overfeeding	Reevaluate nutritional prescription Cycle TPN Avoid overfeeding calories Consider administering carnitine

ECG = electrocardiogram; PN = parenteral nutrition; TPN = total parenteral nutrition.

associated with another focus or multiple infectious foci that cause bacteremia and seed the catheter.

Management of patients with catheter infection depends on their clinical condition. With extremely ill patients with high fevers who are hypotensive or who have local signs of infection around the catheter site, the catheter should be removed, its tip cultured, and peripheral and central venous blood cultures obtained. The organisms that grow from the catheter tip are the same as the ones that are identified in the peripheral blood culture and typically greater than 10^3 organisms are grown from cultures of the catheter tip.

Specific therapy should be initiated against the primary source in patients in whom a source of infection, other than the catheter tip, is present. Peripheral blood cultures should be obtained and blood cultures should not be taken from the central venous catheter port dedicated for PN because this increases the risk of contaminating the line. If the infection resolves, central venous feedings can be continued. If a secondary source is not identified and the symptoms persist, the catheter should be removed and its tip should be cultured. If the culture of the catheter tip returns positive or if the index of suspicion is high, appropriate antibiotic therapy is initiated. Central venous feeding can be resumed, maintaining euglyemia.

Occasionally, the situation arises in which a site of infection, other than the catheter, is identified, but signs and symptoms persist despite what is assumed to be adequate therapy. Again, if blood cultures are positive, the safest course of action may be to remove the catheter. If peripheral blood cultures are negative, the catheter may be changed over a guidewire and the catheter tip cultured to determine if it was contaminated. Central venous feedings may be continued during this interval if the patient is stable. If the catheter tip returns positive, a new catheter should be inserted at a different site. Changing the central venous catheter over a guidewire can also facilitate the diagnosis of primary catheter infections. Changing the site of catheter location, rather than guidewire exchange, is recommended in patients in whom infection is suspected.

OTHER COMPLICATIONS

Common complications, their etiologies, and treatments are outlined in Table 5. Prolonged administration of PN can result in altered hepatic function and changes in liver pathologic conditions that can lead to liver failure. One to 2 weeks after initiating PN, transaminases may be elevated, but this often resolves without any change in the composition of PN or rate of administration. However, in patients receiving long-term PN (>20 days), prolonged elevations of alkaline phosphatase followed by elevated levels of serum transaminases can occur, even after therapy is discontinued.

Serum levels of alkaline phosphatase and bilirubin initially remain normal, but they rise in many patients who receive long-term PN. Patients who do not receive lipids in the PN solution have more frequent and severe hepatic abnormalities, most likely due to higher carbohydrate loads. Excess glucose increases insulin secretion, which stimulates hepatic lipogenesis and results in hepatic fat accumulation. Fatty infiltration is the initial histopathologic change; it is readily reversible and might not be accompanied by altered liver function tests.

Longer PN therapy may be associated with cholestasis, cholelithiasis, steatosis, and steatohepatitis and can progress to active chronic hepatitis, fibrosis, and eventual cirrhosis. The management of PN-related liver dysfunction is summarized in Box 3.

Complications are minimized and nutritional therapy maximized when the care of patients who require specialized nutritional support is supervised by a nutrition support team. Ideally, the nutrition support team consists of a pharmacist, dietitian, nurse, and physician.

REFERENCES

ASPEN Board of Directors: Guidelines for the use of parenteral and enteral nutrition in adult and pediatric patients. JPEN J Parenter Enteral Nutr 2002;26(1 suppl):1SA-138SA.

Bistrian BR, McCowen KC: Nutritional and metabolic support in the adult intensive care unit: Key controversies. Crit Care Med 2006;34:1525-1531.

Butler SO, Btaiche IF, Alaniz C: Relationship between hyperglycemia and infection in critically ill patients. Pharmacotherapy 2005;25:963-976.

Heyland DK, Dhaliwal R, Drover JW, et al: Canadian clinical practice guidelines for nutrition support in mechanically ventilated, critically ill adult patients. JPEN J Parenter Enteral Nutr 2003;27:355-373.

Heyland DK, Dhaliwal R, Suchner U, Berger MM: Antioxidant nutrients: a systematic review of trace elements and vitamins in the critically ill patient. Intensive Care Med 2005;31:327-337.

Heyland DK, MacDonald S, Keefe L, Drover JW: Total parenteral nutrition in the critically ill patient: A meta-analysis. JAMA 1998;280:2013-2019.

Kochevar M, Guenter P, Holcombe B, et al: ASPEN statement on parenteral nutrition standardization. JPEN J Parenter Enteral Nutr 2007;31:441-448.

McClave SA, Chang W-K, Dhaliwal R, Heyland DK: Nutrition support in acute pancreatitis: A systematic review of the literature. JPEN J Parenter Enteral Nutr 2006;30:143-156.

Novak F, Heyland DK, Avenell A, et al: Glutamine supplementation in serious illness: A systematic review of the evidence. Crit Care Med 2002;30:2022-2029.

O'Grady NP, Alexander M, Dellinger EP, et al: Guidelines for the prevention of intravascular catheter-related infections. MMWR Recomm Rep 2002;51(RR-10):1-29.

Parenteral Fluid Therapy for Infants and Children

Method of
Jeremy N. Friedman, MB, ChB, and Carolyn E. Beck, MD, MSc

One could dedicate an entire textbook to the subject of parenteral fluid therapy for infants and children. For the purposes of this article we have chosen to focus on three main issues that confront us, as clinicians, on a daily basis. The first question is what types of intravenous fluids are most appropriate to provide maintenance requirements in children? The second question is how best to assess dehydration. This is extremely common in pediatrics and absolutely critical if appropriate fluid therapy is to be instituted. Finally, when and how should intravenous fluid be used in the management of the dehydrated patient? Unfortunately, many of these issues remain controversial and have not been satisfactorily resolved. As general pediatricians we provide you with some practical, simple, and general principles to guide your approach to parenteral fluid therapy.

Maintenance Fluids

FLUID REQUIREMENTS

Hospitalized children often require intravenous fluids, necessitating that physicians have an approach to their requirements—both

---

BOX 3 Management of Parenteral Nutrition–Related Liver Dysfunction

Have the patient eat, if possible.
Avoid administering large amounts of glucose or protein calories.
Supply lipid emulsions (up to 30% of total calories).
Cycle the parenteral nutrition, infusing for 10-12 hours per day.
Reevaluate caloric needs; reduce caloric intake if liver dysfunction persists.

TABLE 1 Maintenance Fluid Requirements*

Weight (kg)	100/50/20 Rule (Daily Requirements)	4/2/1 Rule (Hourly Requirements)
0-10	100 mL/kg/d	4 mL/kg/h
11-20	1000 mL + 50 mL/kg/d for every kg 11-20	40 mL + 2 mL/kg/h for every kg 11-20
>20	1500 mL + 20 mL/kg/d for every kg >20	60 mL + 1 mL/kg/h for every kg >20

*Assuming normal renal function and usual insensible losses.

TABLE 3 Source of Electrolyte-Free Water

IV Solution	Tonicity	Na (mmol/L)	EFW (%)
D_5W/0.9% NaCl	Isotonic	154	0
D_5W/0.45% NaCl	Hypotonic	77	50
D_5W/0.2% NaCl	Hypotonic	34	78

Abbreviation: EFW = electrolyte-free water.

fluid composition and volume—at their fingertips. While seemingly second nature to many clinicians, the prescription of IV fluids is in fact complex and requires a solid foundation for safe and effective practice.

Maintenance fluid requirements are deep-rooted in pediatric history, dating back to calculations proposed by Holliday and Segar in 1957. These requirements are based on their study of caloric expenditure in healthy children, resulting in the "100/50/20" rule (closely approximated by the "4/2/1" rule) commonly cited today (Table 1). Applying these rules, a 12-kg toddler requires 1100 mL per day by the 100/50/20 rule, or 44 mL per hour by the 4/2/1 rule, values which are almost equivalent.

Maintenance fluids are designed only to replace, or input, naturally occurring output when oral fluids are contraindicated or not tolerated. Output includes urinary losses, in addition to insensible water loss from the skin and lungs. If renal function is abnormal, maintenance fluids by definition do not apply; in this case, fluid requirement is better estimated by calculating insensible water loss (Table 2) and adding it to urine output and any other significant losses (e.g., diarrhea, nasogastric suction). Similarly, factors such as raised body temperature increase insensible water losses and need to be considered when determining appropriate fluid volume.

ELECTROLYTE REQUIREMENTS

Sodium

In the same 1957 paper, Holliday and Segar proposed maintenance sodium requirements for children to be 30 mmol/L. This requirement translates to the use of a hypotonic saline solution for maintenance fluids, equivalent to 0.2% NaCl in 5% dextrose in water (D_5W). Although this solution, or similar hypotonic composites, continues to be widely used in pediatric practice, there is good reason to question its appropriateness.

Holliday's water requirements were based on caloric expenditure in healthy children, and electrolyte composition was derived from that of human and cow's milk. The recommended sodium concentration is less than the average dietary salt intake, and the guideline fails to account for impaired water excretion, an important factor in hospitalized children. Several case reports have raised concern about the routine use of hypotonic solutions in hospitalized children, because reports of potentially fatal hyponatremia have come to light. Factors implicated in the development of hyponatremia include the action of antidiuretic hormone (ADH) preventing water excretion as well as the input of electrolyte-free water (EFW).

There are several reasons for ADH secretion to be elevated in hospitalized children. Apart from osmotic forces, stimuli for ADH release include malignancies, central nervous system disorders (including meningitis), pulmonary disorders (including pneumonia), and several medications, including commonly used drugs such as morphine sulfate (morphine). Additionally, nonspecific symptoms such as pain, nausea, and stress, as well as a postoperative state and hypovolemia, all result in an increase in ADH. Given the illness of hospitalized children in the 21st century, it is rare to care for a patient who does not have at least one of these risk factors for elevated ADH, making water retention an essential consideration in the prescription of IV fluids.

With respect to EFW, the routine use of hypotonic maintenance fluids provides the major source for hospitalized patients. There is 154 mmol/L of sodium in 0.9% NaCl (normal saline), which is isotonic with respect to the cell membrane. Ringer's lactate provides a similar sodium concentration. Solutions with less sodium content are hypotonic (Table 3). Holliday's historic prescription of 0.2% NaCl contributes a large degree of EFW (78%). This contribution of free water via IV fluids, compounded by an impaired ability to excrete water, place the hospitalized child at risk for developing acute hyponatremia. Consequently, IV solutions that are less hypotonic, or even isotonic, are starting to be used in pediatric hospital wards.

Potential risks of using isotonic fluids as maintenance solutions include fluid overload in children with an impaired ability to excrete sodium and hypernatremia in patients with renal concentrating defects, significant water loss, or prolonged fluid restriction. In the absence of these factors, the risks of isotonic fluids are largely theoretical.

Potassium

Maintenance potassium requirements have similarly been derived at 20 mmol/L. In most clinical situations, maintenance potassium should be added to the IV solution. Exceptions include uncertainty regarding the patient's renal function, poor urine output, or any other risk factors for hyperkalemia. In these scenarios, the addition of potassium is not advised, and renal function and electrolytes should be closely monitored. Ongoing losses of potassium (e.g., diarrheal losses) or other reasons for hypokalemia (e.g., prolonged use of albuterol (salbutamol [Ventolin])) can require higher concentrations of potassium, along with appropriate electrolyte monitoring.

GLUCOSE

Dextrose should routinely be added to maintenance fluids as a carbohydrate source when children are in a fasting state in order to provide some calories (albeit minimal) and prevent ketosis. Generally, a child with normal glucose metabolism requires a 5% dextrose solution (D_5W), which can be safely combined with either hypotonic or isotonic solutions. Unlike sodium, glucose can freely cross the cell membrane and thus does not contribute to the osmotic force.

TABLE 2 Insensible Fluid Losses by Body Surface Area

Insensible Losses	Body Surface Area (m²)
400 mL/m² BSA/d (spontaneously breathing) 300 mL/m² BSA/d (ventilated) 500-600 mL/m² BSA/d (neonates)	$\sqrt{\dfrac{Height(cm) \times Weight(kg)}{3600}}$

Abbreviation: BSA = body surface area.

METHOD FOR PRESCRIBING MAINTENANCE FLUIDS: A PRACTICAL APPROACH

No prospective studies have evaluated the risks or benefits of hypotonic versus isotonic IV fluids. Clearly, the routine use of 0.2% saline requires reconsideration, and it is likely inappropriate for use in pediatric wards. A case-control study by Hoorn and colleagues, the most rigorous on the topic to date, recommends that isotonic fluids be used perioperatively as well as in children with a plasma sodium less than 138 mmol/L.

Practically, a decision regarding IV fluid composition must be made on a case-by-case basis. The choice may be viewed as a prescription, taking details about the patient, the clinical scenario, and the baseline laboratory values into account, and monitoring and reevaluating the child's fluids and electrolytes on a regular basis. Rather than following strict rules, judgment is required for each patient. The following scenarios provide some guidance about IV fluid composition.

A normal sodium value ($\geq$136 mmol/L) in a patient who is relatively well should lead one to consider half-normal saline (0.45% NaCl) in D_5W a good choice. This solution provides more sodium (and contributes less EFW) than 0.2% saline while still providing the patient with some free water. A second patient with the same sodium value, however, might require a different fluid prescription. For example, a child with a low-normal sodium of 137 mmol/L in the clinical context of severe pain, meningitis, or pneumonia—all risk factors for elevated ADH—is likely a good candidate for an isotonic solution such as 0.9% NaCl in D_5W. If this same patient presented with a sodium of 132 mmol/L, 0.9% NaCl in D_5W should almost certainly be instituted. In any of these solutions, 20 mmol/L of potassium could be added provided that the patient's urine output is appropriate and no other risk factors for hyperkalemia are present.

With respect to the surgical patient, the recent literature would suggest that isotonic fluids (0.9% NaCl in D_5W, Ringer's lactate) be routinely used in the perioperative period. Postoperatively, approximately 1% of patients develop a serum sodium less than 130 mmol/L. The development of hyponatremia in this clinical context is not surprising, given the multiple factors placing these patients at risk for increased ADH secretion, namely, pain, nausea, stress, narcotic medications, and volume depletion.

A NOTE ABOUT VOLUME

Provided that a patient has normal renal function and usual insensible losses, maintenance fluid guidelines may be followed, estimated by the rules noted in Table 1. It is crucial to note, however, that in studies examining the question of IV fluids in children, excess fluid volume—greater than maintenance requirements—was an important factor associated with development of acute hyponatremia. Often clinicians prescribe maintenance IV fluids when the child is unwell and not taking anything by mouth. In most cases, when the patient's clinical condition improves, oral intake is initiated. Be mindful that oral fluid is hypotonic and can add significantly to the patient's free water load.

To prevent the development of hyponatremia and its significant clinical consequences in these children, IV fluid prescriptions should be reevaluated on a regular basis, taking oral intake into account and adjusting the IV volume to maintain an appropriate total fluid intake.

Rehydration

ASSESSMENT OF DEHYDRATION

Gastroenteritis and Dehydration

Acute gastroenteritis accounts for more than 1.5 million outpatient visits, 10% of all pediatric hospitalizations (200 000), and approximately 300 deaths per year in the United States. This pales in comparison with the estimated 30% of worldwide deaths among infants and toddlers, amounting to 8000 children younger than 5 years dying per day, from diarrhea and dehydration in the developing world. Young children with diarrhea are more prone to dehydration than older children and adults because of their higher body surface–to–volume ratio, a higher metabolic rate, and smaller fluid reserves. In addition, they are often dependent on others to provide fluid. Viruses, primarily rotavirus, are responsible for 70% to 80% of infectious diarrhea in the developed world. There are also many other causes of dehydration not involving diarrhea, including poor oral intake (e.g., stomatitis), increased insensible losses (e.g., fever, tachypnea), and renal losses (e.g., diabetes mellitus, diabetes insipidus).

Classification of Dehydration

The American Academy of Pediatrics (AAP) classifies dehydration as mild (3%-5% fluid deficit), moderate (6%-9%), and severe ($\geq$10%). The first signs of dehydration are believed to appear when the fluid deficit is 3% to 4%. Dehydration can be further classified based on the serum sodium concentration. Isotonic dehydration (Na 130-150 mmol/L) accounts for the vast majority, and hypotonic (Na <130 mmol/L) and hypertonic (Na >150 mmol/L) dehydration account for less than 5% of the total cases. Inaccurate assessment of dehydration can result in permanent injury and death if fluid deficits are underestimated, and overestimation likely leads to unnecessary interventions and inappropriate use of resources.

Accuracy of Historic Factors and Physical Examination

Traditional teaching regarding the assessment of dehydration is empiric and based on clinical experience (Table 4). The gold standard for measuring dehydration is considered to be acute body weight change over the course of the illness. Unfortunately, this information is seldom available due to a lack of an accurate pre-illness weight.

Steiner and colleagues recently performed a systematic review of the literature on the precision and accuracy of history, physical

TABLE 4 Signs Associated with Dehydration

Symptom	Minimal or No Dehydration (<3% Loss of Body Weight)	Mild to Moderate Dehydration (3%-9% Loss of Body Weight)	Severe Dehydration ($\geq$10% Loss of Body Weight)
General appearance	Normal	Thirsty, restless or lethargic, but irritable when touched	Drowsy, limp, cold, sweaty $\pm$ comatose
Urine output	Normal	Decreased	Minimal
Breathing	Normal	Normal to increased	Deep and increased
Heart rate	Normal	Increased	Increased
Systolic blood pressure	Normal	Normal or low	Low
Mucous membranes	Moist	Sticky	Dry
Eyes	Normal	Slightly sunken	Very sunken
Tears	Normal	Decreased	Absent
Skin turgor	Instant recoil	<2 sec	>2 sec
Capillary refill	Normal	Normal to prolonged	Prolonged >2 sec

TABLE 5 A Dehydration Score

Characteristic	0	1	2
General appearance	Normal	Thirsty, restless, lethargic, but irritable when touched	Drowsy, limp, cold, sweaty, ± comatose
Eyes	Normal	Slightly sunken	Very sunken
Mucous membranes (tongue)	Moist	Sticky	Dry
Tears	Present	Decreased	Absent

examination, and laboratory tests in identifying dehydration in children younger than 5 years. They found that historic factors have only moderate sensitivity as a screening test for dehydration. Duration, frequency, and quantity of vomiting, diarrhea, and urination only give a rough estimate of the risk of dehydration. Signs of dehydration (see Table 4) on physical examination are generally imprecise and tend to show only fair to moderate agreement among examiners. Capillary refill time had the best measurement properties, with a sensitivity of 0.60 (95% CI, 0.29-0.91) and specificity of 0.85 (95% CI, 0.72-0.98) for detecting 5% dehydration. The absence of sunken eyes and dry mucous membranes was also found to be potentially clinically useful in decreasing the likelihood of 5% dehydration.

A prospective cohort study by Gorelick and colleagues in an urban U.S. pediatric emergency department evaluated 10 clinical signs of dehydration and found that any two or more of four factors:

- Capillary refill >2 sec
- Dry mucous membranes
- Absent tears
- Abnormal general appearance

indicate a fluid deficit of at least 5%. This subset of four factors predicted dehydration as well as the entire set.

In addition, a clinical dehydration scale has been developed by Friedman and coworkers using formal measurement methodology. A score of 0 reflects no dehydration, and a maximum score of 8 reflects severe dehydration as per Table 5.

Eliciting Signs of Dehydration

As is true in the physical examination of any young child, *opportunism* is the operative word! Start with the least-invasive part, which involves observing the child's overall appearance and interaction with the caregiver. This also allows you to record the respiratory rate over a 30-second period, looking for hyperpnea suggesting a metabolic acidosis. To assess capillary refill time, sufficient pressure should gradually be applied to blanch the palmar surface of the distal fingertip, and then immediately released. Less than 1.5 to 2 seconds for restoration of normal color is considered normal. The examining room should be at a warm ambient temperature. Autonomic nervous system abnormalities or extremes in patient temperature can affect measurement. Dryness of the mucous membranes is best assessed by examination of the tongue because the lips are often dry in mouth breathers and in children with conditions other than dehydration. If the child does not cry during your examination, the presence of tears may need to be inquired about on history. Skin turgor is usually assessed by pinching a small skin fold on the lateral abdominal wall at the level of the umbilicus. This is then released, and return to its normal position is classified as immediate, slightly delayed, or prolonged. False negatives can be seen in hypernatremia and obese children, and malnutrition can cause false positive results. Although decreased blood pressure and severe tachycardia should be examined for, they are late signs and only tend to become evident in severe dehydration.

Remember that the degree of dehydration may be underestimated in hypertonic dehydration as a result of the movement of water from the intracellular to the extracellular space, which helps to preserve the intravascular volume. In hypotonic dehydration the opposite occurs, and an overestimation of dehydration can result.

Usefulness of Blood Tests

There is a tendency to want to use blood test results to help in the assessment of dehydration because they are perceived to be more reliable than the features on history and physical examination. Unfortunately their usefulness has not been supported by data in the literature. In his systematic review, Steiner reviewed six studies that looked at blood urea nitrogen (BUN), BUN-to-serum creatinine ratio, and acidosis in children. The only laboratory measurement that seemed to be helpful was serum bicarbonate. A normal serum bicarbonate concentration of more than 17 mEq/L reduced the likelihood of 5% dehydration.

Why are the laboratory findings so unhelpful? A number of reasons have been suggested. In cases of isolated vomiting or nasogastric drainage, either a metabolic alkalosis can result from gastric acid losses or a metabolic acidosis can result from volume contraction and lactic acidosis. Volume depletion without renal insufficiency should cause a disproportionate rise in the BUN with little or no change in creatinine. This is caused by increased passive reabsorption of urea in the proximal tubule as a result of appropriate renal conservation of sodium and water. But BUN results may be misleading because children with gastroenteritis can have decreased protein intake during their illness, which can cause hypouremia. Not knowing the child's baseline BUN means that it could double but still remain in the normal range. Finally, if dehydration is rapid, BUN, which is a waste product that builds up gradually with decreased renal excretion, might not have the chance to increase significantly.

What Are the Lessons for the Clinician?

Acute change in weight is the best indicator of dehydration. If a child was seen the day before with a weight of 10 kg and returns the next day with a weight of 9 kg, then by definition the child is 10% dehydrated. Unfortunately, this information is not often available, and based on current data, the empiric classification systems suggested in the past are not particularly accurate or reliable. There are more than 30 different potential tests for assessing dehydration but no conclusive way to approach this.

A general classification of a child's dehydration status as none (<3% fluid deficit), some (mild to moderate—3%–9% fluid deficit), or severe (≥10%) is a useful starting point. Having some awareness of the diagnostic usefulness of individual tests allows you to focus on those that have been shown to correlate best with the presence (or absence) of dehydration. Signs of dehydration start to become evident at 3% to 4% fluid deficit. As a single sign, delayed capillary refill seems to have the highest predictive value but can be influenced by a number of factors, including the examination technique and ambient temperature. Groups of signs can simplify and even improve diagnostic precision. For example, any two out of abnormal capillary refill, abnormal general appearance, dry mucous membranes, and reduced tears increase the likelihood of moderate dehydration sixfold.

Commonly obtained laboratory tests are generally not particularly helpful and therefore not usually indicated unless severe dehydration is suspected or other diagnoses requiring testing are being entertained. Of the laboratory tests, a serum bicarbonate greater than 17 mEq/L is the most useful because it means that the child is approximately one fifth as likely to have moderate dehydration. Intuitively, it makes sense that blood tests (e.g., bicarbonate, electrolytes, BUN, creatinine, glucose) should be drawn at the time of IV placement in children with dehydration sufficiently severe to require IV rehydration or in those whose assessment or diagnosis remains unclear after a complete history and physical examination, when they can be used as an adjunctive tool. Current AAP guidelines do not recommend blood tests as part of the assessment of children with diarrhea and mild dehydration.

FLUID MANAGEMENT OF THE DEHYDRATED CHILD

A number of decisions need to be made by the clinician once the degree of dehydration has been assessed. The first decision is whether to try oral rehydration therapy (ORT) or move immediately to placement of an IV line for parenteral therapy. The next decision is exactly how much fluid and how fast to give it. Finally, if using parenteral therapy, which is the most appropriate solution?

Does the Child Require Intravenous Therapy?

Quantifying the extent of a child's dehydration accurately is critical in deciding whether the child is safe to be managed at home, requires observation during ORT, or needs to receive immediate IV fluid therapy. Mild or moderate dehydration caused by gastroenteritis can be treated with ORT if the child is able to orally replace fluid losses. Parenteral fluid therapy (or on occasion, ORT by nasogastric tube) is recommended for children with severe dehydration or those who cannot replace the estimated fluid deficit or ongoing losses orally, for example, because of ongoing vomiting. Although ORT is the recommended treatment for acute gastroenteritis with dehydration, it is used in less than 30% of cases in the United States for which it is indicated. Three quarters of pediatric emergency medicine providers, who classified themselves as very familiar with the AAP recommendations for ORT, reported nearly exclusive use of IV fluids for moderately dehydrated children. Some feel that ORT is too time consuming in a busy outpatient setting, and others feel that rapid IV rehydration therapy might break the vomiting cycle more quickly, allowing more rapid discharge home.

Management with Oral Rehydration Therapy

Absorption of water in the small bowel is mediated by the cotransport of sodium and glucose. Different varieties of ORT are available, based on slight variations in the composition of sodium, chloride, carbohydrate, and osmolality. They have been shown in numerous randomized, controlled trials to be as effective as IV rehydration and to have fewer complications in the management of children with diarrhea and dehydration. Fruit and bubblegum flavors have been added to combat the salty taste, and frozen flavored ice pops are also available. Vomiting is not a contraindication to the use of ORT, and children who are truly dehydrated seldom refuse to drink it.

Children who have no or minimal signs of dehydration can continue with their regular age-appropriate diet, with ORT to compensate for ongoing diarrhea or vomiting losses. Using ORT in mildly to moderately dehydrated children requires 50- to 100 mL/kg given quickly over 3 to 4 hours until the child appears clinically rehydrated. Fluid can be given by spoon, syringe, or cup beginning with 5 mL every few minutes and gradually increasing as tolerated. Gut rest is not indicated, with the goal to quickly return the child to an age-appropriate unrestricted diet after rehydration has been accomplished. Breast-feeding should not be interrupted, and full-strength formula is usually tolerated. Fluid losses from vomiting and diarrhea need to be recorded and replaced on an ongoing basis. An empiric amount of 5 to 10 mL/kg for each watery stool or 2 mL/kg for each emesis has been suggested.

The nasogastric route is an option that should be considered if a slow, steady rate would be helpful (e.g., if the child is vomiting) or if there is refusal to drink (e.g., stomatitis). Children who are not improving with ORT and those who have extremely high losses need to be reassessed carefully on an ongoing basis and remain under careful observation. These children and those who do not tolerate ORT, have a poor suck, have depressed mental status, or are severely dehydrated group require IV rehydration.

Studies of mortality caused by acute diarrhea in the United States have identified prematurity, young maternal age, black race, and rural residence as risk factors for suboptimal outcome. This should be factored in when deciding on length and degree of observation before discharge.

CURRENT DIAGNOSIS

- Acute change in weight is the best indicator of dehydration, hence the importance of frequent monitoring of weight in children with potential dehydration.
- Signs of dehydration are generally imprecise but start to become evident at 3% to 4% fluid deficit.
- Delayed capillary refill (>2 seconds) seems to have the highest predictive value for dehydration. Any two or more out of delayed capillary refill, dry mucous membranes, absent tears, and abnormal general appearance increases the likelihood of moderate dehydration sixfold.
- Laboratory values are generally unhelpful in assessing dehydration and are not indicated unless IV rehydration is necessary. Of the laboratory tests, the most useful is the serum bicarbonate; a normal bicarbonate (>17 mEq/L) decreases the likelihood of moderate dehydration approximately fivefold.

Intravenous Therapy for Dehydration: How Much and How Fast?

The total volume of fluid required has three components: rehydration requirements to replace the deficit of salt and water, maintenance requirements to maintain euvolemia, and replacement of ongoing losses.

Rehydration Requirements (Deficit Therapy)

Step 1 is to restore cardiovascular stability with a rapid bolus of 20 mL/kg over 10 to 30 minutes. Different from providing maintenance fluids, rehydration should always be achieved using isotonic fluids (normal saline or Ringer's lactate), to effectively restore the extracellular fluid volume. Always remember to order fluid on a per-kilogram basis, which differs from the practice in adults, where it may be safe to order by the liter. The child with mild dehydration might not need a bolus, but the severely dehydrated child might require multiple boluses until the pulse, perfusion, and mental status return to normal. Generally, if a child is continuing to show signs of dehydration after 60 mL/kg of isotonic fluid resuscitation, a critical care unit should be consulted and the institution of inotropic therapy considered. Serum electrolytes, bicarbonate, BUN, creatinine, and glucose are usually drawn at the time of the IV start, although rehydration should commence immediately because the laboratory results will not change the initial fluid management.

Step 2 is to calculate the child's fluid deficit based on weight loss or your clinical assessment of dehydration (see previous section). AAP guidelines recommend using a formula of 50 mL/kg deficit for mild dehydration (3%-5% fluid deficit) and 100 mL/kg for moderate dehydration (6%-9% fluid deficit). Subtract the amount of fluid given by bolus from the total amount of rehydration fluid required in 24 hours. In isotonic (Na 130-150 mmol/L) and hypotonic (Na < 130 mmol/L) dehydration, you can give one half of this volume divided over 8 hours, with the other one half over the next 16 hours, or simply divide the total amount required by 24 for a simplified continuous IV rate. Either way, you should aim to rehydrate over 24 hours. As an example, a 10-kg infant who is believed to be 10% dehydrated will require 1000 mL over 24 hours. The baby receives 200 mL as a bolus and then needs 400 mL over the next 8 hours and a further 400 mL over the following 16 hours to account for the rehydration requirement.

For most patients, half-normal saline in D_5W with KCl 20 mEq/L is an appropriate fluid to use. Potassium is usually not included in the intravenous fluids until the child voids. In the less common scenario of hypertonic dehydration (Na >150 mmol/L), the rehydration

CURRENT THERAPY

- Individualize IV orders for children based on the clinical scenario, baseline laboratory results, and frequent reassessments, with particular attention to the concentration of sodium in your prescribed solution. The traditional use of 5% dextrose in 0.2% NaCl is increasingly being questioned, with consideration required for the use of 5% dextrose in half-normal saline or normal saline in certain scenarios.
- Mild or moderate dehydration can be treated with oral rehydration therapy (ORT), which is currently underused in this setting in the United States.
- Appropriate IV therapy for dehydration requires separate consideration of rehydration and maintenance requirements, as well as replacement of ongoing losses.
- IV fluid therapy calculations are really just approximations, and the child's clinical response is far more important. It is therefore imperative to have regular monitoring of clinical signs, urine output, weight, overall fluid balance, and in certain cases serum electrolytes.

period should be extended over 48 hours so as not to decrease the serum sodium concentration by more than 0.5-1 mmol/hour, to minimize the risk of cerebral edema. Repeated serum sodium measurements will initially be required every 4 to 6 hours until normalizing.

Maintenance Requirements

Step 3 is to calculate maintenance requirements as described earlier and add to the rehydration requirement to come up with an hourly rate. As an example, the 10-kg child previously described requires 40 mL/hour of maintenance fluids, which would be added to the initial rehydration requirement of 50 mL/hour (400 mL over 8 hours) for a total of 90 mL/hour in the first 8 hours. For the next 16 hours this is decreased to 40 mL/hour plus 25 mL/hour (400 mL over 16 hours) for a total of 65 mL/hour. Following return to a euvolemic state, and assuming no ongoing losses, normal maintenance fluid volume may be resumed. Remember to account for oral fluid intake as the patient improves.

Replacement Requirements

Step 4 is to calculate replacement requirements. If ongoing stool losses are a factor, they must be accounted for in the IV fluid prescription. Volume of stool loss is normally about 5 mL/kg/day. With diarrhea this can increase dramatically to 200 mL/kg/day or more. It is easy to see how rapidly a small infant can become dehydrated if these ongoing losses are not being consistently recorded and replaced. If possible, the stool losses should be measured by weighing the diaper and replacing with 1 mL of fluid for each 1 mL of stool. If this is not possible to record, then an estimate of 5 to 10 mL/kg per stool has been suggested as a rough guide. Depending on how rapidly the losses are occurring, this can be calculated every 4 to 6 hours. As an example, if our dehydrated child had three stools over 4 hours for a total of 200 mL, then a further 50 mL/hour (200 divided by 4) is added to the 90 mL/hour (which comprises the rehydration and maintenance components) for a total of 140 mL/hour.

A Note on Rapid Rehydration

The preceding approach to the dehydrated child requiring IV fluids adheres to classic pediatric teaching, where circulation is restored via an isotonic fluid bolus, and electrolyte abnormalities are corrected and deficits replaced over a 24-hour period. There is an increasing interest in an alternative approach, termed *rapid rehydration*. The principle here is to rapidly and fully restore the extracellular fluid volume, usually using 40 to 60 mL/kg of an isotonic solution over a few hours. Theoretically, hospital admission is averted because the patient is discharged home with oral feedings successfully resumed in an 8- to 24-hour period. Although potentially an important method, rapid rehydration has not yet been prospectively studied and should be used with appropriate caution. Its safety and efficacy, including patients' urine and serum electrolytes, hydration, and accompanying clinical status, have yet to be determined. Further study is needed to clarify the optimal rapid rehydration regime, as well as its safety.

Monitoring Requirements

It is essential to remember that the fluid therapy calculations for maintenance IV therapy, rehydration, and replacement are all approximations. There is no formula that works in all cases, so therapy must be individualized. The clinical response to therapy is far more important than any calculations, and there is no substitution for frequent clinical and laboratory monitoring. Regular monitoring of any patient on IV fluids should include:

- General appearance, signs of dehydration, heart rate, respiratory rate, blood pressure
- Urine output, urine specific gravity
- Overall fluid balance
- Daily weights
- Electrolytes (if initially abnormal or at risk, e.g., significant ongoing losses)

Euvolemic patients receiving maintenance fluids should maintain their weight and urine output, achieve a balanced fluid status, and have normal electrolytes, with particular attention to the serum sodium.

A previously dehydrated child who is clinically improving demonstrates weight gain, a positive fluid balance, and increasing urine output with decreasing urine specific gravity. In this patient, consideration should be given to decreasing the intravenous fluids and moving toward ORT and normalizing the diet. Conversely, if the steps are followed as outlined and the child still looks dehydrated, continues to lose weight, remains in negative fluid balance, or has poor urine output, then consider further bolus therapy and increasing the intravenous fluid rate.

REFERENCES

Centers for Disease Control and Prevention: Managing acute gastroenteritis among children: Oral rehydration, maintenance, and nutritional therapy. MMWR Recomm Rep 2003;52(No. RR-16):1-8.

Friedman JN, Goldman RD, Srivastava R, Parkin PC: Development of a clinical dehydration scale for use in children between 1 and 36 months of age. J Pediatr 2004;145:201-207.

Gorelick MH, Shaw KN, Murphy KO: Validity and reliability of clinical signs in the diagnosis of dehydration in children. Pediatrics 1997;99(5):E6.

Halberthal M, Halperin ML, Bohn D: Acute hyponatraemia in children admitted to hospital: Retrospective analysis of factors contributing to its development and resolution. BMJ 2001;322:780-782.

Holliday MA, Segar WE: The maintenance need for water in parenteral fluid therapy. Pediatrics 1957;19:823-832.

Hoorn EJ, Geary D, Robb M, et al: Acute hyponatremia related to intravenous fluid administration in hospitalized children: An observational study. Pediatrics 2004;113:1279-1284.

Steiner MJ, Dewalt DA, Byerley JS: Is this child dehydrated? JAMA 2004;291:2746-2754.

SECTION 9

The Endocrine System

Acromegaly

Method of
Moises Mercado, MD

Acromegaly is a disorder resulting from an excessive secretion of growth hormone (GH), with a prevalence of 40 to 60 cases per million and an annual incidence of 3 to 4 per million.

Physiology, Biochemistry and Regulation of the GH/IGF-1 Axis

GH secretion is regulated at the hypothalamus (Fig. 1). The pulsatile secretion of GH-releasing hormone (GHRH) stimulates somatotroph proliferation and GH gene transcription, whereas somatostatin, which is secreted tonically, inhibits GH synthesis. These two hypothalamic signals result in the pulsatile secretion of pituitary GH, with most pulses occurring during the night. GH is also stimulated by ghrelin, a hypothalamic and gastrointestinal orexigenic hormone that binds specific receptors in the somatotroph known as GH-secretagogue receptors. GH exerts its actions through a specific membrane receptor located predominantly in the liver and cartilage. One molecule of GH interacts with two molecules of GH receptor, resulting in functional dimerization and conformational changes that lead to the phosphorylation of several kinases and eventually the interaction with target genes such as the insulin-like growth factor (IGF)-1 gene.

IGF-1 is closely related to proinsulin and circulates in plasma bound to six binding proteins (IGFBPs) that are synthesized and released by the liver. IGFBP3 is the most important of these binding proteins and is also GH dependent; it forms a heterotrimeric complex composed of BP3, IGF-1, and the acid-labile subunit (ALS). IGF-1 is responsible for most of the trophic and growth-promoting effects of GH. Blood levels of IGF-1 are increased during puberty, coinciding with the acceleration of somatic growth, and decline with aging. Malnutrition, poorly controlled type 1 diabetes, hypothyroidism, and liver failure all result in diminished IGF-1 concentrations. IGF-1 is the main player in GH negative feedback regulation and it acts at both the pituitary and the hypothalamic levels. Glucose regulates GH release by increasing (hypoglycemia) or decreasing (hyperglycemia) somatostatin synthesis in the hypothalamus. Exercise and amino acids such as arginine also stimulate GH secretion.

Etiopathogenesis of Growth Hormone–Secreting Tumors

The molecular pathogenesis of pituitary tumors includes the inactivation of tumor suppressor genes, the activation of oncogenes, and the trophic effect of factors such as the hypothalamic releasing hormones. Approximately 40% of GH-producing tumors in whites harbor somatic point mutations of the α subunit stimulatory G protein coupled to the GHRH receptor (GSPα mutations). This molecular alteration causes constitutive activation of the GHRH receptor, resulting in an increased transcription of the GH gene and the promotion of somatotroph proliferation. Acromegalic patients whose tumors harbor GSPα mutations usually have a more benign clinical course and appear to be more susceptible to management with somatostatin analogues. Nonwhite acromegalic populations, including persons of Japanese, Korean, and Mexican heritage, have a much lower prevalence of GSPα mutations.

Other molecular events should be present in GSPα-negative somatotrophinomas. Menin is a protein encoded by a tumor suppressor gene located on the short arm of chromosome 11. Inactivating mutations of menin are the molecular basis of type 1 multiple endocrine neoplasia (MEN1); however, GH-secreting tumors occurring out of this context do not have such genetic abnormalities. Inactivating mutations of other putative tumor-suppressor genes located relatively close to the menin locus have been described in several kindreds with familial acromegaly; however they do not seem to play an important oncogenic role in the sporadic form of the disease. Other genetic alterations such as underexpression of GADD 45γ (growth arrest and DNA damage-inducible protein) and overexpression of the securing molecule PTTG (pituitary tumor transforming gene) have also been shown to be involved in the molecular pathogenesis of acromegaly.

In more than 90% of cases, acromegaly is caused by a sporadic pituitary adenoma. In approximately 70% of these patients, these benign epithelial neoplasms are larger than 1 cm in diameter and are known as *macroadenomas*, whereas one third of the patients harbor lesions smaller than 1 cm or *microadenomas*. One third of the patients have tumors that cosecrete GH and prolactin (PRL) (mammosomatoroph cell adenomas). Real pituitary GH-secreting carcinomas, with documented metastasis as the irrefutable malignancy criterion, are exceedingly rare. On rare occasions, acromegaly results from GHRH-secreting neuroendocrine tumors, usually located in the lungs, thymus, or endocrine pancreas. In this scenario, the ectopically produced GHRH leads to hyperplasia of the somatotroph, with the consequent excessive production of GH. Even less common are GH-secreting tumors arising in ectopic pituitary tissue, usually located in the sphenoid sinus. A case of GH-secreting lymphoma has been reported.

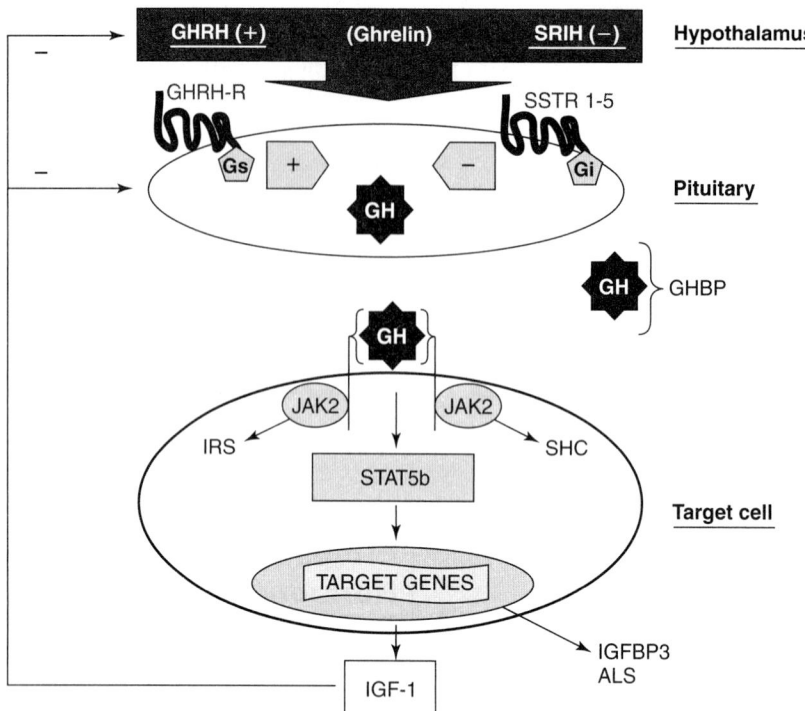

FIGURE 1. GH is regulated positively by GHRH and negatively by somatostatin. Fifty percent of circulating GH is bound to the GH binding protein, which represents the extracellular portion of the GH receptor. One molecule of GH dimerizes two molecules of GH receptor, and the ensuing signal transduction results in IGF-1 synthesis and secretion, which exerts negative feedback on GH secretion at the hypothalamic and pituitary levels. ALS = acid-labile subunit; GH = growth hormone; GHRH = growth hormone–releasing hormone; IGF = insulin-like growth factor; IGFBP3 = insulin-like growth factor binding protein 3; IRS = insulin receptor S; SRIH = somatostatin; SSTR = somatostatin receptor.

Clinical Manifestations

Acromegaly develops insidiously over many years. An 8- to 10-year delay in diagnosis has been estimated from the beginning of the first symptom. Clinical characteristics are often attributed to aging. Symptoms and signs can be divided into those resulting from the compressive effects of the pituitary tumor and those that are a consequence of the GH and IGF-1 excess.

LOCAL TUMOR EFFECTS

Headache results from an increase in intracranial pressure and from the effects of GH itself; it is usually described as a dull pain that persists throughout the day. Occasionally, large tumors invading laterally into the cavernous sinuses give rise to cranial nerve syndromes, usually third and sixth. Visual field defects are relatively common with macroadenomas extending superiorly and compressing the optic chiasm. This usually results in different combinations of bitemporal homonymous hemianopia or quadrontopia.

CONSEQUENCES OF THE GH/IGF-1 EXCESS

Skeletal Growth and Skin Changes

A GH excess developing before the pubertal closure of epiphyseal bone leads to an acceleration of linear growth, and this results in gigantism. Once the patient is in adulthood, the GH/IGF-1 excess results in acral enlargement, which is manifested by increases in ring and shoe sizes as well as enlargement of the nose, supracilliary arches, frontal bones and mandible. There is thickening of soft tissues of the hands and feet; hands are fleshy and bulky and the heel pad is increased. The skin is thickened due to the deposition of glycosaminoglycans and excessive collagen production. Hyperhydrosis and seborrhea occur in 60% of patients; skin tags (previously associated with colon cancer) and acanthosis nigricans are common.

Musculoskeletal System

Generalized arthralgias are present in the majority (80%) of patients. Degenerative osteoarthritis is more common than in the general population. Paresthesias of the hands and feet and a proximal painful myopathy are often reported. Nerve entrapment syndromes such as the carpal tunnel syndrome occur in nearly one half of patients.

Cardiovascular System

Arterial hypertension is found in 30% of patients, and when associated with diabetes it contributes to the increased mortality rate of the disease. Hyperaldosteronism with low renin levels and the resulting sodium retention play an important role in the pathogenesis of hypertension, but other contributors such as an increased sympathetic tone are also present. Echocardiographic findings include left ventricular and septal hypertrophy with varying degrees of diastolic dysfunction. Symptomatic cardiac disease develops in 15% of patients and is usually due to coronary artery disease, heart failure, and arrhythmias. Although the existence of an acromegalic cardiomyopathy is still controversial, there are patients without hypertension and with angiographically normal coronaries, who develop severe congestive heart failure, in whom histologic evidence of subendocardial, subepicardial and myocardial fibrosis and necrosis has been documented.

Respiratory Abnormalities

The majority of patients with acromegaly are affected by loud snoring. A significant fraction of these have sleep apnea (with both central and obstructive components) with significant drops in oxygen saturation, which can be complicated by arrhythmias, daytime somnolence, and chronic fatigue.

Abnormalities in Glucose Metabolism

Chronic GH hypersecretion creates a state of insulin resistance, and glucose intolerance has been reported in 30% to 50% of patients with acromegaly; the percentage with fasting hyperglycemia can be close to 30%, depending on the population. Hyperglycemia has correlated with GH concentrations in some studies and with IGF-1 levels in others.

Abnormalities in Lipid Metabolism

The classic lipid profile consists of diminished total cholesterol, along with elevated triglyceride concentrations. Intermediate-density lipoprotein (IDL) particles and Lipoprotein(a) might also be elevated, and there is a higher percentage of the more atherogenic type II low-density lipoprotein (LDL).

Bone and Calcium Metabolism

Acromegaly is associated with hypercalciuria and hyperphosphatemia. High serum 25-hydroxyvitamin D_3 and urinary levels of hydroxyproline can be found, reflecting a state of increased bone turnover. Cortical bone mineral density is elevated, whereas trabecular bone mass is diminished.

Neoplasia

Retrospective studies suggested that colonic adenomatous polyps and adenocarcinoma were more frequent in acromegalic patients than in the general population. Prospective studies have demonstrated that the risk, albeit smaller than previously thought, is real and probably justifies screening colonoscopy in these patients. Patients with uncontrolled acromegaly have a higher risk of recurrence of premalignant polyps and a higher mortality rate from colon cancer compared with subjects with biochemically controlled disease and the general population.

Associated Endocrine Abnormalities

A euthyroid goiter is often found but seldom requires specific treatment. Hypopituitarism occurs variably, depending on the size and extension of the tumor and whether the patient has undergone surgery or radiation therapy. Hypogonadotropic hypogonadism is the most common pituitary deficiency, occurring in 20% of patients. A decreased libido is a common presenting complaint in both male and female patients with acromegaly; women often have menstrual and ovulatory disturbances and men complain of impotence.

Although an elevated PRL is common, it does not always reflect cosecretion of this hormone by the somatotrophinoma, but rather an interruption of the descending dopaminergic tone by the tumor compressing the pituitary stalk. Central hypocortisolism and hypothyroidism are less common.

GH-secreting pituitary adenomas are the second, after prolactinomas, pituitary tumor occurring in the context of MEN1 (multiple parathyroid adenomas, pituitary adenoma, and pancreatic islet cell tumors). Acromegaly can also develop in patients with the McCune–Albright syndrome (polyostotic fibrous dysplasia, café au-lait-spots, and endocrinopathies such as sexual precocity and autonomous thyroid nodules).

Mortality

Life expectancy in patients with acromegaly is decreased by about 10 to 15 years, and the standardized mortality ratio is 1.5 to 2. Most patients die of cardiovascular causes, followed by cerebrovascular events, respiratory abnormalities, and neoplastic diseases. Hormonal control has a definite impact on survival. Lowering serum GH to less than 2.5 ng/mL results in reduction of the mortality rate to levels comparable with the general population. These safe GH levels were obtained using old radioimmunoassays, and there are no equivalent studies using ultrasensitive GH assays. IGF-1 levels have not been as good as GH as independent predictors of mortality. Other factors associated with an increased mortality include advanced age and the presence of hypertension and diabetes.

Biochemical Diagnosis

Due to the pulsatile nature of GH secretion, random determinations of this hormone are not useful in the diagnosis of acromegaly. The gold standard for the diagnosis is the measurement of GH after an oral glucose load of 75 g; current guidelines state that suppression to less than 0.3 ng/mL (using ultrasensitive assays), reliably excludes the diagnosis. Situations associated with decreased suppression of GH by glucose include puberty, pregnancy, use of oral contraceptives, uncontrolled diabetes, and renal and hepatic insufficiency.

IGF-1 levels reflect the integrated concentrations over 24 hours of GH and correlate well with clinical activity. Blood IGF-1 concentrations decrease with age, reflecting the parallel decline of the somatotropic axis. There is a gender difference in IGF-1 (premenopausal women have lower levels than age-matched male subjects). Other conditions that lower IGF-1 levels include malnutrition, uncontrolled diabetes, and hepatic and renal failure. Normal ranges for IGF-1 should be established in each particular center based on age and sex. The determination of other GH-dependent peptides such as IGFBP3 and ALS has not proved to be superior to IGF-1.

Imaging

Pituitary magnetic resonance imaging (MRI) with gadolinium enhancement allows visualization of lesions as small as 2 or 3 mm in diameter. High-resolution computed tomography (CT) is a reasonable alternative, although it is much less sensitive. An ectopic source of GHRH should be suspected when the MRI is completely normal. In these rare cases, serum GHRH should be measured and the ectopic tumor should be sought, usually with high-resolution CT of the chest and abdomen.

 CURRENT DIAGNOSIS

Clinical

- Headaches, visual field defects
- Coarse features, increased size of hands (rings) and feet (shoes)
- Thick, oily skin, skin tags, acanthosis nigricans
- Arthralgias, osteoarthritis
- Paresthesias, carpal tunnel syndrome
- Hypertension, arrhythmia, heart failure
- Glucose intolerance, diabetes, hypertrygliceridemia
- Snoring, sleep apnea
- Risk of colon polyps or colon cancer

Biochemical

- Glucose-suppressed growth hormone >0.3 ng/mL by ultrasensitive assays or >1 ng/mL by old radioimmunoassays
- Elevated age- and sex-matched insulin-like growth factor 1
- Other growth hormone–dependent peptides: insulin-like growth factor binding protein 3, acid-labile subunit

Imaging

- Computed tomography
- Magnetic resonance imaging

Treatment

The decision as to what therapeutic modality should be used has to take into account medical issues (cardiopulmonary comorbidities, size, and extension of the tumor) as well as the local characteristics of the treating center. The latter refers to the availability of pituitary surgeons and radiotherapeutic technologies as well as the economic feasibility of pharmacologic therapy.

SURGERY

Transsphenoidal surgery has been the traditional treatment for acromegaly and achieves biochemical cure (normalization of IGF-1 and a glucose-suppressed GH <1 ng/mL) in 80% to 90% of microadenomas. Cure rates for macroadenomas are much lower (40%-50%), and invasive lesions have a very slight chance (<10%) of being cured by surgery. Even though surgery often fails to achieve a full biochemical cure, debulking the pituitary adenoma relieves optic chiasm compression and can result in a sufficient decrement of tumor mass (and therefore of GH production) to allow better results with either pharmacologic or radiotherapeutic regimens.

PHARMACOLOGIC THERAPY

Somatostatin analogues are the most commonly used medical treatment for acromegaly. Somatostatin inhibits GH secretion and somatotroph cell growth via its interaction with five different somatostatin receptor (SSTR) subtypes. The development of long-acting somatostatin analogues such as octreotide (Sandostatin) and lanreotide (Somatuline) overcame the pharmacologic difficulties of native somatostatin (short half-life, rebound GH secretion, and need for IV administration) and resulted in a more potent inhibition of GH secretion. The most commonly used preparations are intramuscular octreotide LAR (long-acting repeatable) and subcutaneous lanreotide autogel, which are administered every 4 weeks. Doses of octreotide LAR, the only somatostatin analogues available in the United States, range from 10 to 40 mg. Octreotide and lanreotide have very high affinities for SSTR-2 and to a lesser extent SSTR-5, which are precisely the most commonly expressed somatostatin receptors in GH-secreting adenomas.

When used after surgery has failed, somatostatin analogues can achieve a safe and a normal IGF-1 in 50% to 60% of patients. Primary treatment with somatostatin analogues is increasingly being used in patients with invasive tumors, when cardiopulmonary contraindications are present, and more recently as a result of the patient or treating physician's preference. In these settings, biochemical success rates (achievement of safe GH levels and normalization of IGF-1) have ranged between 50% and 80%, and more than 80% report significant relief of symptoms. Tumor shrinkage occurs in 70% of primarily treated patients. Overall, treatment success is directly related to the abundance of SSTR-2 and SSTR-5 in the tumor. Lower pretreatment GH levels are also associated with a better response to somatostatin analogues. Side effects of somatostatin analogues, including nausea, abdominal pain, alopecia, and biliary sludge, occur in 20% of subjects.

Pegvisomant is a GH mutant that prevents functional dimerization of the GH receptor, thus acting as an antagonist. Its use results in normalization of IGF-1 in more than 90% of patients, while increasing GH levels. Concern about adenoma growth due to the abolition of IGF-1 negative feedback on the tumoral somatotroph, prevents its use in patients with very large lesions in close proximity to the optic chiasm. Transient elevations of liver aminotransferases can occur, although this seldom requires drug discontinuation. Pegvisomant does not compromise insulin secretion, as somatostatin analogues do. GH-receptor antagonists are expensive and should not be used as primary treatment; they are currently indicated in patients who are intolerant or have failed somatostatin analogue therapy.

Few patients respond marginally to difficult-to-tolerate large doses of bromocriptine. Newer dopamine agonists, such as cabergoline, are better tolerated and more efficacious, particularly in tumors that cosecrete PRL. Combination treatment with cabergoline and octreotide appears to be promising in cases resistant to somatostatin analogues.

RADIATION THERAPY

Both external-beam radiotherapy and radiosurgery are indicated in patients with persistent disease and a demonstrable tumor remnant who are either intolerant or resistant to pharmacologic treatment. Biochemical success occurs in 20% to 60% and requires many years to become apparent. Hypopituitarism, involving at least two axes, develops in more than 50% of patients within 10 years. Serious adverse effects such as brain necrosis and optic nerve damage seldom occur with the currently used techniques that minimize radiation to the normal surrounding tissues.

CURRENT THERAPY

- If a pituitary surgeon is available: Transsphenoidal surgery for microadenomas, intrasellar macroadenomas, and debulking or decompressing surgery in invasive macroadenomas
- Somatostatin analogues as secondary treatment for patients failing surgery or waiting for radiotherapy effect to occur and as a primary treatment for patients with inaccessible lesions, contraindications for surgery, or preference
- Dopamine agonists: Bromocriptine (Parlodel) is ineffective; cabergoline (Dostinex)[1] may be added to patients resistant to somatostatin analogues
- Growth hormone receptor antagonists: Pegvisomant (Somavert) for patients resistant or intolerant to somatostatin analogues and who have tumors >5 mm from the optic chiasm
- Radiotherapy for patients resistant or intolerant to pharmacologic therapy, with clinically and biochemically active disease and a tumor remnant on MRI
- Radiosurgery might be better than external-beam radiotherapy

---

[1]Not FDA approved for this indication.

REFERENCES

Bevan JS: Clinical review: The antitumoral effects of somatostatin analog therapy in acromegaly. J Clin Endocrinol Metab 2005;90:1856-1863.

Colao A, Ferone D, Marzullo P, Lombardi G: Systemic complications of acromegaly: Epidemiology, pathogenesis and management. Endocr Rev 2004;25:102-152.

Espinosa-de-Los-Monteros AL, Sosa E, Cheng S, et al: Biochemical evaluation of disease activity after pituitary surgery in acromegaly: A critical analysis of patients who spontaneously change disease status. Clin Endocrinol 2006;64:245-249.

Freda P: Current concepts in the biochemical assessment of the patient with acromegaly. Growth Horm IGF Res 2003;13:171-184.

Freda P, Katznelson L, van der Lely AJ, et al: Long-acting somatostatin analog therapy of acromegaly: A meta-analysis. J Clin Endocrinol Metab 2005;90:4465-4473.

Growth Hormone Research Society; Pituitary Society: Biochemical assessment and long term monitoring in patients with acromegaly: statement from a joint consensus conference of the Growth hormone Research Society and the Pituitary Society. J Clin Endocrinol Metab 2004;89:3099-3102.

Holdaway IM, Rajasoorya RC, Gamble GD: Factors influencing mortality in acromegaly. J Clin Endocrinol Metab 2004;89:667-674.

Kopchick JJ, Parkinson C, Stevens EC, Trainer PJ: Growth hormone receptor antagonists: Discovery, development, and use in patients with acromegaly. Endocr Rev 2002;23:623-646.

Melmed S: Acromegaly. N Engl J Med 2006;355:2558-2573.
Melmed S, Casanueva F, Cavagnini F, et al: Consensus statement: Medical management of acromegaly. Eur J Endocrinol 2005;153:737-740.
Vance ML, Laws ER: Role of medical therapy in the management of acromegaly. Neurosurgery 2005;56:877-885.

Adrenocortical Insufficiency

Method of
Carl D. Malchoff, MD, PhD

Adrenal insufficiency is a life-threatening disorder that is 100% treatable by timely therapy. Because the clinical presentation is nonspecific and the prevalence is low (about 120 per 1 million persons in Western countries), the diagnosis may be overlooked. Recognition of clinical settings that predispose to adrenal insufficiency can alert the astute physician to consider this disorder when confronted with the nonspecific clinical presentation. The diagnosis is confirmed by biochemical testing that exploits endocrine physiology.

Adrenal insufficiency refers to decreased cortisol (hydrocortisone) production. Aldosterone production is low in primary adrenal insufficiency and normal in secondary adrenal insufficiency. Isolated aldosterone deficiency most often occurs in hyporeninemic hypoaldosteronism and is not discussed in this article.

Endocrine Physiology

The adrenal cortex produces both cortisol (a glucocorticoid) and aldosterone (a mineralocorticoid). Cortisol maintains cardiac output, vascular resistance, and hepatic glucose output. Shock and death can occur without adequate glucocorticoids. Aldosterone modulates renal sodium reabsorption in exchange for potassium excretion. Hyperkalemia is caused by aldosterone deficiency.

Cortisol production is controlled by a simple closed feedback loop. The anterior pituitary gland secretes adrenocorticotropic hormone (ACTH), which stimulates adrenal cortisol production. Cortisol inhibits ACTH release to complete the closed feedback loop. A more complex feedback loop controls aldosterone production, which is stimulated directly by angiotensin II. Angiotensin II is generated from angiotensin I, which itself is a proteolytic product of angiotensin substrate that has been cleaved by the enzyme renin. The juxtaglomerular complex of the kidney releases renin in response to low blood pressure. Aldosterone stimulates the distal tubule to transport sodium from the glomerular filtrate back into the vasculature in exchange for potassium. Water accompanies sodium, producing increases in vascular volume and blood pressure that complete the closed feedback loop.

Etiology

In primary adrenal insufficiency the adrenal glands are no longer capable of producing adequate amounts of cortisol and aldosterone (Box 1). In secondary adrenal insufficiency, the pituitary gland or hypothalamus is damaged, and decreased cortisol production is secondary to decreased ACTH release from the anterior pituitary. A familiarity with the causes of primary and secondary adrenal insufficiency will help the physician recognize the settings in which adrenal insufficiency can occur.

In developed countries, primary adrenal insufficiency is most commonly caused by autoimmune destruction of the adrenal glands. The leading cause in underdeveloped countries might still be tuberculosis.

BOX 1 Etiology of Adrenal Insufficiency

- Adrenal disorders (primary adrenal insufficiency)
- Autoimmune disorders: Autoimmune polyglandular syndromes types 1 and 2
- Infections with granulomatous response (tuberculosis, histoplasmosis, others)
- Adrenal hemorrhage
  - Meningococcemia and, less commonly, in other causes of sepsis
  - Anticoagulation
  - Severe stress
  - Antiphospholipid syndrome
- Adrenoleukodystrophy
- Amyloidosis
- Congenital adrenal hyperplasia
- Adrenal hypoplasia (developmental disorders)
- AIDS-associated infections: Cytomegalovirus
- Pharmaceuticals: Metyrapone (Metopirone), mitotane (Lysodren), aminoglutethimide (Cytadren), etomidate (Amidate), ketoconazole (Nizoral)

Autoimmune polyglandular syndrome (APS) type 2 is most familiar to physicians treating adult patients. This disorder tends to be familial, although the genetics are complex (polygenic). It is associated with type 1 diabetes and Hashimoto's disease. Other autoimmune disorders occur with lower frequency, and autoimmune hypoparathyroidism is not associated with adrenal insufficiency in APS type 2, as it is in APS type 1.

APS type 1 is a mendelian disorder with recessive inheritance caused by mutations of the *AIRE* gene that can regulate immune tolerance in the adrenal cortex and parathyroid tissues. Nearly all patients develop the triad of adrenal insufficiency, hypoparathyroidism, and mucocutaneous candidiasis before adulthood. Other less common manifestations include malabsorption, primary hypogonadism in female patients, and alopecia.

Primary adrenal insufficiency was first described in the mid 1800s in the setting of tuberculosis, and infiltrative destruction of the adrenal glands was observed at autopsy. Other infectious disorders that can infiltrate and destroy the adrenal glands include histoplasmosis, cryptococcosis, and blastomycosis. Hemorrhagic adrenal destruction may be caused by meningococcemia or sepsis from other bacterial infections, by anticoagulation, by the antiphospholipid syndrome and even by severe physical stress alone. Malignancies such as breast, kidney, and lung cancers often metastasize to the adrenal glands, where they manifest as large adrenal masses on imaging studies. However, metastases to the adrenal glands usually do not impair adrenal function, although this should be confirmed by biochemical testing.

Inherited disorders causing adrenal insufficiency can cause hyperplasia or hypoplasia of the adrenal gland or they can cause gradual adrenal gland destruction due to failure to metabolize toxic substances. Adrenal insufficiency with adrenal hyperplasia is caused by defects in the enzymes that convert cholesterol to cortisol and usually manifests in the neonatal period. These disorders are collectively referred to as *congenital adrenal hyperplasia;* increased ACTH production causes the adrenal glands to become hyperplastic, even though they produce inadequate amounts of cortisol. Deficiency of the 21-hydroxylase enzyme is the most common cause, although defects can occur at any step in cortisol synthesis. Neonatal adrenal hypoplasia occurs when genes required for normal adrenal development are defective.

Adrenoleukodsytrophy is an X-linked recessive disorder caused by the failure to oxidize long-chain fatty acids. Both neurologic deficits and adrenal insufficiency progress over time due to the toxicity of long-chain fatty acid accumulation. Metyrapone (Metopirone), aminoglutethimide (Cytadren), and mitotane (Lysodren) are used to treat cortisol excess and can produce adrenal insufficiency.

In addition, high-dose ketoconazole (Nizoral) can cause adrenal insufficiency.

Secondary adrenal insufficiency is usually permanent when caused by tumors of the pituitary gland, pituitary irradiation, or traumatic section of the pituitary stalk. However, the defect may be partial. Reversible secondary adrenal insufficiency is commonly caused by long-term high-dose glucocorticoid therapy that suppresses the hypothalamus and pituitary gland. However, this is a slow process, and complete recovery takes about 1 year. Hypophysitis can spontaneously resolve.

Clinical Presentation

Adrenal insufficiency can manifest as an acute crisis or as a slowly progressive illness. In either case, the presentation is often nonspecific, and the clinical context can alert the physician to the diagnosis. It has been suggested that sepsis and other severe illnesses commonly cause a relative adrenal insufficiency, but this remains controversial.

Acute adrenal crisis manifests with hypotension and often fever. It can occur in a patient with untreated adrenal insufficiency who is subjected to physical stress. Although it is well known to occur in meningococcemia, it can also occur in the setting of sepsis caused by other organisms. Severe illness alone can cause adrenal hemorrhage and adrenal crisis. Adrenal insufficiency should be considered in any patient in the intensive care unit with the sudden onset of fever and hypotension.

The presentation of chronic adrenal insufficiency includes anorexia, weight loss, fatigue, abdominal pain, diarrhea, hyperpigmentation, orthostatic hypotension, hyponatremia, and hyperkalemia. Nearly 100% of subjects have anorexia and weight loss, although there are rare exceptions. Weight gain due to hypothalamic obesity can occur following resection of a craniopharyngioma or other hypothalamic lesion, even in the setting of adrenal insufficiency. The differential diagnosis of unexplained weight loss should include adrenal insufficiency. Electrolyte abnormalities are a useful clue but are not always present. Hyperkalemia occurs in about 60% of subjects with primary adrenal insufficiency and does not occur in secondary adrenal insufficiency. Hyponatremia occurs in about 80% of subjects with primary adrenal insufficiency and 60% of subjects with secondary adrenal insufficiency. Although hypoaldosteronism contributes to hyponatremia in primary adrenal insufficiency, antidiuretic hormone (ADH) is the major cause of hyponatremia. Both hypotension and low cortisol concentrations stimulate its production. Hyperpigmentation occurs only in primary adrenal insufficiency.

It has been proposed that relative adrenal insufficiency occurs frequently in sepsis and other severe illnesses. This is controversial. The increase in serum cortisol concentration following stimulation with cosyntropin (Cortrosyn) is often diminished in sepsis and other severe illnesses, suggesting a relative adrenal insufficiency. Alternatively, this finding can indicate that cortisol production is already maximally stimulated in the sickest patients.

One large multicenter study sought to distinguish between these possibilities by random prospective assignment of septic patients to treatment with stress doses of glucocorticoids plus mineralocorticoids versus placebo. Although there was a small statistical benefit of glucocorticoid treatment in subjects with a diminished response to cosyntropin, the study was flawed by the use of etomidate (Amidate) to sedate some patients. Etomidate is a short-acting anesthetic that inhibits cortisol production. When letters brought this to the attention of the study's authors, they declined the opportunity to reanalyze their results with the etomidate-treated subjects excluded from the analysis. Therefore, it is possible that the benefit of glucocorticoids was limited to subjects with iatrogenic adrenal insufficiency.

No general recommendation can be made concerning the use of stress doses of glucocorticoids in patients with sepsis, and this decision is left to the discretion of the treating physician. The exception is in the patient with meningococcemia, who should always receive stress doses of glucocorticoids, because meningococcemia carries a significant risk of adrenal hemorrhage. Glucocorticoid doses that exceed stress doses may be harmful in sepsis.

After the diagnosis of adrenal insufficiency is established, it is necessary to distinguish between primary and secondary adrenal insufficiency. The 8:00 AM plasma ACTH concentration is greater than 100 pg/mL (22 pmol/L) in primary adrenal insufficiency. If a diagnosis of primary adrenal insufficiency is made, then the adrenal glands should be imaged to help determine the cause, and in boys and young men the diagnosis of adrenoleukodystrophy should be excluded by measuring circulating very-long-chain fatty acids. In secondary adrenal insufficiency the pituitary gland and hypothalamus should be imaged by magnetic resonance imaging (MRI).

Biochemical Diagnosis

Biochemical confirmation of adrenal insufficiency often requires dynamic testing (Box 2). The normal responses to these tests are established in healthy persons and might not be completely applicable to critically ill patients, especially those with low cortisol-binding globulin.

Although unstimulated serum cortisol concentrations are usually not diagnostic, an 8:00 AM serum cortisol concentration less than 3 μg/dL (83 nmol/L) is diagnostic of adrenal insufficiency, and a random serum cortisol concentration greater than 23 μg/dL excludes adrenal insufficiency.

Dynamic testing with insulin-induced hypoglycemia is generally considered the gold standard for diagnosing adrenal insufficiency. However, the test requires skill and experience to perform, is contraindicated in ill patients, and is relatively contraindicated in patients older than 50 years, in patients with coronary artery disease, and in patients with seizure disorders. Dynamic testing with synthetic $ACTH_{1-24}$ (cosyntropin) is rapid, safe, and usually accurate. It will diagnose primary adrenal insufficiency and long-standing secondary adrenal insufficiency. There are two versions of this test: a standard (high-dose) test that employs a 250-μg cosyntropin dose and a low-dose test that employs a 1-μg cosyntropin dose. There is debate as to which version has greater sensitivity and specificity, but generally they lead to similar conclusions.

BOX 2   Biochemical Testing

Standard High-Dose ACTH Stimulation Test

The serum concentration of cortisol is measured 60 min following IV or IM administration of 250 μg cosyntropin (Cortrosyn). Although the normal response is probably >23 μg/dL (635 nmol/L), adrenal function is considered adequate if the response is >20 μg/dL (550 nmol/L).

Low-Dose ACTH Stimulation Test

The serum cortisol concentration is measured 60 min following IV administration of 1 μg cosyntropin diluted in normal saline. The minimum normal response is reported by various investigators to be 18-22 μg/dL (500-600 nmol/L).

Insulin-Induced Hypoglycemia Test

This test is more sensitive than cosyntropin testing in the setting of recent-onset secondary adrenal insufficiency. Under the supervision of an endocrinologist or other experienced physician, regular insulin (0.1-0.15 U/kg) is administered intravenously. Serum glucose and cortisol concentrations are measured at 0, 10, 20, 30, 45, 60, and 90 min following the injection. If adequate hypoglycemia is attained (serum glucose <40 mg/dL; 22 mmol/L), then the serum cortisol concentration will increase to 20 μg/dL (500 nmol/L) or greater in normal persons.

Unfortunately, the normal stimulated ranges for each of the different cortisol assays are not well established in most laboratories. Studies have shown considerable variations between different assays for cortisol being performed in the same laboratory. Therefore, the normative data developed in one laboratory might not be applicable to another. A cortisol response of 20 µg/dL (550 nmol/L) or greater at 1 hour following intravenous or intramuscular administration of 250 µg of cosyntropin generally is believed to indicate adequate adrenal function, although the lower normal limit may be 23 µg/dL (635 nmol/L). Various normal values are given for the 1-µg cosyntropin test, and some clinicians have attempted to normalize the cosyntropin response at 30 minutes following the injection rather than 60 minutes.

No test is perfect, and it may be useful to have an experienced endocrinologist assist with the interpretation of borderline results. It is generally considered unnecessary to obtain a basal cortisol concentration, but some, especially those who argue that there is a relative adrenal insufficiency of severe illness, contest this.

For persons with suspected adrenal crisis, it is appropriate to begin dexamethasone (Decadron) before testing for adrenal reserve. Dexamethasone does not cross-react in the immune-based cortisol assays, and, for the first 72 hours of therapy it will not influence the maximum cortisol response to cosyntropin stimulation.

Treatment

The treatment of adrenal insufficiency depends on the presentation (Box 3). It is usually divided into the extremes: treatment of hypotensive adrenal insufficiency crisis and treatment of otherwise healthy persons with adrenal insufficiency. Some patients fall between these two extremes.

Hypotensive adrenal crisis is treated with stress doses of intravenous glucocorticoids, intravenous normal saline with 5% dextrose, vasoconstricting agents necessary to maintain blood pressure, plus antibiotics if infection is suspected. Maximum cortisol production is about 200 mg/day, so that replacement with 50 to 100 mg hydrocortisone (Sozlu-Cortef) IV every 6 hours is appropriate. Because hydrocortisone is an effective mineralocorticoid at these high doses and because there are no intravenous mineralocorticoids available, this is the treatment of choice in hyperkalemic patients. In critically ill patients, treatment with stress doses of glucocorticoids should not be withheld pending the results of adrenal function tests. If the patient is not hyperkalemic, then treatment with IV dexamethasone is appropriate at 2 mg IV every 12 hours, and dynamic testing can be performed during therapy.

Glucocorticoid therapy for otherwise healthy subjects with adrenal insufficiency is titrated to the lowest glucocorticoid dose at which the patient feels well. This is often a total of 20 mg/day of hydrocortisone divided into two to four doses a day. For convenience reasons, some patients prefer prednisone. The equivalent total daily dose of prednisone is about 5 mg/day as a single dose or divided into two doses a day. Dexamethasone has a half-life that varies between patients and with other medications taken by the patients. It should be avoided unless poor patient compliance is the overwhelming reason for choosing an agent with a long half-life. Patients with mild or partial adrenal insufficiency due to pituitary disease might not require glucocorticoid therapy daily, but only at times of stress.

Mineralocorticoid replacement is required for primary adrenal insufficiency but not for secondary adrenal insufficiency. Fludrocortisone (Florinef) is the only agent available, and it is not available in a parenteral preparation. The replacement dose is titrated to that which maintains the upright plasma renin activity in the normal range, and this is usually about 0.1 mg/day.

The patient should wear a medical alert tag that indicates the diagnosis of adrenal insufficiency.

BOX 3 Treatment of Adrenal Insufficiency

Adrenal Crisis
- Administer 1 L normal saline with 5% dextrose IV as fast as possible, and then continue as long as necessary to maintain blood pressure and urine output.
- Immediately administer stress doses of glucocorticoids IV, either hydrocortisone (Solu-Cortef) 50 mg q6h or dexamethasone (Deltasone) 2 mg q12h.
  - Use hydrocortisone to treat hyperkalemia.
  - Use dexamethasone if diagnostic testing will be performed.
- Vasoconstrictors are administered as necessary to maintain blood pressure.

Adrenal Insufficiency in an Otherwise Healthy Patient
- Glucocorticoids
  - Hydrocortisone at 20 mg/d or the lowest tolerated dose divided two to four times a d *or* prednisone at 5 mg/d or the lowest tolerated dose divided one to two times a d.
  - Dexamethasone at 0.5 mg/d is usually avoided due to variable metabolism. However, it may be useful for poorly compliant patients.
- Mineralocorticoid
  - Fludrocortisone (Florinef) 0.1 mg/d and titrated to maintain the plasma renin activity in the normal range
- Androgen
  - Dehydroepiandrosterone (DHEA)[7] at 50 mg/d to women, although not all experts agree that it is necessary.
  - Indications for continued use are improved sense of well-being and improved sexual satisfaction.

---

[7]Available as a dietary supplement.

 CURRENT DIAGNOSIS

- Acute adrenal insufficiency with crisis manifests with hypotension and often fever.
- Chronic adrenal insufficiency without crisis manifests with weight loss and anorexia.
- Primary adrenal insufficiency develops in the setting of disorders affecting the adrenal glands. These include autoimmune disorders, granulomatous diseases, meningococcemia, anticoagulation, and certain pharmaceutical agents.
- Secondary adrenal insufficiency develops in the setting of pituitary disorders.
- Hyponatremia occurs in both primary and secondary adrenal insufficiency.
- Hyperpigmentation occurs in primary adrenal insufficiency but not in secondary adrenal insufficiency.
- Dynamic testing is often necessary to establish the diagnosis. The insulin-induced hypoglycemia test is the gold standard, but this cumbersome test can often be avoided by use of a cosyntropin stimulation test.
- Both the standard high-dose (250 µg) cosyntropin stimulation test and the low-dose (1 µg) stimulation test are useful.
- Some experts contend that a relative adrenal insufficiency in sepsis and other acute illnesses occurs commonly, but this has not been proved.

CURRENT THERAPY

- Acute adrenal insufficiency with hypotensive crisis should be treated with IV glucocorticoids at stress doses, normal saline with 5% dextrose, plus vasoconstrictors as needed to maintain blood pressure. If necessary, initiate therapy before establishing the diagnosis.
- A stress dose of hydrocortisone (Solu-Cortef) is 50-100 mg q6h, and a stress dose of dexamethasone is 2 mg q12 h. The former should be used in the setting of hyperkalemia, and the latter should be used if diagnostic testing will be performed.
- Glucocorticoid therapy of chronic adrenal insufficiency in an otherwise healthy patient is approximately 20 mg/d hydrocortisone (Cortef) divided in 2 to 4 doses, or prednisone 5 mg/d divided in 1 to 3 doses. The dose is titrated to the lowest tolerated by the patient.
- Dexamethasone (Decadron) has a variable half-life and is difficult to dose correctly for chronic use.
- In primary adrenal insufficiency, fludrocortisone (Florinef) is titrated to a normal upright plasma renin activity, and this is usually about 0.1 mg/dL.
  - A medical alert tag serves as an important reminder to emergency medical personnel of this potentially fatal disorder.
  - Dehydroepiandrosterone (DHEA) may be helpful in women with adrenal insufficiency.

Dehydroepiandrosterone (DHEA)[7] at doses of about 50 mg/day has been used to treat women with adrenal insufficiency. Dehydroepiandrosterone is a weak, naturally occurring adrenal androgen that is available without prescription. Some, but not all, double blind prospective studies suggest that it increases sexuality and a feeling of well-being in women with adrenal insufficiency. Potential complications include androgen-dependent hair growth and acne.

During minor illness, less than maximal glucocorticoid doses are usually satisfactory. The glucocorticoid dose is usually doubled when a patient develops a viral syndrome with a fever greater than 38.5°C (101°F). Increased glucocorticoid replacement doses are not required during pregnancy, but they are used transiently at delivery. Parenteral glucocorticoids are indicated for adrenal insufficiency patients with vomiting.

---

[7]Available as a dietary supplement.

REFERENCES

Abdu TAM, Elhadd TA, Neary R, et al: Comparison of the low dose short synacthen test (1 mg), the conventional dose short synacthen test (250 mg), and the insulin tolerance test for the assessment of the hypothalamo-pituitary-adrenal axis in patients with pituitary disease. J Clin Endocrinol Metab 1999;84:838-843.
Annane D, Sebille V, Charpentier C, et al: Effect of treatment with low doses of hydrocortisone and fludrocortisone on mortality in patients with septic shock. JAMA 2002;288:862-871.
Annane D, Sebille V, Troche G, et al: A 3-level prognostic classification in septic shock based on cortisol levels and cortisol response to corticotropin. JAMA 2000;283:1038-1045.
Dickstein G, Shechner C, Nicholson W, et al: Adrenocorticotropin stimulation test: Effects of basal cortisol level, time of day, and suggested new sensitive low dose test. J Clin Endocrinol Metab 1991;72:773-778.
Mayenknecht J, Diederich S, Bahr V, et al: Comparison of low and high dose corticotropin stimulation tests in patients with pituitary disease. J Clin Endocrinol Metab 1998;83:1558-1562.
Minneci PC, Deans KJ, Banks SM, et al: Meta-analysis: The effect of steroids on survival and shock during sepsis depends on the dose. Ann Int Med 2004;141:47-56.
Oelkers W: Adrenal insufficiency. N Engl J Med 1996;335:1206-1243.
Oelkers W, Diedrich S, Bahr V: Diagnosis and therapy surveillance in Addison's disease: Rapid adrenocorticotropin (ACTH) test and measurement of plasma ACTH, renin activity, and aldosterone. J Clin Endocrinol Metab 1992;75:259-264.
Sprung CL, Annane D, Keh D, et al: CORTICUS Study Group. Hydrocortisone therapy for patients with septic shock. N Engl J Med 2008;358:111-124.

Cushing's Syndrome

Method of
Kathryn G. Schuff, MD

The diagnosis of Cushing's syndrome is one of the most difficult but potentially most important that can be made in a patient. The consequences of pathologic hypercortisolism are significant, and excess mortality and morbidity improve with cure of the disease. Although the evaluation and management often involve specialty referral, the primary care provider plays a pivotal role in suspecting the diagnosis and initiating the workup.

Clinical Presentation

Although traditionally considered a rare disease with an incidence of 1 to 2 per 100,000, more recently Cushing's syndrome has been reported to occur in up to 3% to 4% of the obese, uncontrolled diabetic population. The classic presentation (moon facies, purple striae, central obesity) is uncommonly seen, and the presentation more commonly overlaps that of polycystic ovary syndrome, the metabolic syndrome, and depression. Given the nonspecific presentation, health care providers should have a low threshold for screening patients for the disease. More specific features (Table 1) that should prompt evaluation include difficult-to-control diabetes mellitus or hypertension, unexplained osteoporosis, and menstrual irregularities. In addition, physical signs that are disquieting include facial rounding, plethora, supraclavicular fat pad filling, central obesity, thin skin (including

TABLE 1 Clinical Features of Cushing's Syndrome (In Order of Decreasing Specificity)

Feature	Sensitivity (%)	Specificity (%)
Hypokalemia (K^+ <3.6)	25	96
Ecchymoses	53	94
Osteoporosis	26	94
Weakness	65	93
Diastolic blood pressure ≥105 mm Hg	39	83
Red or violaceous striae	46	78
Acne	52	76
Central obesity	90	71
Hirsutism	50	71
Plethora	82	69
Oligomenorrhea	72	49
Generalized obesity	60	38
Abnormal glucose tolerance	88	23

spontaneous ecchymoses), and proximal muscle weakness, particularly if a change in appearance can be demonstrated. Children exhibit poor linear growth, generalized obesity, and menstrual irregularities. The etiologies of hypercortisolism are varied (Box 1) and include both pathologic etiologies causing subclinical and overt Cushing's syndrome as well as pseudo-Cushing's syndrome, which is temporary, nonpathologic hypercortisolemia caused by concurrent medical or psychiatric illness.

SUBCLINICAL CUSHING'S SYNDROME

Subtle hypothalamic-pituitary-adrenal (HPA) axis abnormalities and autonomy have been demonstrated in 5% to 20% of patients with incidentally discovered adrenal masses. These patients do not exhibit frank signs, symptoms, or biochemical abnormalities of Cushing's syndrome, and thus this entity is termed subclinical Cushing's syndrome. However, there are higher rates of hypertension, impaired glucose tolerance, and diabetes in these patients, which often improve with removal of the lesion, and a higher prevalence of cardiovascular dysfunction. Although this syndrome is considered a very mild form of Cushing's syndrome, there appears to be a low rate of progression to overt Cushing's syndrome, and therapeutic decisions must be individualized.

Diagnostic Evaluation

EXOGENOUS GLUCOCORTICOIDS

Cushing's syndrome caused by exogenous glucocorticoid use can be obvious, but careful investigation for unsuspected or surreptitious use must be undertaken in all patients. Infrequently recognized culprits are intraarticular, epidural, topical (inhaled, intranasal, and dermal), and naturopathic preparations. Variations in the metabolic clearance of synthetic glucocorticoids can lead to markedly prolonged glucocorticoid exposure and development of Cushing's syndrome. Detection of the synthetic glucocorticoid may require tandem mass spectrometry evaluation.

BOX 1 Etiologies of Hypercortisolism

- Pseudo-Cushing's syndrome (nonpathologic hypercortisolism)
    - Acute/chronic medical illness
    - Psychiatric illness
    - Alcoholism
- Subclinical Cushing's syndrome (subtle hypercortisolism without features of overt Cushing's syndrome)
    - Adrenal adenoma (incidentaloma)
    - Adrenal macronodular hyperplasia (rare)
    - Pituitary corticotroph adenoma (rare)
    - Aberrant receptor expression (rare)
- Cushing's syndrome (pathologic hypercortisolism)
    Exogenous glucocorticoid use
        Oral glucocorticoids (prednisone, dexamethasone [Decadron], hydrocortisone [Cortef])
        Topical glucocorticoids (inhaled, intranasal, dermal)
        Injected glucocorticoids (articular, periarticular, intramuscular)
        Naturopathic preparations
    Endogenous glucocorticoid production
        ACTH-dependent
            Pituitary corticotroph adenoma
                MEN1 (rare, also includes hyperparathy-roidism and pancreatic islet cell tumors)
            Pituitary corticotroph hyperplasia (some because of ectopic CRH)
            Ectopic ACTH syndrome
                Oat-cell lung carcinoma
                Foregut carcinoid tumors (bronchial, thymic, splenic)
                Pheochromocytoma
                Medullary thyroid carcinoma
                Islet cell tumors
        ACTH-independent
            Adrenal adenoma
            Adrenocortical carcinoma
            Rare: micronodular hyperplasia
            Macronodular hyperplasia
                Aberrant receptor expression (gastric inhibitory peptide—food responsive, 5-hydroxytryptamine, angiotensin II, interleukin-1, luteinizing hormone and human chorionic gonadotropin, vasopressin, β-adrenergic)
                Pigmented micronodular hyperplasia (Carney's triad)
                Adrenal rests
                McCune-Albright (activating mutations)

Abbreviations: ACTH = adrenocorticotropic hormone; CRH = corticotrophin-releasing hormone; MEN1 = multiple endocrine neoplasia, type 1.

 CURRENT DIAGNOSIS

- The clinical presentation of Cushing's syndrome is nonspecific and overlaps that of other more common diseases such as polycystic ovary syndrome, the metabolic syndrome, and depression.
- Signs and symptoms more specific for Cushing's syndrome include unexplained osteoporosis, muscle weakness, spontaneous ecchymoses, hypokalemia, central obesity, and plethora. Children present with growth failure, generalized obesity, and menstrual irregularities.
- A stepwise approach to the diagnosis helps avoid pitfalls in the interpretation of diagnostic tests. The first step is to confirm the diagnosis of Cushing's syndrome. The second step is to determine if the patient has ACTH-dependent or ACTH-independent disease. The final step is to determine if the ACTH source is eutopic (from the pituitary gland) or ectopic (the ectopic ACTH syndrome).
- The 1 mg ON dex test is easy to perform and has good sensitivity for diagnosing Cushing's syndrome. However, because of its poor specificity, confirmatory testing with measurement of urine free cortisol, midnight serum or salivary cortisol or the dex-CRH test is required.
- Random or CRH-stimulated ACTH levels greater than 10 pg/mL indicate ACTH-dependent disease.
- Biochemical testing is inadequate for distinguishing pituitary tumors from the ectopic ACTH syndrome. Jugular venous sampling has a high positive predictive value, but if negative, inferior petrosal or cavernous sinus sampling with CRH stimulation is required.
- Pituitary MRI is positive in only approximately one half of patients with corticotroph adenomas.

Abbreviations: ACTH = adrenocorticotropic hormone; CRH = corticotrophin-releasing hormone; dex = dexamethasone; MRI = magnetic resonance imaging; 1 mg ON dex test = 1 mg overnight dexamethasone suppression test.

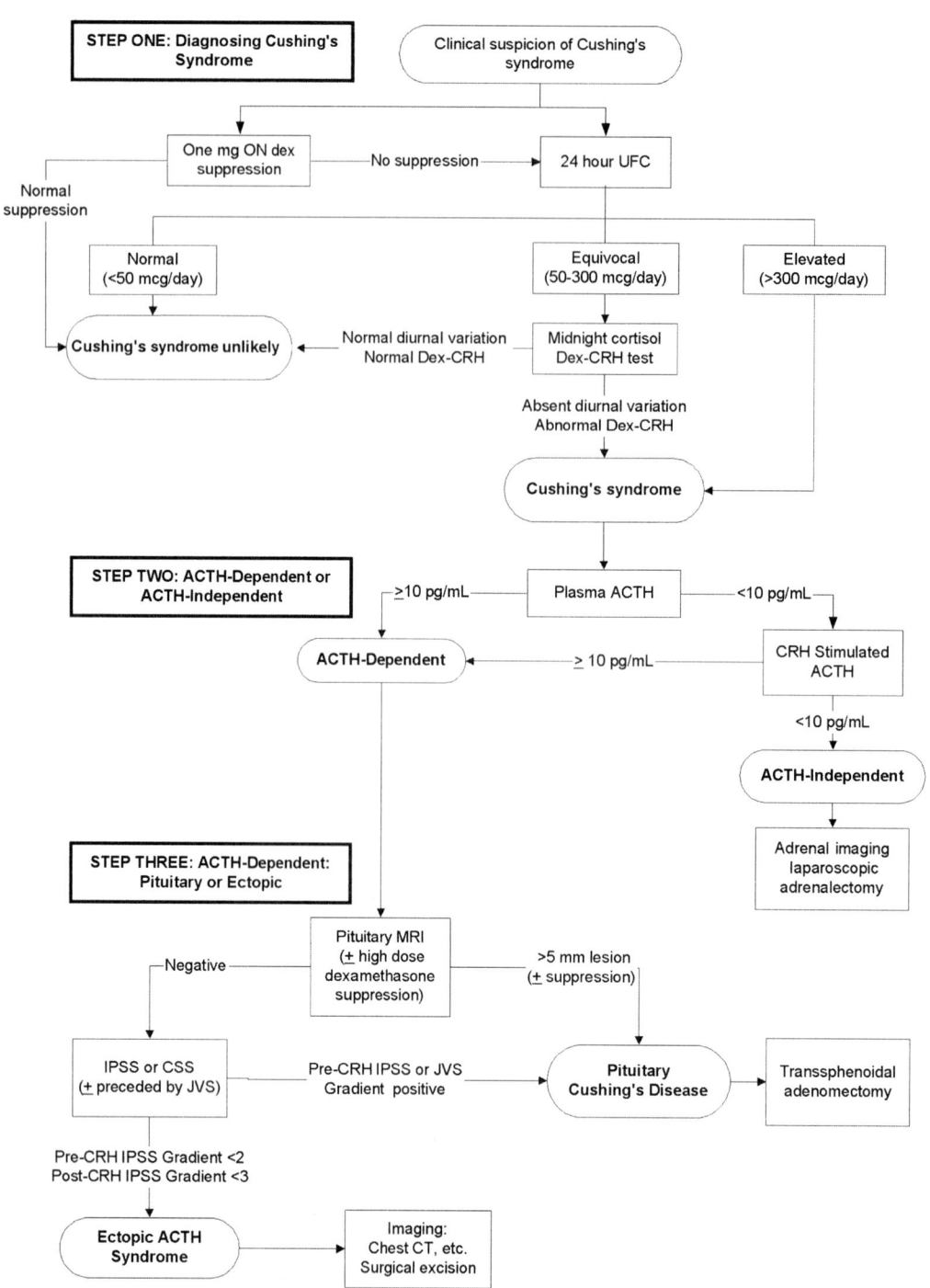

FIGURE 1. Stepwise approach to the diagnosis and differential diagnosis of Cushing's syndrome. ACTH = adrenocorticotropin; CRH = corticotrophin-releasing hormone; CSS = cavernous sinus sampling; CT = computed tomography; dex = dexamethasone; IPSS = inferior petrosal sinus sampling; JVS = jugular venous sampling; MRI = magnetic resonance imaging; ON = overnight; UFC = urine-free cortisol.

ENDOGENOUS HYPERCORTISOLISM

Evaluation of suspected endogenous hypercortisolemia must follow a stepwise approach (Figure 1). The first step is to make the diagnosis of Cushing's syndrome. The second step is to determine if the abnormal cortisol secretion is adrenocorticotropic hormone (ACTH)-dependent (from either a pituitary adenoma (Cushing's disease) or the ectopic ACTH syndrome) or ACTH-independent (primary adrenal disease). Finally, in ACTH-dependent Cushing's syndrome, the health care provider must distinguish pituitary sources of ACTH from the ectopic ACTH syndrome. Proceeding in the evaluation in a stepwise approach is critical for correct interpretation of test results because the premise of many of the tests is that preliminary biochemical diagnoses have been confirmed. For example, Cushing's syndrome must be confirmed before the ACTH level can be interpreted. In addition, because of the high prevalence of incidental pituitary and adrenal lesions and the finding of nodular adrenal disease in some cases of Cushing's disease caused by pituitary adenomas, imaging should not be performed until the biochemical diagnoses have been established. Finally, as many as 15% of patients with Cushing's syndrome will have intermittent hypercortisolemia, and care must be taken that the evaluation is performed when the patient is symptomatic or has documented hypercortisolism.

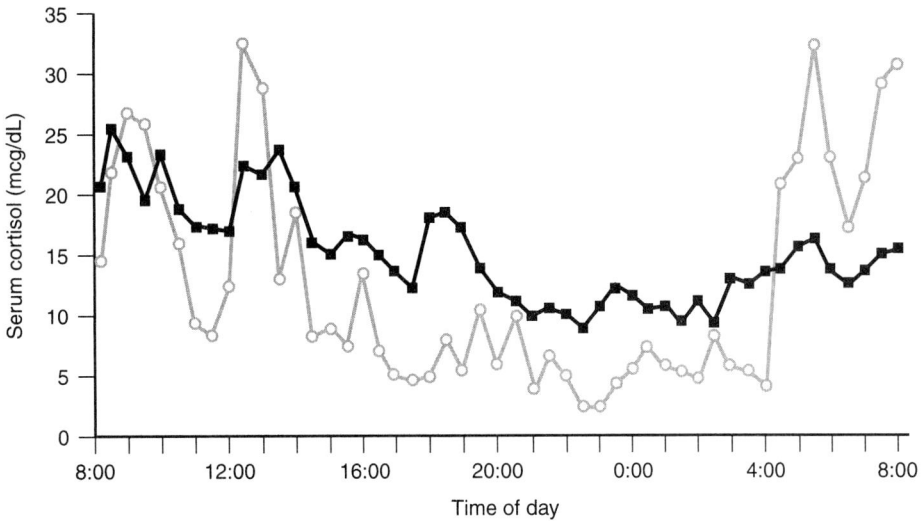

FIGURE 2. Diurnal rhythm of cortisol secretion is lost in Cushing's syndrome. Serum cortisol levels were measured every 30 minutes over 24 hours in a patient with proven Cushing's syndrome *(closed squares)* and a patient with pseudo-Cushing's syndrome *(open circles)*. Urine free cortisol (UFC) was mildly elevated in both patients (Cushing's syndrome, 75 mg/day; pseudo-Cushing's syndrome, 76 μg/day). Loss of diurnal variation in cortisol secretion is seen in the patient with Cushing's syndrome, whereas the patient with pseudo-Cushing's syndrome demonstrated normal diurnal variation with low serum cortisol levels (2.2 μg/dL) at midnight. (Data courtesy of Dr. Mary H. Samuels.)

STEP ONE: DIAGNOSE CUSHING'S SYNDROME

The first step in the evaluation is to establish the diagnosis of Cushing's syndrome by demonstrating pathologic hypercortisolism, either by measuring cortisol overproduction, abnormal HPA regulation, or absent diurnal variation. We recommend four tests for this purpose: the 1 mg overnight dexamethasone suppression (1 mg ON dex) test, measurement of 24-hour urine-free cortisol (24-hour UFC) excretion, assessment of diurnal variation with a midnight serum or salivary cortisol level, and the dexamethasone-suppressed corticotrophin-releasing hormone stimulation (dex-CRH) test.

One Milligram Overnight Dexamethasone Suppression Test

The 1 mg ON dex test has sensitivity sufficiently high to exclude the diagnosis of Cushing's syndrome; however, it lacks sufficient specificity to confirm the diagnosis, with false-positive rates from 5% to 30%. The test is simple to perform and involves administering 1 mg of dexamethasone (Decadron) by mouth at 11 PM. The serum cortisol at 8 AM the next morning should be less than 5 μg/dL; more strict criteria require suppression to less than 2.5 or 3 mg/dL. A simultaneous dexamethasone (Decadron) level can detect false positives that occur in patients taking medications that accelerate dexamethasone (Decadron) metabolism (phenytoin [Dilantin], phenobarbital [Luminal], rifampin [Rifadin], and primidone [Mysoline]). False positives may also be seen with estrogen therapy and tamoxifen (Nolvadex).

Measurement of 24-Hour Urine-Free Cortisol Excretion

Because of the high false-positive rate, an abnormal 1 mg ON dex test must be confirmed, usually by measurement of 24-hour UFC excretion. Alternatively, a 24-hour UFC measurement may be the initial step in the evaluation. As shown in Figure 1, marked elevations in 24-hour UFC (>300 μg/day) confirm the diagnosis, but intermediate levels require additional evaluation. Because of potential problems with incomplete collections and intermittent hypercortisolemia, creatinine should be measured in the specimen, and normal 24-hour UFC excretion should be demonstrated on 2 or 3 occasions before the diagnosis of Cushing's syndrome is excluded. Acute medical illness can cause marked elevations in 24-hour UFC, false positives can occur with high urine volumes, and carbamazepine (Tegretol) can cross-react in the high-pressure liquid chromatography (HPLC) assay.

Midnight Serum or Salivary Cortisol Levels

Loss of the diurnal rhythm in cortisol secretion is a characteristic feature in Cushing's syndrome (Figure 2). Demonstration of a midnight serum cortisol greater than 7.5 μg/dL distinguishes patients with Cushing's syndrome from normal and pseudo-Cushing's patients with high sensitivity and specificity. More recent improvements in the salivary cortisol assay allow collection of a saliva sample at home, avoiding the logistic difficulties in arranging a blood draw at night. Cut-off values for salivary cortisol measurements vary by assay, but normal suppression is generally between less than 0.2 and 0.55 μg/dL.

Dexamethasone-Suppressed Corticotropin-Releasing Hormone Stimulation Test

The dex-CRH test detects the relative resistance to dexamethasone (Decadron) suppression and over-responsiveness to ovine corticotropin-releasing factor (oCRH [Acthrel]) in various tumors. It improves on the poor specificity of the 1 mg ON dex test with a higher dose of dexamethasone (Decadron), 0.5 mg by mouth every 6 hours starting at 12 PM and ending at 6 AM on the second day. Because this dose of dexamethasone (Decadron) will suppress many pituitary adenomas, sensitivity of the test is retained by administration of oCRH (Acthrel)[1] 100 μg intravenously at 8 AM on the final day followed by cortisol and ACTH levels every 15 minutes for 1 hour. A plasma cortisol greater than 1.4 μg/dL distinguishes patients with Cushing's syndrome from those with pseudo-Cushing's with high accuracy.

STEP TWO: ACTH-DEPENDENT OR ACTH-INDEPENDENT DISEASE

Once the diagnosis of Cushing's syndrome has been established, the next step is to determine if the abnormal cortisol secretion is dependent on ACTH. A random ACTH level greater than 10 pg/mL confirms ACTH-dependent disease. However, because ACTH is secreted in a pulsatile, episodic fashion and is rapidly degraded, a low ACTH

---

[1]Not FDA approved for this indication.

level must be confirmed by lack of stimulation to more than 10 pg/mL by oCRH (Acthrel),[1] 100 µg intravenously. When ACTH independent disease is confirmed, we then proceed with adrenal imaging, usually with high-resolution (3- to 5-mm sections), computed tomography (CT) to evaluate primary adrenal disease.

STEP THREE: DISTINGUISH PITUITARY FROM ECTOPIC SOURCES OF ACTH

Once ACTH-dependent disease has been confirmed, the health care provider must determine the source of excess ACTH secretion. Approximately 90% of patients have a pituitary corticotroph adenoma as the source of ACTH. A number of biochemical tests exist to distinguish pituitary from ectopic sources, the most accurate of which is the high-dose dexamethasone suppression test. This test involves comparison of a baseline 24-hour UFC with one collected during the second day of dexamethasone (Decadron) 2 mg by mouth every 6 hours for eight doses. Although failure to suppress more than 90% from the baseline UFC has been reported to have 100% specificity for identifying ectopic tumors, the sensitivity of this test is poor, and there have been subsequent reports of lower specificity. Because of this, we do not rely on biochemical testing. Rather, once ACTH-dependent disease is confirmed, we perform magnetic resonance imaging (MRI) of the pituitary gland. In approximately one half of patients, a definite tumor is identified, and we then proceed with transsphenoidal adenomectomy. However, another reasonable strategy is to proceed with pituitary surgery only if both MRI and high-dose dexamethasone testing suggests a pituitary tumor.

If a tumor is not definitely identified, inferior petrosal or cavernous sinus sampling with oCRH stimulation is required to localize the ACTH source. Finding a central (cavernous sinus or petrosal sinus) to peripheral ratio of more than 2.0 before oCRH or greater than 3.0 after oCRH is highly accurate for identifying a pituitary source of ACTH. In addition, a pre-oCRH lateralization (right to left or left to right) ratio more than 1.4 suggests the intrapituitary location of the tumor. Sampling must be performed by experienced personnel, and the accuracy of the test is highly dependent on oCRH administration, symmetric catheter placement, symmetric flow through the venous sinuses, and hypercortisolemia at the time of testing. In addition, it is critical that the diagnosis of Cushing's syndrome and ACTH-dependence be confirmed before proceeding with sampling. Normal individuals and patients with pseudo-Cushing's syndrome have inferior petrosal sinus sampling (IPSS) results that falsely suggest a pituitary tumor. Patients with ACTH-independent disease (primary adrenal disease) with low but measurable ACTH levels can have IPSS results that falsely suggest either a pituitary tumor or the ectopic ACTH syndrome.

Recently, internal jugular venous sampling has been evaluated as a less invasive alternative to petrosal sinus sampling. A jugular to peripheral ratio of greater than 1.7 before oCRH or more than 2.5 after oCRH indicate a pituitary source with high accuracy. Nondiagnostic ratios are unreliable and should be further evaluated with inferior petrosal or cavernous sinus sampling.

If sampling suggests an ectopic source of ACTH, imaging is then performed to locate the tumor, starting with high resolution CT or MRI of the chest. If those areas are unrevealing, neck, abdomen, and pelvis CT are performed. Octreotide scanning may be helpful but only rarely identifies an abnormality not already seen on anatomic imaging. Often, the culprit lesion is not seen at initial imaging, but becomes apparent on serial studies performed every 6 to 12 months.

Although IPSS is highly accurate, occasional false-negative and rare false-positive results have been reported. In situations where IPSS ratios indicate the ectopic ACTH syndrome but no ectopic tumor can be found, distinguishing a truly occult ectopic ACTH-producing tumor from a false-negative IPSS is extremely difficult. Review of the response of peripheral ACTH levels to oCRH stimulation should be done, because pituitary adenomas have significantly more robust responses than ectopic tumors. Repeat IPSS and consideration of pituitary exploration are appropriate, particularly if the ACTH response to oCRH, biochemical testing, and/or MRI are consistent with a pituitary adenoma.

Therapeutic Interventions

EXOGENOUS GLUCOCORTICOID USE

Once identified, the treatment for iatrogenic Cushing's syndrome is straightforward but often difficult because of the therapeutic benefit of pharmacologic glucocorticoids. Tapering the steroid needs to occur gradually, with close monitoring of the underlying disease process and optimization of nonsteroid therapeutics. Alternate-day dosing regimens may assist in HPA axis recovery but may be limited by the underlying disease process. Patients should wear Medic Alert identification until the taper is completed and normal HPA function is demonstrated.

ENDOGENOUS CUSHING'S SYNDROME

The therapeutic intervention in essentially all etiologies of endogenous Cushing's syndrome is surgical resection of the autonomous tumor or tissue, except for the case of lung carcinomas causing the ectopic ACTH syndrome, where therapy is tailored to the stage of the cancer. Postoperatively, all patients are treated with stress doses of glucocorticoids, tapering quickly to doses approximately twice physiologic replacement, usually hydrocortisone (Cortef)[1] 20 mg by mouth twice or three times daily. Further slow taper is done over the next several months as tolerated by cortisol withdrawal symptoms and recovery of the HPA axis. A morning serum cortisol level less than 2 µg/dL on the second postoperative day is highly predictive of surgical cure; patients with low but detectable serum cortisol levels, such as less than 5 µg/dL, have varying cure rates. Periodic morning cortisol levels and cosyntropin (Cortrosyn)[1] stimulation testing assess recovery of the HPA axis during and after the glucocorticoid taper.

Cushing's Disease

Transsphenoidal adenomectomy is recommended for the vast majority of patients with pituitary tumors, except where extensive cavernous sinus involvement indicates a transfrontal approach. Intraoperative ultrasound or MRI can assist in the localization of tumors. If a tumor is not identified at surgery, hemihypophysectomy based on preoperative MRI and/or IPSS or CSS lateralization ratios may result in cure. Often, tumors are not identified on pathology, because they are semiliquid and "lost" during suctioning.

Mortality and morbidity are generally low in experienced centers, but complications can include cerebrospinal fluid leaks, meningitis, visual impairment, hypopituitarism, hemorrhage, venous thromboembolism, and death. Careful monitoring for abnormalities in vasopressin secretion postoperatively is required, both for diabetes insipidus and the syndrome of inappropriate antidiuretic-hormone secretion. Testing of pituitary function including free T4, IGF-1 with possible growth hormone stimulation testing and testosterone levels or menstrual history is performed at 6 weeks postoperatively.

Even in experienced hands, long-term cure of hypercortisolemia is difficult, with initial success rates reported from 68.5% to 91% and relapse rates of up to 15% over a 10-year period. Cure rates are worse for macroadenomas or invasive tumors and second surgeries, reported at 40% to 55%. Even with biochemical cure and improvement in symptoms, studies show persistent compromise in quality of life.

Primary Adrenal Disease

The laparoscopic approach has essentially replaced open surgery with similar mortality, morbidity, and operative times; and shorter

---

[1] Not FDA approved for this indication.

postoperative recovery, hospital stays, and decreased acute and chronic pain. The laparoscopic approach is not used in cases of adrenocortical carcinoma or patients with coagulopathy, previous surgery or trauma. Lesion size was previously a limitation, but with increasing experience appears to no longer be a significant factor. Unilateral adrenalectomy is indicated for adrenal adenomas and adrenocortical carcinomas; the rare nodular hyperplasias are treated with bilateral surgery. Adrenalectomy is curative for adrenal adenomas and hyperplasia, but carcinomas are often advanced at presentation and generally have a poor prognosis. Adrenolytic therapy with mitotane (Lysodren) may be necessary to control hypercortisolemia and tumor growth in carcinomas postoperatively.

Secondary Therapy for Failed Pituitary Surgery or Occult Ectopic Tumors

If transsphenoidal surgery fails to resolve the hypercortisolemia, patients can be offered pituitary irradiation. If a lesion can be targeted, stereotactic radiosurgery with a linear accelerator (LINAC) system, gamma-knife system, or proton beam system offers lower radiation exposure to surrounding normal tissue and theoretically more effective higher doses to the residual tumor than conventional fractionated radiation therapy. Time to control of hypercortisolemia is variable, reported from 6 to 36 months, requiring interim control of hypercortisolemia by either medical therapy or adrenalectomy. Complications of radiation therapy include hypopituitarism, rare optic neuropathy, and rare (and debated) induction of second tumors and brain necrosis. The risk of Nelson's syndrome (rapid and aggressive growth of corticotroph tumors after adrenalectomy) may be lessened with radiation therapy.

Alternatively, and in the cases of ectopic tumors remaining occult, bilateral adrenalectomy can be performed offering immediate control of hypercortisolemia. Both glucocorticoid and mineralocorticoid (fludrocortisone [Florinef] 0.1 mg by mouth once or twice daily) replacement are generally required. Glucocorticoids are tapered as described above to physiologic doses of hydrocortisone (Cortef)[1] 20 to 30 mg by mouth daily in single or divided doses. Continued surveillance with imaging is required, because of the risk of development of Nelson's syndrome and the occasional, locally invasive, and rarely metastatic potential of ectopic tumors.

Medical Management of Hypercortisolemia

Medical management of hypercortisolemia has an inadequate efficacy and side-effect profile for primary or long-term use. However, it has a very important role in temporizing the pathologic effects of long-standing Cushing's syndrome in preparation for surgical treatment and while awaiting definitive cure from radiation therapy. Strategies include medications (Table 2) that block glucocorticoid synthesis, inhibit pituitary ACTH secretion, or block glucocorticoid action. None of the agents that inhibit ACTH release is very effective but might be useful in combination therapy. The most effective medications are those that block glucocorticoid synthesis including

---
[1]Not FDA approved for this indication.

TABLE 2 Drugs Used in the Medical Therapy of Cushing's Syndrome

Medication	Mechanism of Action	Typical Dosage	Reported Efficacy	Common Toxicities
Steroid Biosynthesis Inhibitors				
Ketoconazole (Nizoral)[1]	Blocks multiple steps in cortisol synthesis	200-1200 mg/d	70%	Hepatotoxicity, gynecomastia, nausea, edema, rash
Metyrapone (Metopirone)[1]	Blocks 11β-hydroxylase	500-6000 mg/d	85%	Hirsutism, acne, lethargy, dizziness, ataxia, edema, nausea, rash
Aminoglutethimide (Cytadren)	Blocks cholesterol to pregnenelone conversion	750-2000 mg/d	>60% Useful additive to metyrapone	Lethargy, somnolence, dizziness, rash, fever, nausea, anorexia, hypothyroidism
Mitotane (o, p′-DDD, Lysodren)[1]*	Blocks side-chain cleavage Adrenolytic	500-12,000 mg/d	83%	Gastrointestinal, impaired mentation, dizziness, hyperlipidemia, gynecomastia, transient rash, hepatotoxicity
ACTH Release Inhibitors				
Cyproheptadine (Periactin)[1]	Impairs ACTH secretion	24 mg/d	30%-50%	Somnolence, hyperphagia, weight gain
Bromocriptine (Parlodel)[1]	Impairs ACTH secretion	3.75-30 mg/d	25%-42%	Nausea, dry mouth, postural hypotension
Octreotide (Sandostatin)[1]	Inhibits ACTH release	100-600 μg/d	Limited experience, additive to ketoconazole	Diarrhea, gallstones
Valproic acid (Depakene)[1]	Potentiates GABA inhibition of CRH and ACTH release	1-2 g/d	Limited experience, additive to metyrapone	Sedation, nausea, hepatotoxicity, pancreatitis
Glucocorticoid Receptor Antagonist				
Mifepristone (RU-486, Mifeprex)[1]	Glucocorticoid receptor antagonist	10-25 mg/kg/d	Limited experience	Nausea, vomiting, irregular menses

[1]Not FDA approved for this indication.
*FDA approved for treatment of adrenocortical carcinoma.
Abbreviations: ACTH = adrenocorticotropic hormone; CRH = corticotropin-releasing hormone; GABA = gamma-aminobutyric acid.

CURRENT THERAPY

- Treatment for Cushing's syndrome is primarily surgical and targeted to the pathologic lesion.
- Transsphenoidal adenomectomy is recommended for pituitary-dependent Cushing's disease, but has a long-term success rate of only 60% to 80%.
- Laparoscopic adrenalectomy has replaced open approaches in the management of primary adrenal lesions except for adrenocortical carcinoma, and for second-line treatment after failed pituitary surgery or failure to localize an occult ectopic tumor.
- Definitive secondary treatments for failed pituitary surgery include pituitary irradiation and bilateral adrenalectomy.
- Medical therapy for Cushing's syndrome is difficult, and reserved for surgical failures awaiting benefit from radiation therapy or in preparation for surgical therapy.

ketoconazole[1] (Nizoral), metyrapone[1] (Metopirone), and mitotane[1,*] (o,p'DDD, Lysodren). These are usually dosed to partially block cortisol production, suppressing it into the normal range. Alternatively, complete adrenal blockade with replacement hydrocortisone can be attempted. Finally, very limited experience with blockade of the glucocorticoid receptor with mifepristone (Mifeprex)[1] has shown clinical efficacy. Because glucocorticoid levels are unaffected, titration of this medication must be done on clinical grounds.

---

[1]Not FDA approved for this indication.
*FDA approved only for adrenocortical carcinoma.

REFERENCES

Bochicchio D, Losa M, Buchfelder M: Factors influencing the immediate and late outcome of Cushing's disease treated by transsphenoidal surgery: A retrospective study by the European Cushing's disease survey group. J Clin Endocrinol Metab 1995;80:3114-3120.

Hammer GD, Tyrrell JB, Lamborn KR, et al: Transsphenoidal microsurgery for Cushing's disease: Initial outcome and long-term results. J Clin Endocrinol Metab 2004;89:6348-6357.

Ilias I, Chang R, Pacak K, et al: Jugular venous sampling: An alternative to petrosal sinus sampling for the diagnostic evaluation of adrenocorticotropic hormone-dependent Cushing's syndrome. J Clin Endocrinol Metab 2004;89:3795-3800.

Leinung MC, Zimmerman D: Cushing's disease in children. Endocrinol Metab Clin North Am 1994;23:629-639.

Mahmoud-Ahmed AS, Suh JH: Radiation therapy for Cushing's disease: A review. Pituitary 2002;5:175-180.

Nieman LK: Medical therapy of Cushing's disease. Pituitary 2002;5:77-82.

Oldfield E, Doppman J, Nieman L, et al: Petrosal sinus sampling with and without corticotropin-releasing hormone for the differential diagnosis of Cushing's syndrome. N Engl J Med 1991;325:897-905.

Papanicolaou DA, Mullen N, Kyrou I, Nieman LK: Nighttime salivary cortisol: A useful test for the diagnosis of Cushing's syndrome. J Clin Endocrinol Metab 2002;87:4515-4521.

Reincke M: Subclinical Cushing's syndrome. Endocrinol Metab Clin North Am 2000;29:43-56.

Yanovski J, Cutler G, Chrousos G, Nieman L: Corticotropin-releasing hormone stimulation following low-dose dexamethasone (Decadron) administration. JAMA 1993;269:2232-2238.

Diabetes Insipidus

Method of
Jennifer Kelly, DO, and
Arnold M. Moses, MD, FACP, FACE

General Principles of Treating Central (Neurogenic) Diabetes Insipidus

The hormonal treatment of diabetes insipidus is accomplished using the synthetic nanopeptide desmopressin (1-deamino [8-D-arginine] vasopressin; DDAVP). Arginine vasopressin (AVP) is the natural hormone of humans. Desmopressin is a synthetic analogue of AVP that does not constrict smooth muscle and has a longer antidiuretic action than does the natural hormone. Because of its lack of vasoactivity, desmopressin can be used without precipitating angina, abdominal cramps, or headaches. It can also be used to treat diabetes insipidus during pregnancy because it resists inactivation by placental vasopressinase. The available preparations of vasopressin are listed in the table above. The durations of antidiuretic responses to the different preparations are listed in Table 1.

For most patients with diabetes insipidus, the treatment of choice is intranasal desmopressin (100 μg/mL). Two delivery systems are available: a nasal (rhinal) tube, which the patient uses to blow measured amounts (0.05-0.2 mL) into the nose, and a compression pump system, which delivers 0.1 mL (see Current Therapy). Treatment is usually initiated with 10 μg of intranasal desmopressin. Patients are instructed to repeat this dose when polyuria recurs. Some patients respond better if the hormone is administered on a more defined schedule. The dose administered can be increased or decreased in accordance with the patient's response. Patients should be told to drink only when they are thirsty.

Some patients prefer to start therapy with oral desmopressin; others can be switched to the oral preparation when absorption of

CURRENT DIAGNOSIS

Central diabetes insipidus (DI) can be diagnosed as follows:
1. Ensure urine volume is increased to ≥3 L/day in adults.
2. Rule out glycosuria (dipstick will suffice).
3. Measure serum sodium concentration during ad libitum fluid intake.
4. If the serum sodium concentration is *above* normal while urine osmolality is *less than* 300 mOsm per kilogram of water, injection of desmopressin (DDAVP) at least doubles the urine osmolality in patients with central DI. If the urine osmolality response is less, the patient may have nephrogenic DI.
5. If the serum sodium concentration is *normal* while urine osmolality is *less than* 300 mOsm per kilogram of water, additional procedures, including a water deprivation or saline infusion test, may be required. Refer to an experienced specialist.
6. Magnetic resonance imaging to detect the presence or absence of the pituitary hyperintense signal may be helpful in differentiating central DI from primary polydipsia. Plasma arginine vasopressin levels do *not* differentiate these two polyuric conditions.

CURRENT THERAPY

Trade Name	Chemical Composition	Concentration	Size	Pharmaceutical Company
Intranasal Preparations				
Desmopressin Rhinal Tube	Desmopressin acetate	100 µg/mL	2.5-mL bottle with rhinal tube delivering sprays of 10–20 µg	Ferring
DDAVP Rhinal Tube	Desmopressin acetate	100 µg/mL	2.5-mL bottle with rhinal tube delivering sprays of 10–20 µg	Aventis
DDAVP Nasal Spray	Desmopressin acetate	100 µg/mL	5.0-mL bottle with spray pump delivering 50 sprays of 10 µg each	Aventis
Oral Preparation				
DDAVP Tablets	Desmopressin acetate	Not applicable	0.1-mg, 0.2-mg tablets	Aventis
Injectable Preparations (Subcutaneous, Intravenous)				
DDAVP Injection	Desmopressin acetate	4 µg/mL	1.0, 10.0 mL/vials	Aventis
Pitressin Injection	Arginine vasopressin	20 U/mL	1 mL/vial	Monarch
Arginine Vasopressin Injection	Arginine vasopressin	20 U/mL	0.5, 1, and 10 mL/vials	American Regent

Caution: Stimate Nasal Spray (desmopressin acetate) is marketed by Aventis Pharmaceuticals in a 2.5-mL nasal spray bottle. It is designed for treating bleeding disorders and contains 1.5 mg/mL desmopressin. Stimate can be confused easily with the less concentrated preparations of desmopressin acetate that are used for treating diabetes insipidus.

the intranasal form is decreased in the presence of nasal congestion. The starting dose of the tablet is usually 0.05 mg (half of a 0.1-mg tablet) twice per day. The maintenance dose is gradually adjusted to provide an adequate limitation of water turnover. The daily oral dose may range from 0.1 to 1.2 mg in divided doses. We do not currently recommend the use of nonhormonal agents such as chlorpropamide (Diabinese),[1] clofibrate,[1,2] or carbamazepine.[1]

In the uncooperative or unconscious patient with diabetes insipidus, desmopressin should be injected subcutaneously, usually starting with 0.5 or 1.0 µg (see Table 1 for duration of action). Subcutaneous AVP is sometimes used in patients with acute onset of diabetes insipidus after head trauma or neurosurgical procedures. Its short duration of action might help prevent water intoxication in patients receiving poorly monitored intravenous fluids. As with desmopressin, it is safest to administer subsequent doses of AVP when polyuria reappears.

As long as untreated patients with diabetes insipidus are conscious, retain normal thirst, and have enough fluid to drink, they seldom become dehydrated. However, severe dehydration with extremely high serum sodium concentrations may occur acutely when patients with untreated diabetes insipidus do not receive adequate fluids (orally or intravenously).

The most common and important problem in the hospitalized patient with diabetes insipidus is iatrogenic hyponatremia. Particularly when it occurs rapidly, hyponatremia may cause severe neurologic problems. Hyponatremia in this setting is caused by overhydration (only rarely does sodium loss contribute) in patients receiving vasopressin and can be prevented by allowing patients to self-regulate their oral intake of fluids whenever possible. When such self-regulation is not feasible because the patient is obtunded, has a defective thirst mechanism, or cannot drink, extreme care must be taken in ordering intravenous fluids to prevent hyponatremia. The patient can be maintained in an antidiuretic state by giving vasopressin when the urine becomes dilute. The intravenous fluid should

TABLE 1 Mean Time That Urine Remains Hypertonic in Adults with Diabetes Insipidus*

Route of Administration	Amount Administered	Mean Duration of Action (hr)
Intranasal desmopressin	10 µg (0.1 mL)	12
	15 µg (0.15 mL)	16
	20 µg (0.2 mL)	20
Subcutaneous or intravenous desmopressin	0.5 µg	10
	1.0 µg	14
	2.0 µg	18
	4.0 µg	22
Oral desmopressin	0.1 mg	6–8
	0.2 mg	8–12
	0.4 mg	16–20
Subcutaneous arginine vasopressin	5 U	4

*Note: Onset of antidiuretic action of subcutaneous or intravenous preparation is 30–45 minutes. Onset of antidiuretic effect of tablets is about 60 minutes.

---
[1] Not FDA approved for this indication.
[2] Not available in the United States.

consist largely of 5% dextrose in water with amounts of normal saline gauged to replace daily urinary sodium losses. The volume of intravenous fluid for every 8-hour period should replace 8-hour urine volumes plus estimated 8-hour insensible losses and fluid losses through perspiration and other routes. The amount of intravenous fluid should be adjusted according to plasma sodium, blood urea nitrogen, and creatinine levels. If hypernatremia occurs, the amount of intravenous fluids should be increased accordingly.

If a major decrease in serum sodium concentration occurs, intravenous fluids should be temporarily discontinued, and, if necessitated by clinical manifestations, the patient should be given 200 to 300 mL of 3% saline, perhaps with 40 mg of furosemide (Lasix) intravenously. Temporary discontinuation of vasopressin should also be considered. To emphasize, the patient with central diabetes insipidus whose fluid intake is maintained intravenously presents a major medical problem and must be followed up carefully to maintain normonatremia.

Pregnancy is associated with significant alterations in water metabolism. The osmotic threshold for secretion of vasopressin is lowered and the threshold for thirst reduced, with a resulting decrease in plasma osmolality by about 10 mOsm per kilogram of water. A deficiency of plasma vasopressin can also result from increased degradation of the hormone by placental vasopressinase. This disorder is referred to as *gestational diabetes insipidus* because the symptoms of diabetes insipidus occur only during pregnancy and remit soon after delivery. An underlying subclinical deficiency in vasopressin secretion may also be involved. Gestational diabetes insipidus is treated successfully with desmopressin, which is not degraded by vasopressinase. The dose of desmopressin should be about the same as that used in the nonpregnant state, but the normal range for serum sodium is about 5 mEq/L lower.

Principles of Treating Specific Problems

THE ALERT PATIENT WITH INTACT THIRST

When antidiuretic therapy is initiated in the alert patient with diabetes insipidus, the patient must consciously avoid excessive drinking for at least several days. By that time, the thirst mechanism usually adapts to the more normal urine volume. However, some patients must be reminded to avoid excessive drinking, which causes the syndrome of inappropriate antidiuresis. Thirst may be perceived with normal or low serum sodium concentration because of a dry mouth, as might occur with mouth breathing, anticholinergic drugs, β-adrenergic blockers, or cigarette smoking. An occasional patient is hyperdipsic because of increased circulating angiotensin II levels or from hypothalamic involvement, as may occur with sarcoidosis involving the hypothalamus. Use of ice instead of liquids may help limit fluid intake.

THE ALERT PATIENT WITH ADIPSIA

The alert patient with adipsia presents a difficult management problem in the hospital and particularly after the patient is discharged from the hospital. Because of the loss of thirst perception, normal serum sodium concentration is maintained only with great difficulty. The patient and family must closely and continuously monitor the patient's intake and output of fluids, body weight, and vital signs. Serum sodium concentration and blood urea nitrogen, uric acid, and creatinine levels should be checked often. Such a patient must always relate fluid intake to volume of urine plus fluid losses through perspiration and the gastrointestinal tract. Failure to properly monitor these patients may allow their condition to go unrecognized until they develop severe dehydration. This may require the infusion of normal saline to restore pulse and blood pressure and then water orally or dextrose in water intravenously. Appropriate antidiuretic therapy should be instituted along with the fluids.

THE CONFUSED, OBTUNDED, OR UNCONSCIOUS PATIENT

When confused, obtunded, or unconscious, such as postoperatively or after head trauma, the patient with diabetes insipidus is monitored in the same ways described for the alert patient with adipsia. The only major difference is that vasopressin must be given by injection or infusion and the fluids given intravenously. In the presence of hypernatremia and associated hypovolemia, normal saline is required to help restore pulse and blood pressure to normal. Otherwise, patients with hypernatremia should be treated with dextrose in water (see later) while antidiuretic therapy is instituted and maintained.

Postoperative hypernatremia should be prevented by the early recognition of diabetes insipidus before, during, and after surgery and by avoidance of osmotic diuretic use during surgery. The patient should be switched to oral fluids as soon as possible, and the adequacy of the patient's thirst mechanism to control fluid intake appropriately should be evaluated. Diabetes insipidus that occurs postoperatively or after head trauma may be variable (biphasic or triphasic), and frequently the diabetes insipidus is transient. Therefore, hormonal treatment should be withheld periodically to determine whether the symptoms of diabetes insipidus recur. After 6 months of diabetes insipidus, remission is very unlikely.

Special Problems of Fluid Balance

THE HYPERNATREMIC PATIENT

Hypernatremia in patients with diabetes insipidus is usually associated with normal total body sodium. The hypernatremia is due to loss of free water by way of the kidneys, but losses from the skin and lungs can aggravate the problem. Alterations in the composition of water and solutes in the brain cells may contribute to the symptoms of hypernatremia. An abrupt increase in plasma sodium concentration causes more severe symptoms than does a gradual rise to the same sodium level.

The goal of treating hypernatremia in patients with diabetes insipidus is restoration of normal plasma volume and tonicity. Desmopressin should be injected to maintain concentrated urine. If the patient has circulatory disturbances due to hypovolemia, isotonic saline should be given until systemic hemodynamics are stabilized. In fact, isotonic saline is relatively hypotonic to plasma in patients with severe hypernatremia and simultaneously corrects both volume and water deficits. After volume deficits are corrected, the hypernatremia can be treated intravenously with 5% dextrose in water, or water can be given by mouth if the patient is able to drink.

The water deficit in these patients can be calculated on the basis of the serum sodium concentration and on the assumption that 60% of body weight is water. For example, if the patient's usual weight is 75 kg, total body water would normally be 75 kg × 0.6 = 45 L. If the serum sodium value is 154 mEq/L, the patient has a 10% deficit of water (154 − 140) ÷ 140 and theoretically requires 4.5 L of water to correct the deficit. Continuing losses of water must also be replaced. Despite inaccuracies, including the assumption that body water is always 60% of the body weight and the postulate that water is lost uniformly throughout all body cells, this approach provides an approximate value that can be used in planning therapy. The major problem is determining the appropriate rate at which to lower serum sodium concentration to normal. Because seizures or even fatal cerebral edema may occur when serum sodium concentration is lowered rapidly, the best recommendation is to correct the hypernatremia over 48 to 72 hours and at a rate not exceeding 0.5 to 2.0 mEq/L/hr. As total body water expands, the serum sodium concentration may fall proportionately. Serum electrolyte values should be monitored frequently to ensure an appropriate response.

Treatment of the hypernatremia due to water loss, as occurs in untreated patients with diabetes insipidus, must also address associated electrolyte abnormalities and underlying medical and surgical conditions. An example is the patient with diabetes insipidus with coexisting hyperglycemia. In this case, the "corrected" serum sodium concentration should be used to calculate the water deficit. Slightly low or abnormal serum sodium concentrations in the presence of high serum glucose often result, when corrected, in hypernatremic values. The corrected serum sodium concentrations can be calculated by increasing the sodium concentration by 1.5 mEq/L for every 100 mg/dL increment in the serum glucose concentration above 100 mg/dL. For example, in a patient with a sodium level of 138 mEq/L and a glucose level of 700 mg/dL, the corrected serum sodium concentration is 138 + (1.5 × 6), or 147 mEq/L.

THE HYPONATREMIC PATIENT

Hyponatremia in diabetes insipidus occurs almost exclusively in patients who are overhydrated orally or parenterally while they are being treated with desmopressin. The severity of hyponatremia correlates closely with the magnitude of fluid overload. The amount of excessive body water can be calculated using the same approach as described for hypernatremia. Rarely, the hyponatremia is aggravated by large amounts of sodium in the urine, probably related to increased levels of atrial natriuretic peptide and glomerular filtration rate and inhibition of aldosterone. The hyponatremia due to natriuresis in the water-overloaded patient can be corrected only partially with saline infusions, because the natriuresis continues until the hypervolemic state is corrected. Hyponatremia can be caused or aggravated by adrenal or thyroid insufficiency.

A large body of literature on the appropriate rate at which to correct hyponatremia is available. Rapidly occurring (acute) and marked hyponatremia can be lethal and should be treated urgently. Under these conditions, and when neurologic symptoms are severe, initial therapy should raise the serum sodium concentration by 1 to 2 mEq/L/hr regardless of the duration of the electrolyte abnormality. Most authorities agree that the rate of change in serum sodium concentrations should not exceed 12 to 20 mEq/L/day. However, in patients with chronic hyponatremia, correction of serum sodium concentration approximating this rate occasionally causes serious, even fatal complications by inducing central pontine myelinolysis.

Fluid restriction is adequate for treatment of the asymptomatic mildly hyponatremic patient. Urine should be analyzed every 4 to 8 hours for volume and osmolality, and fluid replacement should be ordered in relation to *urine volume*. Remember that insensible fluid losses of about 600 mL of free water per day occur in the usual adult. *It is **NOT** appropriate to write for a fixed amount of fluid replacement.* Plasma sodium concentration should be checked frequently and fluid replacement adjusted accordingly. The complaint of thirst by a water-restricted patient should not be ignored. Long-term management is usually less disruptive by adjusting fluid intake than by discontinuing hormonal therapy and allowing the patient to "break through." Alternatively, when the patient has symptomatic or severe hyponatremia (serum sodium concentration <115 mEq/L in chronic hyponatremia or 125 mEq/L in acute hyponatremia), intravenous furosemide (Lasix), may help by causing the excretion of urine that is slightly hypotonic or isotonic. After injection of 40 mg or more of furosemide, 100 mL of 3% saline should be infused in the first hour. This rate should be decreased or discontinued subsequently if symptoms have ameliorated or if the plasma sodium concentration has increased by more than 2 mEq/L in that hour. Infusion of more than a total of 250 mL of 3% saline is rarely necessary.

PREPARATION FOR DIAGNOSTIC TESTS OR TREATMENT

Special care must be taken when patients with treated diabetes insipidus are subjected to certain "standard protocols" associated with many diagnostic and therapeutic procedures. These protocols require the patient to be either fluid restricted, as for preparation for intravenous pyelography, or hydrated, as for intravenous administration of chemotherapy. Tests requiring that a patient receiving no oral fluids should be performed with adequate intravenous hydration matched to the patient's urine output. Intravenous fluids should be started from the time the patient is no longer able to take oral fluids and can be discontinued when oral fluids are again allowed. In contrast, patients receiving antidiuretic therapy for diabetes insipidus should not be made to "force fluids" beyond the amounts determined by thirst or be subject to hydration orders at rates not related to urine output. If high urine flow rates are needed, the patient's antidiuretic therapy must be discontinued. Oral or intravenous fluids can then be given to match the large urine volumes. Sometimes, it may be appropriate (to obtain more precise timing of a diuresis) to continue antidiuretic therapy and administer intravenous furosemide. Close monitoring of serum sodium levels will greatly assist in determining the status of fluid balance in these situations.

Nephrogenic Diabetes Insipidus

Nephrogenic diabetes insipidus is characterized by resistance of the kidney to the antidiuretic action of vasopressin. This disorder is often hereditary, caused by inactivating mutations of the V2 receptor or of the vasopressin-regulated water channel protein aquaporin 2. Standard doses of desmopressin or AVP do not decrease the polyuria. The urine volume can be decreased by 25% to 40% by severe solute restriction and by further inducing hypovolemia with thiazide diuretics. Rarely, very high doses of desmopressin may be effective in females. Occasionally, acquired nephrogenic diabetes insipidus resolves by eliminating the underlying cause (i.e., treating the hypercalcemia or hypokalemia or discontinuing lithium therapy). Nephrogenic diabetes insipidus due to long-term lithium therapy may persist after discontinuation of lithium. Treatment of lithium-induced nephrogenic diabetes insipidus is limited to a low-sodium diet and possibly diuretics. Treatment may reduce urine volume by up to 30% or 40%. Caution must be taken because solute restriction, especially with a diuretic, may lead to lithium toxicity.

REFERENCES

Adrogue HJ, Madias NE: Hypernatremia. N Engl J Med 2000;342:1493-1499.
Gross P: Treatment of severe hyponatremia. Kidney Int 2001;60:2417-2427.
Moses AM, Clayton B, Hochhauser L: Use of T1-weighted MR imaging to differentiate between primary polydipsia and central diabetes insipidus. AJNR Am J Neuroradiol 1992;13:1273-1277.
Moses AM, Moses LK, Notman D, Springer J: Antidiuretic responses to injected desmopressin, alone and with indomethacin. J Clin Endocrinol Metab 1981;52:910-913.
Moses AM, Scheinman SJ, Oppenheim A: Marked hypotonic polyuria resulting from nephrogenic diabetes insipidus with partial sensitivity to vasopressin. J Clin Endocrinol 1984;59:1044-1049.
Rose BD, Post TW: Clinical Physiology of Acid-Base and Electrolyte Disorders, 5th ed, New York, McGraw-Hill, 2001, pp 716-719, 764-775.

Primary Hyperparathyroidism and Hypoparathyroidism

Method of
John P. Bilezikian, MD

Primary Hyperparathyroidism

INCIDENCE AND GENERAL CHARACTERISTICS

Primary hyperparathyroidism (PHPT) is a relatively common endocrine disease with an incidence as high as 1 in 500 to 1 in 1000. The high visibility of PHPT today marks a dramatic change from several generations ago when it was considered rare. The increased

TABLE 1 Differential Diagnosis of Hypercalcemia
Primary hyperparathyroidism
Malignancy
Other endocrinopathies
Hyperthyroidism
Pheochromocytoma
Adrenal insufficiency
VIPoma
Medications
Lithium
Thiazides
Thyroid hormone
Vitamin D
Vitamin A
Granulomatous diseases
Familial hypocalciuric hypercalcemia
Immobilization

incidence is undoubtedly due to widespread use of the multichannel autoanalyzer. PHPT occurs in individuals of all ages but occurs most frequently in the sixth decade of life. Women are affected more often than men by a ratio of 3:1. PHPT in children is an unusual event. It might be a component of one of several endocrinopathies with a genetic basis, such as multiple endocrine neoplasia (MEN), type I or II. PHPT is caused by excessive secretion of parathyroid hormone (PTH) from one or more parathyroid glands. A benign, solitary adenoma is found in 80% of patients. Less commonly, in 15% to 20% of subjects, all four glands are hyperplastic. Four-gland parathyroid disease may occur sporadically or in association with the MEN syndromes. The most uncommon presentation of PHPT is parathyroid cancer, occurring in less than 0.5% of patients with PHPT.

DIFFERENTIAL DIAGNOSIS

The major diagnostic distinction to be made is between PHPT and malignancy, the other most common cause of hypercalcemia. These two etiologies account for more than 90% of all patients with hypercalcemia (Table 1). A much longer, complete list of potential causes of hypercalcemia is considered after these two etiologies are ruled out or if there is reason to believe that a different cause is likely. Today, PHPT presents most often as an asymptomatic disorder. In contrast, malignancy-associated hypercalcemia is usually found at a later stage of the malignant process and is associated with symptoms. Besides a major difference in clinical presentation between these two most common causes of hypercalcemia, the PTH immunoassay is a helpful distinguishing point. In patients with PHPT, the PTH level will be elevated or in the upper range of normal, whereas in malignancy, the PTH level is invariably suppressed.

PATHOPHYSIOLOGY, MOLECULAR GENETICS, AND PATHOLOGY

The pathophysiology of PHPT relates to the loss of normal feedback control of PTH by extracellular calcium. Why the parathyroid cell loses its normal sensitivity to calcium is not known. Genetic abnormalities that could be linked to sporadic parathyroid tumors have been described. A rearrangement of the cyclin D1/(PRAD1) proto-oncogene has been seen in some patients with PHPT. The rearrangement associates the PTH gene with the growth promoter cyclin D1. Only a small number of parathyroid tumors have been demonstrated to harbor this defect. Tumor suppressors, such as the gene associated with MEN-I, have generated interest, as have potential abnormalities in the gene for the calcium-sensing receptor. Although the gene for the calcium receptor has been implicated in familial hypocalciuric hypercalcemia and neonatal severe hyperparathyroidism, there is little evidence for this genetic abnormality in the sporadic form of PHPT. Even the vitamin D receptor has been implicated in pathogenetic abnormalities associated with parathyroid neoplasia.

The typical parathyroid adenoma is an enlarged, oval-shaped, smooth, red-brown gland. A visible rim of normal yellow-brown parathyroid tissue is sometimes seen. The typical parathyroid adenoma is between 300 and 500 mg, much larger than a normal gland that generally weighs 35 to 50 mg. Microscopically, the parathyroid adenoma consists of a network of cells arranged alongside a capillary network, resembling classic endocrine microanatomy. Fat cells are reduced or absent. The form of PHPT characterized by four-gland hyperplasia is seen grossly as enlarged glands that may be of equal size. Microscopically, solid masses of chief cells are seen in the absence of fat cells. In contrast to the adenoma, in which a rim of normal tissue can sometimes be seen, normal tissue is absent in hyperplastic disease.

SIGNS AND SYMPTOMS

PHPT is associated classically with skeletal and renal complications. In severe cases, the skeleton can be involved in a process called *osteitis fibrosa cystica*. Subperiosteal resorption of the distal phalanges, tapering of the distal clavicles, a "salt and pepper" appearance of the skull, bone cysts, and brown tumors of the long bones are all overt manifestations of hyperparathyroid bone disease. This form of hyperparathyroid bone disease is now most unusual, occurring in fewer than 5% of patients with PHPT. Much less severe, but nevertheless significant, skeletal involvement in PHPT is detected by dual energy x-ray absorptiometry (see later). Similar to the reduced incidence of gross skeletal disease, the kidney is also involved in PHPT much less commonly than before. From an incidence of approximately 33% in the 1960s, most series place the incidence of nephrolithiasis now to be no more than 15% to 20%. Nephrolithiasis, nevertheless, is still the most common complication of PHPT. Other renal features of PHPT include diffuse deposition of calcium–phosphate complexes in the parenchyma (nephrocalcinosis). The frequency of this complication is unknown. Hypercalciuria (daily calcium excretion of >250 mg in women or >300 mg in men) is seen in 30% to 40% of patients. PHPT may be associated with a reduction in creatinine clearance, in the absence of any other cause. Classic associations exist between PHPT and other organs, such as the neuromuscular system, the gastrointestinal tract, and the cardiovascular and articular systems, but such panopleistic features of PHPT are rarely seen today. More vexing are nonspecific elements associated with PHPT, such as easy fatigability, a sense of weakness, and a feeling that the aging process is advancing faster than it should be. This is sometimes accompanied by an intellectual weariness and a sense that cognitive faculties are less sharp. Whether these nonspecific features of PHPT are truly part of the disease process, reversible upon successful parathyroid surgery, remains under active investigation.

CLINICAL FORMS OF PRIMARY HYPERPARATHYROIDISM

Asymptomatic PHPT with serum calcium levels within 1 mg/dL above the upper limits of normal is the most common clinical presentation. Most patients do not have specific complaints and do not show evidence of any target organ complications. In parts of the world where severe vitamin D deficiency is common, more symptomatic PHPT is seen. Unusual clinical presentations of PHPT include MEN-I and MEN-II, familial PHPT not associated with any other endocrine disorder, familial cystic parathyroid adenomatosis, jaw tumor syndrome, and neonatal PHPT. Another presentation of PHPT is being described, namely, in individuals with normal serum calcium concentrations but elevated PTH levels. Potential secondary causes of elevated PTH levels are considered but have not been found. It is considered likely that these patients represent the earliest stage of PHPT, when there is glandular overproduction of hormone, before hypercalcemia becomes evident.

DIAGNOSIS AND EVALUATION

Hypercalcemia and elevated levels of PTH establish the diagnosis. The serum phosphorus concentration tends to be in the lower range of

CURRENT DIAGNOSIS

Primary Hyperparathyroidism

- Most common cause of hypercalcemia.
- Diagnosis established by elevated serum calcium concentration and parathyroid hormone level that is frankly elevated or is in the upper range of normal.
- In some patients, the parathyroid hormone level is elevated but the serum calcium concentration is normal.

Hypoparathyroidism

- Much less common than primary hyperparathyroidism.
- Most often due to destruction or removal of the parathyroid glands.
- Diagnosis is established by hypocalcemia and low parathyroid hormone levels.

---

normal. Serum alkaline phosphatase activity may be elevated. More specific markers of bone formation (bone-specific alkaline phosphatase, osteocalcin) and bone resorption (urinary deoxypyridinoline, N or C-telopeptide of collagen) tend to be in the upper range of normal. In some patients, the actions of PTH in altering renal acid-base handling leads to a small increase in the serum chloride concentration and a concomitant small decrease in the serum bicarbonate concentration. Urinary calcium excretion, when elevated, is not generally excessively high. The circulating 25-hydroxyvitamin D concentration is low, and the 1,25-dihydroxyvitamin D concentration is high in some patients.

ROLE OF BONE MASS MEASUREMENT

Dual-energy x-ray absorptiometry shows a pattern of skeletal involvement that is consistent with the physiologic actions of PTH, that of eroding cortical bone while sparing cancellous sites. The typical patient with PHPT shows reductions in bone density that are most marked in the distal third of the forearm, a cortical site, with much less involvement of the lumbar spine, a cancellous site. The hip region, a mixture of cortical and cancellous bone, shows changes

CURRENT THERAPY

Primary Hyperparathyroidism

- When symptoms are present, parathyroid surgery is indicated.
- In the absence of symptoms, surgery is recommended if any one of five criteria are met (see Table 2).
- Preoperative localization testing prior to surgery has become routine.
- Medical management is reserved generally for those who do not meet surgical criteria.
- Prudent use of calcium, hydration, and ambulation is encouraged.
- Pharmacologic agents, such as bisphosphonates and calcimimetics, show promise.

Hypoparathyroidism

- Acute management of hypocalcemia is a medical emergency and requires intravenous administration of calcium.
- Chronic treatment is based upon adequate calcium, vitamin D, and, in some cases, the active vitamin D metabolite 1,25-dihydroxyvitamin D.

---

that are intermediate between changes in the forearm and the lumbar spine.

TREATMENT

Localization Tests Prior to Surgery

Imaging of abnormal parathyroid tissue is accomplished most accurately with technetium-99m sestamibi. Sestamibi is taken up by both thyroid and parathyroid tissue, but it persists in the parathyroid glands. Various approaches to the use of technetium-99m sestamibi include using the imaging agent alone, and thereby depending upon a difference in uptake kinetics between thyroid and parathyroid tissue, or in combination with iodine 123 (^{123}I). Some believe that use of dual isotopic methods provides better definition of the thyroid from which the image obtained with sestamibi can be subtracted. Even more sophisticated approaches have been developed using sestamibi imaging with single-photon emission computed tomography. Ultrasound, computed tomography, and magnetic resonance imaging are also used to localize abnormal parathyroid tissue. Invasive localization tests with arteriography and selective venous sampling for PTH are used when noninvasive studies have not been successful. In the past, parathyroid imaging was reserved for patients who had undergone neck surgery. With greater success in parathyroid imaging and the increasing popularity of minimally invasive parathyroid surgery, preoperative imaging is becoming routine in all patients.

SURGERY

PHPT is cured when abnormal parathyroid tissue is removed. Asymptomatic patients are advised to have surgery if they meet current guidelines (Table 2). Symptomatic patients are always advised to undergo parathyroid surgery. At the present time, a number of different surgical procedures can be performed. The standard four-gland parathyroid gland exploration is performed under general or local anesthesia. The single adenoma is removed, and the other glands are ascertained to be normal but not removed. In the case of multiglandular disease, the approach is to remove all tissue except for a remnant that is left in situ or autotransplanted in the nondominant forearm. A popular recent advance in parathyroid surgery is the minimally invasive parathyroidectomy. This procedure depends upon preoperative localization by an imaging technology and confirmation of the success of parathyroid surgery with intraoperative PTH measurements. The circulating PTH level should fall to less than 50% of the preoperative value within minutes after removal of the parathyroid adenoma. Minimally invasive parathyroid surgery, this latter approach, has become a standard for many parathyroid surgeons now.

MEDICAL MANAGEMENT

In patients who do not meet surgical guidelines or who, for other reasons, will not undergo parathyroid surgery, the following medical principles apply. Adequate hydration and ambulation are always encouraged. Thiazide diuretics are to be avoided because they may lead to worsening hypercalcemia. Dietary intake of calcium should be

---

TABLE 2 Guidelines for Surgical Management of Asymptomatic Primary Hyperparathyroidism*

Serum calcium >1 mg/dL above normal
Hypercalciuria >400 mg/day
Reduced creatinine clearance by >30%
Reduced bone density below T score of −2.5 at any site
Age <50

*These guidelines are meant only for asymptomatic patients with primary hyperparathyroidism. For patients who are symptomatic (i.e., kidney stones, fractures), surgery is recommended unless there are extenuating medical circumstances.

moderate, avoiding both high- and low-calcium diets. Low-calcium diets theoretically could fuel abnormal parathyroid tissue to secrete more PTH. High-calcium diets could be detrimental by worsening hypercalcemia, especially if the 1,25-dihydroxy vitamin D level is elevated. Monitoring with biannual measurements of the serum calcium and annual measurement of bone mass by dual-energy x-ray absorptiometry are recommended. In patients whose 25-hydroxyvitamin D level is low, careful replacement seems reasonable. The serum calcium concentration must be monitored to guard against the potential for worsening hypercalcemia in some patients.

Oral phosphate will lower the serum calcium concentration in PHPT by approximately 0.5 to 1 mg/dL, but concerns about ectopic calcium–phosphate deposition limit its utility. Prior to the results of the Women's Health Initiative, estrogen was an option in postmenopausal women. The serum calcium concentration would fall by about 0.5 mg/dL; estrogens are no longer advised for this specific reason. Preliminary observations suggest that raloxifene, a selective estrogen receptor modulator, may have calcium-lowering effects similar to those of estrogen in postmenopausal women with PHPT.

The bisphosphonate alendronate (Fosamax) has shown promise in patients with PHPT. Lumbar spine bone density improves by as much as 5% in the first year of therapy. Neither the serum calcium concentration nor the PTH level falls significantly. Patients who will not undergo parathyroid surgery but in whom lumbar spine bone density is reduced may benefit from bisphosphonate therapy.

An early clinical experience with hyperparathyroid postmenopausal women has shown that, in principle, a calcimimetic can significantly reduce PTH and serum calcium levels in patients with the disease. By binding to a site on the calcium-sensing receptor, the calcimimetic increases the affinity of the calcium receptor for extracellular calcium. The result is an increase in intracellular calcium and thus reductions in PTH synthesis and secretion. Even though the drug has not yet been approved for use for PHPT in the United States, early data are promising. The serum calcium concentration typically becomes normal and remains within normal limits for as long as the drug is used. Interestingly, the serum PTH level falls only modestly and continues to be elevated despite correction of the hypercalcemia by the drug.

Hypoparathyroidism

Hypoparathyroidism is much more uncommon than is PHPT. It results from the destruction, removal, or dysfunction of all parathyroid tissue.

ETIOLOGY

The most common causes of hypoparathyroidism are neck surgery and an autoimmune process (Table 3). Surgical hypoparathyroidism can follow the operation by many years and can occur after any neck surgery. Autoimmune destruction of the parathyroid glands can occur in an isolated fashion or in connection with a variety of polyglandular syndromes. The two major forms are type I (multiple endocrine gland failure along with candidiasis, pernicious anemia, and/or alopecia) and type II (with adrenal or thyroid failure and/or diabetes mellitus). Activating mutations of the calcium-sensing receptor or of the parathyroid gene itself can be associated with hypoparathyroidism. Parathyroid gland destruction is rarely due to infiltration of the glands by iron, copper, granulomas, or malignancy. In severe magnesium deficiency, parathyroid secretion is impaired along with a peripheral resistance to the actions of PTH. Mild hypoparathyroidism can become symptomatic in the presence of a potent bisphosphonate such as alendronate.

CLINICAL FEATURES

Increased neuromuscular irritability is the clinical hallmark of hypoparathyroidism. Features of hypoparathyroidism can range from mild paresthesias around the mouth, fingers, and toes to muscle cramping, and, at their worst, carpal, pedal, or laryngospasm.

TABLE 3 Causes of Hypoparathyroidism

Parathyroid gland destruction
Postsurgical
Autoimmune
Sporadic
Polyglandular syndromes
Activating antibodies against the calcium-sensing receptor
Infiltration
Iron, copper
Malignancy
Granulomatous
Genetic
Activating mutations of the calcium-sensing receptor
Inactivating mutations in the PTH gene
DiGeorge syndrome
Impaired secretion and/or action of PTH
Hypomagnesemia
Pseudohypoparathyroidism

Abbreviation: PTH = parathyroid hormone.

Central nervous system seizure activity is also seen as a severe manifestation of hypocalcemia. These symptoms are due, in part, to the actual serum calcium level but also to the rate at which the serum calcium level falls. Rapid declines in the serum calcium concentrations are more likely to be associated with symptoms than to situations in which the serum calcium concentration has fallen gradually. If respiratory or metabolic alkalosis is present, symptoms can worsen because the partition between bound and free calcium is shifted to the bound state when the blood pH rises. Signs of hypocalcemia include the Chvostek sign (evoked facial nerve irritability), the Trousseau sign (carpal spasm when the blood pressure cuff is inflated to pressures above systolic), and a prolonged QT interval on the electrocardiogram. When severe hypocalcemia is present, impaired cardiac contractility, unresponsive to inotropic agents until the hypocalcemia is corrected, has been reported. Pseudopapilledema and subcapsular cataracts can be seen. In some individuals, hypoparathyroidism is detected only by an asymptomatic reduction in the serum calcium concentration. Pseudohypoparathyroidism is a group of genetic disorders of the PTH receptor/G-protein transduction system responsible for PTH action. In the type I variant, subjects have a classic phenotype (Albright's hereditary osteodystrophy) with short stature, brachydactyly, subcutaneous and basal ganglia calcifications, rounded facies, shortened neck, seizures, and below-average intelligence. Other endocrine glands, such as the thyroid and gonads, can also be dysfunctional. In the type II form of pseudohypoparathyroidism, PHT resistance is present in the absence of the clinical phenotype.

DIAGNOSIS

Hypocalcemia and an elevated serum phosphorus concentration in association with absent PTH levels confirm the diagnosis of hypoparathyroidism. In pseudohypoparathyroidism, PTH levels are elevated, reflecting the PTH-resistant state, but otherwise the biochemical findings of hypocalcemia and hyperphosphatemia are similar to those of hypoparathyroidism. The urinary calcium concentration is usually not elevated because the filtered load of calcium is low, but actually renal handling of calcium is impaired in this setting because of the lack of PTH. Such individuals have an increase in urinary calcium for the given filtered calcium load, even though the actual amount of urinary calcium excretion might not be excessive.

TREATMENT

The goals of treatment are to establish a serum calcium concentration that is not associated with symptoms or signs and to prevent long-term complications of hypocalcemia. Acute, symptomatic hypocalcemia is a medical emergency and must be treated urgently. The management of chronic hypocalcemia follows a different set of guidelines.

Acute Management

The initial approach is to infuse intravenously 1 to 2 ampules of calcium gluconate (90-180 mg of elemental calcium), diluted in 50 to 100 mL of 5% dextrose over a 10- to 15-minute period. If the acute symptoms are not quickly ameliorated, another 1 to 2 ampules can be administered. To raise the serum calcium concentration further, but more gradually, an infusion of 15 mg/kg of calcium gluconate in 1 L of 5% dextrose over 8 to 10 hours will raise the serum calcium concentration by 2 to 3 mg/dL. Because 1 ampule of calcium gluconate contains 90 mg of elemental calcium, 9 to 11 ampules of calcium gluconate are required for an average-size adult (60-70 kg). The serum calcium concentration should be monitored frequently. If the hypocalcemia is due to magnesium deficiency, these measures are also appropriate while magnesium is being replaced. Acute administration of magnesium without calcium will not immediately correct hypocalcemia because peripheral resistance to PTH, one component of hypocalcemia induced by magnesium deficiency, is not corrected for several days. Intravenous replacement of magnesium is 2.4 mg/kg, up to 180 mg, over a 10-minute period or a continuous infusion of 576 mg of magnesium over 24 hours.

Chronic Management

Oral calcium supplementation is required in virtually all patients. The amount varies but is generally in the range of 1 to 3 g in divided doses. The carbonate or citrated form of calcium is most commonly used. Calcium carbonate is generally preferred because it contains the highest amount of elemental calcium. When calcium preparations are given with meals, both the carbonate and the citrated form of calcium are equally bioavailable. The presence of food obviates the need for gastric acid when calcium carbonate is used.

Most patients also require vitamin D. The amount of ergocalciferol (vitamin D_2) or cholecalciferol (vitamin D_3) ranges from 25,000 to 200,000 IU daily (1.25-10 mg). These large amounts are required because the absence of PTH and hyperphosphatemia both limit the amount of vitamin D that ultimately is converted to 1,25-dihydroxyvitamin D, the active metabolite in the kidney. Because activation of vitamin D is impaired, much more vitamin D is required. There is no impairment of the first activation step in the liver, namely, from vitamin D to 25-hydroxyvitamin D, the storage form. Because there is no impairment in this step, large amounts of 25-hydroxyvitamin D can accumulate in fat tissues. At times and unpredictably, these stores can be mobilized and lead to hypercalcemia. Sometimes, the hypercalcemia is severe, requiring emergent treatment. Other times, a simple adjustment in the amount of calcium and/or vitamin D is sufficient. In any event, patients receiving large doses of vitamin D should always be regularly monitored for serum calcium concentrations approximately every 3 to 6 months.

Although many patients with hypoparathyroidism can be adequately managed with oral calcium and vitamin D, other patients also require therapy with 1,25-dihydroxyvitamin D, the active metabolite of vitamin D. 1,25-Dihydroxyvitamin D is used in addition to, but not in place of, vitamin D because 1,25-dihydroxyvitamin D alone does not provide for smooth control. Perhaps this is because 1,25-dihydroxyvitamin D is not stored to any appreciable extent in fat tissue. The half-life of 1,25-dihydroxyvitamin D is as short as 6 hours. Therefore, patients managed without parent vitamin D but with 1,25-dihydroxyvitamin D as the only source of vitamin D are more likely to have unpredictable fluctuations in serum calcium concen-tra-tion. The amount of 1,25-dihydroxyvitamin D ranges from 0.5 to 1.0 μg/day. Some patients require more. Enhanced gastrointestinal absorption of calcium with 1,25-dihydroxyvitamin D can lead to hypercalciuria because in hypoparathyroidism there is no PTH to facilitate calcium reabsorption in the renal tubule. Urinary calcium should be checked on a regular basis. If hypercalciuria occurs, the dose of 1,25-dihydroxyvitamin D and/or vitamin D should be adjusted downward.

In this situation, a thiazide diuretic such as hydrochlorthiazide[1] can be used to reduce urinary calcium excretion. In pseudohypoparathyroidism, hypercalciuria is less likely to occur because PTH is present and does have some renal effects in reabsorbing filtered calcium.

Another reason for variability in the control of serum calcium concentration in hypoparathyroidism is a change in medications. For example, if a thiazide or loop diuretic is started for hypertension, the serum calcium concentration may increase or decrease, respectively. Glucocorticoids can lead to a reduction in the serum calcium concentration because glucocorticoids interfere with vitamin D action in the gastrointestinal tract. Bile-sequestering resins can interfere with vitamin D absorption. Midcycle changes in estrogen levels in premenopausal women can lead to altered control.

Hypoparathyroidism is one of the few endocrine disorders for which the replacement hormone, namely, PTH, is not yet available, but it is being studied in some clinical trials.

---

[1] Not FDA approved for this indication.

REFERENCES

Arnold A, Shattuck TM, Mallya SM, et al: Molecular pathogenesis of primary hyperparathyroidism. J Bone Miner Res 2002;17(Suppl. 2):N30-N36.
Bilezikian JP, Silverberg SJ: Management of asymptomatic primary hyperparathyroidism. N Engl J Med 2004;350:1746-1751.
Bilezikian JP, Silverberg SJ: Primary hyperparathyroidism. In Favus M (ed): Primer on the Metabolic Bone Diseases and Disorders of Calcium Metabolism, 5th ed. Washington DC, American Society for Bone and Mineral Research, 2003, pp 230-235.
Bilezikian JP, Brandi ML, Rubin M, Silverberg SJ: Primary hyperparathyroidism: new concepts in clinical, densitometric, and biochemical features. J Int Med 2005;257:6-17.
Bilezikian JP, Potts JT, El-Hajj Fuleihan G, et al: Summary statement from a workshop on asymptomatic primary hyperparathyroidism: A perspective for the 21st century. J Bone Miner Res 2003;17(Suppl. 2):N2-N11.
Khan AA, Bilezikian JP, Kung AWC, et al: Alendronate in primary hyperparathyroidism: a double-blind, randomized, placebo-controlled trial. J Clin Endocrinol Metab 2004;89:3319-3325.
Marx SJ: Hyperparathyroid and hypoparathyroid disorders. N Engl J Med 2000;343:1863-1875.
Miller PD, Bilezikian JP: Bone densitometry in asymptomatic primary hyperparathyroidism. J Bone Miner Res 2002;17(Suppl. 2):N98-N102.
Peacock M, Bilezikian JP, Klassen PS, et al: Cinacalcet hydrochloride maintains long-term normocalcemia in patients with primary hyperparathyroidism. J Clin Endocrinol Metab 2005;90:135-141.
Silverberg SJ, Bilezikian JP: Clinical presentation of primary hyperparathyroidism in the United States. In Bilezikian JP, Marcus R, Levine MA, eds: The Parathyroids, 2nd ed. San Diego, CA, Academic Press, 2001, pp 349-360.
Silverberg SJ, Bilezikian JP: "Incipient" primary hyperparathyroidism: A "forme fruste" of an old disease. J Clin Endocrinol Metab 2003; 88:5348-5352.
Stock JL, Marcus R: Medical management of primary hyperparathyroidism. In Bilezikian JP, Marcus R, Levine MA (eds): The Parathyroids, 2nd ed. San Diego, CA, Academic Press, 2001, pp 459-474.

Primary Aldosteronism

Method of
Nathaniel Winer, MD

The combination of hypertension, hypokalemia, inappropriate kaliuresis (urinary potassium excretion of 40 mEq/day), nonsuppressible aldosterone secretion, and suppressed plasma renin activity was first described by Jerome Conn more than 50 years ago.

Excessive aldosterone secretion leads to increased renal tubular sodium reabsorption, extracellular fluid volume expansion, and hypertension. Urinary potassium loss results in hypokalemia. Peripheral edema is usually not observed because countervailing mechanisms, including atrial natriuretic peptide release, prevent further volume expansion.

Subtypes

The most common causes of primary aldosteronism are bilateral adrenal hyperplasia (idiopathic hyperaldosteronism [IHA]) and unilateral aldosterone-producing adenoma (APA) (Box 1). Primary adrenal hyperplasia (PAH), characterized by predominantly unilateral micro- or macronodular hyperplasia of the adrenal glomerulosa, and adrenal cortical carcinoma are relatively rare causes of primary aldosteronism.

Glucocorticoid-remediable aldosteronism (GRA, dexamethasone-suppressible hyperaldosteronism, or familial hyperaldosteronism, type I), is a rare, dominantly inherited form of primary aldosteronism, often diagnosed in early childhood or adolescence, and associated with an increased incidence of cerebral aneurysms. The disorder results from a chimeric gene whose product (located ectopically in the adrenal fasciculata) has actions of both aldosterone synthase and 11β-hydroxylase. In GRA aldosterone secretion is regulated by adrenocorticotropic hormone (ACTH), rather than by angiotensin II. Consequently, aldosterone parallels the diurnal variation of ACTH rather than changes in sodium balance, resulting in chronic mineralocorticoid excess and hypertension. Genetic testing of peripheral blood leukocyte DNA is a highly sensitive and specific method of diagnosing GRA.

Familial hyperaldosteronism (FH II), due to either IHA or APA, is reported to be more common than GRA, but its genetic basis remains to be determined.

The prevalence of primary aldosteronism increases with the degree of hypertension and with resistant hypertension (blood pressure inadequately controlled on 3 or more antihypertensive agents). Patients with primary aldosteronism are at greater risk for cardiovascular events compared with those with comparable blood pressure levels. Primary aldosteronism is also associated with greater arterial wall thickness, central artery stiffness, and albumin excretion than in age-matched controls. Blocking the actions of aldosterone with spironolactone improves survival in older persons with congestive heart failure.

Diagnosis

SCREENING

In 1981, the ratio of plasma aldosterone concentration (PAC) to plasma renin activity (PRA) was introduced as a screening test for primary aldosteronism. Since then, the prevalence rate of primary aldosteronism has increased from less than 0.5% to the current 4.6% to 13%. Newly diagnosed cases have increased more than 10-fold. The fraction of IHA cases has risen from 40% to 60%, APA cases have declined from more than 70% to 35%, and the incidence of hypokalemia has decreased from 80% to 20%.

BOX 1   Subtypes of Primary Aldosteronism

Bilateral adrenal hyperplasia (IHA) (60%)
Aldosterone-producing adenoma (APA) (35%)
Unilateral adrenal hyperplasia (2%)
Aldosterone-producing adrenocortical carcinoma (<1%)
Glucocorticoid-remediable aldosteronism (GRA) (<1%)
Ectopic aldosterone-producing adenoma or carcinoma (<1%)
Famillial hyperaldosteronism (FH type II) (rare)

 CURRENT DIAGNOSIS

- Primary aldosteronism is the most common form of secondary hypertension, affecting 4.6% to 13% of persons with hypertension.
- The criterion for a positive screening test for primary aldosteronism is an ambulatory morning plasma aldosterone concentration–to–plasma renin activity (PAC/PRA) ratio >20 and a PAC >15 μg/dL.
- Confirmation of primary aldosteronism requires urinary excretion of aldosterone >12 μg/day after oral salt-loading or PAC >10 μg/dL after intravenous infusion of 2 L of normal saline over 4 hours.
- The distinction between the most common subtypes of primary aldosteronism, aldosterone-producing adenoma, and idiopathic hyperaldosteronism, is best made by adrenal vein sampling for aldosterone and cortisol.

The morning PAC/PRA ratio has more than 90% sensitivity and specificity. PAC/PRA is unaffected by posture and antihypertensive drugs, except for amiloride (Midamor) and the mineralocorticoid receptor antagonists, spironolactone and eplerenone, which must be discontinued for at least 6 weeks before testing. Angiotensin-converting enzyme inhibitors, angiotensin receptor blockers, and diuretics may be continued; because these agents stimulate renin secretion, suppressed PRA makes underlying primary aldosteronism more likely. Inappropriate elevation of PAC in the face of suppression of renin secretion by adrenergic blockade with β-blockers or central α_2-agonists is consistent with primary aldosteronism. In hypokalemic patients, raising serum potassium levels into the mid-normal range with potassium supplementation increases PAC and optimizes PAC/PRA. Box 2 lists clinical settings in which screening should be performed in patients with hypertension.

CONFIRMING THE DIAGNOSIS

Techniques to confirm the diagnosis of primary aldosteronism evaluate the effect of volume expansion on the suppressibility of PAC or urinary aldosterone.

Oral Salt Loading

Patients whose hypertension and hypokalemia have been controlled ingest a high-sodium diet for 3 days and take supplementary sodium chloride tablets if necessary to achieve a sodium excretion greater than 200 mmol/day. Because high dietary sodium intake can increase potassium excretion, serum potassium must be monitored and replaced as needed. On day 3, aldosterone >12 μg and sodium

---

BOX 2   Indications to Screen for Primary Aldosteronism

Hypertension and hypokalemia, spontaneous or diuretic induced
Resistant hypertension
Blood pressure: systolic ≥160 mm Hg or diastolic ≥100 mm Hg
Juvenile hypertension
Family history of early-onset hypertension or hemorrhagic strokes
Adrenal incidentaloma

>200 mmol in a 24-hour urine collection indicates autonomous adrenal function.

Intravenous Saline Infusion

Unlike normotensive patients, patients with primary aldosteronism fail to show suppression of PAC with saline infusion. After overnight fasting, 2 L of normal saline are infused over a 4-hour period. Preexisting left ventricular dysfunction or renal dysfunction can increase the risk for acute volume overload. Postinfusion PAC in normotensive subjects is less than 5 µg/dL, whereas patients with primary aldosteronism do not suppress below 10 ng/dL. Patients with IHA might have PAC between 5 and 10 ng/dL.

Fludrocortisone Suppression

Fludrocortisone (Florinef) acetate 0.1 mg every 6 hours for 4 days is given with sodium chloride 2 g 3 times daily with meals, while monitoring blood pressure and serum potassium daily. Confirmation of primary aldosteronism requires morning upright PAC to be 6 ng/dL on day 4. The association of QT dispersion and left ventricular dysfunction with fludrocortisone testing has discouraged its use.

DETERMINING THE SUBTYPE

Subtype diagnosis is important because unilateral adrenalectomy corrects hypokalemia and improves or normalizes blood pressure in up to 60% of patients with APA or PAH, whereas surgery in IHA or GRA is usually ineffective.

Adrenal Computed Tomography

In a patient younger than 40 years who has primary aldosteronism and a 1- to 2-cm unilateral, hypodense, single adenoma, unilateral adrenalectomy should be considered, because nonfunctioning incidental adrenal masses are less common in younger patients. However, because adrenal computed tomography (CT) often fails to reveal adenomas smaller than 1 cm, or might show small bilateral macro- or microadenomas, minimal thickening of adrenal limbs, or nonfunctioning adrenal masses in older persons, further testing may be indicated. Patients with high-probability APA are likely to be younger, more hypertensive, and more often hypokalemic, and they have higher aldosterone levels than those with IHA.

Adrenal Vein Sampling

Because adrenal CT is unreliable in differentiating APA from IHA, adrenal vein sampling is necessary in patients who have high-probability APA and seek potential surgical cure of hypertension. Aldosterone and cortisol are measured in blood samples obtained from the adrenal veins and inferior vena cava (IVC). Cosyntropin (Cortrosyn) infusion stabilizes cortisol secretion, maximizes the adrenal vein-to-IVC cortisol gradient, and stimulates aldosterone secretion from an adenoma. A post-cosyntropin adrenal vein-to-IVC cortisol ratio of 10:1 confirms appropriate catheter positioning.

Because cortisol secretion is similar from each adrenal gland, the aldosterone-to-cortisol (A/C) ratio is used as a marker of the dilution of the aldosterone concentration by venous blood. Adrenal vein A/C ratios of 4:1 (affected vs contralateral adrenal) are consistent with unilateral aldosterone excess (APA or PAH), whereas ratios of 3:1 indicate bilateral aldosterone hypersecretion.

Because the right adrenal vein is short and angles superiorly, angiographers inexperienced in adrenal vein catheterization may be unsuccessful in cannulating the right adrenal vein. However, in the absence of a right adrenal vein sample, if the left adrenal vein A/C ratio is significantly lower than that of the IVC, a right adrenal source of the aldosterone excess is likely (Fig. 1). Pharmacologic treatment should be considered in clinical settings in which adrenal vein sampling is not available or experience in performing the procedure is lacking.

[131]I-19-iodocholesterol adrenal scintigraphy, posture stimulation testing, and measurement of plasma 18-hydroxycorticosterone levels have largely been abandoned because of lack of sensitivity.

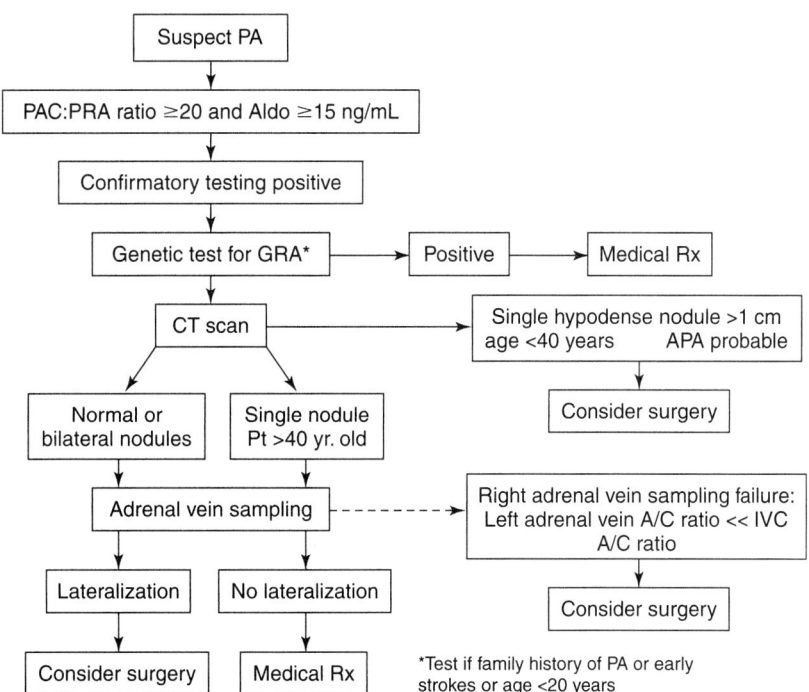

FIGURE 1. Diagnostic algorithm for primary aldosteronism. Note that with adrenal vein catheterization, even in the absence of a blood sample from the right adrenal vein, a right adrenal source of excessive aldosterone would seem likely if the A/C ratio is markedly lower in the left adrenal vein than in the IVC. A/C = aldosterone-to-cortisol ratio; Aldo = aldosterone; APA = aldosterone-producing adenoma; CT = computed tomography; GRA = glucocorticoid-remediable aldosteronism; IVC = inferior vena cava; PA = primary aldosteronism; PAC:PRA = ratio of plasma aldosterone concentration to plasma renin activity; Pt = patient; Rx = prescription.

CURRENT THERAPY

- Unilateral laparoscopic adrenalectomy is the procedure of choice for patients with aldosterone-producing adenoma (APA) who seek potential cure of hypertension.
- Patients with idiopathic hyperaldosteronism and those with APA who are not candidates for surgery should be treated with either spironolactone (Aldactone) or eplerenone (Inspra).[1] The latter agent is less likely to cause gynecomastia, erectile dysfunction, and loss of libido in men and menstrual abnormalities in women.

[1]Not FDA approved for this indication.

Treatment

The goal of treatment is not only to normalize elevated blood pressure and hypokalemia but also to protect against the adverse cardiovascular effects of aldosterone excess.

SURGERY

For APA and PAH, unilateral laparoscopic adrenalectomy is preferred over laparotomy because of lower morbidity and shorter hospitalization stays. Preoperative correction of hypokalemia with potassium supplements or mineralocorticoid receptor antagonists, or both, decreases surgical risk; however, these agents should be withdrawn postoperatively to prevent hyperkalemia. PAC should be determined 1 to 2 days after surgery to confirm biochemical cure. Short-term fludrocortisone and a liberal sodium intake may be required in the 5% of patients who develop hyperkalemia after surgery.

PHARMACOLOGIC TREATMENT

Patients with IHA and GRA and those with APA who are not treated surgically should receive mineralocorticoid receptor antagonists. Traditionally, spironolactone is started at 12.5 to 25 mg/day and titrated to 400 mg/day, if necessary, to raise serum potassium into the high-normal range without oral potassium supplementation. Normalization of elevated blood pressure can take 1 to 2 months, after which spironolactone may be tapered.

Spironolactone, by blocking testosterone receptors and stimulating progesterone receptors, can cause gynecomastia, erectile dysfunction, and decreased libido in men and menstrual abnormalities in women. Eplerenone[1] is a selective mineralocorticoid receptor antagonist that has relatively weak binding affinity for testosterone and progesterone receptors. Because eplerenone has a shorter half-life than spironolactone and may be 25% to 50% less potent on a weight basis, its starting dose is 25 mg twice daily. Patients with IHA often require addition of a thiazide diuretic, because hypervolemia can cause resistance to antihypertensive drug therapy.

Treatment of patients with GRA requires treatment with physiologic doses of a shorter-acting glucocorticoid, such as prednisone or hydrocortisone. A mineralocorticoid receptor antagonist may be equally effective and can obviate the potential adverse effects of steroid therapy, especially in children.

[1]Not FDA approved for this indication.

REFERENCES

Calhoun DA, Nishizaka MK, Zaman MA, et al: Hyperaldosteronism among black and white subjects with resistant hypertension. Hypertension 2002;40:892-896.
Hiramatsu K, Yamada T, Yukimura Y, et al: A screening test to identify aldosterone-producing adenoma by measuring plasma renin activity. Results in hypertensive patients. Arch Intern Med 1981;141:1589-1593.
Litchfield WR, Anderson BF, Weiss, et al: Intracranial aneurysm and hemorrhagic stroke in glucocorticoid-remediable aldosteronism. Hypertension 1998;31:445-450.
Mulatero P, Stowasser M, Loh KC, et al: Increased diagnosis of primary aldosteronism, including surgically correctable forms, in centers from five continents. J Clin Endocrinol Metab 2004;89:1045-1050.
Sawka AM, Young WF, Thompson GB, et al: Primary aldosteronism: Factors associated with normalization of blood pressure after surgery. Ann Intern Med 2001;135:258-261.
Winer N: Mineralocorticoid hypertension. In Re RN, DiPette DJ, Schriffrin EL, Sowers JR (eds): Molecular Mechanisms in Hypertension, NewYork, Informa Healthcare, 2006; pp 123-131.
Young WF: Primary aldosteronism: Renaissance of a syndrome. Clin Endocrinol 2007;66:607-618.
Young WF Jr: Minireview: Primary aldosteronism—changing concepts in diagnosis and treatment. Endocrinology 2003;144:2208-2213.
Young WF, Stanson AW, Thompson GB, et al: Role for adrenal venous sampling in primary aldosteronism. Surgery 2004;136:1227-1235.

Hypopituitarism

Method of
Mary Lee Vance, MD

Definition

Hypopituitarism is target endocrine gland failure because of insufficient hypothalamic or pituitary hormone stimulation of the target gland or tissue. Loss of hypothalamic or pituitary hormone production may cause secondary adrenal insufficiency, secondary hypothyroidism, secondary gonadal failure, growth hormone (GH) deficiency, and/or diabetes insipidus (DI), alone or in combination. Regardless of the etiology, replacement of glucocorticoid and thyroid hormone is necessary to sustain life; replacement of gonadal steroids, GH, and antidiuretic hormone is necessary for normal function and for prevention of morbidity. Loss of all pituitary function is termed *panhypopituitarism;* loss of one or more pituitary hormones is termed *partial hypopituitarism.*

Etiology

The most common cause of hypopituitarism is a pituitary lesion (pituitary adenoma, craniopharyngioma, Rathke's cleft cyst) or infiltrative disease (lymphocytic hypophysitis, sarcoidosis, metastatic tumor) (Table 1). In general, the larger the pituitary lesion, the greater the likelihood of loss of pituitary function. Infiltrative disease often causes permanent loss of pituitary function. Selective removal of a pituitary adenoma, taking care to avoid damage to remaining normal pituitary tissue, may result in recovery of pituitary function.

Hypopituitarism also occurs as a result of any type of pituitary radiation for a pituitary lesion, total brain radiation for a brain lesion, or head and neck radiation for carcinoma (the radiation field often involves the pituitary gland). Head trauma may cause loss of pituitary function, occurring in up to 36% of patients studied. Less commonly, developmental defects of the hypothalamus or pituitary cause loss of pituitary function.

TABLE 1 Causes of Hypopituitarism

Hypothalamic Disease
- Histocytosis
- Eosinophilic granuloma
- Sarcoidosis
- Hypothalamic tumor (gangliocytoma, hamartoma, optic nerve glioma, third-ventricle tumor)
- Metastatic tumor
- Congenital midline defects

Pituitary Disease
- Pituitary adenoma
- Craniopharyngioma
- Rathke's cleft cyst
- Pilocytic astrocytoma
- Infiltrative disease (giant cell granuloma, sarcoidosis, lympho-cytic hypophysitis, lymphoma, plasmacytoma, metastatic tumor)
- Chordoma with pituitary involvement
- Parasellar/suprasellar meningioma
- Pituitary apoplexy (hemorrhage into pituitary adenoma, post-partum hemorrhage)
- Congenital pituitary hypoplasia

Radiation
- Cranial
- Pituitary
- Head/neck

Infection
- Tuberculosis
- Mycoses

Miscellaneous
- Head trauma
- Empty sella
- Carotid-cavernous aneurysm

Diagnosis

The diagnosis of pituitary deficiency is often straightforward but sometimes requires a definitive stimulation test to assess hypothalamic-pituitary-adrenal function and GH reserve. In a patient who presents with a large pituitary lesion, the most critical determination is the need for glucocorticoid and thyroid hormone replacement before recommending surgical resection or medical treatment (macroprolactinoma). A subnormal morning serum cortisol or subnormal free thyroxine (FT$_4$) concentration indicates the need for immediate replacement. In a patient who has undergone pituitary surgery, it is important to review the operative note to assess the amount of resection and to make an estimate of remaining pituitary gland (unfortunately, this estimate is not always mentioned in the operative report).

A history of frequent nocturia, polyuria, and excessive thirst is indicative of DI. Diabetes insipidus most commonly occurs in patients with a craniopharyngioma, Rathke's cleft cyst, or infiltrative disease such as lymphocytic hypophysitis or sarcoidosis. An extensive surgical resection in a patient with one of the aforementioned lesions involving the pituitary stalk indicates a high probability of permanent DI. Extensive surgical resection may also damage the pituitary stalk and cause DI. Serum sodium concentration is usually normal in these DI patients who have normal thirst sensation. Serum osmolality usually is normal; urine osmolality usually is low. The diagnosis of DI is made clinically for a patient with a pituitary lesion and does not usually require a formal water deprivation test. A subnormal morning serum cortisol or FT$_4$ level concentration requires prompt glucocorticoid or thyroxine replacement.

A patient who has a large pituitary lesion commonly has loss of some or all anterior pituitary hormone production. This loss is less common in a patient with a small pituitary lesion but requires evaluation and replacement as indicated. In general, a stimulation test to assess for hypothalamic-pituitary-adrenal function to determine the need for cortisol replacement and for GH deficiency should be conducted after surgical removal of the lesion. Recovery of pituitary function after surgical removal of the lesion may occur but is not common; approximately 6% of patients have recovery of some pituitary function after surgery. Postoperative or postradiation assessment should include clinical history (menses in premenopausal women, sexual function in men, symptoms of hypothyroidism, adrenal insufficiency, DI) and basal and dynamic endocrine testing.

A subnormal morning serum cortisol concentration (without administration of steroid for 2-3 days) is usually adequate to diagnose secondary adrenal insufficiency; the serum ACTH concentration may be low or in the normal range. A normal morning serum cortisol concentration does not provide information regarding the ACTH-cortisol response to stress; the definitive study is an insulin hypoglycemia test in which the serum glucose concentration decreases to 40 mg/dL or less and the serum cortisol concentration increases to 18 μg/dL or greater to exclude secondary impaired hypothalamic-pituitary-adrenal reserve. This test is also the most rigorous test of GH reserve to determine the need for GH replacement (stimulated serum GH concentration <5 ng/mL indicates GH deficiency). Cortisol stimulation with ACTH (Cortrosyn stimulation test) may be misleading in patients with recent ACTH deficiency in whom the cortisol response is normal but the ACTH response to stress is impaired. For this reason, an ACTH stimulation test should not be performed in the immediate postoperative period. It is prudent to wait 4 to 6 weeks after surgery before performing this test.

A subnormal serum FT$_4$ concentration, often in the setting of a "normal" serum thyroid-stimulating hormone (TSH) concentration (not normal for a low FT$_4$), indicates the need for thyroid hormone replacement.

SECONDARY GONADAL FAILURE

The diagnosis of secondary gonadal failure is straightforward. Chronic amenorrhea in a premenopausal woman indicates gonadotropin insufficiency. In premenopausal women, serum LH and FSH concentrations are typically either low or "normal"; the estradiol level is usually low or in the follicular phase range. In men, a low serum testosterone concentration indicates gonadal insufficiency; a low serum testosterone concentration but LH and FSH concentrations within the "normal" range indicate secondary gonadal failure.

GROWTH HORMONE DEFICIENCY

The diagnosis of GH deficiency is more complicated, usually requiring a stimulation test. In a patient with three or four other pituitary hormone deficiencies, the probability of GH deficiency is 96% and 99%, respectively. Three or four pituitary hormone deficiencies and a serum IGF-1 concentration less than 84 μg/L reliably predicted GH deficiency in more than 95% of patients. Despite this finding, many third-party payers (insurance companies) require the results of a stimulation test confirming GH deficiency because of the cost and misuse of GH. The most rigorous test for determining GH deficiency is the insulin hypoglycemia test; the next "best" test is the

---

 CURRENT DIAGNOSIS

- Diagnosis is biochemical in association with clinical features. Diagnosis may require a stimulation test to determine the need for replacement of glucocorticoid, growth hormone, or both.
- Initial patient evaluation should include measurement of concentrations of early-morning serum cortisol, adrenocorticotropic hormone (ACTH), FT$_4$, gonadotropins (luteinizing hormone [LH], follicle-stimulating hormone [FSH]), insulin-like growth factor-1 (IGF-1), and testosterone (in men); menstrual history should be obtained from premenopausal women.

arginine–growth hormone-releasing hormone test. Other tests of GH reserve, such as arginine or clonidine, are less reliable.

Treatment

Treatment of hypopituitarism requires replacement of all hormone deficiencies with adjustment of hormone doses based on both hormone levels and clinical response. Optimal hormone replacement is the goal. Optimal hormone replacement often requires a great deal of time and effort; "one dose" is not suitable for all patients.

Glucocorticoid replacement exemplifies the "art of medicine": no blood test accurately assesses the adequacy or insufficiency of a glucocorticoid dose. In general, a daily dose of hydrocortisone (Cortef) 15 mg on awakening and 5 mg at 6 PM or prednisone 5 mg on awakening and 2.5 mg at 6 PM should be adequate replacement. However, patients who gain weight on this regimen may feel well with a lower dose of hydrocortisone 10 mg on awakening and 5 mg at 6 PM or only 5 mg of prednisone on awakening. Rarely, a patient receiving hydrocortisone replacement requires dosing three times daily. Glucocorticoid replacement with dexamethasone is discouraged because of the long biologic half-life and cumulative effect causing symptoms of Cushing's syndrome and bone loss. Mineralocorticoid therapy (fludrocortisone [Florinef]) is not required in a patient with secondary adrenal insufficiency because mineralocorticoid (aldosterone) secretion is not regulated chronically by pituitary ACTH secretion. Patients should be instructed to double the glucocorticoid dose during intercurrent illness (such as flu, urinary tract infection) and to always wear a medical alert necklace or bracelet.

THYROID HORMONE REPLACEMENT

Thyroid hormone replacement with L-thyroxine (Synthroid, Levoxyl) should be monitored by measuring FT_4, not TSH. Because the TSH level in patients with hypopituitarism is often low, basing hormone replacement therapy on TSH level could result in an inappropriate reduction of the thyroid hormone dose. In healthy patients with no history of coronary artery disease or angina, a beginning dose of 0.088 or 0.1 mg daily is reasonable, with dose adjustment after 1 month of therapy according to the serum free T_4 concentration and clinical response. Thyroid hormone replacement in the elderly or in patients with coronary artery disease should be initiated with a small dose (e.g., 0.025 mg/day) and gradually increased to achieve a normal serum FT_4 concentration.

GONADAL STEROID REPLACEMENT

Gonadal steroid replacement in men is most often accomplished physiologically with either a testosterone gel (AndroGel) or a testosterone patch (Androderm) that delivers a physiologic dose over 24 hours. Intramuscular testosterone, testosterone enanthate (Delatestryl), and testosterone cypionate are not physiologic and often result in supraphysiologic levels soon after injection and subphysiologic levels before the next injection. Depending on the interval after injection, intramuscular testosterone may cause mood swings, including irritability and depression. This formulation may cause erythrocytosis and elevated hemoglobin and hematocrit levels. If the patient must use the intramuscular formulation, hemoglobin and hematocrit levels should be monitored periodically. A buccal formulation of testosterone (Striant) is available and requires multiple daily doses; irritation of the gums may occur. Men should undergo a prostate examination and determination of serum prostate-specific antigen concentration yearly. Testosterone replacement does not cause prostate cancer but may promote growth of an undiagnosed carcinoma. Premenopausal women should receive cyclic estrogen and progesterone replacement for its beneficial effect on bone physiology and libido and for prevention of hot flashes. This can be accomplished with an oral contraceptive or cyclic estradiol and progesterone treatment. Annual gynecologic and breast examinations are necessary.

CURRENT THERAPY

- All hormone deficiencies require replacement. Optimal replacement often requires dose adjustments.
- Dose adjustments should be made at appropriate intervals (e.g., after 6 weeks of thyroid hormone or GH replacement).
- Dose adjustments may be necessary in pregnancy (thyroid hormone) or with addition of estrogen (growth hormone).
- Growth hormone replacement is not approved during pregnancy.

HORMONE REPLACEMENT FOR DIABETES INSIPIDUS

Hormone replacement for DI with desmopressin acetate (DDAVP) can be administered as an oral formulation or as a nasal spray. Because the duration of biologic activity varies among patients, the beginning dose should be low (0.1-mg tablet at bedtime), and dose frequency should be changed according to the duration of activity. Some patients are controlled with a single bedtime dose, whereas others require dosing two or three times daily. The patient can sense when the effect of desmopressin wears off because of frequent urination and return of increased thirst.

GROWTH HORMONE REPLACEMENT

Growth hormone (Genotropin, Humatrope, Norditropin, Nutropin) replacement is indicated in GH-deficient adults. The recommendation is to begin with a small dose (0.3 mg/day by subcutaneous injection) and then titrate the dose every 4 to 6 weeks according to the serum IGF-1 level and symptoms. An optimal serum IGF-1 level is at the middle or a little above the middle of the age-adjusted normal range. Women usually require a higher final dose than do men, and women receiving oral estrogen replacement usually require a higher final dose to achieve an optimal serum IGF-1 level than do women not receiving oral estrogen. Patients should be informed that a beneficial effect on energy, endurance, body composition, and serum lipid levels may not be noted for several months (6 months or more). Patients receiving GH replacement should be monitored every 6 months with a serum IGF-1 measurement, to determine the adequacy of the dose, and yearly serum lipid measurements.

Summary and Conclusions

Loss of pituitary function is common in patients with a hypothalamic or pituitary lesion, resulting either from the lesion or the treatment; these patients require regular monitoring and treatment as indicated. Patients who have undergone pituitary or cranial radiation therapy are always at risk for developing a new pituitary deficiency. Knowing if, or when, a new pituitary deficiency will occur is not possible, thus emphasizing the need for regular endocrine assessment. Optimal hormone replacement is similar to the best possible management of a patient with diabetes mellitus—frequent monitoring and adjustment of hormone doses based on hormone measurements and clinical response. The goal is accurate diagnosis and optimal replacement to prevent risk of premature mortality. With hormone replacement, a patient can lead a normal and productive life.

REFERENCES

Cook DM, Ludlam WH, Cook MB: Route of estrogen administration helps to determine growth hormone (GH) replacement dose in GH-deficient adults. J Clin Endocrinol Metab 1999;84:3956-3960.

Hartman ML, Crowe BJ, Biller BM, et al: Which patients do not require a GH stimulation test for the diagnosis of adult GH deficiency? J Clin Endocrinol Metab 2002;87:477-485.

Kelly KF, Gonzalo IT, Cohan P, et al: Hypopituitarism following traumatic brain injury and aneurysmal subarachnoid hemorrhage: A preliminary report. J Neurosurg 2000;93:743-752.

Lieberman SA, Oberoi AL, Gilkison CR, et al: Prevalence of neuroendocrine dysfunction in patients recovering from traumatic brain injury. J Clin Endocrinol Metab 2001;86:2752-2756.

Vance ML: Hypopituitarism. N Engl J Med 1994;330:1651-1662.

Hyperprolactinemia

Method of
Lisa B. Nachtigall, MD,
and Beverly M. K. Biller, MD

Hyperprolactinemia is the most common of all pituitary disorders. The prevalence of hyperprolactinemia is 0.4% of an unselected normal adult population. Prolactinomas are the most common cause of hyperprolactinemia, with an estimated prevalence of 500 per million people. Although high prolactin levels occur in men and women with equal frequency, prolactinomas are four times more common in women. In women, prolactinomas are usually microadenomas (tumors <1 cm). However, in men most prolactin-secreting tumors are macroadenomas (tumors >1 cm).

Normal Physiology of Prolactin Secretion

The primary known physiologic role of prolactin is to facilitate lactation in postpartum women. Prolactin is normally secreted in a pulsatile fashion by the lactotroph cells of the anterior pituitary. Sleep, food, exercise, stress and suckling are physiologic stimulators of prolactin release, and prolactin levels are normally high during pregnancy and lactation. Prolactin is unique among pituitary hormones because its regulation is primarily through tonic inhibitory control. Hypothalamic dopamine is the major negative regulator of prolactin and inhibits its release by binding to dopamine receptors on lactotrophs. Physiologic and pathologic causes of excessive prolactin secretion are summarized in Box 1.

Clinical Manifestations

Suppression of gonadotropin-releasing hormone by prolactin can cause hypogonadotropic hypogonadism, and this can lead to bone loss in both men and women. In women, hyperprolactinemia often manifests as galactorrhea, primary or secondary amenorrhea, oligmenorrhea, or infertility. Galactorrhea is less common in men with hyperprolactinemia, but gynecomastia can occur. Men might present with decrease in libido, sexual dysfunction, or infertility. Patients with large sellar tumors can present with headaches or visual field abnormalities as a result of dural stretching or optic chiasm compression. Hypopituitarism can also occur if the normal gland is compromised by a large mass.

BOX 1 Causes of Hyperprolactinemia

Physiologic
Food intake
Lactation
Nipple stimulation
Physical stress
Pregnancy
Sleep

Pituitary—Hypothalamic Disorders
Acromegaly
Infiltrative disorders of the sellar, suprasellar or hypothalamic region
Prolactinoma
Other pituitary tumors
Radiation, surgery, or trauma causing damage of the pituitary stalk or suprasellar region
Sellar or suprasellar masses such as tumors, cystic lesions, and aneurysms

Pharmacologic
Antihypertensives (α-methyldopa, verapamil [Calan])
Metoclopramide (Reglan)
Opiates
Protease inhibitors
Psychotropics (antipsychotics and antidepressants)
Recreational drugs (cocaine and marijuana)

Other Pathologies
Chest wall lesions (trauma, surgery, herpes zoster)
Liver failure
Polycystic ovary syndrome
Primary hypothyroidism
Renal insufficiency
Seizures

Diagnosis

The diagnosis of hyperprolactinemia is based on an elevated serum level of prolactin. A repeat sample should be obtained for confirmation of hyperprolactinemia before proceeding with further evaluation. If an elevated serum prolactin level is confirmed, possible nonpituitary causes must be considered as shown in Box 1. Primary hypothyroidism, pregnancy, renal and hepatic insufficiency, and other miscellaneous causes of hyperprolactinemia should be excluded in the appropriate clinical context. In addition, it is

CURRENT DIAGNOSIS

- Confirm high prolactin with repeat sample (consider diluting sample in larger tumors to rule out hook effect).
- Exclude medication, pregnancy and primary hypothyroidism, renal and liver failure (obtain liver function tests, blood urea nitrogen, creatinine, human chorionic gonadotropin and thyroid-stimulating hormone).
- Obtain head magnetic resonance image.
- For macroadenoma, evaluate for hypopituitarism (consider screening for gonadotropin hormone cosecretion with immunoglobulin F1 level).
- For compression of optic chiasm, obtain visual field examination.

TABLE 1 Properties of Dopamine Agonists

Drug*	FDA Approved	Ergot Derived	5-HT$_{2B}$ Agonist	Half-life (h)	Dose Range[†]
Bromocriptine (Parlodel)	Yes	Yes	No	12-14	1.25-15 mg/d
Cabergoline (Dostinex)	Yes	Yes	Yes	63-69	0.25-2.0 mg/wk (orally)
Quinagolide (Norprolac, Prodelion)[2]	No	No	No	17	25-150 µg/d

[2]Not available in the United States.
*In general, side effects prompting discontinuation of therapy were less common in patients receiving cabergoline than in those receiving bromocriptine. All of these drugs have the common side effects of nausea, vomiting, and constipation, fatigue, headache, and orthostatic hypotension.
[†]Rarely, patients with large prolactinomas require much higher doses.

important to review medications carefully, because there are many that cause hyperprolactinemia.

If these causes are excluded, then pituitary-protocol head magnetic resonance imaging (MRI), with gadolinium if the patient does not have renal failure, should be performed. Macroprolactinomas are usually associated with prolactin levels greater than approximately 100-200 ng/mL. If the prolactin level is less than 100 ng/mL in a patient whose MRI shows a pituitary mass greater than 1 cm, the mass is unlikely to be prolactinoma, and other etiologies should be considered.

Any mass compressing the hypothalamic or pituitary stalk can interrupt the tonic inhibition of prolactin by dopamine, causing a rise in prolactin secretion. The primary purpose of head imaging is to exclude the possibility of a large mass causing hyperprolactemia through stalk compression. It is prudent to recognize and diagnose other abnormalities such as craniopharyngiomas, meningiomas, and metastatic disease, as well as cysts, abscesses, or other lesions that can cause an elevated prolactin and masquerade as a prolactinoma (see Box 1), because these lesions do not respond to dopamine agonist therapy and require other therapeutic interventions.

In cases of a large tumor with only modest prolactin elevation, prolactin should be measured in dilution to exclude the rare possibility that extremely high prolactin levels are masked by a laboratory artifact, commonly termed *hook effect.*

Treatment

MEDICAL THERAPY

Dopamine agonists are the first-line therapy for hyperprolactinemia. In the United States, the ergot-derived dopamine agonists bromocriptine (Parlodel) and cabergoline (Dostinex) are the FDA-approved agents for treating hyperprolactinemia. These drugs reduce prolactin and decrease tumor size. In one large study of women with hyperprolactinemia, cabergoline normalized prolactin levels in 83% and bromocriptine normalized prolactin levels in 59%. Amenorrhea resolved in 93% of cabergoline-treated women and 84% of bromocriptine-treated women.

In Canada and Europe, a non–ergot-derived dopamine agonist, quinagolide (Norprolac, Prodelion),[2] is available with efficacy similar to bromocriptine. Cabergoline has been shown to be effective in some patients resistant to bromocriptine or quinagolide. The properties of these dopamine agonists are shown in Table 1. Pergolide (Permax),[1] another ergot-derived dopamine agonist, with proved efficacy in the treatment of hyperprolactinemia, had been FDA approved for the treatment of Parkinson's disease. However, pergolide was removed from the market in 2007 because of evidence of cardiac valve disease associated with high doses of this agent in patients with Parkinson's disease and is no longer available.

Studies in Parkinson's disease patients receiving high doses of cabergoline (>3 mg/day) also revealed an association with cardiac valve disease, but this association was not demonstrated in Parkinson's disease patients receiving bromocriptine in high doses in the same studies. There are six published series to date evaluating the association of valvulopathy in hyperprolactinemic patients receiving cabergoline at lower doses. One of these studies reported an increase in moderate tricuspid regurgitation and the others showed no or mild valvular regurgitation. However, conceptually, the theory that activation of serotonin-2β receptors is involved in the development of valve pathology suggests that bromocriptine and quinagolide[2] may be less likely to cause valve damage than cabergoline and pergolide (see Table 1).

In patients with psychiatric disorders, all of the dopamine agonists should be avoided completely or used in select cases with great caution, under close psychiatric supervision, because they can worsen the psychiatric disorder and can counteract the effects of dopamine antagonists used to treat psychosis.

Microadenomas

Indications for medical treatment of hyperprolactinemia are listed in the Current Therapy box. Women with microadenomas who are asymptomatic, have regular menstrual periods, and do not wish to conceive may be observed with careful MRI follow-up and clinical evaluation and do not require specific therapy unless there is progression. Acne, hirsutism, and bothersome galactorrhea are relative indications for a trial of dopamine-agonist therapy. Patients with oligo- or amenorrhea are treated to prevent bone loss associated with estrogen deficiency. Treatment of hyperprolactinemia, which restores menses in women (or is associated with normalizing testosterone in hypogonadal men) has been shown to improve bone mass. In such patients with amenorrhea, who do not desire fertility, estrogen-containing contraceptives may be used to regulate the menstrual

[2]Not available in the United States.

CURRENT THERAPY

Indications for Medical Therapy
- Macroadenoma
- Hypogonadism
- Infertility
- Acne and/or hirsutism*
- Bothersome galactorrhea*
- Possibly headaches (controversial)*

Indications for Surgery[†]
- Intolerance to dopamine agonists
- Dopamine agonists ineffective
- Apoplexy or hemorrhage within tumor
- Patients on psychiatric medications
- Predominantly cystic macroadenoma

*Relative indication.
[†]If tumor mass is a concern.

[2]Not available in the United States.
[1]Not FDA approved for this indication.

cycle and replace estrogen, although their efficacy in preventing bone loss in hyperprolactinemia has not been proved.

If fertility is desired, bromocriptine is advised because there are more safety data available regarding this agent than with cabergoline during pregnancy. Dopamine agonists are typically stopped as soon as conception is detected. Asymptomatic pregnant patients with stable microadenomas do not routinely require visual field testing, prolactin testing, or MRI during pregnancy because the risk of clinically significant tumor progression is 1% or less.

Macroadenomas

Most macroprolactinomas should be treated to prevent further tumor growth. If the optic chiasm is compressed, causing visual field loss, dopamine-agonist therapy remains the treatment of choice but requires more immediate and careful monitoring. Within the first few weeks of initiating therapy, visual fields should be obtained to assess responsiveness. Surgery is usually considered if vision does not improve or deteriorates. When large macroadenomas are treated with dopamine agonists, rarely apoplexy or CSF leak occurs as the large tumors begin to infarct or regress.

In patients with macroadenomas who seek fertility, surgical resection is sometimes considered before conception, particularly if an expert pituitary surgeon is available, because larger tumors have a greater chance of growing during pregnancy. If prolactinomas cause visual problems during pregnancy, bromocriptine may be initiated, although no dopamine agonist is approved for use in pregnancy. Asymptomatic pregnant women are monitored with visual fields and not treated medically unless visual field changes develop.

SURGERY

The indications for surgery are listed in the Current Therapy box. As might be expected, surgery is more effective in curing hyperprolactinemia in microprolactinomas than in macroprolactinomas, but the success rate is highly dependent on the pituitary expertise of the surgeon.

RADIATION

Radiation therapy is rarely needed and is generally reserved for invasive macroprolactinomas in patients who do not respond to or cannot tolerate dopamine agonists and in whom surgery is ineffective or contraindicated. Radiation might not reverse hyperprolactinemia but usually stops the tumor from growing. Approximately 50% of patients develop at least one pituitary hormone deficiency within 10 years after receiving radiation therapy.

Long-Term Management

It has been shown that after a period of adequate tumor shrinkage and normalization of prolactin levels, such that no tumor remnant remains visible on MRI, medical therapy may be safely withdrawn with careful follow-up. Therefore, an attempt to taper off medication may be appropriate in patients whose prolactin levels are normal and in whom no tumor is visible. After withdrawal of therapy, ongoing follow-up with clinical evaluation, MRI, and prolactin assessment should continue at regular intervals. When dopamine-agonist therapy is withdrawn, patients with residual tumor on MRI are at higher risk for recurrent hyperprolactinemia. Detection of recurrence is an indication to resume therapy with a dopamine agonist.

Summary

It is important to evaluate the etiology of hyperprolactinemia and treat any potential causative disorder. In patients confirmed to have a prolactinoma, consideration should be given to whether treatment is indicated. Dopamine-agonist therapy is very effective in most patients with this disorder.

REFERENCES

Biller BMK, Luciano A, Crosignani PG, et al: Guidelines for the diagnosis and treatment of hyperprolactinemia. J Reprod Med 1999;44(12):1075-1084.
Biller BMK, Molitch ME, Vance ML, et al: Treatment of prolactin-secreting macroadenomas with the once-weekly dopamine agonist cabergoline. J Clin Endocrinol Metab 1996;81:2338-2343.
Bogazzi F, Buralli S, Manetti L, et al: Treatment with low doses of cabergoline is not associated with increased prevalence of cardiac valve regurgitation in patients with hyperprolactinaemia. Int J Clin Pract 2008; Epub ahead of print.
Colao A, Di Sarno A, Cappabianca P, et al: Withdrawal of long-term cabergoline therapy for tumoral and nontumoral hyperprolactinemia. N Engl J Med 2003;349(21):2023-2033.
Colao A, Di Sarno A, Sarnacchiaro FC, et al: Prolactinomas resistant to standard dopamine agonists respond to chronic cabergoline therapy. J Clin Endocrinol Metab 1997;82:876-883.
Colao A, Galderisi M, Di Sarno A, et al: Increased prevalence of tricuspid regurgitation in patients with prolactinomas chronically treated with cabergoline. J Clin Endocrinol Metab 2008; Epub ahead of print.
Lancellotti P, Livadariu E, Markov M, et al: Cabergoline and the risk of valvular lesions in endocrine disease. Eur J Endocrinol 2008;159:1-5.
Kars M, Pereira A, Bax J, Romijn J: Cabergoline and cardiac valve disease in prolactinoma patients: Additional studies during long-term treatment are required. Eur J Endocrinol 2008;159:363-367.
Miller KK, Klibanski A: Amenorrheic bone loss. J Clin Endocrinol Metab 1999;84:1775-1783.
Molitch ME: Management of prolactinomas during pregnancy. J Reprod Med 1999;44(12):1121-1126.
Schade R, Andersohn F, Suissa S, et al: Dopamine agonists and the risk of cardiac-valve regurgitation. N Engl J Med 2007;356(1):29-38.
Schlechte J, Dolan K, Sherman B, et al: The natural history of untreated hyperprolactinemia: A prospective analysis. J Clin Endocrinol Metab 1989;68:412-418.
Vallette S, Serri K, Rivera J, et al: Long-term cabergoline therapy is not associated with valvular heart disease in patients with prolactinomas. Pituitary 2008; Epub ahead of print.
Wakil A, Rigby A, Clark A, Atkin S: Low dose cabergoline for hyperprolactinaemia is not associated with clinically significant valvular heart disease. Eur J Endocrinol 2008;159:R11-R14.
Webster J, Piscitelli G, Polli A, et al: A comparison of cabergoline and bromocriptine in the treatment of hyperprolactinemic amenorrhea. N Engl J Med 1994;331:904-909.
Zanettini R, Antonini A, Gatto G, et al: Valvular heart disease and the use of dopamine agonists for Parkinson's disease. N Engl J Med 2007;356(1):39-46.

Hypothyroidism

Method of
Mona Shimshi, MD, and Terry F. Davies, MD

Hypothyroidism

NORMAL THYROID HORMONE PHYSIOLOGY

The major active thyroid hormone is triiodothyronine (T_3), which is produced either directly by the thyroid gland or peripherally from thyroxine (T_4) by a process of deiodination. Thyroid hormone synthesis and secretion is under the pituitary control of thyroid-stimulating hormone (TSH). Serum T_4 and T_3 exert negative feedback at the anterior pituitary thyrotroph cell, thus controlling TSH release.

In the normal thyroid gland, the ratio of T_4 to T_3 is approximately 15:1, but in the peripheral circulation the amount of T_3 is very much increased. The majority of this additional T_3 is produced in a wide variety of peripheral tissues, particularly the liver and muscles, by the conversion of T_4 to T_3 by a family of deiodinase enzymes. Type 1 5'-monodeiodinase is responsible for most of the T_3 in the circulation and also converts T_4 to rT_3 (reverse T_3). The Type 2 5'-deiodinase enzyme is primarily responsible for local and intracellular production of T_3, especially within the thyrotroph, and maintains a constant level of intracellular T_3 so important, for example, to the central nervous system. A reduction in circulating T_4 causes an increase in the type 2 enzyme in order to maintain this constant level of T_3. The type 3 5'-deiodinase enzyme is the major T_3 and T_4 inactivating enzyme. It protects the tissues from local thyroid hormone excess and is the enzyme primarily responsible for catalyzing the inner ring deiodination of T_4 and T_3. These enzymes are polymorphic and their efficiency varies from person to person.

Thyroid hormones, particularly T_4, are bound to serum proteins such as thyroxine-binding globulin and, therefore one should measure the total or the active free hormone levels. Note that the half-life of T_4 is approximately 6 to 7 days, whereas the half-life of T_3 is only 1 day.

DIAGNOSIS OF THYROID FAILURE

Reference ranges for individual serum total T_4 and T_3 levels are narrow, compared with significantly wider group reference ranges for a population, making the measurement of thyroid hormone levels a relatively insensitive tool for detecting abnormalities. This also applies to measurement of the free thyroid hormones. In contrast, the response of pituitary TSH to minor changes in thyroid hormone levels in a given person is logarithmic, indicating that serum TSH assessment is a superior tool for detecting changes in thyroid hormone output. Hence, an increase in serum TSH is a highly sensitive indicator of hypothyroidism and a decrease in serum TSH is a highly sensitive indicator of hyperthyroidism.

One of the difficulties in discussing hypothyroidism is the definition of the normal TSH range. Since the advent of improved immunoassay techniques for measuring TSH levels, the concern has changed from accurately reproducing the TSH level to greater concern over the normal TSH range. In a population that contains persons at risk for developing hypothyroidism, for example by including patients with antibodies to thyroid peroxidase and a family history of hypothyroidism, the upper limit of TSH was defined as 4.5 or 5.5 µU/mL. However, when one uses a population that does not include such persons known to be at increased risk for developing thyroid disease, the upper limit of TSH is 3.0 µU/mL. The 3.0 µU/mL is now considered by some to be the upper limit of normal in young healthy individuals. TSH, like many pituitary hormones, exhibits a diurnal variation in its pattern of secretion. It is at its lowest level between 9 AM and noon and at its highest level from 8 PM until midnight. In some euthyroid persons, the differences are significantly different, and in patients with any degree of hypothyroidism the differences may become even more exaggerated. Therefore, it is helpful if TSH levels are checked at similar times, and preferably between 9 AM and noon, when they are at their lowest levels.

ETIOLOGY

Hypothyroidism is most commonly due to a primary decrease in production of thyroid hormone by the thyroid gland itself (Box 1). An obvious cause would be that the patient has had thyroid surgery or received radioiodine ablation therapy. However, iodine deficiency remains the most common cause of primary hypothyroidism worldwide, especially in the developing world.

In the United States, autoimmune thyroid disease (AITD), in the form of Hashimoto's thyroiditis, is the most common cause of hypothyroidism. Autoimmune hypothyroidism is due to T cell–mediated apoptosis of thyroid cells. Tissue damage is reflected by the development of serum thyroid peroxidase antibodies (anti-TPO) and thyroglobulin antibodies (anti-Tg), which can themselves be cytotoxic and contribute to the further destruction of the thyroid cells. This results in the subsequent elevation of serum TSH levels. The presence of thyroid autoantibodies is a useful clinical marker of susceptibility to clinical thyroid failure, which progresses at a rate of 2% to 5% per year when TSH levels are borderline. Autoimmune thyroid disease can also be associated with other autoimmune diseases, including other endocrine diseases, such as type 1 diabetes mellitus, Addison's disease, and the polyglandular autoimmune syndromes.

BOX 1 Example Causes of Hypothyroidism

Primary Hypothyroidism
Autoimmune (Hashimoto's thyroiditis)
Iodine deficiency (primarily Asia, Africa, Latin America)
Congenital causes: Organ defects, thyroid hormone resistance, TSH receptor defects

Thyroid Ablation
Radioiodine treatment
Surgery
External irradiation

Transient Hypothyroidism
Subacute thyroiditis
Postpartum thyroiditis
Sick euthyroid syndrome

Central Hypothyroidism (Hypothalamic or Pituitary)
Tumors: Pituitary adenoma, craniopharyngioma
Pituitary apoplexy
Radiation
Infiltrative diseases: Sarcoidosis, tuberculosis
Hypophysitis

Medications
Inhibition of synthesis: Antithyroid drugs (e.g., methimazole [Tapazole]) or propylthiouracil
Iodine excess
Amiodarone (Pacerone, Cordarone)
Lithium (Lithobid)
Inhibition of thyroid hormone action: Anticonvulsants in susceptible people
Precipitation of autoimmune thyroid disease: Interferons
Sunitnib chemotherapy agent
Changes in thyroid-binding globulin levels:
- Increased: Estrogens, tamoxifen (Soltamox), methadone (Dolphine), heroin
- Decreased: Androgens, glucocorticoids

Changes in T_4 absorption
Calcium, iron, aluminum hydroxide gels, sulcrafate (Carafate), resin binders, e.g., cholestyramine (Questran)
Diets high in soy

TSH = thyroid-stimulating hormone.

A number of medications are known to affect thyroid function, either by increasing or decreasing thyroid hormone clearance, presenting high iodine loads, or inducing thyroid-specific T cells and antibodies (see Box 1). Transient hypothyroidism can occur due to subacute thyroiditis or postpartum Hashimoto's disease and during the recovery phase of the sick euthyroid syndrome. Rarely, secondary hypothyroidism may be due to pituitary or hypothalamic disorders that can result in TSH or TSH-releasing hormone (TRH) deficiency.

PREVALENCE

Up to 25 million Americans have an underactive thyroid gland, which remains undiagnosed in almost one half of these people. Women are six to eight times more likely than men to develop such thyroid failure. AITD also runs in families, and the incidence of hypothyroidism increases with age. By age 60 years, as many as 20% of women and 9% of men will have developed an underactive thyroid.

SIGNS AND SYMPTOMS

Thyroid hormones are the primary regulator of the body's metabolism. The signs and symptoms of hypothyroidism are, therefore, multisystemic and are summarized in Box 2.

BOX 2 Signs and Symptoms of Hypothyroidism

Metabolic
Mild weight gain
Elevated cholesterol
Increased sensitivity to insulin
Sleepiness

Cardiovascular
Slowed heart rate
Decreased cardiac output

Muscular (Skeletal)
Muscle weakness
Decreased energy
Increased fatigability

Skin
Dry, scaly skin
Loss of hair

Psychiatric
Impaired concentration
Depression
Fatigue
Lethargy

Gynecologic
Irregular menses
Infertility
Menorrhagia

Gastrointestinal
Constipation
Iron-deficiency anemia
Macrocytic anemia

Ears, Nose, and Throat
Hoarseness of voice
Deepening of voice

Severe Hypothyroidism
Accumulation of hyaluronic acid and water resulting in nonpitting edema
Pericardial and pleural exudative effusions
Periorbital edema

TREATMENT

T$_4$ Therapy

The treatment that most closely mimics normal thyroid physiology is replacement using levothyroxine (T$_4$) (Synthroid, Levoxyl). The absorbed T$_4$ is then converted by the deiodinase enzymes to the active hormone T$_3$. A normal TSH level is the target of this replacement. As discussed earlier, the definition of a normal TSH level varies. For replacement patients we use 0.5 to 3.0 μU/mL, and we generally teach patients that their TSH level should be 1.0.

The average T$_4$ full-replacement dose for adults is 1.6 μg/kg/day. However, the degree of remaining thyroid reserve greatly influences the required amount of T$_4$ and can change considerably with time. Patients who are otherwise healthy and without concurrent illnesses or risk factors for coronary artery disease (CAD) can be started near the full calculated replacement dose. Patients who are elderly or who have CAD or other comorbid risk factors should not be started at dosages greater than 12.5 to 25 μg/day. Therapy is then guided by evaluation of the TSH level at 4- to 6-week intervals.

Replacement in patients who are older than 65 years should be calculated using a more cautious algorithm irrespective of their medical history. Checking T$_4$ levels sooner than 4 weeks can be helpful in confirming that the patient is taking and absorbing the T$_4$ replacement medication but will not be helpful in assessing the final dose needed for adequate replacement, because it takes 4 weeks for TSH to normalize on a new thyroid dose.

Patients who are pregnant might need an increase in preconception T$_4$ intake as high as 50%, and women who initiate estrogen as an oral contraceptive or in the postmenopausal period, while taking T$_4$, might also require an increase in dose.

T$_4$ supplements should be taken on an empty stomach 1 hour before or 2 hours after a meal, and 1 hour before or 3 to 4 hours after taking other medications. Many medications and nutrients affect absorption of T$_4$ (see Box 1). Note, therefore, that intravenous replacement of T$_4$ in patients who cannot take oral medications should contain only 70% to 80% of the calculated oral dose.

Alternatives to T$_4$ Therapy

The majority of clinical studies have failed to show a physiologic or clinical benefit to using T$_3$ (Cytomel) alone or in adding T$_3$ to T$_4$ supplementation in hypothyroid patients. Thyroid hormone preparations that contain T$_3$ or the addition of T$_3$ supplements to T$_4$ therapy are, therefore, currently not recommended. T$_3$ has a short half-life and causes early peaks and then plummets in the same day, requiring twice- or thrice-daily dosing. T$_4$ supplementation and its subsequent conversion to T$_3$ provides physiologically stable levels of both T$_4$ and T$_3$.

Thyroid hormone should also not be replaced with dessicated thyroid preparations (e.g., Armour Thyroid, Nature-Throid, Westhroid, Bio-Throid). These compounds are made from beef or pork thyroid glands and contain thyroglobulin and both T$_4$ and T$_3$. The ratio of T$_4$ to T$_3$ is variable from one preparation to the next and reflects the intrathyroid ratio rather than that of the peripheral circulation. These preparations are, therefore, highly unnatural although they claim otherwise, and patients often run low TSH levels and intermittent high T$_3$ values.

Thyroid Hormone Bioequivalency

In October 2006, the Endocrine Society, the American Association of Clinical Endocrinology, and the American Thyroid Association (ATA) presented to the FDA their concerns about the methods used for testing the bioequivalence of different commercial thyroid hormone preparations.[4] Many patients and practitioners noticed over the years that switching from one T$_4$ brand to another, which was considered equivalent by their standards of bioequivalency testing, led to failures in treating patients with hypothyroidism. Hormones would become either underreplaced or overreplaced, as judged by serum TSH levels, on doses of thyroid hormones that had previously controlled the levels very well. The only difference was a change in the brand. The FDA does not incorporate the TSH level into its pharmacokinetic testing when declaring different brands of T$_4$ replacement bioequivalent, and as of the date of writing has so far refused to do so. Therefore, we recommend that all patients should be maintained on the same brand of T$_4$ replacement and not subjected to different brands or different generic preparations. Using generic versions of T$_4$, or changing commercial brands, in our experience creates unstable replacement regimens requiring costly re-equilibration and retesting strategies.

Subclinical Hypothyroidism

DEFINITION

Subclinical hypothyroidism is defined as an elevated TSH level associated with total and free T$_4$ and T$_3$ levels within the normal range. Usually the TSH in such patients falls between 4.0 and 10.0 μU/mL.[5]

PREVALENCE

The prevalence of patients in the general population with TSH levels between 4.0 and 10.0 μU/mL is typically 5% to 10%. With advancing age this increases, and in women older than 60 years, it can be greater than 20% of the population. Numerous studies have shown that once the diagnosis of subclinical hypothyroidism is made, and TPO antibodies are present, patients develop overt hypothyroidism at the rate of about 5% per year.

SCREENING

In the controversial meetings of the Consensus Panel on Subclinical Hypothyroidism convened, but not endorsed, by the Endocrine Societies and the American Thyroid Association, there were differences in opinions on whom should be screened for this condition within the general population, whether or not all women contemplating pregnancy or in their first trimester of pregnancy should be screened, and whether or not patients with TSH levels less than 10.0 µU/mL should be treated.

The ATA now recommends screening of both men and women beginning at age 35 years and then every 5 years afterward. The American College of Physicians only recommends screening women older than 50 years who present with symptoms consistent with subclinical hypothyroidism. These approaches totally ignore the pregnant population.

TREATMENT

During the Consensus Panel Meeting on Subclinical Hypothyroidism, there were also differences of opinion on which patients should be treated, and no consensus exists to this day. Much of this controversy arises from the quality of the outcomes data related to the treatment of such patients. Although such data remain incomplete, we interpret the evidence as sufficient to warrant treatment of these patients. We believe that once the diagnosis of subclinical hypothyroidism is confirmed by repeat testing within 1 to 3 months, and that causes such as subacute thyroiditis and recovery from nonthyroidal illness have been ruled out as causes of the elevated TSH levels, it is appropriate and safe to treat many such patients to a normal TSH level of 1.0 µU/mL.

OUTCOMES

Two important studies have become available concerning the impact of subclinical hypothyroidism. The first is a prospective study of 3121 cardiac patients with subclinical hypothyroidism, subclinical hyperthyroidism, and low T_3 syndrome. These patients were followed for a mean follow-up of 32 months. Hazard ratios (HRs) for cardiac death were higher in subclinical hypothyroidism (HR, 2.40; 95% confidence interval [CI], 1.36-4.21; $P = 0.02$). Survival from cardiac events was lower, and overall mortality was higher in patients with subclinical hypothyroid patients than in euthyroid patients. In a second report of a prospective study, patients with subclinical hypothyroidism, followed for 12 years, with a TSH level of 10 to 20 mU/L, had a significantly higher incidence of heart failure than patients who were euthyroid or had TSH levels between 4.5 mU/L and 9.9 mU/L. These studies strongly suggest that subtle thyroid failure can have deleterious cardiac effects.

Because thyroid function affects Ca^{2+} influx to the myocardium, it stands to reason that treatment might improve function. In fact, the majority of studies, although small in patient number, have shown clinical improvement in surrogate markers of cardiac function: improvement in actual ventricular function, endothelial function, and lipid profiles. In terms of the effects on mortality, the data remain unclear, although a Japanese population showed a survival advantage in treated men with subclinical hypothyroidism. However, one study of patients older than 85 years has also suggested that such elderly patients with subclinical hypothyroidism who were untreated might actually have an advantage in terms of survival.

Hence, except for patients with an unstable cardiac status, or the very elderly, we feel that subclinical hypothyroidism should be treated, because the treatment of a reliable patient is unlikely to have any harmful effects. In patients with an unstable cardiac status, subclinical hypothyroidism may be watched carefully.

Special Situations

SECONDARY HYPOTHYROIDISM

Secondary hypothyroidism often occurs in the setting of damage to the pituitary gland or hypothalamus. TSH elevation and reduction in this setting are not reliable measures of adequate T_4 replacement. The free T_4 must be corrected to the normal range, ignoring the TSH value. In this setting it is imperative to be certain that the patient does not have coexisting glucocorticoid deficiency. Often it is important to treat with replacement glucocorticoids in order to avoid adrenal insufficiency because the cortisol clearance is enhanced when thyroid hormone is supplemented.

MYXEDEMA COMA

Myxedema coma is a medical emergency. Even with prompt diagnosis the mortality can be as high as 30%. The mean age of patients is approximately 75 years.

Myxedema coma can be precipitated by hypothermia, infection, myocardial infarction, respiratory depression, or blood loss. Often patients have undiagnosed hypothyroidism or have discontinued their medication. Physical signs of hypothyroidism are usually obvious. Usually a high-dose treatment regimen is used in such patients, such as T_4 300 to 500 µg IV followed by 100 µg daily. Some practitioners advocate T_3 10 to 20 µg IV every 4 hours.

Respiratory support and slow rewarming are also essential. Signs of infection may be obscured. Treatment of hyponatremia and hypoglycemia may be necessary as well. Adrenal replacement of hydrocortisone (Cortef) with 50 to 100 mg every 8 hours is advocated.

PREGNANCY

Screening

Only confused recommendations have appeared for screening women planning pregnancy and during the first trimester of pregnancy, except in populations known to be at high risk for developing hypothyroidism, such as in patients with type 1 diabetes mellitus or other autoimmune diseases. However, we recommend screening all pregnant and prepregnant patients for hypothyroidism. A recent study showed that patients at high risk for developing hypothyroidism during their first trimester will be identified if screened, but if the entire population is not screened, then 30% of patients who develop primary hypothyroidism during their first trimester will be missed.

The Endocrine Society has published their recommendations for screening of thyroid dysfunction in pregnancy. This states that although the benefits of universal screening for thyroid dysfunction (primarily hypothyroidism) might not be justified by the current evidence, we recommend case finding among the following groups of women at high risk for thyroid disease by measurement of TSH:

- Women with a history of hyperthyroid or hypothyroid disease, postpartum thyroiditis, or thyroid lobectomy
- Women with a family history of thyroid disease
- Women with a goiter
- Women with thyroid antibodies (when known)
- Women with symptoms or clinical signs suggesting thyroid underfunction or overfunction, including anemia, elevated cholesterol, and hyponatremia
- Women with type 1 diabetes
- Women with other autoimmune disorders
- Women with infertility who should have screening with TSH as part of their infertility work-up
- Women with previous therapeutic head or neck irradiation
- Women with a history of miscarriage or preterm delivery

Postpartum thyroid studies are recommended at 3 and 6 months for patients at risk for thyroid disease.

Treatment

Pregnancy increases the dosage requirements of T_4 replacement for several different reasons. Estrogen causes an increase in the serum thyroxine-binding globulin level, which increases T_4 binding requirements; there is an increased transfer of T_4 to the fetus; and T_4 clearance itself is increased. During the first trimester, normal TSH levels are low or may be suppressed, and the upper limit if normal TSH in pregnancy is considered to be 2.5 μU/mL.

Hypothyroidism in pregnancy is associated with increased obstetric and fetal risks. A recent study suggests that T_4 supplementation starting in the first trimester in patients who have positive TPO antibodies regardless of the baseline TSH level had reduced obstetric complications, miscarriages, and premature deliveries.

For normal intellectual development of the child, it is also essential that the mother be euthyroid during the pregnancy. Therefore, thyroid status in the woman treated with T_4 replacement should be monitored each month. In contrast to the nonpregnant woman, the treatment of subclinical hypothyroidism in pregnancy is endorsed by all clinical societies.

TRANSIENT HYPOTHYROIDISM

Postpartum thyroiditis (a variant transient form of Hashimoto's thyroiditis) and subacute thyroiditis, typically manifests with hyperthyroidism as the thyroid cells undergo apoptosis, and this is then followed by a transient hypothyroid state. Postpartum thyroiditis might affect 10% of all pregnancies. At particular risk are patients with thyroid antibodies in the first trimester of pregnancy, patients with type 1 diabetes mellitus, and patients with a previous history of postpartum thyroiditis.

Postpartum thyroiditis typically develops 3 to 12 months following delivery. Most cases of hypothyroidism following the hyperthyroid phase are transient. Whether or not to treat the hypothyroidism is often, therefore, a clinical decision based on how symptomatic the person is. If one chooses to treat, one may choose to treat with a lower than full replacement dose, making it easier to monitor recovery to the euthyroid state. If one treats with a complete replacement dose, the thyroid supplement has to be stopped completely after 6 to 8 weeks to see if there is recovery.

In people with painful or painless subacute thyroiditis, the treatment scenario is essentially the same. Following the hyperthyroid phase, transient hypothyroidism typically develops. Whether or not to treat the person with a T_4 supplement and at what dose is a clinical decision depending on symptoms.

EUTHYROID SICK SYNDROME

A variety of metabolic abnormalities contribute to a syndrome of abnormal thyroid function tests commonly observed in sick patients. Typically the serum T_3 levels are low as an isolated observation, but the T_4 levels can also fall dramatically as the condition of the patient deteriorates. Serum TSH may be normal or modestly suppressed or even increased. A strong case has been made for the treatment of such patients with thyroid hormone replacement. However, this view is controversial, has not been satisfactorily subjected to controlled trials, and is a view we do not share at this time.

REFERENCES

Abalovich M, Amino N, Barbour LA, et al: Management of thyroid dysfunction during pregnancy and postpartum: An Endocrine Society Clinical Practice Guideline. J Clin Endocrinol Metab 2007;92:S1-S47.
American Thyroid Association; Endocrine Society; American Association of Clinical Endocrinologists: Joint statement on the U.S. Food and Drug Administration's decision regarding bioequivalence of levothyroxine sodium. Thyroid 2004;14(7):486.
Andersen S, Pedersen KM, Bruun NK, Laurberg P: Narrow individual variations in serum T4 and T3 in normal subjects: A clue to the understanding of subclinical thyroid disease. J Clin Endocrinol Metab 2002;87:1068-1072.
Andersen S, Bruun NH, Pedersen KM, Laurberg P: Biologic variation is important for interpretation of thyroid function tests. Thyroid 2003;13:1069-1078.
Casey BM: Subclinical hypothyroidism and pregnancy. Obstet Gynecol Surv 2006;61:415-420.

de Groot LJ: Nonthyroidal illness syndrome is a manifestation of hypothalamic–pituitary dysfunction, and in view of current evidence, should be treated with appropriate replacement therapies. Crit Care Clin 2006;22:57-86, vi.
De Jong FJ, Peeters RP, Den HT, et al: The association of polymorphisms in the type 1 and 2 deiodinase genes with circulating thyroid hormone parameters and atrophy of the medial temporal lobe. J Clin Endocrinol Metab 2007;92:636-640.
Gussekloo J, Van EE, De Craen AJ, et al: Thyroid status, disability and cognitive function, and survival in old age. JAMA 2004;292:2591-2599.
Iervasi G, Molinaro S, Landi P, et al: Association between increased mortality and mild thyroid dysfunction in cardiac patients. Arch Intern Med 2007;167:1526-1532.
Imaizumi M, Akahoshi M, Ichimaru S, et al: Risk for ischemic heart disease and all-cause mortality in subclinical hypothyroidism. J Clin Endocrinol Metab 2004;89:3365-3370.
Negro R, Formoso G, Mangieri T, et al: Levothyroxine treatment in euthyroid pregnant women with autoimmune thyroid disease: Effects on obstetrical complications. J Clin Endocrinol. Metab 2006;91:2587-2591.
Rodondi N, Cappola A, Cornuz J, et al: Subclinical thyroid dysfunction, cardiac function, and the risk of congestive heart failure: The Cardiovascular Health Study American Thyroid Association Annual Meeting. Thyroid 2007;17(Suppl 1):S1-S73.
Surks MI, Ortiz E, Daniels GH, et al: Subclinical thyroid disease: Scientific review and guidelines for diagnosis and management. JAMA 2004;291:228-238.
Vaidya B, Anthony S, Bilous M, et al: Detection of thyroid dysfunction in early pregnancy: Universal screening or targeted high-risk case finding? J Clin Endocrinol Metab 2007;92:203-207.
Wartofsky L, Van ND, Burman KD: Overt and "subclinical" hypothyroidism in women. Obstet Gynecol Surv 2006;61:535-542.

Hyperthyroidism

Method of
Peter A. Singer, MD

Hyperthyroidism encompasses a heterogeneous group of disorders, all of which have two features in common. Firstly, all of the types of hyperthyroidism include a β-adrenergic-mediated symptom complex of varying degrees of severity characterized by symptoms of nervousness, heat intolerance, irritability, palpitations, and increased bowel motility, with frequency of movements. Secondly, hyperthyroidism is associated with the catabolic effects of excess circulating levels of thyroid hormone; such effects can include weight loss, fatigue, muscle weakness, increased appetite, and bone loss. The symptoms and signs of hyperthyroidism depend on a number of variables, including levels of circulating thyroid hormone, duration of disease, the age of the patient, and concurrent illnesses.

Hyperthyroidism can be classified according to the capacity of the thyroid gland to trap radioactive iodine (Box 1). Disorders with increased radioiodine uptake have thyroid gland autonomy (with the exception of thyroid-stimulating hormone [TSH]-secreting pituitary tumors) and require specific treatment, whereas those with suppressed radioiodine uptake include conditions that are usually self-limited and might require only symptomatic treatment.

Physical examination of the hyperthyroid patient generally reveals a person who is somewhat anxious and has a rapid pulse. In the elderly, atrial fibrillation is common, and many elderly patients have widened pulse pressure, warm skin, and palpable thyroid gland findings, depending on the underlying etiology. Examination of the eyes in all types of hyperthyroidism might show eyelid retraction, which is mediated by β-adrenergic stimulation. Infiltrative ophthalmopathy is seen almost exclusively in patients with thyrotoxic Graves' disease.

BOX 1 Causes of Hyperthyroidism*

Hyperthyroidism with Elevated RAIU
- Graves' disease
- Toxic multinodular goiter
- Toxic adenoma
- TSH-secreting pituitary tumor
- Hydatiform mole
- Choriocarcinoma
- Pituitary resistance to thyroid hormone

Hyperthyroidism with Low RAIU
- Factitious
- Subacute granulomatus thyroiditis
- Subacute lymphocytic (postpartum or sporadic)
- Amiodarone-induced thyroiditis
- Iodine-induced hyperthyroidism
- Radiation-induced thyroiditis
- Metastatic functioning follicular tumor
- Struma ovarii

*In probable decreasing order of frequency.
Abbreviations: RAIU = radioactive iodine uptake; TSH = thyroid-stimulating hormone.

Diagnosis

Because many of the symptoms of hyperthyroidism may be compatible with some nonthyroid disorders, such as anxiety or the perimenopausal state, TSH, should be measured in patients in whom hyperthyroidism is suspected. TSH suppressed in hyperthroidism, although in patients with rare TSH-secreting pituitary tumors, TSH levels may be normal or even slightly elevated. TSH levels may be suppressed in hospitalized patients, especially those who are seriously ill or who are receiving pharmacologic doses of glucocorticoids or dopamine, thus limiting the usefulness of serum TSH measurements in such patients.

A suppressed TSH level in patients suspected to have hyperthyroidism should be complemented with a serum free thyroxine (T_4) or its estimate to confirm the diagnosis. Patients with normal thyroid hormone levels and suppressed TSH concentrations have what is termed *subclinical hyperthyroidism*, a disorder usually free of overt symptoms of hyperthyroidism.

After the diagnosis of hyperthyroidism is confirmed, its etiology should be determined by obtaining a thyroid radioactive iodine uptake. Patients with obvious Graves' disease (such as those with infiltrative ophthalmopathy or large goiters with bruits), may forgo the radioactive iodine uptake test. It is important, however, to differentiate between Graves' disease and low radioactive iodine uptake conditions, which usually are self-limited.

In addition to the radioactive iodine uptake, a scan may be helpful in establishing the diagnosis in patients with suspected toxic multinodular goiter, a condition encountered more commonly nowadays due to increasing immigration into the United States from endemic goiter regions.

Treatment

Because approximately 80% of patients with hyperthyroidism in the United States have thyrotoxic Graves' disease, most of the comments in this article pertain to that disorder. Among patients with high radioactive iodine-uptake hyperthyroidism, only Graves' disease may be associated with remission following the use of thionamide drugs.

DEVELOPING A TREATMENT STRATEGY

General Measures and Patient Education

Essential in the early management of Graves' hyperthyroidism is emphasizing to the patient that strict adherence to the treatment regimen is essential in alleviating symptoms and restoring health. Persons with hyperthyroidism commonly tend to be impatient, likely due to their symptoms, and it must be stressed that compliance with treatment advice is essential for a successful outcome. If family members or friends accompany the patient to the appointment, it is helpful to make them familiar with the treatment plan as well.

Initial Treatment of Symptoms

Because many of the symptoms of hyperthyroidism are related to enhanced β-adrenergic stimulation, I routinely employ β-adrenergic-blocking drugs, although mild symptoms might not warrant their use. I prefer propranolol (Inderal),[1] even though it must be given approximately every 6 hours to be completely effective. Propranolol's relatively short half-life makes this agent preferable, because patients learn to titrate their own medication, depending on their symptoms. As patients improve during the course of thionamide therapy (see later), they can omit more doses of propranolol.

The usual starting dose of propranolol[1] is between 20 and 40 mg approximately every 6 hours (or four times a day), and the desired target heart rate is approximately 80 beats per minute. Some physicians prefer longer acting β-blockers, such as atenolol (Tenormin),[1] which may be given as a single daily dose. In patients in whom compliance may be problematic, or in those who prefer once-daily dosing, atenolol 50 to 100 mg a day is an excellent alternative. Other long-acting β-blockers are nadolol (Corgard)[1] and metoprolol (Lopressor).[1] Long-acting β-blockers are cardioselective and are not contraindicated in patients with coexisting asthma, as propranolol is.

CURRENT DIAGNOSIS

Symptoms of Graves' Hyperthyroidism

- Emotional lability
- Eye irritation, photophobia, diplopia
- Fatigue
- Heat intolerance
- Increased appetite
- Increased frequency of bowel movements
- Increased perspiration
- Menstrual irregularities
- Muscle weakness
- Nervousness
- Palpitations
- Shortness of breath
- Sleep disturbances
- Weight loss

Signs of Graves' Hyperthyroidism

- Diffuse goiter
- Eye stare
- Hyperreflexia
- Infiltrative dermopathy (~5%)
- Proptosis
- Proximal muscle weakness
- Systolic hypertension
- Tachycardia
- Thyroid bruit
- Warm, smooth skin
- Widened pulse pressure

---
[1]Not FDA approved for this indication.

CURRENT THERAPY

Treatment Modality	Advantages	Disadvantages
Thionamide drugs	Chance of remission Relatively inexpensive	Relapse (40%) Side effects (5-10%)
Surgery	Rapid, permanent cure	Surgical complications (hypocalcemia, recurrent nerve injury ~1%-3%) Hypothyroidism
Radioactive iodine	Permanent cure	Expensive Hypothyroidism

In my experience, patients who are treated with adequate doses of β-adrenergic blocking drugs have significant relief of symptoms within a few days after the medication is initiated.

Reduction of Serum Thyroid Hormone Levels

Unfortunately, there have been few advances in the management of hyperthyroidism in recent years. Treatment basically consists of lowering the concentrations of serum thyroxine (T_4) and triiodothyronine (T_3), which may be accomplished either with thionamide drugs or with ablative therapy, either radioiodine or surgery. In the United States, radioiodine ablation with ^{131}I is the preferred method of treatment of most practicing endocrinologists. Indeed, in a survey of thyroid experts completed in 1991, 69% of respondents chose radioiodine as the primary form of therapy for a prototypic 43-year-old woman with uncomplicated Graves' disease. Only 1% of physicians recommended surgery, and 30% selected thionamide drugs as the primary form of therapy. The responses were in sharp contrast to thyroid experts in both Europe and Japan, where a similar survey revealed that the majority of physicians favored thionamide drugs as the primary form of therapy. The rationale provided by physicians in the United States who selected radioiodine therapy was the fact that the remission rate following 1 to 2 years of thionamide drugs was only approximately 30%.

Before recommending a specific type of therapy for a patient with Graves' disease, it is essential that the patient be aware of the benefits and pitfalls of each type of treatment.

THIONAMIDE DRUG THERAPY

Initial Treatment

Currently, there are two thionamide drugs available for clinical use in the United States, methimazole (MMI, Tapazole) available in 5-mg and 10-mg tablets, and propylthiouracil (PTU) available in 50-mg tablets. Both agents inhibit the synthesis of thyroid hormone by blocking organification of iodine. PTU also inhibits peripheral conversion of T_4 to T_3, although clinically this may be more of a theoretical than a practical advantage.

I generally prefer MMI, rather than PTU, because of its longer biological half-life and its potency. For uncomplicated hyperthyroidism, MMI may initially be given 2 to 3 times a day in a total dose of 20 to 30 mg, whereas PTU is usually administered 3 to 4 times a day in a total dose of 300 to 400 mg. When biochemical euthyroidism is achieved, usually after 6 to 8 weeks of therapy, MMI may be given once a day, or PTU twice a day, and the total dose may be halved. The relative simplicity of using MMI versus PTU can render it more suitable for patients in whom compliance may be difficult. It must be stressed to the patient that omitting medication doses can result in a rebound of the hyperthyroid state, because the intrathyroid deficiency of iodine produced by thionamide drugs results in more avid trapping of exogenous iodide.

In general, I obtain serum T_4 and T_3 levels about 6 to 8 weeks after initiating thionamide drug therapy to ensure adequacy of treatment response. If there has been little clinical or biochemical improvement, the likeliest scenario is that doses of medication are being omitted. A serum TSH provides no additional information at this point, because TSH suppression is common for up to 3 or 4 months after euthyroidism has been achieved. Patients with very large goiters and fairly severe hyperthyroidism often take somewhat longer than 6 to 8 weeks to become euthyroid and can require larger doses of MMI (e.g., 40 mg/day) or PTU (e.g., 400-600 mg/day).

I stress to patients that any improvement with thionamide drugs can take several weeks, and I recommend that they defer, if possible, making definitive decisions regarding long-term thionamide versus ablative therapy until they have improved to the extent that they are better able to make more reasoned choices. I always discuss the various forms of treatment of hyperthyroidism with patients during our first appointment, however, and reiterate the options after they have improved.

Although the overall remission rate of patients treated with thionamide drugs in the United States is approximately 30%, some patients are more likely than others to go into remission. Patients with mild hyperthyroidism, small goiters, and a negative family history for hyperthyroidism are more likely to respond favorably, as are patients who respond quickly to thionamide drugs in terms of thyroid gland shrinkage and biochemical improvement. Conversely, patients with severe thyrotoxicosis and those with a strong family history of Graves' disease infrequently go into remission. Some clinicians have advocated serologic markers, such as thyroid-stimulating immunoglobulin or anti-TPO antibodies, to predict the likelihood of remission, but there has been no confirmation of their usefulness for such a purpose.

Continuing Treatment

I reevaluate patients taking thionamide drugs approximately every 3 months, and in addition to the clinical examination, I obtain a serum free T_4 (estimate) and TSH. If hypothyroidism occurs while on medication, I often add levothyroxine (Synthroid) rather than reduce the dose of thionamide drug. Most patients can be maintained euthyroid on 20 mg of MMI and 0.1 mg of levothyroxine taken in a single daily dose. If PTU is employed, it usually must be given twice daily.

Combined therapy with thionamide drugs and levothyroxine resulted in a considerable amount of controversy several years ago, following the publication of an article from a Japanese group of researchers who reported that 98% of patients taking both MMI and levothyroxine achieved remission. The researchers maintained serum TSH levels in the suppressed range and theorized that TSH inhibition with levothyroxine resulted in less stimulation of antigen release. Unfortunately, their findings have not been confirmed in subsequent studies, either in Japan or elsewhere. Some physicians, however, have reported improved remission rates following longer durations of thionamide administration, of up to 10 years. The practical aspects of such prolonged therapy however, might be open to question.

Side Effects of Thionamide Drugs

The most common allergic side effects of thionamide drugs range from mild maculopapular rashes to urticarial eruptions and occur in approximately 5% of patients. Allergic reactions usually do not occur until 2 to 4 weeks after initiation of therapy. Mild symptoms may be managed with antihistamines, although complete resolution of itching and rash is uncommon. Therefore, I routinely switch patients from the type of medication they are taking (e.g., MMI) to PTU. Approximately 20% of patients are also allergic to the other thionamides, preventing their continued use.

The most serious side effect of thionamide drugs is agranulocytosis, and although it is rare (0.2%-0.5% of patients), it is potentially fatal. It is usually manifested by fever and symptoms of infection, such as a severe sore throat. Patients must be instructed that if they develop fever and signs and symptoms of infection, they must stop the thionamide drug and call their physician immediately. A white blood cell count and differential must be performed, and if agranulocytosis is diagnosed, hospital admission is required. Successful reversal of agranulocytosis, sometimes employing granulocyte colony stimulating factor (G-CSF), should occur within a few days to a week.

Some physicians obtain periodic white blood cell (WBC) counts, although this practice is probably unnecessary because the WBC does not predict agranulocytosis. Nevertheless, before initiating therapy with thionamide drugs, it is helpful to have a baseline WBC because leukopenia is common in patients with Graves' disease, and if a subsequent WBC is obtained, it is useful for comparison.

Other potential side effects of antithyroid drugs include arthralgias and, rarely, hepatitis. Hepatitis is also potentially fatal.

Stopping Antithyroid Drug Therapy

If therapy with thionamide drugs is used to induce remission, an endpoint of therapy should be determined. I usually treat for 12 to 18 months and then discontinue the thionamide agent. Patients are reevaluated approximately 4 to 6 weeks later, and a serum TSH is obtained. If the serum TSH is suppressed during thionamide therapy, the likelihood of remission is poor. If the patient is euthyroid at 4 to 6 weeks, the next visit is scheduled for approximately 3 months later and at increasing intervals thereafter, but at intervals no longer than 1 year.

Most relapses of hyperthyroidism occur within the first year after stopping thionamide drugs, but they can occur at any time. If relapse occurs, a second course of thionamide drugs does not appear to increase the likelihood of remission, and ablation with radioiodine is then recommended. Some patients, however, prefer to take antithyroid drugs for several, or even many years and often can be maintained on a very small dose of thionamide drug (e.g., 2.5-5 mg/day of MMI). Although such extended therapy is not my preference, there is no absolute contraindication to it. Patients on such a regimen need to be instructed that periodic follow-up, perhaps every 3 to 6 months, is necessary.

RADIOACTIVE IODINE THERAPY

Therapy with radioiodine (^{131}I) is the preferred method of treatment for hyperthyroidism among other thyroid specialists practicing in the United States. Radioiodine has distinct advantages: It is effective, relatively inexpensive, and predictable, and it appears to be free of side effects other than the development of hypothyroidism. Radioiodine has been used to treat hyperthyroidism for approximately 45 years in the United States, and careful follow-up has failed to show an increased incidence of cancer in patients so treated or in genetic defects in offspring of ^{131}I-treated patients. Radioiodine is contraindicated during pregnancy, which should be ruled out in women of childbearing age before its administration. In addition, women who are breast-feeding should not be treated with radioiodine, because the isotope can recirculate in breast milk for up to several weeks after administration.

Selection of Radioiodine Dose

Some clinicians advocate administering a ^{131}I dose that is sufficient to control hyperthyroidism without resulting in hypothyroidism. Various strategies have been employed over the years in an effort to achieve this goal, but they generally have failed. Therefore, I prefer administering a dose large enough to result in hypothyroidism, which usually occurs within 3 to 6 months after ^{131}I administration. A dose of 15 mCi of ^{131}I is usually sufficient to achieve this goal, but the appropriate dose depends on the radioactive iodine uptake and size of the thyroid gland. A 24-hour radioactive iodine uptake should be measured before the treatment dose is administered to ensure that adequate quantities of ^{131}I will be absorbed by the thyroid. A dose of 100-150 fCi/g of thyroid tissue is generally an adequate ablative dose. Some patients are resistant to an initial dose of ^{131}I and require a second or even third treatment. In my experience, male patients, Asians, and patients with large goiters appear to require larger or additional doses. If patients continue to be hyperthyroid 6 months after an initial treatment with ^{131}I, a second dose is administered.

Before administering radioiodine, I usually pretreat patients with thionamide drugs until they are euthyroid, because depletion of thyroid hormone from the thyroid prevents release of excess of thyroid hormone from the gland, thereby preventing exacerbation of hyperthyroidism. This is especially important for older patients or those with cardiovascular risk factors. Antithyroid drugs should be discontinued 3 to 5 days before radioiodine treatment. Patients receiving ^{131}I without having been pretreated with antithyroid drugs (for example, patients who are allergic to thionamides) benefit from administration of propranolol[1] or other β-blockers after treatment, because their underlying hyperthyroidism may be transiently exacerbated by ^{131}I-induced thyroiditis.

Follow-up after Radioiodine Treatment

I usually evaluate patients approximately 6 weeks following radioiodine administration in order to assess the clinical and biochemical responses. If the thyroid gland has not decreased in size by 6 weeks, a beneficial response from radioiodine is unlikely. If patients are euthyroid at 6 weeks, they return 4 to 6 weeks later, and if they are hypothyroid by that time, levothyroxine therapy is begun. If patients are still euthyroid (or hyperthyroid) 3 months after therapy, they are reevaluated in another 3 months. Nearly all patients are hypothyroid by 6 months after radioiodine treatment, and those who are still hyperthyroid require another treatment dose.

As experience with radioiodine has increased over the years, age limits for patients believed to be appropriate for treatment have decreased. It appears to be safe to treat teenagers with radioiodine, although I defer treatment in those who have not completed linear growth. There is little concern for developing thyroid nodularity in teenagers following ^{131}I treatment provided ablative doses are administered.

Radioiodine Treatment and Graves' Ophthalmopathy

Some clinicians think the administration of ^{131}I to patients with Graves' ophthalmopathy can worsen the eye disease and administration of pharmacologic amounts of glucocorticoids for a period of one month to 6 weeks following radioiodine treatment will lessen the likelihood of this occurrence. The data concerning efficacy of steroids are not conclusive, however. I believe that patients with moderate symptoms and signs of eye disease should be evaluated by an ophthalmologist with expertise in Graves' ophthalmopathy before administration of ^{131}I. Indeed, it is often helpful to involve the ophthalmologist in the care of patients with ophthalmopathy, regardless of the type of treatment for hyperthyroidism.

---

[1]Not FDA approved for this indication.

SURGERY

Surgery for Graves' hyperthyroidism is infrequently employed in the United States. Candidates for such treatment include children and teenagers, especially those who have difficulty complying with antithyroid drugs. Other indications include patients with very large goiters, especially those likely to be resistant to radioiodine because of large goiter size. In addition, surgery is the only choice for patients who are allergic to thionamide drugs and who refuse to take radioiodine. Surgery is also indicated for pregnant patients who are allergic to thionamide drugs (see later). Patients who have a coexistent thyroid nodule suspicious for cancer on fine-needle aspiration should be treated surgically.

Before surgery, it is preferred to render the patient euthyroid with thionamide drugs. Some surgeons prefer to administer exogenous iodides for 10 days before surgery. Exogenous iodides produce benefit both by inhibiting thyroid hormone release and by decreasing thyroid gland vascularity. Potassium iodide or Lugol's solution, 10 drops in a glass of water daily for 10 days, is sufficient.

Patients electing to undergo thyroidectomy should be made aware that permanent hypothyroidism will most likely result and that they will require the same type of follow-up as those treated with radioiodine. If insufficient thyroid tissue is removed, persistent or recurrent hyperthyroidism will result, which will necessitate radioiodine ablation.

Although surgery has the advantage of being rapidly curative, it also has potential complications. One is injury to the recurrent laryngeal nerve and the other is the possibility of permanent hypoparathyroidism. In skilled hands, these complications occur no more than 1% to 3% of the time, yet these potential risks must be explained fully to the patient beforehand.

Other Forms of Hyperthyroidism

TOXIC NODULAR GOITER

Toxic multinodular goiter increases in prevalence with increasing age. In elderly persons it is a more common cause of hyperthyroidism than is Graves' disease. The diagnosis should be documented with a radioactive iodine uptake and thyroid scan. Patients with toxic multinodular goiter will not go into remission on thionamide drugs, limiting definitive treatment to either radioiodine or surgery.

Before radioiodine is employed in elderly patients, thionamide drugs should be administered to minimize the risk of exacerbating hyperthyroidism. Radioiodine is the treatment of choice for most patients with toxic multinodular goiter, although surgery may be preferred for patients with especially large glands or with symptoms of compression who are good operative risks. If radioiodine is used for treatment of toxic nodular goiter, the dose required is usually greater than that employed for Graves' disease.

A single thyroid nodule producing hyperthyroidism occurs much less often than toxic multinodular goiter, and it generally occurs in persons younger than those with multinodular goiter. Although radioiodine is commonly employed for such patients, surgery is usually recommended for patients younger than 25 to 30 years.

HYPERTHYROIDISM AND PREGNANCY

Hyperthyroidism during pregnancy can lead to adverse outcomes both for mother and fetus. Adequate control of hyperthyroidism during pregnancy is essential. Either MMI or PTU may be used during pregnancy, but most clinicians favor PTU because it does not cross the placenta as easily as does MMI. For hyperthyroidism that is difficult to control, or if the patient is allergic to antithyroid drugs, thyroidectomy should be performed during the second trimester. β-Adrenergic blocking agents may be given safely during pregnancy to control symptoms.

Patients who continue to be treated with thionamide drugs during pregnancy should have a thyroid-stimulating immunoglobulin level drawn during the last trimester to predict the possible occurrence of neonatal hyperthyroidism. Hyperthyroid pregnant patients should be followed carefully at least every 4 to 6 weeks, and close communication should be maintained between the endocrinologist and obstetrician. It is advisable to use the lowest dose of thionamide drug that maintains maternal euthyroidism.

THYROID STORM

Thyroid storm (or crisis) is characterized by severe manifestations of hyperthyroidism, fever, and altered mental status. The disorder is usually precipitated by a concurrent illness.

Early recognition and treatment of thyroid storm are essential because it is life threatening. Patients must be managed in the intensive care unit, and, in addition to general supportive measures and treatment of concurrent illness, aggressive pharmacologic management of the hyperthyroidism is necessary. Either MMI or PTU may be used, although PTU has the potential advantage of reducing production of T_3 from T_4. A dose of 150 mg of PTU every 6 hours or 15 to 20 mg of MMI every 8 hours is usually sufficient. For patients unable to take medication orally, MMI may be crushed and given by nasogastric tube or may be prepared by the pharmacy as a rectal suppository.

In addition to thionamide drugs, exogenous iodides should be administered. Iopanoic acid may be used for this purpose, because it not only inhibits thyroid hormone release but also has the advantage of being a potent inhibitor of T_4 to T_3 conversion. A dose of 500 mg to 1 g orally daily is sufficient. However it is not currently available in the United States. Alternatively, iodine can be administered in the form of Lugol's solution or saturated solution of potassium iodide, 10 drops in water three times daily, or sodium iodide, 500 mg intravenously every 12 hours. It is essential to administer the first dose of thionamide drug a few hours before administration of iodides to prevent further organification of iodide with resultant additional thyroid hormone production. Some clinicians also use pharmacologic doses of glucocorticoids to further inhibit T_4 to T_3 conversion, although the clinical efficacy of this treatment has not been shown convincingly.

β-Blocking agents, preferably propranolol,[1] are essential in the management of thyroid storm and may be given either orally or intravenously. If the latter route is used, 1 mg every 5 to 10 minutes is given intravenously until the heart rate is less than 100 bpm. Once adequate control of the heart rate is achieved, oral propranolol may be given, and doses of 160 mg or more every 6 hours are not uncommon. Heart failure, which may be due in part to uncontrolled tachycardia, must be treated with adequate digitalis. If diuretics[1] are used, they must be administered very cautiously, because patients with thyroid storm are peripherally vasodilated and can suffer vascular collapse if conventional doses of diuretics are given. Plasmapheresis has been described as a treatment for thyroid storm, although I have neither used it nor seen it employed.

---

[1]Not FDA approved for this indication.

REFERENCES

Auer J, Scheibner P, Mische T, et al: Subclinical hyperthyroidism is a risk factor for atrial fibrillation. Am Heart J 2001;142:838-842.
Baldini M, Gallazzi M, Orsatti A, et al: Treatment of benign nodular goiter with mildly suppressive doses of L-thyroxine: Effects on bone mineral density and on nodule size. J Intern Med 2002;251:407-414.
Bauer DC, Ettinger B, Nevitt MC, Stone KL: Risk for fracture in women with low serum levels of thyroid-stimulating hormone. Ann Intern Med 2001;134:561-568.
Charkes ND: The many causes of subclinical hyperthyroidism. Thyroid 1996;5:391-396.
Cooper DS: Antithyroid drugs. N Engl J Med 1984;311:1353-1362.
Cooper DS: Antithyroid drugs and radioiodine therapy: A grain of (iodized) salt. Ann Intern Med 1994;121:612-614.
Cooper DS: Treatment of thyrotoxicosis. In Braverman LE, Utiger RD, (eds): Werner and Ingbar's The Thyroid: A Fundamental and Clinical Text, 7th ed, Philadelphia, Lippincott-Raven, 1996, pp 708-734.

Cooper DS: Antithyroid drugs for the treatment of hyperthyroidism caused by Graves' disease. Endocrinol Metab Clin North Am 1998;27:225-247.

Franklyn JA: The management of hyperthyroidism. N Engl J Med 1994;130:1731-1738.

Franklyn JA: Drug therapy: The management of hyperthyroidism. N Engl J Med 1994;330:1731-1738.

Klein I, Becker D, Levey G: Treatment of hyperthyroid disease. Ann Inter Med 1994;121:281-288.

Klein I, Ojamaa K: Cardiovascular manifestations of endocrine disease. J Clin Endocrinol Metab 1992;75:339-342.

McIver B, Morris JC: The pathogenesis of Graves' disease. Endocrinol Metab Clin North Am 1998;27:73-89.

Mestman JH: Hyperthyroidism and pregnancy. Best Pract Res Clin Endocrinol Metab 2004;18:267-288.

Motomura K, Brent GA: Mechanisms of thyroid hormone action. Endocrinol Metab Clin North Am 1998;27:1-23.

Papi G, Pearce EN, Braverman LE, et al: A clinical and therapeutic approach to thyrotoxicosis with thyroid-stimulating hormone suppression only. Am J Med 2005;118:349-361.

Roti E, Minelli R, Salvi M: Management of hyperthyroidism and hypothyroidism in the pregnant woman. J Clin Endocrinol Metab 1996;81:1679-1682.

Sawin CT: Thyroid dysfunction in older persons. Adv Intern Med 1991;37:223-249.

Sawin CT, Geller A, Wolf P, et al: Low serum thyrotropin concentrations as a risk factor for atrial fibrillation in older persons. N Engl J Med 1994;331:1249-1252.

Singer PA, Cooper D, Levy E, et al: Treatment guidelines for patients with hyperthyroidism and hypothyroidism. JAMA 1995;273:808-812.

Surks MI, Chopra I, Mariash C, et al: American Thyroid Association guidelines for use of laboratory tests in thyroid disorders. JAMA 1990;263:1529-1532.

Torring O, Tallstedt L, Wallin G, et al: Graves' hyperthyroidism: Treatment with antithyroid drugs, surgery, or radioiodine a prospective, randomized study. J Clin Endocrinol Metab 1996;81:2986-2993.

Wing DA, Millar LK, Koonings PP, et al: A comparision of propylthiouracil versus methimazole in the treatment of hyperthyroidism in pregnancy. Am J Obstet Gynecol 1994;170:90-95.

Thyroid Cancer

Method of
Richard A. Prinz, MD, and Emery Chen, MD

Thyroid cancer is the most common malignancy of the endocrine system. It affects more women than men by a ratio of 3:1. The National Cancer Institute (NCI) estimates that in 2008, 37,340 new cases of thyroid cancer were diagnosed in the United States and 1590 patients will die of thyroid cancer.

From 1997 to 2004, the incidence of thyroid cancer has increased by about 6% per year. This may be due, in part, to the frequent use of imaging modalities that have been detecting increasing numbers of incidental thyroid nodules. The mortality associated with thyroid cancer has not increased appreciably despite its rising incidence. The biological behavior of thyroid cancers, as a group, covers a broad spectrum. The overall 5- and 10-year survival rates of patients with papillary thyroid cancer, the most common type, remain approximately 97% and 90% respectively. Patients with anaplastic thyroid cancer, the least common type, rarely survive beyond 1 year.

The five subtypes of thyroid cancer are papillary, follicular, Hürthle cell, medullary, and anaplastic. Surgery is the initial treatment for all of these; however, the extent of surgery and subsequent adjuvant therapy depend on the clinical features and characteristics of each type.

Causes and Risk Factors

The causes of most sporadic forms of thyroid cancer remain unclear. Persons who have a family history of thyroid cancer or are older than 40 years are at greater risk for developing the disease. The incidence of malignancy in thyroid nodules is higher in children than adults, varying from 15% to 20% versus 5% to 6%, respectively.

The link between prior radiation exposure of the thyroid gland and cancer is clear. In the past, children and adults were sometimes treated with radiation for acne, fungal infections of the scalp, enlarged thymus, tonsils and adenoids, and other benign conditions. Numerous studies have linked these treatments to a higher risk of developing thyroid cancer, especially in patients with a thyroid nodule where the likelihood may be as high as 30% to 50%. Population studies of those affected by the Chernobyl accident showed a dramatic spike in the incidence of thyroid cancer, especially in children. Radiation exposure in adulthood carries a lesser risk of developing thyroid cancer than in children but it is still higher than in the general population.

A diet low in iodine is a risk factor for follicular thyroid cancer, the most common type of thyroid cancer in parts of the world where iodine deficiency is endemic. A low-iodine diet also seems to increase the risk of papillary thyroid cancers in those exposed to radiation.

Diagnosis

Most patients with thyroid cancer present with a nodule, which is extremely common in the general population. Sonographic screening of populations without thyroid disease shows that 33% of adults have at least one thyroid nodule. The number of detected nodules increases with age, with the highest prevalence in the seventh decade. Cancer is rare, occurring in 5% to 6% of those with a palpable thyroid nodule.

The best way to determine the nature of a thyroid nodule is by fine needle aspiration (FNA) for cytology. Some cancers are diagnosed after surgical excision for presumed benign disease (an indeterminate nodule, symptomatic multinodular goiter, or Graves' disease). These occult thyroid cancers are of uncertain biological behavior. Retrospective studies with long-term follow-up suggest that death resulting from papillary or follicular thyroid cancers detected in this fashion is uncommon with appropriate treatment.

Evaluation of a patient with a thyroid nodule (Box 1) should include a detailed review of their risk factors and symptoms, and a thorough neck examination that notes the characteristics of the nodule, and the presence or absence of cervical lymphadenopathy. Serum thyroid stimulating hormone (TSH) level should be measured to determine the patient's thyroid function. If the patient is euthyroid or hypothyroid by clinical evaluation or by having a normal or high TSH level, we proceed directly to FNA biopsy. We also start these

---

BOX 1   Risk Factors, Signs, and Symptoms Associated with Thyroid Cancer

Risk Factors
Head and neck irradiation
Family history of thyroid cancer
Low-iodine diet

Signs
Hard, fixed mass in a thyroid lobe
Cervical lymphadenopathy
Rapidly enlarging thyroid mass

Symptoms
Generally asymptomatic except in advanced disease
New onset of dysphonia, dyspnea, or dysphagia
Pressure or pain is unusual

CURRENT DIAGNOSIS

- A history of thyroid irradiation or family history of thyroid cancer increases the likelihood that a patient with a thyroid nodule will have thyroid cancer.
- Thyroid nodules in children are more likely to be cancers.
- Plasma thyroid-stimulating hormone level should be measured to assess thyroid function.
- A hyperfunctioning thyroid nodule is unlikely to harbor a malignancy.
- Ultrasound evaluation of the thyroid and neck can aid in the diagnosis and treatment of thyroid cancer.
- Fine needle aspiration (FNA) biopsy is the gold standard diagnostic test to detect most thyroid cancers.
- Follicular and Hürthle cell neoplasms require thyroid lobectomy because histopathologic evidence of capsular or vascular invasion is required to diagnose malignancy.

patients on a TSH-suppressive dose of levothyroxine (Synthroid), beginning with 25 μg daily and titrating it to a TSH level just below 1 mIU/L to halt or reverse the growth of the nodule. However, there is no consensus as to the effectiveness of this approach. If the TSH level is suppressed below normal, a thyroid scan can determine if the nodule is a hyperfunctioning adenoma. Increased isotope uptake confirms a toxic or hot nodule. The risk of a hot nodule harboring a malignancy is less than 1%. We recommend thyroid lobectomy for definitive treatment of toxic adenomas; others favor radioiodine if the adenoma is less than 4 cm in diameter.

FNA biopsy is the gold standard test to separate benign disease from malignant disease. This can be guided by direct palpation of the nodule or with ultrasound to increase accuracy. It is a rapid, safe, sensitive, and inexpensive test that can be performed in the office and is well tolerated by patients. Its false-positive rate of 1% to 2% and false-negative rate of 2% to 5% have been well validated.

There are four possible cytopathologic results from an FNA biopsy specimen: malignant, benign, suspicious or indeterminate, and nondiagnostic. Treatment options for the first two possibilities are clear. Malignant lesions mandate thyroidectomy. Benign lesions should be followed unless they are associated with symptoms or growth while under observation. In addition, we recommend a second FNA biopsy in 6 to 12 months to decrease the possibility of a false-negative result.

Suspicious or indeterminate lesions are mainly follicular and Hürthle cell neoplasms. These encapsulated tumors can be either benign or malignant. The differentiation cannot be made on the cytologic appearance of individual or even clusters of cells. The diagnosis of malignancy can only be made by finding direct tumor invasion into the capsule or vasculature. Therefore, thyroid lobectomy with definitive histologic examination of the specimen is recommended. There is conflicting evidence about the accuracy of intra-operative frozen section evaluation to guide surgical treatment. We use it because it is available and can be helpful when the pathologist makes a diagnosis of malignancy, but quite often the diagnosis must be deferred to permanent sections. If the final pathologic diagnosis reveals malignancy, a second procedure for completion thyroidectomy is recommended. For Hürthle and follicular neoplasms larger than 4 cm, total thyroidectomy is advised because of the greater risk of cancer. If the FNA is nondiagnostic, a repeat aspiration should be performed under ultrasound guidance. Patients with nodules that continue to yield nondiagnostic results should be offered thyroidectomy to clarify the diagnosis.

Histologic Classification, Treatment, and Prognosis

Cytology and management of thyroid tumors are shown in Table 1.

PAPILLARY CANCER

Papillary thyroid cancers are the most common form of thyroid cancer, accounting for approximately 80% of thyroid malignancies. They typically appear as hard, white nodules on gross examination. They are characterized microscopically by cuboidal cells with intranuclear cytoplasmic inclusions, nuclear grooves, prominent nuclei with marginated chromatin (Orphan Annie eyes), and round collections of calcium (psammoma bodies). Generally, the tumors are not encapsulated, but if they are, it is usually a good prognostic sign. Multicentric disease is common in papillary cancers, occurring in up to 85% of patients.

The cancer spreads early within the thyroid gland and through the lymphatics of the central and lateral neck. Cervical lymph node metastases occur in 30% to 40% of patients. Hematologic spread to the lungs and bones is usually found only in advanced disease.

The best treatment for papillary thyroid cancer is total thyroidectomy followed by radioiodine ablation and TSH suppression. Central and lateral modified radical neck dissections should be performed when there are nodal metastases in these compartments. Some surgeons advocate routine central compartment lymph node sampling or dissection, which can upstage papillary thyroid cancers without substantially increasing operative morbidity. External beam radiation is reserved for those rare patients who cannot tolerate an operation, have recurrent disease not amenable to resection or who do not concentrate radioiodine, or for treatment of bony metastases. Overall 10-year survival after suitable treatment is greater than 90%.

FOLLICULAR CANCER

Follicular thyroid cancers macroscopically appear as a firm, solitary nodule that is usually encapsulated. Microscopically, they have a well-formed follicular structure composed of well-differentiated cells that are indistinguishable from their benign counterpart, follicular adenoma.

TABLE 1 Fine Needle Aspiration Cytology and Associated Management

FNA Cytology Result	Diagnosis	Treatment
Benign	Benign nodule	Observation with repeat FNA in 6-12 mo
Malignant	Papillary, medullary, or anaplastic thyroid cancer	Total thyroidectomy with TSH suppression and ± adjuvant radioiodine
Indeterminate or suspicious	Follicular or Hürthle cell neoplasm	Thyroid lobectomy; return to surgery for completion thyroidectomy if final pathology shows cancer
Nondiagnostic	N/A	Repeat FNA with ultrasound guidance; Lobectomy if still nondiagnostic

FNA = fine needle aspiration; N/A = not applicable; TSH = thyroid-stimulating hormone.

CURRENT THERAPY

- Total thyroidectomy is the initial treatment for most thyroid cancers.
- Therapeutic neck dissections are performed when evidence of lymph node involvement exists.
- Radioactive iodine and thyroid-stimulating hormone suppression are effective adjuvant therapies in patients with well-differentiated thyroid cancers.
- When final pathology proves a follicular or Hürthle cell neoplasm to be malignant, completion thyroidectomy is recommended if only a lobectomy has been performed.
- Patients with medullary thyroid cancer should be screened for pheochromocytoma, which should be treated before thyroidectomy.
- External beam irradiation and multidrug chemotherapy are adjuvant therapies for patients with anaplastic thyroid cancer.
- Most thyroid cancer patients require long-term follow-up after treatment.

Diagnosis of malignancy requires histologic confirmation of vascular or capsular invasion. Metastases are hematogenous, and lymphatic spread develops late in the disease.

The optimal management for a preoperative diagnosis of follicular neoplasm smaller than 4 cm is thyroid lobectomy and isthmusectomy. If there is histologic evidence of malignancy at operation, a total thyroidectomy should be performed followed by radioactive iodine therapy and TSH suppression. If the diagnosis must be deferred to permanent sections and the final pathology identifies a follicular thyroid cancer, a second procedure for a completion thyroidectomy followed by radioiodine is usually recommended. Lymph node dissection is rarely indicated and is reserved for patients with clinical evidence of nodal metastases. The 10-year survival rate following appropriate treatment is approximately 75% to 85%.

HÜRTHLE CELL CANCER

The American Thyroid Association and the World Health Organization classify Hürthle cell carcinomas, which account for up to 5% of thyroid malignancies, as a subtype of follicular thyroid cancer. Hürthle cell cancers are often more aggressive than the typical follicular cancer, with an increased likelihood of multicentricity and lymphatic spread and a decreased tendency to concentrate radioactive iodine. Microscopically, the eosinophilic granular cytoplasm, large clear nuclei, and trabecular architecture distinguish them from typical follicular thyroid cancers.

Treatment is the same as that described for follicular thyroid cancers. Some surgeons recommend routine central-compartment lymph node sampling or dissection due to the tumor's propensity for lymphatic spread, but there is no consensus on this because good evidence of benefit is lacking. The overall 10-year survival is approximately 60% to 70% following treatment.

MEDULLARY CANCER

Medullary thyroid carcinomas (MTCs) arise from the parafollicular C-cells. These neuroendocrine cells typically secrete calcitonin and can also secrete carcinoembryonic antigen (CEA), which can be used as tumor markers for both diagnosis and monitoring response to treatment. MTCs make up approximately 5% of thyroid cancers.

Grossly, MTC appears as a hard, unencapsulated nodule in the thyroid gland. Microscopically, the tumor's round, polyhedral, and spindle-shaped cells form a variety of patterns that range from trabecular to glandlike. Sheets of amyloid are also commonly found. MTCs tend to metastasize early through the lymphatics but can also spread through the bloodstream to the liver and lungs.

MTC is usually sporadic but approximately 25% are familial. Familial MTC is an autosomal dominant disorder due to mutations in the RET (rearranged during transfection) proto-oncogene. Identification of RET mutations in family members should prompt consideration for early prophylactic thyroidectomy to avert the certain development of medullary thyroid cancer. This is usually done between the ages of 6 months and 10 years, depending on the aggressiveness of the specific RET mutation.

MTC is also one of the endocrinopathies, along with pheochromocytoma and hyperparathyroidism, that make up the multiple endocrine neoplasia (MEN) type 2 syndromes. Patients with MTC should be screened for pheochromocytoma before thyroidectomy. If pheochromocytoma is present, it should be removed before thyroidectomy.

There is widespread agreement that total thyroidectomy with routine central compartment lymph node dissection is the best treatment for MTC. A lateral neck dissection is reserved for patients with clinically involved lymph nodes in the jugular chain. Radioiodine therapy is not an option because parafollicular cells do not take up iodine. Therapy with tyrosine kinase receptor inhibitors that selectively target pathways for tumor growth and angiogenesis is under investigation.

The overall 10-year survival after treatment is approximately 70% to 80% when the disease is confined to the thyroid gland and 30% to 40% when distant metastases are present.

ANAPLASTIC CANCER

Anaplastic thyroid cancers are exceptionally aggressive and lethal. They result in more than one half the deaths attributed to thyroid malignancy every year. They are rare, accounting for up to 2% of all thyroid cancers.

Anaplastic thyroid cancers arise from dedifferentiation of papillary thyroid cancer and usually manifest as a rapidly growing central neck mass. Most patients are elderly, with locally advanced disease and nodal and distant metastases at presentation.

The three main conditions that can occur in a similar fashion are Riedel's thyroiditis, thyroid lymphoma, and parapharyngeal sarcoma. FNA cytology is often insufficient to establish a firm diagnosis and early open wedge biopsy may be needed.

Aggressive therapy with surgery, radiation, and chemotherapy is recommended. However, complete surgical resection is usually not possible, and there is no effective chemotherapy. Tracheostomy should be considered for impending obstruction rather than prophylaxis. Prognosis is poor and median survival varies from 2 to 12 months. One-year survival after multimodality therapy is less than 3%.

Follow-up

Papillary, follicular, and Hürthle cell thyroid cancers are grouped together and referred to as *well-differentiated thyroid cancers* (WDTC). They are all derived from thyroid follicular cells, respond well to surgical and adjuvant therapies, and are associated with generally favorable outcomes (Table 2). A small minority of patients, however, eventually succumbs to WDTC.

Many prognostic factors have been used to classify patients with WDTC into high-risk and low-risk groups. They include the patient's age and sex, tumor size and extent of invasion or metastasis, and completeness of surgical resection. Using these prognostic factors, several scoring systems were devised to reliably predict individual patient prognosis. Among the first was the AGES scoring system (*a*ge, histologic *g*rade of the tumor, *e*xtrathyroidal invasion and distant metastases, tumor *s*ize), which was later refined to the MACIS scoring system (*m*etastases, *a*ge, *c*ompleteness of resection, extrathyroidal *i*nvasion, tumor *s*ize). The DeGroot classification consists of class I (intrathyroidal), class II (cervical node metastases), class III (extrathyroidal extension), and class IV (distant metastases) groups. The AMES system (*a*ge, *m*etastases, *e*xtrathyroidal invasion, primary tumor *s*ize) is easy to use, but does not accurately distinguish low-risk

TABLE 2 Long-Term Follow-Up

Type	Tumor Marker(s)	Imaging	Frequency
WDTC	Tg (basal and stimulated with ↑TSH levels)	Neck U/S, ^{131}I whole body scan	6-12 mo or when Tg >10 ng/mL
Medullary	Calcitonin, CEA	CT of neck, thorax, abdomen; consider PET scan	6-12 mo or when calcitonin is newly elevated
Anaplastic	None	Neck U/S	1-3 mo

CEA = carcinoembryonic antigen; CT = computed tomography; PET = positron emission tomography; Tg = thyroglobulin; TSH = thyroid stimulating hormone; U/S = ultrasound; WDTC = well-differentiated thyroid cancer.

from high-risk patients with FTC. Arguably the most widely used is the TNM staging system (*t*umor size, *n*odal status, distant *m*etastases). None of the scoring systems can be used to guide the extent of surgical resection because the only factors known preoperatively are age and sex.

The rate of recurrence in low-risk patients with WDTC is about 10%, whereas in high-risk patients it is about 45%. Among the low-risk patients who have a recurrence, 33% to 50% die from their disease. Traditionally, radioactive iodine whole body scans (WBS) have been performed every 6 to 12 months to detect recurrent disease. However, the usefulness of serum thyroglobulin assays combined with routine neck ultrasound has decreased the need for frequent WBS.

Serum thyroglobulin is a useful marker for follow-up of patients with WDTC, because most of these tumors synthesize thyroglobulin. After successful treatment, thyroglobulin levels should be undetectable. Thyroglobulin levels that are elevated more than 10 ng/mL in the absence of thyroglobulin antibodies indicate residual thyroid tissue or persistent or recurrent thyroid cancer. Further imaging studies are then used to localize the residual tissue or cancer. For medullary thyroid cancer, elevated serum calcitonin or CEA levels after thyroidectomy should prompt appropriate imaging studies to localize persistent or recurrent disease. Persistent and recurrent disease that is detectable with imaging should be resected if it can be done with minimal morbidity.

There are no useful tumor markers for anaplastic thyroid cancer.

Summary

Thyroid cancer is increasing in frequency. The majority of thyroid cancers are slow growing and indolent, but a small minority can be aggressive and fatal. Thyroid cancer treatment depends on the characteristics of each histopathologic type. FNA biopsy can be useful in detecting the presence and type of thyroid cancer prior to the initiation of therapy. Thyroidectomy is the first step in the successful treatment of most thyroid cancers; however, the extent of surgery and subsequent adjuvant therapy varies with the subtype of thyroid cancer. Serial measurement of tumor markers coupled with neck imaging studies is useful in the long-term follow-up of patients treated for thyroid cancer.

REFERENCES

Ball DW: Medullary thyroid cancer: Therapeutic targets and molecular markers. Curr Opin Oncol 2007;19:18-23.
Chabre O, Piolat C, Dyon JF: Childhood progression of hereditary medullary thyroid cancer. N Engl J Med 2007;356:1583-1584.
Cooper DS, Doherty GM, Haugen BR, et al: Management guidelines for patients with thyroid nodules and differentiated thyroid cancer. Thyroid 2006;16:109-142.
D'Avanzo A, Ituarte P, Treseler P, et al: Prognostic scoring systems in patients with follicular thyroid cancer: A comparison of different staging systems in predicting the patient outcome. Thyroid 2004;14:453-458.
Fialkowski EA, Moley JF: Current approaches to medullary thyroid carcinoma, sporadic and familial. J Surg Oncol 2006;94:737-747.
Kebebew E, Clark OH: Differentiated thyroid cancer: "Complete" rational approach. World J Surg 2000;24:942-951.
Kim AW, Maxhimer JB, Quiros RM, et al: Surgical management of well-differentiated thyroid cancer locally invasive to the respiratory tract. J Am Coll Surg 2005;201:619-627.
Lang BH, Lo CY: Surgical options in undifferentiated thyroid carcinoma. World J Surg 2007;31:969-977.
Mazzaferri EL, Robbins RJ, Spencer CA, et al: A consensus report of the role of serum thyroglobulin as a monitoring method for low-risk patients with papillary thyroid carcinoma. J Clin Endocrinol Metab 2003;88:1433-1441.
Pacini F, DeGroot LJ: Thyroid neoplasia. In DeGroot LJ, Jameson JL, eds: Endocrinology, 5th ed, Philadelphia, Saunders, 2006, pp 2147-2180.
Phitayakorn R, McHenry CR: Follicular and Hürthle cell carcinoma of the thyroid gland. Surg Oncol Clin N Am 2006;15:603-623.
Sanders EM Jr, Livolsi VA, Brierley J, et al: An evidence-based review of poorly differentiated thyroid cancer. World J Surg 2007;31:934-945.

Pheochromocytomas

Method of
Pierre-François Plouin, MD

Pheochromocytomas (PHs) and functional paragangliomas (PGLs) are neoplasms of chromaffin tissue that synthesize catecholamines. Most of these tumors appear in the adrenal medulla (PH proper), but 10% to 20% arise in extra-adrenal chromaffin tissue (PGL). In descending order of frequency, functional PGL can develop in the Zuckerkandl body (located at the root of the upper mesenteric artery), the sympathetic plexus of the urinary bladder, the kidneys, and the heart, sympathetic ganglia in the mediastinum, the head, or the neck. Most head and neck PGLs are nonfunctional. Patients with familial diseases can have bilateral PH or PH plus functional or nonfunctional PGL.

The prevalence of PH and functional PGL is about 0.1% in patients with hypertension and 4% in patients with incidentally discovered adrenal masses or incidentalomas. Their incidence in the general population is less than 1 per 100,000 persons per year. The lifetime incidence of PH and PGL is high in familial syndromes affected by these tumors: 1% to 5% in neurofibromatosis type 1 (NF1), 15% to 20% in von Hippel–Lindau (VHL) disease, 30% to 50% in multiple endocrine neoplasia type 2 (MEN-2), and probably more than 50% in *SDHB* and *SDHD* gene mutation carriers.

Presentation

The increase in catecholamine production in patients with PH and functional PGL causes symptoms (mainly headaches, palpitations, and excessive sweating) and signs (mainly hypertension, weight loss, and diabetes) that reflect the effects of catecholamines on α- and β-adrenergic receptors. Signs and symptoms are varying and often paroxysmal due to the variable and disorderly release of catecholamines by the tumor. The typical presentation is a combination of variable hypertension with paroxysmal symptoms, either occurring spontaneously or provoked by abdominal pressure during anteflexion, micturition, or defecation.

The diagnosis of PH or PGL can be delayed for several reasons. First, these tumors are rare. Second, hypertension may be absent for long periods because active catecholamines can be converted into biologically inactive metanephrines within the tumor. Third, the symptoms and signs are nonspecific and are common to both the tumoral (in PH and PGL) and neuronal (during stress) release of catecholamines. For these reasons, the mean time from the onset of hypertension, when present, to diagnosis of the tumor exceeds 3 years. Indeed, the tumor is often discovered fortuitously during diagnostic testing for symptoms or clinical conditions not related to adrenal disease.

Presymptomatic diagnosis during the exploration of incidentalomas currently accounts for 25% of all cases. Presymptomatic diagnosis is also possible in patients with phenotypic evidence or a family history of a genetic disease associated with PH or PGL.

Diagnosis

LABORATORY TESTING

Biochemical investigation for PH or PGL is offered to hypertensive patients reporting bouts of headaches, palpitations, and sweating, those with hypertension resistant to treatment, and those with incidentalomas or with a familial disease conferring a predisposition to PH or PGL (Figure 1). The positive diagnosis of PH and functional PGL is based on the quantification of plasma or urinary metanephrines (metanephrine itself and normetanephrine), because this test is more sensitive than the quantification of urinary vanillylmandelic acid excretion or plasma concentrations of catecholamines, neuropeptide Y, or chromogranin A. The relative merits of the various determinations of plasma and urinary metanephrines are summarized in Table 1.

Patients undergoing biochemical tests for PH or PGL should be given instructions enabling them to obtain an accurate 24-hour sample of acidified urine (for urine testing) and should be told to avoid tricyclic antidepressants and acetaminophen (paracetamol,

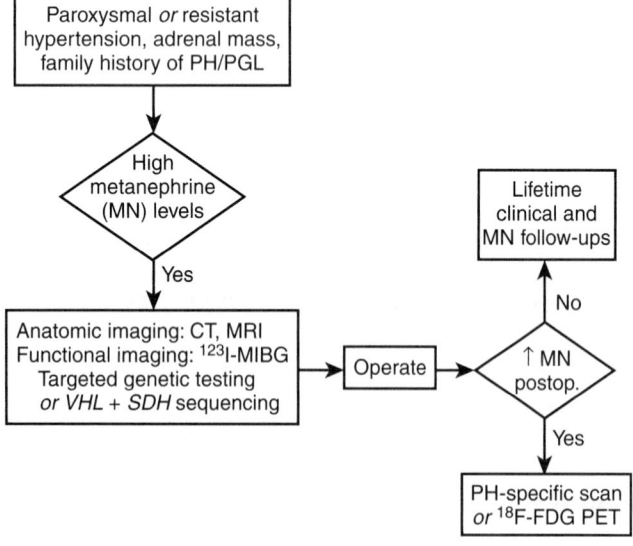

FIGURE 1. Algorithm for the initial management and long-term follow-up of patients with pheochromocytomas (PH) and secreting paragangliomas (PGL). *Abbreviations:* CT = computed tomography; ^{18}F-FDG PET = ^{18}F-fluorodeoxyglucose positron-emission tomography; MIBG = ^{123}I-metaiodobenzylguanidine; MRI = magnetic resonance imaging.

Tylenol) for 5 days, because these drugs can cause false-positive results in plasma metanephrine tests. Because accurate plasma or urinary metanephrine assays are readily available, there is no need to subject patients to the hazards of pharmacologic provocative or suppression tests.

IMAGING

Preoperative imaging tests are designed to locate the tumor and to determine whether it is single or multiple, adrenal or ectopic, benign or malignant, and isolated or present with other neoplasms in the context of familial syndromes. The combination of anatomic imaging studies based on computed tomography (CT) or magnetic resonance imaging (MRI) and radionuclide imaging studies yields a sensitivity of almost 100% for the diagnosis of catecholamine-producing tumors. CT is the most commonly used anatomic imaging technique, but MRI is preferred for children and pregnant patients.

Functional imaging with ^{123}I-metaiodobenzylguanidine (MIBG) should be carried out when possible, because ^{131}I-MIBG scintigraphy is less sensitive. Labetalol (Trandate, Normodyne) and antipsychotic drugs should be withdrawn for several days before the investigations because they reduce MIBG uptake. If no MIBG uptake is observed, mostly in cases of nonfunctional PGL, additional investigations by scintigraphy with nonspecific ligands such as somatostatin receptor scintigraphy or ^{18}F-fluorodeoxyglucose positron-emission tomography (^{18}F-FDG PET) should be carried out.

In addition to the primary tumor, imaging tests can disclose lymph node, bone, liver, or pulmonary metastases, thereby establishing the presence of malignant PH or PGL.

Differential Diagnosis

Catecholamine-secreting tumors mimic paroxysmal conditions with hypertension or cardiac rhythm disorders, particularly panic attacks, in which sympathetic activation linked to anxiety reproduces the signs and symptoms of PH. Plasma and urinary metanephrine concentrations are usually normal in these conditions. Acute cardiovascular events, such as myocardial infarction, pulmonary edema, and stroke, also induce an increase in catecholamine levels that may be sustained for several days and are associated with an increase in plasma or urinary metanephrine concentration. The diagnosis of PH or secreting PGL is excluded in these cases by the normalization of metanephrine levels 10 days after the onset of the event.

Genetic Counseling

Before 2000, three different familial and syndromic diseases were known to result in PH or PGL: MEN-2 due to *RET* gene mutations, VHL disease due to *VHL* gene mutations, and NF1 due to *NF1* mutations. The overall incidence of familial PH or PGL was estimated at 10%. The recent identification of mutations in the *VHL*, *SDHB*, and *SDHD* genes in patients with apparently sporadic tumors has increased estimates of the incidence of an underlying genetic disease in patients with PH or PGL to 20% to 25%. Familial cases are more likely to be bilateral and recurrent than sporadic cases. Carriers of *SDHB* mutations have a high risk of malignant primary tumor or metastatic recurrence. Genetic screening should therefore be offered to most patients with PH or PGL (Figure 2).

Targeted genetic testing should be offered to patients with phenotypic signs consistent with or a family history of MEN-2, VHL disease, or hereditary PGL. Phenotypic signs of MEN-2 include medullary thyroid cancer and hyperparathyroidism, signs of VHL disease include hemangioblastomas and renal or pancreatic tumors, and signs of hereditary PGL include head and neck PGLs and family history in the paternal branch. In patients with an apparently sporadic PH or PGL, priority should be given to analysis of the *VHL*, *SDHB*, and *SDHD* genes. In patients with bilateral PH, the *RET* and *VHL* should be analyzed first. Identification of a causative mutation in one affected patient should lead to presymptomatic genetic testing of the

TABLE 1 Advantages and Limitations of Determining Metanephrine and Normetanephrine in Urine or Plasma

Determinations*	Advantages	Limitations
Urinary-free and conjugated MN and NMN	Easy determination, widely available Integration of 24-h secretion Sensitivity enhanced by use of the MN+NMN-to-creatinine ratio	Need for an acidified 24-h urine collection
Plasma-free and conjugated MN and NMN	Long half-life, high concentration (25 × higher than free MN and NMN)	Includes sulfate-conjugated MN and NMN produced in the GI tract High in cases of renal failure
Plasma-free MN and NMN	Reflects tumor release of MN and NMN and the conversion of epinephrine and norepinephrine into MN and NMN Provides the best combination of sensitivity and specificity	Unstable, low concentration, technically demanding Acetaminophen-containing drugs can give false-positive results

*All these tests have sensitivities exceeding 90%.
Abbreviations: GI = gastrointestinal; MN = metanephrine; NMN = normetanephrine.

family, because early detection of small tumors in persons deemed to be at risk can reduce the morbidity of the disease. Screening for *NF1* gene mutations is feasible but rarely carried out, because the NF1 phenotype (multiple café-au-lait spots, neurofibromas, Lisch nodules, and axillary and inguinal freckling) is sufficiently clear for diagnosis of the condition in adults.

Treatment

TREATMENT OBJECTIVES

PH and functional PGL carry risks of hypersecretion and tumor growth. Surgery aims to eliminate both risks. The consequences of hypersecretion should be carefully managed before and during surgery. Primary tumor resection does not eliminate the risk of tumor persistence (in malignant tumors) or tumor recurrence (mostly in genetic diseases).

PREOPERATIVE MANAGEMENT

Blood pressure (BP) should be normalized, whenever possible, before surgery, because the incidence of perioperative complications has been consistently linked to preoperative BP. Given the variability of BP in PH or PGL, it may be useful to determine 24-hour ambulatory BP. Antihypertensive regimens aim to reduce mean office BP to less than 140/90 mm Hg or 24-hour ambulatory BP to less than 125/80 mm Hg. However, the total abolition of hypertensive paroxysms is not currently possible, and patients should undergo surgery after 1 to 2 weeks of preparation.

BP control requires α- and β-adrenergic antagonists. Because most PHs and PGLs secrete predominantly norepinephrine, an α-agonist, α-adrenergic antagonists are the cornerstone of hypertensive control. Noncompetitive α-blockers, such as phenoxybenzamine (Dibenzyline), bind covalently to α-receptors, causing an irreversible blockade. They allow stable BP control, but they increase the risk of hypotension during tumor removal and the immediate postoperative period. Competitive α-blockers, such as prazosin (Minipress) are more suitable. The initial dose of prazosin can induce a sharp drop in BP, so the dose should be gradually increased from 0.5 to 5 mg three times a day. α-Adrenergic blockade generally gives rise to tachycardia secondary to catecholamine β-receptor stimulation. This requires the subsequent addition of a β-blocker, such as 25 to 100 mg atenolol (Tenormine) daily.

If adrenergic blockade proves insufficient to control BP, then a dihydropyridine may also be administered. Arrhythmia prevention is based on β-blockade and the careful correction of hypokalemia: The chronic excess of catecholamine causes secondary hyperaldosteronism, resulting in an increase in potassium loss. The sodium intake of patients should not be restricted and diuretics should not be used.

ANESTHESIA AND SURGERY

Anesthesia and surgery in patients with PH or PGL may be complex and involve large and acute variations in BP and heart rate. Almost every possible anesthetic technique has been advocated. Perioperative safety relies primarily on correct preoperative pharmacologic control and the referral of patients to centers with extensive experience in treating the disease.

Large variations in BP and heart rate can occur during induction, intubation, peritoneal incision, and tumor handling and devascularization. Radial artery pressure and the electrocardiogram (ECG) should be monitored continuously. I generally use intravenous infusions of nicardipine (Cardene) 0.1 to 1[3] mg/min to control BP and intravenous esmolol (Brevibloc) loading infusion of 0.5 mg/kg/min over 1 minute to control arrhythmia.

Laparoscopic surgery has supplanted open surgery in the management of most cases of PH and intra-abdominal PGL. Adrenal cortex–sparing surgery may be carried out by laparoscopy in patients with hereditary forms of PH.

Postoperative and Long-term Follow-up

Plasma or urinary metanephrine concentration should be determined 10 days after surgery, to check for normalization. If metanephrine

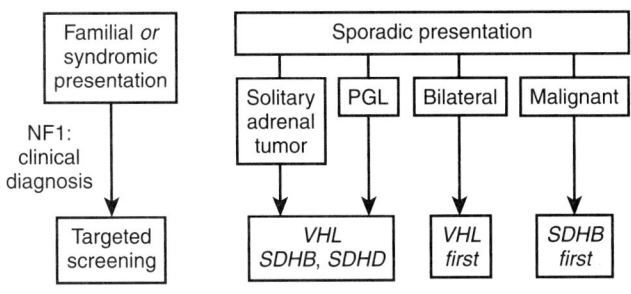

FIGURE 2. Suggested genetic screening in patients with pheochromocytomas (PH) and secreting paragangliomas (PGL). *Abbreviation:* NF1 = neurofibromatosis type 1.

---

[3]Exceeds dosage recommended by the manufacturer.

CURRENT DIAGNOSIS

- Most patients with symptomatic PH or functional PGL are hypertensive. Blood pressure typically rises when symptoms are present (mostly headaches, palpitations, and sweating).
- Presymptomatic diagnosis has become common in patients with incidentally discovered adrenal masses (incidentalomas) and in relatives of patients with symptomatic PH.
- The diagnosis of PH or functional PGL is based on the determination of metanephrines.
- Most catecholamine-secreting tumors arise in the adrenal glands (PH proper) and are easily detected by computed tomography or magnetic resonance imaging. Patients might also harbor extra-adrenal primary tumors (PGL) or distant metastases. Adrenal imaging should therefore be combined with whole-body meta-iodobenzylguanidine scintigraphy.
- One in four patients with PH or PGL has germline mutations conferring a predisposition to catecholamine-secreting tumors. The identification of a causative mutation should lead to presymptomatic genetic testing in the family.

Abbreviations: PGL = paraganglioma; PH = pheochromocytoma.

concentrations remain high, ^{123}I-MIBG scintigraphy should be performed. This technique can detect distant metastases whose MIBG uptake was masked by the primary tumor's higher metabolic activity before surgery. No MIBG uptake might occur in dedifferentiated metastases, and nonspecific radionuclide imaging may be required (see Figure 1).

Because PH and PGL can recur, patients undergoing surgery for PH or PGL should have lifelong follow-up, with checkups at least once yearly, including BP measurement and plasma or urinary metanephrine determination. In a cohort of patients undergoing surgery for PH or PGL, the 10-year probability of recurrence—defined as the reappearance of the disease after eradication of the tumor had been confirmed by negative biochemical and imaging tests—was 16%. Patients with recurrences were younger, had larger tumors, and were more likely to have familial disease or bilateral or extra-adrenal PGL than patients with no recurrence. Recurrences were malignant in one in two patients.

CURRENT THERAPY

- Patients with catecholamine-secreting tumors should be referred to centers with extensive experience in the anesthetic and surgical management of the disease.
- Blood pressure should be normalized before surgery, using α-adrenergic and possibly β-adrenergic antagonists.
- Most PHs and many PGLs can be resected laparoscopically.
- Adrenal cortex–sparing surgery is feasible in patients with bilateral PH.
- PH and PGL can recur. Patients should be subject to life-long follow-up, with checkups at least yearly, including blood pressure measurement and metanephrine determination.

Abbreviations: PGL = paraganglioma; PH = pheochromocytoma.

Malignant PH or PGL is compatible with prolonged survival, with symptom-free intervals lasting from months to decades. In 54 patients with malignant PH or PGL followed at my center, the 5-year and 10-year probabilities of survival were 0.75 and 0.52, respectively.

In cases of small recurrences with an accessible vascular pedicle, surgical excision may be preceded or replaced by therapeutic embolization. In cases in which soft-tissue or skeletal metastases are too widespread for surgery or embolization, several palliative therapies may be considered. Pharmacologic treatment aimed at the long-term blockade of catecholamine synthesis with α-methyl-*p*-tyrosine (Demser) 1 to 4 g/day in divided doses can improve the patient's quality of life, but it has no effect on tumor progression. Conventional radiotherapy can provide effective palliation in cases of painful metastases. Metabolic radiotherapy with ^{131}I-MIBG and chemotherapy can provide clinical, hormonal, and, in some cases, tumoral improvement.

REFERENCES

Diner EK, Franks ME, Behari A, et al: Partial adrenalectomy: The National Cancer Institute experience. Urology 2005;66:19-23.
Eisenhofer G, Bornstein SR, Brouwers FM, et al: Malignant pheochromocytoma: Current status and initiatives for future progress. Endocr Relat Cancer 2004;11:423-436.
Ilias I, Pacak K: Current approaches and recommended algorithm for the diagnostic localization of pheochromocytoma. J Clin Endocrinol Metab 2004;89:479-491.
Lenders JW, Pacak K, Walther MM, et al: Biochemical diagnosis of pheochromocytoma: Which test is best? JAMA. 2002;287:1427-1434.
Plouin PF, Duclos JM, Soppelsa F, et al: Factors associated with perioperative morbidity and mortality in patients with pheochromocytoma: Analysis of 165 operations at a single center. J Clin Endocrinol Metab 2001;86:1480-1486.
Plouin PF, Gimenez-Roqueplo AP: The genetic basis of pheochromocytoma: Who to screen and how? Nat Clin Pract Endocrinol Metab 2006;2:60-61.
Prys-Roberts C: Phaeochromocytoma: Recent progress in its management. Br J Anaesth 2000;85:44-57.

Thyroiditis

Method of
Anthony P. Weetman, MD, DSc

Thyroiditis simply means inflammation of the thyroid gland, and it arises from a number of different causes. Clinically these are best classified by the tempo of inflammation: acute, subacute, or chronic. Mild to moderate focal thyroiditis, in which there is a patchy infiltration of the thyroid gland by lymphocytes, is so common (in ~15% of all autopsy specimens) that it has little clinical significance; in only a small fraction of such patients does disease progress to a chronic thyroiditis and destruction of thyroid tissue. Similarly, a focal thyroiditis is often found adjacent to (or even within) benign or malignant neoplasms of thyroid.

Acute Thyroiditis

BACKGROUND

Acute (suppurative) thyroiditis is a rare condition caused by a suppurative infection of the thyroid through the bloodstream, lymphatics, trauma, a persistent thyroglossal duct, or most commonly, extension from nearby infection. The latter typically arises through the piriform sinus, an anomalous remnant of the fourth branchial pouch, usually on the left side. This is the main cause of acute

CURRENT DIAGNOSIS

- Thyroiditis can be classified as acute, subacute, or chronic, with pain as a hallmark of the first two types.
- Silent thyroiditis occurs after pregnancy or following drug treatment.
- A combination of thyroid function testing and thyroid peroxidase antibody measurement, supplemented by erythrocyte sedimentation rate and thyroid radionuclide uptake is sufficient to establish a diagnosis in most cases.
- Thyrotoxicosis in patients with thyroiditis is transient, and subsequent hypothyroidism should be anticipated.

CURRENT THERAPY

- Antibiotics and subsequent surgery are generally required for acute bacterial thyroiditis.
- Most patients with subacute thyroiditis can be managed with nonsteroidal antiinflammatory drugs; around one third require a short course of prednisolone.
- Thyrotoxicosis following destructive thyroiditis is treated with propranolol (Inderal)[1]; antithyroid drugs are useless in this setting.
- Levothyroxine (Synthroid, Levoxyl) remains the treatment of choice for chronic thyroiditis associated with hypothyroidism.

[1]Not FDA approved for this indication.

thyroiditis in children and young adults; a long-standing goiter, degeneration in a carcinoma, and immunosuppression are additional risk factors.

Virtually any bacterium can cause acute thyroiditis. The most common are *Staphylococcus aureus*, *Streptococci* species, *Klebsiella pneumoniae*, and *Escherichia coli*. In immunosuppressed patients, including those with AIDS, unusual organisms can invade the thyroid, including *Aspergillus*, *Candida*, and *Coccidioides* species and *Pneumocystis jiroveci*. In rare instances, tuberculosis can affect the thyroid, but the picture then is usually one of subacute thyroiditis.

The dominant clinical features are pain in the thyroid radiating to the ear, tenderness and erythema over the gland, fever, dysphagia, respiratory symptoms, and malaise. Features of septicemia may be present, as may lymphadenopathy and a local thrombophlebitis. The differential diagnosis for thyroid pain includes subacute and, rarely, chronic thyroiditis, hemorrhage into a cyst, and lymphoma. Clinical features help in the diagnosis, and simple investigations usually confirm the clinical suspicion.

TREATMENT

Treatment is with high-dose antibiotics selected on the basis of the microbiology results from fine-needle aspiration biopsy. Surgical drainage of any abscess is indicated when pus cannot be fully removed by aspiration. Complications of acute thyroiditis include tracheal obstruction, retropharyngeal abscess, mediastinitis, and internal jugular venous thrombosis. Any piriform sinus should be located (usually by barium swallow study 2 months after the acute episode) and excised to prevent a recurrence; a thyroid lobectomy is usually needed for this.

Subacute Thyroditis

BACKGROUND

Subacute thyroiditis (de Quervain's, viral, or granulomatous thyroiditis) has a variable incidence, depending on region. In North America the incidence is 5 cases per 100,000 population per year. It is possible that it is overlooked in areas of apparently low incidence. Three times more women are affected than men, with a median incidence around the age of 45 years, and HLA-B35 is a predisposing genetic factor.

Many viruses have been implicated, especially Coxsackievirus, influenza, measles, mumps, and Epstein–Barr virus. There is no need to attempt identification serologically.

The main clinical features are a painful and tender goitrous thyroid with fluctuating thyroid hormone levels. The pain can be in one or both thyroid lobes. Occasionally, a nodular form can be detected on palpation.

Patients usually have a phase of thyrotoxicosis (caused by release of stored hormone from the damaged gland) lasting up to 4 weeks, followed by a phase of hypothyroidism of 1 to 3 months and then recovery. Many patients describe a prodromal phase of systemic upset or upper respiratory tract infection. The diagnosis is confirmed by the high erythrocyte sedimentation rate (ESR) and low isotope uptake.

TREATMENT

Mild cases do not require treatment except analgesics, usually nonsteroidal antiinflammatory drugs. Severe disease (around one third of cases) warrants treatment with prednisolone at a dose of 30 to 40 mg/day initially. Depending on the clinical response and sedimentation rate, this is gradually tapered after 1 to 2 weeks so that steroids are stopped after 4 to 6 weeks. Patients' thyroid function should be monitored closely (every 1 to 2 weeks).

During a phase of symptomatic thyrotoxicosis, propranolol (Inderal),[1] 20 to 40 mg three to four times a day, is useful for controlling the symptoms. Antithyroid drugs (methimazole [Tapazole], propylthiouracil [PTU]) are not effective in this situation. Subsequent symptomatic hypothyroidism is treated with levothyroxine (Synthroid, Levothroid, Levoxyl) 50 to 100 μg/day, but this should be withdrawn after 6 to 8 weeks because the phase is typically transient. However, patients with preexisting thyroid abnormalities can develop permanent hypothyroidism after subacute thyroiditis (5%-10% of cases), and therefore full recovery of thyroid function must be established by testing.

Recurrences occur in around 5% of cases and are dealt with in the same way as the initial attack, although prolonging prednisolone treatment by 2 to 4 weeks may be useful.

Silent Thyroiditis

A similar pattern of subacute thyroid dysfunction without thyroid pain is called *silent thyroiditis*. This has an autoimmune etiology and occurs most distinctly 3 to 6 months after pregnancy in women with thyroid peroxidase antibodies before delivery. Treatment for thyroid dysfunction is again with propranolol for thyrotoxicosis and levothyroxine for the usually transient hypothyroidism; steroids are not needed. Thyroxine treatment is discontinued 1 year after delivery and the TSH is checked after 6 weeks to verify the patient is euthyroid.

Postpartum thyroiditis is a risk factor for the development of future permanent hypothyroidism. Affected women should therefore be screened annually for this and should be warned that the disease may well recur in future pregnancies. The appropriateness of screening all pregnant women for thyroid peroxidase antibodies in the first trimester is not yet clear except in women with type 1 diabetes mellitus, who are at particular risk of developing postpartum thyroiditis. In such women, the presence of thyroid antibodies before delivery should lead to careful monitoring of postpartum thyroid function.

[1]Not FDA approved for this indication.

Chronic (Autoimmune) Thyroiditis

BACKGROUND

Hypothyroidism caused by autoimmunity affects approximately 1% of women and 0.1% of men. However, there is a much higher prevalence of subclinical autoimmune thyroiditis shown by the presence of sustained, elevated circulating thyroid-stimulating hormone (TSH) levels with normal free thyroxine levels, with or without accompanying thyroid peroxidase or thyroglobulin antibodies. This condition often comes to light during screening for nonspecific symptoms such as fatigue or weight gain.

Some patients have a goiter of variable size that is usually hard and often irregular (bosselated); this is Hashimoto's, or goitrous, thyroiditis. At the opposite end of the pathologic spectrum is atrophic thyroiditis or primary myxedema in which the thyroid is replaced by fibrous tissue and the only clinical sign of the destructive process is the development of hypothyroidism. These patients may have antibodies that block the TSH receptor, but these are neither frequent nor unique in atrophic thyroiditis.

TREATMENT

Overt hypothyroidism resulting from chronic thyroiditis is treated with levothyroxine. There is no role normally for thyroid extract or for liothyronine (triiodothyronine, T_3) supplementation (Thyrolar, liotrix) or substitution (Cytomel), inasmuch as levothyroxine is converted smoothly and physiologically to T_3, whereas the short half-life of liothyronine leads to peaks and troughs of circulating T_3. Several recent trials have failed to confirm initially promising results from the addition of triiodothyronine to levothyroxine, and such current formulations of treatment can lead to excessive T_3 levels, with the potential for adverse effects on bone and the heart.

In otherwise healthy patients younger than 60 years with overt hypothyroidism, I start levothyroxine at 50 to 100 μg a day, but in those older than 60 years or with ischemic heart disease, the usual starting dose is 12.5 to 25 μg a day, increasing every 2 weeks by 25-μg increments. In all cases, the aim is to normalize the TSH level, although rarely this proves impossible in patients whose angina is worsened by thyroxine replacement. Propranolol[1] or other β-blockers help minimize this adverse effect.

If the TSH is maintained in the reference range, there are no adverse effects. I check TSH levels only 2 to 3 months after changing dose because it can take this length of time for symptoms and TSH levels to normalize. The same applies if the commercial preparation of levothyroxine is changed. Once the desired dose is achieved, TSH levels need to be checked only annually. It is unusual for patients to need more than 200 μg of levothyroxine a day. In my experience an elevated (and usually fluctuating) TSH level in patients taking higher doses usually indicates poor compliance, although malabsorption syndromes and certain drugs—such as colestipol (Colestid), cholestyramine sucralfate (Questran), ferrous sulfate (Feosol), aluminum hydroxide (Amphojel), phenytoin (Dilantin), activated charcoal (CharcoAid), rifampicin (rifampin, Rifadin), and hormone replacement therapy—can interfere with absorption or metabolism.

There is controversy about the optimal management of subclinical hypothyroidism. The risk of progression to overt hypothyroidism is highest in patients with both an elevated TSH and positive thyroid antibodies, and in my view it is worth treating these patients and those whose TSH is higher than 10 mU/L with levothyroxine (usually 25-50 μg initially) from the outset. In those with an elevated TSH but no thyroid antibodies, one option is a 3-month trial of levothyroxine, and if any symptomatic improvement occurs, to continue with this. If there is no improvement or the patient chooses not to have treatment, an annual check of thyroid function should be arranged to deal with the risk of progression to overt hypothyroidism.

The goiter of Hashimoto's thyroiditis usually shrinks with levothyroxine. Surgery is only rarely needed to control the goiter. Any focal irregularity in the goiter raises the suspicion of malignancy; such hard nodules are sometimes found in Hashimoto's thyroiditis and should be investigated, initially by aspiration biopsy. Pain suggests lymphoma, which is a rare complication of autoimmune thyroiditis. Very rarely is the thyroid tender in uncomplicated Hashimoto's thyroiditis, and this may be associated with an elevated ESR. Corticosteroids may be used but are sometimes unhelpful, and surgery may be needed in extreme cases.

Drug-Induced Thyroiditis

Autoimmune thyroiditis can be precipitated by lithium, excess iodide, or recombinant cytokines such as interferon (IFN)-α, interleukin-2, and granulocyte-macrophage colony-stimulating factor (GM-CSF). Such patients usually have thyroid peroxidase and other thyroid antibodies before treatment, and screening for these, as well as measuring serum TSH, should be undertaken before starting these drugs. Regular monitoring of TSH thereafter is also indicated.

Thyroxine replacement should be given and adjusted to maintain a normal TSH level. Treatment with amiodarone (Cordarone), lithium, and IFN-α can be continued. Amiodarone can cause both hypothyroidism, readily managed by levothyroxine, and thyrotoxicosis, the latter resulting either from a destructive process or from excess iodide supply that precipitates hyperthyroidism. Amiodarone-induced thyrotoxicosis can be very difficult to manage and necessitates specialist advice. Corticosteroids, potassium perchlorate, antithyroid drugs, and even surgery might be needed to control the disease, whereas stopping amiodarone has no immediate impact because of the long half-life of the drug. A painful but transient thyroiditis can occur 1 to 2 weeks after radioiodine for hyperthyroidism. It responds to simple analgesics, or corticosteroids if severe.

Riedel's Thyroiditis

Riedel's thyroiditis is a rare condition of unknown etiology that is caused by fibrosis of the thyroid, leading to a woodlike, hard mass often extending outside the thyroid and involving any of the adjacent structures. There is an association with idiopathic fibrosis elsewhere (retroperitoneum, orbit, mediastinum, biliary tree, lung). The condition is often detected because of suspicion of thyroid malignancy. Aspiration biopsy typically yields no specimen, and diagnosis requires open biopsy. Thyroxine is useful only if there is hypothyroidism, and corticosteroids are ineffective. The condition runs an unpredictable course, with a slow progression in many cases, and surgery should be reserved only for patients with esophageal or tracheal compression. Tamoxifen (Soltamox)[1] treatment 20 mg twice daily has been successful in individual cases; due to the rarity of the disease, there have been no controlled trials of treatment.

---

[1]Not FDA approved for this indication.

REFERENCES

Basaria S, Cooper DS: Amiodarone and the thyroid. Am J Med 2005;118: 706-714.

Escobar-Morreale HF, Botella-Carretero JI, Escobar del Rey F, Morreale de Escobar G: Treatment of hypothyroidism with combinations of levothyroxine plus liothyronine. J Clin Endocrinol Metab 2005;90:4946-4954.

Fatourechi V, Aniszewski JP, Fatourechi GZ, et al: Clinical features and outcome of subacute thyroiditis in an incidence cohort: Olmsted County, Minnesota, study. J Clin Endocrinol Metab 2003;88:2100-2105.

Jung YJ, Schaub CR, Rhodes R, et al: A case of Riedel's thyroiditis treated with tamoxifen: Another successful outcome. Endocr Pract 2004;10:483-486.

Nicholson WK, Robinson KA, Smallridge RC, et al: Prevalence of postpartum thyroid dysfunction: A quantitative review. Thyroid 2006;16:573-582.

Surks MI, Ortiz E, Daniels GH, et al: Subclinical thyroid disease: Scientific review and guidelines for diagnosis and management. JAMA 2004;291:228-238.

Weetman AP: The thyroid gland and disorders of thyroid function. In Warrell DA, Cox TM, Firth JD, Benz EJ (eds): Oxford Textbook of Medicine, Vol 2. Oxford, Oxford University Press, 2003, pp 209-224.

SECTION 10

The Urogenital Tract

Bacterial Infections of the Male Urinary Tract

Method of
John N. Krieger, MD

Urinary tract infections (UTIs) include a wide clinical spectrum whose common denominator is bacterial invasion of the genitourinary organs and tissues. Any portion of the urinary tract may be involved from the renal cortex to the urethral meatus. UTI can predominate at a single site, such as the bladder (cystitis), prostate (prostatitis), epididymis (epididymitis), kidneys (pyelonephritis), or perinephric space (perinephric abscess). When any of its parts has become infected, the entire urinary tract is placed at risk for bacterial invasion.

The great majority of UTIs occur by the ascending route. Bacteria from the fecal flora colonize the perineum and then ascend via the urethra to involve the bladder, the ureter, and the kidneys. On occasion, hematogenous dissemination can result in bacterial seeding of the urinary tract. Classic examples of such hematogenous infection are genitourinary tuberculosis or staphylococcal infection of a renal cyst (historically known as a *renal carbuncle*). On rare occasions, the urinary tract may be involved by infection from contiguous structures. For example, patients with diverticulitis or appendicitis occasionally develop abscesses or fistulae that involve the urinary tract.

Distinguishing Complicated from Uncomplicated Infections

The first step in evaluating a patient is to distinguish uncomplicated (medical) infections from complicated (surgical) infections. An uncomplicated UTI occurs in the absence of underlying structural, functional, or neurologic disorders of the urinary tract. Uncomplicated UTIs usually respond promptly to appropriate antimicrobial therapy. Anatomic evaluation and imaging studies are seldom indicated in patients with uncomplicated UTIs.

In contrast, complicated UTIs occur when the urinary tract has been repeatedly invaded by bacteria, leaving residual inflammation or—in cases accompanied by obstruction—stones, foreign bodies, or neurologic conditions that interfere with urinary drainage. Antimicrobial therapy alone is markedly less effective in complicated UTIs than in uncomplicated UTIs. Managing patients with complicated infections often requires anatomic evaluation and imaging studies. An important differential point is that patients with complicated UTIs tend to have persistence of bacteria within the urinary tract in the face of antimicrobial agents to which the bacteria appear to be sensitive in laboratory tests. Often, it is necessary to correct an underlying obstructive lesion or voiding problem to clear the infection.

The ideal goal of UTI therapy is total elimination of the infecting organism from the urinary tract. This is a realistic goal for patients with uncomplicated UTIs. However, achieving this goal can prove difficult in patients with complicated UTIs whose underlying abnormalities cannot be corrected. For example, it is often impossible to achieve long-standing resolution of bacteriuria in patients who require indwelling catheters or who have functional obstruction of their voiding mechanisms. In such cases, resolution of symptoms directly related to UTI is the only practical therapeutic goal.

Natural History

During infancy, the incidence of symptomatic UTIs is higher in boys than in girls. In part, this has been related to male circumcision status. It appears that bacteria can adhere to the prepuce of uncircumcised boys, providing access to the urinary tract. Neonatal circumcision appears to reduce the UTI rate in boys by about 90%. After the neonatal period, symptomatic UTIs in boys and men are distinctly uncommon until middle age. This contrasts dramatically with UTI rates in girls and women, who experience increasing rates of both symptomatic and asymptomatic infections with a marked increase following initiation of sexual activity, then a continued gradual rise with increasing age. Asymptomatic bacteriuria is also distinctly unusual in male patients compared with female patients.

Well-documented UTIs in boys mandate thorough urologic investigation. This is because of the high prevalence of structural urinary tract abnormalities in boys with UTIs. Often, UTI represents the key diagnostic presentation for major abnormalities of the urinary tract. For example, vesicoureteral reflux of urine, posterior urethral valves, and other major structural abnormalities often manifest initially with bacterial UTIs. Early diagnosis and appropriate therapy offer the best chance for preservation of maximal renal function. Unfortunately, the developing kidneys are very susceptible to continued renal scarring, which may be progressive despite appropriate treatment.

Structural urinary tract abnormalities remain a major cause of renal failure in children. Morbidity may be minimized by appropriate evaluation and therapy. Our choice for evaluation of a boy with a urinary tract infection is the combination of renal ultrasound to evaluate the upper urinary tract plus a voiding cystourethrogram to evaluate the lower urinary tract. Voiding cystourethrography should be obtained after resolution of the initial infection, because dilation of the upper urinary tract may be exaggerated after a recent UTI.

Because UTIs are unusual in young men, there are few well-done natural history studies in this population. In young men with UTIs who have no obvious neurologic or structural abnormalities, sexual intercourse, particularly among homosexual men or heterosexual men who practice insertive anal intercourse, may be a risk factor. The overall contribution of these practices to bacterial UTIs in men is uncertain.

Traditional urologic teaching is to carry out a thorough evaluation for structural abnormalities in such patients, including radiographic studies and cystourethroscopy. However, our published experience suggests that previously healthy college-age men with well-documented UTIs have a low rate of structural genitourinary tract abnormalities. A uroflow study and postvoid residual urine determination by ultrasound are adequate to screen for structural abnormalities in young men whose UTIs resolve. We reserve cystoscopy for patients whom we determine to be at risk for significant abnormalities on the basis of these screening studies and a thorough physical examination. The other major risk factors for UTIs in men are instrumentation of the urinary tract and bacterial prostatitis.

Diagnosis and Localization

Accurate diagnosis is prerequisite for appropriate UTI therapy. Therefore, we recommend culture and sensitivity testing of urine specimens from any male patient with symptoms or signs suggesting a UTI. In patients who do not have obstructive lesions, stasis, stones, or foreign bodies, recurrent and persistent bacterial UTIs are often related to bacterial prostatitis. Segmented localization cultures can be used to differentiate cystitis and urethritis from bacterial prostatitis. The procedure should be carried out at a time when the patient does not have bacteriuria.

My procedure for lower urinary tract localization is outlined briefly. After cleaning the glans with sterile water, the first-void urine (initial 5-10 mL of voided urine) is collected in a sterile container. Next, a midstream specimen is obtained. The patient is asked to stop voiding. Prostatic fluid is expressed by digital rectal prostate massage. The post–prostate massage urine (next 5-10 mL voided after the massage) is then collected. Culture and sensitivity testing are then carried out on each of these four specimens. It is critical to ensure that the clinical microbiology laboratory is aware of the purpose of these studies so that they will evaluate low concentrations of uropathogens that may be present in the localization cultures.

Diagnosis of chronic bacterial prostatitis can be made if the post–prostate massage urine specimen or the expressed prostatic secretion contains a 10-fold or greater increase in the concentration of the uropathogen compared with that in the first-void urine specimen. In patients with well-documented bacterial prostatitis, the causative organism is identical to the uropathogen causing recurrent UTI episodes.

It is important to recognize that only a small minority of men presenting with symptoms of prostatitis fit into the acute or chronic bacterial prostatitis categories. The great majority of patients with symptoms of prostatitis are classified in the chronic prostatitis/chronic pelvic pain category. In contrast to the recognized benefit of therapy for patients with acute and chronic bacterial prostatitis, the role of antimicrobial therapy and other treatments has not been defined for men with symptoms of chronic prostatitis/chronic pelvic pain syndrome.

Treatment

There are three keys to successful UTI therapy. First, eliminate or control predisposing factors, if possible. For example, we are often asked to manage resistant urinary infections in long-term care patients with indwelling catheters. One approach is to change their bladder management from a chronic indwelling catheter to an intermittent self- or assisted-catheterization program. Other examples include removal or correction of obstructing lesions, stones, or strictures to improve drainage of the urinary tract. These measures may be successful in eliminating the focus of infection, even with no antimicrobial therapy. Second, eradicate the infection as soon as possible to prevent colonization of the prostate and other structures. Third, ensure resolution of the UTI by obtaining cultures during or immediately after therapy and at follow-up 1 to 2 months after therapy.

UNCOMPLICATED INFECTIONS

Uncomplicated infections generally manifest with symptoms of bacterial cystitis, such as the combination of urinary frequency, urgency, dysuria, nocturia, suprapubic discomfort, low-back pain, or hematuria. Systemic symptoms of fever, chills, and rigor are absent. Urine culture confirms the diagnosis, with *Escherichia coli* being the most common pathogen. Uncomplicated infections, including those introduced by a single or short course of indwelling urethral catheterization, generally respond promptly to a short course of antimicrobial therapy. The infection can persist and become difficult to eradicate if the prostate becomes colonized or if the patient has a stone or structural abnormality of the urinary tract. Thus, an effort should be made to eliminate predisposing factors while routine therapy is guided by in vitro susceptibility tests.

CURRENT DIAGNOSIS

- UTIs include a wide clinical spectrum.
- Infection at any site in the urinary tract places the entire system at risk.
- The critical clinical issue is to distinguish uncomplicated (medical) from complicated (surgical) infections.
- Anatomic evaluation and imaging studies are seldom indicated for patients with uncomplicated UTIs.
- Well-documented UTIs in boys require thorough urologic investigation because of the high prevalence of structural urinary tract abnormalities.
- We recommend culture and sensitivity testing of urine specimens for any male patient with symptoms or signs suggesting a UTI.
- In contrast, we discourage routine screening urine cultures in long-term care patients who have no localizing signs or symptoms suggesting a UTI.

UTI = urinary tract infection.

CURRENT THERAPY

- The optimal goal of therapy is to eliminate the infecting organism from the urinary tract.
- Antimicrobial therapy alone is less effective for patients with complicated UTIs than for patients with uncomplicated UTIs.
- Managing patients with complicated UTIs often requires anatomic evaluation and imaging studies.
- For patients with complicated UTIs it is often necessary to eliminate or control predisposing factors.
- Rapid eradication of the infection can limit the potential for infection of adjacent structures.
- Ensure elimination of the infection by repeating urine cultures.
- A prolonged course of antimicrobial therapy may prove necessary for patients with persistent infections.

UTI = urinary tract infection.

TABLE 1 Oral Antimicrobial Agents Prescribed for Urinary Tract Infections in Men

Agent	Dosage
Fluoroquinolones	
Ciprofloxacin (Cipro)	250-500 mg bid
Ciprofloxacin (CiproXR)	500-1000 mg qd
Lomefloxacin (Maxaquin)	400 mg qd
Levofloxacin (Levaquin LEVA-pak)	500-750 mg qd
Ofloxacin (Floxin)	200-400 mg bid[3]
Norfloxacin (Noroxin)	400 mg bid
Combination Agents	
Trimethoprim-sulfamethoxazole (Bactrim, Septra, Bactrim DS, Septra DS)	160 mg trimethoprim, 800 mg sulfamethoxazole bid
Amoxicillin-clavulanate (Augmentin)	500-875 mg amoxicillin, 125mg clavulonate bid
Other Antimicrobials	
Nitrofurantoin (Macrobid)	50-100 mg bid
Nitrofurantoin (Macrodantin)	50-100 mg qid

[3]Exceeds dosage recommended by the manufacturer.

I prefer oral therapy with one of the agents listed in Table 1. In the Pacific northwest, bacteria causing urinary tract infections have developed substantial resistance to trimethoprim-sulfamethoxazole (Bactrim). Therefore, I usually initiate empiric therapy with a quinolone. Nitrofurantoin (Macrodantin) remains highly effective and is an attractive alternative drug. In general, I recommend that the duration of therapy be at least 2 weeks, although only limited data address this point in male patients.

COMPLICATED INFECTIONS

Patients with systemic signs or those with a history of structural or neurologic abnormalities merit anatomic and functional investigation of the urinary tract. Antimicrobial therapy alone might fail to cure infection and urosepsis can develop unless there is specific management of the underlying problem. My initial choice for evaluating these patients is either computed tomography (CT) with contrast or an excretory urogram with postvoid film. If a renal or retroperitoneal abscess is suspected, computed tomographic scanning has proved superior to the other modalities for diagnosis. In contrast, I prefer transrectal ultrasound for evaluation of possible prostatic abscesses.

Prolonged courses of therapy are indicated for patients with persistent infections, Often, I have used 3 to 4 months of therapy in this situation. In patients with chronic bacterial prostatitis, elderly patients, or those in nursing homes, continuous therapy may be necessary to suppress bacteriuria, even though eradication can prove impossible. Thus, for patients with recurrent or complicated infections, I recommend an attempt to eradicate the focus of infection, following thorough evaluation of the urinary tract. The therapy is usually with the drugs listed in Table 1. My first choice for curative therapy is usually a quinolone. For patients with persistent or frequently relapsing infections, I consider long-term therapy (months or years) using low dosages of antimicrobial drugs for prophylaxis or suppression. In this situation, my choice is usually either trimethoprim-sulfamethoxazole (Bactrim) or nitrofurantoin (Macrodantin).

PROSTATITIS

Acute and chronic bacterial prostatitis can manifest with local urinary tract symptoms characteristic of bacterial cystitis or with systemic signs and symptoms. Acute bacterial prostatitis can manifest with the sudden onset of chills, fever, malaise, and low back and perineal pain, as well as difficulty with urination. On rectal examination, the prostate is tense and exquisitely tender. Excessive palpation can induce septicemia.

For patients who require hospitalization, my initial choice is the combination of a β-lactam drug and an aminoglycoside until the results of antimicrobial sensitivity testing are available. Following parenteral therapy, the patient is managed with continued antimicrobial therapy for at least 4 weeks, usually employing a quinolone. Patients with acute bacterial prostatitis usually respond well to a variety of antimicrobial agents that penetrate an acutely inflamed prostate. Many of these agents are not effective in chronic bacterial prostatitis.

In contrast to acute bacterial prostatitis, chronic bacterial prostatitis is often insidious in onset. Patients usually have recurrent symptomatic UTIs and, sometimes, recurrent episodes of acute prostatitis. Between symptomatic episodes, patients may be totally asymptomatic. Diagnosis depends on the localization cultures described earlier. Treatment must be prolonged, because diffusion of many antimicrobial agents into the uninflamed prostate is poor.

My initial choice is usually a quinolone, with trimethoprim-sulfamethoxazole (Septra, Bactrim) as a second-choice agent. Carbenicillin indanyl sodium (Geocillin) is also approved for this indication, but it has not been particularly effective in my hands.

It is important to avoid confusing bacterial prostatitis with chronic prostatitis/chronic pelvic pain syndrome. This is the most common category of symptomatic prostatitis. A critical distinguishing point is that patients with chronic prostatitis/chronic pelvic pain syndrome do not have bacteriuria and they have negative bacterial localization cultures.

LONG-TERM CARE PATIENTS

My approach to managing UTI differs in long-term care patients, including those with incontinence and indwelling urinary catheters or other devices. In such patients, chronic asymptomatic bacterial colonization should not be treated. It is impossible to sterilize the urine permanently in such men. Furthermore, resistant organisms will likely emerge, making subsequent therapy difficult. I treat such patients only if they develop acute symptoms referable to the urinary tract or before genitourinary tract procedures. I strongly recommend against obtaining screening cultures in long-term care patients because these cultures often lead to unnecessary therapy that selects resistant bacterial flora. Further, there is evidence that bacterial colonization with relatively benign strains can inhibit establishment of symptomatic infections caused by more virulent bacteria.

REFERENCES

Abarbanel J, Engelstein D, Lask D, et al: Urinary tract infection in men younger than 45 years of age: Is there a need for urologic investigation? Urology 2003;62:27-29.

Andrews SJ, Brooks PT, Hanbury DC, et al: Ultrasonography and abdominal radiography versus intravenous urography in investigation of urinary tract infection in men: Prospective incident cohort study. BMJ 2002;324:454-456.

Bjerklund Johansen T: Diagnosis and imaging in urinary tract infections. Curr Opin Urol 2002;12:39-43.

Craig JC, Knight JF, Sureshkumar P, et al: Effect of circumcision on incidence of urinary tract infection in preschool boys. J Pediatr 1996;128:23-27.

Griebling TL: Urologic diseases in America project: Trends in resource use for urinary tract infections in men. J Urol 2005;173:1288-1294.

Hummers-Pradier E, Ohse AM, Koch M, et al: Urinary tract infection in men. Int J Clin Pharmacol Ther 2004;42:360-366.

Johansen TE: The role of imaging in urinary tract infections. World J Urol 2004;22:392-398.

Krieger JN, Nyberg L Jr, Nickel JC: NIH consensus definition and classification of prostatitis. JAMA 1999;282:236-237.

Krieger JN, Ross SO, Simonsen JM: Urinary tract infections in healthy university men. J Urol 1993;149:1046-1048.

Naber KG: Levofloxacin in the treatment of urinary tract infections and prostatitis. J Chemother 2004;16(Suppl 2):18-21.

Nicolle LESHEA Long-Term-Care Committee: Urinary tract infections in long-term-care facilities. Infect Control Hosp Epidemiol 2001;22:167-175.

Sunden F, Hakansson L, Ljunggren E, et al: Bacterial interference—is deliberate colonization with *Escherichia coli* 83972 an alternative treatment for patients with recurrent urinary tract infection? Int J Antimicrob Agents 28 Suppl 2006;1:S26-S29.

Ulleryd P, Zackrisson B, Aus G, et al: Selective urological evaluation in men with febrile urinary tract infection. BJU Int 2001;88:15-20.

Wagenlehner FM, Naber KG: Current challenges in the treatment of complicated urinary tract infections and prostatitis. Clin Microbiol Infect 2006;12(Suppl 3):67-80.

Urinary Tract Infections in Women

Method of
Burke A. Cunha, MD

General Concepts

Urinary tract infections (UTIs) are common in adult women. The two major clinical manifestations of UTIs in adult women are cystitis or pyelonephritis. Young adult women may also present with so-called dysuria pyuria syndrome (abacteriuric cystitis), previously known as acute urethral syndrome, as outpatients. Hospitalized compromised female hosts with cystitis may be complicated by bacteremia or ascending infection. Renal abscess may complicate pyelonephritis in normal or compromised female hosts.

Cystitis Versus Pyelonephritis

The therapeutic approach to UTIs in adult women depends on accurate localization of the site of infection in the urinary tract. The most common clinical problem is differentiating cystitis from pyelonephritis. Patients with acute bacterial cystitis present with dysuria and frequency, which may or may not be accompanied by suprapubic discomfort or lower back pain. The fever accompanying cystitis is ≤ to 38.9°C (102°F) and is not usually associated with chills. The clinical manifestation of cystitis is confirmed by finding pyuria and significant bacteriuria, (i.e., $\geq 10^6$ CFU/mL) in such patients. The urinalysis in acute cystitis is not usually accompanied by microscopic hematuria.

Staphylococcus saprophyticus is the only uropathogen in the ambulatory setting that is responsible for the majority of cases of UTIs accompanied by microscopic hematuria. Microscopic hematuria in a urinalysis in a patient with an apparent UTI should be carefully observed and should disappear after therapy of the UTI. If the microscopic hematuria disappears, then the physician can safely assume it was related to the UTI. Particularly in elderly patients, if the microscopic hematuria persists after eradication of the UTI, then the patient should be investigated for a bladder or renal source of the microscopic hematuria.

Dysuria-Pyuria Syndrome

In sexually active young women, dysuria-pyuria syndrome manifests with the symptoms of cystitis but with negative urine cultures, or if organisms are cultured, they are present in low numbers (i.e., *E coli*) ($\leq 10^3$ CFU/mL). Most cases of dysuria-pyuria syndrome are caused by *Chlamydia trachomatis*. In patients with dysuria-pyuria syndrome, if the urine is cultured for *Chlamydia*, cultures are frequently positive.

Catheter-Associated Bacteriuria (CAB)

Hospitalized patients with indwelling Foley catheters often acquire bacteriuria as a function of time that the Foley catheter is in place. Pyuria is often in the urine of patients with indwelling Foleys because the catheter elicits inflammation of the urinary tract. The presence of pyuria and bacteriuria in a patient with an indwelling Foley suggests either UTI or CAB. The majority of such patients are asymptomatic and afebrile. More than 95% of the time these patients have colonization of the urinary tract without infection. The urinalysis in patients with indwelling Foley catheters is helpful if either bacteria without pyuria or pyuria without bacteria is demonstrated. Bacteriuria without pyuria signifies colonization of the urinary tract, whereas pyuria without bacteriuria indicates inflammation of the urinary tract. In non–Foley catheter patients, the presence of pyuria plus significant bacteriuria is diagnostic of a UTI. This is not the case with CAB. As mentioned in the setting of the Foley catheter, bacteriuria plus pyuria almost always represents colonization and not a UTI.

Benign Bacteriuria of the Elderly

In elderly female patients, varying degrees of relaxation of the pelvic musculature are common. Patients often have varying degrees of cystocele of rectocele, which changes anatomic relationship and the angularity of the urethra as it enters the bladder and predisposes to colonization of the bladder urine by the introital flora, such as coliform flora derived from the colon. For this reason, elderly female patients often have bacteriuria with few or no symptoms of a UTI. The presence of bacteriuria/pyuria is often discovered on a routine urinalysis obtained as part of either admission laboratory work or an outpatient workup/screening test battery. The presence of bacteriuria/pyuria in an elderly female patient without underlying genitourinary (GU) disease or impaired host defenses has been appropriately termed *benign bacteriuria of the elderly*; it has been shown that these patients do not go on to have symptomatic UTIs, ascending infection (e.g., pyelonephritis/renal abscess), or bacteremia from the urinary tract.

Recurrent Urinary Tract Infections: Reinfection Versus Relapse

Most UTIs in women are acute. CAB is often incorrectly considered a chronic UTI because in most cases it represents colonization rather than infection. Recurrent UTIs are chronic in the sense that they persist over a long period of time, but are really episodic infections. However, the approach to recurrent UTIs is based on determining whether the recurrence is on the basis of reinfection or relapse. The reinfection variety of recurrent UTIs is defined as a recurrent UTI because of different organisms being cultured during each UTI episode. The relapse form of recurrent UTIs is defined as demonstrating the same organism during repeated bouts of UTIs. The reinfection form of recurrent UTIs is usually because of rapid colonization of the vaginal introitus/entry into the urethra, usually following sexual intercourse. The relapse variety of recurrent UTI by the same organism recovered during each episode suggests an underlying structural abnormality of the GU tract. The correct diagnostic approach to recurrent UTIs because of relapse is a thorough investigation of the GU tract from the urethra to the kidneys, which determines a possible source for the focus for the organisms to periodically reappear as a relapsing UTI. Relapse UTIs cannot be successfully approached therapeutically without correcting the underlying condition predisposing to relapse (i.e., bladder calculi, kinked ureters, renal stones, renal abscesses).

Acute Pyelonephritis

Acute pyelonephritis is most common in pregnancy and as a complication of an ascending infection from cystitis/GU instrumentation. An acute episode of pyelonephritis may occur in patients who have chronic pyelonephritis; the acute episode is superimposed on the chronic condition. Renal abscess may complicate acute and chronic pyelonephritis. Renal cortical abscesses are often caused by gram-positive cocci (e.g., staphylococci acquired hematogenously), whereas medullary abscesses are usually caused by aerobic gram-negative bacilli (e.g., coliforms or enterococci).

Acute pyelonephritis may be differentiated from cystitis by the presence of unilateral costovertebral angle (CVA) tenderness (otherwise unexplainable) and a temperature of $\geq 38.9°C$ (102°F). Bilateral pyelonephritis is unusual, and the presence of bilateral CVA tenderness should suggest an alternative diagnosis. Pyelonephritis is often bilateral pathologically, but clinically it is almost always unilateral in its presentation with CVA tenderness. The urinalysis in pyelonephritis is the same as in cystitis, for example with significant pyuria/bacteriuria in addition to the findings suggestive of pyelonephritis. The clinical presentation of renal abscess may resemble pyelonephritis if CVA tenderness is present, but this is not an invariable finding. The urinalysis in renal abscess may reveal pyuria and bacteria if the abscess is medullary but only pyuria if the renal abscess is cortical. Renal imaging studies are usually unnecessary in cystitis or pyelonephritis. If there is confusion regarding the presence or absence of chronic pyelonephritis, then a computed tomography/magnetic resonance imaging (CT/MRI) scan of the abdomen or renal ultrasound is appropriate.

Chronic Pyelonephritis

Chronic pyelonephritis results in shrunken and distorted kidneys with a distorted collecting system. If the patient presents with *chronic pyelonephritis* and has kidneys of normal or large size, then an alternate explanation should be sought. The only way to diagnose a renal abscess with certainty is with renal imaging studies. For this purpose,

---

CURRENT DIAGNOSIS

- Acute uncomplicated cystitis is the most common type of UTI in adult women.
- The initial peak incidence of cystitis occurs with sexual intercourse and gradually increases through adulthood.
- Cystitis may occur as a single event or may be recurrent because of reinfection or relapse.
- Cystitis is usually caused by coliform or enterococci from the fecal flora or by *Staphylococcus saprophyticus* from the skin flora.
- Clinically, cystitis is marked by low-grade fever ($\leq 38.9°C$ [102°F]) with lower abdominal/suprapubic discomfort, and/or dysuria.
- *Staphylococcus aureus*, *Streptococcus pneumoniae*, groups A, C, G streptococci, and *Bacteroides fragilis* are not uropathogens in cystitis.
- In elderly women, *cystitis* manifests as pyuria and bacterluria without fever or dysuria, which is termed *benign bacteriuria of the elderly*.
- A variant of cystitis, the so-called *dysuria/pyuria syndrome*, is also known as *abacteriuric cystitis*.
- Dysuria/pyuria syndrome, most common in young adult women, manifests as cystitis, but urine cultures are negative for bacteria or uropathogens such as *Escherichia coli* are present in low numbers. *Chlamydia trachomatis* is frequently isolated if the urine is cultured for *Chlamydia*.
- Pyelonephritis in women may occur as an uncommon complication of cystitis or during pregnancy.
- It is not possible to predict the uropathogen of cystitis from clinical features except for *S. saprophyticus*.
- *S. saprophyticus* cystitis is characterized by a fishy urine odor, microscopic hematuria, and an alkaline urinary pH.
- Cystitis with alkaline urine suggests infection secondary to *S. saprophyticus*, *Ureaplasma urealyticum*, or a struvite stone with associated infection caused by a urea-splitting organism such as *Proteus*.
- Microscopic hematuria is common with *S. saprophyticus* cystitis but is uncommon with other uropathogens. If a patient with cystitis and microscopic hematuria fails to promptly resolve with antimicrobial therapy, work up the patient for a bladder/renal neoplasm or renal TB.
- The diagnosis of cystitis in women is made by demonstrating pyuria and significant bacteriuria ($\geq 10^6$ col/mL) in the setting of cystitis symptoms.
- Cystitis symptoms with gross hematuria should suggest a viral hemorrhagic cystitis or a renal lesion.
- Pyuria without bacteriuria indicates urinary tract inflammation. Persistent pyuria without bacteriuria should suggest interstitial cystitis or renal TB.
- With cystitis, the specific gravity of the urine is not decreased in contrast to pyelonephritis where the specific gravity is decreased.
- Urinary concentration returns to normal with treatment in pyelonephritis.
- Pyelonephritis may be differentiated from cystitis by the presence of fever $\geq 38.9°C$ (102°F) and otherwise unexplained unilateral CVA tenderness.
- The urine analysis/culture findings in pyelonephritis and cystitis are the same. Bacteremia frequently occurs with pyelonephritis but is not a feature of cystitis in normal hosts.
- Nonleukopenic compromised hosts, such as diabetes mellitus, systemic lupus erythematosus, multiple myeloma, cirrhosis, and so on, with cystitis may be complicated by pyelonephritis or bacteremia.
- Pyelonephritis is caused by the same uropathogens that cause cystitis; however, *S. saprophyticus* occurs only in cystitis.
- Acute pyelonephritis clinically improves unless complicated by renal abscess.
- Clinically, pyelonephritis is almost always unilateral, but pathophysical findings may be bilateral.
- Bilateral CVA tenderness should suggest an alternate diagnosis.
- In pyelonephritis, radiologic studies typically show unilateral renal involvement characterized by cortical scarring, medullary abnormalities, and renal shrinkage.
- Bilateral, normal-sized, or enlarged kidneys should suggest an alternate diagnosis to pyelonephritis.

Abbreviations: CVA = costovertebral angle; TB = tuberculosis; UTI = urinary tract infection.

CURRENT THERAPY

- Virtually all cases of initial uncomplicated cystitis will resolve spontaneously with or without treatment. No urine analysis/culture is needed with the initial episode of cystitis.
- For the dysuria of cystitis, phenazopyridine (Pyridium), which has no antibacterial properties but relieves pain and relative urinary obstruction from muscle spasm, may be used. Relief of spasm promptly clears the bacteriuria.
- Recurrent cystitis of the reinfection variety is because of different uropathogens with each episode that the urine is cultured. Reinfection is related to vaginal introital colonization following sexual intercourse and may be treated with a postcoital/HS of an appropriate antibiotic.
- Although the initial attack of cystitis resolves in virtually all patients without treatment, those who prefer to treat may use single-dose therapy with nitrofurantoin (Macrodantin), TMP-SMX (Bactrim), or amoxicillin (Amoxil).
- Cystitis in a nonleukopenic compromised host (discussed previously) should be treated for 1 to 2 weeks to prevent bacteremia/ascending infection, such as pyelonephritis/renal abscess.
- Ampicillin should be avoided because of its high resistance potential. Amoxicillin should be used instead, which has not been associated with resistance and is effective against the common coliforms and enterococci (*Enterococcus faecalis*).
- Nitrofurantoin has no resistance potential, is effective against all common uropathogens and all enterococci, such as *E. faecalis* (non-VRE) and *Enterococcus faecium* (VRE). Nitrofurantoin (Macrodantin) is useful in cystitis or catheter-associated bacteremia but is not to be used in pyelonephritis/bacteremia.
- Recurrent UTI of the relapse variety is caused by the same uropathogen with each occurrence. The problem in relapse UTIs is not therapeutic but diagnostic. Relapsing UTIs have an underlying structural abnormality or ureteral shunts that do not permit antimicrobial therapy to be effective.
- The treatment of pyelonephritis is with IV or PO antibiotics, depending on the severity of the clinical manifestation. Treatment is for 2 to 4 weeks with an effective antibiotic.
- For pyelonephritis, parenteral agents useful against coliforms are cephalosporins, aztreonam (Azactam), aminoglycosides, TMP-SMZ (Bactrim), or renally eliminated quinolones. Against enterococci (most of which are non-VRE), parenteral ampicillin, antipseudomonal penicillins, and meropenem (Merrem) are useful.
- Oral antibiotics useful against coliform causes of pyelonephritis include renally eliminated quinolones, amoxicillin (Amoxil), antipseudomonal penicillins, or TMP-SMZ (Bactrim).
- Linezolid (Zyvox) may be used for pyelonephritis caused by enterococci (non-VRE), amoxicillin (Amoxil), or for VRE.
- Patients with acute pyelonephritis become afebrile/nearly afebrile within 72 hours with or without treatment. Persistence of high fevers for greater than 72 hours should be considered as representing a renal abscess until proved otherwise.

Abbreviations: HD = half dose; IM = intramuscular; IV = intravenous; TMP-SMZ = trimethoprim-sulfamethoxazole; UTI = urinary tract infection; VRE = vancomycin-resistant *Enterococcus*.

---

the CT/MRI of the kidneys is vastly superior in picking up small lesions than is the renal ultrasound. For the purposes of excluding a renal abscess, a negative renal ultrasound should never be used to rule out the diagnosis. A negative renal ultrasound should always be followed with a renal CT/MRI of the kidneys if a renal abscess is in the differential diagnosis.

Therapeutic Considerations

ACUTE CYSTITIS

The initial episode of acute complicated cystitis in a normal host without GU abnormalities/preexisting renal disease need not be treated with antimicrobial therapy. Usually treatment with phenazopyridine (Pyridium), which has no antibacterial effect, is sufficient to relieve bladder spasm and the relative urine obstruction because of the bladder spasm, and the bacteria will spontaneously clear itself without antimicrobial therapy. Repeated episodes of acute cystitis should have appropriate diagnostic studies, for example a urinalysis and urinary culture with sensitivities with each episode to differentiate reinfection from relapse. If cystitis occurs in a nonleukopenic compromised host (e.g., with diabetes mellitus, systemic lupus erythematosus, multiple myeloma, cirrhosis, etc.), then a seven-day course of therapy is recommended with an oral agent such as nitrofurantoin (Macrodantin), trimethoprim-sulfamethoxazole (TMP-SMX) (Bactrim), fosfomycin (Monurol), or amoxicillin (Amoxil). Ampicillin should be avoided because of its resistance potential with coliform bacteria.

DYSURIA-PYURIA SYNDROME

The dysuria-pyuria syndrome because of *Chlamydia* should be treated with a two-week course of doxycycline (Vibramycin). Patients unable to tolerate doxycycline (Vibramycin) may be treated with a macrolide for the same period of time. A grossly hemorrhagic cystitis suggests a viral etiology for which no specific therapy is available. Patients with cystitis and microscopic hematuria are often infected with *S. saprophyticus*.

Fortunately, *S. saprophyticus* is susceptible to a wide range of antibiotics and virtually any agent selected to treat a UTI will be effective. Antimicrobial resistance has not been a problem in *S. saprophyticus* UTIs. Chronic interstitial cystitis is not an infectious disorder and therefore antimicrobial therapy is unnecessary.

CATHETER-ASSOCIATED BACTERIURIA

CAB in hospitalized patients who are normal hosts without structural abnormalities need not be treated, because virtually all of these patients are colonized and not infected. CAB in nonleukopenic compromised hosts (with diabetes mellitus, systemic lupus erythematosus, multiple myeloma, cirrhosis, and so forth), should be treated to prevent ascending infection/bacteremia from the lower urinary tract. Such individuals should be treated with an oral agent such as amoxicillin (Amoxil), nitrofurantoin (Macrodantin), or TMP-SMX (Bactrim) for 1 to 2 weeks.

Nonleukopenic compromised hosts with enterococci CAB are best treated with oral nitrofurantoin (Macrodantin), which is effective against enterococcal strains such as E. faecalis (non-vancomycin-resistant Enterococcus [non-VRE]) as well as E. faecium [VRE]). Enterococcus faecalis strains may also be treated with oral amoxicillin (Amoxil). These instances represent prophylaxis/early therapy because the majority of patients who are nonleukopenic-compromised hosts will have colonization of the urinary tract prior to catheterization or rapidly develop it soon thereafter. Therefore, prevention of ascending infection/bacteremia is the primary aim of therapy in patients with CAB who are compromised on the basis of their host defenses or GU tract abnormalities (e.g., ureteral stents).

ACUTE PYELONEPHRITIS

Acute pyelonephritis may be caused by aerobic gram-negative bacilli, such as coliforms or enterococci (almost always E. faecalis). The empirical treatment of pyelonephritis is based on a Gram stain of the urine, which, if the diagnosis is pyelonephritis, will show significant pyuria and a single predominant organism. In a patient with presumed pyelonephritis, the absence of bacteria in the Gram stain of the urine in an acutely ill patient essentially eliminates the diagnosis of pyelonephritis from further consideration, and an alternate explanation for the patient's fever and CVA tenderness should be sought (e.g., renal imaging studies).

Because acute pyelonephritis is often accompanied by bacteremia (urosepsis), parenteral agents may be used initially followed by oral agents; or in mild-to-moderate cases, oral agents may be used for the entire course of therapy. The parenteral agents useful in the treatment of acute pyelonephritis because of aerobic gram-negative bacilli include aminoglycosides, aztreonam (Azactam), antipseudomonal penicillin (e.g., ticarcillin [Ticar]), piperacillin (Pipracil), or a renally excreted respiratory quinolone. Patients presenting with acute pyelonephritis, who have streptococci in the Gram stain of the urine indicating enterococci, may be treated empirically with ampicillin and antipseudomonal penicillin, ticarcillin (Ticar), piperacillin (Pipracil), or meropenem (Merrem). In the rare instance where there is enterococcal urosepsis complicating acute pyelonephritis because of VRE, then linezolid (Zyvox), quinupristin-dalfopristin (Synercid), or daptomycin (Cubicin) may be used. In patients presenting with acute pyelonephritis where a Gram stain is unobtainable or unavailable, then empirical coverage for both aerobic gram-negative bacilli and enterococci (E. faecalis), may be achieved with antipseudomonal penicillins, nonrenally eliminated respiratory quinolones, or meropenem (Merrem). After the organism responsible for the pyelonephritis is subsequently identified by urine/blood culture, then the patient may be switched to one of the agents mentioned. Similarly, if the patient is shown to have enterococci as the cause of the urosepsis, it may be treated initially as non-VRE, as indicated previously in the article. Patients with pyelonephritis are usually treated for 1 to 2 weeks.

Particularly in critically ill patients, initial therapy is often started parenterally. Patients may be switched to an oral agent as soon as the patient clinically defervesces or treated entirely by an oral agent for the duration of therapy. The ideal oral antibiotic has the same spectrum as its parenteral counterpart and has excellent bioavailability; blood/tissue levels are approximately the same after intravenous/oral (IV/PO) administration. For example, by giving 1 g of amoxicillin (Amoxil) every 8 hours, the same blood/tissue levels are achieved as by giving ampicillin by intramuscular injection (IM). Nonrenally eliminated respiratory quinolones, such as levofloxacin (Levaquin) and gatifloxacin (Tequin), achieve the same blood and tissue levels when given either by the IV or PO route. This permits completion of therapy at home and does not require 2 to 4 weeks of inpatient hospitalization for intravenous drug therapy. There is some rationale for treating acute pyelonephritis for an extended period, such as 2 to 4 weeks, to prevent chronic pyelonephritis.

CHRONIC PYELONEPHRITIS

Patients with chronic pyelonephritis are a therapeutic challenge because of the distorted intrarenal architecture and decreased blood supply to the kidney, which limits access of white blood cells (WBCs), impairs host defenses, and limits penetration of the antibiotic into the infected/diseased areas of the kidney. Treatment of chronic pyelonephritis should be based on susceptibility testing of the isolates that are present in the urine. In chronic pyelonephritis, bacteriuria is intermittent but is present over a long period of time and will persist after short or inadequate treatment. The antibiotic selected should be effective against the isolate recovered from the urine in patients with chronic pyelonephritis and possess the ability to penetrate into diseased kidneys. The ideal oral agents for therapy are TMP-SMX (Bactrim), doxycycline (Vibramycin), or a nonrenally eliminated respiratory quinolone.

RENAL ABSCESS

Acute pyelonephritis treated appropriately results in a rapid defervescence of temperature and decrease in CVA tenderness within 72 hours. If the temperature does not decrease after 72 hours of appropriate therapy, suggest a renal abscess until proved otherwise. Renal abscesses should be treated for the presumed organism based on the location of the abscess by renal imaging studies. If sensitivities from an isolate available from the urine or percutaneous aspiration of the abscess are unavailable, then empirical treatment directed against aerobic gram-negative bacilli for medullary abscesses is indicated. Treatment is the same as for pyelonephritis except is more prolonged and should be given until the abscess is drained or it resolves. For cortical abscesses in the absence of culture and sensitivity data, antibiotic therapy should be directed against Staphylococcus aureus and E. faecalis, and treated in the same manner as pyelonephritis but for an extended period of time. Acute pyelonephritis with or without acteremia is usually treated for 7 days.

RECURRENT UTIs

Reinfection may be treated with nitrofurantoin (Macrodantin), TMP-SMX (Bactrim), or amoxicillin (Amoxil) as a single postcoital dose. Therapeutic approach to relapse is to remove the underlying condition responsible for perpetuating the bacteriuria. Antimicrobial therapy may be selected based on the susceptibility of the organism, but antimicrobial therapy alone will not eradicate the relapsing form of recurrent UTI.

REFERENCES

Cunha BA: Clinical concepts in the treatment of urinary tract infections. Antibiotics for Clinicians 1999;3:88-93.

Cunha BA: Nosocomial catheter-associated urinary tract infections. Hosp Physician 1986;22:13-16.

Cunha BA: *Staphylococcus saprophyticus* urinary tract infections. Intern Med 1985;6:82-89.

Cunha BA: Single-dose therapy of urinary tract infections. Hosp Physician 1983;19:35-37.

Cunha BA: Urosepsis in the Critical Care Unit. In: Cunha BA (ed): Infectious Diseases in Critical Care Medicine, 2nd ed. Informa Healthcare USA, Inc., New York, NY, pp. 527-534.

Cunha BA: Antibiotic Essentials, 6th ed., Physicians Press, Royal Oak, MI, pp. 79-85.

Cunha BA: Urinary tract infections: Therapy. Postgrad Med 1981;70:149-157.

Hooton TM: The current management strategies for community-acquired urinary tract infection. Infect Dis Clin North Am 2003;17:303-332.

Kahan E, Kahan NR, Chinitz DP: Urinary tract infection in women—Physician's preferences for treatment and adherence to guidelines: A national drug utilization study in a managed care setting. Eur J Clin Pharmacol 2003;59:663-668.

Kraft JK, Stamey TA: The natural history of symptomatic recurrent bacteriuria in women. Medicine (Baltimore) 1977;56:55.

Meiland R, Geerlings SE, Hoepelman LI: Management of bacterial urinary tract infections in adult patients with diabetes mellitus. Drugs 2002;62:1859-1868.

Miller LG, Tang AW: Treatment of uncomplicated urinary tract infections in an era of increasing antimicrobial resistance. Mayo Clin Proc 2004;79:1048-1053.

Nicolle LE: Urinary tract infection: Traditional pharmacologic therapies. Am J Med 2002;113(Suppl 1A):35S-44S.

Nicolle LE, Ronald AR: Recurrent urinary tract infection in adult women: Diagnosis and treatment. Infect Dis Clin North Am 1987;1:793.

Ronald AR, Conway B: An approach to urinary tract infection in women. Infection 1992;20(Suppl 3):S203.

Schaeffer AJ, Stuppy BA: Efficacy and safety of self-start therapy in women with recurrent urinary tract infections. J Urol 1999;161:207.

Wong ES, McKevitt M, Running K, et al: Management of recurrent urinary tract infections with patient administered single-dose therapy. Ann Intern Med 1985;102:302.

BOX 2 Colony Count Criteria for Urinary Tract Infection in Children

- If suprapubic aspiration is performed any growth is significant for UTI
- If catheterization of female is performed, greater than 1000 CFU/mL is significant for UTI
- If clean-void urine is performed, greater than 10,000 CFU/mL in pure culture is suggestive; >100,000 CFU/mL is highly likely.
- Growth of two or more species suggests contamination, but does not exclude true infection. Repeat the culture.

Bacterial Infections of the Urinary Tract in Girls

Method of
Candice E. Johnson, MD, PhD

Urinary tract infections (UTIs) are bacterial infections of any mucosal surface of the urinary tract including the urethra, the bladder, the ureters, and the renal calyces, as well as the renal parenchyma (Box 1). The best indicator for differentiating clinical pyelonephritis from cystitis is fever higher than 38.5°C (101.3°F). The classification of UTIs by anatomic location is complicated by the ascending nature of virtually all these infections. Thus, a girl with pyelonephritis usually has cystitis and urethritis simultaneously. Box 2 gives the colony count criteria generally accepted for clinical use, although research studies are usually more stringent.

Epidemiology and Pathogenesis

Approximately 2.2% of girls will have a UTI in the first 24 months of life. In the first year of life, most UTIs in females are febrile and may be hard to diagnose. Because of this difficulty, girls younger than 36 months with no source of fever should have a urine culture and urinalysis obtained. Unfortunately, the sensitivity of a standard urinalysis is only 82%, although it is 92% specific. For unknown reasons, the prevalence of UTI is much higher in white compared with African American girls, with Hispanics having a rate between the two groups.

Risk factors for UTI include:

- A history of recurrent UTI in the mother
- Family history of vesicoureteral reflux (VUR)
- Dysfunctional voiding patterns
- Constipation

Cleanliness and methods of wiping with toilet paper are not risk factors. In girls, an "unstable bladder" is the main cause of dysfunctional voiding. An unstable bladder has strong contractions at volumes 50% to 75% of capacity. These contractions cause both frequency and incontinence, and girls may sit on their feet to attempt to prevent voiding (Vincent's curtsy). In the most severe cases the girl tightens the external sphincter during bladder contraction, and this leads to high bladder pressure. A thickened and trabeculated bladder often occurs as well as VUR.

Diagnosis

A high index of suspicion is needed to diagnose all UTIs, especially those in infants and toddlers. In addition to fever, manifesting symptoms include anorexia and emesis, abdominal pain, fussiness, neonatal jaundice, poor weight gain, enuresis, and hematuria.

Urine should be collected only by catheter or suprapubic aspiration until the child is toilet trained, because urine bags have contamination rates of up to 50%. Box 2 shows the colony counts that best differentiate real UTIs from contamination.

Urinalysis continues to be performed in most laboratories by a dipstick combined with spun urine sediment. This continues despite studies since 1983 showing that unspun urine counted in a hemocytometer is more sensitive and specific. In a private office, the dipstick results for leukocyte esterase, nitrites, and hematuria are sufficient to decide on empirical treatment of girls. Urine cultures should still be sent, even with a negative dipstick, because, unlike adult women, radiologic workups may be needed for confirmed UTIs in girls.

Treatment of Afebrile Urinary Tract Infection

Treatment of a girl with an afebrile UTI (cystitis or lower tract) is straightforward, requiring only a knowledge of national and local antibiotic resistance rates. *Escherichia coli* causes more than 90% of cystitis in girls, with other Enterobacteriaceae and *Staphylococcus saprophyticus* comprising the remainder. *E. coli* is resistant to amoxicillin (Amoxil) more than 50% of the time, so this is not appropriate initial therapy. Rates of resistance to trimethoprim (Proloprim) and sulfonamides are highest in the Pacific Coast states, and rates of

---

BOX 1 Classification of Urinary Tract Infections

- **Urethritis:** Dysuria, frequency or enuresis, accompanied by pyuria, but colony count of 10^3/mL of urine or less.
- **Cystitis:** Afebrile UTI. Dysuria, frequency or enuresis with colony count of at least 10^4/mL of urine. Hematuria may be present, but casts, flank pain, temperature more than 38.5°C (101.3°F) and systemic toxicity are absent.
- **Clinical pyelonephritis:** Febrile UTI ($\geq$38°C [100.4°F]), usually accompanied by flank and abdominal pain. The colony count is usually greater than or equal to 10^5/mL of urine except with *Staphylococcus saprophyticus* or enterococci. Cystitis symptoms may also be present.
- **Proved pyelonephritis:** Shows evidence of acute inflammation on radiologic evaluation by CT, ultrasound, or radionuclide scan.

Abbreviations: CT = computed tomography; UTI = urinary tract infection.

first-generation cephalosporin resistance vary widely. Drugs that retain high sensitivity rates are the second- and third-generation cephalosporins and nitrofurantoin (Macrodantin). Box 3 provides doses of commonly used drugs, and amoxicillin is preferred if the organism is sensitive.

Treatment of Febrile Urinary Tract Infection

Unlike the majority of viral and bacterial infections, a single kidney infection may cause permanent damage (i.e., renal scarring) if not treated rapidly and with effective antibiotics. In 1999, outpatient management of febrile UTIs was demonstrated to be effective in a study of 306 children under 24 months of age. A 2004 study in Montreal of 291 patients who were 3 months to 5 years of age showed that at least 75% of febrile children with UTI could be managed in a day treatment center (DTC). These children had a mean of 3.5 visits to the DTC for intravenous gentamicin (Garamycin), followed by an oral antibiotic to complete 10 days

---

BOX 3 Antibiotic Choices for the Treatment of Urinary Tract Infections

Oral
- Trimethoprim (Primsol oral solution)—8-12 mg/kg/day divided every 12 hours (max dose 320 mg).
- Trimethoprim-sulfamethoxazole (TMP/SMX) (Bactrim, Septra)—8-12 mg of TMP component divided every 12 hours (max dose 320 mg).
- Amoxicillin (Amoxil)—children <40 kg: 40 mg/kg/day divided every 12 hours; children >40 kg: 875 mg every 12 hours.
- Cephalosporins:
  Cefprozil (Cefzil)[1]—30 mg/kg/day divided every 12 hours (max dose 1 g/day).
  Cefixime (generic only)—infants and children: 8 mg/kg/day divided every 12 hours; adolescents and adults: 400 mg/day divided every 12-24 hours.
  Cefdinir (Omnicef)[1]—Infants and children (older than 6 months to 12 years): 14 mg/kg/day divided every 12 hours (max dose 600 mg/day).
  Cephalexin (Keflex)—25-50 mg/kg/day divided every 6 to 8 hours (max dose 4 g/day).
- Nitrofurantoin (Macrodantin) for afebrile infections only—5-7 mg/kg/day divided every 6 hours; children older than 12 years and adults, 300 mg every 12 hours or 600 mg every 24 hours.

Parenteral
- Gentamicin (Garamycin)—5-6 mg/kg/day divided every 8 hours or 5 mg/kg as a single dose every 24 hours (with measured levels after third dose).
- Trimethoprim-sulfamethoxazole (Bactrim, Septra) at 8 mg/kg/day of the TMP component, divided every 12 hours.
- Cephalosporins:
  Ceftriaxone (Rocephin)—50 mg/kg/day once every 24 hours.
  Ceftazidime (Fortaz)—100-150 mg/kg/day divided every 8 hours; (max dose 600 mg)
  Cefotaxime (Claforan)—50-150 mg/kg/day divided every 6-8 hours. (max dose 12 grams/day)
- Fluoroquinolones are not approved for under age 18 years, but may be required for resistant organisms.

[1]Not FDA approved for this indication.

CURRENT DIAGNOSIS

- A high level of suspicion is required in all febrile infants.
- Boys outnumber girls 10:1 in the neonatal period.
- Girls are at highest risk for UTI when younger than 12 months of age and again at 3 to 5 years of age.
- Urine for culture should not be obtained with a bag, but requires a catheterization or suprapubic aspiration, if the child is not toilet trained.
- The colony count cutoff to define a UTI differs with the method used for collection.
- With a negative urinalysis, febrile UTI becomes much less likely, but an afebrile UTI cannot be ruled out.

Abbreviations: UTI = urinary tract infection.

---

of treatment. Successful treatment was seen in 97% of the UTI episodes, and all first UTIs were evaluated by renal sonography and cystography at the DTC.

Because the DTC concept is not widely available for children in the United States, Figure 1 shows a suggested decision tree that does not use a DTC. Inpatient management is recommended for infants younger than 8 weeks as they do not absorb oral antibiotics predictably. Box 4 lists other variables to consider in deciding on inpatient versus outpatient treatment. Antibiotic choices are given in Box 3. Duration of symptoms before presentation is very important, because renal scarring was seen in British studies after as few as 5 days of delayed diagnosis.

Once on antibiotic therapy, defervescence may be expected in approximately 68% of children younger than 2 years by 24 hours and in 89% by 48 hours. The 11% who remain febrile at 48 hours were no more likely to have renal abscesses or hydronephrosis than the others, and they may be discharged after sensitivities are known. It is convenient to the family to perform the cystogram, if indicated, during hospitalization and it greatly improves compliance.

Prophylaxis

There is expert agreement that further prospective studies of antibiotic prophylaxis for childhood UTI are needed. In adult women, the cost-to-benefit ratio favors prophylaxis with three or more UTIs per year. In children, because young age is the major risk for renal scarring, studies are lacking, but expert opinion favors 6 months of prophylaxis after a febrile UTI, with or without VUR. Guidelines from the American Urological Association also suggest

---

CURRENT THERAPY

- Outpatient therapy of febrile UTIs is usually appropriate in infants older than 2 months of age.
- A single dose of intramuscular ceftriaxone (Rocephin) will cover the first 24 hours after diagnosis when emesis is most likely to occur and antibiotic sensitivities are unknown.
- Febrile girls should be seen between 36 and 48 hours after diagnosis to assess clinical improvements and check urine culture results.
- A voiding cystogram remains essential for febrile girls younger than 5 years of age and all boys.

Abbreviations: UTI = urinary tract infection.

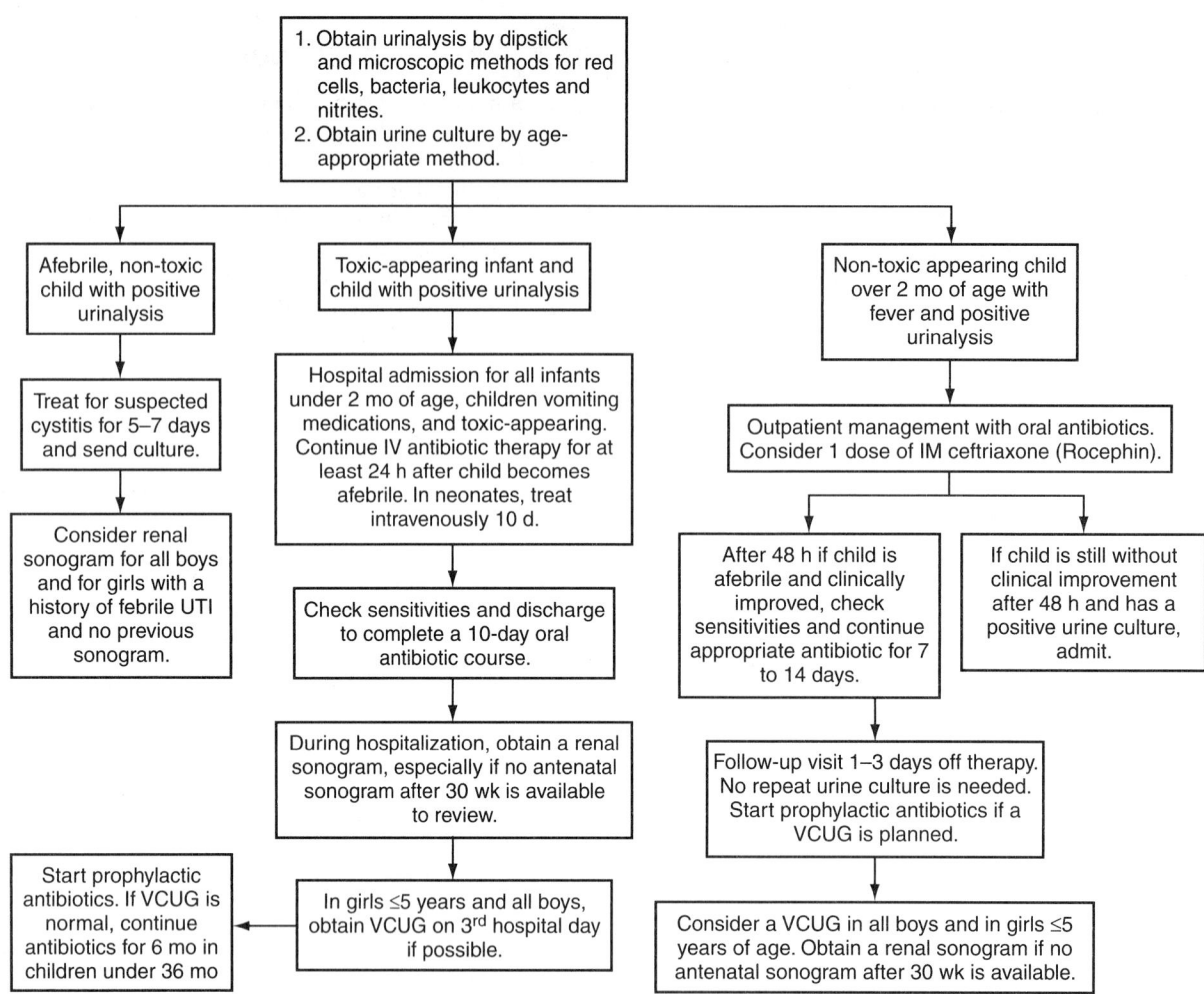

FIGURE 1. Treatment of suspected urinary tract infection in children younger than 13 years old.

BOX 4 Proposed Criteria for Hospitalization of Children With Febrile Urinary Tract Infection

- Sufficient emesis is present to prevent oral therapy.
- Family is judged likely to be noncompliant with antibiotics or follow-up appointments.
- Toxic or ill-appearing child which is suggestive of sepsis.
- Age is younger than 2 months.
- Prolonged duration of symptoms exists (>5 days).
- Renal scarring or impaired renal function is known to be present.
- Diabetes, AIDS, sickle cell, or other serious chronic disease is present.

prophylaxis for all children with VUR, but the Swedish experts suggest stopping at age 24 months in boys and 5 years in girls. Table 1 lists suggested agents. Unfortunately, the choice of antibiotic is becoming limited as trimethoprim (Proloprim) resistance rates rise.

Radiologic Evaluation

No area of childhood UTI evaluation is as controversial as determining which children merit sonography, radionuclide scans, and cystograms. Two recent studies have helped clarify these issues, and several professional academies have agreed on guidelines for febrile children younger than 2 years of age (Pediatrics, Family Practice, Emergency Physicians, Urological, and College of Radiology). These associations recommend a renal sonogram and a voiding cystogram soon after the first febrile UTI. Figure 2 indicates that the initial

TABLE 1 Prophylactic Antibiotics for Childhood Urinary Tract Infections

Drug	Dose	Timing	Side Effects
Trimethoprim-sulfamethoxazole (TMP-SMX) (Bactrim)	2 mg/kg of TMP component (up to 40 mg)	Bedtime	Rash in ~6%
Nitrofurantoin (Macrodantin capsules 25, 50, or 100 mg preferred over oral suspension)	1-2 mg/kg/d up to 100 mg	Bedtime	Vomiting, abdominal pain
Trimethoprim (Primsol oral solution 50 mg/mL or 100 mg tablets)	2 mg/kg up to 40 mg	Bedtime	Rash in ~1%

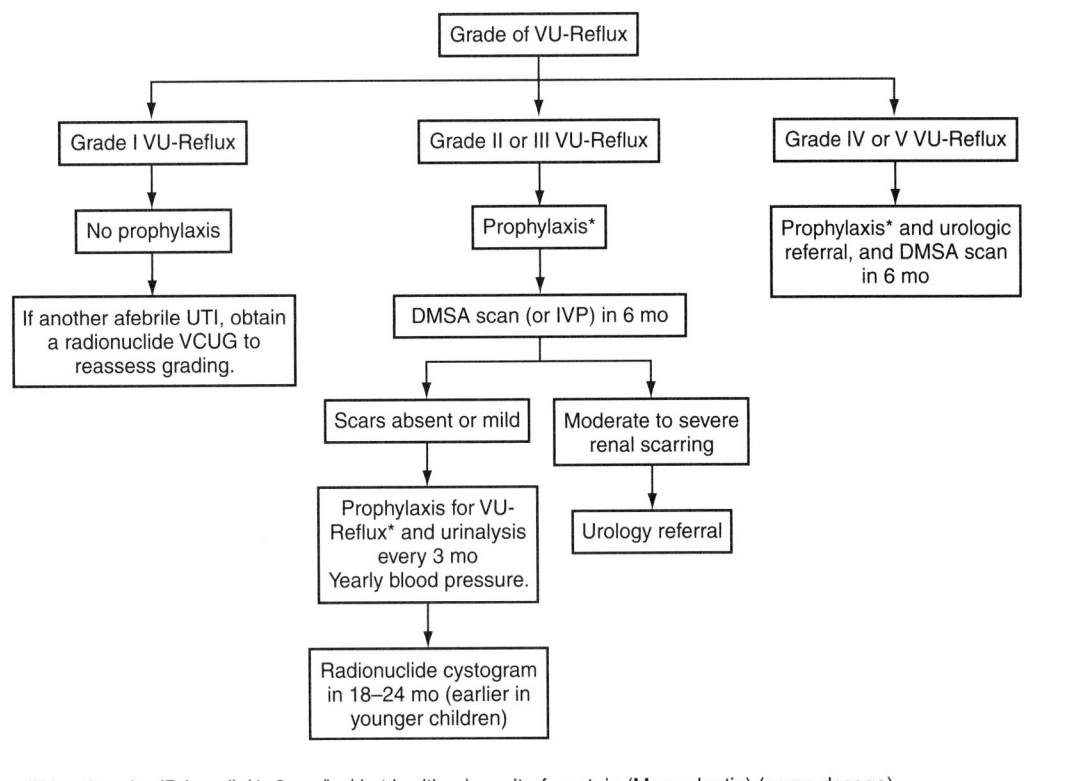

FIGURE 2. Radiologic management of a child with vesicoureteral reflux.

cystogram should be a standard fluoroscopic examination to permit accurate grading of VUR. Follow-up cystograms may be radionuclide studies, which carry less risk of gonadal radiation.

Hoberman and colleagues also question the value of the initial renal sonogram. In a cohort of 309 febrile children who had paired dimercaptosuccinic acid (DMSA) radionuclide renal scans and sonography performed within 48 hours of diagnosis, neither study changed management. All had an antenatal sonogram after 30 weeks of gestation, and anomalies were presumably corrected before UTI could occur. The argument in favor of doing this painless and medically safe study is that children with "dilating reflux" (i.e., grades III-V) would be identified, and the doctor could track down these children if they fail to keep an appointment for a cystogram. In other words, in the absence of a cystogram, a sonogram with hydronephrosis or pelvic caliectasis *will* change management. In the patient with no health insurance who cannot afford both studies, the more important study is the voiding cystogram, not the sonogram.

REFERENCES

Abelson Storby K, Osterlund A, Kahlmeter G: Antimicrobial resistance in *Escherichia coli* in urine samples from children and adults: A 12 year analysis. Acta Paediatr 2004;93:487-491.

Bollgren I: Antibacterial prophylaxis in children with urinary tract infection. Acta Paediatr 1999;(Suppl 431):48-52.

Gauthier M, Chevalie I, Sterescu A, et al: Treatment of urinary tract infections among febrile young children with daily intravenous antibiotic therapy at a day treatment center. Pediatrics 2004;114:469-476.

Hellerstein S: Urinary tract infections in children. Infections in Medicine 2002;19:554-560.

Hoberman A, Charros M, Hickey RW, et al: Imaging studies after a first febrile urinary tract infection in young children. N Engl J Med 2003;348(3):195-202.

Hoberman A, Wald ER, Hickey RW, et al: Oral versus initial intravenous therapy for urinary tract infections in young febrile children. Pediatrics 1999;104(1):79-86.

Jakobsson B, Esbjorner E, Hansson S: Minimum incidence and diagnostic rate of first urinary tract infection. Pediatrics 1999;104(2 Pt):222-226.

Johnson CE: Dysuria. In: Kliegman RM, Greebaum LA, Lye PS, (eds): Practical Strategies in Pediatric Diagnosis and Therapy, 2nd ed. Philadelphia, WB Saunders, 2004, pp 397-411.

Lin D-S, Huang F-Y, Chiu N-C, et al: Comparison of hemocytometer leukocyte counts and standard urinalysis for predicting urinary tract infections in febrile infants. Pediatr Infect Dis J 2000;19:223-227.

Lowe LH, Patel MN, Gatti JM, Alon US: Utility of follow-up renal sonography in children with vesicoureteral reflux and normal initial sonogram. Pediatrics 2004;113:548-550.

Roberts KB: A synopsis of the American Academy of Pediatrics' practice parameter on the diagnosis, treatment, and evaluation of the initial urinary tract infection in febrile infants and young children. Pediatr Rev 1999;20(10):1-4.

Rushton HG: Urinary tract infections in children: Epidemiology, evaluation, and management. Pediatr Clin North Am 1997;44(5):1133-1169.

Childhood Incontinence

Method of
*Christine Geers, MSN, CPNP, and
Andrew Kirsch, MD*

Definition and Terminology

Incontinence is a common complaint in pediatrics and can produce major anxiety and stress in the child and the family. Incontinence as defined by the International Children's Continence Society (ICCS) is the involuntary wetting at an inappropriate time and place in a

> **BOX 1 Terminology of Incontinence**
>
> Continuous: Not in discrete portions
> Enuresis: While sleeping
> Intermittent: In discrete portions

child 5 years old or older. Incontinence can be differentiated as continuous incontinence, intermittent incontinence, and enuresis (Box 1). Continuous incontinence refers to the continuous leakage of urine, not in discrete portions. It often indicates malformation or iatrogenic damage. Intermittent incontinence is the leakage of urine in discrete portions, during day, night, or both. The term *enuresis*, which was previously used for any type of incontinence, is now designated to intermittent urinary incontinence while sleeping, synonymous with (intermittent) nocturnal enuresis. The term is used regardless of whether daytime incontinence or other lower urinary tract symptoms are also present. "Nocturnal" may be added for extra clarity (see Box 1). To identify the etiology of the incontinence in a child, it is important to understand bladder function.

Normal Voiding Patterns

It is not very well understood how children accomplish bowel and bladder control. Generally speaking, bowel control is achieved before bladder control. Bladder control during the day is achieved before control at night. This entire process of toilet training is accomplished anywhere between 24 months and 5 years of age. The infant bladder empties by pure reflex activity when the bladder reaches functional bladder capacity. Bladder function involves two distinct phases: urine storage and urine release.

This process is regulated by the autonomic nervous system. The sympathetic system is responsible for bladder storage and the parasympathetic system is responsible for the emptying phase. During the storage phase, the bladder has to be able to maintain a stable bladder pressure as urine volume increases. Bladder capacity or voided volume can be estimated by:

$$\text{Volume (mL)} = [30 + (\text{age in year} \times 30)]$$

This formula applies until age 12 years, after which the estimated volume is set at 390 mL constant volume. Urinary incontinence during this phase can be caused by small bladder capacity or decreased elasticity due to bladder wall thickening or fibrosis. Malfunctioning of the urinary sphincter system during this phase can also cause urinary incontinence.

The release or voiding phase is an active process involving bladder contraction and relaxation of the pelvic floor muscle followed by reflexive opening of the bladder neck and external urethral sphincter. Any disturbance in the neurologic pathway can interrupt this process and lead to incontinence.

Daytime Incontinence

ETIOLOGY

Urinary incontinence can be divided into neurogenic and non-neurogenic causes (Box 2). Neurogenic incontinence can result from a defect in the neural tube, generally referred to as *spinal dysraphism*. Ninety-five percent of children with spina bifida experience abnormal innervation of the bladder, and urinary incontinence is a common finding. Other pathologies that can cause alteration in the neurophysiologic pathway of bladder function include spinal cord injury, spinal cord or brain tumors, and herniated disk or stroke (less common in children). Incontinence can also be due to areflexic or hyperreflexic detrusor activity.

> **BOX 2 Etiology of Incontinence**
>
> **Neurogenic**
> Brain tumor
> Herniated disk
> Spinal dysraphism
> Spinal cord injury
> Stroke
>
> **Non-neurogenic**
> *Anatomic*
> Bladder exstrophy
> Ectopic ureteroceles
> Ectopic ureters
> Epispadias
> Labial adhesions
> Posterior urethral valves
> Urogenital sinus malformation
> Vaginal reflux
>
> *Functional*
> Dysfunctional voiding
> Giggle incontinence
> Overactive bladder
> Stress incontinence
> Underactive bladder
> Urge incontinence
> Voiding postponement

Non-neurogenic causes of incontinence include anatomic and functional disorders. Anatomic pathology always manifests with chronic and daily incontinence. These children are never dry. Included in this category are structural abnormalities such as posterior urethral valves, ectopic ureteroceles, bladder exstrophy, urogenital sinus malformation, epispadias, ectopic ureters, vaginal reflux, and labial adhesions. Most of these structural abnormalities are repairable by surgical intervention.

Functional causes have to be considered in the absence of any neurologic or anatomic evidence for the incontinence. The ICCS recommends using the term *lower urinary tract dysfunction* to refer to the many conditions that lead to urinary incontinence. An estimated 40% of patients presenting to the urology practice have lower urinary tract dysfunction. Included in this category are overactive bladder, urge incontinence, voiding postponement, underactive bladder, dysfunctional voiding, giggle incontinence, and stress incontinence (see Box 2). All these dysfunctions include either failure to store or failure to empty. Most of the lower urinary tract dysfunctions occur secondary to poor voiding habits.

The child presents with urinary urgency or incontinence, or both. These manifestations are believed to be due to overactive detrusor contractions. The child experiencing these contractions feels a sudden urgency and learns to counteract this sensation with voluntary pelvic floor contractions and holding maneuvers. This can ultimately lead to true dysfunctional voiding. These children are also at higher risk for developing urinary tract infections due to reflux of potential uropathogens from the distal urethra.

Other findings in these children include hesitancy, described as having difficulty initiating a urinary stream. Urinary frequency might also be present but is not in itself a diagnostic component for overactive bladder. These children can experience a transient increase in bladder pressure (as seen on a urodynamic study), which can lead to bladder wall thickening, poor bladder compliance, decreased capacity, ineffective bladder emptying, and ultimately further bladder overactivity.

A child with urge incontinence suffers from a sudden feeling of urinary urgency followed by urinary incontinence. This is a common finding in children with a diagnosis of an overactive bladder.

Voiding postponement applies to children who habitually delay voiding despite the sensation of bladder fullness. A common manifestation is incontinence. Some children, however, may be asymptomatic. Parents often notice posturing or other characteristic behavior to suppress the urgency, such as squatting and pressing their heels into the perineum (Vincent's curtsy), crossing the legs, or tip-toeing.

Underactive bladder is a "condition afflicting patients with a low voiding frequency and the need to raise intraabdominal pressure in order to void." This replaces the term lazy bladder. These children might only void once or twice a day. The bladder capacity is usually large and with each void a large volume is eliminated. Incontinence occurs due to overfill and can be precipitated by physical activity. A voiding cystourethrogram (VCUG) usually shows moderate to large postvoid residual. Urodynamics show decreased sensation with filling, low bladder pressures, and interrupted urinary flow pattern due to decreased detrusor activity and Valsalva maneuver with voiding.

Dysfunctional voiding is one of the most commonly encountered problems in pediatric urology. The term is much misused. According to the ICCS, it refers to the habitual contraction of the urethral sphincter during voiding, as observed on uroflow study (staccato-type uroflow pattern). This may also be referred to as sphincter–detrusor dyssynergia. On imaging studies, the proximal urethra is dilated, and a narrowing is apparent at the membranous urethra. This is also referred to as *spinning top urethra*. In general practice, the term dysfunctional voiding is used to encompass symptoms of urge incontinence, infrequent voiding, delayed voiding, infrequent voiding, and incomplete bladder emptying. Hallmark symptoms of dysfunctional voiding include incontinence and urinary tract infections.

Giggle incontinence is not a commonly encountered form of incontinence, but it can be very anxiety producing. Children, almost exclusively girls, with giggle incontinence lose the entire contents of their bladder during giggling or laughing. The bladder function is completely normal during all other times.

Another less common form of incontinence in pediatrics is stress incontinence, which is associated with increased abdominal pressure. Stimulants such as methylphenidate (Ritalin)[1] have been shown to improve symptoms, but scientific studies are still needed to support this treatment.

EVALUATION

History

Obtaining a thorough history plays a major role in identifying the cause of the incontinence.

Urinary symptoms should be assessed, including urgency, frequency, posturing, dysuria, hematuria, and urinary tract infections. Every aspect of urinary incontinence is elicited, including volume and frequency of incontinence and any identifiable triggers (situation or activity) associated with the incontinence. A beneficial adjunct to obtaining an accurate history is an elimination diary. The patient can complete this before the office visit. Optimal recording includes the number of voids, voided volumes, quantity and frequency of any incontinence, and bowel habits in regard to size, consistency, and frequency of the bowel movements.

The character of the stream is assessed. Ideally, the stream is forceful, sustained, and without deflection. Achievement of developmental milestones is important to rule out that the incontinence is due to intellectual or behavioral delay. A diet history should especially focus on type and amount of fluid intake and the average fiber consumption. Psychosocial history is significant in identifying any situational stressor and establishing level of motivation in parent and child.

Physical Examination

Palpate the abdomen for any masses such as a distended bladder, large amount of stool, and enlarged kidneys. The lower back should be inspected for any signs suggesting neurologic abnormalities, such as pigmented or hairy patch, sacral dimple or sinus, sacral agenesis, and asymmetry of gluteal creases. The rectum is examined for tone and fissures. The genital examination includes inspection of urethral meatus, labia, and vaginal introitus. The neurologic examination should include observation of gait and balance. Eliciting reflexes and strength of lower extremities can further assist in ruling out spinal cord involvement.

Diagnostic Studies

A urinalysis is indicated to rule out urinary tract infection, diabetes mellitus, diabetes insipidus, or other organic causes for the incontinence.

Uroflowmetry in conjunction with ultrasonography is easy to perform and noninvasive. It is helpful in establishing efficiency of voiding.

Most children with incontinence are effectively treated based on history and physical examination only. Invasive studies, such as a VCUG and urodynamic study, are reserved for children who have shown no improvement with conservative treatment or who have obvious signs that the incontinence is not related to a functional cause. MRI of the spine may be indicated if signs of a neuropathic disorder are present.

TREATMENT

The treatment plan discussed here does not include treatment for children with incontinence due to anatomic or neurologic pathology. Bladder retraining is the major focus in the treatment.

Behavior Modification

Therapy is individualized according to the etiology of the incontinence. Because most children with incontinence have poor voiding patterns, treatment is directed at improving elimination habits. The child is usually started on a frequent voiding schedule of every 2 to 3 hours. Children who have a history of postponing voiding have a misconception of bladder fullness and therefore have to be sent to void whether they feel the need to urinate or not. Relaxing during voiding rather than straining is encouraged.

If the child is known to have postvoid residual, double-voiding is implemented. The child voids initially, then waits 1 minute and voids a second time to eliminate any remaining urine.

Positive reinforcement in the form of sticker charts for compliance and having successful dry days plays a major motivating role in the treatment program.

Urinary incontinence can be an effect of constipation and often improves once constipation has resolved. Constipation is treated with increased dietary fiber, increased fluid intake, and sometimes administration of polyethylene glycol 3350 (Glycolax), an osmotic laxative.

Pharmacotherapy

If conservative measures fail to produce any improvement, pharmacotherapy may be indicated (Table 1).

One commonly used class is the anticholinergics, which are effective in blocking the muscarinic receptors, thus exhibiting a musculotropic relaxant effect on the detrusor muscle. This allows increased bladder capacity, decreased frequency of uninhibited contractions, and delaying the initial desire to void. These include oxybutynin chloride (Ditropan) 0.2 mg/kg (maximum 5 mg per dose) two ro three times daily, tolterodine (Detrol)[1] 0.02 mg/kg two or three times daily, and hyoscyamine (Levsin Drop) 0.25-1 mL two or three times daily.

α-Blockers have been successfully used in children with functional outlet obstruction. They include terazosin hydrochloride (Hytrin)[1] 1 mg at bedtime and doxazosin mesylate (Cardura)[1] 0.5 mg at bedtime. These drugs facilitate bladder emptying.

Physical Therapy

Biofeedback therapy aims at changing learned behavior by teaching children awareness of their pelvic floor muscles. The goal of the treatment is to provide children with the ability to relax and contract the pelvic floor muscles.

TABLE 1 Pharmacotherapy to Treat Incontinence

Drug	Dose	Effect
Oxybutynin chloride (Ditropan)	0.2 mg/kg (max 5 mg) bid-tid	Antispasmodic on smooth muscle: Decreased contractions, increased capacity, delayed desire to void
Exybutynin extended release (Ditropan XL)	5-10 mg qd	
Tolterodine (Detrol)[1]	0.02 mg/kg bid-tid	Antispasmodic on smooth muscle: Decreased contractions, increased capacity, delayed desire to void
Tolterodine extended release (Detrol LA)[1]	2-4 mg qd	
Hyoscyamine (Levsin Drop)	0.25-1 mL bid-tid	Antispasmodic on smooth muscle
Terazosin hydrochloride (Hytrin)[1]	1 mg qhs	α-Blocker, relaxes smooth muscle of bladder neck, facilitates bladder emptying
Doxazosin mesylate (Cardura)[1]	0.5 mg qhs	α-Blocker, relaxes smooth muscle of bladder neck, facilitates bladder emptying
Desmopressin (DDAVP)	Oral: 0.2-0.6 mg PO qhs Intranasal: 1 spray (10 µg) each nostril qhs initially	Used to treat nocturnal enuresis Promotes reabsorption of water in the kidneys
Imipramine (Tofranil)	10-25 mg qhs (max, 2.5 mg/kg/d)	Used to treat nocturnal enuresis Mechanism of action is unknown

[1]Not FDA approved for this indication.

Sacral nerve stimulation is used in the adult population, but very limited data are available on use in children. This treatment aims at stimulating the sacral nerves that influence the bladder, sphincter, and pelvic floor during voiding.

Nocturnal Enuresis

Nocturnal enuresis is the involuntary loss of urine during sleep. It can be grouped into primary and secondary nocturnal enuresis. Primary enuresis implies that the enuresis has been present since birth. Secondary enuresis refers to enuresis that started after being dry for 6 months or more. Further grouping of enuresis includes monosymptomatic primary enuresis, nonmonosymptomatic primary enuresis, monosymptomatic secondary enuresis, and nonmonosymptomatic secondary enuresis. Monosymptomatic implies that there are no daytime urinary symptoms present. Nonmonosymptomatic is used when children have daytime symptoms such as urinary frequency, urgency, incontinence, holding maneuvers, and infrequent voiding.

EPIDEMIOLOGY

Nocturnal enuresis affects 5 to 7 million children in the United States. Twenty-three percent of all 5-year-old children still wet the bed; the percentage decreases to 7% to 10% in 8-year-olds and 1% to 2% in 17-year-olds. The ratio of enuresis is 2:1 in boys versus girls. Forsythe and Redmond report a spontaneous cure rate of 14% to 16% annually. Even though the exact cause of nocturnal enuresis is not known, several theories try to explain the etiology of enuresis.

ETIOLOGY

A genetic component has been identified. Bakwin showed that there is a 44% chance of developing enuresis if one parent has a history of enuresis and a 77% risk if both parents have a history of enuresis.

Children who are described by their parents as deep sleepers are thought to wet the bed because they are unaware of bladder distention and uninhibited bladder contractions during sleep. Sleep apnea caused by upper airway obstruction has also been linked to enuresis.

Gross and Dornbush found that enuresis was more prevalent in children with delayed motor and language development. Delayed maturity of the central nervous system can prevent the child from inhibiting bladder contractions.

It is believed that some children have increased urine production during sleep due to a decreased production of antidiuretic hormone (ADH). The nocturnal urine production exceeds their daytime functional bladder capacity, and enuretic episodes occur.

Symptoms of daytime voiding dysfunction are a common finding in patients with enuresis. Eighty percent of children with daytime incontinence wet the bed.

Psychosocial stressors, such as relocation, death in the family, parental separation or divorce, new baby born to the family, trauma, or sexual and physical abuse are believed to cause regressive behavior, which often includes enuresis.

Even though it is not scientifically proved, some literature suggests that certain dietary products can increase the likelihood of enuresis, including carbonated beverages, citrus, caffeine, and milk or milk products.

TREATMENT

After careful history taking, physical examination, and diagnostic studies, a treatment plan is formulated.

Pharmacotherapy

Medications that have shown to be effective in treating enuresis include desmopressin (DDAVP), imipramine (Tofranil), and, less commonly, anticholinergics (see Box 1).

Desmopressin is an analogue to ADH and reduces urine production. It is used in a dose of 0.2 to 0.6 mg at bedtime. Due to risk of water intoxication, oral fluid intake has to be eliminated 2 hours before taking the medication. Desmopressin reduces enuresis by 40% to 70% and has a relapse rate as high as 80% to 100%.

Imipramine, a tricyclic antidepressant, given at a dose of 0.5 to 1.5 mg/kg/day (maximum 50 mg/day or 2.5 mg/kg/d). The exact mechanism of action is unclear; however, changes in sleep cycle or a mild anticholinergic effect are postulated. Success rate is 50%. Possible side effects are more significant than with DDAVP and include mood alteration, daytime sedation, arrhythmias, and hypotension.

Conditioning

Treatment with an alarm system has a 70% success rate. The enuresis alarm has a sensor that attaches to the underwear. When the sensor comes in touch with urine, the alarm is set off. Motivation plays an important role in the success of the alarm. The alarm has a lower relapse rate than medication does.

Whether the child suffers from daytime or nighttime incontinence, it is important for parents to understand that the problem is not resolved within days or weeks. Parents might have to be reminded that it took several years of poor voiding habits to develop incontinence. In general, we believe that it takes one half the time of the time the child exhibited poor voiding habits to see complete resolution.

REFERENCES

Baskin LS, Kogan BA: Handbook of Pediatric Urology. Philadelphia, Lippincott Williams & Wilkins, 2005.
Herndon ACD, Joseph, DB: Urinary incontinence. Pediatr Clin North Am 2006;53(3):1-11.
Homsy YL, Austin PF: Dysfunctional voiding disorders and nocturnal enuresis. In: Belman AB, King LR, Kramer SA (eds): Clinical Pediatric Urology, 4th edition, Informa Healthcare, 2001, pp 345-365.
Nevéus T, Läckgren G, Tuvemo T, et al: Enuresis—background and treatment. Scand J Urol Nephrol Suppl 2000;(206):1-44.
Nevéus T, Von Gontard A, Hoebeke P, et al: The standardization of terminology of lower urinary tract function in children and adolescents: Report from the Standardisation Committee of the International Children's Continence Society. J Urol 2006;176(1):314-324.
Nichelson L, Smith DP: Dysfunctional elimination syndrome: where constipation, daytime urinary problems and bedwetting merge. Advance for Nurse Practitioners, 27-31, March 2007.
Schulman SL, Berry AK: A simple step-wise approach to the child with daytime wetting. Contemporary Urology 2007;19-29.

Urinary Incontinence

Method of
E. Ann Gormley, MD

Urinary incontinence is a significant problem that affects millions of Americans. Patients may not report incontinence to their primary care providers because of embarrassment or misconceptions regarding treatment. Because incontinence is often treatable, it behooves the health care professional to identify patients who might benefit from treatment. Given that the treatment of incontinence varies depending on the etiology, the aim of evaluation is to identify the etiology.

Etiology

Urinary incontinence is generally the result of either bladder or urethral dysfunction (Table 1). Incontinence also may result from a nonurologic cause and is usually reversible when the underlying problem is treated (Table 2). More uncommon causes of incontinence are urinary fistulae and ectopic ureteral orifices.

BLADDER DYSFUNCTION

Bladder dysfunction causes urge or overflow incontinence. *Urge incontinence* occurs when the bladder pressure is sufficient to overcome the sphincter mechanism. Elevated bladder or detrusor pressure tends to open the bladder neck and urethra. An elevation in detrusor pressure may occur from intermittent bladder contractions (detrusor overactivity) or because of an incremental rise in pressure with increased bladder volume (poor compliance). Detrusor overactivity may be idiopathic, or it may be associated with a neurologic disease (detrusor overactivity of neurogenic origin). Detrusor overactivity is common in the elderly and may be associated with bladder outlet obstruction. Poor bladder compliance results from loss of the viscoelastic features of the bladder or because

TABLE 1 Etiology of Incontinence

Bladder Dysfunction
1. Urge incontinence
   - Detrusor overactivity
     - Idiopathic
     - Neurogenic origin
   - Poor compliance
2. Overflow incontinence

Urethral Dysfunction
3. Stress incontinence
   - Anatomic
   - Intrinsic sphincter deficiency

of a change in neuroregulatory activity. The patient with urge incontinence may appreciate a sudden sensation to void but then is unable to suppress the urge fully. In severe cases, the patient may not be aware of the sensation of needing to void until he or she is actually leaking. The amount of leakage in patients with urge incontinence is variable, depending on the patient's ability to suppress the contraction. Patients with urge incontinence will often have frequency and nocturia in addition to urgency and urge incontinence. They may also have nocturnal enuresis.

Overactive bladder is a newer term that describes patients with frequency and urgency with or without urge incontinence.

Overflow incontinence occurs at extreme bladder volumes or when the bladder volume reaches the limit of the bladder's viscoelastic properties. The loss of urine is driven by an elevation in detrusor pressure. Overflow incontinence is seen in the case of incomplete bladder emptying caused by either obstruction or poor bladder contractility. Obstruction is rare in women but can result from severe pelvic prolapse or following surgery for stress incontinence. Patients with overflow incontinence complain of constant dribbling, and they may also describe extreme frequency.

URETHRAL-RELATED INCONTINENCE

Urethral-related incontinence, or *stress incontinence*, occurs because of either urethral hypermobility or intrinsic sphincter deficiency (ISD). Incontinence associated with urethral hypermobility has been called *anatomic incontinence* because the incontinence is due to malposition of the sphincter unit. Displacement of the proximal urethra below the level of the pelvic floor does not allow for transmission of abdominal pressure that normally aids in closing the urethra. Some women with mobility of the bladder neck or urethra do not experience incontinence. ISD was initially believed to occur after failure of one or more operations for stress incontinence. Other causes of ISD include myelodysplasia, trauma, and radiation. Some authors have theorized that all incontinent patients must have an element of ISD in order to actually leak. The patient with stress incontinence leaks urine with any sudden increase in abdominal pressure. In patients with severe ISD, the increase in abdominal pressure required to cause leakage is small, so patients may leak urine with minimal activity.

Evaluation of the Incontinent Patient

The evaluation of the incontinent patient includes a history, physical examination, laboratory tests, and possibly urodynamic testing. The onset, frequency, severity, and pattern of incontinence should be sought, as well as any associated symptoms such as frequency, dysuria, urgency, and nocturia. Incontinence may be quantified by asking the patient if he or she wears a pad and how often the pad is changed. Obstructive symptoms, such as a feeling of incomplete emptying, hesitancy, straining, or weak stream, may coexist with incontinence, particularly in males and in female patients with

TABLE 2 Transient Causes of Incontinence (*DIAPPERS*)

Cause	Comment
Delirium	Incontinence may be secondary to delirium and will often stop when acute delirium resolves.
Infection	Symptomatic infection may prevent a patient from reaching the toilet in time.
Atrophic vaginitis	Vaginitis may cause the same symptoms as an infection.
Pharmacologic	
• Sedatives	Alcohol and long-acting benzodiazepines may cause confusion and secondary incontinence.
• Diuretics	A brisk diuresis may overwhelm the bladder's capacity and cause uninhibited detrusor contractions, resulting in urge incontinence.
• Anticholinergics	Many nonprescription and prescription medications have anticholinergic properties. Side effects of anticholinergics include urinary retention with associated frequency and overflow incontinence.
• α Adrenergics	Tone in the bladder neck and proximal sphincter is increased by α-adrenergic agonists and can cause urinary retention, particularly in men with prostatism.
• α Antagonists	Tone in the smooth muscles of the bladder neck and proximal sphincter is decreased with α-adrenergic antagonists. Women treated with these drugs for hypertension may develop or have an exacerbation of stress incontinence.
Psychological	Depression may be occasionally associated with incontinence.
Excessive urine production	Excessive intake, diabetes, hypercalcemia, congestive heart failure, and peripheral edema can all lead to polyuria, which can lead to incontinence.
Restricted mobility	Incontinence may be precipitated or aggravated if the patient cannot get to the toilet quickly enough.
Stool impaction	Patients with impacted stool can have urge or overflow urinary incontinence and may also have fecal incontinence.

From Resnick NM: Urinary incontinence in the elderly. Med Grand Rounds 1984;3:281-290.

CURRENT DIAGNOSIS

Urge Incontinence

Symptoms
- Urgency
- Frequency
- Nocturia
- Unable to reach the toilet with urge

Stress Incontinence

Symptoms
- Leakage with physical activity

Signs
- Bladder neck mobility
- Positive stress test

Mixed Incontinence

Symptoms
- Urgency
- Frequency
- Nocturia
- Unable to reach the toilet with urge
- Leakage with physical activity

Signs
- Bladder neck mobility
- Positive stress test

Overflow Incontinence

Symptoms
- Frequency
- Nocturia
- Urgency
- Leakage with physical activity

Signs
- High postvoid residual

previous incontinence procedure, cystoceles, or poor detrusor contractility. Female patients should be asked about symptoms of pelvic prolapse, such as recurrent urinary tract infection, a sensation of vaginal fullness or pressure, or the observation of a bulge in the vagina. All incontinent patients should be asked about bowel function and neurologic symptoms. Response to previous treatments, including drugs, should be noted. Important features of the history include previous gynecologic and urologic procedures, neurologic problems, and past medical problems. A list of the patient's current medications, including over-the-counter medications, should be obtained.

Although the history may define the patient's problem, it may be misleading. Urge incontinence may be triggered by activities such as coughing, so according to the patient's history, he or she seems to have stress incontinence. A patient who complains only of urge incontinence may also have stress incontinence. Mixed incontinence is very common; at least 65% of patients with stress incontinence have associated urgency or urge incontinence.

A complete physical examination is performed, with emphasis on the neurologic assessment and on the abdominal, pelvic, and rectal examinations. In females, the condition of the vaginal mucosa and the degree of urethral mobility are determined. Simple pelvic examination with the patient supine is sufficient to determine if the urethra moves with straining or coughing. The degree of movement is not as important as the determination of whether movement occurs. The presence of associated pelvic organ prolapse should be noted because it can contribute to the patient's voiding problems and may have an impact on diagnosis and treatment. A rectal examination in both males and females includes the evaluation of sphincter tone and perineal sensation.

A urinalysis is performed to determine if there is any evidence of hematuria, pyuria, glucosuria, or proteinuria. A urine specimen is sent for cytologic examination if there is hematuria and/or irritative voiding symptoms. The urine is cultured if there is pyuria or bacteriuria. Infection should be treated prior to further investigations or interventions. Hematuria consisting of more than three red cells per high-power field warrants further investigation.

A postvoid residual (PVR) should be measured either with pelvic ultrasound or directly with a catheter. A normal PVR is less than 50 mL, and a PVR greater than 200 mL is abnormal. A significant PVR urine may reflect either bladder outlet obstruction or poor bladder contractility. The only way to distinguish outlet obstruction from poor contractility is with urodynamic testing.

Urodynamic testing is used to accurately diagnose the etiology of a patient's incontinence; however, many patients can be successfully treated without urodynamic testing. The purpose of urodynamic testing is to examine compliance, diagnose stress incontinence, and rule out obstruction as a cause of either overflow or urge incontinence. Urodynamic testing should ideally be performed prior to invasive therapies and certainly in patients who are undergoing repeat procedures following failed procedures.

Treatment of Urinary Incontinence

URGE INCONTINENCE

Patients with urge incontinence need to understand that they leak urine because their bladder contracts with little or no warning. The first line of treatment is timed voiding. Often, reminding patients to void every 1 to 2 hours during the day, before they get an urge to void, will result in them staying dry. Other behavioral interventions, such as modification of fluid intake, avoidance of bladder irritants, and bladder retraining, where the patient attempts to consciously delay voiding and to increase the interval between voids, may also have a role in the treatment of urge incontinence.

Anticholinergics are the mainstay of medical therapy in achieving continence. The side effects of anticholinergics include urinary retention, dry mouth, constipation, nausea, blurred vision, tachycardia, drowsiness, and confusion. They are contraindicated in patients with narrow-angle glaucoma. Anticholinergics are also used to decrease bladder pressure in patients with poor compliance. Anticholinergics are combined with clean intermittent catheterization in patients who have a significant PVR prior to treatment and in patients who develop retention while taking anticholinergics.

Patients with intractable detrusor overactivity may require surgical intervention, consisting of neuromodulation with a sacral nerve stimulator or various forms of bladder augmentation.

The primary goal in caring for the patient with poor compliance is treating the high bladder pressure. Complete bladder emptying with clean intermittent catheterization combined with anticholinergics will often lower bladder pressure to a safe range. Some patients may require a combination of anticholinergics and α agonists. Bladder augmentation is required when medical management fails.

OVERFLOW INCONTINENCE

Overflow incontinence is treated by emptying the bladder. If the cause of overflow is obstruction, then relieving the obstruction should lead to improved emptying. Anatomic obstruction in males derives from either urethral stricture disease or prostatic obstruction. Depending on the severity of urethral stricture disease, the patient may require urethral dilation, internal urethrotomy, or urethroplasty. Prostatic obstruction may be treated in a variety of ways, but transurethral resection remains the gold standard. If a woman is obstructed from previous surgery or from pelvic prolapse, she may benefit from urethrolysis or surgical correction of the prolapse. Clean intermittent catheterization is an option in the obstructed patient who does not want or could not tolerate further surgery.

The patient with overflow incontinence secondary to poor detrusor contractility is best treated with clean intermittent catheterization.

Indwelling catheters are not an optimum treatment modality for treatment of incontinence. All patients with indwelling catheters will have infected urine, which predisposes them to bladder calculi and ultimately to squamous cell carcinoma of the bladder. Any foreign object in the bladder can cause or exacerbate elevated bladder

CURRENT THERAPY

Urge Incontinence

Behavioral Changes
- Avoidance of bladder irritants
- Timed voiding
- Pelvic muscle exercises

Anticholinergics—Antimuscarinics—Nonselective for M3 Receptor
- Propantheline (Pro-Banthine)[1] 7.5 to 30 mg orally, three to five times daily
- Tolterodine (Detrol LA) 4 mg orally, daily
- Trospium (Sanctura) 20 mg orally, two times daily
- Solifenacin (Vesicare) 5-10 mg orally, daily

Anticholinergics—Antimuscarinics—Selective for M3 Receptor
- Darifenacin (Enablex) 7.5-15 mg orally, daily

Anticholinergics—Antimuscarinics/Smooth Muscle Relaxants
- Oxybutynin
- Regular (Ditropan) 2.5-5 mg orally, one to three times daily
- Extended-release (Ditropan XL) 5-30 mg orally, daily
- Transdermal (Oxytrol) 3.9-mg patch, twice per week
- Hyoscyamine (Levsin) 0.125-0.375 mg orally, two to four times daily

Anticholinergics/α Agonist—For Urge or Mixed Incontinence
- Imipramine (Tofranil)[1] 10-25 mg, once to three times daily

Stress Incontinence

Behavioral Changes
- Weight loss
- Quitting smoking
- Pelvic muscle exercises

α Agonists
- Pseudoephedrine (Sudafed)[1] 30-60 mg, up to four times daily

Surgery
- Anatomic
  - Retropubic suspensions
    - Burch
    - Marshall-Marchetti-Krantz
  - Slings
  - Pubovaginal
  - Midurethral
  - Obturator
- Intrinsic Sphincter Deficiency
  - Slings
    - Pubovaginal
    - Midurethral
    - Obturator
  - Artificial sphincter
  - Submucosal Injections with Bulking Agents
  - Collagen (Contigen)
  - Carbon-coated zirconium oxide beads (Durasphere)
  - Ethylene vinyl alcohol copolymer (Tegress)

---

[1]Not FDA approved for this indication.

pressure that is associated with hydronephrosis, ureteral obstruction, renal stones, and eventually renal failure.

STRESS INCONTINENCE

The amount of incontinence and how it affects the patient often determines the aggressiveness of treatment. The patient who is severely restricted because of severe leakage with minimal movement may not want to try medical therapy but may opt for surgical treatment, whereas the patient who leaks small amounts infrequently may choose conservative treatment. Pelvic floor exercises can improve anatomic stress urinary incontinence by augmenting closure of the external urethral sphincter and by preventing descent and rotation of the bladder neck and urethra. To benefit from the exercises, women must be taught to do the exercises properly, and they must do them. Adjuncts to learning pelvic floor exercises include weighted vaginal cones, a perineometer, and electrical stimulation.

α Agonists such as phenylpropanolamine[1] and pseudoephedrine (Sudafed)[1] can be used for treatment of stress incontinence. The bladder neck and proximal urethra have abundant α receptors. Activation of these receptors by α agonists leads to an increase in smooth muscle tone. The usual dose is twice daily, but some women who are incontinent with exercise may benefit from taking an α agonist 1 hour before exercise. Tricyclic antidepressants, such as imipramine (Tofranil),[1] have both α-agonist and anticholinergic properties.

Surgical therapy for stress incontinence is indicated when a patient does not wish to pursue nonsurgical therapy, or if such therapy has failed. The type of surgical therapy depends on the diagnosis. Patients who have anatomic stress incontinence can benefit from a variety of surgical repairs that restore the bladder neck to its normal retropubic position or improve urethral support. Patients with ISD usually have a well-supported bladder neck. These patients require a procedure that will close or coapt the proximal urethra. Coaptation may be achieved with a variety of bulking agents that are injected into the bladder neck or proximal urethra. A pubovaginal sling is the ideal procedure for the patient with both ISD and anatomic stress incontinence, as a sling will coapt the proximal urethra and restore the bladder neck to its normal location.

Synthetic midurethral slings are ideal for the patient with anatomic stress incontinence who wishes surgery with minimal recovery time. In one of the rare randomized surgical trials for stress incontinence, the result with tension-free vaginal tape has been shown to be comparable to that of a Burch colposuspension at 6, 12, and 24 months. The newest sling is a transobturator sling that is placed transversely underneath the urethra from one obturator foramina to the other. The advantage of this sling is that the retropubic space is avoided, with low risk of bladder, bowel, and major vessel injury.

Randomized trials comparing midurethral or transobturator slings to pubovaginal slings have not been performed.

MIXED INCONTINENCE

Stress and urge incontinence often coexist. Burgio et al. advocate pelvic muscle exercises with biofeedback for treatment of stress and urge incontinence. Behavioral therapy can result in a reduction in incontinence episodes and patient-perceived improvement.

Imipramine (Tofranil)[1] is beneficial in patients with mixed (stress and urge) incontinence. The recommended dose is 10 to 25 mg, three times daily.

Seventy percent of patients with combined incontinence (stress and urge) will be relieved of urge incontinence following a procedure for stress incontinence. Patients whose urge incontinence does not respond to anticholinergics preoperatively may have a good response to anticholinergics once their stress incontinence is treated. Box 1 provides an overview of treatments.

---

[1]Not FDA approved for this indication.

BOX 1 Overview of Treatments

Behavioral Changes
- Avoidance of bladder irritants
- Weight loss
- Quitting smoking
- Pelvic muscle exercises

Medical Therapy
- α Agonists
  - Stress incontinent patients
  - Mixed incontinent patients
- Anticholinergics
  - Urge incontinent patients
- Anticholinergics/α agonists
  - Mixed incontinent patients

Surgical Therapy
- Stress incontinent patients
- Rare patients with urge incontinence

REFERENCES

Blaivas JG, Groutz A: Urinary incontinence: Pathophysiology, evaluation, and management overview. In Walsh PC, Retik AB, Vaughan ED Jr, Wein AJ (eds): 8th ed., Campbell's Urology, vol 2, Philadelphia WB Saunders, 2002, p 1027.

Burgio KL, Locher JL, Goode PS, et al: Behavioral vs drug treatment for urge urinary incontinence in older women: A randomized controlled trial. JAMA 1998;280:1995-2000.

Leach GE, Dmochowski RR, Appell RA, et al: Female Stress Urinary Incontinence Clinical Guidelines Panel summary report on surgical management of female stress urinary incontinence. The American Urological Association. J Urol 1997;158:875.

Ward KL, Hilton P: A randomized trial of colposuspension and tension-free vaginal tape (TVT) for primary genuine stress incontinence: 2 year follow-up. Int Urogynecol J Pelvic Floor Dysfunct 2001;12(Suppl. 2):S7-S8.

Epididymitis

Method of
John N. Krieger, MD

Epididymitis is the inflammatory reaction of the epididymis to infection or to local trauma. Epididymitis causes major morbidity, accounting for more than 600,000 visits to physicians per year in the United States. Acute epididymitis is responsible for more days lost from military service than any other disease and is responsible for 20% of urologic admissions in the military. A survey of ambulatory patients documented epididymitis as a cause of 1 in 345 visits (0.3%), representing the fifth most common urologic condition, after prostatitis, urinary tract infections, urinary stones, and sexually transmitted infections.

Clinical Presentation

Painful swelling of the scrotum is the characteristic clinical presentation. In most patients the pain and swelling are unilateral. The onset may be acute over 1 or 2 days or more gradual. Pain can radiate along the spermatic cord or into the lower abdomen. Symptoms of cystitis or urethritis are common. Dysuria or irritative lower urinary tract symptoms are characteristic. Many sexually active men have a urethral discharge. Thus, particular attention should be directed to eliciting a history of genitourinary tract disease or sexual exposure. Some men may have only a nonspecific finding of fever or other signs of infection. This is especially common in hospitalized men who have had urinary tract manipulation or catheterization and may be obtunded by medication.

Tender swelling can occur in the posterior aspect of the scrotum. Usually, the swelling is unilateral and is often accompanied by erythema of the scrotal skin. Early in the course, swelling may be localized to one portion of the epididymis. However, the swelling often progresses to involve the ipsilateral testis, producing an epididymo-orchitis. At this point it is difficult to distinguish the testicle from the epididymis within the inflammatory mass. Scrotal examination reveals the characteristic inflammatory hydrocele caused by secretion of fluid between the layers of the tunica vaginalis. Urethral discharge may be apparent on inspection or on stripping of the urethra.

Ideally, evaluation for urethritis should be done before the patient voids because micturition can make mild urethritis difficult or impossible to detect. The nursing staff should be taught to instruct patients with urogenital tract complaints not to void until after the physical examination. This is a common problem when we are asked to consult on patient management in the emergency department or in primary care settings. Patients with no sexual risk factors or evidence of urethritis should have microscopic evaluation of their midstream urine.

Pathogenesis

Acute epididymitis occurs when uropathogens overcome the host defenses of the male lower genitourinary tract to establish infection of the epididymis. Most cases result from retrograde ascent of organisms through the urethra, prostate, ejaculatory duct, and vas deferens to reach the epididymis. Structural or functional abnormalities of the lower urinary tract increase the risk of epididymitis.

The risk factors for epididymitis vary substantially in different patient populations. In children and older men, anatomic abnormalities are critical risk factors for development of epididymitis. These include congenital anatomic abnormalities, such as an ectopic ureter draining into the vas deferens in children, and acquired anatomic abnormalities, such as bladder outflow obstruction in older men. In contrast, most sexually active younger men with epididymitis have normal urinary tracts. Thus, urologic investigations are indicated in children and older men with epididymitis but are seldom needed for management of epididymitis in young sexually active men.

Infections of the urethra, bladder, or prostate are important risk factors for development of epididymitis. In children and older men, the most common organisms are the typical bacteria that cause urinary tract infections, especially *Escherichia coli*, other enterics, and pseudomonads. In sexually active men, the most common pathogens are *Chlamydia trachomatis* and *Neisseria gonorrhoeae*. Men who practice insertive anal intercourse are also at risk for epididymitis caused by *E. coli* and other enteric bacteria. In addition to the usual causative organisms, immunocompromised patients are at higher risk for epididymitis caused by mycobacteria and fungi.

Diagnosis and Treatment

ACUTE EPIDIDYMITIS

Most patients with acute epididymitis can be considered in two categories, nonspecific bacterial epididymitis or sexually transmitted epididymitis. Unusual patients develop epididymitis after genital trauma or with disseminated infections.

Clinical evaluation begins with a history, with specific attention to eliciting recognized risk factors, and a thorough physical examination. Initial laboratory tests include urinalysis, culture, and sensitivity testing for men with presumed nonspecific bacterial epididymitis.

CURRENT DIAGNOSIS

History

- Exposure to sexually transmitted infection
- Urologic abnormalities or genitourinary tract instrumentation
- Symptoms of dysuria or urethral discharge

Physical Examination

- Pain or swelling on palpation of the epididymis
- Inflammatory hydrocele
- Scrotal skin erythema
- Urethral discharge
- Abnormal genitourinary tract anatomy
- Elevated temperature

Laboratory Studies

- Urethral swab specimen or first-void urine for pyuria
- Midstream urine for evidence of bacteriuria or pyuria
- Urine culture and sensitivity testing
- Samples for evaluation of sexually transmitted infections, as appropriate
- Doppler scrotal ultrasound may be helpful to differentiate epididymitis from testicular torsion or tumor

Men at risk for sexually transmitted epididymitis should also have a gram-stained urethral smear, culture for *N. gonorrhoeae*, and testing for *C. trachomatis*. In the latter group, serologic testing is also recommended for syphilis and for HIV infection.

CURRENT THERAPY

Age Younger than 35 Years with No History of Allergy

- Czeftriaxone (Rocephin) 250 mg IM once
  plus
- Doxycycline (Vibramicin) 100 mg PO bid for 10 days
  or
- Azithromycin (Zithromax) 1 g PO as a single dose

Age Older than 35 Years or Patient with a History of Allergy to Cephalosporins or Tetracyclines

- Ofloxacin (Floxin) 300 mg PO bid for 10 days
  or
- Levofloxacin (Levaquin) 500 mg PO qd for 10 days

All Patients

- Anti-inflammatories
- Decreased activity
- Scrotal elevation
- Pain control

Follow-up

- Failure to improve within 3 days: Reevaluate initial diagnosis and therapy
- For persistent swelling and tenderness after therapy, consider:
  - Testicular tumor
  - Abscess
  - Testicular infarction
  - Tuberculosis
  - Fungal epididymitis

NONSPECIFIC BACTERIAL EPIDIDYMITIS

Infection with coliform or *Pseudomonas* species is the most common cause of epididymitis in men older than 35 years. In most series, gram-negative rods caused more than two thirds of cases of bacterial epididymitis. However, gram-positive cocci are also important pathogens and constituted the most common organisms in other reports.

Patients with bacterial epididymitis often have underlying urologic pathology or have a history of genitourinary tract manipulation. Epididymitis can occur weeks or rarely months after genitourinary tract surgery or urethral catheterization. Epididymitis constitutes a special risk for men who undergo urinary tract surgery or instrumentation while they are bacteriuric. Acute and chronic bacterial prostatitis represent other important predisposing conditions for development of bacterial epididymitis.

Medical management is appropriate for most patients with bacterial epididymitis. Typical patients are managed as outpatients. Initial empiric treatment is initiated with agents appropriate for both gram-negative rods and gram-positive cocci pending urine culture and sensitivity results. Fluoroquinolones represent our first choice for management of nonspecific epididymitis in outpatients. Agents of choice include ofloxacin (Floxin) and levofloxacin (Levaquin). Ciprofloxacin (Cipro) represents a reasonable alternative quinolone. In areas where the rate of bacterial resistance is low, trimethoprim-sulfamethoxazole (TMP-SMX; Bactrim, Septra) represents another reasonable alternative. Initial empiric therapy may be changed, if necessary, after culture results are available. A standard course of therapy is 10 days. More prolonged therapy may be needed for select patients such as those with evidence of bacterial prostatitis, whose antimicrobial therapy is continued for 6 to 12 weeks.

Indications for hospitalization include systemic symptoms, such as leukocytosis and fever, complications, or associated medical conditions. In these severe cases, parenteral antimicrobial therapy is used until the patient defervesces. Choices for empiric therapy of severe cases include the combination of an aminoglycoside plus either a β-lactam agent or a third-generation cephalosporin. After resolution of the acute systemic infection, therapy is continued with oral agents, guided by the culture and sensitivity results.

Nonspecific measures are worthwhile, including bedrest, scrotal elevation, analgesics, and local ice packs. A spermatic cord block with bipuvicaine (Marcaine) may be helpful for managing severe pain. We recommend urologic evaluation, because structural or functional abnormalities are common among men and boys with nonspecific bacterial epididymitis.

SEXUALLY TRANSMITTED EPIDIDYMITIS

Sexually transmitted epididymitis is most common in young men. *C. trachomatis* and *N. gonorrhoeae* are the major pathogens. In most series, *Chlamydia* was identified as the most common cause of epididymitis in younger, sexually active populations. For example, in our institution, *C. trachomatis* infections were documented in 17 (50%) of 34 cases of epididymitis in men younger than 35 years but in only 1 (6%) of 16 cases of epididymitis in men older than 35 years. In the past, these patients were considered to have "idiopathic" nonspecific epididymitis. Sexually transmitted *E. coli* infection also occurs among men who are the insertive partners during anal intercourse.

Often patients with chlamydial epididymitis do not complain of urethral discharge. However, 11 (65%) of 17 patients with epididymitis caused by *Chlamydia* had demonstrable discharge. In most cases, the discharge was scant and watery, characteristic of nongonococcal urethritis. The median interval from the last sexual exposure was 10 days and ranged from 1 to 45 days. Thus, urethral *C. trachomatis* may be carried for long periods before overt epididymitis develops.

In the preantibiotic era, epididymitis occurred in 10% to 30% of men with gonococcal urethritis. However, in current series, *N. gonorrhoeae* was identified in 16% of men with epididymitis in military populations and in 21% of men with epididymitis in civilians younger than 35 years. Many patients with epididymitis do not have a history of urethral discharge, and a discharge may be demonstrable in only 50% of such patients. Diagnosis depends on a high index of clinical suspicion, evaluation for presence of urethritis (which may be asymptomatic), appropriate cultures, or antigen detection tests.

Empiric therapy is recommended before culture results are available. Appropriate therapy includes coverage for both *N. gonorrheae* and *C. trachomatis* infections. The first choice regimen is the combination of ceftriaxone (Rocephin) plus doxycycline (Vibramycin) for 10 days. Allergic patients are treated with one of the quinolone regimens described earlier. Alternatives for coverage of *N. gonorrhoeae* include cefixime (Suprax), ciprofloxacin, ofloxacin, levofloxacin, or spectinomycin (Trobicin). Azithromycin (Zithromax) represents an effective alternative for coverage of *C. trachomatis*. Nonspecific measures are helpful, including bedrest, scrotal elevation, analgesics, and local ice packs. A spermatic cord block with bipuvicaine can reduce the need for analgesics in men with severe pain.

Patients should be evaluated for other sexually transmitted infections, and treatment of sexual partners is important. Patients should be instructed to avoid intercourse until symptoms have resolved completely and to refer all sex partners within the previous 60 days for evaluation and treatment. Underlying genitourinary tract abnormalities are uncommon in this population. Thus, a complete urologic work-up is indicated rarely for patients with uncomplicated sexually transmitted epididymitis.

UNCOMMON CAUSES

Tuberculous epididymitis is the most common manifestation of genital tuberculosis in men, with orchitis and prostatitis less common. The usual symptom is heaviness or swelling. Scrotal swelling with bead-like enlargement of the vas deferens is characteristic. Chronic draining scrotal sinuses can occur. The systemic mycoses rarely cause epididymitis; blastomycosis is the most common pathogen and can also cause a draining sinus through the scrotal wall. Men with HIV infection and uncomplicated epididymitis should receive the same treatment as those without HIV. However, fungal and mycobacterial causes of epididymitis are more common among patients who are immunocompromised.

In the pediatric population, epididymitis can occur with congenital anatomic abnormalities, such as ectopic ureter or posterior urethral valves. Epididymitis occasionally occurs after testicular trauma. Many of these men have evidence of genitourinary tract infections with organisms outlined earlier, but occasional men develop traumatic epididymitis that is not associated with positive cultures or inflammation. We also described an unusual syndrome of noninfectious epididymitis associated with amiodarone (Cordarone) therapy for refractory ventricular arrhythmias. Rare patients develop epididymitis as a complication of collagen vascular disorders, such as Wegener's granulomatosis or Behçet's disease.

Differential Diagnosis

Severe inflammation can lead to an enlarged indurated epididymis that is indistinguishable from the testicle. This can present difficulties in the differential diagnosis of epididymitis from testicular torsion or testicular cancer. Normally, the epididymis lies posterior to the testis. This demarcation is often preserved in cases of epididymitis. Reactive hydrocele formation can render palpation of intrascrotal structures difficult. Although transillumination often identifies hydroceles, color-flow Doppler ultrasonography is my preferred imaging study when the diagnosis is in doubt.

Acute epididymitis must be distinguished from testicular torsion at the initial evaluation because uncorrected torsion results in testicular death within 24 hours. Men with swelling and tenderness that persist after completing therapy should be reevaluated for testicular cancer, tuberculosis, or fungal epididymitis.

Complications

Most patients experience relief of their symptoms within 48 hours. However, swelling and discomfort can persist for weeks or months following eradication of the infecting organism. In some cases, the epididymis remains enlarged or indurated indefinitely. Such men can develop chronic epididymitis, which is characterized by pain and occasionally by recurrent swelling.

Bacterial epididymitis may be an important focus of organisms causing both local morbidity and bacteremia in men with indwelling transurethral catheters. Genitourinary tract complications of acute epididymitis include testicular infarction, scrotal abscess, pyocele of the scrotum, a chronic draining scrotal sinus, chronic epididymitis, and infertility. Ultrasonography, particularly color-flow Doppler ultrasonography, is useful for the differential diagnosis of complicated cases. Surgery may be necessary for complications of acute epididymal infections.

REFERENCES

Centers for Disease Control and Prevention: Sexually transmitted diseases treatment guidelines, 2006. MMWR Morb Mortal Wkly Rep 2006;55:1-94.

Collins MM, Stafford RS, O'Leary MP, Barry MJ: How common is prostatitis? A national survey of physician visits. J Urol 1998;159:1224-1228.

Furuya R, Takahashi S, Furuya S, et al: Is seminal vesiculitis a discrete disease entity? Clinical and microbiological study of seminal vesiculitis in patients with acute epididymitis. J Urol 2004;171:1550-1553.

Karmazyn B, Steinberg R, Kornreich L, et al: Clinical and sonographic criteria of acute scrotum in children: A retrospective study of 172 boys. Pediatr Radiol 2005;35:302-310.

Krieger JN: Sexually transmitted diseases. In Tanagho EA, McAninch JW, (eds): Smith's Urology, 16th ed.. New York: Lange Medical Books/McGraw-Hill, 2004, pp 245-255.

Mittemeyer BT, Lennox KW, Borski AA: Epididymitis: A review of 610 cases. J Urol 1966;95:390-392.

Naber KG, Bergman B, Bishop MC, et al: EAU guidelines for the management of urinary and male genital tract infections. Urinary Tract Infection (UTI) Working Group of the Health Care Office (HCO) of the European Association of Urology (EAU). Eur Urol 2001;40:576-588.

Nickel JC, Siemens DR, Nickel KR, Downey J: The patient with chronic epididymitis: Characterization of an enigmatic syndrome. J Urol 2002;167:1701-1704.

Nickel JC, Teichman JM, Gregoire M, et al: Prevalence, diagnosis, characterization, and treatment of prostatitis, interstitial cystitis, and epididymitis in outpatient urological practice: The Canadian PIE Study. Urology 2005;66:935-940.

Stehr M, Boehm R: Critical validation of colour Doppler ultrasound in diagnostics of acute scrotum in children. Eur J Pediatr Surg 2003;13:386-392.

Primary Glomerular Diseases

Method of
Manuel Praga, MD, and
Enrique Morales, MD

Clinical Presentation And Diagnosis

The clinical manifestations of primary glomerular diseases are very variable, ranging from asymptomatic urinary abnormalities to severe forms of rapidly progressive glomerulonephritis. The different clinical presentations are summarized and defined in Box 1.

Most milder forms of glomerular diseases are diagnosed by a positive dipstick test for microhematuria or proteinuria. All these patients should have quantitative estimations of proteinuria (24-hour proteinuria or protein-to-creatinine ratio in a random sample of urine), urinary microscopic examination, and serum creatinine. Glomerular disorders can be the renal manifestation of systemic diseases of different causes (e.g., malignancies, infections, autoimmune disorders), as discussed later. Therefore, medical history and physical examination should carefully investigate data suggesting such diseases. In addition to general laboratory analysis and assessment of renal morphology (renal echography), more specific determinations should be performed in all patients with suspected glomerular diseases: protein electrophoresis, serum levels of immunoglobulins, serum complement fractions C3 and C4, antinuclear antibody (ANA), anti-DNA antibodies, antineutrophilic cytoplasmic antibodies (ANCA), and tests for hepatitis B virus (HBV), hepatitis C virus (HCV), and HIV infections.

Renal biopsy is the conclusive method for establishing the diagnosis and classification of primary glomerular disorders. Indications for renal biopsy include the nephrotic syndrome in

---

BOX 1 Clinical Presentations of Glomerular Diseases

Nephrotic Syndrome
- Proteinuria >3.5 g/d in adults and >40 mg/h/m² in children
- Hypoalbuminemia
- Hyperlipidemia
- Edema

Nephritic Syndrome
- Hypertension
- Oliguria
- Edema
- Hematuria (usually macroscopic)
- Red cell casts
- Non-nephrotic proteinuria
- Mild and nonprogressive GFR decrease

Rapidly Progressive Glomerulonephritis
- Acute or subacute progressive worsening of renal function
- Hematuria (usually macroscopic)
- Red cell casts
- Proteinuria (usually <3.5 g/d)
- Blood pressure often normal

Persistent Asymptomatic Urinary Abnormalities
- Non-nephrotic proteinuria (<3.5 g/d in adults and <40 mg/h/m² in children)
- Persistent microscopic hematuria

Recurrent Macroscopic Hematuria
- Bouts of gross hematuria, usually triggered by infections
- Persistent microhematuria between the episodes of gross hematuria

Chronic Renal Insufficiency
- Persistent proteinuria and/or microhematuria
- Hypertension
- Small kidneys

Hypocomplementemia

The C3 and C4 fractions of serum complement are characteristically reduced in some types of glomerular diseases. This is an important clue for diagnosis

Abbreviation: GFR = glomerular filtration rate.

adults (except cases attributed to diabetic nephropathy) and steroid-resistant nephrotic syndrome in children, rapidly progressive nephritis, persistent nephritic syndrome with deteriorating renal function, and, usually, recurrent macroscopic hematuria. The need for renal biopsy in patients with asymptomatic urinary abnormalities should be individualized. The most characteristic pathologic findings of the main primary glomerulonephritis are summarized in Box 2, and their commonest clinical presentations are summarized in Box 3.

BOX 2 Main Histologic Findings of Primary Glomerular Diseases

Minimal Change Disease
- Normal glomeruli on light microscopy
- Negative immunofluorescence and diffuse effacement of epithelial foot processes on electron microscopy

Focal and Segmental Glomerulosclerosis
- Focal (some glomeruli) and segmental (parts of affected glomeruli) scarring of the glomerular tuft

Membranous Nephropathy
- Thickening of glomerular capillary walls with projections of glomerular basement membrane ("spikes")
- Subepithelial immune deposits detected by immunofluorescence and electron microscopy

Membranoproliferative Glomerulonephritis
- Increase of mesangial cells and mesangial matrix
- Widening (double contoured appearance) of capillary loops
- IgG, C3, and IgM on immunofluorescence and subendothelial (type I) or intra-GBM (type II) deposits on electron microscopy

IgA Nephropathy
- Predominant deposition of mesangial IgA on immunofluorescence
- Proliferation of mesangial cellularity and mesangial matrix on light microscopy
- Mesangial electron-dense deposits on electron microscopy

Acute Postinfectious (Diffuse Proliferative) Glomerulonephritis
- Marked hypercellularity due to mesangial and endothelial cell proliferation and glomerular influx of neutrophils
- Hump-like subepithelial dense deposits on electron microscopy

Crescentic Glomerulonephritis
- Cellular or fibrocellular crescents in a variable percentage of glomeruli
- Immunofluorescence pattern distinguishes the main three types:
  - Type I: Linear IgG staining of the GBM (anti-GBM disease)
  - Type II: Granular deposits along GBM (immune complex deposition)
  - Type III: Negative immunofluorescence (pauci-immune glomerulonephritis)

Abbreviations: GBM = glomerular basement membrane; Ig = immunoglobulin.

CURRENT DIAGNOSIS

- Clinical presentations of glomerular diseases range from asymptomatic urinary abnormalities (proteinuria, microhematuria) to severe forms of rapidly progressive glomerulonephritis (gross hematuria, edema, acute renal function worsening, hypertension).
- Secondary causes of glomerular disease should be excluded by means of history, physical examination, and appropriate laboratory tests.
- Renal biopsy establishes the diagnosis and classification of primary glomerular diseases.

Treatment

CONSERVATIVE THERAPY

Hypertension is a common finding in patients with primary glomerulonephritis. Current guidelines recommend blood pressure targets lower than 130/80 mm Hg in these patients and lower than 125/75 mm Hg in patients with proteinuria greater than 1 g/24 hours. Any antihypertensive drug or drug combinations are useful, and they

---

BOX 3 Commonest Presentations of the Main Primary Glomerular Diseases

Minimal Change Disease
- Nephrotic syndrome

Focal and Segmental Glomerulosclerosis
- Nephrotic syndrome in more than two thirds of patients
- Non-nephrotic proteinuria in the remaining patients
- Renal insufficiency (20%-40%), hypertension (50%), and microhematuria (40%)

Membranous Nephropathy
- Nephrotic syndrome in >80% of patients
- Non-nephrotic proteinuria in the remaining patients

Membranoproliferative Glomerulonephritis
- Nephrotic syndrome in 50%
- Nephritic syndrome in 20%-30%
- Asymptomatic urinary abnormalities in 20%-30%
- Hypocomplementemia is common.

IgA Nephropathy
- Asymptomatic urinary abnormalities (microhematuria ±proteinuria) in >75%
- Intercalated recurrent or isolated episodes of macroscopic hematuria in >40%
- Nephritic or nephrotic syndrome in <10%

Acute Postinfectious Glomerulonephritis
- Nephritic syndrome
- Hypocomplementemia

Crescentic Glomerulonephritis
- Rapidly progressive glomerulonephritis

Abbreviation: Ig = immunoglobulin.

CURRENT THERAPY

- Appropriate treatment should be instituted as early as possible.
- Blood pressure should be lower than 130/80 mm Hg (<125/75 mm Hg in patients with proteinuria >1 g/24h).
- Angiotensin-converting enzyme inhibitors and angiotensin receptor blockers are indicated in most cases of chronic proteinuric glomerular diseases due to their antiproteinuric, antihypertensive, and renoprotective effects.
- Specific therapy of primary glomerular diseases includes steroids, anticalcineurinic agents, and cytotoxics. Due to the potential risks of these therapies, the likelihood of progression and the presence of chronic irreversible parenchymal damage must be carefully assessed.
- Primary or idiopathic glomerular diseases comprise a wide variety of glomerular histologic lesions, with different clinical presentations and variable prognosis. Although some entities portend a favorable long-term prognosis, a considerable fraction of untreated patients who have other glomerular entities reach end-stage renal failure.

should be selected on the basis of the patient's characteristics. However, blockade of the renin-angiotensin system either with an angiotensin-converting enzyme inhibitor (ACEI) or an angiotensin receptor blocker (ARB) should be the main basis of antihypertensive treatment because of their demonstrated renoprotective effect (slowing or preventing loss of renal function) in patients with chronic renal diseases. The beneficial effects of ACEIs and ARBs appear to be similar and are also observed in proteinuric patients with normal blood pressure. Renal protection induced by ACEIs and ARBs is closely related to the significant reduction in proteinuria that these agents induce. The level of proteinuria is the best way to monitor the efficacy of ACEIs and ARBs. Recent studies in primary glomerular diseases have shown that a combination of ACEI and ARB is more beneficial in terms of renal protection and proteinuria decrease than either drug alone. Serum creatinine and potassium should be monitored after ACEI and ARB therapy is initiated, particularly in patients with reduced renal function.

Hyperlipidemia is a common finding in patients with glomerular diseases, particularly in those with the nephrotic syndrome. Prospective clinical studies have demonstrated that treatment of hyperlipidemia decreases proteinuria and prevents renal function loss. Statins such as atorvastatin (Lipitor) (10-40 mg after the evening meal) are the most commonly used lipid-lowering drugs. A level of LDL cholesterol lower than 100 mg/dL is recommended. Weight loss in obese patients induces a significant reduction in proteinuria, and smoking should be strictly forbidden, because smoking is associated with a more rapid progression toward renal failure in any type of renal disease.

All these measures (blood pressure lowering, treatment with ACEIs and ARBs, treatment of hyperlipidemia, weight loss, cessation of smoking) are also beneficial for the global cardiovascular risk that is significantly higher in proteinuric patients (mainly in those with renal insufficiency) than in the normal population.

The complications of the nephrotic syndrome require specific treatment. Edema is usually managed with a low-sodium diet plus furosemide (Lasix) in doses carefully adjusted to the severity of edema. Daily weight measurement is very important, because excessive diuretic doses can lead to volume depletion and functional worsening of renal function. In resistant cases, combinations of different types of diuretics (furosemide plus a thiazide diuretic, or furosemide plus a potassium-sparing diuretic such as spironolactone [Aldactone])

in patients with hypokalemia) are needed. More severe cases require albumin infusions followed by high-dose intravenous furosemide (although intravenous albumin [Albuminar][1] increases proteinuria) or even removal of fluids by hemodialysis. Nephrotic patients are at increasing risk for thrombotic events. Prophylactic treatment (subcutaneous low-molecular-weight heparin) is indicated in conditions of high risk, such as immobilization.

SPECIFIC THERAPY

Box 4 summarizes the immunosuppressive treatment of primary glomerular diseases.

Minimal Change Disease

Minimal change disease (MCD) is most common in children but also causes 10% to 15% of nephrotic syndrome in adults. Corticosteroid therapy is a very effective treatment for MCD. For children, the dose of prednisone is 60 mg/m^2/day and for adults 1 mg/kg/day (up to 80 mg/day). About 75% of patients respond (complete proteinuria disappearance) within 2 weeks, and more than 90% respond within 8 weeks, but adults show in general a slower response than children. Initial steroid dose is continued for 4 weeks and then changed to alternate-day prednisone (40 mg/m^2 on alternate days) or to daily prednisone, slowly tapering off over 6 to 10 weeks. Keeping patients on steroids for more than 3 months is associated with a lower 1-year relapse rate.

Up to 75% of children and many adults have nephrotic syndrome relapses. Isolated relapses are re-treated with steroids as in the first episode. Frequent relapsers (two or more relapses within a 6-month period) are treated with a low-dose steroid course plus cyclophosphamide (Cytoxan) (1.5-2 mg/kg/day) or chlorambucil (Leukeran)[1] (0.1-0.2 mg/kg/day) in an 8-week course. After these short-term cytotoxic courses, a considerable fraction of patients remain free of proteinuria for prolonged periods, with a low rate of serious complications. Longer or repeated courses can induce severe side effects and are not recommended.

The response of steroid-dependent patients (reappearance of the nephrotic syndrome during or immediately after steroid withdrawal) to cytotoxics is poorer than that of frequent relapsers. Steroid-dependent patients and frequent relapsers unresponsive to cytotoxics are commonly treated with cyclosporine (Neoral)[1] given in an initial dose of 3-4 mg/kg in two divided doses, then adjusting for serum levels of 100-175 ng/mL. Most steroid-dependent patients transform into cyclosporine-dependent, and the risk of cyclosporine-induced nephrotoxicity should be considered. Mycophenolate mofetil (MMF, CellCept)[1] (600 mg/m^2/12 h in children, 500-1000 mg/12 h in adults) is a very useful alternative. Rates of response and relapse are similar to those of cyclosporine, but tolerance is better and there is no risk of nephrotoxicity. Therapy with cyclosporine or MMF if the patient responds is continued for up to 12 months before slow and careful tapering.

Less than 10% of MCD patients are steroid resistant. Because most of them subsequently have focal segmental glomerulosclerosis (FSGS) on biopsy, their therapeutic approach is the same as for FSGS.

Focal and Segmental Glomerulosclerosis

Causes of secondary FSGS (obesity, reflux nephropathy, reduction in renal mass) should be carefully excluded. Treatment with an ACEI or ARB (or both) is the first option in patients with non-nephrotic proteinuria or in patients with nonaggressive nephrotic syndrome (proteinuria <5 g/day, serum albumin >3 g/dL, normal renal function), mainly if hypertension coexists. Patients with severe nephrotic syndrome or nephrotic proteinuria after ACEI or ARB introduction should be treated with prednisone 1 mg/kg/day. Several retrospective studies have shown that steroid treatment maintained for at least 6 months is followed by more than 50% partial or complete

---

[1]Not FDA approved for this indication.

BOX 4 Immunosuppressive Treatment of Primary Glomerular Disease

Minimal Change Disease

First Line
- Steroids

Second Line
- Cytotoxics (frequent relapsers)
- Anticalcineurinics or mycophenolate mofetil (CellCept)[1] (steroid-dependent)

Focal Segmental Glomerulosclerosis

First Line
- Steroids
- ACEIs
- ARBs

Second Line
- Anticalcineurinics
- Mycophenolate mofetil[1]

Membranous Nephropathy

First Line
- Anticalcineurinics
- Steroids plus cytotoxics
- ACEIs
- ARBs

Second Line
- Mycophenolate mofetil
- Intramuscular ACTH (Synacthen)[1,2]
- Rituximab (Rituxan)[1]

Membranoproliferative Glomerulonephritis
- Steroids
- ACEIs
- ARBs

IgA Nephropathy

First Line
- ACEIs
- ARBs

Second Line
- Steroids
- Fish oil
- Cytotoxics

Acute Postinfectious Glomerulonephritis
- Conservative therapy

Crescentic Glomerulonephritis

Type I (anti-GBM)
- Steroids
- Cyclophosphamide (Cytoxan)[1]
- Plasmapheresis

Types II and III
Induction
- Steroids
- Cyclophosphamide[1]
- Plasmapheresis in severe acute renal failure

Maintenance
- Low-dose steroids
- Azathioprine (Imuran)[1]

[1]Not FDA approved for this indication.
[2]Not available in the United States.
Abbreviations: ACEI = angiotensin-converting enzyme inhibitor; ACTH = adrenocorticotropic hormone; ARB = angiotensin receptor blocker; GBM = glomerular basement membrane; Ig = immunoglobulin.

---

remissions. However, in responsive patients, proteinuria starts to decrease after 2 to 3 months of treatment.

If proteinuria did not show significant changes within this period, introduction of an anticalcineurinic agent together with steroid tapering is recommended. Cyclosporine (doses and blood levels as in MCD) has been the most commonly used drug, and prospective studies have shown more than 70% partial or complete remission after 6 months of treatment. Tacrolimus (Prograf)[1] (0.05-0.10 mg/kg/day in two divided doses, then adjusted for serum levels of 4-7 ng/mL) is proved to be effective in some cyclosporine-resistant FSGS cases.

In patients with complete or partial response to cyclosporine or tacrolimus, these drugs should be maintained at the lowest effective doses for at least 1 year before slowly tapering off. In some patients resistant to steroids and cyclosporine, or in those with mild degrees of renal insufficiency, MMF[1] (same doses as in MCD) has decreased proteinuria and stabilized renal function for prolonged periods. Sirolimus (Rapamune)[1] has induced complete (19%) or partial (38%) remission in a series of 21 steroid-resistant FSGS patients in a recent open-label trial.

About 20% to 25% of children with aggressive forms of FSGS have mutations in the genes coding for several podocyte proteins, mainly podocin. Most of these patients are unresponsive to any kind of treatment.

Membranous Nephropathy

More than one third of MGN patients have a spontaneous remission, and most remissions take place during the first 2 years of the disease. Conservative therapy should be maintained during the first 9 to 12 months, unless renal function starts to deteriorate. ACEIs or ARBs, or both, can induce partial remission (non-nephrotic proteinuria) in a considerable percentage of cases.

In patients with an aggressive presentation (massive nephrotic syndrome and deteriorating renal function) a 6-month course of alternating monthly prednisone 0.5 mg/kg/day with a month of chlorambucil[1] 0.2 mg/kg/day is recommended. Other clinicians simultaneously use prednisone starting with 1 mg/kg/day and tapering off over 6 months plus chlorambucil 0.15 mg/kg/day for 14 weeks. Another regimen is prednisone 0.5 mg/kg/day every other day for 6 months plus cyclophosphamide[1] 1.5 mg/kg/day for 12 months.

In patients maintaining normal renal function and persistent nephrotic proteinuria beyond 9 to 12 months, immunosuppressive therapy should be initiated, mainly in the presence of markers of poor outcome, which include male gender, older age, and proteinuria persistently higher than 8 g/day after ACEI or ARB treatment. Alternating prednisone and chlorambucil (as indicated earlier), prednisone and cyclophosphamide, and cyclosporine[1] 3-4 mg/kg/day, targeting blood levels of 100-175 ng/mL are beneficial, inducing complete or partial remission in most patients.

---

[1]Not FDA approved for this indication.

[1]Not FDA approved for this indication.

Side effects (diabetes, bone necrosis, infections) are more serious with steroids plus cytotoxic treatments; trimethoprim-sulfamethoxazole (TMP-SMX, Bactrim) (80 mg/400 mg/day) should be concurrently administered for *Pneumocystis jiroveci* prophylaxis. Cyclosporine, administered for 6 months, is followed by approximately 50% of recurrences after drug withdrawal.

No studies comparing anticalcineurinic and cytotoxics have been published for MGN. Tacrolimus,[1] another anticalcineurinic agent, can also induce partial response in more than 80% of treated patients, although recurrence after withdrawal is the same (50%) as with cyclosporine. A recent randomized pilot trial reported that tetracosactide (Synacthen),[1,2] an analogue of ACTH (1 mg IM twice a week for 1 year) induced remissions in the same percentage as a regimen of steroids plus cyclophosphamide.

Uncontrolled studies reported that MMF[1] (1000-2000 mg/day) reduced proteinuria and stabilized renal function in some MGN patients unresponsive to other therapies. Rituximab (Rituxan),[1] a monoclonal antibody against CD20 B-lymphocytes, has reduced proteinuria in a pilot study.

Membranoproliferative Glomerulonephritis

The incidence of idiopathic membranoproliferative glomerulonephritis (MPGN) has progressively decreased over the last decades, being currently an uncommon disease in developed countries. Most cases of MPGN are now secondary to HCV infection and concurrent cryoglobulinemia. No prospective studies about the treatment of idiopathic MPGN have been carried out in the last several years. Uncontrolled series of patients suggested that prolonged (>2 years) prednisone treatment is beneficial in terms of proteinuria reduction and renal survival. Prospective randomized trials with aspirin[1] and dipyridamole (Persantine)[1] showed a significant reduction in proteinuria some decades ago, but later analysis did not demonstrate long-term benefits on renal survival.

Conservative therapy, including ACEIs and ARBs, should be prescribed in all cases. In patients with the nephrotic syndrome after an observation period or in those with more aggressive presentations (deteriorating renal function, crescents), a 6- to 12-month course of prednisone could be indicated. Some small series of patients suggested that cyclophosphamide[1] is effective in aggressive cases of MPGN, but conclusive evidence is lacking.

Immunoglobulin A Nephropathy

As in all types of primary glomerular diseases, the aggressiveness of therapeutic approaches in patients with immunoglobulin A (IgA) nephropathy should be graded according to the severity of the presentation. In patients with microhematuria and normal renal function, only regular follow-up is required. If slowly increasing proteinuria appears, an ACEI or ARB, or a combination of both drugs, should be started, even in the absence of hypertension, targeting for proteinuria less than 1 g/day and blood pressure lower than 125/75 mm Hg.

In patients with increasing proteinuria greater than 1-1.5 g/day in spite of these measures, other therapies should be contemplated. Steroids were proven to be beneficial in patients with normal renal function and proteinuria greater than 1 g/day in a prospective randomized trial: methylprednisolone (Solu-Medrol) pulses, 1 g/day for 3 days in the beginning of months 1,3, and 5, and oral prednisone 0.5 mg/kg every other day for 6 months reduced proteinuria and increased renal survival in comparison with untreated patients.

Treatment with fish oil supplements[1] in this type of patient remains controversial. Although eicosapentaenoic acid (1.8 g/day) or docosahexaenoic acid (1.2 g/day) demonstrated beneficial effects in some trials, these effects were not reproduced in others.

In patients with more aggressive presentations (proteinuria and deteriorating renal function), a prospective trial demonstrated that prednisone 40 mg/day tapering to 10 mg/day within 2 years plus cyclophosphamide[1] 1.5 mg/kg/day for 3 months followed by azathioprine (Imuran)[1] 1.5 mg/kg/day for at least 2 years significantly improved renal survival in comparison with untreated patients.

After initial suggestions of the benefits of MMF[1] 1000 to 2000 mg/day in IgA nephropathy patients unresponsive to other therapies, recent prospective and controlled trials have failed to demonstrate these good results, although the number of study subjects was small and many of them had advanced renal insufficiency.

Acute Postinfectious (Diffuse Proliferative) Glomerulonephritis

As in MPGN, the incidence of diffuse proliferative glomerulonephritis has drastically decreased in recent years in developed countries. The prognosis is generally good, and signs and symptoms of the disease (nephritic syndrome) resolve sporadically within 2 to 6 weeks in a great majority of cases. Treatment should be focused on adequate control of blood pressure, salt restriction, and diuretics to prevent fluid excess and the risks of cardiac failure. The triggering infection should be investigated and treated if it has not disappeared spontaneously.

Some patients present with more aggressive courses, developing progressive renal insufficiency. In these cases, crescents involving a large proportion of glomeruli can be observed in a second biopsy. No controlled studies have been carried out in these aggressive cases, but some series of patients recommend high-dose intravenous pulse steroid, followed by oral prednisone 1 mg/kg/day, tapering off over 2 to 3 months. There is no evidence that more aggressive immunosuppressive therapy is beneficial.

Crescentic Glomerulonephritis

Treatment of crescentic glomerulonephritis (CGN) should be promptly instituted because of the rapid transformation of cellular crescents into irreversible fibrotic crescents that collapse the glomerular tufts. Prognosis of type I (anti-GBM disease) CGN is poorer than that of types II and III, particularly in the presence of oligoanuria, dialysis requirement, or a large fraction of glomeruli with crescents.

Treatment of type I CGN includes steroids, cyclophosphamide,[1] and plasmapheresis. Pulse intravenous methylprednisolone (500-1000 mg daily for 3-4 days) is followed by oral prednisone (1 mg/kg/day for 3-4 weeks, then slowly tapering off over 6 months). Oral cyclophosphamide (2 mg/kg/day) is usually maintained for 2 to 3 months. Plasmapheresis (daily or alternate-day 4-liter exchanges) using albumin as replacement fluid or fresh frozen plasma if bleeding risk is high, is usually performed for 2 to 3 weeks. The duration of plasmapheresis, as well as the intensity and the duration of immunosuppressive therapy, should be guided by the clinical status and the titers of anti-GBM antibodies. In patients without pulmonary hemorrhage and with very advanced renal involvement (massive presence of glomerular fibrotic crescents), aggressive immunosuppression is not indicated.

The precise etiology of type II CGN (e.g., systemic lupus erythematosus, cryoglobulinemia) should be identified and the therapy guided by the diagnosis. If no apparent diagnosis is available, treatment is similar to that for type III (pauci-immune) CGN.

Induction treatment of type III CGN consists of steroids (oral prednisone, 1 mg/kg/day for 3-4 weeks, slowly tapered to a maintenance dose of 10-20 mg), and intravenous monthly pulses of cyclophosphamide (initial dose 0.5 to 1 g/m^2, adjusted for renal function and age), which has proved to be as effective and less toxic than oral administration. Once remission is achieved (recovery of renal function, absence of extrarenal symptoms), usually within 3 to 6 months, cyclophosphamide is replaced by azathioprine[1] 1 to 2 mg/kg/day for 12 to 18 months plus prednisone 5 to 10 mg daily or every other day. Positive titers of ANCA, particularly p-ANCA, can indicate more prolonged, low-dose, maintenance treatment, because the risk of

---

[1]Not FDA approved for this indication.
[2]Not available in the United States.

[1]Not FDA approved for this indication.

recurrence is high. Plasmapheresis (similar to that in type I CGN) is proven to add benefits in type III CGN manifesting with severe renal failure. Although not tested in prospective trials, MMF[1] (1500-3000 mg/day) has been shown effective and well tolerated, even as induction therapy in some series of patients.

REFERENCES

Cattran DC, Appel GB, Hebert LA, et al: A randomized trial of cyclosporine in patients with steroid-resistant focal segmental glomerulosclerosis. Kidney Int 1999;56:2220-2226.

Cattran DC, Appel GB, Hebert LA, et al: Cyclosporin in patients with steroid-resistant membranous nephropathy: A randomized trial. Kidney Int 2001;59:1484-1490.

Jayne D, Rasmussen N, Andrassy K, et al: A randomized trial of maintenance therapy for vasculitis associated with antineutrophil cytoplasmic autoantibodies. N Engl J Med 2003;349:36-44.

Nakao N, Yoshimura A, Morita H, et al: Combination treatment of angiotensin-II receptor blocker and angiotensin-converting-enzyme inhibitor in non-diabetic renal disease (COOPERATE): A randomized controlled trial. Lancet 2003;361:117-124.

Ponticelli C, Altieri P, Scolari F, et al: A randomized study comparing methylprednisolone plus chlorambucil versus methylprednisolone plus cyclophosphamide in idiopathic membranous nephropathy. J Am Soc Nephrol 1998;9:444-450.

Pozzi C, Bolasco PG, Fogazzi GB, et al: Corticosteroids in IgA nephropathy: A randomised controlled trial. Lancet 1999;13:883-887.

Praga M, Gutiérrez E, González E, et al: Treatment of IgA nephropathy with ACE inhibitors: A randomized and controlled trial. J Am Soc Nephrol 2003;14:1578-1583.

Torres A, Domínguez-Gil B, Carreño A, et al: Conservative versus immunosuppressive treatment of patients with idiopathic membranous nephropathy. Kidney Int 2002;61:219-227.

Pyelonephritis

Method of
Patricia D. Brown, MD

Acute pyelonephritis (APN) is a urinary tract infection (UTI) that involves the renal parenchyma, also referred to as *upper tract UTI*. Most episodes of APN occur as a result of ascending infection from the bladder; patients with APN might or might not have symptoms of concomitant cystitis. Rarely, pyelonephritis occurs secondary to hematogenous seeding of the kidney as a result of infection elsewhere, most commonly endocarditis due to *Staphylococcus aureus* or disseminated fungal infection.

Epidemiology

Surprising little is known about the epidemiology of APN. Similar to cystitis, APN (and hospitalization for APN) is more common in women than men; men have been reported to have higher in-hospital mortality. In contrast to cystitis, risk factors for pyelonephritis are not well defined. One recent study of nonpregnant women 18 to 49 years of age found risk factors for APN included factors known to be risk factors for acute cystitis, including frequency of sexual intercourse, recent UTI, diabetes, and maternal UTI history. The incidence of bacteremia in patients with APN is reported to be 11% to 53% in various studies; risk factors for bacteremia are not well established.

Similar to lower UTI, APN can be further classified into complicated or uncomplicated infection. The factors that make an episode of APN a complicated UTI are outlined in Box 1.

BOX 1   Factors Associated with Complicated Pyelonephritis

- Diabetes
- Foreign body (catheter, stent)
- Health care–associated infections
- Immunocompromise
- Incomplete voiding (detrusor muscle dysfunction due to neurologic disease or medications)
- Infections due to multidrug-resistant pathogens
- Obstruction (including stones)
- Pregnancy
- Recent history of instrumentation
- Renal transplant recipient
- UTI in a male patient
- Vesicoureteral reflux

Abbreviation: UTI = urinary tract infection.

Clinical Presentation

The classic presenting features of APN include abrupt onset of fever, flank pain, and costovertebral angle tenderness with or without symptoms of lower UTI including dysuria, urgency, and frequency. Unfortunately, there is no single constellation of signs or symptoms that is pathognomonic for APN. When localization studies have been performed on patients with symptoms of acute cystitis, 30% to 50% have been shown to have APN. Women who present with symptoms that have been present more than 7 days and those with a recent history of UTI are more likely to have APN. Flank pain is reported in approximately one half of patients with APN but also occurs in almost 20% of patients with cystitis. Fever is present in one half of patients with APN, but less than 5% of patients with cystitis. Nausea, vomiting, and diarrhea occur commonly in patients with APN, and gastrointestinal (GI) symptoms can dominate the presenting complaints.

In general, patients who present with lower urinary tract symptoms or laboratory evidence of urinary tract infection accompanied by fever, flank pain or tenderness, or signs of systemic toxicity, such as GI symptoms, should be treated for APN.

The diagnosis can be particularly challenging in the frail elderly patient, because symptoms such as frequency, urgency, and incontinence are often chronic in this patient population and unrelated to active UTI. Change in mental status may be the only presenting complaint. Because the prevalence of bacteriuria in this patient population is high, particularly among those with chronic indwelling catheters, UTI must be a diagnosis of exclusion.

Acute pelvic inflammatory disease can have a presentation similar to APN. Pelvic examination should be performed on all sexually active women to exclude this diagnosis.

The differential diagnosis of APN is outlined in Box 2.

Diagnosis

Urinalysis, ideally with microscopic examination, using a clean-catch, midstream specimen, should be performed in all patients with suspected APN. Pyuria is a key finding in the diagnosis of UTI, and the absence of pyuria is strong evidence against a diagnosis of APN. Direct microscopic examination under high power of the urinary sediment from a centrifuged specimen should reveal more than 10 leukocytes per high-powered field. The presence of white blood cell (WBC) casts is highly specific for localization of the infection to the kidney, but it is inadequately sensitive to exclude the diagnosis of APN. The dipstick test for leukocyte esterase is used as a rapid screening test to detect significant pyuria; the sensitivity is reported to be 75% to 96%, with a specificity of 94% to 98%. Because of the lower

BOX 2	Differential Diagnosis of Acute Pyelonephritis

- Appendicitis
- Cholecystitis
- Diverticulitis
- Gastroenteritis
- Herpes zoster
- Musculoskeletal pain, including vertebral disorders
- Ovarian cysts, tumors
- Pancreatitis
- Perforated viscus
- Pelvic inflammatory disease
- Pneumonia
- Renal stones, renal vein thrombosis, renal infarction

range of the reported sensitivity of the dipstick test, microscopic examination to exclude significant pyuria should be obtained in patients with suspected APN.

The presence of nitrite in the urine, detected by a dipstick test, has a reported sensitivity of 35% to 85% and a specificity of 92% to 100% for UTI. Microscopic examination of a Gram-stained, centrifuged urine specimen revealing at least one bacterium per oil-immersion field correlates with more than 10^5 colony-forming units (cfu)/mL of bacteria, with a sensitivity of 95%. Although this is the standard definition of significant bacteriuria, it has been shown that women with UTI can have levels of bacteriuria as low as 10^2 cfu/mL.

Although the microbiology of APN has remained predictable, significant changes in antimicrobial susceptibility patterns have occurred. Therefore, in contrast to recommendations for acute uncomplicated cystitis, a urine culture should be obtained in all patients with suspected APN. The need to obtain blood cultures has been debated, because blood cultures rarely yield a pathogen different from what was isolated from the urine. Bacteremia has been reported in 11% to 53% of patients hospitalized with APN. Bacteremic patients have a longer length of stay, and one recent report suggests that this is due to a longer time to resolution of fever. Many experts continue to recommend that blood cultures be obtained as part of the diagnostic evaluation of patients who are ill enough to require hospitalization; blood cultures are not necessary for those who will be managed as outpatients.

CURRENT DIAGNOSIS

- Abrupt onset of fever, flank pain, and costovertebral angle tenderness with or without symptoms of cystitis are classic presenting features.
- Patients with lower UTI symptoms or laboratory evidence of UTI accompanied by flank pain, fever, or signs of systemic toxicity such as GI complaints should be managed as having APN.
- Urinalysis with microscopic examination should be performed in all patients with suspected APN. Absence of pyuria is strong evidence against the diagnosis.
- A urine culture should be obtained in all patients with APN. Blood cultures should be obtained in those who are hospitalized.
- Patients should be categorized into those with uncomplicated and those with complicated infections.

Abbreviations: APN = acute pyelonephritis; GI = gastrointestinal; UTI = urinary tract infection.

The role of diagnostic imaging in the management of APN is discussed later. In some cases with an atypical presentation, imaging may be helpful to confirm the diagnosis of APN. In this setting, pre- and postcontrast computed tomography (CT) is the imaging procedure of choice in adults.

Microbial Etiology

Most cases of APN are caused by *Escherichia coli*. Other enterobacteriaceae, including *Klebsiella* species and *Proteus* species, are also occasionally implicated. Other gram-negative pathogens such as *Pseudomonas, Serratia, Enterobacter,* and *Acinetobacter* should be considered in health care–associated infections. *Enterococcus* is an uncommon pathogen in community-acquired infections, but it must be considered in health care–associated infections, including vancomycin-resistant enterococci. Other gram-positive pathogens include *Streptoccocus agalactiae* and *Staphylococcus* species. Although a common cause of acute cystitis in young women, *Staphylococcus saprophyticus* is a rare cause of pyelonephritis; the finding of *Staphylococcus aureus* in a urine culture should always prompt a search for an extrarenal source of infection that might have served as a source of hematogenous seeding. A Gram stain of the urine is a simple and rapid test to exclude a gram-positive pathogen as the etiology of APN and guide the initial selection of empiric therapy.

The emergence of resistance to trimethoprim-sulfamethoxazole (TMP-SMX [Bactrim]) among *E. coli* has had a major impact on the approach to initial empiric antimicrobial therapy for APN. It is clear that the prevalence of resistance varies depending on geographic region, and clinicians often do not have access to meaningful local resistance data. Recent reports of increasing fluoroquinolone resistance among uropathogens are of great concern, although overall resistance rates in North America remain low.

Treatment

The first decision in the management of patients with APN is whether or not the patient requires hospitalization. Although prospective randomized trials are lacking, several retrospective studies as well as several prospective nonrandomized trials suggest that outpatient management is safe for many patients. Hospitalization should be considered for patients who cannot tolerate oral intake or who have severe pain or signs of severe sepsis. A strategy of initial management in the emergency department or an observation unit with an initial dose of parenteral antibiotic therapy, intravenous fluids, and symptomatic treatment of nausea and pain may be used in select

CURRENT THERAPY

- Hospitalization is recommended for patients unable to tolerate oral intake, those with severe pain, and those with signs of severe sepsis. Hospitalization is generally recommended for patients with complicated infections and for all pregnant women.
- Parenteral regimens for hospitalized patients include an aminoglycoside, third-generation cephalosporin, or fluoroquinolone, with oral switch therapy selected on the basis of culture and susceptibility data.
- Initial empiric therapy for outpatients is a fluoroquinolone.
- Imaging is not recommended for patients with uncomplicated infections. Pre- and postcontrast computed tomographic scans should be obtained in those who fail to respond within 72 hours to appropriate antibiotic therapy.

patients to avoid hospital admission. Patients who will be treated as outpatients should have a stable social situation and the ability to contact the physician and return promptly if their symptoms worsen. Hospitalization is generally recommended for patients with complicated infections. Most experts believe that pregnant women with APN should always be hospitalized.

There are surprisingly few prospective randomized trials of the treatment of pyelonephritis. For patients who require hospitalization, parenteral therapy with an aminoglycoside, a third-generation cephalosporin, or a fluoroquinolone is recommended. At my institution, we discourage fluoroquinolones for this indication because there are other effective alternatives and we wish to minimize the use of these very broad-spectrum agents in the hospital setting. Although resistance to TMP-SMX among uropathogenic *E. coli* appears to have leveled off and might actually be decreasing, this agent should not be used for empiric therapy of APN.

If a gram-positive pathogen is suspected or suggested by the results of urine Gram stain, ampicillin or ampicillin-sulbactam (Unasyn) with or without an aminoglycoside can be used. Patients should receive intravenous therapy until they are clinically improving and able to reliably tolerate oral intake; oral therapy can be chosen based on the results of urine culture and susceptibility data. TMP-SMX, a fluoroquinolone, and ampicillin are all potential candidates for oral switch therapy. The narrowest spectrum, least expensive agent to which the isolated pathogen is susceptible should be chosen. Despite in vitro susceptibility data, first- and second-generation cephalosporins have a poor track record in the treatment of APN and are generally not recommended, with the exception of pyelonephritis in pregnancy.

Bacteremic patients might take longer to respond but do not require more prolonged parenteral therapy. The total duration of therapy for pyelonephritis is generally 14 days. Seven days of therapy with a fluoroquinolone for uncomplicated APN has been shown to be effective. Longer courses of therapy may be required for select patients with complicated pyelonephritis. For outpatients, initial empiric therapy with a fluoroquinolone is recommended, with adjustment of therapy, if needed, based on the results of urine culture. All of the currently available fluoroquinolones can be used, with the exception of moxifloxacin (Avelox), which does not achieve adequate levels in the urine. Although it is useful in the treatment of cystitis, norfloxacin (Noroxin) is not recommended for the treatment of APN because it does not achieve sustained tissue or serum levels. Suggested antimicrobial dosing regimens for APN are outlined in Box 3.

Imaging

Imaging is generally not needed in patients with uncomplicated APN. For patients with complicated infections (e.g., history of stones, prior renal surgery), renal ultrasound with abdominal plain films is considered an acceptable alternative to excretory urography. For patients with diabetes or other immunocompromise and for patients who fail to respond after 72 hours of appropriate antibiotic therapy, pre- and postcontrast CT is the imaging procedure of choice.

Follow-up

Most patients will respond to appropriate antibiotic therapy. Follow-up urine cultures to document microbiological response are not recommended in patients who have responded clinically.

REFERENCES

Foxman B, Klemstine KL, Brown PD: Acute pyelonephritis in US hospitals in 1997: Hospitalization and in-hospital mortality. Ann Epidemiol 2003;13:144-150.

Pappas PG: Laboratory in the diagnosis and management of urinary tract infections. Med Clin North Am 1991;75:313-325.

Sandler CM, Amis ES Jr, Bigongiari LR, et al: Imaging in acute pyelonephritis. American College of Radiology. ACR appropriateness criteria. Radiology 2000;215(suppl):677-681.

Scholes D, Hooton TM, Roberts PL, et al: Risk factors associated with acute pyelonephritis in healthy women. Ann Intern Med 2005;142:20-27.

Talan DA, Stamm WE, Hooton TM, et al: Comparison of ciprofloxacin (7 days) and trimethoprim-sulfamethoxazole (14 days) for acute uncomplicated pyelonephritis in women: A randomized trial. JAMA 2000;283:1583-1590.

Warren JW, Abrutyn E, Hebel JR, et al: Guidelines for antimicrobial treatment of uncomplicated acute bacterial cystitis and acute pyelonephritis in women. Clin Infect Dis 1999;29:745-758.

BOX 3 Antimicrobial Therapy for the Management of Acute Pyelonephritis

Parenteral Regimens

- Ampicillin 2 g q4h-q6h
- Ampicillin-sulbactam (Unasyn) 3 g q6h
- Ceftriaxone (Rocephin) 1-2 g q24h
- Ciprofloxacin (Cipro) 400 mg q12h
- Gentamicin (Garamycin) 3-5 mg/kg q24h
- Levofloxacin (Levaquin) 250-500 mg q24h

Oral Regimens

- Amoxicillin 500 mg q8h
- Ciprofloxacin 500 mg q12h
- Ciprofloxacin XR 1000 mg q24h
- Levofloxacin 250 mg q24h
- Trimethoprim-sulfamethoxazole DS (Bactrim DS) 160/800 mg q12h

---

Trauma to the Genitourinary Tract

Method of
Richard Santucci, MD, and Theodore Barber, MD

In the United States, trauma remains the leading cause of death in persons younger than 45 years; morbidity and mortality secondary to trauma are significant international health problems. Approximately 10% of all victims of major trauma have a genitourinary (GU) injury.

When assessing a patient for possible GU trauma, as with assessment of all trauma victims, initial evaluation should proceed according to the ABCDE mnemonic (*a*irway, *b*reathing, *c*irculation, *d*isability, *e*xposure), with an AMPLE history (*a*llergies, *m*edication, *p*ast medical history, *l*ast meal, *e*vents surrounding injury) obtained if the patient is verbal, or from the family (if possible) if not. It is important that the evaluating physician understands both the mechanism (including projectile trajectory in the case of penetrating trauma) and extent of the injury, because this knowledge will guide subsequent treatment. Assessment of GU trauma requires judicious use of laboratory tests (including urinalysis), radiologic imaging, and urologic consultation in patients thought likely to require surgical intervention.

Renal Injuries

The kidneys are the most common location of trauma to the GU tract. Hematuria is the best indicator of traumatic GU injury. However, in some rare injuries such as renal vascular injuries, hematuria can be absent. When assessing for GU bleeding, it is recommended that the first aliquot of urine be used, because later samples

TABLE 1 AAST Organ Injury Severity Scale for the Kidneys	
Type	Description
Grade I	
Contusion	Microscopic or gross hematuria; urologic studies normal
Hematoma	Subcapsular, nonexpanding; no parenchymal laceration
Grade II	
Laceration	Parenchymal depth <1 cm and no urinary extravasation
Hematoma	Nonexpanding perirenal hematoma confined to retroperitoneum
Grade III	
Laceration	Parenchymal depth >1 cm without collecting system rupture No urinary extravasation
Grade IV	
Laceration	Parenchymal laceration, extending through cortex, medulla, and collecting system
Vascular	Main renal artery or vein injury with contained hemorrhage
Grade V	
Laceration	Kidney completely shattered
Vascular	Avulsion of hilum, devascularizing kidney

AAST = American Academy for the Surgery of Trauma.

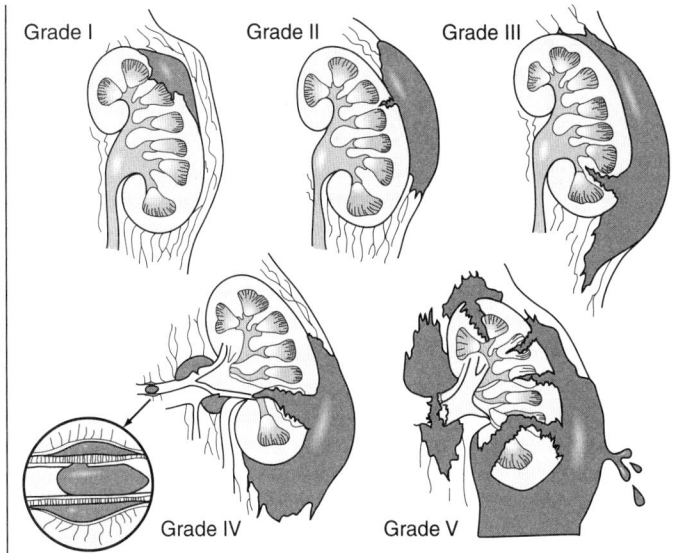

FIGURE 1. Classification of renal injuries by grade. (From McAninch JW, Santucci RA, Renal and ureteral trauma. In Wein AJ, Kavoussi LR, Novick AC (eds): Campbell-Walsh Urology, 9th ed. Philadelphia: Saunders, 2007, p 1276.)

may be diluted secondary to diuresis from intravenous resuscitation fluids. Following examination of the patient and assessment for hematuria, appropriate imaging studies should be performed. Absolute indications for imaging include blunt trauma with gross hematuria or microscopic hematuria (>5 red blood cells per high-power field [RBC/HPF]) and shock (systolic blood pressure [BP] <90 mm Hg), all penetrating injuries with gross or microscopic hematuria, and deceleration injuries.

Computed tomography (CT) remains the gold standard for imaging renal injuries, and often rapid spiral CT is employed. With CT scanning, it is critical that delayed images be obtained 10 minutes after contrast injection to allow opacification of the collecting system. Following CT scanning, the degree of renal injury can be graded according to the American Academy for the Surgery of Trauma (AAST) guidelines (Table 1, Fig. 1). Ultrasound has gained acceptance as an additional tool for the rapid evaluation of abdominal trauma, but it remains unable to clearly assess renal injuries and should not be used. Should a patient require emergent surgical exploration, single-shot intraoperative excretory urography (2 mg/kg IV contrast given 10 minutes before flat-plate abdominal x-ray) may be performed in lieu of CT.

CURRENT DIAGNOSIS

- Computed tomography (CT) scans with contrast and delayed images must be obtained for proper assessment and staging of renal and ureteral injuries.
- Any patient with a questionable bladder injury should undergo either plain-film cystography or CT cystogram.
- Retrograde urethrography is necessary in any patient with suspected urethral injury before attempting instrumentation.
- Female patients with pelvic trauma should undergo a thorough pelvic examination.

Significant injuries requiring surgical exploration occur in approximately 2% of blunt renal trauma cases but in the majority of gunshot wounds. Grades I to III injuries are most likely amenable to nonoperative management with a regimen of hospital admission and bedrest until the hematuria resolves. Even though grades IV and V injuries more often require exploration, they too can often be conservatively managed.

The absolute indication for surgical exploration is hypotension secondary to blood loss from a renal injury. Relative indications include persistent renal bleeding (>2 units/day), urine extravasation plus a devitalized segment, bilateral renal artery thrombosis, or injury to a solitary kidney.

Complications from renal trauma are also seen after the acute injury resolves. Patients with persistent urinary extravasation can require either a ureteral stent or percutaneous nephrostomy tube. Delayed renal bleeding is best treated by a return to bedrest and intravenous hydration, with angiography and embolization reserved for those who fail conservative therapy. In the case of renal abscess formation, percutaneous drainage with later surgical drainage for nonresponders is the preferred method of management.

Ureteral Injuries

Ureteral injuries account for less than 1% of all urologic trauma, but they are often associated with a significant degree of morbidity and mortality, mostly due to significant associated injuries. Although hematuria is a hallmark for GU injury, up to 50% of patients with ureteral injuries fail to demonstrate this finding. Delayed ureteral injury is suggested by the triad of fever, leukocytosis, and generalized peritoneal signs, but anuria, leakage of urine from the wound, and hydronephrosis should also raise suspicion for ureteral injury.

When ureteral injury is suspected, an abdominal and pelvic CT with contrast should be performed as outlined for the evaluation of renal trauma. Delayed images allow contrast to extravasate from the ureters, providing an optimal chance to visualize any injury. If time, or the extent of injury, do not allow a CT to be performed, an intra-operative one-shot intravenous pyelogram may be obtained instead.

Once a ureteral injury is suspected, a urologist should be consulted for further management. Given the tenuous blood supply to the ureters, surgical intervention is often required, which may include stent placement, open surgical repair, or, in the case of severe associated injury, ureteral ligation and percutaneous nephrostomy tube placement with delayed reconstruction. Although contusions

CURRENT THERAPY

- Most renal injuries can be managed nonoperatively.
- Ureteral and urethral injuries often require urologic intervention.
- Intraperitoneal bladder ruptures should be repaired surgically.
- Extraperitoneal bladder ruptures are typically managed with catheter drainage.
- Early operative intervention is imperative in instances of testicular injury.
- Primary closure of vaginal lacerations is strongly recommended.

secondary to blunt trauma account for most "minor" ureteral injuries, healing of even partial injuries can be associated with stricture or breakdown and can require delayed surgical intervention.

Bladder Injuries

Blunt bladder injuries are usually found in association with other severe injuries due to the bladder's retropubic location. Up to 10% of traumatic pelvic fractures are associated with bladder rupture. However, in children, the bladder is an almost entirely abdominal organ and can be ruptured without pelvic fracture. When assessing for bladder injury, it is critical to check for concomitant urethral injury.

Bladder injuries are classified as either intraperitoneal (Fig. 2) or extraperitoneal (Fig. 3). Injury should be suspected in the presence of hematuria, failure of the urethral catheter to return urine, and inability of the patient to void. Diagnosis is confirmed either via retrograde cystography (plain abdominal x-ray obtained after instillation of at least 350 mL of contrast into the bladder by gravity) with both anteroposterior and oblique images or CT scan of the pelvis (following infusion of 350 mL of contrast diluted 1:6 with saline).

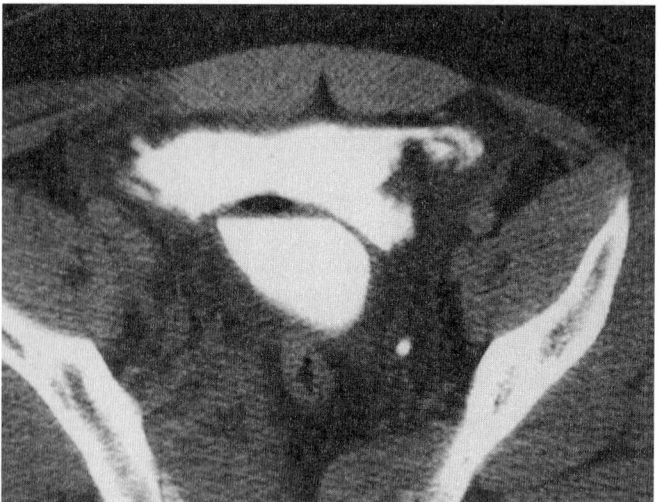

FIGURE 3. Computed tomographic cystogram showing extraperitoneal bladder rupture.

Once the injury is diagnosed, treatment for each type of injury varies. Intraperitoneal bladder ruptures require surgical closure for several reasons: They are often much larger than suggested by radiologic imaging (average size, 6 cm), they are associated with persistent urinary leakage when conservative management is attempted, and persistent urinary leakage causes peritonitis, which can be fatal. In the case of extraperitoneal rupture, conservative treatment is the rule, although surgical intervention might ultimately be required due to bony fragments projecting into the bladder, planned surgical repair of a pelvic fracture (to prevent hardware contamination), or other associated intraabdominal injuries.

With either type of bladder rupture, a catheter is left in place for 10 to 14 days, after which cystography is repeated before the catheter is removed. In addition to catheter placement for extraperitoneal bladder ruptures, antibiotic prophylaxis should be instituted on the day of injury and continued until 3 days after the catheter is removed. Repaired intraperitoneal bladder ruptures require that antibiotics be administered for 3 days perioperatively.

Urethral Injuries

Classically, the male urethra is divided into anterior and posterior segments by the urogenital diaphragm. Posterior urethral injuries are overwhelmingly associated with pelvic fractures. Blood at the urethral meatus is the most common physical finding associated with urethral injuries and is found in 37% to 93% of patients.

If urethral disruption is suspected, immediate retrograde urethrography (RUG) should be performed (Fig. 4). If urethral disruption is demonstrated, the patient requires surgical placement of a suprapubic catheter or an attempt at endoscopic catheter placement. Once a urethral catheter has been placed, it is recommended that the catheter remain in place for 4 to 6 weeks, after which a voiding cystourethrogram (VCUG) is obtained. If no extravasation is seen, the catheter may then be discontinued.

Anterior urethral injuries are rare, most often isolated, and largely involve the bulbar urethra (straddle injuries). As with posterior urethral injuries, a RUG should be performed all cases of penetrating trauma if there is associated blood at the urethral meatus or if the patient is unable to void. In cases of minor injury (contusion or partial disruption), a urethral catheter may be able to be placed. With major urethral injury, suprapubic diversion with delayed repair is necessary.

Female trauma victims require a thorough vaginal examination, because female GU injuries can be subtle in their presentation and are

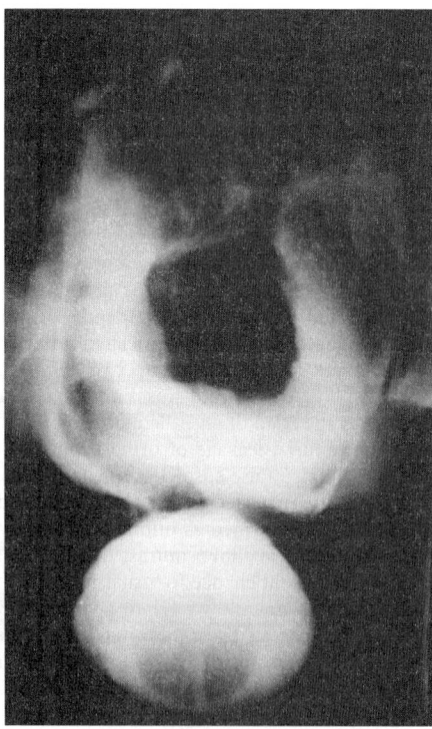

FIGURE 2. Plain cystogram showing an intraperitoneal bladder rupture.

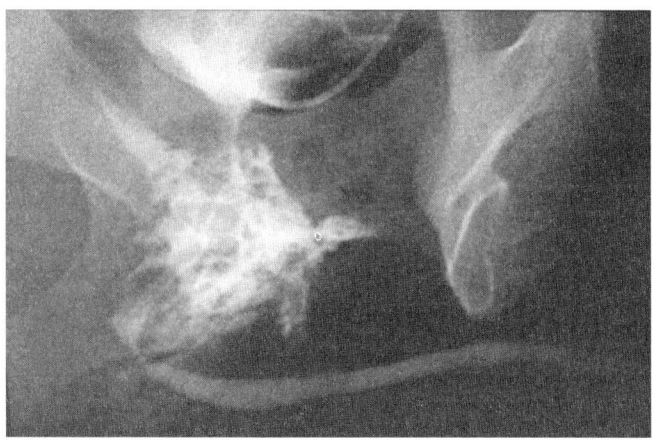

FIGURE 4. Retrograde urethrogram showing urethral disruption.

often missed. Due to the short length of the female urethra, these injuries carry a high risk of urethral sphincter injury, incontinence, and urethrovaginal fistula formation. Thus, immediate repair, if possible, is favored.

External Genital Trauma in Male Patients

Penile injuries may be divided into three main categories: soft-tissue, penetrating, and amputation. Penile fracture is the most commonly reported blunt injury to the penis and typically manifests with a classic history of a sustained blow to the erect penis followed by a popping sound and immediate detumescence. On physical examination, penile swelling and ecchymosis are nearly always present. It is important for the examining physician to be alert to the possibility of associated urethral injury. Once penile fracture has been diagnosed and an assessment for urethral injury performed, immediate repair of the fractured corpora and any associated urethral injury is recommended.

Isolated penile soft tissue injuries are rare. As with any skin wound, initial treatment of a penile soft tissue wound involves irrigation, débridement of necrotic tissue, and use of appropriate antimicrobial agents. Clean, uninfected wounds may be closed primarily after irrigation and débridement, but old or infected wounds should be treated with wet-to-dry dressing changes and antimicrobial prophylaxis against probable pathogens. Skin grafting may be required if the amount of skin lost from the penis is too excessive to allow primary closure. In the case of the unfortunate patient who catches his penis in his trouser zipper, a local anesthetic penile block should be administered and a single attempt made to open the zipper. If this fails, a pair of metal snips may be used to cut the zipper, or a pair of surgical clamps can be used to pull the zipper apart tooth by tooth.

Management of penetrating penile injuries combines treatment modalities for both penile fracture and soft tissue injury. As in the case of penile fracture, primary surgical closure of any corporal disruption is recommended. Once the corpus has been repaired, the skin wound should be treated as any other penile soft tissue injury. For injury to deep structures (e.g., posterior urethra), a staged repair with a suprapubic tube is most suitable.

The most common cause of penile amputation is self-mutilation, often in patients with a history of psychiatric illness. If possible, the severed portion of the penis should be retrieved and an attempt made at reimplantation. If the severed portion of the penis cannot be found or cannot be reimplanted, operative débridement and formalization of the penile stump are necessary.

The testicles are surrounded by the tough tunica albuginea and as a result, a significant amount of force is required to cause rupture of the tunica. However, up to 50% of patients who suffer a direct blow to the testicle have testicular rupture. In addition, the intratesticular parenchymal blood vessels are delicate and rupture easily, causing hematoma formation. The diagnosis of testicular rupture is complicated by the fact that there are no specific symptoms indicating testicular rupture. Diagnosis is best made by thorough physical examination and judicious use of ultrasound imaging.

Treatment for testicular injury is guided by a low threshold for surgical exploration, especially in the case of penetrating injury. Any patient with an equivocal physical examination, significant hematocele, intratesticular hematoma, or frank rupture of the tunica should undergo surgical exploration. Early exploration is advocated in an attempt to preserve testicular hormonal production and spermatogenesis.

Scrotal injuries without testicular involvement may be managed in a fashion similar to that for any other skin wound: irrigation, followed by either primary closure (for clean wounds) or dressing changes and healing by secondary intention (for contaminated or extensive wounds). Scrotal skin defects of up to 50% may be closed primarily. Skin grafting is reserved for more extensive skin loss.

REFERENCES

Gomez RG, Ceballos L, Coburn M, et al: Consensus on genitourinary trauma, consensus statement on bladder injuries. BJU Int 2004;94:27-32.

Lynch TH, Martínez-Piñeiro L, Plas E, et al: EAU guidelines on urological trauma. Eur Urol 2005;47:1-15.

McAninch JW, Santucci RA: Renal and ureteral trauma. In Wein AJ, (ed): Campbell-Walsh Urology, 9th ed. Philadelphia, Saunders, 2007, pp 1274-1292.

Morey AF, Rozanski TA: Genital and lower urinary tract trauma. In Wein AJ, (ed): Campbell-Walsh Urology, 9th ed, Philadelphia, Saunders, 2007, pp 2649-2662.

Santucci RA, McAninch JW, Safir M, et al: Validation of the American Association for the Surgery of Trauma organ injury severity scale for the kidney. J Trauma 2001;50:195-200.

Prostatitis

Method of
Andrea Gallina, MD, Umberto Capitanio, MD, and Pierre I. Karakiewicz, MD

The clinical entity termed *prostatitis* affects 2% to 10% of men during their lifetime. Moreover, prostatitis symptoms are the most common cause for urologic consultation in men 50 years of age. The definition of prostatitis includes a large variety of clinical and nonclinical entities with a common underlying background. To standardize the diagnostics and the therapeutic approaches, the National Institutes of Health (NIH) proposed a classification system of prostatitis syndromes. It consists of four categories that reflect the wide variety of clinical manifestations of this syndrome (Box 1).

Category I: Acute Bacterial Prostatitis

Acute bacterial prostatitis affects 2% to 5% of prostatitis patients. It typically represents an ascending infection of the prostate with uropathogenic bacteria (*Escherichia coli, Klebsiella* spp., *Enterobacter* spp., *Serratia marcescens, Pseudomonas aeruginosa*). The classic presentation includes systemic (fever, chills and malaise) and local symptoms. Local symptoms consist of dysuria and perineal and prostatic pain, and they may be associated with complete or partial bladder outlet obstruction (urinary frequency, incomplete emptying, urgency, hesitancy, or retention). The onset may be sudden. The severity of systemic symptoms determines the need for hospitalization.

> **BOX 1 National Institutes of Health Classification of Prostatitis**
>
> **Category I**
> - Acute bacterial prostatitis
>
> **Category II**
> - Chronic bacterial prostatitis
>
> **Category III**
> - Chronic nonbacterial prostatitis/chronic pelvic pain syndrome (CP/CPPS)
>   - III A: Inflammatory CP/CPPS
>   - III B: Noninflammatory CP/CPPS
>
> **Category IV**
> - Asymptomatic inflammatory prostatitis

On history, recent urinary tract infections and urologic instrumentation (e.g., prostate biopsies, urinary catheters) should be ruled out. A gentle digital rectal examination (DRE) (to avoid local or systemic exacerbation of symptoms) assesses the extent of tenderness (acute infection), and rules out masses (abscess formation or associated prostatic or nonprostatic lesions). Postvoid residual is best assessed ultrasonically, because passage of catheters should be avoided. Presence of significant residual (>20% of voided volume) represents a relative indication for catheter drainage. Size 14 F or smaller catheters represent a valid alternative for suprapubic drainage. Urinalysis, midstream specimen for urine culture, and blood cultures (if systemic symptoms are present) complete the assessment.

Patients with systemic symptoms usually require hospitalization. Intravenous antibiotics (ampicillin and gentamicin) and hydration represent the mainstay of therapy. Ciprofloxacin and levofloxacin are alternatives if allergies or other contraindications exist. Once the patient is afebrile for 24 hours or according to blood culture results, oral fluoroquinolones or trimethoprim-sulfamethoxazole (TMP-SMX) may be initiated. Persistent fever and symptoms after 48 hours of IV antibiotic therapy can indicate an abscess formation, which may be identified with computed tomography (CT), magnetic resonance imaging (MRI), or transrectal ultrasonography. Antibiotic-refractory prostatic abscesses might require drainage with transurethral prostatic resection. Periprostatic abscesses may be drained transrectally.

Category I prostatitis represents a complicated urinary tract infection (UTI). Once symptoms have subsided and antibiotic therapy has been completed, a careful investigation of the upper and lower urinary tract is in order to identify any potentially predisposing causes. Imaging studies (ultrasound, CT, MRI), cystoscopy, and urodynamic studies can reveal an underlying cause, such as prostatic hypertrophy with urinary retention, bladder stone or diverticulum, or urethral stricture, among others.

Category II: Chronic Bacterial Prostatitis

NIH category II prostatitis is defined as a chronic or persistent pathogenic infection (culture proven) of the prostate without systemic symptoms. It accounts for 2% to 5% of patients with prostatitis. It is characterized by intermittent episodes of cystitis-like urinary symptoms, which only rarely involve appreciable discomfort or pain. Recurrent infectious episodes are highly suggestive of chronic bacterial prostatitis, especially if the same pathogen is documented in either a midstream urine specimen or a postprostatic massage urine specimen. *E. coli* (which represents 80% of the infectious agents), *Klebsiella* species, *P. aeruginosa*, and *Proteus* species represent the most commonly seen pathogens.

History and physical and laboratory examinations are virtually the same as those for category I prostatitis. The more protruded nature of category II prostatitis requires 4 to 8 weeks of antimicrobials (fluoroquinolones or TMP-SMX). This therapy is effective in 60% to 80% of patients. However, in cases of recurrent infections, long-term (3-6 months) antibiotic therapy is an alternative treatment. Other modalities have been investigated (for example intraprostatic injection of antibiotics) but have met with limited success.

Category III: Chronic Nonbacterial Prostatitis/Chronic Pelvic Pain Syndrome

Category III prostatitis (CP/CPPS) accounts for 90% to 95% of prostatitis cases and is the most challenging subgroup. Symptoms include pelvic or perineal (or both) pain or discomfort, as well as urinary or ejaculatory symptoms. Pain may be perineal, suprapubic, coccygeal, rectal, urethral, or testicular or scrotal. Urinary frequency, dysuria, urgency, or incomplete emptying and ejaculatory pain affect a significant proportion of patients. Ejaculatory pain suggests worse prognosis. Presence or absence of inflammatory cells in the ejaculate distinguishes between category IIIA (inflammatory) and category IIIB (noninflammatory) prostatitis. However, the clinical presentation and therapeutic approaches are the same for these two groups, and the reliability of this distinction is suboptimal. Only in up to 5% of patients is a pathogen successfully isolated from urine or semen.

The clinical heterogeneity of category III prostatitis and the absence of a diagnostic marker add complexity to the classification and treatment of this syndrome. A multifactorial etiology, which includes infectious, traumatic, inflammatory, hormonal, neurologic, and psychological triggers, is the most likely cause.

DIAGNOSIS

The evaluation of patients with category III prostatitis should include a detailed history (focusing on previous infections, trauma, surgery, or neurologic problems). It should be complemented with the NIH Chronic Prostatitis Symptom Index (NIH-CPSI) questionnaire, which is a standardized assessment of the type and severity of symptoms. Physical examination should include the same elements as in categories I and II prostatitis. Urine analysis and midstream culture are mandatory. Urinary cytology is recommended to rule out irritative symptoms of bladder cancer. Urine flow rate and residual urine determination can also help in the diagnostic work-up. In rare instances, abdominal, pelvic, or neurologic imaging, urodynamic studies, cystoscopy, or prostate-specific antigen testing may be useful.

In most men, the disease has a protracted natural history. Symptom severity predicts recurrence in 30% of men, and previous symptoms predict recurrence in 50% of men. Unfortunately, in most category III prostatitis patients, the cause of pelvic pain cannot be identified. Thus, the diagnosis of CP/CPPS remains a diagnosis of exclusion.

TREATMENT

Several treatments have been investigated and studied for category III prostatitis, with mixed results (Figure 1). These include α-blockers, antibiotics, nonsteroidal anti-inflammatory drugs (NSAIDs), and pentosan polysulfate, among others.

Mehik's group tested the efficacy of an α-blocker, alfuzosin (Uroxatral)[1] 5 mg, against placebo for symptom relief in 70 patients. At 6 months, the pain score was lower in the alfuzosin group ($P = 0.02$). Similar results were obtained by Cheah and colleagues in a cohort of 86 patients treated with terazosin (Hytrin),[1] with dose escal-ation from 1 to 5 mg/day compared with placebo. The α-blocker significantly improved the quality of life and

---
[1]Not FDA approved for this indication.

CURRENT DIAGNOSIS

Category I (Acute Bacterial Prostatitis)

- History
- Physical examination (including gentle DRE)
- Urinalysis
- Urine culture
- Blood cultures (if systemic symptoms are present)
- Postvoid residual

Category II (Chronic Bacterial Prostatitis)

- History
- Physical examination
- Urinalysis
- Urine culture
- Postprostatic massage urine culture
- Evaluation of complicated UTI (optional)

Category III (Chronic Pelvic Pain Syndrome)

- History
- Physical examination
- NIH-Chronic Prostatitis Symptom Index (NIH-CPSI) questionnaire
- Urinalysis
- Midstream culture
- Optional tests (cytology, urine flow, postvoid residual, etc)

Category IV (Asymptomatic Inflammatory Prostatitis)

- No further evaluation

Abbreviations: DRE = digital rectal examination; NIH = National Institutes of Health; UTI = urinary tract infection.

CURRENT THERAPY

Category I (Acute Bacterial Prostatitis)

- Admission
- Intravenous antibiotics (ampicillin or gentamicin)
- Bladder drainage, if urinary retention
- Oral antibiotics for 3 to 4 weeks (fluoroquinolones or TMP-SMX)

Category II (Chronic Bacterial Prostatitis)

- Outpatient treatment
- Antibiotics for 4 to 8 weeks (fluoroquinolones or TMP-SMX)
- Long-term antibiotic therapy

Category III (Chronic Pelvic Pain Syndrome)

- Antibiotics for 4 to 6 weeks (fluoroquinolone or TMP-SMX)
- α-Blockers (e.g., tamsulosin [Flomax],[1] alfuzosin [Uroxatral],[1] terazosin [Hytrin][1])
- Anti-inflammatory medications
- Finasteride (Proscar),[1] pentosan polysulfate (Elmiron),[1] and phytotherapies (e.g., cernilton,[7] quercetin[7])
- Nonpharmacologic therapies (biofeedback, pelvic floor training, thermal treatments)
- Repeat treatment if relief is noted.
- Combine therapies if partial relief is noted.

Category IV (Asymptomatic Inflammatory Prostatitis)

- No treatments

[1]Not FDA approved for this indication.
[7]Available as dietary supplements.
Abbreviation: TMP-SMX = trimethoprim-sulfamethoxazole.

---

significantly reduced pain at 14 weeks ($P = 0.03$). Nickel and colleagues randomized 58 men younger than 55 years to 0.4 mg tamsulosin (Flomax)[1] or placebo. At 45 days, tamsulosin significantly reduced symptoms. However, these benefits were not always replicated, especially in pretreated men.

A 4- to 6-week trial of antibiotics is one of the key management options for patients with category III prostatitis, despite absence of benefit in placebo-controlled trials. Lack of efficacy at 6 and 12 weeks was shown by Nickel's group, who randomized 80 patients with category III prostatitis to either levofloxacin or placebo for 6 weeks. Alexander's group recapitulated these findings with ciprofloxacin.

NSAIDs were tested in a placebo-controlled trial of 161 patients. Rofecoxib (Vioxx) (50 mg) significantly improved pain and NIH-CPSI scores. It has been withdrawn from the market.

Pentosan polysulfate (Elmiron)[1] was tested in a placebo-controlled, randomized trial of 100 men. Three daily 100-mg doses of Elmiron for 16 weeks resulted in a significant improvement in NIH-CPSI quality-of-life scores.

Several other therapeutic approaches are available. These include prostatic massage, which should be considered once or twice weekly, in men who report some degree of symptom relief. Finasteride (Proscar)[1] 5 mg daily and phytotherapy (e.g., cernilton[7] and quercetin[7]) showed some, albeit limited, efficacy. Tricyclic antidepressants

[1]Not FDA approved for this indication.

[1]Not FDA approved for this indication.
[7]Available as dietary supplements.

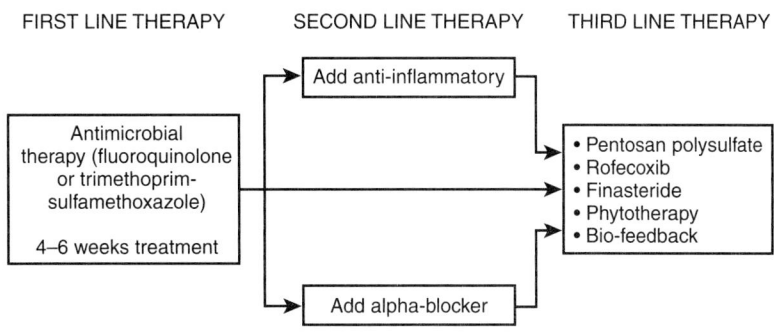

FIGURE 1. Management of NIH category III prostatitis.

(amitriptyline [Elavil][1]), anticholinergics (oxybutynin [Ditropan][1]), anticonvulsants, lifestyle changes (e.g., nutrition, stress reduction), biofeedback, pelvic floor training, and thermal therapy reduced symptoms in some category III prostatitis patients. The use of allopurinol has been reported to alleviate symptoms of CP, but further evaluation is required. Similarly, biofeedback, acupuncture, electromagnetic stimulation, immune and neuromodulating agents, muscle ralaxants and pudendal nerve modulation have been suggested. Although invasive procedures have been advocated for CP/CPPS patients, surgery (including transurethral resection, microwave thermotherapy, or needle ablation) should be considered only as last therapeutic options. The multitude of trials addressing CP/CPPS patients emphasizes the high failure rate (~66%) of sequential monotherapy. It suggests the need for structured assessment of multimodality approaches.

Category IV: Asymptomatic Inflammatory Prostatitis

Category IV prostatitis is defined as incidental observation of leukocytes in prostatic secretions or tissue obtained during evaluation for other disorders, (e.g., leukocytes noted in prostate biopsies performed for elevated prostate-specific antigen [PSA]). Epidemiologic studies estimate the prevalence of category IV prostatitis to be as high as 32.2% in a population of men with elevated PSA levels. Category IV prostatitis needs no further evaluation or treatment.

Acknowledgments

Pierre I. Karakiewicz is partially supported by the Fonds de la Recherche en Santé du Québec, the Centre hospitalier de l'Université de Montréal (CHUM) Foundation, the Department of Surgery, and Les Urologues Associés du CHUM.

---

[1]Not FDA approved for this indication.

REFERENCES

Clemens JQ, Meenan RT, O'Keeffe-Rosetti MC, et al: Prevalence of prostatitis-like symptoms in a managed care population. J Urol 2006;176(2):593-596.

Dimitrakov JD, Kaplan SA, Kroenke K, et al: Management of chronic prostatitis/chronic pelvic pain syndrome: an evidence-based approach. Urology 2006;67(5):881-888.

Fowler JE Jr: Antimicrobial therapy for bacterial and nonbacterial prostatitis. Urology 2002;60(6 Suppl):24-26.

Habermacher GM, Chason JT, Schaeffer AJ: Prostatitis/chronic pelvic pain syndrome. Annu Rev Med 2006;57:195-206.

Krieger JN, Egan KJ, Ross SO, et al: Chronic pelvic pains represent the most prominent urogenital symptoms of "chronic prostatitis." Urology 1996;48(5):715-721.

Krieger JN, Nyberg L Jr, Nickel JC: NIH consensus definition and classification of prostatitis. JAMA 1999;282(3):236-237.

Krieger JN, Ross SO, Riley DE: Chronic prostatitis: Epidemiology and role of infection. Urology 2002;60(6 Suppl):8-12.

Litwin MS, McNaughton-Collins M, Fowler FJ Jr, et al: The National Institutes of Health chronic prostatitis symptom index: Development and validation of a new outcome measure. Chronic Prostatitis Collaborative Research Network. J Urol 1999;162(2):369-375.

Nickel JC: Treatment of chronic prostatitis/chronic pelvic pain syndrome. Int J Antimicrob Agents 2008;31:S112-S116.

Pontari MA, Ruggieri MR: Mechanisms in prostatitis/chronic pelvic pain syndrome. J Urol 2004;172(3):839-845.

Rothman I, Stanford JL, Kuniyuki A, Berger RE: Self-report of prostatitis and its risk factors in a random sample of middle-aged men. Urology 2004;64(5):876-879.

Schaeffer AJ, Datta NS, Fowler JE Jr, et al: Overview summary statement: Diagnosis and management of chronic prostatitis/chronic pelvic pain syndrome (CP/CPPS). Urology 2002;60(6 Suppl):1-4.

Wagenlehner FM, Weidner W, Sorgel F, Naber KG. The role of antibiotics in chronic bacterial prostatitis. Int J Antimicrob Agents 2005;26(1):1-7.

Benign Prostatic Hyperplasia

Method of
Gopal H. Badlani, MD, and
Matthew E. Karlovsky, MD

Epidemiology

Bladder outlet obstruction (BOO) secondary to benign prostatic hyperplasia (BPH) is one of the most common medical conditions in older men and represents up to a 40% clinical risk for urinary retention in a man's lifetime. It is the most prevalent condition in the aging male, affecting 14 million men in the United States, with an annual cost of $4 billion to treat. Age and normal androgenic function are two of the better established risk factors. Whereas BPH is rare before the age of 40, the prevalence of histologic BPH at autopsy is 50% by 60 years of age and 90% by 85 years of age. Approximately 40% of males 70 years of age or older have lower urinary tract symptoms (LUTS) secondary to BPH, and with age, the prevalence increases. Symptomatically, approximately 25% of 55-year-old men experience decreased urinary flow rate and other symptoms of BPH. By 75 years of age, the appearance of this symptom increases to 50%. Age, however, is not a causative factor of BOO. Although the risk for developing symptoms from BPH doubles for each decade of life between 60 and 90 years of age, clinical symptoms of the individual patient do not necessarily progress with age. BPH is more commonly diagnosed because of increased life expectancy and a greater tendency today to seek medical advice at an earlier disease stage.

Normal androgenic function is required for development of BPH. Both androgenic and estrogenic hormonal stimulation can induce prostatic hypertrophy. Other factors, such as race, sexual activity, smoking, socioeconomic status, vasectomy, alcohol intake, and diet, have been implicated in BPH development. Identifying men at clinical risk for BPH and its progression has clinical usefulness in selecting the appropriate intervention when necessary.

Pathophysiology

The pathophysiology of BPH is poorly understood because no direct correlation can be made between prostatic glandular enlargement and the symptomatology of BPH. Because the condition is rare in those younger than 40 years of age and does not develop in castrated men, it is accepted that BPH development requires aging and functional testes for androgen production. BPH is believed to originate in the transitional zone of the prostate, which surrounds the prostatic urethra between the bladder neck and the verumontanum, and is progressive.

Both a static and a dynamic component are involved in BPH development. The static component relates to epithelial and stromal cell proliferation in the prostatic transitional zone (TZ); enlargement is evident as median or lateral lobe hypertrophy. Proliferation is induced by testosterone and its biologically active conversion product, dihydrotestosterone. Conversion of testosterone to dihydrotestosterone occurs via the enzyme 5α-reductase. Two forms of this enzyme have been described, type 1 and type 2. Type 1 is present in liver, skin, and other organs. Type 2 is present in urogenital tissues. Individuals lacking 5α-reductase type 2 do not develop genitalia and prostates.

Conversely, the dynamic component relates to prostatic smooth muscle. High concentrations of $α_1$-adrenergic receptors occur in the prostatic capsule and bladder neck. An increase in smooth muscle tone is responsible for increased urethral resistance and pressure. Pharmacologic blockade with $α_1$ antagonists blocks prostatic smooth muscle contraction and decreases urethral resistance and pressure, subsequently relaxing the dynamic component of BPH.

Symptoms

The diagnosis of BPH is presumptive, based on symptoms. These symptoms, commonly referred to as lower urinary tract symptoms (LUTS), are not specific for BPH. LUTS include frequency, retention, intermittency, decreased force of stream (FOS), straining, urgency, and nocturia. Individuals with LUTS should be carefully assessed to determine the cause, to confirm diagnosis of BPH, and to exclude other bladder and prostate processes. Normal prostate size on digital rectal examination (DRE) does not rule out a diagnosis of BPH because palpable prostate size does not correlate with degree of obstruction or severity of LUTS. However, the odds of having moderate to severe symptoms are five times higher for men with enlarged prostates compared with those with normal prostates. Symptoms of BPH are difficult to assess and quantify, yet they are the keys to proper diagnosis and treatment. Because the vast majority of procedures performed for BPH are to provide symptomatic relief, it is necessary to quantify the level of interference in the quality of life of the patient. Assessment of interference on quality of life can be reliably accomplished using the well-validated International Prostate Symptom Score (IPSS) (Figure 1). Symptoms based on overall score are classified as mild (0 to 7), moderate (8 to 19), and severe (20 to 35). The subjective impact of these symptoms on overall quality of life must also be taken into account. The patient with a severe-range IPSS may feel the symptoms are less bothersome than a patient with a lower IPSS, and this subjective impact on quality of life can direct therapeutic options.

Name: Date:

	Not at all	Less than 1 time in 5	Less than half the time	About half the time	More than half the time	Almost always	Your score
Incomplete emptying Over the past month, how often have you had a sensation of not emptying your bladder completely after you finish urinating?	0	1	2	3	4	5	
Frequency Over the past month, how often have you had to urinate again less than two hours after you finished urinating?	0	1	2	3	4	5	
Intermittency Over the past month, how often have you found you stopped and started again several times when you urinated?	0	1	2	3	4	5	
Urgency Over the past month, how difficult have you found it to postpone urination?	0	1	2	3	4	5	
Weak stream Over the past month, how often have you had a weak urinary stream?	0	1	2	3	4	5	
Straining Over the past month, how often have you had to push or strain to begin urination?	0	1	2	3	4	5	

	None	1 time	2 times	3 times	4 times	5 times or more	Your score
Nocturia Over the past month, how many times did you most typically get up to urinate from the time you went to bed until the time you got up in the morning?	0	1	2	3	4	5	

Total IPSS score	

Quality of life due to urinary symptoms	Delighted	Pleased	Mostly satisfied	Mixed—about equally satisfied and dissatisfied	Mostly dissatisfied	Unhappy	Terrible
If you were to spend the rest of your life with your urinary condition the way it is now, how would you feel about that?	0	1	2	3	4	5	6

FIGURE 1. International prostate symptom score (IPSS).

Diagnosis

Diagnosis of BPH relies on an accurate medical history eliciting the specific voiding complaints, as well as quantification of these symptoms using the IPSS. Other possible causes of LUTS also must be ruled out, including urinary tract infection (UTI), urolithiasis, diabetes, urethral stricture, overactive or neurogenic bladder, prostate/bladder cancer, or congestive heart failure. Medications that can exacerbate obstructive symptoms include tricyclic antidepressants, anticholinergic agents, diuretics, narcotics, and first-generation antihistamines and decongestants. Physical examination should include DRE for prostatic abnormalities, such as palpable nodules, induration or irregularities of malignancy, or infection. On DRE, the posterior lobes, not the transition zone, are palpable. Abdominal examination may detect a suprapubic or low abdominal mass in a patient with BPH-induced retention. The American Urological Association and the American Cancer Society recommend all men older than age 50 receive an annual prostate-specific antigen (PSA) serum level to screen for prostate cancer. In black men or men with a family history of prostate cancer in a first-degree relative, PSA screening should begin at 40 years of age or younger. The normal range for PSA is up to 4.0 μg/mL. Other valuable laboratory data include urinalysis to rule out infection or hematuria, a serum creatinine level to determine renal function, and urine cytologic studies if irritative voiding symptoms are present. More sophisticated studies, such as urinary flow rate, postvoid residual, and pressure flow urodynamic studies, are appropriate for evaluation of men with more severe symptoms (IPSS >8) or with more complex comorbidities. These tests are often used to determine baseline function prior to initiation of therapy or to determine subsequent response to therapy. In patients who fail medical therapy, urodynamic pressure-flow studies and cystoscopy may be appropriate to evaluate the need for operative intervention and to rule out other urologic pathologies. Cystoscopy is also reserved for situations in which invasive treatment is strongly considered. If watchful waiting or noninvasive therapies are appropriate, invasive diagnostic tests are usually not necessary. The variables of importance of disease progression in an artificial neural network analysis were PSA, obstructive symptom score, and transitional zone volume. The Olmsted County study showed risk progression of acute urinary retention (AUR) with age. Overall, a 60-year-old man has a 23% chance of AUR if he survives the next 20 years. The average annual change in prostate volume was 1.6% for all ages. The annual increase was not significantly related to baseline age but was significantly related to baseline prostate volume.

Treatment

WATCHFUL WAITING

Indications for treatment of BPH rely, in large part, on the subjective nature of the symptoms. For the majority of patients with BPH, symptoms are not severe or bothersome enough to warrant long-term medical or surgical intervention. Men with an IPSS of less than 8 are usually treated with expectant management. Advising the patient toward lifestyle modifications, such as minimizing evening fluid intake, avoiding caffeine, and avoiding decongestants, anticholinergics, and other medications that impair voiding, often provides an effective resolution of symptoms. In a study of 556 men with moderate symptoms of BPH comparing outcomes following transurethral resection of the prostate (TURP) with watchful waiting for more than 3 years, 8% of men randomized to TURP and 17% of men with watchful waiting failed treatment. Treatment failure with watchful waiting was mostly because of high postvoid residuals and significant increases in IPSS symptoms. Patients who respond poorly to watchful waiting have multiple medical and surgical options for treatment of BPH.

α_1-ADRENERGIC BLOCKING AGENTS

The α_1-adrenergic antagonists have been shown in numerous randomized placebo-controlled trials to be safe and effective in the treatment of BPH. The most commonly prescribed α_1-adrenergic blockers appear to have similar safety profiles and clinical efficacy and are the common first approach for urologists. Terazosin (Hytrin) and doxazosin (Cardura) were the first α antagonists available for treatment of BPH; however, orthostatic hypotension was a significant concern, requiring careful dose titration. Tamsulosin (Flomax), a highly selective α-blocker, does not induce orthostatic hypotension and so does not require dose titration. Overall, the most common side effects include headaches, dizziness, asthenia, and drowsiness. Sexual side effects are limited to retrograde ejaculation. Alfuzosin (Uroxatral), a newer nonspecific α-blocker, has minimal vasoactive or retrograde ejaculation side effects. Table 1 provides a list for medication dosing and schedules.

5α-REDUCTASE INHIBITION

Finasteride (Proscar) and dutasteride (Avodart) are 5α-reductase inhibitors (type 1 and type 1/2, respectively) that block conversion of testosterone to dihydrotestosterone, the androgen involved in development of BPH. These medications represent the paradigm for androgen suppression of BPH. They have their greatest therapeutic effect in men with prostates greater than 40 g, and treatment for 6 months or more is usually required for a clinical response. The first randomized, multicenter, double-blind, placebo-controlled trial investigating the efficacy of finasteride demonstrated significant improvements in maximum flow rate and decreased prostatic volume. Since then, further studies have confirmed a reduced risk of acute urinary retention and surgical intervention with finasteride use. Finasteride can reduce BPH-associated hematuria. It is effective as adjuvant therapy, following other treatments, and as neoadjuvant therapy prior to minimally invasive therapy. Adverse effects include decreased libido, ejaculatory dysfunction, and gynecomastia. In the patient being monitored for prostate cancer with PSA testing, finasteride therapy must be taken into account when interpreting PSA values; finasteride decreases PSA values by 50%, leading to a false-negative result.

Efficacy of Medical Therapy

The Medical Therapy of Prostate Symptoms (MTOPS) study evaluated the efficacy of doxazosin and finasteride to determine if medical

TABLE 1 Common Medications for Benign Prostatic Hyperplasia

Medication	Class	Dose	Schedule
Alfuzosin (Uroxatral)	α-1 Blocker	10 mg	Once daily
Doxazosin (Cardura)	α-1 Blocker	1-8 mg, titrated	Once daily at bedtime
Tamsulosin (Flomax)	α-1a Blocker	0.4 mg	Once daily
Terazosin (Hytrin)	α-1 Blocker	1-10 mg, titrated	Once daily at bedtime
Dutasteride (Avodart)	5-α Reductase inhibitor	0.5 mg	Once daily
Finasteride (Proscar)	5-α Reductase inhibitor	5 mg	Once daily

therapy delays or prevents disease progression. At 4 years, combination therapy was most effective for reducing risk of clinical progression (AUR) and improving symptom score and urinary flow rate. Fina-steride and combination therapy significantly reduced the risk of AUR and invasive therapy over 4 years. Monotherapy with either medication reduced symptom score and improved flow significantly, but to a lesser degree than combination therapy. Doxazosin delayed time to progression of AUR and invasive therapy but not the risk. Without treatment, the risk of BPH progression was 20% more during the trial. Risk factors for progression include baseline prostate volume (>40 g) and higher serum PSA value (>2 μg/mL).

Phytotherapy

Saw palmetto (*Serenoa repens*)[1,2] extract is the most popular phytotherapeutic agent. Its likely mechanism is inhibition of 5α-reductase. A recent meta-analysis of numerous randomized trials using saw palmetto described a mild to moderate improvement in flow and LUTS; however, because of small study sample, varying products, short treatment times, and varying outcomes, these study conclusions are difficult to interpret. Other popular preparations are African plum (*Pygeum africanum*)[1,2] and South African star grass (*Cynodon nlemfuësis*).[1,2] The former has been shown to have several in vitro effects, such as antiestrogen effects, leukotriene blockade, and inhibition of fibroblast growth factors. The latter has been shown in vitro to increase plasminogen activators, as well as to stimulate release of transforming growth factor-β, an inducer of apoptosis, yet these in vitro effects have not been shown to occur in vivo. A meta-analysis of four clinical trials of South African star grass extract, β-sitosterol, concluded that β-sitosterol improved urologic symptoms and flow rates in men.

There is no standard of care for management of patients using phytotherapy. Nor have the long-term safety effects been established. Patients should be cautioned that doses, efficacy, side effects, and drug interactions with phytotherapy are unknown. For the patient refusing medical therapy of α-blockers and 5α-reductase inhibitors, phytotherapy may be attempted as long as the patient understands the limitations of these agents. If retention, UTI, calculi, or decreased renal function occurs, phytotherapy should be discouraged and more aggressive medical and surgical management undertaken.

Minimally Invasive Therapies

The most commonly employed surgical procedure, and the gold standard for BPH, is transurethral resection of the prostate (TURP), involving endoscopic resection of the obstructive component of the prostate. TURP is highly effective, improving symptoms in up to 95% of patients. Common complications include inability to void postoperatively, clot retention, incontinence, impotence, and retrograde ejaculation. A number of new minimally invasive therapies have been developed to reduce the complications associated with TURP, as well as provide alternatives for the unfavorable surgical candidate. Most minimally invasive therapies use energy, such as radio waves, laser, ultrasound, microwaves, or electrical current.

Transurethral incision of the prostate (TUIP) involves endoscopic placement of one to two incisions into the prostate and capsule to reduce urethral constriction. This procedure is highly effective on prostate glands less than 30 g and is well documented and safe, with efficacy comparable with TURP. TUIP is associated with a 78% to 83% improvement of symptoms. Because TUIP is associated with fewer retrograde ejaculations, less morbidity, and a reoperation rate of less than 1% in 10 years, this procedure is the treatment of choice for small gland BPH in men concerned with fertility and ejaculation.

In transurethral needle ablation (TUNA), low-level energy is transferred by radiofrequency to the prostate, creating a well-defined necrotic lesion within the prostatic parenchyma while preserving the urethral mucosa. A cystoscope-like instrument with two needles set at 90 degrees from each other ablates tissue in 3 to 5 minutes when needles reach temperatures of 27° to 38°C (80° to 100°F). Urethral and rectal temperatures are also vigorously monitored as the device adjusts. Preliminary studies show an increase in peak flow and a decrease in symptom score following TUNA, with no major complications. Transient urinary retention is reported in 10% to 40% of patients. In a prospective study, TURP was superior to TUNA in increasing flow rates but demonstrated comparable improved symptoms at 1 year postoperatively. Transurethral microwave thermotherapy (TUMT) heats prostatic transitional zone tissue to between 60° and 80°C (140° to 176°F), inducing tissue damage. Thermotherapy preferentially destroys smooth muscle by coagulative necrosis while water-conductive cooling of the urethral mucosa preserves periurethral tissues. Although prospective studies indicate that TURP produces more pronounced urinary improvements versus TUMT, thermotherapy consistently improves symptom scores by 75% and increases peak flow rates by 75%. Furthermore, TUMT is a procedure done under local anesthesia. Retrograde ejaculation and urinary retention with prolonged catheterization occurs in greater than one third of patients.

Ultimately, therapeutic decisions depend in large part on symptom scores. Men with low symptom scores without bother are appropriately managed through watchful waiting. As scores increase, or if progression with clinical morbidity develops, more aggressive management is appropriate.

REFERENCES

Bhargava S, Canda AE, Chapple CR: A rational approach to benign hyperplasia evaluation: Recent advances. Curr Opin Urol 2004;14:1-6.
Djavan B, Waldert M, Ghawidel C, Marberger M: Benign prostatic hyperplasia progression and its impact on treatment. Curr Opin Urol 2004;14:45-50.
Fong YK, Milani S, Djavan B: Role of phytotherapy in men with lower urinary tract symptoms. Curr Opin Urol 2005;15:45-48.
Hoffman RM, MacDonald R, Monga M, Wilt TJ: Transurethral microwave thermotherapy vs. transurethral resection for treating benign prostatic hyperplasia: A systematic review. BJU Int 2004;94:1031-1036.
Walsh PC, Retik A, Vaughan D (eds): Campbell's Urology, 8th ed. Philadelphia, Saunders Elsevier Science, 2002.

Erectile Dysfunction

Method of
Luciano Kolodny, MD

The term *erectile dysfunction* (ED) is relatively new, having replaced *impotence* approximately a decade ago. ED is defined as the "inability of the male to attain or maintain an erection sufficient for satisfactory sexual intercourse." ED affects millions of men worldwide with implications that go far beyond sexual activity alone. ED is now recognized as a sentinel event in cardiovascular disease, diabetes mellitus (DM), and depression. It can also be damaging to interpersonal relationships and self-esteem.

Epidemiology

The Massachusetts Male Aging Study is one of the pivotal studies on the prevalence of ED. Between 1987 and 1989, men between the ages of 40 and 70 years received questionnaires inquiring about several aspects of their sexual health. Of the 1790 men who received the questionnaires, 1290 responded. They revealed that 52% of them had some degree of dysfunction, 17% with minimal, 25% with moderate, and almost 10% with complete absence of erectile function.

---

[1]Not FDA approved for this indication.
[2]Available as a dietary supplement.

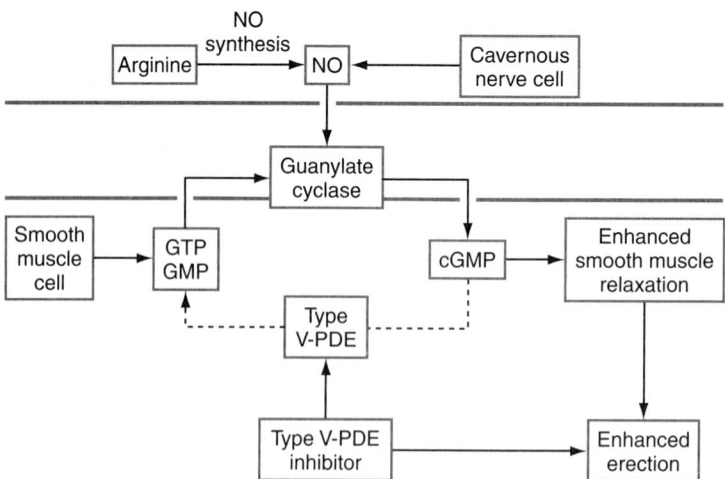

FIGURE 1. The biochemical process involved in erections and the mechanism of action of sildenafil citrate (Viagra). The cavernous nerves (S2-S4) innervate the penis and release NO. NO stimulates the production of cGMP in the smooth muscle cells of the penis. cGMP is directly responsible for increasing smooth muscle relaxation, which leads to increased arterial inflow and an erection. When cGMP is metabolized by PDE5, the penis undergoes detumescence. Sildenafil citrate (Viagra) inhibits PDE5 and increases the available cGMP, thereby leading to an enhanced erection. cGMP = cyclic guanosine monophosphate; NO = nitric oxide; PDE5 = phosphodiesterase 5.

It also showed the extremely detrimental link between coronary artery disease (CAD), DM, and ED. A few years later another group used the same patient database and followed up on these subjects. The risk of ED was 26 cases per 1000 men annually, which increased with age, lower education, DM, heart disease, and hypertension.

Physiology of Erection

The penile erection requires intact vascular, neuronal, and hormonal systems. The intricate details of this process are beyond the scope of this article, but in summary, after any sensorial stimulation, which can be visual, tactile, auditory, or olfactory, nitric oxide (NO) and other neurotransmitters are released at the cavernous nerve terminals. The endothelial cells then release vasoactive relaxing factors, which lead to vasodilatation of the penile blood vessels and increased blood flow. As blood flow increases, compression of the subtunical venular plexuses will substantially decrease venous outflow and finally cause the penis to change from flaccid to erect (Figure 1).

NO is the principal neurotransmitter involved in penile erection, but other vasoactive substances such as vasoactive intestinal peptide, neuropeptide Y, calcitonin gene-related peptide (CGRP), substance P, and serotonin also play roles. High levels of intrapenile NO facilitate the relaxation of intracavernosal trabeculae, thereby maximizing blood flow and penile erection. Nonadrenergic, noncholinergic neurons have been found to release NO, leading to increased production of cyclic guanosine monophosphate (cGMP). Through a series of reactions, cGMP will lead to relaxation of the smooth muscle, directly impacting the ability to go from a flaccid to an erect penile state. The return from erect to flaccid requires the hydrolysis of cGMP to guanosine monophosphate (GMP) by phosphodiesterase 5 (PDE5) (see Figure 1).

Testosterone and Erectile Function

Testosterone provides intrapenile nitrous oxide synthase (NOS), which has an important role in enhancing the production of NO, subsequent local vasodilatation, and penile erection. There is no correlation between serum testosterone levels and the degree of ED. However, hypogonadal men may experience significantly reduced libido. Hypogonadism is associated with decreased self-esteem, depression, osteoporosis, insulin resistance, increased fat mass, decreased lean body mass, and cognitive dysfunction.

Pathophysiology of Erectile Dysfunction

ED can be classified as psychogenic, organic (hormonal, vascular, drug-induced, or neurogenic), or mixed psychogenic and organic. Up to 80% of ED cases have an organic origin. The most common cause of ED is vascular disease (Box 1).

Atherosclerosis is the most common cause of vasculogenic ED, whereas endothelial damage is the most common mechanism. Aging is a well-known risk factor for ED, and it is hypothesized that there are alterations in the levels of NO that occur as a consequence of the aging endothelium. Additionally, chronic illness, depression, and lack of a sexual partner are all prevalent in this age population.

Chronic tobacco use is a major risk factor for the development of vasculogenic ED because of its effects on the vascular endothelium. Additionally, blood nicotine levels rise after smoking, which increases sympathetic tone in the penis and leads to nicotine-induced, smooth-muscle contraction in the cavernosal body. Chronic smoking also leads to decreased penile NOS activity and neuronal NOS content.

DM is a major risk factor for ED. In the Massachusetts Male Aging Study, the diabetic subset had a threefold increased prevalence of ED compared with nondiabetic subjects (28% versus 9.6%). In the same study, the overall incidence rate of ED was 26 cases per 1000 man-years in nondiabetics and 50 cases per 1000 man-years in the diabetic population. The pathogenesis of ED in the diabetic patient is related to accelerated atherosclerosis, alterations in the corporal erectile tissue, and neuropathy.

Hypertension is another major risk factor for ED. Whether ED in patients with hypertension is related to the disease itself or to the use of antihypertensive medications has been debated for years. In a study looking at 104 subjects, the differences in incidence or severity of ED were minor between distinct types of antihypertensive medications or the number of agents being used simultaneously. This favors the concept that antihypertensive agents as well as the disease itself contribute to the appearance of ED. There are, however, classes of antihypertensive medications that are notorious for their negative impact on erectile function such as thiazides and β-blockers. The only β-blocker not associated with significant incidence of ED is carvedilol (Coreg).

> **BOX 1 Classification of Erectile Dysfunction**
>
> **Endocrine**
> - Hypogonadism
> - Hyperprolactinemia
>
> **Drug Induced**
> - β-Blockers
> - Calcium channel blockers
> - Alcohol
> - Nicotine
> - Antiandrogens
> - Cocaine
> - Heroin
> - Marijuana
> - Cimetidine
> - Metoclopramide
> - Antidepressant medications
> - Antipsychotic medications
>
> **Vascular**
> - Coronary artery disease
> - Peripheral vascular disease
> - Hypertension
> - Diabetes mellitus
>
> **Psychogenic**
> - Depression
> - Performance anxiety
>
> **Neurogenic**
> - Spinal cord injury
> - Neuropathy (diabetic, hypertensive)
> - Cerebrovascular disease
> - Radical prostatectomy
> - Pelvic surgery
>
> **Multifactorial**
> - Aging
> - End-stage renal disease
> - Pelvic trauma (neurogenic and vasculogenic)
> - Diabetes mellitus (neurogenic, vasculogenic, drug induced)

> **BOX 2 Tools Used to Quantify Erectile Dysfunction Severity**
>
> Tools used in the quantification of the severity of erectile dysfunction (ED) include the International Index of Erectile Function (IIEF), the Sexual Encounter Profile (SEP), and the Global Assessment Question (GAQ).
>
> **International Index of Erectile Function**
> The IIEF is a standardized questionnaire designed to measure ED and detect treatment-related changes. It is a 15-item questionnaire addressing five different domains: erectile function, orgasmic function, sexual desire, intercourse satisfaction, and overall satisfaction. The IIEF is the most frequently used efficacy measurement employed in ED drug trials. Using a scale from 1 (never/almost never) to 5 (almost always/always), men grade each domain. It is very sensitive and specific, and has been validated in 20 languages to assess treatment-related changes in sexual function. The questions 1-5 and 15 are used to quantify erectile dysfunction severity and are as follows:
>
> 1. How often were you able to get an erection during sexual activity?
> 2. When you had erections with sexual stimulation, how often were your erections hard enough for penetration?
> 3. When you attempted sexual intercourse, how often were you able to penetrate (enter) your partner?
> 4. During sexual intercourse, how often were you able to maintain your erection after you had penetrated (entered) your partner?
> 5. During sexual intercourse, how difficult was it to maintain your erection to completion of intercourse?
> 15. How do you rate your confidence that you could get and keep an erection?
>
> And it is scored as follows:
> | | |
> |---|---|
> | 26-30 | Normal ED |
> | 22-25 | Mild ED |
> | 17-21 | Mild to moderate ED |
> | 11-16 | Moderate ED |
> | ≤10 | Severe ED |
>
> **Sexual Encounter Profile**
> SEP is a five-question survey provided to patients with ED in clinical studies of oral therapies. The survey is completed after each sexual attempt. The questions are as follows:
>
> 1. Were you able to achieve at least some erection?
> 2. Were you able to insert your penis into your partner's vagina?
> 3. Did your erection last long enough to have successful intercourse?
> 4. Were you satisfied with the hardness of your erection?
> 5. Were you satisfied with the overall sexual experience?
>
> Answers to questions 2 and 3 are the ones most often used in the literature.
>
> **Global Assessment Questions**
> GAQ is usually administered at the end of the treatment period during efficacy studies.
> Question 1: Has the treatment taken during the study improved your erections?
> Question 2: If yes, has the treatment improved your ability to engage in sexual activity?
> This is very subjective, and its responses tend to be valued less than SEP and IIEF.

Hyperlipidemia is another etiologic factor for ED. It is believed to contribute to ED by its relationship to endothelial dysfunction. One study showed that decreasing total cholesterol to less than 200 mg/dL by using atorvastatin (Lipitor) led to significant improvement of ED as measured by the International Index of Erectile Function (IIEF).

ED may be a sentinel manifestation of vascular disorders. In a study of 980 subjects seeking ED advice, 18% were suffering from undiagnosed hypertension, 16% had DM, 5% had ischemic heart disease, 15% had benign prostatic hyperplasia, 4% had prostate cancer, and 1% had depression. ED can itself be an independent marker for CAD. In addition, the extent of CAD correlates with the prevalence of ED.

Quantification of the Severity of Erectile Dysfunction and Improvement

There are several tools designed to assess the severity of ED, as well as to measure the efficacy of different treatments. We discuss three different measures, the IIEF, the Sexual Encounter Profile (SEP), and the Global Assessment Question (GAQ) (Box 2).

PATIENT HISTORY

When assessing sexual dysfunction, it is important to inquire about a number of issues:

1. Differentiate between decreased libido and ED: assess whether the patient has one or both
2. Tobacco use: type, amount, duration
3. Alcohol intake
4. History of depression or anxiety disorder
5. Presence of social/relationship stressors
6. Ability to have erections while masturbating versus when with partner
7. List of all prescription, over-the-counter, and herbal medications
8. Knowledge of whether nocturnal erections are present
9. History of drug use: marijuana, cocaine, other recreational drugs
10. History of genitourinary trauma
11. History of prostatic disease, or possible related symptoms
12. History of hypertension, hyperlipidemia, CAD, peripheral vascular disease, cerebrovascular disease
13. History of DM
14. History of spinal cord injury
15. History of penile plaques: possible Peyronie's disease
16. Frequency of intercourse or attempted intercourse
17. Ability to ejaculate

PHYSICAL EXAMINATION

The physical examination should include a careful testicular examination to assess testicular size, asymmetries, presence of hernias, or varicoceles. Additionally, a digital rectal examination to assess the prostatic size, consistency, and presence of nodules is warranted. Penile inspection and palpation should be performed, with special attention to possible fibrotic plaques. Palpation and auscultation of femoral arteries for possible bruits is another important part of the examination.

LABORATORY STUDIES

Laboratory workup on a patient with ED should include total and bioavailable testosterone levels drawn in the morning, prolactin, prostate-specific antigen, fasting glucose, and fasting lipid panel. Further studies may be warranted depending on the results of the aforementioned.

Management of Erectile Dysfunction

The landscape of ED was revolutionized with the introduction of sildenafil citrate (Viagra), the first oral medication for the treatment of this condition. Since then, oral agents have become the preferred mode of treatments by patients in surveys worldwide. There are three oral agents that inhibit PDE5 currently on the market:

1. Sildenafil citrate (Viagra)
2. Vardenafil (Levitra)
3. Tadalafil (Cialis)

All three drugs work by inhibiting PDE5, which maintains intracavernosal levels of cGMP, subsequently producing vasodilatation and penile erection (see Figure 1).

SILDENAFIL CITRATE (VIAGRA)

Sildenafil citrate (Viagra) is an orally active, potent, and selective inhibitor of cGMP-specific PDE5. The predominant phosphodiesterase isoform in the penile tissue is type 5. The selectivity of sildenafil citrate (Viagra) for PDE5 is approximately 4000-fold greater than its selectivity for phosphodiesterase 3 (PDE3), the isoform involved in the control of cardiac contractility. Sildenafil citrate (Viagra) is absorbed rapidly after oral administration, with an absolute bioavailability of 40%. The time of maximal (T-max) plasma after oral dosing in the fasting state is between 30 and 120 minutes. A high-fat meal increases the time to peak plasma concentration by 60 minutes and reduces the peak plasma concentration by 29%. The half-life of the drug is from 3 to 5 hours. Sildenafil citrate (Viagra) is metabolized by hepatic microsomal cytochrome P450 isoenzyme 3A4 for the most part. Cytochrome P450 3A4 inhibitors, cimetidine (Tagamet), erythromycin, ketoconazole (Nizoral), and protease inhibitors may retard the metabolism of sildenafil citrate (Viagra).

The recommended dose is from 25 to 100 mg as needed approximately 1 hour before sexual activity. In some individuals, the onset of activity may be seen as early as 11 to 19 minutes, but this is not the norm. The usual starting dose is 50 mg.

The maximum recommended dose is 100 mg, and the maximum dosing frequency is once daily. A starting dose of 25 mg can be considered for patients older than age 65 years as well as for patients with severe hepatic cirrhosis or severe renal impairment.

There are more than two dozen, randomized, double-blind, placebo-controlled studies involving this agent. It produces positive results regardless of the etiology of ED. It has been studied in patients with DM, CAD, postcoronary artery bypass graft (post-CABG), spinal cord injury, depression, hypertension, prostate cancer post-prostatectomy, benign prostate enlargement post-transurethral resection of the prostate (TURP), patients on hemodialysis, as well as recipients of renal transplants. Results vary according to the underlying condition causing ED in the first place, ranging from 50% to 85%.

The most common side effects of sildenafil citrate (Viagra) include vasodilatory effects such as headaches, flushing, and nasal congestion caused by hyperemia of the nasal mucosa, as well as dyspepsia. Up to 30% of patients may get at least one side effect. Another side effect that presents on occasion is blurred or blue-green vision because of inhibition of phosphodiesterase 6 (PDE6) in the retina. It is absolutely contraindicated in men taking long-acting or short-acting nitrate drugs, and men taking any form of nitrates should be informed about the dangerous interaction.

Do not prescribe sildenafil citrate (Viagra) to patients with unstable CAD who need nitrates. Assess the need for ordering treadmill testing in select patients. Initial monitoring of blood pressure (BP) after the administration of sildenafil citrate (Viagra) may be indicated in men with complicated congestive heart failure (CHF). α-Blockers should not be used in combination with sildenafil citrate (Viagra) because of possible orthostatic hypotension.

VARDENAFIL (LEVITRA)

Vardenafil (Levitra) is a highly potent inhibitor of PDE5. It was approved for use in the United States in late 2003. It is a more selective PDE5 inhibitor than sildenafil citrate (Viagra). The absorption of vardenafil (Levitra) is delayed by a fatty content of more than 30% in a meal. However, that does not seem to affect its effectiveness in different trials. The half-life of vardenafil (Levitra) is 4.4 to 4.8 hours, and the clinical effectiveness may be as long as 12 hours. The time for maximum plasma concentration is between 42 and 54 minutes. The first trial using the agent included 580 patients, excluding patients with spinal cord injury, radical prostatectomy, hypogonadism, thyrotoxicosis, or DM.

The successful rates of intercourse were 71% to 75% on patients taking 5 or 10 mg at a time. Those taking 20 mg had a success rate of 80%. The placebo groups had an average success rate of 30%.

Vardenafil (Levitra) has been tested in patients with type 2 DM; 452 patients were enrolled in a double-blind, placebo-controlled trial. The success rate in the vardenafil (Levitra) group ranged from 57% to 72%.

In a different study involving 736 subjects including men with DM and stable CAD, the success rates were 28% for the placebo group, 65% for those taking 5 mg, 80% for those taking 10 mg, and 85% for the 20-mg group.

Patients who were unresponsive to sildenafil citrate (Viagra) at a dose of 100 mg on several attempts were given vardenafil (Levitra) in doses of 10 and 20 mg (proved in trial). Vardenafil (Levitra) produced statistically and clinically significant results compared with placebo in men who were historically unresponsive to sildenafil citrate (Viagra). The dose that offers the best clinical results is 20 mg. It should not be taken more than once every 24 hours. Safety studies have shown no deleterious effects with long-term daily use of this drug for up to 12 months.

The most common side effects include headaches (10% to 21%), flushing (5% to 13%), rhinitis (9% to 17%), and dyspepsia (1% to 6%) because vardenafil (Levitra) does not inhibit PDE6. Unlike sildenafil citrate (Viagra), it does not produce problems of blurred vision or blue-green visual disturbances. The same warning regarding the use of nitrates as sildenafil citrate (Viagra) applies to vardenafil (Levitra). Patients taking vardenafil (Levitra) may use α-blocking agents with caution.

TADALAFIL (CIALIS)

The third oral agent of this class is tadalafil (Cialis). It has a half-life of 17.5 hours, with two thirds of patients experiencing clinical benefits of this drug up to 36 hours after its use. The clinical onset of action occurs in less than 1 hour. There is no interaction between food and alcohol on the absorption of the drug.

There have been numerous phase II and III studies in Europe, Canada, and the United States using doses of 2, 5, 10, and 25 mg of the drug in comparison with placebo. The average success rates on these studies averaged 17% for placebo, 51% for the 2-mg dose, and 80% for the other doses, as well as up to 88% on the 25-mg dose in one study. In one study looking at 216 subjects with type 2 DM, improved erections were reported in 56% to 64% of the patients.

A recent article looking at all the previously published patient data showed that among 2102 men studied in 11 randomized placebo-controlled trials lasting 12 weeks, each mean improvement in IIEF at 20 mg of tadalafil (Cialis) was 8.6. Mean positive Sexual Encounter Profile Diary Question 3 (SEP3) response was 68% versus 31% in placebo groups. Mean GAQ was 84% versus 33% in placebo group.

In a multicenter, randomized, double-blind, crossover study looking at 181 men who received either sildenafil citrate (Viagra) or tadalafil (Cialis), 73% (132) preferred tadalafil (Cialis) at 20 mg instead of sildenafil citrate (Viagra) at 50 or 100 mg.

The most clinically effective dose of tadalafil (Cialis) is 20 mg. It should be taken at least 30 minutes before intercourse. It may be used with caution in patients using α-blocking agents. Nitrates are absolutely contraindicated for use in patients taking tadalafil (Cialis). The most common side effects include headaches, dyspepsia, back pain, rhinitis, and flushing. There are no visual side effects reported.

APOMORPHINE (UPRIMA)[1]

Apomorphine (Uprima)[1] is a potent emetic that acts on central dopaminergic receptors. The stimulation of central dopaminergic receptors transmits excitatory signals down the spinal cord to the sacral parasympathetic nucleus, stimulating activity of the sacral nerves supplying the penis. It has been used successfully in up to 67% of patients when administered through a sublingual preparation. Subcutaneous injections[2] of apomorphine (Uprima)[1] produce almost a 100% erectile response, but nausea and vomiting are limiting factors to this mode of administration.

The most common side effects are headache, nausea, and dizziness. Rare syncopal episodes have been reported.

PHENTOLAMINE (REGITINE)

Phentolamine (Regitine) is an α_1- and α_2-adrenergic receptor antagonist.

The sympathetic system via the release of noradrenaline (NA) is the primary determinant of cavernosal smooth muscle contraction and detumescence. A relative predominance of NA-induced contraction over NO-induced smooth muscle relaxation may contribute to ED.

In large phase III studies, 55% to 59% of patients receiving 40 and 80 mg were able to achieve vaginal penetration. Adverse effects include nasal congestion (10%), headaches (3% to 5%), dizziness (3% to 5%), tachycardia (3%), and nausea.

TRAZODONE (DESYREL)[1]

Trazodone (Desyrel)[1] is a serotonin reuptake inhibiting agent. Its action in ED is believed to be the result of central serotonergic and peripheral α-adrenolytic activity. The efficacy of trazodone is poorly demonstrated; however, it may have a place in those with performance anxiety. Side effects include drowsiness, insomnia, headaches, and weight loss.

DIETARY SUPPLEMENTS AND ERECTILE DYSFUNCTION

Yohimbine[1] is an α_2-adrenoreceptor antagonist with short duration of action. It is administered orally, and it is believed to have a central effect at adrenergic receptors in brain centers associated with libido and penile erection. A meta-analysis of seven studies established that it is superior to placebo, although results can be very erratic. Side effects include palpitations, tremors, and anxiety. Yohimbine should *not* be recommended as part of the management of ED.

A study with 60 patients who had failed papaverine[1] injections (50 mg or less) were treated with an extract of *Ginkgo biloba*, 60 mg for 12 to 18 months. After 6 months, 50% of the patients reported improvement in erectile function. A placebo-controlled randomized trial using 240 mg of *Ginkgo biloba* extract daily for 24 weeks in patients with vasculogenic ED did not demonstrate significant differences between the groups.

L-Arginine[1] is an amino acid that is the precursor to NO. Three small studies are looking at this drug. There are encouraging results in one study.

Zinc is found in high concentrations in seminal fluid. Anecdotal reports of improvement in ED.

ALPROSTADIL (PROSTAGLANDIN E1, CAVERJECT, MEDICATED URETHRAL SYSTEM FOR ERECTION)

Prostaglandin E1 (PGE_1) exerts a number of pharmacologic effects including systemic vasodilatation, inhibitory actions on platelet aggregation, and relaxation of smooth muscle. PGE_1 binds to PGE receptors and causes a relaxation response mediated by cyclic adenosine monophosphate (cAMP). It can be administered intracavernosally or intraurethrally.

It has been used in combination with papaverine,[1] and the combination was superior to PGE_1 alone. The intracavernosal administration seems to be more effective than transurethral (medicated urethral system for erection [MUSE]). MUSE should be administered in 1-mg doses, applied intraurethrally. Responses to intracavernosal injections (Caverject) as high as 80% may be expected in patients with organic ED with a dose of 20 μg, and much lower to MUSE (35% to 43%). Injections are given with 27- to 30-gauge needles. The administration of PGE_1 is usually relegated as an alternative in patients who have contraindications to the use of phosphodiesterase 5 (PDE5) inhibitors. The possible side effects include penile fibrosis, priapism, urethral bleeding, hypotension, or syncopal episodes.

Papaverine[1] is a nonspecific phosphodiesterase inhibitor that increases cAMP and cGMP levels in penile erectile tissue. It produces smooth muscle relaxation and vasodilatation. It decreases the resistance to arterial inflow and increases the resistance to venous outflow. It is highly effective in psychogenic and neurogenic ED but not vasculogenic. It has been commonly used in combination with

---

[1]Not FDA approved for this indication.
[2]Not available in the United States.

[1]Not FDA approved for this indication.

CURRENT DIAGNOSIS

- The risk factors for ED include tobacco, alcohol, and drug use, as well as DM, hypertension, hyperlipidemia, and prostate disease.
- ED is widely prevalent, and incidence sharply increases with age.
- ED is a cardiovascular sentinel event, and its occurrence warrants a cardiac workup.
- The workup of ED should include checking testosterone levels, prolactin, glucose, and lipid levels.
- First-line therapies include the use of PDE5 inhibitors such as sildenafil citrate (Viagra), vardenafil (Levitra), and tadalafil (Cialis).

Abbreviations: DM = diabetes mellitus; ED = erectile dysfunction; PDE5 = phosphodiesterase 5.

CURRENT THERAPY

- PDE5 Inhibitors
  Sildenafil citrate (Viagra) 25-100 mg
  Vardenafil (Levitra) 10-20 mg
  Tadalafil (Cialis) 10-20 mg
- Alprostadil (PGE[1])Intracavernosal injections (Caverject) 20 µg
  Intraurethral application (MUSE) 1-mg pellet
- Papaverine injections[1] 30-60 mg
- Agents not yet approved for use by the FDA:
  Apomorphine (Uprima)[1] 3, 4, 6 mg
  Phentolamine (oral)[1] 40, 60, 80 mg

[1]Not FDA approved for this indication.
Abbreviations: MUSE = medicated urethral system for erection; PDE5 = phosphodiesterase 5; PGE[1] = prostaglandin E1.

phentolamine (Regitine). Major side effects include priapism, corporeal fibrosis, and possible elevation of liver transaminases.

Moxisylyte chlorohydrate[2] is an α-blocking agent. In a study where 156 subjects received either alprostadil or moxisylyte in a dose-escalating fashion, alprostadil had much better success rates (46% versus 81%).

Chlorpromazine (Thorazine)[1] is useful when given in combination with alprostadil or papaverine. It has α-blocking properties, and it is cheaper than phentolamine (Regitine).

Decreased concentration of vasoactive intestinal polypeptide (VIP)* has been reported in the penile tissue of men with ED. VIP is believed to play a role in the erectile process. It is ineffective when administered alone but can be quite effective in combination with phentolamine (Regitine). In a small study of 52 subjects with organic ED, 100% of them achieved an erection sufficient for intercourse. Further studies into the effectiveness of VIP may be needed.

PENILE PROSTHESES

This surgical approach used to be quite common before the advent of oral agents. The use of prostheses is still a suitable alternative for those who are unresponsive to less invasive treatments. Prostheses can be classified as rod, one-piece inflatable, two-piece inflatable, and three-piece inflatable. Postsurgical infections and malfunctions are the most common complications. Patients are usually satisfied with the results of prosthetic placement.

Vacuum Constrictive Device

Vacuum constrictive device is a plastic cylinder that is placed over the penis and connected to a pump that creates a partial vacuum. After achieving penile rigidity, a band is placed around the base of the penis to maintain the erection. This is a safe, noninvasive, and effective method of treating ED. It requires an understanding partner and the quality of the erection is not ideal; but patients are usually satisfied.

Testosterone

Patients who have low testosterone levels may benefit substantially from replacement. Men may expect significant improvements in libido, self-esteem, and overall energy levels. Additionally, testosterone is necessary for NO generation in the penile tissue.

The different testosterone preparations include injections such as testosterone enanthate (Delatestryl), cypionate (Depo-Testosterone) given as an intramuscular (IM) injection in doses of 100 to 200 mg, every 2 weeks on average. They also include transdermal testosterone patches (Androderm and Testoderm, 5 mg/d) or transdermal gel (AndroGel 5-g packets, one daily; or Testim 1% testosterone gel, one packet daily). Testosterone gel preparations provide physiologic replacement of testosterone and are preferred more than depot IM injections.

Future Trends

In the next few years we will see a sharp rise in the use of combination drugs, such as PDE5 inhibitors and apomorphine (Uprima),[1] PDE5 inhibitors and phentolamine (Regitine), and combinations of PDE5 inhibitors and intraurethral and intracavernosal agents. ED will be recognized universally as a cardiovascular sentinel event and also as a risk factor for vascular disease in general.

[1]Not FDA approved for this indication.

REFERENCES

Archer SL: Potassium channels and erectile dysfunction. Vascul Pharmacol 2002;38:61-71.
Burchardt M, Burchardt T, Baer L, et al: Hypertension is associated with severe erectile dysfunction. J Urol 2000;164(10):1188-1191.
Carson CC, Rajfer J, Eardley I, et al: The efficacy and safety of tadalafil: An update. BJU Int 2004;93:1276-1281.
Crowe SM, Streetman DS: Vardenafil treatment for erectile dysfunction. Ann Pharmacother 2004;38:77-85.
Feldman HA, Goldstein I, Hatzichristou DG, et al: Impotence and its medical and psychosocial correlates: Results of the Massachusetts Male Aging Study. J Urol 1994;151(1):54-61.
Jackson G, Betteridge J, Dean J, et al: A systematic approach to erectile dysfunction in the cardiovascular patient: A consensus statement—Update 2002. Int J Clin Pract 2002;56(9):663-671.
Jaynat D, Shepherd MD: Evaluation and treatment of erectile dysfunction in men with diabetes mellitus. Mayo Clin Proc 2002;77(3):276-282.
Johannes CB, Araujo AB, Feldman HA, et al: Incidence of erectile dysfunction in men ages 40 to 69 years old: Longitudinal results from the Massachusetts Male Aging Study. J Urol 2000;163(2):460-463.
Kirby M, Jackson G, Betteridge J, et al: Is erectile dysfunction a marker for cardiovascular disease? Int J Clin Pract 2002;55(9):614-618.
Lue TF: Drug therapy: Erectile dysfunction. N Engl J Med 2000;342(24):1802-1813.
Michelakis E, Tymchak W, Archer S: Sildenafil: From the bench to the bedside. CMAJ 2000;163(9):1171-1175.
NIH Consensus Development Panel on Impotence: Impotence (NIH Consensus Conference). JAMA 1993;270(1):83-90.
Padma-Nathan H: Intra-urethral and topical agents in the management of erectile dysfunction. In Carson CC III, Kirby RS, Goldstein I (eds): Textbook of Erectile Dysfunction. Oxford, Isis Medical Media, 1999, pp 323-326.

*Investigational drug in the United States.
[1]Not FDA approved for this indication.
[2]Not available in the United States.

Rhoden EL, Teloken C, Mafessoni R, et al: Is there any relation between serum levels of testosterone and the severity of erectile dysfunction? Int J Impot Res 2002;14:167-171.

Shokeir AA, Alserafi MA, Mutabagani H: Intracavernosal versus intraurethral alprostadil: A prospective randomized study. BJU Int 1999;83:812-815.

Spahn M, Manning M, Juenemann KP: Intracavernosal therapy. In Carson CC III, Kirby RS, Goldstein I (eds): Textbook of Erectile Dysfunction, Oxford Isis Medical Media, 1999, pp 345-353.

Sullivan ME, Thompson CS, Dashwood MR, et al: Nitric oxide and penile erection: Is erectile dysfunction another manifestation of vascular disease? Cardiovasc Res 1999;43:658-665.

Acute Renal Failure

Method of
Kevin Schroeder, MD

Epidemiology and Definitions

Acute renal failure (ARF), increasingly called acute kidney injury, is a clinical syndrome that can include decreased urine output, retention of nitrogenous metabolic waste products normally excreted by the kidney, retention of sodium and extracellular fluid resulting in peripheral and sometimes central edema, and various electrolyte and acid-base disturbances that may be associated with elevations in the blood urea nitrogen (BUN) and serum creatinine concentrations. Typically these changes occur rapidly over hours to days. Acute renal failure may further be described by the decrement in urine output: polyuric failure, indicating greater than 3 L urine output per 24 hours; nonoliguric failure, indicating 0.4 to 3L urine output per 24 hours; oliguric failure, indicating less than 400 mL urine output per 24 hours; and anuric failure, with less than 50 mL urine output per 24 hours.

Currently accepted definitions of ARF include a rise in the serum creatinine concentration by more than 0.5 mg/dL or a relative increase in the serum creatinine concentration by more than 25% for patients with preexisting chronic kidney disease (CKD) and a reduction in the glomerular filtration rate (GFR) by 50%. Note that these definitions are very operational and based on laboratory data readily available to practicing physicians, but consensus regarding a single, more sensitive measure of ARF is lacking.

Traditionally, ARF has been subclassified mechanistically into three categories. *Prerenal azotemia* refers to conditions that cause a fall in GFR because of reduced glomerular perfusion pressure. *Intrinsic renal failure* refers to conditions that directly damage any of the four main structural components of the kidney, including the afferent and efferent arterioles, glomeruli, tubules, and interstitium. *Postrenal failure* commonly refers to any condition that causes obstruction of either the upper or lower urinary tract. From a practical standpoint, clinicians must also consider the situation in which ARF occurs (in an ambulatory patient, at hospital admission, during hospitalization, or after discharge) and the rapidity of deterioration, because some diagnoses are more likely depending on the clinical context.

The reported incidence of ARF varies by clinical situation and patient population, occurring in about 2% of all inpatient admissions. Varying definitions of disease and methodologic characteristics of epidemiologic studies also affect the reported incidence. General surgical patients undergoing nonemergent, noncardiac surgery had ARF at a reported incidence of 0.8%, and critically ill surgical patients undergoing noncardiac surgery experienced ARF at a rate nearly 80 times higher. Several scoring systems have been developed to predict the risk of ARF in patients undergoing cardiac surgery, which can vary from 5% to 25%. General medicine patients can experience ARF during a hospitalization at a rate of up to 7%, but the incidence may be in the 30% to 50% range for patients in critical care units. It may be possible that the true incidence of ARF in the United States will increase substantially as the baby boom generation enters its seventh decade.

Despite advances in medical technology, pharmacotherapeutics, and dialysis modalities in the critical care setting, mortality associated with ARF remains largely untouched at 20% to 80%. Recent studies have detected an increased mortality with even a slight rise in serum creatinine (increase <0.5 mg/dL). ARF adds to length of stay by about 4 days and can easily increase the cost of admission by more than $10,000.

Classification

Causes of ARF (Box 1) are elucidated chiefly from the history and physical examination. In particular, the history should focus first on symptoms causing volume depletion, second on symptoms relating to obstruction, and third on systemic symptoms including unexplained malaise, weight loss, fever, sinopulmonary bleeding, joint pain or swelling, rashes, myalgias, and neuropathies. All these factors must be considered in light of the patient's comorbid conditions, especially cardiovascular disease, hypertension, diabetes, liver disease, and peripheral vascular disease. Medications including antihypertensives, diuretics, analgesics, and over-the-counter supplements should be reviewed carefully. The physical examination serves to confirm the patient's volume status (e.g., frank hypotension or orthostatic change in blood pressure with tachycardia), to identify signs of cardiovascular disease and cardiopulmonary decompensation, to assess the status of the urinary bladder, and to detect signs of systemic disease. In addition to routine serum chemistries, BUN, and serum creatinine levels, all patients with nonanuric ARF must have a urinalysis. The clinician must observe the urine sediment for the presence of protein, blood, dysmorphic red cells, and cellular and noncellular casts. Finally, for oliguric patients, calculation of the fractional excretion of sodium (FE_{Na}) might prove useful. Serologic testing regarding acute glomerulonephritis should be obtained when the history and physical examination suggest sufficient pretest probability.

PRERENAL AZOTEMIA

Prerenal azotemia is the most common cause of ARF among patients admitted to general medicine services. It is commonly observed in cases of volume depletion or decreased effective arterial blood volume. These include profuse emesis or diarrhea, hemorrhage, and overzealous diuresis, especially in the face of poor oral intake. In these cases, peripheral and central edema is often absent. Decompensated CHF, decompensated cirrhosis leading to the hepatorenal syndrome, and the nephrotic syndrome all lead to effective decreases in circulating arterial volume. Commonly, patients with these conditions have peripheral edema and sometimes central edema with low albumin states. In the former case, diuretics often improve not only the heart failure but also the renal dysfunction concomitantly. Recalling the principles of vascular autoregulation (Fig. 1), the clinician must realize that the kidneys of elderly patients and patients with chronic hypertension are especially susceptible to intravascular volume changes. This is particularly true when patients are medicated with angiotensin converting enzyme inhibitors and angiotensin receptor blockers, nonsteroidal antiinflammatory drugs and cyclooxygenase-2 inhibitors, and calcineurin inhibitors, all of which effectively paralyze the kidney's ability to regulate glomerular perfusion.

Typical laboratory findings in prerenal azotemia include an elevated BUN:creatinine ratio (>20:1) and a FE_{Na} of less than 1%. However, if the patient had been taking diuretics, the FE_{Na} may be falsely elevated. Metabolic alkalosis and hypokalemia might or might not be present. The urinalysis is expected to show a high specific gravity with no blood, no protein, and bland sediment except maybe a few hyaline casts. Clinically, pure prerenal azotemia often responds quickly to restoration of euvolemia with increased urine output and a falling

> **BOX 1 Causes of Acute Renal Failure**
>
> **Prerenal Azotemia**
> *Effective Arterial Blood Volume and Hypotension*
> Emesis or diarrhea
> Hemorrhage
> Nephrotic syndrome
> Sepsis
> Third spacing
> - Acute abdomen
> - Bowel infarct
> - Burns
> - Cirrhosis or hepatorenal syndrome
> - *Clostridium difficile* colitis
> - Pancreatitis
> - Peritonitis
> - Postoperative abdomen
>
> *Pump Failure*
> - Acute myocardial infarction
> - Congestive heart failure
> - Tamponade
>
> *Overmedication*
> - Anesthetics
> - Diuretics
> - Nonsteroidal antiinflammatory drugs (including cyclooxygenase-2 inhibitors)
>
> **Intrinsic Acute Renal Failure**
> *Acute Tubular Necrosis*
> Toxins
> - Aminoglycosides
> - Cyclosporine (Neoral)
> - Ethylene glycol
> - Heavy metals
> - Hemoglobinuria
> - Iodinated dye
> - Myoglobinuria
> - Nonsteroidal antiinflammatory drugs (including cyclooxygenase-2 inhibitors)
> - Pentamidine (Pentam)
> - Tumor lysis syndrome
> Ischemia
> - Cardiovascular surgery
> - Dissection
> - Embolism
>
> - Severe hypotension
> - Trauma
> Septic
> - Gram-positive or gram-negative sepsis
>
> *Interstitial Nephritis*
> Allopurinol (Zyloprim)
> Antibiotics
> - Cephalosporins
> - Penicillins
> - Rifampin (Rifadin)
> - Sulfonamides
> Diuretics
> Nonsteroidal antiinflammatory drugs
> Phenytoin (Dilantin)
>
> *Macrovascular Disease*
> Atheroembolic disease
> Malignant hypertension
>
> *Microvascular Disease*
> HELLP syndrome
> Hemolytic-uremic syndrome and thrombotic thrombocytopenic purpura
> Hepatorenal syndrome
> Rapidly progressive glomerulonephritis
> Vasculitis
>
> **Postrenal Obstruction**
> *Intratubular Obstruction*
> Crystals
> Myeloma casts
>
> *Ureteral Obstruction*
> Ligation
> Retroperitoneal fibrosis
> Stones/papillae
> Tumor compression
>
> *Bladder Outlet Obstruction*
> Anticholinergic medicines
> Benign prostatic hyperplasia
> Diabetic autonomic dysfunction
> Stones and papillae
> Urethral valves
>
> ---
> HELLP = hemolysis, elevated liver enzymes, low platelets.

creatinine within 24 hours. Therapy for prerenal azotemia should be aimed at restoring clinical euvolemia and eliminating the cause of the azotemia. Infusion of isotonic saline is the norm, with supplemental oral rehydration where possible, and use of colloids or blood products when needed. In the case of decompensated left heart failure with pulmonary embarrassment, it is often necessary to employ an inotrope (e.g., dobutamine [Dobutrex]) in combination with a diuretic, whereas with hepatorenal syndrome, combinations of midodrine (Proamatine)[1] and octreotide (Sandostatin)[1] have been employed with some success.

Intrinsic renal failure may be subdivided into diseases that affect the renal microvasculature, glomeruli, tubules, and interstitium. Although the pharmacologic effects of certain medications (e.g. angiotensin-converting enzyme inhibitors [ACEIs] and nonsteroidal antiinflammatory drugs [NSAIDS]) directly affect the renal microvasculature, renal dysfunction associated with their use physiologically produces a prerenal picture. However, cholesterol emboli syndrome and small vessel vasculitis represent two diseases whose impact on the renal microvasculature is pathologic. In the former case, cholesterol-laden debris dislodged from the abdominal aorta or aortic arch showers distal vascular beds. The classic scenario involves a patient who, having recently undergone an endovascular procedure, presents with abdominal colic, ARF, livedo reticularis, and evidence of ischemic toes. Depending on the size of the embolus, the patient can have frank intestinal or renal infarction or an acutely ischemic lower extremity, necessitating emergent intervention. Eosinophiluria and hypocomplementemia may be noted. The elevation in creatinine can progress in a stepwise fashion for several days to weeks after the original event. Magnetic resonance imaging (MRI) can show evidence of wedge-shaped infarcts in the renal parenchyma. Optimal therapy with regard to antiplatelet agents versus anticoagulants remains uncertain.

---
[1]Not FDA approved for this indication

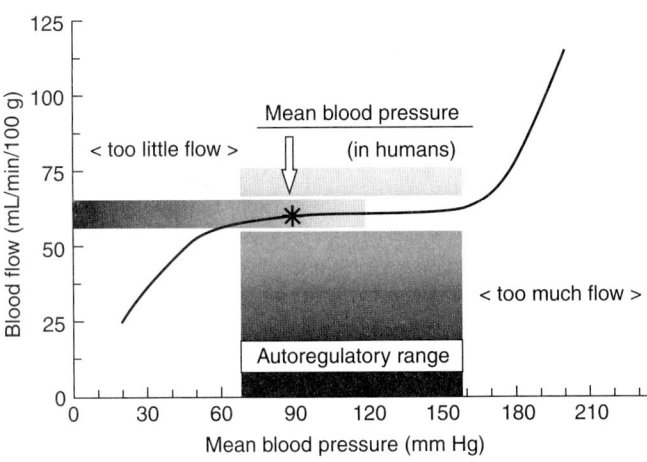

FIGURE 1. Principle of vascular autoregulation.

GLOMERULAR DISEASE

Glomerular disease accounts for roughly 10% of ARF among hospitalized patients. The hallmarks of rapidly progressive acute glomerulonephritis (RPGN) include an active urine sediment (dysmorphic red blood cells (RBCs) and cellular casts), hypertension, some edema, and a rapid decline in renal function over days. World Health Organization (WHO) class IV systemic lupus erythematosus (SLE) nephritis, anti-neutrophil cytoplasmic antibodies (ANCA)-mediated disease, and anti-GBM (glomerular basement membrane) disease are examples. Serologic testing is often useful, but a renal biopsy is almost always indicated for definitive diagnosis. Treatment usually involves some combination of corticosteroids and cytotoxic medications. Because of the severe increase in morbidity and mortality when these diseases are untreated, RPGN should be considered a medical emergency, with prompt attempts to diagnose and treat. It is important to recognize that whereas diseases that primarily manifest as the nephritic syndrome commonly cause ARF, entities associated more with a nephrotic-syndrome picture—including membranous disease, minimal change disease, or focal sclerosis—can certainly produce ARF as well. This usually occurs in the setting of massive nephrotic-range proteinuria (10-20 g/24 hours) and associated marked hypoalbuminemia.

ACUTE TUBULAR NECROSIS

Acute tublar necrosis (ATN) accounts for fully 50% of ARF among hospitalized patients; depending on the scenario, this figure can rise to as much as 75%. ATN has three common causes: ischemic, toxic, and septic. ATN has been described by its phases: Injury, during which time the insult causes direct damage to the tubules, is manifested as a progressive increase in the serum creatinine and possibly the development of oliguria. In the plateau phase, the creatinine, urinary output, and volume status are relatively stable. Recovery is marked by a spontaneous decline in serum creatinine and increase in urinary output, perhaps even into a polyuric range. The time course of ATN from injury to recovery is variable. Depending on the severity of the injury and the preexistence of renal disease, ATN can reverse within 1 to 3 weeks, although a small percentage of patients with ATN remain dialysis dependent after months. ATN is typically associated with a loss of urinary concentration, elevated urinary sodium excretion, and an elevated FE_{Na} of greater than 2%. The BUN and creatinine tend to rise proportionally. The urinary sediment can reveal tubular epithelial cell casts that have a coarsely granular or muddy brown appearance.

Ischemic ATN typically occurs during periods of prolonged hypotension and represents an evolution of prerenal azotemia. Ischemic ATN is commonly observed to varying degrees after cardiovascular and major orthopedic or trauma surgery. Careful attention must be paid to urine output and volume status. High-dose diuretics may be employed to avoid pulmonary edema, and if a suboptimal response is seen, the dosage should be doubled after the first dose. Patients who rapidly become oliguric have a high mortality rate, which is unaffected by diuretics and can therefore require early initiation of dialysis. Specific risk factors for developing ischemic ATN in the postoperative setting include advanced age (older than 70 years), preexisting CKD, diabetes, emergent surgery, preexisting vascular disease, and the need for valvular, particularly aortic valve, heart surgery in addition to bypass grafting. The degree and duration of intraoperative hypotension as well as time spent on cardiopulmonary bypass can also play roles.

Toxic ATN is proximal tubular cell death as a consequence of drugs or other endogenous chemicals. Drugs that classically cause toxic ATN include aminoglycosides, amphotericin B (Fungizone), radiocontrast, platinum-based chemotherapy, and NSAIDs. Endogenous chemicals known to cause toxic ATN include uric acid, myoglobin, and heme. Clinically, it is worthwhile noting that although the onset of ATN after a single dose of NSAID or iodinated radiocontrast material may be rapid (24-72 hours) especially in volume-depleted patients, in the case of aminoglycosides the onset of injury may be a bit slower, consistent with cumulative dose exposure. In general, ATN is best avoided by limiting the dose of potentially toxic medications (e.g., once-daily dosing of aminoglycosides), maintenance of adequate volume status, and close attention to the serum creatinine and urinary output.

In the case of radiocontrast agents, low osmolar and isosmolar agents are thought to be less toxic, and dose limitation (or elimination) to less than 100 mL are helpful strategies. Although prospective randomized, controlled trial data are inconclusive, and meta-analyses are equivocal, in cases of elective contrast exposure it remains common practice at many centers to administer N-acetylcysteine (Mucomyst)[1] in a dosage of 600 mg orally every 12 hours on the day before and the day of exposure. This, along with intravenous fluid administration for up to 6 hours before elective procedures (some authors use bicarbonate-containing solutions) seem to be reasonably safe, low-cost measures that can offer some protection against ATN in patients with known renal disease. After contrast-enhanced procedures, serum creatinine should be measured daily in hospitalized patients and at 48 hours after the procedure in outpatients.

Septic ATN often manifests in the critical care setting in patients with multisystem organ failure. Patients are typically hypotensive with either gram-positive or gram-negative bacteremia and anuria, often with severe acidemia. Unlike patients with prerenal azotemia whose urine output responds to volume resuscitation, patients with septic ATN do not produce urine in response to substantial volume resuscitation (Table 1). The clinical picture is difficult to distinguish from ischemic ATN because the two disease processes can coexist. Clinically, ischemic and toxic ATN are thought to show signs of resolution within 14 days of removal of the insult, whereas the sequelae of septic ATN can persist for one or several months after the infection requiring prolonged hospitalization and dialysis support. Mortality in this setting can be as high as 80%, and patients who survive their initial illness are particularly susceptible to nosocomial infections, catheter-related bacteremia, and malnutrition.

INTERSTITIAL DISEASE

Interstitial disease represents the third most common cause of ARF among hospitalized patients after prerenal azotemia and ATN. Acute interstitial nephritis is usually the effect of either drugs or pyelonephritis. In the case of medications, key diagnostic points include a delayed onset after medication exposure, as much as 7 days, and the co-incidence of fever and a central rash in about 30% of patients. The diagnosis may be suspected in the presence of sterile pyuria, eosinophiluria, and eosinophilia. Because the disease is of nonglomerular and nontubular origin, the urine sediment should be relatively bland, with minimal hematuria or proteinuria. Renal biopsy confirming the presence of increased numbers of eosinophils in the interstitium

---

[1] Not FDA approved for this indication

TABLE 1 Laboratory Differentiation of Prerenal Azotemia from Acute Tubular Necrosis

	Result	
Test	Prerenal Azotemia	Acute Tubular Necrosis
U_{Na}	<10-20	>40
FE_{Na}	<1	>1
Urine SG	>1.020	<1.010
BUN:Cr	>20:1	≈10:1
Fe_{Ur}	>60:1	<20:1
$U_{Cr}:P_{Cr}$	>40:1	<10:1

BUN = blood urea nitrogen; Cr = creatinine; FE_{Ur} = fractional excretion of urea; FE_{Na} = fractional excretion of sodium; SG = specific gravity; $U_{Cr}:P_{Cr}$ = ratio of urine creatinine to serum creatinine; U_{Na} = urine sodium.

remains the gold standard. Antibiotics that are particularly notorious for causing acute interstitial nephritis include penicillins, particularly methicillin (Staphcillin); sulfa-containing drugs; rifampin (Rifadin); and quinolones. Typically, cessation of the suspected agent results in improved renal function within 5 days; however, in severe, prolonged cases, a course of corticosteroids can hasten improvement. Importantly, if the patient is re-exposed to the offending agent, acute interstitial nephritis can develop much more rapidly.

OBSTRUCTIVE DISEASE

Obstructive renal disease, although relatively uncommon, should be highly suspected in any patient with otherwise unexplained anuria, especially in those with a known pelvic malignancy or recent pelvic surgery. Obstruction of the lower tract and bladder outlet is more prevalent among elderly men with prostatic hypertrophy and diabetics with autonomic nervous dysfunction. Upper-tract obstruction can be seen in cases of retroperitoneal fibrosis, uroepithelial malignancy, and nephrolithiasis. Certain systemic processes including tumor lysis syndrome, myeloma cast nephropathy, and ethylene glycol overdose can all cause an intratubular obstruction due to massive crystal and cast deposition within the kidney.

Clinically, obstruction of the bladder outlet may be diagnosed and treated via placement of a Foley catheter. Bladder scans, ultrasounds, and measurement of the pre- and postvoid residual bladder volumes are also important but not always immediately necessary. Bilateral upper tract obstruction requires intervention in the form of bilateral percutaneous nephrostomy tubes or internal double-J stent placement via cystourethroscopy. Patients with severe obstruction may be significantly hyperkalemic at presentation, requiring prompt treatment. Fortunately, if the obstruction is relieved in a timely fashion, the hyperkalemia usually dissipates without emergent dialysis.

CURRENT DIAGNOSIS

- Prerenal azotemia may be associated with a BUN-to-creatinine ratio >20:1 and a FE_{Na} <1%.
- Intrarenal ARF (ATN) may be associated with a BUN-to-creatinine ratio <20:1 and a FE_{Na} >1%.
- Postrenal ARF can manifest with frank anuria.
- Follow the trends of serum chemistries, BUN, creatinine, and urine output on a daily basis.

ARF = acute renal failure; ATN = acute tubular necrosis; BUN = blood urea nitrogen; FE_{Na} = fractional excretion of sodium.

Treatment

Management of hospitalized patients is generally supportive. Specific measures include a thorough daily review of the medication list to ensure that all possible toxic medications have been eliminated and that all drugs excreted via the kidneys have been dose adjusted for the level of renal dysfunction. The patient's volume status should be assessed frequently, with appropriate adjustments in intravenous fluids or diuretics. Similarly, electrolytes, BUN, and creatinine should be checked daily. In general, hospitalized patients should remain hospitalized until the clinical course has at least stabilized and close outpatient follow-up is ensured. Outpatients with acute renal failure can require urgent hospitalization if the cause is not immediately apparent and reversible, or if significant hyperkalemia or volume overload exists, or if the patient has significant comorbidities.

The decision to initiate renal replacement therapy is made by the nephrologist on a patient-by-patient basis. Some absolute clinical indications for dialysis exist, such as severe hyperkalemia; peaked T waves or prolongation of the QRS complex by electrocardiogram; volume overload or acidosis refractory to medical therapy; certain intoxications or electrolyte abnormalities; and symptomatic uremia with pericarditis, neurologic changes, or bleeding diatheses. Depending on the clinical setting, the two most common are hyperkalemia and volume overload; rarely will the nephrologist let ARF with either of these conditions progress to the point of cardiac arrhythmia or intubation undialyzed.

Patients who require urgent or emergent dialysis can typically be dialyzed via standard intermittent hemodialysis. This method is more effective for acute correction of electrolyte, toxin, and acid–base aberrations as well as pulmonary edema. Controversy exists as to the proper dose of dialysis for patients with ARF, particularly those in the critical care setting. Clinical practice varies by center, but studies have shown a survival benefit favoring daily hemodialysis to keep the BUN less than 100 mg/dL.

Continuous renal replacement therapy (CRRT) or continuous veno-venous hemofiltration is usually reserved for critically ill patients, particularly those with hypotension requiring vasopressor support or those with sufficiently poor cardiac performance and volume overload who cannot tolerate acute intravascular volume shifts associated with conventional hemodialysis.

Acute peritoneal dialysis, although certainly a viable modality, is practiced much less commonly in the United States partly due to the widespread availability of hemodialysis.

Emerging Issues

In clinical practice, the diagnosis and treatment of ARF rest on the ability to recognize it in a timely fashion. The two universally available indicators—urinary output and serum creatinine measurement—are limited in their sensitivity and specificity; however, new urinary and plasma biomarkers are emerging that can allow earlier identification of ARF. Urinary neutrophil gelatinase–associated lipocalin (NGAL), kidney injury molecule-1 (KIM-1), and interleukin-18 (IL-18), in combination with plasma

CURRENT THERAPY

- Hemodynamic support and maintenance of euvolemic state
- Correction of electrolyte and acid–base imbalances
- Removal of all offending agents and correction of underlying causes
- Adjustment of all medications for decreased glomerular filtration rate
- Renal replacement when needed on an individual basis

NGAL and cystatin C measurements, are all currently being evaluated in ARF clinical trials. These assays hold the promise of earlier detection and perhaps more specific anatomic localization of the injury within the kidney. Whether these biomarkers are used alone, serially, or in combination as an acute kidney injury panel remains to be seen as they transition from primarily clinical trial–based application to widespread clinical use. Questions regarding their ability to help predict which patients with ARF will spontaneously recover renal function and which will require dialysis remain to be answered.

Nephrotoxicity associated with gadolinium-containing contrast media has risen to the front of discussion among radiologists and nephrologists. Originally thought to be non-nephrotoxic, gadolinium has been implicated in a number of well-documented cases. Perhaps more striking are the mounting reports of gadolinium-related nephrogenic systemic fibrosis, which is characterized by brawny epidermal fibrotic plaques developing over several weeks after exposure. It is important to recognize that other organs including the subcutaneous tissues, skeletal musculature, lungs, and heart may be involved. Although the pathogenesis of this disease has not been fully elucidated, epidemiologically, 90% of cases have been described among end-stage renal disease patients requiring dialysis, and fully 10% have occurred among patients with CKD stages 3 and 4. Because there is no cure for this disease and its clinical consequences are potentially devastating, clinicians now must consider the risk-to-benefit ratio of exposing a patient to gadolinium-enhanced MRI procedures and weigh that risk against the well-established risk of iodinated contrast used in CT scans.

REFERENCES

Coca SG, Peixoto AJ, Garg AX, et al: The prognostic importance of a small acute decrement in kidney function in hospitalized patients: A systematic review and meta-analysis. Am J Kidney Dis 2007;50(5):712-720.

Dennen P, Parikh CR: Biomarkers of acute kidney injury: Can we replace serum creatinine? Clin Nephrol 2007;68(5):269-278.

Devarajan P: Proteomics for biomarker discovery in acute kidney injury. Semin Nephrol 2007;27(6):637-651.

Eachempati SR, Wang JC, Hydo LJ, et al: Acute renal failure in critically ill surgical patients: Persistent lethality despite new modes of renal replacement therapy. J Trauma 2007;63(5):987-993.

Greenberg A, Cheung A, Coffman T, et al (eds): Primer on Kidney Diseases, 2nd ed. San Diego: Academic Press, 1998.

Johnson J, Feehally J: Comprehensive Clinical Nephrology, 1st ed. St Louis: Mosby, 2000.

Kheterpal S, Tremper KK, Englesbe MJ, et al: Predictors of postoperative acute renal failure after noncardiac surgery in patients with previously normal renal function. Anesthesiology 2007;107(6):892-902.

Nagle PC, Warner MA: Acute renal failure in a general surgical population: Risk profiles, mortality, and opportunities for improvement. Anesthesiology 2007;107(6):869-870.

Rakel R, Bope E (eds): Conn's Current Therapy 2007. Philadelphia: Elsevier, 2007.

Chronic Renal Failure

Method of
Jeffrey A. Kraut, MD

Chronic renal failure is defined as a reduction in glomerular filtration rate (GFR) below the normal values of approximately 120 to 130 mL/minute developing over months to years. Its incidence has increased significantly over the last several years, but this probably reflects more accurate estimations of GFR. However, there is an increased prevalence of type II diabetes mellitus, a frequent cause of renal disease, in Western societies that could contribute to a higher incidence of chronic renal failure. When renal failure is severe (GFR <10 mL/minute), renal replacement therapy, either dialysis or renal transplantation, is required to preserve life. However, even before several renal failure ensues, the presence of chronic renal failure has an important impact on organ function and can contribute to the development of significant electrolyte derangements, important hormonal abnormalities, and anemia. Also, its presence can alter the metabolism and therefore the blood concentrations and tissue concentrations of drugs administered for the treatment of various diseases. Moreover, a reduced GFR is associated with an increased risk of death, increased incidence of cardiovascular events, and hospitalizations independent of known risk factors or a history of cardiovascular diseases. Finally, the mortality of several surgical procedures is substantially increased by the presence of chronic renal failure. Therefore, detecting and treating patients with chronic renal failure is extremely important.

Causes of Chronic Renal Failure

Many disorders can cause chronic renal failure. However, epidemiologic studies indicate that diabetes mellitus and hypertension account for the majority of cases (>60%). Chronic glomerulonephritis, polycystic kidney disease, obstructive uropathy, and ischemic nephropathy caused by atherosclerotic renal artery stenosis are less common, but important causes of renal impairment. The latter disorder is postulated to be more frequent than previously believed and is an important undiagnosed cause of chronic renal impairment.

Recent studies have indicated that a reduction in GFR occurs with aging in the absence of factors known to produce renal injury such as hypertension or diabetes. Indeed, the average GFR of subjects in the 8th decade of life in one large study was 40 to 50 mL/minute. Pathologic examination of these individuals, when available, may reveal only benign nephrosclerosis.

Importantly, because a majority of individuals older than 60 years of age have lower muscle mass, the reduced GFR is not accompanied by a rise in serum creatinine concentration. Therefore, renal failure is not detected unless the physician considers other variables such as the patient's age and muscle mass in assessing GFR (see the following section).

Approach to the Diagnosis of Chronic Renal Failure

The first step in the diagnosis of chronic renal failure is, of course, to detect a reduction in GFR. In the past, estimations of GFR were based on the measurement of serum creatinine concentration alone. In adults, the normal serum creatinine ranges between 0.6 and 1.3 mg/dL. Individuals with values greater than this are said to have renal failure. However, there is a wide range of normal values. Also, creatinine production, which is dependent on muscle mass, is a critical variable affecting serum creatinine concentration. Thus, a large group of individuals with reduced muscle mass can have serum creatinine values within the normal range, but a decreased GFR. The most common situation in which this paradox is encountered is in the elderly and in individuals with malignancy or chronic liver disease.

Precise measurement of GFR is accomplished by calculating the clearance of creatinine in a timed urine collection, generally 24 hours in duration:

$$\text{Creatinine clearance (mL/minute)} = U_{cr} \text{ (mg/dL)} \times \text{volume (mL)}/S_{cr} \text{ (mg/dL)}/1440.$$

where U_{cr} = urine creatinine concentration,

S_{cr} = plasma creatinine concentration

However, timed urine collections are often inaccurate because of errors in collection. Moreover, as renal function progresses and serum creatinine rises, or in the presence of nephrotic range proteinuria, GFR tends to be overestimated by creatinine clearance. Most recently, formulas derived from studies of large groups of patients—such as those by Cockroft and Gault and the Modification of Diet in Renal Disease (MDRD) in which GFR was correlated with other factors (e.g., body weight, age, and serum albumin)—are sufficiently accurate to use for clinical purposes:

$$\text{Cockroft} - \text{Gault: CrCl (mL/minute)} = \{(140 - \text{age}) \times \text{wt} \times [1 - (0.15 \times \text{gender})]\}/(0.814 \times \text{Scr})$$

$$\text{MDRD: GFR} = 170 \times [\text{PCr}]^{-0.999} \times [\text{Age}]^{-0.176} \times [0.762 \text{ female}] \times [1.180 \text{ if patient is black}] \times [\text{SUN}]^{-0.170} \times [\text{Alb}]^{+0.318}$$

Once renal function is depressed, the physician determines whether this represents acute or chronic renal failure. When previous measurements of GFR are available, it is relatively easy to determine if the renal failure is chronic in nature. However, if these studies are not available, demonstration that the kidneys are small in size (less than 8 to 9 cm when they are normally approximately 10 to 12 cm) by renal ultrasound will confirm the chronicity of the disease. Evidence of increased echogenicity reflecting augmented fibrous deposits is also suggestive of chronic disease. However, several disorders associated with chronic renal failure have normal kidney size such as diabetes mellitus, polycystic kidney disease, and amyloidosis. Therefore, normal kidney size does not exclude chronic renal failure. If individuals have normal kidney size, the presence of anemia and/or certain abnormalities of divalent ion metabolism can also suggest the disease is chronic in nature.

Once impaired renal function is recognized, measurements of blood urea nitrogen (BUN), sodium, potassium, chloride, bicarbonate, hemoglobin and hematocrit, and calcium and phosphorus are obtained. A urinalysis is obtained looking for increased excretion of protein, presence of blood in the urine, and abnormal cellular elements. In patients with diabetes, studies to find microalbuminuria (albumin urine concentrations less than 300 mg per day) are important to detect the early stages of renal disease. A 24-hour or spot urine protein and creatinine determination to assess the urine's protein-to-creatinine ratio is obtained to quantitate the amount of protein being excreted. Urine protein excretion in excess of 3.5 g daily indicates the presence of glomerular pathology, whereas interstitial disease is characterized by values below 2 g. However, urine protein excretion can vary with glomerular disease so values below 3.5 g are still consistent with this diagnosis. Assessment of urine protein excretion is important for diagnostic purposes, but also because urine protein excretion is often followed to assess effectiveness of therapy.

Obstruction uropathy, an important cause of chronic renal failure and exacerbation of renal failure, can be excluded in the majority of cases by ultrasound of the kidneys. Doppler ultrasound of the renal arteries performed at the same time is helpful in excluding obstruction of the renal arteries. The necessity of obtaining other diagnostic studies such as measurement of serum complement, blood and urine eosinophils, serum and urine and protein electro-phoresis, antiglomerular basement membrane antibodies, anti–double-stranded DNA (dsDNA) antibodies, hepatitis B and C antibodies, sedimentation rate, and HIV studies depends on the context of the renal failure.

Finally, a renal biopsy may be required in certain situations to make a definitive diagnosis. Because treatment of specific diseases can vary, making a precise pathologic diagnosis can be extremely important for proper management. Unfortunately, once the renal failure is moderate to severe in nature, renal pathologic examination may not always be helpful in determining the cause.

Clinical and Laboratory Abnormalities in Chronic Renal Failure

Because the kidney plays a critical role in the regulation of the serum concentrations of sodium, potassium, bicarbonate, chloride, calcium, and phosphorus as well as the levels of hemoglobin and hematocrit, blood pressure and extracellular volume, chronic renal injury can lead to derangements in these parameters as summarized in Table 1.

HYPONATREMIA AND HYPERNATREMIA

The kidney plays an essential role in excreting water by producing a dilute urine (less than 1/6 plasma osmolality) or retaining water by producing a concentrated urine (three to four times plasma osmolality). The ability to concentrate or dilute the urine in the majority of cases is usually retained until GFR falls to less than 30% of normal, and therefore hyponatremia or hypernatremia are uncommon until that time. If the disease is primarily interstitial in nature, alterations in urine concentrating ability can appear prior to significant reductions in GFR. However, even with higher levels of GFR the patient can be at risk for either of these electrolyte abnormalities should they ingest large quantities of fluid or be deprived of appropriate fluid intake.

HYPERKALEMIA

The kidney plays the most critical role in the regulation of potassium balance. Adaptive changes in renal tubular function and possible colonic function enable the kidney to maintain serum potassium within the normal range until GFR falls below 20% to 25% of normal (serum creatinine of 4 mg/dL or greater). Recent studies indicate a tendency for elevations in serum potassium to appear at even modest reductions in GFR (<60 mL/min).

 CURRENT DIAGNOSIS

The following lists the optimal care of patients with chronic kidney disease:
- Test for albuminuria and estimate glomerular filtration rate using MDRD formula yearly for early diagnosis and stratification of CKD.
- If possible, determine cause of kidney disease.
- Initiate treatment to delay or prevent progression of disease including use of converting enzyme inhibitors and/or angiotensin receptor blockers to reduce BP to less than 130/80 mm Hg and urine protein excretion to as low as possible but at least less than 1 g/24 hours.
- Control or prevent biochemical or clinical abnormalities including those of serum potassium, serum bicarbonate, serum phosphorus, parathyroid hormone, and hemoglobin.
- Evaluate patients for presence of and treat important co-morbid conditions, particularly heart disease.
- If the GFR is less than 30 mL/min, consider referral to a nephrologist.

Abbreviations: BP = blood pressure; CKD = care of patients with chronic kidney disease; GFR = glomerular filtration rate; MDRD = modification of diet in renal disease.

TABLE 1 Clinical and Electrolyte Abnormalities Noted With Chronic Renal Failure

Clinical or Laboratory Disorder	GFR or Stage of Renal Failure*
Hypertension	GFR <60 mL/min (stage 3)
Hyponatremia or hypernatremia	GFR <30 mL/min (stage 4)
Hyperkalemia*	GFR <30 mL/min (stage 4)
Hyperphosphatemia*	GFR <30 mL/min (stage 4)
Metabolic acidosis	GFR <30 mL/min (stage 4)
Anemia	GFR <60 mL/min (stage 3)
Uremic symptoms Nausea, vomiting, disturbances in sleep	GFR <15 mL/min (stage 5)

*Descriptions of the various stages are presented in the text. These electrolyte abnormalities can be seen at higher levels of GFR.
Abbreviations: GFR = glomerular filtration rate.

When disease of the kidney involves the medullary portion or hormonal derangements such as hyporeninemic hypoaldosterinism are present, hyperkalemia can be observed prior to significant declines in GFR. In addition, patients with even moderate renal failure have a reduced reserve to eliminated potassium and therefore can develop hyperkalemia if potassium load is increased dramatically.

METABOLIC ACIDOSIS

A fall in plasma bicarbonate concentration in association with a reduced blood pH (metabolic acidosis) is frequently observed when GFR falls below 20% to 25% of normal. The acidosis results from acid excretion falling below acid production leading to positive proton balance. Recent studies have documented that a tendency to the development of metabolic acidosis can be seen with mild reductions in GFR (<60 mL/min).

The electrolyte pattern seen with the metabolic acidosis of renal failure is often of the high anion gap variety, but frequently a hyperchloremic (normal anion gap) or combined anion gap and hyperchloremic pattern can be observed. The degree of acidosis is usually mild to moderate with plasma bicarbonate concentration ranging from 12 to 22 mEq/L. Of interest, at any given level of GFR, the acidosis is often not progressive, but plasma bicarbonate concentration remains stable unless renal function declines further or there is an increment in acid production.

ABNORMAL DIVALENT IN METABOLISM

Serum phosphorus is regulated by the kidney but in most cases remains within the normal range until GFR falls below 20% to 25% of normal. This stabilization of serum phosphorus is attributed to increased tubular excretion of phosphorus as a result of increased parathyroid hormone secretion. As with potassium and bicarbonate, recent studies demonstrate a tendency for elevation in serum phosphorus can be observed with mild renal failure (<50 to 60 mL/min). Serum calcium is usually in the normal range, but varies reciprocally with serum phosphorus. Because of derangements in divalent ion metabolism bone disease with increased tendency to fractures and disordered soft tissue structures can be observed.

Hyperparathyoridism is a common occurrence in patients with renal failure, the values usually being higher with a greater degree of renal impairment. The elevated PTH values are usually induced by hypocalcemia, although increased serum phosphorus concentrations independent of serum calcium values can also play a role. The increased parathyroid hormone levels can induce damage to bone and soft tissue structures, but also may affect other functions such as cardiac function and the production of red blood cells.

ANEMIA

The kidney is the source of erythropoietin, the hormone that regulates bone marrow production of red blood cells. Thus, with the development of renal impairment, there is a fall in red blood cell production. A fall in red cell survival also contributes to development of anemia. Anemia generally appears when GFR falls below 60 mL/minute. There is a rough correlation between the severity of renal failure and the degree of anemia: the more severe the renal failure the greater the degree of anemia. However, this relationship is not invariable, and many patients have only mild reductions in hemoglobin and hematocrit.

Anemia initially was believed to contribute only to changes in oxygen delivery. However, recent studies show that anemia can contribute to the genesis of left ventricular hypertrophy and other cardiomyopathies noted with chronic renal failure and can raise mortality in patients with chronic renal failure.

HYPERTENSION

Recent studies emphasize the importance of the kidneys in the regulation of blood pressure, and the bulk of patients with diabetes or other glomerular disease will develop hypertension in the course of their renal failure. In many instances, hypertension does not develop until GFR is below 40% to 50% of normal. The type of renal disease underlying chronic renal failure appears to be important, as hypertension is less common with pyelonephritis. Hypertension might be observed earlier in the course of renal failure, however, in patients with polycystic kidney disease or ischemic nephropathy. Because hypertension is one of the most critical factors in the genesis of cardiovascular disease and can accelerate the progression of renal failure, careful attention of control of hypertension is important.

VOLUME OVERLOAD

Salt retention often accompanies chronic renal failure even when GFR is not severely compromised. The degree of salt retention can be profound if significant albuminuria with resultant hypoalbuminemia is seen and is more severe as GFR falls below 20% to 25% of normal. Salt retention is a critical factor in the development of hypertension and can promote congestive heart failure.

Symptoms and Signs of Renal Failure

Patients with chronic renal failure are often asymptomatic with little evidence of disease other than laboratory abnormalities until late in the course of renal failure. If anemia is present, patients may complain of fatigue; and if significant elevations in parathyroid hormone levels are noted, bone pain, ruptured tendons or other disorders of soft tissue structures can be noted. Once moderate to severe renal failure appears, symptoms of the electrolyte abnormalities can be observed. Hyperkalemia, if severe, can lead to arrhythmias or heart block and muscle weakness. Metabolic acidosis can contribute to fatigue. Anemia can contribute to fatigue and changes in mentation and physical stamina. Weight loss related to metabolic acidosis and or retention of various uremic toxins may occur. Sexual dysfunction characterized by reduced libido and reduced fertility are common with moderate to severe renal failure.

Once severe renal failure develops (stage 4 or 5), the uremic syndrome can be observed characterized by a decreased appetite, nausea, vomiting, and subtle changes in mental status including changes in sleep patterns. However, even with severe renal failure many patients feel surprisingly well.

Management of Chronic Renal Failure

STAGING OF CHRONIC RENAL FAILURE

As noted earlier, within the last several years, a great deal of effort has been expended into developing guidelines for the evaluation, monitoring, and treatment of patients with chronic renal failure. To this end, experts working with the National Kidney Foundation have divided chronic renal failure into different states based on measurements or estimations of GFR. The value of staging to the physician is that the studies necessary to monitor patients and the complications of chronic renal failure are often different depending on the stage of renal failure.

Stage 0 (GFR Greater Than 90 mL/minute With Risk Factors for Renal Disease)

Patients at stage 0 have increased risk for development of chronic renal failure, such as those with diabetes or hypertension but who have GFR greater than 90 mL/minute in the absence of proteinuria or urinary sedimentary abnormalities. These patients should have their blood pressure and diabetes controlled. Estimates of GFR should be obtained approximately every 6 months from measurement of serum creatinine, and qualitative tests for urine protein excretion should be obtained. In diabetics measurement of microalbumin should also be obtained. Because control of disease may forestall progression glycosylated hemoglobin (HbA1C) values should also be obtained.

Stage 1 (GFR Greater Than 90 mL/minute With Albuminuria)

Once evidence of renal damage is obtained, as reflected by microalbuminuria or proteinuria, but GFR is either normal or increased, patients are said to be in stage 1. These individuals should be monitored more closely and strict attention must be given to maintain blood pressure below 130/80. Furthermore, angiotensin converting enzyme inhibitor (ACEI) or angiotensin receptor blocker (ARB) should be given to prevent evolution of microalbuminuria to full-blown proteinuria (see the following). No clinical or laboratory abnormalities are observed at this stage.

Stage 2: Mild Renal Failure (GFR 60 to 90 mL/minute)

When GFR is mildly reduced to values from 60 to 90 mL/minute, patients are in stage 2. These patients should also be carefully monitored and blood pressure tightly controlled. If diabetes is present, strict attention to maintaining HbA1C within recommended guidelines should be given. Again, it is rare at this stage for any significant clinical abnormalities other than hypertension to be present.

Stage 3: Moderate Renal Failure (GFR 30 to 59 mL/minute)

When GFR ranges between 30 to 59 mL/minute, patients are in stage 3. At this point hypertension may appear, mild abnormalities in serum phosphorus might be observed, and anemia can be seen. Also in some patients an elevation in serum potassium can be noted, particularly if they are ingesting a relatively high potassium diet. These patients need to be followed more closely, and it is recommended that patients at the lower end of this stage (i.e., close to 30 mL/min) be monitored by a nephrologist.

Stage 4: Moderate to Severe (GFR from 15 to 29 mL/minute)

Once GFR falls to values from 15 to 29 mL/minute, patients have severe renal failure, or stage 4 disease. At this level of GFR, significant electrolyte abnormalities such as metabolic acidosis, hyperkalemia, and hyperphosphatemia are frequent. Anemia is common and the patient may begin to note reductions in appetite and have a fall in muscle mass. However, there is great variability in the appearance of symptoms or laboratory derangements.

Stage 5: Severe (GFR Less Than 15 to 29 mL/minute)

When GFR falls below 15 mL/minute, severe electrolyte abnormalities are often present, anemia is common. Clinical symptoms can develop. Renal replacement therapy, either dislysis or transplantation, is usually required at this stage.

Recommendations for treatment of patients are summarized below. The frequency of patient visits, of course, largely depends on the complications of renal disease present and co-morbid conditions. Therefore, these are only general recommendations for frequency of examination.

When patients are in stage 0, they should be seen once per year for renal evaluation. When GFR remains normal or elevated, but proteinuria is present, renal evaluation should be performed every 6 months. When stage 3 develops, we usually repeat renal evaluation every 3 months. Patients in stage 4 are seen more frequently, usually at the minimum of once per month. Patients with end-stage disease require renal replacement therapy.

GENERAL APPROACH TO TREATMENT OF CHRONIC RENAL FAILURE

Treatment of chronic renal failure can be divided into the modalities that are specific to the underlying disorder and those that are used to treat all patients with chronic renal failure. Thus, patients with systemic lupus erythematosus or other immune-mediated or inflammatory disease may benefit from treatment with steroids and immunosuppressive agents. Treatments specific for individual disorders are beyond the scope of this article.

The physician treating the patient with renal failure has two goals: preventing or delaying progression of renal failure, and alleviating the electrolyte and hormonal abnormalities that can lead to symptoms or complications of the disease. Understanding the methods to accomplish the former requires knowledge of those factors that are integral to progression of the disease.

FACTORS CAUSING PROGRESSION OF CHRONIC RENAL FAILURE

It has been recognized for several years that once renal failure has developed, renal function can decline at a predictable rate in the absence of further insults to the kidney. Essential to the optimal approach used to treat chronic renal failure, therefore, is an understanding of those factors that can cause progression of renal failure, including:

- Systemic and intraglomerular hypertension
- Glomerular hypertrophy
- Intrarenal precipitation of calcium and phosphorus
- Hyperlipidemia
- Altered metabolism of prostanoids
- Metabolic acidosis
- Anemia
- Tubulointerstitial disease
- Proteinuria

Intraglomerular Hypertension and Glomerular Hypertrophy

As nephrons are lost, changes are induced in the kidney to preserve GFR such as renal vasodilatation, an increase in glomerular capillary pressure, and an increment in size of individual glomeruli raising wall stress. These adaptive mechanisms probably induce damage by causing endothelial cell damage with detachment of epithelial cells allowing enhanced flux of water and solutes that might cause narrowing of capillary lumens. Also, strain on mesangial cells causes them to produce cytokines and extracellular matrix with resultant expansion of the mesangium and glomerular sclerosis.

Proteinuria

Although proteinuria has traditionally been a marker of glomerular injury, with greater amounts of urinary protein excretion being associated with more severe injury, recent studies indicate that proteinuria, can induce mesangial and tubular damage. Therefore, treatments to reduce proteinuria, may be beneficial in limiting further renal damage.

Tubulointerstitial Disease

Some component of tubulointerstitial disease is generally found in individuals with chronic renal failure even when the primary process affects the glomerulus. It has been postulated that the tubulointerstitial disease can produce atrophy of tubules or obstruction destroying individual nephrons. Even when tubular inflammation is treated, progressive scarring can continue unabated. Thus, treatments designed to reduce interstitial fibrosis may be important for preventing progression of disease. At present, only experimental drugs not available for human use have been examined for this purpose.

Hyperlipidemia

Hyperlipidemia is frequently observed in disorders associated with nephrotic range proteinuria, but is also noted in a large percentage of the general population without renal disease. Experimental evidence obtained from animal studies shows hyperlipidemia can promote progression of renal failure. Thus, loading with cholesterol augments renal injury and treatment with cholesterol-lowering drugs slows the rate of progression. This effect is synergistic to that achieved by lowering blood pressure.

The mechanisms underlying the effects of lipids are not well understood, but possible explanations include mesangial lipid deposition leading to glomerular injury or tubular injury. A few studies performed in human subjects have demonstrated benefit from lipid lowering on the progression of renal injury, although they are not conclusive. Because patients with chronic renal failure have a high prevalence of cardiovascular disease, it is reasonable to inititate therapy with statin drugs to lower serum cholesterol and lipid levels.

Calcium-Phosphate Deposition

A rise in serum phosphorus, usually seen at the later stages of renal failure, can lead to precipitation of calcium phosphate in the renal interstitium. The deposits can then induce an inflammatory response producing interstitial fibrosis and tubular atrophy. Some have indicated that the deposits may form prior to detectable elevations in serum phosphorus concentrations.

Increased Glomerular Prostaglandin Production

An increment in glomerular prostaglandin production has been found in several studies of chronic renal failure. The increased prostanoids produce renal vasodilatation and a rise in intraglomerular pressure, factors that augment progression of disease.

METABOLIC ACIDOSIS

Metabolic acidosis commonly develops in the course of chronic renal failure. In response to the acidosis, ammonia production per residual functioning nephron is augmented. It has been postulated that the increased local production of ammonia in some way induces tubulointerstitial damage. This issue remains controversial, as some studies do not support this possibility.

SPECIFIC TREATMENT MEASURES

Treatment of patients with chronic renal failure should be designed to ameliorate those factors that can cause progression of renal injury, treat or prevent important complications, and normalize important laboratory abnormalities that contribute to symptoms of the disease.

Measures Designed to Reduce the Rate of Progression of Renal Failure

CONTROL OF SYSTEMIC AND INTRAGLOMERULAR HYPERTENSION

Experimental and human studies demonstrate that control of systemic hypertension can slow the rate of progression of renal disease substantially. Recent evidence indicates that target blood pressure levels should be lower than recommended for the general population (<130/80). Control of hypertension with the use of myriad agents can benefit the patient with renal failure. However, as indicated previously, reduction in intraglomerular hypertension may be the most important factor underlying the benefits from blood pressure control. Therefore, when possible, treatment with ACEIs, ARBs, or the combination of these agents should be first-line antihypertensive therapy in these patients. Patients who do not tolerate these drugs might benefit from administration of non-dihydropyridine calcium channel blockers. In patients with proteinuria, even if blood pressure is controlled or they are normotensive, the doses of ACEIs or ARBs should be raised to levels even greater than recommended to reduce urine protein excretion to levels less than 500 mg. This reduction in proteinuria is the most optimal in protecting the kidney.

Potentially serious complications with ACEIs or ARBs include acute reduction in GFR and hyperkalemia. If these complications occur, a reduction in dose or even discontinuation of these agents might be required. It is recommended that these agents be continued even when GFR is less than 20 mL/min. Given the potential severity of these complications, patients should be monitored closely.

PROTEIN RESTRICTION

The benefits of protein restriction in preventing progression are unclear, but it has suggested that reducing protein intake to 0.8 to 1.0 g/kg body weight of high biologic value is beneficial. Others have indicated that 0.6 g/kg body weight should be used. In patients with substantial proteinuria, the quantity of protein recommended will have to be adjusted to prevent hypoalbuminemia. Once patients reached later stage 4, protein restriction may be useful to prevent expression of uremic symptoms. Reducing protein intake will have the added benefit of decreasing acid, potassium, and phosphate production.

CONTROL OF LIPIDS

Control of cholesterol with statins may help prevent progression and should reduce the burden of cardiovascular disease, which remains the most lethal disorder for patients with chronic renal failure. Adherence to the newly proposed aggressive recommendation appears reasonable.

Measures Designed to Treat Significant Laboratory Abnormalities

ANEMIA

Patients with renal anemia should be treated with erythropoietin (Procrit). Although this requires subcutaneous injection once per week, newer, long-lasting forms (darbepoetin [Aranesp]) enable

CURRENT THERAPY

The recommendations for the treatment of patients with renal failure is as follows:

Recommendation	Goal
Control BP	130/80 mm Hg
Reduce proteinuria by administering angiotensin converting enzyme inhibitors or angiotensin receptor blockers. In some cases both agents may have to be given concomitantly.	Decrease urine protein excretion as low as possible but at least less than 1 g per day.
Control phosphate concentrations with phosphate binders with noncalcium containing binders when possible.	Serum phosphate <4.5 mg/dL
Maintain vitamin D by admininistration of ergocalciferol	Maintain 25 OH D levels at 30 ng/mL by administration of ergocalciferol
Prevent hyperparathyroidism with vitamin D or calcimimetics.	Maintain PTH <150 pg/mL
Correct anemia with erythropoietin and iron replacement as needed.	Maintain Hg between 11 and 12 mg/dL
Administer diuretics to control hypertension and volume overload.	Maintain euvolemia when possible
Control serum potassium with dietary restriction, diuretics, and/or potassium exchange resin as necessary.	Maintain serum potassium <5.0 mEq/L
Keep protein intake at 0.6 to 0.8 g/kg body weight per day.	Slow progression of renal disease while preventing protein depletion
Control metabolic acidosis with administration of sodium citrate (Citra pH).	Maintain serum HCO$_3$ >20 mEq/L

Abbreviations: BP = blood pressure; HCO$_3$ = bicarbonate; Hg = mercury; PTH = parathyroid hormone.

---

patients to be treated every 3 weeks. Because iron stores need to be repleted for anemia to be successfully treated, these should be monitored and iron given. Because of the vagaries of ferritin measurements, we use serum iron and iron binding capacity with the goal of maintaining saturation above 20% and near 30%. At present, the target hemoglobin and hematocrit varies between 11 mg/dL and 12 mg/dL 33 and 36, respectively. Given the recent concern about vascular complications with EPO therapy, the clinican must be vigilant in preventing Hg values from exceeding 12 gm/dL.

METABOLIC ACIDOSIS

Controversy exists as to the target value of bicarbonate for patients with chronic renal failure. Some experts recommend raising plasma bicarbonate to levels above 20 mEq/L, whereas others recommend complete normalization of plasma bicarbonate. To properly raise plasma bicarbonate concentration, the deficit should be calculated from the formula:

Desired − prevailing level of plasma bicarbonate
× 50% body weight = Total bicarbonate deficit.

The deficit should be corrected slowly over several days.

Because patients experience gas when the base is given as bicarbonate, the base is usually administered as Shohl's solution sodium citrate,* the citrate being metabolized to bicarbonate in the liver. Each milliliter of Shohl's solution represents 1 mEq of the base.

DIVALENT ION METABOLISM

Serum phosphorus is controlled by administration of phosphate binders usually starting with calcium citrate (Citracal) or acetate (PhosLo). If these are not successful or if patients have elevated serum calcium levels, then sevelamar (Renagel) or lanthanum (Fosrenol) can be used alone or in combination with calcium binders. Physicians should aim to maintain serum phosphorus levels below 5 mg/dL and keep serum calcium phosphorus product below 60.

Parathyroid hormone (PTH) levels should be maintained below 150 pg/mL, or less depending on stage; levels associated with proper bone remodeling but not to values observed in patients without kidney disease. Suppression of parathyroid hormone secretion can be achieved by administration of various vitamin D analogues. The recent recognition of the calcium-sensing receptor and development of calcimimetic drugs that are extremely effective in lowering PTH secretion may make using vitamin D compounds obsolete in the future.

Low 25 OH D levels have been documented in a large number of individuals both with and without renal failure. In patients with renal impairment this can contribute to the abnormal 1,25 OH vitamin D levels. Measurement of 25-hydroxy vitamin D levels should be obtained in all patients with CKD and EGFR <60 mL/min. If levels are below 30 ng/mL they should be supplemented with ergocalciferol sufficient to maintain levels above this level.

HYPERKALEMIA

As this is the most serious electrolyte disorder encountered, patients should be monitored closely. Serum potassium concentrations should be maintained below 5 mEq/L. If hyperkalemia develops during treatment with ACEIs or ARBs, the doses of these agents should be reduced or discontinued. Diuretic administration, often given for control of hypertension, can help control hyperkalemia, but if it should develop, particularly when GFR falls below 20% of normal, it can be treated with the potassium exchange resin, sodium polystyrene sulfonate (Kayexalate).

ELEVATED BLOOD UREA NITROGEN CONCENTRATION

The precise solutes that are retained, which are important for the pathogenesis of the uremic syndrome, are not clear. However, BUN is a marker for other retained solutes and is roughly correlated with development of uremic symptoms. When the BUN is greater than 100 mg/dL and serum creatinine concentration is greater than 8 mg/dL uremic symptoms may develop. These symptoms will often abate merely with protein restriction and reduced production of these compounds. Protein restriction is usually not instituted until GFR is less than 15% to 20% of normal. Prior to that time, it is important to maintain protein intake to keep serum albumin within the normal range.

---

*Investigational drug in the United States.

VOLUME OVERLOAD

Because salt retention is an essential component of the development of hypertension and underlies volume overload, diuretic administration is usually necessary in the treatment of chronic renal failure. Thiazides frequently used in the treatment of hypertension or volume overload in subjects with normal renal function may not be efficacious once GFR is less than or equal to 33% of normal. Therefore, loop diuretics, such as furosemide (Lasix) or a combined loop and proximal tubule diuretic such as metolozone (Zaroxolyn), are generally indicated. Because the effectiveness of both agents requires access to the tubule lumen, the effective dose is often higher than in those with normal renal function. Once patients are in stage 4 renal failure, use of diuretics is hampered by worsening of renal failure and often must be used cautiously.

REFERENCES

Beco JA, Bansal VK: Medical nutrition therapy in chronic kidney failure: Integrating clinical practice guidelines. J Am Diet Assoc 2004;104:404-409.

Clase CM, Garg AX, Kiberd BA: Prevalence of low glomerular filtration rate in nondiabetic Americans: Third National Health and Nutrition Examination Survey (NHANES III). J Am Soc Nephrol 2002;13.

Cleveland DR, Jindal KK, Hirsch DJ, et al: Quality of pre-referral care in patients with chronic renal insufficiency. Am J Kidney Dis 2002;40:30-36.

Curtin RB, Becker B, Kimmel PL, Schatell D: An integrated approach to care for patients with chronic kidney disease. Semin Dial 2003;16:399-402.

Djamali A, Kendziorski C, Brazy PC, Becker BN: Disease progression and outcomes in chronic kidney disease and renal transplantation. Kidney Int 2003;64:1800-1807.

KDOQI Clinical practice guidelines and clinical practice recommendations for diabetes and chronic kidney disease. Am J Kidney Dis 2007;49:S1-S154.

Kopple JD: National Kidney Foundation K/DOQI clinical practice guidelines for nutrition in chronic renal failure. Am J Kidney Dis 2001;37:S66-S70.

Maschio G, Alberti D, Janin G, et al: Effect of the angiotensin-converting-enzyme inhibitor benazepril on the progression of chronic renal insufficiency. N Engl J Med 1996;334:939-945.

Tonelli M, Gill J, Pandeya S, et al: Slowing the progression of chronic renal insufficiency. Can Med Assoc J 2002;166:906-907.

Malignant Tumors of the Urogenital Tract

Method of
Michael S. Cookson, MD, and
Sam S. Chang, MD

CARCINOMA OF THE PROSTATE

Carcinoma of the prostate is the most common solid malignancy in men and the second leading cause of male cancer mortality in the United States. In 2005, it was estimated there would be 232,090 new cases and 30,350 deaths from prostatic cancer alone. The incidence of prostatic carcinoma increases with age, and this is anticipated to continue to increase for the next 25 years in direct relationship to the aging U.S. population. A familial pattern is identified, and prostatic carcinoma is more common in African Americans than in the white population. A high-fat diet is implicated as a contributing factor in some studies. Hereditary prostatic carcinoma has been identified in approximately 9% of patients and may account for as much as 40% of the early age of onset cancers. In fact, the hereditary prostate cancer gene (HPC1) was identified on the long arm of chromosome 1 and is thought to be intimately related to the development of carcinoma of the prostate.

Diagnosis

More than 95% of prostatic cancers are adenocarcinomas. Prostatic carcinoma can be identified at autopsy in more than 75% of individuals older than 80 years, yet clinically the risk of being diagnosed is estimated at one in six men. Thus, there is a large discrepancy between the microscopic presence of the disease and clinically significant disease. Most men with early-stage prostatic cancer have no disease-related symptoms. Prostatic cancer and benign prostatic hypertrophy (BPH) may occur simultaneously, but there is no apparent causal relationship. Obstructive voiding symptoms or hematuria may be present. Patients with advanced disease may present with pelvic pain, ureteral obstruction, or bone pain from distant metastasis.

Early detection has allowed more patients to be identified with lower stage clinical disease, and as a result, such men have had higher recurrence-free survival rates after treatment. Recommendations from groups such as the American Urologic Association and American Cancer Society generally include annual screening with serum prostate-specific antigen (PSA) determination and a digital rectal examination (DRE) for all men older than 50 years and for all African American men and men with a family history of prostatic cancer starting at 40 years of age. These recommendations are not uniformly accepted; the U.S. Public Health Service Task Force does not endorse screening for prostatic cancer because of a lack of convincing prospective data that screening has an impact on the prostatic cancer death rate. The goal of screening is to detect clinically significant prostatic cancer in individuals with at least 10 years of life expectancy.

Serum PSA is specific for the prostate but is secreted by both benign and malignant prostatic epithelial cells. PSA may be elevated in men with prostatitis, BPH, or prostatic cancer. PSA values differ somewhat depending on the assay used. In general, a level of less than 4.0 µg/mL is considered normal, and in younger men, a value of greater than 2.5 ng/mL may be considered abnormal. Approximately 25% of prostatic carcinoma may occur despite what is considered a normal PSA level, and in some studies, the incidence of prostatic carcinoma is 15% even when the PSA is less than 2 µg/mL.

Serum PSA occurs in several forms, with the majority bound to a alpha-1-antichymotrypsin and another portion that is unconjugated or free in serum. The relative proportion of the two forms can be used to improve the specificity of PSA testing. A greater proportion of free PSA is seen in men with BPH compared to those with prostatic cancer. In general, the lower the percentage of free fraction, the

---

CURRENT DIAGNOSIS

Carcinoma of the Prostate

- Average-risk patient offered screening with PSA and DRE at 50 years of age
- High-risk patients with strong family history or African Americans at age 45 years
- Patients with an elevated PSA or abnormal DRE referred for discussion regarding risks, benefits, and alternatives to biopsy of the prostate
- Diagnosis made with transrectal ultrasound-guided biopsy of the prostate
- Staging with bone scan for patients with high-grade tumors (Gleason grade 4 or 5), PSA levels >20 µg/mL, elevated alkaline phosphatase levels, or bone pain

---

Abbreviations: DRE = digital rectal examination; PSA = prostate-specific antigen.

more likely it is to reflect a diagnosis of cancer, with a percentage of less than 25% most commonly associated with prostatic cancer as compared to higher percentages. Newer tests such as complexed PSA are being used to improve the specificity of PSA testing.

Most often, transrectal ultrasonography (TRUS) is used for imaging and as a guide for biopsy of the prostate. TRUS can distinguish the zonal anatomy of the prostate and is an accurate measure of the size of the prostate. Prostatic cancers typically are located in the peripheral zone and may have a hypoechoic pattern. Because of its lack of sensitivity and specificity, TRUS is not used as a screening test.

The grading of prostatic carcinoma is based on the degree of differentiation of the tumor. This provides important prognostic information. Most often, the Gleason grading system is used. Tumors with a Gleason score of 2 to 4 are usually considered to be well differentiated; 5 to 7, moderately differentiated; and 8 to 10, poorly differentiated. Prognosis is strongly linked to grade and Gleason score. Most cancers found through early detection or screening programs are of an intermediate grade (Gleason score 5 to 7).

Staging of prostatic cancer defines the local, regional, and distant extent of disease. The TNM staging system is used to allow categorization of nonpalpable tumors detected because of PSA or ultrasound abnormalities (stage T1c). The primary staging modality for local disease is DRE. Serum PSA levels correlate only roughly with disease extent. However, bone metastasis is quite uncommon in patients with a PSA of less than 20 μg/mL. Radionucleotide bone scanning is the most sensitive method for detection of bone metastases. Bone scan in the absence of symptoms is not required routinely if the PSA value is less than 10 μg/mL and a Gleason sum of less than or equal to 7. Computed tomography (CT) scanning is not routinely used because grossly positive nodes are detected rarely with clinically localized tumor.

Lymph node staging is important in selecting patients for therapy. CT scanning may show enlarged lymph nodes in patients with high-volume or high-grade primary tumors. Laparoscopic pelvic lymphadenectomy is feasible and can provide adequate sampling of the pelvic lymph nodes among those patients not selecting surgery. More commonly, lymph node dissection is performed through an open incision immediately prior to radical prostatectomy.

Treatment

The optimal therapy for localized prostatic cancer is controversial and must be individualized. For men with a life expectancy of less than 10 years, observation alone may be appropriate. Also, some men choose active surveillance rather than initial treatment but later opt for treatment when clinical evidence indicates worsening disease. Surgery and radiation therapy are the most commonly used treatments. For organ-confined tumors, the 15-year disease-free survival rates are greater than 90% for patients treated with surgery. Moreover, the survival outcome is similar after radiation therapy or surgery; however, randomized comparisons among similarly staged patients are lacking. Brachytherapy involves the use of radioactive seeds (iodine 125 or palladium 103) placed into the prostate. This is also a valid option, with similar long-term disease-free survival in low- and intermediate-risk patients. High-dose radiation (HDR) therapy is also an emerging treatment option that allows high doses of radiation therapy to be administered in a relatively short period of time. Cryotherapy (i.e., freezing of the prostate) is also approved in the treatment of men with prostatic carcinoma, but long-term outcomes are not available.

Radical prostatectomy (RP) may be performed via an open surgical approach or by a laparoscopic technique. Most commonly, it is performed via open surgery through a retropubic approach, although some are performed through a perineal incision. Laparoscopic and robot-assisted RPs are being performed with a reduction in blood loss and seemingly comparable oncologic results as compared to open surgery. These minimally invasive techniques may have the potential for improved functional outcomes. In patients who were sexually active before therapy, potency can be retained in nearly 40% to 70% by preservation of the neurovascular bundles. In patients with organ-confined disease, there is an excellent prognosis, with a life expectancy similar to men without prostatic cancer. In patients with positive surgical margins or positive lymph nodes, adjuvant radiation and hormonal therapy may be used, respectively.

Serum PSA should be undetectable after radical prostatectomy because all PSA-producing cells are removed. After radiation therapy, superior results are achieved in patients in whom the PSA level decreases to less than 1 μg/mL. An increasing serum PSA is evidence of tumor recurrence. There is controversy about when to initiate hormonal therapy in men with a rising PSA level after treatment, although several studies suggest early hormonal therapy may be of benefit among those with more aggressive tumors.

Prostatic cancer is a partially androgen-dependent disease. Therefore, the primary treatment for metastatic carcinoma of the prostate is androgen deprivation. Suppression of serum testosterone can be achieved by orchiectomy. Alternatively, medical therapy may be considered. Luteinizing hormone-releasing hormone (LHRH) analogues effectively suppress testosterone to the castrate range within 1 month of administration. LHRH analogues are associated with few serious side effects but do cause vasomotor hot flashes in approximately two thirds of patients. Loss of libido and impotence are also a consequence of treatment.

The median response to hormonal therapy in patients with metastatic disease is approximately 18 to 24 months. After that time, disease progression often occurs and ultimately progresses to death. Once the cancer fails to respond to hormonal therapy, the patient usually dies of the disease, although survival rates of greater than 40 months are reported. Recently, published trials have documented improved survival with docetaxel (Taxotere) chemotherapy among patients with androgen-independent prostatic cancer (AIPC) treatments. In addition, mitoxantrone (Novantrone) is now approved for palliative relief for symptomatic bone pain from AIPC. Radiation can also be effective palliation for isolated sites of bone metastasis. The mechanisms through which prostatic carcinoma escapes hormonal control and achieves androgen independence is an area of intense research.

TUMORS OF THE RENAL PARENCHYMA

Malignant tumors of the renal parenchyma are either primary or metastatic. Among the primary renal lesions, the tumors may be either malignant or benign. The most common malignant tumor is renal cell carcinoma (RCC), whereas other tumor types such as

---

CURRENT THERAPY

Carcinoma of the Prostate

- Treatment is generally offered to men with at least a 10-y life expectancy.
- Treatment options for clinically localized T1c and T2 tumors include active surveillance/watchful waiting, radiation therapy (both external and brachytherapy), and surgery (open and laparoscopic).
- Treatment for locally advanced tumors T3/T4 include surgery and external radiation in combination with androgen-deprivation therapy (ADT).
- Treatment for patients with metastatic disease N1–2 or M1 is generally palliative with ADT.
- Follow-up includes symptom checks with history, physical examination, and PSA monitoring every 6 months for 2 years and then annually. Any abnormalities may be more fully evaluated with appropriate imaging.

Abbreviations: PSA = prostate-specific antigen.

papillary, collecting duct carcinoma, medullary carcinoma, and sarcomas occur infrequently. The most common benign renal tumors are angiomyolipomas and oncocytomas, the latter of which is often indistinguishable from malignant lesions on radiographic imaging. Metastatic lesions such as lung, breast, and ovary may occur, and lymphoma may be present in the kidney.

RENAL CELL CARCINOMA

RCC is the most common primary neoplasm of the kidney and accounts for greater than 85% of all primary renal cancers. In the United States, an estimated 36,160 new cases are diagnosed, and approximately 12,660 patients die of the disease each year. Renal cell carcinoma represents approximately 3% of all adult malignancies. It is a tumor that usually occurs in adults between 40 and 60 years of age, although it is reported in younger age groups. It has a 2:1 male-to-female preponderance and a well-documented association with von Hippel-Lindau disease.

RCCs arise from the proximal convoluted tubules. The most consistent chromosomal changes in RCC are deletions and translocations of the short arm of chromosome 3. No specific agent is implicated as the cause of RCC. Tobacco smoking poses an approximately twofold relative risk for developing kidney cancer. Patients with end-stage renal disease (ESRD) with acquired cystic disease of the kidney (ACDK) have an increased risk of RCC as well. Of these patients, RCC develops in 1% to 2%, with younger dialysis patients having the greatest risk. Renal ultrasound is recommended in these patients annually, with CT scans for more complex cysts.

Diagnosis

Hematuria is the single most common sign associated with renal cell carcinoma; it occurs in 29% to 60% of cases. Flank pain and a palpable mass occur next most frequently, but the classic triad of hematuria, flank pain, and a palpable abdominal mass is reported in only 10% of cases. Other common signs and symptoms are fever, anemia, and elevated sedimentation rate. Although serum lactate dehydrogenase and alkaline phosphatase may be elevated, there are no reliable tumor markers for RCC. RCCs can present only with nonspecific symptoms such as weight loss, fever, or weakness. Most, however, are asymptomatic and are detected incidentally on radiographic imaging.

TNM staging is currently the most commonly used system to determine the extent of the primary lesion, involvement of contiguous structures, vascular involvement, and whether the tumor has metastasized. It allows for a distinction between venous involvement and nodal invasion and stratifies the extent of each stage. RCCs often involve the renal vein and vena cava and may even extend into the right atrium. Five-year survival rates for stages T1N0M0 (less than 7 cm) and T2N0M0 (more than 7 cm) are 80% to 90%, for stages T3N0M0 40% to 60%, and N1–3 and M1 are 10% to 20%.

CURRENT DIAGNOSIS

Renal Cell Carcinoma

- Hematuria is the single most common sign; occurring in up to 60% of cases. Flank pain and palpable mass occur next most frequently, but the classic triad of hematuria, flank pain, and a palpable abdominal mass occurs in only 10%. Other common signs and symptoms are fever, anemia, and elevated sedimentation rate.
- Most are asymptomatic and detected incidentally on radiographic imaging (renal ultrasound, computed tomography scan, or magnetic resonance imaging).

Treatment

Radical nephrectomy is the primary treatment of RCC. This classic procedure removes the kidney en bloc within Gerota's fascia along with the ipsilateral adrenal gland and lymph nodes. Radical nephrectomy traditionally is performed as an open procedure (flank, transabdominal, or thoracoabdominal incision). Radical nephrectomy has evolved, with adrenalectomy performed for upper pole tumors, very large tumors, or lesions that directly extend into the adrenal gland. If the RCC extends into the inferior vena cava, open as compared to laparoscopic nephrectomy is usually the preferred approach. Rarely, cardiopulmonary bypass is needed to remove the entire tumor thrombus, which is particularly important for those thrombi that extend above the level of the diaphragm. Laparoscopic radical nephrectomy, both hand assisted and pure laparoscopic, is equally efficacious as compared to open surgery and is potentially less morbid, allowing patients a faster recovery.

A partial nephrectomy is performed in patients with solitary kidneys, in those with bilateral RCC, and in patients with compromised renal function. It is also generally agreed that partial nephrectomy or tumor enucleation may be used in patients with lesions 4 cm or less and a normal contralateral kidney, with local recurrence rates less than 5%. Like radical nephrectomy, laparoscopic techniques are emerging as viable alternatives to open surgical removal. In addition, there is an emergence of minimally invasive approaches that will likely compete with partial nephrectomy in the near future. These include radiofrequency ablation and cryotherapy, which may effectively treat smaller lesions under radiologic guidance, thus reducing or eliminating the need for surgery.

Up to 25% of patients initially seen with symptoms have metastatic disease. Sites of metastasis in decreasing frequency include the lungs, lymph nodes, liver, bone, and adrenal gland. Chemotherapy and radiation have little to no survival benefit, with

CURRENT THERAPY

Renal Cell Carcinoma

- Treatment for resectable masses is almost always surgical—either radical or partial nephrectomy. Both radical and partial nephrectomy may be done via an open or laparoscopic approach.
- Partial nephrectomy is performed in patients with solitary kidneys, bilateral renal cell carcinoma, and compromised renal insufficiency. Partial nephrectomy or enucleation may be used in patients with lesions ≤4 cm and a normal contralateral kidney, with local recurrence rates of <5%.
- Minimally invasive approaches that are emerging include radiofrequency ablation and cryotherapy, which may effectively treat smaller lesions under radiologic guidance, thus reducing or eliminating the need for surgery.
- Up to 25% of patients have metastatic disease at diagnosis. Sites of metastasis in decreasing frequency include the lungs, lymph nodes, liver, bone, and adrenal gland.
- Chemotherapy and radiation have little to no survival benefit, with radiation only palliating painful metastasis.
- The mainstay of treatment is immunotherapy with 5-year survival rates of 10%–20%.
- Emerging evidence suggests an improved survival for those undergoing nephrectomy prior to immunotherapy.

radiation only palliating painful metastasis. The mainstay of treatment is immunotherapy, with 5-year survival rates of 10% to 20%. Emerging evidence suggests an improved survival in those undergoing nephrectomy prior to immunotherapy.

BENIGN RENAL TUMORS

Benign solid tumors of the kidney are encountered occasionally. An angiomyolipoma can usually be diagnosed by the characteristic appearance of fat within the lesion on CT scan. An angiomyolipoma may occur as an isolated phenomenon or in association with tuberous sclerosis. Tuberous sclerosis is a disease characterized by mental retardation, epilepsy, and adenoma sebaceum. Approximately 50% of patients with tuberous sclerosis develop angiomyolipomas, and many are bilateral and multifocal. The management of angiomyolipomas is controversial. In asymptomatic lesions smaller than 4 cm, observation with annual imaging is reasonable. In patients with an acute bleeding episode, angioinfarction may be used to stabilize the patient. In symptomatic lesions or lesions greater than 4 cm, surgical excision is considered the standard therapy.

Oncocytomas are benign renal tumors that account for between 5% and 10% of solid renal lesions. Renal oncocytomas are more difficult to differentiate from RCCs but usually are round, of uniform density, and may have a central scar or spoke-wheel appearance on CT scan. From a practical standpoint, renal oncocytomas are a pathologic diagnosis, and characteristic masses should be considered to be malignant until proven otherwise. Histologically, they are characterized by eosinophilic granular cells. The cell of origin is thought to be that of distal renal tubules.

Metastatic Renal Lesions

Lung cancer is the most common solid tumor to metastasize to the kidney, although lymphoma and ovarian, bowel, and breast tumors are also seen. Lymphoma of the kidney is almost always a metastatic manifestation of a systemic disease, and therefore surgical treatment is rarely indicated in the absence of symptoms. However, approximately 15% of renal lymphomas present as solitary masses. It is a challenge to differentiate these tumors from renal cell carcinoma preoperatively.

CURRENT DIAGNOSIS

Benign Renal Tumors

- Angiomyolipomas are diagnosed by the characteristic appearance of fat within the lesion on computed tomography (CT) scan.
- Angiomyolipomas may occur as an isolated phenomenon or in association with tuberous sclerosis.
- Tuberous sclerosis is characterized by mental retardation, epilepsy, and adenoma sebaceum. Approximately 50% of patients with tuberous sclerosis develop angiomyolipomas, and many are bilateral and multifocal.
- Oncocytomas are benign renal tumors that account for between 5% and 10% of solid renal lesions.
- Oncocytomas are more difficult to differentiate from RCC but usually are round and of uniform density; they may have a central scar or spoke-wheel appearance on CT scan.
- Oncocytomas are a pathologic diagnosis characterized by eosinophilic granular cells. These masses should be considered malignant until proven otherwise.

CURRENT THERAPY

Benign Renal Tumors

- The management is controversial. In asymptomatic lesions <4 cm, observation with annual imaging is reasonable.
- In patients with acute bleeding, angioinfarction may stabilize the patient. In symptomatic lesions or lesions >4 cm, surgical excision is considered standard therapy.

TUMORS OF THE RENAL PELVIS/URETER

Tumors of the renal pelvis account for approximately 10% of all renal tumors and approximately 5% of all urothelial tumors. Ureteral tumors are even less common, representing approximately 25% of upper tract urothelial tumors. Ureteral tumors are three times more common in men than in women and twice as common in whites as in blacks. Cigarette smoking is strongly associated with an increased risk of developing upper tract transitional cell carcinomas. Additionally, analgesic abuse and cyclophosphamide are associated with an increased risk.

The risk of upper tract tumors is approximately 4% among patients with bladder cancer. However, in patients with carcinoma in situ and high-grade urothelial lesions, the risk may approach 20% with long-term follow-up. Conversely, patients with upper tract tumors have a 40% to 70% risk of developing bladder cancer. Therefore, patients with upper tract tumors should undergo periodic surveillance cystoscopy. The incidence of bilateral upper tract tumors

CURRENT DIAGNOSIS

Tumors of the Renal Pelvis/Ureter

- Renal pelvic tumors account for 10% of all renal tumors and approximately 5% of all urothelial tumors.
- Ureteral tumors are even less common, occurring approximately 25% of the incidence of renal pelvic tumors.
- These tumors are three times more common in men than in women.
- Cigarette smoking is strongly associated with an increased risk. Additionally, analgesic abuse and cyclophosphamide are implicated.
- Most common presenting symptom is hematuria.
- Diagnostic workup usually includes an IVP and cytologic examination of the urine followed by cystoscopy.
- Cytologic examination of the urine may give a false-negative result in up to 85% of patients with a low-grade lesion.
- 50%–75% of patients have a filling defect on IVP. The differential diagnosis includes a tumor, blood clot, fungal ball, sloughed papilla, and radiolucent stone.
- The risk of upper tract tumors is approximately 4% among those patients with bladder cancer. In patients with CIS and high-grade lesions, the risk may approach 20%.
- Patients with upper tract tumors have a 40%–70% risk of developing bladder cancer.

Abbreviations: CIS = carcinoma in situ; IVP = intravenous pyelogram.

is 2% to 5%. In addition to transitional cell carcinomas, squamous cell carcinomas and adenocarcinomas are included in the differential diagnosis; particularly in a patient with a history of recurrent urinary tract infections or staghorn calculi.

Diagnosis

As with renal cell carcinomas, the most common presenting symptom of tumors of the renal pelvis/ureter is hematuria. In patients with normal renal function, the diagnostic workup usually includes an intravenous pyelogram (IVP) and urine cytologic examination followed by cystoscopy. However, it must be kept in mind that a voided urine cytologic examination may be falsely negative in up to 85% of patients with a low-grade lesion. Approximately 50% to 75% of patients have a filling defect on IVP. The differential diagnosis includes a tumor, blood clot, fungal ball, sloughed papilla, and radiolucent stone. A retrograde ureteropyelogram may be helpful in documenting the persistence of the filling defect; however, ureteroscopy with biopsy or brushings may be diagnostic. In renal pelvic defects, a noncontrast CT scan with 3-mm cuts through the kidney is usually able to differentiate a stone from a soft-tissue mass because even radiolucent stones on standard urography are opaque on CT scan. The TNM system is recommended for staging.

Treatment

Patients with low-grade, low-stage lesions do well with conservative or radical treatment. Patients with intermediate- or high-grade tumors are best managed with aggressive surgical resection. Solitary low-grade and low-stage upper ureteral tumors may be managed with segmental resection. Similar distal ureteral tumors can be managed with distal ureterectomy and ureteroneocystostomy. Treatment of high-grade and high-stage tumors is nephroureterectomy with removal of a cuff of the bladder at the ureteral orifice because of the high incidence of ipsilateral ureteral orifice and bladder involvement. This can be accomplished through a single extended flank or midline incision but is often performed through two incisions. Currently, hand-assisted laparoscopic nephroureterectomy is the preferred surgical approach, allowing for complete tumor removal through a single incision and offers the advantage of quicker convalescence. Successful endoscopic management including percutaneous and retrograde approaches is reported in selected cases.

CURRENT THERAPY

Tumors of the Renal Pelvis/Ureter

- Low-grade, low-stage lesions do well with conservative or radical treatment.
- Intermediate- or high-grade tumors are best managed with aggressive surgical resection.
- Solitary low-grade and low-stage upper ureteral tumors may be managed with segmental resection. Similar distal ureteral tumors can be managed with distal ureterectomy and ureteroneocystostomy.
- High-grade and high-stage tumors are treated by nephroureterectomy with removal of a cuff of bladder at the ureteral orifice.
- Hand-assisted laparoscopic nephroureterectomy is the preferred surgical approach, allowing for complete tumor removal through a single incision and often quicker convalescence.

CARCINOMA OF THE BLADDER

Transitional Cell Carcinoma of the Bladder

Bladder carcinoma is the fifth most common malignancy in the United States with more than 63,210 new cases annually. It is almost three times more common among men than women, in whom it is the fourth most common cancer. Because of frequent recurrences, particularly among patients with superficial tumors, bladder cancer is the second most prevalent cancer. Bladder cancer is the fifth most common cause of cancer deaths among men. It is approximately four times more prevalent among cigarette smokers and is associated with known carcinogens including occupational exposures such as those of rubber and oil refinery workers. In addition, patients treated with cyclophosphamide (Cytoxan) have up to a ninefold increased risk of developing bladder cancer. This is believed to be secondary to acrolein, a urinary metabolite of cyclophosphamide.

Approximately 90% of bladder malignancies are transitional cell carcinomas. Of these, 70% of tumors are papillary, 10% are sessile, and 20% are mixed. Approximately 20% to 25% of noninvasive tumors progress to muscle invasion during follow-up. However, of patients with muscular invasive bladder cancer, approximately 80% to 90% have invasion at the time of initial presentation. A strong correlation exists between tumor grade and stage; most well-differentiated tumors are superficial and most poorly differentiated tumors are invasive. Carcinoma in situ (CIS) is a poorly differentiated transitional cell carcinoma that is confined to the urothelium. CIS may be found as a solitary or multifocal process and is found in association with invasive carcinoma in approximately 25% of cases. It is associated with a poor prognosis. Between 10% and 20% of patients treated with cystectomy for diffuse CIS are found to have microscopic muscle-invasive disease.

Diagnosis

Gross painless hematuria is a common presenting sign of bladder cancer. However, approximately 20% of patients may present with only microscopic hematuria. Irritative voiding symptoms such as frequency and urgency may also suggest a malignancy, particularly CIS. Patients suspected of bladder cancer should undergo an evaluation of their upper tracts (IVP or CT scan), cystoscopy, and cytologic examination of the urine. Transurethral biopsy or resection confirms the diagnosis.

CURRENT DIAGNOSIS

Carcinoma of the Bladder

- Painless, gross hematuria is the most common presenting symptom.
- 20% may present with only microscopic hematuria.
- Irritative voiding symptoms such as frequency and urgency may also suggest a malignancy, particularly CIS.
- Patients suspected of bladder cancer should undergo an evaluation of their upper tracts (IVP or CT scan), cystoscopy, and cytologic examination of the urine.
- Transurethral biopsy or resection confirms the diagnosis.
- 90% of bladder cancers are transitional cell carcinoma, and 80% are nonmuscle invasive (superficial) at presentation.

Abbreviations: CIS = carcinoma in situ; CT = computed tomography; IVP = intravenous pyelogram.

Treatment

Management of bladder carcinoma depends on tumor stage. The TNM system is recommended for staging. For most superficial bladder carcinomas, transurethral resection of the tumor is often the only treatment required. However, for CIS or high-grade superficial tumors, tumors that involve the lamina propria (stage T1), and rapidly recurrent tumors, treatment with intravesical agents such as thiotepa (Thioplex), doxorubicin (Adriamycin), and mitomycin C (Mutamycin)[1] or intravesical bacillus Calmette-Guérin (BCG, Tice) may be indicated.

---

[1]Not FDA approved for this indication.

CURRENT THERAPY

Carcinoma of the Bladder

- Treatment depends on tumor stage.
- Superficial bladder (Ta) cancers are managed with transurethral resection.
- CIS or high-grade stage Ta, tumors that involve the lamina propria (stage T1), and recurrent tumors are managed with transurethral resection and intravesical therapy such as thiotepa (Thioplex), doxorubicin (Adriamycin), and mitomycin C (Mutamycin)[1] or intravesical bacillus Calmette-Guérin (BCG, Tice).
- Bladder surveillance is mandatory because the recurrence rate in the bladder may be as high as 50% at 5 years.
- Surveillance protocols include cystoscopy and urinary cytologic examinations every 3 months for the first year, every 4 months for the second year, semiannually in year 3, and annually thereafter.
- Periodic evaluation of the upper tracts should be performed as well.
- In superficial tumors that progress in stage or fail conservative therapy and in those that invade the bladder muscle (stages T2–3), a radical cystectomy and urinary diversion is the treatment of choice.
- Urinary diversion may be either incontinent (conduit) or continent (orthotopic or continent cutaneous).
- Five-year survival rates are 85%–60% after cystectomy for stages T2a and T2b, respectively. For stage T3a and T3b tumors, the 5-year survival decreases to 60% and 40%, respectively, whereas patients with node-positive disease have a 5-year survival of <30%.
- Patients with T2–T4 disease may be offered either neoadjuvant or adjuvant chemotherapy. There have been reports of modest survival advantages (<10%) using MVAC in the neoadjuvant setting.
- Patients with M1 disease are generally treated with chemotherapy as well.
- The standard regimen over the past decade has been methotrexate (Trexall),[1] vinblastine (Velban),[1] doxorubicin (Adriamycin), and cisplatin (Platinol) (MVAC); however, durable complete response rates are <15%.
- Newer agents such as gemcitabine (Gemzar) along with cisplatin appear to offer similar response rates and reduced toxicity.

---

[1]Not FDA approved for this indication.
Abbreviations: CIS = carcinoma in situ.

Bladder surveillance is mandatory because the recurrence rate in the bladder may be as high as 50% at 5 years. Surveillance protocols include cystoscopy and urinary cytologies every 3 months for the first year, every 4 months for the second year, semiannually in year 3, and annually thereafter. Periodic evaluation of the upper tract should be performed to rule out the presence of carcinoma of the bladder in that area.

The risk of progression to muscle invasive disease is relatively low (less than 10%) for stage Ta tumors but increases as tumor stage advances (stage T1) or with high-grade lesions. For superficial tumors that progress in stage or fail conservative therapy, and in those that invade the bladder muscle (stage T2 to T3), a radical cystectomy is the treatment of choice. In addition, a thorough lymphadenectomy is performed at the time of surgery; there have been reports of improved survival based on the completeness of the dissection.

Each year there are an estimated 13,180 deaths in the United States from bladder cancer. Five-year survival rates are approximately 85% to 60% after cystectomy for stages T2a and T2b, respectively. For stage T3a and T3b tumors, the 5-year survival decreases to 60% and 40%, whereas patients with node-positive disease have a 5-year survival of less than 30%. Adjuvant chemotherapy is generally offered to patients at high risk for failure (pathologic stages T3b, T4, and N1/2 disease). The standard regimen over the past decade has been methotrexate (Trexall),[1] vinblastine (Velban),[1] doxorubicin (Adriamycin), and cisplatin (Platinol) (MVAC); however, durable complete response rates have been less than 15%. There have been recent reports of modest survival advantages (less than 10%) using MVAC in the neoadjuvant setting. Newer agents such as gemcitabine (Gemzar)[1] along with cisplatin appear to offer similar response rates and reduced toxicity.

Urinary diversion may be accomplished with an ileal or colon conduit, which requires wearing a collection appliance. A continent cutaneous diversion may be created; most often using the right colon with a tapered and a catheterizable efferent limb of ileum (Indiana pouch) or with creation of a nipple valve (Koch pouch). Approximately 50% of cystectomy patients undergo continent diversion. An orthotopic neobladder allows creation of a reservoir using detubularized ileum or colon with direct anastomosis to the urethra. With the development of orthotopic urinary diversion, functional status and quality of life among patients following cystectomy has improved significantly.

Adenocarcinoma of the Bladder

Adenocarcinomas account for less than 2% of bladder cancers. They are classified into three groups: primary bladder, urachal, and metastatic. Most adenocarcinomas are poorly differentiated and invasive. They are commonly associated with cystitis glandularis rather than CIS. Adenocarcinomas also are found in association with bladder augmentations. Adenocarcinoma is the most common type of cancer in patients with bladder exstrophy. Radical cystectomy with pelvic lymphadenectomy is the treatment of choice.

Squamous Cell Carcinoma of the Bladder

Squamous cell carcinoma accounts for approximately 6% of bladder cancers in the United States but more than 75% of bladder cancers in Egypt. Chronic bladder inflammation, as occurs with chronic indwelling Foley catheters, recurrent bladder infections, or bladder diverticula, is associated with an increase risk of squamous cell carcinoma. Approximately 80% of squamous cell carcinomas in Egypt are associated with *Schistosoma haematobium* infestation. These cancers are known as bilharzial bladder cancers and occur in atients 10 to 20 years younger than those affected with transitional cell carcinoma. The prognosis for squamous cell carcinoma is

---

[1]Not FDA approved for this indication.

CURRENT DIAGNOSIS

Urethral Carcinoma

- Urethral carcinoma is the only urologic malignancy that is more common in females than males.
- 50% of cases are associated with urethral stricture.
- May present as hematuria, obstructive voiding, or a palpable mass.
- Transurethral biopsy is usually required for diagnosis.

generally poor, and radical cystectomy is the standard treatment for patients who are surgical candidates. Chemotherapy, particularly regimens used in transitional cell carcinoma, is not effective in squamous cell carcinoma. The benefit of neoadjuvant radiation therapy prior to radical cystectomy is unproved in patients with squamous cell carcinoma with the possible exception of bilharzial cancers.

URETHRAL CARCINOMA

Diagnosis

Urethral carcinoma is the only urologic malignancy that is more common in women than men. It usually occurs after 60 years of age. Although the etiology remains undetermined, approximately 50% of cases are associated with urethral stricture. A patient should be evaluated for urethral carcinoma when a urethral mass is palpable, obstruction does not respond to conventional stricture management, a urethral abscess and/or fistula occurs, hematuria is present, or inguinal adenopathy becomes evident. The treatment of the primary tumor is surgical excision. Urethrectomy is performed via a perineal incision. Proximal tumors of the bulbar urethra are managed with cystoprostatectomy and en bloc urethrectomy.

Although the etiology of female urethral carcinoma remains obscure, there is an association with urethral malakoplakia and urethral caruncles. Most patients are white and older than 50 years. The usual presenting symptom is a papillary or fungating urethral mass and hematuria.

Treatment

For tumors of the proximal urethra or in cases of extension into adjacent structures, cystectomy with en bloc urethrectomy and anterior vaginectomy along with pelvic lymphadenectomy are usually required. Radiation therapy also provides local control in selected cases. In advanced cases, multimodality treatment with chemotherapy

CURRENT THERAPY

Urethral Carcinoma

- Treatment of the primary tumor is surgical excision and varies based on location and stage of tumor.
- In men, urethrectomy is performed via a perineal incision.
- Proximal tumors of the bulbar urethra are managed with cystoprostatectomy and en bloc urethrectomy.
- Among women, tumors of the proximal urethra or, in cases of extension, into adjacent structures, cystectomy with en bloc urethrectomy and anterior vaginectomy along with pelvic lymphadenectomy are usually required.
- Radiation therapy is also reported to provide local control in selective cases.

CURRENT DIAGNOSIS

Penile Cancer

- Squamous cell carcinoma of the penis occurs most commonly in the sixth decade.
- Symptoms are related to ulceration, necrosis, suppuration, and hemorrhage of the penile lesion.
- Clinical evaluation of patients with penile cancer includes physical examination with palpation of the inguinal region, liver function tests, chest radiograph, computed tomography of the abdomen and pelvis, and bone scan.

and either surgical excision or radiation therapy provides the best chance for cure, although to date no specific regimen has emerged as standard treatment.

PENILE CANCER

Diagnosis

Penile cancer is relatively rare in the United States. Poor personal hygiene and retained phimotic foreskin are implicated in the etiology of penile carcinoma. Penile cancer is extremely rare in men circumcised at birth. Squamous cell carcinoma of the penis occurs most commonly in the sixth decade. The symptoms are related to ulceration, necrosis, suppuration, and hemorrhage of the penile lesion. The clinical evaluation of patients with penile cancer includes physical examination with palpation of the inguinal region, liver function tests, chest radiograph, CT of the abdomen and pelvis, and bone scan.

CURRENT THERAPY

Penile Cancer

- Small penile cancers limited to the prepuce can be treated by circumcision alone.
- Partial penectomy with at least a 1-cm margin of normal tissue is used to treat smaller (2–5 cm) distal penile tumors. The remaining penis should be long enough to permit voiding in the standing position. The 5-year cure rate for patients treated with partial penectomy is 70%–80%.
- Larger distal penile lesions or proximal tumors require total penectomy and perineal urethrostomy. If the scrotum, pubis, or abdominal wall is involved, radical en bloc excision may be necessary.
- Many have inguinal lymphadenopathy at presentation. However, inguinal lymph node enlargement before excision of the primary tumor may be the result of infection and not metastatic disease. Thus, clinical assessment of the inguinal region should be delayed 4–6 wk, during which time the patient is treated with antibiotics.
- If inguinal lymphadenopathy persists or develops, there is a high likelihood of metastatic disease, and ilioinguinal lymphadenectomy should be performed. The procedure is performed on the contralateral side if the initial side contains tumor and could be simultaneously performed or staged.
- Radiation of the primary tumor and regional lymph nodes is an alternative to surgery in patients with small (≤2 cm) low-stage tumors.

Treatment

The TNM stage is based primarily on depth of invasion and usually dictates treatment. Small penile cancers limited to the prepuce can be treated by circumcision alone. Partial penectomy with at least a 1-cm margin of normal tissue is used to treat smaller (2 to 5 cm) distal penile tumors. The remaining penis should be long enough to permit voiding in the standing position. The 5-year cure rate for patients treated with partial penectomy is 70% to 80%. Larger distal penile lesions or proximal tumors require total penectomy and perineal urethrostomy. If the scrotum, pubis, or abdominal wall is involved, radical en bloc excision may be necessary.

Many patients have inguinal lymphadenopathy at presentation. However, inguinal lymph node enlargement before excision of the primary tumor may be the result of infection and not metastatic disease. Clinical assessment of the inguinal region thus should be delayed 4 to 6 weeks during which time the patient is treated with antibiotics. If inguinal lymphadenopathy persists or develops, there is a high likelihood of metastatic disease, and ilioinguinal lymphadenectomy should be performed. However, if inguinal lymphadenopathy resolves, prophylactic lymph node dissection may not be necessary. Radiation of the primary tumor and regional lymph nodes is an alternative to surgery in patients with small (2 cm or less) low-stage tumors.

TESTICULAR CANCER

Malignant disease of the testes can be divided into germinal neoplasms, which includes seminomatous and nonseminomatous germ cell tumors (NSGCTs) and secondary neoplasms. Ninety-five percent of tumors originating in the testis are germ cell tumors. Fewer than 10% of all germ cell tumors arise from extragonadal primary sites. The mediastinum and retroperitoneum are the most common extragonadal sites. Testicular cancer, although relatively rare, represents the most common malignancy in men in the 15- to 35-year-old age group, with 8010 new cases occurring annually.

Testicular cancer has become one of the most curable solid neoplasms and serves as a paradigm for the multimodal treatment of malignancies. The dramatic improvement in survival resulting from the combination of effective diagnostic techniques, improved tumor markers, effective multidrug chemotherapeutic regimens, and modifications of surgical technique has led to a decrease in patient mortality from greater than 50% before 1970 to less than 10% currently.

Germ cell tumors are seen principally in the white population. Recent data show a ratio of approximately 5:1 in white versus black individuals, and a report from the U.S. military showed a relative incidence of 40:1. The cause of germ cell tumors is unknown. Familial clustering is observed, particularly among siblings. Cryptorchidism and Klinefelter's syndrome are predisposing factors in the development of germ cell tumors arising from the testis and mediastinum, respectively. Orchidopexy performed before puberty may not reduce the risk of germ cell tumors but improves the ability to observe the testis.

Diagnosis

A painless testicular mass is pathognomonic of a primary testicular tumor. This occurs in a minority of patients. The majority of testicular tumors present with diffuse testicular pain, swelling, hardness, or some combination of these findings. Because infectious epididymo-orchitis is more common than a testicular tumor, a trial of antibiotics is often undertaken. If testicular discomfort does not abate or the findings do not revert to normal within 2 to 4 weeks, testicular sonography is indicated. A radical inguinal orchiectomy with ligation of the spermatic cord at the internal ring is required for all patients with suspected testicular tumors.

Regional metastasis first appears in the retroperitoneal lymph nodes below the renal vessels. Right testicular tumors usually metastasize to nodes between the aorta and inferior vena cava (interaortocaval nodes), and left testicular tumors to nodes lateral to the aorta (para-aortic). Left supraclavicular adenopathy and pulmonary nodules may occur with or without retroperitoneal disease. CT scan of the abdomen and pelvis and chest radiography are required. Lymph nodes in the primary lymphatic drainage areas (landing zones) of their respective affected testicle that measure between 1 and 2 cm are involved by germ cell tumors in approximately 70% of cases. CT imaging of the chest is required if mediastinal, hilar, or lung parenchymal disease is suspected.

CURRENT DIAGNOSIS

Testicular Cancer

- Testicular cancer, although relatively rare, represents the most common malignancy in males in the 15- to 35-year-old age group, with 8010 new cases annually.
- Usually presents as a painless enlarging testicular mass.
- Malignant disease of the testes can be divided into germinal neoplasms, which includes seminomatous and nonseminomatous germ cell tumors, and secondary neoplasms.
- 95% of tumors originating in the testis are germ cell tumors. Fewer than 10% of all germ cell tumors arise from extragonadal primary sites. The mediastinum and retroperitoneum are the most common extragonadal sites.
- Testicular cancer is one of the few neoplasms associated with accurate serum markers, β-hCG, and AFP.

Treatment

Testicular cancer is one of the few neoplasms associated with accurate serum markers, human β-chorionic gonadotropin (β-hCG), and α-fetoprotein (AFP). These accurate tumor markers allow careful follow-up and intervention earlier in the course of disease. AFP production is restricted to NSGCTs, specifically embryonal carcinoma and yolk sac tumor. Patients with an increased AFP and the finding of pure seminoma on pathologic examination of the orchiectomy specimen should be treated as a NSGCT. Increased serum concentrations of β-hCG may be observed in both seminomatous and nonseminomatous tumors. Increased concentrations of β-hCG are seen in 40% to 60% of patients with metastatic NSGCT and 15% to 20% of patients with metastatic seminomas. A third serum marker, lactate dehydrogenase, is less specific but has independent prognostic value in patients with advanced germ cell tumors. Serum lactate dehydrogenase concentrations are also increased in approximately 60% of patients with NSGCT and 80% of those with seminomatous germ cell tumors.

Increased concentrations of α-fetoprotein, β-hCG, or both without radiographic or clinical findings imply active disease and are sufficient reason to initiate treatment if likely causes of false-positive results are ruled out. The serum half-lives of α-fetoprotein and β-hCG are 5 to 7 days and 30 hours, respectively. Slow clearance suggests residual active disease.

Histologically, seminoma is the most common germ cell tumor, and it is initially considered to be good risk because of its favorable response to treatment. Therapy for low-stage (stages 1, 2a, or 2b) seminomas following radical inguinal orchiectomy is irradiation to the retroperitoneal and ipsilateral pelvic lymph nodes. Relapse recurs in approximately 4% of patients with stage 1 seminomas and 10% of patients with stage 2a or 2b seminomas. Chemotherapy cures more than 90% of patients who have a relapse after radiation therapy. Thus, approximately 99% of patients with low-stage seminomas are cured.

NSGCTs include embryonal cell carcinoma, choriocarcinoma, yolk sac carcinoma, teratoma, and mixed germ cell tumors. The rate of cure for patients with NSGCTs in clinical stage 1 exceeds 95%.

CURRENT THERAPY

Testicular Cancer

- A radical inguinal orchiectomy with ligation of spermatic cord at the internal ring is required for all patients with suspected testicular tumors.
- Once a diagnosis is made, serum tumor markers are determined before, during, and after treatment.
- Radiographic staging is performed with a CT scan of the chest/abdomen/pelvis.
- Histologically, seminoma is the most common germ cell tumor, and is initially considered good risk because of its generally favorable response to treatment. Therapy for low-stage (stage 1, 2a, or 2b) seminomas following radical inguinal orchiectomy is irradiation to the retroperitoneal and ipsilateral pelvic lymph nodes. Relapse occurs in approximately 4% of patients with stage 1 seminomas and 10% of patients with stage 2a or 2b seminomas. Chemotherapy cures >90% of patients who have a relapse after radiation therapy. Thus, approximately 99% of patients with low-stage seminomas are cured.
- NSGCTs include embryonal cell carcinoma, choriocarcinoma, yolk sac carcinoma, teratoma, and mixed germ cell tumors. The rate of cure for patients with NSGCTs in clinical stage 1 exceeds 95%.
- Surveillance and RPLND are both standard treatment options for this group of patients. Twenty percent of clinical stage 1 NSGCT patients have lymph node involvement, and those with vascular invasion or predominance of embryonal cell carcinoma are at increased risk (50%).
- RPLND is a major abdominal operation in which lymph nodes from the retroperitoneum are removed from the renal hilum down to the level of the common iliac artery, with lateral margins being confined by the ureters.
- Patients found to have node-positive disease are generally recommended for chemotherapy with usually two cycles.
- Patients with persistently increased concentrations of AFP, β-hCG, or both but without other clinical evidence of disease following orchiectomy usually have systemic disease and are treated with chemotherapy.

Testicular Cancer

- Initial chemotherapy is required in approximately one third of patients with germ cell tumors. Because relapse is frequent in patients with clinical stage 2c disease or in patients with primary retroperitoneal or mediastinal seminomas who receive radiation alone, these patients are treated initially with chemotherapy. Patients also receive initial chemotherapy if they have stage 3 NSGCTs or multifocal retroperitoneal lymph node involvement, lymph nodes >3 cm in diameter, or tumor-related back pain.
- Postchemotherapy RPLND is usually reserved for residual masses (>3 cm) in patients after treatment for seminoma. In NSGCT, the need for postchemotherapy RPLND is controversial. Some advocate surgery in all patients with initial bulky retroperitoneal disease, whereas others advocate observation rather than surgery in patients with >90% shrinkage of retroperitoneal nodes, no residual nodes >1.5 cm, and no teratomatous elements in the primary tumor.
- Owing in part to the multimodality approach to these tumors, 90%–95% of patients are ultimately cured of their disease.

Abbreviations: AFP = α-fetoprotein; β-hCG = β-chorionic gonadotropin; CT = computed tomography; NSGCT = nonseminomatous germ cell tumor; RPLND = retroperitoneal lymph node dissection.

Twenty percent of patients with stage 1 tumors with no lymphatic or vascular invasion or invasion into the tunica albuginea, spermatic cord, or scrotum are discovered to have regional lymph node or distant metastasis. Surveillance and nerve-sparing retroperitoneal lymph node dissection (RPLND) are both standard treatment options for this group of patients. If patients have stage 1 disease confined to the testes, attention must be paid to the surgical pathology. In any patient with embryonal histology or the presence of lymphovascular invasion or extension beyond the tunica albuginea, RPLND is recommended. The rationale for this treatment stems from a 30% relapse rate in stage 1 patients with these findings.

RPLND is a major abdominal operation in which lymph nodes from the retroperitoneum are removed from the renal hilum down to the level of the common iliac artery, with lateral margins confined by the ureters. In the past, this procedure resulted in lack of ejaculation and infertility in 100% of patients. By performing a modified-template RPLND, the contralateral area of aorta below the inferior mesenteric artery is not manipulated. This maneuver serves to preserve the confluence of sympathetic fibers along the aorta that are responsible for ejaculation, with a 60% to 88% rate of preservation of ejdculation and no reports of recurrence for stage 1 disease. Patients with persistently increased concentrations of α-fetoprotein, β-hCG, or both but without other clinical evidence of disease following orchiectomy usually have systemic disease. These patients should undergo three or four cycles of standard chemotherapy rather than surgery.

Patients with stage 2 NSGCTs are treated initially with either RPLND or chemotherapy depending on the extent of the disease, serum tumor marker concentrations, and the presence or absence of tumor-related symptoms. Asymptomatic patients with solitary retroperitoneal lymph nodes less than 3 cm in diameter as assessed by CT imaging generally undergo retroperitoneal lymph node dissection, whereas bulky stage 2 disease (more than 5 cm) undergo initial chemotherapy. Recurrences within the retroperitoneum are rare after a properly performed operation.

Adjuvant chemotherapy is an important consideration when any lymph node is more than 2 cm in diameter, at least six nodes are involved, or there is extranodal invasion. The majority of patients in this group who relapsed did not receive adjuvant chemotherapy. Although the rate of cure is the same when chemotherapy is withheld until relapse, patients who received adjuvant therapy require fewer cycles of chemotherapy and avoid additional surgery.

Initial chemotherapy is required in approximately one third of patients with germ cell tumors. Because relapse is frequent in patients with clinical stage 2c disease or in patients with primary retroperitoneal or mediastinal seminomas who receive radiation alone, these patients are treated initially with chemotherapy. Patients also receive initial chemotherapy if they have stage 3 NSGCTs or multifocal retroperitoneal lymph node involvement, lymph nodes more than 2 cm in diameter, or tumor-related back pain.

Postchemotherapy RPLND is usually reserved for residual masses (more than 3 cm) in patients after treatment for seminoma. In NSGCT, the need for postchemotherapy RPLND is controversial. Some groups advocate surgery in all patients with initial bulky retroperitoneal disease, whereas others advocate observation rather than surgery in patients with greater than 90% shrinkage of retroperitoneal nodes, with no residual nodes greater than 1.5 cm, and with no teratomatous elements in the primary tumor. There is no debate, however, concerning the need for removal of any significant postchemotherapy residual mass.

The first combination chemotherapy regimens containing cisplatin (Platinol), vinblastine (Velban), and bleomycin (Blenoxane) resulted in complete remission in 70% to 80% of patients with metastatic germ cell tumors. Subsequent studies show that prolonged maintenance chemotherapy was unnecessary, and vinblastine was replaced by etoposide (Vepesid), which is less toxic and probably more efficacious. Serious adverse effects of combination chemotherapy include neuromuscular toxic affects, death from myelosuppression for bleomycin-induced pulmonary fibrosis, and Raynaud's phenomenon.

Leydig cell tumors make up between 1% and 3% of all testicular tumors. Although the majority of cases are recognized in men between

20 and 60 years of age, approximately a fourth are reported before puberty. The prognosis for Leydig cell tumors following radical inguinal orchiectomy is good because of their generally benign nature.

Gonadoblastoma is a rare tumor occurring almost exclusively in patients with some form of gonadal dysgenesis. Gonadoblastomas constitute approximately 0.5% of all testicular neoplasms and occur in all age groups from infancy to beyond 70 years, although the majority occur in individuals younger than 30 years. Radical orchiectomy is the first step in therapy. The high incidence of bilaterality (50%) mandates a contralateral gonadectomy when gonadal dysgenesis is present. The prognosis is excellent for patients with gonadoblastoma.

The most common secondary neoplasm of the testis and the most frequent of all testicular tumors in patients older than 50 years is lymphoma. The median age is approximately 60 years of age. As with lymphomas elsewhere, patients with poorly differentiated lymphocytic types tend to survive longer than those with the histocytic type. Survival is poor with bilateral disease and among patients presenting with lymphoma at other sites who later experience a testicular tumor relapse. However, among those patients with disease apparently confined to the testis, survival appears to be good.

REFERENCES

Carver BS, Sheinfeld J: Germ cell tumors of the testis. Ann Surg Oncol 2005;12:871.
Cohen HT, McGovern FJ: Renal-cell carcinoma. N Engl J Med 2005;353:2477.
Cooperberg MR, Moul JW, Carroll PR: The changing face of prostate cancer. J Clin Oncol 2005;23:8146.
Jemal A, Murray T, Ward E, et al: Cancer statistics, 2005. CA Cancer J Clin 2005;55:10.
Stein JP, Lieskovsky G, Cote R, et al: Radical cystectomy in the treatment of invasive bladder cancer: Long-term results in 1,054 patients. J Clin Oncol 2001;19:666.

Urethral Stricture Disease

Method of
Mahreen Hussain, BSc (Hons), MRCS, and
Tamsin J. Greenwell, MD

Definition

Urethral stricture disease covers a spectrum of pathology ranging from post-traumatic ischemia to postgonococcal inflammation, the end results of which are scarring and narrowing of the urethral lumen.

Pathogenesis

The first identifiable pathologic feature of urethral stricture disease is a change in the lining of the urethra from pseudostratified columnar epithelium to squamous epithelium. Squamous epithelium lacks elasticity. Consequently, tiny cracks develop, allowing urine to escape through the urethra into the surrounding tissues, which leads to inflammation and scarring.

Anatomy

The male urethra is approximately 20 cm long and is divided into five specific anatomic sections. The prostatic urethra leads to the membranous urethra, which passes through the pelvic floor and the external urethral sphincter. Together they make up the posterior urethra. The anterior urethra lies within the corpus spongiosum of the penis. It consists of the bulbar (38-40 Fr) and penile portions, ending distally with the navicular fossa, which at 26 Fr is the narrowest part of the urethra.

The duality of the blood supply to the urethra ensures that ischemia does not ensue following surgical repair requiring detachment of the urethra proximally or distally. The deep penile structures receive their arterial supply from the common penile artery, the terminal branch of the internal pudendal artery. The common penile artery gives off several branches that include the bulbourethral, cavernosal, and deep dorsal penile arteries. The corpus spongiosum receives a dual blood supply via anastomoses between the deep dorsal penile artery and urethral artery branches in the glans.

Etiology

Urethral strictures occur secondary to scarring caused by inflammation, infection, or trauma. The most common cause worldwide of anterior urethral strictures is gonococcal infection, but in the developed world anterior urethral strictures are most commonly idiopathic (probably consequent to prior unidentified infection or trauma) followed by iatrogenic from urethral catheterization and instrumentation or following repair of hypospadias. Fall-astride injuries or perineal blunt trauma related to cycling or sports can also cause anterior urethral strictures; presentation may be late, with voiding difficulties.

Trauma is the commonest cause of posterior urethral stricture formation. During pelvic fracture from blunt trauma, the bulbomembranous junction is the most likely area be injured because it may be sheared from the more rigidly fixed prostatic apex, or bony injury can disrupt the attaching puboprostatic ligaments and allow upward dissociation of the prostate. Iatrogenic injury is a rarer cause of stricture in the posterior urethra and most commonly occurs following radical prostatectomy or transurethral resection of the prostate.

Lichen sclerosis et atrophicus (balanitis xerotica obliterans) is a chronic inflammatory condition of unknown etiology (possibly related to *Borrelia* infection). It is more common in uncircumcised men and leads to scarring of the foreskin and glans and, in a significant minority, anterior urethral stricture.

Other rare causes of stricture disease include urethral ischemia following coronary artery bypass surgery and urethral carcinoma. True congenital strictures, although extremely rare, are due to inadequate fusion of the anterior and posterior urethra. The most common sites are the fossa navicularis and membranous urethra.

CURRENT DIAGNOSIS

- Diagnosis can be made on symptoms alone, including reduced flow rate, reduced ejaculatory force, urinary tract infections, and retention.
- All patients should be assessed with a flow rate and ascending and descending urethrogram.
- Cystoscopy should only be performed if a malignant cause is suspected or if the decision has been made to treat the stricture endoscopically.
- It is important to differentiate between posterior (mostly membranous) and anterior (bulbar or penile) strictures, because the treatments and prognoses differ.
- It is important to assess erectile function preoperatively because erectile dysfunction is not only a side effect of surgery but also can affect the outcome of stricture surgery if it is present preoperatively.

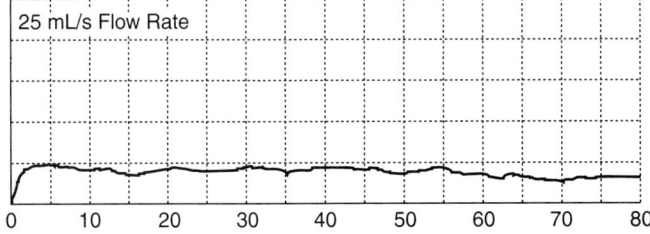

FIGURE 1. A typical urinary flow trace from a man with a urethral stricture.

Acquired strictures in children are usually iatrogenic following hypospadias repair or are secondary to pelvic fractures. The long-term outcomes tend to be worse in children because they have no prostate to protect their urethra during trauma and have immature neurovascular bundles, which are easily damaged.

Diagnosis and Investigation

A detailed focused history should be taken. Common symptoms include poor stream, frequency, hesitancy, straining and, incomplete emptying of the bladder. Some also complain of nocturia and a reduction of ejaculatory force. Symptoms may be due to the presence of a urinary tract infection secondary to urinary stasis, which may in turn lead to prostatitis or epididymo-orchitis. Less commonly, patients present with acute urinary retention and might require suprapubic catheterization.

Completion of the International Prostate Symptom Score questionnaire can give a more objective assessment of the severity of the symptoms and allow early detection of stricture recurrence during follow-up. It is best to document the patient's preoperative erectile function because this can affect the outcome of or be affected by stricture surgery.

A thorough examination of the external genitalia can reveal lichen sclerosis et atrophicus at the meatus or the foreskin. Epididymo-orchitis and prostatitis can be diagnosed by the presence of tender testes or a tender prostate on digital rectal examination, with or without fever. A brief review of the buccal mucosa and posterior auricular region might also prove useful if the use of free graft is a possibility.

A midstream urine specimen is sent to exclude a urinary tract infection. Baseline renal function blood tests are sent if indicated, and a flow rate (Fig. 1) and postvoid residual volume are documented. An ascending and descending urethrogram is always performed to identify the exact number, location, and extent of the stricture(s).

A renal tract ultrasound scan may be performed if upper tract damage is suspected. A Doppler ultrasound of the penile arteries after intracavernosal prostaglandin injection is obtained preoperatively in all men with erectile dysfunction who have suffered urethral injury as a consequence of pelvic fracture.

Treatment

There are two main treatment options: endoscopic or open.

The endoscopic procedures include urethral dilation, performed under local or general anesthetic, direct vision internal urethrotomy (DVIU), and insertion of a urethral stent. For first-time short (<0.5 cm) bulbar strictures, both dilation and DVIU offer cure in up to 50% of cases when cure is defined as stricture-free status at 48 months after the procedure. For recurrent, multiple, or longer strictures and strictures in other locations, these procedures are never curative and provide palliation only. If the first urethrotomy or dilation fails, the patient should be offered the options of urethroplasty or further dilation or DVIU followed by clean intermittent self-catheterization (CISC).

CURRENT THERAPY

- Therapy is endoscopic or open.
- Endoscopic therapy is palliative (in the majority) or curative (<0.5 cm bulbar stricture).
- Endoscopic treatment is used for urethral dilation, direct visual internal urethrotomy, urethral stent, and clean intermittent self-catheterization.
- Open treatment is used for urethroplasty. The type depends on site, number, length, and etiology of the stricture.
- Anastomotic urethroplasty is the procedure of choice where possible.
- Substitution urethroplasty may use a free graft or a tissue flap on a pedicle.

A good case can be made for primary urethroplasty. For short bulbar urethral strictures, urethroplasty has an 80% to 90% 10-year success rate versus a 50% 4-year success rate with dilation or DVIU. A second urethrotomy only cures 25% of those in this good-outcome group. A third urethrotomy is palliative only and can extend the stricture, adversely affecting the outcome of a potential future urethroplasty.

Dilation and DVIU can cause urinary tract infection, sepsis, and bleeding. Longer strictures or extrabulbar strictures are virtually never cured by dilation or urethrotomy—and the patient must therefore perform CISC or have urethroplasty.

Urethral stents had been popularized in the past as a minimally invasive cure for urethral stricture disease. There are two main types: permanent (UroLume wall stent) and removable (thermoexpandable Memokath). These stents work best in urethras with minimal scarring and spongiofibrosis. At best, stents provide long-term stricture control in less than 50% and cause significant side effects such as post-micturition dribble, urethral discomfort, stent migration, and reduced ejaculatory volume, making them unsuitable for young, fit men. Removal of a stent (in particular, the wall stent) can be complex and require extensive reconstructive surgery. Long-term outcome studies of urethral stents suggest that their real use is in stricture management in the elderly, the infirm, and those who refuse urethroplasty and run into difficulties with dilation or DVIU.

Strictures may be repaired with either an anastomotic or substitution urethroplasty as a one- or two-stage procedure. The choice of procedure depends on the stricture site and the length and number of strictures. Cure rates vary depending on the stricture etiology, site, and length, which in turn dictate the type of urethroplasty performed.

The anastomotic repair is a single-stage procedure. It has an excellent long-term success rate (80%-90% at 10 years) and a lower complication rate, and it is the procedure of choice in short bulbar (<1.0 cm) and prostatomembranous (any length) strictures. The strictured area is completely excised and the two healthy ends of urethra widely spatulated and anastomosed. A four-stage transperineal progression approach is used in a stepwise fashion to ensure a tension-free anastomosis for bulboprostatic strictures. Very occasionally, a combined abdominoperineal approach is used for very long bulboprostatic strictures.

Longer bulbar urethral strictures are treated using an augmented free graft anastomotic urethroplasty, which allows stricture excision and is suitable for strictures shorter than 2.0 cm or a Barbagli dorsal onlay free graft patch urethroplasty for strictures longer than 2.0 cm. Restricturing usually results from ischemia; the 5-year restricture rate is 10% to 25%. The long-term results of substitution urethroplasty compare less favorably with those of anastomotic repair. This primarily reflects the increased severity of the underlying stricture disease—site, length and etiology—and to a lesser degree might reflect the fact that a urethral tissue substitute is never as good as native urethra.

For substitution in the bulbar urethra, a dorsal or ventral stricturotomy and patch with flap (penile) or free graft (buccal mucosal or post auricular) may be performed as a single-stage procedure. Dorsal stricturotomy results in less bleeding than ventral stricturotomy, because the thinnest part of the corpus spongiosum is incised. It also allows rigid fixation and hence support of free grafts or flaps. Access is more difficult for patch placement following dorsal than ventral stricturotomy. Penile or scrotal skin flaps can be used; however, there is a higher rate of pouch formation with flaps compared with free grafts in this situation. Ventral stricturotomy is the preferred procedure for repairing complex strictures and in highly scarred or ischemic tissues where the blood supply is poor, when a penile or scrotal skin flap is the patch of choice.

Penile strictures always require some form of substitution urethroplasty. Anastomotic urethroplasty is generally inadvisable due to the development of chordee on erection after excision of even the shortest strictures. A local penile skin flap is easier and as effective as a graft, and the ventral approach is easier and as effective as the dorsal approach for uncomplicated penile strictures: the Orandi urethroplasty. The 5-year stricture-free rate is 80% to 85%. This is lower than that seen following bulbar and prostatomembranous urethral stricture repair, probably because penile urethral strictures are longer and often tighter and more complex, and the penile urethra is more mobile and hostile to successful graft or flap take.

Longer penile strictures due to lichen sclerosis et atrophicus or following previous surgery for hypospadias may be best served with a staged approach, with excision of the severely diseased urethra and a two-stage circumferential repair. In lichen sclerosis et atrophicus, buccal mucosal graft should be used because lichen sclerosis rapidly recurs in genital skin grafts, it recurs with time in extragenital skin grafts, and it has been reported in only one or two cases of buccal mucosal graft in the literature. The comparatively low restricture rate at 5 years (15%-25%) results from having adequate tissue for both tubularization and subsequent skin closure without tension and an adequate-caliber urethrostomy. There is a significant revision rate after the first and second stages, which is a reflection of the extent and severity of the stricture disease in the penile urethra.

The restricture rates at 3 years when urethroplasty is the primary treatment are about 8%. When urethroplasty is performed after previous endoscopic treatment, the restricture rate at 3 years is 12%, and when it is performed after previous failed urethroplasty it is 18%. This makes a good case for offering patients urethroplasty as the primary treatment for urethral stricture disease as opposed to endoscopic therapies; however, the side effects must be taken into account. These include a 20%-30% temporary erectile dysfunction rate (up to 12 months), a 1%-11% permanent erectile dysfunction rate (penile urethra, 1%; bulbar urethra, 2%; prostatic urethra, 11%), a 75% postmicturition dribble rate, and a 2% wound infection rate.

Future Directions

The search for an ideal urethra substitute could lie within the realms of tissue engineering. What better substitute than native urethra itself? Free grafts currently serve their purpose well but are not without the complications of the additional procedure required for graft retrieval, donor site morbidity, and possible prolonged hospital stay.

Materials such as laboratory-grown acellular collagen matrix provide an attractive alternative, particularly because short-term follow-up suggests excellent results. Foreskin epidermal cells have been used to seed an acellular collagen matrix, which appears to be an adequate replacement for urethral epithelium. Obviously, medium- and long-term follow-ups need to be scrutinized. These grafts are all essentially free grafts and liable to the same short-term and long-term complications as the currently available autologous grafts. It may be, however, that duration of success can be enhanced with true urethral replacement.

Biodegradable urethral stents such as the helical mesh stent appear to be useful in treating recurrent stricture disease, especially when they are inserted immediately following DVIU. However, although the stent becomes covered by epithelium and is bioabsorbed, it does not cause scar shrinkage. Still, it might help patients avoid a urethral catheter and unacceptable postoperative urinary retention caused by edema secondary to DVIU. Ideally a bioactive biodegradable stent would be developed that could modulate periurethral fibrosis and formation of urethral scar tissue.

REFERENCES

Barbagli G, Selli C, Tosto A, Palminteri E: Dorsal free graft urethroplasty. J Urol 1996;155:123-126.

Chen F, Yoo JJ, Atala A: Experimental and clinical experience using tissue regeneration for urethral reconstruction. World J Urol 2000;18:67-70.

Fu Q, Deng C, Liu W, Cao Y: Urethral replacement using epidermal cell-seeded tubular acellular bladder collagen matrix. BJU Int 2007;99:1162-1165.

Greenwell TJ, Venn SN, Mundy AR: Changing practice in anterior urethroplasty. Br J Urol 1999;83:631-635.

Harriss D, Beckingham IJ, Lemberger RJ, Lawrence WT: Long-term results of intermittent low-friction self catheterisation in patients with recurrent urethral strictures. Br J Urol 1994;74(6):790-792.

Heyns C, Steenkamp J, De Kock ML, Whitaker P: Treatment of male urethral strictures: Is repeated dilatation or internal urethrotomy useful? J Urol 1998;160:356-358.

Hussain M, Greenwell TJ, Shah PJR, Mundy AR: The long-term outcome of UroLume Wallstents in the treatment of recurrent urethral stricture disease. BJU Int 1994;7:1037-1039.

Matanhelia SS, Salaman R, John A, Mathews PN: A prospective randomized study of self-dilation in the management of urethral strictures. J R Coll Surg Edinb 1995;40:295-299.

Orandi A: One stage urethroplasty. Br J Urol 1968;40:717-719.

Steenkamp J, Heyns C, De Kock M: Internal urethrotomy versus dilatation as treatment for male urethral strictures: A prospective, randomised comparison. J Urol 1997;157:98-101.

Tammela TL, Talja M: Biodegradable urethral stents. BJU Int 2003;92:843-850.

Venn SN, Mundy AR: Early experience with the use of buccal mucosa for substitution urethroplasty. Br J Urol 1998;81:738-740.

Wood DN, Andrich DE, Greenwell TJ, Mundy AR: Standing the test of time—the long term results of urethroplasty. World J Urol 2006;24(3):250-254.

Renal Calculi

Method of
Sujeet S. Acharya, MD, and
Glenn S. Gerber, MD

Nephrolithiasis is a common condition affecting 5% to 10% of the U.S. population. Roughly 2 million patients a year present with kidney stones on an outpatient basis, an increase of 40% from 1994. Stone disease results in pain, loss of time at work, and medical costs in excess of $2 billion a year. Nephrolithiasis is more common in the industrialized world, but with changes in dietary habits, the incidence is increasing worldwide.

Epidemiology

Most kidney stones occur in patients between 20 and 50 years old, with peak onsets of disease between the third and fifth decades of life. Patients with recurrent stones often have their first case of nephrolithiasis in their teens or 20s. The recurrence rate of urinary calculi is roughly 50% within 5 years.

In general, male patients are more commonly affected with kidney stones than female patients by a ratio of 2:1. Stones due to infection (struvite stones), however, are more common in women than in men.

About 6% of men have onset of disease after age 50 years, compared with 25% in female patients. Stones caused by metabolic or hormonal defects and stone disease in children occur equally between the sexes.

Kidney stones are more prevalent in whites, Latin Americans, and Asians than in African Americans and Native Americans. Geographic variation influences frequency as stones are more common in hot and dry areas.

Pathophysiology

Supersaturation of urine by constituents such as calcium oxalate and uric acid is necessary for stone formation. If the concentration of an ion reaches a level beyond which it is not soluble, it has reached the level of supersaturation. Crystals and foreign bodies in the bladder serve as nidi for ions from the supersaturated urine to form microscopic lattice structures. These then increase in size by crystal growth and aggregation. Three quarters of renal calculi contain calcium. The majority of the rest contain uric acid. Cystine, struvite, and other stones occur less often.

Although geography, fluid intake, and diet influence the rate of calculi formation, metabolic derangements and heredity are the major causes of kidney stones. Hypercalciuria, whether absorptive, resorptive, or renal, is the most commonly noted metabolic abnormality. Absorptive hypercalciuria is the most common of the three forms of hypercalciuria. Severe (type 1) absorptive hypercalciuria has excess calcium in the urine independent of diet, whereas the calciuria of mild (type 2) absorptive hypercalciuria normalizes on a calcium-restricted diet. Renal hypercalciuria is caused by impaired renal tubular reabsorption of calcium. To balance calcium losses from urine, parathyroid function increases and eventually causes further mobilization of calcium from bone and increased intestinal absorption. As a result, patients with renal hypercalciuria have normal serum calcium. Resorptive hypercalciuria results from primary hyperparathyroidism, causing both serum and urine calcium levels to be high (Table 1).

Other causes of calcium stones include hyperuricosuria (dietary causes, overproduction), hyperoxaluria (enzyme defects, increased vitamin C, inflammatory bowel disease [IBD], bowel resection), gout, and decreased urine levels of the stone inhibitors citrate and magnesium.

Urate stones result from hyperuricosuria (malignancy, myeloproliferative states, glycogen storage disease) and from the net alkali deficit and dehydration during chronic diarrhea states. Cystine stones result from an autosomal recessive disorder in cystine metabolism, leading to cystinuria. Struvite stones result from urinary tract infection with urea-splitting organisms such as *Proteus* and *Klebsiella* species. These cause the formation of magnesium-ammonium-phosphate crystals, which can rapidly coalesce to form stones.

TABLE 1 Hypercalciuric States

Test	Type 1 AH	Type 2 AH	RH	Resorptive
Serum				
Calcium	Normal	Normal	Normal	Elevated
Phosphorus	Normal	Normal	Normal	Low
PTH	Normal	Normal	Elevated	Elevated
1,25(OH)$_2$D$_3$	Normal	Normal	Elevated	Elevated
Urinary Calcium				
Fasting urine	Normal	Normal	Elevated	Elevated
24-h restricted*	Elevated	Normal	Elevated	Elevated
Post-Ca^{2+} load†	Elevated	Elevated	Elevated	Elevated

*Urine while patient is on a diet restricted in calcium (400 mg/day) and sodium (10 mEq/day).
†Four-hour urine collection after an oral bolus of 1 g calcium.
Abbreviations: 1,25(OH)$_2$D$_3$ = vitamin D3; AH = absorptive hypercalciuria; PTH = parathyroid hormone; RH = renal hypercalciuria.

CURRENT DIAGNOSIS

- Nephrolithiasis affects 5% to 10% of the U.S. population, male patients more than female patients.
- The majority of renal calculi contain calcium.
- Patients usually have pain, nausea, vomiting, fever, dysuria, or hematuria.
- Physical findings include costovertebral angle and/or abdominal tenderness.
- Laboratory tests should include urinalysis, complete blood count, and chemistry profile.
- Recurrent stone formers should undergo metabolic evaluation including a 24-hour urine collection. This helps in classifying their nephrolithiasis and directs their long-term therapy.
- The standard means to evaluate for a suspected kidney stone is noncontrast computed tomography.

Diagnosis

HISTORY AND PHYSICAL EXAMINATION

Patients with urinary calculi present with pain, fever, dysuria, or hematuria. Stones passing into the ureter cause acute obstruction, with proximal urinary tract dilation and are associated with renal colic. Renal colic is marked by cramping, severe flank pain, nausea, and vomiting. While the stone moves distally through the ureter, pain moves from the flank to the abdomen, then to the groin, and finally the scrotal or labial area.

Staghorn calculi are kidney stones occupying the renal pelvis and the calyceal system. These stones are often asymptomatic, and when they do manifest it is usually with hematuria and infection rather than with acute onset of pain. Uncommonly, patients with asymptomatic bilateral obstruction present with renal failure.

During the history it is important to ask about the quality, location, and duration of pain. Prior history of urinary tract infections, urinary calculi, and their management should be noted as well. Other areas useful in stone management include past medical history (hyperparathyroidism), dietary habits, fluid consumption, medications, family history of calculi, loss of renal function, and history of solitary or transplanted kidney.

On physical examination, significant costovertebral angle tenderness is quite common and often moves to the abdomen as the stone migrates. Patients rarely present with peritoneal signs, which is important in distinguishing renal colic from other sources of flank and abdominal pain.

LABORATORY STUDIES

The initial studies useful for stone patients include urinalysis (with or without culture), complete blood count (CBC), and a chemistry profile. Urinalysis evaluates the urine for hematuria and infection and can also assess for pH and crystals (Table 2). An elevated white blood cell (WBC) count indicates renal or systemic infection. A decreased red blood cell (RBC) count and hemoglobin indicate a chronic disease state or significant ongoing hematuria.

A chemistry profile including serum electrolytes, creatinine, calcium, phosphorus, uric acid, and PTH is necessary to assess a patient's renal and metabolic functions. Acidosis and elevations in serum calcium or urate can help reveal the etiology of the stone(s). The same can be said for alterations in PTH or phosphorus. Finally, an acute significant rise in creatinine from baseline can indicate urgent or emergent surgical intervention to relieve obstruction. This is especially true in patients with a solitary kidney or baseline renal dysfunction.

Patients who are recurrent stone formers and high-risk first-time stone formers (patients younger than 30 years and those with renal

TABLE 2 Crystal Shapes in Kidney Stones

Stone Crystal	Shape under Microscope
Calcium oxalate dihydrate	Envelope or bipyramidal
Calcium oxalate monohydrate	Dumbbell or hourglass
Calcium phosphate apatite	Amorphous
Cystine	Hexagonal
Struvite	Coffin lid
Uric acid	Rhomboid
	Irregular plates or rosettes
	Amorphous

failure, struvite stones, multiple stones, intestinal disease, or solitary or transplanted kidney) warrant a more extensive laboratory evaluation, including a 24-hour urine collection. The 24-hour urine collection measures calcium, uric acid, creatinine, sodium, oxalate, citrate, pH, and volume. Elevation of the 24-hour excretion rate of calcium, oxalate, or uric acid indicates predisposition to stone formation. Other tests include the 24-hour urine collection after 1 week of a diet restricted in calcium, sodium, and oxalate; the fasting urine study; and the calcium load study (Table 3).

IMAGING STUDIES

Several imaging modalities can evaluate patients with kidney stones. The plain abdominal x-ray is very useful in assessing total stone burden, size, shape, and location of urinary calculi. On these films, calcium-containing stones are radiopaque, but pure uric acid, indinavir-induced, and cystine calculi are relatively radiolucent.

A renal sonogram not only determines the presence of a stone but also detects the presence of hydronephrosis and hydroureter. A stone seen on ultrasound, but not on radiograph, may be a uric acid or cystine stone.

Intravenous pyelogram (IVP) is the standard study for determining size and location of calculi, as well as providing anatomic and functional information. Disadvantages of an IVP are that it is labor intensive, it involves injection of contrast, and it requires bowel preparation for optimal results.

A helical computed tomography (CT) scan without contrast is the most sensitive imaging technique for kidney stones and is at present the standard means for evaluating patients suspected to have calculi. Even stones radiolucent on plain films (except indinavir-induced stones) are seen on a CT scan. Advantages of a CT scan are that it can identify other pathologies, it is a quick study, and it avoids administration of contrast. Disadvantages of a CT scan are that it cannot evaluate renal function and that it is relatively more expensive than IVP.

The renal tomogram is helpful in finding small stones in the kidneys, especially in obese patients.

Treatment

MEDICAL CARE

Medical care encompasses emergency management of renal calculi and long-term therapy to dissolve stones and to prevent stones from forming. Once renal colic is diagnosed in the emergent setting, it is important to evaluate for obstruction and infection. Obstruction in

TABLE 3 Classification of Nephrolithiasis

Category	General Features	Urine Study Findings
Hypercalciuria		
Absorptive hypercalciuria	Normal serum calcium Normal serum phosphorus	Hypercalciuria: Urine calcium > 200 mg/24 h Type 1: Hypercalciuria independent of diet Type 2: Normocalciuria with low-calcium diet
Renal hypercalciuria	Normal serum calcium Normal serum phosphorus Increased PTH and Vitamin D (2° hyperparathyroidism)	Hypercalciuria independent of diet
Resorptive hypercalciuria	Hypercalcemia Hypophosphatemia Increased PTH and Vitamin D (1° hyperparathyroidism)	Hypercalciuria independent of diet
Other Causes		
Cystinuria		Urine cystine > 250 mg/d
Gouty diathesis	Calcium, uric acid, or mixed stones	Persistently acidic urine (pH <5.5)
Hyperoxaluria	Main cause is enteric Dehydration and low urine citrate due to acidosis contribute	Urine oxalate >45 mg/d Oxalate >80 mg/d: primary or enteric Oxalate 45-80 mg/d: dietary causes
Hyperuricosuria	Normal serum calcium	Urine uric acid >600 mg/24 h Normal urinary calcium and oxalate Normal fasting and calcium load responses Calcium stones with urine pH >5.5
Hypocitraturia	Associated with distal RTA Complete and incomplete forms Associated with calcium stones	Urine citrate <640 mg/d Hypercalciuria
Hypomagnesuria	Often dietary	Urine magnesium <50 mg/d Associated with hypocitraturia, low urine volume
Infection stones		Alkaline urine due to bacterial urease Often hypercalciuria, hypocitraturia
Low urine volume		Urine volume <1 L/d Stone formers should aim for >2 L/d
No abnormality	3%-5% of stone population Normal serum calcium Normal serum PTH	Normal urine volume, pH, calcium, citrate, uric acid, magnesium, and oxalate

Abbreviations: PTH = parathyroid hormone; RTA = renal tubular acidosis.

CURRENT THERAPY

- In the absence of infection and upper urinary tract obstruction, a kidney stone can be managed by analgesics, anti-inflammatory medicines, and antiemetics.
- Drugs that allow ureteral relaxation, such as tamsulosin (Flomax),[1] facilitate passage of stones 5 mm or smaller.
- The most important factor in preventing stone recurrence is to increase fluid intake so urine output is at least 2 L/day.
- Dietary restrictions, thiazide diuretics, and potassium citrate therapy depend on the type of stone being treated.
- Minimally invasive methods of treating kidney stones such as extracorporeal shock-wave lithotripsy, ureteroscopy, and percutaneous nephrostolithotomy are employed more often than open surgery.

[1]Not FDA approved for this indication.

TABLE 4 Summary of Medical Expulsive Therapy

Medicine	Dose
Analgesic	
Hydrocodone w/acetaminophen (Vicodin)	1-2 tablets (5/500 mg) PO q4-6h prn pain
Ibuprofen (Advil, Motrin)	600-800 mg po q8h prn pain
Ketorolac (Toradol)	30 mg IV q6h prn pain
Morphine sulfate	1-2 mg IV q2-4h prn pain
Antiemetic	
Metoclopramide (Reglan)[1]	10-20 mg PO or IV q6h prn nausea[3]
Prochlorperazine (Compazine)	5-10 mg PO q6-8h prn nausea
Ureteral Relaxation	
Nifedipine extended release (Procardia XL)[1]	30 mg PO qd
Tamsulosin (Flomax)[1]	0.4 mg PO qd
Terazosin (Hytrin)[1]	4 mg PO qd

[1]Not FDA approved for this indication.
[3]Exceeds dosage recommended by the manufacturer.

the absence of infection can be managed with analgesics (narcotics or nonsteroidal anti-inflammatory drugs [NSAIDs]) and other forms of medical expulsive therapy. Infection in the absence of obstruction can initially be managed with antibiotics. If neither obstruction nor infection are present, then a trial of analgesics and other medical measures to assist in stone passage can be started. NSAIDs such as ketorolac (Toradol), α-blockers like tamsulosin (Flomax),[1] and calcium channel blockers such as nifedipine (Procardia)[1] have ureter-relaxing effects, but their results in published studies are mixed (Table 4).

Stones are more likely to pass if their diameter is 5 mm or less. Patients should increase fluid intake to increase their urine output, and they should be prescribed antiemetics as necessary. Limit medical expulsive therapy to 10 days, and if outpatient treatment fails, refer the patient to a urologist. If obstruction and infection coexist, then the upper urinary collecting system must be decompressed.

In preventing stones from recurring, the most important factor is for the patient to increase fluid intake so that urine output is at least 2 L per day. Excessive salt, oxalate, and protein intake should be avoided. Dietary calcium should only be restricted if indicated by 24-hour urine collection and metabolic evaluation. Empiric dietary restriction of calcium is not necessary in most patients, and it can have adverse effects on bone mineralization, especially in women and in patients with osteoporosis.

In the absence of sufficient intestinal calcium to bind oxalate, oxalate absorption and hyperoxaluria increase. This can, in fact, increase stone formation in patients with calcium oxalate calculi. Dietary calcium should be restricted to 600 to 800 mg/day in patients with diet-responsive hypercalciuria who form calcium stones. For stone-specific management, see Table 5.

SURGICAL CARE

The indications for surgery are pain, infection, and obstruction. Contraindications to definitive stone manipulation include uncorrected bleeding diathesis and pregnancy (relative contraindication). Treatment for most renal calculi is noninvasive (e.g., lithotripsy); open surgical excision is limited to isolated atypical cases. In an obstructed and infected collecting system secondary to a stone, emergent relief of obstruction is necessary by ureteral stent or percutaneous nephrostomy placement.

Nearly 85% of kidney stones requiring intervention are treated with extracorporeal shock-wave lithotripsy (ESWL). Shocks are generated via an electrohydraulic, electromagnetic, or piezoelectric source and are focused on the calculus. As the stone is hit by the shockwave, it breaks into smaller fragments that can pass in the urine. ESWL is less successful if the stone is larger than 1.5 cm or is in the lower pole of the kidney. In these cases, fragmentation does take place, but due to either the large volume of fragments or their location, the fragments do not pass completely. Cystine stones do not fragment well with ESWL. Do not perform ESWL in pregnant patients or if there is ureteral obstruction distal to the stone.

Ureteroscopic management is the second most common management option. Either a flexible or rigid endoscope is passed into the bladder and up the ureter to visualize the stone. The stone is either extracted with a grasper or basket device or is fragmented via laser, ultrasonic, or electrohydraulic lithotripsy. Commonly, a ureteral stent is placed at the end of the procedure to prevent obstruction secondary to ureteral spasm or edema.

Percutaneous nephrostolithotomy (PCNL) affords fragmentation and removal of large stones from the kidney and ureter, particularly after failed ESWL. Percutaneous access to the kidney is achieved, and a sheath with a 1-cm lumen allows use of larger and more powerful lithotrites. Due to its morbidity, PCNL is generally reserved for large or complex stones that are refractory to management by ureteroscopy or ESWL.

CONSULTATIONS

Consultation with a urologist is recommended when stones are present in the settings of infection and obstruction. Referral is required when medical management fails, for stones refractory to outpatient management, and for stones that do not pass spontaneously.

Follow-up

The postoperative course after minimally invasive stone removal usually consists of discomfort, which is best handled with oral pain medications. If pain continues or worsens, it is important to evaluate for complications such as infection, ureteral obstruction, and hemorrhage. Repeat urine cultures and imaging should be performed to assess for ureteral obstruction or perforation. Antibiotic choice is dictated by urine culture results.

A follow-up examination with abdominal x-ray is often sufficient after uncomplicated stone removal. In patients with stones having unusual characteristics and after difficult or complicated procedures, imaging evaluating renal drainage (IVP, ultrasound, CT scan) may be important.

[1]Not FDA approved for this indication.

TABLE 5 Summary of Medical Treatment by Stone Type

Treatment	Dose	Comments
Absorptive Hypercalciuria		
Diet restriction		May be sufficient for type 2 AH
Thiazide diuretic (e.g., hydrochlorozide [Hydrodiuril])	Various doses	Not ↑ intestinal absorption
		Causes hypercalciuria
		Inexpensive
		Effect decreases with time
		Give potassium supplement
Sodium cellulose phosphate (Calcibind)	10-15 g PO qd	Binds calcium in gut
		Can also cause hypomagnesemia (binds in gut) and 2nd-degree hyperoxaluria)
Renal Hypercalciuria		
Thiazide diuretic (e.g., hydrochlorozide [Hydrodiuril])	50 mg PO bid	Increase calcium reabsorption in distal tubule
		↓ extracellular volume → ↑ proximal tubule reabsorption
Chlorthalidone (Hygroton)[1]	50 mg PO qd	2nd-degree hyperparathyroidism corrected, thus normalizing intestinal calcium reabsorption
		Avoid triamterene (Dyrenium) because of risk of triamterene stones
Resorptive Hypercalciuria		
Parathyroidectomy		Best chance for improvement of disease
		Thiazides are contraindicated because they worsen hypercalcemia
Hyperuricosuria		
Diet restriction		Restriction of purines
Allopurinol (Zyloprim)	200-600 mg PO qd	
Potassium citrate (Urocit-K)	30-90 mEq/d divided tid-qid with food	Complexes calcium and inhibits urate-induced crystallization
Gouty Diathesis		
Potassium citrate	30-90 mEq/d divided tid-qid with food	Increase urinary pH to >5.5
		Avoid increasing urinary pH to >7.0 or risk calcium phosphate stones
Hyperoxaluria		
Calcium citrate	150 mg PO qd	Binds oxalate in gut, preventing absorption
		Raises urinary pH and urine citrate levels
		Add thiazide if hypercalciuria develops
Hypocitraturia		
Potassium citrate	30-90 mEq/d divided tid-qid with food	Same therapy whether hypocitraturia is due to distal RTA or chronic diarrhea or is idiopathic
		Large doses (120 mEq/d[3]) may be needed for severe acidosis
Cystinuria		
High fluid intake		Try to reduce urine cystine to <200-300 mg/L
Potassium citrate	30-90 mEq/d divided tid-qid with food	Aim to increase urine pH to >6.5-7.0
D-Penicillamine (Cuprimine)	125 mg PO qod	Increases cystine solubility
		Associated with the nephrotic syndrome, dermatitis, and pancytopenia
Infection Stones		
Various antibiotics		Control infection
Acetohydroxamic acid (Lithostat)	250 mg PO tid	Works by inhibiting urease of struvite stone-forming organisms

[1]Not FDA approved for this indication.
[3]Exceeds dosage recommended by the manufacturer.
Abbreviations: AH = absorptive hypercalciuria; HCTZ = hydrochlorothiazide; RTA = renal tubular acidosis.

In patients older than 40 years who have a single stone that passed either spontaneously or after intervention, follow-up for recurrent stones is generally not necessary. These patients have a low recurrence risk, especially if they maintain increased fluid intake. For patients at risk for recurrence, annual radiograph or ultrasound and 24-hour urine analyses are adequate.

REFERENCES

Menon M, Resnick MI: Urinary lithiasis: Etiology, diagnosis, and medical management. In Walsh PC, Retik AB, Vaughan ED, et al (eds): Campbell's Urology, 8th ed. Philadelphia: WB Saunders, 2002, 3229-3305.

Preminger GM: Medical management of urinary calculus disease. Part 1: Pathogenesis and evaluation. AUA Update Series, lesson 5. 1995;14:37-44.

Preminger GM: Medical management of urinary calculus disease. Part 2: Classification of metabolic disorders and selective medical management. AUA Update Series, lesson 5. 1995;14:45-52.

Stoller MLS, Bolton DM: Urinary stone disease. In Tanagho EA, McAninch JW (eds): Smith's General Urology, 15th ed. New York: McGraw-Hill, 2000, pp 291-321.

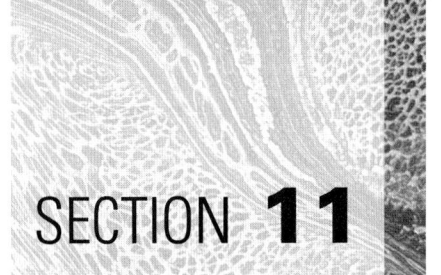

SECTION 11

The Sexually Transmitted Diseases

Chancroid and Granuloma Inguinale

Method of
Mark Tyndall, MD

Genital ulcer disease (GUD) due to chancroid and granuloma inguinale are found primarily in resource-poor settings outside of some isolated outbreaks. The limited availability of diagnostic testing and the overlap in the clinical presentation of the most common GUD pathogens, have made the epidemiology of both chancroid and granuloma inguinale difficult to capture. The associations between GUD, circumcision status, and enhanced HIV transmission have major implications for the HIV epidemic in some countries. Despite the paucity of reliable data around GUD in general, the incidences of chancroid and granuloma inguinale appear to be waning globally.

Chancroid

Haemophilus ducreyi is the gram-negative bacillus that causes chancroid. The association between chancroid and HIV transmission has made the control and potential eradication of chancroid all the more compelling. The disproportional infection rate seen among men (as high as 25:1 when compared with women) is consistent with the transmission dynamics. The setting for endemic chancroid is where high numbers of female commercial sex workers (CSW) are transmitting the infection to their male sex partners. The women generally have poor access to medical services, prevention information, and timely antimicrobial treatment. Therefore, interventions to disrupt this pattern of transmission should focus on providing diagnosis and treatment as part of a comprehensive health program for women who sell sex.

Chancroid is a painful progressive genital infection that causes significant morbidity. Patients often present with severe disease due to lack of medical services and effective antibiotic treatment. The initial papules can appear within hours of the sexual exposure and quickly ulcerate. The common site of infection for men is beneath and around the foreskin as well as the penis shaft. For women, the ulcers commonly occur on the labial surfaces, although vaginal and cervical lesions may be present and go unnoticed. The irregular borders, deep ulcerations, purulent exudate at the ulcer base, bubo formation, and severe pain on contact are characteristic, but studies have shown that the clinical diagnosis can be challenging. Herpes simplex infection with or without secondary bacterial infection is the pathogen that most commonly mimics chancroid. Although standard culture techniques can successfully isolate *H ducreyi*, the lack of adequate laboratory facilities in many regions has led to the adoption of syndromic-based approaches to the management of GUD.

The recommended treatment for chancroid has remained relatively unchanged since trimethoprim-sulfamethoxazole (Bactrim) resistance was identified. Some studies, however, have shown reduced cure rates among HIV-positive and uncircumcised men. At the very least, intensive post-treatment follow-up is required for these patients. Randomized clinical trials to update treatment recommendations, especially in areas with high rates of HIV, are needed. The increased use of azithromycin (Zithromax) for GUD as well as other sexually transmitted infections might have a dramatic impact on the prevalence of chancroid.

CURRENT DIAGNOSIS

Chancroid

- Lesions begin as papules within hours of sexual exposure and develop into painful ulcers with irregular borders and a purulent ulcer base.
- They often occur under the foreskin in uncircumcised men.
- Up to 50% of cases are associated with localized painful lymphadenopathy, which can form pus-filled inguinal buboes.
- Pathogens may be cultured on chocolate media, but in most regions empiric therapy is used following syndromic diagnostic algorithms.

Granuloma Inguinale

- Lesions begin as papules that ulcerate and form beefy red painless ulcers with raised edges that bleed on contact.
- Healing may be associated with scarring and lymphatic damage, leading to elephantiasis in the most severe cases.
- Diagnosis is clinical in most cases, although the visualization of intracellular Donovan bodies in monocytes from tissue smears can be done, and tissue cultures have been used in specialized laboratories.

CURRENT THERAPY

Chancroid

- Azithromycin (Zithromax) 1 g orally in a single dose
- Ceftriaxone (Rocephin)[1] 250 mg IM in a single dose
- Ciprofloxacin (Cipro)[1] 500 mg orally bid for 3 days
- Erythromycin (Ery-Tab)[1] 500 mg orally tid for 7 days

Granuloma Inguinale

- Doxycycline (Vibramycin) 100 mg orally bid for at least 3 weeks or until ulcers are healed
- Azithromycin (Zithromax)[1] 1 g orally once per week for at least 3 weeks
- Ciprofloxacin (Cipro)[1] 750 mg orally bid for 3 weeks
- Erythromycin (Ery-Tab)[1] 500 mg orally qid for at least 3 weeks
- Trimethoprim-sulfamethoxazole (Bactrim)[1] one double-strength (160 mg/800 mg) tablet PO bid for at least 3 weeks.

[1]Not FDA approved for this indication.

Granuloma Inguinale (Donovanosis)

Klebsiella granulomatis is the intracellular gram-negative bacterium that causes granuloma inguinale. This bacterium was formerly known as *Calymmatobacterium granulomatis*. It is found sporadically in select populations in Brazil, Papua New Guinea, Australia, and parts of Africa and the Caribbean. There is some evidence that the incidence of granuloma inguinale is decreasing, but the published data are scarce.

Although the presentation of the ulcer disease is very characteristic, the lack of access to diagnostic testing can lead to underdiagnosis. Further, the chronic nature of the infection results in treatment failure due to inadequate antimicrobial coverage.

The infection begins as painless papules that eventually break down into beefy red ulcers that bleed easily on contact. In male patients the lesions occur primarily on the shaft of the penis and around the foreskin, and in female patients the lesions are found on the labia and fourchette. In more advanced disease the cervical lesions can mimic carcinoma of the cervix. It is also not uncommon to develop secondary bacterial infections that can alter the clinical presentation. Inguinal involvement is common, and healing may be associated with severe scarring and lymphatic damage. In the most-severe cases, elephantiasis is the end result, with serious physical and social consequences.

The diagnosis is usually made clinically because *K. granulomatis* is difficult to culture. Diagnosis may also be made by visualizing Donovan bodies in monocytes from a tissue crush preparation or biopsy, although this is not widely available.

The approach to treatment is based largely on clinical experience and the use of antimicrobials with known activity against gram-negative organisms because few controlled treatment trials have been conducted. The most important component of therapy is an extended duration. The recommendations call for at least 3 weeks of therapy, but longer duration is often required depending on the clinical response. Relapse can occur up to 18 months following what was presumed to be successful therapy.

REFERENCES

Bong CT, Bauer ME, Spinola SM: *Haemophilus ducreyi*: Clinical features, epidemiology, and prospects for disease control. Microbes Infect 2002; 4(11):1141-1148.
Gupta S, Kumar B: Donovanosis in India: Declining fast? Int J STD AIDS 2002;13(4):277.
Malonza IM, Tyndall MW, Ndinya-Achola JO, et al: A randomized, double-blind, placebo-controlled trial of single-dose ciprofloxacin versus erythromycin for the treatment of chancroid in Nairobi, Kenya. J Infect Dis 1999;180(6):1886-1893.
Morse SA, Trees DL, Htun Y, et al: Comparison of clinical diagnosis and standard laboratory and molecular methods for the diagnosis of genital ulcer disease in Lesotho: Association with human immunodeficiency virus infection. J Infect Dis 1997;175(3):583-589.
O'Farrell N. Donovanosis. Sex Transmit Infect 2002;78:452-457.
Paz-Bailey G, Rahman M, Chen C, et al: Changes in the etiology of sexually transmitted diseases in Botswana between 1993 and 2002: Implications for the clinical management of genital ulcer disease. Clin Infect Dis 2005; 41(9):1304-1312.
Sturm PD, Moodley P, Govender K, et al: Molecular diagnosis of lymphogranuloma venereum in patients with genital ulcer disease. J Clin Microbiol 2005;43(6):2973-2975.
Tyndall MW, Agoki E, Plummer FA, et al: Single dose azithromycin for the treatment of chancroid: A randomized comparison with erythromycin. Sex Transm Dis 1994;21(4):231-234.
Tyndall M, Malisa M, Plummer FA, et al: Ceftriaxone no longer predictably cures chancroid in Kenya. J Infect Dis 1993;167(2):469-471.
Weiss HA, Thomas SL, Munabi SK, Hayes RJ: Male circumcision and risk of syphilis, chancroid, and genital herpes: A systematic review and meta-analysis. Sex Transm Infect 2006;82(2):101-109.

Gonorrhea

Method of
Khalil Ghanem, MD, PhD

Gonorrhea is caused by the gram-negative diplococcus *Neisseria gonorrhoeae*, an obligate parasite of humans that has no other natural host and to which no other animal is naturally susceptible. Nearly 358,366 cases in the United States were reported to the Centers for Disease Control and Prevention (CDC) in 2006, a slight increase from the previous year. This number is likely an underestimate because many cases are asymptomatic and others go unreported. Rates of gonorrhea in the United States declined sharply starting in the 1970s following the institution of gonorrhea control programs. It remains, however, the second most commonly reported communicable disease. Worldwide, more than 60 million new cases are estimated to occur every year.

In 2006 the gonorrhea rate among women in the United States was 124.3 and the rate among men was 116.8 cases per 100,000 population; the rate among African Americans was 18 times greater than the rate for whites; this is a decrease from 2001, when there was a 26-fold difference. Risk factors for infection include young age, unprotected intercourse, multiple sexual partners, new sexual partners, and sexual activity associated with illicit drug use. Gonococcal infection increases the rate of HIV transmission five-fold.

N. gonorrhoeae infects noncornified epithelia including urethral, endocervical, rectal, oropharyngeal, and conjunctival cells. It is transmitted through contact with infected secretions, most often sexually, although vertical transmission from mother to infant is well described. Sexual transmission is efficient: A man who has intercourse 2.5 times with an infected female partner has a 22% chance of becoming symptomatically infected.

Clinical Manifestations

Asymptomatic urethral infections occur in at least 10% of men and asymptomatic cervical infections occur in about 40% to 50% of women. More than 50% of rectal and up to 90% of pharyngeal gonorrhea in both men and women may be asymptomatic. These numbers highlight the importance of a thorough sexual history in all at-risk patients.

In men, urethritis is the most common manifestation of gonococcal infection. Urethral discharge and dysuria are the most common symptoms, occurring 2 to 5 days following exposure. Acute epididymitis, manifesting as unilateral scrotal pain, is the most common local complication. In young men, 30% of cases of acute epididymitis are due to N. gonorrhoeae. Rarely, cellulitis, lymphangitis, or periurethral abscesses complicate local infections. Differential diagnosis of urethritis in men includes Chlamydia trachomatis, Mycoplasma genitalium, and T. vaginalis infections.

Among women, the most common manifestation of local gonococcal infection is cervicitis, which tends to occur 5 to 10 days after exposure. In symptomatic women, common complaints include a vaginal discharge, dysuria, and genital itching. Concomitant infection of the urethra can occur in up to 90% of women and accounts for some of these symptoms. N. gonorrhoeae can also infect Skene's and Bartholin's glands. The differential diagnosis of cervicitis includes C. trachomatis, T. vaginalis, M. genitalium, herpes simplex virus, and bacterial vaginosis.

An important complication of gonococcal infections in women is pelvic inflammatory disease (PID). PID is the result of ascending infection involving the uterus, fallopian tubes, ovaries, or peritoneum. Sequelae of PID include infertility, ectopic pregnancy, and chronic pelvic pain. All women presenting with cervicitis should undergo a bimanual examination. The diagnosis of PID is made when one or more of the following signs are present: uterine tenderness, cervical motion tenderness, or adnexal tenderness.

Among men and women with rectal gonorrhea, those who are symptomatic might complain of rectal discharge, pain, and tenesmus. Most cases of rectal gonorrhea in men are due to receptive anal intercourse; in women, some cases may be due to perineal contamination. The differential diagnosis includes C. trachomatis (including lymphogranuloma venereum strains), Treponema pallidum, and herpes simplex virus infections. Most cases of pharyngeal gonorrhea are asymptomatic; when signs and symptoms are present, they can include acute pharyngitis, tonsillitis, and cervical lymphadenopathy.

The pharynx may be the only infected site in up to 10% of patients. Thus, a careful history, including oral–genital contact, is warranted. Conjunctivitis is rare in adults and usually is a result of self-inoculation from anogenital infections.

Disseminated gonococcal infections (DGI) occur in up to 2% of untreated patients. Certain gonococcal strains are more likely to cause DGI. Although patients are bacteremic, many appear nontoxic. Symptoms and signs can include fevers, myalgias, arthralgias, asymmetric polyarthritis, and a characteristic dermatitis consisting of a small number (<30) of skin lesions on the distal extremities, which begin as papules and progress to pustules and ulcerations. Rarely, meningitis and endocarditis occur.

Vertical transmission to neonates can result in ophthalmia neonatorum, sepsis, arthritis, meningitis, rhinitis, vaginitis, urethritis, and inflammation at the sites of fetal monitoring. Gonococcal infections diagnosed in preadolescent children are highly suspicious for sexual abuse.

Diagnosis

Gram stain of urethral discharge among symptomatic men is 90% sensitive and 95% specific. It is only 70% sensitive in asymptomatic men. Endocervical Gram stain is only 50% to 70% sensitive. Culture (usually on Thayer–Martin medium) is 95% sensitive in symptomatic men and slightly less so for asymptomatic men and women (~80%-90%). The sensitivity of culture in detecting gonococcal infections from urine is low. Culture is the most common test used to diagnose pharyngeal and rectal infections and is the only FDA-approved test to diagnose gonococcal infections in children. Antibiotic susceptibility testing can only be performed on cultured specimens.

Nonamplified molecular tests (e.g., GenProbe Pace II) are currently the most common tests used in the United States The sensitivity is 85% to 90% and their specificity greater than 95%. They can only be performed on urethral or endocervical specimens. Nucleic acid amplification tests (e.g., polymerase chain reaction or transcription-mediated amplification) are highly sensitive (>95%) and specific (>95%), and most can be performed on urethral and cervical specimens, in addition to urine and self-collected vaginal swabs. They are not FDA approved for pharyngeal and rectal specimens, although increasing data suggest that they have excellent sensitivity and specificity in detecting pharyngeal infections. Serologic tests exist and have been used for epidemiologic studies, but they should not be used for diagnosis. All patients tested for gonorrhea should also be tested for C. trachomatis, syphilis, and HIV.

Antimicrobial Resistance and Therapy

For 40 years, penicillin was the drug of choice for treating gonorrhea. Tetracyclines were also highly effective. By the 1980s, widespread resistance to both of these classes rendered them all but useless. Subsequently, drug resistance to aminoglycosides, spectinomycin,[2] macrolides, trimethoprim-sulfamethoxazole (Bactrim)[1], and fluoroquinolones has made the treatment of gonorrhea more challenging.

Fluoroquinolone-resistant Neisseria gonorrhoeae (FQRNG) strains emerged in the 1990s, and high rates have been reported in Asia, Africa, and the Middle East. In the United States, rates of FQRNG have been increasing. In April 2007, the CDC recommended that fluoroquinolones not be used to treat gonococcal infections in the United States.

Box 1 summarizes the current CDC recommendations for treating uncomplicated and complicated gonococcal infections. Since 1997, there have been no reports of ceftriaxone-resistant strains in the United States Thus, cephalosporins are currently the most reliable and only recommended first-line agents to treat gonorrhea. Ceftriaxone (Rocephin) is given intramuscularly and is effective for infections at all sites. Cefixime (Suprax) is effective for anogenital infections, but it might have lower efficacy than ceftriaxone for pharyngeal infections. Cephalosporins are safe to use in pregnancy. Additionally, patients should be treated for presumed C. trachomatis coinfection unless it is ruled out. All sexual contacts (in the preceding 60 days) of index patients should be treated.

In penicillin-allergic patients, treatment of gonorrhea has become more challenging. Initially, spectinomycin was recommended as a second-line agent. Currently, spectinomycin is no longer available in the United States. Spectinomycin has less than 80% efficacy in treating pharyngeal gonococcal infections.

Alternative agents include a single dose of azithromycin (Zithromycin) 2 g orally. The gastrointestinal side effects associated with this high dose and fear of increasing drug resistance resulted in the CDC's dropping it as a second-line agent in its 2006 treatment guidelines. However, if tolerated by the patient, this regimen has excellent activity against anogenital and pharyngeal infections. Azithromycin has been used in pregnant women without evidence of teratogenicity.

To prevent gonococcal ophthalmia neonatorum, 1% silver nitrate aqueous solution, 0.5% erythromycin ophthalmic ointment (Ilotycin), or 1% tetracycline ophthalmic ointment should be instilled into the eyes of all newborns. Treatment of gonococcal ophthalmia requires hospitalization, evaluation for evidence of disseminated infection, and ceftriaxone (Rocephin) 25 to 50 mg/kg IM or IV for one dose.

Several drugs are currently being tested for the future treatment of gonorrhea. These include cefpodoxime (Vantin), ertapenem (Invanz),[1] telithromycin (Ketek),[1] tigecycline (Tygacil),[1] and newer-generation fluoroquinolones (e.g. gemifloxacin [Factive][1]). None are currently recommended by the CDC.

---

[1]Not FDA approved for this indication.
[2]Not available in the United States.

> **BOX 1** The 2006 CDC Recommended Treatment Options For Complicated And Uncomplicated Gonorrhea
>
> **Uncomplicated Infections of the Cervix, Urethra, and Rectum***
> Ceftriaxone (Rocephin) 125 mg IM × 1
> or
> Cefixime (Suprax) 400 mg PO × 1
> plus
> Treatment for *Chlamydia trachomatis* if not ruled out:
> Azithromycin (Zithromax) 1g PO × 1
> or
> Doxycycline (Vibramycin) 100 mg PO bid × 7 days
>
> **Infections of the Pharynx**
> Ceftriaxone (Rocephin) 125 mg IM × 1
> plus
> Treatment for *C. trachomatis* if not ruled out
>
> **Epididymitis**
> Ceftriaxone (Rocephin) 250 mg IM × 1
> plus
> Doxycycline (Vibramycin) 100 mg PO bid × 10 days
>
> **Gonococcal Conjunctivitis**
> Ceftriaxone (Rocephin) 1 g IM × 1
>
> **Disseminated Gonococcal Infections**[†]
> Ceftriaxone (Rocephin) 1 g IM or IV q24h
>
> ---
> *Alternative agents include Spectinomycin 2 g IM × 1, if available.
> [†]Should be treated with parenteral regimen until 24 h after clinical improvement; may complete a 7-day course of therapy with oral cefixime.

Prevention and Screening

Abstinence from sexual intercourse is the single most reliable method of preventing infection. Male condoms, when used correctly and consistently, are highly efficacious at preventing infection. Diaphragms can help prevent gonococcal infections in women. To date, there have not been any successful vaccine candidates.

The CDC does not recommend universal screening for *N. gonorrhoeae*. High-risk women (multiple sexual partners, illicit drug use, past history of gonorrhea or other sexually transmitted infection, commercial sex worker, inconsistent condom use) should be screened. High-risk pregnant women should be screened during the first prenatal visit. Repeat testing during the third trimester for those at continued risk is recommended.

REFERENCES

Centers for Disease Control and Prevention: Update to CDC's sexually transmitted diseases treatment guidelines, 2006: Fluoroquinolones no longer recommended for treatment of gonococcal infections. MMWR Morb Mortal Wkly Rep 2007;56(14):332-336.

Cook RL, Hutchison SL, Ostergaard L, et al: Systematic review: Noninvasive testing for *Chlamydia trachomatis* and *Neisseria gonorrhoeae*. Ann Intern Med 2005;142:914-925.

Newman LM, Moran JS, Workowski KA: Update on the management of gonorrhea in Adults in the United States. Clin Infect Dis 2007;44: S84-S101.

Peterman TA, Tian LH, Metcalf CA, et al: High incidence of new sexually transmitted infections in the year following a sexually transmitted infection: A case for rescreening. Ann Intern Med 2006;145:564-572.

Workowski KA, Berman SM: Sexually transmitted diseases treatment guidelines, 2006. MMWR Recomm Rep 2006;55(RR-11):1-94.

Nongonococcal Urethritis

Method of
John N. Krieger, MD

Urethritis is defined as inflammation of the urethra and is commonly caused by urogenital infection. Urethritis is classified as either gonococcal, in patients whose inflammation is caused by *Neisseria gonorrhoeae*, or nongonococcal (NGU), in patients with inflammation that is not related to infection with *N. gonorrhoeae*.

Clinical Presentation

More than 4 million NGU cases are estimated to occur among men in the United States every year. Urethritis is characterized by symptoms of urethral discharge and dysuria, often accompanied by increased urinary frequency or pruritus. Signs of urethritis include urethral discharge that can occur spontaneously or after stripping of the urethra, erythema, and urethral tenderness.

Although the clinical presentation varies, the incubation of NGU averages 7 to 14 days from exposure to an infected partner. Typically the onset is gradual, with mild dysuria and mucoid discharge. In some high-risk populations, up to 50% of infections are asymptomatic.

Etiology

NGU should be considered infectious until proven otherwise. Most infectious cases of urethritis are sexually transmitted.

Chlamydia trachomatis remains the most important pathogen, accounting for 15% to 40% of NGU cases. The prevalence of *C. trachomatis* is lower in older patients and in referral populations. Other infectious causes of NGU include *Mycoplasma genitalium*, *Trichomonas vaginalis*, and herpes simplex virus. The etiologic roles are less well defined for other infectious agents including *Ureaplasma urealyticum*, enteric bacteria, anaerobes, and *Candida* species. Occasionally, patients with other urologic conditions (e.g., prostatitis, urethral stricture disease, or, rarely, bacterial urinary tract infection) present with symptoms of NGU. Other unusual causes of NGU include chemical, allergic, and autoimmune processes.

Diagnosis

It is important to document the presence of urethral inflammation. This may be done by finding mucoid or mucopurulent discharge on physical examination or by diagnostic testing. The Gram stain is the preferred rapid diagnostic test. Urethral inflammation may also be documented by a positive leukocyte esterase test on first-void urine or by finding pyuria on microscopic examination of the first-void urine sediment.

Diagnostic testing for both *N. gonorrhoeae* and *C. trachomatis* organisms is strongly recommended. Specific etiologic diagnosis may guide therapy and can improve compliance and partner notification. These infections are both reportable to state health departments. Patients at risk for *N. gonorrhoeae* and *C. trachomatis* should receive appropriate counseling and should receive testing for HIV and syphilis. Clinical evaluation and treatment of sex partners are critical for preventing complications and interrupting sexual transmission. Pathogens responsible for NGU are associated with cervicitis, pelvic inflammatory disease, and tubal infertility.

The Gram stain is the preferred rapid diagnostic test for evaluating urethritis because it provides high sensitivity and specificity. Gonococcal infection can be established by documenting the presence of white blood cells (WBCs) containing intracellular gram-negative diplococci. Presence of gram-negative rods should raise the suspicion for enteric bacteria.

CURRENT DIAGNOSIS

- Documenting urethral inflammation is critical for diagnosis of urethritis. One or more of the following techniques can provide documentation:
  - Physical examination showing urethral discharge, either present spontaneously at the meatus or after stripping the urethra. This discharge may be either mucoid or purulent in character.
  - Gram stain of urethral exudate showing five or more WBCs per oil immersion field ($\times 1000$). The Gram stain is the preferred rapid diagnostic test.
  - Urine leukocyte esterase dip stick test positive on first-void urine
  - First-void urine sediment microscopic examination demonstrating 10 or more WBCs per high-power field ($\times 400$).

Abbreviation: WBC = white blood cell.

CURRENT THERAPY

Recommended Regimens

- Azithromycin (Zithromax) 1 g PO in a single dose
- Doxycycline (Vibramycin) 100 mg PO bid × 7 days

Alternative Regimens

- Erythromycin base (E-Mycin, ERYC, E-Base) 500 mg PO qid × 7 days
- Erythromycin ethylsuccinate (EES) 800 mg PO qid × 7 days
- Ofloxacin (Floxin) 300 mg PO bid × 7 days
- Levofloxacin (Levaquin)[1] 500 mg PO qd × 7 days
- If an erythromycin regimen is the only possibility and the patient cannot tolerate high-dose schedules, then one of the following regimens should be considered.
- Erythromycin base (E-Mycin, ERYC, E-Base) 250 mg PO qid × 14 days
- Erythromycin ethylsuccinate (EES) 400 mg PO qid × 14 days

[1]Not FDA approved for this indication.

Confirmatory tests should be employed to identify a specific etiology. *N. gonorrhoeae* and *C. trachomatis* can be detected using culture, DNA hybridization tests on a urethral specimen, or nucleic acid amplification tests on a urethral or urine specimen. Because of their increased sensitivity, nucleic acid amplification tests are recommended for diagnosing chlamydial infection. For urine testing, 10 to 15 mL of first-void urine is collected then evaluated using nucleic acid amplification testing.

Diagnostic tests for the genital mycoplasmas (*M. genitalium*, *U. urealyticum*, and other genital mycoplasmas) are available in research settings. Such tests are usually unavailable for routine clinical use. *T. vaginalis* may be cultured, but specific media are necessary for isolation. To increase sensitivity, cultures of both a urethral swab sample and a urine specimen are recommended.

Treatment

If gonorrhea cannot be ruled out by Gram stain of urethral secretions, potentially noncompliant patients should be treated for both gonorrhea and chlamydial infection. Both azithromycin (Zithromax) and doxycycline (Vibramycin) are highly effective for treating chlamydial NGU. Azithromycin also provides convenient single dosing and the opportunity for directly observed therapy. Doxycycline is inexpensive but requires twice-daily dosing for a full week. Alternatives include erythromycin and fluoroquinolones regimens.

For patients with erratic health care–seeking behavior in whom poor compliance is anticipated, azithromycin offers the easiest administration. Further, *M. genitalium* appears to respond better to macrolides than to tetracyclines. Patients should be advised to abstain from sex until therapy is completed, symptoms have resolved, and sex partners have been treated.

Follow-up

Routine follow-up is not recommended for patients whose symptoms resolve after therapy. Patients with persistent or recurrent symptoms should return for reevaluation.

Symptoms alone should not prompt a second course of therapy unless the patient has documented urethritis or a positive test for a urogenital pathogen. Patients should return for evaluation and treatment if their symptoms persist or recur after completion of therapy. Patients with NGU should refer all sex partners in the past 60 days for evaluation and treatment.

Chronic Urethritis

Chronic urethritis is defined as persistent or recurrent urethritis within 6 weeks following treatment. An estimated 20% to 40% of NGU cases do not respond to first-line therapy. Although up to 20% of men with chlamydial NGU develop chronic urethritis, up to 50% of men with nonchlamydial NGU develop chronic urethritis. Noncompliance and reinfection are important considerations. Other causes include organisms that do not respond to the standard treatment regimens, such as *T. vaginalis*, tetracycline-resistant mycoplasmas, viral etiologies, and other bacteria.

Up to 30% of NGU has no identifiable infectious etiology. These cases can involve allergy and postinfectious immunologic responses. Before administering therapy, presence of urethral inflammation should be documented. Patients with persistent or recurrent urethritis who did not comply with therapy or who had exposure to an untreated sex partner should be re-treated with the initial drug regimen. Otherwise, recommended treatment regimens include metronidazole (Flagyl),[1] 2 g orally in a single dose, plus either erythromycin base (E-Base), 500 mg orally four times a day for 7 days, or erythromycin ethylsuccinate (EES), 800 mg orally four times a day for 7 days.

Complications

For infected men, complications of untreated NGU include epididymitis in less than 3% of cases and, rarely, Reiter's syndrome. Patients with a history of NGU also appear to be at increased risk for developing chronic prostatitis/chronic pelvic pain syndrome.

Female sex partners are at risk for pelvic inflammatory disease, tubal infertility, and ectopic pregnancy. Prompt and appropriate therapy and treatment of sexual partners decrease the risk of complications substantially.

REFERENCES

Aydin D, Kucukbasmaci O, Gonullu N, Aktas Z: Susceptibilities of *Neisseria gonorrhoeae* and *Ureaplasma urealyticum* isolates from male patients with urethritis to several antibiotics including telithromycin. Chemotherapy 2005;51:89-92.

[1]Not FDA approved for this indication.

Bradshaw CS, Tabrizi SN, Read TR, et al: Etiologies of nongonococcal urethritis: Bacteria, viruses, and the association with orogenital exposure. J Infect Dis 2006;193:336-345.

Centers for Disease Control and Prevention: Screening tests to detect *Chlamydia trachomatis* and *Neisseria gonorrhoeae* infections. MMWR Recomm Rep 2002;51(RR-15):3-19.

Centers for Disease Control and Prevention: Sexually transmitted disease treatment guidelines 2002. MMWR Recomm Rep 2002;51(RR-6):30-42.

Deguchi T, Yoshida T, Miyazawa T, et al: Association of *Ureaplasma urealyticum* (biovar 2) with nongonococcal urethritis. Sex Transm Dis 2004; 31:192-195.

Falk L, Fredlund H, Jensen JS: Symptomatic urethritis is more prevalent in men infected with *Mycoplasma genitalium* than with *Chlamydia trachomatis*. Sex Transm Infect 2004;80:289-293.

Geisler WM, Yu S, Hook EW 3rd: Chlamydial and gonococcal infection in men without polymorphonuclear leukocytes on Gram stain: Implications for diagnostic approach and management. Sex Transm Dis 2005;32:630-634.

Jensen JS: *Mycoplasma genitalium:* The aetiological agent of urethritis and other sexually transmitted diseases. J Eur Acad Dermatol Venereol 2004;18:1-11.

Kaydos-Daniels SC, Miller WC, Hoffman I, et al: The use of specimens from various genitourinary sites in men, to detect *Trichomonas vaginalis* infection. J Infect Dis 2004;189:1926-1931.

Leung A, Eastick K, Haddon LE, et al: *Mycoplasma genitalium* is associated with symptomatic urethritis. Int J STD AIDS 2006;17:285-288.

O'Mahony C: Adenoviral non-gonococcal urethritis. Int J STD AIDS 2006; 17:203-204.

Ozgül A, Dede I, Taskaynatan MA, et al: Clinical presentations of chlamydial and non-chlamydial reactive arthritis. Rheumatol Int 2006;26:879-885.

Pontari MA, McNaughton-Collins M, O'Leary P, et al: A case-control study of risk factors in men with chronic pelvic pain syndrome. BJU Int 2005; 96:559-565.

Swygard H, Sena AC, Hobbs MM, Cohen MS: Trichomoniasis: Clinical manifestations, diagnosis and management. Sex Transm Infect 2004;80:91-95.

Taylor SN: *Mycoplasma genitalium.* Curr Infect Dis Rep 2005;7:453-457.

Taylor-Robinson D, Gilroy CB, Thomas BJ, Hay PE: *Mycoplasma genitalium* in chronic non-gonococcal urethritis. Int J STD AIDS 2004;15:21-25.

Yasuda M, Maeda S, Deguchi T: In vitro activity of fluoroquinolones against *Mycoplasma genitalium* and their bacteriological efficacy for treatment of *M. genitalium*–positive nongonococcal urethritis in men. Clin Infect Dis 2005;41:1357-1359.

Syphilis

Method of
Mrunal Shah, MD

One of the oldest infections known, syphilis dates back more than 500 years. It was known as "The Great Pox" because of its skin manifestations; in contrast to the "small pox" seen around the same time. Studies were done before the use of antibiotics, which is where most of our natural history information comes from. The most recent epidemic occurred in 1990 (20.3 cases per 100,000 population) and has fallen steadily each year since. In the year 2000, the rate was at an all time low of 2.2 cases per 100,000 population. This was a 9.6% drop since 1999. The Centers for Disease Control and Prevention (CDC) hopes to eradicate the disease completely by 2005, but this may be difficult.

Peak ages are 30 to 39 years of age in men and 20 to 24 years of age in women. African Americans have always had higher incidences than whites. In the 1990s, it was 60:1, but the incidence has since declined to 30:1.

Microbiology

Treponema pallidum is the bacterium responsible for causing syphilis. It is very small and cannot be detected by ordinary microscopy, a feature that complicates diagnosis. The organism can be seen with darkfield microscopy, a technique that uses a special condenser to cast an oblique light. This allows visualization of a corkscrew-shaped organism with tightly wound spirals. This organism is extremely sensitive to penicillin, as is discussed later in the article. It has a very slow doubling rate, therefore requiring longer courses of treatment.

Pathophysiology

T. pallidum initiates infection when it gains access to subcutaneous tissues through microabrasions that can occur during sexual intercourse. Even though it has a slow doubling time (30 hours), it escapes host immune defenses and leads to the initial ulcerative lesion, the chancre. These can be seen anywhere around the genitalia including the cervix, perianal and rectal areas, and the oral mucosa. Regional lymphadenopathy also can be seen. As the host immune system fights the initial infection, *T. pallidum* is disseminated throughout the host. This is known as latency, as the patient will have no symptoms. There is also vertical spread in utero or during delivery, which is why prenatal panels include screening tests for syphilis.

Clinical Manifestations

The initial clinical manifestation is also called *primary* syphilis. This usually consists of a painless chancre at the site of inoculation. Primary syphilis represents a local infection, but it quickly becomes systemic with widespread dissemination of the spirochete. Because it is painless, most people do not seek medical attention. Even without treatment, the chancre will resolve in 4 to 6 weeks. It is this painlessness that helps separate it from herpes simplex virus (genital herpes) and *Haemophilus ducreyi* (chancroid).

In approximately weeks to months after the resolution of the chancre, patients will develop *secondary* syphilis, which includes systemic symptoms of rash, fever, headache, malaise, anorexia, and diffuse lymphadenopathy. The rash typically involves the palms and soles but can also include mucosal surfaces. Many patients do not realize that they had these lesions. These symptoms usually resolve spontaneously but can relapse for up to 5 years.

After symptoms resolve, and for up to many years later, the disease goes into *latent* syphilis, which is characterized by a lack of symptoms but seropositive test results. This can be separated into early and late latent phases based on being potentially infectious in the early phase. This is defined by the United States Public Health Service (USPHS) as infection of 1 year's duration or less. Anything longer is late latent.

Finally, for the next 1 to 30 years, untreated patients have a 25% to 40% risk of developing *late* or *tertiary* syphilis. It may involve many tissue types, so the spectrum of disease can be very confusing. Moreover, patients need not have had symptoms of primary or secondary syphilis prior to developing late syphilis. Tissues involved include cutaneous (gumma formation), cardiovascular (aortic disease), and central nervous system (CNS) (tabes dorsalis, meningitis, neurosyphilis) diseases (Table 1).

Diagnosis

The quickest, most direct method of diagnosing primary and secondary syphilis is direct visualization of the spirochete of moist lesions by means of darkfield microscopy. This is difficult and requires using laboratories that perform a high volume of sexually transmitted disease analyses. In general, a moist lesion should be cleaned with saline (not iodine because of bacteriocidal effect). Then, using gauze, the lesion should be unroofed. Any serosanguineous material should be collected on a dry slide for examination.

More common is serologic testing that can be done in most laboratories. The two most common screening tests are rapid plasma reagin (RPR) and the Venereal Disease Research Laboratory (VDRL) test. These tests are designed to test for IgM and IgG

TABLE 1 Clinical Manifestations and Treatment of Syphilis

Stage	Clinical Manifestation	Treatment
Primary	Painless ulcer (chancre), adenopathy	Benzathine penicillin G (Bicillin LA), 2.4 million U IM × 1
Secondary (weeks to months)	Rash, mucocutaneous lesions, adenopathy, hepatitis, arthritis, glomerulonephritis, condyloma lata	Benzathine penicillin G, 2.4 million U IM × 1
Latent	Asymptomatic	
Early (<1 year)		Benzathine penicillin G, 2.4 million U IM × 1
Late		Benzathine penicillin G, 2.4 million U IM weekly × 3
Tertiary (late) 1-30 years		
Cutaneous	Gummatous lesions	Benzathine penicillin G, 2.4 million U IM weekly × 3
Cardiovascular	Aortic aneurysm, aortic insufficiency	Benzathine penicillin G, 2.4 million U IM weekly × 3
CNS	Neurosyphilis, tabes dorsalis, Argyll-Robertson pupils, paresis, seizures, subtle psychiatric manifestations, dementia; may be asymptomatic	Aqueous crystalline penicillin G, 18-24 million U/d given as 3-4 million units IV q4h for 10-14 days or Procaine penicillin (Wycillin), 2.4 million U qd with probenecid 500 mg PO qid for 10-14 days

Abbreviations: CNS = central nervous system; IM = intramuscularly; IV = intravenously; PO = orally; qd = daily; qid = 4 times per day.
Adapted from the CDC: Guidelines for the treatment of STDs. MMWR Morb Mortal Wkly Rep 2002;51(RR-06):1-80.

antibodies against a cardiolipin-cholesterol-lecithin antigen. Positive tests are reported as a dilutional titer. False positives are less than 1:4, whereas higher titers (1:16 to 1:128) are found in secondary and early latent syphilis. This titer is important as a benchmark to follow treatment. Lack of expected decreases in titer indicate inadequate treatment, false-positive result, re-infection, or late-stage therapy.

Before treatment, a positive screening test needs to be confirmed with specific *T. pallidum* antigen testing, such as the fluorescent treponemal antibody absorption test (FTA-ABS). These tests are expensive and have a high false-positive rate, making them unsuitable as screening tests. They also remain positive for life in most people.

Newer molecular tests include the use of polymerase chain reaction (PCR), which can be used to detect multiple organisms. It has high sensitivity and specificity and can distinguish among *H. ducreyi*, herpes simplex virus, and *T. pallidum*. This test is very expensive and is likely to be available only in specialized laboratories, for now.

The most significant morbidity of syphilis occurs during the tertiary phase and includes neurosyphilis. *T. pallidum* can be found in the cerebrospinal fluid (CSF) during primary and secondary phases, but it usually resolves on its own. Those patients who have an abnormal CSF during the latent phase are at higher risk for symptomatic neurosyphilis, making it helpful to distinguish asymptomatic neurosyphilis. The CDC recommends that CSF testing be done whenever there is clinical evidence of neurosyphilis or vision changes, active tertiary syphilis, treatment failure, or HIV infection. CSF-VDRL is highly specific, but, unfortunately, very insensitive (as low as 30%) and therefore can rule in but cannot exclude neurosyphilis.

Although the HIV epidemic showed a resurgence of syphilis, it is controversial as to what diagnostic changes occurred in testing. Several studies show contradictory information; one shows that there was an increase in the false-positive rates, whereas a second study showed a decrease in true-positive rates, and a third study showed higher false negatives. In any case, testing should still be performed as in non-HIV patients and followed accordingly.

Pregnancy poses only increased risk, including perinatal death, premature delivery, low birth weight, congenital anomalies, and active congenital syphilis of the neonate. Physical examination and serologic testing should be performed in any female considering pregnancy or during initial antepartum testing at least. Treatment, discussed below, should be given as if the patient is not pregnant.

Treatment

In all stages, the main reason for treatment is to prevent progression and spread of the disease. Historic treatments included mercury, salvarsan (an arsenic derivative), fever therapy, and malarial injection. Today's treatment has been in use since 1943, since the introduction of penicillin. Because there has been no reported resistance, penicillin remains the treatment of choice, so much so that penicillin-allergic patients have undergone desensitization therapy in order to receive it. Although penicillin G, given parenterally, is the preferred drug, the preparation used (benzathine, procaine, crystalline), dosage, and duration of therapy depend on stage and clinical manifestations (see Table 1). Oral penicillin is not considered appropriate for treatment. Alternative treatments could include doxycycline (Vibramycin), tetracycline, erythromycin, or ceftriaxone (Rocephin).[1]

Once treatment is started, physicians should be aware of a potential complication called the Jarisch-Herxheimer reaction. It is an acute, febrile reaction accompanied by headache and myalgias, which represents treponemal cell death and release of toxins. It peaks within 2 hours and subsides within 24 hours, and is most common in primary and secondary disease.

Follow-up of Treated Patients

Any patient with syphilis diagnosed at any stage should get testing for HIV and should be retested in 3 to 6 months if a member of a high-risk population. After treatment, repeat serologic testing should be done at 6 and 12 months and titers at 24 months. If there is not at least a fourfold decrease in 6 months, there is likely treatment failure. A lumbar puncture should be done to rule out neurosyphilis, and retreatment with three weekly injections of 2.4 million units of benzathine penicillin (Bicillin LA) is recommended unless there is evidence of neurosyphilis.

Partners of patients with syphilis should also be notified and treated. In primary disease, any partner within the previous 3 months should be identified. Empiric treatment is recommended unless there is good follow-up and serologic surveillance.

---

[1]Not FDA approved for this indication.

Contraception

Method of
Linda Roethel, MD, and
Samuel Sandowski, MD

Contraceptives were not always easily available or legal in the United States. In the early 20th century Margaret Sanger devoted her life to fighting for reproductive freedom for women. In 1914, she coined the term *birth control*, and in 1921 she founded the American Birth Control League, which led to today's Planned Parenthood Federation. Even now, with many more contraceptive options available, approximately one half of the pregnancies in the United States are unintended, and about one half of those end in induced abortions. This occurs even though 54% of women with an unintended pregnancy used contraception in the month that they conceived. To minimize unintended pregnancies, appropriate, correct, and consistent use of birth control are essential.

Natural Family Planning and Fertility Awareness Methods

Natural family planning is also known as fertility awareness. The couple avoids intercourse or uses a barrier method of contraception during the woman's fertile days. Knowing the woman's fertile days can also help a couple achieve a pregnancy. In the United States, more than one half a million couples use natural methods of family planning for contraception. It is based on a 6-day window of fertility, the 5 days before ovulation and the day of ovulation. The peak fertile days are the 2 days preceding ovulation. Identifying the 6-day window of fertility can be difficult, because it can vary from cycle to cycle.

There are a variety of methods that a woman can use to identify her fertile time. Combining methods increases efficacy but at the cost of increasing complexity.

The various methods of identifying the window of fertility are based on the calendar (or rhythm), cervical mucus, basal body temperature, or hormonal monitoring devices. Natural family planning can be an effective contraceptive if used correctly and consistently. For calendar-based methods, the pregnancy rate is 11 to 18 pregnancies per 100 woman-years. When combining cervical mucus monitoring with a hormonal monitoring device, the pregnancy rate was reduced to 2.1 pregnancies per 100 woman-years with perfect use and 14.2 pregnancies with imperfect (typical) use.

Advantages of natural family planning include absence of side effects or health risks. For some, this method is chosen for religious or moral reasons. It is inexpensive, unless hormonal monitoring devices are used.

Hormonal Methods

ESTROGEN–PROGESTIN COMBINATIONS

Oral contraception (OC) is at present the most popular form of reversible contraception in the United States, with more than 12 million users of hormonal OC. Of women born since 1945, approximately 80% have had some experience with OC. Perfect use failure rates are less than 1%.

The majority of present-day combination oral contraceptives (COCs) contain 20 to 35 μg ethinyl estradiol (EE), which provides cycle control, resulting in regular, predictable bleeding episodes, mimicking menses. It also minimizes breakthrough bleeding. The progestin ranges from 0.1 to 1.0 mg daily and provides ovulation suppression by preventing the luteinizing hormone surge. Progestin also provides endometrial protection. Progestins used today include norgestrel, levonorgestrel (LNG), norgestimate, desogestrel, and drospirenone. To lower the total dose of progestin even further, triphasic COCs vary the dose of progestin over the 3 weeks of active pills. This decreases side effects while still maintaining the contraceptive efficacy.

The traditional package of COCs contains 21 days of active pills followed by 7 days of inert pills. Withdrawal bleeding occurs during the week of inert pills. COCs are also available as 24 days of active pills followed by 4 days of inactive pills. This reduces the number of days of withdrawal bleeding, improves contraceptive effectiveness, and reduces adverse effects. Extended preparations provide 84 days of active pills containing 30 μg of EE and 0.15 mg of LNG, followed by 7 days of inert pills (Seasonale) or 7 days of pills containing 10 μg of EE (Seasonique). With this preparation, the woman has extended cycles of amenorrhea with withdrawal bleeding every 3 months.

COC pills are started on the first day of a woman's menses or as a Sunday start, the first Sunday after the start of a woman's menses. Sunday starts allow withdrawal bleeding to occur during the week and not on the weekend. If COC are started off cycle, pregnancy testing, emergency contraception, or backup contraception, depending on the individual circumstance, should be considered.

Other advantages of COCs include control of menstrual abnormalities, decreased blood loss, decreased iron-deficiency anemia, decreased dysmenorrhea, decreased benign breast disease, and decreased incidence of endometrial and ovarian cancers. Low-dose COCs (30 μg of EE) are safe for healthy, nonsmoking perimenopausal women, 40 to 50 years of age.

Adverse effects of COCs include thromboembolism, pulmonary embolism, headache, breast tenderness, and nausea. As the dose of hormones decreases, the risk of adverse effects decreases, but the risk of breakthrough bleeding increases. With continued use, the incidence of breakthrough bleeding decreases.

Contraindications to COCs include breast-feeding, smoking by women older than 35 years, uncontrolled hypertension, history of cerebrovascular disease, myocardial infarction or angina, serious heart valve problems, history of venous thromboembolism (including pulmonary embolism), certain inherited blood clotting disorders, diabetes with vascular disease, history of breast or liver cancer, history of migraine with aura, undiagnosed abnormal genital bleeding, prolonged bedrest, and pregnancy.

Combination hormonal contraception, in the United States, is also available as a transdermal patch and an intravaginal ring. Both are longer-acting hormonal contraception, with less failure due to better compliance.

Ortho Evra is a transdermal hormonal contraceptive patch, which contains 20 μg of EE and 150 μg norelgestromin. It is applied weekly for 3 weeks. The fourth week is patch-free, resulting in estrogen withdrawal bleeding. This cycle is then repeated. The contraindications are the same as COCs. The advantages are also similar, but include better compliance. The adverse effects are the same as for COCs but also include skin irritation and a risk of venous thromboembolism that is twice that with COCs.

An intravaginal ring that releases 15 μg of EE and 120 μg of etonogestrel daily is available as NuvaRing. It is also a first-day or Sunday start, as with COC. The ring is a flexible intravaginal device, effective for 3 weeks, then removed. After a 7-day ring-free period, during which time estrogen withdrawal bleeding occurs, a new intravaginal ring is placed. It avoids the daily fluctuations of hormone levels that are seen with COCs. There is less irregular bleeding and better cycle control compared with COCs. The advantages, adverse effects, and contraindications are similar to those for COCs.

PROGESTIN ONLY

Progestin only pills (POPs), also known as minipills, are available. They are less commonly prescribed than COCs, but are effective. POPs contain 0.35 mg norethindrone (Micronor). They affect ovulation and blunt, but not eliminate, the midcycle luteinizing hormone peaks. POPs also increase cervical mucus viscosity, preventing sperm from ascending the cervical canal, and make the endometrium unfavorable for implantation.

POPs are started on the first day of a menstrual period and are taken continuously, without hormone-free days. Because of their short half-life, it is important that each pill be taken at the same time each day. If a woman is more than 3 hours late in taking a pill or forgets a pill, she should resume POP as soon as possible, and use a nonhormonal backup form of contraception for at least 48 hours.

The most common adverse effect of POP is menstrual changes, such as short cycles, spotting or breakthrough bleeding, and amenorrhea. Enlarged ovarian cysts are also more common in POP users, which tend to enlarge and regress over time.

POP are safe for a number of women who cannot use COCs. They can be used in women who are breast-feeding and in smokers older than 35 years. They are acceptable in the clinical setting of vascular disease associated with diabetes or lupus, coronary artery disease, congestive heart failure, cerebrovascular disease, complicated migraine headaches, increased risk of thromboembolism, diabetes, lipid disorders including hypertriglyceridemia, or when COCs cause unacceptable side effects.

Progestin-based contraception is also available as an injection give every 3 months and as an intrauterine device that is effective for 5 years.

Depot-medroxyprogestrerone acetate (DMPA) is available as 150 mg/1 mL intramuscular injection (Depo-Provera) and 104 mg/0.65 mL subcuntaneous injection (Depo-Sub Q Provera 104). Both are administered during the first 5 days of a normal spontaneous mentrual period, and repeated every 3 months (13 weeks). They suppress ovulation completely. When administered properly, no backup method is needed, even with the first cycle. Under this regimen, perfect use failure rate is 0.3% and a typical use failure rate is 3% during the first year of use. The adverse effects of DMPA are similar to those of POP, but it causes more irregular breakthrough bleeding initially, and then with time more amenorrhea, compared with POP. Because DMPA suppresses estradiol production, there is a decline in bone mineral density. It is regained rapidly after DMPA is discontinued. Studies comparing former DMPA users and women who never used DMPA showed no deficit in bone mineral density. DMPA is appropriate in the same clinical settings as POP.

Previously, implantable forms of hormonal contraception, such as Norplant[2] were popular. Currently, none is available in the United States.

Intrauterine Devices

In the United States at present, two intrauterine devices (IUDs) are approved. One is a copper-coated IUD, ParaGard, effective for 10 years. The other is a progestin-releasing IUD, Mirena, which releases 20 μg/day of levonorgestrel and is approved for 5 years of continuous use. Both are modifications to a T-shaped polythylene frame.

The ideal candidate for an IUD is a parous woman who is in a stable monogamous relationship and at low risk for sexually transmitted diseases (STDs) or pelvic inflammatory disease (PID). Either IUD type is acceptable for perimenopausal women. They can be used by nulliparous women, but there is a higher rate of spontaneous expulsion of the IUD.

Insertion of either type of the IUD is best within 7 days of the onset of menses to minimize an undiagnosed pregnancy. If the IUD is inserted at another time, pregnancy should be ruled out. If it is inserted during the luteal phase, another form of contraception, such as condoms, should be used until the next menses. Additionally, STDs such as gonorrhea and chlamydia need to be identified before an IUD is inserted.

The copper IUD has been available in the United States since 1988. It is approved for 10 years of continuous use, but it may be effective for as long as 12 years. The copper interferes with sperm motility and creates an environment that is spermicidal. Its typical effectiveness is 99.2% during the first year. Adverse effects include increased menstrual bleeding and dysmenorrhea. It is contraindicated with pregnancy, unexplained vaginal bleeding, and a lifestyle that increases risk for STDs and PID. It cannot be used by women with a copper allergy or Wilson's disease.

Mirena, the progestin IUD, available since 2000 in the United States, is currently approved for 5 years of continuous use, but it may be effective as long as 7 years. It works by thickening the cervical mucus, making it difficult for sperm to pass. It also thins the endometrial lining, making it unfavorable to implantation. In some women, it might also prevent ovulation. Initially, the progestin IUD causes increased spotting and breakthrough bleeding, but then it can reduce bleeding and dysmenorrhea. Because of this, it has been used as a treatment for menorrhagia, dysfunctional uterine bleeding, and leimyomas. Its contraindications are similar to those for other progestin products and the copper IUD. It can, however, be used by women who have a copper allergy or Wilson's disease.

Barrier Methods and Spermicides

Male condoms were used by the Egyptians in 1000 BCE and were made of fabric. Today, they are made of latex, polyurethane, or natural membranes, such as lamb cecum. Latex condoms, invented in the 1880s, and polyurethane condoms, introduced in 1995, offer protection against pregnancy, as well as HIV and a number of other STDs. These include gonorrhea, chlamydia, mycoplasma, trichomonas, hepatitis, cytomegalovirus, and herpes. Natural-membrane condoms do not protect against HIV and possibly other STDs. Male condoms, when used correctly, have a failure rate of about 15%. They are available without a prescription.

The female condom is made of polyurethane. It can be inserted up to 8 hours before intercourse and is removed afterward. When used properly, it has a failure rate of approximately 21%. It is less effective than male condoms as a barrier to semen. It is available without a prescription.

Currently, three models of diaphragms are available, two made of latex and one made of silicone. The correct size needs to be determined by a health care provider, and it is available by prescription. The diaphragm, with a spermicide, can be inserted intravaginally up to 6 hours before intercourse and must be left in place at least 6 hours afterward; it must not be left in place for more than 24 hours total. It has a pregnancy rate of 16% to 20% during the first year of typical use. Contraindications are history of toxic shock syndrome and latex allergy (for the latex models).

Less common, but also available, are Lea's shield and the cervical cap, FemCap. Both require a prescription and are meant to be used with a spermicide.

Nonoxynol-9 (Conceptrol, K-Y Plus, Semicid) is the spermicide available in the United States. It is available without a prescription and comes in a number of forms including foams, creams, gels, films, suppositories, and tablets. They can be combined with other forms of contraception, such as barrier methods. Nonoxynol-9 does not offer protection against STDs and might reduce protection against HIV.

Available also is a soft polyurethane foam cushion, Today Sponge, containing nonoxynol-9. It is available without a prescription and has a failure rate of 32% in parous women and 16% in nulliparous women.

All these contraceptive methods are acceptable forms for perimenopausal women.

Sterilization

Sterilization as a method of contraception is available for both women and men. Among women and men using contraception, sterilization increases as a choice with age, but more so for women than men. For women ages 25 to 29 years using contraception, 15% choose bilateral tubal ligation. At 40 to 44 years of age, 51% of women using contraception choose sterilization. For men 40 to 44 years old, 18% using contraception choose vasectomy.

Approximately 750,000 tubal ligations are performed annually in the United States. It is the predominant choice of contraception for women desiring permanent contraception. Bilateral tubal sterilization can be done by a variety of techniques via a laparascopic approach, either postpartum or as outpatient ambulatory surgery. Sterilization can be accomplished by removing part of the fallopian tubes, or the tubes can be ligated with clips, rings, coils, or plugs or via coagulation-induced blockage (electrical or chemical).

Female sterilization via a hysteroscopic approach, using a microinsert, Essure, was approved by the FDA in 2002. Transcervical placement of the microinsert can be done as an outpatient office procedure without surgical incision or general anesthesia and with less postprocedure pain. The microinsert is placed in the proximal

---
[2]Not available in the United States.

portion of the fallopian tube, where it elicits a benign tissue response that results in the anchoring of the device and ultimate occlusion of the tubes by 3 months after insertion.

Regret over sterilization is more common in women sterilized before or at 30 years of age. In women sterilized when they are older than 30 years, regret over the procedure is about 6%. Tubal sterilization is an acceptable form of contraception for the perimenopausal woman.

Male sterilization, also known as vasectomy, is the only permanent male contraception. It is important that the man be educated that sterilization is not intended to be reversible. Vasectomy is safer, easier, and less expensive than female sterilization. It is a minor surgical procedure that blocks the vas deferens that carry sperm. Sperm are therefore prevented from getting into the ejaculated fluid. Azoospermia takes about 3 to 6 months after the procedure. Until azoospermia is confirmed, another form of contraception is needed.

Vasectomy has a failure rate of about 9.4 per 1000 at 1 year and 11.3 per 1000 at years 2, 3, and 5. Approximately one half of failures occur within the first 3 months, when backup contraception is recommended and before semen analysis to confirms azoospermia.

Studies have shown that vasectomy has no effect on cardiovascular, prostate, testicular, or neoplastic disease or on circulating hormone and sexual function.

Emergency Contraception

In the United States, there are currently two types of emergency contraception available: the emergency contraceptive pill (ECP; Plan B) and the copper IUD (ParaGard). The ECP consists of two pills, with 750 µg of the progestin levonorgestrel per pill. Commonly referred to as *the morning after pill*, and known as Plan B, it is available without a prescription to women at least 18 years of age. A prescription is required for girls younger than 18 years. A previous combination emergency contraceptive pill, Preven, is no longer available, because Plan B was found to be safe, to have fewer side effects, and to be more effective.

CURRENT THERAPY

- About one half of the pregnancies in the United States are unintended.
- Approximately one half of these unintended pregnancies are electively aborted.
- Contraceptives that require less-frequent user action have typical use failure rates that approach perfect-use failure rates.
- Oral contraceptives are the most popular type of reversible contraception in the United States.
- Combination estrogen–progestin contraception is available as pills, patch, and intravaginal ring.
- Progestin-only pills are suitable for many women for whom estrogen is contraindicated.
- The intrauterine device is available as two types: Copper-coated (ParaGard) and progestin-releasing (Mirena).
- Many of the barrier methods can be combined with a spermicide for increased efficacy.
- Sterilization, both female and male, is a permanent form of contraception.
- For those who choose natural family planning and fertility awareness, a variety of methods can be used, alone or in combination.
- Progestin emergency contraception (Plan B) is now available without a prescription.

Plan B works before fertilization to inhibit, delay, or blunt the luteinizing hormone surge or to inhibit follicle rupture, thereby delaying or inhibiting ovulation. It is most effective if started by 72 hours (3 days) after unprotected intercourse, but it can be offered and still have some effect up to 120 hours (5 days) after unprotected intercourse. Its efficacy is up to 94% if used within 5 days of unprotected intercourse.

Most common adverse effects with ECP are nausea (18%) and vomiting (4%). Other adverse effects of progestin are also possible, but they are less common because of the short course of treatment. ECP can effect the next menstrual period in timing and duration of flow. The only absolute contraindication to ECP is pregnancy.

Another option for emergency contraception is the copper IUD.[1] It can be inserted up to 120 hours (5 days) after unprotected intercourse. It works as a spermicide and prevents implantation. It does not, however, disrupt an already implanted embryo. Adverse effects and contraindications are the same as for the copper IUD when used for normal indications. It is more effective than ECP.

After using emergency contraception, menses is expected within 3 weeks. If this does not occur, pregnancy must be excluded.

---

[1]Not FDA approved for this indication

REFERENCES

Anderson FD, Hait H: A multicenter, randomized study of an extended cycle oral contraceptive. Contraception 2003;68:89-96.
Audet M, Moreau M, Koltun WD, et al: Evaluation of contraceptive efficacy and cycle control of a transdermal contraceptive patch vs an oral contraceptive. JAMA 2001;285:2347-2354.
Bjarnadóttir R, Tuppurainen M, Killick SR: Comparison of cycle control with a combined contraceptive vaginal ring and oral levonorgestrel/ethinyl estradiol. Am J Obstet Gynecol 2002;186:389-395.
Brunton J, Beal M: Current issues in emergency contraception: An overview for providers. J Midwifery Womens Health 2006;51:457-463.
Collins G, Herbst S, Aqua KA: Permanent sterilization for the 21st century using the hysteroscopic approach. Surg Technol Int 2004;13:115-119.
Cullins V: The state of contraceptive care in the United States today: Perspectives from the Planned Parenthood Federation of America. Manag Care Interface 2006;19(Suppl A):5-10, 20.
Fehring R: New low- and high-tech calendar methods of family planning. J Midwifery Womens Health 2005;50:31-38.
Fehring R, Schneider M, Raviele K, Barron ML: Efficacy of cervical mucus observations plus electronic hormonal fertility monitoring as a method of natural family planning. J Obstet Gynecol Neonatal Nurs 2007;36:152-160.
Galvão L, Oliveira L, Díaz J, et al: Effectiveness of female and male condoms in preventing exposure to semen during vaginal intercourse: A randomized trial. Contraception 2005;71:130-136.
Hansen L, Saseen J, Teal SB: Levonorgestrel-only dosing strategies for emergency contraception. Pharmacotherapy 2005;27:278-284.
Herdiman J, Nakash A, Beedham T: Male contraception: past, present and future. J Obstet Gynaecol 2006;26:721-727.
Himmerick K: Enhancing contraception a comprehensive review. JAAPA 2005;18:26-33.
Jain J, Jakimiuk AJ, Bode FR, et al: Contraceptive efficacy and safety of DMPA-SC. Contraception 2004;70:269-275.
Jamieson D, Costello C, Trussell J, et al: The risk of pregnancy after vasectomy. Obstet Gynecol 2004;103:848-850.
Johnson BJ: Insertion and removal of intrauterine device. Am Fam Physician 2005;71:95-102.
Kailas NA, Sifakis S, Koumantakis E: Contraception during perimenopause. Eur J Contracept Reprod Health Care 2005;10:19-25.
Kaunitz A: Beyond the pill: New data and options in hormonal and intrauterine contraception. Am J Obstet Gynecol 2005;192:998-1004.
Kaunitz A: Revisiting progestin-only OCs. Contemporary OB/GYN 1997; 42:91-92, 97-98, 101, 104.
Linn E: Hormonal contraceptive methodology and historical review. Int J Fertil 2005;50:88-96.
Masimasi N, Sivanandy MS, Thacker HL: Update on hormonal contraception. Cleve Clin J Med 2007;74:186-198.
Mosher WD, Martinez GM, Chandra A, et al: Use of contraception and use of family planning services in the United States: 1982-2002. Adv Data 2004;(350):1-46.
Narrigan D: Women's barrier contraceptive methods, poised for change. J Midwifery Womens Health 2006;51:478-485.

SECTION 12

Diseases of Allergy

Anaphylaxis and Serum Sickness

Method of
Stephen F. Kemp, MD

Anaphylaxis

Anaphylaxis, an acute and potentially lethal multisystem allergic reaction, is virtually unavoidable in medical practice. Health care professionals must be able to recognize the signs of anaphylaxis, treat an episode promptly and appropriately, and be able to provide preventive recommendations. Epinephrine, which should be administered immediately, is the drug of choice for acute anaphylaxis.

Anaphylaxis is not a reportable disease, and both its morbidity and mortality are probably underestimated. A variety of statistics on the epidemiology of anaphylaxis have been published, but the lifetime risk per person in the U.S. is presumed to be 1% to 3%, with a mortality rate of 1%.

There is no universally accepted definition of anaphylaxis. An international and interdisciplinary group of representatives and experts from thirteen professional, governmental, and lay organizations proposed the following working definition: "Anaphylaxis is a serious allergic reaction that is rapid in onset and may cause death." Clinically, anaphylaxis is considered likely to be present if any one of the following three criteria is satisfied within minutes to hours: Acute onset of illness with involvement of skin, mucosal surface, or both, and at least one of the following: respiratory compromise, hypotension, or end-organ dysfunction; two or more of the following occurring rapidly after exposure to a likely allergen: involvement of skin or mucosal surface, respiratory compromise, hypotension, or persistent gastrointestinal symptoms; hypotension develops after exposure to a known allergen for that patient: age-specific low blood pressure or decline of systolic blood pressure of greater than 30% compared with baseline. In clinical practice, however, waiting until the development of multiorgan symptoms is risky because the ultimate severity of anaphylactic reaction is difficult to predict from the outset.

Anaphylaxis has varied clinical presentations, but respiratory compromise and cardiovascular collapse cause the most concern because they are the most frequent causes of fatalities. Urticaria and angioedema are the most common manifestations (more than 90% in retrospective series) but may be delayed or absent in rapidly progressive anaphylaxis. The previous severity of anaphylaxis is not predictive of the severity of a future reaction. The more rapidly anaphylaxis occurs after exposure to an offending stimulus, the more likely the reaction is to be severe and potentially life threatening. Anaphylaxis often produces signs and symptoms within 5 to 30 minutes, but reactions sometimes may not develop for several hours.

PATHOPHYSIOLOGY

The chemical mediators that cause anaphylaxis are preformed and released from granules (histamine, tryptase, and others) or are generated from membrane lipids (prostaglandin D_2, leukotrienes, and platelet-activating factor) by the activated mast cell or basophil.

Tryptase is concentrated selectively in the secretory granules of all human mast cells. Its plasma levels during mast cell degranulation correlate with the clinical severity of anaphylaxis but need not be elevated in all forms of anaphylaxis (e.g., food-associated anaphylaxis).

Histamine exerts its pathophysiologic effects via both H_1 and H_2 receptors. Erythema (flushing), hypotension, and headache are mediated by both H_1 and H_2 receptors, whereas tachycardia, pruritus, bronchospasm, and rhinorrhea are associated with H_1 receptors alone.

Increased vascular permeability during anaphylaxis can produce a shift of 35% of intravascular fluid to the extravascular space within 10 minutes. This shift of effective blood volume causes compensatory catecholamine release, activates the renin-angiotensin-aldosterone system, and stimulates production of endothelin-1.

Mast cells accumulate at sites of coronary plaque erosion and rupture and they may contribute to coronary artery thrombosis. Because antibodies attached to mast cells can trigger mast cell degranulation, some investigators suggest that anaphylaxis may promote plaque rupture.

AGENTS THAT CAUSE ANAPHYLAXIS

Cause and effect often is confirmed historically in subjects who experience recurrent, objective findings of anaphylaxis upon

CURRENT DIAGNOSIS

- Cutaneous: urticaria, angioedema, diffuse erythema, generalized pruritus
- Respiratory: tachypnea, bronchospasm, laryngeal or tongue edema, dysphonia
- Cardiovascular: tachycardia, bradycardia, hypotension, angina, cardiac arrhythmias
- Gastrointestinal: nausea, emesis, diarrhea, abdominal cramps, dysphagia
- Other: rhinitis, conjunctivitis, uterine cramps, headache, dizziness, syncope, blurred vision, seizure

TABLE 1 Representative Agents That Cause Anaphylaxis

IgE dependent:
- Foods (such as peanuts, tree nuts, and crustaceans)
- Medications (such as antibiotics)
- Venoms (fire ants, yellow jackets, others)
- Allergen extracts
- Latex
- Exercise (where food or medication dependent)
- Hormones

IgE independent:
- Nonspecific degranulation of mast cells and basophils
  - Opioids
  - Muscle relaxants
  - Idiopathic
  - Physical factors
    - Exercise
    - Cold, heat
- Disturbance of arachidonic acid metabolism
  - Aspirin and other nonsteroidal anti-inflammatory drugs (NSAIDs)
- Immune aggregates
  - Intravenous immunoglobulin
- Cytotoxic
  - Transfusion reactions to cellular elements (IgM, IgG)
- Multimediator complement activation/activation of contact system
  - Radiocontrast media
  - Angiotensin-converting enzyme (ACE) inhibitor administered during renal dialysis with selected dialysis membranes
  - Protamine (possibly)

Psychogenic

Modified and abridged from Kemp SF, Lockey RF: Anaphylaxis: A review of causes and mechanisms. J Allergy Clin Immunol 2002;110:341-348.

inadvertent reexposure to the offending agent. Diagnostic testing, where appropriate, may confirm the presence of specific IgE and/or the degranulation of mast cells and basophils.

Virtually any agent capable of activating mast cells or basophils may potentially precipitate anaphylactic or anaphylactoid reactions. Table 1 lists common causes of anaphylaxis classified by pathophysiologic mechanism. Idiopathic anaphylaxis, anaphylaxis with no identifiable cause, has accounted for approximately a third of cases in most retrospective studies of anaphylaxis. However, of 601 patients evaluated more than two decades in a university-affiliated practice (the largest retrospective series), 59% of subjects were deemed to have idiopathic anaphylaxis.

Idiopathic anaphylaxis remains a diagnosis of exclusion, however. Serial histories and diagnostic tests for foods, spices, and vegetable gums occasionally identify a specific culprit in subjects previously presumed to have idiopathic anaphylaxis. The most common identifiable causes of anaphylaxis are foods, medications, insect stings, and immunotherapy injections. Anaphylaxis to peanuts and/or tree nuts causes the greatest concern because of its life-threatening severity, especially in subjects with asthma, and the tendency for subjects to develop lifelong allergic responsiveness to these foods.

RECURRENT ANAPHYLAXIS

Depending on the report, recurrent (biphasic) anaphylaxis occurs in 1% to 20% of subjects who experience anaphylaxis. Signs and symptoms experienced during the recurrent phase of anaphylaxis may be equivalent to or worse than those observed in the initial reaction and may occur 1 to 72 hours (most within 8 hours) after apparent remission. Thus, it may be necessary to monitor subjects up to 24 hours after apparent recovery from the initial phase. Observation periods after apparent recovery from the initial phase should be individualized and based on such factors as comorbid conditions and distance from the patient's home to the closest emergency facility, particularly because there are no reliable predictors of biphasic anaphylaxis

DIFFERENTIAL DIAGNOSIS

Several systemic disorders share clinical features with anaphylaxis. The vasodepressor (vasovagal) reaction probably is the condition most commonly confused with anaphylactic reactions. In vasodepressor reactions, however, urticaria is absent, dyspnea is generally absent, the blood pressure is usually normal or elevated, and the skin is typically cool and pale. Tachycardia is the rule in anaphylaxis. Bradycardia may be underrecognized in anaphylaxis, however. Brown and others conducted sting challenges in 19 subjects known to be allergic to jack jumper ants (*Myrmecia*). All eight subjects who became hypotensive developed bradycardia after an initial tachycardia.

Systemic mastocytosis, a disease characterized by mast cell proliferation in multiple organs, usually features urticaria pigmentosa (brownish macules that transform into wheals upon stroking them) and recurrent episodes of pruritus, flushing, tachycardia, abdominal pain, diarrhea, syncope, or headache. Other diagnostic considerations include myocardial dysfunction, pulmonary embolism, foreign body aspiration, acute poisoning, and seizure disorder.

MANAGEMENT OF ANAPHYLAXIS

Table 2 outlines a sequential approach to management. Assessment and maintenance of airway, breathing, circulation, and mentation are necessary before proceeding to other management steps. Subjects are monitored continuously to facilitate prompt detection of any treatment complications. The recumbent position is strongly recommended. In a retrospective review of prehospital anaphylactic fatalities in the United Kingdom, the postural history was known for 10 individuals. Four of the 10 were associated with assumption of an upright or sitting posture and postmortem findings consistent with "empty heart" and pulseless electrical activity.

Epinephrine is the treatment of choice for acute anaphylaxis. Aqueous epinephrine 1:1000 dilution, 0.2 to 0.5 mL (0.01 mg/kg in children; maximum dose, 0.3 mg) administered intramuscularly every 5 minutes, as necessary, should be used to control symptoms and sustain or increase blood pressure. Comparisons of intramuscular injections to subcutaneous injections during acute anaphylaxis are not available. However, absorption is more rapid and plasma levels are higher in asymptomatic individuals who receive epinephrine intramuscularly in the anterolateral thigh.

All subsequent therapeutic interventions depend on the initial response to epinephrine and the severity of the reaction. Development of toxicity or inadequate response to epinephrine injections indicates that additional therapeutic modalities are necessary.

The α-adrenergic effect of epinephrine reverses peripheral vasodilation, which alleviates hypotension and also reduces angioedema and urticaria. It may also minimize further absorption of antigen from a sting or injection. The β-adrenergic properties of epinephrine increase myocardial output and contractility, cause bronchodilation, and suppress further mediator release from mast cells and basophils.

Fatalities during witnessed anaphylaxis usually result from delayed administration of epinephrine and from severe respiratory and/or cardiovascular complications. *There is no absolute contraindication to epinephrine administration in anaphylaxis.*

Oxygen should be administered to subjects with anaphylaxis who require multiple doses of epinephrine, receive inhaled β_2 agonists, have protracted anaphylaxis, or have preexisting hypoxemia or myocardial dysfunction.

Antihistamines (H_1 and H_2 antagonists) support the treatment of anaphylaxis. However, these agents act much slower than epinephrine and should never be administered alone as treatment for anaphylaxis. Antihistamines thus should be considered as *second-line* treatment.

Systemic corticosteroids have no role in the acute management of anaphylaxis because even intravenous administration of these agents may have no effect for 4 to 6 hours after administration. Although corticosteroids traditionally are used in the management of anaphylaxis, their effect has never been evaluated in placebo-controlled trials. Corticosteroids administered during anaphylaxis might provide additional benefit for patients with asthma or other conditions recently treated with corticosteroids.

TABLE 2 Management of Anaphylaxis

Immediate intervention:
- Assessment of airway, breathing, circulation, and adequacy of mentation.
- Administer aqueous epinephrine 1:1000 dilution, 0.2–0.5 mL (0.01 mg/kg in children; maximum dose, 0.3 mg) *intramuscularly* q5 min, as necessary, to control symptoms and blood pressure.

Possibly appropriate, subsequent measures depending on response to epinephrine:
- Place subject in recumbent position and elevate lower extremities.
- Establish and maintain airway.
- Administer oxygen.
- Establish venous access.
- Use normal saline IV for fluid replacement.

Specific measures to consider after epinephrine injections, where appropriate:
- An epinephrine infusion might be prepared. Continuous hemodynamic monitoring is essential (see reference for specific details).
- Diphenhydramine (Benadryl). Note: In the management of anaphylaxis, a combination of diphenhydramine and ranitidine (Zantac)[1] is superior to diphenhydramine alone.
- For bronchospasm resistant to epinephrine, use nebulized albuterol (Proventil).
- For refractory hypotension, consider dopamine (Intropin), 400 mg in 500 mL D_5W, administered IV at 2–20 μg/kg/min titrated to maintain adequate blood pressure. Continuous hemodynamic monitoring is essential.
- Where use of β-blockers complicates therapy, consider glucagon,[1] 1–5 mg (20–30 μg/kg; maximum: 1 mg in children), administered IV over 5 min followed by an infusion, 5–15 μg/min. Aspiration precautions should be observed.
- For patients with a history of asthma and for those who experience severe or prolonged anaphylaxis, consider methylprednisolone (Solu-Medrol) (1.0–2.0 mg/kg/d).
- Consider transportation to the emergency department or an intensive care facility.

Interventions for cardiopulmonary arrest occurring during anaphylaxis:
- High-dose epinephrine and prolonged resuscitation efforts are encouraged, if necessary, because efforts are more likely to be successful in anaphylaxis where the subject (often young) has a healthy cardiovascular system (see reference for specific details).

Observation and subsequent outpatient follow-up:
- Observation periods after apparent resolution must be individualized and based on such factors as the clinical scenario, co-morbid conditions, and distance from the patient's home to the closest emergency department. After recovery from the acute episode, patients should receive epinephrine syringes (EpiPen or TwinJect) and be instructed in proper technique. Everyone postanaphylaxis requires a careful diagnostic evaluation in consultation with an allergist-immunologist.

[1]Not FDA approved for this indication.
Abbreviation: IV = intravenous.
Modified from Lieberman P, Kemp SF, Oppenheimer J, etal (chiefs eds). Joint Task Force on Practice Parameters. The diagnosis and management of anaphylaxis: An updated practice parameter. J Allergy Clin Immunol 2005;115:S483-S523.

TABLE 3 Preventive Measures for Subjects with Anaphylaxis

General measures:
- Obtain thorough history to diagnose life-threatening food or drug allergy.
- Identify cause of anaphylaxis and those individuals at risk for future attacks.
- Provide instruction on proper reading of food and medication labels, where appropriate.
- Patient should avoid exposure to antigens and cross-reactive substances.
- Manage asthma and coronary artery disease optimally.

Specific measures for high-risk subjects:
- Individuals at high risk for anaphylaxis should carry self-injectable syringes of epinephrine (EpiPen or TwinJect) at all times and receive instruction in proper use with placebo trainer.
- Individuals should wear a Medic Alert bracelet or chain.
- Other agents for β-adrenergic antagonists, angiotensin-converting enzyme (ACE) inhibitors, tricyclic antidepressants, and monoamine oxidase inhibitors should be substituted whenever possible.
- Agents suspected of causing anaphylaxis should be administered slowly, supervised, and orally if possible.
- Where appropriate, use specific preventive strategies, including pharmacologic prophylaxis, short-term challenge and desensitization, and long-term desensitization.

Modified from Kemp SF: Anaphylaxis: Current concepts in pathophysiology, diagnosis, and management. Immunol Allergy Clin N Am 2001;21:611-634.

Numerous cases of unusually severe or refractory anaphylaxis are reported in subjects receiving β-blocking agents. Greater severity of anaphylaxis observed in usual doses of epinephrine administered during anaphylaxis to subjects taking β-blockers may not produce the desired clinical response. In such situations, both isotonic volume expansion and glucagon[1] administration are recommended. Glucagon may potentially reverse refractory hypotension and bronchospasm because it bypasses the β-adrenergic receptor and directly activates adenyl cyclase.

Persistent hypotension despite epinephrine injections should first be treated with intravenous crystalloid solutions. Saline is generally preferred. One to 2 L of normal saline might need to be administered to adults at a rate of 5 to 10 mL/kg in the first 5 minutes. Children should receive up to 30 mL/kg in the first hour. Large volumes (e.g., 7 L) are often required.

Vasopressors should be administered if epinephrine injections and volume expansion fail to alleviate hypotension. Dopamine (Intropin) frequently increases blood pressure while maintaining or enhancing renal and splanchnic perfusion. These agents would not be expected to work as well in patients already maximally vasoconstricted by their internal compensatory response to anaphylaxis.

PREVENTION OF ANAPHYLAXIS

Table 3 outlines the basic principles for the prevention of future anaphylactic episodes in high-risk individuals. An allergist-immunologist can provide comprehensive professional advice on these matters.

All subjects at high risk for recurrent anaphylaxis should carry epinephrine syringes and know how to administer them. An EpiPen (Dey Laboratories) is a spring-loaded, pressure-activated syringe with a single 0.3 mg dose (1:1000 dilution) of epinephrine. It is easy to use and injects through clothing. An EpiPen Jr, which delivers 0.15 mg (1:2000 dilution) epinephrine, is appropriate for children weighing less than 30 kg. The TwinJect (Verus Pharmaceuticals) is a prefilled, pen-sized, epinephrine auto-injector with two doses of either 0.3 or 0.15 mg.

Serum Sickness

Serum sickness is a clinical syndrome of fever, malaise, and urticarial and/or morbilliform cutaneous eruption that is often preceded by generalized erythema and pruritus. Arthralgias or arthritis (mainly large joints), neuropathy, lymphadenopathy, nephritis, abdominal pain (emesis or melena are possible), or vasculitis (cutaneous or systemic) may occur in some cases. Cutaneous vasculitis, also known as hypersensitivity vasculitis, is often manifested by palpable purpura, which most commonly are found on the lower extremities of ambulatory individuals or on the sacral or gluteal region of patients with restricted mobility. These purpura reflect vascular leakage from inflamed postcapillary venules. Systemic vasculitis may occur in association with autoimmune diseases, infection, or malignancy.

Many agents may produce serum sickness or serum sickness–like reactions (Table 4). *Serum sickness* classically refers to the immune

---

[1]Not FDA approved for this indication.

TABLE 4 Representative Agents That Cause Serum Sickness

Medications: β-lactam antibiotics, sulfonamides, ciprofloxacin (Cipro), metronidazole (Flagyl), rifampin (Rifadin), allopurinol (Zyloprim), carbamazepine (Tegretol), phenytoin (Dilantin), fluoxetine (Prozac), bupropion (Wellbutrin), methimazole (Tapazole), propylthiouracil, thiazide diuretics, captopril (Capoten), propranolol (Inderal), verapamil (Calan), streptokinase (Streptase), others Heterologous (animal-derived) antisera:
- Horse: snake and spider venom, tetanus, botulism, diphtheria
- Horse or rabbit: anti-lymphocyte globulin

Mouse: monoclonal antibodies (muromonab-CD3 [Orthoclone OKT3], rituximab [Rituxan], infliximab [Remicade])
Homologous (human-derived) antisera: cytomegalovirus, hepatitis B, rabies, tetanus, perinatal RH₀(D)

complex syndrome caused by immunization with heterologous serum proteins (often equine or murine). The most frequent cause is immune complex-mediated drug hypersensitivity. A serum sickness–like drug reaction generally develops 6 to 21 days after the culprit medication is started, but it can occur within 12 to 48 hours in previously sensitized individuals.

PATHOGENESIS AND LABORATORY ABNORMALITIES

Healthy individuals regularly generate low levels of circulating immune complexes, which are either excreted by the kidneys or extracted in the liver and spleen by monocytes and macrophages. It is hypothesized that serum sickness results when a drug (hapten) binds to plasma protein and antibodies are generated in response to the drug-protein complex. Complement activation occurs when large quantities of soluble antigen-antibody (immune) complexes fix to vascular endothelial receptors. Complement fragments attract and activate neutrophils, which release proteases that induce tissue injury. The urticaria in serum sickness probably results from immune complex necrotizing vasculitis and complement activation that induces mast cell degranulation. IgE-dependent mechanisms likely are also contributory in some individuals. Laboratory abnormalities include elevated erythrocyte sedimentation rate, leukopenia (acute phase), occasional plasmacytosis, and decreased total hemolytic complement (CH50), C3, and C4. Slight albuminuria, hyaline casts, and microscopic hematuria may also occur.

TREATMENT

Stoppage of the culprit agent, when identified, is recommended. Serum sickness is usually self-limited and rarely life threatening when the offending drug or protein is stopped or removed. Symptoms generally improve over 2 to 4 weeks as patients clear their immune complexes. Evidence-based treatment recommendations for serum sickness are very limited. Long-acting, less-sedating H₁ antihistamines such as cetirizine (Zyrtec), desloratadine (Clarinex), fexofenadine (Allegra), or loratadine (Claritin) generally control urticaria. Systemic corticosteroids (e.g., prednisone, 0.5 to 1.0 mg/kg/day) may help severe symptoms. Fever and arthralgias typically resolve within 48 to 72 hours of treatment, and the formation of new cutaneous eruptions usually ceases within the same time frame. Antihistamine therapy is continued for 1 week after apparent resolution of symptoms and then slowly discontinued. Skin testing with heterologous antisera is performed routinely to avoid anaphylaxis to future administration of heterologous serum.

REFERENCES

American Heart Association in collaboration with International Liaison Committee on Resuscitation: 2005 American Heart Association guidelines for cardiopulmonary resuscitation and emergency cardiovascular care. Anaphylaxis. Circulation 2005;112(Suppl 4):143-145.
Brown SGA, Blackman KE, Stenlake V, Heddle RJ: Insect sting anaphylaxis: Prospective evaluation of treatment with intravenous adrenaline and volume resuscitation. Emerg Med J 2004;21:149-154.
Kemp SF, Lockey RF: Anaphylaxis: A review of causes and mechanisms. J Allergy Clin Immunol 2002;110:341-348.
Lieberman P: Biphasic anaphylactic reactions. Ann Allergy Asthma Immunol 2005;95:217-226.
Lieberman P, Kemp SF, Oppenheimer J, et al: (chief eds). Joint Task Force on Practice Parameters. The diagnosis and management of anaphylaxis: An updated practice parameter. J Allergy Clin Immunol 2005;115:S483-S523.
Project Team of the Resuscitation Council (UK): Emergency medical treatment of anaphylactic reactions. J Accid Emerg Med 1999;16:243-247.
Pumphrey RSH: Fatal posture in anaphylactic shock. J Allergy Clin Immunol 2003;112:451-452.
Pumphrey RSH: Fatal anaphylaxis in the UK, 1992–2001. Novartis Found Symp 2004;257:116-128.
Sampson HA, Muñoz-Furlong A, Campbell RL, et al: Second symposium on the definition and management of anaphylaxis: Summary report—second National Institute of Allergy and Infectious Disease/Food Allergy and Anaphylaxis Network symposium. J Allergy Clin Immunol 2006;117:391-397.
Simons FER, Gu X, Simons KJ: Epinephrine absorption in adults: Intramuscular versus subcutaneous injection. J Allergy Clin Immunol 2001;108:871-873.
Simons FER, Roberts JR, Gu X, Simons KJ: Epinephrine absorption in children with a history of anaphylaxis. J Allergy Clin Immunol 1998;101:33-37.
Wener M: Serum sickness and serum sickness-like reactions. In: Rose BD (ed): UpToDate, www.uptodateonline.com, Version 16.1 (current through November 2007), Wellesley, Ma.

Asthma in Adolescents and Adults

Method of
Michael Schatz, MD, MS

Asthma is an extremely common chronic medical condition that causes substantial morbidity among its sufferers. In addition to discomfort, asthma can cause sleep disruption, missed school and work, limitations of recreational activities, and acute episodes requiring emergency hospital care. Although the past 30 years have seen the introduction of increasingly effective and convenient medications, recent surveys continue to suggest that asthma remains suboptimally controlled in the majority of patients. The purpose of this article is to describe an approach to assessment and therapy that leads to optimal asthma control. It is based on the recently released National Asthma Education and Prevention Program (NAEPP) Expert Panel Report 3: Guidelines for the Management of Asthma (http://www.nhlbi.nih.gov/guidelines/asthma/asthgdln.pdf).

Diagnosis

The first step in evaluating a patient with asthma is to confirm the diagnosis. This is particularly important in patients with atypical symptoms or a poor response to asthma therapy. Asthma is confirmed by the demonstration of reversible airways obstruction, which most commonly is an increase in forced expiratory volume in 1 second (FEV₁) by 12% or more and at least 200 cc after an inhaled bronchodilator. For some patients, 2 to 4 weeks of chronic inhaled asthma therapy or 2 weeks of oral corticosteroid therapy is necessary to demonstrate reversibility. The latter is particularly important in adults with a history of smoking in whom chronic obstructive pulmonary disease (COPD) is a diagnostic consideration. In patients with normal pulmonary function, asthma can also be confirmed by means of methacholine (Provocholine) or exercise challenge.

Particularly important masqueraders of asthma include vocal cord dysfunction, panic attacks, hyperventilation, and cough due to postnasal drip, reflux, or angiotensin-converting enzyme (ACE) inhibitor therapy. All of these can also coexist with asthma, so their presence does not exclude asthma. Even when these conditions coexist with asthma, their diagnosis and appropriate therapy usually reduce the patient's respiratory symptoms.

Assessment

Assessment of asthmatic patients involves assessment of past severity, identification of aggravating factors, and definition of current status regarding treatment and clinical severity or control.

PAST SEVERITY

Asthma can be a mild, infrequent illness or a daily severe one. Certain severity markers identify patients who are more likely to experience severe exacerbations or to have symptoms that are more difficult to control and who thus require more careful surveillance. These include histories of asthma hospitalization, especially requiring intensive care or intubation, past requirement for oral corticosteroids, and exacerbation by aspirin or other NSAIDs. In patients with prior severe exacerbations, the rapidity of the onset of the exacerbation should be ascertained.

AGGRAVATING FACTORS

Factors that appear to trigger asthma symptoms should be assessed because they may be targets for avoidance therapy. Certain aspects of the patient's *environment* that can contribute to asthma triggering should be specifically ascertained, including occupational exposures, age of the home, pets, carpeting, visible mold, passive smoke, and cockroach exposure. Patients with persistent asthma should have in vitro or skin tests to identify *allergic sensitization* to pollens, house dust mites, mold spores, animal dander, and cockroaches that can contribute to the maintenance of asthma inflammation or can trigger episodes. The presence of *comorbidities* that can aggravate asthma, including cigarette smoking, obesity, rhinitis, sinusitis, reflux, and COPD, should be identified and treated. Finally, *psychosocial factors* to assess include a history or symptoms of anxiety or depression, attitudes toward asthma and asthma therapy, adherence to therapy, and social support. These may be targets for therapy or may be necessary to understand in order to create an effective therapeutic plan and therapeutic alliance.

CURRENT STATUS

Assessment of the current therapy the patient is actually taking is necessary for understanding the asthma's severity and to appropriately initiate or change therapy. It is particularly important to determine if the patient is taking long-term control medications, such as inhaled corticosteroids, long-acting β-agonists, leukotriene modifiers, cromolyn (Intal), nedocromil (Tilade), or theophylline (Theo-Dur). If the patient is not taking controllers, *severity* should be assessed, as described in Table 1,

TABLE 1 Classifying Asthma Severity and Initiating Treatment in Patients 12 Years and Older Not Currently Taking Long-Term Control Medications

		Classification of Severity*		
			Persistent	
Components of Severity	Intermittent	Mild	Moderate	Severe
Impairment				
Symptoms	≤2 d/wk	>2 d/wk but not daily	Daily	Throught the d
Nighttime awakenings	≤2 ×/mo	3-4×/mo	>1×/wk but not nightly	Often 7×/wk
Short-acting β₂-agonist use for symptom control (not prevention of EIB)	≤2 d/wk	>2 d/wk but not daily, and not more than 1 time on any d	Daily	Several times per d
Interference with normal activity	None	Minor limitation	Some limitation	Extremely limited
Lung function†	Normal FEV₁ between exacerbations FEV₁>80% predicted FEV₁/FVC normal	FEV₁ >80% predicted FEV₁/FVC normal	FEV₁ >60% but <80% predicted FEV₁/FVC reduced 5%	FEV₁ <60% predicted FEV₁/FVC reduced >5%
Risk				
Exacerbations requiring oral systemic corticosteroids	0-1/y‡	≥2/y‡ ──→		
		←────── Consider severity and interval since last exacerbation. ──────→		
		Frequency and severity may fluctuate over time for patients in any severity category.		
		Relative annual risk of exacerbation may be related to FEV₁.		
Recommended Step for Initiating Treament§				
Initiation	Step 1	Step 2	Step 3¶	Step 4 or 5¶
Follow-up	In 2-6 wk, evaluate level of asthma control and adjust therapy accordingly.			

*Level of severity is determined by assessment of both impairment and risk. Assess impairment domain by patient's/caregiver's recall of previous 2-4 weeks and spirometry. Assign severity to the most severe category in which any feature occurs.
†See Table 3 for normal FEV₁/FVC.
‡At present, there are inadequate data to correspond frequencies of exacerbations with different levels of asthma severity. In general, more frequent and intense exacerbations (e.g., requiring urgent, unscheduled care, hospitalization, or ICU admission) indicate greater underlying disease severity. For treatment purposes, patients who had ≥ 2 exacerbations requiring oral systemic corticosteroids in the past year may be considered the same as patients who have persistent asthma, even in the absence of impairment levels consistent with persistent asthma.
§See Table 6 for treatment steps. The stepwise approach is meant to assist, not replace, the clinical decision making required to meet individual patient needs.
¶And consider short course of oral systemic corticosteroids.
Abbreviations: EIB = exercise-induced bronchospasm; FEV₁ = forced expiratory volume in one second; FVC = forced vital capacity; ICU = intensive care unit.
Data from the National Asthma Education and Prevention Program (NAEPP) Expert Panel Report 3: Guidelines for the Management of Asthma.

TABLE 2 Assessing Asthma Control and Adjusting Therapy in Patients 12 Years and Older

Components of Control	Classification of Control*		
	Well Controlled	**Not Well Controlled**	**Very Poorly Controlled**
Impairment			
Symptoms	≤2 d/wk	>2d/wk	Throughout the d
Nighttime awakenings	≤2x/mo	1-3x/wk	≥4x/wk
Short-acting β_2-agonist use for symptom control (not prevention of EIB)	≤2 d/wk	>2 d/wk	Several times per d
Interference with normal activity	None	Some limitation	Extremely limited
FEV_1 or peak flow	>80% predicted or personal best	60%-80% predicted or personal best	<60% predicted or personal best
Validated Questionnaires[b]			
ACQ	≤0.75[†]	≥1.5	N/A
ACT	≥20	16-19	≤15
ATAQ	0	1-2	3-4
Risk			
Exacerbations requiring oral systemic corticosteroids	0-1/y	≥2/y[a]	→
Progressive loss of lung function	Evaluation requires long-term follow-up care		
Treatment-related adverse effects	Medication side effects can vary in intensity from none to very troublesome and worrisome. The level of intensity does not correlate to specific levels of control, but it should be considered in the overall assessment of risk.		
Recommended action for treatment[‡]	Maintain current step. Regular follow-up at every 1-6 mo to maintain control. Consider step down if well controlled for ≥3 mo	Step up 1 step and reevaluate in 2-6 wk. For side effects, consider alternative treatment options	Consider short course of systemic oral corticosteroids. Step up 1-2 steps and reevaluate in 2 wk. For side effects, consider alternative treatment options

*The level of control is based on the most severe impairment or risk category. Assess impairment domain by patient's recall of previous 2-4 weeks and by spirometry or peak flow measures. Symptom assessment for longer periods should reflect a global assessment, such as inquiring whether the patient's asthma is better or worse since the last visit.
[†]ACQ values of 0.76-1.4 are indeterminate regarding well-controlled asthma.
[a]At present, there are inadequate data to correspond frequencies of exacerbations with different levels of asthma control. In general, more frequent and intense exacerbations (e.g., requiring urgent, unscheduled care, hospitalization, or ICU admission) indicate poorer disease control. For treatment purposes, patients who had ≥2 exacerbations requiring oral systemic corticosteroids in the past year may be considered the same as patients who have not-well-controlled asthma, even in the absence of impairment levels consistent with not-well-controlled asthma.
[b]Validated questionnaires for the impairment domain (the questionnaires do not assess lung function or the risk domain). Minimal important difference. 0.5 for the ACQ, 1.0 for the ATAQ, not determined for the ACT.
[‡]See Table 3 for treatment steps. The stepwise approach is meant to assist, not replace, the clinical decision making required to meet individual patient needs. Before a step up in therapy, review adherence, inhale technique environmental control, and comorbid conditions. If an alternative treatment option was used in a step, discontinue it and use the preferred treatment for that step.
Abbreviations: ACQ = Asthma Control Questionnaire; ACT = Asthma Control Test; ATAQ = Asthma Therapy Assessment Questionnaire; EIB = exercise-induced bronchospasm; FEV_1 = forced expiratory volume in one second; N/A = not applicable.
Data from the National Asthma Education and Prevention Program (NAEPP) Expert Panel Report 3: Guidelines for the Management of Asthma.

CURRENT DIAGNOSIS

- Confirm the diagnosis by demonstrating an increase in FEV_1 by 12% or more after asthma therapy.
- Assess past severity by a history of exacerbations requiring hospitalization, intubation, or oral corticosteroids.
- Identify environmental exposures, allergic sensitization, and comorbidities that may be aggravating asthma.
- Assess current *severity* in patients not taking long-term control medications and assess *control* in patients who are taking long-term control medications based on symptom frequency, nocturnal awakenings, rescue therapy use, activity limitation, spirometry, and recent exacerbation history.

Abbreviation: FEV_1 = forced expiratory volume in 1 second.

based on symptom frequency, nocturnal awakenings, rescue therapy use, activity limitation, spirometry, and exacerbation history. If the patient is already taking controllers, *control* should be assessed (Table 2). Normal FEV_1/FVC (forced vital capacity) by age is shown in Table 3.

Long-Term Management

The goals of long-term management are to achieve and maintain well-controlled asthma. Both nonpharmacologic and pharmacologic therapy must be considered.

NONPHARMACOLOGIC THERAPY

The first tenet of nonpharmacologic therapy in the long-term management of asthma is *education*. Patients need to understand the inflammatory pathophysiology of asthma and the relationships among airway inflammation, bronchospasm, and symptoms. Patients should be informed that the cause of asthma is unknown and there is no cure

TABLE 3 Normal FEV₁/FVC by Age

Age Range (y)	Normal FEV₁/FVC (%)
8-19	85
20-39	80
40-59	75
60-80	70

Abbreviations: FEV₁ = forced expiratory volume in one second; FVC = forced vital capacity.
Data from the National Asthma Education and Prevention Program (NAEPP) Expert Panel Report 3: Guidelines for the Management of Asthma.

---

but that triggers can be identified and asthma can be controlled. They should receive education regarding self-assessment, either based on symptoms or peak flow monitoring, and regarding the recognition of early signs of an impending exacerbation.

The next step is to discuss and agree on the *goals of therapy*. The NAEPP has defined the following goals:

- Prevent chronic and troublesome daytime and nighttime symptoms.
- Maintain optimal pulmonary function for that patient.
- Maintain normal activity, including work, school, leisure activity, and exercise.
- Prevent recurrent exacerbations, especially those requiring urgent medical visits.
- Provide pharmacotherapy with minimal or no adverse effects.
- Achieve patient and family satisfaction with asthma care.

The physician should let the patient know that these are the expectations of optimal management and confirm that those are the patient's goals as well.

A very important component of nonpharmacologic therapy is reduction of relevant *environmental triggers*. Information should be given regarding environmental control of pollen, mite, mold, animal dander, and cockroach antigens (Box 1) that appear to be relevant based on the history and results of skin or in vitro specific IgE tests. Inhalant allergen *immunotherapy* should be considered for patients who have persistent asthma when there is clear evidence of a relationship between symptoms and exposure to an allergen to which the patient is sensitive.

Finally, *psychosocial* issues should be considered and addressed. For many patients, the education and therapeutic alliance described earlier adequately addresses psychosocial concerns. For other patients, poor past adherence requires identifying the barriers to adherence and finding solutions together. Resources for patients with poor social support should be identified. Clinically significant anxiety or depression that can make asthma harder to control should be treated.

PHARMACOLOGIC STEP THERAPY

The main principle of asthma pharmacologic step therapy is to add therapy in steps until control is achieved (step up) and decrease therapy in reverse steps (step down) to established the lowest effective dose necessary to maintain control.

There are two types of asthma medications: quick-relief medications (Table 4) and long-term control medications (Table 5). Systemic corticosteroids can be used either short-term to treat an exacerbation (see Table 4) or as long-term maintenance therapy for patients with severe disease (see Table 5). The generally recommended steps of pharmacologic therapy are shown in Table 6. Definitions of low, medium, and high dose inhaled corticosteroids for each of the available preparations are given in Table 7. At each therapeutic step level, the NAEPP Expert Panel has indicated *preferred* medications, which generally identify medications with the best balance of efficacy and safety in clinical trials for patients at that level of severity. However, these recommendations are based on population data and must be tailored to individual patient needs, circumstances, and responsiveness to therapy.

BOX 1 Measures to Control Environmental Factors that Can Make Asthma Worse

Allergens
Reduce or eliminate exposure to the allergen(s) the patient is sensitive to:

Animal Dander
- Remove animal from house or, at a minimum, keep animal out of the patient's bedroom and keep the bedroom door closed.

House-dust Mites
- Recommended
  - Encase mattress in a special dust-proof cover
  - Encase pillow in a special dust-proof cover or wash it weekly in hot water.
  - Wash sheets and blankets on the patient's bed in hot water weekly. Water must be hotter than 130°F to kill the mites. Cooler water used with detergent and bleach can also be effective.
- Desirable
  - Reduce indoor humidity to 60% or less.
  - Remove carpets from the bedroom.
  - Avoid sleeping or lying on cloth-covered cushions or furniture.
  - Remove carpets that are laid on concrete.

Cockroaches
- Keep all food out of the bedroom.
- Keep food and garbage in closed containers.
- Use poison baits, powders, gels or paste (e.g., boric acid). Traps can also be used.
- If a spray is used to kill cockroaches, stay out of the room until the odor goes away.

Pollens (from Trees, Grass, or Weeds) and Outdoor Molds
- Try to keep windows closed
- If possible, stay indoors, with windows closed, during periods of peak pollen exposure, which are usually during the midday and afternoon.

Indoor Mold
- Fix all leaks and eliminate water sources associated with mold growth.
- Clean moldy surfaces.
- Dehumidify basements if possible.

Tobacco Smoke
- Advise patients and others in the home who smoke to stop smoking or to smoke outside the home.
- Discuss ways to reduce exposure to other sources of tobacco smoke, such as from daycare providers and the workplace.

Indoor and Outdoor Pollutants and Irritants
- if possible, do not use a wood-burning stove, kerosene heater, fireplace, unvented gas stove, or heater
- Try to stay away from strong odors and sprays, such as perfume, talcum powder, hair spray, paints, new carpet, or particle board.

Data from the National Asthma Education and Prevention Program (NAEPP) Expert Panel Report 3: Guidelines for the Management of Asthma.

TABLE 4 Usual Dosages for Quick-Relief Medications for Patients 12 Years and Older

Medication	Dosage Form	Adult Dose	Comments
Inhaled Short-Acting β_2-Agonists (SABA)			
Metered-Dose Inhaler		*Applies to all four SABAS*	
Albuterol CFC	90 μg/puff, 200 puffs/canister	2 puffs 5 min before exercise	An increasing use or lack of expected effect indicates diminished control of asthma.
Albuterol HFA (Proventil, Ventolin)	90 μg/puff, 200 puffs/canister	or	Not recommended for long-term daily treatment. Regular use exceeding 2 d/wk for symptom control (not prevention of EIB) indicates the need for additional long-term control therapy
Pirbuterol CFC (Maxair)	200 μg/puff, 400 puffs/canister	2 puffs q4-6h prn	
Levalbuterol HFA (Xopenox)	45 μg/puff, 200 puffs/canister		Differences in potencies exist, but all products are essentially comparable on a per puff basis.
			May double usual dose for mild exacerbations.
			For levalbuterol, should prime the inhaler by releasing 4 actuations prior to use. For HFA, periodically clean HFA activator, as drug may block/plug orifice.
			Nonselective agents (epinephrine [Primatene Mist], isoproterenol [Isopro Aerometer], metaproterenol [Alupent]) are not recommended due to their potential for excessive cardiac stimulation, especially in high doses.
Nebulizer Solutions			
Albuterol (Accuneb, Proventil)	0.63 mg/3 mL 1.25 mg/3 mL 2.5 mg/3 mL 5 mg/mL (0.5%)	1.25-5 mg in 3 mL saline q4-8h prn	May mix with budesonide (Pulmicort) inhalant suspension, cromolyn (Intal) or ipratropium (Atrovent) nebulizer solutions.
			May double the dose for severe exacerbations.
Levalbuterol (R-albuterol) (Xopenex)	0.31 mg/3 mL 0.63 mg/3 mL 1.25 mg/0.5 mL 1.25 mg/3 mL	0.63 mg-1.25 mg q8h prn	Compatible with budesonide (Pulmicort) inhalant suspension. The product is a sterile-filled, preservative-free, unit-dose vial.
Anticholinergics			
Metered-Dose Inhalers			
Ipratropium HFA (Atrovent)	17 μg/puff, 200 puffs/canister	2-3 puffs q6h	Multiple doses in the emergency department (not hospital) setting provide additive benefit to short-acting beta agonists
			Treatment of choice for bronchospasm due to beta blocker
			Dose not block EIB
			Reverses only cholinergically mediated bronchospasm; does not modify reaction to antigen
			May be alternative for patients who do not tolerate short-acting beta-agonist
			Evidence is lacking for anticholinergics producing added benefit to β_2 agonists in long-term control asthma therapy.
Ipratropium with albuterol (Combivent)	18 μg/puff of ipratropium bromide and 90 μg/puff of albuterol 200 puffs/canister	2-3 puffs q6h	
Nebulizer Solutions			
Ipratropium bromide	0.25 mg/mL (0.025%)	0.25 mg* q6h	
Ipratropium bromide with albuterol (DuoNeb)	0.5 mg/3 mL ipratropium bromide and 2.5 mg/3 mL albuterol	3 mL q4-6h	Contains EDTA to prevent discoloration of the solution. This additive does not induce bronchospasm.
Systemic Corticosteroids			
Methylprednisolone (Medrol)	2, 4, 6, 8, 16, 32 mg tab	Short course (burst): 40-60 mg/d as single or 2 divided doses for 3-10 d	Short courses (bursts) are effective for establishing control when initiating therapy or during a period of gradual deterioration. Action may be begin with-in an hour. The burst should be continued until symptoms resolve. This usually requires 3-10 d but can require longer. There is no evidence that tapering the dose following improvement prevents relapse in asthma exacerbations.
Prednisolone (Delta-Cortef, Prelone)	5 mg tabs, 5 mg/5 mL, 15 mg/5 mL		
Prednisone (Deltasone, Orasone)	1, 2.5, 5, 10, 20, 50 mg tabs; 5 mg/mL, 5 mg/5 mL		
Repository Injection			
Methylprednisolone acetate (Depo-Medrol)	40 mg/mL 80 mg/mL	240 mg[2,†] IM once	May be used in place of a short burst of oral steroids in patients who are vomiting or if adherence is a problem.

[2]Exceeds dosage recommended by the manufacturer.
*0.5 mg per package insert.
†80-120 mg per package insert.
Abbreviations: CFC = chlorofluorocarbon; EIB = exercise-induced bronchospasm; HFA = hydrofluoroalkane; PEF = peak expiratory flow; tab = tablet.
Data from the National Asthma Education and Prevention Program (NAEPP) Expert Panel Report 3: Guidelines for the Management of Asthma.

TABLE 5 Usual Dosages for Long-Term Control Medications for Patients 12 Years and Older

Medication	Dosage Form*	Adult Dose	Comments
Systemic Corticosteroids			
Methylprednisolone (Medrol)	2, 4, 8, 16, 32 mg tab	7.5-60 mg qd in a single dose in AM or qod as needed for control	For long-term treatment of severe persistent asthma, administer single dose in AM either daily or on alternate d (alternate-day therapy may produce less adrenal suppression).
Prednisolone (Delta-Cortef, Prelone)	5 mg tab 5 mg/5 mL, 15 mg/5 mL	Short-course (burst) to achieve control, 40-60 mg/d as single or 2 divided doses for 3-10 d	Short courses (bursts) are effective for establishing control when initiating therapy or during a period of gradual deterioration. There is no evidence that tapering the dose following improvement in symptom control and pulmonary function prevents relapse.
Prednisone (Deltasone, Orasone)	1, 2.5, 5, 10, 20, 50 mg tab 5 mg/mL, 5 mg/5 mL		
Inhaled Long-Acting β_2-Agonists			Should not be used for acute symptoms relief or exacerbations. Use only with ICS.
Salmeterol (Serevent)	DPI 50 µg/blister	1 blister q12h	Decreased duration of protection against EIB may occur with regular use.
Formoterol (Foradil)	DPI 12 µg/single-use capsule	1 cap q12h	Each cap is for single use only; additional doses should not be administered for at least 12 h. Caps should be used only with the Aerolizor inhaler and should not be taken orally.
Inhaled Combined Medications			
Fluticasone and salmeterol (Advair)	DPI 100 µg/50 µg, 250 µg/50 µg, or 500 µg/50 µg HFA 45 µg/21 µg 115 µg/21 µg 230 µg/21 µg	1 inhalation bid; dose depends on level of control	100/50 DPI or 45/21 HFA for patients not controlled on low-to-medium dose ICS 250/50 DPI or 115/21 HFA for patients not controlled on medium-to-high dose ICS
Budesonide and formoterol (Symbicort)	HFA MDI 80 µg/4.5 µg 160 µg/4.5 µg	2 inhalations bid; dose depends on level of control	80/4.5 for patients not controlled on low-to-medium dose ICS 160/4.5 for patients not controlled on medium-to-high dose ICS
Inhaled Cromolyn and Nedocromil			
Cromolyn (Intal)	MDI 0.8 mg/puff	2 puffs qid	One dose before exercise or allergen exposure provides effective prophylaxis for 1-2 h. Not as effective for EIB as SABA. 4-6 wk trial of cromolyn or nedocronil may be needed to determine maximum benefit Dose by MDI may be inadequate to affect hyperresponsiveness Once control is achieved, the frequency of dosing may be reduced.
	Nebulizer 20 mg/ampule	1 amp qid	
Nedocromil (Tilade)	MDI 1.75 mg/puff	2 puffs qid	
Leukotriene Modifiers			
Leukotriene Receptor Antagonists			
Montelukast (Singulair)	4 mg or 5 mg chewable tab 10 mg tab	10 mg qhs	Montelukast exhibits a flat dose-response curve. Doses >10 mg do not produce a greater response in adults
Zafirlukast (Accolate)	10 or 20 mg tab	40 mg/d (20 mg tab bid)	For zafirlukast: Administration with meals decreases bioavailability; take at least 1 h before or 2 h after meals. Zafirlukast is a microsomal p450 enzyme inhibitor that can inhibit the metabolism of warfarin. Doses of this drug should be monitored accordingly Monitor for signs and symptoms of hepatic dysfunction.
5-Lipoxygenase Inhibitor			
Zileuton (Zyflo)	600 mg tab	2400 mg daily (600 mg qid)	Monitor hepatic enzymes (ALT). Zileuton is a microsomal p450 enzyme inhibitor that can inhibit the metabolism of warfarin and theophylline. Doses of these drugs should be monitored accordingly

Continued

TABLE 5 Usual Dosages for Long-Term Control Medications for Patients 12 Years and Older—cont'd

Medication	Dosage Form*	Adult Dose	Comments
Methylxanthines Theophylline (Slophyllin, Theobid, TheoDur)	Liquids, sustained-release tab, cap	Starting dose 10 mg/kg/d up to 300 mg max Usual max 800 mg/d	Adjust dosage to achieve serum concentration of 5-15 µg/mL at steady-state (≥48 h on same dosage). Due to wide interpatient variability in theophylline metabolic clearance, routine serum theophylline level monitoring is essential. Patient should be told to discontinue if they experience symptoms of toxicity Various factors (diet, food, febrile illness, age, smoking, and other medications) can affect serum concentration
Immunomodulators Omalizumab (Anti-IgE)	Subcutaneous (SQ) injection 150 mg/1.2 mL following reconstitution with 1.4 mL sterile water for injection	150-375 mg SQ every 2-4 wk, depending on body weight and pretreatment serum 1 gE level	Do not administer more than 150 mg per injection site Monitor patient following injections; be prepared and equipped to indentify and treat anaphylaxis that may occur Whether patients will develop significant antibody titers to the drug with long-term administration is unknown

*See Table 7 for estimated comparative daily dosages for inhaled corticosteroids.
Abbreviations: ALT = alanineaminotransferase; amp = ampule; cap = capsule; DPI = dry powder inhaler; EIB = exercise-induced bronchospasm; HFA = hydrofluoroalkane; ICS = inhaled corticosteroid; LABA = long-acting β2-agonist; max = maximum; MDI = metered-dose inhaler; SABA = short-acting β2-agonist; tab = tablet.
Data from the National Asthma Education and Prevention Program (NAEPP) Expert Panel Report 3: Guidelines for the Management of Asthma.

All patients with asthma should have an action plan that describes their pharmacologic self-management. Aspects of pharmacologic self-management include the maintenance medication schedule, rescue therapy doses for increased symptoms, when and how to increase control medication therapy, when and how to use prednisone, how to recognize a severe exacerbation, and when and how to seek urgent or emergency care. Control medications should be increased with an upper respiratory infection or with symptoms requiring more than two doses of rescue therapy in 12 hours. Although doubling the dose of inhaled corticosteroids does not appear to generally be sufficient to provide clinical benefit under these circumstances, higher-fold increases may be effective (e.g., three- or fourfold increases). The increased dose of control medications should be maintained at least until increased symptoms resolve. Prednisone is usually needed for patients with incomplete or temporary responses to adequate doses of β-agonists (4 puffs with a spacer, waiting at least 1 minute between puffs), substantial interference with sleep every night, requirement for 12 or more puffs of β-agonist in a 24-hour period, or a peak flow less than 60% predicted. Home treatment of exacerbations is further discussed later.

For patients not on long-term control medications, assess *severity* and select the level of treatment that corresponds to the patient's level of severity (see Table 1). Persistent asthma is most effectively controlled with daily long-term control medications, specifically anti-inflammatory therapy. For patients receiving long-term control medications, identify their current *step of therapy*, based on what they are actually taking (see Table 6), and their level of *control* (see Table 2). In general, step up one step for patients whose asthma is not well controlled. For patients with very poorly controlled asthma, consider increasing by two steps, a course of oral corticosteroids, or both. Before increasing pharmacologic therapy, consider adverse environmental exposures, poor adherence, or comorbidities as targets for intervention. For patients with troublesome or debilitating side effects from asthma therapy, explore a change in therapy.

TABLE 6 Stepwise Approach For Managing Asthma in Patients 12 Years and Older[a]

Step	Preferred Therapy	Alternative Therapy
1	Short-acting β-agonist prn.	—
2	Low-dose ICS	Cromolyn (Intal), LTRA, nedocromil (Tilade), theophylline (Theo-Dur)
3	Low-dose ICS *plus* LABA or Medium-dose ICS	Low-dose ICS *plus* LTRA *or* theophylline *or* zileuton (Zyflo)
4	Medium-dose ICS *plus* LABA	Medium-dose ICS *plus* LTRA *or* theophylline *or* zileuton
5	High-dose ICS *plus* LABA Consider omalizumab (Xolair) for patients who have allergies	—
6	High-dose ICS *plus* LABA *plus* oral corticosteroid[b] Consider omalizumab for patients who have allergies	—

Abbreviations: ICS = inhaled corticosteroid; LABA = long-acting β agonist; LTRA = leukotriene receptor antagonist.
[a]The stepwise approach is meant to assist, not replace, the clinical decision making required to meet individual patient needs.
[b]In step 6, before oral corticosteroids are introduced, a trial of high-dose ICS +LABA+either LTRA, theophylline or zilecton may be considered, although this approach has not been studied in clinical trials.
Data from the National Asthma Education and Prevention Program (NAEPP) Expert Panel Report 3: Guidelines for the Management of Asthma.

Follow-up

Patients whose asthma is not controlled should be seen every 2 to 6 weeks (depending on their initial level of severity or control) until control is achieved. Once control is achieved, follow-up contact at 1- to 6-month intervals is recommended. These checkups should ensure continued control, identify other changes in the patient's status, and update the patient's action plan.

TABLE 7 Estimated Comparative Daily Dosages for Inhaled Corticosteroids for Patients 12 Years and Older

Drug	Dosage Form	Daily Dose Low (µg)	Medium (µg)	High (µg)
Beclomethasone HFA (QVAR)	40 or 80 µg/puff	80–240	>240–480	>480
Budesonide DPI (Pulmicort)	90, 180, or 200 µg/inhalation	180–600	>600–1,200	>1,200
Flunisolide (AeroBid)	250 µg/puff	500–1,000	>1,000–2,000	>2,000
Flunisolide HFA (AeroSpan)	80 µg/puff	320	>320–640	>640
Fluticasone-HFA (Flovent HFA, Flovent Diskus)	MDI: 44, 110, 220 µg/puff DPI: 50, 100, 250 µg/inhalation	88–264 100–300	>264–440 >300–500	>440 >500
Mometasone DPI (Asmanex)	200 µg/inhalation	200	400	>400
Triamcinolone acetonide (Azmacort)	75 µg/puff	300–750	>750–1500	>1500

Abbreviations: DPI = dry powder inhaler; HFA = hydrofluoroalkane.
Data from the National Asthma Education and Prevention Program (NAEPP) Expert Panel Report 3: Guidelines for the Management of Asthma.

When well-controlled asthma has been maintained for at least 3 months, a step down in therapy can be considered to determine the minimal amount of medication required to maintain control or reduce the risk of side effects. Reduction in therapy should be gradual because asthma can deteriorate at a highly variable rate and intensity. Doses of inhaled corticosteroids may be reduced about 25% to 50% every 3 months to the lowest dose possible to maintain control. Most patients with persistent asthma relapse if inhaled corticosteroids are totally discontinued.

Patients should be encouraged to contact their asthma physician for signs of loss of asthma control, such as nocturnal symptoms, increasing β-agonist use, or activity limitation. The Expert Panel recommends consultation with an asthma specialist if the patient has difficulties achieving or maintaining control of asthma, immunotherapy or omalizumab (Xolair) is being considered, the patient requires step 4 care or higher, or the patient has had an exacerbation requiring hospitalization.

Treatment of Exacerbations

Asthma exacerbations are acute or subacute episodes of progressively worsening shortness of breath, cough, wheezing, or chest tightness associated with decreases in expiratory airflow.

HOME MANAGEMENT

Patients' action plans should direct their home therapy of asthma exacerbations according to the following recommendations.

CURRENT THERAPY

- Nonpharmacologic therapy includes asthma education (especially regarding inhaler technique, self-monitoring, and self-management), reduction in environmental triggers, addressing any relevant psychosocial issues, and immunotherapy for select patients.
- Preferred step therapy for long-term asthma management is (in order): low-dose inhaled corticosteroids; medium-dose inhaled corticosteroids or low-dose inhaled corticosteroids plus long-acting β-agonists; medium-dose inhaled corticosteroids plus long-acting β-agonists; high-dose inhaled corticosteroids plus long-acting β-agonists; and oral prednisone.
- Asthma exacerbations should be treated with high-dose inhaled β-agonists and early use of systemic corticosteroids.

Initial therapy should be with inhaled short-acting β-agonists (2-6 puffs by metered-dose inhaler [MDI] or nebulizer). This may be repeated in 20 minutes. With a good response (minimal or no symptoms and peak expiratory flow (PEF) ≥80% predicted or personal best), the patient may continue β-agonists every 3 to 4 hours for 24 to 48 hours. If repeated β-agonists are needed, a short course of oral corticosteroids should be considered.

With an incomplete response to initial therapy (persistent wheezing and dyspnea and PEF 50% to 79% predicted or personal best), oral corticosteroids should be added, β-agonists should be repeated, and the clinician should be contacted that day.

With a poor response (marked wheezing and dyspnea at rest, PEF <50% predicted or personal best), oral corticosteroids should be added, the β-agonist should be repeated immediately, and the patient should call the clinician and usually proceed to the emergency department. For signs of severe distress (e.g., difficulty talking in full sentences, diaphoresis, drowsiness, confusion, or cyanosis), 911 should be called. Patients with histories of rapid-onset severe exacerbations should have self-injectable epinephrine (Epipen)[1] at home to use at the onset of increased symptoms.

EMERGENCY DEPARTMENT AND HOSPITAL MANAGEMENT

Assessment should rapidly determine the severity of the exacerbation based on intensity of symptoms, signs (heart rate, respiratory rate, use of accessory muscles, chest auscultation), peak flow (unless the patient is too dyspneic to perform), and pulse oximetry. Treatment should begin immediately following recognition of an exacerbation severe enough to cause dyspnea at rest, peak flow less than 70% predicted or personal best, or pulse oximetry oxygen saturation less than 95%. While treatment is being given, a brief focused history and physical examination pertinent to the exacerbation can be obtained.

In patients with *mild-moderate exacerbations* (PEF >40% predicted), initial therapy is oxygen to achieve oxygen saturation greater than 90% and inhaled short-acting β-agonist by nebulizer or MDI (4-8 puffs) with holding chamber, which may be repeated up to three times in the first hour. Oral corticosteroids (prednisone 40-80 mg) are recommended if there is no immediate response to therapy or if the patient had been recently treated with oral corticosteroids.

In patients with *severe exacerbations* (PEF <40% predicted), initial therapy is oxygen as above, inhaled high-dose short-acting β-agonist (e.g., albuterol 5 mg) and ipratropium (0.5 mg) by nebulizer every 20 minutes or continuously for 1 hour, and oral or intravenous corticosteroids (prednisone or methylprednisolone 80 mg).

Repeated assessments of symptoms, signs, PEF, and oxygen saturation determine the responsiveness of the exacerbation to therapy. Such assessments should be made in patients presenting with severe

---

[1]Not FDA approved for this indication.

exacerbations after the initial bronchodilator treatment and in all patients after three doses of bronchodilator therapy (60-90 min after initial treatment). In patients who are improving, short-acting β-agonists may be repeated every hour until a good response is achieved (no distress, PEF >70%). When this response is sustained at least 60 minutes after the last treatment, the patient may usually be discharged on a course of oral corticosteroids (generally prednisone 40-60 mg for 5-10 days), initiation or continuation of medium-dose inhaled corticosteroids, and arrangement for outpatient follow-up.

In patients who are not improving with the above therapy, adjunctive therapy, such as with intravenous magnesium sulfate[1] (2 g) or heliox, may be considered. Intubation and mechanical ventilation may be required for patients with respiratory failure in spite of treatment.

Summary

Asthma is a very common problem with the potential to cause substantial interference with quality of life. Although there is no cure for asthma, asthma can be well controlled in the majority of patients with proper management and an effective patient-physician relationship. I hope that the method described herein for assessing and managing asthma will help physicians help their patients to achieve well-controlled asthma.

---

[1]Not FDA approved for this indication.

Asthma in Children

Method of
Gerald B. Kolski, MD, PhD

Asthma is the most common cause of significant childhood morbidity. This includes school absenteeism, hospitalizations, emergency department visits, and acute care visits. Its prevalence has been increasing throughout the 1990s and into this century. An estimated 5 million children younger than 15 years have asthma as identified by the National Health Interview Survey of 2003. According to this survey, the prevalence of asthma in the general population is somewhere between 6% and 10%. Prevalence in inner-city populations and especially in African Americans is closer to 14% to 15%. Pediatricians and family practitioners are often reluctant to make the diagnosis because of difficulty with giving prognostic information to parents. Wheezing during the first few years of life can often be associated with acute viral infections, especially respiratory syncytial virus (RSV) and rhinovirus (RV). Longitudinal studies suggest there are three patterns to wheezing in children. There are a group of children who wheeze during infancy associated with viral infections, a second group that wheeze during infancy and also as they get older, and a third group that only develops wheezing later after sensitization with allergens. Because of these groups it is oftentimes difficult to give prognostic information to parents until you have seen the pattern that a child will follow.

Despite tremendous improvement in medications and treatments for asthma, deaths from asthma continue to occur. Most recently, however, the mortality rates seem to have leveled off or decreased slightly.

One theory for the high prevalence of asthma is the "hygiene hypothesis." Studies done in homogeneous populations in Europe and Scandinavian countries have noted less asthma and allergies in rural populations versus those that live in urban environments. Attempts have been made to correlate this with endotoxin exposure during infancy and/or infections during this period of time that turn on immune responses that do not promote allergies. This concept favors an immune response, which postulates that certain infections and endotoxin exposure promote a T_H1 T cell response in which interferon gamma and interleukin(IL)-2 predominate, whereas a lack of these infections promotes a T_H2 response where there is an IL-4, IL-13, and IL-5 predominance with increased IgE production.

Pathophysiology

Over the last several decades the idea that reversible bronchoconstriction is the main element in asthma has changed. It has become apparent that in addition to bronchoconstriction there is considerable inflammation involving increased mucus production, inflammatory cell infiltrates, and airway thickening. With longitudinal studies it has become apparent that there may in fact be some fibrosis that leads to "airway remodeling." The increased inflammatory infiltrates lead to increasing airway reactivity characterized by hyperresponsiveness to various stimuli. The inflammatory cell infiltrates can include eosinophils, lymphocytes, basophils, neutrophils, and macrophages depending on the stimulus. Unchecked inflammation is believed to be the cause of the fibrosis. Clearly it is important to try and identify the triggers in an individual patient that are causing the inflammation as well as treating the inflammation.

Differential Diagnosis

Determining the cause of wheezing in infancy can often be difficult. During the first year of life if the wheezing is associated with a viral infection, a diagnosis of bronchiolitis is often made. A clinical response to bronchodilators might be helpful in assessing whether this is going to be a child with asthma. Recurrent wheezing in an atopic child with a strong family history of asthma would strongly suggest that the child has underlying asthma. An association with eczema and/or other allergic manifestations might also be suggestive of asthma. Because of the difficulty in doing pulmonary functions during the first few years of life, clinical assessment is the key. In addition to asthma, Table 1 lists the other diagnoses that have to be considered. Cystic fibrosis, gastroesophageal reflux disease, and foreign body aspiration probably are the most common diagnoses that have to be entertained. Recurrent infiltrates should make you worry about immune deficiencies including hypogammaglobulinemia and ciliary defects such as immotile cilia syndrome.

Diagnostic tests such as a sweat test, immunoglobulins, skin or radioallergosorbent assay test (RAST), barium swallow, bronchoscopy, or chest radiograph may be indicated.

In older children asthma may be diagnosed by doing pulmonary functions. Spirometry can often be done in the office and can be a reproducible way to measure the extent of airway disease in known asthmatics as well as diagnostic by looking at pre- and postbronchodilator responses. The forced expiratory volume at 1 second (FEV_1) is often thought to be a measure of large airway obstruction. The FEF_{25-75} or expiratory flow between the 25th and 75th percentile of the forced vital capacity (FVC) is often thought to be a measure of small airway disease. A 15% increase in FEV_1 pre- and

TABLE 1 Differential Diagnosis of Wheezing

Infants	Older Children
Laryngomalacia	Asthma
Tracheomalacia	Cystic fibrosis
Vascular rings	Gastroesophageal reflux disease
Subglottic stenosis	Foreign body aspiration
Airway congenital masses	Airway tumors
Gastroesophageal reflux	Viral infections (RSV, adenovirus)
Bronchiolitis	Tuberculosis
Pneumonia	

Abbreviations: RSV = respiratory syncytial virus.

postbronchodilator or 25% increase in FEF_{25-75} is thought to be diagnostic of asthma. Inhalation challenges with methacholine (Provocholine) or histamine are often used to measure airway reactivity in experimental studies. Bronchoconstriction with these inhalation challenges can determine the degree of airway hyperreactivity. Similar results can also be obtained with exercise challenges or cold air challenges. These tests are often used to diagnose asthma in children whose pulmonary functions at baseline are not significantly depressed. In children with asthma, peak expiratory flow rates (PEFRs) are often used to monitor the asthma as well as the management. This test is effort dependent.

Key Diagnostic Points Consistent with Asthma

- Recurrent wheezing responding to bronchodilators
- Coughing or wheezing shortly after exercise
- Pulmonary functions that show obstruction responding to bronchodilators
- Strong family history of asthma
- Associated allergic symptoms including seasonal rhinitis, eczema, or urticaria

History

Once a diagnosis of asthma is made, it is important to determine the trigger for this individual's asthma symptoms or exacerbations. The history is very important in determining treatment. Box 1 lists the most common causes for asthma exacerbations.

The most common perennial allergens are dust mites, cockroaches, mold, and pets. In the inner cities, cockroaches and dust mites are very common causes for allergic sensitization. They are extremely common and very difficult to control. Dust mites need moisture and thus are much more common in humid areas. With increased humidity, molds also can play a significant role. Children are often treated with humidifiers or vaporizers for upper respiratory infections, which may exacerbate dust mite and mold exposure. In drier climates, pets, especially indoor animals, are often exacerbating causes. Recent studies have indicated that more than two or three pets decreased the likelihood of sensitization, whereas an isolated pet is more likely to be associated with the development of allergy. This may have to do with endotoxin and the previously discussed hygiene hypothesis.

Children who only have difficulty with their asthma in the spring and fall may have sensitization to the pollens. This is very regional and often associated with being outdoors. Pollination and dissemination is most problematic with dry windy days. Keeping the windows closed at night as well as air conditioning may benefit individuals with seasonal allergies. These children may need medications at particular times of the year but not throughout the year. Airway reactivity often continues even 4 to 6 weeks after the allergen is no longer present.

Children who have trouble with viral infections may also have increased reactivity from perennial or seasonal exposures that exacerbate the asthma with infection. It is often helpful to reduce allergy exposure in these individuals so as to reduce their response to viral infections. Parents may be alerted to signs of upper respiratory infection so that they can increase asthma treatment at those times.

At all times cigarette smoke causes increased mucus production as well as decreases mucociliary clearance. Children with asthma thus are especially prone to having difficulty around cigarette smoke. During infancy, cigarette smoke exposure is associated with a two- to threefold increase in risk of asthma as well as upper respiratory infections, ear infections, and pneumonia. Smoking during pregnancy is also associated with a sustained decrease in infant pulmonary functions. Smoke is a form of indoor air pollution. Outdoor air pollution, especially small particles, ozone, nitrogen dioxide, and sulfur dioxide, all can be exacerbating factors in asthma.

Exercise is associated with asthma exacerbations because of the inhalation of cold dry air. Exercise is often associated with mouth breathing. The nose normally moisturizes, filters, and warms the air. Nasal congestion secondary to allergies, viral infections, or nasal obstruction can all lead to more difficulty with exercise as well as with breathing cold dry air at any time.

Weather changes are often a problem secondary to what is in the air or the changes in temperature of the air. Children who have trouble with weather changes are often responding to changes in pollen distribution or other allergens or irritants.

Children who have reflux as the exacerbating cause of their asthma often have difficulty at night when they lie down, shortly after meals, or when ingesting very acidic substances. Often there will be considerable coughing and if the child is old enough to talk some significant heartburn. Reflux is often worse when the asthma is a problem because the lower esophageal sphincter tone decreases with hyperinflation at that time.

Children with sensitivity to aspirin or nonsteroidal anti-inflammatory drugs (NSAIDs) often have associated sinusitis, nasal polyps, and profuse rhinorrhea with aspirin exposure. It often goes undiagnosed until adulthood. Nasal polyps should always raise this possibility in addition to a diagnosis of cystic fibrosis.

Sinusitis can be associated with significant exacerbations of asthma. Often treating the sinusitis treats the asthma exacerbation. Purulent nasal discharge for 5 to 7 days associated with significant coughing and maxillary tenderness may be suggestive of underlying sinusitis. In children with allergic rhinitis, complications of sinusitis often occur.

In all children with asthma it is very important that you try and assess severity of disease. There should be questions asked about whether the patient has ever been intubated or had an intensive care unit admission. In addition questions about recent use of oral corticosteroids should be asked to determine the recent course of asthma. Children with underlying seizure disorders are also important to identify because they are at greater risk for mortality. Signs of mental illness or depression should also be noted because this predisposes children to significant morbidity and mortality.

 CURRENT DIAGNOSIS

- Always focus on the ABCs (airway, breathing, and circulation).
- Start prescription early and aggressively (titrate β-agonist to effect).
- Reevaluate frequently (try to avoid intubation at all cost).
- Lack of wheezing is not always a good thing.
- Plan ahead in case things go bad.
- Ensure adequate hydration.

BOX 1 Asthma Triggers

- Allergies: perennial or seasonal
- Viral infections
- Irritants, especially cigarette smoke and air pollution
- Exercise
- Weather changes
- Gastroesophageal reflux
- Medications including aspirin and nonsteroidal anti-inflammatory drugs (NSAIDs)
- Sinusitis

Physical Examination

In examining a patient with asthma, the complete physical is extremely helpful. Children with skin findings of eczema or hives associated with an exacerbation of asthma may often lead to a search for an allergy exposure that is responsible for symptoms. Nasal examination may show boggy turbinates suggestive of allergy or erythematous turbinates suggestive of infection. Purulent discharge associated with sinus tenderness may suggest sinusitis. Nasal polyps should also be looked for to ascertain whether the patient may have underlying cystic fibrosis or aspirin-sensitive asthma. Enlarged tonsils and adenoids may predispose to mouth breathing and exacerbate underlying asthma. Examination of the chest may show whether there is a pectus suggesting chronic disease or whether there is hyperinflation with a barrel chest. Supraclavicular, intercostal, and subcostal muscular activity give information as to the work of breathing. The cardiac examination should focus on heart rate as well as any sign that might indicate this is cardiac wheezing instead of asthma. Abdominal examination is important to evaluate any signs of liver or spleen enlargement that might indicate evidence of pulmonary hypertension or cardiac disease. Examination of the extremities is important to look for clubbing and/or cyanosis. The neurologic exam is especially important acutely to ascertain whether the patient is having any change in mental status secondary to hypoxia.

Treatment

Treatment for asthma has changed considerably since the mid 90's. The chronic management of asthma has focused on assuring that the patient functions as normally as possible with the following goals of asthma management:

- No nocturnal asthma
- Full exercise activity
- No emergency department visits or hospitalizations
- No lost time from school or work
- No or minimal side effects from medication

Asthma treatment has focused on the anti-inflammatory nature of the disease to eliminate long-term damage to the lungs. Asthma treatment has followed the National Heart, Lung, and Blood Institute (NHLBI) guidelines with assessment of asthma severity and management based on the classifications (Table 2). We developed a color-coded questionnaire that gives an indication of asthma control.

CURRENT THERAPY

- **Severe:** ABCs, oxygen, monitors, POX, IV, isotonic fluids to maintain volume.

Start with (consider SC epinephrine if really tight):

- Albuterol, 0.5% inhalation solution, 0.5 mL (<20 kg), 0.75 mL (>20 kg) q20min × 3 (may give as mini-Nebs or start continuous at 2–3 mL/h). After initial stabilization patient will likely need q2h Nebs or continuous albuterol.
- Methylprednisolone (Solu-Medrol), 2 mg/kg IV (maximum, 125 mg) then start 1 mg/kg q6h (maximum, 80 mg/dose).
- Ipratropium bromide (Atrovent), 250 μg (<5 y), 500 μg (>5 y) × 2, then q4h.

If minimal improvement:

- Magnesium sulfate,[1] 45 mg/kg IV over 20 min (maximum, 2 g).

If still severe, consider terbutaline drip:

- Terbutaline (Brethine), 2–10 μg/kg loading dose, then start infusion at 0.1–0.4 μg/kg/min (maximum, 6 μg/kg/min). **Needs pediatric intensive care unit (PICU).**

At any time if minimal air entry, use:

- Epinephrine (1:1000), 0.01 mL/kg SC (maximum, 0.3 mL) or
- Terbutaline, 0.01 mg/kg SC (maximum, 0.25 mg)

Note: Adequate volume can be critical in maintaining circulatory volume (preload), so use volume freely. Also buffering with THAM for severe acidosis can be useful. These two strategies may help you avoid intubation.

If you really need to intubate (impending respiratory failure), use atropine, 0.02 mg/kg IV (minimum, 0.1 mg (maximum, 1 mg); ketamine (Ketalar), 1–2 mg/kg IV; or vecuronium (Norcuron), 0.1–0.2 mg/kg IV.

- **Moderate:** ABCs, POX, oxygen, monitors. ± IV

Start with

- Albuterol, 0.5 mL (<20 kg), 0.75 mL (>20 kg) q20 min × 3 (may start with mini Nebs or continuous). Then patient will likely need q2h Nebs or continuous albuterol (2 mL/h <10 kg, 3 mL/hr >10 kg)
- Ipratropium bromide, 250 μg (<5 y), 500 μg (>5 y) × 2, then q4h
- Prednisone, 2 mg/kg (maximum, 80 mg) if tolerating PO or
- Methylprednisolone, 2 mg/kg (maximum, 80 mg) (continue steroids for 5 d, 2 mg/kg/d)

If minimal improvement:

Consider magnesium sulfate as above.

- **Mild:** ABCs, POX

Start with

- Albuterol Nebs or MDI with spacer q2–4h
- Prednisolone, 2 mg/kg loading dose (maximum, 80 mg), then 2 mg/kg/d divided bid × 5 d

For mild to moderate exacerbation, discharge home may be considered if patient shows good improvement, is no longer dyspneic or hypoxic, tolerates Nebs q4h, and has good supervision at home.

CXR: Consider for a first-time wheezer; a condition other than asthma (i.e., FB); a febrile child with clinical signs of pneumonia; or no clinical improvement or worsening condition (pneumothorax, pneumomediastinum).

Continuous albuterol: To calculate the total amount of albuterol and normal saline, remember that the total amount of solution per hour must equal 30 mL.

Example: For a child >10 kg, the albuterol dose for continuous Nebs is 3 mL/h so you need to add 27 mL of NSS to run for 1 h (to set it up for 4 h, total mL = 120 with 12 mL albuterol + 108 mL NSS).

---

[1]Not FDA approved for this indication.

Abbreviations: ABCs = airway, breathing, and circulation; CXR = chestradiograph; FB = foreign body; IV = intravenous; Nebs = nebulized; NSS = normal saline solution; POX = pulse oximter; SC = subcutaneous; THAM = tromethamine.

TABLE 2 Stepwise Approach for Managing Asthma in Children

Classify Severity: Clinical Features Before Treatment or Adequate Control			Medications Required to Maintain Long-Term Control
	Symptoms/Day	*PEF or FEV$_1$*	
	Symptoms/Night	*PEF Variability*	*Daily Medications*
Step 4 Severe persistent	Continual Frequent	<60% >30%	**Preferred treatment:** • High-dose inhaled corticosteroids, *and* • Long-acting inhaled β$_2$-agonists (combination preferred) *and*, if needed, • Corticosteroid tablets or syrup long term (2 mg/kg/d, generally do not exceed 60 mg/d). (Make repeat attempts to reduce systemic corticosteroids and maintain control with high-dose inhaled corticosteroids.)

Step 3
Moderate persistent
	Daily
	>1 night/wk
		>60% – <80%
		>30%
			• **Preferred treatment:**
			  • Low- to medium-dose inhaled corticosteroids.
			• **Alternative treatment** (listed alphabetically):
			  • Increase inhaled corticosteroids within medium-dose range
			  or
			  • Low to medium–dose inhaled corticosteroids and either leukotriene modifier or theophylline.
			
			If needed (particularly in patients with recurring severe exacerbations):
			• **Preferred treatment:**
			  • Increased inhaled corticosteroids within medium-dose range and add long-acting inhaled β$_2$-agonists (combination inhaler preferred).
			• **Alternative treatment** (listed alphabetically):
			  • Increase inhaled corticosteroids within medium-dose range, and add either leukotriene modifier or theophylline.

Step 2
Mild persistent
	>2/wk but <1/d
	>2 nights/mo
		>80%
		20% – 30%
			• **Preferred treatment:**
			  • Low-dose inhaled corticosteroids.
			• **Alternative treatment** (listed alphabetically):
			  • Cromolyn (Intal).
			  • Leukotriene modifier.
			  • Nedocromil (Tilade) *or* sustained-release theophylline (Slo-bid Gyrocaps) to serum concentration of 5–15 µg/mL.

Step 1 Mild intermittent	<2d/wk <2 nights/mo	>80% <20%	• **No daily medication needed.** • Severe exacerbations may occur, separated by long periods of normal lung function and no symptoms. A course of systemic corticosteroids is recommended.

Note: Children <5 y cannot do adequate peak flows.

Quick relief
All patients
- Short-acting bronchodilator: 2–4 puffs short-acting inhaled β$_2$-agonists as needed for symptoms.
- Intensity of treatment depends on severity of exacerbation; up to 3 treatments at 20-min intervals or a single nebulizer treatment as needed. Course of systemic corticosteroids may be needed.
- Use of short-acting β$_2$-agonists >2 times/wk in intermittent asthma (daily, or increasing use in persistent asthma) may indicate the need to initiate (increase) long-term-control therapy.

↓ **Step down**
Review treatment q1–6 mo; a gradual stepwise reduction in treatment may be possible.

↑ **Step up**
If control is not maintained, consider step up.
First, review patient medication technique, adverse effects from medications.

Notes:
The stepwise approach is meant to assist, not replace, the clinical decision-making required to meet individual patient needs.
Classify severity: Assign patient to most severe step in which any feature occurs (PEF is percentage of personal best; FEV$_1$ is percentage predicted).
Gain control as quickly as possible (consider a short course of systemic corticosteroids); then step down to the least medication necessary to maintain control.
Minimize use of short-acting inhaled β$_2$-agonists. Overreliance on short-acting inhaled β$_2$-agonists (e.g., use of approximately 1 canister/mo even if not using it every day) indicates inadequate control of asthma and the need to initiate or intensify long-term control therapy.
Provide education on self-management and controlling environmental factors that make asthma worse (e.g., allergens and irritants).
Refer to an asthma specialist if there are difficulties controlling asthma or if step 4 care is required. Referral may be considered if care at level step 3 is required.

Continued

TABLE 2 Stepwise Approach for Managing Asthma in Children—cont'd

Usual Dosages for Long-Term-Control Medications

Medication	Dosage Form	Child Dose
Systemic Corticosteroids		
Methylprednisolone (Medrol)	2-, 4-, 8-, 16-, 32-mg tablets	0.25–2 mg/kg daily in single dose in AM or qod as needed for control
Prednisolone (Prelone) (Orapred)	5-mg tablets 5 mg/5 mL, 15 mg/5 mL	Short-course "burst": 1–2 mg/kg/d, maximum
Prednisone (Orasone)	1-, 2.5-, 5-, 10-, 20-, 50-mg tablets: 5 mg/5 mL, 5 mg/mL	60 mg/d for 3–10 d
Long-Acting β_2-agonists		
(*Do not use for symptom relief or for exacerbations.*)		
Salmeterol (Serevent)	DPI 50 µg/blister	1 blister q12h
Formoterol (Foradil)	DPI 12 µg/single-use capsule	1 capsule q12h
Combine Medication		
Fluticasone/salmeterol (Advair)	DPI 100, 250, or 500 µg/50 µg	1 inhalation bid; dose depends on severity of asthma
Budesonide/formoterol	80 or 160/4.5	
Mast Cell Stabilizer		
Cromolyn (Intal)	MDI 800 µg/puff Nebulizer 20 mg/ampule	1–2 puffs tid–qid 1 ampule tid–qid
Nedocromil (Tilade)	MDI 1.75 mg/puff	1–2 puffs bid–qid
Leukotriene Modifiers		
Montelukast (Singulair)	4- or 5-mg chewable tablet 10-mg tablet	4 mg qhs (2–5 y) 5 mg qhs (6–14 y) 10 mg qhs (>14 y)
Zafirlukast (Accolate)	10- or 20-mg tablet	20 mg daily (5–11 y) (10-mg tablet bid)
Methylxanthines		
(*Serum monitoring is important.*)		
Theophylline (Slo-Phyllin)	Liquids, sustained-release tablets and capsules	Starting dose 10 mg/kg/d; usual maximum: <1 y: 0.2 (age in wks) + 5 = mg/kg/d >1 y: 16 mg/kg/d

Estimated Comparative Daily Dosages for Inhaled Corticosteroids

Drug	Low Daily Dose	Medium Daily Dose	High Daily Dose
Beclomethasone HFA (QVAR) 40 or 80 µg/puff	80–160 µg	160–320 mcg	>320 µg
Budesonide DPI (Pulmicort) 200 µg/inhalation	200–400 µg	400–800 mcg	>800 µg
Budesonide inhalation suspension for nebulization (Pulmicort Respules)	0.5 mg	1.0 mg	2.0 mg
Flunisolide (AeroBid) 250 µg/puff	500–750 µg	1000–1250 µcg	1250 µg
Fluticasone (Flovent) MDI: 44, 110, or 220 µg/puff DPI: 50, 100, or 250 µg/inhalation	88–176 µg 100–200 µg	176–440 µg 200–400 µg	>440 µg >400 µg
Triamcinolone acetonide (Azmacort) 100 µg/puff	400–800 µg	800–1200 µg	>1200 µg
Mometasone fumarate (Asmanex) 220 mg	220 µg	440 µg	880 µg

Abbreviations: DPI = daily permissible intake; FEV_1 = forced expiratory volume at 1 second; MDI = metered-dose inhaler; PEF = peak expiratory flow (rate).

The new guidelines for 2008 put out by NHLBI focus on asthma control and asthma control questionnaires.

Medications

Asthma medications are classified according to medications that are used for acute relief of symptoms called *relievers* and those that are used for chronic control of symptoms characterized as *controllers*. This classification was established to give patients a better understanding of the role of their individual medications. It is also a better way to educate patients as to why they have to continue to take medications even when they are not having symptoms. It is important to discuss these individual classifications and medications for both acute and chronic management.

RELIEVERS

Various bronchodilators are used for acute management of asthma. These bronchodilators are predominantly β-agonists such as albuterol (Proventil), pirbuterol (Maxair), levalbuterol (Xopenex), and terbutaline (Brethine) that are selective for β_2-receptors. Table 3 gives the generic as well as trade names for these medications. The short-acting β-agonists are used for acute relief in most

TABLE 3 Medications for the Acute Relief of Symptoms

Generic β-agonist	Brand Name*
Albuterol	Ventolin, Ventolin HFA, Proventil HFA, Proventil
Pirbuterol	Maxair, Maxair Autohaler
Terbutaline	Brethaire, Brethine, Bricanyl
Metaproterenol	Alupent
Levalbuterol	Xopenex

*Many of these drugs are available in liquid, tablet, inhalation aerosol, as well as metered-dose inhalers.
Albuterol is also available in an inhaler in combination with ipratropium bromide (Combivent).

circumstances. In children anticholinergics such as ipratropium bromide (Atrovent) are often used in the emergency department and hospital setting acutely but are rarely given chronically. Chronic use of β-agonists is avoided because of a decrease in effectiveness as well as an increase in airway reactivity with their chronic use. With chronic use there is also a decrease in both the number and affinity of β-receptors for these bronchodilators. The affinity as well as number of β-receptors is increased with the use of corticosteroids.

In the management of acute episodes of asthma, an algorithm is used (see Current Therapy box). β-agonists are given either by nebulizer or inhaler. In addition to albuterol, a selective stereoisomer levalbuterol (Xopenex) is also available but is more expensive. This isomer may cause fewer side effects and have a slightly longer duration of action. In the acute setting, treatments are often given every 20 minutes times three and then are continued every 2 to 3 hours for hospitalized patients. In critical situations, albuterol may also be given continuously. It is during the acute situation where ipratropium bromide is beneficial for the first 24 to 48 hours of treatment. It can be given by nebulizer every 4 to 6 hours.

Injectable epinephrine is still recommended especially in the acute attack if it is thought to be secondary to allergies or anaphylaxis. It also can be used in the acute situation to make sure that inhaled drugs can reach the lower airway.

Magnesium sulfate[1] is used intravenously in severe asthmatics for its bronchodilator properties to prevent intubation or respiratory failure. This is outlined again in the acute management algorithm (Current Therapy box).

Theophylline (Theolair) was often the mainstay of asthma management in the 1980s, but its toxicity and the difficulty in having to monitor levels has reduced its use. Nausea, vomiting, abdominal pain, and an increase in hyperactivity often lead to noncompliance. With the selective β-agonists their use has been minimal. They can be used for chronic management in patients to decrease corticosteroid need.

Oral or systemic corticosteroids are always indicated in acute management of episodes of asthma exacerbation. The usual recommended starting dose is 2 mg/kg and should be continued during the episode. Prolonged use of corticosteroids may require a taper, but a short course of 4 to 5 days does not usually require a taper. Any patient who was admitted for an acute exacerbation of asthma should go home on a controller with an action plan for future attacks.

In the chronic management of asthma, albuterol is still the mainstay of acute attacks, pre-exercise, and for any reduction in peak flow or pulmonary functions. Albuterol (Proventil or Ventolin) is usually given by metered-dose inhaler and for most patients it is recommended that it be given with a spacer. Spacers increase the deposition in the lower airway and increase the effectiveness of inhaled drugs. In the chronic management of asthma, the NHLBI guidelines recommend that if albuterol is being used more than two or three times a week a step up in controller medications is suggested (Table 2).

CONTROLLERS

Inhaled corticosteroids are established as the mainstay of chronic management of asthma. Various preparations are available either by dry powder inhaler or metered-dose inhaler. Table 2 outlines the doses and route. Side effects of growth suppression and decreases in bone mineralization are dose related as well as preparation dependent. Individuals on any of the corticosteroids need to have their growth monitored and also to have instructions on mouth rinsing after inhalation to reduce fungal colonization in the oropharynx.

Leukotriene antagonists are available in oral preparations. These offer some advantage in pediatric patients in that they do not require good inhalation technique and can be given once a day. This may improve compliance and offer benefit in asthma as well as allergic rhinitis. They are not as effective as inhaled corticosteroids but offer some benefit in mild disease or as an adjunct to inhaled corticosteroids.

Cromolyn (Intal) and nedocromil (Tilade) are available as inhaled medications. Both of these drugs are mast cell stabilizers and appear to be most effective in allergic patients. These drugs should be taken three to four times a day, which makes their compliance more difficult. There are no significant side effects to these medications, however, and they are used in children because of their safety profile. They are used primarily in the mildest of patients and as pretreatment before allergy exposure.

Long-acting β-agonists are characterized as controllers, but these medications cannot be taken as anti-inflammatory agents. They have an increased risk of mortality when taken alone. For this reason only the preparations that are in combination with inhaled corticosteroids should be used in children. The drug preparations contain varying doses of inhaled corticosteroid with one standard dose of long-acting β-agonist.

Oral corticosteroids have been used for asthma since they were developed. They were used for patients with severe or chronic asthma before inhaled steroids were available. Because oral corticosteroids have significant side effects they should be used with caution. Prolonged use of systemic steroids leads to adrenal suppression, osteoporosis, and growth suppression. With prolonged use the dose should be reduced gradually. Inhaled corticosteroid effects can be similar to the systemic corticosteroids, especially if they are used at doses higher than recommended.

OMALIZUMAB

Omalizumab (Xolair) is a monoclonal antibody that is humanized and was developed against IgE. It is expensive and requires monthly injections. It is most effective when allergies are the main trigger for asthma. It is also used in patients with severe anaphylaxis.[1] It is indicated for children with moderate to severe persistent asthma that is exacerbated by significant documented allergies. Because it is nonspecific it does not reduce specific allergies and cannot be used in patients who have no significant atopy.

IMMUNOSUPPRESSIVE AGENTS

Various experimental studies in patients with chronic steroid-dependent asthma have used immunosuppressive agents such as methotrexate[1] (Trexall), IV gammaglobulin[1] (Gamimune N), and anti-inflammatory monoclonal antibodies against cytokines. None of these produced dramatic results and none is available or can be recommended at this time.

IMMUNOTHERAPY

Specific injections of extracts of allergens to which the patient is allergic is effective for allergic rhinitis that is secondary to certain allergens. Therapy with allergy extracts is effective for pollens, and by reducing allergic rhinitis symptoms it can affect nasal breathing and therefore benefit asthma. Because of the risk of reactions to

---
[1]Not FDA approved for this indication.

immunotherapy it should be used cautiously when the patient is having significant asthma symptoms at the time of injection. Studies in Europe suggest that in the future sublingual immunotherapy may be effective. Well-documented studies in this country have not been done and it is not approved as an FDA procedure.

Education and Environmental Control

Education of the individual asthmatic is important. Action plans in which treatment of acute episodes is outlined is recommended. Parents and patients should be taught about the patient's triggers as well as steps they should take to increase or decrease their medications depending on symptoms. Environmental precautions such as dust mite avoidance, focusing on reducing humidity, and limiting tobacco smoke exposure have had some success. Pet avoidance has not worked unless the pet is totally eliminated.

The NHBLI Guidelines as put forth in NAEPP Expert Panel 3 has been updated. It focuses on asthma control and uses asthma control questionaries.[1] In addition, it recommends that asthmatics on being discharged from the hospital or after being seen by their primary care physician be sent home with an action plan. In addition to assessing severity of asthma and outlining an action plan, a risk assessment is suggested with an emphasis on removing triggers, controlling the environment, and assessing comorbidities. The characteristic of the new guidelines focuses on the severity at the initial assessment, but in subsequent evaluations focuses on assessing control. The recommendation is to step up treatment if there is inadequate control and step down on treatment if it can be achieved with continued excellent control. Periodic assessment and monitoring are recommended, especially using spirometry, when possible.

REFERENCES

Castro-Rodriguez JA, Holberg CJ, Wright AL, Martinez FD: A clinical index to define risk of asthma in young children with recurrent wheezing. Am J Respir Crit Care Med 2000;162:1403-1406.

National Institutes of Health/National Heart, Lung, and Blood Institute: NAEPP expert panel report 2: Guidelines for the diagnosis and management of asthma. Publication no. 97-4051, Bethesda, Md, The Institutes, 1997.

National Institutes of Health/National Heart, Lung, and Blood Institute: NAEPP expert panel report 3: Guidelines for the diagnosis and management of asthma. Publication no. 08-4051, Bethesda, Md, The Institutes, 2007.

O'Connor GT: Allergen avoidance in asthma: What do we do now? J Allergy Clin Immunol 2005;116:26-30.

Romagnani S: Immunologic influences on allergy and the TH1/TH2 balance. J Allergy Clin Immunol 2004;113:395-400.

Spahn JD, Szefler SJ: Childhood asthma: New insights into management. J Allergy Clin Immunol 2002;109:3-13.

---

[1]Not FDA approved for this indication.

Allergic Rhinitis

Method of
Linda Cox, MD

Allergic rhinitis is the most prevalent of the allergic diseases, affecting up to 40 million Americans and 10% to 25% of the population worldwide. However, this figure is likely an underestimate of its prevalence because many patients do not recognize rhinitis as a disease and therefore do not seek medical attention. There has been an increasing prevalence of allergic rhinitis in the past few decades, particularly in developed countries. The prevalence of allergic rhinitis varies by age, with the frequency increasing from childhood into adulthood. Symptoms of allergic rhinitis develop before the age of 20 years in 80% of patients, and up to 40% of children suffer from allergic rhinitis. Allergic rhinitis is one of the top ten reasons for visiting primary care clinics.

Allergic rhinitis is sometimes trivialized because it is not potentially life-threatening and generally it is not a severe disease. However, it can significantly affect school performance, work productivity, and overall quality of life. In addition, the economic burden of allergic rhinitis both in terms of direct medical costs (e.g., medication, office visits) and indirect costs due to absenteeism and presenteeism (i.e., loss of work and school productivity), can be very significant. In the United States, allergic rhinitis causes approximately 3.5 million lost work days and 2 million lost school days annually, and it ranks fifth among the chronic conditions in terms of overall economic burden. In a recent survey, the estimated combined indirect and direct medical costs were $271 per employee, which would amount to a total of approximately $10 billion for the estimated 40 million Americans with allergic rhinitis.

Classification

There are currently two methods of classifying allergic rhinitis. One method is based on frequency and severity, and the other is based on the cause. Both classification systems are recognized and commonly used by allergy specialists.

TYPE OF AEROALLERGEN

The older method classifies allergic rhinitis by type of aeroallergen: seasonal versus perennial. Aeroallergens are often identified as indoor or outdoor allergens. Outdoor allergens such as pollen grains or mold spores are generally seasonal. For the most part, flowering plants are not allergenic because they are pollinated by insects and not by wind, and thus they are not airborne in sufficient quantities to sensitize people.

Seasonal allergen patterns can vary with the geographic location. Depending on the region, trees tend to pollinate earliest, beginning in late winter and early spring. The grass season follows, generally beginning in May and continuing through July, with longer seasons in the southern states; in some warmer climates (e.g., Hawaii and southern Florida), grass pollinates all year. Weeds usually begin in mid-August and continue to pollinate until the first frost. The weed season is also extended in the warmer climates. Mold and fungi can be seasonal (mid-summer) or perennial depending on the geographic location.

In addition to being an outdoor allergen, some molds and fungi can be significant indoor allergens, especially in environments with significant water damage or high humidity and poor ventilation. The most common indoor perennial allergens are produced by dust mites, cockroaches, dogs, and cats. Dog and cat allergens have been found in virtually every household in one large survey of U.S. houses. Cockroach sensitization and levels have been linked with asthma severity, a common comorbid condition. Dust mites, a common cause of allergic respiratory disease, can be found in most indoor environments unless the humidity is less than 50% because they cannot survive in arid conditions.

Indoor allergens are generally perennial but they can have seasonal peaks as well: cat and dog dander in late winter, cockroaches in summer, and dust mites in late summer to early fall. It is estimated that 20% of all cases of allergic rhinitis are seasonal, 40% are perennial, and 40% are a combination of perennial allergic with seasonal exacerbations.

SEVERITY AND FREQUENCY

The other rhinitis classification method uses a system similar to the commonly used for asthma classification: mild or moderate/severe and intermittent or persistent (Box 1). This method was developed by the Allergic Rhinitis and its Impact on Asthma Workshop Group (ARIA), an international workgroup. One of the rationales for the

> **BOX 1 ARIA Classification Of Allergic Rhinitis**
>
> *Intermittent* means that the symptoms are present:
> - Less than 4 days a week *or*
> - For less than 4 weeks
>
> *Persistent* means that the symptoms are present:
> - More than 4 days a week *and*
> - For more than 4 weeks.
>
> *Mild* means that none of the following items is present:
> - Sleep disturbance
> - Impairment of daily activities or leisure or sport activities
> - Impairment of school or work
> - Troublesome symptoms
>
> Moderate to severe means that one or more of the following items are present:
> - Sleep disturbance
> - Impairment of daily activities or leisure or sport activities
> - Impairment of school or work
> - Troublesome symptoms
>
> ARIA = Allergic Rhinitis and its Impact on Asthma Workshop Group.

ARIA workgroup discarding the "seasonal" and "perennial" classification is that an aeroallergen (e.g., grass pollen) that occurs seasonally in one region can be detected throughout the year (perennially) in another geographic area. According to the ARIA classification, *intermittent rhinitis* is defined as having symptoms less than 4 days per week for less than 4 weeks, and *persistent rhinitis* is defined as having symptoms more than 4 days per week for more than 4 weeks a year. The rhinitis is further classed by severity, with mild being no impairment of daily activities or sleep impairment and moderate–severe defined as having significant impairment in both as well as other troublesome symptoms.

Pathogenesis

The allergic reaction involves complex interactions between many components of the immune system. Immunoglobulin E (IgE), an antibody produced by plasma cells found beneath the mucosal surfaces of the eyes, upper and lower airways, and the gastrointestinal tract, is a key component of the allergic reaction. Two helper T cell (TH) profiles direct the allergic pathway: TH2 (the allergy profile), which produces the cytokines interleukin (IL)-4, IL-5, and IL-13, and TH1 (nonallergic), which produces interferon (IFN)-γ and IL-2. The TH2 cytokines IL-4 and IL-13 cause a class switching in B cells that leads to the production of IgE, and IL-5 promotes eosinophil activation and longevity. Dysregulation of the T-cell profiles leads to an imbalance and a predominance of the TH2-induced cytokines and subsequent IgE production and allergic inflammation.

IgE binds specific high-affinity receptors on basophils in the circulation and mast cells in various tissues. IgE can become sensitized to an allergen from prior exposure to the allergen. On re-exposure, the allergen binds the sensitized IgE molecule on the basophil or mast cell surface. If the allergen binds and cross-links two IgE antibodies, a series of signals is sent to the basophils or mast cells, leading to activation and degranulation. There is subsequent release of several preformed and postactivation-induced vasoactive mediators such as histamine, tryptase, leukotrienes, and prostaglandins, as well as several chemokines and cytokines that can induce immediate and delayed symptoms. The allergic reaction can have two phases: an early phase, with symptoms beginning minutes after cell activation and mediator release, and the late phase, beginning 4 to 12 hours after the initial allergic reaction.

The mediators histamine, tryptase, and the leukotrienes cause many of the immediate allergic symptoms that in the nose can manifest as sneezing, itching, rhinorrhea, and nasal congestion. During the immediate reaction, chemotactic factors are released that recruit inflammatory cells such as basophils, eosinophils, and T lymphocytes, which cause the late-phase reaction and may be associated with a recrudescence of symptoms. The early and late phases can be easily distinguished if there is a single exposure to the allergen (e.g., a cat-allergic patient visiting a house with a cat). However, with persistent allergen exposure (e.g., to dust mites) the late-phase inflammatory process is ongoing, producing chronic symptoms, and the immediate reaction would not be as apparent. Chronic allergic inflammation can increase sensitivity and lower the threshold for an allergen to induce an allergic reaction: For example, at the end of ragweed season it takes considerably less ragweed to induce symptoms compared with the beginning of the season. This phenomenon is referred to as *priming*.

Comorbid Conditions

Several other respiratory conditions are often linked with allergic rhinitis. Asthma, sinusitis, otitis media, and conjunctivitis are some common comorbid conditions associated with allergic rhinitis. Approximately 20% of allergic rhinitis patients have asthma, and 60% to 78% of asthma patients have allergic rhinitis. Some studies suggest the frequency of allergic rhinitis in asthmatic patients is as high as 99%. In most cases, allergic rhinitis precedes the onset of asthma, with the asthma developing within 2 years of the allergic rhinitis diagnosis. Up to 40% of patients with sinusitis have allergic rhinitis, and this number rises to 80% in people with bilateral sinusitis.

Some studies suggest that up to 30% of persons with chronic otitis media have allergic rhinitis. In children, the relationship between otitis media and allergic rhinitis is much stronger, with some studies reporting that allergic rhinitis was present in 40% to 50% of children referred for ear tube placement.

Nasal polyps are inflammatory tissue that can complicate allergic rhinitis by causing obstruction, which can lead to infectious sinusitis due to the impediment in sinus drainage. It has been estimated that 10% to 15% of patients with allergic rhinitis have nasal polyps. However, nasal polyps are rarely seen in children and generally indicate another condition, such as cystic fibrosis.

Conjunctivitis symptoms are very common in patients in allergic rhinitis, but epidemiologic studies often fail to evaluate eye symptoms, so there is likely underestimation of the link between conjunctivitis and allergic rhinitis. Some studies combine the two conditions in the term *allergic rhinoconjunctivitis*.

Sleep disturbances are very common in allergic rhinitis patients. Nasal obstruction can cause sleep-disordered breathing, and it has been estimated that 57% of adult patients and 88% of pediatric patients with allergic rhinitis have sleep disturbances.

Differential Diagnosis

Allergic rhinitis is a very common cause of rhinitis. However, because approximately 50% of patients with rhinitis do not have allergic rhinitis, other potential causes must be considered (Box 2).

The symptoms of allergic rhinitis—sneezing, clear rhinorrhea, and congestion—are very similar to those of the common cold (rhinovirus infection). It may be particularly difficult to diagnose allergic rhinitis in young children because frequent viral upper respiratory tract infections are not unexpected in this population.

A form of nonallergic rhinitis referred to as *irritant rhinitis* is as common as allergic rhinitis. It is characterized by an increased susceptibility to irritants (nonallergenic triggers), which results in the release of inflammatory mediators similar to that seen with an allergic reaction. This form of rhinitis has also been referred to as *vasomotor rhinitis*, implying that the etiology is a neurovascular imbalance, but the mechanism for irritant-induced rhinitis is not fully understood. A variant of irritant rhinitis called *gustatory rhinitis*

> **BOX 2 Differential Diagnosis of Rhinitis**
>
> Allergy is a very common cause of rhinitis. However, approximately 50% of patients with rhinitis do not have allergic rhinitis, so other potential causes must also be considered.
>
> **Nonallergic Rhinitis**
> Infectious
> - Acute
> - Chronic
>
> Nonallergic rhinitis with eosinophilia syndrome (NARES)
> Irritant-induced rhinitis (sometimes referred to as vasomotor rhinitis)
> - Chemicals or irritants
> - Cold air
> - Emotional factors
> - Exercise
> - Food (gustatory rhinitis)
>
> **Occupational Rhinitis**
> Caused by protein and chemical sensitizers; IgE mediated
> Caused by chemical sensitizers (e.g., diisocyanates); immune mechanism uncertain
> Caused by irritants
>
> **Other Rhinitis Syndromes**
> Atrophic rhinitis
> Ciliary dyskinesia syndrome
> Hormone-induced syndromes
> - Hypothyroidism
> - Menstrual cycle
> - Pregnancy rhinitis
>
> Drug-induced syndromes
> - Antihypertensive therapy
> - Aspirin and other nonsteroidal antiinflammatory drugs
> - Oral contraceptives
> - Rhinitis medicamentosa
> - Other drugs
>
> **Conditions that Can Mimic Symptoms of Rhinitis**
> Structural or mechanical factors
> - Adenoidal hypertrophy
> - Choanal atresia
> - Deviated septum or septal wall anomalies
> - Foreign bodies
> - Hypertrophic turbinates
> - Nasal tumors
>   - Benign
>   - Malignant
>
> Inflammatory or immunologic factors
> - Midline granuloma
> - Nasal polyposis
> - Sarcoidosis
> - Wegener's granulomatosis
>
> Cerebrospinal fluid rhinorrhea

is characterized by rhinorrhea while eating. A common misconception is that gustatory rhinitis is caused by food allergens, but the cause is likely the same as irritant rhinitis and can involve an aberrant neurologic–vascular reflex that results in the production of nasal secretions.

Hormonal factors such as hypothyroidism and pregnancy can lead to increased nasal congestion. Some medications can produce rhinitis symptoms, such as the older hypertensive medications (e.g., methyldopa [Aldomet], reserpine) and aspirin. Chronic use of topical α-adrenergic agonists can lead to rebound hyperemia and progressively worsening nasal congestion, a phenomenon known as *rhinitis medicamentosa*. Another relatively uncommon condition that mimics allergic rhinitis is *nonallergic rhinitis eosinophilic syndrome* (NARES). It is similar to allergic rhinitis in terms of its inflammatory features (nasal eosinophilia) but is distinct in that no specific cause (i.e., allergen) is identified.

Diagnosis

HISTORY

A careful history usually suggests the diagnosis of rhinitis. A thorough general medical history should include questions specific to the rhinitis symptoms, including information on seasonal pattern (or lack of one), chronicity, response to medications, possible precipitating factors, environment, occupation, and family history. The history should also focus on potential comorbid conditions such as asthma and sinusitis. Most patients with allergic rhinitis develop their symptoms before the age of 20 years, but allergic rhinitis can develop at any age, including infancy and old age. The frequency of symptoms should be noted and whether they are daily, episodic, seasonal or perennial. The duration and severity of the symptoms should also be determined. Manifesting symptoms can vary considerably, with some patients complaining primarily of sneezing and rhinorrhea and others presenting with nasal congestion (stuffiness) as their primary symptom.

Symptoms related to blockage of the airways include frequent sore throats, dryness of the mouth and oropharynx, a nasal quality to the voice, and snoring. Consistent obstruction on one side is not typical of allergic rhinitis and suggests a polyp, foreign body, structural problem (e.g., septal deviation), or, rarely, a tumor. Hyposmia and anosmia are most often associated with nasal polyps or severe disease, although these symptoms can also be the result of viral respiratory tract infection.

The history can provide some clues to the causative allergen: acute symptoms during house cleaning or vacuuming suggest dust mite sensitivity or mold sensitivity; symptoms exacerbated by harvesting, mowing, or leaf raking, activities that lead to mold spore dispersal, suggest mold sensitivity.

A positive family history makes it more likely that an allergy will develop, but the pattern of inheritance has not been established and a negative family history does not rule out the diagnosis of allergic rhinitis. The response to previous medications can assist in establishing the diagnosis: A good response to antihistamines favors an allergic process, whereas a favorable response to nasal corticosteroids can be seen in a number of conditions.

EXAMINATION

Physical examination of the head can reveal some findings characteristic of allergic rhinitis. A transverse crease in the skin of the lower third of the external nose can be seen in children, who chronically thrust the palm of the hand upward or sideways against the tip of the nose in response to itchiness or rhinorrhea, a movement commonly referred to as the *allergic salute*. Dennie's lines are folds under the eyes caused by edema. Dark discoloration under the eyes, referred to as *allergic shiners*, is caused by venous engorgement resulting from the nasal congestion. Nasal turbinates appear edematous (boggy), with a pale bluish hue, the appearance believed to be pathognomonic of allergic rhinitis. However pale, boggy turbinates can be seen in nonallergic rhinitis patients and, likewise, the turbinates of an allergic person may be erythematous and not pale blue. Lymphoid hyperplasia can be visualized in the posterior pharynx of some allergic rhinitis patients, and this effect is referred to as *cobblestoning*. In children, chronic mouth breathing caused by nasal obstruction can cause several facial features: high arched palate, elevation of the upper lip, and overbite (malocclusion).

DIAGNOSTIC TESTING

Although the clinical history can suggest the diagnosis, allergy diagnostic testing is needed to confirm the diagnosis. Allergy diagnostic testing is a means to identify a particular allergen-specific IgE. Testing methods include skin testing and in vitro tests.

Two types of skin test methods are commonly used: percutaneous and intradermal. The percutaneous method (prick) involves introducing a small amount of allergen into the skin by making a small puncture with a device that has been coated with the allergen extract. The intradermal method involves injecting a small amount of allergen (0.02-0.05 mL) under the skin. The latter method is considerably more sensitive than the percutaneous or in vitro test, but the increased sensitivity is offset by a lower specificity (higher false-positive rate). After the allergen is introduced into the skin, a localized allergic reaction, manifesting as a wheal and flare, occurs within 15 minutes if allergen-specific IgE is present.

Several types of laboratory assays can measure allergen-specific IgE, but their accuracy, precision, and quantitative ability can vary significantly. The first in vitro assays, Phadebas and Phadezym radioallergosorbent tests (RASTs), were designed to minimize false-positive results, which resulted in a high number of false-negative tests (low sensitivity). A modified RAST was developed in 1979 that improved the sensitivity with a slight decrease in specificity, but the sensitivity was still less than the percutaneous skin test. A newer technology, the ImmunoCAP assay, significantly improved the sensitivity without a change in specificity compared with the older methods. However, the costs of the in vitro allergy tests are, in general, greater than the costs of the allergy skin tests, and the test results are not immediately available, as they are with allergy skin testing. The percutaneous skin test is considered the most specific and cost-effective method for allergy diagnostic testing.

The clinical history can direct the selection of allergens for testing, and the number of allergens tested varies depending on the patient's symptom pattern and exposure history: seasonal, perennial, perennial with seasonal exacerbations, occupation, and so on.

Treatment

PHARMACOTHERAPY

The treatment of allergic rhinitis can include environmental avoidance measures, pharmacotherapy, and allergen immunotherapy. Pharmacotherapy is the most common mode of treatment, although it is not always the most effective. Allergic symptoms will not be controlled after the pharmacotherapy is discontinued because none of the available medications to treat allergic rhinitis has a disease-modifying effect.

H_1 antihistamines are probably the most commonly prescribed and over-the counter (OTC) medications for allergic rhinitis (Table 1). Antihistamines are most effective against the symptoms of sneezing, itching, and rhinorrhea but are not very effective against nasal congestion. Many of the oral first-generation H_1 antihistamines are available as OTC preparations. Limitations of the first-generation antihistamines are sedation and anticholinergic effect (mucosal dryness). The sedative properties of first-generation antihistamines include drowsiness and performance impairment. In the majority of states in the United States, patients taking sedating antihistamines are legally considered impaired. These sedative and anticholinergic effects are undesirable and potentially dangerous risks associated with first-generation antihistamines. Second-generation antihistamines have the advantage of being less anticholinergic and causing little or no sedation. For this reason, second-generation antihistamines have a safety advantage and are preferred for treating allergic rhinitis. There is currently one nasal antihistamine available in the United States, azelastine (Astelin) and one nasal combination mast cell stabilizer and antihistamine (Patanase).

Leukotriene receptor antagonists were initially approved by the U.S. Food and Drug Administration (FDA) for use in asthma, but montelukast (Singulair) was later approved for allergic rhinitis therapy as well. A recent systematic review and meta-analysis showed these agents to be as effective as antihistamines and inferior to nasal corticosteroids in improving symptoms and quality of life in patients with seasonal allergic rhinitis.

Nasal corticosteroids are the most effective medication class in controlling symptoms of allergic rhinitis (Table 2). A meta-analysis showed superiority of nasal corticosteroids over antihistamines in controlling rhinitis symptoms, and another meta-analysis demonstrated superiority of intranasal corticosteroids over topical antihistamines. In clinical studies, nasal corticosteroids have been shown to be more effective than nasal cromolyn (Nasalcrom), leukotriene receptor antagonists, and the combination of an antihistamine and leukotriene antagonists. Adverse side effects are minimal with nasal corticosteroids, but nasal irritation and bleeding can occur, and nasal

TABLE 1 Antihistamines

Drug	Availability	Usual Adult Dose
First-Generation Antihistamines		
Brompheniramine (Lodrane XR, LoHist 12 Hours, others)	OTC	4 mg q4-6 h ER: 12 mg q12h
Chlorpheniramine (Chlor-Trimeton, others)	OTC	4 mg q4-6h ER: 12 mg q12h
Clemastine (Tavist, others)	OTC	1.34-2.68 mg q12h
Cyproheptadine hydrochloride (Periactin, generic)	Prescription	4 mg up to tid
Diphenhydramine (Benadryl, others)	OTC	25-50 mg q4-6h
Hydroxyzine[1] (Atarax, Vistaril, generic)	Prescription	25-100 mg q6-8h
Triprolidine/pseudoephrine (Actifed Cold & Allergy)	OTC	1 tablet q6h
Second-Generation Antihistamines		
Acrivastine (Semprex)	Prescription	8 mg tid
Acrivastine/pseudoephedrine (Semprex-D)	Prescription	8/60 mg qid
Azelastine (Astelin)	Prescription	1-2 sprays per nostril bid
Cetirizine (Zyrtec)	OTC	5-10 mg qd
Cetirizine/pseudoephedrine (Zyrtec-D)	Prescription	5 mg/120 mg bid
Desloratadine (Clarinex)	Prescription	5 mg qd
Fexofenadine (Allergra)	Prescription	60 mg bid or 180 mg qd
Fexofenadine/pseudoephedrine (Allegra-D 12)	Prescription	60/120 mg bid
Loratadine (Claritin, Alavert, others)	OTC	10 mg qd
Loratadine/pseudoephedrine (Claritin-D 12, Alavert-D, Claritin-D 24, others)	OTC	5/120 mg bid 10/240 mg qd
Xyzol	Prescription	5 mg qd

[1]Not FDA approved for this indication.
ER = extended release; OTC = over the counter;

TABLE 2 Nasal Corticosteroids and Other Nasal Sprays

Drug	Dose
Nasal Corticosteroids	
Beclomethasone (Beconase AQ)	1-2 sprays in each nostril bid
Budesonide (Rhinocort Aqua)	1-4 sprays each nostril qd
Ciclesonide (Omnaris)	2 sprays in each nostril qd
Flunisolide 0.025% nasal solution (Nasarel Spray)	2 sprays in each nostril bid
Fluticasone furoate (Veramyst)	2 sprays in each nostril qd
Fluticasone propionate (Flonase, generic)	2 sprays in each nostril qd or 1 spray in each nostril bid
Mometasone furoate monohydrate (Nasonex)	2 sprays in each nostril qd
Olopatadine hydrochloride (Patanase)	2 sprays in each nostril bid
Triamcinolone acetonide (Nasacort AQ)	1-2 sprays in each nostril qd
Other Nasal Sprays	
Azelastine (antihistamine) (Astelin)	2 sprays in each nostril bid
Cromolyn sodium (mast cell inhibitor) (OTC) (Nasalcrom)	1 spray in each nostril qid
Ipratropium bromide (anticholinergic) (Atrovent 0.03% or 0.06%, generic)	2 sprays in each nostril tid
Oxymetazoline (decongestant) (Afrin, others)	Varies with product; generally 1-2 sprays in each nostril bid × ≤3 d Longer use than 3 d can result in rebound nasal congestion

septal perforation, presumably caused by topical vasoconstriction, has been rarely reported.

Concern over systemic side effects of nasal corticosteroids is generally not warranted. It is unusual for adult patients to develop systemic side effects after taking nasal corticosteroids in recommended doses. Studies of newer corticosteroid preparations at recommended and moderate doses given once daily demonstrate minimal systemic corticosteroid effect on the hypothalamic–pituitary–adrenal axis, as assessed by morning cortisol concentrations, cosyntropin stimulation, and 24-hour urinary free cortisol excretion. This is most likely related to the lower bioavailability of the newer preparations after intranasal administration. In children, an effect of nasal corticosteroids on growth has been demonstrated in some preparations, although an effect on the hypothalamic–pituitary–adrenal axis has not been demonstrated, and no reduction in bone density or other systemic effects has been reported.

An anticholinergic topical preparation, ipratropium bromide (Atrovent 0.03% or 0.06% nasal spray), may be useful for rhinitis associated with significant rhinorrhea. It is probably more effective for nonallergic irritant rhinitis such as cold air–induced rhinitis, gustatory rhinitis, or the profuse rhinorrhea associated with viral respiratory tract infections. Ipratropium has no effect on nasal congestion. Methscopolamine (Pamine, Pamine Forte) is an oral quaternary ammonium anticholinergic used as a drying agent and found primarily in combination with antihistamines such as chlorpheniramine and decongestants such as phenylephrine (Dallergy, Hista-Vent DA, Pre-Hist-D).

Cromolyn (Nasalcrom), a mast cell stabilizer, can be used as a topical nasal spray for allergic rhinitis, but the recommended dosing of every 4 hours for optimal efficacy may be difficult for most patients to comply with.

The use of oral and nasal decongestants is problematic in terms of potential adverse side effects, such as hypertension, tachycardia, and cerebrovascular accidents. Phenylpropanolamine was removed from the U.S. market after an increased association with hemorrhagic stroke in women was found. Adverse side effects and concerns about misuse or overuse have led to limitation on access to pseudoephedrine, which is available as a nonprescription behind-the-counter medication. Phenylephrine is the decongestant found in most combination products. Overuse of topical decongestants like phenylephrine (Neo-Synephrine) and oxymetazoline (Afrin) results in well-described rebound nasal congestion and repeated use can cause rhinitis medicamentosa.

The use of saline nasal washes is highly recommended. This modality is especially useful in patients with complicating chronic sinusitis. Commercially available products for nasal irrigation include a squeeze bottle with premixed packets of sodium chloride and baking soda (Neilmed), premixed sodium chloride solutions (Ocean Spray), and nasal adapter for an irrigation system (Water-Pik with Grossan adapter; Hydromed). Nasal washes also can be performed with a rubber ear syringe and a homemade saline solution: 1 teaspoon of table salt and a pinch of baking soda mixed in a pint of warm water.

AVOIDANCE AND ENVIRONMENTAL CONTROLS

Complete allergen avoidance should result in resolution of the allergic disease, but this is difficult to accomplish for most allergens. Avoidance of outdoor aeroallergens can only be achieved by remaining indoors with the windows shut. Pollen-allergic persons should be instructed to stay indoors during high pollen counts and immediately shower after being outdoors for an extended period of time.

Complete avoidance of indoor allergens may be equally difficult. Pets can be removed from the home, but it can take many months for airborne animal dander allergens to subside to the level of a non–pet owner's home. In addition, a recent survey of more than 800 U.S. homes found measurable cat and dog dander in all of the homes, and a significant percentage had levels high enough to sensitize (induce allergies) and to precipitate an asthma attack in persons who were already sensitized to cat or dog allergens. Many pet owners will not remove an allergenic animal. In these instances, it should be recommended that the animal not be allowed in the bedroom and the central heating or air-conditioning vents should be closed off in that room to prevent recirculation of the animal dander. A HEPA (high-efficiency particulate air) filtration device might help reduce airborne pet dander levels. Washing the cat twice a week has also been shown to reduce airborne cat dander levels.

Carpet is a large reservoir for many indoor allergens, and allergen-control measures should include carpet removal. Controlling indoor humidity at 50% makes the environment less habitable for molds and dust mites. Washing the bedding at least once a week in hot water (130°F or 55°C) kills dust mites. Encasing bedding with covers impermeable to dust mite allergens can reduce exposure to dust mites. However, studies on the efficacy of allergen-impermeable encasings in reducing allergic symptom have yielded conflicting results.

Cockroach control is very difficult to achieve. Approaches to the elimination of cockroaches are based on eliminating suitable environments by removing food sources and by restricting access to water and access and entry ports through caulking and sealing cracks in the plaster work and flooring. Studies have shown that aggressive measures that include professional extermination can reduce cockroach numbers, but no studies have evaluated the effect of cockroach eradication on rhinitis. Measures for avoiding indoor mold are similar to those for controlling exposure to cockroaches and dust mites: maintaining indoor humidity at 50%, sealing water leaks, and removing carpet. Additionally, live Christmas trees and plants are not recommended. However, there are no controlled studies showing that these measures are effective in benefiting allergic rhinitis patients.

SPECIFIC ALLERGEN IMMUNOTHERAPY

Allergen immunotherapy is currently the only immune-modifying treatment for allergic disease. Numerous controlled studies have demonstrated the efficacy of specific allergen immunotherapy in the treatment of allergic rhinitis.

Allergen immunotherapy may be unique in that it is both a treatment for a disease and the only intervention that can potentially modify the allergic disease. Allergen immunotherapy can produce long-term clinical remissions after it is discontinued, whereas this sustained benefit is not seen after discontinuing pharmacologic treatment. Allergen immunotherapy can also prevent allergic rhinitis from progressing to asthma and can prevent new allergen sensitizations from developing. The efficacy appears to be dose dependent, and the immunologic mechanisms responsible for the clinical efficacy of immunotherapy are still being elucidated.

Immunologic changes associated with immunotherapy include inducing T-regulatory cells, increasing allergen-specific IgG4, increasing IL-10 production, and down-regulating the TH2 response. The disadvantages of allergen immunotherapy include risk of adverse events and the time required because it is recommended that subcutaneous immunotherapy be administered in a medical facility. Risks of immunotherapy include large local reactions and mild systemic reactions such as rhinnorrhea or sneezing. Serious adverse reactions from immunotherapy injections, including death, do occur, but they are very rare.

Effective immunotherapy has been associated with significant improvements in symptom and medication scores and quality of life measures, as well as in objective parameters such as organ provocation challenge and immunologic changes in cell markers and cytokine profiles. Allergen immunotherapy should be considered for patients who have symptoms of allergic rhinitis or rhinoconjunctivitis after natural exposure to allergens and who have demonstrable evidence of specific IgE antibodies to clinically relevant allergens.

The decision to begin allergen immunotherapy depends on the degree to which symptoms can be reduced by avoidance and medication, the amount and type of medication required to control symptoms, and the adverse effects of medications. The severity and duration of symptoms should also be considered. Time lost from work or school, emergency department or physician office visits, work or school performance, and response to pharmacotherapy are important objective indicators of allergic disease severity. The impact of the patient's symptoms on quality of life and responsiveness to other forms of therapy, such as allergen avoidance or medication, should also be considered. Unacceptable adverse effects of medications, the patient's desire to avoid long-term pharmacotherapy, and comorbid medical conditions such as asthma or sinusitis should also be factors in the decision to begin allergen immunotherapy.

Patients with allergic asthma and allergic rhinitis should be managed with a combined aggressive regimen of allergen avoidance and pharmacotherapy; these patients may also benefit from allergen immunotherapy. Immunotherapy is likely more cost-effective than pharmacotherapy over time.

Currently, subcutaneous immunotherapy is the only route with an FDA-approved formulation. Sublingual immunotherapy (SLIT) is a method in which the allergen is administered in a liquid or dissolvable tablet under the tongue and held for approximately 2 minutes before swallowing. Pharmacokinetic studies indicate that the allergen is not absorbed systemically from the sublingual mucosa; it appears to be absorbed locally in the sublingual mucosa, where a small percentage can be found up to 20 hours later. This mode of treatment has been used with increasing frequency in Europe over the past 20 years, and in parts of Europe, such as Italy and France, approximately 80% of the new allergen immunotherapy prescriptions are for sublingual immunotherapy. Published studies suggest that high doses are required to achieve clinical efficacy and that the magnitude of improvement might not be as great as with subcutaneous immunotherapy.

Conclusion

Pharmacotherapy is the most commonly used therapeutic modality in allergic rhinitis. Inhaled corticosteroids are the most effective class of medications for allergic rhinitis. Antihistamines are most effective against the symptoms of rhinorrhea, itchiness, and sneezing but tend not to be as effective as congestion. Second-generation antihistamines are preferable because they are associated with less sedation and fewer anticholinergic adverse effects. Antileukotrienes might also be effective as an add-on therapy to nasal corticosteroid or combination nasal corticosteroid and antihistamine regimens. Allergen avoidance is recommended, but it may be difficult to achieve for many allergens. Allergen immunotherapy is currently the only disease-modifying treatment for allergic disease. In contrast to pharmacotherapy, it can lead to long-lasting clinical remission after treatment is discontinued and can prevent the progression of the allergic disease.

REFERENCES

Bousquet J, Van Cauwenberge P, Khaltaev N, et al: Allergic rhinitis and its impact on asthma. J Allergy Clin Immunol 2001;108:S147-S334.

Calderon MA, Alves B, Jacobson M, et al: Allergen injection immunotherapy for seasonal allergic rhinitis. Cochrane Database Syst Rev 2007;(1):CD001936.

Cox LS, Li J, Nelson H, Lockey R: Allergen Immunotherapy: A practice parameter second update. J Allergy Clin Immunol 2007;in press.

Cox LS, Linnemann DL, Nolte H, et al: Sublingual immunotherapy: A comprehensive review. J Allergy Clin Immunol 2006;117:1021-1035.

Lanier B: Allergic rhinitis: Selective comparisons of the pharmaceutical options for management. Allergy Asthma Proc 2007;28:16-19.

Nathan RA: The burden of allergic rhinitis. Allergy Asthma Proc 2007;28:3-9.

Passalacqua G, Durham S: Allergic rhinitis and its impact on asthma update: Allergen immunotherapy. J Allergy Clin Immunol 2007;119:881-891.

Ross RN, Nelson HS, Finegold I, et al: Effectiveness of specific immunotherapy in the treatment of allergic rhinitis: An analysis of randomized, prospective, single- or double-blind, placebo-controlled studies. Clin Ther 2000;22:342-350.

Williams PB, Ahlstedt S, Barnes JH, et al: Are our impressions of allergy test performances correct?. Ann Allergy Asthma Immunol 2003;91:26-33.

Wood RA, Phipatanakul W, Hamilton RG, Eggleston PA, et al: A comparison of skin prick tests, intradermal skin tests, and RASTs in the diagnosis of cat allergy. J Allergy Clin Immunol 1999;103:773-779.

Allergic Reactions to Drugs

Method of
Donald McNeil, MD

Drug allergic reactions fall under the broader category of adverse drug reactions (ADRs), which also include toxic drug effects, drug interactions, drug intolerance, and, finally, allergic (or immunologic) drug reactions. Adverse drug reactions are common and often result in only trivial consequences. Some may be severe and life-threatening, and may result from both allergic and nonallergic causes.

The incidence of adverse drug effects is unknown but estimates of 20% of hospital admissions are not unreasonable. A skin rash is the most common manifestation; more importantly, however, severe life-threatening reactions occur, of which only a small portion have an allergic etiology. Most drug reactions are the result of unknown mechanisms. Drug intolerance, drug overdose, and side effects of drugs, as well as drug interactions, all play a significant role. These reactions should be considered both common and predictable.

Although allergic drug reactions are potentially severe, they are also the least common and least predictable. Allergic drug reactions are given particular attention because of the unpredictable, costly, and severe consequences that occasionally arise.

Several mechanisms may play a role in the underlying etiology of immunologic drug reactions. Immediate IgE-mediated reactions represent the classic allergic reaction. This is well characterized and the best understood, but other mechanisms also exist, for example, a

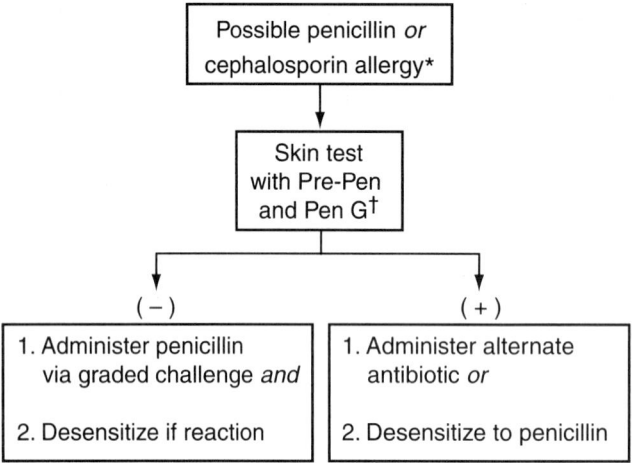

FIGURE 1. Penicillin allergy evaluation.

cytotoxic reaction in which drug-induced antibodies result in hemolytic anemia. Another example is immune complex formation resulting in organ damage. This is commonly referred to as a "serum sickness" reaction and is characterized by fever, rash, and arthralgia beginning 2 to 4 weeks after initiation of drug. Finally, a delayed-type hypersensitivity reaction occurs when drug-specific T-lymphocytes react. This completes the picture of the four types of immunologic-mediated drug reactions according to the original Gell and Coombs classification. These are referred to as Type I, II, III, or IV reactions, respectively.

Cutaneous reactions comprise the most frequent type of allergic drug reaction. Approximately 94% cause a morbilliform rash and only 5% cause an urticarial reaction. Idiosyncratic reactions are still the most likely cause for a rash and occur much more frequently than a true drug-induced allergic reaction. Ampicillins in conjunction with a viral hepatitis or sulfa drugs taken in the AIDS population are common examples.

Both allergic and nonallergic reactions are known to be associated with severe reactions, including fatalities. Contrast media agents, allergic extracts, anesthetics, and antibiotics are the most commonly implicated drugs. Penicillin remains the most common cause of fatal drug reactions and accounts for up to 75% of these severe drug reactions in the United States.

An allergy to penicillin is the most frequently reported, but as many as 90% of patients labeled "penicillin allergic" are able to tolerate penicillin. This allergy is often mislabeled because of underlying illness or interaction between antibiotic and illness. Unfortunately one third to half of vancomycin (Vancocin) prescriptions in hospitals are given because of a history of "penicillin allergy." This raises the incidence of drug-resistant bacteria because of broad-spectrum antibiotic overuse. The economic impact of treating antibiotic-resistant infections is roughly $4 billion annually.

Pathophysiology

Some drugs are capable of reacting in the body without further alteration in chemical structure, whereas others must first be metabolized to become immunogenic. Many drugs are too small to be immunogenic alone and are incapable of eliciting an immune allergic response. These drugs require binding to a high-molecular-weight protein followed by antigen processing and presentation by the macrophage in the presence of major histocompatibility complex (MHC)-specific antigen to appropriate T-cell receptors.

Penicillin is capable of inducing an allergic reaction in more than one manner. Benzylpenicilloyl, the major penicillin determinant, is able to produce a strong antigenic response. A commercially available product, benzylpenicilloyl-polylysine (PPL) (Pre-Pen), provides the means to reproduce the same allergic response by simple skin testing. Minor determinants are metabolic derivatives of penicillin that may also produce an immune response. The diagnostic capabilities of a penicillin allergy are strengthened by including some measure of the allergic response to the minor determinants when skin testing is conducted for penicillin (Figure 1).

Patients with a history of penicillin allergy but negative skin testing to PPL and the minor determinants rarely experience allergic reactions on re-exposure. If they should occur, these are not fatal, but rather mild and self-limited.

PPL alone will potentially miss a significant percentage of allergic reactions to penicillin. Allergy testing with fresh benzylpenicillin G, aged penicillin (reconstituted more than 24 hours) as well as skin testing with the specific penicillin in question will greatly enhance the likelihood of uncovering of penicillin allergy in a patient with a positive history.

Cephalosporins do not provide the same degree of certainty with respect to an allergic evaluation. Cross-reactivity with penicillin allergy patients is known to exist, and although uncommon, it is also unpredictable. To err on the side of safety, a patient with a known penicillin allergy should not be treated with a cephalosporin. A patient with a previous cephalosporin reaction with a negative penicillin skin test cannot safely receive penicillin or another cephalosporin unless further diagnostic measures are taken. This patient may be allergic to a side chain on the cephalosporin that has not been identified by penicillin skin testing. Others recommend a graded oral challenge using a cephalosporin with a different side chain. The latter should be done realizing that standardized procedures have not been developed for this and therefore false negative results may occur.

Successful desensitization to penicillin has permitted a similar approach with other drugs. If the drug in question is required, either intravenous or oral drug administration is possible by incremental doses given usually every 15 minutes. A 10,000-fold dilution of the initial dose is usually sufficient to begin, followed by higher doses, 2-fold or greater. The vital signs are monitored throughout the procedure with timely medical intervention if problems arise.

Sulfonamides typically cause cutaneous reactions, infrequently in healthy individuals but extremely common in AIDS patients. Reactions may be relatively benign in nature such as urticaria or

> **BOX 1 Graded Challenge**
>
> 1. Cautious administration of medications to patient not likely allergic to drug.
> 2. Not to be considered equivalent to desensitization.
> 3. Used when insufficient evidence available to exclude drug allergy.
> 4. Medication administered in incremental doses beginning at 1:100 dilution of final dose.
> 5. Adequate medical resources exist to treat allergic reaction.

fixed-drug eruption, but may also cause more serious reactions (Stevens-Johnson syndrome, toxic epidermal necrolysis). A variety of mechanisms may exist, alone or in combination, using IgE antibody response, T-lymphocytes, and inflammatory cytokines. Because of our inadequate understanding of these mechanisms, there are no universally acceptable means of evaluating sulfonamide hypersensitivity. Unless there has been previously severe reaction, a graded challenge with the drug in question is considered a reasonable alternative (Box 1). Although a theoretical risk exists between sulfonamides and drugs with sulfonamide derivatives (diuretics, COX-2 inhibitors), little data show this is actually true.

Radiographic contrast media (RCM) produce an anaphylactoid reaction by an unknown mechanism. Conventional RCM is hypertonic. The newer nonionic RCM with lower osmolarity are associated with fewer anaphylactoid or allergic-like reactions. Complement system activation, which is capable of causing histamine release, is thought to be the method by which this reaction occurs.

In the continuum of adverse drug effects with suspected hypersensitivity, exposure to *aspirin* and other nonsteroidal anti-inflammatory drugs (NSAIDs) rarely exhibits features that are IgE mediated and allergic in nature, and are more often nonimmunologic mediated. A non–IgE-mediated event must still be approached with caution because the consequences are potentially life-threatening.

More commonly, NSAIDs are associated with the asthma triad syndrome associated with nasal polyps or rhinitis, and severe asthma. This is not an allergic drug reaction, but it represents a largely unrecognized subpopulation of asthmatics who will benefit by avoiding the use of NSAIDs.

The antibiotic *vancomycin* (Vancocin) causes a reaction referred to as *red man syndrome*. Histamine and other mast cell mediators are released, but not through vancomycin-induced IgE antibody (rare cases have been reported). Most, but not all, cases of the red man syndrome are related to the rate of the infusion, and most will subside once the medication is stopped. A graded challenge with the drug or a full course of desensitization usually permits resumption of treatment.

Angiotensin-converting enzyme (ACE) inhibitors are well known to be associated with cough and angioedema, but like NSAIDs, the mechanism is unknown. Newer ACE inhibitors have been described to cause similar reactions but at a much lower incidence. The symptoms of cough and angioedema may continue to recur for several months and up to a year after the discontinuation of the drug.

As seen from the discussion above, IgE-mediated allergic drug reactions represent only a portion of immune-mediated drug reactions. To assist in the diagnosis, a 7- to 10-day delay in the appearance of the drug reaction after initial treatment or immediate reactivation on re-exposure suggests an immunologic etiology. Oftentimes, only the history will provide this index of suspicion. Confirmation by positive skin testing with the drug in question is highly predictive of IgE-mediated hypersensitivity.

Attempts to label reactions as either IgE- or non–IgE-mediated may prove to be costly, time-consuming, and of no immediate benefit. Non-IgE reactions are capable of eliciting changes in vital signs, pulmonary function, and cutaneous effects similar to anaphylaxis and are referred to as anaphylactoid. These need to be regarded with the same degree of caution as IgE-mediated reactions. Narcotics, radiographic contrast media, and chemotherapeutic agents may directly affect mast cell mediator release with the consequences listed above. Antihistamines and corticosteroids given prior to administration of these drugs are usually sufficient to prevent a reoccurrence, or at least to minimize these reactions.

Drug desensitization is indicated for those patients with positive skin tests who must receive the drug, but should not be assumed to be universally safe or protective. Some chemotherapeutic agents, such as etoposide (VePesid) and teniposide (Vumon), have a much higher incidence of anaphylactoid reactions. Readministration of these drugs in the face of a previous reaction and in spite of prophylactic measures often leads to disappointing results.

Current biologic response modifier agents, as well as others soon to arrive, are associated with adverse reactions. Monoclonal antibodies, T- and B-cell inactivators, and others may prove to have adverse immunologic effects that will only become more apparent with the experience of increased use.

Evaluation of Drug Allergy in Practice

The importance of a reliable history in a medical evaluation is never more evident than during the initial workup of a suspected drug allergy. The timing of exposure, with the first allergic reaction occurring within days of the priming dose or immediately upon re-exposure, strongly points to an allergic etiology. Multiple exposures to the same drug on previous occasions do not preclude an allergic reaction de novo. Similarly, a previous history of an allergic drug reaction does not by itself predict a reoccurrence on re-exposure. The allergic diathesis may wane over time for drugs just as it may occur for other allergens.

Armed with this suggestive drug history and clinical findings such as a rash, fever, bronchospasm, or anaphylaxis, the evaluation becomes more straightforward. In the appropriate clinical setting, eosinophilia will also support a drug-allergic reaction.

Avoiding the implicated drug may be the simplest approach because confirmation of the diagnosis with appropriate skin testing is often unavailable. (Standardized skin testing exists only for penicillin, but even this does not provide 100% reliability.) Skin testing with the drug is questionable, but using both a positive and negative control of histamine and saline may still provide useful information. A positive skin test would certainly discourage use of this drug unless adequate precautions were taken.

If a non–life-threatening history of a reaction exists and the drug cannot be appropriately substituted, the option exists for a graded oral challenge to confirm the diagnosis. This should not be considered to be the same as desensitization because it involves higher doses and exposure over a shorter period of time than would be considered safe in a truly allergic individual. A challenge such as this should be conducted in suitable medical facilities under close medical supervision.

If the drug in question has been shown to cause an allergic reaction but still must be used, then a carefully monitored drug desensitization program should be considered. Under medical supervision, the drug should be administered orally or intravenously beginning with doses that are tenfold more dilute than the final strength. Incrementally higher doses of the drug should be administered every 15 minutes, increasing the dose twofold each time.

Drug-induced skin reactions are common and warrant particular attention. Early recognition is necessary to avoid an incorrect diagnosis and to institute appropriate interventional measures as soon as possible.

The following points will assist the physician in arriving at a correct diagnosis. The *timing of the onset* of the reaction in relation to the time the drug was given provides an important clue. Often signs and symptoms develop 1 to 2 weeks after time of initial drug exposure. Symptoms may develop rapidly on repeat exposure. *Pruritic urticarial lesions* strongly suggest an adverse drug reaction. A *symmetrical or truncal distribution* or a rash that occurs only in sun-exposed areas (polymorphous light eruption) also supports an ADR finding.

TABLE 1 Drugs Used to Treat AIDS/HIV

Drug	Reaction
Zidovudine, AZT (Retrovir)	Hyperpigmentation
Zalcitabine, ddC (Hivid)	Oral ulcers
Abacavir (Ziagen)	Severe rash/anaphylaxis
Nevirapine (Viramune)	Toxic epidermal necrolysis
Foscarnet	Urethral ulceration
Trimethoprim-sulfamethoxazole (TMP-SMX) (Bactrim)	Morbilliform rash or erythema multiforme

The morphology of the reaction is helpful, although many types occur (lichenoid, morbilliform, eczematous). The histopathology of the lesion on skin biopsy may reveal eosinophils, which may also be detected in the peripheral blood.

Drugs that commonly cause ADRs tend to be antibiotics. The most common is the morbilliform rash when ampicillin is given in the presence of a viral infection such as infectious mononucleosis or cytomegalovirus. Rarely is this IgE mediated and it should not be regarded as a basis for a history of penicillin allergy. It should also be noted that not all ADRs are caused by prescription medications. A patient may fail to disclose over-the-counter medications that might be responsible (e.g., St. John's wort).

The *response to treatment* may aid in the recognition of an ADR. An incomplete response to topical steroids is typical of an ADR and systemic steroids may turn out to be the therapy of choice. Finally, the *response to withdrawal* of drug may range from a rapid recovery to slow clearing over many weeks, but a favorable response nonetheless.

Table 1 lists several drugs used to treat AIDS/HIV that are worthy of mention. Not all should be considered to be an allergic cause of ADR.

A careful and systematic approach to the patient with a suspected drug allergy will provide valuable information for both the immediate and the long-term management of the patient. A suspected drug allergy that is disproved will facilitate good medical care because unnecessary expense and the risk of further sensitizing the patient to a new medication will be spared if the patient is not allergic. On the other hand, a positive screen for a suspected drug allergy will result in a safe alternative. It should be emphasized, however, that neither a family history of a drug allergy nor a patient requesting a "test" for a possible drug allergy without other reason is an indication for further drug allergy evaluation because of the risk of false-negative results.

Allergic Reactions to Insect Stings*

Method of
David B. K. Golden, MD

Insect bites and stings normally cause temporary localized swelling, redness, pain, and itching. Allergic swelling can also result from insect bites or stings, but stinging insects of the order Hymenoptera can cause anaphylaxis. Allergic reactions to stings from honeybees, vespids (yellow jackets, hornets, wasps), and ants (imported fire, harvester, jack jumper), are caused by IgE antibodies directed against the protein allergens in the venoms (but not in the bodies or saliva) of these insects. Yellow jacket and hornet venoms are almost identical and are partially cross reactive with wasp venoms, but honeybee venom and fire ant venom are each unique. Commercial venom vaccines are available for honeybee, yellow jacket, yellow hornet, white-faced hornet, and *Polistes* wasps (ALK Laboratories; Hollister-Stier Laboratories). For fire ant sting allergy, imported fire ant whole body extract is the only commercial available material. Although it contains sufficient venom allergens for diagnostic use and for immunotherapy, evidence indicates that venom is superior.

Allergic reactions may be localized or systemic. Large local reactions have a late-phase inflammatory mechanism that progresses for 24 to 48 hours after the sting, causing a painful induration that is often larger than 6 inches in diameter and lasts for 5 to 10 days. A large local reaction to a sting can mimic laryngeal edema (from a sting in the mouth or throat) or cellulitis (lymphangitic drainage from the reaction on an extremity). Systemic reactions are immediate hypersensitivity reactions with manifestations distant from the site of the sting, which can include any one or more of the signs or symptoms of anaphylaxis including urticaria, angioedema, flushing, throat or chest tightness, dyspnea, dizziness, or hypotensive shock. The reported frequency of 40 fatal reactions per year in the United States is certainly an underestimate. Elevated serum tryptase and venom-specific IgE antibodies are reported in postmortem blood samples in cases of unexpected death in young individuals. Half of fatal reactions occurred in persons with no prior history of reactions to stings, and most occur in individuals older than 45 years. The population at risk is greater than generally appreciated: 3% of adults in the United States have a history of a systemic allergic reaction to insect stings, and more than 20% have IgE antibodies to venom allergens detectable in the skin or blood.

Diagnosis

A detailed history provides the most important diagnostic information. The exact features and time course of the reaction can distinguish large local, systemic, and nonallergic reactions. Objective signs and documented clinical observations are more reliable than subjective descriptions. Venom-specific IgE antibodies can be demonstrated by skin testing or serologic methods (radioallergosorbent assay test [RAST]) but must be interpreted in the context of the clinical history. Skin testing with the five Hymenoptera venoms (or fire ant whole body extract) is recommended for patients who have had systemic allergic reactions to a sting but is not required for large local reactions. Skin tests are performed with superficial intradermal injection of 0.02 mL of each venom at concentrations starting at 0.001 µg/mL and increasing incrementally up to 1.0 µg/mL, if needed, until a positive wheal and flare reaction is elicited. Diagnostic laboratory measurement of venom-specific IgE antibodies (RAST) may be useful when skin testing is inconclusive or cannot be performed but is less sensitive than skin testing. The venom RAST is positive in 10% of affected patients with negative skin tests, and conversely, the RAST is negative in 20% of patients with positive skin tests. A positive venom skin test in an individual with no history of sting

CURRENT DIAGNOSIS

- History of systemic allergic reactions to sting
- Positive venom skin tests or radioallergosorbent assay test (RAST)
- Degree of test reaction not correlated with severity of sting reaction
- Low risk if previous large local sting reactions
- Low risk in children with mild systemic reactions
- Quality of life and frequency of exposure a consideration

---

*This work was supported by National Institutes of Health (NH) grant A108270.

TABLE 1 Clinical Recommendations Based on History of Sting Reactions, Age, and Results of Venom Skin Test (or RAST)

Reaction to Previous Sting	Skin Test (or RAST)	Risk of Systemic Reaction	Clinical Recommendation
No reaction	Positive	10%–15%	Avoidance
Large local	Positive	5%–10%	Avoidance
Cutaneous systemic	Positive: child	5%–10%	Avoidance
	Positive: adult	15%–20%	Venom immunotherapy
Anaphylaxis	Positive	30%–60%	Venom immunotherapy
	Negative	5%–10%	Repeat skin test/RAST

Abbreviations: RAST = radioallergosorbent assay test.

reaction is associated with a 17% frequency of systemic reaction to a subsequent sting. The level of sensitivity on skin test or RAST predicts the frequency but not the severity of the sting reaction. The risk of anaphylactic reaction to stings is increased with β-blocker medication, and with elevated baseline serum tryptase.

Assessing the risk of a systemic reaction to a future sting is based on the detailed history of previous reactions, the presence of venom-specific IgE antibodies, and the known natural history of the condition (Table 1). In adults with positive venom skin tests and a prior history of systemic reactions, the risk of systemic reaction is 30% to 60%, with the higher risk in patients with the most severe reactions (airway obstruction, unconsciousness) and the lower frequency in patients who had cutaneous systemic signs (urticaria, angioedema) and/or mild dizziness or throat tightness. The risk declines with time, but remains at 15% to 20% even after 20 to 30 years. The risk of systemic reaction is known to be low in the general population and in some subgroups of sensitized individuals (Table 2). The majority of affected children (16 years and younger) have had systemic reactions limited to skin manifestations, including generalized hives and angioedema of the face or lips but with no tongue or throat swelling and no dyspnea or hypotension. In these children, subsequent stings cause no systemic reaction in 90%, mild cutaneous systemic reactions in 5%, and more severe systemic reaction in less than 5% of cases. Patients with large local reactions generally have strongly positive venom skin tests but have only a 5% risk of systemic reaction to future stings.

Treatment and Avoidance of Sting Reactions

Local sting reactions can be treated symptomatically with ice and oral antihistamines. Large local reactions may require a burst of oral prednisone (e.g., 40 to 60 mg the first day, tapering over 4 to 7 days) but almost never require antibiotic treatment. Systemic reactions generally require the intramuscular administration of epinephrine (1:1000), 0.3 mg in an adult (0.01 mg/kg in children), with the availability of oxygen, intravenous fluids, or airway support if needed. Corticosteroids have no benefit in the acute stage, but despite a lack of supporting evidence are often administered in the hope of preventing late-phase manifestations. The patient should be monitored for 3 to 6 hours because more than 20% of severe cases develop biphasic or protracted anaphylaxis. Any patient judged to have a risk for anaphylaxis to future stings should have a prescription for an epinephrine injection kit and detailed instructions on when to use or not use it. Commercial kits include the EpiPen (0.3 mg epinephrine) and EpiPen Jr (0.15 mg epinephrine) (Dey Laboratories) and the Twinject (two doses of either 0.15 or 0.3 mg epinephrine) (Sciele Pharma, Inc.). Such individuals should also be referred to a specialist for evaluation and discussion of risks and treatment options. Sting-allergic patients should avoid nesting areas, trash receptacles, eating or drinking outdoors, lawn mowing, or going barefoot.

Prevention of Sting Reactions (Venom Immunotherapy)

Systemic reactions to insect stings can be prevented with up to 98% efficacy with venom immunotherapy. The indications for therapy are simply a positive history (of systemic reaction to stings) and positive venom skin tests (or RAST), although the severity of previous reactions and the patient's age at the time are also important variables (Table 3). Venom immunotherapy, and therefore skin testing, is not considered necessary for low-risk patients because more than 90% will never have a systemic reaction, such as in patients with large local reactions and in children with cutaneous systemic reactions.

Venom immunotherapy should begin with all of the venoms giving a positive skin test and follows a dose schedule described in the product package insert (ALK Laboratories; Hollister-Stier Laboratories). Injections are generally administered weekly for 8 to 26 weeks to achieve the full maintenance dose of 100 μg of each venom. More rapid treatment is not associated with more frequent adverse reactions. This dose is then repeated every 4 weeks for at least 1 year, then every 6 weeks for 1 to 2 years, and every 6 to 8 weeks thereafter. During immunotherapy, systemic reactions occur in 5% to 15% of cases, with variable degrees of urticaria, airway obstruction, or hypotension. The majority of such reactions are mild, but some require aggressive treatment for anaphylaxis. Venom injections also cause large local reactions in many patients during the first few months of therapy, but they

TABLE 2 Considerations in Stopping Venom Immunotherapy

Severity/pattern of systemic reaction
Age (child/teen, adult, senior)
Skin tests/RAST (persistent strong)
Time/duration of venom immunotherapy
Systemic reaction during venom immunotherapy
 (to injection or sting)
Quality of life/exposure

Abbreviation: RAST = radioallergosorbent assay test.

 CURRENT THERAPY

- Epinephrine Autoinjector (EpiPen or Twinject) and avoidance strategies for low-risk patients is suggested.
- Venom immunotherapy is for high-risk patients.
- Venom immunotherapy is up to 98% effective.
- Most patients can discontinue venom immunotherapy after 5 years.
- Highest risk patients may need indefinite venom immunotherapy.

TABLE 3 Patients with Low Risk for Anaphylaxis

Minimal (<5%)	General adult population
	Patients on venom immunotherapy
	Children with cutaneous systemic reactions
Low (5%–10%)	Large local reactors
	Discontinued venom immunotherapy after 5 y

are not predictive of systemic reactions and should not interfere with attaining the full recommended dose. All adverse reactions are much less common during maintenance treatment. The frequency of systemic reactions is similar with venom immunotherapy and immunotherapy with inhalant allergens. Periodic monitoring of venom skin test or RAST sensitivity is recommended every 2 to 5 years to determine possible early discontinuation of therapy. The level of venom-specific IgG antibodies is correlated with clinical protection and may be measured during the first 3 years of venom immunotherapy, especially to determine whether protection is adequate with single-venom therapy and when maintenance intervals are extended. Some patients require higher doses for full protection.

The duration of venom immunotherapy remains a matter of judgment. The product package insert advises that venom immunotherapy should be continued indefinitely. Some experts advocate stopping treatment if skin tests (or RAST) become negative, but this occurs in only 25% of patients treated for 5 years and in 60% of those treated for 7 to 10 years. When venom immunotherapy is stopped after at least 5 years of maintenance treatment, the chance of reaction to a sting is 10% for each sting that occurs, even 10 to 15 years after stopping even if there are uneventful intervening stings and even if skin tests become negative. The cumulative risk of reaction is 15% to 20% more than 10 years after discontinuing treatment. The risk of a very severe reaction exists primarily in patients who had such a reaction prior to treatment, and they should therefore consider remaining on therapy indefinitely. Other high-risk patients who should consider continuing treatment beyond 5 years include those who had a systemic reaction during treatment whether to an injection or a sting. The relapse rate is also higher in honeybee allergic patients, as is the frequency of systemic reactions to venom injections and the failure rate for reaction to stings during therapy. Both the relapse rate and the level of venom-specific IgE (or skin test) are higher in patients who stop therapy after only 3 years compared to 5 years. Some investigators have suggested that lower risk patients (e.g., children with reactions of any severity and adult patients with mild reactions) might be able safely to stop after 3 years of treatment, but there are limited data published about this.

REFERENCES

Bernstein JA, Kagan SL, Bernstein DI, Bernstein IL: Rapid venom immunotherapy is safe for routine use in the treatment of patients with Hymenoptera anaphylaxis. Ann Allergy 1994;73:423-428.

Freeman TM: Hypersensitivity to Hymenoptera stings. N Engl J Med 2004;351:1978-1984.

Freeman TM, Highlander R, Ortiz A, Martin ME: Imported fire ant immunotherapy: Effectiveness of whole body extracts. J Allergy Clin Immunol 1992;90:210-215.

Golden DBK: Insect sting allergy and venom immunotherapy: A model and a mystery. J Allergy Clin Immunol 2005;115:439-447.

Golden DBK, Kagey-Sobotka A, Norman PS, et al: Outcomes of allergy to insect stings in children with and without venom immunotherapy. N Engl J Med 2004;351:668-674.

Golden DBK, Kwiterovich KA, Kagey-Sobotka A, et al: Discontinuing venom immunotherapy: Outcome after five years. J Allergy Clin Immunol 1996;97:579-587.

Golden DBK, Marsh DG, Kagey-Sobotka A, et al: Epidemiology of insect venom sensitivity. JAMA 1989;262:240-244.

Hamilton RG: Diagnostic methods for insect sting allergy. Curr Opin Allergy Clin Immunol 2004;4:297-306.

Hoffman DR: Fatal reactions to Hymenoptera stings. Asthma Allergy Proc 2003;24:1-5.

Hunt KJ, Valentine MD, Sobotka AK, et al: A controlled trial of immunotherapy in insect hypersensitivity. N Engl J Med 1978;299:157-161.

Moffitt JE, Golden DBK, Reisman RE, et al: Stinging insect hypersensitivity: A practice parameter update. J Allergy Clin Immunol 2004;114:869-886.

Stafford CT: Hypersensitivity to fire ant venom. Ann Allergy Asthma Immunol 1996;77:87-95.

SECTION 13

Diseases of the Skin

Acne Vulgaris and Rosacea

Method of
*Steven R. Feldman, MD, PhD, and
Alan B. Fleischer, Jr., MD*

Acne and rosacea are common conditions that share a propensity to cause red follicular papules of the face. Nonetheless, they are distinct disorders.

Acne is associated with comedones, a noninflammatory plugging of follicular orifices. Comedones may become inflamed, at least partially due to the inflammatory activity induced by the action of bacterial skin flora (*Pityrosporum* species) on lipids produced by sebaceous glands. There is a distinct tendency toward development of acne nodules with scarring.

The pathogenesis of rosacea is less well understood. Vascular dilatation and inflammation are important components of the process, with prominent flushing and blushing. Although telangiectasia can become permanent, scarring is rare. Another feature distinguishing rosacea from acne is a tendency for ocular involvement.

Acne Vulgaris

CLINICAL FEATURES

Acne is a common disorder of teenagers and young adults but occurs in middle age as well. The manifestations of acne are diverse. The face is characteristically involved, and the upper trunk is involved in some patients. The individual lesions can consist of comedones, inflammatory papules, pustules, and deeper inflammatory nodules mistakenly termed *cysts*. There might or might not be resulting scarring. Genetics contributes to the pattern of involvement. Environmental exposures seem less important, although some oil-based cosmetic products can induce acne comedones.

TREATMENT

Treatments for acne address several different components of the pathogenesis of the disorder. Topical retinoids appear to have a primary effect on normalizing keratinization of the follicular ostia, reducing comedones and inflammatory papules and pustules. Topical and oral antibiotics reduce bacteria counts on the skin and can have intrinsic anti-inflammatory activity. Hormonal treatments in women reduce the production of sebaceous gland lipids. Oral retinoids (isotretinoin in particular), the most effective therapy for acne, reduces sebaceous gland activity as well.

There are no well-established evidence-based guidelines for acne treatment. There are, however, generally accepted patterns of treatment based on the type and extent of the clinical lesions. At its simplest, topical retinoids are the foundation of treatment because of their effect on comedones, the primary lesion of acne, as well as their effect on inflammatory acne papules and pustules. With increasing microbial resistance, retinoid agents work independently of direct effects on skin flora and are excellent long-term agents. Topical antibiotics, prescribed singly, in combination with antimicrobial products, or in combination with topical retinoids, are used for superficial inflammatory lesions. Oral antibiotics are used when the inflammation and potential scarring are more severe. Hormonal treatment (in the form of oral contraceptives) is used for female patients when the acne is unresponsive to both topical retinoids and topical and oral antibiotics or if there are menstrual abnormalities that suggest the acne is secondary to a primary hormonal process.

Topical Retinoids

Topical retinoids are used for nearly all patients with acne because of their comedolytic effect and their activity on papules and pustules, as well as to spare the use of antibiotics in an age of growing antibiotic resistance. The first topical retinoid was topical tretinoin (Retin-A). It is available in cream, gel, solution, and newer slow-release particle vehicles. The main side effect of topical retinoids is the potential for drying and irritation of the skin. This is less of a problem with lower strengths of topical tretinoin (0.025% and 0.05% cream) and more of a problem with the stronger strengths (0.01% and 0.025% gel and the 0.1% cream). The drying effect may be beneficial for patients who feel their skin is too oily.

Topical tretinoin is easily oxidized and photodegraded. With the growing use of benzoyl peroxide as an anti-acne treatment, there is greater concern about the liability of topical tretinoin. Topical adapalene (Differin) gel or cream can be used as an alternative. It is equally effective as tretinoin, but it has far less potential to cause irritation. Less irritation can lead to greater compliance. It also is a robust molecule that is stable when combined with other agents, including benzoyl peroxide. Topical tazarotene (Tazorac) is another retinoid that is more effective than tretinoin and adapalene, but it is much more irritating than the other agents.

Adapalene and tazarotene may be used at any time of the day, but tretinoin should be used at night because of its photodegradation. This recommendation probably started with topical tretinoin because of the potential for photoinactivation of tretinoin.

Topical Antimicrobial Agents

The most widely used topical antimicrobial agent is benzoyl peroxide. This biocide is available in a wide variety of inexpensive and expensive over-the-counter and prescription acne products. Benzoyl peroxide is very effective at reducing bacterial counts on the skin, and it is probably far more effective than the traditional topical antibiotics such as erythromycin (Akne-Mycin), clindamycin (Cleocin), and sulfacetamide (Klaron).

Benzoyl peroxide (in 2.5%-10% formulations) is often used in conjunction with topical retinoids or with other topical antibiotics. Combined use of benzoyl peroxide with topical erythromycin (Benzamycin) or clindamycin (BenzaClin) helps prevent development of bacterial strains resistant to the antibiotics. A combined benzoyl peroxide–erythromycin product was once widely used, but it needed to be kept refrigerated, and had a short shelf life. Newer benzoyl peroxide–clindamycin preparations (Benzaclin, Duac) are more stable, can be used once or twice daily, and have excellent efficacy.

All benzoyl peroxide products bleach clothing, bed linens, and towels. Not all vehicles are appropriate for all patients, and excellent vehicle choices can enhance compliance and clinical outcomes.

Topical azelaic acid is a useful adjunct, especially in the 15% gel formulation (Finacea). It is antimicrobial and anti-inflammatory, and it can promote pigmentary normalization. Azelaic acid can be simultaneously combined with many other agents and does not appear to be subject to microbial resistance.

A combination clindamycin–tretinoin product is now available in the United States (Ziana). Topical dapsone (Aczone) has also been approved by the FDA but is not currently marketed. Sulfacetamide is occasionally used and many forms are available (e.g., Klaron), either alone or combined with precipitated sulfur. Sulfacetamide chemically reacts with benzoyl peroxide, and these two agents should not be used simultaneously.

Oral Antibiotics

Oral antibiotics remain widely used for acne, sometimes for short courses, other times for more prolonged periods. There are growing efforts to limit the course of these drugs in order to limit side effects and antibiotic resistance. Commonly used antibiotics include tetracycline (Sumycin), doxycycline (Doryx), minocycline (Dynacin), and erythromycin.

Of these, minocycline may be the most effective, although it has potential for uncommon and rare side effects. Common side effects include vestibular symptoms; rare ones include altered cutaneous pigmentation and lupus-like syndromes. Minocycline, in extended-release tablets (Solodyn), is the only FDA-approved antibiotic for acne treatment and has fewer vestibular side effects than other agents. This agent has an established dose-response relationship and is most effective with least toxicity at 1 mg/kg/day. It is available in 45-mg, 90-mg, and 135-mg doses.

None of the tetracycline agents should be used during pregnancy or in children younger than 12 years, because tetracycline can stain developing teeth. Erythromycin may be used in these situations; however, there are often poor gastrointestinal tolerance and marginal efficacy. Other antibiotics such as cephalexin (Kelex),[1] ampicillin,[1] or trimethoprim-sulfamethoxazole (Bactrim)[1] are alternatives that are occasionally used.

Birth Control Pills

Oral contraceptives are somewhat effective antiacne treatments that can be used in women. Three products (Tri-Cyclen, Estrostep, and Yaz) are FDA approved for the treatment of acne. The former two are combinations of norethindrone acetate and ethinyl estradiol, although other formulations are probably also effective. Yasmin and Yaz, for instance, have an effective antiandrogenic agent, drospirenone, combined with the ethinyl estradiol. Oral contraceptives should be considered as a treatment for moderate to severe acne in women (along with topical agents and oral antibiotics) before isotretinoin is used. If effective, it can spare the need to expose a woman of childbearing potential to the teratogenic isotretinoin. If this approach is not effective, the woman will already be taking an oral contraceptive when isotretinoin is started.

---

[1]Not FDA approved for this indication.

Isotretinoin

Isotretinoin (Accutane, Sotret, and others) is a highly effective oral agent that can cure even very severe acne. It is given in doses of 0.5 to 2.0 mg/kg/day for 4 to 5 months. It is a potent teratogen and must be used with great caution in women of childbearing potential. Although evidence is lacking, it has been reported to cause depression in rare instances, and true informed consent is required. Other potential side effects include hair loss, decreased night vision, xerophthalmia, epistaxis, cheilitis, xerosis, arthralgias, hepatic dysfunction, and elevated cholesterol and triglycerides. Oral retinoids should not be used in conjunction with tetracycline agents because of the possible increased risk of pseudotumor cerebri.

Behavioral Issues

Perhaps the most important environmental exposure affecting acne is behavioral: patients' tendency to pick at their acne lesions, resulting in excoriation, infection, and scarring. Psychological fixation on facial appearance is not uncommon. Patients often perceive that their follicular ostia (pores) are too large. They can manipulate their skin, resulting in excoriated lesions that mimic acne. This type of acne is not uncommon and is termed acne excoriée. The severity and extent of the lesions vary. Some patients have few lesions, others have many with considerable scarring.

Treatment of acne excoriée is difficult. Some patients respond to the suggestion that they "are spreading the infection by manipulating the skin." For other patients with more severe psychological issues, oral psychotropic medication and psychotherapy may be warranted.

Another key factor affecting outcomes of acne treatment is adherence. Patients' adherence to even short-term oral medication regimens is often poor. Adherence to topical treatment is generally worse, and adherence to chronic topical treatment is probably severely limited. Involvement of the patient in treatment planning, choosing regimens of limited complexity, and psychological interventions to promote better adherence can lead to improved treatment outcomes. Whenever possible, agents that can be administered in combination and may be used once daily are likely to promote compliance and increase efficacy.

Rosacea

DIAGNOSIS AND DIFFERENTIAL DIAGNOSIS

Rosacea is a common cause of a red face in adults. It must be distinguished from other conditions causing a red face, particularly seborrheic dermatitis, irritant dermatitis, and lupus. Seborrheic dermatitis, another common condition, is typically more scaly than rosacea. Seborrheic dermatitis involves the scalp (a cause of dandruff), eyebrows, nasal bridge, nasolabial and melolabial folds, and central chest. Rosacea does not typically have scale or scalp involvement of seborrhea and typically involves the cheeks and nose, sparing the fold in between. Irritant dermatitis may be confused as well, because rosacea patients report burning and stinging. Lupus is a far less common disorder and may be associated with scarring lesions of the face or a malar pattern of erythema.

CLASSIFICATION

Rosacea is divided into four subtypes, papulopustular, erythematotelangiectatic, phymatous, and ocular. Papulopustular rosacea responds best to topical and oral therapies, ocular disease responds best to oral therapy, and erthematotelangiectatic and phymatous types respond best to physical modalities. None of these subtypes or treatment modalities is mutually exclusive. Rosacea patients with papulopustular and erythematotelangiectatic subtypes should receive counseling about gentle cleansing and use of moisturizers and sunscreens, because these improve outcomes.

TREATMENT

Topical Antibiotics

Most patients with papulopustular rosacea benefit from topical antibiotic therapies. There are three agents in widespread use: metronidazole, azelaic acid, and sodium sulfacetamide and sulfur preparations. Metronidazole is widely used and is available in gel, lotion (Metrolotion), and cream (Metrocream) for twice-daily use at 0.75%, and cream (Noritate) and gel (Metrogel) for once-daily use at 1%. The gel vehicle is likely the preferred for facial use, and this is a generally well-tolerated agent. The 1% product offers the advantage of single daily dosing. Some patients report mild irritation from the use of these agents. Topical azelaic acid 15% (Finacea) gel is more effective than metronidazole gel 0.75%, but appears to be equal in effectiveness to metronidazole 1% gel. Like metronidazole, it can cause mild irritation and appears slightly more irritating than metronidazole.

Sodium sulfacetamide and sulfur compounds are available as washes and topical gels and may be additional agents that can improve outcomes in treating rosacea. One product, with sodium sulfacetamide 10% and 5% sulfur with sunscreen (Rosac) was found to be at least as effective as metronidazole cream 0.75%. Small reports of the efficacy of topical clindamycin and erythromycin appear in the dermatology literature.

As with acne therapy, combinations of topical agents are more effective than monotherapy. Thus, combinations of metronidazole, azelaic acid, and sodium sulfacetamide and sulfur compounds in various combinations and permutations improve outcomes. Most patients, when counseled about appropriate use of combinations of products, with good soap-free cleansing and moisturizing products, can tolerate these agents.

Oral Antibiotics

Oral tetracycline agents are commonly used to treat rosacea. Some employ antimicrobial doses such as tetracycline 500 mg twice daily or doxycycline 100 mg twice daily. Then the dose is tapered to the lowest dose that maintains control of the disease. A sub-antimicrobial dose doxycycline product (Oracea) has been FDA approved as a rosacea treatment. This product reduces the inflammation of rosacea and can help prevent development of organisms resistant to the antibiotic. When oral therapies are employed, efficacy of topical therapies is increased, which can decrease the need for or duration of the systemic agent.

Isotretinoin

Isotretinoin is an effective agent in treating papulopustular rosacea, and lower doses than those employed for acne can be highly effective. With increasing difficulty in using isotretinoin due to the iPLEDGE program, physicians might find other therapeutic alternatives more appealing.

CURRENT DIAGNOSIS

Acne

- Determine the type of acne: Comedonal, inflammatory (papules and pustules), nodulocystic, excoriée.
- Scarring indicates need for more intensive treatment.
- In female patients, is there menstrual irregularity to suggest endocrinopathy?

Rosacea

- Determine the type of rosacea: Papulopustular, erythematotelangiectatic, phymatous.
- Ocular involvement (itching, irritation, or redness) indicates need for oral treatment.
- Scaling of the eyebrows and nasal folds suggests seborrheic dermatitis

CURRENT THERAPY

Acne

- Topical retinoids are used as a foundation in acne treatment to eliminate the comedones that start the disease process.
- Topical benzoyl peroxide, often in combination with topical clindamycin, is highly effective at reducing skin bacterial counts without risk of bacterial resistance.
- Oral antibiotics may best be used in short courses to control inflammatory acne.
- Oral contraceptives can be used in women with resistant disease as an acne treatment prior to starting isotretinoin.
- Controlling patients' tendency to excoriate the face is difficult, yet may be necessary to reduce the severity of the lesions.
- Adherence to topical treatments is poor, especially in the setting of chronic illness. Careful attention should be focused on maximizing patients' adherence to the treatment regimen.

Rosacea

- Papulopustular rosacea is the form most responsive to medical treatment.
- Topical metronidazole (Flagyl), azelaic acid (Finaca), and sulfacetamide (Klaron) are the most common topical rosacea treatments.
- Oral antibiotics add further benefit and are usually needed for patients with ocular rosacea.
- rythematotelangiectatic rosacea and rhinophyma respond best to physical modalities (laser ablation of blood vessels and surgery, respectively).

Physical Modalities

Although there has been a report of a series of patients with erythematotelangiectatic rosacea responding well to azelaic acid 15% gel, most patients are likely to require optical vascular destructive modalities, including vascular laser or intense pulsed light. These approaches often require multiple treatment sessions, but they do decrease erythema, flushing and blushing, and telangiectasia. Phymatous disease responds well to surgical approaches, including use of high-frequency electrosurgery with a wire loop, CO_2 laser, or scalpel surgery.

REFERENCES

Gollnick H Cunliffe W, Berson D, et al: Global Alliance to Improve Outcomes in Acne: Management of acne: A report from a Global Alliance to Improve Outcomes in Acne. J Am Acad Dermatol 2003;49(1 suppl):S1-S37.

James WD: Clinical practice. Acne. N Engl J Med 2005;352(14):1463-1472.

Leyden JJ, Shalita A, Thiboutot D, et al: Topical retinoids in inflammatory acne: A retrospective, investigator-blinded, vehicle-controlled, photographic assessment. Clin Ther 2005;27(2):216-224.

Leyden JJ, Thiboutot DM, Shalita AR, et al: Comparison of tazarotene and minocycline maintenance therapies in acne vulgaris: A multicenter, double-blind, randomized, parallel-group study. Arch Dermatol 2006; 142(5):605-612.

Margolis DJ, Bowe WP, Hoffstad O, Berlin JA: Antibiotic treatment of acne may be associated with upper respiratory tract infections. Arch Dermatol 2005;141(9):1132-1136.

Ozolins M, Eady EA, Avery AJ, et al: Comparison of five antimicrobial regimens for treatment of mild to moderate inflammatory facial acne vulgaris in the community: Randomised controlled trial. Lancet 2004;364(9452): 2188-2195.

Sanchez J, Somolinos AL, Almodovar PI, et al: A randomized, double-blind, placebo-controlled trial of the combined effect of doxycycline hyclate 20-mg tablets and metronidazole 0.75% topical lotion in the treatment of rosacea. J Am Acad Dermatol 2005;53(5):791-797.

Thevarajah S, Balkrishnan R, Camacho FT, et al: Trends in prescription of acne medication in the U.S.: Shift from antibiotic to non-antibiotic treatment. J Dermatolog Treat 2005;16(4):224-228.

Hair Disorders

Method of
Thomas N. Helm, MD

Hair has no vital physiologic function, but hair is important to our self-image and influences our concept of beauty and aesthetics. Hair disorders may be classified as problems of hair loss, too much hair, or hair shaft abnormalities (Box 1).

Hair growth changes over time. When we are born, we have fine hairs over our bodies known as *lanugo hairs*. The lanugo hair is shed, and terminal hairs develop. On the scalp, terminal hairs have an active hair matrix situated in the fat that gives rise to a hair shaft surrounded by an inner root sheath and an outer root sheath. The outer root sheath is continuous with the surrounding epidermis. The hair matrix is very metabolically active, and mitotic figures are encountered on histologic examination. The human scalp has more than 100,000 hairs.

Hairs go through various well-defined stages of growth. At any time, hairs on the scalp are in different phases. The active growth phase is known as the anagen phase. The anagen phase usually lasts approximately 3 to 5 years. After this, hair growth ceases, and there is an upward retraction of the hair shaft. A hyaline basement membrane surrounds the hair root. The hair then enters the telogen phase. Telogen hairs are shed after approximately 3 months; when examined grossly, telogen hairs have a nonpigmented bulb at the end. About 10% of hairs at any one time are in the telogen phase, and almost 90% of hairs are in the anagen phase. Approximately 2% of hairs are in the catagen phase, which represents a transitional stage between the anagen and telogen phases.

When a patient presents with a hair abnormality, a number of questions need to be assessed. These include the pattern of remaining hairs, the duration of the hair problem, and the presence or absence of symptoms such as itching, discomfort, and any associated skin lesions (Box 2). The presence or absence of scarring on biopsy also helps with classification.

Noninflammatory Diffuse Hair Loss

ACUTE TELOGEN EFFLUVIUM

One of the most common causes of diffuse noninflammatory hair loss is telogen effluvium. Telogen effluvium represents an abnormality of the hair growth cycle. Hairs in an anagen phase abruptly switch into the telogen mode. Six to 16 weeks after a triggering insult, a precipitous hair shed is noted. From 30% to 40% of scalp hair can be lost. Clinical findings may be very impressive or relatively subtle.

Common culprits for telogen effluvium include major surgery, childbirth, crash diets, nutritional deficiencies, malabsorption, systemic disease, thyroid abnormalities, iron deficiency, and drugs. The most common types of drugs implicated include β-blockers, birth control pills, calcium channel blockers, nonsteroidal antiinflammatory agents, retinoids, salicylates, and angiotensin-converting enzyme inhibitors. Many other drugs can at times cause telogen effluvium (Box 3).

BOX 1   Classification of Hair Disorders

Noninflammatory Hair Loss
Patterned
- Androgenic alopecia
- Hair shaft abnormalities
- Traction

Nonpatterned
- Alopecia areata
- Androgen effluvium (toxic exposure)
- Secondary syphilis
- Telogen effluvium

Inflammatory Hair Loss
Scarring
- Acne keloidalis
- Autoimmune blistering disease
- Central centrifugal scarring alopecia
- Infections (e.g., dissecting cellulitis of the scalp)
- Lichen planopilaris
- Lupus erythematosus
- Neoplasms
- Trauma

Nonscarring
- Alopecia areata
- Psoriasis
- Secondary syphilis
- Tinea captis

Too Much Hair
Ethnic and racial hair growth
Hirsutism due to androgenic excess

Hair Shaft Abnormalities
Bubble hair
Ectodermal dysplasia
Exogenous injuries to the hair
Genetic abnormalities
Irregularities of the hair shaft
Monilethrix
Pseudomonilethrix
Trichorrhexis nodosa
Trichothiodystrophy

Telogen effluvium gradually subsides over several months and hair regrows. Many patients have a regrowth of fine hairs in areas of shedding but might still be bothered because the new hairs are of little cosmetic value. Patients must be reassured that with time, adequate hair growth will take place. If history and examination are not helpful in identifying an underlying cause, screening laboratory studies may be indicated (Box 4).

CHRONIC TELOGEN EFFLUVIUM

A telogen effluvium that lasts longer than 6 months is classified as chronic telogen effluvium. Chronic effluvium primarily affects middle-aged women, is idiopathic, and needs to be distinguished from

---

BOX 2   Points to Consider When Evaluating Hair Loss

Duration of hair loss
Pattern of hair loss
Associated symptoms (e.g., redness or itching)
Associated skin lesions

BOX 3	Medicines that Can Cause Telogen Effluvium

Angiotensin-converting enzyme inhibitors
Anticoagulants
Anticonvulsants
Antithyroid drugs
β-Blockers
Birth control pills
Calcium channel blockers
Cholesterol-lowering agents
Cimetidine (Tagamet)
Lithium
Nonsteroidal antiinflammatory agents
Retinoids
Salicylates

androgenic alopecia. Patients complain of sudden onset of hair loss and demonstrate a fluctuating course that involves the entire scalp. A scalp biopsy processed by horizontal sectioning can help differentiate this type of hair loss from female-pattern hair loss.

ANAGEN EFFLUVIUM

Anagen effluvium represents an abrupt cessation of anagen hair growth. Immediate hair loss occurs, and there is usually complete recovery once the triggering factor is removed. The most common example of this is the hair shedding encountered after treatment with a chemotherapeutic agent. Methotrexate (Rheumatrex), vinblastine, vincristine (Vincasar), doxorubicin (Adriamycin), daunorubicin (Cerubidine), cytarabine (Tarabine), cyclophosphamide (Cytoxan), bleomycin (Blenoxane), and etoposide (VePesid) are common culprits. Poisoning with arsenic, bismuth, borax, or thallium can also give rise to an anagen effluvium.

Instead of hairs switching from the anagen to the telogen phase, anagen hairs abruptly stop growing because of the metabolic effect on the hair matrix, and hairs are shed. When hairs are examined under the microscope, they have a jagged or tapered end (pencil-point hairs). Hair loss is noted over the entire scalp, but hairs that are not in an active anagen phase (e.g., eyelashes and eyebrows) are spared. Once the triggering cause is removed, hair regrowth can be expected. It can take several months for adequate regrowth to occur.

Anagen effluvium in the pediatric age group needs to be distinguished from the loose anagen syndrome. Loose anagen syndrome is a congenital defect in the hair follicle inner root sheath. Hairs are easily shed even with brushing or pulling and seem not to grow because of the consistent shedding. No treatment is available for this structural problem, although in some affected persons the condition seems to improve at puberty.

PATTERNED NONINFLAMMATORY HAIR LOSS

The most common cause of patterned hair loss is androgenic alopecia. *Androgenic alopecia* is a term for hair loss that is genetically predetermined. In androgenic alopecia, hair follicles are exquisitely sensitive to circulating androgens, and in predetermined areas, such as the crown and vertex of the scalp, progressive miniaturization of hair follicles occurs. Terminal hairs are transformed into vellus hairs in areas of hair thinning. Sebaceous lobules might increase in size, and biopsy reveals miniaturized follicles in the skin.

In men, hair thinning begins after puberty. Approximately one fourth of men aged 25 years have some degree of clinically apparent androgenic alopecia. Bitemporal recession and balding over the vertex are most common. Coarse hairs can develop at the temples and along the sideburns and are referred to as *whisker hairs.* In women, the frontal hair line is often spared and there is loss of hair in the crown area. In many instances there is a strong family history of baldness.

The treatment for androgenic alopecia is difficult. Topical minoxidil solution (Rogaine) has been shown to be of benefit. Two percent minoxidil can be applied twice daily and stimulates the development of terminal hairs and androgenic anagen phase. Finasteride (Propecia), at a dosage of 1 mg daily, has also been shown to stimulate hair growth in men. Finasteride is helpful in preventing further hair loss and yields significant clinical improvement when compared with placebo in maintaining terminal hair counts. Finasteride can lower prostate-specific anagen (PSA) levels, and care must be taken to screen patients to ensure that no underlying prostatic problem is overlooked in men taking this therapy. The current recommendation is that the PSA level be doubled to give a more accurate reflection of the true value in patients taking finasteride. Other treatment options that may be of value include oral spironolactone (Aldactone) and surgical approaches, such as hair transplantation surgery. Persons with darker or curly hair seem to benefit more from surgical approaches.

When hair loss in women is associated with signs of androgen excess (e.g., acne, weight gain, menstrual irregularities), evaluation is warranted to evaluate the possibility of underlying endocrinopathy, such as polycystic ovary disease, adrenal hyperplasia, or androgen-producing tumors of the ovaries. Laboratory studies that should be considered include determination of free and total testosterone levels, dehydroepiandrosterone sulfate, and cortisone levels and perhaps a dexamethasone (Decadron) suppression test.

Some hair shaft abnormalities, such as autosomal-dominant monilethrix, cause hairs to break easily. This may be associated with more pronounced hair loss of the vertex area and can mimic androgenic alopecia.

Inflammatory Hair Loss

Inflammatory hair loss can be evaluated and classified into scarring and nonscarring varieties. Often, scarring can be identified clinically, but sometimes scarring and destruction of follicular units can be only ascertained by biopsy. Biopsy is therefore very helpful when inflammatory hair loss is suggested. Hair loss is typically patchy and irregular.

NONSCARRING INFLAMMATORY HAIR LOSS

Alopecia areata is a common and yet idiopathic cause of inflammatory nonscarring hair loss. Alopecia areata manifests as smooth areas of hair loss that are often round or oval. Areas are asymptomatic but occasionally may be associated with mild itching or discomfort. No redness is noted on the skin, nor do pustules develop. The most important differential diagnosis for alopecia areata is fungal infection of the scalp, which is usually associated with scaling, erythema, and pustule formation. Biopsy or culture will help clarify the diagnosis.

Alopecia areata may be associated with other autoimmune abnormalities, such as autoimmune thyroid disease and vitiligo, as well as connective tissue diseases, such as lupus erythematosus. Most cases of alopecia areata do not require treatment. Most localized lesions remit on their own.

When lesions are more widespread, intralesional injections of corticosteroids are of greatest benefit in stimulating regrowth. Intralesional triamcinolone acetonide (Kenalog) at concentrations of 2.5 to 5.0 mg/mL may be administered every 3 to 4 weeks with a small-gauge needle as an intradermal injection. Topical corticosteroids

BOX 4	Laboratory Studies for Telogen Effluvium

Complete blood cell count
Ferritin level
Free testosterone level
Serum dehydroepiandrosterone sulfate level
Serum electrolyte level
Thyroid-stimulating hormone level

may be of value, and other topical agents that may be of benefit in some instances include anthralin, squaric acid dibutylester, and minoxidil.

Systemic agents will lead to hair regrowth but are not advised because they are toxic when used for long-term therapy. If hair growth is established and these agents are withdrawn, hair loss occurs, and patients can develop a dependency on these medicines. Because alopecia areata itself does not lead to any serious medical consequence, it is difficult to justify the long-term administration of a medication with many known serious side effects.

Traction Alopecia

Traction alopecia results from injury to the scalp from hair styling (e.g., cornrow braids) and other types of braiding practices or from wearing gear on the scalp, such as audio headphones. Rubbing and friction over time can cause damage to the hair shaft and impair hair growth.

Trichotillomania

Some persons under psychological duress pull, rub, or pick at the hair incessantly, leading to hair breakage and hair injury. In these instances, hair shaft fragments may be found in the dermis and are surrounded by an inflammatory infiltrate. Early on in this process is nonscarring, which can be reversed. If the trichotillomania is long-standing, permanent damage to the hair shaft can result.

Identifying and avoiding the underlying cause may be of value. In children younger than 6 years, it is often a self-limited psychological problem. In adults, trichotillomania is usually related to severe psychological problems requiring psychiatric referral.

Tricyclic antidepressants such as clomipramine (Anafranil), fluoxetine (Prozac), pimozide (Orap),[1] or newer agents such as topiramate (Topamax)[1] may be required to control this manifestation of obsessive-compulsive disorder.

Psoriasis and Inflammatory Skin Diseases

Although most dermatoses on the scalp are not associated with substantial hair loss, psoriasis and seborrheic dermatitis, as well as other dermatoses, may be associated with a temporary shedding of hair. The mechanism is not entirely clear but might relate to a telogen effluvium stimulated by the underlying dermatosis. Other cutaneous clues help in establishing a diagnosis. For example, in cases of psoriasis, scaly plaques may be found over the extensor surfaces and behind the ears.

INFLAMMATORY SCARRING HAIR LOSS

Infections

Tinea infection is the most common cause of inflammatory hair loss in children. Dermatophytes such as *Trichophyton rubrum*, *T. tonsurans*, and *Microsporum audouinii* infect the skin and then move down the hair shaft, where they destroy hair follicles. Hair can break off and give a black-dot appearance. Pustules and erythema develop, and the hair loss progresses. If the process is not controlled early on, the inflammatory infiltrate can lead to permanent damage of the hair follicle and lasting hair loss. Boggy and edematous suppurative areas of tinea infection are referred to as *kerion*. Biopsy or culture will help establish the diagnosis.

Topical antifungal agents are not efficacious for tinea capitis because reliable penetration is not achieved around the hair follicle. Oral agents such as griseofulvin (Gris-PEG), ketoconazole (Nizoral), itraconazole (Sporanox),[1] fluconazole (Diflucan),[1] and terbinafine (Lamisil) are all of value. In children, the greatest experience has been with the use of fluconazole elixir[1] or itraconazole elixir.[1] Itraconazole is, however, not FDA approved at this time for use in children. In adults, other infectious etiologies, such as secondary syphilis, can mimic tinea capitis and should be considered in the differential diagnosis.

Dissecting Cellulitis of the Scalp

Dissecting cellulitis is a disorder most common in African Americans. The cause is not known, but use of topical oils and scalp treatments may predispose to the development of pustules and abscesses that spread underneath the skin surface, damaging hairs. If this is not appropriately treated early on, lasting hair loss develops. Incision and drainage, use of oral antibiotics such as tetracycline (Sumycin) or ampicillin, and use of isotretinoin (Accutane)[1] can all be of value.

Acne Keloidalis

Acne keloidalis is a common cause of scarring alopecia, especially in African Americans. Patients develop follicle-based papules and pustules on the nape of the neck, which results in areas of alopecia with keloid scars. Treatment with topical or intralesional steroids, topical retinoids, and oral antibiotics can demonstrate limited efficacy. In severe cases, extensive surgery has been used.

Lupus Erythematosus

Cutaneous lupus can manifest itself in many different ways. Acute lupus manifests as a malar rash, and chronic lupus (discoid lupus erythematosus) manifests as erythematous scaly plaques with atrophy and hair loss. Biopsy reveals thickening of the basement membrane zone and increased mucin in the skin as well as destruction of follicular units.

Early on, topical corticosteroids can arrest the inflammatory process. Using sunscreens and sun protection is important because sun stimulates the development of discoid lupus. In cases in which topical treatments are not effective, antimalarials such as hydroxychloroquine (Plaquenil)[1] or chloroquine (Aralen)[1] are of value. Systemic corticosteroids may be warranted in extensive cases of discoid lupus when widespread scarring must be prevented.

Lichen Planopilaris

Lichen planopilaris is a variant of lichen planus. This idiopathic condition may be associated with lichen planus elsewhere on the body or can manifest simply as oval, pink-red to violaceous papules and plaques on the scalp. Lichen planopilaris can lead to lasting hair loss. A probable variant of lichen planopilaris involving the frontal scalp and occasionally the eyebrows has been called *frontal fibrosing alopecia*. The treatment is similar to that for cutaneous lupus. Topical corticosteroids, intralesional corticosteroids, and hydroxychloroquine[1] are the mainstays of therapy.

Central Centrifugal Scarring Alopecia

Scarring alopecias often exhibit overlapping features. The most common type of scarring alopecia has been called *central centrifugal scarring alopecia*. Patients develop hair loss in the central portion of the crown that progresses centrifugally. Central centrifugal scarring alopecia encompasses scarring alopecias that have been classified as pseudopelade, tufted folliculitis, folliculitis decalvans, and follicular degeneration syndrome in the past. Scarring alopecias are usually very difficult to treat, and the focus of treatment should be on limiting the disease progression. A variety of therapeutic agents such as topical and systemic steroids, oral antibiotics, and antimalarials have been tried with limited success.

Miscellaneous

Occasionally, metastases or follicular involvement with lymphoma manifest with alopecia. Biopsy is critical in establishing the diagnosis in unusual situations or when unusual clinical presentations occur.

---

[1]Not FDA approved for this indication.

Too Much Hair

ETHNIC VARIATION

Many patients present with the complaint of excessive body or facial hair. Often this relates to ethnic variation. Asians have relatively little facial and body hair, whereas persons from Middle Eastern countries have a greater degree of body hair. Often reassurance is all that is required. Unfortunately, because of the high premium placed on good looks and the image presented in the media, the beauty of less body and facial hair in women is emphasized in our culture and many people seek treatment. Treatment of unwanted hair consists of electrolysis, in which galvanic current is used to damage the hair bulb of unwanted follicles and impede further hair growth. Laser hair removal is also effective, but it is generally more expensive.

HIRSUTISM

If there is increased body hair in a woman in a pattern more typical of a man, the diagnosis of hirsutism is likely. Androgen-dependent growth occurs on the upper lip, chin, cheeks, central chest, and lower abdomen. This may be associated with virilization, such as masculine body habitus, clitoral hypertrophy, and amenorrhea. The dehydroepiandrosterone sulfate and testosterone levels may be increased. Excessive secretion of androgens from the ovary or adrenal glands can occur, or there may be excessive stimulation by pituitary tumors. Polycystic ovary disease (Stein–Leventhal syndrome) is associated with hirsutism in almost one half of cases. Cushing's disease, acromegaly, and prolactin-secreting adenomas are all possible culprits as well.

If appropriate testing has ruled out serious underlying pathology, then wax, depilatories, and epilation by laser treatment may all be considered. Spironolactone (Aldactone)[1] and cyproterone acetate[2] are also useful agents.

Hair Shaft Abnormalities

ACQUIRED HAIR SHAFT ABNORMALITIES

Split ends, hair breakage, and damage can occur through the many cosmetic treatments given to hair. Frequent use of hair dryers can cause damage to the hair shaft in which hairs have bubbles within them (bubble hair deformity). Exposure to ultraviolet light, detergents, and other factors can also lead to the development of split ends. Rarely, hair shaft abnormalities such as uncombable hair may be acquired. Identifying the causes of hair shaft abnormality and avoidance of these traumatic insults to the hair lead to improvement in many cases.

HEREDITARY HAIR SHAFT DISORDERS

Hereditary hair shaft disorders are uncommon but important to recognize. Some disorders, such as Menkes' kinky hair disorder, are associated with defects in copper metabolism and are associated with hypothermia, seizures, and early death. Trichothiodystrophy represents an abnormality in the sulfur bond formation in hairs and is associated with brittle hairs that break and can have a spangled appearance or a twisted architecture when analyzed under the microscope. Microscopic examination of hair shafts by a dermatopathologist or dermatologist allow accurate diagnosis. No treatments are likely to be of value in these hereditary abnormalities.

Conclusion

Many abnormalities of hair growth and development are encountered in clinical practice. Identifying the pattern and history allows accurate diagnosis in the overwhelming majority of cases. Nonscarring patterned loss is likely to be due to androgenic alopecia. Localized nonscarring hair loss may be due to alopecia areata. The presence of pustules and broken hairs suggests an infectious etiology.

REFERENCES

Hordinsky MK: Medical treatment of noncicatricial alopecia. Semin Cutan Med Surg 2006;25(1):51-5.
Nield LS, Keri JE, Kamat D: Alopecia in the general pediatric clinic: Who to treat, who to refer. Clin Pediatr 2006;45(7):605-612.
Price VH: Treatment of hair loss. N Engl J Med 1999;341(13):964-973.
Ross EK, Tan E, Shapiro J: Update on primary cicatricial alopecias. J Am Acad Dermatol 2005;53(1):1-37.
Sellheyer K, Bergfeld WF: Histopathologic evaluation of alopecias. Am J Dermatopathol 2006;28(3):236-259.
Silverberg NB: Helping children cope with hair loss. Cutis. 2006;78(5):333-6.
Stough D, Stenn K, Haber R, et al: Psychological effect, pathophysiology, and management of androgenetic alopecia in men. Mayo Clin Proc 2005;80(10):1316-1322.

Cancer of the Skin

Method of
Lucile E. White, MD, and Murad Alam, MD

Based on prognostic factors, skin cancers are usually classified as melanoma or non–melanoma skin cancers. Non–melanoma skin cancers include squamous cell carcinoma (SCC) and basal cell carcinoma (BCC). BCCs are the most common form of cancer in the United States, with more than 800,000 cases diagnosed in 1999. If a patient has a history of one BCC, the risk of developing another BCC within 3 years is 10 times greater than for patients who have never had skin cancer. Actinic keratoses are a common, premalignant lesion in patients with light skin. Estimates vary, but several studies suggest that 0.1% to 10% of actinic keratoses develop into SCCs. In 1999, there were more than 200,000 SCCs in the United States. Risk factors for developing non–melanoma skin cancer are exposure to ultraviolet radiation, fair skin and hair, immunosuppression, and genetic susceptibility.

Clinical Features

Early skin cancer can resemble other benign skin conditions such as acne, skin trauma, or scars. If a lesion has been present for more than 6 weeks and the patient cannot recall recent or distant trauma to the area, then the lesion warrants a biopsy.

There are several types of BCCs with various clinical morphologies. Nodular BCC is the most common type and usually appears as a pink, shiny papule similar to an acne lesion without the purulence. Telangiectasias may be seen within the papule on close inspection. Superficial BCCs often appear as shiny, pink, thin patches or plaques and may be mistakenly overlooked as a scar. Morpheaform BCCs can also appear as shiny scarlike thin or atrophic areas of skin. Morpheaform BCCs have the highest rate of recurrence due to their penetrating and irregular spread patterns on histopathology. If BCCs are not treated, they can ulcerate and penetrate through the underlying tissue.

Actinic keratoses are essentially precancerous lesions. They usually appear as an erythematous area with overlying scale. Often, because erythema can be mild with these lesions, these rough lesions are more noticeable on physical examination while running the fingers over the rough, affected skin. Patients might tolerate these lesions for longer than necessary because they simply attribute them to a small area of dry skin.

---

[1]Not FDA approved for this indication.
[2]Not available in the United States.

CURRENT DIAGNOSIS

- Skin cancer can resemble other benign skin conditions such as acne, skin trauma, or scars.
- Actinic keratoses are precancerous lesions that can appear as an erythematous area of skin with varying amounts of overlying scale.
- Squamous cell carcinoma can appear as erythematous skin with overlying scale or crust that bleeds easily.
- Basal cell carcinoma can appear as a pink, shiny papule, a pink, shiny thin patch, or a scarlike thin area of skin.

SCCs often appear as erythematous skin with overlying scale that bleeds easily. On mucosal areas, the scale may be absent. Keratoacanthoma is a well-differentiated form of SCC that appears as a dome-shaped erythematous papule with keratotic or scaling center.

Treatment

ACTINIC KERATOSES

Some actinic keratoses have been reported to undergo spontaneous remission, but because they can be precursors to SCC, and because whether a lesion remits or progresses is unpredictable, these lesions are usually treated. Treatment with liquid nitrogen, known as *cryotherapy*, is the most common form of treatment for isolated lesions. Response rates vary based on the technique: 39% of lesions cleared with freezing times of less than 5 seconds, and 83% of lesions cleared with freezing times longer than 20 seconds. The most common side effect of cryotherapy is hypopigmentation in the area that was treated.

Topical treatments can be used for patients with many lesions in a localized area. Such topical treatments consist of topical chemotherapy or immune system up-regulators.

Imiquimod (Aldara) 5% cream is an immune system up-regulator that is FDA approved for treating actinic keratoses. Imiquimod is applied once daily, 2 or 3 days a week, for 16 weeks. In randomized, blinded, controlled trials, the medication has complete clearance rates of 27% to 57% and partial clearance rates ranging from 37% to 72%. A second course of imiquimod can increase complete and partial clearance rates to 54% and 61%, respectively.

Fluorouracil (Efudex) is a topical chemotherapy medication. Fluorouracil is available in 5%, 1%, and 0.5% cream and solution formulations. In a study comparing 5% with 0.5% cream, the complete clearance rate of 43% was the same for both concentrations. It is important to note that the degree of inflammation during treatment correlates with lesion clearance. This topical medication is applied once or twice a day for 2 to 6 weeks depending on the formulation

CURRENT THERAPY

- Actinic keratoses can be treated with cryotherapy, topical therapy, or photodynamic therapy.
- Basal cell and squamous cell carcinomas are most commonly treated with excision or Mohs' micrographic surgery.
- Mohs' surgery is indicated for tumors larger than 2 cm, tumors with poorly defined margins, tumors with aggressive histologic morphology, recurrent tumors, or tumors around the ears, nose, mouth, or eyes, which have a higher risk of recurrence.
- Radiation therapy is usually reserved for patients who cannot tolerate a local excision.

and treatment site. If intense vesiculation occurs, a contact allergy should be suspected and the treatment should be discontinued. Diclofenac sodium (Solaraze) can also be applied over large areas of actinic keratoses and is reported to cause less irritation than fluorouracil.

A new modality for treating actinic keratoses is photodynamic therapy. Photodynamic therapy entails applying a topical photosensitizer to the skin. The precancerous lesions are more sensitive to this medication, and when light in the blue spectrum is applied to the treated area, the chemical is activated, destroying the precancerous cells.

SQUAMOUS CELL AND BASAL CELL CARCINOMAS

Squamous cell carcinoma may be difficult to distinguish from an advanced actinic keratosis, and if an actinic keratosis does not resolve with liquid nitrogen, a biopsy should be performed to rule out an SCC. Excision with standard technique or Mohs' micrographic surgery is the current standard of care for cutaneous SCC. Mohs' surgery provides same-day microscopic margin control to ensure that a tumor is completely removed while preserving healthy tissue. Mohs' micrographic surgery is the treatment of choice for tumors with high recurrence rates such as the areas around the ears, nose, mouth, or, eyes. Mohs' surgery is also used for tumors larger than 2 cm, with poorly defined margins, aggressive histologic morphology, or tumors that recur.

Basal cell carcinomas are also most commonly treated with standard excision or Mohs' micrographic surgery, although Mohs' surgery has a lower recurrence rate (1%-2%) than standard excision (3%-8%). Other treatment options that do not provide assurance of tumor clearance include electrodessication with curettage, with an 8% recurrence rate, and radiation, with a 7% recurrence rate. Radiation therapy is often reserved for patients who are not candidates for surgery because the risk of recurrence is higher and the treatment is more expensive than surgical options.

Prevention and Screening

In patients who develop recurrent BCCs, approximately two thirds of tumors recur within 3 years of initial treatment; thus, regular monitoring of patients with non–melanoma skin cancer is suggested. Most physicians prefer to have patients with a recent history of non–melanoma skin cancer return for complete skin examinations at least every 6 months. Reducing sun exposure and wearing sunscreen should also be advised for patients who have had skin cancer.

REFERENCES

Alam M, Ratner D: Cutaneous squamous-cell carcinoma. N Engl J Med 2001;344:975-983.
Jorizzo J, Dinehart S, Matheson R, et al: Vehicle-controlled, double-blind, randomized study of imiquimod 5% cream applied 3 days per week in one or two courses of treatment for actinic keratoses on the head. J Am Acad Dermatol 2007;57:265-268.
Korman N, Moy R, Ling M, et al: Dosing with 5% imiquimod cream 3 times per week for the treatment of actinic keratosis: Results of two phase 3, randomized, double-blind, parallel-group, vehicle-controlled trials. Arch Dermatol 2005;141:467-473.
Lebwohl M, Dinehart S, Whiting D, et al: Imiquimod 5% cream for the treatment of actinic keratosis: Results from two phase III, randomized double-blind, parallel group, vehicle-controlled trials. J Am Acad Dermatol 2004;50:714-721.
Loven K, Stein L, Furst K, et al: Evaluation of the efficacy and tolerability of 0.5% fluorouracil cream and 5% fluorouracil cream applied to each side of the face in patients with actinic keratosis. Clin Ther 2002;24: 990-1000.
Marcil I, Stern RS: Risk of developing a subsequent nonmelanoma skin cancer in patients with a history of nonmelanoma skin cancer: A critical review of the literature and meta-analysis. Arch Dermatol 2002;136:1524-1530.
Miller DL, Weinstock MA: Nonmelanoma skin cancer in the United States: Incidence. J Am Acad Dermatol 1994;30:774-778.

Rowe DE, Carroll RJ, Day CL: Long-term recurrence rates in previously untreated (primary) basal cell carcinoma: Implications for patient follow-up. J Dermatol Surg Oncol 1989;15:315-328.
Salasche SJ: Epidemiology of actinic keratoses and squamous cell carcinoma. J Am Acad Dermatol 2000;42:4-7.
Szeimies RM, Gerritsen MJP, Gupta G, et al: Imiquimod 5% cream for the treatment of actinic keratosis: Results from a phase III, randomized, double-blind, vehicle-controlled, clinical trial with histology. J Am Acad Dermatol 2004;51:547-555.
Thai KE, Fergin P, Freeman M, et al: A prospective study of the use of cryosurgery for the treatment of actinic keratoses. Int J Dermatol 2004;43:687-692.
Thissen MR, Neumann MH, Schouten LJ: A systematic review of treatment modalities for primary basal cell carcinomas. Arch Dermatol 1999;135:1177-1183.

Cutaneous T-Cell Lymphomas (Mycosis Fungoides and Sézary's Syndrome)

Method of
Christiane Querfeld, MD, Timothy M. Kuzel, MD, and Steven T. Rosen, MD

Cutaneous T-cell lymphomas (CTCLs) clinically and biologically represent a heterogeneous group of non-Hodgkin's lymphoma with clonal proliferation of skin-homing malignant T-lymphocytes. CTCLs are characterized by a prolonged clinical course with a different clinical behavior and outcome compared to their systemic counterpart. However, disease progression can involve lymph nodes, peripheral blood, and visceral organs with a less-favorable prognosis. Features of the different types of CTCL are recognized in the new revised European Organization for Research and Treatment of Cancer (EORTC) and World Health Organization (WHO) classification for primary cutaneous lymphomas, which distinguish indolent types such as mycosis fungoides (MF) from aggressive types such as Sézary's syndrome (SS).

The most common types of CTCL, MF and SS, represent monoclonal T-helper memory lymphomas. MF and SS are predominantly diseases of older patients, with a male predominance of approximately 2:1 and age-adjusted ratio of African Americans to whites of 1:1.7. A recent update on epidemiologic features of CTCL and trends in incidence from nine population-based U.S. cancer registries that constitute the Surveillance, Epidemiology, and End Results Program (SEER-9) differed from those of previous reports. The incidence of CTCL has risen consistently since 1973, with an overall annual age-adjusted incidence of 6.4 cases per million that overall represented 3.9% of all non-Hodgkin's lymphomas in these population-based studies.

It has been suggested that the condition results from persistent antigen stimulation, with an increased risk for the development of CTCL in patients exposed to chemicals or pesticides; however, recent studies on the subject produced controversial results. Patients with MF and SS are at significantly increased risk for developing a second primary lymphoma, especially Hodgkin's disease.

Cutaneous lymphomas include other entities such as adult T-cell leukemia/lymphoma (ATLL), which is etiologically associated with human T-lymphotropic virus (HTLV)-1. The chronic smoldering form is often associated with skin lesions resembling MF. Lymphomatoid papulosis (LyP) and anaplastic large T-cell lymphoma (ALCL) belong to the CD30+ lymphoproliferative disorders. Their common phenotypic hallmark is the CD30+ T-lymphocyte that morphologically resembles Reed–Sternberg cells. Cutaneous ALCL rarely carries the t(2;5) translocation and is usually anaplastic large-cell lymphoma kinase (ALK) negative. Both appear to have a favorable clinical course. Subcutaneous panniculitis-like T-cell lymphoma is a cytotoxic T-cell lymphoma that involves the subcutaneous tissue, mimicking panniculitis. The heterogeneous group of peripheral T-cell lymphoma includes provisional entities such as cutaneous aggressive CD8+ cytotoxic T-cell lymphoma, cutaneous γ/δ T-cell lymphoma, and the cutaneous CD4+ small to medium pleomorphic T-cell lymphoma. Other hematologic neoplasms such as the Epstein–Barr virus (EBV)-associated extranodal natural killer (NK)/T-cell lymphoma, nasal type, and the EBV-negative blastic NK-cell lymphoma commonly present in the skin with or without concurrent extracutaneous manifestations.

Clinical and Pathologic Features

MF has numerous clinical and histologic variants. Besides the classic Alibert–Bazin type of MF, three major variants have been recognized in the new WHO–EORTC classification including granulomatous slack skin, which is characterized by the development of folds of lax skin; folliculotropic MF, characterized by involvement of hair follicles with or without mucin, often leading to alopecia; and pagetoid reticulosis, which manifests as a solitary psoriasiform patch with intraepidermal involvement of atypical (pagetoid) T-cells typically expressing a CD4-CD8+ phenotype. MF is typified by the development of patches, plaques, or tumors. Most patients remain in clinical stages limited to the skin; however, a small percentage progress to the tumor or erythrodermic stages, which have an estimated 5-year survival rate of only 40%.

SS is the erythrodermic and aggressive variant of CTCL. It has a leukemic component, characterized by circulating, atypical malignant T-lymphocytes with cerebriform nuclei (Sézary cells), erythroderma, and often lymphadenopathy. Severe pruritus, ectropion, alopecia, and palmoplantar keratoderma are common associated features. Patients with SS have an unfavorable prognosis with an estimated 5-year survival of 15%.

Several histologic features are useful in establishing a diagnosis of MF and SS. In most cases, it consists of an upper dermal band–like lymphocytic infiltrate with atypical lymphocytes, variable findings of inflammatory cells, and epidermal involvement with solitary cells or small clusters of malignant lymphocytes (Pautrier's microabcesses). Tumor lesions express more diffuse and deep infiltrates with diminished epidermotropism. Biopsies from erythrodermic MF or SS often lack these features; therefore, the presence of a dominant T-cell clone is an important diagnostic criterion. Procedures based on polymerase chain reaction (PCR) are the most sensitive to detect clonality and represent an important adjuvant procedure, in association with histopathology and immunophenotyping, to support the clinical diagnosis. With disease progression, the malignant lymphocytes can undergo large cell transformation and can disseminate to blood, lymph nodes, and visceral organs.

In cases of classic MF and SS, the neoplastic lymphocytes bear a T-helper/memory cell and often lose the CD5, CD7 and/or CD26 antigen in advanced stages. Recently, CD158k, a major histocompatibility class I antigen receptor, was found to be selectively expressed on circulating and cutaneous malignant T cells from SS patients, which might represent a new phenotypic marker. Aberrant T-plastin expression was also found in Sézary cells. Patients with advanced-stage MF and SS show an imbalance between helper T-cell type 1 (Th1) and Th2, with a predominant type 2 immune response characterized by increased cytokine production of interleukin (IL)-4, IL-6, and IL-10 and decreased interferon-gamma (IFN-γ) and IL-2, resulting in an impaired cell-mediated immunity. In advanced stages, the number of reactive cytotoxic CD8+ T cells and dendritic cells, which are characteristic in early patch stage cutaneous lesions, tend to decrease with increase of neoplastic CD4+ T cells.

It is not clear what mechanisms are adopted by the malignant T lymphocytes to proliferate and to escape immune surveillance. Immune dysregulation is demonstrated by the constitutive phosphorylation of STAT-3 in neoplastic T cells. These cells can express the activation markers CD45RO and the IL-2α receptor (CD25) that has provided a target for biological therapy with denileukin diftitox. Naturally occurring regulatory T cells (Tregs) also express the CD25 molecule. They suppress the activity of other immune cells, thus maintaining immunologic tolerance. Tregs account for 5% to 10% of CD4+ T cells in peripheral blood. Features of Tregs appear

CURRENT DIAGNOSIS

Early Stage Mycosis Fungoides

- Clinical: Persistent patches or plaques in non–sun-exposed areas
- Histopathologic: Epidermotropism, Pautrier's microabsesses, atypical lymphocytes, bandlike infiltrate
- Immunophenotypic: $CD4^+$, $CD8^-$ phenotype (skin)
- Molecular: Clonal T-cell receptor gene rearrangement (skin)

Advanced Stage Mycosis Fungoides Sézary's Syndrome

- Clinical: Generalized erythroderma, lymphadenopathy
- Immunophenotypic: $CD4^+$, $CD8^-$ phenotype (blood), loss of $CD5^-$ and/or $CD7^-$
- Molecular: Clonal T-cell receptor gene rearrangement (blood)
- Laboratory: Sézary cells, elevated lactate dehydrobenase

to play a role in the immunosuppression of advanced stages, but their role in CTCL is still controversial.

Etiology, Molecular Biology, and Molecular Genetics

Many factors have been implicated in the etiology of CTCL including microbiological, environmental, or occupational theories, but none has yet been verified. Previous studies on the pathogenesis have revealed acquired oncogene abnormalities such as diminished expression of the tumor suppressor gene transforming growth factor (TGF)-β receptor II, *Fas*, *p15*, and *p16* and overexpression of *JUNB* on peripheral malignant $CD4^+$ T lymphocytes, suggesting that they may be crucial in the pathogenesis of CTCL. Comparative analyses of clonal lymphocytes derived from SS patients reveal aberrations in signaling pathways by the signal transducer and activator of transcription (STAT) family and by impaired CD40 and CD40L interaction. Complementary DNA (cDNA) microarray analysis, a novel technique for genomic analysis in tumors, has been used to rapidly screen for genomic imbalances and to globally show oncogene changes in MF and SS. A recent study showed that the antiapoptotic T-cell oncogene *Twist* and the growth-promoting tyrosine kinase receptor EpH4 were among the highly and selectively expressed genes in malignant T-lymphocytes. CTCL is characterized by the accumulation of genetic mutations during disease progression. Molecular cytogenetic studies have identified common regions of chromosomal deletion and amplification, involving structural rearrangements of chromosomes 1, 2, 6, 9, 14, and 16 and numerical abnormalities of 6, 8, 10, 11, 13, 17, and 21.

The molecular events involved in the pathogenesis of MF and transformation of the tumor and tumor cells during disease progression remain elusive. Controversial data on frequency and prognostic value of microsatellite instability in the progression of MF have been reported. One group identified microsatellite instability consistent with deficits in DNA repair in a large number of biopsies from patients with MF with a higher prevalence in tumor stages. Promoter hypermethylation leading to tumor-suppressor gene inactivation appeared to be associated with disease progression. In contrast, a recent longitudinal study did not find any microsatellite instability and correlated with a normal mismatch repair gene expression.

BOX 1 Tumor–Node–Metastasis–Blood Classification for Mycosis Fungoides and Sézary's Syndrome

T (Skin)

T1
Limited patch/plaque (<10% of BSA)

T2
Generalized patch/plaque (>10% of BSA)

T3
Tumors

T4
Generalized erythroderma

N (Nodes)

N0
No clinically abnormal peripheral lymph nodes

N1
Clinically abnormal peripheral lymph nodes

NP0
Biopsy performed, not CTCL

NP1
Biopsy performed, CTCL

LN0
Uninvolved

LN1
Reactive lymph node

LN2
Dermatopathic node, small clusters of convoluted cells (<6 cells/cluster)

LN3*
Dermatopathic node, small clusters of convoluted cells (>6 cells/cluster)

LN4*
Lymph node effacement

M (Metastases to Viscera)

M0
No visceral metastasis

M1
Visceral metastasis

B (Blood Metastases)

B0
Atypical circulating cells not present (<5%)

B1
Atypical circulating cells present (>5%)

---

*Pathologically involved lymph nodes.
BSA = body surface area; CTCL = cutaneous T-cell lymphomas.

TABLE 1 Stage Classification for Mycosis Fungoides and Sézary's Syndrome

Stage	Tumor (T)	Node (N)	Node Biopsy (NP)	Metastasis (M)
IA	1	0	0	0
IB	2	0	0	0
IIA	1/2	1	0	0
IIB	3	0/1	0	0
III	4	0/1	0	0
IVA	1–4	0/1	1	0
IVB	1–4	0/1	0/1	1

Staging and Prognostic Factors

The recommended staging system is the TNMB (tumor, node, metastasis, blood) that considers the extent of skin involvement, presence of lymph node or visceral disease, and detection of Sézary cells in the peripheral blood (Box 1 and Table 1). Routine evaluation should include complete physical examination, complete blood count with differential and Sézary cell assessment, chemistry panel with lactate dehydrogenase, skin biopsy for histology, immunophenotyping and gene rearrangement studies, and lymph node biopsies in cases with enlarged nodes at presentation. Diagnosis in early stages of MF has been improved due to advances in T-cell receptor (TCR) gene rearrangement techniques with increased sensitivity and specificity. Imaging studies should be reserved for patients with clinical and laboratory findings suggesting systemic disease or prominent lymphadenopathy. Patients with T1 disease have a normal life expectancy, whereas patients with increased tumor burden have a significantly decreased survival. The median survival time of patients who develop extracutaneous disease is approximately 25 months.

Several studies have attempted to identify clinical, biological, histopathologic, or immunophenotypic characteristics that can predict outcome. So far, the main prognostic factors identified in MF and SS are the type and extent of skin involvement, extracutaneous manifestation of the disease, initial response to treatment, histologic large cell transformation, high serum level of lactate dehydrogenase, and detection of a cutaneous or peripheral blood T-cell clone. A high Sézary cell count, loss of T-cell markers, blood eosinophilia, chromosomal abnormalities in T cells, and high serum concentration of soluble α chain of the IL-2 receptor (sIL-2R) are also independently associated with a poor outcome. The presence of cytotoxic CD8$^+$ T-lymphocytes in the dermal infiltrate and the density of epidermal Langerhans cells greater than 90 cells/mm^2 is associated with a better prognosis.

Treatment

EARLY-STAGE DISEASE

The treatment of MF and SS is stage-dependent and regarded as palliative, so no definitive curative treatment strategies are available at present. Patients with early-stage CTCL are ideally treated with topical agents such as nitrogen mustard, carmustine (BiCNU), retinoids, rexinoids, narrowband ultraviolet light B (NB-UVB), photochemotherapy with psoralens and UVA (PUVA), and total skin electron-beam irradiation. Multiagent chemotherapy regimens used early in the course demonstrate no survival benefit.

Two recent retrospective studies have supported this approach. Kim and colleagues reported on 203 patients with MF and SS clinical stages I to III treated with topical nitrogen mustard. Relapse-free rates in T1 at 2 and 5 years were 74% and 54%, respectively, and in T2, 54% and 29%, respectively. Most relapses occurred within 2 years. Querfeld and colleagues reported on long-term remissions of patients with early stage disease treated with PUVA. Depending on T stage,

 CURRENT THERAPY

Topical
- Nitrogen mustard
- Phototherapy
- Retinoids
- Radiation
- Steroids

Systemic Chemotherapy
- CHOP and CHOP-like
- Gemcitabine (Gemzar)[1]
- Nucleoside analogue: Pentostatin (Nipent)[1]
- Pegylated doxorubicin (Adriamycin)
- Temozolomide (Temodar)[1]

Biological Therapy
- Denileukin diftitox
- ECP
- Histone deacetylases
- IFN-α

Stem Cell Transplant
- Allogeneic transplant
- Mini-allogeneic transplant

Combined Therapy
- Bexarotene (Targretin) plus phototherapy
- ECP plus IFN-α
- ECP plus bexarotene
- IFN-α plus bexarotene
- IFN-α plus phototherapy

Investigational Therapy
- Antibodies: Alemtuzumab (Campath),[1] zanolimumab (HuMax-CD4)[8]
- Immunomodulatory therapy: Lenalidomide (Revlimid)[1]
- Cytokines (IL-12, IFN-γ)
- Vaccination strategies

CHOP = cyclophosphamide, doxorubicin, vincristine,[1] and prednisone; ECP = extracorporeal phototherapy; IFN = interferon.
[1]Not FDA approved for this indication.
[8]Orphan drug in the United States.

30% to 50% of patients remain disease-free after 10 years, but based on the occurrence of late relapses, a permanent cure is not suggested.

Our current approach for early-stage patients is topical monotherapy. If patients fail to respond, we switch to a different topical therapy. Our first-line treatment for early-stage patients is PUVA or NB-UVB therapy. However, in cases of refractory early stages we consider combination therapy such as PUVA or NB-UVB with low-dose systemic bexarotene or IFN-α.

Phototherapy

Since 1974, PUVA therapy has been widely used in treating psoriasis, vitiligo, and other skin disorders. 8-Methoxypsoralen (8-MOP), after oral ingestion, becomes activated when exposed to UVA light. UVA (320–400 nm), with its peak emission wavelength between 330 and 340 nm, penetrates the skin approximately 1 to 2 mm into the mid-dermis. The combination is thought to act at the nuclear level of cells, inhibiting DNA and RNA synthesis through formation of mono- or bifunctional thymine products, induction of gene mutations, or sister chromatid exchanges. Initial exposure times of patients are limited to the phototype according to the Fitzpatrick grading system, the ability to tan, and the patient's history of sunburns. The initial UVA dosage is approximately 0.5 J/cm² and is increased per treatment as tolerated or up to the minimal erythema dose. Therapy is typically given three times a week until complete remission is achieved. Additional maintenance therapy can be administered while gradually reducing PUVA from once a week to once every 4 to 6 weeks to maintain longer remission times.

It is extremely effective at clearing patch and plaque disease, with successfully reapplied courses in relapsed patients. Several studies confirmed the efficacy of this treatment with reported complete remissions in up to 71.4% of patients. Long-term remissions of more than 8 years have been reported in patients with early-stage MF. Disease-free survival rates for stage IA at 5 and 10 years were 56% and 30%, respectively, and for stage IB/IIA 74% and 50%, respectively. The most common reported acute side effects are erythema, pruritus, and nausea, which are usually mild at presentation and generally manageable with dose adjustments of UVA or psoralens or dose interruptions. Long-term exposure is associated with an increased risk for developing chronic photodamage and skin cancer. Results of two multicenter, dose-randomized evaluations of oral low-dose bexarotene (75 mg or 150 mg daily for 24 weeks) and PUVA in patients with stage IB-IIA have shown a response rate similar to that for PUVA monotherapy, but the results were achieved with lower cumulative energy. Folliculotropic MF is often less responsive to PUVA. Combined treatment with low-dose bexarotene or IFN-α may be considered in such cases.

NB-UVB is considered less carcinogenic and may be an alternative treatment option in early-stage MF. In three small retrospective analyses, patients with clinical stage IA or IB and parapsoriasis and treated with NB-UVB showed complete remission rates between 54.2% and 83%. However, remission times were short and a maintenance schedule has been difficult to establish.

Topical Nitrogen Mustard

Many investigators have demonstrated the efficacy of topical nitrogen mustard (Mustargen) in early-stage MF with occasional long-term remissions of more than 8 years. Updates on 203 patients with MF treated with topical nitrogen mustard demonstrated its efficacy with reported complete remission rates of 76% to 80% for patients with stage IA disease and 35% to 68% for those with stage IB disease. The median duration of remission was short at 12 months, although less than 10% of patients developed progression to a higher stage. Skin clearance required 6 months or longer and was followed by maintenance therapy; however, there was no evidence that prolonged maintenance was beneficial. Only 11% of patients maintained complete remission after 10 years. The most common side effect was irritant contact dermatitis and hypersensitivity reaction. No secondary malignancies related to therapy were reported. Topical nitrogen mustard was equally effective when used after disease relapses.

Topical Retinoids

Topical retinoid application may be an effective approach in early stage MF. They exert their effects through two basic types of nuclear receptors, the retinoic acid (RAR) and rexinoid (RXR) receptor family. No comparison of different retinoids has been evaluated. Bexarotene 1% gel, a new rexinoid, was approved by the FDA as a therapy for stages IA through IIA MF. In a dose-escalating trial of bexarotene from 0.1% to 1.0%, the complete remission rate was 21%, with a 63% overall response rate. The median duration of remission was 24 months. A multinational phase III study of patients with refractory or persistent early stage MF, treated with 1% bexarotene gel in a dose- and frequency-escalating fashion, demonstrated an overall response rate of 54%, with complete remission in 10%. The median duration was less favorable at 7 months. Reported events were mostly localized skin irritation.

Total Skin Electron Beam Treatment

Total skin electron beam treatment (TSEBT) is a treatment in which ionizing radiation is administered to the entire skin surface penetrating at least 4 mm into the dermis. The standard total dose is 36 Gy delivered with electrons of at least 4 MeV energy and fractionated over 8 to 10 weeks. Techniques including dynamic rotation, six-field, or regional patch treatments are used to administer the electron beam. Published data of therapeutic efficacy of total skin electron beam therapy (TSEB) from centers with extensive experience show 40% to 98% complete remission rates among patients from stage IA to IB, with approximately 50% of patients with clinical stage IA and 25% of patients with clinical stage IB remaining in long-term remission. TSEB treatment in early stages remains controversial because of its potential toxicity. Side effects can be significant and consist of erythema, edema, scaling, ulceration, and irreversible loss of skin adnexae. TSEB may be repeated for palliative effects, although at reduced doses. Adjuvant therapy including PUVA, photopheresis, and IFN-α can improve the duration of response.

ADVANCED-STAGE DISEASE

Treatment goals in advanced stages should be to reduce tumor burden, to relieve symptoms, to delay disease progression, and to preserve quality of life. In particular, SS is known to be refractory to most therapies, and historically no treatment has been demonstrated to significantly modify the natural course of this disease. Approaches to treatment include spot radiation for single or localized skin tumors, mono- or polychemotherapy, extracorporeal photopheresis, IFN-α, oral retinoids, monoclonal antibodies, recombinant toxins, combinations of these, and high-dose chemotherapy with allogeneic bone marrow transplant (see Table 1). Nonrandomized clinical trials have not suggested that any one treatment is preferable. Treatment choice should be made with the patient's preference and the practitioner's skill in mind. The toxicity of treatment should not outweigh the cosmetic and functional disability of the disease.

Systemic Chemotherapy

Single-agent and combination chemotherapies in advanced or refractory MF and SS have been associated with high response rates but short durations. Their use is limited to palliation of symptoms. Options include single-agent or multiagent chemotherapy including steroids, methotrexate, chlorambucil (Leukeran), vincristine (Oncovin),[1] doxorubicin (Adriamycin), cyclophosphamide (Cytoxan), etoposide (Vepesid),[1] and alkylators. A combination regimen including cyclophosphamide, doxorubicin, vincristine,[1] and prednisone (CHOP) or CHOP-like therapy has been shown to achieve higher response rates of approximately 70% to 80% compared with 25% to 35% for monotherapy.

Among single-agent chemotherapies, liposomal doxorubicin (Doxil), pentostatin (Nipent), and gemcitabine (Gemzar) are reported to be particularly effective. Pegylated liposomal doxorubicin was empirically tested in MF and SS patients and showed an overall response rate of 80%, with complete remission in 6 of 10 patients (60%). More recent published multicenter data of pegylated doxorubicin in 34 patients with recurrent or recalcitrant CTCL revealed a response rate of 88.2%. Twenty-seven patients (79.4%) achieved complete remission, with a median duration of 12 months, ranging from 9.5 to 44 months. Adverse effects were generally mild compared with other chemotherapy regimens.

Gemcitabine,[1] a pyrimidine antimetabolite with a low-toxicity profile, was evaluated in a phase II study for advanced and relapsed patients with MF or peripheral T-cell lymphoma. The compound was intravenously administered on days 1, 8, and 15 of a 28-day schedule at a dose of 1200 mg/m² for a total of three cycles. The reported overall response rate for 21 patients with MF and SS was 70% with complete remission in 10% of patients and only mild hematologic toxicities observed.

Treatment with Temozolomide (Temodar),[1] an oral alkylating agent, appears to be effective in patients with MF and SS. Patients with MF and SS, who have been shown to have low levels of the DNA repair enzyme O^6 alkylguanine DNA alkyltransferase (AGT) that

---

[1]Not FDA approved for this indication.

inhibits the drug activity. Preliminary data reported a response in 5 of 19 patients with MF and SS (26%) with a median duration of 4 months. Response rate correlated with low levels of AGT. Patients with high AGT expression did not respond to treatment.

Biological Therapies

Increased understanding of the pathophysiology of the disease has led to attempts to develop agents that can augment the host antitumor response to selectively target the malignant cells.

Retinoids

Retinoids have been used therapeutically since the early 1980s and the benefits of some derivatives such as isotretinoin, etretinate, and acitretin have been confirmed in several small monotherapy studies. Response rates ranged from 44% to 67%, with complete remission rates from 21% to 35% and median response duration around 8 months. Common effects consisted of skin and mucous membrane dryness.

The FDA has approved oral bexarotene (Targretin), a novel synthetic rexinoid, for treating refractory or relapsed CTCL. In two multicenter phase II and III clinical trials in early and advanced stages of CTCL patients, reported response rates in early stages were between 45% and 54%. An overall response rate in 94 patients with advanced disease was only 4% complete responders and a median duration of 10 months.

The recommended dose of 300 mg/m^2 daily is associated with significant side effects such as hyperlipidemia, hypothyroidism, and cytopenias. Retrospective comparison data suggest that there may be little difference in efficacy between bexarotene and agents such as all-*trans* retinoic acid (RAR-specific retinoid), but clear differences in toxicity exist.

New insights into the immunomodulatory function of retinoids with potential augmentation or reconstitution of T$_H$1 response suggest opportunities for combined treatment with IFN-α, denileukin diftitox, or phototherapy.

Interferon-α

IFN-α (Roferon-A, Intron-A) is one of the most widely used first-line treatments and probably the most effective single agent in the treatment of CTCL. It is generally given as long-term therapy, although the optimal dose and duration in CTCL have not been established. IFN-α is initiated at low doses between 1 and 3 million IU (MU) three times weekly with gradual escalation to 9 to 12 MU daily or as tolerated. Th1 cytokines support cytotoxic T-cell mediated immunity, and it has been speculated that IFN-α maintains or enhances a Th1-cell population balance for an effective cell-mediated response to malignant T-lymphocytes.

Bunn and colleagues first reported in 1984 the treatment of advanced and heavily pretreated patients with MF and SS with IFN-α. There was an overall response rate of 45%. Papa and colleagues achieved response rates between 70% for advanced stage disease and 80% for early-stage disease. Olsen and colleagues tested 3 MU versus 36 MU daily of IFN-α2a in 22 patients with clinical stage I to IV MF and SS; an overall response rate of 38% was observed in those treated with low doses compared to 79% with high doses.

Side effects are dose related and are most commonly flulike symptoms. Depression, cytopenias, or impaired liver function tests occur with chronic administration. The development of neutralizing antibodies has been associated with IFN-α therapy, with variable impact on response rates. The combination therapy with IFN-α and PUVA results in higher response rates and shows superiority to other interferon combinations.

Kuzel and colleagues reported on 39 patients with progressive disease treated with combined IFN-α/PUVA with an overall response rate of 92% and complete remission in 62% of patients and a median duration of 28 months. The combination abrogated the development of neutralizing antibodies.

IFN-α modified with a polyethylene glycol (PEG) chain has a longer half-life compared with standard IFN-α and is typically given once weekly. PEG-IFN-α has demonstrated improved efficacy and tolerability compared with standard IFN-α in other cancers. A recent case study provided evidence that PEG-IFN-α might demonstrate a favorable alternative to traditional IFN-α.

Extracorporeal Photochemotherapy

Extracorporeal photochemotherapy or photopheresis (ECP) was originally designed as a modified PUVA treatment. Circulating mononuclear cells are separated by a leukapheresis-based method, mixed with 8-MOP (UVADEX), exposed to UVA light (1-2 J/cm^2) that activates the 8-MOP, causing cross-linking of DNA, and reinfused to the patient. One suggested mechanism of action is induction of apoptosis in circulating malignant T lymphocytes, with subsequent release of tumor antigens, leading to a systemic antitumor response against the malignant T cell clone.

ECP has been found to affect dendritic cells to produce Tregs. Immunosuppressive cytokines, such as TGF-β and IL-10, released in response to the uptake of apoptotic cells, can induce the development of tolerogenic dendritic cells that remain immature and increase immune tolerance toward the acquired antigen. Still, the relative importance of these findings for the treatment of CTCL is not clear.

Treatment is empirically given on two consecutive days every 14 to 28 days. It usually takes several months to see an improvement and is especially beneficial for erythrodermic MF and SS with circulating neoplastic T cells. Reported response rates are 36% to 64% for patients with advanced disease. Optimal candidates for ECP are patients with SS with modest tumor burden and circulating neoplastic cells and almost normal counts of circulating CD8$^+$ T lymphocytes. Treatment of patients with plaques and tumors has not been as effective.

Monoclonal antibodies

The developments of T-lymphocyte–specific monoclonal antibodies might add to the treatment of MF and SS. Monoclonal antibodies can mediate antitumor effects through three major mechanisms: intrinsic cytotoxic activity, antibody-dependent cellular cytotoxicity, and activation of complement-dependent cytolysis.

Alemtuzumab is a humanized monoclonal IgG$_1$ antibody that targets the CD52 antigen that is abundantly expressed on normal and malignant B and T lymphocytes but not on hematopoietic stem cells. It is FDA approved for treating chronic lymphocytic leukemia. A multicenter European study on alemtuzumab in low-grade non-Hodgkin's lymphoma included 8 patients with heavily pretreated relapsed or refractory MF and SS with reported overall response rate of 50% and complete remission in two patients (25%).

A recently published phase II trial of alemtuzumab in 22 patients with advanced MF and SS demonstrated a clinical response in 55% of cases, with 32% complete remissions; the most impressive results were demonstrated in SS patients. Median response duration was 12 months. Alemtuzumab was administered at a dose of 30 mg three times per week after using an initial dose-escalating regimen.

The compound is associated with significant hematologic toxicities and infectious complications consisting of reactivation of cytomegalovirus, herpes zoster, miliary tuberculosis, and pulmonary aspergillosis. Cytopenias and prolonged immunosuppression require prophylactic antibiotic, antiviral, and antifungal treatments and potential support with granulocyte colony-stimulating factor (G-CSF). An ongoing clinical phase II trial with alemtuzumab for advanced stages of CTCL shows efficacy particularly in patients with erythrodermic CTCL.

Targeted Modalities

Denileukin Diftitox

Recombinant toxins are proteins made by genetic engineering consisting of a toxin fused to a ligand that binds selectively to a target cell. The recombinant fusion protein denileukin diftitox (DAB389-IL-2, Ontak), composed of diphtheria toxin coupled to human IL-2, is FDA approved for use in advanced and refractory CTCL. It targets the intermediate and high-affinity IL-2R on malignant T-lymphocytes. Once bound to the IL-2R, it is internalized by endocytosis with subsequent inhibition of adenosine diphosphotase–ribosyltransferase and subsequent inhibition of protein synthesis with induction of apoptosis.

Response rates to denileukin diftitox in patients with relapsed and refractory MF and SS range from 30% to 37%. Response correlates with improved quality of life. Adverse effects including acute infusion-related events such as fever, rash, chills, dyspnea, and hypotension, and later effects such as myalgias, elevated serum transaminases, and vascular leak syndrome (VLS) have been reported. VLS occurred in 27% of patients, which may be diminished by premedication with steroids.

Bexarotene is known to up-regulate the expression of the high-affinity form of IL-2R in malignant lymphocytes, thus enhancing the susceptibility of leukemia cells to denileukin diftitox. A phase II study with bexarotene combined with denileukin diftitox using escalating doses of bexarotene up to 300 mg/m^2 has shown an overall response rate of 57% in mostly relapsed and refractory CTCL patients with manageable toxicities. All patients, however, have been premedicated with dexamethasone (Decadron).

Histone Deacetylase Inhibitors

Hyperacetylation of tumor-suppressor genes results in chromatin compaction and inactivation of genes that is often observed in various hematologic malignancies and solid tumors. These genes are silenced by histone deacetylases (HDACs), which remove acetyl groups from histones, which form complexes with DNA (nucleosome). HDAC inhibitors can restore the expression of tumor suppressor or cell cycle regulatory genes, or both, by increasing the acetylation of histones.

SAHA (suberoylanilide hydroxamic acid, vorinostat [Zolinza]) is an oral inhibitor of histone acetylase and histone deacetylase regulatory enzymes and was approved in 2006 for treating patients with CTCL who had progressive, persistent, or recurrent disease and who were taking or had taken two systemic therapies, one of which must be bexarotene. The overall response rate was modest, with partial responses seen in 8 out of 33 patients (24.2%); no complete responders were observed. Median time to progression was short at 148 days. Intriguingly, this study showed that about one half of the patients with CTCL experienced significant pruritus relief with vorinostat therapy and, hence, a marked improvement in their quality of life. The most common serious toxicities (Grades 3 and 4) were thrombocytopenia, anemia, dehydration, vomiting, hypotension, infection, sepsis, pulmonary embolism, and deep venous thrombosis, which were reversible on discontinuation of the drug.

Peripheral Stem Cell Transplantation

Autologous stem cell transplantation after high-dose chemotherapy has yielded disappointing results. Despite reported complete remissions in the majority of patients treated, relapses occurred rapidly. Allogeneic transplants are known to achieve much more durable complete remissions, most likely due to an immune-mediated graft-versus-lymphoma (GVL) effect. Response durations as far as 6 years after transplant have been reported, suggesting that it may be a curative option. It does, however, carry a higher risk of treatment-related mortality, including life-threatening infections and graft-versus-host disease (GVHD). Reduced-intensity (mini) allogeneic transplants potentially offer a GVL effect with lesser toxicities related to the conditioning regimen.

Investigational Approaches

CD4 Antibodies

Therapeutic effects of a chimeric (mouse–human) anti-CD4 antibody had been observed as an active agent in MF and SS as early as in 1991. Zanolimumab (HuMax-CD4)[8] is a fully human anti-CD4 (IgG$_1$) monoclonal antibody that targets the CD4 receptor expressed on T-helper memory cells.

The efficacy and safety of zanolimumab in patients with refractory CTCL have been assessed in two multicenter, prospective, open-label, uncontrolled clinical phase II studies. Patients received 17 weekly infusions of zanolimumab (early-stage patients: 280 and 560 mg; advanced-stage patients: 280 and 980 mg). Overall response rates using the physician's global assessment were seen in 36% to 55% of early-stage patients and in 30% to 38% of advanced-stage patients, with a median response of 81 weeks. Higher response rates were achieved with greater doses in early and advanced stages. Adverse events reported most often included low-grade infections and eczematous dermatitis.

Immunomodulatory Therapy

Lenalidomide (Revlimid), an oral immunomodulatory thalidomide analogue, is currently being used in clinical trials to treat various hematologic malignancies and solid tumors. The immunomodulatory properties such as T-cell costimulation with induction of T_H1 cytokine production and cytotoxic activity along with antiangiogenic, antiproliferative, and proapoptotic properties provided the rationale to use this agent in patients with MF and SS. Preliminary data from an ongoing phase II trial have shown efficacy in heavily pretreated patients with advanced MF and SS with mild toxicities.

Vaccine Therapy

Therapeutic vaccination against MF and SS requires the characterization of tumor-specific epitopes, activation of dendritic cells for tumor antigen processing, and generation of a cytotoxic CD8$^+$ T-cell response. One strategy uses the complete remission as a target to develop a TCR idiotype vaccine, but this is complicated by the variability of TCR-α and TCR-β chains. It was observed by Berger and colleagues that extracorporeal photopheresis induces apoptosis in malignant T cells and maturation of immature dendritic cells, with presentation of tumor-specific antigens leading to a cytotoxic CD8$^+$ T-cell response. These findings have led to the development of transimmunization that induces transfer of tumor-specific antigens to dendritic cells, initiating an immunization against the malignant T cells. Dendritic cell–based vaccines have shown efficacy in animal models. Cytosine–phosphate–guanosine oligodeoxynucleotides (CpG ODN), added as immunoadjuvant in dendritic cell–based vaccinations, might enhance tumor-specific immune responses.

Conclusion

At present, there is no cure for this disease, and stage-dependent therapy is the best approach. Treatment goals are disease palliation, improvement of survival, and improvement of quality of life. Given the nature of the disease and despite initial responses to standard therapy, all patients eventually relapse. Immunomodulatory regimens in patients should be used initially in patients with all stages of MF and SS to reduce the need for cytotoxic therapies with more damaging side effects. Investigational strategies continue to be developed to improve outcomes.

REFERENCES

Duvic M, Talpur R, Ni X, et al: Phase 2 trial of oral vorinostat (suberoylanilide hydroxamic acid, SAHA) for refractory cutaneous T-cell lymphoma (CTCL). Blood 2007;109:31-39.

Kim YH, Duvic M, Obitz E, et al: Clinical efficacy of zanolimumab (HuMax-CD4): Two phase 2 studies in refractory cutaneous T-cell lymphoma. Blood 2007;109:4655-4662.

Kim YH, Liu HL, Mraz-Gernhard S, et al: Long-term outcome of 525 patients with mycosis fungoides and Sézary syndrome: Clinical prognostic factors and risk for disease progression. Arch Dermatol 2003;139:857-866.

Kuzel TM: Systemic chemotherapy for the treatment of mycosis fungoides and Sézary syndrome. Dermatol Ther 2003;16:355-361.

---

[8]Orphan drug in the United States.

Kuzel TM, Roenigk HH Jr, Samuelson E, et al: Effectiveness of interferon alfa-2a combined with phototherapy for mycosis fungoides and the Sézary syndrome. J Clin Oncol 1995;13:257-263.

Querfeld C, Kuzel TM, Guitart J, Rosen ST: Treatment approaches to cutaneous lymphomas. In Sekeres MA, Kalaycio ME, Bolwell BJ (eds): Clinical Malignant Hematology. New York: McGraw–Hill, 2006.

Querfeld C, Nagelli LV, Rosen ST, et al: Bexarotene in the treatment of cutaneous T-cell lymphoma. Expert Opin Pharmacother 2006;7:907-915.

Querfeld C, Rosen ST, Kuzel TM, et al: Long-term follow-up of patients with early-stage cutaneous T-cell lymphoma who achieved complete remission with psoralen plus UV-A monotherapy. Arch Dermatol 2005;141:305-311.

Rosen ST, Querfeld C: Cutaneous T-Cell Lymphomas: Mycosis Fungoides and Sézary Syndrome. A Guide for the Community Oncologist. Manhasset, NY: CMP Medica, 2006.

Willemze R, Jaffe ES, Burg G, et al: WHO–EORTC classification for cutaneous lymphomas. Blood 2005;105:3768-3785.

Papulosquamous Eruptions

Method of
*Gary S. Chuang, MD, and
Alice Gottlieb, MD, PhD*

The papulosquamous eruptions are cutaneous disorders that share a primary morphologic feature forming patches and plaques with scales. This article discusses some of the most common papulosquamous eruptions, including psoriasis, seborrheic dermatitis, lichen planus, tinea corporis, tinea versicolor, and pityriasis rosea (Box 1).

Psoriasis

Psoriasis is a chronic inflammatory cutaneous disorder characterized by well-demarcated, erythematous plaques covered with dry, silvery scales. The lesions are typically found on the scalp, the extensor surfaces of the extremities, the periumbilical area, and the nails. These lesions can also be associated with symptoms including itching, pain, or burning. Early lesions typically occur as small erythematous macules, which are covered with thin scales and increase in size by extension or by coalescence with neighboring lesions. New lesions can occur at sites of trauma (Koebner's phenomenon). When the adherent scales are peeled off, pinpoint bleeding can occur (Auspitz's sign). The nail involvement can manifest as pitting, oil spot, or distal onycholysis (detachment of the nail plate from the nail bed).

Psoriasis is one of the most common cutaneous disorders, afflicting approximately 2% of the general population in the United States. The mean age at onset is around 27 years, but the disease can occur from infancy to old age. Although the precise etiology of psoriasis remains elusive, a combination of genetic predisposition, immune response, and environmental triggers appear to be significant.

Both environmental and external factors have been known to influence psoriasis. Guttate psoriasis has been known to occur after some acute infections, such as streptococcal pharyngitis. Stress has been shown to be positively correlated with severity of the disease. Psoriasis may be induced or exacerbated by β-blockers, lithium, antimalarials, angiotensin-converting enzyme (ACE) inhibitors, interferons, and withdrawal from systemic steroids.

From 5% to 42% of the patients with psoriasis develop psoriatic arthritis. The most common clinical pattern of psoriatic arthritis is oligoarthritis, with swelling and tenosynovitis of one or a few hand joints, which represents 70% of patients with psoriatic arthritis. Incorporating a review of the musculoskeletal system and assessment of joint mobility during the evaluation of a psoriasis patient is crucial. Several studies have found that patients with severe psoriasis are predisposed to develop the metabolic syndrome, with increased cardiovascular risks such as diabetes, hypertension, hypertriglyceridemia, hyperlipidemia, and obesity. Whether psoriasis patients are at increased risk for lymphoma remains controversial.

TREATMENT

Topical Therapy

For patients with plaque-type psoriasis with a limited or localized form of psoriasis, a combination of topical treatment modalities such as corticosteroids, vitamin D analogues, coal tar, topical immunomodulators, tazarotene (Tazorac), anthralin, and salicylic acid is recommended.

The initial treatment would include at least one topical corticosteroid. A mid- to potent steroid such as triamcinolone (Kenalog) ointment is suitable for application to plaque-type psoriasis on the trunk and extremities. Triamcinolone can be initially be applied to the thick plaques of psoriasis on the trunk twice daily for 2 weeks, then continued as pulse application on the weekends to reduce the side effects of prolonged steroid use. The ointment form of corticosteroid has the best penetration for plaque-type psoriasis on the trunk. On the scalp, corticosteroids in propylene glycol, gel, foam, and spray bases are preferred. Patients with more brittle hair might desire ointment or oil-based preparations. For the face and the intertriginous area, mid- to low-potency steroid may be used.

Another class of topical medication for plaque-type and scalp psoriais is the vitamin D analogue calcipotriene (Dovonex) in ointment, cream, or solution. It works through inducing epidermal differentiation, inhibiting keratinocyte proliferation, and suppressing local cellular immunity. Calcipotriene is a nonsteroidal topical medication and is not associated with the side effects of corticosteroids. It may be used as monotherapy or as a steroid-sparing adjunct to a high-potency corticosteroid. A typical regimen for plaque-type psoriasis on the trunk and extremities includes applying calcipotriene to the affected area on the body twice daily during the weekday and a class I steroid during the weekend. Calcipotriene may also be used to treat the face and intertriginous area, which are highly vulnerable to atrophy induced by topical corticosteroid.

Tazarotene is a vitamin A–derived topical medication that acts by binding to the retinoic acid receptor, which modulates epidermal differentiation and proliferation of keratinocytes. The tazarotene gel or cream may be used for mild to moderate plaque-type psoriasis in combination with a topical steroid. It is important for the medication

---

BOX 1 Papulosquamous Differentials

Uniform Scales

Cutaneous lupus erythematous (subacute)
Drug eruption
Lichen planus
Mycosis fungoides
Pityriasis rubra pilaris
Pityriasis lichenoides chronica
Psoriasis and parapsoriasis
Seborrheic dermatitis
Secondary syphilis
Tinea versicolor

Annular Scales

Cutaneous lupus erythematous (subacute)
Erythema annulare centrifugam
Lichen planus
Pityriasis rosea
Porokeratosis
Secondary syphilis
Tinea corporis

to be applied at night because it is not photostable. Most patients experience mild location irritation with tazarotene, but the irritation improves with prolonged use and may be diluted with coapplication of petroleum jelly. One concern is that patients can form psoriatic lesions in retinoid-induced dermatitis, as part of the Koebner phenomenon of psoriasis. Also, because retinoids are photosensitizers, patients should be cautioned about increased photosensitivity. Female patients of childbearing potential should be warned about the teratogenic potential of retinoids and use contraception. If a patient becomes pregnant while on tazarotene, the medication should be stopped immediately

Crude coal tar and tar extracts have long been used to treat psoriasis. Tar is safe and effective against psoriasis and has very few side effects. The tar products are available in gels, cream, ointment, shampoo, and bath oil. Tar shampoo is still widely used to treat scalp psoriasis. The limited side effect of tar is related to the staining and unpleasant odor of tar products.

Topical calcineurin inhibitors, such as tacrolimus (Prograf)[1] and pimecrolimus (Elidel),[1] are used off-label to treat thin psoriasis lesions on the face and intertriginous area, which are prone to developing atrophy or acneiform eruption with topical steroid. The topical calcineurin inhibitors are not suitable for large plaque-type psoriasis due to low penetrance.

Keratolytic agents such as salicylic acid and urea are useful additions to the treatment of thick large-plaque psoriasis. The keratolytics are particularly useful in débriding the thick scales of psoriasis, thus allowing a greater absorption of other topical therapies, particularly topical steroids. Young children and patients with renal or hepatic disease can absorb high systemic levels of salicylic acid and are not ideal candidates for salicylic acid therapy. In combination therapy, the prescribing physician needs to be aware that salicylic acid blocks ultraviolet (UV) light and inactivates calcipotriene in concurrent application.

Phototherapy

In most cases, sun exposure improves psoriasis. UVB in broadband or narrowband spectrums is the most common form of phototherapy. UVB spectrum delivers light in the range of 290 to 320 nm. Narrowband UVB phototherapy, delivering monochromatic light in between 305 and 315 nm, has been shown to be superior to broadband UVB.

A history of improvement with sun exposure is a positive prognosticator for good response. Patients are typically treated three times a week. The UVB phototherapy may be used in synergy with other topical agents including topical steroid, tar, calcipotriene, and tazarotene and systemic therapy such as oral retinoid and methotrexate. Although studies have not shown that UVB phototherapy is associated with increased risk of skin cancer, the long-term safety is not known at this time.

With psoralen plus UVA (PUVA), patients receive high-intensity long-wave UVA radiation (range of 320-400 nm) 2 hours after ingesting 8-methoxypsoralen. Patients are usually treated twice a week. PUVA is very effective, even in severe psoriasis. Although PUVA therapy is very effective, oral psoralen is associated with photosensitivity and cataracts. Patients should wear protective eyewear during sun exposure.

PUVA therapy is a risk factor for developing skin cancer, including squamous cell carcinoma and melanoma. Men treated with PUVA without covering genitals are predisposed to developing squamous cell carcinomas of the penis and scrotum. PUVA use is also associated with increased numbers of melanoma. Prior history of arsenic exposure can increase the risk of squamous cell carcinoma in patients on PUVA. It is becoming more evident that the skin-cancer risk may be related to the cumulative PUVA exposure. Thus, PUVA therapy is increasingly used in combination with other systemic therapies like oral retinoid.

Patients who have severe hepatic or renal impairment, who have photosensitivity disorders, or who are childbearing should not be on PUVA therapy.

Systemic Therapy

Methotrexate is one of the most commonly used systemic agents for psoriasis. Methotrexate works as a folic acid antagonist to block dihydrofolic acid reductase, which blocks DNA synthesis. Methotrexate is appropriate for moderate to severe plaque-type psoriasis, erythrodermic acute pustular psoriasis, and psoriatic arthritis. The medication is given as a single weekly oral dose of 5 to 30 mg[3] in one dose or in three divided doses taken 12 hours apart.

It is very important to rule out hepatic or renal impairment, which can decrease clearance and increase toxicity. Methotrexate is contraindicated in alcohol abuse, liver cirrhosis, pregnancy, lactation leukopenia, thrombocytopenia, active infection, immunodeficiency, anemia, and colitis. Baseline laboratory tests of liver function profile, complete blood count, platelet count, hepatitis serology (B and C), HIV antibody, and urinalysis should be checked at baseline and routinely. Liver biopsy is recommended for psoriatic patients taking methotrexate. The first biopsy should be obtained at the methotrexate cumulative dose of 1.0 to 1.5 g and repeated every subsequent 1.5 to 2.0 g until a total of 4.0 g is reached. The frequency then changes to every 1.0 to 1.5 g of cumulative dose.

Patients taking methotrexate commonly complain of gastrointestinal upset, including nausea and vomiting, which can be reduced by taking oral folic acid supplementation 1 mg daily. Trimethoprim-sulfamethoxazole (Bactrim) must be avoided due to the increased risk of potentially life-threatening bone marrow suppression when used in combination with methotrexate.

Cyclosporine (Neoral, Gengraf) is a highly effective systemic immunosuppressive agent that down-modulates the proinflammatory cytokines in psoriatic skin. Doses of cyclosporine at 2 to 5[3] mg/kg/day produce rapid clearing. The medication is contraindicated in patients with a history of hypertension because the risk of renal impairment is increased. Short-term therapy up to 6 months is ideal when possible, because long-term treatment with cyclosporine is associated with nephropathy.

Blood pressure and serum creatinine level should be measured at baseline and during routine follow-up. A baseline complete blood count, liver function tests, renal function tests, magnesium, uric acid, and lipid profile are also recommended. Patients should be warned about the possible side effects of malaise, nausea, headache, tremor, hypertrichosis, and gingival hyperplasia associated with cyclosporine. Because cyclosporine is metabolized by the hepatic cytochrome P-450 3A4 system, medication that competes for or induces this P-450 isoform can increase or decrease the cyclosporine concentration in the blood, respectively.

Retinoids have been known to inhibit epidermal proliferation and inhibit the expression of keratin 16 and the enzyme transglutaminase, resulting in inhibition of cornified envelope formation. Acitretin (Soriatane) is a metabolite of etretinate with a shorter half-life and similar efficacy. However, while taking acitretin, patients need to avoid alcohol. Acitretin becomes esterified to etretinate, which has a longer half-life. Acitretin can be use as a monotherapy or in combination with phototherapy for plaque-type psoriasis. When treating women of childbearing potential, the patient must be properly counseled and cautioned that retinoids are potent teratogens.

Biologicals

Several systemic biological therapies have been developed and investigated in the past several years. These have been shown to have good efficacy in psoriasis and psoriatic arthritis. Biologicals are made in living organisms and include antibodies, fusion proteins, and recombinant cytokines. At the time of publication, several tumor necrosis factor (TNF)-α blockers have received regulatory approval from the FDA for

---

[1]Not FDA approved for this indication.

[3]Exceeds dosage recommended by the manufacturer.

TABLE 1 Biological Agents for Treating Psoriasis and Psoriatic Arthritis

Agent	Biological Structure	Mechanism of Action	Route	FDA Monitoring	Pregnancy Category
Alefacept (Amevive)	LFA-3 and IgG1 fusion protein	Block T-cell activation and proliferation	IM	CD4; hold if <250/μL	B
Efalizumab (Raptiva)	Monoclonal Antibody to CD11a	Block T-cell activation and trafficking	SC	Platelet count	C
Infliximab (Remicade)	Chimeric antibody to TNF-α	Blocks TNF-α	IV	TB screening	B
Entanercept (Enbrel)	TNF receptor and IgG1 fusion protein	Blocks TNF-α	SC	None	B
Adalimumab (Humira)	IgG1 monoclonal Antibody to TNF-α	Blocks TNF-α	SC	TB screening, anti-dsDNA antibody if suspect SLE	B

dsDNA = double-stranded DNA; Ig = immunoglobulin; LFA = leukocyte-function associated; SLE = systemic lupus erythematosus; TB = tuberculosis; TNF = tumor necrosis factor.

treatment of psoriasis or psoriatic arthritis, or both. These include infliximab (Remicade), etanercept (Enbrel), and adalimumab (Humira). Alefacept (Amevive) and efalizumab (Raptiva) target T cells and are approved for treating moderate to severe psoriasis only (Table 1).

The TNF-α blockers, as a class of immunomodulators, share common side effects and require similar laboratory work-ups before and during treatment. Common side effects include injection-site reactions, cough and respiratory symptoms, infections, and headaches. More serious side effects include hypersensitivity reactions, infusion reactions (with infliximab), worsening of congestive heart failure (CHF), invasive fungal infections, and a lupus-like syndrome. There is an increased risk of flaring of central nervous system (CNS) demyelinating disease. The TNF-α blockers can increase the risk of reactivating hepatitis B and cause elevation of liver transaminases. Patients are at increased risk for acquiring opportunistic infection or reactivating tuberculosis. There is also a concern for increased risk of developing lymphoma while on the TNF-α blocker treatment.

Contraindications include hypersensitivity, CHF (New York Heart Association class III or IV). TNF-α blockers can be used in conjunction with methotrexate. Tuberculosis skin testing is required before initiating infliximab and adalimumab, and it is recommended before initiating etanercept. Complete blood count, baseline antinuclear antibodies, liver function tests, and hepatitis B and C screening are suggested for all TNF-α blockers.

Infliximab

Infliximab is a chimeric (75% human and 25% murine) monoclonal antibody that binds and blocks TNF-α, which has been shown to play a role in rheumatoid arthritis, Crohn's disease, ankylosing spondylitis, psoriasis, and psoriatic arthritis. Infliximab is given as a weight-based IV infusion of 5 mg/kg over 2 hours at weeks 0, 2, and 6 weeks and then every 8 weeks. Many dermatologists use infliximab in combination with low doses of methotrexate to prevent loss of response and infusion reactions. Infliximab has also been shown to induce rapid and effective improvement in psoriasis and psoriatic arthritis.

In clinical trials, psoriasis patients are assessed based on Psoriasis Area Severity Index (PASI), which is a combined measurement of the redness, thickness, and scales of psoriasis weighed by body surface area of involvement. A 75% reduction in the PASI score is denoted as PASI 75. In one study, 80% of patients treated with infliximab achieved at least a 75% improvement from baseline (PASI 75), and 57% achieved at least a 90% improvement (PASI 90). The improvements were maintained through week 24 and week 50.

The pregnancy category is B and lactation safety is not known.

Etanercept

Etanercept is another anti-TNF-α agent that comprises a fusion protein of Fc of human immunoglobulin (Ig)G1 and the extracellular TNF-α receptor. The medication binds to soluble TNF and blocks the interaction with cell surface receptor. The dosing for psoriasis is given as 50 mg SC twice a week for 12 weeks and then 50 mg SC weekly. For psoriatic arthritis, the dose is 50 mg SC once weekly. In clinical studies, 47% of patients achieved PASI 75 at 3 months and 54% at 6 months. Of patients achieving a PASI 75 at 3 months with 50 mg SC injections twice weekly for 3 months, 77% maintained their improvement at month 6 with 25 mg SC weekly. Etanercept has been shown to be effective in psoriatic arthritis and can be used in conjunction with methotrexate. The pregnancy category is B and lactation safety is not known.

Adalimumab

Adalimumab is a human IgG1 monoclonal antibody against soluble and transmembrane TNF-α. It binds to TNF-α and blocks its interaction with cell surface TNF receptor. Adalimumab is given as a 40-mg SC injection over 3 to 5 minutes every 2 weeks for 12 weeks. Adalimumab is effective for psoriatic arthritis, but it is not yet approved for psoriasis. In one study, 53% pf patients taking 40 mg adalimumab every other week, 80% of patients taking adalimumab weekly, and 4% of patients taking placebo achieved PASI 75 at 12 weeks after the start of treatment. Responses were sustained for 60 weeks. Adalimumab can be used in conjunction with methotrexate, steroids, salicylates, and NSAIDs. The pregnancy category is B and lactation safety is not known.

Efalizumab and Alefacept

Another class of biologicals, which includes efalizumab and alefacept, directs at blocking the effects of T cells.

Efalizumab is a humanized form of murine antibody directed against CD11a of LFA1, inhibiting T-cell activation, cutaneous trafficking, and adhesion to keratinocytes through blocking the LFA-1 and ICAM-1 binding. The dosing for efalizumab is weight based, which can be more effective in obese patients. The dosing is 0.7 to 1.0 mg/kg SC self-injection for the first week. In clinical trials, 22% to 39% of patients achieved PASI 75 and 52% to 61% achieved PASI 50 at 12 weeks. Of the patients achieving PASI 75 at 12 weeks, 77% maintained their improvement through a second 12-week treatment period. A rebound effect is seen with discontinuation in nearly 14% of patients. Atypical psoriasis flares can be seen during treatment as well. The median time to relapse is 60 to 80 days. Patients need to be checked for platelet count at baseline and during follow-up for 3 months, because efalizumab is associated with thrombocytopenia. Patients need to be warned about rebound flare in both psoriasis and psoriatic arthritis. The pregnancy category is C and it is unsafe to take during lactation.

Alefacept is another fusion protein of human LFA-3 and the Fc portion of the IgG1, which acts by inhibiting the T-cell activation and proliferation by blocking the interaction between LFA-3 and CD2 interaction. The inhibition of CD2 results in selective apoptosis of T cells. Alefacept is given as a 15-mg weekly IM injection in the medical office for a total 12-week course. Lymphopenia has been well documented in some patients taking alefacept. The FDA requires checking a CD4 level at the baseline and then weekly. If the CD4 count falls below 250, alefacept should be held.

In clinical trials, 21% of patients achieved PASI 75 and 42% achieved PASI 50 at week 14. Most patients maintained at least a PASI 50 through the 3-month observation period. Serious adverse effects include lymphopenia, malignancies, serious infections, hypersensitivity, increased transaminase levels (rare), and cardiovascular events. Use should be discontinued if CD4 drops below 250 cells/μL until the level returns to >250 cells/μL. Precautions should be taken if the patient has an infection, has a history of malignancy, or has received live vaccines. The pregnancy category is B and lactation safety is not known.

Seborrheic Dermatitis

Seborrheic dermatitis is a common inflammatory disorder that is characterized by chronic, superficial scaling on an erythematous base with predilection for locations on the body rich in sebaceous glands, including the scalp, eyebrows, eyelids, and nasolabial creases. Typical lesions are well-defined pink plaques with powdery scale distributed in the eyebrows, glabella, nasolabial fold, and postauricular area. The condition can be associated with intense pruritus. The scales often have a yellow, greasy appearance. Seborrheic dermatitis can also be found in the groin and gluteal creases. In this area, the appearance often overlaps with that of inverse psoriasis. In fact, many of these patients have an overlap of the two conditions, appropriately called sebopsoriasis or seborrhiasis. Seborrheic dermatitis in the infant is characterized by yellow or brown scaling lesions covering the scalp, which is also known as cradle cap.

The etiology of the seborrheic dermatitis is thought to be related to the presence of lipophilic yeast *Pityrosporum ovale*, with increased density of the yeast correlated with severity of the disease. Seborrheic dermatitis may be associated with or worsened by other medical conditions. Patients with HIV infection and AIDS have an increased prevalence of seborrheic dermatitis than the general population. Parkinson's disease is often associated with severe refractory seborrheic dermatitis involving the scalp and face.

The first-line treatment for mild seborrheic dermatitis is the over-the-counter shampoos containing tar, selenium sulfide, or zinc pyrithione. Patients are instructed to apply the shampoo and lather on the affected area including the scalp, face, and trunk daily until the condition is under control. Once the disease is under control, patients can continue to use the shampoo once or twice weekly for maintenance. For seborrheic dermatitis not controlled with the shampoo, 2% ketoconazole (Nizoral) cream or shampoo, which is active against the lipophilic yeast *Pityrosporum ovale*, can be used daily on the affected area. For severe seborrheic dermatitis, topical corticosteroid cream such as 1% to 2.5% hydrocortisone or desonide cream can be applied once or twice daily to keep the condition under control. Topical corticosteroids should not be used as a maintenance regimen to prevent steroid-induced rosacea. Steroid-sparing agents, such as topical calcineurin inhibitors, are often used in place of topical corticosteroids with good effects. Topical tacrolimus (Protopic) and pimecrolimus (Elidel) are both effective when applied to the affected area once or twice daily. In patients infected with HIV, lithium succinate ointment (Efalith) has been effected for facial seborrheic dermatitis.

Lichen Planus

Lichen planus is a common pruritic inflammatory disease of the skin, mucous membranes, and hair follicles, characterized by purple, flat-topped polygonal papules that can coalesce and form a large plaque. The surface is usually smooth but can be dry, with scant, adherent scale. The surface can include gray or white streaks (Wickham's striae) across the lesions. The condition has a predilection for the wrist flexors, trunk, medial thigh, shins, dorsal hands, and glans of the penis. The prominent feature of the disease is the severe pruritus. New lesions can occur on areas of trauma (Koebner's phenomenon).

Nails, mucous membrane, and genital involvement are common. Nail changes, such as ridging and splitting, are commonly associated with lichen planus. Lichen planus on the mucous membrane can ulcerate, which causes severe pain and discomfort in the patient. Oral lichen planus can involve any portion of the mouth, but most commonly the buccal mucosa (90%) and gingiva (50%). Oral lichen planus has been associated with metal allergy, especially to dental filling materials such as mercury, gold, and palladium. Oral and vulvovaginal lichen planus does not appear to increase the risk of developing squamous cell carcinoma. Lichen planus occurring on the scalp, also known as lichen planopilaris, can cause scarring alopecia.

Hepatic abnormality has been associated with lichen planus, such as hepatitis C virus (HCV), HBV immunization, and primary biliary cirrhosis.

Isolated lichen planus lesions can be treated with superpotent topical corticosteroid or intralesional steroid injections. Application of clobetasol (Temovate) 0.05% ointment twice daily can be used on isolated lesions with good response. Widespread lesions can require systemic corticosteroids, but the relapse rate is high. Other oral immunosuppressive agents are also effective. Cyclosporine and mycophenolate mofetil (Cellcept)[1] can induce remission in severe cases of cutaneous and oral lichen planus. Phototherapy, including narrow-band UVB, UVA1, and PUVA, has been shown to be effective as a steroid-sparing adjunct therapy. For oral lesions, the superpotent steroids in ointment, orabase, or gel form are very useful. Application of clobetasol in orabase twice daily to the affected oral mucosa is a good initial treatment. For the erosive lichen planus of the oral and genital mucosa, topical tacrolimus 0.1% ointment is also very effective. Patients should be warned that they might experience some burning sensation with topical tacrolimus.

Tinea Corporis

Tinea corporis is a common papulosquamous disorder caused by infection of the superficial dermatophyte on the skin other than the scalp, beard area, face, hands, feet, and groin. This form of dermatophytosis is characterized by well-circumscribed annular, erythematous scaly plaques. The scales are most prominent on the advancing edge of the plaque, giving them the colloquial name *ringworm*. The lesions can widen to form larger plaques or rings of several centimeters in diameter. Immunosuppressed patients are most susceptible to widespread tinea infection. In the United States, *Tinea rubrum*, *Microsporum canis*, and *Trichophyton mentagrophytes* are the most common causes.

The diagnosis is made by scraping scales of the lesion with a No. 15 blade and placing the scales in the center of a microscope slide with KOH. The finding of branching pseudohyphae clinches the diagnosis. Alternatively, the skin scraping can be cultured in a suitable medium.

Localized disease can be treated with topical antifungal creams, such as miconazole (Monistat-derm), clotrimazole (Lotrimin AF), econazole (Spectazole), ketoconazole (Nizoral), and terbinafine (Lamisil). Most antifungal creams can be applied to the affected area twice daily for 2 to 4 weeks. The combination of antifungal with a potent corticosteroid often produces widespread tinea and fungal folliculitis and should be discouraged. Extensive tinea corporis can require systemic therapy with griseofulvin (Gris-PEG) 500 to 1000[3] mg/day for 4 to 6 weeks. Patients should be instructed to take griseofulvin with whole milk or ice cream to improve absorption. Alternatively, terbinafine at 250 mg/day for 1 to 2 weeks, itraconazole 200 mg/day for 1 week, or fluconazole 150 mg once weekly for 4 weeks are also effective.

---

[1]Not FDA approved for this indication.
[3]Exceeds dosage recommended by the manufacturer.

Tinea Versicolor (Pityriasis Versicolor)

The causative agent for tinea versicolor was known as *Malassezia furfur*, which has been more recently classified as *Pityrosporum orbiculare*. The organism is part of the commensal flora of the human skin, which causes skin lesions during the hyphal growth phase. Tinea versicolor is characterized by hypopigmented or hyperpigmented scaly macules on the trunk and upper arms. The skin lesions have a predilection for sebum-producing areas of the body such as the sternum, chest, back, abdomen, neck, and intertriginous areas. Tinea versicolor occurs more commonly during the summer. The hypopigmented tinea versicolor may be more apparent in dark-skinned people and can persist for weeks or months after the dermatophyte is cleared.

Diagnosis is done by scraping the scales overlying each individual lesion and staining the scraping on the slide with KOH. In microscopy, the scraping shows short, fungal hyphae and a large number of spores, which are commonly referred to as *spaghetti and meatballs*.

Topical treatments with selenium sulfide shampoo or lotion, imidazoles, triazoles, ciclopirox olamine, zinc pyrithione are reported to be very helpful. Selenium sulfide shampoo or zinc pyrithione shampoo can be very effectively when applied daily for 4 weeks. The patient is instructed to use the shampoo to lather the scalp and affected area of the body once daily for 4 weeks, each time leaving the lather on the affected area for about 5 minutes. Then, the patient washes away the lather. After the active lesions are clear, the shampoos can be used monthly to reduce colonization.

For severe and resistant cases, oral ketoconazole 400 mg once a month is very effective. Alternatively, oral itraconazole 200 mg once a day for 7 days is also effective. Patients should be educated that the hypo- and hyperpigmentation will take time to resolve and is not a sign of treatment failure.

Pityriasis Rosea

Pityriasis rosea is an acute inflammatory eruption characterized by coalescing salmon-colored papules and plaques. The individual plaques are oval or circinate and covered with a crinkled scaly surface, which can desquamate or form a collaret of scale. The lesions have a characteristic arrangement of a long axis of the lesion running parallel to the skin tension line. The eruption is typically generalized, affecting mostly the trunk, and sparing the sun-exposed surfaces of the body. The eruption may be preceded by a single larger lesion known as a *herald patch*. Usually the generalized eruption occurs after the involution of the herald patch. The eruption then resolves spontaneously after 3 to 8 weeks.

Pityriasis rosea is thought to be caused by active replication of the human herpes virus (HHV)-6 and HHV-7 in mononuclear cells of the lesional skin. The incidence of pityriasis rosea is highest between the ages of 15 and 40 years and is most common during the seasons of spring and autumn. Women are more commonly affected than men.

As the disease mimics the course of a viral exanthema, no therapy is required for most asymptomatic patients. UVB in erythema exposure appears to expedite the involution of the lesion. Pruritus sometimes causes discomfort in patients. Corticosteroid ointment and creams such as triamcinolone 0.1% ointment applied to the affected lesions twice daily for 2 weeks appear to provide symptomatic relief.

REFERENCES

Boehncke WH, Prinz J, Gottlieb AB: Biologic therapy for psoriasis. A systematic review. J Rheumatol 2006;33(7):1447-1451.

Gottlieb AB, Mease PJ, Mark Jackson J et al: Clinical characteristics of psoriatic arthritis and psoriasis in dermatologists' offices. J Dermatolog Treat 2006;17(5):279-287.

Schwartz RA, Janusz CA, Janniger CK: Seborrheic dermatitis: An overview. Am Fam Physician 2006;74(1):125-130.

Thomas VD, Yang FC, Kvedar JC: Biologics in psoriasis: A quick reference guide. Am Acad Dermatol 2005;53(2):346-351.

Zhang AY, Camp WL, Elewski BE: Advances in topical and systemic antifungals. Dermatol Clin 2007;25(2):165-183.

Connective Tissue Disorders

Method of
John Varga, MD, Susan Manzi, MD, MPH, and Gabriella Lakos, MD, PhD

Systemic lupus erythematosus (SLE), scleroderma (or systemic sclerosis), and the inflammatory myopathies are distinct but related idiopathic autoimmune connective tissue diseases. Each of these diseases is associated with significant morbidity and mortality. Each is characterized by considerable clinical heterogeneity and a chronic and unpredictable clinical course, often with remissions and relapses. Each is more common in women than men and associated with progressive damage to multiple organs. Prominent target organs include the skin, the cardiovascular system, the lungs, and the musculoskeletal system; in SLE, the brain and the kidneys are also affected. At the tissue level, inflammation and progressive scarring are prominent. Furthermore, each of these diseases is associated with high levels of autoantibodies in the circulation. Autoimmunity, a hallmark of connective tissue diseases, reflects a fundamental breakdown in immunologic self-tolerance. Although the connective tissue diseases have no cure, many effective treatment options are currently available. Because of their clinical heterogeneity, protean multiorgan systemic manifestations, and chronic and unpredictable course, the evaluation and management of patients with connective tissue diseases present unique challenges.

Systemic Lupus Erythematosus

Chronic inflammation and immune dysregulation characterize SLE. The precise etiology is unknown but likely results from a combination of genetic, hormonal, and environmental factors. The spectrum of manifestations in SLE is quite broad and the time course extremely variable. Some patients develop life-threatening irreversible organ damage, whereas the most incapacitating condition in others may be fatigue. Therapy should be tailored to the individual patient and designed not only to suppress disease activity but also to alleviate symptoms as well. Patients with SLE are optimally managed by a team of specialists that may include, in addition to the rheumatologist, a dermatologist, nephrologist, cardiologist, psychiatrist, psychologist, pulmonologist, gastroenterologist, orthopedic surgeon, and physical therapist.

Although a definitive cure for SLE remains elusive, recent advances, both nonpharmacologic and pharmacologic, have significantly improved survival and quality of life. According to Manzi, established treatments fall into four main categories: nonsteroidal anti-inflammatory drugs, antimalarial agents, corticosteroids, and cytotoxic and immunosuppressive agents. Choosing an appropriate treatment regimen requires careful thought in light of the complexity and marked clinical heterogeneity of the disease and the potential long-term side effects of the drugs used. Consultation with a rheumatologist or other subspecialist with expertise in lupus is recommended.

GENERAL PRINCIPLES OF THERAPY

As patients become more information savvy, the role of health professionals in patient education becomes crucial. Physicians and their staff should assist patients in evaluating the flow of information

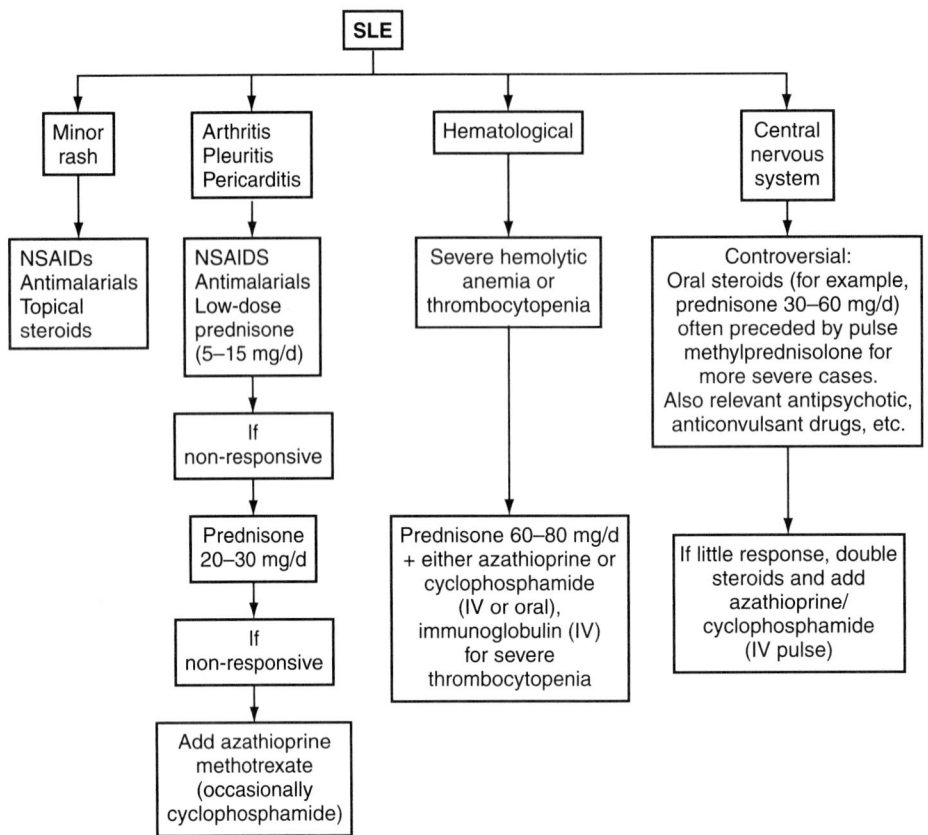

FIGURE 1. Management of nonrenal lupus. (Adapted from Ioannou Y, Isenberg DA: Current concepts for the management of systemic lupus erythematosus in adults: A therapeutic challenge. Postgrad Med J 2002;78:599-606.)

available through modern technology such as the Internet. A patient may be alarmed by hearing or reading about worst-case scenarios. Reassurance that the manifestations and course of disease vary considerably may ease this anxiety. Providing information about support groups may also be helpful. Moreover, physicians should recognize and address the psychological impact that a diagnosis of a chronic, potentially serious disease may have on a previously healthy individual.

Although not life-threatening, fatigue is a challenge for many SLE patients. Physicians should search for contributing factors such as hypothyroidism, fibromyalgia, or depression and must emphasize the importance of adequate rest. Overexposure to ultraviolet (UV) radiation may cause systemic disease flares in addition to skin rashes. Photosensitive patients should avoid excessive exposure to sunlight and wear protective clothing and sunscreen (SPF [sun protection factor] of 35) routinely. Certain prescription drugs, including sulfa drugs and other antibiotics, can exacerbate photosensitivity as well as other lupus disease activity.

Unexplained fever should not be ignored because lupus patients are susceptible to infections. To minimize this risk, physicians should exercise caution when prescribing immunosuppressive agents and corticosteroids and consider influenza and pneumococcal immunizations. Because a disease flare during pregnancy poses risk to the fetus, pregnancies in women with lupus are considered high risk. High-dose estrogen contraceptives should generally be avoided, particularly in patients with increased risk of blood clots; low-dose estrogen, progesterone-only pills, or other effective means of contraception should be considered. Planning pregnancies during periods of disease remission and careful monitoring of both the mother and fetus can improve the chances for healthy outcomes.

Other considerations in the general management of patients with SLE include their increased risk of cardiovascular disease and osteoporosis. Patients should be screened for these conditions and be advised to adopt a cardioprotective lifestyle and take measures to ensure their bone health. These actions include smoking cessation, moderate intake of alcohol, heart-healthy diet, adequate intake of dietary calcium and vitamin D, and regular weight-bearing exercise. Although no definitive link is established between SLE and malignancy, routine gynecologic testing and breast examinations should be performed.

NONSTEROIDAL ANTI-INFLAMMATORY DRUGS

Although nonsteroidal anti-inflammatory drugs (NSAIDs) do not have disease-modifying properties in SLE, they are used to treat fever, pleuritis, pericarditis, and musculoskeletal complaints (Figure 1). Because SLE patients may take NSAIDs for long periods of time, consideration should be given to gastroprotective agents. Furthermore, the potential adverse effects of these drugs on the kidney, liver, and central nervous system may be confused with worsening disease activity. Table 1 lists the general recommendations for monitoring NSAIDs and other commonly used agents in SLE.

ANTIMALARIAL AGENTS

Antimalarial agents are frequently prescribed in the treatment of SLE. The most commonly used are hydroxychloroquine (Plaquenil)[1] and chloroquine (Aralen).[1] Antimalarials are regularly used in the management of cutaneous and musculoskeletal manifestations, constitutional symptoms, and in some cases serositis. Antimalarials may be used in combination when one agent by itself is ineffective because their actions can be synergistic. A particular benefit of antimalarial agents is their steroid-sparing effect. Hydroxychloroquine[1] (200 to 400 mg daily) is generally well tolerated, but it may take 6 to 8 weeks for the benefit to become apparent. Because of potential ophthalmologic toxicity, patients should have an ophthalmologic examination when they begin treatment and every 6 to 12 months

---

[1]Not FDA approved for this indication.

TABLE 1 Standard Drug Therapies in Systemic Lupus Erythematosus and Recommended Monitoring Strategies

Drug	Toxicities Requiring Monitoring	Baseline Evaluation	System Review	Laboratory
Salicylates, nonsteroidal anti-inflammatory drugs	Gastrointestinal bleeding, hepatic toxicity, hypertension	CBC, creatinine, urinalysis, AST, ALT	Dark/black stool, dyspepsia, nausea/vomiting, abdominal pain, shortness of breath, edema	CBC yearly, creatinine yearly
Hydroxychloroquine	Macular damage	None unless patient is over 40 y of age or has previous eye disease	Visual changes	Funduscopic and visual fields q 6-12 mo
Glucocorticoids	Hypertension, hyperglycemia, hyperlipidemia, hypokalemia, osteoporosis, avascular necrosis, cataract, weight gain, infections, fluid retention	BP, bone densitometry, glucose, potassium, cholesterol, triglycerides (HDL, LDL)	Polyuria, polydipsia, edema, shortness of breath, BP at each visit, visual changes, bone pain	Urinary dipstick for glucose q 3-6 mo, total cholesterol yearly, bone densitometry yearly to assess osteoporosis
Azathioprine	Myelosuppression, hepatotoxicity, lymphoproliferative disorders	CBC, platelet count, creatinine, AST or ALT	Symptoms of myelosuppression	CBC and platelet count q 1-2 wk with changes in dose (q 1-3 mo thereafter), AST yearly, PAP test at regular intervals
Cyclophosphamide	Myelosuppression, myeloproliferative disorders, malignancy, immunosuppression, hemorrhagic cystitis, secondary infertility	CBC and differential and platelet count, urinalysis	Symptoms of myelosuppression, hematuria, infertility	CBC and urinalysis monthly; urine cytology and PAP test yearly for life
Methotrexate	Myelosuppression, hepatic fibrosis, cirrhosis, pulmonary infiltrates, fibrosis	CBC, chest radiograph within past year, hepatitis B, C serology in high-risk patients, AST, albumin, bilirubin, creatinine	Symptoms of myelosuppression, shortness of breath, nausea/vomiting, oral ulcer	CBC and platelet count, AST or ALT, and albumin q 4-8 wk, serum creatinine, urinalysis
Mycophenolate mofetil	Myelosuppression, gastrointestinal	CBC and differential and platelet count, creatinine, AST, ALT	Symptoms of myelosuppression, nausea, diarrhea	CBC and platelet count q 1-2 wk with changes in dose (q 1-3 mo thereafter), AST, ALT, creatinine q 1-3 mo.

Abbreviations: ALT = alanine transaminase; AST = aspartate transaminase; BP = blood pressure; CBC = complete blood count; HDL = high-density lipoprotein; LDL = low-density lipoprotein.
Adapted from Manzi S: Treatment of systemic lupus erythematosus. In Klippel JH, Stone J, Weyand C, Crofford LJ (eds): Primer on the Rheumatic Diseases. Atlanta, Arthritis Foundation, 2001, pp 346-352.

thereafter. Although it is unclear whether antimalarials prevent major organ disease, they do have lipid-lowering and possible antiplatelet activities.

CORTICOSTEROIDS

Corticosteroids are used to treat a broad spectrum of lupus manifestations. Oral administration of 5 to 30 mg of prednisone daily in single or divided doses is effective in treating constitutional symptoms, cutaneous disease, arthritis, and serositis. Once immediate relief is achieved, their dose is often tapered while slower-acting agents such as antimalarials or immunomodulatory therapy are added. For more serious organ involvement, such as nephritis, central nervous system or hematologic abnormalities, or systemic vasculitis, prednisone at higher doses (1 to 2 mg/kg) daily or parenteral corticosteroid preparations in equivalent doses are given. Pulses of methylprednisolone (1000 mg) can be given for 3 consecutive days in severe situations. According to Ionnaou and Isenberg, the infusion should be given over several hours to minimize the risk of reactions such as joint pain, flushing, headache, or tachycardia. Although high-dose corticosteroids may be required to preserve major organ function, patients who require such aggressive treatment over extended periods are subjected to highly unfavorable side effects, including emotional lability, weight gain, hypertension, hyperlipidemia, diabetes, glaucoma, risk of infection, avascular necrosis of bone, and osteoporosis. It is recommended that treating physicians attempt to taper corticosteroids to discontinuation or to a minimal dose administered daily or on alternate days once disease activity is controlled.

CYTOTOXIC AGENTS

Aggressive therapy with cytotoxic agents is required for patients with severe disease involving major organs. In general, such therapy should be administered by specialists aware of the potential dangers involved. Cyclophosphamide (Cytoxan)[1] and azathioprine (Imuran),[1] are the agents most commonly prescribed. Methotrexate (Rheumatrex),[1] mycophenolate mofetil (CellCept),[1] and intravenous immunoglobulin (IVIG)[1] also show promising results.

Cyclophosphamide

According to Ortmann and Klippel, cyclophosphamide[1] is the drug of choice for treating most forms of lupus nephritis (Figure 2). Glucocorticoids in combination with intravenous bolus regimens of cyclophosphamide (0.5 to 1.0 g/m²) is more effective than glucocorticoids alone in preserving renal function. Cyclophosphamide[1] appears to be most effective in diffuse proliferative lupus nephritis, although it may also be useful in membranous nephropathy. Less severe forms of lupus nephritis are commonly treated with corticosteroids alone; however, physicians should be prepared to administer immunosuppressive agents if more severe nephritis develops or if patients develop unacceptable side effects from corticosteroids. Renal biopsy is helpful in determining the therapy of choice. Regardless of the type of immunosuppressant used, it is necessary to control blood pressure effectively to prevent irreversible organ damage. Cyclophosphamide[1] is also effective in nonrenal manifestations of SLE, such as cytopenia, central nervous system disease, pulmonary hemorrhage, and vasculitis.

Cyclophosphamide[1] has numerous undesirable side effects. Nausea, vomiting, hair loss, infertility, and bone marrow suppression are the most common. Gastrointestinal toxicity can be minimized with the administration of antiemetics, and hair loss is normally reversible when treatment is discontinued. Older age and cumulative dose appear to be the major risk factors for infertility. Adjusting the dose of cyclo-phosphamide[1] can often regulate leukopenia, which typically peaks 8 to 12 days after intravenous administration. Patients on cyclophosphamide[1] are also at increased risk for infections, particularly herpes zoster. Bladder carcinoma can develop even

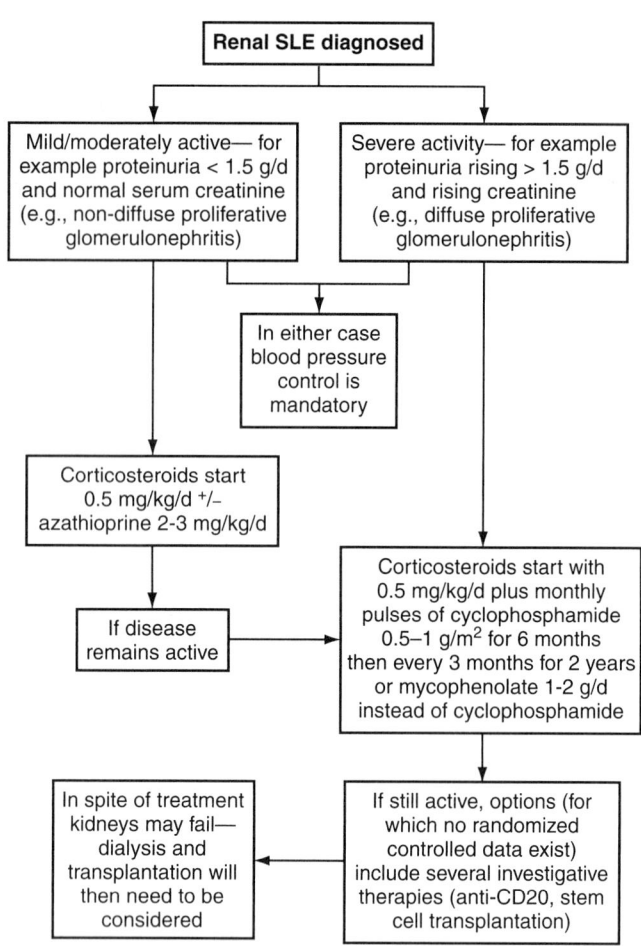

FIGURE 2. Management of renal lupus. (Adapted from Ioannou Y, Isenberg DA: Current concepts for the management of systemic lupus erythematosus in adults: A therapeutic challenge. Postgrad Med J 2002;78:599-606.)

years after cyclophosphamide[1] therapy has stopped; thus urinalysis, urine cytology, and cystoscopy are indicated in patients with hematuria.

Azathioprine (Imuran)

Azathioprine[1] can be used for lupus nephritis, as a steroid-sparing agent in patients with nonrenal manifestations, and in patients at low risk for progressive renal failure. Azathioprine[1] is generally started at 50 mg daily and increased by 25 mg per week to a maintenance dose of 2 to 3 mg/kg daily. Azathioprine[1] is generally better tolerated than cyclophosphamide[1]; however, bone marrow, hepatic, and gastrointestinal toxicity are common.

Methotrexate (Rheumatrex)

Much evidence supports the effectiveness of methotrexate in rheumatoid arthritis, but very few controlled studies have been conducted in SLE. Evidence suggests that methotrexate at 15 to 20 mg per week is effective in controlling cutaneous and articular manifestations. Because side effects are common at high doses, methotrexate[1] is currently used primarily as a steroid-sparing agent in milder SLE.

Mycophenolate Mofetil (CellCept)

Mycophenolate mofetil[1] (500 to 1000 mg twice daily) appears to be effective for lupus nephritis. In one small study, it was effective in

---

[1]Not FDA approved for this indication.

reducing proteinuria and improving serum creatinine in severe lupus nephritis refractory to cyclophosphamide. A recent randomized, open-label, noninferiority trial supports the notion that MMF appeared to be as effective as intravenous cyclophosphamide in inducing short-term remission of lupus nephritis with a better safety profile. The role of MMF in improving long-term outcomes of lupus nephritis remains unknown. An ongoing larger, multicenter, randomized, controlled trial will examine the effectiveness of MMF compared with intravenous cyclophosphamide during induction, and MMF compared with azathioprine during the maintenance phase. MMF is a promising addition to the armamentarium for treatment for lupus nephritis, particularly in young women of childbearing potential when there are concerns of infertility.

Intravenous Immunoglobulin

Intravenous immunoglobulin (IVIG)[1] is used most commonly for the treatment of refractory thrombocytopenia. Platelet counts rise rapidly following initiation of treatment at 400 mg/kg daily. Similar doses have produced improvements in arthritis, nephritis, fever, mucocutaneous manifestations, and immunologic parameters. Patients with SLE-associated IgA deficiency should be treated with alternative therapies. Common side effects of IVIG include fever, myalgia, arthralgia, and headache; rarely, aseptic meningitis and thromboembolism can occur.

Immunoablation and Autologous Stem Cell Transplantation

The rationale behind immunoablation with cyclophosphamide, followed by stem cell transplantation, is to "rescue" bone marrow of the patient with autologous stem cell transplantation after receiving a high myeloablative dose of cyclophosphamide. In addition, a high-dose cyclophosphamide regimen is purported to reset the naive immune response in the bone marrow stem cells by destroying the autoreactive lymphocytes. In the retrospective analysis of 53 patients with refractory SLE who underwent immunoablation and autologous stem cell transplantation, the European group found a remission rate based on a reduction of SLE disease activity index (SLEDAI) to less than 3 in 66% of these patients. However, the one-year transplant-related mortality was high, at 12%. A recent open-label study demonstrated a reduction in disease activity by nonmyeloablative autologous hematopoietic stem cell transplantation in patients with refractory SLE. The long-term risk/benefit ratio of this treatment modality remains unclear.

Novel Therapies

Moving away from "global" immunosuppression by traditional drug therapies for SLE, "designed" therapeutics of the future provide improved efficacy and lower toxicity by targeting specific steps in the pathogenesis of SLE while preserving immunocompetence. Many of the novel therapeutics are being developed and studied currently in clinical trials. Some of the promising novel therapies are discussed in the following overview.

B-CELL DEPLETION

Rituximab and epratuzumab are two antibody-based agents, which target a specific cell-surface antigen on B cells and result in B-cell depletion. Rituximab is a chimeric monoclonal antibody that binds CD20 on the surface of B cells. It is the first monoclonal antibody therapy approved by the FDA for the treatment of non-Hodgkin's lymphoma and, more recently, rheumatoid arthritis. In open-label clinical studies, rituximab has been shown to be beneficial in the treatment of patients with SLE. Various dosing regiments have been used to achieve complete B-cell depletion. A multicenter randomized placebo-controlled (Phase II/III) trial has begun to study the efficacy of rituximab in patients with moderate to severe lupus flares. Another similar Phase III trial will study the efficacy of rituximab in the treatment of lupus nephritis in adult patients. (Epratuzumab is a human monoclonal antibody that targets CD22 on B cells. In an open-label Phase II trial, epratuzumab showed efficacy in patients with SLE, despite causing only modest B-cell depletion.)

INHIBITION OF B-CELL SURVIVAL

B-cell activating factor (BAFF)/B-cell stimulator (BlyS) modulates B-cell survival and maturation, and is a member of the TNF superfamily. Belimumab is a human BAFF monoclonal antibody that recognizes BlyS and reduced B-cell proliferation and differentiation in animal models. A Phase II clinical trial revealed that belimumab performed better than placebo at reducing lupus disease activity in a subset of SLE patients with elevated anti-dsDNA antibodies and low serum C3. A Phase III trial is currently under way.

INHIBITION OF COSTIMULATORY INTERACTIONS

Abatacept is a fusion protein of CTLA4-Ig that binds to B7 molecules (CD80/CD86) on dendritic cells and blocks the binding of costimulatory molecules CD80 and CD86 with CD28 on T cells, thereby interrupting signals required for the activation of naive T cells and their downstream effects on B-cell activation. This drug has been approved by the FDA for the treatment of rheumatoid arthritis. Multicenter clinical trials are currently under way in SLE.

CYTOKINE BLOCKADE

TNF-α inhibitors (etanercept, infliximab, and adalimumab) have been very successful in the treatment of rheumatoid arthritis and psoriatic arthritis. A small open-label study of infliximab in SLE showed significant improvement in patients with refractory nephritis, despite a parallel increase in levels of anti-dsDNA antibodies. However anti-TNF-α therapy has been associated with autoantibody production, specifically anti-dsDNA antibodies, in patients with various autoimmune conditions. Anti-TNF-α therapy has also been associated with several cases of demyelinating disease. Controlled clinical trials are needed to determine the long-term safety and efficacy of this therapy in SLE.

Interleukin 6 (IL-6) is another proinflammatory cytokine secreted predominantly by macrophages, and tocilizumab is a humanized monoclonal antibody against IL-6 receptor (IL-6R) that suppresses IL-6 signalling mediated by both membranous and soluble IL-6R. The results of an open-label trial of IL-6 blockade are not yet available.

Elevated serum levels of interferon-α are found in patients with SLE. More recent studies showed a striking interferon-α signature on gene expression in peripheral blood mononuclear cells of patients with SLE compared with those of controls. Interferon-α modulation may be another promising therapeutic target for use in the treatment of SLE.

There is an explosion of new potential drug therapies for lupus currently being testing in clinical trials. The complexity of lupus suggests that a variety of therapeutic options will be needed to successfully treat this disease.

Scleroderma/Systemic Sclerosis

Scleroderma, or systemic sclerosis (SSc), is a chronic connective tissue disease characterized by evidence of widespread vascular injury, autoimmunity, fibroproliferative process, and variable clinical course. Localized sclerodermas (morphea and linear scleroderma) are distinct from SSc, occur more frequently in children, and are not associated with internal organ involvement. According to Mayes and colleagues, median survival in SSc is 11 years. Survival is determined by the

---

[1] Not FDA approved for this indication.

> **BOX 1 Prominent Organ Involvement in Systemic Sclerosis (SSc)**
>
> - Skin (inflammation, induration and tethering; hyper- and hypopigmentation, calcinosis)
> - Lungs (alveolitis and pulmonary fibrosis; pulmonary arterial hypertension)
> - Heart (restrictive cardiomyopathy, pericarditis)
> - Peripheral vascular (mucocutaneous telangiectasia, Raynaud's phenomenon, digital ulcers and infarction, watermelon stomach, male erectile dysfunction)
> - Gastrointestinal tract (see Box 4)
> - Muscle (myositis)
> - Joints (contractures, arthralgia, tendon friction rubs)

> **BOX 3 Potentially Disease-Modifying Interventions for Systemic Sclerosis (SSc)**
>
> - Immunomodulatory
> - Cyclophosphamide* (intermittent intravenous or daily oral)
> - Mycophenolate Mofetil§
> - Azathioprine*
> - High-dose immunosuppressive therapy with autologous stem cell rescue¶
> - Methotrexate§
> - Photophoresis*
> - Antifibrotic
> - D-Penicillamine§
> - Mycophenolate§
> - Interferon-γ¶
> - Anti-transforming growth factor-β antibody¶
>
> *Efficacy supported by randomized clinical trial.
> §Efficacy equivocal; not supported by randomized clinical trial.
> ¶Experimental treatment.

extent of internal organ involvement. Prominent target organs include the skin, lungs, heart, kidneys, and gastrointestinal tract (Box 1). SSc has substantial clinical heterogeneity. Based on the constellation of clinical and laboratory findings present, patients are subclassified as "limited cutaneous SSc" or "diffuse cutaneous SSc" (Box 2). These two subtypes predict distinct patterns of organ involvement, clinical course, and survival. Some patients with SSc show features of overlap with other autoimmune diseases and manifest sicca syndrome, arthritis, myositis, or thyroiditis.

GENERAL PRINCIPLES OF THERAPY

In light of the clinical heterogeneity of SSc and its variable course, treatment must be individualized according to the unique needs of each patient; some need early aggressive intervention, whereas others need a conservative symptom-based approach with close monitoring. According to Bryan and colleagues, predictors of poor outcome include older age onset (>60 years of age), anemia, evidence of significant cardiac or pulmonary involvement, tendon friction rubs, and the presence of antitopoisomerase antibodies. In general, therapies fall into two groups: those that target the underlying pathophysiologic process, and those that alleviate or reverse target organ complications. Because major internal organ involvement develops early, disease-modifying interventions should be considered before tissue damage becomes established. Because SSc is invariably a multisystem disease, a coordinated approach to evaluation and management by an integrated multidisciplinary team including a rheumatologist, pulmonologist, cardiologist, gastroenterologist, vascular or orthopedic surgeon, and physical therapist is desirable. Patients should also be given the opportunity to participate in controlled clinical trials on novel therapeutic agents.

DISEASE-MODIFYING THERAPIES

To date, no therapy is shown conclusively to be disease modifying in SSc. Nonetheless, based on historical or anecdotal evidence or empirical considerations, many agents are used widely in an attempt to reverse or halt the progression of the immunologic, vascular, and fibrotic damage (Box 3). In light of the potential toxicities associated with these therapies and their lack of proven benefit, decisions regarding their use must be considered carefully. In patients with limited SSc and stable disease, organ-based treatments directed toward specific complications of the disease (see later) are generally more appropriate than these generalized disease-modifying treatment strategies.

ORGAN-BASED TREATMENT APPROACHES

Therapy for Skin Involvement

Skin induration can be progressive and widespread in diffuse cutaneous SSc, whereas it is generally not prominent in limited cutaneous form. Extensive skin involvement often, but not invariably, predicts severe internal organ involvement. In diffuse SSc, skin induration generally peaks in the first 2 to 4 years of SSc, after which it regresses with spontaneous softening. In early disease, inflammation of the skin dominates, with edema, erythema, and pruritus. Patients at this stage benefit form antihistamines such as hydroxyzine (Atarax),[1] 25 mg at bedtime. Low-dose glucocorticoids such as prednisone,[1] 5 mg daily, provide substantial symptomatic relief for inflammation in early SSc but should be used with caution in light of the increased risk of scleroderma renal crisis (see later); patients taking low-dose prednisone[1] should be instructed to monitor their blood pressure daily. Digital ulcers can be managed using Duoderm[1] application to promote healing and topical povidone-iodine (Betadine)[1] solution for cleansing.

> **BOX 2 Clinical Features of Systemic Sclerosis (SSc) Subsets**
>
> - Limited cutaneous SSc
>   - Limited extent of skin induration (distal extremities and face); no truncal skin involvement; slowly progressive
>   - Prominent vascular involvement (cutaneous telangiectasia, Raynaud's phenomenon, digital ulcers; pulmonary hypertension)
>   - Calcinosis cutis
>   - Antibodies to centromere
> - Diffuse cutaneous SSc
>   - Progressive and diffuse skin induration; truncal involvement frequent
>   - Pulmonary fibrosis
>   - Scleroderma renal crisis
>   - Antibodies to topoisomerase-I

---

[1]Not FDA approved for this indication.

Therapy for Vascular Involvement

Raynaud's Phenomenon and Its Complications

Widespread damage of small and medium-sized peripheral blood vessels is virtually universal in SSc. Endothelial cell injury is associated with release of vasoconstrictors such as thromboxane and endothelin 1 (ET1), impaired production of vasodilators such as nitric oxide and prostacyclin, and platelet aggregation and thrombosis. What starts out as a reversible dysfunction of vascular smooth muscle often progresses to irreversible structural alterations characterized by intimal layer proliferation, medial hypertrophy, and adventitial fibrosis. Reduced blood flow and repeated episodes of ischemic reperfusion in the digits, kidneys, lungs, heart, and other involved organs cause tissue ischemia, progressive vascular damage, and fibrosis.

Cold-induced Raynaud's phenomenon is the most common presenting problem in SSc and may precede other manifestations of the disease by years. Repeated and increasingly severe Raynaud's episodes lead to digital ischemia, resulting in painful ulcers and nonhealing pitting scars and, in extreme cases, digital infarction and gangrene. Patients should be counseled to stop smoking and to avoid cold exposure, which triggers vasoconstriction; not only the hands but the whole body should also be kept warm. Mild Raynaud's phenomenon can be effectively treated with orally active vasodilators (Table 2) and treatment is most commonly started with calcium channel blockers. Infection complicating digital ulcers should be treated aggressively with antibiotics; such ulcers may take months to heal and may progress to osteomyelitis. The ET1 receptor blocker bosentan (Tracleer),[1] 125 mg twice daily, is effective in preventing digital ulcers. Patients with impending digital infarction may respond to intravenous epoprostenol (Flolan),[1] 0.5 to 6 µg/kg body weight per minute for 6 to 24 hours, or nonpharmacologic interventions such as sympathetic ganglion blockade and surgical digital sympathectomy. The role of statin drugs, antioxidants such as tocopherol (vitamin E)[1] (400 IU daily), and diets rich in fish oils in preventing vascular damage in Raynaud's phenomenon are not yet adequately studied.

Pulmonary Arterial Hypertension

Pulmonary arterial hypertension (PAH), which occurs in at least 15% of SSc patients, has a major impact on survival. PAH may complicate interstitial pulmonary fibrosis or may occur in the absence of parenchymal lung disease; the latter is indistinguishable from primary (idiopathic) and familial pulmonary hypertension. Because PAH may be asymptomatic until advanced, it was historically underdiagnosed in SSc. Moderately severe PAH is associated with exertional dyspnea, chest pain, and syncope; right-sided heart failure is seen in late-stage disease. Emphasis must be placed on early preclinical recognition of PAH. A combination of pulmonary function testing and Doppler echocardiography is appropriate for screening and should be performed yearly. Right heart catheterization is the gold standard for determining pulmonary arterial pressures and cardiac index and for excluding pulmonary embolism.

Several new classes of agents provide at least short-term symptomatic and hemodynamic improvement in PAH. Patients with New York Heart Association functional class III or IV symptoms (ordinary activity causing dyspnea, chest pain, or near syncope) should start an orally active ET1 receptor blocker such as bosentan (Tracleer). In addition, warfarin anticoagulation (to achieve an INR [international normalized ratio] of 1.5 to 2.0), low-flow oxygen therapy, diuretics, and digitalization are generally indicated. Patients who fail to respond to ET1 antagonists may benefit from parenteral prostacyclin analogues such as inhaled iloprost (Ventavis), every 2 hours up to 45 µg daily, or continuous infusions of subcutaneous treprostinil (Remodulin) 1.25 µg/kg per minute, or intravenous epoprostenol (Flolan), 2 to 10 µg/kg per minute. A major limitation of these therapies is their cost, now exceeding $30,000 per year. Furthermore, because of their short half-lives, prostacyclin analogues must be administered by continuous infusion or frequent inhalations. Epoprostenol requires long-term ambulatory central venous catheterization, which may be complicated by line sepsis and pump failure with potentially catastrophic consequences. Combinations of a prostacyclin analogue together with an ET1 antagonist or a phosphodiesterase type 5 inhibitor such as sildenafil (Viagra),[1] up to 50 mg three times daily, appear to be well tolerated and provide added benefit. Surgical options for patients unresponsive to pharmacologic therapies include atrial septostomy and lung transplantation. In light of the complexity involved, the evaluation and management of PAH in SSc patients should be coordinated by specialized centers having appropriate expertise.

Therapy for Interstitial Lung Disease

Some degree of interstitial lung disease is present in most patients with SSc and is a leading cause of death. The extent and progression of pulmonary fibrosis are major determinants of outcome. Combined with pulmonary function testing, high-resolution computed tomography (HRCT) scan of the chest is more sensitive for interstitial lung disease screening than chest radiography. A ground-glass appearance generally correlates with active inflammation (alveolitis). Patients with alveolitis may benefit from cyclophosphamide (Cytoxan)[1] (orally up to 50 mg daily, or intravenously as pulse therapy up to 1000 mg/m^2 monthly) to stabilize lung function. Low-dose prednisone[1] (up to 20 mg daily) is often used in combination with cyclophosphamide. The optimal duration of cyclophosphamide[1] treatment is uncertain, but some experts recommend at least a year. General supportive measures include pneumococcal vaccination and yearly influenza immunization, avoidance of smoking, prevention of gastroesophageal reflux, nasal oxygen supplementation, and bronchodilators. Respiratory tract infections should be treated with empirical antibiotics. For selected patients with progressive respiratory decline, lung transplantation remains an option.

Therapy for Gastrointestinal Tract Involvement

Gastrointestinal involvement is common, can be extensive, and significantly contributes to the morbidity of SSc. Gastroesophageal reflux may be associated with dyspepsia, dysphagia, and regurgitation and can lead to chronic esophagitis and its complications (Box 4). Reflux should be managed by elevating the head of the bed, eliminating triggers such as chocolates, alcohol, and tobacco, and restricting food intake before going to sleep. Most patients require long-term

---

[1]Not FDA approved for this indication.

TABLE 2 Oral Vasodilator Therapy for Raynaud's Phenomenon in Systemic Sclerosis

Agent	Dose
Calcium Channel Blockers	
Nifedipine (Procardia)	10-30 mg three times daily
Diltiazem (Cardizem)	30-120 mg three times daily
Amlodipine (Norvasc)	5-20 mg daily
Felodipine (Plendil)	2.5-10 mg daily
Angiotensin II Receptor Antagonists	
Losartan (Cozaar)	25-100 mg daily
Valsartan (Diovan)	80-320 mg daily
Sympatholytic Agents	
Prazosin (Minipress)	1-5 mg daily
Doxazosin (Cardura)	1-16 mg daily
Nitroglycerin	2% ointment topically once daily

Adapted from Wigley FM: Raynaud's phenomenon. N Engl J Med 2002;347(13):1001-1008.

> **BOX 4 Gastrointestinal Tract Complications of Systemic Sclerosis (SSc)**
>
> - Esophageal dysmotility leading to dysphagia and chronic gastroesophageal reflux; dyspepsia, esophagitis, strictures, ulcers, pulmonary aspiration; Barrett's esophagus and esophageal adenocarcinoma
> - Watermelon stomach with upper gastrointestinal bleeding
> - Gastroparesis and small bowel hypomotility
> - Blind loop syndrome with malabsorption, weight loss, diarrhea
> - Large bowel pseudo-obstruction
> - Colonic perforation
> - Pneumatosis cystoides intestinalis

treatment with proton pump inhibitors such as omeprazole (Prilosec)[1] in doses sufficient to suppress reflux symptoms (up to 160 mg daily). Prokinetic agents such as metoclopramide (Reglan)[1] (10 mg four times daily) or erythromycin[1] (250 mg three times daily) may be effective for gastroparesis. Chronic diarrhea and malabsorption caused by small bowel bacterial overgrowth can be treated with periodic courses of tetracycline[1] (500 mg four times daily) or metronidazole (Flagyl)[1] (500 mg three times daily). Some patients benefit from subcutaneous octreotide injections (Sandostatin,)[1] (50 mg one to four times daily). Nutritional assessment and support are important aspects of management. Gastric vascular ectasia (watermelon stomach) is frequent in SSc and causes recurrent occult gastrointestinal bleeding. It can be effectively treated with laser argon ablation.

Therapy for Renal Involvement

Scleroderma renal crisis, which develops in up to 15% of patients with SSc, was uniformly fatal in the pre–angiotensin-converting enzyme(ACE)[1] inhibitor era. Risk factors include progressive skin induration, male sex, and glucocorticoid use. Renal crisis characteristically manifests with an abrupt rise in blood pressure, frequently associated with retinal hemorrhages, and occasionally with seizures and pulmonary hemorrhage, microangiopathic hemolysis, and rapidly progressive oliguric renal insufficiency. The key to controlling this dreaded complication of SSc is early recognition. Accordingly, high-risk patients should monitor their blood pressure daily, and if there is a rise in blood pressure, a new onset of proteinuria, or a rise in creatinine, patients should be hospitalized for close monitoring and aggressive management. Some patients (<10%) develop scleroderma renal crisis in the absence of hypertension. Treatment with increasing doses of ACE inhibitors such as captopril (Capoten)[1] (up to 200 mg daily) should be started immediately. The creatinine may continue to rise even on ACE inhibitor therapy[1] and with adequate blood pressure control. Despite aggressive treatment, progressive renal insufficiency may ensue, necessitating dialysis. Nevertheless, up to 40% of patients may ultimately recover adequate renal function to discontinue dialysis. There is insufficient evidence to support prophylactic use of ACE inhibitors[1] in SSc.

Polymyositis/Dermatomyositis

Idiopathic inflammatory myopathies (IIM) include adult and childhood dermatomyositis (DM), polymyositis (PM), myositis associated with malignancy or other connective tissue diseases, and inclusion body myositis (IBM) (Table 3). Although the etiology of IIM is unknown, the presence of cellular infiltrates in the muscle provides strong evidence for an immune mechanism of muscle damage. In DM, the main immune effector response appears to be humoral and directed against the microvasculature, whereas in both PM and IBM, cytotoxic CD8$^+$ T cells and macrophages invade and destroy muscle fibers. Inflammatory myopathies are characterized by progressive symmetric weakness of the proximal muscles, causing difficulty walking, standing, and lifting objects. In DM, a characteristic erythematous rash on the face, eyelids, neck, upper chest, and back is seen. Muscle biopsy is helpful in differentiating PM/DM from drug-induced myopathies and from endocrine and metabolic myopathies. Myositis-specific anti-bodies may be of prognostic value; patients with Jo-1 or other anti–aminoacyl-tRNA autoantibodies are at high risk for interstitial lung disease (ILD) and show poor response to therapy. The levels of serum creatine kinase (CK) are useful in assessing disease activity. Involvement of the gastrointestinal muscles can lead to dysphagia. Patients with new myositis and especially adults with dermatomyositis, should be carefully screened for malignancy.

GENERAL PRINCIPLES OF THERAPY

Immunosuppressive therapies are the primary treatment for the IIM. Early intervention is crucial to prevent irreversible muscle damage. Because long-term administration of high doses of corticosteroids is associated with significant morbidity, a second-line agent such as methotrexate[1] or azathioprine[1] should be introduced early. Intravenous Ig therapy,[1] cyclophosphamide (Cytoxan),[1] and cyclosporine (Neoral)[1] are also used with some benefit. Rehabilitative and physical therapeutic interventions are essential to complement pharmacologic therapy. Although PM and DM can usually be controlled by immunosuppressive agents, the treatment of IBM remains unsatisfactory.

Corticosteroids

Prednisone[1] (1 mg/kg daily) is effective as initial therapy in the majority of the cases. In patients with rapidly progressive myositis or extramuscular manifestation such as ILD, intravenous pulse methylprednisolone[1] (1 g daily for 3 days) may be used. Both muscle

---

[1]Not FDA approved for this indication.

TABLE 3 Clinical Characteristics of Idiopathic Inflammatory Myopathies

Dermatomyositis	Polymyositis	Inclusion	Body Myositis
Female to male	2:1	1:1	1:3
Age (y)	10-80	30-60	50-70
Muscle atrophy	Frequent	Rare	Frequent
Skin rash	Yes	No	No
Lung disease	Frequent	Frequent	
Dysphagia	Frequent	Rare	Rare
Arthralgia	Frequent	Rare	No
Malignancy	5%-17%	Rare	No

BOX 5	Rationale for Using a Second-Line Immunosuppressive Agent in Idiopathic Inflammatory Myopathy (IIM)

- Increased risk of corticosteroid-related side effects (diabetes mellitus, osteoporosis)
- Disease relapse after corticosteroid tapering attempts jeopardy
- Corticosteroid complications (myopathy)
- Severe or progressive myositis
- Serious extramuscular manifestations
- Lack of efficiency of corticosteroid as a single agent

strength and functional status and serum levels of CK should be checked regularly. Clinical improvement usually follows a fall in CK levels. Prednisone at 10 mg daily may be needed for 6 to 12 months. Progressive weakness in the face of declining CK levels suggests steroid myopathy.

Other Immunosuppressive Agents

In patients who fail to respond to corticosteroids, azathioprine[1] (2 mg/kg daily) or methotrexate[1] (20 mg weekly) may be used. Box 5 shows the indications for using second-line agents. Blood cell counts and liver functions should be closely monitored. Intermittent bolus IVIG (up to 2 g/kg infused every 4 to 8 weeks) may also be effective in some steroid-resistant DM patients and for severe esophageal involvement.

Treatment of Extramuscular Manifestations

Alveolitis and ILD are frequent complications. Some experts recommend high-dose daily corticosteroids in combination with a second-line immunosuppressive agent (cyclophosphamide,[1] azathioprine,[1] or cyclosporine[1]) early in the treatment. Skin rash can be effectively treated with hydroxychloroquine (Plaquenil)[1] (200 to 400 mg daily). Patients with severe proximal dysphagia may need a feeding tube to prevent aspiration and malnutrition.

Rehabilitative Measures

The goal of physical therapy is to preserve existing muscle function and to prevent muscle atrophy and joint contractures. Bedridden patients should receive passive exercise, stretching, and massage. As muscle strength improves, resistive exercise followed by an active aerobic conditioning regimen can be introduced. Proximal oropharyngeal dysphagia should be managed by speech therapy.

---

[1]Not FDA approved for this indication.

CURRENT DIAGNOSIS

- Protean manifestations in multiple organs
- Marked clinical heterogeneity
- Unpredictable, often remitting-relapsing clinical course
- Diagnosis based on characteristic constellations of clinical and laboratory features (criteria)
- Accurate diagnosis, specific subset, and stage of disease must be established

CURRENT THERAPY

- Prompt diagnosis and early intervention are desirable.
- Treatment strategies must be individualized.
- Treatment plan must consider both short-term symptom control and long-term strategies.
- Both organ-based and disease-modification approaches are used.
- Immunosuppression is often complicated by side effects.
- Management by a multispeciality team of experts is desirable.

REFERENCES

Bryan C, Knight C, Black CM, Silman AJ: Prediction of five-year survival following presentation with scleroderma: Development of a simple model using three disease factors at first visit. Arthritis Rheum 1999; 42(12):2660-2665.
Dalakas MC: High-dose intravenous immunoglobulin in inflammatory myopathies: Experience based on controlled clinical trials. Neurol Sci 2003; 24(Suppl 4):S256-S259.
Ionnaou Y, Isenberg DA: Current concepts for the management of systemic lupus erythematosus in adults: A therapeutic approach. Postgrad Med J 2002;78:599-606.
Isenberg DA, Allen E, Farewell V, et al: International consensus outcome measures for patients with idiopathic inflammatory myopathies. Development and initial validation of myositis activity and damage indices in patients with adult onset disease. Rheumatology (Oxford) 2004;43(1):49-54.
Manzi S: Treatment of systemic lupus erythematosus. In Klippel JH, Stone J, Weyand C, Crofford LJ (eds): Primer on the Rheumatic Diseases, Atlanta: Arthritis Foundation, 2001, pp 346-352.
Mayes MD, Lacey JV Jr, Beebe-Dimmer J, et al: Prevalence, incidence, survival, and disease characteristics of systemic sclerosis in a large US population. Arthritis Rheum 2003;48(8):2246-2255.
Oddis CV: Idiopathic inflammatory myopathies: A treatment update. Curr Rheumatol Rep 2003;5(6):431-436.
Ortmann RA, Klippel JH: Update on cyclophosphamide for systemic lupus erythematosus. Rheum Dis Clin North Am 2000;26:363-375.
Ramirez A, Varga J: Pulmonary arterial hypertension in systemic sclerosis: Clinical manifestations, pathophysiology, evaluation, and management. Treat Respir Med 2004;3(6):339-352.
Wigley FM: Raynaud's phenomenon. N Engl J Med 2002;347(13):1001-1008.

Cutaneous Vasculitis

Method of
Manisha J. Patel, MD, and
Joseph L. Jorizzo, MD

Vasculitis refers to inflammation and necrosis of blood vessels. It can be local or systemic and may be primary or secondary to another disease process. In patients with systemic involvement, the kidneys, gastrointestinal (GI) tract, or peripheral nerves may be involved. The classic cutaneous manifestation of small-vessel vasculitis is palpable purpura; the clinical manifestation greatly depends on the size and type of the vessel affected.

Clinical Presentation

The typical primary skin lesion of small-vessel cutaneous vasculitis (CV) is palpable purpura with lesions ranging in size from 1 mm to

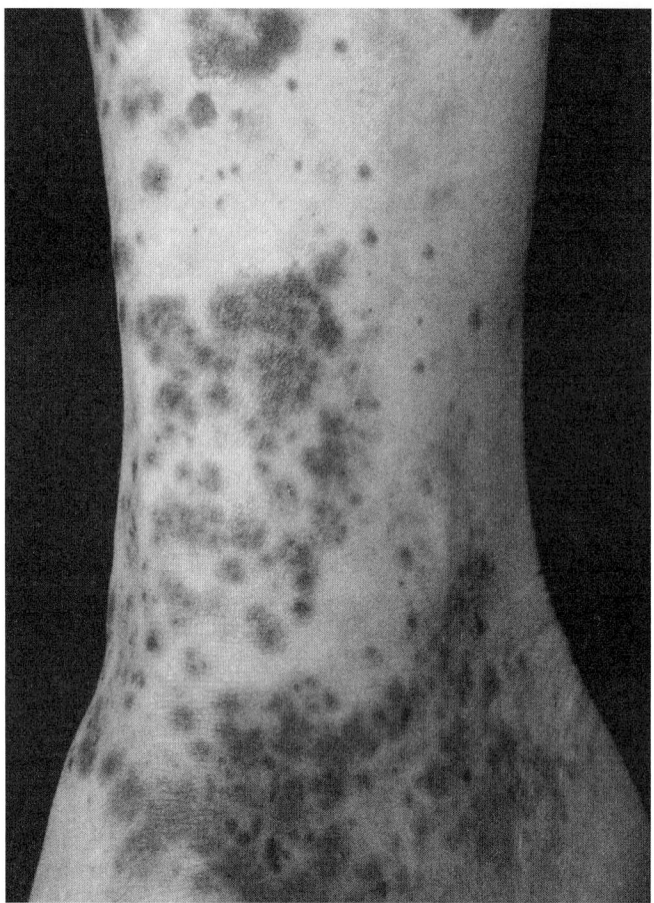

FIGURE 1. Small-vessel cutaneous vasculitis. Palpable purpura and early central necrosis are seen on the distal lower extremity. (Courtesy of Dr. Kelly Barham, Wake Forest University School of Medicine, Winston-Salem, NC.)

several centimeters (Figure 1). The lesions arise as a simultaneous *crop* and result from the exposure to an inciting stimulus. Usually macular in the early stages, lesions may progress to wide array of lesions including, papules, nodules, vesicles, plaques, bullae, or pustules. Secondary findings include ulceration, necrosis, and postinflammatory hyperpigmentation. Other cutaneous findings include livedo reticularis, edema, and urticarial lesions. Lesions most commonly occur on dependent areas, such as ankles and lower legs or other areas prone to stasis.

Although normally asymptomatic, local symptoms may include pruritus, pain, or burning. Systemic symptoms including fever, arthralgias, myalgias, anorexia, or GI pain should raise the suspicion that the CV may be associated with a systemic vasculitis.

Typically 50% of all patients with CV experience an acute or transient course, 30% develop chronic disease, and 20% experience relapsing disease. The percentage of patients with CV who have systemic involvement of one or more systems depends on the subspecialty of the series authors and the definition of systemic involvement. Most patients presenting to dermatologists do not have significant systemic involvement, excluding arthralgias, myalgias, fever, and serum sickness-like symptoms. It is best to consider that every patient with small-vessel CV may have systemic disease; this mandates a careful history, physical examination, and laboratory evaluation. Table 1 summarizes the key steps in evaluating suspected small-vessel CV and highlights the assessment for possible systemic involvement.

Histopathology

The hallmark histopathologic pattern of small-vessel CV is leukocytoclastic vasculitis. The histologic specimen shows an infiltration of neutrophils within and around blood vessel walls; leukocytoclasia (degranulation and fragmentation of neutrophils leading to the production of nuclear dust); fibrinoid necrosis of the damaged vessel walls; and necrosis, swelling, and proliferation of the endothelial cells. New clinical lesions should be selected for biopsy because specimens taken too late (i.e., older than 48 hours) may show the pathology of repair more than of the initial injury. Direct immunofluorescence microscopic studies on fresh lesions frequently demonstrate perivascular deposits of IgM or activated third component of complement (C3) in the superficial dermal papillary vessels. One exception is the deposition of IgA in patients with Henoch-Schönlein purpura. Documenting leukocytoclastic vasculitis in biopsy specimens is essential to confirming the diagnosis.

Etiology

Small-vessel CV is considered to be an aberrant immune complex response that is usually triggered by an infection, exposure to a drug, or association with an autoimmune disease; most etiologic factors identified have been incriminated by association rather than by direct demonstration. Between 50% and 60% of patients have no identifiable cause. Of the approximately 50% of patients in whom a cause is identifiable, 20% are associated with infections; and another 20% are thought to be triggered by an exposure to a drug. Bacterial infections associated with CV include streptococcus, staphylococcus, and gram-negative organisms. Several viral agents include HIV, hepatitis B and C, herpes simplex virus (HSV), and influenza. Suspected medications include antibiotics (penicillins, sulfonamides), anticonvulsants, isoniazid (Laniazid), oral contraceptives, and thiazides. Less than 5% of patients have underlying connective tissue disease. There have been patients with small-vessel CV reported rarely in patients with malignancies, especially Hodgkin's disease, mycosis fungoides, and adult T-cell lymphoma.

Differential Diagnosis

Not all dermatoses associated with purpura are a result of vasculitis. In the differential diagnosis of vasculitis, be aware of disorders that may present with livedo or infarcted lesions secondary to vascular occlusion disorders. Some examples of vaso-occlusive disorders include cryoglobulinemia, cholesterol emboli, Sneddon's syndrome, septic emboli, and malignant atrophic papulosis (Degos' disease). The histopathology in these disorders results from either initially occlusive or mediation by antiphospholipid antibodies, and therefore, falls into the category of microvascular occlusion. The differential diagnosis also includes trauma, coagulopathies, and thrombocytopenia. Purpuras secondary to coagulopathies and thrombocytopenia are noninflammatory and often nonpalpable; they can be distinguished promptly on histologic and laboratory testing.

Given the wide array of systemic diseases that can be associated with small-vessel CV, it is important to carefully evaluate each patient for coexistent disease; the first manifestation of large-vessel vasculitis is often small-vessel disease.

 CURRENT DIAGNOSIS

- Clinical spectrum of lesions ranging from purpura to palpable purpura, urticarial lesions, or ulcers: concentrated on dependent areas
- Small-vessel CV involves postcapillary venules only
- Histologic finding: leukocytoclastic vasculitis
- Pathogenesis: circulating immune complexes, neutrophils, cytokines, and adhesion molecules

Abbreviation: CV = cutaneous vasculitis.

TABLE 1 Evaluation of Suspected Small Vessel Cutaneous Vasculitis

Confirming Histopathologic Correlation	Assessing the Extent of the Disease	Establishing Etiology
Punch biopsy early lesion	General • Myalgia • Arthralgia • Fever	Infection • Bacterial • Viral • Fungal • Acid-fast bacilli • Other
Incisional biopsy for suspected larger vessel vasculitis	Renal involvement (acute and chronic renal failure) • Proteinuria • Hematuria Nervous system • Central or peripheral • Diffuse or local findings	Drugs Diseases associated with immune complexes • Connective tissue/autoimmune diseases • Malignancy (especially myelodysplastic) • Inflammatory bowel disease
	Musculoskeletal involvement • Nonerosive polyarthritis Gastrointestinal system • Abdominal pain (colicky, nausea, vomiting, diarrhea) • Gastrointestinal bleeding (melena or hematemesis) Pulmonary involvement • Pleural effusion • Pleuritis • Hemoptysis Pericardial involvement (myocardial angiitis or pericarditis) • Pericardial effusion Ocular involvement (retinal vasculitis) • Conjunctivitis • Keratitis Other	Idiopathic (50%)

Modified from Barham KL et al: Rook's Textbook of Dermatology, 7th ed. Oxford, Blackwell Publishing, 2004.

HENOCH-SCHÖNLEIN PURPURA

Henoch-Schönlein purpura (HSP) deserves specific mention given its history and frequent occurrence. Heberden first described a single patient with HSP in 1801. Johann Schönlein and Eduard Henoch elucidated features in the mid-19th century as a tetrad of palpable purpura, arthritis, and GI and renal involvement. Henoch-Schönlein purpura is defined by the Chapel Hill Consensus Conference as a vasculitis affecting small vessels, involving deposition of IgA immune complexes that characteristically involves the skin, GI system, and glomeruli with or without arthralgia or arthritis. Approximately 30% of cases follow an upper respiratory infection. The clinical outcome is excellent with fewer than 10% of patients developing chronic disease. A small percent of patients will develop persistent renal or GI disease requiring systemic immunosuppressive therapy.

URTICARIAL VASCULITIS

Another important subtype of small-vessel CV is urticarial vasculitis. Urticarial vasculitis is a chronic disorder consisting of episodic urticarial and/or angioedematous lesions lasting longer than 24 hours that histologically manifest features of leukocytoclastic vasculitis. Urticarial vasculitis may range from patients with only urticarial skin lesions to those with urticarial vasculitis associated with hypocomplementemia with some systemic features; this meets criteria for systemic lupus erythematosus. Patients with urticarial vasculitis may also have underlying autoimmune connective tissue diseases, infections (hepatitis B and C), neoplastic processes, or medications as underlying etiologic factors. Treatment is directed at underlying etiologies and/or follows the same therapeutic ladder as for small-vessel CV (Table 2).

Treatment

Because small-vessel CV is generally self-limited, treatment is often unnecessary except for symptomatic relief. When possible, identification and removal of a causative agent (e.g., infection, drug, chemicals, food) should be accomplished. Removal of an inciting agent is

CURRENT THERAPY

- Small-vessel CV is generally self-limited; treatment is often unnecessary except for symptomatic relief, which may be achieved with leg elevation, gradient support stockings, nonsteroidal anti-inflammatory drugs, and antihistamines.
- Skin manifestations alone may be managed with agents such as colchicine and dapsone.
- Systemic treatment is advised for patients with significant systemic manifestations or those with significant cutaneous ulceration.

Abbreviation: CV = cutaneous vasculitis.

TABLE 2 Therapeutic Ladder for Small-Vessel Cutaneous Vasculitis

	Double-Blind Studies	Case Series	Case Reports
Skin lesions alone	Colchicine[1]	Nonsteroidal anti-inflammatory drugs Dapsone[1]	Supportive therapy • Antihistamines • Pentoxifylline (Trental)[1] • Hydroxychloroquine (Plaquenil)[1] • Thalidomide (Thalomid)[1] • Low-dose weekly methotrexate (Rheumatrex)[1]
Ulcerative skin lesions alone		Prednisone[1]	
Systemic disease	Interferon-α and ribavirin (Rebetron) (if associated with hepatitis C) 3 million units 3/wk and 1000 mg/d, respectively	Prednisone[1] Azathioprine (Imuran)[1] 1–2.5 mg/kg/d PO as single dose or divided in half	Mycophenolate mofetil (CellCept)[1] 500–2000 mg PO bid Cyclosporine (Neoral, Sandimmune)[1] 2.5 mg/kg/d PO divided in half qd; after 4 wk, dose may be increased 0.5 mg/kg/d at 2-wk intervals; maximum of 4 mg/kg/d
		Cyclophosphamide (Cytoxan)[1] pulsed dosing regimen, 40–50 mg/kg IV in divided doses over 2–5 d *or* 10–15 mg/kg IV q 7–10 d *or* 3–5 mg/kg IV 2/wk	• IV gammaglobulin (Gammagard)[1] • Extracorporeal immunomodulation • Biologic agents: infliximab (Remicade),[1] etanercept (Enbrel)[1] (TNF-α inhibitors) • Rituximab (Anti-CD20)[1]
	Methotrexate (Trexall)[1] 7.5–15 mg once a week*		

*There is no study associated with this drug.
[1]Not FDA approved for this indication.
Abbreviations: IV = intravenously, TNF-α = tumor necrosis factor-α.
Modified from Barham KL et al: Rook's Textbook of Dermatology, 7th ed. Oxford, Blackwell Publishing, 2004.

occasionally followed by rapid resolution of the lesions and no other treatment is indicated; otherwise, local and systemic therapies are recommended. Symptomatic improvement may be achieved with leg elevation, gradient support stockings, nonsteroidal anti-inflammatory drugs, and antihistamines.

Small-vessel CV with persistent palpable purpura without significant internal organ complications may respond to treatment with oral colchicine[1] in doses of 0.6 mg two to three times daily. Dosing is limited by GI symptoms. This therapy is supported by anecdotal reports, but a statistically significant difference was not confirmed in a randomized controlled trial. Dapsone[1] (50 to 200 mg per day) has also been used in patients only having skin involvement.

Systemic treatment is advised for patients with small-vessel CV who have significant systemic manifestations or significant cutaneous ulceration. However, almost no double-blind, placebo-controlled prospective trials exist. Table 2 describes a therapeutic ladder for small-vessel CV. The medications discussed in Table 2 have not been FDA approved for this indication. Oral corticosteroids (Prednisone[1] 0.5 to 1 mg/kg per day) are indicated for progressive, symptomatic nodular, vesicular, or ulcerating purpura as well as systemic involvement. Once the patient's symptoms have stabilized, prednisone should be tapered gradually over 3 to 6 weeks because a rapid taper can lead to clinical disease rebound.

Small-vessel CV can manifest clinically with a spectrum of cutaneous lesions; palpable purpura is the classic presentation. The hallmark histologic appearance is a leukocytoclastic vasculitis. There is a presumed immune complex mediated pathogenesis. The therapeutic approach requires elimination of the cause (drugs, chemicals, infection) when possible. In most patients, only the skin is involved and can be treated with supportive measures. The most important step in evaluation is the full workup to find etiology and extent (systemic involvement) of the disease process. Skin manifestations alone may be managed with nonsteroidal anti-inflammatory drugs, gradient support stockings, colchicine, and dapsone. Systemic treatment is advised in small-vessel CV with significant systemic manifestations or those with significant cutaneous ulceration.

[1]Not FDA approved for this indication.

REFERENCES

Fiorentino DF: Cutaneous vasculitis. J Am Acad Dermatol 2003;48(3):311-340.
Gonzalez-Gay MA, Garcia-Porrua C, Pujol RM: Clinical approach to cutaneous vasculitis. Curr Opin Rheumatol 2005;17(1):56-61.
Lamprecht P: TNF-alpha inhibitors in systemic vasculitides and connective tissue diseases. Autoimmun Rev 2005;4(1):28-34.
Lotti T, Ghersetich I, Comacchi C, Jorizzo JL: Cutaneous small-vessel vasculitis. J Am Acad Dermatol 1998;39(5 Pt 1):667-687.

Diseases of the Nails

Method of
Nathaniel Jellinek, MD

Overview

The nail plate in humans has many functions. It facilitates scratching; it is used as a tool, a weapon, and a form of adornment (to the cost of approximately $6 billion per year in the United States); and most importantly it supports the underlying distal phalanx and soft tissue to maximize fine touch and manual dexterity.

The nail unit consists of the nail plate, an underlying nail bed, a germinative nail matrix, proximal and lateral nail folds, a cuticle and distal hyponychium (Fig. 1). The matrix exists under the proximal nail fold, beginning just distal to the insertion of the dorsal extensor tendon, and extends distally under the nail plate beyond the cuticle as the crescent-shaped lunula. The lunula is usually most apparent on the thumbnail, less so on each consecutive finger. The nail bed is contiguous with the matrix, tightly adherent to the overlying plate,

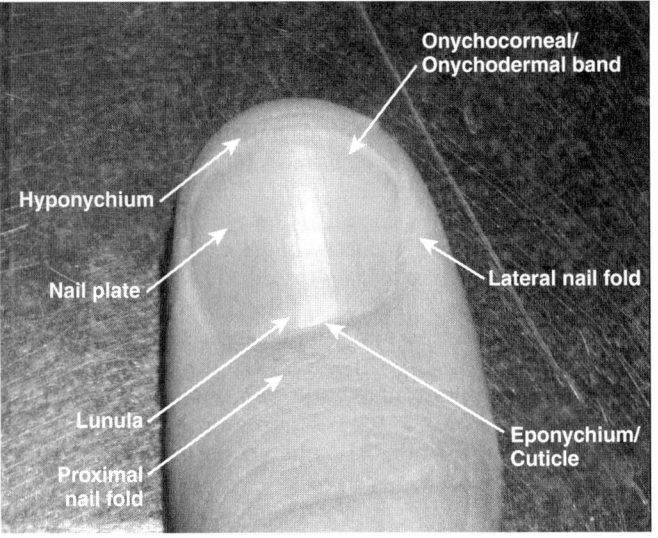

FIGURE 1. Surface anatomy of the nail.

to which it is connected in a tongue-and-groove pattern, ending distally at the onychocorneal (or onychodermal) band, the distal-most attachment point between the bed and plate. The onychocorneal band region provides the ventral barrier of the nail unit. When it is breached, onycholysis results.

Dorsally and laterally, the nail folds provide an anatomic barrier to the nail unit. When they are breached, moisture, yeast, bacteria, and contact irritants and allergens penetrate the normal barrier and cause paronychia, acute and chronic.

An understanding of normal nail anatomy facilitates comprehension of the pathology discussed here.

Lichen Planus

CLINICAL FEATURES AND DIAGNOSIS

Lichen planus is an inflammatory disorder that can involve the skin, hair, nails, and mucous membranes. Nail disease can accompany skin or mucosal disease or can manifest as isolated nail disease. It is characterized histologically by lichenoid inflammation and can involve any or all of the nail subunits. Onychorrhexis, longitudinal striations in the nail plate, and nail plate thinning or fragility, result from nail matrix involvement. Onycholysis (nail lifting) and nail thickening are caused by hyponychium and nail bed involvement. Nail pain can herald the onset of bullous lichen planus of the nail. This represents an urgent problem, because permanent scarring of the nail bed and matrix can result, manifesting clinically as dorsal pterygium. It is crucial to check all patients with suspected nail lichen planus with a complete skin and oral mucosal examination for lesions.

TREATMENT

Overt, repetitive, and incidental trauma to the nail apparatus worsens the nail disease and makes it more resistant to treatment (the Koebner phenomenon.) The Koebner and Koebner-like phenomena are important in the diathesis of lichen planus. Therefore, trauma, contact irritants, and moisture must be minimized or avoided. The nails should be kept short. Intralesional triamcinolone 2.5 to 5 mg/mL monthly for several months and occasionally systemic corticosteroids may be required in more severe cases or with scarring.

 CURRENT DIAGNOSIS

Brittle Nails

- Brittle nails are present in approximately 20% of the North American population
- They are more common in women, those who use nail cosmetics, and persons >50 years old
- Diagnose with subjective complaint of brittle nails with observation of onychorrhexis (longitudinal nail plate ridging) and onychoschizia (lamellar splitting of nail plate

Onychomycosis

- Make an objective diagnosis with KOH, culture or clipping for periodic acid–Schiff
- Onychomycosis is much more common on the toenails than the fingernails
- The most common organisms are *Trichophyton rubrum* or *Trichophyton mentagrophytes*
- *Candida* only rarely causes onychomycosis. It is primarily a colonizer in the setting of barrier breakdown of the nail apparatus
- Nondermatophyte molds (such as *Aspergillus, Fusarium, Penicillium* spp) are unusual causes of onychomycosis in the United States. Repeat tests showing the same organisms and ruling out other causes are mandated before initiating treatment

Primary Onycholysis and Chronic Paronychia

- Primary onycholysis and chronic paronychia are diagnoses of exclusion. Onychomycosis, psoriasis, lichen planus, and drug reactions all must be ruled out before diagnosis.
- Both are more common on the fingernails than the toenails, in women, in adults, in those who use nail cosmetics, or and those who have recurrent exposure to moisture or chemicals.
- Both primary onycholysis and chronic paronychia represent breakdown in the normal barrier of the nail apparatus. Onycholysis results from breakdown of the onychocorneal band or nail bed–nail plate connection. Chronic paronychia results from breakdown of the cuticle and nail folds.
- In both scenarios, moisture, contact irritants, contact allergens, colonizing yeast, and bacteria invade the exposed nail apparatus and contribute to a cycle of inflammation.

Ingrown Nails

- Common risk factors include incorrect nail cutting, wide feet, narrow-toed shoes, lateral plate malalignment, and lateral nail fold hypertrophy.
- Neonates and infants demonstrate distal nail ingrowing, which is separate in pathogenesis and treatment from the disease in adolescents and adults.
- Ingrown nails can be graded on a scale from I to III, with I being erythema and swelling with drainage from the nail fold and III being associated with exuberant overgrowth of granulation tissue over and around the ingrown nail plate.

CURRENT THERAPY

Brittle Nails

- Treatment is frustrating and represents the limitations in our understanding of disease pathogenesis.
- Oral biotin, 2-3 mg (2000-3000 μg) (Appearex) daily, dosed for 4-6 months and then discontinued, is a reasonable trial. Patients will notice an effect during this period if it has helped, then may continue to treat if it is helpful.
- Topical moisturizers (petrolatum) or humectant agents (12% ammonium lactate, 20% urea) might help those with hard brittle nails.

Onychomycosis

- Topical treatment is disappointing, except in cases of superficial white onychomycosis.
- Oral treatment should be reserved for patients with symptomatic disease or who are at risk for complications (diabetics, immunosuppressed, at risk of secondary bacterial cellulitis).
- Oral treatment is more successful than topical treatment. Terbinafine (Lamisil) 250 mg Po qd × 90 days in adults is the first-line treatment. Itraconazole (Sporanox), dosed daily or pulsed 1 week per month, is the next most successful agent.
- Patients are at high risk for recurrence. Post-treatment prevention of tinea pedis is important to prevent reinfection.

Primary Onycholysis and Chronic Paronychia

- It is important not to misdiagnose the presence of yeast (especially *Candida*) as a primary infection or pathogen. It almost always represents a colonizer. Treatment of the yeast is therefore secondary.
- Avoidance is the mainstay of treatment. Avoid all wet work and exposure to acids, bases, and chemicals by wearing cotton gloves under heavy-duty vinyl gloves. Avoid all nail cosmetics and nail manipulation except for regular plate trimming. No nail salon. Keep the plate trimmed to its proximal-most attachment point. Avoid obvious triggers and traumas to the nail apparatus.
- It can take up to 6 months for the nail apparatus to normalize.

Ingrown Nails

- Infantile disease: Warm soaks followed by massage of the nail and distal phalangeal tuft.
- Adolescent and adult disease: Correct nail plate cutting and shoes. For mild disease, twice daily cold soaks, topical steroids, 20% to 40% topical urea cream (Keralac, Carmol), and cotton wisps or dental floss under the aggravating part of the lateral nail plate will decrease inflammation, improve symptoms, and normalize the nail plate without surgery.
- For more advanced cases, twice-daily warm soaks, oral antibiotics (with signs of infection), followed by lateral plate avulsion and lateral matricectomy (either chemical or surgical).

Onychomycosis

CLINICAL FEATURES AND DIAGNOSIS

Approximately one half of all doctor visits relating to nail complaints are for onychomycosis. It is not only the most common nail diagnosis, however; it is also the most common misdiagnosis, and even experienced nail clinicians might not make an accurate diagnosis up to 50% of the time. It is therefore crucial to confirm the diagnosis by potassium hydroxide, fungal culture, or clipping for periodic acid–Schiff analysis before initiating any therapy, with its inherent risks and costs.

In the United States, 80% to 90% cases of onychomycosis are caused by dermatophyte fungi, most commonly *Trichophyton rubrum* or *Trichophyton mentagrophytes*. The tendency to acquire these infections appears to be inherited in an autosomal dominant fashion with incomplete or variable penetrance. The infection usually begins with tinea pedis; the nail barrier between plate and hyponychium or nail fold is compromised, often through repetitive trauma, and fungus enters the nail apparatus.

There are four main types of onychomycosis: distal and lateral subungual onychomycosis (DLSO, most common), occasionally leading to total dystrophic onychomycosis (TDO), superficial white onychomycosis (SWO), and proximal subungual onychomycosis (PSO). SWO is the most straightforward to diagnose; scraping the surface yields abundant fungi for examination. DLSO and TDO are best diagnosed by acquiring the proximal-most area of involved nail plate and subungual debris; this occasionally involves aggressive paring by the practitioner to remove the distal nail plate and debris, with lower diagnostic yield. PSO may be a marker for systemic immunosuppression and is therefore important to diagnose. A nail plate punch biopsy is the most direct and accurate way to make this diagnosis of the latter.

Candida only rarely causes onychomycosis. This fact is widely misunderstood, probably because *Candida* is commonly found as a colonizing organism in conditions such as primary onycholysis and chronic paronychia. The unusual situation of primary *Candida* onychomycosis is limited to those with inherited chronic mucocutaneous candidiasis or severe immunosuppression. The presence of this organism in the setting of onychomycosis should arouse doubt rather than confirm the diagnosis. In most cases, it is a colonizer rather than a pathogen.

The presence of an underlying disease with nail manifestations (such as psoriasis or lichen planus) does not rule out the concomitant presence of onychomycosis and can cause barrier breakdown of the nail apparatus, facilitating secondary fungal infection.

TREATMENT

Oral treatment should be reserved for patients who have symptomatic disease or who are at risk for complications, such as diabetics and immunocompromised patients, who are at risk for secondary bacterial cellulitis.

Confirm the diagnosis. The presence of *Candida* or nondermatophyte mold is unusual in the United States. Tests should be repeated and other diagnoses should be entertained before diagnosing onychomycosis and initiating treatment. If a dermatophyte is found, systemic terbinafine (Lamisil) offers the best systemic choice. Systemic itraconazole (Sporanox) is the next most effective agent and can be dosed in a pulsed fashion (off label) or daily like terbinafine. Topical ciclopirox (Loprox) clears the nails in less than 10% of cases; other topical agents are equally ineffective.

Because a person is often genetically predisposed to acquire onychomycosis, once the disorder is cleared by a systemic agent, then topical agents must be used indefinitely, with the goal being to avoid subsequent cases of tinea pedis. Powders and lotions are available over the counter and may be used on a regular basis.

Brittle Nails

CLINICAL FEATURES AND DIAGNOSIS

A simplistic view, but perhaps representing the best of our understanding about brittle nails, is that hard brittle nails are caused and worsened by too little moisture, and that soft brittle nails are associated with too much moisture. Both may be worsened by irritants. Older persons tend to have dry brittle nails, analogous to skin in the aging population. Although up to 20% of North Americans have brittle nails, our understanding of the pathogenesis is limited.

Brittle nails are diagnosed when subjective and objective criteria are met. Patients must complain of nail fragility and easy breaking with clinical signs of onychorrhexis (longitudinal ridging), onychoschizia (lamellar splitting), and occasionally dull, lusterless plate appearance.

TREATMENT

Biotin (vitamin H or B_7) 2 to 3 mg (often dosed as 2000-3000 µg) [gkuo2][3],[7] taken once daily improves brittleness in some cases. It is helpful to have the patient take this water-soluble vitamin for 4 to 6 months, then discontinue it for a several months to evaluate for improvement, worsening, or no change. This initial trial therapy can prevent continued cost to the patient if he or she notices no improvement and then worsening when taking and discontinuing the vitamin, respectively. Irritant avoidance is also helpful. Application of petrolatum at bedtime under light white cotton gloves (apply ointment after soaking the nail in water for 5 minutes) increases the moisture content of the nail plate. Topical humectant agents include over-the-counter 12% ammonium lactate cream and 10% to 20% urea preparations.

Ingrown Nails

CLINICAL FEATURES AND DIAGNOSIS

Ingrown nails represent a foreign body reaction of the nail plate in the lateral nail fold. It is more common on toenails, particularly the great toenails, than fingernails. Predisposing factors include wide feet, ill-fitting or narrow-toed or high heeled shoes, lateral plate malalignment, hypertrophic lateral nail folds, cutting the nails incorrectly in a half-circle instead of straight across, and possibly hyperhidrosis. Secondary infection can occur after the plate pierces the nail fold skin.

In adolescents and adults, the nail fold embedding and spicule formation tends to be lateral, whereas in neonates and young children the embedding tends to be distal. The former group is predisposed to multiple episodes of ingrowing; procedural treatment is recommended and often required. The latter group often responds to conservative treatment; surgery is only occasionally required.

TREATMENT

Correct nail cutting and appropriate shoes are the main treatment. For mild disease, use of twice-daily cold soaks, topical steroids, 20% to 40% topical urea cream, and cotton wisps or dental floss under the aggravating part of the lateral nail plate can decrease inflammation, improve symptoms, and normalize the nail plate without requiring surgery. For more advanced cases, twice-daily warm soaks, oral antibiotics (with signs of infection), followed by lateral plate avulsion and lateral matricectomy (either chemical or surgical) represent standard of care. Infantile disease responds to warm soaks followed by massage of the nail and distal phalangeal tuft.

[3]Exceeds dosage recommended by the manufacturer.
[7]Available as a dietary supplement.

Subungual Hematoma

CLINICAL FEATURES AND DIAGNOSIS

Blood under the nail plate can appear red or black. Because the physiologic blood-metabolizing enzymes are not found in the nail plate, blood trapped between the plate and bed is not metabolized to the same evolving brown- and green-colored metabolites in the nail, and instead stays red-black and grows out with the nail plate. Nail plate growth is slow, approximately 3 mm/month for fingernails and about one half that rate for toenails, so that growing out of the hematoma will take several months and may be difficult to appreciate without photographs or serial measurements.

Diagnosis is usually straightforward. In ambiguous presentations, a urinalysis reagent strip efficiently and accurately tests for subungual blood. However, nail tumors are often preceded or first recognized after trauma, and they might even bleed spontaneously. Therefore, the presence of blood does not rule out a concomitant neoplasm.

TREATMENT

Any hematoma involving more than 50% of the nail plate carries a significant risk of underlying distal phalangeal fracture, and an x-ray should be ordered. For relief of acute symptomatic subungual hematomas, digital anesthesia followed by trephination using a sterilized hot paper clip, punch, #11 blade, or nail drill provides rapid relief and confirms the diagnosis. For most cases, however, no treatment is indicated, and the blood will grow out distally with the nail plate, albeit slowly.

Psoriasis

CLINICAL FEATURES AND DIAGNOSIS

Psoriasis commonly involves the nails in patients with cutaneous disease and occasionally occurs as a disease isolated to the nail unit. In those with psoriatic arthritis, nail disease is over-represented, and may be present up to 90% to 95% of the time. Like lichen planus, psoriasis can involve any part of the nail unit; hyponychium and nail bed involvement manifest as onycholysis and subungual hyperkeratosis and a red nail bed or oil drop (salmon patch) change.

Nail pitting occurs from proximal matrix psoriasis, where parakeratotic columns lose attachment from the superficial plate, leaving a narrow depression behind in the nail plate. Any patient with these signs should have a detailed history (looking for family history) and complete skin examination, with particular attention given to the scalp, external auditory meatus, postauricular crease, umbilicus, intergluteal fold, groin, and flexural areas. Even without these helpful cutaneous signs, the combination of three nail signs is highly suggestive of nail psoriasis. In ambiguous cases, a nail clipping or nail bed biopsy can provide additional diagnostic information.

TREATMENT

Overt, repetitive, and incidental trauma to the nail apparatus worsens the nail disease and makes it more resistant to treatment (the Koebner phenomenon.) Therefore, it is important to keep the nails trimmed short, use no nail cosmetics or artificial nails, and avoid aggressive nail manicuring or débridement of nail bed hyperkeratosis.

Topical treatment may be applied with a variety of agents, many of which represent off-label uses: corticosteroids, 5-fluorouracil (Efudex, Carac),[1] calcipotriene (Dovonex), tazarotene (Tazorac), cyclosporine (Sandimmune), and urea (Keralac, Carmol). Topical treatment is low risk but generally disappointing. Intralesional injection of triamcinolone 2.5 to 5 mg/mL is effective and can be dosed on a monthly basis and gradually tapered until the nails are free of disease; this therapy can provide a period of remission from nail disease. Systemic agents (methotrexate (Trexall), cyclosporine, or

[1]Not FDA approved for this indication.

injectable therapies) used for severe psoriasis and psoriatic arthritis are inappropriate to use off label for isolated nail disease; however, in the case of widespread disease, they often improve concomitant nail psoriasis. Systemic corticosteroids, as with all forms of psoriasis, are contraindicated and can provoke an outbreak of widespread pustular (von Zumbush) psoriasis.

Primary (Simple) Onycholysis

CLINICAL FEATURES AND DIAGNOSIS

Onycholysis means separation of nail plate from nail bed or nail folds and represents a ventral or lateral break in the normal nail barrier. It can be graded from stage 1 (minimal involvement) to stage 4 or 5 (maximal involvement). The longer onycholysis is present, the less likely it is to resolve as the nail bed can pathologically cornify and develop a granular layer.

The most common causes are trauma and contact irritants or moisture. Other causes include psoriasis and onychomycosis; whereas onychomycosis tends to involve the toenails only and manifests with yellow nails, onycholysis nearly always involves the fingernails and demonstrates classic physical signs. Primary onycholysis usually involves the fingernails, and might involve only one nail. Women, those who use nail cosmetics, and persons with prolonged irritant or moisture contact, are all at highest risk.

Monodactylous onycholysis should always raise the possibility of an underlying neoplasm. Yeast is commonly cultured but is usually an opportunistic colonizer rather than a pathogenic organism. Hence the presence of *Candida* does not mean a diagnosis of onychomycosis, but secondary colonization in the setting of onycholysis.

TREATMENT

Nails must be kept short. Patients must practice a strict irritant and moisture avoidance regimen, including avoidance of all nail cosmetics and artificial nails. They should use heavy cotton gloves for dry work and light cotton gloves under vinyl gloves for wet work. A topical antifungal solution, lotion, or lacquer may be added as an adjuvant agent but is considered secondary after the avoidance regimen. For monodactylous cases, x-ray and biopsy should always be considered.

Primary (Simple) Chronic Paronychia

CLINICAL FEATURES AND DIAGNOSIS

Chronic paronychia may be defined as inflammation of one or more nail folds, usually the proximal fold, lasting 6 weeks or longer. It represents a dorsal or lateral (or both) barrier breakdown of the nail unit, compared with onycholysis on the ventral of the nail plate. In both situations, irritants and moisture contribute to a chronic irritant contact dermatitis and yeast colonization. Women, persons who use nail cosmetics or work in the food industry, and persons with prolonged irritant or moisture contact are at risk. As with onycholysis, patients with single-digit involvement or refractory cases who fail to respond to treatment should bring to mind the possibility of an underlying neoplasm, and a biopsy is warranted.

TREATMENT

The same principles apply to treatment of chronic paronychia as for onycholysis. An irritant and moisture avoidance regimen, combined with an antifungal solution as an adjuvant, is central to therapy. Nail cosmetics and nail manipulation, with an orange stick, for example, are forbidden. A topical corticosteroid agent may be used to decrease inflammation for 3 to 4 weeks initially, combined with the avoidance regimen. Refractory cases might respond to intralesional corticosteroids 2.5 to 5 mg/mL or occasionally a surgical saucerization of the proximal nail fold.

REFERENCES

Daniel CR 3rd, Daniel MP, Daniel J, et al: Managing simple chronic paronychia and onycholysis with ciclopirox 0.77% and an irritant-avoidance regimen. Cutis 2004;73(1):81-85.
de Berker D: The physical basis of cosmetic defects of the nail plate. J Cosmet Dermatol 2002;1(1):35-42.
de Berker D: Management of nail psoriasis. Clin Exp Dermatol 2000; 25(5):357-362.
Gupta AK, Tu LQ: Onychomycosis therapies: Strategies to improve efficacy. Dermatol Clin 2006;24(3):381-386.
Haneke E: Ingrown and pincer nails: evaluation and treatment. Dermatol Ther 2002;15:148-158.
Rounding C, Bloomfield S: Surgical treatments for ingrowing toenails. Cochrane Database Syst Rev 2005(2):CD001541.
Tosti A, Piraccini BM: Treatment of common nail disorders. Dermatol Clin 2000;18(2):339-348.
van de Kerkhof PC, Pasch MC, Scher RK, et al: Brittle nail syndrome: A pathogenesis-based approach with a proposed grading system. J Am Acad Dermatol 2005;53(4):644-651.

Keloids

Method of
Carol Drucker, MD

When injured skin heals with excessive scar tissue, keloids or hypertrophic scars form. Keloids are distinguished from hypertrophic scars by growing beyond the borders of the original wound and rarely spontaneously regressing. Both can itch, but keloids tend to be more symptomatic with sensations of itch, pain, and pulling. Keloids are more common in African Americans, Latin Americans, and Asians, but they can occur in any race. Hormonal changes in pregnancy can also increase the incidence.

Clinical Features

Keloids are characterized by uncontrolled synthesis and excessive deposition of collagen and glycoprotein. Whether increased synthesis or decreased resorption of collagen due to reduced generation of collagenase or direct enzyme inhibition is responsible is unclear. The combination of both mechanisms must be considered. The keloidal keratinocytes stimulate the underlying fibroblasts. The fibroblasts respond by increasing the expression of and signaling by transforming growth factor (TGF)-β.

Hypertrophic scars are common at places of increased tension such as the upper back and mid chest. They rise above the surface of the skin, can be firm, red, and itchy, but they tend to gradually improve spontaneously within 2 years.

Keloids are more aggressive. They do not necessarily occur at areas of tension; they can occur on earlobes at pierce sites or on the chest from acneiform papules. Keloids can become large and unsightly and may be very painful. After a time of stability, increased itching usually signifies impending growth.

 CURRENT DIAGNOSIS

- Overgrown scar extends beyond margins of injury
- Can occur months to years after injury
- Does not spontaneously regress
- Can undergo quiescent periods followed by more growth
- Can manifest with symptoms of itch, pain, burn, pulling

Treatment

One must be wary of the first reflex to excise the unsightly mass, because a larger, more problematic keloid can form in its place. Many modalities have been advocated for treating keloids. Each treatment is discussed separately, but most are used in combinations, and most keloids require more than one treatment. If a treatment is not achieving desired results, alternative approaches are undertaken.

INTRALESIONAL STEROIDS

Intralesional steroids are the usual first-line monotherapy and adjuvant treatment after surgical excision. Corticosteroids inhibit α-macroglobulin, which inhibits collagenase, and further proliferation of fibroblasts is probably reduced by steroid-induced suppression of endogenous vascular endothelial growth factor. Depending on the size and density of the keloid, strength of triamcinolone acetonide suspension can range from 10 to 40 mg/mL.

A series of injections is needed. The first injection is more difficult to infiltrate due to the density of the keloid. Local anesthesia may be needed or the steroid can be mixed with xylocaine with epinephrine. Subsequent injections, even if the keloid does not look or feel grossly different, usually are easier to administer. Injections should be given at 2- to 3-week intervals.

The overlying skin can atrophy, flattening can be irregular, and depigmentation can occur, so the continuation of treatment depends on results of decreasing symptoms and improving cosmetic results.

LIQUID NITROGEN

Liquid nitrogen has been used as monotherapy and adjuvant therapy. Freezing keloids causes cellular and microvascular damage followed by selective tissue necrosis, leading to tissue flattening. Thaw cycles of 20 to 30 seconds should be repeated every 2 to 3 weeks for 2 to 12 weeks. Side effects include hypo- and depigmentation and atrophy. Some first freeze the keloid with liquid nitrogen and allow it to thaw and become slightly edematous before injecting intralesional steroids, especially for the early injections. The edema facilitates injection and more even spread of the steroid.

SILICONE

Silicone has been shown to soften, flatten, blanch, increase elasticity, and decrease pruritus and pain of keloids. A number of commercial silicone elastomer products are available to treat keloids. These can be used on early healing wounds to help prevent keloids, on established keloids, and adjunctively with intralesional steroids and other modalities. The sheeting is worn over the keloid for 12 to 24 hours daily.

CURRENT THERAPY

- Intralesional steroids
- Liquid nitrogen
- Silicone
- Onion extract
- Pressure
- Bleomycin (Blenoxane)[1]
- Mitomycin C (Mutamycin)[1]
- 5-Flourouracil (Adrucil)[1]
- Interferon-α (Intron A)[1]
- 5% Imiquimod (Aldara)[1]
- Excision with adjunctive treatment
- Radiation therapy
- Laser or light therapy

[1]Not FDA approved for this indication.

ONION EXTRACT

Disagreement exists over the effectiveness of onion extract (Mederma) on keloids. At least one study does show it to be better than silicone at reducing the redness and suggests it be used in conjunction with silicone sheets.

PRESSURE

Pressure helps more in preventing keloids, especially the recurrence after excision than in the treatment of an existing keloid. The most common application of this method is in earlobe keloids, where pressure earrings are used as a part of the therapeutic regimen.

BLEOMYCIN

Bleomycin (Blenoxane)[1] has been used successfully to treat keloids by multiple superficial puncture technique and intralesional technique. In the first technique, three applications by multiple superficial puncture are given at 15-day intervals, and a fourth treatment is given 2 months later. With this treatment, 80% showed satisfactory flattening of the keloid, 88% had complete relief of the pruritus, and only 14% had recurrences.

Intralesional Bleomycin, 1 unit/mL diluted with normal saline to 0.1% or less has been reported effective in keloids that have not responded to intralesional steroid treatment.

MITOMYCIN C

Mitomycin C (Mutamycin)[1] inhibits fibroblast proliferation and interferes with the ability of fibroblasts to produce a scar, without causing changes in epithelialization. Studies have shown success with slightly varying protocols, but satisfactory results have been achieved by removing the keloid with shave and aluminum chloride hemostasis, then applying mitomycin C 1 mg/mL for 3 minutes, with application repeated every 3 weeks.

5-FLUOROURACIL

5-Fluorouracil (5-FU) (Adrucil)[1] is a pyrimidine analogue that inhibits the proliferation of fibroblasts and has shown promising results in clinical reports. Intralesional injections are started three per week; as results are seen, injections can be given weekly. 5-FU is used at a concentration of 50 mg/mL and limited to 50 to 150 mg per treatment. It may be mixed with 0.1 mL of triamcinolone acetonide (10 mg/mL) or other combinations to achieve an adjunctive effect of the two drugs. Systemic side effects have not been observed. Local pain and purpura at the injection site, temporary hyperpigmentation, and temporary ulcerations have been reported.

INTERFERON-α-2B

Interferon-α-2b (IFN-α-2b)[1] (Intron A) has antiproliferative and antifibrotic properties. Treatment by IFN-α-2b injected into the keloid twice a week, and triamcinolone injected into the keloid every 2 weeks, has produced satisfaction with results. Debate exists over the superiority of IFN-α-2b as postsurgical monotherapy compared with intralesional steroids, and adverse systemic side effects are possible with interferon, such as flulike symptoms. Further studies are needed.

IMIQUIMOD

Imiquimod 5% (Aldara)[1] induces cytokine production, leading to down-regulation of collagen synthesis. When applied 7 days after suture are removed from keloid excisions and then every other night for 8 weeks, an especially low recurrence of keloids was accomplished in areas of less tension. Imiquimod has also shown promising

[1]Not FDA approved for this indication.

results when applied after shaving of keloids. Side effects are limited to local irritation and dyspigmentation.

EXCISION WITH ADJUVANT THERAPY

Excision alone usually results in a recurrent keloid, which is often larger than the original lesion. Therefore, excision is combined with other modalities to decrease recurrences. Intralesional steroids are used, sometimes several times before the surgery and then after the surgery to try to prevent the recurrence. Pressure earrings are a common adjunct after removal of earlobe keloids.

RADIATION THERAPY

One of the best-documented adjunctive treatments to excision of keloids is x-ray therapy. Several different protocols for administering radiation have been used, and the surgeon should work with the radiation therapist when planning the keloid excision.

LASER THERAPY

Laser and other light modalities are used to treat keloids, with the target being the vasculature of the overgrown scar. These include pulsed dye laser, erbium YAG (yttrium–aluminum–garnet) laser, photodynamic therapy, and intense pulsed light. The intensity, number, and duration of pulses and the number of treatments vary depending on the modality and on the size, shape, and color of the keloid. Patients should be referred to a practitioner well versed in the use of these methodologies.

REFERENCES

Aggarwal H, Saxena A, Lubana PS, et al: Treatment of keloids and hypertrophic scars using bleomycin. J Cosmet Dermatol 2008;7:43-49.
Bailey JNR, Waite AE, Clayton WJ, et al: Application of topical mitomycin C to the base of shave-removed keloid scars to prevent their recurrence. Br J Dermatol 2007;156:682-686.
Berman B, Perez OA, Konda S, et al: A review of the biologic effects, clinical efficacy, and safety of silicone elastomer sheeting for hypertrophic and keloid scar treatment and management. Am Soc Dermatol Surg 2007;33:1291-1302.
Chuangsuwanich A, Gunjittisomram S: The efficacy of 5% imiquimod cream in the prevention of recurrence of excised keloids. J Med Assoc Thai 2007;90:1363-1367.
Hosnuter M, Payasli C, Isikdemir A, et al: The effects of onion extract on hypertrophic and keloid scars. J Wound Care 2007;16:251-254.
Karsai S, Roos S, Hammes S, et al: Pulsed dye laser: What's new in non-vascular lesions? J Eur Acad Dermatol Venereol 2007;21:877-890.
Lee JH, Kim SE, Lee AY: Effects of interferon-alpha 2b on keloid treatment with triamcinolone acetonide intralesional injection. Int J Dermatol 2008;47:183-186.
Nanda S, Reddy BS: Intralesional 5-fluorouracil as a treatment modality of keloids. Dermatol Surg 2004;30:54-56.
Speranza G, Sultanem K, Muanza T: Descriptive study of patients receiving excision and radiotherapy for keloids. Int J Radiat Oncol Biol Phys 2008;71:1465-1469.

Verrucae (Warts)

Method of
Carol Drucker, MD

Warts, verrucous papules caused by more than 100 known subtypes of human papillomavirus (HPV), can occur on any skin or mucosal surface at any age. In some, the HPV is recognized by the host immune system, which mounts a response and the papules spontaneously clear. Some persist, and many patients seek medical

CURRENT DIAGNOSIS

Verrucae Vulgaris

- Verrucous-surfaced papule
- Disrupts normal skin lines
- Pinpoint black or brown dots of thrombosed dermal papillary capillaries
- May be painful to direct pressure

Verrucae Plana (Flat Warts)

- May be multiple, small, flat-topped papules
- Unusually on the face, legs or hands
- Pink or light brown
- Can be linear due to spread from surface scratch

Unusually Large or Recalcitrant Warts, Rule Out:

- Squamous cell carcinoma
- Amelanotic melanoma

treatment for them. Remedies suggested vary from laser surgical destruction to hypnosis, but no one treatment consistently works.

Contagion and Pathophysiology

The HPV virus is inoculated on the skin surface by direct contact with the virus, usually skin to skin. However, HPV is a nonenveloped double-stranded DNA virus; it can live on fomites (inanimate objects) and can be transferred without direct person-to-person contact.

HPV is gaining medical significance as more subtypes are being identified as oncogenic. Two HPV vaccines are available. Cervarix targets HPV-16 and HPV-18, which are responsible for 70% of cervical cancers. Gardasil, a quadrivalent vaccine, targets HPV-16 and HPV-18 plus HPV-6 and HPV-11, types responsible for more than 80% of genital warts. It is also effective in preventing vulvar and vaginal neoplasia. In addition to alleviating painful and unsightly lesions, the treatment of warts is becoming medically important in cancer prevention. Biopsy should be done on larger or unusually recalcitrant warts to rule out squamous cell carcinoma.

Immunosuppressed patients can have increased numbers of warts, multiple subtypes of HPV, increased difficulty eradicating them, and increased cancerous transformation of them, making these patients especially challenging.

Treatment

Whenever there are many treatments available for a disease, there is not one good treatment. Treating warts can be frustrating to physician and patient alike, often requiring a series of painful treatments and typically including recurrences, costly methods, and not always great results. Treatments can be combined and used in conjunction with each other. Few-evidence based studies support any particular treatment. Randomized, controlled studies are needed. The treatment or treatments chosen depend on many factors, including location of the wart, age of the patient, availability of equipment, and other variables. Approach to wart treatment can be considered in three broad categories: physical destruction, stimulation of the immune system, and miscellaneous.

PHYSICAL DESTRUCTION

Liquid Nitrogen

Probably the most common treatment offered for warts, liquid nitrogen ($-196°C$ [$-320°F$]) is sprayed or applied with a cotton swab to

CURRENT THERAPY

Physical Destruction
- Liquid nitrogen
- Curettage and dessication
- Light treatment
- Antimitotics
- Acids
- Cantharidin (Cantharone)[1,2]

Stimulation of the Immune System
- Imiquimod 5% (Aldara)[1]
- Candida antigen,[1] dinitrochlorobenzene[2]
- Interferon[1]

Miscellaneous
- Duct tape occlusion
- Hypnosis
- Home remedies

[1]Not FDA approved for this indication
[2]Not available in the United States

the wart for 30 seconds or longer to freeze the visibly involved tissue and 1 to 2 mm around it. Many repeat this process. As the tissue thaws, there is necrosis of the frozen cells, often blister or blood blister formation, and sloughing and healing of the treated skin in 7 to 10 days. More than one treatment may be needed to eliminate the wart; recurrence is not uncommon. The freeze is variably painful and can leave a scar.

Dessication and Curettage

The wart may be physically removed and the base cauterized for hemostasis and to decrease chances of residual or recurring lesion. Local anesthetic is necessary. If no specimen is needed for pathology, the verrucous papule may be cauterized first, which can allow it to be more easily curetted off the base, with further cauterization and curettage to ensure clearance of all visible lesions. A scar usually results. Local recurrence is possible.

Laser or Light Destruction

Pulsed dye laser (PDL) and Erbium YAG (yttrium–aluminum–garnet) lasers target the vascular structure of the wart and have been successful at removal. The CO_2 laser can also destroy the infected tissue with success. Visible light in two modalities has been used in warts: intense pulsed light (IPL) also targets the vascular supply of the viral lesions. Photodynamic therapy (PDT)[1] has shown varying degrees of success; 5-aminolaevulinic acid is applied, which renders the wart photosensitive, and the wart is exposed to red light. A series of treatments is usually needed for the laser and light therapies, special equipment and expertise using it are necessary, and recurrences are possible.

Antimitotics

Bleomycin (Blenoxane),[1] 5-flurouracil(5-FU [Efudex, Carac]),[1] and tretinoin (Retin A),[1] antimitotic drugs, have all been used against verrucae. Intralesional injection of bleomycin 0.1 mL of 1 unit/mL in 0.1% solution with normal saline can be an effective way to treat recalcitrant warts. The injection can be painful. In days after the injection, the wart usually turns dark and hard, or it can form a blood blister. Within 2 to 3 weeks the necrotic skin can be peeled off. Repeat treatment at 2- to 3-week intervals may be necessary.

[1]Not FDA approved for this indication.

Side effects include Raynaud's phenomenon in a treated digit and nail dystrophy, discoloration, or even loss of the nail after treatment of periungual warts. Bleomycin should be used with caution on fingers and toes.

Topical 5-FU can be applied nightly to warts. Tretinoin can be used alone or can be added to 5-FU to increase effectiveness. Flat warts on the legs, beard area, and hands are especially suited to this approach. Irritation can develop.

Acids

Salicylic acid (e.g., Compound W, Occlusal HP), trichloracetic acid (Tri-Chlor), and bichloracetic acid are used alone or with intermittent paring or freezing and paring to more gradually eradicate either larger warts or warts in stubborn or difficult locations, such as periungual or plantar areas. The number and frequency of treatments depend on the aggressiveness of each treatment. The salicylic acids are available over the counter and can be used by the patient without medical consultation. Trichloroacetic and bichloroacetic acids are used with paring or with paring plus cryosurgery every 2 to 3 weeks by the physician. Treatment can be painful.

Cantharidin

Cantharidin (Cantharone)[1,2] extract of blister beetles is very useful in treatment of warts in children. The physician applies it with precision to the wart and the patient washes it off 1 to 6 hours later. It is painless to apply, but painful blisters can develop within 24 hours. This pain rarely lasts more than 1 day. On return to the office in 3 to 4 weeks, most children do not associate the painful response with the painless application of the liquid and easily allow re-treatment.

STIMULATION OF THE IMMUNE SYSYTEM

Interferon

All interferons[1] have anti-HPV activity, and they have been used for cutaneous and anogenital warts. Partial and total remissions have been achieved with topical, intralesional, and systemic administration.

5% Imiquimod (Aldara)[1]

Used alone or in conjunction with almost any of the other wart treatment modalities, 5% imiquimod cream is an immune modulator that induces interferon production at the site of application, stimulating reaction to the HPV. It can be used in between freezes or paring and acid treatments. On mucosal surfaces, it may be used alone. It is applied 3 nights a week on mucosal surfaces and as often as nightly on thickly keratinized skin.

Candida Antigen and Dinitrochlorobenzene

Multiple warts present a special challenge. *Candida* antigen[1] and dinitrochlorobenzene[2] (DNCB) are useful particularly in this situation.

A sensitizing dose of *Candida* antigen 0.1 mL is placed intradermally on the upper inner arm and in the largest or most assessable wart. The patient is told that the arm will probably get red and then itch and react within a few days to a week. The treated wart might or might not react much with the first treatment. Some physicians prefer to see a reaction on the arm, indicating successful sensitization, before treating the warts. At 4 to 6 weeks, the reaction may be slight in the wart: peeling, decrease in size, drier white surface. Treat as many lesions as possible with 0.1 mL *Candida* antigen again, and repeat every 4 to 6 weeks until all warts have cleared. Later treatments can cause stronger, sometimes painful, reactions in digital or periungual warts due to swelling and pressure of a

[1]Not FDA approved for this indication.
[2]Not available in the United States.

pronounced response. Successful treatment rarely requires injection into each wart.

Similarly, DNCB 2% to 3% is applied to the upper inner arm to sensitize the patient and is then applied to the warts at concentrations of 0.03% to 2% weekly.

MISCELLANEOUS

Duct Tape Occlusion

Duct tape applied over warts to occlude them for periods of 2 to 3 weeks has been reported to induce regression, especially in plantar warts. Some theorize maceration can lead to immune recognition of the virus.

Hypnosis

Hypnosis has worked on warts over the ages. In some cases, referral to a psychiatrist who uses therapeutic hypnosis can help with recalcitrant warts.

Anecdotal Home Remedies

"Rub the wart with a half a potato and bury the potato in the backyard on a full moon night"—and the wart disappears. This and hundreds, of other anecdotal stories abound of successful wart treatments ordered by aunts, uncles, and other wart warriors. It has not worked in my practice.

REFERENCES

Bernard H: Established and potential strategies against papillomavirus infections. J Antimicrob Chemother 2004;53:137-139.
Clifton MM, Johnson SM, Roberson PK, et al: Immunotherapy for recalcitrant warts in children using intralesional candida antigens. Pediatre Dermatol 2003;20:268-271.
Gibbs S, Harvey I: Topical treatments for cutaneous warts. Cochrane Database Syst Rev 2006(1):CD001781.
Price NM: Bleomycin treatment for verrucae. Skinmed 2007;4:166-171.
Schellhaas U, Gerber W, Hammes S, Ockenfels HM: Pulsed dye laser treatment is effective in the treatment of recalcitrant viral warts. Dermatol Surg 2008;34:67-72.
Stender IM, Na R, Fogh H, et al: Photodynamic therapy with 5-aminolaevulinic acid or placebo for recalcitrant foot and hand warts: Randomized double-blind trial. Lancet 2000;355:963-966.
Urman CO, Gottlieb AB: New viral vaccines for dermatologic disease. J Am Acad Dermatol 2008;58:361-370.

Condyloma Acuminatum (Genital Warts)

Method of
Karl R. Beutner, MD, PhD,
and Alice N. Do, DO

Genital warts are the most common manifestation of infection of the genital area with the human papilloma virus (HPV). Genital HPV infection is the most common viral sexually transmitted disease. Approximately 1% of the general population has genital warts at any time.

Proliferation of HIV-infected keratinocytes results in a genital wart. More than 100 genotypes of HPV exist. Low-risk HPV types 6 and 11 cause genital warts. High-risk HPV, most often types 16 and 18, are commonly associated with squamous cell carcinoma (SCC) in situ, also known as bowenoid papulosis or vulvar intraepithelial neoplasia of the external genital area, as well as abnormal Papanicoulaou (Pap) smears including in situ and invasive SCC of the cervix. In immunocompetent hosts, in situ SCC of the skin rarely, if ever, evolves into invasive SCC. Genital skin appears not to be as susceptible to the oncogenic potential of HPV as are the transformation zones of the uterine cervix and the anal canal.

Diagnosis is clinical, so identification of various presentations of genital warts involves understanding the different genital skin types that influence wart morphology. Three types of genital skin are fully keratinized hair-bearing, fully keratinized non–hair-bearing, and partially keratinized non–hair-bearing. The later appears moist and is often mistakenly referred to as mucous membranes. However, there are no mucus glands, and it appears moist because it is partially keratinized.

Treatment can be directed by skin type and wart morphology. The four morphologic types of genital warts are:

1. Cauliflower-type, or condyloma acuminatum
2. Smooth papular type, which are skin-colored, dome-shaped, 1 to 4 mm papules
3. Keratotic type, which may mimic seborrheic keratoses or common warts
4. Flat type, which are slightly raised.

Condyloma acuminatum occurs most commonly on moist, partially keratinized skin, whereas the smooth papular and keratotic types are seen most frequently on fully keratinized areas; the flat type is seen on all types of genital skin.

Genital warts may appear on the penile shaft, scrotum, perineum or perianal areas, labia, vulva, or pubic area, or in the crural folds. They can also be found in the urethra or bladder or in the oral cavity. The oral cavity should also be examined in patients being evaluated for genital warts.

Biopsy is usually unnecessary to confirm a clinical diagnosis of external genital warts. However, a biopsy should be considered when lesions are atypical, pigmented, ulcerated, indurated, or fixed to underlying tissue; fail to respond to treatment or worsen during treatment; frequently recur; exhibit individual (noncoalescent) warts larger than 1 cm in diameter; or are suspicious for malignancy. Biopsy should also be considered when diagnosis is unclear.

Acetowhitening to aid in diagnosis of external genital warts is no longer recommended because it lacks adequate specificity and sensitivity.

Differential diagnosis includes lichen planus, skin tags, seborrheic keratoses, molluscum contagiosum, condyloma latum, pearly penile papules, sebaceous glands, lichen nitidus, Crohn's disease, and SCC in situ.

Treatment

Genital warts may spontaneously resolve or persist. Discuss expectations of therapy with patients. The goal is to eliminate symptoms, namely visible wart lesions, rather than to address HPV infection. Rather than a treatment, a course of therapy is required to achieve a wart-free state. It is unknown whether wart elimination will decrease or eliminate the patient's infectivity to current or future sexual partners. Even after proper treatment, recurrence is due to latent HPV in the surrounding normal tissue, and not necessarily due to reinfection. Once two individuals are infected with the same HPV type, they will not continue to reinfect one another. Any given treatment carries a 40% to 75% change of clearing and a 25% to 50% chance of recurrence. Recurrence is responsible for a prolonged course for the patient. Treatment failure is commonly caused by improper selection or use of a therapeutic modality. At the present time, all treatments are comparable in effectiveness.

Choice of Treatment

Selection of treatment is influenced by wart morphology, anatomic site, total wart area, wart count, clinician's experience, and patient

CURRENT DIAGNOSIS

Diagnosis of genital warts requires their identification on physical exam. The clinician should become adept at recognizing the various morphologies of genital warts, which are influenced by the overlying genital skin type.

External Wart Morphology	Description	Skin Type
Condyloma acuminatum	Coalescent cauliflower-like plaques	Moist/partially keratinized
Smooth papular	Skin-colored, dome-shaped, 1 to 4 mm papules	Fully keratinized
Keratotic	Discrete, warty papules	Fully keratinized
Flat type	Slightly raised, flat-topped papules	Moist/partially keratinized or fully keratinized

CURRENT THERAPY

Treatment modalities can be divided into either provider-administered or patient-applied therapies. The choice of therapy will depend on skin type, wart quantity, and location.

Treatment	Mechanism	Good Choice for	Poor Choice for	Procedure
Provider administered				
Cryotherapy	Direct tissue destruction	• Small, flat, few warts • Dry or moist warts • Pregnancy OK	• Large wart areas (> 10 cm^2)	• Liquid nitrogen applied on a large, loosely wound piece of cotton on a wooden stick; or with a cryoprobe, by the spray technique • Freeze the wart and 1- to 2-mm surrounding border
Podophyllin resin	Arrest in mitosis leading to tissue necrosis	• Moist warts	• Dry wart areas • Do not exceed 10 cm^2 treatment area • Not for pregnancy	• Use a cotton tip and apply a thin layer to wart and allow to air-dry before the patient assumes a normal anatomic position • Leave on overnight and avoid washing, bathing, and sexual contact • Repeat treatment 1 week later, as needed
TCA (Tri-Chlor)[1]	Chemical coagulation of wart proteins	• Small, moist, few warts • Pregnancy OK	• Large wart areas (> 10 cm^2) • Dry warts	• Apply sparingly to the lesion, being careful not to let the solution run onto normal skin • Repeat weekly or every other week, as needed
Surgery	Direct removal of lesions	• Large or small treatment areas • Rectal lesions OK • Pregnancy OK	• Bleeding disorders	• Superficial tangential scissor excision, electrodesiccation, hot cautery, curettage, or CO$_2$ laser may be used
Patient applied				
Podofilox (Condylox)	Arrest in mitosis → tissue necrosis	• Moist warts	• Do not exceed 10 cm^2 treatment area • Not for pregnancy • Poor compliance	• Apply bid for 3 days following by a 4-day treatment-free period • Repeat weekly cycles four to six times, as needed
Imiquimod (Aldara)	Immunomodulator	• Moist warts	• Large wart areas (> 10 cm^2) • Dry warts • Poor compliance	• Apply every other night on moist warts or intertriginous areas, or every night on dry warts • May be used for up to 16 weeks, as tolerated

[1]Not FDA approved for this indication.
Abbreviations: TCA = trichloroacetic acid.

preference. Not all patients respond equally well to all modalities. Proper matching of patient with modality will usually shorten treatment duration. Pregnancy and immunosuppression are associated with larger and more numerous genital wart lesions. Certain treatment modalities are more appropriate in pregnancy. Immunosuppressed patients do not respond as well to therapy and have a high recurrence rate. These patients have a higher incidence of SCC. Have a plan or set protocol, particularly when a limited number of modalities are available. In general, if after three to four treatments with a given therapy a clinically significant response is not seen, or if after six treatments no clearance is achieved, the treatment modality should be changed and the diagnosis should be re-evaluated.

TREATMENT MODALITIES

Current treatments are divided into provider-administered and patient-applied therapies. Provider-administered therapies include cryotherapy, podophyllin resin (Podocon-25), trichloroacetic acid (Tri-Chlor)[1], and surgery. Patient-applied therapies allow the patient greater control and include podofilox (Condylox) and imiquimod (Aldara). However, these require good compliance and that the patient be able to view and reach the warts.

PROVIDER-ADMINISTERED THERAPIES

Cryotherapy

Cryotherapy works well for small, flat, few warts in dry or moist areas. It can be used on the penile shaft and vulva with little scarring. It can be used during pregnancy. It is not recommended for large wart areas, which can be quite painful and cause wound-care issues. A small, tightly wound cotton swab (Q-tip) that holds inadequate amounts of liquid nitrogen cannot effectively freeze a wart. Apply liquid nitrogen with a large, loosely wound piece of cotton on a wooden stick or with a cryoprobe.

A few small warts can be frozen without an anesthetic. Patients with more warts should be offered local anesthesia, with either injection of 1% lidocaine[1] or topical application of a eutectic mixture of 2.5% lidocaine and 2.5% prilocaine (EMLA cream).[1] Freeze the wart and 1- to 2-mm surrounding border. For larger warts, two freeze-thaw cycles are effective. How *hard* to freeze the warts can be learned with experience.

Cryotherapy requires proper training. Complications are rare but inexperienced clinicians often underfreeze areas, reducing efficacy. Overfreezing increases pain and the probability of scarring and other complications. Warn patients about post-treatment pain and blistering.

Podophyllin Resin

Podophyllin resin (Podofin, Podocon-25, Podofilm) is from the plant species *Podophyllum peltatum* or *Podophyllum emodii*. This resin contains podofilox (podophyllotoxin), 4-dimethylpodophyllotoxin, α-peltatum, and β-peltatum, which cause cellular mitotic arrest and lead to tissue necrosis. It is a good choice for moist warts and up to a 10 cm^2 surface area. It is ineffective in dry areas, such as the scrotum, penile shaft, and labia majora.

Podophyllin resin lacks a standardized preparation, but it is commonly used as a 10% to 25% solution in tincture of benzoin. Use a cotton tip and apply a thin layer directly to the wart and allow to air dry before the patient assumes a normal anatomic position. Traditionally, patients were advised to wash off podophyllin 2 to 4 hours after application, but benzoin is water insoluble and cannot be removed simply with soap and water. Another ill-advised but not uncommon practice is to create a *barrier* around the wart with Vaseline or K-Y jelly, and apply podophyllin resin to the central wart. Body temperature thins the barrier, which mixes with the podophyllin resin, and spreads over the entire area, creating an impressive irritant reaction. I advise patients to leave the podophyllin resin on overnight and avoid washing, bathing, or sexual contact until the next day. Local side effects include erythema, pain, and irritation. Systemic side effects are caused by increased toxic absorption and are associated with large treatment area (>10 cm^2) or allowing the resin to absorb for an extended time. Avoid podophyllin resin in pregnancy.

Trichloroacetic Acid (Tri-Chlor)[1]

Trichloroacetic acid ([TCA] Tri-Chlor)[1] chemically coagulates warts and adjacent skin. Use for small, few, moist warts. TCA[1] can be used during pregnancy. Although 30% to 70% solutions are employed, the optimal concentration is undetermined. Use extreme caution with the higher concentrations, which can be highly caustic. Apply sparingly to lesions, being careful not to let the solution run onto normal skin. Treatment can be repeated weekly, or every other week, as needed. TCA[1] can be neutralized, if needed, with soap and sodium bicarbonate.

Surgery

Surgery renders the patient wart free with a single visit. It is a good choice for limited or large treatment areas. There is no clearly superior surgical modality. Selection of a surgical approach depends on clinician experience and availability of equipment. Good results can be achieved with superficial tangential scissors, electrodesiccation, hot cautery, curettage, or CO_2 laser.

PATIENT-APPLIED THERAPIES

Podofilox

The major active lignin in podophyllin resin is podofilox, available as a 0.5% solution or gel (Condylox). Apply to warts twice daily for 3 days followed by a treatment-free period of 4 days. Repeat this cycle four to six times to achieve wart clearance. A maximum of 10 cm^2 should be treated, and podofilox should be avoided in pregnancy.

Imiquimod

Imiquimod (Aldara) is a 5% cream, applied three times weekly at bedtime to moist wart areas. Dry and nonintertriginous areas may respond better to daily application. It can be used for up to 16 weeks. As imiquimod stimulates an inflammatory response, however, local irritation, burning, and ulceration are expected side effects and are similar to those seen with other modalities.

5-Fluorouracil

5-Fluorouracil creams (Carac, Effudex),[1] used previously for genital warts, are no longer recommended because of side effects, uproven efficacy, and the availability of other treatments.

Transmission and Prevention

HPV is a sexually transmitted disease (STD). Educate patients to tell sexual partners that they have this infection. Condoms may decrease transmission but do not completely prevent infection. Asymptomatic partners can harbor a subclinical infection, and examination for genital warts is appropriate if lesions are suspected. It is unknown whether treatment of genital wart lesions eliminates infectivity. Discuss the oncogenic potential of HPV types associated with bowenoid papulosis. Women with external genital warts or whose male partners have lesions should have a Pap smear and remain in the system for monitoring for cervical cancer. Investigations for other STDs should be done if suspected.

Acquiring an STD carries a negative social stigma and emotional trauma. Patients often fear discovery and rejection and feel guilty and victimized. They view themselves as less sexually desirable, enjoy sex

---

[1]Not FDA approved for this indication.

less, and have concerns about transmission. Teaching and educational materials are available from the American Social Health Association (1-919-361-8422).

REFERENCES

Beutner KR, Richwald GA, Wiley DJ, et al: External genital warts: Report of the American Medical Association consensus conference. Clin Infect Dis 1998;27:796-806.

Beutner KR, Wiley DJ, Douglas JM, et al: Genital warts and their treatment. Clin Infect Dis 1999;28(Suppl 1):S37-S56.

Habif TP: Sexually transmitted viral infections. In Hodgson S, Cook L (eds): Clinial Dermatology, A Color Guide to Diagnosis and Therapy, 4th ed, Philadelphia: Mosby, 2004, pp 336-342.

Odom RB, James WD, Berger TG: Viral diseases. In Fathman EM, Geisel EB, Salmo A (eds): Andrews' Diseases of the Skin, Clinical Dermatology, 9th ed. Saunders: WB Philadelphia, 2000, pp 541-591.

Melanocytic Nevi

Method of
*Jane M. Grant-Kels, MD, and
Michael Murphy, MD*

Melanocytic nevi, or moles, are benign neoplasms composed of melanocytes. Melanocytic nevus cells are derived from melanocytes. Compared with melanocytes, nevus cells are not dendritic, are larger, and contain more abundant cytoplasm, often with coarse melanin granules. Nevus cells tend to aggregate into groups or nests. Melanocytic nevi are extremely common and can be found on almost everyone, anywhere on the cutaneous surface. This article discusses the most common types of melanocytic nevi: acquired melanocytic nevi, recurrent melanocytic nevi, halo melanocytic nevi, congenital melanocytic nevi, blue nevi, Spitz nevi, and dysplastic melanocytic nevi.

Acquired Melanocytic Nevi

Acquired melanocytic nevi are subdivided into junctional, compound, and intradermal types based on the location of the nevus cells. By definition, these lesions are not present at birth but can begin to appear in early childhood, usually after 6 to 12 months of age. Peak ages of appearance of melanocytic nevi are 2 to 3 years of age in children and 11 to 18 years in adolescents. Although nevi can appear at any age, it is relatively unusual for new melanocytic nevi to develop in middle-aged or older adults. With time, nevi can spontaneously regress. Consequently, patients in their ninth decade of life usually demonstrate few melanocytic nevi. An average white adult has 10 to 40 melanocytic nevi, but African Americans have far fewer, averaging only 2 to 8.

The number and location of melanocytic nevi have been shown to be associated with sun exposure, immunologic factors, and genetics. Consequently, melanocytic nevi are most numerous on the sun-exposed skin of the head, neck, trunk, and extremities, but they are only rarely found on covered areas such as the buttocks, female breasts, and scalp. Evidence suggests that patients with an increased number of melanocytic nevi (>50) might have an increased risk of melanoma.

Melanocytic nevi appear in a sequential fashion. Junctional melanocytic nevi arise during childhood as flat, dark macules. Histologically, an increase in single or nests of melanocytes are located at the dermoepidermal junction. With time, some of the junctional nests of melanocytes migrate into the dermis (compound melanocytic nevi). Clinically, compound melanocytic nevi are elevated and less heavily pigmented than junctional melanocytic nevi. Ultimately, all of the nevus cells migrate into the dermis (intradermal melanocytic nevi), resulting in the development of a tan or skin-colored dome-shaped papule. Melanocytic nevi can be flat or elevated and even polypoid, papillomatous, or verrucous and can demonstrate a range of color from skin-tone to black, but they are characteristically uniform in color, symmetrical, well marginated, and usually smaller than 6 mm in diameter.

All melanocytic lesions of clinical concern should be examined with a dermatoscope, a hand-held instrument with a magnified lens and a light source similar to an ophthalmoscope. This instrument allows evaluation of colors and microstructures not visible to the naked eye, helps distinguish whether pigmented lesions are melanocytic or nonmelanocytic, and helps distinguish whether melanocytic pigmented lesions are likely to be malignant. Used by an experienced dermatologist with proper training, the dermatoscope improves diagnostic accuracy by 20% to 30%.

It is unnecessary to surgically remove all melanocytic nevi because they are benign neoplasms of melanocytes. However, indications for removal include ABCD (*a*symmetry, irregular *b*order, variegation or change in *c*olor, or change in *d*iameter), symptoms (e.g., pruritus), evidence of inflammation or irritation, cosmetic issues, and patient anxiety. Melanocytic nevi on acral, genital, or scalp skin that appear benign do not require surgical removal. Shave biopsies are appropriate therapy for lesions considered clinically benign. However, if a lesion is being removed because of concern regarding the possibility of malignancy, an excisional biopsy (biopsy of choice) or incisional biopsy (including punch or deep scoop) that extends to the subcutaneous tissue is indicated. All melanocytic lesions should be submitted to a dermatopathologist for histologic review. A history of recent sun exposure or trauma should be conveyed to the dermatopathologist because such external trauma can induce reactive atypical histologic findings.

Recurrent Melanocytic Nevi

Recurrent melanocytic nevi are melanocytic nevi that have previously been incompletely removed (either iatrogenically or traumatically) and have recurred weeks to months later. Irregular brown pigmentation is clinically noted within the scar site. If the original biopsy demonstrated a benign melanocytic nevus, re-treatment is unnecessary unless the aforementioned indications are present. However, these nevi can demonstrate pseudomelanomatous histologic features. Therefore, if the repigmented area is excised, the dermatopathologist should be notified of the clinical history and, if possible, the slides from the original biopsy should be obtained and reviewed to ensure that the lesion is not histologically misdiagnosed.

Halo (Melanocytic) Nevi

Halo (melanocytic) nevi are melanocytic nevi in which a white rim or halo has developed. This phenomenon most commonly occurs around compound or intradermal nevi and is histologically associated with a dense, bandlike inflammatory infiltrate. The white halo area is histologically characterized by diminished or absent melanocytes and melanin. Approximately 20% of patients with halo nevi also exhibit vitiligo.

Although a halo can develop around many lesions in the skin, the most important differential diagnosis is between a halo nevus and melanoma with a halo. The halo and the central melanocytic nevus of halo nevi are symmetrical, round or oval, and sharply demarcated. Halo nevi most commonly occur in adolescence as an isolated event, but approximately 25% to 50% of affected persons have two or more.

The clinical course of halo nevi is variable. With time, the halo can repigment while the central nevus persists. Alternatively, the melanocytic nevus can regress completely and leave a depigmented macule that can persist or repigment over months or years.

Halo nevi do not require surgical excision unless atypical clinical features suggest the possibility of an atypical melanocytic lesion. It is

CURRENT DIAGNOSIS

Benign Melanocytic Lesions

- Symmetrical
- Sharply demarcated border
- Uniform color
- Diameter usually ≤6mm and stable

Malignant Melanocytic Lesions

- Asymmetrical
- Poorly circumscribed border
- Variegated in color
- Diameter often ≥10mm and increasing (changing or evolving)

CURRENT THERAPY

- Acquired melanocytic nevus: No treatment is required unless the lesion is asymmetrical or has an irregular border, change or variegated in color, or change in diameter. Symptomatic lesions should be biopsied.
- Recurrent melanocytic nevus: No treatment required if the original biopsy was benign.
- Halo melanocytic nevus: No treatment, but excision is recommended if atypical clinical features are identified.
- Congenital melanocytic nevus: Removal based on melanoma risk, cosmetics, and functional outcome. If not excised, routine follow-up with the use of photography, dermoscopy, and computer assistance is recommended.
- Blue nevus: No treatment, but excision is recommended if atypical clinical features are identified
- Spitz nevus: If clinically unusual, a complete excisional biopsy is recommended.
- Dysplastic nevus: If only one lesion is present, excision is recommended. Patients with many dysplastic nevi require close surveillance with removal of any lesion suspicious for melanoma.

advisable (particularly in adults, in whom halo nevi are less common) to perform a complete cutaneous examination with and without the aid of a Wood's lamp to rule out any associated atypical pigmented or regressed lesions. All patients should be warned to use sunscreens or protective clothing because of the increased risk of sunburn in the depigmented halo region.

Congenital Melanocytic Nevi

By definition, congenital melanocytic nevi are present at birth. Arbitrarily, they have been classified into small (<1.5 cm), medium (1.5-20 cm) and large (>20 cm) lesions. Terms such as *bathing trunk* or *garment-type* nevi refer to CMN that cover a significant portion of the cutaneous surface.

The approximate incidence of small congenital nevi is 1% of all live births. Large congenital nevi are rare and reported in only 1 in 20,000 births. Histologically, some congenital nevi have distinguishing histologic features (melanocytic nevi cells that extend into the deeper dermis as well as the subcutis and melanocytic nevi cells arranged periadnexally, angiocentrically, within nerves, and interposed between collagen bundles). However, these features have been identified in some acquired melanocytic nevi and are absent in some congenital nevi (especially small ones). In addition, the history obtained from the patient or their parents is often inaccurate. Consequently, it can be very difficult in some cases to distinguish a small congenital nevus from an acquired nevus.

Congenital nevi can give rise to dermal or subcutaneous nodular melanocytic proliferations. The vast majority of these lesions, particularly in the neonatal period, are biologically benign, despite a worrisome clinical presentation and atypical histologic features. Genetic analysis has shown that benign melanocytic proliferations within congenital nevi express aberrations qualitatively and quantitatively different from those seen in melanoma.

The primary significance of congenital nevi is related to the potential risk for progression to melanoma. Essentially, the larger the nevus, the greater the risk of progression to melanoma. Historically, even small nevi were estimated to exhibit a lifetime melanoma risk of 5%. However, recent prospective studies suggest that small and medium congenital nevi are associated with a low risk that may approximate the risk of acquired nevi. Conversely, large congenital nevi have a lifetime risk of melanomatous progression of approximately 6.3%. Up to two thirds of melanomas that arise in these giant congenital nevi have a nonepidermal origin, thus making clinical observation for malignant change difficult. Approximately 50% of these melanomas occur in the first 5 years of life, 60% in the first decade, and 70% before 20 years of age. Patients with large congenital nevi, especially those that involve posterior axial locations (head, neck, back, or buttocks) and are associated with satellite congenital nevi, are at increased risk for neurocutaneous melanosis (melanosis of the leptomeninges).

For large congenital nevi that involve a posterior axial location, magnetic resonance imaging (MRI) is indicated. If clinical symptoms or MRI indicate neurocutaneous melanosis, excision of the large nevus should be postponed until 2 years of age (the median age of neurologic symptoms). Patients with neurocutaneous melanosis have a greater than 50% mortality rate within 3 years. The risk and morbidity of multiple, staged excisions of a large congenital nevus might not be appropriate in these patients. All other large congenital nevi should be excised as soon as general anesthesia is considered a relatively safe event. Other issues that need to be considered before undertaking staged excisions include cosmetic issues, functional outcome, and psychosocial issues. The staged excisions are usually started after 6 months of age for nevi on the trunk and extremities and later for those on the scalp to allow closure of the fontanelle. If removal is not undertaken, follow-up with monthly self-examination, photography, dermoscopy, confocal laser microscopy, and computer assistance are recommended.

For small congenital nevi, routine excision is not always recommended because the risk of melanoma is lower, and if it occurs, it usually arises within the epidermis after puberty. If the lesions are not excised, follow-up by alternating visits to a dermatologist and primary care physician along with serial photography are indicated. Inasmuch as small congenital nevi typically enlarge with the growth of the child and can change in appearance with time, educating families on benign, predictable changes in contradistinction to potentially alarming changes is extremely important. If a lesion enlarges or changes suddenly or if parental anxiety or cosmetic issues arise, excision should then be contemplated for even small congenital nevi. Elective excision is best done when the patient is approximately 8 years old. With the use of topical anesthetic cream EMLA (eutectic mixture of local anesthetics: 2.5% lidocaine plus 2.5% prilocaine) or topical 4% lidocaine (ELA-Max), children of this age are usually cooperative and unscathed by the procedure.

Blue Nevi

Blue nevi occur primarily on the face and scalp, in addition to the dorsal surfaces of the hands and feet, as well-circumscribed, slightly raised or dome-shaped bluish papules that are usually less than 1 cm in diameter. Although these lesions are usually acquired in childhood and adolescence, rare congenital lesions have been reported. Histologically, blue nevi demonstrate a combination of intradermal spindle or dendritic melanin-pigmented melanocytes and melanophages with dermal fibrosis. The blue appearance of these lesions is a function of both the depth of the melanin in the dermis and the Tyndall phenomenon: longer wavelengths of light penetrate the deep dermis and are absorbed by the lesional melanin, and shorter wavelengths (e.g., blue) are reflected back. Blue nevi that are clinically stable and that do not demonstrate atypical features do not require removal.

Spitz Nevi

Nevi of large spindle and epithelioid cells (Spitz nevi) are relatively uncommon. In Australia, an annual incidence of 1.4 per 100,000 people has been recorded. Most Spitz nevi are noted in children and adolescents: One third occur before the age of 10 years, one third between the ages 10 to 20 years, and one third past the age of 20 years. Rarely, lesions can occur in patients older than 40 years. Seven percent of SN have been reported as congenital.

Four clinical types of SN are recognized: light-colored soft Spitz nevi that can resemble a pyogenic granuloma; light-colored hard Spitz nevi that can resemble a dermatofibroma; dark Spitz nevi that must be distinguished from other melanocytic lesions, including melanoma; and disseminated or agminated Spitz nevi. Spitz nevi are typically smaller than 6 mm in diameter and dome shaped, with a smooth pink or tan surface and sharp borders. Although they can occur anywhere on the cutaneous surface except mucosal or palmoplantar areas, they are most commonly seen on the face (especially in children) and legs (especially in women). Spitz nevi in adults are usually more heavily melanized than those in children.

Dermatoscopy or epiluminescent microscopy (examination of lesions with enhanced light and a dermatoscope) helps magnify the images in vivo and can assist in establishing the clinical diagnosis of some Spitz nevi. Histologically, the lesion can demonstrate features similar to those of melanoma, which earned the lesion its original designation by Sophie Spitz as a melanoma of childhood. Because Spitz nevi can be histologically difficult to distinguish from melanoma, if a biopsy is performed on a lesion because of parental, cosmetic, or transitional concern, complete excision with clear margins is recommended. Spitz nevi show fundamental genomic differences compared with MM, consistent with the generally benign behavior of these lesions. Spitz nevi typically demonstrate no or only a very restricted set of chromosomal aberrations (i.e., 11p gain in a subset of Spitz nevi).

Dysplastic Melanocytic Nevi

Dysplastic melanocytic nevi, or Clark's nevi, or nevi with architectural disorder and cytologic atypia can occur sporadically as an isolated lesion or lesions or as part of a familial autosomal dominant syndrome. When such lesions occur sporadically, they are considered a marker for a patient who is at increased risk of melanoma (6% risk versus an approximate 0.6% risk in the normal white population in the United States). In association with a family history or personal past medical history of melanoma, patients with dysplastic melanocytic nevi should be considered to have a significant risk of melanoma. One first-degree family member with melanoma is associated with a lifetime risk of melanoma of 15% for the patient with dysplastic melanocytic nevi. Two or more first-degree family members with melanoma place a patient with dysplastic melanocytic nevi at a lifetime risk of developing melanoma that approaches 100%. Less commonly, dysplastic melanocytic nevi can progress to melanoma. Such progression has been documented by serial photography. However, these data are confounded by the fact that clinically and histologically, dysplastic melanocytic nevi may be difficult to distinguish from an early melanoma.

Dysplastic melanocytic nevi are clinically distinguished from common acquired melanocytic nevi by a diameter usually larger than 6 mm, irregular border, asymmetry, and variable color with possible shades of brown, red, pink and black; DMN can be flat with or without a raised center (fried egg appearance). The lesions begin to appear in mid childhood and early adolescence. New lesions can appear throughout the patient's life. In addition to the back and extremities, these lesions can occur on sun-protected areas, including the scalp, buttocks, and female breasts. Dysplastic melanocytic nevi can be few or numerous, with hundreds of lesions.

Histologically, dysplastic melanocytic nevi show both architectural disorder: extension of the junctional component beyond the dermal component (shouldering); bridging between adjacent rete ridges; papillary dermal concentric and lamellar fibroplasia; and a variable lymphocytic infiltrate with vascular ectasias. They also show cytologic atypia of melanocytes: increased nuclear size, hyperchromasia, dispersion or variation of nuclear chromatin patterns, and presence of nucleoli. Although there is some discordance in the histologic grading of dysplastic melanocytic nevi among expert dermatopathologists, there is some evidence to support the use in clinical practice of a two-tier grading system: Grade A are dysplastic melanocytic nevi with mild or moderate cytologic atypia and grade B are dysplastic melanocytic nevi with severe cytologic atypia. Firstly, the probability of a having personal history of melanoma in any given dysplastic melanocytic nevi patient correlates with the grade of cytologic atypia in dysplastic melanocytic nevi. In addition, the presence of severe cytologic atypia in dysplastic melanocytic nevi correlates with a significantly greater risk of melanoma development (19.7%) compared with moderate (8.1%) or mild (5.7%) cytologic atypia.

Management of these patients is difficult. Dysplastic melanocytic nevi are not uncommon. Reportedly, as many as 4.6 million people in the United States have one or more sporadic dysplastic melanocytic nevi. Familial dysplastic melanocytic nevi are estimated to involve 50,000 patients in the United States. The risk of melanoma for these patients is probably on a continuum and correlated with their family history of melanoma or dysplastic melanocytic nevi, personal history of melanoma, number of acquired melanocytic and dysplastic lesions, and history of sun exposure. Removal of all dysplastic melanocytic nevi would be inappropriate inasmuch as the chance of any single lesion becoming malignant is small.

Management includes patient education and total body photography for comparison at future skin examinations. Patients should avoid the sun and use sun screens and protective clothing. These patients should have regular biannual or quarterly examinations of the entire integument, including the oral, genital, and perianal mucosa, the scalp, and an ophthalmologic examination. Comparison with the previous total body photographs and use of the dermatoscope can be helpful. Any lesions that are suspicious for melanoma should be excised. Examination of first-degree family members (parents, siblings, and children) of patients with melanoma or dysplastic melanocytic nevi is recommended to identify other persons at high risk.

REFERENCES

Arumi-Uria M, McNutt NS, Finnerty B: Grading of atypia in nevi: correlation with melanoma risk. Mod Pathol 2003;16:764-771.

Bauer J, Bastian BC: Distinguishing melanocytic nevi from melanoma by DNA copy number changes: Comparative genomic hybridization as a research and diagnostic tool. Dermatol Ther 2006;19:40-49.

Bett BJ: Large or multiple congenital melanocytic nevi: Occurrence of cutaneous melanoma in 1008 persons. J Am Acad Dermatol 2005;52:793-797.

de Snoo FA, Kroon MW, Bergman W, et al: From sporadic atypical nevi to familial melanoma: Risk analysis for melanoma in sporadic atypical nevus patients. J Am Acad Dermatol 2007;56:748-752.

Ferrara G, Soyer HP, Malvehy J, et al: The many faces of blue nevus: A clinicopathologic study. J Cutan Pathol 2007;34:543-551.

Krengel S, Hauschild A, Schafer T: Melanoma risk in congenital melanocytic naevi: a systematic review. Br J Dermatol 2006;155:1-8.

Naeyaert JM, Brochez L: Dysplastic nevi. N Engl J Med 2003;349:2233-2240.

Park HK, Leonard DD, Arrington JH 3rd, Lund HZ: Recurrent melanocytic nevi: Clinical and histologic review of 175 cases. J Am Acad Dermatol 1987;17:285-290.

Tromberg J, Bauer B, Benvenuto-Andrade C, Marghoob AA: Congenital melanocytic nevi needing treatment. Dermatol Ther 2005;18:136-150.

Melanoma

Method of
*Jennifer L. DeFazio, MD, and
Ashfaq A. Marghoob, MD*

Melanoma, a malignancy derived from melanocytes, is the sixth most common cancer in the United States. Although 95% of melanomas originate on the skin and mucous membranes, primary melanoma can also develop in extracutaneous sites such as the eyes, gastrointestinal tract, and leptomeninges.

Epidemiology

It is estimated that in 2008, in the United States there were 62,480 new cases of invasive melanoma, 54,020 new cases of in situ melanoma, and 8420 deaths from melanoma. The age-adjusted incidence of melanoma is approximately 23 per 100,000 men and 15 per 100,000 women. Although the incidence of virtually every other malignancy in the United States is declining, the incidence of melanoma continues to increase. The lifetime risk of developing invasive melanoma for a person born in 2007 is estimated to be 1 in 49 for men and 1 in 73 for women, which is 30 times higher than the risk for a person born in 1930.

Melanoma often strikes young to middle-aged persons. The mean age at diagnosis is approximately 52 years, which is approximately 10 years younger as compared with the other common cancers. It is more common in fair-skinned persons, with white populations having an approximate 10- to 20-fold increased risk for cutaneous melanoma compared with black populations.

Risk Factors

The risk factors for developing cutaneous melanoma are shown in Box 1. The risk factors can be classified into environmental factors, genetic factors, and host factors.

Diagnosis

Early detection remains the cornerstone in improving outcome. The education of the public and health care professionals about the

BOX 1 Risk Factors for Melanoma

Environmental Factors
Residing at a low latitude or in a sunny climate
Intense intermittent UV exposure (including tanning salon use)
Sunburns
Immunosuppression

Genetic Factors
Skin type: Tans poorly, burns easily
Fair skin, blond or red hair, light eyes
Personal history of skin cancer or family history of melanoma
Xeroderma pigmentosum

Phenotypic Factors (Genes and Environment)
Evidence of chronic sun damage: Freckles, solar elastosis, keratoses
Clinically atypical or histologically dysplastic nevi
Increased total number of nevi

CURRENT DIAGNOSIS

- ABCDEs of melanoma include:
  - A: Asymmetry of the lesion
  - B: Border irregularity
  - C: Color variation within a lesion
  - D: Diameter ≥6 mm (pencil eraser head)
  - E: Evolving or changing characteristics of a lesion
- Other signs and symptoms: bleeding, pruritus, ulceration, or ugly duckling sign (lesion that looks different from surrounding nevi)
- Dermoscopy can aid in the early detection of melanoma
- Suspected lesions should be biopsied with a full thickness excision

warning signs of melanoma has contributed significantly to the timely detection of most melanomas. In fact, more than 80% of melanomas are diagnosed while localized to the skin, with survival rates of 99%.

The patient's history is very important in helping to detect skin cancer. Patient perception of new, changing, and symptomatic lesions should prompt close examination. The visual examination of the entire cutaneous surface remains paramount in helping to detect melanoma. Many melanomas display characteristics of *a*symmetry, *b*order irregularity, *c*olor variability, and a large *d*iameter (≥6 mm). Unfortunately, most nodular and amelanotic melanomas lack these characteristic ABCD features. However, these melanomas can be detected based on change. In fact, change, which includes new, changing, and *e*volving lesions, is the most sensitive indicator of melanoma. These five characteristics are conveniently referred to as the *ABCDEs* of melanoma.

The *ugly duckling sign* relies on the concept that most nevi in one person will resemble each other. A lesion that deviates from this pattern can be a harbinger for melanoma and should alert the physician to further evaluate the lesion. Comparative recognition strategies such as comparing lesions with previously obtained baseline images (i.e., total body photography) has enhanced our ability to detect subtle changes within lesions that prove to be melanoma. Visual aids, such as a magnifying glass, may be used to help evaluate skin lesions. A great advance in our ability to recognize the primary morphology of melanoma and differentiate it from other skin lesions is dermoscopy.

The dermatoscope is a hand-held instrument with a transilluminating light source and a 10× magnification lens. It allows the observer to visualize structures in the epidermis and papillary dermis that are otherwise not visible to the unaided eye. Criteria have been developed to aid in the diagnosis of both benign and malignant lesions. The features commonly seen in melanoma are listed in Box 2. It has been well documented that experienced dermoscopists have an increased sensitivity, specificity, and diagnostic accuracy for melanoma. This results in fewer melanomas being missed, while at the same time avoiding the unnecessary biopsy of many benign lesions.

BOX 2 Dermoscopic Structures Commonly Seen in Melanoma

Atypical network, branched streaks
Streaks, pseudopods
Atypical dots, globules
Negative network
Off-center blotch
Blue-white veil, peppering over macular areas (regression structures)
Blue-white veil over raised areas
Atypical vascular structures
Peripheral light brown structureless areas

If melanoma is suspected, a full-thickness excisional biopsy of the entire lesion with narrow margins is the preferred biopsy method. The lesion should be sent for histopathologic assessment, and the pathologist should be requested to step-section the lesion. A full-thickness biopsy that is adequately step-sectioned allows accurate measurement of tumor thickness, a critical factor for management and prognosis.

Subtypes of Melanoma

The four most common subtypes of melanoma are superficial spreading, nodular, acral lentiginous, and lentigo maligna melanoma. Each has a different etiology, growth rate, and set of mutations.

Superficial spreading is the most common subtype, accounting for approximately 70% of all melanomas diagnosed. This subtype of melanoma is often associated with a precursor dysplastic nevus or congenital melanocytic nevus. Superficial spreading melanoma is most often found on the back in men and the back and legs in women.

Nodular melanoma is the second most common subtype of melanoma. In comparison, invasive superficial spreading and lentigo maligna melanomas vertical growth rates were estimated to be less than 0.14 mm/month.

Acral lentiginous melanoma by definition occurs on the soles, palms, or subungual area. Lentigo maligna melanoma is most commonly found on chronically sun-exposed skin of the head and neck in older persons. Lentigo maligna melanomas usually develop over a course of many years.

Other less-common variants of melanoma include amelanotic, desmoplastic, mucosal, and verrucous melanoma.

Staging and Prognosis

As mentioned earlier, tumor thickness is a strong prognostic indicator and is one of the main factors influencing staging, treatment, and management. Breslow thickness is the depth of a melanoma measured from the granular layer of the epidermis to the deepest component of the tumor. The Clark classification reports a tumor's anatomic level of invasion into tissue. Level I tumor is confined to the epidermis. At level II, the tumor begins to invade the papillary dermis, at level III the tumor fills the papillary dermis, at level IV it invades the reticular dermis, and level V is invasion of the subcutaneous tissues.

The American Joint Commission on Cancer (AJCC) devised a staging classification system based on Breslow thickness, Clark's level (T1 melanomas only), lymph node involvement, and presence or absence of distant metastases (Table 1). It includes tumor ulceration as a prognostic factor. Ulceration portends a poorer prognosis for all invasive melanomas, regardless of depth. Other prognosticators of poorer outcome include head or neck location, older age, male gender, high mitotic rate, regression, and vascular invasion. The 5- and 10-year survival rates are provided in Table 1.

TABLE 1 AJCC Melanoma Staging and Survival Rates (2002)

Stage	TNM	Histology	5-Year Survival	10-Year Survival
0	Tis N0 M0	Melanoma in situ	100%	100%
IA	T1a N0 M0	≤1 mm without ulceration and Clark level II/III	95%	88%
IB	T1b N0 M0	≤1 mm with ulceration or Clark level IV/V	91%	83%
	T2a N0 M0	1.01-2.0 mm without ulceration	89%	79%
IIA	T2b N0 M0	1.01-2.0 mm with ulceration	77%	64%
	T3a N0 M0	2.01-4.0 mm without ulceration	79%	64%
IIB	T3b N0 M0	2.01-4.0 mm with ulceration	63%	51%
	T4a N0 M0	>4 mm without ulceration	67%	54%
IIC	T4b N0 M0	>4 mm with ulceration	45%	32%
IIIA	T1-4a N1a M0	Any thickness primary without ulceration and a single micrometastatic regional node	70%	63%
	T1-4a N2a M0	Any thickness primary without ulceration and 2-3 microscopic regional nodes	63%	57%
IIIB	T1-4b N1a M0	Any thickness primary with ulceration and a single micrometastatic regional node	53%	38%
	T1-4b N2a M0	Any thickness primary with ulceration and 2-3 microscopic regional nodes	50%	36%
	T1-4a N1b M0	Any thickness primary without ulceration and a single macrometastatic regional node	59%	48%
	T1-4a N2b M0	Any thickness primary without ulceration and 2-3 macrometastatic regional nodes	46%	39%
	T1-4a/b N2c M0	Any thickness primary with/without ulceration and in-transit metastases or satellite lesions without nodal involvement		
IIIC	T1-4b N1b M0	Any thickness primary with ulceration and a single microscopic regional node	29%	24%
	T1-4b N2b M0	Any thickness primary with ulceration and 2-3 macrometastatic regional nodes	24%	15%
	T1-4b N3 M0	Any thickness primary with/without ulceration and 4 or more micro/macrometastatic nodes, or matted nodes, or in-transit metastases or satellite lesions with metastatic nodes	27%	18%
IV	T1-4b Nany M1a	Distant skin, subcutaneous, or nodal metastases	19%	16%
	T1-4b Nany M1b	Lung metastases	7%	3%
	T1-4b Nany M1c	All other visceral metastases	10%	6%

AJCC = American Joint Committee on Cancer.
Adapted from Balch C, Buzaid A, Soong S, et al: Final version of the American Joint Committee on Cancer staging system for cutaneous melanoma. J Clin Oncol 2001;19:3635-3648.

Work-up and Treatment

Malignant melanoma in situ (MMIS), deemed stage 0, has a 100% 5-year survival rate. Current recommendations for the treatment of MMIS are excision to subcutaneous fat with at least 5-mm margins of uninvolved skin. For melanomas less than 1 mm in thickness, the current recommendation is excision to fascia with 1.0-cm margins. Melanomas with a thickness of 1 to 4 mm are usually excised to fascia with 2-cm margins. Breslow thickness greater than 4 mm can be excised to fascia with margins of at least 2 cm. Because the aim of the excision is to completely remove the primary tumor, it is acceptable under certain circumstances to excise melanoma with narrower margins if the anatomic location or other factors preclude a wider excision.

Patients who have melanomas 1 mm or thicker and who have no clinical evidence of lymphadenopathy are candidates for sentinel lymph node biopsy (SLNB), which is usually performed at the time of the definitive excision of the primary melanoma. Sentinel lymph node biopsy is used as a staging tool because it provides information regarding regional lymph node involvement, which is a strong predictor of survival. Patients who have a positive sentinel node are offered a complete lymph node dissection and adjuvant therapy. Although lymph node dissection with or without adjuvant therapy after a positive SLNB appears to prolong disease-free survival, it remains unclear whether overall survival is improved. Regarding adjuvant therapy, the only FDA-approved medication in this setting is interferon alfa-2b (Intron A), which is usually administered for 1 year. Although interferon alfa-2b improves relapse-free survival in a small fraction of patients treated, the evidence for improvement in overall survival is variable. Significant side effects can be experienced, including flulike symptoms such as fever, chills, muscle aches, malaise, and depression. Given the limited efficacy and the side-effect profile, many physicians offer patients the option to enroll in investigative adjuvant clinical trials.

In patients with clinical lymphadenopathy or in-transit metastases (stage IIIB/IIIC), the work-up usually entails a fine needle aspiration or open biopsy of the lymph node. The presence of cutaneous in-transit metastasis is usually confirmed via a skin biopsy. Patients presenting with evidence of distant metastatic disease (stage IV), which is often established via imaging studies (computed tomography, magnetic resonance imaging, positron emission tomography, or ultrasound), usually undergo fine needle aspiration or open biopsy to confirm suspected distant spread. Stage IV disease portends a poor prognosis. Treatment is variable based on extent of metastatic disease. Box 3 lists available therapies for advanced or metastatic disease.

Follow-up

After the diagnosis and treatment of melanoma, frequency of follow-up varies based on depth of the melanoma and lymph node status.

CURRENT THERAPY

- Early detection is essential for improved outcome.
- The melanoma should be excised with appropriate margins based on the histologic depth.
- When excising melanomas of ≥1 mm, sentinel lymph node biopsy can be performed to determine regional lymph node involvement.
- Dissection of the lymph node basin can be offered to patients with micronodal or macronodal metastases.
- Adjuvant therapy should be considered for stage III disease.
- Stage IV treatment depends on location and extent of metastatic disease. It ranges from surgical resection to chemotherapy and biological therapy to radiation therapy.

BOX 3 Therapies for Advanced or Metastatic Melanoma

Excision of isolated metastatic lesions
Hyperthermic isolated limb perfusion (melphalan[1])
Radiation therapy for localized disease
Dacarbazine or temozolomide[2]–based chemotherapy
Interferon alfa-2b
High-dose interleukin-2
Anti CTLA-4[3]
Clinical trials

CTLA = cytotoxic T-lymphocyte antigen.
[1]Not FDA approved for this indication
[8]Orphan drug in the United States.

The follow-up is structured with the goal of helping to detect recurrence, metastasis, and new primary melanomas as early as possible.

The most common areas to which melanoma metastasizes are the skin, lymph nodes, lungs, liver, and brain. These metastases usually appear within 5 years. In addition, patients with melanoma are at high risk for developing subsequent new primary melanomas and nonmelanoma skin cancers. Thus, these patients should be under lifelong cutaneous surveillance and should be encouraged to perform periodic skin self-examinations to help detect new melanomas at an early and curable stage.

In general, those with melanoma less than 1 mm receive a physical examination every 3 months for the first year, then every 6 to 12 months until the fifth year. After the fifth year these patients are followed annually. Those with melanomas larger than 1 mm undergo a physical examination every 3 months for 1 to 2 years, then every 6 months until the fifth year, followed by annual examinations thereafter.

The follow-up visits for all patients should include a thorough history, review of systems, complete skin examination, and examination of the lymph nodes. In addition, patients at high risk for metastatic disease should also have their lungs and liver examined. Suspicious findings on the history or physical examination should direct the physician to obtain appropriate imaging studies, laboratory studies, or biopsies to further investigate. Evidence to support the use of routine imaging and laboratory studies in asymptomatic patients with a normal physical examination remains controversial and is left to the discretion of the physician.

REFERENCES

Balch C, Buzaid A, Soong S, et al: Final version of the American Joint Committee on Cancer staging system for cutaneous melanoma. J Clin Oncol 2001;19:3635-3648.

Berwick M, Wiggins C: The current epidemiology of cutaneous malignant melanoma. Front Biosci 2006;11:1244-1254.

Freedberg I, Eisen A, Wolff K: Fitzpatrick's Dermatology in General Medicine. New York: McGraw-Hill, 2-3.

Grin C, Kopf A, Welkovich B, et al: Accuracy in the clinical diagnosis of malignant melanoma. Arch Dermatol 1990;126:763-766.

Howe HL, Wu X, Ries LA, et al: Annual report to the nation on the status of cancer, 1975-2003: Featuring cancer among U.S. Hispanic/Latino populations. Cancer 2006;107(8):1711-1742.

Jemal A, Siegel R, Ward E, et al: Cancer statistics, 2008. CA Cancer J Clin 2008;58:71-96.

Kittler H, Phehamberger H, Wolff K, Binder M: Diagnositic accuracy of dermoscopy. Lancet Oncol 2002;3(3):159-165.

Liu W, Dowling JP, Murray WK, et al: Rate of growth in melanomas: Characteristics and associations of rapidly growing melanomas. Arch Dermatol 2006;142(12):1638-1640.

Marghoob A, Braun R, Kopf A: Atlas of Dermoscopy, London: Taylor & Francis, 2005.

Markovic SN, Erickson LA, Rao RD, et al: Malignant melanoma in the 21st century. Part 1: Epidemiology, risk factors, screening, prevention, and diagnosis. Mayo Clin Proc 2007;82(3):364-380.

National Comprehensive Care Network: Clinical Practice Guidelines in Oncology- v.2. 2007, Melanoma. Available at: http://www.nccn.org/professionals/physician_gls/PDF/melanoma.pdf (accessed June 6, 2008).

Rigel D, Friedman R, Dzubow L, et al: Cancer of the Skin, Philadelphia: Saunders, 2005.

Premalignant Lesions

Method of
Donald Clemons, MD

Premalignant Lesions

Premalignant lesions of the skin are those that, if left untreated, can evolve into malignant invasive and potentially metastasizing tumors. With early treatment, these lesions can be managed and the threat of malignancy averted. These premalignant diseases include actinic keratosis (AK), actinic cheilitis, Bowen's disease, bowenoid papulosis, porokeratosis, and nevus sebaceus.

Nonmelanoma skin cancer's worldwide economic and health implications are enormous, because it is the most prevalent form of cancer. However, it is also one of the most preventable cancers and, in early stages, relatively easy to diagnose and treat. We must educate our patient population to not only recognize and seek treatment for these early manifestations but to also act as public health advocates regarding modification of behavioral patterns of our at-risk population.

Premalignant lesions are most commonly located on chronic sun-exposed and sun-damaged skin in lighter-skinned individuals who easily burn, have light hair color, have blue or green eyes, and freckle. Both genetic and extrinsic factors are responsible for the development and progression of these lesions. Chronically damaged skin, such as burn scars and long-standing ulcers, infections, and areas having received ionizing radiation are also more likely to develop malignant transformation. Other factors placing patients at increased risk include chronic arsenic exposure and immunosuppression as seen in the elderly, organ transplant recipients, HIV-infected individuals, and patients receiving systemic steroid therapy. This large subset of patients is more likely to rapidly develop malignant transformation and show aggressive behavior in their lesions. They should be closely monitored and considered for long-term prophylactic care.

Actinic Keratosis

Actinic keratosis, a form of squamous cell carcinoma (SCC) in situ, is usually found on photo-damaged skin and is characterized clinically by rough adherent scale on an erythematous nonindurated occasionally friable and tender base. The background is usually telangiectatic with areas of dyspigmentation. Hyperpigmented and atrophic variations can be seen. They may be palpated easier than visualized but can progress to thickened hyperkeratotic plaques. Rapidly enlarging lesions or those that are excessively hyperkeratotic or indurated should be biopsied to rule out malignant progression to SCC. Histologically, AKs are characterized by a partial thickness disordered windblown maturation of atypical epidermal keratinocytes and a thickened compact stratum corneum. The hair acrotrichium and sweat duct acrosyringium are spared involvement and no invasion is seen. The epidermis can be thickened or atrophic.

TREATMENT OF ACTINIC KERATOSIS

Treatment can be by physical disruptions or chemically applied methods. Among the physical methods, liquid nitrogen cryosurgery

CURRENT DIAGNOSIS

Actinic keratosis
- Tender, rough adherent scale on erythematous base
- Background of photo-damaged skin
- Suspect SCC if indurated or hyperkeratotic

Actinic cheilitis
- Protuberant lower lip mucosa, fair skin, photo damage
- Often history of pipe or chewing tobacco use
- Up to 25% metastatic incidence with invasion

Bowen's disease
- Erythematous sharply demarcated plaque with variable scale
- Involves hair follicles
- Frequently recurs if inadequately treated
- May affect genital mucosal skin

Bowenoid papulosis
- Clinically indistinguishable from warts
- Genital skin
- Histologically indistinguishable from Bowen's disease
- Associated with HPV-16

Porokeratosis
- Papules or annular plaques with thin peripheral collarette of scale
- Discrete or linear
- Sun damaged skin or palms or soles
- Coronoid lamella seen histologically

Nevus sebaceus
- Perpetual elevated often inapparent plaques usually on head or neck
- Postpubertal evolve into yellow-orange papillomatous plaques devoid of hair
- Malignancies are usually low grade

Abbreviations: HPV-16 = human papilloma virus type 16; SCC = squamous cell carcinoma.

is most commonly used. Care must be taken to adequately freeze and destroy the lesion yet minimize significant pigment alteration or scarring. The length of the freeze time will vary by size, thickness, and location of the tumor, ethnic skin color, and concomitant systemic illness such as lupus erythematosus or cryoglobulinemia.

Light curettage, medium-depth chemical peels, and dermabrasion can be used for more extensive lesions. Carbon dioxide (CO_2) and Er:YAG (erbium:yttrium-aluminum-garnet) lasers, although more expensive and having more potential complications, are effective methods of treatment. Surgical excision is usually reserved for clinically suspicious discrete lesions or treatment recalcitrant lesions.

The topically applied chemical methods include topical tretinoin (Retin-A, Differin, Tazorac[1]), fluorouracil cream or solution (Efudex, Fluoroplex, Carac), diclofenac sodium gel (Solaraze), imiquimod cream (Aldara), or 20% aminolevulinic acid (ALA) (Levulan) with photodynamic therapy. Tretinoin[1] cream or gel is applied daily to photo-damaged skin indefinitely. Results are usually not clinically evident for 4 to 6 months of therapy. Side effects of dryness and scaling can be improved by judicious use of medication; moisturizers; and initially alternate- or every-third-day therapy, gradually increasing as tolerated. Ultraviolet A (UVA) and ultraviolet B (UVB) blocking sunscreens are critical to retard further skin damage.

---
[1]Not FDA approved for this indication.

CURRENT THERAPY

Actinic keratosis
- Cryotherapy, light curettage, dermabrasion, or chemical peels
- Topical or systemic tretinoin (Retin-A), fluorouracil (Efudex), diclofenac (Solaraze), imiquimod (Aldara), or PDT

Actinic cheilitis
- Cryotherapy, fluorouracil, imiquimod
- Vermilionectomy, laser, PDT

Bowen's disease
- All methods used for actinic keratosis
- Excision to include Mohs' surgery

Bowenoid papulosis
- Same as Bowen's
- Imiquimod may be treatment of choice

Porokeratosis
- Cryosurgery, salicylic plaster and fluorouracil, topical tretinoin[1]
- Imiquimod

Nevus sebaceus
- Watchful waiting with appropriate biopsies
- Excision

---

[1]Not FDA approved for this indication.
Abbreviations: PDT = photodynamic therapy

Fluorouracil can be found in a 0.5%, 1%, or 5% cream or 1% solution and is applied once or twice daily for up to 8 weeks as tolerated. It is highly effective; but side effects of redness, pain, erosion, and allergic reaction may limit its usefulness. Side effects often persist for weeks after therapy has ceased. Diclofenac gel is applied twice daily for 2 to 3 months; although better tolerated clinically, it is expensive, requires compliance, and can have side effects similar to fluorouracil as well as photosensitive and anticoagulative effects. Imiquimod cream 0.5% is a new class of immunomodulator drug that is applied once daily 2 to 5 times per week for 4 to 6 weeks.[2] It can cause erythema, scaling, and erosion but is usually relatively painless and resolves as the lesions clear. It is expensive but may offer more long-term clearing and may be effective against concomitant superficially invasive cancers.

Topical photodynamic therapy (PDT) is the most recent addition to the treatment arm. After acetone pretreatment, 20% ALA (Levulan) is applied and allowed to incubate for 1 to 3 hours. It is activated by a light source such as a blue light, an intense pulsed light, or a long pulse dye laser causing destruction of individual lesions and cosmetic improvement of photo-damaged skin. One to three treatments at 3-week intervals are needed. The therapy is expensive, requires equipment, causes 24- to 36-hour photosensitivity, and is variably uncomfortable. This therapy is also highly effective, and cosmetic downtime is lessened. Lack of scarring or dyspigmentation and less noncompliance issues combined with superior cosmetic photo-damage repair make this a useful alternative treatment. Hypertropic extremity lesions can be pretreated for 5 days with fluorouracil before PDT.

Oral tretinoin (acitretin)[1] 25 mg or 0.4 mg/kg/day as tolerated can be an effective treatment for chronic AKs in immunosuppressed individuals minimizing the progression to invasive SCC. Benefits cease with disruption of therapy.

---

[1]Not FDA approved for this indication.
[2]Exceeds dosage recommended by the manufacturer.

Actinic Cheilitis

Actinic cheilitis (leukokeratosis or leukoplakia of the lip) usually occurs on the lower lip mucosa. Predisposing factors include chronic photodamage, fair skin, protuberant lower lip, and pipe or chewing tobacco use. This disease is essentially AK, and much of what was previously discussed about AK applies here. Unfortunately, the incidence of invasion is higher and the subsequent chance of metastatic spread may approach 25%. Clinically, actinic cheilitis can appear as a tender whitish plaque adherent to the mucosa. Erosion, induration, and erythema should be evaluated further because these are often signs of invasion; a biopsy of the most clinically affected area may be necessary to rule invasion out.

TREATMENT OF ACTINIC CHELITIS

Treatment is often accompanied by pain, discomfort, erosion, and slow healing. The most commonly used method of treatment is liquid nitrogen spray. If fluorouracil or imiquimod (Aldara) are used, only 2 to 3 weekly applications may be tolerated; treatment may be necessary for 6 to 8 weeks with erosion persisting for many weeks afterward.

Surgical advancement of normal mucosa (vermilionectomy) with removal of affected tissue or CO_2 laser ablation can be performed, but these procedures are technically difficult and potentially scarring. Recently, another form of photodynamic therapy using 20% ALA incubated for 2 to 3 hours followed by activation with a pulse dye laser 595 nm long pulsed has been reported very effective with minimal discomfort and erosive side effects. This therapy might be an alternative treatment, if this laser is available.

Bowen's Disease

Bowen's disease is a form of SCC in situ that differs histologically from AK by involving the full thickness of the epidermis to include involvement of the hair follicle acrotrichium. Because of hair follicle involvement, superficial treatments that are effective on actinic keratosis often fail when treating Bowen's disease. Recurrence as well as development of invasive squamous cell carcinoma may occur. Bowen's disease occurring on non–sun-exposed hair-bearing skin is suggestive of arsenic exposure; concomitant lymphoreticular or gastrointestinal malignancies may develop. Bowen's disease on mucosal surfaces of the penis or labia (erythroplasia of Queyrat) has a higher incidence of invasion and metastasis (20% to 30%) and, therefore, should be managed more aggressively and closely monitored. Clinically, these lesions appear as an erythematous sharply demarcated plaque with light to moderate scale on sun-damaged skin. It can often be mistaken for eczema or psoriasis. On mucosal surfaces, it may be more indurated and velvety. Care must be taken to ensure that there is no involvement of the urethral meatus.

TREATMENT OF BOWEN'S DISEASE

Treatment modalities include aggressive liquid nitrogen therapy, topical fluorouracil (Efudex) two times a day for 6 to 8 weeks[2], and curettage; but there is a significant risk of recurrence on hair-bearing skin. Topical imiquimod (Aldara) 3 to 5 times weekly for 6 to 8 weeks may be more effective, especially on mucosal skin, but long-term cure rates are uncertain. Simple excision, or Mohs' surgery, probably affords the most effective and curative method available; but there is significant potential for scarring and may result in a mutilating procedure on genital skin.

Bowenoid Papulosis

Bowenoid papulosis represents SCC in situ on genital skin associated primarily with human papilloma virus type 16 (HPV-16) that can

---

[2]Exceeds dosage recommended by the manufacturer.

progress to invasive SCC. Clinically, these lesions are indistinguishable from common warts, or condyloma acuminatum, and present as tan or reddish-brown papules or plaques. Histologically, viral changes are absent and show classic features of Bowen's disease.

TREATMENT OF BOWENOID PAPULOSIS

The same treatment modalities used in Bowen's disease are effective; although imiquimod may be the treatment of choice to cure additional clinically inapparent or distal lesions on cervix or vaginal mucosa. Daily application 3 times weekly[2] for 8 weeks has shown cure. In addition, PDT activated by a Diode laser and topical cidofovir (Vistide)[1] may also have use in recalcitrant lesions.

Porokeratosis

Porokeratosis presents as papules or annular plaques, which may be discrete or linear and occur on photo-damaged skin or on palms or soles. Clinically, they show central flattening and a peripheral fine thin collarette of scale and may show centrifugal spread. These lesions may be congenital or acquired and are represented by five distinct variants with several types sometimes present in one patient. They may evolve into invasive SCC. Histologically, they are all characterized by having a thin angled parakeratotic column over a focus of dyskeratotic cells without a granular cell layer (coronoid lamella), which represents the advancing margin.

TREATMENT OF POROKERATOSIS

Successful treatment of these lesions is often difficult. Hard cryosurgery is effective but may scar. Topical tretinoin[1] 0.1% gel daily for 4 months or a combination of salicylic acid plaster pads (Mediplast)[1] in the morning and fluorouracil in the afternoon or evening has been successful. Topical 5% imiquimod 3 times weekly for at least 3 weeks may be used as well as topical or systemic fluorouracil, as tolerated.

Nevus Sebaceus

Nevus sebaceus is a congenital hamartoma of infancy comprised of immature sebaceous, follicular, and apocrine elements. Following puberty, benign pilosebaceous and apocrine tumors may develop as well as low-grade malignant neoplasms. Rarely, aggressive malignant sebaceous and apocrine carcinomas have been reported. Clinically, they are slightly elevated often inapparent linear plaques most often present on the head or neck. At puberty, they evolve into yellow-orange plaques devoid of hair with a velvety or papillomatous surface.

TREATMENT OF NEVUS SEBACEUS

Treatment is by surgical excision or watchful waiting. Large lesions can be removed by staged excisions. Development of nodules or ulcerations should be biopsied to rule out tumor development.

---

[1] Not FDA approved for this indication.
[2] Exceeds dosage recommended by the manufacturer.

REFERENCES

Dereli T, Ozyurt S, Ozturk G: Porokeratosis of Mibelli: Successful treatment with cryosurgery. J Dermatol 2004;31(3):223-227.
Jones E, Korzenko A, Kriegel D: Oral isotretinoin in the treatment and prevention of cutaneous squamous cell carcinoma. J Drugs Dermatol 2004; 3(5):498-502.
Jorrizo J, Carney P, Ko W, et al: Treatment options in the management of actinic keratosis. Cutis 2004;74(6s):9-15.
Villa A, Berman B: Immunomodulators for skin cancer. J Drugs Dermatol 2004;3(5):533-539.

Bacterial Infections of the Skin

Method of
Philip S. Barie, MD, MBA, and
Soumitra R. Eachempati, MD

The U.S. Food and Drug Administration (FDA) classifies skin and soft tissue infections as uncomplicated or complicated infections. Uncomplicated skin and soft tissue infections are those that are superficial or self-limited, such as cellulitis, impetigo, erysipelas, furunculosis, carbunculosis, and small abscesses. They may require only incision and drainage (without antibiotics) or oral antibiotics (without drainage). Hospitalization is rarely necessary.

Complicated skin and soft tissue infections involve deeper tissues, require major surgical intervention, or occur with medical comorbidities, specifically renal insufficiency, diabetes mellitus, or arterial insufficiency. Examples of complicated skin and soft tissue infections include large abscesses, diabetic foot infections, some postoperative surgical site infections, infected decubitus ulcers, and necrotizing soft tissue infections.

Cellulitis

Cellulitis is an acute pyogenic infection of the dermis and subcutaneous tissues, most commonly complicating a breach of lower extremity skin integrity. The infected tissue is warm, erythematous, edematous, and tender. The differential diagnosis of cellulitis includes both infectious and inflammatory conditions, including insect bites, acute gout, deep venous thrombosis, drug reactions, pyoderma gangrenosum (characteristic of inflammatory bowel disease or collagen vascular disease), and metastatic carcinoma.

Important clues to etiology include recent trauma, physical activity, water contact, and human or animal bites. Cellulitis can also manifest a deeper infection (e.g., subjacent osteomyelitis). Bloodstream infection is a rare cause after meningococcal, pneumococcal, or staphylococcal bacteremia. *Pseudomonas* bacteremia can cause skin lesions in neutropenic patients.

The clinical diagnosis of cellulitis is made based on circumstances and the appearance of the lesion; neither imaging studies nor cultures have a high diagnostic yield. Needle aspiration yields an organism only about 30% of the time. Punch biopsies of skin have a higher yield, but the invasiveness is seldom justified, because empiric therapy is usually successful in uncomplicated cases. Radiologic studies are unnecessary unless a deep-seated infection cannot be excluded by examining the patient.

Most cases of cellulitis are caused by gram-positive cocci, either *Staphylococcus aureus* or streptococci, and are characterized by diffuse or poorly circumscribed lesions. Oral β-lactam antibiotics active against methicillin-sensitive *S. aureus* are the treatments of choice unless the patient has systemic signs (e.g., fever, chills), medical comorbidity, or a rapidly spreading lesion, any of which indicate initial intravenous therapy. Choices for parenteral therapy include penicillin G (for erysipelas; see later), cefazolin, nafcillin or ceftriaxone (Rocephin) (Box 1). If methicillin-resistant *S. aureus* (MRSA) is suspected or the patient is allergic to penicillin (anaphylactoid reaction), vancomycin (Vancocin) or linezolid (Zyvox) may be chosen.

MRSA skin infections require particular mention. Increasingly observed among patients without recent health care contact, community-acquired MRSA (CA-MRSA) has emerged as a major pathogen among outpatients. About 75% of infections caused by CA-MRSA involve skin; it is now the predominant cause of skin infections in patients presenting to emergency departments.

Outbreaks of CA-MRSA have been associated with groups of people in close proximity, including prison inmates, sports teams, military recruits, and children in daycare centers. Direct contact

BOX 1 Recommendations for Diagnosis and Treatment of Skin and Soft Tissue Infections

Level I

Impetigo
Mupirocin (Bactroban) is the best topical agent and is equivalent to oral systemic antimicrobials when lesions are limited in number. Patients who have numerous lesions or who do not respond to topical therapy should receive an oral antimicrobial agent. Penicillin or penicillinase-resistant penicillin are treatments of choice for nonbullous lesions. Penicillin or first-generation cephalosporin is recommended for bullous lesions.

Erysipelas
Penicillin is the treatment of choice for streptococcal infection. Penicillinase-resistant penicillin or a first-generation cephalosporin is recommended if staphylococci are suspected.

Cellulitis
Penicillinase-resistant penicillin or first-generation cephalosporin are the treatments of choice, unless resistant organisms are common in the community. Use clindamycin (Cleocin) or vancomycin for penicillin-allergic patients.

Cutaneous Abscess
Incision and drainage is the treatment of choice.

Furunclosis
Recurrent furunculosis may be treated with mupirocin to the anterior nares (for chronic staphylococcal carriers) or clindamycin 150 mg/d for 3 months.

Methicillin-resistant Staphylococcus Aureus
Linezolid (Zyvox), daptomycin (Cubicin), and vancomycin have excellent efficacy in skin or soft tissue infection in general and in particular those caused by MRSA.

Necrotizing Soft Tissue Infection
Surgical intervention is the major therapeutic intervention

Polymicrobial Necrotizing Soft Tissue Infection
Ampicillin-sulbactam (Unasyn) plus ciprofloxacin (Cipro) plus clindamycin is the treatment of choice for community-acquired infection

Monomicrobial Necrotizing Soft Tissue Infection
Clindamycin-penicillin combination therapy is the treatment of choice.

Level II

Furunculosis
Attempt to eradicate the staphylococcal carrier state among colonized persons.

Polymicrobial Necrotizing Soft Tissue Infection
A variety of antimicrobials directed against aerobic gram-positive and gram-negative bacteria and anaerobes may be used in mixed necrotizing infection.

Monomicrobial Necrotizing Soft Tissue Infection
Consider intravenous immunoglobulin (IVIg) therapy. Penicillin-clindamycin combination therapy is the treatment of choice for infections caused by Clostridium perfringens.

Animal Bites
Oral amoxicillin-clavulanate (Augmentin) or intravenous ampicillin-sulbactam or ertapenem (Invanz) should be administered to non–penicillin-allergic patients because of suitable activity against Pasturella multocida. Acceptable alternative regimens include piperacillin-tazobactam (Zosyn), imipenem-cilastatin (Primaxin), and meropenem (Merrem).

Level III

Cutaneous Abscess
Gram stain, culture, and systemic antibiotics are rarely necessary.

Furuncle
Systemic antibiotics are usually unnecessary absent fever or extensive surrounding cellulitis.

Animal Bites
First-generation cephalosporins, penicillinase-resistant penicillin, macrolides, and clindamycin should be avoided as therapy because of poor activity against P. multocida.

Human Bites
Intravenous ampicillin-sulbactam or cefoxitin (Mefoxin) are the treatments of choice for non–penicillin-allergic patients. A hand surgeon should evaluate clenched-fist injuries for penetration into synovium, joint capsule, or bone.

Surgical Site Infection
Suspicion of possible surgical site infection does not justify use of antibiotics without a definitive diagnosis and the initiation of other therapies, such as opening the incision. All infected surgical incisions should be opened.

MRSA = methicillin-resistant Staphylococcus aureus.

---

with skin is a definite risk factor, as are shared personal hygiene items (e.g., towels, soap). Other at-risk patients are young children and persons of lower socioeconomic status.

Skin infections caused by CA-MRSA have a characteristic appearance that can raise suspicion of the diagnosis. The lesions are usually superficial and well-demarcated, often with a necrotic center (Fig. 1). For uncomplicated lesions, incision and drainage alone or topical mupirocin (Bactroban) ointment or chlorhexidine solution (BactoShield 2) may be sufficient therapy. The antimicrobial susceptibilities of CA-MRSA in vitro include macrolides, clindamycin (Cleocin), and trimethoprim and sulfamethoxazole (TMP-SMX); TMP-SMX is most reliable orally. Macrolide-inducible clindamycin resistance has been associated with treatment failures; therefore, caution is advised in using clindamycin for therapy. If antibiotic therapy is required, TMP-SMX is preferred.

Erysipelas

Erysipelas, a form of cellulitis, is distinguished by two factors: raised lesions above the level of surrounding skin and a sharp demarcation between infected and normal skin. Most infections remain superficial. Erysipelas is most common among young children and older adults. The etiologic agent is almost always group A streptococci or rarely other streptococci or S. aureus. Penicillin is the treatment of choice unless staphylococci are suspected (see Box 1).

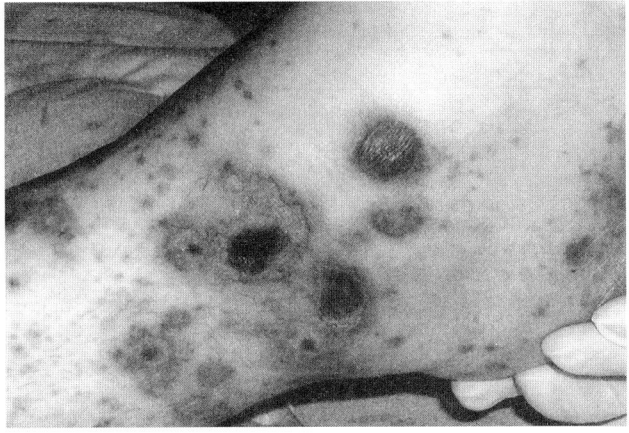

FIGURE 1. Necrotizing skin lesion characteristic of community-associated methicillin-resistant *Staphylococcus aureus* infection.

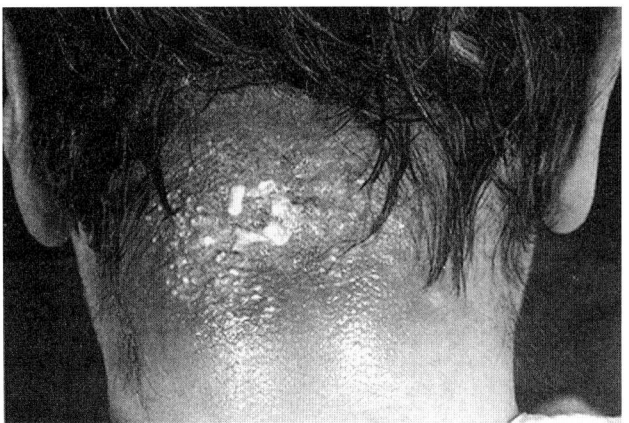

FIGURE 3. Several furuncles have coalesced to form a spontaneously draining carbuncle on the nape of the neck. Formal incision and drainage is necessary.

Impetigo

Impetigo consists of discrete purulent lesions that are nearly always caused by β-hemolytic streptococci or *S. aureus* (Fig. 2). Impetigo is most common among economically disadvantaged children in warm climates (summertime in temperate climates). Organisms colonize unbroken skin as a prelude to impetigo, emphasizing personal hygiene in the pathogenesis. Inoculation by minor trauma occurs subsequently. Impetigo usually invades exposed skin, primarily of the face and extremities. The lesions are usually multiple and may be bullous (*S. aureus*) or nonbullous. A deeply ulcerated form of impetigo is known as ecthyma.

A penicillinase-resistant penicillin or first-generation cephalosporin is preferred for therapy, but cases caused by CA-MRSA are on the increase. Topical therapy with mupirocin is equivalent to therapy with oral antibiotics (see Box 1).

Cutaneous Abscess

Cutaneous abscesses can infect dermis and subcutaneous tissue. These lesions are usually painful, tender, and fluctuant, with a central pustule and surrounding erythema and edema. These infections are typically polymicrobial, with pure culture of *S. aureus* isolated in only one quarter of cases. Epidermoid cysts (erroneously called sebaceous cysts) can contain skin flora in the soft keratinous, cheesy center, even when not inflamed. Inflammation usually results from cyst rupture, with extrusion of cyst contents into surrounding tissue, rather than infection per se. Treatment of cutaneous abscesses is incision and drainage, with mechanical destruction of intracavitary loculations (see Box 1). Gram stain, culture, or systemic antibiotics are rarely necessary absent systemic signs or severe immunocompromise.

Furuncles (boils) are infected hair follicles, usually caused by *S. aureus*. Suppuration extends through the dermis to subcutaneous tissue, forming a small abscess. This contrasts with folliculitis, also an inflammation of hair follicles, where inflammation is more superficial and pus is present in the epidermis. Furuncles can appear anywhere on hair-bearing skin. Infection of several adjacent follicles can coalesce into a carbuncle, with multiple draining sites (Fig. 3). Carbuncles have a predilection to form on the dorsum of the neck in patients with diabetes mellitus.

Small furuncles may be treated with moist heat to promote spontaneous drainage; antibiotics are rarely necessary. Some patients are also subject to recurrent episodes of furunculosis, for which nasal carriage of staphylococci is a strong predisposing factor. Intranasal 2% mupirocin ointment twice daily for 5 days each month can reduce recurrences by one half. Oral clindamycin 150 mg/day for 3 months is even more successful, reducing recurrences by 80%.

Hidradenitis Suppurativa

Hidradenitis suppurativa is a chronic acneiform infection of the cutaneous apocrine glands that involves adjacent subcutaneous tissue and fascia of the axillae, groin, or wherever apocrine glands are concentrated, such as the areola, the intramammary cleft, gluteal folds, perineum, circumanal area, or infraumbilical skin. Ingrown hairs are a predisposing factor; the incidence is highest in women with curly hair. Hot weather, excessive perspiration, and obesity may be aggravating factors.

Obstructed apocrine gland secretion leads to trapped secretions, superimposed bacterial growth, and extravasation into surrounding tissue, causing subcutaneous inflammation and infection. As suppuration progresses, cellulitis can develop. The condition manifests most commonly as painful, tender, firm, nodular lesions in one or both axillae and can resemble folliculitis or furunculosis. Nodules can drain spontaneously, then heal slowly over 2 to 4 weeks, with or without surgical drainage. Remissions may be prolonged, but recurrences are common, and some patients are afflicted continuously. Patients with chronic affliction can manifest fibrosis that results in unsightly scarring.

Incision and drainage may be helpful for fluctuant nodules that have not opened spontaneously. Antibiotics are indicated if cellulitis or fever is present. In severe or intractable cases, excision of the pathologic tissue with split-thickness skin grafting offers the best chance for cure.

Prevention includes minimized heat exposure and consequent perspiration. Obese patients should lose weight. Constrictive clothing

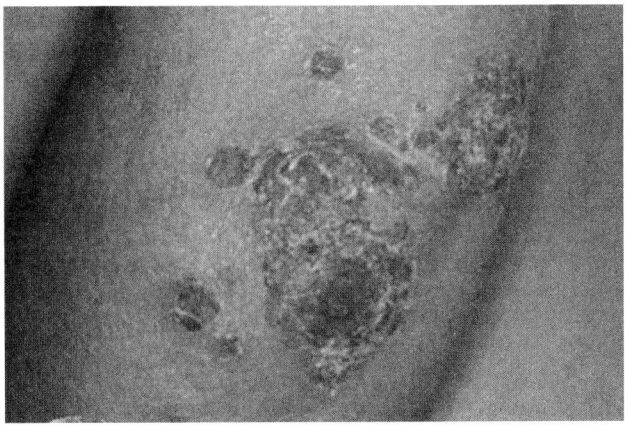

FIGURE 2. Staphylococcal impetigo.

and frictional trauma to affected skin should be avoided, as should underarm antiperspirants and deodorants. Affected hair-bearing areas should be kept shaved to prevent re-ingrowth of hair.

Diabetic Foot Infection

Diabetic foot infections usually begin in ulcerated skin, either from abrasions or ischemia. Skin ulcers are common in diabetic patients because of vascular insufficiency and peripheral sensory neuropathy. Two thirds of patients with diabetic foot infection present with peripheral arterial disease, and the prevalence of sensory neuropathy is about 80%.

Although most diabetic foot infections remain superficial, as many as 25% of such infections spread contiguously to involve subcutaneous tissue or bone (osteomyelitis). Recurrent infections are common, and 10% to 30% of affected patients eventually come to amputation. Acute diabetic foot infections in untreated patients are usually monomicrobial, caused most commonly by *S. aureus*; even when it is not the only isolate, it is usually part of the flora of mixed infections. Serious infections requiring hospitalization are more likely to be mixed infections, including both aerobic and anaerobic gram-negative bacilli.

Infections affect the forefoot most commonly, especially the toes and the metatarsal heads on the plantar surface. Systemic signs (uncommon in diabetic foot infection, even with limb-threatening infection), purulent drainage, or at least two local signs of inflammation (e.g., calor [warmth], rubor [redness], dolor [pain or tenderness], or tumor [induration]) suggest infection. Metabolic abnormalities (e.g., hyperglycemia, ketoacidosis, hyperosmolar state) can provide a clue. More than one half of patients do not have fever, leukocytosis, or an elevated erythrocyte sedimentation rate (ESR). Whenever the diagnosis of diabetic foot infections is considered, aggressive management is indicated because these infections sometimes progress rapidly.

Intravenous antibiotics are indicated for patients with systemic illness, severe infection, intolerance of oral antibiotics, or pathogens that are not susceptible to oral agents. After improvement, oral antibiotic therapy may be appropriate. Most initial therapy is empiric, directed at common pathogens. Empiric coverage for gram-positive bacteria (staphylococci and streptococci) is almost always required; prospective trials indicate that gram-positive monotherapy is equivalent to broad-spectrum therapy. Effective agents for therapy of diabetic foot infections in clinical trials include cephalosporins, β-lactamase inhibitor combination antibiotics, fluoroquinolones, clindamycin, carbapenems, vancomycin, and linezolid. Anaerobic coverage should be considered for necrotic or foul-smelling wounds. If the patient responds to empiric therapy, a broad-spectrum regimen should be narrowed when microbiology data become available. If the patient does not respond, the possibility of fastidious organisms missed by culture should be reconsidered, or surgery may be needed.

The optimal duration of therapy for diabetic foot infection has not been determined. A 1-week course of therapy is sufficient for most mild infections, whereas up to 2 weeks may be necessary for serious infections. Adequate débridement, resection, or amputation can shorten the duration of therapy. Surgical revascularization to improve blood flow to the ischemic, infected foot may be a crucial determinant of outcome.

Surgical Site Infection

Surgical site infections complicate about 3% of surgical procedures. Numerous factors determine whether a patient will develop a surgical site infection, including factors contributed by the patient, the environment, and the treatment (Box 2). The risk of surgical site infection increases with the number of risk factors. Diabetes mellitus and obesity are each estimated to double the risk of surgical site infection.

The microbiology of surgical site infection depends on the type of operation, with an increased likelihood of gram-negative bacilli after gastrointestinal surgery or infrainguinal vascular surgery. Most surgical site infections are caused by gram-positive cocci that are commensal skin flora, including *S. aureus*, *Staphylococcus epidermidis*, and *Enterococcus* species.

Surgical patients should be assessed before elective surgery for correctable risk factors. Open skin lesions should heal beforehand. The patient should be free of bacterial infections of any kind, and should quit smoking, preferably 1 month before surgery. The patient must not be shaved the night before, considering that the risk of surgical site infection is increased by shaving. Obese patients should lose as much weight as is safely possible. Malnourished patients can reduce the risk of surgical site infection significantly with as little as 5 days of enteral nutritional supplementation.

Preoperative administration of prophylactic antibiotics is of proved benefit in many circumstances. However, only the incision itself is protected, and antibiotics are not a panacea. Antibiotic prophylaxis is indicated for most clean-contaminated and contaminated (or potentially contaminated) operations. Antibiotic prophylaxis for clean surgery is controversial. Where bone is incised (e.g. craniotomy, sternotomy) or a prosthesis is inserted, antibiotic prophylaxis is generally indicated. A first-generation cephalosporin is preferred for most noncolon operations, and clindamycin should be used for penicillin-allergic patients. The optimal time to give parenteral antibiotic prophylaxis is within 1 hour before the time of incision. Antibiotics given sooner are ineffective. Single-dose preoperative prophylaxis is often sufficient, but 24- to 48-hour regimens (the latter for cardiac surgery) have become standard.

There is one constant in the management of established surgical site infection: Incise and drain the incision. Adequate drainage is essential not only to control the infection but also to diagnose and treat any associated conditions, such as necrosis that requires débridement, fascial dehiscence or evisceration, or subfascial drainage that

---

BOX 2 Risk Factors for the Development of Surgical Site Infections

Patient Factors
Ascites (for abdominal surgery)
Chronic inflammation
Corticosteroid therapy (controversial)
Diabetes mellitus
Extremes of age
Hypocholsterolemia
Hypoxemia
Obesity
Peripheral vascular disease (for lower extremity surgery)
Postoperative anemia
Prior site irradiation
Recent operation
Remote infection
Skin carriage of staphylococci
Skin disease in the area of infection (e.g., psoriasis)
Undernutrition

Environmental Factors
Contaminated medications
Inadequate disinfection or sterilization
Inadequate skin antisepsis
Inadequate ventilation

Treatment Factors
Drains
Emergency procedure
Hypothermia
Inadequate antibiotic prophylaxis
Oxygenation (controversial)
Prolonged preoperative hospitalization
Prolonged operative time

could signal a deeper infection or fistula. Antibiotic therapy is not required for uncomplicated surgical site infections that are opened and drained adequately. Likewise, if antibiotic therapy is unwarranted, then culture and susceptibility testing of wound drainage can be omitted. Antibiotics may be indicated if there is systemic evidence of toxicity or cellulitis that extends more than 2 cm beyond the incision. Coverage against gram-positive cocci is indicated in most circumstances.

Necrotizing Soft Tissue Infection

Necrotizing soft tissue infections are dangerous, but fortunately they are also uncommon. Danger exists because of rapid progression and much systemic toxicity. Necrotizing soft tissue infections are also dangerous because of their rarity; initial manifestations can be subtle, increasing the possibility of delayed diagnosis. Although most presentations are obvious, a necrotizing soft tissue infection must always be considered whenever a patient presents with severe pain, particularly of the perineum or an extremity, that is out of proportion to any physical findings. There may be no obvious portal. Gas in soft tissues is helpful but unreliable if absent. Delayed definitive therapy is the major risk factor for mortality; therefore, familiarity is crucial for anyone (e.g., surgeon, emergency physician, primary care physician) who might encounter an early presentation. True necrotizing soft tissue infections cannot be treated successfully with antibiotics alone, so timely surgical consultation is mandatory. Even with optimal therapy, mortality is approximately 25% to 30%.

Approximately 80% of necrotizing soft tissue infections are polymicrobial, with bacteria acting synergistically to promote dissemination and increase toxicity. Monomicrobial necrotizing soft tissue infections are most commonly caused by *S. pyogenes*, with *Clostridium perfringens* also relatively common. Polymicrobial necrotizing soft tissue infections are caused by aerobic gram-positive and -negative bacteria and anaerobes. *Escherichia coli* and *Bacteroides fragilis* are the most common aerobic and anaerobic isolates, respectively.

The diagnosis of necrotizing soft tissue infection is based primarily on the history and physical examination. One notable early characteristic is severe pain that is disproportionate to local physical findings. Inspection of the overlying skin may yield few early clues. Characteristic features include edema and tenderness that extend beyond the margin of erythema, skin vesicles or bullae, crepitus, and the absence of lymphangitis and lymphadenitis. As infection progresses, cutaneous anesthesia and necrosis develop along with systemic manifestations of sepsis. A white blood cell (WBC) count greater than $14,000 \times 10^9$ and a serum sodium concentration lower than 135 mEq/dL together have high sensitivity (>80%) for the diagnosis of necrotizing soft tissue infection, and these results should be alarming in the appropriate clinical context. Other prediction rules with comparable accuracy have been reported.

If the diagnosis is not obvious by physical examination and laboratory testing, radiographic studies may be obtained. Plain radiographs can demonstrate soft tissue gas in the absence of crepitus, but it is usually a late finding. Computed tomography is sensitive for the presence of soft tissue gas, and it can also demonstrate asymmetrical edema of tissue planes (a nonspecific finding). However, imaging must not delay the operative management of the patient.

Surgical management of necrotizing soft tissue infection is a true emergency. Delayed operative débridement is the single most important factor influencing morbidity and mortality. Once the diagnosis is made, tissue salvage and patient survival can only be achieved by prompt widespread débridement. Antibiotics are a necessary adjunct and must be started immediately.

Empiric antibiotics must be effective against a broad range of potential pathogens (gram-positive cocci, gram-negative bacilli including *Pseudomonas*, and anaerobes). Monotherapy can be achieved with a carbapenem or piperacillin-tazobactam (Zosyn); ampicillin-sulbactam (Unasyn) now has questionable activity against many gram-negative bacilli. Clindamycin in a high dosage may be preferable to penicillin G for streptococcal infections because of in vitro evidence that clindamycin inhibits toxin production. Metronidazole (Flagyl) is preferred for therapy of polymicrobial necrotizing soft tissue infection because of better anaerobic coverage. Polymicrobial combination therapy that includes vancomycin is now popular, especially considering that nearly 60% of *S. aureus* strains are now MRSA. All identified pathogens should be treated. The duration of therapy must be individualized, but most necrotizing soft tissue infections require a minimum of 10 days of therapy.

REFERENCES

Attanoos RL, Appleton MA, Douglas-Jones AG: The pathogenesis of hidradenitis suppurativa: A closer look at apocrine and apoeccrine glands. Br J Dermatol 1995;133:254-258.

Barie PS, Eachempati SR: Surgical site infections. Surg Clin North Am 2005; 85:1115-1135.

Frazee BW, Lynn J, Charlebois ED, et al: High prevalence of methicillin-resistant *Staphylococcus aureus* in emergency department skin and soft tissue infections. Ann Emerg Med 2005;45:311-320.

Fridkin SK, Hageman JC, Morrison M, et al: Active Bacterial Core Surveillance Program of the Emerging Infections Program Network. Methicillin-resistant *Staphylococcus aureus* disease in three communities. N Engl J Med 2005;352:1436-1444.

Hirshmann JV: Impetigo: Etiology and therapy. Curr Clin Top Infect Dis 2002;22:42-51.

Lipsky BA: Medical treatment of diabetic foot infections. Clin Infect Dis 2004;39(Suppl 2):S104-S114.

National Nosocomial Infections Surveillance (NNIS) System report, data summary from January 1992 through June 2004, issued October 2004. Am J Infect Control 2004;232:5470-485.

Stevens DL, Bisno AL, Chambers HF, et al: Practice guidelines for the diagnosis and management of skin and soft-tissue infections. Clin Infect Dis 2005;41:1373-1406.

Swartz MN: Cellulitis. N Engl J Med 2004;350:904-912.

Wong CH, Khin LW, Heng KS, et al: The LRINEC (Laboratory Risk Indicator for Necrotizing Fasciitis) score: A tool for distinguishing necrotizing fasciitis from other soft tissue infections. Crit Care Med 2004;32:1535-1541.

Herpes Simplex Virus Types 1 and 2

Method of
Angela Yen, MD, and Silonie Sachdeva, MD

Etiology and Epidemiology

Herpes simplex virus types 1 and 2 (HSV-1/HHV-1 and HSV-2/HHV-2) belong to the family Herpesviridae and the subfamily Alphaherpesvirinae. The two viruses cause clinically indistinguishable mucocutaneous findings. Classic clinical manifestations are grouped or clustered vesicles and erosions on an erythematous base, often with secondary crusting. Predilection for the mucocutaneous surfaces is the rule, with perioral and anogenital surfaces most commonly affected. HSV-1 is the most common culprit of orofacial HSV, which typically occus at and around the oral surfaces. The etiology of most genital herpes infections is HSV-2 (70%-90%), although recent reports demonstrate an increasing incidence associated with HSV-1 (10%-30%).

HSV-1 seropositivity is approximately 90% worldwide in adults 20 to 40 years old, with an estimated one third of the world's population able to transmit the virus during periods of viral shedding at any time. Despite the high worldwide seropositivity, only 20% to 40% of infected persons have a history of lesions, translating to a high number of infected persons unaware of their ability to transmit disease.

In the past 2 decades, there has been an alarming increase in the seroprevalence of HSV-2 in the United States, with approximately 1.6 million persons acquiring primary genital HSV annually. An estimated 25% to 30% of women and 20% of men in the United States are infected with HSV-2. Factors associated with the transmission of genital herpes include the number of lifetime sexual partners, the age of greatest sexual activity, black or Hispanic race, lower socioeconomic status, female gender, homosexuality, and HIV infection.

Pathogenesis

HSV types 1 and 2 are transmitted primarily through direct contact with active lesions, contaminated saliva, semen, or cervical secretions. More commonly, transmission occurs in patients without active disease, in whom subclinical or asymptomatic viral shedding occurs. Following viral replication at the mucocutaneous site of contact, viral nucleocapsids travel by retrograde axonal flow to the dorsal root ganglia and establish latency until reactivation. Latent virus has been recovered from trigeminal, sacral, and vaginal ganglia both ipsilateral and contralateral to the clinical lesion. Reactivation accounts for repeated episodes of viral shedding that result in further transmission or dissemination of disease. Many instances of reactivation are spontaneous, but others are due to physical or emotional stress, fever, exposure to ultraviolet light, compromised skin barrier function (abrasion or other trauma), immune suppression, menses, or fatigue.

Clinical Features

HERPES SIMPLEX

HSV infections are variable in clinical expression, and most cases are in fact subclinical. In primary infections, a prodrome of fever, malaise, and lymphadenopathy as well as tingling, burning, or localized pain may be present. These symptoms are followed days later by the development of characteristic painful and grouped papules, vesicles, ulcers, or erosions on an erythematous base with secondary crusting and re-epithelialization. Lesions typically heal within 7 to 10 days without scarring. Recurrent outbreaks may be preceded by prodromal symptoms and are characterized by subsequent lesions that are decreased in number, severity, and duration.

Orofacial labialis, also known as herpes labialis, is the most common manifestation of HSV infection. Worldwide, 20% to 30% of children older than 5 years are seropositive for HSV-1. Primary infection with HSV-1 typically manifests as herpetic gingivostomatitis in children and young adults. Sore throat and fever develop, as well as painful vesicles and erosions on the tongue, palate, gingiva, buccal mucosa, and lips. Edema, pain, and ulceration can cause associated dysphagia, anorexia, and drooling. Young adults might have an associated pharyngitis and mononucleosis-like syndrome. In men, herpetic folliculitis of the beard area can occur and is often mistaken for a bacterial infection due to its pustular appearance. Prodromal symptoms and recurrent episodes are historical clues to the diagnosis.

Primary genital herpes infection, usually due to HSV-2 infection, produces an exquisitely painful erosive balanitis, vulvitis, or vaginitis. Involvement of the cervix, buttocks, and perineum with associated lymphadenopathy may be seen in women. Associated fever, dysuria, urinary retention, or aseptic meningitis can occur, in decreasing order of frequency, in 10% to 20% of affected female patients. Involvement of the glans penis or shaft is typical in men. Recurrent disease may be subclinical or less severe. Resolution occurs within 1 week in recurrences versus 2 to 3 weeks in primary infection. The severity of the primary infection correlates with the frequency of recurrences. Prodromal symptoms of tingling or burning can precede episodes of reactivation, with lesions typically occurring at the site of initial manifestation.

Eczema herpeticum, also known as Kaposi's varicelliform eruption, is a widespread dissemination of HSV that occurs in patients with atopic dermatitis, burns, or other underlying skin conditions. Painful monomorphous and crusted papules or vesicles develop over mucocutaneous surfaces including the face, extremities, or trunk. Secondary bacterial infection may be present and often hinders diagnosis. The presence of pain and grouped lesions are clues to the diagnosis.

Herpetic whitlow is HSV infection of a digit, most commonly observed in children and medical professionals due to direct contact or autoinoculation of HSV-1 or HSV-2.

Herpes gladiatorum occurs in contact-sport athletes such as wrestlers. Direct contact with active lesions or areas of asymptomatic shedding in an infected person underlies this condition, which is most commonly seen on the head, neck, or proximal trunk.

HSV keratitis is a major cause of blindness worldwide, most often due to infection with HSV-1. Clinical manifestations are unilateral or bilateral keratoconjunctivitis with eyelid edema, photophobia, and preauricular lymphadenopathy. Fundic examination reveals branching dendritic lesions. Complications include corneal ulceration, scarring, globe rupture, and blindness.

HSV encephalitis most often affects the temporal lobe and manifests with bizarre behavioral changes and altered mental status. Fever and focal neurologic deficits may be present. Mortality is significant at 70%, and long-term sequelae are often observed. Mollaret's meningitis (benign recurrent aseptic meningitis) has been reported with herpes simplex virus type 2.

HSV in HIV patients is often severe and may be chronic. Bone marrow and solid organ transplant patients, as well as chemotherapy patients, are also vulnerable. Atypical clinical manifestations include large verrucous papules or plaques, pustules, ulcers, widespread distribution, and visceral organ involvement.

Neonatal HSV continues to be an important public health concern, with most instances transmitted by mothers unaware of their HSV-2 infection. The incidence of perinatal transmission of neonatal herpes infection has been reported at 1 in 3200 births. The risk of transmission is highest in women with first-episode genital herpes at or near the time of delivery. Acute hemorrhagic edema of infancy has also been reported with herpes simplex type 1 stomatitis. Associated neonatal morbidity and mortality are high. Disseminated disease with liver, adrenal, or encephalopathic involvement are poor prognostic indicators.

HERPES ZOSTER

Varicella zoster virus (VZV/HHV-3) is the cause of varicella (chickenpox) and herpes zoster (shingles). A widespread, pruritic vesicular eruption is highly characteristic. Following transmission via airborne droplet or direct contact with vesicular fluid, replication and viremia ensue. Epidermal invasion results from virus transmigration from the endothelial cells. VZV eventually establishes latency in the dorsal root ganglia via mechanisms similar to HSV.

Before the introduction of live attenuated varicella vaccine, more than 90% of children in the United States contracted the primary infection, varicella, before the age of 10 years. Since the advent of the vaccine, an overall decrease in incidence approaching 87% was observed between 1995 and 2000. The greatest decline in varicella incidence has been observed in preschool children, which correlates with reduction in the number of hospitalizations for varicella. Reports of outbreaks of varicella in highly immunized groups has shown a milder disease course with fewer lesions and with fewer complications and systemic symptoms than the disease among previously unvaccinated children, providing support for ongoing efforts aimed at universal immunization in children in the United States.

Herpes zoster occurs in up to 20% of people infected with VZV and can occur at any time after the primary varicella infection. In its classic form, it is recognized by a dermatomal distribution of blisters. This eruption is due to reactivation of VZV from latently infected sensory ganglia and is most commonly observed in immunocompetent persons older than 50 years with a known prior history of varicella. Younger adults or children with herpes zoster typically experience a primary varicella infection relatively early, typically within the first year of life. A prodrome of pain, pruritus, tingling, tenderness, or hyperesthesia often precedes the classic sensory dermatomal vesicular eruption. Pain that persists for more than 1 month after resolution of the herpes zoster rash is known as *postherpetic neuralgia*, a complication that is often chronic and refractory to treatments. The effect of the varicella vaccine on the incidence of postherpetic neuralgia appears to be unclear, with different studies showing an increase or a decrease in the incidence of this complication. Other complications include secondary bacterial infection, ophthalmic zoster, meningoencephalitis, pneumonitis, and hepatitis.

Ophthalmic zoster is a serious complication that occurs in 5% to 10% cases, with an associated significant risk of blindness. Vesicles or crusted papules along the nasal tip, sidewall, or base is known as *Hutchinson's sign* and signifies involvement of the nasociliary branch of the trigeminal nerve. This clinical presentation is an indication for immediate empiric antiviral therapy and ophthalmology referral, because varicella zoster virus is also the leading cause of acute retinal necrosis. Von Szily reaction can also occur with herpetic keratitis in one eye and contralateral retinal necrosis.

Severe or disseminated herpes zoster (>20 vesicles outside the primarily involved dermatome) is most often observed in the immunosuppressed population. Atypical clinical manifestations such as crusted, verrucous papules and plaques may also be noted.

Diagnosis

HERPES SIMPLEX

Viral culture, serology, direct immunofluorescence, and molecular techniques are available laboratory tests for diagnosing HSV infection. Viral culture is a useful method of diagnosis in first-time genital outbreaks or a few mucocutaneous lesions. The cell culture technique is most reliable at the onset of symptoms, before healing or crusting of the vesicular lesions. False-negative results can occur, especially in lesions that are already healing.

Direct fluorescent antibody staining of vesicle base scrapings is 95% diagnostic and can be used to distinguish VZV from HSV. In one study, direct immunofluorescence and culture were shown to be equally sensitive at 88% in detecting HSV, whereas direct immunofluorescence was four times more sensitive (100% vs 18%) as culture in the case of VZV.

The gold standard of serologic diagnosis is the Western blot, which is 99% sensitive and 99% specific for HSV antibodies. To distinguish between HSV-1 and HSV-2, type-specific serologic assays based on type-specific glycoproteins from HSV-1 and HSV-2 are available and approved by the FDA.

The Tzanck smear offers a rapid and useful bedside test of HSV infection and relies on the identification of multinucleated giant cells in vesicular scrapings. However, this test does not differentiate among HSV-1, HSV-2, or VZV.

On histopathologic examination, characteristic ballooning degeneration of keratinocytes, spongiosis or frank vesiculation, and nuclear molding may be observed. Intranuclear inclusion bodies might also be present.

Polymerase chain reaction (PCR) of the cerebrospinal fluid is the test of choice for HSV infections of the central nervous system.

HERPES ZOSTER

A thorough history and physical examination are critical in the diagnosis and often prompt initial antiviral therapy. The Tzanck smear can aid in prompt diagnosis, but it does not distinguish between HSV and VZV. Similar limited information may be provided by histopathologic specimens of lesional skin. Direct fluorescent antibody, viral culture, serology, and PCR can all distinguish between HSV and VZV. Viral culture is the most specific, albeit a less-sensitive test. PCR is the test of choice for detecting VZV in the cerebrospinal fluid. Serologic tests have limited usefulness because most of the population is seropositive.

Treatment

HERPES SIMPLEX

Both topical and systemic antiviral treatments are useful in managing orolabial herpes in immunocompetent persons. Oral valacyclovir (Valtrex) 2 g orally taken twice in one 24-hour period, as well as topical 1% penciclovir (Denavir) decrease the duration of pain, clinical lesions, and viral shedding.

Systemic antiviral agents are the agents of choice for treating primary and recurrent genital herpes (Table 1). Three highly effective and well-tolerated antivirals include acyclovir (Zovirax), valacyclovir, and famciclovir (Famvir). All have been shown to shorten the duration, severity, pain, and period of viral shedding for initial and recurrent genital herpes infections. Because they inhibit only actively replicating viral DNA, these medications are not useful for treating

TABLE 1 Systemic Antiviral Therapy for Herpes Simplex Virus and Varicella Zoster Virus

Infection	Treatment
First Episode of Genital Herpes	
Acyclovir (Zovirax)	400 mg PO tid × 7-10 d
Acyclovir	200 mg PO 5×/d × 7-10 d
Famciclovir (Famvir)	250 mg PO tid × 7-10 d
Valacyclovir (Valtrex)	1 g PO bid × 7-10 d
Recurrent Episode of Genital Herpes	
Acyclovir	400 mg PO tid × 5 d
Acyclovir	200 mg PO 5×/d × 5 d
Acyclovir	800 mg PO bid × 5 d
Famciclovir	125 mg PO bid × 5 d
Valacyclovir	500 mg PO bid × 3-5 d
Valacyclovir	1.0 g PO bid × 5 d
Valacyclovir	2.0 g PO bid × 1 d
Chronic Suppressive Therapy	
Acyclovir	400 mg PO bid
Famciclovir	250 mg PO bid
Valacyclovir	500 mg PO q (<10 outbreaks per y)
Valacyclovir	1.0 g PO qd (≥10 outbreaks per y)
Recurrent Orolabial or Genital HSV in Immunosuppressed Patients	
Acyclovir	400 mg PO tid × 5-10 d
Acyclovir	200 mg 5×/d × 5-10 d
Acyclovir	5 mg/kg IV q8h × 7-10 d
Famciclovir	500 mg PO bid × 5-10 d
Valacyclovir	1.0 g PO bid × 5-10 d
Chronic Suppressive HSV Therapy in Immunosuppressed Patients	
Acyclovir	400-800 mg PO bid or tid
Famciclovir	500 mg PO bid
Valacyclovir	500 mg PO bid
Varicella Zoster Virus Infection	
Varicella	
Acyclovir	20 mg/kg (800 mg maxdose) PO qid × 5 d
Zoster	
Acyclovir	800 mg PO 5×/d × 7-10 d
Famciclovir	500 mg PO tid × 7 d
Valacyclovir	1 g PO tid × 7 d
Adult Immunosuppressed Patients	
Acyclovir	10 mg/kg IV 18h × 7-10 d
Pediatric Immunosuppressed Patients	
Acyclovir	10 mg/kg IV q8h × 7-10 d

HSV = herpes simplex virus.

latent infection. To treat recurrent genital herpes, a single 1000 mg dose of famciclovir twice in one day, and to treat recurrent labial herpes, a single 1500 mg dose of famciclovir have been tried and found to be effective in recent trials.

Intravenous acyclovir is reserved for neonatal HSV infection, severe HSV infections in immunocompromised hosts, and HSV patients with systemic complications.

For neonatal herpes simplex, treatment is with high-dose intravenous acyclovir (60 mg/kg/day in three divided doses) for 14 to 21 days. Prophylaxis in infants can be accomplished by cesarean delivery when women have active lesions at the onset of labor. Neonates delivered through an infected birth canal should be screened between 24 and 48 hours of age with viral cultures of the eyes, nasopharynx, mouth, and rectum. If results are positive, they should be treated with acyclovir even if they are asymptomatic. Suppressive acyclovir therapy beginning at 36 weeks of gestation is often prescribed for women with frequent recurrences of genital herpes. Women with a first episode of HSV during any stage of pregnancy should be treated with a 7- to 14-day course of an antiviral agent.

Immunosuppressed persons require more aggressive management with oral or intravenous antivirals until complete mucocutaneous clearing is observed. For patients with more than six outbreaks per year, chronic suppressive therapy is indicated and is associated with a 95% reduction of asymptomatic viral shedding (see Table 1).

Acyclovir-resistant HSV and VZV are increasing in incidence, especially in the immunosuppressed. Most commonly, a mutation in thymidine kinase is responsible. Antivirals that are thymidine kinase dependent are not effective in such cases. Alternative antivirals include foscarnet (Foscavir)[1] and cidofovir (Vistide).[1]

An alum and monophosphoryl lipid A–adjuvanted subunit glycoprotein D2 vaccine has demonstrated activity in the prevention of HSV-2 infection and disease in HSV-uninfected women and is currently in phase III clinical trials.

HERPES ZOSTER

Early treatment with antiviral agents is critical for herpes zoster, and empiric therapy is warranted (see Table 1). Acyclovir, valacyclovir, and famciclovir are FDA approved for herpes zoster and result in decreased VZV duration and pain. Adequate pain control with narcotics or other appropriate agents are required. Intravenous acyclovir is the treatment of choice for herpes zoster in patients with complications or immunosuppression.

A live, attenuated VZV vaccine (Zostavax) has been developed and recently approved by the FDA for preventing herpes zoster in persons 60 years and older.

Postherpetic neuralgia correlates with active viral replication at the dorsal root ganglion and poses a difficult therapeutic challenge. Both famciclovir and valacyclovir are effective at reducing the duration and pain. Low-dose tricyclic antidepressants[1] and gabapentin (Neurontin)[1] are also shown to be effective in reducing pain and sleep disturbances. Narcotics, analgesics, capsaicin, biofeedback, and nerve blocks are other options.

Related Pathogens

HUMAN PARVOVIRUS B19

A small, single-stranded DNA virus and member of the family Parvoviridae, human parvovirus B19 is transmitted through respiratory droplets, with peak infection rates noted in 4- to 15-year-olds. Human parvovirus B19 is responsible for several clinical syndromes including the benign childhood exanthem known as erythema infectiosum, or fifth disease. Less commonly, purpuric eruptions or severe complications including aplastic anemia and hydrops fetalis can occur. It has also been found to be associated with chronic fatigue syndrome and Henoch–Schönlein purpura.

Classic clinical manifestations of erythema infectiosum include low-grade fever and mild upper respiratory symptoms that occur 2 to 3 days before onset of the easily recognized slapped-cheeks erythema over the bilateral malar cheeks, with circumoral pallor. A pink lacy or reticular eruption over the trunk and extremities shortly follows. Duration is 7 to 14 days and occurs without scarring or long-term sequelae. Adolescents and other susceptible persons can present with arthralgias or arthritis. Persistent parvovirus B19 infection can lead to carpal tunnel syndrome. Severe disease is only seen in immunosuppressed patients, including pregnant women.

Papular purpuric stocking-and-glove syndrome is also associated with acute B19 infection and is most common in young adults in the spring. Burning and pruritus are associated with this infection. Fetal B19 infection can result in fetal hydrops, anemia, spontaneous miscarriage, or stillbirth.

Diagnostic confirmation of B19 infection may be confirmed by detection of serum anti-B19 IgM antibody. Polymerase chain reaction assays may also be used. Symptomatic management of most B19 infections is adequate. Patients with arthralgia can require nonsteroidal antiinflammatory drug treatment. Patients in transient aplastic crisis can require erythrocyte transfusions while the marrow recovers. Chronic red cell aplasia, if severe, can require intravenous immune globulin therapy. This treatment can improve anemia symptoms, but it can precipitate a rash or arthropathy. A vaccine has been developed but is not yet available. Affected fetuses can require in utero blood transfusions. Nucleic acid amplification techniques may be employed to identify and quantify B19 contamination in human blood and plasma derivatives to prevent iatrogenic transmission of parvovirus.

HAND, FOOT, AND MOUTH DISEASE

Hand foot and mouth disease is a common benign exanthem of childhood, characterized by a palmoplantar vesicular eruption and stomatitis. Common causal agents are Coxsackievirus A16 (CV-A16) and human enterovirus 71 (HEV71), but other enteroviruses, including CV-A5 and CV-A10, can also cause it. When caused by CV-A16 infection, it is usually a mild disease. Enteroviruses can cause more serious disease such as meningoencephalitis and myocarditis. Occasional myocarditis can be caused by Coxsackievirus A16 infection.

Transmission is via the oral–oral or fecal–oral route. A prodrome of malaise, low-grade fever, anorexia, abdominal pain, or upper respiratory symptoms can occur. Oval-shaped erythematous macules progress to small vesicles on the palms, soles, tongue, buccal mucosa, palate, and tonsillar pillars. Rarely, buttocks and perineal surfaces are involved. The vesicles evolve into yellow-gray ulcerations with peripheral erythema in the same distribution. Children are particularly infectious until the blisters have disappeared.

Self-limited resolution occurs without scarring. Treatment is symptomatic. In hand, foot, and mouth disease outbreaks, collecting swabs from the throat plus one other site—vesicles, if these are present (at least two should be swabbed), or the rectum if there are no vesicles—is helpful in diagnosis. Vesicle swabs give a high diagnostic yield. Use of Microchip, reverse-transcription polymerase chain reaction, and culture methods can help to detect enterovirus infection in pediatric patients.

POXVIRUSES

Molluscum Contagiosum

Molluscum contagiosum is caused by the molluscipox genus of Poxviridae, a family of large, brick-shaped double-stranded DNA viruses. Children, sexually active adults, and immunosuppressed persons are the most common hosts, and transmission is via direct contact or fomites. In children, molluscum contagiosum is a common, benign, self-limited eruption characterized by numerous scattered dome-shaped pearly papules with central umbilication that show

---

[1]Not FDA approved for this indication.

predilection for the face, trunk and skin folds. Children with atopic dermatitis are at risk for an increased number of molluscum lesions. Henderson–Patterson bodies (intracytoplasmic inclusion bodies) may be demonstrated by lesional scrapings and aid in the diagnosis. Treatment is not required, although numerous modalities including topical cantharidin, curettage, electrodessication, cimetidine, topical tretinoin, topical cidofovir, and chemical peels are available. Similar cutaneous findings are observed in sexually active adults, although the distribution favors the perineal areas, lower abdomen, and thighs in this population. Immunosuppressed persons exhibit atypical, larger eroded papules or plaques that are often widespread and deforming in this patient group. For recalcitrant molluscum contagiosum lesions, 5-aminolevulinc acid and photodynamic therapy can be used.

Orf and Milker's nodules

Orf, or ecthyma contagiosum, is caused by a parapoxvirus endemic in sheep and goats. Direct contact with infected animals or fomites results in transmission to humans. The clinical presentation is typically on the dorsal digits or hands, with single or multiple 1.5- to 5.0-cm discrete plaques or nodules. Initial lesions typically progress through several stages, including maculopapular, targetoid, nodular, regenerative, papillomatous and regressive lesions before eventually healing 35 to 40 days later. Diagnosis is by history and physical examination. Treatment is symptomatic. Cidofovir[1] in the therapy and short-term prophylaxis of orf can be used. Vaccination of sheep with the recombinant library provides protection against challenge with virulent orf virus and can be used to prevent infection.

Milker's nodule (bovine papular stomatitis) is a clinical entity similar to orf and arises from a closely related parapoxvirus transmitted from infected cattle. Physical manifestations are indistinguishable from those of orf. The condition is benign and self-limited. Treatment is supportive.

---

[1]Not FDA approved for this indication.

REFERENCES

Armstrong GL, Schillinger J, Markowitz L: Incidence of herpes simplex virus type 2 infection in the United States. Am J Epidemol 2001;153:91-99.
Centers for Disease Control and Prevention: Sexually transmitted diseases treatment guidelines 2002. MMWR Morb Mortal wkly Rep 2002; 51(RR-6):1-80.
Douglas MW, Johnson RW, Cunningham AL: Tolerability of treatments for postherpetic neuralgia. Drug Safety 2004;27(15):1217-1233.
Freij BJ: Management of neonatal herpes simplex virus infections. Indian J Pediatr 2004;71:921-926.
Holcomb K, Weinberg JM: A novel vaccine (Zostavax) to prevent herpes zoster and postherpetic neuralgia. J Drugs Dermatol. 2006;5:863-866.
Langtry LAA, Ostlere AS, Hawkins DA, Staughton RCD: The difficulty in diagnosis of cutaneous herpes simplex virus infection in patients with AIDS. Clin Exp Dermatol 1994;19:224-226.
Mahnert N, Roberts SW, Laibl VR, et al: The incidence of neonatal herpes infection. Am J Obstet Gynecol 2007;6:55-56.
Miron D, Lavi I, Kitov R, Hendler A: Vaccine effectiveness and severity of varicella among previously vaccinated children during outbreaks in day-care centers with low vaccination coverage. Pediatr Infect Dis J 2005; 24(3):233-236.
Spruance SL, Bodsworth N, Resnick H, et al: Single-dose, patient-initiated famciclovir: A randomized, double-blind, placebo-controlled trial for episodic treatment of herpes labialis. J Am Acad Dermatol 2006;55:47-53.
Stalkup JR, Yeung-Yue K, Brotjens M, Tyring SK: Human herpesviruses. In Bolognia JL, Jorizzo JL, Rapini RP, eds: Dermatology. London: Mosby, 2003, pp 1245-1253.
Takahashi M: Effectiveness of live varicella vaccine. Expert Opin Biol Ther 2004;4(2):199-216.
Vázquez M: Varicella zoster virus infections in children after the introduction of live attenuated varicella vaccine. Curr Opin Pediatr 2004; 16:80-84.

Parasitic Diseases of the Skin

Method of
Philip D. Shenefelt, MD, MS

Parasitic afflictions of the skin are caused by protozoa, helminths, and arthropods. Table 1 lists cutaneous parasites, their geographic distribution, parasitic diseases, and their treatment. Although a number of cutaneous parasites occur primarily in the tropics, world travel exposes increasing numbers of persons from temperate climates to these pathogens. Travel history and recreational or occupational history are important when cutaneous findings indicate that parasitic skin disease is in the differential diagnosis.

Protozoa

AMEBIASIS

Cutaneous amebiasis caused by *Entamoeba histolytica* is rare and occurs by direct inoculation from feces or an abscess. The lesion typically is an irregular painful ulcer on the perineum, buttock, or abdomen. Trophozoites may be found in the ulcer or stool. Metronidazole (Flagyl) 750 mg PO every 8 hours for 5 to 10 days is recommended, followed by iodoquinol (Yodoxin) 650 mg 3 times daily for 20 days to eliminate the intestinal source.

LEISHMANIASIS

Cutaneous leishmaniasis is transmitted by the bite of an infected sandfly, with several *Leishmania* species involved. The lesion is an ulcer with elevated border and central crater.

Polymerase chain reaction (PCR) diagnostic tests on tissue are highly sensitive and specific and capable of identifying the species. Sodium stibogluconate pentavalent antimony (Pentostam)[5] 20 mg/kg/day IV or IM daily for 21 to 28 days is available from the Centers for Disease Control and Prevention (CDC) Drug Service.

TRYPANOSOMIASIS

Chagas' disease, caused by *Trypanosoma cruzi*, often is clinically unapparent on the skin but can manifest as Romaña's sign (unilateral eyelid edema and conjunctivitis) or a chagoma (an erythematous indurated subcutaneous nodule). This occurs at the bite site from an infected reduviid bug. Early treatment is important to prevent late sequelae of cardiomyopathy or gastrointestinal involvement. Nifurtimox (Lampit)[5] is available through the CDC Drug Service, and is given 8 to 10 mg/kg/day PO in four divided doses for 120 days.

African sleeping sickness is transmitted by the bite of the tsetse fly infected with *Trypanosoma bruci* var *gambiense* or *rhodesiense*. About one half of patients develop an initial 2- to 5-cm erythematous nodule surrounded by a white halo at the bite site 5 to 15 days after the bite. An evanescent macular eruption can occur weeks to months later. Early treatment is very important to prevent central nervous system involvement. For *Trypanosoma bruci* var *gambiense*, eflornithine (Ornidyl),[2] available from the World Health Organization, is given at 400 mg/kg IV in 4 divided doses for 2 weeks followed by 300 mg/kg/day PO for 3 to 4 weeks. Suramin sodium (Antrypol),[5] available from the CDC Drug Service, can be used to treat either *Trypanosoma bruci* var *gambiense* or *rhodesiense*. The dosage is a 100-mg test dose followed by 20 mg/kg to a maximum of 1 g IV on days 1, 3, 7, 14, and 21.

---

[2]Not Available in the United States.
[5]Investigational drug in the United States.

TABLE 1 Cutaneous Parasites, Parasitic Diseases, and Their Treatment

Causative Organism	Geographic Distribution	Cutaneous Manifestations	Recommended Treatment
Protozoa			
Entamoeba histolytica	Worldwide	Amebiasis cutis	Metronidazole (Flagyl) 750 mg PO q8h × 5-10 d
Leishmania species	Africa, Asia, Middle East, Central and South America	Cutaneous leishmaniasis	Sodium stibogluconate (Pentostam)[5] 20 mg/kg/d IV or IM × 21-28 d
Trypanosoma cruzi	Central and South America	Chagas' disease	Nifurtimox (Lampit)[5] 8-10 mg/kg/d in 4 doses × 120 d
Trypanosoma bruci	Africa	Trypanosomal chancre or macular eruption	Eflornithine[1] or suramin[5]
Helminths			
Ancyclostoma braziliense	Worldwide	Cutaneous larva migrans	Topical 10%-15% thiabendazole suspension (Mintezol) bid × 2d Ivermectin* (Stromectol)[1] 200 µg/kg
Ancyclostoma duodenale Necator americanus	Africa, Asia, Mediterranean Central and South America Southeastern North America	Ground itch, dew itch	Mebendazole (Vermox) 100 mg PO q12h × 3 d
Dracunculus mediensis	Asia, Africa, Middle East	Guinea worm	Surgical removal
Loa loa	Africa	Calabar swellings	Diethylcarbamazine (Hetrazan) 6 mg/kg/d × 21 d
Onchocerca volvulus	Africa, Central and South America	Onchodermatitis River blindness	Ivermectin* 150 µg/kg q6-12mo
Schistosoma species	Africa, Asia, Middle East, Caribbean, South America	Schistosomiasis Cercarial dermatitis Swimmer's itch	Praziquantel (Biltricide) 20 mg/kg bid or tid × 1 d
Strongyloides	Worldwide Stercoralis	Larva currens, urticaria	Ivermectin* 200 µg/kg PO
Wuchereria bancrofti Brugia species	Asia, Africa, Caribbean, South America	Lymphatic filariasis, elephantiasis	Diethylcarbamazine (Hetrazan) 6 mg/kg/d PO × 6-12 d
Arthropoda			
Dermatobia hominis	Worldwide	Myiasis botflies	Surgical removal
Pediculus humanus Phthirus pubis	Worldwide	Head lice, body lice, pubic lice	1% permethrin (Nix Creme Rinse) × 10 min, repeat in 1 wk
Sarcoptes scabiei	Worldwide	Scabies	5% permethrin cream or ivermectin[1],* 200 µg/kg PO
Tunga penetrans	Central and South America Africa	Tungiasis	Surgical removal

[1]Not FDA approved for this indication.
[5]Investigational drug in the United States.
*Ivermectin is officially indicated only for onchocerciasis and gastrointestinal strongyloidiasis.

Helminths

CREEPING ERUPTION (CUTANEOUS LARVA MIGRANS)

Cutaneous larval migrans, or creeping eruption, occurs when the larvae of the cat and dog hookworm, *Ancyclostoma braziliense*, penetrate skin in contact with the ground. The infestation usually occurs in warm, moist, sandy areas such as the beach, playgrounds, sandboxes, and under houses. Within a few hours of contact, an erythematous papule appears at the site of skin penetration. In a day or two, pruritic erythematous serpiginous tracks develop. They usually progress at 1 to 2 cm per day. The larvae are accidental intruders and usually die within a few weeks, although some persist for up to a year with cycles of remission and exacerbation.

Small numbers of lesions can be treated with ethyl chloride or liquid nitrogen freezing. Larger numbers can be treated topically with thiabendazole 10% to 15% (Mintezol) suspension applied two times a day until the lesions have resolved. Oral thiabendazole (Mintezol) 25 to 50 mg/kg/day in two divided doses up to a maximum of 1.5 g/day for patients weighing more than 70 kg may be given for 2 consecutive days after weighing the benefits with the potential adverse reactions. Oral ivermectin (Stromectol)[1] 200 µg/kg PO in a single dose is a good alternative.

Patients should be instructed in preventive measures. Minimizing contact with the ground, covering sandboxes when not in use, and draping the ground with plastic before performing work in areas frequented by domestic animals help to prevent further exposure.

DRACUNCULIASIS

Dracunculiasis occurs when the larvae are swallowed inside infested water fleas. *Dracunculus mediensis*, the Guinea worm, can be extracted by winding them around a small stick as they emerge from the subcutaneous tissues. Metronidazole 250 mg PO 3 times daily for 10 days reduces inflammation and facilitates removal of the worm.

LOIASIS

Migratory angioedema, called Calabar swellings, and worms visible in the scleral conjunctiva typify the cutaneous manifestation of *Loa loa*. Transmission is by infected tabanid fly bite. Treatment is with diethylcarbamazine (Hetrazan) 8 mg/kg/day PO in three divided doses for 21 days.

LYMPHATIC FILARIASIS

Elephantiasis occurs as a late sequela of lymphatic channel obstruction by *Wuchereria bancrofti* or *Brugia* species, which are transmitted by infected mosquito bite. Microfilarae may be visible in blood samples viewed under the microscope. Treatment is with diethylcarbamazine (Hetrazan) 6 mg/kg/day PO in three divided doses for 6 to 12 days.

---

[1]Not FDA approved for this indication.

ONCHODERMATITIS

Pruritic dermatitis and subcutaneous nodules are characteristic of *Onchocerca volvulus* infections. Transmission is by the blackfly. These tend to occur adjacent to the rivers where the blackfly larvae develop, hence the name *river blindness* for the ocular manifestations. Microfilarae may be visible in blood samples viewed under the microscope. Treatment with ivermectin (Stromectol) 150 µg/kg PO every 6 to 12 months keeps the microfilaria under control. The adult worms are resistant to this treatment, hence the need for ongoing suppression of the microfilariae.

SCHISTOSOMIASIS

Skin exposure to contaminated water is the cause of schistosomiasis. The duck snail schistosome causes cercarial dermatitis or swimmer's itch, with pruritic erythematous papules that last 5 to 7 days. Infection with the nonhuman species of *Schistosoma* is self-limited, not requiring treatment. Human snail schistosomiasis can be treated with praziquantel (Biltricide) 20 mg/kg 2 or 3 times in a single day.

LARVA CURRENS

Strongyloides stercoralis often causes a serpiginous eruption similar to cutaneous larval migrans, but migration is much more rapid, up to 10 cm/day. It is often accompanied by diarrhea and proximal bowel infection. Ivermectin (Stromectol) 150 to 200 µg/kg PO as a single dose is very effective for both the bowel and cutaneous involvement.

UNCINARIAL DERMATITIS

The human hookworms *Ancyclostoma duodenale* and *Necator americanus* cause dew itch or ground itch similar to cutaneous larval migrans, but the larvae penetrate venules, exit into the lungs, ascend the trachea, are swallowed, attach to the small intestine, and mature. Treatment is with mebendazole (Vermox) 100 mg PO every 12 hours for 3 days.

Arthropods

MYIASIS

Human myiasis can occur with *Dermatobia hominis* or one of several other species of the botfly, screwworm fly, or flesh fly. These diptera deposit eggs on the skin, and the larvae burrow into the skin, creating an erythematous pruritic papule with a central punctum within which the tip of the larval abdomen periodically appears. Occlusion of the central punctum with petroleum jelly can force the larva to emerge to avoid suffocation. Otherwise, diagnosis and treatment are accomplished by surgical extirpation.

PEDICULOSIS

Human lice are of three types. *Phthirus pubis*, the pubic louse or crab louse, prefers the pubic hair but can be found on body and axillary hair, eyebrows, eyelashes, and occasionally the occipital scalp. *Pediculus humanus* var *capitus*, the head louse, and var *corporis*, the body louse, are elongate and fast-moving. The head louse prefers the scalp, and the body louse hides in seams in clothing. The eggs or nits of the pubic and head louse are cemented to the bases of hairs, and those of the body louse are laid on clothing, especially in seams. Nits remain viable for up to a month. They hatch and evolve into adults within 2 or 3 weeks. Spread occurs from one person to another by close contact or sharing a bed or clothing. The louse bite results in a red pruritic macule with a central hemorrhagic center.

Pediculosis Pubis

Crab lice are identified by their characteristic shape and slow movement. They are difficult to see unless one looks closely. The nits also can be seen attached to the bases of hairs. In addition to the pubic hair, the body hair, axillary hair, eyebrows, eyelashes, and occipital scalp should also be examined. Pruritus and excoriations are common, and secondary impetiginization can supervene. Scattered bite sites may be seen on the skin near hairs.

Permethrin 5% cream (Elimite) should be applied to the affected areas as a lotion for 10 minutes, then showered off. Alternatively, lindane (Kwell, Gamene) shampoo should be applied to the affected areas for 5 to 10 minutes, then showered off. A fine-toothed nit comb may be used to remove nits by combing the hairs. The treatment may be repeated once in 5 to 7 days. Eyelash infestations may be treated with careful mechanical removal of nits and lice using a fine forceps. Alternatively, petrolatum may be applied in a thick layer twice a day for a week. Clothing and bedding should be laundered in hot soapy water and mechanically dried for at least 20 minutes. Close contacts should be treated if infested.

Pediculosis Capitis

Head lice move quickly, so one must be alert for sudden movement when parting the hair. The nits are easier to find. The areas of heaviest nit involvement typically are at the occipital scalp. Nits are attached at the bases of hairs. Pruritus with excoriations is usually present. Secondary impetiginization may occur. Because head lice are highly contagious in children, all closely associated children should be treated.

Permethrin (Nix) is effective as a single-dose treatment. It is applied after shampooing and toweling dry. After 10 minutes it is rinsed out with water. A nit comb is used to remove nits.

Pyrethrin piperonyl butoxide liquid (Rid) is applied to dry hair and then shampooed out after 10 minutes. Because it is less effective as an ovacide, treatment should be repeated once in a week. Nits should be removed using a nit comb.

Lindane (Kwell, Gamene) shampoo has poor ovacidal activity. It is applied in contact with the scalp and hair for 4 minutes, then removed by shampooing. Nit combing must be thorough. Repeat treatments may be necessary.

Pediculosis Corporis

Body lice are most commonly found on vagabonds or in wartime. Because the louse lives in the seams of clothing, it is not often observed on the skin. Typical feeding sites are on the trunk and buttocks. The resulting red papules are often extensively excoriated. Secondary impetiginization is common. Nits and lice should be sought in the seams of clothing for diagnosis.

Laundering or dry cleaning the clothes and bedding kills the lice and nits. After the skin is cleansed with soap and water, pruritus may be treated with topical corticosteroid creams and oral antihistamines.

SCABIES

Scabies is a skin infestation by the mite *Sarcoptes scabiei*. The mite lives and breeds in the stratum corneum. Usually the human host does not notice the initial exposure infestation until several weeks have passed. Sensitization to the mite or its scybellae (fecal droppings) then results in intense pruritus, accentuated at night. Reinfestation results in pruritus usually within a day. Because of the asymptomatic initial phase of infestation, close contacts of a scabies patient should be treated even if not symptomatic. A successfully treated patient can continue to experience pruritus for a couple of weeks after treatment.

The distribution of scabies on the body typically involves the fingerwebs, wrists, ankles, elbowes, axillae, waistline, under the breasts and on the nipples in women, umbilicus, genitalia, and buttocks. Typically, lesions are small red papules, often excoriated. Secondary impetiginization can supervene. Uncommonly, nodules can appear on the genitalia, groin, or axilla. Vesicles can occur, especially in children. A pathognomonic lesion, the burrow, can sometimes be identified as a tiny line on a fingerweb or lateral finger. Lesions do not ordinarily occur above the neck except in infants and toddlers.

If the reaction to scabies has been partially suppressed by topical or systemic corticosteroids, scabies incognito can occur and be difficult to recognize. At the other extreme, a mentally retarded or debilitated or immunocompromised patient can have thick crusted areas and thousands of mites, even burrowing into the fingernails. This condition is known as *Norwegian* or *crusted scabies.*

A presumptive diagnosis of scabies can be made from the clinical presentation. To confirm the diagnosis, using a number 15 scalpel blade dipped in mineral oil, one should scrape several lesions down almost to the point of pinpoint bleeding and transfer the scrapings to a drop of mineral oil on a clean glass slide. After placing a cover slip over the specimen, one then examines the slide under a microscope using the 10× or 40× objective. Finding the mite, its eggs, or its scybellae (droppings) clinches the diagnosis. Treatment of scabies is generally quite effective. To prevent reinfestation, asymptomatic close contacts should be treated simultaneously. Bedsheets and all clothing worn in the past 3 days should be laundered in hot soapy water or dry cleaned.

Permethrin 5% (Elimite) cream is applied from the neck down and left on overnight for 8 to 12 hours. Reapplication after 5 days is often advisable. If used on infants and toddlers, it should be applied to the head and scalp also.

Lindane 1% (Kwell, Gamene) lotion is applied from the neck down and left on overnight for 8 to 12 hours. Reapplication after 5 days is often advisable. Lindane should usually be avoided in infants, pregnant women, and epileptics due to its neurotoxicity. Up to 40% of scabies mites may be resistant to lindane.

Precipitated sulfur 6% in petrolatum is applied daily for 3 consecutive days without removal or bathing during the 3-day time interval. Treatment of infants and toddlers should include the face and scalp. This agent is preferred for infants, toddlers, and pregnant women due to its minimal toxicity.

Oral ivermectin[1] 200 μg/kg PO single dose may be useful for crusted scabies or scabies in an immunocompromised host.

TUNGIASIS

Infestation by the burrowing female flea, *Tunga penetrans*, typically manifests as an erythematous papule with a central black spot. Location is usually on the foot. Diagnosis is confirmed and treatment is accomplished by surgical removal of the embedded flea.

---

[1]Not FDA approved for this indication.

Fungal Diseases of the Skin

Method of
Rebecca Lewis Kelso, MD,
and Sharon S. Raimer, MD

Dermatophytes may be distinguished by their genera and typical environmental hosts. The most common genera to cause superficial dermatophyte infection of skin include *Epidermophyton, Microsporum,* and *Trichophyton.* Dermatophytes may be anthropophilic, infecting humans as the primary host; zoophilic, with animals as the primary host; or geophilic, with soil as the primary host. When infecting humans, dermatophytes are dependent on the stratum corneum for growth and nutrition, which confines them to a superficial infection aside from very rare cases of dissemination.

Diagnosis

Dermatophyte infection may be readily diagnosed in an office setting. Perhaps the most rapid method of diagnosis involves the scraping of scales onto a glass slide with a No. 15 blade, placing a drop of potassium hydroxide (KOH) onto the specimen, and placing a coverslip on top. In the case of tinea unguium, a small curette may be used to obtain subungual keratin debris from the proximal portion. If a dermatophyte is present, septated hyphae may be seen traversing the scales under light microscopy. In the case of tinea versicolor, both yeast and hyphae forms are seen with a "spaghetti and meatballs" appearance. Dermatophyte infections can also be diagnosed by fungal culture or, in the case of tinea unguium, periodic acid–Schiff (PAS) staining of a nail clipping. Use of a topical antifungal medicine prior to scraping can yield a false-negative result.

Dermatophyte Infections of the Skin

DIAGNOSIS

Dermatophyte infections of the skin may be classified by body site involved.

Tinea corporis involving the neck, trunk, or extremities typically appears clinically as slightly erythematous scaly patches with central clearing and an elevated advancing border. This pattern gives rise to the term *ringworm.*

Tinea pedis typically appears as scaling of the plantar aspect of the feet, classically involving the third toe web space. Maceration may also be present, and hyperhidrosis is believed to be a contributing factor. *Trichophyton rubrum* is the usual organism. The infection can involve the entire foot in a moccasin pattern. If *Trichophyton mentagrophytes* is the inciting agent, vesicles and bullae can predominate in a more inflammatory clinical pattern. Tinea pedis warrants examination for scaling of one hand, because patients sometimes have "two foot one hand syndrome."

Tinea cruris occurs more often in men on the medial aspects of the thighs, with sparing of the scrotum and penis. This is particularly seen in men who live in hot, humid environments or who wear tight clothing.

Tinea barbae describes involvement of the beard area and may be characterized by nodular or superficial pustular forms. Sparing of the upper lip is characteristic. Majocchi's granuloma is an erythematous plaque with perifollicular pustules often found on glabrous skin, particularly on the shins or wrists. Clinical distinction of these two forms of dermatophytes is important, because involvement of the hair follicles necessitates systemic antifungal therapy.

TREATMENT

Treatment for uncomplicated cutaneous tinea infection is best accomplished by applying a cream from the allylamine or benzylaminegroups, such as terbinafine (Lamisil) cream twice daily, butenafine (Mentax) cream once daily, or naftifine (Naftin) cream once daily for a minimum of 2 weeks. Other treatment options include the topical azoles, which have lesser activity against tinea infections but do have higher efficacy for candidal infections, or ciclopirox (Loprox).

For tinea barbae, Majocchi's granuloma, or extensive tinea corporis, oral therapy is indicated. In these cases, terbinafine 250 mg orally once daily for 2 weeks is one recommended treatment. The other treatment of choice is griseofulvin (Grifulvin V), which is given 500 mg twice daily for the microsized formula or 250 mg twice daily for the ultramicrosized, formula, for 4 weeks.

Other options include oral itraconazole (Sporanox) or fluconazole (Diflucan).[1]

---

[1]Not FDA approved for this indication.

CURRENT DIAGNOSIS

Tinea Corporis
- Erythematous scaly patches with elevated borders and central clearing

Tinea Cruris
- Erythematous scaly patches in the groin with elevated borders and central clearing
- Typically spares the scrotum

Tinea Pedis
- Erythematous scaly patches on the plantar aspects of the feet
- Third web space is most commonly infected
- Can have extensive moccasin pattern or bullous pattern

Tinea Barbae
- Pustules or nodules in the beard region
- Spares the upper lip

Majocchi's Granuloma
- Erythematous plaque with perifollicular pustules
- Commonly on shins or wrists

Tinea Capitis
- Erythematous scaly patches on scalp with or without alopecia
- Pustules may be present

Tinea Unguium
- Thickened, dystrophic nails
- Evaluate for concomitant tinea pedis infection

Tinea Versicolor
- Hypo- or hyperpigmented slightly scaly patches
- Typically involves back and chest; can extend to upper arms
- In fair-skinned patients, lesions can appear erythematous

Cutaneous Candidiasis
- Erythematous papules, typically in intertriginous areas
- Might have satellite lesions
- In men with groin involvement, can extend to involve the scrotum

Nondermatophyte Infections of the Skin

DIAGNOSIS

Superficial infection may be caused by yeasts. In particular, *Candida albicans*, although often a commensal organism on the skin can overgrow under certain conditions such as warmth, moisture, or occlusion. Candidal infections of the skin typically manifest in beefy erythematous papules that can become confluent, typically in intertriginous areas such as skin folds. Satellite pustules may be present around the periphery. In contrast to tinea cruris, candidal infections of the groin often involve the scrotum. Pityriasis (tinea) versicolor, caused by *Malassezia furfur*, also can cause superficial skin infection. Clinically, hypopigmented or hyperpigmented slightly scaly patches are seen, typically on the back, chest, and arms. In patients with fair skin, the patches may be erythematous. As with *Candida albicans*, infections are seen more commonly in warm, humid environments.

TREATMENT

Patients with cutaneous candidiasis should be encouraged to keep involved areas dry. Clotrimazole 1% (Lotrimin) cream applied twice a day for 2 weeks is recommended and may be combined with hydrocortisone cream 1% in equal parts for areas of intertrigo. Treatment of tinea versicolor may be accomplished by applying ketoconazole shampoo 2% (Nizoral) for 15 minutes, then washing off, repeating in 1 week and then in 1 month. Alternatively, patients may take a single oral dose of ketoconazole 400 mg. Patients who are predisposed to tinea versicolor are likely to have a recurrence, so periodic application of ketoconazole shampoo as prophylactic therapy may be of great value.

Onychomycosis

DIAGNOSIS

Fungal infection of the nail (tinea unguium) manifests with thickening and dystrophy of the nail. Usually, the infection is due to *T. rubrum* or *T. mentagrophytes* or, less commonly, yeasts or molds. Likelihood of infection increases with advanced age, diabetes mellitus, immunosuppressive states, poor peripheral circulation, and smoking.

TREATMENT

Successful treatment of onychomycosis usually requires oral antifungal therapy. Treatment regimens include terbinafine 250 mg daily for 3 months for toenail infections or for 6 weeks for fingernail infections. Alternatively, itraconazole may be given in pulsed doses of 200 mg twice daily for 1 week per month for 2 months for fingernail infection and for 3 months for toenail infection. Therapeutic considerations must include the risk of hepatotoxicity and potential drug interactions with other medicines, and appropriate laboratory tests should be ordered. However, treatment may be warranted in those with recurrent tinea pedis, because onychomycosis can act as a reservoir of infection.

Tinea Capitis

DIAGNOSIS

Tinea capitis occurs most commonly in children. It may manifest as erythematous scaly patches, generally with patchy hair loss. Pustules and boggy, tender plaques (kerion) are seen occasionally. Infection is most commonly due to *Trichophyton tonsurans* or, less commonly, *Microsporum canis*. Identification of the fungus via culture is ideal, because it can affect the treatment choice.

TREATMENT

Although griseofulvin is the only FDA-approved treatment for tinea capitis, for infections caused by *T. tonsurans*, a 2-week course of terbinafine[1] yields high cure rates. For infections caused by *M. canis*, griseofulvin given daily for 8 weeks is the treatment of choice (see the Current Therapy box for medication dosages). As with all oral antifungal medicines, appropriate blood tests should be ordered and potential drug interactions should be considered.

Considerations in HIV/AIDS Patients

Although candidiasis and therefore intertrigo (macerated candidal infections of intertriginous areas) are common in patients with

---
[1] Not FDA approved for this indication.

CURRENT THERAPY

- Encourage patients to keep areas dry.
- Consider medicated powders such as miconazole 2% (Zeasorb AF) once the skin is clear.

Complicated* Cutaneous Tinea Infection

SYSTEMIC

- Griseofulvin (Grifulvin V) 500 mg bid for ultramicrosized, 250 mg bid for microsized × 4 wk

or

- Itraconazole (Sporanox) 100 mg bid × 2 wk

or

- Fluconazole (Diflucan)[1] 150 mg/wk × 4 wk

or

- Terbinafine (Lamisil) 250 mg/d × 2 wk

Uncomplicated Cutaneous Tinea Infection

TOPICAL

- Butenafine (Mentax) cream qd × 2 wk

or

- Terbenafine cream qd × 2 wk

or

- Naftifine (Naftin) cream qd × 2 wk

ALTERNATIVE

- Oxiconazole (Oxistat) cream qd × 2-4 wk

or

- Ketoconazole (Nizoral) cream qd × 2-4 wk

or

- Econazole (Spectazole) cream qd × 2-4 wk

Tinea Capitis

SYSTEMIC

- Adult: Terbinafine 250 mg qd × 2 wk[1,3]

Infections due to Microsporum canis

- Griseofulvin microsized 1000 mg/d × 8 wk

or

- Griseofulvin ultramicrosized 500-750 mg/d

SYSTEMIC (PEDIATRIC)

- Griseofulvin microsized liquid 20-25 mg/kg/d[3] × 6-8 wk

or

- Griseofulvin ultramicrosized 15-20 mg/kg/d[3] × 6-8 wk

or

- Terbinafine[1] 62.5 mg (¼ tab) qd × 2 wk for children weighing ≤14 kg

or

- Terbinafine[1] 125 mg (½ tab) qd × 2 wk for children weighing 14-28 kg

or

- Terbinafine[1] 250 mg qd × 2 wk for children weighing ≥28 kg

TOPICAL

- Recommend concomitant therapy with medicated shampoo for several months: ketoconazole shampoo 2% or ciclopirox (Loprox) or selenium sulfide (Selsun Blue) at least twice weekly

Tinea Unguium

SYSTEMIC

- Terbinafine 250 mg/d × 3 mo (toenails) or 6 weeks (fingernails)

ALTERNATIVE

- Itraconazole 200 mg bid for 1 wk per mo × 3 mo (toenails) or × 2 mo (fingernails)

Tinea Versicolor

TOPICAL

- Ketoconazole shampoo 2%. Apply to affected areas for 15 min, then rinse off, repeat in 1 wk, then repeat monthly

ALTERNATIVE

- Selenium sulfide (Selsun) lotion (2.5%) applied qhs and washed off in AM × 7 d

SYSTEMIC

- Ketoconazole 400 mg PO × 1 dose

Cutaneous Candidiasis

TOPICAL

- Clotrimazole (Lotrimin) cream bid × 2-4 wk

or

- Ketoconazole cream qd × 2-4 wk
- For intertriginous areas, consider combination with equal parts 1% hydrocortisone cream

SYSTEMIC

- Fluconazole 150 mg PO weekly × 2-4 wk

---

*Severe, recalcitrant, extensive, or involving hair follicle.
[1]Not FDA approved for this indication.
[3]Exceeds dosage recommended by the manufacturer.

HIV/AIDS, opportunistic dermatophyte infections do not occur any more frequently than in HIV-negative patients. However, they can manifest with more severe clinical disease, such as extensive moccasin-pattern tinea pedis, onychomycosis without interdigital tinea pedis, and Majocchi's granuloma. If highly active antiretroviral therapy (HAART) is given early on, and the CD4 count is 500/mL or more, there is no difference in frequency of tinea infections. If HAART is given later in the disease, and the CD4 count is greater than 100/mL, the tinea infection might improve or clear without any specific antifungal treatment. There is no difference in epidemiology or causative organisms. It is believed that perhaps the lack of an increase in tinea infections in HIV-positive patients in industrialized nations is due to frequent oral treatment with azoles or terbinafine for invasive candidal or fungal infection, which coincidentally provides prophylaxis against dermatophyte infection.

Treatment of HIV/AIDS patients can require a longer course of treatment or possibly oral therapy. For early disease, with a CD4 count of 500/mL or greater, for cutaneous tinea infections, treatment may include terbinafine 250 mg orally once a day for 7 days or for 2 weeks for advanced disease with CD4 count of less than 100/mL. Alternative treatment is itraconazole 200 mg orally once a day for 7 days for tinea corporis or tinea cruris, and twice a day for tinea pedis. Immunosuppressed patients might require topical therapy in conjunction with oral therapies, as well as prophylaxis once the infection is cleared. Prophylactic measures for all patient populations include eliminating any shoes that might have fungal residua, avoiding walking barefoot in public places, and using antifungal powder in shoes.

REFERENCES

Adams BB: Tinea corporis gladiatorum. J Am Acad Derm 2002;47(2):286-290.
Foster KW, Gannoum MA, Elewski BE: Epidemiologic surveillance of cutaneous fungal infection in the U.S. from 1999-2002. J Am Acad Dermatol 2004;50:748-752.
Gupta AK, Chaudhry M, Elewski B: Tinea corporis, tinea cruris, tinea nigra, and piedra. Dermatol Clin 2003;21(3):395-400.
High W: Combating superficial cutaneous fungal infections. Prac Dermatol 2006;36-42.
Johnson RA: Dermatophyte infections in HIV disease. J Am Acad Dermatol 2000;43(5 suppl):S135-S142.
Milliken LE: Role of oral antifungal agents for treatment of superficial fungal infections in immunocompromised patients. Cutis 2001;68(1 suppl):6-14.
Roberts DT, Taylor WD, Boyle J: Guidelines for treatment of onychomycosis. Br J Dermatol 2003;148:402-410.

Diseases of the Mouth

Method of
Carl M. Allen, DDS, MSD

A wide variety of disease processes other than dental caries and periodontal disease affect the oral region. These diseases may be classified based on the etiopathogenesis of the disease (e.g., viral, neoplastic); the clinical form of the lesions (e.g., plaque, vesicle, ulcer); or the anatomic region affected (e.g., lips, buccal mucosa). The clinical form and anatomic region are particularly useful for the clinician confronted by an unknown lesion. An accurate diagnosis is the most important aspect of patient management because treatment is predicated on diagnosis. The lesions that tend to affect certain oral mucosal sites preferentially are listed here according to their frequency; space limitations prohibit discussion of rare entities.

Generalized Oral Involvement

Xerostomia is the subjective feeling of a dry mouth. In most instances, it is caused by any of a variety of medications (antihypertensives, antihistamines, psychoactive drugs), and withdrawal or substitution of the medication may be helpful. A smaller number of patients may have xerostomia secondary to autoimmune destruction of the salivary gland tissue (Sjögren's syndrome) or caused by radiation therapy of the head and neck region. Such patients may develop a number of problems. The mucosa is not as well lubricated and becomes susceptible to traumatic ulceration. The dry environment predisposes the individual to the erythematous or angular cheilitis forms of oral candidiasis. If the patient has natural teeth, a marked increase in dental caries is noted.

A number of over-the-counter artificial saliva substitutes, in both liquid and gel form, are available to help manage the symptoms of dryness. Oral ulcerations should be managed conservatively using a protective hydroxypropylcellulose medication (Zilactin),[1] applied as often as necessary. Oral candidiasis can be treated with any of several antifungal medications, although those with high sucrose content, such as nystatin pastilles (Mycostatin Oral Pastilles), should probably be avoided in dentulous patients because these agents could contribute to caries activity. A prescription-strength topical fluoride preparation, such as 1.1% neutral sodium fluoride gel (PreviDent), should be used daily by patients who have natural teeth to prevent dental decay. Application of the topical fluoride is best performed at night after brushing the teeth and before retiring. Several drops of the fluoride gel should be placed on the toothbrush and gently massaged onto the surfaces of the teeth next to the gum tissue.

Lips

COMMON CONDITIONS

Fordyce's Granules

Fordyce's granules, a variation of normal anatomy, are heterotopic sebaceous glands seen in more than 80% of adults. They occur as 1-mm yellow-white submucosal dots distributed on the lateral upper lip and the buccal mucosa. No treatment is indicated because of the completely benign nature of the condition.

Angular Cheilitis

Angular cheilitis is characterized by inflammation of the corners of the mouth, accompanied by fissuring and sometimes scaling. This condition was thought to be caused by B vitamin deficiency, but the vast majority of these lesions are now thought to be caused by a low-grade infection of *Candida albicans*, with or without *Staphylococcus aureus*.

These lesions can be easily treated with a topical antifungal agent such as nystatin-triamcinolone cream (Mycolog-II Cream). Another alternative is iodoquinol-hydrocortisone cream (Vytone Cream),[1] which is both antifungal and antibacterial but must be used externally. Either medication should be applied three to four times daily for at least 1 week. With recurrence, a careful search for an intraoral source of infection may be indicated, and the possibility of HIV infection may need to be ruled out. Angular cheilitis with associated intraoral candidiasis requires treatment. Topical agents include clotrimazole troches (Mycelex Oral Troches) and nystatin pastilles, each dissolved in the mouth four to five times daily for 7 to 10 days. Systemic therapy with fluconazole (Diflucan) may be more convenient for some patients because it is given orally, 200 mg the first day, followed by 100 mg daily for the next 6 days.

Herpes Labialis

Recurrent herpes labialis affects approximately 25% of the population. Reactivation of the virus is usually triggered by sun (ultraviolet light) exposure, with many patients experiencing an itching or tingling sensation in the prodromal phase. A cluster of vesicles then develops on the vermilion zone of the lip or on perioral skin, rupturing within 1 to 3 days and leaving a crusted area that resolves after a few more days.

No curative therapy exists for this condition, and treatment results may be difficult to interpret because of the strong placebo effect in some instances. High sun protection factor (SPF) sun-blocking agents significantly reduce the frequency of episodes triggered by exposure to ultraviolet light. Low-dose acyclovir (Zovirax)[1] or valacyclovir (Valtrex)[1] may prevent attacks if it is taken continuously (400 mg twice daily; 1 g per day, respectively), but attacks resume as usual once the medication is stopped. Systemic valacyclovir, 2-g doses 12 hours apart given during the prodromal phase, reduces lesion formation in a subset of individuals affected by this condition. Topical acyclovir ointment shows no benefit in double-blind, placebo-controlled trials in immunocompetent patients, whereas topical penciclovir cream (Denavir) has only a modest effect on the course of the lesions.

Melanotic Macule

Melanotic macule, a solitary lesion, usually develops on the vermilion zone of the lips, but it may be seen intraorally. The lesion occurs as a

---
[1]Not FDA approved for this indication.

1- to 5-mm macule that exhibits a uniform, well-demarcated brown to black color.

If the patient indicates the lesion has been present for several years and has not observed any change in size or color, no treatment is indicated unless the patient is concerned about cosmetic appearance. If changes in the lesion are recent, excisional biopsy is indicated to rule out the possibility of an early melanoma.

Actinic Keratosis (Cheilitis)

Actinic keratosis is a premalignant process affecting the lower vermilion zone of the lip of fair-skinned adults with a history of chronic sun exposure. The lesions have a scaly texture and ill-defined margins.

Excision, by either scalpel or laser, or cryosurgery is indicated for treatment. Excision is often accomplished by vermilionectomy, in which the entire vermilion zone is removed as a strip for histopathologic examination. The labial mucosa is then advanced over the resulting defect. When topical chemotherapy with fluorouracil (Efudex) is used, dysplastic epithelial cells persist histologically. All patients with sun-damaged lips should be advised to use a sunscreen with high SPF, applied particularly to the lower lip when sun exposure is anticipated.

UNCOMMON CONDITIONS
Squamous Cell Carcinoma

The malignancy of squamous cell carcinoma affects the lower vermilion zone, typically arising in a preexisting actinic keratosis. Such lesions usually have a relatively slow, steady growth, with a roughened or ulcerated surface. The diagnosis should be established by biopsy. Wide surgical excision, obtaining at least a 1-cm margin of normal tissue, is usually adequate treatment because these lesions are rather indolent and do not metastasize until relatively late in their course.

Reactive Cheilitis

Patients may present occasionally with a complaint of fissured, painful lips. Evaluation of the problem should include a history of onset, duration, and use of medications and cosmetics. Lipstick and artificially flavored cinnamon products may produce a contact cheilitis. Isotretinoin (Accutane) often causes exfoliative cheilitis. Solitary chronic lip fissures, which usually occur in the winter months, may respond to topical antibiotic preparations, with surgical excision reserved for resistant lesions. Many cases of reactive cheilitis appear to be factitial, although patients may be reluctant to admit their habit of licking and nibbling at the vermilion zone. Constant moistening of the lips also predisposes the individual to a superimposed candidal infection, which exacerbates the inflammatory symptoms, and petrolatum-based lip balms may contribute to the problem by trapping moisture and thereby promoting the growth of yeast.

Telangiectasias

Superficial dilated blood vessels may occur on the vermilion zone of the lips as an isolated finding or, if multiple, as a component of either hereditary hemorrhagic telangiectasia or CREST (calcinosis, Raynaud's phenomenon, esophageal dysfunction, sclerodactyly, and telangiectasias) syndrome. Patients should be evaluated to distinguish between these two entities because their prognoses are different. Treatment of the telangiectatic lesions can be performed by laser excision, cryotherapy, or electrodesiccation.

Labial Mucosa

COMMON CONDITIONS
Mucocele

The mucocele represents a collection of extravasated mucin within the submucosal connective tissue caused by the disruption of a minor salivary gland duct by minor trauma. Most mucoceles develop on the lower labial mucosa, appearing suddenly as a painless, soft, bluish, circumscribed swelling. A cycle of swelling, breaking, and swelling again is typical. Surgical excision of the mucous deposit and the associated gland usually is necessary for resolution of the problem.

Varix

The varix, similar to varicose veins of the leg, is seen on the labial mucosa, lips, buccal mucosa, and tongue of patients older than 50 years. Patients usually describe the gradual onset of a painless purplish or bluish nodule.

Generally, no treatment is indicated. If the lesion is a cosmetic problem or if it occurs in areas likely to be traumatized, the varix may be treated by surgical excision or cryotherapy.

Aphthous Ulcer (Canker Sore)

The aphthous ulcer is perhaps one of the most misdiagnosed, mismanaged, and misunderstood of all oral diseases. Most authorities believe that aphthous ulcers are immunologically induced. No convincing scientific data link the process to viral infection. Furthermore, studies suggesting the lesions are associated with certain foods or vitamin deficiencies have not been duplicated. Several mechanisms may initiate the abnormal immune response leading to focal destruction of the oral mucosa. The lesions are typically recurrent, ranging from 1 to 24 episodes per year. The most common form of aphthous ulcer is the minor aphthous ulcer, manifesting as a 1- to 10-mm ulceration with an erythematous periphery and smooth borders. From one to five ulcers may develop simultaneously. Aphthous ulcers are located on movable mucosa, not mucosa bound to periosteum, a situation directly opposite to recurrent intraoral herpes. The patient typically reports pain that seems out of proportion to the size of the lesion. With no treatment, minor aphthae heal within 5 to 10 days. Patients with frequent attacks should be questioned regarding ocular complaints or genital ulcerations to rule out Behçet's syndrome. Infrequently, aphthous-like oral ulcerations may be a manifestation of Crohn's disease as well.

Topical application of a relatively strong corticosteroid, such as fluocinonide (Lidex Gel),[1] betamethasone dipropionate (Diprolene Gel),[1] or clobetasol (Temovate Gel),[1] is most effective in controlling the lesions. For optimum response, small amounts of the medication should be applied as a thin film often (four to five times daily) and as early in the course of the lesion as possible.

UNCOMMON CONDITIONS
Major Aphthous Ulcers

Major aphthae are debilitating oral lesions that resemble minor aphthae, except they are much larger (ranging up to 3 cm), and they persist for periods of up to 6 weeks before healing. Topical application of fluocinonide,[1] betamethasone dipropionate,[1] or clobetasol[1] usually controls this process. If the lesions are in the posterior segments of the mouth, betamethasone syrup (Celestone Syrup),[1] used as a mouth rinse and swallowed (10 mL after meals and at bedtime for 7 to 10 days), often provides relief.

Herpetiform Aphthous Ulcers

Herpetiform aphthous ulcers resemble primary herpetic gingivostomatitis, and they can be distinguished from that condition by their history of recurrence. Herpetiform aphthae are most effectively treated with one of the topical corticosteroid preparations or rinses described earlier.

Angioedema

Angioedema is thought to occur because of localized release of histamine from mast cells. Most cases are sporadic and harmless.

---

[1] Not FDA approved for this indication.

The lips are most frequently affected, followed by the tongue. A tingling sensation usually precedes the sudden onset of rather dramatic, nontender swelling. The overlying skin appears normal, and the patient is otherwise asymptomatic; these features should help distinguish this condition from cellulitis associated with a dentoalveolar abscess. With no treatment, the condition resolves in 24 to 48 hours; however, oral antihistamine therapy seems to speed resolution. Attacks are commonly recurrent, and the precipitating factor is often difficult to identify. A rare hereditary form, caused by a deficiency of C1 esterase inhibitor, can be life-threatening if the laryngeal tissues are involved. With persistent swelling, biopsy may be indicated to rule out relatively rare conditions such as orofacial granulomatosis (cheilitis granulomatosa, Melkersson-Rosenthal syndrome).

Buccal Mucosa

COMMON CONDITIONS

Linea Alba

The oral linea alba merely represents a mild thickening of the epithelium along the plane of occlusion in dentate patients. The extent to which it is evident varies tremendously from patient to patient. No treatment is indicated for this completely benign condition.

Leukoedema

Leukoedema is considered a variation of normal. Clinically, it has a whitish, filmy, almost opalescent appearance, usually affecting the buccal mucosa. Stretching the mucosa causes the white appearance to diminish greatly or disappear completely. The surface epithelial cells histologically are edematous but otherwise normal, and no treatment is necessary for this benign condition.

Cheek-Chewing

Cheek-chewing is a harmless chronic habit. Although the anterior buccal mucosa is the most common site, the labial mucosa and lateral tongue may also be affected. A white, ragged alteration of the mucosa is seen clinically. Actual ulceration is uncommon because only the outer layers of the epithelium (which have no nerve fibers) are nibbled. The patient usually admits to the habit if questioned. This habit is completely benign and requires no further management once it is identified.

Fibroma (Irritation Fibroma, Focal Fibrous Hyperplasia)

The fibroma represents an accumulation of dense collagenous connective tissue at a site of irritation. For this reason, most of these lesions are found on the buccal mucosa. The lesion appears clinically as a sessile, dome-shaped, smooth-surfaced nodule. Patients may complain because they bite the lesion inadvertently.

Because this lesion cannot be definitively differentiated clinically from a wide array of other neoplasms, excisional biopsy is generally indicated. Recurrence is uncommon.

Lichen Planus

Lichen planus is an immunologically mediated condition of unknown cause that affects adults. The oral lesions manifest in two patterns: reticular and erosive. The reticular pattern is more common and usually seen bilaterally on the posterior buccal mucosa, occurring as white fine interlacing lines or papules. The gingivae and the tongue may also be affected. The erosive form of the condition is symptomatic because of the presence of ulcerations. These ulcerations usually have a central yellow-white area of fibrin surrounded by an erythematous halo and radiating white striae.

Reticular lichen planus requires no treatment. In 20% of cases, candidiasis is present, which should be treated with an antifungal agent. Erosive lichen planus can usually be managed effectively with the more potent topical corticosteroids such as fluocinonide,[1] betamethasone dipropionate,[1] or clobetasol.[1] Application of a thin film of medicationto the lesional areas, four to five times daily, often resolves the ulcers within a few days. Other conditions, such as epithelial dysplasia, lichenoid amalgam reactions, contact stomatitis, lichenoid drug reactions, and systemic lupus erythematosus, may mimic lichen planus clinically; biopsy is thus warranted if classic clinical features are not present. Malignant transformation of reticular lichen planus is not thought likely, although erosive lichen planus could possibly be premalignant. Affected patients should be reevaluated periodically for evidence of significant mucosal change, with rebiopsy performed if necessary.

UNCOMMON CONDITIONS

Verrucous Carcinoma

Verrucous carcinoma is a relatively low-grade malignancy of surface epithelial origin. It appears as a diffuse, white, rough-surfaced, spreading plaquelike lesion affecting the buccal mucosa, palate, or alveolar process in patients over 65 years of age.

Treatment is complete surgical excision, via scalpel or laser, with evaluation of the lesional tissue histopathologically because 25% of verrucous carcinomas may contain foci of routine squamous cell carcinoma. The prognosis is generally good because this lesion does not metastasize.

Oral Mucosal Cinnamon Reaction

The oral mucosal cinnamon reaction affects the buccal mucosa, the lateral tongue, and gingivae. The lesions appear as diffuse areas of mucosal erythema with varying degrees of superimposed white plaques and, less commonly, ulceration. Such lesions may be mistaken clinically for lichen planus, candidiasis, leukoplakia, or erythroplakia. Discontinuing the artificially flavored cinnamon product (usually chewing gum) resolves the lesions within 1 week. The diagnosis can be confirmed by challenging the oral mucosa with the offending agent, although patients are often reluctant to do so after their lesions clear.

Hard Palate

COMMON CONDITIONS

Torus

Palatal tori are common developmental lesions representing a benign accumulation of dense bone in the midline posterior hard palate region. The diagnosis can be made clinically because no other condition manifests as a bony hard midline palatal mass. No treatment is necessary for this benign process, although denture construction may be hampered. Removal of the torus by an oral surgeon is recommended in that situation.

Denture Stomatitis

Denture stomatitis is almost invariably associated with a maxillary removable denture worn 24 hours per day. The palatal mucosa directly beneath the denture appears red, although it is asymptomatic. The redness is confined to the denture-bearing mucosa.

In many cases, simply having the patient remove the denture at night may resolve the palatal erythema. If the patient has a complete upper denture, it can be soaked in a mild sodium hypochlorite solution (Clorox) (1 teaspoon in 8 ounces of water) each night for a week to disinfect it. (Note: Chrome-cobalt metal denture frameworks should not be soaked in Clorox; severe corrosion will result and ruin the denture.) Because denture stomatitis is a benign and asymptomatic condition, treatment need not be a top priority.

---

[1]Not FDA approved for this indication.

Inflammatory Papillary Hyperplasia

Inflammatory papillary hyperplasia (IPH) (denture papillomatosis) is seen almost exclusively in patients who wear ill-fitting complete upper dentures. The lesions appear as multiple, erythematous 1- to 2-mm papules typically confined to the palatal vault area. These papules are composed of dense fibrous connective tissue that has accumulated secondary to chronic irritation in the superficial mucosa.

Treatment of this benign process is somewhat controversial. Some prosthodontists prefer to have these lesions surgically removed prior to constructing a new denture, although this procedure may not be necessary in every case.

UNCOMMON CONDITIONS

Recurrent Intraoral Herpes

Recurrent intraoral herpes is much less common than aphthous ulcerations, a condition with which it is frequently confused. Recurrent intraoral herpes affects only the hard palate and the attached gingiva (the paler firm gum tissue directly adjacent to the teeth). Most patients experience mild symptoms and may give a history of recurrent episodes. Lesions appear as a cluster of 1- to 2-mm shallow ulcerations that heal within 1 week. Generally no treatment is necessary, although the patient should be cautioned that virus is being shed from the lesion.

Salivary Gland Tumors

The posterior hard palate/anterior soft palate region is the most common site for the development of intraoral salivary gland neoplasia. This type of lesion presents as a slowly growing, rubbery firm, nontender mass that may or may not be ulcerated. The clinical appearance does not distinguish benign from malignant tumors, so a biopsy should be obtained that includes a margin of normal adjacent tissue. Approximately 50% of these tumors are pleomorphic adenomas, whereas the remainder represent mucoepidermoid carcinoma, polymorphous low-grade adenocarcinoma, adenoid cystic carcinoma, or acinic cell carcinoma. Complete excision is recommended for the pleomorphic adenoma, including overlying mucosa and underlying periosteum. The malignancies should be treated with a much more aggressive surgical approach, depending on the histologic type, the extent of bone involvement, and the size of the lesion. Adjunctive radiation therapy may be indicated for adenoid cystic carcinoma and high-grade mucoepidermoid carcinoma.

Soft Palate/Tonsillar Pillars

COMMON CONDITIONS

Papilloma

The squamous papilloma is the most common benign epithelial neoplasm that affects the oral mucosa, typically occurring as a solitary exophytic growth with numerous finger-like or frondlike projections on its surface. The soft palate/tonsillar pillar region is the most common site for the papilloma, and its color may range from pink to white.

Excisional biopsy, including the base of the lesion, should be performed. For those lesions of the posterior soft palate, periodic observation may be appropriate, particularly if the patient is experiencing no symptoms and the lesion is clinically characteristic.

UNCOMMON CONDITIONS

Pemphigus Vulgaris

Pemphigus vulgaris is an immunologically mediated condition characterized by the formation of vesicles and bullae secondary to attack of desmosomal complexes of the surface epithelium by autoantibodies. The condition usually is first seen intraorally, with painful, erosive lesions distributed diffusely on the oral mucosa. The soft palate is a primary site of involvement. Diagnosis should be established by light microscopy with direct and indirect immunofluorescence studies. Systemic immunosuppressive therapy is necessary to control this condition addressed in other areas of the text.

Tongue

COMMON CONDITIONS

Coated and Hairy Tongue

Coated and hairy tongue represents the accumulation of excess keratin on the filiform papillae of the dorsal tongue, resulting in the formation of elongated filamentous strands that superficially resemble hairs. Contrary to the description in numerous textbooks, this condition is not caused by an overgrowth of yeast.

No treatment is required, but if the patient is concerned about the appearance of the tongue, gentle daily débridement with a tongue scraper or the edge of a spoon assists in removing the accumulations of dead keratinized cells.

Fissured Tongue

Fissured tongue is essentially a variation of normal that usually develops sometime after the first decade of life. The patient may be concerned about the appearance of the tongue, but no symptoms are associated with the condition. The extent and pattern of fissuring can vary, and no treatment is indicated.

Benign Migratory Glossitis (Erythema Migrans, Geographic Tongue)

Benign migratory glossitis, a condition of unknown etiology, is seen in approximately 2% of the population. Most patients are asymptomatic, with lesions detected on routine examination. The dorsal tongue exhibits one or more well-demarcated zones of papillary atrophy that are surrounded, at least partially, by yellow-white slightly raised linear serpentine borders. The lesions typically resolve in one area and move to another, appearing in various stages of resolution and activity concurrently.

Because this is a benign condition, treatment is usually unnecessary. Approximately 5% of patients complain of sensitivity to hot or spicy foods when their lesions are active, but usually they do not require treatment. With severe symptoms, topical fluocinonide (Lidex Gel)[1] or one of the other stronger topical corticosteroids, applied as a thin film to the lesions several times daily, seems to reduce the discomfort.

Traumatic Ulcer

The traumatic ulcer occurs most frequently on the lateral tongue, buccal mucosa, and overlying bony prominences such as tori and exostoses. Most of these lesions are associated with relatively little pain. The traumatic ulcer manifests clinically as a defect covered by creamy white fibrin. Although most of these lesions heal within a week or so, some tend to persist, developing a rolled margin and peripheral induration.

Often no treatment is required because of the minimal degree of discomfort and the rapid healing time. If the patient complains of tenderness when eating salty or acidic foods, a protective medication (Zilactin) can be applied as needed. Topical corticosteroids should probably not be used because they may delay healing in this situation. If an ulcer is present for longer than 2 weeks, with or without previous treatment, a biopsy is mandatory to rule out malignancy. A possible exception to this rule might be those ulcers overlying tori because they are notoriously difficult to resolve.

---

[1]Not FDA approved for this indication.

Burning Tongue Syndrome (Idiopathic Glossopyrosis)

The burning tongue syndrome seems to affect postmenopausal women predominantly. The patient often reports the rather sudden onset of a sensation that feels like the tongue was scalded. Symptoms are usually localized to the anterior tongue, although the labial mucosa and anterior hard palate may also be affected. Clinically, the mucosa appears normal. If mucosal erythema is identified, a variety of conditions should be ruled out, including candidiasis, anemia, local trauma, and erythema migrans. A culture for *Candida albicans* should be performed. If the workup shows no evidence of these conditions, a diagnosis of burning tongue syndrome can be made. Because there is no medically proven therapy, no specific treatment exists. The numerous suggested treatments in the literature have generally not been examined in controlled trials, and their efficacy is typically no more than that of the placebo effect. Reassuring patients this is a harmless condition, nothing more than a nuisance, and that the condition often resolves spontaneously after a period of months or years is usually sufficient.

UNCOMMON CONDITIONS

Squamous Cell Carcinoma

The lateral/ventral tongue is one of the most common sites for squamous cell carcinoma. In the early stages, the lesion is relatively asymptomatic, which underscores the importance of a regular and thorough oral mucosal examination. Slight thickening or nodularity within a white or red plaque frequently heralds the onset of invasion. As the lesion grows, the surface becomes ulcerated and symptoms of pain and tenderness develop. On palpation, squamous cell carcinomas are usually firm and show infiltrative borders. Biopsy is mandatory because other chronic ulcerative processes, such as chronic traumatic ulcer, deep fungal infections, mycobacterial infections, Wegener's granulomatosis, and other malignancies, may have a similar clinical presentation.

Treatment consists of wide surgical resection or radical radiation therapy, or both, depending on a number of factors. Prognosis is directly related to the tumor stage, although, in general, these patients do poorly because their lesions are not diagnosed until the later stages.

Hairy Leukoplakia

Hairy leukoplakia is an HIV-related lesion, significant because it often heralds a rapid decline in the patient's immune status. The lesion affects the lateral borders of the tongue, usually bilaterally, appearing as white plaques with vertical streaks. Sometimes the degree of keratinization may be great enough to produce hairlike projections, hence the name. Because this is otherwise a benign condition, no treatment is necessary. Hairy leukoplakia is caused by Epstein-Barr virus, thus medications used against other herpes viruses, such as acyclovir (Zovirax),[1] valacyclovir (Valtrex),[1] and dihydroxypropoxymethyl guanine (DHPG) (ganciclovir [Cytovene]),[1] may produce transient resolution.

Herpes in the Immunocompromised Host

With an immunocompromised host, the normal rules governing the location of the lesions of recurrent herpes are not applicable. The virus is not contained by the host, as in the normal individual, and the result is the formation of large, shallow, painful ulcerations with slightly elevated serpentine or scalloped margins. The diagnosis should be established by exfoliative cytology or viral culture, and treatment should be instituted immediately with systemic acyclovir, orally or intravenously, depending on the severity of the clinical infection.

---
[1]Not FDA approved for this indication.

Macroglossia

Macroglossia is the term used to describe enlargement of the tongue. Among the more frequent causes of macroglossia are hemangiomas and lymphangiomas. Hemangiomas are usually present at birth or develop shortly thereafter, with the tongue the most common site. These lesions are typically red or purple in color. If no compromise in function of the involved tissue is seen, treatment should be delayed until the child is older than 6 years of age because many of these lesions regress spontaneously. For those lesions that do not regress, argon laser excision is the optimal therapy. Other methods of management include cryotherapy and sclerosing agents.

Lymphangiomas affecting the oral tissues often exhibit a characteristic so-called frog-egg or tapioca-pudding surface morphology because of the dilated lymphatic vessels that are close to the surface. Treatment is surgical excision, although the decision to treat may depend on the size and site of the lesion. Recurrence rates as high as 40% are reported in some series of cases.

Other causes of macroglossia are much less common and include amyloidosis as well as benign and malignant tumors. Biopsy would be indicated to establish a diagnosis prior to treatment planning.

Floor of the Mouth

COMMON CONDITIONS

Leukoplakia

Leukoplakia is a clinical term that should be applied only to those white patches of the oral mucosa that cannot be wiped off and cannot be diagnosed as any other condition clinically. Leukoplakia is considered a premalignant condition and usually diagnosed in the sixth and seventh decades of life. Clinically, the condition appears as a well-defined white plaque that may show varying degrees of redness. The most worrisome sites of involvement include areas prone to cancer development, such as the lateral tongue, floor of the mouth, and the tonsillar pillar region.

Ideally, treatment is complete removal with microscopic evaluation of the excised specimen. Cryotherapy and laser excision may be used, but tissue may be rendered unsuitable for histopathologic examination. More concern should be given to leukoplakias found in nonsmokers, in high-risk areas for oral cancer, in lesions with a red component, in multifocal lesions, or those found in patients 20 to 50 years of age. If complete excision is accomplished, 30% of leukoplakias still recur, so careful follow-up with rebiopsy is indicated.

Sialolithiasis

Sialolithiasis (salivary duct stones) may appear with symptoms or be discovered on routine examination. The classic presentation is sudden painful unilateral swelling of the involved salivary gland occurring at mealtime. Most stones involve the submandibular gland, and these can be palpated as a hard submucosal mass in the floor of the mouth. Treatment usually involves surgical removal of the stone with repositioning of the salivary duct opening proximally. Sialography should then be performed to assess the function of the gland, and if it appears abnormal, it should probably be removed to prevent subsequent episodes of chronic recurrent sialadenitis.

UNCOMMON CONDITIONS

Erythroplakia

The premalignant lesion of erythroplakia represents the nonkeratinized version of leukoplakia. Erythroplakia appears as a well-demarcated, velvety red plaque that is typically asymptomatic. Dysplastic changes are likely, and treatment should consist of complete removal by the most expedient means.

Squamous Cell Carcinoma

The clinical appearance of squamous cell carcinoma at this site is similar to that of the lateral tongue, as is the treatment.

Alveolar Process/Gingiva

COMMON CONDITIONS

Mandibular Tori/Exostoses

Mandibular tori/exostoses are benign developmental lesions that consist of dense, viable bone. Mandibular tori are located on the lingual surface of the mandible in the premolar region, whereas exostoses occur on the alveolar process in other sites. Radiographic evaluation of any asymmetric bony swelling is indicated, and the exostosis should appear as a well-defined radiopacity. Generally, no treatment is necessary unless the bony outgrowths interfere with denture construction, in which case surgical removal is indicated.

Amalgam Tattoo

The amalgam tattoo is produced by the iatrogenic implantation of dental amalgam into the oral soft tissues. Amalgam tattoos are usually macular and range in color from gray to blue to black or brown. Periapical radiographs often show the fine radiopaque metallic particles.

No treatment is necessary if the diagnosis can be made definitively from the radiograph. If no radiopacity is seen, biopsy is generally indicated to rule out a relatively rare oral melanocytic process such as a nevus or melanoma.

Dental Sinus Tract (Parulis)

The lesion of the dental sinus tract (parulis) represents a proliferation of granulation tissue at the drainage site of a sinus tract originating form the apical root portion of a nonvital tooth. Clinically, the parulis appears as an erythematous papule on the alveolar mucosa. Symptoms of pain may wax and wane. Treatment consists of either extraction or endodontic therapy for the offending tooth, and the prognosis is good.

Acute Necrotizing Ulcerative Gingivitis (Trench Mouth, Vincent's Infection)

Acute necrotizing ulcerative gingivitis is a disease produced by bacteria that are normal inhabitants of the oral microflora. The condition, which occurs in the third or fourth decade of life, is associated with poor oral hygiene, poor diet, and stress. College students are especially vulnerable during final examinations, and the condition may be seen in HIV-positive patients as well. Patients invariably present with a complaint of painful, foul-smelling gingivae. Examination shows punched-out ulceration of the interdental papillae. Acute necrotizing ulcerative gingivitis is frequently confused with primary herpes, which also is associated with pain and ulceration, but the punched-out interdental papillae are not seen in herpes infection.

Débridement, often requiring topical or local anesthesia, or both, is very important. This should be combined with systemic antibiotic therapy, such as tetracycline,[1] 250 mg every 6 hours, or potassium penicillin V, 500 mg every 6 hours. HIV-infected patients should also use chlorhexidine (Peridex) mouth rinse twice daily to prevent recurrence of acute necrotizing ulcerative gingivitis. For non-HIV patients, the prognosis is reasonably good, assuming they improve their diet and oral hygiene status.

Primary Herpetic Gingivostomatitis

Primary herpetic gingivostomatitis is caused by the initial exposure of the patient to herpes simplex virus, usually type I. Most of these infections occur during childhood, but occasionally an individual escapes contact with the virus until adulthood. Patients present with fever, cervical lymphadenopathy, malaise, and oropharyngeal pain. Examination of the oral mucosa reveals multiple shallow ulcerations distributed diffusely throughout the mouth, although the gingivae are often markedly affected. The gingival involvement is different from that of acute necrotizing ulcerative gingivitis, in that the interdental papillae do not show the punched-out ulcerations with the herpetic infection.

Patients should be managed symptomatically with analgesics, antipyretics, and topical anesthetics as indicated. Dehydration is sometimes a problem if oral pain prevents intake of fluids. Having the patient rinse with 5 mL of viscous lidocaine (Xylocaine Viscous) or dyclonine HCl (Dyclone) prior to meals provides temporary relief. Systemic acyclovir (Zovirax)[1] or valacyclovir (Valtrex)[1] may have a significant impact on the course of this disease if given during the first few days of the infection.

Inflammatory Fibrous Hyperplasia (Denture Epulis, Epulis Fissuratum, Denture Fibroma)

Inflammatory fibrous hyperplasia is caused by low-grade irritation from an ill-fitting denture. Clinically, the lesions are seen as smooth-surfaced sessile masses that appear to arise from the mucosa of the alveolar process or vestibule. Sometimes a groove or fissure runs lengthwise across the lesion, corresponding to the denture flange. Ulceration of the surface may be seen.

Surgical excision of the lesion is indicated prior to construction of new dentures. If the lesion is removed and the patient continues to wear the old denture, inflammatory fibrous hyperplasia recurs, but it is a completely benign process that does not undergo malignant transformation.

UNCOMMON CONDITIONS

Pyogenic Granuloma, Peripheral Giant Cell Granuloma, and Peripheral Ossifying Fibroma

Pyogenic granuloma, peripheral giant cell granuloma, and peripheral ossifying fibroma are benign gingival lesions probably initiated by chronic irritation in most instances. Although they are histologically distinctive, their clinical appearance and biologic behavior are similar. All of these lesions appear as sessile, dome-shaped masses that develop mainly on the gingiva (although pyogenic granuloma may be seen on any surface). They range from pink to reddish purple in color and are often ulcerated. Excisional biopsy is recommended to rule out the less likely possibility of metastatic neoplasm, which may clinically appear very similar. A recurrence rate of 15% can be expected for each of these lesions.

Generalized Gingival Hyperplasia

Generalized gingival hyperplasia usually develops as a side effect of medication: phenytoin (Dilantin), calcium channel blocking agents, or cyclosporine (Sandimmune). Only 30% to 50% of patients receiving one of these drugs show the diffuse gingival enlargement, which is usually related to the level of oral hygiene of the patient. If the drug cannot be discontinued or substituted, periodic periodontal surgery with reinforcement of oral hygiene instruction can usually control the problem. Rarely such enlargement may be associated with any of several genetic syndromes. These patients typically require periodic surgical reduction of the gingival tissues by a periodontist. Generalized gingival hyperplasia may also be a manifestation of myelomonocytic leukemia, although these patients usually complain of other signs and symptoms related to their leukemic state. Biopsy and appropriate hematologic evaluation are necessary to establish a diagnosis.

Desquamative Gingivitis

Desquamative gingivitis is a descriptive term for a reaction pattern that affects the gingival tissues of adults. Patients complain of red, tender gingival mucosa that has a tendency to slough with minor

---

[1]Not FDA approved for this indication.

manipulation. Vesicles may sometimes be reported. This condition must be biopsied for light microscopic evaluation as well as direct immunofluorescence studies because it invariably represents one of several distinct entities: erosive lichen planus, cicatricial pemphigoid, linear IgA disease, pemphigus vulgaris, or chronic ulcerative stomatitis. Once the definitive diagnosis is established, the patient can be managed appropriately.

REFERENCES

Neville BW, Damm DD, Allen CM, Bouquot JE: Oral and Maxillofacial Pathology, 3rd ed, Philadelphia: Elsevier Science, 2008.
Neville BW, Day TA: Oral cancer and precancerous lesions. CA Cancer J Clin 2002;52:195-215.
Regezi JA, Sciubba JJ, Jordan RCK: Oral Pathology. Clinical Pathologic Correlations, 4th ed, Philadelphia: Elsevier Science, 2003.
Sapp JP, Eversole LR, Wysocki GP: Contemporary Oral and Maxillofacial Pathology, 2nd ed, Philadelphia: Elsevier Science, 2004.
Scully C, Gorsky M, Lozada-Nur F: The diagnosis and management of recurrent aphthous stomatitis: A consensus approach. J Am Dent Assoc 2003;134:200-207.

Venous Leg Ulcers

Method of
*Jaymie Panuncialman, MD, and
Vincent Falanga, MD*

Background

Chronic venous ulceration is associated with considerable morbidity and is costly to treat. The prevalence of this condition is increasing due to our aging population. Although venous ulcers rarely lead to amputation, the socioeconomic impact of this disease is substantial. Twenty-two percent of patients develop venous ulcers by the age of 40 years. Disability related to venous ulcers results in loss of productive work hours estimated at 2 million workdays per year. Venous ulcers lead to decreased mobility and loss of independence in the elderly, further reducing their quality of life. The goals of venous ulcer treatment are to decrease healing time and to prevent recurrence.

Pathophysiology

The fundamental problem in venous ulcers is venous hypertension. The veins of the lower extremity are divided into the superficial and deep venous system, which are connected by perforator veins. Veins have one-way valves to ensure that blood flows proximally from the extremities and back to the heart. The valves act in concert with the contraction of the leg muscles. This pumping action (the calf muscle pump) results in a pressure differential that allows blood from the superficial venous system to drain into the deep venous system through the series of perforators. Venous hypertension is defined as a failure of the pressure in the deep veins to decrease with ankle movement and lower extremity exercise. Venous hypertension may be the result of valve dysfunction, obstruction of the veins due to stenosis or thrombosis, or failure of the calf muscle pump function, as seen in patients with limited ankle joint motion. The sustained pressure in the venous system leads to changes in the microcirculation.

It is postulated that the compromised microcirculation caused by venous hypertension has important consequences at the molecular and cellular levels, including abnormal fibrin deposition, macromolecular leakage, and trapping of growth factors, wound fluid and electrolyte abnormalities, and oxygen radical formation. The altered microenvironment in the wound bed can also lead to the accumulation of resident cells that are unresponsive to stimulatory signals important for wound healing.

Clinical Features

Patients with chronic venous ulcers often complain of leg aching and swelling, which is worse at the end of the day and is relieved by leg elevation. In contrast, the pain in arterial disease is worse with leg elevation and relieved when the legs are in a dependent position. Most patients have risk factors predisposing them to venous insufficiency, including heredity, multiple pregnancies, obesity, leg trauma or surgeries, and a previous history of a deep venous thrombosis. The ulcerations are generally painful, and the pain is not directly correlated to the size of the ulcer. Difficult to heal venous ulcers are associated with duration longer than 6 months, size greater than 5 cm^2, history of previous surgeries for venous disease, location at or below the malleolus, and presence of severely indurated skin (lipodermatosclerosis).

Patients with venous ulcers are highly sensitive to topically applied agents and should be evaluated carefully for allergic contact dermatitis. Patients are commonly allergic to neomycin, latex, lanolin, fragrance, and preservatives. The dermatitis is often persistent and does not resolve easily, even weeks after discontinuing the offending agent.

The ulcers are generally irregular in size, shallow and not involving tendons or bone, and located in the gaiter area, that is from the midcalf to the ankle. Venous ulcers can occur in other locations on the leg, but not on the plantar surface or above the midcalf. Black eschars are very rare, and the surface of the ulcer is often covered with a fibrinous or exudative component. A sign suggesting venous insufficiency is dependent edema improved with leg elevation. There is also hyperpigmentation, scaling, and inflammation of the skin, referred to as *venous stasis dermatitis*. *Lipodermatosclerosis* is the woody induration of the skin involving the lower leg circumferentially, resulting in an inverted champagne bottle appearance. *Atrophie blanche* refers to the ivory white areas of skin studded with tiny blood vessels and is not specific for venous disease.

Diagnosis

The diagnosis of venous ulceration is largely based on the clinical features and the exclusion of arterial disease or inflammatory ulcers. When indicated, a biopsy of the ulcer can help in excluding malignancy, vasculitis, or conditions due to small vessel occlusion

CURRENT DIAGNOSIS

- Venous leg ulceration diagnosed mainly on clinical presentation.
- Swelling and aching pain relieved by elevation are symptoms of venous insufficiency.
- Skin findings suggesting venous insufficiency are varicosities, hyperpigmentation, scaling, lipodermatosclerosis, and atrophie blanche.
- Venous ulcers occur mainly on the gaiter area and are shallow and clean based.
- Ankle–brachial pressure index (ABI) between 0.7 and 1.1 helps exclude significant arterial insufficiency, but the test is unreliable in diabetic patients.
- Duplex ultrasound is a standard test in visualizing venous anatomy and function.
- Tests for coagulation parameters should be done in young patients with deep venous thrombosis and ulceration.
- A wound biopsy is warranted in longstanding ulcers to exclude malignancy.

(cryoglobulinemia, cryofibrinogenemia). Using Doppler testing to measure the systolic blood pressure at the ankle and brachial artery allows determination of the ankle–brachial pressure index (ABI), which is between 0.7 and 1.1 in the absence of arterial disease. The ABI is not reliable in patients with diabetes because of poor compressibility of blood vessels. In that case, referral to a vascular laboratory for color duplex scanning, measurements of venous reflux, toe pressures, and pulse volume recordings may be required.

The venous duplex ultrasound is considered a standard test of noninvasive evaluation of chronic venous disease. It is a means to directly visualize the anatomy of the deep and superficial venous systems as well as valve function. Venous insufficiency is measured by reflux, which is the time in seconds that there is retrograde blood flow through the veins. A reflux time longer than 1.0 second is considered significant. An abnormal reflux does not prove that the ulcer is venous, but the results from this test may be used as a guide to determine if surgical intervention might benefit a patient unresponsive to optimal medical therapy. When venous ulcers occur in younger patients, procoagulative conditions such as factor V Leiden mutation should be excluded.

Treatment

A treatment algorithm for venous leg ulcers is shown in Figure 1.

Compression therapy is the standard and accepted treatment for venous ulceration. It reduces the edema and redirects some blood flow from the superficial to the deep venous systems. However, this does not correct venous hypertension. High compressive bandages exerting 30 to 40 mm Hg at the ankle are more effective than low compression. Among different high-compression systems there is no current consensus that one is better than the other. Elastic compression (long-stretch bandages) is preferred over nonelastic or short-stretch bandages (Unna's boot), which are probably effective only in ambulatory patients; in ambulatory patients, the calf muscles can press against the rigid or semirigid bandage during walking.

CURRENT THERAPY

- Properly applied compression therapy is the cornerstone of treatment.
- Patient compliance is key to compression therapy.
- Exercise to improve calf muscle function should be emphasized.
- Dressings are useful for débridement, for controlling exudate, and for decreasing the bacterial burden.
- Pentoxifylline (Trental) should be used, and preferably at the higher dose of 800 mg three times a day.[3]
- Bioengineered skin can accelerate healing, particularly in hard-to-heal ulcers.
- Traditional skin grafting and minimally invasive venous surgery may be considered in select patients unresponsive to medical management.

[3]Exceeds dosage recommended by the manufacturer.

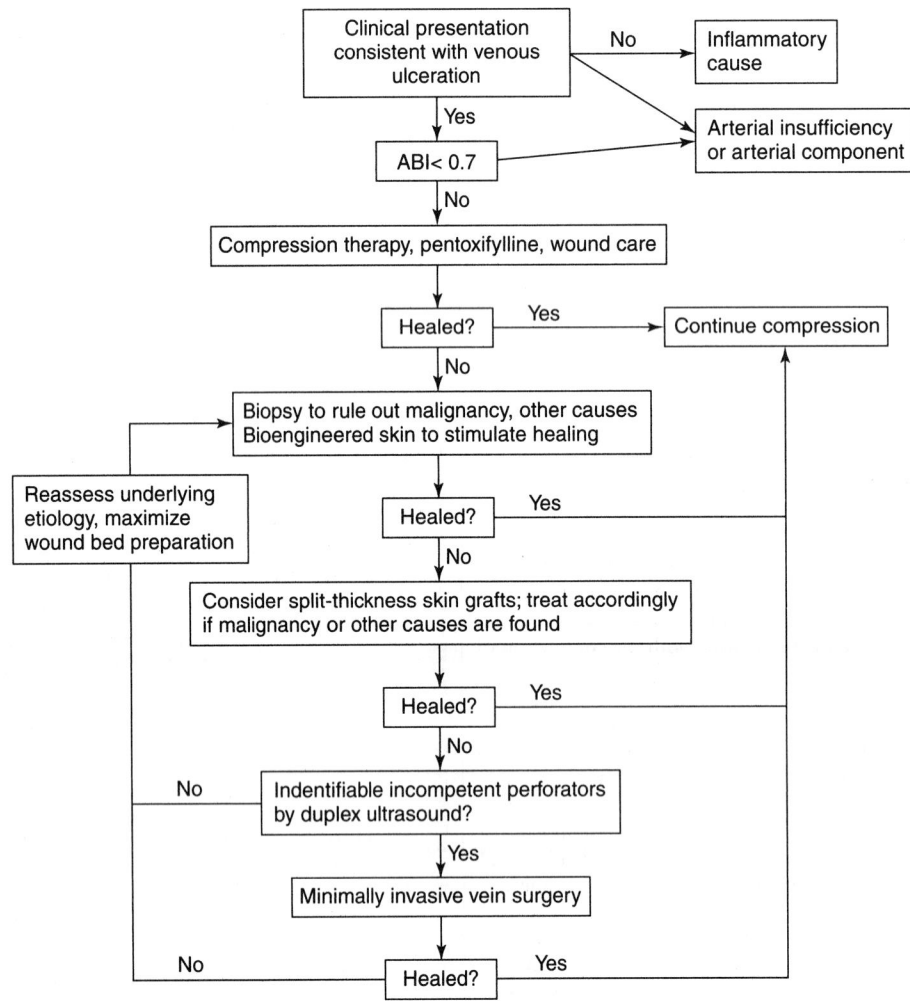

FIGURE 1. Treatment algorithm for venous leg ulcers. ABI, ankle–brachial pressure index.

Exercise plays a role in improving calf muscle function and should be part of the therapeutic regimen. Patients will be using compression for the rest of their lives. Difficulty wearing compression bandages, need for trained health care workers to apply them, and controlling drainage underneath the bandage are problems that decrease patient compliance. These factors must be taken into consideration when prescribing compression treatment for the patient.

No particular wound dressing has been shown to increase wound closure or time to heal in venous ulcers; possibly such studies have not been powered adequately for this important outcome.

Dressings have properties that are useful adjuncts in treating venous ulcers. Slow-release antiseptic dressings (with silver or iodine) are often useful in controlling bacterial burden. Many moisture-retaining dressings improve pain and may be used for autolytic débridement. Foams and calcium alginates have high absorptive capacities and can maintain a moist environment. Hydrocolloids are absorptive and can be useful, whereas film dressings are not absorptive and are much less used in treatment. In general, it is better to avoid adherent dressings, and therefore foams and alginates are preferred. Enzymatic débridement with collagenase (Santyl) can be helpful, and surgical débridement is sometimes required. Débridement is useful in removing necrotic tissue and bacteria and in preparing the wound for advanced treatments, such as bioengineered skin.

In spite of adequate compression therapy, 50% of venous ulcers will fail to heal. Pentoxifylline (Trental) at doses of 800 mg three times a day[3] has been shown to decrease time to heal. This is a higher dose than is normally prescribed, but one that was found effective in a multicenter controlled trial. Application of bioengineered skin, consisting of a living bilayered construct, has been found effective and is approved for use by the FDA. The mechanisms of bioengineered skin are unknown, but this treatment might provide the wound with an appropriate repertoire of cytokines and growth factors. The effectiveness of bioengineered skin is greatly improved by wound bed preparation steps to minimize the bacterial burden, decrease exudate and edema, and develop healthy granulation tissue.

If in spite of these interventions the wound still has not healed, other options are conventional split-thickness grafting or surgical intervention to tie incompetent perforators, as for example with subfascial endoscopic perforator vein surgery (SEPS). SEPS is also helpful in severe lipodermatosclerosis, even in the absence of ulceration. SEPS has been reported to accelerate healing in some cases and might have some benefit in decreasing ulcer recurrence. Malignancy must be considered in ulcers that do not heal. Thus, a wound edge biopsy in nonhealing ulcers may be required. Occasionally, the ulcer is not venous in etiology, and other diagnostic considerations must be entertained. Once an ulcer heals it is imperative that compression therapy be continued.

It is important to monitor the percentage change in ulcer area to assess healing. Wound tracings and digital photography provide objective ways to monitor healing. An ulcer that does not heal or show significant healing within 4 weeks should prompt a clinician to reevaluate and consider advanced therapies. In a satisfactory situation, the edges of the wound should move inward by 0.7 cm a week or faster. This rate of healing should be evident by 4 weeks and has been correlated with ultimate wound closure.

---

[3]Exceeds dosage recommended by the manufacturer.

REFERENCES

Barwell JR, Davies CE, Deacon J, et al: Comparison of surgery and compression with compression alone in chronic venous ulceration (ESCHAR study): Randomised controlled trial. Lancet 2004;363(9424):1854-1859.

Brem H, Kirsner RS, Falanga V: Protocol for the successful treatment of venous ulcers. Am J Surg 2004;188(1A Suppl):1-8.

Cavorsi J, Vicari F, Wirthlin DJ, et al: Best-practice algorithms for the use of a bilayered living cell therapy (Apligraf) in the treatment of lower-extremity ulcers. Wound Repair Regen 2006;14(2):102-109.

Elias SM, Frasier KL: Minimally invasive vein surgery: Its role in the treatment of venous stasis ulceration. Am J Surg 2004;188(1A Suppl):26-30.

Fletcher A, Cullum N, Sheldon TA: A systematic review of compression treatment for venous leg ulcers. BMJ 1997;315(7108):576-580.

Jull A, Waters J, Arroll B: Pentoxifylline for treatment of venous leg ulcers: A systematic review. Lancet 2002;359(9317):1550-1554.

Eberhardt RT, Raffetto JD: Chronic venous insufficiency. Circulation 2005; 111(18):2398-2409.

Falanga V, Brem H, Ennis WJ, et al: Maintenance debridement in the treatment of difficult-to-heal chronic wounds. Osteotomy Wound Management. In press.

Phillips T, Machado F, Trout R, et al: Prognostic indicators in venous ulcers. J Am Acad Dermatol 2000;43(4):627-630.

Pressure Ulcers

Method of
David R. Thomas, MD

A pressure ulcer is the visible evidence of pathologic changes in blood supply to the dermal and underlying tissues, usually because of compression of the tissue over a bony prominence.

A differential diagnosis of ulcer type is critical to treatment. Chronic ulcers of the skin include arterial ulcers, venous stasis ulcers, diabetic ulcers, and pressure ulcers. Pressure ulcers generally appear in soft tissue over a bony prominence. A classic presentation aids the diagnosis. For example, arterial ulcers occur in the distal digits or over a bony prominence, diabetic ulcers occur in regions of callus formation, and venous stasis ulcers occur on the lateral aspect of the lower leg. However, atypical presentations may occasionally obscure the etiology. The treatment of these various etiologies differs considerably. This discussion is limited to the treatment of pressure ulcers and should not be used to treat other types of ulcers.

Seven principles of management guide treatment of pressure ulcers. The chief cause of these ulcers is pressure applied to the tissues that compromises blood flow. Therefore, the first treatment principle is to relieve pressure. Pressure relief can be obtained by positioning the patient frequently at a fixed interval to relieve pressure over the compromised area. Turning and positioning may be difficult to achieve because of a patient's self-positioning or medical treatments that interfere with the ability to position the patient. Because of this difficulty, a number of medical devices are designed in an attempt to relieve pressure. These devices can be classified as static or dynamic. Static devices include air-, gel-, or water-filled containers that reduce the tissue–surface interface. Dynamic devices use a power source to fill compartments with air that support the patient's weight or alternate the pressure on different areas of the body. Choose a static device when the patient has good bed mobility. Choose a dynamic device when the patient cannot self-position in bed.

At the present time, results of reported clinical trials do not favor one device over another. The choice should be based on durability, ease of use, and patient comfort. A simple check for so-called bottoming out should be done for all devices. Your hand should be inserted palm upward under the patient's sacrum between the device and the bed surface. If there is not an air column between the patient and the bed surface, the device is ineffective and should be changed. No device is effective in reducing heel pressure, the second

CURRENT DIAGNOSIS

- Differentiate among pressure, diabetic, venous stasis, and arterial ulcers.

CURRENT THERAPY

Seven Principles of Pressure Ulcer Therapy

- Relieve pressure.
- Assess pain.
- Assess nutrition and hydration.
- Remove necrotic debris.
- Maintain a moist wound environment.
- Encourage granulation and epithelial tissue formation.
- Control infection.

most common site for pressure ulcers. Bridging with pillows is effective in reducing heel pressure in immobile patients; patients with high bed mobility may require boot devices to elevate the heel off the bed surface. Patients who fail to improve or who have multiple pressure ulcers should be considered for a dynamic-type device, such as a low-air-loss bed or air-fluidized bed.

The second principle of pressure ulcer therapy is to assess pain. Pressure ulcers do not always result in pain, particularly in insensate patients. However, some pressure ulcers do result in pain and should be treated aggressively. Oral or parenteral pain medications should be used to control symptoms.

The third principle of ulcer therapy is to assess nutrition and hydration. Pressure ulcers occur in sicker individuals in whom nutrient intake may be reduced by coexisting illness. Increased intake of protein (1.2 to 1.5 g/kg/day) is associated with higher healing rates. Achievement of high protein intake may be difficult because of anorexia of aging or anorexia associated with coexisting diseases. Adequate calories, adjusted for stress (30 to 35 kcal/kg/day), should be prescribed. Adequate dietary intake should provide adequate vitamins and minerals. No difference in healing rates is associated with supertherapeutic doses of vitamin C or zinc. If adequate dietary intake is compromised, a supplemental vitamin/mineral prescription at RDA (recommended daily allowance) doses should be considered. Adequate hydration can be maintained by 30 mL/kg/day of water. The decision to institute enteral feeding in patients with pressure ulcers who are unable to maintain adequate oral intake should not be undertaken lightly. The decision to use enteral feeding must consider the patient's wishes, overall goal of care, and the complications of enteral feeding. In several studies, the long-term result of enteral feeding was associated with poorer outcomes in patients with pressure ulcers.

The fourth principle of pressure ulcer management requires removing necrotic debris. Phagocytosis removes necrotic debris naturally. Accelerating the rate of removal may shorten healing time. Options include sharp surgical débridement, mechanical débridement with gauze dressings, application of exogenous enzymes, or autolytic débridement under occlusive dressings. Choose surgical débridement if the ulcer is infected. Surgical débridement is the fastest method but may remove some viable tissue, cause discomfort, and is the most expensive method, especially if done in an operating room. Applying moist gauze that is allowed to adhere to the ulcer bed by drying is a form of débridement. When the dry dressing is removed, nonselective tissue removal occurs. This method can be associated with discomfort, may delay healing while débridement is in progress, and is often defeated when the dressing is remoistened before removal. Enzymatic débridement can digest necrotic material. Three enzymatic preparations are available in the United States: collagenase, papain/urea, and papain/urea combined with chlorophyll. Enzyme preparations are nonselective, possibly resulting in some damage to fibroblasts, epithelial cells, or granulation tissue. Enzymatic débridement is slower, can be associated with discomfort, and should be limited in duration until a clean wound bed is obtained. Autolytic débridement is achieved by allowing autolysis under an occlusive dressing. Both enzymatic and autolytic débridement may require 2 to 6 weeks to achieve a clean wound bed. A total of five clinical trials did not show that enzymatic agents increased the rate of complete healing in chronic wounds compared to control treatment. Unless clinically infected, heel ulcers are better left undebrided because they occur in poorly vascularized tissues.

The fifth principle of pressure ulcer management is to maintain a moist wound environment. Maintaining a moist wound environment is associated with more rapid healing rates compared to dressings that are allowed to dry. Continuously moist saline gauze is the historical standard dressing for stage II through IV pressure ulcers. Care must be taken to change the gauze frequently to prevent drying because this may delay healing. Newer wound dressings provide a low moisture vapor transmission rate (MVTR), a measure of how quickly the dressing allows drying. A MVTR of less than 35 g of water vapor per square meter per hour is required to maintain a moist wound environment. Woven gauze has a MVTR of 68 g/m^2/hour, and impregnated gauze has a MVTR of 57 g/m^2/hour. By comparison, hydrocolloid dressings have a MVTR of 8 g/m^2/hour. Dressings with low MVTR provide a healing environment that encourages granulation tissue formation and epithelialization.

The use of occlusive-type dressings is more cost effective than gauze dressings primarily because of a decrease in nursing time for dressing changes. A meta-analysis of five clinical trials comparing a hydrocolloid dressing with a dry dressing demonstrated that treatment with a hydrocolloid dressing resulted in a statistically significant improvement in the rate of pressure ulcer healing (odds ratio: 2.6).

Occlusive dressings can be divided into broad categories of polymer films, polymer foams, hydrogels, hydrocolloids, alginates, and biomembranes. Each has advantages and disadvantages. No single agent is perfect. The choice of a particular agent depends on the clinical circumstances. Nonpermeable polymers can be macerating to normal skin. Polymer films are not absorptive and may leak, particularly when the wound is highly exudative. Most films have an adhesive backing that may remove epithelial cells when the dressing is changed. Hydrogels are hydrophilic polymers that are insoluble in water but absorb aqueous solutions and are available in amorphous gels or sheet dressings. They are poor bacterial barriers and are nonadherent to the wound. Because of their high specific heat, these dressings are cooling to the skin, aiding in pain control and reducing inflammation. Most of these dressings require a secondary dressing to secure them to the wound. Hydrocolloid dressings are complex dressings similar to ostomy barrier products. They are impermeable to moisture and bacteria and highly adherent to the skin. Hydrocolloid dressings have an accelerated healing of 40% compared to moist gauze dressings. Hydrocolloid dressings are particularly suited for areas subject to urinary and fecal incontinence. Their adhesiveness to surrounding skin is higher than some surgical tapes, but they are nonadherent to wound tissue and do not damage epithelial tissue in the wound. The adhesive barrier is frequently overcome in highly exudative wounds. Hydrocolloid dressings cannot be used over tendons or on wounds with eschar formation. Alginates are complex polysaccharide dressings that are highly absorbent in exudative wounds. This high absorbency is particularly suited to exudative wounds. Alginates are nonadherent to the wound, but if the wound is allowed to dry, damage to the epithelial tissue may occur with removal. Alginates may be used under other dressings to absorb exudate. The biomembranes are very expensive and not readily available.

Stages I and II pressure ulcers can be managed with a polymer film or hydrocolloid dressing. Stages III and IV dressings may require a wound filler, such as a calcium alginate or an amorphous hydrogel, to obliterate dead space and decrease anaerobic colonization.

Vacuum-assisted closure is used in both acute and chronic wounds. Only two randomized, controlled trials in pressure ulcers are reported. In both trials, vacuum-assisted closure was equivalent to treatment with a hydrogel or moistened gauze.

Electrotherapy is used for stages III and IV pressure ulcers unresponsive to conventional therapy. Several clinical trials suggest that electrotherapy is likely to be marginally effective. Hyperbaric oxygen, ultrasound, infrared, ultraviolet, and low-energy laser irradiation have insufficient data to recommend their use currently. No data support the use of a systemic vasodilator, hemorheologics, serotonin inhibitors, or fibrolytic agents in the treatment of pressure ulcers.

Topical agents such as zinc, phenytoin,[1] aluminum hydroxide,[1] honey, sugar, yeast, aloe vera gel, or gold[1] were not effective in clinical trials.

Because the theory of augmenting ulcer healing under the newer dressings suggests that wound fluid contains favorable healing factors, it is important not to change the dressings too frequently. Unless the wound fluid seeps from under the dressing, it should not be changed more often than every 3 to 7 days.

The sixth principle of pressure ulcer treatment is to encourage granulation tissue formation and promote reepithelialization. Growth factors show promising early results, but the data do not suggest accelerated healing of pressure ulcers. It is important not to affect granulation and epithelial tissue negatively. A number of wound cleaners and antiseptics are toxic to fibroblasts and epithelial tissues, including benzalkonium chloride, povidone-iodine solution (Betadine), Dakin's solution, hydrogen peroxide, Granulex, Hibiclens, and pHisoHex. The use of these agents in a pressure ulcer should be limited to use in infected ulcers and strictly limited in duration.

The seventh principle of pressure ulcer management is to control infection. Quantitative microbiology alone is a poor predictor of clinical infection in chronic wounds. All pressure ulcers are colonized with bacteria, usually from skin or fecal flora. The presence of microorganisms alone (colonization) does not indicate an infection in pressure ulcers. The diagnosis of infection in chronic wounds must be based on clinical signs: erythema, warmth, pain, edema, odor, fever, or purulent exudate. In the presence of clinical signs of infection, enteral or parenteral antibiotics should be used. In ulcers that are not progressing toward healing, an empirical trial of topical antimicrobials may be considered, although the data are inconclusive.

---

[1] Not FDA approved for this indication.

REFERENCES

Thomas DR: The role of nutrition in prevention and healing of pressure ulcers. Geriatr Clin North Am 1997;13:497-512.
Thomas DR: Are all pressure ulcers avoidable? J Am Med Dir Assoc 2001;2:297-301.
Thomas DR: Improving the outcome of pressure ulcers with nutritional intervention: A review of the evidence. Nutrition 2001;17:121-125.
Thomas DR: Issues and dilemmas in managing pressure ulcers. J Gerontol Med Sci 2001;56:M238-M340.
Thomas DR: Prevention and management of pressure ulcers. Rev Clin Gerontol 2001;11:115-130.
Thomas DR: The promise of topical nerve growth factors in the healing of pressure ulcers. Ann Intern Med 2003;139:694-695.
Thomas DR: Management of pressure ulcers. J Am Med Dir Assoc 2006; 7:46-59.

Atopic Dermatitis

Method of
Mark Boguniewicz, MD

Atopic dermatitis is a common, chronically relapsing inflammatory skin disease often associated with respiratory allergy. In the United States, up to 17% of school-age children are affected and more than 50% of patients with atopic dermatitis develop asthma and allergic rhinitis. Atopic dermatitis is associated with abnormalities in skin barrier function including increased transepidermal water loss, increased levels of endogenous proteolytic enzymes, and reduced ceramide levels. Epidermal changes contribute to increased allergen absorption into the skin and microbial colonization.

Mutations in the filaggrin *(FLG)* gene, located in the epidermal differentiation complex on chromosome 1q21, have been shown to result in loss of expression of filament-aggregating protein (filaggrin) involved in formation of the epidermal barrier. *FLG* mutations were also shown to be a major risk factor for asthma associated with atopic dermatitis. Although significant progress has been made in the understanding of atopic dermatitis, the relationship of genetic, epidermal, environmental, and immunologic components in this disease remain to be fully elucidated.

Atopic dermatitis can result in significant morbidity, leading to school absenteeism, occupational disability, and emotional stress. Management requires a comprehensive approach that includes recognizing and avoiding triggers, skin hydration and maintenance of an intact skin barrier, optimal use of topical antiinflammatory therapy, addressing skin infection and colonization by microbial organisms, attenuating the itch–scratch cycle, dealing with behavioral aspects of the disease, and educating patients and caregivers.

Diagnosis

Atopic dermatitis has no pathognomonic skin lesions or unique laboratory parameters. The diagnosis is based on the presence of major and associated clinical features. Major features include pruritus, a chronically relapsing course, typical morphology and distribution of the skin lesions (facial and extensor aspects of extremities in infants and young children, flexural involvement in older patients,) and a personal or family history of atopic disease. The presence of pruritus is essential to the diagnosis of atopic dermatitis.

Complicating Features

Patients with atopic dermatitis often have nonspecific hand dermatitis that is aggravated by repeated wetting, especially in an occupational setting. Atopic keratoconjunctivitis is always bilateral, with itching, burning, tearing, and copious mucoid discharge. It is commonly associated with eyelid dermatitis and chronic blepharitis and can result in visual impairment from corneal scarring. Keratoconus is a conical deformity of the cornea resulting from persistent rubbing of the eyes.

Patients with atopic dermatitis are susceptible to colonization and infection with a variety of microbial organisms that may be due to a T_H2-type cytokine–mediated antimicrobial peptide deficiency of keratinocytes. The most common organism complicating atopic dermatitis is *Staphylococcus aureus*, which can be cultured from the skin of more than 90% of patients with atopic dermatitis, compared with only 5% of normal subjects. The high rate of *S. aureus* colonization in atopic dermatitis may be associated with colonization of the nares, with the hands serving as the vector of transmission. Most *S. aureus* produce toxins that act as superantigens, interacting with much greater numbers of cells than conventional antigens, which in turn results in significant skin inflammation. Recurrent staphylococcal pustulosis can be a significant problem in atopic dermatitis; however, invasive *S. aureus* infections occur rarely and should raise the possibility of an immunodeficiency, such as hyper-IgE (immunoglobulin E) syndrome.

Dissemination of herpes virus results in eczema herpeticum. When it involves the periocular area, it should be treated as an ocular emergency. Even patients with quiescent disease can develop eczema vaccinatum, a potentially lethal complication of smallpox vaccine. The opportunistic yeast *Malassezia sympodialis* (previously termed *Pityrosporum ovale*) has been associated with a predominantly head-and-neck distribution of atopic dermatitis.

Psychosocial Aspects

Patients with atopic dermatitis often have psychosocial issues that can exacerbate their illness. Patients often respond to stress or frustration with pruritus and scratching. Stimulation of the central nervous system can intensify cutaneous vasomotor and sweat responses and contribute to the itch–scratch cycle. Scratching may be associated with significant secondary gain or with a strong component of habit. Of considerable importance, sleep disturbance is common and significantly affects the quality of life of patients and their families.

Differential Diagnosis

The differential diagnosis of atopic dermatitis includes immunodeficiencies such as Wiskott–Aldrich syndrome, an X-linked recessive disorder characterized by eczematous rash, thrombocytopenia, and humoral and cellular immune abnormalities.

Immune dysregulation, polyendocrinopathy, enteropathy, X-linked (IPEX) syndrome is associated with dermatitis, enteropathy, type 1 diabetes, thyroiditis, hemolytic anemia, and thrombocytopenia resulting from mutations of *FOXP3*, a gene located on the X chromosome that encodes a DNA-binding protein required for development of regulatory T cells.

Hyper-IgE syndrome is an autosomal dominant multisystem disorder characterized by recurrent deep-seated bacterial infections, including cutaneous cold abscesses and pneumonias due primarily to *S. aureus*.

Scabies is an intensely pruritic skin disease; however, linear lesions, distribution in the genital and axillary areas and diagnostic skin scrapings help differentiate it from atopic dermatitis.

In adults, contact dermatitis, either irritant or allergic is common. Typical distribution can point to a suspected contactant, although allergic contact dermatitis should be confirmed by patch testing.

In adults with new onset eczematous rash, without obvious etiology, especially in those without a history of childhood eczema or atopic diseases such as asthma, cutaneous T-cell lymphoma needs to be ruled out. Ideally, biopsies should be sent from three separate sites to increase the yield in identifying abnormal Sézary cells. An eczematous rash can be seen also in patients with AIDS.

Triggers of Atopic Dermatitis

Skin hyperreactivity is an important feature of atopic dermatitis. Changes in the environment, which might not affect normal persons, can trigger the itch sensation in patients with atopic dermatitis and set off the itch–scratch cycle. resulting in a flare of eczema. A variety of factors can irritate atopic skin. Patients' abnormal skin barrier can facilitate entry of irritants, allergens. and microbes into the skin where they can interact with cells of the immune system. Eliminating known triggers of atopic dermatitis is an important part of managing the patient's disease.

IRRITANTS

Extremes of temperature, excessive washing without use of moisturizers, and exposure to soaps, detergents, and chemicals can contribute to skin irritation.

ALLERGENS

Controlled allergen challenges have demonstrated that foods and inhalant allergens can trigger atopic dermatitis in a subset of sensitized patients. The most common food allergens are milk, egg, peanut, soy, wheat, fish, and tree nuts. Environmental allergens such as dust mites and animal danders can also trigger atopic dermatitis. It is important to understand that positive allergy skin or blood tests do not necessarily identify clinically relevant allergic triggers.

INFECTIOUS AGENTS

Microbial organisms including bacteria, primarily *S. aureus*, viruses such as herpes simplex virus, molluscum contagiosum. and yeast such as *M. sympodialis* can all contribute to skin inflammation in atopic dermatitis as discussed earlier.

EMOTIONAL STRESS

Stress can activate immune cells, which effect cutaneous inflammatory responses. Behavioral modification or biofeedback can help with chronic itching and scratching. Counseling and patient and family support organizations can also be helpful.

Treatment

Successful management requires proper diagnosis; hydration and repair of the damaged skin barrier; identification and elimination of exacerbating factors, including irritants and allergens; appropriate use of topical antiinflammatory medications; control of pruritus and infections; evaluation of psychosocial aspects of the disease; and education (Fig. 1).

HYDRATION AND BARRIER REPAIR

The best way to reestablish the skin's barrier function is to soak the affected area or bathe for approximately 10 minutes in warm water and then immediately apply an occlusive agent to retain the absorbed water and prevent evaporation. Baths may need to be taken several times a day during flares of atopic dermatitis, although showers may be adequate for patients with mild disease.

The use of an effective emollient, especially when combined with hydration therapy, helps to restore and preserve the stratum corneum barrier and can decrease the need for topical steroids. Moisturizers are available as lotions, creams, and ointments and many are available in 1-pound jars. Lotions contain more water than creams and may be more drying because of an evaporative effect. Lotions and creams can cause skin irritation secondary to added preservatives and fragrances. Vegetable shortening (Crisco) can be used if an inexpensive moisturizer is needed. Petroleum jelly (Vaseline) is an effective occlusive when used to seal in water after bathing. Several newer nonsteroidal creams (Atopiclair, MimyX) marketed as medical devices require prescriptions.

IDENTIFICATION AND ELIMINATION OF EXACERBATING FACTORS

An important component in managing atopic dermatitis is to reduce skin irritation, which decreases the urge to scratch. Patients should apply moisturizer whenever the skin feels dry or itchy, wash all new clothes before wearing to remove formaldehyde and other irritating chemicals, add a second rinse cycle to ensure removal of residual laundry detergent, and wear garments that allow air to circulate freely. Keeping fingernails short helps prevent damage from scratching. Use of sedating antihistamines at bedtime can reduce the itching sensation through tranquilizing and sedative effects. Patients should also be instructed to use sunscreen with an SPF of 15 or higher on a regular basis and avoid getting sunburned. Patients should shower or bathe immediately after swimming in a chlorine pool using a mild cleanser to remove residual chemicals, then apply a moisturizer.

Proper testing and challenges should be done in a controlled environment under supervision to determine which allergens contribute to a patient's atopic dermatitis. Patients should avoid only proven allergens rather than be on unnecessarily restrictive diets or activities. When chemicals are suspected allergens, patch testing may be useful in evaluation.

TOPICAL ANTIINFLAMMATORY MEDICATIONS

Topical corticosteroids reduce inflammation and pruritus and are effective for both the acute and chronic components of atopic dermatitis. They are available in formulations ranging from extremely high- to low-potency preparations. High-potency steroids include clobetasol (Temovate), betamethasone dipropionate (Diprolene) 0.05%,

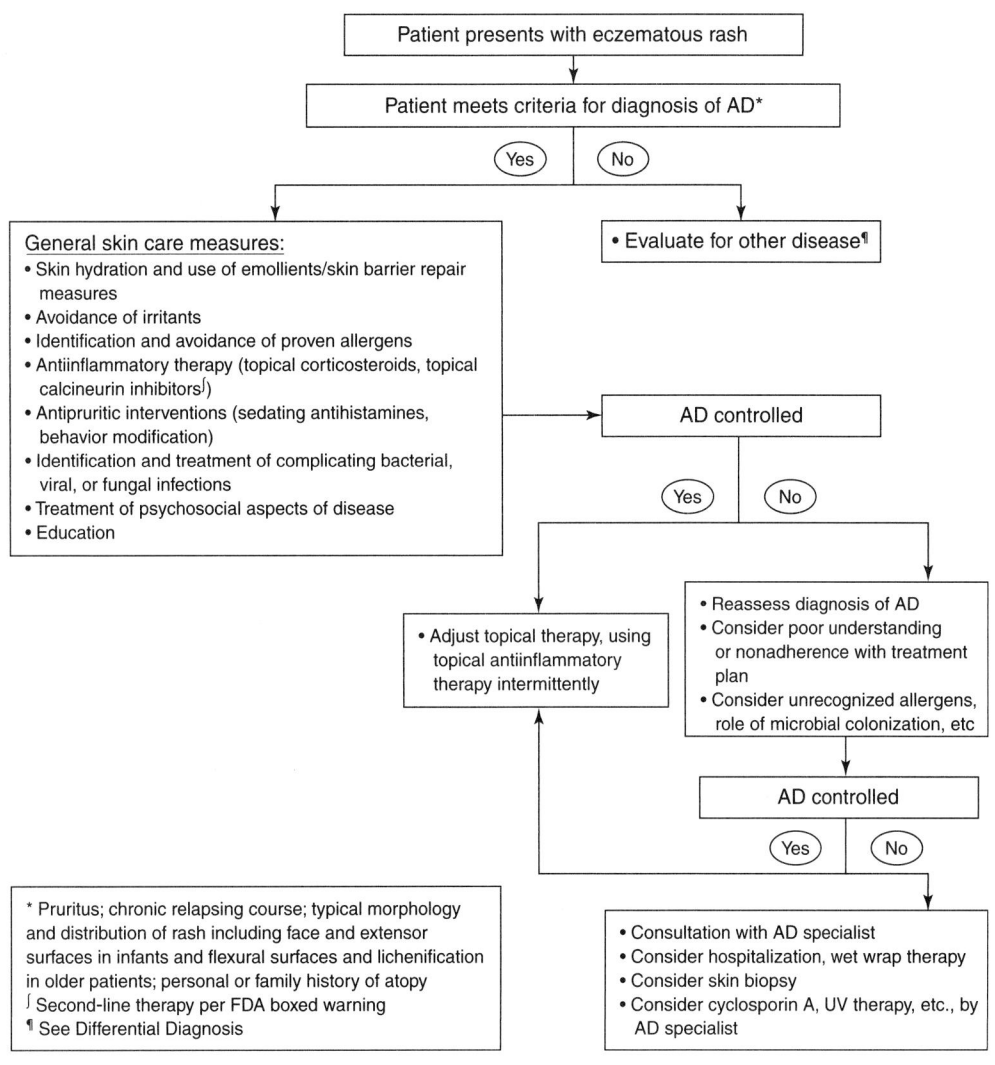

FIGURE 1. Approach to the patient with atopic dermatitis. AD = atopic dermatitis; UV = ultraviolet light.

and fluocinonide (Lidex) 0.05%. Mid-potency steroids include triamcinolone (Kenalog) 0.1%, fluocinolone (Synalar) 0.025%, fluticasone (Cutivate) 0.05/0.005%, and mometasone (Elocon) 0.1%. Low-potency steroids include desonide (Desonate) 0.05% and alclometasone (Aclovate) 0.05%. Patients might incorrectly assume that the potency of their prescribed steroid is based solely on the percentage stated after the compound name (e.g., that hydrocortisone 2.5% is more potent than fluocinonide 0.05%) and may apply the preparations incorrectly.

Choice of a particular product depends on the severity and distribution of skin lesions, although in general, high-potency steroids should only be used on thickened areas of the hands and feet and only low-potency preparations should be used on the face, groin, or axillae. Topical steroids with pediatric indications include fluticasone 0.05% cream and desonide 0.05% hydrogel for up to 28 days in children 3 months of age or older, fluticasone lotion for children 12 months and older, and mometasone 0.1% cream and ointment for children 2 years and older. Topical steroids are available in a variety of bases, including ointments, creams, lotions, solutions, gels, and oil, and there is no need to compound them. Ointments are most occlusive and as a rule provide better delivery of the medication while preventing evaporative losses. Creams may be better tolerated than ointments in a humid environment. Inadequate prescription size is often a cause of treatment failure, especially with widespread, chronic disease. Note that approximately 30 g of medication are required to cover the entire body of an average adult. In addition, patients or caregivers often delay using topical steroids due to concerns about side effects. Once-daily treatment with topical fluticasone or mometasone can help with patient adherence.

Topical calcineurin inhibitors (TCIs) are nonsteroidal immunomodulators. Because treatment with TCIs is not associated with skin atrophy, they are particularly useful for treating the face and intertriginous regions. A fairly common side effect is transient burning of the skin, although rarely patients complain of prolonged burning or stinging. Currently, tacrolimus (Protopic) ointment 0.03% is approved for intermittent treatment of moderate to severe atopic dermatitis in children ages 2 years and older, tacrolimus ointment 0.1% for intermittent treatment of moderate to severe atopic dermatitis in adults, and pimecrolimus (Elidel) cream 1% is approved for intermittent treatment of patients ages 2 years and older with mild to moderate atopic dermatitis. Although there is no evidence of a causal link between cancer and the use of TCIs, the FDA has issued a boxed warning for tacrolimus ointment 0.03% and 0.1% (Protopic, Astellas) and pimecrolimus cream 1% (Elidel, Novartis) because of a lack of long-term safety data (see U.S. package inserts). The new labeling states that these drugs are recommended as second-line treatment and their use in children younger than 2 years is currently not recommended. Ongoing surveillance has not shown a trend to increased infections, impaired immune responses, or malignancies.

ANTI-INFECTIVE MEASURES

Systemic antibiotic therapy may be needed for secondary infection, most commonly due to *S. aureus*. Semisynthetic penicillins or first- or second-generation cephalosporins for 7 to 10 days are usually effective. Erythromycin-resistant organisms are fairly common, making macrolides less useful. Maintenance antibiotic therapy should be avoided due to colonization by methicillin-resistant *S. aureus* (MRSA). Topical mupirocin (Bactroban) applied three times daily to affected areas for 7 to 10 days may be effective for localized areas of involvement, and twice-daily nasal mupirocin for 5 days can reduce nasal carriage of *S. aureus*.

Bathing may also reduce colonization by *S. aureus*. Although antibacterial cleansers are effective in reducing bacterial skin flora, they can cause significant skin irritation. Dilute bleach baths together with nasal mupirocin have been recommended by some dermatologists to reduce skin infections in patients with recurrent MRSA (⅛-½ cup of household bleach per *full* tub of water). Care should be taken not to cause severe skin irritation due to incorrect proportion of bleach to water. Topical steroids and TCIs can also decrease *S. aureus* colonization.

Patients with disseminated eczema herpeticum usually require treatment with systemic acyclovir (Zovirax).[1] Recurrent cutaneous herpetic infections can be controlled with daily prophylactic oral acyclovir. Superficial dermatophytosis and *M. sympodialis* infections can be treated with topical or, rarely, systemic antifungal drugs.

ANTIPRURITIC MEASURES

Systemic first-generation antihistamines such as diphenhydramine (Benadryl) or hydroxyzine (Vistaril) and anxiolytics can have beneficial tranquilizing and sedative effects and should be used primarily in the evening to avoid daytime drowsiness. Second-generation antihistamines are less effective for treating atopic dermatitis–associated pruritus. Topical antihistamines and anesthetics should be avoided because of potential sensitization.

RECALCITRANT DISEASE

Systemic steroids should be avoided in the management of a chronic, relapsing disorder such as atopic dermatitis. The dramatic improvement observed with systemic steroids may be followed by significant flare of atopic dermatitis after discontinuation. If a short course of oral corticosteroids is given, topical skin care should be intensified to suppress rebound flaring of atopic dermatitis. Wet-wrap dressings using a layer of wet clothing (e.g., wet pajamas or long underwear, tube socks) with dry clothing (e.g. sweatsuit, socks) on top can reduce inflammation and pruritus and act as a barrier to trauma from scratching. The face can be covered by wet gauze with dry gauze over it and secured in place with an elastic bandage. Dressings may be removed when they dry, or they may be rewetted. They are often best tolerated at bedtime. Overuse of wet dressings can result in chilling, maceration of the skin or, infrequently, secondary infection. Because this approach can be somewhat labor intensive, it should be reserved for acute exacerbations of atopic dermatitis along with selective use in areas of resistant lesions. The package inserts for TCIs recommend that they not be used under occlusive dressing.

Patients who have erythroderma or severe disseminated disease resistant to first-line therapy might need to be hospitalized. Placing the patient in a controlled environment with intense education and supervised therapy usually results in rapid and marked clinical improvement. In this setting, patients can also undergo appropriately controlled challenges to help identify potential triggering factors and address stressors. Patients requiring further therapy including oral cyclosporin A (Neoral),[1] mycophenolate mofetil (Cellcept),[1] or UV light therapy should be referred to an atopic dermatitis specialist.

---

[1]Not FDA approved for this indication.

REFERENCES

Akdis CA, Akdis M, Bieber T, et al: Diagnosis and treatment of atopic dermatitis in children and adults: European Academy of Allergology and Clinical Immunology/American Academy of Allergy, Asthma and Immunology/PRACTALL Consensus Report. J Allergy Clin Immunol 2006;118:152-169.
Boguniewicz M, Schmid-Grendelmeier P, Leung DYM: Atopic dermatitis. J Allergy Clin Immunol 2006;118:40-43.
Fonacier L, Spergel J, Charlesworth EN, et al: Report of the Topical Calcineurin Task Force of the American College of Allergy, Asthma and Immunology and the American Academy of Allergy, Asthma and Immunology. J Allergy Clin Immunol 2005;115:1249-1253.
Hanifin JM, Paller AS, Eichenfield L, et al: Efficacy and safety of tacrolimus ointment treatment for up to 4 years in patients with atopic dermatitis. J Am Acad Dermatol 2005;53:S186-S194.
Leung DYM, Boguniewicz M, Howell M, et al: New insights into atopic dermatitis. J Clin Invest 2004;113:651-657.
Paul C, Cork M, Rossi AB, et al: Safety and tolerability of 1% pimecrolimus cream among infants: Experience with 1133 patients treated for up to 2 years. Pediatrics 2006;117:e118.
Zuberbier T, Orlow SJ, Paller AS, et al: Patient perspectives on the management of atopic dermatitis. J Allergy Clin Immunol 2006;118:226-232.

Erythema Multiforme, Stevens-Johnson Syndrome, and Toxic Epidermal Necrolysis

Method of
Anne Marie Tremaine, MD, and
Stephen K. Tyring, MD, PhD

Previously, erythema multiforme, Stevens-Johnson syndrome (SJS), and toxic epidermal necrolysis (TEN) were considered part of a continuous spectrum of disease. There is now evidence that erythema multiforme is distinct from SJS and TEN, which do appear to be a disease spectrum. The etiologies, clinical findings, clinical severity, histologic findings, and prognosis of erythema multiforme differ from SJS and TEN (Table 1). In contrast to mild and self-limited erythema multiforme, SJS and TEN are more severe, with diffuse mucosal and epidermal involvement that requires early diagnosis, immediate medical attention, and often hospitalization for supportive care. In all three diseases, elimination of any precipitating factors is critical to the clinical outcome.

Erythema Multiforme

Erythema multiforme is an acute, self-limited, often recurrent, but typically mild cutaneous inflammatory disease that usually requires only symptomatic care. It is characterized by the sudden onset of a symmetrical erythematous eruption with primarily an acral distribution. The *typical target lesion* is the hallmark of this disease, but erythema multiforme actually has an evolving eruption. Erythema multiforme manifests with fixed (lasting longer than 24 hours) erythematous flat macules, which rapidly progress to erythematous raised papules, and then develop a pale or dusky central zone with edema or bulla formation (*raised atypical target lesion*). Some of the lesions progress to regular, round lesions with three distinct zones of color. These *typical target lesions* possess a dusky core with a pale edematous halo surrounded by an erythematous border. The lesions continue to appear for 24 to 72 hours but then regress spontaneously within 1 to 4 weeks, usually without sequelae.

CLASSIFICATION

Erythema multiforme is categorized into erythema multiforme minor and erythema multiforme major. Erythema multiforme minor lacks

CURRENT DIAGNOSIS

- Typical target lesion has three concentric zones of color: palpable round red lesion with a dusky center and a pale halo.
- Atypical target lesion has two concentric zones of color: palpable round red lesion with central edema or bulla.

Erythema Multiforme

- Symmetrical erythematous acral eruption with target lesions
- Mucosal involvement variable, oral only
- Self-limited, resolves spontaneously within 1 to 4 weeks
- Most commonly associated with herpes simplex virus types 1 and 2 and *Mycoplasma pneumoniae*

Stevens-Johnson Syndrome and Toxic Epidermal Necrolysis

- Severe mucocutaneous disease
- Extensive mucosal involvement; mouth, eyes, and genital mucosa
- Prodrome of fever and constitutional symptoms
- Atypical target lesions
- Epidermal necrosis
- Require supportive therapy and often hospitalization
- Most commonly associated with adverse drug reactions

BOX 1 Reported Etiologies of Erythema Multiforme

Bacteria
Chlamydia psittaci
Mycobacterium
Mycoplasma pneumoniae*
Salmonella

Fungi
Histoplasma capsulatum

Viruses
Coxsackievirus
Cytomegalovirus
Epstein–Barr virus
Hepatitis virus
Herpes simplex virus (types 1 and 2)*
HIV
Parapoxvirus
Parvovirus
Varicella zoster virus

Drugs
Anticonvulsants
Nonsteroidal anti-inflammatory
Sulfonamides and other antibiotics

Miscellaneous Causes
Inflammatory bowel disease
Lupus erythematous
Poison ivy

*The most common causes.

---

bullous lesions, has mild or absent mucosal involvement, and is asymptomatic. Mucosal involvement of the lips, buccal mucosa, and tongue is common with erythema multiforme major, and patients can have bullous lesions and complain of pain or pruritus.

ETIOLOGY

The precipitating causes of erythema multiforme are listed in Box 1, but the most common etiology is herpes simplex virus (HSV) types I and II, followed by *Mycoplasma pneumoniae*. Erythema multiforme is seen 1 to 10 days after the appearance of recurrent HSV outbreak, which explains the recurrent nature of erythema multiforme itself. HSV DNA has been detected in the erythema multiforme lesions and it is currently believed to be secondary to the HSV-specific host immune response.

TREATMENT

Elimination of the Etiologic Factor

Finding and eliminating the etiologic trigger is of utmost importance in erythema multiforme. Most cases of erythema multiforme result from an infection, which must be treated on diagnosis.

In recurrent herpes-associated erythema multiforme, a 5-day course of either oral acyclovir (Zovirax) 200 mg five times daily or 400 mg three times daily, a 3-day course of oral valacyclovir (Valtrex) 500 mg two times daily, or a 1-day, two-dose schedule of famciclovir (Famvir) 1000 mg tablets should be initiated at the first prodromal symptom. Antivirals are not effective if initiated after the development of either the HSV outbreak or the erythema multiforme lesion.

Oral erythromycin (EES, Erythrocin, E-mycin) 500 mg four times daily for 7 to 10 days or oral azithromycin (Zithromax) 500 mg on day 1 and then 250 mg daily for 4 days are treatment options for *Mycoplasma pneumoniae*.

There have been attempts to treat acute erythema multiforme with prednisone (Deltasone),[1] dapsone,[1] thalidomide (Thalomid),[1]

---

[1]Not FDA approved for this indication.

TABLE 1 Comparing Erythema Multiforme, Stevens-Johnson Syndrome, and Toxic Epidermal Necrolysis

Feature	Erythema Muliforme	Stevens-Johnson Syndrome	Toxic Epidermal Necrolysis
Characteristic lesion	Symmetrical, erythematous, typical target lesions	Extensive symmetrical bullous lesions, atypical target lesions	Painful erythema with rapid progression to sheets of necrosis, atypical target lesions
Distribution	Acral	Face and trunk	Face and trunk
Symptoms	Often none	Present	Present
Mucosal involvement	Minimal to none, oral only	Present	Multiple sites present
Etiology	Infectious	Drug	Drug
Prodrome	Absent	Present	Present
Body surface area	N/A	<10%	>30%
Treatment	Usually unnecessary (self-limited)	Necessary	Necessary

CURRENT THERAPY

Erythema Multiforme

- Eliminate acute herpes simplex virus infection with oral therapy
  - Valacyclovir (Valtrex) 500 mg bid × 3 days
  - Famciclovir (Famvir) 1000 mg bid × 1 day
  - Acyclovir (Zovirax) 200 mg 5× daily × 5 days or 400 mg tid × 5 days
- Initiate treatment at onset of first prodromal symptom but not after HSV or erythema multiforme lesion appears.
- Prevent recurrent HSV infection with suppressive antiviral therapy for a minimum of 6 months. (Also try suppressive antiviral therapy for patients with recurrent erythema multiforme of unknown etiology)
  - Valacyclovir (Valtrex) 500 mg qd-bid
  - Famciclovir (Famvir) 250 mg bid
  - Acyclovir (Zovirax) 400 mg bid
- Reduce/avoid triggers
  - UV light exposure
  - Emotional stress
  - Tight clothing
  - Hot tubs
  - Local trauma

Stevens-Johnson Syndrome and Toxic Epidermal Necrolysis

- Eliminate/or prevent etiologic factors
  - Immediately stop suspected drug(s)
  - Avoid exposure to causative drug and chemically related agents
  - Treat *Mycoplasma pneumoniae* infection if present.
- Provide supportive care (see below)
- Stop progression of epidermal necrosis
  - Administer high-dose IVIg:[1] 1 g/kg/day × 3 consecutive days (total dose 3 g/kg). Adjust dose for renal insufficiency; lower the daily dose and lengthen the duration of treatment.
  - Discontinue IVIg once disease progression ceases, or if there is no clinical response in 3 to 6 days.

Supportive Care

- Early referral to intensive care or burn unit
- Intravenous fluid replacement
- Soft diet, liquid diet, or tube feeds
- Systemic treatment for pain and pruritus
- Respiratory and physical therapy
- Use of proper bed and bedding

Wound Care

- Limit dressing changes to once daily, to minimize trauma and further epithelial detachment
- Cover detached areas with petrolatum and gauze until re-epithelialization occurs
- Closely monitor for signs of secondary infection, culture when indicated, and initiate treatment with the appropriate antibiotic coverage
- Keep intact skin dry
- Keep sterile procedures
- Gently débride crust
- Apply daily antibiotic ointment around the ears, nose, and mouth

Mouth Care

- Use sterile saline mouthwash every 2 hours
- Give symptomatic pain relief with topical anesthetics, such as dyclonine, viscous lidocaine, or a 1:1 mixture of Kaopectate and elixir of diphenyhydramine (Benadryl) swish

Eye Care

- Arrange immediate ophthalmologic consult and frequent ophthalmic follow-up
- Use topical steroids to decrease ocular inflammation
- Use ophthalmic lubricants to hydrate the ocular surface and wash away inflammatory particles
- Use topical antibiotics for prophylaxis against infection
- Perform lysis of adhesions

IVIg = intravenous immunoglobulin.

---

cyclosporine (Neoral),[1] mycophenolate mofetil (CellCept),[1] interferon-α,[1] and azathioprine (Imuran); however, very few controlled studies have evaluated these systemic therapeutic options for the treatment of acute erythema multiforme.

Symptomatic Care

Oral and topical antihistamines, oral analgesics, and topical anesthetics can provide symptomatic relief. Topical antivirals and corticosteroids are not beneficial. More detailed information for the care of skin and mouth erosions is addressed in the following section.

Prevention

The common association between recurrent HSV infection and erythema multiforme makes suppressive HSV therapy a possible option to lessen the frequency and severity of episodic erythema multiforme as well as HSV. Oral suppressive treatment options include valacyclovir 500 mg once or twice daily, famciclovir 250 mg twice daily, or acyclovir 400 mg twice daily for 6 months or longer. Avoidance of triggers, such as sun exposure, tight clothing, hot tubs, emotional stress, and local trauma, is also useful to decrease the number of recurrences. Because asymptomatic subclinical HSV episodes can trigger erythema multiforme, patients with recurrent erythema multiforme of unknown etiology might benefit from a course of suppressive antivirals.

Stevens-Johnson Syndrome and Toxic Epidermal Necrolysis

SJS and TEN are acute, severe mucocutaneous diseases that are most often the result of an adverse drug reaction. Both are associated with a 1- to 3-day prodrome of constitutional symptoms, fever, sore throat, and cutaneous pain before onset of the eruption.

CLINICAL PRESENTATION

SJS is characterized by sudden onset of erosions of the mucous membranes (lips, buccal mucosa, and conjunctivae) in association with an extensive blistering eruption with primarily facial and truncal distributions. The eruption begins with erythematous flat macules (*macule with or without blister*), which often develop a dusky core and can progress to bullae with epidermal necrosis. When two zones of concentric color are present, the lesion is described as a *flat atypical target lesion*. Up to 10% of the patient's body surface area (BSA) can have epidermal detachment. Painful conjunctival erosions can lead to photophobia, conjunctival and corneal scarring, dry eyes, and permanent vision loss. Oral mucosal erosions are also painful and result in characteristic hemorrhagic-crusted lips. SJS is most often linked with an adverse drug reaction, but infectious etiologies are possible, especially *Mycoplasma pneumoniae*.

TEN is characterized by widespread (>30% BSA involvement) full-thickness necrosis and sloughing of the epidermis. Patients with 10% to 30% BSA involvement are classified as having SJS-TEN overlap. The eruption begins with painful, symmetrical ill-defined erythematous macules and patches on the face and trunk, which rapidly progress to bullae and sheetlike areas of epidermal necrosis. Alternatively, TEN may begin as coalescing erythematous or violaceous macules that develop bullae. Nearly all patients have mucosal involvement including the oropharynx, conjunctivae, and genital mucosa. In extreme cases of TEN the erosion extends down to the epithelium in the esophagus and the respiratory tract.

ETIOLOGY

More than 100 drugs have been associated with SJS and TEN, but the classes of drugs most commonly associated with these diseases (Box 2) include anticonvulsants, antibiotics, nonsteroidal antiinflammatory drugs, antiretroviral drugs, barbiturates, antifungals, and allopurinol. The greatest risk for SJS and TEN is during the initial use of a drug, but each class is slightly different. The greatest risk for antibiotics is 7 to 21 days after drug initiation; for most anticonvulsants, the risk is highest during the first 2 months.

The mechanism of tissue injury in SJS and TEN is not completely understood although it is believed to be a result of uncontrolled keratinocyte apoptosis mediated by Fas/Fas ligand, tumor necrosis factor (TNF)-α, cytotoxic T cells, or impaired ability to detoxify drug metabolites. The apoptotic cells accumulate faster than can be cleared by the phagocytes in the epidermis. Quickly, the numerous cells become necrotic, leak their intracellular contents, and initiate an inflammatory response.

BOX 2 Drugs With the Highest Risk of Stevens-Johnson-Syndrome/Toxic Epidermal Necrolysis

Anticonvulsants
Carbamazepine (Tegretol)
Chlormezanone[2]
Lamotrigine (Lamictal)
Phenobarbitol
Phenytoin (Dilantin)
Valproic acid (Depakote)

Anti-infectives
Aminopenicillins
Antiretroviral drugs
Cephalosporins
Imidazole
Quinolones
Sulfonamides
Tetracycline

Miscellaneous
Allopurinol (Zyloprim)
Barbiturates
Nonsteroidal antiinflammatories (Oxicams)

---

[2]Not available in the United States.

TREATMENT

Elimination of Etiologic Factors

The initial step in a therapeutic response to SJS and TEN is to discontinue any potential causative drugs as soon as possible. Mortality decreases with early diagnosis and discontinuation of the offending agent before early blister formation. It is also important in SJS to treat any infections that are diagnosed. In addition, avoidance of all unnecessary medications is useful to prevent further complications.

Intervention with Systemic Therapy to Stop Progression

Supportive care is of utmost importance in both of these conditions, but the indication for the use of systemic therapy in SJS and TEN is highly controversial because there are no controlled trials to document efficacy of any intervention. Systemic therapy would be beneficial because SJS and TEN are such devastating diseases with high mortality rates. Glucocorticoids have been used for a long time but their use remains controversial. There is little evidence-based medicine to support their use, and previous studies indicate that patients had increased morbidity, prolonged hospitalization, and mortality after treatment with systemic glucocorticoids. The rest of the treatment options come from case reports and small uncontrolled studies and include medications such as oral cyclosporine (Sandimmune),[1] high-dose intravenous cyclophosphamide (Cytoxan),[1] plasmapheresis, interferon-α,[1] thalidomide,[1] and N-acetylcystine.[1] The thalidomide trials were discontinued because of the significant increase in mortality in the thalidomide treatment arm. Systemic therapies should be discontinued once disease progression ceases or if no clinical response is noted within 3 to 6 days to minimize the risk of associated complications.

High-dose intravenous immunoglobulin (IVIg)[1] appears to inhibit keratinocyte apoptosis by blocking the binding of Fas to the Fas ligand, and thus is currently the most promising and widely advocated systemic therapy available. In the initial landmark pilot study, 10 TEN patients treated with IVIg demonstrated rapid cessation of disease progression and 100% survival. Subsequently, a multitude of case reports and uncontrolled studies reported overall safety and efficacy of IVIg. The current IVIg dosage recommendations are 1 g/kg/day for 3 days (total dose of 3 g/kg). Doses less than 2 g/kg appear to be insufficient. A randomized, placebo-controlled trial of IVIg in TEN has yet to be carried out and will be difficult to do, given the rarity of the disease and the ethical issues of placebo use in a disease with high morbidity and mortality.

Supportive Care

Supportive care is crucial to the management of SJS and TEN, and hospitalization is often essential. In mild cases of SJS, only supportive care is needed. The extensive epidermal and mucosal necrosis and detachment lead to abnormal barrier function causing fluid, electrolyte, and protein loss. Patients are also at increased risk for infection, impaired thermoregulation, altered immune status, and increased energy expenditure. The patients require support via fluid, electrolyte, and calorie replacement, as well as physical and respiratory therapy. Special beds and bed linens are required. The mortality rate is 25% to 40%, and sepsis is the leading cause of death.

Close monitoring is vital for these patients. Early referral of severe cases to an intensive care unit or burn unit decreases mortality. Poor outcome can be predicted by a TEN-specific severity of illness score (Box 3) and correlates with the mortality present within the first 24 hours after admission to an intensive care unit. Once the patient is in the unit, attempts must be made to guard against iatrogenic infections by stopping all systemic steroids, avoiding indwelling lines and catheters, following sterile procedures at all times, and limiting antibiotic use to specific culture-proved infections.

---

[1]Not FDA approved for this indication.

> **BOX 3   SCORTEN: A Severity of Illness Score Predictive of Mortality in Toxic Epidermal Necrolysis**
>
> Number of risk factors indicates mortality risk: 0-1 risk factor is associated with a 3% mortality, which increases to 12% with 2 risk factors, 35% with 3 risk factors, 58% with 4 risk factors, and 90% with 5 or more risk factors.
> Age >40 years
> Presence of malignancy
> Initial epidermal detachment of >10% body surface area
> BUN >10 mmol/L
> Glucose >14 mmol/L
> HCO$_3$ <20 mmol/L
> Heart rate >120 bpm
>
> BUN = blood urea nitrogen.

Wound Care

The essence of wound care in SJS and TEN is minimal manipulation. Once-daily wound care is performed to minimize further epidermal detachment, and it includes covering detached areas with petrolatum and gauze until re-epithelialization occurs, keeping intact skin dry, gently débriding crust, and applying antibiotic ointment around the ears, nose, and mouth. Lesions should be closely monitored for signs of secondary infection, cultured when indicated, and treatment should be initiated with the appropriate antibiotic coverage. Oral antihistamines and analgesics can provide relief for pruritic or painful lesions. Topical steroids are not beneficial.

Mouth Care

Good oral hygiene, in patients with oral mucosa involvement, is crucial to minimizing infection and discomfort. Sterile saline mouthwash every 2 hours provides cleansing and gentle débridement. Symptomatic pain relief can be provided with topical anesthetics, such as dyclonine, viscous lidocaine, or a 1:1 mixture of Kaopectate and elixir of diphenhydramine[1] swish. Depending on the severity of the oral involvement, a liquid or soft diet may be better tolerated, whereas in severe cases more aggressive nutritional support, such as tube feeding, might be required.

Eye Care

Sixty percent of patients with erythema multiforme, SJS, or TEN have ocular involvement. The potential for permanent vision changes warrants immediate ophthalmologic consultation and frequent ophthalmic follow-up. Corticosteroid eyedrops are used in moderation to decrease the ocular inflammation, ophthalmic lubricants hydrate the ocular surface and wash away inflammatory particles, and topical antibiotics lower the risk of infection and are often administered on a prophylactic basis. Patients with ocular adhesions require daily lysis to lower the chance of late complications.

Patient Education

Patients should be counseled on the causative agent of their disease and the importance of avoiding this agent and related compounds in the future.

---

[1]Not FDA approved for this indication.

REFERENCES

Bachot N, Revuz J, Roujeau J-C: Intravenous immunoglobulin treatment for Stevens–Johnson syndrome and toxic epidermal necrolysis: A prospective noncomparative study showing no benefit on mortality or progression. Arch Dermatol 2003;139:33-36.
Cartotto R, Mayich M, Nickerson D, Gomez M: SCORTEN accurately predicts mortality among toxic epidermal necrolysis patients treated in a burn center. J Burn Care Res 2008;29:141-146.
Chang Y-S, Huang F-C, Tseng S-H, et al: Erythema multiforme, Stevens–Johnson syndrome, and toxic epidermal necrolysis: Acute ocular manifestations, causes, and management. Cornea 2007;26:123-129.
French LE, Prins C: Erythema multiforme, Stevens–Johnson syndrome, and toxic epidermal necrolysis. In Bolognia JL, Jorizzo JL, Rapini RP (ed): Dermatology, 2nd ed. London: Mosby, 2008, pp 287-300.
Huff JC, Weston WL, Tonnessen M: Erythema multiforme: A critical review of characteristics, diagnostic criteria, and causes. J Am Acad Dermatol 1983;8:763-775.
Kerob D, Assier-Bonnet, Esnault-Gelly P, Bland F, Saiag P: Recurrent erythema multiforme unresponsive to acyclovir prophylaxis and responsive to valacyclovir continuous therapy. Arch Dermatol 1998;134:876-877.
Papuet P, Pierard GE: Erythema multiforme and toxic epidermal necrolysis: A comparative study. Am J Dermatopathol 1997;19:127-132.
Prins C, Kerdel FA, Padilla S, et al: Treatment of toxic epidermal necrolysis with high-dose intravenous immunoglobulins: Multicenter retrospective analysis of 48 consecutive cases. Arch Dermatol 2003;139:26-32.
Roujeau J-C, Kelly JP, Naldi L, et al: Medication use and the risk of Stevens–Johnson syndrome or toxic epidermal necrolysis. N Engl J Med 1995;333:1600-1607.
Tatnall FM, Schofield JK, Leigh IM: A double-blind, placebo-controlled trial of continuous acyclovir therapy in recurrent erythema multiforme. Br J Dermatol 1995;132:267-270.
Viard I, Wehrli P, Bullani R, et al: Inhibition of toxic epidermal necrolysis by blockade of CD95 with human intravenous immunoglobulin. Science 1998;282:490-493.
Wehrli P, Viard I, Bullani R, et al: Death receptors in cutaneous biology and disease. J Invest Dermatol 2000;115:141-148.

Bullous Diseases

Method of
Craig N. Burkhart, MD, MS,
David S. Rubenstein, MD, PhD,
and Luis A. Diaz, MD

Bullous Pemphigoid

OVERVIEW

Bullous pemphigoid is an autoimmune blistering disease in which basal keratinocyte hemidesmosomal proteins are targeted by immunoglobulin (Ig)G autoantibodies, resulting in complement activation and neutrophil recruitment. Neutrophil proteases lead to subepidermal vesicles. Bullous pemphigoid is most commonly a generalized cutaneous disease affecting persons in the sixth to seventh decade. Nevertheless, localized, mucosal, pediatric, and young adult cases have been described.

Before pursuing treatment, the clinician must distinguish bullous pemphigoid from other blistering dermatoses such as erythema multiforme, epidermolysis bullosa acquisita, bullous systemic lupus erythematosus, and linear IgA disease. This is accomplished by histology, direct and indirect immunofluorescence, antigen-specific enzyme-linked immunosorbent assay (ELISA), and clinical history.

TREATMENT

Localized and Nonaggressive Disease

Less-aggressive, localized forms of bullous pemphigoid are amenable to conservative therapy. For instance, ultrapotent topical corticosteroids, such as clobetasol (Temovate) cream or ointment two or three

CURRENT DIAGNOSIS

- All bullous diseases are diagnosed by combining clinical, histologic, and immunologic findings.
- The pemphigoid group is characterized by subepidermal bullae and autoantibodies to hemidesmosomal and hemidesmosome-related proteins.
- The pemphigus group is characterized by intraepidermal bullae and autoantibodies to desmosomal proteins.
- Clinical features such as scarring, mucosal involvement, pattern of cutaneous disease, and systemic findings are used to subclassify disease within the pemphigoid and pemphigus groups.

CURRENT THERAPY

- Localized nonscarring disease may be managed with topical corticosteroids alone.
- Progressive, scarring, or generalized disease requires early institution of systemic immunosuppressants.
- Close follow-up is required because all forms of immunosuppression are commonly complicated by side effects.
- Response to therapy is guided primarily by clinical findings.

times daily, can control localized disease without any systemic medications. Dapsone[1] may be used when topical corticosteroids are ineffective (Table 1). Therapy is begun at 50 mg/day for the first week. If no significant drop in the red or white blood cell count is detected, the dose is increased at weekly intervals by 50 mg a day until the disease responds or a maximum of 200 mg/day (100 mg twice daily) is reached. Once the disease is under control (as evidenced by the absence of new blister formation), the dapsone dose is decreased to the minimum that allows disease control. If no response is achieved within 6 weeks of reaching the maximum dose, then the patient is considered unresponsive to dapsone as a single agent.

Tetracycline (Sumycin)[1] and niacinamide[1] can also be effective for a nonaggressive or localized bullous pemphigoid, although in our hands its use has been unrewarding. Therapy is begun with tetracycline 500 mg four times daily and niacinamide 500 mg three times daily. If no new lesions develop after 1 month, the medications are slowly tapered. Baseline liver function tests (LFTs) should be obtained before and 1 month after initiation of therapy. Patients should be clinically monitored for signs of pseudotumor cerebri, photosensitivity, and hepatotoxicity. Gastric distress from tetracycline can be managed by decreasing its dose or changing to doxycycline (Doryx)[1] or minocycline (Dynacin).[1] Gastric distress and flushing from niacinamide require reducing its dose.

Aggressive and Generalized Disease

Because of their rapid onset of action, systemic corticosteroids are the first-line treatment of choice for aggressive, generalized bullous pemphigoid. Prednisone is begun at 1.0 mg/kg every morning and increased incrementally to 2.0 mg/kg in nonresponding patients. After 2 to 4 weeks in which no new blisters develop, the daily prednisone dose can be tapered by 5 mg every 2 to 4 weeks. At 30 mg/day, switch to alternate-day dosing by reducing the first day's dose by 2.5 mg every 2 weeks while maintaining the second day's dose at 30 mg/day. In the absence of recurrence, tapering of the second day's dose is then continued by 2.5 mg every 2 weeks. Patients on chronic prednisone should be followed for signs of infection, adrenal suppression, hypertension, diabetes, glaucoma, atherosclerosis, peptic ulcer disease, and osteoporosis.

Adjunctive therapies are initiated when bullous pemphigoid fails to respond rapidly to systemic prednisone and to limit side effects from chronic systemic corticosteroid use. The most commonly used agents are dapsone,[1] azathioprine (Imuran),[1] cyclophosphamide (Cytoxan),[1] mycophenolate mofetil (CellCept),[1] and methotrexate[1] (see Table 1). These agents are coadministered with systemic corticosteroids. Once disease has been under control for 6 weeks, the steroid-sparing agent is maintained at its current dose, and the systemic corticosteroid is tapered as above. After the corticosteroid taper is complete, the patient should remain on adjuvant therapy for an additional 3 to 6 months before discontinuing therapy.

Azathioprine and mycophenolate mofetil are excellent first-line adjuvants due to their great effectiveness and low toxicity when compared with other agents. Thiopurine methyltransferase (TPMT) levels may be helpful in guiding initial dosing (Table 2). If TPMT levels are not available, initiating therapy at a low dose (50 mg/day) and rechecking a complete blood count (CBC) with differential with every dosage increase (see Table 1) reduces the risk of severe myelosuppression. The most common side effect of mycophenolate mofetil, gastric distress, may be avoided by initiating therapy at 500 mg/day before titrating to its effective dose. Gastric distress can also occur with methotrexate and is minimized by supplementing folate (1 mg/day) on the 6 days of the week that methotrexate is not dosed.

Additional therapeutic options in treatment-resistant patients include plasmapheresis, intravenous immunoglobulin (IVIg),[1] and tumor necrosis factor α (TNF-α) antagonists.[1] All TNF-α antagonists should be avoided in patients with a personal or family history of demyelinating central nervous system disorders, uncontrolled congestive heart failure, or active infections. IVIg (400 mg/kg/day) appears effective, is relatively safe, and has few side effects; however, prohibitive cost can prevent its widespread use.

Cicatricial Pemphigoid

OVERVIEW

Also known as *mucous membrane pemphigoid*, cicatricial pemphigoid is a group of chronic, progressive, scarring autoimmune diseases that result from subepidermal blisters of mucosal surfaces or skin, or both. Pathogenic autoantibodies attach to hemidesmosomal proteins or proteins that link the hemidesmosome to anchoring fibrils. Cicatricial pemphigoid typically manifests with painful mucosal erosions and ulcerations of the oral cavity or irritation and scarring of the eyes. Involvement of other mucosal epithelia, including nasal, laryngeal, esophageal, urogenital, and anogenital, can cause significant morbidity from scarring and stenosis. Cicatricial pemphigoid can be clinically distinguished from bullous pemphigoid, which less commonly involves mucosal surfaces and does not cause scarring, and epidermolysis bullous acquisita, which occurs on trauma-prone surfaces and heals with scars and milia. Before initiating therapy, a diagnosis of cicatricial pemphigoid should be confirmed by histology and by direct and indirect immunofluorescence studies.

TREATMENT

The high morbidity associated with scarring in cicatricial pemphigoid requires an aggressive approach. Patients should be screened for signs and symptoms of ocular (conjunctivitis or burning, gritty, or dry sensations), laryngeal (hoarseness or dysphonia), and esophageal (dysphagia) involvement. If any of these signs or symptoms are present, early referral to the appropriate specialist (ophthalmologist, otolaryngologist, or gastroenterologist) is warranted.

---

[1]Not FDA approved for this indication.

TABLE 1 Steroid-Sparing Agents

Medication	Contraindications	Baseline Labs	Initial Dose	Titration	Renal Dosing	Maximum Dose	Routine Labs	Important Side Effects	Long-Term Risks
Dapsone[1]	G6PD deficiency, Sulfonamide allergy	G6PD, CBC with differential, LFTs, BUN, creatinine	50 mg p.o. q.d.	Increase every wk by 50 mg	Data not available	200 mg/d	CBC with differential Weekly x 1 mo Monthly x 5 mo Then q6mo	Hemolysis, Methemoglobinemia, Gastric distress, Agranulocytosis, Dapsone hypersensitivity syndrome, Hepatitis	Peripheral neuropathy
Azathioprine (Imuran)[1]	TPMT deficiency	TPMT level, CBC with differential, LFTs, BUN, creatinine	50-100 mg PO qd	Increase every 4-6 wk by 0.5 mg/kg/d	Cl_{Cr} 10-50 mL/min: 75% of normal dose; Cl_{Cr} <10 mL/min: 50% of normal dose	2.5 mg/kg	CBC with differential, LFTs, BUN, creatinine Weekly x 1 mo Biweekly x 1 mo Then bimonthly	Gastric distress, Myelosuppression, Hepatitis, pancreatitis	Hematologic malignancy
Cyclophosphamide (Cytoxan)[1]	Neutropenia, Active infection, Bladder cancer, History of hemorrhagic cystitis, Pregnancy	CBC with differential, BUN, creatinine, urinalysis	1-2 mg/kg/d	Increase every 4-6 wk	Cl_{Cr} <10 mL/min: 75% of normal dose	2.5 mg/kg/d	CBC with differential, BUN, creatinine urinalysis Biweekly	Hemorrhagic cystitis, myelosuppression	Transitional cell carcinoma of the bladder
Mycophenolate mofetil (Cellcept)[1]	Active peptic ulcer disease, HGPT deficiency (Lesch–Nyhan syndrome), Pregnancy	CBC with differential, BUN, creatinine, urine pregnancy test	500-1000 mg PO bid	Increase every 2-4 wk	Cl_{Cr} <25 mL/min: avoid dosing >2000 mg/d	3000 mg/d	CBC with differential Weekly x 1 mo Biweekly x 2 mo Then monthly	Myelosuppression, Gastric distress	Lymphoma
Methotrexate[1]	Cirrhosis, Active hepatitis, Alcoholism, Severe renal disease	CBC with differential, LFTs, BUN, creatinine	2.5 mg PO x 1	Increase every 2-4 wk by 2.5 mg	Cl_{Cr} 51-80 mL/min: 70% of dose; Cl_{Cr} 10-50 mL/min: 30% of dose; Cl_{Cr} <10 mL/min: avoid	15 mg/wk	CBC with differential, LFTs, BUN, creatinine Weeks 1, 2, 4, 8, and 12 Then q3mo	Gastric distress, Myelosuppression, Pneumonitis	Cirrhosis, Lymphoma

[1]Not FDA approved for this indication.
BUN = blood urea nitrogen; CBC = complete blood count; Cl_{Cr} = creatinine clearance; G6PD = glucose-6-phosphate dehydrogenase; HGPT = hypoxanthine-guanine phosphoribosyltransferase; LFT = liver function test; TPMT = thiopurine methyltransferase.

TABLE 2 Recommended Azathioprine Dosing

TMPT Level (U/mL of RBC Lysates)	Azathioprine Dose
<5.0	none
5.0-13.7	0.5 mg/kg
13.7-19.0	1.5 mg/kg
>19.0	2.5 mg/kg

RBC = red blood cell; TPMT = thiopurine methyltransferase.

Localized Cutaneous and Oral Disease

Disease localized to the skin or oral mucosa alone is occasionally controlled with local therapies. Ultrapotent corticosteroids (clobetasol), in an ointment or cream for application to the skin or in a gel or orabase for application to the oral mucosa, may be effective when applied two or three times daily. Alternatively, perilesional triamcinolone (usually 5-10 mg/mL suspension) to a maximum dose of 40 mg/mL can be injected every 4 weeks.

Unresponsive, Ocular, and Systemic Disease

Patients who fail to respond to local measures or who present with ocular or systemic disease require systemic therapy. Dapsone[1] is a highly effective first-line agent for cicatricial pemphigoid (see Table 1). If no response is obtained within 4 to 6 weeks, or if there are signs or symptoms of disease progression, systemic corticosteroids (1-2 mg/kg/day) should be initiated. Adjunctive agents (see Table 1) are added to gain better control of the disease and to aid in weaning from systemic corticosteroids. When these modalities fail, other modalities such as plasmapheresis and IVIg[1] may be tried.

Surgical repair of ocular deformities, laryngeal stenosis, or esophageal stenosis should be delayed until the disease is under good control to prevent further, surgically induced scarring. Increasing the dose of immunosuppressive medications in the perioperative period can also improve surgical outcomes.

Pemphigus Vulgaris

OVERVIEW

Pemphigus is a group of autoimmune blistering diseases in which autoantibodies against desmoglein 3 (desmosomal glycoprotein) induce loss of cell–cell adhesion in the epidermis (acantholysis). The two major variants are pemphigus vulgaris and pemphigus foliaceous. Pemphigus vulgaris produces suprabasal splitting and pemphigus foliaceous produces upper epidermal splitting. The mechanism by which pemphigus vulgaris IgG induces blister formation is incompletely understood, but it might include proteinase activation, steric hindrance, or activation of transmembrane signaling.

The typical clinical presentation is a middle-aged (40 to 60 years) individual with painful erosions in the mouth. Patients can have coexistent cutaneous blisters and erosions or involvement of other mucosal surfaces (pharyngeal, laryngeal, esophageal, ocular, anal, or genital). Pemphigus vulgaris limited to mucosa is termed *mucosal pemphigus vulgaris*. Pemphigus vulgaris affecting the mucosa and skin is termed *mucocutaneous pemphigus vulgaris*. Before initiating treatment, the diagnosis of pemphigus vulgaris should be confirmed by histology, direct and indirect immunofluorescence, and antigen-specific ELISAs.

TREATMENT

Treatment of pemphigus vulgaris is guided in the short term by clinical findings and in the long term by laboratory findings.

---

[1]Not FDA approved for this indication.

Systemic therapy should be initiated immediately alone or in combination with immunosuppressive agents. Once blistering stops and erosions have healed, indirect immunofluorescence titers are used to guide steroid and immunosuppressant tapering. Immunosuppression should only be tapered when patients are clinically in remission and indirect immunofluorescence titers are stable or decreasing. As a practical rule, we must educate the patient that the therapy will last for several months or years and that the response to therapy in individual patients is unpredictable.

Systemic corticosteroids (prednisone 1.0-2.0 mg/kg/day) are used first. If the disease fails to respond rapidly to systemic steroids (no new bullae or erosions within 1-2 weeks), adjuvant therapy should be initiated (see Table 1). As with bullous pemphigoid, azathioprine[1] and mycophenolate mofetil[1] are first-line adjuvants and titrated in the same manner as described for bullous pemphigoid. Azathioprine and mycophenolate mofetil are also effective as monotherapy in mild cases. As opposed to bullous pemphigoid, however, methotrexate,[1] tetracycline[1] plus niacinamide[1], and single-agent dapsone[1] are ineffective for pemphigus vulgaris. Tapering steroids and immunosuppressive agents should be very slow and gradual, we find the schedule described for bullous pemphigoid therapy is very useful in our patients.

Adjuvant IV immunoglobulins, TNF-α antagonists (etanercept [Enbrel][1] 50 mg subcutaneously twice weekly with prednisone), IVIg, plasmaphoresis, and rituximab (Rituxan)[1] (anti-CD20 chimeric monoclonal antibody) may be tried. In the future, medications targeting specific intracellular signaling events important in cell–cell adhesion may be used. For example, several p38 mitogen-activated protein kinase (MAPK) inhibitors are currently in phases II and III clinical trials for other inflammatory disorders and might show promise in the treatment of pemphigus vulgaris.

Pemphigus Foliaceus

OVERVIEW

Pemphigus foliaceus is a form of pemphigus in which superficial epidermal vesicles form as a result of the binding of pathogenic IgG autoantibodies against desmoglein 1, a desmosomal glycoprotein. Due to the superficial location of epidermal splitting, patients usually present with crusted, scaling plaques on the face, scalp, and upper trunk of middle-aged adults. Unlike pemphigus vulgaris, mucosal surfaces are uninvolved and patients generally have a better prognosis. As with all bullous diseases, histology, direct and indirect immunofluorescence, and confirmatory antigen-specific ELISA should be obtained before initiating therapy.

TREATMENT

Pemphigus foliaceous is managed in a very similar manner to pemphigus vulgaris. Due to the generally milder and more insidious course, topical corticosteroids (clobetasol ointment twice daily) are often used as first-line agents for localized disease. Nevertheless, disease that is widespread or resistant to local therapy requires systemic prednisone combined with steroid-sparing agents at the same dosing as used for bullous pemphigoid and pemphigus vulgaris (see Table 1).

Acknowledgment

This work was supported in part by National Institutes of Health grants T32 AR007369, RO1 AR32081, and RO1 AR32599 (Luis A. Diaz); and RO1 AI49427 (David S. Rubenstein).

---

[1]Not FDA approved for this indication.

REFERENCES

Berkowitz P, Hu P, Liu Z, et al: Desmosome signaling. Inhibition of p38MAPK prevents pemphigus vulgaris IgG-induced cytoskeleton reorganization. J Biol Chem 2005;280(25):23778-23784.

Berkowitz P, Hu P, Warren S, et al: p38MAPK inhibition prevents disease in pemphigus vulgaris mice. Proc Natl Acad Sci U S A 2006;103(34):12855-12860.

Korman NJ: Bullous pemphigoid. The latest in diagnosis, prognosis, and therapy. Arch Dermatol 1998;134:1137-1141.

Liu Z, Diaz LA, Troy JL, et al: A passive transfer model of the organ-specific autoimmune disease, bullous pemphigoid, using antibodies generated against the hemidesmosomal antigen, BP180. J Clin Invest 1993;92:2480-2488.

Mutasim DF: Management of autoimmune bullous diseases: Pharmacology and therapeutics. J Am Acad Dermatol 2004;51(6):859-877.

Nousari HC, Griffin WA, Anhalt GJ: Successful therapy for bullous pemphigoid with mycophenolate mofetil. J Am Acad Dermatol 1998;39:497-498.

Snow JL, Gibson LE: The role of genetic variation in thiopurine methyltransferase activity and the efficacy and or side effects of azathioprine in dermatologic patients. Arch Dermatol 1995;131:193-197.

Yosipovitch G, Hoon TS, Leok GC: Suggested rationale for prevention and treatment of glucocorticoid-induced bone loss in dermatologic patients. Arch Dermatol 2001;137:477-481.

Contact Dermatitis

Method of
Peter C. Schalock, MD, and
Kathryn A. Zug, MD

Eczema is well described by the word's Greek roots, with "ek" meaning "out or over" and "zein" meaning "to boil." Thus, this boiling over pattern of superficial inflammatory skin diseases of the skin is one of the most common reaction pattern seen by dermatologists. Pruritus is the most characteristic skin sensation associated with eczema.

Irritant Contact Dermatitis

Contact dermatitis (CD) is caused by exogenous substances coming into contact with the skin. Irritant contact dermatitis (ICD) is the most common form of CD, caused by frequent or chronic exposure to an irritating substance. ICD will eventually occur in any person exposed to these irritating substances in sufficient concentration. This type of reaction is the most common form of occupational skin disease and is a problem for many individuals worldwide. The most common location for ICD is the hands. Other locations commonly involved are the palms, fingers, and dorsal web spaces. As opposed to allergic contact dermatitis, the dorsal hands are most often spared from dermatitis.

Allergic Contact Dermatitis

Two types of immune reactions are seen in allergic contact dermatitis (ACD): type I immediate-type hypersensitivity and type IV delayed-type hypersensitivity. Immediate-type reactions are most commonly caused by animal or plant proteins that are able to bind to mast cells and cause mast cell degranulation, leading to an urticarial or anaphylactic reaction. The most commonly recognized cause of this type of immediate hypersensitivity is natural rubber latex proteins. Allergy to these proteins is caused by exposure to products containing natural rubber latex, especially rubber gloves. Type IV allergy is caused by substances that are taken up by Langerhans cells in the epidermis and processed and presented to T cells in the regional lymph node, thus creating memory T cells that are capable of reacting the next time the individual is exposed to the substance. The delayed reaction is due to the time needed to mount the immune response. Frequent culprits are urushiol (poison ivy/oak), topical antibiotics, nickel, and formaldehyde/formaldehyde-releasing preservatives.

Diagnosis

Evaluation for the etiology of CD reactions depends upon the type of allergy sought. Evaluation for type I immediate-type allergy is different than for type IV delayed-type reactions. Testing for type I allergy can be achieved by in vivo and in vitro methods. Prick testing can be performed for panels of suspected allergens. For the prick test, the skin on the flexor forearm or other area is cleaned, and a small amount of a pure dilution of the suspect protein is placed on the skin. The skin is pricked using a sterile lancet, and the patient is observed for a wheal and flare reaction. Histamine should also be used as a positive control. This type of testing can elicit an anaphylactic type of reaction and should be performed with caution. Many allergens that elicit a type I reaction can also be tested by the allergen-specific immunoglobulin E antibody test or radioallergosorbent assay test (RAST).

Type IV allergy is best evaluated by patch testing. A patch test is made with hypoallergenic tape to which Finn chambers (small metal chambers) or IQ Ultra chambers (Chemotechnique Diagnostics, Vellinge, Sweden) are placed with a purified potential allergen. The patches are placed most often on the patient's upper back and left for 48 hours. The patches are then removed, the locations of the allergens marked, and the initial reading performed. The patient is seen again in another 48 hours for the final reading. Two readings are preferable to allow assessment of some reactions that appear after the patch has been removed and of some reactions initially thought to be positive that may actually have been irritant reactions. Patch testing technique has been described in detail by Corey.

Once the patient's sensitivities are determined, the information is useful to help educate the patient regarding avoidance of the offending allergen. There is no "cure" for ACD. The Contact Allergen Replacement Database available through the American Contact Dermatitis Society is a useful tool for helping patients avoid their allergens (available at: www.contactderm.org). The patient can enter each allergen into the database, and a list of products free of the allergens is generated.

In the United States, only the 23 thin-layer rapid-use epicutaneous (TRUE) test allergens are Food and Drug Administration (FDA) approved for use. A multitude of other allergens for patch testing are available in Europe. Chemotechnique AB (Malmo, Sweden) and Hermal (Reinbek, Germany) both manufacture many standard and specialty series of allergens. Patch testing with an expanded series of allergens can be useful in identifying relevant allergens. TRUE test allergens encompass 1.4% of the more than 3700 known allergens, although 28% of patients are fully evaluated with this panel. By expanding the series to the 65 standard allergens used by the North American Contact Dermatitis Group (NACDG), 50.2% of relevant allergies are identified. Although use of the TRUE test may be a good starting point for evaluation of ACD, an expanded panel of allergens with additional testing for suspected agents to which the patient may have contact gives a much greater return on testing.

CURRENT DIAGNOSIS

Type I Allergy

- Prick test
- Use test (perform with caution)
- Radioallergosorbent assay test (RAST) for specific allergens

Type IV Allergy

- Patch test using a broad panel of allergens and patient's personal care products most helpful
- Repeated open application test (ROAT)/use test

Treatment

Treatment of CD hinges upon four premises: education of the patient regarding skin care and the etiology of the dermatitis, postexposure skin care, strict avoidance of the offending allergen(s), and pharmacologic therapy of active dermatitis. Patients educated on the basics of good skin care and on the cause of their ICD and ACD had less dermatitis than did those without intervention. For patient with ICD and ACD, postexposure skin care plays an important role in treatment. ICD can play a role in the development and perpetuation of ACD by allowing greater penetration of allergens. Good skin care, such as the use of appropriate barrier creams, bland emollients, and avoidance of wet work or macerating gloves, can decrease skin irritation and transepidermal water loss. Good skin care and prevention of irritation should be an integral part of preventing and treating ACD.

In cases of mild to moderate dermatitis, a medium- or high-potency topical steroid, such as triamcinolone acetonide (Aristoco A) 0.1% or desoximetasone (Topicort) 0.25%, can be used two to three times daily for monotherapy. For widespread cases, a 1-lb (454 g) jar of generic triamcinolone acetonide 0.1% is preferable. Ointments are preferable to creams because the water and preservatives present in creams may worsen the irritant reaction. Simple, greasy lubricants, such as Aquaphor or Vaseline, should be used every time the body or hands are washed or appear dry. Widespread dermatitis will often improve rapidly with open wet dressings preceded and followed by a topical corticosteroid cream. For hand dermatitis, use of the steroid or of Vaseline under cotton gloves can be helpful, either for short periods or overnight. For sensitive areas such as the face and genitalia, topical calcineurin inhibitors can be useful. Either tacrolimus (Protopic) 0.1% ointment or pimecrolimus (Elidel) 1% cream twice daily can be used. For more severe cases of dermatitis, topical therapy and a corticosteroid taper can be helpful in alleviating the patient's symptoms as well as calming the dermatitis. Short prednisone tapers (i.e., "dose packs") will not always be adequate, with the patient flaring after the short taper is finished. Using prednisone in a 4-week course with 7-day tapering steps, such as 60-40-20-10 mg, can be helpful in breaking the cycle of chronic inflammation and excoriation/pruritus. Open wet dressings with application of topical corticosteroid before and after can diminish dermatitis quickly. For patients with severe pruritus, especially at night, hydroxyzine (Atarax) 10 to 50 mg orally or doxepin[1] (Sinequan) 10 to 20 mg orally at bedtime can be helpful.

Conclusion

Contact dermatitis is a broad diagnosis encompassing both immediate- and delayed-type hypersensitivities. Testing can be helpful in characterizing specific allergens and in guiding the patients as to which substances to avoid to prevent dermatitis. The RAST or prick test is useful for determining immediate-type hypersensitivity and patch testing for delayed-type allergy. TRUE tests will fully evaluate 28% of patients. Broadening the screen with other allergens, such as the NACDG panel, can be useful for defining ACD in patients with dermatitis. Treatment of CD consists of topical steroids, open wet dressings, moisturization, topical calcineurin inhibitors, and infrequently oral corticosteroids.

---

[1]Not FDA approved for this indication.

REFERENCES

Bauer A, Kelterer D, Stadeler M, et al: The prevention of occupational hand dermatitis in bakers, confectioners and employees in the catering trades. Preliminary results of a skin prevention program. Contact Dermatitis 2001;44:85-88.

Corey G: Applying patch tests from a technician's or nurse's point of view. Am J Contact Dermat 1993;4:175-181.

Kalimo K, Kautiainen H, Niskanen T, Niemi L: "Eczema school" to improve compliance in an occupational dermatology clinic. Contact Dermatitis 1999;41:315-319.

Saripalli YV, Achen F, Belsito DV: The detection of clinically relevant contact allergens using a standard screening tray of twenty–three allergens. J Am Acad Dermatol 2003;49:65-69.

Pruritus Ani and Vulvae

Method of
Brenda L. Bartlett, MD

Pruritus ani is defined as localized pruritus of the anus and perianal skin. This condition affects 1% to 5% of the population with a 4:1 predominance seen in male patients. The majority of those affected are between the ages of 30 and 70 years of age. Similarly, pruritus vulvae is localized pruritus of the vulva, which may be as common and debilitating as pruritus ani. Patients with either of these conditions note that symptoms tend to be worse at night and can develop lichenification due to repetitive trauma. The evaluation, differential diagnosis, and treatments for pruritus ani and pruritus vulvae are similar.

Etiology

Acute-onset anogenital pruritus is most often due to infection, irritant and contact dermatitis, and hemorrhoids. Infection should be ruled out in the evaluation of acute itching and should include a vaginal smear for *Candida*, *Trichomonas*, and *Gardnerella* in female patients. Although bacterial vaginosis (caused by *Gardnerella*) is not inherently pruritic, pruritus can result form excessive cleansing in attempt to relieve the characteristic malodor associated with bacterial vaginosis. *Candida* infection can be intensely pruritic, and recurrent candidiasis is common. Vaginal cultures in female patients and anal cultures in both sexes should be considered. Risk factors for candidiasis include use of antibiotics, use of steroids or other immune

---

> **CURRENT THERAPY**
>
> - Strict avoidance of the offending allergen(s) and pharmacologic therapy for active dermatitis.
> - Patient education on good skin care and prevention of irritation.
> - Simple, greasy lubricants, such as Aquaphor or Vaseline, should be used every time the body or hands are washed or appear dry.
> - Groin or face dermatitis: Tacrolimus (Protopic) 0.1% ointment or pimecrolimus (Elidel) 1% cream twice daily
> - Mild to moderate dermatitis: Medium- or high-potency topical steroid such as triamcinolone acetonide (Aristocort A) 0.1% or desoximetasone (Topicort) 0.25% bid-tid for monotherapy.
>   - Widespread dermatitis: Generic triamcinolone 0.1% cream (454-g jar) bid-tid
>   - Pruritus: Hydroxyzine (Atarax) 10-50 mg PO bid–tid PRN
> - Severe Dermatitis
>   - Prednisone in a 4-week course with 7-day tapering steps, such as 60-40-20-10 mg
>   - Open wet dressings with topical steroid application

suppressants, HIV infection, and estrogen therapy. When infection is suspected, cultures of secretions and skin scrapings are indicated. In the pediatric population, pinworm infection must be considered as a cause of pruritus ani.

The etiology of chronic anogenital pruritus can be more challenging to elucidate. Although infection can exacerbate chronic itching, it is rarely the cause except for chronic infections such as HSV or HPV. Underlying skin disease is responsible for the majority of chronic anogenital pruritus with eczema, lichen simplex chronicus (LSC), and lichen sclerosis (LS) among the most common. *Lichen simplex chronicus* refers to local thickening of the skin secondary to repeated episodes of itching and scratching. LSC is identified by a leathery, scaly texture and accentuation of normal skin lines. Irritable nerve endings in LSC lesions trigger an itch-scratch-itch cycle that typically continues long after the initial insult has resolved. Less-common dermatoses that can cause anogenital pruritus include psoriasis and lichen planus. These dermatoses have been responsible for pruritus ani and pruritus vulvae; however, other factors exist that are more specific to pruritus ani.

Primary, or idiopathic, pruritus ani is anal pruritus in the absence of an underlying pathology; it accounts for 25% to 95% of reported cases. Several factors have been identified that can contribute to primary pruritus ani. Patients with idiopathic pruritus ani have been found to have abnormal transient internal sphincter relaxation and early incontinence on saline incontinence tests. Minimal anorectal dyskinesia can lead to seepage of feces, which induces intense pruritus on contact with the anus due to the presence of bacterial endopeptidases (trypsin, kzinase). Pruritus due to fecal incontinence is then exacerbated by excessive or vigorous cleansing. Dietary factors such as excessive caffeine intake (due to a decrease in resting anal canal pressure), spicy foods, foods containing histamine such as tomatoes, and food allergens have been implicated along with psychogenic factors. Drugs can also cause pruritus ani; colchicine and quinidine are among the most common.

Secondary pruritus ani is a symptom related to a preexisting pathology. In addition to infection and dermatoses, proctologic causes include anal fissures or fistulas (12%), hemorrhoids (internal and external, 20%), and cancers of the colon, rectum, and anus (20%).

Clinical Features and Diagnosis

Anogenital pruritus can have an insidious onset, and patients can have symptoms for months or years before seeking medical attention. Clinical findings vary from normal-appearing skin to localized erythema to severe irritation with crusting, lichenification, and ulceration. In addition to a physical examination, evaluation should also include a complete history and psychiatric screening because anxiety and depression have been identified as aggravating factors. Patch testing should also be considered to rule out allergic contact dermatitis, which could be a result of irritating substances in soaps and feminine hygiene products or, more commonly, from repeated exposure to topical medications.

Further work-up may be required in certain circumstances. Cases of pruritus ani that are refractory to standard treatment may require a rectosigmoidoscopy or colonoscopy to evaluate for colon or anorectal pathologies such as hemorrhoids or cancer. Patients with loose stools on chronic antibiotics may undergo pH testing. A pH of 8 to 10 might indicate a *Lactobacillus* deficiency. In the setting of visible skin changes, a biopsy should be considered

CURRENT DIAGNOSIS
- Examination for skin disease
- Microscopic examinations and cultures for infection
- Careful history including contacts and irritants

BOX 1 Treatment of Anogenital Pruritus

Nonspecific Measures
Patient education and reassurance
Careful evaluation for infection and dermatoses
Elimination of irritants: excessive cleansing, infection, nighttime scratching, unnecessary topical medications and lubricants
Nighttime sedation
Sitz baths, cool compresses
Topical anesthetics: topical lidocaine (Xylocaine) jelly 2% or ointment 5%; pramoxine (Summer's Eve Anti-itch gel). Topical benzocaine (Vagisil) and diphenhydramine (Benadryl) should be avoided.

Specific Measures
Itching Secondary to Infection
Acute pruritus: Treat with standard therapy
Chronic pruritus: Evaluate for concomitant dermatosis; infection treated and suppressed long enough for skin to heal and itching to respond to therapy for concomitant process.

Itching Secondary to Dermatoses
Lichen sclerosis: Clobetasol propionate (Temovate) ointment two times daily until skin texture is normal, then three times weekly for life (prepubertal girls occasionally experience remission at puberty; boys remit after circumcision). Or (less effective and concern regarding squamous cell carcinoma), continuous tacrolimus (Protopic) 0.1%, two times daily.
Eczema or lichen simplex chronicus: Clobetasol propionate ointment twice daily until skin is normal and itching is controlled, then taper use to three times weekly, twice weekly, once weekly, then off. Restart if itching flares or recurs. Or (less effective), tacrolimus (Protopic) or pimecrolimus (Elidel), twice daily.

Itching without Objective Signs
Treated as eczema or lichen simplex chronicus with clobetasol propionate for presumed subtle eczema or lichen simplex chronicus
Address anxiety or depression
Gradual increase of the following medications:
- Amitriptyline (Elavil), up to 150 mg at bedtime
- Venlafaxine (Effexor), up to 150 mg extended release per day in patients with normal renal function
- Gabapentin (Neurontin),[1] up to 3600 mg[3] per day for neuropathic pain in patients with normal renal function
- Pregabalin (Lyrica), up to 300 mg per day in patients with normal renal function

---
[1]Not FDA approved for this indication.
[3]Exceeds dosage recommended by the manufacturer.

---

to differentiate among genital dermatoses such as psoriasis, lichen planus, or lichen sclerosis and to rule out malignancies such as intraepithelial neoplasia or carcinoma in situ and extramammary Paget's disease.

Treatment

Treatment depends on the etiology (Box 1). Primary pruritus ani might respond to sitz baths and cool compresses. Good personal hygiene is of importance in pruritus ani and pruritus vulvae, but patients should be advised to avoid excessive cleansing. Symptomatic relief of mild cases can usually be achieved with the use of a low-potency corticosteroid cream or ointment (class VI to VII) such as

CURRENT THERAPY

- Careful evaluation for underlying etiologies
- Specific therapies for all appropriate underlying etiologies
- Specific therapy continued long enough for the skin to heal and the itch–scratch cycle to cease
- Patient education regarding the chronic and recurrent nature of itching and the role of irritants
- Consideration of neuropathy and anxiety or depression in patients without observable disease who are resistant to topical corticosteroid treatment

triamcinolone acetonide 0.025% (Aristocort A cream) or hydrocortisone 2.5% ointment (Hytone).

Nearly all dermatoses, whether acute or chronic, can be treated with an ultrapotent topical corticosteroid such as clobetasol propionate 0.05% cream (Temavate) or halobetasol propionate 0.05% ointment (Ultravate); ointments tend to be less irritating than creams or gels. Short-term, twice-daily application produces rapid, safe control of symptoms. The frequency of application or the potency of the corticosteroid may be tapered once itching is controlled. In chronic cases, immunomodulators such as tacrolimus (Protopic) or pimecrolimus (Elidel) might need to be considered to eliminate the risk of atrophogenesis, which is often seen in prolonged treatment with corticosteroids. However, immunomodulators are slow in onset and produce burning with application. A study by Lysy and colleagues in 2003 showed that topical capsaicin[1] 0.006% cream is a safe and highly effective treatment for severe intractable pruritus ani and may also be considered for treatment.

Secondary anogenital pruritus requires treatment of the underlying disorder. Acute itching due to infection can generally be cleared rapidly and definitively by treating the infection. When no identifiable etiology exists, antidepressants and anxiolytics may be indicated because the pruritus might be psychogenic. Patients and physicians alike are inclined to use antihistamines for relief of all itching. These are ineffective because antihistamines do not have inherent anti-itch properties and generally are useful only for histamine-mediated pruritus seen in urticaria. However, the sedative properties of antihistamines can provide some relief by acting as a sleep aid and subsequently decreasing scratching.

It is important that patients be educated about the possibility of recurrence of pruritus regardless of the etiology. A recurrence does not imply misdiagnosis or a failure of treatment but rather a need for sufficient duration of therapy to allow complete skin healing and cessation of the itch–scratch cycle.

---

[1]Not FDA approved for this indication.

REFERENCES

Alan A, Ambrose NS, Silverman S: Physiological study of pruritus ani. Br J Surg 1987;74:576-579.
Aucoin E J: Pruritus ani. Postgrad Med 1987;82(7):76-80.
Daniel GL, Longo WE, Vernava AM, 3rd: Pruritus ani. Causes and concerns. Dis Colon Rectum 1994;37(7):670-674.
Hagermark O: Itch mediators. Semin Dermatol 1995;14(4):271-276.
Handa Y, Watanabe O, Adachi A: Squamous cell carcinoma of the anal margin with pruritus ani of long duration. Dermatol Surg 2003;29(1):108-110.
James WD, Berger TG, Elston DM: Pruritus and neurocutaneous dermatoses. In James WD, Berger TG, Elston DM (ed): Andrews' Diseases of the Skin Clinical Dermatology, 10th ed. Philadelphia: Saunders, 2006, pp 54-56.
Lieberman DA: Common anorectal disorders. Ann Intern Med 1984;101(6):837-846.
Lysy J, Sistiery-Ittah M, Israelit Y, et al: Topical capsaicin—a novel and effective treatment for idiopathic intractable pruritus ani: A randomised, placebo controlled, crossover study. Gut 2003;52:1323-1326.
Petros JG, Rimm EB, Robillard RJ: Clinical presentation of chronic anal fissures. Am Surg 1993;59(10):666-668.
Powell FC, Perry HO: Pruritus ani: Could it be malignant? Geriatrics 1985;40(1):89-91.
Rohde H: Routine anal cleansing, so-called hemorrhoids, and perianal dermatitis: Cause and effect? Dis Colon Rectum 2000;43(4):561-563.
Weisshaar E, Kucenic MJ, Fleischer AB Jr, et al: Pruritus and dysesthesia. In Bolognia JL, Jorizzo JL, Rapini RP (eds): Dermatology. London: Elsevier, 2003.
Zuccati G, Lotti T, Mastrolorenzo A, et al: Pruritus ani. Dermatol Ther 2005;18(4):355-362.

Urticaria and Angioedema

Method of
Aron J. Gewirtzman, MD

With a high lifetime incidence in the general population (reportedly 10%-25%), urticaria and angioedema are among the most common afflictions seen in primary care, allergy, and dermatology clinics. These similar conditions are vascular reactions of the skin characterized by wheals in the dermis (urticaria) or deeper swellings of the dermis or the subcutaneous or submucosal tissues (angioedema). Avoiding the underlying cause is the simplest and most effective therapy, but unfortunately most cases of chronic urticaria have no identifiable trigger. In these cases, treatment is guided through understanding of the pathophysiologic mechanisms involved in the development of urticarial lesions and reversing them through systematic pharmacology.

The multiple variants of urticaria and angioedema can be differentiated by time course and by nosological classification (Box 1). Urticarial lesions are by definition transient, with individual pruritic wheals appearing and persisting for up to 24 hours. Crops of wheals often recur sporadically but subside within the same 24-hour time period. Lesions lasting longer than 24 hours are potentially concerning for urticarial vasculitis, although this condition typically produces lesions lasting 36 to 48 hours. Once it has been established that a patient's lesions are indeed urticarial, duration is the next most important factor to assess. Cases that resolve within 6 weeks of onset are labeled *acute urticaria*. Daily episodes of urticaria or angioedema that last more than 6 weeks are termed *chronic*.

Urticaria is caused by fluid leakage and edema in vessels of the dermis, and the edema of angioedema is caused by vessels in the skin below the dermis. Unlike urticaria, lesions of angioedema often involve mucosa. Itch, a symptom almost always associated with urticaria, is variably found with angioedema, which can instead manifest with pain and tenderness.

CURRENT DIAGNOSIS

- Lesions of urticaria are transient, appearing and persisting for up to 24 hours at a time.
- Urticaria causes wheals in the dermis; angioedema occurs below the dermis and often involves mucosa.
- Cases that resolve within 6 weeks of onset are acute. Daily episodes of urticaria and/or angioedema that last more than 6 weeks are chronic.
- The hallmark symptom of urticaria is itch, whereas angioedema may be more painful and/or more tender.
- History is the most important component in evaluating potential causes of urticaria and angioedema.

BOX 1 Causes of Urticaria and Angioedema

Immunologic

Type I (IgE mediated)
- Foods: Peanuts and legumes, tree nuts, fish, shellfish, eggs, milk, soy, wheat
- Medications: Penicillins, cephalosporins, aspirin, NSAIDs
- Insect bites and stings
- Aeroallergens: Dust mites, pollens, molds, animal dander

Type II (cytotoxic antibody-mediated): Transfusion reaction

Type III (antigen-antibody mediated): Serum sickness reaction

Nonimmunologic

Physical urticaria: Dermatographism, cholinergic, delayed-pressure, vibratory, exposure to sun, water, or temperature extremes

Pseudoallergic
- Direct mast cell releasers: opiates, vancomycin
- Indirect reactions: Aspirin, radiocontrast media, NSAIDs, ACE-Inhibitors
- Foods containing high levels of histamines: Strawberries, tomatoes, cheese, shellfish

Autoimmune disease: Hashimoto's thyroiditis, rheumatic disease (e.g., systemic lupus erythematosis or vasculitis)

Hereditary: C1-inhibitor deficiency (hereditary angioedema)

Idiopathic (diagnosis of exclusion)

ACE = angiotensin-converting enzyme; NSAID = nonsteroidal antiinflammatory drug.

Adapted from Dibbern DA Jr: Urticaria: Selected highlights and recent advances. Med Clin North Am 2006;90(1):187-209; and Muller BA: Urticaria and angioedema: A practical approach. Am Fam Physician 2004;69(5):1123-1128.

Evaluation

ACUTE URTICARIA

A thorough history is the most important component in evaluating urticaria. Such historical details that should be explored include foods and medications (including over-the-counter products and herbal supplements), recent travel, infections, occupational exposure, and exposure to physical stimuli. Approximately 50% of new cases have an etiology that can be inferred from a detailed history and elimination trials of the potential offending agents. The majority of new-onset urticaria cases (up to 80% by some estimations) resolve within 2 weeks.

Foods and medications are the most common identifiable causes of acute urticaria, and patients are often suspicious of such exposures as the source of their symptoms. An elimination or addition diet can be used to test for a possible offending agent, but it is necessary to allow a period of 2 to 3 days between each modification to distinguish between the normal variation in disease activity and the true sensitivity to a medication or dietary component. If an agent is found to reproducibly cause urticaria in a patient, it should of course be avoided in the future.

In acute urticaria, it is rarely useful to perform thorough laboratory testing that can be invasive and costly, particularly because most cases are short lived. These tests may be appropriate for certain cases of chronic urticaria.

CHRONIC URTICARIA

Urticaria persisting for longer than 6 weeks is frustrating for both patients and caregivers. As with acute urticaria, a thorough history is the most important aspect of the evaluation, because the condition might not improve without eliminating the causative agent. Unfortunately, the numerous potential triggers make chronic urticaria a diagnostic dilemma. In the past, the true etiology of chronic urticaria was determined in less than 25% of cases, with the remainder being termed *chronic idiopathic urticaria*, a diagnosis of exclusion. Recent findings suggest that up to 25% to 45% of patients previously thought to have idiopathic urticaria might in fact have autoimmune urticaria.

In evaluating the underlying cause of chronic urticaria, it is prudent to perform only laboratory tests that are indicated from the history and physical examination, because it is rare that a trigger will be uncovered using a shotgun approach. Potentially useful tests include a complete blood count with differential; leukocytosis can indicate an infection, and eosinophilia could point to helminthic infestation or atopy. Erythrocyte sedimentation rate can screen for inflammatory or occult neoplastic processes. Autoimmune disease may be discovered by testing for antinuclear antibodies, rheumatoid factor, or serum complement. Serum cryoglobulins can point to cold-induced urticaria, although a challenge test by placing an ice cube to the forearm for 5 to 20 minutes is a less invasive method to test for this particular cause.

The various physical urticarias (including dermatographism, cholinergic urticaria, heat and cold urticaria, solar urticaria, and vdelayed pressure urticaria) can ultimately be confirmed through provocative challenges. Dermatographism, in which localized edema or wheals occur following stroking of the skin, can be reproduced by stroking or scratching the skin and evaluating the area minutes later. Cholinergic urticaria is produced by the action of acetylcholine on the mast cell and can be reproduced by exercise or a methacholine skin test. The provocative test for adrenergic urticaria, attributable to norepinephrine, is the intradermal administration of 3 to 10 ng of norepinephrine. Temperature extremes can cause urticaria. The test for cold urticaria is discussed earlier, and heat urticaria may be tested by heating a cylinder to 50 to 55°C and applying it to the skin for 30 minutes. Delayed pressure urticaria may be reproduced by placing a 15-lb weight to the skin for 20 minutes and re-inspecting the area several hours later.

Approximately 50% of chronic urticaria remits within 1 year, but 20% of patients continue to have urticaria for more than 20 years.

ANGIOEDEMA

Angioedema shares many triggers with urticaria, and once again a thorough history is the most important aspect of the evaluation. However, in addition to allergic and physical causes, angioedema can also be due to an autosomal dominant inheritance. Hereditary angioedema is characterized by recurrent episodes of potentially life-threatening angioedema and is caused by a deficiency of C1 inhibitor. Deficiency of the C1 inhibitor allows release of bradykinin and subsequently induces edema formation.

 CURRENT THERAPY

- If a cause can be identified, the trigger should be avoided whenever possible.
- Antihistamines are the cornerstone of pharmacologic therapy for both urticaria and angioedema.
- Nonsedating H_1-receptor blockers should be used for initial therapy, followed by the addition of sedating H_1-receptor blockers, H_2-receptor blockers, and leukotriene modifiers if symptoms are uncontrolled.
- Steroids might provide some relief for refractory cases but should not be used long term.
- Angioedema of the larynx is life-threatening and can require epinephrine, intubation, or tracheostomy.

Initial therapy: Second-generation H₁-receptor antagonist

Symptoms not adequately controlled

Add first-generation sedating H₁-receptor antagonist at night

Symptoms remain uncontrolled

Add H₂-receptor antagonist or leukotriene modifier

Symptoms remain severe

Add oral corticosteroid as a short-term measure

Symptoms persist

Consider cyclosporine (Neoral),[1] mycophenolate mofetil (Cellcept),[1] IVIg,[1] plasmapheresis, azathioprine (Imuran),[1] or methotrexate (Trexall)[1]

[1] Not FDA approved for this indication

FIGURE 1. Progression of treatment for urticaria. IVIg, intravenous immunoglobulin. (Adapted from Muller BA: Urticaria and angioedema: A practical approach. Am Fam Physician 2004;69(5):1123-1128.)

Treatment

URTICARIA

Regardless of the underlying trigger, the wheal formation, vasodilation, and erythema of urticaria are caused by release of mediators such as histamine and prostaglandins from cytoplasmic granules from mast cells. When the trigger cannot be isolated or avoided, several pharmacologic therapies have been found useful in treating acute and chronic urticaria.

The mainstay of pharmacologic treatment are the second-generation (nonsedating) H₁ antihistamines, such as loratadine (Claritin)[1] 10 mg daily, cetirizine (Zyrtec) 10 mg daily, fexofenadine (Allegra) 60 mg twice daily, or desloratadine (Clarinex) 5 mg daily. Antihistamines are generally safe and have few significant adverse effects or drug interactions. It is common to exceed the FDA-approved dose recommendations for severely affected patients. Antihistamines are most effective when given on a scheduled basis rather than treating symptomatically, particularly for chronic urticaria. Often, the addition of a sedating antihistamine, such as diphenhydramine (Benadryl) 25 to 50 mg or hydroxyzine (Atarax) 50 mg, is given at night to aid patients who have difficulty sleeping due to itching. Because blood vessels in the skin have both H₁ and H₂ histamine receptors, the addition of H₂-receptor antagonists such as ranitidine (Zantac)[1] 75 to 150 mg daily can often help when combinations of H₁-receptor antagonists fail.

The tricyclic antidepressant doxepin (Sinequan),[1] 25 mg tid, antagonizes both H₁ and H₂ receptors and is therefore an option as monotherapy. The leukotriene modifiers, such as monteleukast (Singulair)[1] 5 mg daily, are another class of medications that have a role in a select group of patients who fail antihistamines alone, but these should be only used in addition to antihistamines.

Patients who are unresponsive to these classes of medications might benefit from a brief course of systemic steroids. In addition to suppressing multiple facets of the cellular and humoral immune system, steroids block arachidonate metabolism, thus preventing formation of leukotrienes and prostaglandins. Steroids should be used with caution because their side effects are multiple and well known, but they may be helpful as a short-term measure. A course of 40 mg of prednisone (Sterapred) daily tapered over 2 to 4 weeks can be attempted, but extended use of steroids for urticaria is contraindicated. Unfortunately, urticaria often recurs as soon as the medication is tapered.

Steroid-sparing medications such as cyclosporine (Neoral)[1] 2.5 to 5 mg/kg/day and mycophenolate mofetil (CellCept)[1] 1000 mg twice a day for 12 weeks have also shown promise in the treatment of urticaria refractory to antihistamines. Other therapeutic options include azathioprine (Imuran),[1] methotrexate (Trexall),[1] intravenous immune globulin,[1] and plasmapheresis. See Figure 1 for a simplified algorithm for treating urticaria.

ANGIOEDEMA

Most cases of angioedema are treated similarly to urticaria, beginning with antihistamines and progressing to glucocorticoids or steroid-sparing medications if necessary. In emergency situations such as angioedema of the larynx, 0.3 mg intramuscular injection of a 1:1000 solution of epinephrine (EpiPen) is indicated, because it reverses vascular

---

[1] Not FDA approved for this indication.

permeability in addition to its bronchodilatory effects. Angioedema of the larynx can require intubation or tracheotomy.

Hereditary angioedema tends not to respond to the medicines that are the mainstay of treatment for other forms of urticaria and angioedema. Currently available treatments for acute attacks of hereditary angioedema include fresh frozen plasma (2 units IV) and anabolic androgens such as danazol (400-600 mg PO daily in 2-3 divided doses). Prophylaxis has been attempted using danazol 200 mg orally three times daily or FFP before procedures that could bring about hereditary angioedema. Although not currently available, C1-inhibitor concentrate (500 units) has been shown to successfully and consistently relieve severe abdominal or subcutaneous attacks and laryngeal edema. C1-inhibitor concentrate has also been shown to be effective for short-term prophylaxis.

REFERENCES

Clarke P: Urticaria. Aust Fam Physician 2004;33(7):501-503.
Dibbern DA Jr: Urticaria: selected highlights and recent advances. Med Clin North Am 2006;90(1):187-209.
Farkas H, Jakab L, Temesszentandrasi G, et al: Hereditary angioedema: A decade of human C1-inhibitor concentrate therapy. J Allergy Clin Immunol 2007;120(4):941-947.
James WD, Berger TG, Elston DM (ed): Andrews' Diseases of the Skin Clinical Dermatology, 10th ed. Philadelphia: Saunders, 2006, pp 149-156.
Jauregui I, Ferrer M, Montoro J, et al: Antihistamines in the treatment of chronic urticaria. J Investig Allergol Clin Immunol 2007;17(Suppl 2):41-52.
Kaplan AP, Greaves MW: Angioedema. J Am Acad Dermatol 2005;53(3):373-388.
Muller BA: Urticaria and angioedema: A practical approach. Am Fam Physician 2004;69(5):1123-1128.
Shahar E, Bergman R, Guttman-Yassky E, Pollack S: Treatment of severe chronic idiopathic urticaria with oral mycophenolate mofetil in patients not responding to antihistamines and/or corticosteroids. Int J Dermatol 2006;45(10):1224-1227.
Vena GA, Cassano N, Colombo D, et al: Cyclosporine in chronic idiopathic urticaria: A double-blind, randomized, placebo-controlled trial. J Am Acad Dermatol 2006;55(4):705-709.
Wedi B, Raap U, Kapp A: Chronic urticaria and infections. Curr Opin Allergy Clin Immunol 2004;4(5):387-396.
Zuraw BL: Current and future therapy for hereditary angioedema. Clin Immunol 2005;114(1):10-16.

Pigmentary Disorders

Method of
*Robert A. Schwartz, MD, MPH,
and Camila K. Janniger, MD*

Cutaneous pigmentation protects humans from harmful ultraviolet light radiation. It results from many factors, including carotenoids and hemoglobin, with the number, size, type, and distribution pattern of melanosomes being an important determinate. Melanin produced in epidermal melanocytes is the principal pigment of concern, although the lipochrome carotene, when ingested in excessive amounts, can produce a yellow-orange coloration that can be mistaken for jaundice. However, hypothyroidism, diabetes mellitus, hepatic diseases, anorexia nervosa, and renal diseases can produce carotenemia unassociated with the ingestion of carotene. Similarly, deposition of some medications or their metabolites produce discoloration. A correct diagnosis is mandatory.

Pigmentary disorders represent a wide variety of diseases, including tinea versicolor, acanthosis nigricans, Addison's disease, melanoma, onchocerciasis, mycosis fungoides, tuberous sclerosis and leprosy, the latter a reason for the social stigma of depigmentation in much of the world.

Superficial melanin tends to be seen as tan or brown, whereas deeper deposits often produce a gray or blue-gray hue due to the Tyndall light-scattering effect. Wood's lamp examination can aid in this distinction, showing epidermal melanin, which absorbs it, to appear darker than dermal melanosis, in which light scattering makes the patches less prominent. In general, epidermal melanosis is more amenable to therapy. Both types may be present. In addition, the Wood's lamp long wavelength ultraviolet blacklight examination may be valuable for hypopigmentation in separating total pigment loss from partial forms, detecting the yellowish-green fluorescence of some patches of tinea versicolor, and visualizing 1- to 10-cm depigmented spots (Fitzpatrick patches) on light-complexioned babies with tuberous sclerosis.

Patient education and realistic expectations are critical. All skin products should be first tested by limited application to noncosmetically sensitive normal skin and evaluated at 24 and 48 hours. In addition, effective sunscreens or sunblocks should be employed whenever tretinoin, psoralens, or hydroquinone is used. Therapy for the disorders discussed here is usually directed at improvement rather than cure. Thus, the results may be modest but are usually not permanent, and repeat courses of therapy may be necessary.

The risk of side effects needs to be stressed. Tretinoin and hydroquinone can produce irritant or allergic dermatitis. Hydroquinone has recently come under regulatory scrutiny, in part because it can induce exogenous ochronosis, a permanent blue-black hyperpigmentation at the site of application after prolonged and extensive use, which should be avoided. Some hydroquinone products contain sodium metabisulfite, a sulfite that can cause allergic reactions, sometimes life-threatening, which are more common in asthmatics than in nonasthmatics.

New medications are being developed for hyperpigmentation, in part as a response to concern about the safety of hydroquinone. They include kojic acid, mandelic acid, azelaic acid, bearberry extract, licorice extract, mulberry extract, and arbutin. Kojic acid is a chelation agent produced by several species of fungus, especially *Aspergillus oryzae*, and normally used as a food additive and preservative, a skin-whitening agent in cosmetics, a plant-growth regulator, and a chemical intermediate. It can be employed alone or in combination with hydroquinone. However, kojic acid can be problematic in terms of its chemical stability and its potential negative effects on the skin.

Hyperpigmentation Disorders

MELASMA

Clinical Findings

Melasma (chloasma) is a common cutaneous disorder characterized by patchy hyperpigmentation of the face, occasionally the neck, and rarely the forearms. There are three main patterns: centrofacial, malar, and mandibular. It occurs most commonly in women taking oral contraceptives or in those who are pregnant (mask of pregnancy) and rarely in women with ovarian tumors, but it can also be evident in adolescent girls, boys in puberty, men, and nonpregnant women. Hormonal and genetic factors are important; people of lineages from South Asia, China, and Latin America have a propensity for melasma. It tends to darken on solar exposure and fade during winter without it. Hydantoin use can induce a similar eruption.

Treatment

In melasma, epidermal pigmentation, often tan and appearing to darken on Wood's lamp examination due to epidermal melanin absorption, tends to respond to hydroquinone, whereas bluish grey dermal pigmentation is much less responsive. Tri-Luma cream (fluocinolone acetonide 0.01%, hydroquinone 4%, tretinoin 0.05%) is a good approach. It needs to be used together with an appropriate sunscreen, ideally a sunblock such as Lydia O'Leary's Covermark. Tri-Luma cream is indicated for short-term and intermittent long-term treatment of moderate to severe melasma. A combination of hydroquinone 4% cream containing sunscreen (Solaquin Forte) applied twice daily and 0.1% tretinoin gel (Renova)[1] applied at night for

---

[1]Not FDA approved for this indication.

TABLE 1 Sunscreens

Brand Name	Sunscreen Type	Characteristics
Bull Frog QuikGel	Chemical sunscreen	Greaseless vehicle, waterproof
Coppertone Sport	Chemical sunscreen	Waterproof, reduced eye stinging
Durascreen 30	Combination chemical and physical sunscreen	Wide spectrum of UV protection, thicker vehicle
Olay Complete	Chemical sunscreen, physical blocker	Elegant vehicle, wide spectrum of UV protection
Ombrelle 30	Chemical sunscreen	Water-resistant, fragrance-free, wide spectrum of UV protection

4 to 6 months can produce substantial lightening, but also can cause irritation, especially when first applied. A similar product is hydroquinone 4% and retinol, EpiQuin Micro, a high-technology effort that is worth trying. Another combination formulation is AlphaquinHP (hydroquinone 4% cream with glycolic acids and sunscreens).

Tretinoin 0.1% cream alone can fade the spots somewhat, but treatment is often protracted. Applying tretinoin cream every other night for the first 2 to 3 weeks and then increasing the frequency of application to nightly can minimize the irritation. Azelaic acid (Azelex)[1] 20% cream applied twice daily with or without 0.1% tretinoin gel for 6 months may also bleach the patches. It can also be combined with hydroquinone 4% cream, both agents to be applied twice daily. The value of azelaic acid for melasma may be enhanced by the use of sequential therapy with it and a potent topical steroid.

It is critical that hormonal therapy, if in use, be discontinued and sun exposure be avoided diligently during therapy. Some hydroquinone products, such as Solaquin Forte, contain sunscreens. All patients with melasma should also use an additional sunscreen agent after treatment. The product should have a sun protection factor (SPF) of at least 15. Water-resistant products are preferred in those who exercise outdoors or sweat heavily (Table 1). If not otherwise contraindicated, oral vitamins C and E supplements may be slightly beneficial.

SOLAR LENTIGO

Clinical Findings

Solar lentigines (also called senile lentigines or liver spots) occur in most elderly light-complexioned persons of European or East Asian heritage. A majority by age 60 years may be affected, although lentigines often occur in younger people with marked solar exposure. They begin as tiny macules on the face, shoulders, or dorsal hands, expanding and coalescing into uniformly brown patches, often with an irregular configuration. Solar lentigo has no malignant potential, but it takes clinical experience to distinguish it from lentigo maligna, an early melanoma.

Treatment

Tretinoin 0.05% emollient cream (Renova)[1] applied sparingly once daily, might gradually work. Bleaching creams containing hydroquinone or azelaic acid[1] function slowly and incompletely in most cases. The addition of tretinoin cream can improve the results somewhat. Tri-Luma cream[1] (flucinolone acetonide 0.01%, hydroquinone 4%, tretinoin 0.05%) is more effective, but it needs be used together with an appropriate broad-spectrum sunscreen of SPF 30 or higher.

---
[1]Not FDA approved for this indication.

A combination of mequinol 2% and tretinoin 0.01% has been FDA approved for solar lentigines, marketed as Solagé. It should not be used in women of childbearing potential or in patients using other potentially phototoxic oral or topical medications. A comprehensive ultraviolet light avoidance plan needs to be employed. Another combination formulation is AlphaquinHP (hydroquinone 4% cream with glycolic acid and sunscreen).

Liquid nitrogen cryotherapy is effective using a superficial freeze (light pressure with dipped cotton swab for 5-7 seconds), but post-therapy hypopigmentation can occur. Mid-depth trichloroacetic acid or glycolic acid chemical peels can lighten or eradicate multiple lesions in a single sitting. The Nd-YAG laser, Q-switched ruby laser, photodynamic therapy, or resurfacing CO_2 laser, can also be effective.

DRUG-INDUCED HYPERPIGMENTATION

Clinical Findings

Many medications can produce abnormal skin, nail, or oral pigmentation as a result of either deposition of the drug or its metabolites or a drug-induced stimulation of epidermal melanogenesis (Table 2). Some reactions require or are enhanced by ultraviolet light exposure. These color alterations range from tan to slate gray to blue-black. Drugs such as 5-fluorouracil (Adrucil), gold, silver, and amiodarone (Cordarone) produce preferential darkening in sun-exposed sites. Other medications such as zidovudine (Retrovir), bleomycin (Blenoxane), doxorubicin (Adriamycin), chloroquine (Aralen), and cyclophosphamide (Cytoxan) also cause pigmented bands in the nails. Minocycline (Minocin; Dynacin) can produce brown-gray discoloration in old acne scars, hyperpigmented patches on the anterior legs, and a generalized brown-gray discoloration.

Treatment and Prevention

In most instances, the dyspigmentation that appears with drugs slowly fades in months to years after the drug has been discontinued. However, certain medications such as gold and topical hydroquinone can be responsible for irreversible color changes. The use of sunscreens is encouraged in patients with photo-enhanced drug-induced hyperpigmentation to minimize additional pigment production.

POSTINFLAMMATORY HYPERPIGMENTATION

Clinical Findings

This is probably the most common cause of altered skin coloration. This acquired excess of pigment represents the sequelae of a variety of skin disorders, traumas, therapeutic interventions, infections,

TABLE 2 Medication-Induced Pigmentary Abnormalities

Medication	Clinical Characteristics
Amiodarone (Cordarone)	Gray discoloration in sun-exposed sites
Busulfan (Myleran)	Generalized increased skin color resembling Addison's disease
Doxorubicin (Adriamycin)	Pigmented nail bands and palmar creases
Estrogen (Premarin)	Melasma
5-Fluorouracil	Increased pigment in sun-exposed sites
Gold (Myochrysine)	Permanent blue-gray color in sun-exposed areas
Hydroxychloroquine (Plaquenil)	Brown or gray discoloration of the shins, trunk
Levodopa plus carbidopa (Sinemet)	Diffuse hyperpigmentation
Minocycline (Minocin)	Gray pigment in old scars and/or on the legs or a generalized muddy color
Zidovudine (AZT) (Retrovir)	Nail pigmentation, diffuse Addison's-like pigmentation

allergic reactions, mechanical injuries, burns, reactions to medications, phototoxic reactions, and inflammatory diseases, and requires that the underlying process be effectively treated. This results in melanin being released into the dermis, where it is phagocytized by macrophages. This pigment can remain indefinitely and cause macular hyperpigmentation. Superficial melanin tends to be seen as tan or brown, whereas deeper deposits often produce a gray or blue-gray hue.

Treatment

One should attempt to effectively treat underlying skin disorders, avoiding the inciting reaction, regardless of etiology. This includes manual manipulation when applicable. Topical tacrolimus 0.03% ointment (Protopic)[1] twice a day for 3 months is now our first choice, because it is also therapy for many of the underlying concerns. Patients should avoid cosmetics. Topical tretinoin 0.1% gel may be effectively employed every other day for 2 weeks and continued nightly as tolerated.

If the pigment is superficial, the areas can be lightened somewhat with the agents noted earlier for melasma. They do not work well in deep dermal melanosis. A combination of hydroquinone 4% cream containing sunscreen (Solaquin Forte) applied twice daily and 0.1% tretinoin gel (Retin-A)[1] applied at night for 4 to 6 months can produce substantial lightening. Daily use of sunscreens with a sun protection factor of 15 or greater is essential. Tri-Luma cream (flucinolone acetonide 0.01%, hydroquinone 4%, tretinoin 0.05%) is another option, which needs to be used together with an appropriate sunscreen. Other choices are hydroquinone 4% cream combined with hyaluronic acid, 10% glycolic acid, and the sunscreens avobenzone, oxybenzone, and octocrylene as Glyquin-XM. The combination can cause irritation when first used. Applying tretinoin cream every other night for the first 2 to 3 weeks and then increasing the frequency of application to a nightly treatment program can minimize the irritation. Tretinoin alone can fade the spots somewhat, but treatment is often protracted. Laser therapy is ineffective in most cases. Sunscreens are helpful to minimize increased pigmentation in sites that are already too dark.

A common concern in the dark complexioned acne vulgaris patient is postinflammatory acne hyperpigmentation, often accentuated by manipulating the papules or pustules. The naturally occurring dicarboxylic acid, azelaic acid, in a 20% cream (Azelex) applied as a thin film twice a day, is a good choice for moderately severe comedonal and inflammatory acne and for the hyperpigmentation itself. However, for both purposes its onset of action is somewhat slow. In addition, it can cause annoying stinging, itching, and burning which usually desists with continued use. Its adverse effects include hypopigmentation and the possible initiation of vitiligo. It is a pregnancy category B drug, and safety in patients younger than 12 years is not established.

ACRAL ACANTHOSIS NIGRICANS

Acral acanthosis nigricans (acral acanthotic anomaly), a distal form of acanthosis nigricans, is a disorder seen relatively commonly as velvety hyperpigmented plaques in dark-complexioned persons. It is particularly prominent over the elbows, knees, knuckles, and dorsal surfaces of the feet in otherwise healthy persons. Axillae and other intertriginous regions appear normal. Tretinoin cream at bedtime alone can fade the eruption somewhat after prolonged treatment.

Hypopigmentation Disorders

VITILIGO

Clinical Findings

Milk white patches of idiopathic vitiligo affect about 1% to 2% of the general population worldwide without racial, sexual, or regional differences. However, they are more pronounced and easily visualized in darker-complexioned people, and visibility is enhanced by a tendency of some patches to be surrounded by borders of hyperpigmentation. Because vitiliginous patches do not tan, ultraviolet light exposure also emphasizes them when adjacent skin tans normally.

Vitiligo reflects total destruction of all melanocytes within the affected epidermis. The hair within vitiligo becomes white if hair bulb melanocytes are destroyed. Vitiligo is most often seen on the face, backs of the hands and wrists, in the axillae and umbilicus, and on the genitalia. It tends to be especially prominent around body orifices: eyes, nostrils, mouth, nipples, umbilicus and genitalia. It begins as small patches and enlarges peripherally, with new lesions appearing occasionally. It can coalesce into large patches or remain localized. Evolving lesions may be hypopigmented initially, especially in dark complexioned persons. Vitiligo can also appear on the arms, elbows, and knees at sites of trauma or sunburn (Koebner's phenomenon). Striking generalized vitiligo after dermatitis medicamentosa might also reflect this circumstance in a predisposed patient.

Nonsegmental vitiligo is about three times more common than segmental vitiligo; the latter is generally more common in children. Segmental vitiligo tends to have an early onset, spreads rapidly into the involved dermatome, stabilizes within 2 years, and persists throughout life. The initial involvement is usually solitary. The face is the most common site; trigeminal is the commonest dermatome. Nonsegmental vitiligo typically has new patches appearing throughout life and shows a persistent degree of symmetry in early as well as advanced lesions. Patients should also be evaluated for possible coexisting thyroid disease, as well as for a wide range of other occasionally associated autoimmune disorders. Some consider the white halo surrounding the halo nevus and the halo melanoma to represent a type of vitiligo. Halo nevi are not unusual in adolescent girls using birth control pills.

Chemical-induced vitiligo may be caused by industrial germicidal phenolic cleansers, rubbers, and plastics. Therapy must begin by terminating such exposure.

Treatment

There are multiple options but no reliable therapy. Patients might find a psychological benefit from cosmetic cover-ups, such as Dermablend or Covermark, even if no therapy is desired after patient education that vitiligo will not go away spontaneously and that medical therapy might not be effective. Topical dyes and self-tanning products, such as Vitadye stain and sun-free tanning products containing dihydroxyacetone, such as Chromelin Complexion Blender, are also good. Regardless, sunscreen use, if it is not already incorporated into one of these agents, is important, because skin with vitiligo is more likely to sunburn than skin with normal pigmentation, and can ultimately develop skin cancer.

Successful therapy is initially reflected by perifollicular repigmentation after about 3 months, which enlarges as melanocytes migrate laterally. Thus, if vitiligo is on the vermilion borders of the lips, distal fingers, or penile shaft, or has white hair extruding from it, the patient should be advised that medical therapy will not be successful. In that case, surgical repigmentation techniques such as thin-split section grafts or minigrafts of autologous skin or autologous cultured melanocytes into large vitiliginous dermabraded patches would be necessary for stable vitiligo, although the Koebner phenomenon might limit this approach.

Topical tacrolimus 0.03% ointment (Protopic)[1] twice a day for 3 months is now our first choice, because cutaneous atrophy and telangiectasia are a risk with topical steroids. For a child with localized vitiligo, our next approach is a topical steroid. In children younger than 10 years, hydrocortisone valerate 0.2% cream daily on the face or desonide 0.05% cream daily to the trunk or extremities may be good. For facial and genital vitiligo, use 0.05% fluorcinonide cream (Lidex).[1] Elsewhere, clobetasol propionate cream (Temovate)[1] has been employed in patients as young as 5 years of age, with the

---
[1]Not FDA approved for this indication.

best results in facial lesions of dark-complexioned patients, in whom progressive repigmentation continues after discontinuing therapy. Vitiligo might respond on the face but rarely does so on the hands, elbows, and knees. One can use this steroid for 3 to 4 months, evaluating monthly and stopping if there is evidence of cutaneous atrophy or telangiectasia.

Photochemotherapy for vitiligo is sometimes beneficial in the highly motivated, because response is often partial and can take years. For localized vitiligo, the topical psoralen methoxsalen (Oxsoralen lotion 0.01%) is applied 30 minutes before UVA exposure (PUVA), although blistering can be a problem. Widespread vitiligo requires oral methoxypsoralen 0.6 mg/kg administered 90 minutes before UVA exposure three times a week for 3 to 4 months before perifollicular spots become evident. We do not recommend phototherapy for children younger than 12 years. Vitiligo might respond on the face but rarely does so on hands, elbows, and knees. Narrowband UVB by itself is another option and is photochemotherapy using natural sunlight. Patients should be warned that phototherapy has hazards, including the risk of cancer.

If vitiligo involves more than 50% to 75% of the skin, a permanent depigmentation (chemical vitiligo) may be induced, to provide uniform coloration. Generalized permanent bleaching can be achieved with monobenzyl ether of hydroquinone 20% cream (Benzoquin) twice a day for 6 to 12 months or longer for adults with generalized vitiligo. Hyperpigmentation from acquired ochronosis is a risk with this therapy, potentially exacerbating the cosmetic problem.

IDIOPATHIC GUTTATE HYPOMELANOSIS

Clinical Findings

Idiopathic guttate hypomelanosis is a common benign condition of unknown etiology in which asymptomatic oval or angular 2- to 3-mm or larger white macules develop. They are persistent, are most numerous on the anterior lower extremities, and tend to increase in incidence with age so that elderly persons can have hundreds of them.

Treatment

Therapy is usually unsatisfactory. Tretinoin 0.1% gel used for 4 to 6 months can partially restore skin color in affected areas. Cryotherapy with liquid nitrogen may be tried; a gentle 5-second light freeze is sometimes beneficial. Intralesional triamcinolone acetonide 3 mg/mL occasionally is beneficial.

PITYRIASIS ALBA

Clinical Findings

Pityriasis alba is a relatively common disorder of hypopigmented macules that appears most commonly on the faces of preadolescent children and occasionally young adults. It may be the manifesting complaint or an incidental finding. It is a benign, chiefly cosmetic defect that is more prominent in, and problematic for, dark-skinned persons. The etiology of pityriasis alba is not known precisely, although it has been linked with atopy, and it is thought by some to be a postinflammatory reaction in atopic dermatitis. It is usually evident as round to oval hypopigmented macules, 0.5 to 5 cm or more in diameter, with generally well defined but irregular borders. Macules are chiefly on the face (forehead and malar ridges) but occasionally on the shoulders, upper arms, or legs. There are often two or three, but this can vary from one to twenty or more. Some become confluent.

Initially there is a pink patch with an elevated, slightly erythematous border, which may be slightly pruritic. After a few weeks the erythema fades, leaving a whitish macule, which may be covered with a fine, adherent scale. The late stage is a smooth hypopigmented macule. Repigmentation usually occurs in months to years. Macules in all three stages can occur simultaneously, or all may be in the same stage. The lesions are often most apparent in summer, due to tanning of the surrounding skin. On rare occasions, mycosis fungoides has hypopigmented macules resembling pityriasis alba. Therefore, long-standing patches unresponsive to therapy might require biopsy.

Treatment

An emollient or bland lubricant, such as petrolatum, may be useful in masking scale; no therapy is overwhelmingly successful. Repigmentation can be sometimes accelerated by the use of a mild to medium strength nonfluorinated topical steroid such as hydrocortisone 1% cream or desonide 0.05% cream. Mild peeling agents may be used with or without these topical steroids. More-potent steroids, such as triamcinolone acetonide 0.1% cream and hydrocortisone valerate 0.2% cream, are recommended for nonfacial lesions. Topical tretinoin 0.1% gel applied every other evening may also be useful.

REFERENCES

Huggins RH, Janniger CK, Schwartz RA: Childhood vitiligo. Cutis 2007; 79:277-280.

Lacz NL, Vafaie J, Kihiczak NI, Schwartz RA: Postinflammatory hyperpigmentaiton: a common and often troubling disorder. Int J Dermatol 2004; 43:362-365.

Schwartz RA, Fernández G, Kotulska K, Józwiak S: Tuberous sclerosis complex: advances in diagnosis, genetics, and management. J Am Acad Dermatol 2007;57:189-202.

Schwartz, RA, Kihiczak NI: Postinflammatory hyperpigmentation. eMedicine Dermatology [Journal serial online]. 2008. Available at: http://emedicine.com/derm/topic876.htm Last accessed August 18, 2008.

Sinha S, Schwartz RA: Juvenile acanthosis nigricans. J Am Acad Dermatol 2007;57:502-508.

Sunburn

Method of
Warwick L. Morison, MD

Sunburn is a common problem, particularly in fair-skinned white persons, caused by excessive exposure to ultraviolet (UV) radiation from sunlight or artificial sources such as sunlamps. When induced by sunlight, it is mainly due to UVB (280-320 nm) radiation plus a smaller contribution from UVA (320-400 nm) radiation. Sunburn is also described as erythema and it appears 3 to 4 hours after exposure, reaches a maximum at 12 to 18 hours, and usually settles after 72 to 96 hours. In severe reactions with blistering, complete resolution can take a week or more.

Sunburns are graded as pink, red, and blistering. In contrast, thermal burns are graded by degree (first, second, and third), but this classification should not be applied to sunburns because thermal burns have quite different sequelae, such as scarring and death, which are extremely rare consequences of a sunburn. Keratoconjunctivitis, or ocular sunburn, can also be caused by UV radiation and it follows a similar time course.

There are two facets to management of sunburn: prevention and treatment. Because there is no effective treatment for an established sunburn, most emphasis should be placed on prevention.

Prevention

Skin color and the capacity of a person to tan will determine how important it is for an individual person to take preventive measures. However, even dark-skinned people can sunburn provided the exposure dose is sufficiently high. Skin color, past history of sunburn, and likely exposure should therefore be used as a guide in advising people about protection. Protection from sunlight is often equated with use of sunscreens, but this approach is too narrow, and protection should consist of a package of measures: avoiding overexposure to sunlight, using sunscreens, and wearing protective clothing.

CURRENT DIAGNOSIS

- Sunburn appears 3 to 4 hours after exposure to sunlight or an artificial source of UV radiation such as a sunlamp.
- The redness of skin is diffuse and continuous, unlike rashes, which are often discontinuous.
- Sunburns are graded as pink, red, and blistering.

CURRENT THERAPY

- Prevention is the best approach to management and consists of a package of measures: avoiding over-exposure, using sunscreens, and wearing protective clothing.
- Treatment of a sunburn consists of cool baths and use of moisturizing creams.
- Topical and systemic corticosteroids do not alter the course of a sunburn.

AVOIDANCE OF EXPOSURE

Simple avoidance of excessive exposure to a threshold dose of UV radiation is often the best advice for fair-skinned people. Scheduling outdoor activities for before 10 AM and after 4 PM will avoid the peak UV irradiance period and still permit enjoyment of the outdoors. This advice should be accompanied by several warnings. Sitting in the shade or under a beach umbrella only reduces exposure by about 70%. A cloudy day is often the setting for the worst sunburns because even complete white cloud cover reduces UV exposure by only about 50%.

Clothing is not always an effective protector. If it is possible to see through a fabric, UV radiation can also penetrate to a significant extent. The geographic location of exposure must also be considered because UV radiation may be twice as intense at the equator as compared with much of continental North America.

SUNSCREENS

There is now a great number of sunscreens on the market, and they contain numerous active ingredients. If this is not enough to cause confusion, some are not even labeled as sunscreens: sunblocks and tanning lotions are other terms. However, the informed physician need only know four properties of a sunscreen: the sun protection factor (SPF), the spectrum of protection, the base, and whether or not it is water resistant.

The SPF is a index of the amount of protection provided by the sunscreen. For example, a fair-skinned person who normally begins to sunburn after a 10-minute exposure to sunlight should be able to tolerate up to 150 minutes of exposure after application of an SPF 15 sunscreen.

There are several provisos for this statement. To provide the stated protection, a sunscreen must be applied 10 minutes before exposure to allow binding to skin proteins to occur, and it must be applied in an adequate amount. Several studies have shown that under ideal circumstances in which sunscreen is supplied freely and the subject is observed while making the application, most people only use one half the required amount. Ordinary use probably provides much less protection. As a rough guide, one ounce of sunscreen is necessary to cover a 70-kg adult in a bathing suit; in other words, a four ounce bottle of sunscreen only provides four applications.

Sunscreens vary in the amount of the solar spectrum for which they provide protection. All sunscreens provide protection against UVB radiation and the shorter end of UVA radiation. Some sunscreens claim to provide broad-spectrum protection against UVB and UVA radiation and contain avobenzone or titanium dioxide to protect against the longer wavelengths in the UVA spectrum. Ecamsule (Mexoryl SX), a recently approved sunscreen active, provides good absorption in the middle of the UVA spectrum so that a sunscreen containing this, avobenzone, and octocrylene, an absorber of UVB radiation, provides very good broad-spectrum protection.

The base of a sunscreen is also important because it often determines whether or not a sunscreen will be used. Men usually prefer alcohol-based lotions because they dry quickly and leave a dry and nongreasy film. Women usually prefer lotions or creams because they give a moisturizing feel to the skin.

Finally, a sunscreen may be labeled water resistant or very water resistant. Because almost all outdoor pastimes involve perspiring or contact with water, a very water-resistant sunscreen should be selected.

A fair-skinned person should always use a sunscreen with an SPF 15 or higher. People who tan well and never burn are probably adequately protected with an SPF of 8 to 10. People with black or brown skin probably do not need sunscreens except for extreme occupational or social exposure.

A few myths should be dismissed. There is no effective oral sunscreen. Many have been tested and all have failed. Self-tanning preparations are not sunscreens. They do provide the appearance of a tan and are safe to use but they provide no significant protection against UV radiation.

PROTECTIVE CLOTHING

There has been significant progress in recent years in the development, testing, and classification of UV-protective clothing. Akin to the SPF for sunscreens, such clothing is labeled with an ultraviolet protective factor (UPF), and a fabric with a UPF of 50 blocks transmission of 98% of UV radiation. A hat with a 3-inch brim all around completes the package of protection.

PROTECTIVE TANNING

The proliferation of suntan parlors has generated a lot of interest in protective tanning, with much misinformation provided by the commercial interests involved. Little scientific information is available to provide a guide as to whether protective tanning is of any value in preventing the long-term hazards of excessive exposure to sunlight, namely skin cancer and premature aging of the skin. Certainly, preventive tanning using multiple suberythemal doses of UV radiation can prevent sunburn, but the cost in terms of chronic damage is unknown.

Most tanning salons claim to use only UVA radiation in their tanning beds, but this claim is false. All so-called UVA tanning beds emit some UVB radiation, the most damaging wavelengths, and in addition, UVA radiation, especially in large doses can produce the same damaging effect as UVB radiation. Furthermore, a UVA-induced tan is not very protective and at most has an SPF of 6 to 8.

A person who tans well and never burns might gain some protection from sunlight by preventive tanning without incurring too much damage. However, the risk-to-benefit ratio for people who do sunburn is probably very unfavorable.

Treatment

When a person has a sunburn, general supportive measures are the only approach to treatment. Cold compresses and cool baths with bath oil provide some relief. Frequent application of moisturizing creams help alleviate dryness. Blistering of the skin can lead to secondary infection and require use of an antibiotic cream. Rarely, an extremely severe sunburn necessitates hospitalization and management as a thermal burn.

Topical corticosteroids reduce erythema by causing vasoconstriction, but this effect is temporary and does not reduce epidermal damage. Systemic corticosteroids, even in very large doses, do not alter the course of a sunburn. Nonsteroidal antiinflammatory drugs, if given at the time of exposure or beforehand, reduce the degree of erythema over the first 24 hours but do not change epidermal damage. Of course, few people lying on the beach anticipate an excessive exposure, so they are unlikely to embark on such preventive measures.

SECTION 14

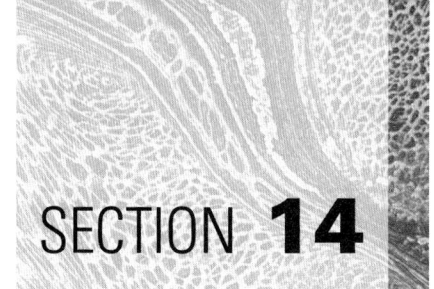

The Nervous System

Alzheimer's Disease

Method of
Monica Peterson Gordon, MD, and
L. Jaime Fitten, MD

Definition and Clinical Presentation

Alzheimer's disease (AD) is a progressive, neurodegenerative disorder characterized by a gradual decline of cognitive processes, such as memory, language, judgment, behavior, and global functioning. According to the *Diagnostic and Statistical Manual of Mental Disorders, Fourth Edition (DSM-IV, 2000)*, dementia of the Alzheimer's type is the development of multiple cognitive deficits manifested by both memory impairment and one or more cognitive disturbances, such as aphasia, apraxia, agnosia, and disturbance in executive functioning. The deficits must cause significant impairment in social or occupational functioning and represent a decline from previous levels of functioning and cannot be due to psychiatric, systemic, substance-induced states, or delirium that cause cognitive impairment or produce the dementia syndrome. Other more detailed, research-oriented criteria also have been developed by the National Institute of Neurological and Communicative Disorders and Stroke and the Alzheimer's Disease and Related Disorders Association (NINCDS-ADRDA, 1984).

Alzheimer's disease has a gradual onset often beginning after age 60 years but most commonly after age 70 years. The rarer familial forms can have an onset as early as the fourth decade of life. Recent studies suggest that an isolated, mild but progressive forgetfulness, in the absence of functional or other cognitive impairment, signals a preclinical stage of the disease in a high percentage of cases and has been referred to as *mild cognitive impairment* of the amnestic type. Typically, AD has a 10- to 12-year progressive course. In its early stage, the disease is characterized by a declarative memory deficit that makes it difficult for patients to learn new information or recall recently experienced events. During this stage, language deficits are not always immediately apparent; however, a degree of word finding difficulty may exist. In addition, minor difficulties with visuospatial and drawing skills may be found. Mild executive dysfunction or subtle personality changes, such as reduction in spontaneity and initiative, may be present. Variations in mood may occur. As the disease progresses, memory deficits become more profound, and most of the patient's capacity for new memory formation is lost. Access to old memories becomes increasingly impaired. Language and other cognitive deficits become more pronounced, with clear evidence of aphasia, apraxia and agnosia. The ability to manipulate concepts is lost, and thought becomes increasingly simple and concrete. During this phase, patients usually begin to exhibit behavioral and psychiatric symptoms, such as agitation, wandering, and irritability. They may experience circadian abnormalities, such as sleep cycle reversal. They may also develop psychotic symptoms such as persecutory delusions, and auditory or visual hallucinations. In the advanced stages, patients have more profound cognitive and memory deficits such that meaningful communication even at its basic level may be difficult. The loss of autonomy and the emergence of difficult to manage behavioral and psychiatric symptoms during this stage frequently lead to institutionalization. Patients invariably need full assistance for their activities of daily living and may be incontinent. Motor disturbances and difficulty walking emerge, and the patient becomes bed or chair bound in the end stages of the illness (Table 1).

Although AD accounts for more than 50% of dementias in the United States and Europe, other dementing conditions must be included in the differential diagnosis. The second and third most commonly occurring dementias are dementia with Lewy bodies and vascular dementia. Dementia with Lewy bodies can be characterized by symptoms of global cognitive impairment, including memory, and earlier neuropsychiatric disturbance than occurs in AD, with the appearance of visual hallucinations and parkinsonism. In vascular dementia, executive dysfunction is more prominent than in AD, and memory difficulties may be minimal early in the course of the illness. In contrast to AD, in which behavioral and psychiatric symptoms appear later in the progression of the illness, in vascular dementia these symptoms may appear earlier in the course. However, more than one etiologic factor may exist in patients with dementia. At autopsy, neuropathologic findings of concomitant AD and cerebrovascular disease have been reported in the brain tissue of 7% to 25% of patients who received a diagnosis of probable AD. Comorbid AD and dementia with Lewy bodies could account for as many as 20% of patients diagnosed with dementia. The frontotemporal group of dementias has a much lower incidence. These dementias occur earlier in life by a decade or two from the typical appearance of AD and often present initially with behavioral disturbances such as disinhibition, inappropriateness, apathy, and executive dysfunction. Other cognitive functions and memory become clearly impaired later in the disease process. Depression may, at times, be accompanied by cognitive impairment, producing a dementia-like clinical impression (Table 2). Elements of a diagnostic evaluation for AD are given in Table 3.

Epidemiology

An estimated eighteen million people worldwide currently suffer from AD. This number is expected to double within the next

TABLE 1 Stages of Alzheimer's Disease

Stage	Mild	Moderate	Severe
Folstein Mini Mental State Examination (MMSE) Score	20–29	10–19	0–9
Symptoms	Memory impairment evident Early language problems (e.g., word-finding difficulty) Decreased insight and scope of judgment Early mood and personality changes Withdrawal from more demanding activities May need assistance with some instrumental ADLs	Unable to learn or recall new information Worsening long-term memory and recall Language, orientation, executive and other cognitive functions impaired Development of behavioral and psychiatric disturbances Sleep disturbance common Requires help with most all instrumental ADLs	Major, broad cognitive deterioration Loss of language; mutism Motor disturbances and unstable gait Dysphagia, frequent weight loss Poor basic ADLs to complete dependence Progresses to bedridden state Institutionalization common

Abbreviation: ADL = activity of daily living.

25 years. The current prevalence of AD in the United States has been estimated between 1.1 and 4.8 million cases. Although symptoms of the disease usually appear after age 60 years, the incidence of AD increases sharply and steadily after age 70 years. It has been estimated that nearly half of all people 85 years and older have some form of dementia. The National Institutes of Health estimates that, if the current trend continues, 8.5 million Americans will have AD by the year 2030.

Research has shown that the major risk factor for AD is age. Other risk factors include genetics (presenilin-1 and presenilin-2, apolipoprotein E4 status, Down syndrome), female gender, lack of education, head trauma, and myocardial infarction. The influences of presenilin on AD are based on the autosomal dominant forms of the disease, which account for 1% to 2% of all cases and result from missense mutations of genes that encode the amyloid precursor protein APP (chromosome 21) or proteolytic enzymes that cleave APP (chromosomes 1 and 14). Such mutations are associated with an increased production of β-amyloid peptide (Aβ) and result in early-onset AD. Apolipoprotein E (ApoE) status has been suggested as a risk factor for typical AD (chromosome 19). ApoE is a protein involved in cholesterol transport and has three alleles: e2, e3, and e4. Homozygous individuals who carry two ApoE e4 alleles have an increased probability of developing AD by age 85 years and do so about 10 years earlier than individuals carrying the other allelic variants. Possible mechanisms are ApoE e4 enhancement of β-amyloid deposition and amyloids reduced clearance from extracellular space.

Pathology

The brains of AD patients are atrophic with ventricular and sulcal enlargement. Histologic specimens are significant for progressive neuronal loss, β-amyloid deposition with formation of senile and neuritic plaques, and intraneuronal neurofibrillary tangles. Early changes are most abundant in the mesial temporal lobe (entorhinal cortex, hippocampus). With disease progression, parietal and frontal association areas become involved. Primary sensorimotor cortex involvement is last. The current prevailing hypothesis of AD pathogenesis contends that the initial pathogenic event is extraneuronal and intraneuronal accumulation of a misfolded protein, amyloid β-peptide, which initiates a pathogenic cascade that results in neurotoxicity, neural dysfunction, and neuronal death and culminates in the clinical syndrome of AD.

Treatment and Management of Cognitive Symptoms

More than 30 years ago, researchers first showed decreased cholinergic markers, such as choline acetyltransferase, in the cortex of AD patients. Others subsequently demonstrated loss of basal forebrain cholinergic neurons innervating neocortex and hippocampus in AD patients. These collective findings were the basis of a cholinergic hypothesis of AD that resulted in efforts to treat AD through a variety of cholinergic interventions. Cholinesterase inhibitor (ChE-I) therapy in use today evolved from those early efforts and received FDA approval based on its good tolerability and modest efficacy. ChE-Is are believed to increase acetylcholine signaling in damaged cortical areas where neurodegeneration has occurred. Three ChE-Is are in use today: donepezil (Aricept), rivastigmine (Exelon), and galantamine (Razadyne). Tacrine (Cognex), the ChE-I first approved in 1993, is rarely used today because of its hepatoxicity. In blinded controlled studies, donepezil treatment resulted in cognitive and global functioning benefits for up to 1 year in patients with mild to moderate AD. Patients treated with rivastigmine for 6 months also showed improvement in cognitive and global functioning. Well-controlled

TABLE 2 Causes of Dementia Syndrome

Causal Condition	Approximate Incidence*
Common	
• Alzheimer's disease	50%–70%
• Dementia with Lewy bodies	15%
• Vascular dementia	10%
• Alzheimer's disease and vascular dementia (mixed dementia)	10%
• Depression	5%–10%
Less Common	
• Toxic-metabolic disorders	<5%
• Parkinson's disease	<5%
• Frontotemporal dementias	<5%
• Infections	<3%
• Space-occupying lesions	<3%
• Other neurodegenerations	<2%
• Immune inflammatory	<1%
• Prion diseases	<1%

*Considerable geographic variation has been reported.

TABLE 3 Elements of a Dementia Evaluation

Historical Information
- Symptoms (onset, duration of cognitive, psychiatric, behavioral, and personality changes).
- Functional status (driving, cooking, finances, social contacts, other basic and instrumental activities of daily living).
- Past history (medical, neurologic, psychiatric, social functioning, family history of major medical and neuropsychiatric disorders).
- Medications.

Mental Status Examination
- Evaluation of behavior at interaction, mood, thought content and process, psychosis, insight, and judgment, as well as cognitive evaluation that includes orientation, attention, memory, language, calculations, visuospatial abilities, executive functions.
- Folstein Mini Mental State Examination and the Clock Drawing Test are useful brief instruments.
- Neuropsychologic testing is occasionally indicated in some cases for diagnostic clarity.

Review of Symptoms
- Falls, constipation, urinary incontinence, sensorial deficits, dentition, pain, sleep difficulties.

Physical and Neurologic Examination
Laboratory evaluation
- Complete blood cell count, standard chemistry panel, vitamin B_{12}, folate, thyroid-stimulating hormone, neurosyphilis treponemal screen (e.g., *Treponema pallidum* hemagglutination assay), urinalysis.
- Additional tests may be indicated under specific circumstances.

Neuroimaging
- Magnetic resonance imaging frequently used for exclusion of other conditions and for diagnostic clarity
- Positron emission tomography may be indicated when frontotemporal dementia is in the differential diagnosis.

---

trials of galantamine in AD have shown comparable cognitive gains for patients treated for 5 to 6 months. More recent work has indicated that ChE-Is appear to reduce the rate of cognitive decline for periods of 6 months to 1 year or possibly longer, rather than producing a significant cognitive improvement after the start of therapy. All three agents have comparable efficacy, although their side-effect profiles and dosing schedules vary (Table 4).

Donepezil (Aricept) has an elimination half-life of about 70 hours, needing only once-daily dosing. A starting dose of 5 mg/day is given orally for 4 to 6 weeks. The dose is then increased to a maximum of 10 mg/day as tolerated. Donepezil is taken with or without food but preferably in the morning because vivid dreams may disturb sleep in some patients. Rivastigmine (Exelon) is given twice daily because of its shorter elimination half-life. Dosing starts at 1.5 mg twice daily and is titrated upward slowly, every 2 weeks, to a maximum of 6 to 12 mg/day. If rivastigmine is taken with food and titration occurs in 1.5-mg twice daily increments over 4-week intervals, cholinergic side effects are reduced. Dose reduction is suggested in patients with renal or hepatic impairment. Galantamine (Razadyne) also requires twice-daily dosing. Starting dose is 4 mg twice daily. After 4 weeks, the dose is slowly augmented over several weeks to a maximum of 12 mg twice daily if tolerated. Dose reduction is advised in patients with moderate renal or hepatic impairment. The total dose should not exceed 16 mg/day. Galantamine is contraindicated in patients with severe hepatic or renal impairment.

The side effects of all ChE-Is are similar. However, some agents may be better tolerated than others. The most common side effects are nausea, vomiting, diarrhea, anorexia, weight loss, vivid dreams,

TABLE 4 Pharmacologic Treatment of Cognitive Impairment

Medication	Disease Stage	Recommended Dose	Half-Life	Main Side Effects	Hepatic Cytochrome P-450 Metabolism
Donepezil (Aricept)	Mild to moderate	Start 5 mg qd for 4–6 wk then increase to 10 mg as tolerated	70 hr	Nausea, diarrhea, insomnia, hypertension/hypotension, bradycardia, urinary obstruction	Partial inhibition by ketoconazole, quinidine Induction by carbamazepine
Galantamine (Razadyne, previously Reminyl)	Mild to moderate	Start 4 mg bid for 4 wk and taper slowly to a maximum of 12 mg bid	7 hr	Nausea, vomiting, diarrhea, bradycardia, syncope Contraindicated in severe hepatic or renal disease	Partial inhibition by ketoconazole, paroxetine Clearance reduced by fluoxetine, quinidine, amitriptyline
Rivastigmine (Exelon)	Mild to moderate	Start 1.5 mg bid and increase slowly every 2 wk to a final dose of 6–12 mg/day	1.5 hr	Dizziness, vomiting, headache, diarrhea, anorexia, abdominal pain; titrate slowly with hepatic or renal disease	Not affected by a wide variety of commonly used medications
Memantine (Namenda)	Moderate to severe	Start 5 mg qd and after 1 wk can be increased in 5-mg increments to a maximum of 20 mg daily	60–80 hr	Hypertension, constipation, dizziness, hallucinations, headache, Stevens-Johnson syndrome	Predominantly renal metabolism and clearance

insomnia, and muscle cramps. Donepezil appears to have a lesser frequency of gastrointestinal side effects than do galantamine or rivastigmine. In all three agents, these side effects tend to be dose related and transient. The vagotonic effects of ChE-I therapy can cause bradycardia. Therefore, patients with a history of sick sinus syndrome, supraventricular tachycardia, congestive heart failure, and acute coronary artery disease should be monitored. The patient's ability to tolerate side effects is a major factor affecting medication adherence. However, an optimal ChE-I medication trial should consist of at least 3 to 4 months of treatment at the maximally tolerated dose prior to discontinuation of therapy for inadequate response, because that period of time is needed to establish that the patient has continued to deteriorate at the expected nontreated rate. If the patient does not respond to one ChE-I, another can be tried.

In 2003, memantine (Namenda), a noncholinergic-related N-methyl-D-aspartate (NMDA) receptor antagonist, was approved by the FDA for treatment of moderate to severe AD based on the results of two controlled studies involving more than 600 moderately to severely demented AD patients. The first 28-week study involved memantine alone versus placebo. Results demonstrated that memantine treatment was of moderate benefit to patients in terms of both cognitive and functional measures. For 12 weeks, cognition remained stable in the memantine group then declined afterward; however, significantly less impairment was noted at endpoint in the memantine group than in the placebo group. The second study evaluated memantine in AD patients already receiving donepezil. The patients treated with donepezil plus memantine showed a modest but better therapeutic effect in cognition sustained from baseline than did the donepezil with placebo group. Treatment of mildly demented AD patients with memantine has produced less robust results, and memantine is not currently FDA approved for this use (see Table 4).

Memantine should be started at 5 mg once daily for 1 week. It can be increased in 5-mg increments per week to a maximum dose of 20 mg/day. It is then best given 10 mg twice daily. Memantine is generally well tolerated and can be taken with or without food. Because of its partial renal clearance, dosage reduction is recommended for patients with significant renal insufficiency. Potential side effects include headache, agitation, confusion, constipation, dizziness, hallucinations, and insomnia. Memantine can be used as monotherapy in patients with moderate to severe AD who do not respond to or tolerate ChE-Is. A decreased rate of cognitive decline for a period of time, as with ChE-Is, appears to be the main therapeutic effect. Best use of memantine may be in combination with a ChE-I, as benefits of the combination appear to be superior to that of either drug used alone.

Treatment of Behavioral and Psychiatric Symptoms

Patients with AD frequently develop behavioral and psychiatric symptoms in addition to cognitive impairments. These symptoms become more prominent as the disease progresses and often lead to institutionalization. When dementia is well established, patients commonly develop some form of agitation (excessive purposeless activity), either motoric or verbal, during the day or evening hours. They may become intermittently irritable and aggressive with family members. Nearly half will develop psychosis, either as hallucinations (auditory or visual) or simple delusions of infidelity or persecution, such as believing someone is stealing from them. They may manifest apathy (loss of motivation) and disordered mood with symptoms of depression, anxiety, and irritability. Optimal management is both nonpharmacologic and pharmacologic.

NONPHARMACOLOGIC MANAGEMENT

Often patients are confused and agitated as a consequence of temporal-spatial disorientation and need to be reassured and redirected with regularity. Environmental cues, such as the posted date and visible familiar objects and pictures of loved ones, may help.

Agitated and/or aggressive behavior may be exacerbated by environmental triggers, such as insufficient (e.g., poor daytime lighting) or excessive (too much activity) sensorial stimulation. These elements can and should be adjusted. It is important to educate the patient, family, and staff (if the patient is institutionalized) regarding target behavioral symptoms and the environmental and behavioral techniques useful in their management. Implementation of a management plan can then proceed with better consistency and effectiveness wherever the patient resides. Managing AD patients is a large burden for caregivers. According to studies, caregivers have a 52% prevalence of psychiatric symptoms compared with 15% to 20% in the general population. As part of an overall management plan, caregivers will need support through reassurance, education, and referral to important community resources, such as the Alzheimer Association, caregiver support groups, day care centers, and social or legal services.

PHARMACOLOGIC TREATMENT

Pharmacologic management of behavioral and mood symptoms depends on accurate analysis of problem moods and behaviors and should be individualized. Broadly speaking, depression and anxiety are managed with newer antidepressants (selective serotonin reuptake inhibitors [SSRIs], mirtazapine [Remeron], trazodone [Desyrel]). Dementia-related psychotic symptoms and aggression are treated with atypical antipsychotics. Pure agitation without aggression can be treated with trazodone,[1] buspirone[1] (BuSpar), SSRIs,[1] or anticonvulsants.[1] Newer studies also suggest that cholinesterase inhibitors and memantine (Namenda) may be helpful in the management of this condition. Certain benzodiazepines are occasionally a useful adjunct for short-term treatment of anxiety-driven agitation or anxiety with depression (Table 5).

Depressive symptoms requiring treatment (e.g., withdrawal, appetite loss, worsening sleep, negativism, irritability, somatization) are more common than the classic major depressive syndrome in demented AD patients. Because of their safety profile, tolerability, and efficacy, newer antidepressants, such as the SSRIs or venlafaxine (Effexor; 50–300 mg/day) and mirtazapine (15–45 mg/day), are the mainstay of treatment. The SSRIs have comparable efficacy, but agents with low drug–drug interactions and low side-effect profiles, such as citalopram (Celexa; 10–60 mg/day) and sertraline (Zoloft; 50–200 mg/day), are preferred. Onset of action of the antidepressants may require 1 to several weeks. Patience and dose adjustments are needed. Treatment of the first episode of depression should last 1 year at the therapeutic dose before the antidepressant is tapered off. In a patient with a history of episodes of depression, therapy should be maintained indefinitely. It is useful to match the side-effect profile of the antidepressant with the patient's main symptoms. For example, for an inactive, withdrawn patient, an activating antidepressant such as venlafaxine or sertraline may be useful. On the other hand, for an anxious patient who is not sleeping or eating well, a calming agent that enhances appetite and can increase evening sedation, such as mirtazapine, may be a preferable initial choice.

The newer antidepressants are also effective in treating anxiety and irritability, both of which commonly occur in AD, although the onset of action of these agents may not be immediate. When relief of anxiety is needed more quickly, a benzodiazepine of moderately short duration of action, such as oxazepam (Serax; 15 mg/day) or lorazepam (Ativan; 1–2 mg/day), can be initiated at the same time an antidepressant at low dose is started. Over a period of 2 to 3 weeks, as the antidepressant dose is titrated upward, the benzodiazepine is tapered off to reduce exposure to possible benzodiazepine side effects, such as memory loss, falls, confusion, and behavioral disinhibition. The antidepressant should now exert a greater anxiolytic effect. For patients with mild anxiety, trazodone[1] (25–200 mg/day) or buspirone (BuSpar) can be tried.

The newer, atypical antipsychotics are helpful in treating psychosis alone and psychosis associated with aggression/agitation. These medications have demonstrated some utility in treating irritability and

---

[1]Not FDA approved for this indication.

TABLE 5 Pharmacologic Treatment of Behavioral and Mood Symptoms

Medication	Indication	Recommended Dose	Main Side Effects	Caution
Antidepressants				
Citalopram (Celexa)	Depression, agitation,[1] irritability,[1] anxiety[1]	10–60 mg/day	Headache, nausea, hyponatremia, insomnia, diarrhea, somnolence	
Sertraline (Zoloft)	Depression, agitation,[1] irritability,[1] anxiety[1]	50–200[3] mg/day	Headache, nausea, hyponatremia, insomnia, diarrhea, somnolence	Adjust dose in hepatic impairment
Mirtazapine (Remeron)	Depression, agitation,[1] irritability,[1] anxiety[1]	15–45[3] mg/day	Somnolence, increased appetite, arrhythmia, hypercholesterolemia agranulocytosis	
Venlafaxine (Effexor)	Depression, agitation,[1] irritability,[1] anxiety[1]	50–300 mg/day	Hypertension, hyponatremia, nausea, headache, nervousness, dizziness	
Trazodone (Desyrel)	Agitation alone,[1] mild anxiety,[1] insomnia[1]	25–200 mg/day	Somnolence, dizziness, headache, nausea, priapism, orthostasis	
Antipsychotics				
Haloperidol (Haldol)	Acute psychosis with agitation or aggression[1]	0.25–3 mg/day, IM, if oral dosing not possible	Hypertension, hypotension, tachycardia, movement disorders	Parkinsonism, tardive dyskinesia, neuroleptic malignant syndrome
Quetiapine (Seroquel)	Subacute or chronic psychosis without or with agitation or aggression[1]	25–200 mg/day PO	Weight gain, dizziness, headache, agitation, sedation	QT_c prolongation possible, glucose intolerance, increased stroke risk? Monitor
Risperidone (Risperdal)	Subacute or chronic psychosis without or with agitation or aggression[1]	0.25–2 mg/day PO	Hypotension, hyperglycemia, insomnia, agitation, headache, weight gain, extrapyramidal symptoms	QT_c prolongation possible, glucose intolerance, increased stroke risk? Monitor
Olanzapine (Zyprexa)	Subacute chronic psychosis without or with agitation or aggression[1]	Start 2.5–5 mg/day PO, increase by 2.5 mg/wk to a maximum of 10–15 mg/day	Hyperglycemia, headache, agitation, dizziness, dyspepsia, hypotension, weight gain, somnolence	QT_c prolongation possible, glucose intolerance, type 2 diabetes mellitus?, increased stroke risk? Monitor
Anticonvulsants				
Divalproex (Depakote)	Aggression with or without agitation or irritability[1]	Start 125 mg/day and may increase slowly to a maximum of 1500 mg/day	Liver toxicity, pancreatitis, thrombocytopenia, somnolence, dizziness, diarrhea, tremors, nausea, vomiting	Adjust dose for hepatic and renal impairment
Benzodiazepines and Other Anxiolytics				
Lorazepam (Ativan)	Anxiety	1–2 mg/day	Memory impairment, sedation, dizziness, falls	For short-term use only while concomitant antidepressants are titrated to effectiveness
Oxazepam (Serax)	Anxiety	15 mg/day	Hepatic dysfunction, leukopenia, dizziness	For short-term use only while concomitant antidepressants are titrated to effectiveness
Buspirone (BuSpar)	Anxiety, agitation only[1]	30–60 mg/day	Dizziness, sedation	

[1]Not FDA approved for this indication.
[3]Exceeds dosage recommended by the manufacturer.

CURRENT DIAGNOSIS

Criteria	Description
Intellectual functioning	Development of multiple cognitive deficits, including memory impairment plus one or more of the following attributes: ■ Aphasia (language disturbance) ■ Agnosia (impaired recognition) ■ Apraxia (impaired motor activity) ■ Executive dysfunction (difficulties in planning and organization)
Functional capacity	Cognitive deficits cause significant impairment in social, occupational, or usual activities of daily living and represent a significant decline from a previous level of functioning.
Course of symptoms	Symptoms have a gradual or insidious onset, and patient experiences a continuous cognitive decline.
Absence of delirium	Cognitive deficits do not occur solely during the course of delirium.
Other neurologic and medical conditions excluded	Cognitive defects described are not caused by other central nervous system disorders that cause progressive deficits in memory and cognition (e.g., cerebrovascular disease, Huntington's or Parkinson's disease, subdural hematoma, normal-pressure hydrocephalus, brain tumor) or by systemic conditions known to cause the dementia syndrome (e.g., hypothyroidism, vitamin B_{12} or folic acid deficiency, hypercalcemia, neurosyphilis, HIV infection)
Psychiatric conditions excluded	Disturbance is not caused by another major psychiatric disorder (e.g., schizophrenia, major depression, substance abuse)

CURRENT THERAPY

- If delirium, acute psychosis, depression, or major aggression/agitation is present initially, treat this condition first and then re-evaluate.
- If no acute psychosis, depression, or major behavioral perturbation is evident, treat cognitive symptoms with a memory enhancer such as a ChE-I or memantine (Namenda; an N-methyl-D-aspartate receptor antagonist) as appropriate for disease stage.
- Mild Alzheimer's disease: ChE-I—donepezil (Aricept), galantamine (Razadyne), or rivastigmine (Exelon).
- Moderate Alzheimer's disease: ChE-I and/or memantine (Namenda).
- Severe Alzheimer's disease: ChE-I and/or memantine.
- Consider nonpharmacologic interventions for behavioral and mood problems.
- Treat persistent psychiatric and behavioral symptoms as follows:
  - Acute psychosis with agitation/aggression: Haloperidol[1] (Haldol)
  - Subacute, chronic psychosis with or without aggression/agitation: Atypical antipsychotic
  - Depression, irritability: Second generation non-TCA antidepressant
  - Agitation alone: Trazodone[1] (Desyrel), second generation non-TCA antidepressant, nonpharmacologic intervention
  - Anxiety: Atypical antidepressant with or without short-term benzodiazepine, trazodone,[1] or buspirone[1] (BuSpar)
  - Insomnia: Trazodone,[1] short-term only benzodiazepine, or similar hypnotic

---
[1]Not FDA approved for this indication.
Abbreviation: ChE-I = cholinesterase inhibitor.

aggression but not agitation alone. Patients with acute psychosis who are unable to take oral medication may respond to haloperidol (Haldol) intramuscularly 0.25 to 3 mg/day, although side effects are more prominent with this conventional antipsychotic. Patients with subacute and chronic psychotic symptoms can be treated with oral risperidone[1] (Risperdal; 0.25–2 mg/day), quetiapine[1] (Seroquel; 25–200 mg/day), or olanzapine[1] (Zyprexa; 2.5–15 mg/day). Movement disorders, such as parkinsonism and tardive dyskinesia, are less frequent with atypical antipsychotics than with conventional ones. In addition to the use of atypical antipsychotics for aggression with psychosis, aggression alone or with irritability can be treated with SSRIs having low drug–drug interactions, such as citalopram[1] (Celexa; 10–60 mg/day) or sertraline[1] (Zoloft; 50–200 mg/day), with mirtazapine[1] (Remeron; 7.5–45 mg/day), or with anticonvulsants, such as divalproex[1] (Depakote; 125–1500 mg/day). Persistent male sexual aggression may benefit from treatment with medroxyprogesterone[1] (Depo-Provera) intramuscularly 150 mg biweekly or monthly. Agitation alone without psychosis or aggression may respond to environmental adjustments in combination with trazodone[1] (25–200 mg/day), buspirone[1] (30–60 mg/day), or a ChE-I. Apathy may improve in some patients with standard doses of ChE-Is.

Caution is necessary when prescribing most medications to the elderly because of their sensitivity to adverse reactions. Specifically, newer antipsychotic medications can cause QT_c prolongation, weight gain, hyperlipidemia, increased glucose resistance, and type 2 diabetes mellitus. They have even been associated with a possible small increase in stroke or death risk in exposed demented populations, although additional prospective studies are needed to reach more definitive conclusions. When prescribing atypical antipsychotics to patients with a vulnerable cardiac or metabolic status, a baseline and treatment electrocardiogram, lipid panel, chemistry panel, and weight measurement should be performed, with subsequent monitoring as indicated.

In refractory patients, combination therapies may be necessary, and in such cases pharmacologic agents belonging to different classes should be combined. However, certain cautions should be observed. Only one change should be introduced at a time, and lower initial doses should be used. Avoid olanzapine (Zyprexa) and clozapine

---
[1]Not FDA approved for this indication.

(Clozaril) in patients with diabetes. The following combinations are best avoided: clozapine (Clozaril) and carbamazepine (Tegretol); ziprasidone (Geodon) and tricyclic antidepressants; conventional antipsychotics and fluoxetine (Prozac); and conventional antipsychotics and lithium, divalproex (Depakote), or lamotrigine (Lamictal). However, divalproex and risperidone (or haloperidol) is an acceptable combination. Key therapeutic points are summarized in Current Therapy.

Sleep Disorders

Method of
David N. Neubauer, MD

In recent years there has been increasing recognition of the high prevalence and significant consequences of sleep disorders and the effects of insufficient sleep. The National Sleep Foundation estimates that about 70 million Americans have problems with their sleep. Research has documented various medical and psychiatric comorbidities with sleep disorders and how sleep disturbances can increase the risk of other disorders. While the number of sleep specialists and sleep disorder centers continue to grow, primary care medicine remains the frontline in the clinical evaluation and treatment of sleep disorders. This chapter provides a broad overview of the common sleep disorders encountered in clinical practice. Sleep-disordered breathing is covered in greater detail in the article on Sleep Apnea.

The foundation of understanding sleep disorders is an appreciation of the two primary processes normally regulating the sleep-wake cycle. A *homeostatic* sleep drive determines the amount of sleep we need for alertness and vigilance during our waking hours. For most individuals, a daily sleep total of approximately 8 hours is ideal. Insufficient sleep, whether acute or chronic, leads to increased sleepiness. The ability to achieve sufficient sleep at night and subsequent wakefulness throughout the daytime and evening is optimized by the *circadian* process, which is coordinated through the suprachiasmatic nucleus in the anterior hypothalamus with input from the photoperiod. The circadian process generates maximum arousal in the evening to offset the homeostatic sleepiness that evolves throughout the day. These two processes together promote sustained wakefulness for about 16 hours and sleep for about 8 hours in synchrony with the day-night cycle.

The homeostatic and circadian processes describe the normal pattern of alertness and sleepiness, but they also may help explain clinical problems associated with insufficient sleepiness (insomnia) and excessive sleepiness. Daytime or evening napping reduces the homeostatic sleep drive available to promote sleep onset and maintenance during a desired nighttime sleep period. This may lead a patient to complain of insomnia. Difficulty falling asleep and remaining asleep also may result from attempts to sleep outside the normal photoperiod-reinforced circadian zone of increased sleep propensity. Sleep difficulty associated with shift work is a typical example.

Symptoms of Sleep Disorders

The evaluation of patients with sleep difficulties should begin with a thorough history of their sleep-related symptoms. How long has it been a problem? Is it intermittent, or a daily or nightly problem? What time of the day or night do the symptoms occur? Are there obvious precipitants or consequences? Is there impairment in normal functioning? What have been the typical sleep-wake hours for the individual, and what is the current pattern? Are there medical or psychiatric disorders or medications that might be influencing the sleep-related symptoms? Input from a bed partner or other informant can be invaluable. Having patients maintain sleep logs can offer a concise view of the patterns of their sleep disturbances and help demonstrate the effects of treatment strategies. Questionnaires and scales (e.g., Epworth Sleepiness Scale, Pittsburgh Sleep Quality Index) can be useful for screening patients for possible sleep disturbances.

Symptoms of sleep disorders may include an inability to sleep at desired times (insomnia), an inability to remain fully awake and attentive at desired times (excessive sleepiness), snoring and fluctuations in breathing patterns during sleep, uncomfortable sensations prior to sleep onset, abnormal movements before and during sleep, and abnormal behaviors emanating from sleep (parasomnias). Although insomnia, excessive daytime sleepiness, and parasomnias are the primary symptom clusters, individual patients may experience overlapping symptoms. For instance, sleep-disordered breathing can be associated with disrupted nighttime sleep and excessive daytime sleepiness.

Insomnia

Insomnia is difficulty falling asleep or remaining asleep when people expect to be able to sleep and when there is an opportunity for them to be in bed sleeping. An insomnia disorder persists for at least 1 month and is associated with daytime impairment. Insomnia affects about 30% of the general adult population intermittently and about 10% on a chronic basis. Insomnia is a problem for more than half of patients with chronic medical conditions. Insomnia may occur idiopathically or may result from distressing circumstances; psychological conditioning; environmental factors; jet lag and shift work schedules; medication effects; and medical, psychiatric, and sleep disorders.

Treatment of insomnia may require multiple strategies that involve correction of sleep hygiene problems, bedtime routine and schedule modifications, cognitive and other psychotherapeutic techniques, strategically timed exposure to bright light, and use of medications. Additionally, optimizing the management of comorbid conditions (e.g., major depression, chronic pain, sleep-disordered breathing, and congestive heart failure) may be necessary for sleep quality improvements. General sleep hygiene recommendations are listed in Table 1. Delaying bedtime may help patients spending excessive frustrating wakeful time in bed. Cognitive therapy techniques may be especially helpful for the patients who catastrophize about their sleep problems.

Significant advances in the pharmacologic treatment of insomnia have been made in recent years. Patients may experience improved sleep with sedating medications prescribed for comorbid conditions (e.g., antidepressants). The medications indicated for treatment of

TABLE 1 Sleep Hygiene Recommendations

- Try to maintain a regular sleep-wake schedule.
- Avoid afternoon or evening napping.
- Allow yourself enough time in bed for adequate sleep duration (e.g., 11 PM to 7 AM).
- Develop a relaxing evening routine for the hours approaching bedtime.
- Spend some idle time reflecting on the day's events before going to bed. Make a list of concerns and how some might be resolved.
- Reserve the bed for sleep and sex. Do not do homework, pay bills, or engage in serious domestic discussions in bed.
- Avoid evening alcohol.
- Avoid caffeine in the afternoon and evening.
- Minimize annoying noise, light, or temperature extremes.
- Consider a light snack before bedtime.
- Exercise regularly, but not late in the evening.
- Do not try harder and harder to fall asleep. If you are unable to sleep, do something else out of bed and in another room, if possible.
- Avoid smoking.

TABLE 2 Medications Indicated for Treatment of Insomnia

Medication	Available Doses (mg)	Duration of Action
Hypnotic		
Benzodiazepines:		
Estazolam (ProSom)	1, 2	Intermediate-long
Flurazepam (Dalmane)	15, 30	Long
Quazepam (Doral)	7.5, 15	Long
Temazepam (Restoril)	7.5, 15, 22.5, 30	Intermediate
Triazolam (Halcion)	0.125, 0.25	Short-intermediate
Nonbenzodiazepines:		
Eszopiclone (Lunesta)	1, 2, 3	Intermediate
Zaleplon (Sonata)	5, 10	Very short
Zolpidem (Ambien)	5, 10	Short
Zolpidem (Ambien CR) extended-release	6.25, 12.5	Short-intermediate
Melatonin Receptor Agonist		
Ramelteon (Rozerem)	8	Short

insomnia (Table 2) include both traditional benzodiazepines and newer nonbenzodiazepine hypnotics. All of these hypnotics function through enhancing the inhibitory responses of γ-aminobutyric acid (GABA)-A receptors. The newer medications have pharmacokinetic and pharmacodynamic characteristics that improve their safety profile. Ramelteon (Rozerem), a nonsedating, selective melatonin receptor agonist that targets activity of the circadian system, also is approved for treatment of insomnia.

The duration of action of the newer generation hypnotics ranges from the very short-acting zaleplon (Sonata) to the progressively longer-acting zolpidem (Ambien), extended-release zolpidem (Ambien CR), and eszopiclone (Lunesta). The pattern of patients' sleep disturbances influences the selection of hypnotics. Exclusive sleep-onset difficulty may be treated adequately with a very short-acting medication; however, most insomnia patients have combined difficulty falling asleep and maintaining sleep. Accordingly, moderately short-acting medications that do not cause residual morning sedation generally are optimal.

Until recently, all prescription sleep-promoting medications were approved for short-term treatment of insomnia; however, beginning in 2005 the FDA began approving sleep-promoting agents simply for treatment of insomnia without the implied short-term restriction. Whereas the majority of patients taking hypnotic medications require help with their sleep only for limited periods of time, others with chronic insomnia have experienced continued improvement in nighttime sleep and daytime functioning with longer-term nightly or intermittent hypnotic use. All of the currently approved benzodiazepine receptor agonist hypnotics remain Schedule IV controlled substances. In contrast, ramelteon (Rozerem) is not classified as a controlled substance.

Circadian Rhythm Disorders

Although the circadian system typically promotes nighttime sleep from approximately 10 to 11 PM until about 6 to 7 AM, many individuals have long-standing tendencies to experience either earlier or later sleep propensity zones. An individual's circadian phase can contribute to complaints of insomnia or excessive sleepiness, although this influence often is not recognized. Adolescents and young adults are more likely to have later sleep propensities, whereas elderly individuals tend to have an earlier onset and offset of sleepiness. People with an *advanced sleep phase* are early birds; they become sleepy earlier in the evening and then are unable to sleep later in the morning. They may complain of persistent early morning awakening as well as daytime fatigue and sleepiness. Night owls with a *delayed circadian phase* have difficulty falling asleep early and tend to sleep later in the morning. This can represent a significant clinical problem. Patients may report sleep-onset insomnia or excessive daytime sleepiness, particularly during the morning hours. Melatonin receptor agonists given prior to bedtime also may help advance and stabilize the sleep onset and morning awakening times for delayed sleep phase patients. Evening bright light exposure may help patients with a long-term predisposition for early evening sleepiness and bothersome early morning awakening. Conversely, bright light exposure upon awakening may help those with a night-owl pattern.

Excessive Daytime Sleepiness

Excessive sleepiness during waking hours is a major public health problem most evident in associated workplace and vehicular accidents, injuries, and fatalities. Excessively sleepy patients typically complain of sleepiness for major portions of the day and report a high propensity for falling asleep during sedentary activities. In severe cases, patients may fall asleep while driving, conversing, or attending important meetings. Chronic sleepiness may lead to educational, occupational, and social difficulties. The most common cause of excessive sleepiness is insufficient sleep, whether due to work schedules or lifestyle choices. Sedating medications and other substances can lead to excessive sleepiness. Emerging evidence suggests that sleep deprivation may contribute to metabolic and immune impairment, even in healthy young individuals.

Patients complaining of difficulty remaining awake during the daytime should be evaluated at a sleep center unless there is an obvious and reversible cause. Sleep laboratory testing includes the standard nighttime polysomnography and possibly a series of daytime nap opportunities that objectively assess sleep onset latency and sleep stages. The key sleep disorders associated with excessive daytime sleepiness are narcolepsy, hypersomnolence disorders, and sleep-disordered breathing. To a limited extent, insomnia and other disorders causing frequent arousals and awakenings, or awakenings with difficulty returning to sleep, may contribute to daytime sleepiness. The latter might include restless legs syndrome, periodic limb movement disorder, and parasomnias.

Narcolepsy

Although *narcolepsy* is the classic disorder of excessive sleepiness, it affects only about 0.05% of the population. It is characterized by persistent sleepiness and difficulty maintaining attention. Symptoms typically begin to evolve by the late teens and continue through life. In addition to disturbed daytime wakefulness and nighttime sleep, narcolepsy patients have symptoms reflecting dysregulation of the characteristics of rapid eye movement (REM) sleep. *Cataplexy* is the loss of postural muscle tone that occurs during waking and is precipitated by heightened emotion, such as anxiety or laughter. The effects may range from a barely noticeable jaw drop to the patient lying on the ground awake but unable to move for up to several minutes. *Sleep paralysis* occurs at the transition to sleep when a person becomes aware of a complete inability to move any muscles voluntarily. It resolves spontaneously within minutes. Cataplexy and sleep paralysis both involve the intrusion of the normal paralysis that accompanies REM sleep; however, it occurs at an abnormal time. Narcolepsy patients also are more likely to experience *hypnagogic hallucinations*, which are dreamlike experiences occurring at sleep onset. Sleep laboratory testing confirms the diagnosis.

Treatment of narcolepsy begins with the establishment of therapeutic goals, typically including maximizing attention and alertness during certain hours of the day, along with the elimination of cataplexy. Narcolepsy patients should be careful to allow sufficient hours for nighttime sleep, as sleep deprivation will exacerbate their symptoms. Scheduled brief naps and periods of increased physical activity during the daytime may be very helpful. Most narcolepsy patients will require pharmacotherapy to enhance daytime alertness.

Modafinil (Provigil) may be adequate for some patients; however, many will respond best to amphetamine medications. Antidepressants (e.g., venlafaxine[1] [Effexor]) may reduce cataplexy. Sodium oxybate (Xyrem), which is taken in two nighttime doses, has been shown to improve nighttime sleep, reduce cataplexy, and increase daytime alertness in narcolepsy patients.

Hypersomnolence Disorders

In addition to narcolepsy, various central nervous system processes can cause persistent sleepiness that interferes with daytime functioning. Patients with hypersomnolence may sleep for extended periods and nap during the day, but they still never feel fully alert and refreshed. This condition may be idiopathic, or it may be related to head trauma, viral infections, encephalitis, tumors, and neurodegenerative disorders. As with narcolepsy, stimulants represent the primary treatment approach but often are less reliable in providing significant benefit for these patients.

Sleep-Disordered Breathing

This topic is covered in greater detail in the article on Sleep Apnea. *Sleep-disordered breathing* involves fluctuations in airflow during sleep. Most commonly it is due to an obstructive process involving an abnormal collapsibility of the upper airway, which may result in recurrent episodes of hypopneas and apneas. Alternately, it may involve a decreased respiratory drive associated with central mechanisms, as can occur with congestive heart failure with a prolonged circulation time. Sleep apnea can cause frequent arousals that undermine sleep quality and lead to excessive sleepiness during the daytime.

Restless Legs Syndrome and Periodic Limb Movements

Although the primary discomfort of restless legs syndrome (RLS) occurs prior to sleep, it is considered a sleep disorder because it is associated with delayed and disrupted sleep and because the irresistible urge to move the legs follows a circadian pattern with increasing symptoms as bedtime approaches. As the condition worsens over time, the sense of restlessness may begin earlier in the afternoon or morning. The discomfort is most bothersome when patients are at rest. Moving the legs offers only very brief relief. In severe cases, patients often experience such intense restlessness that they are unable to sleep for long periods and often will pace until exhaustion finally allows sleep. During sleep, about 80% of RLS patients exhibit periodic limb movements. In some patients, these involuntary jerking movements occur frequently and cause arousals that further undermine sleep quality. Occasionally patients have periodic limb movements during sleep without the pre-sleep restlessness.

Although RLS often occurs idiopathically, there also is a significant familial component. Other risk factors are iron deficiency, peripheral neuropathies, renal failure, and use of certain medications, including most antidepressants, sedating antihistamines, and centrally acting dopamine antagonists. Pregnancy may be associated with a temporary worsening of symptoms.

Iron supplementation may be beneficial for RLS patients with low ferritin levels (<50 ng/mL). Otherwise, the first-line approach consists of dopamine agonists, such as ropinirole (Requip) and pramipexole (Mirapex). Selected patients may benefit from opiates (e.g., propoxyphene[1] [Darvon] and methadone[1] [Dolophine]), benzodiazepines (e.g., clonazepam[1] [Klonopin]), or gabapentin[1] (Neurontin).

---

[1]Not FDA approved for this indication.

CURRENT DIAGNOSIS

- Patient should be screened routinely for problems associated with sleep and wakefulness.
- Ask patients and bed partners about difficulty falling and staying asleep, movements and behaviors during sleep, and snoring and breathing irregularities during sleep.
- The most common sleep disorders encountered in primary care settings are insomnia, sleep-disordered breathing, and restless legs syndrome. Parasomnia, narcolepsy, and other hypersomnolence disorders are relatively uncommon.
- Excessive sleepiness is a potentially dangerous condition that should be evaluated aggressively. Sleep laboratory testing is appropriate for cases not easily explained by sleep deprivation.

Parasomnias

Behaviors and other symptoms emanating from sleep are considered *parasomnias*. Although most parasomnias are relatively benign, occasionally injuries to patients or bed partners result from these behaviors. Evaluation of patients with parasomnias should include a consideration of sleep-disordered breathing as a possible precipitant to the abnormal behaviors. Most parasomnias can be categorized according to their association with non-REM or REM sleep.

Slow-wave sleep, classified as non-REM stages 3 and 4, generally occurs during the first few hours of sleep. Children have the most slow-wave sleep, and the amount declines with age. Compared with other sleep stages, it is most difficult to awaken from these stages. *Sleep terrors*, *sleepwalking*, *sleep-related eating disorder*, and *confusional arousals* all represent incomplete awakenings. Often people experiencing these parasomnias have no recollection of them the following morning. These parasomnias may be exacerbated by sleep insufficiency when there is an increase in slow-wave sleep intensity during recovery sleep. Sleep terrors may be especially dramatic. When they are frequent or involve dangerous behaviors, then treatment with a benzodiazepine receptor agonist may be appropriate.

REM sleep is associated with the most intense dreaming experiences and markedly decreased skeletal muscle tone. It occurs intermittently throughout the night but for the longest periods during the last few hours of the night. *Nightmares* are distressing awakenings

CURRENT THERAPY

- Patients with persistent insomnia may benefit from improved sleep hygiene measures, cognitive-behavioral therapy, and pharmacologic agents.
- Sleep-promoting medications approved by the Food and Drug Administration include benzodiazepine and nonbenzodiazepine hypnotics, and a selective melatonin receptor agonist.
- Iron supplementation may benefit patients with restless legs syndrome and low ferritin levels. Otherwise, dopamine agonists are the first-line treatment.
- Narcolepsy can be treated with central nervous system stimulants, rapid eye movement suppressants, and sodium oxybate (Xyrem).
- Parasomnia behaviors should be treated when they frequently disrupt sleep or represent a danger to the patient or bed partners.

from REM sleep with the awareness of frightening dream content. *REM sleep behavior disorder*, which is more common among elderly individuals, involves an incomplete muscle paralysis during REM sleep leading patients to move during REM sleep. Patients seem to be acting out intense dream experiences. The results can be dangerous because patients may thrash about in bed, fall out of bed, or even attack bed partners before awakening. Bedtime clonazepam[1] (Klonopin) has been the standard treatment; however, recent studies suggest melatonin[1] also may be beneficial.

Summary

Sleep disorders can have a significant impact on a patient's quality of life and on comorbid conditions. Initial screening for sleep-wake cycle disturbances is as simple as asking patients how they are sleeping and whether they feel awake and alert throughout the daytime. Most sleep disorders can be identified with a thorough history in a primary care setting; however, consultation with a sleep specialist and sleep laboratory testing may be helpful in the evaluation and management of complex insomnia, hypersomnia, and parasomnia patients.

---

[1]Not FDA approved for this indication.

REFERENCES

The International Classification of Sleep Disorders: Diagnostic & Coding Manual, ICSD-2, 2nd ed. Westchester, IL: American Academy of Sleep Medicine, 2005.
Chokroverty S: Sleep Disorders Medicine: Basic Science, Technical Considerations, and Clinical Aspects. Boston: Butterworth-Heinemann, 1994.
Earley CJ: Clinical practice: Restless legs syndrome. N Engl J Med 2003;348:2103-2109.
Kryger MH, Roth T, Dement WC: Principles and Practice of Sleep Medicine, 4th ed. Philadelphia: Elsevier/Saunders, 2005.
Mahowald MW, Bornemann MC, Schenck CH. Parasomnias. Semin Neurol 2004;24:283-292.
Neubauer DN: Understanding Sleeplessness: Perspectives on Insomnia. Baltimore: Johns Hopkins University Press, 2003.
Reid KJ, Zee PC: Circadian rhythm disorders. Semin Neurol 2004;24:315-325.
Thorpy M: Current concepts in the etiology, diagnosis and treatment of narcolepsy. Sleep Med 2001;2:5-17.

Intracerebral Hemorrhage

Method of
J. Claude Hemphill III, MD, MAS

Spontaneous nontraumatic intracerebral hemorrhage (ICH) accounts for 10% to 15% of acute stroke in most case series. It is consistently associated with a high mortality rate (usually around 40%) and is more likely to result in death or major disability than cerebral infarction or subarachnoid hemorrhage (SAH). Currently, without an approved treatment of proven benefit, recent clinical trials have helped to define surgical indications and suggest new interventions for ICH.

Epidemiology and Etiology

Of the 700,000 strokes occurring annually in the United States, more than 70,000 are ICH (Box 1). ICH is more common among minority groups, including Asians and African Americans. Whether this represents a genetic predisposition or a result of less access to preventive health care is not completely clear. The average age of ICH patients is younger than for ischemic stroke, and only 20% of ICH patients are functionally independent a year after their stroke.

BOX 1   Etiologies of Primary Intracerebral Hemorrhage

Common
Arteriovenous malformations
Cerebral amyloid angiopathy
Chronic hypertension
Coagulopathy (warfarin-related)
Drugs of abuse (cocaine, methamphetamine)

Rare
Cerebral vasculitis
Coagulopathy (von Willebrand's)
Moyamoya syndrome

HYPERTENSION

Hypertension remains the most common, and most treatable, cause of acute ICH. At least 60% of ICH is caused by the chronic effects of hypertension on the small penetrating arteries of the brain. Typical sites of hypertensive ICH are the basal ganglia (especially the putamen), the thalamus, the pons, and the cerebellum. An ICH occurring in other locations (e.g., lobar ICH) or in a young person without a prior history of hypertension should prompt a diagnostic evaluation for other causes of ICH. Aggressive treatment of hypertension prevents a substantial portion of ICH from occurring in the first place, and this is the mainstay of primary and secondary prevention for ICH.

CEREBRAL AMYLOID ANGIOPATHY

Cerebral amyloid angiopathy (CAA) is an increasingly recognized cause of primary intracerebral hemorrhage, especially lobar ICH. Occurring almost exclusively in patients older than 65 years, CAA is associated with dementia and recurrent lobar ICH, especially in carriers of the apolipoprotein E ε4 gene allele. Magnetic resonance imaging (MRI) using gradient echo sequences can demonstrate prior microhemorrhages and is a useful diagnostic test in the setting of lobar hemorrhage in older patients. There is currently no treatment for CAA.

COAGULOPATHY, VASCULAR MALFORMATIONS, AND DRUGS OF ABUSE

Warfarin (Coumadin)-related ICH is increasing in incidence and accounts for 5% to 15% of ICH. Mortality from warfarin-related ICH is substantially higher than for noncoagulopathic ICH. Additionally, hematoma expansion is even more common in the setting of an elevated international normalized ratio (INR) (<1.4) and can continue for up to a day after ICH onset unless coagulopathy is corrected back to normal.

Vascular malformations are a relatively uncommon cause of ICH, but they account for a substantial portion of young patients with ICH and for ICH in patients without hypertension. Arteriovenous malformations (AVMs), cavernous malformations, dural arteriovenous fistulas (dAVFs), and saccular aneurysms can all cause acute ICH.

Diagnostic evaluation with MRI and magnetic resonance angiography (MRA) is recommended in patients with lobar hemorrhage and in patients younger than 45 years without an obvious other cause. CT angiography (CTA) is increasingly being used instead of MRA. Diagnostic catheter angiography remains the gold standard for AVMs and dAVF, but it does not detect cavernous malformations.

Because the ICH hematoma can obscure a small vascular anomaly, delayed MRI after hematoma resorption (2-3 months) may be necessary. Primary and metastatic tumors can bleed, mimicking primary ICH, and therefore a delayed MRI is useful if there is no other systemic evidence of a tumor.

Sympathomimetic drugs of abuse are an increasing cause of ICH, especially in younger patients. A urine toxicology screen for cocaine and methamphetamine should be a routine part of the ICH work-up in all patients. A positive toxicology screen is not necessarily ultimately diagnostic because these drugs can precipitate hemorrhage from an underlying vascular anomaly such as an AVM or aneurysm.

Numerous other less common etiologies of ICH exist, including cerebral vasculitis, moyamoya syndrome, and secondary hemorrhage into an arterial or venous infarct. Many times the pattern of hemorrhage on head CT scan or other associated findings on physical or laboratory examination provides clues to one of these less common etiologies.

Diagnosis

Patients with ICH present with what appears to be an acute stroke, although level of consciousness is often more diminished than with ischemic stroke. An urgent head CT scan is an essential part of the diagnostic evaluation of all acute stroke patients. Noncontrast head CT scanning has traditionally been performed, but recent studies suggest that the addition of contrast may be useful, because contrast extravasation predicts mortality, likely due to hematoma enlargement. Also, CTA can be performed concurrently to evaluate for an underlying vascular anomaly.

A rapid coagulation panel (prothrombin time [PT], INR, and partial thromboplastin time [PTT]) should be obtained in all patients, as should a urine toxicology screen. Because history may be limited at the time of initial evaluation, these laboratory tests can provide unexpected clues as to etiology and identify urgent interventions needed.

The importance of early hematoma expansion is now recognized in ICH. Previously, enlargement of an ICH was believed to indicate systemic coagulopathy or underlying AVM, but it is now recognized that a significant portion of all ICH patients will suffer early hematoma expansion. Hematoma expansion tends to happen early in the clinical course, with hematomas enlarging by at least one third in 30% to 40% of patients who present within 3 hours of symptom onset. Hematoma expansion to this degree is usually associated with neurologic deterioration.

Numerous studies have identified a range of clinical and neurologic imaging factors that predict outcome. The ICH Score (Table 1) is one simple clinical grading scale that can be used to risk stratify patients for 30-day mortality based on age, Glasgow Coma Scale score, hematoma volume and location, and presence of intraventricular hemorrhage on CT scan.

CURRENT DIAGNOSIS

- Obtain an emergency head CT scan immediately on hospital arrival.
- Extravasation on contrast CT might predict hematoma expansion.
- Check INR and determine if the patient is on anticoagulant therapy.
- Obtain history: Check for hypertension, dementia, prior stroke.
- MRI, MRA, CTA, or angiography for patients younger than 45 years or with lobar ICH.

Abbreviations: CT = computed tomography; ICH = intracerebral hemorrhage; INR = international normalized ratio; MRA = magnetic resonance angiography; MRI = magnetic resonance imaging.

Treatment

The revised 2007 guidelines from the Stroke Council of the American Heart Association address numerous aspects of ICH management, with the recognition that there is limited evidence to guide many of these treatments (Table 2).

INITIAL EVALUATION AND TRIAGE

Because level of consciousness is often diminished in acute ICH patients, early attention to airway protection is essential to avoid aspiration and hypoxia. Intubation may be necessary. Most patients with acute ICH should be managed in an intensive care unit for at least 24 hours.

BLOOD PRESSURE MANAGEMENT

Most patients with ICH are acutely hypertensive, sometimes to very extreme levels. The 2007 ICH guidelines recommend lowering the blood pressure to achieve a mean arterial pressure (MAP) less than 110 mm Hg or a combined blood pressure less than 160/90. The guidelines also recommend maintaining a cerebral perfusion pressure (CPP) of 60-80 mm Hg in patients with elevated intracranial pressure (ICP). Lowering blood pressure to limit hematoma expansion is intuitively appealing, but studies of the influence of high blood pressure on hematoma expansion have had conflicting results. Prior concerns that blood pressure lowering might create perihematoma ischemia appear largely unfounded. Clinical trials are currently under way in the United States and Australia to determine whether acute blood pressure lowering improves outcome after ICH.

SURGICAL HEMATOMA EVACUATION

Prior studies of ICH hematoma evacuation have included no more than 100 patients. Thus, the recent completion and publication of the results of the STICH (Surgical Trial in Intracerebral Haemorrhage)

TABLE 1 The ICH Score

Component	ICH Score Points
Glasgow Coma Scale Score*	
3-4	2
5-12	1
13-15	0
ICH Volume (mL)†	
≥30	1
<30	0
Intraventricular Hemorrhage‡	
Yes	1
No	0
Infratentorial Origin of ICH	
Yes	1
No	0
Age (years)	
≥80	1
<80	0
Total	**0-6**

*GCS score on discharge from the emergency department.
†ICH volume on the initial CT scan was calculated using the ABC/2 method, where A is the greatest diameter of the hemorrhage (by CT scan), B is the diameter 90 degrees to A, and C is the CT slice thickness (cm) times the approximate number of CT slices that include hemorrhage.
‡Presence of any intraventricular hemorrhage on initial CT.
Abbreviations: CT = computed tomography; GCS = Glasgow Coma Scale; ICH = intracerebral hemorrhage.

CURRENT THERAPY

- Remember the ABCs (airway, breathing, circulation).
- Reverse warfarin (Coumadin) coagulopathy immediately with a prothrombin complex concentrate or recombinant factor VIIa (NovoSeven); also give fresh-frozen plasma and vitamin K.
- Lower blood pressure to mean arterial pressure less than 110 mm Hg or combined blood pressure less than 160/90.
- Surgery for cerebellar hemorrhage and possibly lobar hemorrhage.
- Clinical monitoring for re-bleeding or neurologic worsening for the initial 24 hours.
- Do not use corticosteroids.

study represent a major step both in understanding the role of surgical hematoma evacuation and in demonstrating that large clinical trials in intracerebral hemorrhage can be undertaken.

The STICH study was a randomized, controlled trial designed to test the hypothesis that early surgical evacuation in supratentorial spontaneous intracerebral hemorrhage was superior to initial conservative treatment. Overall, 1033 patients from 27 different countries were randomized. About one half of patients had lobar intracerebral hemorrhage and one half had deep (thalamic or basal ganglia) hemorrhages. At 6 months, there was no difference in the fraction of patients with good functional outcome (early surgery 26%, initial conservative treatment 24%; $P = 0.4$) and no difference in mortality (early surgery 36%, initial conservative treatment 37%; $P = 0.7$). However, 26% of the patients randomized to initial conservative treatment underwent surgical hematoma evacuation later in their hospital course based on the discretion of their treating surgeon. The subgroup of STICH patients with lobar hematomas within 1 cm of the cortical surface had a strong trend toward better outcome with surgical evacuation, and the new STICH II trial is examining surgical evacuation in this group of patients.

STICH included only patients with supratentorial ICH. Cerebellar hemorrhages are considered by most to be surgically appropriate lesions, despite the lack of a randomized trial studying this group of patients. The 2007 ICH guidelines recommend surgery for deteriorating patients with cerebellar hemorrhages larger than 3 cm.

TABLE 2 Highlights of the 2007 Intracerebral Hemorrhage Treatment Guidelines

Management Issue	Recommendations
Blood pressure	Maintain MAP < 110 mm Hg or BP < 160/90
Surgical hematoma evacuation	Cerebellar ICH >3 cm Consider lobar ICH in young patient if deteriorating Structural lesions (e.g., AVM)
Intracranial pressure (ICP) monitoring	Treat elevated ICP with analgesia and sedation, osmotic diuretics, CSF drainage. Maintain CPP 60-80 mm Hg.
Anticonvulsants	Consider prophylaxis
Glucocorticoids	No
Temperature	Maintain normothermia

Abbreviations: AVM = arteriovenous malformation; GCS = Glasgow Coma Scale; ICH = intracerebral hemorrhage; MAP = mean arterial pressure.

PREVENTING HEMATOMA EXPANSION

The safety and efficacy of recombinant factor VIIa (NovoSeven)[1] were tested in a randomized, blinded, placebo-controlled phase II study of patients with acute ICH. Hematoma growth (the primary study outcome measure) was significantly less in the patients who received recombinant factor VIIa (pooled across three doses tested, $P = 0.01$). Three-month mortality (secondary outcome) was significantly less in those treated with recombinant factor VIIa (18% vs. 29%; pooled $P = 0.02$), and functional outcome was better as well. However, a recently completed phase III trial of recombinant factor VIIa in ICH did not demonstrate clinical benefit despite less hematoma growth compared with placebo.

COAGULOPATHY-RELATED INTRACEREBRAL HEMORRHAGE

Because of the especially high risk of ongoing hematoma expansion and increased morbidity and mortality in the setting of warfarin-related ICH, immediate correction of coagulopathy (to an INR ≤ 1.4) is absolutely essential. Studies have demonstrated that protocols that use only fresh-frozen plasma (FFP) and vitamin K (Phytonadione) might not reverse coagulopathy sufficiently fast. International guidelines recommend prothrombin complex concentrate (PCC) in addition to FFP and vitamin K. There are also reports of the successful use of recombinant factor VIIa in this setting.

OTHER MANAGEMENT ISSUES

The use of prophylactic anticonvulsants is controversial. Some advocate administration in all ICH patients or just in lobar hemorrhage, and others treat with anticonvulsants only after a seizure. Prior small trials of corticosteroids in ICH suggested no benefit and an increase in systemic complications. Deep venous thrombosis prophylaxis is essential. Use of sequential compression devices (SCDs) and stockings should be instituted at hospital admission; subcutaneous heparin or heparinoids are likely safe to administer 72 to 96 hours after ICH onset, unless the patient has an intracranial pressure monitor in place, in which case they may be deferred in favor of SCDs.

---

[1]Not FDA approved for this indication.

REFERENCES

Becker KJ, Baxter AB, Bybee HM, et al: Extravasation of radiographic contrast is an independent predictor of death in primary intracerebral hemorrhage. Stroke 1999;30:2025-2032.

Broderick J, Connolly S, Feldmann E, et al: Guidelines for the management of spontaneous intracerebral hemorrhage in adults: 2007 update: A guideline from the American Heart Association/American Stroke Association Stroke Council, High Blood Pressure Research Council, and the Quality of Care and Outcomes in Research Interdisciplinary Working Group. Stroke 2007;38:2001-2023.

Brott T, Broderick J, Kothari R, et al: Early hemorrhage growth in patients with intracerebral hemorrhage. Stroke 1997;28:1-5.

Hemphill JC 3rd, Bonovich DC, Besmertis L, et al: The ICH score: A simple, reliable grading scale for intracerebral hemorrhage. Stroke 2001;32:891-897.

Kothari RU, Brott T, Broderick JP, et al: The ABCs of measuring intracerebral hemorrhage volumes. Stroke 1996;27:1304-1305.

Mayer SA, Brun NC, Begtrup K, et al: Recombinant activated factor vii for acute intracerebral hemorrhage. N Engl J Med 2005;352:777-785.

Mendelow AD, Gregson BA, Fernandes HM, et al: Early surgery versus initial conservative treatment in patients with spontaneous supratentorial intracerebral haematomas in the international surgical trial in intracerebral haemorrhage (STICH): A randomised trial. Lancet 2005;365:387-397.

Qureshi AI, Tuhrim S, Broderick JP, et al: Spontaneous intracerebral hemorrhage. N Engl J Med 2001;344:1450-1460.

Ischemic Cerebrovascular Disease

Method of
Hans-Christoph Diener, MD

Stroke is the third most common cause of mortality after coronary heart disease and malignancies. Stroke is the most common cause of permanent disability.

Epidemiology and Etiology

The incidence of transient ischemic attack (TIA), defined as focal neurologic deficits lasting less than 24 hours, is 50 per 100,000 population per year. The incidence of ischemic stroke varies between 150 and 500 per 100,000 population per year. Stroke is more prevalent in the elderly. About 80% of strokes are due to cerebral ischemia, 15% to cerebral hemorrhage, and 5% to subarachnoid hemorrhage or dural sinus or venous thrombosis.

Investigations

The prior history is most important in the differential diagnosis of TIA. The typical feature of cerebral ischemia is the sudden onset of focal neurologic symptoms. The history should also reveal vascular risk factors such as hypertension, diabetes mellitus, smoking, and high cholesterol and vascular diseases such as coronary heart disease, atrial fibrillation (AF), and peripheral arterial disease. The neurologic examination allows the clinician to assign neurologic deficits to supply areas of cerebral arteries.

Doppler- and duplex sonography, including transcranial ultrasound, can identify stenoses and occlusions of extra- and intracranial arteries that are greater than 50%. Duplex sonography in addition visualizes atherosclerotic plaques and intima-media thickness. Computed tomography (CT) has a high sensitivity for detecting intracerebral and subarachnoid hemorrhage. CT might be normal or show only subtle changes in acute ischemic stroke. CT can also reveal the pathophysiology of an ischemic stroke depending on the pattern of ischemia. Territorial infarction is usually due to arterioarterial embolization, whereas watershed infarctions are seen in patients with high degree stenosis or occlusion of the internal carotid artery (ICA). Lacunar infarcts are small infarcts in the white matter of the brain. Cardiac emboli lead to multiple infarctions in different vascular territories.

Magnetic resonance imaging (MRI) is more sensitive than CT, notably in the acute phase of an ischemic stroke. Diffusion-weighted MRI identifies ischemia within minutes after a stroke, whereas the combination of perfusion-weighted and diffusion-weighted MRI is able to disclose the penumbra, an area of brain with potential salvageable brain tissue. CT or MR angiography (CTA, MRA) can be performed in the acute phase of stroke and can show stenoses or occlusions of brain-supplying arteries. Angiography can identify patients who are candidates for endarterectomy or stenting with balloon angioplasty.

Lumbar puncture should be performed in cases of a typical history suggesting subarachnoid hemorrhage with negative CT and in cases of suspected meningoencephalitis.

Risk Factors

Risk factors for stroke are (in decreasing importance) age, hypertension, cardiac disease (AF), diabetes mellitus, smoking, high cholesterol, and alcohol abuse. Less-significant risk factors are race, sex, obesity, physical inactivity, snoring, elevated C-reactive protein (CRP), and high homocysteine. Important concomitant diseases are coronary heart disease, peripheral arterial disease, and asymptomatic carotid or vertebral stenosis.

Pathophysiology and Clinical Signs and Symptoms

Arterioarterial emboli are generated on the irregular surface of ruptured plaques. The most prevalent site of plaques is the carotid bifurcation. Indicators for arterioarterial emboli are systemic atherosclerosis (coronary heart disease, peripheral arterial disease), hypertension, smoking, diabetes mellitus, and large-vessel disease identified by ultrasound or CTA or MRA. Plaques are identified by duplex sonography.

Local thrombosis happens at atherosclerotic plaques in medium or small brain arteries and leads to vessel occlusion. Occlusion of large and medium-size arteries leads to territorial infarction; occlusion of small penetrating vessels leads to lacunar strokes. Lacunar strokes are characterized by pure motor hemiparesis, pure hemisensory deficit, ataxic hemiparesis, or clumsy hand plus dysarthria.

Hemodynamically induced infarctions result from a sudden occlusion of a major artery or a high-degree of stenosis in combination with a sudden drop in blood pressure. Indicators for this stroke mechanism (large-vessel disease) are high-degree stenosis or occlusion of major arteries shown by ultrasound or CTA or MRA; recurrent TIAs within the territory of a single brain-supplying artery (e.g., amaurosis fugax), in particular in the early morning or after intake of blood pressure–lowering drugs; and stroke at nighttime.

Strokes from cardiac sources are due to emboli arising in the atrium (atrial fibrillation), cardiac valves (endocarditis, rheumatic heart disease, and artificial heart valves), the ventricle (acute myocardial infarction, heart failure), or a patent foramen ovale (PFO) with atrial sepal aneurysm. Indicators for cardiac embolisms are absence of plaques on duplex sonography, atrial fibrillation, TIA or stroke with symptoms indicating different vascular territories, and secondary hemorrhagic transformation of ischemic area in CT.

Rare causes of stroke are arteritis, arterial dissection, sinus–venous thrombosis, and drug abuse.

Symptoms

Ischemic strokes in the territory of the middle cerebral artery lead to contralateral hemiparesis, hemisensory loss, and in some patients to hemianopia. Affection of the dominant hemisphere leads to aphasia, ischemia of the nondominant hemisphere to dysarthria, and neglect. Ischemia in the anterior cerebral artery leads to contralateral proximal weakness of the leg, aphasia, or loss of initiative. Posterior cerebral artery (PCA) ischemia results in hemianopia and headache. Bilateral PCA ischemia (usually cardioembolic) results in cortical blindness and severe short-term memory loss. Occlusion of the vertebral artery leads to Wallenberg's syndrome, consisting of ipsilateral Horner's syndrome, hoarseness, hiccup, dysphasia, nystagmus, ipsilateral limb ataxia, and ipsilateral sensory loss for pain and temperature in the face and contralateral in the body. Basilar artery occlusions may begin with fluctuating symptoms of hemi-, para- or tetraparesis followed by dysarthria, dysphagia, nystagmus, and progressive loss of consciousness.

Transient Ischemic Attack

TIAs are characterized by focal neurologic deficits lasting less than 24 hours. Isolated vertigo and loss of consciousness should generally not be considered TIA. Most TIAs last less than 10 minutes. From 30% to 40% of TIA patients will suffer a stroke in the next 5 years. The risk after a TIA is highest within the next 48 hours. This explains the urgent need to identify the underlying pathophysiology and to initiate secondary prevention as early as possible. Advanced age, symptoms lasting longer than 10 minutes, hypertension, and diabetes are predictors of stroke after a TIA.

The neurologic examination shows the reversibility of neurologic deficits. MRI shows diffusion deficits in up to 40% of all patients with TIA. Ultrasound examination, electrocardiogram, and echocardiography are performed to identify the potential source of cerebral ischemia. In cases of a noncardioembolic source of embolism, secondary prevention is initiated with antiplatelet drugs (for details see later). Patients with a cardiac source of embolism (e.g., atrial fibrillation) are orally anticoagulated with warfarin (Coumadin). Anticoagulation is initiated as soon as a cerebral hemorrhage is ruled out. Vascular risk factors are identified and treated. In patients with significant stenosis (>70%) of extracranial arteries and life expectancy beyond 5 years, endarterectomy or stenting should be considered. Intracranial stenosis leading to recurrent TIAs despite treatment with antiplatelet drugs might benefit from stenting, followed by dual antiplatelet therapy with clopidgrel (Plavix) and aspirin.

Ischemic Stroke

Patients with ischemic stroke experience sudden focal neurologic deficits lasting longer than 24 hours. Mortality following ischemic stroke is 20% to 30% due to brain edema and secondary complications such as aspiration pneumonia, deep venous thrombosis and pulmonary embolism, sepsis, or heart failure. Predictors for poor outcome are initial loss of consciousness, age older than 70 years, hemiplegia with forced eye deviation, prior stroke, and concomitant coronary heart disease.

The reduced blood flow leads to neural and glial death in the core of the infarct. The core of the stroke area is surrounded by the penumbra, with diminished cerebral blood flow and damaged neurons and glia with the potential to survive. The best strategy to rescue this tissue is recanalization. Ischemia triggers a complex cascade of release of excitatory amino acids, Ca^{2+} influx, and release of intracellular calcium and production of free radicals. Neuroprotective therapy aiming at interrupting these processes has failed so far in human stroke.

The first diagnostic procedure after physical and neurologic examination is CT or MRI to exclude cerebral hemorrhage. Indirect signs of cerebral ischemia can be seen in CT within 2 to 3 hours. Diffusion-weighted MRI shows ischemia immediately also in areas in which CT is difficult due to artifacts such as the posterior fossa. CT or MR angiography can identify significant stenosis or occlusion of brain-supplying arteries. Diffusion- and perfusion-weighted MR imaging allows the clinician to detect the penumbra and can identify patients who qualify for either systemic or local thrombolysis beyond the 3-hour window.

Patients with acute stroke should be admitted to a dedicated stroke unit. Stroke unit care decreases mortality and permanent severe disability by 20%. In the initial phase after a stroke, treatment aims at keeping or bringing physiologic parameters into the normal range. Prospective studies showed a negative effect on outcome of too low or high blood pressure, sudden drop of blood pressure, increased blood glucose, increased temperature, fluid loss, or hypoxia. Blood pressure increases in the acute phase of stroke and returns to normal or prior levels after a few days. Therefore, only very high blood pressure values exceeding 220/110 mm Hg should be treated. The following approach is recommended although not proved by randomised trials.

Systolic blood pressure should be maintained between 120 and 200 mm Hg. Increased blood glucose should be lowered with insulin. Increased temperature is lowered by acetaminophen or cooling blankets. Infections leading to fever are treated with antibiotics. Po_2, O_2 and heart rhythm ae monitored. Prophylactic measures against deep venous thrombosis in patients with paretic leg or immobilization include low-molecular-weight heparin, heparin, stockings, and physical therapy. Early mobilization, physical therapy, speech therapy, occupational therapy, and neuropsychological therapy are performed as needed depending on the neurologic deficits.

CURRENT DIAGNOSIS

- History suggests ischemic or hemorrhagic stroke.
- Neurologic examination shows focal deficits.
- Perform CT or MRI to rule out hemorrhage and to identify pathophysiology of cerebral ischemia.
- DW MRI and PW-MRI imaging are used to select candidates for thrombolysis.
- Doppler or duplex sonography or CT angiography or MR angiography to identify stenosis or occlusion of brain-supplying arteries.

CT = computed tomography; DW = diffusion weighted; MRI = magnetic resonance imaging; PW = perfusion weighted.

The only specific therapy in acute ischemic stroke is systemic thrombolysis with recombinant tissue plasminogen activator (rtPA [Activase]). The most important contraindications are cerebral bleeds, severe stroke, age older than 80 years, recent surgery, coagulation disorders, and blood pressure higher than 180 mm Hg. Thrombolysis is effective in anterior and posterior circulation strokes. The most dangerous complication is cerebral hemorrhage, which occurs in about 5% of all patients. Based on the results of DW- and PW-MR imaging, some centers use thrombolysis off-label in the time window beyond 3 hours, when penumbra is still present. Specialized centers might alternatively perform local thrombolysis via microcatheter with urokinase (Abbokinase)[1] or rtPA (Activase)[1] or use thrombus extraction devices such as the Merci retriever.

Stroke in the posterior fossa can lead to occlusive hydrocephalus, requiring the insertion of a shunt. In space-occupying cerebellar infarctions, craniectomy of the posterior fossa and resection of the ischemic brain tissue are necessary. Malignant middle cerebral artery infarction in patients younger than 60 years can be treated by hemicraniectomy. This procedure dramatically reduces mortality (from 80% to 30%) but might increase morbidity in surviving patients. The use of corticosteroids or hemodilution or the systemic use of streptokinase (Streptase) is ineffective or even damaging.

Secondary Prevention

Patients who had a TIA or ischemic stroke are at high risk for a recurrent cerebrovascular event or for myocardial infarction or sudden death. Secondary prevention in patients with a noncardiac source of stroke is performed by the combination of low-dose acetylsalicylic acid (ASA) (2 × 25 mg ASA) plus extended-release dipyridamole (2 × 200 mg) (Aggrenox). This combination is superior to ASA monotherapy and does not lead to an increase in severe bleeding complications. Patients who cannot tolerate ASA, patients with peripheral arterial disease, and patients with multivessel atherosclerotic disease should be treated with clopidogrel 75 mg. Patients with a cardiac source of embolism should be treated with oral anticoagulation. An international normalized ratio (INR) of 2.0 to 3.0 offers the best balance between preventive action (avoiding strokes) and severe bleeding complications.

Patients with isolated PFO and cryptogenic stroke have no increased stroke risk compared with patients without PFO and should be treated with antiplatelet drugs. Patients with PFO in combination with atrial septal aneurysm have an increased stroke risk and should be treated with oral anticoagulation or percutaneous PFO closure.

Patients with large-vessel disease and high-degree stenosis of the internal carotid artery should be treated by either carotid endarterectomy or stenting with angioplasty. Recent studies indicate that

---

[1]Not FDA approved for this indication.

CURRENT THERAPY

- Patients with acute stroke should be admitted to a stroke unit and physiologic variables should be controlled.
- Perform systemic thrombolysis with rtPA (Alteplase [Activase]) in patients with symptoms <3 hours and exclude bleeding with CT or MRI.
- Initiate antiplatelet therapy in patients with atherothrombotic stroke or TIA.
- Initiate oral anticoagulation (INR 2.0-3.0) in patients with cardiac source of embolism.
- Perform endarterectomy or stenting and balloon angioplasty in patients with high-degree stenosis of brain-supplying arteries.

CT = computed tomography; INR = international normalized ratio; MRI = magnetic resonance imaging; rtPA = recombinant tissue plasminogen activator; TIA = transient ischemic attack.

surgery has a lower short-term risk and a lower restenosis rate. Stented patients are treated for 3 to 6 months with dual antiplatelet therapy (clopidogrel plus ASA). Carotid procedures are only effective when performed with a complication rate of less than 6% and within 4 weeks after the ischemic event.

In addition, vascular risk factors have to be treated. angiotensin-converting enzyme inhibitors in combination with diuretics and angiotensin receptor blockers are most effective in treating hypertension. Atorvastatin (Lipitor) has shown stroke-preventive action in secondary prevention compared with placebo in patients with hypercholesterolemia.

REFERENCES

Adams HP: Principles of Cerebrovascular Disease. New York: MacGraw-Hill, 2006.
Adams HP, Jr., del Zoppo G, Alberts MJ, et al: Guidelines for the early management of adults with ischemic stroke: a guideline from the American Heart Association/American Stroke Association Stroke Council, Clinical Cardiology Council, Cardiovascular Radiology and Intervention Council, and the Atherosclerotic Peripheral Vascular Disease and Quality of Care Outcomes in Research Interdisciplinary Working Groups: The American Academy of Neurology affirms the value of this guideline as an educational tool for neurologists. Stroke 2007;38(5):1655-1711.
CAPRIE Steering Committee. A randomised, blinded trial of clopidogrel versus aspirin in patients at risk of ischaemic events (CAPRIE). Lancet 1996;348:1329-1339.
Diener HC, Cuhna L, Forbes C, et al: European Stroke Prevention Study 2. Dipyridamole and acetylsalicylic acid in the secondary prevention of stroke. J Neurol Sci 1996;143:1-13.
The ESPRIT Study Group. Aspirin plus dipyridamole versus aspirin alone after cerebral ischaemia of arterial origin (ESPRIT): Randomised controlled trial. Lancet 2006;367:1665-1673.
Hacke W, Donnan G, Fieschi C, et al: Association of outcome with early stroke treatment: Pooled analysis of ATLANTIS, ECASS, and NINDS rt-PA stroke trials. Lancet 2004;363:768-774.
Hankey G: Stroke Treatment and Prevention. Cambridge, UK: Cambridge University Press, 2005.
Messe S, Silverman I, Kizer J, et al: Practice parameter: Recurrent stroke with patent foramen ovale and atrial septal aneurysm: report of the Quality Standards Subcommittee of the American Academy of Neurology. Neurology 2004;62:1042-1050.
Rothwell PM, Eliasziv M, Gutnikov SA, et al: Analysis of pooled data from the randomized controlled trials of endarterectomy for symptomatic carotid stenosis. Lancet 2003;361:107-116.
Sacco RL, Adams R, Albers G, et al: Guidelines for prevention of stroke in patients with ischemic stroke or transient ischemic attack: A statement for healthcare professionals from the American Heart Association/American Stroke Association Council on Stroke: Co-sponsored by the Council on Cardiovascular Radiology and Intervention: The American Academy of Neurology affirms the value of this guideline. Circulation 2006;113(10):e409-e449.
Vahedi K, Hofmeijer J, Juettler E, et al: Early decompressive surgery in malignant infarction of the middle cerebral artery: A pooled analysis of three randomised controlled trials. Lancet Neurol 2007;6(3):215-222.

Rehabilitation of the Stroke Survivor

Method of
Richard D. Zorowitz, MD

Stroke remains one of the most serious neurologic problems in the United States today. It is the leading cause of serious, long-term disability in the United States and is the leading reason for admission to nursing homes or extended-care facilities. Approximately 5.5 million stroke survivors live in the United States. Of patients who survive a stroke past 30 days, 50% are still alive after 7 years, and 33% live 12 years or more. The estimated cost of stroke totals $57.9 billion per year, of which $20.6 billion is lost in productivity due to mortality and morbidity.

Comprehensive rehabilitation can improve the functional abilities of the stroke survivor, despite age and neurologic deficit, and decrease long-term patient care costs. Although motor recovery occurs in predictable patterns (Box 1) and can plateau 3 to 6 months after stroke, functional recovery can continue for up to several years. Approximately 80% of stroke survivors can benefit from rehabilitation in acute, subacute, skilled nursing, day hospital, outpatient, or home care environment. Ten percent of patients achieve complete spontaneous recovery within 8 to 12 weeks, and 10% of patients receive no benefit from any treatment. Intensive post-stroke rehabilitation significantly improves functional outcomes and increases the likelihood of returning to the community. Yet, larger, more comprehensive studies are needed to determine what aspects of rehabilitation work and why rehabilitation works.

Stroke rehabilitation involves a transdisciplinary, holistic approach that addresses medical, functional, and psychosocial issues. The team can include a physiatrist (i.e., physician specializing in rehabilitation), rehabilitation nurse, physical therapist, occupational therapist, speech-and-language pathologist, social worker, psychologist, vocational counselor, family, and the patient. Therapy uses components of conventional methods and neurophysiologic theories (Box 2). As the team meets periodically and evaluates the stroke survivor, functional gains are documented and short- and long-term goals are set. The stroke survivor often meets with the team to review functional progress, to confirm discharge plans, and to discuss any problems. The family participates in therapy sessions in preparation for overseeing patient care at home.

Researchers are gaining a better understanding of the physiologic basis of functional recovery. Growth factors may be responsible for enhanced recovery of sensorimotor function within the first month after stroke. Functional imaging (e.g., functional magnetic resonance imaging, single-photon-emission computed tomography, positron-emission tomography) and transcranial magnetic stimulation demonstrate that neurons not usually used during normal movement (i.e., areas surrounding infarcts, in ipsilateral homologous sites, and in supplementary motor areas) are activated during rehabilitation activities. Medications such as dextroamphetamine (Dexedrine),[1] methylphenidate (Ritalin),[1] and levodopa–carbidopa (Sinemet)[1] appear to modify noradrenergic or dopaminergic systems, thus

---
[1]Not FDA approved for this indication.

> **BOX 1 Synergy Patterns of Motor Recovery**
>
> **Upper Extremity**
> *Flexor*
> Shoulder flexion, adduction, internal rotation
> Elbow flexion
> Wrist flexion
> Finger flexion
>
> *Extensor*
> Shoulder extension
> Elbow extension
> Wrist extension
> Finger extension
>
> **Lower Extremity**
> *Flexor*
> Hip flexion, adduction
> Knee flexion
> Ankle dorsiflexion
>
> *Extensor*
> Hip extension
> Knee extension
> Ankle plantar flexion

facilitating motor recovery and initiation or quality of movement or speech.

Mobility and Locomotion

Probably the most important priority of the stroke survivor is ambulation. Prerequisites for ambulation include the ability to follow commands; adequate trunk control for sitting and standing; minimal or no contractures of the hip flexor, knee flexor, and ankle plantar flexor muscles; and adequate muscle strength to stabilize the hip and knee joints. The hip extensor muscles are the most important muscles used in ambulation because they provide stability to the hip and knee.

> **BOX 2 Techniques of Stroke Rehabilitation**
>
> Biofeedback: Modifies function using volitional control and auditory, visual, sensory cues
> Brunnstrom method: Facilitate synergistic movement
> Constraint-induced movement therapy (CIMT): Forces use of affected extremity
> Conventional: Range of motion, strengthening; compensatory strategies, mobility training, activities of daily living training
> Cortical stimulation: Submaximal electrical stimulation of cortex during therapy
> Electrical stimulation: Random or coordinated contraction of muscles
> Motor learning: Improves the smoothness and accuracy of movement
> Neurodevelopmental therapy (Bobath NDT): Suppress synergistic movement, facilitate normal movement
> Partial weight support: Ambulation training using a treadmill and harness system to decrease body weight
> Proprioceptive neuromuscular stimulation (Knott and Voss [PNF]): Suppress normal movement, facilitate defined mass movement
> Rood method: Modify movement with cutaneous sensory stimulation
> Treadmill training

Gait training begins by teaching transfers to the bed, mat, and wheelchair. The patient must be able to bear weight consistently on the affected extremity. Standing balance must be maximized using visual, proprioceptive, or labyrinthine cues. The patient is taught the most optimal gait pattern in and out of the parallel bars, and on stairs, ramps, and curbs. Orthoses (braces) and assistive devices are used to correct gait deviations and can decrease energy expenditure during gait. There is no difference in the amount of energy used with plastic or metal orthoses. Harnesses to provide partial body weight support can help promote motor recovery and increase velocity of gait.

Falls during transfers or ambulation can be a disincentive to attaining mobility goals or can produce frank injury, such as hip fracture. Falls are most common in stroke survivors with right-hemisphere lesions that result in hemineglect, anosagnosia, and impulsivity. Other factors, such as use of psychotropic drugs, severity of disability as reflected by urinary incontinence, or decline in mental status, are associated with falls. Stroke survivors who are more likely to fall also may be more depressed, may be less socially active, and have more stressed caregivers.

Stroke survivors who have limited or no ability to ambulate can require wheelchairs for mobility. The seat should be narrow enough to allow operation of the hand rim with the unaffected arm, and it should be low enough to allow propulsion with the unaffected leg. Arm rests should permit seating at tables. Arm rests and leg rests should be removable to make transfers easier. Lightweight or electric chairs may be issued to patients with cardiac or other severely debilitating conditions.

Activities of Daily Living

Stroke survivors usually do not place the same degree of importance on activities of daily living (ADLs) as they place on ambulation. Yet, in many cases, teaching ADLs may be more difficult than teaching ambulation because the affected upper limb is less functional than the affected lower limb. Performance of ADLs requires visual, cognitive, perceptual, and coordination skills in addition to range of motion, motor strength, and sensation. Occasionally, tendon lengthening or transfer procedures can improve functional status by correcting muscle imbalance, spasticity, or instability. Apraxia, poor memory skills, left hemineglect, or loss of sensory function can render the affected arm useless. Poor prognostic factors for upper-extremity function include onset of upper-extremity movement longer than 4 weeks after the stroke, absence of voluntary hand movement longer than 6 weeks, prolonged flaccid period, and severe proximal spasticity.

Patients can be taught one-handed techniques to perform feeding, grooming, dressing, bathing, and writing with the nondominant unaffected limb. The affected limb can be trained to stabilize or give gross assistance. The unaffected arm can be immobilized, thus forcing the affected arm to be more active in function activity. Trials of submaximal cortical stimulation during therapy can help to facilitate movement. Adaptive equipment augments the abilities of the hemiplegic patient in feeding, bathing, dressing, and grooming. Velcro closures and straps can allow easier donning and doffing of clothing, splints, and slings. Occupational therapists can fabricate devices customized to the needs of the patient and are limited only by their imaginations and technical skills.

Driving is an important goal for some stroke survivors. Occupational therapists administer predriving evaluations that test basic cognitive skills needed for driving: memory, spatial organization, attention, concentration, and reaction times. Driving skills are tested in simulators or behind the wheel with licensed instructors. Adaptive aids, such as spinner knobs and accelerator extenders, may be incorporated to compensate for motor deficits. Three fourths of stroke survivors with left-hemisphere lesions are able to pass a driving test, but 50% of stroke survivors with right-hemisphere lesions fail driving tests due to cognitive and perceptual deficits.

Approximately one third of stroke survivors younger than 65 years are able to return to work. To return to work, patients with left-hemisphere strokes must demonstrate adequate verbal, cognitive, and language skills, and patients with right-hemisphere strokes must have adequate ambulation skills, use of the left upper extremity, and abstract reasoning skills. Vocational assessments can include neuropsychological and driving evaluations, functional capacity evaluations, work hardening, and on-site evaluations.

Speech and Language Disorders

Speech and language disorders may be diagnosed by formal testing and by conversational interaction. Impaired content of speech suggests aphasia or cognitive-communication impairment. Aphasias are characterized by decreased word finding or syntax, word substitutions, and errors in understanding conversational questions or statements. Aphasias are classified as nonfluent, fluent, or global. Nonfluent aphasia (Broca's, transcortical motor) is characterized by a slow, telegraphic style of delivery. Fluent aphasia (Wernicke's, conduction, anomic, transcortical sensory) is characterized by rapid style with paraphasias or neologisms. Global aphasias involve all modes of speech and may be fluent or nonfluent.

Cognitive-communication impairments usually are associated with right-hemisphere dysfunction. They are characterized by decreased concentration, attention, memory, and orientation; confusion; confabulation; concrete or irrelevant thinking; or vague language. Associated functional problems can include unilateral neglect, constructional and dressing apraxias, anosognosia, and impairments in safety awareness and judgment.

Impaired acoustic features of speech can indicate apraxias or dysarthrias. Apraxias are characterized by inconsistent errors either in programming the positioning of the speech musculature (oral) or in sequencing muscle movements for articulation of volitional speech (verbal). Dysarthric stroke survivors present with consistent errors in articulation, decreased normal resonance or phonation, or problems with volume or breath control.

Therapy generally focuses on teaching compensatory strategies and self-correction of errors. Exercises of the oral, lingual, buccal, and laryngeal musculature can increase physiologic support for speech. Facilitation techniques are thought to recruit right-hemisphere areas that enhance verbal output. Alternative communication techniques and augmentative communication devices may be used as long as apraxia and comprehension deficits do not interfere with their use. Family education is essential to increase the awareness of the deficits and discuss prognosis. Global aphasia usually has a poor prognosis, but patients with conduction aphasia and anomia often have a complete recovery. The prognosis of apraxic stroke survivors is improved when oral apraxia and aphasia are absent. Persistent cognitive-communication problems can cause an otherwise independent patient to require 24-hour supervision.

Common Medical Complications

Every stroke survivor admitted to the rehabilitation unit must be considered for secondary prophylaxis of stroke. Aspirin or aspirin with extended-release dipyridamole (Aggrenox) remains the standard treatment for completed thrombotic or lacunar strokes. Warfarin (Coumadin) is the appropriate treatment after embolic strokes or when significant hypercoagulable states are identified. Clopidogrel (Plavix) may be chosen for patients who have recurrent strokes and are on aspirin therapy or when warfarin therapy is contraindicated. Cholesterol-lowering agents also have demonstrated direct stroke-prophylaxis properties. Antihypertensive therapy should be initiated 7 to 10 days after stroke. Diabetes mellitus should be strictly controlled using insulin or oral agents, or both. Folate[1] is used as adjunctive therapy in strokes resulting from hyperhomocysteinemia. Secondary prophylaxis of hemorrhagic stroke includes control of etiologic factors, such as hypertension or hypercoagulable states. All stroke survivors should stop smoking.

Deep venous thrombosis (DVT) occurs in 30% to 60% of stroke survivors. Clinical signs and symptoms, such as pain, swelling, and warmth of the extremities, are at best marginally diagnostic. Clinical suspicion should be raised in the nonambulatory hemiplegic stroke survivor. Noninvasive testing, such as duplex ultrasonography and impedance plethysmography, is a routine part of diagnosis. Stroke survivors at risk for DVT should be given compression stockings, pneumatic compression, and low-dose subcutaneous or low-molecular-weight heparin. Prophylaxis may be discontinued once the stroke survivor is ambulating consistently in or out of the parallel bars. Treatment of DVT includes anticoagulation for at least 3 months or, if anticoagulation is contraindicated, insertion of an inferior vena cava filter.

Proper positioning of the stroke survivor will prevent numerous complications. Positioning in the bed and wheelchair can prevent both flexion contractures and traction neuropathy. Dependent patients should be turned every 2 hours in bed. Wheelchair seats should be provided with appropriate cushions to decrease the incidence of pressure sores. Affected extremities can be elevated with pillows, footrests, and elevated arm rests to prevent edema. Retrograde massage or placement of a compression glove can prevent or reduce edema of the affected hand.

Stroke can disinhibit the reflex mechanisms for emptying the bowels, and sensation or cognitive impairments can prevent control of defecation. Diets should include adequate fluids and fiber. Patients should be toileted after meals to take advantage of the gastrocolic reflex. Stool softeners and bowel stimulants may be prescribed as necessary. Patients who remain incontinent might require a suppository or enema every 1 or 2 days to prevent incontinence at socially inappropriate times. Persistent bowel incontinence lasting longer than 4 weeks usually is a poor predictive indicator.

A variety of voiding disorders may be observed after stroke. Reversible causes, such as urinary tract infection, fecal impaction, and reduced mobility, should be evaluated and treated. Postvoid residuals should be measured by ultrasonography or catheterization to assess the degree of bladder emptying. Symptoms of urinary incontinence, frequency, and urgency should be noted. Patients with voiding dysfunction should be referred for urodynamic studies to characterize the voiding disorders and to determine appropriate intervention. Toileting every 2 to 4 hours during the day and fluid restriction after dinner can prevent incontinence in many patients. External catheters may decrease the incidence of enuresis. Intermittent or indwelling catheterization may be indicated in patients with areflexic bladders.

Swallowing dysfunction, or dysphagia, occurs in up to one third of patients with cortical or brainstem lesions. Dysphagia should be suspected in patients with impaired cognition, nasal regurgitation, coughing, gurgly voice, or impaired cough associated with absence of bilateral gag reflex. Following evaluation by a speech-and-language pathologist, a videofluorographic swallowing study of liquids, purees, and solids can be undertaken to identify swallowing disorders and organize a treatment plan. Changes in diet, head positioning, or other compensatory strategies may be incorporated to prevent aspiration pneumonitis. Stimulation of the anterior faucial arches can help to initiate an impaired or absent pharyngeal swallow. Non-oral feedings by gastrostomy or jejunostomy may be necessary if oral caloric intake is not adequate to meet nutritional needs.

Almost three fourths of stroke survivors experience at least one episode of shoulder pain within the first year after stroke. Shoulder pain most commonly is correlated with limited range of motion, especially external rotation. Other causes of shoulder pain include brachial plexopathy, shoulder trauma, bursitis, tendinitis, adhesive capsulitis, rotator cuff tear, heterotopic ossification, and complex regional pain syndrome. A diagnosis often may be determined from a physical examination alone, but radiographs, electromyography, bone scans, or magnetic resonance imaging can support clinical findings. Pain may be relieved with appropriate use of nonsteroidal antiinflammatory drugs, corticosteroids, tricyclic antidepressants, antiepileptic medications, narcotics, electrical nerve stimulation, muscle or nerve blocks, local injections, or sympathectomy. Range of motion exercises, along with proper positioning of the limb using orthoses and supports, have been credited with a decrease in the number of pain complaints.

Another type of post-stroke pain is known as the *post-stroke central pain syndrome*, which usually occurs as a result of a lesion in the thalamus. The sensation of thalamic pain consists of a burning

---

[1]Not FDA approved for this indication.

CURRENT THERAPY

- Every stroke survivor should be considered for a rehabilitation program, whether as an inpatient, as an outpatient, or at home.
- Care following acute stroke should be delivered in a setting where rehabilitation care is formally coordinated and organized.
- Rehabilitation therapy should start as early as possible, once medical stability is reached.
- Every stroke survivor should participate in a secondary stroke prevention program, including risk factors (e.g., hypertension, diabetes mellitus, hyperlipidemia, coronary artery disease, smoking) and secondary complications (e.g., deep venous thrombosis, pressure sores, bowel and bladder dysfunction)
- Patients with depression or with severe, persistent, or troublesome tearfulness should receive a trial of antidepressant medication if no contraindication exists.
- Outpatient rehabilitation services should be continued in the setting where they can most appropriately and effectively be carried out. This is based on medical status, function, social support, and access to care.

or other unpleasant sensation when an area on the body is stimulated. The most common treatments available today include antidepressant medications, such as tricyclics, selective serotonin reuptake inhibitors, or selective serotonin and norepinephrine reuptake inhibitors, and antiepileptic medications (e.g., phenytoin [Dilantin],[1] carbamazepine [Tegretol],[1] gabapentin [Neurontin][1]), mexiletine (Mexitil),[1] and narcotics. Nondrug modalities that can relieve post-stroke central pain include transcutaneous electrical nerve stimulators (TENS) or dorsal column stimulators.

Spasticity is a common complication that results from enhanced excitatory synaptic input, reduced inhibitory synaptic input, or changes in intrinsic electrical properties of the neuron. Modalities used to treat spasticity include ice, electrical stimulation of antagonist muscles, and splinting. Dantrolene (Dantrium) reduces spasticity peripherally by reducing the release of calcium from the sarcoplasmic reticulum of muscle cells. Tizanidine (Zanaflex) is a central α_2-receptor agonist that decreases the release of excitatory amino acids in spinal motor neurons. Oral baclofen (Lioresal) does not have a role in cerebral spasticity. Diazepam (Valium) is unsuitable for patients with cerebral spasticity due to its sedating properties. Phenol[1] or botulinum toxin[1] (type A [Botox] or type B [Myobloc]) injections can inhibit spasticity in individual or groups of muscles for up to 3 to 6 months. Intrathecal baclofen (Lioresal Intrathecal) has a role in stroke survivors with severe spasticity. If contractures inhibit function or cause significant pain, tendon releases or transfers can reestablish normal joint alignment. When surgery is performed to release contractures, spasticity management must be initiated postoperatively to prevent recurrence of contractures.

Mood disorders commonly affect stroke survivors. Depression can occur in 25% to 79% of stroke survivors, but less than 5% receive psychotherapeutic or medical intervention. Depression may be related to mourning the loss of function or to the alteration of function of catecholamine-containing neurons. Stroke survivors also can develop involuntary emotional expression disorder (IEED), characterized by episodes of involuntary and inappropriate laughing, crying, irritability, anger, frustration, or aggressive behavior as a result of neurologic disease. Treatment includes dextromethorphan with quinidine (Neurodex).[5]

---
[1]Not FDA approved for this indication.
[5]Investigational drug in the United States.

Issues of sexual functioning rarely are addressed with stroke victims. Patients generally are fearful of causing another stroke from sexual activity. Cardiac limitations should be discussed, and medications should be reviewed. Couples should be encouraged to experiment with sexual techniques and positions and to communicate their needs to each other.

Continuity of Care

Physiatric care should be provided throughout the continuum of rehabilitation care. Patients should return to their primary care practitioners for routine medical care, but they should be seen by a physiatrist 1 month following discharge and periodically thereafter. Blood pressure and weight should be measured, and medications should be reviewed. Progress of mobility and ADLs should be reviewed and validated by a family member. Psychosocial issues should be discussed. All equipment should be inspected, and the patient should be able to demonstrate his or her home exercise program. A neurologic examination should be performed, including gait with appropriate assistive devices and orthoses. Most importantly, time should be allowed for questions. Good communication between the physiatrist and the patient and family will facilitate optimal care and provide the patient with the opportunity to reach his or her maximal functional potential.

REFERENCES

Albers GW, Amarenco P, Easton JD, et al: Antithrombotic and thrombolytic therapy for ischemic stroke: The seventh ACCP conference on antithrombotic and thrombolytic therapy. Chest 2004;126:483S-512S.
American Heart Association: 2006 Heart and Stroke Statistical Update. Dallas, TX: American Heart Association, 2005.
Bates B, Choi JY, Duncan PW, et al: Veterans Affairs/Department of Defense clinical practice guideline for the management of adult stroke rehabilitation care. Executive summary. Stroke 2005;36:2049.
Büller HR, Agnelli G, Hull RD, et al: Antithrombotic therapy for venous thromboembolic disease. The seventh ACCP conference on antithrombotic and thrombolytic therapy. Chest 2004;126:401S-428S.
Hackett ML, Anderson CS, House AO: Interventions for treating depression after stroke. Cochrane Database Syst Rev 2004;(3):CD003437.
Pollock A, Baer G, Pomeroy V, Langhorne P: Physiotherapy treatment approaches for the recovery of postural control and lower limb function following stroke. Cochrane Database Syst Rev. 2007. Jan 24(1):CD001920.
Stroke Unit Trialists' Collaboration: Organised inpatient (stroke unit) care for stroke. cochrane Database Syst Rev 2007;(4):CD000197.
VA/DoD Clinical Practice Guideline Working Group: Management of Stroke Rehabilitation. Office of Quality and Performance publication 10Q CPG/STR-03. Washington, DC: Veterans Health Administration 2003.

Seizures and Epilepsy in Adolescents and Adults

Method of
Erik K. St. Louis, MD, and Mark A. Granner, MD

Epilepsy is a common public health problem afflicting approximately 2.5 million Americans and 30 million persons worldwide. Epilepsy is equally prevalent between the sexes until older age, where the increased incidence of epilepsy in elderly men mirrors that of cerebrovascular disease.

Epilepsy was recognized in antiquity, described by Hippocrates as "the falling sickness." The etymology of epilepsy stems from the Greek *epilepsia*, "to be seized or taken hold of," derived from the erroneous belief and unfortunately persistent stigma that epileptic seizures result from supernatural or spiritual, rather than medical causes. Such historical misunderstandings, coupled with limited availability of effective treatments, have instilled fear of epilepsy for centuries in patients, their families and caregivers, and society. Fortunately, an evolving medical understanding of epilepsy and its many causes and imitators has enabled improved diagnostic testing and an ever-expanding palette of effective, tolerable antiepileptic drug and surgical therapies over the last three decades. All clinicians should be familiar with epilepsy not only because of its prevalence, but because its treatments are increasingly adopted for a wide variety of neurologic and psychiatric conditions including migraine, pain, and mood disorders.

Seizures and Epilepsy Defined

An epileptic seizure is a sudden, transient alteration in behavior caused by an abnormal, excessive neuronal discharge in the cerebral cortex. Everyone has a seizure threshold and holds the potential to have a seizure. Only a small subset of the population, however, experiences spontaneous seizures or develops epilepsy. The lifetime prevalence of experiencing a single seizure is approximately 10%, but only approximately 30% of incipient seizures recur and become epilepsy.

Seizures are most often provoked by an extrinsic (systemic) or intrinsic (brain) factor. Table 1 lists the causes of provoked seizures. An individual may have recurrent provoked seizures without developing epilepsy. In most cases, a provoked seizure does not recur when the provoking factor is successfully corrected, avoided, or removed. The tendency toward recurrent provoked seizures speaks either to the root cause (e.g., recurrent episodes of alcohol withdrawal seizures) or to a heightened sensitivity to seizures in the individual (e.g., a lower than average seizure threshold).

Epilepsy is characterized by recurrent, unprovoked seizures. The prevalence of epilepsy in the general population is approximately 1%. The principal clinical symptoms and signs of epilepsy include ictal (during a seizure), postictal (immediately following seizure termination), and interictal (between seizure episodes) manifestations. Behavioral alterations accompanying epileptic seizures are diverse, ranging from subjective feelings reported by the patient, to objectively witnessed behavioral arrest, unresponsiveness, or involuntary movements. The nature of the ictal behavioral disturbance depends on the location of seizure onset in the brain and its pattern of propagation.

Diagnosis of Seizure Type and Epilepsy Syndrome

A seizure is only a symptom of brain dysfunction, and the seizure type is not in itself an etiologic diagnosis. A diversity of underlying causative pathologies may result in identical phenotypes of clinical seizure behavior and electroencephalographic (EEG) manifestations. The patient's prognosis and treatment are directed by a diagnosis of the underlying epilepsy syndrome, which incorporates an understanding of the cause of the seizures as well as the clinical and EEG characteristics. Epilepsy syndromes are regarded as idiopathic, symptomatic, or cryptogenic.

The International League Against Epilepsy (ILAE) has created consensus terminology defining different seizure types and, in parallel, descriptions of epilepsy syndromes. Diagnosis of ILAE seizure type and epilepsy syndrome is based on electroclinical criteria, including the description of seizure behavior and EEG manifestations. Most experts now also use neuroimaging to diagnose the most likely seizure type and epilepsy syndrome. The seizure type and epilepsy syndrome diagnoses are crucial steps in the approach to the patient with epilepsy because this information determines the patient's prognosis, which type of antiepileptic drug (AED) therapy is indicated, and whether surgical therapies can potentially be offered if AEDs are ineffective.

TABLE 1 Common Causes of Provoked Seizures

Drugs of Abuse
Alcohol
- Severe acute alcohol intoxication
- Alcohol withdrawal

Amphetamine and methamphetamine
Cocaine
Lysergic acid diethylamide (LSD)
Phencyclidine

Iatrogenic (Prescription Drugs)
Antibiotics
- High-dose intravenous penicillin
- Imipenem

Antiarrhythmic agents
- Lidocaine (Xylocaine)
- Procainamide (Pronestyl)
- Propafenone (Rythmol)

Insulin overdose
Pain medications
- Opiate analgesics, especially meperidine (Demerol)
- Tramadol (Ultram)

Psychotropic drugs
- Antidepressants
  - Clomipramine (Anafranil)
  - Bupropion (Wellbutrin)
- Antipsychotics
  - Clozapine (Clozaril)

Stimulants
- Amphetamines mixed (Adderall), methylphenidate (Ritalin)

Infection
Brain abscess
Cerebritis
- Lyme disease
- Neurosyphilis

Encephalitis
- Cytomegalovirus
- Herpes simplex virus type 1
- Varicella-zoster virus
- West Nile virus

Acute meningitis
- Bacterial
- Fungal
- Viral

Metabolic Disorders
Hypocalcemia
Hypoglycemia
Hyperglycemia
- Nonketotic hyperosmolar state
- Diabetic ketoacidosis

Hypomagnesemia
Hyponatremia
Hypernatremia
Hypophosphatemia

Herbal Products
Guarana
Ma Huang

The two principal varieties of epileptic seizures are partial (also known as focal or localization-related) and generalized seizures. Partial seizures begin in one brain region, whereas generalized seizures have their onset simultaneously in both cerebral hemispheres. Differentiating epileptic seizure type and syndrome is often difficult in new-onset epilepsy. Many partial seizures present clinically as a secondarily generalized tonic–clonic seizure without focal features, and patients usually present for evaluation after only one or a few seizures have occurred, so the full spectrum of their epilepsy is not yet apparent.

Partial seizures are subclassified as simplex, complex, and secondarily generalized seizures. A simple partial seizure is restricted at onset to one focal cortical region and does not impair consciousness. Simple partial seizures are synonymous with the term *aura* and involve autonomic, gustatory, cognitive, somatosensory, or involuntary motor activity depending on where they begin in the brain.

TABLE 2 Typical Partial Seizure Characteristics According to Region of Seizure Onset

	Simple Partial	Complex Partial	Secondary Generalized
Frontal	Focal clonic motor or none	Amnestic Automatisms Hypermotor common	Frequent
Temporal	Mesial (none possible) • Autonomic • Dysmnesic 　• Déjà vu 　• Jamais vu • Gustatory Lateral/posterior neocortical 　Auditory 　Complex visual	Amnestic Automatisms	Less frequent
Parietal	Somatosensory or none	Amnestic Automatisms	Frequent
Occipital	Simple visual or none	Amnestic Automatisms	Frequent

When a simple partial seizure propagates beyond the initial seizure focus, it may evolve into a complex partial or secondarily generalized seizure. A complex partial seizure is defined by the feature of altered consciousness (although often not full loss of consciousness) and may involve behavioral arrest, blank staring, oral automatisms such as chewing or swallowing, limb automatisms including aimless fumbling movements of the hands, and amnesia. A complex partial seizure may or may not be preceded by an aura, and it may propagate to the whole brain to become a generalized tonic–clonic seizure. There may be considerable variability of behavioral characteristics between different patients with partial seizures or even within a given patient (although a patient's personal seizures tend to be rather monomorphic). Table 2 provides a summary of characteristic auras and behavioral manifestations of partial seizures according to the region of seizure onset. An EEG during a partial seizure usually demonstrates focal rhythmic activity overlying the region of seizure onset.

Generalized seizures involve simultaneous seizure onset in both cerebral hemispheres. By definition, consciousness is impaired from seizure onset, although myoclonic seizures may be too brief to detect an alteration in consciousness. Absence seizures, frequently confused with complex partial seizures because both were previously (and unfortunately) referred to as petit mal seizures, are brief episodes (typically less than 10 seconds) of behavioral arrest, staring with unresponsiveness, and oral or limb automatisms. Absence seizures lack an aura or postictal state. Tonic seizures involve symmetric tonic posturing of the extremities and, if prolonged, may have prominent autonomic instability. Atonic (also known as astatic) seizures involve loss of tone and may lead to falls. Generalized tonic–clonic seizures involve an initial phase of tonic posturing, generally lasting less than 20 seconds, followed by symmetric clonic movements of the limbs for 1 to 3 minutes. Ictal EEG during generalized seizures demonstrates generalized epileptiform patterns of repetitive spike-wave discharges, polyspikes, or background attenuation.

The accurate diagnosis of an epilepsy syndrome in each patient is an important tenet in epilepsy care; whereas diagnosis of the habitual seizure type describes the ictal seizure characteristics, an epilepsy syndrome diagnosis reaches further, inferring knowledge of the underlying etiology and therefore determining the prognosis and most appropriate therapy. Despite rigorous diagnostic testing, many times the epilepsy syndrome remains ambiguous in new-onset epilepsy cases.

Partial seizures and their associated epilepsy syndromes are most common in adolescents and adults, representing approximately 70% of all epilepsy in these age groups. Most partial epilepsy is related to known acquired etiologies such as head injury, cerebrovascular disease, or tumors. Conversely, idiopathic or cryptogenic partial epilepsies and idiopathic generalized epilepsies are often inherited. The basis of inherited epilepsies is a rapidly evolving field. Many of the known gene effects relate to ion channelopathies.

The Differential Diagnosis of Paroxysmal Spells

The differential diagnosis of epilepsy is wide. Numerous paroxysmal non-neurologic and neurologic disorders may closely mimic the behavioral alterations of an epileptic seizure. Table 3 differentiates commonly confused seizure types and nonepileptic paroxysmal spells by behavioral characteristics, duration, and usual ictal EEG findings. Although most of these conditions are reviewed elsewhere in this text, psychological mimicry of epilepsy is particularly common. Psychogenic nonepileptic spells (also known as pseudoseizures) are most often an expression of a conversion disorder with subconsciously motivated spells of behavioral unresponsiveness or unusual movements that may closely resemble epileptic seizures. Psychogenic spells, however, frequently involve behavioral characteristics of eye closure, nonphysiologic patterns of movements, prominent pelvic thrusting, prolonged duration (often over 5 to 10 minutes), lack of stereotypy between episodes, and failure to respond to antiepileptic drugs. Because true epileptic seizures may also share all of these characteristics, the diagnosis of psychogenic nonepileptic spells is necessarily a diagnosis of exclusion and requires diagnostic ictal video-EEG monitoring for confirmation.

Clinical Approach to the Patient with Seizures

The fundamental goals in epilepsy care are both diagnostic and therapeutic: to understand the underlying cause of epilepsy and determine the epilepsy syndrome when possible; to strive for seizure freedom without adverse side effects of treatment whenever feasible (or, at the very least, to minimize disabling, injurious seizures and limit adverse effects); and to identify and treat interictal co-morbidities in epilepsy.

THE INTERICTAL STATE IN SEIZURES AND EPILEPSY

Recent studies have shown that quality of life in epilepsy is largely determined by the interictal state. Although reducing seizure burden is an integral determinant of patient quality of life, interictal mood disorders such as depression or bipolar affective disorder, cognitive impairments, and adverse effects of antiepileptic drugs more often affect how patients feel on a daily basis between their seizure episodes, and have great impacts on perceived quality of life. Physicians should thus proactively inquire regarding altered mood and adverse affects in patients with epilepsy. The approach to new-onset seizures and

TABLE 3 Differentiating Epileptic Seizures from Nonepileptic Spells

	Premonitory Symptoms	Behavioral Characteristics	Duration	Postictus Symptoms	Ictal EEG Findings
Absence seizure	None	Staring, automatisms	<10 sec	None	Generalized 3-Hz spike wave
Partial complex seizure	Aura variable; if sensory march, brief over 10–30 sec	Staring, automatisms, posture often preserved	30–180 sec	Common; amnesia, aphasia, sleepiness, ± incontinence	Focal rhythmic activity
Generalized tonic–clonic seizures	Aura variable	Sequence of tonic limb posturing for 10 sec, then clonic movements	1–3 min	Invariable; frequently amnesia, sleep, incontinence, tongue biting	Repetitive spikes (tonic phase); spike wave (clonic phase)
Psychogenic nonepileptic spells (pseudoseizures)	Variable	Variable; behavioral unresponsiveness Nonstereotypy, and unusual movements common	Variable; may be prolonged (>10 min)	Variable; often none	None, other than movement artifact
Syncope	Common; lightheadedness	Falling, eye closure, variable convulsive movements, incontinence	Minutes	None to brief confusion; no postical amnesia	Suppression
Migraine	Prolonged; sensory march over minutes	"Positive" symptoms (e.g., tingling paresthesias)	20–30 min	None	Slowing/suppression
Transient ischemic attack (TIA)	Sensory march rapid (<10 sec)	More often "negative" (e.g., anesthetic numbness, weakness)	Variable; <1 h	None	Slowing/suppression
Sleep disorders: Cataplexy	Emotional provocation	Behavioral sleep	Minutes	None	REM stage sleep
Parasomnias	None	Arousal from sleep, confusion, dream enactment	Minutes	Brief confusion	Onset in REM/NREM sleep

Abbreviations: EEG = electroencephalogram; NREM = nonrapid eye movement (sleep); REM = rapid eye movement (sleep).

---

chronic care of the patient with established epilepsy is now considered.

THE SINGLE SEIZURE AND NEW-ONSET EPILEPSY

The focus during the approach to new-onset seizures is different than in chronic epilepsy. The emphasis for new-onset seizures is prompt diagnosis of the underlying cause because it is imperative to ensure there is no symptomatic etiology requiring further diagnosis or therapy (e.g., brain mass or vascular malformation). Diagnostic tests also help determine the epilepsy syndrome diagnosis and judge the prognosis for future seizure recurrence.

After an apparent single seizure, the physician should take a detailed history from the patient and any available collateral historians about the presenting event. Although serum laboratory values are frequently obtained after a first seizure, these tests actually have little value in the diagnosis of most uncomplicated first seizures in adolescents and adults. Electrolytes and complete blood count may assure overall general health and serve as a baseline prior to contemplation of antiepileptic drug therapy. A serum or urine drug screen is often appropriate to exclude drug abuse or intoxication as a cause of provoked seizures in adolescents and adults.

The two most important diagnostic tests in the initial evaluation of new-onset seizures are a magnetic resonance image (MRI) of the brain and an EEG; the former provides a measure of structure and the latter a complementary measure of function. A computed tomography (CT) of the head is insufficient to disclose subtle epileptogenic pathology in the brain. The only reason to obtain a head CT after a new-onset seizure is for emergency exclusion of acute neurologic catastrophes requiring urgent attention, such as cerebral hemorrhage or infarction. If a patient has recovered to baseline and neurologic examination is normal, head CT can often be deferred if a definitive brain MRI and neurologic consultation may be obtained promptly (i.e., within 1 week following the seizure). If there is a question of head or neck trauma, head CT should be performed emergently, and cervical radiographs may be necessary. EEG is particularly valuable when brain MRI is normal because it may disclose functional evidence for a heightened epileptogenic potential by demonstrating interictal epileptiform discharges that help determine risk of seizure recurrence after a single seizure or diagnose the epilepsy syndrome when there have been recurrent spells.

Additional diagnostic studies such as ictal video-EEG monitoring, positron emission tomography (PET) of the brain, magnetoencephalography (MEG), and neuropsychological testing may be used later in the course of a patient's evaluation if empirical medical therapy is unsuccessful and if surgical candidacy is questioned, but they are of generally limited value in new-onset seizure disorders. V-EEG is appropriate when psychogenic nonepileptic spells are the suspected diagnosis to exclude epilepsy and to allow prompt triage to appropriate psychological care, thereby sparing the patient from an errant diagnosis and the potential risks of unnecessary antiepileptic drug therapy.

The risk of seizure recurrence following a single seizure is approximately 30% when both MRI and EEG are normal. Multiple seizures occurring over a single day should still be considered as a single seizure episode. The risk of recurrence following a second remote seizure is variable, ranging from roughly 50-80%. Evidence is conflicting on the precise prognostic value of an abnormal EEG following a first seizure, but most experts consider EEG abnormalities to raise the risk of seizure recurrence substantially, especially when the EEG shows generalized epileptiform discharges.

Following a second unprovoked seizure, most experts diagnose epilepsy and recommend treatment. Treatment may be considered even following a first seizure if a structural cortical lesion is found because the risk of seizure recurrence is more than 50% in such instances, or if the patient leads a lifestyle where a second seizure would be highly undesirable (such as dependency on driving or a risky occupation).

All patients with new-onset epilepsy must be counseled regarding safety and driving. All patients with consciousness-impairing seizures should be instructed to avoid work, hobbies, or sports activities exposing them to heightened risk of personal injury until seizures are controlled for at least 3 to 6 months. Driving is a critical personal and public safety concern with legal implications to both patient and physician. Because laws vary between states, clinicians must ensure intimate familiarity with the law governing epilepsy in their own jurisdiction and counsel patients appropriately, then document their discussion in the medical record. A few states require physicians to report epilepsy patients.

CHRONIC EPILEPSY CARE AND DETERMINATION OF REFRACTORY EPILEPSY

The approach to the patient with chronic epilepsy is to determine whether the epilepsy is benign or refractory (also known as medically intractable, pharmacoresistant). Following from the tenet in new-onset epilepsy evaluation, determination of the patient's epilepsy syndrome directs the choice of AED therapy most likely to control seizures successfully and allows prognosis for future remission or commitment to long-term AED therapy. Symptomatic or cryptogenic partial or generalized epilepsies and juvenile myoclonic epilepsy rarely remit and usually require long-term AED treatment. Idiopathic partial epilepsy or unclassified epilepsy syndromes more frequently remit after 2 to 5 years of treatment, suggesting future AED withdrawal is worth considering. Drug withdrawal is a complicated decision that is best made in consultation with a neurologist.

Determination of the epilepsy syndrome is more readily achieved during longitudinal continuity of care, given information derived from observations of seizure episodes and further opportunities to obtain interictal or ictal EEG recordings. With repeated or prolonged interictal EEG recording, the yield of identifying interictal epileptiform discharges increases. However, even after repeated outpatient EEGs, or with intensive inpatient V-EEG recording, approximately 20% of those with eventually proven epilepsy lack definite interictal EEG abnormalities. It is important to realize that the diagnosis of epilepsy remains at heart a clinical determination. The absence of abnormalities on MRI or interictal laboratory EEGs does not exclude an epilepsy diagnosis. If MRI or EEG has not been performed prior to evaluation, it is helpful to begin with these investigations to determine the patient's epilepsy syndrome and to exclude symptomatic pathology. Inpatient V-EEG is the gold standard for establishing a diagnosis of epilepsy and should be considered when patients are refractory to one to two empirical AED treatment trials. Even if a patient has infrequent seizures while maintained on AED therapy, admitting patients to an epilepsy monitoring unit allows an opportunity for withdrawal of medication in a safe, carefully supervised environment with a goal of increasing seizure frequency so that one or more habitual clinical seizures may be recorded. Ambulatory EEG or outpatient V-EEG are also available at many centers but have lower yield, given limitations of the inability to withdraw AEDs safely, to conduct behavioral testing or capture video, and to accomplish a technically adequate recording.

Patients continuing to experience breakthrough seizures may have refractory epilepsy. Just more than 10% of patients who have an efficacy failure on their first AED ever become seizure free during future AED trials, suggesting the need for vigilance toward achieving the clinical goals of seizure freedom without AED side effects. If a patient fails to achieve seizure freedom following one to two AED monotherapy trials, referral to a comprehensive epilepsy center should be strongly considered to permit appropriate seizure classification and consideration of surgical options.

Approximately one-third of those with epilepsy, approximately 750,000 in the United States, have medically refractory epilepsy (i.e., epilepsy that is resistant to AEDs with continued breakthrough seizures and intolerable AED adverse effects). Those afflicted with refractory epilepsy consistently report lower quality of life for multiple reasons, including lost productivity at work or school, inability to drive, self-injury, and the fear of living with the constant uncertainty of when their next seizure may occur. Even more alarming, growing evidence indicates that patients with refractory epilepsy are at a heightened risk for mortality from sudden unexplained death in epilepsy (SUDEP). Even in patients who are well controlled on their drug treatment, approximately half of those surveyed are not satisfied with their current regimen of AEDs, in most instances because of unpleasant or disabling drug-related side effects. A determination of refractory epilepsy from breakthrough seizures or intolerable AED adverse effects should be made relatively early in the course of treatment to permit other potentially more effective care options to be considered. Because of the limitations of current AEDs, both patients and their physicians may be lulled into a dangerous complacency by the desperation of chronic refractory epilepsy, perhaps figuring that any further efforts toward improvement of the situation will prove futile. However, given the severe morbidity and potential mortality of refractory epilepsy, clinicians must aspire beyond the status quo of a so-called acceptable seizure burden and educate their patients that intensive evaluation may lead to more effective treatment for their seizures. Patients who may benefit from referral to a comprehensive epilepsy center include those with these situations:

- An uncertain diagnosis of spells (i.e., the diagnosis of epilepsy is still in question)
- Failure to achieve complete seizure control
- Adverse effects on current AED therapy
- Injury from their seizures
- Lost productivity at work or school because of seizures or adverse effects
- A complicated regimen of concurrent medications and/or other confounding medical, psychiatric, or psychosocial conditions

Epilepsy Therapies

The goals of all epilepsy therapies are to achieve seizure freedom without adverse effects of treatment. Choosing between the numerous options available for epilepsy treatment can be daunting for physicians and patients alike. The last two decades have seen the release of a number of newer AEDs into clinical use, many of which offer improved tolerability and safety profiles. Another advent is vagus nerve stimulation (VNS), the first device using the novel approach of electrical stimulation in epilepsy approved by the Food and Drug Administration (FDA). Centers offering expert evaluation for epilepsy surgery have also become more widely available.

Guidelines for choosing among epilepsy therapies are currently lacking. Until evidence-based guidelines are developed, optimal therapeutic triage must be highly individualized by synthesizing available data, clinical wisdom, and the patient's preference.

All AEDs have the potential to cause dose-related neurotoxic adverse effects. Fortunately, these may be obviated in most patients by dose reduction or substituting for a better tolerated AED.

ANTIEPILEPTIC DRUG THERAPY

Table 4 itemizes specific AEDs with accompanying information on clinical spectrum of uses, pharmacokinetics, typical dosing and blood levels, and cardinal adverse effects. There are currently no clear evidence-based algorithms to guide the temporal sequencing of different AED trials. Nonetheless, common treatment principles

TABLE 4 Properties of the AEDs

	Spectrum of Effect	Daily Adult Dosage/Interval	Usual Level (µg/mL)	Adverse Effects	Idiosyncratic Toxicities	Interactions
Older AEDs						
Carbamazepine (Tegretol)	Partial	400–1600+ mg (bid-qid)	4–12+	Diplopia, dizziness, ataxia, hyponatremia	Yes	Bidirectional (AEDs, OC, AC, many)
Ethosuximide (Zarontin)	Absence	500–1500+ mg (bid)	40–100+	Nausea, sedation	Yes	Unidirectional
Phenobarbital	Partial	90–180+ mg (qd)	15–40	Sedation, psychomotor slowing	Yes	Bidirectional (AEDs, OC, AC, many)
Phenytoin (Dilantin)	Partial	200–400+ mg (qd–bid)	8–20+	Sedation, dizziness, ataxia, gingival hyperplasia	Yes	Bidirectional (AEDs, OC, AC, many)
Primidone (Mysoline)	Partial	500–1500+ mg (bid–tid)	5–12 (measure phenobarbital)	Sedation, psychomotor slowing	Yes	Bidirectional (AEDs, OC, AC, many)
Valproate (Depakene)	Broad	750–2500+ mg (qd–tid)	50–100+	Nausea, tremor, hair loss, weight gain	Yes	Bidirectional (AEDs)
Newer AEDs						
Felbamate (Felbatol)	Broad	1800–4800+ mg (bid–tid)	30–100+	Irritability, insomnia, weight loss	Yes	Bidirectional (AEDs, OC, AC)
Gabapentin (Neurontin)	Partial	900–3600+ mg (tid–qid)	4–20++	Sedation, dizziness, weight gain	No	None
Lacosamide	Partial (? Broad)	200–600 mg	?	Sedation, fatigue	? (None in clinical trials)	None known
Lamotrigine (Lamictal)	Broad	300–600+ mg (qd–bid)	1–20+	Dizziness, rash	Yes	Bidirectional (AEDs, OC)
Levetiracetam (Keppra)	Broad	1000–3000++ mg (bid)	5–40++	Sedation, dizziness	No	None
Oxcarbazepine (Trileptal)	Partial	600–3600+ mg (bid)	10–40+ (MHD)	Sedation, dizziness	Yes	Bidirectional (AEDs, OC)
Pregabalin (Lyrica)	Partial	150–600+ mg (bid)	2–10	Sedation, dizziness, weight gain	No	None
Retigabine	Partial	600–1200+	?	Dizziness, somnolence, confusion, incoordination	?	?
Tiagabine (Gabitril)	Partial	16–64 mg (bid–tid)	100–300 µg/mL	Sedation, weight gain	No	Unidirectional
Topiramate (Topamax)	Broad	100–600+ mg (qd–bid)	10–20+	Sedation, cognitive complaints, paresthesias, weight loss, rare nephrolithiasis	No	Bidirectional (AEDs, OC at high doses)
Vigabatrin (Sabril)	Partial/ infantile spasms	2000–4000+mg/d	?	Somnolence, fatigue, weight gain, behavioral disturbances	Visual field deficit	Unidirectional
Zonisamide (Zonegran)	Broad	100–600+ mg (qd–bid)	10–40+	Sedation, paresthesias, weight loss, rare nephrolithiasis	Yes	Unidirectional

Notes: AED = antiepileptic drug; + = higher doses/levels often additionally effective, as tolerated; ++ = considerably higher doses/levels sometimes additionally effective in intractable patients, as tolerated; MHD = 10, 11 Monohydroxy derivative active metabolite of oxcarbazepine. Interactions: Unidirectional indicates that other AEDs or drugs may affect this AED; bidirectional indicates that other drugs may affect this AED, and this AED affects other drugs; OC = oral contraceptives, AC = anticoagulants; many = many other non-AEDs.
? = Available information incomplete and based on pre-marketing published data from clinical trials.

underlie the choosing, dosing, sequencing, and monitoring of AED therapy in epilepsy care. Here are several basic principles:

- Choose AED therapy appropriate for the epilepsy syndrome.
- Consider patient characteristics and co-morbidities when choosing AEDs.
- Employ AED monotherapy at the lowest effective dosage to achieve seizure freedom.
- Reserve AED polytherapy (combining two or more AEDs) for refractory patients and minimize total drug load to limit adverse effects.
- Treat according to the patient's clinical response, not the AED level.
- Monitor for long-term complications of older AED therapy and consider withdrawal of therapy when appropriate.
- Choose affordable AED therapy.

Choosing an AED appropriate for the patient's epilepsy syndrome is an important tenet of epilepsy care. AEDs have different spectrums of efficacy for various seizure types within epilepsy syndromes. Some AEDs are narrow in their spectrum of efficacy, whereas others are broader, treating a variety of different seizure types well. Broad-spectrum AEDs may be favored when the epilepsy syndrome diagnosis is ambiguous because they offer potential efficacy against most seizure types and have less potential to aggravate some epilepsy syndromes. To some degree, the spectrum of efficacy of an AED is related to its postulated mechanism of action. AEDs that chiefly antagonize sodium channel ionophores or promote γ-aminobutyric acid (GABAergic) neurotransmission are generally most effective in partial-onset seizures, whereas drugs that combine these and other mechanisms of action may have broader efficacy in primary generalized seizure types.

Evidence from prospective, blinded, randomized clinical trials is only available for certain AEDs for monotherapy use. Gabapentin (Neurontin), oxcarbazepine (Trileptal), and lamotrigine (Lamictal) possess randomized controlled trial evidence for monotherapy treatment of partial-onset seizures, and topiramate (Topamax) has evidence for monotherapy use in new-onset epilepsy. All older AEDs and other newer AEDs have either comparator trial or anecdotal monotherapy evidence. All marketed newer AEDs have randomized controlled trial evidence for use as adjunctive treatment in partial-onset seizures, whereas older AEDs have comparator trial evidence.

Patient characteristics and co-morbidities may affect the choice of an AED. For example, weight is an important consideration. Valproate (Depakene), pregabalin (Lyrica), and carbamazepine (Tegretol) may contribute to weight gain, whereas topiramate (Topamax) and zonisamide (Zonegran) may include weight loss among their adverse effect profile. The patient with both epilepsy and migraine might favor topiramate or valproate, drugs that are efficacious for both conditions.

In general, AED monotherapy is just as effective—or more effective—than polytherapy. Monotherapy limits the potential for adverse effects and drug interactions. AED dosing must be individualized to achieve optimal results. Our strategy is to titrate the AED toward a target dose that has proven effective for most individuals in clinical studies and in our experience. Dose adjustment can then be made in the event of adverse drug reactions or recurrent seizures. If the endpoint of seizure freedom is preserved, maintaining a lower but clinically therapeutic AED dosage is entirely acceptable. If a patient continues to experience breakthrough seizures, raising the AED dose to the maximal dose tolerated is sometimes necessary, although recent evidence demonstrates that only a minority of patients become seizure free when dosed above the usual therapeutic range, so a practical viewpoint of treatment futility should be realized when patients experience frequent breakthrough seizures despite adequate AED dosages. Therapeutic change should be made when seizure freedom is not maintained at AED doses effective for most patients. Overlapping AEDs in transitional polytherapy (where the baseline AED is maintained at the current dose to limit breakthrough seizures, the newly added AED is titrated to a protective dose, then the original drug is tapered and discontinued) is the preferred method when introducing a new AED monotherapy. Abruptly stopping the existing AED increases the risk of seizures (and perhaps status epilepticus), whereas introducing the new AED too rapidly may induce adverse effects that taint the patient's perception of what could be an effective therapy.

Many medically refractory epilepsy patients require chronic polytherapy. Overall, only a small minority of refractory patients can be rendered seizure free with AED polytherapy, but they may benefit substantially by reduction of seizure burden. Although no good evidence for specific AED polytherapy combinations exists, augmenting monotherapy with an AED offering a different or complementary mechanism of action may be considered. Great care must be taken to avoid excessive drug dosing and drug–drug interactions. Initiating and maintaining AED polytherapy is difficult and requires oversight by a neurologist with extensive knowledge of clinical pharmacology.

AED dosing should be adjusted to achieve the clinical goals of seizure freedom without adverse effects. This may indeed be a delicate balancing act for some patients because all AEDs have the potential to cause dose-related so-called neurotoxic adverse effects. Fortunately, adverse effects may be obviated in most patients by dose reduction or substituting for a better tolerated AED.

Philosophies on the use of AED blood level monitoring differ, but most agree that blood levels should in most cases be considered only a guideline to treatment. AED levels should not be perceived as an absolute indication for altering AED dosing, divorced from clinical judgment of the patient's seizure control or adverse effects. Blood-level monitoring can help guide therapy, but so-called therapeutic levels are derived from treatment of populations. An individual patient may require a lower or higher intensity of AED therapy to achieve optimal results. For example, some patients develop breakthrough seizures even at supratherapeutic or toxic levels, others may experience adverse effects within the usual therapeutic range, whereas some patients become seizure-free on levels in a subtherapeutic range. The danger of overreliance on AED blood levels is twofold: levels may lead both physicians and patients to a false sense of therapeutic adequacy or may lead to errant manipulation of AEDs in patients who require no adjustments. Typical clinical scenarios where clinicians should obtain AED levels include the following:

1. After reaching steady-state administration of an AED, to establish a patient's individual personal baseline against which future comparisons can be made in event of breakthrough seizures.
2. While titrating individual AEDs in complex polypharmacy regimens, when drug interactions may influence either the new adjunctive AED or baseline antiepileptic and other medications.
3. Adjusting for alterations in AED metabolism during aging, disease states, and during each trimester of pregnancy when AED levels can fluctuate substantially based on altered drug absorption, metabolism, protein binding, and clearance. With some heavily protein-bound drugs, especially phenytoin (Dilantin), obtaining free drug levels is necessary to discern the biologically active fraction of the drug, especially in chronically or critically ill patients.
4. When trying to determine the AED responsible for adverse effects in a patient receiving polytherapy.

In summary, AED levels are most useful when testing a clinical hypothesis. We discourage the use of routine or scheduled levels, an exception being chronic phenytoin therapy in institutionalized patients (where zero-order kinetics from nonlinear hepatic metabolism may lead to drug accumulation and toxicity).

With chronic AED therapy, intermittent blood testing for monitoring of liver function tests and hematologic functions is reasonable although not of proven value. The highest risk of idiosyncratic reactions associated with AEDs such as serious rash, hepatotoxicity, and hematologic dyscrasias is during the first 6 to 12 months of therapy and extremely rare thereafter. There is, however, mounting concern that patients on chronic maintenance therapy with older AEDs are at risk for osteopenia and osteoporosis. Any enzyme-inducing AED (carbamazepine [Tegretol], phenytoin [Dilantin], phenobarbital, primidone [Mysoline], and oxcarbazepine [Trileptal]) has the potential to decrease bone density. Valproate (Depakote) may also lead to decreased bone density. Chronic phenytoin exposure is of particular concern, given its rare association with cosmetic adverse effects including gingival hyperplasia (which may be severe enough to warrant repeated gingivectomies), peripheral neuropathy, and irreversible cerebellar ataxia. Considering AED withdrawal in appropriate candidates or transition to another newer AED therapy without such untoward effects is often reasonable.

AED cost is a crucial social issue that may trump all other medical principles in selection and maintenance of AED therapy in patients who lack adequate medical insurance. Choosing expensive AEDs that a patient cannot afford may erode the patient's adherence to treatment and trust in the physician. Insurance and financial status must therefore be considered, so that available resources (i.e., indigent federal- or state-sponsored insurance or corporate pharmaceutical assistance programs) can be summoned if a prohibitively expensive newer AED is the best therapeutic choice. Some of the patents of newer AEDs will expire by publication of this book, leading to increased availability of generic drug formulations that could reduce the impact of medication cost, but the pharmacokinetic reliability of these generic formulations must also be established before their widespread use is recommended.

Withdrawal from chronic AEDs is a difficult consideration in the older adolescent or adult with epilepsy because seizure recurrence may impact driving and work abilities. In general, it is worthwhile to consider an attempt at withdrawing AED therapy when the patient has been seizure free for an arbitrary period between 2 and 5 years. Available data suggest that approximately 25% to 70% of patients experience seizure recurrence with AED withdrawal. The decision to withdraw AED therapy must be discussed in the context of the patient's lifestyle and responsibilities because driving and work considerations may be paramount and trump the medical prognosis. Neurologic consultation should be strongly considered when AED withdrawal is contemplated.

EPILEPSY SURGERY

Evaluation for epilepsy surgery should be strongly considered in patients with refractory partial epilepsy. A syndrome particularly amenable to surgical intervention is mesial temporal-lobe epilepsy (MTLE), characterized by medically refractory complex partial seizures, often a history of complex febrile seizures in infancy, and hippocampal sclerosis on brain MRI.

Resective surgery for epilepsy has been performed for over a century, and advances in EEG and neuroimaging have increased the widespread application of epilepsy surgery. A pivotal clinical trial established the clear superiority of anterior temporal lobectomy over medical therapy for chronically refractory MTLE in carefully selected patients.

Identification of potential candidates for epilepsy surgery remains the biggest challenge for tertiary care epilepsy centers. Some have estimated that nearly 75,000 potential surgical candidates in the United States remain under care in primary care settings with ongoing seizures, yet only 3000 or fewer surgical procedures for epilepsy are performed annually.

Potential candidates for resective epilepsy surgery have refractory epilepsy with ongoing seizures that have been resistant to at least two to three appropriately administered AEDs. The precise seizure burden meriting an aggressive, invasive approach remains a subject of conjecture, but even one to two consciousness-impairing seizures annually may be highly disabling in patients who aspire to work and drive.

The basic approach in epilepsy surgery involves identification and precise localization of the epileptogenic zone, the region of the brain that is necessary and sufficient to cause clinical seizures; determining whether the patient possesses appropriate functional reserve for safe removal of that seizure focus; and subsequent operative resection of this area.

A variety of investigations must be performed at specialized comprehensive epilepsy centers to determine if epilepsy surgery would be effective and safe for an individual patient. The most useful and important initial investigations are a high-resolution volumetric brain MRI (with thin cut coronal plane acquisition perpendicular to the hippocampal long axis) and inpatient prolonged ictal V-EEG monitoring that permits intimate correlation and offline, post hoc detailed analysis of the ictal behavior and EEG to localize the patient's habitual clinical seizures. Additional techniques that help localize the epileptic focus preoperatively include functional imaging techniques such as single photon emission computed tomography (SPECT) and PET, magnetoencephalography, and neuropsychological testing. An intracarotid sodium amytal test is necessary in most patients to lateralize memory functions accurately and estimate functional reserve prior to surgery. In some cases, invasive EEG recording with surgically implanted subdural or parenchymal strips or grids of electrodes is necessary to confirm the seizure focus precisely and allow mapping of eloquent functional cerebral cortex to reduce operative morbidity.

When a structural epileptogenic mesial temporal brain lesion evident on MRI is concordant with well-localized habitual clinical seizures by ictal V-EEG, there is a 60% to 90% chance that surgery will produce seizure freedom. Resection in neocortical epilepsies offers a 30% to 80% chance of achieving a seizure-free outcome, depending largely on whether a MRI lesion concordant with the seizure focus is present. Surgical efficacy contrasts with a 5% or less chance that additional AED therapy will render the refractory patient seizure free. Favorable seizure outcome must be balanced with a 3% or less risk of major morbidity (i.e., hemorrhage, infection, stroke, memory, language, or hemianopic visual field deficit) incurred by surgery. Risk may be higher in extratemporal epilepsy surgery for postoperative motor, sensory, and visual deficits, depending on the location of the seizure focus. Memory or language deficits may occur in temporal lobe operations.

OTHER ALTERNATIVE THERAPIES

Some patients with refractory partial epilepsy are not suitable epilepsy surgical candidates because of diffuse or unlocalizable epileptic foci, whereas others may choose not to undergo brain surgery despite suitable candidacy. In these cases, other options may still exist.

The vagus nerve stimulator (VNS) is the only electrical device currently approved as an adjunctive treatment for partial-onset seizures. A battery-operated generator and programmable computerized stimulator are placed surgically in a subcutaneous pocket on the left anterior chest. The device looks much like a cardiac pacemaker and has electrical leads connected to the left vagus nerve in the neck. Once implanted, the device is programmed by means of a radiofrequency wand in the physician's office and provides a small electrical current to the nerve at preset intervals and amounts. The patient also has the opportunity to trigger a stronger current to attempt to abort or lessen an oncoming seizure by means of a magnet that is passed externally over the device.

The efficacy of VNS for seizure reduction is roughly comparable to that of AEDs; approximately 40% of patients experience a 50% or greater reduction in their seizures, and up to 15% of patients become seizure free. Although there are no current evidence-based guidelines for the best timing of VNS placement, we reserve VNS for patients who are not resective surgery candidates or who refuse surgery and those who have failed most older and newer AEDs. In addition to reducing seizure burden, VNS may improve a patient's quality of life by improving alertness, mood, and memory. Predictors of which patients are most likely to benefit from VNS, and the optimal dosing of the device once it is implanted, are yet to be defined in prospective clinical trials. Additional neurostimulation therapies are being evaluated. The efficacy and safety of more specific neurostimulation modalities such as deep brain and cortical stimulation therapies are currently being evaluated in large randomized clinical trials. Two recent randomized controlled trials of transcranial magnetic stimulation (TMS) have yielded conflicting findings concerning efficacy; one study targeting patients with MRI-visible cortical malformations demonstrated TMS efficacy for seizure reduction.

Specialized diets may be a useful adjunctive treatment for epilepsy. The best studied of these is the ketogenic diet, a high-fat, low-protein, low-carbohydrate diet that induces systemic ketosis, which has an antiepileptogenic effect on the brain. The ketogenic diet is most often successfully used in children, but it may also be tried in adolescents and adults. Unfortunately, unless rigid compliance is assured, the ketogenic diet produces little benefit and, in general, most adolescents and adults have limited tolerance of the diet. However, highly motivated and desperately refractory epilepsy patients may benefit from the ketogenic diet. An alternative that is often more tolerable, but not yet robustly studied, is the modified Atkins diet, a high-fat, moderate-protein, low-carbohydrate diet that induces mild ketosis.

Identifying and treating seizure aggravators is an important consideration. Recent studies have suggested that obstructive sleep apnea syndrome (OSAS) is a frequent co-morbidity in refractory epilepsy, and nasal central positive airway pressure in patients with refractory epilepsy and co-morbid OSAS may lead to seizure reduction. Primary sleep disorders such as restless legs syndrome and periodic limb movements of sleep may fragment sleep and worsen seizure burden in patients with refractory epilepsy. If a primary sleep disorder is suspected, a diagnostic polysomnogram should be ordered, and aggressive treatment for the sleep disorder should be initiated.

Although most complementary and alternative therapies in epilepsy have not been rigorously studied, a variety of behavioral stress reduction techniques, meditation, yoga, or naturopathic treatments may be considered. Most of these therapies have few risks and occasionally benefit individual patients. Botanical extracts for epilepsy therapy that possess potent in vitro antiepileptogenic properties and wide therapeutic windows are currently being investigated as another avenue of therapy for refractory patients.

STATUS EPILEPTICUS: IDENTIFICATION AND MANAGEMENT

Status epilepticus is a prolonged, unremitting epileptic seizure that constitutes a medical emergency. Until the last decade, status epilepticus was defined as a seizure lasting 30 minutes or longer (from onset through the end of the ictal period, exclusive of the postictal recovery phase that may in itself last well over 30 minutes). However, more recent data suggest that most seizures that self-terminate do so by 3 minutes after onset, indicating that longer lasting seizures are unlikely to stop without intervention.

Status epilepticus may be convulsive or nonconvulsive. Status epilepticus frequently begins with a prolonged generalized tonic–clonic or partial motor seizure, followed by a minimally convulsive or nonconvulsive phase with or without subtle motor features such as facial or eyelid twitching, or nystagmus. Status epilepticus thus evolves in a manner analogous to a lethal cardiac dysrhythmia, proceeding from clinically overt convulsive movements toward an eventual electromechanical dissociative state where the epileptic seizure continues as a subclinical electrographic discharge evident only during EEG monitoring.

Management of status epilepticus begins with securing the airway, respiration, and circulation and placement of two large-bore intravenous catheters for drug administration and fluid resuscitation. Obtaining a stat glucose is appropriate before rapid administration of thiamine, followed by intravenous dextrose (to avoid Wernicke encephalopathy in malnourished patients). If intravenous access is not readily available, rectal diazepam (Diastat) or intramuscular fosphenytoin (Cerebyx) can be used. Rectal diazepam is also useful in the out-of-hospital treatment of prolonged seizures or seizure clusters in adolescents and adults, potentially obviating escalation into status epilepticus and preventing an emergency department visit.

Initial pharmacotherapy of status epilepticus begins with intravenous lorazepam (Ativan) given at 2 mg/minute to a goal of 0.1 mg/kg (or 8 mg total) with cautious respiratory monitoring, then loading with phenytoin (Dilantin) at 20 mg/kg, given no faster than 50 mg/minute to avoid hypotension, with ECG and hemodynamic monitoring. Phenytoin should be given through a dedicated peripheral intravenous line because of potential for cardiotoxicity and to avoid precipitation by other drugs. Intravenous phenytoin, a highly insoluble alkaline solution, may lead to substantial soft-tissue toxicity (including the much feared purple-glove phenomenon). An alternative is fosphenytoin, which may be administered at up to 150 mg/min, and is not associated with tissue injury if extravasation occurs.

The success of treatment of status epilepticus can be measured clinically, but if the patient remains unresponsive after the convulsive movements stop, an urgent EEG may be needed to exclude nonconvulsive status epilepticus. Refractory status epilepticus can be treated with midazolam (Versed),[1] propofol (Diprivan),[1] pentobarbital (Nembutal), sodium pentothal (Thiopental), or phenobarbital.[1] Case series reports suggest that intravenous valproate and levetiracetam may also be tried. An advantage of short-acting agents such as midazolam and propofol is the rapidity with which pharmacologically induced coma can be reversed to examine the patient, whereas valproate and levetiracetam offer the advantage of avoiding hemodynamic or respiratory complications. An expanding armamentarium for status epilepticus is expected, in that intravenous forms of the novel drug lacosamide and the older AED, carbamazepine, are currently being developed.

Conclusion

Epilepsy is characterized by recurrent, spontaneous seizures. Epilepsy has many causes and represents a collection of syndromes that have varying natural histories and responses to therapy. Diagnosis is based on the history and may be supported by physical examination. The two most important investigations in initial evaluation of the patient with new-onset seizures or epilepsy are high-resolution brain MRI and EEG. There are many mimickers of epilepsy requiring careful differential diagnosis. When confronted with spells of an uncertain type, evaluation with VEEG may secure the correct diagnosis.

The past decade has seen tremendous expansion in available AED therapies, many of which are more tolerable and safer for long-term use. Choice of AED in an individual patient depends on the epilepsy syndrome, consideration of available efficacy evidence, patient characteristics and co-morbidities, and cost. AED monitoring should reinforce, and not replace, clinical judgment. Chronic complications of certain older AEDs may include osteopenia, adverse cosmetic effects, weight gain, and neuropathy. Withdrawal of AEDs in selected seizure-free patients or transition to AEDs without chronic toxicities should be considered in such instances.

Unfortunately, despite advances in available AEDs, more than a third of patients with epilepsy are refractory. Early determination of refractory epilepsy and triage to intensive diagnostic and therapeutic resources at a comprehensive epilepsy care center is critical. Epilepsy surgery may render carefully selected patients seizure free, and VNS is a viable alternative when surgery is not possible, leading to reduced seizure burden and improved quality of life. Physicians should approach their patients with epilepsy with enthusiasm and hope for effecting an improvement in their condition.

---

[1]Not FDA approved for this indication.

REFERENCES

French JA, Kanner AM, Bautista J, et al: Efficacy and tolerability of the new antiepileptic drugs: I. Treatment of new-onset epilepsy: Report of the Therapeutics and Technology Assessment Subcommittee and Quality Standards Subcommittee of the American Academy of Neurology and the American Epilepsy Society. Neurology 2004;62(8):1252-1260.

French JA, Kanner AM, Bautista J, et al: Therapeutics and Technology Assessment Subcommittee of the American Academy of Neurology; Quality Standards Subcommittee of the American Academy of Neurology; American Epilepsy Society. Efficacy and tolerability of the new antiepileptic drugs: II. Treatment of refractory epilepsy: Report of the Therapeutics and Technology Assessment Subcommittee and Quality Standards Subcommittee of the American Academy of Neurology and the American Epilepsy Society. Neurology 2004;62(8):1261-1273.

Kwan P, Brodie MJ: Early identification of refractory epilepsy. N Engl J Med 2000;342(5):314-319.

St. Louis EK, Gidal BE, Henry TR, et al: Conversions between monotherapies in epilepsy: Expert consensus. Epilepsy and Behavior 2007;11(2):222-234.

Wiebe S, Blume WT, Girvin JP, Eliasziw M: A randomized, controlled trial of surgery for temporal-lobe epilepsy. N Engl J Med 2001; 345:311-318.

Epilepsy in Infants and Children

Method of
Mary Zupanc, MD

Epilepsy is defined as two or more unprovoked seizures. A seizure is the result of an abnormal synchronous depolarization of a group of neurons. The clinical manifestations of a seizure depend on where in the brain the discharges begin and how they spread.

Epilepsy is a common medical condition, occurring in 0.5% to 1% of all children. Each year 150,000 children and adolescents in the United States have a single unprovoked seizure. One fifth of those, or 30,000, eventually develop epilepsy. The highest incidence of epilepsy is during the first year of life.

Appropriate classification of epilepsy is the cornerstone of therapy. Most children with epilepsy are seizure-free with the use of one antiepileptic drug (AED) without side effects. Some epileptic children, approximately 15%, have medically refractory seizures.

Classification

In any evaluation of a child who might have had a seizure, the first job of the physician is to determine whether the event was indeed an epileptic seizure or some other paroxysmal event. The history is the key to differentiating between these episodes and epileptic seizures.

There are many different types of paroxysmal events in children that can mimic seizures (Box 1). For example, pallid or cyanotic breath-holding spells can result in brief generalized tonic–clonic seizures. Pallid breath-holding spells are precipitated by excitement, surprise, or trivial head trauma, resulting in an exaggerated vasovagal event with concomitant bradycardia and central nervous system (CNS) ischemia. If the event is sufficiently prolonged, the child might have a brief seizure. Cyanotic breath-holding spells, on the other hand, are prolonged crying episodes, often stimulated by frustration or anger, resulting in an involuntary inability to breathe, with concomitant cyanosis, decreased oxygen concentration, and hypercapnia. This is typically followed by a brief loss of consciousness; sometimes a brief generalized tonic–clonic seizure follows. These episodes must be distinguished from the unprovoked seizures characteristic of epilepsy. Breath-holding spells do dissipate in the preschool years and do not need to be treated with AEDs.

Other paroxysmal events that can resemble seizures include motor tics; vasovagal syncope; shuddering attacks, a rare condition associated with tremor or shuddering of the upper trunk and shoulders with no alteration of consciousness, occurring in young toddlers and preschoolers; confusional migraines, which can mimic complex partial seizures; sleep disturbances; gastroesophageal reflux, which sometimes produces tonic posturing and can resemble tonic seizures (Sandifer's syndrome); and paroxysmal choreoathetosis or dystonia. There are also patients who have pseudoseizures. Their events can mimic seizures; sometimes they cannot be distinguished from clinical epileptic seizures without performing closed-circuit television electroencephalographic monitoring. Children with pseudoseizures often have complex psychosocial situations and may be victims of either physical or sexual abuse.

If it is determined that a child most likely has epilepsy, the primary physician must determine the appropriate seizure classification and epilepsy syndrome in order to make intelligent decisions with respect to diagnostic studies, treatment, and prognosis. The International League Against Epilepsy has established the International Classification of the Epilepsies and Epileptic Syndromes. This system is used as the foundation for decision making.

In the classification of epilepsy, seizures are divided into two categories, generalized and partial (Box 2). *Generalized seizure* indicates that the clinical seizure does not contain any focal features. Electrographically, the electroencephalogram (EEG) demonstrates generalized spike, polyspike, or sharp wave discharges (or some combination of these) without localizing features over both hemispheres. Clinical seizures of this type are myoclonic, tonic (episodes of tonic posturing), atonic (drop attacks), absence (formerly petit mal), and tonic–clonic (old terminology, grand mal). On the other hand, *partial seizures* are events that begin focally in one part of the brain. The clinical manifestations depend on where in the brain the epileptic discharge begins. A simple partial seizure is a seizure in which there is no associated alteration of consciousness. A simple partial seizure can constitute the aura that patients often refer to before they have more recognizable clinical seizures. As the electrical discharges progress, simple partial seizures typically transform into complex partial seizures. Complex partial seizures are defined as focally generated seizures that are associated with an alteration of consciousness. These seizures can, and often do, generalize to become generalized tonic–clonic seizures. Examples of simple partial seizures include olfactory hallucination, abdominal queasiness, déjà vu, jamais vu, or a tingling sensation in the hands. An example of a complex partial seizure is a paroxysmal episode that begins with staring, drooling, lip smacking automatism, and confusion, lasting 1 to 2 minutes.

In addition to seizure classification, the clinician should be aware of the International Classification of Epilepsy Syndromes. The epilepsy syndromes are determined by further classifying epileptic seizures on the basis of age at onset; seizure type; family history; risk

---

BOX 1 Nonepileptic Events that can be Mistakenly Diagnosed as Epilepsy in Children

Benign paroxysmal vertigo
Breath-holding spells
- Classic (cyanotic)
- Pallid

Paroxysmal choreoathetosis or dystonia
Syncope
Migraine, especially acute confusional
Pseudoseizures
Shuddering spells
Sleep disorders
Tics

BOX 2 Classification of Epileptic Seizures

Partial Seizures

Simple partial seizures
- With motor signs, such as focal clonic activity
- With somatosensory or special-sensory symptoms such as lateralized numbness, tingling, visual or auditory hallucinations, abnormal odors or smells
- With automatic symptoms or signs such as tachycardia, diaphoresis
- With psychic symptoms such as fear, anxiety, déjà vu, jamais vu, confusion

Complex partial seizures
- With simple partial seizures (aura) at onset
- With impairment of consciousness at onset

Partial seizures evolving to secondarily generalized seizures

Generalized Seizures

Absence seizures
Myoclonic seizures
Clonic seizures
Tonic seizures
Tonic–clonic seizures
Atonic seizures

factors for epilepsy; associated neurodevelopmental delays; neuroimaging results; EEG data, both ictal and interictal; other diagnostic tests, such as lumber puncture and metabolic testing; and physical examination. This information can more specifically identify an epileptic condition, resulting in more appropriate management and predictions with respect to prognosis.

Epilepsy Syndromes

The classification of epilepsy syndromes differentiates generalized, localization-related, and undetermined epileptic syndromes, in addition to special syndromes (Box 3). These syndromes are classified into *idiopathic*, implying normal neurologic status and a genetic predisposition; *symptomatic*, implying an underlying lesion or other CNS pathologic condition; and *cryptogenic*, implying that the epileptic condition is probably symptomatic but the exact cause cannot be pinpointed.

GENERALIZED EPILEPSY SYNDROMES

Examples of idiopathic generalized epilepsy syndromes include childhood absence epilepsy, juvenile absence epilepsy, and juvenile myoclonic epilepsy. Childhood absence epilepsy is probably genetically linked to juvenile absence epilepsy and juvenile myoclonic epilepsy. These epilepsy syndromes are most likely different phenotypic expressions of the same gene. These children have normal neurologic examinations and tend to have above-average intelligence. Depending on the age at onset, children and adolescents with these epilepsy syndromes can have a varied clinical manifestation: absence, myoclonic, or generalized tonic–clonic seizures.

Childhood and Juvenile Epilepsy

Childhood absence epilepsy accounts for 2% to 8% of all cases of childhood epilepsy. The age at onset is during elementary school age, and the peak is at 6 to 7 years of age. The seizure semiology is characterized by absence seizures, which are brief episodes of staring, often accompanied by eyelid fluttering, facial clonic activity, or upper extremity myoclonus. These seizures are very brief, lasting only 2 to 10 seconds, occurring multiple times per day and without a concomitant postictal phase. Absence seizures can be induced by hyperventilation. If the epilepsy begins before 9 years of age, the risk of having comorbid generalized tonic–clonic seizures is only 16%. If the epilepsy begins later, the risk of generalized tonic–clonic seizures is close to 50%. Myoclonic seizures are rare.

Juvenile absence epilepsy is associated with absence seizures and generalized tonic–clonic seizures. The age at onset is prepubertal, usually between 10 and 15 years of age. Absence seizures occur in all patients; generalized tonic–clonic seizures occur in almost 80%.

With juvenile myoclonic epilepsy, the age at onset is typically during adolescence, between 12 and 18 years of age. The characteristic clinical symptom is early morning sudden myoclonic jerks of the shoulders and arms. Ninety percent of patients have generalized tonic–clonic seizures, and 33% have absence seizures.

The interictal EEG in all cases demonstrates generalized spike and slow-wave discharges. With the earlier onset, the generalized spike and slow-wave discharges are at 3 cycles per second (cps). With juvenile myoclonic epilepsy, the generalized discharges consist of generalized polyspike, spike, and slow-wave discharges at 4 to 5 cps.

The treatment for these three epilepsy syndromes is similar. Valproate (Depakote) is the drug of choice for patients with both absence and generalized tonic–clonic seizures, except in girls of reproductive age (see later). Ethosuximide (Zarontin) can be used if the patient is having only absence seizures. Preliminary clinical research indicates that lamotrigine (Lamictal) may be very effective in these epilepsy syndromes. Lamotrigine is approved as adjunctive therapy for generalized tonic–clonic seizures in children older than 2 years. Topiramate (Topamax) also shows promise in treating generalized tonic–clonic seizures and myoclonus but not with absence seizures. Levetiracetam (Keppra)[1] is also being studied to determine its efficacy with respect to absence seizures. Levetiracetam is approved as adjunctive therapy for myoclonic seizures in juvenile myoclonic epilepsy in adolescents 12 years and older. Levetiracetam is also approved as adjunctive therapy for primary generalized tonic clonic seizures in the idiopathic generalized epilepsy syndromes in children and adolescents 6 years and older.

The prognosis varies, depending on the age at onset. Juvenile myoclonic epilepsy requires lifelong treatment because of the high rate of relapse when AED therapy is discontinued. On the other hand, childhood absence epilepsy has a much better prognosis, with more than 50% of patients outgrowing their epilepsy by the age of puberty.

Infantile Spasms

Another generalized epilepsy syndrome is infantile spasms. The incidence of infantile spasms is 1 in 4000 to 6000 live births. The peak age at onset is 4 to 6 months. The seizures are characterized by flexor or extensor (or both) myoclonic spasms, usually occurring in clusters after the infant awakens in the morning or from a nap.

Infantile spasms can be divided into three categories: symptomatic, cryptogenic, and idiopathic. Improvements in neuroimaging and metabolic testing now enable better identification of a specific etiology for infantile spasms. Some of the most common causes of symptomatic infantile spasms include tuberous sclerosis (approximately 25% of patients with tuberous sclerosis have infantile spasms); malformations of cortical development, such as Aicardi's syndrome or malformations in the posterior quadrants of the brain; chromosomal abnormality, one of the most common abnormalities is trisomy 21; inborn errors of metabolism, aminoacidopathies, or mitochondrial cytopathies; asphyxia; meningitis or encephalitis; and trauma.

Interictally, the EEG demonstrates a hypsarrhythmia pattern. This is a markedly abnormal pattern with high amplitude slowing at 1 to 3 cps and multifocal polyspike, spike, and slow-wave discharges.

BOX 3 Classification of Epileptic Syndromes

Localization Related (Focal, Local, Partial)
Benign rolandic epilepsy
Benign occipital epilepsy
Idiopathic
Symptomatic

Generalized

Idiopathic, Age Related
Benign idiopathic convulsions
Benign myoclonic epilepsy in infancy
Benign neonatal familial convulsions
Childhood absence epilepsy
Epilepsy with tonic–clonic seizures on awakening
Juvenile absence epilepsy
Juvenile myoclonic epilepsy

Idiopathic and/or Symptomatic
Epilepsy with myoclonic–astatic seizures
Epilepsy with myoclonic absences
Infantile spasms (West's syndrome)
Lennox–Gastaut syndrome
Symptomatic: early myoclonic encephalopathy

Focal or Generalized (Not Known)
Acquired epileptic aphasia (Landau–Kleffner syndrome)
Epilepsy with continuous spike waves during slow-wave sleep
Neonatal seizures
Severe myoclonic epilepsy in infancy

---

[1] Not FDA approved for this indication.

According to the new practice parameter published by the American Academy of Neurology, the mainstay of treatment for infantile spasms in the United States is corticotropin (ACTH [HP Acthar]).[1] It demonstrates "probable" efficacy, using current evidence-based medicine. The mechanism of action for ACTH remains unclear, but this drug does affect CNS concentration of various biogenic amines and increases γ-aminobutyric acid (GABA)-receptor affinity. It also reduces corticotropin-releasing hormone (CRH), which is elevated in patients with infantile spasms and is a potent proconvulsant. In Europe and Canada, vigabatrin (Sabril),[5] a structural analogue of GABA, is the drug of choice in treating infantile spasms, particularly in children with tuberous sclerosis. Vigabatrin appears to be about 89% to 90% effective in eliminating infantile spasms in children with tuberous sclerosis and infantile spasms. Vigabatrin has not been approved by the FDA because of reports of retinal changes and peripheral visual constriction after long-term use of this drug. Other drugs that have questionable efficacy (due to inadequate evidence) in treating infantile spasms include the benzodiazepines, valproate, zonisamide (Zonegran),[1] topiramate,[1] lamotrigine,[1] and felbamate (Felbatol).[1] The principal deterrent in the use of valproate in these children is the risk of hepatotoxicity.

Lennox–Gastaut Syndrome

Lennox–Gastaut syndrome (LGS) is another generalized epilepsy syndrome, predominantly confined to children. The criteria for the diagnosis of LGS include generalized, multiple seizure types, including tonic, atonic, absence, and myoclonic seizures; an electrographic signature of generalized slow spike and wave discharges at 1½ to 2½ cps; and cognitive impairment. The degree of cognitive impairment is correlated with the underlying substrate of epilepsy and seizure control. As with infantile spasms, LGS can be divided into categories of symptomatic, cryptogenic, and idiopathic. In 30% of patients, infantile spasms evolve to LGS. Therefore, it follows that the two epileptic syndromes have similar underlying etiologies. This epileptic syndrome is often medically intractable.

Relatively few AEDs have been shown to be effective in treating LGS. The ketogenic diet is one of the oldest known treatments for pediatric epilepsy and status epilepticus. It remains a reasonable alternative therapy for LGS. The ketogenic diet consists of a high ratio of fats to carbohydrates and protein. Every piece of food must be carefully weighed and measured for fat, carbohydrate, and protein content so that the proper ratios are maintained. Any deviation from the diet can result in a loss of ketosis and renewed seizures. The exact mechanism by which the ketogenic diet provides seizure control remains unknown. It is presumed that the ketones have anticonvulsant properties. One third to one half of children with LGS have an excellent response to the ketogenic diet, with either a significant reduction in or complete elimination of seizures. Phenobarbital[1] and phenytoin (Dilantin),[1] in part because of their sedative effects, have never been shown to be effective in treating LGS.

The introduction of valproate in the late 1970s provided one of the first effective antiepileptic drugs in treating LGS, based on empiric evidence. There has never been a double-blind, placebo-controlled trial of valproate in treating LGS. The only AEDs that do have evidence to support their use in treating LGS are felbamate, topiramate, and lamotrigine. Felbamate, released in 1993, showed great promise in treating LGS. Unfortunately, it has been associated with an increased risk of aplastic anemia and liver failure. The risk of aplastic anemia is now known to be highest in women with known autoimmune disorders; it has never been reported in a child younger than 13 years. The collective risk is 20 to 207 per million patients treated with this drug. The risk of hepatotoxicity is no greater than that of any of the other AEDs. Felbamate is reserved for patients with severe, intractable epilepsy. It is probably the most effective AED in treating LGS. The benzodiazepines are occasionally helpful in patients with LGS, but only if given intermittently to abort seizure clusters. Otherwise they are too sedating, and many patients develop tachyphylaxis.

LOCALIZATION-RELATED EPILEPSIES

The localization-related epilepsies can also be divided into two categories: symptomatic and idiopathic. The symptomatic localization-related epilepsies are the result of an underlying CNS abnormality, such as tumor, stroke, encephalomalacia from head trauma, hemorrhage, or malformation of cortical development. It is thought that the idiopathic epilepsies have an underlying genetic predisposition.

The most common epilepsy syndrome of childhood is an idiopathic localization-related epilepsy (benign rolandic epilepsy or benign epilepsy of childhood) associated with central-temporal spikes (BECTS). It accounts for 24% of all epileptic seizures in children between the ages of 5 and 14 years. It is genetically determined, probably autosomal dominant with variable penetrance and age-limited expression. The children are neurologically normal. The seizure semiology is characterized by sensorimotor symptoms and clonic activity in the face, arm, or leg, usually with associated hypersalivation and speech arrest. The seizure frequency varies, but typically seizures are rare. They are usually nocturnal, occurring in children in the early morning hours before they awaken or soon after they fall asleep. One known precipitating factor is sleep deprivation.

In benign rolandic epilepsy, the interictal EEG demonstrates drowsiness and sleep-activated central temporal spikes that can be asymmetrical or have a wide field spread. AEDs are seldom used in patients with rare seizures. They may be indicated for patients who are experiencing more frequent seizures that disrupt sleep, school performance, or psychosocial well-being. This epilepsy condition is outgrown in virtually 100% of patients by the time of adolescence.

SPECIAL SYNDROMES

Neonatal Seizures

Neonatal seizures are commonly the result of hypoxic–ischemic injury, hypoglycemia, or hypocalcemia in the perinatal period. Sepsis can also result in seizures. Three rare causes of neonatal seizures include pyridoxine dependency, folinic acid deficiency, and glucose transporter deficiency.

Pyridoxine dependence causes seizures unresponsive to AEDs. It is related to an insufficient production of GABA, a primary inhibitory neurotransmitter. The glucose transporter deficiency is characterized by a low cerebrospinal glucose concentration. There is an enzymatic defect in glucose transport that disrupts facilitative diffusion of glucose across the blood–brain barrier. The seizure semiology is different from that in older children and adolescents. Because of the primitive synaptic network, neonatal seizures can be quite subtle. Examples of neonatal seizures include eye deviation with apnea or multifocal clonic activity. Neonates do not have generalized tonic–clonic seizures, although they can have tonic seizures. There is controversy over whether or not the bicycling movements and lip-smacking seen in neonates are subtle seizures or "brainstem release" phenomena.

The most important therapeutic intervention in neonatal seizures is recognition of the underlying cause, followed by its prompt treatment. This can, in itself, abort any further seizure activity without the use of chronic AEDs. A pyridoxine[1] challenge and treatment with folinic acid (Leucovorin)[1] should be given to any neonate with intractable seizures. For status epilepticus in neonates, the most effective initial therapy is 20 mg/kg of phenobarbital given twice if necessary. Fosphenytoin (Cerebyx)[1] [mc1] at 20 mg/kg can also be used if the phenobarbital is ineffective. However, even when both of these medications have been given for neonatal status epilepticus, the success rate is only 67%. Preliminary studies indicate that intravenous lidocaine (Xylocaine)[1] may be effective for refractory neonatal seizures. The benzodiazepines are less effective in neonates than in older

---

[1]Not FDA approved for this indication.
[5]Investigational drug in the United States.

[1]Not FDA approved for this indication.

infants and children because the GABA receptors are excitatory in neonates, not inhibitory.

Febrile Seizures

Febrile seizures denote a special developmental seizure disorder that is not highly correlated with the development of epilepsy. By definition, a febrile seizure is a generalized tonic–clonic seizure occurring in a child between the ages of 6 months and 5 years and associated with a high fever not related to an underlying CNS infection. Simple febrile seizures carry a low risk of epilepsy (only 1%-2%) compared with the general population's risk of 0.5% to 1%. There is an underlying genetic predisposition, with a positive family history in one third of first-degree relatives. The risk of febrile seizure recurrence is quite high, with 33% of children having at least one recurrence. If a child is younger than 12 months at the time of the first febrile seizure, the risk of recurrence is 50%.

If the history is clear, no diagnostic studies need to be performed, with the exception of a lumbar puncture in infants younger than 18 months. The physician should design the work-up in response to the most likely cause of the fever. If meningitis is suspected at all, a lumbar puncture should be performed. This is particularly true in infants younger than 18 months who present with high fever, because they might not have reliable clinical signs and symptoms of meningismus.

Although phenobarbital[1] was once used to prevent febrile seizure recurrence, this is no longer the standard of care. There is no evidence to suggest that phenobarbital treatment decreases the risk of the development of epilepsy. Furthermore, the side effects of phenobarbital in these children are significant, with more than 40% exhibiting hyperactivity, aggressive behavior, impulsivity, poor attention and concentration, or sleep disturbance. Oral or rectal diazepam (Valium, Diastat) therapy can be given to prevent recurrence of febrile seizures in predisposed children. The dosage of oral diazepam[1] is 0.33 mg/kg every 8 hours during the course of the febrile illness. This medication can produce side effects including sedation and irritability. The dosage of rectal diazepam for patients 2-5 years of age is 0.5 mg/kg. It is usually reserved for febrile seizure recurrence and prolonged febrile seizure (>5 min).

The prognosis for febrile seizures is excellent. Very few children develop epilepsy (1%-2%). Those who have a greater risk for developing epilepsy include children with focal or prolonged febrile seizures, children with a family history of epilepsy, and children with developmental delays and abnormal neurologic examinations. These risk factors suggest that an underlying substrate of epilepsy already exists and that the seizure threshold was simply lowered by the fever.

Landau–Kleffner Syndrome

Landau–Kleffner syndrome (acquired epileptic aphasia) is a poorly understood syndrome that is characterized by a regression in expressive and receptive language in association with an epileptiform EEG, either focal or multifocal. Overt clinical seizures occur in more than 70% of patents; in the remaining 30%, the only ictal manifestation is the deterioration in speech and language. The diagnosis of Landau–Kleffner syndrome is determined solely on the basis of clinical symptoms and EEG finding. Twenty-four-hour EEG monitoring may be helpful in establishing the diagnosis because there is generally activation of the epileptiform discharges during sleep.

The underlying pathophysiology of Landau–Kleffner syndrome remains unknown. The treatment of this syndrome is controversial, in part related to our poor understanding of this disorder. The goal of therapy is normalization of the EEG and improvement in speech and language, although it has still not been determined if the epileptiform discharges produce the symptoms of Landau–Kleffner syndrome or if they simply represent an epiphenomenon. AEDs are used, particularly valproate (Depacon). Steroid therapy has also been tried with some reported success. In refractory cases, multiple subpial transections have been performed over the epileptogenic zone, with only a few reported cases in the literature. A multicenter, double-blind, placebo-controlled treatment trial is needed to determine appropriate and effective therapies. The prognosis for this disorder is variable.

Some clinicians have broadened the definition of Landau–Kleffner syndrome to include children with developmental aphasia and underlying epileptiform EEGs. As a result, some children with autism have been treated with AEDs and even steroids to see whether there would be an improvement in clinical symptoms. This remains an area of considerable controversy. Again, are the epileptiform discharges producing the clinical symptoms or are the epileptiform abnormalities merely an epiphenomenon pointing to an underlying, poorly understood CNS disorder?

Assessment

Appropriate classification of a paroxysmal event is the initial step in the evaluation of a child with a suspected seizure. The history is the key to the diagnosis. Care must be taken to elicit possible precipitating factors and risk factors for epilepsy. Precipitating factors that result in provoked seizures include an underlying CNS infection or head trauma. With breath-holding spells, as mentioned earlier, frustration, anger, surprise, excitement, or trivial head trauma can provoke a spell sometimes followed by a brief generalized tonic–clonic seizure. The risk factors for epilepsy include history of encephalitis or meningitis; history of significant head trauma—associated loss of consciousness, concussion, skull fracture, prolonged coma, or penetrating injury; history of a prolonged febrile seizure lasting longer than 20 minutes; developmental delays; abnormal neurologic examination; and history of asphyxia.

The seizure semiology and its evolution are also very helpful in determining the portion of the brain where the epileptogenic focus resides. Specifically, if the patient typically senses a funny taste or feels queasy before the episode of staring, drooling, and lip smacking automatism, one can surmise that the epileptogenic zone probably resides in either one of the temporal lobes. If the epileptogenic focus is near the sensorimotor cortex, the patient might first experience numbness and tingling in the contralateral extremity followed by rhythmic clonic activity of this same extremity as the epileptogenic discharges spread. Forced head version is a reliable indicator of a contralateral frontal epileptogenic focus.

Home videos of paroxysmal events have proved helpful in appropriately classifying both epileptic and nonepileptic events. An EEG—both awake and asleep—is especially helpful. The presence of focal or generalized epileptiform discharges in the context of an appropriate clinical history is usually sufficient for making the appropriate diagnosis. However, a normal awake and asleep EEG does not exclude the diagnosis of epilepsy, particularly in the face of a compelling history. If the epileptiform discharges are infrequent or deep-seated in the mesial temporal structures, the EEG might not reflect the underlying epileptogenic zone. Untreated generalized epilepsies, however, almost invariably are associated with generalized spike and slow-wave discharges on routine EEGs. Prolonged closed-circuit television EEG monitoring is reserved for patients whose diagnosis is unclear or whose seizures are sufficiently intractable to warrant an evaluation for epilepsy surgery.

If epilepsy is confirmed, depending on the nature of the epilepsy syndrome, further diagnostic studies may be necessary. If the diagnosis is clearly a known benign generalized epileptic syndrome such as childhood absence epilepsy, no further tests are needed and the child can begin AED therapy. If the diagnosis is a localization-related epilepsy, a neuroimaging study is indicated, preferably magnetic resonance imaging (MRI). Computed tomography is inadequate for detecting the underlying substrates of epilepsy. If the epilepsy is thought to be the result of an underlying encephalopathy, metabolic testing and a chromosomal analysis might also need to be performed. In addition, the neurocutaneous syndromes, particularly tuberous sclerosis, are associated with epilepsy. In 25% of patients with tuberous sclerosis, the initial apparent symptom is infantile spasms.

---

[1]Not FDA approved for this indication.

Treatment

Epilepsy is a condition characterized by recurrent seizures. It is not necessary to treat the patient after the first seizure. The chance of seizure recurrence after the first seizure is approximately 30% to 40%. If the EEG demonstrates temporal epileptiform discharges or generalized spike and slow-wave discharges, the chance of recurrence is much higher, bordering on 90%. If a child has a second seizure, the risk of continued seizures is also much higher. Antiepileptic medication is generally recommended after a second seizure. There are exceptions to this, particularly if a benign epilepsy syndrome is identified (e.g., benign rolandic epilepsy). There are also epilepsy syndromes that are malignant. When these are identified, treatment should begin without delay, regardless of the seizure frequency.

When antiepileptic drug therapy is discussed, it is important to recognize the seizure type as well as the epileptic syndrome. This is the single most important criterion in making a decision about antiepileptic medication. There are basic principles to remember in choosing AED therapy:

- AED monotherapy is effective in most patients and avoids undesirable drug interactions.
- AEDs should be titrated slowly and only to the point of seizure control, if possible.
- Seizure control should not be achieved without trying to avoid side effects. If side effects develop, attempts should be made to reduce the dosage, change to a sustained-release formulation, or change AEDs.
- Drug compliance is enhanced when medication is given once or twice daily. Therefore, sustained-release medication should always be considered.
- Therapeutic blood levels are determined on the basis of trough levels and represent a statistical range of efficacy. They are not absolute levels.

The last few years have seen a rapid escalation in the marketing of AEDs. The drugs of choice for partial seizures now include a broad range of AEDs, including carbamazepine (Tegretol; Carbatrol [extended-release formulation]), oxcarbazepine (Trileptal), gabapentin (Neurontin), lamotrigine, topiramate, valproate, levetiracetam, zonisamide (not approved for children <16 years), phenobarbital, and phenytoin (Tables 1 and 2). The new AEDs have all been approved by the FDA as adjunctive therapy in treating partial seizures in adults. Topiramate has received approval for treating partial seizures in children as young as 2 years. Lamotrigine has been approved for treating both partial seizures and generalized tonic–clonic seizures, as adjunctive therapy, in children ages 2 or older. Levetiracetam is approved as adjunctive therapy for partial seizures and for myoclonic seizures. Phenobarbital and phenytoin are not currently being prescribed by pediatric neurologists nearly as often as they were in the past 10 years.

ANTIEPILEPTIC DRUGS

Carbamazepine

Carbamazepine is still the most widely used AED in treating partial seizures. Its mechanism of action is similar to that of phenytoin. Both drugs work by inhibiting the high-frequency repetitive firing of voltage-dependent sodium channels. Carbamazepine is generally tolerated well but should be introduced slowly. This reduces the risk of toxicity and enhances compliance. Autoinduction of carbamazepine metabolism via the cytochrome P-450 enzyme system occurs within the first month of therapy, often necessitating an increase in the total dosage of carbamazepine. If at all possible, once the dosage has been adjusted, attempts should be made to change to a sustained-release preparation. Carbamazepine is available in a liquid formulation, chewable tablets, tablets, a sustained-release preparation, and sustained-release sprinkle capsules.

The toxic side effects of carbamazepine include dizziness, diplopia, sedation, ataxia, and nausea. Rare idiosyncratic reactions include aplastic anemia and hepatic dysfunction. Transient leukopenia occurs in 10% of children, usually during the first month of therapy.

Allergic rash occurs in about 8% to 10% of patients; cases of Stevens-Johnson syndrome have been reported. Other rare side effects include irritability and dystonia. The antibiotic erythromycin alters the kinetics of carbamazepine, resulting in significant increases in carbamazepine levels.

Before carbamazepine therapy is initiated, a baseline complete blood cell count with differential and liver function tests should be obtained. These studies should be repeated monthly for the first 3 months of therapy or if there are signs or symptoms of liver dysfunction or blood dyscrasias.

Oxcarbazepine

Oxcarbazepine is related to carbamazepine and is approved as adjunctive therapy in treating localization related epilepsy. It does not induce the cytochrome P-450 enzyme system and is not metabolized to 10,11-epoxide, the known metabolite of carbamazepine thought to be responsible for teratogenicity and for many of carbamazepine's toxic side effects. It is formulated as a liquid (300 mg/5 mL suspension) or in pills (150 mg; 300 mg; 600 mg). It can be given twice daily. It has the same mechanism of action as carbamazepine and can produce the same side effects with toxicity. Patients can develop hyponatremia with this medication.

Valproate

Valproate is a broad-spectrum AED demonstrating efficacy for both partial and generalized seizures. Its mechanisms of action include reduction of T-type calcium channel currents, modulation of sodium channels, and, possibly, enhancement of GABA activity, the primary inhibitory neurotransmitter. Valproate comes in several formulations, including the liquid valproic acid, sodium divalproex tablets; and sodium divalproex sprinkle capsules.

The most common side effects of valproate include an increase in appetite with concomitant weight gain and tremor. Rarely, valproate causes an encephalopathy with sedation and cognitive impairment. Occasionally, this is due to hyperammonemia. At other times, the exact mechanism remains unclear. With high doses, tremor, transient alopecia, and thrombocytopenia (with easy bruising and bleeding) can occur. Another rare side effect of valproate is pancreatitis.

The most publicized and serious side effect of valproate is hepatotoxicity. There have been fatalities. The highest risk group is children younger than 2 years who have developmental delays and abnormal neurologic examination and who are on multiple AEDs. The risk of hepatic failure in these children is estimated at 1 in 500. The hepatotoxicity is an idiosyncratic reaction, is not dose related, and occurs in the first 6 months of therapy. The initial signs and symptoms of liver dysfunction are sedation, nausea, vomiting, and anorexia. Most pediatric neurologists and researchers agree that these cases of fatal hepatotoxicity probably occur in children with an underlying defect in the β-oxidation of fatty acids. Carnitine is an essential cofactor in this process. Therefore, carnitine supplementation[1] at 30 to 100 mg/kg/day is recommended for any child younger than 2 years. It is thought that carnitine provides protection against liver toxicity, aiding β-oxidation by bringing fatty acids across the mitochondrial membrane and binding to toxic valproate metabolites.

Literature has implicated valproate in the development of polycystic ovary syndrome. This syndrome is associated with infertility, dyslipidemia, and insulin-resistant diabetes mellitus. The exact mechanism by which this occurs is still being investigated, but the risk of polycystic ovaries, hyperandrogenism, and anovulatory menstrual cycles is definitely increased in women with epilepsy who are taking valproate. In addition, because of these findings and its teratogenic effects (increased risk of neural tube defects and possible neurocognitive effects in the fetus), the American Academy of Neurology and the American Epilepsy Society have both stated that valproate is relatively contraindicated in women with epilepsy who are in the reproductive age.

---

[1]Not FDA approved for this indication.

A baseline complete blood cell count with differential and liver function studies should be obtained before initiating valproate therapy. During the first 6 months of therapy; these blood parameters should be followed monthly or more often if signs and symptoms warrant a closer check.

Gabapentin

Gabapentin is one of the newer AEDs that is sometimes used in treating partial seizures. Its mechanism of action remains largely unknown although it is structurally related to GABA. Gabapentin has not been shown to be effective in treating generalized epilepsies. Gabapentin does not come in a chewable tablet but is available in an oral solution and in tablet and capsule form.

One of the biggest advantages of gabapentin is the lack of drug interactions. It is generally safe and tolerated well. There are no known fatal side effects. In the pediatric population, irritability, aggressiveness, agitation, and other behavioral side effects have been reported, particularly in children with underlying encephalopathy.

Unlike other AEDs, gabapentin is not metabolized by the liver, does not induce the cytochrome P-450 enzyme system, and is not highly protein bound. It is excreted via the kidneys.

Lamotrigine

Lamotrigine was released in 1994. The best known mechanisms of action for lamotrigine include an inhibition in the release of glutamate and an effect on voltage-sensitive sodium channels. It has been approved as adjunctive therapy for treating partial seizures and for treating generalized tonic–clonic seizures. It is probably another broad-spectrum AED, effective in treating partial and generalized seizures. Clinical research is ongoing to determine its efficacy in treating generalized epilepsies. Lamotrigine comes in several formulations including tablets and chewable dispersible tablets.

Lamotrigine has been associated with an allergic rash. Patients who take a combination of valproate and lamotrigine are at highest risk for an allergic rash. Valproate inhibits the metabolism of lamotrigine, resulting in an increase in the half-life from 12 to 72 hours. Therefore, the level of lamotrigine escalates considerably if valproate is added; the required dosage of lamotrigine when taken in combination with valproate is only 2 to 3 mg/kg/day as opposed to 4.5-7.5 mg/kg/day.[3] When lamotrigine therapy is initiated, the dosage must be increased very slowly, especially when it is used in combination with valproate. If a rash is reported, the patient should be seen immediately because the rash can progress rapidly. Patients who have reported skin allergies to other drugs, especially to carbamazepine, are also at high risk for an allergic rash from lamotrigine.

Other less common side effects of lamotrigine include dizziness, headaches, diplopia, sedation, and movement disorders, including choreoathetosis and dystonia. Positive behavioral side effects, including antidepressant effects, have been reported with lamotrigine.

Topiramate

Topiramate is another broad-spectrum AED. Topiramate appears to have a variety of mechanisms of action, including inhibition of voltage-sensitive sodium channels, enhancement of the inhibitory action of GABA, modest inhibitory effects on glutamate receptors, and weak inhibition of carbonic anhydrase. Drug interactions are minimal. It comes in several formulations including tablets and sprinkle capsules.

The major side effect of topiramate is cognitive dysfunction, including dysnomia, slowing of cognitive processing, and poor memory. These side effects can be minimized by a slow titration process, waiting to increase the dosage until habituation has taken place. Rare patients have an idiosyncratic reaction to topiramate, becoming encephalopathic on very small dosages of this medication. Topiramate can also cause renal stones, probably a result of its inhibition of carbonic anhydrase. Therefore, it should be used with caution in patients who are on the ketogenic diet or who have kidney dysfunction. Patients should be kept well hydrated.

Tiagabine

Tiagabine (Gabatril) is another antiepileptic drug that has been approved as adjunctive therapy by the FDA for treating partial seizures (for those $\geq$12 years of age). Its mechanism of action is via the inhibition of GABA reuptake in the synaptic cleft. There are no known drug interactions. It is formulated in pills only.

The major side effects of tiagabine include lethargy, irritability, aggressive behavior, dizziness, headache, and tremor. It is 96% protein bound and is metabolized by the liver.

Levetiracetam

Levetiracetam is also one of the newer antiepileptic medications. It has a novel mechanism of action that probably involves the synaptic vesicle protein. Levetiracetam has been approved as adjunctive therapy for partial seizures in children and adolescents 4 years and older, for myoclonic seizures in juvenile myoclonic epilepsy in adolescents 12 years and older, and for generalized tonic–clonic seizures in primary generalized epilepsy in children and adolescents 6 years and older.

Levetiracetam has no drug interactions; it is not toxic to the bone marrow or to the liver. It is excreted via the kidneys. Its major side effect is irritability and agitation. This is most prominent in those children who are already behaviorally disinhibited. Levetiracetam comes in a liquid preparation (500 mg/5 mL) or in tablets of 250 mg, 500 mg, 750 mg, or 1000 mg.

Zonisamide

Zonisamide is related to topiramate, with respect to its mechanisms of action. It is approved as adjunctive therapy in partial seizures in children and adolescents at least 16 years of age. In Japan, it is commonly used for myoclonic seizures associated with mitochondrial disorders. Preliminary studies indicate possible efficacy with infantile spasms,[1] myoclonic seizures,[1] and absence seizures.[1]

Its major side effects include lethargy, irritability, cognitive slowing, renal stones, and oligohidrosis. Therefore, it should be used with caution in patients who are on the ketogenic diet or who have kidney dysfunction. Patients should be kept well hydrated. Zonisamide comes in 25-mg, 50-mg, and 100-mg capsules.

ALTERNATIVES TO ANTIEPILEPTIC DRUGS

The ketogenic diet as a treatment for epilepsy has been known since biblical times. It was rediscovered in the modern era by Dr. Haddow Keith from the Mayo Clinic, who observed in a 1921 newsletter that children with status epilepticus usually experienced cessation of seizure activity once they were in ketosis. The ketogenic diet again fell out of favor with the advent of phenobarbital and phenytoin as AEDs. It has recently been repopularized by the Johns Hopkins Medical Center.

In appropriately chosen cases, the ketogenic diet can eliminate seizures in one third of patients and can decrease seizure frequency by more than 50% in another third, but it lacks efficacy in the final third. Patients with LGS have the best chance of responding to this diet. The diet requires that every piece of food and medicine be analyzed with respect to fat, carbohydrate, and protein content. All food and drink must be weighed and measured with respect to calories and type of food. The diet can be very difficult for children who already have dietary preferences.

The vagal nerve stimulator (VNS) has been approved by the FDA for use as adjunctive therapy in treating medically refractory, localization-related epilepsy in adults and children older than 12 years. The vagal nerve stimulator is a pacemaker, implanted in the chest pocket below the clavicle, that delivers pulses from a bipolar electrode connected to the vagus nerve. The exact mechanism of action remains an

---

[3]Exceeds dosage recommended by the manufacturer.

[1]Not FDA approved for this indication.

TABLE 1 Summary of Commonly Used Antiepileptic Drugs (Established Drugs)

Drug	Indications	Maintenance Dosage (mg/kg/d)	Starting Dosage	Half-Life (h)	Therapeutic Range (ug/mL)	Common Side Effects	Serious Idiosyncratic Side Effects
Carbamazepine (Tegretol)	Partial Partial w/secondary general, primary general, tonic–clonic	10-20	5-10 mg/kg/d	8-25	8-12	Diplopia, lethargy, blurred vision, ataxia, incoordination	Rashes, hepatic dysfunction, pancreatitis, aplastic anemia, leukopenia
Ethosuximide (Zarontin)	Absence	15-40; most children require 15-20	<6 y: 10 mg/kg/d >6 y: 250 mg/d	25-40	40-100	Gastrointestinal distress, hiccups, lethargy	Rashes, leukopenia, pancytopenia, systemic lupus erythematosus
Phenobarbital	Partial Partial w/secondary general, primary general, tonic–clonic	<1 y: 5-6 >1 y: 4-6 Teenagers, adults: 1-3	Same as maintenance	40-70	15-40	Irritability, hyperactivity, lethargy	Rashes
Phenytoin (Dilantin)	Partial Partial w/secondary general, primary general, tonic–clonic	5 (might need higher doses in children <5-6 y)	Same as maintenance	Depends on concentration	10-20	Lethargy, dizziness, ataxia, gingival hypertrophy, hirsutism	Rashes, hepatic dysfunction, lymphadenopathy, blood dyscrasias
Primidone (Mysoline)	Partial Partial w/secondary general, primary general, tonic–clonic	12-25	<6 y: 50 mg qhs <12 y: 100 mg qhs[3] >12 y: 100-125 mg qhs[3]	5-8 (phenobarbital 40-70)	5-12	Irritability, hyperactivity, lethargy, nausea	Rashes
Valproic Acid (Depakene)	Partial Partial w/secondary general, primary general, tonic–clonic Absence Myoclonic Tonic Atonic	15-60	5-15 mg/kg/d; incr by 10-15 mg/kg/d every 2 wk Max dosage 60 mg/kg/d	4-14	60-100	Lethargy, weight gain or loss, hair loss, tremor	Hepatic dysfunction, pancreatitis, anemia, thrombocytopenia

[3] Exceeds dosage recommended by the manufacturer.

TABLE 2 Summary of Commonly Used Antiepileptic Drugs (New Drugs)

Drug	Indications	Maintenance Dosage (mg/kg/d)	Starting Dosage	Half-Life (h)	Therapeutic Range (mg/mL)	Common Side Effects	Serious Idiosyncratic Side Effects
Felbamate (Felbatol)	Partial Partial w/secondary general Tonic Atonic	30–45, max 90[3]	15 mg/kg/d; incr in 10-mg/kg increments to 60 mg/kg/d[3] if necessary	13–24	30–100 (not well established)	Anorexia, insomnia, somnolence, tics	Aplastic anemia, hepatoxicity, rashes
Gabapentin (Neurontin)	Partial Partial w/secondary general	20–60[3]	10 mg/kg/d, incr in 5-mg/kg increments	5–8	Not established 2–6	Lethargy, dizziness, irritability	None
Lamotrigine (Lamictal)	Partial Partial w/secondary general Generalized tonic–clonic	5–15[3]; dosage depends on other drugs used: w/enzyme inducers, use 10–15; w/valproate, use 2–3	12.5–25 mg/d; incr slowly; be cautious in patient on valproate	15–60 (highly dependent on concomitant AEDs)	Not established 5–15	Rashes, lethargy, irritability, movement disorder	Rashes
Levetiracetam (Keppra)	Partial Partial w/secondary general Myoclonic	30–60	10 mg/kg/d, incr in 10-mg/kg increments	6–8	3–40	Agitation, behavioral disinhibition	None
Oxcarbazepine (Trileptal)	Partial Partial w/secondary general	30–60	15 mg/kg/d[3], incr by 10–15 mg/kg increments	8–10	10–35	Hyponatremia, somnolence, lethargy, dizziness, blurred vision	Rash
Tiagabine (Gabitril)	Partial Partial w/secondary general (approved for ≥12 y)	0.5–1; dosage depends on other drugs used: w/enzyme inducers, use 0.7–1.5; w/o enzyme inducers, use 0.3–0.4	0.1 mg/kg/d; incr weekly by 0.1 mg/kg/d	3–13	Not established 5–70 ng/mL	Lethargy, confusion, mental dullness, difficulties with concentration	None
Topiramate (Topamax)	Partial Partial w/secondary general	5–10[3]	1–2 mg/kg/d; incr weekly by 1 mg/kg/d	12–60	5–20	Irritability, hyperactivity, cognitive slowing, weight loss, renal stones, metabolic acidosis, oligohidrosis	Rash
Zonisamide (Zonegran)	Partial Partial w/secondary general (approved for ≥16 y)	5–10	2 mg/kg/d, incr by 1–2 mg/kg	48–65	10–40	Irritability, cognitive slowing, weight loss, renal stones, oligohidrosis	Rash

[3] Exceeds dosage recommended by the manufacturer.
AED = antiepileptic drug; incr = increase.

enigma. The VNS influence over the EEG is probably mediated by the solitary tract nucleus–parabrachial nucleus ceruleus–thalamic pathways with concomitant cortical projections. High stimulation of the vagus nerve appears to result in EEG desynchronization, with the full effects gradually being seen over 6 months to 1 year.

Side effects include bleeding, infection, voice alteration or hoarseness when the VNS cycles on, cough, throat pain, dyspepsia, and nausea. There are no reports of cardiac arrhythmias with this device.

Preliminary research on the VNS in patients with symptomatic generalized epilepsies such as LGS indicates significant efficacy, especially over time.

IMMUNOTHERAPY

Immunotherapy has been used in treating a variety of rare and unusual epileptic syndromes, such as Rasmussen's syndrome and Landau–Kleffner syndrome. Rasmussen's syndrome is characterized by progressive hemiparesis, associated cognitive decline, and epilepsia partialis continua. Studies have suggested that autoimmune mechanisms play a role in the pathogenesis of Rasmussen's syndrome. The syndrome affects only one hemisphere. Immunotherapy appears to result in a transient improvement in seizure control.

Steroids are also used in treating infantile spasms and Landau–Kleffner syndrome, as described earlier.

EPILEPSY SURGERY

The five most important questions that must be asked before the consideration of a presurgical evaluation are as follows: is this an epileptic syndrome that is most likely going to continue without resolution? Are the epileptic seizures having a significant impact on the child's development or quality of life? Have the seizures been intractable to a variety of AEDs? Is the epileptogenic zone identifiable? Can the epileptogenic zone be resected without unacceptable neurologic deficits?

Certain children are possible candidates for epilepsy surgery. It can be effective for children with nonlesional localization-related epilepsy in whom standard AED therapy—two to three AEDs—has failed and in children with lesional localization-related epilepsy—the presence of a tumor or other structural lesion, whether or not controlled with AEDs. Children with catastrophic epilepsies in whom the continuation of the epileptic encephalopathy and clinical seizures would result in substantial morbidity in terms of development and quality of life can benefit from surgery. Examples include patients with infantile spasms; Sturge–Weber syndrome with progressive hemiparesis and intractable seizures; Rasmussen's syndrome with progressive encephalopathy, seizures, and hemiparesis; and malformations of cortical development (e.g., hemimegalencephaly). Surgery can be effective for children with medically refractory generalized or multifocal epilepsies in whom the clinical presentation, seizure semiology, EEG findings, MRI of the brain, or other ancillary tests suggest an underlying focal generator for the epileptic condition. Children with intractable generalized epilepsy who have tonic or atonic seizures may be candidates for corpus callosotomy.

The presurgical evaluation must consist of a multidisciplinary approach. The concept of convergence is very important. The identification of the epileptogenic zone requires the confluence of data accumulated by the medical history, seizure semiology, physical examination, EEG interictal and ictal MRI of the brain, and the newer neuroimaging techniques. One technique is MRI of the brain with thin contiguous cuts and FLAIR sequencing (fluid-attenuated inversion recovery technique, i.e., T2-weighted imaging with the cerebrospinal fluid signal subtracted out). Ictal SPECT scan determines cerebral blood flow using radiotracers. These compounds rapidly cross the blood–brain barrier and record the cerebral blood flow at the time of injection. Observations made a century ago document that there is increased cerebral blood flow at the site of the epileptogenic focus during an ictal event. The SPECT scan can, therefore, provide one with a snapshot of the epileptogenic zone. It becomes increasingly accurate if the ictal SPECT scan is subtracted from the interictal SPECT scan and coregistered with the MRI study, a technique termed SISCOM. Interictal positron-emission tomography (PET) scan is another noninvasive functional imaging technique used to identify cerebral metabolic rates using a radioisotope designed to measure glucose metabolism. Interictally, the epileptogenic zone is hypometabolic. Other experimental technologies include MRI (looking at dynamic metabolism of the brain), magnetoencephalography (looking at the flux of magnetic fields in the brain), and functional MRI mapping.

The type of epilepsy surgery performed depends on the localization of the epiletogenic zone. Some of the more common surgical procedures include temporal lobectomy with amgydalohippocampectomy, focal cortical resection, hemispherectomy, implantation of a VNS, corpus callosotomy, and multiple subpial transaction (a technique employed over eloquent cortex that one chooses not to resect because of the potential loss of functional tissue).

Epilepsy surgery can be very effective in eliminating seizures in carefully chosen patients. For example, if a patient has mesial temporal sclerosis and seizures emanating from the temporal lobe, the chance of surgery's producing a seizure-free outcome is as high as 85% to 90%.

REFERENCES

Baumann RJ, Duffner PK: Treatment of children with simple febrile seizures: The AAP practice parameter. Pediat Neurol 2000;23(1):11-17.

Donat JF: The age-dependent epileptic encephalopathies. J Child Neurol 1992;7:7-21.

Dreifuss FE, Rosman NP, Cloyd JC, et al: A comparision of rectal diazepam gel and placebo for acute repetitive seizures. N Engl J Med 1998;26:1869-1875.

Freeman JM, Vining EP, Pillas DJ, et al: The efficacy of the ketogenic diet-1998: A prospective evaluation of intervention in 150 children. Pediatrics 1998;102(6):1358-1363.

Genton P, Dravet C: Lennox–Gastaut syndrome and other childhood epileptic encephalopathies. In Engel J Jr, Pedley TA (eds): Epilepsy: A Comprehensive Textbook, vol 3. Philadelphia: Lippincott-Raven, 1997, pp 2355-2366.

Glauser TA, Pellock JM, Bebin EM, et al: Efficacy and safety of levetiracetam in children with partial seizures: An open-label trial. Epilepsia 2002; 43(5):518-524.

Hirtz D, Berg A, Bettis D, et al: Practice parameter: Treatment of the child with a first unprovoked seizure. Neurology 2003;60:166-175.

Levisohn PM: Safety and tolerability of topiramate in children. J Child Neurol 2000;15(Suppl 1):S22-S26.

Loiseau P: Benign focal epilepsies of childhood. In Wyllie E (ed): The Treatment of Epilepsy: Principles and Practice. Philadelphia: Lea and Febiger, 1993, 503-512.

Mackay MT, Weiss SK, Adams-Webber T, et al, for the American Academy of Neurology and Child Neurology Society: Practice parameter: medical treatment of infantile spasms. Report of the American Academy of Neurology and the Child Neurology Society. Neurology 2004; 62(10):1668-1681.

Messenheimer J, Ramsay RE, Willmore LJ, et al: Lamotrigine therapy for partial seizures: A multicenter, placebo-controlled, double-blind, cross-over trial. Epilepsia 1994;35:113-121.

Morrell MJ: Reproductive and metabolic disorders in women with epilepsy. Epilepsia 2003;44(Suppl 4):11-20.

Murphy JV; Pediatric VNS Study Group. Left vagal nerve stimulation in children with medically refractory epilepsy. J Pediatr 1999;134:563-566.

Nordli DR, Bazil CW, Sheuer ML, Pedley TA: Recognition and classification of seizures in infants. Epilepsia 1997;38:553-560.

Shinnar S, Pellock JM, Berg AT, et al: Short term outcomes of children with febrile status epilepticus. Epilepsia 2001;42(1):47-53.

Tharp BR: Neonatal seizures and syndromes. Epilepsia 2002;43(Suppl 3):2-10.

Trevathan E: Seizures and epilepsy among children with language regression and autistic spectrum disorders. J Child Neurol 2004;19(Suppl 1):S49-S57.

Zupanc ML: Infantile spasms. Expert Opin Pharmacother 2003;4(11):2039-2048.

Zupanc ML: Early Onset Epilepsy. Pediatric Neurology Continuum: Lifelong Learning in Neurology. American Academy of Neurology, Lippincott Williams and Wilkins, Philadelphia, Sept. 1999.

Zupanc ML: Neuroimaging in the evaluation of children and adolescents with intractable epilepsy. I: MRI and substrates of epilepsy. Pediatr Neurol 1997;17:19-26.

Attention-Deficit/Hyperactivity Disorder

Method of
*Christopher Kratochvil, MD, and
Martin Wetzel, MD*

Overview

Attention-deficit/hyperactivity disorder (ADHD) is a common and impairing disorder with a prevalence of 3% to 7% in children and 4% in adults. Once ADHD is identified, highly effective treatment is available that can dramatically improve functioning. Screening for ADHD should be part of every patient's mental health assessment (Boxes 1 and 2).

ADHD can manifest as inattentive subtype or hyperactive/impulsive subtype, but most often it manifests as combined subtype. Due to the more subtle presentation of inattentive symptoms, in many children with inattentive subtype, ADHD is never diagnosed or is diagnosed later than other subtypes. Therefore, providers should screen for ADHD of all subtypes when evaluating children with academic or behavioral problems.

It is important to note that at all ages mental concentration is dynamic. ADHD patients might initially sit still and focus at the beginning of a novel situation, but as the novelty declines, ADHD symptoms often increase. The salience level or degree of emotion associated with activities can lead to tremendous variability in an ADHD patient's ability to focus from moment to moment.

Approximately 60% of children with ADHD continue to experience symptoms of ADHD severe enough to impair functioning in adulthood. Adults with ADHD suffer economically and emotionally, yet ADHD is diagnosed in less than 20% of adults with this common condition.

Diagnosis

There is no validated laboratory or radiologic test to diagnose ADHD; the gold standard remains a thorough diagnostic interview with collateral information. All evaluations for ADHD should also include past medical history, family history, and social history. ADHD is often comorbid, so a comprehensive assessment is necessary. Refer for neuropsychological testing when specific learning disabilities are suspected or when learning problems continue despite treatment. Laboratory or neurologic testing is generally not indicated if the medical history is unremarkable.

CHILDREN AND ADOLESCENTS

Children with hyperactive/impulsive subtype ADHD are often identified at a very early age due to the overt presentation of their symptoms. The preschool or kindergarten setting is commonly a backdrop where the restlessness, impulsivity, and disruptions of ADHD are observed in marked contrast to peers. There is a continuum of symptom severity however, and clinicians should understand normal

---

BOX 1 Diagnosis of Attention-Deficit/Hyperactivity Disorder

Six (or more) persistent symptoms of inattention that are maladaptive and (in children) inconsistent with developmental level for at least 6 months.
- Has difficulty sustaining attention
- Has difficulty organizing
- Avoids activity requiring sustained attention
- Has difficulty completing projects
- Misplaces items
- Is easily distracted
- Is forgetful
- Has difficulty listening when spoken to directly
- Makes frequent careless mistakes or shows poor attention to detail

Six (or more) persistent symptoms of hyperactivity-impulsivity that are maladaptive and (in children) inconsistent with developmental level for at least 6 months.
- Fidgeting
- Difficulty staying seated
- Excessive and inappropriate running or climbing (children); feeling restless (adolescents and adults)
- Difficulty playing or relaxing quietly
- On the go or driven by a motor
- Excessive talking
- Blurts out answers to questions
- Difficulty waiting to take turns
- Interrupting or intruding

Some of these symptoms caused impairment before age 7 years.
Impairment due to ADHD symptoms in two or more settings such as school, work, home, or peer relationships.
Clear evidence of clinically significant impairment in social, academic, or occupational functioning.
Symptoms not exclusively due to another mental or medical disorder.

Adapted from *Diagnostic and Statistical Manual of Mental Disorders*, fourth edition (text revision) (DSM-IV TR) criteria.

BOX 2 Additional Diagnostic Aids

Children and Adolescents
ADHD-IV Rating Scale: http://www.guilford.com/cgi-bin/cartscript.cgi?page=pr/dupaul2.htm&dir=pp/adhdr&cart_id=914119.11682
NICHQ Vanderbilt Assessment Scale for ADHD: http://www.nichq.org/NR/rdonlyres/076CE716-5ABD-4CB5-8E0F-8C847D63ED65/2971/03VanAssesScaleParentInfor.pdf

Adults
Adult Self-Report Scales: http://www.med.nyu.edu/psych/assets/adhdscreen18.pdf
Canadian ADHD Resource Alliance Adult ADHD Assessment Guideline: http://www.caddra.ca
Wender Utah Rating Scale: http://168.144.150.122/Wender%20Utah%20Rating%20Scale%20checklist.pdf

---

CURRENT DIAGNOSIS

- ADHD should be diagnosed using a comprehensive diagnostic interview, using collaborating information as available.
- ADHD often persists from childhood to adulthood, although symptom presentations can change.
- ADHD is often comorbid with additional psychiatric disorders.

ADHD = attention-deficit/hyperactivity disorder.

development before diagnosing ADHD. The assessment of symptoms and impairment should include home, social, and academic settings.

Children with inattentive subtype ADHD are often identified in the later school years compared with other subtypes. A high-IQ child who is eager to please might be older when exhibiting overt impairment or distress due to inadequate coping skills to meet increasing demands. Adolescents can appear depressed or anxious as a cumulative consequence of untreated ADHD symptoms.

There are high rates of comorbid psychiatric diagnoses in children with ADHD. Up to two thirds of children with ADHD have one additional mental health or learning disorder. Identification and treatment of comorbid psychiatric disorders can improve ADHD outcomes. The most common comorbid diagnosis is oppositional defiant disorder (54%-84%), followed by learning or language disabilities (35%) and anxiety or mood disorders (33%). Fifteen to nineteen percent of older children with untreated ADHD smoke; untreated ADHD children are twice as likely to use illicit drugs compared with controls.

ADULTS

Adults typically have more symptoms of inattention than hyperactivity. Childhood histories commonly reveal underachievement or adequate performance with a great deal of effort. School and work records and interviews with family members can help confirm the diagnosis.

Up to 80% of ADHD adults also have a second major comorbid psychiatric disorder (including substance abuse). Many receive mental health treatment for these comorbid illnesses, yet their ADHD remains undiagnosed. All psychiatric conditions should be addressed as the patient and clinician mutually decide on symptom significance to guide treatment priorities.

The initial diagnostic evaluation should confirm that the symptoms of ADHD are not attributable to other psychiatric conditions. For example, anxiety, depression, and ADHD can all result in poor concentration and psychomotor agitation. However, other psychiatric diagnoses often have relatively distinct episodes of onset and remission, whereas ADHD is persistent and more apt to be lifelong. For a comprehensive assessment, consider screening with an instrument such as the Psychiatric Review of Systems (http://www.aafp.org/afp/981101ap/carlat.html).

Treatment

Treatment of ADHD has three components: education, individualized medication titration (in combination with other therapies if indicated), and regular monitoring and adjustment of treatment. For some patients, the ADHD diagnosis can itself be extremely therapeutic, explaining years of symptoms and providing hope for a successful intervention. Education for the patient and family can facilitate acceptance of the diagnosis and provide a rationale for treatment. An empathetic initial assessment with educational support also promote adherence. Clinicians should have a well-rehearsed

---

BOX 3 Resources for Physicians, Patients, and Families

American Academy of Child and Adolescent Psychiatry:
  http://www.aacap.org
American Association of Pediatrics: http://www.aap.org
Children and Adults with Attention Deficit/Hyperactivity
  Disorder: http://www.chadd.org
National Institute of Mental Health:
  http://www.nimh.nih.gov
National Resource Center on ADHD:
  http://www.help4adhd.org
Attention Deficit Disorder Association:
  http://www.add.org

 CURRENT THERAPY

- Treatment for ADHD begins with education
- ADHD pharmacotherapy is safe, effective, and often fundamental to treatment success
- Medication management includes individualized titration to optimize response and tolerability, with regular monitoring and adjustments as needed
- ADHD treatment can be enhanced with nonpharmacologic interventions

ADHD = attention-deficit/hyperactivity disorder.

---

explanation of the diagnosis and treatment options and provide supplementary material to reinforce the discussion (Box 3). Specific needs should be addressed regarding school and workplace accommodations.

Decades of research support the safety and efficacy of ADHD pharmacotherapy for children, with more recent research demonstrating safety and efficacy in adolescents and adults as well. Behavioral therapy has demonstrated benefit alone and as an augmentation to medication treatment for children. Cognitive therapy has been shown to positively augment medication treatment for adults. There is growing interest in neurofeedback for ADHD but very limited research. Similarly, various exercises have been reported to be helpful but data are limited. Despite numerous anecdotal reports, no diets, supplements, or herbs have been researched adequately to recommend for ADHD treatment.

PREPARING FOR PHARMACOLOGIC THERAPY

A medication pretreatment assessment should include a physical examination, including height, weight, blood pressure, and pulse. If there is a history of tics, monitor and document tic activity at each visit. Review all over-the-counter and prescription medications, including herbal preparations and caffeine. If the patient has a history of preexisting heart disease or family history of early-age sudden death, refer to cardiology for evaluation. If there is a history of glaucoma, refer to ophthalmology for evaluation before medication treatment.

Pharmacologic Therapy

Medications for ADHD (all approved for children, some approved for adults) are shown in Table 1.

Stimulants

Stimulants are the most common pharmacotherapy for ADHD, so clinicians should be familiar with dosing, duration, and management of side effects of these medications.

Begin with the lowest dose and titrate upward weekly until the patient experiences no further benefit from increased doses or all target symptoms have resolved, the patient experiences intolerable side effects, or higher doses produce no consistent benefit.

Stimulants should be dispensed immediately on awakening, and maximum effectiveness can take up to an hour. Pills should be taken with water because acidic drinks, such as orange juice, when combined with stimulants, can interfere with consistent absorption. Adequate duration of symptom control can require combinations of long-acting and short-acting preparations.

The most common side effects from stimulant medication are reduced appetite, weight loss, problems sleeping, headaches, stomach pain, and irritability. These are often temporary and usually can be managed by reducing the dose or switching medication. Rare but serious potential side effects include psychotic or manic symptoms,

TABLE 1 Current FDA-Approved Medications for ADHD

Medication	Starting Dose	Approved Daily Maximum
Mixed amphetamine salts tablets (Adderall)	3-5 y: 2.5 mg >6 y: 5 mg	40 mg
Mixed amphetamine salts extended-release capsules* (Adderall XR)	5 mg	6-12 y: 30 mg ≥13 y: 20 mg
Oros methylphenidate extended-release tablets (Concerta)	18 mg	Child: 54 mg Adolescent: 72 mg
Methylphenidate transdermal system (Daytrana)	10 mg patch	30 mg
Methamphetamine hydrochloride tablets (Desoxyn)	5 mg	25 mg
Dextroamphetamine spansule capsules and tablets (Dexedrine)	3-5 y: 2.5 mg >6 y: 5 mg	40 mg
Dexmethylphenidate tablet (Focalin)	2.5 mg	20 mg
Dexmethylphenidate extended-release capsules* (Focalin XR)	Child: 5 mg Adult: 10 mg	20 mg
Methylphenidate extended-release capsules (Metadate CD)	10 mg	60 mg
Methylphenidate oral solution (Methylin)	5 mg	60 mg
Methylphenidate chewable tablets (Methylin)	5 mg	60 mg
Methylphenidate tablets (Ritalin)	5 mg	60 mg
Methylphenidate sustained-release tablets (Ritalin SR)	20 mg	60 mg
Methylphenidate extended-release capsules (Ritalin LA)	10 mg	60 mg
Atomoxetine capsules* (Strattera)	10 mg bid	Lesser of 1.4 mg/kg or 100 mg

*FDA approved for adults.

aggression, long-term suppression of growth, serious cardiovascular events, and dependence.

Atomoxetine

Atomoxetine (Strattera) is a nonstimulant approved for treating ADHD in children and adults. Titration is similar to that for stimulants, gradually as tolerated, with the package insert describing increases at the earliest of every 3 days in children and every 2 weeks in adults. Onset of symptom improvement may be gradual.

The most common side effects of atomoxetine are nausea, reduced appetite, weight loss, and (particularly in men older than 40 years) urinary hesitancy or retention. Rare but serious potential side effects include suicidal ideation, severe liver injury, serious cardiovascular events, and psychotic or manic symptoms.

MONITORING

During medication initiation and titration, patients should be closely monitored. Throughout treatment, all patients taking medication should have vital signs recorded, and children should have height and weight recorded. Visit frequency depends on treatment response and tolerability. Usually several visits are necessary before the patient and physician agree that maximum benefit has been achieved.

Once stabilized, patients should be seen at a minimum of several times per year. Patients and families should be made aware that response to medication can fluctuate over time with maturity, environmental change, new comorbidities, or changing pharmacotherapy. Patients can require ADHD treatment for long periods (potentially lifelong). Frequent changes in doses, formulations, and scheduling of dosing are not typically necessary. It is generally accepted that ADHD can enter natural remission.

In cases of poor treatment response, assess adherence, ensure medication is administered first thing in the morning with water, and optimize the dose. If symptoms emerge later in the day as medication effect declines, consider changing to a longer-acting preparation, using additional dosing, or adding a short-acting medication. Reevaluate for comorbid conditions including substance abuse, anxiety disorders, mood disorders, learning disorders, sleep disorders, and history of brain injury or toxin exposures. Consider adding cognitive behavior therapy. Consider different ADHD pharmacotherapy agents.

Fostering a clinical relationship of flexibility and ongoing communication includes collaborating on choices of medication, whether to take medication on weekends or holidays, adequate duration of effect, and how well patients can adhere to multiple doses per day. It is also important to understand the patient's and family's expectations regarding the evaluation for ADHD and the anticipated outcomes of treatment.

ADHD is a common disorder, and the informed clinician can safely and effectively bring significant relief to those in need of treatment.

REFERENCES

Barkley RA: Attention-Deficit Hyperactivity Disorder: A Handbook for Diagnosis and Treatment. New York: Guilford Press, 2006.
Biederman J: Attention-deficit/hyperactivity disorder: A selective overview. Biological Psychiatry 2005;57:1215-1220.
Chatfield J; American Academy of Pediatrics: AAP guideline on treatment of children with ADHD. Am Fam Physician 2002;65:726, 728.
Culpepper L: Primary care treatment of attention-deficit/hyperactivity disorder. J Clin Psychiatry 2006;67(Suppl 8):51-58.
Faraone SV, Biederman J, Spencer T, et al: Diagnosing adult attention deficit hyperactivity disorder: Are late onset and subthreshold diagnoses valid? Am J Psychiatry 2006;163(10):1720-1729.
Kessler RC, Adler L, Barkley R, et al: The prevalence and correlates of adult ADHD in the United States: Results from the national comorbidity survey replication. Am J Psychiatry 2006;163(4):716-723.
MTA Cooperative Group: A 14-month randomized clinical trial of treatment strategies for attention-deficit/hyperactivity disorder. Multimodal treatment study of children with ADHD. Arch Gen Psychiatry 1999;56:1073-1086
Pliszka S: AACAP Work Group on Quality Issues. Practice parameter for the assessment and treatment of children and adolescents with attention-deficit/hyperactivity disorder. J Am Acad Child Adolesc Psychiatry 2007; 46:894-921.

Gilles de la Tourette Syndrome

Method of
Cathy L. Budman, MD

Gilles de la Tourette syndrome, or Tourette's syndrome, is an inherited neuropsychiatric disorder of childhood onset characterized by the presence of repetitive, nonrhythmic, stereotypic movements and vocalizations (tics) that wax and wane in severity and change in location.

In 1825, Jean Itard first described the ticcing and cursing symptoms of the 26-year-old Marquise de Dampierre, noting the peculiar contrasts between her peculiar disinhibited behavior and her otherwise preserved intellect and propriety. Sixty years later this association of tics with behavioral symptoms, including obsessions, compulsions, mood lability, and phobias was again described by the French neurologist Gilles de la Tourette, after whom this disorder is named. The complex interplay of neurologic, psychological, and environmental influences on tics contributes to the wide variation in their severity, form, frequency, and intensity. Once believed to be rare, it is now clear that milder cases of Tourette's syndrome are common, often unrecognized, and commonly misdiagnosed.

Clinical Features

Historically, tic symptoms have been classified as either motor or vocal, depending on whether sounds are produced via moving air through the nose, mouth, or throat. Tics are further subclassified as either simple or complex.

Simple motor tics are characterized by repetitive, sudden, brief, isolated movements of a single muscle group. Examples include eye blinking, facial grimacing, and head jerking. Slower, sustained tonic movements, such as neck twisting and abdominal or buttock tensing, also occur and are called *dystonic tics*.

Complex motor tics consist of more coordinated, complicated movements involving several muscle groups such as twirling around, squatting, and hopping. Certain complex motor tics such as touching, tapping, smelling, copropraxia (obscene gestures), and echopraxia (mimicking others' movements) may be confused with volitional behavior or compulsions.

Simple vocal tics include a variety of inarticulate noises and sounds ("ooh" "tsk" "eh"), as well as throat clearing and humming. Although technically a simple motor tic, repetitive sniffing is also included in this category. Such symptoms might go unnoticed or be misattributed to seasonal allergies or nervous habits.

Complex vocal tics are phonic ejaculations with linguistic meaning, consisting of full or truncated words. Complex tics include echolalia (repeating the words of others), palilalia (repeating one's own words), and coprolalia (involuntary utterance of obscene words). Although coprolalia is a dramatic and distressing symptom, it occurs in only a minority of people with Tourette's syndrome and is certainly not necessary for establishing the diagnosis.

The tic itself is often experienced as an irresistible urge, a psychic itch that can usually be suppressed temporarily but at the expense of a buildup of inner tension relieved only by the tic. Because tics can be suppressed for minutes to hours at a time, the term *involuntary* is not completely accurate; tics are actually unvoluntary in nature, that is, the movement relieves the tension. *Premonitory symptoms*, characterized by patterns of uncomfortable somatic sensations such as pressure, tickle, or warmth that are localized to specific body regions, often precede the tic performance and may be more distressing and distracting than the tic itself.

Tics are increased by excitement, anxiety, fatigue, and concurrent medical illness but are often attenuated while the ticquer is performing absorbing activities. Tics typically occur in bouts: Periods of tic exacerbation can last days or weeks followed by other periods during which tics are relatively diminished or even absent. Tic symptoms also classically change in type and location over time, often progressing in a rostral-caudal fashion. Hence, episodes of repetitive eye blinking or facial grimacing can occur for several weeks, disappear for a period, then be replaced by repetitive head shaking or shoulder shrugging. This classic waxing-waning course, change in tic character, and capacity for temporary tic suppression contribute to the delay in Tourette's syndrome diagnosis.

Natural History and Epidemiology

Although Tourette's syndrome has been identified worldwide in all ethnic groups and appears to be uniformly distributed across socioeconomic classes, it occurs 3 to 4 times more frequently in male patients than in female patients. It is currently estimated that Tourette's syndrome affects 0.5% to 1% of school-age children. Most tics manifest between ages 2 and 18 years, with an average age of tic onset at 6 to 7 years. Tics tend to peak in severity between ages 11 and 12 years, just before puberty, and in most cases they diminish by late adolescence or early adulthood. Tic severity in early childhood is not a good predictor of later tic persistence. However, the presence of severe tics in late adolescence appears associated with persistent tic symptoms into adulthood.

Some adults with Tourette's syndrome report several years, even decades, of relative tic quiescence or remission that are curiously punctuated by sudden, unexpected episodes of tic exacerbations in mid-life or later life. The explanations and risk factors for such recurrences are not clear and may be related to a combination of physiologic, psychological, and environmental factors. In the majority of Tourette's cases, however, it is not tic symptoms per se that most negatively affect quality of life but the presence and persistence of associated comorbid psychiatric conditions.

Differential Diagnosis

At this time there is no biological marker or test that can be performed to confirm the diagnosis of Tourette's syndrome. Hence, physicians must rely on a careful, detailed history of symptoms and on clinical examination, employing the *Diagnostic and Statistical Manual of Mental Disorders*, fourth edition (text revision) (DSM-IV TR) diagnostic criteria.

Primary tic disorders generally have an onset before age 18 years and cannot be attributed to the direct physiologic effects of a substance or general medical condition (Box 1).

The primary tic disorders include chronic motor or vocal tic disorder, transient tic disorder, Tourette's disorder, and tic disorder not otherwise specified (TDNOS). Chronic motor or vocal tic disorders differ from Tourette's syndrome in that either motor or vocal tics, but not both, are present for longer than 1 year. Transient tic disorder is diagnosed when the duration of tic symptoms is less than 1 year. Tourette's disorder (used interchangeably with the term Tourette's syndrome) is characterized by motor and one or more vocal tics that have been present at some time during the illness, although not necessarily concurrently, and a course of tics that occurs nearly every day or intermittently throughout a period of more than 1 year. The category of tic disorder not otherwise specified is reserved for tic phenomena that do not meet diagnostic criteria for a specific primary tic disorder, such as, for example, tics that occur with an onset after age 18 years or tics that first occur following a severe head trauma.

Primary tics must be distinguished from other stereotypic repetitive movement disorders, such as myoclonus, tardive dyskinesia, and dystonias (e.g., blepharospasm, torticollis) (Box 2). Stereotypic movements (stereotypies) associated with mental retardation, psychosis, autism, or congenital blindness or deafness may be difficult to distinguish from motor tics, and tics and sterotypies often co-occur in this population. The tendency to wax and wane in severity, change in location, and presence in context of other typical tic symptoms can be helpful in differentiating these two phenomena.

Secondary tics can result from infection, head trauma, carbon monoxide poisoning, and illegal substance abuse and can also occur in a number of neurologic disorders including Huntington's disease, Parkinson's disease, progressive supranuclear palsy, neuroacanthocytosis, Meige's syndrome, startle disorders, and developmental basal ganglia syndrome. An intriguing and highly controversial theory posits that some cases of Tourette's syndrome or obsessive-compulsive disorder (OCD) are immune-mediated secondary to

---

BOX 1   DSM-IV TR Classification of Tic Disorders

- Tourette's disorder
- Chronic motor and vocal tic disorder
- Transient tic disorder
- Tic disorder not otherwise specified

Abbreviation: DSM-IV TR = *Diagnostic and Statistical Manual of Mental Disorders,* fourth edition (text revision).

> **BOX 2 Differential Diagnosis of Tics**
>
> **Abrupt**
> - Myoclonus chorea
> - Paroxysmal dyskinesia
> - Seizure
>
> **Premonitory Symptoms**
> - Dystonia
> - Restless legs
>
> **Suppressibility**
> - All hyperkinesias
>
> **Increased Distraction or Focus**
> - Akathisia
> - Chorea
> - Psychogenic hyperkinesias
>
> **Decreased Stress or Relaxation**
> - Most hyperkinesias
>
> **Present during Sleep**
> - Myoclonus seizures
> - Periodic movements

> **BOX 3 Pharmacologic Management of Tics**
>
> **Antihypertensives**
> - Clonidine (Catapres)[1]
> - Guanfacine (Tenex)[1]
>
> **Atypical Antipsychotics**
> - Aripiprazole (Abilify)[1]
> - Olanzapine (Zyprexa)[1]
> - Quetiapine (Seroquel)[1]
> - Risperidone (Risperdal)[1]
> - Ziprasidone (Geodon)[1]
>
> **Neuroleptics**
> - Fluphenazine (Prolixin)[1]
> - Haloperidol (Haldol)
> - Pimozide (Orap)
>
> ---
> [1]Not FDA approved for this indication.

group A β-hemolytic streptococci (GABHS) infection. The PANDAS (*p*ediatric *a*utoimmune *n*europsychiatric *d*isorders *a*ssociated with *s*treptococcal infection) hypothesis proposes that antibodies produced against GABHS cross-react with critical brain tissues, leading to a characteristically explosive onset or exacerbations of tic symptoms. However, there is currently conflicting basic science and clinical evidence both supporting and refuting the PANDAS hypothesis, and apart from treating culture-positive streptococcal infections with a course of antibiotics, no specific interventions are yet recommended outside research settings.

Treatment

In the majority of Tourette's syndrome cases, tic symptoms tend to be mild and medication intervention is not necessary. Psychoeducation for patients, family members, peers, and school staff about Tourette's syndrome and its associated psychiatric disorders, appropriate modifications of the educational environment, and psychotherapy to improve adaptive functioning are the recommended initial therapeutic interventions for such cases. Pharmacotherapy should be considered once it has been determined that the tics are functionally disabling and not remediable by psychosocial interventions. The goal in treating tics is generally to achieve a satisfactory *attenuation* (not elimination) of tic symptoms with the minimum, and tolerable, medication side effects (Box 3).

α₂-ADRENERGIC RECEPTOR AGONISTS

Initial medication for tic intervention typically employs an α₂-adrenergic receptor agonist at a therapeutic dosage for a 4- to 6-week trial.

Clonidine (Catapres)[1] is started at 0.05 mg at bedtime and increased by 0.05-mg increments every few days to a maximum of 0.4 to 0.6 mg total daily, divided in a three- or four-times-daily dosing schedule. Many responders take 0.05 to 0.1 mg three or four times daily. Sedation and dry mouth are the most commonly encountered adverse effects. Transdermal clonidine[1] is an alternative dosing form, particularly for children who cannot swallow pills, but this formulation can cause skin irritation and is impractical during summer months.

Guanfacine (Tenex)[1] has the advantages of once- or twice-daily dosing and is usually less sedating. It is initiated at 0.5 to 1 mg at bedtime and increased by 0.5-mg increments every few days to a maximum daily dosage of 4 mg, which is split into a twice-a-day dosing schedule (e.g., 0.5-2.0 mg bid). When clonidine or guanfacine is to be discontinued, the drug should be tapered over 7 to 10 days to prevent withdrawal phenomena, such as tachycardia or rebound hypertension.

ATYPICAL ANTIPSYCHOTICS

The newer atypical antipsychotics have generally supplanted the conventional antiypsychotics as second-line tic suppressants due to their improved adverse-effects profile. With the atypical antipsychotics, extrapyramidal effects—drug-induced parkinsonism, akathisia, tardive dyskinesia, and acute dystonic reactions—are reduced. However, these agents can cause significant extrapyramidal side effects too, particularly at higher doses. Furthermore, there is increasing evidence that these agents can cause the metabolic syndrome as well as untoward endocrine effects in adults and children.

The atypical neuroleptics can generally be given in a single bedtime dose. Atypical antipsychotics with reported tic-suppressing actions include risperidone[1] (Risperidal) 0.25 to 4 mg/day, olanzapine[1] (Zyprexa) 2.5-15 mg/day, and ziprasidone[1] (Geodon) 20-120 mg/day. Case reports have described tic-suppressant efficacy with the atypical antipsychotics aripiprazole[1] (Abilify) and quetiapine[1] (Seroquel). Significant weight gain is a common and problematic side effect with most of these agents and that can be limited somewhat by strict diet control and increased physical activity.

CONVENTIONAL ANTIPSYCHOTICS

When the atypical antipsychotics are ineffective or not tolerated, a trial of a conventional antipsychotic may be indicated. Pimozide (Orap) is an effective tic suppressant that appears to be better tolerated than haloperidol (Haldol). It is initiated at 0.5 mg daily and can be titrated up to approximately 6 mg total daily dosage. Common extrapyramidal side effects associated with dopamine-2 receptor blockade as well as a propensity toward prolongation of the QT interval on cardiac conduction (which is further worsened when combined with other medications that cause QT prolongation) can limit its use.

Haloperidol (Haldol) remains one of the most commonly employed conventional neuroleptics for treating tics, although most patients stop using it because of its unacceptable side effects.

---

[1]Not FDA approved for this indication.

BOX 4 Other Treatments for Tics
• Substituted benzamides: Tiapride[2], sulpiride[2] • Nicotine: Nicotine patch (Nicoderm CQ)[1] • Dopamine agonists: Pergolide (Permax)[1] • Dopamine depleters: Tetrabenazine (Nitoman)[2] • Botulinum toxin type A[1] (Botox) for dystonic tics
[1]Not FDA approved for this indication. [2]Not available in the United States.

Haloperidol is initiated at 0.25 mg daily at bedtime. When the patient can continue taking it, a favorable tic response usually occurs with 3 mg/day or less.

If haloperidol is unsuccessful either due to lack of efficacy or excessive side effects, one can then switch to another conventional neuroleptic.

OTHER TREATMENTS

Other medication strategies for suppressing tics are listed in Box 4. These agents have not been studied as extensively as the conventional and atypical antipsychotics, but in general they have a somewhat milder side-effect profile.

Although most medication interventions are nonspecific in their abilities to suppress tics, focal intramuscular injections of botulinum toxin (Botox)[1] have been used to treat patients with painful dystonic tics and might offer a unique possibility to target a specific tic.

If these preliminary attempts to attenuate tic symptoms are not successful, consultation and possibly referral to an experienced Tourette's syndrome specialist should be considered.

Associated Psychiatric Disorders

Although tic symptoms contribute to the colorful, sometimes dramatic presentation of Tourette's syndrome, careful clinical assessment and treatment intervention for comorbid psychiatric disorders and psychosocial problems are of paramount concern. Comorbid psychiatric disorders such as obsessive-compulsive disorder (OCD), attention-deficit/hyperactivity disorder (ADHD), affective disorders (depression, bipolar spectrum disorders, non-OCD anxiety disorders), and impulse-control disorders are commonly encountered when treating Tourette's syndrome in the clinical setting. Recent studies have demonstrated that up to 50% of outpatients with Tourette's syndrome suffer from behavioral and emotional symptoms that would meet threshold criteria for a comorbid psychiatric disorder. Because distress and impairment caused by psychiatric comorbidities in Tourette's syndrome often surpass those caused by tics, active screening and specific treatment of associated emotional and behavioral symptoms are of paramount importance.

Such complex Tourette's syndrome cases often necessitate a referral to a specialist with expertise in the treatment of Tourette's syndrome and its psychiatric comorbidities. Cognitive behavior therapy (CBT), parent skills training, social skills training, family therapy, and anger management training are important nonpharmacologic interventions for Tourette's syndrome associated psychiatric disorders. (Zinner's article gives an excellent overview of the management of Tourette's syndrome and its psychiatric comorbidities.)

[1]Not FDA approved for this indication.

REFERENCES

American Psychiatric Association: Diagnostic and Statistical Manual of Psychiatric Disorders, 4th ed, text revision. Washington, DC: American Psychiatric Association, 2000.
Coffey B, Park K: Behavioral and emotional aspects of Tourette syndrome. Neurol Clin 1997;15:277-289.
Jankovic J: Botulinum toxin in the treatment of tics associated with Tourette's syndrome. Neurology 1993;43(suppl 2):A310.
Jankovic J, Stone L: Dystonic tics in patients with Tourette's syndrome. Mov Disord 1991;6:248-252.
Kurlan R, Behr J, Medved L, et al. Severity of Tourette's syndrome in one large kindred: Implication for determination of disease prevalence rate. Arch Neurol 1987;44:268-269.
Kurlan R, Lichter D, Hewitt D: Sensory tics in Tourette's syndrome. Neurology 1989;39:731-734.
McMahon WM, Leppert M, Filloux F, et al: Tourette symptoms in 161 related family members. Adv Neurol 1992;58:159-165.
Robertson M: Tourette syndrome, associated conditions and the complexities of treatment. Brain 2000;32:436-447.
Scahill LD, Leckman JF, Marek KL: Sensory phenomena in Tourette's syndrome. Adv Neurol 1995;65:273-280.
Swedo SE, Leonard HL, Garvey M, et al: Pediatric autoimmune neuropsychiatric disorders associated with streptococcal infections: Clinical description of the first 50 cases. Am J Psychiatry 1998;155:264-271.
Tanner CM: Epidemiology. In Kurlan R (eds): Handbook of Tourette's Syndrome and Associated Tic and Behavioral Disorders. New York: Marcel Dekker, 2005, pp 399-410.
The Tourette Syndrome Classification Study Group: Definitions and classification of tic disorders. Arch Neuol 1993;50:1013-1016.
Zinner SH: Tourette syndrome: Much more than tics. Contemp Pediatr 2004;21:38-49.

Headache

Method of
R. Michael Gallagher, DO

Headache is a disturbing and sometimes fearsome affliction that has plagued humankind throughout recorded history. It often is debilitating and particularly disturbing to the sufferer because the pain is located in the head, the very center of the body's cognitive and control functions. With its accompanying pain and debilitating symptoms, stress can mount and the headache can become all consuming.

Headache is experienced by all age groups from young children to the elderly. It is more common than asthma, diabetes, mental illness, and rheumatoid arthritis. In fact, the World Health Organization identifies severe migraine, along with psychosis and quadriplegia, as "one of the most debilitating chronic conditions." Although the majority of Americans experience tension-type headaches at some time in their lives, approximately 30 million experience migraine headache: 13% of women and 6% of men, predominantly in their most productive years between the ages of 13 and 55 years. Prepubescent boys and girls suffer equally; however, boys often outgrow their migraine attacks as they mature, and they are less subjected to hormonal influences. Smaller percentages of people, by comparison, suffer with other chronic headaches, such as cluster headache and chronic daily headache.

No sure diagnostic tests are available to differentiate headache types. The headache condition can progress over time in frequency, severity, and debilitation. Each sufferer can be different and may require a detailed evaluation and individualized treatment plan; more frequent or prolonged attacks often necessitate a more comprehensive treatment plan. Thus, the headache problem can be a challenge for both the sufferer and the clinician.

During the 20th century, dramatic advancements were made in medicine. Longevity and quality of life improved for many individuals. Unfortunately, for headache sufferers, most of these advances were for maladies that killed or maimed rather than for non–life-threatening conditions. It was not until the 1960s that even a reasonable preventive medication, propranolol (Inderal), was introduced, and by the 1980s only a handful of medications were available for wide use. Physicians had to improvise with medications and treatments that were originally designated for other medical conditions.

In the late 1980s and 1990s, epidemiologic, psychosocial, and pharmacologic research resulted in an increase in available headache information and treatment possibilities. The development of the triptans, serotonin agonists, brought a new awareness to both physicians and sufferers. Today, seven triptans and two relatively new preventive medications are available. In spite of this, a minority of migraine sufferers use these options, and more than 50% continue to self-treat without benefit of professional care.

In the past, patients wanted the physician to believe their headache problem was real. They hoped that they would be taken seriously and that the physician would make a sincere attempt to help them. The headache patient has changed. The headache sufferer who seeks treatment today is more knowledgeable and interested in rapid relief and tolerability of medication.

Evaluation and Diagnosis

An accurate diagnosis is essential for effective management of patients with the more commonly encountered headaches. Because no biologic markers or diagnostic tests exist to determine headache type, the history is the single most important element in the evaluation of the headache patient. Various headache types sometimes have similar initial presentations, or patients may suffer with more than one type of headache (e.g., migraine and tension-type headache), which can be confusing at first, but the careful history usually differentiates the headache type. In general, little in the way of diagnostic testing is needed unless a physical cause is suspected. Some physicians prefer to perform simple laboratory tests to establish a baseline for medication toleration and monitoring as necessary (Table 1).

The headache complaint on occasion can be a sign of a more serious medical condition, such as a tumor, infection, or aneurysm. For this reason, the clinician always must be cautious and diligent in establishing an accurate and timely diagnosis. Certain so-called red flags in the history require immediate attention. These include any complex of symptoms or history that does not fit a typical headache type; report of a significant neurologic deficit; significant or prolonged neurologic deficit with aura; late-onset migraine (patient older than 30 years); sudden onset of a new head pain without history of similar headaches; changes in headache character; headache associated with elevated temperature; or completely unresponsive attacks in the absence of analgesic or caffeine overuse. When any of these symptoms are present or physical examination reveals significant findings, further diagnostic evaluation with imaging studies and consultation is imperative.

The appropriate headache patient evaluation includes a thorough history, physical examination with special attention to the head and the neurologic, cardiovascular, and musculoskeletal systems, and diagnostic tests when appropriate. The history should include headache onset, location, pain character (e.g., pressure, throb), frequency, duration, associated symptoms, aura or prodrome, triggers, previous treatment, and family history. Certain clues in the history may lean toward the diagnosis of migraine, such as motion sickness, absence of headache during pregnancy, and headache relationship to menses, sun glare, oversleep, fatigue, fasting, foods, or alcohol.

Various diagnostic screening questionnaires and tools have been developed over the years to assist busy clinicians in establishing the diagnosis of migraine. Most are long and cumbersome and do not easily become a part of routine patient evaluation. A simple three-question screener for migraine is helpful for generalist clinicians. A "yes" answer to all three questions indicates a strong possibility of the migraine diagnosis:

1. Do you experience headaches severe enough to see a physician?
2. Are your headaches accompanied by other symptoms?
3. Are your headaches intermittent (i.e., nondaily)?

Note: This screener should not be substituted for a complete history; it should be used only for screening purposes.

TENSION-TYPE HEADACHE

Tension-type headache (TTHA) is the most common of headaches and first was believed to be caused by sustained muscle contraction of the neck, jaw, scalp, or facial muscles. However, it is now thought that the sustained muscle contraction can, in fact, be an epiphenomenon to possible central disturbances rather than a primary process. Evidence suggests that altered levels of serotonin, substance P, and neuropeptide Y in the serum or platelets of patients with TTHA are responsible.

TTHA is characterized by intermittent or persisting bilateral pain, usually described as a squeezing pressure or a bandlike sensation around the head. Most patients experience their symptoms in the frontal, temporal, or occipital areas of the head. Location frequently varies with the attack, and tightness of the neck and shoulders is common. Intensity varies greatly. The attacks can last from hours to days, and in some extreme cases they may last for months. Aura, nausea, photophobia and phonophobia, and incapacitation are not typically associated with TTHA.

Many TTHA sufferers easily recognize the origin of their attacks. TTHA typically results from emotional upset, periods of stress, and major life changes. Anxiousness, poor adaptation skills, and anxiety

TABLE 1 Current Diagnosis

Symptoms	Frequency	Duration
Tension-Type Headache		
Bilateral variable pain	Variable	Hours to days
Squeezing or bandlike	Often related to known precipitant	
Tightness of head and shoulders		
Migraine Headache		
Unilateral mostly	1–6 mo	Hours to days
Throbbing or constant pain	Sometimes cyclic	
Nausea, vomiting		
Photophobia/phonophobia		
Fluid disturbances		
Mood changes		
Can be associated with aura		
Cluster Headache		
Unilateral severe boring pain	Multiple daily	45–90 min
Ipsilateral lacrimation, scleral injection, rhinorrhea	Near-daily	Cycles of attacks
Eyelid droop		
Restlessness		

CURRENT DIAGNOSIS

- Seizures may be partial (focal or localization-related) or generalized in onset. Clinical history, EEG, and imaging data assist the clinician in determining the seizure type and epilepsy syndrome.
- The most important initial diagnostic tests for evaluating new-onset epilepsy in adolescents and adults are high-resolution brain magnetic resonance imaging and EEG.
- In refractory epilepsy or spells of an uncertain type, the patient should be referred for video-EEG monitoring to document and localize the seizure type.

BOX 1 Migraine Dietary Triggers

- Dairy: Ripened cheese (cheddar, brie, camembert, half-cup of sour cream)
- Meats: Processed lunch meats, hot dogs, sausage, bologna, salami, chicken liver
- Fish: Pickled or dried herring
- Grains: Sourdough bread
- Fruits: Bananas, raisins, figs, avocado, half-cup limit of citrus
- Vegetables: Broad and fava beans, onions, snow peas
- Other: Chocolate, nuts, peanut butter, pickled foods, Chinese food with monosodium glutamate (MSG)
- Beverages: Most wines and alcohol, 200-mg daily limit of caffeine
- Additives: MSG, soy sauce, meat tenderizers, aspartame, sulfites, garlic

and depression often are present. Physical causes, such as degenerative joint disease, trauma to the head or neck, poor posture, or temporomandibular joint dysfunction, also can precipitate attacks. Persons older than 50 years are prone to excessive muscle contraction because of arthritis of the neck and jaw, poor posture, or stress. TTHA that is consistently precipitated by tension or pathology of the neck frequently is referred to as a *cervicogenic headache*. In contrast to migraine headache, TTHA is more likely to begin in later life.

MIGRAINE HEADACHE

Migraine headache is a familial disease characterized by unilateral or bilateral paroxysmal headache lasting hours to days. Adult women experience attacks more than men by a ratio of 3:1. Children and the elderly experience migraine equally. Attacks occur from as infrequently as one or two per year to several times weekly. Associated symptoms usually occur and frequently include throbbing, nausea, vomiting, photophobia, phonophobia, fluid retention, and mood changes.

The two basic types of migraine headache are *migraine with aura* (previously called classic migraine) and *migraine without aura* (previously called common migraine). Migraine with aura is preceded by an aura, a transient neurologic symptom that usually is visual, such as scotoma, teichopsia, tunnel vision, or visual field deficit, lasting 10 to 30 minutes. However, aura can manifest as any neurological deficit. Migraine without aura is more commonly experienced and comes on gradually or is present on awakening from sleep. In some patients, these headaches are associated with a nonspecific prolonged prodrome, such as mood changes, food cravings, or fluid retention hours before the pain.

The underlying cause of migraine headache is not clearly established, and various theories are proposed. Migraine appears to be of genetic origin and to be an inflammatory disease that causes disturbances in serotonin use and activity. Strong evidence indicates the migrainous attack originates in the central nervous system by stimulation of the locus ceruleus and dorsal raphe nuclei. Resultant changes alter cerebral and extracranial blood flow, activate the trigeminovascular system, and cause vascular dilation, neurogenic inflammation, and pain. Various precipitants are known, and many sufferers report that migraine attacks frequently are associated with menstruation or are triggered by foods containing vasoactive amines, strong odors, too much or too little sleep, sun glare, stress, altitude, weather changes, exertion, or fasting (Boxes 1 and 2, Table 2).

Some physicians classify migraine according to its precipitant or description (e.g., menstrual migraine, exertional migraine, coital migraine, cervicogenic migraine, cyclic migraine, acephalic migraine). Regardless, the fundamentals of evaluation and treatment are the same.

CLUSTER HEADACHE

The cause of cluster headache is unknown, and little credible research is available. Various possibilities or theories are suggested and include, but are not limited to, disturbances in histamine production or use; hypothalamic biorhythm dysfunction; or serotonin and neurotransmitter mechanisms similar to those of migraine. Some authorities consider cluster headache one of the most severe pain conditions known to humankind.

Cluster headache predominantly affects men, with a male-to-female ratio of 6:1. It occurs in well under 0.5% of the population. Onset later in life (after age 30 years) is common, and patients sometimes report head injury or a traumatic event occurring months before onset. Attacks occur on a daily or near-daily basis for weeks or months at a time and mysteriously disappear for months to years regardless of treatment, only to recur and cycle again. Although nonspecialist physicians only occasionally encounter the patient with cluster headaches, it is important to consider cluster headaches in the differential diagnosis.

The typical patient with a cluster headache experiences relatively brief attacks (45–90 minutes) of horrible unilateral head pain associated with ipsilateral lacrimation, scleral injection, rhinorrhea, or eyelid droop. The hallmark of the syndrome is its associated symptoms and its severe and intense pain. During attacks, most cluster patients move about, trying unsuccessfully to get more comfortable, similar to renal colic, in contrast to migraine sufferers, who prefer to lie quietly in a dark quiet room. Few triggers are identified, and alcohol almost always precipitates an attack during a cluster "on" cycle. A rare form of cluster headache, chronic cluster, does not cycle and continues on a daily or near-daily basis without cessation.

Treatment

The doctor–patient relationship frequently is the key to successful treatment in the headache patient. Although to some this statement

BOX 2 Migraine Triggers

- Altitude
- Alcohol
- Caffeine withdrawal
- Fluorescent or flickering lights
- Sun glare
- Weather changes
- Stress, stress letdown
- Foods
- Skipping meals
- Smoky environment
- Noisy environment
- Strong odors
- Lack of sleep, oversleep
- Exertion
- Hormonal changes

TABLE 2 Current Therapy

Headache Type	PRN	Prophylaxis
Tension	OTC*	Stress/precipitant avoidance
	NSAIDs	Stretching
	Muscle relaxants	Warm packs
	Combination analgesics	Relaxation techniques
		NSAIDs
		Muscle relaxants
		Antidepressants
Migraine	NSAIDs*	Biofeedback
	Triptans*	β-Blockers*
	Ergotamine*	Divalproex sodium*
	Dihydroergotamine*	Topiramate*
	Isometheptene*	TCA antidepressants
	Combination analgesics	Calcium channel blockers
Cluster	Oxygen	No alcohol
	Triptans	Calcium channel blockers
	Dihydroergotamine	Divalproex sodium
	Ergotamine	NSAIDs
		Lithium
		Steroids

*FDA indication.
Abbreviations: NSAID = nonsteroidal anti-inflammatory drug; OTC = over-the-counter; TCA = tricyclic antidepressant.

seems an obvious truism, its importance cannot be overemphasized. Patients who experience frequent, near-daily, or daily headaches invariably require a comprehensive treatment program that necessitates good communication. Anxious patients sometimes do not comprehend medical explanations or instructions; busy doctors sometimes do not have or take the time to ensure that the patient understands.

The two elements of headache treatment are *abortive treatment*, directed at attacks once they have begun, and *prophylactic treatment*, directed at preventing or reducing the frequency of attacks. In general, the abortive approach is used for patients who suffer infrequent attacks and for those who experience breakthrough attacks while undergoing prophylactic therapy. Prophylactic therapy should be instituted when headaches are frequent, when headaches are unresponsive to abortive medication, or when there are contraindications to abortives (Table 2).

Headache treatment can include nonpharmacologic measures, such as physical exercise, stretching, stress avoidance, relaxation exercises, biofeedback, manipulation, massage, or cold/warm packs. Pharmacologic therapies can include a vast array of medications from over-the-counter (OTC) drugs to prescription drugs such as triptans, other vasoconstrictors, β-blockers, antiepileptic agents, antidepressants, nonsteroidal anti-inflammatory drugs (NSAIDs), analgesics, muscle relaxants, anxiolytics, and others.

Treatment, whether prophylactic or abortive, should follow a definite plan incorporating the clinician and patient into a team focused on reducing the headache frequency, severity, and disability. As mentioned earlier, impressions and physical findings should be explained to the patient in as much detail as necessary to ensure the patient's complete understanding. The complexity of the headache condition needs to be explained, emphasizing its chronicity, rather than its curability, and that the goal of treatment is disease control.

The comprehensiveness of the treatment plan depends on the frequency of the patient's attacks. The more frequent and severe the attacks, the more detailed plan may be necessary. Patients experiencing infrequent attacks (e.g., once or twice monthly) may require only an abortive medication and little else. Patients with more frequent attacks may benefit from dietary restrictions, psychosocial intervention, biofeedback relaxation training, manipulation, and physical modality intervention, in addition to medication.

TENSION-TYPE HEADACHE TREATMENT

TTHA often is associated with emotional stress and muscle strain or tension of the shoulders and neck. Simple self-administered measures, such as stress avoidance, stretching, warm packs, or relaxation techniques, can be helpful in reducing or relieving attacks. More comprehensive professional intervention, such as manipulation, physical therapy, local injections, or biofeedback training, are considerations for more frequent or severe cases.

Prophylactically, the use of OTC or prescription medications can be considered in addition to nonmedicinal measures for reducing the frequency and duration of attacks. NSAIDs, muscle relaxants, or antidepressants (tricyclic antidepressant [TCA], selective serotonin reuptake inhibitor [SSRI]), at the lowest effective doses, are more commonly used.

Daily use of the longer-acting NSAIDs, such as naproxen[1] (Naprosyn) or celecoxib[1] (Celebrex), in the appropriately screened patient over a 2- to 3-week period, can be an effective preventative. TCAs, such as nortriptyline[1] (Pamelor) or amitriptyline[1] (Elavil), in low doses at night over 1 to 3 months, are frequently effective, especially in patients with anxiety or mild depression. The SSRI drugs, such as fluoxetine[1] (Prozac) or sertraline[1] (Zoloft), similarly can be useful. The muscle relaxant cyclobenzaprine[1] (Flexeril), at low doses, with a similar mechanism to the TCAs, can be administered at night for limited periods. Other muscle relaxants occasionally can be effective. Potential side effects can limit the use of NSAIDs (gastrointestinal irritation) and the TCAs (fatigue and weight gain).

Abortive or symptomatic treatment of TTHA can include simple OTC medications (e.g., aspirin or acetaminophen), NSAIDs (short-acting), muscle relaxants, combination analgesics, and, in some cases, opioid or opioidlike drugs. Caution should be exercised in prescribing potentially habituating drugs. Daily or near-daily use of analgesics can lead to analgesic rebound headache, Medication Overuse Headache, which can compound the patient's headache problem.

Botulism toxin[1] (Botox) reportedly is helpful in the treatment of tension-type and migraine headache, but controlled studies are limited. In this treatment, a diluted solution of botulism toxin is injected into various muscles of the face, scalp, neck, or shoulders. Because this treatment frequently is used in headache specialty and pain centers, simultaneous comprehensive measures and medication may contribute to positive results. Side effects from botulism toxin are low when injected properly.

MIGRAINE TREATMENT

Migraineurs are unique individuals, and the effectiveness and tolerance of medications can vary from patient to patient. Medication changes, combinations of medications, and trial and error may be necessary in the early stages of treatment.

Nonmedicinal measures for migraine sufferers include biofeedback stress reduction, caffeine and dietary restrictions, regimentation of meals and sleep, rest, exercise, stretching, and avoidance of work or activity overload. Limiting caffeine to less than 200 mg/day is important to prevent the caffeine headache (rebound headache) in most patients. Elimination of vasoactive foods, such as chocolate, aged cheese, and processed meats, and avoidance of fasting for more than 4 hours can be helpful for patients with more frequent attacks (Table 3). Regular exercise and stretching, planned relaxation, regular sleep schedules, and following a healthy lifestyle are frequently included in a comprehensive treatment regimen. In some patients, especially children and adolescents, biofeedback stress reduction or psychotherapeutic intervention may be necessary.

---

[1]Not FDA approved for this indication.

TABLE 3 Triptans

Medication	Brand Name	Half-life	Form/Strength
Sumatriptan	Imitrex	1.5 hr	Oral: 25, 50, 100 mg; NS: 20 mg; injection: 6 mg, 4 mg
Naratriptan	Amerge	6 hr	Oral: 2.5 mg
Zolmitriptan	Zomig	3 hr	Oral: 2.5, 5 mg; Melt: 2.5, 5 mg; NS: 5 mg
Rizatriptan	Maxalt	2–3 hr	Oral: 5, 10 mg; Melt: 10 mg
Almotriptan	Axert	3–4 hr	Oral: 6.25, 12.5 mg
Frovatriptan	Frova	25 hr	Oral: 5 mg
Eletriptan	Relpax	4 hr	Oral: 20, 40 mg

[1]Not FDA approved for this indication.
Abbreviations: Melt = oral disintegrating; NS = nasal steroid.

The more commonly used medications for prophylaxis are β-blockers, calcium channel blockers, antiepileptics (neurostabilizers), and the antidepressants. Treatment should be continued for a 4- to 8-week trial before discontinuation for ineffectiveness. Determination of which medication to use depends on comorbidities, interactions with concomitant medications, and tolerability.

β-Blockers such as propranolol (Inderal) and timolol (Blocadren) are nonselective and are approved by the Food and Drug Administration (FDA) for migraine prevention. Other β-blockers, such as nadolol[1] (Corgard), metoprolol[1] (Lopressor), and atenolol[1] (Tenormin), also can be effective. The mechanism of action in migraine is not wholly understood, but it is thought to involve anxiolytic effects as well as vascular changes and stabilization. The usual dosage is recommended (e.g., timolol 10–30 mg/day, propranolol 120–160 mg/day), and many consider the nighttime dose the more significant.

Calcium channel antagonists are well tolerated in general and can be as effective as the β-blockers. They are believed to alter serotonin release and inhibit platelet serotonin uptake and release within the brain. Verapamil[1] (Calan) is considered the more effective and is commonly recommended to patients. Dosage can vary from 120 to 480 mg/day. Nimodipine[1] (Nimotop) is equally effective, but it is rarely used in the United States because of its high cost.

Antiepileptic medications such as phenytoin[1] (Dilantin) and carbamazepine[1] (Tegretol) have been prescribed for migraine prevention over the years, with mixed results. Their use is now limited with the advent of newer, more easily tolerated agents, such as divalproex sodium (Depakote) and topiramate (Topamax).

Divalproex sodium is effective in reducing migraine attacks and is particularly useful in patients with coexisting head injury, seizure disorders, and bipolar disorders. It is thought to improve inhibitory and excitatory amino acid imbalance in the brain. It is best to start with a lower dose and to gradually increase as needed and tolerated. The dosage of 500 to 1000 mg/day is more frequently prescribed. A commonly experienced side effect is sedation, which can sometimes be used to the patient's advantage when anxiolytic effects are needed.

Topiramate is the most recent preventive medication approved by the FDA for migraine prophylaxis. It has multiple mechanisms of action, but its exact mechanism in migraine headache is unknown. Its effectiveness is believed to involve sodium ion channel stabilization, calcium ion channels, GABA (γ-aminobutyric acid) receptors, and neuronal membrane stabilization. The average daily dose is variable and ranges from 30 to 100 mg/day. A most unusual side effect of weight loss or appetite suppression can be used to the patient's advantage in preventing weight gain, which frequently accompanies migraine prophylactic medications.

The TCAs can be useful in patients who experience frequent attacks and in those who experience anxiety and depression. The TCAs inhibit synaptic reuptake of serotonin, thereby reducing neuron firing and release of neurotransmitters. Starting with a low dose in the evening and titrating up to efficacy and tolerability is recommended. Significant anticholinergic and sedation effects sometimes limit their use. The SSRIs[1] are reported helpful in some patients, but their use in migraine prevention is limited.

In general, prophylactic medications should be taken for 6 to 8 weeks to determine efficacy. If effective, a course of 4 to 6 months is recommended before an attempt is made to discontinue medication.

A variety of abortive treatment options are available for migraine sufferers. Although the triptans (Table 3) have generated much interest and are frequently prescribed, other medications continue to be used, including ergotamine and its derivatives, isometheptene, and NSAIDs. Many of the abortive medications carry significant prescribing limitations that must be taken into consideration. Vasoconstrictor medications are contraindicated in patients with cardiovascular or peripheral vascular disease. NSAIDs should not be used in those with gastrointestinal or bleeding disorders. As with all medications, the clinician must consider appropriate prescribing, contraindications, and side-effect information.

The vasoconstrictor ergotamine is available in oral, rectal (Ergocaff PB), and sublingual forms (Ergomar). Ergotamine has a relatively long half-life and duration of action (up to 3 days) and should be used no more frequently than every 4 to 5 days to avoid ergotamine rebound headache. The ergot derivative dihydroergotamine (DHE-45, Migranal NS) is available for intramuscular (IM), subcutaneous (SC), intravenous (IV), and intranasal use. IV dihydroergotamine (DHE-45) sometimes is used for intractable migraine (status migrainosus) in emergency departments and inpatient settings. The intranasal form (Migranal) is an effective treatment when administered correctly by the patient. Unfortunately, dihydroergotamine is not absorbed by the gastrointestinal tract, and, unlike other abortive nasal sprays, any swallowed medication will be wasted. Dihydroergotamine has a low headache recurrence rate of approximately 12%. All forms of ergotamine and dihydroergotamine are more effective when taken early in attacks.

Isometheptene is used in combination with dichloralphenazone and acetaminophen (Midrin, Duradrin). It is slow acting and more effective when taken early in attacks and when used for attacks preceded or accompanied by stress and muscle tension of the neck. Although isometheptene is considered less potent than ergotamine and triptans, it is preferred by many patients whose headaches have features of both migraine and TTHA.

At the present time, seven serotonin agonists (triptans) are approved for abortive migraine treatment in the United States (see Table 3). As a category, the triptans are approximately 65% to 70% effective in published clinical trials. Their similarities are greater than their differences, but each triptan is not necessarily effective for all patients, and familiarity with their differences can be helpful to the treating physician. Half-life, onset and duration of action, adverse events, tolerability, recurrence of headache, and routes of administration may vary and allow the physician to match the medication to the individual patient. For example, a slower onset of action and longer-lasting triptan may be appropriate for slow-onset, longer-lasting migraine attacks.

Like other treatments, oral triptan tablets are more effective in the early phases of migraines. It is thought that peripheral sensitization—allodynia—is a sign of later phase migraine, and treating the attack before this phenomenon occurs is important. When treatment is delayed or the patient awakens with severe migraine, the injection, nasal spray, or rapidly acting triptans may be more beneficial. Although triptans as a group are very effective, recurrence of headache, after initial relief,

---

[1]Not FDA approved for this indication.

requiring retreatment is common and can be as high as 40%. The recurrence rate tends to be less with triptans having a longer half-life.

The ergots and triptans are contraindicated in patients with ischemic heart disease, uncontrolled hypertension, and cerebrovascular disease. Physicians initially were extremely cautious about recommending triptans to their patients when the triptans were first introduced in the United States. However, significant human exposure to the triptans has revealed that catastrophic myocardial infarction or serious ischemia is rare. Chest pain following triptan use affects a small percentage of patients, and because the significance of this finding is not clear, refraining from future triptan use in these patients is recommended.

Sumatriptan (Imitrex), the first triptan approved in the United States, is available in nasal spray (20 mg), SC (6 mg, 4 mg), and oral formulations (25, 50, 100 mg). Its half-life is approximately 1.5 hours, and its duration of action is less than 4 hours. The injectable form produces rapid relief in 70% to 80% of patients, and it appears to be the most effective of all the available triptan forms. Conversely, it appears to cause the most side effects, and, for this reason, it should be used only for the more severe attacks. The oral forms are more favorable with regard to adverse effects, and their effectiveness is similar to that of other triptans (approximately 65%). Because of sumatriptan's short half-life and duration of action, recurrence of headache is common, necessitating repeat dosing.

Zolmitriptan (Zomig) is available in 2.5- and 5-mg oral and oral disintegrating tablets (ZMT) and as a 5-mg nasal spray. The efficacy of oral zolmitriptan is approximately 65% and that of the nasal form is 70%. The half-life of oral zolmitriptan is 3 hours, and its duration of action is longer than the nasal form, which improves on the need to re-medicate. The nasal spray has a biphasic absorption curve, which accounts for its favorable adverse effect profile over the 5-mg oral tablet.

Naratriptan (Amerge) was the first to be approved of the gradual-onset, longer-acting triptans. It is available as oral 2.5-mg tablets and has a half-life of 6 hours. Naratriptan is well tolerated by patients and often is used by patients with slow-onset migraine. Some specialists prescribe daily naratriptan for limited periods for treatment of menstrual or intractable migraine attacks.

Rizatriptan (Maxalt) is available as oral 5- and 10-mg tablets and as an oral disintegrating form (MLT). It has a relatively rapid onset of action and a favorable one-dose 2-hour response rate. Patients who are undergoing concomitant treatment with propranolol should take the lesser 5-mg rizatriptan dose because of higher resultant rizatriptan plasma levels.

Almotriptan (Axert) is available in 6.25- and 12.5-mg tablets. It has a half-life of 3.5 hours and, because of a broad T_{max} (time of maximal concentration) range of 1.4 to 3.8 hours, a relatively rapid onset of action. Almotriptan has favorable adverse effect and headache recurrence profile. Chest pain symptoms after almotriptan use are similar to placebo in clinical trials.

Frovatriptan (Frova) is a long-acting triptan available in 2.5-mg oral tablets. It has the longest half-life of 25 hours and a favorable recurrence rate. Frovatriptan is frequently used for treatment of menstrual migraine and for attacks of longer duration. Some specialists prescribe daily frovatriptan for a limited period for menstrual and prolonged migraine attacks.

Eletriptan (Relpax) is the most recently approved triptan. It is available in 20- and 40-mg oral tablets and has a half-life of nearly 5 hours. Eletriptan has a relatively rapid onset but a longer duration of action and a favorable recurrence rate. In studies, some patients who were unresponsive to other triptans responded to eletriptan.

Various attempts have been made to compare triptans. Head-to-head trials mostly have compared one triptan to sumatriptan. A meta-analysis of 53 clinical trials published in 2001 compared the efficacy, recurrence, duration of action, and tolerability of all available triptans. Almotriptan and eletriptan were rated favorably across the major parameters of onset of action, efficacy, adverse events, and recurrence. In spite of efforts to adjust for variations in protocols and placebo response, specialists reached no clear consensus as to the validity or value of the meta-analysis or the preferability of one triptan over another.

NSAIDs frequently are recommended for treatment of acute migraine and can be effective when taken early. Their effects on the physiology of pain, inflammation, and platelets are believed to be the mechanisms responsible. Some physicians recommend taking a NSAID with the first dose of a triptan for added efficacy. Various agents are used, but none of the rapid-acting NSAIDs appears to have significant efficacy superiority. OTC ibuprofen (Motrin) and aspirin, in combination with caffeine and acetaminophen (Excedrin Migraine), is approved by the FDA for treatment of migraine.

Symptomatic treatment of pain may be necessary in patients who do not respond to recommended abortive treatment. Any effective analgesic can be appropriate, provided it is used infrequently and not on a daily or near-daily basis. In general, the more effective analgesics have anti-inflammatory and sedative properties.

CLUSTER HEADACHE TREATMENT

Cluster headache is one of the more unusual pain conditions occasionally encountered by physicians. Pain onset is rapid, and the duration of the attack is brief. For this reason, prophylactic treatment usually is the most practical. Abortive prescriptions frequently are given, but, for the most part, the cluster attack is resolving by the time medication is absorbed.

Nonmedicinal prophylactic measures are extremely limited. The reduction of cigarette smoking, the addressing of individual stress and hostility issues when appropriate, and the complete cessation of alcohol consumption during cluster periods should be part of any treatment program. Prophylactic medications include the calcium channel blockers verapamil[1] (Calan) and nimodipine[1] (Nimotop), the neurostabilizers valproate[1] (Depakote) and topiramate[1] (Topamax), various NSAIDs, ergotamine,[1] lithium[1] (Eskalith), cyproheptadine (Periactin) and, in extreme cases, short intervals of steroids.[1] These medications are used in average therapeutic doses, and combinations of medications are commonly needed (Table 4). The preventatives should be used during the cluster cycle and discontinued during off-cycle periods.

Abortive treatment is less preferred for cluster headache, as noted previously. However, inhalation oxygen via facial mask at 6 L terminates cluster attacks in 75% to 80% of sufferers within 12 minutes. Other possibilities include sumatriptans (Imitrex) SC or nasal spray,[1] zolmitriptan (Zomig ZMT) nasal spray,[1] ergotamine (Ergomar) sublingual, or dihydroergotamine injection (DHE-45) or nasal spray[1] (Migranal). The occasional patient reports relief with the oral triptans or analgesics. When triptans, ergotamine, or analgesics are used, appropriate prescribing and frequency guidelines should

---

[1]Not FDA approved for this indication.

TABLE 4 Cluster Headache Prophylactic Medications

Medication	Brand	Average Daily Dose
Verapamil[1]	Calan, Isoptin, Verelan	240–420 mg
Divalproex[1]	Depakote	500–1500 mg
Topiramate[1]	Topamax	50–200 mg
Indomethacin[1]	Indocin	100–150 mg
Naproxen[1]	Naprosyn	1000–1500 mg
Lithium[1]	Lithobid	600–1200 mg*
Ergotamine[1]	Bellergal[1]	1 tablet bid[†]
Prednisone[1]	—	100 mg, decrease to 0
Cyproheptadine	Periactin	8–16 mg

[1]Not FDA approved for this indication.
*With serum level monitoring.
[†]Ergotamine 0.6 mg with phenobarbital 40 mg and 0.2 mg L-alkaloids of belladonna.

be followed. In general, with the exception of oxygen, daily as-needed medications should be avoided.

Headache continues to present a challenging problem for clinicians as well as for suffering patients. In spite of recent treatment advances and more public awareness, millions continue to needlessly endure pain and debilitation. At first glance, the headache problem appears complex and difficult when, in actuality, most sufferers experience straightforward, easily diagnosed headaches. The interested generalist or specialist who takes the time to elicit a careful history can establish the headache diagnosis and direct a simple treatment plan that can make a tremendous difference in the headache sufferer's life.

REFERENCES

Astin JA, Ernst E: The effectiveness of spinal manipulation for the treatment of headache disorders: A systematic review of randomized clinical trials. Cephalalgia 2002;22:617-623.

Diamond ML, Dalessio DJ (eds): Diamond and Dalessio's The Practicing Physician's Approach to Headache, 5th ed. Philadelphia: WB Saunders, 1999.

Ferrari MD, Roon KI, Lipton RB, et al: Oral triptans (serotonin 5HT-IB/ID-agonists) in acute migraine treatment: A meta-analysis of 53 trials. Lancet 2001;358:1668-1675.

Gallagher RM, Kunkel R: Migraine medication attributes important for patient compliance: Concerns about side effects may delay treatment. Headache: J Head Face Pain 2003;43:36-43.

Goadsby PJ, Lipton RB, Ferreri MD: Migraine current understanding and treatment. N Engl J Med 2002;346:257-270.

Silberstein SD, Lipton EB, Dalessio DJ: Wolff's Headache and Other Head Pain, 7th ed. New York: Oxford University Press, 2001.

Vernon H, McDermaid C, Hagino C: Systematic review of randomized clinical trials of complementary/alternative therapies in the treatment of tension-type and cervicogenic headache. Complement Ther Med 1999;7:142-155.

Viral Meningitis and Encephalitis

Method of
Mark J. Abzug, MD

Viral meningitis is the most common cause of aseptic meningitis, an inflammatory process involving the meninges in which usual bacterial etiologies cannot be identified. Encephalitis is an inflammatory process that affects the brain parenchyma, typically producing more severe illness. Many viral infections of the central nervous system produce inflammation of both the meninges and brain tissue (meningoencephalitis). Encephalitis may result from acute viral invasion of the brain and a concomitant inflammatory response or from a postinfectious, autoimmune process characterized by demyelination following a viral illness or vaccination (acute disseminated encephalomyelitis). The majority of the approximately 8000 to 13,000 cases of aseptic meningitis and approximately 20,000 cases of encephalitis reported annually in the United States are caused by viral infections.

Clinical Features

Regardless of etiology, most cases of viral meningitis present similarly. Infants and young children display nonspecific symptoms, such as fever, irritability, lethargy, anorexia, and emesis. More specific findings suggestive of meningeal inflammation, such as nuchal rigidity, bulging fontanelle, and photophobia, are often absent. In older children and adults, nuchal rigidity and photophobia, along with fever, headache, and emesis, are more frequent. Focal neurologic findings and seizures are uncommon presenting findings in viral meningitis, although approximately 10% of children hospitalized with viral meningitis may develop acute complications such as obtundation, seizures, increased intracranial pressure, and inappropriate antidiuretic hormone secretion. Illness can last up to 1 to 2 weeks, with protracted headache not uncommon in adults.

Encephalitis is distinguished from meningitis by a change in sensorium and/or by focal neurologic findings. In younger children, encephalitis typically presents with irritability and/or lethargy, often after a febrile illness. Older children may manifest headache, disorientation, unusual behavior, abnormal speech, bizarre movements, and disorientation in addition to fever, nausea, emesis, myalgias, and photophobia. Generalized or, less commonly, focal neurologic abnormalities, including seizures and motor deficits, may be present. Progression to extreme lethargy, stupor, or coma may ensue.

Etiology

In recent studies, a specific etiologic agent was identified in 55% to 70% of presumed cases of viral meningitis and in only 25% to 65% of cases of encephalitis despite thorough investigation. The list of implicated viruses is extensive (Table 1). Enteroviruses (EVs) are the most common cause of both viral meningitis and encephalitis of proven etiology. Other important agents include arboviruses (transmitted by arthropod vectors such as mosquitoes or ticks), herpes simplex virus (HSV), influenza virus, Epstein-Barr virus, varicella-zoster virus, adenovirus, and rabies virus.

Diagnosis

Important diagnostic clues may come from history (respiratory or gastrointestinal symptoms, family exposures, seasonality, prevalent diseases, travel, animal and insect exposure, and recreational activities) and physical examination (see Table 1). The presence of a rash may suggest specific agents, such as varicella-zoster virus or EVs. Whereas identification of a mucocutaneous vesicle in a neonate may be key to the diagnosis of HSV infection, cold sores in older children and adults are *not* predictive of HSV encephalitis. The combination of findings of encephalitis and myelitis in the same patient is suggestive of infection with an EV (especially EV 71), West Nile virus, or Japanese encephalitis virus. Although focal signs are present in the majority of older children and adults with HSV encephalitis, the positive predictive value of focal findings for HSV is low.

Examination of the cerebrospinal fluid (CSF) is indicated in suspected meningitis or encephalitis unless contraindicated by concern for a space-occupying lesion or increased intracranial pressure. CSF in viral meningitis typically has a low-grade pleocytosis (100–1000 white blood cells [WBCs]/mm^3, range <100 to ≥2000 WBC/mm^3). Polymorphonuclear leukocytes may predominate early, with the profile becoming mononuclear within 8 to 48 hours. In general, CSF protein is normal or slightly increased, and the glucose concentration is normal or slightly decreased, although exceptions occur. The CSF in encephalitis typically has a predominantly mononuclear pleocytosis, increased protein, and normal glucose, although CSF may be normal in 3% to 5% or more of cases, especially early in the course. Certain viruses, including influenza and parvovirus B19, typically cause encephalopathies characterized by the absence of pleocytosis.

Imaging and electroencephalography (EEG) are useful adjuncts, particularly for encephalitis. Magnetic resonance imaging generally has better sensitivity than does computed tomography, especially early in disease. Characteristic imaging findings may suggest specific pathogens (see Table 1), and imaging can exclude alternative diagnoses; for example, a parameningeal focus or tumor. EEG is the most sensitive tool for confirming encephalitis and can distinguish infection from metabolic encephalopathy.

Viral culture, polymerase chain reaction (PCR), and serology are the major techniques for specific virologic diagnosis. Sensitivity of CSF viral culture is better for meningitis than for encephalitis.

TABLE 1 Epidemiology and Clinical Features of Viral Meningitis and Encephalitis

Enteroviruses
Epidemiology
- Most common proven cause of viral meningitis and encephalitis (up to 85%–95% of viral meningitis and 80% of viral encephalitis).
- Majority of meningitis and encephalitis occurs in children <1 year old; incidence of meningitis exceeds that of encephalitis.
- Epidemic in warm seasons in temperate climates.
- Poliovirus infection decreased with widespread immunization.
- Enterovirus 71 frequently occurs in regional outbreaks, e.g., Asia since the late 1990s. Severe disease occurs primarily in children <5 years old.

Clinical Features
- Meningitis and severe encephalitis more common in younger children, especially neonates. Encephalitis may be part of systemic illness in newborns.
- Encephalitis typically generalized, although focal seizures and other abnormalities may occur, especially in neonates.
- May have biphasic febrile course; meningeal and encephalitic symptoms occur during second phase.
- Rash (macular, maculopapular, petechial, vesicular), enanthem, conjunctivitis, respiratory symptoms, pleurodynia, pericarditis, myocarditis, diarrhea, myalgias may accompany.
- Chronic meningoencephalitis with waxing and waning neurologic symptoms and high fatality rate occur in hypogammaglobulinemic patients.
- Enterovirus 71 associated with hand-foot-and-mouth disease, herpangina, and neurologic disease (meningitis, brainstem encephalitis, myelitis/acute flaccid paralysis, Guillain-Barré syndrome).
  - Signs of brainstem encephalitis include myoclonic jerks, tremors, ataxia, cranial nerve palsy, limb weakness, altered consciousness, seizures, increased intracranial pressure.
  - Imaging reveals high-intensity lesions in the midbrain, brainstem, and spinal cord anterior horn cells and ventral roots.
  - Pulmonary edema/hemorrhage, cardiac failure, shock may develop rapidly.

Herpes Simplex Virus
Epidemiology
- ~1%–3% of viral meningitis.
  - Predominantly associated with primary type 2 HSV genital infection and less frequently with primary type 1 HSV genital infection, nonprimary HSV genital infection (either type), or without recent genital disease.
  - Mollaret's meningitis (recurrent, benign aseptic meningitis) mostly associated with type 2 infection without signs of genital infection and occasionally with type 1 HSV or with Epstein-Barr virus.
- ~10%–20% of encephalitis in the United States.
  - Encephalitis primarily due to type 2 HSV in neonates and type 1 HSV in older age groups.
  - Encephalitis occurs in ~50% of neonatal HSV infections.
  - ~33%–50% of non-neonatal HSV encephalitis is caused by primary HSV infection and ~50%–67% is caused by HSV reactivation.
  - Most common focal viral encephalitis in nonepidemic settings; most common sporadic fatal encephalitis.

Clinical Features
- Neonatal encephalitis characterized by seizures (focal and generalized), lethargy, irritability, tremors, anorexia, temperature instability, bulging fontanelle.
  - Central nervous system–only disease frequently begins in temporal lobe and then becomes bitemporal.
  - Encephalitis with disseminated disease more commonly is diffuse.
- Non-neonatal encephalitis characterized by fever and focal encephalitis with necrosis and hemorrhage.
  - Tropism for temporal lobe: Aphasia, anosmia, temporal lobe seizures, other focal findings.
  - Findings include headache, emesis, altered consciousness, bizarre behavior, personality changes, disorientation, ataxia, hallucinations, hemiparesis.
  - Focal findings are not always present; bilateral disease, widespread disease, or brainstem encephalitis may occur.
  - Elevated red blood cell count may be present in CSF; CSF protein levels may be normal early and increase over time.
  - Focal abnormalities on imaging studies, especially involving one or both temporal lobes, are suggestive of HSV disease. However, focal disease may occur with other viruses, other regions of the brain may be affected by HSV, and imaging may be normal in early HSV.
  - Temporal lobe focality on electroencephalography, especially with periodic lateralizing epileptiform discharges, is characteristic of HSV but is not specific.
  - Rapid progression is common; however, atypical and mild, slowly progressive cases are increasingly being reported.

Arboviruses
Epidemiology
- ~5% of viral meningitis and important cause of encephalitis.
- Prevalent during warm and/or wet seasons; incidence related to mosquito or tick exposure.
- Leading agents in the United States:
  - West Nile virus: U.S. outbreaks since late 1990s; July to December predominance. Lower incidence and severity in children. Risk factors for severe neurologic disease include older age and immune compromise.
  - La Crosse virus: Central, eastern United States. Incidence of encephalitis approximately equal to that of meningitis; affects children more than adults.
- St. Louis encephalitis virus: Central, western, southern United States. Incidence of encephalitis less than that of meningitis; lower incidence and severity of encephalitis in children.
- Japanese encephalitis virus: Most common cause of epidemic encephalitis worldwide; causes encephalitis more than meningitis. Prevalent in Asia and Australia; affects children more than adults.
- Other important viruses
  - Eastern equine encephalomyelitis virus: Causes encephalitis more than meningitis.
  - Western equine encephalomyelitis virus: Causes encephalitis more than meningitis.
  - Venezuelan equine encephalomyelitis: Causes encephalitis more than meningitis.
  - Colorado Tick Fever virus: Rocky Mountains; tickborne. Meningitis in up to 18% of cases; encephalitis uncommon.
  - Powassan, Rocio, Murray Valley, Kyasuma Forest, Jamestown Canyon, California encephalitis, tickborne encephalitis, Ilheus, Snowshoe Hare, Rift Valley viruses.

TABLE 1 Epidemiology and Clinical Features of Viral Meningitis and Encephalitis—cont'd

Clinical Features
- West Nile virus
  - ~20% of infections are symptomatic; West Nile fever in majority of these infections.
  - Neurologic illness in ~1/150 infected; of these, meningitis in ~30% and encephalitis in ~65%. Neurologic manifestations also include acute asymmetrical flaccid paralysis, polyradiculitis, transverse myelitis, Guillain-Barré syndrome, optic neuritis, and chorioretinitis.
  - Encephalitis is characterized by altered consciousness, cranial nerve palsies (brainstem involvement), generalized or focal motor deficits (weakness, tremor, myoclonus), movement disorders, sensory deficits, and ataxia. Focal temporal lobe disease may mimic HSV. Case fatality rate ~10%.
  - Fever, emesis, maculopapular rash (especially in children) frequently accompany neurologic disease.
- Japanese and Eastern equine encephalitides
  - Thalamic, midbrain, basal ganglia, brainstem lesions characteristic.

Influenza Virus
Epidemiology
- Rare cause of meningitis.
- Cause of 8%–10% of encephalitis.
  - More commonly associated with influenza A than with influenza B.
  - Encephalitis may be acute or postinfectious.
  - Acute necrotizing encephalopathy reported primarily in 1- to 5-year-old children in Asia since the late 1990s.
- Neurologic spectrum includes Reye's syndrome (influenza B), myelitis, Guillain-Barré syndrome.

Clinical Features
- Acute necrotizing encephalopathy
  - Fever, altered consciousness, prolonged seizures; rapid progression to coma.
  - Elevated CSF protein, usually without pleocytosis.
  - Magnetic resonance imaging: Bilateral thalamic lesions and multifocal symmetrical lesions (brainstem, putamina, medulla, periventricular white matter, cerebellum).
  - Mortality ~30%; severe sequelae among survivors.

Varicella-Zoster Virus
Epidemiology and Clinical Features
- Chickenpox associated with cerebellar ataxia, meningitis, encephalitis, postinfectious encephalitis/ADEM, transverse myelitis, Guillain-Barré syndrome.
- Zoster associated with encephalitis, granulomatous hemiparesis, myelitis, cranial neuritis (including Bell's palsy). Neurologic complications may occur with rash, weeks to months after rash or without rash (especially in immune-compromised patients).

Epstein-Barr Virus
Epidemiology and Clinical Features
- Neurologic complications occur in 1%–5% of primary infections.
- Etiology of 2%–5% of acute viral encephalitis.
- Spectrum includes meningitis, encephalitis, ADEM, cranial nerve palsy (including Bell's palsy), transverse myelitis, and Guillain-Barré syndrome. Alice in Wonderland syndrome, consisting of visual seizures with metamorphopsia, may accompany encephalitis.
- Neurologic disease more frequent in immune compromised hosts.
- Typical features of infectious mononucleosis, atypical lymphocytosis, and heterophile antibody often absent in Epstein-Barr virus neurologic syndromes.

Cytomegalovirus
Epidemiology and Clinical Features
- Encephalitis primarily in congenitally infected neonates and immune-compromised hosts.
- Insidious progression.

Human Herpesvirus 6
Epidemiology and Clinical Features
- Meningoencephalitis occasionally occurs with primary infection.
- Increased incidence of encephalitis in immune-compromised hosts.
- Confusion, headache, seizures may accompany encephalitis; disease may be focal and mimic HSV encephalitis.

Adenovirus
Epidemiology and Clinical Features
- Neurologic spectrum includes acute encephalitis, postinfectious encephalitis, Reye's syndrome-like encephalopathy, and transient encephalopathy.
  - Acute encephalitis is characterized by seizures, CSF pleocytosis, and severe disease.
  - Transient encephalopathy is characterized by obtundation, normal CSF, and complete recovery within several days.

Lymphocytic Choriomeningitis Virus
Epidemiology and Clinical Features
- Transmission by rodent secretions.
- Meningitis and encephalitis more commonly occur in developing countries.
- Spectrum includes encephalitis, hydrocephalus, transverse myelitis.

Human Immunodeficiency Virus
Epidemiology and Clinical Features
- Transient meningitis and, more rarely, encephalitis may accompany primary infection (acute retroviral syndrome).
- Chronic infection may be associated with subacute encephalopathy (loss of developmental milestones in young children, dementia).
- Acute encephalitis may accompany treatment failure during chronic infection (uncommon).

Continued

TABLE 1 Epidemiology and Clinical Features of Viral Meningitis and Encephalitis—cont'd

Rabies Virus
Epidemiology and Clinical Features
- Relatively uncommon in United States; major sources are bats, raccoons, foxes, skunks.
- Important cause of encephalitis in developing countries; important sources are dogs and cats.
- Incubation period can vary from weeks to months to years. Pain, pruritus, or paresthesias at bite wound is followed by prodromal fever and anxiety and then by encephalitis.

Measles, Mumps, Rubella Viruses
Epidemiology and Clinical Features
- Meningitis occurs in ~30% of measles infections; measles also causes acute encephalitis, postinfectious encephalitis, and delayed subacute sclerosing panencephalitis.
- Mumps was the leading cause of meningitis in the prevaccine era.
- Meningitis and encephalitis due to each virus dramatically decreased with widespread immunization in developed countries.

Other Viral Agents
- Parainfluenza virus, respiratory syncytial virus, human metapneumovirus, rhinovirus, coronavirus, parvovirus B19, rotavirus, encephalomyocarditis virus, hepatitis C virus, simian herpes B virus, human T-lymphotropic virus, JC virus, Lassa fever virus, yellow fever virus, Hendra virus, Nipah virus, Australian bat Lyssavirus.

Acute Disseminated Encephalomyelitis
Epidemiology
- Implicated in 10%–15% of cases of encephalitis in the United States.
- Increased incidence in infants and children.
- Onset days to weeks after respiratory tract infection (influenza, enteroviruses, measles, mumps, rubella, *Mycoplasma pneumoniae*, and others), gastroenteritis (rotavirus), and other infections (HSV, Epstein-Barr virus, varicella-zoster virus, human herpesvirus 6, cytomegalovirus).
- History of preceding infection or vaccination elicited in up to two thirds of cases.
- Winter–spring predominance in some series.

Clinical Features
- Diffuse, often multifocal symptoms reflecting regions of brain affected. Spectrum includes motor deficits, cranial nerve palsies, optic neuritis, cerebellar ataxia, altered consciousness, psychosis, seizures, transverse myelitis, peripheral neuritis.
- Multifocal, asymmetrical demyelinating lesions in imaging studies, with predilection for white matter.
- CSF cytology may be normal or show pleocytosis; CSF protein elevated in 50%–70%.
- Typically monophasic; occasionally relapses occur.
- Acute hemorrhagic leukoencephalitis is a rare entity representing the fulminant end of the spectrum. It primarily affects young adults and is characterized by seizures, coma, cerebral edema, and a rapid, often fatal course.

Abbreviations: ADEM = acute disseminated encephalomyelitis; CSF = cerebrospinal fluid; HSV = herpes simplex virus.

Sensitivity reaches 65% to 75% for EVs, and CSF culture may be positive in young infants lacking pleocytosis. CSF culture is positive in 25% to 40% of neonates with HSV encephalitis but in less than 2% of older children and adults. CSF PCR is generally more sensitive than culture in both meningitis and encephalitis. CSF PCR for EVs has greater than 95% sensitivity and specificity. Sensitivity and specificity of CSF PCR for HSV are between 75% and 100% in neonatal HSV encephalitis and 91% and 98% in older children and adults with HSV encephalitis. Importantly, HSV PCR may be falsely negative within the first 3 to 4 days of illness in up to 25% of cases; repeat testing 4 to 7 days later is generally positive. In many viral encephalitides, viral cultures, antigen detection tests, and PCR of non-CSF specimens have better yields than do CSF culture and PCR (e.g., throat and stool/rectum for EV 71, for which CSF culture and PCR are more often negative, and respiratory specimens for influenza, adenovirus, and other respiratory viruses). Detection of serum and CSF antibodies can be performed for many viruses (e.g., most arboviruses and lymphocytic choriomeningitis virus), frequently requiring acute and convalescent specimens. Serum and CSF IgM assays can be diagnostic for West Nile virus, Japanese encephalitis virus, Epstein-Barr virus, and EV 71. A brain biopsy should be considered in a patient with symptoms that are progressive or do not improve, with an uncertain diagnosis, and with a focal, accessible lesion.

Treatment

The mainstay of therapy for viral meningitis and encephalitis is supportive care. In patients in whom there is difficulty distinguishing between bacterial and viral meningitis (e.g., young children, especially those younger than 1 year), hospitalization and parenteral antibiotics (e.g., vancomycin [Vancocin] plus a third-generation cephalosporin such as cefotaxime [Claforan] or ceftriaxone [Rocephin]) are administered until bacterial cultures are negative and/or an alternative diagnosis is made. Additionally, newborns or other immune-compromised patients with EV meningitis may require supportive therapy for severe disseminated disease (e.g., hepatitis, coagulopathy, or myocarditis). A presumptive diagnosis of viral meningitis can often be made in older children and adults who are not very ill based on clinical and CSF examination (low-grade pleocytosis with mononuclear predominance initially or 8–24 hours later, normal to slightly depressed glucose concentration, normal to slightly increased protein level). Lumbar puncture may alleviate symptoms such as headache, irritability, and emesis. Therefore, in older children and adults, hospitalization and/or empirical antibiotic treatment are indicated for patients who appear ill, including those requiring parenteral hydration and/or analgesics, those in whom viral and bacterial infection cannot be readily distinguished, and those who manifest findings of encephalitis. Presumptive therapy for *Mycobacterium tuberculosis* may be indicated if the exposure history, clinical presentation, CSF examination, and imaging findings are suggestive of this agent.

There are few proven specific antiviral therapies for meningitis and encephalitis. Acyclovir[1] (Zovirax) can hasten recovery from HSV meningitis, although HSV meningitis without encephalitis generally has an excellent outcome without antiviral treatment. Valacyclovir[1] (Valtrex) and famciclovir[1] (Famvir) are also available for oral therapy of HSV meningitis associated with genital HSV in immune-competent patients.

For children and adults with encephalitis, empirical therapy with acyclovir (30 mg/kg/day up to 45–60 mg/kg/day intravenously divided every 8 hours) should generally be initiated pending

---

[1]Not FDA approved for this indication.

CURRENT DIAGNOSIS

Differential diagnosis of viral meningitis and encephalitis is broad and includes:
- Bacteria: *Streptococcus pneumoniae, Neisseria meningitidis, Haemophilus influenzae, Listeria monocytogenes, Mycobacterium tuberculosis, Borrelia burgdorferi, Mycoplasma pneumoniae, Mycoplasma hominis, Bartonella henselae,* syphilis, leptospirosis, brucellosis, rickettsial and ehrlichial infections
- Parasites: Neurocysticercosis, toxoplasmosis, amebic encephalitis
- Fungi: *Cryptococcus neoformans, Coccidioides immitis*
- Parameningeal focus: Brain abscess or subdural or epidural empyema
- Kawasaki disease
- Sarcoidosis
- Autoimmune disease: Systemic lupus erythematosus, cerebral vasculitis, Wegener's granulomatosis, Hashimoto's disease
- Medication-induced meningitis: Nonsteroidal anti-inflammatory drugs, sulfa antibiotics, immune globulin, cytosine arabinoside (Cytarabine), muromonab-CD3 (Orthoclone OKT3), carbamazepine (Tegretol)
- Metabolic derangements: Inborn errors of metabolism, leukodystrophy, uremia, hepatic encephalopathy, Reye's syndrome
- Cerebrovascular hemorrhage and/or infarct
- Malignancy
- Drug toxicity (e.g., neuroleptic malignant syndrome)
- Toxins

Historical information may suggest specific etiologic viruses:
- Respiratory symptoms: Influenza virus, adenovirus, other respiratory viruses
- Gastrointestinal symptoms: Rotavirus
- Family exposure: Influenza virus, EV
- Seasonality and prevalent diseases in the community: EV, West Nile virus, other arboviruses, influenza virus, other respiratory viruses
- Travel to areas with endemic or epidemic disease: West Nile virus, EV 71, Japanese encephalitis virus, other arboviruses
- Animal exposure: Rabies virus, lymphocytic choriomeningitis virus
- Mosquito exposure: West Nile virus, other arboviruses
- Tick exposure: Colorado tick fever virus, Powassan virus
- Recreational activities: Spelunking-associated bat exposure and rabies infection, hiking-associated mosquito and tick exposure and arbovirus infection

Useful laboratory evaluations for viral meningitis and encephalitis include CSF examination, imaging (especially magnetic resonance imaging), and electroencephalography. Imaging abnormalities may suggest certain pathogens (see Table 1). CSF PCR, serum IgM assays, and viral culture/antigen detection/PCR of mucosal specimens are especially useful specific diagnostic tests.

- CSF PCR is a more sensitive technique than viral culture for detection of viruses such as EVs; HSV; varicella-zoster virus, cytomegalovirus, human herpesvirus 6, Epstein-Barr virus, and JC virus in immune-compromised patients; measles virus; parvovirus B19; and human immunodeficiency virus. CSF PCR for other viruses, such as adenovirus, influenza virus, and arboviruses (including West Nile virus), have low or variable sensitivity. PCR of saliva has high sensitivity for rabies virus (other testing includes immunostain of a nape of neck biopsy, corneal impression, buccal mucosa, or brain tissue).
- The etiology of encephalitis is elusive in many cases. Extensive investigations ultimately are able to identify a specific etiologic agent in only 25% to 65% of cases.

Abbreviations: CSF = cerebrospinal fluid; EV = enterovirus; PCR = polymerase chain reaction.

---

diagnostic studies, particularly in the presence of fever and any evidence of focal neurologic abnormality (clinical examination, imaging, or electroencephalography). Treatment for 14 to 21 days* is indicated if HSV infection is confirmed or if clinical and diagnostic findings are strongly suggestive in the absence of other proven etiologies; a 21-day course is generally favored for more severe disease. Acyclovir (60 mg/kg/day intravenously divided every 8 hours) should be presumptively administered to newborns with encephalitis with focal or generalized findings. Treatment of proven or highly suspect neonatal HSV encephalitis is generally continued for 21 days and until an end-of-therapy CSF PCR is negative, although proof that extending therapy until the PCR is negative is beneficial is lacking. Whether higher doses (60 mg/kg/day) or longer courses (21 days) confer additional benefit outside the neonatal period is not established. Relapse within the first 1 to 3 months after therapy of neonatal and childhood/adult HSV encephalitis has been reported with variable incidence, in some cases correlated with lower daily dose and treatment duration. Whether relapses reflect active viral replication or an immune-mediated phenomenon is controversial, although CSF PCR positivity in some cases suggests the former.

Whether encephalitis associated with varicella-zoster virus is due more often to direct viral infection or an immune-mediated parainfectious process is not established. Thus, although acyclovir is frequently used for varicella-zoster virus encephalitis, including cerebellar ataxia, the role of antiviral therapy is unproven. Ganciclovir (Cytovene) and foscarnet (Foscavir) are used for meningoencephalitis in immune-compromised hosts caused by cytomegalovirus and human herpesvirus 6.

Pleconaril (Picovir) is an experimental agent that has been studied for treatment of EV meningitis and encephalitis, including chronic meningoencephalitis in hypogammaglobulinemic patients, with some evidence of benefit; however, the agent is not currently available. Intraventricular, intrathecal, and intravenous administration of immune globulin[1] have been used to suppress or stabilize chronic EV meningoencephalitis in immune-compromised patients. The mainstays of management of severe EV 71 neurologic disease are close monitoring, fluid restriction, osmotic diuretics, and cardiorespiratory support. Various agents, including pleconaril, interferon α,[1] intravenous immune globulin, and corticosteroids have been tried, but none has been proven to be effective.

---

*Exceeds duration recommended by the manufacturer.

[1]Not FDA approved for this indication.

CURRENT THERAPY

- General supportive measures for patients with severe meningitis or encephalitis include:
  - Analgesics for headache, antiemetics, intravenous fluids and medications for patients with depressed consciousness, anticonvulsants for seizures, provision of a quiet environment
  - Intensive care for severely ill patients, including tracheal intubation for airway protection, respiratory support, cardiorespiratory monitoring
  - Mild fluid restriction for cerebral edema or inappropriate antidiuretic hormone secretion
  - Head of bed elevation, hyperventilation, osmotic (mannitol) and loop diuretics, and control of temperature, pain, and seizures for increased intracranial pressure
- Specific antiviral agents available for meningoencephalitis include acyclovir (Zovirax) for HSV and varicella-zoster virus, ganciclovir (Cytovene) for cytomegalovirus and human herpesvirus 6, foscarnet (Foscavir) for cytomegalovirus and human herpesvirus 6, amantadine (Symmetrel) for susceptible influenza A, rimantadine (Flumadine) for susceptible influenza A, and oseltamivir (Tamiflu) for influenza A and B.
- Rehabilitative therapy and neurodevelopmental follow-up are frequently necessary after the acute phase of encephalitis regardless of the etiologic agent.
- Prognosis for viral meningitis is generally favorable without long-term sequelae, although fatigue, decreased concentration, and irritability may last for several weeks.
- Prognosis for viral encephalitis is variable and may be difficult to predict, especially early in the course of illness. In general, a worse prognosis is associated with extremes of age (infants <1 year and older adults), specific etiologies (HSV, enterovirus 71, West Nile virus, Japanese encephalitis virus, rabies), more severe illness (lower Glasgow Coma Scale) and extensive brain involvement, and, in the case of HSV, longer duration prior to initiation of treatment.

Abbreviation: HSV = herpes simplex virus.

Influenzal encephalitis is frequently treated with oral antivirals, including amantadine (Symmetrel) for influenza A (if susceptible), rimantadine (Flumadine) for influenza A (if susceptible), and oseltamivir (Tamiflu) for influenza A and B; corticosteroids and immune globulin[1] have also been tried. However, none of these agents has been proven to be effective for influenzal encephalitis. A combination of antiviral treatment, corticosteroids, and intravenous immune globulin has been suggested to reduce mortality due to influenzal acute necrotizing encephalopathy. There currently are no established therapies for West Nile virus encephalitis. Ribavirin (Rebetol),[1] interferon, high-titer immune globulin, and corticosteroids have been used, and therapeutic trials are currently ongoing. No specific therapies have been proven to be effective for encephalitis due to other arboviruses or for rabies; successful use of coma-inducing therapy plus the antivirals ribavirin and amantadine was reported in one patient with rabies encephalitis. Corticosteroids, intravenous immune globulin, and plasmapheresis have been used for acute disseminated encephalomyelitis, but efficacy trials have not been performed.

REFERENCES

Beaman MH, Wesselingh SL: Acute community-acquired meningitis and encephalitis. Med J Aust 2002;176:389-396.
Chang L, Hsia S, Wu C, et al: Outcome of enterovirus 71 infections with or without stage-based management: 1998-2002. Pediatr Infect Dis J 2004;23:327-331.
Glaser CA, Gilliam S, Schnurr D, et al: In search of encephalitis etiologies: Diagnostic challenges in the California encephalitis project, 1998-2000. Clin Infect Dis 2003;36:731-742.
Huang C, Morse D, Slater B, et al: Multiple-year experience in the diagnosis of viral central nervous system infections with a panel of polymerase chain reaction assays for detection of 11 viruses. Clin Infect Dis 2004;39:630-635.
Kennedy PGE: Viral encephalitis: causes, differential diagnosis, and management. J Neurol Neurosurg Psychiatry 2004;75(Suppl 1):i10-i15.
Kimberlin DW: Herpes simplex virus infections of the central nervous system. Semin Pediatr Infect Dis 2003;14:83-89.
Rotbart HA: Viral meningitis. Semin Neurol 2000;20:277-292.
Watson JT, Gerber SI: West Nile virus: A brief review. Pediatr Infect Dis J 2004;23:355-358.
Weitkamp J, Spring MD, Brogan T, et al: Influenza A virus-associated acute necrotizing encephalopathy in the United States. Pediatr Infect Dis J 2004;23:259-263.
Whitley RJ, Gnann JW: Viral encephalitis: Familiar infections and emerging pathogens. Lancet 2002;359:507-514.
Willoughby RE Jr, Tieves KS, Hoffman GM, et al: Survival after treatment of rabies with induction of coma. N Engl J Med 2005;352:2508-2514.

Multiple Sclerosis

Method of
Robert J. Fox, MD

Multiple sclerosis (MS) is a recurrent, chronic demyelinating disorder affecting the central nervous system (CNS): the brain, spinal cord, and optic nerves. MS affects approximately 400,000 people in the United States and 2.5 million worldwide.

The pathology of MS classically has been thought to involve primarily CD4+ helper T cells directed against the myelin sheath around axons. However, recent studies have suggested an important role of CD8+ cytotoxic T cells, monocytes, and even antibody-producing B cells in the pathogenesis of MS. MS was originally thought to only affect the myelin sheath that surrounds and protects nerve fibers, but studies have identified significant neuronal injury and atrophy early in the disease course.

The accumulation of tissue injury over time makes MS the most common nontraumatic cause of neurologic disability among young adults. The development of effective therapies that slow the progression of tissue damage and physical disability emphasizes the importance of accurate diagnosis and early treatment.

Symptoms and Classification

There are two general types of clinical symptoms associated with MS: clinical relapses and gradual progression of disability. Clinical relapses are acute or subacute in onset, typically developing over several days or weeks and stabilizing or resolving over several weeks to months. Symptoms can include any neurologic function but typically involve blurry or double vision, numbness, weakness, or dyscoordination. Relapses usually have no precipitants, although infections are sometimes associated with relapses. Clinical relapses herald the onset of the relapsing–remitting form of MS (RRMS), which accounts for about 85% of MS patients.

---
[1]Not FDA approved for this indication.

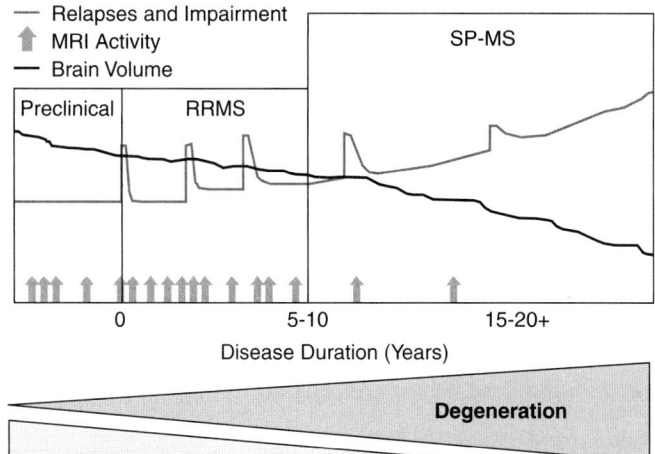

FIGURE 1. Typical clinical and MRI course of multiple sclerosis. MRI activity (vertical arrows) indicates an inflammatory lesion measured on brain MRI. MRI activity typically is more frequent than clinical relapses (spikes in clinical disability). Loss of brain volume, or atrophy, is measured on MRI and indicates permanent tissue damage. The early inflammatory activity is thought to be replaced later by a neurodegenerative process. MRI = magnetic resonance imaging; MS = multiple sclerosis; SP = secondary progressive; RR = relapsing–remitting. (Adapted from Fox RJ, Bethoux F, Goldman MD, Cohen JA: Multiple sclerosis: Advances in understanding, diagnosing, and treating the underlying disease. Cleve Clin J Med 2006;73(1):91-102.)

After 10 to 20 years of RRMS, clinical relapses become relatively infrequent, being replaced by gradually progressive neurologic symptoms (Fig. 1). This form of the disease most commonly manifests as a myelopathy involving the legs and later the arms, with progressive weakness, numbness, spasticity, and lack of coordination. This later stage of MS is called *secondary progressive MS* (SPMS), indicating that it has followed an initial relapsing–remitting form of the disease. SPMS is thought to represent an accelerated degenerative process, initiated during the relapsing–remitting stage of the disease. Current disease-modifying therapies are most effective in the RRMS stage, with little efficacy in SPMS.

Gradually progressive symptoms may also be the initial manifesting symptoms of the disease, a form of disease called *primary progressive MS* (PPMS). PPMS accounts for about 10% of MS patients and, similar to SPMS, has limited treatment options to slow progressive disability.

In about 2% to 4% of patients, inflammation is limited to the optic nerves and spinal cord and is called neuromyelitis optica, or Devic's disease. Brain involvement is unusual in this form of the disease, appearing as large, atypical lesions extending from the surface of the ventricles. Spinal cord involvement extends over many segments, sometimes involving the entire length of the spinal cord. Pathology shows necrotic destruction of nervous tissues, which explains the significant residual neurologic disability persisting after clinical episodes. Recent studies have identified the aquaporin-4 water ion channel as the autoimmune target in neuromyelitis optica, and many clinicians now differentiate neuromyelitis optica as a disease separate from MS.

Diagnosis

The diagnosis of MS is made through an assimilation of clinical history, neurologic examination, and paraclinical studies. Diagnostic criteria have shifted over time, but the basic elements remain unchanged: identification of multiple episodes of demyelination, disseminated in both time and space throughout the central nervous system, with other etiologies excluded. The most basic scenario is two episodes of demyelination affecting two different areas of

 CURRENT DIAGNOSIS

Recurrent CNS Demyelination, Disseminated in Time and Space

- Dissemination demonstrated clinically or on MRI
- Typical lesion on brain or spine MRI
- Inflammatory CSF (when needed)
- Visual evoked potentials (when needed)

MRI Lesions

- Periventricular
- Perpendicular to the lateral ventricle
- Corpus callosum
- Subcortical white matter
- Deep white matter (nonspecific)
- Hypointense on T1 images
- Gadolinium-enhancing lesions
- Posterior fossa, particularly cerebellum
- Spinal cord

CNS = central nervous system; CSF = cerebrospinal fluid; MRI = magnetic resonance imaging.

the central nervous system and leaving findings on neurologic examination. For example, transverse myelitis (inflammation of the spinal cord) and optic neuritis (inflammation of the optic nerve), the onset of each separated by at least one month, would fulfill the diagnostic criteria if objective findings were observed during the episodes or afterward. Transverse myelitis can leave hyperreflexia, and optic neuritis can leave disc pallor on fundoscopy or delayed visual evoked potentials. Two episodes of optic neuritis or transverse myelitis also fulfill criteria, so long as the two episodes involve different eyes or different regions of the spinal cord.

Current diagnostic criteria also allow the diagnosis to be made after a single episode of demyelination, often called a clinically isolated syndrome (Table 1). Dissemination can be fulfilled through magnetic resonance imaging (MRI) studies, with different requirements for dissemination in time and space. Dissemination in space requires a minimum number of lesions seen on brain and spine MRI. Dissemination in time requires an MRI 3 months or more after the onset of the clinically isolated syndrome showing either a gadolinium-enhancing lesion at a location different from the location of the initial event or a new T2 lesion (seen on T2-weighted MRI scan) compared with an MRI done at least 1 month after the initial event.

Brain MRI has taken on an increasingly important role in both the diagnosis and management of MS. Typical MS lesions are located in the periventricular white matter, as well as the subcortical white matter and posterior fossa (cerebellum) (Figs. 2 and 3). Lesions involving the deep white matter are also typical of MS, but they are relatively nonspecific, being seen commonly in patients with vascular risk factors, migraine, or even just normal aging. MS lesions are typically round or ovoid and often oriented perpendicular to the lateral ventricles—Dawson's fingers. These perpendicular lesions are best seen on sagittal T2-weighted imaging, such as fluid-attenuated inversion recovery (FLAIR) MRI. Also adding to the specificity of MS diagnosis is gadolinium enhancement and lesions in the spinal cord, although there are no pathognomic findings on MRI for MS (Fig. 4).

The diagnosis of PPMS requires 1 year of progressive symptoms and a combination of MRI findings and inflammatory cerebrospinal fluid studies. Proposed diagnostic criteria for neuromyelitis optica require optic neuritis, acute myelitis, and two of the following three supportive criteria: contiguous spinal cord lesion extending at least 3 vertebral segments, brain MRI not meeting diagnostic criteria for MS, and positive neuromyelitis optica immunoglobulin G (NMO-IgG) serology.

Evaluation of cerebrospinal fluid used to be an essential element in the diagnostic evaluation of MS, but its limited sensitivity and

TABLE 1 2005 Revision to the McDonald Diagnostic Criteria for Multiple Sclerosis

Clinical Presentation	Additional Data Needed for Diagnosis
Two or more attacks; objective clinical evidence of two or more lesions	None, although brain MRI is recommended to confirm diagnosis
Two or more attacks; objective clinical evidence of one lesion	Dissemination in space, demonstrated by: MRI* or Two or more MRI lesions consistent with MS plus positive CSF (oligoclonal bands or elevated IgG index) or A second clinical attack at a different site
One attack; objective clinical evidence of two or more lesions	Dissemination in time, demonstrated by: MRI† or A second clinical attack
One attack; objective clinical evidence of one lesion (clinically isolated syndrome)	Dissemination in space, demonstrated by: MRI* or Two or more MRI lesions consistent with MS plus positive CSF (oligoclonal bands or elevated IgG index) or A second clinical attack at a different site plus Dissemination in time, demonstrated by: MRI† or A second clinical attack
Insidious neurologic progression suggesting MS (primary progressive MS)	One year of neurologic progression and two of the following: Positive brain MRI (9 T2 lesions or ≥4 T2 lesions with positive visual evoked potentials) Positive spinal cord MRI (≥2 focal T2 lesions) Inflammatory CSF (oligoclonal bands or elevated IgG index)

*MRI criteria for dissemination in space require three of the following: ≥1 gadolinium-enhancing lesion or ≥9 T2 hyperintense lesions in the brain or spine; ≥1 one infratentorial brain lesion or spine lesion; ≥1 juxtacortical lesion; ≥3 periventricular lesions.
†MRI criteria for dissemination in time requires either gadolinium-enhancing lesion ≥3 months after the onset of the initial clinical event and in a different site corresponding to the initial event or a new T2 lesion compared with a reference scan done at least 30 days after the onset of the initial clinical event.
CSF = cerebrospinal fluid; IgG = immunoglobulin G; MRI = magnetic resonance imaging; MS = multiple sclerosis.
Adapted from Polman CH, Reingold SC, Edan G et al: Diagnostic criteria for multiple sclerosis: 2005 revisions to the "McDonald Criteria." Ann Neurol 2005;58:840-846.

specificity and the widespread availability of MRI have reduced the importance of cerebrospinal fluid studies. Currently, cerebrospinal fluid is useful when there are only a few lesions on brain MRI or in the diagnosis of primary progressive MS.

Evoked potential studies are used to evaluate neural transmission, which is impaired within demyelinated tissue. Visual evoked potentials are useful in either confirming previous optic neuritis or identifying a previous subclinical episode of optic neuritis. Auditory brainstem and somatosensory evoked potentials can also detect impaired neural transmission, but their poor sensitivity and specificity significantly reduce their usefulness.

Although MS is a diagnosis of exclusion, the recognition of classic MRI changes have helped improve diagnostic accuracy. Many symptoms of MS overlap with other disorders, such as the fatigue, numbness, paresthesias, and pain seen in fibromyalgia and chronic fatigue syndrome. In contrast to MS, these nonspecific symptoms tend to

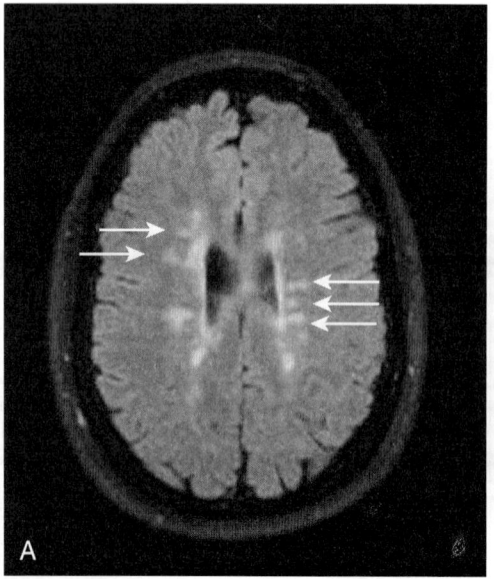 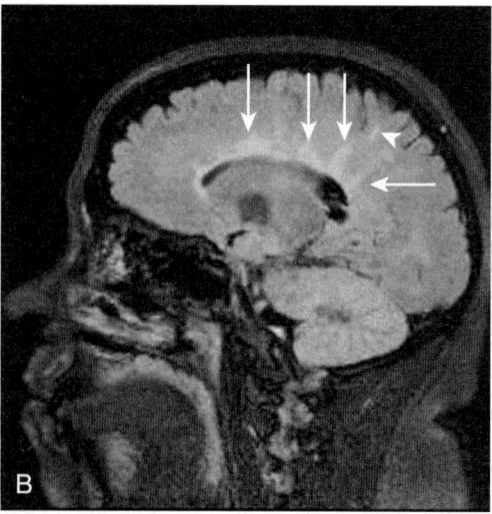

FIGURE 2. Axial (**A**) and sagittal (**B**) FLAIR MR images of the brain, illustrating the periventricular nature of demyelinating lesions (arrows), often perpendicular to the lateral ventricle. A subcortical lesion can also be seen (arrowhead in **B**). FLAIR = fluid-attenuated inversion recovery.

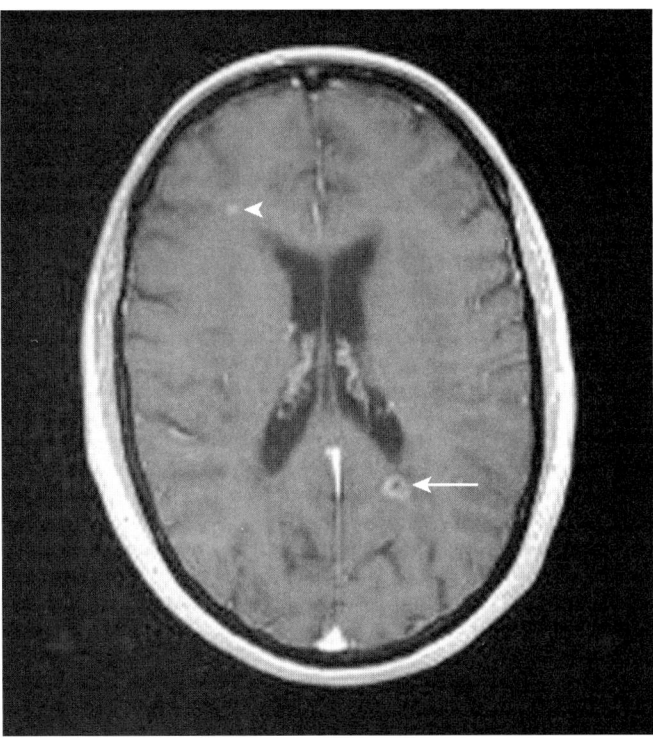

FIGURE 3. Axial post-gadolinium T1 MRI of the brain, illustrating areas of active inflammation. The *arrow* indicates a ring-enhancing lesion, which usually represents reactivation of an old multiple sclerosis lesion. The *arrowhead* indicates a homogeneous enhancing lesion, which usually represents a new focus of inflammation.

wax and wane over hours and days and to migrate through different parts of the body. The diagnosis of MS should be made only with extreme caution in patients with these relatively nonspecific symptoms, particularly in the absence of objective neurologic findings.

Similarly, T2 hyperintensities on brain MRI are relatively common, being seen in up to 7% of healthy adults. These nonspecific lesions are typically located in the deep frontal and parietal white matter, sparing the periventricular region, corpus callosum, cerebellum, temporal lobe, and spinal cord. Brain MRIs from patients with vascular risk factors (smoking, hypertension, diabetes) and migraine headaches commonly have these nonspecific findings. Despite their commonness, radiology reports typically include demyelination in the differential diagnosis, which leads to needless referrals and work-ups. In a patient without specific neurologic symptoms or findings on neurologic examination, these nonspecific findings need no further evaluation.

Differential Diagnosis

When MS manifests in a classic fashion—multiple discrete episodes of CNS inflammation, disseminated in time and space, with periventricular T2 lesions and gadolinium enhancement—the differential diagnosis is very limited. There are no required exclusionary tests, although many clinicians would consider blood tests for antinuclear antibodies (ANA), vitamin B_{12}, and (where geographically indicated) Lyme serology. When the presentation is atypical, the differential diagnosis is extremely broad, including a wide variety of other inflammatory disorders, infections, metabolic disorders, and neoplastic disorders. Atypical presentations of MS should be a red flag that prompts careful consideration of other etiologies. MS remains a diagnosis of exclusion, requiring continuing vigilance for alternative diagnoses. Recognition of neuromyelitis optica is important because its long-term treatments are different from those for typical RRMS.

Treatment

Treatment of MS can be divided into three broad categories: treatment of relapses, long-term disease-modifying medications, and symptomatic management. These three treatment pathways should be considered in parallel, with the clinical picture driving the priority for different pathways. Treatment of progressive MS is limited and typically focuses on symptomatic management, optimizing current neurologic functioning. Devic's disease also requires a different treatment approach.

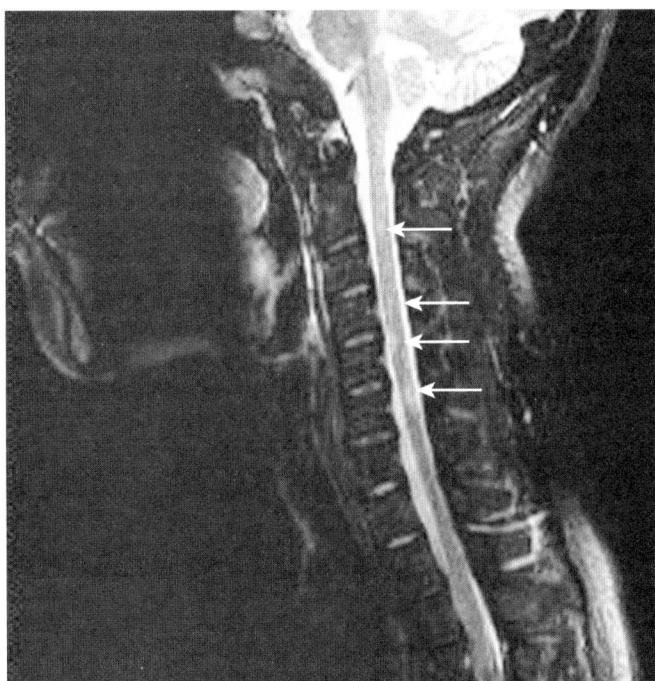

FIGURE 4. Sagittal short tau inversion recovery (STIR) MRI of the cervical spinal cord, illustrating demyelinating lesions *(arrows)*.

 CURRENT THERAPY

Clinical Relapse

- Evaluate for infections
- Methylprednisolone (Solu-Medrol)

Long-term Disease Therapy

- Interferon-β-1
- Glatiramer acetate (Copaxone)
- Mitoxantrone (Novantrone)
- Natalizumab (Tysabri)

Symptomatic Therapy

- Medications
- Physical therapy
- Assistive devices
- Psychotherapy

RELAPSES

The development of acute or subacute neurologic symptoms suggests active inflammation within the CNS. Most clinical relapses recover spontaneously, regardless of treatment. Two lines of evidence argue for treating clinical relapses with corticosteroids. First, controlled trials have found that treatment with corticosteroids hastens recovery from relapse, although final level of clinical recovery is not improved with corticosteroids. Second, pathologic studies have found more than 10,000 transected axons/mm^3 in areas of active inflammation. This irreversible axonal injury argues for aggressive curtailment of inflammation to minimize permanent tissue injury.

Therefore, most clinicians treat a clinical relapse with a course of corticosteroids. A typical relapse treatment regimen is 3 days of 1 g/day intravenous methylprednisolone (Solu-Medrol), with or without an oral prednisone taper. Treatments of up to 5 days are sometimes used with severe relapses or when a second course is needed for the same relapse. Typical side effects include emotional lability (particularly irritability), fluid retention, increased appetite, and metallic taste. Hypokalemia and hyperkalemia are also occasionally seen. Corticosteroids are relatively well absorbed and tolerated when orally administered, although comparator trials with intravenous formulations have not yet been reported.

Low or moderate doses of oral corticosteroids are used by some clinicians, particularly for mild relapses. The Optic Neuritis Treatment Trial suggested that low-dose steroids were associated with a shorter interval to the next attack, compared with placebo. Accordingly, high-dose corticosteroids are preferred wherever possible. Oral administration of high doses of corticosteroids is a reasonable administration option for patients in whom intravenous administration is not possible.

Treatment of a relapse should also include evaluation and treatment of infection. Infections can precipitate a relapse and can prevent later recovery. Bladder infections are the most common infection needing treatment. Patients reporting an incomplete response to a treatment with corticosteroids should also be evaluated for infection.

Recovery from a clinical relapse usually starts within a couple days of corticosteroid initiation and continues for many months. When relapses do not respond sufficiently to corticosteroid treatment, plasma exchange or immune globulin (Gammagard)[1] should be considered.

Relapse treatment has traditionally targeted clinical symptoms. However, active inflammation is sometimes observed as multiple gadolinium-enhancing lesions on MRI in patients without any symptoms. The severe tissue injury observed in pathologic studies of active inflammation suggest that this MRI relapse would benefit from a course of corticosteroids.

LONG-TERM DISEASE

Currently, there are six long-term disease-modifying therapies approved throughout the world for the treatment of relapsing forms of MS, as well as several other treatments that have some data supporting their efficacy. All of these treatments are only partially effective when assessed in large groups of patients, although in individual patients, disease may be completely controlled by any of these therapies. All approved treatments are given by either injection or infusion, and each has its own specific side effects. The four injection therapies (three interferon-β-1 preparations, and glatiramer acetate [Copaxone]) are standard first-line treatments for RRMS. The chemotherapy mitoxantrone (Novantrone) and the monoclonal antibody natalizumab (Tysabri) are reserved for patients who fail or are intolerant to the injectable therapies (Table 2).

INTERFERON-β-1

The same endogenous cytokine made by the body to fight viral infections is produced in vitro for exogenous administration in MS. Originally used when MS was hypothesized to be caused by a viral infection, its precise mechanism of action in MS is not fully understood. Three interferon-β-1 therapies are available. All three were found in phase III clinical trials to similarly reduce the rate of clinical relapses by 31% to 32% compared with placebo. All three preparations led to a robust reduction in new lesions on brain MRI. Where properly powered placebo-controlled trials were performed, sustained progression of disability was also reduced by interferon-β-1 treatment.

Common side effects of interferon-β-1 therapy include flulike symptoms and transient transaminitis and bone marrow suppression. Flulike symptoms are relieved by nonsteroidal antiinflammatory drugs (NSAIDs). Interferon therapies are given in the evening, so that patients can sleep through the flu symptoms. The long-acting NSAID naproxen (Aleve) is particularly helpful, because its dosing schedule provides full overnight efficacy. Periodic monitoring of liver and bone marrow function is recommended but rarely leads to discontinuation of interferon therapy. Other possible side effects include depression and worsening of preexisting weakness, spasticity, pain, and headaches.

One interferon-β-1 preparation is given by intramuscular injection: interferon-β-1a (Avonex), taken once weekly. The other two interferon-β-1 preparations are given by subcutaneous injection: interferon-β-1a (Rebif), given thrice weekly; and interferon-β-1b (Betaseron), given every other day. Injection site reactions can be seen with the subcutaneous preparations, rarely leading to abscess formation.

GLATIRAMER ACETATE

Glatiramer acetate is a random polypeptide 80 to 120 amino acids in length, derived using the four amino acids contained in brain proteins thought to be an common autoimmunogenic target in MS. First developed to induce an animal model of MS, its surprising protective effect led to successful clinical trials in MS. Similar to the interferon therapies, glatiramer acetate therapy is associated with a 29% reduction in the rate of clinical relapses and significant reduction in new brain lesions on MRI.

Common side effects of glatiramer acetate are primarily injection-site reactions. There are no associated flulike symptoms or hepatic or bone marrow disturbance. About 10% of patients treated with glatiramer acetate report a systemic reaction involving transient flushing, chest pain, palpitations, anxiety, and dyspnea shortly after injection. This reaction usually lasts only several minutes and is not thought to be related to cardiac ischemia. The reaction is always self-limited, and treatment discontinuation is not necessary.

OPTIMAL INITIAL TREATMENT

As suggested by their similar efficacy in separate placebo-controlled trials, open-label comparison studies have generally found the four injectable therapies to have relatively comparable efficacies. A few head-to-head studies suggested that the more frequently administered subcutaneous interferon-β-1 preparations might have slightly greater efficacy than the less-frequently administered intramuscular interferon-β-1 preparations. In one trial, this advantage was limited to the first 6 months of therapy, after which the efficacies were similar. This difference may be explained by the development of anti-interferon antibodies, which are much more common with subcutaneous interferon-β-1 (25%-35%) than intramuscular interferon-β-1 (2%-4%). These antibodies typically develop in the first 6 to 24 months of treatment and have been shown to abrogate both the biological effect and therapeutic benefit of interferon-β-1. In addition, bone marrow and hepatic toxicity is greater in subcutaneous interferon-β-1 preparations, most likely due to their higher amount of administered interferon.

Early MRI studies suggested that interferon-β-1 therapy had a greater reduction in the development of new brain lesions than glatiramer acetate, leading many clinicians to suspect greater clinical efficacy from interferon-β-1 therapy, too. However, two separate

---

[1] Not FDA approved for this indication.

TABLE 2 Side Effects and Complications of Common Therapies Used in Multiple Sclerosis

Side Effects and Complications	Comments
Corticosteroids	
Insomnia	Over-the-counter sleep aids, short-acting benzodiazepines
Altered mood: irritability, restlessness, rarely mania	
Fluid retention	Minimize salt intake
Potassium depletion (rare)	Increase dietary potassium (bananas, orange juice)
Indigestion	H$_2$-blockers; avoid NSAIDs
Metallic taste	Candy might help
Interferon-β1	
Flulike symptoms (myalgias, chills, fever, headache)	Start at low (Rebif) or partial (Avonex, Betaseron) dose and gradually escalate to full dose over 1-2 mo
	Long-acting NSAIDs, e.g., naproxen (Aleve)
	Changing to powder formulation (Avonex preparation only)
Hepatic and bone marrow irritation	Periodic blood test monitoring
Skin reactions (subcutaneous preparations only)	Allow medication to warm to room temperature before injection
	Witch hazel (*Hamamelis* water) or diphenhydramine cream (Benadryl)
	Lidocaine 2.5% + prilocaine 2.5% cream (EMLA)
	Ice site before and after injection
	Occasionally causes abscess
Worsened preexisting conditions, such as depression, spasticity, pain	Targeted symptomatic management
	Consider changing to non-interferon therapy
Glatiramer acetate (Copaxone)	
Skin reactions, pain	Allow medication to warm to room temperature before injection
	Witch hazel or diphenhydramine cream
	Lidocaine 2.5% + prilocaine 2.5% cream (EMLA)
	Ice site before and after injection
	Administer after a hot shower
Self-limited postinjection systemic reaction: chest tightness, dyspnea, palpitations, flushing, anxiety	Always self-limited
	Does not need treatment discontinuation
Mitoxantrone (Novantrone)	
Cardiotoxicity	Monitor with echocardiogram or MUGA scan before every dose
Leukemia	May be seen years after treatment is discontinued
Natalizumab (Tysabri)	
Hypersensitivity reaction: rash, pruritus, dyspnea	May be seen up to 1 h after infusion is complete
	Immediately and permanently discontinue treatment
Progressive multifocal leukoencephalopathy	Clinical vigilance for changes in personality or cognition, weakness, ataxia
	Further evaluate with brain MRI and cerebrospinal fluid, if indicated.

EMLA = eutectic mixture of local anesthetics; MRI = magnetic resonance imaging; MUGA = multiple uptake gated acquisition; NSAID = nonsteroidal antiinflammatory drug.

---

head-to-head studies comparing glatiramer acetate to two different interferon-β-1 preparations failed to show significant differences between the treatments in primary and secondary endpoints.

Altogether, these studies suggest that all four of the injectable therapies have relatively similar efficacies, and any of them are reasonable first-line treatment for relapsing MS. The choice of therapy should be driven by individual patient preferences, such as frequent (every 1-3 days) subcutaneous versus less frequent (weekly) intramuscular injections, tolerance for skin reactions, and potential aggravation of preexisting conditions. Ongoing symptoms such as weakness, spasticity, depression, and pain syndromes suggest use of glatiramer acetate over interferon-β-1.

ADVANCED THERAPIES

Mitoxantrone

A synthetic anthracenedione, mitoxantrone intercalates into the DNA, causing cross-linking and strand breaks. It also interferes with RNA and topoisomerase II, an enzyme involved in DNA repair. The cytocidal effects of mitoxantrone lead to bone marrow suppression and immunosuppression. It is given by infusion once every 3 months. Controlled clinical trials found that mitoxantrone reduces clinical relapses and progressive disability. Mitoxantrone is approved for use in worsening RRMS or SPMS, although clinical experience has found its efficacy in SPMS is limited to very early SPMS, when active inflammation persists. Mitoxantrone is blue, which leads to a transient bluish discoloration of sclera, urine, and occasionally nail beds. Alopecia, nausea, leukopenia, and menstrual irregularities are also seen.

The main safety concerns with mitoxantrone are cardiotoxicity and leukemia. Decreased cardiac ejection fraction is observed in a cumulative dose-dependent fashion, requiring an echocardiogram or multiple uptake gated acquisition (MUGA) scan before every dose and limiting total exposure to 120 mg/m^2. Reduction of ejection fraction by 10% from baseline or below 50% suggests ongoing cardiotoxicity. Secondary acute myeloid leukemia is also a complication of mitoxantrone therapy, with a prospective 5-year study finding an incidence of 2.5%. This toxicity has led some clinicians to use a short course as an induction agent. One clinical trial found that three monthly infusions followed by standard injectable MS therapy quickly controlled disease while minimizing total exposure to mitoxantrone. Nonetheless, the significant risks of mitoxantrone have rendered its use uncommon in the treatment of MS.

Natalizumab

α4-Integrin is an adhesion molecule on circulating leukocytes that mediates an important step in leukocytes, leaving the circulation and entering into the brain in response to inflammation. Natalizumab is a monoclonal antibody blocking α4-integrin. Natalizumab is administered by 1-hour intravenous infusion every 4 weeks. Controlled trials found natalizumab reduces clinical relapses by 68% compared with placebo, slows the progression of disability by 42%, and reduces the development of new brain lesions by 92%, all of which is significantly greater than that seen with any of the injectable therapies.

Natalizumab is generally well tolerated, with few side effects. One significant safety concern with natalizumab is infusion hypersensitivity reactions. Infusion hypersensitivity reactions occur within 2 hours of the start of infusion and include urticaria, pruritus, and rigors. Therefore, a 1-hour clinical observation is required after completion of every 1-hour infusion.

The other significant safety concern with natalizumab is progressive multifocal leukoencephalopathy (PML), a rare, destructive brain infection caused by the ubiquitous JC virus, which is carried by most adults. The estimated incidence of PML in natalizumab-treated patients is 1 per 1000 over 18 months of therapy. Immune reconstitution is the only treatment with demonstrated efficacy in PML, so it is hoped that the accelerated clearance of natalizumab by plasma exchange can help MS patients who develop PML secondary to natalizumab treatment. Recognition of PML led to the development of a control system for natalizumab distribution. Patients, prescribing physicians, dispensing pharmacies, and infusion centers are required to register in the Tysabri Outreach Unified Commitment to Health (TOUCH) Program, which will help ensure appropriate use of the medication and monitor for PML and other possible opportunistic infections.

OTHER IMMUNOMODULATORY THERAPIES

Given the limited number of disease-modifying treatment options available for this lifelong disease, many other immunomodulating therapies have been used to treat MS. Oral weekly methotrexate (Trexall)[1] and bimonthly pulse corticosteroids are sometimes used for long-term therapy when standard injectable therapies do not sufficiently control disease, although a recent controlled trial showed them to be only marginally effective. Short-term (6-12 months) courses of monthly cyclophosphamide (Cytoxan)[1] have been used for several decades, but a controlled clinical trial showed only modest efficacy, which disappeared after treatment was stopped. Azathioprine (Imuran)[1] and mycophenolate mofetil (Cellcept)[1] are occasionally used, although their efficacy is supported only by small, mostly uncontrolled studies.

Rituximab (Rituxan)[1] is a monoclonal antibody that destroys B cells for 6 months or more following each course of treatment. Despite theories that MS is a T cell–mediated disease, a 6-month phase II trial of rituximab found that this anti–B cell therapy reduced MRI lesion activity by 91% and relapse rate by 56%.

In addition, several dozen new and old immunomodulating therapies are in various stages of development for the treatment of MS. These therapies include both oral and infusion treatments and target all forms of the disease, from clinically isolated syndrome to primary and secondary progressive MS. Many of these treatments should become available over the next several years.

DISEASE MONITORING

MS clinicians generally agree that MS therapies should be started immediately on the diagnosis of active RRMS. However, optimal monitoring and management of MS patients while they are receiving therapy, particularly regarding when to change therapies, are more controversial. Just as MRI has taken on an important role in the diagnosis of MS, MRI has also taken an important role in the assessment of response to therapy. The familiar mantra "treat the patient, not the scan" is being replaced by recognition that MRI scans provide significant insight into disease activity. For example, recent studies found that new brain lesions on MRI are a stronger predictor of future disability than clinical relapses. There remains a significant disconnect between the total amount of injury on brain MRI and clinical disability, but measures of disease activity (gadolinium-enhancing lesions and new T2 lesions) have a stronger association with progressive clinical disability.

---

[1]Not FDA approved for this indication.

Several factors should be weighed when assessing the efficacy of long-term disease-modifying therapy: frequency of clinical relapses, recovery from clinical relapses, progressive disability over time, and MRI activity. Over the course of 1 year, a single, mild relapse with good recovery would generally not merit a change in therapy. However, multiple mild relapses or a moderate to severe relapse with poor recovery would suggest that current therapy is inadequate.

Brain MRI can be used to confirm the clinical impression of disease activity. Although MRI does not always show new or enhancing lesions at the time of a clinical relapse, multiple relapses in the context of a stable MRI should raise the suspicion for an alternative diagnosis. Recurrent infections and emotional distress are two common causes of symptoms that mimic an MS clinical relapse.

The proper performance of MRI is crucial to accurate assessment of the MS disease state. Standard guidelines include sagittal FLAIR, axial FLAIR, T2-, and T1-weighted images, as well as T1-weighted images 5 or more minutes after gadolinium contrast injection. Because an important goal of monitoring MRI studies is to compare with previous images, MRIs should be performed using contiguous, nongapped slices. Ideally, imaging should be performed at the same imaging center over time so that comparable images are obtained and historical comparison can be performed by the radiologist. Multiple new or enhancing lesions over time suggest that current therapy is suboptimal in controlling disease activity. New brain lesions outnumber spine lesions by about 10 to 1, and new spine lesions typically cause clinical symptoms. Therefore, surveillance imaging is typically limited to brain MRI with and without gadolinium.

SYMPTOM MANAGEMENT

MS can cause a wide range of symptoms, affecting motor, sensory, coordination, gait, sphincter, sexual function, and psychiatric spheres. These symptoms can cause significant morbidity through impairment in quality of life and daily function. There are effective treatments for almost all of these symptoms, and symptomatic management should be part of routine management of MS patients (Box 1). Effective symptom management extends beyond medication alone, often involving physical or occupational therapy, psychotherapy, exercise and stretching programs, and the collaboration of other specialists such as urology and physical medicine and rehabilitation.

Special Clinical Circumstances

PROGRESSIVE MULTIPLE SCLEROSIS

Underlying both primary and secondary progressive forms of MS is thought to be a neurodegenerative process, for which no current therapies have demonstrated clinical efficacy. When active inflammation is present, as demonstrated by a clinical relapse or gadolinium-enhancing lesion, immunomodulating therapies can be partially effective. In the absence of active inflammation, numerous clinical trials have shown that immunomodulating therapies are ineffective, often causing only troublesome side effects. Intermittent pulses of corticosteroids can sometimes slow the progressive course of MS, which is often measured by patients through self-report of ambulatory function. Treatment of progressive MS should focus on symptomatic management, targeting spasticity, gait stability and mobility, pain, and sphincter dysfunction. Vigilance should be maintained for other contributing conditions, such as mechanical compressive myelopathy (disc herniation), vitamin B_{12} deficiency, and thyroid disorder.

NEUROMYELITIS OPTICA

Acute treatment of neuromyelitis optica is no different from that of a standard MS relapse. A rebound return of symptoms is common after the course of corticosteroids is complete, so prolonged prednisone taper over weeks or months can be helpful. Neuromyelitis optica typically does not respond to the standard long-term MS injectable therapies interferon-β-1 and glatiramer acetate. Azathioprine (Imuran)[1] 2-3 mg/kg/day is often effective in controlling disease,

> **BOX 1 Symptomatic Management of Multiple Sclerosis**
>
> **Weakness**
> Exercise program
> Assistive devices: Ankle foot orthotic, cane, rolling walker
>
> **Spasticity**
> Stretching program twice daily
> Baclofen (Lioresal) 5-20 mg bid-qid
> Tizanidine (Zanaflex) 2-8 mg bid-qid
> Gabapentin (Neurontin)[1] 100-600 mg bid-qid
> Clonazepam (Klonopin)[1] 0.5-4 mg qhs
> Diazepam (Valium) 2-10 mg qhs
> Intrathecal baclofen pump
> Botulinum toxin type A (Botox) injection (for focal spasticity)
>
> **Neuropathic Pain and Paresthesias**
> Gabapentin (Neurontin)[1] 100-600 mg bid-qid
> Amitriptyline (Elavil)[1] 25-150 mg qhs
> Nortriptyline (Pamelor)[1] 25-150 mg qhs
> Phenytoin (Dilantin)[1] 150-300 mg daily-bid
> Carbamazepine (Tegretol)[1] 200-400 mg tid
> Duloxetine (Cymbalta)[1] 20-60 mg daily or divided bid
>
> **Fatigue**
> Routine exercise program
> Good sleep hygiene
> Amantadine (Symmetrel)[1] 100 mg bid
> Modafinil (Provigil)[1] 100-200 mg qd-bid
> Methylphenidate (Ritalin)[1] 10-20 mg bid-tid
>
> **Depression**
> Psychotherapy
> SSRIs, such as citalopram (Celexa) 20-60 mg daily, fluoxetine (Prozac) 20-80 mg daily, or paroxetine (Paxil) 20-50 mg daily
> SNRIs, such as venlafaxine (Effexor) 37.5-225 mg/d divided bid-tid, duloxetine (Cymbalta) 20-60 mg daily or divided bid
> Bupropion (Wellbutrin SR) 100-400 mg/day divided bid
>
> **Urinary Frequency, Urgency, and Incontinence**
> Tolterodine (Detrol) 1-2 mg po bid (watch for acute retention)
> Oxybutynin (Ditropan) 2.5-5 mg bid-qid (watch for acute retention)
> Intermittent straight catheterization
> Diverting suprapubic catheter
>
> **Recurrent Urinary Tract Infections**
> Nitrofurantoin (Macrodantin) 100 mg qhs
> Diverting suprapubic catheter
>
> **Constipation**
> Bulk-forming agents
> Stool softeners
> Laxatives
>
> **Sexual Dysfunction**
> Phosphodiesterase 5 inhibitors: sildenafil (Viagra) 50-100 mg, tadalafil (Cialis) 10-20 mg, vardenafil (Levitra) 10-20 mg
> Estrogen replacement: oral, topical, vaginal ring
> Psychotherapy to improve communication
> Avoidance of exacerbating medications (e.g., if using SSRIs, use bupropion [Wellbutrin] instead)
> Devices: Mechanical vibrators and vacuum devices
>
> **Tremor**
> Very difficult to treat
> Sometimes responds to levetiracetam (Keppra)[1] 500-1000 mg bid
>
> **Tonic Spasms**
> Spasms 10-60 seconds in duration, usually affecting the unilateral face, arm, and leg, without altered consciousness
> Carbamazepine extended release (Tegretol XR)[1] 100-300 mg bid
> Phenytoin extended release (Dilantin)[1] 100-300 mg daily
>
> ---
> [1]Not FDA approved for this indication
> SNRI = serotonin-norepinephrine reuptake inhibitor; SSRI = selective serotonin reuptake inhibitor.

and case series have found rituximab (Rituxan)[1] is also effective. Discovery of a common pathogenic antibody against aquaporin-4 ion channels has led many clinicians to use plasma exchange as treatment for acute relapses and as long-term maintenance therapy.

PREGNANCY

MS typically starts in the third or fourth decade, making it commonly coincident with pregnancy. Observational studies found that MS often becomes quiescent during pregnancy, but then rebounds shortly following pregnancy. None of the long-term disease-modifying therapies is recommended for use during pregnancy, although glatiramer acetate is probably the best choice for patients who need treatment to continue during pregnancy. Clinical relapses with significant functional impairment can be treated with a course of methylprednisolone, and intermittent immune globulin[1] can be used as a maintenance therapy.

Long-term disease-modifying therapies are also not recommended while breast-feeding. Immune globulin[1] is again a treatment option. Low doses of corticosteroids diffuse freely in and out of breast milk within a few hours of administration, leaving little being passed on to the infant 4 hours after administration. However, no studies have been done with the very high doses of methylprednisolone typically used in MS. Therefore, breast milk should be pumped and discarded out to 24 hours after completion of a course of intravenous methylprednisolone.

MULTIPLE SCLEROSIS IN THE OLD AND YOUNG

MS can be seen in both children and the elderly, although both are uncommon. The formal diagnostic criteria were intended to be applied to persons ages 10 to 59 years, but they can be used in younger and older patients. Treatment options for children and adolescents are similar to those for adults, except that current FDA regulations prohibit use of natalizumab in patients younger than 18 years. Relapse recovery is generally very good in children and adolescents, but gradually progressive disability is common by the third or fourth decade. Therefore, aggressive treatment and monitoring are recommended.

---
[1]Not FDA approved for this indication.

The diagnosis of MS in the older adult is complicated by the increased frequency of other neurologic disorders, as well as nonspecific T2 lesions commonly seen on brain MRI. MS in persons beyond the seventh decade is typically a gradually progressive myelopathy, but some patients present with active inflammation requiring immunomodulating therapy.

REFERENCES

Francis GS, Rice GP, Alsop JC: Interferon beta-1a in MS: Results following development of neutralizing antibodies in PRISMS. Neurology 2005;65(1):48-55.
Hauser SL, Waubant E, Arnold DL, et al: B-cell depletion with rituximab in relapsing-remitting multiple sclerosis. N Engl J Med. 2008;358(7):676-688.
Kappos L, Weinshenker B, Pozzilli C, et al: Interferon beta-1b in secondary progressive MS: A combined analysis of the two trials. Neurology 2004;63(10):1779-1787.
Lennon VA, Wingerchuk DM, Kryzer TJ, et al: A serum autoantibody marker of neuromyelitis optica: Distinction from multiple sclerosis. Lancet 2004;364(9451):2106-2112.
Polman CH, O'Connor PW, Havrdova E, et al: A randomized, placebo-controlled trial of natalizumab for relapsing multiple sclerosis. N Engl J Med 2006;354(9):899-910.
Polman CH, Reingold SC, Edan G, et al: Diagnostic criteria for multiple sclerosis: 2005 revisions to the "McDonald Criteria". Ann Neurol 2005;58:840-846.
Rudick RA, Lee JC, Simon J, et al: Defining interferon beta response status in multiple sclerosis patients. Ann Neurol 2004;56(4):548-555.
Trapp BD, Peterson J, Ransohoff RM et al: Axonal transection in the lesions of multiple sclerosis. New Eng J Med 1998;338:278-285.
Yousry TA, Major EO, Ryschkewitsch C, et al: Evaluation of patients treated with natalizumab for progressive multifocal leukoencephalopathy. N Engl J Med 2006;354(9):924-933.

Myasthenia Gravis and Related Disorders

Method of
Jenice Robinson, MD, and Milind J. Kothari, DO

Myasthenia gravis (MG) is a relatively uncommon disease of the postsynaptic neuromuscular junction (NMJ). Most patients with myasthenia have an acquired immunologic abnormality, but other uncommon inherited forms of myasthenia may result from structural abnormalities of the NMJ. The following discussion focuses on acquired (autoimmune) MG.

The physiologic abnormality in autoimmune MG results from the reduction in concentration of the nicotinic acetylcholine receptor (AChR) on the endplates of somatic muscles at the NMJ. Although the cause of the disorder is unknown, the pathogenesis of autoimmune MG is now well understood. Two antigens have been described: AChR and muscle-specific receptor tyrosine kinase (MuSK). Antibodies against AChR are found in 80% to 90% of patients with MG. Antibodies against MuSK are found in 40% of the remaining patients. Strong evidence supports the role of antibodies in the pathogenesis of MG. Anti-AChR antibodies cause disruption of myotubes in culture and cause myasthenic symptoms when transferred to experimental animals. Removal of anti-AChR antibodies results in clinical improvement. The thymus plays an important but incompletely understood role in MG.

Clinical Features

The hallmark of MG is fluctuating or fatigable weakness. MG presents with ocular symptoms of ptosis or diplopia in 60% of patients. Diplopia may not fluctuate, and an ocular misalignment may appear fixed. This presentation may mimic a neuropathy of the third, fourth, or sixth cranial nerves, or an internuclear ophthalmoplegia. Abnormalities of pupillary function should not be present in MG. Patients may present initially to an optometrist or ophthalmologist for these problems. Ocular symptoms eventually develop in almost all patients with MG. Presenting symptoms are bulbar (dysarthria, dysphagia, or facial weakness) in 10%, leg weakness in 10% to 20%, and generalized weakness in 10%. Symptoms often worsen with exercise and improve with rest. Symptoms are often most prominent late in the day. Weakness in MG arises from fluctuating strength of the voluntary muscles and always causes a functional deficit, such as an inability to hold the arms above the head when washing the hair or leg weakness resulting in sudden falls. If a patient has only generalized fatigue or tiredness, MG is unlikely. Chronic pain and sensory complaints are not features of MG. Respiratory dysfunction is the initial presenting symptom in only 1% of patients but, if present, requires admission to the hospital for monitoring and treatment because respiratory failure may occur rapidly. Weakness in MG can be worsened by infection, physical stress such as surgery, emotional stress, and medications. Medications that reportedly worsen strength in MG are listed in Table 1.

The prevalence of MG is estimated to be 14 per 100,000 people. MG may present at any age, but the most common ages of onset are in the second and third decades in women and in the seventh and eighth decades in men. In the past MG was more common in women than men, but with aging of the population, MG now is more common in men. Associated autoimmune diseases, such as thyroid disease, rheumatoid arthritis, lupus, and pernicious anemia, are present in 5% to 10% of patients. Approximately 10% of MG patients have an associated thymoma, and 50% to 70% of patients have thymic hyperplasia. Familial occurrence of autoimmune MG is rare, although the incidence of autoimmune diseases in first-degree relatives of patients with MG may be increased.

TABLE 1 Medications Reported to Exacerbate Myasthenia Gravis

Antibiotics
Aminoglycosides, ampicillin sodium, ciprofloxacin hydrochloride (Cipro), erythromycin, imipenem (Primaxin), kanamycin sulfate (Kantrex), pyrantel (Antiminth), chloroquine (Aralen)

Cardiovascular Agents
β-Blocking agents (propranolol hydrochloride [Inderal], oxprenolol hydrochloride[2] [Trasicor], timolol maleate [Blocadren]), procainamide (Procanbid), verapamil hydrochloride (Calan), propafenone hydrochloride (Rythmol), quinidine
Penicillamine (Cuprimine)
Corticosteroids (transiently when initiating therapy)
Magnesium salts and lithium carbonate (Eskalith)
Phenothiazine antipsychotics
Phenytoin sodium (Dilantin)

Neuromuscular Blocking Agents
Vecuronium bromide (Norcuron), succinylcholine chloride (Anectine)

Ocular Drugs
Timolol maleate (Timoptic), proparacaine hydrochloride (Alcaine), tropicamide (Mydriacyl)

Anticholinergic Agents
Trihexyphenidyl hydrochloride (Artane)
Acetazolamide (Diamox)

[2]Not available in the United States

Diagnosis

An accurate diagnosis prior to initiating treatment for MG is crucial. A critical assessment of the patient's symptoms is the most important initial step in evaluation. The differential diagnosis of MG is quite limited in most patients. Disorders that may mimic MG are listed in Table 2.

All patients suspected of having MG should undergo testing consisting of a complete blood count (CBC), erythrocyte sedimentation rate, thyroid-stimulating hormone and thyroxine levels, rheumatoid factor concentration, and liver and renal profiles. Autoimmune thyroid disease may mimic or accompany MG. In addition to excluding other diagnoses, these tests are important because treatments of MG may have adverse effects on the bone marrow, liver, and kidneys.

The role of specific testing for MG is to confirm the clinical diagnosis. For a patient with ptosis, the ice test is easy and convenient. A small amount of ice is placed over the ptotic lid for a few minutes. Improvement of the ptosis with cooling is suggestive of a defect of neuromuscular transmission. Further testing should then be pursued.

EDROPHONIUM CHLORIDE (TENSILON) TEST

The edrophonium (Tensilon) test is readily available, but the result may be invalid if the test is not properly performed. A defined clinical endpoint is needed, and vague patient reports of improvement in strength are not acceptable. Cranial nerve deficits, such as ptosis, dysconjugate gaze, and limitation of extraocular movements, provide the most reliable endpoints. The test should be performed in a location where syncope, hypotension, or respiratory failure can be managed, as these complications can rarely occur in supersensitive individuals. Atropine sulfate 0.4 mg should be available in case of symptomatic bradycardia. An intravenous line is often started for the test, although some practitioners use a butterfly needle for administration. Edrophonium 10 mg (1 mL) is drawn up in a syringe. The strength or maximum excursion of the target muscles is assessed immediately prior to administration of the edrophonium. A 2-mg (0.2-mL) test dose is given to ensure that the patient is not supersensitive to the drug. If no respiratory or cardiac side effects occur, 3 mg (0.3 mL) of edrophonium is given. Re-examination of the target muscle is performed. If no definite improvement is observed at 60 seconds, the remaining 5 mg (0.5 mL) of edrophonium is given. If unequivocal improvement in the strength of the target muscle occurs within 60 seconds of administration of a dose of edrophonium, the test is considered positive. Edrophonium 10 mg will not weaken normal muscles, but the full dose may induce weakness in a patient with a defect in neuromuscular transmission. For this reason, the medication should be given in the manner described so that any improvement in muscle strength is not missed.

The edrophonium (Tensilon) test is positive in more than 90% of patients with MG, but a positive result is not specific for MG. Positive edrophonium tests have been reported in patients with the Lambert-Eaton myasthenic syndrome, motor neuron disease, lesions of the oculomotor nerves, and conditions affecting the extraocular muscles.

ANTIBODY TESTING

Acetylcholine receptor antibodies (AChR-Ab) are present in 90% of patients with generalized MG and in approximately 50% to 60% of patients with ocular myasthenia. They are the most specific test

---

 CURRENT DIAGNOSIS

- Hallmark of MG is fluctuating or fatigable weakness.
- Initial symptom is ptosis or diplopia in 60% of patients.
- Generalized fatigue or tiredness alone is not a symptom of MG.
- Diagnostic evaluation includes:
    - Laboratory evaluation: Thyroid-stimulating hormone level, complete blood count, erythrocyte sedimentation rate, rheumatoid factor, liver and renal function studies
    - Edrophonium chloride (Tensilon) test: >90% sensitivity, but be certain to choose a defined clinical endpoint (e.g., improvement in ptosis)
    - Antibody testing: Send AChR binding antibodies first. Binding antibodies are found in ~90% of patients with generalized MG, and 50% with ocular MG. If negative, send AChR modulating antibodies. If both are negative, send muscle-specific receptor tyrosine kinase antibody.
- All patients with suspected MG should undergo chest computed tomography with contrast for thymoma
- If antibodies are negative or if searching for evidence of generalized MG in a patient with pure ocular symptoms, obtain electromyography with repetitive nerve stimulation. This test result is abnormal in >70% of patients with generalized MG but is less sensitive in patients with pure ocular symptoms
- If diagnosis remains unclear, refer to neuromuscular specialist.

Abbreviations: AChR = acetylcholine receptor; MG = myasthenia gravis.

TABLE 2 Clinical Presentations and Diagnostic Considerations in Myasthenia Gravis

Site of Predominant Weakness	Alternative Diagnoses
Ocular	Brainstem and cranial nerve disorders due to processes such as neoplasm, stroke, and multiple sclerosis
	Horner syndrome
	Oculopharyngeal muscular dystrophy
	Kearns-Sayre syndrome
	Graves' disease
	Congenital myasthenia
	Botulism (if symptom onset is acute)
	Miller-Fischer variant of GBS
Bulbar	Brainstem and multiple cranial nerve dysfunction due to processes such as neoplasm, stroke, and multiple sclerosis
	Bulbar-onset ALS
	Obstructive lesion of the oropharynx or laryngeal lesion
	Botulism (if symptom onset is acute)
Proximal extremity weakness	Inflammatory myopathies (e.g., polymyositis, dermatomyositis)
	LEMS
	GBS
	Periodic paralysis
Isolated respiratory weakness	Acid maltase deficiency
	ALS
	Polymyositis
	LEMS
	Myotonic dystrophy
Isolated neck weakness	ALS
	Inflammatory myopathies
	Paraspinous myopathy

Abbreviations: ALS = amyotrophic lateral sclerosis; GBS = Guillain-Barré syndrome; LEMS, Lambert-Eaton myasthenic syndrome.

for MG. False-positive results can occur but are rare. Antibody levels are not predictive of the severity of MG in an individual patient.

Three different tests for AChR-Ab are available commercially: binding, modulating, and blocking antibodies. The binding antibody is the antibody most commonly found in MG and should be tested first. If the test result is negative, a modulating antibody test should be performed because this may be positive in a small number of patients who do not have binding antibodies. The blocking antibody titer adds little additional diagnostic value and is not generally indicated.

Recently, antibodies against muscle-specific receptor tyrosine kinase (MuSK-Ab) have been described in approximately 40% of patients with "seronegative" MG. Evidence indicates that MuSK is involved in the proper distribution of AChR at the muscle endplate, and some evidence indicates that MuSK-Abs are pathogenic in these patients. The MuSK-Ab test is commercially available. Patients with MuSK-Ab are almost always seronegative for AChR-Ab. For this reason, the MuSK-Ab test should be sent only if the patient has already been tested for AChR-Ab and is seronegative. MG in patients with MuSK-Ab may have a different natural history and response to treatment, and this is an area of active investigation. Patients with MuSK-Ab are more likely to be young women and present with bulbar, neck, or respiratory symptoms. Edrophonium (Tensilon) testing is less likely to yield a positive result. Whether thymectomy should be performed in patients with MuSK-Ab is unclear.

Striational antibodies are a marker for thymoma, although false-positive and false-negative results are common. Chest computed tomography (CT) with contrast to evaluate for possible thymoma is indicated for all patients diagnosed with MG. The added value of performing striational antibodies has not been definitely demonstrated.

ELECTROPHYSIOLOGIC TESTING

Electrophysiologic testing is indicated for evaluation of possible MG if the AChR-Ab test is negative. In antibody-positive patients, electrophysiologic testing is often not necessary unless the test is being performed to evaluate for evidence of generalized disease in those with purely ocular symptoms. Typically, routine nerve conduction studies and needle electromyography (EMG) are normal. These tests are performed to ensure that other disorders of the peripheral nerves or muscles are not present. Repetitive nerve stimulation (RNS) is then performed if the study was ordered to evaluate for an NMJ disorder. RNS has a sensitivity of approximately 50% to 60% in all patients with MG, with a higher yield in patients with generalized MG and a lower yield in patients with pure ocular MG. RNS of the spinal accessory and facial nerves may increase the yield of testing. It should be emphasized that abnormal RNS is not specific for MG, and routine nerve conduction studies and needle EMG must be performed to exclude other conditions. Single-fiber EMG (SFEMG) is a highly specialized and demanding technique with a sensitivity of approximately 90% to 95% in patients with MG. SFEMG is abnormal in many neuromuscular diseases and therefore should be performed only in the correct clinical context and after a routine EMG with RNS has been performed. Because of the demanding nature of the study, SFEMG is usually performed by a neuromuscular specialist.

OTHER INVESTIGATIONS

Currently all patients diagnosed with MG should undergo a CT scan of the chest with contrast to evaluate for an associated thymoma. Routine chest radiography or determination of antistriational antibodies is not an adequate substitute.

Prognosis

The natural history of MG is highly variable. Ocular symptoms are the presenting symptoms in approximately 50% to 60% of MG patients. Weakness subsequently develops in other muscles in most patients. Weakness remains restricted to the extraocular muscles for the entire course of MG in 15% to 20% of patients (pure ocular myasthenia). Patients with initial ocular involvement typically develop weakness in other muscles within the first year of having the disease. If no generalized symptoms develop after 2 years, subsequent generalization is unlikely. The maximal weakness from MG occurs within the initial 3 years of symptoms in 70% of patients. Mortality from MG is now low because of advances in critical care; however, quality of life is often affected by MG. Long-lasting remission occurs spontaneously in approximately 10% to 15% of patients if no immunosuppressive agents are used. Spontaneous remissions may be more frequent in patients with pure ocular myasthenia.

Treatment

CHOLINESTERASE INHIBITORS AS FIRST-LINE THERAPY

Cholinesterase inhibitors (ChEIs) are first-line therapy in all patients with MG. The commonly available ChEIs are listed in Table 3. Acetylcholinesterase (AChE) is anchored in the synaptic cleft on the postsynaptic membrane. AChE normally cleaves acetylcholine (ACh) released from the presynaptic nerve terminal, which normally prevents repeat binding of ACh to the AChR. ChEIs reduce the hydrolysis of ACh and increase the amount of ACh available at the postsynaptic membrane. ChEIs used for treatment of MG are reversible inhibitors of AChE and cause few central nervous system side effects because they do not cross the blood–brain barrier efficiently.

TABLE 3 Commonly Available Cholinesterase Inhibitors

Medication	Route of Administration	Unit Dose	Average Dose (Adult)	Children's Dose
Pyridostigmine bromide tablet (Mestinon)	Oral	60-mg tablets, double-scored for splitting	30–60 mg every 4–6 hours, maximum 120 mg every 3 hours	1 mg/kg every 4–6 hours
Pyridostigmine bromide syrup	Oral	12 mg/mL	30–60 mg every 4–6 hours	1 mg/kg every 4–6 hours
Pyridostigmine bromide sustained-release (Mestinon Timespan)	Oral	180-mg tablet (not crushable)	1 tablet at bedtime	—
Pyridostigmine bromide	Intravenous	5 mg/mL ampules	1/30 of usual oral dose, i.e., 1–2 mg every 3–4 hours	—
Neostigmine bromide (Prostigmin)	Oral	15-mg tablets	7.5–15 mg every 3–4 hours	
Edrophonium (Tensilon)	Intravenous		Used for diagnosis	Used for diagnosis

CURRENT THERAPY

Be certain of the diagnosis
- Ocular symptoms only or mild weakness: Cholinesterase inhibitors
- Moderate to severe weakness:
  - Cholinesterase inhibitors, and
  - Thymectomy for patients younger than 60 years (with complete removal of the gland)
- If symptoms are uncontrolled with cholinesterase inhibitors, use immunosuppression:
  - Prednisone if urgent or severe
  - Azathioprine[1] (Imuran) or mycophenolate mofetil[1] (CellCept)
    - As a steroid-sparing agent to facilitate prednisone taper
    - Prednisone fails to elicit patient response
    - Prednisone contraindicated
    - Excessive prednisone side effects
- Plasma exchange or intravenous immune globulin[1]
  - Myasthenic crisis
  - Preoperative (i.e., before thymectomy)
- If the above measures fail:
  - Refer to neuromuscular specialist

[1]Not FDA approved for this indication.

Absorption from the gastrointestinal tract is inefficient, and oral bioavailability is low.

Pyridostigmine bromide (Mestinon) is the most widely used ChEI. Onset of action is within 15 to 30 minutes of an oral dose, with peak action at 1 to 2 hours and gradual wearing off at 3 to 4 hours. All ChEI medications have muscarinic side effects, including cramping, diarrhea, salivation, lacrimation, and bradycardia. For this reason, the medication should always be introduced in low dose, preferably on the weekend. Pyridostigmine tablets are double scored and can be easily split. Start the patient with a half tablet (30 mg) of pyridostigmine once daily in the morning. The dose is then increased by a half tablet each day to a dose of a half tablet (30 mg) four times daily. Subsequently, the dose can be increased further to a full tablet (60 mg) four times daily. If necessary for symptom relief, pyridostigmine can be increased to a maximum dose of 120 mg every 3 to 4 hours, but 60 mg every 4 hours usually provides optimum benefit. If a patient has weakness while eating, pyridostigmine doses can be timed to be taken 1 hour before meals. If a patient has significant weakness upon awakening, the extended-release formulation of pyridostigmine (Mestinon Timespan) can be given at bedtime; however, absorption is too unpredictable for daytime use. If a patient requires parenteral dosing of medications, intravenous pyridostigmine is given at 1/30 the oral dose (usually 1–2 mg intravenously) every 3 to 4 hours.

When symptoms are not controlled with 60 to 120 mg of pyridostigmine every 4 hours, possible initiation of an immunosuppressive agent must be discussed fully with the patient. Most patients with generalized MG will require immunosuppressive treatment in order to induce a remission of symptoms. Pyridostigmine is often initially very effective, but therapeutic efficacy usually gradually diminishes. The immunosuppressive agents used in MG are corticosteroids, azathioprine[1] (Imuran), mycophenolate mofetil[1] (CellCept), cyclosporin A[1] (Neoral), and cyclophosphamide[1] (Cytoxan). Each of these agents is discussed separately in Table 4. Important considerations are the clinical severity of the MG, the patient's perception of his or her disability, any coexisting medical conditions, as well as the patient's age, gender, and overall lifestyle. For example, a physically active patient will be less tolerant of weakness than a patient with a sedentary lifestyle.

[1]Not FDA approved for this indication.

TREATMENT OF PURE OCULAR MYASTHENIA GRAVIS

From 15% to 20% of patients with MG have only visual symptoms for the entire course of their disease. Visual symptoms in patients with MG result from ptosis or ocular misalignment. Approximately 50% of patients will experience significant relief of visual symptoms with ChEIs alone and will be satisfied with their treatment. The effect on symptoms should be clear within 1 month of beginning pyridostigmine (Mestinon) therapy. In general, pyridostigmine provides significant relief of ptosis and is less helpful for ocular misalignment.

Among the 50% of patients who achieve significant control of ocular symptoms using pyridostigmine, this may be the only treatment necessary. If symptoms are not controlled, the patient's perception of his or her disability and lifestyle are very important to treatment. A patient who is unable to work because of visual misalignment will require further treatment. Nonpharmacologic options for symptom management include eyelid taping or eyelid crutches for ptosis and eye patching for ocular misalignment.

If the patient requests further treatment, prednisone[1] can be started at 10 mg/day, with an increase of 5 mg every other day until a dose of 40 to 60 mg/day is reached. This dose should be continued for approximately 1 month. The vast majority of patients will improve. At 1 month, a taper at 5 mg/wk can be started; at 20 mg the taper should be slowed to improve the chances of maintaining remission.

The role of corticosteroids in the treatment of pure ocular MG is controversial. Some data suggest that corticosteroids decrease the chance of developing generalized MG. However, corticosteroids have many undesired effects. In general, corticosteroids are used for ocular myasthenia only when the symptoms are significant to the patient and are uncontrolled by ChEIs.

CORTICOSTEROIDS

Corticosteroids are usually the first-line immunosuppressive agent. After 6 weeks of treatment with a corticosteroid, approximately 90% of patients have improvement in symptoms. Approximately 30% of patients treated with prednisone obtain remission, and 50% experience marked improvement. Paradoxically, 50% of patients have an initial increase in weakness during the first weeks of treatment with corticosteroids. The reasons for this effect are not well understood. Some practitioners begin treatment at the full therapeutic dose of prednisone 60 to 80 mg/day, with careful monitoring for increased weakness. If weakness worsens, the patient may require hospitalization and treatment with plasma exchange or intravenous immune globulin[1] (IVIG; Gamimune N). Others begin treatment at a lower dose with a gradual increase to the target dose over 1 month with the goal of avoiding the initial worsening of strength. An example of this method begins with a dose of prednisone 20 mg once daily. The dose is increased by 5 mg every third day until the target dose of 60 to 80 mg/day is reached. Alternate-day dosing with a target dose of 100 to 120 mg every other day can also be used. When beginning prednisone, calcium, vitamin D, and a bisphosphonate medication should be started at the same time unless a contraindication is present. This is appropriate because most patients will require long-term therapy with prednisone.

A clinical effect is typically seen within 6 weeks. If a remission is achieved, the full dose should be maintained for 6 weeks, followed by a slow taper. Initially the daily prednisone dose can be decreased by 5 mg/month. When the daily dose reaches 30 mg/day, the taper should be slowed, with further decreases in dose of 2.5 mg/month. Clinical exacerbations are frequent when the daily dose of prednisone reaches 20 to 30 mg/day, and a slower taper may prevent this problem. If an exacerbation occurs, the daily prednisone dose should be increased by 5 to 10 mg. The new dose can be maintained for 6 weeks, followed by a slower taper. Some practitioners use alternate-day dosing, with tapering from an initial dose of 100 to 120 mg every other day.

[1]Not FDA approved for this indication.

TABLE 4 Oral Immunosuppressive Agents Used on Myasthenia Gravis

Medication	Starting Dose	Therapeutic Dose	Time to Clinical Effect	Laboratory Monitoring	Side Effects	Advantages
Prednisone[1]	60–80 mg daily (see text)	60–80 mg daily (or 120 mg every other day)	Days to weeks	May need to follow blood glucose level; follow bone density every 6 mo	Many serious long-term side effects (see text); always start with calcium 1500 mg/day and vitamin D 400 IU/day; may also require bisphosphonate	Short time to clinical effect; long clinical experience in MG; not teratogenic; relatively safe in pregnancy; no increase in malignancy
Azathioprine[1] (Imuran)	50 mg daily	2–3 mg/kg/day in divided doses	4–12 mo	CBC, LFT weekly as dose increased; may then check once per month; if WBC <2500, stop azathioprine	~10% fever, nausea, abdominal pain during first weeks of treatment; increased risk of malignancy with long-term use; teratogenic	Long clinical experience; predictable; fewer long-term side effects than prednisone
Mycophenolate mofetil[1] (CellCept)	500 mg twice daily	1000–1500 mg twice daily	2–6 mo	CBC monthly, but significant myelosuppression is uncommon	Diarrhea; risk of malignancy with long-term use is currently unclear; should not be used in pregnancy because safety is unknown; clinical experience in MG is limited—randomized study is ongoing	Usually well tolerated; few serious side effects; faster onset of clinical effect than azathioprine
Cyclosporine[1] (Sandimmune, Neoral)	3–5 mg/kg/day in divided doses	3–5 mg/kg/day in divided doses	2–6 mo	Renal function, trough cyclosporine levels, electrolytes monthly; follow blood pressure	Significant renal toxicity is common and is a frequent reason to stop the drug; hypertension; should not be used in pregnancy; many drug interactions; use only under guidance of neuromuscular specialist	Faster onset of clinical effect than azathioprine
Cyclophosphamide[1] (Cytoxan)	25 mg/day orally; parenteral administration may be used in severe, refractory MG	2–5 mg daily		CBC monthly	Significant myelosuppression, hemorrhagic cystitis, risk of opportunistic infections; increased risk of malignancy; absolutely contraindicated during pregnancy; use only under guidance of neuromuscular specialist	May be effective in patients refractory to other treatments

[1]Not FDA approved for this indication.
Abbreviations: CBC = complete blood count; LFT = liver function test; MG = myasthenia gravis; WBC = white blood cell count.

Long-term use of corticosteroids is associated with serious complications, including osteoporosis, fractures, medication-induced diabetes mellitus, obesity, glaucoma, cataracts, gastric and duodenal ulcers, anxiety or depression, myopathy, opportunistic infections, and avascular necrosis of the large joints. Most patients are not able to completely discontinue prednisone and require a minimum dose to maintain improvement of their MG. The decision to start a steroid-sparing agent is often not clear-cut. In general, if a patient has more than one relapse when tapering off steroids, therapy with a steroid-sparing agent should be considered. If a patient does not have a remission with steroids, combined therapy with a steroid-sparing agent should be considered. In the older patient population, treatment with a steroid-sparing agent should be considered early in the course. In a young patient, particularly a woman in her childbearing years, steroid-sparing drugs should be avoided when possible because of teratogenicity and the increased risk of lymphoma with long-term use of these agents.

OTHER IMMUNOSUPPRESSIVE AGENTS

Azathioprine[1] (Imuran) has been extensively used in MG, usually as a steroid-sparing medication. Azathioprine is an inhibitor of purine synthesis and therefore affects rapidly dividing cell populations, such as lymphocytes. A large double-blind, randomized study demonstrated improvement in steroid tapering with the use of azathioprine. The major drawback of azathioprine is that a clinical effect may not be seen until 12 months. Side effects are less common than with steroids. Approximately 10% of patients have an idiosyncratic reaction in the first weeks of therapy, with fever, nausea, vomiting, and abdominal pain. Symptoms resolve with cessation of the drug but usually recur if azathioprine is restarted. Azathioprine may cause leukopenia or thrombocytopenia, vomiting, or hepatic dysfunction. Mild leukopenia occurs in 25% of patients but is usually not significant. Elevation of hepatic enzyme levels occurs in 5% of patients but is usually reversible with cessation of the drug. The risk of lymphoma increases slightly after 10 years of use. Azathioprine is potentially teratogenic and should be avoided in women of childbearing age. The initial dose is 50 mg/day (or 1 mg/kg/day). The dose is increased over a few months until the therapeutic dose of 2 mg/kg/day in divided doses is reached. CBC with differential and liver function tests initially should be tested weekly and monthly after the target dose has been reached. Leukopenia may develop even after several years of treatment. If the white blood cell count drops below 2500 cells/mm^3 or the absolute neutrophil count below 1000 cells/mm^3, the drug should be stopped. Overall, approximately 50% of patients improve with azathioprine therapy. Relapse after discontinuation of azathioprine occurs in more than 50% of patients.

Mycophenolate mofetil[1] (CellCept) is a newer immunosuppressant that inhibits proliferation of T and B lymphocytes by blocking de novo purine synthesis. Lymphocytes are selectively affected because they are unable to use the purine salvage pathway. The major advantages of mycophenolate are its relatively fast onset of clinical effect and its favorable side-effect profile. Side effects are usually mild and nclude diarrhea, abdominal pain, nausea, peripheral edema, and mild leukopenia. The long-term risk of malignancy with use of mycophenolate is unclear; however, an elderly MG patient who developed primary central nervous system lymphoma in association with mycophenolate use has been recently reported. Treatment trials of patients with MG are ongoing. Some practitioners use mycophenolate to induce remission without the concomitant use of steroids. Others use mycophenolate only as a steroid-sparing agent in steroid-dependent patients. The standard starting dose is 500 mg twice daily. The therapeutic dose for treatment of MG is 1000 to 1500 mg twice daily. Significant myelosuppression is uncommon; however, a monthly check of CBC with differential is standard practice.

Cyclosporine[1] (Sandimmune, Neoral) is an inhibitor of T-helper cell function through blockade of calcineurin-mediated cytokine signaling. Cyclosporine is of limited use for treatment of MG because of renal toxicity. Cyclosporine is used for cases of severe MG when steroids and azathioprine are not tolerated or are ineffective. The standard dosage for treatment of MG is 3 to 5 mg/kg/day in divided doses. Anecdotally, a lower target dose of 2 mg/kg/day may decrease the incidence of renal insufficiency while still achieving clinical improvement. A clinical effect is usually seen within the first 6 months of treatment. Renal function and trough cyclosporine levels should be followed monthly. Creatinine levels greater than 50% of the pretreatment levels are an indication to stop the drug. A rise in creatinine level typically occurs after several years of use. Hypertension is a frequent side effect, and blood pressure must be monitored regularly. In general, this medication should be used for treatment of MG under the guidance of a neuromuscular specialist.

Cyclophosphamide[1] (Cytoxan) is an alkylating agent that acts on DNA, inhibiting cell proliferation. Cyclophosphamide has limited use in MG because of multiple serious toxicities. Cyclophosphamide is used in patients with severe MG when steroids and azathioprine are ineffective or not tolerated. It appears effective at inducing remission when used in this manner. Cyclophosphamide has been used in combination with steroids for patients with severe disease who have not responded to steroids alone. The risk of side effects from cyclophosphamide is high. Cyclophosphamide may cause severe bone marrow suppression, severe opportunistic infections, bladder toxicity, and increased risk of neoplasm. Cyclophosphamide is a chemotherapeutic agent at higher doses, and parenteral high-dose administration has occasionally been used for patients with refractory, severe MG. In general, this medication should be used for treatment of MG only under the guidance of a neuromuscular specialist.

SHORT-TERM IMMUNOTHERAPY: PLASMA EXCHANGE AND INTRAVENOUS IMMUNE GLOBULIN

Plasma exchange (i.e., plasmapheresis) is a well-established intervention that produces short-term clinical improvement in patients with MG. Plasmapheresis is typically used in a MG patient with rapid worsening of weakness or myasthenic crisis. Plasma exchange treatments may be performed prior to an elective surgical procedure, such as thymectomy, to decrease the likelihood of a myasthenic exacerbation. Rarely a patient is refractory or intolerant of all long-term therapies and requires periodic plasma exchange on an ongoing basis. Typical treatment of a myasthenic exacerbation consists of five exchanges of 3 to 4 L each over a period of approximately 2 weeks. The effect is rapid and improvement is seen within days of starting therapy, but the effect is short lived. Typically the beneficial effects of plasma exchange last only a few weeks. Central venous access, typically with a large-bore catheter, is required. Complications of plasma exchange are usually related to the vascular access. Patients are at risk for significant iatrogenic infections, particularly because many of these patients are undergoing long-term therapy with immunosuppressive agents. Hematoma at the site of line placement, pulmonary embolism from venous thrombosis, electrolyte imbalance, pneumothorax, and hypotension during plasma exchange treatments can occur.

IVIG[1] is used for identical indications as plasma exchange. The standard dose is 400 mg/kg/day for 5 days. The only large, randomized study of IVIG in MG found IVIG equivalent to plasmapheresis for treatment of myasthenic crisis. Some practitioners anecdotally believe plasma exchange produces more rapid improvement in strength. The advantages of IVIG are that it is generally more widely available than is plasmapheresis, and it does not require central venous access. The most common side effects are headache and transient flulike symptoms. However, IVIG may cause volume overload, vascular events such as ischemic stroke, and venous thrombosis. IVIG should be used with caution in patients with risk factors for these conditions. IVIG cannot be used in patients with IgA deficiency,

---

[1]Not FDA approved for this indication.

a relatively frequent condition. An IgA level must be determined prior to the first IVIG treatment to avoid a potentially serious allergic reaction. Anecdotally, some patients refractory to IVIG will have a good response to plasma exchange.

THYMECTOMY

Thymectomy has been standard therapy for treatment of MG for more than 50 years, but it has never been evaluated in a large, prospective, randomized controlled trial. Thymectomy appears to be effective in improving the course of MG in patients without thymoma. If a thymoma is present, thymectomy is mandatory. The procedure is not a cure for MG, but it appears to increase the likelihood of clinical remission, particularly if performed within the first year of symptom onset. Approximately 75% of patients appear to receive some benefit from the procedure, but the effect may be apparent only after several years. Thymectomy appears to be more effective in younger patients, which may reflect the involution of the thymus with aging. Patients younger than 60 years with moderate to severe MG are candidates for thymectomy. Patients with pure ocular myasthenia do not usually undergo thymectomy unless a thymoma is suspected. Thymic tissue may be present throughout the neck and the mediastinum. The majority of surgical centers perform a combined transsternal–transcervical exposure with en bloc removal of the thymus to ensure complete removal of the gland. Incomplete resections have been followed by persistent symptoms that were later relieved by removal of residual thymus at reoperation. Referrals for thymectomy should be made to an experienced surgeon willing to perform a maximal resection. In the days preceding thymectomy, patients often undergo plasma exchange to decrease the likelihood of an exacerbation due to the surgery. The surgery involves sternotomy and a 4- to 6-week convalescence. Serious complications are uncommon when the surgery is performed at an experienced center by anesthesiologists and neurologists familiar with the perioperative management of MG.

TREATMENT OF MYASTHENIC CRISIS

A myasthenic crisis is an exacerbation of MG producing respiratory weakness or profound muscle weakness. Myasthenic crisis is a neurologic emergency. Patients with worsening weakness should undergo tests including chest radiograph, blood and urine cultures, CBC with differential, and serum chemistries to screen for concurrent infections. The patient's medication list should be scrutinized and any recent additions or changes noted. Patients occasionally increase their ChEI dose to toxic levels without consulting their physician, resulting in increased muscle weakness and a "cholinergic crisis." This event is relatively uncommon, but recent consumption of ChEI must be determined in all myasthenic patients with increasing weakness. Signs of cholinergic crisis include abdominal cramps, diarrhea, nausea and vomiting, excessive secretions, and miotic pupils; these are not characteristics of myasthenic crisis. If cholinergic crisis is a consideration, the ChEI must be stopped. A patient in myasthenic crisis should be admitted to an intensive care unit if any signs of respiratory failure are present because respiratory deterioration may occur quickly. The vital capacity and peak negative inspiratory force should be followed as measures of respiratory strength. As a rule, elective intubation should be performed when the vital capacity falls below 15 mL/kg and peak negative inspiratory force below −20 cm H_2O. Arterial blood gas measurements do not accurately reflect the degree of respiratory muscle weakness in MG. P_{CO_2} and p_{O_2} measurements may be normal until just prior to respiratory collapse. While a patient is ventilated, it is reasonable to discontinue pyridostigmine (Mestinon) because this medication may increase respiratory secretions. Any immunosuppressive agents should be continued. If the patient is a new-onset myasthenic, it is appropriate to begin prednisone therapy 60 to 80 mg/day while the patient is ventilated. Options for improving strength during crisis are plasma exchange treatments and IVIG (discussed earlier). Readiness for weaning from the ventilator can be assessed using the vital capacity and peak negative inspiratory force measurements. Weaning from the ventilator may otherwise be performed according to standard protocols. Once the patient is successfully extubated, treatment with ChEIs can be resumed. A treatment plan to prevent future myasthenic crises should be developed.

Other Issues

TRANSIENT NEONATAL MYASTHENIA

Transient neonatal myasthenia occurs in 10% of infants of mothers with autoimmune MG. Following delivery, the infant has a weak cry or suck, appears floppy, and may require mechanical ventilation. The symptoms result from maternal antibodies transferred across the placenta to the infant in utero and resolve within a few weeks. Infants with severe weakness can be treated with oral pyridostigmine 1 to 2 mg/kg every 2 hours.

LAMBERT-EATON MYASTHENIC SYNDROME

Lambert-Eaton myasthenic syndrome (LEMS) is an uncommon autoimmune disorder of the presynaptic NMJ. LEMS is characterized by fluctuating proximal extremity weakness. Symptoms typically include difficulty walking, standing up from a chair, and climbing stairs. Patients may complain of autonomic symptoms, such as dry mouth, blurry vision, anhidrosis, or constipation. Unlike MG, in LEMS ptosis, diplopia, dysphagia, and dysarthria are usually not prominent. Respiratory failure may occur but is uncommon. Patients may report improvement in muscle strength after sustained activity. Other frequent symptoms include myalgias, muscle stiffness, paresthesias, and a metallic taste in the mouth.

On examination, patients typically have proximal muscle weakness, more prominent in the lower extremities. The objective weakness may be less than expected given the patient's symptoms. Characteristically, muscle stretch reflexes are absent. Sustained muscle grip strength often increases over the first several seconds (Lambert's sign).

LEMS is a paraneoplastic syndrome in 60% of patients, most often due to a small cell carcinoma of the lung. In patients without malignancy, LEMS is often associated with other autoimmune conditions. Male patients older than 40 years are more likely to have an associated malignancy, whereas patients without malignancy are more often young women. All patients with suspected LEMS should undergo a thorough evaluation for malignancy, however. If no malignancy is found, the evaluation should be repeated at regular intervals. Presentation of LEMS may antedate the discovery of a malignancy by up to 2 years.

LEMS is believed to result from autoantibodies against the presynaptic voltage-gated calcium channels of cholinergic nerve terminals. At the NMJ, decreased release of acetylcholine from the presynaptic nerve terminal results in muscle weakness. The cholinergic nerve terminals of the autonomic nervous system are also affected. Seventy-five percent of patients with LEMS have detectable serum IgG antibodies against voltage-gated P/Q calcium channels. The diagnosis of LEMS should always be confirmed by electrophysiologic studies. Nerve conduction studies reveal diffusely low compound motor action potential (CMAP) amplitudes with normal sensory responses. RNS shows a CMAP decrement with slow rates of stimulation but marked increment of the CMAP response after brief exercise. A similar increment is seen with fast rates of RNS.

In LEMS with an associated malignancy, treatment of the malignancy may lead to improvement of LEMS symptoms. For symptomatic treatment, some patients achieve improvement with use of ChEIs such as pyridostigmine (Mestinon). 3,4-Diaminopyridine (DAP) increases release of ACh from the presynaptic nerve terminal by decreasing potassium conductance. 3,4-DAP is not approved by the Food and Drug Administration (FDA) for use in the United States. In countries where 3,4-DAP is approved, it represents the first-line symptomatic therapy for LEMS. The typical starting dose is 10 mg every 4 to 6 hours. In patients with disabling symptoms, immunosuppressive therapies such as long-term corticosteroids, plasma exchange treatments, and IVIG[1] can be used.

[1] Not FDA approved for this indication.

REFERENCES

Chaudry V, Cornblath DR, Griffin JW, et al: Mycophenolate mofetil: a safe and promising immunosuppressant in neuromuscular diseases. Neurology 2001;56:94-96.

Drachman DB: Myasthenia gravis. N Engl J Med 1994;330:1797-1810.

Gajdos PH, Chevret S, Clair B, et al: Clinical trial of plasma exchange and high-dose intravenous immunoglobulin in myasthenia gravis. Ann Neurol 1997;41:789-796.

Jaretzki A, Steinglass KM, Sonett JR: Thymectomy in the management of myasthenia gravis. Semin Neurol 2004;24:49-62.

Kaminski HJ (ed): Current Clinical Neurology: Myasthenia Gravis and Related Disorders, Totowa, NJ: Humana Press, 2002.

Katirji B, Kaminski HJ: Electrodiagnostic approach to the patient with suspected neuromuscular junction disorder. Neurol Clin 2002;20:557-586.

Palace J, Newsom-Davis J, Lecky B: A randomized double-blind trial of prednisolone alone or with azathioprine in myasthenia gravis. Neurology 1998;50:1778-1783.

Pascuzzi RM, Coslett HB, Johns TR: Long-term corticosteroid treatment of myasthenia gravis: Report of 116 patients. Ann Neurol 1984;15:291-298.

Richman DP, Agius MA: Treatment of autoimmune myasthenia gravis. Neurology 2003;61:1652-1661.

Saperstein DS, Barohn RJ: Management of myasthenia gravis. Semin Neurol 2004;24:41-48.

Seybold ME, Drachman DB: Gradually increasing doses of prednisone in MG. N Engl J Med 1974;290:81-84.

Vincent A, Leite MI: Neuromuscular junction autoimmune disease: Muscle specific kinase antibodies and treatments for myasthenia gravis. Curr Opinion Neurol 2005;18:519-525.

Trigeminal Neuralgia

Method of
Ronald F. Young, MD

Trigeminal neuralgia (TN) is one of the most devastating pain conditions that people endure. The pain is frequently misdiagnosed as being of dental or paranasal sinus origin. Unnecessary dental procedures, such as root canals and extractions or sinus surgery, are often performed in misguided attempts to treat the pain. The condition is also referred to as *tic douloureux* because of the sudden facial grimacing that may be seen as a reaction to the pain. The illness is estimated to affect about 1 in 20,000 people and becomes more frequent with advancing age. TN may be of primary (idiopathic) origin or secondary origin due to a variety of structural conditions, such as tumors (meningiomas and vestibular schwannomas in particular), multiple sclerosis (MS), vascular malformations, and cysts of the posterior cranial fossa. The exact etiology of TN is still debated, but it is generally accepted that most cases of idiopathic TN are due to compression of the trigeminal nerve root near its entry into the brainstem at the pons by adjacent blood vessels, most commonly arteries. Such compression is thought to result in segmental demyelination due to the constant pulsatile forces directed against the nerve root. The underlying pathology is thought to be related to the aging process wherein arteries (particularly the superior cerebellar artery) that normally course superior to, but not in contact with, the nerve root gradually come into contact and then compress and distort the nerve root as a result of constant pulsatile pressure. Such pressure causes localized demyelination and loss of the normal insulating function of the myelin. Ephaptic or nonsynaptic transmission and abnormal local depolarization are then postulated to result in ectopic impulse generation. Such impulses are thought to activate nerve fibers in the trigeminal nerve root that generate the pain of TN. Ephaptic transmission is also thought to account for the "triggering" of pain by usually innocuous stimuli, such as lightly touching the face or brushing the teeth.

Diagnosis

In spite of modern technology, TN is a diagnosis based almost exclusively on the medical history. Neither laboratory nor imaging studies establish the diagnosis conclusively, although properly formatted magnetic resonance imaging (MRI) scans recently have been thought to contribute to the correct diagnosis if they demonstrate arterial compression of the trigeminal nerve root. Three aspects of the history are critical to the diagnosis: (1) the type of pain, (2) the location of the pain, and (3) the factors that trigger or activate the pain. The pain of TN is sharp, sudden, severe, and brief in character, usually lasting only a few seconds but often occurring in repeated bursts. The pain is often described as feeling like an electric shock or ice pick jabbing into the face. Pains that are of longer duration and described as burning, aching, boring, or like pressure are not typical of TN; when such symptoms are described, an alternative diagnosis should be considered. The pain of TN is confined within one or more of the major three peripheral divisions of the trigeminal nerve: the first division encompassing the anterior two thirds of the scalp, the forehead, the eye, and the upper portion of the nose; the second division encompassing the edges of the nares, the upper lip and cheek, the upper teeth, gums, and mucosal lining of the mouth; and the third division encompassing the skin over the mandible, including the lower lip as well as the lower teeth, gums, and anterior two thirds of the tongue. Pain that is located in the mastoid or occipital region, deep within the ear canal, extending below the edge of the mandible onto the neck or traversing the midline is not trigeminal in origin. TN is almost exclusively a unilateral condition. Bilateral pain is estimated to occur in less than 1% of cases; when bilateral, the pain on the two sides is often different with regard to the age of the patient at onset and the location of the pain. Most cases of bilateral TN occur in patients with MS wherein the pain is due to demyelination in the trigeminal nerve root secondary to an MS plaque. One of the most characteristic historical features of TN is the triggering of jabs or jolts of pain by stimuli that usually are innocuous. Such triggers include a variety of light mechanical stimuli, such as touching the face lightly, brushing the teeth, talking, attempting to eat and drink, and even a light breeze blowing against the face. Light, gentle stimuli are often more effective in eliciting the pain than are more forceful ones. Facial pain, even severe pain, probably is not TN if trigger phenomena are not described. The time course of TN is marked by unexplained, erratic exacerbations and remissions that may last days, weeks, months, or even years. The exacerbations tend to be less severe and shorter in duration at the onset of the illness and tend to become more severe and longer in duration and marked by shorter interval remissions as the illness persists over time. Patients who complain of persistent, unremitting facial pain, often with durations of weeks, months, or even years, probably do not suffer from TN. TN is often misdiagnosed as being of dental or paranasal sinus origin, but

CURRENT DIAGNOSIS

- Sudden, sharp, severe pain on one side of the face
- Confined to the cutaneous or intraoral distribution of the trigeminal nerve
- Triggered by otherwise innocuous stimulation of the face or mouth
- Usually due to arterial compression of the trigeminal nerve root but may be due to multiple sclerosis, tumors, or vascular malformations

conversely other forms of facial pain are often misdiagnosed as TN. Most commonly misdiagnosed is so-called atypical facial pain. Such pain, often seen in young or middle-aged women but seen in men as well, usually is described as a strong, unremitting pressure or burning sensation that encompasses an area of the head and/or neck outside of the distribution of the trigeminal nerve, unassociated with trigger phenomena, often of prolonged durations (years), and usually unresponsive to a variety of medical interventions. Patients with atypical facial pain often express feelings of depression and hopelessness. Such pain is unresponsive to surgical intervention, and ill-advised surgical procedures often aggravate the pain and may leave the patient with new medical problems due to complications of the surgical procedures.

Physical Examination

In classic, or idiopathic, TN due to vascular compression of the trigeminal nerve root, the physical examination is usually completely unremarkable. Specifically, at least by the usual clinical examination techniques, facial sensation including the corneal reflex is normal. When loss of facial sensation to innocuous or painful stimuli is detected, a structural cause of TN should be sought. Tumors, vascular malformations, and MS are usually accompanied by other abnormal neurologic examination findings, including double vision, unilateral hearing loss, and facial weakness. MRI scanning is recommended in all patients with a suspected diagnosis of TN because even in some cases of TN caused by structural lesions, the examination may be normal, and the diagnosis of TN may be strengthened if an MRI scan demonstrates arterial compression of the trigeminal nerve root. Occasionally, an MRI scan discloses a completely unexpected cause of TN, such as a tortuous vertebrobasilar artery complex compressing the nerve root or even a large contralateral tumor or cyst displacing the brainstem. Such findings may radically alter any surgical recommendations made for treatment of TN. Patients who are unable to undergo MRI scanning because they have a cardiac pacemaker, for instance, should undergo thin-section computed tomography scanning, which cannot detect arterial vascular compression and small tumors but can detect larger tumors, vascular malformations, and vertebrobasilar artery compression.

Treatment

MEDICAL TREATMENT

The anticonvulsant family of drugs is the mainstay of medical treatment of TN. Carbamazepine (Tegretol) and oxcarbazepine (Trileptal)[1] are the best drugs for initial medical treatment of TN. Both should be started in relatively low doses, for example, 100 to 200 mg once or twice daily and then increased gradually and slowly until either satisfactory control of the pain or intolerable side effects occur. Such side effects include drowsiness, weakness, difficulty with recent memory, and unsteadiness of gait. Older patients are particularly sensitive to such side effects, and the initial dose and maximum tolerable dose are usually lower in older patients, particularly those in their 70s and older. From 5 to 7 days should elapse between dosing increments in order to allow development of a stable blood level of medication. Additional increments of 100 to 200 mg/day are recommended. Laboratory tests of serum levels of the medications are of little or no help in the treatment of TN. In order to establish a consistent blood level of these medications and to provide the best chance for achieving lasting pain relief with minimum side effects, counseling of the patient by the physician regarding the correct dosing regimen is essential. Patients often regard these medications as analgesics and vary the dosage on an as-needed basis, some days taking little or no medication and other days taking large amounts. Because of their pharmacokinetics, these medications must be taken

[1]Not FDA approved for this indication.

CURRENT THERAPY

- Usually responds to oral anticonvulsant medications, such as carbamazepine (Tegretol) or oxcarbazepine (Trileptal).[1]
- Early radiosurgical treatment offers a good chance of curing the illness with minimal side effects.
- Microvascular decompression is the most effective surgical treatment of TN, but it is associated with the greatest risk of serious complications.

[1]Not FDA approved for this indication.

in a consistent dosage on a daily basis in order to maximize the chance of success. It is surprising how hard it may be for patients to understand and adhere to such a regimen, but maintaining the regimen is essential for successful pain relief. Gabapentin (Neurontin)[1] has become popular for the treatment of TN, but experience indicates it is a secondary medication only. It may be useful when pain control cannot be achieved with carbamazepine (Tegretol) or oxcarbazepine (Trileptal) or when those medications cannot be tolerated because of side effects. Other potential second-line medications include a variety of other anticonvulsants (e.g., lamotrigine [Lamictal],[1] phenytoin [Dilantin][1]) as well as baclofen (Lioresal) A variety of toxicities, including liver dysfunction, bone marrow suppression, and allergic reactions, may accompany use of these medications, so appropriate laboratory surveillance should be performed per manufacturers' recommendations.

SURGICAL TREATMENT

In the past, surgery was reserved for patients who did not respond to medical management of TN because the medication was ineffective or the side effects or toxicities were intolerable. However, some studies suggest that the longer the illness persists, the smaller the chance for lasting successful surgical relief of the pain. Many patients considered the potential side effects and complications of the surgical procedures unacceptable, and neurologists often referred patients for surgical procedures only as a last resort. With the advent of radiosurgery as a viable, successful, and safe surgical treatment of TN, consideration of surgical intervention earlier rather than later in the disease course may be better. Microvascular decompression (MVD) is the most effective, yet most dangerous, of the surgical procedures for TN. About 90% of patients will achieve immediate relief of TN after MVD, but this success rate drops to about 75% in long-term follow-up. MVD is the only surgical procedure that treats the putative cause of TN, namely, vascular compression of the trigeminal nerve root. In the MVD procedure, a small posterior fossa craniotomy is performed. The trigeminal nerve root is visualized using the operating microscope, any compressing vessels are dissected free of the nerve, and future contact is prevented by placing a shock-absorbing material, usually shredded Teflon felt, between the vessel and the nerve. Fatal complications may occur in up to 1% of patients undergoing the MVD procedures. From 15% to 20% of patients who undergo MVD experience some complication of the procedure, such as cerebellar edema, brainstem infarction, subdural and epidural hematomas, facial paralysis, unilateral hearing loss, cerebrospinal fluid leakage, meningitis, and infection. Percutaneous procedures (e.g., radiofrequency electrocoagulation, glycerol rhizolysis, balloon compression) are considerably safer than MVD, but loss of facial sensation usually accompanies such procedures. Loss of facial sensation should be avoided in order to prevent secondary complications such as anesthesia dolorosa and loss of the corneal reflex with subsequent corneal ulceration or loss of vision. The initial success rate is

[1]Not FDA approved for this indication.

about 90% with the percutaneous procedures, but recurrences are frequent. Serious side effects, such as meningitis, brain abscess or hematoma, and carotid artery to cavernous sinus fistulas, occasionally occur. One of the attractive features of percutaneous procedures is that they can be repeated fairly easily if pain recurs. Radiosurgery is gaining increased acceptance as a surgical method for treating TN. Although considered a form of surgery, the procedure is accomplished without an incision, instead using either gamma rays (Gamma Knife, Elekta, Inc.) or high-energy x-rays (linear accelerator [LINAC]) that are focused on the trigeminal nerve root adjacent to the brainstem. The treatment is planned using MRI or computed tomography scanning, and the radiation is guided to the target at the trigeminal nerve root in such a way as to avoid injury to adjacent structures. The procedure provides pain relief in about 60% of patients with TN without the need for medication; another 15% to 20% of patients experience pain relief with small tolerable doses of medication. Radiosurgery is attractive to patients and referring physicians because of the ease of performing the procedure and the minimum risk of side effects. Radiosurgery is a destructive form of treatment of TN, but the degree of damage to the nerve root is usually minimal enough that normal facial sensation is maintained. Permanent losses of facial sensation may occur in as few as 5% of patients treated with radiosurgery, depending on the dose of radiation used for the treatment. Drawbacks of radiosurgery include delayed onset of pain relief after treatment (usually a few months) and recurrences. Radiosurgery can be repeated in the event of initial failure of the treatment or in case of recurrence after an initially successful treatment. The reasonable success rate, the ease of performance of the procedure, and the minimal risk of side effects make radiosurgery a treatment that can be recommended early in the treatment of TN, once the diagnosis has been well established, because it may provide permanent cure of the disease with minimal risk.

REFERENCES

Bagheri SC, Fairhdvash F, Perciaccante VJ: Diagnosis and treatment of patients with trigeminal neuralgia. Am Dent Assoc 2004;135:1713-1717.

Kres B, Schindler M, Rasche D, et al: MRI volumetry for the preoperative diagnosis of trigeminal neuralgia. Eur Radiol 2005;15:1344-1348.

Liu JK, Apfelbaum RI: Treatment of trigeminal neuralgia. Neurosurg Clin North Am 2004;15:319-334.

Shetter AG, Aabramisk JM, Speiser BL: Microvascular decompression after gamma knife surgery for trigeminal neuralgia: intraoperative findings and treatment outcomes. J Neurosurg 2000;102(Suppl.):259-261.

Young RF: Stereotactic procedures for facial pain. In Apuzzo M (ed): Brain Surgery: Complication Avoidance and Management. New York: Churchill Livingstone, 1993, pp 2097-2114.

Young RF: Radiosurgery versus microsurgery for trigeminal neuralgia: current techniques in neurosurgery. In Salcman M (ed): Current Medicine. New York: Springer, 1998, pp 35-43.

Young RF, Vermeulen SS, Grimm P, et al: Gamma knife radiosurgery for treatment of trigeminal neuralgia: Idiopathic and tumor related. Neurology 1997;48:608-614.

Young RF, Vermeulen SS, Posewitz A: Gamma knife radiosurgery for treatment of trigeminal neuralgia. Stereotact Funct Neurosurg 1998;70:192-199.

Bell's Palsy (Idiopathic Acute Peripheral Facial Paralysis)

Method of
W. Cooper Scurry, Jr., MD, Jon E. Isaacson, MD, and Fred G. Fedok, MD, FACS

Epidemiology

Facial nerve paralysis has an extensive differential diagnosis but is most commonly idiopathic (Box 1). Although most facial paralysis is of unknown etiology, more serious causes are ruled out by careful evaluation. Each case requires cautious management to avoid secondary sequelae such as eye exposure.

Facial nerve paralysis that is rapid in onset and idiopathic in origin is referred to as *Bell's palsy*. The Scottish surgeon Charles Bell first identified and described the motor function of the facial nerve in 1821. Facial nerve paralysis that is gradually worsening in nature or has a known cause such as trauma or tumor should not be referred to as Bell's palsy.

The incidence of Bell's palsy is 20 to 30 cases per 100,000 persons per year. This condition accounts for 60% to 75% of all cases of unilateral facial paralysis. Approximately 40,000 cases occur in the United States each year, and one in 60 people will be affected during their lifetime. Bell's palsy can occur at any age; however, the median age at onset is 40 years, and the incidence is highest in people older than 70 years. Men and women are affected equally, and left and right sides are affected equally as well. Pregnant women are at significantly increased risk for developing Bell's palsy, and patients with diabetes mellitus and hypertension are at a slightly increased risk.

Pathogenesis

The facial nerve (cranial nerve VII) leaves the brainstem and enters the temporal bone of the skull via the internal auditory canal. On exiting the internal auditory canal, and throughout the temporal bone, the facial nerve travels through the bony fallopian canal. This represents the longest intraosseous course of any of the cranial nerves. The labyrinthine segment of the nerve runs through the narrowest

---

BOX 1 Differential Diagnosis of Acute Facial Nerve Paralysis

- Bell's palsy
- Herpes zoster (Ramsay Hunt syndrome)
- Guillain-Barré syndrome
- Autoimmune disease
- Lyme disease
- HIV
- Kawasaki disease
- Trauma (temporal bone fracture, facial injury)
- Otitis media (acute, chronic, cholesteatoma)
- Sarcoidosis
- Melkersson-Rosenthal syndrome
- Diabetes mellitus
- Hypertension
- Sjögren's syndrome
- Eclampsia
- Amyloidosis
- Parotid tumor
- Vestibular schwannoma
- Malignancy

CURRENT DIAGNOSIS

- Acute-onset facial paresis is evaluated with a full head and neck and neurologic physical examination as soon as possible to establish the extent of facial weakness and determine a House-Brackmann score.
- History and physical examination include evaluation of the affected eye.
- All facial paresis patients need full audiometric testing.
- If a patient with facial paralysis demonstrates no improvement at 2 to 3 months, appropriate imaging is obtained.

portion of the fallopian canal, measuring only 0.6 mm. It is at this segment where inflammation and swelling of the nerve against the bony confines of the canal lead to ischemia and subsequent neural conduction block.

Although Bell's palsy has been a synonym for idiopathic facial paralysis, a viral etiology was first suggested by McCormick in 1972. In 1996, Murakami's group identified DNA fragments of herpes simplex virus type 1 (HSV-1) in the perineural fluid of 11 of 14 patients undergoing facial nerve decompression surgery during the acute phase of an illness.

Not only have scientific experiments demonstrated evidence for a viral etiology, but recent clinical work also shows an advantage to the use of antivirals in the treatment of Bell's. In a double-blind study of 99 Bell's palsy patients treated with either acyclovir-prednisone or placebo-prednisone, Adour reported on the superior final outcome of acyclovir-prednisone compared with prednisone alone. Other studies regarding the benefit of antivirals in the management of Bell's palsy are ongoing and include a 500-patient randomized, controlled trial in Scotland that finished enrolling patients in June 2006.

Clinical Evaluation

Patients with Bell's palsy present to a variety of caregivers. The most important aspect of the evaluation is obtaining a clear history, whether in an emergency department, primary care setting, or subspecialty setting. The provider needs to ascertain the time of onset and whether the paresis is getting better or worse. If the paralysis is complete, one should determine how long it took to evolve to completion. Bell's palsy usually manifests over only hours to days. A slowly progressive paralysis that worsens over weeks to months is not Bell's palsy and should be worked up otherwise. One should rule out a history of malignancies of the head and neck in patients with Bell's palsy. Cutaneous malignancies of the face, scalp, and auricle are especially pertinent.

Seventy percent of Bell's palsy patients will have had a preceding viral-type illness such as an upper respiratory tract infection. Other symptoms accompanying facial paralysis include otalgia, paresthesias, cephalgia, dysgeusia, and phonophobia. The facial nerve also carries parasympathetic nerve fibers and thus Bell's palsy patients might have decreased saliva and tear production ipsilateral to their palsy. Other history questions should be asked to help rule out other etiologies of a facial nerve paralysis such as Lyme disease, Ramsay Hunt syndrome, and Melkersson-Rosenthal syndrome.

A thorough head and neck examination is performed in each patient presenting with facial paralysis. Palpation of the neck and parotid is performed to rule out a mass impinging the facial nerve. Such a mass might be palpated over the mastoid bone, the parotid gland, or in the soft tissues of the face on the affected side. A complete cranial nerve examination is performed in addition to a general neurologic examination. If, on examination, the patient with facial paralysis exhibits sparing of the upper face, a central etiology such as an infarct or tumor should be considered and a contralateral central process must be ruled out by imaging.

The House-Brackmann scale provides a unique scoring system for assessing facial weakness, allowing interphysician communication (Box 2). Though the scale has inherent weaknesses, it is the most universally acknowledged scale for the description of facial nerve function.

The diagnosis of Bell's palsy is strictly clinical and does not require any imaging or further testing in its initial presentation. Most patients show signs of significant recovery within 6 weeks. Patients with Bell's palsy that has not shown some return of facial function by 3 months should undergo imaging. A gadolinium-enhanced magnetic resonance imaging (MRI) study images the entire nerve, highlights inflammation of the facial nerve, and rules out other lesions. A dedicated temporal bone computed tomography (CT) demonstrates superior bone detail and often complements MRI. Because significant sensorineural hearing loss in the presence of facial nerve paralysis

---

BOX 2   House-Brackmann Facial Nerve Grading System

Grade I: Normal Function
- Normal facial function in all areas

Grade II: Mild Dysfunction
- Gross
  - Slight weakness noticeable on close inspection
  - Might have very slight synkinesis
- At rest
  - Normal symmetry and tone
- Motion
  - Forehead: Moderate to good function
  - Eye: Complete closure with minimum effort
  - Mouth: Slight asymmetry

Grade III: Moderate Dysfunction
- Gross
  - Obvious but no disfiguring difference between the two sides
  - Noticeable but no severe synkinesis, contracture, and/or hemifacial spasm
- At rest
  - Normal symmetry and tone
- Motion
  - Forehead: Slight to moderate movement
  - Eye: Complete closure with effort
  - Mouth: Slightly weak with maximum effort

Grade IV: Moderately Severe Dysfunction
- Gross
  - Obvious weakness and/or disfiguring asymmetry
- At rest
  - Normal symmetry and tone
- Motion
  - Forehead: None
  - Eye: Incomplete closure
  - Mouth: Asymmetric with maximum effort

Grade V: Severe Dysfunction
- Gross
  - Only barely perceptible motion
- At rest
  - Asymmetry
- Motion
  - Forehead: None
  - Eye: Incomplete closure
  - Mouth: Slight movement

Grade VI: Total Paralysis
- No movement

suggests the possibility of Ramsay Hunt syndrome or a skull base tumor, all facial paresis patients should undergo full audiometric testing.

Electrical testing is a controversial topic in the work-up of Bell's palsy. Although some authors rely heavily on electrical testing to stratify patients in treatment algorithms, few practitioners regularly order testing. Electrical testing, specifically electroneurography (ENog), is performed by stimulating the facial nerve as it exits the temporal bone at the stylomastoid foramen. ENog measures the peripheral muscle compound action potential response to an electrically evoked stimulus of the facial nerve on the paralyzed side as compared with the action potential on the normal side of the face. Patients should be sent for ENog between days 3 and 14 after developing a complete facial paralysis. Greater than 90% nerve degeneration by ENog combined with no voluntary motor unit potentials detectable on electromyography (EMG) leads some surgeons to recommend surgical decompression.

Treatment

Treatment of Bell's palsy is controversial and has historically varied from expectant management, to multiple medical therapies, to intracranial surgical decompression of various portions of the fallopian canal. Studies describing the natural history of Bell's palsy established that 71% of untreated patients recover completely and an additional 13% achieve near-normal function. Empiric treatment of all patients who present with Bell's palsy has been widely adopted because there is no ideal test to predict which patients will recover completely.

PHARMACOLOGIC THERAPY

Many studies support the use of steroids to counteract the facial nerve swelling documented during decompression surgery. A randomized, double-blind, placebo-controlled trial demonstrated a higher rate of recovery of facial function among 35 patients treated with prednisone as compared with 41 patients given placebo. Meta-analyses have also substantiated the use of steroids to improve outcomes for patients with Bell's palsy. Steroid therapy consists of a starting dose of 1 mg/kg (or 60-80 mg) of oral prednisone[1] for 7 days and then tapering (Figure 1).

---

[1] Not FDA approved for this indication.

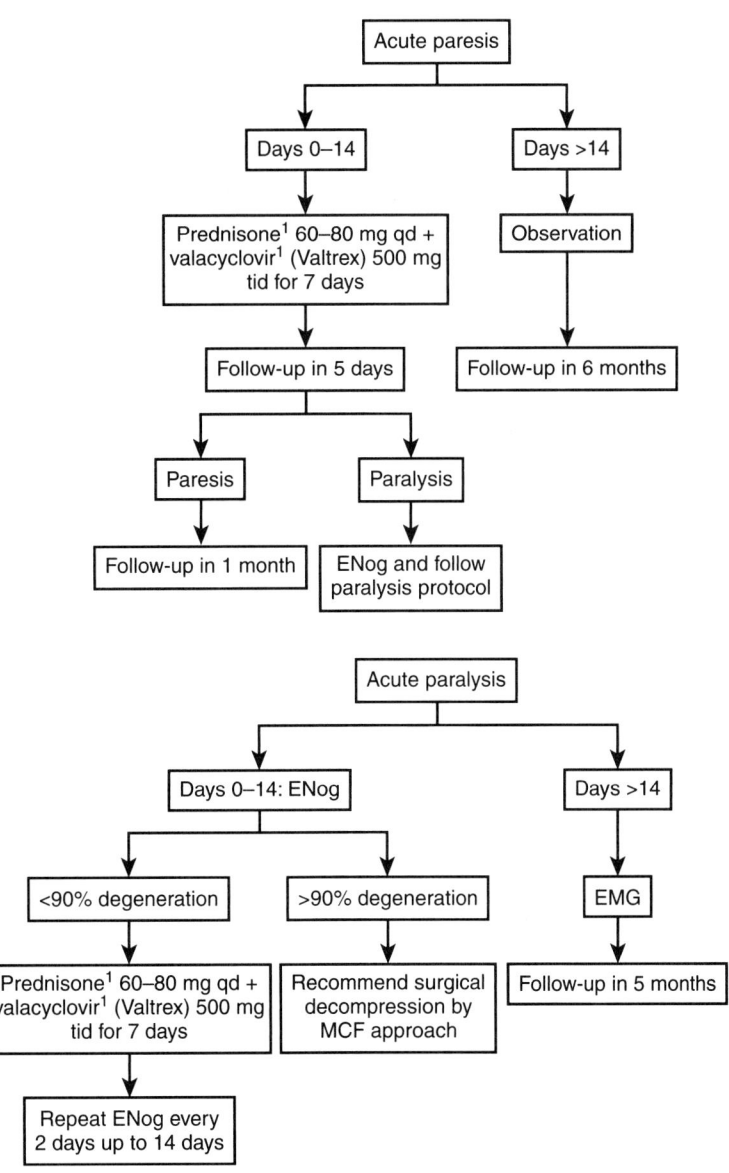

FIGURE 1. Algorithm for management of acute idiopathic facial palsy. *Abbreviations:* EMG = electromyography; ENog = electroneurography; MCF = middle cranial fossa.

CURRENT THERAPY

- On the diagnosis of Bell's palsy, administration of prednisone[1] (start 1 mg/kg) for 1 week then tapered and valacyclovir (Valtrex)[1] (500 mg) daily for 1 week is recommended.
- Three days after the onset of acute facial paralysis, electroneurography (ENog) is performed. If before day 14 after acute facial paralysis ENog demonstrates greater than 90% nerve degeneration, referral for discussion of surgical decompression is warranted.
- Eye care for the patient with facial paresis or paralysis consists of frequent (hourly) daytime ocular artificial tear (Refresh) drops and nighttime use of ocular ointment and a protective moisture chamber.

[1]Not FDA approved for this indication.

Since the establishment of the herpes simplex virus as the likely etiologic agent in the pathogenesis of Bell's palsy, many have sought to demonstrate the clinical efficacy of antiviral therapy. Although antiviral therapy for Bell's palsy makes clinical sense, no study has yet firmly established clear evidence for its benefit. Grogan and Gronseth and the Quality Standards Subcommittee of the American Academy of Neurology have recently summarized the roles of steroids, acyclovir[1] (Zovirax), and surgery for Bell's palsy in an evidence-based review. They conclude that early treatment with acyclovir in combination with prednisone is *possibly* effective to improve facial functional outcomes with Level C evidence. Early treatment with oral steroids is *probably* effective with Level C evidence. A typical regimen for antiviral therapy in the treatment of Bell's palsy is to prescribe valacyclovir[1] 500 mg three times per day for 1 week.

In addition to treatments proposed to facilitate the recovery of facial motion, medical therapies must also be prescribed to prevent damage to an exposed eye. Eye care for the patient with facial paresis or paralysis consists of frequent (hourly) daytime ocular artificial tear drops (Refresh) and nighttime use of ocular ointment and a protective moisture chamber.

SURGICAL THERAPY

Beginning in 1982, surgeons at the University of Iowa, University of Michigan, and Baylor University began prospectively enrolling patients meeting their criteria for surgical decompression. Patients with greater than 90% denervation by ENog and no voluntary motor unit potentials detectable on EMG testing were offered middle cranial fossa facial nerve decompression. In 1999, their study compared the outcomes at 7 months for these patients with control patients with similar electrical findings who elected steroid therapy. The results of this study demonstrated that 91% of the surgical patients achieved a good result (House-Brackmann score of I or II), whereas only 42% of patients electing medical therapy achieved a good result.

The Gantz study emphasizes the importance of the middle cranial fossa approach for decompression surgery to allow appropriate exposure of the narrowest portion of the fallopian canal. Furthermore, the study points out the importance of following ENog with EMG, which demonstrates nerve regeneration, with polyphasic potentials predicting good prognosis. No patients in the Gantz study received antiviral therapy.

One of the management difficulties in the care of Bell's palsy is that the surgical specialist rarely sees the patient within the first 2 weeks (see Figure 1). Decompression surgery for Bell's palsy is not routinely offered by all neurologic surgeons. According to the Grogan and Granseth report, there is insufficient evidence to make recommendations regarding the use of facial nerve decompression to improve facial functional outcomes.

Permanent facial nerve paralysis is a physically and emotionally debilitating condition. Fortunately, most cases of facial nerve paralysis manifest as virally induced, short-lived Bell's palsy from which greater than 80% of patients regain satisfactory facial function. Determining which patients fail to regain full facial nerve function remains the most difficult aspect in the management of these patients. All patients must be carefully managed to prevent the sequelae of exposure keratopathy. Patients who remain debilitated by facial paralysis are candidates for facial reanimation procedures.

Acknowledgments

Thank you to Lisa McCully of the Department of Surgery at the Hershey Medical Center for preparation of our algorithm.

Thank you to Dr. Bruce Gantz of the University of Iowa for permission to modify and publish their algorithm from the Acute Facial Paralysis (Bell's Palsy) chapter in the 2006 edition of *Conn's Current Therapy*.

REFERENCES

Adour KK, Ruboyianes JM, Von Doersten PG, et al: Bell's palsy treatment with acyclovir and prednisone compared with prednisone alone: A double-blind, randomized, controlled trial. Ann Otol Rhinol Laryngol 1996;105:371-378.

Adour KK, Wingerd J: Idiopathic facial paralysis (Bell's palsy): Factors affecting severity and outcome in 446 patients. Neurology 1974;24:1112-1116.

Austin JR, Peskind SP, Austin SG, et al: Idiopathic facial nerve paralysis: A randomized double blind controlled study of placebo versus prednisone. Laryngoscope 1993;103:1326-1333.

Gantz BJ, Rubinstein JT, Gidley P, et al: Surgical management of Bell's palsy. Laryngoscope 1999;109:1177-1188.

Gilden DH: Clinical practice: Bell's palsy. N Engl J Med 2004;351:1323-1331.

Grogan PM, Gronseth GS: Practice parameter: Steroids, acyclovir, and surgery for Bell's palsy (an evidence-based review): Report of the Quality Standards Subcommittee of the American Academy of Neurology. Neurology 2001;56:830-836.

House JW, Brackmann DE: Facial nerve grading system. Otolaryngol Head Neck Surg 1985;93:146-147.

Murakami S, Mizobuchi M, Nakashiro Y, et al: Bells palsy and herpes simplex virus: Identification of viral DNA in endoneurial fluid and muscle. Ann Intern Med 1996;124:27-30.

Peitersen E: Bell's palsy: The spontaneous course of 2,500 peripheral facial nerve palsies of different etiologies. Acta Otolaryngol Suppl (Stockh) 2002:4-30.

Schirm J, Mulkens PS: Bell's palsy and herpes simplex virus. APMIS 1997;105:815-823.

Scurry WC Jr, Isaacson JE, Fedok FG: New-onset facial paralysis and undiagnosed recurrence of cutaneous malignancy: Evaluation and management. Am J Otolaryngol 2006;27:139-142.

Parkinsonism

Method of
Rajesh Pahwa, MD, and Kelly E. Lyons, PhD

Clinical Features

Parkinsonism is a clinical syndrome with the cardinal motor signs of bradykinesia, rigidity, tremor and postural instability. A diagnosis of parkinsonism requires the presence of at least two of the four cardinal

[1]Not FDA approved for this indication.

features. Other motor features can include hypomimia, decreased blink rate, speech difficulties including hypophonia and dysarthria, micrographia, no or reduced arm swing, shuffling and short steps, freezing, festination, difficulty turning in bed, and stooped posture or kyphosis. Common autonomic features include orthostatic hypotension, dysphagia, constipation, urinary frequency and urgency, incontinence, nocturia, sexual dysfunction, and thermoregulatory dysfunction. Sensory symptoms such as anosmia, visual difficulties, pain, and paresthesias can also occur with parkinsonism. Sleep disturbances including insomnia, fragmented sleep, excessive daytime sleepiness, vivid dreaming, and an increased incidence of sleep disorders are common. Finally, neuropsychiatric disturbances such as anxiety, depression, dementia, and psychosis are often seen with parkinsonism.

Differential Diagnosis

There are many possible causes of parkinsonism (Box 1). Diagnosis is based primarily on clinical examination, medical history, family history and past and current medication use. The most common cause of parkinsonism is Parkinson's disease (PD). PD is a slowly progressive neurodegenerative disease generally with unilateral onset. It is estimated that 0.03% of the general population, 3% older than 65 years and 10% older than 80 years develop PD, with an estimated 50,000 new cases diagnosed each year.

 CURRENT DIAGNOSIS

Cardinal Motor Signs

- Bradykinesia
- Postural instability
- Rigidity
- Tremor

Autonomic Dysfunction

- Cardiovascular (e.g., orthostatic hypotension)
- Gastrointestinal (e.g., dysphagia, drooling, constipation, delayed gastric emptying)
- Sexual (e.g., erectile dysfunction, decreased desire and arousal)
- Thermoregulatory (e.g., hyperhydrosis)
- Urologic (e.g., increased frequency and urgency, incontinence, nocturia)

Neuropsychiatric Dysfunction

- Anxiety
- Depression
- Dementia
- Psychosis

Sensory Dysfunction

- Olfactory disturbance (e.g., anosmia)
- Pain
- Paresthesia
- Visual disturbances (e.g., abnormal eye movements, blurred or double vision)

Sleep Dysfunction

- Excessive daytime sleepiness
- Insomnia or fractionated sleep
- Sleep disorders (e.g., REM behavior disorder, sleep apnea, restless legs syndrome)

REM = rapid eye movement.

PD is a clinical diagnosis based on the presence of two of three cardinal symptoms of bradykinesia, rigidity, and tremor with a positive response to carbidopa/levodopa (Sinemet). Several features suggest a diagnosis of a form of parkinsonism other than PD (Table 1). The most common features include a poor response to levodopa, falling as an early symptom, symmetrical onset of symptoms, rapid progression, lack of tremor, and early autonomic symptoms such as urinary incontinence and symptomatic orthostatic hypotension.

PARKINSON-PLUS SYNDROMES

The Parkinson-plus syndromes, progressive supranuclear palsy (PSP), multiple system atrophy (MSA), corticobasal degeneration (CBD), and dementia with Lewy bodies (DLB), can be difficult to differentiate from PD and are often, especially early in the disease course, misdiagnosed as PD.

PSP is a slowly progressive neurodegenerative disease occurring after the age of 40 years; however, the disease course is generally more rapid than that of PD. It can manifest with bradykinesia, rigidity, hypomimia, hypophonia and postural instability with falling, often in the first year. The onset of PSP is often symmetrical, minimal to no rest tremor is observed, and the response to levodopa is poor. As the disease progresses, vertical gaze limitations and other eye movement abnormalities along with dysarthria and dysphagia generally occur. Neck rigidity is usually greater than limb rigidity, and the neck can be held in an extended posture. Frontal dementia and apathy are also commonly seen with PSP.

MSA is a neurodegenerative disorder with various combinations of parkinsonian, autonomic, cerebellar, and pyramidal signs. The disease course is generally more rapid than that of PD, and it generally affects people in their 50s and 60s. It is estimated that 80% of MSA patients have predominantly parkinsonian (MSA-P) features and 20% have predominantly cerebellar features (MSA-C). Autonomic symptoms most commonly include orthostatic hypotension, urinary incontinence or partial bladder emptying, and erectile dysfunction. Parkinsonian features can include bradykinesia, rigidity, postural instability, and tremor. In addition, orofacial dystonia, antecollis, and a jerky postural tremor can occur. MSA generally responds poorly to levodopa; an initial response may be observed, but it is rarely sustained. Cerebellar features include gait and limb ataxia, ataxic dysarthria, and sustained gaze-evoked nystagmus.

BOX 1 Causes of Parkinsonism

Degenerative Disorders

Parkinson's disease (sporadic and familial)
Parkinson-plus syndromes
- Progressive supranuclear palsy (PSP)
- Multiple system atrophy (MSA)
- Corticobasal degeneration (CBD)
- Dementia with Lewy bodies (DLB)

Other Degenerative Disorders

Hallervorden–Spatz disease
Huntington's disease
Lubag (X-linked dystonia–parkinsonism)
Neuroacanthocytosis
Parkinsonism–ALS–dementia complex of Guam
Spinocerebellar ataxias
Wilson's disease

Secondary Parkinsonism

Drug-induced
Infectious (e.g., Creutzfeld–Jakob disease)
Metabolic (e.g., parathyroidism)
Structural (e.g., hydrocephalus, trauma, tumor)
Toxin-induced
Vascular

ALS = amyotrophic lateral sclerosis.

TABLE 1 Features Indicating a Form of Parkinsonism Other than Parkinson's Disease

Feature	Possible Diagnosis
Acute onset	Vascular, drug or toxin-induced, psychogenic
Alien limb	Corticobasal degeneration
Apraxia	Corticobasal degeneration
Ataxia	Multiple system atrophy
Autonomic disturbances (early in disease course)	Multiple system atrophy
Dementia	Dementia with Lewy bodies
Gaze palsies	Progressive supranuclear palsy, corticobasal degeneration, multiple system atrophy, dementia with Lewy bodies
Hallucinations (unrelated to drug use)	Dementia with Lewy bodies
Pyramidal signs	Multiple system atrophy, vascular
Postural instability (early in disease course)	Progressive supranuclear palsy, multiple system atrophy
Symmetrical onset	Progressive supranuclear palsy, multiple system atrophy
Stepwise worsening	Vascular
Tremor minimal or absent	Progressive supranuclear palsy, vascular
Young-onset (<40 y of age)	Drug induced, Wilson's disease

BOX 2 Medications that Can Cause Parkinsonism

Antipsychotics
Acetophenazine (Tindal)[2]
Chlorpromazine (Thorazine)
Chlorprothixene (Taractan)
Fluphenazine (Permitil, Prolixin)
Haloperidol (Haldol)
Loxapine (Loxitane)
Mesoridazine (Serentil)
Molindone (Moban)

Antiemetics
Metoclopramide (Reglan)
Ondansetron (Zofran)

Miscellaneous
Amiodarone (Cordarone)
Amoxapine (Asendin)
Divalproex (Depakote)
Lithium (Eskalith)
Olanzapine (Zyprexa)
Perphenazine (Trilafon)
Perphenazine + amitriptyline (Etafron, Triavil)
Procaine (Novocain)
Prochlorperazine (Compazine)
Promethazine (Phenergan)
Risperidone (Risperdal)
Thioridazine (Mellaril)
Thiothixene (Navane)
Trifluoperazine (Stelazine)
Trifluopromazine (Vesprin)
Ziprasidone (Geodon)

[2]Not available in the United States.

CBD is a progressive, asymmetric disorder affecting persons in their 60s and 70s. The cortical signs include cortical sensory loss, alien limb phenomenon, apraxia, frontal release reflexes, visual or sensory hemineglect, cognitive dysfunction, and dysphasia. The basal ganglia signs include akinesia, rigidity, action or postural tremor, limb dystonia, athetosis, postural instability, falling, and orolingual dyskinesia. Additional signs include hyperreflexia, impaired ocular motility, dysarthria, focal reflex myoclonus, blepharospasm, and dysphagia. CBD does not respond to levodopa.

DLB can be difficult to differentiate from PD dementia (PDD). In general, if the dementia and motor features occur within a year of each other, a diagnosis of DLB rather than PDD is made. DLB results in a progressive decline in cognition that is severe enough to interfere with activities of daily living. It is not uncommon to see fluctuations in cognition with significant variability in attention and alertness and recurrent visual hallucinations. Motor symptoms consistent with parkinsonism are also present. Additional supportive features include frequent falling, syncope, transient loss of consciousness, delusions, REM sleep behavior disorder, and depression. In DLB, the response to levodopa is variable, but few patients have the strong positive response seen in PD.

DRUG-INDUCED PARKINSONISM

Drug-induced parkinsonism occurs in 20% to 40% of patients taking dopamine-blocking agents. The most common offenders are antipsychotics and antiemetics, although other miscellaneous drugs have been reported to cause drug-induced parkinsonism (Box 2). Drug-induced parkinsonism generally has a subacute, asymmetrical onset and can resolve without discontinuation of the offending agent; however, it is best if the offending agent can be stopped. It also tends to be more common and more severe in older persons. Anticholinergics can be helpful with drug-induced symptoms in some patients, as can dopaminergic drugs; however, these drugs can worsen nausea and hallucinations.

Treatment

Although there are multiple treatment options that can improve PD symptoms, there is no known treatment for the other forms of parkinsonism. Often the same medications that are used for PD are tried for other forms of parkinsonism without significant improvement in symptoms. Occasionally, MSA initially responds to PD medications; however, the response is not sustained. In fact, a dramatic and sustained response to antiparkinsonian therapy usually confirms the diagnosis of PD. Symptomatic medical or surgical therapy is the basis of the management of PD. There is increasing attention being focused on the management of nonmotor symptoms of PD such as dementia, depression, psychosis, dysautonomia, and sleep disturbances.

MEDICATIONS

Currently available PD medications include carbidopa/levodopa, monoamine oxidase type B (MAO-B) inhibitors, dopamine agonists, catechol-O-methyl transferase (COMT) inhibitors, anticholinergics, and the antiviral drug amantadine (Symmetrel).

Levodopa

Dopamine is one of the main neurotransmitters that is reduced in PD, and treatment to date has focused on restoring or manipulating this neurotransmitter. Oral dopamine is metabolized and cannot be used as treatment in PD. Levodopa, which is the precursor of dopamine, is considered the gold standard for the symptomatic

CURRENT THERAPY

- Dopamine precursor (levodopa)
- MAO-B inhibitors
- Dopamine agonists
- COMT inhibitors
- Amantadine
- Anticholinergics

COMT = catechol-*O*-methyl transferase; MAO = monoamine oxidase.

treatment of PD. Orally administered levodopa is mainly absorbed in the upper gastrointestinal tract. Levodopa is metabolized in the periphery mainly to dopamine by aromatic amino acid decarboxylase (AAAD) and to 3-*O*-methyldopa (3-OMD) by the COMT enzyme. Once levodopa crosses the blood–brain barrier, it is converted to dopamine intraneuronally.

Orally administered levodopa is almost completely absorbed from the gut. Due to metabolism by AAAD and COMT, less than 5% of an oral dose of levodopa crosses the blood–brain barrier. Hence, levodopa is combined with carbidopa, an AAAD inhibitor. Because carbidopa does not cross the blood–brain barrier, it does not inhibit the conversion of levodopa to dopamine in the brain. The half-life of levodopa is approximately 50 minutes, but when administered with carbidopa it increases to 90 minutes. Approximately 70 to 100 mg of carbidopa is required to saturate peripheral decarboxylase to reduce the peripheral side effects of dopamine, such as nausea and vomiting.

Levodopa improves all the cardinal motor features of PD including tremor, bradykinesia, and rigidity. It is the most efficacious medication for PD. Levodopa does not generally improve nonmotor symptoms such as depression or dementia, nor does it improve axial motor symptoms such as speech or swallowing difficulties, freezing of gait and postural instability.

Carbidopa/levodopa is available in dosages of 10/100 mg, 25/100 mg, and 25/250 mg tablets. The initial dose of carbidopa/levodopa is generally one 25/100 mg tablet three times per day. It is advisable to initiate carbidopa/levodopa slowly, starting with one half of a 25/100 mg tablet twice a day for 1 week and then increasing by one-half tablet daily until symptoms are well controlled. Carbidopa/levodopa is also available in an orally dissolvable formulation (Parcopa). This formulation is available in the same strengths as immediate-release carbidopa/levodopa and has similar safety and efficacy. It is particularly useful in patients with swallowing difficulties.

There is also a controlled-release formulation of carbidopa/levodopa (Sinemet-CR) in doses of 25/100 mg and 50/200 mg. This formulation is generally started with 25/100 mg/day and increased to a typical dose of 25/100 mg three times per day or 50/200 mg twice a day. Controlled-release preparations are not as well absorbed, and the bioavailability is 20% to 30% lower than standard preparations. These formulations do not provide any major advantage over the standard formulations.

One of the biggest limitations to the long-term use of levodopa is the development of motor fluctuations and dyskinesia. Approximately 50% of PD patients develop these motor complications after 5 years of levodopa use. Motor fluctuations include end-of-dose wearing-off and random on/off phenomena. When levodopa is initiated, patients generally have a stable control of PD symptoms during the day. However, over a period of months to years, they experience improvement in the PD symptoms for only a few hours after levodopa ingestion and the effects of the drug wear off before the next dose, which is required before the symptoms improve again. This is known as *end-of-dose wearing off*. As the disease progresses, the number of hours of benefit with each dose of levodopa decreases and the patient often requires multiple doses throughout the day. Random on/off fluctuations are rapid transitions (over seconds) between the on state (when the PD symptoms are under good control) and off state (when PD symptoms are present), and these are usually unpredictable and not unrelated to the timing of levodopa dose.

Dyskinesia is another long-term motor complication of levodopa therapy. Dyskinesia involves involuntary movements such as chorea, dystonia, and ballismus. The most common types of dyskinesia are peak-dose dyskinesia, wearing-off dystonia, and diphasic dystonia/dyskinesia. Peak-dose dyskinesia is the most common form of dyskinesia and occurs when dopamine levels are at their peak. These movements consist of involuntary choreiform movements of the arms, legs, trunk, and head. Wearing-off dystonia is the painful dystonic movements that occur when dopamine levels are low, usually between levodopa dosing, in the middle of the night, or early in the morning before levodopa is taken. Diphasic dystonia/dyskinesia is uncommon and occurs when dopamine levels are rising or falling.

Common acute adverse effects with carbidopa/levodopa include nausea, vomiting, somnolence, and orthostatic hypotension. Other side effects include skin rash, diaphoresis, cardiac arrhythmias, and pedal edema. Psychiatric side effects include confusion, vivid dreams, nightmares, hallucinations, and delusions.

Dopamine Agonists

Dopamine agonists are drugs that directly stimulate the postsynaptic dopamine receptors. After levodopa, dopamine agonists are the most efficacious symptomatic therapy for PD. Dopamine agonists were initially used as an adjunctive therapy to levodopa; however, currently they are increasingly used as both initial monotherapy and as adjunctive therapy. Studies have demonstrated that initial use of dopamine agonists as monotherapy for PD delays the onset of motor fluctuations and dyskinesia. Dopamine agonists also reduce off time in PD patients on levodopa therapy with motor fluctuations.

Commonly used dopamine agonists include pramipexole (Mirapex) and ropinirole (Requip and Requip XL). Other dopamine agonists include bromocriptine (Parlodel), pergolide (Permax),[2] apomorphine (Apokyn), and the rotigotine transdermal system (Neupro).

Bromocriptine

Bromocriptine is an ergoline dopamine agonist and was the first dopamine agonist approved for use in the United States in 1978. Bromocriptine is mainly a D_2 agonist with weak D_1 antagonist properties. It is rapidly absorbed: Its half-life is between 3 and 8 hours and the peak drug plasma levels are reached in 1 to 2 hours. Due to the risk of ergot-related side effects, bromocriptine is rarely used in clinical practice. It is generally started at 1.25 mg once per day and titrated over several weeks to a maximum dose of 10 to 40 mg/day divided into three or four doses.

Pergolide

Pergolide is an ergot-derived dopamine agonist that was recently withdrawn from the United States market due to concerns of cardiac valvular fibrosis. Patients previously exposed to pergolide might be at risk and should undergo echocardiogram screening.

Pramipexole

Pramipexole is a nonergot dopamine agonist approved for use as monotherapy and adjunctive therapy in PD. Pramipexole mainly acts on the D_2, D_3, and D_4 dopamine receptors. It has a half-life of 8 to 12 hours and reaches peak drug plasma concentration in approximately 2 hours. Pramipexole is excreted in the urine mostly unchanged. It is initiated at 0.125 mg three times per day and slowly increased over several weeks to a maximum dose of 1.5 mg three times per day (Table 2).

---

[2]Not available in the United States.

TABLE 2 Dopamine Agonist Titration Schedules

Week	Pramipexole (Mirapex)	Ropinirole (Requip)	Ropinirole Extended Release (Requip XL)
1	0.125 mg tid	0.25 mg tid	2 mg qd
2	0.25 mg tid	0.5 mg tid	4 mg qd
3	0.5 mg tid	0.75 mg tid	6 mg qd
4	0.75 mg tid	1.0 mg tid	8 mg qd
5	1.0 mg tid	1.5 mg tid	12 mg qd
6	1.25 mg tid	2.0 mg tid	16 mg qd
7	1.5 mg tid	2.5 mg tid	20 mg qd
8		3.0 mg tid	24 mg qd
Maximum	1.5 mg tid	8.0 mg tid	24 mg qd

Ropinirole

Ropinirole is also a nonergot dopamine agonist approved for both monotherapy and adjunctive therapy in PD. It has affinity for the D_2 family of dopamine receptors and no effect on the D_1 or D_5 dopaminergic receptors. The plasma half-life of ropinirole is approximately 6 hours, and peak drug plasma concentrations occur in 1 to 2 hours. Ropinirole is initiated at 0.25 mg three times per day and gradually increased over several weeks to a maximum dose. An of 8 mg three times per day. An extended release formulation, ropinirole extended release (Requip XL) is also available, allowing once daily dosing (see Table 2).

Rotigotine

Rotigotine was the first transdermal PD medication approved for use in the United States; however, it was withdrawn from the market in 2008 due to manufacturing issues. It is a nonergot dopamine agonist currently approved for early PD. It mainly acts on the D_3, D_2, and D_1 receptors but also has action on the D_4 and D_5 receptors. It is continuously absorbed over 24 hours with stable plasma levels and a half-life of 5 to 7 hours. Rotigotine is initiated at 2 mg per 24 hours and over a period of 3 weeks can be increased to a maximum of 6 mg per 24 hours (see Table 2). The patch is changed daily. The transdermal patch is applied to different body locations, which should change daily, avoiding application to a previous location for at least 14 days to reduce the incidence of skin reactions.

Apomorphine

Apomorphine is approved for advanced PD as a rescue therapy for severe off periods. It is the only subcutaneous injection for PD available in the United States. It is a nonergot, fast-acting dopamine agonist with a high affinity for D_4 receptors, moderate affinity for D_2, D_3, D_5 receptors, and low affinity for D_1 receptors. Apomorphine is rapidly absorbed in 10 to 60 minutes, has a half-life of approximately 40 minutes, and provides an effect for up to 90 minutes. It can be given every 2 hours; however, there are limited data for use exceeding five times per day. A test dose of 2 mg (0.2 mL) is given under medical supervision during an off state, and the dose is titrated by 0.1 mL increments up to a maximum single dose of 0.6 mL.

Apomorphine is an emetic and can cause severe nausea and vomiting; therefore, an antiemetic such as trimethobenzamide (Tigan)[1] should be used for 3 days before administration and for at least 6 weeks after administration of apomorphine. Due to severe hypotension and possible loss of consciousness, apomorphine should not be used with 5-HT_3 antagonists like ondansetron (Zofran), granisetron (Kytril), dolasetron (Anzemet), palonosetron (Aloxi), and alosetron (Lotronex).[11]

---

[1]Not FDA approved for this indication.
[11]Required to enroll in the manufacturer's prescribing program.

Adverse Effects

All dopamine agonists have similar side effects except for the long-term risks of pulmonary fibrosis, retroperitoneal fibrosis, and cardiac valvular fibrosis associated only with the ergot dopamine agonists. Adverse effects may be dose and time dependent, and they often occur when therapy is initiated. Common adverse effects include nausea, vomiting, dizziness, somnolence, insomnia, peripheral edema, and orthostatic hypotension. Central adverse effects are mainly psychiatric such as hallucinations, confusion, mood changes, depression, irritability, euphoria, vivid dreams, sleep disturbances, inappropriate sexual behavior, delusions, agitation, and paranoid psychosis. There have been reports of patients falling asleep during activities of daily living, including while operating motor vehicles, and of impulsive disorders like gambling, eating, shopping, and sexual behavior with dopamine agonists.

Catechol-*O*-Methyl Transferase Inhibitors

COMT inhibitors are drugs that increase the half-life of levodopa by reducing its metabolism. Using COMT inhibitors with levodopa prolongs the action of individual doses of levodopa. Tolcapone (Tasmar) and entacapone (Comtan) are both specific and reversible inhibitors of COMT, and they increase the area under the levodopa plasma concentration/time curve. At therapeutic doses, entacapone only acts peripherally and does not affect central COMT activity. Tolcapone can pass the blood–brain barrier and block central COMT in addition to its peripheral actions.

Tolcapone

Tolcapone (Tasmar) has a half-life of approximately 2 to 3 hours, and the time to maximum plasma concentration is approximately 2 hours. It is initiated at 100 mg three times a day and increased to 200 mg three times a day if needed. Tolcapone should always be used with levodopa.

The majority of the adverse effects related to tolcapone are dopaminergic in nature. Dyskinesia, nausea, hallucinations, insomnia, anorexia, and orthostatic hypotension are common. These adverse effects are usually improved by reduction in the levodopa dose. Diarrhea as an adverse effect usually begins at 6 to 12 weeks but can appear as early as 2 weeks after tolcapone is started. If the diarrhea is bothersome, therapy must be discontinued. Urine discoloration is a harmless side effect that occurs in less than 10% of patients.

Significant increases in liver enzymes have been reported, and after FDA approval, there were three cases of fatal liver injury reported with the use of tolcapone. This led to strict guidelines regarding the use of tolcapone: it may only be used in PD patients who have tried all other antiparkinsonian medications, and serum ALT and AST should be tested at baseline, every 2 to 4 weeks for the first 6 months, and then as clinically indicated. Tolcapone should be discontinued if the patient does not have a response or if there is a two times increase in the upper limit of ALT and AST.

Entacapone

Entacapone (Comtan) is approved for the management of motor fluctuations in PD. Its half-life is approximately one half hour (0.4-0.7 hours). It reduces the peripheral metabolism of levodopa and prolongs the levodopa half-life from 1.3 to 2.4 hours. It is initiated at 200 mg with each dose of levodopa for a maximum of eight doses per day.

The side effects of entacapone are similar to those of tolcapone and mostly related to increased dopaminergic stimulation. Dyskinesia, nausea, vomiting, and hallucinations are the most commonly seen dopaminergic adverse effects. These side effects can usually be reduced or eliminated by decreasing the levodopa dose. There is no known hepatotoxicity associated with entacapone and no requirement for liver enzyme monitoring.

Carbidopa/Levodopa/Entacapone

The triple combination carbidopa/levodopa/entacaopone (Stalevo) is available in four different combinations: Stalevo 50 (carbidopa 12.5 mg/levodopa 50 mg/entacapone 200 mg), Stalevo 100 (carbidopa 25 mg/levodopa 100 mg/entacapone 200 mg), Stalevo 150 (carbidopa 37.5 mg/levodopa 150 mg/entacapone 200 mg) and Stalevo 200 (carbidopa 50 mg/levodopa 200 mg/entacapone 200 mg). This triple combination is indicated in PD patients as a substitute for immediate-release carbidopa/levodopa and entacapone previously administered separately. It can also replace immediate-release carbidopa/levodopa (without entacapone) in patients experiencing end-of-dose wearing-off who are taking 600 mg or less of levodopa and are not having dyskinesia. The adverse effects are similar to those seen with carbidopa/levodopa and entacapone used separately.

Monoamine Oxidase B (MAO-B) Inhibitors

Selegiline (Eldepryl), orally disintegrating selegiline (Zelapar), and rasagiline (Azilect) are the MAO-B inhibitors available in United States. They are selective irreversible MAO-B inhibitors. MAO-B inhibitors increase the half-life of levodopa by blocking the metabolism of dopamine by MAO.

Selegiline

Selegiline is an irreversible MAO-B inhibitor and has an elimination half-life of approximately 2 hours. However, because the drug irreversibly inhibits MAO-B, the therapeutic benefits are lost after the enzyme is regenerated. The major plasma metabolites of selegiline are N-desmethylselegiline (the only metabolite with MAO-B inhibiting properties), L-amphetamine, and L-methamphetamine. Selegiline is approved as an adjunct treatment to levodopa; however, it is also used as monotherapy in early disease. The typical dose is 5 mg with breakfast and lunch.

Selegiline is generally well tolerated. The most common adverse effects include nausea, dizziness, insomnia, constipation, excessive sweating, confusion, hallucinations, dry mouth, and orthostatic hypotension. When used as an adjunct to levodopa therapy, an increase in dyskinesia can occur, as well as increases in other levodopa-related side effects. As the dose of selegiline is increased, its selectivity to inhibit MAO-B is decreased, and inhibition of MAO-A can also occur.

Orally Disintegrating Selegiline

The orally disintegrating selegiline tablet is available for oral administration (not to be swallowed) in the strength of 1.25 mg. It is approved for use in advanced PD with motor fluctuations. The initial dose is 1.25 mg a day, which can be increased to 2.5 mg per day if clinically indicated. Selegiline disintegrates within seconds after placement on the tongue and is rapidly absorbed. The pregastric absorption of orally disintegrating selegiline and the avoidance of first-pass metabolism results in higher concentrations of selegiline and lower concentrations of its metabolites compared with the 5-mg swallowed selegiline tablet. Side effects are similar to those reported with selegiline tablets. There are no data on the use of orally disintegrating selegiline as monotherapy in PD.

Rasagiline

Rasagiline is an irreversible MAO-B inhibitor. It is rapidly absorbed and reaches peak plasma concentrations in approximately 1 hour. Its half-life is approximately 3 hours, but because it irreversibly inhibits MAO-B, the therapeutic benefit is not dependent on its half-life. It is approved as monotherapy in early disease (1 mg/day) and in PD patients with advanced disease experiencing motor fluctuations (0.5 mg/day, which can be increased to 1 mg/day as needed).

The most commonly observed adverse events with rasagiline monotherapy were flu syndrome, arthralgia, depression, dyspepsia, and falls. As an adjunct to levodopa, the common adverse effects included dyskinesia, accidental injury, weight loss, postural hypotension, vomiting, anorexia, arthralgia, abdominal pain, nausea, constipation, dry mouth, rash, ecchymosis, somnolence, and paresthesia.

Contraindications

Although MAO inhibitors used in the treatment of PD are specific MAO-B inhibitors, at higher than recommended doses or as an idiosyncratic reaction, MAO-A can also be inhibited. Hence, certain medications should not be used with these medications: analgesics such as meperidine (Demerol), tramadol (Ultram), methadone (Dolophine, Methadose), and propoxyphene (Darvon); the antitussive agent dextromethorphan (found in many over-the-counter cough medicines); St. John's wort, mirtazapine (Remeron), and cyclobenzaprine (Flexeril); sympathomimetic amines, including amphetamines as well as cold products and weight-reducing preparations that contain vasoconstrictors (e.g., pseudoephedrine, phenylephrine, phenylpropanolamine,[2] and ephedrine[2]); and other MAO inhibitors.

Anticholinergics

Anticholinergics were the first class of drugs used for the treatment of PD. They work mainly on the muscarinic acetylcholine receptors. The exact mechanism of action of anticholinergics is unclear. It is believed that there is antagonism between the effects of dopamine and acetylcholine in the basal ganglia and that anticholinergics work by correcting the disequilibrium between striatal dopamine and acetylcholine activity.

A number of anticholinergics are available. They are generally well absorbed after oral administration and usually require dosing two or three times a day. The commonly used anticholinergics for PD include biperiden (Akineton), trihexyphenidyl (Artane), benztropine (Cogentin), and procyclidine (Kemadrin). Anticholinergics should be started at low doses and increased very slowly. Anticholinergics are mildly beneficial in the management of PD and mainly help tremor without significantly affecting bradykinesia or rigidity. Anticholinergics are mainly used in young patients due to safety concerns.

Anticholinergics are contraindicated in patients with narrow-angle glaucoma, tachycardia, prostate hypertrophy, gastrointestinal obstruction, and megacolon. Common side effects include blurring of vision, nausea, constipation, urinary retention, and dry mucous membranes in the mouth and eyes. Acute confusion, hallucinations, psychosis, and sedation can occur. All central adverse effects are more likely to occur in patients with advanced age and in patients with impaired cognitive function.

Amantadine

Amantadine (Symmetrel) was initially marketed as an antiviral agent but was reported to be helpful for tremor, rigidity, and bradykinesia in PD. Since then, the efficacy of amantadine both as monotherapy and in combination with levodopa in the treatment of PD has been demonstrated. There are several modes of action of amantadine, but the exact mechanism in PD is unknown. Presynaptically, amantadine enhances the release of stored catecholamines from dopaminergic terminals and inhibits the reuptake process. Postsynaptically, amantadine exerts a direct effect on dopamine receptors. In addition, it is believed that amantadine has anticholinergic effects and N-methyl-D-aspartate (NMDA) glutamate receptor blockade.

Amantadine is quickly absorbed, with peak blood levels 2 to 4 hours after an oral dose. It should be used with caution in patients with impaired renal function and should not be used in patients with renal failure. The usual dose is 200 to 300 mg/day in divided doses. In early PD, amantadine has mild antiparkinsonian benefits on tremor, bradykinesia, and rigidity. In advanced PD, amantadine has been reported to be efficacious in improving dyskinesia. Common side effects include dizziness, anxiety, impaired coordination, insomnia,

---

[2]Not available in the United States.

and nervousness. Nausea and vomiting occur in 5% to 10% of patients. In some patients, pedal edema and livedo reticularis can be bothersome and can lead to discontinuation of therapy.

DEEP BRAIN STIMULATION

When motor fluctuations and dyskinesia cannot be adequately controlled with medications, surgery may be an option for appropriate patients. Deep brain stimulation (DBS) involves implanting a stimulating electrode into the brain. There are three possible DBS targets for treating PD. DBS of the thalamus results in marked improvement in tremor but does not improve bradykinesia, rigidity, or drug-induced dyskinesia and only minimally improves activities of daily living. DBS of the globus pallidus interna improves all of the cardinal symptoms of PD (tremor, rigidity, bradykinesia) and markedly reduces dyskinesia. DBS of the subthalamic nucleus is the most commonly performed DBS procedure for PD and results in improvements in all the cardinal motor symptoms of PD, motor fluctuations, and dyskinesia, while allowing a substantial decrease in antiparkinsonian medications.

Candidates for Deep Brain Stimulation

Thalamic stimulation is rarely used for PD and may be recommended for patients who have disabling, medication-resistant tremor with minimal signs of bradykinesia and rigidity. Patients who have levodopa-responsive PD and medication-resistant motor fluctuations and dyskinesia are appropriate candidates for pallidal or subthalamic stimulation. For DBS procedures, patients should not have significant cognitive, psychiatric, or behavioral problems, such as dementia or severe depression.

Adverse Events

In general, all DBS procedures have similar adverse effects. These adverse effects can be categorized as surgical, device-related, and stimulation-related complications. The experience of the neurosurgeon and proper patient selection generally reduce the occurrence of adverse events. Serious surgical complications can occur in 1% to 2% of patients and include intracranial bleeds, strokes, and seizures. Infections have been reported in 5% to 8% of patients. Device-related events can occur in up to 25% of patients. These include lead reposition due to incorrect placement, lead displacement, erosion of the skin over the lead or the extension, breakage of the lead or the extension, or malfunction of the implanted pulse generator. Adverse effects related to stimulation depend on the location of the electrode and the stimulus intensity, and they usually improve with stimulation adjustments.

MANAGEMENT

Early Disease

Multiple options are available in initiating therapy in a patient with newly diagnosed PD. Anticholinergics are rarely used due to concerns of adverse effects. In a young patient with tremor-predominant symptoms, anticholinergics might be considered. Patients with mild symptoms are occasionally initially treated with amantadine. However, if a patient has functional impairment, rasagiline or selegiline, dopamine agonists, or levodopa are initiated. Rasagiline is a milder agent and may be used in patients with mild PD symptoms. If the symptoms are causing significant functional disability, in young patients, dopamine agonists such as ropinirole, ropinirole extended release, or pramipexole are initiated. In older patients, especially those with cognitive impairment, levodopa is initiated. As the disease progresses, patients often end up on combination therapy.

Advanced Disease

There are multiple treatment options for patients on levodopa who develop motor fluctuations. These include increasing the dose or dosing frequency of levodopa and providing adjunctive therapy with dopamine agonists, COMT inhibitors, or MAO-B inhibitors. Often, patients end up taking medications from each of these classes. Amantadine is the only drug reported to improve dyskinesia. If motor fluctuations and dyskinesia cannot be managed with medications, DBS may be considered in some patients.

REFERENCES

Litvan I: Atypical Parkinsonian Disorders: Clinical and Research Aspects. Totowa, NJ: Humana Press, 2005.
Miyasaki JM, Martin W, Suchowersky O, et al: Practice parameter: Initiation of treatment for Parkinson's disease: An evidence-based review. Neurology 2002;58:11-17.
Olanow CW, Watts RL, Koller WC: An algorithm (decision tree) for the management of Parkinson's disease (2001): Treatment guidelines. Neurology 2001;56(suppl 5):S1-S88.
Pahwa R, Factor SA, Lyons KE, et al: Practice parameter: Treatment of Parkinson disease with motor fluctuations and dyskinesia (an evidence-based review). Neurology 2006;66:983-995.
Pahwa R, Lyons KE: Handbook of Parkinson's Disease, 4th ed. New York: Informa Healthcare, 2007.
Suchowersky O, Reich S, Perlmutter J, et al: Practice parameter: Diagnosis and prognosis of new onset Parkinson disease (an evidence-based review). Neurology 2006;66:968-975.

Peripheral Neuropathies

Method of
Kerrie Schoffer, MD, FRCPC

Disorders of the peripheral nerve system (PNS) include pathology affecting the spinal cord roots (radiculopathies), the dorsal root ganglia (neuronopathies), the brachial, lumbar, and sacral plexuses (plexopathies), and the terminal nerve (mononeuropathies) or nerves (polyneuropathies). They are among the most common and challenging problems in medical practice, with literally hundreds of conceivable causes. An organized diagnostic approach consists of first categorizing the neuropathy based on clinical and electrophysiologic assessments and then performing a tailored diagnostic evaluation. However astute the diagnostician, the cause of a neuropathy might not found in up to 20% of patients.

Anatomy

Four types of fibers are found in the PNS: motor, large fiber sensory, small fiber sensory, and autonomic. Motor fibers extend peripherally to the neuromuscular junction of their respective muscles and have their cell bodies in motor neurons located in the spinal cord. Conversely, sensory fibers receive information from peripheral sensory receptors and transfer this to cell bodies in the dorsal root ganglia, located near, but outside, the spinal cord. Large, myelinated sensory fibers supply information regarding position and vibration. Small myelinated axons, composed of autonomic and sensory fibers, are responsible for light touch, pain, temperature, and parasympathetic and sympathetic information.

Damage can occur to the cell bodies (neuronopathy), nerve fibers (axonopathy), or to the surrounding myelin sheath (myelinopathy). Myelinopathies principally affect only the coating around the nerve, and an axonopathy results in degeneration of both the axon and myelin. The most distal segments usually degenerate first, in a process termed *Wallerian degeneration*, resulting in a dying-back neuropathy and a stocking and glove clinical pattern. Neuronopathies affect either the motor neuron or dorsal root ganglion and result in degeneration of both peripheral and central processes.

Five-Step Approach to Neuropathies

When evaluating neuropathy, the differential diagnosis can be limited by asking five key questions:

- What is the *fiber type* involved (motor, large sensory, small sensory, autonomic, combination)?
- What is the *pattern of distribution* (distal or proximal, symmetric or asymmetric)?
- What is the *temporal course* (acute, chronic, progressive, stepwise, relapsing remitting)?
- Are there any *key features* pointing to a specific etiology?
- What is the *pathology* (axonal, demyelinating)?

FIBER TYPE

The PNS produces symptomatology in only two ways: negative symptoms (weakness, numbness), which reflects loss of nerve signaling; or positive symptoms (tingling, burning) due to inappropriate spontaneous nerve activity. Box 1 lists symptoms and signs that suggest localization to the peripheral nerves and point specifically to motor, sensory, or autonomic involvement. When inquiring about symptoms, it is important to ask the patient to be as specific as possible. Many patients simply describe an area as numb when, in fact, they are experiencing tingling or even weakness.

A detailed motor examination should include inspection for atrophy, particularly in the distal extensor digitorum brevis and first dorsal interosseous muscles, and for fasciculations (visible twitches of muscle), which are best seen using tangential light. Strength should be tested against resistance, as well as with active maneuvers such as walking on the heels and toes to assess distal strength, and rising from a squatting position to examine proximal muscles. Facial muscles should also be tested. When assessing deep tendon reflexes, ensure the reflex is truly absent by asking the patient to concurrently perform a Jendrassic maneuver (pulling against interlocking fingers) or clench the jaw. Note that the reflex arc consists of large-diameter afferent sensory input as well as motor nerve output, so that dysfunction of either can impair reflexes. Tone is sometimes reduced in peripheral nerve diseases.

On sensory examination, sensation should be tested with a pin and a 128-Hz vibratory tuning fork, beginning at the big toe level and moving progressively more proximal. Likewise, position testing should begin distally, with fingers placed on the lateral sides of the big toe and progressively smaller movements tested. Severe loss of position sense can result in athetoid movements of the fingers when the eyes are closed (pseudoathetosis) or a positive Romberg's sign. Temperature can be tested informally by placing a cold tuning fork on the skin. Foot injuries may be apparent with severe sensory loss.

Other important signs include high arches and hammertoe deformities, which suggest a long-standing neuropathy causing differences in muscular force. Demyelinating neuropathies, amyloidosis, and leprosy can cause nerve thickening, which is felt best in the dorsal cutaneous nerve of the foot or the great auricular nerve. Superficial nerves, such as the ulnar nerve at the elbow, can be palpated when appropriate. Postural blood pressure should be assessed for a blood pressure drop more than 20 mm Hg systolic or more than 10 mm Hg diastolic, following 5 minutes of supine rest at a minimum, to test autonomic functioning.

Several other levels of the nervous system can mimic symptoms of PNS disease. Myelopathy and motor neuron disease can manifest with weakness similar to motor neuropathies, although upper motor neuron features such as spasticity and increased reflexes are clues. Myopathies can also cause weakness, but usually more proximal than distal and without any sensory impairment. Isolated sensory involvement should be a red flag that the dorsal root ganglia may be the site of involvement rather than the peripheral nerve, particularly important because neuronopathies have a limited differential.

BOX 1 Signs and Symptoms of Peripheral Nervous System Disease by Fiber Type

Motor
- Cramps
- Fasciculations
- Hyporeflexia
- Hypotonia
- Muscle atrophy
- Myokymia
- Pes cavus
- Weakness

Large Fiber Sensory
- Decreased vibration and position
- Hyporeflexia
- Pins and needles
- Tingling
- Unsteady gait, especially at night or with eyes closed

Small Fiber Sensory
- Burning
- Decreased pain sensation
- Decreased temperature sensation
- Jabbing

Autonomic
- Decreased or increased sweating
- Heat intolerance
- Impotence
- Postural hypotension
- Urinary retention

PATTERN OF DISTRIBUTION

The pattern of distribution should be classified in two ways: symmetric or asymmetric and distal or proximal. Putting this together with the fiber type, six patterns of PNS disorders can be appreciated, with specific differentials (Table 1).

The symmetric distal sensorimotor neuropathy (pattern 1) manifests in a stocking-and-glove distribution and is the most common type of polyneuropathy. Once the level of the upper calves is reached, fibers of the same length in the fingertips begin to be affected. Sensorimotor polyneuropathies that affect both the distal and proximal nerves (pattern 2) should alert the physician to think of inflammatory neuropathies, such as Guillain-Barré syndrome (GBS) and chronic inflammatory demyelinating polyneuropathy (CIDP).

Asymmetric patterns (pattern 3) are often a result of trauma or compression, such as that seen in mononeuropathies, radiculopathies, and plexopathies. A pattern that affects multiple anatomically separated nerves is termed *mononeuritis multiplex* and is usually the result of a more diffuse process, such as diabetes or vasculitis.

Predominant motor neuropathies (pattern 4) are often proximal, such as diabetic amyotrophy. An exception is lead neuropathy, which affects motor fibers in a distal radial and peroneal distribution. Pure sensory neuropathies (pattern 5) are more likely to be distal, with the exception of a rare few such as Tangier disease, which manifests with a bathing-suit pattern. Neuropathies with autonomic impairment have a limited differential (pattern 6).

Additionally, involvement of the cranial nerves is only seen in a few causes of neuropathy. GBS, CIDP, Lyme disease, sarcoidosis, HIV-associated neuropathy, and Tangier disease are examples.

TEMPORAL COURSE

Acute neuropathies are relatively rare and suggest an etiology such as GBS, acute intermittent porphyria, ischemia, toxins (thallium toxicity), drugs, or infections (diphtheric neuropathy). Subacute onset (>8 weeks)

TABLE 1 Causes of Neuropathy by Pattern Type

Causes	Potentially Useful Tests
Sensorimotor	
Symmetric and Distal	
Metabolic disorders	OGTT, LFT, creatinine, TSH, vitamin B$_{12}$
Hereditary disorders (CMT)	EMG/NCS
Infections (HIV, leprosy)	HIV test, review of medical and social history
Toxins (drugs, alcohol, arsenic, thallium)	
Symmetric and Proximal and Distal	
Inflammatory neuropathies (GBS, CIDP)	EMG/NCS, CSF
Asymmetric	
Mononeuropathy, radiculopathy, plexopathy	EMG/NCS
Mononeuritis multiplex Vasculitis	ANA, RF, ESR, ANCA, nerve bx
Diabetes	OGTT
HIV	HIV test
Multifocal CIDP	CSF
Rare: Porphyria, leprosy, HNPP	
Pure Motor	
Proximal	
Diabetic amyotrophy	OGTT
MMNCB	EMG/NCS
Motor variants of GBS, CIDP, MGUS	CSF, SPE, IF
Lymphoma	CBC
Distal	
Rare: Lead toxicity, porphyria	
Pure Sensory	
Neuropathies	
Nonsystemic vasculitis neuropathy	Nerve bx
Chronic gluten enteropathy	Antigliadin antibodies
Vitamin E deficiency	Vitamin E level
Distal, demyelinating, symmetric neuropathy	SPE, IF
Rare: Primary biliary cirrhosis, Crohn's disease	
Neuronopathies	
Paraneoplastic neuronopathy	Anti-Hu/CV2, Imaging
Sjögren's syndrome	Lip biopsy
HIV-related sensory neuronopathy	HIV test
Miller Fisher variant	EMG/NCS
Drugs (see Box 4)	Medication review
Autonomic	
Diabetes	OGTT
GBS	EMG/NCS
Paraneoplastic sensory neuropathy	Anti-Hu, CV2, imaging
HIV-related neuropathy	HIV test
Vincristine (Oncovin)	Medication review
Thiamine deficiency	Alcohol history
Rare: Porphyria, hereditary autonomic neuropathy, amyloidosis	

Abbreviations: ANA = antinuclear antibodies; ANCA = antineutrophilic cytoplasmic antibodies; bx = biopsy; CBC = complete blood count; CIDP = chronic inflammatory demyelinating polyneuropathy; CMT = Charcot-Marie-Tooth disease; CSF = cerebrospinal fluid; EMG/NCS = electromyography/nerve conduction studies; ESR = erythrocyte sedimentation rate; GBS = Guillain-Barré syndrome; HIV = human immunodeficiency virus; HNPP = hereditary neuropathy with liability to pressure palsies; IF = immunofixation; LFT = liver function tests; MGUS = monoclonal gammopathy of unknown significance; MMNCB = multifocal motor neuropathy with conduction blocks; OGTT = oral glucose tolerance test; RF = rheumatoid factor; SPE = serum protein electrophoresis; TSH = thyroid-stimulating hormone.

---

is seen in nutritional deficiencies, metabolic neuropathies, paraneoplastic syndromes, and CIDP. A chronic course is typical of hereditary neuropathies, a stepwise pattern can be seen in mononeuropathy multiplex, and a relapsing-remitting course occurs with intermittent exposure to a toxin or drug and in CIDP.

KEY SIGNS

Sometimes, there is a key classic feature on history or examination that significantly narrows the differential immediately. Box 2 includes a checklist of items for inquiry and observation during assessment of neuropathy.

BOX 2 Key Diagnostic Features

Medical History
- Connective tissue disease
- Diabetes
- Renal disease
- Thyroid disease

Surgical History, Trauma
- Compression neuropathies

Medication History
- Drug-induced neuropathy

Family History, High Arches
- Inherited neuropathy

Nutrition, Alcohol Use
- Alcoholic neuropathy
- Vitamin deficiency

Occupational Exposures
- Toxic neuropathy

History of Weight Loss
- Amyloidosis
- HIV
- Malignancy

Recent Infection, Travel
- Diptheria
- Guillain-Barré syndrome
- HIV
- Leprosy
- Lyme disease

Dry Eyes and Mouth
- Sarcoidosis

Severe Pain
- Amyloidosis
- Diabetes
- Guillain-Barré syndrome
- HIV
- Vasculitis

Skin Lesions
- Anaesthetic patches (leprosy)
- Bullous lesions (porphyria)
- Hyperpigmentation (osteosclerotic myeloma)
- Mee's lines (arsenic or thallium poisoning)
- Orange tonsils (Tangier disease)
- Angiokeratomas (Fabry's disease)

PATHOLOGY AND THE ROLE OF NEUROPHYSIOLOGY

Nerve conduction studies (NCSs) and electromyography (EMG) are highly specialized tests that are performed principally by neurologists. NCSs electrically activate peripheral nerves at particular sites and then assess for abnormal transmission from the stimulation point to the final muscle response. EMG involves placing a small needle into the muscle to observe both the sound and appearance of the muscle at rest and with motor units firing. Because NCSs can only be performed at points where the nerve is superficial (most often distal), EMG is needed to assess for more proximal damage such as radiculopathy. EMG can also rule out other mimics of PNS disease, such as myopathy.

For the general physician, the most important thing is being able to interpret the results of these tests. Often, a report will be received back such as: "There is evidence of a symmetric distal axonal sensorimotor neuropathy." An NCS/EMG study should be able to specify the distribution and if motor or sensory fibers are involved. Autonomic and small sensory fibers are not tested well by EMG, so the diagnosis of these types of neuropathies is often clinical or requires more specialized testing. Thus, a normal NCS/EMG does not rule out neuropathy.

A further feature that electrophysiology can add is whether the pathology is demyelinating or axonal. Demyelination is characterized by slowed conduction velocity, temporal dispersion of the muscle action potential, and conduction block. Hereditary demyelinating neuropathies, such as Charcot-Marie-Tooth disease, do not show the latter two features, which are only seen in acquired neuropathies. Axonal disease is characterized by modest slowing of velocities, and more marked reduction in the amplitudes of the muscle and sensory action potentials. On EMG, there are fibrillations within 3 weeks of the neuropathic injury, indicating spontaneous firing of denervated muscle. Enlarged and prolonged motor unit potentials indicate subsequent regeneration, which occurs after several weeks to months.

Demyelination has a limited differential (Box 3), and often a better prognosis, because myelin can start to regenerate within a few days. Axonal regeneration proceeds at a far slower rate of 1 to 3 μm/day, and nerves with proximal lesions must go a long distance to reinnervate their muscle and might never reach their goal.

Investigations

Once the neuropathy has been subclassified, investigations for the specific causes in that pattern class should be undertaken (see Table 1). Several recent papers suggest that 2-hour oral glucose tolerance testing (OGTT) is the best test for glucose intolerance due to the relatively low sensitivity of serum glucose levels and glycosylated hemoglobin (HbA1c). Likewise, vitamin B_{12} levels have a low sensitivity, and serum metabolites methylmalonic acid (MMA) and homocysteine (Hcy) should be measured in patients with a result less than 300 pg/mL to improve diagnostic accuracy. These metabolites can be falsely increased with hypovolemia, renal insufficiency, hypothyroidism, and increased age, but a return to normal levels 1 to 2 weeks after beginning replacement therapy indicates this is the cause. The combination of elevated gastrin and anti–parietal cell antibodies may be used to diagnose pernicious anemia. The yield of general testing for other vitamin deficiencies in polyneuropathy is relatively low.

Antinuclear antibodies (ANA) probably are usually only significant in the context of suggestive features (abrupt onset, mononeuropathy multiplex pattern, arthralgia or arthritis, fevers, rash, or renal abnormalities) because they are positive in about 3% of normal patients. However, referral to a rheumatologist should be considered with a very high titer (>1:1280).

The erythryocyte sedimentation rate (ESR) is often elevated, especially in older patients. Rates greater than 70 mm/hour tend to be more meaningful, particularly with a mononeuritis multiplex pattern.

Serum protein electrophoresis lacks sensitivity, and immunofixation should be ordered if there is high suspicion of a paraproteinemia. If an elevated monoclonal antibody is found, a 24-hour urine test for Bence Jones proteinuria, skeletal survey, CBC, renal function tests, and serum calcium should be ordered. If the M protein is greater than 2.5 g/dL or if abnormalities are detected on these tests, referral to a hematologist for bone marrow aspiration is required. Polyclonal antibodies are not associated with neuropathy.

If there is suspicion of amyloidosis, a rectal, abdominal fat, or sensory nerve biopsy can be undertaken. Sural nerve biopsy is reserved for difficult diagnostic situations because it causes a permanent area of numbness with possible dysesthesias over the biopsied area. Suspicion of vasculitis is the most common indication, but pathology can also be seen in leprosy and with tumor infiltrate.

In approximately 20% of patients, an underlying cause of neuropathy is not found. These patients are said to have a cryptogenic sensory or sensorimotor neuropathy. A distinct clinical picture has emerged, most commonly of a patient in the sixth or seventh decade, manifesting with distal dysesthesias and possibly with mild weakness and sensory ataxia. These patients tend not to develop significant disability, and treatment is mainly for neuropathic pain.

CURRENT DIAGNOSIS

- The five-step approach to classify neuropathies based on fiber type, pattern of distribution, temporal course, pathology, and key features allows a tailored diagnostic evaluation.
- Electrodiagnostic testing provides a useful adjunct to the clinical evaluation.
- The cause of neuropathy might not be found in 20% of patients, but there are treatments for several known etiologies, as well as specific medications to treat neuropathic pain.

BOX 3 Demyelinating Neuropathies

- Charcot-Marie-Tooth disease
- Hereditary neuropathy with liability to pressure palsies
- Inflammatory neuropathies
- Monoclonal gammopathies and paraproteinemias
- Multifocal motor neuropathy with conduction block
- Neuropathies caused by drugs such as amiodarone (Cordarone) and suramin[2]
- Neuropathies caused by infections (diptheria) or toxins (arsenic)

[2]Not available in the United States.

Treatment

MONONEUROPATHIES

The most common cause of mononeuropathy is nerve compression, and surgical treatment is often a consideration for these patients. The four most common locations are median neuropathy at the wrist (carpal tunnel syndrome), ulnar neuropathy at the elbow, peroneal neuropathy at the fibular head, and facial nerve palsy (Bell's palsy).

Carpal tunnel syndrome manifests with pain and numbness principally in the first three digits, although it is often poorly localized. Classic features include pain at night and shaking out the hand to relieve pain. For milder symptoms, a nighttime splint, which prevents wrist flexion and high pressure in the carpal tunnel, is often helpful.

Local corticosteroid injections can provide relief, and surgical decompression has a very high success rate.

Ulnar neuropathy manifests with numbness of the fourth and fifth digits and wasting of the interosseous muscles, often with pain localized to the elbow. Peroneal neuropathies manifest with foot drop and numbness on the dorsum of the foot. In both cases, avoidance of pressure over the nerve often leads to improvement. Surgery might improve symptoms, but less reliably so than carpal tunnel surgery.

Bell's palsy is an inflammatory rather than compressive process, presumably due to a viral etiology. Treatment is controversial, but early (within 14 days) use of prednisone[1] 60 mg daily, decreasing by 10 mg steps every 2 days, along with acyclovir (Zovirax)[1] 800 mg five times daily for 7 days has been advocated. About 15% of patients have residual facial weakness.

GUILLAIN-BARRÉ SYNDROME

GBS often begins following gastroenteritis with *Campylobacter jejuni*, or an upper respiratory tract infection, due to a presumed autoimmune response directed against myelin. The incidence is 1 or 2 per 100,000 persons per year. Characteristic features are ascending weakness, areflexia, and sensory and autonomic symptoms progressing over a few days up to 4 weeks. Facial diplegia and pain can occur. Electrophysiology shows acute demyelination with conduction blocks, and cerebrospinal fluid (CSF) reveals an increase in protein with a cell count of less than 5 white blood cells (cytoalbuminologic dissociation) in more than 80% of patients after 2 weeks. A CSF pleocytosis of more than 10 lymphocytes/mm^3 should alert the physician to another cause such as sarcoidosis, Lyme disease, or early HIV.

The Miller-Fisher variant is characterized by specific clinical features of sensory ataxia, areflexia, and ophthalmolplegia. *C. jejuni* infection has been correlated with more severe variants, such as acute motor axonal neuropathy (AMAN) and acute motor and sensory axonal neuropathy (AMSAM), which damage axons in addition to myelin. *C. jejuni*–related GBS correlates with anti-GM1 antibodies, although they are not prognostic or specific. Recovery can take months to years. Only 20% of patients are left without residual deficit. About 5% to 10% have significant persistent disability, and the mortality rate is 5%.

During early treatment, patients might require admission to intensive care, with close monitoring of pulmonary function tests for respiratory compromise. Diaphragmatic weakness correlates with neck flexion and extension and shoulder abduction. The patient should be intubated when the forced vital capacity (FVC) declines to less than 15 mL/kg or when negative inspiratory flow (NIF) is less than −20 to −30. Monitoring of the cardiac rhythm is important due to dysautonomia.

The preferred treatment is intravenous immunoglobulin (IVIg)[1] at a dose of 0.4 g/kg/day for 5 days. This is generally well tolerated, and adverse side effects such as myalgia, headache, or flu-like symptoms often resolve with a reduced infusion rate. If IVIg is contraindicated (renal failure, IgA deficiency), plasmapheresis can be initiated with four alternate-day exchanges over 7 to 10 days for a total of 200 to 250 mL/kg. Both plasmapheresis and IVIg continue to work for several weeks after the treatment period, but if patients experience a secondary worsening after successful treatment, a second dose may be initiated. Steroids were reviewed recently by a Cochrane systematic review and were not found to be of benefit in GBS.

CHRONIC INFLAMMATORY DEMYELINATING POLYNEUROPATHY

This neuropathy is pathologically similar to GBS, but progression is longer than 8 weeks, often with a relapsing-remitting course. Symmetric distal and proximal weakness and sensory impairment, hyporeflexia, and cytoalbumingergic dissociation in the CSF is the classic presentation, although there are variants.

Treatment is either IVIg[1] or prednisone. IVIg is given initially at 0.4 g/kg/day for 5 days, then the dose and frequency are reduced over time. Prednisone is given 1 mg/kg/day until improvement, followed by a slow tapering of 5 mg every 2 to 3 weeks over a period of months. Response is usually seen within 4 weeks. Refractory patients have been treated with repeated plasmapheresis treatments or immunosuppressive therapy with cyclosporine (Sandimmune).[1]

MULTIFOCAL MOTOR NEUROPATHY

Multifocal motor neuropathy (MMN) is not a common disorder but is important not to mistake for motor neuron disease because it has a very different prognosis and treatment. Patients present with progressive asymmetric distal weakness, often of the arm, without sensory loss and with less atrophy than would be expected for the degree of weakness. Unlike motor neuron disease, there are no upper motor neuron signs. It is different from multifocal acquired demyelinating sensory and motor neuropathy (MADSAM), an asymmetric variant of CIDP, in that loss of reflexes and weakness involves only the affected limb, there is a relatively normal CSF protein concentration, and sensory nerve conduction studies are normal. Diagnosis is supported by finding conduction blocks in sites not usually associated with compression. The GM1 antibody is elevated in 60% of cases. Repeated treatments with IVIg[1] or cyclophosphamide (Cytoxan)[1] are common choices. Rituximab (Rituxan),[1] a monoclonal antibody, has also been used. Prednisone classically worsens the condition.

DIABETIC NEUROPATHY

Diabetes is one of the most common causes of neuropathy. Patients can present with a symmetric distal neuropathy, autonomic proximal diabetic neuropathy, mononeuritis multiplex, compressive and cranial neuropathies, and trunk polyradiculopathies.

The distal symmetric sensory polyneuropathy (DSPN) correlates with the duration of the diabetes, control of hyperglycemia, and presence of retinopathy and nephropathy. The exact etiology is unknown, but theories include a metabolic process involving aldose reductase, ischemic damage, or an immunologic disorder. Typical symptoms include lancinating pains or burning, worse at night, and possible dysautonomia. Atrophy may be noted in the foot muscles, but severe weakness is atypical. NCS may be normal because small fibers are primarily affected. Treatment includes blood sugar control to limit progression and symptom control for neuropathic pain. Gabapentin (Neurontin)[1] and tricyclic antidepressants are common choices (see later). Drugs such as QR-333, a topical compound that contains quercetin, a flavonoid with aldose reductase–inhibitor effects, are being investigated specifically for diabetic neuropathy.

Autonomic neuropathy is treated symptomatically, with fludrocortisone (Florinef)[1] 0.1 mg/day for orthostatic hypotension, metoclopramide (Reglan) 10 mg before meals for gastroparesis, and sildenafil (Viagra) 25 mg 1 hour before sexual intercourse for impotence.

Proximal diabetic neuropathy (diabetic amyotrophy) manifests typically with unilateral pain in the anterior thigh followed by stepwise progression over weeks to months of quadriceps weakness, atrophy of the proximal leg muscles, and a reduced knee reflex, with occasional contralateral leg involvement. The erythrocyte sedimentation rate (ESR) may be elevated and CSF protein mildly increased (120 mg/dL on average). NCS and EMG reflect multifocal active axonal damage (fibrillations) to the lumbar plexus and roots. Small retrospective studies have reported that IVIg[1] and other forms of immunosuppressive therapy are effective in treating patients with proximal diabetic neuropathy. A short course of corticosteroids (prednisone[1] 50 mg/day for 1 week, then tapering by 10 mg/week) can be used to ease pain in severe cases, with close monitoring of the glucose level, but overall prognosis is quite good, ranging from 1 to

---

[1]Not FDA approved for this indication.

18 months of recovery phase (mean of 6 months) and partial or complete restoration of strength in approximately 70% of patients.

PARAPROTEINEMIC NEUROPATHIES

Multiple myeloma, Waldenström's macroglobulinemia, cryoglobulinemia, osteosclerotic myeloma (POEMS syndrome), and monoclonal gammopathy of unknown significance (MGUS) are associated with monoclonal antibodies directed at PNS components, such as myelin-associated glycoprotein (MAG). Neuropathies associated with an immunoglobulin (Ig)M monoclonal protein (approximately 60%) are typically distal, demyelinating, and symmetric, whereas IgG (30%) and IgA (10%) gammopathies can be axonal or demyelinating. In terms of treatment, the distal demyelinating neuropathy of IgM paraproteinemias tends to be treatment refractory. IgG and IgA gammopathies can mimic the demyelination pattern seen in CIDP, and patients with any antibody and this pattern should receive immunotherapy as recommended for CIDP (see earlier). Axonal neuropathies and IgM, IgG, or IgA gammopathies have a less clear relationship and are typically not responsive to treatment.

HEREDITARY NEUROPATHIES

Charcot-Marie-Tooth (CMT) disease is among the most common of genetic neuromuscular disorders, and more than 30 genes have been identified. Clues are a history of difficulty running in childhood, high arches, hammertoes, ankle weakness, and nerve hypertrophy developing in teenage years. Depending on the subtype, the neuropathy may be axonal or demyelinating, but the most common type (CMT-1) is caused by an autosomal dominant gene encoding peripheral myelin protein 22 and is easily diagnosed by the relatively uniform slowing on nerve conduction velocities (<25% of lower limits of normal). Patients have a mild course and remain ambulatory throughout life in most cases.

Hereditary neuropathy with liability to pressure palsies (HNPP) is another dominantly inherited neuropathy in which patients have recurrent episodes of isolated mononeuropathies, typically affecting, in order of decreasing frequency, the common peroneal, ulnar, radial, and median nerves. Most attacks are sudden onset, painless, and followed by complete recovery. There is no treatment other than preventive measures.

TOXIC AND NUTRITIONAL NEUROPATHIES

Treatment of toxic and nutritional neuropathies involves detection and removal of the underlying cause. A thorough review of medications, occupational exposures, and nutritional risk factors is essential (Box 4). Drug toxicity is much more common than environmental toxicity. Incidence of neuropathy does not always correlate with the dosage and duration of exposure. For instance, amiodarone neuropathy has been reported with dosages as low as 200 mg/day and durations as short as 1 month. Symptoms might not improve, or might even worsen, for several weeks after the drug is stopped before improvement starts, a phenomenon known as *coasting*.

Cisplatin can cause a neuropathy that overlaps in symptomatology with paraneoplastic sensory neuronopathy, and dapsone is associated with a motor axonopathy. Gold neuropathy can have prominent myokymia and can mimic GBS.

Specific treatments for drug-induced neuropathies include cyanocobalamin (vitamin B_{12})[1] for nitrous oxide neuropathy and pyridoxine (vitamin B_6)[1] for hydralazine and isoniazid neuropathies. Excessive vitamin B_6 can also *cause* a neuropathy. Glutamine[7] and vitamin E[1] 300 mg twice a day has shown promise for paclitaxel neuropathy, and neuroprotective agents such as nerve growth factor are being investigated for cisplatin-induced neuropathy. Tacrolimus can cause a CIDP-like neuropathy that responds to IVIg[1] or plasmapheresis.

---

[1]Not FDA approved for this indication.
[7]Available as a dietary supplement.

One of the most common nutritional neuropathies is caused by thiamine deficiency and is associated with alcohol consumption of at least 100 g per day. Patients present with burning feet, and early alcohol abstinence and treatment with thiamine denotes better chance of recovery. Vitamin B_{12} deficiency is vital not to miss and can manifest with a subacute combined degeneration, whereby patients have a superimposed myelopathy and neuropathy (spasticity but reduced reflexes). Sudden-onset symptoms, particularly in the feet and hands simultaneously, are also suggestive.

BOX 4 Causes of Toxic and Nutritional Neuropathies

Drug Toxins

Axonal
- Colchicine
- Dapsone
- Disulfiram
- Ethambutol
- Hyralazine
- Isoniazid
- Metronidazole
- Nitrofurantoin
- Nitrous oxide
- Nucleosides
- Paclitaxel
- Phenytoin
- Tacrolimus
- Vincristine

Demyelinating
- Amiodarone (Cordarone)
- Chloroquine (Aralen)
- Gold
- Suramin[2]

Neuronopathy
- Cisplatin (Platinol-AQ)
- Pyridoxine (vitamin B_6)
- Thalidomide (Thalomid)

Environmental Toxins
- Acrylamide (plastics)
- Allyl chloride (insecticides)
- Arsenic
- Carbon disulfide (cellophanes)
- Ethylene glycol (antifreeze)
- Ethylene oxide (sterilizer)
- Hexacarbons (glue)
- Lead
- Mercury
- Methyl bromide (fumigant)
- Organophosphates (insecticides)
- Thallium (pesticides)
- Trichloroethylene (drycleaning)
- Vacor (rodenticide)

Vitamin Deficiencies
- B_1 (alcoholism)
- B_3 (alcoholism)
- B_6 (isoniazid use)
- B_{12} (vegans, pernicious anemia)
- E (cholestasis and abetalipoproteinemia)

---

[2]Not available in the United States.

TABLE 2 Select Neuropathic Pain Medications

Drug	Dosage	Side Effects
Amitriptyline (Elavil)[1]	10 mg/d, increasing weekly by 10 mg, up to 150 mg/d	Dry mouth, sedation, urinary retention, cardiac arrhythmias, orthostatic hypotension, constipation, weight gain Contraindications: cardiac arrhythmias, CHF, recent MI, narrow angle glaucoma, urinary retention
Capsaicin (Zostrix)	0.075% cream applied tid to qid	Sneezing, coughing, rash, skin irritation
Carbamazepine (Tegretol)[1]	100 mg bid, increasing by 100 mg weekly Max: 1200 mg/d	Somnolence, dizziness, nausea, gait changes, urticaria, hyponatremia, pancytopenia, hepatic dysfunction Obtain baseline and 6-wk CBC and LFT
Gabapentin (Neurontin)[1]	300 mg on d 1, 600 mg on d 2, 900 mg on day 3 Max: 3600 mg/d.	Sedation, fatigue, dizziness, confusion, tremor, weight gain, peripheral edema, headache Reduce dose in renal insufficiency
Lamotrigine (Lamictal)[1]	25 mg at night for 2 wk, increasing weekly by 25-50 mg Max: 400 mg/d	Severe rash (especially if increased too quickly), dizziness, unsteadiness, drowsiness, diplopia
Tramadol (Ultram)	50 mg bid Titrate 50 mg every 3-7 d, using a tid or qid schedule Max: 100 mg qid	Constipation, headache, nausea Risk of seizures with neuroleptics and antidepressants Reduce dose with hepatic or renal dysfunction

[1]Not FDA approved for this indication.
Abbreviations: CBC = complete blood count; CHF = congestive heart failure; LFT = liver function test; max = maximum; MI = myocardial infarction.

METABOLIC AND INFECTIOUS NEUROPATHIES

Peripheral neuropathy can complicate renal failure, hypothyroidism, biliary cirrhosis, porphyria, Tangier disease, Fabry's disease, and mitochondrial diseases.

Early in the course, HIV can manifest as a GBS-like syndrome, although with CSF pleocytosis. This typically responds to IVIg[1] and plasmapheresis. In later stages, patients might develop a distal symmetric polyneuropathy, although it is important to determine if this might be due to nucleoside reverse transcriptase inhibitors, nutritional deficiency, or infection. Cranial neuropathies, sensory neuronopathy, lumbosacral polyradiculopathies, and mononeuritis multiplex also occur.

Leprosy is the most common treatable neuropathy worldwide. Tuberculoid leprosy leads to hypopigmented patches with loss of pain and temperature sensation. Lepromatous leprosy, a more severe form seen in immunosuppressed persons, can cause ulnar, common peroneal, and facial neuropathies. Treatment involves a long-term multidrug regimen of dapsone and rifampin (Rifadin).[1]

Herpes zoster can cause a postherpetic neuralgia, defined as pain persisting for more than 6 weeks after the rash appears. Early treatment with acyclovir (Zovirax) (800 mg five times daily for 7 days) can reduce the duration of the acute phase. Chronic discomfort is treated with medications for neuropathic pain (see later).

Lyme disease, caused by *Borrelia burgdorferi*, begins with erythema migrans, followed by multifocal peripheral and cranial neuropathies, particularly facial diplegia. CSF lymphocytic pleocytosis plus serologic demonstration of *B. burgdorferi* infection on serum or CSF are the diagnostic features. Early stages are treated with a 3-week course of doxycycline[1] 100 mg twice daily, and intravenous penicillin G[1] should be given in the late stages.

CARCINOMATOUS NEUROPATHY

Tumors can cause neuropathy by compression, metastatic spread, paraneoplastic antibodies, hemorrhage, and treatment with chemotherapy or radiation therapy. A distal sensorimotor neuropathy is associated with many different tumors and seldom precedes tumor diagnosis. Pathogenesis can include toxic, nutritional, and immunologic causes. A sensory neuronopathy is less common, but often precedes tumor diagnosis, thus warranting a careful work-up. Lung, breast, ovary, and gastrointestinal tract cancers are the most likely associated types. Imaging and paraneoplastic antibodies (particularly anti-Hu and anti-CV2, most commonly associated with lung cancer) may help in making the diagnosis. Treatment focuses on the underlying neoplasm.

VASCULITIC NEUROPATHY

Vasculitis can be primary (polyarteritis nodosa, Wegener's granulomatosis, Churg-Strauss syndrome, microscopic polyangitis) or secondary (connective tissue diseases, systemic infections, drug reactions). It classically manifests with a painful mononeuritis multiplex with asymmetric patchy features, reflecting multifocal ischemic damage. If the patient's vasculitis is restricted to the PNS, serologic testing for these disorders is often negative. In this case, a sural nerve biopsy might reveal fibrinoid necrosis and perivascular inflammation.

Treatment needs to be carefully undertaken with intravenous methylprednisolone (Solu-Medrol)[1] for 3 days followed by oral prednisone. In many cases, other immunosuppressive drugs are eventually used.

Neuropathic Pain

Often pain is the most predominant and distressing feature of neuropathy. Several classes of medications can be tried (Table 2), although it is important to counsel the patient that complete abolition of pain is unlikely. A trial period should be for at least 6 to 8 weeks before concluding that the patient does not respond. A combination of agents with different mechanisms can have an advantage over monotherapy for the nonresponsive patient.

First-line treatment is generally with tricyclic antidepressants. Serotonin and noradrenaline reuptake inhibitors such as amitriptyline[1] (Elavil), imipramine[1] (Tofranil), and clomipramine[1] (Anafranil) may be marginally more effective than those with relatively selective noradrenergic effects such as desipramine and nortriptyline. However, nortriptyline and desipramine are less sedating. Selective serotonin reuptake inhibitors appear to be less effective. Second-line antidepressants include venlafaxine[1] (Effexor), bupropion[1] (Wellbutrin), and the recently approved duloxetine (Cymbalta), which have the advantage of better tolerability due to less muscarinic, histaminergic, and α-adrenergic affinity.

The typical next class of medications to try is the antiepileptics. Gabapentin[1] is a common choice and is generally well tolerated. Pregabalin (Lyrica) is a newer related agent that, unlike gabapentin, exhibits linear pharmacokinetics and can be initiated at a therapeutic

---
[1]Not FDA approved for this indication.

dose without a long titration. Second-line choices include lamotrigine[1] (Lamictal), carbamazepine[1] (Tegretol), and topiramate[1] (Topamax). Valproate[1] (Depacon) and zonisamide[1] (Zonegran) have limited evidence, and phenytoin[1] (Dilantin) can cause neuropathy. Oxcarbazepine[1] (Trileptal), like carbamazepine, slows the recovery rate of voltage-activated sodium channels, but it also inhibits high-threshold N-type and P/Q-type calcium channels and reduces glutamatergic transmission. As a result, it can modulate both peripheral and central neuropathic pain pathways, and several studies into its efficacy are under way.

Topical creams, such as capsaicin (Zostrix), an extract of chili, can be tried. Capsaicin works by depleting substance P and can temporarily worsen pain by causing a burning sensation. Lidocaine[1] (Xylocaine) can be also used topically.

Other agents for severe neuropathies include opioid agents, such as tramadol (Ultram), which has low-affinity binding for μ-opioid receptors coupled with mild inhibition of norepinephrine and serotonin reuptake. Slow-release opioids, such as oxycodone (OxyContin) 30 to 60 mg/day, can help, and risk of addiction is low in this population. Glutamate antagonists, such as dextromethorphan[1] (Delsym), have shown benefit in some studies, as has mexiletine[1] (Mexitil), a class IB antiarrhythmic agent and oral analogue of lidocaine. Nonpharmacologic therapies, such as transcutaneous electrical nerve stimulation (TENS) and acupuncture, might also provide adjunctive relief.

---

[1]Not FDA approved for this indication.

REFERENCES

Donofrio PD, Albers JW: AAEM minimonograph 34: Polyneuropathy: Classification by nerve conduction studies and electromyography. Muscle Nerve 1990;13:889-903.

Dworkin RH, Backonja M, Rowbotham MC, et al: Advances in neuropathic pain: Diagnosis, mechanisms, and treatment recommendations. Arch Neurol 2003;60:1524-1534.

Grant I, Benstead TJ: Differential Diagnosis of Peripheral Neuropathy. In Dyck PJ, Thomas PK (eds): Peripheral Neuropathy. Philadelphia: Saunders, 2005.

Poncelet AN: An algorithm for the evaluation of peripheral neuropathy. Am Fam Physician 1997;57(4):755-764.

Stewart JD: Focal peripheral neuropathies. New York: Raven, 1993.

Management of Head Injuries

Method of
Todd W. Vitaz, MD

Traumatic brain injury (TBI) most commonly results from motor vehicle crashes (MVC) and typically affects males in the 2nd through 4th decades of life. These sudden random acts can have long-lasting effects on the patient and family, but these events also impact society as a whole when a young, viable working-age individual becomes suddenly disabled and dependent on the care of others. TBI has no regard for age or gender, however, and can be seen in infants as a result of nonaccidental trauma as well as in geriatric patients following falls. The management of these patients can become extremely complicated and often requires the close interaction of numerous different health care providers ranging from trauma, orthopedic, and neurologic surgeons to nurses, social workers, speech, occupational, and physical therapists. Unfortunately, current interventions are still limited to the avoidance or minimization of secondary injury and rehabilitative intervention. However, when these patients are managed with aggressive, comprehensive, multidisciplinary approaches, the outcomes at times can be rewarding.

TBI can be categorized based on numerous factors. Most commonly it is differentiated based on mechanism and injury type (closed versus penetrating), whether it has occurred with or without systemic injuries (isolated versus multisystem), and the severity (mild, moderate, severe). The Glasgow Coma Scale (GCS) (Table 1), which was initially developed as a prognostic indicator following closed head injury, has become the principal triage tool for evaluating these patients. Patients are scored based on their best response in each of the three categories (eye opening, verbal responses, and motor score) and then subdivided into mild (13 to 15), moderate (9 to 12), and severe (3 to 8). One caveat to this assessment tool is that it can be affected by numerous alterations: hypoxia, hypotension, hypothermia, intoxication, infection, and other metabolic derangements, which are commonly seen in the trauma population.

TABLE 1 Glasgow Coma Scale

Best Motor Score	Best Verbal Response	Best Eye Opening
6 Obeys commands	5 Normal speech	4 Spontaneous
5 Localizes to pain	4 Confused	3 To voice
4 Withdraws to pain	3 Inappropriate words	2 To pain
3 Flexor posturing	2 Incomprehensible sounds	1 No eye opening
2 Extensor posturing	1 No verbal response	
1 No motor reponse	Intubated patients receive a 1 with the suffix T added to score	

Pathology

Another common classification system following TBI is based on pathophysiologic findings. Concussion commonly occurs following mild or moderate TBI as the result of transient (typically seconds to minutes) neurologic dysfunction in the setting of a normal computed tomography (CT) scan. Brief loss of consciousness, commonly with amnesia regarding the event, is not uncommon and is often associated with nausea, vomiting, headache, dizziness, and transient visual obscuration. These symptoms may persist for several hours to weeks as part of the *postconcussive syndrome* and, in rare instances, especially following repetitive injury, these alterations may become long-lasting. As a result of these persistent problems, in addition to a better understanding of the neurocognitive effects following this type of injury, there has been an enormous emphasis placed on their prevention (see text following).

Skull fractures may occur in isolation or be associated with other types of brain injuries. They are commonly classified based on whether they are open (overlying laceration) or closed, linear or comminuted, nondepressed or depressed. Skull fractures occur either as the result of a large force directed to a small area (i.e., depressed skull fracture following a blow to the head with a golf club) or when larger forces are dissipated throughout the skull resulting in fracture through the weakest area (linear fractures through frontal skull base, petrous, or squamous temporal bone). Linear fractures are commonly associated with raccoon eyes (frontal skull base fractures), Battle's sign (posterior skull base fracture), cerebrospinal fluid leak (otorrhea or rhinorrhea) or olfactory, facial or acoustic nerve injury (amnesia, facial palsy, sensorineuronal deafness).

In addition, temporal bone fractures may also be associated with epidural hematomas (EDHs). These extra-axial blood clots are most commonly caused by laceration of the middle meningeal artery and result in accumulation of *high-pressure arterial bleeding* in the potential space between the dura and skull. EDHs are more commonly seen in younger individuals probably because of the decreased skull thickness and lack of adhesions between the skull and dura mater in this population. Commonly, these lesions appear on CT scan as lens-shaped, extra-axial hematomas most often in the temporal region and can be rapidly expansive secondary to the high-pressure arterial bleeding. The clinical course in these patients is classically described by a brief loss of consciousness from the initial concussion, followed by a "lucid interval" in which the patient may be awake and alert, which then gives way to another episode of decreased mental status that may be rapidly progressive and associated with signs of brain stem compression (flexor or extensor posturing, dilated nonreactive pupil). EDHs are usually treated surgically unless they are extremely small and constitute one of the few true neurosurgical emergencies where mere minutes may make an enormous difference in the patient's outcome.

Unlike EDHs, subdural hematomas (SDHs) are often associated with other types of brain injury and thus typically involve an altered level of consciousness (LOC) from the onset. SDHs are typically caused by bleeding from bridging veins that get torn when the brain moves within its cerebrospinal fluid (CSF) buffer while the veins remain tethered at their dural insertions; however, other causes such as venous or arterial hemorrhage from a brain laceration also exist. CT scanning reveals that these lesions commonly appear more crescent-shaped but never cross the dural boundaries (falx or tentorium). Unlike the high-pressure EDHs, SDHs typically expand at a slower rate but still cause devastating neurologic dysfunction from compression of the underlying brain. In addition mortality rates tend to be higher with worse outcome for SDH as a result of the common underlying brain injury. Once again these extra-axial clots frequently require surgical evacuation unless they are small and fail to have substantial compression on the underlying brain, where they are managed with serial imaging and close neurologic observation. In patients for whom a small SDH is not treated surgically, the physician must remain cognizant of the fact that a small proportion of these will increase in size between 1 and 4 weeks following the trauma and can be a cause of delayed deterioration or increased headache and new neurologic findings.

Intraparenchymal hematomas occur quite commonly following TBI and can be either hemorrhagic or nonhemorrhagic. These lesions range in size from 1 to 2 mm, up to several centimeters, and can cause a full range of symptoms and neurologic findings based on their location, size, and degree of compression on surrounding structures. Just like extra-axial hematomas, these lesions may increase in size and commonly coalesce or mature and *blossom* during the first 12 to 24 hours following the trauma. In addition, larger hematomas incite an inflammatory reaction in the surrounding brain resulting in increased edema around the lesion, which may result in increases in the intracranial pressure (ICP) (commonly seen on postinjury days [PIDs] 3 to 7). Management of these lesions depends on their size, location, and associated findings and ranges from serial observation and repeat imaging, surgical evacuation of the hematoma, or decompressive craniectomy with or without lobectomy.

The final category of pathologic abnormalities following TBI occurs as the result of shear injury to the axons themselves, called diffuse axonal injury (DAI). This is caused by either acceleration and deceleration or rotational forces to the axons resulting in micro- or macroscopic areas of injury and axonal transection. Most commonly this is encountered in the setting where a patient clinically has signs of a severe TBI, often with a GCS score less than 6; however, the CT scan is either unimpressive or shows only small areas of petechial hemorrhage. In addition ICP recording typically shows normal or only slightly elevated values. Magnetic resonance imaging (MRI) is commonly used in this subset of patients and can be used as a predictive indicator for determining the severity of injury, especially if CT is negative. MRI commonly shows areas of increased intensity on fluid attenuation inversion recovery (FLAIR) and T2-weighted sequences in the brainstem, diencephalon, deep white matter tracts, or corpus callosum. Recovery following this type of injury is variable and depends more on the injury location (reticular activating system of brainstem versus supratentorial white matter tracts) rather than the injury volume.

In addition to these abnormalities, patients with TBI are also at risk for damage to the spinal cord and vertebral and carotid arteries. Thus, patients with altered LOC should be assumed to have spinal instability and possible spinal cord injury (SCI); they should remain immobilized until the absence of these can be confirmed. The incidence of carotid and vertebral artery injury associated with severe TBI is unknown, but patients with facial or cervical fractures and those with soft tissue neck or chest injury (seat belt sign) have been found to be at higher risk. The appropriate screening for and treatment of these injuries have become a topic of intense debate in recent years but should be suspected in a patient with focal neurologic findings without identifiable cause on other imaging.

INTRACRANIAL PRESSURE AND THE MONROE-KELLIE DOCTRINE

Regardless of the pathophysiologic type of injury, the end result commonly is the generation of increases in the ICP, which can then lead to secondary brain injury. ICP dynamics are easily understood if one considers the principles of the volume pressure relationships outlined by the Monroe-Kellie doctrine. The basis of this principle resides on the fact that the skull is a fixed and rigid volume; because of this any changes to the volume of its contents will directly affect the pressure within this rigid space. In simplest terms the intracranial cavity contains blood, water, and tissue. Blood may be intravascular (IV) or extravascular (EV) in the case of extra-axial blood clots; water includes not only cerebrospinal fluid, which may build up in cases of hydrocephalus, but also edema following traumatic injuries; brain parenchyma typically compromises the tissue component but in select instances tumors or cysts may also fall into this category.

As increases in any or all three of these categories occur, the pressure inside the cranial cavity increases proportionally. At first compensatory changes occur, which accommodate for these increases, resulting in only mild pressure changes; however, eventually a critical volume is reached where the compensatory mechanisms are saturated, resulting in rapid and dramatic pressure changes. The following scenario illustrates these principles. A patient is involved in a motor vehicle crash and suffers a head injury with a small epidural hematoma. Initially he is awake and alert without any focal neurologic findings. The epidural hematoma creates an increase in the EV blood component of the Monroe-Kellie doctrine; however, compensatory changes in intracranial CSF volume result in decreases in the water component, thus preventing significant changes in ICP. However, the hematoma continues to enlarge, causing increases in ICP exhibited clinically by slow deterioration in the patient's level of consciousness. The patient is now intubated and mildly hyperventilated causing vasoconstriction, therefore decreasing the intravascular blood component and reducing ICP with an improvement in the patient's neurologic condition. Unfortunately, as the operating room (OR) is being prepared, the patient suffers a rapid decrease in his level of conscious, becoming unresponsive with flexor posturing and a nonreactive pupil. Although the hematoma has expanded at a constant rate over time, the rapid change in the patient's condition

---

CURRENT DIAGNOSIS

Classification of Head Injuries

- Closed versus penetrating
- Isolated versus multisystem injuries
- Severity
    - Mild (GCS 13-15)
    - Moderate (GCS 9-12)
    - Severe (GCS 3-8)

Pathologic Findings with Closed Head Injuries

- Skull fractures
- Epidural hematomas
- Subdural hematomas
- Parenchymal contusions
- Intraparenchymal hematomas
- Diffuse axonal injury

is the result of him reaching the critical point where all compensatory mechanisms have been exhausted, thus causing profound rapid changes in the patient's ICP.

Treatment of Elevated Intracranial Pressure

Acute changes in ICP result in altered LOC, and at times other localizing neurologic findings such as *blown* (dilated, nonreactive) pupils and flexor or extensor posturing, and such findings may be the sign of impending herniation and death without immediate intervention. In a patient without a ventricular drain already in place, hyperventilation is the most rapid mechanism for acutely lowering elevated ICP. Currently, aggressive hyperventilation ($Pco_2 < 30$) is recommended only for short durations in cases of impending cerebral herniation while patients are being stabilized. As stated previously, hyperventilation causes vasoconstriction, which reduces intravascular blood within the cranial vault and almost instantaneously lowering ICP. However, several studies have now shown that the routine use of aggressive hyperventilation in the management of patients with severe closed head injury (CHI) results in decreased outcomes because of hypoxic injury and possible stroke caused by the sustained hyperventilation. Our current practice is to maintain Pco_2 values between 35 and 38 with controlled ventilation in all patients with severe CHI; because of this we leave all these patients intubated and mechanically ventilated until their ICPs normalize and all other therapies are withdrawn.

Adequate sedation and pain control are also important elements of ICP control. Patients who are restless and agitated will have higher ICPs than similar patients who are resting quietly in bed. Another important point is the prevention of venous congestion. This occasionally is evident in cervical collars, which are fastened too tight or with the use of trach ties that are wrapped too tightly around the neck to hold the endotracheal tube in place.

Several medications are available for the treatment of elevated ICP with the most common one being mannitol. Although this agent acts as an osmotic diuretic and helps pull excess interstitial fluid into the vascular space and thus lower ICP, there are several other hypothetical mechanisms that probably also increase its efficacy such as increasing RBC flexibility, decreasing RBC and platelet clumping in small arterioles and capillaries, and increasing intravascular volume, thus improving cardiac function. Other diuretics such as furosemide (Lasix)[1] or urea (Ureaphil) may also be used but have less dramatic effects on ICP. Hypertonic saline (NaCl 3% to 5%)[1] has also been used more recently by some physicians and has been shown to have many of the same effects as mannitol.

CSF diversion is one of the simplest, quickest acting methods for decreasing ICP especially if a ventricular drain is already in place. The emergent surgical evacuation of mass lesions such as large epidural, subdural, or intraparenchymal hematomas is also extremely effective for controlling ICP, and in many instances it is also life-saving. However, in some instances, underlying brain injury or stroke from prolonged brain compression may be exhibited as massive intraoperative brain swelling and in these instances may necessitate that the bone flap be left off (craniectomy).

Management of Severe Closed Head Injury

The current recommendations of the Brain Trauma Foundation Guidelines for the management of closed head injuries call for the placement of ICP monitors in all patients who fall into the severe category (GCS score < 9). At our institution we routinely place combination intraventricular monitors and drains in all patients with a postresuscitation GCS score of less than 7. Monitors are inserted into

---

[1]Not FDA approved for this indication.

 CURRENT THERAPY

Management of Elevated Intracranial Pressure
- Prevention of venous engorgement
- CO_2 control (mild hyperventilation)
- Sedation and pain control
- Cerebrospinal fluid drainage
- Mannitol
- Lasix
- Hypertonic saline
- Decompressive craniectomy
- Pentobarbital coma

---

patients with a GCS score of 7 to 9 on an individual basis depending on whether there are distracting reasons, such as intoxication, to cause the altered LOC. If patients are intubated and not following commands but are purposeful in their movements, we will sometimes elect not to place a ventriculostomy and follow the patient's clinical course over several hours. Other factors include CT findings and the need to go to the operating room during the acute period for the treatment of other life-threatening injuries, age, or for heavy sedation secondary to other injuries or pulmonary problems. At times patients in this GCS range will be given 6 to 12 hours and treated medically to see whether or not they improve prior to placement of an ICP monitor.

Once an ICP monitor and drain have been placed elevations in ICP are treated in a systematic order. Target values include attempts to keep ICP less than 15 to 20 and cerebral perfusion pressure (CPP) greater than 60. Low CPP (CPP = mean arterial blood pressure [MAP] − ICP) is caused by either elevated ICP or low MAP. For patients with low MAP or uncontrolled ICP, vasopressors may be used to increase blood pressure (BP) and central venous pressure. At the University of Louisville, dopamine (Intropin) is used as a first line agent, followed by phenylephrine (Neo-Synephrine) and norepinephrine (Levophed) in refractory cases. ICP elevations are initially treated with adequate sedation and pain control, such as midazolam (Versed),[1] propofol (Diprivan), and/or morphine (Lioresal),[1] to prevent agitation and elevated airway pressures, which can further increase ICP and intermittent CSF diversion. In cases where this fails to control ICP, mannitol is then added to the treatment protocol along with more continuous CSF diversion and finally chemical paralysis. Mannitol is administered as a bolus infusion in doses ranging from 0.25 to 1.0 mg/kg body weight every 4 to 8 hours with the endpoints being either ICP control or measured serum osmolarity greater than 315 mOsmL.

Patients who continue to have sustained increases in their ICP despite these interventions are considered to have refractory ICP and at our facility are considered for one of two potential salvage treatments. Pentobarbital (Nembutal)[1] coma has been used successfully on occasion in young patients without mass lesions to decrease the metabolic demands of the brain during these periods of sustained ICP. Patients need to be chosen wisely for this therapy because it carries enormous risks in addition to the possibility of preserving the patient in a long-term, nonfunctional, persistent vegetative state. Initiation of pentobarbital (Nembutal)[1] coma causes severe hypotension, and patients almost always require the use of pressors in addition to volume expansion. At our facility we also place all of these patients on a Rotorest bed in an attempt to minimize the pulmonary complications that frequently occur with the use of this technique.

The second salvage therapy is decompressive craniectomy. This procedure involves the removal of a significant area of skull, typically almost an entire hemisphere or both frontal regions with opening of the dura. This permits the injured swollen brain to herniate through the opening and is the only intervention that increases the volume of

---

[1]Not FDA approved for this indication.

the intracranial compartment, thereby reducing pressure. In addition this technique allows for the evacuation of large hemorrhagic contusions, or in cases of extreme ICP elevations it can be coupled with either frontal or temporal lobectomy. Once again, patients must be selected carefully for this intervention. Decompressive craniectomy is used much more frequently than pentobarbital (Nembutal)[1] coma at our institution. We use this strategy for patients with elevated ICP—more than 30 to 40 for more than 30 minutes—or a significant change in neurologic condition that is nonresponsive to all other interventions. In order for either of these two salvage approaches to be effective, they must be used at the first signs of refractory ICP prior to the occurrence of complications such as ischemic infarcts or brainstem compression or hemorrhage.

Patients treated with decompressive craniectomies are at risk for significant alterations in CSF dynamics that may result in delayed deterioration. Signs of hydrocephalus either in the form of ventriculomegaly or extra-axial or interhemispheric CSF fluid collections will be evident in 50% to 80% of these patients. When necessary these patients will be treated with external ventricular or subdural drains followed by early cranioplasty (replacement of the bone plate). In many instances these changes will resolve following cranioplasty and therefore avoid the need for ventriculoperitoneal shunting, with its associated risks and complications.

All patients with abnormal head CT scans (regardless of GCS score) are treated with close neurologic observation most commonly in an intensive care unit (ICU) setting, serial CT scans (4 to 6 hours later and on PID 1), and placed on 7 days of phenytoin (Dilantin). Temkin and colleagues showed that patients with post-traumatic intracranial hemorrhage were at increased risk of suffering seizures in the acute period; treatment with antiepileptics beyond 7 days did not decrease the risk of these patients from developing epilepsy or delayed seizures but there were increased risks associated with side effects from medication administration. Patients who experience a seizure following CHI (with the exception of acute post-traumatic seizures) should be maintained on antiepileptics for at least 3 to 6 months and possible indefinitely depending on their clinical condition and EEG results. Patients with acute post-traumatic seizures (within the first several minutes following the event) are not felt to be at increased risk for developing further seizures and receive the routine 7-day treatment. At the University of Louisville we have found that changing phenytoin dosing to a weight-based schedule (15 mg/kg load, 2 mg/kg every 8 hours unless elderly [$\geq$70 years old], then 2 mg/kg every 12 hours) increases the chance of achieving a therapeutic dose earlier in the treatment course and lowers the costs of monitoring these agents.

Finally, the treatment of these patients requires a tight-knit group of specialists and ancillary service providers with open communication channels. We have found that the use of a time-independent phased outcome clinical pathway helps maximize the level of patient care and maintain cost-effectiveness. By using such an approach all routine interactions are initiated at the time of admission and each care provider has a clear role and responsibility; one of the most important aspects of this system is the creation of a clinical coordinator whose responsibility includes ensuring that all aspects of patient care and family education are completed at the appropriate intervals. We believe another key component of this is our philosophy toward early feeding (prior to PID 3) and early tracheotomy and percutaneous endoscopic gastrostomy (PEG) feeding tube placement in a majority of these individuals (PID 4). We have shown that such an aggressive approach to these issues helps reduce infectious complications and minimizes length of ICU stay.

Treatment of Mild and Moderate Traumatic Brain Injury

In many circumstances patients with moderate TBI are treated almost as though they had severe TBI, with the exception of invasive ICP monitoring. Many patients will be intubated at the time of admission and require sedation and adequate pain management. This can be difficult because it is of utmost importance to maintain the ability to perform serial neurologic examinations. Therefore, we commonly use a combination of propofol (Diprivan) infusions and intermittent morphine (Lioresal)[1] injections in these patients, thereby allowing hourly assessment of neurologic function. We have found that a subset of patients (older than age 45 years, multisystem trauma, presence of early pneumonia) with moderate TBI requires more aggressive treatment with early tracheostomy and PEG tube placement and at times ICP monitors.

The subset of patients with moderate TBI who are not intubated at the time of admission are also watched closely in the ICU. Once again, close monitoring of neurologic function and vigorous pulmonary toilet is of key importance because some patients may be lethargic and are at risk of pulmonary decompensation. We have found ipratropium (Atrovent)[1] and albuterol (Proventil)[1] nebulizers and early mobilization minimize pulmonary problems. Patients with progressive lethargy, worsening neurologic function, hypoxia, hypercapnia, or the inability to protect their airways are intubated and placed on mechanical ventilation. Once again, patients unable to tolerate a diet by PID 3 have a nasogastric feeding tube placed to allow for early enteral nutritional support; however, PEG tubes are not placed until later in the hospital course in the predischarge phase because many patients in this category will improve throughout their hospitalization and be able to tolerate an oral diet by the time of discharge.

Patients with mild TBI are treated over a much wider continuum, ranging from discharge from the emergency room (ER) with appropriate adult supervision to observation in the ICU to immediate surgical treatment of surgical mass lesions. The two most important factors in determining treatment algorithms for these patients are presence or absence of abnormal CT findings and neurologic function, with associated symptoms such as nausea, vomiting, dizziness, or visual problems. Headache is a common complaint in all of these patients and must be taken in context with other complaints and imaging results. Patients with severe headaches, dizziness, and vomiting (postconcussive syndrome) may commonly require a brief hospital stay to allow for delayed imaging and at least partial resolution of some of the complaints.

Early and Delayed Neurologic Changes

Any patient suffering a significant neurologic injury requires close neurologic monitoring. Although most patients remain unchanged or show gradual improvement in the early phases, a small percentage will show signs of neurologic deterioration. At first these signs may be subtle (agitation, mild increase in lethargy, protracted vomiting); but eventually they may become more profound and can be precursors to impending neurologic demise and death. When these changes are the result of either expanding mass lesions or increases in ICP, treatment instituted in the early phases is more likely to be more successful compared to instances when interventions are performed under conditions associated with cerebral herniation syndromes. Thus any patient showing persistent signs of neurologic decline should be promptly evaluated by a physician and many may also require repeat CT scanning.

However, not all neurologic changes are the result of changes in ICP or expansion of mass lesions, and such irregularities may be caused by a long list of other metabolic or neurologic conditions. Some of the more common causes are seizures, strokes (especially from carotid or vertebral dissections), electrolyte imbalances, hypoxia, hypercarbia, fever, excess sedation, or drug and/or alcohol withdrawal.

---

[1]Not FDA approved for this indication.

Concussions and Sports-Related Injuries: Return to Play Guidelines

Over the past 2 decades, the knowledge regarding the detrimental effects of repetitive mild head injuries has led to intense public debate concerning whether athletes should be allowed to return to play following such injuries. Concussions are not uncommon among participants of competitive sports including football, hockey, baseball, and soccer. Concerns regarding the full negative impact of repetitive, almost innocuous injury have led many youth soccer leagues to ban or modify rules regarding *heading* of the ball. In addition, other concerns exist following more severe concussions such as development of other life-threatening neurologic injuries such as subdural or epidural hematomas, development of the double-impact syndrome (rapid uncontrolled increases in ICP following sequential minor traumas), and the long-term neuropsychological impact of these injuries. As a result of these concerns, the guidelines concerning when and if an athlete should be allowed to return to play have undergone modification since development of the earlier criteria. Because of these frequent changes, readers are encouraged to check with their local medical agencies or recent publications and Internet sources if faced with these issues. In short, if a player loses consciousness or has persistent symptoms (>15 to 20 minutes), they should not be allowed to return to play on that day or even not for 1 to 2 weeks following the complete resolution of all symptoms. It should also be stressed that an individual may have a concussion without loss of consciousness and that concussion is defined as any transient change in mental status. To this end many organizations including the National Football League have developed a sideline neuropsychological screening test that can often help illustrate these deficits even when the athlete appears normal.

Restorative Therapies

Patients suffering any type of TBI can have long-lasting cognitive, psychological, and emotional dysfunction in addition to their functional and neurologic deficits. Although most people assume that the resolution of decreased alertness and consciousness symbolizes resolution of the overall neurologic injury, this is not the case in most patients. In our series of patients with moderate TBI, we found that almost 50% of patients at median follow-up of 27 months complained of persistent emotional or cognitive problems that interfered with their lifestyle despite the fact that they all were discharged from the hospital with a GCS score of 14 to 15. Long-term speech and cognitive therapies as well as individual, group, and family counseling will be helpful for many of these patients.

In the late hospital and early rehabilitative stages, numerous pharmacologic agents may be helpful to overcome some of the neurologic side effects following TBI. Patients with autonomic storms (intermittent episodes of diaphoresis, tachycardia, fever, agitation) may respond to adrenergic antagonists such as clonidine (Catapres)[1] or propanolol (Inderal),[1] in addition to volume resuscitation, morphine (Lioresal),[1] baclofen,[1] and bromocriptine (Parlodel).[1] Patients with hypoarousal are treated with amantadine[1] (Symmetrel), 100 mg at 8 am and 12 pm, and bromocriptine,[1] 5 to 15 mg every day. Trazodone (Desyrel), 50 to 100 mg at bedtime, may be helpful in restoring sleep-wake cycles, whereas risperidone (Risperdal),[1] olanzapine (Zyprexa),[1] and quetiapine (Seroquel)[1] may be helpful to control agitation and combativeness during the subacute recovery phases.

Future Considerations

The previously mentioned treatment strategies include what is considered common practice at the University of Louisville; however, newer, more aggressive treatments and monitoring capabilities are always being developed. Some of the newer monitoring systems under development include cerebral oximetry measurements (frequently through invasive indwelling catheters) or cerebral microdialysis systems, in which continuous assessments are performed to determine the concentrations of critical markers such as lactate in the brain or CSF. Both of these methods provide physiologic feedback for the metabolic environment of the brain, are sensitive enough to predict changes in regional oxygenation, and have been found to be correlated with outcomes in small nonrandomized studies.

REFERENCES

Brain Trauma Foundation: Management and Prognosis of Severe Traumatic Brain Injury. New York: Brain Trauma Foundation, 2000.

Mcilvoy L, Spain DA, Raque G, et al: Successful incorporation of the Severe Head Injury Guidelines into a phased-outcome clinical pathway. J Neurosci Nurs 2001;33(2):72-78, 82.

Miller PR, Fabian TC, Bee TK, et al: Blunt cerebrovascular injuries: Diagnosis and treatment. J Trauma 2001;51(2):279-286.

Temkin NR, Dikmen SS, Wilensky AJ, et al: A randomized, double-blind study of phenytoin for the prevention of post-traumatic seizures. N Engl J Med 1990;323:497-502.

Vitaz TW, McIlvoy L, Raque GH, et al: Development and implementation of a clinical pathway for severe traumatic brain injury. J Trauma 2001;51(2):369-375.

Vitaz TW, McIlvoy L, Raque GH, et al: Development and implementation of a clinical pathway for spinal cord injuries. J Spinal Disord 2001;14(3):271-276.

Vitaz TW, Jenks J, Raque GH, Shields CB: Outcome following moderate traumatic brain injury. Surg Neurol 2003;60(4):285-291.

Traumatic Brain Injury in Children

Method of
Stephen R. Deputy, MD

Traumatic brain injury (TBI) is one of the leading causes of death and disability among children, adolescents, and young adults. An estimated 185 per 100,000 children (ages 0 to 14 years) and 550 per 100,000 adolescents (ages 15 to 19 years) are hospitalized each year for TBI. The etiology of TBI varies depending on the age of the patient, with younger children more likely to be injured from falls and pedestrian injuries, and adolescents more often injured in motor vehicle accidents and assaults. Inflicted TBI (shaking-impact syndrome of infancy) is the leading cause of injury-related deaths in children younger than 4 years of age and accounts for 80% of deaths from head trauma in children younger than 2 years of age.

Types and Severity of Head Injury

Closed head injury is the most common type of TBI seen in children. Forces from rapid deceleration are applied diffusely throughout the brain and consciousness is frequently impaired. *Open head injuries*, in which the dura is breached, are caused by focal penetrating forces, and the risk of post-traumatic epilepsy is relatively high.

Primary brain injury is caused by the mechanical forces of the trauma itself. Diffuse axonal injury is an example of primary brain injury. During rapid deceleration, angular forces applied to the head cause the brain to rotate about its center of gravity. Shifting regions of differing densities within the brain itself result in shearing along

---

[1]Not FDA approved for this indication.

planes such as the gray-white junction, corpus callosum, and brainstem. The shearing of axons effectively serves to "disconnect" the cortex from the brainstem and consciousness becomes impaired. Translational (straight-line) forces applied to the head produce impact-loading contact phenomena, resulting in focal injuries to the scalp, skull, and brain, such as lacerations, skull fractures, cerebral contusions, and epidural hematomas. *Subdural hematomas* may occur because of tearing of fragile dural bridging veins during rapid decelerations.

Secondary brain injury follows and is the consequence of primary injury. Examples include hypoxic-ischemic injury (secondary to low cerebral perfusion pressure or anoxia), disrupted cerebral autoregulation, seizures or status epilepticus, diffuse cerebral edema, hydrocephalus, and raised intracranial pressure. The goal of treatment for TBI is to reduce or prevent secondary brain injury from occurring because the primary brain injury has already happened at the time of trauma and cannot be altered.

The severity of TBI can be broken down into mild, moderate, and severe. *Mild* TBI is defined as head trauma with an initial Glasgow Coma Scale (GCS) score of 13 to 15. *Moderate* TBI occurs with an initial GCS score of 9 to 12. *Severe* TBI occurs with an initial GCS score of 8 or less. The GCS is modified for use in infants under the age of 36 months (Table 1).

Special attention should be given to those infants with TBI who do not show evidence of external facial or head trauma and who may not be presented by their caregivers as having a history of head injury. The *shaking-impact syndrome* is usually found in infants younger than 3 years of age with a peak incidence in infants younger than 1 year of age. Presenting symptoms include irritability, lethargy, or coma, apnea or breathing irregularities, and seizures. Retinal hemorrhages may be found in from 65% to 95% of these patients and should be actively looked for with a dilated funduscopic examination in any case where head trauma is suspected. Computed tomography (CT) imaging most commonly shows evidence of acute or remote subdural hematomas with or without evidence of cerebral infarction. Workup should include a skeletal survey to look for evidence of skull, posterior rib, or long bone fractures of different healing stages. Infants may be more susceptible to shaking-impact syndrome given their relatively large head size compared to their underdeveloped neck musculature. Infants also have thinner skulls, and translational forces may cause more severe contusions. Relatively longer subdural veins that bridge the infant's enlarged subarachnoid spaces can be easily lacerated from angular forces, resulting in subdural hematomas.

Management of Traumatic Brain Injury in Children

MILD TRAUMATIC BRAIN INJURY

Mild TBI accounts for more than 90% of all pediatric admissions for TBI. Children in this category should have a GCS score of 15 upon arrival to the emergency room, no focal neurologic deficits, and no signs of increased intracranial pressure (ICP). These children may have had a brief loss of consciousness (less than 1 minute), amnesia for the event, an immediate impact seizure, vomiting, or lethargy (as long as the GCS score is 15 during the evaluation). Children without loss of consciousness or amnesia may be observed or sent home with competent caregivers without performing neuroimaging studies. Vigilance for any change in the child's neurologic status should be maintained for up to 72 hours after the injury. If there has been a brief loss of consciousness or amnesia for the event, the risk of intracranial hemorrhage is still relatively low, and it is up to the discretion of the treating physician whether CT imaging is warranted.

Clinical predictors of intracranial hemorrhage are less reliable for children under the age of 2 years, and nonaccidental trauma also comes into consideration in this age group. Therefore, most children under the age of 2 years with TBI should undergo CT imaging followed by careful observation.

MODERATE TRAUMATIC BRAIN INJURY

Patients who fall within the moderate category generally need more intensive monitoring and medical management to avoid secondary brain injuries. As with all critical illness, attention should first be paid to following the ABCs (airway, breathing, circulation).

Airway

Patients with a GCS score of 9 or greater usually do not require endotracheal intubation for airway protection, although they should be kept NPO (nothing by mouth) in case of clinical deterioration.

Breathing

Hypoxemia and hypoventilation may increase ICP, so supplemental oxygen by nasal cannula may be helpful.

Circulation

It is important to avoid hypotension to maintain adequate cerebral perfusion pressure (CPP). Isotonic intravenous fluids should be provided with care to avoid fluid overload, hypoglycemia, or hyperglycemia. Careful attention should be paid to fluid and sodium balance because these patients may be at risk for developing diabetes insipidus. Likewise, the head of the bed should be raised to 30 degrees and the patient's head kept midline to optimize venous return from the cranium to the right side of the heart. Sedation with short-acting sedatives (propofol [Diprivan] or midazolam [Versed]) or opioids may be necessary to avoid agitation, which can also reduce venous return to the heart.

Early post-traumatic seizures are fairly rare in children with moderate TBI. The need for empirical anticonvulsant therapy in this group remains controversial and should be reserved for those patients in whom raised intracranial pressure is of concern. Likewise, empirical use of mannitol has little clinical support for this group.

TABLE 1 Glasgow Coma Scale for Children

Score	Eyes Open	Best Verbal Response	Best Verbal Response	Best Motor Response (<36 mo)	Best Motor Response (<36 mo)
6	—	—	—	Follows commands	Normal spontaneous movements
5	—	Oriented and converses	Coos and babbles	Localizes pain	Withdraws to touch
4	Spontaneously	Confused	Irritable to pain	Withdraws to pain	Withdraws to pain
3	To verbal commands	Inappropriate words	Cries to pain	Flexor posturing	Flexor posturing
2	To painful stimuli	Nonspecific sounds	Moans to pain	Extensor posturing	Extensor posturing
1	None	None	None	No response	No response

SEVERE TRAUMATIC BRAIN INJURY

Patients in the severe group are at the highest risk for secondary brain injuries. The following additional interventions are recommended.

Airway

By definition, these patients have a GCS score of 8 or lower and require endotracheal intubation for airway protection.

Breathing

Hyperventilation with a goal Pco_2 of 26 to 30 mm Hg should be performed only if there is impending brainstem herniation or to bridge the gap until more definitive neurosurgical intervention can be performed to lower intracranial pressure. The benefit of hyperventilation is generally short lived (1 to 24 hours) and may worsen local ischemia following trauma or acute stroke.

Circulation

In the setting of suspected raised intracranial pressure, the goal of fluid and blood pressure management should be to maintain the cerebral perfusion pressure greater than 50 to 70 mm Hg. Recall that CPP equals MAP (mean arterial blood pressure) minus ICP. Because children generally have a lower MAP than adults, it is not always necessary to provide vasopressor therapy to keep the CPP above 70 mm Hg unless there is evidence of raised ICP. Invasive intracranial pressure monitoring should be considered if the GCS score is lower than 8 or in the setting of elevated ICP to optimize CPP.

Other Techniques to Lower Intracranial Pressure

NEUROSURGICAL

Obvious mass lesions, such as hydrocephalus, subdural and epidural hematomas, and contused cortical tissue should be surgically evacuated whenever feasible. CT scanning is able to identify most of these surgical lesions. Decompressive craniectomy is now used more frequently to relieve pressure when multifocal contusions or diffuse cerebral edema is present. As mentioned earlier, ICP monitoring is usually warranted for all severe TBI patients.

OSMOTHERAPY

Mannitol (20% solution) may be given as an initial bolus of 0.5 to 1 g/kg. Repeat doses of 0.25 to 0.5 g/kg are given every 6 to 8 hours as needed to maintain the serum osmolality and sodium levels to less than or equal to 320 mOsmL and 150 mEq, respectively. Osmotic diuretics should be used with caution in patients with renal insufficiency. The beneficial effects occur within minutes, peak at 1 hour, and last 4 to 24 hours. Potential disadvantages include worsening of focal cerebral edema in areas where the blood-brain barrier is disrupted.

CURRENT DIAGNOSIS

- Children under the age of 2 years with traumatic brain injury (TBI) may require neuroimaging because clinical predictors of intracranial hemorrhage are less reliable in this age group.
- Children under the age of 1 year presenting with lethargy, irritability, apnea, or seizures should be evaluated with computed tomography (CT) imaging and a dilated funduscopic examination to rule out shaking-impact syndrome.

CURRENT THERAPY

- Children with mild TBI and a GCS score of 15 at presentation can usually be observed clinically without the need for neuroimaging.
- The goal of treatment for TBI is to minimize *secondary* brain injury.
- In the setting of raised ICP, it is important to maintain CPP above 50 to 70 mm Hg.
- Early post-traumatic seizures are relatively frequent in open head injury and in severe TBI. They should be empirically treated in any patient in whom raised ICP is a concern.
- Direct intracranial pressure monitoring should be considered in any TBI patient with a GCS score of 8 or less.

Abbreviations: CPP = cerebral perfusion pressure; ICP = intracranial pressure; GCS = Glasgow Coma Scale; TBI = traumatic brain injury.

BARBITURATES

Sedating agents may lower ICP by reducing pain as well as by making the brain metabolically less active. Pentobarbital is given as a loading dose of 5 to 20 mg/kg, followed by a continuous infusion of 1 to 4 mg/kg per hour. Continuous EEG monitoring to maintain a burst suppression pattern is warranted with this therapy. Potential disadvantages include systemic hypotension and a long half-life that may interfere with the declaration of brain death.

ANTICONVULSANT THERAPY

Children with severe TBI are at a high risk for early post-traumatic seizures, which can further elevate the ICP. It is generally recommended empirically to load these children with 20 mg/kg of intravenous phenytoin (Cerebyx). Maintenance therapy can be achieved with 5 mg/kg per day divided every 8 hours with target blood levels of 10 to 20 mg/dL.

HYPOTHERMIA

More centers are including hypothermia as an option for patients with elevated ICP not responsive to medical or surgical management. The best method of cooling (i.e., whole body versus head only) and the optimal core temperature are not established for children.

Of note, apart from neurosurgical interventions, none of the techniques just described are shown definitively to reduce morbidity or mortality in children with severe TBI.

REFERENCES

Annegers JF, Grabow JD, Grover RV, et al: Seizures after head trauma: A population study. Neurology 1980;30:683-689.
Bruce DA, Zimmerman RA: Shaken impact syndrome. Pediatr Ann 1989;18:482-494.
Committee on Quality Improvement, American Academy of Pediatrics: The management of minor closed head injury in children. Pediatrics 1999;104(6):1407-1415.
Deputy SR: Shaking-impact syndrome of infancy. Semin Pediatr Neurol 2003;10(2):112-119.
Kraus JF, Nourjah P: The epidemiology of uncomplicated brain injury. J Trauma 1988;28:1637-1643.
Schutzman SA, Barnes P, et al: Evaluation and management of children younger than two years old with apparently minor head trauma: Proposed guidelines. Pediatrics 2001;107:983-993.

Brain Tumors

Method of
*Ashwatha Narayana, MD, Eve S. Ferdman, BA,
and Shahzad Raza, MD*

Primary brain tumors will account for an estimated 21,800 new cases that will be diagnosed and 13,810 deaths for the year 2008 in the United States. Several histopathologically different tumors arise in the brain, reflecting the diversity of phenotypically distinct cells within the central nervous system (CNS) that have a capacity for neoplastic transformation. Gliomas, the most common tumors, are considered first in this article, followed by a description of many of the principles of brain tumor management. Then less common tumors are briefly presented, and the article closes with a discussion about managing metastatic brain tumors.

Gliomas

INCIDENCE

Malignant gliomas make up 35% to 45% of primary brain tumors, and of these, nearly 85% are glioblastoma multiforme. The incidence of anaplastic astrocytoma peaks in children younger than 10 years of age and then remains constant in each subsequent decade of life. In contrast, the incidence of glioblastoma multiforme increases dramatically after the age of 40 years. Low-grade astrocytomas make up 5% to 15% of primary brain tumors and 67% of low-grade gliomas. The remainder of low-grade gliomas are mixed oligoastrocytomas (19%) and oligodendrogliomas (13%). Unlike their malignant counterparts, low-grade gliomas are most common between the ages of 20 and 40 years and rarely occur after the age of 50 years.

GENETICS AND ETIOLOGY

Genetic abnormalities are demonstrated for 50% to 75% of adult astrocytomas. It is hypothesized that p53 gene mutations are associated with the transition to grade II tumors. Malignant progression to anaplastic astrocytoma is associated with loss of heterozygosity (LOH) for chromosomes 9p, 13q, or 19q and CDK4 gene amplification. Subsequent LOH on chromosome 10 and amplification of the epidermal growth factor receptor genes characterize further progression to glioblastoma multiforme. A second, p53-independent, pathway that leads more directly to glioblastoma multiforme development is also described.

Losses of genetic information from chromosomes 1p and 19q are commonly seen in oligodendroglioma specimens, whereas losses on 17p and p53 gene mutations are notably less frequent, suggesting that early events in their oncogenesis are distinct from those associated with astrocytic tumors.

Although some environmental factors are linked with brain tumor development, they do not appear responsible for most brain tumors. Radiation-induced gliomas are reported, mainly in children with acute leukemia who received prophylactic cranial irradiation and chemotherapy. The hereditary syndromes associated with an increased risk of brain tumors include neurofibromatosis type 1 and neurofibromatosis type 2, tuberous sclerosis, Li-Fraumeni syndrome, familial polyposis, Turcot's syndrome, Gardner's syndrome, and von Hippel-Lindau disease.

PATHOLOGY

CNS tumors are generally classified as follows (Table 1):

- Gliomas
- Neuronal/glioneuronal neoplasms
- Embryonal neoplasms
- Meningeal neoplasms
- Miscellaneous nonglial neoplasms

Reliance on a pathologic classification of brain tumors is a requisite for treatment. Indeed, histopathology is more important than anatomic staging in determining the clinical behavior and prognosis of these tumors. Neuropathologists do not all agree on a uniform classification system for astrocytic gliomas. The World Health Organization system, which divides astrocytic tumors into four grades—from grade I, corresponding to pilocytic astrocytomas, to grade IV, corresponding to the glioblastoma multiforme—is used more often.

Low-grade astrocytomas are well-differentiated tumors that display increased cellularity compared with normal brain tissue and have mild to moderate nuclear pleomorphism (Figure 1). The cytoplasmic processes that extend from the astrocytes contain a characteristic filamentous protein, glial fibrillary acidic protein (GFAP), which provides an immunohistochemical marker for these tumors. Over time, at least 50% of these tumors transform into more anaplastic lesions. The characteristic histopathologic features of anaplastic astrocytomas include moderate hypercellularity, moderate cellular and nuclear pleomorphism, variable mitotic activity, and microvascular proliferation. The presence of tumor necrosis is the hallmark that distinguishes anaplastic astrocytoma from glioblastoma multiforme (Figure 2).

Oligodendrogliomas, in contrast, are composed of small uniform cells with round central nuclei and distinct cytoplasmic borders. Formalin fixation causes a perinuclear halo that produces a "fried egg" or "honeycomb" appearance. The cells lack fibrillary cytoplasmic processes. Calcification is a frequent feature.

CLINICAL PRESENTATION

The presenting symptoms and signs of brain tumors include those associated with a mass effect and increased intracranial pressure and those that are focal. The most common presenting symptom with gliomas is headache. Approximately two thirds of adult patients with low-grade astrocytomas and 20% of patients with malignant tumors present with seizures but are otherwise neurologically intact. Others exhibit a slowly progressive neurologic syndrome consisting of headache, vomiting, motor deficit, visual or sensory loss, language disturbance, or personality change. Symptoms may be present for months or years before the diagnosis is made.

ROUTES OF SPREAD

The most common route of spread for gliomas is through local extension. As they enlarge, malignant gliomas extend directly into adjacent lobes and disseminate along anatomically defined nerve fiber pathways. Multicentric gliomas are found in less than 5% of patients. Dissemination by seeding through the CPF pathways occurs in approximately 10% of cases but is usually a late event. Metastases rarely arise outside the CNS.

DIAGNOSTIC STUDIES

Computed tomography (CT) and magnetic resonance imaging (MRI) play indispensable roles in the management of brain tumors. CT is a reliable screening and diagnostic method for suspected supratentorial brain tumor lesions. MRI, now more frequently used in patients with malignant brain tumors, is the screening procedure of choice for diagnosing and localizing tumors in the brainstem, posterior fossa, and spinal cord. Ordinary astrocytomas appear as diffuse, poorly defined, low-density, nonenhancing lesions. Approximately 40% of ordinary astrocytomas enhance, and calcification is found in 10% of cases. Although the majority of malignant gliomas enhance with contrast media, as many as 30% of anaplastic astrocytomas present as nonenhancing lesions. In both low-grade and malignant gliomas, parenchymal infiltration by isolated tumor cells may be present in regions of T2-weighted abnormality that appear normal on CT (Figures 3 and 4). Positron emission tomography (PET), single-photon emission computed tomography (SPECT) with thallium-201 (^{201}Tl), and magnetic resonance spectroscopy (MRS) are other imaging approaches used in brain tumor management.

TABLE 1 Histopathology of Brain Tumors

Major Classification	Variants	WHO Grade
Gliomas		
Astrocytic: circumscribed	Pilocytic astrocytoma	I
	Subependymal giant cell astrocytoma (SEGA)	I
	Pleomorphic xanthoastrocytoma (PXA)	II
Astrocytic: diffuse	Astrocytoma	II
	Anaplastic astrocytoma	III
	Glioblastoma multiforme	IV
Oligodendroglial	Oligodendroglioma	II
	Anaplastic oligodendroglioma	III
Mixed gliomas	Oligoastrocytoma	II
	Anaplastic oligoastrocytoma	III
Ependymal	Subependymoma	I
	Myxopapillary ependymoma	I
	Ependymoma	II
	Anaplastic ependymoma*	III
Choroid plexus	Choroid plexus papilloma	I
	Choroid plexus carcinoma*	III
Cranial and Peripheral Nerve Tumors	Schwannoma	I
Neuronal and Glioneuronal Tumors	Gangliocytoma/ganglioglioma	I–III
	Desmoplastic infantile ganglioma (DIG)	I
	Dysplastic cerebellar gangliocytoma	I
	Central neurocytoma	I
	Dysembryoplastic neuroepithelial tumor	I
	Paraganglioma	I
Pineal Parenchymal Tumors (PPTs)	Pineocytoma	II
	PPT with intermediate differentiation	III
	Pineoblastoma	IV
Embryonal Tumors	Medulloepithelioma*	IV
	Primitive neuroectodermal tumor (PNET),* including medulloblastoma and variants*	IV
	Atypical teratoid/rhabdoid tumor (AT/RT)	IV
	Cerebral neuroblastoma/ganglioneuroblastoma	IV
	Ependymoblastoma*	IV
	Olfactory neuroblastoma (esthesioneuroblastoma)	IV
Meningeal Tumors	Meningioma	I
	Atypical meningioma	II
	Anaplastic (malignant) meningioma	III
Germ Cell Tumors	Hemangiopericytoma†	II–III
	Germinoma	NA
	Mature teratoma	NA
	Nongerminomatous germ cell tumors	NA
Tumors of the Sellar Region	Craniopharyngioma: adamantinomatous	I
	Craniopharyngioma: papillary	I
Hemopoietic Neoplasms	Primary central nervous system lymphoma (PCNSL)	NA
	Secondary lymphoma/leukemia	NA
	Histiocytic tumors and histiocytoses	NA
Secondary Tumors/Metastases	Carcinomas and sarcomas	NA

*Indicates those tumors with a tendency to disseminate throughout the central nervous system (CNS).
†The origin of hemangiopericytoma is uncertain.
Abbreviations: WHO = World Health Organization; NA = not applicable.

STAGING

No accepted staging system exists for primary brain tumors. The American Joint Committee on Cancer proposed a staging scheme for primary brain tumors based on tumor size and metastases as well as tumor grade. Because this system was not generally adapted to clinical use, it was subsequently removed.

PROGNOSTIC FACTORS

Age, histologic appearance, Karnofsky performance score (KPS), mental status, duration of symptoms, neurologic functional class, extent of surgery, and radiation dose are identified as significant partitioning covariates in clinical trials. This information is important for correctly interpreting the results of studies comparing different treatment regimens and for assessing the potential of new therapeutic methodologies.

STANDARD THERAPEUTIC APPROACHES FOR GLIOMAS

Surgery

The combination of surgery, radiation therapy, and chemotherapy represents the standard approach to the treatment of gliomas. The

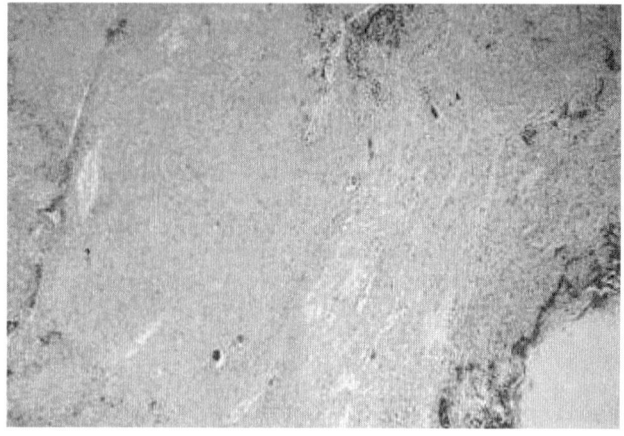

FIGURE 1. Low-grade astrocytoma showing mildly increased cellularity with uniform cells and nuclei.

goals of surgery are to provide a histologic diagnosis, to alleviate intracranial hypertension and focal neurologic deficits because of a mass effect, and to permit rapid corticosteroid dose tapering. Pilocytic astrocytomas are relatively well circumscribed, and 60% to 80% are amenable to total removal. Resection of the more common diffuse astrocytomas is limited by the lack of clear demarcation between the infiltrating tumor and normal brain tissue. Evidence suggests that patients with more complete resections live longer and have an improved functional status compared with those who undergo a biopsy or partial resection only. Advances in neurosurgery, including diagnostic ultrasound, lasers, ultrasonic tissue aspirators, cortical mapping, functional imaging, and computer-assisted stereotactic laser techniques, have improved the ability of neurosurgeons to radically remove intracranial tumors.

Radiation Therapy

Limited radiation fields are used for the treatment of gliomas. Three-dimensionally designed complex treatment plans with multiple fields are used whenever appropriate to limit the high-dose volume and to minimize the risk of long-term radiation sequelae. Doses of 50.4 to 54 Gy are usually recommended for low-grade gliomas and 59.4 to 60 Gy for high-grade gliomas. Rapid fractionation schemes (such as 30 to 36 Gy) may be appropriate for some elderly or poor performance status patients with glioblastoma multiforme who have relatively short survival expectancies.

In low-grade gliomas, the role of radiation therapy is debatable. Although it improves disease-free survival, overall survival is not

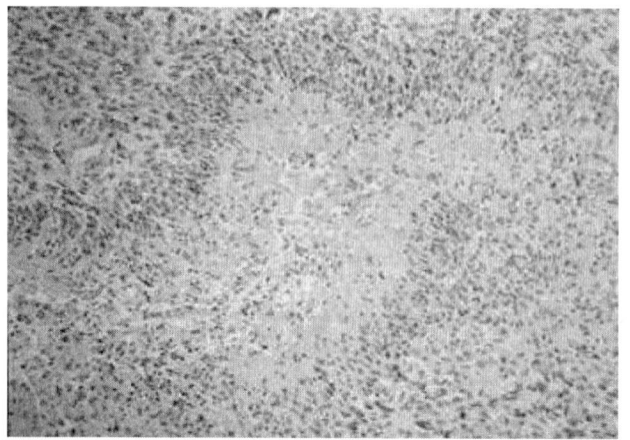

FIGURE 2. Glioblastoma multiforme with the hallmark features of necrosis with peripheral pseudopalisading of neoplastic nuclei.

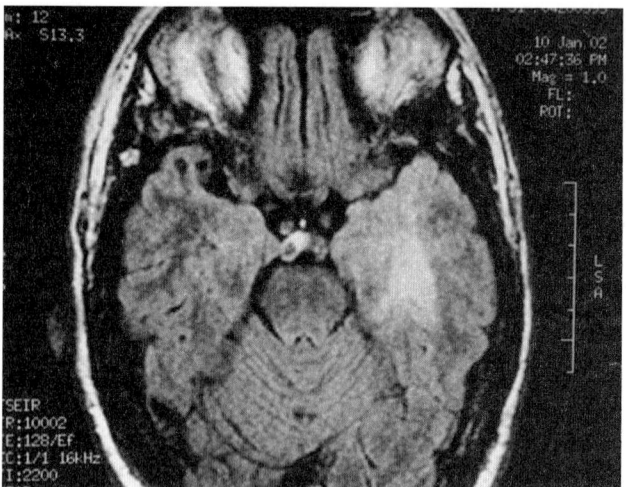

FIGURE 3. Axial magnetic resonance imaging scan of low-grade astrocytoma of left temporal lobe.

altered, indicating that deferring postoperative therapy is an option for selected group of patients. Evidence also indicates that lower doses of radiation therapy are probably as effective as higher doses of radiation for low-grade gliomas.

Randomized trials provide seminal evidence that external beam irradiation favorably affects the outcome of malignant gliomas. These trials demonstrate both a significant survival advantage and ability to maintain a full or partial working capacity for irradiated patients.

Chemotherapy

Chemotherapy has little established role in adult low-grade astrocytomas, but adjuvant chemotherapy is part of the standard therapeutic regimen for malignant gliomas. The addition of chemotherapy to radiation therapy improves the 1-year survival by 10% and the 2-year survival by 8.6%. The nitrosoureas, especially BCNU (N,N'-bis(2-chloroethyl)-N-nitrosourea, carmustine), are the most active single agents. No benefit of chemotherapeutical agents such

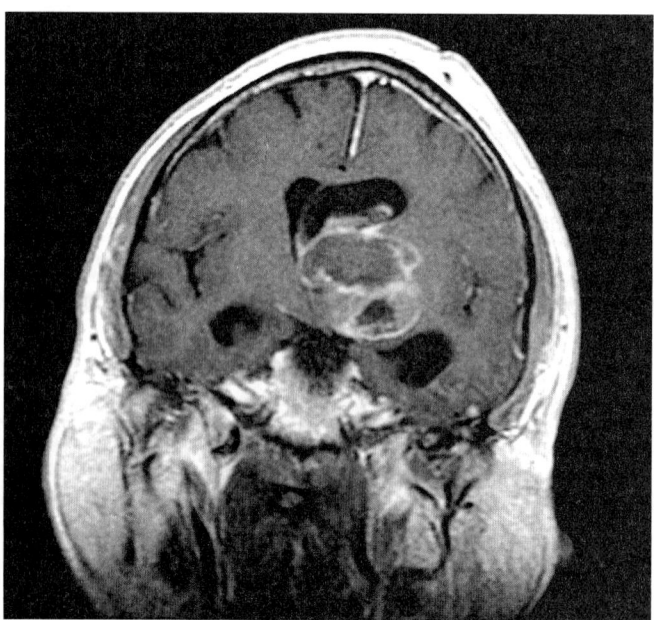

FIGURE 4. Coronal magnetic resonance imaging scan of high-grade astrocytoma of left internal capsule and brainstem region.

as tirapazamine, topotecan (Hycamtin), paclitaxel (Taxol), B-IFN (Avonex), and thalidomide (Thalomid) is noted when used with standard radiation in clinical trials. Temozolomide (Temodar) is an alkylating agent that demonstrates an improvement in survival by an additional 2 to 3 months when given concurrently with radiation in high-grade gliomas. Anaplastic oligodendrogliomas are chemosensitive tumors. PCV (procarbazine, lomustine [CCNU], and vincristine) chemotherapy regimens produce response rates of 50% to 75% in both recurrent and newly diagnosed anaplastic oligodendrogliomas. Unfortunately, improved response to chemotherapy does not translate into improved survival for these tumors.

Some of the newer biologic agents explored today in gliomas include anti-angiogenic agents, tyrosine kinase inhibitors, matrix metalloproteinase inhibitors, and antitenascin antibodies.

Outcome

The 5-year recurrence-free survival rates of patients with low-grade astrocytomas or mixed oligoastrocytomas who undergo total or radical subtotal tumor resection range from 52% to 95%. The median survival times for high-grade gliomas using conventional radiation therapy alone or with chemotherapy consistently range from 9 to 14 months. The median survival for patients with glioblastoma multiforme is 10 to 12 months, whereas the 3-year survival rate is only 6% to 8%. The median survival for patients with anaplastic astrocytoma is 36 months, and the 3-year survival rate is approximately 50%.

Uncommon Primary Brain Tumors

PRIMARY CENTRAL NERVOUS SYSTEM LYMPHOMA

Primary CNS lymphomas (PCNSLs) represent approximately to 2% to 5% of all intracranial neoplasms. During the decade from 1985 to 1994, the incidence had increased in both the AIDS and immunocompetent general population by fivefold. However, over the past 10 years, with the introduction of more effective anti-retroviral therapy, the incidence has decreased significantly. PCNSLs most frequently arise in the supratentorial paraventricular region of the brain. Multifocal tumors are present at diagnosis in 25% to 50% of immunocompetent patients and in 60% to 80% of AIDS patients. Cytologic examination of CPF reveals malignant cells in up to two thirds of immunocompetent patients and in nearly all AIDS patients. The neoplastic cells are similar to those of non-Hodgkin's lymphoma arising in extranodal sites. Single or multiple uniformly contrast-enhancing lesions in the paraventricular regions, basal ganglia, thalamus, or corpus callosum on MRI are characteristic findings.

The role of surgery is to establish a tissue diagnosis only. Primary CNS lymphomas respond dramatically to corticosteroid therapy. At least 90% of patients improve clinically, whereas 40% of lesions shrink considerably. Methotrexate-based chemotherapy and whole-brain irradiation with corticosteroids is the standard treatment for PCNSL. Recommended doses range from 36 to 45 Gy. Several reports document improved survival when chemotherapy is added to radiation therapy. The outcome is better with high-dose methotrexate-based regimens, often combined with intrathecal chemotherapy.

Survival times for primary CNS lymphoma with no treatment or steroids alone are approximately 1 to 4 months. The median survival for radiotherapy alone varies from 12 to 20 months. Median survival times for treatment programs that include high-dose methotrexate-based chemotherapy range from 33 to 42 months.

EPENDYMOMA

Ependymomas represent approximately 5% of all intracranial gliomas. The incidence peaks at 5 years and again at 34 years of age. Approximately 60% to 70% of ependymomas arise in the infratentorial brain. Ependymomas are separated into low-grade and high-grade lesions. The 5-year survival for low-grade tumors ranges from 60% to 80%, whereas it varies from 10% to 47% for high-grade tumors. Supratentorial ependymomas generally have a poorer prognosis than their infratentorial counterparts.

Most ependymomas cannot be completely excised because of their location and growth characteristics. Postoperative irradiation improves local tumor control and survival and is an accepted part of the standard treatment for these tumors. Although most ependymomas are slow growing, others are more aggressive and may disseminate throughout the CSF pathways. Current therapy for high-grade ependymomas after surgical debulking is with local fields to a dose of 59.4 Gy. The value of chemotherapy in adults with ependymomas and anaplastic ependymomas is not well defined.

BRAINSTEM GLIOMA

Brainstem gliomas account for less than 2% of brain tumors. Children constitute approximately two thirds of the reported cases. Diagnostic imaging is sufficient for the majority of the cases. The role of surgery is minimal and limited to biopsy only if there are questions about the diagnosis. Radiation therapy alone by conventional fractionation to 54 Gy in symptomatic or large brainstem lesions is recommended. Chemotherapy does not show any benefit in the management of brainstem gliomas. The median survival time is 9 to 12 months.

MEDULLOBLASTOMA

Medulloblastoma accounts for a third of pediatric brain tumors and is the most common tumor arising in the posterior fossa in children. It arises from the roof of the fourth ventricle or from the vermis. The presenting symptoms include headache, vomiting, and imbalance. On microscopic examination, small blue undifferentiated cells are noted consistent with primitive neuroectodermal tumor. CSF involvement is noted in 25% to 40% of the patients. Five-year survival rates range from 50% to 80%, and 10-year rates vary from 40% to 55%.

Surgery involves maximal resection of the tumor. Radiation therapy to the entire craniospinal axis is essential. The dose to the craniospinal axis is 23.4 to 36 Gy. A boost of 18 to 31.4 Gy is given to the posterior fossa to bring the total to 54 Gy. The role of chemotherapy is to decrease the craniospinal radiation dose and to improve the survival in poor-risk patients. Combinations of vincristine, CCNU, and *cis-* platinum are used.

Brain Metastases

EPIDEMIOLOGY

Metastases to the brain occur in as many as 30% of patients with systemic cancer and represent the most common type of intracranial tumor. Brain metastases exert a profound effect on the quality and length of survival, and despite the best current management, they represent the direct cause of death in 25% to 30% of affected patients. Melanoma and carcinomas of the lung, breast, and colorectum have a higher propensity to metastasize to the brain. Approximately 50% of patients present with a solitary lesion. Most brain metastases, particularly those that arise from primary sites other than the lung, occur at a late stage when metastatic dissemination is present elsewhere in the body.

STANDARD TREATMENT APPROACHES

Because the majority of patients with metastatic brain lesions have or will soon develop widely disseminated disease, treatment is dictated by the need to achieve immediate short-term palliation and the desire for durable symptom-free remission. The median survival of patients with symptomatic brain metastases is approximately 1 month without treatment and 2 months with corticosteroid administration. Survival is longer and the quality of life better if brain metastases are treated.

Corticosteroids

Corticosteroids rapidly ameliorate many symptoms of brain metastasis and should be used at the onset for all symptomatic patients. Symptomatic but stable patients can begin with approximately 16 mg of dexamethasone daily in two to four divided doses. Patients who are receiving whole-brain irradiation should receive steroids for at least 48 hours before treatment. Steroid tapering may begin during week 2 of radiotherapy. For patients receiving 16 mg of dexamethasone, the drug should be tapered by 2 to 4 mg every fifth day.

Surgery

Surgery establishes the diagnosis of metastatic brain disease when it is uncertain and serves as a treatment for single metastases. Surgery can provide better local control and immediate relief of neurologic signs and symptoms because of a mass effect. Surgically treated patients also live longer, have fewer recurrences of cancer in the brain, and enjoy a better quality of life compared with those treated by radiotherapy alone. Only 10% of patients are ideal candidates for surgical extirpation, however.

Whole-Brain Radiation Therapy

Radiotherapy is the appropriate treatment for most patients with brain metastases, including those with multiple lesions and those with single metastases who are not candidates for surgery. The standard approach is to treat the whole brain to 30 Gy in 10 daily fractions over 2 weeks. Depending on the symptom, the response rate varies from 70% to 90%. Neurologic function is improved overall in 50% of patients. The median survival with radiation therapy is 4 to 6 months. Overall, 75 to 80% of remaining life is spent in an improved or stable neurologic state.

Stereotactic Radiosurgery

Stereotactic radiosurgery (SRS) is an excellent alternative to surgical extirpation of solitary and multiple brain metastases. The procedure involves the delivery of a single large dose of radiation to a small volume of the brain region under stereotactic frame guidance. Recently, data from a large randomized trial show that addition of SRS to whole-brain radiation therapy improves both the survival and the quality of life in patients with limited brain metastases. Although surgery and SRS have never been compared directly in a clinical trial, local control, survival, and quality of life in selected patients seem comparable in retrospective trials.

Chemotherapy

Chemotherapy can be considered in selected patients who progress locally after whole-brain irradiation. Systemic chemotherapy shows a response rate of 25% to 50%. Temozolomide shows promise both as an adjuvant to whole-brain radiation therapy and in patients who fail radiation therapy.

REFERENCES

Andrews DW, Scott CB, Sperduto PW, et al: Whole brain radiation therapy with or without stereotactic radiosurgery boost for patients with one to three brain metastases: Phase III results of the RTOG 9508 randomised trial. Lancet 2004;363:1665-1672.

Deangelis LM, Hormigo A: Treatment of primary central nervous system lymphoma. Semin Oncol 2004;31:684-692.

Henson JW, Gaviani P, Gonzalez RG: MRI in treatment of adult gliomas. Lancet Oncol 2005;6:167-175.

Jemal A, Tiwari RC, Murray T, et al: Cancer statistics, 2004. CA Cancer J Clin 2004;54:8-29.

Kleihues P, Cavenee WK: Pathology and Genetics: Tumours of the Nervous System, 2nd ed. Lyon, France: IARC Press, 2000, pp 6-7.

Narayana A, Leibel SA: Primary and metastatic brain tumors in adults. In Leibel SA, Philips TL (eds): Textbook of Radiation Oncology, 2nd ed., Philadelphia: WB Saunders, 2004, pp 463-496.

Patchell RA, Tibbs PA, Regine WF, et al: Postoperative radiotherapy in the treatment of single metastases to the brain: A randomized trial. JAMA 1998;280:1485-1490.

Reifenberger G, Collins VP: Pathology and molecular genetics of astrocytic gliomas. J Mol Med 2004;82:656-670.

SECTION 15

The Locomotor System

Rheumatoid Arthritis

Method of
Eric L. Matteson, MD, MPH

Rheumatoid arthritis (RA) is a common chronic disease of the immune system characterized by polyarthritis and a variety of systemic features. It often leads to articular cartilage and bone damage, physical dysfunction, and work disability. The disease affects 1% to 2% of persons worldwide, typically developing in the fourth to sixth decades, with predominance among women of approximately 2.5:1. RA may be associated with extra-articular inflammatory features, including fatigue, subcutaneous nodules, pleuritis and pericarditis, interstitial lung disease, vasculitis, and Sjögren's syndrome. Patients with RA have excess mortality due principally to extraarticular disease and increased atherosclerotic cardiovascular disease. Other concerns in RA patients are listed in Box 1.

Steady decline in joint function caused by progressive cartilage damage, bone erosions, and tendon rupture as well as systemic features are responsible for work disability rates among patients with RA that are more than 50% within 10 years of disease onset. Joint damage begins early, and bone erosions are detectable within 2 years of disease onset in as many as 70% of patients. In some patients, RA progresses rapidly, leading to early work disability if effective therapy is not started to control the inflammatory response and joint damage.

Initial treatment of the polyarthritis is with a combination of nonsteroidal anti-inflammatory agents (NSAIDs) and when needed corticosteroids to provide sufficient time to confirm the persistence of joint inflammation and complete the diagnostic evaluation. Disease-modifying antirheumatic drugs (DMARDs) are then added, because over the long term they lessen joint damage and disability. DMARDs (Box 2) are defined by the ability to reduce the signs and symptoms as well as slow the progression of joint damage, as measured by radiographic changes in the amount of bone erosions and joint space narrowing.

Prompt DMARD treatment is critical to improve disease control and outcome. The goals of treatment include:

- Early diagnosis and intervention
- First-line therapy with DMARDs that reduces progressive joint damage followed by adding to or changing DMARDs if disease activity persists
- Management of comorbidities such as disease- and treatment-related osteoporosis

DMARDs that can be used effectively alone or in combination represent an important advance in treatment. Still, RA remains a chronic illness, usually requiring lifelong anti-inflammatory and immunomodulating treatment to limit joint damage and minimize disability (see Box 2).

Diagnosis

In the absence of a definitive diagnostic test, the diagnosis of RA is based on clinical features and supportive laboratory tests. The American College of Rheumatology (ACR) 1987 criteria require at least four of seven features to be present for longer than 6 weeks to classify a patient as having RA for the purpose of clinical research (Table 1). The ACR criteria are highly sensitive (95%) but only modestly specific (75% to 89%) for making the clinical diagnosis of RA in patients with established disease.

Characteristic radiographic lesions are only present in up to 70% of patients within the first 2 years of disease. Recently, both musculoskeletal ultrasound (US) and magnetic resonance imaging (MRI)

BOX 1 General Medical Concerns in Rheumatoid Arthritis

- Infection
  - Immunizations
  - Prompt treatment of infections
  - Tuberculosis and hepatitis screenings
- Lifestyle
  - Control of blood pressure (corticosteroids, NSAIDs, cyclosporine, extraarticular disease all contribute to hypertension)
  - Control of lipids
  - Smoking cessation
- Prevention of GI bleeding
  - Antacids
  - Coxibs where appropriate
  - H_2-blockers
  - Proton pump inhibitors
  - Avoid NSAIDs whenever possible
- Osteoporosis treatment and prevention (osteoporosis is common in rheumatoid arthritis)
  - Calcium 1200-1500 mg/day
  - Vitamin D 400 IU/day
  - Consider an antiresorptive agent such as a bisphosphonate for all patients on long-term corticosteroids, including men
- Moisturization for patients with sicca symptoms

BOX 2 Drugs Used to Treat Rheumatoid Arthritis

Traditional DMARDs
- Azathioprine (Imuran)
- Cyclosporine (Neoral)
- Gold (intramuscular or oral) (Myochrysine, Auranofin)
- Hydroxychloroquine (Plaquenil)
- Leflunomide (Arava)
- Methotrexate (Trexall)
- Minocycline (Dynacin)
- Sulfasalazine (Azulfidine)

Biological Response Modifiers
- Anti B-cell therapy: Rituximab (Rituxan)
- Anti-TNF monoclonal antibodies
  - Adalimumab (Humira)
  - Infliximab (Remicade)
- Soluble TNF receptor
  - Etanercept (Enbrel)
- IL-1 receptor antagonist
  - Anakinra (Kineret)
- T-cell signaling inhibitor: Abatacept (Orencia)

Abbreviations: DMARD = disease-modifying antirheumatic drug; IL = interleukin; TNF = tumor necrosis factor.

TABLE 1 American College of Rheumatology Criteria for Rheumatoid Arthritis Diagnosis*

Criterion	Definition
Morning stiffness	In and around joints, lasting at least 1 h before maximal improvement
Arthritis in at least three joint areas	Simultaneously involved by soft tissue swelling or fluid observed by a physician
Arthritis of hand joints	At least one area swollen: wrist, MCP, PIP
Symmetric arthritis	Simultaneous involvement of the same joint areas on both sides of the body Bilateral involvement of PIPs, MCPs, or MTPs acceptable without absolute symmetry
Rheumatoid nodules	Subcutaneous nodules over bony prominences, extensor surfaces, or in extraarticular regions observed by a physician
Serum rheumatoid factor	Abnormal amounts by any method for which the result has been positive in <5% of normal control subjects
Radiographic changes	Typical of RA on posteroanterior hand and wrist radiographs, which must include erosions or unequivocal bony decalcification localized or most obvious adjacent to involved joints (osteoarthritis changes alone do not qualify)

Abbreviations: MCP = metacarpophalangeal; MTP = metatarsalphalangeal; PIP = proximal interphalangeal; RA = rheumatoid arthritis.
*Patient must satisfy four of the seven criteria listed. Criteria 1 through 4 must be present for at least 6 weeks.

have been shown to detect erosive lesions early in the disease course, in many cases before they are evident on plain radiographs. Antibodies to cyclic citrullinated peptides (anti-CCP) detected in serum aid the diagnosis. They are more specific but less sensitive for the diagnosis of RA than serum rheumatoid factor (RF). The presence of RF or anti-CCP increases the diagnostic sensitivity for RA to more than 80%; the presence of both increases diagnostic sensitivity to more than 95%.

Primary care providers play an important role in the diagnosis of RA. Recognition of inflammatory arthritis and prompt referral to rheumatologists lead to early initiation of effective joint-protective therapies. Early inflammatory polyarthritis might not always meet diagnostic criteria for RA; however, approximately 30% of these cases of undifferentiated arthritis ultimately evolve into RA (see Table 1).

The importance of early accurate diagnosis of RA has grown with evidence that early DMARD therapy can alter the natural history of the disease. Strategies using single or a combination of initial DMARD therapies are employed. Studies of initial combinations of traditional DMARDs such as methotrexate (Trexall), sulfasalazine (Azulfidine), and hydroxychloroquine (Plaquenil) have shown that early introduction of combination therapy with and without corticosteroids improves long-term radiographic outcomes. The more intensive use of DMARDs, especially methotrexate and the biological response modifiers, has lessened disability and improved survival in patients with RA. Treatment with the more aggressive use of DMARDs has resulted in a decreasing need for joint surgery in recent years.

Treatment

THERAPEUTIC GOALS

Successful treatment of RA is predicated on reductions in symptomatic joint pain and swelling, relief of joint stiffness, return of lost function, and prevention of joint damage (Figure 1). Clinically, response to therapy can be determined by examining joints for tenderness and swelling, obtaining laboratory measures of inflammation (erythrocyte sedimentation rate [ESR] and C-reactive protein [CRP]), and assessing patient-reported outcomes using questionnaires, such as the Health Assessment Questionnaire (HAQ), or visual analogue scales of global well-being. Long-term therapy goals include reducing joint damage (joint erosions and joint space narrowing), missed work days, delaying disability, and decreasing early mortality (see Figure 1).

Both short- and long-term goals can be reached using DMARDs, which reduce joint inflammation and retard the development of radiographic joint damage. The most commonly used DMARD, methotrexate, has a long track record of efficacy and acceptable toxicity and is often the treatment with which other agents or regimens are compared. Other DMARDs used previously for the treatment of RA, such as gold salts, penicillamine (Cuprimine), azathioprine (Imuran), and cyclophosphamide (Cytoxan),[1] are rarely used today because of either relatively poor efficacy or excessive toxicity.

Biological response modifiers (BRMs) have been a major advance in RA therapy for many patients with RA, with improved safety and efficacy profiles. The Current Therapy box summarizes the current treatment approaches to RA. Box 3 summarizes drug therapy for RA.

METHOTREXATE

Methotrexate (MTX) is a purine antimetabolite that reduces symptoms of joint inflammation and decreases radiographic joint damage in patients with RA. MTX is the most common anchor DMARD. It is generally well tolerated. Most patients still use the drug after 5 years of treatment.

Side effects may be minor, including nausea, diarrhea, mucosal ulcerations, and alopecia. Serious complications include hepatotoxicity and bone marrow suppression. Hepatotoxicity is typically characterized by fibrosis and cirrhosis, which occur rarely with frequent monitoring for possible toxicity. Minor toxicities are an infrequent

---

[1] Not FDA approved for this indication.

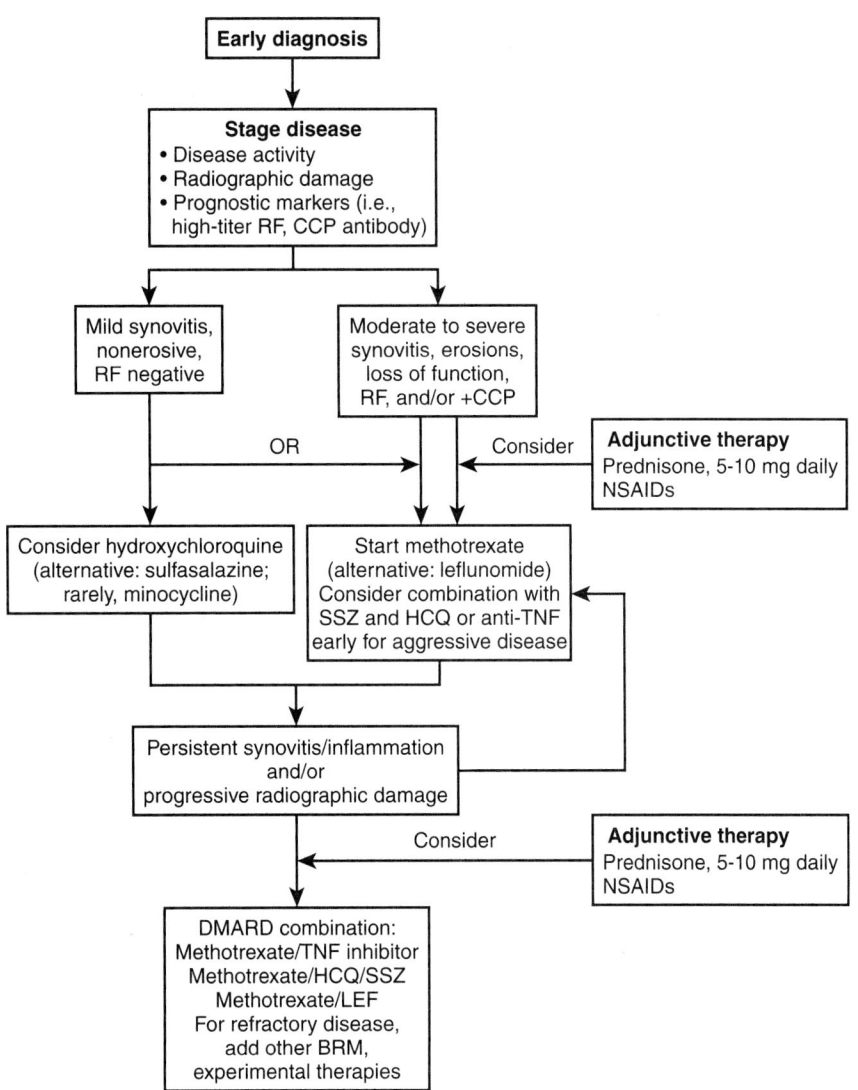

FIGURE 1. This flow diagram illustrates key decision points for rheumatoid arthritis therapy and has been adapted from the recommendations of the American College of Rheumatology. *Abbreviations:* BRM = biological response modifier; CCP = anticyclic citrullinated antibody; DMARD = disease-modifying, antirheumatic drug; HCQ = hydroxychloroquine; LEF = leflunomide; MTX = methotrexate; NSAID = nonsteroidal anti-inflammatory drug; RA = rheumatoid arthritis; RF = rheumatoid factor; SSZ = sulfasalazine; TNF = tumor necrosis factor. (From the American College of Rheumatology Subcommittee on Rheumatoid Arthritis Guidelines: Guidelines for the management of rheumatoid arthritis: 2002 update. Arthritis Rheum 2002;46:328-323.)

cause of MTX discontinuance and can often be managed with folic acid supplementation or by switching from oral to parenteral administration. ACR guidelines recommend monitoring hepatic transaminases and serum albumin at 4- to 8-week intervals and reserving liver biopsy for an otherwise unexplained decrease in albumin or persistent or recurrent elevation of transaminases.

MTX-induced pneumonitis is rare. It typically develops early after initiation and is characterized by cough, dyspnea, and fever. Chest radiographs reveal diffuse interstitial changes. Pneumonitis should be managed by immediately discontinuing the drug and considering corticosteroid treatment in severe cases. Pneumonitis often recurs with rechallenge; therefore, patients experiencing this complication should be treated with an alternative DMARD. MTX is contraindicated in patients with impaired renal function, because delayed clearance increases drug levels and, hence, the risk of side effects.

MTX is administered in once-weekly doses. It is important to maximize the beneficial effects of MTX by titrating to 20 to 25 mg[3]

---

[3]Exceeds dosage recommended by the manufacturer.

per week, because lower doses are often less effective. There has been little additional benefit observed in patients treated with doses greater than 25 mg per week; however, toxicities become more common at these higher doses. Folic acid (folate), generally 1 mg daily, reduces the occurrence and frequency of some toxicities (Table 2).

INHIBITORS OF TUMOR NECROSIS FACTOR-α

TNF-α is a pleiotropic cytokine expressed by activated T lymphocytes and macrophages. It upregulates production of other proinflammatory cytokines, including interleukin 1 (IL-1) and IL-6, matrix metalloproteinases, and reactive oxygen intermediates, that provoke inflammation and injure articular cartilage and bone. In addition, TNF-α is an important promoter of immune-competent cells including receptor activation of nuclear factor-κB ligand (RANK ligand) expression that leads to differentiation and activation of osteoclasts. In RA, osteoclasts are responsible for articular bone loss characterized by erosions and osteopenia. TNF-α also has a role in the differentiation of synoviocytes into a fibroblastic phenotype that confers invasive, tumor-like qualities on these cells. Fibroblast-like synoviocytes

> **BOX 3   Drug Therapy for Rheumatoid Arthritis**
>
> **Control of Symptoms: Pain and Swelling, Loss of Function**
>
> *NSAIDs and Other Analgesics as Needed*
> - Consider patient age, sex, past medical history (GI bleeding, etc.).
> - Consider cost and convenience (dosing frequency).
> - These are not disease modifying.
>
> *Corticosteroids*
> - Oral.
>   - It is controversial whether corticosteroids are disease modifying. In general, less is better.
>   - Severe polyarticular disease: 2-15 mg/d, often in divided doses (e.g., 2 mg tid). Use split dosing because of the short half-life of the anti-inflammatory effect of oral steroids. It is desirable but often not possible to avoid continuous corticosteroid therapy.
>   - Serious systemic disease (vasculitis, scleritis): 40-60 mg/d, tapering according to response.
> - Intraarticular for single recalcitrant joints.
>
> **Control of Disease with DMARDs**
> DMARDs may be used with NSAIDs. Corticosteroids may be given if needed.
>
> *Initiating DMARD Therapy*
> - Start DMARD therapy as soon as the diagnosis is strongly suspected or established.
>   - Mild disease: MTX is preferred; hydroxychloroquine and sulfasalazine are also useful.
>   - Moderate disease: MTX or leflunomide (±hydroxychloroquine, sulfasalazine, others). Use bridge therapy: Initially treat with a combination of DMARDs ±corticosteroids, tapering off steroids and DMARDs as disease is better controlled. Biological response modifiers may be considered at this point.
>   - Severe or recalcitrant disease: Combination therapies of two or three DMARDs. Add biological response modifier therapy; consider experimental therapies.
> - In general, the effect of DMARDs is apparent in 1 to 4 wk (BRMs) to 1 to 2 mo (MTX, leflunomide). It can take 3 to 6 mo to know whether hydroxychloroquine or sulfasalazine are effective.
> - Add to or change DMARDs within 3 to 4 mo of initiating therapy if there has not been an adequate response.
>
> *Tapering DMARD Therapy*
> - Rheumatoid arthritis is a chronic condition. The goal of therapy is long-term disease control and prevention of joint and organ damage. DMARDs can only infrequently be stopped without disease recrudescence.
> - When symptoms are well controlled, taper corticosteroids, then taper the NSAIDs (or use NSAIDs on an as-needed basis).
> - Continue with DMARD therapy indefinitely. If the patient does well and has no signs of active disease for 6 to 12 mo, the DMARD therapy can be carefully tapered.
> - If the patient is doing well on combination DMARD therapy, attempt to taper one of these drugs. MTX is often viewed as anchor therapy and generally is continued long term if the patient is on baseline MTX.
> - If a patient is on combination therapy, consider tapering one of the DMARDs if the patient has been in remission for at least 6 mo.
> - DMARD therapy should not be completely discontinued until a patient has been in complete remission for at least 1 y on treatment. Even then, a very few patients with bona fide, seropositive rheumatoid arthritis remain in treatment-free remission.
>
> **Extra-articular Disease**
> - Serositis, vasculitis, and scleritis require systemic corticosteroids and might require immunosuppressive agents such as cyclophosphamide[1] or cyclosporine.
> - Consider BRMs, especially anti-B-cell therapy, for severe extraarticular disease (scleritis, pneumonitis, vasculitis).
>
> [1]Not FDA approved for this indication.
> *Abbreviations:* BRM = biological response modifier; DMARD = disease-modifying antirheumatic drug; MTX = methotrexate; NSAID = nonsteroidal anti-inflammatory drug.

form the synovial pannus, a tumor-like mass unique to rheumatoid joints that invades and damages cartilage.

Clinical studies of several TNF-inhibiting agents have demonstrated the therapeutic benefits of TNF blockade on RA disease activity and joint damage. The three TNF-inhibiting drugs approved for the treatment of RA—etanercept (Enbrel), infliximab (Remicade), and adalimumab (Humira)—appear similarly efficacious for the treatment of this disease, but they have not been directly compared in clinical trials. Many clinical trials have compared treatment using TNF inhibitors and MTX to placebo-control patients on MTX alone. In these trials, 40% to 60% of patients on anti-TNF agents met ACR-20 criteria for improvement at week 20 (Box 4). Approximately 10% to 20% of patients improved even more, reaching ACR-70 criteria.

The TNF-blocking agents are generally well tolerated. However, an increased risk of reactivation of latent tuberculosis has led to the recommendation in the United States and certain other countries that a purified protein derivative (PPD) skin test should be performed before the patient begins taking a TNF inhibitor. A chest radiograph should be obtained in patients with a history of tuberculosis exposure, positive PPD, or emigration from countries where tuberculosis is endemic. Patients who have a positive PPD or history

TABLE 2 Disease-Modifying Antirheumatic Drug Monitoring

DMARD	Tests	Interval
Methotrexate (MTX, Trexall)	Hepatic transaminases, serum creatinine, CBC, albumin	Baseline and every 4-8 wk
	CXR, HBV and HCV serology, β-hCG	Baseline
Leflunomide (Arava)	Hepatic transaminases, serum creatinine, CBC, albumin, HBV and HCV serology, β-hCG	Baseline
	ALT	Monthly for 6 mo, then every 6-8 wk
	Hepatic transaminases, serum creatinine, CBC, albumin	Every 6-8 wk
TNF inhibitors: etanercept (Enbrel), infliximab (Remicade), adalimumab (Humira)	PPD, CXR (if positive PPD, emigration from TB-endemic country, or TB exposure history), CBC	Baseline, thereafter undetermined
Sulfasalazine (Azulfidine)	CBC, hepatic transaminases, creatinine	Baseline and then every 2 wk for 1-3 mo, then every 4 wk for 3 mo, then every 12 wk
Hydroxychloroquine (Plaquenil)	Ophthalmologic evaluation: visual acuity and retinal function tests	Baseline and then yearly
Cyclosporine (Neoral)	Serum creatinine, hepatic transaminases, CBC, potassium, BP	Baseline and then every 2 wk until dosage is stable, then every mo
Azathioprine (Imuran)	CBC, hepatic transaminases, creatinine	Baseline and then every 2 wk for 2-3 mo, then monthly for 3 mo, then every 2-3 mo
Anakinra (Kineret)	CBC	Baseline, then undetermined
Rituximab (Rituxan)	CBC, screen PPD, CXR, HBV and HCV serology	Baseline, then undetermined
Abatacept (Orencia)	CBC, screen PPD, CXR, HBV and HCV serology	Baseline, then undetermined

Abbreviations: ALT = alanine aminotransferase; BP = blood pressure; CBC = complete blood count; CXR = chest radiograph; DMARD = disease-modifying antirheumatic drug; G6PD = glucose-6-phosphatase deficiency; HBV = hepatitis B virus; hCG = human chorionic gonadotropin; HCV = hepatitis C virus; PPD = purified protein derivative; TB = tuberculosis.

---

of tuberculosis should be treated with appropriate therapy before initiating anti-TNF agents.

Clinical trials of TNF inhibitors in patients with advanced congestive heart failure and multiple sclerosis suggest that these conditions may be exacerbated by these drugs. Demyelinating syndromes have been reported rarely in association with therapeutic TNF blockade. TNF inhibitors have been associated in trials with a slight increase in minor infections (primarily upper respiratory), although concerns about increased overall risk of infection with TNF therapy remains undefined. Postmarking surveillance suggests that infections with organisms that promote granulomatous inflammatory responses, such as histoplasmosis, coccidioidomycosis, and listeriosis might occur more often in patients treated with TNF inhibitors. There have been rare reports of lupus-like syndromes characterized by rash, serositis, and development of antinuclear and anti–double-stranded DNA autoantibodies.

Three TNF-inhibiting agents are commercially available. Etanercept is a soluble TNF-receptor type II (p75)-to-Fc fusion protein. Infliximab is a chimeric human-to-mouse monoclonal anti-TNF antibody, and adalimumab is a fully human anti-TNF monoclonal antibody. Etanercept (Enbrel) is administered by a subcutaneous injection at a dose of 25 mg twice weekly or 50 mg once weekly. Adalimumab is administered subcutaneously at a dose of 40 mg every 2 weeks. Infliximab is given as an intravenous infusion. Standard initial dosing for infliximab calls for 3 mg/kg to be given at 0, 2, and 6 weeks, followed by regular infusions at 8-week intervals. The dosage may vary among patients from 3 to 10 mg/kg, and the interval may be adjusted between 4 and 8 weeks, depending on the patient's clinical response.

Although TNF inhibitors may be used as monotherapy, more commonly, they are added to MTX or other DMARD therapy to improve disease control and possibly reduce some antibody formation, especially with infliximab. However, clinical trials in early RA suggest that combining MTX with a TNF inhibitor may be more effective than either therapy alone.

OTHER DISEASE-MODIFYING ANTIRHEUMATIC DRUGS

Other DMARDs may be used alone or in combination to treat RA. Some traditional DMARDs such as gold and D-penicillamine are now rarely used because of poor efficacy and toxicity. In some cases of mild RA, agents such as hydroxychloroquine or minocycline (Dynacin)[1] may be useful. Hydroxychloroquine is an antimalarial drug that may be used alone in early and mild RA or as part of a combination regimen (see Box 3). It is typically prescribed at doses of 5 to 7.5 mg/kg/day (200-400 mg daily). The primary serious side effect, although rare, is retinal toxicity, so routine (at least annual) ophthalmologic evaluation is suggested. Gastrointestinal side effects and skin rashes can also occur.

Leflunomide (Arava) is a pyrimidine antimetabolite that has been shown in clinical trials to be as efficacious as MTX. The recommended starting dose is 20 mg/day. The dose may be reduced to 10 mg/day when used in combination with MTX or if the starting dose is not tolerated. Leflunomide side effects are typically observed

---

BOX 4 American College of Rheumatology Criteria for Improvement in Rheumatoid Arthritis

- Requires 20% improvement in the following two:
  - Tender joint count (68 joints)
  - Swollen joint count (66 joints)
- Requires 20% improvement in each of the first three:
  - Patient assessment of pain (10 cm visual analogue scale)
  - Patient assessment of disease activity (10 cm visual analogue scale)
  - Physician global assessment of disease activity (10 cm visual analogue scale)
  - Patient assessment of physical function (HAQ score)
  - Serum CRP or erythrocyte sedimentation rate

Abbreviations: CRP = C-reactive protein; HAQ = Health Assessment Questionnaire; RA = rheumatoid arthritis.

---

[1] Not FDA approved for this indication.

beginning 2 to 4 weeks after starting treatment. The most important serious toxicities are hepatoxicity and cytopenias. Therefore, laboratory monitoring (see Table 2) of hepatic transaminases and a complete blood count should be performed at 4- to 8-week intervals. Some patients develop hypertension and peripheral neuropathy related to the drug. Leflunomide is an alternative to MTX as a first-line DMARD in patients intolerant of MTX or with mild renal insufficiency. Leflunomide may be used in combination with TNF inhibition.

Other DMARDs include sulfasalazine and cyclosporine (Neoral). With respect to efficacy, these agents are comparable with MTX as monotherapy, and they improve control of synovitis when combined with MTX. Sulfasalazine treatment is started at 500 mg twice daily and may be titrated gradually to 3.0 gm/day,[3] divided in two or three doses. Gastrointestinal toxicity can limit the dose. Interval monitoring for hepatotoxicity and cytopenias is also required (see Table 2). Cyclosporine is used at doses of 100 to 400 mg a day depending on body weight and tolerance. It is started at 2.0 to 2.5 mg/kg/day in two divided doses. It may be titrated to 4.5 to 5 mg/kg/day,[3] but the dose may be limited by hypertension or renal toxicity. Long-term side effects such as nephrotoxicity and hirsutism make it difficult for most patients to maintain therapy with cyclosporine for long periods.

Gold salts are now infrequently initiated for RA and have a generally unfavorable efficacy and safety profile. Many patients are forced to discontinue gold because of side effects that include cytopenia, nephropathy, and cutaneous hypersensitivity.

Anakinra (Kineret), a recombinant IL-1 receptor antagonist (IL-1ra), is a biological agent that blocks the proinflammatory activities of IL-1. IL-1 shares many of the proinflammatory actions of TNF-α in promoting the symptoms of arthritis and joint damage in RA. Anakinra is a naturally occurring anti-inflammatory molecule that competes with soluble IL-1β for binding to cells expressing the IL-1 receptor type 1. It reduces joint pain and swelling when administered in combination with MTX to patients with RA that is refractory to MTX monotherapy. Anakinra is given by self-administered daily subcutaneous injection (100 mg/day). Many patients develop local injection site reactions, but these are self-limited and usually subside over time. Anti-TNF agents are generally preferred over anakinra for reasons of efficacy and safety. The costs of all BRMs are substantial.

Azathioprine and cyclophosphamide are traditional cytotoxic agents that have demonstrated efficacy in RA, but their use is limited by toxicity. Cyclophosphamide in particular is usually reserved for life-threatening, extraarticular manifestations of RA such as interstitial lung disease or vasculitis.

ABATACEPT

Abatacept (Orencia; CTLA-4Ig) is a recombinant fusion protein that blocks T-cell activation by means of signaling inhibition. T-cell activation requires two signals, the first of which is related to antigen presentation through a major histocompatibility complex peptide and the second of which acts by binding of a T-cell costimulatory receptor to the antigen presenting cell (APC). This costimulatory signal occurs by CD28-CD80/86 (B7) binding to the ligand on the APC. With T-cell activation, cytotoxic T-lymphocyte associated antigen (CTLA-4) becomes expressed, leading to deactivation of T-cells. Competitive binding of CTLA-4 to CD80 and CD86 prevents this interaction between CD28 and CD80, thereby interfering with the second costimulatory signaling required for T-cell activation.

Studies of abatacept have demonstrated significant improvement in ACR20 responses used in patients with refractory disease. The drug is administered by 30-minute infusion, with the second infusion given at 2 weeks following the first infusion, then at 4 weeks following the first infusion, and then every 4 weeks thereafter. The dose is 500 to 1000 mg per infusion, depending on body weight. Side effects include hypersensitivity and possible increased risk of infections. It is not clear whether the drug predisposes to malignancy. Drug monitoring is, as yet, undefined. The drug may be used with conventional DMARDs but should not be used with other biological response modifiers.

RITUXIMAB

Rituximab (Rituxan) is a chimeric murine/human monoclonal antibody directed against the CD20 antigen on B-lymphocytes, leading to B-cell lysis. Like T cells, B cells play an important role in the pathophysiology of rheumatoid arthritis and are important to T-cell activation, cytokine production, and production of rheumatoid factor. Rituximab use results in prompt depletion of peripheral B-lymphocytes, which can remain depleted for months and even years following therapy. Standard treatment in rheumatoid arthritis is an initial dose of rituximab at 1000 mg given at 2-week intervals. Patients often require re-treatment after a varying amount of time, generally after 6 months. The B cells may be peripherally depleted even with recrudescence of disease, so they have not been useful parameters to follow for disease remission or recrudescence.

Rituximab is usually administered together with methotrexate. Acute infusion reactions can occur; methylprednisolone (Solu-Medrol), 100 mg IV is recommended 30 minutes before each infusion to reduce the probability and severity of infusion reactions. Rituximab can lead to severe hypersensitivity reactions and possibly infections. However, serious infections have not been demonstrated to be more common in rituximab-treated patients than in placebo-treated patients.

COMBINATION THERAPY

Although many patients' disease appears to be well controlled using a simple DMARD, persistent synovitis or progressive radiographic joint damage is common with such an approach. The current treatment paradigm favors a rapid step-up strategy, which calls for the addition of a second or third DMARD if synovitis persists despite adequate dosing with a single DMARD (see Box 3). One approach is to add a TNF inhibitor to MTX. Another approach is triple therapy, which consists of sulfasalazine and hydroxychloroquine in addition to MTX. Biologic response modifiers should not be combined with each other. Available data suggest that combination therapy improves radiographic and functional outcomes for patients with RA inadequately controlled with a single DMARD.

CORTICOSTEROIDS

Corticosteroids are potent anti-inflammatory agents used since 1948 for controlling signs and symptoms of synovitis in RA. The use of corticosteroids in RA is limited by the side effects associated with long-term therapy and by concerns about their effectiveness as true DMARDs. For short periods, higher doses (0.25-0.5 mg/kg/day) may be used to control severe flare-ups of arthritis (see Box 3). However, corticosteroids are most commonly used in low daily doses (5 to 10 mg/day) as bridge treatment while a concomitantly administered DMARD takes effect or as adjuvant therapy to control persistent symptoms in patients with DMARD-refractory disease.

In clinical studies, low-dose corticosteroids can reduce the number of radiographic erosions that develop early after disease onset. These doses are rarely sufficient to completely control synovitis and are, therefore, most commonly used in conjunction with traditional DMARDs or biological agents. Low-dose corticosteroids are generally well tolerated, but complications, particularly osteoporosis and diabetes, are possible and the patient should be carefully monitored for them. Intraarticular injection of corticosteroids is useful for managing individual inflamed joints or joints responding slowly to systemic therapies.

NONSTEROIDAL ANTI-INFLAMMATORY DRUGS

NSAIDs are widely used to reduce pain, swelling, and stiffness in joints affected by RA. Although NSAIDs are useful adjunctive agents, they are not considered disease-modifying drugs. Traditional NSAIDs inhibit cyclooxygenase (COX) enzymes and thereby block the conversion of arachidonic acid into prostaglandins, molecules that can stimulate

---
[3]Exceeds dosage recommended by the manufacturer.

CURRENT THERAPY

- The goals of therapy are the control of symptoms, prevention of joint destruction and loss of function, and prevention and management of disability.

Classes of Agents

- Analgesics and NSAIDs, including aspirin and coxibs
- Second-line or slow-acting antirheumatic drugs (DMARDs)
  - Synthetic DMARDs
    - Hydroxychloroquine, methotrexate, sulfasalazine, gold, azathioprine, leflunomide
  - Biological response modifiers
    - TNF-antagonists: adalimumab, etanercept, infliximab
    - IL-1 receptor antagonist: anakinra
    - T-cell signaling inhibitor abatacept
    - B-cell depletion: rituximab
  - Others
    - Experimental and chemotherapeutic agents including cyclophosphamide, cyclosporine;
    - Minocycline
    - D-Penicillamine[1] and gold now rarely used
  - Glucocorticosteroids

Treatment Strategy: Early in the Disease

- Proper diagnosis is essential
- Physical modalities
  - Physical therapy, occupational therapy consultation
  - Joint protection and functional enhancement
  - Splints, orthotics, adaptive and adequate footwear, adaptive devices
  - Range-of-motion exercises for affected joints
  - Appropriate stretching, strengthening, and conditioning exercises
- Disease education
  - Disease treatment and prognosis
  - Vocational and avocational counseling
  - Lifestyle and family counseling
  - Self-esteem
  - Home modifications

[1]Not FDA approved for this indication.
Abbreviations: coxib = selective cyclooxygenase-2 inhibitor; DMARD = disease-modifying antirheumatic drug; GI = gastrointestinal; IL = interleukin; NSAID = nonsteroidal anti-inflammatory drug.

inflammation. There are two major forms of COX enzymes, COX-1 and COX-2. COX-1 is expressed constitutively in the gastric mucosa, where it functions to protect the stomach from luminal acid secretion, and in the kidney, where it serves to maintain renal perfusion. COX-2 is expressed at sites of inflammation and is also expressed constitutively in the kidney.

Traditional NSAIDs, which block the function of both COX-1 and COX-2, have anti-inflammatory effects, but they also produce gastrointestinal toxicity that can manifest as gastritis, peptic ulcers, and hemorrhage, or enteritis. NSAID toxicity may be significantly reduced by proton pump inhibitor therapy. NSAIDs that specifically antagonize COX-2 activity, termed *coxibs* (celecoxib [Celebrex]), have anti-inflammatory efficacy similar to that of the nonselective NSAIDs, but they cause less gastrointestinal toxicity. The gastrointestinal benefits of coxibs may be reduced by the concurrent use of aspirin. Coxibs have a variable propensity to increase the risk of cardiovascular and cerebrovascular events.

Summary

The effectiveness of RA treatment has improved dramatically with recent advances in early diagnosis, the development of less toxic and more effective disease-modifying treatments, and more intensive DMARD regimens that control persistent synovitis and progressive radiographic damage. Recognition of the impact of associated disorders including osteoporosis and atherosclerotic disease, in addition to appropriate therapeutic intervention for these disorders, will likely result in improved morbidity and mortality rates among patients with RA. Most patients today are able to live productively with RA because of the timely use of effective DMARDs, including BRMs, to control the signs and symptoms of disease. The future holds an improved diagnostic and therapeutic armamentarium, which promises to afford even better disease control and less disability.

REFERENCES

Arnett FC, Edworthy SM, Bloch DA, et al: The American Rheumatism Association in 1987 revised criteria for the classification of rheumatoid arthritis. Arthritis Rheum 1988;31:315-324.

Emery P, Fleischmann R, Filipowicz-Sosnowska A, et al: The efficacy and safety of rituximab in patients with active rheumatoid arthritis despite methotrexate treatment: Results of a phase IIB randomized, double-placebo-controlled, dose-ranging trial. Arthritis Rheum 2006;54:1390-1400.

Fries JF, Williams CA, Morfeld D, et al: Reduction in long-term disability in patients with rheumatoid arthritis by disease-modifying antirheumatic drug–based treatment strategies. Arthritis Rheum 1996;39:616-622.

Genovese NC, Becker JC, Schiff M, et al: Abatacept for rheumatoid arthritis refractory to tumor necrosis factor alpha inhibition. N Engl J Med 2005;353:1114-1123.

Kremer JM, Genovese MC, Cannon GW, et al: Concomitant leflunomide therapy in patients with active rheumatoid arthritis despite stable doses of methotrexate: A randomized, double-blind, placebo-controlled trial. Ann Intern Med 2002;137:726-733.

Landewe RB, Boers M, Verhoeven AC, et al: COBRA combination therapy in patients with early rheumatoid arthritis: Long-term structural benefits of a brief intervention. Arthritis Rheum 2002;46:347-356.

Lee D, Schur PH: Clinical utility of the anti-CCP assay in patients with rheumatic diseases. Ann Rheum Dis 2003;62:870-874.

Matteson EL: Extraarticular features of rheumatoid arthritis and systemic involvement. In MCHochberg, AJSilman, JSSmolen, et al, editors: Rheumatology, ed 3rd ed., Edinburgh, Mosby 2003, pp 781-792.

O'Dell JR, Haire CE, Erickson N, et al: Treatment of rheumatoid arthritis with methotrexate alone, sulfasalazine and hydroxychloroquine, or a combination of all three medications. N Engl J Med 1996;334:1287-1291.

St. Clair EW, Wagner CL, Fasanmade AA, et al: The relationship of serum infliximab concentrations to clinical improvement in rheumatoid arthritis: Results from ATTRACT, a multicenter, randomized, double-blind, placebo-controlled trial. Arthritis Rheum 2002;46:1451-1459.

van Everdingen AA, Jacobs JW, Siewertsz Van Reesema DR, Bijlsma JW: Low-dose prednisone therapy for patients with early active rheumatoid arthritis: Clinical efficacy, disease-modifying properties, and side effects: A randomized, double-blind, placebo-controlled clinical trial. Ann Intern Med 2002;136:1-12.

Juvenile Idiopathic Arthritis

Method of
Terry L. Moore, MD

Juvenile rheumatoid arthritis (JRA), now mainly known by the International League of Associations of Rheumatologists (ILAR) classification as juvenile idiopathic arthritis (JIA), is a protean disorder whose variable modes of onset and patterns of disease course are accompanied by a myriad of diverse signs, symptoms,

CURRENT DIAGNOSIS

- Diagnose early and treat aggressively.
- Reduce inflammation and symptoms.
- Suppress joint activity and reduce erosions to prevent disability.
- Establish a team approach with pediatric rheumatologist, ophthalmologist, physical therapist, and occupational therapist.

and manifestations. JIA affects approximately 250,000 children in the United States. No distinct race predilection is noted at this time. It is the most common disease cause of children missing school in the United States. It is also the second leading cause of eye pathology in children. JIA presents a difficult diagnostic problem because of its lack of specific serologic abnormalities. This represents a dual problem to a clinician in that it makes it difficult to establish an early diagnosis of JIA when the clinical picture is not clear, and even after the diagnosis is established, it is difficult to know when the disease has remitted or an exacerbation is beginning. The diagnosis of JIA is usually made clinically. Serologic studies can be informative, but in the past no routine laboratory tests have been diagnostic.

Diagnostic criteria for JIA include children younger than 16 years with persistent arthritis of one or more joints for at least 6 weeks. Arthritis is defined as swelling of a joint or limitation of motion with heat, pain, and tenderness.

JIA Subtypes

These are the seven basic subgroups or categories of JIA:

1. **Polyarthritis (RF positive)**: 19S IgM rheumatoid factors (RF) are present in the peripheral blood on testing and usually anticyclic citrullinated peptide antibodies (αCCP Ab). This group is manifested by arthritis in five or more joints in the first 6 months of disease. The joints most commonly affected are peripheral joints, including the knees, ankles, wrists, and fingers, but all synovial joints can become involved. There may also be an associated tendonitis. The classical joints involved are predominantly the metacarpophalangeal (MCP) and proximal phalangeal (PIP) joints producing fusiform-shaped swelling of the fingers. The knees are usually the first joints to limit function. They may exhibit deformity and flexion contractures. Polyarthritis (RF positive) is seen in approximately 5% to 10% of the children with JIA. The incidence of this type increases with age with the highest incidence found in adolescent females. The disease course in these children is generally believed to be one of a lifelong constantly active, or recurrent, relapsing pattern. It is associated with subcutaneous nodules and a higher incidence of vasculitis than the other forms of JIA. Radiograph films may show erosions with greater frequency than other forms of arthritis in children and may be helpful in diagnosis. Antinuclear antibodies (ANA) are present in approximately 80%.
2. **Polyarthritis (RF negative)**: This group by definition also has arthritis in five or more joints involved during the first 6 months; however, RF testing is negative, but αCCP Ab may be present. The disease pattern is similar to that of the RF-positive polyarthritis group. The course of these patients may be long term; however, most improve over a period of time. This type of onset occurs in approximately 20% to 30% of children with JIA. This type also shows female predominance.
3. a. **Oligoarthritis (pauciarthritis) with iridocyclitis** (inflammation of the iris and ciliary body in the posterior uveal tract of the eye): Oligoarthritis is manifested by arthritis of one or more joints involved in the first 6 months, but less than five joints. This type of onset is seen in approximately 50% of children with JIA and again shows female predominance. The most common children presenting are younger than 4 years at onset and have ANA present on testing. The ANA positivity is found in approximately 90% of the children developing chronic iridocyclitis. This group has a very good prognosis with little residual joint damage. There may be occasional asymmetric growth and leg length differences that develop; however, the process usually produces no long-term abnormalities. Approximately 50% of these children develop some type of iridocyclitis. Most children with iridocyclitis are easily controlled with anti-inflammatories such as naproxen, local steroid drops, or mydriatics (dilators). Therefore, any child being considered for a diagnosis of JIA requires frequent slit-lamp examinations by an ophthalmologist. b. **Extended oligoarthritis**: This type has an oligoarticular onset and then becomes more widespread, developing polyarthritis with five or more joints involved after the first 6 months of disease.
4. **Enthesitis related**: This category is predominantly seen in males who may later develop sacroiliitis and ankylosing spondylitis. This type of onset is associated with an enthesitis such as Achilles tendonitis or arthritis of the lower extremities again involving fewer than five joints in the first 6 months. The large joints, such as knees, ankles, hips, and sacroiliac joints, are usually involved. Anterior uveitis may be associated. The onset type is predominantly male, usually from 8 to 14 years of age, and may progress on to true ankylosing spondylitis. It is seen in approximately 10% to 15% of children with JIA. There is a high incidence of familial predisposition in these patients with an 80% to 95% occurrence of the HLA-B27 antigen found. Sacroiliitis is often present on radiographs before symptoms develop and precedes the development of real limitation of motion of the spine.
5. **Systemic arthritis**: Initially seen with daily temperatures rises usually late afternoon from normal to exceeding 39°C (103°F) in an intermittent, spiking pattern. This usually occurs for more than 2 weeks. The onset of this type may include a salmon-colored, transient skin rash, lymphadenopathy, splenomegaly, hepatomegaly, pleuritis, pericarditis, or abdominal pain. It is seen in approximately 20% of children with JIA. RF, αCCP Ab, and ANA are usually negative, but white blood cell counts may exceed 30 to 40,000/mm³. Erythrocyte sedimentation rate (ESR) and C-reactive protein (CRP) are elevated and anemia may rapidly develop. This group also shows a male predominance. Approximately 50% of children develop an oligoarticular pattern and remit quickly, but many of the children go on to develop a long-term symmetric polyarthritis. This type of onset causes the most consternation in the diagnosis because it may mimic severe localized infections, sepsis, or neoplasms, such as lymphomas or leukemias.
6. **Psoriatic arthritis**: Arthritis and psoriasis or dactylitis with nail pitting and onycholysis. Usually there is a first-degree relative with a psoriasis. RF is negative.
7. **Other arthritis**: Children with arthritis of unknown cause that persists for at least 6 weeks and does not fulfill criteria for any of the other categories or fulfills criteria for more than one of the other categories.

JIA Evaluation

The workup on a JIA patient includes a complete blood count (CBC) that may show an anemia, leukocytosis, and thrombocytosis in systemic onset. ESR and CRP are quite high in systemic and polyarticular disease but may be minimally elevated or normal in oligoarticular disease. RF is only positive in the late-onset polyarticular patients and αCCP Ab also mainly appears in this group but may be seen in a small number of RF-negative polyarticular and oligoarticular patients. ANA are found in the polyarticular group and also in the oligoarticular group, associated with the presence of iridocyclitis. Other immunologic testing and liver, muscle, and kidney function

---

[3]Exceeds dosage recommended by the manufacturer.

tests should be in the normal range. Radiographs should be performed of involved joints looking for periarticular demineralization, joint space narrowing, and/or erosions.

JIA Prognosis

The course and outcome of JIA is generally good, however, the disease needs to be treated early and aggressively to prevent asymmetrical skeletal development, osteopenia, chronic eye disease, or systemic manifestations. Approximately 75% of the children do well long term, with the oligoarticular group rarely having any residual damage. Approximately 25%, usually found in the polyarthritis and systemic groups, develop continuous arthritis with some long-term disability.

JIA Therapy

The therapy of JIA begins with the use of physical and occupational therapy (PT/OT). The object of PT is to strengthen muscles, improve range of motion, and decrease the impact loading on the joints. The object of OT is to improve body mechanics, posture, and other modalities to decrease any kind of impact loading on the joints. Medical therapy begins with the judicious use of nonsteroidal anti-inflammatory drugs (NSAIDs). Oligoarthritis patients are usually placed on a NSAID, usually naproxen (Naprosyn), at a dosage of 10 to 20 mg/kg in two divided doses. Naproxen has an advantage over other NSAIDs in that it comes in both a tablet and a liquid form at 125 mg/5 mL and has a long half-life so it can be given in two doses, which is more amenable to taking before and after school for compliance. The other nonsteroidal in tablet form generally used is tolmetin sodium (Tolectin) at a dosage of 20 to 30 mg/kg in three to four divided doses. One other medication, meloxicam (Mobic), comes in a tablet and a liquid form. It has an advantage of a long half-life and can be given once daily at dosages of 0.125 to 0.25 mg/kg. The liquid form is 7.5 mg/5 mL. Two other medications are approved for the use of children with JIA including aspirin (dosages of 80 to 120 mg/kg in four divided doses) and ibuprofen at 30 to 40 mg in three or four divided doses. A liquid preparation comes at 100 mg/5 mL. Other NSAIDs recently used in trials in JIA but not Food and Drug Administration (FDA) approved include nabumetone (Relafen),[1] at 30 mg/kg. This medication has an advantage in that it is only once a day and also can be used in a liquid form by crushing the tablet and dissolving in warm water. Other agents are occasionally used such as oxaprozin (Daypro), at 10 to 20 mg/kg in one to two doses; fenoprofen (Nalfon), at 40 to 50 mg/kg three to four times per day; diclofenac sodium (Voltaren), 20 to 40 mg/kg twice to three times per day; sulindac (Clinoril), 4 to 6 mg/kg in a twice daily dosage; or celecoxib (Celebrex), a cyclooxygenase-2 (COX-2) inhibitor, at 4 to 6 mg/kg in two doses. Laboratory studies including CBC, urinalysis, and comprehensive metabolic panel should be drawn every 4 months to monitor medication toxicity.

Children who have erosions on radiograph or show more aggressive disease at time of onset, usually those with polyarthritis, with systemic disease with polyarthritis, or with very aggressive oligoarticular disease, benefit greatly by combination therapy to reduce long-term disability. This means being aggressive with therapy in the first 2 years of disease. The first 2 years of disease are the period in which the most erosions and joint damage occurs. Combination therapy has become the standard of care of patients with JIA. The most common combination is the use of two or more of the disease-modifying antirheumatic agents (DMARDs), which include methotrexate (MTX), hydroxychloroquine (Plaquenil) [HCQ], or some of the new biologic preparations. MTX, a purine inhibitor, in dosages of 10 to 20 mg/m^2 once weekly along with folic acid at 400 µg to 1 mg daily is a very efficacious DMARD with little toxicity. MTX can be given orally or by intramuscular (IM) or subcutaneous (SC) injection. Orally, the liquid preparation at 25 mg/mL can be given in 0.1 mL/2.5 mg increments from 5 mg (0.2 mL) to 20 mg (0.8 mL) or in pill form of 2.5 mg tablets from 5 mg (2 tablets) to 20 mg (8 tablets) once per week. Dosages more than 20 mg should always be administered IM or SC. These children, however, do need to be monitored monthly to every 6 weeks with CBC, urinalysis, and liver and kidney function tests to monitor the medication toxicity. The combination of MTX and HCQ is the most common with the addition of HCQ in dosages of 6 mg/kg as an excellent adjunct along with the NSAID. Eye exams every 6 months to monitor HCQ toxicity are indicated. MTX is also monitored once a year with a chest radiograph and also if any cough is present. The toxicities of these medications are relatively minimal in patients with JIA. Other DMARDs, although not approved by the FDA in children, are cyclosporine (Neoral)[1] at 2.5 to 3 mg/kg, intramuscular gold[1] at a dosage of 1 mg/kg weekly for 20 weeks, and sulfasalazine (Azulfidine) (SSZ) at doses of 50 mg/kg beginning at 500 mg per day and up to 2 g twice a day.[3] These are used with efficacy in JIA patients. Also, leflunomide (Arava)[1], a pyrimidine synthetase inhibitor, is effective in children. It also has liver toxicity, so it should be monitored like MTX. Abdominal complaints such as diarrhea are the most common side effects. The drug has a long half-life and potential teratogenicity, so it should be used with caution in females of childbearing age. Recently, the use of biologics or anticytokines in JIA has brought about a great deal of improvement in some of the patients. One medication is etanercept (Enbrel) at 0.4 mg/kg SC two times per week or 0.8 mg/kg SQ once per week. It has brought about marked improvement in many patients with long-standing polyarthritis. Efficacy has been sustained for up to 10 years now. This medication has caused marked decrease in joint swelling, tenderness, decreased sedimentation rate, and marked improvement in fatigue. The mechanism of action is that of blocking tumor necrosis factor (TNF), a cytokine that increases the inflammatory response in joints. Etanercept is produced to function like the p75 receptor for TNF. It binds to TNF and keeps it from binding to its own receptor and increasing the inflammatory response. It is well tolerated with the main side effect injection site reactions. TNF blockers can exacerbate an underlying tuberculosis infection, so before starting the medication a chest radiograph and purified protein derivative (PPD) skin test should be performed and then yearly while on the medication. Its counterpart, infliximab (Remicade), a chimeric monoclonal antibody to TNF, though not FDA approved, also is very efficacious in JIA. It is used as an intravenous (IV) preparation at 3 mg/kg given at baseline, 2 weeks, 6 weeks, and 8 eight weeks thereafter in an IV infusion over a 2-hour period. The dosage may be increased to 5 to 8 mg/kg and the interval shortened to every 4 to 6 weeks if needed. This agent markedly decreases the inflammatory response. It has mainly been used in older children with polyarticular disease. Recently, also now FDA approved, a fully humanized monoclonal antibody to TNF, adalimumab (Humira) is given at 20 mg SC every 2 weeks for children 15 to 20 kg and at 40 mg

---

[1]Not FDA approved for this indication.

CURRENT THERAPY

- Anti-inflammatory agents (NSAIDs: naproxen [Naprosyn], ibuprofen [Advil], tolmetin [Tolectin], meloxicam [Mobic]) and intra-articular steroids for oligoarticular disease
- Disease-modifying agents (methotrexate [Rheumatrex], hydroxychloroquine [Plaquenil], sulfasalazine [Azulfidine], etc.) and/or biologics (etanercept, adalimumab, abatacept) for polyarticular and systemic disease

Abbreviation: NSAIDs = nonsteroidal anti-inflammatory drugs.

---

[1]Not FDA approved for this indication.
[3]Exceeds dosage recommended by the manufacturer.

SC every 2 weeks for children greater than 30 kg. Also, studies are being run on the interleukin (IL)-1 receptor antagonist, Anakinra (Kineret), in children. It is given daily at 1 to 2 mg/kg SC up to 100 mg SC per day. This medication shows a more favorable response in children with systemic-onset than with polyarticular or oligoarticular disease. A high number of children experience injection site reactions. Also, recently FDA approved for children is abatacept (Orencia), which blocks T-cells from proliferating and producing inflammatory cytokines. It is given as an IV infusion at 10 mg/kg on days 1, 15, and 30 and then monthly. Other biologic medications are in trials, including an IL-6 receptor antagonist (tocilizumab)[2] in systemic onset JIA, anti-B cell therapy (rituximab) (Rituxan), and an IL-1 trap medication (rilonacept).

Prednisone still may be used in severe systemic disease to control fever, rash, and/or other systemic manifestations in dosages of 1 to 2 mg/kg. The possibility of long-term side effects such as growth retardation, avascular necrosis, osteoporosis, weight gain, and acneiform lesions from steroids make their long-term use tentative in children. If disease is controlled, steroids should be tapered. Steroid eye drops may be used at times for severe iridocyclitis or orally in those patients with severe eye disease. Intra-articular (IA) steroids may be used in all onset-types if one or more joints are severely involved at one point in time. Local injections of 10 to 40 mg of triamcinolone hexacetonide may provide symptomatic relief in one specific joint. In the long course of the disease, other immunosuppressives such as cyclophosphamide (Cytoxan), azathioprine (Imuran), and chlorambucil (Leukeran)[1] are used in certain cases of severe systemic or polyarthritis, but the use of these has waned with the new biologic medication.

The use of PT and OT is indicated at the first onset of disease. The child, after being evaluated, is sent to PT for instructions in the use of moist heat to the joints such as hot packs, the judicial use of rest, and two to three periods each day of passive or active assisted exercises performed by the patient or aided by the parent. Splints that protect joints may be prescribed to decrease the development of deformities. Splints can be made out of lightweight plastic that is molded while warm to fit the child in the desired position. The wrists and knees are the most amenable to splinting, but finger splints may hold the entire hand in slight dorsiflexion to decrease ulnar drift. If flexion contractures occur, splints can be used to hold the joint in maximum extension. The use of OT begins with the instructions for the patient in posture, body mechanics, improvement in activities of daily living, and instructions in joint protection. These instructions help the patient learn to protect and not increase the impact loading on the joints. Exercises are important in all stages of the care of the child with arthritis. During appearance of disease activity, excessive exercises exacerbate the inflammation. In these stages, passive range of motion exercise should maintain range of motion along with active assistive exercise. As joints improve and the inflammation is reduced, the exercise should be increased to a more active form. Resistive and strengthening exercises should be introduced along with isometric exercises to help provide muscle tone. Swimming or hydrotherapy or water aerobics for exercise may greatly aid in improving muscle strength. The use of regular cycling exercises may also be helpful. If the child has a lot of morning stiffness in the hands, the use of paraffin baths may be of great help, and the use of Theraputty to squeeze and improve muscle strength in the hands is indicated.

In conclusion, children with JIA should be diagnosed as soon as possible and treated aggressively. It is not a benign condition if left partially treated or untreated. Early treatment prevents further disease progression, maintains range of motion of the joints, and promotes normal growth and development. Combination therapy of NSAIDs, DMARDs, and/or biologics should be used early in those patients identified with aggressive disease. The team approach of the pediatric rheumatologist, ophthalmologist, and physical and occupational therapists will best benefit the JIA patient for a good long-term outcome.

---

[2]Not available in the United States.
[1]Not FDA approved for this indication.

REFERENCES

Cassidy JT, Petty RE: Chronic arthritis. In Cassidy JT, Petty RE (eds): Textbook of Pediatric Rheumatology. Philadelphia, WB Saunders 2005, pp 206-341.

Kietz DA, Pepmueller PH, Moore TL: Therapeutic use of etanercept in polyarticular course juvenile rheumatoid arthritis over a two-year period. Ann Rheum Dis 2002;61:171-173.

Lovell D, Giannini EH, Reiff A, et al: Etanercept in children with polyarticular juvenile rheumatoid arthritis. N Engl J Med 2000;342:763-769.

Low JM, Chauhan AK, Kietz DA, et al: Determination of anti-cyclic citrullinated peptide antibodies in sera of patients with juvenile idiopathic arthritis. J Rheumatol 2004;31:1829-1833.

Moore TL: Immunopathogenesis of juvenile rheumatoid arthritis. Curr Opin Rheumatol 1999;11:377-383.

Petty JE, Southwood TR, Manners P, et al: International League of Associations for Rheumatology classification of juvenile idiopathic arthritis; Second revision, Edmonton, 2001. J Rheumatol 2004;31:390-392.

Syed RH, Gilliam BE, Moore TL: Rheumatoid factors and anticyclic citrullinated peptide antibodies in pediatric rheumatology. Curr Rheumatol Rep 2008;10:156-163.

Wallace CA, Huang B, Bandeira M, et al: Patterns of clinical remission in select categories of juvenile idiopathic arthritis. Arthritis Rheum 2005;52:3554-3562.

Ankylosing Spondylitis

Method of
Finbar D. O'Shea, MB, MRCPI, and
Robert D. Inman, MD

Ankylosing spondylitis (AS) is a chronic inflammatory rheumatic disease characterized by inflammatory back pain due to sacroiliitis and spondylitis, restricted spinal mobility due to the formation of syndesmophytes, and often peripheral arthritis, enthesitis, and acute anterior uveitis (iritis). Symptoms commonly begin in late adolescence and early adulthood. With an estimated prevalence of 0.9% in northern European white populations, AS is a significant health burden to the community.

AS has long been a therapeutic challenge for the clinician. Exercise and nonsteroidal anti-inflammatory drugs (NSAIDs) have been the mainstays of symptom control for decades, but there has until recently been a dearth of effective disease-modifying treatments. The advent of biological treatments (specifically anti–tumor necrosis factor [TNF] agents) is currently revolutionizing the management of AS.

AS belongs to a group of related diseases termed *spondyloarthropathies* (SpA), which also comprises conditions such as arthritis/spondylitis associated with psoriasis, arthritis/spondylitis associated with inflammatory bowel disease, reactive arthritis, and undifferentiated spondyloarthritis (uSpA). They share many clinical manifestations and an association with human leukocyte antigen (HLA)-B27. The SpA group as a whole is one of the most common rheumatic diseases, with a prevalence of up to 1.9%, and this makes them at least as common as rheumatoid arthritis. The most common subgroups of SpA are AS and uSpA. It appears that all SpA subsets can progress to full-blown AS.

Diagnosis

DIFFICULTIES AND DELAYS IN DIAGNOSIS

Among the inflammatory rheumatic diseases there is a long delay between the onset of symptoms and the time of diagnosis for AS; in several studies an average duration of about 7 years has been reported. The mean age at onset of symptoms is in the mid-20s,

| BOX 1 | Modified New York Criteria for Ankylosing Spondylitis |

Clinical Criteria

- Low back pain and stiffness for more than 3 months that improves with exercise but is not relieved by rest
- Limitation of motion of the lumbar spine in both the lateral and frontal planes
- Limitation of chest expansion relative to normal values correlated for age and sex

Radiographic Criterion

- Sacroiliitis, grade ≥2 bilaterally or grade 3 to 4 unilaterally

Note: *The condition is definitely AS if the radiographic criterion is associated with at least 1 clinical criterion.*

 CURRENT DIAGNOSIS

- Screen all patients younger than 40 years who have back pain longer than 3 months for features of IBP. IBP features include:
  - Early morning stiffness longer than 30 min
  - Improved back pain with exercise, not rest
  - Nocturnal pain, especially the second half of the night
  - Alternating buttock pain
- Screen for history of psoriasis, inflammatory bowel disease, iritis and any family history of these conditions
- Search for restriction in spinal mobility
  - Forward flexion (Schober's test)
  - Lateral spinal flexion
  - Chest expansion
- AP pelvic x-ray if IBP suspected for presence or absence of sacroiliitis
- If conventional radiography is not diagnostic and clinical suspicion remains, consider MRI (STIR sequence required). MRI allows direct visualization of inflammation in the spine and sacroiliac joints before conventional radiography shows any abnormality.

Abbreviations: AP = anteroposterior; IBP = inflammatory back pain; MRI = magnetic resonance imaging; STIR = short T1 inversion recovery.

---

thus at the normally most productive time of life. If AS is undiagnosed and untreated, or not treated effectively, continuous pain, stiffness, and fatigue are the consequences. Furthermore, a potentially progressive loss of spinal mobility and function cause a reduction in the quality of life and an increase in direct and indirect medical costs.

There are two major reasons for the long delay in the diagnosis of AS. First, the established classification criteria for AS, which date back more than 20 years, rely on the combination of clinical symptoms plus unequivocal radiographic sacroiliitis of at least grade 2 bilaterally or grade 3 unilaterally (see Box 1 for the modified New York criteria for the diagnosis of AS). The radiographs are often normal when symptoms arise, and it usually takes several years for definite radiographic sacroiliitis to evolve. Second, there is no unique clinical symptom or laboratory test to make the diagnosis of AS; thus it is a huge challenge to attempt to identify the estimated 5% of patients with SpA (including AS) among the great number of patients with chronic low back pain seen by the primary care physician.

Efforts have been made to try to address these issues. MRI has been used successfully to detect the presence of spinal and sacroiliac inflammation in early disease. However, until MRI detection of sacroiliitis is shown to be sensitive and specific for early AS, and until the availability of MRI greatly improves, most clinicians are left with plain radiography as the diagnostic test.

CLINICAL FEATURES

Choosing clinical parameters for screening patients for underlying AS is attractive because their determination is not expensive. The clinical symptom of inflammatory back pain has been suggested as a cardinal symptom for AS for years, and assessment requires neither laboratory testing nor x-ray. It has been estimated that when symptoms of inflammatory back pain are present in a patient with chronic low back pain, the post-test probability for this patient of having axial SpA is 14%.

Recent refinement of these clinical features has identified a new set of criteria for inflammatory back pain. The new criteria consist of morning stiffness for longer than 30 minutes, improvement in back pain with exercise but not with rest, awakening because of back pain during the second one half of the night only, and alternating buttock pain. These features were defined by a study that sought to identify the most sensitive and specific combination of parameters for inflammatory back pain using a cohort of patients with an established diagnosis of AS. Fulfillment of at least two of these four parameters yielded a sensitivity of 70% and a specificity of 81%, with a positive likelihood ratio of 3.7. If at least three of the four parameters were fulfilled, the positive likelihood ratio increased to 12.4. However, how these discriminating features perform in a large non-specific back pain population has yet to be examined.

Treatment

Until recently, the treatment options for AS were limited. Regular physiotherapy and treatment with NSAIDs were the only available options. Approximately one half of AS patients are adequately managed with this regimen. However, conventional disease-modifying antirheumatic drugs, which are effective in other chronic inflammatory diseases such as rheumatoid arthritis, have only a very limited effect on spinal inflammation. Local injections of corticosteroids can be used effectively if inflammation is confined to a small number of joints. Thus, although an early and accurate diagnosis has been recognized as important in these patients, this seemed less urgent for many physicians because of the lack of therapeutic options.

This treatment approach has now changed. NSAIDs should probably be taken more regularly once a diagnosis has been made. Tumor necrosis factor (TNF) blockers offer an exciting new possibility for effective treatment and possibly for arresting disease progression. It has recently been shown that the anti-TNF agents infliximab (Remicade), etanercept (Enbrel), and adalimumab (Humira) have a prompt and robust effect on almost all aspects of active disease—most notably pain and fatigue, but also function, spinal mobility, peripheral arthritis, enthesitis, bone density, and acute inflammation as reflected by acute-phase reactants and MRI. In studies using these three compounds, a 50% improvement of the disease activity could be demonstrated in about one half of the treated patients whose disease had proved refractory to NSAIDs and physiotherapy. In 72% of patients with a disease duration of less than 10 years there was at least 50% improvement of the Bath AS Disease Activity Index (BASDAI), clearly higher than patients with a longer disease duration. This finding supports the essential need for early diagnosis.

Recent studies have shown a sustained response among AS patients with the anti-TNF agents superior even to that seen in rheumatoid arthritis. Short- to medium-term data show them to be well tolerated. On the basis of the MRI changes, it is believed that the

CURRENT THERAPY

- Physical therapy and a regular stretching program are important in all AS patients.
- NSAIDs are first-line therapy.
- Use a second NSAID even if the first has not achieved control of symptoms.
- Consider local corticosteroid injection if few joints involved.
- Ongoing disease activity is best reflected by the Bath Ankylosing Spondylitis Disease Activity Index (BASDAI). If the patient scores at least 4 out of 10 despite a full trial of two NSAIDs, an anti-TNF agent should be considered.

Abbreviations: NSAID = nonsteroidal anti-inflammatory drug; TNF = tumor necrosis factor.

anti-TNF agents will have a positive effect on long-term radiographic progression; however, this has yet to be proved.

Infliximab and adalimumab are monoclonal antibodies directed against the proinflammatory cytokine TNF-α. Etanercept is a fusion protein of the p75 TNF receptor linked to the Fc portion of an immunoglobulin (Ig) G1 molecule that binds and inactivates TNF-α. Inflixiamb is administered intravenously in three loading doses and then every 8 weeks at a dose of 3 to 5 mg/kg. Etanercept is administered subcutaneously once weekly (50-mg injection). Adalimumab is administered subcutaneously every other week (40-mg injection). All three agents appear to have similar efficacy and tolerability. The most serious potential side effect with any of these agents is infection, specifically tuberculosis (TB). This has been greatly minimized by screening for any evidence of latent TB infection with a chest x-ray and a TB skin (PPD) test before commencing these agents. The issue of altered rates of malignancies with these agents in AS has not been resolved and is being addressed with monitoring of biologics registries in several countries.

Prognosis and Long-Term Outcomes

AS is a chronic condition with no predictable pattern of progression, and the disease does not follow a single defined course. Although many outcomes are possible, findings from previous prospective studies suggest that a pattern of AS emerges within the first 10 years of disease. About 74% of patients who had mild spinal restriction after 10 years did not progress to severe spinal involvement. In contrast, 81% of patients who had severe spinal restriction had been severely restricted within the first 10 years. What differentiates the rapid progression group has not been completely resolved. Hip involvement has repeatedly been shown to be an indicator of more severe disease. Other predictors of a poor outcome include a raised erythrocyte sedimentation rate (ESR), poor response to NSAIDs and peripheral oligoarthritis. Cigarette smoking is associated with worse clinical, functional, and radiologic outcomes. Early age at onset has been recently shown to be associated with a worse prognosis.

Men are afflicted with AS approximately 2 to 3 times more often than women. The disease pattern also varies by sex. The spine and pelvis are more commonly affected in men. In contrast, women have less severe involvement of the spine and more symptoms in the knees, ankles, and hips. It has been shown that women have a later age at onset. It was previously believed that women also had milder disease than men, but this view has been questioned recently.

With the advent of new effective therapies for AS, it has become important to identify predictors of response to these agents. This is important because the anti-TNF agents are expensive for the health care system and have potential side effects for the patient. It has been shown that younger patients with shorter disease duration, raised acute phase markers, and a higher disease activity at initiation do better. However, it has also been shown that patients with long-standing disease and established radiographic changes can also respond to these agents, and these patients should be also afforded a trial if conventional treatments have proved inadequate.

REFERENCES

Davis JC, van der Jeijde DM, Braun J, et al: Sustained durability and tolerability of etanercept in ankylosing spondylitis for 96 weeks. Ann Rheum Dis 2005;64(11):1557-1562.
Maksymowych WP, Landewe R: Imaging in ankylosing spondylitis. Best Pract Res Clin Rheumatol 2006;20(3):507-519.
Rudwaleit M, van der Heijde D, Khan MA, et al: How to diagnose axial spondyloarthritis early. Ann Rheum Dis 2004;63:535-543.
Rudwaleit M, Metter A, Listing J, et al: Inflammatory back pain in ankylosing spondylitis: A reassessment of the clinical history for application as classification and diagnostic criteria. Arthritis Rheum 2006;54(2):569-578.
Sieper J, Braun J, Rudwaleit M, et al: Ankylosing spondylitis: An overview. Ann Rheum Dis 2002;61(suppl 3): iii8-iii18.
Sieper J, Rudwaleit M: Early referral recommendations for ankylosing spondylitis (including pre-radiographic and radiographic forms) in primary care. Ann Rheum Dis 2005;64:659-663.
Sieper J, Rudwaleit M, Khan MA, Braun J: Concepts and epidemiology of spondyloarthritis. Best Pract Res Clin Rheumatol 2006;20(3):401-417.
Stone M, Warren RW, Bruckel J, et al: Juvenile-onset ankylosing spondylitis is associated with worse functional outcomes than adult-onset ankylosing spondylitis. Arthritis Rheum 2005;53(3):445-451.
van der Heijde D, Dijkmans B, Geusens P, et al: Efficacy and safety of infliximab in patients with ankylosing spondylitis: Results of a randomized, placebo-controlled trial (ASSERT). Arthritis Rheum 2005;52(2):582-591.
van der Heijde D, Kivitz A, Schiff MH, et al: Efficacy and safety of adalimumab in patients with ankylosing spondylitis: Results of a multicenter, randomized, double-blind, placebo-controlled trial. Arthritis Rheum 2006;54(7):2136-2146.
van der Linden S, Valkenburg HA, Cats A: Evaluation of diagnostic criteria for ankylosing spondylitis: A proposal for modification of the New York criteria. Arthritis Rheum 1984;27(4):361-368.
Zochling J, van der Heijde D, Burgos-Vargas R, et al: ASAS/EULAR recommendations for the management of ankylosing spondylitis. Ann Rheum Dis 2006;65:442-452.

Temporomandibular Disorders and Orofacial Pain

Method of
Richard Ohrbach, DDS, PhD, and Jeffrey Burgess, DDS, MSD

Temporomandibular disorder (TMD) and orofacial pain include pain in the oral, facial, or head regions. TMD is a collection of conditions that affect the muscles of mastication, the temporomandibular joint (TMJ), or both. The primary symptom is pain localized most often in the muscles of mastication or the preauricular area. Associated pain symptoms can involve the ear or cervical area and often include headache. The other major symptoms include limitation in jaw functioning (e.g., restriction in range of motion, difficulty with mastication) or noises or altered functioning in the TMJ.

In contrast, orofacial pain disorders are *not* typically associated with alterations in mandibular function but extend diagnostically across the disciplines of neurology, otolaryngology, psychiatry, and dentistry. The pain complaint is primarily located within the orofacial area, but the distribution (as well as underlying pathology) can extend beyond the orofacial area in either a caudal or cephalad direction. Contrasting TMDs and orofacial pain disorders, diagnostic distinctions are generally clear given a careful history. Many of the orofacial pain disorders represent diagnostic red flags for the TMDs.

Epidemiology

TMDs are relatively common; estimated U.S. prevalences are about 12% for TMD-related pain (6 months' duration) and about 8% for a diagnosed TMD requiring treatment. Any of the three major characteristics of a TMD (pain, limitation in motion, joint noise) occur in 5% to 50% of the population, and treatment-seeking appears to be primarily related to pain severity and limited jaw functioning. The modal patient is 18 to 45 years old, and the prevalence is much lower for late adolescents, the middle-aged, and elderly; women present for treatment 4 to 7 times more often than men, whereas the population gender prevalence is only 2:1. Emerging evidence suggests that genetic sensitivity for pain is a primary risk factor for TMD, and hormonal factors might account for the gender disparity, although an explanatory mechanism remains absent.

The orofacial pain conditions, excluding toothache and sinusitis, are much less common. Orofacial pain manifesting as facial migraine variants is probably less common than migraine headache but are also probably underdiagnosed.

Clinical Features and Diagnosis

Psychosocial factors are central in the diagnosis and treatment for the TMDs and are presumed to also play a role in the treatment of orofacial pain disorders when they have become chronic (i.e., at least 3-6 months in duration) or refractory to initial treatment. Thus, a dual-axis approach including biomedical and biobehavioral aspects is standard.

BIOMEDICAL EVALUATION

History

The pain history includes: assessment of pain location, referral patterns, quality (e.g., ache, throb, burning, electrical), duration (e.g., brief, hours, days, months), temporal (e.g., intermittent, paroxysmal, recurrent, constant), patterning (e.g., morning, evening, during sleep), modifying factors (e.g., cold, chewing, head or body movement), and associated symptoms (e.g., dysesthesia, photophobia, phonophobia). A pain description that appears atypical should not be discounted but approached carefully because it can reflect multiple diagnoses or etiologies: central (e.g., intracranial), nonfacial (e.g., cardiac, oncologic, neck), or biobehavioral etiology.

A past or present history of TMJ noises such as clicking, popping, or crepitus may be important. A distinct click or pop occurring in the TMJ might suggest internal derangement of the disk, but nonpainful TMJ noise is considered to be benign, self-limited, and not needing intervention. In contrast, significant TMJ dysfunction involves intermittent or persistent locking for longer than 24 hours. Crepitus suggests degenerative disease. A history of intermittent joint noise (click or pop) followed by sudden opening limitation, pain, absence of noise, and severe opening deviation suggest nonreducing disk displacement and can be treated acutely. Chronic nonreducing disk displacement, ruled out by magnetic resonance imaging (MRI), might or might not be symptomatic and is significant only if opening continues to be limited.

Orofacial trauma involving jaw fracture is typically associated with acute malocclusion and severe pain at the fracture site; it might also be associated with limited jaw opening and lateral movement, and the patient may be able to partially occlude the teeth. TMJ intracapsular injury is more complex, if not controversial, and assessment of function takes priority. Complaint of progressive change in the bite, such as an opening between the posterior or anterior teeth, can indicate the presence of significant joint (e.g., rheumatoid or degenerative) or endocrine (e.g., acromegaly) disease. A perceived malocclusion (in the absence of objective evidence of such) coupled with facial or head pain suggests the presence of a myofascial or dysesthesia condition.

Physical Examination

Physical examination includes vital signs, general inspection of the head, and otologic and cranial nerve examination. Palpation of the neck, including the musculature, is also recommended because pain can be referred from this region to the cranium. Lack of published criteria for performing neck muscle palpation can limit its reliability and validity, and results should be interpreted cautiously, particularly in the absence of accompanying history. It is generally accepted that if pain in the head is being caused by the neck musculature, repeated palpation of identified trigger points should reproduce the phenomena. Neurophysiologic linkage between masticatory and cervical muscles during function can support a causal relationship between regional pain disorders; referred pain can also produce overlap.

A standardized examination (e.g., Research Diagnostic Criteria, RDC/TMD) has become the norm for TMD assessment, in part to prevent overdiagnosis. Although initially intended as a more reliable research instrument, the RDC is also time efficient in the clinical setting. Jaw opening is reliably measured with a millimeter ruler, and less than 35 mm is generally considered limited for both male and female patients. Jaw opening is evaluated for deviation and for disk movement by the application of light pressure over the TMJs. A stethoscope is probably more reliable for detection of crepitus. For palpation, 2 pounds of pressure to the primary extraoral masticatory muscles and 1 pound to the TMJs and the intraoral muscles appear to have appropriate sensitivity and specificity. The teeth, mucosa, and posterior pharynx should always be evaluated. Excessive tooth wear indicates past or present parafunctional behavior. Although TMD is not generally associated with malocclusion, malocclusion may be significant in certain circumstances.

Panography is sufficient for initial screening of maxillomandibular pathology and may be the only imaging necessary for most patients. CT is useful for confirming the diagnosis and extent of disease with suspected developmental abnormalities, neoplasm, trauma or fracture, sinus pathology, degenerative disease, chronic infection (e.g., osteomyelitis), and TMJ ankylosis. MRI of the TMJs should be ordered when jaw locking does not respond to initial treatments. SPECT, although not specific, can be helpful with suspected inflammatory disorders. Orofacial pain problems, depending on history and examination findings, often warrant greater use of regional imaging and laboratory and serologic assessment.

BIOBEHAVIORAL EVALUATION

Chronic TMD is similar to other chronic pain conditions such as headache and back pain with respect to psychophysiologic mechanisms, coping, behavioral manifestations, and impact. In contrast,

---

CURRENT DIAGNOSIS

- Primary symptoms of TMD are pain localized to the face and temple area coupled with some limitation in mandibular function; the clinical examination confirms limitation of mobility, interference in function, and regional pain from movement or palpation.
- Pain history supports the diagnosis of orofacial pain disorders, and examination is used to rule out other possible diagnoses.
- For these primarily pain disorders, biobehavioral factors are also assessed.

these aspects can require less consideration in diagnosis and management of acute TMDs. Orofacial pain problems appear to be independent of these processes with respect to diagnosis, but they can become relevant in treatment when the orofacial pain disorder has become more persistent or refractory.

TMD characteristics shared with other chronic musculoskeletal pain disorders include poor correspondence between subjective complaints of pain and suffering versus the identifiable pathophysiology; impact of psychosocial stress in effecting nonfunctional increases in muscle activity; more frequent distress and greater difficulty in coping, which may be either a premorbid style or emerging from the chronic pain; greater prevalence of clinically diagnosable depression, anxiety, or somatization, the latter referring to the reporting of multiple somatic problems simultaneous with significant life disarray; disruption in usual performance at home, work, or school; and frequent health care visits, previous treatment successes now no longer effective, medication abuse, pursuing treatments that are exclusively somatic, and avoiding biobehavioral treatments. These similarities suggest that the following four domains be evaluated as potential yellow flags (summarized in Box 1).

Subjective Aspects of the Condition

The *pain complaint* should be evaluated for its relationship to relevant anatomy and physiology, which factors (physical, psychosocial) alter it, and what activities have been altered due to it. *Treatment history* should be evaluated with respect to which types of treatments were successful or unsuccessful, whether there was a preponderance or avoidance of any particular type (e.g., medications, behavioral treatment), whether there was premature abandonment of a treatment, and what factors were involved with resuming treatment when prior treatment-seeking was intermittent. The patient's *explanatory model* should be explored regarding the origin of the problem, the meaning of the symptoms, and the role of physical versus psychological treatments, with respect to etiology, maintenance, and exacerbation of the problem.

BOX 1 Diagnostic Yellow Flags For Temporomandibular Disorder and Chronic Orofacial Pain

Subjective
Pain complaint: Anatomic correlates, whether altered by physical or psychosocial factors, and behavioral consequences.
Treatment history: Types of treatment previously effective or not, adherence, triggers for treatment cycles
Illness explanatory model: Symptom origin and meaning, expected outcome of physical or psychological treatments
Receptiveness to psychological referral

Behavior
Oral parafunctional behavior
Covariance of symptoms with other behavior

Psychological Status
Depression and anxiety
Somatization and somatoform disorders
Spectrum of nonspecific physical symptoms

Psychosocial Status
Activities of daily living
Mastication and speech
Social interaction
Intimate behavior

Referral for biobehavioral treatment should be considered at the outset rather than waiting until all physical diagnostic or therapeutic approaches have been tried and *then* referring the patient to a psychologist or psychiatrist. That latter approach to intervention gives the implicit message that the pain was initially real but, with the failure of treatment, has become imaginary. A patient with a rigid explanation that the problem is completely of physical origin is often highly reluctant, perhaps even resistant, to consider a biobehavioral perspective, and such patients have been reinforced to hold such views by repeated evaluations that are somatically focused and that exclude the biobehavioral domain.

Behavior

Oral parafunctional behavior during the waking state often indicates response to psychosocial stress. Psychosocial stress can also affect the related cervical muscles and contribute to the pain. Other potentially important behaviors, such as whether changes in pain are associated with specific home or work situations, are often best assessed via a self-report diary containing columns for the desired information coupled with specific instructions and follow-up by the physician. For example, a patient who reports no linkage of symptomatology to daily events (especially when the pain is daily and purportedly unchanging) might, after maintaining a diary for a week, report a very different symptom picture.

Psychological Status

Psychological status includes depression, anxiety, and somatization. These can be assessed through a standard clinical interview or standardized questionnaires such as the Symptom Checklist (SCL)-90R. Other measures can be used for depression and anxiety, but the SCL-90R is perhaps the best current tool for assessing the continuum underlying nonspecific physical symptoms. All TMD patients should receive the same screening evaluation in order to more consistently identify changes in psychological status that often escape detection by clinical interview.

The question is the extent and manner in which changes in psychological status manifest in this particular patient and contribute to the pain-related suffering, and whether to refer the patient for more specialized evaluations through referral to either a clinical psychologist or psychiatrist who specializes in chronic pain. Depression is common in the TMD population, is often comorbid with elevated anxiety, and responds to treatment (either pharmacologic or behavioral), which often alters the reported pain as well.

Somatization as a formal disorder is rare, but as a continuum it is present surprisingly often, and when present it can significantly influence treatment outcome and increase doctor shopping and treatment-seeking behaviors.

Psychosocial Status

Interference in psychosocial function (activities of daily living, mastication and speech, social interaction, oral intimate behavior) and increased health care use lead to a worse prognosis.

DIAGNOSTIC INTEGRATION

For the TMDs, a dual-axis system—the physical diagnosis and the biobehavioral implications for treatment—has been used for 20 years. The dual-axis system is probably applicable to orofacial pain disorders. One common practice is to escalate diagnostic testing for the physical disorder without equal consideration of the biobehavioral domain; both areas should be investigated equally from the outset.

TEMPOROMANDIBULAR DISORDERS

The most common TMDs are described in Box 2. Not included in this box are some potential disorders not yet well described in the

> **BOX 2** Temporomandibular Disorders: Diagnostic Criteria
>
> **Group I: Muscle Disorders**
> I. Myofascial pain (pain in the muscles of mastication)
> Pain or ache at rest or during function in the jaw, temples, face, preauricular area, inside the ear, *plus*
> Palpation pain in at least three of 20 muscle sites
> - Posterior, middle, anterior temporalis
> - Origin, body, insertion of masseter
> - Stylohyoid, digastric, lateral pterygoid, temporalis tendon)
> Palpation pain must be at least present on the side of pain complaint
>
> **Group II: Disk Displacements**
> Disk displacement with reduction
> - Reciprocal clicking in the TMJ
>   - Click on both opening and closing or a click on either opening or closing
>   - Click during lateral or protrusive excursions
> Disk displacement without reduction, with limited opening
> - Report of significant limitation of mandibular opening *plus*
> - Maximum unassisted opening ≤35 mm *plus*
> - Passive stretch increases opening 4 mm or less beyond unassisted opening *plus*
> - Contralateral excursion <7 mm and/or uncorrected deviation to the ipsilateral side on opening *plus*
> - Absence of joint sounds, or presence of joint sounds not meeting criteria for disk displacement with reduction
> Disk displacement without reduction, without limited opening
> - Report of significant limitation of mandibular opening *plus*
> - Maximal unassisted opening >35 mm *plus*
> - Passive stretch increases opening at least 5 mm *plus*
> - Contralateral excursion ≥7 mm *plus*
> - Presence of joint sounds not meeting criteria for disk displacement with reduction *plus*
> - If joint imaging is requested, it should image the disk in closed and open mouth positions with arthrography or MRI
>
> **Group III: Arthralgia, Arthritis, Arthrosis**
> Arthralgia (pain in the joint)
> - Pain in one or both joint sites during palpation *plus*
> - One or more self-reports of pain in the region of the joint, pain in the joint during maximum unassisted or assisted opening, or lateral excursions *plus*
> - Absence of coarse crepitus
> Osteoarthritis of the TMJ (inflammatory changes in the joint)
> - Arthralgia (see above) *plus*
> - Coarse crepitus in the joint or joint imaging showing erosions, sclerosis of condylar head or articular eminence, or flattening of the joint surfaces
> Osteoarthrosis of the TMJ (remodeling of the articulating surfaces)
> - Absence of arthralgia *plus*
> - Coarse crepitus or joint imaging showing joint changes
>
> Data from Dworkin SF, LeResche L: Research diagnostic criteria for temporomandibular disorders: Review, criteria, examinations and specifications, critique. J Craniomandib Disord 1992;6:301-355.

literature and without clear inclusion criteria: muscle contracture, spasm, splinting, inflammatory disease (synovitis), and ligamentous injury (perforation, tearing).

OROFACIAL PAIN DISORDERS

Orofacial pain differential diagnosis is confounded by the anatomic complexity and potential for noncranial referral. In patients with chronic orofacial pain, the diagnosis may be further complicated by multiple overlapping diagnoses and emergence of biobehavioral factors.

Facial pain conditions are presented in Table 1. Of the many intracranial problems causing facial pain, cerebellar pontine angle meningioma (versus neuralgia or pulpal pathology) should be considered when there is paroxysmal pain plus patient description of dysesthesia (i.e., tingling or numbness) confirmed by cranial nerve examination. Other conditions associated with neuralgia-like pain include cranial tumor (e.g., epidermoid, metastatic, brainstem glioma), acoustic neuroma, nasopharyngeal carcinoma, vascular lesions (e.g., arteriovenous malformation), scleroderma, and Paget's disease. Neuralgia-like pain can also follow orthognathic and third molar surgery in a small number of cases.

Neurovascular problems presenting diagnostic difficulty include the atypical migraine variants, paroxysmal hemicrania, cluster-tic syndromes, temporal arteritis, carotodynia, and chronic cluster where pain may be perceived in the mid-face, cheek, or temple. The epidemiology, precipitating factors, and associated symptoms assist in differentiating between these conditions. For example, patients with nonchronic cluster are typically men ages 18 to 40 years, and ipsilateral nasal discharge, lacrimation, conjunctival injection, and facial flushing occurs with pain. Patients with temporal arteritis, in contrast, are typically older men or women who report pain and feeling ill, and the pain location and scalp hyperpathia in conjunction with muscle palpation tenderness could be misdiagnosed as a TMD.

Atypical neurogenic conditions including neuralgias and deafferentation syndromes can be confused with pain of odontogenic or intracranial etiology. Orofacial pain associated with TMD must be differentiated from tension headache; the migraine variants; odontogenic pain caused by pulpal or periapical pathology (abscess); neurovascular or inflammatory headache with facial involvement; lesions of the parotid, ear, nose, and pharynx; and pain referred from the cervical musculature. A TMD diagnosis does not rule out non-TMD pain conditions. With traumatic injury, the differential diagnosis must contend with overlapping of multiple conditions causing pain.

Treatment

BIOMEDICAL TREATMENT

The management of TMD varies depending on the pain history and presence of biobehavioral factors but generally consists of treatments used in managing other musculoskeletal conditions as listed in Box 3. Normally, TMD is self-limited and symptoms can be effectively reduced with assurance, accurate information regarding the disease and prognosis, instructions regarding behavior modification,

> **CURRENT THERAPY**
>
> - Temporomandibular disorder is managed using symptomatic treatments according to a rehabilitation model for orthopedic type problems, and pharmacotherapy provides the primary management route for orofacial pain disorders.
> - Behavioral management for pain disorders is included as indicated.

TABLE 1 Orofacial Pain Disorders: Characteristics and Differential Diagnosis

Condition	Pathognomonic Pain Characteristics	Pathognomonic Nonpain Characteristics	Differential Diagnosis
Intracranial			
Aneurysm	Throbbing with rapid increase in severity worsened with exertion	Neurologic signs, gastrointestinal upset	Odontogenic pathology, TMD, sinus disease, Tolosa–Hunt syndrome, migraine
Cerebellar pontine angle tumor	Constant ache exacerbated by head movement or coughing. Neuralgia-like pain	Dysesthesia, paresthesia	Trigeminal neuralgia, odontogenic pathology
Neurovascular (Throbbing, Midface or Temporal)			
Migraine variant*	Pain intensity exacerbated by physical activity or triggered by stress or alcohol	Autonomic dysfunction, somatosensory hyperesthesia	Common migraine, Chiari malformation, Tolosa–Hunt syndrome, Raeder's syndrome
Chronic paroxysmal hemicrania	3- to 5-min paroxysms, 5-20 episodes/day, pain-free intervals between paroxysms; no known trigger. Unremitting form: daily at least for 1 y. Remitting form: daily for days to months, with remissions and recrudescence	Responsive to Indomethacin (Indocin)	Cluster headache, neuralgia, sinusitis, odontogenic pain
Cluster headache[†]	Burning or sharp, unilateral, eye region	Nocturnal episodes, Horner's facial flushing, tearing, conjunctival injection	Atypical cluster, cluster-tic syndrome,[†] sinusitis, odontogenic pain, atypical migraine, chronic paroxysmal hemicrania (remitted form)[†]
Atypical cluster headache[†]	Throbbing, bilateral, not eye region	Not nocturnal, infrequent ocular or nasal signs	Same as cluster; chronic paroxysmal hemicrania (unremitted form)[†]
Temporal arteritis	Burning, associated claudication	Scalp allodynia, hyperesthesia, pain in maxillary teeth, positive sedimentation rate	Migraine, sinusitis, odontogenic pain, TMD
Neurogenic			
Neuralgia (trigeminal, glossopharyngeal)	Stabbing or electrical quality, paroxysms triggered by trivial sensation in associated distribution, duration of seconds with complete remission between episodes	Absence of sensory or reflex deficit by neurologic testing	Tumor (epidermoid, metastatic), brainstem glioma, acoustic neuroma, nasopharyngeal carcinoma, vascular lesion, CT disease, Paget's disease, syphilis, toxins, MS
Postherpetic	Distribution of V3, burning/ache with allodynia (cold), dysesthesia	Preceded by vesicular disease	Odontogenic pain, post trauma, jaw surgery
Other			
Odontogenic pathology (pain in jaw, teeth, midface)	Pain with chewing, intraoral hot or cold	Caries, exposed cementum or dentin, mucosal swelling, acute malocclusion	Neurogenic, neurovascular pain, TMD, sinusitis
Stylohyoid process syndrome[†]	Deep throbbing pain (mandible or throat region) evoked by swallowing or head turning or by palpation of stylohyoid ligament or carotid trunk	Dizziness	TMD, glossopharyngeal neuralgia, carotid arteritis, tonsillitis, parotitis, osteomyelitis
Salivary disease (pain in cheek, inferior mandible)	Pain with introduction of food or drink, sour taste	Associated swelling in region of gland with resolution and recrudescence	TMD, odontogenic pathology
Sinus pathology (pain in midface)	Constant or intermittent ache aggravated by postural change involving head movement; maxillary tooth pain	Facial flushing, positive imaging	Migraine variants, odontogenic pathology TMD

*Classic and common migraine should also be considered in the differential when TMD or craniofacial pain is located in or refers to the temporal region.
[†]Per taxonomy from the International Association for the Study of Pain, 2nd edition
MS = multiple sclerosis; TMD = temporomandibular disorder.

and short-term use of medications. If parafunctional behavior such as nail biting, daytime tooth clenching, gum chewing, or habitual jaw popping are identified, they should be managed. Because habitual behavior is often stress related, the environmental factors that initiate or perpetuate the activity should be explored.

Pharmacologic management includes use of analgesics, nonsteroidal antiinflammatory drugs (NSAIDs), anxiolytics, muscle relaxants, and occasionally corticosteroids. Antidepressants, specifically the tertiary tricyclics (e.g., amitriptyline (Elavil)[1], nortriptyline (Pamelor)[1]), are especially useful for TMD because in addition to analgesic activity, they improve sleep and can suppress sleep bruxism; dosages are typically in the range of 10 to 25 mg at bedtime. In contrast, the SSRI antidepressants have been linked to increased

---
[1]Not FDA approved for this indication

BOX 3	Initial Symptomatic Treatment For Temporomandibular Disorder

Jaw rest and pain-free chewing for 14 days
Nonsteroidal antiinflammatory drugs at clinical dosage for 7–14 days
Cyclobenzaprine (Flexeril), 5–10 mg hs, or diazepam (Valium) 5 mg hs, for 7–14 days
Monitor red flags (see Table 1)
Monitor yellow flags (see Box 1)
Monitor symptom response at 2–4 weeks and determine whether other diagnostic tests or biobehavioral factors warrant further investigation
Refer to appropriate specialist if symptoms are not responding appropriately

sleep bruxism and could aggravate TMD unless combined with sleep medication.

Narcotic analgesics are discouraged in cases other than trauma because other approaches are generally available, but aggressive analgesics are important. NSAIDs are particularly effective for managing acute joint and muscle pain; dosages at the maximum recommended level should be considered. If one drug is ineffective, additional trials with others is appropriate. To prevent abuse, muscle-relaxant medication such as cyclobenzaprine (Flexeril) or anxiolytics such as diazepam (Valium) should be prescribed using a time-dependent administration. Therapeutic benefit may be increased by coupling these drugs with physical medicine intervention or a treatment contract.

In the patient with severe joint inflammation, pain relief is facilitated with corticosteroid (dexamethasone (Decadron) delivered via iontophoresis, injection (4-8 mg), or by mouth (40-60 mg tapered over 7-10 days).

If trigger points are identified in the masticatory muscles, 0.5% procaine in isotonic saline or isotonic saline alone can be delivered via local injection. Dry needling of trigger points can also be efficacious.

Physical therapy can reduce symptoms in TMD but should be prescribed carefully in order to avoid dependence. The main modality with proved efficacy is repetitive active or passive jaw exercises; physical therapy modalities are commonly used, but efficacy data are poor. A home program in which the patient opens slowly in the midline 10 times, three times a day, coupled with thermal agents may be as useful in reducing pain as physical therapy. Active jaw stretching is contraindicated with acute nonreducing disk displacement. Continuous passive jaw movement may be helpful following TMJ surgery and in cases of chronic nonreducing disk displacement and osteoarthritis.

Intraoral appliances (splints, orthotics, nightguards), used historically to treat TMD, are constructed of soft or hard acrylic, fit over maxillary or mandibular teeth, and can protect the joint(s) in cases of trauma or TMJ injury or assist in controlling sleep bruxism. No additional benefit is gained with the appliance for sleep bruxism by repositioning the jaw. Intraoral appliances are an active treatment that can alter the occlusion; hence, this treatment should only be used by a knowledgeable clinician. Orthodontics, dental reconstruction, and bite adjustment are unlikely to cause greater symptom reduction than reversible treatment, are expensive, and create additional risks that might outweigh any long-term benefits. They are appropriate therapies only when symptoms are confounded by dental pathology or significant tooth loss.

At present, the use of botulinum toxin to treat orofacial pain associated with TMD is not well supported by randomized, controlled trials.

Arthrocentesis for acute locking TMJs involves joint lavage coupled with corticosteroids and appears to be useful. Arthroscopic surgery, in addition to irrigating the joint, allows visualization of the superior synovial space, débridement of minor adhesions, and biopsy. Arthroscopic surgery is not useful for changing disk position in cases of locking, but it can increase associated hypomobility. Arthrotomy or open joint surgery may be helpful for fibrous ankylosis, suspected neoplasm, and severe osteoarthritis.

TMJ surgery for internal derangements (displacement without reduction) should be approached rarely and generally only if jaw disability is high and after failure of standard office treatments coupled with sufficient treatment adherence. In sum, surgery should be considered if identifiable disease has failed medical management and disability is increasing. Independent of surgical indications, refractory pain warrants additional medical (e.g., neurosurgical, neurologic) and biobehavioral assessment.

The treatment of orofacial pain is predicated on the identified pathology, clinical diagnosis and, if chronic, biobehavioral components. For most orofacial pain conditions not involving frank pathology, initial therapy is pharmacologic. Specific therapies, including drug protocols, are outlined in the specific disease chapters (e.g., migraine and variants, neuralgias, odontogenic disease, mucosal diseases). Adjunctive therapy can include biobehavioral, nutritional, and preventive treatments and, in limited cases, surgery such as for trigeminal neuralgia.

BIOBEHAVIORAL TREATMENT

Although acute orofacial pain disorders may be appropriately treated with medical management, chronic orofacial pain disorders as well as both acute and chronic TMDs are best managed, like all chronic pain conditions, using a rehabilitation approach. More reliance is placed on the patient acquiring self-management skills, including pain-coping behavior, cognitive skills, adaptive responses to emotional states, and managed medications.

Biobehavioral treatments are effective and based on two fundamental aims: change the perception of the pain, and modify the action pattern. Similar to its impact in back pain and headache, a single psychoeducational session for TMD pain reduces pain-related interference at 1-year follow-up. Relaxation and biofeedback have clear beneficial effects in reducing both the psychophysiologic activation generally present with TMD pain and in promoting general self-regulation.

Premorbid psychosocial characteristics often influence the patient's adherence in using these two methods, and these characteristics often become the focus of the biobehavioral therapy. In that case, biobehavioral therapy focuses on the interactions among emotional reactivity, pain, suffering, and coping. Rapid improvement in general functioning as well as in pain can be observed in as few as six sessions when the patient is motivated. Motivation, in turn, is often influenced by the character of the referral and the patient's relationship with his or her primary physician. These approaches appear to have significant and enduring benefits compared with the usual clinical treatment for TMD.

Very little is known about which aspect of treatment—medical or biobehavioral—is responsible for changes in clinical symptoms. Thus, multimodal approaches are recommended, because we do not currently understand which patient will respond to which treatment. Before escalating either diagnostic intervention or treatment within the biomedical domain, the biobehavioral domain should be equally included at the outset and its diagnostic or treatment escalation should proceed in parallel with that in the biomedical domain. Outcome assessment has almost exclusively been focused on physical parameters and not psychosocial ones. We suspect that failure to incorporate the biobehavioral domain into treatment results in greater likelihood of relapse if not increased invasiveness of treatment in certain patients.

For orofacial pain disorders, biobehavioral treatments have been poorly studied and used. Although their role is likely small for the acute orofacial pain disorder, it is also likely that biobehavioral approaches for TMD are just as useful for chronic or refractory orofacial pain disorders.

REFERENCES

Cheung LK, Lo J: The long-term effect of transport distraction in the management of temporomandibular joint ankylosis. Plast Reconstr Surg 2007;119:1003-1009.
Clark GT, Stiles A, Lockerman LZ, Gross SG: A critical review of the use of botulinum toxin in orofacial pain disorders. Dent Clin North Am 2007;51:245-261.
DiFabio RP: Physical therapy for patients with TMD: A descriptive study of treatment, disability, and health status, J Orofac Pain 1998;12:124-135.
Dworkin SF, LeResche L: Research diagnostic criteria for temporomandibular disorders: Review, criteria, examinations and specifications, critique. J Craniomandib Disord 1992;6:301-355.
Herman CR, Schiffman EL, Look JO, Rindal DB: The effectiveness of adding pharmacologic treatment with clonazepam or cyclobenzaprine to patient education and self-care for the treatment of jaw pain upon awakening: A randomized clinical trial. J Orofac Pain 2002;16:64-70.
Johansson CB, Samuelsson N, Dahlstrom L: Utilization of pharmaceuticals among patients with temporomandibular disorders: A controlled study. Acta Odontol Scand 2006;64:187-192.
Ohrbach R: Biobehavioral therapy. In Laskin DM, Greene CS, Hylander WL (eds): TMDs: An Evidence-Based Approach to Diagnosis and Treatment. Hanover Park, IL, Quintessence Publishing 2006, pp 391-403.
Schiffman EL, Look JO, Hodges JS, et al: Randomized effectiveness study of four therapeutic strategies for TMJ closed lock. J Dent Res 2007;86:58-63.
Truelove E, Huggins KH, Mancl L, Dworkin SF: The efficacy of traditional, low-cost and nonsplint therapies for temporomandibular disorders: A randomized controlled trial. J Am Dent Assoc 2006;137:1099-1107.

Bursitis, Tendinitis, Myofascial Pain, and Fibromyalgia

Method of
Kevin Deane, MD

Bursitis, tendinitis, myofascial pain, and fibromyalgia are considered part of a spectrum of soft tissue pain syndromes that are commonly evaluated in primary care settings. In many cases, bursitis, tendinitis, and regional myofascial pain are focal entities associated with trauma or overuse injuries; however, they can also occur in the setting of systemic disease or result from underlying abnormalities of joints, nerves, or muscle. They can be self-limited or can require local or systemic therapy for resolution. Unlike bursitis, tendinitis, and regional myofascial pain, fibromyalgia is a diffuse pain syndrome of unknown etiology. It can be a primary diagnosis or can be associated with other diseases. In most cases, all of the soft tissue pain disorders can be diagnosed by a good history and physical examination, and additional diagnostic tests are rarely needed.

Bursitis

Bursae are closed saclike structures that act to protect overlying soft tissue from bony structures. The causes of bursitis vary by the location of the bursa. Common causes of olecranon or prepatellar bursitis are trauma (acute or repetitive), infection, crystal disease, or systemic inflammatory diseases such as rheumatoid arthritis. Bursitis of other areas such as subacromial, ischial, trochanteric, and medial knee (pes anserine) are usually due to abnormal mechanics and trauma, although inflammatory disease can also cause bursitis in these areas.

The most common symptoms of bursitis are pain and associated loss of range of motion, which are often worse when activities that strain the bursa are performed. Swelling and redness are commonly

CURRENT DIAGNOSIS

Bursitis

- Common causes
    - Trauma (acute or chronic)(may be hemorrhagic if the patient is anticoagulated)
    - Infection (usually superficial bursae: olecranon, prepatellar)
    - Crystal disease (gout, pseudogout)
    - Systemic inflammatory disease (rheumatoid arthritis)
    - Abnormal mechanics or impingement (subacromial, trochanteric, and pes anserine bursitis)
- Common sites
    - Upper extremity: Olecranon bursitis (student's elbow), subacromial bursitis, scapulothoracic bursitis
    - Hip/pelvis: ischial bursitis (weaver's bottom), trochanteric bursitis, iliopsoas bursitis
    - Lower extremity: Prepatellar bursitis (housemaid's knee), pes anserine bursitis, semimembranous or gastrocnemius bursitis (sometimes referred to as a Baker's cyst), retrocalcaneal bursitis, metatarsophalangeal bursitis (often associated with hallux valgus deformity)
- Common physical findings
    - Localized tenderness, swelling, warmth, or redness.
    - Often increased tenderness with active range of motion.
    - If signs of inflammation are present, aspiration to evaluate for infection or crystals may be necessary.

Tendinitis

- Common areas
    - Upper extremity: Abductor pollicis longus and extensor pollicis brevis in the wrist at the base of the thumb (de Quervain's tenosynovitis), lateral epicondylitis (tennis elbow), medial epicondylitis (golfer's elbow), bicipital tendinitis, rotator cuff tendinitis
    - Lower extremity: Patellar tendinitis (jumper's knee), Achilles tendinitis, great toe metatarsophalangeal joint (bunion)
- Common techniques to identify specific areas
    - de Quervain's tenosynovitis: Finkelstein's test
    - Bicipital tendinitis: Speed's test
    - Rotator cuff tendinitis: Shoulder abduction to 90 degrees, external/internal rotation
    - Lateral epicondylitis: Wrist dorsiflexion against resistance
    - Medial epicondylitis: Wrist flexion against resistance

Fibromyalgia

- Classification Criteria (see Box 1)
    - History of widespread pain.
    - Pain in 11 of 18 tender point sites on digital palpation.
- Common coexisting symptoms or disorders
    - Symptoms: Soft tissue pain and tender points, poor sleep, chronic fatigue, dry eyes and mouth, subjective joint swelling, paresthesias, palpitations, cognitive dysfunction, headaches, skin symptoms including flushing, abnormal sweating, cold sensitivity
    - Disorders: Tension and migraine headaches, irritable bowel syndrome, temporomandibular joint pain, dysmenorrhea, chronic pelvic pain, bladder syndromes (interstitial cystitis, chronic bladder pain), depression, anxiety, chronic fatigue syndrome

seen with the more superficial bursae at the olecranon and prepatellar regions. In some cases of chronic olecranon or prepatellar bursitis, swelling may be the only symptom. For deeper structures such as the subacromial, ischial, and trochanteric bursae, pain and limited motion are the most common symptoms. On examination, the bursae are usually tender when compressed. This can require direct palpation for more superficial bursae (olecranon, prepatellar, trochenteric), and anatomic positioning for deeper bursae (subacromial, iliopsoas).

Diagnostic aspiration of the bursa is often needed if signs of inflammation are present (fever, warmth, redness, marked tenderness, or swelling). Fluid should be sent for Gram stain and culture, cell count and differential, and crystal analysis. Bursal fluid normally has few nucleated cells in it. A bursal fluid white blood cell (WBC) count greater than $1000/mm^3$ represents significant inflammation, and thus infection, crystal disease, or systemic inflammatory disease should be considered.

Imaging is required in the evaluation of bursitis if there is a possibility of an underlying bony abnormality or foreign body or to clarify the diagnosis, such as distinguishing subacromial bursitis from rotator cuff injury or tendinitis. In addition, because of the large number of bursae in the hip and pelvis region (>14) and their relatively deep location, MR imaging of the hip or pelvis may be required to verify that symptoms are attributable to a bursitis and not other causes. Severe prepatellar or olecranon bursitis can be difficult to distinguish from knee or elbow arthritis. Often aspiration of the bursa along with a careful examination that distinguishes the joint from overlying soft tissue can help decide the point, although specialist evaluation or imaging is sometimes necessary.

Treatment options for bursitis depend to some extent on the location and etiology of the bursitis. Traumatic superficial bursitis benefits from avoidance of injury, local application of ice, occasional drainage with subsequent compression wrap to prevent recurrence, and, if appropriate from a general medical standpoint, therapy with nonsteroidal antiinflammatory drugs (NSAIDs), which can be systemic or topical. In refractory cases, local corticosteroid injection or surgical removal of the bursa may be indicated. If infection is present, serial aspirations or surgical drainage should be performed, and adequate antibiotics should be administered, usually for a minimum of 14 days due to the avascular nature of bursae.

For deeper bursae, some of the same treatment strategies apply: avoidance of injury, local application of heat or ice, NSAIDs, and corticosteroid injection. In addition, identification and management of underlying causes of deeper bursitis such as gait abnormalities or limb length discrepancy with trochanteric bursitis or abnormal shoulder girdle mechanics in subacromial bursitis is important, and referrals to physical therapy for strengthening and correction of abnormal motion are often necessary to prevent recurrent symptoms. In some cases, surgical management of causative factors is necessary. Finally, underlying disorders that are contributing to bursitis such as hyperuricemia or rheumatoid arthritis, should be identified and managed appropriately.

Tendinitis

Tendons are formed of collagen and provide connections between muscle and bone. To enhance their movement, they are typically enclosed in a sheath lined with cells similar to those found in the synovium.

Tendinitis develops when mechanical or inflammatory injury damages the tendon or sheath, causing rupture and swelling into the tendon itself (usually mechanical injury) or swelling and inflammation along the sheath (usually inflammatory injury). Trauma or overuse injuries are the most common causes of tendinitis. However, systemic inflammatory diseases including infection (e.g., disseminated gonorrhea and Lyme disease), crystal disease, and autoimmune diseases such as rheumatoid arthritis, scleroderma, and seronegative spondyloarthropathies can also lead to tendinitis and should be considered, especially in patients presenting with recurrent or unusual tendinitis or systemic features. Fluoroquinolone antibiotics have also been associated with spontaneous tendinitis and rupture.

Patients with tendinitis typically present with pain with range of motion and activity. The pain is usually maximal with weight loading or extreme ranges of motion. Limitation of motion is often present, and in the case of flexor tendinitis of the hand, a finger can trigger or lock in the flexed position. Rupture of a tendon can result in loss of motion. With superficial tendons, patients might also complain of swelling over the affected area.

The examiner should initially have the patient recreate the symptomatic movements, with the patient pointing with one finger to the most symptomatic area if possible. Further examination should then focus to identify the abnormal tendon. Recording the range of motion with active movement is an important aspect of the examination for tendinitis to ensure that no tendon rupture is present. A careful history and physical examination should be performed to ensure no systemic process is present. In particular, rheumatoid arthritis or scleroderma can manifest with tendinitis crepitans, where there is a grating sensation with tendon movement, and occasionally an audible tendon rub or squeak is heard.

To diagnose tendinitis in deeper structures or when rupture is suspected (for example, the patient's inability to abduct the shoulder), imaging may be required. Certain types of tendinitis, such as rotator cuff tendinitis or suspected inflammatory tendinitis, are best visualized with MRI with intravenous or intraarticular contrast, and these types cof examinations should be ordered after specialist consultation.

Treatment for tendinitis initially consists of avoiding straining activities, applying ice, and taking NSAIDs. In some cases, local injection of corticosteroid can speed resolution of inflammation. The risk of tendon rupture after corticosteroid injection is low, but it can be decreased further by using appropriate doses of corticosteroids, by avoiding direct tendon injection, and by having the patient avoid significant strain of the tendon for 1 to 2 weeks after injection. In cases of tendinitis related to traumatic injury or in athletes, specialist consultation may be necessary before injection of corticosteroids because risk of tendon rupture is higher in these settings.

In certain types of tendinitis (lateral epicondylitis, de Quervain's tenosynovitis) splinting may be helpful. To prevent recurrent tendinitis, physical or occupational therapy to improve the mechanics of the tendon use are often helpful. Extracorporeal shock wave therapy has been approved by the FDA for treatment of some tendon disorders, although more data are needed to determine efficacy. In refractory cases of tendinitis, or in cases of suspected infection or tendon rupture, surgical intervention may be necessary.

Regional Myofascial Pain

Regional myofascial pain is typically a pain syndrome in a focal region of the body and is usually from a source other than specific bursae, tendons, bones, or joints. Plantar fasciitis is a better understood type of regional myofascial pain, although it is often categorized as a tendinitis. The source of regional myofascial pain is likely a combination of muscle or soft tissue and nerve irritation from multiple causes including trauma, overuse, or nerve injury. There may be a clear inciting factor (e.g., thigh pain after a long horseback ride or hike), although in some cases there is no distinguishable inciting event or injury.

Patients with regional myofascial pain present with focal areas of pain. They may also report altered sensation in the area including a feeling of burning or stinging, or they have limitations in movement due to pain or spasm in the area. Examiners should make sure to determine what actions or movements worsen symptoms or if there have been recent focal movements that might have led to injury (for example, excessive use of the arm with manual labor such as hammering). On examination, there may be diffuse tenderness in a localized area, or more focal trigger points. The movement mechanics of the involved area need to be observed; for example, abnormal gait from a leg-length discrepancy or lumbar spine disease can lead to myofascial pain over the lateral thigh. Also, examination should focus on possible underlying causes for the regional pain such as nerve injury or degenerative disease. Focal inflammatory processes such as infection or myositis are causes of localized pain and need to be considered in patients with regional myofascial pain; these might require laboratory studies or imaging to identify.

Treatment includes identification and avoidance of the inciting event, if possible, or physical therapy to improve local mechanics. Local heat or ice or NSAID therapy may also be of benefit, and local tissue injection with anesthetic may be helpful as well. Referral to a physical medicine specialist may be necessary for refractory cases. If an underlying disorder (such as degenerative joint disease) is suspected, treatment for this may be indicated. For plantar fasciitis, in addition to ice and NSAID therapy, patients might benefit from soft shoe inserts, stretching exercises, and corticosteroid injection for refractory cases. Because steroid injections increase the risk of plantar fascia rupture or fat pad atrophy, these should only be administered by trained health care providers.

BOX 1 American College of Rheumatology's 1990 Classification Criteria for Fibromyalgia*

For classification purposes, patients will be said to have fibromyalgia if both criteria are satisfied. Widespread pain must have been present for at least 3 months. The presence of a second clinical disorder does not exclude the diagnosis of fibromyalgia.

History of Widespread Pain

Definition: Pain is considered widespread when all of the following are present: pain in the left side of the body, pain in the right side of the body, pain above the waist, and pain below the waist. In addition, axial skeletal pain (cervical spine or anterior chest or thoracic spine or low back) must be present. In this definition, shoulder and buttock pain is considered as pain for each involved side. Low back pain is considered lower segment pain.

Pain in 11 of 18 Tender Point Sites on Digital Palpation

Definition: Pain, on digital palpation, must be present in at least 11 of the following 18 sites:
- Occiput: Bilateral, at the suboccipital muscle insertions
- Low cervical: Bilateral, at the anterior aspects of the intertransverse spaces at C5-C7
- Trapezius: Bilateral, at the midpoint of the upper border
- Supraspinatus: Bilateral, at origins, above the scapula spine near the medial border
- Second rib: Bilateral, at the second costochondral junctions, just lateral to the junctions on upper surfaces
- Lateral epicondyle: Bilateral, 2 cm distal to the epicondyles
- Gluteal: Bilateral, in upper outer quadrants of buttocks in anterior fold of muscle
- Greater trochanter: Bilateral, posterior to the trochanteric prominence
- Knee: Bilateral, at the medial fat pad proximal to the joint line

Digital palpation should be performed with an approximate force of 4 kg (force required to blanch nail bed).

For a tender point to be considered positive, the patient must state that the palpation was painful. "Tender" is not to be considered painful.

---
*Wolfe F, Smythe HA, Yunus MB, et al: The American College of Rheumatology 1990 Criteria for the Classification of Fibromyalgia. Report of the Multicenter Criteria Committee. Arthritis Rheum 1990;33(2):160-172.

Fibromyalgia Syndrome

Fibromyalgia is a chronic, diffuse pain syndrome. Fibromyalgia can be considered primary if no other significant musculoskeletal disorder exists. It is considered secondary if it is found in the setting of confirmed systemic disease such as rheumatoid arthritis, systemic lupus erythematosus, or osteoarthritis.

The main features of fibromyalgia are diffuse soft tissue pain and poor sleep or fatigue. However there can be multiple other symptoms present. Pain and disability can range from mild to severe. Fibromyalgia affects women 10 times more than men and increases in prevalence in older populations, with estimates of prevalence of approximately 2% in 20-year-olds increasing to 8% in 70-year-olds.

The etiology of fibromyalgia is unknown. However, based on current understanding, it likely results from a complex interaction between genetic, psychosocial, environmental, and biochemical factors leading to abnormal pain regulation and possibly abnormal autonomic nervous system function.

The American College of Rheumatology's 1990 Classification Criteria for fibromyalgia is shown in Box 1. This scheme requires that 11 of 18 tender points be present for diagnosis; however, many health care providers make a diagnosis of fibromyalgia in diffuse pain syndromes even if patients do not have 11 tender points. The presence and degree of sleep disturbance and fatigue should also be assessed in fibromyalgia. Patients with primary fibromyalgia may have joint tenderness on examination, but not true swelling or deformity; also they should have normal strength. If swelling or deformity of joints or weakness is noted, diagnoses other than fibromyalgia need to be considered.

There is no laboratory test to confirm fibromyalgia; however, routine laboratory testing including compete blood counts, comprehensive metabolic panels, thyroid function testing, and markers of inflammation should be normal in fibromyalgia patients. Caveat: Many diseases can manifest with symptoms similar to fibromyalgia, and these should be considered in the initial assessment, although laboratory testing for these diseases is not routinely recommended unless evidence for them is present on history and physical examination (Box 2).

Once the diagnosis of fibromyalgia has been made, treatment for fibromyalgia should initially focus on patient education regarding fibromyalgia. Patients can be informed that fibromyalgia is a valid

---

BOX 2 Diseases That Can Mimic or be Associated With Fibromyalgia

Autoimmune Disease
Inflammatory myopathy or myositis
Polymyalgia rheumatica
Rheumatoid arthritis, systemic lupus erythematosus, Sjögren's syndrome
Seronegative spondyloarthropathies

Infections
Hepatitis C
Lyme disease

Metabolic Disease
Celiac disease
Hemachromatosis
Hypothyroidism or hyperthyroidism
Vitamin D deficiency (controversial)

Other Diseases
Degenerative joint disease (including spinal degeneration with nerve injury)
Hypermobility syndromes
Peripheral nerve injury or neuropathy
Sleep disorders (apnea, periodic limb movement, restless legs syndrome)

CURRENT THERAPY

Bursitis
- Traumatic
  - Identification and removal of mechanical causes
  - Rest, ice, nonsteroidal antiinflammatory therapy (including topical antiinflammatories)
  - Compression to prevent recurrence of fluid accumulation
  - Aspiration or injection
- Infectious
  - Drainage of affected bursa either by serial aspiration or surgical incision
  - Appropriate antibiotics (usually 14 days)
- Crystalline
  - Antiinflammatory therapy or aspiration or injection
  - Consider systemic therapy for crystalline disease
- Systemic inflammatory disease
  - Aspiration or injection
  - Management of underlying disease
- Recurrent bursitis can require surgical removal of the bursa or physical or occupational therapy to avoid repetitive mechanical stress leading to bursal inflammation
- The dose of corticosteroids for bursal injection varies by location. Typically, 40 mg of methylprednisolone (Solu-Medrol) or triamcinolone (Kenalog) is used for deeper areas including subacromial bursitis or trochanteric bursitis; 20 mg of these agents can be used for more superficial bursae. There may be a higher risk of fat atrophy and skin hypopigmentation with superficial use of fluorinated corticosteroids such as triamcinolone acetonide.

Tendinitis
- Identify and remove contributory factors. Treatment can include physical therapy or occupational therapy
- Rest, ice or heat, nonsteroidal antiinflammatory agents, topical analgesics or antiinflammatories, splinting
- Local corticosteroid injection if initial measures fail to control symptoms: 10-20 mg of methylprednisolone or equivalent for small tendons (de Quervain's tenosynovitis or flexor tendons of the fingers); 20-40 mg of methylprednisolone or equivalent for larger tendons (epicondylitis or rotator cuff tendinitis)
  - Avoid direct tendon injection because of risk of rupture if this occurs
  - Surgical therapy for infectious tendinitis or refractory cases

Fibromyalgia
- Establish the diagnosis and identify and treat related conditions (mood disorder, sleep abnormalities)
- Patient education
- Physical modalities
  - Exercise: aerobic and strengthening; graded increases in activity level to avoid flares of fatigue and pain
  - Sleep hygiene
  - Touch therapies
  - Cognitive behavior therapy
- Pharmacologic therapy (see Box 3)
  - Begin with low-dose tricyclic antidepressant or cyclobenzaprine (Flexeril).[1]
  - If no effect, may switch to or add another agent or consider specialty evaluation.
- Specialist evaluation
  - Rheumatology, physical medicine/rehabilitation psychiatry, pain management, or sleep specialist consultation might be necessary.
  - Consider consultation if diagnosis is unclear, comorbid conditions are suspected, additional medications are needed, or the patient has severe disability.

---

diagnosis and that the disease likely results from problems with pain processing. Patients can be encouraged that no study has shown increased mortality directly due to fibromyalgia. For further information, patients can be directed to the Arthritis Foundation or websites supported by universities or reputable foundations.

In general, if patients can be managed as part of a multidisciplinary treatment team outcomes may be improved. Cognitive-behavior therapy focusing on management of pain may be helpful. Underlying mood disorders such as anxiety or depression should be identified and treated.

Patients should be encouraged to get regular exercise, which includes aerobic as well as muscle-strengthening activities. Warm-water pool therapy to reduce impact may be beneficial in some patients. Maintaining exercise programs for fibromyalgia patients can be difficult, because many patients perceive that exercise worsens their pain and fatigue. However they can be counseled to start slow and at a low level of activity, gradually increase their activity levels (5%-10% every 2-4 weeks) as their fitness level improves. Stretching and toning exercises such as yoga or Pilates are helpful in some patients. Also, therapies such as massage, biofeedback, transcutaneous stimulation, acupuncture or acupressure can also be helpful in some patients. Trigger point injections with anesthetics have been tried for fibromyalgia, but there are few data regarding their benefit.

Medications for fibromyalgia may be used at the time of diagnosis or if other modalities have not resulted in sufficient improvement (Box 3). Multiple medications have been postulated to improve symptoms in fibromyalgia, but many of these have not been rigorously studied or showed no benefit. However, several medications have been shown to be beneficial, especially agents that act as neuromodulators. In particular, agents that act centrally and improve sleep such as tricyclic antidepressants[1] and cyclobenzaprine (Flexeril)[1] have been beneficial, although their use may be limited by side effects and loss of efficacy over time. Other neuroactive medications including selective serotonin reuptake inhibitors[1] and serotonin-norepinephrine reuptake inhibitors[1] have been tried and in some cases found beneficial in fibromyalgia. The anticonvulsants gabapentin (Neurontin)[1] and pregabalin (Lyrica) may also be useful. The use of long-term opiates in fibromyalgia is controversial, and most physicians avoid prescribing them because they have not been shown in controlled studies to be significantly beneficial. Preliminary studies using hormone modulation and anticonvulsant therapy are encouraging, but more data are needed before these agents can be widely used in fibromyalgia. Systemic steroids should not be used to treat primary fibromyalgia.

The role of mental illness in the development of fibromyalgia is unclear; however, many patients with fibromyalgia meet criteria for mood disorders, including depression and anxiety. Thus, patients with fibromyalgia should be formally assessed for mental illness and

---

[1]Not FDA approved for this indication.

> **BOX 3 Pharmacologic Therapy for Fibromyalgia***
>
> **Initial Therapy**
> Begin with low-dose tricyclic antidepressant or cyclobenzaprine (Flexeril).[1] If the medication has no effect, you may switch to or add an agent from section B or consider specialty evaluation.
> A. Evidence of benefit shown in more than one randomized, controlled trial
>   - Amytriptyline (Elavil)[1] 25-50 mg at bedtime
>   - Cyclobenzaprine[1] 5-10 mg at bedtime, may be dosed during day
> B. Evidence of benefit shown in one randomized, controlled trial or positive results from multiple nonrandomized, controlled trials:
>   - Tramadol (Ultram), with or without acetaminophen (Tylenol)
>   - Selective serotonin reuptake inhibitors: fluoxetine
>   - Dual-reuptake inhibitors: venlafaxine (Effexor),[1] duloxetine (Cymbalta)[1]
>   - Anticonvulsants: gabapentin (Neurontin),[1] pregabalin (Lyrica)
>   - Pramipexole[1]
> C. Limited or no evidence of benefit:[1]
>   - Benzodiazepines
>   - Corticosteroids
>   - Dehydroepiandrosterone (DHEA)
>   - Dextromethorphan
>   - Guaifenesin
>   - Melatonin
>   - Nonsteroidal antiinflammatory agents
>   - Opiates
>   - Thyroid hormone (in absence of hypothyroidism)
>
> **Specialist Evaluation**
> Consider a specialist evaluation (rheumatology, physical medicine or rehabilitation, psychiatry, pain management, sleep specialist) if the diagnosis is unclear, comorbid conditions are suspected, additional medications are needed, or the patient has severe disability.
>
> ---
> [1]Not FDA approved for this indication.
> *Adapted from Goldenberg DL, Burckhardt C, Crofford L. Management of fibromyalgia syndrome. JAMA 2004;292:2388-2395.[8]

treated appropriately. If there is a history of emotional, physical, or sexual abuse, patients might need special counseling and management.

In general, patients with fibromyalgia continue to have pain, and management is an ongoing process. Predictors for a better prognosis (long-term employment, satisfying life) include a patient's willingness to engage in physical activity and a patient's belief that the pain is not damaging and that the patient has some control over the pain.

Summary

Soft-tissue pain disorders are common complaints in medical practice, and health care providers need to be well versed in the diagnosis and management of bursitis, tendinitis, myofascial pain syndromes, and fibromyalgia. In most cases, these diagnoses can be made by careful history and physical examination. For bursitis, tendinitis, and regional myofascial pain syndromes, treatment usually includes identification and removal of inciting factors, rest, ice or heat, and systemic or topical antiinflammatory agents. Local anesthetic or corticosteroid injections can be used for more resistant cases.

Fibromyalgia is a diffuse pain syndrome that can require long-term therapy, which should include patient education, an exercise program and pharmacologic therapy.

REFERENCES

Borg-Stein J, Simons DG: Focused review: Myofascial pain. Arch Phys Med Rehabil 2002;83(3 Suppl 1):S40-S47, S8-S9.
Goldenberg DL, Burckhardt C, Crofford L: Management of fibromyalgia syndrome. JAMA 2004;292(19):2388-2395.
Paige NM, Nouvong A: The top 10 things foot and ankle specialists wish every primary care physician knew. Mayo Clin Proc 2006;81(6):818-822.
Rees JD, Wilson AM, Wolman RL: Current concepts in the management of tendon disorders. Rheumatology (Oxford) 2006;45(5):508-521.
Small LN, Ross JJ: Suppurative tenosynovitis and septic bursitis. Infect Dis Clin North Am 2005;19(4):991-1005, xi.
Wilson JJ, Best TM: Common overuse tendon problems: A review and recommendations for treatment. Am Fam Physician 2005;72(5):811-818.
Wolfe F, Ross K, Anderson J, et al: The prevalence and characteristics of fibromyalgia in the general population. Arthritis Rheum 1995;38(1):19-28.
Wolfe F, Smythe HA, Yunus MB, et al: The American College of Rheumatology 1990 Criteria for the Classification of Fibromyalgia. Report of the Multicenter Criteria Committee. Arthritis Rheum 1990;33(2):160-172.

Osteoarthritis

Method of
David H. Neustadt, MD

Osteoarthritis (OA) (degenerative joint disease) is the most commonly encountered rheumatic disorder and the major cause of disability and reduced activity after 50 years of age. Radiographic evidence of OA is found in up to 85% of people older than 65 years. Autopsies indicate evidence of OA in weight-bearing joints of almost all persons by the age of 45 years.

In spite of the evidence of pathologic changes of OA found in Java and Neanderthal human skeletons and dinosaur skeletons, OA was confused with rheumatoid arthritis (RA) until the turn of the 20th century. It is characterized pathologically by involvement of cartilage, varying from fissures and microfibrillations in early disease to erosive destruction in advanced disease. Weight-bearing or shearing forces are transmitted to the subchondral bone, leading to sclerosis, cyst formation, and bone remodeling. Osteophytes (spurs) develop at the margins of joints, and new cartilage proliferates over these bony spurs.

An inflammatory component is present in most patients with symptomatic OA. The traditional belief that OA is simply a wear-and-tear condition associated with the stress of advancing years is not tenable. This mistaken belief is considered the major reason for the relatively slow progress of cartilage and bone research and investigation into the etiology and pathogenesis of OA. During the past decade, much new knowledge on cartilage, including metabolic changes, genetic mutations, metalloproteinases, and possible diagnostic biomarkers and inflammatory mediators, has fostered considerable excitement and interest in new approaches for the prevention, monitoring, and treatment of OA.

Although the cause of OA is unknown, contributing factors include heredity, trauma, overweight, overuse of joints, and aging. OA may be classified into primary (idiopathic) and secondary forms. Secondary OA results from trauma or repetitive overuse of a specific joint; in an inflammatory form of arthritis such as RA, repeated attacks of gout, or septic arthritis; developmental problems such as congenital dysplasia of a hip or slipped capital femoral epiphysis; or

CURRENT DIAGNOSIS

- Enhanced understanding and knowledge of the pathogenesis of osteoarthritis have led to increasing optimism for the 20 to 30 million osteoarthritis sufferers in the United States.
- Osteoarthritis is now known to involve inflammatory mechanisms, not mechanical wear and tear, as believed in the past.

BOX 2 Measures to Protect Knees

Avoid knee bending when weight bearing
Avoid steps when possible
Use high chair or high stool
Use elevated toilet seat
Use cane, crutches, or walker for prolonged walking
Do isometric quadriceps muscle-strengthening exercises

---

metabolic and miscellaneous causes including hemophiliac arthropathy, ochronosis (alkaptonuria), and osteonecrosis. Thus, OA may be considered a (final) common pathway resulting from a host of many different problems.

Joints commonly affected in OA include the large weight-bearing and frequently used joints, such as the hips and knees, spine, distal interphalangeal (DIP) joints (Heberden's nodes), and trapeziometacarpal (carpometacarpal thumb base) and first metatarsophalangeal joint (bunion). Joints often spared in OA include the metacarpals, the wrists, the shoulders, and the ankles (except in ballet dancers).

Clinical Features

The onset of OA is insidious, and the course is slowly progressive. Clinical features include variable pain and mild stiffness, with associated limited motion; bony enlargement with or without tenderness; synovitis of the knees; and functional impairment with malalignment (varus or valgus deformities) when advanced involvement of the knees or hips develops. There are no specific laboratory abnormalities or specific (disease) markers of the disease, except in ochronosis.

Radiographs and other imaging procedures demonstrate evidence of OA, manifested chiefly by a narrowed joint space (loss of cartilage), osteophyte formation, and secondary subchondral sclerosis. There may be a poor correlation between symptoms and underlying abnormal structural findings on x-ray images. Special subsets of OA and significant associated conditions include inflammatory (cystic erosive) OA, calcium pyrophosphate dihydrate disease (chondrocalcinosis), and diffuse idiopathic skeletal hyperostosis (DISH).

Treatment

The optimal management program for OA should be individualized to the specific problems and clinical syndromes presented by each patient (Box 1).

GENERAL CONSIDERATIONS

Realistic reassurance that the patient does not have a serious, potentially crippling disease such as RA and adequate understanding of what to expect are of paramount importance for successful management. Education of the patient is the basic foundation of the treatment program. The updated OA booklet provided by the National Arthritis Foundation is an available useful supplement to education. Involving spouses and other family members in coping skills training may be helpful. Understanding the patient's problem permits reasonable delegation of responsibilities for chores and engaging in activities. Patients and spouses who are better informed about the disease and its outlook are generally better able to cope with the condition. Cognitive behavior techniques can help patients confront the variability of symptoms, the effects of rest and exercise, and emotional aspects.

PROPHYLACTIC MEASURES

Reducing the impact of the load and shearing force on an osteoarthritis joint not only can diminish symptoms but also can retard progression of the disease. Explaining the biomechanical factors enables the patient to understand the need for rest and protection of the affected joints. Weight reduction by dietetic means is strongly encouraged for the obese patient. Protective and preventive measures for the knee include avoiding weight-bearing knee bending, stair climbing, jogging, and prolonged walking. Knee loading during weight bearing can be avoided by using a high chair or stool, elevated toilet seat, knee supports or braces, and walking devices (Box 2).

NONPHARMACOLOGIC THERAPY

The most important aspect is specific instructions for balanced rest and exercise (preferably at home). Exercises should be mainly isometric (nonmovement), such as quadriceps muscle strengthening, stretching, and range-of-motion exercises.

Instructions should be given for joint protection with measures to conserve energy and on the use of any needed assistive aids, such as canes, crutches, walkers, splints, back supports and braces, cervical supporting collars, and proper shoes with any needed modifications and orthotics.

Heat modalities should be prescribed in the form of hot showers or tub soaks, hot packs such as a Bed Buddy (microwavable cervical collar or back wrap), and a warm pool for water aerobic exercises. These measures ameliorate discomfort and facilitate the exercise program. Diathermy, short wave, and ultrasound methods are relatively expensive and of questionable benefit. The use of a hot tub or whirlpool bath, especially after exercise or work, may be of palliative benefit.

Job and recreational activities must be assessed and modified if necessary to avoid overuse of affected joints. Sexual counseling may be needed, especially in some patients with severe knee, hip, or back involvement.

PHARMACOTHERAPY

The basic program of education and reassurance of the patient, joint rest and protection, and physical measures can control symptoms in some patients with early mild OA. Many patients, however, require drug therapy. Although no available drugs predictably reverse or halt the inexorable progression of the disease, the drugs do reduce pain and inflammation, enhancing the patient's quality of life.

BOX 1 Comprehensive Management Program for Osteoarthritis

Education of the patient and family
Coping measures: Rest and modification of activities of daily living
Measures to reduce joint loading
Physical therapy, occupational therapy, assistive devices
Pharmacotherapy
Intraarticular therapy (steroids, hyaluronan)
Surgery

CURRENT THERAPY

- Although there is no cure for osteoarthritis, coping strategies including simple measures such as weight reduction and modification of activities to reduce stress and load on the joints should be emphasized.
- Pharmacotherapy includes acetaminophen (Tylenol), other simple analgesics, and judicious use of nonsteroidal antiinflammatory drugs. Opioids should be avoided.
- When usual medical measures fail to control the pain of osteoarthritis, intraarticular injections of a corticosteroid is the next step.
- A painful effusion is the major indication for arthrocentesis, aspiration, and if fluid is not infectious, instillation of a corticosteroid preparation.
- After a corticosteroid injection for knee osteoarthritis, increased therapeutic response results if a postinjection rest regimen is imposed. The patient remains in bed or at rest for 3 days and then uses walking devices (cane or crutches) for 2 to 3 weeks.
- The main factors that influence the therapeutic response from a series of hyaluronan injections are the extent of loss of cartilage and severity of the osteoarthritis disease in the affected knee.
- Total knee and hip replacement procedures are considered when nonoperative management fails to adequately control symptoms and pain.

Analgesics

Some patients with OA have minimal inflammation and can be managed with analgesics alone. Analgesic agents (non-narcotic) currently available include acetaminophen (Tylenol), propoxyphene (Darvon), and tramadol (Ultram). Effective dosages of acetaminophen are 1.0 to 1.3 g administered every 8 hours or three or four times daily (do not exceed 4 g/day). Adverse effects are rare, but caution must be exercised in patients who have preexisting renal or liver conditions. Propoxyphene is effective, especially in combination with acetaminophen (Darvocet-N 100), and may be given in a dosage of 1 tablet every 4 to 6 hours for supplementary analgesia. Side effects are usually minimal, with the patient occasionally intolerant because of nausea or lightheadedness. Tramadol can be given in 50-, 100-, 200-, or 300-mg tablets up to two to three times daily for pain relief (do not exceed 400 mg of immediate-release tablets per day or 300 mg of extended-release tablets per day). These drugs are generally well tolerated, and nausea, vomiting, and dizziness are the most common adverse effects. A combination preparation, Ultram 37.5 plus acetaminophen (Ultracet), is available. I advise avoiding regular use of opioids. Opioids may be needed occasionally for intense pain, but the benefits are limited owing to the common gastrointestinal adverse events and the potential for addiction.

Antiinflammatory Agents

A much-discussed report compared acetaminophen 4 g/day with ibuprofen (Advil, Motrin) 1200 to 2400 mg/day, in OA of the knee. The clinical results demonstrated no significant difference in efficacy among the three treatment groups. Critical analysis of this comparative study, however, discloses a short duration of the treatment trial (4 weeks) and a relatively low antiinflammatory dosage (up to 2400 mg) of ibuprofen. In my experience and that of many others, pain in OA patients is often not adequately controlled with pure analgesics, whereas nonsteroidal antiinflammatory drugs (NSAIDs) in adequate dosage can provide significant clinical improvement.

Nonacetylated salicylates are widely used in OA. Compounds currently available include salsalate, choline magnesium trisalicylate, and magnesium salicylate. These agents are weak prostaglandin (cyclooxygenase) inhibitors, thus avoiding the anticlotting effect and potential adverse effect on the gastrointestinal tract and kidneys. Side effects are relatively uncommon and minor with nonacetylated salicylates when administered in a dosage of 1 to 1.5 g twice daily. Gastrointestinal and cardiovascular problems have not been reported. Salicylism with ototoxicity is a rare side effect.

If simple analgesics and salsalate fail to provide adequate relief, one of the many currently available NSAIDs may be selected for a therapeutic trial. Clinical trials with naproxen, diclofenac, and sulindac showed significantly greater improvement of the NSAID when compared with high-dose acetaminophen. The chief limiting factor in the use of NSAIDs is the possible induced gastric pathologic changes, disturbed renal function, and potential increased cardiac events.

Cost and compliance also must be given consideration. Many of the NSAIDs are now available in dosage forms that can be given once or twice daily, which helps overcome the compliance problem.

Currently available NSAIDs are all similar in their proposed mechanism of action but vary considerably in their pharmocokinetics, dosage, clinical response, and side effects. The variability of the effects of different NSAIDs in patients is significant and unpredictable. All NSAIDs are metabolized in the liver, except two available compounds, sulindac (Clinoril) and nabumetone (Relafen), which are prodrugs that are not converted to active drugs until after absorption and hepatic biotransformation. The prodrug effect might partially spare the gastrointestinal tract and also produces less suppression of renal prostaglandins. Etodolac (Lodine) reportedly has fewer gastric complications, and endoscopy does not demonstrate the typical gastric erosions found in the gastric mucosa of the majority of patients taking older NSAIDs.

Concomitant prophylactic use of misoprostol (Cytotec) has been recommended to protect gastric mucosa in patients with a previous history of peptic ulcer or gastrointestinal bleeding. Unfortunately, misoprostol causes cramps and diarrhea in a relatively high percentage of patients. A gastroprotective agent, such as a proton pump inhibitor, will reduce the risk of gastrointestinal adverse effects.

The question of potential deleterious effect on cartilage versus chondroprotective properties by various NSAIDs remains controversial.

Cyclooxygenase 2 Inhibitors

Prostaglandin synthesis in humans is catalyzed by two enzyme forms of cyclooxygenase: cyclooxygenase 1 (COX-1) and cyclooxygenase 2 (COX-2).

COX-1 is constitutively expressed and is considered responsible for suppression of physiologic functions including gastric mucosal protection. In contrast, COX-2 is induced by inflammatory mediators and is responsible for inflammation without any significant effect on the gastric mucosa. The development of agents that selectively inhibit the COX-2 pathway without significant gastrointestinal adverse effects was considered an extremely important advance.

Currently only one COX-2–specific inhibiting NSAID is FDA approved and available. Celecoxib (Celebrex) is equivalent to the older nonselective NSAIDs with regard to therapeutic effectiveness, but the risk of gastrointestinal toxicity and adverse effects on platelet aggregation is lessened. The risk of renal side effects is probably comparable with that of the conventional NSAIDs. A trial assessing the effect of celecoxib on cardiovascular events found a slightly higher risk of cardiovascular events but chiefly only at higher doses (400 mg/day or greater). Celecoxib can be used with low-dose aspirin (81 mg) daily and anticoagulants including warfarin (Coumadin).

INTRAARTICULAR INJECTIONS

Corticosteroids

After many years of controversy concerning intraarticular corticosteroid therapy in OA, there is now consensus that this form of therapy is of considerable value when it is indicated and skillfully administered. Although early on it is still preferable to attempt to control symptoms by simple measures with oral therapy, rather than by local injection, when faced with relatively acute painful conditions such as synovitis of the knee or inflamed Heberden's nodes, quick and sometimes lasting relief can be obtained with intrasynovial steroid injection. This form of treatment is considered an adjunct to a conventional management program.

A painful knee effusion is the most common indication for arthrocentesis followed by a local corticosteroid injection. The remote potential deleterious effect of instability developing in the knee can be avoided by giving injections at infrequent intervals and prescribing a strict postinjection rest regimen. Specific instructions are given to the patient to refrain from weight-bearing activity for 3 days, except getting up for meals and going to the bathroom. The patient is advised to reduce loading of the injected knee by using a cane or crutches with a three-point gait during weight bearing for 2 to 3 weeks after the procedure. This rest regimen delays escape of the steroid suspension from the joint cavity and promotes a longer duration of response to the injection. I have observed numerous patients with OA of the knee associated with large recurrent synovitis who had been given three to five or more local injections with only transient benefit. When a strict postinjection rest program was imposed, these patients obtained substantial improvement in the duration of the effect, and some achieved indefinite "cures." The remote risk of introducing infection from the procedure is minimized by adhering to a meticulous aseptic technique.

Another important indication for arthrocentesis and intraarticular steroid therapy is OA associated with crystal synovitis due to calcium pyrophosphate dihydrate disease (CPPD) or pseudogout. Diagnosis is confirmed by radiographic findings of chondrocalcinosis and polarized microscopic identification of the specific crystals in the fluid. Treatment, including aspiration and administration of intraarticular steroids, is usually successful in controlling the acute synovitis.

Hyaluronans (Hyaluronic Acid, Hyaluronate)

Intraarticular hyaluronan, approved by the FDA in 1997 as a new procedure for clinical use in OA of the knee, represents a valuable addition to the therapeutic armamentarium for the treatment of OA. The clinical use of intraarticular hyaluronan in painful OA of the knee was introduced in Europe in the 1990s. The mechanism of action of hyaluronate is termed *viscosupplementation* in an effort to restore normal viscoelastic properties to the pathologically altered synovial fluid. Other possible beneficial effects include protection of the chondrocytes, antiinflammatory effects, and improvement of the mechanics of joint motion.

Numerous preparations of FDA approved hyaluronan preparations are in wide use in the United States. Initially, all hyaluronans were extracted from rooster combs. Table 1 lists the more common hyaluronans that are available for injecting knee osteoarthritis. The hyaluronan products are injected in a series of three, four, or five at weekly intervals in accordance with the patient's response. All the hyaluronans are highly purified natural preparations except Hylan G-F20, which is cross-linked with added formaldehyde and vinyl sulfone in an effort to increase retention in the joint cavity. Effectiveness and duration of improvement are similar with all the products. Undesirable complications and adverse effects are limited to rare local mild pain, with the exception of the cross-linked Hylan G-F20, which can cause a severe acute inflammatory reaction (SAIR, or pseudoseptic reaction) in approximately 2% to 8% of patients injected with the product.

Newer hyaluronan products are non–animal-derived preparations that are developed from biological fermentation of streptococcal origin. Until recently, these hyaluronans have been available only in Europe. One of these products (Euflexxa) has been approved by the FDA for use in the United States. This preparation would be especially useful in the rare patient who is allergic to avian products. Hyaluronan therapy has been studied in other specific joints including the hip, shoulder, ankle, and first carpometacarpal joints. Approval from the FDA is expected. Drawbacks of intraarticular hyaluronan include difficulty injecting and limited response in patients with extreme obesity and severe advanced osteoarthritis of the knee (grade 4 Kellgren classification). Re-treatment with intraarticular hyaluronic acid 1 year after the first series is safe and effective in patients whose initial course of therapy was successful. A new hyaluronan preparation (Monovisc) has been developed, containing 4 or 5 times the amount of hyaluronan used in the usual knee injection, which is given in a series of 3 or 4 weekly injections. The approach, if effective, would simplify the procedure, especially for "needle shy" patients. The treatment is available in Europe but is not FDA approved as yet for use in the United States.

JOINT LAVAGE AND ARTHROSCOPY

Lavage of the arthritic knee may be performed with arthroscopic visualization. The authors of a recent double-blind sham-controlled evaluation concluded that "most, if not all" of the effects of tidal irrigation seem to be attributable to a placebo effect. Arthroscopy permits inspection of the joint cavity. Associated abnormalities such as ligamentous and meniscal tears can be observed in conjunction with osteoarthritis. Calcified loose bodies can be removed, and débridement can be carried out.

TREATMENT OF CYSTIC EROSIVE (INFLAMMATORY) OSTEOARTHRITIS

Cystic erosive OA is the genetically determined clinical syndrome manifested by the lumpy-bumpy fingers with involvement of the DIP joints (Heberden's nodes) and proximal interphalangeal joints (Bouchard's nodules). It rarely causes significant pain except during the early developing stage. It is important to strongly reassure the patient that this is not a serious crippling disease, emphasizing the distinction of the knobby nodes from the swelling of the synovitis of RA. However, if the thumb base joint (trapeziometacarpal, first carpometacarpal) is involved, abduction splinting or local injection may be necessary for relief of pain.

Occasionally, when OA of the fingers is symptomatic, warm soaks; application of an analgesic balm, such as triethanolamine, after the warm soaks; and the wearing of spandex gloves during sleep at night are sometimes useful. When a digital node is inflamed, local instillation of a few drops of a corticosteroid suspension often provides prompt relief.

If symptoms persist, a cautious trial with one of the topical analgesic pepper plant creams (capsaicin) such as Zostrix may be worthwhile. Capsaicin is an inhibitor of substance P, the neuropeptide pain mediator. The topical cream is safe, and a local burning or transient stinging sensation during application is the only troublesome adverse effect. The stinging diminishes with use after a few days.

NEW APPROACHES

Disease-Modifying Drugs

The purpose of the investigational disease-modifying drugs is to play a role in either enhancing the biosynthesis of cartilage matrix or preventing enzymatic degradation and inhibiting catabolic cytokine

TABLE 1 Some Common FDA-Approved Hyaluronans and Their Molecular Weights

Product	MW (kD)	Dose (Weekly)
Hylan G-F20 (Synvisc)	5000-6000	3 × 16 mg
High-molecular-weight hyaluronan (Orthovisc)	1000-2900	3-4 × 30 mg
Sodium hyaluronate (Hyalgan)	500-720	3-5 × 20 mg
Sodium hyaluronate (Supartz)	620-1200	5 × 25 mg
1% Sodium hyaluronate (Euflexxa)*	2400-3600	3 × 20 mg

*Derived from biological fermentations.

activity in an attempt to induce cartilage repair and restore joint homeostasis.

Tetracycline (Sumycin)[1] and its congeners (doxycycline (Vibramycin),[1] minocycline (Dynacin)[1]) have shown evidence of inhibiting enzymatic degradation of cartilage, including that by stromelysin, collagenase, and gelatinase, in dog, guinea pig, and rabbit models of OA. A proposed long-term clinical trial in human subjects is in progress.

Hydroxychloroquine (Plaquenil)[1] and chloroquine (Aralen)[1] have been administered successfully for many years in RA and systemic lupus erythematosus. Recently, anecdotal and retrospective uncontrolled studies have reported the efficacy of hydroxychloroquine in retarding the progression of inflammatory (cystic) erosive OA. It has been suggested that the beneficial action of hydroxychloroquine is due to its inhibitory effects on lysosomal enzymes and the secretion of interleukin-1. Experience thus far suggests that this agent may be promising in inflammatory OA.

Other novel therapeutic approaches that are under study but lack conclusive significant data at this time include insulin-like growth factors, transforming growth factor-β, and glucosamine, a proteoglycan component and a growth factor for cartilage. In an ongoing study, an antinerve growth factor antibody, fully humanized, effectively reduces pain and improves function in subjects with knee osteoarthritis. Undesirable effects so far are minor, including a rare transient mild peripheral neuritis.

Chondrocyte Transplantation

Chondrocyte transplantation was initially developed and carried out in Sweden for localized cartilage damage resulting from trauma in young subjects. A subsequent report described relatively successful treatment of 23 patients who had chondral defects of the knee and were given autologous chondrocyte transplantation combined with periosteal grafting. The expectation that the procedure will "cure" OA lesions remains an unmet possibility for the future. Regeneration of articular cartilage is a complex process and will require long-term evaluation of the function of the new cartilage and prospective controlled clinical studies to confirm the value of the procedure.

Gene Therapy

Gene therapy is an exciting new technology that holds promise for the future but requires considerable further investigation and refinement. Techniques to introduce gene transfer in conjunction with autologous cultured chondrocytes are being explored.

Glucosamine and Chondroitin Sulfate

Glucosamine[7] and chondroitin[7] sulfate are over-the-counter nutraceuticals (dietary supplements) that have considerable anecdotal data touting their symptom-modifying effects. Some reports have suggested that glucosamine can retard or modify structural changes of OA, but convincing evidence for this effect is lacking. The drugs are well tolerated and have no significant adverse effects. Recently published studies have no evidence or significant data demonstrating that either of these preparations used alone or in combination prevents or reduces pain in osteoarthritis of the knee. Further observations with long-term randomized, double-blind studies are needed to confirm any value of these popular but unproved medications.

SURGERY

When appropriate medical (nonoperative) management fails to adequately control pain, and functional disability significantly interferes with lifestyle, surgical options should be considered.

Available procedures include osteotomy for joint malalignment (varus knee deformities); arthroscopy, especially for specific lesions such as calcified loose bodies or meniscal tears; and arthrodesis (fusion) for unstable joints, when joint replacement is not indicated or declined. Arthrodesis may be the optimal procedure in young, overweight, active patients with severe OA involving a single knee.

Partial or total arthroplasty, especially total knee and hip replacement, may be carried out in patients in whom medical management fails to adequately control symptoms. An estimated 125,000 total hip replacements, most of which are for OA, are performed each year in the United States. Total knee replacement (total knee arthroplasty) is an increasingly gratifying operation for advanced knee OA. Innovative approaches and new techniques, including the development of minimal invasive procedures (MIS), bodes well for the future.

REFERENCES

Mandell BF, Lipani J: Refractory osteoarthritis. Differential diagnosis and therapy. Rheum Dis Clin North Am 1995;21:163-178.

Neustadt DH: Intra-articular injections for osteoarthritis of the knee. Cleve Clin J Med 2006;73:897-910.

Neustadt DH: Current approach to therapy for osteoarthritis of the knee. Louisville Med 2004;51:341-343.

Neustadt DH, Altman RD: Intra-articular therapy. In Moskowitz RW, Howell DS, Goldberg VM, et al (eds): Osteoarthritis, Diagnosis and Medical/Surgical Management, 4th ed. Philadelphia, Lippincott, Williams & Wilkins 2007, pp 287-301.

Poole AR, Howell DS: Etiopathogenesis of osteoarthritis. In Moskowitz RW, Howell DS, Goldberg VM, et al (eds): Osteoarthritis, Diagnosis and Medical/Surgical Management, 4th ed. Philadelphia, Lippincott, Williams & Wilkins 2007, pp 27-49.

Sharma L, Kapoor D, Issa S: Epidemiology of osteoarthritis. In Moskowitz RW, Howell DS, Goldberg VM, et al (eds): Osteoarthritis, Diagnosis and Medical/Surgical Management, 4th ed. Philadelphia, Lippincott, Williams & Wilkins 2007, pp 1-26.

Steinbrocker O, Neustadt DH: Aspiration and Injection Therapy, Arthritis and Musculoskeletal Disorders: A Handbook on Technique and Management. Hagerstown MD, Harper & Row 1972.

Polymyalgia Rheumatica and Giant Cell Arteritis

Method of
Gideon Nesher, MD

Diagnosis

GIANT CELL ARTERITIS

Giant cell arteritis (GCA) involves the major branches of the aorta, with a predilection for the extracranial branches of the carotid artery, such as the temporal arteries. The aorta itself may also be involved. GCA is often associated with polymyalgia rheumatica (PMR), a syndrome of bilateral aching and stiffness of the shoulder girdle and sometimes the neck and hip girdle. More commonly, PMR occurs as an isolated disease, without GCA. Both GCA and PMR occur in persons older than 50 years. Women are more commonly affected. Their clinical features and laboratory abnormalities are presented in Box 1.

Color duplex ultrasonography of the temporal arteries can aid in the diagnosis of GCA. A recent meta-analysis concluded that when the pretest probability of GCA is low, negative results of ultrasonography practically exclude GCA. It appears that ultrasonography better serves to rule out GCA, but a positive test needs to be confirmed by temporal artery biopsy. However, because GCA affects the vessels

---

[1]Not FDA approved for this indication
[7]Available as a dietary supplement

BOX 1 Clinical and Laboratory Features of Giant Cell Arteritis

Common

Headache, scalp tenderness
Prominent temporal arteries
Jaw claudication
Systemic symptoms: Fever, malaise, fatigue, anorexia, and weight loss
Polymyalgia rheumatica
Elevated erythrocyte sedimentation rate and C-reactive protein, anemia of inflammation, thrombocytosis, elevated alkaline phosphatase

Uncommon

Vision loss, diplopia, and other ophthalmic manifestations
Stroke, transient ischemic attacks and other neuropsychiatric manifestations
Vestibuloauditory manifestations (hearing loss, tinnitus)
Scalp or tongue infarction
Aortic arch syndrome, aortic valve insufficiency, aortic aneurysm and dissection.
Peripheral neuropathies
Respiratory symptoms (cough, sore throat, hoarseness)
Involvement of other arteries (e.g., coronary, femoral)

 CURRENT DIAGNOSIS

Giant Cell Arteritis

- Typical clinical manifestations include headache, tenderness over temporal arteries, jaw claudication, polymyalgia rheumatica, acute vision loss, and low-grade fever in an elderly patient.
- Laboratory markers of inflammation include elevated erythrocyte sedimentation rate and C-reactive protein, anemia of inflammation, and thrombocytosis.
- Color duplex ultrasonography of the temporal arteries can aid in diagnosis. When the pretest probability is low, negative results of ultrasonography practically exclude giant cell arteritis.
- Temporal artery biopsy showing vasculitis, often with giant cells, confirms the diagnosis. In cases with negative biopsy, rule out other conditions and rely on the clinical presentation and laboratory abnormalities, together with the typical prompt response to glucocorticoid therapy.

Polymyalgia Rheumatica

- Bilateral aching of the shoulder girdle, sometimes the neck and hip girdle, in an elderly patient, is typical. Morning stiffness is a prominent feature. Onset may be acute or gradual.
- Polymyalgia rheumatica may be isolated or associated with giant cell arteritis.
- Laboratory markers of inflammation include elevated erythrocyte sedimentation rate and C-reactive protein, sometimes anemia of inflammation.
- Prompt response to low-dose glucocorticoid therapy is typical and is sometimes used to confirm the diagnosis.

focally, histologic examination is normal in about 15%. A threshold size of 1 cm of temporal artery specimen is associated with increased diagnostic yield. It is preferable to perform the biopsy before therapy, but in most cases therapy should not be delayed pending the biopsy or its results (see later). There may be histologic signs of arteritis even after 2 to 4 weeks of treatment.

There are no criteria to determine whether GCA is present when temporal arteries biopsy is negative. The American College of Rheumatology (ACR) criteria for the classification of GCA can assist in diagnosis (Table 1). However, classification criteria work

TABLE 1 Suggested Criteria for the Diagnosis of Polymyalgia Rheumatica and Classification of Giant Cell Arteritis

Feature	PMR — Bird et al	PMR — Chuang et al	GCA — American College of Rheumatology
Age (y)	>65	>50	>50
Onset and duration	Onset <2 wk	Duration >1 mo	Not required
Area of pain	Shoulders	Two areas out of neck or torso, shoulders or proximal arms, hips, or proximal thighs	Headache (new onset)
Tenderness	Upper arms	Not required	On palpation of TA, or decreased pulsation of TA
Morning stiffness	>1 h	>30 min	Not required
Other features	Weight loss, depression	Not required	TA biopsy: vasculitis with mononuclear-cell infiltrates, often with giant cells
Erythrocyte sedimentation rate	>40 mm/h	>40 mm/h. If ESR is not elevated, look for other evidence to support the diagnosis	>50 mm/h
Requirements for diagnosis	≥3 criteria: sensitivity, 92%; specificity, 80%	All criteria must be present	≥3 criteria: sensitivity, 93%; specificity, 91%.

ESR = erythrocyte sedimentation rate; GCA = giant cell arteritis; PMR = polymyalgia rheumatica; TA = temporal artery.
Bird HA, Esselinckx W, Dison ASJ, et al: An evaluation of criteria for polymyalgia rheumatica. Ann Rheum Dis 1979;38:434-439.
Chuang TY, Hunder GG, Ilstrup DM, Kurland LT: Polymyalgia rheumatica: A 10-year epidemiologic and clinical study. Ann Intern Med 1982;97:672-680.
Hunder GG, Bloch DA, Michel BA, et al: The American College of Rheumatology 1990 criteria for the classification of giant cell arteritis. Arthritis Rheum 1990;33:1122-1128.

best in studying groups of patients and less well when used for diagnosing individual cases. Meeting classification criteria is not equivalent to making the diagnosis in individual patients; the diagnosis should be based on all clinical and laboratory findings.

POLYMYALGIA RHEUMATICA

There is no single diagnostic test for PMR, but sets of diagnostic criteria have been suggested by several groups of investigators. Two commonly used sets of criteria are presented in Table 1.

There is a wide range (4%-31%) of reported frequency of GCA in patients presenting with PMR. The two conditions can ocur together but are sometimes separated by long intervals, and either one can appear first. Aside from the typical features of GCA (see Box 1), severe systemic symptoms, severe degrees of anemia, thrombocytosis and ESR elevation, and poor clinical response to prednisone 15 to 20 mg/day with persistent abnormalities in laboratory parameters of inflammation all suggest GCA in patients presenting with PMR symptoms. In such cases, temporal artery ultrasonography or biopsy should be performed to rule out GCA.

Treatment

Glucocorticoids are the treatment of choice for both PMR and GCA (Boxes 2 and 3). Symptoms typically begin to abate within 1 to 3 days of commencing therapy. This dramatic improvement is characteristic of both PMR and GCA. Prompt treatment is crucial in GCA to prevent irreversible complications of acute vision loss and stroke.

Levels of erythrocyte sedimentation rate (ESR) and C-reactive protein (CRP) do not always correlate with disease activity. Elevation of their levels while the patient is asymptomatic is not an indication to increase the dose of prednisone. In such cases, it is preferable to slow the rate of dose tapering and continue to watch closely for recurrence of symptoms. The dose should be increased if symptoms recur, even when ESR or CRP remain within the normal range.

The average duration of treatment is 2 to 3 years, but in some patients it is necessary to continue low doses of prednisone (5-10 mg/day) for longer periods. Relapses are experienced by 25% to 65% of patients, mostly during the first year of treatment or after discontinuation of glucocorticoids. Most relapses are mild, but some GCA patients develop vision loss or stroke while tapering glucocorticoid dosage or after discontinuing therapy.

Glucocorticoid-related adverse effects can become a source of great morbidity. No steroid-sparing agent has been proved widely effective. Thus, the preferred approach to limit side effects is to use the lowest dose possible for the shortest period of time while avoiding disease relapses.

Low-dose aspirin (100 mg/day) has been shown to significantly decrease the rate of vision loss and stroke during the course of glucocorticoid therapy, probably mediated by its antiplatelet effect.

CURRENT THERAPY

- Glucocorticoids are the treatment of choice for both giant cell arteritis and polymyalgia rheumatica. No steroid-sparing agent is proved to be widely effective thus far.
- Rapid improvement of clinical manifestations following treatment initiation is characteristic.
- Prompt treatment is crucial in giant cell arteritis to prevent irreversible complications of acute vision loss and stroke. Addition of low-dose aspirin can further prevent these complications.
- The average duration of treatment is 2 to 3 years. Relapses are common but often mild.

BOX 2 Guidelines for Glucocorticoid Therapy in Giant Cell Arteritis*

Starting Daily Dose of Prednisone

40-60 mg for 2-4 weeks

Patients with vascular ischemic complications (stroke, vision loss) or imminent ischemic complications (transient ischemic attacks, amaurosis fugax, diplopia) are treated initially with higher prednisone doses (up to 120 mg) or 500-1000 mg/day of intravenous methyprednisolone (Solumedrol) for 3 consecutive days in an attempt to prevent additional ischemic complications. Starting with such high doses of intravenous methylprednisolone for 3 days also can allow more rapid tapering of oral glucocorticoids.

Tapering and Maintenance

Reduce by 5-10 mg every 2-4 weeks until dose is 20 mg
Then reduce by 2.5-5 mg every 2-4 weeks until the dose is 10 mg
Then reduce by 1 mg every month

If symptoms recur, increase the dose to the previous level or slightly above it for several weeks, then resume tapering. In case of recurrent ischemic symptoms, restart treatment with a full dose.

Additional Therapies

Aspirin 100 mg/d (decreases the rate of vision loss and stroke),
Calcium, vitamin D, and bisphosphonates (to prevent osteoporosis)

---

*Individual cases vary greatly. The exact doses and the duration of treatment should be adjusted to the needs of the individual patient, considering both disease manifestations and glucocorticoid adverse effects. According to this schedule, treatment may be completed in 1-2 years

---

BOX 3 Guidelines for Glucocorticoid Therapy in Polymyalgia Rheumatica*

Starting Daily Dose of Prednisone

15-20 mg for 2-4 weeks

Tapering and Maintenance

Reduce by 2.5-5 mg every 2-4 weeks until the dose is 10 mg
Then reduce the dose by 1 mg every month

If symptoms recur, increase the dose to the previous level or slightly above it for several weeks, then resume tapering.

Additional Therapies

Calcium, vitamin D, and bisphosphonates (to prevent osteoporosis)

---

*Individual cases vary greatly. The exact doses and the duration of treatment should be adjusted to the needs of the individual patient, considering both disease manifestations and glucocorticoid adverse effects. According to this schedule, treatment may be completed in about 1 year

Aortic complications in the thoracic segment (aneurysms, dissection) can occur late in the course of GCA, sometimes after the completion of treatment. It is advisable that all GCA patients have evaluation of the thoracic aorta during the follow-up period and after completing treatment.

REFERENCES

Bird HA, Esselinckx W, Dison ASJ, et al: An evaluation of criteria for polymyalgia rheumatica. Ann Rheum Dis 1979;38:434-439.

Chuang TY, Hunder GG, Ilstrup DM, Kurland LT: Polymyalgia rheumatica: A 10-year epidemiologic and clinical study. Ann Intern Med 1982;97:672-680.

Hachula E, Boivin V, Pasturel-Michon U, et al: Prognostic factors and long-term evolution in a cohort of 133 patients with giant cell arteritis. Clin Exp Rheumatol 2001;19:171-176.

Hunder GG, Bloch DA, Michel BA, et al: The American College of Rheumatology 1990 criteria for the classification of giant cell arteritis. Arthritis Rheum 1990;33:1122-1128.

Karassa FB, Matsagas MI, Schmidt WA, Iannidis JP: Meta-analysis: Test performance of ultrasonography for giant cell arteritis. Ann Intern Med 2005;142:359-369.

Mazlumzadeh M, Hunder GG, Easley KA, et al: Treatment of giant cell arteritis using induction therapy with high-dose glucocorticoids: A double-blind, placebo-controlled, randomized prospective clinical trial. Arthritis Rheum 2006;54:3310-3318.

Nesher G, Berkun Y, Mates M, et al: Low-dose aspirin and prevention of cranial ischemic complications in giant cell arteritis. Arthritis Rheum 2004;50:1332-1337.

Nesher G, Rubinow A, Sonnenblick M: Efficacy and adverse effects of different corticosteroid dose regimens in temporal arteritis: A retrospective study. Clin Exp Rheumatol 1997;15:303-306.

Proven A, Gabriel SE, Orces C, et al: Glucocorticoid therapy in giant cell arteritis: Duration and adverse outcomes. Arthritis Rheum 2003;49:703-708.

Weyand CM, Fulbright JW, Evans JM, et al: Corticosteroid requirements in polymyalgia rheumatica. Arch Intern Med 1999;159:577-584.

Osteomyelitis

Method of
Luca Lazzarini, MD

BOX 1   The Cierny-Mader Staging System for Osteomyelitis

Anatomic Type
- Stage 1: medullary osteomyelitis
- Stage 2: superficial osteomyelitis
- Stage 3: localized osteomyelitis
- Stage 4: diffuse osteomyelitis

Physiologic Class
- A: normal host
- B: compromised host
- Bs: systemically compromised
- Bl: locally compromised
- C: treatment worse than the disease

Factors Affecting Host Status
- Systemic
  Malnutrition
  Renal and hepatic failure
  Diabetes mellitus
  Chronic hypoxia
  Immune disease
  Malignancy
  Extremes of age
  Immunosuppression
- Local
  Chronic lymphedema
  Venous stasis
  Major vessel compromise
  Arteritis
  Extensive scarring
  Radiation fibrosis
  Small-vessel disease
  Neuropathy
  Tobacco use

Osteomyelitis is a complex disease often associated with high morbidity and considerable health care costs. This condition can be classified by duration (acute or chronic), pathogenesis (hematogenous or contiguous spread), site, extent, and by the type of patient (infant, child, adult, or compromised host). The Waldvogel classification system subdivides osteomyelitis as being either hematogenous or secondary to a contiguous focus of infection. Contiguous focus osteomyelitis has been further subdivided into osteomyelitis with or without vascular insufficiency. An alternative to the Waldvogel classification system has been developed by Cierny and Mader. The Cierny-Mader staging system is based on the anatomy of the bone infection and the physiology of the host (Box 1). The anatomic types of osteomyelitis are medullary (stage 1), superficial (stage 2), localized (stage 3), and diffuse (stage 4). Stage 1 infection is confined to the medullary surface of the bone. Hematogenous osteomyelitis and infected intramedullary rods are examples of this anatomic type. Stage 2 is a contiguous focus infection occurring when an exposed infected necrotic surface of bone lies at the base of a soft tissue wound. Stage 3 is usually characterized by a full-thickness, cortical sequestration that can be removed surgically without compromising bony stability. Stage 4 is a through-and-through process that usually requires an intercalary resection of the bone to arrest the disease process. Further, the patient is classified as an A, B, or C host. An A host represents a patient with normal physiologic, metabolic, and immunologic capabilities. The B host is either systemically compromised, locally compromised, or both. When the morbidity of treatment is worse than that imposed by the disease itself, the patient is given the C host classification. This classification system aids in the understanding, diagnosis, and treatment of bone infections in children and adults (Table 1).

Etiology

In hematogenous osteomyelitis, a single pathogenic organism is almost always recovered from the bone. In infants *Staphylococcus aureus*, *Streptococcus agalactiae*, and *Escherichia coli* are most frequently isolated from blood or bones. However, in children more than 1 year of age, *S. aureus*, *Streptococcus pyogenes*, and *Haemophilus influenzae* are most commonly isolated. The incidence of *H. influenzae* infection decreases after age 4 years. However, the overall incidence of *H. influenzae* as a cause of osteomyelitis is decreasing because of the new *H. influenzae* vaccine now given to children. In adults, *S. aureus* is the most common organism isolated. Multiple organisms are usually isolated from the infected bone in contiguous focus osteomyelitis. *S. aureus* remains the most commonly isolated pathogen. However, gram-negative bacilli and anaerobic organisms are also frequently isolated. Other microorganisms, such as mycobacteria and fungi, can be involved as well.

Clinical Manifestations

SIGNS AND SYMPTOMS

Hematogenous osteomyelitis in children may present with acute signs of infection including abrupt fever, irritability, lethargy, and local signs of inflammation. However, 50% of children present with

TABLE 1 Principal Antibiotics Used in the Initial Intravenous Treatment of Osteomyelitis

Staphylococci, methicillin sensitive	Nafcillin (Unipen) 2 g q4-6h (+ rifampin [Rifadin][1] 600 mg qd PO)
Staphylococci, methicillin resistant	Vancomycin (Vancocin) 1 g q12h (+ rifampin [Rifadin][1] 600 mg qd PO)
Streptococci	Penicillin[1] 2 MU q4h
Anaerobes, gram-positive	Clindamycin[1] (Cleocin) 900 mg q8h
Anaerobes, gram-negative	Metronidazole[1] (Flagyl) 500 mg q8h
Enterobacteriaceae, Pseudomonas	Ciprofloxacin (Cipro) 400 mg q12h

[1]Not FDA approved for this indication.
Abbreviations: PO = orally; q = every; qd = every day.

vague complaints, including pain of the involved limb of 1 to 3 months in duration and minimal, if any, temperature elevation.

Adults with hematogenous osteomyelitis usually present with vague complaints consisting of nonspecific pain and few constitutional symptoms lasting 1 to 3 months. However, acute clinical presentations with fever, chills, swelling, and erythema over the involved bone(s) are occasionally seen. The source of bacteremia may be from a trivial skin infection or from a more serious infection such as acute or subacute bacterial endocarditis. Hematogenous osteomyelitis that involves either long bones or vertebrae is an important complication of injection drug abuse.

Patients with contiguous focus osteomyelitis often present with localized bone and joint pain, erythema, swelling, and drainage around the area of trauma, surgery, or wound infection. Signs of bacteremia such as fever, chills, and night sweats may be present in the acute phase of osteomyelitis, but not in the chronic phase.

The sedimentation rate is usually elevated, reflecting chronic inflammation, but the leukocyte count is usually normal. The chronic disease is usually either not progressive or slowly progressive. If a sinus tract becomes obstructed, the patient may present with a localized abscess and or an acute soft tissue infection. A sedimentation rate that returns to normal during the course of therapy is a favorable prognostic sign.

MICROBIOLOGY

The diagnosis and determination of the etiology of long bone osteomyelitis rests on the isolation of the pathogen(s) from the bone lesion or blood or joint culture. Except in hematogenous osteomyelitis, where positive blood or joint fluid cultures may suffice, antibiotic treatment of osteomyelitis should be based on meticulous cultures of bone taken at débridement surgery or from deep bone biopsies. If possible, cultures should be obtained before antibiotics are initiated. Sinus tract cultures are unreliable for predicting which organisms will be isolated from infected bone; however, those growing *S. aureus* show a positive correlation with bone cultures.

RADIOLOGY

In hematogenous osteomyelitis, radiographic changes usually correlate with the destructive process and are usually seen when at least 50% to 75% of the bone matrix is destroyed. This happens at least 2 weeks after the infection was initiated. The earliest radiologic changes are swelling of the soft tissue, periosteal thickening and/or elevation, and focal osteopenia. Radiographic improvement may lag behind clinical recovery, even when the patient is receiving appropriate antimicrobial therapy. In contiguous focus osteomyelitis, the radiographic changes are subtle, often found in association with other nonspecific radiographic findings, and require a careful clinical correlation to achieve diagnostic significance. Computed tomography (CT) may play a role in the diagnosis of osteomyelitis. Increased marrow density occurs early in the infection, and intramedullary gas has been reported in patients with hematogenous osteomyelitis. The CT scan can also help identify areas of necrotic bone and assess the involvement of the surrounding soft tissues. One disadvantage of this study is the scatter phenomenon, which occurs when metal is present in or near the area of bone infection. Magnetic resonance imaging (MRI) has been recognized as a useful modality for diagnosing the presence and scope of musculoskeletal infection. The resolution of MRI makes it useful in differentiating between bone and soft tissue infection, often a problem with radionuclide studies. Radionuclide scans may be obtained when the diagnosis of osteomyelitis is ambiguous or to help gauge the extent of bone and soft tissue inflammation.

Treatment

Therapy of osteomyelitis is both surgical and medical and includes adequate drainage and débridement, obliteration of dead space, soft tissue coverage, and specific antimicrobial treatment. If the patient is a compromised host, an effort is made to correct or improve the host defect.

ANTIBIOTIC TREATMENT

According to the results of animal studies, the optimal duration of antibiotic treatment is 4 to 6 weeks. The time needed for bone revascularization after débridement surgery is approximately 3 weeks. Shorter durations are probably successful when the infection is superficial (stage 2) and a complete débridement is performed and when ablative surgery (amputation above the infected region) is performed.

Antibiotic treatment for osteomyelitis is traditionally administered by the intravenous (IV) route. To reduce hospitalization and health care costs, outpatient IV therapy is currently used. This modality of administration reduces treatment cost and improves patient quality of life.

Antistaphylococcal penicillins (nafcillin [Unipen],[1] oxacillin [Prostaphlin][1]) are used for the treatment of methicillin-sensitive staphylococcal osteomyelitis. A first-generation cephalosporin, cefazolin (Ancef), is effective in the treatment of staphylococcal

---
[1]Not FDA approved for this indication.

CURRENT DIAGNOSIS

- Clinical signs
- Plain radiographs
- CT, NMR, and bone scans obtained in selected cases
- Cultures from sinus tract are unreliable
- Perform bone biopsy for culture and histology whenever possible

Abbreviations: CT = computed tomography; NMR = nuclear magnetic resonance.

CURRENT THERAPY

- Stabilization (if needed) and surgical débridement
- Antibiotic treatment of 4 to 6 weeks after surgical débridement
- Select antimicrobial according to in vitro sensitivity tests; consider toxicity, allergy, costs
- Antibiotic suppressive therapy in selected cases

osteomyelitis. The glycopeptides vancomycin (Vancocin)[1] and the oxazolidinone antibiotic linezolid (Zyvox)[1] are used to treat methicillin-resistant staphylococcal osteomyelitis. Several third- and forth-generation cephalosporins, such as cefotaxime (Claforan)[1] or cefepime (Maxipime)[1] can be used to treat osteomyelitis because of gram-negative bacilli.

Oral antibiotics have also been successfully used to treat osteomyelitis. Several oral drugs, such as clindamycin (Cleocin),[1] rifampin (Rifadin),[1] cotrimoxazole (Bactrim),[1] and fluoroquinolones (e.g., ciprofloxacin [Cipro] and levofloxacin [Levaquin][1]) are currently used in the treatment of osteomyelitis. Clindamycin (Cleocin), a lincosamide antibiotic active against most gram-positive bacteria, possesses an excellent bioavailability and is currently used orally, after an initial IV treatment of 2 weeks. Oral therapy using quinolones for gram-negative organisms is used in adult patients with osteomyelitis. The current quinolones have variable *S. aureus* and *Staphylococcus epidermidis* coverage. Pediatric patients should not be given the quinolone class of antibiotics because of possible damage to cartilage.

The initial treatment of most cases of osteomyelitis usually starts on an empirical basis. After cultures are obtained, a parenteral antimicrobial regimen is begun, covering the clinically suspected pathogens. Once the organism is identified, different antibiotics can be selected by appropriate sensitivity methods. If possible, antibiotics should not be initiated until the results of the bone bacterial culture and sensitivities are known.

ANTIBIOTIC TREATMENT BY CIERNY-MADER STAGE

Stage 1 osteomyelitis in children usually responds to antibiotics alone. Stage 1 osteomyelitis in adults is more refractory to therapy and is usually treated with antibiotics and surgery. The patient is treated for 4 to 6 weeks with appropriate antimicrobial therapy, dated from the initiation of therapy or after the last major débridement surgery. If after 48 hours there is no clinical improvement, surgical treatment may be needed in conjunction with another 4-week course of antibiotics.

In stage 2 osteomyelitis shorter courses of antibiotics, such as 2 weeks, are usually given. In stages 3 and 4 osteomyelitis the patient is treated with 4 to 6 weeks of antimicrobial therapy dated from the last major débridement surgery. This long treatment is needed because even when all necrotic tissue has been adequately débrided, the remaining bed of tissue must be considered contaminated with the responsible pathogen(s).

SUPPRESSIVE ANTIBIOTIC THERAPY

When surgical treatment of osteomyelitis is not feasible, a long-term antibiotic therapy is usually given to control the disease and to prevent flare-ups. Oral antibiotics are usually used. Suppressive therapy has been studied extensively in the setting of infected orthopedic implants. The efficacy of suppressive treatment in osteomyelitis without implants has not been determined. Suppressive therapy is usually administered for 6 months. If recurrence of the infection occurs after discontinuation, a new, culture-directed suppressive regimen is begun and administered indefinitely.

SURGICAL TREATMENT

Surgical treatment of osteomyelitis includes adequate drainage, extensive débridement of all necrotic tissue, obliteration of dead spaces, adequate soft tissue coverage, and restoration of an effective blood supply.

Adequate débridement may leave a large bony defect termed *dead space*. The goal of dead space management is to replace dead bone and scar tissue with vascularized tissue. Local tissue flaps or free flaps may be used to fill dead space. An alternative technique is to place cancellous bone grafts beneath local or transferred tissues where structural augmentation is necessary. Antibiotic-impregnated acrylic beads may be used to sterilize and temporarily maintain dead space. The beads are usually removed within 2 to 4 weeks and replaced with a cancellous bone graft. The most commonly used antibiotics in beads are vancomycin (Vancocin),[1] tobramycin,[1] and gentamicin.[1] Because beads act as a biomaterial surface to which bacteria adhere, infection associated with the use of beads has been described.

If movement is present at the site of infection, measures must be taken to achieve permanent stability of the skeletal unit. Stability may be achieved with plates, screws, rods, and/or an external fixator. External fixation is preferred more than internal fixation because of the tendency of medullary rods to become secondarily infected and to spread the extent of the infection. The Ilizarov fixator is a type of external fixator that allows reconstruction of segmental bone defects and difficult infected nonunions. The technique is used for difficult cases of osteomyelitis when stabilization and bone lengthening is necessary.

Adequate soft tissue coverage of the bone is often necessary to arrest osteomyelitis. Small soft tissue defects may be covered with a split thickness skin graft. In the presence of a large soft tissue defect or with an inadequate soft tissue envelope, local muscle flaps and free vascularized muscle flaps may be placed in a one- or two-stage procedure. Local muscle flaps and free vascularized muscle transfers improve the local biologic environment by bringing in a blood supply important in host defense mechanisms, antibiotic delivery, and osseous and soft tissue healing.

---

[1]Not FDA approved for this indication.

REFERENCES

Cierny G, Mader JT, Pennick JJ: A clinical staging system for adult osteomyelitis. Contemp Orthop 1985;10:17-37.
Lew DP, Waldvogel FA: Osteomyelitis. Lancet 2004;364:369-379.
Shuford JA, Steckelberg JM: Role of oral antimicrobial therapy in the management of osteomyelitis. Curr Opin Infect Dis 2003;16:515-519.
Simpson AH, Deakin M, Latham JM: Chronic osteomyelitis. The effect of the extent of surgical resection on infection-free survival. J Bone Joint Surg Br 2001;83:403-407.

Common Sports Injuries

Method of
Dennis Y. Wen, MD

Participation in sports and exercise, whether for recreation or competition, is a common activity in our society and has many health-related benefits. However, injuries do occur as a result of sports participation. Several of the more common sports injuries are discussed in this article, along with some conditions that are considered sports-related but that occur quite commonly in nonsporting populations.

Knee Injuries

When evaluating a patient with a knee complaint, it is useful to establish whether the condition resulted from a traumatic injury, such as a twisting episode, or began insidiously without any specific trauma. The differential diagnosis for traumatic versus nontraumatic injuries involves different conditions. Traumatic injuries include fractures of the femur, tibia, patella, or fibula; anterior cruciate ligament (ACL) tears; posterior cruciate ligament (PCL) tears; medial collateral

---

[1]Not FDA approved for this indication.

CURRENT DIAGNOSIS

- A thorough history covering mechanism of injury, or lack of injury, should be sought.
- Many physical examination tests and maneuvers require practice and experience to determine significance of findings but can assist in diagnosis.
- Selective use of imaging can further enhance the diagnostic process.

ligament (MCL) tears; patellar dislocations and subluxations; meniscal tears; and other less common injuries. Nontraumatic causes of knee symptoms include patellofemoral pain, osteoarthritis, patellar tendinosis, Osgood–Schlatter syndrome, and other conditions.

Most significant fractures around the knee result in inability to bear weight, along with swelling in the area of the fracture, such as a large effusion for intraarticular fractures. Plain radiographs, or sometimes advanced studies with magnetic resonance imaging (MRI) for more subtle fractures such as subtle growth plate injuries in children, generally depict the injury. These fractures often require specialized care, and consultation with an orthopedist is recommended for most of these injuries.

ACL tears are a fairly common injury encountered in sports, and they often occur concurrently with meniscal tears or MCL tears. The mechanism involves twisting of the knee, often into a valgus position with the knee near extension. Often the patient hears or feels a pop or snap. Immediate swelling (within hours), which consists of hemarthrosis, usually occurs. Because the ACL, once torn, will not heal again, continued instability or buckling of the knee occurs, mainly with twisting or pivoting motions.

Several physical examination findings have been described to evaluate for ACL deficiency, but the Lachman maneuver is thought to be the most reliable, with increased translation of the tibia with respect to the femur and the lack of a solid endpoint. Treatment can be operative or nonoperative, depending on the level of instability, as well as the desired activity level of the patient. For most young active persons, surgical reconstruction of the ACL is the preferred treatment option. Older or less active persons may do well with nonoperative intervention consisting of physical therapy and possibly a derotation-type knee brace.

PCL tears are not nearly as common as ACL tears. The mechanism usually involves either a posteriorly directed force against the proximal tibia while the knee is flexed or a hyperextension injury. An effusion might or might not be present. Similarly, instability might or might not be present. The posterior drawer test can demonstrate increased posterior translation of the tibia with or without a solid endpoint. Many isolated PCL tears can be treated nonoperatively with rest and physical therapy, but success depends on the activity level of the patient. Operative intervention with graft reconstruction is usually recommended for higher-level athletes and those with concomitant injuries to the posterolateral corner.

MCL tears are quite common in sports, usually related to a valgus stress to the knee. Unless associated injury occurs to the ACL or PCL, effusion is usually absent, but local swelling over the MCL may be noted. Usually the patient can localize the pain to the medial side of the knee, and direct palpation of the MCL demonstrates tenderness. Valgus stress testing of the knee reproduces pain, and laxity of the MCL may be noted. Management of isolated MCL injuries (not associated with an ACL tear) is conservative, consisting of rest, local application of ice, and physical therapy. Knee strengthening and gradual recovery of motion are emphasized. For associated ACL injuries, subsequent surgical reconstruction of the ACL may be necessary after the MCL heals.

Dislocation or subluxation of the patella can occur from a twisting injury. Pain and tenderness can occur on the medial side of the patella due to tearing of the medial patellofemoral ligament, or it can occur on the lateral side of the patella from the patella shearing against the lateral femoral condyle, or both. An effusion is usually present, and the lateral patellar instability can be reproduced with the patellar apprehension test, during which the examiner pushes the patella laterally while slowly flexing the knee from an extended position. Standard treatment is conservative and includes initial immobilization with the knee extended along with isometric strengthening exercises performed with the knee in extension. However, many experts now recommend early surgical repair of the medial patellofemoral ligament.

Meniscal injuries occur commonly, usually from twisting, and can be associated with other injuries such as ACL tears. Some degenerative meniscal tears can develop in older patients with minimal or no trauma. An effusion may be present. Direct tenderness over the menisci is the most reliable diagnostic mode. Some meniscal tears heal spontaneously or at least become asymptomatic over time. Those that remain symptomatic often require either surgical repair or partial resection. Often, difficult decisions arise between recommending conservative treatment for a few weeks versus early surgical intervention.

The most common nontraumatic cause of knee pain is patellofemoral pain, also known as anterior knee pain syndrome. This can affect almost any age group. The actual etiology of the pain remains unclear. The examination can reveal tenderness along the medial or lateral patellar facets or it can be entirely normal. Treatment consists of physical therapy, concentrating on strengthening of the quadriceps muscles. Temporarily decreasing the level of activity may be necessary.

Although knee osteoarthritis is not usually caused by sports participation, the symptoms can inhibit full participation in sports and exercise. Treatment usually begins conservatively with analgesic medications and physical therapy. Intraarticular injections of either corticosteroid or hyaluronic acid derivatives (viscosupplementation) can also be helpful. Surgical arthroplasties are indicated for recalcitrant cases.

The etiology of patellar tendinosis (jumper's knee) is unknown but has now clearly been documented to have no inflammatory component. Many cases are recalcitrant to treatment, but conservative management with physical therapy is standard.

In preadolescents and adolescents, Osgood–Schlatter syndrome is quite common, manifesting with a painful, tender swelling of the tibial tubercle. Conservative treatment of this self-limited condition with relative rest and physical therapy usually controls symptoms adequately.

Lower Leg Pain

Exercise-related lower leg (shin) pain most commonly results from the nonspecific entity of shin splints or tibial stress fractures, although other entities such as compartment syndromes exist. Although the true pathology of shin splints is unknown, diffuse tenderness over the medial cortex of the tibia usually indicates this condition. Temporary rest along with a course of physical therapy is usually recommended for shin splints, although studies documenting their efficacy are lacking. More localized tenderness over the tibia can indicate a stress fracture, which is treated with a more prolonged

CURRENT THERAPY

- For many sports-related injuries, an initial course of physical therapy is helpful, sometimes even if the exact diagnosis is unclear.
- Many sports-related injuries do not have a true inflammatory component, and therefore prescribing antiinflammatory medications is not always necessary.
- Most nontraumatic sports injuries, with the exception of stress fractures, do not require complete rest; some modified activity can usually be instituted.

period of rest, possibly including crutches. Plain radiographs along with a bone scan or MRI may be needed to define a stress fracture and to distinguish it from shin splints.

Ankle Injuries

Ankle sprains are one of the most common sports injuries, and the vast majority occur from an inversion mechanism. Treatment of these inversion sprains is directed at protecting the injured lateral ligaments while limiting the amount of swelling. Compression along with ice can be helpful. Partial immobilization with bracing offers protection while allowing some beneficial ankle motion. Strengthening and proprioceptive exercises can be initiated by a physical therapist as symptoms allow. The majority of cases of inversion sprains can be successfully treated conservatively, although a few cases require late surgical intervention.

External rotation ankle injuries, commonly known as *high ankle sprains*, tend to be more serious. Associated fractures of the fibula or tibial malleolus, along with disruption of the tibiofibular syndesmosis, can occur, often necessitating operative intervention.

The etiology of Achilles tendinosis is unknown and is often difficult to treat. Standard management consists of relative rest and physical therapy. The treatment of an acute rupture of the Achilles tendon remains controversial. Advantages and disadvantages to nonoperative cast treatment versus immediate surgical repair exist, with advocates for each.

Shoulder Injuries

The shoulder is extremely complex and remains incompletely understood. Shoulder pain and injuries are very common, both among sports participants as well as sedentary persons. The majority of shoulder conditions arise without trauma and consist of some combination of rotator cuff dysfunction, microinstability, and cuff impingement. These conditions can occur in athletes using an overhead throwing motion, but they can also occur in other persons. Pain with overhead motions, along with positive impingement tests and tests of rotator cuff function on physical examination, usually lead to the diagnosis.

The treatment for this broad category of cuff dysfunction and impingement is conservative. Temporary avoidance of overhead positions of the shoulder along with a physical therapy program directed toward strengthening of the rotator cuff can be helpful. For symptoms refractory to physical therapy, subacromial injections of anesthetics and corticosteroids often allow further improvement. For recalcitrant cases, surgical subacromial decompression with or without rotator cuff repair is usually recommended.

Injuries to the cartilaginous labrum of the shoulder (known as SLAP (superior labral anterior and posterior) lesions can occur either traumatically or nontraumatically. The diagnosis is often difficult to establish because the signs and symptoms overlap with those for rotator cuff and impingement pathology. If a SLAP lesion is suspected, a rehabilitation program similar to that for rotator cuff problems can be initiated. Magnetic resonance arthrograms might depict the injury. Cases that fail conservative treatment with physical therapy can require surgical repair.

Anterior dislocation or subluxation of the glenohumeral articulation usually occurs from an indirect trauma that levers the humeral head out anteriorly from its usual position within the glenoid fossa. Numerous reduction methods have been described, most with high success rates, but often requiring sedation and intravenous analgesia. Following successful reduction of the shoulder, the traditional treatment has consisted of a period of immobilization, possibly followed by physical therapy. However, numerous studies have documented the lack of efficacy of immobilization and therapy in terms of reducing future redislocation rates, especially in young patients. There now exists a growing trend favoring early surgical repair of the anterior labral and glenohumeral ligament complex, which appears to greatly reduce the rates of redislocation.

Injuries to the acromioclavicular joint occur traumatically, usually as a result of a fall onto the lateral tip of the shoulder. Pain and tenderness localized to the acromioclavicular joint corroborate the diagnosis. A step-off deformity can also be seen and palpated. Unless severe displacement of the clavicle with respect to the acromion occurs, treatment is usually conservative, consisting of analgesics, local ice, and use of a sling. Although opinions differ, some surgeons now recommend operative intervention for markedly displaced injuries.

Most fractures of the clavicle occur in the middle third of the bone. The mechanism of injury can be similar to that producing an acromioclavicular joint injury, usually a fall onto the shoulder. Displacement is almost always present on radiographs, but treatment is usually conservative, with either use of a sling or clavicle strap, along with local ice and analgesics. Fractures occurring in either the proximal third or distal third are potentially more complicated and can require referral for specialized care.

In adolescents and preadolescents, overuse injuries can occur involving the proximal humeral physis, often as a result of constant throwing, known as Little Leaguers' shoulder. Shoulder pain along with local tenderness over the humeral growth plate should raise suspicion of this injury. Rest and refraining from throwing, often for a prolonged period (months), is the usual treatment for this potentially serious condition.

Elbow Injuries

One of the most common maladies at the elbow is lateral epicondylosis, commonly known as tennis elbow. Although this is usually considered a sports injury, it occurs more often in the nonsporting population. The pathology involves degenerative fibrosis of a wrist extensor tendon, for which the etiology is unknown. Tenderness localized to the lateral epicondyle, and reproduction of pain and weakness with resisted extension of the wrist with the elbow in an extended position, helps confirm the diagnosis. Lateral epicondylosis can often be refractory to treatment, but the management usually consists of some combination of relative rest, counterforce bracing, and physical therapy. Local injections can also offer relief of pain, but often the effects are transient. Surgical débridement is generally reserved for recalcitrant cases.

The throwing motion can place a great deal of stress on the elbow, mostly as a result of valgus overload, which places a distraction stress on the medial side of the elbow. Specifically, the ulnar (or medial) collateral ligament (UCL), which provides most of the stability to the medial elbow, can be injured. Tears of the UCL can occur traumatically from sudden valgus stress, or the UCL can slowly become attenuated from repetitive valgus overload from throwing. Medial elbow pain along with laxity to valgus stress testing can suggest the diagnosis. In adolescents, physeal injuries to the medial humeral epicondyle can occur. Treatment initially involves rest and perhaps modification to the throwing technique, but many complete UCL tears require surgical reconstruction if high-level throwing is again desired.

Wrist and Hand Injuries

Scaphoid bone injuries occur during sports as well as nonsports activities. Usually these result from a fall onto an extended wrist, but other mechanisms exist. Most scaphoid fractures occur at the waist, or middle third, of the bone. Radial-sided wrist pain along with tenderness at the scaphoid waist in the anatomic snuff box should raise suspicion. Radiographs can demonstrate the fracture, but they may be normal. Treatment involves immobilization with a thumb spica cast. Many experts recommend long-arm casting, at least initially, followed by short-arm thumb spica casting. Prolonged casting (8-12 weeks) may be necessary. Due to the high rate of delayed union or nonunion, some surgeons now recommend initial surgical repair as an alternative to prolonged casting.

If initial radiographs are normal and suspicion is still high for a scaphoid fracture, advanced imaging with either a bone scan or MRI may be indicated. Alternatively, thumb spica casting for 1 to 2 weeks, followed by repeat examination and radiographs, can confirm the diagnosis.

One common finger injury is the mallet deformity of the distal interphalangeal (DIP) joint. This results from axial load with a forced flexion component to the DIP joint (a type of jammed finger). The patient is unable to actively extend the DIP joint. Whether a purely ligamentous injury to the extensor tendon occurs or a small avulsion of the dorsal base of the distal phalanx occurs, treatment with a splint to maintain complete extension of the DIP joint for 6 to 8 weeks usually provides adequate results.

Injury to the thumb metacarpophalangeal (MCP) ulnar collateral ligament (UCL), known as gamekeeper's or skier's thumb, can occur from a fall onto the thumb, producing hyperextension of the MCP joint and tearing the UCL. Local tenderness, along with laxity to stress testing of the UCL, confirm the diagnosis. Partial tears of the UCL (minimal laxity to stress testing) can be treated by a thumb spica splint or cast. A complete tear (gross laxity to stress testing) usually requires surgical intervention.

Concussions

Concussions are quite common in certain sports, especially football, and result from an angular acceleration force applied to the head. Transient confusion and a feeling of being dazed occur, usually without loss of consciousness. Restricting the patient from further brain insults until spontaneous recovery occurs is the cornerstone of treatment. Several guidelines exist to assist the clinician in deciding the length of restriction from sports, but none are based on any scientific data. The common theme for the various recommendations is that no athlete should be returned to sports unless completely asymptomatic.

REFERENCES

Beynnon BD, Johnson RJ, Abate JA, et al: Treatment of anterior cruciate ligament injuries, part I. Am J Sports Med 2005;33:1579-1602.

Daniel DM, Stone ML, Dobson BE, et al: Fate of the ACL-injured patient: A prospective outcome study. Am J Sports Med 1994;22:632-644.

Fulkerson JP: Diagnosis and treatment of patients with patellofemoral pain. Am J Sports Med 2002;30:447-456.

Herring SA, Bergfeld JA, Boland A, et al: Concussion (mild traumatic brain injury) and the team physician: A consensus statement. Med Sci Exerc Sports 2005;37:2012-2016.

McFarland EG, Selhi HS, Keyurapan E: Clinical evaluation of impingement: What to do and what works. J Bone Joint Surg Am 2006;88:432-441.

Pijnenburg ACM, van Dijk CN, Bossuyt PMM, Marti RK: Treatment of ruptures of the lateral ankle ligaments: A meta-analysis. J Bone Joint Surg Am 2000;82:761-773.

Wen DY: Current concepts in the treatment of anterior shoulder dislocations. Am J Emerg Med 1999;17:401-407.

SECTION 16

Obstetrics and Gynecology

Antepartum Care

Method of
Kirk D. Ramin, MD, and
Jessica P. Swartout, MD

Antepartum Care

Ideally, antepartum care commences 3 months before actual conception with the recommendation that women who are sexually active and not using contraception should begin taking daily multivitamin or folic acid supplements. The most convincing trials of this were performed in Europe and China when it was concluded that women of reproductive age should take multivitamin supplements containing 0.4 mg of folate daily. Women with histories of children with neural tube defects or other anomalies should increase this dose to 4 mg of folate in the periconceptional period to reduce risks of recurrence.

Preconception counseling should also include an accurate assessment of preexisting maternal medical conditions. This is the ideal time to stress changes in factors that respond to early intervention: quitting smoking, refraining from alcohol or drug abuse, treating gum disease, and avoiding teratogens. Alcohol is a known teratogen. Immunization status should be reviewed and vaccines should be administered as appropriate. Special consideration is given to patients with thyroid disease. Concern focuses on associations with low intelligence quotients (IQs) in children conceived by hypothyroid mothers. Patients with diabetes should be counseled that the increased risk of birth defects is directly related to the level of glucose control at conception.

High-risk obstetric referrals may be offered to women with potential for obstetric complications suggested by conditions listed in Box 1. Identification of the high-risk patient is critical to avoiding adverse outcomes.

In most cases, a woman's pregnancy is a normal event that is complicated by potentially dangerous disease in a minority of cases. The physician who manages pregnant patients must follow the normal changes that occur during antepartum care, so that abnormalities can be recognized and treated appropriately. Additionally, routine prenatal care offers multiple opportunities for patient education, primary intervention, and appropriate monitoring of the low-risk pregnancy in the setting of the family and community. For some women, antepartum care is part of their own continuum in a long-term primary care relationship with caregivers.

Timeline of Routine Antepartum Care

FIRST VISIT AND EARLY CARE

History

After pregnancy is confirmed, it is extraordinarily important to determine the duration of pregnancy and the estimated date of confinement (EDC). Further care is heavily predicated on this estimate. The history begins with ascertaining the first day of the last menstrual period and calculating the EDC by assuming duration of pregnancy averages 280 days (40 weeks).

The documentation of prior obstetric history includes prior complications, route of delivery, and estimated birth weights. Maternal medical disorders are often exacerbated by pregnancy; cardiovascular, renal, and endocrine disorders require evaluation and counseling concerning possible treatments required. A history of previous gynecologic surgery, including cesarean delivery, is important to consider. A family history of twinning, diabetes mellitus, familial disorders, or hereditary disease is relevant.

Current medications (prescription and nonprescription) are reviewed. Certain prescription medications are known teratogens and should be discontinued. Examples include isotretinoin (Accutane), tetracycline (Sumycin), quinolone antibiotics (ciprofloxacin [Cipro], levofloxacin [Levaquin]), and warfarin (Coumadin). Angiotensin-converting enzyme (ACE) inhibitors should not be used during the second and third trimesters, and the FDA has recently raised doubt about their use in the first trimester.

BOX 1 Potential Indications for High-Risk Referral

- Current disease involving renal, cardiac, or endocrine systems
- Fetal anomalies
- History of preterm delivery
- Incompetent cervix
- Isoimmunization
- Known carrier of genetic disorder
- Multiple gestation
- Placenta previa after 28 weeks
- Prior intrauterine fetal demise or stillbirth
- Systemic diseases such as hypertension, diabetes, or asthma
- Third-trimester bleeding

According to the approved label, ACE inhibitors are labeled pregnancy category C for the first trimester and pregnancy category D during the second and third trimesters. On June 8, 2006, the FDA issued an alert that infants whose mothers had taken an ACE inhibitor during the first trimester had an increased risk of major congenital malformations.

Honest discussion of substance abuse (alcohol, tobacco, and illicit drugs) is an integral part of the patient interview. Counseling patients about smoking cessation is vital in early pregnancy. Smoking increases the risk of fetal death or damage in utero. It is also associated with increased risk of placental abruption and placenta previa, each of which put both mother and child at risk.

Examination

Physical examination begins with a thorough general examination to assess maternal well-being including body mass index (BMI) and blood pressure (BP). The BMI is calculated by dividing weight in kilograms by height in meters squared. The BMI of a patient is categorized as underweight (under 19.8), normal weight (19.8 to 25), overweight (25 to 30), or obese (over 30). A brief fundoscopic examination might reveal signs of hypertension-induced changes.

Breast examination may be significant for changes in pregnancy that result from hormonal responses by the mammary ducts. These changes include engorgement and vascular prominence, occasionally resulting in mastodynia. Enlargement of areolar sebaceous glands (Montgomery's tubercles) occurs between 6 and 8 weeks' gestation.

A pelvic examination is performed with attention to the adequacy of pelvis and evaluation for adnexal masses. Numerous changes in the pelvic organs occur in pregnancy. For example, congestion of the pelvic vasculature (Chadwick's sign) causes bluish discoloration of the vagina and cervix. Softening of the cervix due to increased vascularity of the cervical tissue (Goodell's sign) can occur as early as 4 weeks. The uterus is palpable at the pubic symphysis at 8 weeks.

Portable devices using Doppler effect will reliably detect fetal heart tones at a rate of 120 to 160 beats per minute as early as 8 weeks.

Laboratory Studies

Routine laboratory studies ordered at the first visit include complete blood count (CBC) with differential, ABO and Rh typing, red cell antibody screen, rubella immunoglobulin (Ig)G, hepatitis B surface antigen (HBsAg), syphilis serology, and HIV 1 and HIV 2 antibody screens. Patients may refuse HIV testing, but all patients are counseled and offered the option for screening. A Papanicolaou (Pap) smear is performed in conjunction with cultures for chlamydia and gonorrhea.

A midstream urinalysis checks for the presence of protein or glucose. A microscopic examination of the urine is performed to rule out infection or asymptomatic bacteriuria. A baseline 24-hour urine protein collection and serum creatinine should be collected from all patients with hypertension, diabetes, or other preexisting renal disease.

Other Studies

Special-purpose studies are also considered in early gestation. First-trimester screening with nuchal translucency should be offered to all women older than 35 years between 11 and 14 weeks. The first-trimester screen uses the nuchal translucency and maternal serum-free β–human chorionic gonadotropin (hCG) and pregnancy-associated plasma protein A (PAPP-A) and detects up to 85% of Down syndrome and trisomy 18 cases.

Chorionic villus sampling (CVS) may be offered at 10 to 13 weeks to women older than 35 years, to those with abnormal first-trimester screens, and to those with abnormal pedigrees. From this, placental tissue may be subjected to chromosomal, metabolic, or DNA study. CVS cannot be used for diagnosis of neural tube defects, because this requires measuring alpha fetoprotein (AFP) levels in maternal serum at a later date.

Patients with tuberculosis exposure may be assessed for active tuberculosis with skin testing (if not vaccinated with bacille Calmette-Guérin [BCG]) and chest x-ray. Serologic assessment for toxoplasmosis, cytomegalovirus, and varicella immunity is not routinely indicated.

Screening for genetic disorders may be undertaken if concern exists based on racial or ethnic background (hemoglobinopathies, β-thalassemia, α-thalassemia, Tay-Sachs disease) or familial background (cystic fibrosis, fragile X, Duchenne's muscular dystrophy).

Follow-up

Follow-up visits are scheduled once monthly until 28 weeks' gestation, and then patients are followed twice monthly until 36 weeks. Visits are then scheduled at weekly intervals until delivery. At each visit, weight gain, edema, BP, fundal height, Leopold's maneuvers, and fetal heart tones are recorded. Because BP tends to decrease during the second trimester, increases of 30 mm Hg systolic or 15 mm Hg diastolic over first trimester pressures are abnormal. Interval history includes questions about diet, sleeping patterns, and fetal movement. Warning signs such as bleeding, contractions, leaking of fluid, headache, or visual disturbances are reviewed.

15 TO 18 WEEKS' GESTATION

Alpha Fetoprotein Testing

Maternal serum AFP testing is offered for all pregnancies at 16 to 18 weeks as a means of screening for open neural tube defects or chromosomal trisomy. In pregnancy, AFP is produced in sequence by the fetal yolk sac, the fetal gastrointestinal tract, and the fetal liver. AFP in the maternal serum occurs via placental exchange and transamniotic diffusion.

High levels of AFP are associated with various fetal anomalies including neural tube defects, multiple gestations, and ventral wall defects. Unexplained elevation of AFP has been associated with poor fetal growth, fetal loss, and preeclampsia. In cases with unexplained elevation of AFP, maternal and fetal surveillance should be increased. Low levels of AFP are associated with increased risk of Down syndrome.

The interpretation of this test depends on the gestational age; even if timed correctly, it is known to have a moderate level of false-positive results. Expanded serum markers of AFP, unconjugated estriol, inhibin A, and β-hCG are available to more accurately screen for Down syndrome, but detection is only about 60%, and false-negative results remain at 5%.

Amniocentesis

A more certain diagnosis is available via ultrasound-guided transabdominal amniocentesis at 16 to 18 weeks. Chromosomes from fetal cells are subjected to fluorescent in-situ hybridization (FISH) analysis, which detects trisomies 13, 18, 21, and abnormal numbers of sex chromosomes.

Physical Findings

Interval changes in the physical examination now include the start of colostrum secretion, which can begin as early as 16 weeks' gestation.

Chloasma is darkening of the skin over the forehead, bridge of the nose, or cheekbones and is more obvious in those with dark complexions. It can begin to manifest at this time, and is intensified by exposure to sunlight. Darkening of the skin in the areolae and nipples becomes more accentuated. A darkened line appears in the lower midline of the abdomen from the umbilicus to the pubis (linea nigra). The basis of these changes is stimulation of melanophores by increased melanocyte-stimulating hormone.

At 15 to 20 weeks, abdominal enlargement can appear more rapid as the uterus rises out of the pelvis and into the abdomen.

18 TO 20 WEEKS' GESTATION

Physical Findings

The mother might detect fetal movements (quickening) at around 20 weeks. The uterus is palpable at 20 weeks at the umbilicus, and ballottement reveals a fetus floating in amniotic fluid. Measurements that are 2 cm smaller than expected for week of gestation are suspicious for oligohydramnios, intrauterine growth restriction, fetal anomaly, or abnormal fetal lie. Conversely, measurements 2 cm larger than expected can indicate multiple gestation, polyhydramnios, or fetal macrosomia. These rules apply for the gestational ages of 18 to 32 weeks. Either condition can be fully evaluated with ultrasound examination.

Laboratory Studies

Increased surveillance for preeclampsia includes testing for urine protein in patients with BP greater than 140/90 mm Hg or in those with weight gains greater than 3 pounds/week. Evaluation is also necessary for clinical signs of upper extremity edema, right upper quadrant tenderness, headaches, or vision changes. Proteinuria of more than 300 mg in 24 hours can indicate renal dysfunction or the onset of preeclampsia.

Ultrasonography

Sonography has long established itself as the single most useful technology in monitoring pregnancy and diagnosing complications. It is for this reason that basic level ultrasound is offered at 18 to 20 weeks to evaluate growth, placentation, amniotic fluid volume, and fetal anatomy. If earlier dating of the pregnancy is uncertain, this is an opportunity to confirm or refute prior estimates. If anomalous conditions are discovered, more comprehensive ultrasonography becomes necessary.

28 WEEKS' GESTATION

Physical Findings

New physical examination findings at this time include the onset of stretch marks (striae) of the breasts and abdomen. These are caused by separation of underlying collagen tissue, a response to increased adrenocorticosteroid. The ligamentous structures of the pelvis also undergo slight but definite relaxation of the joints, a progesterone effect. As the uterus enlarges, it often rotates to the right. Fundal size roughly correlates with the estimated gestational age at 26 to 34 weeks. Braxton Hicks contractions, characterized as painless uterine tightening, increase in regularity. The fetal outline can be easily palpated through the maternal abdominal wall.

Laboratory Studies

A CBC for anemia and a 1-hour glucose tolerance test (after ingestion of 50 g of glucose) is scheduled to detect patients at risk for developing gestational diabetes. If the screening test is abnormal, a 3-hour test is performed to confirm the diagnosis. Two or more abnormal values on this test are considered diagnostic of gestational diabetes mellitus.

A repeat Rh antibody is checked at this time in Rh-negative mothers. Those who remain unsensitized in the third trimester receive a first dose of Rho(D) immune globulin (RhoGAM) to prevent maternal isoimmunization to fetal red blood cells. A 300 μg dose is sufficient for 15 mL of red cells (equivalent to 30 mL of whole blood).

Follow-up

Return visits at 2-week intervals are now initiated, and the patient is oriented to the labor and delivery ward. Precautions are given regarding the onset of conditions listed in Box 2. The onset of any of these should prompt immediate medical attention.

36 WEEKS' GESTATION

Physical Findings

Patients might complain of increased vaginal discharge at this time in their pregnancy, a physiologic consequence of hormone stimulation. The discharge consists mainly of epithelial cells and cervical mucus and is treated with reassurance. Discharge accompanied by itching, burning, or malodor should be evaluated and treated accordingly, however.

BOX 2 Warning Signs and Symptoms Prompting Medical Attention

- Burning with urination
- Chills or fever
- Prolonged vomiting or inability to keep liquids down
- Pronounced decrease in fetal movements
- Rhythmic cramping pains (>6/h)
- Rupture of membranes
- Severe abdominal, pelvic, or back pain
- Signs of preeclampsia (headache, edema, right upper quadrant pain)
- Vaginal bleeding

Laboratory Studies

Vaginal and rectal cultures are collected to evaluate for the presence of group B streptococcus (GBS) at 35 to 37 weeks. GBS organisms are implicated in preterm labor, amnionitis, endometritis, and wound infection. If cultures are positive, the patient will be given antibiotic prophylaxis during active labor in efforts to protect the newborn against vertical transmission, resulting in newborn sepsis.

Follow-up

Follow-up visits are planned on a weekly basis with emphasis on weight gain, BP, and signs of preeclampsia. Review of precautions regarding infection, pregnancy loss, and symptoms of preeclampsia completes the visit.

POST-TERM GESTATION

About 3% to 12% of pregnancies continue beyond 43 weeks of gestation and are considered post-term. Although some of these may be due to inaccurate dating, some patients clearly progress to excessively long gestations that are a significant risk to the fetus. Increased antepartum surveillance by cervical examination, fetal heart rate testing (see the discussion of contraction stress testing), and biophysical profile should be initiated between 41 and 42 weeks. Even if fetal testing is reassuring, patients with reliable dating greater than 41 weeks are candidates for induction of labor.

Common Concerns of the Antenatal Period

BLEEDING

About one half of pregnant women experience some form of bleeding during the pregnancy; often this is benign. Patients also have a heightened awareness of symptoms that previously may have gone unnoticed in the nonpregnant state. Efficient and competent evaluation, followed by compassion and reassurance when prudent, allays many fears and provides clear direction. Spotting due to bleeding at the implantation site occurs from the time of implantation (about 6 days after fertilization) until 29 to 35 days after the last menstrual period in many women. Some women have unexplained cyclic bleeding throughout pregnancy. Usually, cardiac activity on ultrasound and appropriate β-hCG levels confirm a viable early pregnancy. First-trimester bleeding in lieu of these findings may be a sign of spontaneous miscarriage or ectopic pregnancy. Vaginal bleeding in late pregnancy is covered in other articles.

NAUSEA

Nausea is a common symptom that occurs in most pregnancies. It is heightened before 14 weeks' gestation and is largely benign. The etiology is not well understood but likely is related to elevating levels of β-hCG. Its moniker "morning sickness" is misleading, because nausea of pregnancy can occur at any time during the day.

Aggravating factors vary with the individual patient; success varies with interventions designed to reduce symptoms.

Uncomplicated nausea may be responsive to small nonfatty portions at mealtime. Pyridoxine (vitamin B_6)[1] tablets 12.5 mg twice a day or doxylamine (Unisom)[1] 12.5 mg twice a day are safe in pregnancy and may be helpful. Antiemetic drugs in the outpatient setting are a measure of last resort.

Inability to control protracted vomiting in conjunction with clinical dehydration can require hospitalization for intravenous fluids and treatment of hyperemesis gravidarium. Extreme nausea and vomiting or nausea and vomiting that persists beyond 18 to 20 weeks' gestation may be signs of multiple gestation, thyroid disease, or molar pregnancy.

NUTRITION AND WEIGHT GAIN

The mother's nutrition is a vital factor in the development of the fetus from preconception through the postpartum period. Therefore, the pregnant woman should be advised to eat a balanced diet and should be informed of the additional 300 kcal/day needed during pregnancy. The American College of Obstetricians and Gynecologists (ACOG) recommends a target weight gain of 10 to 12 kg (22-27 lb) during pregnancy. They also advise that underweight women might need to gain more and obese women should gain less. Nutritional requirements for protein are 80 g/day, for calcium are 1500 mg/day, for iron are 30 mg/day, and for folate are 0.4 mg/day (4 mg/day in some cases). Patients with seizure disorders managed with valproic acid (Depakene) or carbamazepine (Tegretol) are also at risk and might benefit from the higher dose of folate.

HEARTBURN

Heartburn in the form of reflux esophagitis is caused by the enlarging uterus displacing the stomach and by progesterone's relaxation of the lower esophageal sphincter. Treatment consists of taking antacids, decreasing exacerbating factors such as spicy foods, eating more frequently but in smaller quantities, limiting eating before bedtime, and taking H_2-receptor inhibitors.

URINARY SYMPTOMS

Urinary frequency, nocturia, and bladder irritability are common complaints due to progesterone-mediated relaxation of smooth muscle and subsequent altered bladder function. Later in pregnancy, urinary frequency becomes even more prominent from pressure on the bladder by the enlarging uterus and the fetal presenting parts, such as when the fetal head descends into the pelvis.

Dysuria, however, is often a sign of infection that requires antibiotic treatment. Bacteriuria combined with urinary stasis from altered bladder function predisposes the patient to pyelonephritis. Although simple urinary tract infections are treated on an outpatient basis, pyelonephritis remains the most common nonobstetric cause for hospitalization during antenatal care.

Patients with a diagnosis of pyelonephritis require hospitalization, aggressive fluid replacement, and IV antibiotics until they remain afebrile for longer than 24 hours. Close monitoring of maternal respiratory status is important because these women are at risk for acute respiratory distress syndrome (ARDS). All patients should complete a 10-day course of antibiotic treatment. After treatment has been completed, suppressive therapy should be continued until delivery.

INFECTION

Two infections of special note are HIV and bacterial vaginosis (BV). HIV transmission to the newborn can be reduced significantly with appropriate infectious disease and maternal-fetal medicine specialty management. Appropriate treatment of BV in women at high risk for preterm delivery or recurrent loss can significantly reduce either of these untoward outcomes. Debate exists as to whether or not low-risk women should be screened.

Chlamydia trachomatis is an obligate intracellular bacterium and is the most common sexually transmitted bacterial infection in women of reproductive age. It may be associated with urethritis, mucopurulent cervicitis, and acute salpingitis, or it may be clinically silent. Perinatal transmission is clearly associated with neonatal conjunctivitis (leading to blindness) and pneumonia and is likely associated with preterm delivery, premature rupture of membranes, and perinatal mortality. Diagnosis is confirmed by polymerase chain reaction (PCR) during routine screening. Doxycycline should be avoided in pregnancy, and erythromycin is associated with gastrointestinal upset, so treatment with azithromycin is often appropriate.

Gonococcal infection is associated with concomitant chlamydia infection in about 40% of infected pregnant women. It is usually limited to the lower genital tract, including the cervix, urethra, and periurethral or vestibular glands. Because of an association between gonococcal cervicitis and septic spontaneous abortion, and because preterm delivery, premature rupture of membranes, and postpartum infection are more common with gonococcal infection, routine cultures are appropriate at the first antenatal visit. Because some strains have rendered some β-lactam drugs ineffective for therapy, the recommendation for uncomplicated gonococcal infection is intramuscular ceftriaxone 125 mg.

Vaginosis due to *Candida albicans* can become symptomatic with caseous white discharge and vaginal itching or burning, and it may be associated with red satellite lesions on the vulva. Marked inflammation of the vagina and introitus may be noted. Topical application of over-the-counter antifungal creams such as miconazole nitrate (Monistat) or nystatin (Mycostatin) is generally helpful in controlling the imbalance of vaginal flora.

Cytomegalovirus is a ubiquitous DNA herpes virus that is transmitted horizontally between humans by droplet infection. It is transmitted vertically from mother to fetus and is the most common cause of perinatal infection. The virus becomes latent after primary infection, with periodic reactivation and viral shedding. Infection is usually clinically silent. Many of the affected infants have died from infection, and most of the survivors have severe handicaps, including mental retardation, blindness, and deafness. Serious sequelae are more common among primary infections. The syndrome of congenital cytomegalovirus infection includes low birth weight, microcephaly, intracranial calcifications, chorioretinitis, mental and motor retardation, sensorineural deficits, hepatosplenomegaly, jaundice, hemolytic anemia, and thrombocytopenic purpura. Confirmation of primary infection is suggested by a fourfold increase of IgG titers in paired acute and convalescent sera or by detecting IgM cytomegalovirus antibodies. There is no effective therapy for maternal infection.

Human parvovirus B19 causes erythema infectiosum, or fifth disease. This is a single-stranded DNA virus that is heralded by the appearance of clinical findings of bright red macular rash and accompanying arthralgias. Acute infection is confirmed by IgM-specific antibody and can prompt adverse pregnancy outcomes, including spontaneous miscarriage and fetal death.

Rubella, also known as German measles, is directly responsible for spontaneous miscarriage and severe congenital malformations. Although large epidemics of rubella are nonexistent in the United States because of immunization, the disease can still affect the up to 25% of susceptible women. Absence of rubella antibody indicates susceptibility. Vaccination involves an attenuated live virus (MMR) and therefore is avoided in pregnancy. Vaccination of nonpregnant susceptible women (including those during the postpartum period) and hospital personnel continues to be the mainstay of therapy. Detection by IgM-specific antibody confirms recent infection. Congenital rubella syndrome (CRS) is a severe example of antenatal infection and includes one or more of the conditions listed in Box 3.

Varicella-zoster virus, the etiologic agent of childhood chickenpox, is a DNA herpes virus that remains latent in the dorsal root ganglia and may be reactivated years later to cause herpes zoster or shingles. Infection early in pregnancy can lead to severe congenital malformations including chorioretinitis, cerebral cortical atrophy, hydronephrosis, and cutaneous and bony leg defects.

---

[1]Not FDA approved for this indication.

BOX 3 Conditions Associated with Congenital Rubella Syndrome

- Central nervous system defects (meningoencephalitis)
- Chromosomal abnormalities
- Chronic diffuse interstitial pneumonitis
- Eye lesions
  - Cataracts
  - Glaucoma
  - Microphthalmia
- Heart disease
  - Patent ductus arteriosus
  - Septal defects
  - Pulmonary artery stenosis
- Hepatic dysfunction
  - Hepatitis
  - Hepatosplenomegaly
  - Jaundice
- Osseous changes
- Retarded growth
- Sensorineural deafness
- Thrombocytopenia and anemia

Varicella-zoster immunoglobulin (VZIg) 125 U/10 kg can attenuate varicella infection if given within 96 hours.

Genital herpes simplex virus (HSV) may be confirmed by tissue culture if active lesions are present; in this event, cesarean delivery is indicated because the fetus is at risk for acquiring the virus during passage through the birth canal. Oral or topical acyclovir can improve symptoms. If no lesions and no prodromal symptoms are present, vaginal delivery is recommended.

Trichomonas vaginalis can be found in 20% to 30% of pregnant patients, but only a small number complain of discharge or irritation. This flagellated, oval, motile organism can be seen on normal saline wet prep and is evident clinically by presence of a foamy or greenish discharge accompanied by multiple cervical petechiae. Treatment is oral metronidazole.

Prenatally acquired infection caused by the protozoan parasite *Toxoplasma gondii* can result in the presence of abnormalities such as microcephalus or hydrocephalus at birth, development of jaundice with hepatosplenomegaly or meningoencephalitis in early childhood, or delayed appearance of ocular lesions such as chorioretinitis in later childhood. Exposure to the parasite is through eating undercooked meat, gardening in soil that is potentially contaminated by mammalian feces, or cleaning a cat's litter box.

VARICOSE VEINS

Pressure by the enlarged uterus on venous return from the legs and progesterone-mediated vasodilation can lead to prominent varicosities and edema of the legs or vulva. Any concern for deep vein thrombosis should be ruled out by examination for erythema, edema, cords, or tenderness. Doppler ultrasound may be indicated in equivocal findings of the lower extremities. Benign varicosities almost invariably return to normal after delivery, thus limiting the need for intervention in the antepartum period. Edema of the lower extremities is common, responds to elevation, and must be differentiated from facial or hand edema accompanying preeclampsia. Hemorrhoids are manifestations of the varicosities of the rectal veins. Treatment focuses on stool softeners, sitz baths, and over-the-counter topical preparations.

CONSTIPATION

Bowel transit time and relaxation of intestinal smooth muscle are both increased due to progesterone effects, resulting in overall slowing of bowel function. If pronounced, this can lead to constipation. Dietary management of this condition is centered around recommendations for increased fluids and high-fiber foods. Enemas and laxatives are avoided.

UPPER EXTREMITY DISCOMFORT

Periodic numbness and tingling of the fingers is due to exacerbations of carpal tunnel compression exacerbated by tissue edema. Splinting of the affected hand at night is indicated, with anticipation of resolution during postpartum diuresis.

CURRENT DIAGNOSIS

- Pregnancy evaluation should begin 3 months before conception with optimization of underlying medical conditions and commencement of prenatal vitamins with 400 μg of folic acid.
- Preconception counseling with a specialist in high-risk pregnancies should be considered in all patients with underlying medical conditions, if possible.
- The first prenatal visit should include a review of the medical and obstetric histories, current medications, herbal remedies, and tobacco, alcohol, and drug use.
- Prenatal laboratory studies should be done at the first visit after a pregnancy is confirmed with a urine pregnancy test. These studies include hemoglobin, platelet count, type and screen, rubella status, and hepatitis B testing. All women should be offered screening for HIV. High-risk patients should be screened for hepatitis C, gonorrhea, and chlamydia.
- Genetic screening should be offered based on ethnic background and family history.
- Both first-trimester screening (nuchal translucency combined with maternal serum PAPP-A/free β-hCG) and second-trimester quadruple screen should be offered to all patients. These tests aid in diagnosis of chromosome abnormalities. If a patient opts for a first-trimester screen, it is important to perform an AFP screen in the second trimester to screen for neural tube defects.
- Appropriate weight gain in pregnancy depends on maternal BMI before pregnancy. In patients with a normal BMI, a 25- to 35-pound weight gain is recommended. Underweight patients are encouraged to gain 30 to 40 pounds, and overweight patients are encouraged to gain no more than 25 pounds.
- Prenatal visits should begin at 8 to 12 weeks' gestation and continue monthly until 24 weeks. Visits should then be every 2 weeks until 36 weeks and then weekly. Each visit should include assessment of maternal weight, BP, urinalysis for protein and glucose, fundal height measurement, documentation of fetal heart tones, and review of symptoms of preterm labor and preeclampsia.
- All patients should undergo a glucose challenge test at 24 to 28 weeks. This is done by administering a 50-g load of glucose and obtaining a serum sample 1 hour after administration. A level greater than 140 mg/dL is considered abnormal, and a 3-hour glucose tolerance test is indicated. If a woman demonstrates abnormalities in two of the four values, gestational diabetes is diagnosed.

Abbreviations: AFP = alpha fetoprotein; BMI = body mass index; BP = blood pressure; hCG = human chorionic gonadotropin; PAPP-A = pregnancy-associated plasma protein A.

CURRENT THERAPY

- Administration of the inactivated influenza vaccine (Fluzone, Fluvirin, Fluvarix) is recommended in all pregnant patients, regardless of trimester, who will be pregnant during the flu season.
- Folic acid supplementation should begin before conception. The recommended dose is 400 µg daily. In patients with a previous pregnancy complicated by a neural tube defect, 4 mg daily is recommended to prevent recurrence of a neural tube defect.
- Pyelonephritis requires hospitalization and IV antibiotics in all pregnant patients. IV antibiotics should be continued until the patient is afebrile for longer than 24 hours. Oral antibiotics should then be commenced to complete a 10-day course. All patients should continue on suppressive antibiotic therapy until delivery.
- All patients with HIV should be treated with antiretroviral therapy regardless of gestation. Intrapartum zidovudine is recommended for all patients with HIV.

BACKACHE AND PELVIC DISCOMFORT

Endocrine relaxation of ligamentous structures coupled with an offset center of gravity create exaggerated spinal curve, joint instability, and compensatory back pain. Most women experience some form of this discomfort as pregnancy progresses. Advice given for improvements in posture, local heat, acetaminophen, and massage may be helpful. Minimizing the time spent standing can have a positive effect. Round ligament pain usually occurs during the second trimester and is described as sharp bilateral or unilateral groin pain. It may be exacerbated by change in position or rapid movement and might respond to similar measures. These routine aches and pains of pregnancy must be differentiated from rhythmic cramping pains originating in the back. The latter may be a sign of preterm labor requiring appropriate evaluation.

LEG CRAMPS

Leg cramps in the form of recurrent muscle spasms in pregnancy are believed to be due to lower levels of serum calcium or higher levels of serum phosphorus. The calves are most commonly involved and attacks are more frequent at night and in the third trimester. There are no data from controlled trials to show benefit over placebo for treatment targeted toward reduced phosphate and increased calcium or magnesium intake. Local heat, putting the affected muscle on stretch, acetaminophen, and massage can be helpful in acute events.

INTERCOURSE

In general, intercourse is considered safe in pregnancy. The exception to this rule is found in patients who are experiencing uterine bleeding, or postcoital cramps, and spotting. It may be wise to avoid intercourse in couples who are at risk for special circumstances. Firmer recommendations can be made in instances of placenta previa or known rupture of membranes; in these instances intercourse should not occur.

DENTAL CARE

Ideally, women should have dental care completed before conception. However, dental procedures under local anesthesia may be carried out at any time during the pregnancy. Use of nitrous oxide inhalants is to be avoided, however. Long procedures should be postponed until the second trimester. Antibiotics are given for dental abscesses and in cases of rheumatic heart disease or mitral valve prolapse.

X-RAYS, IONIZING RADIATION, AND IMAGING

The adverse effects of ionizing radiation are dose dependent, but there is no single diagnostic procedure that results in a dose of radiation high enough to threaten the fetus or embryo. Diagnostic radiation of less than 5000 mrad is considered by ACOG to have minimal teratogenic risk, and if medically indicated, x-ray imaging may be performed safely. For example, patients may undergo chest x-rays as indicated; a dose of 0.05 mrad is typical exposure. Patients receiving dental x-rays are additionally protected by a lead apron. Still, the need for x-ray films should be evaluated for risks and potential benefits in the individual pregnant patient to conservatively protect the mother and fetus from theoretical genetic or oncogenic risk. MRI is considered safe due to its mechanism of action, which is a nonionizing form of radiation. Radioactive iodine (^{131}I) is contraindicated in pregnancy.

IMMUNIZATION

Live virus vaccines must be avoided during pregnancy because of possible effects on the fetus. These include measles, mumps, rubella (MMR) and yellow fever (VF-Vax). The risks to the fetus from the administration of rabies vaccine (RabAvert, IMOVAX) are unknown. The varicella vaccine (Varivax) is not recommended in pregnancy.

Diphtheria and tetanus toxoid (Td) may be administered in pregnancy if exposure to pathogens is likely. The hepatitis B vaccine (Engerix B, Recombivax HB) series is safe and may be given in pregnancy to women at risk. The inactivated influenza vaccine (Fluzone, Fluvirin, Fluvarix) is also recommended in all women during any trimester they will be pregnant during the flu season.

Tests of Fetal Well-Being

A primary goal in antepartum care is the competent management of patient care extended to both mother and baby in order to reduce the risk of fetal demise after 24 weeks, ensure optimal conditions for term delivery after 37 weeks, and intervene for evolving conditions threatening the well-being of either patient. Any pregnancy that may be at increased risk for antepartum fetal compromise is a candidate for tests of fetal well-being performed weekly, beginning at 28 to 32 weeks. Some conditions requiring antepartum testing are listed in Box 4.

NONSTRESS TEST

The nonstress test consists of fetal heart rate monitoring in the absence of uterine contractions. A reactive tracing is one in which heart rate accelerations of 15 bpm above the baseline of 120 to 160 bpm are of at least 15 seconds' duration. Two of these accelerations must be observed in a 20-minute period. False-positive nonreactive tracings are more common before 28 weeks' gestation.

CONTRACTION STRESS TEST

The requirements for a reactive tracing are combined with tocodynamometer recordings of three contractions of 40 seconds or more duration in a 10-minute period. If no contractions are present, they may be induced via nipple stimulation or intravenously administered

---

BOX 4 Conditions that Prompt Further Testing

- Decreased fetal movements
- Fetal growth restriction
- Hypertensive disorders
- Insulin-dependent diabetes mellitus
- Multiple gestation with discordant fetal growth
- Oligohydramnios or polyhydramnios
- Post-term pregnancy
- Prior loss or stillbirth

TABLE 1 Possible Results of the Contraction Stress Test

Result	Description
Negative	No late decelerations
Positive	Late decelerations follow 50% of contractions
Equivocal	Intermittent or variable decelerations
Unsatisfactory	<3 contractions in 10 minutes

oxytocin. Relative contraindications to this test are preterm premature rupture of membranes, classic uterine incision scar, placenta previa, and unexplained vaginal bleeding. The results of the contraction stress test are categorized in Table 1.

BIOPHYSICAL PROFILE

The biophysical profile consists of a nonstress test with ultrasound observations. A total of ten points is given for the following elements (two points each):

- Reactive nonstress test
- Presence of fetal breathing movements of 30 seconds or more in 30 minutes
- Fetal movement defined as three or more discrete body or limb movements within 30 minutes
- Fetal tone defined as one or more episodes of fetal extremity extension and return to flexion
- Quantification of amniotic fluid volume, defined as a pocket of fluid that measures at least 2 cm by 2 cm

Antepartum Hospitalization

Pregnant patients with complications requiring hospitalization are admitted to a high-risk antepartum floor in close proximity to the labor and delivery area. Specialists in maternal-fetal medicine are intimately involved in the care plans of these patients.

REFERENCES

American College of Obstetricians and Gynecologists: Compendium of Selected Publications. Atlanta: American College of Obstetricians and Gynecologists, 2007.
Carpenter MW, Coustan DR: Criteria for screening tests for gestational diabetes. Am J Obstet Gynecol 1982;144(7):763-773.
Centers for Disease Control and Prevention: Influenza: Information for Health Professionals. Available at http://www.cdc.gov/flu/ (accessed July 13, 2007).
Cunningham FG, Leveno KL, Bloom SL, et al: Williams Obstetrics, 22nd ed. New York: McGraw-Hill, 2005.
Lopez A, Dietz VJ, Wilson M, et al: Preventing congenital toxoplasmosis. MMWR Recomm Rep 2000;49(RR-2):59-68.
Wald NJ, Rodeck C, et al: First and second trimester antenatal screening for Down's syndrome. The results of the Serum, Urine and Ultrasound Screening Study. J Med Screen 2003;10(2):56-104.

Ectopic Pregnancy

Method of
Gary H. Lipscomb, MD

In the United States, the incidence of ectopic pregnancies has increased dramatically during the last several decades. Commonly cited risks include prior pelvic inflammatory disease (PID), previous tubal surgery, intrauterine device (IUD) use, previous ectopic pregnancy, ovulation induction and in vitro fertilization, progestin-containing contraceptives, smoking, previous abdominal surgery, in utero diethylstilbestrol (DES) exposure, and previous induced abortion.

A high degree of suspicion is necessary for the early diagnosis of an ectopic pregnancy. Almost all ectopic pregnancies have episodes of vaginal bleeding or lower abdominal pain prior to rupture. Such patients are appropriate candidates to evaluate for ectopic pregnancy. Figure 1 illustrates a diagnostic algorithm that is useful in efficiently coordinating and interpreting the tests used in the diagnosis of ectopic pregnancy.

Diagnosis

Serum progesterone levels are helpful as an initial screening test for ectopic pregnancy. Levels higher than 25 ng/mL are associated with ectopic pregnancy in only 1% to 2% of cases; levels less than 5 ng/mL are associated with a nonviable pregnancy (either intrauterine or ectopic) more than 99% of the time. If progesterone levels are not readily available in a timely manner, however, human chorionic gonadotropin (hCG) levels alone may be used.

Levels of hCG rise in an essentially linear fashion until after 41 days of gestation. By this gestational age, an intrauterine pregnancy (IUP) should be seen on ultrasound. In 85% of normal pregnancies, hCG doubles approximately every 2 days, rising at least 66% in 48 hours. However, 15% of normal IUPs rise less than this in 48 hours. Conversely, 15% of ectopic pregnancies rise more than 66%. But a rise of less than 50% is associated with an abnormal pregnancy 99.9% of the time.

Because the interassay variability of hCG is 15%, a change of less than this amount is considered a plateau. Plateaued levels are the most predictive of ectopic pregnancy. The use of a urine pregnancy test to rule out the possibility of phantom hCG is strongly recommended prior to surgical or medical treatment. This phenomenon, caused by heterophilic serum antibodies, produces false-positive hCG levels usually less than 1000 IU/L.

The sonographic identification of an intrauterine gestational sac essentially excludes an ectopic pregnancy. A viable IUP should always be visualized at an hCG titer of 2000 IU/L by transvaginal scan and by 6500 IU/L with transabdominal ultrasound. An adnexal mass, in a patient with a presumed ectopic pregnancy and hCG levels less than 2000 IU/L, should not automatically be assumed to be an ectopic without the presence of a yolk sac, fetal pole, or cardiac activity. Such masses are frequently corpus luteum cysts associated with an early IUP.

Except in the rare case of heterotopic pregnancy, the identification of chorionic villi in uterine contents essentially eliminates the diagnosis of ectopic pregnancy. The use of dilation and curettage (D&C) also eliminates giving methotrexate unnecessarily to a patient with a failed IUP.

CURRENT DIAGNOSIS

- Screening for symptomatic patients or those with risk factors
- Diagnostic algorithm to coordinate testing
- hCG titers every 48 hours
- Ultrasound at hCG level of 2000 mIU/mL
- D&C for inappropriate hCG rise (<50% in 48 hours) below 2000 mIU/mL

Abbreviations: D&C = dilation and curettage; hCG = human chorionic gonadotropin.

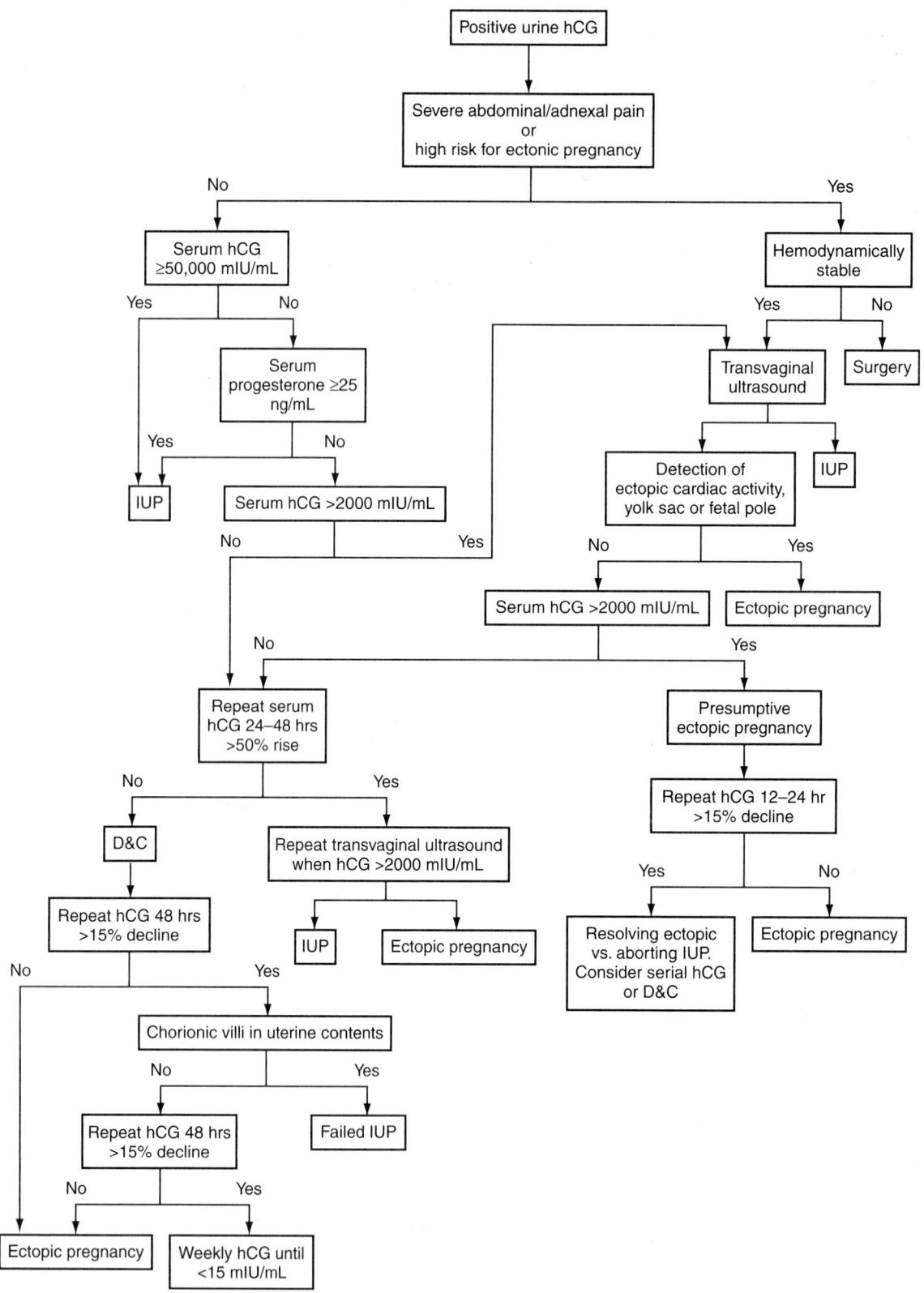

FIGURE 1. University of Tennessee Diagnostic Algorithm. D&C = dilation and curettage; hCG = human chorionic gonadotropin.

A D&C is particularly important in patients with hCG titers below the discriminatory zone of ultrasound. In these patients, the appropriate use of hCG doubling times and serum progesterone levels is necessary to avoid interrupting a viable IUP. Patients with hCG titers that plateau (less than 15% change) or an hCG rise of less than 50% in 48 hours should undergo D&C to differentiate between a failed IUP and an ectopic pregnancy. Villi is absent on final histology in up to 50% of these cases. Because only the presence of villi is diagnostic, those without villi require serial hCG titers. While awaiting final histologic pathology, hCG titers are also followed. As noted in the ectopic algorithm, a serum hCG drawn after D&C is followed by a repeat level in 12 to 24 hours. Rising or inappropriately falling levels after D&C are considered diagnostic of an ectopic pregnancy.

CURRENT THERAPY

- Surgery: treatment of choice for unstable patients
- Methotrexate success: correlation with hCG levels
- Multidose methotrexate: 1 mg/kg body weight IM alternate days with leucovorin 0.1 mg/kg IM until hCG declines 15%
- Multidose treatment follow-up: daily hCG until decline, then weekly
- Single-dose methotrexate: 50 mg/m^2 based on actual body weight
- Single-dose treatment follow-up: hCG on days 1, 4, 7, then weekly if 15% decline between days 4 and 7

Abbreviations: hCG = human chorionic gonadotropin; IM = intramuscularly.

Laparoscopy remains the gold standard for the diagnosis of ectopic pregnancy. It should be employed in any patient with suspected ectopic rupture, unreliable patients, or any others suspected of ectopic pregnancy for which the diagnostic algorithms are inappropriate.

Treatment

Surgery is the classic treatment for ectopic pregnancy and remains the treatment of choice in hemodynamic unstable patients, those desiring no further pregnancies, or those who are unsuitable or unwilling to risk medical therapy.

Medical therapy with methotrexate[1] is an acceptable option to surgical therapy. Reported success rates range from 75% to 96%, with an average of approximately 90%. Whether a multidose or single-dose methotrexate protocol is most effective remains debatable, but single-dose methotrexate is the most popular because of its ease of use and low incidence of side effects.

Contraindications to medical therapy remain ill defined, but Boxes 1 and 2 note frequently used contraindications. The hCG level is the single factor most predictive of failure. With hCG levels of 5000 to 9999, success rates fall to approximately 87%, further dropping to 82% for levels 10,000 to 14,999 and 68% if more than 15,000. These levels can be used to counsel patients about the risk of failure.

MUITIDOSE METHOTREXATE

Intramuscular methotrexate, 1 mg/kg of actual body weight, alternating with citrovorum rescue factor (Leucovorin), 0.1 mg/kg, is given daily and continued until a 15% decline in two consecutive daily hCG titers. Human chorionic gonadotropin levels are then followed weekly. A repeat course of methotrexate/citrovorum is given if levels fall to less than 15% or rise between two consecutive hCG titers.

[1] Not FDA approved for this indication.

BOX 1 Generally Accepted Contraindications to Medical Therapy

White blood count <1500 cells/mL
Alanine aminotransferase (ALT) >twice upper limit normal
Creatinine >twice upper limit normal
Ectopic size >4 cm
Ectopic size >3.5 cm if cardiac activity present the upper limit of normal, hemodynamically unstable
Immunocompromised status

BOX 2 Relative Contraindications to Medical Therapy

Ectopic cardiac activity*
Serum hCG level >15,000[†]

*Controversial; however, when corrected for hCG level, no longer a risk factor.
[†]Acceptable if patients are counseled on failure rate.
Abbreviation: hCG = human chorionic gonadotropin.

SINGLE-DOSE METHOTREXATE PROTOCOL

Methotrexate, 50 mg/m^2 based on actual body weight, is given intramuscularly. The day methotrexate is given is considered day 1. A repeat hCG is performed on days 4 and 7. If there is an appropriate decline, hCG levels are followed weekly. If the hCG level declines less than 15% between days 4 and 7, a second dose of methotrexate is given and the protocol restarted at a new day 1. Although this protocol is referred to as "single-dose methotrexate," approximately 20% of patients require more than one treatment cycle.

In conclusion, the incidence of ectopic pregnancy has reached epidemic proportions in the United States. Nevertheless, the mortality associated with this disease is steadily declining. This decline is primarily because of earlier diagnosis that allows treatment prior to rupture. This earlier diagnosis is the result of improved assays for progesterone, hCG, transvaginal ultrasound, and the use of diagnostic algorithms that do not require the use of laparoscopy. Once diagnosed, numerous treatment options are now available, including the option of medical therapy. Future developments ideally will provide for an even earlier diagnosis as well as data on the optimum candidates for each form of treatment.

REFERENCES

Brenaschek G, Rudelstorfer R, Csaicsich P: Vaginal sonography versus serum human chorionic gonadotropin in early detection of pregnancy. Am J Obstet Gynecol 1988;158:608-612.
Kadar N, Freedman M, Zacher M: Further observation on the doubling time of human chorionic gonadotropin in early asymptomatic pregnancy. Fertil Steril 1980;54:783-787.
Lipscomb GH, McCord ML, Huff G, et al: Predictors of success of methotrexate treatment in women with tubal ectopic pregnancies. N Engl J Med 1999;341:1874-1878.
Lipscomb GH, Stovall TS, Ling FW: Nonsurgical treatment of ectopic pregnancy. N Engl J Med 2000;343:1325-1329.
Stovall TS, Ling FW, Buster JE: Nonsurgical diagnosis and treatment of tubal pregnancy. Fertil Steril 1990;54:537-538.
Stovall TG, Ling FW, Gray LA, et al: Methotrexate treatment of unruptured ectopic pregnancy: A report of 100 cases. Obstet Gynecol 1991;77:749-753.

Vaginal Bleeding in Late Pregnancy

Method of
Jami Star Zeltzer, MD

Vaginal bleeding in late pregnancy complicates approximately 6% of pregnancies and is associated with increased maternal and fetal morbidity and mortality. Excluding labor, the most likely causes are placenta previa and placental abruption, followed by uterine rupture and vasa previa; less common etiologies include trauma, cervical lesions, and coagulopathy. The primary focus in obstetric hemorrhage, regardless of cause, is maternal hemodynamic assessment and stabilization. Given the extraordinary blood flow to the uterus at term (600 to 800 mL/min), exsanguination can occur rapidly. Additionally, redistribution of maternal blood flow may lead to fetal hypoxia.

Early maternal signs of hemodynamic compromise include tachycardia and tachypnea; later, hypotension, weakened pulses, and oliguria ensue, along with evidence of fetal compromise. Further decompensation can ultimately result in the death of both mother and fetus. Guidelines for restoration of maternal circulating volume are approximately 3 mL of intravenous crystalloid, (i.e., normal saline or Ringer's solution) per 1 mL of blood lost (often underestimated). Laboratory evaluation includes a complete blood count, blood type, and crossmatch; in the setting of thrombocytopenia (less than 100,000 platelets), coagulation studies (prothrombin time [PT], partial thromboplastin time [PTT], fibrinogen, fibrin degradation products [FDPs]) are recommended. Packed red blood cells, fresh-frozen plasma, platelets, and/or cryoprecipitate are given to maintain maternal hemoglobin near 10 g/dL and correct coagulopathy (unlikely if whole blood is observed to clot in less than 8 minutes). Additional measures include administration of oxygen, lateral displacement of the uterus and, rarely, vasopressors. Fetal evaluation and treatment, including consideration of delivery, follow stabilization of the mother.

Placenta Previa

Placenta previa, or the implantation of the placenta adjacent to or covering the internal os, complicates approximately 0.5% of all deliveries. The degree of placenta previa may be:

- Complete (internal os covered entirely)
- Partial (portion of internal os covered)
- Marginal (placental edge at cervix or less than 2 cm away)
- Low lying (not a true previa, where the placental edge implants in the lower uterine segment but doesn't reach the cervix)

Box 1 lists the risk factors. The pathophysiology appears to involve endometrial damage, with resulting limitation of healthy uterine tissue for implantation.

The hallmark symptom is painless vaginal bleeding, presumably initiated by development of the lower uterine segment. Usually, this occurs by 29 to 30 weeks of gestation, although in approximately 33% of cases, there is no bleeding until labor. The first bleed may be self-limited, but rebleeding complicates approximately 60% of cases. The diagnosis is often made in the absence of symptoms on routine ultrasound. The incidence of placenta previa is 5% to 10% in midgestation; this resolves in most cases with development of the lower uterine segment (*placental migration*). When asymptomatic, expectant management is appropriate, although vaginal precautions after 28 weeks' gestation may be advised.

When a patient presents with third-trimester bleeding, speculum exams are contraindicated until placenta previa is ruled out. The most accurate method of diagnosis is transvaginal ultrasound, which is safe in experienced hands; transperineal or transabdominal ultrasound carry greater risks of false-positive and false-negative results.

BOX 1   Risk Factors for Placenta Previa

- Advancing maternal age
- Ethnic background (increased in Asians)
- Multiparity
- Multiple gestation
- Previous curettage
- Prior cesarean section (increases with number of sections)
- Prior placenta previa
- Smoking

Observation in the hospital is recommended following a bleed, during which time approximately 50% of patients will deliver. Steroids are indicated for enhancement of fetal lung maturation. Tocolysis can be administered if the mother and fetus are stable, but betasympathomimetics should be avoided in order to minimize cardiovascular effects. Outpatient management is acceptable if bleeding ceases, as long as the patient is compliant and has ready access to a hospital. Serial ultrasound assessment is recommended because there is an increased risk of intrauterine growth restriction. Transfusion should be offered to maintain hemoglobin greater than 10 mg/dL.

Urgent delivery by cesarean section is indicated when there is ongoing maternal hemorrhage or evidence of fetal compromise. In the stable patient, a planned cesarean section can be performed at 35 to 36 weeks, generally after an amniocentesis is performed to confirm fetal lung maturity. Vaginal delivery may be attempted if delivery is imminent, or with marginal previa, although a double setup for emergent cesarean section is advised. In the setting of fetal demise, vaginal delivery is preferable.

Placenta previa predisposes to postpartum hemorrhage, either from atony of the lower uterine segment or inability to remove the placenta because of absence of the decidua basalis. The most common form of this latter condition is placenta accreta, where the trophoblast adheres to the myometrium. Less common forms include placenta increta (the trophoblast invades the myometrium) and placenta percreta (trophoblast invades uterine serosa and/or adjacent organs). The primary risk factor for placenta accreta is the number of previous cesarean sections, with an incidence approaching 40% in patients with two prior cesarean sections and a placenta previa. Other risk factors include age, parity, and history of curettage. Color Doppler ultrasound and magnetic resonance imaging (MRI) are helpful but not always definitive for diagnosis. If placenta accreta is suspected, preparations can be made for scheduled delivery with trained personnel and blood products available. At delivery, the placenta should be left in place if a cleavage plane cannot be developed easily. Cesarean–hysterectomy is often required for hemostasis, although conservative management, including preoperative and intraoperative selective embolization and/or use of methotrexate, has been reported. With placenta percreta, bladder invasion may require cystoscopy and urologic repair.

Placental Abruption

Abruption of the placenta, or separation of the normally implanted placenta before birth, complicates 1% to 2% of pregnancies. Bleeding into the decidua basalis, with subsequent separation of varying amounts of placental tissue from the endometrium, may result in fetal compromise and/or demise. The exact pathophysiology is unclear. Box 2 lists the risk factors.

Vaginal bleeding in the second half of pregnancy is assumed to be caused by placental abruption, once placenta previa and other rare causes are ruled out. Concealed hemorrhage, present in 10% to 20% of cases, can complicate the diagnosis. Abdominal pain, back pain, uterine contractions (often described as low amplitude, high frequency), hypertonus, uterine tenderness, and/or idiopathic premature labor may be present. While ultrasound can identify placenta previa, it cannot be relied upon to definitively diagnose abruption, as clot is sonographically visible in less than 50% of cases. The differential diagnoses include uterine rupture, appendicitis, and chorioamnionitis, as well as other causes of abdominal pain.

Most commonly, bleeding is not profuse and, if the episode is self-limited, expectant management of a preterm gestation includes observation, serial fetal growth assessment, fetal well-being testing, and steroid therapy to accelerate fetal lung maturation. With ongoing significant blood loss, stabilization of the mother, fetal assessment, and laboratory evaluation are indicated. Coagulopathy is rare in the absence of fetal demise. If tocolysis is required, betasympathomimetics should be avoided, as they may mask maternal cardiovascular decompensation.

Vaginal delivery is appropriate if mother and fetus are stable. Amniotomy may decrease extravasation of blood into the

BOX 2 Risk Factors for Placental Abruption

- Chorioamnionitis
- Cocaine use
- Ethnic background (highest in blacks)
- Hypertension
- Male fetal gender
- Multiple gestation
- Parity
- Polyhydramnios (rapid decompression at membrane rupture and/or therapeutic amniocentesis)
- Preterm premature rupture of membranes
- Previous cesarean section
- Smoking
- Trauma, including domestic violence
- Unexplained elevated second trimester alpha-fetoprotein
- Uterine anomalies/short umbilical cord

BOX 4 Uterine Rupture

Risk Factors
Previous cesarean section (especially classical)
Use of oxytocin, prostaglandins, or misoprostol
Multiparity
Midforceps application
Breech version/extraction
Placental abruption
Shoulder dystocia
Placenta percreta
Müllerian duct anomalies
History of pelvic radiation

Differential Diagnoses
Appendicitis
Biliary colic
Pancreatitis
Peptic ulcer disease
Intestinal obstruction
Ovarian torsion
Placental abruption
Urinary tract disorders

myometrium by head compression. Not uncommonly, effacement will precede dilatation; oxytocin (Pitocin) is acceptable for labor dysfunction. In the event of an intrauterine demise, vaginal delivery is preferred. Acute hemorrhage requires immediate cesarean delivery, with blood and coagulation factor replacement as needed.

Potential complications of abruption include hemorrhagic shock, disseminated intravascular coagulation (unlikely unless there is greater than 2000 mL blood loss and/or fetal demise), ischemic necrosis of maternal organs (especially kidney), and Couvelaire uterus (extravasation of blood into uterine muscle). Recurrence is approximately 5% to 15%, increasing with each subsequent event. There are no known preventive measures other than correcting modifiable risk factors. Research into the association between thrombophilia and abruption is ongoing, but in absence of other risk factors, a workup for hypercoagulability may be considered.

Vasa Previa

Vasa previa is a rare condition (estimated 1 in 2500 deliveries) in which fetal blood vessels cross over the membranes in advance of the presenting part. This is most often associated with velamentous insertion of the umbilical cord (vessels reach the placenta after coursing through the membranes rather than by direct insertion); Box 3 lists the risk factors. Vasa previa carries a profound risk of fetal mortality from exsanguination, particularly at the time of membrane rupture (fetal blood volume at term is approximately 250 mL). Even in the absence of bleeding, vessel compression may result in compromise of the fetal circulation.

Signs include hemorrhage, as well as fetal heart rate abnormalities. A high index of suspicion is required, and advances in imaging techniques (color Doppler, transvaginal ultrasound) make prenatal diagnosis possible. If there is unexplained bleeding, an Apt test or Kleihauer-Betke test can identify fetal red blood cells. If the diagnosis of vasa previa is strongly suspected at term, or if hemorrhage is significant, prompt cesarean delivery is recommended, followed by neonatal resuscitation.

BOX 3 Risk Factors for Vasa Previa

- Bilobed placenta
- In vitro fertilization
- Low-lying placenta
- Multiple pregnancy
- Succenturiate lobe
- Velamentous insertion of umbilical cord

Uterine Rupture

Most often reported following prior cesarean section, uterine rupture can also occur in an unscarred uterus (1 in 8000 to 1 in 15,000 deliveries). This phenomenon implies complete separation of the uterine wall (as compared to uterine dehiscence), with or without expulsion of the fetus. Box 4 lists risk factors and differential diagnoses.

Common signs and symptoms include abdominal pain/tenderness and vaginal bleeding; additional complaints include epigastric or shoulder pain, abdominal distention, and constipation. The fetal tracing may show sudden variable decelerations or abrupt and prolonged bradycardia, often accompanied by recession of the presenting part. Maternal and fetal morbidity and mortality are high, particularly with delayed diagnosis. Treatment is urgent cesarean delivery, with repair of the uterus and/or hysterectomy as needed. Repeat cesarean section is advised in the future because of the risk for recurrence.

Hypertensive Disorders of Pregnancy

Method of
Baha M. Sibai, MD

Management of preeclampsia depends on the severity of the disease process, gestational age at onset, and maternal and fetal well-being. Hypertensive disorders are the most common medical complications of pregnancy, with a reported incidence ranging between 5% and 10%. These disorders are the second leading cause of maternal death in the United States and a leading cause of perinatal mortality and morbidity worldwide. The clinical manifestations in some of these disorders are usually similar (e.g., hypertension, generalized edema, proteinuria, hematuria, renal insufficiency); however, they can result from different underlying causes, including essential hypertension, gestational hypertension, preeclampsia, renal disease, or connective tissue disease.

Hypertension is the hallmark for the diagnosis of these disorders. Therefore, in caring for pregnant women with hypertension, it is

TABLE 1 Hypertensive Disorders of Pregnancy

Clinical Findings	Chronic Hypertension	Gestational Hypertension	Preeclampsia	Renal Disease
Time of onset of hypertension	<20 wk	Usually after 33 wk	<20 wk	Usually before 20 wk
Degree of hypertension	Mild or severe	Mild	Mild or severe	Usually severe
Proteinuria*	Absent	Absent	Usually present	Usually severe
Serum urate <5.5 mg/dL (0.33 mmol/L)	Rare	Absent	Present in almost all cases	Variable
Hemoconcentration	Absent	Absent	Present in severe disease	Present in some conditions
Thrombocytopenia	Absent	Absent	Present in severe disease	May be present[†]
Serum creatinine ≥1.2 mg/dL	Absent	Absent	Rare	Usually present
Hepatic dysfunction	Absent	Absent	Present in severe disease	Absent

*Defined as ≥300 mg in a 24-h urine collection.
[†]Present in hemolytic–uremic syndrome and patients with lupus nephritis.

important to differentiate among gestational hypertension, chronic hypertension, preeclampsia, and silent renal disease (Table 1). In general, maternal and perinatal outcomes are usually good in those who have either mild essential chronic hypertension or gestational hypertension. In contrast, maternal and neonatal complications are increased among pregnant women who have secondary chronic hypertension, renal disease, or severe preeclampsia.

Definitions and Classification

The terminology used to describe the hypertensive disorders of pregnancy and the definitions used to diagnose hypertension in pregnancy have been confusing and inconsistent. Some of these terms, such as *pregnancy-induced hypertension*, are vague and broad, whereas others, such as *pregnancy-associated hypertension*, are nonspecific. In addition, a variety of classifications have been proposed by the American College of Obstetricians and Gynecologists, the International Society for the Study of Hypertension in Pregnancy, and the Working Group on High Blood Pressure in Pregnancy. In general, all current definitions and classification schemes have certain pitfalls as they relate to clinical diagnosis and management. In this review, hypertensive disorders are divided into three major categories: chronic hypertension, gestational hypertension, and preeclampsia (see Table 1).

Chronic Hypertension

The incidence of chronic hypertension in pregnancy ranges from 1 to 5%, depending on the woman's age, body mass index, and ethnic origin. The etiology and severity of chronic hypertension are important considerations in the management of pregnancy. Chronic hypertension is subdivided into two categories: primary (essential) and secondary. Primary hypertension is by far the most common cause of chronic hypertension seen during pregnancy (90%). In 10% of the cases, chronic hypertension is secondary to one or more underlying disorders such as renal disease (glomerulonephritis, interstitial nephritis, polycystic kidneys, renal artery stenosis), collagen vascular disease (lupus, scleroderma), endocrine disorders (diabetes mellitus with vascular involvement, phoechromocytoma, thyrotoxicosis, Cushing's disease, hyperaldosteronism), or coarctation of the aorta.

For management and counseling purposes, chronic hypertension in pregnancy also is categorized as either low risk or high risk. The patient is considered to be at low risk when she has mild essential hypertension without any organ involvement. Blood pressure criteria are based on blood pressure measurements at the initial visit regardless of whether patients are on antihypertensive medications. A patient who initially is classified as low risk early in pregnancy can become high risk if she later develops severe hypertension or in the event of preeclampsia or fetal growth restriction.

DIAGNOSIS

The diagnosis of chronic hypertension during pregnancy is usually based on either a history of hypertension before pregnancy or blood pressure elevations to at least 140/90 mm Hg before 20 weeks' gestation. The diagnosis is more severe when definite evidence of hypertension is documented before conception, particularly when antihypertensive agents have been prescribed.

The diagnosis of chronic hypertension may be difficult in pregnant women in whom the blood pressure before pregnancy is not known. During normal pregnancy, blood pressure progressively decreases from the first trimester, reaching a nadir at 14 to 24 weeks' gestation, with a gradual return to prepregnancy levels during the third trimester. As a result of these physiologic changes in blood pressure during the second trimester, many women with actual chronic hypertension before pregnancy have normal blood pressure readings before 20 weeks' gestation. The majority of these women subsequently develop increased blood pressure during the third trimester, and thus gestational hypertension or preeclampsia is erroneously diagnosed.

In the nonpregnant state, hypertension is classified as mild, moderate, or severe on the basis of either systolic or diastolic blood pressure readings. In pregnancy, it is easier to classify chronic hypertension. Mild hypertension is systolic pressure between 140 and 159 mm Hg or diastolic pressure between 90 and 109 mm Hg, or both. Severe hypertension is systolic pressure at least 160 mm Hg or diastolic pressure at least 110 mm Hg, or both. In pregnancies complicated by chronic hypertension, perinatal outcome is adversely affected mostly because of superimposed preeclampsia. The diagnosis of superimposed preeclampsia should be made on the basis of

CURRENT DIAGNOSIS

- In women with chronic hypertension, the diagnosis of preeclampsia requires new-onset proteinuria (>0.5 g/24 h) and/or severe central nervous system symptoms or thrombocytopenia.
- Gestational hypertension is defined as onset of elevation of blood pressures (systolic ≥140 mm Hg or diastolic ≥90 mm Hg) after 20 weeks of gestation on at least two occasions at least 6 hours apart, but within 1 week of each other.
- Preeclampsia is defined as gestational hypertension plus proteinuria (≥300 mg/24 h).
- HELLP syndrome is diagnosed in the presence of preeclampsia plus hemolysis, elevated liver enzymes, and low platelet count (<100,000/mm³).

TABLE 2 Drug Therapy for Hypertension In Pregnancy*

Drug	Daily Oral Dose	Indications	Comments
Methyldopa (Aldomet)	750-4000 mg[3] in 3 or 4 divided doses	First drug of choice in chronic hypertension	Safety to the fetus and long-term effects on the infant well studied
Labetalol (Normodyne, Trandate)	300-2400 mg in 3 or 4 divided doses	Second or an alternative drug in chronic hypertension Initial drug to treat severe hypertension in preeclampsia	Limited data regarding long-term effects on infant
Nifedipine (Procardia)	40-120 mg in 4 divided doses	Second or an alternative drug in chronic hypertension Drug of choice to control blood pressure in severe preeclampsia both antepartum and postpartum	Limited data regarding long-term effects on infant
Thiazide diuretics (hydrochlorothiazide)	25-50 mg in 2 divided doses	Patients with salt-sensitive chronic hypertension and those with evidence of left ventricular diastolic dysfunction	Can cause plasma volume depletion To be discontinued if superimposed preeclampsia or poor fetal growth develops

[3]Exceeds dosage recommended by the manufacturer.
*All other drugs that are used in nonpregnancy are either rarely indicated or contraindicated to treat hypertension in pregnancy.

exacerbated hypertension plus the development of new-onset proteinuria (at 0.5 g/24 hours). In women with renal disease, proteinuria and elevated uric acid values may already be present from early in pregnancy. In such women, the diagnosis of superimposed preeclampsia may be difficult. I recommend establishing the diagnosis on the basis of onset of thrombocytopenia or symptoms such as persistent headaches, visual abnormalities, or epigastric pain.

MATERNAL AND PERINATAL RISKS

Women with pregnancies complicated by chronic hypertension are at increased risk for the development of superimposed preeclampsia and abruptio placentae. The reported rates of preeclampsia with mild hypertension range from 15% to 25%. The rate of preeclampsia in women with severe chronic hypertension averages 30% to 50%. One study examined the rate of superimposed preeclampsia among 763 women with chronic hypertension who were observed prospectively at several medical centers in the United States. The overall rate of superimposed preeclampsia was 25%. The rate was not affected by maternal age, race, or presence of proteinuria early in pregnancy. However, the rate was significantly greater in women who had hypertension for a least 4 years (31% vs 22%), in those who had had preeclampsia during a previous pregnancy (32% vs 23%), and in those whose diastolic blood pressure was 100 to 110 mm Hg when compared with those whose diastolic blood pressure was less than 100 mm Hg at baseline (42% vs 24%).

TREATMENT

Management of the patient with chronic hypertension should begin before conception to establish the etiology as well as the severity of the hypertension. Attention should be paid to the degree and duration of the hypertension, presence of associated medical disorders (cardiac, renal, diabetes, connective tissue disease), presence of target organ damage (left ventricular disease), type and number of antihypertensive drugs required to control maternal blood pressure, and outcome in previous pregnancies. In addition, attention should be paid to maternal diet, social habits (drugs, alcohol, smoking), and activity. Based on this assessment, the patient is then classified as having low-risk hypertension (essential hypertension without associated medical disorders or target organ involvement) or high-risk hypertension (patients with severe hypertension and those with target organ damage or associated medical disorders). Patients with primary renal disease with renal insufficiency (serum creatinine concentration >1.4 mg per dL) and hypertension and those with severe hypertension requiring multidrug therapy should be informed about the risks to the fetus and the potential for renal failure during pregnancy.

The use of angiotensin-converting enzyme inhibitors and angiotensin-receptor blocking drugs during pregnancy is associated with fetal growth restriction, oligohydramnios, neonatal renal failure, and neonatal death. In addition, chronic use of atenolol (Tenormin) during pregnancy has adverse effects on placental function and fetal growth. Therefore, women receiving such medications should be switched to different agents before conception. Some of the drugs that are believed relatively safe for use in pregnancy are listed in Table 2. In addition, the adverse effects of illicit drugs, alcohol, and smoking on maternal blood pressure as well as on the fetus should be emphasized, and the woman should be encouraged to discontinue their use before conception.

Early onset of prenatal care and careful antepartum supervision with proper fetal testing are the keys for a successful outcome of pregnant women with chronic hypertension. At the time of the first prenatal visit, it is important to determine gestational age and confirm an estimated date of confinement, which are important to monitor fetal growth and for timing of delivery. Most patients have low-risk chronic hypertension and thus have a favorable maternal and perinatal prognosis without the use of antihypertensive drugs.

Fetal testing should include an ultrasound examination every 4 weeks to monitor fetal growth and amniotic fluid starting at 32 weeks and nonstress testing starting at 34 to 36 weeks' gestation. The patient should be carefully monitored for the development of superimposed preeclampsia or abnormal fetal growth. The onset of either of these

---

CURRENT THERAPY

- Pregnant women with essential hypertension and without target organ damage require antihypertensive therapy only once systolic blood pressure (BP) is above 159 mm Hg and/or diastolic BP is above 104 mm Hg.
- Pregnant women with target organ damage should receive medications to keep systolic BP below 140 mm Hg and/or diastolic BP below 90 mm Hg.
- Labetalol (Normodyne), nifedipine (Procardia), α-methyldopa (Aldomet), and diuretics can be safety used during pregnancy.
- Delivery is the ultimate cure for women with preeclampsia.

complications requires either hospitalization or frequent antenatal testing.

Timing for delivery should be individualized according to each particular situation. Delivery is indicated at or beyond 37 weeks' gestation in those who develop either superimposed preeclampsia or abnormal fetal test result or growth, whereas pregnancy can usually continue until cervical ripening or until 40 weeks' gestation in women not requiring antihypertensive medications and who have normal fetal growth.

Women with high-risk chronic hypertension require more frequent antenatal visits and earlier onset of fetal testing. In addition, these women require the use of antihypertensive drugs to keep systolic blood pressure below 140 mm Hg and diastolic pressure below 90 mm Hg.

PHARMACOLOGIC TREATMENT

The indications for and the benefits of antihypertensive drugs in the management of chronic hypertension in pregnancy remain unclear. Therefore, the decision to initiate drug therapy in a woman with chronic hypertension should take into account the severity of the hypertension, the response in maternal blood pressure during the second trimester, the potential risk of damage to target organs, and the presence or absence of preexisting cardiovascular disease.

My experience indicates that maternal blood pressure spontaneously decreases to normotensive values during pregnancy in nearly 50% of women with mild uncomplicated chronic hypertension. In addition, the results of the largest prospective randomized trial conducted to date by me revealed no beneficial effects from antihypertensive drugs in the management of these pregnancies. It is my policy to discontinue or not to initiate antihypertensive drugs in all women with uncomplicated mild hypertension (low risk) at the time of their first prenatal visit. Only 15% of these women subsequently require drug therapy because of exacerbated severe hypertension.

Antihypertensive drugs are continued or initiated in all women considered to have high-risk chronic hypertension and in those whose diastolic blood pressure at time of first prenatal visit is at least 105 mm Hg (Korotkoff's 5). The initial drug of choice is labetalol (Trandate) because its safety during pregnancy has been documented in clinical trials. The daily dosage and indications for drugs recommended for use during pregnancy are summarized in Table 2.

Gestational Hypertension

Gestational hypertension is defined as the development of high blood pressure without other symptoms of preeclampsia after 20 weeks' gestation in a previously normotensive woman. Persistent elevation in blood pressure to at least 140/90 mm Hg on at least two separate occasions more than 4 hours apart is the hallmark for the diagnosis of this disorder. In clinical practice, the majority of women with hypertensive disorders of pregnancy fit this diagnosis.

In some women, gestational hypertension may be only an early manifestation of preeclampsia, whereas in others it may be an early sign of unrecognized chronic hypertension. In general, this diagnosis is made late in the third trimester, during labor, or immediately postpartum. As a result, pregnancy outcome in these women is invariably good without drug therapy.

However, about 20% of these pregnancies may progress to preeclampsia and will be at slightly increased risk for fetal growth restriction (5%-10%), abruptio placentae (0.6%-0.8%), and eclampsia (development of convulsions, 0.1%). Thus, in those who have a ripe cervix for induction (Bishops' cervical score ≥6) at 38 weeks' gestation labor should be induced for delivery. For those remote from term (>37 weeks), management should include restricted activity with rest at home, close observation of maternal blood pressure and urine protein level, and instructions regarding symptoms of preeclampsia. Fetal evaluation with nonstress testing should begin at the time of diagnosis and be repeated as needed. Ultrasound examination is required to evaluate fetal growth and amniotic fluid.

BOX 1 Clinical Findings Consistent with Severe Preeclampsia

Severe hypertension plus proteinuria
Mild hypertension plus severe proteinuria (>5 g/24 h)
Cerebral dysfunction
Persistent headaches or visual symptoms
Changes in mental status
Convulsions
Acute renal failure or oliguria (<500 mL/24 h)
Thrombocytopenia (<100,000/mm^3)
Documented microangiopathic hemolysis
Severe epigastric pain plus liver dysfunction
Onset of pulmonary edema

Preeclampsia

Preeclampsia has traditionally been defined as the occurrence of hypertension, edema, and proteinuria after 20 weeks' gestation in a previously normotensive woman. In general, preeclampsia is diagnosed in the presence of gestational hypertension plus proteinuria. It is classified as mild or severe primarily on the basis of the degree of elevation in blood pressure (similar to chronic hypertension), the degree of proteinuria (greater or less than 5 g in a 24-hour urine sample), or both. However, emphasis on either hypertension or proteinuria can minimize the clinical importance of other disturbances in various organ systems that make preeclampsia severe (Box 1).

PATHOGENESIS AND PATHOPHYSIOLOGY

Preeclampsia is a disorder of unknown etiology that is peculiar to human pregnancy. Many theories regarding its cause have been suggested in the past centuries, but none has withstood the test of time.

One of the earliest abnormalities noted in women with preeclampsia is failure of the second wave of trophoblast invasion into the spiral arteries of the uterus. As a result of this defect in placentation, there is failure of the normal cardiovascular adaptations (increased plasma volume and reduced systemic vascular resistance) that are characteristic of normotensive pregnancies. In established preeclampsia, both cardiac output and plasma volume are reduced, whereas systemic vascular resistance is increased.

These abnormalities are usually present in women with severe disease. These changes result in reduced perfusion of the placenta, kidneys, liver, and brain. Other major pathophysiologic abnormalities include endothelial dysfunction with resultant vasospasm, altered vascular permeability, activation of the coagulation systems, altered prostanoids ratio, and abnormal nitric oxide production. An imbalance in angiogenic factors includes reduced placental growth factor and VEGF with increased soluble Flt-1 and endoglin.

PREVENTION

Prevention of preeclampsia requires knowledge of its etiology as well as the availability of methods for prediction of those at risk. Numerous clinical, biophysical, and biochemical tests have been proposed for predicting preeclampsia. Most of the available methods for prediction suffer from poor sensitivity and poor positive predictive values. As a result, most clinical trials on prevention have used patients with risk factors that increase the incidence for this disorder (Box 2).

For many years, salt restriction and diuretic drugs have been used to prevent preeclampsia. The only randomized trial of a low-salt diet in pregnancy did not demonstrate such a benefit. In addition, a meta-analysis of nine randomized trials comprising more than 7000 subjects regarding the use of diuretics in pregnancy revealed a decrease in the incidence of edema and hypertension but not in the incidence of preeclampsia.

BOX 2 Risk Factors for Preeclampsia

Nulliparity
Obesity and insulin resistance
Pregnancies after donor insemination, oocyte, or embryo donation
Multiple gestations
Family history of preeclampsia
Multifetal gestation
Preeclampsia–eclampsia in previous pregnancy
Chronic hypertension or renal disease
Insulin-dependent diabetes mellitus
Evidence of fetal growth restriction in current pregnancy
Presence of thrombophilia
Connective tissue disease
Persistent proteinuria in current pregnancy
Relative hypertension in association with symptoms
Abruptio placentae in current pregnancy
Abnormal Doppler velocimetry
Hydropic degeneration of the placenta

The results of a review of early studies in women at risk for preeclampsia suggested that low doses of aspirin[1] (50-150 mg/day) reduced the incidence and severity of preeclampsia. In contrast, several large multicenter and multinational randomized trials in nulliparous women and women at varying degrees of risk for preeclampsia found minor beneficial effects in the aspirin-treated women. In addition, a trial supported by the National Institute of Child Health and Development found no reduction in the incidence of preeclampsia with the administration of aspirin in women with chronic hypertension, multifetal gestation, previous history of preeclampsia, or insulin-dependent diabetes. However, a recent meta-analysis of published studies suggested that low-dose aspirin prophylaxis in women at risk reduces the rate of preeclampsia by 10% compared with no treatment.

The results of epidemiologic studies suggested an inverse association between dietary calcium intake and the incidence of preeclampsia–eclampsia in certain populations. However, the results of a large, randomized, double-blind trial in 4589 nulliparous women performed by the National Institute of Child Health Development found no such benefit. In contrast, a meta-analysis of published trials regarding calcium supplementation[1] in pregnancy reported that calcium reduces the rate of hypertensive disorders during pregnancy only in women with very low calcium intake. On the other hand, an evidence-based review by the FDA concluded that the relationship between calcium and risk of preeclampsia is highly unlikely.

Increased oxidative stress is suggested as an important pathophysiologic abnormality before to onset of preeclampsia. One early trial found that supplementation with antioxidant vitamins C[1] and E[1] early in pregnancy reduced the rate of preeclampsia in women at risk for this complication. In contrast, the results of two large multicenter trials using supplementation with vitamins C and E in women identified at risk revealed no reduction in rates of preeclampsia.

TREATMENT

Early diagnosis, close medical supervision, and timely delivery are the key steps in the management of preeclampsia. The ultimate goals of treatment must always be safety of the mother first and then the delivery of a live infant who will not require intensive and prolonged neonatal care. Therefore, once the diagnosis is established, subsequent management should be based on the initial evaluation of maternal and fetal conditions. On the basis of the results of this evaluation, a decision is then made regarding hospitalization, expectant management, or delivery. This decision should depend on the severity of the disease process, maternal condition and desire, gestational age, fetal status according to tests of fetal well-being, and presence of labor or rupture of membranes.

Mild Preeclampsia

Women with preeclampsia require close observation for early detection of sudden worsening of the disease process. Women with mild preeclampsia at term (≥ 37 weeks) should be considered for delivery, particularly if the cervix is favorable for induction or if they have labor or rupture of the membranes. Women who are remote from term can be managed expectantly provided that they receive close maternal and fetal evaluation.

Figure 1 is an algorithm for the management of mild preeclampsia. This evaluation can be performed in the hospital if possible. Outpatient management may be considered if compliance is expected to be good, symptoms are absent, hypertension and proteinuria are mild, and the result of fetal testing is normal.

Regardless of the management strategy chosen, the woman should have evaluation of blood pressure, weight, urinary protein excretion, platelet count (twice a week), liver enzymes (twice a week), and symptoms of worsening preeclampsia, and she should be encouraged to have relative rest. In addition, the fetus should be monitored with serial ultrasound examinations for growth and quantity of amniotic fluid (every 3 weeks) and with the nonstress test (once or twice per week). During this management, the patient must be educated about immediately reporting labor, vaginal bleeding, abdominal pain, and symptoms of worsening preeclampsia. If there is evidence of disease progression in either mother or fetus, hospitalization or delivery is indicated.

The role and benefits of antihypertensive drugs in the management of mild preeclampsia are unclear. The results of several randomized trials revealed conflicting findings. Few of these trials revealed reduced frequency of progression to severe disease and premature delivery with drug therapy. However, the results of a recent meta-analysis of large randomized trials conducted by me found no clear benefit to drug treatment in women with mild preeclampsia. Thus, I do not recommend drug therapy for these women.

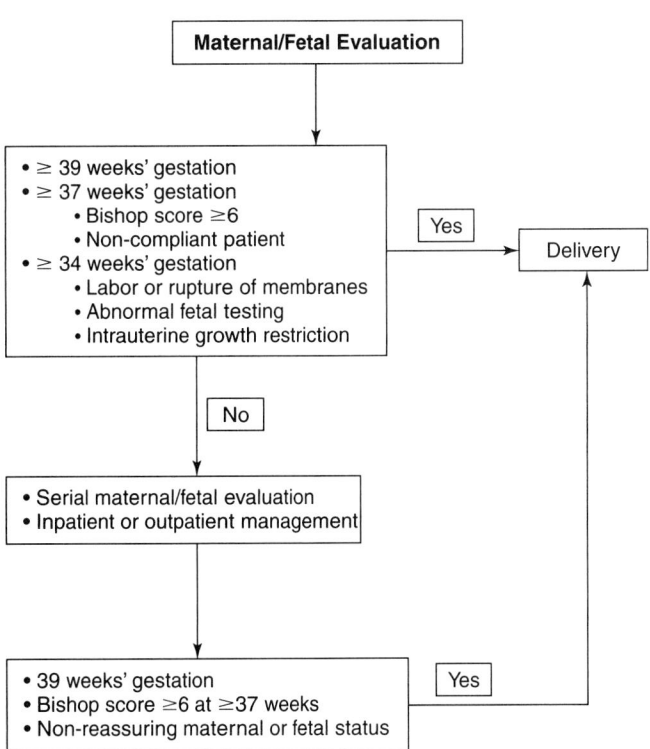

FIGURE 1. Management of mild hypertension and preeclampsia.

---

[1] Not FDA approved for this indication

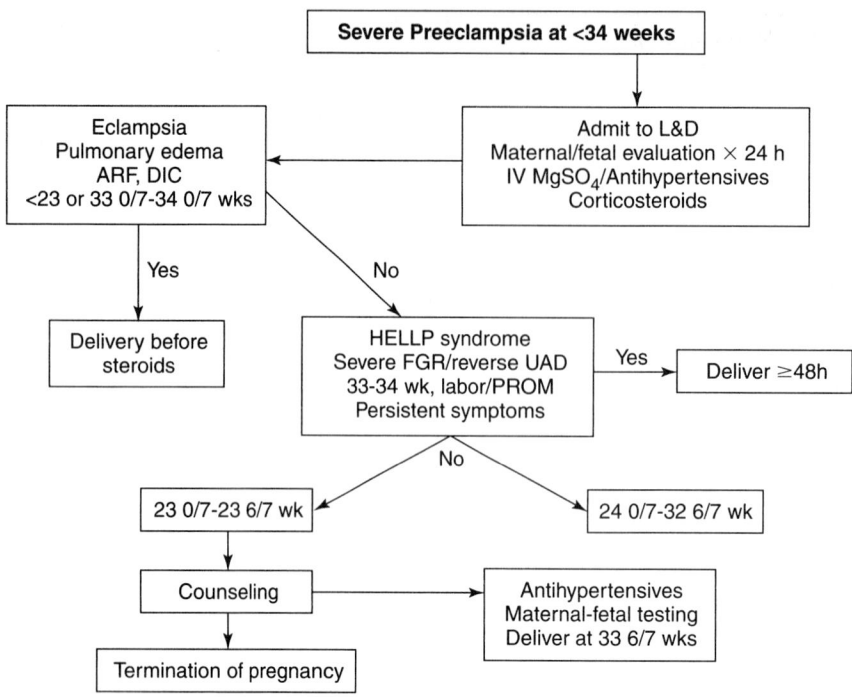

FIGURE 2. Management of severe preeclampsia at less than 34 weeks' gestation. ARF = acute renal failure; DIC = disseminated intravascular coagulation; FGR = fetal growth restriction; HELLP = hemolysis, elevated liver enzymes, and low platelets; L&D = labor and delivery; PROM = premature rupture of membranes; UAD = uterine artery Doppler. (Adapted from Sibai BM, Barton JR: Expectant management of severe preeclampsia remote from term: patient selection, management, and delivery indications. Am J Obstet Gynecol 196:514.e1-514.e9, 2007.)

Severe Preeclampsia

Severe preeclampsia may be rapidly progressive, resulting in sudden deterioration in the status of both the mother and fetus; thus, prompt hospitalization is required. Prompt delivery is clearly indicated when there is imminent eclampsia, multiorgan dysfunction, or fetal distress or when fetal gestational age is 34 weeks or more. Early in gestation, however, prolongation of pregnancy with intensive monitoring at a tertiary care facility may be indicated to improve neonatal survival and reduce short-term and long-term neonatal morbidity (Figure 2). The benefits of this management have been documented in several studies.

However, such management entails risks to both mother and fetus and thus requires extensive maternal counseling as well as daily evaluation of both maternal and fetal conditions. Women who have a sustained diastolic blood pressure of at least 110 mm Hg receive either labetalol or nifedipine in doses as described in Table 2. The aim of drug therapy is to keep the mean arterial pressure below 126 mm Hg (but not less than 105 mm Hg) and the diastolic pressure below 105 mm Hg (but not less than 90 mm Hg). These thresholds are important for both maternal and fetal safety.

HELLP Syndrome

Some patients with preeclampsia develop laboratory evidence of *h*emolysis, *e*levated *l*iver enzymes, and *l*ow *p*latelets, or HELLP syndrome (Box 3). Several of the signs, symptoms, and laboratory abnormalities that constitute this syndrome may be confused with similar findings that are usually present in a number of distinct medical and surgical disorders. This is particularly true when the manifestations develop remote from term.

CLINICAL FINDINGS

One of the major problems with early detection of HELLP syndrome lies in its clinical presentation, because patients can present with nonspecific symptoms or subtle signs of preeclampsia. Patients can present with various signs and symptoms, none of which is diagnostic of preeclampsia and all of which may be found in patients with severe preeclampsia–eclampsia without HELLP syndrome. From 30% to 90% of patients have right upper quadrant or epigastric pain, nausea, or vomiting. Most patients give a history of malaise for the past few days before presentation, and some have nonspecific viral syndrome–like symptoms. Headaches are reported by 33% to 61% of the patients, and visual changes are reported in approximately 17% of patients. A subset of patients with HELLP syndrome present with symptoms related to thrombocytopenia, such as bleeding from mucosal surfaces, hematuria, petechial hemorrhages, or ecchymosis.

Although most patients have hypertension (82%-88%), it may be only mild in 15% to 50% of patients and absent in 12% to 18%. Most patients (86%-100%) have proteinuria by dipstick examination; however, it was reported to be absent in 13% of patients in the two largest series.

BOX 3 Recommended Criteria for HELLP Syndrome

Hemolysis (at least two of these)
- Peripheral smear (schistocytes, burr cells)
- Serum bilirubin ($\geq$1.2 mg/dL)
- Low serum haptoglobin
- Severe anemia unrelated to blood loss

Elevated liver enzymes
- AST or ALT at least twice upper level of normal
- LDH at least twice upper level of normal*

Low platelets (<100,000/mm^3)

---
*Also elevated in severe hemolysis
ALT = alanine aminotransferase; AST = aspartate aminotransferase; HELLP = hemolysis, elevated liver enzymes, and low platelets; LDH = lactate dehydrogenase.

These pregnancies are associated with substantial maternal and perinatal morbidity. Thus, the presence of HELLP syndrome requires immediate hospitalization and consideration for delivery within 48 hours, depending on gestational age and maternal condition. These women also require close monitoring for at least 48 hours after delivery because of the risks of pulmonary edema, renal failure, and continued hemolysis and thrombocytopenia. Differential diagnosis for these women should include the hemolytic–uremic syndrome, thrombotic thrombocytopenic purpura, acute fatty liver of pregnancy, and exacerbation of lupus.

Intrapartum and Postpartum Management

Women with preeclampsia should have close observation during labor and delivery and postpartum, with special attention to fluid intake and output, level of blood pressure, and cerebral symptoms. The primary objective of this management is to prevent cerebral complications (encephalopathy, convulsions, or hemorrhage), pulmonary edema, and renal failure. The threshold for treatment of blood pressure is a sustained diastolic blood pressure of 110 mm Hg or more. Other experts recommend mean arterial pressure greater than 125 mm Hg. The initial treatment of choice is hydralazine (Apresoline) given intravenously in 5- to 10-mg bolus doses to be repeated as needed every 20 minutes for up to a cumulative total of 25 to 30 mg. Alternative drugs could also include labetalol (Trandate) (20-40 mg) intravenous doses to be repeated every 10 minutes for up to a cumulative dose of 220 mg or nifedipine (Procardia) 10 to 20 mg orally.

Mode of Delivery

There are no randomized trials comparing optimal methods of delivery in women with gestational hypertension or preeclampsia. A plan for vaginal delivery should be attempted for all women with mild disease and for most women with severe disease, particularly those beyond 30 weeks of gestation. The decision to perform cesarean delivery should be based on fetal gestational age, fetal condition, presence of labor, and cervical Bishop score. In general, the presence of severe preeclampsia or eclampsia is not an indication for cesarean delivery. It is appropriate to consider cesarean delivery for all women with severe preeclampsia earlier than 30 weeks of gestation who are not in labor and whose Bishop score is less than 5. Similar consideration for cesarean delivery is given to those with severe preeclampsia plus fetal growth restriction if the gestational age is less than 32 weeks in the presence of an unfavorable Bishop score.

Women with preeclampsia have an increased risk for convulsions during labor. The risk is highest in women with severe preeclampsia remote from term, those with cerebral symptoms, and those with HELLP syndrome. Therefore, intravenous magnesium sulfate should be given prophylactically during labor and after delivery to all women with preeclampsia. I recommend a loading dose of 6 g for a period for 15 to 20 minutes, followed by a maintenance dose of 2 g/h after delivery. The efficacy of magnesium sulfate in preventing and treating eclamptic convulsions has been proved in randomized trials.

Occasionally, preeclampsia worsens after delivery or develops for the first time within 1 week after delivery. In addition, some women with the HELLP syndrome continue to show deterioration in their laboratory findings or in renal function for several days after delivery. Therefore, close maternal observation should continue beyond delivery. The use of invasive hemodynamic monitoring is rarely indicated in the management of women with severe preeclampsia.

REFERENCES

ACOG Committee on Practice Bulletins—Obstetrics: ACOG Practice Bulletin. Diagnosis and management of preeclampsia and eclampsia. Obstet Gynecol 2002;99:159-167.

Askie LM, Duley L, Henderson-Smart DJ, Stewart LA, on behalf of the PARIS Collaborative Group: Antiplatelet agents for prevention of preeclampsia. Lancet 2007;369:1791-1798.

Conde-Agudelo A, Villar J, Lindheimer M: World Health Organization systematic review of screening tests for preeclampsia. Obstet Gynecol 2004;104:1367-1391.

Sibai BM: Chronic hypertension in pregnancy. Obstet Gynecol 2002;100:369-377.

Sibai BM: Diagnosis and management of gestational hypertension and preeclampsia. Obstet Gynecol 2003;102:181-192.

Sibai B, Kekker G, Kupferminc M: Pre-eclampsia. Lancet 2005;365:785-799.

Sibai BM: Diagnosis, controversies, and management of the syndrome of hemolysis, elevated liver enzymes, and low platelet count. Obstet Gynecol 2004;103:981-991.

Sibai BM, Barton JR: Expectant management of severe preeclampsia remote from term: Patient selection, management, and delivery indications. Am J Obstet Gynecol 2007;196:514. e1-e9.

Postpartum Care

Method of
Brenda Stokes, MD

The postpartum period, or puerperium, is the time immediately after birth when the uterus returns to its normal size. It starts with the delivery of the placenta and ends 6 weeks after birth. This chapter reviews specific concerns and problems that arise in the postpartum period.

Postpartum Hemorrhage

The World Health Organization defines postpartum hemorrhage as 500 mL or more of blood loss in the first 24 hours after delivery. Postpartum hemorrhage occurs in approximately 30% to 40% of all deliveries. It continues to be a major cause of maternal morbidity and mortality in both developed and developing countries.

Early recognition and treatment are essential in preventing complications from postpartum hemorrhage. The amount of blood loss following a delivery is difficult to measure accurately. It is typically estimated by visual inspection. Brisk vaginal bleeding following birth should trigger an investigation for its etiology.

The etiology of postpartum hemorrhage is shown in Box 1. Uterine atony is the most common cause of immediate postpartum hemorrhage. Once brisk bleeding is identified, a careful examination for the cause is performed. Palpation of the uterine fundus is done to assess the tone of the uterus. Bimanual uterine massage both confirms and treats uterine atony. The medications listed in Table 1 are oxytocics used to control vaginal bleeding due to uterine atony. Emptying the bladder with catheterization is useful to keep the uterus contracted. Surgical methods are considered if medications and uterine massage fail to control the bleeding. A careful inspection of the vagina and cervix for lacerations needs to be done. Manual curettage of the uterus can be performed immediately postpartum under appropriate anesthesia.

BOX 1 Etiology of Postpartum Hemorrhage
Uterine atony
Lacerations
Retained products of conception
Coagulation disorders

TABLE 1 Medications Used in the Treatment of Postpartum Hemorrhage

Medication	Dosage	Route	Dosing Interval	Cautions and Contraindications
Oxytocin (Pitocin)	10 units IM, 10-40 units/1000 mL IV fluids	IV, IM	One dose IM, IV rate as needed to control bleeding	Hypersensitivity to drug or class
Carboprost tromethamine (Hemabate)	250 µg	IM	Every 15-90 min up to 2 mg total	Active cardiac, pulmonary, liver, or renal disease
Methylergonovine (methergine)	0.2 mg	IM, oral	Every 2-4 h up to 5 doses IM, oral tid-qid for 3-7 d	Hypertension

Breast-Feeding

Breast-feeding has many benefits for both the infant and mother. Breast milk provides the proper nutrition for the infant and protection against certain infectious diseases. Breast-feeding enhances maternal infant bonding and can delay ovulation.

Mothers need support for initiation and continuation of breast-feeding. Both social and professional support systems are invaluable resources for lactating mothers.

Common breast-feeding problems include sore nipples, breast engorgement, blocked milk ducts, and infections. Sore nipples are usually due to improper latch-on of the infant during feeding. This will improve after correction of the latch-on. Breast engorgement usually responds to emptying the breasts by feeding or pumping.

Blocked milk ducts can be confused with infections. A blocked milk duct appears as a localized area of tenderness and erythema in one breast. It responds to warm compresses and gentle massage to express the breast milk and unclog the duct. Mastitis manifests as an erythematous, tender, hard area on one breast. Most women have systemic symptoms, such as fever and chills. Narrow-spectrum antibiotics can be used in most cases. Breast-feeding should be continued on both breasts. If the mother is unable to breast-feed, both breasts should be emptied by a breast pump. A breast abscess can develop as a complication of mastitis and must be surgically drained.

Nutrition and Activity

There are no dietary restrictions in healthy women in the postpartum period. Lactating women need to increase the protein, calories, and calcium in their diet. Physical activity is recommended in pregnancy and should be continued in the postpartum period. Less active women tend to retain more weight at 1 year postpartum than active women.

Puerperal Infections

Uterine infection, which is referred to as *endometritis*, is a common cause of puerperal fever. It is more common following a cesarean delivery. Diagnosis is made from history and physical examination. Fever is the typical manifesting symptom. Uterine tenderness is usually present. Endometritis is a polymicrobial infection. Broad-spectrum intravenous antibiotics are required for treatment. Intravenous antibiotics should be continued for 24 hours after defervescence. Oral antibiotics are not needed following the initial intravenous antibiotics. Complications of endometritis include pelvic infections, pelvic abscess, and septic pelvic thrombophlebitis.

Contraception

Postpartum contraception needs to be addressed with every patient because most will become sexually active before the traditional 6-week postpartum visit. The choice of contraception depends on patient preference, desire for future fertility, and clinical considerations. Table 2 lists methods of postpartum contraception and precautions specific to the postpartum period.

Medical Complications

Hypertension and preeclampsia can occur in the postpartum period with persistently elevated blood pressures. Blood pressure is highest 3 to 6 days postpartum. According to a 2005 Cochrane review of trials for treatment and prevention of postpartum hypertension, there are no reliable data to guide its treatment. Significantly elevated blood pressures should be treated as indicated. Evaluation for preeclampsia should be performed postpartum when suspected based on typical symptoms.

Peripartum cardiomyopathy can occur any time from the last month of pregnancy to 5 months postpartum. Diagnosis is made when heart failure develops during this time with no other identifiable cause or preexisting heart failure. Echocardiography is used to document left ventricular systolic dysfunction.

Gestational diabetes complicates approximately 2% to 14% of all pregnancies. Postpartum glucose tolerance testing in gestational diabetics is recommended by the American College of Obstetricians and Gynecologists and the American Diabetes Association. This can be completed at the 6-week postpartum visit.

Other medical problems that can occur in the postpartum period include venous thromboembolic disease, urinary retention,

CURRENT DIAGNOSIS

- Recognize and treat postpartum hemorrhage early.
- Uterine atony is the most common cause of immediate postpartum hemorrhage.
- Return to normal diet and physical activity can occur just after birth.
- Endometritis is the most common cause of puerperal fever.
- Screen for postpartum depression several times throughout the postpartum period.
- Address postpartum contraception early after delivery.

CURRENT THERAPY

- Postpartum hemorrhage usually responds to uterine massage and oxytocics.
- Social and professional support systems are key factors in successful continuation of breast-feeding.
- Oral antibiotics are not necessary after intravenous treatment of endometritis.
- All methods of contraception are acceptable choices postpartum with a few special considerations.

TABLE 2 Methods of Postpartum Contraception

Method of Contraception	When to Start	Precautions in Postpartum Period
Barrier Methods: Condoms, Diaphragm, cervical cap	At the resumption of sexual activity	Diaphragm or cervical cap will need to be refitted about 6 wk postpartum
Progesterone-only pills (Micronor), injectable (Depo-Provera), or implant (Implanon)	Any time after 24 h postpartum	Pills need to be taken the same time every d Can cause irregular prolonged bleeding postpartum Does not interfere with lactation
Combined oral contraceptive pills, patch (Ortho-Evra), or vaginal ring (NuvaRing)	4 wk postpartum	Decreases breast milk production Not advised if high risk of thromboembolic disease
Intrauterine device or system, progesterone containing (Mirena) or copper T (ParaGard)	Immediately postpartum or 6 wk postpartum	Increased risk of expulsion if inserted immediately postpartum Not advised if high risk of infection or previous ectopic pregnancy
Sterilization: Male or female (transabdominal or transcervical (Essure))	Male anytime, but ideally during the antepartum period. Female after delivery but before hospital discharge or 6 wk postpartum	Future fertility not desired Requires surgery Transcervical sterilization is an outpatient procedure but requires follow-up testing
Lactational amenorrhea method	Can be effective if exclusively breastfeeding up to 6 mo	Not reliable Ovulation can resume at any time
Natural family planning	After onset of first menses	None

and other infections. These should be identified and treated as appropriate based on the patient's symptoms.

Mood Disorders

Postpartum depression is a common problem that can negatively affect both the mother and infant. Early diagnosis and treatment are important to prevent any negative effects on the child or mother. It is important to screen for depression several times during the postpartum period. The baby blues is very common in the first week after birth and resolves without treatment. Symptoms in patients at high risk for postpartum depression or those that persist after the first week should be treated.

Treatment of postpartum depression should be individualized. Treatment consists of social support and counseling with or without medications. A Cochrane systematic review in 2001 shows that professional or social support for the mother with postpartum depression results in a reduction in depression at 25 weeks after birth. Antidepressants may be used in the postpartum period but might need to be adjusted during lactation.

Postpartum psychosis is uncommon but potentially dangerous for the mother and infant. The risk of suicide and homicide is high. Inpatient treatment is recommended for postpartum psychosis.

REFERENCES

Dennis CL, Creedy D: Psychosocial and psychological interventions for preventing postpartum depression. Cochrane Database Syst Rev 2004;(4):CD001134.
French LM, Smaill FM: Antibiotic regimens for endometritis after delivery. Cochrane Database Syst Rev 2004;(4):CD001067.
Grimes DA, Schulz KF, Van Vliet H, et al: Immediate post-partum insertion of intrauterine devices. Cochrane Database Syst Rev 2001;(2):CD003036.
Jansen AJG, van Rhenen DJ, Steegers EAP, Duvekot JJ: Postpartum hemorrhage and transfusion of blood and blood components. Obstet Gynecol Surv 2005;60:663-671.
Magee L, Sadeghi S: Prevention and treatment of postpartum hypertension. Cochrane Database Syst Rev 2005;(1):CD004351.
Olson CM, Strawderman MS, Hinton PS, Pearson TA: Gestational weight gain and postpartum behaviors associated with weight change from early pregnancy to 1 year postpartum. Int J Obes Relat Metab Disord 2003; 27:117-127.
Ray KL, Hodnett ED: Caregiver support for postpartum depression. Cochrane Database Syst Rev 2001;(3):CD000946.
Ro A, Frishman WH: Peripartum cardiomyopathy. Cardiol Rev 2006;14: 35-42.
Russell MA, Phipps MG, Olson CL, et al: Rates of postpartum glucose testing after gestational diabetes mellitus. Obstet Gynecol 2006;108:1456-1462.
Committee on Health Care for Underserved Women; Committee on Obstetric Practice: Breastfeeding: Maternal and infant aspects. Int J Gynaecol Obstet 2001;74:217-232.

Resuscitation of the Newborn

Method of
O. D. Saugstad, MD, PhD

Of the approximately 130 million infants born worldwide every year 4 to 7 million (3%-5% of all births) need some kind of resuscitation at birth. Of these, 4 million suffer from birth asphyxia. One million of these children will die and an equal number develop sequelae. Approximately 1.6 million stillbirths occur annually due to intrauterine asphyxia. In the United States, it has been reported that 5% of all newborn infants require basic life support in the delivery room or nursery, constituting 200,000 newborn infants in the United States alone. In Western Europe, figures are similar.

There is therefore no doubt that a large number of newborn infants require resuscitation at birth both in industrialized and low-income countries. As most deliveries throughout the world still occur at home without authorized health care personnel present, it is also important to develop simple resuscitation routines.

Indications for Resuscitation

The decision to resuscitate or not is based on clinical judgment. By observing breathing movements, tone, color, and (not least) heart rate, indications may be found whether the infant is in need of resuscitation or not. According to the American Heart Association and American Academy of Pediatrics (AHA/AAP), every time a child is delivered, the following four questions should be answered: Is amniotic fluid clear of meconium? Is the baby breathing or crying? Is there a good muscle tone? Was the baby born at term? If the answer is "no"

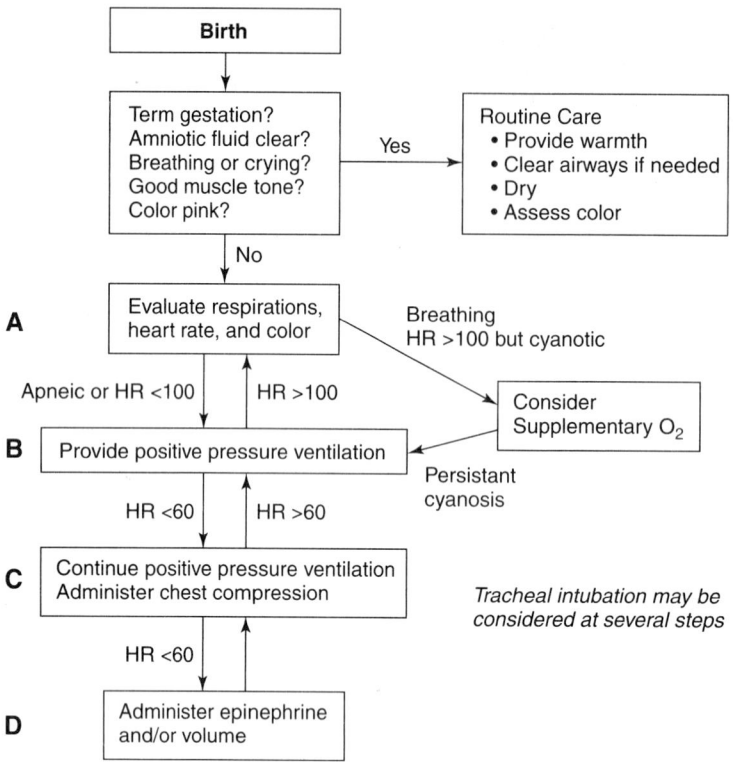

FIGURE 1. The ABCD algorithm for newborn resuscitation. A: Airways. B: Breathing. C: Circulation. D: Drugs. HR = heart rate. (Adapted from The International Liaison Committee on Resuscitation (ILCOR) Consensus on Science With Treatment Recommendations for Pediatric and Neonatal Patients: Neonatal resuscitation. Pediatrics 2006;117:e978-e988.)

to any of these questions, resuscitation should be considered. In the former guidelines, a fifth question was included: Is the color pink? Recent data have, however, indicated that a newborn baby does not necessarily need to be pink the first few minutes of life. In fact, there are indications this may be harmful, and this question therefore was removed from the most recent guidelines (Figure 1).

Guidelines for Resuscitation

There are several sets of international guidelines for newborn resuscitation. The World Health Organization published their guidelines for basic newborn resuscitation in 1998, and it is applicable for most children around the world. The International Liaison Committee on Resuscitation (ILCOR) guidelines from 1999 are widely used internationally; these guidelines were renewed in 2005. AHA/AAP have, in close collaboration with ILCOR, produced their own guidelines. A number of countries also have their own national guidelines, modifying the ILCOR guidelines.

AHA/AAP has published an extensive textbook with CD-ROM demonstrations. These guidelines emphasize a practical approach, and ILCOR has striven to be as evidence based as possible.

Selection of Risk Cases

It is important to anticipate infants at risk. The antepartum and intrapartum histories often help in predicting which infants will need resuscitation. Fetal-movement counting, nonstress testing, fetal biophysical profile, electronic fetal monitoring, and scalp pH measurement all contribute to an identification of infants at risk for low Apgar scores and need for resuscitation. Electronic fetal heart monitoring combined with scalp pH determinations improves the specificity; however, sensitivity is low. In spite of these measures, the need for resuscitation often cannot be foreseen, and 20% to 50% of the infants requiring resuscitation have no identifiable risk factors; therefore, at every delivery, the physician should be prepared for a possible intervention.

Most deliveries are uneventful and the adaptation to extrauterine life occurs smoothly.

Only in some infants should more vigorous resuscitation procedures be carried out. Most of these can be performed with bag and face mask, but in some newborn infants, endotracheal intubation and more sophisticated treatment and observation are needed.

Resuscitation is teamwork, and at least one person trained in resuscitation and one assistant should attend the delivery. Optimally, two trained persons should actually perform the resuscitation and one should assist. Team members should identify themselves, and it should be clear who is the team leader. Each order should be stated clearly and repeated by the recipient.

Initial Stabilization and Evaluation

ABCD for resuscitation is the same whatever size of the patient. Airways should be cleared and the infant positioned correctly. Breathing should be stimulated or performed. Circulation should be assessed by heart rate and skin color. Drugs should be administered if needed, which is rare. Approximately 30 seconds are available to assess whether one should move from one stage to the next.

Resuscitation follows five steps:
1. Assess the baby's response to birth.
2. Keep the baby warm and position the baby correctly and keep airways clear. Stimulate to breathe by drying.
3. Establish effective ventilation by bag and mask or, in some, by endotracheal intubation.
4. Provide chest compression.
5. Administer medications.

Every newborn infant needs to go through the first step, stabilization, and almost everyone the second, drying and warming.

A few—approximately 5%—need the third, bag and mask resuscitation. Of these, very few term or near-term infants need endotracheal intubation. The fourth step, chest compression, is needed in approximately 1% to 3% of those needing bag and mask resuscitation, one or two per 1000 deliveries. The fifth and final stage is giving drugs and volume expansion, which today is easy because basically only one drug, epinephrine (adrenaline), is required in less than 1 per 1000 births. Volume expansion is even more rarely needed, perhaps 1 in 12,000 term or near-term infants. Volume expansion should be performed with normal saline or, in case of acute blood loss, a blood transfusion.

RESPONSE TO BIRTH

As soon as the infant is delivered, a clock is started, and during the transport to the resuscitation table, the personnel should make a preliminary opinion regarding the seriousness of the situation. The respiratory efforts are assessed, the heart rate is recorded, and color is noted. Heart rate should, after the short initial stabilization, be monitored more precisely. Bradycardia combined with no respiratory efforts or gasping are warnings for immediate intervention. Central cyanosis indicates insufficient oxygenation; pallor may be a sign of reduced cardiac output, anemia, hypovolemia, hypothermia, or acidosis. Apgar scoring is not performed before 1 minute of life, and in addition it takes some time. It therefore in itself should never be used as a criterion for resuscitation.

INITIAL STABILIZATION

Most infants require only to be delivered into a warm room where they can be dried immediately. The cord should be cut with sterile equipment and the breathing pattern should be observed. The mother herself is most often the best caregiver and provider of warmth, food, and protection from infections.

Heat loss should be prevented, and this is one important reason why deliveries should be performed in a warm delivery room. The newborn should be quickly dried with towels, giving particular attention to the drying of the head, and swept into preferably prewarmed towels or other linens. It is recommended that the infant be placed supine under a radiant heater on a table designed for resuscitation with the baby's head toward the person performing resuscitation.

Airways

Airways are secured both by suctioning and by positioning the infant correctly in the supine position. Airways are best opened with the head in the sniffing position; overextension should be avoided. Tactile stimulation is performed by gently rubbing the baby's back; do not shake the baby and do not waste time stimulating an apneic child.

There is no justification for the practice of routine suctioning in the mouth and pharynx or gastric suctioning, not even after cesarean section, because such suctioning can be harmful. However, occasionally the mouth, nose, and pharynx should be suctioned to clear airways. Remember that the mouth should be suctioned before the nose to prevent aspiration if the newborn should gasp when his or her nose is suctioned.

Breathing

According to a recent study from the United Kingdom, bag and mask ventilation was performed in 2.6% of all deliveries in 2000. This was a decrease from 3.9% in 1988.

Clinical judgment for when to initiate ventilation should be based on heart rate, breathing efficiency and color, and tone. However, the formal indications are very simple: If the newborn is apneic, or if breathing movements are insufficient, or if the heart rate is less than 100 bpm, or if the newborn is breathing with a heart rate greater than 100 bpm but is persistently cyanotic, ventilation should be started.

Apneic infants with a heart rate faster than 100 bpm probably have primary apnea, and they often require tactile stimulation and a few inflations with a bag and mask only. Apnea and heart rate less than 100 bpm might represent secondary apnea, and ventilation should be initiated. In most of these cases, the heart rate improves and spontaneous ventilation quickly develops. Ventilation, when needed, should start as soon as possible, preferably not later than 30 seconds after birth.

The recommended rate of ventilation according to the AHA/AAP is 40 to 60 breaths per minute. Inflation pressure of 30 cm H_2O or even greater is occasionally needed. The best way to monitor successful ventilation is to follow the heart rate, which should be rapidly increasing, and improvements in color and muscle movements. Observations of the movements of the chest wall, in present guidelines, is classified as a secondary sign of efficient ventilation. The pulse very quickly picks up during a successful resuscitation procedure, for instance increasing 20 bpm or more during the first 30 seconds of ventilation. At least three quarters of asphyxiated infants have spontaneous breathing after these initial steps are established. In aerated lungs, correct bag and mask ventilation provides tidal volumes of 5 to 15 mL.

After adequate ventilation has been established for 15 to 30 seconds, the heart rate should be recorded for 10 seconds. If the heart rate is at least 100 bpm and spontaneous respirations are established, positive pressure ventilation may be discontinued. If the heart rate is greater than 60 bpm and improving, ventilation should continue. If the heart rate is less than 60 bpm and not improving, assisted ventilation is continued and external heart massage is started. A self-inflating bag, a flow-inflating bag, or a T-piece resuscitator may be used.

Endotracheal Intubation

Endotracheal intubation is necessary when bag and mask ventilation is not efficient to normalize the heart rate and establish spontaneous respiration. If chest compression does not quickly improve heart rate or if prolonged assisted ventilation is anticipated, endotracheal intubation should be carried out. A newborn infant without any heart beat or respiratory movement should also be promptly intubated, because bag and mask ventilation probably is not very efficient. Some infants in secondary apnea also need intubation, and the most immature infants, who often do not have enough muscle strength for their respiratory drive to be sufficient, should be intubated. The new guidelines recommend that exhaled CO_2 be monitored for confirmation of tracheal tube placement by, for instance, a colorimetric detector.

Endotracheal intubation is rare in term infants. In a study from the United Kingdom it was carried out in approximately 1 per 1000 deliveries.

Oxygen Supplementation

High concentration of supplemental oxygen (80%-100%) has usually been recommended by most textbooks and guidelines dealing with newborn resuscitation. There was, however, no scientific basis for such recommendations. New studies have shown that even the most depressed newborn infants seem to be adequately resuscitated with room air when assessed by response in the neonatal period. Several meta-analyses, now including seven studies with approximately 2000 enrolled newborn infants in need of resuscitation, have shown that early recovery is faster if resuscitation is carried out with ambient air instead of 100% O_2, because time to first breath was registered 30 seconds earlier; heart rate at 90 seconds and 5-minute Apgar score were higher. More importantly, neonatal mortality is significantly reduced in babies resuscitated with 30% to 40% in room air. A 30-second delay in establishing first breath and therefore adequate heart rate means that more infants, according to present guidelines, will go through more aggressive resuscitation if 100% oxygen is used instead of room air. For this reason, 100% oxygen should be avoided in routine newborn resuscitation.

The new ILCOR guidelines leave it open as to which oxygen concentration one should start out with: "There is insufficient information to recommend for or against the use of any specific inspired oxygen concentration during and immediately after resuscitation." In the next sentence, however, they support the use of 100% O_2 if available. Consequently Australia, Canada, and Sweden, in their recent national guidelines, start out with room air. In the United States there has been more hesitation, and up to now it has been recommended to start out with 100% O_2 and then quickly reduce the Fio_2 according to the response. However, pure oxygen is used more and more rarely in the United States for newborn resuscitation. However, the AHA/AAP guidelines have been modified in this respect, because oxygen is no longer recommended during the initial 30 seconds of stabilization.

If room-air resuscitation is not successful within 90 seconds, we have supplemented with oxygen. In such cases, it probably is optimal to monitor the arterial oxygen saturation by pulse oximetry. The oxygen supply in all delivery units should have a blender, so that the oxygen concentration can be adjusted to the requirement. If supplemental oxygen is justified, it is recommended to start with 30% to 60% oxygen and adjust according to the clinical response and, if possible, oxygen saturation should be measured by pulse oximetry.

Circulation

Chest compression is rarely needed and is not included for basic newborn resuscitation. If bradycardia persists with a heart rate of less than 60 bpm and no signs of improvement after 30 seconds of adequate ventilation, chest compressions should be carried out. This is needed in 0.5 to 1 per 1000 term or near term births and 2-10% in preterm.

Chest compression should always be carried out simultaneously with adequate ventilation. A synchronized chest compression and ventilatory rate of 3:1, giving 90 compressions and 30 breaths per minute, is recommended. An adequately performed resuscitation with chest compressions obviously requires at least two trained persons.

Heart rate should be assessed after 30 seconds of well-coordinated chest compressions and ventilation. When the spontaneous pulse rate has reached 60 bpm, chest compression should be discontinued and positive pressure ventilation should be continued at a rate of 40 to 60 breaths per minute.

Drugs

When oxygenation is established through an adequate ventilation of the asphyxiated infant, it is extremely rare that drugs are needed.

Epinephrine (adrenalin) was, in one study, indicated in 1 in 1200 deliveries. It is indicated in asystole or in sustained bradycardia (<60 bpm) in spite of a minimum of 30 seconds of adequate ventilation and oxygenation and another 30 seconds of coordinated chest compressions and ventilations. Epinephrine (1:10 000 solution) is given as a bolus as rapidly as possible, preferably intravenously (or intratracheally) at a dose of 0.01 to 0.03 mg/kg (0.1-0.3 mL/kg), which may be repeated every 3 to 5 minutes if needed. Bradycardia due to insufficient ventilation technique should be corrected by adequate ventilation before administering epinephrine.

Hypovolemia is rare, and in one study, volume infusion was administered in 1 in 3000 deliveries; however, hypovolemia was found in only 25% of these. Thus, hypovolemia is an extremely rare event occurring in only 1 in 10,000 near-term or term infants.

Hypovolemic shock should be suspected if there is pallor, delayed capillary refill, weak pulses, and persistently low heart rate or if circulatory status does not improve in response to the treatment steps described earlier. Shock may be treated with repeated transfusions of volume expanders, usually 10 mL/kg. As volume expanders, normal saline or Ringer's lactate are recommended. The volume expander may be given over 5 to 10 minutes and repeated. Albumin or other plasma substitutes are no longer recommended. Blood volume expanders during acute resuscitation are only indicated when there are unmistakable signs of shock with evidence of acute blood loss, including fetal–maternal hemorrhage. For blood loss, O-negative blood cross-matched with the mother's blood is given. Avoid giving rapid boluses of volume expanders or hyperosmolar solutions to premature newborn infants.

Sodium bicarbonate, tris(hydroxymethyl)aminomethane (THAM), and naloxone have no routine place in newborn resuscitation.

Meconium Aspiration

If the amniotic fluid is meconium-stained, there is no evidence that suctioning the oropharynx before the thorax is delivered has any beneficial effects. There are today no indications that an infant with thick meconium-stained amniotic fluid benefits from routine intubation and suctioning. It is therefore no longer recommended that suctioning of the nose, mouth, and posterior pharynx be carried out thoroughly before delivery of the shoulder and thorax. However if the child is nonvigorous, the trachea should be suctioned. If the child is vigorous, the mouth and nose are suctioned only and resuscitation proceeds as required.

Vigorous is defined as a newborn having strong respiratory efforts, good muscle tone, and a heart rate faster than 100 bpm.

Preterm Infants

There are no or very few studies on optimal resuscitation of premature infants. This means that even the extremely premature newborn infants are resuscitated according to the guidelines and principles established for term and near-term infants. Recent studies have shown that cardiorespiratory resuscitation of very premature neonates in the delivery room is not futile, and a more active approach seems therefore to be established. It is also clear that preterm infants need intervention more often than near-term or term newborn infants. In one study in the United States, 5% of babies with birth weights between 500 and 1500 g needed chest compression, and 4% received epinephrine.

Those with a gestational age of less than 28 weeks should be put into a plastic bag to keep warm. They often need to be intubated and given surfactant, and in some centers they are immediately extubated, the INSURE approach. Ventilation should be carried out using a positive end expiratory pressure of 5 to 6 cm H_2O. These infants should be handled as gently as possible. Avoid rapid boluses of fluid and quick changes in body positions.

Preliminary data indicate that the extremely-low-birth-weight infant in need of resuscitation should be given a brief exposure of oxygen; for instance, start out with 30% O_2 to get an adequate heart rate response. More data are needed before firmer recommendations for these tiny infants are given.

Withholding and Withdrawing Resuscitation

In some cases, resuscitation should be withheld. Infants with malformations incompatible with life and extremely preterm infants should not be routinely resuscitated. Many centers do not resuscitate newborn infants with a gestational age of less than 23 weeks. According to many guidelines and my opinion, the following conditions represent contraindications to newborn resuscitation: anencephaly, bilateral renal agenesis, spinal muscular atrophy type I (Werdnig–Hoffmann disease) with neonatal onset, trisomy 13, trisomy 18, and other diseases and conditions not compatible with survival beyond the neonatal period or infancy. I resuscitate and try to stabilize all infants with a gestational age of 23 weeks or more.

Often, neither the exact diagnosis nor the gestational age is known at birth. A liberal policy of resuscitation is recommended whenever doubt about the care of the individual infant exists. This allows the doctor to collect more information about the clinical status and prognosis of the child. This also allows one to inform the parents so that they can become prepared and perhaps participate in the discussion and decisions about subsequent therapy. In the new ILCOR guidelines, if the heart rate fails to increase after 10 minutes of resuscitation, the physician may consider stopping the resuscitation.

Postresuscitation Care

After a successful resuscitation, heat loss should be prevented. The child should be labeled and frequently checked with regard to breathing efforts, respiratory rate, color, and heart rate, signs of birth injury, or malformations. If the resuscitation was brief and the situation was not too dramatic, the newborn could be monitored in the nursery provided adequate respiration is established. The child should be placed so that skin-to-skin contact with the mother is obtained. However, this depends on the local conditions and the possibilities for adequate observation by a trained observer.

Even if the infant is not in need of artificial ventilation following resuscitation, the child is often brought to the intensive care unit for further close follow-up, which includes monitoring of the heart rate, ventilation, determination of arterial pH and blood gases, treatment of any hypotension with volume expanders or pressors, appropriate fluid therapy, and treatment of any seizures. Any hypoglycaemia or hypocalcemia should be corrected. Breast-feeding should be encouraged, if possible, as soon as 1 hour after birth. If the resuscitation was unsuccessful and the child died, the parents need a close follow-up.

Hypothermia Therapy

Although the new ILCOR guidelines do not recommend it, many centers have introduced moderate hypothermia as a protective treatment. Hypothermia should be induced in a controlled way. It is, however, extremely important to avoid hyperthermia because it can augment any brain injury in severe asphyxia.

Documentation

It is useful if one attending person observes and immediately writes down the procedures followed. A thorough documentation in the medical record of all observations and actions and names of the participants is required before the resuscitation is complete. Each institution should keep records documenting the condition and procedures carried out at birth.

Every institution that provides deliveries must develop its own standards for newborn resuscitation and a plan of action should exist. The personnel should gain and maintain skills in newborn resuscitation by training using manikins, and an evaluation of the training is necessary.

REFERENCES

Escrig R, Arruza L, Izquierdo I, et al: Achievement of targeted saturation values in extremely low gestational age neonates resuscitated with low or high oxygen concentrations: a prospective, randomized trial. Pediatrics 2008;121:875-881.

Finer NN, Horbar DH, Carpenter JH and the Vermont Oxford Network: Cardiopulmonary resuscitation in the very low birth weight infant: The Vermont Oxford Experience. Pediatrics 1999;104:428-434.

International Liaison Committee on Resuscitation (ILCOR) Consensus on Science With Treatment Recommendations for Pediatric and Neonatal Patients: Neonatal resuscitation. Pediatrics 2006;117:e978-e988.

Kattwinkel J (ed): Textbook of Neonatal Resuscitation 5th ed. Elk Grove Village Ill: American Academy of Pediatrics and American Heart Assocation, 2005.

Little M, Järvelin M-R, Neasham DE, et al: Factors associated with fall in neonatal intubation rates in the United Kingdom — prospective study. Br J Obst Gynaecol 2007;114:156-164.

Rabi Y, Rabi D, Yee W: Room air resuscitation of the depressed newborn: A systematic review and meta-analysis. Resuscitation. 2007;72:353-363.

Saugstad OD: New guidelines for newborn resuscitation. Acta Paediatr 2007;96:333-337.

Saugstad OD, Ramji S, Vento M: Resuscitation of depressed newborn infants with ambient air or pure oxygen: A meta-analysis. Biol Neonate. 2005;87:27-34.

World Health Organization: Basic Newborn Resuscitation: a Practical Guide. Geneva: World Health Organization, 1998.

Wyckoff MH, Perlman JM, Laptook AR: Use of volume expansion during delivery room resuscitation in near-term and term infants. Pediatrics 2005;115:950-955.

Care of the High-Risk Neonate

Method of
Dilcia McLenan, MD

Despite advances in prenatal care and diagnosis, the overall prematurity rate has not changed in the last two decades. The rate remains at 10% to 12% of all births in the United States. Although the overall mortality rate and the short-term morbidity rate have improved with the advances in neonatal care, premature births are still responsible for 75% to 85% of neonatal deaths. Congenital anomalies are associated with 20% to 30% of perinatal deaths. The early identification of the high-risk neonate is essential to improve outcome. The goal is to prevent the development or progression of more serious illnesses and to minimize the risk of both morbidity and mortality.

The definition of the high-risk neonate can be applied in the prenatal, perinatal or postnatal period. Approximately 75% of risk factors affecting the fetus are identified in the prenatal period. Maternal high-risk factors include age, race, socioeconomic status, nutrition and past obstetric history, current pregnancy problems, and maternal drug use. Maternal acute and chronic illness can also adversely affect the fetus. The placenta is considered fetal tissue; all conditions that affect the placenta will also affect the fetus, and vice versa. Fetal factors are limited to genetic conditions (chromosomal and nonchromosomal), and metabolic.

The prenatal diagnosis of the high-risk neonate uses many tools, such as chorionic villus sampling (CVS), amniocentesis, maternal serum screening, and cordocentesis. With the use of cytogenetics, molecular biology, and the fluorescence in situ hybridization, many genetic disorders and infectious conditions can be diagnosed. Fetal ultrasonography is another valuable tool in diagnosing high-risk conditions, including fetal growth abnormalities, which are associated with increased perinatal morbidity and mortality. The Doppler can assess blood velocity in the umbilical and fetal vessels. There is increased morbidity and mortality in fetuses with absent umbilical artery flow or with reverse end diastolic flow. The measurement of the nuchal translucency, done between 10 and 14 weeks of gestation by fetal ultrasound (US) in conjunction with the maternal serum markers, increases the detection rate of Down syndrome and other chromosomal and genetic syndromes, fetal structural malformations, and adverse pregnancy outcome.

Prenatal care facilitates the diagnosis and care of the high-risk neonate through a multidisciplinary approach. This multidisciplinary approach sets the stage for counseling, referrals, and the plan of care pre- and postnatally. When counseling the family, consider the gestational age at diagnosis, effect on maternal outcome and neonatal prognosis with or without therapy, plans for delivery, intrapartum management, and surgical intervention when applicable. General discussion with the parents during the intrapartum period regarding the preterm or high-risk neonate will include such things as anticipated birth weight and gestational age, the need for respiratory support, procedures to be expected, the need for transfusion of blood products, short- and long-term complications of each problem or condition, the need for other specialists, and morbidity and mortality. Involving the neonatologist in the counseling can aid families in making difficult decisions. One should also explain the need for transport, if delivered at a nontertiary care center, and the role the parents will have while their infant is in the neonatal intensive care unit (NICU).

The delivery management of the high-risk neonate is influenced by the factors identified in the antepartum and intrapartum period. In the intrapartum period, neonatal resuscitation facilitates the transition from the intrauterine to the extrauterine life. Approximately 5% to 10% of all newborns need help making this transition; 1% of all newborns need a more extensive intervention. The fetus is dependent on its mother and the placenta for the delivery of oxygen and nutrients as well as removal of carbon dioxide. After the umbilical cord is clamped and cut, the newborn needs to expand its lungs, establishing respirations and convert from a fetal (parallel) to an adult (in series) circulation for a successful transition, and avoid the development of asphyxia.

Resuscitation aims at facilitating the transition and reversing the process of asphyxia by clearing the airway, providing adequate oxygenation and ventilation, ensuring adequate cardiac output, and keeping oxygen consumption to the minimum. These objectives can be achieved by adhering to the initial steps and the four principles of neonatal resuscitation.

Principles of Neonatal Resuscitation

The American Heart Association (AHA) and the American Academy of Pediatrics (AAP) Neonatal Resuscitation Program (NRP) have defined the following principles of neonatal resuscitation:

- **Anticipation.** Risk factors in the antepartum and intrapartum history help identify instances that may potentially require intervention (Box 1).
- **Preparation.** In preparing the area, equipment should be assembled and checked, and drugs should be readied.
- **Availability of qualified personnel.** At every delivery there should be at least one person skilled in neonatal resuscitation whose only responsibility is the newborn; skills include the proper use of the bag and mask. In cases of emergency or if further intervention is needed, additional competent personnel should be immediately available.
- **Organized response to the emergencies—evaluation, decision, and action.** The ABCs (airway, breathing, and circulation) of resuscitation is the order in which assessment and needed intervention will be evaluated. The evaluation assesses the breathing, heart rate, and color, then the decision or diagnosis is made followed by the action or treatment.

TABLE 1 At Birth

Initial Step	Objective
Provide warmth.	Prevent heat loss, maintain oxygen consumption at a minimum, and prevent hypoglycemia.
Position, clear the airway (as necessary).	Establish an airway.
Dry stimulate and reposition.	Initiate breathing and open the airway.

BOX 1 Antepartum/Intrapartum Factors Associated with Potential Asphyxia

Antepartum Factors

Age >35 years
Maternal diabetes
Pregnancy-induced hypertension
Chronic hypertension
Anemia or isoimmunization
Previous fetal or neonatal death
Bleeding in 2nd or 3rd trimester
Maternal infection
Hydramnios
Oligohydramnios
Premature rupture of membranes

Post-term gestation
Multiple gestation
Size-dates discrepancy
Drug therapy, e.g.:
  Lithium carbonate
  Magnesium
  Adrenergic blocking drugs
Maternal substance abuse
Fetal malformation
Diminished fetal activity
No prenatal care

Intrapartum Factors

Emergency cesarean section
Breech or other abnormal presentation
Premature labor
Prolonged rupture of membranes >24 h before delivery
Precipitous labor
Prolonged labor (>24 h)
Prolonged second stage of labor (>2 h)

Nonreassuring fetal heart rate pattern
Use of general anesthesia
Uterine tetany
Narcotics administered to mother within 4 h of delivery
Meconium-stained amniotic fluid
Prolapsed cord
Abruptio placentae; Placenta previa

Note: Keep these factors in mind because they will alert you that depression and possibly asphyxia are potential problems.
From Bloom RS, Cropley C: The AHNAAP Neonatal Resuscitation Program Steering Committee. Textbook of Neonatal Resuscitation. Dallas, TX, 1994, Copyright American Heart Association.

The initial steps of resuscitation provide the support needed to make the transition from the intrauterine to the extrauterine life (Table 1).

Shortcutting these steps prolongs the resuscitation process, increases the risk for asphyxia, and increases the likelihood of morbidity and mortality. In cases where further intervention is needed beyond the initial steps of resuscitation, a thorough evaluation should be done to diagnose conditions that might have contributed to the need for further resuscitation, such as congenital abnormalities of the airway, heart, gastrointestinal (GI) tract, genitourinary (GU) system, or secondary cardiopulmonary disorders. Infants with Apgar scores below 7 at 10 minutes should be admitted to the NICU for further observation and management.

Asphyxia

Asphyxia is the result of prolonged decrease of oxygen delivery to the tissues. During the event, there is redistribution of blood flow to the heart, brain, and adrenals. The continuation of the insult results in bradycardia, impaired gas exchange, and reduced tissue perfusion. These series of events can occur prenatally, intrapartum, or postnatally. In severe cases of asphyxia almost every organ of the body is affected:

- Central nervous system (CNS): hypoxic ischemic encephalopathy
- Cardiovascular: myocardial dysfunction
- Renal: renal dysfunction and or acute renal failure
- GI: liver dysfunction and increased risk of necrotizing enterocolitis
- Hematologic: coagulopathy
- Pulmonary: activation of the mechanisms that cause persistent pulmonary hypertension of the newborn, surfactant (Survanta) deficiency, and meconium aspiration syndrome (MAS)
- Metabolic: acidosis, hypoglycemia, and hypocalcemia

After birth the normal newborn goes through a period of transition that lasts for several hours. During this period the cardiovascular, pulmonary, and sympathetic systems regulate themselves to adjust to extrauterine life. During the transition, abnormalities in color, respirations, heart rate, sleep state, motor activity, GI function, and temperature stability can be identified and will require care in the NICU. Clinical manifestations of abnormal transition include persistent tachypnea, nasal flaring, grunting, retractions, persistent cyanosis, apnea and bradycardia, pallor, temperature instability, blood pressure (BP) instability, lethargy, and other neurologic symptoms.

Postnatal Care

The postnatal care of the high-risk neonate is extremely important. There are interventions and supportive care that are common to the

TABLE 2 Thermoregulation: Types, Mechanisms, and Management

Type/Definition	Mechanism	Prevention
Conduction, transfer of heat from the body core to surface, and object in contact with body.	Cold surfaces, cold objects in contact with the body	Use rubber mattresses, warm blankets, and warm mattresses.
Convection, heat transfer from the body surface to the surrounding air.	Cool rapid air flow, cold oxygen flow	Swaddle using a cap, warm oxygen, and placing infant away from draft. Servo control air or skin incubators, warm room temperature.
Evaporation, moisture on the body surface or respiratory tract evaporates. Major source of heat loss after delivery or during bath. Inversely related to gestational age.	Wet skin, increase of activity, tachypnea, under radiant warmer and phototherapy	Dry infant immediately after birth and bath; increase humidity; use warm soaks and solutions; use polyethylene wraps, warm and humidified oxygen.
Radiation, transfer of heat from the body to surrounding cooler surfaces not in contact with the infant.	Dependent on ambient temperature, air speed and other heat loss mechanisms	Double-wall incubators, radiant warmer, and heat shield.

high-risk neonates to ensure the best possible outcome. These include thermoregulation, nutrition, developmental care, and parental involvement. Notwithstanding, individualized care that will address specific needs of each infant should always be kept in mind.

THERMOREGULATION

Thermoregulation is the balance between heat production and heat loss. It is closely linked to morbidity and mortality. In the neonate, heat loss can exceed heat production because of larger surface area to body mass ratio, decreased subcutaneous (SC) tissue or fat, increased permeability to water and small radius of curvature of exchange surfaces.

The newborn generates heat by nonshivering mechanisms—brown fat, increased muscular activity, flexion, and increased metabolic rate with increased oxygen consumption. The newborn loses heat through conduction, convection, evaporation, and radiation (Table 2).

In the neonate there is always a combination of types and mechanism of heat loss. The prevention of cold stress and hypothermia is critical for intact survival of the neonate (Figure 1).

Heat production is a result of metabolic processes that generate energy by oxidative metabolism of glucose (most efficient in the premature infant), fat, and protein. In the newborn, heat or energy production is low relative to heat or energy losses. Brown adipose tissue generates more energy than any other tissue in the body. The brown adipose tissue cells begin to differentiate by 26 to 30 weeks of gestation and continue to develop until 3 to 5 weeks after birth; they constitute 10% of the adipose tissue in term infants.

Thermoregulation is achieved by providing the appropriate thermal environment to prevent heat loss, hypothermia, and cold stress. The neutral thermal environment (NTE) is an idealized range of ambient temperature at which the body temperature is normal, metabolic rate or oxygen consumption is minimal, and thermoregulation is achieved by basal nonevaporative physical processes. It promotes growth and stability and minimizes heat (energy) and water loss. Newborns have a narrow control range that make them vulnerable to alterations in the thermal environment. The NTE is achieved for the:

- Term infant at 32°C (89.6°F) to 33.5°C (92.3°F)
- Preterm infant greater than 1500 g at 34°C (93.2°F) to 35°C (95°F)
- Preterm infant less than 1500 g at 36.7°C (98.1°F) to 37.3°C (99.1°F)

The two common methods of supporting thermoregulation are the radiant warmer and the incubator (Table 3).

NUTRITION

Proper nutrition is essential for adequate growth, development, and healing. Protein and lipid stores are decreased in the neonate, who has a higher baseline energy requirement compared to children and adults. The low-birth-weight (LBW) infant and the premature infant have even higher baseline requirements. The premature infant has minimal stores of fat and carbohydrates and rapidly develops nutritional deficiencies in calcium, phosphorus, iron trace elements, and vitamins. Nutritional requirements of calories and protein increase even further in the critically ill neonate with overwhelming infections, severe lung disease, and major surgical conditions. These conditions obviate the enteral route of delivering adequate nutrition as well as the immature digestive pathways of the GI tract. In these cases parenteral nutrition is the only option. In premature infants nutritional support is aimed at achieving an intrauterine growth pattern of 15 to 30 g per day. To achieve comparable weight at term-corrected age, compared to a term infant, the daily growth rate would have to be higher to achieve catch-up growth. When there is early positive nitrogen balance, weight loss is less, there is a better rate of growth, and healing and recovery are faster.

With parenteral nutrition the fluid requirement starts at 80 mL/kg per day and increases daily up to 150 mL/kg per day. Infants with increased fluid losses, in addition to their maintenance fluid requirement, will require replacement fluid with specific electrolytes to offset their losses. The caloric requirement varies from 80 kcal to 120 kcal/kg per day. Higher caloric needs of 20% to 30% more are required in the extremely premature infants and in the critically ill neonate. To achieve the expected postnatal growth pattern, the total nonprotein calories requirement should be at least 70 to 105 kcal/kg per day; and the protein intake should be 2.7 to 3.5 g/kg per day of protein for positive nitrogen balance, adequate nitrogen accretion, and good neurodevelopmental outcome. Protein is given in the form of an amino acid solution. These amino acids are the building blocks required for growth, preservation of skeletal muscle protein mass, tissue repair, and appropriate inflammatory response. Protein intake starts at the recommended daily intake of 3 to 4 g/kg per day. Critically ill neonates will also require an increase in protein intake by 10% to 20%.

Calories or energy is given through carbohydrates and fat. Glucose is the carbohydrate used in parenteral nutrition and is the preferred substrate for the brain. It provides 3.4 cal/g of glucose. Fat is given as a 20% lipid emulsion solution, and it provides 2 cal/mL. The use of the lipid emulsion will prevent essential fatty acid deficiency, improve protein use and will not increase significantly CO_2 production or metabolic rate compared to glucose. This is an important factor in infants with chronic lung disease and retention of carbon dioxide. The infusion rate of fat begins at 0.5 g/kg per day and is advanced by 0.5 g daily up to 2 to 3 g/kg per day. Close monitoring of triglycerides is required. A level above 250 mg/dL is considered high, so the rate of infusion should then be cut back. Adequate energy intake will promote or facilitate positive nitrogen balance and nitrogen accretion. Other components of parenteral nutrition are calcium, phosphorus, vitamins, and trace minerals. Sodium and potassium are added based on the serum electrolyte results. Carnitine is added when premature infants are on prolonged parenteral nutrition with no enteral feedings.

THERMOREGULATION

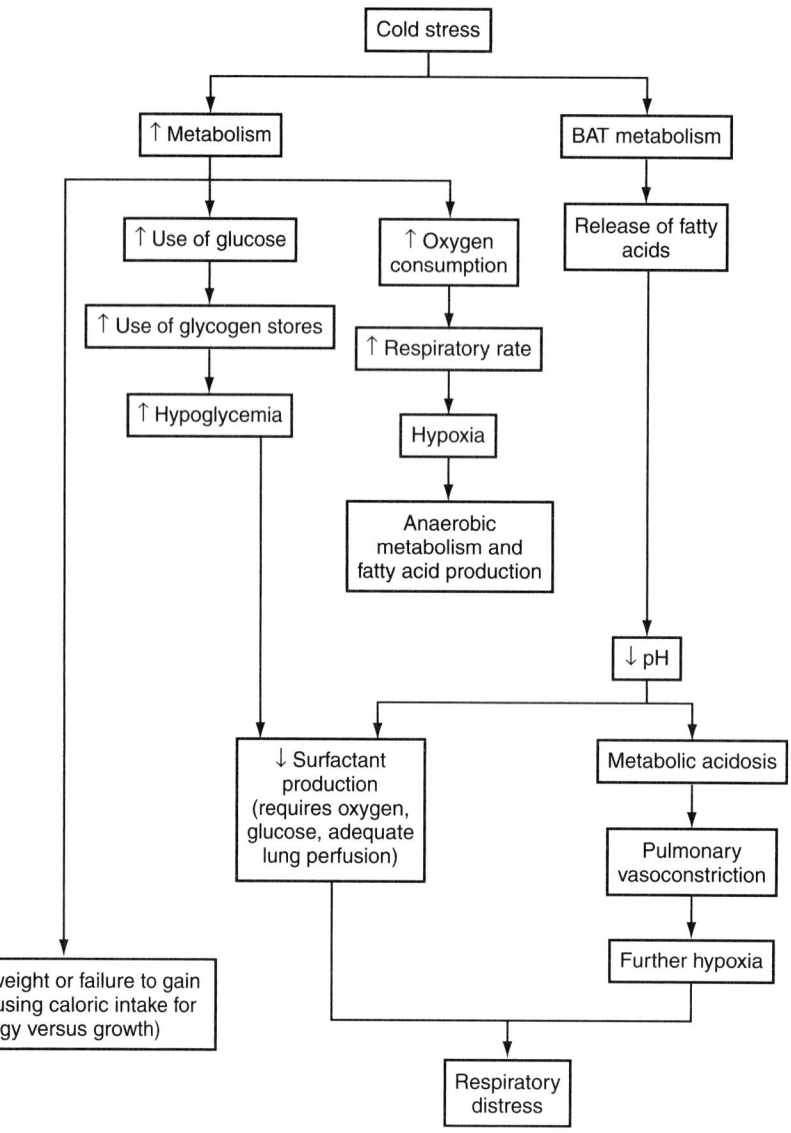

FIGURE 1. Physiologic consequences of cold stress. BAT = Brown adipose tissue.

TABLE 3 Measures to Promote Thermoregulation in Incubators and Radiant Warmers

Bed	Basis	Measures
Incubator	Decrease evaporative water and heat loss	Increase humidity Plastic heat shield Thermal blanket Semiocclusive dressings or emollients
	Reduce radiant and convective losses	Double-walled incubator Heat shield Thermal blanket
Radiant warmer	Promote conductive heat gain	Heated mattress
	Decrease evaporative water and heat loss	Heat shield Plastic wrap Thermal blanket
	Reduce radiant or convective losses	Heat shield Plastic wrap Thermal blanket

Modified from Sinclair, J. (1992). Management of the thermal environment. In J.C. Sinclair and M.B. Brocker (eds). Effective care of the newborn infant. Oxford: Oxford University Press.

The task of providing adequate nutrition is multidisciplinary; the neonatologist, pharmacist, and nutritionist form part of the team. Close metabolic monitoring for glucose, electrolytes, urea, lipids, and acid–base balance is an integral part of the nutritional management of the high-risk neonates. This will help assess and meet nutritional needs as well as monitor for complications such as metabolic acidosis, electrolyte imbalance, cholestatic jaundice, increased triglyceride levels, and infection. When enteral feeding is possible, human milk should be considered. Although it may not provide adequate caloric and protein intake, it has many other assets that are important in promoting healing, neurodevelopment, and protection against infection.

DEVELOPMENTAL CARE

The NICU environment plays a major role in the growth and development of the high-risk neonate and may contribute to the morbidity of these fragile infants. The amount of abnormal sensory stimulus that these fragile beings are exposed to is the source of overwhelming stress at sensitive periods of their development, and in turn will modify their brain development. The cortex of the brain is part of the sensory system, and both deprivation and overstimulation can modify its development. The sensitive period when this occurs is between 28 and 40 weeks of gestation. Therefore the NICU environment is crucial as part of the care of the sick newborn infant. These infants are subject to numerous stress factors, unpleasant procedures, continuously disrupted sleep, frequent noxious oral stimulus, noise, and bright lights. Stress causes autonomic instability, with secretion of cortisol and catecholamines. These hormones in turn interfere with tissue healing and growth.

When considering the NICU environment and the input or stimuli that could be beneficial to these high-risk neonates, one has to take into consideration the in utero environment and how the sensory stimulus would have been perceived in that environment, and the normal development of the sensory system for planned interventions. The hierarchical organization, maturation, and integration of the sensory system is as follows:

- Tactile
- Vestibular
- Gustatory
- Olfactory
- Auditory
- Visual

The visual sensory system is the least mature at term and maturation continues after birth. There is overlapping regarding when a sensory system maturation begins and ends, but there is clear evidence that disruption of one sensory system will affect the maturation of the system that has not yet developed. The same is true when a later sensory system is stimulated earlier than expected.

The interventions that support the development of the sensory system are as follows:

- Minimal handling
- Clustering of care
- Soft swaddling
- Stroking, rocking, and holding when appropriate
- Non-nutritive sucking
- Positioning prone or on the side
- Nesting
- Placing the infant in an infant seat; then swaddle and nest
- Soothing, soft, simple repetitive, and harmonic sounds with limited dynamic range
- Limit ambient light
- Shield eyes and chest from bright lights
- Limit the initial visual stimulus to the human face
- Massage therapy

These suggested interventions should take into consideration the gestational age and the clinical acuity of the high-risk patient. The goal is to improve growth and neurodevelopmental outcome of the high-risk neonate.

PARENTAL INVOLVEMENT

When looking at specific high-risk situations, one can appreciate the scope of support needed by these high-risk neonates from various subspecialists and ancillary health care professionals. One of the things often forgotten is the major role the parents play in the healing and development of their sick infant. Parents have a sense of loss from the time their sick newborn has to be resuscitated and/or is admitted to the NICU. They have a sense of loss for delivering prematurely, for not having a healthy full-term infant, loss of self-esteem, and social status as parents. Involving the parents in the care of their infant will provide some emotional, psychosocial, and spiritual support to the parents. The literature continues to support the need for and the benefits of parental involvement in the NICU as part of the care of the high-risk neonate.

Kangaroo care, or skin-to-skin contact between the parent and the infant, provides sustained multimodal stimulation of tactile, vestibular, proprioceptive, olfactory, and auditory sensory systems. Physiologic benefits such as stable temperature; stable oxygen consumption; higher saturation levels; increased quiet sleep, which lowers cortisol levels resulting in fewer infections; and better growth have been described. It promotes non-nutritive sucking, and there is a better letdown in breast-feeding mothers. Kangaroo care acts as a behavioral organizer or facilitator, decreases motor activity, increases the quiet state in stable preterm infants, and reduces the effect of painful stimuli. These infants are also discharged sooner.

Parents can also participate in massage therapy. It has a calming effect on infants; they express fewer stress behaviors, are more alert, actively respond to face and voice, and show more organized limb movements on the Brazelton behavioral scale. Better weight gain and early discharge have been reported. At 8 months these infants continue to show better weight gain and higher scores on the Bayley Scales of Infant Development.

Conditions Associated With Abnormal Transition

A few conditions associated with abnormal transition are described in the following text.

HYALINE MEMBRANE DISEASE

Hyaline membrane disease (HMD) is the result of surfactant deficiency. Surfactant reduces the surface tension of the alveoli and prevents them from collapsing. This disorder is common to preterm infants. The clinical presentation of HMD is that of respiratory distress characterized by grunting, retractions, and flaring. Grunting is used to maintain the intra-alveoli pressure and prevent it from collapsing. The blood gas typically has hypoxemia and to a lesser degree respiratory acidosis. Radiographically the lungs have a ground glass appearance (this represents microatelectasis) and air bronchograms (the contrast of the air-filled bronchi against the collapse parenchyma). These infants are managed with ventilator support and/or continuous positive airway pressure (CPAP), and surfactant (Survanta) replacement therapy. The use of antenatal steroids has decreased the incidence of HMD and the need for exogenous surfactant in the premature newborn, especially in infants who are 28 weeks' gestation or more.

TRANSIENT TACHYPNEA OF THE NEWBORN

Transient tachypnea of the newborn (TTN) is described as the retention of lung fluid or transient pulmonary edema. In some cases, there may be mild surfactant deficiency. During labor the increased level of prostaglandins causes dilation of the lymphatic vessels in the lungs promoting the absorption of the pulmonary interstitial fluid. After birth, this process is further accelerated by the expansion of the lungs with air-filled alveoli and increased pulmonary circulation. Any delay in this process will result in tachypnea and occasional grunting and flaring. This is common after elective cesarean section. The arterial blood gas shows various degrees of respiratory acidosis and some hypoxemia. The typical chest radiographic findings reveal increased interstitial marking with fluid in the fissure and on occasion pleural effusion. This condition is self-limited, resolving in 1 to 2 days. These infants are managed with oxygen support by hood and rarely require ventilator support.

MECONIUM ASPIRATION SYNDROME

Meconium staining of the amniotic fluid occurs in 10% to 25% of all deliveries. It is seen in fetuses beyond 35 weeks of gestation. Passage of meconium in utero is often the result of a hypoxemic event. Meconium can be aspirated before, during, or after delivery. Once aspirated it can cause obstruction of the airway and pulmonary air leak, chemical pneumonitis and secondary bacterial infection, secondary surfactant deficiency, and pulmonary hypertension of the newborn (PPHN) if hypoxemia persists. After birth, a depressed neonate with poor or no respiratory effort should be intubated and suctioned immediately after being placed under the radiant warmer. This action will clear the airway and prevent aspiration or any further aspiration. The key in preventing meconium aspiration in neonates who did not have in utero aspiration is suctioning of the airway at the perineum by the obstetrician as soon as the head is delivered. The severity of the disease varies. The arterial blood gas pictures vary from mild respiratory acidosis with mild hypoxemia to severe respiratory failure with marked hypoxemia. The classic radiographic finding of the lungs is that of patchy infiltrates throughout the lung fields with areas of hyperlucency; air leak is seen in 10% to 20% of these cases. Postnatal management consists of support to minimize all factors that will perpetuate asphyxia and trigger pulmonary hypertension. Decrease energy loss and oxygen consumption by providing warmth, oxygen, and glucose. Aggressive respiratory support is needed, providing high concentration of oxygen in a hood or through the ventilator. In cases associated with severe PPHN, inhaled nitric oxide (iNO [INO$_{max}$]), and ultimately extracorporeal membrane oxygenation (ECMO) may become part of the management.

PERSISTENT PULMONARY HYPERTENSION OF THE NEWBORN

Persistent pulmonary hypertension of the newborn is the result of severe hypoxemia because of right-to-left shunting through the foramen ovale and ductus arteriosus, without associated structural heart abnormality. The pulmonary hypertension results from increased pulmonary vasoreactivity and increased muscle mass of the pulmonary arterial vessels. The increase in pulmonary smooth arterial muscle mass seen in term infants is triggered by intrauterine stress or hypoxemia. The vasoreactive response seen after birth is caused by alteration of the balance between the circulating pulmonary vasodilator (endothelium-derived relaxing factor or endogenous nitric oxide) and pulmonary vasoconstrictors (endothelin). This vasoreactive response is seen also in preterm and term infants with primary lung disease, such as surfactant deficiency, pneumonia, or MAS. Tachypnea and cyanosis is the clinical presentation. The blood gas has severe hypoxemia and combine metabolic and respiratory acidosis. In primary PPHN, the chest radiograph is normal; in secondary PPHN, it will be characteristic of the disease in question. The diagnosis of PPHN is made with the aid of the echocardiogram, which will exclude structural heart disease, measure the pulmonary artery pressure and resistance and visualize the right-to-left shunts, and tricuspid regurgitation that is commonly present.

The management of neonates with PPHN can be challenging. The goal is to correct the hypoxemia and acidosis, both of which cause pulmonary vasoconstriction. The acidosis can be managed with hyperventilation using conventional or high-frequency ventilator (to achieve a Paco$_2$ close to 30 mm Hg) and/or infusion of sodium bicarbonate to maintain the arterial pH around 7.40. The hypoxemia is more difficult to manage because these infants do not always respond to high concentrations of oxygen with high ventilator support. The Pao$_2$ should be maintained above 80 mm Hg. Concurrent metabolic derangement, such as hypoglycemia and hypocalcemia, and polycythemia should be corrected. The systemic arterial BP should be maintained in the high range of normal. The use of vasopressor agents (dopamine [Intropin] or dobutamine [Dobutrex]) is recommended in achieving this goal, as opposed to volume expansion. The increase in the systemic BP may decrease the right-to-left shunt through the ductus arteriosus and improve pulmonary blood flow and in turn improve the hypoxemia.

When the previously described management fails, the use of iNO at a dose of 20 ppm or less will cause selective pulmonary vasodilatation. Because many infants respond to iNO, the need for ECMO has decreased. Extracorporeal membrane oxygenation is available only in a few medical centers for those cases that fail to respond to maximum ventilator support and iNO.

The Infant with Surgical Conditions

Infants before, during, or after surgery require special consideration regarding management and support of the cardiopulmonary system, thermoregulation, fluid and electrolyte management, nutritional support, and infection control.

GASTROSCHISIS

The combined incidence of omphalocele and gastroschisis is 1:4000 live births. Of these two abdominal wall defects, gastroschisis is the more common. It is a cleft in the abdominal wall to the right of the umbilical cord with herniation of the bowel. The association of other congenital and chromosomal anomalies is rare compared with omphalocele. Common associated problems seen in gastroschisis are malrotation of the bowel, undescended testes, stenosis, and atresia of the bowel, all of which are the result of vascular injury. In 20% of the patients, necrotizing enterocolitis has been reported postoperatively.

Gastroschisis can be diagnosed in the prenatal period. This will allow for proper counseling of the family as well as the plans for intrapartum and postnatal management. The intrapartum and postnatal management consist of preventing further injury to the bowel, temperature stabilization, fluid and electrolyte management, antibiotic therapy, nutritional support, and surgical correction. The exposed bowel is at risk for further circulatory compromise. This may be avoided by having the infant lie on his or her side. Because there is a large surface area exposed to the environment, heat and fluid losses are increased. The bowel should be wrapped in cephalexin (Keflex) soaked in warm normal saline, and then covered with a plastic barrier. The prolonged exposure of the bowel to the amniotic fluid causes a severe inflammatory response that results in ileus. In addition to the increased fluid losses through the exposed bowel, there is intraluminal loss of fluid and electrolyte because of the severe ileus. In these patients 1.5 to 2 times their fluid maintenance is needed for fluid resuscitation. The bowel should be decompressed using a nasogastric or orogastric tube connected to intermittent low suction. Close monitoring of vital signs, intake and output, and serum electrolytes will give indications of the fluid and electrolyte status of these infants.

Nutritional support in infants with gastroschisis is crucial for healing and to decrease morbidity and mortality. Prior to parenteral nutrition, the mortality in these infants was very high, malnutrition and complications associated with infection being major causes. These infants may go for several weeks before enteral feedings can be attempted or tolerated. Early placement of central venous access will facilitate the long-term nutritional support and the overall management. Long-term parenteral nutrition is the key for full recovery of these infants.

The surgical approach considers two options: primary or secondary closure. Secondary closure creates an enclosed hernia, a silo with the bowel content. The bowel is then slowly returned to the abdominal cavity over several days. Antibiotics are continued until the abdominal wall is closed. Primary closure returns the bowel into the abdominal cavity in one step. It is not uncommon, especially with large defects, to have respiratory compromise requiring ventilator support. Be conscious of the need for pain management in these infants, more so in those with respiratory compromise. Other complications seen with primary closure are further bowel compromise with bloody drainage, acidosis, infection, and increased intra-abdominal pressure that causes decrease renal and or central venous perfusion.

CONGENITAL DIAPHRAGMATIC HERNIA

The incidence of congenital diaphragmatic hernia (CDH) is 1:2000 to 5000 live births. This condition can be diagnosed in the prenatal period. When diagnosed in the prenatal period the plan of management begins. The infant should be delivered at a tertiary care center experienced in counseling and treatment of CDH. In these patients, further workup should be done to exclude other malformations of the heart, GI tract, GU system, and CNS and chromosomal anomalies. Associated malformations should be taken into account when counseling the family and when developing the postnatal plan of management. Plans to deliver at term, and at a center where there is a pediatric surgeon, capability for iNO (INO$_{max}$) and ECMO is desired. Once delivered, the infant should be intubated immediately, venous access obtained in case of needed circulatory support, and a nasogastric or orogastric tube placed to decompress the bowel. Bowel distention can further compromise respiration and cardiac function.

The infant should be transferred to the NICU, an arterial line should be placed and blood obtained for blood gas and crossmatch. Obtain a chest and abdominal radiograph to confirm the diagnosis and line placement. An echocardiogram should be done to assess for structural abnormalities of the heart and to estimate the degree of pulmonary hypertension. A head US should be obtained if the infant will be placed on ECMO, because of the risk of intracranial hemorrhage in patients on ECMO.

Skilled ventilator management is important because of the coexisting pulmonary hypertension. Barotrauma and volutrauma should be avoided in these patients. Permissive hypercapnia is permitted once there is adequate preductal oxygenation (preductal oxygenation is measured or obtained from the right upper extremity; the preductal blood perfuses the heart and brain). The highest rates of survival result in patients in whom barotrauma and volutrauma are avoided and permissive hypercapnia is allowed.

A patient is considered unstable or to have failed ventilator support when the pH is <7.25, a peak inspiratory pressure of >30 cm H$_2$O is needed, and preductal saturation is <90% on 60% oxygen. The use of iNO (INO$_{max}$) may be considered in these cases, but the direct effect on pulmonary vascular resistance and right heart function need to be monitored closely. Therapy should be discontinued if no response is demonstrated. Extracorporeal membrane oxygenation is a reasonable choice for patients that have received maximum medical intervention. A venous-venous shunt is preferred unless there is significant cardiac instability.

Surgical correction is done if the infant is stable after the honeymoon period (the first 24 hours). Achievement of 90% survival is possible in a nonselect group of patients with the combination of careful ventilator management, attention to the pulmonary hypertension, delayed surgery, and aggressive early nutrition support. Survival rates are also dependent on the presence or absence of associated abnormalities and their severity. Long-term follow-up beyond the neonatal period is necessary for accurate estimation of morbidity and mortality in patients who are placed on ECMO.

The Extremely Low Birth Weight Infant

A premature infant is a neonate who is delivered before 37 completed weeks of gestation. These infants can be further classified according to their birth weight:

- Low birth weight (LBW) if less than 2500 g
- Very low birth weight (VLBW) if less than 1500 g
- Extremely low birth weight (ELBW) if less than 1000 g

Within the ELBW infants is a subgroup called the micropremie, if birth weight is less than 750 g. The need for intrapartum and postnatal intervention and support is inversely proportional to gestational age as well as the morbidity and mortality associated with these infants. The increased risks for asphyxia, heat and water loss, intraventricular hemorrhage, and respiratory distress increase with decreasing gestational age. In the delivery room, the initial steps of resuscitation will support transition by preventing heat and water loss and asphyxia. The use of surfactant (Survanta) should be considered in ELBW infants. In infants more than 1000 g, surfactant replacement therapy should be done as soon as the neonate presents a clinical picture of surfactant deficiency (HMD). Surfactant should be given with the proper ventilator support and, it is not uncommon to require multiple doses. With delay in therapy the morbidity and mortality associated with HMD increases.

The ELBW infants are a special group within the premature infants because the advances in health care and technology seem to have had less of an impact on this group of infants. The overall morbidity and mortality continue to be comparatively high in these infants and more so in the micropremie or infants less than 27 weeks of gestation. Table 4 lists the common problems faced by the ELBW infants and their management.

TABLE 4 Common Problems and Management of the Extremely Low Birth Weight Infant

Problems	Management
Delivery Room. It is anticipated that a complete team will be needed for resuscitation: neonatal nurse, respiratory therapist, and neonatologist.	Prevent heat loss, provide respiratory support, prevent asphyxia, and avoid trauma. Place under radiant warmer and dry well, use warm blankets and cap. Use bag and mask properly and prompt intubation when needed. Properly position the ETT; avoid high inspiratory pressure with overdistention of the lungs. Follow the ABCs of resuscitation.
NICU. The management in the delivery room and the first hours of life sets the stage for the rest of the NICU care.	In the NICU, the infant is placed under a radiant warmer for easy access and thermoregulation. Connect to all monitors, insert umbilical venous and arterial catheters for fluid management, BP monitoring, and to facilitate blood draw. Obtain chest and abdominal radiograph to assess the severity of lung disease and position of the ETT, venous, and arterial catheters. Cover infant with plastic wrap to decrease evaporative heat and fluid loss. Frequent weighing with a bed scale will estimate hydration status. There should be minimal handling and clustered care in the first week of life.

Continued

TABLE 4 Common Problems and Management of the Extremely Low Birth Weight Infant—cont'd

Problems	Management
Fluid and Electrolytes. The high insensible water loss in the ELBW infant increases the risk for dehydration, hypernatremia, and hyperkalemia	Fluid requirements range from 100 to 150 mL/kg/d, given as D5W with no added electrolytes in the first 24-48 h. Monitoring of the electrolytes and strict I&O will estimate the hydration status. Monitor blood draw and replace with PRBC from a single donor, CMV negative, when 10% of blood volume is removed. Hypernatremia is caused by increased water loss and corrected with increased intake of free water. Risk of hyperkalemia is caused by water loss and increases if there is extravascular blood collection; this is corrected using insulin infusion with glucose, correcting acidosis with sodium bicarbonate, calcium gluconate to stabilize the myocardium, and a cation exchange resin per rectum—sodium polystyrene sulfonate (Kayexalate).
Nutrition. Long-term parenteral nutrition is required in these infants. Good nutritional support is necessary for growth and neurodevelopment.	Beginning early parenteral nutrition within the first 24 h in stable infants will provide a source of energy (glucose), protein to decrease the risk of negative nitrogen balance, calcium, vitamins, and trace minerals. Placement of percutaneous CVC should be done early in the course. Please refer to the section on nutrition in this article for further nutrition management.
CNS. There is an increased risk of developing IVH in unstable infants in the first few days of life.	To prevent IVH, stressful conditions like cold stress, hypoxemia, acidosis swing in BP, and increased intrathoracic pressure should be avoided. Initial US in the first 3 d if unstable and at the end of the first week if stable. Follow-up will depend on findings. Infants with no IVH should have a repeat at 36 weeks postmenstrual age. The use of sedation in the first week of life has not shown significant changes in the incidence of IVH.
Respiratory. HMD is the most common condition. Avoid complications associated with the disease (air leaks and pulmonary emphysema, pulmonary hemorrhage, ICH, and CLD).	Use of exogenous surfactant when indicated and rapid weaning of PIP and O_2 and close monitoring to avoid complications. Blood gas is obtained 10-15 min after each change. Use high ventilator rate and the lowest PIP to maintain saturation 93%-95%, permissive hypercapnia ($Paco_2$ 50-60), mild acidosis (pH 7.25-7.35), and Po_2 50-70 are the goal. When stable, extubate to NCPAP. Apnea is common in these infants; they are treated with caffeine citrate (Cafcit). An initial bolus of 20 mg/kg is given followed by maintenance of 5 mg/kg every 24 h.
Cardiovascular. PDA occurs in >50% of ELBW infants. Appearing when the lung disease is improving, clinically there is increased need for respiratory support associated with desaturation, active precordium, bounding pulses, and wide pulse pressure. The diagnosis is confirmed by echocardiogram. The ductus arteriosus of the preterm responds less to the vasoconstrictive effect of oxygen.	Medical treatment consists of fluid restriction, maintenance of hematocrit around 40%, and the use of indomethacin (Indocin IV). Complications of indomethacin (Indocin IV) are decreased GFR causing fluid retention, and platelet dysfunction (contraindicated in renal failure, bleeding disorders, and low platelets). The dose is 0.2 mg/kg for four doses and a diuretic such as furosemide (Lasix) at 1 mg/kg/dose to try to prevent oliguria. If there is no response, additional dosing or courses can be given. The definitive treatment would be ligation of the ductus. Some centers use prophylactic indomethacin (Indocin IV).
Skin. Underdevelopment of the stratum corneum cause increase transepidermal water loss → dehydration → electrolyte imbalance and evaporative heat loss. Traumatized skin is the port of entry for many infectious organisms. Acceleration of skin maturation occurs after birth over the next 10-14 d.	Use of plastic shields, increased humidity, and topical skin emollient will decrease heat and water loss and may be protective to the skin.
Glucose. Hyperglycemia is secondary to high glucose-infusion rates. When an infant becomes hyperglycemic on a stable glucose-infusion rate, consider infection and or IVH. Early hypoglycemia is common in this group of infants due to poor glycogen stores and immature hormonal adaptation of the endocrine system.	Glucose level should be >40 mg/dL in the first 48-72 h and > 45 mg/dL after 72 h. When hypoglycemic, a bolus of D10W at 200 mg/kg (2 mL/kg) is given. Glucose level is obtained in 30 min, frequent monitoring is continued every 1-3 h, and further boluses are given as needed. Maintenance fluid provides 4-6 mg/kg/min of glucose infusion. This rate of infusion should be increased by 2 mg/kg/min with every need for D10W bolus. Refer to specific text for detailed management.
Calcium. The stores of calcium are limited and the reserves are rapidly depleted after birth.	Higher intake of calcium with adequate phosphorus intake is required for bone formation and growth.
Jaundice. These infants are at increased risk for brain toxicity from high bilirubin levels. High bilirubin level develops due to hepatic immaturity, shorter RBC life span, extravasation of blood, and increased enterohepatic circulation, coupled with lower serum albumin level.	The level that causes toxicity is lower in these infants. A crude method to determine the need for phototherapy at 50% the weight in kg: A 0.9 Kg infant is placed under phototherapy for a bilirubin level of 4.5 mg/dL. Exchange level is determined by the weight, in this case 9 mg/dL. The risk for toxicity increases in the unstable infant, the reason why lower levels should be used when managing. Fluid intake should be increased 15%-20% in infants under phototherapy.

Abbreviations: ABC = airway, breathing, and circulation; BP = blood pressure; CLD = chronic lung disease; CMV = cytomegalovirus; CVC = central venous catheter; ELBW = extremely low birth weight infant; ETT = endotracheal tube; GFR = glomerular filtration rate; HMD = hyaline membrane disease; I&O = intake and output; ICH = intracranial hemorrhage; IV = intravenous; IVH = intraventricular hemorrhage; NCPAP = nasal continuous positive airway pressure; NICU = neonatal intensive care unit; PDA = patent ductus arteriosus; PIP = peak inspiratory pressure; PRBC = packed red blood cells; RBC = red blood cell; US = ultrasound.

CURRENT DIAGNOSIS

- Review of risk factors: antenatal, perinatal, and postnatal
- Assessment of infants in the delivery room: airway, breathing and circulation—respiration, heart rate, and color
- Continued assessment in the nursery: respirations, heart rate, color, temperature, and CNS
- Common problems: pulmonary, circulatory, gastrointestinal, metabolic, surgical, and temperature instability

Abbreviation: CNS = central nervous system.

Special Therapy

Although there are continued attempts to provide care for the ELBW infant, there are infants outside the scope of *viability*—infants with complex congenital malformations, including those labeled as *incompatible with life*, and those whose condition is irreversible and ultimately will lead to death. For such infants, we see the need for comfort care or palliative care. In these situations both the health care professional and parents find themselves in an awkward position. The family remains hopeful based on the perceived information that the health care professional gives, or the family goes through turmoil when interventions seem endless in a situation that they perceive as hopeless.

The decision for palliative care is made through collaboration between the health care team and the parents. The two factual considerations in making the decision for palliative care are pertinent medical facts (diagnosis, response to treatment given, potential response to other treatments, and prognosis) and the human value (what the parents anticipate, expect, and desire for their infant) and what motivates these values in the parents. The values of the health care team involved in the care of the infant are also considered.

CURRENT THERAPY

- Use functioning equipment and qualified personnel in the delivery room: initial steps and ABCs of neonatal resuscitation.
- Provide neutral thermal environment.
- Respiratory and cardiovascular support: oxygen, mechanical ventilation, vasopressor agent (dopamine).
- Infuse bolus of D10W and glucose at 6-8 mg/kg per minute or higher if needed.
- Use phototherapy for early jaundice and the bruised ELBW infant.
- Transfer to appropriate level of care when indicated.
- Monitor closely fluid and electrolytes and decreased IWL. Provide good nutritional support beginning in the first 24 hours and closely monitor for complications and tolerance.
- Provide family-centered care and appropriate environment to promote growth and development.
- Benefit special cases, especially those deemed futile, with a multidisciplinary approach.

Abbreviations: ABC = airway, breathing, and circulation; ELBW = extremely low birth weight; IWL = insensible water loss.

Palliative care, as defined by the World Health Organization (WHO), is care for patients for whom cure is no longer a reasonable expectation or possibility. It is an active and comprehensive management of the entire patient, and not abandonment of care.

Practical considerations that need to be taken into account, and specific components of the palliative care that are appropriate for each individual high-risk neonate, are considered before a specific plan can be put in place. The application of palliative care in the NICU is not only possible, but necessary.

REFERENCES

Aly H: Respiratory disorders in the newborn: Identification and diagnosis. Pediatr Rev 2004;25:201-208.
Avery GB, Fletcher MA, Macdonald MG (eds): Neonatology: Pathophysiology and Management of the Newborn, 5th ed. Philadelphia: Lippincott Williams & Wilkins, 1999, pp 143-173.
Blackburn ST: Maternal, Fetal, and Neonatal Physiology: A Clinical Perspective, 2nd ed. Philadelphia: WB Saunders, 2003, pp 707-730.
Carter BS: Comfort care principles for the high-risk newborn. NeoReviews 2004;e484-e490.
Chescheir NC, Harsen WF: What's new in perinatology. Pediatr Rev 1999;20:57-63.
Downard CD, Wilson JM: Current therapy of infants with congenital diaphragmatic hernia. Semin Neonatol 2003;8:215-221.
Field TM: Stimulation of preterm infants. Pediatr Rev 2003;24:4-10.
Heird WC: Determination of nutritional requirements in preterm infants, with special reference to "catch-up" growth. Semin Neonatol 2001;6:365-375.
Klaus MH, Fanaroff MB: Care of the High-Risk Neonate, 5th ed. Philadelphia: WB Saunders, 2001, pp 195-215.
Kattwinkel J (ed): Neonatal Resuscitation Textbok, 5th ed. American Heart Association, Elk Grove Village, Ill.
Kleinman RE (ed): Pediatric Nutrition Handbook, 5th ed. Philadelphia: WB Saunders, 1999, pp 83-113.
Welch KK, Malone FD: Advances in prenatal screening: Nuchal translucency ultrasonography in the first trimester. NeoReviews 2002;3:e202-e208.
Welch KK, Malone FD: Advances in prenatal screening: Maternal serum screening for Down syndrome. Neoreviews 2002;3:e209-e213.

Normal Infant Feeding

Method of
Meg Begany, RD, CSP, LDN, and Maria Mascarenhas, MBBS

Adequate and appropriate nutrition is especially critical during infancy. Infancy, defined as birth to 1 year of age, is characterized by the period of most rapid growth and development during the life cycle. In addition, recent research shows that nutrition during infancy can influence risk factors for disease at other stages of the life cycle.

Infant Feeding

For the healthy term infant, the suck-swallow and rooting reflexes are present at birth, and thus liquid feedings can be initiated almost immediately following delivery.

BREAST-FEEDING

The American Academy of Pediatrics (AAP) recommends human milk as the feeding of choice for nearly all infants whenever possible and mutually desirable for the mother and infant. Successful lactation and breast-feeding requires a supportive environment for the mother provided by the medical practitioner, including instruction and counseling. The World Health Organization (WHO) Expert Consultation on the Optimal Duration of Exclusive Breastfeeding, which considered the results of a systematic review of the evidence, concluded that human milk is recommended as the exclusive source of nutrition for the first 6 months and continuing human milk in combination with complementary foods until at least 12 months of age. The nutrient needs of the full-term normal birth weight infant can be met by human milk alone, with few exceptions, for the first 6 months if the mother is well nourished. The benefits of breast-feeding over formula feeding are well established and include enhanced maturity and motility of the gastrointestinal tract; maternal–infant bonding; monetary savings; facilitated fat, protein, and carbohydrate digestion and absorption; passive immunity; improved cognitive development; and decreased incidence of otitis media and respiratory and gastrointestinal disease. Further potential benefits, such as lower risk of overweight in children and adults, as well as decreased risk of cardiovascular disease in adulthood, were demonstrated in recent research.

Breast-feeding should be offered as early as possible after birth and then every 2 to 3 hours until satiety for approximately 10 to 15 minutes per breast during the first few weeks. Less frequent feedings may occur once breast-feeding is established. Intervals of more than 5 hours in between breast-feeding should be avoided during the first few weeks, including at night. Adequacy of breast-feeding is demonstrated when the infant has feedings 8 to 12 times per day, at least 6 to 8 wet diapers per day, regular stooling pattern, and is growing along established growth curves.

The composition of breast milk varies from individual to individual, as well as within the same individual, with composition changes occurring with stage of lactation, time of day, maternal diet, and time elapsed since feeding began. Milk production tends to be higher during the daytime, and fat content is increased toward the end of a feeding. On average, breast milk provides approximately 20 calories per ounce.

Contraindications to breast-feeding include maternal infections by organisms known to be transmitted to the infant via breast milk (e.g., HIV); maternal exposure to drugs, foods, or environmental agents that are excreted in human milk and harmful to the infant; and inborn errors of metabolism that are exacerbated by components present in human milk (e.g., galactosemia).

INFANT FORMULA

When a mother chooses not to breast-feed or human milk is not an option, infant formula is an appropriate substitute. Although the composition of infant formula does not exactly duplicate that of breast milk, the composition of infant formulas continues to evolve in an effort to do so. The addition of docosahexaenoic acid (DHA) and arachidonic acid (ARA) is a recent modification to infant formula. Unlike breast milk, infant formulas prior to 2002 contained only the precursor essential fatty acids, linoleic and α-linolenic acids, from which DHA and ARA had to be synthesized. Multiple studies in both preterm and term infants have demonstrated significantly lower levels of DHA and ARA in the erythrocytes of formula-fed infants compared to their breast-fed counterparts. This suggested that infant formula containing only the precursors, α-linolenic acid and linoleic acid, could be ineffective in allowing adequate synthesis of DHA and ARA. Thus multiple studies have been published comparing visual acuity, developmental outcomes, and growth of infants fed DHA and ARA supplemented and unsupplemented formula or breast milk. Some of these studies, but not all, found short-term improvements in visual and cognitive functions in both preterm and term infants. However, no long-term benefits were demonstrated. Although the single supplementation of DHA alone resulted in ARA deficiency status and poor growth in premature infants, the balanced supplementation of both DHA and ARA consistently do not show any adverse effect on growth.

Both iron-fortified and low-iron formulas are commercially available. The AAP has stated that there is no role for the use of low-iron formulas in infant feeding and recommends that all formulas fed to infants be fortified with iron. Well-controlled studies failed to show a benefit, in terms of feeding tolerance, related to the use of low-iron formula. The amount of iron present in iron-fortified formulas meets the iron requirements through the entire first year.

Infant formula should be prepared and stored with careful attention to the manufacturer's guidelines to prevent the risk of bacterial growth.

VITAMIN AND MINERAL SUPPLEMENTATION

The majority of vitamin and mineral requirements for infants are met in full by breast milk or infant formula. Guidelines for supplementation of vitamin K, vitamin D, iron, and fluoride are established. A single dose of vitamin K is typically given to all infants intramuscularly at birth to prevent hemorrhagic disease of the newborn.

For the breast-fed infant, the AAP recommends a supplement of 200 IU of vitamin D by 2 months of age. A multivitamin or tri-vitamin preparation can be used; solitary vitamin D supplements are not practical because of cost and dosing.

The iron requirements for formula-fed infants are met through iron-fortified formula. Although the iron content of human milk is minimal, its bioavailability is high. However, the iron body stores of the breast-fed infant diminish by 4 to 6 months of age, and thus an additional iron source is recommended at this age. Iron needs of the breast-fed infant can be met with the introduction of complementary foods when foods with good sources of iron are included (e.g., meat, fish, iron-fortified cereal, whole grains, and dark leafy green vegetables).

Fluoride supplementation is recommended at 6 months of age for both breast-fed infants and formula-fed infants who receive exclusively ready-to-feed formulas or whose water supply contains less than 0.3 ppm of fluoride.

INTRODUCTION OF COMPLEMENTARY FOODS

At approximately 6 months of age, human milk or infant formula can no longer supply all of an infant's nutrition requirements, and complementary foods are needed to ensure adequate nutrition and growth. It is the micronutrients, rather than energy and protein, which are likely to become lacking. The ability to digest and absorb carbohydrates, proteins, and fats is mature by 6 months of age. Trypsin and chymotrypsin activities increase during the first 4 months of life. Age should not be the only factor in determining the timing of introduction of complementary feeding, but rather the timing should be determined by individual physical and psychological readiness of the infant, as well as rate of maturation of the nervous system, intestinal tract, and kidneys. Before spoon feedings are introduced, the infant should exhibit trunk stability, head control, and disappearance of the extrusion reflex. At approximately 5 to 6 months, an infant is able to indicate a desire for food by leaning forward and opening his or her mouth to indicate hunger and leaning back and turning away to show disinterest or satiety. Muraro et al. state that introduction of complementary feedings prior to 4 months of age is associated with an increased risk of atopic eczema and cow's milk protein allergy. There are presently no controlled studies showing an allergy preventative effect of restrictive diets after 6 months of age. Studies suggest that introducing complementary foods prior to 6 months does not result in increased caloric intake and has no growth advantage because the infant will displace breast milk to maintain the same level of caloric intake. Although it is possible to meet the nutrition needs of the infant solely from infant formula through the entire first year, delay of introduction of solids can lead to feeding aversions and food refusal. All infants need exposure to a variety of tastes, textures, and foods to develop appropriate feeding practices and a wider acceptance of new

CURRENT THERAPY

Infant Formula Composition and Indications

Formula	Examples	Indications	Characteristics
Milk based	Enfamil LIPIL, Similac Advance, Good Start, Good Start DHA & ARA, Enfamil LactoFree LIPIL, Similac Organic Enfamil LactoFree LIPIL, Similac Sensitive Enfamil AR, Similac Sensitive RS (thickens with gastric pH)	Breast milk substitute for term infants	Ready to feed, powder, or liquid concentrate Variable whey-to-casein ratio 20 kcal/oz May contain DHA/ARA
Soy based	Enfamil ProSobee LIPIL, Similac Isomil Advance Good Start Soy DHA & ARA Similac Isomil DF	Breast milk substitute for infants with lactose intolerance or milk protein allergy*	Lactose free; some sucrose free Ready to feed, powder, or liquid concentrate 20 kcal/oz May contain DHA/ARA May contain fiber
Premature (hospital grade)	Enfamil Premature LIPIL, Similac Special Care Advance, Good Start Premature	Breast milk substitute for low-birth-weight hospitalized preterm infants	Low lactose 60:40 whey-to-casein ratio High calcium and phosphorus Contain MCT 20, 24, or 30 kcal/oz Contain DHA/ARA
Human milk fortifiers	Similac Human Milk Fortifier, Enfamil Human Milk Fortifier	Fortification of human milk for low-birth-weight preterm infants	Increase calorie, protein, and vitamin/mineral content of breast milk Contain MCT
Premature transitional	Similac NeoSure Advance, Enfamil Enfacare LIPIL	Breast milk substitute for preterm infants >2.5 kg or discharge formula for preterm infants (used until 6-12 mo corrected age or until catch-up growth is completed)	22 kcal/oz Ready to feed or powder Contain DHA/ARA Vitamin and mineral content between that of term and premature formulas
Hypoallergenic	Nutramigen LIPIL, Nutramigen AA LIPIL	Milk or soy protein allergy	Hydrolyzed protein or free amino acids Ready to feed, powder, or liquid concentrate Sucrose free, lactose free No MCT May contain DHA/ARA
Protein hydrolysate with MCT	Similac Alimentum, Enfamil Pregestimil	Malabsorption Short bowel syndrome Allergy	Lactose free Hydrolyzed protein Contain MCT May contain DHA/ARA Ready to feed or powder
Amino-acid based	Neocate, EleCare	Malabsorption Short bowel syndrome Allergy	Lactose free Free amino acids May contain MCT May contain DHA/ARA Powder only
Fat modified	Monogen Portagen (no longer recommended for infants) Similac Alimentum, Enfamil Pregestimil	Defects in digestion, absorption, or transport of fat	Contain increased % of kcals as MCT
Carbohydrate modified	RCF 3232 A	Simple sugar intolerance	Requires addition of complex carbohydrate to be complete

CURRENT THERAPY—cont'd

FORMULA	EXAMPLES	INDICATIONS	CHARACTERISTICS
Amino acid modified	Multiple products (e.g., Cyclinex, MSUD Analog, Phenyl-Free)	Inborn errors of metabolism	Low or devoid of specific amino acids that cannot be metabolized
Electrolyte modified	Similac PM 60/40	Renal or other disease state requiring low renal solute load	Decreased potassium content Decreased calcium and phosphorus content May be low iron content

*Children allergic to milk protein may also be allergic to soy protein.
Abbreviations: ARA = arachidonic acid; DHA = docosahexaenoic acid; HMF = human milk fortifier; MCT = medium chain triglycerides; MSUD = maple syrup urine disease.

---

foods. In addition to adequate nutrition, the feeding relationship between the infant and caregiver is vital for normal growth and development.

To observe for symptoms of intolerance, only one new food should be introduced every 3 days. Because of its hypoallergenicity, infant rice cereal is often introduced as the first feeding. However, if spoon feeding is initiated at 6 months of age, gastrointestinal and renal development is mature enough to allow feedings from multiple food groups. Despite enhanced bioavailability, breast milk is relatively low in iron and zinc. Because low liver reserves of zinc at birth may predispose some infants to zinc deficiency, similar to the situation for iron, meat may be the ideal first food to provide these nutrients at the levels needed. Dr. Samuel Fomon states that unless there is a strong family history of allergy, introduction of soft-cooked red meats is desirable by 5 to 6 months of age. Furthermore, the proportion of Dietary Reference Intakes that needs to be supplied by complementary foods is highest for iron, zinc, phosphorus, and magnesium. Regardless of the food choice for the first feeding, the consistency should be thin and liquid/pureed. Thinning foods with breast milk or infant formula can enhance acceptability of the food by the infant. Repeated exposure to a new food may be necessary before it is accepted.

By 9 months of age, finely chopped foods and finger foods can be added to the infant's diet. At 12 months of age, rotary chewing is well controlled, and many infants can progress to table foods. Choking hazards that are round and hard, such as grapes, nuts, popcorn, hot dogs, and hard candy, should be avoided.

For the average healthy infant, meals of complementary foods should be provided two to three times per day from 6 to 8 months of age and three to four times per day from 9 to 12 months of age, with addition of nutritious snacks once or twice per day as desired. Vegetarian diets cannot meet nutrient needs at this age unless fortified products or nutrient supplements are provided. Estimates of the energy gap that must be filled by complementary food in industrialized countries is approximately 130 kcal/day at 6 to 8 months, 310 kcal/day at 9 to 11 months and 580 kcal/day at 12 to 23 months of age.

Juice is not a necessary component of the diet and may displace the intake of nutrient-dense breast milk or formula. In addition, offering juice by bottle can contribute to dental caries. If juice is provided, it should be limited to 4 to 8 ounces per day and should not be given prior to 6 months of age.

Whole cow's milk should not be introduced before 12 months of age because of its low iron content, high renal solute load, potential for causing gastrointestinal bleeding, and increased risk of cow's milk protein allergy. Furthermore, cow's milk is a poor source of vitamin C, vitamin E, and essential fatty acids. Breast-fed infants weaned before 12 months of age should receive an iron-fortified infant formula rather than cow's milk.

Nutritional Requirements

Because of the rapid rate of growth and development during infancy, nutrient needs per unit of body weight are very high in comparison to that of the older child or adult. Energy needs for the healthy term infant are 108 kcal/kg from birth to 6 months of age. From 6 to 12 months of age, caloric needs are 98 kcal/kg. The Recommended Daily Allowance (RDA) for protein is 2.2 g/kg from birth to 6 months of age and 1.6 g/kg from 6 to 12 months of age. Caloric distribution during infancy is recommended to be 40% to 50% fat, 7% to 11% protein, and 40% to 55% carbohydrate. The water-to-energy ratio should be 1.5 mL/kcal. Both human milk and infant formulas are models of this distribution. Hydration requirements are met by breast milk or infant formula without further addition of water to the diet, except potentially during periods of illness with fever, diarrhea, or emesis.

Growth

Weight, length, and head circumference should be monitored serially during infancy and plotted on the gender-specific 2000 CDC (Centers for Disease Control and Prevention) Growth Charts. Breast-fed infants tend to gain less weight and usually are leaner than formula-fed infants in the second half of infancy. This difference does not seem to be the result of nutritional deficits but rather infant self-regulation of energy intake.

Obesity is increasing among children in the United States. High rates of weight gain during the first few months of life are associated with obesity in childhood and early adulthood. Optimal nutrition and growth during infancy should be promoted by encouraging healthy eating patterns in the infant to prepare for a healthy lifestyle later in life. Early identification and intervention may be a key component for establishing appropriate weight gain patterns.

Although no consensus exists on universal criteria to define failure to thrive, careful evaluation should occur when weight is less than the 5th percentile or falls more than two major percentiles from a previously established growth channel. In addition, relationship of weight to height must be considered. Prompt intervention with nutritional rehabilitation is essential to prevent illness, growth stunting, cognitive delay, and social and behavioral problems.

For the treatment of either over- or undernutrition, a multidisciplinary team approach involving the physician, dietitian, psychologist, and social worker, along with community services, can often be beneficial and necessary.

In conclusion, infant feeding during the first year of life is a complex process, and guidelines are based on developmental, nutritional, and social factors. Human milk is superior to infant formula and

CURRENT DIAGNOSIS

Expected Growth Velocity during Infancy

Age	Weight Gain (g/d)	Length (cm/mo)	Head Circumference (cm/wk)
0–3 mo	25–35	2.5–3.5	0.3–0.6
3–6 mo	15–21	1.6–2.5	0.2–0.5
6–12 mo	10–13	1.2–1.7	0.1–0.4

should be the feeding of choice for all infants. Although infant formulas do not exactly duplicate breast milk, the composition of infant formulas continues to evolve in an effort to do so. Complementary foods should be introduced at 6 months of age. Cow's milk should not be introduced until 1 year of age. Careful attention should be paid to growth and nutritional status throughout infancy, with prompt attention to any deviation from expected growth patterns.

REFERENCES

American Academy of Pediatrics, Committee on Nutrition: Iron fortification of infant formulas. Pediatrics 1999;104:119-123.
American Academy of Pediatrics, Section on Breastfeeding: Breastfeeding and the use of human milk. Pediatrics 2005;115:496-506.
Dewey KG: Nutrition, growth and complementary feeding of the breastfed infant. Pediatr Clin North Am 2001;48:87-104.
Foman SJ: Feeding normal infants: Rationale for recommendations. J Am Diet Assoc 2001;101:1002-1005.
http://www.cdc.gov/growthcharts
Kleinman RE (ed): Pediatric Nutrition Handbook, 5th ed. Elk Grove Village, Ill: American Academy of Pediatrics, Committee on Nutrition, 2003.
Michaelsen KF: Cows' milk in complementary feeding. Pediatrics 2000;106:1302-1303.
Muraro A, Dreborg S, Halken S, et al: Dietary prevention of allergic diseases in infants and small children. Part III: Critical review of published peer-reviewed observational and interventional studies and final recommendations. Pediatr Allergy Immunol 2004;15:291-307.
PAHO and WHO: Guiding Principles for Complementary Feeding of the Breastfed Child. Washington, DC: Pan American Health Organization and World Health Organization, 2003.
Samour PQ, King K (eds): Handbook of Pediatric Nutrition, 3rd ed. Sudbury, Mass, Jones and Bartlett, 2005.
Slaughter CW, Bryant AH: Hungry for love: The feeding relationship in the psychological development of young children. Permanente J 2004;8:23-29.
WHO Working Group on the Growth Reference Protocol and the WHO Task Force on Methods for the Natural Regulation of Fertility: Growth of healthy infants and the timing, type, and frequency of complementary foods. Am J Clin Nutr 2002;76:620-627.

Diseases of the Breast

Method of
Paniti Sukumvanich, MD, and Patrick Borgen, MD

Benign Diseases of the Breast

Benign diseases of the breast historically are subdivided into proliferative and nonproliferative lesions (Table 1). In a study by Dupont and Page, patients with breast biopsies yielding nonproliferative lesions had no increased risk of subsequent breast cancer. In contrast,

TABLE 1 Benign Diseases of the Breast

	Increase in Breast Cancer Risk
Nonproliferative Lesions	
Mild hyperplasia without atypia	None
Squamous or apocrine metaplasia	None
Duct ectasia	None
Mastitis	None
Cysts	None
Proliferative Lesions	
Fibroadenoma	None
Moderate or florid hyperplasia	Minimal
Microglandular adenosis	Minimal
Sclerosing adenosis	Minimal
Papilloma	Minimal
Atypical ductal hyperplasia	4- to 5-fold
Atypical lobular hyperplasia	5.8-fold

Copyright © 1985 Massachusetts Medical Society. All rights reserved.

proliferative lesions were associated with a minimal to a fivefold increased risk of breast cancer. In clinical practice, of the proliferative lesions, only atypical epithelial lesions increase breast cancer risk significantly. Appropriate treatment and counseling of patients depends on the risk of breast cancer associated with these benign breast diseases.

Nonproliferative Lesions

Nonproliferative lesions comprise mild hyperplasia without atypia, squamous or apocrine metaplasia, duct ectasia, mastitis, and cysts. In the study of 3303 patients by Dupont and Page, only 2.2% of patients with nonproliferative lesions had breast cancer following a benign breast biopsy with a mean follow-up time of 17 years (Figure 1).

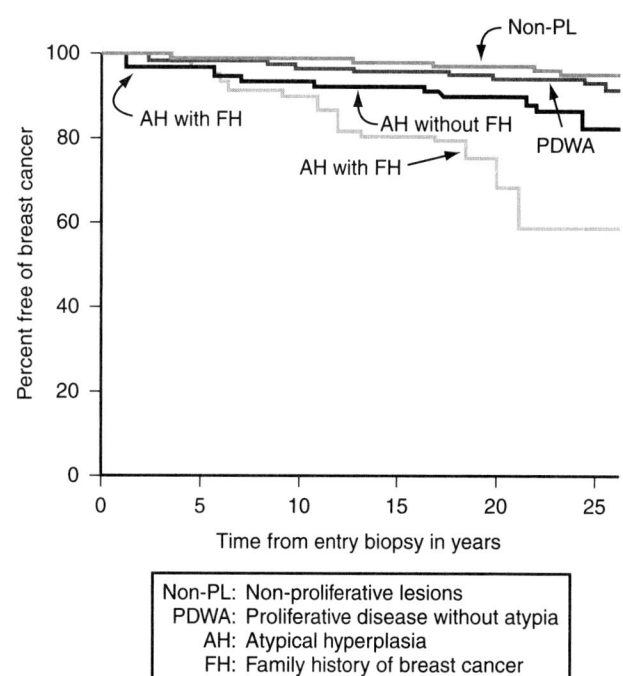

FIGURE 1. Nonproliferative lesions in breast cancer.

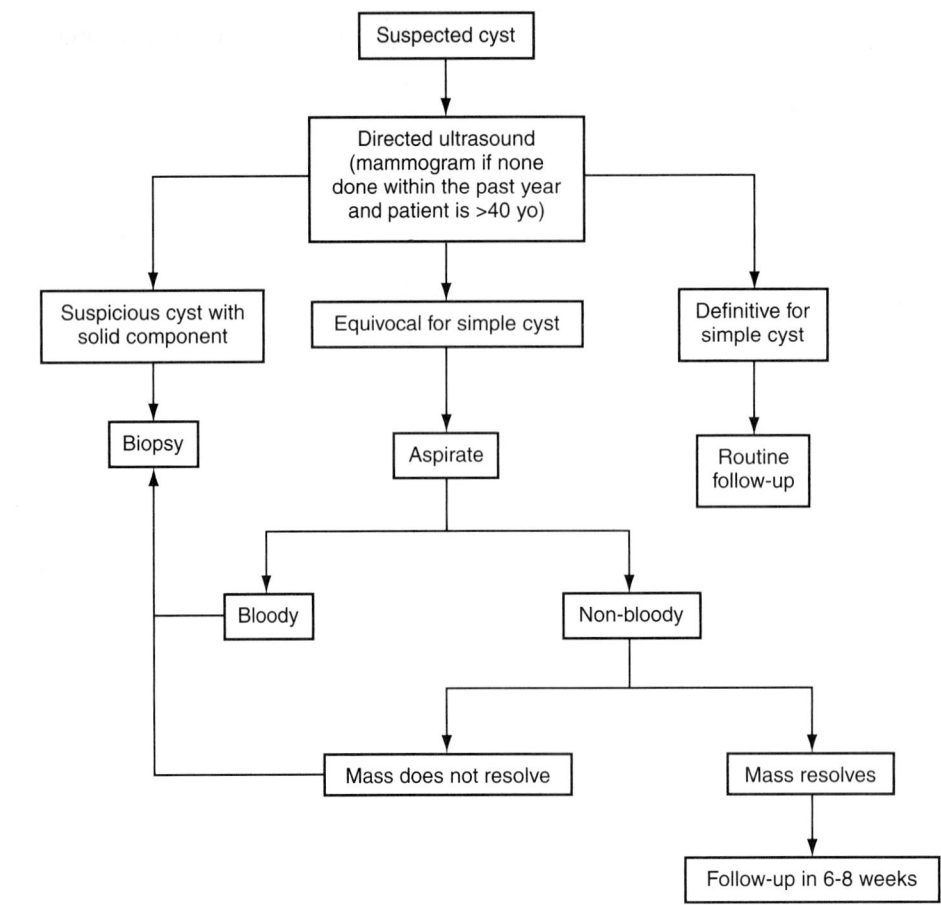

FIGURE 2. Algorithm for the management of suspected cysts.

BREAST CYSTS AND FIBROCYSTIC BREAST DISEASE

Fibrocystic breast disease is a benign process in which generalized microcystic formation with stromal proliferation leads to increased breast nodularity. Cysts within the breast are most common in perimenopausal women 50 to 59 years of age as well as premenopausal women. Postmenopausal women not on hormone replacement therapy are unlikely to develop cysts in their breasts. Benign cysts are often tender and fluctuate in size with the menstrual cycle. Cysts may be detected either on physical examination as a palpable, smooth, mobile nodule or by breast ultrasound. They may appear as a solitary nodule or in a cluster. Ultrasonographic appearance of simple benign cysts is that of an anechoic, round or oval, well-circumscribed mass with posterior enhancement. If the mass has all four criteria, the accuracy of ultrasound is close to 100% for the diagnosis of a simple benign cyst. Cysts that appear complex, with internal echoes, thick septations, and irregular walls, are suspicious for breast carcinoma and should be examined surgically or with an ultrasound-guided biopsy. Confirmation of the diagnosis can be made by fine-needle aspiration (FNA) of the cystic fluid. Bloody fluid may be an indication for a biopsy. In a study of 6782 cyst aspirates, Ciatto and colleagues found that cytologic examination identified atypical cells in 1677 specimens. Of these specimens, only 0.3% of these cases had clinically and radiologically negative intracystic papillomas. Cytologic examination was positive in only 0.1% of these cases. Thus fluid from cyst aspirations are not sent routinely for cytologic examination. Figure 2 describes the management of suspected cysts.

MASTITIS AND DUCT ECTASIA

Mastitis is divided into lactational or nonlactational. Lactational mastitis can occur from the reflux of bacteria into the breast during breast-feeding. The causative bacteria are usually gram-positive cocci. Patients should be treated with antibiotics with the appropriate coverage and can continue to nurse or pump the breast to prevent engorgement. Nursing mothers can continue to breast-feed because the infant is not at risk for infection. Nonlactational (periductal) mastitis can be caused by duct ectasia, which occurs when the milk ducts become congested with secretions and debris, resulting in a periductal inflammation. These patients may present with greenish nipple discharge, nipple retraction, and subareolar noncyclical pain. The treatment of nonlactational mastitis includes broad-spectrum antibiotics to cover for gram-positive cocci and skin anaerobes. Total duct excision and eversion of the nipple may be necessary to treat recurrent periductal mastitis.

Proliferative Benign Breast Diseases

Proliferative breast diseases include moderate or florid hyperplasia, microglandular and sclerosing adenosis, papilloma, fibroadenoma, and atypical ductal and lobular hyperplasia. All proliferative lesions have an increased risk of subsequent breast cancer after biopsy except for fibroadenoma. Overall, with a median follow-up of 17 years, 5.3% of patients with proliferative lesions develop breast cancer. This percentage increases to 12.9% in the presence of atypia (see Figure 1). Patients with moderate or florid hyperplasia, sclerosing adenosis, and solitary papilloma without atypia carry a minimal increase in risk of developing breast cancer over the general population. These patients are not classified as high risk. But the risk of subsequent breast cancer is increased by four- to fivefold in the presence of atypia. Atypical lobular hyperplasia carries a higher risk than atypical ductal hyperplasia, with a relative risk as high as 5.8. This increased risk applies to the contralateral breast because subsequent breast carcinomas are evenly divided between both breasts.

PROLIFERATIVE LESIONS WITH NO INCREASED RISK OF SUBSEQUENT CANCER: FIBROADENOMA

Fibroadenomas are benign tumors commonly found in young women (less than 30 years of age with a peak incidence at 21 to 25 years of age). They are characteristically detected on physical examination as well-circumscribed, rubbery, highly mobile, palpable masses. On mammograms, these lesions may appear as a well-circumscribed mass. Involution of fibroadenomas in the elderly can lead to hyalinization and dense popcorn-like calcification on mammograms. Fibroadenomas pose no increased risk of breast cancer and do not mandate surgical removal unless desired by the patient. Pregnancy can increase the size of these lesions; thus it may be reasonable to remove them prior to a planned pregnancy. Removal may facilitate follow-up, given the inability to follow breast masses adequately during pregnancy. Other types of fibroadenomas include juvenile and giant fibroadenomas. Juvenile fibroadenomas occur in adolescent women and can grow larger than 5 cm in diameter. These lesions are not malignant; given their large size, however, surgical excision may be needed to prevent asymmetry of the breasts. Giant fibroadenomas are large fibroadenomas found in the lactating breast or in the breasts of pregnant patients. These lesions may regress in size once hormonal stimulation subsides. Lesions that remain large can be excised surgically. Fibroadenomas and phyllodes tumors may be linked. Any rapidly enlarging fibroadenoma should be considered for surgical excision to rule out phyllodes tumor because it is difficult clinically to differentiate fibroadenoma from phyllodes tumor.

PROLIFERATIVE LESIONS WITH MINIMAL INCREASED RISK OF SUBSEQUENT BREAST CANCER

Multiple Peripheral Papillomas

Multiple peripheral papillomas are lesions that occur in the peripheral ducts. They most commonly present as a mass but may also present with nipple discharge. Complete excisional removal should be considered to rule out a papillary carcinoma of the breast. Approximately 10% to 33% of patients have subsequent breast cancer; thus close follow-up of these patients is warranted.

Sclerosing and Microglandular Adenosis

Sclerosing adenosis occurs as result of the proliferation of stromal tissue along with small terminal ductules. Often these lesions are picked up incidentally, but they may also present as microcalcifications on mammogram or as a mass (termed *adenosis tumor*). Sclerosing adenosis may be confused with a tubular carcinoma. Staining with immunohistochemical (IHC) markers such as actin, smooth muscle myosin heavy chain p63, or calponin may be helpful in distinguishing between the two lesions because only sclerosing adenosis contains myoepithelial cells. Microglandular adenosis is an uncommon lesion that may be mistaken for tubular carcinoma on histologic examination, and it can increase the patient's subsequent breast cancer risk. Concomitant breast cancer has been reported, so complete surgical excision should be considered for these lesions.

PROLIFERATIVE LESIONS WITH A FOUR- TO FIVEFOLD RISK OF SUBSEQUENT BREAST CANCER: ATYPICAL DUCTAL AND LOBULAR HYPERPLASIA

Atypical ductal and lobular hyperplasia are very similar to their in situ counterparts. These lesions are termed *atypical hyperplasia* because they lack some of the microscopic features of in situ disease. The distinction between atypical hyperplasia and carcinoma in situ is sometimes hard to make. In a study by Rosai, five expert breast cancer pathologists reviewed 17 cases of ductal or lobular lesions.

In no case did all five agree on a diagnosis. Four out of the five were able to agree on a diagnosis in three cases (18%). In one third of the patients, the diagnosis ran the gamut from hyperplasia without atypia to carcinoma in situ. Despite such difficulty, the diagnosis of atypical hyperplasia is on the rise as mammographic screening becomes more popular. Atypical hyperplasia, which is detected secondary to microcalcifications or by serendipity, carries the highest risk of subsequent breast carcinoma among all proliferative lesions of the breast, with a four- to fivefold increased risk over the general population. Atypical lobular hyperplasia carries a higher risk than atypical ductal hyperplasia, with a relative risk as high as 5.8. This risk applies to the contralateral breast as well as the ipsilateral breast. Surgical excision of atypical hyperplasia on a core biopsy is recommended because 20% of patients are found to have breast cancer at time of surgical excision for atypical hyperplasia. It is not necessary to achieve negative margins for these lesions.

OTHER BENIGN BREAST LESIONS: FAT NECROSIS, HAMARTOMA, MONDOR'S DISEASE, RADIAL SCARS, AND PSEUDOANGIOMATOUS STROMAL HYPERPLASIA

Other benign lesions of the breast include fat necrosis, hamartoma, Mondor's disease, radial scars, and pseudoangiomatous stromal hyperplasia (PASH). Trauma to the breast may lead to fat necrosis and can be mistaken for carcinomas on clinical examination. Fat necrosis lesions present clinically as painless, irregular masses with or without associated skin changes such as skin thickening. These lesions can be normal or may have rim calcifications on mammograms. No further treatment is needed when a core biopsy definitively makes the diagnosis of fat necrosis.

Hamartomas are benign lesions that are often picked up on a mammogram. The fatty composition of the mass makes these lesions clinically occult. They can be mistaken for fibroadenomas on mammograms. Hamartomas can be left alone without histologic confirmation if diagnosed definitively on a mammogram.

Mondor's disease is a thrombophlebitis of the superficial breast veins that presents as a palpable tender cord leading to the axilla. In a study of 63 cases, 8 patients (25%) had an underlying malignancy; thus a mammogram should be done to rule out the presence of breast carcinoma.

Radial scars are benign lesions whose etiology is unknown. They are often mistaken for breast carcinoma on mammograms because of their stellate appearance. Radial scars may also mimic breast carcinoma histologically. Staining for myoepithelial cells can help distinguish between invasive carcinoma and a radial scar. Radial scars carry a 1.5-fold increase in risk of subsequent breast carcinoma, so these lesions should be considered markers of future disease.

First described in 1986, PASH is a benign proliferative lesion that may present as an incidental finding or a mobile breast mass. It can occur in all ages and also in men. On a mammogram, PASH appears as a round noncalcified mass. Histologically, PASH may be mistaken for low-grade angiosarcoma. Unlike angiosarcoma, however, there should be no evidence of mitosis or cytologic atypia in PASH specimens. The role of hormones in the pathogenesis of PASH is controversial. Although these lesions tend to occur in young patients or in elderly patients on hormone therapy, most cases tend to be negative for estrogen receptors. The treatment for PASH is complete surgical excision. Approximately 7% of cases recur despite adequate treatment.

Risk Factors for Breast Cancer

An estimated 80% of women in whom breast cancer develops have no documented risk factors or determinants. Risk factors cannot be changed, whereas risk determinants can be altered to decrease a person's risk of subsequent breast cancer. Common risk factors include a familial history of breast cancer, personal breast biopsy history, menarche before 12 years of age, menopause after 55 years of age, increasing age, geographical location, and mutations of the BRCA1 or BRCA2 genes. Women known to have the BRCA1 or BRCA2 genetic mutation have an 85% lifetime risk of breast cancer as well as an increased risk of ovarian cancer. BRCA1 carriers are at a higher risk for developing ovarian cancer than BRCA2 (60% versus 20%, respectively). The risk determinants for breast cancer include reproductive factors such as nulliparity and first pregnancy after the age of 30 years and previous radiation exposure. Previous therapy for lymphoma, especially during adolescence, elevates a woman's risk of subsequent breast cancer.

Screening Techniques

Screening for breast cancer includes mammography, ultrasound, breast self-examination (BSE), and physical examination by a physician. Multiple studies such as the Göthenborg and Malmö trials show a reduction in breast cancer mortality from 30% to 40% in patients 40 to 49 years of age who undergo screening mammograms. A meta-analysis of six randomized trials indicates a 30% reduction in breast cancer mortality in patients 50 to 69 years of age. The sensitivity of mammograms depends on the patient's age and ranges from 53% to 81% in women 40 to 49 years of age to 73% to 81% in patients 50 years of age or older. An estimated 10% to 15% of breast cancer cases are not detectable on screening mammography, thus emphasizing the importance of physical breast examination by a physician and BSE that include both visual inspection and manual examination of the breast. On inspection, signs of breast malignancy include skin or nipple retraction or discoloration, nipple discharge/crusting, or peau d'orange edema of the breast. On palpation, any asymmetric mass of the breast or axilla may be regarded as a potential malignancy that deserves further evaluation.

Current recommendations are for a woman to start performing BSE at 18 years of age, have a yearly physical exam, and initiate annual mammography at 40 years of age. Little data exist on what should be the upper age limit of mammogram screening. Given that breast density decreases with age and breast cancer increases with age, mammograms should be even more sensitive and specific in the older age group. For these reasons, mammograms may be continued in very elderly patients as long as the patient is not suffering from any major co-morbidities. In patients who have a very high risk of breast cancer, such as BRCA carriers, screening should start 10 years earlier than the age of onset of an affected relative or at the age of 35. Kriege screened 1909 patients (including 358 BRCA mutation carriers) who had more than a 15% lifetime risk of developing breast cancer. These patients had a biannual breast exam as well as annual mammogram and breast magnetic resonance imaging (MRI). In this population, mammograms had a sensitivity of 33% with a specificity of 95%. Breast MRI had significantly higher rates of sensitivity and specificity at 80% and 90%, respectively. Given these findings, breast MRI should be a part of the screening exam for these high-risk patients. MRI is recommended as a standard screening test in BRCA heterozygotes. Routine surveillance in high-risk patients includes a 6-month interval alternating between breast MRI and mammograms. Patients with a history of mantle radiation for lymphoma should start annual screening at 25 years of age and biannual screening 10 years after receiving radiation therapy.

Workup of a Breast Mass

DOMINANT PALPABLE MASS

The workup of a dominant palpable breast mass depends on the patient's menopausal status and the degree of suspicion. It is not unreasonable to follow a premenopausal patient with a nonsuspicious mass over one menstrual cycle and then reexamine her. Suspicious lesions present as a hard, nontender, irregular mass or as a mass in a high-risk patient. Palpable masses in postmenopausal patients may also warrant a workup. FNA should not be performed prior to diagnostic imaging because it may result in a hematoma that could obscure the image of the mass. Certain benign lesions on core biopsy should be excised, including lobular carcinoma in situ (LCIS), atypical ductal hyperplasia (ADH), radial scars, sclerosing papillary lesions, columnar cell hyperplasia with atypia, and PASH (Figure 3). Twenty percent of surgeries performed for atypical ductal hyperplasia have concurrent carcinoma in the specimen. Patients with a high-risk proliferative lesion should have close follow-up after surgery including physical examinations. Negative findings on a mammogram do not preclude the diagnosis of cancer because 10% of cancers are occult mammographically. This number drops to 3% when a lesion is occult both mammographically and ultrasonographically. An alternative to core biopsies in younger women is the use of the triple test: a physical exam in conjunction with breast imaging (mammogram or ultrasound) and FNA. When all three components indicate the mass is benign, the negative predictive value is 100%. In a study by Morris, a triple test score assigns points to each component of the test. One point is given for benign findings, 2 points for suspicious findings, and 3 points for malignant findings. When added together, masses with scores of 4 or less are found to be benign. The triple test should only be used in women 40 years of age or younger because the incidence of breast cancer increases dramatically after that cutoff.

MASSES REVEALED ON SCREENING MAMMOGRAMS

The American College of Radiology's classification lexicon, the Breast Imaging Reporting and Data System (BI-RADS), is used in breast imaging (Table 2). BI-RADS 0 means the assessment is incomplete and more workup is needed. BI-RADS 1 indicates a normal mammogram. Mammograms with BI-RADS 2 signify benign findings. Patients with BI-RADS 3 have a 1% to 2% risk of malignancy and should have short-term follow-up with another mammogram in 6 months. BI-RADS 4 indicates the presence of suspicious lesions with a 20% to 40% probability of a malignant lesion. BI-RADS 5 is highly suggestive of cancer with a greater than 95% chance of harboring an underlying malignant lesion. BI-RADS 6, recently added as a category, indicates known malignant disease. BI-RADS 4 and 5 both indicate a biopsy.

A core biopsy via ultrasound guidance may be attempted first. A stereotactic core biopsy should be considered if this is not possible. Stereotactic biopsies may be impossible in patients with lesions that are very superficial or close to the chest wall or in patients with very small breasts that compress to less than 3 cm or who are unable to lie still for the procedure. In such situations, surgical excision with needle localization is warranted. In studies comparing surgical excision to core biopsies, the concordance rate is close to 100%. The surgeon can obviate the need for multiple surgeries in the same patient by performing a core biopsy for diagnosis. High-risk proliferative lesions, such as LCIS, atypical ductal hyperplasia, radial scars, sclerosing papillary lesions, columnar cell hyperplasia with atypia, and PASH, should be considered for an excisional biopsy if the diagnosis is made by a core biopsy.

In Situ Diseases

LOBULAR CARCINOMA IN SITU

Lobular carcinoma in situ (LCIS) should be considered a marker for future breast cancer risk and not an early noninvasive lobular cancer. This disease is most commonly seen in premenopausal women, with a peak incidence in women 40 to 50 years of age. Only 10% of LCIS occurs in postmenopausal women. Unlike ductal carcinoma in situ, LCIS is often found incidentally because typically no clinical or radiologic abnormalities are seen at time of diagnosis. In 50% of patients, LCIS is a multifocal finding. In 30% of patients, it can be found in the contralateral breast. Patients with LCIS are at 8 to 10 times the risk of the general population for subsequent breast cancer. Their overall lifetime risk is as high as 30% to 40% for the development of invasive breast cancer. In a meta-analysis, 15% of patients developed breast cancer in the ipsilateral breast, and 9.3% of patients developed cancer

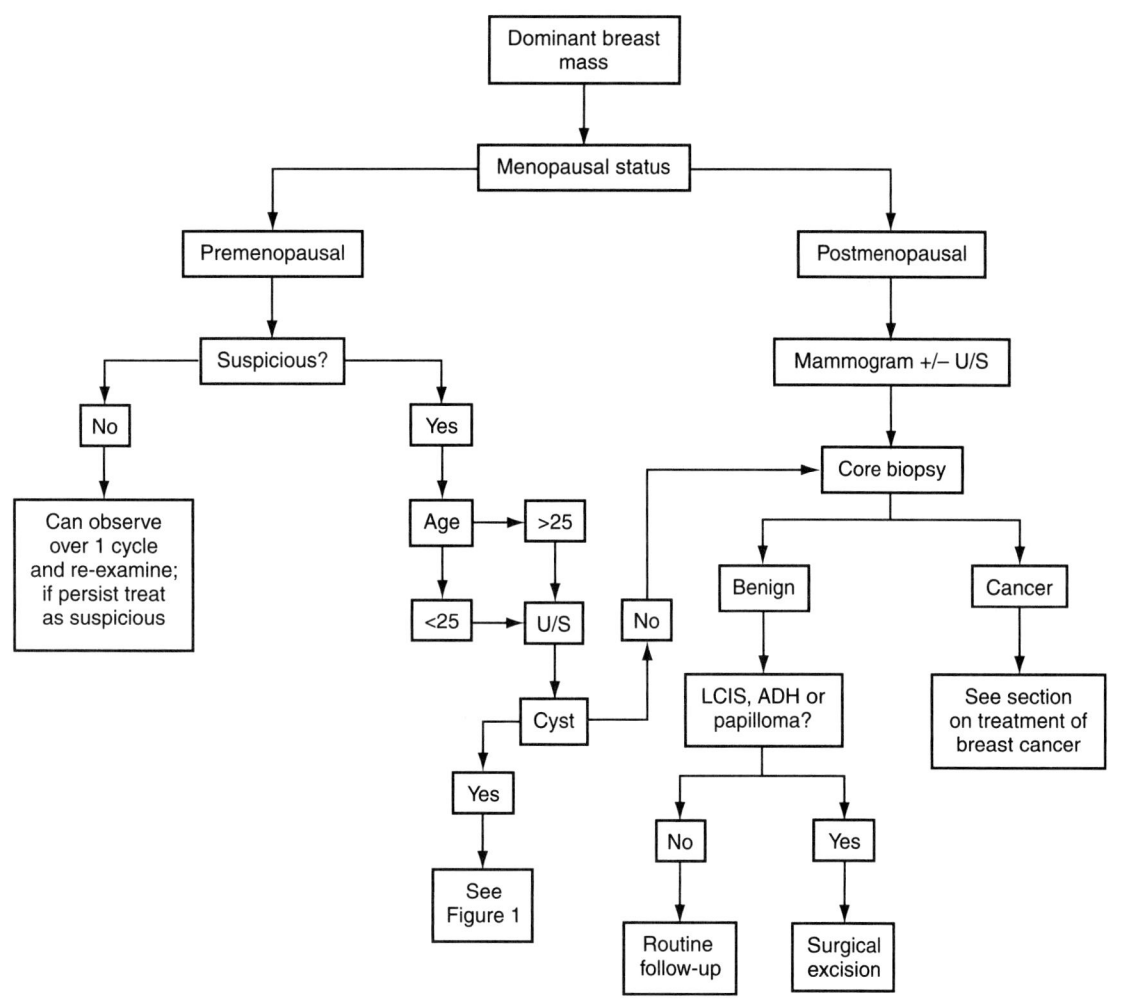

FIGURE 3. Algorithm for workup of a breast mass. ADH = atypical ductal hyperplasia; LCIS = lobular cancer in situ; U/S = ultrasound.

in the contralateral breast. The type of breast cancer can be either ductal or lobular, although the majority is ductal.

DUCTAL CARCINOMA IN SITU

Ductal carcinoma in situ (DCIS), or intraductal carcinoma, is a noninvasive breast cancer and designated stage 0. Historically, DCIS represented only approximately 5% of breast cancer cases, whereas today it constitutes 20% to 30% of all cases. This rise is predominantly attributed to the increasing use of screening mammography because DCIS is most often detected as mammographic microcalcifications. It tends to occur at a later age than LCIS and is not considered a multifocal or bilateral disease. Unlike LCIS, DCIS should be considered a true precursor lesion because if left untreated, approximately 60% to 100% of DCIS cases progress to invasive carcinoma.

TREATMENT FOR IN SITU DISEASE

Lobular Carcinoma in Situ

LCIS should be treated as a marker for increased breast cancer risk. Surgery in an attempt to achieve negative margins is not warranted for LCIS. The NSABP P-1 (the National Surgical Adjuvant Breast and Bowel Project) randomized trial examined the role of tamoxifen (Nolvadex) as a chemopreventive agent in high-risk patients, including those with LCIS. Women taking tamoxifen had a 50% reduction in the subsequent risk of breast cancer without any improvement in overall survival. The main risks of tamoxifen include increased risk of thromboembolic disease and endometrial cancer. The rate of pulmonary embolism was 3 in 1000 patients in the tamoxifen group versus 1 in 1000 in the placebo group. The rate of deep-vein

TABLE 2 BI-RADS Mammography Classification

BI-RADS Category	Definition	Risk of Malignancy	Recommended Follow-Up
0	Incomplete assessment	N/A	Further workup
1	Negative study	N/A	Repeat mammogram in 1 y
2	Benign	N/A	Repeat mammogram in 1 y
3	Probably benign	<2%	Repeat mammogram in 6 mo
4	Suspicious	20%	Biopsy should be considered
5	Highly suggestive of malignancy	90%	Appropriate action should be taken
6	Known biopsy-proven malignancy	N/A	Appropriate action should be taken

Abbreviation: BI-RADS = Breast Imaging Reporting and Data System.

thromboembolism was 5 in 1000 patients in the tamoxifen group versus 3 in 1000 in the placebo group. Endometrial cancer was seen in 9 in 1000 patients in the tamoxifen group versus 3.5 in 1000 in the placebo group. The decision to use tamoxifen as a chemopreventive agent should be made on an individual basis given these side effects. The highest reduction in breast cancer occurred in the LCIS group with a 70% reduction in risk. Despite this, no difference in survival was seen between the tamoxifen and placebo group.

Ductal Carcinoma in Situ

Treatment of DCIS has evolved from simple mastectomy to lumpectomy with radiation therapy. A simple mastectomy is associated with a 1% local recurrence rate. Thus it is still considered a viable option in patients who do not desire or are ineligible for breast conservation therapy (BCT). No difference in survival is seen in patients treated with mastectomy versus BCT. The NSABP B-17 randomized trial examined the role of lumpectomy with and without radiotherapy for the treatment of DCIS. The addition of radiotherapy decreased the recurrence rate from 16.4% to 7% with 8 years of follow-up. More importantly, it decreased the rate of invasive carcinoma from 8% to 2%. The 5-year event-free survival with lumpectomy and radiation is 84%. Limited data support excision alone in small well-differentiated DCIS with surgical margins of at least 1 cm. Silverstein showed in retrospective studies that the recurrence rate in such patients is approximately 4%. Routine axillary lymph node dissection (ALND) is not recommended for DCIS because only 1% of patients have positive axillary nodes. Recent studies, however, show that sentinel lymph node biopsy may have a role in the management of selected patients with DCIS. This is especially true in patients receiving a mastectomy as definitive treatment or if there is a question of microinvasion on the core biopsy. Patients with DCIS and microinvasion can have anywhere from a 3% to 20% incidence of nodal involvement. Indications for a sentinel node biopsy include extensive calcifications, a palpable lesion, patients undergoing mastectomy as treatment for DCIS, and lesions for which the pathology reads "can not rule out microinvasion." Tamoxifen (Nolvadex) can also be considered in cases of DCIS that are estrogen receptor positive. The NSABP B-24 randomized trial examined the utility of tamoxifen in patients treated with lumpectomy and radiotherapy. Ipsilateral tumor recurrences decreased from 13.4% without tamoxifen to 8.2% with tamoxifen. The incidence of invasive cancer was reduced by 47%. No difference in survival was observed between the placebo and the tamoxifen group. Side effects are similar to that of the NSABP P-1 trial.

Invasive Breast Cancer

INCIDENCE

An estimated 1 in 9 women living in the United States if they survive to 90 years of age will develop breast cancer. The average age at diagnosis is 64 years of age and increases along with age.

The American Joint Committee on Cancer TMN (tumor, metastasis, node) system designates breast cancer as stage 0, I, II, III, or IV. This system categorizes breast cancer by its invasive or noninvasive character, tumor size, axillary lymph node status, and the presence of metastatic disease (see Table 2). Overall survival with breast cancer is related to stage (Table 3).

HISTOLOGY

The most common type of infiltrating carcinoma is ductal carcinoma-not otherwise specified (IFDC-NOS), which represents 85% of all invasive breast cancer. Infiltrating lobular carcinoma originates from the lobular structures of the breast and accounts for 15% of all invasive breast cancer. Other less common subtypes represent less than 10% and include tubular, medullary, mucinous, and papillary carcinoma. Additional rare subtypes of breast cancer include inflammatory carcinoma, malignant phyllodes tumor, sarcoma, lymphoma, and Paget disease.

TABLE 3 Overall Survival in Breast Cancer Patients

Stage	10-Year Overall Survival	15-Year Overall Survival
I	74% -95%	64%
II	76%	62%
IIA	81%	72%
IIB	70%	52%
III	50%	40%
IIIA	59%	49%
IIIB	36%	18%
IIIC	36%	18%
IV	18%	18%

Adapted from Rosen PP, et al: J Clin Oncol 1989;355-366; Woodward WA, Strom EA, Tucker SL, et al: Changes in the 2003 American Joint Committee on Cancer staging for breast cancer, dramatically affect stage-specific survival. J Clin Oncol 2003;21:3244-3248.

BREAST CANCER STAGING

In 2003 the American Joint Committee on Cancer (AJCC) revised their staging system on breast cancer. This latest revision stresses the importance of nodal status as a prognostic factor by making several changes in how it is classified within the staging system. Major changes to the staging system include the following:

- Designation is made for isolated tumor cells (ITCs), which are differentiated from micrometastasis and defined as "single tumor cells or small cell clusters not greater than 0.2 mm, usually detected only by IHC (immunohistochemistry) or molecular methods, but which may be verified on H&E (hematoxylin-eosin) stains. ITCs do not usually show evidence of malignant activity, e.g., proliferation or stromal reaction." ITCs are designated as pN0 with modifiers for positive or negative IHC (i−, i+) and molecular findings (mol−, mol+).
- Internal mammary nodes (IMNs) are reclassified based on how they are detected and whether or not there is concomitant axillary lymph node metastasis. Detection of IMNs by sentinel node biopsy alone is classified as pN1b in the absence of positive axillary nodes or pN1c in the presence of positive axillary nodes. Internal mammary nodes detected by imaging studies (excluding lymphoscintigraphy) or by clinical exam are classified as pN2b in the absence of positive axillary nodes or pN3b in the presence of positive axillary nodes.
- Supraclavicular nodal involvement is now reclassified as N3 disease; thus a patient with supraclavicular nodal involvement does not automatically have stage IV disease.
- Infraclavicular nodal involvement is added as N3 disease.
- Axillary lymph node involvement is now classified by the number of nodes involved. Involvement of 1 to 3 axillary nodes is considered pN1 disease. Involvement of 4 to 9 axillary nodes is considered pN2 disease. Involvement of greater than 10 axillary nodes is considered pN3 disease.

Staging of breast cancer can be divided into clinical staging versus pathologic staging. Factors used for clinical staging include the size of the tumor within the breast, presence or absence of pathologically confirmed lymph nodes, and presence or absence of distant metastasis. There are five stages for breast cancer. Stage 0 is defined as the presence of in situ disease only, without evidence of nodal or distant metastasis. Stage I is considered breast cancer confined to the breast, regardless of tumor size. Exception to this general characterization includes tumors with extension to the chest wall or skin or inflammatory breast cancers. These tumors are at least stage IIIB. Stage II is considered a breast cancer of any size with pathologically positive ipsilateral mobile axillary nodes. Stage IIIA is considered a breast cancer of any size with pathologically positive ipsilateral fixed axillary

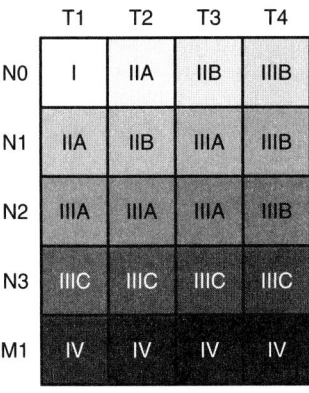

FIGURE 4. Pathologic staging of breast cancer.

nodes or clinically apparent internal mammary nodes in the absence of positive axillary nodes. Also any large tumors (bigger than 5 cm) with any type of positive axillary or internal mammary nodes are considered stage IIIA. Stage IIIB tumors are breast tumors with extension to the skin or chest wall or inflammatory breast cancer. Involvement of the pectoralis major or minor muscle does not constitute chest wall involvement. Stage IIIC tumors are breast cancers of any size with either positive infraclavicular or supraclavicular nodes or positive internal mammary nodes in the presence of positive axillary nodes. Stage IV connotes any breast cancers with distant metastasis (see Figure 3).

Pathologic staging of breast cancer is more complicated and differs from clinical staging in that the number of nodes involved as well as how nodal metastasis is detected are used in stage designation of nodal status (Figures 4 and 5).

SURGICAL TREATMENT OF THE BREAST

A significant paradigm shift in the treatment of breast cancer has occurred over the past several decades. The Halsted paradigm, popularized at the beginning of the 20th century, hypothesized that breast cancer spreads in a contiguous fashion from the breast to the axillary lymph nodes and then to distant sites elsewhere in the body. The Fisher paradigm, which views breast cancer as systemic from very early in the course of the disease, modified this theory; the axillary lymph nodes act not as a barrier but as indicators of disease aggressiveness. Both paradigms are correct and incorrect. At a certain point in the evolution of a breast cancer, the disease changes from a local disease to a systemic disease. The Halsted paradigm promotes more intensive local treatment to eradicate the cancer, whereas the Fisher paradigm promotes less aggressive local treatment with the addition of systemic treatment in most women, even with relatively early disease. Because of this philosophy change and the detection of earlier disease through diligent screening techniques, surgical treatment of breast cancer is progressing toward less radical surgery and more adjuvant therapy, with equal or better outcomes. Recent mammograms of both breasts should be reviewed for any other suspicious lesions. There may be a slight increase in synchronous breast cancer in patients with invasive lobular cancer, although the rate of contralateral breast cancer is equal to that of invasive ductal carcinoma over the lifetime of the patient. The risk of distant metastasis is 25% to 50% in patients with inflammatory breast cancer.

Breast Conservation Therapy

Most small noninvasive and invasive breast cancers are treated by BCT, which consists of wide local excision with negative surgical margins and irradiation of the breast. The NSABP B-06, Milan I and Milan II, as well as other clinical trials, show no statistically significant difference in patient survival with mastectomy or BCT.

The addition of radiation treatment to wide local excision in patients with noninvasive and invasive carcinoma is currently the standard of treatment. The NSABP B-06 randomized trial evaluated local recurrence of small invasive tumors with and without irradiation after lumpectomy. It found that patients who did not undergo radiation therapy had significantly higher rates of local recurrence. With BCT, incidence of recurrence in the treated breast is 7% at 5 years, 14% at 10 years, and 20% at 20 years. Local recurrence rate is much lower in patients treated with mastectomy, with an overall incidence of 5% to 10%. The majority of recurrences occur in the first 3 years after surgery. Contraindications to BCT include tumor of any size that can not be adequately excised with significant

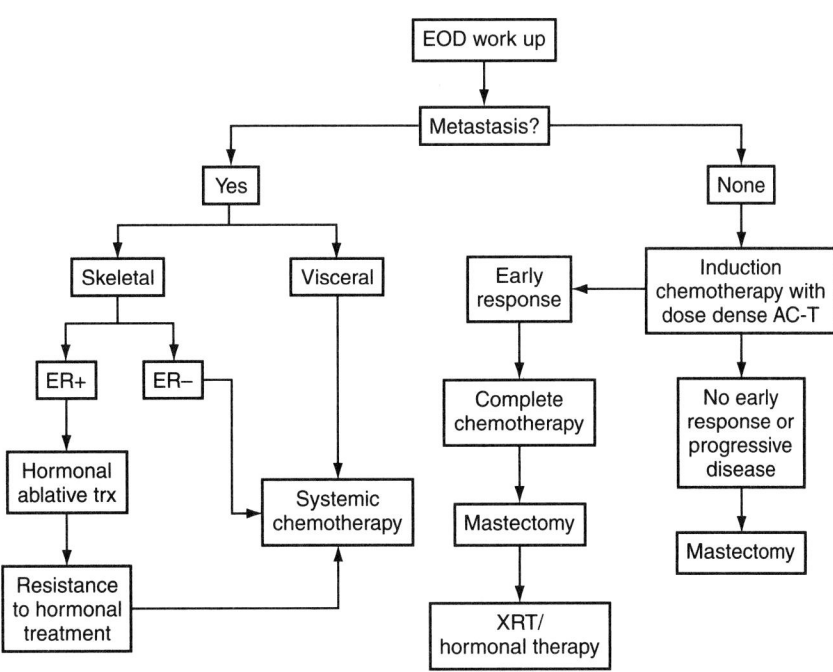

FIGURE 5. Algorithm for treatment of locally advanced breast cancer (LABC). AC-T = Adriamycyin and cyclophosphamide plus Taxol; EOD = extent-of-disease; trx = treatment; XRT = x-radiation therapy.

deformity to the breast, multicentric disease, noncompliant patient, first- or second-trimester pregnant patient, history of significant collagen vascular disease, and history of previous radiation therapy to the chest wall. If both BCT and mastectomy are viable options, the patient's preference should also play a role in the decision to proceed with BCT versus a mastectomy.

MASTECTOMY

A patient with contraindications to breast conservation should have a mastectomy with or without immediate reconstruction. Total mastectomy surgically removes the breast parenchyma, pectoral fascia, nipple, and the areola complex. A modified radical mastectomy includes axillary dissection. A radical mastectomy, rarely done today, includes removal of the pectoralis major and minor muscles and axillary dissection.

BREAST RECONSTRUCTION

Any patient recommended to have a mastectomy should be offered the option of immediate or delayed reconstruction and referred to a plastic and reconstructive surgeon to discuss which techniques are appropriate. One commonly used method of breast reconstruction is a tissue expander breast implant. A tissue expander is placed beneath the pectoralis muscles, and expansions are performed over a period of several weeks to months to stretch the subpectoral pocket to accommodate the permanent implant. The permanent saline or silicone implant is then inserted as a secondary procedure.

Another method of breast reconstruction is the transverse rectus abdominis myocutaneous (TRAM) flap, which involves the transfer of skin, fat, and muscle from the lower part of the abdomen to create a reconstructed breast. This procedure can be performed as a free flap with the arterial and venous supply anastomosed to vessels in the axilla or as a pedicle flap with the arterial and venous supply from the superior epigastric vessels. Other types of flap reconstructions include latissimus dorsi or gluteal flaps. Reconstruction of the nipple and areola is often performed as a later procedure.

SURGICAL TREATMENT OF THE AXILLA

The status of the axilla should be assessed for metastases in any patient with invasive breast cancer for several reasons. The status of the axillary lymph nodes is important in determining the patient's stage of disease. The presence or absence of axillary lymph node metastases is predictive of the prognosis and facilitates decisions by the medical oncology team regarding adjuvant therapy. Relapse-free survival is closely related to the number of lymph nodes that are positive. In a study of 2873 patients, Hilsenbeck found that the relapse-free survival at 5 years was 80% in patients with node-negative disease. This number decreased to 70%, 60%, and 40% with 1 to 3 positive nodes, 4 to 9 positive nodes, and more than 10 positive nodes, respectively. Nodal status is now incorporated into the sixth revision of the AJCC staging system. Surgical removal of metastatic nodes in the axilla significantly decreases the possibility of axillary recurrence. ALND may improve overall survival, but this issue is debated in the medical literature.

Sentinel Lymph Node Biopsy

Axillary dissection traditionally was performed on all patients with invasive breast cancer. Today, sentinel lymphadenectomy, or sentinel lymph node (SLN) biopsy, identifies the first, or sentinel, lymph node or nodes in the axillary chain to receive drainage from the breast cancer and thus the most likely to contain metastases. The SLN biopsy is performed by injecting isosulfan blue dye and/or radioactive isotope to localize the sentinel lymph node.

The sentinel node can be identified in 95% of all cases. Multiple studies show that SLN biopsy can predict accurately the presence of axillary metastases in T1-2 breast cancer with a false-negative rate of 5% and an accuracy rate of 95%. The false-negative rate of SLN biopsy can be decreased to 1% to 3% if any palpable node is removed along with any hot or blue nodes. The SLN biopsy, a less invasive way to assess the status of the axilla, is associated with fewer complications than an axillary node dissection. Areas of controversy in SLN biopsy include T3, palpable suspicious axillary lymph nodes, and previous neoadjuvant therapy. In a study by Specht, 25% of palpable suspicious axillary lymph nodes proved benign on final pathology. Previous axillary dissection is not a strict contraindication per se because 75% of these patients can still have an identifiable sentinel node. The success rate depends on the number of nodes previously removed, with a success rate of 87% when fewer than 10 nodes are removed versus a success rate of 47% when more than 10 nodes are removed. Contraindications to SLN biopsy include T4 breast cancer and pregnancy. SLN biopsy is contraindicated in pregnancy because of the lack of data regarding fetal safety, although computer models suggest the amount of radiation exposure to the fetus is negligible.

Axillary Dissection

Patients who have metastatic cells on SLN biopsy typically undergo complete ALND. Alternatively, if a patient is not a candidate for SLN biopsy, ALND should be considered. Axillary dissection involves the removal of 10 to 30 lymph nodes from the axilla. The potential risk of axillary dissection includes the accumulation of a seroma, ipsilateral arm lymphedema, and numbness around the area of the intercostal brachial innervation if the nerve is sacrificed at the time of surgery. Because of the lifetime increased chance of arm lymphedema and possible infection, patients should avoid any trauma or procedures such as venipuncture or blood pressure measurements on the ipsilateral arm.

Adjuvant Therapy

Adjuvant therapy is used to treat patients with a demonstrable likelihood for the development of metastatic disease. Most medical oncologists consider this risk sufficient in node-negative patients with a tumor diameter of 1 cm or larger and in those with nodal metastases to justify adjuvant chemotherapy or hormonal therapy. Most commonly used cytotoxic regimens include CMF (cyclophosphamide [Cytoxan], methotrexate, and 5-FU [fluorouracil]) for 6 cycles or AC-T for 8 cycles (4 cycles of doxorubicin [Adriamycin] and cyclophosphamide followed by 4 cycles of paclitaxel [Taxol]). There appears to be a slight improvement of 3% in overall survival favoring the anthracycline-containing regimen over the CMF regimens. In the elderly population, the CMF regimen may be easier to tolerate than the AC-T regimens. In a recent study, a dose dense regimen of AC-T results in a slight improvement of disease-free and overall survival. Dose-dense regimen involves giving the chemotherapy in cycles every 2 weeks, with bone marrow support such as G-CSF (Neupogen), as opposed to the traditional cycles every 3 weeks. The improvement in survival is approximately 3%. In the Early Breast Cancer Trialists' Collaborative Group (EBCTCG) meta-analysis, adjuvant chemotherapy appears the most beneficial for women younger than 50 years of age. Combination chemotherapy resulted in the improvement of 10-year-overall survival from 71% in node-negative patients not receiving chemotherapy to 78% in those that did receive chemotherapy. This increase was even more dramatic in node-positive patients, with an improvement of overall survival from 42% to 53%. A much smaller effect was seen in patients older than 50 years of age. In this group of patients, survival was increased from 67% to 69% when node-negative patients not receiving chemotherapy were compared to those receiving chemotherapy. In node-positive elderly patients, improvement in overall survival was also minimal, with an increase of survival from 47% to 49% with chemotherapy.

Hormonal therapy, such as tamoxifen, is a commonly used adjuvant treatment in early breast cancer patients with estrogen receptor–positive tumors. The EBCTCG meta-analysis looking at the role of tamoxifen in the premenopausal patients found that tamoxifen results in an absolute improvement of 10-year overall survival of 5.6% in node-negative patients and 10.9% in node-positive patients. This effect is even greater in the postmenopausal population, with a 26% proportional reduction in 10-year mortality rates. The recommended length of treatment for node-negative patients is 5 years. Additionally, tamoxifen can be used as a chemopreventive agent to decrease the chance of an additional ipsilateral tumor developing in patients undergoing breast conservation or to decrease the possibility of contralateral breast cancer.

More recently, three large randomized trials of aromatase inhibitors, such as anastrozole (Arimidex), exemestane (Aromasin), and letrozole (Femara), was published. In the ATAC (Arimidex, Tamoxifen, Alone or in Combination) trial, patients on anastrozole had a statistically significant longer disease-free interval when compared with patients on tamoxifen alone (hazard ratio of 0.83). No difference in survival was seen between the two groups. In another large study, patients on tamoxifen for 2 to 3 years were randomized to continuing tamoxifen versus switching to exemestane for a total of 5 years of therapy. There appeared to be an improvement in disease-free survival in the aromatase inhibitor arm (hazard ratio of 0.68). No difference in survival was seen, and given the early stoppage and cross-over of patients, no survival data will be obtainable from this study. Yet another large double-blinded randomized trial involved patients who had finished a 5-year course of tamoxifen and were then randomized to receiving letrozole versus placebo. The trial was stopped at a mean follow-up of 2.4 years secondary to a significant improvement in disease-free survival in the letrozole arm (hazard ratio of 0.57). Again, no difference in survival was seen. Aromatase inhibitors are useful only in postmenopausal patients. Premenopausal patients may benefit from an aromatase inhibitor only after ovarian ablation.

Recommendations regarding tamoxifen, aromatase inhibitors, and chemotherapy depend on the clinical judgment of the treating medical oncologist. In general, if adjuvant chemotherapy is given, it should take place prior to the initiation of radiotherapy. Consideration should be given to the likelihood of systemic recurrence based on nodal status, tumor size, and tumor grade. Estrogen receptor positivity of the tumor is predictive of a response to hormonal therapy, and *HER2-neu* may determine the type of appropriate chemotherapy. Another factor is the patient's age and any co-morbid diseases that would decrease the patient's tolerance to a course of chemotherapy.

Surveillance After a Diagnosis of Breast Cancer

Surveillance should continue alter diagnosis and treatment of breast cancer to detect local recurrence or a new primary breast cancer in either the ipsilateral or contralateral breast. The National Comprehensive Cancer Network guidelines recommend that patients continue diligent monthly self-examinations and that a physician perform a physical examination at 6-month intervals to assess for evidence of local recurrence and symptoms of metastatic disease. The ipsilateral arm should be evaluated to detect early signs of lymphedema and initiate appropriate management. Bilateral mammograms should be obtained every year. Bone and computed tomographic scans and other tumor markers should be performed only on patients with symptomatic systemic disease because of the lack of evidence of improved survival with early detection of distant metastases.

Special Topics in Breast Disease

PHYLLODES TUMOR

Phyllodes tumor (cystosarcoma phyllodes) is a fibroepithelial lesion that can be either benign or malignant. It is a rare tumor of the breast accounting for 1% of all cases. The mean age of patients is 54 years of age. These tumors often present as a breast mass on clinical and mammographic examination., and they are considered benign or malignant depending on stromal cellularity, mitotic activity, presence of necrosis, and type of borders. Treatment is complete excision without axillary node dissection. Metastases secondary to malignant phyllodes are hematogenous and primarily travel to the lungs. It is important to obtain negative margins. A mastectomy occasionally may be warranted for large lesions. Patients with malignant phyllodes have an 80% chance of 5-year survival as opposed to more than 95% for benign phyllodes.

NIPPLE DISCHARGE

Nipple discharge can occur at any age and presents as a bloody, serous, or milky discharge. Only 6% to 12% of patients with a nipple discharge are found to have an underlying malignancy. This risk is slightly elevated if the discharge is bloody. The most common cause of serous or serosanguineous nipple discharge is a benign intraductal papilloma. Numerous drugs can also cause nipple discharge, such as phenothiazine, tricyclic antidepressants, reserpine, butyrophenones, cimetidine (Tagamet), verapamil (Calan), metoclopramide (Reglan), thiazides, and hormone replacement therapy. The most common underlying malignancy is DCIS. Ductograms may be useful in locating the papilloma. When the nipple discharge is unilaterally persistent, spontaneous, or postmenopausal, further workup may be considered. Other suspicious nipple discharges are those confined to one duct or that are bloody or serous. In general, the evaluation of nipple discharge should begin with a clinical examination and a mammogram. Cytologic examination of the discharge has a low sensitivity for detection of underlying malignancy and should be not be used in the workup. Treatment consists of a major duct excision.

GYNECOMASTIA

Gynecomastia is the unilateral or bilateral benign enlargement of male breast tissue. The etiology is often related to various substances, including exogenous hormones, cimetidine (Tagamet), thiazides, digoxin, theophylline, phenothiazines, alcohol, and marijuana use; it may also be idiopathic. The main concern is to rule out the diagnosis of male breast cancer. Once breast cancer is excluded, no treatment is indicated. If medication and lifestyle etiologies are eliminated without remission of the gynecomastia, the excess breast tissue may be surgically removed for cosmetic considerations or for breast pain.

MALE BREAST CANCER

Carcinoma of the male breast represents 1% of all breast cancers. Because men are not routinely screened for breast cancer, the diagnosis is often delayed. The most common manifestation of male breast cancer is a painless, firm, subareolar breast mass. The differential diagnosis includes gynecomastia. Breast imaging with mammography and/or ultrasound may be helpful in rendering a diagnosis inasmuch as the appearance of male breast cancer is a stellate, irregular solid mass. Any suspicious breast mass in a male patient should undergo diagnostic biopsy. If a malignancy is diagnosed, standard treatment is mastectomy with assessment of the axillary nodes by SLN biopsy or ALND. Most cases of male breast cancer are estrogen receptor positive, and recommendations for adjuvant chemotherapy or hormonal therapy should be based on criteria similar to those for breast cancer in female patients.

BREAST CANCER IN PREGNANCY

Pregnancy-associated breast cancer represents less than 2% of all breast cancer diagnoses. The breast cancer frequently is diagnosed at a late stage because of the difficulty of examining the breast in pregnant women and the avoidance of mammography during pregnancy. Any suspicious lesion noted during pregnancy should be subjected to biopsy in the same fashion as in a nongravid woman. Radiation therapy should not be administered during pregnancy, so breast conservation is generally contraindicated unless the diagnosis is made within a few weeks of delivery. Surgical treatment with mastectomy and ALND is the standard treatment of breast cancer during pregnancy. Adjuvant chemotherapy can be delivered with selective agents during the second and third trimesters. The prognosis is similar to that of nongravid women in whom breast cancer is diagnosed at a comparable stage.

INFLAMMATORY BREAST CANCER

The classic manifestation of inflammatory breast cancer is erythema, edema, peau d'orange, and color of the breast resembling an infectious process. Malignant cells within the dermal lymphatic vessels of the breast confirm the diagnosis. The usual pathology of the associated carcinoma is IFDC-NOS. Inflammatory carcinoma is a very aggressive type of breast cancer, with over 90% of patients having positive axillary lymph nodes at diagnosis. The recommended treatment is multimodality therapy, with chemotherapy preceding surgery. Surgical treatment is mastectomy followed by radiation therapy and often additional chemotherapy.

LOCALLY ADVANCED BREAST CANCER

Patients with N2 or N3 nodal status or those with four or more positive axillary nodes, T3 or T4 tumors, or involvement of the pectoralis fascia have locally advanced breast cancer (LABC). The recommended treatment for patients is neoadjuvant chemotherapy, which is administered before surgical treatment, although it has no impact on overall survival. An extent-of-disease (EOD) workup should be done in patients with LABC and includes a computed tomography (CT) of the chest, abdomen, and pelvis along with a bone scan. Figure 5 provides an algorithm for the treatment of LABC.

Endometriosis

Method of
David L. Olive, MD

Endometriosis is one of the most common diseases encountered by the practicing gynecologist, yet it is also one of the most vexing. Researchers have been searching for answers to even the most fundamental questions regarding this disease for well over a century; even today huge gaps remain in the understanding of this disorder.

Definition

Endometriosis is defined as the presence of endometrial glands and stroma outside the endometrial cavity and uterine musculature. The requirement for both glands and stroma is an arbitrary standard, and it is unclear whether either component of endometrium alone, if placed ectopically, can result in the symptoms and signs of endometriosis.

Two related diseases are also frequently observed. Adenomyosis is the presence of endometrial glands and stroma within the myometrium. This disorder is epidemiologically and pathogenically distinct from endometriosis, but the resulting symptoms (and medical treatments) are similar. Endosalpingiosis is identical to endometriosis in location and appearance but histologically resembles tubal glands and stroma. This latter abnormality has been poorly studied, and to date, little is known regarding the distinction between endometriosis and endosalpingiosis.

Genetics

Evidence continues to accumulate that endometriosis has a genetic basis. Evidence for this includes familial clustering, concordance in monozygotic twins, and increased prevalence among first-degree relatives. A search was recently undertaken to identify the gene or genes responsible for susceptibility to endometriosis. Although suggestive linkages were discovered, no genes have been firmly identified as instrumental in this disorder. It is hoped, however, that genetic research will eventually uncover information critical to understanding the molecular and cellular basis of this disease.

Pathogenesis

The pathogenesis of endometriosis is a controversial subject inspiring many researchers to investigate it. Over the last 25 years considerable advancement has been made, providing solid clues to the understanding of the disease process. Today, a clear picture is beginning to emerge regarding how women develop endometriosis.

HISTOGENESIS

Leading researchers in the field have proposed numerous theories of histogenesis. The primary theory of histogenesis is transplantation of shed uterine endometrium to ectopic locations. A number of routes of dissemination of the tissue are proposed, including lymphatic dissemination, vascular spread, iatrogenic transplantation, and retrograde menstruation.

A critical aspect of this theory is that cast-off endometrium cells remain viable and capable of implanting. Furthermore, it proposes that the tissue distribution has the capacity to sustain implantation. Considerable research has established that shed endometrial cells are viable in vitro. In vitro studies of endometrial attachment to peritoneum also support the concept of transplantation, attachment, and invasion.

Additional theories of histogenesis include coelomic metaplasia and induction of endometriosis. However, little scientific evidence indicates that either route is a viable etiology of the disease, much less a common method for development.

ETIOLOGY AND MAINTENANCE

Retrograde menstruation is a well-established phenomenon. Data available from women undergoing peritoneal dialysis and laparoscopy at the time of menses suggest that 76% to 90% of women have retrograde flow. This mechanism is considered a critical first step in the initiation of much if not most endometriosis by a wide variety of epidemiologic and anatomic data. However, the majority of women do not have endometriosis. The question that arises is "Why not?"

Because the placement of menstrual debris into the peritoneal cavity happens with each menses, a mechanism must exist to eliminate this tissue. The prime candidate for removal of endometrial cells is cell-mediated cytotoxicity. Deficient cytotoxic response to ectopic endometrium is suggested as a mechanism for allowing implantation and growth. It is also postulated that factors positively affecting growth and maintenance may be altered to enhance the risk of endometriosis. Current evidence suggests that a variety of cytokines, including monocyte chemotactic protein-1, interleukin-8, and regulated on activation, T-cell expressed and secreted (RANTES) are overexpressed in women with endometriosis, resulting in the attraction and activation of macrophages. The source of this cytokine increase could be one or more of several tissues: Endometrium, peritoneal mesothelium, and macrophages themselves could be the primary aberrancy by which this cascade is begun.

Other abnormalities are speculated to promote endometriosis. These include abnormal expression of matrix metalloproteinases and the enzyme aromatase, which could locally produce a hyperestrogenic proimplantation environment. The mechanisms by which these abnormalities may cause disease as well as the source of such alterations are under investigation.

BOX 1 Epidemiology of Endometriosis

Increased risk with:
- Menses >6 d
- More menses

Decreased risk with:
- Increased parity
- Irregular menses
- Oral contraceptives
- Late menarche
- Exercise
- Smoking

Prevalence and Epidemiology

Endometriosis is a disease found almost exclusively in reproductive-age women. The mean age at diagnosis is reported to be from 25 to 29 years, although this figure depends on the diagnostic method. Because traditional diagnosis requires laparoscopy, it is likely that the disease is frequently present in even younger patients for whom many gynecologists do not readily schedule surgery.

Although rare in the premenarcheal female, adolescent endometriosis is a relatively common entity. Endometriosis is found in 47% to 65% of women younger than 20 years with chronic pelvic pain or dyspareunia.

Endometriosis is associated with increased exposure to menstruation typified by earlier menarche, more frequent menses, longer menses, fewer pregnancies, later initial pregnancy, and less breast-feeding. In addition, factors known to decrease the amount of menses or lower estrogen levels also reduce the risk: oral contraceptive use, irregular menses/oligomenorrhea, stress, exercise, and cigarette smoking (Box 1).

Postmenopausal endometriosis seldom occurs; this age group represents only 2% to 4% of all women requiring laparoscopy for endometriosis. The majority of such cases are a sequela to reactivation of disease by hormone replacement therapy; this is not true in all cases.

Clinical Presentation

Endometriosis is associated with a wide array of presenting signs and symptoms, although many women with physical manifestations of the disease remain completely asymptomatic. Commonly, the severity of symptoms does not correlate with the stage of endometriosis; extensive disease sometimes causes only minimal symptoms, and in others, minimal disease can be associated with severe symptoms. Some symptoms may strongly suggest the presence of endometriosis, but none are pathognomonic of this disorder. Because endometriosis most commonly involves the pelvis, infertility, dysmenorrhea, pelvic pain, dyspareunia, and menstrual dysfunction are common clinical presentations. When the ovary is severely involved, an ovarian cyst or pelvic mass may be the initial sign of endometriosis.

Pelvic pain is the most frequent complaint for endometriosis patients. This generally presents as secondary dysmenorrhea, worsening primary dysmenorrhea, dyspareunia, or even noncyclic lower abdominal pain, chronic pelvic pain, and backaches. In addition, pain may be site specific when endometriosis is found in unusual locations outside of the pelvis.

Only rarely are physical findings specific for endometriosis. Localized cul-de-sac and uterosacral ligament tenderness may frequently be detected. Thickened, nodular uterosacral ligaments or rectovaginal masses may be palpable. Adnexal enlargement or tenderness may reflect ovarian involvement. Retroverted fixation of the uterus may be noted with posterior cul-de-sac obliteration by the disease.

Cutaneous manifestations may be present, with apparent lesions on the perineum or vagina, or, less commonly, in the inguinal region, the umbilical area, or at the site of surgical scars. They should be suspected whenever a scar or lesion is associated with cyclical pain, tenderness, swelling, or bleeding.

Diagnosis

The current gold standard for the definitive diagnosis of endometriosis is laparoscopy. However, because of the heterogeneity in appearance of endometriosis lesions, the accuracy of laparoscopic diagnosis is variable and depends on the ability of the surgeon to recognize the disease. Although histologic confirmation would be ideal to ensure the presence of disease, this is infrequently accomplished because of the reticence of surgeons to excise endometriosis lesions.

Ultrasound is most useful for the detection of ovarian endometriomas, although the appearance of a cystic structure with heightened echogenicity is certainly not limited to this form of endometriosis. Structures often confused with endometriomas include corpora lutea, hemorrhagic cysts, unilocular dermoid cysts, and other benign cystic neoplasias. Ultrasound is not currently useful for identifying focal implants.

Magnetic resonance imaging (MRI) demonstrates significant potential in the diagnosis of endometriosis. MRI is clearly of value in diagnosing the ovarian endometrioma, and as technology improves, the potential for detecting peritoneal lesions will increase.

Treatment

MEDICAL THERAPY

The first drug to be approved for the treatment of endometriosis in the United States was danazol (Danocrine), a derivative of testosterone. It was originally thought to produce a pseudomenopause, but subsequent studies have revealed that the drug acts primarily by diminishing the midcycle luteinizing hormone (LH) surge, creating a chronic anovulatory state. The recommended dosage of danazol for the treatment of endometriosis is 600 to 800 mg/day; however, these doses have substantial androgenic side effects such as increased hair growth, mood changes, adverse serum lipid profiles, deepening of the voice (possibly irreversible), and, rarely, liver damage (possibly irreversible and life threatening) and arterial thrombosis. Studies of lower doses as primary treatment for endometriosis-associated pain have been uncontrolled or with small numbers and thus contain information of limited value.

Progestogens are a class of compounds that produce progesterone-like effects on endometrial tissue. A large number of progestogens exist, ranging from those chemically derived from progesterone (progestins), such as medroxyprogesterone acetate (MPA), to 19-nortestosterone derivatives such as norethindrone and norgestrel. The proposed mechanism of action of these compounds causes initial shedding of endometrial tissue followed by eventual atrophy. The most extensively studied progestational agent for the treatment of endometriosis is medroxyprogesterone (dep-subQ Provera 104), which is currently approved by the Food and Drug Administration (FDA) for use in treating endometriosis in

CURRENT DIAGNOSIS

- Symptoms associated with endometriosis are primarily those of pain and infertility, although site-specific symptoms and signs may exist when the disease is in unusual locations.
- The standard for diagnosis is laparoscopic visualization; however, this method has a high false-positive and false-negative rate. The only method to confirm the disease absolutely is excisional biopsy.

CURRENT THERAPY

- Both medical and surgical therapies are efficacious in the treatment of endometriosis-associated pain. It is unclear which offers the better approach.
- Combined medical/surgical therapy may offer an advantage over surgery alone, if the medication is used at least 6 months postoperatively.
- Medical therapy has no role in the treatment of endometriosis-associated infertility.
- Surgical therapy for endometriosis-associated infertility appears to be of value for all stages of disease, but its relative value compared to assisted reproduction is not yet determined.

a depot subcutaneous form. A common side effect is transient breakthrough bleeding, which occurs in 38% to 47% of patients. This is generally well tolerated and, when necessary, can be adequately treated with supplemental estrogen or an increase in the progestogen dose. Other side effects include nausea (0% to 80%), breast tenderness (5%), fluid retention (50%), and depression (6%). A recent approach to treating endometriosis with progestogen is the use of a progestogen-containing intrauterine contraceptive device[1] (Mirena).

The combination of estrogen and progestogen for therapy of endometriosis, the so-called pseudopregnancy regimen, has been used for 40 years. The most commonly used pseudopregnancy regimen today is the oral contraceptive pill[1] (OCP); in fact, it is the most commonly prescribed treatment for endometriosis symptoms. Like progestational therapy, pseudopregnancy is believed to produce initial decidualization and growth of endometrial tissue, followed in several months by atrophy.

Gonadotropin-releasing hormone (GnRH) agonists are analogues of the hormone GnRH. This hypothalamic hormone is responsible for stimulating the pituitary gland to secrete follicle-stimulating hormone (FSH) and LH, two hormones necessary for normal ovarian function. GnRH is secreted in a pulsatile manner; the correct pulse results in stimulation of FSH and LH release, whereas too high or too low a pulse rate results in a decrease in pituitary hormone secretion. GnRH agonists are modified forms of GnRH that bind to the pituitary receptors and remain for a lengthy period. Thus, they are identified by the pituitary as rapidly pulsatile GnRH, and after initial stimulation of FSH and LH secretion, result in a shutdown (down-regulation) of the pituitary and no stimulation of the ovary. The result is a hypoestrogenic state similar to that of menopause, producing endometrial atrophy and amenorrhea. The agonist can be given intranasally (naferelin [Synarel]), subcutaneously (goserelin [Zoladex]), or intramuscularly (IM) (leuprolide acetate [Lupro Depot]), depending on the specific product, with frequency of administration ranging from twice daily to every 3 months. The side effects are those of hypoestrogenism such as transient vaginal bleeding, hot flashes, vaginal dryness, decreased libido, breast tenderness, insomnia, depression, irritability and fatigue, headache, osteoporosis, and decreased skin elasticity; these are dose dependent.

A recent modification of GnRH agonist treatment is to add back small amounts of steroid hormone in a manner similar to that used in the treatment of postmenopausal women. The theory is that the requirement for estrogen is greater for endometriosis than is needed by the brain (to prevent hot flashes), the bone (to prevent osteoporosis), and other tissues deprived of this hormone. With this approach there is an equivalent rate of pain relief with far fewer side effects than GnRH agonist alone. Estrogen as a solitary add-back, however, is less effective and thus not indicated.

---

[1]Not FDA approved for this indication.

SURGICAL THERAPY

Most surgeons performing surgery for endometriosis must choose one of two possibilities: conservative surgery, where the patient's future fertility remains an option, or definitive surgery. The latter procedure generally involves removal of the female gonads, a hysterectomy, or a combination of the two. The general perception is that definitive surgery is more effective over time than conservative treatment, but it must be reserved for patients in whom fertility or continued endocrine function is deemed less important than relief of pain symptoms.

When conservative surgery is desired, the first technical issue confronted is method of access. Traditionally, laparotomy was used for endometriosis surgery. However, recently, most surgeons performing extensive surgery for endometriosis have favored a laparoscopic approach because of improved magnification of disease with a resulting increase in surgical precision.

Surgical destruction of endometriosis lesions can be accomplished in a variety of ways: Excision, vaporization, and fulguration/desiccation have all been used. Excision is generally thought to be the most complete of these techniques, but no comparative trials have assessed the relative efficacy of each approach.

Endometriomas, or ovarian cysts formed from endometriosis, are commonly present in the patient with endometriosis. The ovaries should first be freed of all adhesions when operating on endometriomas. The endometrioma may open spontaneously during this process; if not, incision and drainage is indicated. At this point, the cyst wall may be stripped, excised, or drained.

TREATMENT RESULTS

Medical therapy is effective against endometriosis-associated pain. Placebo-controlled randomized clinical trials (RCTs) have proven that danazol and medroxyprogesterone reduce pain significantly better than no treatment for up to 6 months following discontinuation of the drug. No good data exist for longer follow-up periods. Numerous randomized trials have compared medical therapies to one another. In 15 RCTs comparing danazol to GnRH agonists, no difference was demonstrated between the two as first-line drugs. Similarly, little difference was seen when GnRH agonists were compared to oral contraceptives, progestogens, or gestrinone.

Several trials have addressed the efficacy of combined add-back therapy and GnRH agonist treatment during 6-month treatment periods. In general, pain was relieved as effectively with the combination as with GnRH agonist alone, and it significantly reduced the side effects of the GnRH agonist. The results were similar in three longer trials of approximately 1-year duration (Figure 1). The amelioration of side effects with maintenance of efficacy seems to be even when the add-back therapy is begun during the first month of treatment, suggesting that an add-back-free interval at the beginning of a treatment cycle is unnecessary.

Although the studies just described randomize patients for initial therapy of endometriosis-associated pain, one study examined the value of GnRH agonist in patients failing primary therapy. Ling and colleagues treated women having failed to obtain relief with OCPs with either GnRH agonist or placebo. Those treated with active drug responded significantly better than those given placebo, with more than 80% experiencing pain relief in 3 months (Figure 2). Of interest is the fact that the therapy seemed to be beneficial whether or not endometriosis was seen at laparoscopy.

Most of the established medical therapies used to treat endometriosis have been applied to the problem of subfertility in women with this disease. These medications inhibit ovulation, and thus they are used to treat the disease for a period of time prior to allowing an attempt at conception. Five randomized trials with six treatment arms have compared one of these medical treatments for endometriosis to placebo or no treatment with fertility as the outcome measure. Another eight RCTs compared danazol to a second medication. These latter trials were summarized by a meta-analysis by Hughes et al. and modified by Olive and Pritts to include loss of fertility while on the

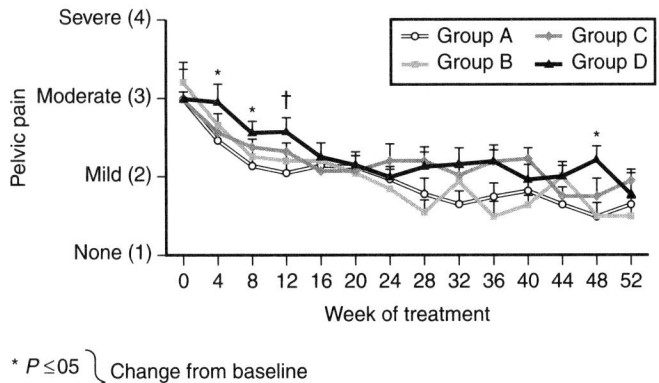

FIGURE 1. Pain relief from gonadotropin-releasing hormone (GnRH) agonist (Group A) and three different add-back therapies. (High dose progestin, low dose estrogen/progestin, higher dose estrogen/progestin). No difference is seen among the groups in the amount of pain relief. (From Hornstein MD, Surrey ES, Weisberg GW, Casino LA: et al: Leuprolide acetate depot and hormonal add-back in endometriosis: A 12-month study. Lupron Add-Back Study Group. Obstet Gynecol 1998;91(1):16-24.)

Study	Medical	No treatment	Relative risk (95% CL)
Bayer	11/37	17/36	0.63 (0.32–1.22)
Fedele	10/35	13/36	0.79 (0.36–1.68)
Telimaa	4/35	5/14	0.32 (0.08–1.24)
Thomas	4/20	4/17	0.85 (0.20–3.69)
Total	29/127	39/103	0.60 (0.39–0.93)

FIGURE 3. Meta-analysis of all randomized trials comparing medical therapy versus no treatment or placebo for endometriosis-associated infertility. Note that the untreated group has a significantly better pregnancy rate.

medications (Figure 3). The data clearly show that medical therapy for endometriosis has not proven to be of value, and in fact may be counterproductive, to the subfertile patient.

Only two studies have investigated surgery for endometriosis-associated pain versus sham surgery. Sutton and colleagues assessed the efficacy of laser laparoscopic surgery in the treatment of pain associated with minimal, mild, or moderate endometriosis. They found that there was no difference in pain at 3 months follow-up, but by 6 months a clear-cut advantage was seen for surgery. Abbott and colleagues evaluated excision of endometriosis versus diagnostic laparoscopy and had nearly identical results at 6 months. Thus, both techniques were proven better than no therapy.

Conservative surgery was used extensively in an attempt to enhance fertility. Most studies, however, are uncontrolled and of poor quality. Two randomized trials were performed to examine the value of ablation of early-stage endometriosis versus sham surgery, with contradictory results. When combined into a meta-analysis, surgical treatment of early-stage endometriosis still appears to provide a significant improvement in pregnancy rates. No such trials exist for more extensive disease; expert opinion would suggest that surgery will enhance fertility but may be inferior to advanced reproductive technologies.

The use of medical therapies for endometriosis is not restricted to their use as stand-alone agents. Clinicians frequently have used drugs in combination with surgical treatment of the disease. Numerous trials have examined the issue of postoperative medical therapy as an effective adjunct for pain. Those that have treated patients for at least 6 months after surgery showed efficacy, but in those studies where only 3 months of postoperative treatment was performed, no benefit was seen. Results are similar for all medications (Table 1).

In summary, endometriosis is an enigmatic disease that has long frustrated clinicians and patients. However, great strides in the understanding of this disorder are being made. The coming years are likely to produce a plethora of new treatment approaches targeting the biologic basis of this disease. In this regard, better understanding will undoubtedly result in renewed hope for the patient suffering from the ravages of endometriosis.

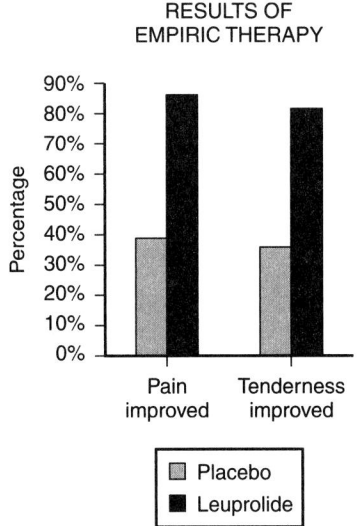

FIGURE 2. Patients with pain relief from empirical gonadotropin-releasing hormone (GnRH) agonist or placebo.

TABLE 1 Postoperative Medical Therapy

Drug	Duration of Treatment	Studies	Findings
OCPs	6 mo	1	NS at 24, 36 mo
Medroxy-progesterone, 100 mg/d	6 mo	1	$p < 0.05$ at 6 mo
Danazol, 600 mg/d	3 mo	1	NS at 6 mo
Danazol, 600 mg/d	6 mo	1	$p < 0.05$ at 6 mo
Danazol, 100 mg/d	6 mo	1	$p < 0.05$ at 24 mo
GnRH-a	3 mo	1	NS at 6 mo
GnRH-a	6 mo	2	$p = 0.008$ at 12 mo

Abbreviations: GnRH = gonadotropin-releasing hormone; NS = no sample; OCP = oral contraceptive pill.

REFERENCES

Abbott JA, Hawe J, Hunter D, et al: Laparoscopic excision of endometriosis: A randomized, placebo controlled trial. Fertil Steril 2004;82:878-884.

Hornstein MD, Surrey ES, Weisberg GW, Casino LA, Lupron Add-Back Study Group: Leuprolide acetate depot and hormonal add-back in endometriosis: a 12-month study. Obstet Gynecol 1998;91:16-24.

Hughes E, Ferorkow D, Collins J, Vandekerckhone P: Ovulation suppression for endometriosis (Cochrane review). The Cochrane Library (issue 1): Oxford, England: Update Software, 2000.

Jacobson TZ, Barlow DH, Koninclex PR, et al: Laparoscopic surgery for subfertility associated with endometriosis. Cochrane Database Syst Rev 2002;(4):CD001398.

Jansen RPS, Russel P: Nonpigmented endometriosis: Clinical, laparoscopic and pathologic definition. Am J Obstet Gynecol 1986;155:1154.

Ling FW: Randomized controlled trial of depot leuprolide in patients with chronic pelvic pain and clinically suspected endometriosis. Obstet Gynecol 1999;93:51-58.

Moghissi KS, Schlaff WD, Olive DL, et al: Goserelin acetate (Zoladex) with or without hormone replacement therapy for the treatment of endometriosis. Fertil Steril 1998;69:1056-1062.

Olive DL, Pritts EA: The treatment of endometriosis: a review of the evidence. Ann NY Acad Sci 2002;955:360-372.

Olive DL, Pritts EA: Treatment of endometriosis. N Engl J Med 2001;345:266-275.

Sampson JA: Perforating hemorrhagic (chocolate) cysts of the ovary. Arch Surg 1921;3:245.

Sutton CJG, Ewen SP, Whitelaw N, Haines P: Prospective, randomized, double-blind, controlled trial of laser laparoscopy in the treatment of pelvic pain associated with minimal, mild, or moderate endometriosis. Fertil Steril 1994;62:696.

Dysfunctional Uterine Bleeding

Method of
Beth W. Rackow, MD, and Aydin Arici, MD

Abnormal uterine bleeding is a common disorder among reproductive-age women. Dysfunctional uterine bleeding, defined as bleeding that occurs with no identifiable anatomic pathology, affects 33% to 50% of women with abnormal bleeding. Normal menstrual bleeding predictably occurs at the end of an ovulatory cycle because of estrogen and progesterone withdrawal, and lasts up to 7 days, with a cycle interval of 21 to 35 days. Any imbalance of either hormone, estrogen or progesterone, may lead to dysfunctional bleeding. Thus bleeding may occur from estrogen withdrawal because of bilateral oophorectomy or the midcycle fall in estrogen prior to ovulation; from estrogen breakthrough, such as with prolonged estrogen stimulation from chronic anovulation; from progesterone withdrawal after a short or long course of progestin therapy; and from progesterone breakthrough in the setting of a high ratio of progesterone to estrogen, such as with estrogen-progestin and progestin-based contraceptives. Dysfunctional uterine bleeding is a diagnosis of exclusion and requires elimination of other congenital and acquired abnormalities.

Evaluation of the woman with abnormal uterine bleeding must consider a broad differential diagnosis that includes a complication of pregnancy, cervical and uterine pathology (polyps, fibroids, adenomyosis, malignancies, chronic endometritis, congenital anomalies), infectious etiologies (sexually transmitted diseases, vaginitis), endocrinopathies (thyroid or androgen disorders, hyperprolactinemia), medications (exogenous hormonal therapy, anticoagulants, antibiotics, glucocorticoids, tamoxifen [Nolvadex], herbal supplements), bleeding diathesis, systemic illness (liver or renal disease), and genital trauma or foreign bodies. A thorough menstrual history is essential and should include details about past and present length of intermenstrual intervals, regularity of menses, volume and duration of bleeding, onset of abnormal bleeding, factors associated with change in bleeding (postcoital, contraceptive method, postpartum, new medical diagnosis, change in weight), and associated symptoms (premenstrual symptoms, dysmenorrhea, dyspareunia, pelvic pain, hirsutism, galactorrhea). A complete medical history, list of medications, and review of systems helps identify any systemic illness or medication effect contributing to the abnormal bleeding. The physical exam should include careful inspection of the external genitalia, vagina, and cervix and a bimanual exam to palpate the uterus and adnexa to assess size, contour, and tenderness.

Laboratory evaluation provides further information. A negative pregnancy test (preferably quantitative) rules out bleeding because of a pregnancy complication. A complete blood count evaluates for anemia and thrombocytopenia, and is important with prolonged or heavy bleeding. A serum progesterone timed to the luteal phase of the cycle determines if the patient is ovulatory; a level greater than 3 pg/mL is consistent with recent ovulation. Endocrine testing includes serum thyroid stimulating hormone, prolactin, testosterone levels, and further evaluation as indicated. Coagulation studies (prothrombin, partial thromboplastin, bleeding time, and von Willebrand's testing) should be performed in adolescents, women with unexplained menorrhagia, and those with a personal or family history concerning for a bleeding disorder. In the setting of a systemic disorder such as chronic liver or renal disease, appropriate testing should be performed.

An endometrial biopsy should be performed in women at high risk for hyperplasia and cancer based on age (35 years and older) and duration of unopposed estrogen exposure. Young women (less than 35 years old) with chronic anovulation, thus prolonged estrogen exposure, should also undergo endometrial biopsy because they can develop endometrial hyperplasia and cancer. If the biopsy (preferably done in the luteal phase) reveals secretory, not proliferative, endometrium, ovulation has occurred. A pap smear, cervical cultures, and wet mount should also be performed as indicated.

A history of regular menstrual cycles with an increasing amount or duration of bleeding, or intermenstrual bleeding, is suggestive of an anatomic cause of abnormal bleeding. Transvaginal ultrasound provides detailed assessment of the uterus and endometrium. Pathology such as leiomyomas and polyps can be identified, and size and location determined. Although an endometrial biopsy may not be necessary if the endometrium is thin (less than 5 mm), clinical suspicion of endometrial pathology takes precedence. Sonohysterography (or saline-infusion sonography) involves ultrasound assessment of the uterus and endometrium while sterile saline distends the uterine cavity. This procedure has high sensitivity and specificity for identifying uterine and endometrial pathology and is comparable to hysteroscopy. Hysteroscopy can simultaneously diagnose and treat intrauterine pathology, but involves an invasive procedure. During assessment of uterine anatomy, it is important to recognize when anatomic abnormalities, such as leiomyomas, are present but not contributing to the bleeding.

Anovulatory Dysfunctional Uterine Bleeding

A menstrual history that reveals irregular, infrequent, unpredictable bleeding, a varying amount and duration of bleeding, and no reliable symptomatology is often sufficient to diagnose anovulatory bleeding. Considered a systemic disorder, anovulatory bleeding occurs because of a variety of endocrinologic, neurochemical, and pharmacologic processes. Estrogen breakthrough is the most common scenario: persistently high estrogen levels stimulate overgrowth of an endometrium that is fragile without the stabilizing, growth-limiting effects of progesterone, and focal areas of the endometrium breakdown, bleed, and subsequently heal because of estrogen effect. This dysfunctional bleeding is common in women with polycystic ovary syndrome or obesity, in postmenarchal adolescents, and in perimenopausal women. Other conditions associated with anovulation include thyroid disorders, hyperprolactinemia, androgen disorders, psychological or physical stress, eating disorders, dramatic weight changes, and insulin resistance.

Management of anovulatory bleeding involves treating both the cause of anovulation and the abnormal bleeding. Progestins are the foundation of this medical therapy. Cyclic progestins stabilize the estrogen-stimulated endometrium and result in withdrawal bleeding after the progestin course. Medications used for a 10-day course every 4 to 6 weeks include medroxyprogesterone acetate (Provera), 5 to 10 mg, and norethindrone acetate (Aygestin), 5 mg. If bleeding does not occur after progestin withdrawal, the woman may also be hypoestrogenic, and further evaluation is indicated. Estrogen-progestin contraceptives are advantageous for women with intermittent ovulation who require contraception, and they also effectively decrease the amount of bleeding. Combined contraceptives are available in pill, patch, and vaginal ring preparations. Medroxyprogesterone acetate (Depo-Provera),[1] 150 mg intramuscularly every 3 months, can also be used to manage anovulatory bleeding, especially if women cannot take combined contraceptives. This therapy may cause irregular bleeding in the first few months, but 50% of women report amenorrhea by 12 months of use. Treatment of prolonged heavy anovulatory bleeding can be achieved with either low-dose monophasic combined contraceptives,[1] one pill twice daily for 5 to 7 days until the bleeding slows or stops, followed by routine daily use if desired, or with a higher-dose course of progestin therapy. Once the heavy bleeding is controlled, further evaluation is warranted.

Estrogen therapy is indicated for the treatment of dysfunctional bleeding with a thinned endometrium because of low estrogen levels or prolonged bleeding. This can be accomplished with conjugated estrogens (Premarin),[1] 1.25 mg, or micronized estradiol (Estrace),[1] 2 mg daily for 7 to 10 days. Similarly, estrogen (a 7- to 10-day course) can be used to treat progestin breakthrough bleeding in the setting of low-dose combined contraceptives or long-acting progestin therapy (medroxyprogesterone acetate [Depo-Provera]).

Ovulatory Dysfunctional Uterine Bleeding

Heavy or prolonged bleeding may occur during ovulatory cycles, and often no specific etiology is identified. Local defects in endometrial hemostasis are implicated. A number of medical and surgical therapies are effective in this situation. Nonsteroidal anti-inflammatory drugs (NSAIDs), such as ibuprofen (Motrin),[1] naproxen (Aleve),[1] or mefenamic acid (Ponstel),[1] decrease menstrual blood loss by inhibiting prostaglandin synthesis, and thus altering the balance of factors required for endometrial hemostasis. NSAIDs may decrease blood loss by 20% to 40%, and should be initiated just prior to the onset of menses and continued for 3 to 5 days. Similarly, combined contraceptives can reduce menstrual flow by 40% to 60%. Another option is the levonorgestrel-releasing intrauterine system (Mirena)[1]; the local progestin effect on the endometrium is profound and can reduce menstrual blood loss by 75% to 90% in women with heavy bleeding. Although cyclic progestins are often ineffective in this setting, a course of progestin (norethindrone acetate, 5 mg three times daily) from days 5 to 26 of the cycle can suppress heavy ovulatory bleeding. Gonadotropin-releasing hormone agonists produce a hypoestrogenic state and thus cause amenorrhea as well as shrinkage of myomas, if present. This therapy is best reserved for short-term management of heavy bleeding and severe anemia prior to a surgical procedure because of its cost and significant side effects such as menopausal symptoms and bone demineralization. Less commonly employed therapies include tranexamic acid (Cyklokapron),[1] an antifibrinolytic agent used in Europe to treat menorrhagia (1 g every 6 hours for the first few days of bleeding), and danazol (Danocrine),[1] a therapy that inhibits ovulation and decreases menstrual blood loss but involves androgenic side effects (200 mg daily).

Intermenstrual bleeding can also occur during ovulatory cycles. This dysfunctional bleeding may be caused by anatomic abnormalities, infection, or the preovulatory decline in estrogen. Conjugated estrogens (Premarin),[1] 1.25 mg, or micronized estradiol (Estrace), 2 mg for 2 to 3 days midcycle or 7 to 10 days for persistent breakthrough bleeding, are effective.

---

[1]Not FDA approved for this indication.

CURRENT DIAGNOSIS

- Detailed medical and menstrual history
- Thorough physical and gynecologic examination
- Pregnancy test for all reproductive-age women
- Determination of ovulatory status by history, laboratory tests
- Laboratory evaluation: complete blood count, endocrine studies, coagulation profile
- Endometrial sampling if high risk for hyperplasia or cancer
- Imaging studies to evaluate anatomy

For patients who fail medical therapy or for those who do not desire future fertility, surgical management is appropriate. The definitive procedure is hysterectomy, but this surgery carries a significant risk of complications and involves longer recovery time. Endometrial ablation by hysteroscopic, thermal, or cryosurgical techniques is a less invasive procedure for the management of abnormal bleeding in women who do not desire future fertility. These techniques can result in significantly reduced bleeding and dysmenorrhea, and even amenorrhea, but approximately 20% of patients require additional procedures. Patients with menorrhagia attributed to uterine myomas can be managed with myomectomy (hysteroscopic, laparoscopic, or abdominal procedures as indicated) or uterine artery embolization. Pregnancy is not recommended after the latter option because little data are available on postprocedure pregnancy outcomes.

Uterine Hemorrhage

Acute heavy bleeding requires high-dose estrogen therapy. Women who need inpatient management should receive conjugated estrogens (Premarin), 25 mg intravenously every 4 hours for 24 hours or until

---

CURRENT THERAPY

- Progestins
    - Cyclic or intermittent use
    - Prolonged therapy
    - Progestin-releasing intrauterine device (IUD) (Mirena)[1]
- Estrogens[1]
    - Intermittent use
    - High-dose course for acute heavy bleeding
- Estrogen-progestin contraceptives[1]
    - Cyclic use
    - High-dose course with taper for heavy bleeding
- Other therapies
    - Nonsteroidal anti-inflammatory drugs[1]
    - Tranexamic acid (Cyklokapron)[1]
    - Danazol (Danocrine)[1]
    - Gonadotropin-releasing hormone agonists
- Surgical options
    - Endometrial ablation
    - Myomectomy
    - Uterine artery embolization
    - Hysterectomy

---

[1]Not FDA approved for this indication.

the bleeding decreases. A Foley catheter balloon (30 cc) can be placed in the uterine cavity to tamponade the bleeding. Additionally, dilation and curettage can be performed to help stop acute uterine hemorrhage. If stable for outpatient management, women can receive conjugated estrogens (Premarin),[1] 1.25 mg, or micronized estradiol (Estrace),[1] 2 mg every 4 to 6 hours for 24 hours, and when the bleeding is controlled, the dose is tapered to once daily for 7 to 10 days. Another effective regimen uses high-dose combination contraceptives[1] (3 to 4 pills daily) until the bleeding is decreased, followed by a taper to 1 pill daily for several weeks. Estrogen therapy should be followed by progestins or combined contraceptives to stabilize the estrogen-stimulated endometrium.

Because dysfunctional uterine bleeding is a diagnosis of exclusion, a thorough history and evaluation, including determination of ovulatory status, is essential. A number of medical and surgical options exist for the management of dysfunctional bleeding. However, treatment failures require further evaluation.

---

[1]Not FDA approved for this indication.

REFERENCES

American College of Obstetricians and Gynecologists: Management of anovulatory bleeding. ACOG Practice Bulletin, no. 14, March 2000.
Bayer SR, DeCherney AH: Clinical manifestations and treatment of dysfunctional uterine bleeding. JAMA 1993;269:1823-1828.
Berek JS (ed): Benign diseases of the female reproductive tract. In Berek JS, ed: Novak's Gynecology, Philadelphia: Lippincott Williams & Wilkins, 2002, pp 351-373.
Farquhar CM, Lethaby A, Sowter M, et al: An evaluation of risk factors for endometrial hyperplasia in premenopausal women with abnormal menstrual bleeding. Am J Obstet Gynecol 1999;181:525-529.
Kouides PA, Conard J, Peyvandi F, et al: Hemostasis and menstruation: Appropriate investigation for underlying disorders of hemostasis in women with excessive menstrual bleeding. Fertil Steril 2005;84:1345-1351.
Munro MG: Dysfunctional uterine bleeding: Advances in diagnosis and treatment. Curr Opin Obstet Gynecol 2001;13:475-489.
Munro MG: Medical management of abnormal uterine bleeding. Obstet Gynecol Clin North Am 2000;27:287-304.
Shwayder JM: Pathophysiology of abnormal uterine bleeding. Obstet Gynecol Clin North Am 2000;27:219-234.
Speroff L, Fritz M: Dysfunctional uterine bleeding. In Clinical Gynecologic Endocrinology and Infertility. Philadelphia: Lippincott Williams & Wilkins, 2005, pp 548-571.

Infertility

Method of
Steven R. Williams, MD

Absence of desired conception despite 12 months of unprotected intercourse generally defines infertility. Historical and physical factors allow the physician to adjust this definition to the individual patient. For example, women with longstanding amenorrhea or known distal hydrosalpinges should consider intervention before 12 months, time has elapsed. However, the couple, 22 years of age, with a negative history can be encouraged to try a bit longer than 12 months before evaluation begins. After 6 months of trying, approximately 45% of couples achieve pregnancy, and after 12 months of trying, approximately 85% will conceive. Pregnancy can occur with sex 6 days before ovulation, although one study found no pregnancies were conceived from sex the day after ovulation. Thus we recommend couples trying for a baby should plan to be active together every other day starting about 6 days before ovulation is expected (cycle day 8) until 2 to 3 days after ovulation has happened (cycle day 18). If the mood were to strike more often, that's fine with us; if the mood strikes less often, we can still be comfortable given the 6-day interval previously described. As in all of medicine, important historical points can guide the direction of the evaluation and treatment of the infertile couple.

Male-factor historical points include fathering past pregnancies or miscarriages, sexual function, urologic or hernia surgery, infections, medications, and tobacco use. Semen analysis remains the most important test for male factor evaluation. The World Health Organization (WHO) reports normal males to have more than 20 million sperm per cc with greater than 50% motility. It is probably best to advise 48 hours of abstinence before collection of the sample. A urologic exam and evaluation is indicated with abnormal counts. Modern in vitro fertilization (IVF) treatments can achieve pregnancies as long as any sperm at all can be isolated, even if that means surgical aspiration. Before pursuing assisted reproduction for severely low counts, genetic testing will be recommended because severely low counts can predict higher rates of cystic fibrosis carrier status, balanced translocation, and perhaps microdeletions of the Y chromosome.

A women's age has a strong correlation with fertility success. Figure 1 compares the live birth rate when IVF patients used their own eggs fertilized with their partner's sperm compared to the rate when young oocyte donor's eggs are fertilized with the IVF patient's partner's sperm and the resultant embryos transferred into the IVF patient's uterus. One must conclude from these data that the majority of the decline in success is related to oocyte quality, as anyone can expect the success of a woman 25 years of age who uses the oocytes from a woman 25 years of age! Follicle-stimulating hormone (FSH) measured on day 3 of the menstrual cycle correlates well with ovarian reserve and is commonly ordered for women more than 30 years of age with infertility. In our office, day-3 FSH values lower than 9 mU/mL are reassuring with respect to ovarian reserve, whereas values greater than 20 mU/mL are rarely associated with future fertility success using that patient's eggs.

Previous full-term deliveries are reassuring, whereas recurrent abortions or preterm deliveries can predict a uterine issue. Pelvic infections, intrauterine device (IUD) use, previous abdominal surgery, dysmenorrhea, or dyspareunia can predict tubal obstruction. This is explored with hysterosalpingography (HSG). After sterile preparation of the cervix, a sterile cannula is inserted, and under fluoroscopic guidance radiograph contrast is injected. The dye reveals the contour of the uterine cavity and displays uterine septa and intracavitary lesions such as fibroids or polyps. It then fills into the fallopian tubes and spills into the abdominal cavity. Most women describe the discomfort of the test as a severe menstrual cramp that

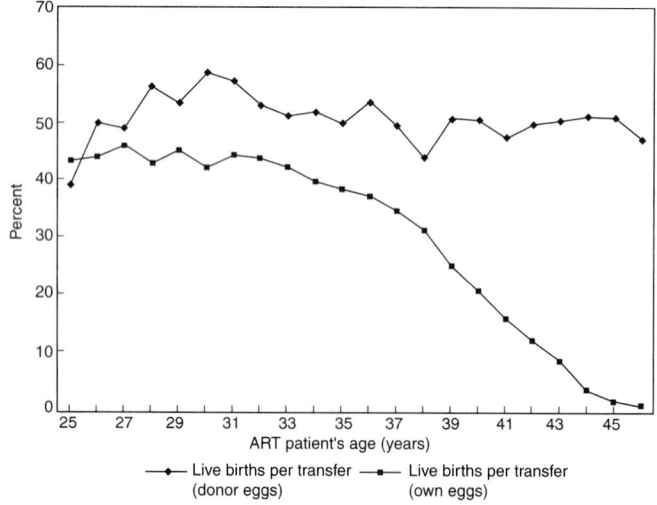

FIGURE 1. Live births per transfer for ART cycles using fresh embryos from own and donor eggs, by ART patient's age, 2002. ART = assisted reproductive technology.

CURRENT DIAGNOSIS

- Medical history can guide fertility testing.
- Simple laboratory and radiograph tests can determine infertility causes.

CURRENT THERAPY

- Clomiphene citrate is a low risk treatment option when indicated.
- Assisted reproduction is delivering more and more babies with fewer multiples.

lasts for several minutes. Pain is reduced by slow injection of the dye, gentle tissue handling, and pretreatment with nonsteroidal anti-inflammatory drugs (NSAIDs). Many authors suggest that the procedure itself has a fertility-enhancing effect. The American College of Obstetricians and Gynecologists (ACOG) suggests prophylaxis with doxycycline (Vibramycin)[1] 100 mg twice daily orally for 5 days after HSG if dilated tubes are demonstrated; no prophylaxis is indicated in a normal study. Abnormal uterine cavities can be further evaluated with saline infusion hysterograms or magnetic resonance imaging (MRI). Many uterine abnormalities can be treated completely with hysteroscopic surgery. Unilateral tubal disease noted on the HSG predicts subtle decreases in future fertility in these women compared with women with normal tubes. Bilateral tubal disease discovered on HSG predicts dramatic declines in fertility. Tubal patency established by HSG does not rule out peritubal adhesions that can affect fertility. Laparoscopy is an outpatient surgical procedure that can be used to further evaluate tubal abnormalities seen on HSG or to look for undetected peritubal adhesions. Laparoscopy also will detect endometriosis.

Endometriosis is noted in approximately 1 in 30 laparoscopies performed for tubal ligation (presumably for fertile women), although one third of women undergoing infertility evaluations will have endometriosis. Surgical treatment of minimal or mild endometriosis does appear to help with subsequent fertility somewhat. A prospective study of infertile women found to have mild or minimal endometriosis noted at laparoscopy showed a 31% preganancy rate in the next 9 months for patients randomized to treatment versus a 17% pregnancy rate in the next 9 months for women randomized to no treatment.

Irregular menstruation generally indicates irregular ovulation and diminished fertility. Even with regular menstruations, serum progesterone measurements in the luteal phase (6 to 8 days after ovulation) should be greater than 10 ng/mL for the "most fertile" of ovulations. If it is not, thyroid and prolactin studies should be ordered and induction of ovulation with clomiphene citrate (Clomid) considered. Clomiphene citrate in a 50-mg dose is taken orally for 5 days starting on menstrual day 3. Serum luteal phase progesterone is drawn 7 days after ovulation and is expected to be greater than 10 ng/dL. If it is, refills for 2 more months of treatment are written. If it is not, we recommend increasing the dose of clomiphene citrate to 100 mg daily for 5 days and repeating the luteal phase progesterone assay. If still not greater than 10 ng/dL, clomiphene citrate at 150 mg daily can be tried. If the patient is still anovulatory, referral to a gynecologist or reproductive endocrinologist is considered. For resistant patients, adjunctive treatments with the clomiphene citrate can include ultrasound monitoring with HCG injections when mature follicles are noted or adding insulin-sensitizing agents or glucocorticoids. Clomiphene ovulation induction yields approximately a 70% ovulation rate and, in young couples, approximately an 8% pregnancy rate per month. One in ten clomiphene citrate pregnancies are twins, although triplets and quadruplets are very rare on this therapy. Side effects of clomiphene citrate include hot flushes, emotional lability, mittelschmerz, headache, and sleep disturbance. Discontinue the drug if the patient experiences severe visual disturbance. Because the majority of clomiphene citrate pregnancies happen early in treatment, referral to reproductive specialists should be considered if the patients is not pregnant after 3 months of treatment.

Gonadotropin ovulation induction is available for women who failed to ovulate using clomiphene citrate or did not conceive on

[1]Not FDA approved for this indication.

that therapy. This medication is the natural hormone used to initiate ovulation; therefore, response and pregnancy rates are better than with clomiphene citrate. Unfortunately, dramatic increases in multiple pregnancy are associated with these medications, and often they are quite expensive. One large study reviewed success and multiple pregnancy rates in patients treated with gonadotropin ovulation induction. The authors concluded the protocols employed with gonadotropin ovulation induction lead to an unacceptably high incidence of higher-order multiple pregnancies and raised the question whether that treatment could be replaced by IVF.

IVF involves induction of ovulation with gonadotropin in hopes of retrieving multiple oocytes. Ovarian response is monitored with pelvic ultrasounds and serum estradiol measurements. When the oocytes are mature, HCG is given to trigger the completion of oocyte development. Then transvaginal ultrasound is used to guide an aspirating needle through the posterior cul-de-sac and into the ovaries for aspiration of the oocytes. The procedure takes approximately 15 minutes under local anesthesia and is often performed in an office setting. Oocytes are then inseminated in the lab with the husband's sperm and cultured. In certain circumstances (vey low sperm count, surgically aspirated sperm, previous failed fertilization) the oocytes can be directly injected with the sperm via intracytoplasmic sperm injection (ICSI). The resultant embryos are then cultured for 2 to 5 days and then transferred into the uterus via a simple transcervical approach. IVF thus allows embryo development without tubal ovarian interaction, making it a great choice for patients with tubal disease or endometriosis. In fact, nothing we can find at laparoscopy that was not discovered by pelvic ultrasound and HSG will affect IVF success (Figure 2). We are developing protocols that reduce the numbers of embryos transferred for couples at high risk for multiple pregnancy to one. I believe that in the future IVF will replace both gonadotropin ovulation induction and the need for laparoscopy for treatment of infertility. The 2001 Centers for Disease Control (CDC) report on assisted reproductive technology (ART) success reported national average live birth rates in the high 30% per cycle start for women younger than 35 years of age. Some individual centers are reporting live birth rates in the 50% range. IVF is a very effective and increasingly safer alternative to older treatments for refractory infertility.

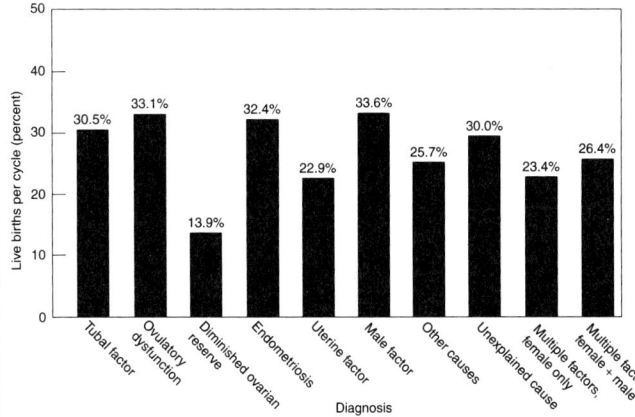

FIGURE 2. Live birth rates among women who had ART cycles using fresh nondonor eggs or embryos, by diagnosis, 2002. ART = assisted reproductive technology.

REFERENCES

American College of Obstetrics and Gynecology: Antibiotic prophylaxis for gynecologic procedures. ACOG Practice Bulletin 2003;23.

Centers of Disease Control: 2002 Assisted reproductive technology success rates, National summary and fertility clinic reports. Atlanta: Center for Disease Control, 2002.

Gleicher N, Oleske DM, Tur-Kaspa I, et al: Reducing the risk of higher order multiple pregnancy after ovarian stimulation with gonadotropins. N Engl J Med 2000;343:2-7.

Jain T, Soules MR, Collins JA: Comparison of basal follicle-stimulating hormone versus the clomiphene citrate challenge test for ovarian reserve testing. Fertil Steril 2004;82:180-185.

Jordan J, Craig K, Clifton DK, et al: Luteal phase defect: The sensitivity and specificity of diagnostic methods in common clinical use. Fertil Steril 1995;63:427-428.

Marcoux S, Maheux R, Berube S: Laparoscopic surgery in infertile women with minimal or mild endometriosis. Canadian collaborative group on endometriosis. N Engl J Med 1997;337:217-222.

Mol BW, Swart P, Bossuyt BM, et al: Is hysterosalpingography an important tool in predicting fertility outcome? Fertil Steril 1997;67:663-669.

Schwabe MG, Shapiro SS, Haning RV Jr: Hysterosalpingography with oil contrast medium enhances fertility in patients with infertility of unknown etiology. Fertil Steril 1983;40:604-606.

Trimbos JB, Trimbos-Kemper GC, Peters AA, et al: Findings in 200 consecutive asymptomatic women, having a laparoscopic sterilization. Arch Gynecol Obstet 1990;247:121-124.

Wilcox AJ, Weinberg CR, Baird DD: Timing of sexual intercourse in relation to ovulation. Effects on the probability of conception, survival of the pregnancy, and sex of the baby. N Engl J Med 1995;333:1517-1521.

Amenorrhea

Method of
Vickie Martin, MD, and Robert L. Reid, MD

Amenorrhea, simply put, is the absence of menses. It can be classified as either primary (when a woman of reproductive age has never had menstruation) or secondary (when amenorrhea occurs after menstruation has been established). There are normal situations in which amenorrhea is expected (physiologic amenorrhea): during pregnancy, during lactation, and at the onset of menopause. Approximately 5% of reproductive-age women experience amenorrhea at times other than these, which warrants investigation. Women with amenorrhea often present with significant apprehension and anxiety. Thus, an appropriate but timely work-up and diagnosis are required. The clinician must have a systematic approach for evaluating such women to ensure that important causes of amenorrhea are identified. As always, a detailed history, a targeted physical examination, and selective use of simple diagnostic tests are required.

Definition

Amenorrhea may be defined as the absence of menstruation for 3 or more months in women with past menses (secondary amenorrhea) or the absence of menarche by the age of 16 years in girls who have never menstruated (primary amenorrhea). Infrequent menstruation, termed *oligomenorrhea*, may have similar causes and also warrants investigation.

Menstrual Cycle

A clear working knowledge of the menstrual cycle and its physiology is mandatory for the clinician in these circumstances. Menstruation normally results when a cascade of hormonal signals from the hypothalamus (gonadotropin-releasing hormone [GnRH]) to cause pituitary release of luteinizing hormone (LH) and follicle-stimulating hormone (FSH). These in turn stimulate the development of an egg-containing ovarian follicle. Estrogen from this follicle results in steady growth of the endometrial lining over a 2-week period (follicular phase). When ovulation occurs, the follicle (now called the corpus luteum) develops the ability to produce a second hormone, progesterone.

The secretion of estrogen and progesterone for the next 2-week period causes the endometrial lining to become lush (decidualized) in preparation for implantation of a pregnancy. If pregnancy fails to occur, the corpus luteum undergoes a spontaneous demise, the endometrium no longer has adequate hormonal support to survive, and the tissue is sloughed synchronously over the next 5 to 7 days as menstrual flow. The final steps of this process require a means of egress for blood, implying a normal uterus with a patent cervix and vagina (the outflow tract).

Etiology

Different classification systems have been employed. One system defines the type of amenorrhea based on the level of FSH in circulation. For example, high FSH levels indicate that the hypothalamus and pituitary are fully functioning but that the ovary is not responding (similar to menopause). The gonadotropin (FSH) levels are high and the ovary (gonad) is not functioning, which is termed *hypergonadotropic hypogonadism*. *Hypogonadotropic hypogonadism* refers to the situation where FSH levels are very low due to some central disturbance of hypothalamic or pituitary function. The problem with this classification is that normal FSH levels are often low and the distinction between hypogonadotropic and eugonadotropic causes of amenorrhea can be difficult.

A simple way to consider causes of amenorrhea is to divide the processes that regulate menstruation (the hypothalamic-pituitary-ovarian axis [HPO axis]) into compartments (Figure 1) and then consider possible contributory factors for disruption of normal processes at each of these levels. Always consider the possibility that amenorrhea may be due to unexpected pregnancy before moving on to a full investigation.

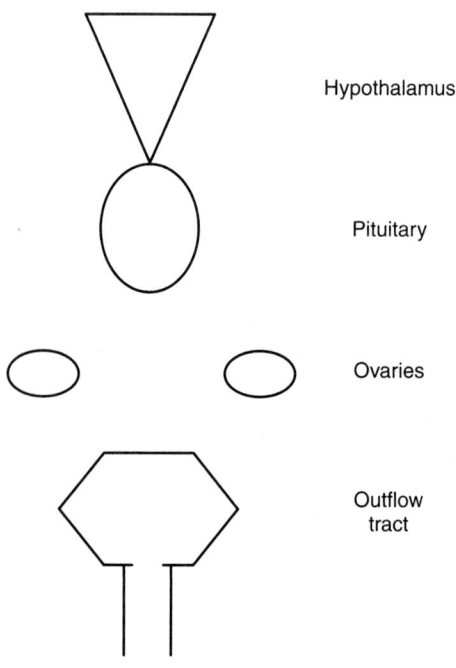

FIGURE 1. The four compartments to consider when evaluating amenorrhea.

HYPOTHALAMIC COMPARTMENT

The hypothalamus integrates a wide variety of signals from the brain and is ultimately responsible for turning on or off the hormonal cascade necessary for triggering ovulatory and menstrual function. In adolescents, the development of breasts (thelarche) between ages 8 and 10 years is usually the first sign that the HPO axis has turned on and first menstruation (menarche) typically follows within 3 to 5 years. All girls with primary amenorrhea by age 14 years, particularly if 5 or more years have passed since the first evidence of pubertal development, warrant careful investigation, because girls with primary amenorrhea on the basis of constitutional delay cannot readily be differentiated on clinical history from the two thirds of patients with primary amenorrhea who have irreversible causes of reproductive failure.

Constitutional Delay

One third of young women presenting with primary amenorrhea have constitutional delay of puberty, meaning that they are undergoing a normal sequence of pubertal development at a rate that falls 2.5 standard deviations behind the mean. Girls with constitutional delay often present between ages 13 and 16 with primary amenorrhea and only early signs of breast development. Investigation reveals low to low-normal levels of gonadotropins and an otherwise negative work-up.

Congenital Causes

A variety of unusual congenital conditions result in hypogonadotropic hypogonadism and primary amenorrhea. These conditions may be caused by deficiency of GnRH production or by abnormalities of the GnRH receptor. A Kallman's-like syndrome has been identified in some affected women who present with anosmia and a complete lack of pubertal development.

Acquired Causes

Acquired diseases can lead the hypothalamus to shut down the reproductive hormonal cascade, resulting in amenorrhea, which may be primary or secondary, depending on when they develop. Nutritional deprivation (including eating disorders), excessive caloric demand due to participation in demanding sports, and extreme psychological stress are common reasons for delayed activation of reproductive processes by the hypothalamus. Less commonly, systemic illnesses, including malabsorption states, active autoimmune diseases, and rare hypoxemic states related to congenital heart malformations or severe anemias (sickle cell disease), can lead to amenorrhea.

PITUITARY COMPARTMENT

Lesions of the pituitary stalk that interrupt normal delivery of GnRH to the pituitary include those resulting from head trauma, rare stalk tumors such as craniopharyngiomas, or from the surgery to remove these.

Pituitary causes of amenorrhea are almost always due to oversecretion of prolactin. Hyperprolactinemia resulting in amenorrhea, if associated with central retro-orbital headache and bitemporal hemianopia, can result from a prolactin-producing tumor.

Other causes of hyperprolactinemia originate outside the pituitary. For example, primary hypothyroidism, breast or chest wall lesions (or piercings) in the T4-6 dermatome, renal failure, and a variety of medications have all been linked to hyperprolactinemia. Medications that can cause hyperprolactinemia include dopamine receptor antagonists (phenothiazines, butyrophenones, thioxanthenes, risperidone, metoclopramide, sulpiride,[2] pimozide), dopamine-depleting agents (e.g., methyldopa, reserpine), H_2-blockers (cimetidine), opiates, and cocaine.

---

[2]Not available in the United States.

Rarely, other pituitary conditions result in amenorrhea. In empty sella syndrome, radiologic examination reveals an apparently empty sella due to pituitary regression from some vascular or other insult. Other conditions include Sheehan syndrome (postpartum pituitary necrosis), pituitary apoplexy (massive pituitary infarction), and radiation-induced hypopituitarism. In each of these situations, amenorrhea is usually part of a larger picture of endocrine disruption.

OVARIAN COMPARTMENT

Depletion of eggs from the ovary before or after puberty results in primary or secondary amenorrhea, respectively. FSH levels are markedly elevated in these cases, as the hypothalamus and pituitary try to elicit follicular development from the unresponsive ovary. Destruction of oocytes by any of several environmental insults, including ionizing radiation, various chemotherapeutic (especially alkylating) agents, and certain viral infections can accelerate follicular atresia.

Primary amenorrhea in a woman with evidence of gonadal failure should elicit a search for a chromosomal abnormality. It is known that two intact X chromosomes are needed for maintenance of ovarian function. A variety of X chromosome structural abnormalities have been identified in women with premature ovarian failure, including complete absence of one X chromosome (Turner's syndrome).

Elevated FSH occurs in association with a normal karyotype. These women have normal 46,XY or 46,XX karyotypes without the phenotypic abnormalities of Turner's syndrome. Those with a Y chromosome should have their gonads removed because of the potential for malignant transformation.

Several rare inherited enzymatic defects also may be associated with premature ovarian failure. These include partial deficiencies in four enzymes in the steroidogenic pathway—17α-hydroxylase, 17,20-desmolase, 20,22-desmolase, and aromatase—and galactosemia.

Premature ovarian failure may be associated with a number of autoimmune disorders. Most commonly associated with thyroiditis, ovarian failure also occurs in women with polyglandular failure, including hypoparathyroidism, hypoadrenalism, and mucocutaneous candidiasis.

Though it is not exclusively an ovarian disorder, it is useful to consider polycystic ovary syndrome (PCOS) in the ovarian compartment for the purpose of completeness in considering possible diagnoses. PCOS is one of the most common causes of secondary amenorrhea. Typically, women suffering from this condition are overweight (although one third have normal body weight) and have clinical features of hyperandrogenism (acne and hirsutism), hyperinsulinism (acanthosis nigricans), and hyperestrogenism (watery cervical mucus). Months of amenorrhea may be punctuated by episodes of heavy and prolonged menstrual bleeding as an estrogen-thickened endometrium sheds irregularly over several weeks.

OUTFLOW TRACT COMPARTMENT

Congenital abnormalities of development of the reproductive outflow tract can cause amenorrhea. Complete absence of a uterus can be due to isolated müllerian agenesis or it can manifest in phenotypic females with a 46,XY karyotype who have complete androgen insensitivity. Developmental abnormalities can include cervical atresia, tranverse vaginal septum, and imperforate hymen. These latter abnormalities may be associated with cyclic menstrual pain in the absence of bleeding (cryptomenorrhea). Similarly, monthly cramps can occur with cervical stenosis following trachelectomy or conization. Uterine synechiae due to a vigorous curettage in the face of a postpartum or postabortion endometritis can result in obliteration of the uterine cavity and secondary amenorrhea with or without monthly menstrual-like cramps.

OTHER CAUSES

Pregnancy must always be considered in a sexually active female patient presenting with secondary amenorrhea. Hormonal suppression of the endometrium can be accomplished with a variety of medications. The progestin component of the cyclic oral contraceptive gradually results in a thinner and thinner endometrium, which can ultimately result in pill-withdrawal amenorrhea. Other medications, including danazol, medroxyprogesterone, and long-acting GnRH agonists can result in amenorrhea.

Diagnosis

HISTORY

A search for clues as to the etiology should start with a personal developmental history in the amenorrheic teen and with a menstrual and reproductive history in the older amenorrheic woman. Events in the 3 to 6 months preceding the onset of amenorrhea are often critical. Rapid weight gain or loss or a marked change in energy expenditure through exercise may be important. Systems review should examine possible disruption to any of the compartments (Box 1). Inquiry about general health, risk of pregnancy, and use of medication (including illicit drugs) is important.

PHYSICAL EXAMINATION

Height, weight, and body mass index (BMI) should be determined. Body habitus often provides an important clue to which patients are amenorrheic due to excessive physical or nutritional stress (eating disorder or malnutrition). In primary amenorrhea, examination for the stage of breast and pubic hair development (Tanner staging) can indicate whether there has been delay or disruption to the entire process of pubertal development. Restriction of later visual fields to examination by confrontation, the presence of galactorrhea, or evidence of recent scars or lesions in the region of the breast (such as zoster) can implicate hyperprolactinemia. The thyroid gland should be palpated and features of hypothyroidism sought. A lower abdominal mass may be due to pregnancy, hematocolpos or hematometra.

The gynecologic examination should be tailored to the patient. The external genitalia should be evaluated for pubic hair, acanthosis nigricans, and clitoral size. The hymen should be visualized; an imperforate hymen usually shows a bluish central bulge.

CURRENT DIAGNOSIS

- Always consider the possibility of pregnancy in any woman presenting with secondary amenorrhea.
- Secondary amenorrhea is most commonly the result of some significant lifestyle change (weight gain or loss, stress, excessive exercise) or illness (with marked weight loss) in the preceding 6 months.
- Obesity and features of androgen excess are most often related to polycystic ovary syndrome (PCOS).
- Because constitutional delay of puberty is found in only one third of girls presenting with delayed menarche, an investigation should be initiated at the time of presentation rather than waiting until the girl is 16 years old (meeting the definitional criteria).
- Primary amenorrhea, particularly with the absence of other features of pubertal development (breasts and pubic and axillary hair) suggests ovarian failure.
- When amenorrhea due to ovarian failure (high FSH) occurs before age 35 years, a karyotype is indicated. If Y chromosome material is identified on karyotype, gonadectomy is required to reduce the risk of malignancy in the gonadal tissues.

BOX 1 A Compartmental Approach to Systems Review

Hypothalamic Compartment
- Changes in temperature regulation, sleep, appetite, thirst
- Headache or visual field defects

Pituitary Compartment
- Central retro-orbital headache, bitemporal hemianopia
- Galactorrhea
- Features of hypothyroidism
- Medications affecting prolactin

Ovary Compartment
- Hot flushes
- Insomnia
- Night sweats
- Vaginal dryness

Outflow Compartment
- Cyclic cramps
- Possibility of pregnancy
- Recent gynecologic procedures (dilation and curettage, cervical laser or conization)

Estrogenization of the tissues (presence of leukorrhea, thickened mucosa, or watery cervical mucus) can be assessed with speculum examination (choosing a speculum size appropriate to the sexual maturity of the patient). Visualization of the cervix in most circumstances is sufficient to rule out an outflow compartment problem.

INVESTIGATIONS

Initial Investigations

Initial investigation for any patient with amenorrhea or oligomenorrhea includes follicle-stimulating hormone (FSH), prolactin (PRL), thyroid stimulating hormone (TSH), and a sensitive pregnancy test if pregnancy is a possibility.

Ultrasonography can be helpful when an internal examination cannot be performed. When a congenital anomaly is considered, magnetic resonance imaging (MRI) can provide more definitive information.

Follow-up Investigations

A low normal FSH in the presence of a normal outflow tract should elicit a more detailed search for hypothalamic disruptors (such as nutritional, physical, or psychological stress). In a patient who has low FSH in conjunction with an elevated PRL and who is not taking medications known to increase PRL and whose TSH is normal, lesions of the hypothalamus or pituitary should be excluded with CT or MRI.

An elevated FSH indicates ovarian failure and should elicit a search for possible explanations such as past surgery, exposure to radiation or chemotherapy, or genetic causes. With an elevated FSH, a karyotype is usually indicated unless there is some obvious cause for loss of ovarian function. If the karyotype reveals any Y chromosome material, then, at the appropriate age, referral to a gynecologist is necessary for counseling and gonadectomy to reduce the risk of gonadoblastoma and dysgerminoma.

Evidence of outflow tract obstruction on pelvic examination or the possibility of cervical stenosis (cyclic dysmenorrhea without bleeding after a cervical surgical procedure such as a loop excision, cone biopsy, or trachelectomy) or Asherman's syndrome (obliteration of the endometrial cavity following a postpregnancy or postabortion dilation and curettage) merits referral to a gynecologist for further assessment and management.

Secondary amenorrhea related to weight gain or obesity, particularly when associated with features of acne and hirsutism, suggests the polycystic ovary syndrome. Management depends on whether the patient is seeking menstrual cycle regulation and relief from hirsutism (cyclic progestational therapy or an oral contraceptive plus an antiandrogen) or pregnancy (weight loss and fertility medication such as clomiphene citrate [Clomid]).

REFERENCES

Rebar RW: Evaluation of amenorrhea, anovulation and abnormal bleeding (March 26, 2006). Available at http://endotext.org/female/female4/femaleframe4.htm (accessed June 15, 2007).

Reid RL: Amenorrhea. In Copeland L, Jarrell J, McGregor J (eds): Textbook of Gynecology, 2nd ed. Philadelphia: : WB Saunders 1997; pp 365-390.

Reindollar R, Lalwani S. Abnormalities of female pubertal development (November 21, 2002). Available at http://endotext.org/female/female2/femaleframe2.htm (accessed June 15, 2007).

Dysmenorrhea

Method of
Laeth S. Nasir, MBBS

Dysmenorrhea, or pain accompanying menses, is a leading cause of morbidity among women and accounts for substantial short-term disability. Prevalence rates among women of reproductive age are reported to be higher than 90%. In some women, dysmenorrhea is significant enough to impair their quality of life to the same extent as health conditions such as angina and osteoarthritis.

Prostaglandin production during menses, resulting in tetanic uterine contractions and ischemia, plays a central role in the production of symptoms. Menstrual fluid from women who suffer from dysmenorrhea contains much higher prostaglandin levels than those who do not. Evidence also suggests that increased stress and cognitive factors such as catastrophic pain are associated with greater menstrual pain intensity.

Primary dysmenorrhea is defined as pelvic pain not associated with macroscopic pelvic pathology; whereas secondary dysmenorrhea is the presence of menstrual pain coexisting with pelvic pathology.

Primary Dysmenorrhea

Primary dysmenorrhea typically presents with the onset of ovulatory cycles, which are present in 80% of adolescents by 4 to 5 years after menarche. The pain is often described as intermittent, cramping suprapubic pain, which may be severe and radiate to the back or inner thighs. Systemic symptoms such as fatigue, malaise, anxiety, dizziness, diarrhea, and nausea and vomiting are frequently present. Symptoms may persist for 48 to 72 hours.

DIAGNOSIS

In patients with primary dysmenorrhea, the history, including gynecologic review of systems, is usually unremarkable. Patients who present with a typical history and unremarkable past medical history do not generally require extensive evaluation at the initial visit. In sexually naive patients, a rectoabdominal exam may provide sufficient information if the clinician feels that an evaluation of the pelvic organs is in order. Patients with an atypical history or who may be at risk for conditions such as pelvic inflammatory disease (PID) should undergo a focused clinical examination, including a pelvic exam with microscopic examination of vaginal fluid. Microbiologic testing and other tests or procedures such as

CURRENT DIAGNOSIS

- Colicky midline suprapubic pain radiates to lower back and thighs.
- Pain begins at onset of menses and lasts 12-72 h.
- May be accompanied by malaise, fatigue, diarrhea, vomiting, and other systemic symptoms.

ultrasound or laparoscopy may be necessary if indicated by elements of the history or physical exam.

TREATMENT

The three major treatment approaches to the management of primary dysmenorrhea are nonsteroidal anti-inflammatory drugs (NSAIDs), hormonal treatment, and complementary therapies. Therapy can be initiated using any of these methods according to patient preferences or the clinical situation. In subsequent follow-up, incomplete response, side effects, or patient preference can lead to combining therapies or changing treatment modalities.

The majority of patients have tried self-care using NSAIDs before coming to the physician. Frequently, however, inappropriately low doses and irregular dose intervals of NSAID are used. The physician often supports patients' self-care efforts through reassurance and modifications of the patient's medication regimen. The goal of NSAID treatment of dysmenorrhea is aimed primarily at preempting the production of prostaglandins. The major principle of treatment is to start the medication prophylactically and use sufficient doses to maximally suppress prostaglandin production. Ideally, the NSAID should be started 24 to 48 hours prior to the onset of expected menses and continued for an additional 24 to 48 hours. Clinicians sometimes recommend an initial loading dose of NSAID, followed by regular doses for the subsequent 24 to 48 hours. In patients without special needs, it is often best to choose the least expensive, most readily available NSAID to start with (Table 1. Suboptimal response to a NSAID may necessitate a trial of a different NSAID class. Traditionally, clinicians have recommended to patients that three cycles be monitored prior to evaluation of regimen efficacy.

Patients who desire contraception and have no contraindications may be candidates for hormonal therapy of dysmenorrhea. Suppression of ovulation leads to a thinning of the endometrial lining of the uterus with subsequent reduction of fluid contents of the uterus during menses. Prostaglandin levels in menstrual fluid are also reduced. Hormonal therapy usually consists of oral contraceptive pill[1] (OCP) or depot-medroxyprogesterone acetate[1] (Depo-Provera). Monophasic OCPs are believed to be more effective than triphasic formulations and hormonal patches in this regard. Women taking OCPs may elect to use the so-called long cycle method by skipping placebo pills and allowing menses to occur once every 3 months. The major disadvantage of this approach is the breakthrough bleeding that occurs in many women.

Rarely, therapies that suppress ovarian function more fully, such as the use of leuprolide acetate (Lupron[1]) or danazol (Danocrine[1]), may be considered. However, these have significant side effects and are very expensive. These should be considered once other causes of dysmenorrhea are ruled out and the cost-benefit ratio against other treatments is evaluated.

---

[1]Not FDA approved for this indication.

CURRENT THERAPY

- Nonsteroidal anti-inflammatory drugs
- Hormonal manipulation
- Complementary therapies

TABLE 1 Nonsteroidal Anti-inflammatory Drugs (NSAIDs) for Treatment of Dysmenorrhea		
Drug	Formulation (mg)	Dosage
Propionic Acids		
Ibuprofen (Motrin, Advil)	200, 400, 600, 800	400 mg q4-6h; max 2400 mg/d
Ketoprofen (Orudis, Oruvail)	12.5, 25, 50, 75, 100	25–50 mg PO q6–8h; max 300 mg/d
Naproxen (Naprosyn)	250, 375, 500	500 mg first dose, then 250 mg q6–8h prn; max 1250 mg/d
Naproxen sodium (Anaprox)	275, 550	550 mg PO first dose, then 275 mg PO q6–8h; max 1375 mg/d
Fenamates		
Mefenamic acid (Ponstel)	250	500 mg first dose, then 250 mg PO q6h prn; max 3 d
Meclofenamate	50, 100	100 mg PO tid; max 300 mg/d for 6 d
Cyclooxygenase-2 (COX-2) Selective Inhibitors		
Celecoxib (Celebrex)	100, 200, 400	400 mg PO first dose, then 200 mg PO bid; may take additional 200 mg on d 1

Abbreviations: max = maximum; PO = orally.

COMPLEMENTARY THERAPIES

Complementary therapies can be subdivided into pharmacologic methods, dietary modification or supplements, and physical modalities. Pharmacologic therapies that are efficacious in reducing symptoms but are infrequently used include nitroglycerin patches[1] (Nitro-Dur) and oral nifedipine[1] (Procardia).

Effective dietary or supplementation interventions are reported to include a low-fat vegetarian diet and an increased intake of omega-3 fatty acids as fish oil (one trial reported significant improvement with consumption of 2 g of fish oil daily). One study reported that 100 mg of thiamine[1] daily was highly effective in reducing dysmenorrhea, but 90 days of treatment was required before an effect was apparent. Two randomized controlled trials reported that 200 international units (IU) twice daily or 500 IU of vitamin E[1] once daily taken starting 48 hours before the onset of menses and continued for a total of 5 days were both effective in reducing symptoms.

A number of physical modalities are reported to be efficacious in the treatment of dysmenorrhea. A randomized, controlled, and blinded trial showed that acupuncture was highly effective in reducing symptoms. Acupressure and high-frequency transcutaneous electrical nerve stimulation (TENS) are also reported to reduce symptoms of cramping and pain significantly. A topically applied heating patch that maintained a temperature of approximately 38.9°C (102°F) for 12 hours a day was found to be as effective as ibuprofen (Advil) in reducing pain.

Although a Cochrane Review found insufficient evidence for benefit, invasive treatments such as nerve blocks, presacral neurectomy, uterosacral nerve ablation, and hysterectomy are rarely used in cases of severe primary dysmenorrhea resistant to conservative treatment.

Secondary Dysmenorrhea

Diagnosis of secondary dysmenorrhea may be made in patients who have significant pain with the onset of menses (when initial cycles are likely to be anovulatory), who develop increasingly severe dysmenorrhea after several years of stable menstrual symptoms, or those who fail to respond to conventional treatments such as NSAIDs or oral contraceptives. A history of atypical pelvic pain pattern such as the onset of pain several days before the onset of menses or persistence of pain after menses resolve is also suggestive of a secondary cause of dysmenorrhea. Common causes of secondary dysmenorrhea include endometriosis, pelvic inflammatory disease (PID), and anatomical abnormalities such as cervical stenosis, endometrial or endocervical polyps, or congenital obstructive müllerian anomalies.

Menstrually exacerbated nongenital causes of pelvic pain such as interstitial cystitis, irritable bowel syndrome, and psychogenic disorders seldom correspond to a history of symptoms in the menstrual cycle.

REFERENCES

ACOG Practice Bulletin Number 11. Medical Management of Endometriosis. December 1999.

Akin MD, Weingand KW, Hengehold DA, et al: Continuous low-level topical heat in the treatment of dysmenorrhea. Obstet Gynecol 2001;97:343.

Helms JM: Acupuncture for the management of primary dysmenorrhea. Obstet Gynecol 1987;69:51.

Proctor ML, Farquhar CM, Sinclair OJ, Johnson NP: Surgical interruption of pelvic nerve pathways for primary and secondary dysmenorrhea. The Cochrane Library, Issue 3. Oxford: Update Software, 2003. Review.

Proctor ML, Roberts H, Farquhar CM: Combined oral contraceptive pill (OCP) as treatment for primary dysmenorrhoea. Cochrane Database Syst Rev 2001;(4):CD002120. Review.

Proctor ML, Smith CA, Farquhar CM, Stones RW: Transcutaneous electrical nerve stimulation and acupuncture for primary dysmenorrhea. Cochrane Database Syst Rev 2002;(1):CD002123Review.

Smith RP: The dynamics of nonsteroidal anti-inflammatory therapy for primary dysmenorrhea. Obstet Gynecol 1987;70:785.

Sulak PJ, Cressman BE, Waldrop E, et al: Extending the duration of active oral contraceptive pills to manage hormone withdrawal symptoms. Obstet Gynecol 1997;89:179.

Wilson ML, Murphy PA: Herbal and dietary therapies for primary and secondary dysmenorrhoea. Cochrane Database Syst Rev 2001;(3):CD002124.

Ziaei S, Faghihzadeh S, Sohrabvand F, et al: A randomised placebo-controlled trial to determine the effect of vitamin E in treatment of primary dysmenorrhea. BJOG 2001;108:1181.

Premenstrual Syndrome

Method of
Ellen W. Freeman, PhD

The premenstrual syndromes (PMS) are characterized by mood, behavioral, and physical symptoms that occur from several days to 2 weeks before menses and remit with the menstrual flow. The term *PMS* as used by clinicians and the general public is generic, imprecise, and commonly applied to numerous symptoms. Included symptoms

---
[1]Not FDA approved for this indication.

range from the mild and normal physiologic changes of the menstrual cycle to clinically significant symptoms that limit or impair normal functioning. In recent years, randomized controlled trials and other well-designed studies have defined diagnostic criteria for PMS and identified effective treatments for this disorder.

Based on scientific evidence at this time, serotonergic antidepressants are considered the primary treatment for clinically significant PMS, and particularly its severe form termed premenstrual dysphoric disorder (PMDD). This review focuses on PMS and its treatment with serotonergic antidepressants. It is not a comprehensive review of all treatments or associated literature. Other recent reviews may guide the reader to further information and other treatments for PMS and PMDD.

Symptoms

Numerous symptoms were traditionally attributed to PMS. This plethora is related in part to the absence of a clear diagnosis that distinguishes PMS from other co-morbid conditions. Many disorders, both physical and psychiatric, are exacerbated premenstrually or occur as a co-morbid disorder with PMS. When a careful diagnosis is made to distinguish PMS from other conditions, a much smaller group of symptoms appear to be typical of the disorder (Box 1).

Mood symptoms are usually the main complaint (irritability, anxiety, tension, mood swings, feeling out of control, depression), but behavioral symptoms (e.g., decreased interest, fatigue, poor concentration, poor sleep) and physical symptoms, most commonly breast tenderness and abdominal swelling, are also present. Several recent studies suggest that irritability is the cardinal symptom of PMS. Although depressive symptoms such as low mood, fatigue, sleep difficulties, and poor concentration are frequent complaints of women with PMS, the growing evidence indicates that PMS is not a simple variant of depression but has distinct mechanisms that differ from those of depressive disorders.

Prevalence

Surveys indicate that PMS is among the most common health problems reported by reproductive-age women. Current estimates from epidemiologic data indicate that approximately 25% of women experience severe and clinically significant premenstrual symptoms, although only 6% to 8% of menstruating women meet the stringent and predominantly dysphoric criteria for PMDD.

Morbidity

The morbidity of PMS is related to its severity, chronicity, and resulting distress that affect work, personal relationships, or daily activities. The level of impairment is significantly above community norms and similar to that of other health problems such as major depressive disorder. Studies consistently demonstrate that the greatest impairment or distress resulting from PMS is in relationships with the partner or children and in the effectiveness of work.

Etiology

The etiology of PMS remains undefined, although the monthly cycling of the reproductive hormones appears to have an essential role in the disorder. While circulating levels of the hormones are in normal range, the dominant theory is that some women have an underlying vulnerability to the normal fluctuations of one or more of these hormones. It is further believed that PMS involves central nervous system–mediated interactions of the reproductive steroids with neurotransmitters. The principal research evidence at this time supports the involvement of reproductive hormones, serotonergic dysregulation, and possibly dysregulation of GABAergic receptor functioning.

Diagnosis

A diagnosis of PMS is determined primarily by the *timing* and the *severity* of the symptoms. These factors, together with an assessment of whether other physical or psychiatric disorders may account for the symptoms, are more important for the diagnosis than the particular symptoms, which are typically nonspecific and must be assessed for their relationship to the menstrual cycle.

Box 2 lists the diagnostic criteria for PMS presented by the American College of Obstetricians and Gynecologists in 2000. These criteria indicate that PMS symptoms must be experienced during the 5 days before menses and abate during the menstrual flow. The symptoms should cause identifiable impairment or distress, be confirmed by prospective reports recorded daily by the woman for at least two menstrual cycles, and not be accounted for by other disorders.

The diagnostic criteria for premenstrual dysphoric disorder (PMDD) are listed in the *Diagnostic and Statistical Manual of Mental Disorders, Fourth Edition (DSM-IV)*. Importantly, the Food and Drug Administration (FDA) has approved medications only for the indication of PMDD and not for the indication of PMS at the present time. The PMDD criteria are intended to diagnose a severe, dysphoric form of PMS and require 5 of 11 listed symptoms including at least one of the mood symptoms. Physical symptoms, regardless of the number, are considered a single symptom in meeting the diagnostic criteria. The 11 PMDD symptoms are depressed mood, anxiety or tension, mood swings, anger or irritability, decreased interest, concentration difficulties, fatigue, appetite change or food

---

BOX 1 Symptoms of Premenstrual Syndrome

Affective
- Irritability
- Anxiety
- Angry outbursts
- Confusion
- Social withdrawal
- Depression

Somatic
- Bloating
- Swelling
- Breast tenderness
- Headache

From American College of Obstetricians and Gynecologists (ACOG) Practice Bulletin 15, 2001.

 CURRENT DIAGNOSIS

- Confirm that symptoms occur premenstrually and abate following menses.
- Confirm that symptoms are clinically significant and impair daily activities and/or cause problems for the woman.
- Obtain a medical history and conduct a physical examination to determine that other disorders are not causing the symptoms.
- Query depression, stress, substance abuse, and other diagnoses that could cause the symptoms.
- Ask the woman to maintain a daily symptom report for two or more menstrual cycles to confirm the reported symptoms and their relation to the menstrual cycle.
- Perform laboratory tests only as needed to confirm general good health or rule out other suspected conditions.

| BOX 2 | Diagnosis of Premenstrual Syndrome |

Presenting symptoms:
- Consistent with premenstrual syndrome
- Restricted to the luteal phase
- Cause impairment or distress
- Not an exacerbation of another disorder
- Confirmed by 2 cycles of daily symptom rating

From American College of Obstetricians and Gynecologists (ACOG) Practice Bulletin 15, 2001.

 CURRENT THERAPY

SSRI	Range Studied (mg)	Mean Dose (mg/d)
Citalopram (Celexa[1])	10–30	20
Escitalopram (Lexapro[1])	10–20	15
Fluoxetine (Prozac,[1] Sarafem*)	10–60	20
Paroxetine (Paxil[1])	10–30	20
Paroxetine-CR* (Paxil-CR)	12.5, 25	NA[†]
Sertraline (Zoloft*)	50–150	75
SNRI		
Venlafaxine (Effexor[1])	37.5–200	112.5

[1]Not FDA approved for this indication
*FDA approved for the indication of premenstrual dysphoric disorder (PMDD).
[†]Not applicable because of fixed-dose study.

cravings, sleep disturbance, feeling overwhelmed, and physical symptoms. At least five of these symptoms must each be severe premenstrually and abate with the menstrual flow. The symptoms must markedly interfere with functioning, be confirmed by daily symptom reports for at least two menstrual cycles, and not be an exacerbation of another physical or mental disorder.

To diagnose PMS, a medical history should be obtained and a complete physical with gynecologic examination performed. PMS is understood to occur in ovulatory menstrual cycles; cycles that are irregular or outside the normal range are an indication for further gynecologic investigation. Co-morbid conditions such as dysmenorrhea, endometriosis, uterine fibroids, pelvic inflammatory disease, thyroid disorders, migraine, diabetes, mood disorders, substance abuse, and numerous other possibilities should be identified. It may be difficult to determine whether the symptoms under investigation are an exacerbation of a co-morbid condition or superimposed on another condition. In either case, the usual recommendation is to treat the ongoing condition first, then reassess and possibly add treatment for the symptoms that arise premenstrually.

No laboratory test identifies PMS and none should be routinely performed for diagnosis. Laboratory tests that indicate or confirm other possible disorders are useful if suggested by the individual woman's symptom presentation or medical findings.

The key diagnostic tool for evaluating premenstrual symptoms is the daily symptom report. The diagnostic criteria for both PMS and PMDD include a daily symptom report that is kept by the woman for at least two menstrual cycles to confirm that the woman's reported symptoms are linked to the menstrual cycle in the requisite pattern. Numerous symptom reports appropriate for this diagnosis are identified in the medical literature on PMS and PMDD. It is important that the ratings indicate the severity of each symptom (and not simply check the presence or absence of symptoms).

It is informative to use two visits for the diagnostic evaluation. Although counterintuitive, seeing the patient following menses when PMS symptoms have abated is instructive. If symptoms are absent, it provides strong evidence for the diagnosis. If symptoms are present in the follicular phase, the type and severity of the symptoms are important diagnostic information for identifying other physical or mental disorders that may be the primary focus of treatment.

Treatment

SELECTIVE SEROTONIN REUPTAKE INHIBITORS

Serotonergic antidepressants are the primary treatment for severe PMS and PMDD at this time. Modulating serotonergic function is consistent with a leading theoretical view that the normal gonadal steroid fluctuations of the menstrual cycle are associated with an abnormal serotonergic response in vulnerable women. A meta-analysis of randomized controlled trials of selective serotonin reuptake inhibitors (SSRIs) in treatment of PMS and PMDD determined that these drugs were an effective first-line therapy, with both a statistically significant and clinically meaningful difference from placebo. The FDA has approved fluoxetine (Sarafem), sertraline (Zoloft), and paroxetine (Paxil) for the indication of PMDD. Other randomized, placebo-controlled, double-blind trials showed efficacy for citalopram (Celexa[1]), venlafaxine (Effexor[1]) (a selective serotonin-norepinephrine reuptake inhibitor [SNRI]), and clomipramine (Anafranil[1]) (a tricyclic antidepressant) for treatment of PMS and PMDD.

Effective doses of SSRIs are consistently at the low end of the dose range for depressive disorders in all reports of PMS and PMDD treatments. Significant response is often seen in the first menstrual cycle of treatment, with smaller increments with or without dose adjustments in the second and third treatment cycles. If there is not sufficient response in the first treated menstrual cycle, the dose should be increased in the next cycle unless precluded by side effects.

Side effects are common with the initiation of an SSRI but are usually transient and abate within 1 to 2 weeks of continued treatment. The most common side effects include headache, nausea, insomnia, fatigue or lethargy, diarrhea, decreased concentration, dizziness, and decreased libido or delayed orgasm. The sexual side effects of SSRIs have received considerable attention, although it is often difficult to determine the extent to which sexual effects are related to the medication or to preexisting conditions. The incidence of decreased sexual interest or delayed orgasm in the few published reports of PMS patients is approximately 9% to 16%, which is notably lower than the rates reported with the use of SSRIs by depressed patients. Another important issue is the lack of any well-controlled clinical trials of SSRI treatment for PMS and PMDD in adolescents. Whether SSRIs are safe and effective for this indication in women younger than 18 years is not demonstrated.

Luteal Phase Dosing

The use of medication only in the symptomatic luteal phase of the menstrual cycle is particularly important in PMS because of the cyclic pattern of the symptoms, which occur only in the premenstrual phase and abate following menses. Efficacy of luteal phase administration of the SSRIs is demonstrated in multiple trials: three large multicenter, randomized, placebo-controlled trials that examined fluoxetine (Sarafem), paroxetine (Paxil), and sertraline (Zoloft); a trial that

[1]Not FDA approved for this indication.

directly compared continuous and luteal phase administration of sertraline; and multiple preliminary studies.

Luteal phase administration of an SSRI is typically initiated 14 days prior to the expected onset of menstrual bleeding and concluded within several days of bleeding, using a taper for increased doses. As with continuous dosing, the SSRI doses are usually at the low end of the dose range.

One preliminary study compared symptom-onset dosing (mean of 6 days before menses) to luteal phase dosing and found no difference between the two dosing regimens in improvement overall, although there was suggestion that women with more severe symptoms may respond better to full luteal phase dosing.

Side effects may be less frequent with an intermittent dosing regimen because they may not occur when not taking the medication. However, some women experience recurring side effects when dosing is resumed, and discontinuation symptoms might also occur with the stop-start dosing pattern. At this time, no systematic data confirm discontinuation symptoms with the intermittent dosing regimen.

Insufficient Response to Selective Serotonin Reuptake Inhibitors

Approximately 60% of PMS and PMDD patients in controlled studies respond well to an SSRI. There are no clear predictors of response. An adequate trial of an SSRI for PMS and PMDD is at least two menstrual cycles at a dose level of demonstrated efficacy, with a third cycle when there is partial response. If a woman has an insufficient response or unacceptable side effects, it is reasonable to try another SSRI. Although the SSRIs are similar in their structure and have similar response rates and side-effect profiles, an individual patient may respond better to one SSRI versus another.

Other approaches to a poor treatment response include augmenting the SSRI with another medication to address the nonresponding symptoms, but there is no systematic information on this in PMS or PMDD treatment. Switching to another class of medication, such as anxiolytics, is suggested, but no data indicate whether nonresponders to SSRIs will respond to another class of medication. Nonresponse may also be related to other co-morbid disorders. A thorough review of the diagnosis and adjustments of the premenstrual doses of medication for both the primary disorder and PMS should be considered before pursuing other treatments.

OTHER TREATMENTS

Hormonal

In spite of the evidence for hormonal involvement in PMS and PMDD, traditional oral contraceptives (OCs) do not show efficacy for the disorder. However, recent data indicate that shortening or omitting the placebo week in the traditional OC pill pack may effectively treat PMS and PMDD. The FDA has approved the oral contraceptive YAZ, a 24/4-day combination pill, to treat PMDD.

Gonadotropin-releasing hormone (GnRH) agonists such as depot leuprolide[1] (Lupron) and buserelin[2] (Suprefact) are effective for PMS and PMDD but are of limited usefulness because of the risks associated with low estrogen levels that result from these treatments. Although add-back therapy using low-lose estrogen and progesterone together with the GnRH agonist did not appear to reduce efficacy in a meta-analysis, there are no definitive data on the safety and efficacy of this approach in long-term treatment. The historic use of progesterone has failed to show efficacy for the mood and behavioral symptoms of PMS in numerous controlled trials.

Anxiolytics

Alprazolam[1] (Xanax) and buspirone[1] (Buspar) showed modest efficacy for PMS in some studies but not others. Although these medications offer an alternative to antidepressants, the response rates appear much lower, and it is not known whether a PMS patient who does not respond to antidepressants will respond to an anxiolytic. The risk of dependency with alprazolam should be considered. Dosing should be strictly limited to the luteal phase, and the patient should have no history of substance abuse.

Nonpharmacologic

Calcium supplementation[1] (600 mg twice daily) reduced PMS symptoms significantly more than placebo. Calcium offers a dietary supplement approach that may be beneficial for some women with PMS, although there are no predictors of which women will respond well to this therapy. Other complementary and alternative therapies may be helpful for some women, but there is no convincing evidence of their efficacy for PMS.

Behavioral treatments that facilitate coping or reduce stress may reduce PMS symptoms. Cognitive-behavioral therapy is effective for PMS, and in one study it was as effective as the SSRI fluoxetine after 6 months of treatment.

TREATMENT DURATION

All published studies of treatment efficacy for PMS and PMDD are based on acute treatment of 2 to 3 months' duration. Several small pilot investigations suggest that PMS symptoms are likely to return within several months after medication is stopped. It also appears that PMS symptoms do not resolve spontaneously but continue for many years. These observations of PMS as a chronic condition and the swift return of symptoms following the cessation of medication suggest that treatment can be expected to be long term; notably, there are no data from long-term maintenance studies at this time.

The SSRIs are currently the first-line treatment for severe PMS and PMDD. Continuous dosing and luteal phase dosing regimens are similarly effective for these disorders when the symptoms are clearly limited to the luteal phase of the menstrual cycle. Hormonal treatments have lacked consistent scientific evidence of their efficacy or safety or both for PMS treatment. Several new oral contraceptives that decrease or omit the placebo interval may provide an effective alternative to antidepressant medications. Preliminary evidence indicates that long-term maintenance of the medication may be required for PMS and PMDD, but currently, there are no studies of the effectiveness, costs, and benefits of long-term treatment.

---

[1]Not FDA approved for this indication.

REFERENCES

ACOG Practice Bulletin: Premenstrual syndrome. Int J Gynecol Obstet 2001;73(2):183-190.

Dell DL: Premenstrual syndrome, premenstrual dysphoric disorder, and premenstrual exacerbation of another disorder. Clin Obstet Gynecol 2004;47(3):568-575.

Dimmock PW, Wyatt KM, Jones PW, O'Brien PM: Efficacy of selective serotonin-reuptake inhibitors in premenstrual syndrome: A systematic review. Lancet 2000;356(9236):1131-1136.

Freeman EW: Luteal phase administration of agents for the treatment of premenstrual dysphoric disorder. CNS Drugs 2004;18(7):453-468.

Girman A, Lee R, Kligler B: An integrative medicine approach to premenstrual syndrome. Am J Obstet Gynecol 2003;188(5 Suppl):S56-S65.

Grady-Weliky TA: Premenstrual dysphoric disorder. N Engl J Med 2003;348(5):433-438.

Halbreich U: The etiology, biology, and evolving pathology of premenstrual syndromes. Psychoneuroendocrinology 2003;28(Suppl 3):55-99.

Johnson SR: Premenstrual syndrome, premenstrual dysphoric disorder, and beyond: A clinical primer for practitioners. Obstet Gynecol 2004;104(4):845-859.

Stevinson C, Ernst E: Complementary/alternative therapies for premenstrual syndrome: A systematic review of randomized controlled trials. Am J Obstet Gynecol 2001;185(1):227-235.

---

[1]Not FDA approved for this indication.
[2]Not available in the United States.

Menopause

Method of
Irina Burd, MD, PhD, Stacey A. Scheib, MD, and Krystene I. Boyle, MD

Menopause is the physiologic process characterized by a marked decrease in the number of oocytes, subsequent follicular depletion, decreased ovarian estrogen secretion, and finally cessation of menses. For 95% of women, menopause occurs between the ages of 45 and 55, with a mean age of 51. Time of menopause is influenced by genetic as well as environmental factors (Box 1). Menopause before age 40 years is considered premature ovarian failure.

Diagnosis

Menopause is defined clinically as 12 months of amenorrhea following the last menstrual period in the absence of other causes. The Staging of Reproductive Aging Workshop (STRAW) has provided a beneficial staging system to help categorize patients (Box 2).

The differential diagnosis for menopause includes thyroid disease, pregnancy, hyperprolactinemia, medications, carcinoid, pheochromocytoma, or underlying malignancy, which are important in considering the diagnosis algorithm (Box 3). Follicle-stimulating hormone (FSH) and estradiol are commonly measured to diagnose menopause and are often misleading because they can fluctuate vastly in the perimenopausal period.

Systemic Manifestations of Menopause

VASOMOTOR SYMPTOMS

Hot flushes are the most common symptom associated with menopause. They are self-limited sensations of generalized heat that last 2 to 4 minutes and vary widely among people and across cultures. Without treatment, they resolve within 1 to 5 years.

SLEEP DISTURBANCES

Sleep disturbances often occur in menopause as a result of hot flushes arousing the woman from sleep. When the hot flushes are treated, sleep usually improves. Persistent sleep disturbances can lead to more serious symptoms such as difficulty concentrating, fatigue, mood disturbances, depression, and other psychological symptoms.

GENITOURINARY SYMPTOMS

Estrogen deficiency leads to atrophy of the urethral and vaginal epithelium. Vaginal atrophy can result in vaginal dryness, itching, irritation, and dyspareunia. The pH in the vagina also increases and, with vaginal atrophy, can lead to recurrent vaginal infections. Decreasing elasticity of the vaginal wall elasticity can result in a shorter and narrower vagina, especially without continued sexual activity. The lack of estrogen affects blood flow to the vagina and vulva, which in turn causes decreased lubrication and neuropathy. These are both reversible with estrogen replacement therapy, especially vaginal therapy.

Incontinence incidence increases with age but has not been clearly associated with menopause. The theory is that atrophy of the urethral epithelium results in diminished urethral mucosal seal, loss of compliance, and irritation. These are believed to contribute to stress and urge incontinence. These patients also report recurrent urinary tract infections; this is probably related to the increase in vaginal pH.

ABNORMAL BLEEDING

Even though most postmenopausal bleeding is due to atrophy, during the perimenopausal period the endometrium may be exposed to unopposed estrogen that can result in anovulatory bleeding or

---

CURRENT DIAGNOSIS

- For women older than 45 years who have menopausal symptoms, no further work-up is necessary unless there are symptoms of hyperthyroidism.
- For women younger than 45 years, proceed with an oligomenorrhea or amenorrhea work-up: Check serum hCG, prolactin, TSH, and FSH.
- Women younger than 40 years should have a complete evaluation for premature ovarian failure.
- Common symptoms of menopause include abnormal bleeding, hot flushes, genitourinary complaints, sleep disturbances, mood disturbances, joint pain, and difficulty concentrating.
- FSH and estradiol levels can be misleading and so should not be used to make the diagnosis.

Abbreviations: FSH = follicle-stimulating hormone; hCG = human chorionic gonadotropin; TSH = thyroid-stimulating hormone.

BOX 1   Factors that Influence the Timing of Menopause

- Alcohol abuse
- Chemotherapy
- Cigarette smoking
- Contraception
- Family history of early menopause
- Galactose consumption
- Obesity
- Parity
- History of pelvic irradiation
- Physiologic and psychological stresses (e.g., living at high altitudes, depression)
- Race
- Shorter cycle length during adolescence
- Type 1 diabetes mellitus

BOX 2   STRAW Staging System

- Perimenopause
  - Stage −2 (early): Variable cycle length (>7 days from normal cycle)
  - Stage −1 (late): ≥2 skipped cycles and amenorrhea interval ≥60 days
- Menopause
  - Stage +1 (early): First 5 years after final menstrual period
  - Stage +2 (late): 5 years after final menstrual period until death

Abbreviation: STRAW = Stages of Reproductive Aging Workshop.

BOX 3 Algorithm for the Diagnosis of Menopause

Older than 45 years
- No symptoms suggestive of hyperthyroidism: No further diagnostic evaluation
- With symptoms suggestive of hyperthyroidism: Check serum TSH, T3, free T4

Younger than 45 years
- Oligomenorrhea or amenorrhea work-up: Check serum hCG, prolactin, TSH, FSH

Younger than 40 years
- Complete evaluation for premature ovarian failure

Abbreviations: FSH = follicle-stimulating hormone; hCG = human chorionic gonadotropin; T3 = triiodothyronine; T4 = thyroxine; TSH = thyroid-stimulating hormone.

BOX 4 Risk Factors for Osteoporosis

Modifiable Risk Factors
- Chronic corticosteroid use
- Cigarette smoking
- Early menopause (before age 45 years)
- High alcohol intake
- High caffeine intake
- Low body weight (<127 pounds)
- Low dietary calcium intake
- Low vitamin D intake
- Premenopausal amenorrhea (>1 y)
- Sedentary lifestyle

Nonmodifiable risk factors
- Dementia
- Family history of osteoporosis
- Poor general health
- White or Asian ethnicity

---

endometrial hyperplasia. If this occurs, endometrial biopsy is needed to rule out endometrial hyperplasia or cancer. A transvaginal ultrasound can also be used as a screening tool first and then be followed by an endometrial biopsy if the endometrial thickness is greater than 4 mm.

MOOD DISTURBANCES

In the Study of Women's Health Across the Nation (SWAN), higher risks of mood symptoms were found in perimenopausal women. The strongest risks of depression associated with menopause are a prior history of depression and premenstrual syndrome. Depression might not be entirely related to the physiology of menopause but may be a result of stressors concomitantly occurring around the time of menopause, such as children leaving home, dealing with aged parents, and midlife adjustment.

MENSTRUAL MIGRAINES

Menstrual migraines are believed to be related to decreased estrogen levels around the time of menses. Because menopause is related to a decrease in estrogen, menstrual migraines can increase in intensity and frequency.

BALANCE AND OSTEOPOROSIS

Estrogen deficiency can have an effect on the central nervous system by impairing balance. Along with osteoporosis, loss of balance remains one of the big causes of fractures in menopausal women. There are multiple risk factors for osteoporosis, modifiable and nonmodifiable (Box 4).

OTHER EFFECTS

Other long-term issues that are believed to be related to menopause include cardiovascular disease and dementia.

Treatment

HORMONE REPLACEMENT THERAPY

Until relatively recently, long-term estrogen and combined estrogen and progestin therapy was routinely given to postmenopausal women. Hormone replacement therapy (HRT) was believed to prevent cardiovascular disease and osteoporosis. The Women's Health Initiative (WHI) was a set of clinical trials, whose results were first published in 2002, that resulted in a dramatic change in clinical practice. The study was designed to see if there was a decrease in cardiovascular risk with conjugated equine estrogen (CEE [Premarin]) in patients without a uterus or in combination with medroxyprogesterone acetate (MPA [Provera]). The CEE-MPA (Prempro) arm of the trial was stopped early after 5 years because of the increased risks for breast cancer, coronary heart disease (CHD) (29%), stroke (41%) and venous thromboembolism (VTE) (33%), even though there was a reduction in risk of hip and vertebral fractures and colon cancer. There was also an increased risk of stroke (39%) and VTE (33%) in the CEE-alone arm after 7-year follow-up, but there was no difference in heart disease.

The Heart and Estrogen/progestin Replacement Studies (HERS I and II trials) looked at secondary prevention in postmenopausal women with known CHD, which showed that there was not a reduction of CHD events with CEE-MPA. Both the WHI and HERS studies revealed an increase in the number of VTEs.

CURRENT THERAPY

- CEE or 17-β estradiol plus MPA, as either continuous or cyclic short-term therapy lasting no more than 5 years is a first-line treatment for vasomotor symptoms in a patient with no contraindications.
- Locally active estrogen-containing compounds are available for treating urogenital symptoms.
- SERMs provide an alternative for treating menopausal symptoms, specifically osteoporosis. Raloxifene has less antiresorptive action than the bisphosphonates (e.g., alendronate) and should be given to patients who do not tolerate bisphosphonates.
- Alendronate increases BMD in the vertebral spine and femoral neck more than raloxifene, but patients taking both alendronate and raloxifene increased their BMD the most.
- More research is needed in the use of androgen replacement in menopause, although some evidence suggests that it might improve libido.

Abbreviations: BMD = bone mineral density; CEE = conjugated equine estrogen; MPA = medroxyprogesterone acetate; SERM = selective estrogen-receptor modulator.

TABLE 1 Treatment of Vasomotor Symptoms

Treatment	Suggested Dose	Possible Side Effects
Hormones		
CEE (Premarin) or 17-β estradiol, plus MPA (Provera), either continuous or cyclic	CEE 0.3 mg/d *or* Estradiol 0.5 mg PO qd *or* Estradiol 0.05 mg patch qd *plus* MPA 2.5 mg/d or for 12-14 d/mo	See text
MPA	20 mg/d[3] oral or 150 mg IM (Depo-Provera)[1] q3 mo	Mood disturbances, breast tenderness, alopecia
Megestrol acetate (Megace)[1]	20 mg bid	Vomiting, diarrhea, flatulence
Selective Serotonin Reuptake Inhibitors		
Paroxetine (Paxil, Paxil CR)[1]	10-20 mg/d or 12.5-25 mg CR/d	Fatigue, dry mouth, nausea, decreased libido
Fluoxetine (Prozac)[1]	20 mg/d	
Venlafaxine (Effexor, Effexor XR)[1]	37.5-75 mg XR/d	
Other Medications		
Gabapentin (Neurontin)[1]	300-900 mg/d	Dizziness, somnolence, peripheral edema
Clonidine (Catapres TTS)[1]	0.1 mg/24 h wk patch	Orthostatic hypotension, drowsiness
Dietary Supplements		
Vitamin E[1]	800 IU/d	Fatigue, weakness, diarrhea
Black cohosh[7]		Gastrointestinal complaints, dizziness
Evening primrose oil[7]		
Other Interventions		
Acupuncture or accupressure		
Exercise		
Lifestyle interventions (e.g., layered clothing, fans, air conditioners)		

[1] Not FDA approved for this indication.
[3] Exceeds dosage recommended by the manufacturer.
[7] Available as a dietary supplement.
Abbreviations: CEE = conjugated equine estrogen; MPA = medroxyprogesterone acetate.

In the WHI Memory Study (WHIMS), with CEE and CEE-MPA there was an increased risk of dementia compared with placebo, but this was in an older postmenopausal population. Epidemiologic studies indicate that estrogen may be neuroprotective if initiated earlier. Therefore, therapy should not initiated after age 65 years.

As a result of these studies and the recommendations of the North American Menopause Society, the only use for estrogen therapy, either alone or combined with progestin, is for control of menopausal symptoms, particularly hot flushes, vaginal dryness, urinary symptoms, joint pain, skin changes, and emotional lability. Studies are inconclusive whether CEE alone or CEE-MPA is beneficial for incontinence. Contraindications to estrogen therapy are a history of endometrial cancer, liver disease, breast cancer, CHD, history of VTE or stroke, or high risk of any of the above. In the Nurses' Health Study, an increased incidence of new onset of asthma that may be dose related and development of systemic lupus erythematosus might result from estrogen therapy.

The absolute risk of an adverse event is extremely low. For a 50-year-old woman on combined estrogen-progestin, estimated risk is 1:1000 at 1 year and 1:200 at 5 years. This absolute risk doubles for a 60 year-old woman. The goal of treatment is a short-term therapy, lasting no more than 5 years. Therapy should be tapered, decreasing by one pill every 1 or 2 weeks, so that there is no rebound in menopausal symptoms.

Progestin should be added to HRT for any woman with a uterus in order to prevent endometrial hyperplasia and cancer. The Postmenopausal Estrogen/Progestin Interventions (PEPI) trial showed a statistically significant reduction in the incidence of simple, complex, and atypical endometrial hyperplasia with CEE-MPA therapy compared with CEE alone. The only recommended progestin at this time is MPA 2.5 mg/day. Alternative progestin doses, less frequent administration, and alternative routes of administration have not been studied and thus might not be able to prevent endometrial hyperplasia or cancer; if these are used, closer endometrial surveillance is necessary.

Women with premature ovarian failure should be given hormonal therapy, and risks and benefits should be reassessed at age 50 years.

More research is needed the in use of androgen replacement in menopause, although some evidence suggests that it might improve libido.

Alternative therapy has been proposed for menopausal symptoms (Table 1 and Box 5).

BISPHOSPHONATES

Bisphosphonates impair osteoclastic bone resorption and are used to treat osteoporosis (Box 6). The most common side effects are bone pain and upper gastrointestinal disorders such as dysphagia, esophagitis, and esophageal or gastric ulcer. They are contraindicated in patients with renal impairment, uncorrected hypocalcemia, or sensitivity to the drug components. There have been no randomized, controlled studies comparing one type of bisphosphonate with another.

BOX 5 Treatment of Urogenital Atrophy Symptoms

- Systemic estrogen therapy alone or combined with progestin
- Estrogen cream (Estrace Vaginal, Premarin Vaginal): 0.5-1 g biw-tiw
- Estradiol vaginal tablet (Vagifem): 1 tablet tiw
- Estrogen-containing vaginal ring (Estring): 1 ring inserted every 3 mo
- Lubricants with intercourse as needed

> **BOX 6 Treatments for Osteoporosis**
>
> **Bisphosphonates**
> - Alendronate (Fosamax) 70 mg/wk or 70-mg oral solution weekly or 10 mg/d
> - Risedronate (Actonel) 35 mg/wk
> - Ibandronate (Boniva) 150 mg/mo or 3-mg injection once every 3 mo
>
> **Selective Estrogen-Receptor Modulators**
> - Raloxifene 60 mg/d

> **BOX 7 ACOG Recommendations for Monitoring Women on Tamoxifen**
>
> - Perform annual gynecologic examinations.
> - Monitor for signs or symptoms of endometrial hyperplasia or cancer.
> - Investigate any abnormal vaginal symptoms.
> - Reassess use if atypical hyperplasia develops and proceed with appropriate gynecologic management.
> - Discontinue tamoxifen after 5 years because benefit has not been demonstrated beyond 5 years of use.
>
> *Abbreviation*: ACOG = American College of Obstetricians and Gynecologists.

SELECTIVE ESTROGEN RECEPTOR MODULATORS

Selective estrogen receptor modulators (SERMs) provide an alternative for treating menopausal symptoms, specifically osteoporosis (Box 6). SERMs bind to the estrogen receptor, but they have tissue-specific properties. The two SERMs that have been studied the most are raloxifene (Evista) and tamoxifen (Nolvadex). Raloxifene's mechanism for tissue-specific activity is not fully clear. Tamoxifen probably works by variable gene expression in different cell types.

Raloxifene

Two major double-blinded, placebo-controlled trials, one in the United States and one in Europe, have looked at raloxifene versus placebo, measuring bone mineral density (BMD), markers of bone turnover, and serum lipid levels. In all treatment arms in both studies, BMD was significantly increased and serum concentrations of both total and low-density lipoprotein (LDL) cholesterol were significantly decreased compared with placebo. In both trials there was no difference in complaints of breast pain or vaginal bleeding and no difference in endometrial thickness.

In the longer-term Multiple Outcomes of Raloxifene Evaluation (MORE) study, there was a relative risk reduction in vertebral fractures but not for nonvertebral fractures. The risk of invasive, but not noninvasive, breast cancer appeared to decrease, most likely due to the antagonistic effect of raloxifene. There was no increase in endometrial cancer. The relative risk of thromboembolic disease was 3.1 compared with placebo, but it appears that the risk is less than that with tamoxifen. There was no difference in cardiovascular events, except there was a decrease in the subset of women at greatest risk.

In a study looking at osteoporosis in postmenopausal women, patients on alendronate (Fosamax) increased their BMD in the vertebral spine and femoral neck more than patients on raloxifene, but patients taking both medications increased their BMD the most. CEE had a better effect on BMD compared with raloxifene in hysterectomized postmenopausal women. Raloxifene has less antiresorptive action than the bisphosphonates (e.g., alendronate) and should be given to patients who do not tolerate bisphosphonates.

Raloxifene significantly increased the occurrence of hot flushes compared with placebo in all the studies. Other side effects of raloxifene noted were influenza-like symptoms, peripheral edema, and leg cramps. It does not appear to affect vaginal symptoms, urinary symptoms, gallbladder disease, cognitive decline, or cataracts.

The recommended starting dose is 60 mg/day.

Tamoxifen

Tamoxifen[1] has demonstrated some benefit for osteoporosis, but estrogen and bisphosphonates have shown a greater increase in lumbar spine BMD. In the National Surgical Adjuvant Breast and Bowel Project (NSABP) P-1 Trial, women on tamoxifen had fewer hip, wrist, and vertebral fractures at 7-year follow-up. In this study there was not a significant difference in the occurrence of cardiovascular events. Total and LDL cholesterol were significantly decreased on tamoxifen.

In combination with adjuvant therapy for estrogen receptor–positive breast cancer, tamoxifen can decrease the risk of recurrence and death and aid those with metastatic disease.

As with raloxifene, patients taking tamoxifen have a greater risk for VTE. This association is found particularly in patients who are concomitantly receiving chemotherapy.

The main difference between raloxifene and tamoxifen is that tamoxifen use is associated with a greater risk of endometrial cancers, especially uterine sarcoma. This risk depended on length of treatment. As a result, the American College of Obstetrics and Gynecologists (ACOG) has recommendations regarding monitoring women taking tamoxifen (Box 7), but these are not evidence based. For prevention, an intrauterine levonorgestrel could be placed. Even though there is evidence to suggest that tamoxifen is effective in preventing and treating osteoporosis, it is not approved by the FDA except for the prevention and treatment of breast cancer.

REFERENCES

American College of Obstetricians and Gynecologists: Tamoxifen and endometrial cancer. ACOG Committee Opinion 232. Washington, DC: American College of Obstetricians and Gynecologists 2000.

American College of Obstetricians and Gynecologists Task Force: Hormone Therapy. Obstet Gynecol 2004;104(suppl 4):S1-S129.

Barnabei VM, Cochrane BB, Aragaki AK, et al: Menopausal symptoms and treatment-related effects of estrogen and progestin in the Women's Health Initiative. Obstet Gynecol 2005;105:1063-1073.

Barrett-Connor E, Cauley JA, Kulkarni PM, et al: Risk-benefit profile for raloxifene: 4-Year data from the Multiple Outcomes of Raloxifene Evaluation (MORE) randomized trial. J Bone Miner Res 2004;19:1270-1275.

Grady D, Herrington D, Bittner V, et al: Cardiovascular disease outcomes during 6.8 years of hormone therapy: Heart and Estrogen/Progestin Replacement Study follow-up (HERS-II). JAMA 2002;288:49-57.

Hulley S, Grady D, Bush T, et al, for the Heart and Estrogen/Progestin Replacement Study (HERS) Research Group: Randomized trial of estrogen plus progestin for secondary prevention of coronary heart disease in postmenopausal women. JAMA 1998;280:605-613.

North American Menopause Society: Treatment of menopause-associated vasomotor symptoms: Position statement of The North American Menopause Society. Menopause 2004;11:11-33.

Soules MR, Sherman S, Parrott E, Rebar R: Executive summary: Stages of Reproductive Aging Workshop (STRAW). Fertil Steril 2001;76:874-878.

Women's Health Initiative Steering Committee: Effects of conjugated equine estrogen in postmenopausal women with hysterectomy. JAMA 2004;291:1707-1712.

Writing Group for the PEPI Trial: Effects of estrogen or estrogen/progestin regimens on heart disease risk factors in postmenopausal women. The Postmenopausal Estrogen/Progestin Interventions (PEPI) Trial. JAMA 1995;273:199-208.

Writing Group for the Women's Health Initiative Investigators: Risks and benefits of estrogen plus progestin in healthy postmenopausal women: Principal results from the Women's Health Initiative randomized controlled trial. JAMA 2002;288:321-333.

---

[1] Not FDA approved for this indication.

Vulvovaginitis

Method of
Christine Hudak, MD

From a medical perspective, it is tempting to consider vulvovaginitis a minor problem. However, to the woman affected, getting relief is quite important. In addition to the immediate physical discomfort and potential risks in pregnancy, those with untreated vaginitis can experience body image issues and sexual problems. Evaluation of vaginitis accounts for more than 10 million office visits a year in the United States, so proper diagnosis and management are essential. This article addresses the most common causes of vaginitis: bacterial vaginosis (40%-50% of cases), candidiasis (20%-25%), and trichomoniasis (15%-20%.) Of these three, only trichomoniasis is sexually transmitted, although all have been associated with other sexually transmitted infections.

Symptoms of vaginitis most commonly include vaginal redness, itching, and discharge that may be malodorous. Trichomoniasis can also cause dysuria, dyspareunia, and postcoital bleeding. Candidal infections can also produce vulvar redness, itching, dysuria, and dyspareunia.

Identifying the etiology of vaginitis is primarily based on patient history, pelvic examination, vaginal pH measurement, and microscopic evaluation of the discharge. Even in expert hands, the sensitivity of a 0.9% normal saline and 10% KOH slide preparations is 50% to 60%. Culture and newer office-based testing options are also available.

Bacterial Vaginosis

Bacterial vaginosis is not an infection but rather a shift in the normal bacterial vaginal flora. There is a decrease of lactobacilli and an overgrowth of *Gardnerella vaginalis, Mycoplasma hominus,* and anaerobes. Factors that are associated with bacterial vaginosis include multiple sex partners, a new sex partner, and douching.

Clinical indicators of bacterial vaginosis include Amsel's criteria: abnormal gray discharge, vaginal pH greater than 4.5, a positive amine test, and more than 20% clue cells on normal saline microscopy. If two or three of the criteria are present, the clinical diagnosis of bacterial vaginosis can be made with a 90% sensitivity and 77% specificity. (The amine test is commonly referred to as the *whiff test* and is positive if the addition of KOH to a sample of the discharge produces a strong fishy odor.) Additional microscopic findings can include a large amount of coccobacillary bacteria and a lack of lactobacilli.

A recent meta-analysis evaluating the accuracy of signs and symptoms of vaginitis to determine etiology found that in patients with the symptom of vaginal odor, the likelihood ratio for having bacterial vaginosis was 1.6 with a sensitivity of 97% and a specificity of 40%. The use of culture for the diagnosis of bacterial vaginosis is not recommended because the organisms in question are all normal vaginal flora. There is also a rapid office test available (QuickVue Advance *G. vaginalis* test) for CLIA (Clinical Laboratory Improvement Admendment) moderately complex labs. Changes suggesting bacterial vaginosis reported on a Papanicolaou (Pap) smear do not require treatment unless the patient is symptomatic.

In addition to causing vaginitis, bacterial vaginosis has also been associated with pelvic inflammatory disease, infections after gynecologic surgery, and acquisition of sexually transmitted infections such as herpes and HIV. Treatment for bacterial vaginosis prior to hysterectomy and abortion decreases the postoperative infection rate.

In pregnant patients, bacterial vaginosis has been associated with premature rupture of membranes (PROM), prematurity, chorioamnionitis, and low birth weight. In symptomatic patients, the treatment of bacterial vaginosis decreases those risks, though the current data do not support screening asymptomatic patients during pregnancy. The exception may be for women at high risk for preterm delivery.

BOX 1 Treatment of Bacterial Vaginosis

Nonpregnant Patients
Recommended Regimens

Metronidazole (Flagyl): 500 mg PO bid × 7 days
Metronidazole gel 0.75% (MetroGel-Vaginal): 1 applicator (5 g) intravaginally qhs × 5 days
Clindamycin cream 2% (Cleocin): 1 applicator (5 g) intravaginally qhs × 7 days

Alternative Regimens

Clindamycin (Cleocin): 300 mg PO bid × 7 days
Clindamycin ovules (Cleocin): 100 g intravaginally qhs × 3 days

Pregnant Patients

Metronidazole (Flagyl): 500 mg PO bid × 7 days
Metronidazole: 250 mg PO tid × 7 days
Clindamycin (Cleocin): 300 mg PO bid × 7 days

Several studies demonstrated that screening and treating asymptomatic pregnant women for bacterial vaginosis decreased the risk of prematurity and PROM, although one study did not show a benefit.

Box 1 summarizes the 2006 Centers for Disease Control and Prevention (CDC) recommendations for treating bacterial vaginosis. Because this is not a sexually transmitted infection, treatment of the partner is not recommended.

Vulvovaginal Candidiasis

Vulvovaginal candidiasis is the second most common etiology of clinical vaginitis. Symptoms of candidiasis are vaginal itching, irritation, a thick white discharge, dysuria, and dyspareunia. With the availability of over-the-counter antifungal treatments, many women self-diagnose and treat their symptoms. Unfortunately, the accuracy of self-diagnosis is not very good. If women have had a prior episode of candidiasis, they correctly identify recurrence 36% of the time. With no prior episode, self-diagnosis accuracy drops to 9%. Women treating themselves empirically for candidiasis can delay treatment of other more serious disorders. Although self-treatment may be a good option for some, it is important for patients to be evaluated by a physician if the initial treatment fails.

Similarly, physicians are not very accurate at making the diagnosis from symptoms and physical examination findings alone. The most predictive signs and symptoms are thick white curdlike discharge and vulvar inflammation. Microscopy with 10% KOH demonstrates blastospores or pseudohyphae and few (if any) leukocytes. Vaginal pH is typically normal in the presence of candidiasis, 4 to 4.5. The sensitivity of microscopy has been estimated at 65% and varies with the experience of the physician.

Most candidiasis is caused by *Candida albicans,* although non-albicans types can also cause symptoms. *Candida* is normal flora in the vagina and so is not a sexually transmitted infection but rather an overgrowth phenomenon like bacterial vaginosis. Culture is typically reserved for women who do not respond to treatment and is especially helpful when identifying non-albicans infections. *Candida glabrata* does not form the typical pseudohyphae seen on microscopy of *C. albicans.*

The CDC divides candidiasis into two categories: complicated and uncomplicated. Patient risk factors for complicated candidiasis include pregnancy, diabetes (or other serious medical conditions) and immunocompromised status. Other characteristics of complicated candidiasis are the suspicion of a non-albicans infection, a severe infection, or infection that recurs four or more times a year. Treatment recommendations are different for complicated and uncomplicated candidiasis. Partners of women with candidiasis do not need to be treated because this is not a sexually transmitted infection. Candidiasis has not been associated with any pregnancy risks.

BOX 2 Treatment of Uncomplicated Vulvovaginal Candidiasis

1-Day Therapy

Fluconazole (Diflucan): 1 150-mg tablet PO
Butoconazole 2% SR cream (Gynazole-1): 1 applicator (5 g) intravaginally × 1
Tioconazole 6.5% cream (Monistat-1, Vagistat-1): 1 applicator (4.6 g) intravaginally × 1
Miconazole 1200 mg suppository (Monistat-1 Combination Pack): 1 suppository intravaginally × 1

3-Day Therapy

Butoconazole 2% cream (Femstat-3, Mycelex 3) 1 applicator (5 g) intravaginally qhs × 3 days
Terconazole 0.8% cream (Terazol-3), 1 applicator (5 g) intravaginally qhs × 3 days
Clotrimazole 200 mg vaginal tablet (Gyne-Lotrimin-3) 1 tablet intravaginally qhs × 3 days
Miconazole 200 mg suppository (M-zole 3 combo pack) 1 suppository intravaginally qhs × 3 days
Terconazole 80 mg suppository (Terazol-3) 1 suppository intravaginally qhs × 3 days

7-Day+ Therapy

Clotrimazole 1% cream (Gyne-Lotrimin 7, Mycelex-7): 1 applicator (5 g) intravaginally qhs × 7-14 days
Miconazole 2% cream Femizol-M, Monistat-7): 1 applicator (5 g) intravaginally qhs × 7 days
Terconazole 0.4% cream (Terazol-7) 1 applicator (5 g): intravaginally × 7 days
Clotrimazole 100 mg tab (Mycelex-7 Combo pack): 1 tab intravaginally qhs × 7 days
Miconazole 100 mg suppository (Monistat 7): 1 suppository intravaginally qhs × 7 days
Nystatin 100,000 U tab: 1 tab intravaginally qhs × 14 days

Boxes 2 and 3 summarize the 2006 CDC recommendations for treatment of candidiasis.

Non-albicans infections such as those caused by *C. glabrata* are only about 50% responsive to the azoles. For azole treatment failure, 600 mg vaginal boric acid capsules[6] can be used daily for 14 days. Topical flucytosine cream[1,6] has also been used successfully in resistant infections. For recurrent candidiasis, maintenance regimens are suggested by the CDC, although there is a high rate of relapse once the medications are discontinued.

---

[1]Not FDA approved for this indication.
[6]May be compounded by pharmacists.

BOX 3 Treatment of Complicated Vulvovaginal Candidiasis

Treatment Regimens

Fluconazole (Diflucan) 100, 150, or 200 mg tablet: 1 tablet PO q 3 days × 3 doses
Topical azole cream, tablet or suppository: 1 dose intravaginally qhs × 7-14 days

Maintenance Regimens

Fluconazole 100, 150, or 200 mg tablet: 1 tablet PO every week × 6 months
Clotrimazole 200 mg suppository (Gyne-Lotrimin 3): 1 suppository intravaginally qhs 2×/week
Butoconazole 2% cream (Femstat-3, Mycelex-3): 1 applicator (5 g) intravaginally qhs × 3 days

---

 CURRENT DIAGNOSIS

- Bacterial vaginosis: pH, >4.5; 20% clue cells, malodorous discharge
- Vulvovaginal candidiasis: pH, 4-4.5; pseudohyphae, blastospores, thick curdlike discharge, vulvar inflammation
- *Trichomonas* vaginitis: pH, >4.5; motile, flagellated trichomonads, many WBCs, yellow discharge, vulvovaginal inflammation

Trichomonas Vaginitis

Trichomoniasis is sexually transmitted and caused by the flagellated protozoan, *Trichomonas vaginalis*. Women may be asymptomatic (as their partners often are) or report symptoms of malodorous yellow-green discharge, itching, dysuria, dyspareunia, and postcoital bleeding.

Diagnosis in women is most commonly made by viewing motile trichomonads microscopically, which has a sensitivity of 60% to 70%. A large number of white blood cells can also be seen on the wet preparation. Vaginal pH is typically higher than normal. Office point-of-care testing kits are available, including the OSOM Trichomonas Rapid Test and the Affirm VP III (the last tests for *T. vaginalis*, *G. vaginalis*, and *C. albicans*). Samples may also be sent for culture of trichomonas, although they are not commonly used clinically.

In men, urethral swab, urine, or semen can be cultured if necessary because the wet preparation and microscopy are not sensitive. Physicians might consider empirically treating the partner to decrease the rate of reinfection.

In pregnant patients, trichomonas infection is associated with harmful outcomes such as PROM, preterm delivery, and low-birth-weight babies. Curiously, studies that have been done to date do not show a decrease in these outcomes when women have been treated. Those studies had some limitations, and there is no current recommendation about the necessity of treatment in pregnancy. However, the most common medication for treatment, metronidazole (Flagyl), is Category B and considered safe for use in all trimesters.

Box 4 summarizes the 2006 CDC recommendations for treatment of *Trichomonas* vaginitis.

Tinidazole (Tindamax) is newly approved in the United States for the treatment of trichomoniasis and is as efficacious as metronidazole. Resistance to metronidazole is estimated to be less than 5%, and this can often be overcome with a higher dose of metronidazole or by treating with tinidazole due to its longer half-life. Topical preparations of metronidazole (MetroGel-Vaginal, Vandazole) are not very successful in treating trichomonas and are not recommended. Follow-up testing is not required for patients who are asymptomatic after treatment.

BOX 4 Treatment of Trichomoniasis

Recommended Regimens

Metronidazole (Flagyl) 2 g PO × 1 dose *or*
Tinidazole (Tindamax) 2 g PO × 1 dose

Alternative Regimen

Metronidazole 500 mg PO bid × 7 days

REFERENCES

ACOG Committee on Practice Bulletins—Gynecology: ACOG Practice Bulletin. Clinical managementgidelines for obstetrician–gynecologists, Number 72, May 2006: Vaginitis. Obstet Gynecol 2006;107:1195-1206.

Anderson, MR, Klink, K, Cohrssen, A: Evaluation of vaginal complaints. JAMA 2004;291(11):1368-1379.

Centers for Disease Control and Prevention Workowski KA, Berman SM: Sexually transmitted diseases treatment guidelines, 2006. MMWR Recomm Rep 2006;55(RR-11):1-94.

Owen, MK, Clenney, TL: Management of vaginitis. Am Fam Physician 2004;70:2125-2132, 2139-2140.

Chlamydia trachomatis

Method of
Catherine Stevens-Simon, MD[*]

The Scope of the Problem

Responsible for more than 3 million infections each year in the United States, *Chlamydia trachomatis* poses a public health problem of epidemic proportions. Because of the large reservoir of undiagnosed, asymptomatic infections, the number of reported cases significantly underestimates the true prevalence of this infection. Nonetheless, *C. trachomatis* is not only the most commonly reported bacterial sexually transmitted disease (STD) in the United States but also the nation's most commonly reported bacterial infection. It is difficult to give meaningful prevalence figures because the proportion of infected individuals depends on the characteristics of the population studied and how they are studied. In addition, whereas passive surveillance systems indicate that the prevalence of this infection has risen precipitously over the last decade, studies conducted at sentinel surveillance sites demonstrate a decline, which suggests that expanded screening, increased reporting, and improved test sensitivity mask a true decrease in prevalence in some sectors of American society. The epidemiologic characteristics and clinical manifestations of chlamydial infections in the United States reflect the fact that most infections are sexually transmitted and that prevalent stereotypes have an affinity for columnar epithelium. Teenage girls are most susceptible to these infections because of the following factors:

- At their age, the columnar epithelium is prominent on the ectocervix.
- Some experience a high level of unprotected, serially monogamous sexual activity with older men whose sexual risk profiles they rarely investigate.

With these two factors combined, teenage girls are at maximal biologic and social risk. Although the national prevalence of chlamydial infections in this population is unknown, school- and clinic-based studies suggest a range of 8% to 26% (compared to 3% to 5% in sociodemographically similar young adult women), with the highest age-specific prevalence reported among adolescents ages 14 to 15 years. Although readily eradicable, the economic and human costs of these infections are staggering. Annual expenditures are estimated to exceed $1.5 billion, with 75% of the cost devoted to treating sequelae of cervical infections that were initially uncomplicated. Because the majority of severe consequences of untreated infections occur in women, and as much as 66.6% of tubal factor infertility and 33.3% of ectopic pregnancies in the United States are attributed to chlamydial infections, it is estimated that every dollar spent on screening and treating asymptomatic young women and their sex partners saves approximately $12. Although this uniquely positions primary health care providers to prevent the costly sequelae of chlamydial infections, given their prevalence among teenagers, expansion of screening and treatment programs to nontraditional settings such as schools, juvenile detention centers, and drug treatment facilities is likely to be a critical component of any national strategy to ontrol this infection.

Clinical Presentation

Chlamydial infections are an excellent example of the dependence of the clinical manifestations of disease on the intrinsic properties of the pathogen and host. In Western industrialized countries, virtually all chlamydial infections are either sexually transmitted or vertically transmitted at birth. They are caused by nonlymphogranuloma venereum stereotypes that have an affinity for columnar epithelium and can only survive by a cytotoxic, replicative cycle that evokes a variable immune response in the host. Hence, in the United States, the endocervix, urethra, rectum, and conjunctiva are preferentially affected, and clinical manifestations range from asymptomatic to florid inflammatory conditions with severe reproductive consequences. *Chlamydia* should be suspected in these populations:

- Women and men with dysuria and pyuria
- Women with dyspareunia; abnormal vaginal discharge; postcoital, irregular menstrual, or breakthrough contraceptive bleeding; and lower abdominal or pelvic pain
- Infants with conjunctivitis or a staccato cough

These signs and symptoms are neither a sensitive nor a specific indication of infection, however. Indeed, because nearly 90% of chlamydial infections are asymptomatic and *C. trachomatis* is isolated from less than 33.3% of women with mucopurulent cervicitis and less than 50% of men with nongonococcal urethritis, such complaints are unreliable predictors of infection. In women, the most common sign is mucopurulent cervicitis, a nonspecific clinical syndrome characterized by erythema, edema, and friability of the ectocervix and purulent endocervical exudate. Mucopurulent cervicitis, however, is also caused by other STDs and noninfectious factors (i.e., cyclical fluctuations in gonadal hormones), which increase the size of the cervical ectropion or the resident population of cervical leukocytes. Other clinical manifestations of lower genital tract chlamydial infections in women include urethritis and bartholinitis. Although pelvic inflammatory disease (PID) is a polymicrobial infection, *C. trachomatis* is also often involved, and, conversely, PID is the most common complication of chlamydial cervicitis. The estimated incidence ranges from 10% to 40% in untrcatcd womcn. Young age and prolonged or recurrent infection significantly increase, whereas treatment of asymptomatic infections significantly decreases both disease severity and sequelae, such as salpingo-oophoritis, perihepatitis (Fitz-Hugh-Curtis syndrome), infertility, ectopic pregnancy, and chronic pelvic pain. Adverse outcomes associated with chlamydial infections during pregnancy include preterm labor, premature rupture of the placental membranes, low-birth-weight delivery, neonatal death, postpartum or postabortal endometritis, and vertical transmission to infants. In the infected infants, 30% to 50% develop conjunctivitis, 15% to 20% develop nasopharyngitis, and 5% to 10% develop pneumonia.

In men, the most common clinical manifestation is urethritis, the symptoms of which typically commence 1 to 3 weeks after exposure and range from mild dysuria to frank penile discharge. Other clinical syndromes in men include epididymitis, prostatitis, acute proctocolitis, and Reiter syndrome (urethritis, conjunctivitis, arthritis, and mucocutaneous lesions). These suppurative complications rarely require inpatient therapy and are far less common than those encountered in women. Nonetheless, sequelae ranging from urethral strictures to infertility do occur. Nongenital clinical manifestations, such as conjunctivitis, tenosynovitis, and arthritis, are uncommon among adults in the United States.

---

[*]Deceased.

Diagnosis and Screening

In the United States, testing for both symptomatic and asymptomatic chlamydial infections is done with ligase chain reaction (LCR), polymerase chain reaction (PCR), and other nucleic acid amplification techniques (NAATs) because they do not require the presence of intact organisms. Urine, cervical, vaginal, or urethral fluids can be used as the analyte for these tests; specimens are stable and easy to transport; and results can be obtained within a day. This is a major advantage over the stringent collection, transport, and 3-day growth period culturing requirements associated with this fastidious organism. Although nonculture assays, non-NAATs, and rapid diagnostic tests capable of making a diagnosis within 30 minutes are available, these assays are too insensitive to be recommended for routine testing.

The signs and symptoms of chlamydial infection are nonspecific and often persist for weeks after documented eradication of the pathogen. Because of this, leukocyte, esterase-positive urine dipsticks, leukocyte-laden vaginal wet mounts, and endocervical Gram stains should be regarded as no more than a trigger for testing. Although concerns about the consequences of underdiagnosis and undertreatment typically overshadow concerns about the consequences of overdiagnosis and overtreatment, therapeutic decisions should not be based on these poorly standardized tests. Indeed, given their low positive predictive value for chlamydial infections, the adverse psychological effects of being diagnosed with an STD, and the serious public health problems that the indiscriminate use of antibiotics creates—even in settings where the prevalence of chlamydial infections is high and patient follow-up is uncertain and in resource-poor clinics where NAATs are unavailable—enthusiasm for the practice of diagnosing chlamydial infections empirically. This must be tempered by the knowledge that to prevent one individual from suffering the sequelae of an untreated infection, hundreds will needlessly suffer the adverse psychosocial consequences of an STD diagnosis. This is true even when the diagnosis is made based on characteristic symptom complexes, suggestive leukocyte esterase urine dipsticks, and/or vaginal wet mounts. Thus, with sensitivities and specificities fluctuating approximately 98% on male urethral and urine specimens as well as on female cervical specimens, NAATs are currently the best chlamydial tests available. However, because the sensitivity of these assays for detecting infections in women is significantly lower when urine (80% to 95%) or patient- or provider-collected vaginal fluid (70% to 85%) is the analyte, endocervical specimens should be used, except in screening situations where it is impractical to perform pelvic examinations. Thus every case diagnosed on a urine or vaginal specimen is a bonus.

CURRENT DIAGNOSIS

- Signs and symptoms are neither a sensitive nor a specific indication of chlamydial infection and often persist for weeks after documented eradication of the pathogen.
  Most chlamydial infections are asymptomatic.
  Chlamydia trachomatis is isolated from less than half of women and men with the most common signs and symptoms (mucopurulent cervicitis and urethritis).
- *Chlamydia* should be suspected in:
  Women and men with dysuria and pyuria.
  Women with dyspareunia, abnormal vaginal discharge, abnormal bleeding, and lower abdominal or pelvic pain; infants with conjunctivitis or a staccato cough
- Routine periodic screening with nucleic acid amplification techniques (NAATs) is the only reliable way to diagnose this infection.

Despite consensus about how to screen, uncertainty continues about whom to screen and how frequently to screen them. Pregnant women and sexually active women younger than 25 years of age are the only groups for whom there is good evidence that the benefits of screening outweigh the harms. Specifically, when prevalence rates exceed 2%, testing and treating these individuals for asymptomatic chlamydial infections is a cost-effective preventive measure that:

- Averts PID and associated medical complications.
- Reduces transmission to sex partners.
- Reduces the risk of acquiring HIV.
- Lowers the prevalence of *Chlamydia* in the community.

It is unlikely that these benefits reflect factors other than screening (i.e., increased condom use) because knowledge of sexual risk behavior adds nothing to predictive algorithms that include age and prior STD history. However, because of the highly infectious nature of this bacterium, the lack of a vaccine, and the failure of the human immune system to build up resistance to the bacteria, reinfection of effectively treated individuals tends to diminish short-term efficacy, making long-term periodic screening a prerequisite of cost efficacy.

The only other caveat is that most cost-effectiveness analyses are based on culture-proven disease and therefore may reflect a larger inoculum than infections diagnosed by NAAT assays, which can detect extremely low levels of viable and nonviable organisms. Thus further research is needed to determine if and how inoculum size affects disease presentation and to define the clinical and public health significance of NAAT-detectable infections. Specifically, studies comparing transmission rates and the clinical consequences of infections that are detected only by NAAT assay versus those that are detected by traditional assays are still needed to prove that routine, periodic, urine-based screening of asymptomatic individuals is a cost-effective way to control chlamydial infections at the population level. Moreover, because identifying infected individuals is only the first step in effective disease control, it is also important to demonstrate that once identified, the majority of these asymptomatically infected individuals and their sex partners can be contacted and treated. The randomized trial data that determine how frequently community members should be screened to lower chlamydial infections at the population level are lacking; however, observational studies consistently indicate that among sexually active teens the median time between first and repeat infections is approximately 6 months. Based on these data, biannual screening seems reasonable for women at this age (older than 25 years). Because the risk of reinfection is inversely related to age, it is unclear if this recommendation should be extended to young adults. Nevertheless, a history of prior infection predicts reinfection regardless of sexual risk behavior, and in women repeat infections are implicated in the pathogenesis of upper genital tract damage. It may be wise, therefore, to rescreen all women who were treated for chlamydial infections at 6-month intervals.

Developing selective screening criteria is a vigorously pursued public health goal. With the exception of age, however, no single demographic or behavioral risk factor or combination of risk factors consistently identifies a group of young, sexually active women who should not be screened. The utility of more selective screening is limited by the high proportion of missed infections.

Parallel evidence to support screening asymptomatic men may be lacking because before the introduction of urine screening men were not routinely tested for chlamydial infection. But because the cost of treating men is lower than the cost of treating women, a greater proportion of infected men are symptomatic than women, and the harm associated with misdiagnoses is not inconsequent, it will undoubtedly be more difficult to justify routine periodic male screening. However, false-negative test results create a reservoir of untreated disease that is likely to contribute disproportionately to the spread of *C. trachomatis*; but the psychosocial consequences of false-positive test results can range from dysphoric feelings and decreased self-esteem to the disruption of romantic relationships and domestic violence. Moreover, if treatment is initiated inappropriately, the adverse effects of drug reactions and bacterial resistance caused by antibiotic overuse must be taken into account. Thus, until more data become available, the United States Preventive Services Task Force recommends symptom-based screening for all men and for women older than 25 years of age who do not exhibit other characteristics associated with a high prevalence of chlamydial infections (i.e., unmarried status, African American race, a history of STDs, a history of new or multiple sex partners, cervical ectopy, and inconsistent condom use).

Treatment

Recommendations for antibiotic treatment of chlamydial infections depend on the clinical syndrome. Box 1 summarizes the options for outpatient therapy of uncomplicated genital tract infections in men and women. However, because humans do not develop a natural immunity to chlamydia, treated patients remain at risk for reinfection. For this reason therapy should not be considered complete until all recent sexual contacts are treated and the patient is counseled about future disease prevention. An estimated 70% of the male partners of women with chlamydial cervicitis are infected, and, conversely, approximately 30% of the female partners of *Chlamydia*-infected men are infected. Treatment is recommended for the most recent sex partner and all other individuals who had sexual contact with the infected person during the 60 days preceding the onset of symptoms or diagnosis. Also, partners should abstain from sexual intercourse for a week after they complete treatment.

CURRENT THERAPY

- Antibiotic treatment is easy to summarize in tabular form but is ineffective if given in isolation of sexual network.
    - Large reservoir of asymptomatically infected partners and potential partners undermines the effectiveness of individual treatments.
    - Half of all chlamydial infections occur in previously-treated persons.
- Therapy is not complete until all recent sexual contacts are treated and patient counseled about disease prevention.
- Prevalence of *Chlamydia trachomatis* in the sexual network is the best predictor of infection.
- Who an individual has sexual intercourse with puts them at higher risk for acquisition of this infection than how they do so.
- For disease prevention—condoms are plan B—plan A is choosing low-risk sexual partners.

BOX 1 *Chlamydia trachomatis*: Recommended Treatment Regimens by Clinical Syndrome

Asymptomatic, cervicitis, urethritis*

- First-choice regimen
- Azithromycin (Zithromax), 1 g orally in a single dose

or

- Doxycycline (Vibramycin), 100 mg orally twice a day for 7 days

Alternative Regimens (One of the Following)

- Erythromycin base (E-Mycin), 500 mg orally four times a day for 7 days
- Erythromycin ethylsuccinate (EES), 800 mg orally four times a day for 7 days
- Ofloxacin (Floxin), 300 mg orally twice a day for 7 days
- Levofloxacin (Levaquin),[1] 500 mg orally for 7 days

Epididymitis

- Ceftriaxone (Rocephin),[1] 250 mg intramuscularly (single dose)

or

- Doxycycline,[1] 100 mg orally twice a day for 7 days

Outpatient Pelvic Inflammatory Disease

- Ceftriaxone, 250 mg intramuscularly (single dose)

plus

- Doxycycline, 100 mg orally twice a day for 14 days
  with or without
- Metronidazole (Flagyl), 500 mg orally twice a day for 14 days

Alternative Regimens

- Ceftriaxone, 250 mg intramuscularly (single dose)

or

- Cefoxitin (Mefoxin), 2 g intramuscularly (single dose)

plus

- Probenecid, 1 g orally

plus

- Doxycycline, 100 mg orally twice a day for 14 days
  with or without
- Metronidazole, 500 mg orally twice a day for 14 days

Inpatient Pelvic Inflammatory Disease[†]

- Cefotetan (Cefotan), 2 g intravenously every 12 hours

or

- Cefoxitin, 2 g intravenously every 6 hours

plus

- Doxycycline,[1] 100 mg orally or intravenously every 12 hours

Alternative Regimens

- Clindamycin, 900 mg intravenously every 8 hours

plus

- Gentamicin,[1] 2 g/kg of body weight loading dose, then 1.5 mg/kg of body weight every 8 hours. Treatment should be continued for 24 to 48 hours after significant clinical improvement occurs and then should consist of oral therapy with doxycycline, 100 mg orally twice a day for 14 days, or clindamycin, 450 mg orally four times a day, for a total of 14 days.

Providers should consult the Centers for Disease Control and Prevention's website at: http://www.cdc.gov/std/treatment/ for up-to-treatment recommendations.
[1]Not FDA approved for this indication.
*Pregnancy: Doxycycline, erythromycin estolate (Ilosone), and ofloxacin are contraindicated, and repeat testing 3 weeks after completion of therapy is recommended because antibiotics may be less efficacious. HIV infection: Patients who have chlamydial infection and who also are infected with HIV should receive the same treatment regimen as those who are HIV-negative.
[†]Studies indicate that the efficacy of inpatient and outpatient treatment is comparable in terms of fertility and other long-term health outcomes. Criteria for inpatient treatment include surgical emergencies, pregnancy, unresponsive to oral antimicrobial therapy, unable to follow or tolerate an outpatient oral regimen, severe illness, nausea and vomiting, or high fever, or tubo-ovarian abscess.

Although patient-delivered partner treatment is as effective as partner notification, partners are more likely to be treated if informed by physicians rather than by the patients. This is because only 65% (approximately) of women with known chlamydial infections refer their sex partners for therapy, and even fewer (approximately 45%) infected men do so. Because the cure rate for single-dose azithromycin (Zithromax) therapy is close to 100% and the medication can easily be administered under medical supervision, a test of cure 3 weeks after treatment—NAATs remain positive for this long despite successful eradication of infection—is only recommended for pregnant women (among whom antibiotic efficacy may be reduced) and when compliance is in doubt.

Approximately 50% of all chlamydial infections occur in previously treated persons. Demographic characteristics, such as age and a past history of chlamydial infection, are better predictors of infection than behavioral risk factors, such as multiple sexual partners and the failure to use condoms consistently. Being involved with a sexual network in which *Chlamydia* is hyperendemic appears to put individuals at greater risk for infection than unsafe sexual behavior in the general population. Hence, to control the spread of *C. trachomatis*, it may be necessary to:

- Extend screening and treatment beyond recent partners to include the group of core transmitters in the infected individual's sexual network.
- Help STD patients learn to choose less risky sex partners by promoting sexual health communication within partnerships.

Although the debate about the content and duration of counseling necessary to achieve this goal is ongoing, there is a growing consensus that brief (5 minutes), personalized (provider-delivered and client-centered) counseling sessions—aimed at personal risk reduction and increasing awareness of partner risk behavior—are more effective than the conventional didactic approach to STD prevention education. They are certainly as effective as more prolonged sessions, which are difficult to conduct in busy public health clinics.

REFERENCES

Aral SO, Hughes JP, Stoner B, et al: Sexual mixing patterns in spread of gonococcal and chlamydial infections. Am J Pub Health 1999;89:825-833.
Biro F, Workowski K, Blythe MJ, Lara-Torre E: NASPAG/JPAG roundtable discussion annual clinical meeting 2003—Philadelphia, PA: Sexually transmitted diseases (STD) treatment guidelines 2002. J Pediatr Adolesc Gynecol 2004;17:143-146.
Cates W Jr: Contraception, unintended pregnancies, and sexually transmitted diseases: Why isn't a simple solution possible? Am J Epidemiol 1996;143:311-318.
Critchlow CW, Wolner-Hanssen P, Eschenbach DA, et al: Determinants of cervical ectopia and cervicitis: Age, oral contraception, specific cervical infection, smoking, and douching. Am J Obstet Gynecol 1995;173:534-543.
Duncan B, Hart G, Scoular A, Bigrigg A: Qualitative analysis of psychosocial impact of diagnosis of *Chlamydia trachomatis*: Implications for screening. BMJ 2001;322:195-199.
Ford CA, Viadro CI, Miller WC: Testing for chlamydial and gonorrheal infections outside of clinic settings. A summary of the literature. Sex Transm Dis 2004;31:38-51.
Kamb ML, Fishbein M, Douglas JM Jr, et al: Efficacy of risk-reduction counseling to prevent human immunodeficiency virus and sexually transmitted diseases: A randomized controlled trial for the Project RESPECT Study Group. JAMA 1998;280:1161-1167.
Peipert JF: Clinical practice. Genital chlamydial infections. N Engl J Med 2003;349:2424-2430.
Rietmeijer CA, Van Bemmelen R, Judson FN, Douglas JM: Incidence and repeat infection rates of *Chlamydia trachomatis* among male and female patients in an STD clinic. Sex Transm Dis 2002;29:65-72.
U.S. Preventive Services Task Force. Screening for chlamydial infection: Recommendations and rationale. Am J Prev Med 2001;20(3S):90-94.

Pelvic Inflammatory Disease

Method of
Adrianne Williams Bagley, MD,
and Maria Trent, MD, MPH

Pelvic inflammatory disease (PID) is a spectrum of disorders characterized by an infection of the female upper genital tract. Organs that may be affected include the uterus (endometritis, parametritis), fallopian tubes (salpingitis), and ovaries (oophoritis, tubo-ovarian abscesses [TOAs]), or the infection may involve the pelvic peritoneum.

Epidemiology

Approximately 800,000 women per year are diagnosed with PID. Up to 20% of cases occur in teenagers. Risk factors associated with development of PID mirror the risk factors that increase the likelihood of acquiring a sexually transmitted infection. These risk factors include having multiple sex partners and inconsistent or incorrect use of condoms. Douching and use of intrauterine devices are also associated with PID. Women with a prior diagnosis of PID are at higher risk of developing future episodes.

Pathophysiology

The infection of the female upper genital tract that characterizes PID is caused by the ascent of infectious organisms from the vagina and cervix. It is postulated that the ascent of organisms may occur more readily during menses because of reflux of blood in the fallopian tubes, and studies show a temporal relationship between menses and the subsequent diagnosis of PID.

The infectious agents most often implicated in PID are the sexually transmitted organisms *Neisseria gonorrhoeae* and *Chlamydia trachomatis*. However, PID may be a polymicrobial infection. Other contributing infectious etiologies include anaerobic bacteria such as Bacteroides and *Peptostreptococcus* species, *Gardnerella vaginalis*, *Haemophilus influenzae*, *Streptococcus* species, *Mycoplasma hominis*, *Ureaplasma urealyticum*, enteric gram-negative bacilli, and cytomegalovirus.

Diagnosis

The diagnosis of PID is made based on clinical assessment; therefore, a detailed history, careful examination, and the use of additional supportive diagnostic tests are warranted. Patients may present with varied nonspecific complaints including lower abdominal pain, vaginal discharge, and irregular menses or bleeding with sexual intercourse. Patients may or may not be febrile, experience vomiting or diarrhea, or have urinary symptoms. The differential diagnosis includes processes that affect not only the reproductive tract but also the gastrointestinal and urinary tracts. The differential diagnosis includes but is not limited to ovarian cyst, endometriosis, dysmenorrhea, ectopic pregnancy, septic or threatened abortion, gastroenteritis, appendicitis, diverticulitis, constipation, inflammatory bowel disease, irritable bowel syndrome, urethritis, cystitis, pyelonephritis, and nephrolithiasis.

The 2006 Centers for Disease Control and Prevention (CDC) guidelines recommend empirical treatment for PID in sexually active women with minimum diagnostic criteria of uterine tenderness, adnexal tenderness, or cervical motion tenderness, in whom no other cause can be identified. Additional supportive criteria may be used to increase the specificity of diagnosis; these criteria include oral temperature greater than 38°C (101°F), abnormal cervical or vaginal

CURRENT DIAGNOSIS

- Pelvic inflammatory disease is a clinical diagnosis.
- The minimum diagnostic criterion is one or more of the following clinical findings: uterine tenderness, adnexal tenderness, *or* cervical motion tenderness in the patient in whom no other cause can be identified.
- The use of additional supportive criteria can increase the accuracy of the diagnosis.

mucopurulent discharge, presence of white blood cells on saline wet mount of vaginal secretions, elevated erythrocyte sedimentation rate (ESR) or Creactive protein (CRP), and documented cervical infection with *N. gonorrhoeae* or *C. trachomatis*. However, if cervical infection with *N. gonorrhoeae* or *C. trachomatis* is not found, these organisms can still be responsible for upper genital tract infection. Additional diagnostic tests may include complete blood cell count (CBC) with differential, urine dipstick or urinalysis, urine culture, and urine pregnancy test. Pelvic ultrasonography should be obtained if there is evidence of a pelvic mass on examination or if there is adnexal tenderness in the setting of high fever, elevated white blood cell count, or elevated CRP or ESR; this constellation of findings may suggest a TOA.

Treatment

Treatment should be initiated promptly for the patient with suspected PID to prevent complications, which include chronic pelvic pain, ectopic pregnancy, and infertility. Antibiotic treatment is broad spectrum to ensure coverage of typical pathogens, namely *N. gonorrhoeae*, *C. trachomatis*, and anaerobes. With prompt appropriate medical treatment, the future reproductive ability of the patient may be protected.

The Current Therapy box outlines the 2006 CDC treatment guidelines for inpatient treatment. Hospitalization for parenteral treatment is reserved for patients for whom surgical causes of abdominal pain cannot be excluded, patients who are pregnant, patients who fail outpatient regimens (unable to follow or tolerate an outpatient regimen, no clinical response to oral antibiotics after 72 hours), patients with severe illness, nausea, vomiting, or high fever, and patients with a TOA. Patients younger than 16 years and those with extenuating social circumstances may also be candidates for inpatient treatment.

Outpatient treatment for PID is appropriate in most cases for patients who do not meet the criteria for hospitalization. Metronidazole (Flagyl) is often included as part of the treatment regimen to provide anaerobic coverage, and it is an appropriate adjunct medication in patients who also have evidence of bacterial vaginosis on saline wet mount.

FOLLOW-UP

Patients treated with outpatient therapy should be reevaluated in 48 to 72 hours to assess response to treatment. At this visit, the medical provider can review medication adherence, readdress partner notification, review the importance of safe sexual practices, discuss related family planning issues, answer questions that the patient may have about the diagnosis, and reexamine the patient to ensure that she is improving on the current therapeutic regimen. Patients who are not improving on oral antibiotics or who have been unable to adhere with the outpatient regimen may need additional diagnostic testing for complications and hospitalization for parental treatment.

Patients being treated for PID should be advised to abstain from sexual intercourse throughout the course of treatment. All sexual partners within the past 60 days should be tested and empirically treated for both *N. gonorrhoeae* and *C. trachomatis*.

CURRENT THERAPY

Inpatient Treatment for Pelvic Inflammatory Disease

Regimen A:
- Cefotetan (Cefotan), 2 g IV q12h, *or* cefoxitin (Mefoxin), 2 g IV q6h, *plus* doxycycline (Vibramycin), 100 mg PO or IV q12h

Regimen B:
- Clindamycin (Cleocin), 900 mg IV q8h, *plus* gentamicin (Garamycin) loading dose: 2 mg/kg IV/IM, followed by maintenance dose: 1.5 mg/kg IV q8h. Single daily dosing may be substituted.

Alternative Regimen:
- Ampicillin/Sulbactam (Unasyn) 3 g IV q6h *plus* doxycycline (Vibramycin) 100 mg PO or IV q12h.

Note: Parenteral therapy for PID should be considered for 24 h following clinical improvement, and patients should be discharged home on an oral course of doxycycline (Vibramycin) 100 mg PO bid, or clindamycin (Cleocin) 450 PO qid to complete 14 d.

Outpatient Treatment for Pelvic Inflammatory Disease

Recommended Oral Regimens:
- Ceftriaxone (Rocephin), 250 mg IM in a single dose, *or*
- Cefoxitin (Mefoxin), 2 g IM in a single dose, with probenecid, 1 g PO in a single dose, *or*
- Other parenteral third-generation cephalosporins (ceftizoxime [Cefizox] or cefotaxime [Claforan]) *plus* doxycycline (Vibramycin), 100 mg PO bid for 14 d, *with or without* metronidazole (Flagyl), 500 mg PO bid for 14 d.

Alternative Oral Regimens:
- Levofloxacin (Levaquin) 500 mg PO once daily for 14 d or ofloxacin (Floxin) 400 mg PO bid for 14 d with or without metronidazole (Flagyl) 500 mg PO bid for 14 d, if the community prevalence and individual risk of gonorrhea are low (see CDC Sexually Transmitted Disease Treatment Guidelines, 2006). Testing for N. gonorrhoeae must be performed prior to treatment. If NAAT test is positive, parental cephalosporin is recommended. If culture is positive for *N. gonorrhoeae*, treatment should be based on antimicrobial susceptibility. If antimicrobial susceptibility cannot be obtained or culture is quinolone resistant *N. gonorrhoeae* (QRNG), parenteral cephalosporin is recommended.

Note: Recommendations from the Centers for Disease Control and Prevention 2006 Sexually Transmitted Diseases Treatment Guidelines are available at http://www.cdc.giv/std/treatment.
Abbreviations: IM = intramuscular; IV = intravenous; PO = orally.

Potential Complications

Short-term complications of PID include TOA and Fitz-Hugh-Curtis syndrome. Patients with TOA require hospitalization for parenteral treatment. Fitz-Hugh-Curtis syndrome is a perihepatitis that may result from spread of *N. gonorrhoeae* or *C. trachomatis* and is characterized by right upper quadrant pain.

Long-term complications of PID include chronic pelvic pain, tubal infertility secondary to scarring, and ectopic pregnancy. Patients with a history of PID have a 6- to 10-fold increased risk of ectopic pregnancy.

Prevention

Primary prevention of PID can be best accomplished by prevention of sexually transmitted infections. Sexually active women should undergo routine screening for gonorrhea and *Chlamydia* and be instructed about the importance of proper condom usage. Secondary prevention can be accomplished with partner notification and empirical treatment using antibiotics with adequate coverage for infections caused by *N. gonorrhoeae* and *C. trachomatis*.

REFERENCES

American Academy of Pediatrics: Pelvic inflammatory disease. In Pickering LK (ed): Red Book: 2003 Report of the Committee on Infectious Diseases, 26th ed. Elk Grove Village, Ill: American Academy of Pediatrics, 2003, pp 468-472.
Centers for Disease Control and Prevention: Sexually transmitted disease treatment guidelines 2006. MMWR 2006;55(No. RR-11):56-61.
Ness RB, Soper DE, Holley RL, et al: Effectiveness of inpatient and outpatient treatment strategies for women with pelvic inflammatory disease: Results from the pelvic inflammatory disease evaluation and clinical health (PEACH) randomized trial. Am J Obstet Gynecol 2002;186(5):929-937.
Rein DB, Kassler WJ, Irwin KL, et al: Direct medical costs of pelvic inflammatory disease and its sequelae: Decreasing, but still substantial. Obstet Gynecol 2000;95(3):397-402.
Shrier LA: Bacterial sexually transmitted infections: gonorrhea, chlamydia, pelvic inflammatory disease, and syphilis. In Emans SJ, Laufer MR, Goldstein DP (eds): Pediatric and Adolescent Gynecology, 5th ed. Lippincott-Raven, 2004, pp 583-598.
Trent MA, Ellen JM, Walker A: Pelvic inflammatory disease in adolescents—care delivery in pediatric ambulatory settings. Pediatr Emerg Care 2005;21(7):431-436.
Trent M, Judy SL, Ellen JM, Walker A: Use of an institutional intervention to improve quality of care for adolescents treated in pediatric ambulatory settings for pelvic inflammatory disease. J Adolesc Health 2006;39(1):50-56.
Update to CDC's sexually transmitted diseases treatment guidelines, 2006: Fluoroquinolones no longer recommended for treatment of gonococcal infections. MMWR Weekly April 13, 2007;56(14):332-336.

Uterine Leiomyomas

Method of
Tod C. Aeby, MD, and Stella Dantas, MD

Epidemiology

Uterine leiomyomas are the most common pelvic tumor in women. They affect approximately 20% of women older than 35 years of age and 40% of women older than 50 years of age, although they are found any time from puberty through menopause. Survey studies involving histologic examination of the uterus suggest they are present in more than 80% of women. Nulliparity, early menarche, and African American ethnicity increase the risk of developing leiomyomas. The incidence among women of African descent is not as high in countries other than the United States, which suggests possible dietary, environmental, and genetic influences on development. Risk is also increased in women with a higher body mass index, presumably because of the increased estrogen production in adipocytes. Pregnancy reduces the risk of developing leiomyomas.

Pathophysiology

The etiology of uterine leiomyomas is not completely understood, but development is thought to be a multistep process. They are benign monoclonal tumors of the smooth muscle of the myometrium that presumably derive from a normal myocyte. Estrogen and progesterone, in concert with local growth factors, lead to a somatic mutation of normal myometrium to a leiomyoma. Some growth factors that cause leiomyoma proliferation are epidermal growth factors, insulin-like growth factors, heparin-binding growth factors, and transforming growth factor-β. Leiomyomas develop during the reproductive years and increase in size during pregnancy. Growth usually ceases in menopause, and leiomyomas then decrease in volume. This supports the theory that estrogen and progesterone promote growth.

Symptoms and Signs

Most uterine leiomyomas are asymptomatic. They are categorized into subgroups based on their anatomic relationship and position in the uterus, and symptoms usually depend on those relationships. They can be subserosal, intramural, submucosal, or pedunculated. The most common symptom is abnormal uterine bleeding, usually menorrhagia, occurring in 30% of women with leiomyomas. The cause of the abnormal bleeding is not totally clear but may be the result of abnormal growth and function of the endometrium near the leiomyoma and local interference with normal physiologic mechanisms for hemostasis.

Pelvic pain and increasing pelvic pressure occur in 30% of women with leiomyomas. Other symptoms include dysmenorrhea, postcoital bleeding, and dyspareunia. Pain can be caused by leiomyomas outgrowing their blood supply and becoming necrotic. This red degeneration is common in pregnancy. Patients may have an increasing abdominal girth and pressure symptoms as a result of large fibroids. Pressure on adjacent organs such as the bladder or bowel can cause urinary frequency and urgency or constipation. Rarely, an enlarged uterus causes a palpable kidney secondary to hydronephrosis from ureteral obstruction. Patients also may be lethargic from anemia secondary to menorrhagia. Leiomyomas may also be associated with infertility, although the relationship is controversial.

A rapidly enlarging uterus should raise concern for malignant transformation. But leiomyosarcomas are extremely rare, occurring in less than 0.1% of women operated on for presumed leiomyomas.

Diagnosis

Uterine leiomyomas are typically diagnosed at pelvic exam when an enlarged and irregularly shaped uterus is noted. Abdominal and transvaginal ultrasound is often helpful in making the diagnosis and in differentiating leiomyomas from adnexal masses or other pelvic pathology. Serial ultrasounds also can be used to monitor their growth. During a pelvic exam, it may not be possible to palpate ovaries next to an enlarged uterus, but an adnexal tumor can be suspected if the mass moves independently of the uterus. Submucosal leiomyomas are diagnosed using saline infusion sonohysterography and hysteroscopy. Definitive diagnosis requires histologic examination.

CURRENT DIAGNOSIS

- Abnormal uterine bleeding, postcoital spotting
- Pelvic pain, pressure, dysmenorrhea and dyspareunia
- Urinary frequency and urgency, constipation
- Lethargy
- Infertility
- Physical findings: Enlarged, irregular, and firm uterus
- Ultrasound: Diagnostic imaging modality of choice
- Saline infusion sonohysterography and/or hysteroscopy: Used to evaluate the uterine cavity

TABLE 1 Comparison of Various Procedures for the Treatment of Symptomatic Uterine Leiomyoma

Therapy	Success Rate	Complication Rate	Possibility of Future Childbearing	Comments
Hysterectomy	100%	40%	No	Recovery time varies depending on the route of removal.
Myomectomy and myolysis	75%	39%	Yes	Can be associated with significant blood loss and can result in an unplanned hysterectomy. Recurrent leiomyomas are common.
Myolysis			Yes	Several methods for myolysis are available, including bipolar electrocautery, laser energy, and cryotherapy.
Uterine artery embolization	77%–91%	5%	Not currently recommended	Complication rates are low but can be severe, including infection, sepsis, and nontarget tissue necrosis. A few deaths have been reported.
Hydrothermal endometrial ablation	91%*	1%-2%	No	Hysteroscopic resection of submucosal leiomyomas, prior to endometrial ablation, improves success rates. Pregnancies have occurred after these procedures, so contraception is still required.

*Best estimate based on limited studies.

Management

For the most part, asymptomatic leiomyoma should be managed expectantly. The approaches to the patient experiencing problems fall into the three general categories of medical management, conservative procedures, and hysterectomy. The choice should be individualized to the patient, based on the severity of her symptoms, her plans for future childbearing, and her personal interest in retaining her uterus. Other causes of abnormal bleeding should be considered.

Current medical therapy is limited to the use of gonadotropin-releasing hormone (GnRH) analogues and antagonists (i.e., leuprolide acetate [Lupron Depot], 3.75 mg monthly; nafarelin acetate [Synarel],[1] 200 μg intranasally twice a day; and goserelin acetate implant [Zoladex],[1] 3.6-mg implant monthly, cetrorelix [Cetrotide]).[1] These expensive medications are shown to decrease the uterine size by up to 65%, allowing for easier or more conservative surgical treatments. The progesterone antagonist mifepristone (Mifeprex)[1] is also effective but not currently available for this purpose in the United States. GnRH therapy has significant side effects, mostly related to the induced hypoestrogenic state. To preserve bone density the duration of therapy must be limited. Additionally, the uterus rapidly returns to its enlarged size when the therapy is discontinued. These medications are a very effective means of inducing amenorrhea to allow for correction of an anemia prior to surgery.

---
[1]Not FDA approved for this indication.

Conservative procedures include myomectomy or myolysis (surgical removal or destruction of the individual fibroids while preserving the uterus), uterine artery embolization, and endometrial ablation. Each of these approaches has different risks, benefits, and complications (Table 1).

Hysterectomy remains the most common treatment for women with symptomatic leiomyoma and offers the advantage of a complete and definitive cure. The uterus can be removed through the vagina (with or without the aid of laparoscopic techniques) or through an abdominal incision. The route of removal largely depends on the size of the uterus, the patient's medical and surgical history, and the experience and preference of her surgeon.

REFERENCES

Buttram VC Jr, Reiter RC: Uterine leiomyomata: Etiology, symptomatology, and management. Fertil Steril 1981;36:433-445.

Felberbaum RE, Germer U, Ludwig M, et al: Treatment of uterine fibroids with a slow-release formulation of the gonadotrophin-releasing hormone antagonist Cetrorelix. Hum Reprod 1998;13(6):1660-1668.

Goldfarb HA: Bipolar laparoscopic needles for myoma coagulation. J Am Assoc Gynecol Laparosc 1995;2(2):175-179.

Lethaby A, Vollenhoven B, Sowter M: Pre-operative GnRH analogue therapy before hysterectomy or myomectomy for uterine fibroids. The Cochrane Database of Systematic Reviews 2001, Issue 2. Article CD000547. DOI: 10.1002/14651858.CD000547.

Parker WH, Fu YS, Berek JS: Uterine sarcoma in patients operated on for presumed leiomyoma and rapidly growing leiomyoma. Obstet Gynecol 1994;83:414.

Pron G, Bennett J, Common A, et al: Ontario Uterine Fibroid Embolization Collaboration Group. The Ontario Uterine Fibroid Embolization Trial: II. Uterine fibroid reduction and symptom relief after uterine artery embolization for fibroids. Fertil Steril 2003;79(1):120-127.

The Hydro ThermAblator system for management of menorrhagia in women with submucous myomas: 12- to 20-month follow-up. J Am Assoc Gynecol Laparosc 2003;10(4):521-527.

CURRENT THERAPY

- Only symptomatic leiomyomas require treatment.
- Medical therapy is for temporizing and making invasive procedures easier or more effective.
- Conservative procedures include myomectomy, myolysis, hydrothermal endometrial ablation, and uterine artery embolization.
- Hysterectomy is the only definitive therapy for leiomyomata.
- Choice of treatment should be made considering the severity of symptoms and respecting the patient's preferences.

Cancer of the Endometrium

Method of
D. Scott McMeekin, MD, and
Tashanna K.N. Myers, MD

> **BOX 1 Histologic Classification of Endometrial Cancers**
>
> - Endometrioid adenocarcinoma (includes adenosquamous carcinoma)
> - Mucinous carcinoma
> - Serous carcinoma
> - Clear cell carcinoma
> - Squamous carcinoma
> - Undifferentiated carcinoma
> - Mixed carcinoma

Epidemiology

Endometrial cancer is the most common gynecologic cancer facing women in the United States. The lifetime risk of endometrial cancer is currently 1 in 38. In 2007, approximately 39,000 women were found to have endometrial cancer, and 7,400 (3%) women died from the disease. Endometrial cancer is the eighth leading cause of cancer death for women in the United States. African American women appear to have a poorer prognosis: Nearly twice than many (1.8:1) African American women die from endometrial cancer than white women.

Endometrial cancer primarily occurs in postmenopausal women, and the average age at onset is 60 years. Only 25% of patients are premenopausal, and of these, only 5% are younger than 40 years.

Etiology

Endometrial cancer is classically divided into two types (Table 1). Type I, the more common form, is associated with estrogen excess and often arises in the background of a precursor lesion, atypical hyperplasia. Type II tumors are rarer and more aggressive, and they arise in a background of atrophic endometrium or polyps.

The etiology is unclear. Despite the broad generalizations of the two categories, molecular and genetic changes differentiate these two groups as well. For example, mutations of *p53* are common in papillary serous tumors and are rare in type I tumors. *PTEN* mutations are common in type I tumors but are rare in papillary serous tumors. Global gene expression profiles also differ between type I and type II tumors.

Increased exposure to endogenous or exogenous estrogen increases the risk of developing type I cancers. Since the 1970s, unopposed estrogen use has been a known risk factor, prompting the routine addition of a progestin in combination with hormone replacement therapy regimens. Endogenous exposure to estrogens associated with obesity or chronic anovulation (polycystic ovary syndrome) are believed to be more common etiologies.

Other factors associated with an increased risk of developing endometrial cancer include late menopause (older than 52 years), nulliparity, diabetes, hypertension, or a diagnosis of complex atypical hyperplasia. In contrast, normal weight, oral contraceptives, progestin use, cigarette smoking, and multiparity have been associated with a decreased incidence of endometrial cancer. Type II tumors account for a small percentage of endometrial cancers, occur in an older population, and account for nearly one half of all relapses. Papillary serous, clear cell, and perhaps, grade 3 tumors fit into the type II category. Tamoxifen (Nolvadex) used in the prophylaxis of, or treatment for, breast cancer is an established risk factor for developing either type I or type II tumors.

Presentation and Diagnosis

Patients with endometrial cancer most commonly present with abnormal bleeding. Papanicolaou (Pap) smears detect only 30% to 50% of endometrial cancers and are not useful for diagnosing endometrial cancer. The diagnosis of endometrial cancer is most commonly made by biopsy. An endometrial biopsy can usually be performed in the office and has greater than 90% diagnostic accuracy. The histologic classification of endometrial cancers is listed in Box 1. Ultrasound has also been used to evaluate abnormal bleeding. Studies show that endometrial cancers are exceedingly uncommon if the endometrial thickness is less than 5 mm on ultrasound in postmenopausal women. Symptomatic patients with a thickened endometrium or patients with persistent bleeding despite a thin lining should have a histologic evaluation.

Currently there is no good screening test for endometrial cancer, and thus there are no screening recommendations. A high degree of suspicion should be maintained for women who have received unopposed estrogens and for patients with vaginal bleeding who are postmenopausal, obese, or taking tamoxifen. Hereditary syndromes (Lynch's) account for 3% to 5% of endometrial cancers and are seen in patients with strong familial histories of hereditary nonpolyposis colorectal, ovarian, and pancreatic cancers.

Staging

Endometrial cancer is surgically staged according to the 1988 criteria established by the International Federation of Gynecology and Obstetrics (FIGO) (Table 2). Staging includes collection of pelvic washings for cytology, a hysterectomy with removal of bilateral fallopian tubes and ovaries, and pelvic and para-aortic lymph node dissection. Controversies currently exist as to who should undergo lymph node dissection (all, some, or few patients), the type of nodal dissection (sampling or complete lymphadenectomy), and when to use adjuvant therapies.

The most important pathologic prognostic indicators include histologic grade, depth of invasion and lymph node status. The Gynecologic Oncology Group (GOG) performed a surgical pathologic study evaluating 621 patients with endometrial cancer and

TABLE 1 Comparison Between Type I and Type II Endometrial Cancers

Factor	Type I	Type II
Clinical Features		
Risk factors	Unopposed estrogen	Age
Race	White > African American	White = African American
Differentiation	Well differentiated	Poorly differentiated
Histology	Endometrioid	PS, CC, Grade 3
Stage	Early	Advanced
Prognosis	Favorable	Poorer
Molecular Features		
Ploidy	Diploid	Aneuploid
k-ras over expression	Yes	Yes
her-2/neu over expression	No	Yes
p53 mutation	No	Yes
PTEN mutation	Yes	No
Microsatellite instability	Yes	No

Abbreviations: CC = clear cell; PS = papillary serous.

CURRENT DIAGNOSIS

- Patients with postmenopausal bleeding warrant endometrial biopsy.
- Patients at risk include those with abnormal bleeding and obesity, chronic anovulation, and unopposed estrogen or tamoxifen (Nolvadex) exposure.
- Office biopsy should be performed when possible, and D&C should be performed if office biopsy is not available or biopsy results are equivocal.
- Malignancy is unlikely if the endometrial stripe/thickness is less than 5 mm on ultrasound.

Abbreviation: D&C = dilation and curettage.

TABLE 3 Estimates of Distribution and Survival of Endometrial Cancer by Stage

Stage	Distribution of Cases (%)	5-year Survival (%)
Stage IA	22	92
Stage IB	37	88
Stage IC	13	78
Stage II	9	72
Stage III	15	53
Stage IV	4	10

demonstrated important associations between grade, depth of myometrial invasion, and nodal involvement. For example, patients with deeply invasive (extending into the outer two thirds of the myometrium) tumors had pelvic nodal metastases between 11% and 34%, depending on tumor grade.

Fortunately, most women with endometrial cancer have stage I disease and have a favorable prognosis (Table 3). The 5-year survival for stage I disease approaches 90%, but the 5-year survival for women with stage IV (abdominal or distant spread) disease is only about 10%.

Treatment

SURGICAL MANAGEMENT

Surgical management continues to evolve. The GOG has recently completed a large prospective trial evaluating the role of laparoscopic hysterectomy and nodal dissection compared with an abdominal approach. The study, evaluating more than 2500 patients, found that laparoscopic management was feasible, and 76% of the time patients randomized to laparoscopy could have the procedure performed without conversion to laparotomy. The numbers of nodes removed and the frequency of finding positive lymph nodes were similar in the two treatment arms. Despite an increased operative time, results showed that laparoscopic surgery resulted in a shorter hospital stay.

The benefits of routine nodal dissection include better stratification of patients into high-, intermediate-, or low risk-categories, reduced use of postoperative therapies for most node-negative patients, and improved identification of a subset of patients with nodal metastases who might benefit from adjuvant therapies. Information from a lymph node dissection is prognostic, but a lymphadenectomy is potentially therapeutic. Today, the more frequent use of nodal dissection has resulted in the less-frequent use of postoperative pelvic irradiation therapy.

Without information on nodal status, physicians and patients must decide whether or not to use postoperative therapies based on perceived risk determined from the hysterectomy findings. Because of this, many have recommended that a second surgery to complete the surgical staging be performed when only a hysterectomy was performed. Laparoscopic restaging is often a feasible approach. The risk of nodal dissection must be balanced by the information provided. Serious complications related to nodal dissection include bleeding and visceral injury, and complications have been reported to occur in less than 2% of surgeries. Lower extremity lymphedema appears to be more common but is rarely severe.

TABLE 2 FIGO (1988) Surgical Staging System for Endometrial Cancer

Stage	Description
IA	Tumor is confined to the endometrium
IB	Tumor is confined to less than one half of the myometrium
IC	Tumor is confined to more than one half of the myometrium
IIA	Cervical involvement is limited to the endocervical glands
IIB	Cervical involvement includes cervical stroma
IIIA	Tumor involves uterine serosa or adnexa or positive peritoneal cytology
IIIB	Vaginal metastases
IIIC	Tumor involves pelvic or para-aortic lymph nodes
IVA	Tumor involves bladder or bowel mucosa
IVB	Distant metastases including intra-abdominal and inguinal lymph node involvement

Abbreviation: FIGO = International Federation of Gynecology and Obstetrics.

CURRENT THERAPY

- Surgical therapy is the mainstay of endometrial cancer treatment. Laparoscopic surgery is increasingly being used.
- Surgical staging, including pelvic and para-aortic lymph node dissection, is recommended.
- The best way to define risk is to identify patients with nodal disease.
- Staging typically requires referral to a gynecologic oncologist.
- Unstaged patients may be considered for a restaging operation.
- Most patients have stage I (uterine-confined) disease.
- Low-risk patients—stages IA and IB, grades 1 or 2—require no additional therapy.
- Intermediate-risk patients—stage IB grade 3 and stage IC grades 1 or 2—require no additional therapy or vaginal cuff brachytherapy.
- High-intermediate-risk patients are those 50 years old with two risk factors or older than 70 years with one risk factor. Risk factors are:
  - Grade 2 or 3 tumor
  - Lymphovascular space involvement
  - Outer one third myometrial invasion
  - Stage I plus papillary serous or clear cell histology
- Treatment of these patients is controversial. There is no clear consensus regarding performing no additional therapy, performing vaginal cuff brachytherapy with or without chemotherapy, or performing pelvic radiation therapy.

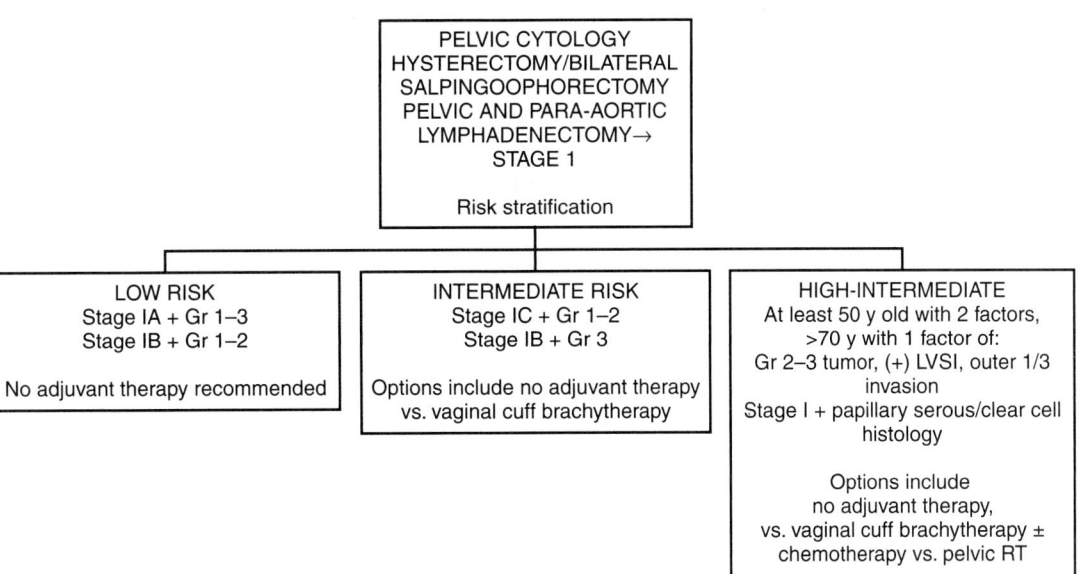

FIGURE 1. Postoperative treatment algorithm used at the University of Oklahoma for surgical staged endometrial carcinoma. Surgical staging allows risk stratification based on pathologic factors. *Abbreviations*: Gr = grade; LVSI = lymphovascular space involvement, RT = radiation therapy.

ADJUVANT THERAPY

Early Stage Disease

Two large trials have evaluated the role of post-operative pelvic radiation in patients with early stage (stage I to occult stage II) endometrial cancer. In the PORTEC trial, 715 patients were randomized to pelvic radiation or surveillance. Lymph node dissection was not performed. Most patients had low-grade tumors (90% grade 1-2), and about 50% had superficial myometrial invasion (<50% invasion). Results showed that although radiation could reduce local and regional recurrences (14% vs. 4% with radiation), 5-year survival was 81% with and 85% without radiation. Similarly, the GOG performed a study with 392 patients with grades 1 to 3 tumors and any amount of myometrial invasion. All patients had a specified lymph node dissection and received either pelvic radiation or no additional therapy. Results showed that radiation reduced local recurrences but did not appreciably affect survival (4-year survival was 92% with radiation, 86% without radiation).

The lack of benefit from pelvic radiation in these studies may be due to the excellent outcomes seen in the low-risk populations enrolled in these studies. For example, in the GOG trial, only 18% of patients had grade 3 tumors, and 31% had deep myometrial invasion. The GOG trial did suggest that a subgroup of patients at higher risk for recurrence could be defined based on age, tumor grade, depth of invasion, and the presence of lymph-vascular space invasion. These high-intermediate risk patients represented one third of the total population but accounted for two thirds of recurrences, suggesting that it might be possible to identify some patients for whom radiation might offer a benefit.

The PORTEC and GOG studies also showed that vaginal cuff recurrences were the most common site of failure without radiation, and authors for both studies suggested that vaginal cuff brachytherapy might be a reasonable alternative to for pelvic radiation. Several studies have demonstrated excellent vaginal cuff control with the use of less toxic and more tolerable vaginal cuff brachytherapy. A proposed treatment algorithm is shown in Figure 1.

Patients with papillary serous and clear cell tumors are believed by many to be at particularly increased risk for recurrence. Extrauterine disease spread is common at initial presentation, making complete surgical staging especially important in these patients. Even patients with stage I disease have a risk of failure near 30% to 50%. Chemotherapy has been increasingly advocated for this group of patients.

Advanced and Recurrent Disease

Radiation therapy (pelvic, pelvic with an extended field to treat para-aortic nodes, and whole abdominal) has been the treatment of choice for patients with disease spread outside of the uterus. Recently, the GOG presented data showing improved progression-free and overall survival when chemotherapy (doxorubicin and cisplatin) was used compared with whole abdominal radiation in patients with stage III or IV disease. As a result, chemotherapy has been increasingly used in first-line management. Combining radiation with chemotherapy is being actively explored in clinical trials.

For patients with bulky advanced or recurrent disease, hormone therapy with progestins has been a long-standing treatment. Patients with grade 1 tumors, or those with estrogen- and progesterone-receptor positive tumors have shown the greatest likelihood of benefit. Chemotherapy has been increasingly integrated in a first-line setting for many patients due to the identification of several active agents. The most active agents include paclitaxel,[1] doxorubicin,[1] and platinum analogues.[1] Combinations of these agents have resulted in improved response rates, and the three-drug paclitaxel plus doxorubicin plus cisplatin regimen has been shown to have improved survival over the two-drug doxorubicin plus cisplatin regimen. Given the advanced age and concurrent medical comorbidities that are seen in patients with endometrial cancer, a careful balance between treatment objectives and toxicity must be made.

Future Directions

Increasing the understanding of endometrial cancer at a genetic and molecular level is a primary goal of current research. This information might provide insights into the prognosis and predict benefits of particular therapies. Targeted biological agents are currently being explored in patients with endometrial cancer, and their use in combination with cytotoxic chemotherapy agents might result in improved outcomes, as seen in other solid tumors such as breast and colon cancers.

---

[1]Not FDA approved for this indication.

REFERENCES

American College of Obstetricians and Gynecologists: ACOG practice bulletin, management guidelines for obstetrician-gynecologists, number 65, August 2005: Management of endometrial cancer. Obstet Gynecol 2005;106:413-425.

Cragun J, Havrilesky L, Calingaert B, et al: Retrospective analysis of selective lymphadenectomy in apparent early-stage endometrial cancer. J Clin Oncol 2005;23:3668-3675.

Creasman W, Kohler M, Odicino F, et al: Prognosis of papillary serous, clear cell, and grade 3 stage I carcinoma of the endometrium. Gynecol Oncol 2004;95:593-596.

Creasman WT, Morrow CP, Bundy BN, et al: Surgical pathologic spread patterns of endometrial cancer. Cancer 1987;60:2035-2041.

Creutzberg C, van Putten W, Koper P, et al: Surgery and post-operative radiotherapy versus surgery alone for patients with stage 1 endometrial carcinoma: Multi-center randomized trial. Lancet 2000;355:1404-1411.

Fleming G, Brunetto V, Cella D, et al: Phase III trial of doxorubicin plus cisplatin with or without paclitaxel plus filgrastim in advanced endometrial cancer: A Gynecologic Oncology Group study. J Clin Oncol 2004;22:2159-2166.

Keys H, Roberts J, Brunetto V, et al: A phase III trial of surgery with or without adjuvant external pelvic radiation therapy in intermediate risk endometrial adenocarcinoma: A Gynecologic Oncology Group study. Gynecol Oncol 2004;92:744-751.

Kilgore LC, Partridge EE, Alvarez RD, et al: Adenocarcinoma of the endometrium: Survival comparisons of patients with and without pelvic node sampling. Gynecol Oncol 1995;56:29-33.

Randall M, Filiaci G, Muss H, et al: Whole abdominal radiotherapy versus combination doxorubicin-cisplatin chemotherapy in advanced endometrial carcinoma: A randomized phase III trial of the Gynecologic Oncology Group. J Clin Oncol 2006;24:36-44.

Straughn JM, Huh WK, Kelly FJ, et al: Conservative management of stage I endometrial carcinoma after surgical staging. Gynecol Oncol 2002;84:191-193.

Cancer of the Uterine Cervix

Method of
Nader Husseinzadeh, MD

Invasive cervical cancer accounts for 2% to 3% of all cancers in women in the United States. Incidence and mortality from cervical cancer have declined dramatically with early detection and treatment of preinvasive disease. It is estimated that approximately 9710 new cases will be diagnosed and 3700 patients died from cervical cancer in 2006 worldwide. Both incidence of and mortality from cervical cancer are second to breast cancer. Cervical cancer is a largely preventable disease with a known causative agent, the human papilloma virus (HPV), especially types 16 and 18.

Epidemiology

Age-specific incidences for white women are lower than those for African American women. Major risk factors for cervical cancer are listed in Box 1.

Some epidemiologic studies have shown that women using oral contraceptives tend to have more sexual contacts. Cigarette smoking has been linked to an increased risk of squamous cell carcinoma, and presence of nicotine byproduct as a carcinogen in cervical mucous or the partner's semen are possible explanations. Reduced risk of cervical cancer is noted in virgins and in women whose sexual partners were circumcised.

BOX 1   Major Risk Factors for Cervical Cancer

- Immunosuppression (e.g., transplant, infection with HIV)
- Multiple pregnancies
- Multiple sexual partners
- Promiscuous sexual activity
- Sexually transmitted disease (herpes simplex virus, chlamydia, and human papillomavirus)
- Smoking
- Sexual activity at a young age

Etiology and Pathogenesis

The etiology of cervical cancer is unknown. Numerous studies have indicated a close association between HPV and cervical cancer.

Although HPV appears to be the causative agent, many other changes at the molecular level have been identified that might not directly involve HPV. The molecular oncogenesis in cervical carcinoma can be explained to a degree by the regulation and function of two viral proteins, E6 and E7. The *E6* gene binds to the *p53* tumor suppressor gene and induces degradation. The *E7* gene binds another tumor suppressor, the retinoblastoma gene *(Rb)*. By binding to it, it functionally inactivates the protein, which like p53, works in cell cycle. There are more than 100 types of HPV, stratified into low-, intermediate-, and high-risk categories based on the strength of their association with invasive lesions. High-risk HPV types exhibit greater inactivation of *p53* and *Rb* genes.

The link between human leukocyte antigens (HLAs) and HPV might help to explain why the same HPV type leads to invasive cancer in one patient but not in another. It has been established that cervical dysplasia in HIV-infected women is associated with higher incidence, more rapid progression, and higher recurrence rates when compared with HIV-negative women.

Staging

Cervical cancer is staged clinically. Surgical-pathologic staging is superior to clinical staging. It provides useful information regarding the extent of disease and status of pelvic and para-aortic lymph nodes (Box 2).

PHYSICAL FINDINGS

The gross appearance of cervical cancer varies depending on whether the lesion is exophytic, endophytic, or ulcerative. Exophytic growths that characteristically bleed on contact are the most common type of cervical cancer. Sometimes the cancer develops entirely within the endocervical canal, manifesting as a hard, indurated, and often barrel-shaped lesion. The cancer can also appear as a small, shallow ulcer.

HISTOPATHOLOGY

Squamous cell carcinoma is the most common type of cervical cancer. Adenocarcinoma and other carcinomas are less common (Box 3).

PATHOPHYSIOLOGY

Cervical cancer in the early stage invades lymphatics in the parametrium and pelvic lymph nodes through tumor emboli. As the primary lesion progresses, the tumor extends to the pelvic side wall laterally, to the bladder base anteriorly, and, less frequently, to the rectum posteriorly.

SPREAD PATTERN

Cervical cancer exhibits three spread patterns. Direct extension is to parametrial tissue and the pelvic wall (ureter), to the bladder and

> **BOX 2 FIGO Staging for Carcinoma of the Cervix**
>
> - Stage 0: Carcinoma in situ, intraepithelial carcinoma
> - Stage 1: The carcinoma is strictly confined to the cervix; extension to the corpus should be disregarded.
>   - Stage IA: Invasive carcinoma diagnosed only by microscopy; all visible lesions, even with superficial invasion, are stage IB.
>   - Stage IA1: Invasion of stroma is less than 3.0 mm^2, and the horizontal spread must not exceed 7.0 mm^2.
>   - Stage IA2: Invasion of stroma is greater than 3.0 mm^2 and not more than 5.0 mm, and the horizontal spread is 7.0 mm or less. Larger lesions should be classified as stage IB.
>   - Stage IB: Clinically visible lesions confined to the cervix or lesions of greater dimensions than Stage IA2
>   - Stage IB1: Clinically visible lesions no greater than 4.0 cm or less in greatest dimension
>   - Stage IB2: Clinically visible lesions greater than 4.0 cm
> - Stage II: The carcinoma extends beyond the cervix but not to the pelvic wall or to the lower one third of the vagina.
>   - Stage IIA: Without parametral invasion, involving upper one half of the vagina
>   - Stage IIB: Tumor with parametrial invasion
> - Stage III: The tumor extends to the pelvic wall or involves the lower one third of the vagina or causes hydronephrosis or nonfunctioning kidney
>   - Stage IIIA: Tumor involves lower one third of the vagina, no extension to the pelvic wall
>   - Stage IIIB: Tumor extends to pelvic wall and/or causes hydronephrosis or nonfunctioning kidney
> - Stage IV: The tumor has extended beyond the true pelvis or has involved the mucosa of the bladder or rectum. A bullous edema does not qualify as a criterion for stage IV disease.
>   - Stage IVA: Tumor spread to adjacent organs (bladder, rectum, or both)
>   - Stage IVB: Distant metastasis
>
> *Abbreviation*: FIGO = International Federation of Gynecology and Obstetrics.

> **BOX 3 Histopathology of Cervical Cancer**
>
> - Squamous cell carcinoma (80%)
> - Nonsquamous carcinoma (15%)
>   - Adenocarcinoma
>   - Adenosquamous carcinoma
>   - Clear cell adenocarcinoma
>   - Glassy cell carcinoma
>   - Small cell (neuroendocrine) carcinoma
> - Other carcinomas (5%)
>   - Choriocarcinoma
>   - Melanoma
>   - Metastatic: uterus (most common), then breast, stomach, and bladder; leukemia and lymphoma are rare
>   - Sarcoma: stromal sarcoma, leiomyosarcoma, mixed mesodermal sarcoma, rhabdomyosarcoma

rectum, or to the uterine corpus and vagina. Lymphatic spread is of two kinds. The primary group involves the paracervical, obturator, hypogastric, and external iliac lymph nodes, and the secondary group involves the common iliac, inguinal, and aortic lymph nodes. Hematogenous spread is to the lung, liver, bone, and brain.

EXAMINATION AND TESTING

The initial work-up includes history and physical examination; chest x-ray, intravenous pyelogram (IVP), or computed tomography (CT); and HIV testing (Box 4). Some centers do not routinely use IVP and CT or cystoscopy and protosigmoidoscopy for early-stage disease because of relatively low yield. In patients who are not candidates for surgery, a CT scan can be helpful in assessing nodal disease. Enlarged lymph nodes should be studied histocytologically by either surgical excision or fine-needle aspiration because of the 5% to 10% false-positive rate of a CT scan. More recently, magnetic resonance imaging (MRI) has been studied for early parametrial and nodal disease. Positron emission tomography (PET) has been reported as useful to predict para-aortic disease. Because of infrequent colon involvement, sigmoidoscopy or barium enema should be restricted to symptomatic patients or those with a positive guiac test.

Treatment

SURGERY AND RADIATION

In general, early-stage cervical cancer can be treated with radical hysterectomy or radiation. However, surgery is preferred for premenopausal women to preserve ovarian function and a functioning vagina following surgery. In patients with high-risk criteria—positive surgical margin, parametrial involvement, and positive pelvic nodes—cisplatin-based chemoradiation is usually recommended. Those with intermediate risk factors such as tumor size greater than 4 cm, deep cervical stromal invasion greater than 50%, or lymphovascular invasion might also benefit from chemoradiation.

Radical trachelectomy is a reasonable alternative treatment for select young patients who desire to maintain their childbearing capacity. The criteria include early-stage cervical cancer with a lesion less than 2 cm, no lymphovascular invasion, and no lymph node metastasis.

Laparascopic-assisted radical vaginal hysterectomy (LARVH), like other surgical procedures, may be considered in select patients with early-stage cervical cancer. Reported advantages are less blood loss, better cosmetic results, shorter hospitalization, and earlier recovery.

CHEMORADIATION THERAPY

Squamous cell carcinoma of the cervix is a chemosensitive malignancy, particularly when cisplatinum-based chemotherapy is being used. In February 1999, the National Cancer Institute published a consensus statement demonstrating superiority of platinum-based chemoradiation compared with radiation alone for locally advanced cervical cancer (stage IIB-IVA), high-risk early-stage cervical cancer (IA2-IIA2), or bulky stage IB cervical cancer (Table 1).

Since then, chemoradiation has become the standard of care, and cisplatinum has shown the best activity as a single agent in cervical cancer, with a 20% to 30% objective response. Tumor cytotoxicity is intensified when cisplatinum is combined with radiation at the same time. Clinical studies have chiefly included neoadjuvant

> **BOX 4 Cervical Cancer Work-up**
>
> - History and physical
> - Chest x-ray
> - Intravenous pyelogram
> - Computed tomography of the abdomen and pelvis
> - Cystoscopy or protosigmoidoscopy
> - Magnetic resonance imaging (possibly)
> - Positron emission tomography (possibly)

TABLE 1 Concurrent Chemoradiation for Cervical Cancer

Reference	Study	FIGO Stages	Patients	Treatment Regimen	Overall Survival
Whitney, et al	GOG 85	IIB-IVA	368	Cisplatin[1]/5-FU[1] + RT	67%
				Hydroxyurea[1] + RT	57%
Rose, et al	GOG 120	IIB-IVA	526	Weekly cisplatin + RT	65%
				Cisplatin/5-FU/hydroxyurea + RT	65%
				Hydroxyurea + RT	47%
Morris, et al	RTOG 9001	IB2-IVA*	388	Cisplatin/5-FU + RT	75%
				RT alone	63%
Keys, et al	GOG 123	IB2[†]	369	Weekly cisplatin + R	83%
				RT	74%
Peters, et al	GOG 109, SWOG 8797	IA2-IIA	243	Cisplatin/5-FU + RT	81%
				RT	71%

[1]Not FDA approved for this indication.
*Stages IB and IIA required positive pelvic nodes or tumor size >5 cm.
[†]Extrafascial hysterectomy followed by chemoradiation or radiation.

References cited in the table:
Keys HM, Bundy BN, Stehman FB, et al: Cisplatin, radiation, and adjuvant hysterectomy compared with radiation and adjuvant hysterectomy for bulky stage IB cervical carcinoma. N Engl J Med 1999;340(15):1154-1161.
Morris M, Eifel PJ, Lu J, et al: Pelvic radiation with concurrent chemotherapy compared with pelvic and para-aortic radiation for high-risk cervical cancer. N Engl J Med 1999;340(15):1137-1143.
Peters WA 3rd, Liu PY, Barrett RJ 2nd, et al: Concurrent chemotherapy and pelvic radiation therapy compared with pelvic radiation therapy alone as adjuvant therapy after radical surgery in high-risk early-stage cancer of the cervix. J Clin Oncol 2000;18(8):1606-1613.
Rose PG, Bundy BN, Watkins EB, et al: Concurrent cisplatin-based radiotherapy and chemotherapy for locally advanced cervical cancer. N Engl J Med 1999;340(15):1144-1153.
Whitney CW, Sause W, Bundy BN, et al.: Randomized comparison of fluorouracil plus cisplatin versus hydroxyurea as an adjunct to radiation therapy in stage IIB-IVA carcinoma of the cervix with negative para-aortic lymph nodes: A Gynecologic Oncology Group and Southwest Oncology Group study. J Clin Oncol 1999;17(5):1339-1348.

Abbreviations: FIGO = International Federation of Gynecology and Obstetrics; 5-FU =5-fluorouracil; GOG = Gynecologic Oncology Group; RT = radiation therapy; RTOG = Radiation Therapy Oncology Group; SWOG = SouthWest Oncology Group.
Data from National Cancer Institute: Concurrent chemoradiation for cervical cancer. Clinical announcement, Washington, DC, February 22, 1999.

chemotherapy or a combination of chemotherapy and radiation when given together.

Although chemoradiation is associated with higher toxicity and increased cost, there is some economic benefit from less disease recurrence and subsequent medical costs.

THERAPY BY STAGE

Stage IA1

Patients with no lymphovascular invasion and tumor invasion to less than 3 mm (stage IA1) have less than 1% risk of nodal metastasis. The decision to proceed with conization versus abdominal or vaginal hysterectomy is based on the patient's desire for childbearing. Women with stage IA1 cancer may be treated by conization alone, provided that all cone margins are free of disease and endocervical curettage is negative. When lymphovascular invasion is present and tumor invasion is less than 3 mm, most physicians prefer modified radical hysterectomy over radiation.

Stage IA2

For patients with stroma invasion more than 3 mm or those with lymphovascular space involvement, the preferred treatment is modified or radical hysterectomy with pelvic lymphadenectomy. Radical trachelectomy with pelvic lymphadenectomy has been performed in women who desire further childbearing, with some women successfully becoming pregnant.

Stage IB

Patients with stage IB1 (tumor size <4 cm) can effectively be treated by radical hysterectomy with or without pelvic or para-aortic lymphadenectomy. Radiation therapy can be used in patients with stage 1A2 or 1B, particularly in those who are not medically suitable for radical surgery.

Treatment for patients with Stage 1B2 (bulky or barrel-shaped lesions) is the same as for stage 1B1. However, many of these tumors extend anatomically beyond the curative isodose curve of the radiation field and have significant central recurrences. Therefore, preoperative radiation therapy followed by extrafascial hysterectomy has been recommended.

Because nodal metastases are present in 20% to 25% of patients with stage 1B2 cervical cancers, para-aortic lymph node dissection should be considered at the time of hysterectomy if the para-aortic nodes were not included in the preoperative radiation fields.

Stage IIA

The optimal treatment for most patients with stage IIA cervical cancer is similar to that for stage 1B: Patients may be treated effectively by radical hysterectomy with pelvic and para-aortic lymphadenectomy and upper vaginectomy, provided that all surgical margins are free of disease. Many authors recommend postoperative whole pelvic radiation for patients with microscopic parametrial invasion, nodal metastasis, and involvement of resection margins. Morbidity from radiation therapy limited to 4500 to 5000 cGy appears acceptable; however, local recurrence is decreased, and the survival advantage, if any, is not known.

Stages IIB to IVA

For patients with locally advanced cervical cancer, primary radiation therapy (external beam and brachytherapy) and concomitant chemotherapy is recommended. Para-aortic nodal involvement is the most important prognostic factor in patients' survival. In the absence of para-aortic nodal metastasis, transposition of both ovaries in young women should be considered.

Elective para-aortic radiation is an alternative to surgical para-aortic lymphadenectomy. The two main methods of radiation for cervical cancer are external beam radiation and brachytherapy. Brachytherapy can be performed by either the intracavity technique or by the interstitial technique, using needles or after-loading catheters. Interstitial brachytherapy is used when cervical cancer cannot be optimally encompassed by intracavity applications.

> **BOX 5 Complications of Radiation Therapy in Cervical Cancer**
>
> **Intestinal**
> - Abdominal cramps, diarrhea
> - Malabsorption
> - Nausea and vomiting
> - Stricture causing bowel obstruction
> - Ulceration, bleeding, and perforation causing rectovaginal fistula
>
> **Urinary**
> - Dysuria and urinary frequency
> - Hematuria that can progress to perforation, causing vesicovaginal fistula or scarring, resulting in smaller bladder capacity and incontinence
> - Ureteral stricture, hydroureter, and hydronephrosis
>
> **Vaginal**
> - Decreased vaginal lubrication
> - Dyspareunia
> - Shortening and stenosis
>
> **Vascular**
> - Fibrosis and thrombosis of pelvic vessels, causing leg edema

Potential complications of radiation therapy can be acute occurring during treatment or they can be delayed, usually occurring 1.5 to 2 years after treatment is completed (Boxes 5 and 6).

Recurrence

It is estimated that approximately 35% of patients with invasive cervical cancer will have recurrent or persistent disease following therapy. Recurrence can be expected in 10% to 20% of patients treated with radical hysterectomy and lymphadenectomy. Most recurrences are distant metastasis involving the lung, bone, abdominal cavity, and supraclavicular lymph nodes.

> **BOX 6 Complications of Radical Hysterectomy in Cervical Cancer**
>
> **Intestinal**
> - Ileus, bowel obstruction
> - Rectal atony, rectal injury
> - Rectovaginal fistula
>
> **Urinary**
> - Bladder atony, bladder injury resulting in vesicovaginal fistula
> - Ureteral injury causing stricture or hydroureter and ureterovaginal fistula
>
> **Vaginal**
> - Dyspareunia
> - Shortening vagina
>
> **Vascular**
> - Vascular injury, deep vein thrombosis, causing leg edema and pulmonary embolism
> - Lymphocyst formation and lymphedema exist but are uncommon

Prognosis for patients with recurrent disease is more favorable in those with a small (<3 cm) central recurrence, no sidewall involvement, and longer disease-free interval.

SURGERY

Patients with central pelvic recurrences after primary treatment with radiation therapy may be salvaged with surgery. Those with small recurrences limited to the cervix or upper vagina can occasionally be treated with modified radical hysterectomy and upper vaginectomy with excellent results. Patients with larger central recurrences or those who have received previous high-dose radiation require pelvic exenteration for salvage therapy.

Recently, more attention has been directed to reconstructive procedures performed at the time of pelvic exenterations to improve quality of life. These include performing continent urinary diversion, primary colon reanastomosis, and vaginal reconstructions with myocutaneous flap.

RADIATION THERAPY

Radiation therapy may be useful in patients with localized central pelvic recurrence after radical hysterectomy or as palliation to control symptoms such as bleeding and pelvic pain.

CHEMOTHERAPY

Cervical cancer is a slow-growing neoplasm with poor response to chemotherapy. Cisplatinum (cisplatin)[1] remains the drug of choice for treating recurrences, although phase II trials are currently examining the efficacies of a broad range of compounds such as topotecan, paclitaxel,[1] and gemcitabine.[1] Combination therapy with agents such as paclitaxel and cisplatinum has been studied in phase II trials of recurrent or advanced squamous cell cancer of the cervix with 12% complete responses and 34% partial responses, although 61% of patients experienced severe neutropenia. Given the palliative nature of chemotherapy in recurrent disease, the quality of life and drug toxicity must be factored into the choice of agents.

The encouraging activity of topotecan plus cisplatin in phase II trials led to the comparison of this combination against single-agent cisplatin in GOG 179. The main goals of this trial were overall response rate, progression-free survival, and quality of life.

GOG 204 is a randomized phase III trial with four treatment arms designed to evaluate the efficacy and tolerability of cisplatin-based doublets in the treatment of primary stage IVB, recurrent, or persistent cervical cancer (Figure 1).

In addition to the exploration of new doublets, the incorporation of biological agents such as erlotinab[1] and bevacizumab[1] into the treatment of cervical cancer are ongoing as GOG phase II multicenter trials.

FOLLOW-UP

Most recurrence occurs in the first 2 years following primary therapy. Therefore, physical examination with nodal assessment, abdominal examination, pelvic examination including rectovaginal examination, and Pap smear should be done at 3-month intervals for the first year, at 4-month intervals for the second year, and at 6-month intervals thereafter. After 5 years, an annual examination appears to be appropriate. Interval chest x-ray and abdominal CT scanning should be considered. Symptoms of pain, bleeding, and gastrointestinal or genitourinary dysfunction should be investigated for possible recurrence.

---

[1]Not FDA approved for this indication.

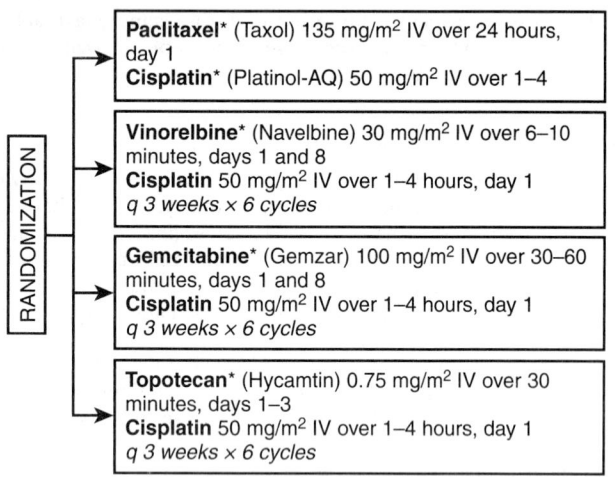

FIGURE 1. Treatment schema of the Randomized Phase III Study of Paclitaxel Plus Cisplatin vs. Vinorelbine Plus Cisplatin vs. Gemcitabine Plus Cisplatin vs. Topotecan Plus Cisplatin in Stage IVB, Recurrent, or Persistent Carcinoma of the Cervix (GOG 204). *Abbreviation:* GOG = Gynecologic Oncology Group.

Special Categories

CARCINOMA OF THE CERVICAL STUMP

Although supracervical hysterectomy is now rarely performed, carcinoma of the cervical stump is still encountered. Stage for stage, it is treated the same as cervical carcinoma of the intact uterus; for early stages, radical cervicectomy and parametrectomy with pelvic and possible para-aortic lymphadenopathy is performed. When radiation therapy is required, the short cervix often limits the amount of intracavitary radiation, therefore requiring higher-dose external irradiation.

INVASIVE CERVICAL CANCER AFTER HYSTERECTOMY

Occasionally, diagnosis of unsuspected invasive cervical cancer is made after a hysterectomy for a benign disease. Those with microinvasive disease do not require additional therapy. Those with invasive cancer confined to the cervix can be treated with radical parametrectomy, upper vaginectomy, and pelvic and para-aortic lymphadenopathy. The alternative is radiation therapy with or without chemotherapy.

INVASIVE CERVICAL CANCER DURING PREGNANCY

Pregnancy does not appear to affect the prognoses of patients with cervical cancer, and the fetus is not affected by maternal cervical cancer. However, the fetus might suffer consequences from treatment.

Patients with microinvasion diagnosed with conization can continue pregnancy until term and deliver vaginally. Before fetal maturity, patients should be treated individually, and the concerns for fetal survival must be weighed against the risk of delayed therapy.

Patients with stages IA2 to IIA can be treated by radical hysterectomy and pelvic lymphadenectomy with the fetus in situ. If the patient does not want to terminate the pregnancy or if she is close to term, then the fetus can be delivered with classic cesarean section followed by radical hysterectomy and pelvic lymphadenectomy.

Patients with larger tumors or locally advanced disease can be treated with chemoradiation. Those close to term or with fetal lung maturity can be delivered by cesarean section and surgical staging followed by chemoradiation. In a patient who declines pregnancy termination, consideration may be given to neoadjuvant chemotherapy to prevent progression of disease and time for fetal lung maturity.

ADENOCARCINOMA OF THE CERVIX

The management of adenocarcinoma of the cervix is similar to that for squamous cell carcinoma. The worse prognosis reported in some cases is attributed to a higher rate of distant metastasis.

Adenocarcinoma In Situ

Adenocarcinoma in situ (ACIS) may be identified from investigation of an abnormal Pap smear. When diagnosed on biopsy, conization is required because ACIS can be diffuse or multifocal and may be associated with underlying adenocarcinoma. The differential diagnosis includes well-differentiated adenocarcinoma (adenoma malignum or minimal deviation adenocarcinoma) and microglandular hyperplasia, which is associated with oral contraceptives and Arias-Stella changes of pregnancy. Simple hysterectomy is the treatment of choice for women who have no desire for further childbearing. Otherwise, cone biopsy may be adequate if the margins are clear and endovervical curettage is negative.

Microinvasive Adenocarcinoma

Patients with stage IA1 can be managed with simple hysterectomy. However, conization can be done for young women who desire to preserve fertility. Therefore, treatment should be individualized according to depth of invasion, margin of resection, and lymphovascular invasion.

Invasive Adenocarcinoma

Invasive adenocarcinoma accounts for approximately 5% to 10% of all cervical carcinomas. Adenocarcinoma has been classified into five subtypes: endocervical, endometrioid, clear cell, adenocystic, and adenosquamous.

Cervical adenocarcinoma usually originates from the endocervical canal. Vaginal bleeding and discharge are the most common symptoms. Endocervical and endometrial curettage are essential in the evaluation of patients if the results of gross examination of the cervix, colposcopy, and cervical biopsy are negative.

The recommended treatment for stage IA2 microinvasion is modified radical hysterectomy and pelvic lymphadenectomy. For stages IB and IIA, radical hysterectomy and pelvic lymphadenopathy are recommended. Adjuvant pelvic radiation should be considered for patients with nodal metastasis, lymphovascular invasion, poorly differentiated tumor, or larger lesions. When radiation is the primary treatment, an adjuvant simple hysterectomy is recommended. Follow-up CEA (carcinoembryonic antigen) and CA-125 (cancer antigen 125) are of value in cervical adenocarcinoma.

Adenosquamous Carcinoma

Adenosquamous carcinoma represents 20% to 30% of cervical adenocarcinomas. Overall 5-year survival and disease-free survival rates are not significantly different from those of other adenocarcinomas.

Clear Cell Adenocarcinoma

In clear cell adenocarcinoma, the tumor occurs in two distinct groups of patients—those younger than 24 years and those older than 45 years. Cancer in the older group is unrelated to diethylstilbestrol (DES) exposure in utero. Unlike uterine clear cell adenocarcinoma, the prognosis is the same as for other adenocarcinomas.

Glassy Cell Carcinoma

Glassy cell carcinoma is a poorly differentiated adenosquamous (or large cell undifferentiated) carcinoma with a moderate amount of cytoplasm and a typical ground glass appearance. The prognosis is poor. Reported survival for stage IB cancer treated with radical hysterectomy was 55%.

Small Cell Carcinoma

Small cell (neuroendocrine) carcinoma is very rare, only 0.6% of cervical cancers. Small cell carcinoma histologically stains for neuroendocrine markers. These cells can synthesize amines and hence are also called amine precursor uptake and decarboxylation (APUD) cells. Small cell carcinoma has a tendency to a higher lymphovascular invasion, resulting in higher recurrence and lower survival because of their propensity for early systemic spread. Chemotherapy is usually recommended in addition to surgery and radiation.

A larger study involving 23 women compared adjuvant chemotherapy with cisplatin,[1] vinblastine,[1] and bleomycin[1] (PVB) against vincristine,[1] doxorubicin,[1] and cyclophosphamide[1] (VAC) alternating with cisplatin[1] and etoposide[1] (PE) after radical hysterectomy. The reported survival was higher in the VAC/PE group (10 of 14) compared with the PVB group (3 of 9), with median follow-up of 41 months.

Chemoprevention and Vaccination

Due to the relatively long premalignant phase of cervical carcinogenesis (5-10 years), some investigators are studying the effect of chemoprevention or vaccination on disease progression. Investigators have focused on the retinoids as chemoprevention agents for cervical dysplasia based on their cell-differentiating properties.

Topical *trans*-retinoic acid[1] (tretinoin) in a randomized phase III clinical trial has been shown to induce regression of mild and moderate dysplasias, but not of severe dysplasias. Other suitable agents for chemoprevention include difluoromethylornithine,[5] beta-carotene,[7] and cyclooxygenase-2 inhibitors.[1]

HPV vaccines are focused on targeting the oncogenic E6/E7 proteins as therapeutic vaccines. These peptide vaccines are designed to stimulate cytotoxic T lymphocytes against specific E6/E7 epitopes. HPV16 and HPV18 together cause about 70% of cervical cancers. It is estimated that 20 million people are infected worldwide and 6.2 million people in the United States get a new infection of HPV each year. Two new vaccines, Gardasil (Merck) and Cervarix[5] (GlaxoSmithKline) reported 100% protection against HPV 16 and HPV 18 infection. To improve that effort, researchers are already working on second-generation vaccines and exploring the possibility of a therapeutic vaccine that could help prevent HPV-related cancers in those who are already being infected by the virus.

---

[1]Not FDA approved for this indication.
[5]Investigational drug in the United States.
[7]Available as dietary supplement.

REFERENCES

Boss EA, van Golde RI, Beerendonk CC, Massuger LE: Pregnancy after radical trachelectomy: A real option? Gynecol Oncol 2005;99(3 suppl 1):S152-S156.
Dargent D, Martin X, Sacchetoni A, Mathevet P: Laparoscopic vaginal radical trachelectomy: A treatment to preserve the fertility of cervical cancer carcinoma patients. Cancer 2000;88:1877-1882.
Delgado G, Bundy B, Zaino R, et al: Prospective surgical-pathological study of disease-free interval in patients with stage IB squamous cell carcinoma of the cervix: A Gynecologic Oncology Group study. Gynecol Oncol 1990;38:352-357.
Giacalone PL, Laffargue E: Neoadjuvant chemotherapy in the treatment of locally advanced cervical carcinoma in pregnancy: A report of two cases and review of issues specific to the management of cervical carcinoma in pregnancy including planned delay of therapy. Cancer 1999;85:1203-1204.
Hopkins MP, Lavin JP: Cervical cancer in pregnancy. Gynecol Oncol 1996;63:293.
Jemal A, Siegel R, Ward E, et al: Cancer statistics, 2006. CA Cancer J Clin 2006;56:106-130.
Jensen PT, Groenvold M, Klee MC, et al: Early-stage cervical carcinoma, radical hysterectomy, and sexual function: A longitudinal study. Cancer 2004;100:97-106.
Lertsanguansinchai P, Lertbutsayanukul C, Shotelersuk K, et al: Phase III randomized trial comparing LDR and HDR brachytherapy in treatment of cervical carcinoma. Int J Radiat Oncol Biol Phys 2004;59:1424-1431.
Plante M, Renaud MC, FranÁois H, Roy M: Vaginal radical trachelectomy: An oncologically safe fertility-preserving surgery: An updated series of 72 cases and review of the literature. Gynecol Oncol 2004;94:614-623.
Roman LD, Felix JC, Muderspach LL, et al: Risk of residual invasive disease in women with microinvasive squamous cancer in a conization specimen. Obstet Gynecol 1997;90:759-764.
Sedlis A, Bundy BN, Rotman MZ, et al: A randomized trial of pelvic radiation therapy versus no further therapy in selected patients with stage IB carcinoma of the cervix after radical hysterectomy and pelvic lymphadenectomy: A Gynecologic Oncology Group Study. Gynecol Oncol 1999;73:177-183.
Steed H, Rosen B, Murphy J, et al: A comparison of laparascopic-assisted radical vaginal hysterectomy and radical abdominal hysterectomy in the treatment of cervical cancer. Gynecol Oncol 2004;93:588-593.

Neoplasms of the Vulva

Method of
Susan A. Davidson, MD

The female external genitalia includes the mons pubis, labia majora, labia minora, clitoris, perineal body, and the structures of the vaginal introitus or vestibule. Whether benign or malignant, vulvar neoplasms are uncommon, occur at all ages, and have varying characteristics. Therefore liberal use of biopsies is usually required for diagnosis and to guide treatment.

Benign Cystic Neoplasms

Benign cystic lesions of the vulva include Bartholin's duct cyst, sebaceous and epidermal inclusion cysts, mucinous cysts, Skene duct cysts, and cysts of the canal of Nuck. Bartholin's duct cyst, located in the posterior labia near the vaginal introitus, is most common. Treatment is usually not required in asymptomatic young women (<40 years). If the cyst is symptomatic or infected, however, drainage by marsupialization or use of a Word catheter, is indicated. Bartholin's gland carcinomas are rare, especially in women younger than 40 years of age. But if the mass feels firm or nodular, it should be biopsied.

Sebaceous and epidermal inclusion cysts are also common. They are prone to infection but rarely malignant. If an infection develops, they should be incised and drained. Mucinous cysts are rare and possibly arise from the minor vestibular glands. They are located anteriorly on the vulva, typically on the inner labia minora. Skene duct cysts are located next to the urethra. Excision of these cysts is necessary only if symptomatic.

Cysts of the canal of Nuck are located in the anterior portion of the labia majora at the termination of the insertion of the round ligament. These cysts represent herniation of the peritoneum through the inguinal canal and contain peritoneal fluid. If symptomatic, excision must be accompanied by closure of the fascial defect to prevent recurrence.

Benign Solid Neoplasms

The benign solid tumors of the vulva include fibromas, myomas, lipomas, hidradenomas, syringomas, myoblastomas, vestibular adenomas, and angiomas, among others. Benign pigmented lesions, such as nevi and seborrheic keratoses, may occasionally be found. Malignancy is rare, but most should be excised for diagnostic and therapeutic purposes.

CONDYLOMA ACUMINATUM

Vulvar condyloma acuminatum is a sexually transmitted verrucous lesion of the vulva caused by human papilloma virus (HPV), most frequently types 6 and 11. These lesions are warty growths that frequently cover large areas of the vulva. Smoking and immunosuppression are risk factors. Representative biopsies should be obtained to document disease and rule out malignancy. Wide local excision can be used for small lesions, although these growths are usually best treated by ablation.

Chemical ablative techniques include topical application of trichloroacetic acid (Tri-Chlor), podofilox (0.5%, Condylox), 5-fluorouracil[1] (1%, Fluoroplex or 5%, Efudex),[1] or imiquimod (5%, Aldara). Podophyllin can be applied twice daily for 3 days, repeated weekly for 4 weeks. Imiquimod can be applied three times per week for up to 16 weeks. Podophyllin and 5-fluorouracil should not be used in women who could become pregnant. Surgical ablative therapies include CO_2 laser vaporization and use of the Cavitron ultrasonic aspirator (CUSA), especially for extensive disease.

Intraepithelial Neoplasms of the Vulva

VULVAR INTRAEPITHELIAL NEOPLASIA

Vulvar intraepithelial neoplasia (VIN) is a dysplastic condition of the squamous epithelium whose incidence is increasing, especially in younger women. Risk factors are HPV types 16 and 18, smoking, and immunosuppression. Symptoms include pruritus (most common), pain, a noticeable lesion, and discoloration. Most patients with HPV-related disease have multifocal lesions including vaginal and cervical dysplasia. The most common location is in the area of the posterior fourchette and perineal body. Typical findings are raised white, gray, red, or mottled lesions; application of 4% acetic acid for several minutes can help identify faint lesions and outline abnormal vascular patterns. Diagnosis of VIN is made by punch biopsies through full thickness of the epithelium to rule out invasion, present in 20% of patients with VIN III (full-thickness dysplasia or carcinoma in situ). Of those patients with invasion, half (10% of VIN III) have invasion more than 1 mm.

Treatment of VIN can be categorized into excisional and ablative therapies. Patients at risk for microinvasion (unifocal disease, raised lesions, older age, and prior radiation) should have the lesion excised completely if possible. Skinning vulvectomy is rarely used because of psychological and sexual consequences related to scarring and disfigurement.

The ablative therapies can be divided into mechanical and chemical. The mechanical method most commonly used is the CO_2 laser, although use of the CUSA is also described. Both can ablate large or multifocal lesions successfully with an excellent cosmetic and functional outcome. The chemical method most commonly used is topical 5-fluorouracil (5%, Efudex).[1] Because of its teratogenic potential, it should not be used in women who could become pregnant. It can be applied on two consecutive nights weekly for 10 weeks. An alternative ablative therapy is use of imiquimod[1] (Aldara), as described earlier. Because of the irritation caused by these topical therapies, many patients have problems with treatment compliance. Residual disease should be excised to rule out invasion.

Patients with VIN frequently have recurrent disease, regardless of the treatment method used (Table 1). Continued smoking increases this risk, so patients should be counseled in smoking cessation. In those patients whose cancers recur and are retreated, subsequent

---
[1]Not FDA approved for this indication.

TABLE 1 Recurrence of Vulvar Intraepithelial Neoplasia III

Treatment Method	% Recurrence
Chemical ablation	20-40
Mechanical ablation	20-40
Wide local excision	
Negative margin	15-25
Positive margin	30-45

5-fluorouracil prophylaxis, with a single application biweekly, is used successfully to minimize further recurrences.

PAGET'S DISEASE

Paget's disease of the vulva is an uncommon condition characterized by a patchy, eczematoid lesion that frequently covers much of the vulva. Most patients are postmenopausal and present with complaints of pruritus. Although Paget's disease is an in situ disease process, 15% to 25% of patients have an underlying malignancy, usually an adenocarcinoma of the apocrine glands but occasionally an invasive Paget's. In addition, up to 30% of patients have a synchronous adenocarcinoma of the breast, colon, rectum, or upper genital tract. Screening for these cancers is therefore recommended. To assess for invasion, the lesion should be excised via wide local excision or simple vulvectomy with at least 5 mm of the adjacent subcutaneous tissue. Achieving negative margin status is frequently difficult. However, the risk of recurrence is approximately 30% whether margins are negative or positive. Thus expectant management, reserving treatment for symptomatic recurrences, is usually recommended.

Invasive Vulvar Lesions

Less than 5% of gynecologic cancers arise on the vulva. Approximately 85% are squamous cell carcinomas. The etiology of this type appears mixed. Up to 50% evolve from VIN III and are usually associated with HPV-16. These women are slightly younger (age 45-52 years). Most arise in older women (mean age 60-69 years), and suggested risk factors include immunosuppression, hypertension, diabetes mellitus, obesity, and chronic vulvar inflammation. Other histologic types are melanomas (5% to 10%), basal cell carcinomas (2% to 3%), adenocarcinomas (1%), and sarcomas (1% to 2%) Most patients present with a combination of symptoms, including pruritus, discomfort, and complaints of a mass. Examination frequently reveals a suspicious lesion, which should be biopsied for diagnosis. Vulvar cancers typically spread by local extension and lymphatic dissemination. Factors that influence dissemination include tumor size (Table 2), depth of invasion (Table 3), lymphovascular space invasion, and tumor grade. Staging is surgical and classified using the tumor, nodes, and metastasis (TNM) system (Box 1) as well as the International Federation of Gynecology and Obstetrics (FIGO) system (Box 2).

TABLE 2 Incidence of Regional Node Metastases by Tumor Diameter

Tumor Diameter (cm)	% Positive Inguinal Nodes
<1	0-15
5-20	
25-35	
35-50	
≥50	≥50

TABLE 3 Incidence of Regional Node Metastases by Depth of Tumor Invasion	
Depth of Invasion (mm)	% Positive Inguinal Nodes
<1	1-5
1-3	10-15
3-5	15-30
5-10	30-45
>10	>40

SQUAMOUS CELL CARCINOMAS AND ADENOCARCINOMAS

Surgical management of squamous cell carcinomas and adenocarcinomas depends on the size, depth of invasion, and location of the lesion. The vulvar lesion is managed with a radical excision. Management of the groins is based on depth of invasion. Lesions with invasion of <1 mm have minimal risk of lymphatic spread and do not require lymphadenectomy. All others require surgical assessment of the lymph nodes. Lesions located in the midline structures require bilateral groin dissection, whereas lateral lesions are managed with ipsilateral groin dissection. This surgical approach is associated with significant morbidity including disfigurement, wound breakdown, and problems with lymphocysts and chronic lymphedema. For patients with very large lesions or lesions in sensitive areas such as the clitoris, preoperative radiation, followed by less radical excision of residual disease, may minimize problems with the vulvar wound. Current investigations are ongoing in the use of sentinel lymph node dissections as a method of minimizing the groin morbidity without sacrificing survival. Positive vulvar margins or metastases to lymph nodes are managed with postoperative radiation. Survival depends on stage at diagnosis (Table 4).

MALIGNANT MELANOMA

Malignant melanoma is the second most common vulvar malignancy. Most patients have disease on the mucosal surfaces of the vulvar introitus, clitoris, and labia minora. The vulvar lesion is treated by radical excision, but management of the groins is controversial. The risk of spread is significant with a tumor thickness greater than 0.75 mm, but survival at 5 years is only approximately

BOX 1	TNM Classification of Vulvar Carcinoma
T	Primary tumor
Tis	Carcinoma in situ
T1	Confined to vulva, diameter ≤2 cm
T2	Confined to vulva, diameter >2 cm
T3	Adjacent spread to urethra, vagina, perineum, or anus (any size)
T4	Infiltration of upper urethral mucosa, bladder, rectum, or bone
N	Regional lymph nodes
N0	No lymph node metastases
N1	Unilateral regional lymph node metastasis
N2	Bilateral regional lymph node metastasis
M	Distant metastases
M0	No clinical metastases
M1	Distant metastasis (including pelvic lymph node metastasis)

Abbreviations: TNM = tumor, node, metastasis.

BOX 2	FIGO Classification (With Corresponding TNM Classification) for Vulvar Carcinoma
Stage I (T1N0M0)	Tumor confined to vulva and/or perineum, 2 cm in greatest dimension; nodes are negative
Stage IA	Stromal invasion no greater than 1 mm
Stage IB	Stromal invasion >1 mm
Stage II (T2N0M0)	Tumor confined to the vulva and/or perineum, >2 cm in greatest dimension; nodes are negative
Stage III	
T3N0M0	Tumor of any size with adjacent spread to the lower urethra and/or the vagina or the anus
T3N1M0	Unilateral regional lymph node metastasis
T2N1M0	
Stage IVA	
T1N2M0	Tumor invades any of the following: upper urethra, bladder mucosa, rectal mucosa, pelvic bone, and/or bilateral regional node metastasis
T2N2M0	
T3N2M0	
T4 any N M0	
Stage IVB	
Any T any N M1	Any distant metastasis including pelvic lymph nodes

Abbreviations: FIGO = International Federation of Gynecology and Obstetrics; TNM = tumor, node, metastasis.

CURRENT DIAGNOSIS

- Most cystic lesions are benign. Excision is reserved for symptomatic cysts and suspicious Bartholin's gland cysts, especially in women older than 40 years of age.
- All solid lesions should be biopsied for diagnostic purposes.
- Multifocal disease requires multiple biopsies to rule out invasive disease.
- Most premalignant and malignant lesions cause pruritus, discomfort, or a noticeable lesion.
- The vagina and cervix in women with dysplastic or malignant vulvar lesions should be evaluated.

TABLE 4 Survival Rate by FIGO Stage for Patients With Invasive Squamous Cell Vulvar Cancer	
FIGO Stage	% Surviving 5 years
I	70-90
II	50-80
III	30-50
IV	10-15

Abbreviation: FIGO = International Federation of Gynecology and Obstetrics.

CURRENT THERAPY

- Benign solid lesions should be excised.
- After ablative treatment of vulvar intraepithelial neoplasia (VIN), excise any residual lesions to rule out occult invasive disease.
- Avoid podophyllin and 5-fluorouracil in women of reproductive potential.
- Rule out synchronous neoplasms in women with Paget's disease.
- Invasion more than 1 mm requires radical excision and lymph node evaluation.

10% with groin node metastases. Some argue against node dissection for this reason. However, given some long-term survivors with modern melanoma therapy, either lymphadenectomy or sentinel lymph node dissection, as is done for other cutaneous melanomas, appears indicated.

VERRUCOUS CARCINOMA

Verrucous carcinoma is a large exophytic tumor that resembles giant condyloma acuminatum. It is a variant of squamous carcinomas but has an excellent prognosis because of the lack of metastases. Verrucous carcinomas have a high tendency to recur and should be managed with radical local excision.

BASAL CELL CARCINOMA

Basal cell carcinomas typically occur in elderly white women, are commonly located on the labia majora, and have characteristics similar to basal cell carcinomas at other sites. Treatment is wide local excision only because metastases are rare. Basal cell carcinomas are prone to local recurrence, however. A malignant squamous component must be ruled out because it should be managed as a squamous cell carcinoma.

SARCOMAS

Leiomyosarcoma is the most common vulvar sarcoma and usually arises in the labia majora. Malignant fibrous histiocytoma is the second most common. Management of these lesions is radical vulvar excision.

REFERENCES

Garland SM: Imiquimod. Curr Opin Infect Dis 2003;16:85-89.
Homesley HD, Bundy BN, Sedlis A, et al: Prognostic factors for groin node metastasis in squamous cell carcinoma of the vulva (a Gynecologic Oncology Group study). Gynecol Oncol 1993;49:279-283.
Krebs HB: The use of topical 5-fluorouracil in the treatment of genital condylomas. Obstet Gynecol Clin North Am 1987;14(2):559-568.
Modesitt SC, Waters AB, Walton L, et al: Vulvar intraepithelial neoplasia III: Occult cancer and the impact of margin status on recurrence. Obstet Gynecol 1998;92(6):962-966.
Phillips GL, Bundy BN, Okagaki T, et al: Malignant melanoma of the vulva treated by radical hemivulvectomy, a prospective study of the Gynecologic Oncology Group. Cancer 1994;73:2626-2632.
Tebes S, Cardosi R, Hoffman M: Paget's disease of the vulva. Am J Obstet Gynecol 2002;187:281-284.
Trimble CL, Trimble EL, Woodruff JD: Diseases of the vulva. In Hernandez E, Atkinson BF (eds): Clinical Gynecologic Pathology. Philadelphia: WB Saunders, 1995, pp 1-90.
Wright VC, Chapman WB: Colposcopy of intraepithelial neoplasia of the vulva and adjacent sites. Obstet Gynecol Clin North Am 1993;20(1):231-255.

Ovarian Cancer

Method of
*Amanda Nickles Fader, MD, and
Jerome Belinson, MD*

Although ovarian carcinoma is only the second most common of the gynecologic malignancies, it is by far the most deadly. According to the American Cancer Society, ovarian cancer will be diagnosed annually in more than 23,000 U.S. women and an estimated 15,000 will die of their disease. Thus, ovarian cancer represents the fifth most common cause of cancer-related death in women in the United States. Although incidence rates have remained stable over the last 2 decades, the overall 5-year survival rate has only slightly improved during this time (from 37% to 44%), primarily due to the lack of effective screening strategies. As a result, more than 75% of ovarian cancers will not be diagnosed until the disease is advanced.

Most primary ovarian tumors are epithelial in origin, the most common subtype of which is papillary serous. The second most common cause of cancer in the ovaries is metastatic disease, especially from breast cancer or Krukenberg tumors (mucin-producing signet-ring cells) from the gastrointestinal tract. Most other histologic subtypes arise from the ovary and include germ cell, sex cord-stromal, and mixed-cell tumors.

The median age of patients with ovarian cancer is 60 years. The cause of epithelial ovarian cancer is still unknown, but most cases occur as a result of sporadic mutations. Risk factors include low parity, high-fat diet, obesity, family history of ovarian or breast cancer, and certain genetic mutations. Multiple pregnancies and the use of oral contraceptives can decrease a woman's risk of developing the disease by as much as 50%, perhaps because of decreased ovulation.

The lifetime risk of ovarian cancer for all U.S. women is about 1.4%, but certain women have a higher risk. Approximately 10% of epithelial ovarian cancers occur as a result of an inherited mutation, and usually arise earlier than ovarian cancers caused by sporadic mutations. Women with one or more first-degree relatives with ovarian cancer have an increased risk of 3% to 5% of developing the disease themselves. Women with known *BRCA1* and *BRCA2* gene mutations have an even greater risk of developing both ovarian and breast cancers. *BRCA1* and *BRCA2* are tumor suppressor genes found on chromosomes 17 and 13, respectively, and are inherited in an autosomal dominant fashion. The lifetime risk of a woman with a *BRCA1* mutation for developing ovarian and breast cancers is 40% and 80%, respectively, and the risk for a woman with a *BRCA2* mutation is 15% and 60%, respectively. Women of Ashkenazi Jewish ancestry have a higher incidence of germ-line mutations in *BRCA1* and *BRCA2* genes.

A second important familial disorder that increases a woman's risk of ovarian and other gynecologic and gastrointestinal cancers is the Lynch II syndrome (hereditary nonpolyposis colorectal cancer syndrome [HNPCC]). It is caused by inherited germ-line mutations in DNA-mismatch repair genes. The lifetime risk of ovarian cancer in HNPCC carriers is 5% to 10%.

Genetic counseling and testing for genetic mutations should be offered to women who have a family history of breast or ovarian cancer in either two first-degree relatives or in a first-degree and a second-degree relative, *BRCA1* or *BRCA2* gene mutations, or HNPCC. Oral contraceptives can be offered to women who desire fertility, and oophorectomy should be considered in high-risk women who have completed their childbearing, because these measures decrease the risk of developing ovarian cancer.

Screening

Screening tests for ovarian cancer remain controversial. Although quite sensitive for diagnosing ovarian cysts and tumors, transvaginal ultrasonography is nonspecific and its use results in unnecessary surgical exploration of a large number of women with benign (and often physiologic) ovarian cysts. Another such screening test is for serum levels of CA-125 (a tumor-associated antigen). Serum levels greater than 35 U/mL are present in 80% of postmenopausal women with ovarian cancer. However, many early-stage ovarian tumors do not cause elevated levels of CA-125, whereas endometriosis, heavy menses, pelvic inflammatory disease, appendicitis, diverticulitis, benign ovarian tumors, and other benign disorders of the gastrointestinal tract may do so. Therefore, the rarity of ovarian cancer coupled with the lack of sensitivity and specificity for these two currently available tests to detect this disease make for an inability to effectively screen for ovarian cancer at this time.

Although screening is not currently recommended for women in the general public, the exception is the 5% to 10% of women who may be affected by a genetic mutation that increases their risk of ovarian cancer. Women with a potentially increased risk of a hereditary ovarian and breast cancer syndrome should be referred to a geneticist as well as a gynecologic oncologist, who can enroll appropriate candidates into an ovarian cancer screening trial and potentially offer them prophylactic surgery. For *BRCA1* or *BRCA2* mutation carriers, decision analysis indicates that prophylactic surgery or chemoprevention leads to better survival than surveillance alone.

Diagnosis

An obstacle to diagnosing ovarian cancer is that the associated symptoms are usually nonspecific and occur relatively commonly in daily life as well as with other benign gynecologic and bowel disorders. Early-stage ovarian carcinoma is usually asymptomatic, and symptoms of late-stage disease are often vague, poorly defined, and might not be severe or specific enough to prompt a woman to seek medical attention. As a result, most cases of ovarian carcinoma are advanced at the time of diagnosis.

Advanced ovarian cancer is typically associated with abdominal distention, nausea, constipation, urinary frequency, anorexia, or early satiety due to the presence of ascites and omental or bowel metastases; dyspnea is occasionally present due to a pleural effusion. The nonspecific nature of these symptoms was illustrated by comparing survey results from women before surgery for a pelvic mass with those who visited a primary care clinic for a variety of medical issues (controls). Bloating was present in 70% of women subsequently found to have ovarian cancer, 49% of those with a benign ovarian mass, and 38% of those seeking primary care. In the control population, symptom prevalence and severity decreased with advancing age, suggesting that in young women, many of these symptoms are related to normal cyclical hormonal changes. Furthermore, ovarian cancer patients were more likely than control patients seeking primary care to have symptoms for a shorter time (onset within a few months rather than a year or more), multiple symptoms (the combination of bloating, increased abdominal girth, and urinary symptoms was present in 44%), and a greater frequency of occurrence and severity of symptoms.

If a physician suspects ovarian cancer, conducting a rectovaginal examination as part of the assessment of the pelvis is extremely important. Such an examination can lead to the discovery of the only palpable sign of ovarian disease, which would reside in the cul-de-sac. A serum CA-125 should also be drawn, and imaging studies with either transvaginal ultrasound or computed tomography of the abdomen and pelvis may be performed to help establish the diagnosis. An ovarian mass that has both solid and cystic features with Doppler flow coursing through the solid areas is concerning for ovarian cancer, especially in postmenopausal women with an elevated CA-125. Finally, if there is any suspicion that a woman may have ovarian cancer, she should be referred to a gynecologic oncologist.

Treatment

SURGERY

Surgery is still the cornerstone in the management of advanced epithelial ovarian cancer. With surgery, the gynecologic oncologist can confirm the diagnosis of ovarian cancer, appropriately stage the cancer, and remove as much disease as possible (primary cytoreduction). Significantly, there is substantial evidence that patients having such surgery performed by gynecologists with a special training in gynecologic oncology have a survival advantage over patients having such surgery performed by general surgeons or general gynecologists. Researchers in a recently published meta-analysis of 81 studies on the effect of maximal cytoreductive surgery on median survival in patients with advanced ovarian carcinoma concluded that referral of patients with apparent advanced ovarian cancer to gynecologic oncologists for primary surgery may be the most efficient effort currently available for improving overall survival.

CHEMOTHERAPY

Standard treatment of ovarian cancer requires not only surgical but also medical strategies. Therapy for newly diagnosed epithelial ovarian cancer is determined primarily by the extent of disease at the time of diagnosis as described in the International Federation of Gynecology and Obstetrics (FIGO) staging system. Women with low-grade stage IA disease can generally be managed with initial surgery and observation alone. However, for most women with stage IA grade 2 disease or greater, careful staging and maximum surgical cytoreduction followed by platinum-based chemotherapy

CURRENT DIAGNOSIS

- Most ovarian tumors are epithelial in origin, and the most common histologic subtype is papillary serous.
- Inherited mutations, such as *BRCA1* and *BRCA2*, cause 5% to 10% of ovarian cancers.
- There are no effective screening tests at this time.
- Symptoms of ovarian cancer are nonspecific.
- Physical examination should include palpation of the abdomen for masses or fluid wave, rectovaginal examination for detection of cul-de-sac lesions, and lung auscultation for pleural effusion.
- Ovarian cancer is associated with elevated serum levels of CA-125 and can appear as a complex mass (with solid and cystic features) on imaging.

CURRENT THERAPY

- Women with a family history of breast or ovarian cancer should be referred to a gynecologic oncologist.
- Refer any woman with suspected ovarian cancer (by physical examination, imaging, or CA-125 criteria) to a gynecologic oncologist.
- The standard of care is adequate surgical staging, optimal cytoreductive surgery, and adjuvant chemotherapy with combination intravenous carboplatin and paclitaxel.
- Cooperative oncology group trials suggest that intraperitoneal chemotherapy is an alternative and promising primary treatment modality.
- Treatment of recurrent disease is based on sensitivity to platinum agents, toxicity, and quality-of-life considerations.

are recommended. The prognostic significance of residual disease before chemotherapy has been demonstrated in many reports, and the maxim that survival is correlated to amount of residual disease is generally accepted.

In the mid 1970s, the standard of care for advanced epithelial ovarian cancer was the combination of cyclophosphamide (Cytoxan) and doxorubicin (Adriamycin), the efficacy of which was established by studies conducted by the Gynecologic Oncology Group (GOG). Chemotherapy for this disease has evolved dramatically since that time, with the most important contribution being the discovery that platinum-containing regimens are highly active against ovarian cancer. Three randomized phase III U.S. trials (GOG 111, OV-10, and ICON 3) support the superiority of platinum therapy (either cisplatin [Platinol AQ] or carboplatin [Paraplatin]) to alternative regimens. The addition of a taxane agent to a platinum compound was further shown to improve disease-free outcomes for ovarian cancer patients, and this combination (most commonly carboplatin and paclitaxel), given intravenously, has now become standard therapy for the first-line treatment of women with advanced epithelial ovarian cancer. For women with stage III or IV disease, response rates approach 90%, with 75% achieving a clinical complete response.

Recent studies examining the role of intraperitoneal (IP) chemotherapy in the treatment of primary ovarian carcinoma suggest that this treatment modality might become the standard of care in the 21st century, because it may be a more effective strategy to treat a cancer that primarily remains confined to the peritoneal cavity throughout its natural course. IP therapy has several advantages for the treatment of ovarian cancer. Placing chemotherapy drugs in the peritoneal cavity takes advantage of the diffusion characteristics of some agents. This technique of dose intensification can allow a several-fold increase in drug concentration in the abdominal cavity compared with systemic IV administration. Depending on the particular drug, the chemotherapy is more slowly absorbed by capillaries, thereby prolonging time of contact with the actual tumor.

Several phase III trials of cisplatin IP[1] chemotherapy as a first-line therapeutic strategy for optimally debulked stage III cancer have been conducted in the last decade. These trials compared chemotherapy administration through IP with IV routes. The best evidence supporting IP chemotherapy is derived from three large multicenter randomized GOG trials. These trials differ in their design but have consistently shown a survival benefit with IP chemotherapy administration. Although toxicities were more commonly seen in the IP arms (catheter complications and increased short-term toxicities), there was no increase in deaths from toxicity, and quality of life measures were similar between the IV and IP arms 1 year after therapy was complete.

Unfortunately, despite the high initial response to platinum-based chemotherapy (80%-90%), most patients with advanced-stage ovarian cancer experience relapse and eventually die of progressive, chemotherapy-resistant disease. However, after recurrence, many patients can be managed in a chronic disease mode by careful selection of therapies and with close monitoring of drug toxicities. The concept of ovarian cancer as a chronic condition has led to a new paradigm in the management of patients with this disease. Prolonged survival with disease is possible in a subset of ovarian cancer patients, and goals of therapy have now become long-term control of disease while minimizing toxicity and maximizing patient quality of life.

Although platinum and paclitaxel remain the standards for primary therapy for ovarian cancer in the United States, many other compounds possess activity against the disease. Patients with a recurrence after a 1-year disease-free interval are typically referred to as *platinum sensitive* and can be re-treated with one or both of the initial drugs. Commonly used second- or third-line agents in the treatment of platinum-resistant recurrent disease include liposomal doxorubicin, gemcitabine, topotecan, and etoposide.[1]

The occurrence of bowel dysfunction due to intraabdominal tumor also commonly adds a management dilemma in patients with recurrent disease, but dietary management (low-residue diets and liquids) can help avert bowel obstruction in these cases.

Considerable effort has been invested in new treatment strategies for ovarian cancer. Current clinical trials continue to investigate novel cytotoxic agents as well as the role of incorporating biological agents with an emphasis on molecularly targeted therapy into the treatment of ovarian and other cancers. Promising biologicals currently under investigation include antiangiogenesis agents that target the vascular endothelial growth factor receptor and agents that target other growth factor receptors commonly overexpressed in human tumors. Moreover, intense investigation to develop new screening strategies is ongoing.

---

[1]Not FDA approved for this indication.

REFERENCES

Armstrong DK, Bundy B, Wenzel L, et al: Gynecologic Oncology Group: Intraperitoneal cisplatin and paclitaxel in ovarian cancer. N Engl J Med 2006;354:34-43.

Bristow RE, Tomacruz RS, Armstrong DK, et al: Survival effect of maximal cytoreductive surgery for advanced ovarian carcinoma during the platinum era: A meta-analysis. J Clin Oncol 2002;20:1248-1259.

Colombo N, Guthrie D, Chiari S, et al: International Collaborative Ovarian Neoplasm trial: A randomized trial of adjuvant chemotherapy in women with early-stage ovarian cancer. J Natl Cancer Inst 2003;95:125-132.

Earle CC, Bodurka D, Bristow RE, et al: Effect of surgeon specialty on processes of care and outcomes for ovarian cancer patients. J Natl Cancer Inst 2006;98(3):172-180.

Goff BA, Mandel LS, Melancon CH, Muntz HG: Frequency of symptoms of ovarian cancer in women presenting to primary care clinics. JAMA 2004;291(22):2705-2712.

Hacker NF, Berek JS, Lagasse LD, et al: Primary cytoreductive surgery for epithelial ovarian cancer. Obstet Gynecol 1983;61:413-420.

International Collaborative Ovarian Neoplasm Group: Paclitaxel plus carboplatin versus standard chemotherapy with either single-agent carboplatin or cyclophosphamide, doxorubicin, and cisplatin in women with ovarian cancer: The ICON3 randomised trial. Lancet 2002;360:505-515.

Jemal A, Siegel R, Ward E, et al: Cancer statistics, 2006. CA Cancer J Clin 2006;56:106-130.

McGuire WP, Hoskins WJ, Brady MF, et al: Cyclophosphamide and cisplatin versus paclitaxel and cisplatin: A phase III randomized trial in patients with suboptimal stage III/IV ovarian cancer. N Engl J Med 1996;334:1-6.

Ozols RF, Bundy BN, Greer BE, et al: Gynecologic Oncology Group: Phase III trial of carboplatin and paclitaxel compared with cisplatin and paclitaxel in patients with optimally resected stage III ovarian cancer: A Gynecologic Oncology Group study. J Clin Oncol 2003;21:3194-3200.

Paulsen T, Kjaerheim K, Kaern J, et al: Improved short-term survival for advanced ovarian, tubal, and peritoneal cancer patients operated at teaching hospitals. Int J Gynecol Cancer 2006;16(suppl 1):11-17.

Pecorelli S, Benedet JL, Boyle P, et al: FIGO Annual Report on the Results of Treatment in Gynecological Cancer, vol 24. J Epidemiol Biostat 2001; 6:1-184.

---

[1]Not FDA approved for this indication.

SECTION 17

Psychiatric Disorders

Alcoholism

Method of
Richard N. Rosenthal, MD

Epidemiology

Alcohol-use disorders are among the most prevalent mental disorders in the population, occurring at frequencies that rival those of mood and anxiety disorders. In any year, almost 8½% of the U.S. population older than 18 years meets criteria for a formal alcohol use disorder (alcohol abuse or dependence), and almost 4% meets criteria for alcohol dependence.

Economic and Medical Sequelae

Alcohol use disorders are important to identify and treat for several reasons. The first is the direct negative impact of chronic heavy alcohol exposure on cognitive, physical, social, and vocational functioning. The second is the well-described long-term medical sequelae of alcohol dependence such as hepatic cirrhosis, pancreatitis, and dementia. Chronic heavy drinking, even in the absence of a formal diagnosis of alcohol dependence, is associated with an increased risk of diabetes mellitus, hypertension, gastrointestinal bleeding, hemorrhagic stroke, and several forms of carcinoma. The third reason for identification and treatment is the public impact of alcohol use disorders, which covers associated traumatic injuries from motor vehicle and job-related accidents, alcohol-related crime, and their associated economic costs. More than $180 billion is lost to the U.S. economy each year due to alcohol-related crime, injury, health care costs, and lost productivity in the workplace.

Screening

SCREENING RATIONALE

Screening for alcohol problems arrays patients on a continuum from abstinence to dependence and is a highly efficient way to identify patients who are at acute risk for the effects of alcohol abuse and dependence as well as those who do not currently meet formal alcohol-related diagnoses but who are at risk for long-term medical and social consequences of heavy alcohol exposure (Box 1). The U.S. Preventative Services Task Force (USPSTF) found that screening could accurately identify patients whose levels or patterns of alcohol consumption do not meet criteria for alcohol dependence but that place them at risk for increased morbidity and mortality. The USPSTF also found good evidence that brief interventions that consist of behavioral counseling and follow-up can reduce alcohol consumption for 6 to 12 months or longer and that the benefits outweigh any potential harms. Thus, it is recommended that alcohol screening and brief interventions be performed in primary care settings to reduce alcohol problems for adults, including pregnant women.

BRIEF SCREENING

Every patient should t5be asked about alcohol use. Because drinking is normative in the United States, if drinking is denied, it is useful to determine if the patient used to drink but has stopped because of a past problem. After determining if a patient currently uses any alcohol, the simplest strategy is to ask about the number of heavy drinking days in the past year, where heavy drinking is defined as more than four drinks for men and more than three drinks for women in one day. If that threshold is reached, which corresponds to at-risk or hazardous drinking, then further evaluation of alcohol-related problems is indicated through the use of screening instruments. A standard drink is the same amount of alcohol contained in different volumes of alcoholic beverages (Box 2).

BOX 1 Current Risk Terms

Abstinence
- No alcohol use

Moderate Drinking
- Men: No more than 2 standard drinks per drinking d
- Women: No more than 1 standard drink per drinking d
- Elderly persons (>65 y): No more than 1 standard drink per drinking d

Risky or Hazardous Drinking
- Men
  - More than 4 standard drinks per drinking d
  - More than 14 standard drinks per wk
- Women
  - More than 3 standard drinks per drinking d
  - More than 7 standard drinks per wk
- Elderly persons (>65 y):
  - More than 3 standard drinks per drinking d
  - More than 7 standard drinks per wk

> **BOX 2 Standard Drinks**
>
> Each equivalent drink contains about 14 g of pure alcohol:
> - 12 oz of beer or wine cooler
> - 8-9 oz of malt liquor
> - 5 oz of wine
> - 3 to 4 oz of fortified wine (e.g., port)
> - 1½ oz of 80-proof distilled spirits (or 1 jigger of liquor before mixing)

The Alcohol Use Disorders Identification test (AUDIT) (Table 1) is a 10-item screen developed by the World Health Organization. Given its length, the AUDIT can be used as a self-report screener that patients can fill out in the waiting area before seeing the clinician. The minimum score is 0 and the maximum score is 40. A score of 8 or more for men or 4 or more for women, adolescents, and persons older than 65 years, like a positive endorsement of any heavy drinking days, indicates the need for further evaluation of alcohol use and an increased risk of an alcohol use disorder. For brevity, the AUDIT-C, a truncated version of the AUDIT consisting of the first three AUDIT questions focused on alcohol consumption, can be used as a part of a waiting-room health history form. A score of 6 or more for men or 4 or more for women on the AUDIT-C indicates a need for further evaluation.

Asking about alcohol consumption during a routine clinical interview is best bundled with other questions about lifestyle and health, such as diet, smoking, and exercise. In addition to giving the patient a pre-examination questionnaire to fill out such as the AUDIT, another screening strategy is to ask the CAGE questions (Box 3) during the clinical examination. A positive answer to any of these questions also indicates the need for further evaluation of alcohol use. Two or more CAGE questions answered affirmatively identifies a patient at high risk for alcohol dependence. Because the CAGE screens for consequences, it is not as sensitive for risky drinking.

There are other question sets that are more sensitive than the CAGE in specific demographic subsets, and these can also be easily asked during a routine history. The five-item TWEAK questionnaire (Table 2) may be a more optimal screening questionnaire for identifying women (including pregnant women) with risky drinking or alcohol-use disorders in racially mixed populations. The CRAFFT (Box 4) is a 6-item question set that has high sensitivity in screening adolescents for alcohol and other substance-abuse problems. For patients older than 65 years, the Short Michigan Alcoholism Screening Test—Geriatric (S-MAST-G) (Box 5) is useful in identifying those at risk for alcohol problems, because these patients might not need the same volumes of alcohol intake as others to develop alcohol-related problems. To complete the initial screening, one should compute the average number of drinks per week by multiplying the days per week on average that the patient drinks by the number of drinks consumed on a typical drinking day.

Laboratory testing for elevations of alanine aminotransferase (ALT), aspartate aminotransferase (AST), γ-glutamyltransferase (GGT), or carbohydrate-deficient transferrin (CDT) have no incremental sensitivity over those of validated screening instruments, and they may be better suited to monitoring patients already in treatment for alcohol-use disorders. The patient must still be asked about quantity and frequency of alcohol use. However, laboratory testing can provide indicators of covert heavy drinking (e.g., elevated GGT and CDT) when the patient does not reveal the extent of alcohol intake.

TABLE 1 Alcohol Use Disorders Identification Test (AUDIT)

Questions	0	1	2	3	4
Consumption (AUDIT-C)					
How often do you have a drink containing alcohol?	Never	Monthly or less	2 to 4 times a mo	2 to 3 times a wk	4 or more times a wk
How many drinks containing alcohol do you have on a typical day when you are drinking?	1 or 2	3 or 4	5 or 6	7 to 9	10 or more
How often do you have five or more drinks on one occasion?	Never	Less than monthly	Monthly	Weekly	Daily or almost daily
Personal Consequences					
How often during the last year have you found that you were not able to stop drinking once you had started?	Never	Less than monthly	Monthly	Weekly	Daily or almost daily
How often during the last year have you failed to do what was normally expected of you because of drinking?	Never	Less than monthly	Monthly	Weekly	Daily or almost daily
How often during the last year have you needed a first drink in the morning to get yourself going after a heavy drinking session?	Never	Less than monthly	Monthly	Weekly	Daily or almost daily
How often during the last year have you had a feeling of guilt or remorse after drinking?	Never	Less than monthly	Monthly	Weekly	Daily or almost daily
How often during the last year have you been unable to remember what happened the night before because of your drinking?	Never	Less than monthly	Monthly	Weekly	Daily or almost daily
Social Consequences					
Have you or someone else been injured because of your drinking?	No		Yes, but not in the last y		Yes, during the last y
Has a relative, friend, doctor, or other health care worker been concerned about your drinking or suggested you cut down?	No		Yes, but not in the last y		Yes, during the last y

Scoring and Interpretation
Add all scores to obtain a total: >8 points for men or >4 points for women indicates a high risk of alcohol use disorder.
AUDIT-C (first three AUDIT questions): >6 points for men or >4 points for women indicates a need for further evaluation.

BOX 3 CAGE Questionnaire

- Have you ever felt that you should *Cut down* on your drinking?
- Have people *Annoyed* you by criticizing your drinking?
- Have you ever felt bad or *Guilty* about your drinking?
- Have you ever taken a drink (*Eye opener*) first thing in the morning to steady your nerves or to get rid of a hangover?

One yes response indicates need for further assessment. Two yes responses indicate risk of an alcohol use disorder.

CDT, which is perturbed less than other indices by nonalcoholic liver disease, may be a more specific and sensitive indicator of heavy drinking.

Diagnosis

Screening can identify those who are at risk for the sequelae of risky or hazardous drinking and who might benefit from a brief intervention conducted in the primary care office, but only a diagnostic evaluation can confirm the clinician's suspicion that the patient's use of alcohol meets syndromal criteria and warrants specific medical and psychosocial treatment beyond the brief intervention. If, during the last 12 months, alcohol has contributed to repeated episodes of failure to fulfill obligations at home, school or work, episodes of increased risk of physical harm, arrests or other legal problems, or recurrent problems with significant others, then the patient has a diagnosis of alcohol abuse, according to *Diagnostic and Statistical Manual of Mental Disorders*, fourth edition (text revision) (DSM-IV TR) criteria (Table 3). The patient has a diagnosis of alcohol dependence if he or she has three or more of the following criteria over a 12-month period: physical tolerance, symptoms of withdrawal, repeatedly drinking more than intended, unsuccessful reduction or quit attempts, increased time drinking or recovering from drinking, reduced time in other pleasurable or important activities, and continued drinking despite physical or psychological problems.

Rates of co-occurring mood and anxiety disorders are especially high among those with alcohol-use disorders. Untreated mood and anxiety disorders tend to have a negative impact on alcoholism recovery. Among treatment-seeking patients in the National Epidemiologic Survey on Alcohol and Related Conditions (NESARC) sample with a current alcohol use disorder, 40% had at least one current independent mood disorder, and more than one third had at least one current independent anxiety disorder. Heavy alcohol intake can also induce symptoms of mood and other mental disorders. To differentiate alcohol-induced symptoms from independent disorders, it is optimal to reassess symptoms of a mental disorder several weeks after cessation or significant reduction of alcohol intake.

 CURRENT DIAGNOSIS

Risky or Hazardous Drinking (Need Further Evaluation)

- Men who drink more than four standard drinks per day or 14 standard drinks per week
- Women and those older than 65 years who drink more than three standard drinks per day or more than seven standard drinks per week
- Drinking concurrent with any medical condition where alcohol is contraindicated

Alcohol Abuse

- Repeated failure to fulfill obligations at home, school or work
- Increased risk of physical harm
- Legal problems or interpersonal problems in any year.

Alcohol Dependence (Three or More in Any Year)

- Cannot cut down or stop
- Decreased time spent in other usual activities
- Drinking despite physical or psychological consequences
- Drinking more than intended
- Physical tolerance
- Preoccupied with drinking
- Withdrawal episodes

Brief Intervention

INTENTION

Although risky or hazardous drinking is not a formal diagnosis, it describes a group with a higher likelihood to develop alcohol problems with risk for accidents, injuries, and social and health problems compared with the general population (see Box 1). Thus, even without a formal diagnosis, it is beneficial to help the patient with risky drinking to change his or her drinking behavior. Several well-described short interchanges between the clinician and the patient, organized under the rubric of *brief interventions*, have been validated in randomized trials as decreasing alcohol intake in those who drink too much but do not have a diagnosis of alcohol dependence. Brief intervention has been demonstrated to reduce weekly alcohol use, frequency of binging, liver enzymes associated with heavy drinking, blood pressure, emergency department visits, hospital days, and psychosocial problems, typically for 6 to 12 months, and to reduce drinking and hospital days at up to 4 years in one study. Because most at-risk patients seen in primary care settings are subsyndromal for alcohol-use disorders, the typical clinical interaction related to alcohol will be that of screening and then a brief intervention for positive cases. The two are typically referred to together under the acronym SBI (screening and brief intervention).

TABLE 2 TWEAK Questionnaire

Feature	Question	Answer	Score
Tolerance	How many drinks does it take before you begin to feel the first effects of alcohol?	≥3	2
Worry	Have your friends or relatives worried or complained about your drinking in the past year?	Yes	2
Eye-opener	Do you sometimes take a drink in the morning when you first get up?	Yes	1
Amnesia	Are there times when you drink and afterward you can't remember what you said or did?	Yes	1
Kut	Do you sometimes feel the need to cut down on your drinking?	Yes	1

Scoring and interpretation: Two or more points indicate a possible alcohol problem.

> **BOX 4 CRAFFT Questionnaire**
>
> - Have you ever ridden in a **C**ar driven by someone (including yourself) who was high or had been using alcohol or drugs?
> - Do you ever use alcohol or drugs to **R**elax, feel better about yourself, or fit in?
> - Do you ever use alcohol or drugs while you are **A**lone?
> - Do you ever **F**orget things you did while using alcohol or drugs?
> - Do your **F**amily or **F**riends ever tell you that you should cut down on your drinking or drug use?
> - Have you ever gotten into **T**rouble while you were using alcohol or drugs?
>
> One yes response indicates need for further assessment. Two yes responses indicate risk of alcohol-use disorder.

The basic intention of a brief intervention is to educate the patient about the risks of heavy alcohol use in such a way as to motivate him or her to reduce weekly alcohol consumption. The standard initial brief intervention takes about 15 minutes and consists of feedback, advice, and goal setting. It can be performed wholly in the primary care setting by the physician or other members of the health delivery team. Including alcohol screening, the USPSTF suggests five As to conducting SBI: *assess* the patient's alcohol consumption with a screening tool and clinical evaluation as indicated; *advise* reduction of alcohol consumption to appropriate levels, including abstinence if indicated; *agree* on individual goals for reducing alcohol use, including abstinence if indicated; *assist* patients in obtaining the motivation, skills, or supports needed to institute changes in drinking; and *arrange* for follow-up support, including specialty treatment referral for dependent patients. The most effective interventions are multi-contact ones that provide ongoing assistance and follow-up.

PROCEDURE

Assess

Screen patients with the AUDIT or with the CAGE, TWEAK, CRAFFT, or S-MAST-G questionnaires as appropriate, and compute average drinks per week.

> **BOX 5 S-MAST-G Questionnaire**
>
> - When talking with others, do you ever underestimate how much you actually drink?
> - After a few drinks, have you sometimes not eaten or been able to skip meals because you didn't feel hungry?
> - Does having a few drinks help decrease your shakiness or tremors?
> - Does alcohol sometimes make it hard for you to remember parts of the day or night?
> - Do you usually take a drink to relax or calm your nerves?
> - Do you drink to take your mind off your problems?
> - Have you ever increased your drinking after experiencing a loss in your life?
> - Has a doctor or nurse ever said that they were worried or concerned about your drinking?
> - Have you ever made rules to manage your drinking?
> - When you feel lonely, does having a drink help?
>
> Two or more yes responses indicate a probable alcohol problem
>
> ---
>
> *Abbreviation:* S-MAST-G = Short Michigan Alcoholism Screening Test—Geriatric.

Advise

Give feedback in the form of expression of concern, direct conclusions, and recommendations. Present medical findings, such as elevated liver enzymes, to back up conclusive statements such as "I'm concerned that your alcohol intake exceeds safe limits." Show the patient information comparing use with population norms and the associated health risks. Educate the patient about how alcohol can lead to medical, psychosocial, and legal consequences. Where possible, link the patient's current symptoms to alcohol use. Recommend appropriate and specific changes in behavior, such as "I strongly recommend you cut down your drinking," or in the case where any drinking places the patient at high risk, "I strongly suggest you quit drinking."

Agree

Determine the patient's readiness to change drinking behavior, such as asking, "Do you think that cutting down on your drinking is something you are willing to talk about?" If the patient is ambivalent, avoid labeling the patient's behavior with a diagnosis at this stage, which can increase resistance to change, but encourage the patient to reflect on the positive reasons for drinking and the negative consequences of drinking. Offer concerns that continued drinking at the same level will impede the patient's achievement of goals such as decreased gastric distress or improved sleep patterns.

Empathic listening is generally more effective than a confrontational approach, and it is useful to express optimism about the patient's capacity to change. Elicit what the patient's concerns are about cutting down or quitting. Avoid arguing or challenging when the patient is unready to change, but schedule a follow-up visit to continue the dialogue and reassess drinking behavior. Restate your commitment to help when the patient is ready and that you remain open to questions.

When the patient concurs that a change in drinking would be beneficial, agree on a specific goal to cut down to particular daily and weekly limits for low-risk drinking or to stop drinking, if indicated, for a specific period of time. The agreement should be recorded and a copy given to the patient both as a reminder and motivator for behavioral change.

Assist

Work with the patient to formulate concrete steps to implement the drinking reduction plan. These steps include how to avoid high-risk drinking situations, how to keep a record of alcohol intake, and who can support the patient in meeting his or her goals. Provide resources in the form of patient educational materials, examples of which can be downloaded from the National Institute of Alcohol Abuse and Alcoholism (NIAAA) web site (www.niaaa.nih.gov).

Arrange

Set up follow-up support and counseling visits or refer patients meeting dependence criteria for specialty treatment. Advise the patient to seek immediate medical treatment if withdrawal symptoms occur.

Treatment

DETOXIFICATION

Put simply, detoxification is medical stabilization that offers an opportunity to engage patients in alcoholism treatment, but it is not in itself treatment for alcohol dependence. Patients who drink more than 250 grams of alcohol daily are likely to experience physiologic withdrawal symptoms on cessation of drinking, but volume is not the only predictor of withdrawal severity. Although often mild, untreated alcohol withdrawal can result in seizures or delirium tremens (DTs), with increased risk of mortality.

TABLE 3 Diagnosis of Alcohol-Use Problems

Criteria	Typical Symptoms and History
Alcohol Abuse (≥1 in the last 12 mo)	
Alcohol has caused or contributed to repeated:	
Failure to fulfill obligations at home, school, or work	Hangovers at work, truancy at school, missing appointments
Episodes of increased risk of physical harm	Drinking and driving, swimming, or operating machinery
Arrests or other legal problems	Public intoxication, DUI or DWI
Problems with significant others	Spousal strife, physical fights
Alcohol Dependence (≥3 in the last 12 mo)	
Development of physical tolerance	Drinks more for the same effect
Episodes of withdrawal syndrome (see below)	Morning shakes, nausea, anxiety
Drinking more than intended repeatedly	Binging episodes
Unsuccessful efforts to cut down or stop drinking	Failed New Year's resolution
Increased time planning for drinking, drinking, or recovering from drinking	Instead of being with kids, spends weekend mornings sleeping in
Reduced time in other pleasurable or important activities	Stopped socializing with friends, withdrew from hobby group
Drinking persists despite physical or psychological problems	Developed depressed mood, but kept on drinking
Alcohol Withdrawal (≥2 within h to d after lowered blood alcohol levels)	
Autonomic hyperactivity	Heart rate ≥100 bpm, diaphoresis
Hand tremor	Hands shake when extended
Insomnia	Difficulty falling asleep
Nausea or vomiting	Feels queasy
Anxiety	Spontaneous report of fear
Psychomotor agitation	Inability to keep still, pacing
Hallucinations or illusions	Reports visual disturbances
Seizures	Tonic-clonic movements

Assessment

The Clinical Institute Withdrawal Assessment—Alcohol Revised (CIWA-Ar) is a public domain scale that scores 10 signs and symptoms of withdrawal by severity ranging from not present to severe (Box 6). A score of less than 8 indicates mild withdrawal, characterized by increased autonomic activity with low-grade anxiety, diaphoresis, agitation, nausea, and elevated blood pressure, temperature, and heart rate. Scores of 8 to 15 indicate moderate withdrawal, and scores of 15 or more indicate more severe withdrawal states. In severe withdrawal, in the context of autonomic hyperarousal, the patient can become disoriented and have a clouded sensorium, the hallmarks of delirium.

Prior history of severe withdrawal, such as DTs, is a reasonable predictor of similar future responses to alcohol withdrawal. Risk for withdrawal delirium is increased if the patient has a heart rate of greater than 120 bpm before treatment, a current infectious disease, withdrawal symptoms in the context of a blood alcohol concentration greater than 100 mg/dL, a prior history of either delirium or seizures, or a high CIWA-Ar score, indicating severe autonomic hyperactivity. Patients who have severe withdrawal symptoms, who are at high risk for seizures, or who have a medical condition likely to be exacerbated by withdrawal, such as type 1 diabetes or coronary artery disease, should have medically supervised inpatient detoxification.

CURRENT THERAPY

All At-Risk Patients

- Assess: Screen patients with standard instruments and compute average standard drinks per week.
- Advise: Give feedback, express concern, present findings and conclusions, and recommend specific behavioral changes.
- Agree: Determine the patient's readiness to change, encourage reflection, listen empathically, elicit patient concerns, avoid arguing, express optimism, set a specific reduction or abstinence goal.
- Assist: Formulate concrete implementation plan, including avoiding high-risk situations, recording alcohol intake, and eliciting family and community support for patient goals.
- Arrange: Set up follow-up visits and refer patients meeting dependence criteria for specialty treatment.

Additionally for Alcohol-Dependent Patients

- Offer or arrange for detoxification if indicated.
- Offer or arrange for specialty alcoholism treatment and/or mutual help groups.
- Offer pharmacotherapy to support maintenance of abstinence: naltrexone, acamprosate, or disulfiram.
- Offer medication management support during follow-up visits.

Pharmacologic Therapy

Alcohol withdrawal is best treated with sedative hypnotic medications that are cross-tolerant with alcohol, such as benzodiazepines. Longer-acting benzodiazepines such as diazepam (Valium) and chlordiazepoxide (Librium) are easier to titrate against withdrawal symptoms and give a gradual offset in plasma concentration, but shorter-acting benzodiazepines such as lorazepam (Ativan)[1] are less likely to oversedate the patient. Rapid-onset benzodiazepines have a higher abuse liability and are generally best avoided. However, patients with severe hepatic impairment (elevated total bilirubin) are best treated with benzodiazepines that are not oxidized by the liver, such as oxazepam (Serax) or lorazepam.

Typical dosing is chlordiazepoxide 50 to 100 mg, diazepam 10 to 20 mg, oxazepam 20 to 40[3] mg, or lorazepam[1] 2 to 4 mg. The typical front-loading style of dosing is to administer medication at the higher end of the dose range every 1 to 2 hours so that the CIWA-Ar score is less than 8 for 24 hours.

With long-acting medications, once symptoms subside, there is often no need to taper doses. The short-acting benzodiazepines and

---
[1]Not FDA approved for this indication.
[3]Exceeds dosage recommended by the manufacturer.

BOX 6 Clinical Institute Withdrawal Assessment of Alcohol Scale, Revised (CIWA-Ar)

Patient: _____ Date: _____ Time: _____ (24 hour clock, midnight = 00:00)
_____

Pulse or heart rate, taken for one minute: _____ Blood pressure: _____ mm Hg
_____

Nausea and Vomiting – Ask "Do you feel sick to your stomach? Have you vomited?" Observation:

0 no nausea and no vomiting
1 mild nausea with no vomiting
2
3
4 intermittent nausea with dry heaves
5
6
7 constant nausea, frequent dry heaves, and vomiting

Tactile Disturbances – Ask "Have you any itching, pins and needles sensations, any burning, any numbness, or do you feel bugs crawling on or under your skin?" Observation:

0 none
1 very mild itching, pins and needles, burning, or numbness
2 mild itching, pins and needles, burning, or numbness
3 moderate itching, pins and needles, burning, or numbness
4 moderately severe hallucinations
5 severe hallucinations
6 extremely severe hallucinations
7 continuous hallucinations

Tremor – Arms extended and fingers spread apart. Observation:

0 no tremor
1 not visible, but can be felt fingertip to fingertip
2
3
4 moderate, with patient's arms extended
5
6
7 severe, even with arms not extended

Auditory Disturbances – Ask "Are you more aware of sounds around you? Are they harsh? Do they frighten you? Are you hearing anything that is disturbing to you? Are you hearing things you know are not there?" Observation:

0 not present
1 very mild harshness or ability to frighten
2 mild harshness or ability to frighten
3 moderate harshness or ability to frighten
4 moderately severe hallucinations
5 severe hallucinations
6 extremely severe hallucinations
7 continuous hallucinations

Paroxysmal Sweats – Observation:

0 no sweat visible
1 barely perceptible sweating, palms moist
2
3
4 beads of sweat obvious on forehead
5
6
7 drenching sweats

Visual Disturbances – Ask "Does the light appear to be too bright? Is its color different? Does it hurt your eyes? Are you seeing anything that is disturbing to you? Are you seeing things you know are not there?" Observation:

0 not present
1 very mild sensitivity
2 mild sensitivity
3 moderate sensitivity
4 moderately severe hallucinations
5 severe hallucinations
6 extremely severe hallucinations
7 continuous hallucinations

Anxiety – Ask "Do you feel nervous?" Observation:

0 no anxiety, at ease
1 mild anxious
2
3
4 moderately anxious, or guarded, so anxiety is inferred
5
6
7 equivalent to acute panic states as seen in severe delirium or acute schizophrenic reactions

Headache, Fullness in Head – Ask "Does your head feel different? Does it feel like there is a band around your head?" Do not rate for dizziness or lightheadedness. Otherwise, rate severity:

0 not present
1 very mild
2 mild
3 moderate
4 moderately severe
5 severe
6 very severe
7 extremely severe

> **BOX 6   Clinical Institute Withdrawal Assessment of Alcohol Scale, Revised (CIWA-Ar)—cont'd**
>
> **Agitation –** Observation:
> 0 normal activity
> 1 somewhat more than normal activity
> 2
> 3
> 4 moderately fidgety and restless
> 5
> 6
> 7 paces back and forth during most of the interview or constantly thrashes about
>
> **Orientation and Clouding of Sensorium –** Ask "What day is this? Where are you? Who am I?"
> 0 oriented and can do serial additions
> 1 cannot do serial additions or is uncertain about date
> 2 disoriented for date by no more than 2 calendar d
> 3 disoriented for date by more than 2 calendar d
> 4 disoriented for place or person
>
> Total CIWA-Ar Score _____
> Rater's Initials _____
> Maximum Possible Score: 67
>
> The CIWA-Ar *is not* copyright and may be reproduced freely. This assessment for monitoring withdrawal symptoms requires approximately 5 minutes to administer.
>
> From Sullivan JT, Sykora K, Schneiderman J, Naranjo CA, Sellers EM: Assessment of alcohol withdrawal: The revised Clinical Institute Withdrawal Assessment for Alcohol scale (CIWA-Ar). Br J Addiction 1989;84:1353-1357.

long-acting benzodiazepines given to patients at high-risk for seizures or DTs are best given on a fixed-dose regimen of four times daily for the first 24 hours, with the patient reassessed 1 to 2 hours after each dose, and additional medication given as needed. On days 2 and 3, 50% of the dose can be given four times daily.

Long-acting barbiturates, such as phenobarbital,[1] can be also used on a fixed-dose regimen of 60 mg every 4 to 6 hours, with a loading dose of 120 mg orally or intramuscularly every hour for acute withdrawal symptoms (e.g., pulse >110 bpm) or a CIWA-Ar score of 10 or more.

Anticonvulsants such as carbamazepine (Tegretol),[1] valproate (Depakote),[1] or gabapentin (Neurontin)[1] have also been used effectively in uncomplicated withdrawal, but they are unproved in preventing withdrawal-related seizures and in treating DTs.

Although phenothiazines and haloperidol are somewhat effective compared with benzodiazepines in reducing withdrawal symptoms such as agitation, they are not as protective against seizures or delirium and thus are not recommended.

Thiamine (Vitamin B_1) supplementation of 100 mg/day for 3 days can counteract the thiamine deficiencies that are common in alcoholic patients.

PSYCHOSOCIAL INTERVENTIONS FOR ALCOHOL DEPENDENCE

In addition to brief interventions for risky alcohol use, the most opportune and practical psychosocial intervention that the primary care office can provide is clinical behavioral support for pharmacotherapy for alcohol dependence. Simply put, medication management support consists initially of feedback to the patient of screening and medical evaluation results and the negative health effects of continued heavy drinking, as in a brief intervention. The patient is then given the basis for the diagnosis of alcohol dependence, the rationale for abstinence, and recommendation for pharmacotherapy. The patient is given information about medication and the appropriate prescriptions and is encouraged to seek community support for sobriety in mutual help groups such as Alcoholics Anonymous or to follow a plan such as Rational Recovery. Follow-up visits consist of assessment of medication side effects, patient adherence to the medication regimen, assessment of abstinence or quantity and pattern of alcohol intake, and assessment of overall functioning. Problems with medication adherence are identified and addressed.

There are evidence-based psychosocial interventions that are typically performed in the context of specialty programs for alcohol dependence, but they can be offered by clinical personnel in the context of the physician's office. Cognitive behavior therapy, network therapy, behavioral family therapy, and motivational interviewing are effective approaches for the treatment of alcohol dependence. Motivational interviewing is especially adaptable for use in primary care settings in that it is an approach to interacting with the alcohol-dependent patient that can be learned quickly and executed by any staff with clinical contact. A motivational enhancement manual can be accessed at the NIAAA web site (http://www.niaaa.nih.gov/)

MEDICATION MANAGEMENT OF ALCOHOL DEPENDENCE

There are currently four FDA-approved medications for the treatment of alcohol dependence. Any of these medications can and should be given concurrently with other interventions such as psychosocial treatment or mutual help groups.

Disulfiram (Antabuse) works by inhibiting the metabolism of ethyl alcohol, causing a buildup of acetaldehyde, a noxious substance, which causes a strong stereotypic aversive response (flushing, diaphoresis, nausea, tachycardia) in the patient. Standard dosing is 250 mg/day (range, 125-500 mg). The major clinical concern with disulfiram is patient noncompliance with the medication regimen. Thus, it is most likely to be effective when there is a concrete method for supporting compliance in place, such as directly observed therapy by a spouse or in a clinic.

More recently, the opioid antagonist naltrexone (ReVia, Depade) was approved for the treatment of alcohol dependence. It is dosed at 50 mg once daily. Naltrexone reduces days of heavy drinking and can reduce alcohol craving. Naltrexone in a long-acting intramuscular formulation (Vivitrol) allows once-monthly dosing (380 mg) and reduces the risk of noncompliance. It reduces heavy drinking overall and helps maintain abstinence in those who are abstinent at initial drug administration. Both oral and IM naltrexone formulations carry FDA black-box warnings related to findings of reversible elevations of liver enzymes at three to six times the standard dosage; however, naltrexone is safe at the recommended dose.

Acamprosate (Campral) is a taurine analogue that has been demonstrated to reduce relapse to any drinking as well as reducing heavy drinking in nonabstinent patients. It is dosed as two 333-mg tablets three times a day to patients who have ceased alcohol intake. It is excreted unchanged through the kidneys and has no interactions with other medications. Side effects are benign, and the most frequent is loose stools, which are mild to moderate and self-limited.

---

[1]Not FDA approved for this indication.

REFERENCES

American Psychiatric Association: Diagnostic and Statistical Manual of Mental Disorders, 4th ed, text revision. Washington, DC, American Psychiatric Association, 2000.
Bertholet N, Daeppen J-B, Wietlisbach V, et al: Reduction of alcohol consumption by brief alcohol intervention in primary care systematic review and meta-analysis. Arch Intern Med 2005;165:986-995.
Bradley KA, Boyd-Wickizer J, Powell SH, Burman ML: Alcohol screening questionnaires in women: A critical review. JAMA 1998;280:166-171.
Chang G, Kosten TR: Detoxification. In Lowinson JH, Ruiz P, Millman RB, Langrod JG (eds): Substance Abuse: A Comprehensive Textbook. Philadelphia, Lippincott Williams & Wilkins, 2004, pp 579-587.
Fleming MF, Mundt MP, French MT, et al: Brief physician advice for problem drinkers: Long-term efficacy and cost-benefit analysis. Alcohol Clin Exp Res 2002;26:36-43.
Grant BF, Stinson FS, Dawson DA, et al: Prevalence and co-occurrence of substance use disorders and independent mood and anxiety disorders: Results from the National Epidemiologic Survey on Alcohol and Related Conditions. Arch Gen Psychiatry 2004;61:807-816.
Knight JR, Sherritt L, Shrier LA, et al: Validity of the CRAFFT substance abuse screening test among adolescent clinic patients. Arch Pediatr Adolesc Med 2002;156(6):607-614.
Maisto SA, Saitz R: Alcohol use disorders: Screening and diagnosis. Am J Addict 2003;12(suppl 1):S12-S25.
McCaul ME, Petry NM: The role of psychosocial treatments in pharmacotherapy for alcoholism. Am J Addict 2003;12(Suppl 1):S41-S52.
National Institute on Alcohol Abuse and Alcoholism: Helping Patients Who Drink Too Much: A Clinician's Guide. Rockville, MD, National Institute on Alcohol Abuse and Alcoholism, 2005. Available at http://pubs.niaaa.nih.gov/publications/Practitioner/CliniciansGuide2005/guide.pdf(accessed June 15, 2007).
Saitz R: Unhealthy alcohol use. N Engl J Med 2005;352:596-607.
Saunders JB, Aasland OG, Babor TF, et al: Development of the Alcohol Use Disorders Screening Test (AUDIT). WHO collaborative project on early detection of persons with harmful alcohol consumption. Addiction 1993;88:791-804.
Sullivan JT, Sykora K. Schneiderman J, et al: Assessment of alcohol withdrawal: The revised Clinical Institute Withdrawal Assessment for Alcohol scale (CIWA-Ar). Br J Addict 1989;84:1353-1357.
U.S. Preventive Services Task Force: Screening and behavioral counseling interventions in primary care to reduce alcohol misuse: Recommendation statement. Ann Intern Med 2004;140:554-556.

Drug Abuse

Method of
Norman S. Miller, MD

Epidemiology

PREVALENCE

Drug abuse and dependence are continuing major causes of death and costly medical morbidity in public health in the United States and throughout the world. Overall, the lifetime prevalence of drug abuse and dependence is 7% in the United States, alcohol dependence is 15%, and comorbid drug and alcohol dependence is 20%. In recent years, the growing trend includes dependent use of prescription medications to add the already high rates of illicit drug abuse and dependence.

The concurrent and collaborative use of drugs with alcohol is common. As many as 80% of alcoholics younger than 30 years use drugs dependently. For instance, 80% of alcoholics are addicted to nicotine and 80% of cocaine addicts are addicted to alcohol. Given the prevalence of drug and alcohol abuse and dependence, the combination of drug and alcohol use constitutes drug abuse and dependence in alarming epidemic proportions.

MORBIDITY AND MORTALITY

Drugs and alcohol cause death in epidemic proportions. Illicit drug use causes 100,000 excess deaths, and nicotine causes 400,000 excess deaths. In addition, drug use and dependence cause major deleterious psychological and social problems, including family dysfunction, domestic and criminal violence, and child abuse (Table 1).

Of central importance, drug and alcohol use and dependence contribute significantly to many of the other leading causes of death, namely, heart disease, cancer, stroke, respiratory disease, accidents, diabetes, Alzheimer's disease, influenza and pneumonia, kidney disease, suicide, liver disease, hypertension, Parkinson's disease, and homicide. Also, drugs and alcohol are toxic to the fetus and contribute significantly to leading causes of infant death, namely, congenital malformations, short gestation and low birth weight, sudden death infant syndrome, maternal complications, accidents, respiratory distress, bacterial sepsis, neonatal hemorrhage, and circulatory diseases.

As a perspective, in 2004, 41,000 deaths were due breast cancer, 652,000 due to heart disease, 150,000 due to stroke, 112,000 due to accidents, 32,000 due to suicide, 17,000 due to homicide, and 73,000 due to diabetes. In 2004, 30,000 deaths were from drug-induced causes: 19,000 in males, and 11,000 in females for all races. For whites, the figures are 27,000 total, 17,000 male, and 10,000 female. For blacks the figures are 3581 total, 2300 male, 1281 female. The category drug-induced causes includes not only deaths from dependent and nondependent use of drugs (legal and illegal) but also poisoning from medically prescribed and other drugs. The category excludes unintentional injuries, homicides, and other causes indirectly related to drug use. In 2004, there were a total of 21,000 alcohol-induced deaths: 16,000 male and 5000 female. For whites, the total was 18,000: 14,000 male and 4000 female. For blacks, the total was 2000: 1700 male and 500 female. The category alcohol-induced causes includes not only deaths from dependent and nondependent use of alcohol but also accidental poisoning by alcohol. It excludes unintentional injuries, homicides, and other causes indirectly related to alcohol use as well as deaths due to fetal alcohol syndrome.

ECONOMIC, MEDICAL, AND TREATMENT COSTS

In economic terms, drug and alcohol abuse cost nearly $300 billion annually in the United States or 25% of the national health care budget, and $34 billion is attributed to direct health care costs for hospitals, treatment programs, residential care, and professional services. In medical terms, drug and alcohol use and addictions are implicated in 25% to 50% of all general hospital admissions and 50% to 75% of psychiatric admissions, and they contribute substantially to medical complications and costs to those admitted to hospitals for other reasons.

In terms of treating pain and suffering from drug abuse and dependence, according to the Treatment Episode Data Set Highlights, 2005, 1,849,548 admissions for drug and alcohol dependence or problems, and nearly one million persons are active in specialized treatment for drug and alcohol problems—29% for drug addiction, 45% for alcoholism, and 26% for both alcoholism and drug addiction—at

TABLE 1 Causes of Death in 1990

Cause	Estimated Number	Total Deaths (%)
Tobacco	400,000	19
Diet or activity patterns	300,000	14
Alcohol	100,000	5
Microbial agents	90,000	4
Toxic agents	60,000	3
Firearms	35,000	2
Sexual behavior	30,000	1
Motor vehicles	25,000	1
Illicit use of drugs	20,000	<1
Total	1,060,000	50

any given time. In growing numbers, over 400,000 patients seek treatment annually for prescription drug dependence or problems.

Clinical Features and Diagnosis

Drug and alcohol disorders are behavioral, brain, and genetic diseases. Importantly, drug and alcohol addictions are not due to moral problems, though their consequences can create moral dilemmas for patients. Unfortunately, attitudes toward drug and alcohol addictions remain ambivalent, and physicians share the ambivalence in their reluctance to consider drug and alcohol disorders as medical problems for which they are responsibility.

Addiction is a definable behavioral syndrome based on brain pathophysiologic changes common to many types of addicting drugs, including alcohol. Central to addiction as a disease is the loss of control over drug and alcohol use that renders the patient a victim of uncontrolled drug use. Although the patient might have initially chosen to use a drug, once addiction is established, the victim has lost choice and is compelled to use drugs despite adverse consequences.

PHARMACOLOGIC TOLERANCE AND WITHDRAWAL

Pharmacologic tolerance is the decreasing effect from a drug or the need to increase the dose to maintain the effect. Importantly, pharmacologic tolerance develops to most drugs. For example, a 10- to 20-fold increase in dose is common for opiates, and a two- to four-fold increase in dose is common for alcohol. Pharmacologic tolerance can be expected as a neurologic adaptation to regular drug and alcohol use over time as the brain and body maintain homeostasis in the presence of the drug. On the other hand, *pharmacologic dependence* is the predictable, stereotypic response to the withdrawal of the drug during elimination after intoxication. Pharmacologic dependence is an expected neurologic adaptation to loss of drug effect and attempt to maintain homeostasis in the absence of the drug.

Each class of drug (alcohol, opiates, stimulants, sedative–hypnotics, tranquilizers) possesses its own known set of signs and symptoms of withdrawal following cessation of drug use (Box 1). Outstanding changes in vital signs are not a regular finding in most drug withdrawals except for alcohol; therefore, vital signs are not particularly useful in the diagnosis and treatment of specific drug withdrawal. Behavioral manifestations are usually more informative of drug withdrawal (and intoxication) than physical findings during drug withdrawal.

Peak periods of duration of withdrawal vary with drug types and half-life of the drug. In general, the shorter half-life leads to shorter withdrawal, and the longer and higher the dose used, the more severe the withdrawal. For instance, opiate and alcohol withdrawal peaks in 3 days, lasts 5 to 7 days, and can be identified by characteristic signs and symptoms. Craving or drive to use drugs is prominent in most drug withdrawals, either consciously or unconsciously in the person undergoing withdrawal. Subjective reports of craving are less reliable than objective manifestations, namely, drug seeking.

EVALUATION

Physicians and other health care professionals are in key positions to assess and treat persons who seek evaluation and treatment for medically related health problems associated with drug and alcohol use and addiction. Well-known medical complications from drug disorders are too numerous to cite but prominently include widespread medical, surgical, and psychiatric diseases. Physicians can fulfill important roles in preventing, managing, and treating drug disorders in their patients, including diagnosis, treatment, referral, and monitoring.

Management of intoxication and withdrawal syndromes is a key service that physicians can provide to reduce morbidity and mortality from drug disorders in their patients. Each drug has a characteristic and predictable intoxication and withdrawal state based on pharmacokinetic and pharmacodynamic principles that require medical

---

BOX 1 Characteristics of Withdrawal

Alcohol
Alcohol Withdrawal
Peak period: 1-3 days
Duration: 5-7 days
Signs: Elevated blood pressure, pulse, and temperature; hyperarousal; agitation; cutaneous flushing; tremors; diaphoresis; dilated pupils; ataxia; disorientation
Symptoms: anxiety, paranoid delusions, illusions, visual and auditory hallucinations

Alcohol Withdrawal Seizures
Onset 12-24 hours

Delirium Tremens
Onset: 72-96 hours
Mortality rate: 30%-50% untreated

Benzodiazepines and Other Sedatives and Hypnotics
Peak period: 2-4 days for short-acting drugs (alprazolam) or 4-7 days for long-acting drugs (clonazepam)
Duration: 4-7 days for short acting; 7-14 days for long acting
Signs: elevated blood pressure, pulse, and temperature; cutaneous flushing; tremors; diaphoresis; dilated pupils; ataxia; disorientation
Symptoms: agitation, anxiety, muscular weakness, delirium

Opiates
Peak period: 1-3 days
Duration: 5-7 days
Signs: drug seeking, mydriasis, piloerection, diaphoresis, rhinorrhea, diarrhea, nausea, vomiting, insomnia, elevated blood pressure and pulse
Symptoms: intense desire for drugs, muscle cramps, arthralgia, anxiety, malaise

Stimulants (Cocaine, Amphetamines, and Derivatives)
Peak period: 1-3 days
Duration: 5-7 days
Signs: behavioral withdrawal, psychomotor retardation, hypersomnia, hyperphagia
Symptoms: depression, anhedonia, suicidal thoughts and behavior, paranoid delusions

---

evaluation and intervention. Unfortunately, in a study of primary care physicians, 94% of physicians failed to list a drug disorder as one of five possible diagnoses when presented with a case describing a patient with early symptoms of an alcohol disorder. Forty-one percent of pediatricians failed to list drug disorders as one of five possible diagnoses when presented with a case describing classic symptoms of drug disorder in a teenager. Twenty percent of physicians considered themselves "very prepared" to diagnose a substance disorder—substantially lower than the 83% who feel "very prepared" to diagnose hypertension, 82% for diabetes, and 44% for depression. Forty-three percent of patients with a drug disorder reported that their physicians never diagnosed the disorder; an additional 10.7% reported their physicians knew about their disorder but did nothing about it. Critically important, almost three quarters of patients reported their primary care physician was not involved in their decision to seek treatment.

Despite these disappointing findings, physicians can use known knowledge and develop skills in the medical treatment of drug disorders. Physicians can be sanguine about what they offer their patients if they know that with proper diagnosis, treatment of withdrawal states, and referral for addiction treatment, between 50% and

90% of their patients can achieve abstinence for 1 year or longer. Management of withdrawal by the physician can be lifesaving and can assist with the progression from diagnosis to recovery. The physician can prescribe medications to reduce morbidity and mortality during intoxication and withdrawal and to increase compliance with psychosocial treatments. In addition, the physician can prescribe medications to patients in the subacute and chronic state to reduce relapse to addicting drugs and maintain patients in the substituted-drug or abstinent state.

Treatment

APPROACHES AND EFFECTIVENESS

Following detoxification, the abstinence-based method is commonly used to treat alcohol and drug addiction (95% of programs surveyed). This method uses cognitive behavior techniques and referral to 12-step recovery programs, such as Alcoholics Anonymous (AA) and Narcotics Anonymous.

One-year abstinence rates of 80% to 90% were achieved when patients participated in weekly continuing care or AA meetings, or both, after discharge from the treatment program. Also, 1-year abstinence rates were associated with reduced rates of medical and psychiatric use.

According to results of a 1992 survey conducted by AA, of those members sober in AA less than 1 year, 41% will attend AA another year. Of those members sober more than 1 year and less than 5 years, 83% will attend AA another year. Of those members sober 5 years or more, 91% will attend AA another year.

Physicians often encounter, in addition to alcohol, other drugs such as nicotine, cannabis, cocaine, opiates, sedative hypnotics and anxiolytics, amphetamines and derivatives, hallucinogens including phencyclidine, inhalants, anticholinergics, and anabolic steroids. Careful assessment, including toxicology and breathalyzer, and management of intoxication and withdrawal from these classes of drugs can be accomplished according to a rational basis for prescribing pharmacotherapies (Box 2). Each class of drug has predictable signs and symptoms for intoxication and withdrawal and responds to medications designed to counteract and suppress withdrawal states. The physician can prescribe in a medically safe and effective manner to promote freedom from these adverse drug effects and improvement in overall health. Drug testing for alcohol and drugs should be conducted simultaneously with ordering a chest x-ray or complete blood count (CBC) in diagnosing and treating other medical conditions.

ALCOHOL

Because many patients addicted to drugs are also using and addicted to alcohol, concurrent diagnosis and treatment of alcohol withdrawal are often necessary. General principles apply for management of withdrawal syndromes and relapse prevention in alcohol and drug dependence (Box 3). In particular, careful attention to assessing and treating alcohol withdrawal is necessary in alcohol use and dependence (Box 4).

NICOTINE

Nicotine is the psychoactive substance that is self-administered in addictive patterns in cigarettes, chewing tobacco, snuff, pipes, and cigars. As with other drugs, persons self-administer nicotine in addictive patterns according to blood levels of nicotine. Nicotine absorption leads to intoxication and produces stimulation and depression. Behavioral and subjective effects include nausea, euphoria, agitation and sedation, and physiologic changes that include increased heart rate, blood pressure, and motor activity. Significant pharmacologic tolerance and dependence develop to these effects over months and within a given day. Acute withdrawal begins within hours, extends over 3 to 5 days, and can last 1 to 2 weeks or more. Nicotine withdrawal produces depressed mood,

---

BOX 2   Medications for Withdrawal

Alcohol Withdrawal

Mild Withdrawal

Diazepam 5-10 mg[3] PO prn q4-6h × 1-3 days
or
Lorazepam[1] 1-2 mg PO prn q4-6h × 1-3 days

Moderate Withdrawal

Diazepam 5-10 mg PO: qid days 1 and 2, tid day 3, bid day 4, once day 5
Lorazepam[1] 2-4 mg PO qid days 1 and 2, 1-2 mg PO qid days 3 and 4, 1 mg PO bid day 5

Severe Withdrawal

Diazepam 10-25 mg[3] PO prn every hour while awake until sedation occurs × 5-7 days
or
Lorazepam[1] 1-2 mg IV prn every hour while awake until sedation occurs × 5-7 days

Benzodiazepines and Other Sedatives and Hypnotics

Short-term taper is 7-10 days, long-term taper is 10-14 days based on dose and duration of use.
Diazepam[1] 5-10 mg PO qid; taper to 5-10 mg PO qd
or
Calculate barbiturate or benzodiazepine equivalence and give 50% of the original dosage; taper (if actual dosage is known before detoxification).
Carbemazepine (Tegretol):[1] 400-1000 mg/day (average dose, 400-600 mg); maintain therapeutic blood level for 1-2 months (4-12 mg/dL)
Vaproic acid (Depakote):[1] 500-1500 mg/day (average dose, 1000-1500 mg); maintain therapeutic blood level for 1-2 months (100-150 mg/dL)

Note: Avoid giving the drug as needed. Adjustments in dosage according to the patient's clinical state may be indicated.

Opiates

Withdrawal can be managed with clonidine[1] for intranasal ulcers and methadone (Dolophin): those motivated to achieve abstinence.

Stimulants (Cocaine, Amphetamines, and Derivatives)

Observation and monitoring for depression and suicidal behavior are advised.
Mild to moderate withdrawal: diazepam[1] 5-10 mg either on a fixed schedule or prn
Severe withdrawal: Therapy may be initiated with antidepressants (SSRIs)

[1]Not FDA approved for this indication.
[3]Exceeds dosage recommended by the manufacturer.

---

insomnia, irritability, anxiety, difficulty concentrating, restlessness, decreased heart rate, and increased appetite.

Eighty percent of smokers express a desire to quit, 35% attempt to quit each year, and less than 5% can stop without interventions. Current interventions for smoking cessation include pharmacologic and behavioral methods to reduce relapse and promote abstinence from nicotine consumption. Nicotine replacement (gum, transdermal patch, nasal spray, inhaler) and antidepressant therapies are the main pharmacologic therapies. However, liability for addictive use of nicotine remains a problem in achieving abstinence from cigarettes.

> **BOX 3** General Principles for Management of Withdrawal Syndromes and Relapse Prevention in Alcohol Dependence
>
> **Alcohol and Drug Withdrawal**
> Best predictor of future withdrawal is past withdrawals
> Withdrawal is stereotypic and predictable for each class of drugs
> Treatment of withdrawal enhances compliance with addiction treatment and relapse prevention
>
> **Relapse to Alcohol and Drugs: General Principles**
> Relapse is remarkably similar for each class of drugs
> Interventions and treatments shift curve up and to the right to increase abstinence for longer durations
>
> **Approach to Diagnosis**
> Confront with knowledge, skill, and evidence
> Show consequences of addictive use
> Maintain concern and nonjudgmental attitude
>
> **Impediments to Diagnosis and Detoxification**
> Denial of drug and alcohol consequences
> Minimalization of drug and alcohol effects
> Rationalization of drug and alcohol use

Nicotine Replacement

Nicotine polacrilex gum (Commit) is nicotine bound to ion-exchange resin. It is available over the counter in 2- and 4-mg doses and taken several per day for 1 to 3 months. The nicotine is absorbed from buccal mucosa, with peak nicotine at 30 minutes. Cessation rates of 20% to 40% for 1 year can be achieved in conjunction with behavioral therapies.

The transdermal patch (Nicoderm CQ) has a lower potential for addictive use because of the controlled sustained release from the skin on the upper body, in doses of 7, 14, and 21 mg. The patch is applied each morning and removed in the evening. Peak concentration of nicotine is achieved in 2 to 6 hours, and steady state is reached in 2 to 3 days after continued patch use. Suggested treatment duration is 8, and cessation rates are doubled at 6-month follow-up.

Nicotine nasal spray (Nicotrol NS) delivers nicotine through nasal mucosa, approximating the absorption profile of cigarette smoking. Nicotine reaches peak levels at 5 minutes, and one to two doses are self-administered per hour. Abstinence rates at 1 year from cigarettes were twice the rates in subjects using placebo. However, potential for addiction is high because nicotine is delivered at steady and pulsating intervals to the brain.

Nicotine inhalers (Nicotrol Inhaler) are used similarly to sprays, with peak absorption at 15 minutes from 80 inhalations per 20 minutes, leading to cigarette cessation rates twice those with placebo at 3 months. However, the inhalers also have high addiction potential.

Bupropion

The antidepressant bupropion (Zyban), in sustained-release form, is given in 150-mg or 300-mg doses over 1 to 2 months. Cigarette smoking may cease at 1 week from starting bupropion, and abstinence rates of twice those with placebo are achieved at 1 year. The risk for seizure is 1 in 1000 smokers. Bupropion is relatively contraindicated in alcohol withdrawal. Bupropion's effectiveness does not appear related to its antidepressant effect because no change in mood was found in studies.

Varenicline

Varenicline (Chantix) contains no nicotine, but it targets the same receptors that nicotine does. Varenicline is believed to block nicotine from these receptors. Studies showed at the end of 12 weeks of varenicline, 44% quit smoking, compared with 30% who quit on bupropion and 17% on placebo. Varenicline combines smoking cessation research with psychological and behavioral therapy for a day-by-day plan to abstain from nicotine. The most common side effects include nausea (30%), trouble sleeping, vivid dreaming, constipation, gas, and vomiting. Starting dose is 0.5 mg daily for 3 days, then 0.5 mg twice daily for 4 days, then 1 mg twice daily for a total of 12 weeks. Varenicline is initiated 1 week before the quit date set in advance.

Other Medications

Other antidepressants such as nortriptyline (Pamelor)[1] were found to be efficacious. The antihypertensive clonidine (Catapres)[1] may be useful in oral or transdermal preparations in 0.1-mg or 0.2-mg patches or doses every 6 hours[3] for 3 to 5 days. Hypotension and sedation are limiting side effects from clonidine.

SEDATIVE HYPNOTICS AND ANXIOLYTICS

Intoxication from this class of drugs (benzodiazepines, barbiturates, ethchlorvynol, meprobamate) includes slowed mental and physical activities, hypotension, bradycardia, and reduced respiratory rate. Prolonged and severe respiratory depression can lead to acidosis, arrhythmias, cardiac arrest, and death. Flumazenil (Romazicon), a benzodiazepine antagonist, can be given intravenously to counter respiratory depression. Withdrawal symptoms from sedative hypnotics and anxiolytics include increased psychomotor activity, anxiety, depression, disorientation, agitation, muscle weakness, tremulousness, hyperpyrexia, diaphoresis, seizures, delirium with visual and auditory hallucinations, hypertension, and tachycardia.

Because benzodiazepines have cross-tolerance and dependence with other drugs in the sedative–hypnotic class but have a lower potential for respiratory depression, they can be substituted to reduce signs and symptoms of withdrawal. Dose equivalents can be calculated for tapering schedule. A long-acting preparation is generally preferred to produce a smooth suppression of withdrawal, but short-acting preparations should be considered when elimination times are delayed (e.g., significant documented liver disease).

> **BOX 4** Medications for Alcohol Withdrawal
>
> Benzodiazepines are recommended for alcohol withdrawal due to their documented efficacy and cross-tolerance and dependence.
> Benzodiazepines are recommended over other sedative-hypnotics because they have a better documented efficacy, a greater margin of safety, and lower abuse potential
> All benzodiazepines are equally effective and can be chosen on the following bases:
> Long-acting agents (e.g., diazepam) may be more effective in preventing withdrawal seizures
> Long-acting agents (e.g., diazepam) can contribute to a smoother withdrawal with fewer rebound symptoms
> Short-acting agents (e.g., lorazepam[1]) might have a lower risk of oversedation (liver disease)
> Certain benzodiazepines (e.g., diazepam) have a higher potential for misuse
> Cost of benzodiazepines varies greatly

---

[1]Not FDA approved for this indication.

[1]Not FDA approved for this indication.
[3]Exceeds dosage recommended by the manufacturer.

TABLE 2 Phenobarbital Equivalents for Treating Benzodiazepine Withdrawal

Benzodiazepine	Phenobarbital (mg) per 30 mg Benzodiazepine
Alprazolam (Xanax)	1
Chlordiazepoxide (Librium)	25
Clonazepam (Klonopin)	2
Clorazepate (Tranxene)	15
Diazepam (Valium)	10
Furazepam (Dalmane)	30
Lorazepam (Ativan)	2
Temazepam (Restoril)	15
Triazolam (Halcion)	0.25-0.50
Quazepam (Doral)	15
Estazolam (ProSom)	2

BOX 5 Clonidine[1] Substitution

Clonidine patch #1 or #2
and/or
Clonidine 0.1 mg PO qid × 2 days
or
Clonodine 0.1-0.2 mg PO q4-6h prn for signs and symptoms of withdrawal × 5-7 days (peak dosages are given days 2 through 4)
Check blood pressure before each dose and do not give medication if patient is hypotensive (systolic blood pressure <90 mm Hg)

[1]Not FDA approved for this indication.

Typically, the longer and higher the use of sedative, hypnotic, and anxiolytic drugs, the greater the duration and dose of taper for the substituted drug. Generally, 50% of the dose is used to begin taper over 7 to 10 days for short-acting preparations and over 10 to 14 days for long-acting preparations, given orally three or four times a day. However, for withdrawal when these medications have been taken over a few years, up to 1 to 2 months may be required for the taper.

Anticonvulsants such as carbamazepine (Tegretol)[1] or valproic acid (Depakote)[1] are effective in conjunction with benzodiazepine taper (conservative approach) or alone in lieu of benzodiazepines. Anticonvulsants are given until therapeutic blood levels are reached, and dose is maintained for 2 to 4 weeks, followed by a taper (Table 2).

OPIATES

Addiction and Withdrawal

Intoxication from all opiates (heroin, narcotic analgesics, and methadone) is similar in producing suppression of the central nervous system (CNS). Psychological responses include initial euphoria followed by apathy, dysphoria, depressed mood and affect, psychomotor agitation or retardation, impaired judgment, impaired social or occupational functioning, drowsiness, slurred speech, and impairments in attention and concentration. Physiologic responses include pupillary constriction, hypotension, constipation, respiratory depression, and cardiovascular collapse in large enough doses.

Symptoms of withdrawal from opiates include dysphoria, nausea, vomiting, muscle aches, lacrimation or rhinorrhea, pupillary dilation, sweating, diarrhea, yawning, fever, insomnia, and intense drive to use more drugs, particularly opiates. The peak period of withdrawal depends on the half-life of the opiate. For heroin the peak withdrawal period is 3 days, for opiate analgesics it can vary from 3 to 7 days, and for methadone (Dolophin) the range is 7 to 14 days. The duration of withdrawal can last to up 7 days for heroin, 7 to 14 days for opiate analgesics, and 14 to 28 days and longer for methadone, depending on the duration of use of the opiate and dose. The longer the use and the higher the dose, the more severe and protracted the withdrawal. Withdrawal from opiates is not generally life threatening except when accompanied by comorbid medical and psychiatric disorders. However, adequate treatment of opiate withdrawal improves compliance with treatments for medical and surgical disorders and treatment for opiate and other drug addictions to reduce relapse to opiates.

Pharmacologic Therapy

Pharmacologic therapies for opiate withdrawal are aimed at reducing the drive or craving for drugs, high levels of agitation, and physiologic and psychological distress accompanying withdrawal. Nonopiate and opiate medications can be used to ameliorate these symptoms; the nonopiate medication is more effective for treating intranasal and oral opiate use and lower dosages, and the opiate medications are more effective for treating intravenous opiate use and higher dosages. However, clonidine[1] can often reduce the symptoms of opiate withdrawal in either instance, particularly when given in an inpatient setting, by 50% to 75%, and more if given in adequate dosages (Box 5).

Clonidine

Typically, a clonidine[1] patch (either #1 or #2 patch) is applied, on day 1, with 0.1 to 0.2 mg, depending on body weight, for 2 to 3 days, until blood levels from the patch reach equilibrium. In addition, clonidine 0.1 mg to 0.2 mg orally four times a day can be given throughout the withdrawal state for up to 1 to 2 weeks, and the clonidine patch may be continued for 2 weeks or longer for protracted withdrawal. Frequent monitoring of blood pressure, pulse, and mental state is indicated because rate-limiting factors include hypotension and sedation from the clonidine. Parameters for withholding clonidine vary with patients, but systolic blood pressures 90 to 100 mm Hg or a pulse of 60 bpm require discontinuation of the patch, and regular dosing; only as-needed use.

Diazepam

Often, because of high levels of agitation and craving for drugs, diazepam (Valium)[1] 5 to 10 mg orally four times a day is given for 2 to 3 days. In addition, diazepam 5 to 10 mg orally four times a day as needed is given to supplement, depending on signs and symptoms of drug withdrawal. As with clonidine, careful monitoring of vital signs and mental state is indicated to avoid hypotension and oversedation, while balancing against the need to suppress withdrawal to enhance compliance with treatments.

Methadone Taper

Methadone for short-term detoxification from opiates is initiated with a test dose of 10 mg, and if the patient tolerates it (no excessive sedation or lowering of vital signs), an additional 10 to 20 mg is given for signs and symptoms of withdrawal in a 24-hour period. Typically, 20 to 30 mg/day for 2 or 3 days is sufficient to suppress most withdrawal symptoms from opiates, but an additional 5 to 10 mg may be given in unusually severe withdrawal. Because the acute withdrawal period only lasts 5 to 7 days, methadone is tapered in 5- to 10-mg increments over 3 to 5 days for duration of approximately 1 week. Clonidine can be initiated during the methadone taper, as outlined earlier, in part or wholly to suppress the withdrawal symptoms from methadone during its taper.

---

[1]Not FDA approved for this indication.

Methadone Maintenance and LAAM

Certain patients may be referred to a methadone maintenance program for chronic substitution therapy with methadone or LAAM (L-α-acetylmethadol). Candidates for opiate maintenance therapy should be screened from the population of opiate users. Generally, detoxification and drug-free addiction treatment should be attempted before commitment to long-term opiate substitution therapy. Methadone and LAAM are opiates, addicting themselves, and studies show favorable results with shorter term therapy and when combined with psychosocial therapies. Effective doses can range from 20 mg/day to more than 100 mg/day, and tolerance develops to methadone, requiring increasing doses. A particular limitation of methadone in the longer term is that relapse rates are substantial to heroin and to use of addicting drugs including benzodiazepines, alcohol, cocaine, and prescription narcotics.

Currently, methadone and LAAM are prescribed in a program setting approved and monitored by the FDA. The Center for Substance Abuse Treatment accredits and monitors methadone and LAAM programs.

Buprenorphine

Buprenorphine (Subutex) is a newer synthetic agonist–antagonist opiate, which means it has both morphine-like activity (40 times more potent than morphine), and naltrexone-like activity (blocks morphine). Major advantages expected are a ceiling effect on overdose because of antagonist properties while still retaining the agonist effect that addicts seek in their addictive use of drugs. Buprenorphine is likely to be effective in treating opiate withdrawal because of its mixed agonist–antagonist properties, but its effectiveness in substitution therapies similar to methadone is less clear. Opiate addicts are likely to prefer methadone with its stronger agonist effects than buprenorphine with its antagonist effects.

Pain and Addiction

We saw a fivefold increase in the incidence of narcotic prescription medication used for nonmedical purposes from between the 1980s and 2000. In 1999, approximately 4 million people were using prescription drugs nonmedically, which is about double the 2.1 million people who use heroin and cocaine.

In 2003, an estimated 6.3 million persons, or 2.7% of the population age 12 years or older, had used prescription psychopharmacologic therapeutic medications nonmedically in the month before being surveyed. This number included 4.7 million persons using pain relievers, predominantly prescription opiate medications, whose sources for the prescriptions were physicians.

In addition, the Drug Abuse Warning Network (DAWN) narcotic analgesic the mentions in the emergency department increased 253%—from 42,857 to 108,320 emergency department visits—between 1995 and 2002. Dependence was the most commonly mentioned motive underlying drug abuse related to opioid mentions (47%), followed by suicide (22%) and psychic effects (15%). Of patients receiving emergency treatment for effects of opioid analgesics, 53% were admitted for treatment, 44% were admitted and released from the hospital, and 3% left against medical advice.

To underscore the growing magnitude of addiction and dependence to opioid analgesics, in 2003 an estimated 415,000 Americans received treatment for pain medication abuse and addiction in that year. Correspondingly, the number of new users of opioid analgesics (as pain relievers) increased from 573,000 in 1990 to 2.5 million in 2000 (55% female).

Increased Sensitivity to Chronic Administration of Opioid Medications

Increased, rather than lowered, pain sensitivity can result from chronic administration of opioid analgesic medications in humans. In one study, patients treated chronically with opiates reported more pain than the matched nonopioid-treated controls. In addition, there was an increased demand for opiates from patients who had received opiates as compared with the matched patients without intraoperative opioid infusion.

These phenomena are different and are distinguished from traditional pharmacologic tolerance (reduced analgesic effect) as increased sensitivity to pain caused by chronic use of opioid medications. Increased sensitivities are described as allodynia, which is a painful response to normally non-noxious stimuli, and hyperalgesia, which is an exaggerated painful response to normally noxious stimuli. Opioid addicts (chronic opiate use) have increased pain sensitivity, and enhancement of pain sensitivity is seen in patients actively maintained in methadone programs.

Addiction to narcotic medications carries with it significant medical morbidity and mortality and is in itself a painful state with components of depression, decreased mental acuity, decreased energy, preoccupation with acquiring narcotics to the exclusion of normal activities, conflict in interpersonal relationships, illicit activities to obtain narcotics and the legal consequences therefrom, aggravation of underlying sources of pain without relief from pain, and lethal overdose, either accidental or from suicidal intent.

COCAINE

Cocaine is a dramatic CNS stimulant that initially produces intense euphoria. The euphoria diminishes with development of tolerance in chronic use, accompanied by increasing levels of anxiety and depression. Potential physical effects from cocaine intoxication include elevated blood pressure and pulse, palpitations and cardiac arrhythmias (possibly life threatening), vasoconstriction and ischemia with consequent angina and cerebrovascular stroke, mydriasis, hyperthermia, seizures, tremulousness, hyperactive reflexes, dry mouth, decreased appetite and weight loss, respiratory arrest, and coma. Common psychological effects include euphoria, anxiety, depression, grandiose thinking, delusions, auditory and visual hallucinations, irritability, stereotypic and compulsive behaviors (sometimes self-inflicted or mutilating), and suicidal and homicidal thinking.

Treatment of acute intoxication is aimed at the agitation, hypertension, tachycardia, delusions, and hallucinations. Pharmacologic therapy includes propranolol (Inderal)[1] in doses to reduce hypertension, 20 to 40 mg two or three times a day or as needed and tolerated; haloperidol (Haldol)[1] 5 to 10 mg as needed, and diazepam (Valium)[1] 5 to 10 mg. Because cocaine has a short half-life (1-2 hours), treatment of intoxication is brief except in cases of extreme overdose. Other supportive measures may be indicated, such as monitoring cardiac and respiratory status.

Cocaine withdrawal characteristically peaks in 2 to 3 days acutely and lasts 5 to 7 days. The major symptoms are anxiety, depression, fatigue and hypersomnia, increased appetite, and generalized malaise. Because the depth of the depression can be severe, evaluation for suicidal risk is often necessary; depression typically lasts only during the acute period of withdrawal. The treatment is supportive because there is no specific medication that suppresses symptoms of cocaine withdrawal.

Because the hallmark of cocaine withdrawal is irritability, sedatives such as diazepam are effective in reducing discomfort and improving compliance. Diazepam[1] 5 to 10 mg four times a day for 2 or 3 days is often sufficient to suppress withdrawal, including craving or desire to use more cocaine. No particular medication is effective in preventing relapse to cocaine, and studies do not support the use of antidepressants in preventing relapse.

AMPHETAMINES AND DERIVATIVES

Amphetamine and its derivatives share characteristics of intoxication and withdrawal similar to those of other stimulants, particularly cocaine. Their half-lives are short acting, and the course of withdrawal is similar to cocaine. Amphetamine drugs include

---

[1]Not FDA approved for this indication.

dextroamphetamine (Dexedrine), methylphenidate (Ritalin), and other CNS stimulants. Amphetamines are highly addicting and produce the greatest propensity for developing addiction when ranked with other addicting drugs. Studies show mortality rates near 90% when animals are allowed to self-administer amphetamines in research paradigms.

Dextroamphetamines and methyphenidate, and similar stimulants, are used to treat attention deficit disorders and other behavior problems. Careful assessment of pattern of use is indicated to determine if therapeutic effects are still present and to what extent addictive use of these medications has developed. Evaluation of other drug use is indicated as a marker for problematic use of these stimulants. Disturbances of mood, affect, and cognition are common and should be assessed in anyone using these medications chronically.

MDMA (3,4-methylenedioxymethamphetamine), known best as Ecstasy, is a potent amphetamine derivative and is highly popular among teenage populations. MDMA is used in many settings but is particularly prevalent in rave parties, where participants use MDMA and other drugs continuously for 24 hours or more. Significant medical and psychiatric complications ensue, particularly physical and mental exhaustion, disrupted concentration and memory, impaired insight and judgment, depersonalization and derealization, mystical experiences, suspiciousness, and frank paranoid delusions. Perceptual disturbances include loss of boundaries, heightened sensory acuity, overvalued attribution of meaning to ordinary objects, belief that usual thoughts are novel and profound, rage reactions, panic dissociative states, depression, and suicidal thinking and behavior.

Acute use of MDMA also produces jitteriness, anxiety, depression, jaw clenching, insomnia, sleep disturbances, seizures, hypertension, hyperthermia, dehydration, renal failure, disseminated intravascular coagulation, and rhabdomyolysis. Long-term consequences can include persistent neurotoxicity, at least in animal studies. Careful assessment of humans is not yet available.

Treatments are directed at the medical and psychiatric complications and can include rehydration, restoring electrolyte balances, sedating with diazepam[1] and haloperidol,[1] and providing a protective and supportive environment during the acute withdrawal period when depression and suicidal thinking may be prominent. Assessment for other drug use, including alcohol, and treatment of withdrawal is mandatory in young populations where multiple drug use is the rule.

CANNABIS

Cannabis is a poorly understood drug whose pharmacologic properties are generally underestimated and rationalized. Marijuana and hashish are obtained from the plant *Cannabis sativa*. The principal psychoactive constituent is tetrahydrocannabinol (THC), which is a hallucinogenic substance responsible for the psychological and physical effects in humans. In acute doses, cannabis produces a general feeling of well-being; relaxation; emotional disinhibition; drowsiness; distortions of perception of time, body image, and distance; increased auditory and visual acuity; and enhanced senses of touch, smell, and taste, as well as body awareness and perceptions. Attention span and ability to process information can be impaired, as well as ability to perform complex motor tasks. Chronic users can display depressed mood and high anxiety levels, including fearfulness and paranoia, misperceptions, and violent and retaliatory behavior. Memory loss and poor judgment often accompany regular and chronic cannabis use, and users are aware of these deficits at times.

Studies have shown negative effects of cannabis intoxication on driving performance of automobiles, by interfering with motor coordination, tracking, perception, and vigilance and that actual performance on the road is impaired. The interaction of alcohol and cannabis intensifies the adverse effects of each drug on driving performance.

Studies also confirm personality changes with prolonged use, characterized by diminished drive, lessened ambition, decreased motivation, apathy, shortened attention span, distractibility, poor judgment, impaired communication skills, loss of effectiveness, introversion, magical thinking, derealization and depersonalization, diminished capacity to carry out complex plans or prepare realistically for the future, a peculiar fragmentation in the flow of thought, habit deterioration, and progressive loss of insight.

Physical effects of acute use include increased heart rate, decreased peripheral resistance and increased peripheral blood flow, hypotension, lightheadedness, orthostatic changes, and injected conjunctiva. Other physical effects include increased appetite, dryness of mouth and throat, reduced sex drive, and headaches. Chronic users develop bronchitis, asthma, sore throat, and chronic irritation of and damage to sensitive mucous membranes in the respiratory tract, impaired gas exchange, increased signs of airway obstruction, and chronic inflammation changes in the lungs.

Withdrawal from cannabis is subtle and definite and includes malaise, craving for cannabis, mild tachycardia and hypertension, anxiety, and depression. Because cannabis is taken up and stored in muscle and fat, the release can be slow over time, and withdrawal symptoms can be protracted over weeks and months. Importantly, patients should be advised that their urine toxicology can be positive in low levels for weeks and months. High levels of THC in the urine suggest recent use; thus, quantification of the amount of THC is important to determine recent use and relapse.

Treatment of cannabis intoxication and withdrawal is supportive and directed at the specific signs and symptoms. Generally, diazepam[1] in usual doses, 5 to 10 mg four times a day, and as needed for agitation over a few days, is sufficient, and use of haloperidol[1] 5 to 10 mg four times a day, and as needed for psychotic and perceptual abnormalities may be indicated. Often, cannabis users have become addicted to cannabis and other drugs and require evaluation for additional drug use, including alcohol, by clinical interview and urine toxicology. Cannabis addicts often respond to addiction treatment, which is necessary for preventing relapse to cannabis and other drugs.

HALLUCINOGENS AND PHENCYCLIDINE

The classification of hallucinogens is a loosely grouped category of drugs related by their ability to produce changes in perceptions, sometimes causing frank hallucinations. The intoxicated state is characterized by alterations in perceptions that affect basically all modalities of sensation, often visual and auditory but less commonly touch and taste. Subtle and marked distortions in time and motion combine to create a sometimes surreal experience for the user, which is an attraction for particularly young users. Clear visual hallucinations of colors and patterns, and even of individuals and objects, accompany intoxication. Also, auditory hallucinations consist of voices and sound clearly audible during drug intoxication.

In sufficient doses, cognitive or memory impairments, disorientation, and confusion often occur. The hallucinogenic experience correlates with changes seen during rapid eye movement (REM) sleep and can account for the dreamlike quality of intoxication. Phencyclidine (PCP) is a prototype drug whose pharmacologic properties are representative of the hallucinogen class of drugs. PCP and the related dissociative anesthetic ketamine are particularly dangerous drugs. Their typical intoxication includes severe impairment in insight and judgment, visual and auditory hallucinations, and paranoid delusions. Users appear hyperactive and can be violent due to the combined effects of PCP.

Because it is an anesthetic, users may be insensitive to pain, which enables them to perform feats of great strength and to break out of restraints, over powering and injuring themselves and others, making them particularly dangerous. On physical examination, intoxicated persons show hypertension, tachycardia, eyelid retraction (wide-eyed stare), dry flushed skin, mydriasis, nystagmus, and hyperreflexia.

Many drugs can be classified in this group and include psychedelics, lysergic acid diethylamide (LSD), mescaline, psilocybin, and dimethyltryptamine. Important commonly used hallucinogens

---

[1]Not FDA approved for this indication.

include PCP, ketamine (Ketalar) and similarly acting arylcyclohexylamines, and anticholinergics, such as scopolamine.

Treatment is directed at the particular constellations of symptoms. Generally, diazepam[1] in usual doses, and higher as needed to sedate agitated users, 20 to 60 mg[3] in a 24-hour period, is given orally or parentally, depending on clinical requirements. Haloperidol[1] may be given for psychotic symptoms in doses ranging from 5 mg to 20 mg in a 24-hour period, orally or intramuscularly. Addition of an anticholinergic medication to offset extrapyramidal effects such as dystonia, tremors, and rigidity, is often indicated. Intoxicated persons can require physical restraints for their protection, particularly if they are out of control and at risk for harm to themselves or others.

INHALANTS

Surveys show that inhalants are the fourth most commonly used drug used by adolescents and young adults. Inhalants are commercially available drugs contained in commonly found products, such as gasoline, adhesives, aerosols, cleaning fluids, paint thinners, and lighter fluid. The chemicals are organic hydrocarbon compounds, which are volatile liquids that form gases when released into air. Young people are particularly attracted to the exhilarating and hallucinogenic properties that they experience on inhaling the gases. Of critical importance is that these products can be bought over the counter in stores without limitations, including glues, butane lighters, gasoline, and food aerosols.

In general, inhalants produce a mixed picture of stimulation and depression and perceptual and mood distortions. In sufficient doses, respiratory depression, sleep, and anesthesia occur. Effects are felt rapidly, rendering the person drowsy and sometimes confused. Memory and cognitive disturbances are common, and at times visual hallucinations and bizarre delusions occur. Long-term use is associated with prolonged neurologic impairments such as cognitive impairments, dysarthria, gait ataxia, nystagmus, loss of hearing and smell, tremors, and cerebral and cerebellar atrophy. Persistent changes occur in personality such as conduct disorders, antisocial personality, and depressive symptoms.

Physical effects, including toxicity, produce increased heart rates, irregular heartbeats, lethal arrhythmias, coughing, inflammation of upper respiratory passages, nosebleeds from chronic irritation in sniffing, respiratory depression, nausea, vomiting, diarrhea, liver failure, and renal failure. Organ damage and death occur, and unexplained death in a youth should trigger consideration of inhalant use.

Treatment is directed at identifying the offending organic solvent, conducting a medical and psychiatric assessment, and prescribing medications aimed at symptoms. Diazepam,[1] haloperidol,[1] and other selected sedative–hypnotics and antipsychotics may be used according to the clinical indications. Evaluation of other drug use including alcohol is essential in populations of young drug users. Referral for acute monitoring of cardiac status and treatment, as well as neurologic and psychiatric evaluations, may be necessary depending on clinical indications.

ANABOLIC STEROIDS

Androgenic anabolic steroids include testosterone, the male sex hormone, and derivatives of testosterone. Body builders and athletes who compete in sports that require strength and power are attracted to the anabolic effects of these steroids. The source of these drugs tends to be the illicit markets, although physicians remain a source, as they are for other drugs. These compounds can be produced in private and illegally operated laboratories.

The effects of the steroids are to develop male characteristics, such as deepening of male voice, increases in penis size and body hair, large muscular development, increased vigor, and a feeling of well-being. The psychological effects include euphoria, anxiety, irritability, aggression, reduced or increased fatigue, insomnia, depression and

---

[1]Not FDA approved for this indication.
[3]Exceeds dosage recommended by the manufacturer.

elation, delirium, psychosis, and suicidal or homicidal effects. The physical effects include cardiomegaly, heart failure, myocardial infarction, and increased blood pressure, thromboembolic events in extremities, nausea, vomiting, and gastric irritation. In women, irregular menstrual periods, and in men, decreases in sperm production, testicle size, and potency are associated with suppression of follicle-stimulating hormone and luteinizing hormone. Women can experience masculinzation from testosterone, and men can experience feminization due to metabolism of testosterone into estrogen. Musculoskeletal problems occur including tendon rupture and premature closure of long bones. Liver toxicity includes enlargement, hepatitis, and cancer of the liver.

Steroids can be used addictively and produce psychiatric complications similar to those of other drugs. Severe paranoia and suicidality are relatively common in chronic, regular users, as well as physical changes. Treatment is directed at eliminating its use and in treating symptoms including sedation and psychosis. Medical and psychiatric evaluations and long-term rehabilitation of addiction, psychiatric, and medical complications may be required.

ANTICHOLINERGICS AND ANTIHISTAMINES

Anticholinergics and antihistamines are commonly prescribed in many branches of medicine and psychiatry for many indications. Their common potential for abuse and addiction for and medical and psychiatric complications are the anticholinergic and antihistaminic effects in a variety of medications. Antidepressants, antipsychotics, antihistamines, and antiextrapyramidal medications contain these properties. These medications can be used addictively and produce significant levels of toxicity including euphoria, compulsive use, sedation, drowsiness, confusion, paranoia, visual hallucinations, delusions, delirium, coma, tachycardia, arrhythmia, hypotension, constipation, fatigue, mydriasis, blurred vision, dry mouth, and sleep disturbances.

Emergencies can result from these drugs, including life-threatening medical and psychiatric conditions. Rapid diagnosis and treatment including intensive monitoring may be required. Pharmacologic treatments are aimed at reducing agitation and psychotic, cardiovascular, gastrointestinal, and neurologic complications. Evaluation of other drug use and psychiatric and medical conditions is often indicated.

Conclusions

Because 25% to 50% of patients with alcohol and drug problems are found in a typical medical practice, physicians must be knowledgeable and skilled in assessing and managing alcohol and drug withdrawal, treating dependence, and referring for abstinence and relapse prevention. Because medical schools and residency training programs often do not provide adequate education and experience in diagnosis and treatment of alcohol and drug dependence and withdrawal, physicians might need to obtain addiction training to understand and apply the principles in this chapter to their practices.

Anxiety Disorders

Method of
Jacqueline Carinhas McGregor, MD

Anxiety disorders are the most common psychiatric disorders in the world among both children and adults. In the United States, 30 million people or approximately one of every four meet the criteria for an anxiety disorder in their lifetimes. It is estimated that the annual cost of anxiety disorders in 1998 dollars was more than

$63 billion. More than half of these costs were due to nonpsychiatric direct medical costs, which include undiagnosed, misdiagnosed, or inadequately treated anxiety disorders. It is clear that much of the emotional and economic burden caused by these disorders could be alleviated by improving diagnosis and treatment.

Genetics, temperament, and life stressors can all be contributors to anxiety disorders. Norepinephrine and serotonin are thought to be the major neurotransmitters involved in mediating anxiety symptoms whereas the sympathetic nervous system also plays an important role. The onset of anxiety disorders can usually be traced to childhood, adolescence, or young adulthood. With the exception of obsessive-compulsive disorder, women are more likely than men to suffer from anxiety disorders. Anxiety disorders occur across racial groups without distinction.

Anxiety is characterized by subjective feelings of worry, dread, or anticipation and can include hypervigilance, excessive negativity, and a myriad of somatic symptoms. These symptoms can include diaphoresis, palpitations, shortness of breath, dizziness, chest pain, tremulousness, gastrointestinal complaints, fatigue, dry mouth, sleep problems, hot flashes, polyuria, and restlessness. Because of the wide variety of physical complaints, underlying organic causes and disorders secondary to substances use must first be ruled out (Box 1). A detailed history of present illness, past medical history, substance history, and review of symptoms is essential. If a patient initially presents with anxiety symptoms in middle or late adulthood, has no family history of anxiety disorders, has no temporally related stressors, and does not respond to psychiatric intervention, a closer investigation of organic causes of anxiety should be undertaken.

In patients describing chest pain, cardiovascular causes such as angina, mitral valve prolapse, arrhythmias, and pulmonary embolism should be ruled out. Pulmonary ailments such as asthma, chronic obstructive pulmonary disorder, and pneumonia should be considered in patients describing shortness of breath. Hyperthyroidism, pheochromocytoma, and Cushing's syndrome are examples of endocrine disorders that can mimic anxiety disorders. Other disorders to consider include anemia, delirium, menopause, and gastroesophageal reflux. Medications such as stimulants (including herbal supplements and caffeine), decongestants, antipsychotics, theophylline, steroids, calcium channel blockers, and anticholinergics should all be considered. Alcohol and illicit drug use or withdrawal are other possible causes of anxiety symptoms.

The most common diagnoses of anxiety disorders include generalized anxiety disorder (GAD), panic disorder, social anxiety disorder, obsessive-compulsive disorder (OCD), posttraumatic stress disorder (PTSD), and specific phobias. Those suffering from anxiety disorders are likely to have another co-morbid psychiatric disorder such as a mood disorder or substance dependence. These patients also have a higher risk for suicidal behaviors. It is important to distinguish anxiety disorders from each other, as well as from other psychiatric disorders because the specific diagnosis may have significant impact on treatment decisions. Simple phobias, for example, are not responsive to medication and require cognitive behavioral intervention. OCD requires significantly higher doses of antidepressants than other disorders. Patients with GAD and panic disorder need lower starting doses of antidepressants to avoid iatrogenically exacerbating their symptoms. In the case of patient with comorbid bipolar disorder, special care should be used with antidepressants to prevent the induction of a manic episode.

Psychotherapeutic interventions are often considered the first line of intervention in anxiety disorders, particularly for patients with mild symptoms, those who prefer nonpharmacologic treatment, and for children. Cognitive behavior therapy (CBT) is a specific type of psychotherapy that combines behavioral therapy with cognitive therapy and has the best evidence-based research supporting its use in anxiety disorders. The behavioral component of CBT includes exposure and ritual prevention whereas the cognitive aspect includes identifying false, irrational thoughts and the automatic responses to them. It is important to find skilled therapists with specialized training in these modalities in order to facilitate helpful referrals.

The pharmacologic treatment of most anxiety disorders usually includes selective serotonin reuptake inhibitors (SSRIs) serotonin-norepinephrine reuptake inhibitors (SNRIs), and/or benzodiazepines. The SSRIs fluoxetine (Prozac) and paroxetine (Paxil) are both potent inhibitors of cytochrome P450 2D6, and significant interactions can occur with other drugs that a patient may be taking. Escitalopram (Lexapro) has the most favorable SSRI side effect profile with the least protein-binding and cytochrome-P450 interactions. The most common side effects of SSRIs are nervousness, insomnia, restlessness, nausea, and diarrhea. Venlafaxine (Effexor) has a lower risk of significant drug interactions compared to the SSRIs; however, patients prescribed venlafaxine (Effexor) should have their blood pressure monitored as it can cause or worsen existing hypertension. Benzodiazepines should be used carefully because of their addictive potential and should be avoided in patients with a history of substance abuse.

As with any drug, it is important to discuss the risk and benefits of medication options with patients before coming to a treatment decision. The dosage of a medication should be carefully titrated to minimize side effects while providing adequate symptom response. The Food and Drug Administration (FDA) issued a labeling change request in October 2004 for a black box warning on antidepressant medications about the *possible* association of SSRIs with suicidality in the treatment of major depressive disorder. The antidepressant side effect of agitation has been known to trigger suicidal behavior in those with or without premorbid depression. A physician should exercise special care in using SSRI medications, especially with those younger than 18 years of age. Frequent follow-up visits are recommended to monitor side effects and treatment response. Three of the most prevalent and burdensome anxiety disorders are GAD, OCD, and panic disorder. The remainder of this article will focus on the diagnosis and treatment of GAD and OCD disorders. Panic disorder is discussed in another article.

Generalized Anxiety Disorder

DIAGNOSIS

According to the *Diagnostic and Statistical Manual of Mental Disorders IV-TR*, individuals with GAD suffer from uncontrollable, excessive anxiety and worry involving several areas of functioning on most days in a 6 month period. It must be associated with three or more of the following symptoms: restlessness, fatigue concentration difficulties, irritability, muscle tension, or sleep problems. The anxiety cannot be the result of another Axis I disorder; it must cause a significant impairment in functioning, and it cannot be due to substance abuse, a medical disorder, or occur exclusively in the context of a mood disorder, psychotic disorder, or pervasive developmental disorder.

BOX 1 Organic Causes of Anxiety Symptoms

Cardiopulmonary	Angina, mitral valve prolapse, pulmonary embolism, COPD, asthma
Endocrine	Hyperthyroidism, pheochromocytoma, Cushing's syndrome, menopause
Gastrointestinal	Gastroesophageal reflux, irritable bowel syndrome, gastritis
Neurologic	Dementia, substance intoxication or withdrawal, seizure disorder, migraine
Medications	Stimulants, herbal supplements, decongestants, steroids, antipsychotics, theophylline, calcium channel blockers, anticholinergics

Abbreviation: COPD = chronic obstructive pulmonary disease.

The 12-month prevalence for GAD is 3.1%, and the lifetime prevalence is close to 5%. Women are twice as likely as men to suffer from GAD. GAD usually develops sometime during late adolescence or early adulthood, its symptoms tend to have a chronic duration, and there is a high incidence of comorbid psychiatric disorders (especially depression) associated with it.

GAD can be difficult for the physician to diagnose because patients can be reluctant to discuss their anxiety or be unable to identify it as the source of their concerns. Patient complaints of fatigue, insomnia, somatic symptoms, or chronic pain should be a signal for the physician to ask more about anxiety symptoms.

TREATMENT

Psychotherapy, pharmacotherapy, and their combination can be successfully used to treat GAD. Psychotherapy, particularly cognitive-behavior therapy and applied relaxation, are effective treatment strategies for GAD. Psychotherapy can be used concomitantly with pharmacotherapy, often with better result than if either were used alone.

There are a variety of psychopharmacologic interventions that can be used for patients with GAD (Table 1). An antidepressant or the 5-HT$_{1A}$ partial agonist, buspirone (BusPar), is considered the first line of drug treatment. Paroxetine (Paxil), escitalopram (Lexapro), and venlafaxine (Effexor) are the only antidepressants that have an FDA indication for GAD, although there is evidence that both imipramine (Tofranil)[1] and sertraline (Zoloft)[1] are effective drugs in the treatment of GAD. SSRIs are usually considered the antidepressant of choice because of their safety and relatively modest side effects. Use tricyclic antidepressants such as imipramine (Tofranil) with care because of their more troublesome side-effect profile, proarrhythmic properties, and potential lethality in overdose. The most commonly noted side effects of buspirone (BusPar) are dizziness, nausea, headache, nervousness, and insomnia. Benzodiazepines can play an important role in the treatment of GAD. It is important to keep in mind the addictive potential of these medications before using them. In the first weeks of treatment with SSRIs, it can be helpful to use benzodiazepines to address acute anxiety symptoms while allowing sufficient time for the SSRI to achieve its effect. As symptoms begin to respond, the physician should consider tapering and discontinuing the benzodiazepine.

After an 8- to 10-week course of treatment with an antidepressant, if there has been an insufficient response at an adequate dose, the clinician should consider switching to or augmenting with another drug (e.g., another antidepressant, buspirone [BusPar] or a benzodiazepine). Patients need significant support and encouragement from their physician to be compliant with daily medication regimes and to continue their medication once they begin to experience symptom relief. There is little data on the length of treatment or whether pharmacologic intervention can prevent future relapse. It is common practice to continue treatment for at least 6 to 12 months after resolution of symptoms before stopping medications. At that time a gradual tapering of the medication dose can be considered.

---

[1]Not FDA approved for this indication.

TABLE 1 Pharmacotherapy in the Treatment of Generalized Anxiety Disorder

Drug	Starting Dose	Target Dose
SSRIs		
Paroxetine (Paxil CR)*	10 mg qd	10–60 mg qd
Escitalopram (Lexapro)*	5–10 mg qd	10–20 mg qd
Sertraline (Zoloft)	12.5–25 mg qd	50–200 mg qd
Fluoxetine (Prozac)	10 mg qd	20–40 mg qd
SNRIs		
Venlafaxine (Effexor XR)*	37.5 mg qam	150–300 mg qam
OTHER		
Buspirone (BusPar)	5 mg bid-tid	10 mg bid to tid

*FDA indication for generalized anxiety disorder (GAD).
Abbreviations: bid = twice daily; qam = every morning; qd = every day; tid = three times daily.
SNRIs = serotonin-norepinephrine reuptake inhibitors; SSRIs = selective serotonin reuptake inhibitors.

Obsessive Compulsive Disorder

DIAGNOSIS

The *Diagnostic and Statistical Manual of Mental Disorders IV-TR* outlines the criteria for OCD as having obsessions and/or compulsions. Obsessions are defined as recurrent, persistent thoughts, impulses, or images that are experienced as intrusive and inappropriate and cause significant distress. They cannot be excessive worries about realistic or reasonable concerns. The individual attempts to ignore the obsessions or counteract them with another thought or action and understands that the obsessions are a product of his or her own mind. Compulsions are defined as repetitive behaviors or mental acts that the individual feels compelled to perform in response to an obsession. The compulsion is aimed at reducing distress or preventing some dreaded event, but is not clearly connected to the distress or event or is clearly excessive. Except in the case of children,

---

CURRENT THERAPY

	First Intervention	Second Intervention	Third Intervention
GAD	CBT	SSRI OR venlafaxine (Effexor) OR buspirone (BusPar) OR	Change to different antidepressant or buspirone (BusPar) OR Augment with a different antidepressant class, buspirone (BusPar), or benzodiazepine
OCD	CBT	High dose SSRI (push to maximum dose in 4 to 8 weeks)	Change to another SSRI or clomipramine (anafranil) OR Augment with atypical antipsychotic

Abbreviations: CBT = cognitive behavior therapy; GAD = generalized anxiety disorder; OCD = obsessive-compulsive disorder; SSRI = selective serotonin reup-take inhibitor.

at some point in the course of the disorder the individual recognizes that the obsessions or compulsions are unreasonable. This last point is important in distinguishing OCD from obsessive compulsive personality disorder. The obsessions or compulsions must cause significant impairment and, if another Axis I disorder coexists, the obsessions and/or compulsions cannot be restricted only to the content of that disorder (e.g., preoccupations with food in the case of an eating disorder, hair pulling in the case of trichotillomania). As in the case of GAD, the symptoms cannot occur because of the effects of a substance or secondary to a general medical disorder.

It is not uncommon for OCD to occur with other psychiatric disorders including major depressive disorder, other anxiety disorders, eating disorders, and tic disorders. In children, streptococcal infections are associated with the development of obsessions and compulsions. Psychotic disorders can have obsessive or compulsive behaviors, but these are typically much more bizarre, and the individual has little insight into his or her behavior. It is also important to consider illnesses that can have OCD-like symptoms such as basal ganglia disorders (e.g., Huntington's disease) or tic disorders.

OCD usually appears in late adolescence or early adulthood and has a waxing and waning course. Unlike other anxiety disorders there is an equal occurrence in males and females. The lifetime prevalence rate of OCD is 2% to 3% of the population. Neuroimaging studies of OCD suggest that there are structural and functional problems in the orbitofrontal-subcortical circuitry.

People with OCD often avoid seeking treatment for their illness. Diagnosis often requires explicit questioning regarding specific behaviors such as perfectionism, rituals, washing, counting, checking, or hoarding. The physicians should also be on the lookout for excessively red or raw hands, recurring request for reassurance about medical illnesses, frequent emergency room visits, or usual repetitive behaviors observed in the examining room such as tic-like motions or tapping.

TREATMENT

There are a variety of treatment approaches that can be used for OCD. As with GAD, psychotherapy can be utilized effectively. There is significant research that supporting cognitive behavioral therapy that incorporates exposure-response prevention is a successful treatment for obsessions and compulsions. In more severe cases of OCD, optimal treatment uses a combination of cognitive behavioral therapy and medication.

Several studies demonstrated the efficacy of SSRIs in OCD. A reasonable trial of SSRIs in OCD can be longer and requires higher doses than what would be expected in GAD or major depressive disorder. Setraline (Zoloft), fluoxetine (Prozac), paroxetine (Paxil), and fluvoxamine (Luvox) are SSRIs with FDA indications for OCD.

For those with an inadequate response to treatment with SSRIs, the clinician should consider changing SSRIs, switching to the tricyclic antidepressant, clomipramine (Anafranil), or to the SNRI, venlafaxine (Effexor).[1] The most common side effects of clomipramine (Anafranil) include dry mouth, sedation, dizziness, and weight gain, however, more serious, less common side effects include hypertension and cardiac arrhythmias. Augmentation with a dopamine agonist such as risperidone (Risperdal)[1] or olanzapine (Zyprexa) has been shown to be an effective treatment approach as has the addition of buspirone (BusPar)[1] or benzodiazepines (Table 2).

There is some evidence to support the use of monoamine oxidase inhibitors (MAOIs) in treatment-resistant OCD, but because of the significant side effects, potential drug and food interactions, and toxicity, they are considered an option only when other medication options have proven unsuccessful. For those who fail psychotherapy and psychopharmacology and continue to have significant functional impairment, transcranial magnetic stimulation and neurosurgery are considered treatments of last resort.

Treatment of OCD can usually be accomplished on an outpatient basis; however, in severe refractory cases, inpatient treatment at a facility that specializes in OCD may be necessary. Whatever treatment strategy is employed, the physician should be mindful of the fact that the patient's family often needs to be involved in the treatment. Families often unknowingly reinforce a patient's OCD behaviors by going along with their rituals or participating in excessive reassurance.

Anxiety disorders are quite common and cause a significant burden to individuals as well as to society. The differential diagnosis of anxiety disorders is quite extensive given that anxiety symptoms are often nonspecific. Anxiety disorders often go undiagnosed or are inadequately treated and are likely to occur together with other psychiatric disorders. Primary care physicians are more likely to have the opportunity to detect anxiety disorders and, in fact treat more of these disorders than mental health care practitioners. Effective treatments for anxiety including psychotherapeutic as well as psychopharmacologic interventions are shown in Box 2.

BOX 2 Helpful Resources for Anxiety Disorders

National Alliance for the Mentally Ill	www.nami.org
National Institute of Mental Health	www.nimh.org
Anxiety Disorders Association of America	www.adaa.org
Obsessive-Compulsive Foundation	www.ocfoundation.org

TABLE 2 Pharmacotherapy in the Treatment of Obsessive-Compulsive Disorder

Drug	Starting Dose	Target Daily Dose
SSRI		
Sertraline (Zoloft)*	25-50 mg qd	100-300 mg[3]
Paroxetine (Paxil CR)*	12.5 mg qd	25-50 mg
Fluoxetine (Prozac)*	10 mg qd	20-60 mg
Fluvoxamine (Luvox)*	25-50 mg qd	100-300 mg
SNRI		
Venlafaxine (Effexor XR)	37.5 mg qam	150-300 mg
TCA		
Clomipramine* (Anafranil)	25 mg qhs	100-300 mg

*FDA indication for obsessive-compulsive disorder (OCD).
[3]Exceeds dosage recommended by the manufacturer.
Abbreviations: qam = every morning; qd = every day; qhs = at bed time.

---

[1]Not FDA approved for this indication.

REFERENCES

American Psychiatric Association: Diagnostic and Statistical Manual of Mental Disorders, 4th ed. text rev. Washington, DC; American Psychiatric Association, 2000.

Baer L, Rauch SK, Ballantine T, et al: Cingulotomy for intractable obsessive-compulsive disorder. Arch Gen Psych 1995;52:384-392.

Borkovec T, Costello E: Efficacy of applied relaxation and cognitive-behavioral therapy in the treatment of generalized anxiety disorder. Journal of Consulting and Clinical Psychology 1993;61(4):611-619.

Food and Drug Administration: FDA labeling change request letter for antidepressant medications, 2004.

Greenberg BD, George MS, Martin DJ, et al: Effect of prefrontal repetitive transcranial stimulation in obsessive-compulsive disorder: A preliminary study. Am J Psychiatry 1997;154:867-869.

Greenberg PE, Sisitsky T, Kessler RC, et al: The economic burden of anxiety disorders in the 1990s. J Clin Psychiatry 1990;60:427-435.

Jenike MA, Baer L, Minichiello WE (eds): Obsessive-compulsive disorders: practical management 3rd ed. St Louis, Mosby, 1998.
Karno M, Golding JM, Sorenson SB, et al: The epidemiology of obsessive-compulsive disorder in five US communities. Arch Gen Psychiatry 1988;45(12):1094-1099.
Kessler RC, McGonagle KA, Zhao S: Lifetime and 12-month prevalence of DSM-III-R psychiatric disorders in the United States. Arch Gen Psychiatry 1994;51(1):8-19.
Kobak KA, Griest JH, Jefferson JW, et al: Behavioral versus pharmacologic treatment of obsessive compulsive disorder: A meta-analysis. Psychopharmacology (Berl) 1998;136:205-216.
Koran LM, Rinhold AL, Elliot MA: Olanzapine augmentation in obsessive compulsive disorder refractory to selective serotonin reuptake inhibitors: An open label case series. J Clin Psychiatry 2000;61:514-517.
Ladouceur R, Dugas MJ, Freeston MH, et al: Efficacy of a cognitive behavioral treatment for generalized anxiety disorder evaluation in controlled clinical trial. J Consult Clin Psychol 2000;68(6):957-964.
Liebowitz MR, DeMartinis NA, Weihs K, et al: Efficacy of sertraline in severe generalized social anxiety disorder: results of a double-blind, placebo-controlled study. J Clin Psychiatry 2003;64(7):785-792.
McDougle CJ, Epperson CN, Pelton GH, et al: A double blind placebo controlled study of risperidone addition in serotin reuptake inhibitor-refractory obsessive compulsive disorder. Arch Gen Psych 2000;57:794-801.
Rickels K, Downing R, Schweizer E, et al: Antidepressant for the treatment of generalized anxiety disorder: a placebo controlled comparison of imipramine, trrazodone, and diazepam. Arch Gen Psychiatry 1993;50:884-895.
Rickels K, Schweizer E: The spectrum of generalized anxiety in clinical practice: The role of short term intermittent treatment. Br J Psychiatry 1998;173(Suppl 34):49-54.
Saxena S, Bota RG, Brody AL: Brain-behavior relationships in obsessive-compulsive disorder. Semin Clin Neuropsychiatry 2001;6(2):82-101.

Bulimia Nervosa

Method of
Pauline S. Powers, MD

Bulimia nervosa is a common disorder with an estimated lifetime prevalence of 1.5% among girls and women and 0.5% among boys and men in the United States. These figures are derived from a replication of the National Comorbidity Survey using current diagnostic criteria. The number of affected persons translates to approximately 2.3 million girls and women and 700,000 boys and men. The number of girls and women afflicted with bulimia is higher than the number with schizophrenia (approximately 1.1% lifetime prevalence or 1.6 million). It is well established that bulimia causes significant role impairment, is often comorbid with other psychiatric disorders, and usually has significant physiologic complications. Thus, bulimia nervosa is a serious illness requiring early effective intervention.

Diagnosis

The current *Diagnostic and Statistical Manual of Mental Disorders*, fourth edition (text revision) (DSM-IV TR) describes the key feature of bulimia as recurrent binge eating associated with inappropriate compensatory behavior.

A binge episode has two required characteristics. The first characteristic for a binge is consumption of an amount of food in a discrete time period that is definitely larger than most people would eat during a similar period of time and under similar circumstances. The second required characteristic is that there is an associated sense of lack of control during the eating episode. Typically, patients are able to distinguish overeating from binge eating because of the feeling that they are unable to stop, or even control the binge.

Self-induced vomiting is the most common compensatory behavior and usually (but not always) promptly follows the binge. Other compensatory behaviors include laxative, diuretic, or enema abuse; exercise; and fasting. Two additional diagnostic criteria for bulimia are that the episodes of binge eating and inappropriate compensatory behavior must occur at least twice weekly for 3 months and that self-evaluation is unduly influenced by body shape and weight.

Two types of bulimia nervosa are described: the purging type (vomiting or misuse of laxatives, diuretics, or enemas) and the nonpurging type (inappropriate use of fasting or exercise to compensate for binge eating).

One of the main problems with the current diagnostic criteria is that the majority of patients who have serious eating disorders that resemble bulimia do not meet strict DSM-IV TR criteria. The frequency criterion for binge eating or compensatory behavior is often not met, or there may be an absence of objective binge episodes. These patients (who technically have a diagnosis of eating disorder not otherwise specified) are usually as psychiatrically and physically ill as patients who meet strict criteria for bulimia nervosa. Similar treatment strategies are usually recommended for patients who have conditions that resemble bulimia but do not meet strict diagnostic criteria.

CURRENT DIAGNOSIS

- Recurrent episodes of binge eating: Consumption of a large quantity of food in a discrete time period that would be considered definitely larger than most people would eat under similar circumstances
- Feeling of loss of control during binge
- Inappropriate compensatory behavior (including self-induced vomiting, laxative or diuretic abuse, fasting, excessive exercise)
- Occurs an average of twice weekly for 3 months
- Body dissatisfaction
- Two types: Purging type (most common) and nonpurging type. Common comorbid psychiatric disorders include affective disorders (depression, bipolar disorder), anxiety disorders (generalized anxiety disorder, social phobia, obsessive compulsive disorder), substance-use disorders (alcohol, cocaine), and borderline personality disorder

Clinical Features

PRESENTING FEATURES

The typical age at onset of bulimia is during adolescence or young adulthood. Girls and women are most often affected, but it is not rare among boys and men. Bulimia nervosa has been diagnosed in children as young as 4 years, and there is a growing literature suggesting that the incidence is increasing among middle-aged women. Although some patients are underweight, most are normal weight or overweight. Because many people who suffer from bulimia are very secretive about their bulimic behavior, the diagnosis can be delayed for decades or perhaps missed altogether. At presentation, patients typically have marked body dissatisfaction and are preoccupied with eating, weight, size, and shape. Mood disturbances are often apparent at the initial interview. A past history of anorexia nervosa is common. Many patients with anorexia nervosa eventually relinquish restrictive eating but then feel compelled to compensate for food consumption with various types of purging behavior. A pattern of binge eating and compensatory behavior develops, with consequent weight gain, and the person then meets the criteria for bulimia nervosa.

COMORBID PSYCHIATRIC DISORDERS

As with other eating disorders, comorbid axis I psychiatric disorders are common. About one half of bulimic patients have an axis I mood or anxiety disorder during their lifetime. The most common are depression, bipolar disorder, generalized anxiety disorder, social phobia, and obsessive–compulsive disorder. About 40% of patients have a substance use disorder, most often alcohol or cocaine abuse or dependence. Typically (but not always) the eating disorder begins first and then, as the disorder is experienced as out of control, the patient uses alcohol as a self-soothing strategy or cocaine as a means of maintaining a lower weight. A history of sexual abuse is common (in the range of 25%), with the majority having had these experiences in childhood. These adverse sexual experiences usually have long-lasting negative effects (both psychological and physiologic) that complicate treatment.

Among the axis II (personality) disorders, borderline personality disorder (BPD) is common and often requires special treatment strategies. Suicide attempts and self-injurious behavior are also common and often difficult to manage. Suicide attempts may be more likely in patients who also have depression, bipolar disorder, or social phobia. Self-injurious behavior may be more likely in patients who have personality disorders or who have harm-avoidant temperaments.

PHYSIOLOGIC COMPLICATIONS

Although some patients can go for years without obvious physical complications, this is not usually the case. Often the patient does not reveal to health care professionals that binge–purge behavior is occurring and thus the cause of various problems might not be detected.

The most immediately dangerous complications affect the heart and brain. Cardiac arrhythmias can occur in association with electrolyte abnormalities (typically hypokalemia) and electrocardiographic changes (particularly a prolonged QT interval). These cardiac arrhythmias can result in supraventricular and ventricular arrhythmias (including torsade de pointes) and infrequently (but often unpredictably) sudden death. These cardiac abnormalities are typically the result of various types of intense purge behavior (particularly self-induced vomiting, laxative and diuretic abuse) but also can occur with restrictive food intake. Brain abnormalities include cognitive impairment, mood disturbances, and seizures. Seizures can occur associated with electrolyte abnormalities (especially hyponatremia) or hypoglycemia.

Other physiologic complications that commonly occur affect the gastrointestinal tract. Dental abnormalities (particularly erosion of the enamel on the lingual surfaces) is common and can progress to cavities and then to very severe infectious problems requiring extensive oral surgery. Enlarged salivary glands are usually not dangerous or painful but often reveal that a patient has relapsed. Gastrointestinal problems include heartburn (and the eventual development of gastroesophageal reflux disorder), delayed gastric emptying, abdominal pain, constipation (particularly in patients who abuse laxatives), and (rarely) esophageal ruptures or bezoars. Patients with alcohol-use disorders often have physiologic complications that overlap with complications from the eating disorder, including liver abnormalities, pancreatitis, and anemia. Patients are also at greater risk for decreased bone density and the emergence of osteopenia or osteoporosis. Patients with a prior history of anorexia nervosa are at particular risk for this complication.

After a complete psychiatric history, medical history, physical examination, and mental status examination have been obtained, basic laboratory testing in all patients with bulimia should include blood chemistry studies (serum electrolytes, blood urea nitrogen, serum creatinine, thyroid-stimulating hormone, and complete blood count), liver enzymes, and urinalysis. In malnourished or severely symptomatic patients, additional laboratory tests should include an electrocardiogram, 24-hour urine for creatinine clearance, and additional serum blood chemistry tests (calcium, magnesium, phosphorus, and ferritin). If the patient has a history of 6 months or more of amenorrhea since menarche, a dual-energy x-ray absorptiometry and serum estrogen in female patients (or serum testosterone in male patients) should be obtained. Other laboratory measures may be required for patients with significant cognitive defects, pancreatitis, or gastrointestinal bleeding.

Treatment

GENERAL STRATEGIES

Key aspects of treatment that are helpful to patients with bulimia are those known to be helpful to most patients.

First, establishment of a cooperative, positive doctor–patient relationship can facilitate the willingness of the patient to accept appropriate treatment and relinquish the shame, guilt, and stigmatization that often accompany the illness. Because the causes of eating disorders are poorly understood and are often inappropriately considered lifestyle choices or failures in personal motivation rather than the illnesses they are, patients are often reluctant to reveal the extent of their difficulties. An empathic physician can provide the needed support that can allow patients to freely report the wide range of difficulties they are encountering. Many patients have seen numerous physicians before they acknowledge the bulimia, and this can be avoided by routinely enquiring about typical symptoms (either directly or via a brief questionnaire).

Second, because many patients require a treatment team, rather than one health care professional, a team leader is necessary. In addition, an established method of communication is required. Sometimes one member of the team can be both team leader and designated communicator, but, for patients with multiple diagnoses, often these roles need to be differentiated and formalized even before treatment begins.

Third, the site of treatment needs to be determined. Although many patients can achieve clinically significant improvements with outpatient treatment alone, many cannot. Those most likely to require residential or inpatient treatment include patients with multiple comorbid psychiatric disorders (especially substance-use disorders) or physiologic complications, or both.

COMMON ACUTELY DANGEROUS PHYSIOLOGIC COMPLICATIONS

Patients with electrolyte abnormalities or hypoglycemia often require hospitalization. The most common acutely dangerous electrolyte abnormality is hypokalemia (often associated with hypochloremia or bicarbonate abnormalities). Supplemental oral potassium chloride (or intravenous fluids with appropriate electrolytes) is prescribed while preventing purging.

Hyponatremia is often the consequence of fluid loading in an effort to assuage hunger without consuming calories. Appropriate

---

CURRENT THERAPY

General Strategies

- Establish a positive doctor–patient relationship.
- Establish a treatment team with a leader and communicator.
- Determine the site of treatment.
- Assess and treat dangerous physiologic complications.

Specific Evidence-Based Treatments

- Cognitive behavior therapy
- Fluoxetine (Prozac) 60 mg daily (adults and older adolescents)

Treat Comorbid Psychiatric Disorders

- Comorbid substance use disorders: Treat substance use disorder first (with 12-step program) or concurrently with eating disorder
- Borderline personality disorder: Dialectical behavior therapy

limitation of fluid intake to approximately 2 L per day must be ensured, often in a controlled hospital setting; some patients require intravenous administration of saline-containing fluids. Patients with hypoglycemia should consume glucose-containing foods or might require intravenous administration of glucose.

These complications are often treated in the emergency department or during very brief hospital stays. However, they indicate a severe or chronic condition that requires intense treatment, often in a specialized structured eating-disorder program and usually for lengthy periods of time.

SPECIFIC EVIDENCE-BASED TREATMENTS

Cognitive behavior therapy (CBT) is a psychotherapy strategy that has been found to be the most effective treatment for adults (and older adolescents) with bulimia. It is based on the theory that the core psychopathology in bulimia is a negative focus on body shape and weight that leads to dysfunctional dieting and unhealthy weight control measures with the eventual development of binge eating and inappropriate compensatory behavior. Treatment is manual based and typically delivered in 16 to 20 individual or group sessions over the course of 4 to 5 months, often with two sessions per week in the initial phase. The treatment includes strategies to reduce cognitive distortions (inaccurate or distorted beliefs that are resistant to logic) and behavioral regimens aimed at re-establishing a regular flexible pattern of eating. The specific strategies and procedures are those recommended by Fairburn and colleagues. When these procedures are strictly followed, 30% to 50% of patients completely remit with CBT. Although many others improve, others drop out of treatment or fail to respond. Relapse is more common among those who have only a partial response to CBT.

Fluoxetine, which is a selective serotonin reuptake inhibitor (SSRI), is the only medication approved by the FDA for bulimia nervosa in adults. It is somewhat less effective than CBT, with about 20% to 30% of patients responding with significant reductions in binge eating and purging. CBT appears to have more enduring benefit, but the long-term benefit of fluoxetine has not been well studied. The dose shown to be effective is 60 mg (higher than typically required for depression), and the benefit in reducing binge eating and purging is unrelated to presence or absence of depressive symptoms. The results of studies using both CBT and fluoxetine have been mixed. Other SSRIs and other classes of antidepressants might also be effective, but most have not been well studied.

A complicating factor is recent concern over a possible increased risk of suicide among adolescents on SSRIs for depression. There is a black box warning on the package insert for fluoxetine warning of possible increased risk of suicide. However, recent reports have found that in a few adolescents with depression there is a temporary increase in suicidal ideation but no completed suicide attempts. Nonetheless, this possibility should be considered in any depressed adolescent patient with bulimia for whom fluoxetine (or any other SSRI) is being considered.

COMORBID SUBSTANCE-USE DISORDERS

A common treatment dilemma is management of the patient with bulimia nervosa and alcohol or cocaine abuse or dependence. Despite the common co-occurrence of bulimia and these disorders, there are very few reports of effective treatment. At present, the general clinical consensus is that alcohol misuse or other substance use disorder should be addressed first (or concurrently) with the eating disorder using the Alcoholic Anonymous (AA) 12-step method. CBT methods for the eating disorder symptoms are used concurrently or following abstinence from the misused substance.

Although many treatment programs use modified 12-step programs to treat eating disorders, the evidence for this is either nonexistent or negative. Programs that focus on abstinence from sugar or starch (a concept loosely based on AA principles) have demonstrated little efficacy, although some patients have found them useful.

COMORBID BORDERLINE PERSONALITY DISORDER

Dialectical behavior therapy (DBT) is based on the theory that people who have experienced invalidating environmental experiences in childhood, and who are also biologically predisposed, can develop abnormal responses to emotional stimulation. These responses include increased frequency and intensity of emotional arousal that takes longer than normal to return to baseline. Common maladaptive responses to this intense emotional arousal include suicidal behavior and self-injury. Because of their lack of early validation, these persons have few adaptive coping responses.

There are two main components of DBT. The first component is individual weekly psychotherapy sessions in which particular problematic behavior is identified and explored in detail including the chain of events that led to the behavior. Possible alternative solutions are reviewed, as well as what kept the patient from using these solutions. The focus is on helping the patient manage emotional situations rather than avoid them. The second component of DBT is a series of weekly group skills training sessions. One promising study has found that using a modified group skills training module for patients with eating disorders (along with individual weekly sessions) is helpful to patients with bulimia.

Prognosis

The prognosis for full recovery from bulimia is poorly understood. bulimia is a relapsing–remitting condition, and the natural course of the illness is unclear. Many patients begin with what appears to be uncomplicated bulimia nervosa (or anorexia nervosa that evolves into bulimia) and subsequently develop other conditions (substance-use disorder or depression) that could be viewed as either self-soothing strategies (substance-use disorders) or complications (e.g., depression) of untreated bulimia. Current evidence indicates that 30% to 50% of adults and older adolescents who receive the recommended form of CBT can have complete cessation of binge eating and purging for at least several years.

REFERENCES

American Psychiatric Association: Diagnostic and Statistical Manual of Mental Disorders, 4th ed, text revision. Washington, DC: American Psychiatric Association, 2000.

Fairburn CG, Cooper Z, Bohn K, et al: The severity and status of eating disorder NOS: Implications for DSM-V. Behav Res Ther 2007;45:1705-1715.

Fairburn CG, Macus MD, Wilson GT: Cognitive-behavioral therapy for binge eating and bulimia nervosa: A comprehensive treatment manual. In Fairburn CG, Wilson GT (eds): Binge Eating: Nature, Assessment and Treatment. New York: Guilford Press, 1993, pp 361-404.

Favaro A, Santonastaso P, Monteleone P, et al: Self-injurious behavior and attempted suicide in purging bulimia nervosa: Associations with psychiatric comorbidity. J Affect Disord 2008;105(1-3):285-289.

Fluoxetine Bulimia Nervosa Collaborative Study Group: Fluoxetine in the treatment of bulimia nervosa. A multicenter, placebo-controlled, double-blind trial. Arch Gen Psychiatry 1992;49:139-147.

Gura T: Lying in Weight: The Hidden Epidemic of Eating Disorders in Adult Women. New York: HarperCollins, 2007.

Hudson JI, Hiripi E, Pope HG, Kessler RC: The prevalence and correlates of eating disorders in the National Comorbidity Survey Replication. Biol Psychiatry 2007;61:348-358.

National Institute for Clinical Excellence: Eating disorders: Core interventions in the treatment and management of anorexia nervosa, bulimia nervosa and related eating disorders. Clinical Guideline 9, January 2004. Available at http://www.nice.org.uk/CG009NICEguideline (accessed June 12, 2008).

Palmer RL, Birchall H, Damani S, et al: A dialectical behavior therapy program for people with an eating disorder and borderline personality disorder—description and outcome. Int J Eating Disord 2003;33:281-286.

Yager J, Devlin M, Halmi K, et al: American Psychiatric Association Practice Guideline for the Treatment of Patients with Eating Disorders, Third Revision. Part A. Am J Psychiatry 2006;163(7 suppl):1-54.

Delirium

Method of
Jonathan M. Flacker, MD

Recognizing Delirium

The clinical presentation of delirium can mimic other acute psychiatric conditions such as mania, anxiety, depression, or psychosis. However, spending large amounts of effort on distinguishing between delirium, dementia, and depression is at best an interesting intellectual exercise; at worst it leads to misidentification of delirium. Nothing about dementia or depression is protective against delirium. Thus, although depression or dementia may be present, the important clinical question becomes "Does this patient have delirium or not?" (Figure 1).

The most useful information in this regard is determining the patient's baseline cognition and functioning prior to the acute changes. Indeed, the only other cognitive condition to exhibit a disturbance in consciousness and such fluctuating symptoms as delirium is dementia with Lewy bodies, which is a chronic and not acute problem. For delirium, perhaps more so than any other medical condition, failure to diagnose is a direct result of failure to consider.

The *Diagnostic and Statistical Manual of Mental Disorders*, fourth edition (text revision) (DSM-IV TR) is helpful in classifying and studying delirium, but for the typical clinician the confusion assessment method (CAM), shown in Box 1 is more useful.

Other common symptoms of delirium may be present such as sleep–wake cycle disturbances, mood lability, psychosis, tremors, and even paranoia. Such symptoms, although important from a management perspective, are not helpful diagnostically.

Recognition of delirium begins in the outpatient setting, where all older patients should have baseline cognitive testing, preferably updated annually. This is analogous to a baseline electrocardiogram (ECG) in cardiac patients. A formal cognitive assessment (such as with a Mini Mental State Exam and CAM) should be performed on hospital admission. When no person is present to give a history, the care team should do their best to establish baseline cognitive function from others such as friends, family, neighbors, and assisted-living or nursing home staff, where available. Once baseline cognition is established, the patient can then be monitored for mental status. In a confused patient, where baseline cannot be established, delirium should be assumed to be present and the patient managed accordingly.

Nondelirious patients should be monitored daily for cognitive changes. To do this one must appreciate the full spectrum of motoric subtypes of delirium: hypoactive, hyperactive, and mixed. Hyperactive delirium (about one third of delirium patients) is not commonly missed because the agitation brings attention to such patients. Hypoactive delirium (also about one third of delirium patients) is harder to recognize in a patient lying in a quiet delirious state. The remaining one third of delirious patients fluctuate between the two extremes.

Prevention

Some patients present with delirium. For such patients prevention is irrelevant; however, the principles of prevention apply to their treatment also. The risk that a particular patient will develop delirium is a combination of patient-related factors such, as advanced age, comorbidity, dementia, alcohol or sedative use, malnutrition, and poor vision or hearing, and illness-related factors, such as bladder catheters, dehydration, fever, fractures, illness severity, infection, and physical restraints. Thus, prevention is targeted to improving the

---

BOX 1 Confusion Assessment Method

Delirium is indicated by the presence of all three of the following:
- Acute onset of a change in cognition: Delirium begins over minutes to hours, not days to weeks.
- Abnormal attention: Spectrum ranges from near somnolence (hypoactive delirium) to extreme agitation (hyperactive delirium).
- Fluctuating symptoms: Cognitive symptoms fluctuate over minutes to hours, not days to weeks.

Plus the presence of one of the following:
- Disorganized thinking: Confused, irrelevant or rambling speech.
- Abnormal level of consciousness: Might range from near-coma to disorganized agitation, but patient clearly is not normally alert.

 CURRENT DIAGNOSIS

- Delirium is an acute brain syndrome characterized by acute onset, abnormal attention, and fluctuating cognition.
- Delirium is best diagnosed at the bedside by the confusion assessment method (CAM).
- Delirium requires an emergent work-up.
- Delirium always has one or more precipitating causes.
- Delirious patients may be hyperactive, hypoactive, or mixed.

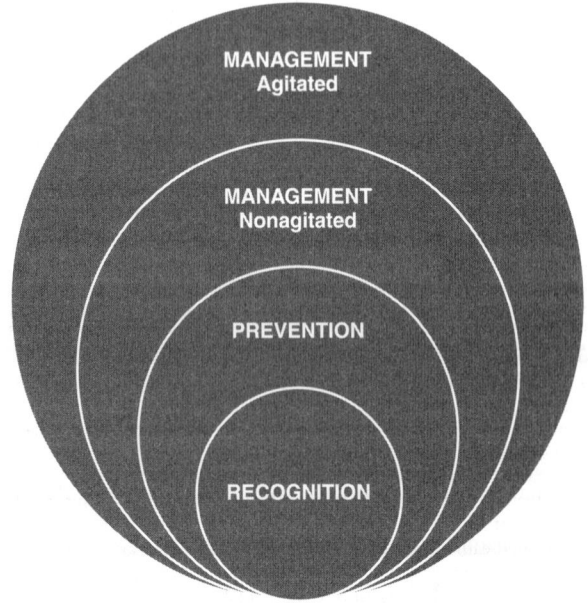

FIGURE 1. The four levels of delirium treatment. At each level as one progresses from recognition to management of agitated delirium, all of the treatment strategies for the previous level are maintained. For example, the treatment of a patient with nonagitated delirium includes all of the treatments for delirium prevention as well as additional therapy for the delirious patient.

modifiable risk factors. This approach has demonstrated efficacy in both medical and surgical patients. Important modifiable contributing factors to delirium include oxygenation, fluid and electrolyte imbalances, regulation of bowel and bladder function, nutritional intake, Foley catheters, mobilization and rehabilitation, orienting communication, use of visual and hearing aids, regulation of sleep–wake cycles, and avoidance of excessive or inappropriate medications.

Some appropriate interventions are not implementable by individual physicians but rather take a change in hospital systems. It is counterproductive, for example, if diphenhydramine (Benadryl) is the standard formulary sleep medication, or if glasses and hearing aids are sent home rather than kept with the patient due to hospital protocol.

Treatment

MANAGING THE NONAGITATED PATIENT

Begin delirium management by implementing all of the prevention measures. Then identify the precipitating factor(s). Delirium always has one or more medical precipitants. New-onset delirium is a red flag that something new and potentially serious is wrong. The list of all potential causes of delirium is composed of the list of all known (and probably some unknown) acute medical illnesses. The key is to recognize that new-onset delirium requires a rapid, thoughtful, thorough work-up.

The approach is simply one of good medical evaluation: vital signs, thorough physical examination, and careful neurologic examination. Select laboratory tests, such as a complete blood count, electrolytes, blood urea nitrogen, creatinine, liver panel, urinalysis and culture, and chest x-ray is a reasonable start. Depending on history and physical findings, or if the diagnosis remains unclear, oxygen saturation, toxicology screens, ammonia level, thyroid function, ECG, and brain imaging may be in order. It is unusual for lumbar puncture or electroencephalography to be needed.

Medications must be reviewed, including herbal and over-the-counter treatments. Raising particular suspicion are medications with anticholinergic, narcotic, or sedative effects. Meperidine (Demerol) is both narcotic and anticholinergic and thus is especially worth avoiding in older patients. Potentially harmful drugs should be removed, or at least doses should be reduced. Preferably a less toxic alternative can be chosen or a nonpharmacologic approach can be implemented. Delirium can result from withdrawal of some medications, including central cholinesterase inhibitors, benzodiazepines, narcotics, stimulants, steroids, and selective serotonin reuptake inhibitors.

Acute infections should be actively sought. While in younger patients infections that affect the central nervous system (CNS) are most common, in older patients CNS infection as the precipitant of the delirium is the exception. The lungs and urinary tract are far more likely to be the sources.

Delirium can be precipitated by the full range of metabolic disturbances, including various endocrine diseases, renal or hepatic failure, and rapid alterations in sodium, calcium, or glucose. Strokes, trauma, and neoplasm can cause delirium, but they rarely do so in the absence of physical examination signs. Interestingly, in the surgical patient, route of anesthesia does not seem to influence the occurrence of delirium. Other commonly overlooked precipitants of delirium are urinary retention and fecal impaction.

Further, one needs to support the patient and protect him or her from iatrogenic complications. The general measures for this are the same as those used to prevent delirium, including attention to volume status, nutritional support, and mobilization. Delirium patients, particularly those with the hypoactive form of delirium, are typically less mobile, which makes DVT prophylaxis and attention to preventing pressure ulcers high-priority items. In stuporous patients, airway protection should be considered to prevent aspiration.

MANAGING THE AGITATED PATIENT

Treating the agitated delirium patient involves all of the measures recommended in the previous levels of treatment. Nonpharmacologic treatments are preferable for mild agitation. This includes encouragement of family or sitters at the bedside, music, massage, and relaxation techniques. Uninterrupted sleep in a quiet room with low-level lighting is desirable. Paranoid delusions and hallucinations are not necessarily indications for medication, and calm, empathic, reassurance should be tried first. Physical restraints are to be avoided as much as feasible.

The significantly agitated delirious patient must have 24-hour visual monitoring by nurses or a sitter. Chemical or physical restraints should be considered only if there is imminent danger of harm to self or others, such as physical injury to staff or threat of self-extubation from required ventilator support. Physical restraints, when used, should be reassessed every few hours and discontinued as soon as possible. Chemical restraints should be reevaluated daily and titrated off as rapidly as possible. Overstimulation should be avoided, although visits from family and other friendly faces can be helpful.

The FDA has yet to approved any medications for the treatment of delirium or its behavioral symptoms. Antipsychotic medications are the mainstay of treatment, and haloperidol[1] in particular has better demonstrated efficacy than benzodiazepines. Starting doses are typically 0.25 to 0.5mg, with reevaluation and additional dosing every 30 to 60 minutes as required. Only in emergency situations should a higher initial dose be used. Although it is effective, haloperidol has risks of extrapyramidal side effects (e.g., parkinsonism, akathisia). Atypical neuroleptics such as risperidone[1] (Risperidol, 0.25-0.5 mg twice a day), quetiapine[1] (Seroquel, 25-50 mg two or three times a day), and olanzapine[1] (Zyprexa, 2.5-5 mg daily) are often used, although they are not as well studied. Although acetylcholinesterase

CURRENT THERAPY

- Aspirin, acetaminophen, and nonsteroidal anti-inflammatory drugs (NSAIDs) are first-line choices in the treatment of mild to moderate pain.
- The treatment of delirium begins with its recognition (see Figure 1).
- Agitation and psychosis are common, and nonpharmacologic approaches are preferred in the absence of immediate danger to the patient or others.
- Antipsychotic medications, including haloperidol (Haldol),[1] risperidone (Risperdal),[1] olanzapine (Zyprexa),[1] quetiapine (Seroquel),[1] and others, are not FDA approved for treating delirium, but they are commonly used. Of these, haloperidol has the best demonstrated efficacy and relative safety for treating symptoms of delirium, particularly agitation and psychosis.
- Benzodiazepines may be used to treat alcohol or benzodiazepine withdrawal or for patients who cannot tolerate antipsychotic medications. They treat agitation much better than they treat psychosis.
- A nonpharmacologic approach to treat delirium involves providing a familiar, structured environment, glasses and hearing aids as needed, and calm environment with orientation cues.
- Delirium may be the most common complication of illness in older persons.

---

[1]Not FDA approved for this indication.

[1]Not FDA approved for this indication.

inhibitors are attractive for theoretical reasons, there is little evidence to support their use.

Bezodiazepines should be used in those who have not responded to neuroleptics, for patients who have preexisting parkinsonism, and for alcohol or benzodiazepine withdrawal. Preferred benzodiazepines include lorazepam (Ativan)[1] (0.25-0.5 mg as an initial dose; reevaluate every 30-60 minutes) and oxazepam[1] (Serax, 10 mg bid-tid as an initial dose).

Course and Prognosis

In two thirds of patients, delirium lasts less than 1 week. In the rest, symptoms last from 2 days to a week. As many as 15% of patients, however, still show signs of delirium 6 months after the episode. Even when treated, delirium delays functional recovery and increases the length of hospital stays, nursing care intensity, and the need for home health services or nursing home placement. All of these factors are worse when there is underlying dementia and when underlying etiologies are not adequately treated.

---

[1]Not FDA approved for this indication.

REFERENCES

Fong HK, Sands LP, Leung JM: The role of postoperative analgesia in delirium and cognitive decline in elderly patients: A systematic review. Anesth Analg 2006;102(4):1255-1266.
Inouye SK: Delirium in older persons. N Engl J Med 2006;354(11):1157-1165.
Meagher DJ: Delirium: Optimising management. BMJ 2001; 322(7279): 144-149.
Pandharipande P, Jackson J, Ely EW: Delirium: Acute cognitive dysfunction in the critically ill. Curr Opin Crit Care 2005;11(4):360-368.
Robertson BD, Robertson TJ: Postoperative delirium after hip fracture. J Bone Joint Surgery Am 2006;88(9):2060-2068.
Young J, Inouye SK: Delirium in older people. BMJ 2007;334(7598):842-846.

Mood Disorders

Method of
Bret R. Rutherford, MD, and
Steven P. Roose, MD

Major Depression

Depressive disorders are highly prevalent and impose significant social and economic burdens on patients and society. Major depression alone affects approximately 15% of people at some point in their lives, resulting in 340 million cases worldwide. Depression is twice as common in women and is prevalent from childhood through late life.

DIAGNOSIS

Diagnosis of major depression is based on a clinical interview. As shown in Box 1, the diagnosis of a major depressive episode requires that the patient have a depressed mood or loss of pleasure or interest in usual activities for a period of at least 2 weeks. Patients may report their depressed mood in different ways, from feeling sad, blue, or

---

BOX 1 DSM Criteria for Major Depressive Episode

Depressed mood most of the day, nearly every day, as indicated by either subjective report or observation made by others
Markedly diminished interest or pleasure in all, or almost all, activities most of the day, nearly every day
Significant weight loss when not dieting or significant weight gain, or decrease or increase in appetite nearly every day
Insomnia or hypersomnia nearly every day
Psychomotor agitation or retardation nearly every day
Fatigue or loss of energy nearly every day
Feelings of worthlessness or excessive or inappropriate guilt nearly every day
Diminished ability to think or concentrate, or indecisiveness, nearly every day
Recurrent thoughts of death, recurrent suicidal ideation without a specific plan, or suicide attempt or a specific plan for committing suicide

---

DSM = *Diagnostic and Statistical Manual of Mental Disorders*, fourth edition (text revision).

---

anxious to numb or not having any feelings. Loss of interest typically manifests in a change in patients' daily activities: They might withdraw socially, cease participating in previously pleasurable pastimes, or socially isolate themselves.

Patients with depression often report changes in appetite, with accompanying weight gain or loss. They might have difficulty falling asleep or staying asleep or wake too early in the morning, or else they might find themselves oversleeping. Depressed persons can experience psychomotor slowing (manifested in slow, mumbled speech with long pauses, slowed thinking, and slow body movements) or agitation (motor restlessness manifested in pacing, wringing hands, or other repetitive movements). Many patients also report having low energy and being more easily fatigued than is usual for them.

Cognitive changes are often observed in patients with depression. Patients can feel worthless or inferior and tend to evaluate external events in unrealistically pessimistic or hopeless ways. Memory and concentration are often affected, and patients might find themselves unable to function at work, making careless mistakes at home, and being more forgetful than usual. Patients might report feeling helpless and that they must push themselves to do activities that previously did not require effort (e.g., bathing, dressing).

In every patient with depression, it is critical to assess for the presence of suicidal thoughts. Clinicians must ask whether patients have had thoughts of death, whether they ever think of harming themselves, and if so, in what ways they have thought of harming themselves. Intent to commit suicide should be evaluated by asking patients whether they intend to carry out a suicidal plan, or if not, what stops them and how close they have come to implementing such a plan in the past. Patients should be asked about their access to lethal means, such as firearms, lethal supplies of medications, and other weapons. If a patient has a history of suicide attempts, careful consideration should be given to discovering the circumstances and stressors precipitating the event, what the patient was thinking as the attempt was made, and the patient's reactions to surviving.

Additionally, clinical and demographic factors placing patients at increased risk for suicide should be carefully assessed and combined with these data to generate a suicide risk assessment. Clinical factors associated with increased suicide risk are the presence of mood or psychotic disorders (psychotic depression having particularly high risk), ongoing substance abuse (especially alcohol), medical illness, global insomnia, anhedonia, anxiety, impulsivity and aggressiveness, hopelessness, recent loss, history of trauma or abuse, a

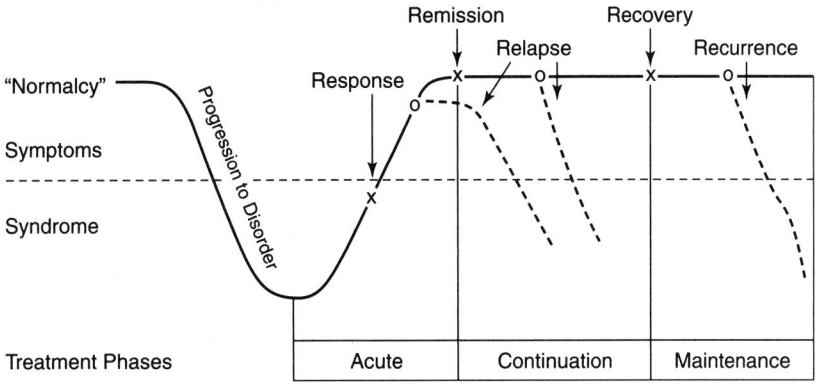

FIGURE 1. Phases of depression treatment. Modified from Kupfer DJ: Long-term treatment of depression. J Clin Psychiatry 1991;52(suppl 5):28-34.

personal history of prior suicide attempts, and a family history of suicide. Demographic risk factors include age older than 65 years, male gender, white race, and divorced or widowed marital status. In summary, clinicians may use the helpful mnemonic SIGECAPS to remember the DSM criteria for depression: sleep, interest, guilt, energy, concentration, appetite, psychomotor agitation or retardation, and suicidality.

In the differential diagnosis of patients with depression, it is critical to rule out medical illness manifesting with depressed mood. Some neurodegenerative conditions (e.g., Alzheimer's disease, Parkinson's disease, Huntington's disease), endocrine disorders (e.g., thyroid, parathyroid, adrenocortical system abnormalities), infectious diseases (e.g., HIV, AIDS), malignancies, and vascular disease (e.g., stroke) can manifest with depressed mood. Patients seeking help at unusual ages or with atypical presentations should be carefully screened for medical problems. For this reason, medical histories and physical examinations must be performed in patients with depression, and a laboratory work-up must be performed including complete blood count, basic metabolic panel, liver function tests, and thyroid function panel,

Although most patients with mood disorder have unipolar depression, the accurate diagnosis of bipolar disorder is essential. Bipolar depression does not respond well to treatment with antidepressants alone, and this can lead to increased frequency of cycling and switches to mania. Bipolar disorder should be specifically ruled out in patients presenting with highly recurrent major depression and in those with family histories of bipolar disorder or postpartum depression.

Ongoing substance abuse or dependence is also important to discover and quantify when treating depression. Although in the past it was widely thought that treatments for depression would be less effective in patients with current drug or alcohol abuse, more recent data have suggested depression may be successfully treated even in the context of heavy substance use. However, treatment can require specific modifications to ensure compliance and safe treatment.

TREATMENT

Phases of Treatment

One major development in the last 20 years regarding the pharmacologic treatment of depression is the shift in treatment goals from response to remission. Response refers to significant improvement in depressive symptoms without complete relief, and it is typically defined in terms of a 50% or more decrease from baseline scores on standardized measurements such as the Beck Depression Inventory (BDI) or the Hamilton Rating Scale for Depression (HRSD). Remission denotes a clinical situation of minimal or no symptoms and return to functional normality, and it is often measured by scores below a certain threshold on standardized measures. The term *recovery* is used to describe a patient in full remission for a period of time.

The goal of treatment has shifted from achieving response to remission in light of greater recognition of the consequences of persistent symptoms: increased risks of relapse and treatment resistance, continued psychosocial limitations and decreased work productivity, cardiovascular morbidity and mortality, and sustained risk of suicide and substance abuse.

With respect to the phases of depression treatment, as shown in Figure 1, the acute phase begins when the patient presents with an episode of major depression. The goal of treatment in this phase is to achieve remission. In the continuation phase, medication treatment is continued at the same dose required to achieve remission for 6 to 9 months to prevent relapse. Maintenance treatment continues indefinitely in patients with recurrent illness to prevent new episodes.

Antidepressant Drugs

Few data are available to guide clinicians in the selection of one particular agent over another, although a patient's personal history of response to a medication, family history of good response, or history of side effects might incline clinicians toward or away from certain agents. Additionally, the presence of significant anxiety comorbid with depression can influence clinicians to choose an agent with a serotoninergic mechanism of action, such as a selective serotonin euptake inhibitor (SSRI) or serotonin–norepinephrine reuptake inhibitor (SNRI). Furthermore, certain medications may be relatively contraindicated in the presence of some medical comorbidities (e.g. tricyclic antidepressants [TCAs] and intraventricular conduction delay).

Selective Serotonin Reuptake Inhibitors

Introduced in the late 1980s, the SSRIs rapidly became the most-prescribed antidepressant class owing to their relative tolerability and safety profiles. There is no consistent evidence that the SSRIs differ in efficacy or side effects. However, some, but not all, SSRIs significantly inhibit the action of hepatic cytochrome P-450 isoenzymes in addition to acting as a substrate for them and therefore have the potential for drug–drug interactions (see Box 2).

The most common side effects of SSRI treatment in the acute phase are gastrointestinal (nausea, vomiting, diarrhea), central nervous system (jitteriness, anxiety, akathisia), and sexual side effects (anorgasmia, erectile difficulty, decreased desire). Long-term treatment can be associated with significant weight gain. A rare but serious complication (and usually happening only when SSRIs are given in combination with another medication that enhances serotonin) is serotonin syndrome. Clinical signs and symptoms of serotonin syndrome include mental status changes (delirium, agitation), autonomic instability (diaphoresis, tachycardia, hyperpyrexia), and neuromuscular symptoms (rigidity, tremor). The combination of SSRIs and MAOIs is contraindicated due to the risk of serotonin syndrome. A major benefit to the SSRIs is that they are relatively safe in overdose.

BOX 2 Table of Substrates, Inhibitors, and Inducers of Cytochrome P-450 Isoenzymes

SUBSTRATES

1A2
clozapine
cyclobenzaprine
omipramine
mexiletine
naproxen
riluzole
tacrine
theophylline

2B6
bupropion
cyclophosphamide
efavirenz
ifosfamide
methadone

2C8

2C19

Proton Pump Inhibitors:
omeprazole
lansoprazole
pantoprazole
rabeprazole

Anti-epileptics:
diazepam
phenytoin
phenobarbitone
amitriptyline
clomipramine
clopidogrel
cyclophosphamide
progesterone

2C9

NSAIDs
diclofenac
ibuprofen
piroxicam

Oral Hypoglycemic Agents:
tolbutamide
glipizide

Angiotensin II Blockers:
NOT candesartan
irbesartan
losartan
NOT valsartan
celecoxib
fluvastatin
naproxen
phenytoin
sulfamethoxazole
tamoxifen
tolbutamide
torsemide
warfarin

2D6

Beta Blockers:
S-metoprolol
propafenone
timolol

Antidepressants:
amitriptyline
clomipramine
desipramine
imipramine
paroxetine

Antipsychotics:
haloperidol
risperidone
thioridazine
aripiprazole
codeine
dextromethorphan
duloxetine
flecainide
mexiletine
ondansetron
tamoxifen
tramadol
venlafaxine

2E1
acetaminophen
chlorzoxazone
ethanol

3A4, 5, 7

Macrolide Antibiotics:
clarithromycin
erythromycin
NOT azithoromycin
telithromycin

Anti-arrhythmics:
quinidine

Benzodiazepines:
alprazolam
diazepam
midazolam
triazolam

Immune Modulators:
cyclosporine
tacrolimus (FK506)

HIV Protease Inhibitors:
indinavir
ritonavir
saquinavir

Prokinetic:
cisapride

Antihistamines:
astemizole
chlorpheniramine

Calcium Channel Blockers:
amlodipine
diltiazem
felodipine
nifedipine
nisoldipine
nitrendipine
verapamil

HMG CoA Reductase Inhibitors:
atorvastatin
cerivastatin
lovastatin
NOT pravastatin
simvastatin
aripiprazole
buspirone
gleevec
haloperidol (in part)
methadone
pimozide
quinine
NOT rosuvastatin
sildenafil
tamoxifen
trazodone
vincristine

INHIBITORS

1A2
cimetidine
fluoroquinolones
fluvoxamine
ticlopidine

2B6
thiotepa
ticlopidine

2C8
gemfibrozil
montelukast

2C19
fluoxetine
fluvoxamine
ketoconazole
lansoprazole
omeprazole
ticlopidine

2C9
amiodarone
fluconazole
isoniazid

> **BOX 2** Table of Substrates, Inhibitors, and Inducers of Cytochrome P-450 Isoenzymes—cont'd
>
> | | | |
> |---|---|---|
> | **2D6**
amiodarone
buprorion
chlorpheniramine
cimetidine
clomipramine
duloxetine
fluoxetine
haloperidol
methadone
mibefradil
paroxetine
quinidine
ritonavir
2E1
disulfiram
3A4,5,7
HIV Protease Inhibitors:
indinavir
nelfinavir
ritonavir
amiodarone
NOT azithromycin | cimetidine
clarithromycin
diltiazem
erythromycin
fluvoxamine
grapefruit juice
itraconazole
ketoconazole
mibefradil
nefazodone
troleandomycin
verapamil
INDUCERS
1A2
tobacco
2B6
phenobarbital
phenytoin
rifampin
2C8 | **2C19**
N/A
2C9
rifampin
secobarbital
2D6
N/A
2E1
ethanol
isoniazid
3A4,5,7
carbamazepine
phenobarbital
phenytoin
ethanol
rifampin
St. John's wort
troglitazone |
>
> Adapted from Flockhart DA. Drug Interactions: Cytochrome P450 Drug Interaction Table. Indiana University School of Medicine (2007). Available at http://www.medicine.iupui.edu/flockhart/clinlist.htm (accessed June 13, 2008)

SSRIs are started at the lowest effective dose and then titrated upward as required for clinical response. There may be a significant delay between starting an SSRI and achieving clinical effect, although some evidence suggests that patients who show benefit in the first 1 or 2 weeks of treatment might have a more positive long-term prognosis. Typical starting dosages are fluoxetine (Prozac) 10 to 20 mg, sertraline (Zoloft) 50 mg, paroxetine (Paxil) 20 mg, citalopram (Celexa) 20 mg, escitalopram (Lexapro) 10 mg, and fluvoxamine 100 mg. Children and adolescents, the elderly, and patients with panic or significant anxiety might require lower starting dosages. Initial doses are maintained for 1 to 2 weeks and then increased weekly as required for clinical benefit to maximum dosages of fluoxetine 80 mg, sertraline 200 mg, paroxetine 60 mg,[3] citalopram 60 mg, escitalopram 20 mg, and fluvoxamine 300 mg.

Serotonin–Norepinephrine Reuptake Inhibitors

SNRIs share the serotonin reuptake inhibition that is a hallmark of the SSRIs while also having strong affinity for the norepinephrine transporter. Venlafaxine appears to have a dual effect, whereby it primarily inhibits the serotonin transporter at lower doses and affects both the norepinephrine and serotonin transporters at doses greater than 150 mg/day. Venlafaxine is typically started at a dose of 37.5 mg daily and increased by 37.5 to 75 mg per week to a maximum of 300 mg daily.

Duloxetine is usually started at a dose of 30 mg daily and raised to 60 mg. If there is no clinical response at 60 mg, the dose could be raised to 120 mg,[3] which has been safely used in clinical and research populations. However, as with all the SSRIs and SNRIs, the benefits of increasing the dose above the minimally effective dose are unproved.

SNRIs share many aspects of their side-effect profile with SSRIs owing to their similar mechanisms of action. However, possibly due to their effects on norepinephrine reuptake, at higher doses these medications can result in mild elevations in blood pressure. For this reason, baseline blood pressures should be documented, followed by ongoing monitoring of blood pressure as long as the patient is taking an SNRI.

Buprorion

The aminoketone buprorion (Wellbutrin) is an interesting antidepressant whose mechanism of action is poorly understood, although it appears to reduce dopamine and norepinephrine reuptake. Buprorion is typically started at 150 mg/day and increased by 150 mg/week to a maximum of 450 mg daily. Some studies have reported that buprorion is less likely to cause manic switching in patients with bipolar disorder. It is also approved as a treatment for smoking cessation and may be a good choice in patients with depression and comorbid nicotine dependence. Typical adverse effects with buprorion include anxiety, insomnia, palpitations, dry mouth, and nausea.

Tricyclics

TCAs include imipramine, amitriptyline (Elavil), desipramine (Norpramin), maprotiline, protiptyline (Vivactil), and doxepin (Sinequan). Despite robust efficacy and the ability to regulate dose by monitoring plasma levels, the TCAs are generally less used due to their higher frequency of troublesome side effects and high mortality rate in overdose. All TCAs bring about norepinephrine transporter

---
[3]Exceeds dosage recommended by the manufacturer.

reuptake inhibition, and some have strong affinity for the serotonin transporter as well. TCAs are well absorbed in the small intestine and reach peak plasma levels 2 to 6 hours after oral administration. Metabolism is by hepatic microsomal enzymes, often to active metabolites. For example, imipramine's primary metabolite is desipramine, and amitriptyline's major metabolite is nortriptyline.

Anticholinergic side effects due to blockade of muscarinic receptors can be significant problems with TCAs. These can include decreased salivation, constipation, urinary retention, blurry vision and mydriasis, tachycardia, and impaired memory and cognition. Sympathomimetic side effects caused by inhibition of norepinephrine reuptake can cause anxiety, tremors, tachycardia, and diaphoresis. α-Receptor blockade can result in postural hypotension and falls in the elderly.

Starting doses for TCAs are generally 50 to 75 mg/day, with the exception of nortriptyline (25-50 mg/day) and protriptyline (10-15 mg/day). Dosages are titrated to achieve a therapeutic plasma level. Nortriptyline is the only TCA known to have a therapeutic window of blood plasma levels, making regular laboratory monitoring helpful. Plasma levels of 50 to 150 ng/mL appear optimal for nortriptyline, and imipramine and desipramine have a curvilinear dose-response curve with optimum blood levels from 150 to 300 ng/mL.

Monoamine Oxidase Inhibitors

Monoamine oxidase inhibitors (MAOIs), the first antidepressants discovered, inhibit the action of monoamine oxidase, which is the enzyme carrying out catabolism of the monoamines. MAO-A is the enzyme subtype located primarily in the brain, and MAO-B is localized to the gut. Enzymatic inhibition is irreversible for most MAOIs, meaning that new MAO enzyme must be synthesized to restore functioning, a process that can take approximately 2 weeks.

The use of MAOIs requires dietary restriction to avoid hypertensive crises. Inhibition of MAO prevents the metabolism of tyramine, which stimulates the release of norepinephrine from sympathetic terminals. Increased norepinephrine levels precipitate hypertension and hypertensive crises, which generally manifest clinically in pounding headaches. Obviously, extensive education about dietary requirements is necessary before patients begin an MAOI (see http://patienteducation.upmc.com/Pdf/MaoiDiet.pdf), and many clinicians supply their patients with 10 mg nifedipine (Adalat) tablets that may be taken in the case of a severe headache.

Phenelzine (Nardil) is started at a dose of 30 mg/daily and increased by 15 mg weekly to a target dose of 45 to 90 mg daily. Tranylcypromine (Parnate) may be started at 10 mg daily and increased by 10 mg weekly to 30 to 60 mg/day. The recent introduction of transdermal selegiline offers the potential for a better-tolerated MAOI with fewer dietary restrictions. This patch is available in 6, 9, and 12 mg/day dosages, with only the latter two appearing to require dietary restrictions on tyramine-containing foods.

Other Antidepressants

Other antidepressant medications have numerous mechanisms of action. Nefazodone exhibits norepinephrine and serotonin reuptake inhibition, while also antagonizing 5-HT$_{2A}$ and α1-receptors. Nefazodone has a black box warning for the risk of liver failure due to the 1 in 250,000 to 300,000 patient-years risk of this outcome. This medication is usually given twice daily starting at 100 mg twice a day. Titration is done at a rate of 100 to 200 mg weekly to reach a maximum of 600 mg total daily. Mirtazapine (Remeron) appears to work through the blockade of α2-autoreceptors on presynaptic noradrenergic neurons and 5-HT$_2$ and 5-HT$_3$ receptors. It can be started at doses of 15 mg daily and increased by 15 mg weekly to a maximum of 45 mg/day. Paradoxically, doses lower than 15 mg daily may be more sedating than doses greater than 15 mg. Trazodone has been associated with penile priapism at a rate of 1 in 6000 to 8000 men. It is started at dosages of 50 to 75 mg/day and increased to a maximum of 400 to 600 mg/day. Currently, it is primarily used at lower doses for its hypnotic effect.

Psychotherapy

A number of specific psychotherapies are effective for treating depression. However, no single psychotherapy has been demonstrated to be superior to another, and many studies have shown nonspecific supportive psychotherapy to be as effective as the specific psychotherapies.

Cognitive Behavior Therapy

Developed by Aaron Beck and his colleagues in the 1960s, cognitive behavior therapy (CBT) is based on the cognitive model of mood disorders, which posits that the way people interpret their experiences influences how they feel and behave. For example, patients with depression typically have negative views of themselves, how others view them, and their future prospects. CBT focuses on identifying and changing these negative cognitions, which cause people to feel depressed or anxious. Patients learn to monitor these automatic thoughts and examine the evidence for and against them, alternative ways of thinking about the situation, and how different ways of thinking might influence the way they feel and behave.

This cognitive work is complemented by behavioral homework assignments, which require patients to keep a log of their daily activities, undertake graded exposure exercises to challenge maladaptive automatic thoughts, and role play new ways of thinking with their therapists. These behavioral experiments help patients develop a better sense of self-efficacy and mastery in addition to providing corrective experiences to counter maladaptive automatic thoughts. CBT is often undertaken one or more times weekly for 12 to 16 weeks, after which continuing meetings or booster sessions may be helpful.

Interpersonal Psychotherapy

Interpersonal psychotherapy (IPT) was developed by Klerman and colleagues in the 1970s to treat depression. IPT begins with a thorough evaluation, diagnosis, and assigning the patient the sick role. Patients' difficulties are then classified into one of four domains: grief, interpersonal role disputes, role transitions, and interpersonal deficits. Specific strategies to address the main problem areas (e.g., facilitate mourning in the case of grief) are then pursued with attention to improving the patient's interpersonal relationships. Termination is addressed explicitly, and the progress made by the patient is reviewed. IPT is usually conducted in 12 to 20 sessions over a 4- to 5-month period and may be individual or in a group.

Psychodynamic Psychotherapy

The overall goal of this psychotherapy is to increase patient's self-awareness, improve personal satisfaction, and resolve difficulties in interpersonal and romantic relationships. This treatment shares a theoretical framework with psychoanalysis, including the concepts of transference, countertransference, resistance, and unconscious conflict. Psychodynamic psychotherapy makes use of the techniques of clarification, confrontation, and interpretation and is usually undertaken at a frequency of one or more times weekly for a period of months or years.

Treatment-Resistant Depression

Many patients with major depression do not experience remission with the first antidepressant medication or course of psychotherapy. Patients are typically considered to have treatment-resistant depression when a minimum of two treatments at adequate dosage and duration have failed. One influential nomenclature for treatment-resistant depression developed by Thase and Rush relies on nonresponse to sequential trials of antidepressants with varying mechanisms of action. Stage I resistance is defined as lack of response to an adequate trial of one antidepressant; stage II resistance is defined as stage I resistance plus failure to respond to a second antidepressant having a different mechanism of action; stage III resistance is stage II resistance plus nonresponse to a tricyclic medication; stage IV resistance is stage III plus nonresponse to an MAOI; and stage V resistance is stage IV followed by nonresponse to electroconvulsive therapy (ECT).

Patients with treatment-resistant depression are among the most disabled persons with major depressive disorder, which itself ranks fourth among diseases worldwide in accounting for disability-adjusted life-years. Persistence of depressive symptoms can lead to continued psychosocial limitations and decreased work productivity, cardiovascular morbidity and mortality, and sustained risks of suicide and substance abuse. Due to the immense burden associated with treatment-resistant depression, there is consensus that the goal of treatment for patients is to achieve remission, defined as a final score of 10 on the HRSD or some comparable scale.

A unique perspective on the use of medications and psychotherapy to treat depression has been provided by the National Institute of Mental Health–sponsored Sequenced Treatment Alternatives to Relieve Depression (STAR*D) study, which is the largest prospective trial for depression ever conducted. Patients presented to one of 41 sites seeking treatment, and inclusion or exclusion criteria were structured so as to promote maximum generalizability. As shown in Figure 2, all 3271 patients received monotherapy with citalopram in level 1, and those whose depressions did not remit were encouraged to proceed with additional trials until remission was achieved. At level 2, patients were allowed to express preference for medication or psychotherapy and for switching treatments or augmenting treatment. Switch options were randomization to bupropion, sertraline, venlafaxine, and CBT; augmentation options were randomization to bupropion, buspirone, or CBT in addition to citalopram. Patients whose depressions still did not remit could be randomized at level 3 to either of two switch options (nortriptyline or mirtazapine) or two augmentation options (adding lithium or triiodothyronine (T_3) to whatever antidepressant they were taking). The final step, level 4, involved randomizing patients to tranylcypromine or the combination of venlafaxine and mirtazapine.

After initial treatment with citalopram, 37% of patients achieved remission. In level 2, patients who switched medications received either sustained-release bupropion up to 400 mg/day, sertraline up to 200 mg/day, or extended-release venlafaxine up to 375 mg/day. Remission rates, as measured by HRSD scores less than 7 on these medications, were 21% for bupropion, 18% for sertraline, and 25% for venlafaxine, which were not significantly different from one another. Augmentation of citalopram was with sustained-release bupropion up to 400 mg/day or buspirone up to 60 mg/day, and remission rates were identical (30% in each). In the level 3 augmentation trial, 16% of patients achieved remission with lithium compared to 25% of patients receiving T_3, which was not a significant difference. However, there was a suggestion that T_3 was better tolerated than lithium. In the level 4 trial, 7% of patients receiving

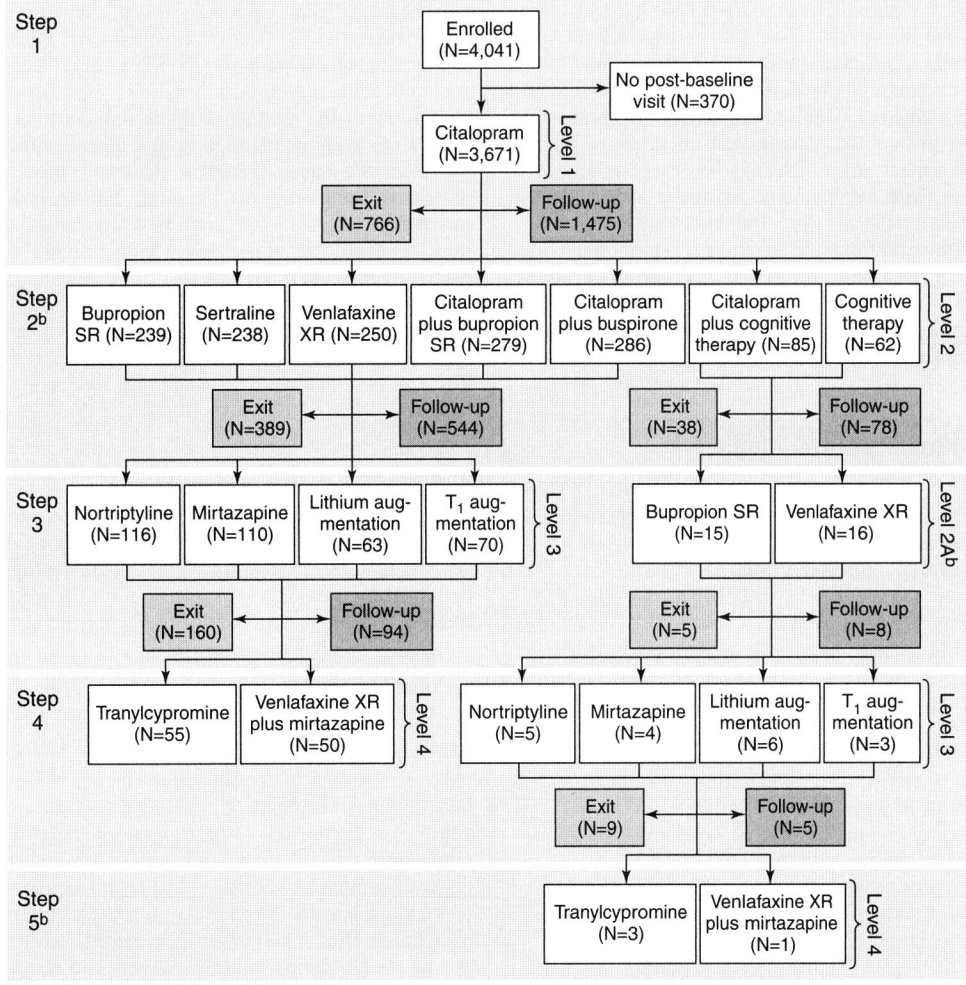

FIGURE 2. Sequenced Treatment Alternatives to Relieve Depression (STAR*D) study design. Adapted from Rush AJ, Trivedi MH, Wisniewski SR, et al: Acute and longer-term outcomes in depressed outpatients requiring one or several treatment steps: A STAR*D Report. Am J Psychiatry 2006;163:1905-1917.

tranylcypromine and 14% of patients receiving combined venlafaxine and mirtazipine remitted, which were not significantly different results.

Brain Stimulation

When patients fail multiple pharmacologic and psychotherapeutic trials, or when rapid control of depressive, manic, or psychotic symptoms is necessary, ECT should be strongly considered. ECT remains a safe and effective treatment for mood disorders, and new protocols for treatment delivery aim to minimize cognitive side effects. Other brain stimulation treatments being studied as possible therapeutic tools include vagal nerve stimulation, deep brain stimulation, transcranial magnetic stimulation, and magnetic seizure therapy.

Bipolar Disorder

Epidemiologic studies show that 0.5% to 1.5% of people suffer from bipolar disorder, although up to 5% of the population might have bipolar spectrum illnesses. Patients usually present with a mood episode in their teens or 20s, and the risk of developing bipolar disorder dramatically decreases after the age of 50 years. Men and women are affected equally, and most persons go on to suffer a chronic course of repeated mood episodes.

DIAGNOSIS

Patients with bipolar spectrum disorders must meet diagnostic criteria for a hypomanic, manic, or mixed episode, and they often have had one or more major depressive episodes in the past. A manic episode is characterized by a period lasting at least 1 week of persistently elevated, expansive, or irritable mood (Box 3). Elevated moods are clearly recognized as excessive by persons close to the patient, and the expansiveness of manic episodes is manifested in much increased enthusiasm for new projects or interpersonal interactions. Patients often have increased self-esteem, which may become psychotic as in grandiose delusions. Most persons experiencing a manic episode demonstrate a decreased need for sleep and increased energy.

Mental status examination of patients who are manic often reveals loud, rapid, poorly interruptible speech of dramatically increased productivity. Patients might report racing thoughts, which are experienced as moving faster than they can articulate or fully understand. Increased goal-directed activity refers to the excessive planning of and participation in activities such as new business ventures, house-cleaning, hypergraphia, and calling people on the telephone. This activity is often coupled with impulsivity and poor judgment, as when patients engage in risky or dangerous activities such as spending sprees, violence, dangerous driving, and substance misuse.

To meet criteria for a manic episode, the impairment due to the mood disturbance must be severe enough to bring about marked difficulty functioning or require hospitalization. Hypomanic episodes are less severe than manic episodes, involving at least 4 days of elevated or irritable mood, fewer accompanying manic symptoms, and less severe functional impairment. Mixed episodes are 1-week periods during which the diagnostic criteria for both a major depressive episode and a manic episode are met. Clinicians may use the mnemonic DIGFAST to easily remember the list of DSM manic symptoms: *d*istractibility, *i*llegal (risky) activities, *g*randiosity, *f*light of ideas, decreased *s*leep, increased goal-directed *a*ctivities, and *t*alkativity.

As in the case of depressive disorders, suicide must be carefully evaluated in patients with bipolar disorder, because their risk of suicide is among the highest of all psychiatric patients. Medical conditions causing the manic, hypomanic, or mixed episode must be carefully ruled out, and other possible diagnoses such as substance induced mood disorders and attention-deficit/hyperactivity disorder must be considered.

TREATMENT
Overview

Bipolar disorder is a chronic illness requiring lifelong management. Therefore, conducting an extensive process of patient education, facilitating treatment compliance, and developing a good therapeutic alliance are of great importance. Clinicians and patients have more information on which to base treatment decisions if continuous monitoring of the patient's mood (whether depressed or euphoric) is conducted using mood journals. Triggers for mood disturbance in each patient (e.g., long plane flight, fight with spouse, use of alcohol) should be carefully attended to and taken seriously when evident.

Given the highly recurrent nature of bipolar disorder and the severity of the disruption it typically causes, most experts agree that maintenance treatment is indicated after an acute manic, mixed, or depressive state resolves. A common practice in preventing future episodes of bipolar disorder is to continue the medication that resolved an acute episode. Many patients with bipolar disorder continue to experience significant symptoms even after they are considered to have remitted from an acute episode of depression or mania. These must be carefully assessed and treated to promote functional recovery and a good quality of life.

Mood Stabilizers

Phases of treatment for bipolar disorder include treatment of acute mania, prevention of mania, treatment of acute depression, and prevention of depression. Available mood-stabilizing agents are generally better in one phase than another, and no treatment is available that treats all phases of bipolar disorder.

Lithium

Lithium has been studied as a treatment for mania since the late 1940s. Several good-quality randomized, controlled trials demonstrate its efficacy in treating acute mania in bipolar patients; there is more limited evidence supporting the efficacy of lithium in patients with acute depression. Lithium appears effective in preventing both manic and depressive episodes, although some studies suggest more limited usefulness for lithium in preventing depression.

Lithium has good oral absorption, reaching peak plasma levels 1 to 3 hours after ingestion. It is excreted renally, which necessitates dosing modifications in older patients and in the setting of medications affecting tubular reabsorption. Lithium's exact mechanism of action is unknown, but it may be related to effects on noradrenergic and dopaminergic transmission or on complex transduction pathways.

BOX 3 DSM Criteria for Manic Episode

Distinct period of abnormally and persistently elevated, expansive or irritable mood, lasting at least 1 week (or any duration if hospitalization is necessary) and accompanied by:
Inflated self-esteem or grandiosity
Decreased need for sleep (e.g., feels rested after only 3 hours of sleep)
More talkative than usual or pressure to keep talking
Flight of ideas or subjective experience that thoughts are racing
Distractibility (i.e., attention too easily drawn to unimportant or irrelevant external stimuli)
Increase in goal-directed activity (at work, at school, or sexually) or psychomotor agitation
Excessive involvement in pleasurable activities that have a high potential for painful consequences (e.g., engaging in unrestrained buying sprees, sexual indiscretions, or foolish business investments)

DSM = Diagnostic and Statistical Manual of Mental Disorders, fourth edition (text revision).

Before a patient starts taking lithium, it is necessary to perform a medical work-up including medical history, physical examination with weight, blood urea nitrogen and creatinine, thyroid-function studies, complete blood count, and pregnancy testing for women of childbearing age. Lithium is usually started between 600 and 1200 mg daily for acute mania, with blood level determination (sampled 12 hours after last dose) after 4 days of treatment. A blood concentration between 0.8 and 1.2 mmol/L is desirable for acute mania, with toxic effects generally starting at blood levels of 1.5 and above. Patients with hypomania or in need of mania prophylaxis are started on lower doses of lithium, 300 to 600 mg daily, and titrated up more slowly to achieve blood levels of 0.6 to 0.8 mmol/L.

Common lithium side effects include nausea, vomiting, fine tremor, diarrhea, polydipsia, and polyuria. These are often transient and can be mitigated by dosage changes and slower titration strategies. Side effects of chronic treatment can include acne, psoriasis, hypothyroidism, and nephrogenic diabetes insipidus. Lithium toxicity is always a serious and potentially fatal condition. Signs and symptoms of toxic blood levels include mental status changes, ataxia, coarse tremor, and bradycardia. Treatment can require renal dialysis.

Anticonvulsants

Anticonvulsants have been used in patients with bipolar disorder since the 1960s, when "kindling" as a shared pathologic process with seizure disorders was purported to be the cause of disordered mood states. Not all anticonvulsants have proved effective for bipolar disorder, and those that have exhibit a wide range of mechanisms of action.

Divalproex sodium (Depakote) was the first anticonvulsant approved to treat acute mania and remains a first-line treatment for preventing and treating mania. However, this medication does not appear as effective for treating and preventing depression. Treatment of acutely manic patients with divalproex is typically begun with an oral loading dose of 15 to 20 mg/kg body weight divided into two or three daily doses, which is then continued for 4 days before checking a drug plasma level. Less urgently ill patients might have fewer side effects with more gradual titrations, starting at 250 to 500 mg daily and titrated up as needed. Blood levels of 50 to 125 mg/L represent the therapeutic range for this medication. Gastrointestinal side effects such as nausea and diarrhea are often observed with divalproex, as are sedation, weight gain, and tremor. Rare but potentially life-threatening adverse effects are hepatic failure, hemorrhagic pancreatitis, and encephalopathy caused by high ammonia levels.

Carbamazepine (Tegretol) has proved efficacy for mania in a number of randomized, controlled trials, but it too is of unclear benefit in treating and preventing depressive episodes. This medication is generally started at 200 to 600 mg daily in divided doses, then increased by 200 mg weekly to therapeutic effect or a maximum of 1600 mg/day. An extended release form of carbamazepine is available that allows once-daily dosing. Therapeutic blood levels for epilepsy are 4 to 12 mg/L. The most commonly observed adverse effects with carbamazepine are nausea, sedation, blurred vision, and ataxia. Rare but serious side effects include hyponatremia due to secretion of inappropriate antidiuretic hormone (SIADH), liver transaminase elevations, aplastic anemia, and rash.

After being used off-label for several years for the prevention and treatment of bipolar depression, lamotrigine (Lamictal) received FDA approval in 2003 as a maintenance treatment for bipolar disorder. It has been shown in multiple randomized, controlled trials to be significantly superior to placebo in bipolar patients with recently resolved depression or mania in delaying the recurrence of a mood episode. Lamotrigine appears to be more effective in preventing episodes of depression than mania. Its value in the treatment of acute depressive episodes is much less clear. An initial randomized, controlled trial of lamotrigine versus placebo in patients with bipolar I depression revealed significant improvement in patients receiving 200 mg of lamotrigine compared with placebo. However, several more recent randomized, controlled trials have failed to replicate this finding, and the usefulness of this medication for patients with acute bipolar depression remains unclear.

Lamotrigine is generally started at doses of 25 mg daily for 2 weeks, followed by 50 mg for 2 weeks, and then 100 mg daily, with future titration of approximately 50 mg every 2 to 4 weeks. This slower titration schedule is thought to be helpful in reducing the risk of treatment-emergent rash, which can occur in up to 10% of patients on lamotrigine, and the rarer but more serious Stevens–Johnson syndrome. In patients who develop a rash and systemic signs such as fever or lymphadenopathy while taking lamotrigine, the medication should be immediately discontinued and the patient should be evaluated in an emergency room. The most common side effects observed with lamotrigine are dizziness, headache, blurred vision, and gastrointestinal distress.

Atypical Antipsychotics

All currently available atypical antipsychotics have now been approved by the FDA for managing acute bipolar mania, and quetiapine (Seroquel) is now appoved for bipolar depression. Many atypicals have proved efficacy as monotherapies for mania but also show improvement versus placebo when added on to other mood stabilizers. Most atypicals have high affinity for dopamine, serotonin, and α-adrenergic receptors, and some have additional high affinity for histamine. The exact mechanism of action of atypical antipsychotics in treating mania is unclear, although those that exert D_2-blocking effects might work by this route. Atypicals shown to be effective in treating depression might work by means of D2 and 5-HT_{2A} blockade.

Olanzapine (Zyprexa) is started at 10 to 15 mg daily and increased to 20 to 30 mg[3] daily as needed to control acute mania. An intramuscular form of olanzapine is also available for use in hospitalized patients with severe agitation. It is administered in a 10-mg dose that can be repeated 2 and 4 hours later for a total daily dose of 30 mg. Concomitant treatment with lorazepam is contraindicated due to reported cases of profound respiratory depression.

Quetiapine is started at 25 to 50 mg twice daily and titrated up as tolerated over the course of 1 to 2 weeks to approximately 600 mg daily. Evidence exists for the use of quetiapine in acute mania, and more recently two randomized, controlled trials have demonstrated significant antidepressant benefits for quetiapine monotherapy of patients with bipolar I or II depression. Apart from olanzapine and quetiapine, very limited evidence exists for the efficacy of other atypical antipsychotics in bipolar depression.

There is good evidence of efficacy for risperidone (Risperdal) as monotherapy for acute mania and as add-on treatment to lithium or an anticonvulsant. Risperidone is generally started at 1 to 2 mg/day in divided doses and titrated up by 1 to 2 mg daily to a range of 4 to 6 mg/day. Risperidone is currently the only atypical antipsychotic available in a long-acting preparation, which is injected intramuscularly[1] to provide slow release of risperidone over 3 weeks. Clinicians may start with 12.5 to 25 mg IM every 2 weeks, with increases of 12.5 mg every 4 weeks as needed up to 50 mg IM every 2 weeks.

Ziprasidone (Geodon) should be started at 40 mg twice daily, given with meals to increase the absorption of medication. Ziprasidone should be titrated up to a total of 160 mg/day within the first week of treatment, because some reports of activation in the lower dosing range have been reported. It is available in an intramuscular[1] form to assist in the management of acute agitation, with 10 to 20 mg given every 2 to 4 hours as needed up to a maximum of 40 mg daily.

Aripiprazole (Abilify) is the newest atypical antipsychotic approved for use in acute mania. As opposed to other atypicals, aripiprazole is a partial agonist at the D2 receptor. It can be started at 10 to 15 mg daily and titrated up over the course of a week to approximately 30 mg daily. An intramuscular form of aripiprazole

---

[3] Exceeds dosage recommended by the manufacturer.
[1] Not FDA approved for this indication.

is now available to treat acute agitation, and this injected is given at a dose of 9.75 mg every 2 hours to a maximum of 30 mg daily.

The most significant category of side effects noted with the use of atypical antipsychotics is weight gain, dyslipidemia, and onset of type 2 diabetes mellitus. Management of patients taking these medications must include monitoring of waist circumference, fasting glucose, weight, and lipid profile.

Conclusions

Unipolar and bipolar mood disorders are often observed in clinical practice and have serious negative psychosocial and health consequences. Treatment must follow a structured approach beginning with comprehensive evaluation and diagnosis, proceeding through informed consent and patient education, and culminating in the initiation of treatment. In addition to several evidence-based psychotherapeutic modalities, numerous antidepressant and mood-stabilizing medications are available in a number of classes for treating depression and mania. The careful use of these treatments may be of considerable benefit for most patients with these disorders.

REFERENCES

Bowden CL, Calabrese JR, Sachs G, et al: A placebo-controlled 18-month trial of lamotrigine and lithium maintenance treatment in recently manic or hypomanic patients with bipolar I disorder. Arch Gen Psychiatry 2003;60:392-400.
Calabrese JR, Bowden CL, Sachs G, et al: A placebo-controlled 18-month trial of lamotrigine and lithium maintenance treatment in recently depressed patients with bipolar I disorder. J Clin Psychiatry 2003;64:1013-1024.
Calabrese JR, Bowden CL, Sachs GS, et al: A double-blind placebo-controlled study of lamotrigine monotherapy in outpatients with bipolar I depression. Lamictal 602 Study Group. J Clin Psychiatry 1999;60:79-88.
Calabrese JR, Keck PE Jr, Macfadden W, et al: A randomized, double-blind, placebo-controlled trial of quetiapine in the treatment of bipolar I or II depression. Am J Psychiatry 2005;162,1351-1360.
Frank E: Treatment outcomes for depression in primary care. Arch Gen Psychiatry 1991;48:851-855.
Greden JF: The burden of disease for treatment-resistant depression. J Clin Psychiatry 2001;62(Suppl 16):26-31.
Judd LL, Paulus MJ, Schettler PJ, et al: Does incomplete recovery from first lifetime major depressive episode herald a chronic course of illness? Am J Psych 2000;157:1501-1504.
Kessler RC, Berglund P, Demler O, et al: The epidemiology of major depressive disorder: Results from the National Comorbidity Survey Replication (NCS-R). JAMA 2003;289:3095-3105.
Kupfer DJ: Long-term treatment of depression. J Clin Psychiatry 1991; 52(suppl 5):28-34.
McGrath PJ, Stewart JW, Fava M, et al: Tranylcypromine versus venlafaxine plus mirtazapine following three failed antidepressant medication trials for depression: A STAR*D report. Am J Psychiatry 2006;163:1531-1541.
Murray CJL, Lopez AD: The Global Burden of Disease: A Comprehensive Assessment of Mortality and Disability from Disease, Injuries, and Risk Factors in 1990 and Projected to 2020, vol 1. World Health Organization. Cambridge, Mass: Harvard University Press, 1996.
Nierenberg AA, Fava M, Trivedi MH, et al: A comparison of lithium and T3 augmentation following two failed medication treatments for depression: A STAR*D report. Am J Psychiatry 2006;163:1519-1530.
Nierenberg AA, Wright EC: Evolution of remission as the new standard in the treatment of depression. J Clin Psychiatry 1999;60(Suppl 22):7-11.
Paykel ES, Ramana R, Cooper Z, et al: Residual symptoms after partial remission: an important outcome in depression. Psychol Med 1995;25:1171-1180.
Thase, ME, MacFadden, W, Weisler, RH, et al: Efficacy of quetiapine monotherapy in bipolar I and II depression: A double-blind, placebo-controlled study (the BOLDER II study). J Clin Psychopharmacol 2006;26:600-609.
Thase ME, Ninan PT: New goals in the treatment of depression: Moving toward recovery. Psychopharmacol Bull 2002;36(Suppl 2):24-35.
Thase ME, Rush HA: Treatment-resistant depression. In Bloom FE, Kupfer DJ (eds). Psychopharmacology, The 4th Generation of Progress New York, Raven, 1995, pp 1081-1098.
Trivedi MH, Rush AJ, Wisniewski SR, et al: Evaluation of outcomes with citalopram for depression using measurement-based care in STAR*D: implications for clinical practice. Am J Psychiatry 2006;163:28-40.

Schizophrenia

Method of
Jeffrey Rado, MD, MPH, and
Philip G. Janicak, MD

Schizophrenia is a chronic, debilitating mental disorder that causes significant morbidity and mortality. It has a lifetime prevalence of approximately 1%. In some studies, men and women are affected equally, but in other studies the incidence, morbid risk, and mortality are higher in men. Men also have an earlier age at onset (late adolescence to early 20s) than women, who present on average 6 years later. Core symptoms include hallucinations (primarily auditory), delusions, disorganization of thoughts and behavior, and deterioration in psychosocial functioning. Most patients require long-term, comprehensive psychosocial treatment combined with antipsychotic medication.

Clinical Presentation

The diagnosis of schizophrenia is based on criteria from the *Diagnostic and Statistical Manual of Mental Disorders*, fourth edition (text revision) (DSM-IV TR). A combination of the characteristic signs and symptoms described later must be present for at least 1 month. The illness is marked by impaired social and occupational functioning, as well as difficulties with interpersonal relationships and self-care. Symptoms cannot be due to the direct physiologic effect of a substance or medical condition.

A broad range of diagnostic syndromes can be involved in the differential diagnosis. These include schizoaffective disorder, bipolar disorder with psychotic features, major depression with psychotic features, delusional disorder, brief psychotic disorder, schizophreniform disorder, neurologic conditions (e.g., brain neoplasm, seizures), delirium, dementia, and psychosis secondary to a general medical condition or substance-induced psychosis.

Course and Prognosis

Schizophrenia can have a variable course. A premorbid or prodromal phase of the illness can include gradual social withdrawal and isolation, bizarre or eccentric behavior, and changes in appearance and hygiene, although more acute onsets are common. The early phase of the illness is typically followed by an overt or insidious onset of psychotic symptoms (e.g., hallucinations, delusions, disordered thoughts and behavior). Early in the clinical course, disease progression is usually punctuated by acute psychotic episodes followed by progressively greater levels of residual impairment. Later stages can have a more stable course (albeit with substantial disability) with fewer exacerbations. Intensity of psychotic symptoms tends to lessen with age. A long-term decline in psychosocial functioning is common and a complete return to premorbid functioning is rare. Social disengagement and chronic unemployment are usual outcomes.

Despite treatment, remission rates are low, and about 40% of patients are noncompliant with treatment after 6 months. Most patients experience multiple relapses and have a higher incidence of comorbid medical conditions (e.g., diabetes, cardiac disease, and substance-use disorders) compared with the general population. Overall, mortality rates are increased due to suicide and morbidity related to medical illness.

Symptom Domains

POSITIVE SYMPTOMS

Hallucinations (i.e., abnormal perceptions in any of the senses) are a predominant feature of schizophrenia. Patients most often report hearing sounds, often single or multiple voices speaking to them or having a conversation. Visual hallucinations involving recognizable objects such as people and animals or unformed shapes or lights also occur but are less common than auditory experiences. Taste, smell (e.g., strange odors), or sensation (e.g., feeling of something moving under the skin) hallucinations usually have an identifiable physical cause. *Command hallucinations* consist of auditory instructions for the patient to carry out specific actions.

Delusions are fixed false beliefs that involve both misperceptions and misinterpretations. These are commonly paranoid in nature but can also have somatic or religious themes. A *delusion of reference* is a belief that specific events (e.g., a news broadcast or radio program) contain a special message intended for the patient and may result in delusionally driven actions. *Thought broadcasting* refers to the experience that one's thoughts can be heard by other people. *Thought insertion* is the belief that thoughts have been placed inside one's head by another party.

COGNITIVE SYMPTOMS

Cognitive dysfunction is a core characteristic of this illness. Impairments can occur in attention, memory, and executive functioning. *Disorganized speech and behavior* are prominent. This can range from vagueness or mild distractibility to derailment (i.e., ideas slip from one theme to another and can be completely unrelated). *Thought blocking* involves the sudden interruption of thought processes. Speech may be illogical, incomprehensible, or incoherent.

NEGATIVE SYMPTOMS

Negative (or deficit) symptoms include affective flattening, alogia, avolition, and anhedonia. All can cause significant functional impairment. *Blunted affect* involves a major reduction in the intensity and variation of expressed emotion, the extreme case being termed *flat affect*. Normal variation in *voice intonation* may be lost. *Poverty of speech* refers to a restricted amount of spontaneous speech, whereas *poverty of content* refers to speech that conveys little information.

Etiology

The etiology of schizophrenia is thought to involve an interaction between *genetic predisposition* involving multiple genes and *environmental influences* early in life. Although monozygotic twins have a concordance rate for schizophrenia of about 50% and first-degree relatives have at least a 10-fold increased risk compared with the general population, the number of susceptibility genes, their mode of transmission, and their identity are unknown. *Neuroimmunovirologic causes* (e.g., current or previous central nervous system (CNS) viral infections, autoimmune reactivity, in utero exposure to maternal infection and influenza) have also been proposed. Epidemiologic studies demonstrate increased risk resulting from *birth and pregnancy complications* (e.g., hypoxia, maternal infection), as well as exposure to a variety of *environmental stressors* (e.g., famine, physical disasters, season of birth). The underlying mechanisms by which these factors increase risk are unclear.

Pathophysiology

Neurodevelopmental as well as neurodegenerative changes in brain structure are implicated in the pathophysiology of schizophrenia. Prefrontal cortical and mesolimbic regions in the brain are the principal neuroanatomic regions of interest. For example, structural and functional brain imaging has demonstrated ventricular enlargement and decreased prefrontal cortical activity. Decreased prefrontal white and gray matter volumes, prefrontal cortical interneuron dysfunction, and disturbed prefrontal metabolism and blood flow have also been reported. Certain changes (e.g., enlarged lateral ventricles and reduced neocortical gray matter volume) are present at the onset of illness, suggesting a neurodevelopmental origin. Other changes (e.g., frontal and temporal gray matter volume reductions) emerge during the course of the illness, suggesting a neurodegenerative component.

The underlying physiology of the disease is thought to partially involve the dopamine system. For example, medications that increase brain dopamine levels (L-dopa, methylphenidate [Ritalin, Concerta], cocaine) can induce psychosis in susceptible persons. Drugs such as antipsychotics that block postsynaptic dopamine receptors in the mesolimbic regions reduce positive symptoms, whereas agents that enhance dopamine transmission in the prefrontal cortex can improve deficit (negative) symptoms as well as some of the cognitive deficits associated with this disorder.

The various antipsychotics differ in terms of which dopamine receptor subtypes (e.g., D_2 vs. D_1) they act on, their potency, and their selectivity for specific brain regions. Other neurotransmitters that have a modulatory effect on dopamine activity have also been implicated. For example, the serotonin system can modulate dopamine activity in critical CNS regions relevant to the symptoms that define schizophrenia. A role for glutamate and its receptors (e.g., N-methyl-D-aspartate [NMDA]) is supported by the ability of phencyclidine (PCP) to produce positive and negative symptoms and by observations of abnormal NMDA receptor binding and messenger RNA (mRNA) expression in the hippocampus of schizophrenic patients. Abnormalities in γ-aminobutyric acid (GABA) interneurons, as well as noradrenergic and cholinergic activity in various brain regions of schizophrenic patients, also implicate these neurotransmitters. For example, the α7 nicotinic cholinergic receptor mediates sensory gating and certain cognitive functions that are compromised in this disorder.

Treatment

Treatment initiation early in the illness course (prodromal phase, first episode) may be associated with a better long-term outcome. A combination of psychosocial and pharmacologic therapies is optimal. In addition to medication, treatment approaches include psychoeducation, social skills training, vocational rehabilitation, and cognitive behavior therapy (CBT). Acute stabilization of psychotic symptoms can require inpatient hospitalization. Once the patient is stable, the goals of long-term management include preventing relapse, minimizing residual psychotic symptoms, improving functional status, and facilitating adherence to treatment.

PSYCHOSOCIAL

Psychoeducation involves the patient and family and consists of illness education, crisis management, emotional support, and

---

CURRENT DIAGNOSIS

- Two or more of the following symptoms persisting for one month: Delusions, hallucinations, disorganized speech, disorganized or catatonic behavior, negative symptoms
- Persistence of some disturbance over a 6-month period
- Significant social or occupational dysfunction
- Symptoms not secondary to substance use, a general medical condition, or another psychiatric disorder (schizoaffective disorder, mood disorder with psychotic features)

CURRENT THERAPY

- Psychosocial therapies include cognitive behavior therapy, social skills training, vocational rehabilitation, and family psychoeducation
- Antipsychotics at onset of symptoms
- Second-generation antipsychotics for first-line treatment
- Regular monitoring of metabolic parameters and other adverse effects

development of coping skills. Social skills training focuses on improving expressive actions and social perceptions through behavioral rehearsal. Vocational rehabilitation includes employment programs in which patients learn skills and are provided with the support necessary to succeed in obtaining and keeping jobs. In this context, CBT (often combined with medication) focuses on a rational examination of psychotic symptoms by challenging the evidence for these experiences and subjecting them to reality testing.

PSYCHOPHARMACOLOGIC

Overview

Seven second-generation antipsychotics (SGAs) (Box 1) are approved in the United States for the treatment of schizophrenia and other psychotic conditions. These agents are thought to work through modulation of dopamine and serotonin receptors, primarily in mesolimbic and mesocortical pathways of the brain. SGAs have less potential to cause extrapyramidal symptoms (EPS) (e.g., pseudoparkinsonism, dystonia, akathisia) and tardive dyskinesia (TD) than do the first-generation antipsychotics (FGAs). SGAs may also prevent relapse more effectively than FGAs and are arguably more effective in treating mood, negative, and cognitive symptoms. Their clinical benefit, however, must be balanced with the risk for adverse events. Common side effects include sedation, orthostatic hypotension, anticholinergic effects, QTc prolongation, increased prolactin levels, weight gain, and metabolic derangements. Most important, antipsychotics should be dosed to maximize clinical efficacy, minimize the risk of adverse events, and improve long-term adherence.

Several large studies have compared the efficacy and adverse events associated with various antipsychotic medications in seminaturalistic settings. The Comparison of Atypicals for First Episode Psychosis (CAFE) trial involved 400 *first-episode* schizophrenic subjects who were randomized to treatment with quetiapine (Seroquel), risperidone (Risperdal) or olanzapine (Zyprexa). The primary outcome measure was treatment discontinuation for any reason (e.g., patient decision, adverse events, inadequate response). Unfortunately, 70% of patients discontinued their medication during the year-long study period regardless of which antipsychotic drug they received.

In the Clinical Antipsychotic Trials of Intervention Effectiveness (CATIE) study (a large trial sponsored by the National Institute of Mental Health), 1460 patients with *chronic* schizophrenia were randomly assigned to treatment with perphenazine (a moderately potent FGA) or to one of four SGAs (olanzapine, risperidone, quetiapine, or ziprasidone) for up to 18 months. As with the CAFE Study, the primary outcome measure was treatment discontinuation. Overall, 74% of patients discontinued the initial treatment to which they were randomly assigned. Surprisingly, there was no substantial difference in outcome between perphenazine and the SGAs. Although olanzapine had the lowest overall discontinuation rate (64%) and longest time (9 months) to discontinuation, it was the most problematic medication in terms of weight gain and metabolic derangements.

Several study design issues make it difficult to draw definitive conclusions from either study. These include inadequate dosing with some agents and exclusion of more difficult patients (i.e., those with TD) from the perphenazine group.

Recommended Pharmacologic Treatment Strategy

At present, most patients are initially treated with an SGA. A benzodiazepine may be added briefly to control agitation. If clinical response is insufficient over 4 to 8 weeks, the patient can be switched to a different SGA or FGA. With significant mood symptoms, a mood stabilizer or antidepressant may be used to enhance response. In patients for whom compliance with daily oral antipsychotic medication is problematic, various long-acting injectable agents (e.g., haloperidol decanoate, fluphenazine decanoate, risperidone microspheres) may be reasonable alternatives. In treatment-resistant patients, several options are available, including clozapine (Clozaril); augmentation of an antipsychotic with mood stabilizers, antidepressants or another antipsychotic; and electroconvulsive therapy. Clozapine has proved efficacy for treatment-refractory patients but is usually a third-line choice due to several black box warnings including a 1% risk of agranulocytosis and the need for frequent monitoring of complete blood count.

In addition to EPS, TD and neuroleptic malignant syndrome (NMS) are two potentially serious adverse effects associated with antipsychotics. TD consists of late-onset buccolinguomasticatory or choreiform movements associated with length of exposure (4% per year) and can result in significant disability. The risk of TD with high-potency FGAs is greater than with SGAs. The symptoms of NMS include fever, muscle rigidity, altered consciousness, and autonomic changes (e.g., fluctuations in vital signs, diaphoresis). In rare cases, it can be fatal.

Weight gain and subsequent metabolic complications secondary to treatment with antipsychotics are of increasing concern. Risk of weight gain, diabetes, and dyslipidemia varies with each agent (Table 1). Recommended guidelines for monitoring and managing metabolic parameters in patients prescribed these agents have been published. To summarize briefly, weight and body mass index (BMI) should be measured at baseline and then monthly for the first 3 months and then quarterly. Waist circumference should be monitored at

BOX 1 Second-Generation Antipsychotics

Aripiprazole (Abilify)
Clozapine (Clozaril)
Olanzapine (Zyprexa)
Paliperidone (Invega)
Quetiapine (Seroquel)
Risperidone (Risperdal)
Ziprasidone (Geodon)

TABLE 1 Metabolic Effects of Second-Generation Antipsychotics

Drug	Weight Gain	Risk for Diabetes	Worsening Lipid Profile
Aripiprazole	+/−	−	−
Clozapine	+++	+	+
Olanzapine	+++	+	+
Quetiapine	++	D	D
Risperidone	++	D	D
Ziprasidone	+/−	−	−

+ = increased effect; − = no effect; D = discrepant results.
Adapted from the American Diabetes Association, American Psychiatric Association et al: Consensus development conference on antipsychotic drugs and obesity and diabetes. Diabetes Care 2004;27(2):596-601.

baseline and followed yearly. Blood pressure and fasting blood glucose should be assessed at baseline, at 12 weeks, and then yearly afterward. Finally, fasting lipid profile should be measured at baseline, at 12 weeks, and every 5 years. Because schizophrenic patients usually do not receive adequate primary medical care, the metabolic risks posed by antipsychotics underscore the need for improved physical monitoring of these patients.

Summary

Schizophrenia is a psychotic disorder characterized by an early age of onset; a chronic, relapsing course; substantial lifelong disability; and varying responses to existing treatments. Optimal therapy consists of combined psychosocial and pharmacologic interventions to manage symptoms while minimizing the long-term negative consequences of the illness and adverse effects of medication.

REFERENCES

American Diabetes Association, American Psychiatric Association et al: Consensus development conference on antipsychotic drugs and obesity and diabetes. Diabetes Care 2004;27(2):596-601.
Dickerson FB, Lehman AF: Evidence-based psychotherapy for schizophrenia. J Nerv Ment Dis 2006;194(1):3-9.
Janicak PG, Davis JM, Preskorn SH, Ayd FJ, Marder SR, Pavuluri M: Principles and Practice of Psychopharmacotherapy, 4th ed. Philadelphia: Lippincott Williams & Wilkins, 2006, pp 69-182.
Marder SR, Essock SM, Miller AL, et al: Physical health monitoring of patients with schizophrenia: Treatment with antipsychotics. Am J Psychiatry 2004;161(8):1334-1349.
Sadock BJ, Sadock VA: Comprehensive Textbook of Psychiatry, 8th ed. Philadelphia: Lippincott Williams & Wilkins, 2005.

Panic Disorder

Method of
Manuel E. Tancer, MD

Panic attacks are time-limited, intense, episodes of anxiety with both somatic and psychological symptoms. The symptoms of a panic attack are listed in Box 1. Importantly, the attack must reach a peak within 10 minutes. Panic attacks do not last all day.

Epidemiology

The National Comorbidity Survey found that 22.7% of the population had experienced at least one panic attack. The diagnosis of panic disorder requires multiple panic attacks or one attack and worry about subsequent attacks. Panic attacks initially appear out of the blue but can become paired with certain places or situations. Interference with daily function and distress is required for the diagnosis of panic disorder. In addition, medical causes for the panic symptoms needs to be excluded. *Agoraphobia* is the term given to avoidance of places. It generally follows the emergence of panic attacks. Panic disorder can occur with or without agoraphobia. Box 2 lists the diagnostic criteria for panic disorder.

Panic disorder without agoraphobia has a lifetime prevalence of 3.7%, and panic disorder with agoraphobia has a lifetime prevalence of an additional 1.1% of the population. Panic disorder tends to start during the 20s and is twice as common in women than men. However, panic disorder can start in childhood and can also emerge in late life.

BOX 1 Diagnostic Symptoms of a Panic Attack

Panic attack is a discrete episode of intense fear or discomfort associated with at least four of the following symptoms and reaching a peak within 10 minutes

Somatic Symptoms
Shortness of breath or smothering feeling
Palpitations, pounding heart, or accelerated heart rate
Chest pain or discomfort
Trembling or shaking
Feeling of choking
Sweating
Nausea or stomach distress
Feeling unsteady, dizzy, lightheaded, or faint
Numbness or tingling sensations
Hot or cold flashes

Psychological Symptoms
Feelings of unreality or of being detached from yourself
Fear of losing control or going crazy
Fear of dying

Etiology and Clinical Features

The somatic symptoms often lead to emergency department or primary care evaluations that are almost always negative. Medications, changes in medications, endocrine abnormalities (hypothyroidism or hyperthyroidism), cardiac conduction or perfusion problems, caffeine, and over-the counter and illicit drug use need to be ruled out before diagnosing panic disorder. Common medications include steroids (e.g., prednisone), oral contraceptives, quinolone antibiotics, and pseudoephedrine (Sudafed). Changes in medications, such as switching from one oral contraceptive to another or reducing the dose of a β-blocker, can lead to anxiety symptoms. Caffeine, as found in carbonated drinks, coffee or tea, or in over-the-counter pain medications, can trigger anxiety attacks in vulnerable people. Cocaine and stimulants such as methamphetamine and methylphenidate (Ritalin) can also trigger panic attacks. Withdrawal from sedatives such as alcohol, barbiturates, or benzodiazepines can lead to anxiety attacks.

Panic disorder should be on the differential for every young adult presenting to the emergency department with chest pain. Reassurance that nothing is wrong is rarely helpful for persons suffering from anxiety attacks. Better to say something like "Your heart seems to be fine. I think you are having an anxiety attack."

BOX 2 Diagnostic Criteria for Panic Disorder

Recurrent unexpected panic attacks, at least one of which has been followed by 1 month (or more) of at least one of the following:
- Persistent concern about having additional attacks
- Worry about the implications of the attack or its consequences (e.g., losing control, having a heart attack, going crazy)
- A significant change in behavior related to the attacks

Agoraphobia might or might not co-occur.
The attack is not due to direct effect of medications, drugs of abuse, or medical conditions.
The attack is not better accounted for by another mental disorder.

CURRENT DIAGNOSIS

- Intense, episodic anxiety attacks with somatic and psychological symptoms
- Symptoms peak within 10 minutes and then dissipate
- Not due to medication(s), drugs of abuse, or underlying medical condition

CURRENT THERAPY

- Pharmacotherapy and cognitive behavior therapy are both effective.
- FDA-approved medications include the antidepressants fluoxetine (Prozac), paroxetine (Paxil), sertraline (Zoloft), and venlafaxine (Effexor) as well as the high-potency benzodiazepines alprazolam (Xanax) and clonazepam (Klonopin).
- Cognitive behavior therapy is a specific type of psychotherapy. It can be conducted by an experienced therapist or by patients using self-help manuals.

Panic disorder often co-occurs with major depression and other anxiety disorders. There is an increased risk of suicide in patients with panic disorder that is not totally explained by depressive symptoms.

Treatment

COGNITIVE BEHAVIOR THERAPY

There is strong evidence that both cognitive behavior therapy and medications are effective in treating panic disorder. Cognitive behavior therapy is a specialized form of psychotherapy and requires training and experience. Experienced cognitive therapists are not easy to find. Fortunately, there is evidence that patients with panic disorder can benefit from self-help manuals. The self-help manuals can also be useful adjuncts to medication treatment. The selection of medication versus cognitive behavior therapy should be determined by patient preference, availability of experienced therapists, and symptom severity (the extent of functional impairment).

Cognitive behavior therapy is based in the theory that panic attacks and avoidant behavior are due to distorted or exaggerated responses to interoceptive cues. Patients with panic symptoms tend to be hyperalert to common bodily symptoms such as palpitations. A panic disorder patient might interpret a palpitation as portending a catastrophic event such as a myocardial infarction. Cognitive behavior therapy involves identifying the cognitive distortions and then using graded exposure therapy to confront and then modify these assumptions. It requires an ability to tolerate the symptoms and a willingness to put oneself in previously uncomfortable situations. Cognitive behavior therapy requires homework and practice; potential patients need to be highly motivated.

PHARMACOTHERAPY

Four antidepressants and two high-potency benzodiazepines are currently FDA-approved for treating patients with panic disorder. Table 1 gives starting doses and dose ranges.

My medication-treatment strategy depends on course of illness, presence of comorbid states, previous medication response, and family history of drug response. Patients with rapidly progressing symptoms or upcoming deadlines (e.g., school examinations) need rapid intervention. Both alprazolam and clonazepam offer rapid relief of anxiety symptoms in most patients. Most experience significant reduction in symptoms within one week. Although benzodiazepines are highly effective, I am reluctant to use them as first-line treatment because of the common comorbid major depression (which is not helped by benzodiazepines) and the issues of benzodiazepine tolerance and dependence. When using one of the benzodiazepines for rapid relief, I simultaneously start an antidepressant with the goal of tapering the benzodiazepine after 4 to 6 weeks.

For the majority of patients with more chronic or milder forms of the illness, I start with an antidepressant alone. Patients with panic disorder are very sensitive to side effects so it is worth spending a few minutes going over possible common side effects. Starting at a very low dose and gradually increasing the dose are prudent.

I treat patients until they are panic or avoidance free for 9 to 12 months and then very gradually start tapering the medication. Symptoms recur in some patients during the discontinuation. Most patients are rapidly helped by resuming the previous medication at the maintenance dose.

Patients should be informed that panic disorder is a chronic-relapsing illness and might or might not recur. Previous episodes of panic attacks are associated with increased rate of relapse.

Other medications, not approved by the FDA, such as other selective serotonin reuptake inhibitors and older antidepressants (such as tricyclic antidepressants and monoamine oxidase inhibitors) may be helpful in cases where FDA-indicated medications fail. However, more complicated cases of treatment-resistant panic disorder should probably be referred to a specialist.

TABLE 1 Pharmacotherapy for Panic Disorder

Drug	Starting Dose	Target Dose
Benzodiazepines		
Alprazolam (Xanax)	0.5 mg tid	4-7 mg/d
Alprazolam sustained release (Xanax-XR)	0.5 mg qd	3-6 mg/d
Clonazepam (Klonopin)	0.25 mg bid	1-4 mg/d
Selective Serotonin Reuptake Inhibitors		
Fluoxetine (Prozac)	5-10 mg/d	20-60 mg/d
Paroxetine (Paxil)	5-10 mg/d	20-60 mg/d
Paroxetine controlled release (Paxil CR)	12.5 mg/d	25-75 mg/d
Sertraline (Zoloft)	25-50 mg/d	50-200 mg/d
Serotonin–Norepinephrine Reuptake Inhibitor		
Venlafaxine (Effexor XR)	37.5 mg/d	75 mg-225 mg/d

Summary

In summary, panic disorder is common and treatable. Unfortunately, most studies have found that most patients in the community are not treated in accordance with treatment guidelines or evidence-based practice.

REFERENCES

American Psychiatric Association: Diagnostic and Statistical Manual of Mental Disorders, 4th ed. Washington, DC: American Psychiatric Press, 2000.

Febbraro GA: An investigation into the effectiveness of bibliotherapy and minimal contact interventions in the treatment of panic attacks. J Clin Psychol 2005;61:763-779.

Furukawa TA, Watanabe N, Churchill R: Combined psychotherapy plus antidepressants for panic disorder with or without agoraphobia. Cochrane Database Syst Rev 2007;(1)CD004364.

Kessler RC, Chiu WT, Jin R, et al: The epidemiology of panic attacks, panic disorder, and agoraphobia in the National Comorbidity Survey Replication. Arch Gen Psychiatry 2006;64:415-424.

Landon TM, Barlow DH: Cognitive-behavioral treatment for panic disorder: Current status. J Psychiatr Pract 2004;10:211-226.

Roy-Byrne PP, Craske MG, Stein MB, et al: A randomized effectiveness trial of cognitive-behavioral therapy and medication for primary care panic disorder. Arch Gen Psychiatry 2005;62:290-2988.

SECTION 18

Physical and Chemical Injuries

Burn Treatment Guidelines

Method of
Barbara A. Latenser, MD

The initial management of the severely burned patient follows guidelines established by the American College of Surgeons (ACS). It is crucial that the patient be managed properly in the early hours after injury because the initial management of a seriously burned patient can significantly affect the long-term outcome. Optimal burn-care criteria have been established and refined by the American Burn Association (ABA) over the past 20 years.

Because of regionalization, it is common for the initial care of the seriously burned patient to occur outside the burn center. Burns are a specialized form of trauma. Therefore, the ABCs (airway, breathing, circulation) are the same as for the trauma patient: airway with cervical spine immobilization if appropriate, breathing, circulation, disability, and exposure. Also, the burn patient could be a victim of associated trauma. It is easy to be sidetracked by the obvious thermal injury. Only after the primary and secondary surveys have been performed should you evaluate the severity of the burn injury. Obtain as much information as possible regarding the incident and about the patient. An easy way to remember the information is the mnemonic AMPLE:

- Allergies
- Medications
- Past medical history
- Last meal
- Events

Universal precautions appropriate for each burn patient must be implemented by every member of the health care team.

The most commonly used guide for making an initial estimate of the second- and third-degree burns is the Rule of Nines (Figure 1). Various anatomic regions are roughly 9% of the total body surface area (TBSA) or multiples thereof. To calculate scattered burn areas, the patient's palm, including fingers, represents approximately 1% of the TBSA. A much more precise estimate of TBSA burn is provided by the Lund-Browder Classification (Figure 2). By drawing in the areas that are burned, the TBSA burn necessary for calculating resuscitation requirements can be determined. The consensus formula for the first 24 hours postburn is:

$$4 \text{ mL lactated Ringer's} \times \text{body weight in kg} \times \text{percent BSA burn}$$

Half the calculated amount is given in the first 8 hours and the rest over the remaining 16 hours. Patients with burns on more than 20% TBSA are prone to gastric dilatation and should have a nasogastric (NG) tube. To determine hourly urine output, a urinary catheter is necessary. Intravenous (IV) morphine sulfate is indicated for control of pain associated with burns. Intramuscular (IM) or subcutaneous (SC) routes of drug administration should not be used as absorption is erratic. To calculate fluid needs, weigh the patient or estimate the preinjury weight. Reliable peripheral veins should be used to establish an IV line. Use vessels underlying burned skin if necessary. If it is impossible to establish peripheral IV access, a central line may be necessary.

The burn wound should be covered with a clean, dry sheet to prevent air currents from causing pain in partial-thickness burns and to decrease fluid losses and hypothermia. Although there are many common topical antimicrobials in use, the optimal dressing prior to burn center transfer is plastic wrap such as Saran Wrap. Topical antimicrobials will just have to be washed off on arrival to the burn center, causing patient discomfort and mechanical trauma to the wound. Cold applications are appropriate only in small burns because they rapidly lead to hypothermia. Ice should never be applied because it will deepen the zone of ischemia in a thermal injury.

Escharotomies and/or fasciotomies are rarely required prior to burn center transfer, unless transfer is delayed beyond 24 hours. Patients most at risk are those with large TBSA burns, circumferential full-thickness burns, and those with electrical injury. Circumferential chest/abdominal burns may restrict ventilatory excursion. A child has a more pliable rib cage and may need an escharotomy earlier than an adult burn. If you are considering performing an escharotomy, confer with the accepting burn physician before proceeding.

So how do you know which patients should be referred to a burn center? To guide your decision making there are currently 10 burn unit referral criteria. You should have a written transfer agreement in place with a referral burn unit. The agreement should specify which patients will be referred, what stabilization is expected, who arranges transportation, and what the patient will need during transport.

Partial-Thickness Burns on More Than 10% Total Body Surface Area

Second-degree or partial-thickness burns involve a variable portion of dermis. The skin may be red, blistered, and edematous. Because sensory nerves are damaged and/or exposed, these wounds are typically extremely painful. Healing time is proportional to the depth of dermal injury. Scarring is minimal if healing occurs in 14 days or less. With closure time beyond 3 weeks, scarring will occur, the degree being greater in darker skinned individuals.

Proper fluid management is critical to the survival of patients with extensive burns. Fluid resuscitation is aimed at maintaining tissue

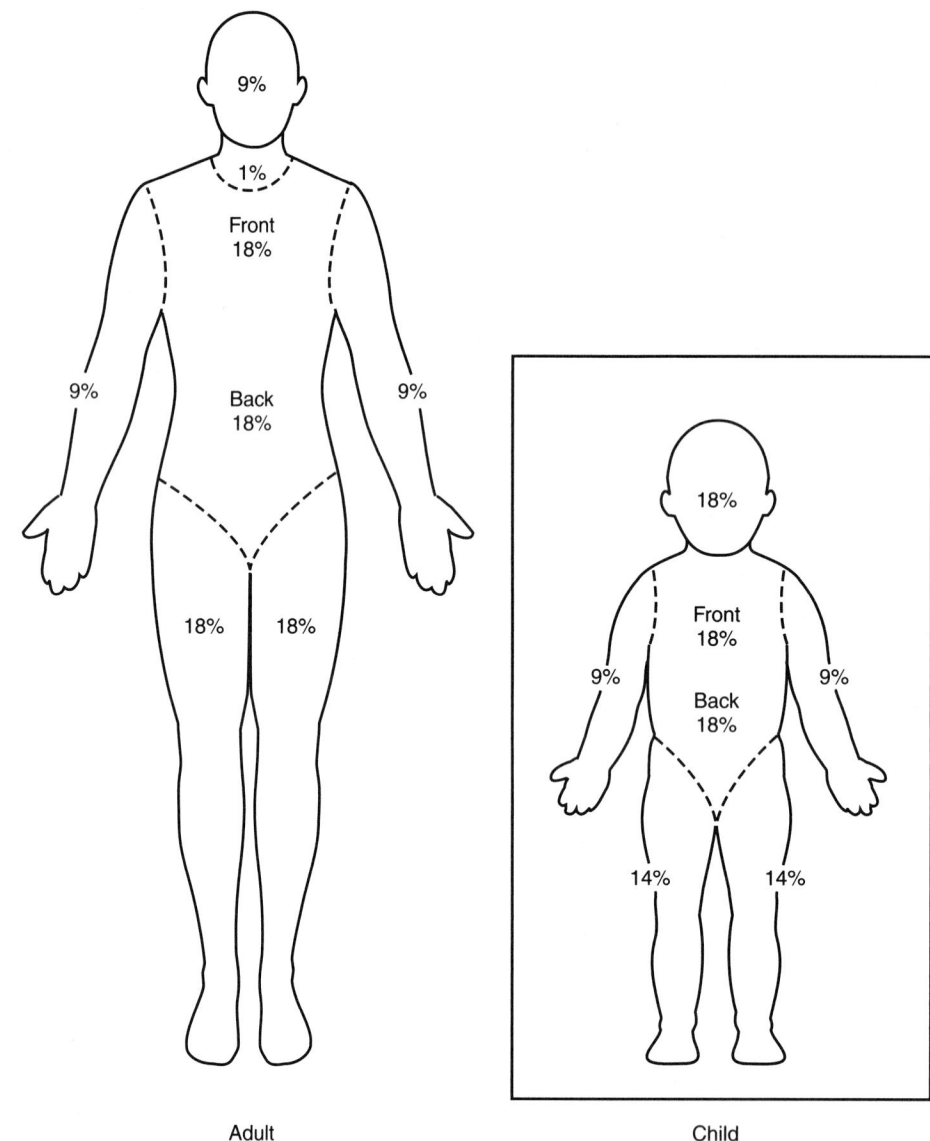

FIGURE 1. Rule of Nines.

perfusion and organ function while avoiding the complications of inadequate or excessive fluid therapy. Shock and organ failure, most commonly acute renal failure, may occur as a consequence of hypovolemia in a patient with an extensive burn who is inadequately resuscitated. The increase in capillary permeability caused by the burn is greatest in the immediate postburn period and diminution in effective blood volume is most rapid at that time. A marked increase in peripheral vascular resistance accompanied by a decrease in cardiac output occurs in the first 18 to 24 hours postinjury.

In the presence of increased capillary permeability, colloid content of the resuscitation fluid exerts little influence on intravascular retention during the initial hours postburn. Crystalloid fluid is the initial resuscitation of burn patients. *Always* remember, estimates are inexact. Each patient reacts differently to burn injury and resuscitation. The actual volume of fluid infused should be varied from the calculated volume as indicated by physiologic monitoring. The patient's general condition reflects the adequacy of fluid resuscitation and should be assessed and reassessed. Mental status, anxiety, and restlessness may be signs of hypoxemia, hypovolemia, or pain.

Although urine output does not guarantee tissue perfusion, it remains the most readily available and generally reliable guide to resuscitation. Adults should produce 0.5 mL/kg per hour of urine. Children should produce 1.0 mL/kg per hour of urine, and infants 12 months or younger should produce 2.0 mL/kg per hour of urine.

Oliguria is most frequently the result of inadequate fluid administration. Diuretics are contraindicated; the rate of resuscitation should be increased. During the first 24 hours, neither the hemoglobin nor the hematocrit is a reliable guide to resuscitation, and using either leads to over-resuscitation.

Measuring blood pressure (BP) by a sphygmomanometer may be misleading in a burned limb with progressive edema formation. As the swelling increases, the signal becomes diminished. If fluid infusion is increased based on this finding, edema formation may be exaggerated. Even intra-arterial monitoring may be unreliable in patients with massive burns because of peripheral vasoconstriction secondary to marked elevation of catecholamines. Heart rate is also of limited usefulness in monitoring fluid therapy. The level of tachycardia depends on the normal heart rate in each child.

Burns That Involve the Face, Hands, Feet, Genitalia, Perineum, or Major Joints

Facial burns are considered a serious injury. The possibility of respiratory tract damage must be considered. Because of the rich blood supply and loose areolar tissue of the face, facial burns are associated

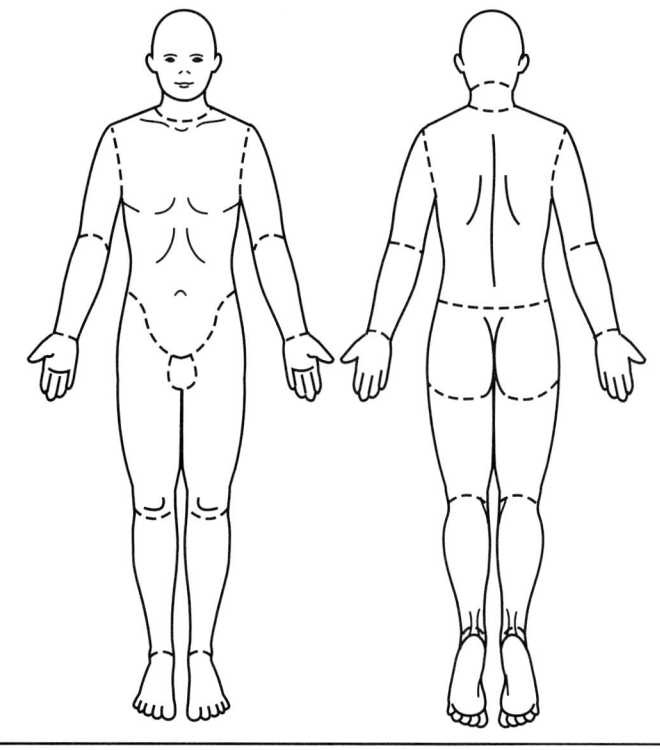

	Birth 1 yr.	1–4 yrs.	5–9 yrs.	10–14 yrs.	15 yrs.	Adult	Burn size estimate
Head	19	17	13	11	9	7	
Neck	2	2	2	2	2	2	
Anterior trunk	13	13	13	13	13	13	
Posterior trunk	13	13	13	13	13	13	
Right buttock	2.5	2.5	2.5	2.5	2.5	2.5	
Left buttock	2.5	2.5	2.5	2.5	2.5	2.5	
Genitalia	1	1	1	1	1	1	
Right upper arm	4	4	4	4	4	4	
Left upper arm	4	4	4	4	4	4	
Right lower arm	3	3	3	3	3	3	
Left lower arm	3	3	3	3	3	3	
Right hand	2.5	2.5	2.5	2.5	2.5	2.5	
Left hand	2.5	2.5	2.5	2.5	2.5	2.5	
Right thigh	5.5	6.5	8	8.5	9	9.5	
Left thigh	5.5	6.5	8	8.5	9	9.5	
Right leg	5	5	5.5	6	6.5	7	
Left leg	5	5	5.5	6	6.5	7	
Right foot	3.5	3.5	3.5	3.5	3.5	3.5	
Left foot	3.5	3.5	3.5	3.5	3.5	3.5	

Total BSAB _____

FIGURE 2. Lund-Browder Classification Burn Size and Diagram.

with extensive edema formation. To minimize this edema, keep the head of the bed elevated at 30°. Cool saline compresses on the face may also help. Careful examination of the eyes should be completed as soon as possible because the rapid onset of eyelid swelling will make this difficult. Fluorescein should be used to identify corneal injury. Chemical burns to the eyes should be rinsed with copious amounts of saline. Burns of the ears require examination of the external auditory canal and ear drum before swelling occurs.

Minor burns of the hands may result in only temporary disability and inconvenience. More extensive thermal injury may cause permanent loss of function. Monitoring the digital and palmar pulses with an ultrasonic flowmeter is the most accurate means of assessing perfusion of the tissues in the hand. The burned extremity should be elevated above the heart to minimize edema formation. Digital escharotomies are not indicated prior to transfer to a burn center. Contact the accepting burn center physician if you are concerned about the extent of the digital injury. As with burns of the upper extremity, it is important to assess the circulation and neurologic function of the feet on an hourly basis.

CURRENT DIAGNOSIS

- Maintain a high index of suspicion
- Remember the ABCs
- Rule out concomitant trauma
- Establish size and depth of burn
- Be wary of chemical and electrical burns, which may be misleading
- Establish resuscitation requirements

Abbreviations: ABC = airway with cervical spine immobilization if appropriate, breathing, circulation, disability, and exposure.

CURRENT THERAPY

- Communicate with your burn center early and often
- Remember the ABCs
- Cover the wound with Saran Wrap
- Prevent hypothermia
- Transport to the burn center

Abbreviations: ABC = airway with cervical spine immobilization if appropriate, breathing, circulation, disability, and exposure.

Third-Degree Burns in Any Age Group

A full-thickness or third-degree burn occurs with destruction of the entire epidermis and dermis, leaving no dermal elements to repopulate. A characteristic initial appearance is a waxy white color. Full-thickness injuries require emergent management. In most cases, treatment of the wound requires surgical skin grafting. Deep partial-thickness and full-thickness burns heal with severe scarring if not treated by surgical excision and skin grafting for optimal recovery. Disfigurement is common, and long-term functional problems can persist for years. There is also a high risk of infection, because an unexcised full-thickness burn behaves like an undrained abscess.

Electric Burns, Including Lightning Injury

Electrical burns can be divided into flash (typical thermal injury) and high-tension injury. The latter, caused by more than 1000 volts, produces clinically characteristic entry and exit wounds. They are usually ischemic, painless, and dry; wounds of entry may appear charred and the exit explosive. Deep-muscle injury may be present even when skin appears normal. Findings that suggest electrical injury include loss of consciousness, paralysis or mummification of an extremity, loss of peripheral pulses, flexor surface burns, myoglobinuria, serum creatine kinase (CK) more than 1000, and cardiopulmonary arrest at the scene. Electrical injuries can produce vascular thrombosis, muscle tetany causing fractures, and internal organ damage. In addition to other interventions, obtain a 12-lead electrocardiogram (ECG), cardiac enzymes, and evaluate the urine for myoglobin. If there is evidence of myoglobin from muscle damage, the urine output should be maintained at 2 mL/kg per hour until the urine grossly clears to prevent acid hematin deposition in the kidney and irreversible renal damage. Compartment pressures must be monitored. If a compartment syndrome develops, contact your burn center physician because fasciotomy may be required. The most serious immediate problem associated with electrical injuries is ventricular fibrillation, asystole, or other dysrhythmias. Life-threatening arrhythmias are treated according to advanced cardiac life support (ACLS) protocols. Survival of contact with voltage greater than 70,000 volts is uncommon.

The approximate electrical potential of a lightning bolt is 20 million volts. Lightning injury can produce an enormous spectrum of clinical symptoms and signs ranging from common (cardiac asystole, respiratory arrest, arborescent markings) to the rare (disseminated intravascular coagulation [DIC], intracerebral hemorrhage). Immediate neurologic manifestations include agitation, amnesia, loss of consciousness, or motor disturbances. The eyes are particularly vulnerable to injury from electrical current, and symptoms closely correlate with the extent of the central nervous system (CNS) injury. Vitreous hemorrhage, iridocyclitis, retinal tear, macular puncture, and retinal detachment have been reported.

Lightning injuries are not usually associated with deep burns but most often with superficial injury to the skin and underlying soft tissue called *ferning*. The feathering type of burn appears as an arborescent, branching skin marking that disappears within a few hours. Pathognomonic of lightning injury, they may be of great diagnostic value in a comatose patient. Often the respiratory arrest lasts longer than the cardiac arrest. Severely injured victims often present in asystole or ventricular fibrillation. Cardiac resuscitation may occasionally be successful; but direct brain trauma as well as blunt trauma, skull fracture, and intracranial injuries, are common in these patients. The prognosis for recovery in this group is usually poor.

Chemical Burns

Health care providers must wear protective clothing when caring for patients with potential chemical injury. The initial appearance of a chemical burn is usually deceptively benign. The severity of a chemical injury is related to the agent, concentration, volume, duration of contact, and mechanisms of action of the agent. Immediate irrigation decreases the concentration and duration of contact, reducing the severity of injury. If the agent is a powder, brush it off and irrigate with water. Irrigation should continue through emergency evaluation in the hospital and in general until evaluation in a burn center, especially for an alkali or if an unknown agent. Neutralizing agents are contraindicated because of the potential for heat generation, thereby giving the patient both a chemical and a thermal injury!

Acid burns are less severe than alkali burns. They are found in many household products including bathroom cleansers, drain cleaners, and swimming pool acidifiers. Tissue is damaged by coagulation necrosis and protein precipitation. Once a layer of eschar is formed, the burning process is self-limiting. The exception to this rule is hydrofluoric acid (HA), which is used to etch glass, make Teflon, and to remove rust. The pathogenesis of tissue damage in HA burns is distinct from other acids. HA readily crosses lipid membranes and has a potent diffusing capacity into the tissues. The molecule releases the freely dissociable fluoride ion, which produces extensive liquefactive necrosis of the soft tissues. Fluoride rapidly binds free calcium in the blood, and death from hypocalcemia may occur. Treatment is intra-arterial calcium gluconate[1] (or calcium chloride)[1] administered until the characteristic *pain out of proportion to the burn* has resolved. Even small areas of contact may result in profound hypocalcemia and death. Cardiac monitoring and frequent serum calcium determinations are indicated.

Alkalis damage tissue by liquefaction necrosis and protein denaturation. Tissue pH abnormalities may persist for 12 hours postburn, allowing deeper spread of the chemical and more severe burns. Examples would include the hydroxides, caustic sodas, and ammonium compounds found in oven cleaners, fertilizer, and cement. Wet cement damages skin in three ways: allergic dermatitis as a reaction to chromate ions, abrasions caused by the gritty nature of the cement,

---

[1]Not FDA approved for this indication.

and as an alkali with a pH of 12.5. The ability of cement to cause such injury is not well recognized, even by professional users. With the increased media interest in do-it-yourself projects, it is likely this problem will increase.

Organic compounds such as creosote and petroleum products produce contact chemical burns as well as systemic toxicity. Gasoline and diesel fuel are petroleum products that may produce a full-thickness burn that initially appears as only partial thickness. Organic compounds cause cutaneous damage by delipidation because of their fat solvent action on cell membranes. After a motor vehicle crash involving petroleum products, always look for petroleum exposure in the lower extremities, back, and buttocks. Systemic effects include elevated liver enzymes and decreased urinary output.

Inhalation Injury

Smoke inhalation injuries are the leading cause of fatalities from burn injuries, accounting for some 80% of all fire-related deaths. The major forms of inhalation injuries are carbon monoxide (CO) toxicity, injury to the upper airway, and pulmonary parenchymal damage. Each has different symptoms and signs, treatment, and prognosis. The compromised airway is protected by tracheal intubation, and respiratory failure is treated with assisted ventilation. Inhalation injury is manifested by the pathology and dysfunction that rapidly become evident in the airways, lungs, and respiratory system after inhaling the products of incomplete combustion. Patients receiving massive fluid resuscitation can develop upper airway edema with subsequent asphyxiation.

Immediate medical attention and diagnosis depend on a high index of suspicion, an appropriate history, careful examination of the upper airway, the presence of clinical symptoms, and suggestive arterial blood gases. An inhalation injury is suspected in any patient with full-thickness facial burns or with any burns combined with a history of being confined within an enclosed space. Other classic signs are soot or carbonaceous sputum, stridor or hoarseness, or blistering of the pharynx or vocal cords. Late signs include grunting, nasal flaring, retractions, wheezes, and rales. Use of prophylactic antibiotics and steroids is discouraged.

The effect of CO poisoning may be exhibited by respiratory symptoms and CNS findings such as altered level of consciousness, seizures, or coma. Cardiovascular effects include diminished cardiac output evidenced by decreased perfusion and hypotension. There is much controversy regarding hyperbaric oxygen therapy, but there are no objective data proving the efficacy of hyperbaric oxygen in CO poisoning. At this time, hyperbaric oxygen treatment for acute CO toxicity should be restricted to randomized prospective studies. The correct treatment is administering 100% oxygen, thereby decreasing the CO half-life from 4 hours to 45 minutes.

Burn Injury in Patients with Preexisting Medical Disorders That Could Complicate Management, Prolong Recovery, or Affect Mortality

Peripheral vascular disease can lead to a decrease in wound blood flow. Diabetes, through high glucose, will impede capillary flow. Optimum control of the blood glucose is needed to optimize blood flow. A local decrease in wound-tissue oxygen tension is recognized to be a major wound-healing impediment because all phases of healing are oxygen dependent, including local infection control. Most common causes are a decrease in systemic blood volume and oxygen delivery, decrease in hemoglobin saturation, eschar on the wound surface, or infection. Treatment modalities need to focus first on correction of systemic abnormalities: correct cardiovascular and lung function, correct large vessel obstructive disease impeding wound flow, aggressive wound debridement, and eliminate tissue exudates. Patients with preexisting cardiac disease are particularly sensitive to fluids and may tolerate the necessary fluid resuscitation poorly.

Any Patient With Burns and Concomitant Trauma (Such as Fractures) in Which the Burn Injury Poses the Greatest Risk of Morbidity and Mortality

In such cases, if the trauma poses the greater immediate risk, the patient may be initially stabilized in a trauma center before being transferred to a burn unit. Physician judgment will be necessary in such situations and should be in concert with the regional medical control plan and triage protocols.

Most burn-trauma publications cite a 5% frequency of burn-trauma patient. Because burn trauma is rare outside of a major conflict or disaster, most centers see only a few patients annually. By definition, child abuse falls into the burn-trauma category. It may be the burn injury that prompts relatives or neighbors to bring the child to the hospital or report the family to authority. The visibility of the injury may instigate corrective action. In a 44-month review we saw 120 cases of burns and trauma. Although motor vehicle crashes (MVCs) can result in fracture, soft tissue, and thermal injury, unique to this burn-trauma population was that the MVC injury was frequently a result of assault. With the graying of America, elder abuse may become a larger societal problem.

Burned Children in Hospitals Without Qualified Personnel or Equipment for the Care of Children

Each year more than 2500 children die and 10,000 more sustain permanent disability from thermal injury. Children are not just little adults! They respond differently than adults to severe trauma, maintaining normal vital signs longer but decompensating rapidly. Because of the smaller cross-sectional diameter of the pediatric airway, it takes much less edema to compromise a pediatric airway. If intubation is required, the most experienced pediatric airway manager should intubate the child because repeated attempts may create sufficient airway edema as to cause obstruction. Anatomical airway differences make intubation by the inexperienced even more difficult.

The greater surface area per unit of body mass of children necessitates the administration of relatively greater amounts of resuscitation fluid. The surface area/body mass relationship of the child also defines a lesser intravascular volume per unit surface area burned. This makes the burned child more susceptible to fluid overload and hemodilution. Hypoglycemia may occur if the limited glycogen stores of the child are rapidly exhausted by the early postburn elevation of circulating levels of steroids and catecholamines. Infants should receive maintenance fluids with 5% dextrose in addition to the resuscitation fluids outlined in the consensus formula. Children younger than 2 years of age have disproportionally thin skin so that exposures that would produce only partial-thickness burns in older patients produce full-thickness injuries. Children have a relatively small muscle mass, hampering intrinsic heat generation. Children younger than 6 months of age are unable to shiver and thus are even more prone to develop hypothermia.

Stress for the burned child not only includes the body surface area (BSA) burn and the pain that is involved but also the separation from parents and loved ones. This escalates especially if the parents were also burned in the fire. Emergency management of each pediatric burn patient requires an individual care plan. Early consultation with the burn center physician is advised.

Burn Injury in Patients Who Will Require Special Social, Emotional, and/or Long-Term Rehabilitative Intervention

Failure to recognize the thermal manifestations of child abuse not only negates protection of the child but predicates potential lethal injury. Awareness of the patterns of abuse, the behavior patterns of the parents, and the physical manifestations will protect the child by early recognition and reporting. Physical child abuse victims frequently present with thermal injuries of varying degrees. The history of injury should correlate with the physical findings. The history also becomes important in identifying repetitious hospital visits for accidental injury. Not infrequently, the hospital visits will be made at different hospitals to avoid disclosure and identification.

The events leading to an injury are extremely important in the initial evaluation of an infant or child. *Always* consider the potential for child abuse. The incidence of child abuse is approximately 10% of all children presenting to an emergency department (ED), with a mortality rate less than 1%. Abused children present with a higher median Injury Severity Score, more severe injuries of the head and integument, longer hospital lengths of stay, and a high mortality rate.

A burn of any magnitude can be a serious injury. Health care providers must be able to assess the injuries rapidly and develop a priority-based plan of care. The plan of care is determined by the type, extent, and degree of burn as well as by available resources.

Burn care is complex. It involves a multisystem assessment and appropriate intervention. The first 24 hours of management are perhaps the most critical for patient survival. Burn centers provide optimal care in a cost-effective, multidisciplinary manner. Every health care provider must know how and when to contact the closest burn center. If the attending physician determines that the patient should be treated at the burn center, the extent of treatment provided at the referring hospital—and the method of transport to the burn center—should be decided in consultation with the burn center physician. A complete list of verified burn centers is available at http://ameriburn.org.

REFERENCES

Advanced Burn Life Support Course, American Burn Association, 625 N. Michigan Ave., Suite 1530, Chicago, IL. 60611. 2001.

American College of Surgeons Committee on Trauma: Resources for optimal care of the injured patient: 1999, Chicago. American College of Surgeons, 1999.

Andrews CJ, Cooper MA, Darveniza M, Mackerras D (eds): Lightning injuries: Electrical, medical, and legal aspects. Boca Raton, Fla, CRC Press, 1992, pp 62-63, 82-85, 88-98, 101-110.

Burd A: Hydrofluoric acid—revisited. Burns 2004;30(7):720-722.

Chang DC, Knight V, Ziegfeld S, et al: The tip of the iceberg for child abuse: The critical roles of the pediatric trauma service and its registry. J Trauma 2004;57(6):1189-1198.

Heimbach DM: Regionalization of burn care: A concept whose time has come. J Burn Care Rehabil 2003;24(3):173-174.

Latenser BA, Iteld L: Smoke inhalation injury. Seminars in Respiratory and Critical Care Medicine. 2001;22(1):13-22.

Luce EA (ed): Clinics in Plastic Surgery. An International Quarterly. Burn Care and Management. Philadelphia. WB Saunders, 2000;27(1):133-143.

Varghese TK, Kim AW, Kowal-Vern A, Latenser BA: Frequency of burn-trauma patients in an urban setting. Arch Surg. 2003;138:1292-1296.

High-Altitude Illness

Method of
James A. Litch, MD, DTMH

Decreased partial pressure of oxygen at high altitude results in pronounced physiologic responses that range from beneficial to pathologic. Slow ascent normally leads to acclimatization. High-altitude illness is a collective term for a cluster of acute clinical syndromes that are a direct consequence of rapid ascent to high altitude above 2500 m. The acute syndromes affecting the brain include acute mountain sickness (AMS) and high-altitude cerebral edema (HACE). The acute syndrome affecting the lung is high-altitude pulmonary edema (HAPE). All unacclimatized sojourners to high altitude are potentially at risk. The characteristic cerebral and pulmonary abnormalities are not subtle, but when unrecognized or ignored, they may progress to death. Each year millions travel to high-altitude locations on every continent, resulting in morbidity and mortality with associated economic consequences.

Normal Acclimatization

It is not uncommon for normal acclimatization of novice healthy visitors to high altitude to cause concern that they are experiencing a health problem. Normal acclimatization includes immediate hyperventilation, shortness of breath with moderate excursion, and a decreased work capacity. These are followed by diuresis, disturbed sleep (including periodic breathing), and peripheral/facial edema. It is important to recognize the signs of normal acclimatization so reassurance and education may be appropriately provided.

Incidence and Risk Factors

Determinants of whether high-altitude illness will occur are individual susceptibility, rate of ascent, altitude reached, and sleep altitude. Incidence rates of AMS reported in literature are difficult to compare because of variability in methodology and rates of ascent. Reported incident figures for AMS following ascent by hiking, vehicle, or flying range from 10% to 40% at 2700 to 3000 m, and from 40% to 95% at 3800 to 4000 m. HACE and HAPE are both far less common than mild AMS, but actual incident rates are unavailable. HAPE can occur as low as 2500 m. HACE is rare below 3600 m. Most cases of HACE and HAPE are preceded by AMS.

Risk factors for altitude illness include a history of previous high-altitude illness, residence at altitude below 1000 m, physical exertion, and preexisting cardiopulmonary conditions. Traveling in a large group presents a risk because a tight itinerary often does not allow time for acclimatization, and members are reluctant to declare symptoms for fear of being left behind. Children appear to carry the same risk for altitude illness as adults, but persons over 50 years of age seem less susceptible, possibly because of a more cautious ascent profile. There appears to be little or no gender difference for AMS, but women may be less susceptible to HAPE. Heavy physical exertion at exceedingly high altitude appears to be an important risk factor for HAPE. Rapid ascent, especially by flying or driving to altitude, places sojourners at risk for altitude illnesses.

Prevention of Altitude Illnesses

Gradual ascent to altitude over several days to allow for acclimatization reduces the likelihood of acute mountain sickness. Ascent rates of less than 300 m per day at altitudes of more than 2500 m is a common recommendation; but individuals will still experience altitude illness when abiding to this recommendation. However, the critical understanding to prevent serious life-threatening altitude illness (HAPE and HACE) is to halt further ascent until symptoms resolve.

Medications are available to help prevent the symptoms of AMS when rapid ascent (<24 hours) to altitudes more than 3000 m is anticipated, or for those with a past history of AMS with a similar ascent profile. These agents are started the evening before ascent and continued for 2 to 3 days. The most commonly used medications are acetazolamide (Diamox) (125 to 250 mg twice a day), acetaminophen[1] (325 mg four times a day), or aspirin[1] (325 mg three times a day). Acetazolamide (Diamox) is particularly useful because it actually improves oxygenation, has a positive impact on the quality of sleep at high altitude, and is effective for periodic breathing that occurs during sleep. However, these medications do not protect against the development of life threatening altitude illness: HAPE and HACE. Other medications have been suggested for use in preventing altitude illness. Randomized double blinded placebo-controlled trails of ginkgo biloba[1] and acetazolamide (Diamox) have shown no benefit from ginkgo biloba over placebo, and reduced incidence and severity of AMS symptoms from acetazolamide (Diamox). Dexamethasone (Decadron),[1] a potent steroid, is generally best avoided as a prevention measure against AMS during ascent so it may be used, if needed, for treatment of HACE along with descent.

Nifedipine (Adalat, Procardia)[1] has been studied for use in prevention of HAPE and found to be of benefit for persons with a history of recurrent HAPE. Studies are underway to evaluate sildenafil citrate (Viagra),[1] an agent that selectively lowers pulmonary artery pressure, in the prevention of HAPE. In addition, inhaled salmeterol (Serevent)[1] has been found effective for the prevention of HAPE in a small group of climbers who had previously shown susceptibility to HAPE. However, these high-risk individuals would do far better with cautious gradual ascent, rather than relying on a medication with limited effect for a life-threatening condition.

Several nonmedication measures that can prevent or ameliorate symptoms of high-altitude illness include the following:

- Begin a high-carbohydrate diet one or two days before the climb and maintain during the ascent
- Adapt plans to realistically reflect the decreased work capacity at high altitude
- Reschedule or slow the ascent should an upper respiratory or other active infection present
- Avoid overexertion during ascent by maintaining a reasonable pace and not overloading with nonessential gear
- Maintain adequate hydration on the climb to offset increased fluid loss at altitude
- Avoid nonessential medications and remedies
- Provide good ventilation for camp stoves used in confined places
- Allow for several days of altitude exposure the week prior to ascent to high altitude

Acute Mountain Sickness and High-Altitude Cerebral Edema

AMS is defined as a headache in the setting of recent altitude gain and typical symptoms which include anorexia, nausea, vomiting, insomnia, dizziness, or fatigue (Current Diagnosis box). Symptoms are nonspecific, and there is an absence of physical findings. The differential diagnosis is extensive and other conditions should be considered (Box 1). Pulse oximetry values may be high, normal, or low for the altitude and do not correlate to severity of symptoms. A careful and detailed history is essential to steer diagnostic decision making. Often in outdoor settings multiple conditions can be present such as AMS and dehydration. Rapid resolution of symptoms during treatment with oxygen is very specific to AMS. Early recognition of AMS is a key principle in remote areas with limited support.

AMS is not life threatening, but ignoring it can be. Progressive neurologic deterioration may occur over hours or days as dangerous collections of fluid develop in the brain leading to HACE. HACE presents with truncal ataxia, confusion, and hallucination in the setting of recent altitude gain. The period of time from initial ataxia and confusion to onset of coma may be as little as 8 to 12 hours. If descent or oxygen supplementation is not accomplished within hours, coma and death can ensue from brain herniation. A presumptive and/or rigid diagnosis of HACE in the setting of progressive neurologic deterioration has led to tragic situations when other life-threatening conditions were actually present (see Box 1). Details of the initial presentation, response to immediate descent/supplemental oxygen, and recognition of additional signs can guide clinical decision making while maintaining a high index of suspicion for other neurologic conditions. Patients with persistent symptoms after descent require prompt evacuation and thorough evaluation. In addition, HAPE may develop concurrently with HACE resulting in shortness of breath while at rest and a further reduction of oxygen delivery to the body.

Definitive diagnosis is available using imaging studies such as CT and MRI. However, these have limited application, because the condition should have greatly improved from oxygen/descent before the opportunity presents to obtain the study. Neuroimaging demonstrates vasogenic edema in individuals with moderate to severe AMS or HACE.

Management of AMS is directed at limiting further hypoxia by halting ascent, and providing additional oxygen should symptoms persist or progress to HACE. Acetazolamide (Diamox) is helpful for the treatment of AMS. For the management of HACE improved oxygenation is the definitive treatment. There are several methods of oxygen delivery: (1) descent, (2) supplemental oxygen via cylinder or concentrator, and/or (3) portable hyperbaric bag. These may be combined or applied in series depending on resources, location, and logistic support. Concomitant pharmacologic treatment with dexamethasone (Decadron)[1] and acetazolamide (Diamox) aid recovery.

BOX 1 Differential Diagnosis of High-Altitude Illnesses

Acute Mountain Sickness and High-Altitude Cerebral Edema
- Alcohol indoxication
- Brain tumor
- CO inhalation
- CNS infection
- Cerebral vascular accident
- Dehydration
- Diabetic ketoacidosis
- Exhaustion
- Hypoglycemia and insulin shock
- Hyponatremia
- Hypothermia
- Migraine
- Narcotics
- Poisoning
- Psychosis
- Sedatives overdose
- Seizures
- Subarachnoid hemorrhage
- Transient ischemic attack

High-Altitude Pulmonary Edema
- Adult respiratory distress syndrome
- Asthma
- Bronchitis
- Congestive heart failure
- Myocardial infarction
- Pneumonia (infection or aspiration)
- Poisoning
- Pulmonary embolus
- Respiratory failure

Abbreviations: CNS = central nervous system; CO = carbon monoxide.

---

[1]Not FDA approved for this indication.

CURRENT DIAGNOSIS

- Acute Mountain Sickness—In the setting of a recent gain in altitude, the presence of headache and at least one of the following: GI symptoms (anorexia, nausea, or vomiting), fatigue or weakness, dizziness or light-headedness, or difficulty sleeping
- High-Altitude Cerebral Edema—In the setting of a recent gain in altitude, the presence of a change in mental status and/or ataxia in a person with AMS, or the presence of both mental status change and ataxia in a person without AMS
- High-Altitude Pulmonary Edema—In the setting of a recent gain in altitude, the presence of at least two of the following symptoms: dyspnea at rest, cough, weakness or decreased exercise performance, chest tightness, or congestion; and two of the following signs: rales or wheezing in at least one lung field, central cyanosis, tachypnea, or tachycardia

*The Lake Louise Consensus on the Definition and Quantification of Altitude Illness.
Abbreviations: AMS = acute mountain sickness; GI = gastrointestinal.

 CURRENT THERAPY

Acute Mountain Sickness
- Halt ascent, do not exceed light activity level, oral hydration.
- Administer acetazolamide (Diamox) 250 mg PO bid.
- Administer analgesics and antiemetics.
- If readily available, administer oxygen 1 to 2 L per minute as needed to resolve symptoms.
- If no improvement after 24 hours, descend to altitude where person last slept without symptoms until fully recovered.

High-Altitude Cerebral Edema
- Administer oxygen 2 to 4 L per minute.
- In remote mountain areas, prepare for immediate descent of at least 600 m by ground or aircraft, and if oxygen unavailable, use portable hyperbaric chamber.
- Monitor at all times, and replenish/maintain hydration as needed.
- Administer dexamethasone (Decadron) 8 mg IM, IV, or PO × 1 dose, then 4 mg q6h.
- Administer acetazolamide (Diamox) 250 mg PO bid.

High-Altitude Pulmonary Edema
- Administer oxygen initially 4 to 6 L per minute, then titrate to keep arterial oxygen saturation more than 90%.
- In remote mountain areas, prepare for immediate descent of at least 600 m by ground or aircraft; and if oxygen unavailable, use portable hyperbaric chamber on incline with head end elevated.
- Sit upright at 45 degree angle, strict rest, and monitor at all times.
- Administer nifedipine (Adalat, Procardia) 10 mg PO initially, then 30 mg extended release q12h *IF* oxygen unavailable *AND* IV fluid resuscitation immediately available.
- Administer salmeterol (Serevent) inhaler, 1 puff bid *OR* albuterol (Proventil) inhaler, 4 to 6 puffs q4h.
- Administer dexamethasone (Decadron) 8 mg IM, IV or PO × 1 dose, then 4 mg q6h *IF* suspect or unsure if HACE is also present.

Abbreviations: bid = twice daily; IM = intramuscular; IV = intravenous; PO = orally; q = every.

Persons with suspected HACE who do not rapidly recover during treatment or those with focal neurologic deficits should be hospitalized and undergo comprehensive neurologic evaluation including magnetic resonance imaging (MRI). The Current Therapy box summarizes management of HACE.

High-Altitude Pulmonary Edema

HAPE is defined as noncardiogenic edema resulting from hypoxia-induced changes in the pulmonary circulation. HAPE is commonly preceded by AMS, and 20% of individuals with HAPE develop HACE. Early symptoms of HAPE include decreased exercise performance beyond that expected for the altitude, often accompanied with a dry cough (see Current Diagnosis Box). Progression is rapid with even minimal continued physical activity without descent. The hallmark of progression requiring prompt action is dyspnea at rest. Rales are present at this stage. Resting pulse oximetry reveals below-normal oxygen saturation for the altitude. Tachypnea and tachycardia beyond that expected for the altitude also are present. Pink, frothy sputum develops late in the illness. Early diagnosis is important because progression of the illness further limits oxygenation and worsens the degree of hypoxemia causing the condition.

HAPE is a life-threatening emergency; immediate improvement in oxygenation is critical to arrest the progression and is the definitive treatment. In medical facilities high-flow supplemental oxygen while at rest and sitting in an upright position should be initiated immediately during the initial assessment of the patient. Response may be assessed by pulse oximetry and resting respiratory rate. Despite prompt improvement during the first few hours of treatment, maintenance of oxygenation (oxygen saturation greater than 90%) with low-flow supplemental oxygen and rest is often required for 2 to 3 days unless descent is achieved. For vacationers to high-altitude resort areas, this oxygen requirement can be maintained outside the hospital using a cylinder or concentrator as an alternative to descent for informed individuals that wish to remain in the locale of family and friends. A continued requirement of high-flow oxygen of 4 to 5 L per minute or more to maintain oxygen saturation greater than 90%, or concurrent HACE, requires hospitalization. Antibiotics are indicated if infection is suspected. Endotracheal intubation and mechanical ventilation are rarely indicated. The differential diagnosis is extensive, and a high index of suspicion for other conditions should be maintained throughout the treatment course (see Box 1).

In remote areas oxygen may be administered by:

- Descent with minimal exertion
- Supplemental oxygen via cylinder or concentrator
- Portable hyperbaric bag placed on an incline to keep the head elevated

Because of a lack of equipment, immediate descent may be the only option available. In late stages more than one oxygen modality may need to be employed concurrently. These efforts place great strain on the limited resources of groups traveling in remote areas. It is common for the shared concern and cooperation among group members (tourists/staff/porters) to disintegrate or for groups to discover that they are woefully unequipped to handle HAPE. As a result fatal outcomes are common when HAPE presents in remote settings.

Pharmacologic treatment is directed at agents that reduce pulmonary artery pressure and thereby may improve oxygenation in HAPE. Medications including nifedipine (Adalat, Procardia),[1] nitric oxide (INO$_{max}$),[1] epoprostenol (Flolan),[1] and sildenafil (Viagra)[1] have been studied for use in treatment of HAPE. Current clinical experience warrants consideration of nifedipine (Adalat, Procardia) as an adjunct treatment for HAPE when immediate supplemental oxygen is unavailable or descent is delayed. Vascular access and intravenous (IV) fluid should be immediately available if nifedipine (Adalat, Procardia) is administered because patients are often intravascularly depleted and risk a severe hypotensive event that could be devastating in the setting of concomitant HACE. Sildenafil citrate (Viagra)[1] can also selectively lower pulmonary artery pressure with less effect on systemic blood pressure, and is under study for the treatment of HAPE. Inhaled β-agonists, salmeterol (Serevent),[1] and albuterol (Proventil)[1] are currently under study for treatment of HAPE because β-agonists increase the clearance of fluid from the alveolar space and might lower pulmonary artery pressure. The Current Therapy Box summarizes the management of HAPE.

Reascent After Altitude Illness

Mild AMS is common and indicative of an ascent rate that is too rapid for a given person. Further ascent should not resume until full resolution of all symptoms. Future trips with similar ascent profiles warrant consideration of prophylaxis with acetazolamide (Diamox).

After episodes of HACE and HAPE resolve fully, reascent has been successful for many patients, some reaching exceptionally high summits. Caution is warranted, however. Persons should be advised to ascend more slowly and to recognize and act appropriately for early signs of altitude illness. Persons with multiple episodes of HAPE may benefit during subsequent ascent from prophylaxis with nifedipine (Adalat, Procardia)[1] and potentially with salmeterol (Serevent)[1] while stressing the value of cautious gradual ascent over medication. Recurrent HAPE or HAPE occurring at altitudes below 3000 m should prompt evaluation to rule out cardiac or pulmonary shunts, valvular disease, or pulmonary hypertension.

---

[1]Not FDA approved for this indication.

REFERENCES

Bartsch P, Merki B, Hofstetter D, et al: Treatment of acute mountain sickness by simulated descent: A randomized controlled trial. BMJ 1993;306:1098-1101.

Chow T, Browne V, Heileson HL, et al: Ginkgo biloba and acetazolamide prophylaxis for acute mountain sickness: A randomized placebo-controlled trial. Arch Intern Med 2005;165:296-301.

Consensus Group: The Lake Louise Consensus on the Definition and Quantification of Altitude Illness. In Sutton JR, Coates G, Houston CS: Hypoxia and Mountain Medicine. Burlington, Vt. Queen City Printers, 1992;327-330.

Litch JA: Endotracheal intubation and mechanical ventilation following respiratory arrest from high altitude pulmonary edema. West J Med 1999;170(3):174-176.

Litch JA, Basnyat B, Zimmerman M: Subarachnoid hemorrhage at high altitude. West J Med 1997;167(3):180-181.

Litch JA, Bishop RA: Re-ascent following resolution of high altitude pulmonary edema (HAPE). High Alt Med Biol 2001;2(1):53-55.

Litch JA, Bishop RA: Oxygen concentrators for the delivery of supplemental oxygen in remote high altitude areas. Wilderness Environ Med 2000;11(3):189-191.

Larson EB, Roach RC, Schoene RB, Hornbein TF: Acute mountain sickness and acetazolamide—Clinical efficacy and effect on ventilation. JAMA 1982;248:328-332.

Oelz O, Maggiorini M, Ritter M, et al: Prevention and treatment of high altitude pulmonary edema by a calcium channel blocker. Int J Sports Med 1992;13(Suppl 1):S65-S68.

Pollard AJ, Niermeyer S, Barry P, et al: Children at high altitude: An international consensus statement by an ad hoc committee of the International Society of Mountain Medicine. High Alt Med Biol 2001;2(3):389-403.

Rabold MB: Dexamethasone for prophylaxis and treatment of acute mountain sickness. West J Med 1992;3:54-60.

Sartori C, Allemann Y, Duplain H, et al: Salmeterol for the prevention of high-altitude pulmonary edema. N Engl J Med 2002;346(21):1631-1636.

Disturbances Due to Cold

Method of
*Frederick K. Korley, MD, and
Jerrold B. Leikin, MD*

Accidental Hypothermia

Hypothermia is classically defined as a reduction in the body's core temperature below 95.0°F (35.0°C). Most reported cases of hypothermia are due to exposure to low ambient temperatures (accidental hypothermia). Other causes of hypothermia include sepsis, severe hypothyroidism, diabetic ketoacidosis, multisystem trauma, and prolonged cardiac arrest.

EPIDEMIOLOGY

Risk factors for developing hypothermia include extremes of age (the elderly might not be able to remove themselves from cold environments, and young children lose heat more rapidly due to their increased total body surface area), major trauma, homelessness, psychiatric illness, and drug and alcohol abuse (Box 1). Cold-related deaths also are reported in military combatants and outdoor winter sports participants. Several drugs and chemicals can predispose to hypothermia (Box 2). Alcohol is the most common intoxicant associated with hypothermia due to its ability to cause cutaneous vasodilation, impairment of shivering, and impairment of adaptive behavior.

Between 1979 and 2002, a total of 16,555 deaths in the United States, an average of 689 per year, were attributed to exposure to low environmental temperatures. In 2002, of the 646 hypothermia-related deaths reported, 66% occurred in male patients, 52% of all decedents were aged 65 years or younger, 45% of the deaths occurred among white male patients, and 14% occurred among black male patients. The states of Alaska, New Mexico, North Dakota, and Montana had the largest overall death rates due to hypothermia in 2002. The lowest recorded core temperature in a pediatric survivor of accidental hypothermia is 57.9°F (14.4°C) and the lowest is 56.7°F (13.7°C) in an adult survivor.

PATHOPHYSIOLOGY

The normal range of human core temperature is 97.5°F (36.4°C) to 99.5°F (37.5°C). Humans are thus warm-blooded and are normally able to maintain their body temperature by heat-generating mechanisms and heat-conserving behavior. These compensatory responses, however, can be overwhelmed under extreme environmental conditions, leading to hypothermia.

The anterior hypothalamus coordinates the nonshivering heat conservation and dissipation mechanisms, and the posterior hypothalamus coordinates shivering thermogenesis. Heat loss usually occurs by four mechanisms: About 55% to 65% of heat is lost by radiation, 25% to 30% by evaporation from the skin and

> **BOX 1** Factors Predisposing to Hypothermia or Frostbite
>
> **Physiologic**
> *Decreased Heat Production*
>   Age extremes (infants, elderly)
>   Dehydration or nalnutrition
>   Diaphoresis or hyperhidrosis
>   Endocrinologic insufficiency
>   Hypoxia
>   Insufficient fuel
>   Overexertion
>   Physical conditioning
>   Prior cold injury
>   Trauma (multisystem or extremity)
>
> *Increased Heat Loss*
>   Burns
> - Dermatologic malfunction
> - Cold infusions
> - Emergency resuscitation
> - Poor acclimatization or conditioning
> - Shock
> - Vascular diseases
>
> *Impaired Thermoregulation*
> - Central nervous system trauma or disease
> - Metabolic disorders
> - Pharmacologic or toxicologic agents
> - Sepsis
> - Spinal cord injury
>
> **Psychological**
> - Fatigue
> - Fear or panic
> - Hunger
> - Intense concentration on tasks
> - Intoxicants
> - Mental status or attitude
> - Peer pressure
>
> **Environmental**
> - Altitude with or without associated conditions
> - Ambient temperature or humidity
> - Duration of exposure
> - Heat loss (conductive, evaporative, radiative, convective)
> - Quantity of exposed surface area
> - Wind chill factor
>
> **Mechanical**
> - Constricting or wet clothing or boots
> - Inadequate insulation
> - Immobility or cramped positioning

respiratory tract, and 10% to 15% by conduction and convection. The amount of heat lost via conduction is markedly increased in cold-water immersion (by about 32 times). Each organ system is affected uniquely by hypothermia.

The Cardiovascular System

One of the initial heat-conserving mechanisms is peripheral vasconstriction to decrease blood flow to the skin. There are also initial increases, in heart rate and blood pressure due to a catecholamine surge. At core temperatures below 82.4°F (28.0°C), bradycardia can occur. The myocardium also becomes irritable, predisposing it to arrhythmias. Atrial arrhythmias can occur with a slow ventricular response and they can precede ventricular arrhythmias and asystole at core temperatures below 77.0°F (25.0°C). The characteristic Osborn or J waves (a hump seen at the QRS-ST junction) may be seen on the electrocardiogram (ECG) at core temperatures below 89.6°F (32.0°C).

The Renal System

Renal blood flow is increased by peripheral vasoconstriction, leading to cold-induced diuresis. Antidiuretic hormone activity is usually inhibited. This results in intravascular volume depletion, subsequent vasodilation, to increase renal blood flow, and ultimately acute renal failure.

The Respiratory System

At core temperatures below 82.4° F (28°C), minute ventilation is reduced; bronchorrhea can occur, with a loss of cough and gag reflexes leading to an increased risk for aspiration. Apnea can then result.

The Central Nervous System

Cerebral metabolism is depressed 6% to 7% per 1°C decrease in core temperature. Cerebrovascular autoregulation remains intact until below 77.0°F (25.0°C), which helps maintain cortical blood flow. Electroencephalographic activity is clearly not prognostic, and it silences around 66.2°F to 68.0°F (19.0°C-20.0°C).

CLINICAL PRESENTATION

Accidental hypothermia is classified as mild at body temperatures of 90°F (32.2°C) to 95°F (35°C), moderate at body temperatures of 82.4°F (28.0°C) to 90°F (<32.2°C), or severe at body temperatures less than 28°C (82.4°F).

In general, a patient's symptoms depend on the severity of the temperature drop. Patients with mild hypothermia can develop vigorous shivering and cold diuresis. Those with moderate hypothermia can have a paradoxical decrease in shivering, slurred speech, hyporeflexia, and confusion. They may have Osborn J waves on the ECG. They are also at risk for intravascular thrombosis. Splanchnic vasoconstriction, gastric erosions, hepatic necrosis, and pancreatitis can occur.

During severe hypothermia, shivering gives way to rigor, minute ventilation decreases, and heart rate and cardiac output decrease. Cardiac instability can be seen at this stage and can manifest in the form of arrhythmias, heart blocks, and eventually asystole. Neurologically, the patient's mental status declines. He or she might attempt to undress (paradoxical undressing) and might respond only to painful stimuli, have decreased gag reflexes, and eventually become apenic. Generally, at about 68.0°F (20.0°C), patients become totally neurologically unresponsive, lose corneal and ocular reflexes, and can have a flat electroencephalograph (EEG).

EMERGENCY DEPARTMENT EVALUATION

Typically, the source of hypothermia is revealed from the patient's history; however, it is very important to rule out secondary causes of hypothermia such as sepsis, hypothyroidism, central nervous system (CNS) lesions, and hypoglycemia among others. All patients arriving in the emergency department with hypothermia need a complete evaluation to rule out traumatic injuries and drug or toxin ingestion or overdose.

As in all resuscitation, attention should be paid to the ABCs (airway, breathing and circulation). Respiratory failure should be treated with endotracheal intubation and mechanical ventilation. Hypotension can be treated initially with warmed fluids. Placing the patient in a warm environment, removing all cold and wet clothes, and remembering to cover up the patient after he or she has been exposed should help avoid further heat loss.

BOX 2 Drugs and Chemicals that Can Cause Hypothermia

Medicinals

Acetaminophen (Tylenol)
Amphotericin B (Fungizone)
Azithromycin (Zithromax)
Baclofen (Lioresal)
Barbituates
Benzodiazepines
β-Adrenergic blocking agents
Bethanechol (Urecholine)
Biperiden (Akineton)
Bromocriptine (Parlodel)
Carbamazepine (Tegretol)
Chloral hydrate (Noctec)
Chlorpromazine (Thorazine)
Clonidine (Catapres)
Colchicine
Diltiazem (Cardizem)
Ethchlorvynol (Placidyl)
Ethyl alcohol
Fenoprofen (Nalfon)
Fluphenazine (Prolixin)
Fosphenytoin (Cerebyx)
Gallium nitrate (Ganite)
Glutethimide (Doriden)[2]
Guanabenz (Wytensin)
Guanfacine (Tenex)
Haloperidol (Haldol)
Heroin
Ibuprofen (Advil, Motrin)
Insulin preparations
Interferon-β-1b (Betaseron)
Lithium (Eskalith, Lithobid)
Loxapine (Loxapac, Loxitane)
Magnesium sulfate
Maprotiline (Ludiomil)
Mefenamic acid (Ponstel)
Methyldopa (Aldomet)
Methyprylon (Noludar)[2]
Moricizine (Ethmozine)

Morphine sulfate
Naphazoline (Naphcon)
Omeprazole (Prilosec)
Oxymetazoline (Afrin)
Phencyclidine
Phenol
Phenytoin (Dilantin)
Pilocarpine (Salagen)
Prazosin (Minipress)
Propoxyphene (Darvon)
Rauwolfia serpentine
Reserpine
Salicylate
Terazosin (Hytrin)
Tetracycline (Sumycin)
Tetrahydrozoline (Visine, Opti-Clear)
Thioridazine (Mellaril)
Tretinoin (Topical) (Retin A)
Tricyclic antidepressants
Valproic acid and derivatives (Depakene)
Zinc sulfate

Nonmedicinals

Acrylamide
Aldicarb
Amitraz
Barium
Bromophos
Carbon disulfide
Carbon monoxide
Chloralose
Chlorfenvinphos
Chloryrifos
Coumaphos
Cyanide
Diazinon
Dichlorvos

Dicrotophos
Dioxathion
Disulfoton
Ether
Ethion
Fensulfothion
Fenthion
Hexachlorobenzene
Hydrogen sulfide
Isopropyl alcohol
Lewisite
Malathion
Methidathion
Methiocarb
Methomyl
Methylparathion
Nickel
Parathion
Profenofos
Pyrimidifen
Sodium azide
Terbufos
Tetraethly pyrophosphate

Biologicals

Ackee fruit poisoning
Ciguatera food poisoning
Delphinium
Lobelia
Marijuana *(Cannabis)*
Monkshood
Nutmeg
Star of Bethlehem *(Hippobroman longiflora)*
Tetrodotoxin food poisoning
White chameleon

---
[2]Not available in the United States.

The temperature should be confirmed by checking a core temperature (e.g., rectal, bladder, or esophageal), using a thermometer capable of recording very low temperatures. Patients should be placed on a cardiac monitor and an ECG should be obtained. Laboratory testing is especially useful in the postresuscitative period when complications begin. Laboratory tests should include a complete blood count (CBC), a chemistry panel, creatine phosphokinase (CPK) to evaluate for rhabdomyolysis, a coagulation profile, blood type and screen, an arterial blood gas (ABG), and a drug screen. A Foley catheter should be placed to access urinary output.

REWARMING STRATEGIES

There are several methods of rewarming. The method of choice usually depends on the severity of hypothermia. During rewarming, the patient should be placed on a cardiac monitor with frequent measurements of blood pressure and temperature (via a rectal probe) for easy detection of complications of rewarming such as rewarming-related hypotension, arrhythmias, and core temperature after-drop.

Passive External Warming

Passive external warming is ideal for patients with mild hypothermia who are otherwise healthy. It uses the patient's endogenous heat production for rewarming and it involves simple, logical passive maneuvers that minimize heat dissipation. When using this method, all wet clothing should be removed, the ambient core temperature should exceed 70.0°F (21.0°C), and the patient should be covered with insulating materials. Patients warmed easily using this method can be safely discharged.

Active External Rewarming

Active external rewarming is controversial. It involves exposing the skin of the patient to exogenous heat sources. Radiant heat, thermal mattresses, electric heating blankets, and forced-air heating blankets are some of the available techniques.

This method has a number of disadvantages. First, burn injuries can occur to the vasoconstricted skin. Second, any sort of immersion can hinder monitoring and other resuscitative activities. Finally and most important, active external rewarming produces a phenomenon called *core temperature after-drop*. This refers to a drop in core temperature as a result of sudden peripheral vasodilation. This causes cold, acidic blood to return to the core. Hypotension and potentially fatal dysrhythmias can result. Focusing on rewarming the trunk only (rather than the trunk and extremities) can prevent these temperature gradients. In general, active external rewarming is used in conjunction with active core rewarming.

CURRENT DIAGNOSIS

- Accidental hypothermia may be classified as mild, moderate, or severe.
- The measured temperature should be the core body temperature.
- The method of rewarming depends on the severity of the temperature drop.
- The complications of rewarming include arrhythmias, rewarming-related hypotension, core temperature after drop, and rhabdomyolysis.
- Patients can only be declared dead after they are warm and dead.

BOX 3 Drugs Displaying Reduced Metabolism or Clearance in Hypothermia

- Atropine
- Digoxin
- D-Tubocurarine
- Fentanyl (Sublimase, Duragesic)
- Gentamicin (Garamycin)
- Lidocaine (Xylocaine)
- Phenobarbital
- Procaine
- Propranolol (Inderal)
- Sulfanilamide (AVC Cream)
- Suxamethonium (Succinylcholine, Anectine)

Active Core Rewarming

Active core rewarming involves techniques to deliver direct heat internally. It should be used in patients with moderate to severe hypothermia. The simplest method entails the administration of heated, humidified oxygen at 107.6°F to 114.8°F (42.0°C-46.0°C) and intravenous saline solution warmed to 109.4°F (43.0°C). Saline should be administered via a central line at 150 to 200 mL/hour. Gastric, bladder, and colonic irrigations have been used but their relatively small surface areas usually limit their effect.

Another method of active core rewarming is pleural irrigation using two large-bore (36 F or greater) thoracostomy tubes. One tube is placed at the midclavicular line and is connected to saline to 107.6°F (42.0°C). The other tube is placed at the posterior axillary line and connected to a chest tube drainage kit.

A more aggressive method of active core rewarming is via peritoneal lavage and dialysis. This can be accomplished using a standard diagnostic peritoneal lavage (DPL) kit and introducing an 8-F catheter into the peritoneum using Seldinger's technique. The crystalloid diasylate should be warmed to 104.0°F to 113.0°F (40.0°C-45.0°C). This method affords the added advantage of allowing the serum potassium level to be adjusted.

The most efficient and physiologic active core rewarming method is via extracorporeal warming or heated cardiopulmonary bypass. This is the method of choice for the most severe cases, patients with severe rhabdomyolysis, and for patients who require cardiopulmonary resuscitation.

Most arrhythmias are corrected by rewarming. Atropine is typically ineffective for associated bradydysrhythmias. Ventricular tachycardia and fibrillation require electrocardioversion and the use of bretylium,[2] if it is available. The safety of amiodarone (Cordarone) in these situations is questionable. Dopamine (Intropin) may be an effective vasopressor. Empiric antibiotics may be given. However, the empiric use of levothyroxine (Synthroid)[1] and corticosteroids may be hazardous. Phenytoin (Dilantin)[1] might have cardiac-depressant qualities in the moderately hypothermic patient. Box 3 demonstrates drugs with possible decreased metabolism or clearance with increase in toxicity in hypothermia.

Indicators of grave prognosis include development of profound hyperkalemia (serum potassium >10 mEq/L), underlying medical conditions, intravascular thrombosis (fibrinogen <59 mg/dL), pH less than 6.5, and a core temperature less than 50.0°F to 53.6°F (10.0°C-12.0°C).

Peripheral Cold Injuries

Peripheral cold injuries span a spectrum ranging from minimal to severe tissue damage. Freezing and nonfreezing syndromes can cause these injuries. Frostnip and frostbite are caused by exposure to freezing temperatures. *Frostnip* refers to the numbness and blue-white discoloration of the face and extremities that occur during exposure to freezing temperatures. It is a precursor to frostbite. It is characterized by reversible skin changes including blanching and numbness with no permanent tissue damage, unlike frostbite. Nonfreezing injuries depend on whether the ambient environment during exposure was wet (trench or immersion foot) or dry (pernio or chilblain).

PATHOPHYSIOLOGY

During exposure to cold temperatures, the core body temperature is preserved to the detriment of the extremities. Frostbite occurs in four stages: prefreeze, freeze-thaw, vascular stasis, and late ischemic stages. The prefreeze phase occurs when the temperature of the extremities falls below 50.0°F (10.0°C) and cutaneous sensation is lost. Vasoconstriction also occurs along with leakage of intracellular fluid into the interstitium. The freeze-thaw phase begins at the freezing point of water (32.0°F or 0°C) with the formation of ice crystals extracellularly. This further enhances the exit of water from the intracellular space under osmotic forces, resulting in cell shrinkage and ultimately damage. During the vascular stasis phase, plasma leakage and formation of ice crystals continue. Arachidonic acid break down products are then released from underlying damaged tissue. Both prostaglandin $F_{2\alpha}$ and thromboxane A_2 produce platelet aggregation, leukocyte immobilization, and vasoconstriction. Endothelial cells are sensitive to cold injury, and the microvasculature becomes distorted and clogged, leading to tissue ischemia. The late ischemic phase is characterized by ischemia, thrombosis, continued shunting, gangrene, autonomic dysfunction, and denaturation of tissue proteins. The tissue can eventually mummify and demarcate more than 60 to 90 days later.

CLINICAL PRESENTATION

The face and ears are the most common sites prone to cold injury, followed by the hands and feet.

Frostnip and Frostbite

Patients with frostnip usually have blanching and numbness of their fingertips. Frostbite has been classified as superficial, affecting the skin and subcutaneous tissue, or deep, affecting the bones, joints, and tendons. When a superficial frostbite is rewarmed, the skin can form a clear blister; however, when a deep frostbite is rewarmed, it can form a hemorrhagic blister. This classification, however, has no therapeutic or prognostic value given that frostbites can initially appear benign. Many weeks can pass before the demarcation between viable and nonviable tissues becomes apparent.

Although no prognostic factors can be entirely predictive, favorable factors include retained sensation, normal skin color, and clear rather than cloudy fluid in the blisters, if present. Poor prognostic features include nonblanching cyanosis, firm skin, and dark,

---

[2]Not available in the United States.
[1]Not FDA approved for this indication.

fluid-filled blisters. Patients can present with pain, numbness, and a clumsy "chunk of wood" sensation in the affected extremity. The pain is initially described as a dull ache and evolves to become a throbbing sensation in about 48 to 72 hours.

Chilblain

Chilblain results from repetitive exposure to cold dry air. It manifests as erythematous or cyanotic lesions often referred to as *cold sores*. These lesions usually develop on exposed surfaces after a delay of 12 to 14 hours and are characterized by pruritus and burning paresthesias. Young women, especially those with Raynaud's phenomenon, are at risk.

Trench Foot and Immersion Foot

Trench foot occurs as a result of prolonged exposure to a damp, cold, nonfreezing environment. It has been classically described among soldiers in World War I, many of whom were confined to cold and damp trenches for prolonged periods. Symptoms include numbness and painful paresthesias that can progress to a throbbing and burning sensation. Initial evaluation reveals a cold, pale extremity, with or without vesicles or bullae.

Immersion foot may be considered the sailor's counterpart to trench foot. It occurs after prolonged immersion in cold water at temperatures above freezing.

TREATMENT

Treatment of frostbite should begin with removing all wet or frozen clothing. For patients with moderate and severe hypothermia as described above, initial resuscitative efforts should be geared toward raising their core temperature. The patient should be moved to a warm environment and all wet clothing should be removed. The frozen extremity should be rewarmed by immersion in circulation water at 104.0°F to 108.0°F (40.0°C-42.0°C) for about 15 to 30 minutes. Given the risks of thermal injury, the frozen parts should not be exposed to direct or dry heat (such as hair dryers, heating pads, or heat lamps). Do not rub or massage the affected area. The process should be continued until the extremity appears warm and well perfused. Due to the pain associated with reperfusion, there may be the temptation to abruptly abort the rewarming process. This can, however, promote further tissue damage. Parenteral analgesic medications (nonsteroidal anti-inflammatory drugs [NSAIDs] and opioids) may be administered as needed to make this process more tolerable.

Almost all authors agree that hemorrhagic blisters should not be débrided because of the risk of secondary desiccation of deep dermal layers, extending the injury. Débriding broken vesicles or bullae is also widely accepted; however, clear, intact vesicles may be broken and débrided or left intact. Topical aloe vera ointment (Dermaide Aloe) (a thromboxane inhibitor) or topical antibiotic ointments may be applied. The injured tissue should be loosely covered with sterile, dry, nonadherent dressing. Hands and feet may be splinted and elevated to reduce edema. Because the damaged tissue is tetanus prone, patients whose tetanus status has not been updated need a tetanus shot (Td).

Adjunctive agents that have been used for their antithrombotic and vasodilative properties with varying success include heparin,[1] steroids,[1] NSAIDs,[1] dimethylsulfoxide (DMSO),[1] nonionic detergents,[1] dipyridamole (Persantine),[1] calcium channel blockers,[1] pentoxifylline (Trental),[1] and phenoxybenzamine (Dibenzyline).

Surgical consultation is appropriate for guiding long-term management, because some patients might need débridement of infections or skin grafts for nonhealing wounds. A sympathetic nerve block can relieve painful and refractory vasospasms.

Chilblain (pernio) may be treated with nifidipine (Procardia)[1] at an oral dose of 20 to 60 mg daily.

---

[1]Not FDA approved for this indication.

 CURRENT THERAPY

Mild Hypothermia: 32.2°C (90°F) to 35°C (95°F)
- Passive external rewarming
  - Remove wet clothing.
  - Ambient temperature should exceed 21.0°C (70.0°F).
  - Cover patient with insulating material.

Moderate Hypothermia: 28°C (82.4°F) to 32.2°C (90°F)
- Active external rewarming
  - Radiant heat
  - Thermal mattresses
  - Electric heating blankets
  - Forced-air heating blankets
- Active core rewarming
  - Warmed humidified oxygen
  - Warmed intravenous saline
  - Bladder, colonic, and gastric irrigation
  - Pleural cavity lavage

Severe Hypothermia: Less than 28°C (82.4°F)
- Aggressive active core rewarming
  - Warmed, humidified oxygen
  - Warmed intravenous saline
  - Bladder, colonic, and gastric irrigation
  - Pleural cavity lavage
  - Peritoneal lavage or dialysis
  - Extracorporeal warming or heated cardiopulmonary bypass

Frostnip
- Gentle rewarming
- Usually self-resolving

Frostbite
- Warm-water immersion
- Débride broken vesicles
- Apply topical aloe vera or antibiotic ointment
- Use NSAIDs for pain
- Update tetanus status

Chilblain
- Gentle rewarming
- Nifidipine (procardia)

Trenchfoot
- Dry the foot
- Gentle rewarming

Abbreviation: NSAID = nonsteroidal anti-inflammatory drug.

SEQUELAE

Late sequelae of frostbite include cold hypersensitivity, numbness, pain, and decreased sensation. This is a result of early neuronal damage and abnormal sympathetic tone. Patients with chronic symptoms should be advised to avoid nicotine and cold exposure while using NSAIDs. Tissue demarcation can occur 60 to 90 days after initial injury. Amputation decisions should be deferred unless there is supervening sepsis or gangrene. The ultimate tissue salvage after a spontaneous slough usually far exceeds the most optimistic initial estimates.

Therapeutic Hypothermia

Therapeutic hypothermia for reducing anoxic brain injury has been increasingly used in clinical practice in post–cardiac arrest states.

The usual scenarios for such a practice are in patients with suspected postanoxic injuries following cardiopulmonary resuscitation, traumatic brain injuries associated with elevation of intracranial pressure, stroke, and various perioperative situations (such as vascular surgery). Hypothermia can reduce the metabolic oxygen utilization rate in the brain by 6% for every 1°C reduction in brain temperature (over 82.4°F or 28°C) due to reduced normal cerebral electrical activity and suppression of chemical reactions (such as free radical and glutamate production along with calcium shifts) associated with reperfusion injury. Cooling is usually initiated within 6 hours following return of spontaneous circulation, with moderate hypothermia (82.4°F to 90°F or 28°C to 32.2°C) for induction. Intravenous cooling techniques (infusion of 30 mL/kg of crystalloid solution at 4°C over 30 minutes) or extracorporeal cooling methods have been used. An intravascular heat-exchange device has also been developed. Shivering is prevented via neuromuscular blockade and sedation. Temperature can be monitored by a bladder temperature probe or through a central pulmonary catheter.

REFERENCES

Aslam AF, Aslam AK, Vasavada BC, Khan IA: Hypothermia: Evaluation, electrocardiographic manifestations, and management. Am J Med 2006; 119(4):297-301.

Bhagat H, Bithal PK, Chouhan RS, Arora R: Is phenytoin administration safe in a hypothermic child? J Clin Neurosci 2006;13:(9):953-955.

Centers for Disease Control and Prevention (CDC): Hypothermia-related deaths—United States, 2003-2004. MMWR Morb Mortal Wkly Rep 2005;54(7):173-175.

Danzl DF: Hypothermia. Semin Respir Crit Care Med 2002;23(1):57-68.

Danzl DF, Pozos RS: Accidental hypothermia. N Engl J Med 1994;331(26):1756-1760.

Ervasti O, Juopperi K, Ketlumen P, et al: The occurance of frostbite and its risk factors in young men. Int J Circumpolar Health 2004;63(1):71-80.

Gilbert M, Busund R, Skagseth A, et al: Resuscitation from accidental hypothermia of 13.7 degrees C with circulatory arrest. Lancet 2000; 355(9201):375-376.

Lloyd EL: Accidental hypothermia. Resuscitation 1996;32:111-124.

McCauley RD, Smith DJ, Robson MC, et al: Frostbite and other cold-induced injuries. In Auerbach PS (ed): Wilderness Medicine: Management of Wilderness and Environmental Emergencies. 3rd ed. St Louis. Mosby, 1995, pp 129-145.

McDonagh DL, Allen IN, Keifer JC, Warner DS: Induction of hypothermia after intraoperative hypoxic brain insult. Anesth Analg 2006;103(1):180-181.

Nolan JP, Morley PT, Vanden Hoek TL, Hickey RW, et al; International Liaison Committee on Resuscitation: Therapeutic hypothermia after cardiac arrest: An advisory statement by the advanced life support task force of the International Liaison Committee on Resuscitation. Circulation 2003;108:118-121.

Ulrich AS, Rathlev NK: Hypothermia and localized cold injuries. Emerg Med Clin North Am 2004;22(2):281-298.

Disturbances Caused by Heat

Method of
John F. Coyle II, MD

Exertional Heat Stroke

Heat stroke is an illness caused by failure of thermoregulation with elevation of core temperature to 40.6°C (105°F) or more, associated with central nervous system dysfunction. Heat stroke is traditionally subdivided into *exertional* and *classic* (or nonexertional) forms.

Exertional heat stroke is a sporadic illness triggered by exercise in warm environmental conditions that add to the thermal load produced by muscular contraction. It mainly strikes manual laborers, soldiers in training, and athletic competitors; indeed, it is the third leading cause of death among high school and college athletes in the United States. Exertional heat stroke may occur at moderate temperatures, especially if humidity is high, but both exertional and classic heat strokes most likely develop in conditions of high heat. The incidence of heat stroke increases exponentially when heat stress exceeds a boundary value. Appearance of the first case should sound an alarm that conditions have become dangerous, and more cases should be anticipated. The typical heat stroke victim is highly motivated, poorly conditioned, obese, and not acclimatized. Fatigue and sleep deprivation are commonly encountered, and recent or ongoing febrile or dehydrating illness increases risk. Dehydration may play a role, especially if severe. The use of certain medicines also increases risk, most notably those that decrease cardiac output (β-blockers), promote dehydration (diuretics), affect hypothalamic control (major tranquilizers, neuroleptics, alcohol), inhibit sweating (anticholinergics, tricyclic antidepressants, antihistamines), or increase thermogenicity (amphetamines, cocaine).

Prevention is the ideal treatment. Because behavior is the most powerful thermoregulatory mechanism, education and empowerment have the greatest preventive potential. To avoid exertional heat stroke, organizers should schedule vigorous exercise in the coolest hours of the day (shortly after dawn or after nightfall, in difficult seasons). Exercise level should be governed by athlete fitness, acclimatization, hydration status, and freedom from intercurrent illness. Clothing should be appropriate for exercise conditions. Medication use that might interfere with effective thermoregulation should be recognized, and medical personnel must be charged with the responsibility for stopping any participant who appears to be decompensating.

Triage of those with exertional heat stroke is highly variable. Runners who are plunged unconscious into an ice water bath at the end of a race often respond promptly to treatment, reawaken, and are sometimes sent home without hospitalization. A less-favorable response necessitates hospital admission.

Classic (Nonexertional) Heat Stroke

Classic (nonexertional) heat stroke usually occurs during heat waves that cause passive warming by exposure to unrelenting hot and humid conditions, afflicting urban dwellers who are elderly, infirm, solitary, and poor. Heat waves tend to be "silent and invisible killers of silent and invisible people." Their housing lacks air-conditioning or they do not use it because of expense or confusion. Alcoholism and chronic illness, especially mental illness, predispose people to heat stroke. Young children are susceptible, reflecting their high surface-to-volume ratio, relatively inefficient sweat glands, and dependent status. Classic heat stroke requires preventive measures at the community level. Those with chronic illness and substance abuse history are at highest risk, and they may be the most difficult to contact. Although ventilation fans are of little help in hot and humid conditions, a few hours spent in air-conditioned rooms each day can significantly reduce the likelihood of heat stroke. Whether this is primarily a physiologic or a sociologic effect is unclear. Patients with classic heat stroke usually respond slowly to treatment and require hospital admission.

Pathophysiology

The pathophysiology of heat stroke is incompletely understood. Although a vast number of runners in a marathon may develop dehydration and a high core temperature, very few proceed to heat stroke. Excessive heat is a noxious agent that causes direct cell injury. The severity of heat stroke is related to the degree and duration of

CURRENT DIAGNOSIS

- Heat stroke often occurs in the first 2 hours of exercise and may occur in so-called moderate heat stress conditions.
- Heat stroke may occur in sedentary urban dwellers during heat waves, especially in the presence of drug or alcohol use, senility, or in young children.
- Abnormal mental status (coma, delirium, agitation, confusion, combativeness) is a constant feature of heat stroke.
- Rectal temperature should be checked immediately. Axillary and aural temperatures may be misleadingly low. A rectal temperature of 40.6°C (105°F) or more is required for diagnosis of heat stroke, but delayed measurement may produce a misleadingly low temperature.
- The trap of proceeding with complex diagnostic procedures (such as computed tomographic scans) before core temperature is assessed and lowered to less than 39°C (102.2°F) should be avoided.
- After cooling measures are instituted, blood samples should be obtained to assess coagulation status, hepatic function, renal function, likelihood of infection, acid-base status, and muscle injury.

CURRENT THERAPY

- Injury because of heat stroke is related to both the magnitude and duration of core temperature elevation.
- After elevated rectal temperature is documented, treatment should not be delayed. In particular, it should not be delayed to start an intravenous line or to carry out advanced testing such as computed tomography or other radiograph study.
- Ideal treatment for heat stroke is cold-water immersion in a low tub, such as a child's wading pool, with the patient's arms, legs, and head hanging out of the tub.
- If low tub immersion is not available, constant flowing of cold water from a tap over the patient with drainage through a slotted Gurney cart in the presence of constant high-velocity electric fanning can be effective.
- Applying ice packs to the axillae, groins, trunk, and as many other skin surfaces as possible can be useful, but this method of cooling is not as efficient as cold-water immersion or constant cold-water flow because of reduced contact surface and limited thermal gradient.
- Rectal temperature should be checked every 5 minutes during cooling. Cooling measures are discontinued when rectal temperature reaches 39°C (102.2°F) to avoid excessive cooling. Clinicians should watch for rebound temperature elevation after cooling is discontinued.
- Clinicians should be prepared to support the patient through multisystem organ failure. Hemorrhage should be treated with transfusion of red blood cells, platelets, fresh-frozen plasma, and clotting factors. Heparin has no role in treatment of this consumptive coagulopathy. Volume expansion may be needed. Prolonged ventilator support and hemodialysis may be required.
- Medications that may be needed are diazepam (Valium), 5 mg intravenously (IV), for seizures; pressors; and mannitol, 0.25 g/kg IV, and furosemide (Lasix), 0.5 to 1.0 mg/kg IV, for renal protection from rhabdomyolysis, but only after adequate volume expansion is achieved.

temperature elevation above 41.6°C (106.9°F). Exercise lowers the thermal threshold for heat stroke because of hormonal effects and competing demands of organ systems as blood flow is directed away from the viscera to the active muscles and the skin. Gut ischemia may result in release of bacterial polysaccharides into the blood. What happens next is a complex interplay of factors including cytokines, bacterial polysaccharides, and heat shock proteins. As endothelial abnormalities accumulate, there is precipitation of a cascade of events including activation of the coagulation system and vascular dilation, resulting in hypotension and coagulation disorders. These events in many respects mimic sepsis.

Because the brain is extremely sensitive to heat stress, the first signs of heat stroke are neurologic. Judgment is impaired, and the chance for self-diagnosis is greatly reduced. After loss of consciousness, muscular activity is markedly diminished, but temperature may remain elevated for hours. Multisystem injury may follow, with the possibility of neurologic, pulmonary, cardiac, hepatic, renal, vascular, hematologic, and immunologic damage. A high percentage of classic heat stroke patients suffer infection within 36 hours of hospital admission.

Treatment

Treatment of heat stroke can be summarized easily:

- Lower rectal temperature immediately to 39°C (102.2°F).
- Support organ systems injured by heat, hypotension, inflammation, and coagulopathy.

There is a *golden hour* after the onset of heat stroke in which therapy can be extremely effective. When treating a patient outside of the hospital, the patient should be moved to a shaded area, clothes removed, and the person covered with water and fanned. When resources become available, the simplest treatment appears to be cold-water immersion in a shallow tub, with patient head, arms, and lower legs outside the tub. The high efficiency of this method comes from two properties of water: It has 25 times the thermal conductivity of air, and it makes perfect contact with all skin surfaces. In addition, the hydrostatic properties of water tend to reduce the risk of hypotension. Other methods of cooling include skin wetting with fanning, application of total-body ice packs (24 ice packs, with special emphasis on the neck, armpits, and groin), or use of a body-cooling unit (evaporation and convection).

Assessment of the patient with presumed heat stroke should be delayed pending initiation of cooling. Determination of rectal temperature, heart rate, and blood pressure can be carried out while the patient is being cooled. Oral and tympanic membrane temperatures cannot be used because they may be misleadingly low. Rectal temperature should be measured every 5 to 10 minutes, and the patient should be removed from cooling when 39°C (102.2°F) is reached, to avoid overshoot hypothermia. Hydration with normal saline or lactated Ringer's solution should be started after initiation of cooling, and most patients require 1 L in the first hour of treatment. Further rehydration needs to be guided by estimated water losses, and in difficult cases placement of a central venous monitoring catheter may be needed. Overhydration may promote cerebral edema, pulmonary edema, and hyponatremia.

Seizures, which occur commonly, should be managed with diazepam (Valium), 5 mg intravenously (IV). Shivering may also be treated with diazepam. The patient must be monitored closely with use of this medication, which occasionally promotes hypotension. Hypotension should be treated with cooling and volume expansion. If blood pressure remains depressed, pressors may be needed. For patients with prolonged exertional heat stroke, mannitol, 0.25 g/kg, or furosemide (Lasix), 0.5 to 1 mg/kg, should be given after volume expansion is carried out to minimize the adverse effects of rhabdomyolysis on renal function.

In patients with severe multiorgan damage, disseminated intravascular coagulation (DIC) is a common finding. Bleeding in DIC should be treated with transfusion of fresh-frozen plasma, cryoprecipitate, and platelet concentrates as needed. There is no role for heparin or thrombolytics in DIC in this setting. Adult respiratory distress syndrome tends to occur in conjunction with DIC, and prolonged ventilator support may be required. Hepatic failure in heat stroke is usually transient. Renal failure may necessitate emergency hemodialysis. No evidence supports use of anti-inflammatory agents or antipyretic agents in heat stroke. Use of strategies that are helpful in sepsis may ultimately find a role in treatment of heat stroke, but such treatments should be considered experimental at this time.

Prognosis can be estimated by time to recovery of consciousness (shorter is better) and elevation of liver enzymes (lactate dehydrogenase [LDH] at 24 hours less than three times normal is a good prognostic sign).

Heat stroke should usually be regarded as an accident, like drowning. The population at highest risk is readily defined, but because of the rarity of this ailment it is difficult to maintain a high level of preparedness for its prevention and treatment. Once encountered, heat stroke must be treated with much the same urgency as cardiac arrest because prompt cooling can sometimes make the crisis little more than an inconvenience. After the process of systemic injury becomes established, heat stroke's cascade of microvascular dysfunction can take on a life of its own, eventuating in a desperate struggle against multisystem failure and a high mortality rate.

REFERENCES

Bouchama A, Knochel JP: Heat stroke. N Engl J Med 2002;346(25):1978-1988.
Crandall CG, Vongpatanasin W, Victor RG: Mechanism of cocaine-induced hyperthermia in humans. Ann Intern Med 2002;136(11):785-791.
Dematte JE, O'Mara K, Buescher J, et al: Near-fatal heat stroke during the 1995 heat wave in Chicago. Ann Intern Med 1998;129(3):173-181.
Eichner ER: Treatment of suspected heat illness. Int J Sports Med 1998;19(Suppl 2):S150-S153.
Epstein Y, Moran DS, Shapiro Y: Exertional heatstroke in the Israeli Defence Forces. In Pandolf KB, Burr RE (eds): Medical Aspects of Harsh Environments. U.S. Defense Dept., Army, Office of the Surgeon General, 2001, pp 281-292. Available free online: http://www.bordeninstitute.army.mil/medaspofharshenvrnmnts/
Gaffin SL, Hubbard RW: Pathophysiology of heatstroke. In Pandolf KB, Burr RE (eds): Medical Aspects of Harsh Environments. U.S. Defense Dept., Army, Office of the Surgeon General, 2001, pp 161-208. Available free online: http://www.bordeninstitute.army.mil/medaspofharshenvrnmnts/
Gardner JW, Kark JA: 2001. Clinical diagnosis, management and surveillance of exertional heat illness. In Pandolf KB, Burr RE (eds): Medical Aspects of Harsh Environments. U.S. Defense Dept., Army, Office of the Surgeon General, 2001, pp 221-279. Available free online: http://www.bordeninstitute.army.mil/medaspofharshenvrnmnts/
Klinenberg E: Review of heat wave: Social autopsy of disaster in Chicago. N Engl J Med 2003;348(7):666-667.
Shephard RJ, Shek PN: Immune dysfunction as a factor in heat illness. Crit Rev Immunol 1999;19(4):285-302.

Spider Bites and Scorpion Stings

Method of
Rachel Haroz, MD, and James R. Roberts, MD

Spider Bites

Most of the approximately 34,000 species of spiders are considered to be venomous, but their short and delicate jaws generally prevent significant human envenomation. Approximately 200 species, however, do possess the ability to envenomate humans, resulting in symptoms ranging from minor to occasionally serious skin lesions to neurotoxicity, systemic illness, multiorgan dysfunction, and death. Spider identification after a bite is desirable but usually impossible. Here we discuss features, symptoms of envenomation, and treatment for bites from the *Loxosceles, Latrodectus*, and tarantula spiders.

LOXOSCELES ENVENOMATION

Relatively small (approximately 1.5 cm in leg span), *Loxosceles* spiders are light brown in color with darker brown markings on their dorsal surface. The most distinctive identifying characteristic appears on the female brown recluse (*L. reclusa*), which is described as violin shaped. Eleven native species of *Loxosceles* exist in the United States in the southern, southwestern, and central states. Most confirmed necrotic arachnidism in the United States is caused by *L. reclusa*. *Loxosceles* spiders have six eyes, which differs from the typical eight eyes found in most other spiders. Females are usually larger than males, which are rarely considered venomous. Considered nonaggressive and nocturnal, most *Loxosceles* bites occur when the spider is inadvertently caught between clothing or bedding and the victim's skin. Perineal and genital bites can occur in outhouses. The bite may be minimally painful or go totally unnoticed.

The initial skin manifestation is a small, erythematous, flat lesion surrounded by a light-colored ring. Within hours to days this lesion becomes bluish with a deepening of the color of the ring and progressing to a blister/bleb. A necrotic eschar with an ulcerative base may develop, which rarely becomes quite extensive. The lesion is minimally painful but often takes several weeks to heal, occasionally requiring extensive débridement or skin grafting. Some ulcerated wounds (approximately 10%) produce permanent scarring. *Loxosceles* venom contains various toxic enzymes, most notably sphingomyelinase D, that contribute to cellular destruction and tissue damage.

Systemic symptoms are rare (1% to 3% of all bites) but may include hemolysis, platelet aggregation, hemoglobinuria, myoglobinuria, maculopapular rash, nausea, vomiting, renal failure, disseminated intravascular coagulation, fever, seizures, coma, and death. These symptoms are more common in children and following South American *Loxosceles* bites.

There is little the clinician can do to affect favorably the course of a *Loxosceles* bite, with the ultimate outcome dependent on the amount and potency of the venom and host factors. Local wound care includes antisepsis, immobilization, and elevation of the affected extremity, cool compresses, appropriate analgesics, antihistamines for itching, and tetanus prophylaxis. Envenomation is difficult to differentiate from infection, but antibiotics may be necessary for secondarily infected wounds. Debridement of necrotic tissue is performed as needed. Delayed excision and wound grafting may be indicated. Once recommended, early wound excision and intrawound steroid injections should be avoided. Several other treatments to ameliorate tissue necrosis are advocated, including dapsone,[1] colchicine,[1] topical nitroglycerin,[1] high-dose vitamin C,[1] electric shock therapy, cyproheptadine

---
[1]Not FDA approved for this indication.

CURRENT DIAGNOSIS

- *Loxosceles* spider bites generally result in local symptoms, whereas *Latrodectus* and scorpion stings have predominantly systemic manifestations, which may be severe.
- The spider or scorpion should be identified if at all possible.
- Not all necrotic wounds are spider bites; therefore a differential diagnosis should be entertained.

CURRENT THERAPY

- Conservative wound care is essential in all envenomations, particularly for a *Loxosceles* spider bite.
- Particular care should be given to the very young, elderly, and patients with co-morbidity. In the setting of significant systemic symptoms, the administration of antivenom, if available, should be considered.
- Patients with ocular symptoms after exposure to a tarantula spider must be promptly referred to an ophthalmologist.
- Supportive care is often more valuable than antivenom administration, particularly considering the relatively high rate of both immediate and delayed hypersensitivity reactions.

(Periactin),[1] and hyperbaric oxygenation, but none has proven effective. Patients exhibiting systemic symptoms should be hospitalized and receive supportive care.

Absent a witnessed attack, a spider bite is usually a clinical diagnosis made by exclusion. *Loxosceles* and other spider bites are overreported and occur far less frequently than suspected by the lay public or diagnosed by clinicians. Outside of the endemic areas, *Loxosceles* bites are highly unlikely. Importantly, if the spider was not positively identified, a differential diagnosis should be entertained. Entities confused with a spider bite include clandestine drug injection (especially cocaine and amphetamines), methicillin-resistant *Staphylococcus aureus* (MRSA) skin infections, early shingles lesions, other bug bites, self-induced trauma, and infectious embolic lesions (such as endocarditis and gonococcemia).

NON-LOXOSCELES NECROTIC ARACHNIDISM

Several other species of spiders in the United States (*Cheiracanthium* species and *Tegenaria agrestis* [hobo] spiders) are associated with necrotic lesions. *Cheiracanthium* spiders are widespread and usually found indoors (e.g., in the folds of curtains or on warm windowsills). They are aggressive night foragers and produce painful, pruritic bites, usually resolving within several days. Their bites rarely result in ulceration and necrosis. Hobo spiders inhabit the Pacific Northwest to where they recently emigrated from Western Europe. They are large, aggressive, and inhabit woodpiles, subfloors, and baseboards. Their bites are usually painless but may lead to multiple ruptured blisters within 1 to 2 days and a necrotic wound. Hobo spider bites are probably responsible for necrotic arachnidism in the colder areas of the United States where the brown recluse spider is not found. Treatment of hobo spider bites is similar to that of *Loxosceles* bites.

LATRODECTUS ENVENOMATION

Latrodectus species (widow spiders) are found worldwide. In the United States, five widow spiders are endemic. These spiders are generally dark with various ventral patterns; the most well known is the red hourglass figure found on the female black widow spider. Females are larger (16- to 20-mm leg span) and more venomous than males. *Latrodectus* spiders generally inhabit outdoor dark spaces and are nonaggressive, but they do bite if provoked. The initial bite may be mildly painful, resulting in a small raised wheal. The neurotoxicity associated with these bites results from α-latrotoxin in the venom that causes a large calcium-dependent presynaptic terminal release of neurotransmitters including norepinephrine, glutamate, acetylcholine, and dopamine. The reuptake of choline is simultaneously inhibited. Symptoms begin approximately 30 minutes to an hour after the bite, and patients can appear quite ill. Muscle cramps and pain spread from the bite site and can be severe. Facial contortion and periorbital swelling, *facies latrodectismica*, may occur. Abdominal rigidity mimicking an acute abdomen, thoracic muscle spasm leading to hypoventilation and respiratory failure, diaphoresis, hypertension, nausea, vomiting, diffuse skin erythema, tremor, priapism, headache, tachycardia, paresthesias, and coma have been described.

Lower extremity pain and diaphoresis, even in upper extremity bites, seem to be characteristic features. Symptoms resolve over 3 to 7 days, and death is rare.

Local wound care includes thorough cleansing, appropriate analgesics, ice application, and tetanus prophylaxis. Severe pain and muscle spasms are treated with intravenous opioids and benzodiazepines. Intravenous calcium, although recommended in the past, is ineffective. *Latrodectus* antivenom (antivenin Lactrodectus mactans) is horse based and may cause anaphylaxis and serum sickness in allergic persons. It should be reserved for patients with severe systemic symptoms or those with potential for complications, such as the elderly, young children, pregnant patients, and patients with severe cardiovascular disease. Patients who manifest refractory pain, autonomic instability, respiratory distress, or significant neurologic changes should be treated with antivenom. The clinical response to antivenom can be dramatic even when administered 24 hours or more after envenomation.

TARANTULAS

Approximately 1500 species of tarantulas are found worldwide, with 40 species endemic to the southwestern United States. Tarantulas are also now popular household pets because many are considered harmless and nonvenomous. Relatively large spiders (18- to 24-cm leg span), tarantulas live in underground burrows and are night foragers. Tarantula envenomations in humans often cause mild pain with some surrounding inflammation, but necrotic wounds and systemic symptoms are rare. Bites in dogs, however, are usually rapidly fatal.

Several tarantula species possess urticating hairs, which they launch to incapacitate their enemy. These hairs may penetrate the human skin and cause intense inflammation or lodge in the cornea leading to keratitis, uveitis, and ophthalmia nodosa, a condition characterized by granulomatous lesions in the cornea. Case reports generally describe patients who developed eye symptoms after cleaning tarantula cages or handling the tarantulas. Treatment involves wound care including cleansing, elevation, and immobilization of the affected extremity, tetanus prophylaxis, and appropriate analgesics. Hairs embedded in the cornea that are readily identified should be removed and the patient promptly referred to an ophthalmologist. Antihistamines and corticosteroids may be necessary for pruritus and inflammation. Patients with ophthalmia nodosa may require prolonged topical corticosteroids. Tarantula owners should be cautioned to wear gloves and eye protection when handling their pets and to wash their hands and avoid any eye rubbing after such interactions.

Scorpion Stings

Scorpions range in size from several millimeters to 15 cm. They have a lobster-like appearance with a small head, two front claws, eight paired legs, and a segmented abdomen ending in a venom-containing

---
[1]Not FDA approved for this indication.

tail consisting of a storage vesicle and a stinger. Scorpions are typically night stalkers and often found hidden under rocks, in shallow burrows, and in shoes, clothing, and cooking pots. Most of the severe envenomations in the United States are caused by stings by *Centruroides exilicauda (sculpturata)*, a small (4 to 7 cm long) yellowish brown scorpion.

Scorpion stings are usually very painful, quickly causing local paresthesias and edema. In adults, this usually resolves in several hours. Systemic effects are usually seen in the elderly and in infants and children. Scorpion venom blocks sodium and potassium channels and causes marked acetylcholine and catecholamine release. This leads to an initial cholinergic toxidrome characterized by the SLUDGE syndrome: salivation, lacrimation, urination, defecation, gastroenteritis, and emesis. Subsequently, catecholamine release leads to anxiety, tachycardia, hypertension, pulmonary edema, confusion, dystonic and myoclonic movements, seizures, ataxia, hyperglycemia, hyperpyrexia, and pancreatitis. Myocardial depression, myocardial infarctions without thrombosis, and ischemic strokes are rarely described.

Wound care should encompass thorough cleansing, elevation and immobilization of the affected extremity, cool compresses, tetanus prophylaxis, and appropriate analgesics. Patients should be observed for a period of 6 hours after the sting for the development of systemic symptoms.

Supportive care is the mainstay of treatment. Sympathetic symptoms should be blunted aggressively. Benzodiazepines, β-blockers, diuretics, digoxin (Lanoxin),[1] and nitroprusside (Nitropress) are successful. Dopamine (Intropin) and dobutamine (Dobutrex) may be necessary for the hypotensive patient, and mechanical ventilation may be required for respiratory failure. Angiotensin-converting enzyme inhibitors, opioids, and nifedipine may be detrimental and should be avoided.

Goat-derived antivenom use is controversial. It is not FDA approved and its availability is limited to the state of Arizona. The incidence of immediate and delayed hypersensitivity is relatively high (3% and 60%, respectively). The antivenom is species specific and must be administered within 1 hour of the exposure. Although helpful with pain, antivenom does not reverse cardiovascular and respiratory compromise because these are secondary to massive catecholamine release.

---

[1]Not FDA approved for this indication.

REFERENCES

Blaikie AJ, Ellis J, Sanders R, et al: Eye disease associated with handling pet tarantulas: Three case reports. BMJ 1997;314:1524-1525.

Clark RF, Wethern-Kestner S, Vance MV, et al: Clinical presentation and treatment of black widow spider envenomations: A review of 163 cases. Ann Emerg Med 1992;21:782-787.

Diaz HJ: The global epidemiology, syndromic classification, management, and prevention of spider bites. Am J Trop Med Hyg 2004;71:239-250.

Hered RW, Spaulding AG, Sanitato JJ, et al: Ophthalmia nodosa caused by tarantula hairs. Ophthalmology 1988;95:166-169.

LoVecchio F, Welch S, Klemens J, et al: Incidence of immediate and delayed hypersensitivity to Centruroides antivenom. Ann Emerg Med 1999;5:615-619.

Mazzei de Davila CA, Davila DF, Donis JH: Sympathetic nervous system activation, antivenin administration and cardiovascular manifestations of scorpion envenomation. Toxicon 2002;40:1339-1346.

Merchant ML, Hinton JF, Geren CR: Effect of hyperbaric oxygen on sphingomyelinase D activity of brown recluse spider (*Loxosceles reclusa*) venom as studied by ^{31}P nuclear magnetic resonance spectroscopy. Am J Trop Med Hyg 1997;56:335-338.

Mold JW, Thompson DM: Management of brown recluse spider bites in primary care. J Am Board Fam Pract 2004;17:347-352.

Saucier JR: Arachnid envenomation. Emerg Med Clin North Am 2004; 22:405-422.

Suntorntham S, Roberts JR, Nilsen GJ: Dramatic clinical response to the delayed administration of black widow spider antivenom. Ann Emerg Med 1994;24:1198-1199.

Swanson DL, Vetter RS: Bites of brown recluse spiders and suspected necrotic arachnidism. N Engl J Med 2005;352:700-707.

Snakebite

Method of
Craig S. Kitchens, MD

The combination of fear of snakes and the unfamiliarity of most physicians with the management of snakebite often leads to an ill-founded perception of danger on the part of practitioners. It should be kept in mind that approximately 10,000 poisonous snakebites in the United States occur every year, yet fewer than 10 victims die.

In the past, treatment was often empirical and shrouded by folklore. Because survival is a near statistical certainty, various therapies including alcohol, application of ice, electric shock therapy, wide surgical débridement, or even providing no therapy have appeared efficacious. Treatment has now evolved from this disorganized state to a scientifically supported therapeutic regimen based on both the availability of antivenin and the experience garnered by large series of patients by clinical investigators. Morbidity and mortality are minimized by appropriate therapy.

Here we discuss care of patients bitten by North American poisonous snakes. In the United States, approximately 95% of poisonous snakebites are inflicted by pit vipers (family Crotalidae), which comprise multiple species of rattlesnakes as well as water moccasins and copperheads. Approximately 1% to 2% of all U.S. snakebites involve coral snakes (family Elapidae). Another 2% to 3% of snakebites are inflicted by exotic poisonous snakes that are either appropriately housed in zoos or owned by professional snake handlers or inappropriately kept as pets by amateurs. Treatment of persons bitten by exotic snakes is beyond the scope of this chapter. It is suggested that in such encounters a Poison Control Center should be consulted because antivenin to treat exotic snake bites is not commercially available in the United States; reputable handlers of such snakes usually have a supply of their own specific antivenin.

Diagnosis

It is of prime importance to know the species of the offending snake because prognosis and treatment both heavily depend on this information. Undue risk should not be assumed by either the victim or others, yet identification of the snake is important and, if possible, the snake should be brought to the treatment facility for identification. The species of snake is actually more important than is its size in terms of prognosis. Primary care practitioners and emergency department personnel should have at least a modicum of information for identification of local poisonous snakes. Bites from the pygmy rattlesnake (*Sistrurus miliarius*) have not resulted in a documented human death, and envenomations by the copperhead (*Agkistrodon contortrix*) and water moccasin (*A. piscivorus*) generally result in moderate envenomation syndromes with death rarely occurring. The Eastern diamondback (*Crotalus adamanteus*), Western diamondback (*C. atrox*), and Mojave rattlesnake (*C. scutulatus*) each have a higher degree of toxicity and indeed account for most of the fatalities in the United States.

The coral snake (*Micrurus fulvius*) accounts for only 1% to 2% of all snakebite cases in North America but has a higher than expected mortality based on its characteristic and severe neurotoxicity. Treatment of coral snake envenomation is not discussed further here. Suffice it to say that the neurotoxicity is the cause of morbidity and mortality from envenomation by the coral snake, usually through aspiration pneumonia and cessation of breathing. Accordingly, these severe manifestations can be attended by respiratory support and the natural history (i.e., without antivenin therapy), which usually is approximately a week before it reverses. Also important regarding coral snake envenomation is the absence of any signs of local pain, swelling, or discoloration, which are characteristic of pit viper envenomation. Patients cannot be assumed to have eluded envenomation by a coral snake because they lack these symptoms. That symptoms

CURRENT THERAPY

- IV access and administer crystalloid as indicated.
- Obtain CBC, PT, PTT, platelet count q6-12h for 1 d, then daily if abnormal.
- Estimate severity of envenomation.
  - Species of snake
  - Age and health status of victim
  - Rate of progression of signs/symptoms
- Administer CroFab as per Table 2.
- Determine tetanus vaccination status.
- Seek consultation from experts or a Poison Control Center, especially if one is treating envenomation for the first few times.

Abbreviations: CBC = complete blood count; IV = intravenous; PT = prothrombin time; PTT = partial thromboplastin time.

are often delayed for 8 to 24 hours must be anticipated, so 1 or 2 days of hospitalization for observation is frequently suggested.

The vast majority (approximately 80%) of envenomations by pit vipers are nonaccidental; that is, they are the result of poor judgment or senseless behavior, often in combination with intoxication with any of various substances. Most snakebite victims not only see and correctly identify the snake as poisonous but feel compelled to play with, taunt, or capture the animal and in the process may well be bitten. Fewer than 20% of snakebites are actually what most persons would call accidental.

Pit vipers are easily recognized by the so-called pit (an infrared heat-detection organ) approximately midway between the nostril and the eye. All North American pit vipers have pupils shaped like those of a cat, as opposed to round pupils characteristic of nonpoisonous snakes (with the exception of the coral snake). Pit vipers have large fangs through which a considerable volume of venom is injected, often deeply, into the victim. Because fangs are continually replaced, there may be one, two, three, or even four fangs at one time that may leave a similar number of puncture wounds.

Pit viper venom is extremely complex, containing a broad range of proteolytic enzymes designed to digest protein, fat, connective tissue, nucleic acids, and other biologic material. It also contains numerous small peptides, which probably accounts for autonomic symptoms such as tachycardia, diaphoresis, diarrhea, and vomiting. There is a great variability in this complex poison with variability not only between species but also within species, and even within a single specimen if it is observed over years. Variability of the venom most likely accounts for the variability of the signs, symptoms, and prognosis in envenomation syndromes because of various species of pit vipers.

For instance, the hematologic abnormalities seen in North American pit viper envenomation occur through certain principles in pit viper venom. The Eastern diamondback rattlesnake contains a thrombin-like enzyme that partially cleaves fibrinogen, clearing it from the circulation, with the concomitant production of huge amounts of fibrin degradation products with only modest thrombocytopenia. The venom of the Western diamondback rattlesnake contains a principle that directly activates plasminogen to plasmin with resulting hyperfibrinolysis. Although through differing mechanisms, bites of each of these rattlesnakes may result in dramatic alterations of the prothrombin time (PT) and partial thromboplastin time (PTT) but little bleeding. Whereas envenomation by the Eastern or Western diamondback rattlesnake produces a minimal elevation of serum creatinine kinase (CK), myonecrosis with marked CK elevations are the hallmark of the canebrake rattlesnake (*C. horridus atricaudatus*) to include a brisk elevation of the CK-MB band yet with negative assays for either troponin I or T consistent with the lack of cardiac muscle myonecrosis. The bite of the Mojave rattlesnake produces myonecrosis similar to that of the canebrake rattlesnake as well as neurologic symptoms but minimal coagulation abnormalities. Severe thrombocytopenia usually refractory to platelet transfusion is seen in envenomation by the timber rattlesnake (*C. horridus horridus*). Thus, one can see that many envenomations have a signature, so to speak, that is slowly being unraveled (Table 1).

Approximately 20% of persons bitten by a positively identified pit viper are fortunate enough not to be envenomated by the snake and are considered to have a "dry bite." For these fortunate victims, the administration of antivenin obviously is not indicated. Dry bites are often deduced by the normality of the patient with the near complete absence of any pain, swelling, or discoloration within 1 to 2 hours of the bite.

Treatment

It is most important to distinguish the severity of the bite to determine the need for and extent of antivenin therapy. Good supportive therapy should be instituted with the establishment of at least one large intravenous (IV) line and the infusion of saline or similar crystalloid for volume and blood pressure indications.

It is difficult to overestimate the importance of sensing the *rate of change of signs and symptoms* in determining the severity of bites. It is of more clinical significance that a patient bitten 20 minutes ago has a

TABLE 1 Distinguishing Clinical Characteristics of Envenomation by Selected *Crotalus* Species

Common Name	Scientific Name	Distribution	Neurologic Symptoms	Coagulopathic Findings	Rhabdomyolysis
Eastern diamondback	*Crotalus adamanteus*	Southeastern United States	+	Prolonged PT/PTT	+
Canebrake	*C. horridus atricaudatus*	Eastern United States	—	—	++++
Mojave	*C. scutulatus*	Desert Southwest United States	+++	—	++++
Timber	*C. horridus horridus*	Eastern United States	—	Prolonged PT/PTT; moderate to severe thrombocytopenia	—

Abbreviations: PT = prothrombin time; PTT = partial thromboplastin time.
— = nil; + = mild; ++ = moderate; +++ = pronounced; ++++ = severe.

CURRENT THERAPY

- Confirm patient was bitten by a venomous snake.
- Determine snake species if possible.
- Evaluate for local signs of envenomation:
  - Pain
  - Swelling
  - Discoloration
- Evaluate for systemic signs of envenomation:
  - Alterations in vital signs
  - Nausea, vomiting, diarrhea, and diaphoresis
  - Fasciculations
  - Coagulation abnormalities
  - Altered mental status

rapidly swelling arm than a patient bitten 3 hours ago has an even larger yet not still enlarging arm. Such a philosophy is also important in judging the efficacy of any administration of antivenin because one cannot expect prior damage to include swelling and discoloration to subside promptly, but rather one determines whether such symptoms cease to progress or progress at such a slow rate that continued therapy may not be indicated. It is clear that the efficacy of the antivenin is a function of the time lapsed since the bite. It is ideal to treat bites that should be treated as soon as possible, and I prefer to initiate administration of antivenin prior to 6 or 12 hours after a bite, and essentially I never initiate treatment after 24 hours because what damage is going to be done is done and cannot be reversed.

Dry bites comprise approximately 20% of snakebites, and there is no evidence of any envenomation either locally or by laboratory evaluation. No treatment is indicated (Table 2).

Minimal envenomations are characterized by pain, swelling, and discoloration that are caused by the dissolution of underlying tissue. In general, there are no systemic signs, symptoms, or laboratory abnormalities, although anxiety is almost universal and, in the case of envenomation for rattlesnakes, notorious for their hematologic manifestations. Laboratory alterations of the coagulation system may be present, but in and of themselves they are not indications, in our experience, for the administration of antivenin.

The primary differentiation between minimal envenomations and *moderate envenomations* is not only the extent but particularly the rate of development and progression of pain, swelling, and discoloration because one may see a doubling of these symptoms within the initial hour of evaluation and care administered to the patient. Such patients should be administered antivenin to halt or lessen such progression. In general, these patients do not have severe alterations of vital signs or laboratory findings, although coagulation abnormalities may be quite dramatic with unclottable PTs and PTTs and modest thrombocytopenia on the order of 30,000 to 100,000/mm^3. Most of these patients are treated with antivenin, especially if they are children, elderly, or have significant co-morbidity.

Essentially all patients with *severe envenomation* are treated with antivenin. These are patients with severe alterations of vital signs, including hypotension, a peculiar unpleasant taste in the mouth, marked diaphoresis, universal diarrhea and vomiting, and frequently a stupor or inattention revealing alterations in mental status. Often the bite is in a highly vascular muscle (thenar, hypothenar, calf, or arm muscle) rather than the comparatively less vascular hand or foot. The coagulation abnormalities may again be quite remarkable. In our experience, most severe envenomations are obviously severe soon after the bite (10 to 30 minutes) with only a very small minority progressing from lesser degrees to severe.

Clinically relevant bleeding is rarely seen despite the marked alterations in coagulation tests. The explanation for this is that with North American pit viper envenomations, thrombin generation is intact so what little fibrinogen and platelets are available are used to maintain effective hemostasis. In other words, this is not disseminated intravascular coagulation (DIC) but chiefly a syndrome whose laboratory values mimic DIC. Exotic snakes may directly activate prothrombin (*Echis* species and *Bothrops* species) and/or factor X (*Vipera* species and *Dispholidus* species) leading to a true DIC with marked organ dysfunction related to thrombosis of organs with subsequent death.

Bleb formation at the site of a bite is not an important sign in and of itself, although it generates much attention.

Compartment syndromes are seen quite rarely, with surgical intervention indicated in only 1% to 5% of envenomated patients. Of interest, marked swelling itself is not often a sign of a compartment syndrome because in a true compartment syndrome, swelling is limited owing to the anatomic restriction by fibrous tissue, such as seen in the lateral anterior compartment of the lower leg or in the palm of the hand. The chief sign for a true compartment syndrome is the intense hardness of these areas and dysfunction of muscles within the compartment.

The administration of fresh-frozen plasma (FFP), platelet concentrates, or other blood products is rarely necessary in North American pit viper envenomation. We advocate a permissive posture with regard to the prolongation of the PT and PTT as long as there is no clinical bleeding. Should bleeding be present, the lack of fibrinogen is best treated with infusions of 8 to 10 bags of cryoprecipitate and monitored by serial determination of the fibrinogen level. This maneuver typically corrects the PT and PTT. Severe thrombocytopenia, implying platelet counts of less than 10,000/mm^3, may well be an indication for platelet transfusion, particularly if an invasive or surgical procedure is planned. It has not been our experience that patients have significant hemorrhage. Leakage of blood into swollen tissues, dilution from crystalloid administration, and hemolysis of red blood cells from hemolysins in the venom account for most decreases in hematocrit values.

TABLE 2 Grades of Severity of Envenomation by Pit Vipers

Grade	Frequency (%)	Initial Findings	CroFab Vials in First 24 H
No envenomation	0–15	No local, systemic, or laboratory abnormalities 2 h after bite	0
Minimal envenomation	20–40	Local and slowly progressive swelling without systemic or severe laboratory abnormalities	0–6
Moderate envenomation	20–40	Rapidly progressive local swelling; systemic symptoms of nausea, vomiting, diarrhea, diaphoresis, fasciculations, moderate hypotension, and moderate hemostatic abnormalities but without bleeding	6–12
Severe envenomation	5–10	Severe systemic symptoms as above plus severe hypotension and lethargy; severe hemostatic abnormalities and possible bleeding	12–24 or more

Emergency management in the field consists primarily of getting the patient to a medical facility. It is there that directed therapy should start. The use of tourniquets, cut-and-suck methodology, electric shock therapy, and the application of ice or administration of alcohol do not work and only serve to delay adequate evaluation and treatment. The victim should be kept calm and at rest during transport to the hospital. It is advised that should ice or tourniquets be in place on arrival at the hospital, it be documented in the report and removed.

The mainstay of treatment for North American pit viper envenomation is Crotalidae polyvalent immune Fab (ovine) antivenin (CroFab), which is an ovine-based preparation of immunoglobulins that is chemically treated so that only the Fab portion of the immunoglobulins is infused because the Fc fragment has been cleaved. Because the Fc fragment accounts for the majority of immunologic reactions, the Fab product appears to be much less allergenic than the prior equine-based product of intact immunoglobulins. Pretreatment skin or conjunctival testing is not required prior to administration of CroFab. Additionally, the smaller Fab molecule appears to give the advantage of facilitated penetration deep into affected tissues, but conversely, it has a rather short half-life of only several hours as opposed to several days with the previously available equine antivenin. This may be problematic in that an envenomation syndrome may appear by all accord to have been controlled with the cessation of the progression of swelling, normalization of vital signs, and the beginning of normalization of laboratory studies, only to have a relapse of these findings a few hours or days after antivenin administration. Readministration (as opposed to the initiation of antivenin administration) may very well be indicated. Because we hold that the defibrination syndrome is so benign in the first place, we do not regard the common reappearance of defibrination and secondary prolongation of the PT and PTT without evidence of clinical bleeding as an independent free-standing reason for antivenin readministration.

CroFab is administered as an IV solution starting slowly to alert for any possible adverse reaction. If such is not encountered, six vials are typically infused over 1 hour. If local and systemic findings cease or slow, the syndrome is deemed to be controlled. If not, two more vials, each over 6 hours, are suggested for a total of 12 vials in the first 24 hours. The rare severe and/or relapsing case may require up to 24 or more vials over several days.

Antibiotics are generally not employed but are indicated in wounds that were manipulated in the field, such as with a knife. Determination of which antibiotic to administer should include anaerobic bacterial coverage. Tetanus vaccination status should be determined and acted on appropriately. The extremities should be cleansed. Many find outlining the edges of the enlarging wound with a pen helpful in following the rate of change of progression of the swelling. We do not advocate determination of intercompartmental pressures routinely. The extremities should be slightly elevated above the level of the heart. The wound should not be covered or bound; it should be easily observable.

In-hospital therapy is usually given in closely monitored areas beginning with the emergency department and progressing to the intensive care unit (ICU), although ICU therapy is not necessarily a standard of care. Patients should be observed closely; particularly victims of coral snake bites or those who are deemed most likely to have dry bites. If signs, symptoms, or other evidence for envenomation do not occur within 24 to 36 hours, the patient can be discharged. We do not hold that all patients need admission to the hospital if it is very clear, within several hours, that envenomation did not occur, or if it did, it was minimal, such as with a pygmy rattlesnake bite. Because our patients typically are intoxicated, that in itself is more often than not a possible reason to keep the patient in the hospital for a day or so.

Nearly all swelling and tissue destruction is transient with North American pit viper envenomation. Edema that results from the dissolution of capillaries and particularly lymphatics may take as long as 1 to 2 months to resolve but may even be permanent in older or debilitated patients. In general, there is a total return of function to the bitten extremity, although a weakness or stiffness may be experienced by some patients for up to a year. A loss of tissue, to include fingers or limbs, is exceptionally rare and usually is accompanied by prehospital use of tourniquets and/or ice, extremely delayed therapy, overaggressive surgical procedures, or neural damage in rare cases where a fasciotomy may have been indicated. Unfortunately, patients who are bitten by snakes tend to retain those habits that led to this envenomation and therefore may be seen again.

REFERENCES

Bond RG, Burkhart KK: Thrombocytopenia following timber rattlesnake envenomation. Ann Emerg Med 1998;31:139-141.
Boyer LV, Seifert SA, Cain JS: Recurrence phenomena after immunoglobulin therapy for snake envenomations: Part 2. Guidelines for clinical management with Crotaline Fab antivenom. Ann Emerg Med 2001;37:196-201.
Carroll RR, Hall EL, Kitchens CS: Canebrake rattlesnake envenomation. Ann Emerg Med 1997;20:45-48.
Dart RC, Hurlbut KM, Garcia R, et al: Validation of a severity score for the assessment of crotalid snakebite in the United States. Ann Emerg Med 1996;27:321-326.
Farstad D, Thomas T, Chow T, et al: Mojave rattlesnake envenomation in southern California: A review of suspected cases. Wilderness Environ Med 1997;8:89-93.
Kitchens CS: Hemostatic aspects of envenomation by North American snakes. Hematol/Oncol Clin North Am 1992;6:1189-1195.
Kitchens CS: From ETOH to FAB: The medicalization of therapy for pit viper envenomation. Trans Am Clin Climatol Assn 2001;112:117-135.
Kitchens CS, van Mierop LHS: Mechanisms of defibrination in humans after envenomation by the eastern diamondback rattlesnake. Am J Hematol 1983;14:345-353.
Kitchens CS, van Mierop LHS: Envenomation by the Eastern coral snake (*Micrurus fulvius fulvius*). A study of 39 victims. JAMA 1987;258:1615-1618.

Marine Poisonings, Envenomations, and Trauma

Method of
Allen Perkins, MD, MPH

The United States has more than 80,000 miles of coastline, and more people are enjoying water-dependent recreation activities such as scuba diving, snorkeling, and surfing. As a consequence, people are more likely to suffer trauma, envenomation, or poisoning related to an encounter with a marine creature, which will come to the attention of a physician. The science of marine medicine is limited; hence, treatment of these conditions is largely based on case reports and expert opinion; very few randomized, controlled studies are available. Misdiagnosis is common, especially when the patient has returned from vacationing or when the patient has been poisoned by improperly handled seafood. This article describes common ailments and injuries occurring as a consequence of direct contact with sea creatures and discusses management and prevention.

Ingestions

CIGUATERA

Epidemiology

Ciguatera poisoning is the most commonly reported marine toxin disease in the world. It is caused by human ingestion of reef fish that have bioaccumulated sufficient amounts of the dinoflagellate Gambierdiscus toxicus, either through direct ingestion or through ingestion of smaller reef fish. Although limited to tropical regions, it is heat and cold tolerant, is lipid soluble, and can survive transport to other areas. The toxin becomes more concentrated as it passes up the food chain; fish such as amberjack, grouper, and snapper pose less of a risk than predatory fish such as barracuda and moray eel. Ciguatera poisoning affects at least 50,000 people worldwide annually, and there are several thousand cases of poisoning in Puerto Rico, the U.S. Virgin Islands, Hawaii, and Florida each year.

Clinical Features

Patients can exhibit a primarily gastrointestinal (diarrhea, abdominal cramps, and vomiting), neurologic (paresthesias, diffuse pain, blurred vision), cardiac (bradycardia), or mixed pattern of symptoms. Additionally, a cold sensation reversal, in which a patient perceives the cold temperatures as a hot sensation and vice versa, occurs in 80% of patients and is considered pathognomonic for ciguatera poison (Box 1).

The attack rate is high. As many as 80% to 100% of people who ingest affected fish develop symptoms depending on the size of the fish and the toxin load. Ingestion of internal organs where the toxin accumulates (e.g., liver, roe) is associated with more severe symptoms, but avoiding these organs is not protective. The symptoms are also related to the number of exposures over time, and patients typically have more severe symptoms with subsequent exposures. There is no age-related susceptibility, and no immunity is acquired through exposure.

Symptoms typically begin 1 to 6 hours after ingestion, although a delay of 12 to 24 hours can occur. Duration is 7 to 14 days, and neurologic symptoms occasionally persist for months to years. Chronic ciguatera syndrome can also occur as a constellation of symptoms such as general malaise, depression, headaches, muscle aches, and dysesthesias in the extremities. Patients with chronic disease report recurrences with ingestion of fish, ethanol, caffeine, and nuts up to 6 months after the acute illness resolves.

BOX 1 Symptom Patterns Associated with Ciguatera Poisoning

Gastrointestinal Pattern

Onset 15 minutes to 24 hours, typically worsens, lasts 1-2 days and resolves
- Nausea and/or vomiting
- Profuse, watery diarrhea
- Abdominal pain

Neurologic Pattern

Onset up to 24 hours after ingestion, commonly nonphysiologic pattern, can last several months
- Numbness and paresthesias
- Vertigo
- Ataxia
- Severe weakness or lethargy
- Severe myalgia
- Decreased vibration and pain sensations
- Diffuse pain pattern
- Cold sensation reversal
- Coma

Cardiovascular Pattern

Onset up to 24 hours after ingestion is uncommon but occurs rapidly
- Bradycardia
- Hypotension
- Cardiovascular collapse

CURRENT DIAGNOSIS

- History of exposure is necessary for diagnosis.
- Ingested toxins can cause unusual symptoms, predominately gastrointestinal.
- Jellyfish envenomation is very painful but almost always self-limited.
- Trauma management follows principles of dirty wounds.
- Specific marine pathogens should be covered if contamination is suspected.

Diagnosis

The diagnosis should be entertained in any patient who has neurologic, gastrointestinal, or cardiac symptoms and a history of ingesting predatory fish within the past 24 hours. The symptom constellation can be similar to other ingestions, such as certain shellfish toxins, and differentiation requires knowledge of the patient's diet for the previous day. Additionally, scombroid and type E botulinum poisoning should be considered, but these are unlikely if the patient did not ingest ill-appearing game. Other poisonings, such as organophosphates, can produce a similar symptom complex. There are no currently available clinical assays to assist in making the diagnosis, which is based on clinical suspicion and knowledge of the patient's diet history.

Treatment

If ciguatera poisoning is suspected soon after ingestion, I would consider gut decontamination with activated charcoal (Actidose-Aqua) because it can reduce the toxin load and subsequent symptoms. Initial symptomatic treatment typically consists of fluid replacement to replace gastrointestinal losses.

Atropine (AtroPen) is used in patients who have bradycardia. Temporary electrical pacing may be used for refractory symptoms, and pressors may be needed in cases of severe hypotension. Neurologic symptoms are problematic because of their extended course as well as their severity. Mannitol (Osmitrol)[1] is often cited as effective in reducing the duration of neurologic symptoms, but I would use it with caution because the only double-blind trial failed to show any benefit. Nifedipine (Procardia)[1] (adult dose 10-20 mg three times daily) shows some theoretical promise in this regard, but there have been no studies in humans at this time. There are many local remedies used throughout the world that are said to be successful, which likely attests to the self-limited course of the ingestion in most cases. Table 1 offers more details regarding treatments currently used for ciguatera poisoning.

Prevention

Prevention is difficult except by avoiding ingestion of affected reef fish. The toxin is not deactivated by cooking, freezing, smoking, or salting. There are no outward signs of ciguatera: The fish look, taste, and smell normal. Although several commercial assays are available, they are neither sensitive nor specific enough to be relied on to prevent ciguatera poisoning.

To decrease the risk of ciguatera poisoning, I recommend the following steps: Avoid warm-water reef fish, especially those caught where ciguatera poisoning is known to occur; avoid moray eel injection; avoid ingesting large game fish; avoid consuming the internal organs; and limit the amount of initial ingestion if you are in an area where ciguatera is known to occur. Additionally, patients travelling to distant locales should be made aware that, although the vast majority

---

[1]Not FDA approved for this indication.

TABLE 1 Treatment for Ciguatera Poisoning

Drug	Dose	Indication
Activated charcoal (Actidose-Aqua)	Children < 1 y: 1g/kg Children 1-12 y: 25-50 g Adults: 25-100 g	Gut emptying and decontamination More effective in first h
Antiemetics (no preference)	Administer per dosing recommendations	Intractable nausea and/or vomiting
Intravenous fluid bolus and infusion (normal saline or Lactated Ringer's as initial)	Per volume replacement protocols	Hypovolemia
Atropine (AtroPen)	0.5-1.0 mg IV every 3-5 min to a maximum dose of 0.04 mg/kg per episode Maximum total dose: 3 mg for adults, 2 mg for adolescents, 1 mg for young children	Bradycardia
Pressors: Dopamine (Intropin), dobutamine (Dobutrex), epinephrine	Varies with clinical response	Hypotension, shock
Antihistamines (no preference)	Administer per dosing recommendations	Pruritis
Mannitol (Osmitrol)[1]	1 g/kg of a 20% solution given IV over several h Adult dose 25-100 g, titrate to urinary output of 100 mL/h	Neurologic symptoms, double-blind study did not show benefit
Amitriptyline (Elavil)[1]	25-75 mg PO bid for patients >25 kg	Pruritis, dysesthesias

[1]Not FDA approved for this indication.

of cases result from direct ingestion, there have been cases of ciguatera passed through sexual contact and through breast milk, so they should be wary of body fluid contact if ciguatoxin is endemic to the area, if for no other reasons.

SCOMBROID

Epidemiology

Scombroid poisoning (also known as histamine fish poisoning) results from improper handling of certain fish between the time the fish is caught and the time it is cooked. In the United States it is most common in Hawaii and California. Improper preservation and refrigeration lead to histamine and histamine-like substances being produced in the dark meat of certain fish through a conversion of histadine to histamine by bacterial decarboxylases. Members of the family Scombridae, such as tuna and mackerel, contain the highest amounts of this substance, but both scombroid and nonscombroid fish have been associated with the disease. The production of toxins requires the introduction of bacteria during the handling process, primarily during storage at high temperatures. It is the total amount of histamine, the presence of other biogenic amines, and individual susceptibility that determine the severity of the symptoms.

Clinical Features

The patient develops a histamine reaction 20 to 30 minutes after ingestion. Symptoms can be cutaneous, gastrointestinal, neurologic, or hemodynamic or any combination of these. Cutaneous (flushing, urticaria and conjunctival injection, and localized edema; gastrointestinal symptoms include dry mouth, nausea, vomiting, diarrhea, and abdominal cramping; neurologic symptoms include severe headache and dizziness; and hemodynamic symptoms include palpitations and hypotension. In severe cases there can be bronchospasm and respiratory distress. These symptoms typically come on rapidly (within several minutes) and last less than 6 to 8 hours. Flushing is the most consistent clinical sign, occurring on exposed areas so it typically resembles sunburn. Diarrhea is also very common, occurring in 75% of symptomatic patients.

Diagnosis

As with ciguatera, the diagnosis is one of history. If the time between ingestion and illness is short and the patient has ingested a type of fish previously implicated in scombroid, then a tentative diagnosis can be made. The diagnosis is often confused with an allergic reaction. It can be distinguished from allergy by the lack of a previous allergic reaction as well as by testing the remaining fish for histamine, although testing is rarely warranted.

Treatment

Treatment is the same as for any histamine reaction, the cornerstone of which is antihistamine. Diphenhydramine (Benadryl) 50 mg for adults and 0.5-1 mg/kg/dose for children, repeated every 4 hours until symptoms abate, is delivered either intravenously or intramuscularly in severe cases and orally for milder cases. For severe cases, cimetidine (Tagamet)[1] 300 mg for adults, 20 mg/kg for children, either orally or intravenously, might be added for more complete histamine-receptor blockade. In cases where ingestion was recent, consider induced emesis using syrup of ipecac: 15 mL for children younger than 12 years or 30 mL otherwise. Most patients require only reassurance, and pharmacologic treatment will be unnecessary. It should be stressed to the patient that this is not an *allergic* reaction to fish, because the histamine is exogenous. Prevention is possible in regions where food storage and preparation are monitored through identification and removal of suspect fish.

OTHER INGESTED TOXINS

In addition to the toxins just discussed, ingestion of certain other marine creatures can lead to problems.

Ingestion of bivalves harvested from contaminated waters has been associated with hepatitis A, Norwalk virus, *Vibrio parahaemolyticus* and *Vibrio vulnificans* infections, the latter two particularly problematic and occasionally fatal in immunocompromised patients. I counsel patients likely to be immunocompromised, including diabetics and those with known liver disease, to avoid uncooked bivalves.

Shellfish are occasionally known to contain one or more of several toxins acquired through bioaccumulation of certain algae. These dinoflagellates tend to bloom in summer months. The symptoms occur immediately after ingestion and last several hours and are typically neurologic or gastrointestinal, or both. The shellfish poisoning syndromes are known as paralytic, neurologic, diarrheal, or amnestic depending on the predominant symptom. The care is typically

---

[1]Not FDA approved for this indication.

supportive. Public health officials typically monitor local mollusk populations fairly carefully and alert the public to possible hazards.

Ingestion of the flesh of certain puffer fish has been associated with tetrodotoxin poisoning. The flesh of the fish (fugu) is considered a delicacy. The toxin builds up in internal organs such as the liver and the roe. If the toxin is ingested, it is likely to be fatal but there are certified chefs who are trained in avoiding the toxin when preparing the dish. Despite this precaution, as many as 50 deaths occur in Japan annually from exposure to this toxin. Avoiding this puffer fish and avoiding the ingestion of certain other exotic animals (such as the blue-ringed octopus) eliminate the risk of acquiring this toxin.

Envenomations

Many marine creatures are venomous, and beachgoers experience clinically significant envenomations with some regularity. Jellyfish and related creatures (Cnidarians), sea urchins (Echinodermata), and stingrays (Chondrichthyes) are some of the more commonly identified marine animals involved with envenomations.

JELLYFISH

These invertebrates have stinging cells called *nematocytes*, which carry nematocysts that continue to function when separated from the larger organism. For example, jellyfish nematocysts can sting if the tentacle is separated and after the jellyfish is dead. The venom is antigenic and causes a reaction of a dermatonecrotic, hemolytic, cardiopathic, or neurotoxic nature. The severity of the reaction depends on several variables, including the number of nematocysts that discharge, the toxicity of the coelenterate involved, and each patient's unique antigenic response.

Clinical Features

Although occasionally fatal as a consequence of an anaphylactic response in the United States and Caribbean, the primary concern in these areas with contact is pain, which is almost always self-limiting. Other less common symptoms include parasthesias, nausea, headaches, and chills. The symptoms may last up to 2 to 3 days. Certain Pacific jellyfish primarily found in the waters around Australia have a more potent toxin and are much more likely to cause death (which is still very uncommon). Additionally, the Irukandji syndrome, which occurs in the Pacific, is a suite of symptoms including muscle spasms, vomiting, hypertension, incessant coughing, and occasionally heart failure and brain hemorrhage. Almost all exposed people, regardless of the geographic location, do not have a severe reaction, and the principles of first aid are primarily the same throughout the world.

Treatment

In my experience, treatment is mostly concerned with limiting pain and neurologic symptoms, because anaphylaxis and other severe reactions are rare, and the following general guidelines can be applied. In the field, either the victim or a companion should remove any visible tentacles. To do so requires using care, with gloves or forceps being optimal to prevent further stings. If a towel is used, any nematocysts remaining on the towel can still discharge. Household vinegar will prevent discharge of the remaining nematocysts on the skin and should be applied liberally when available. If vinegar is not available in the field, salt water can be used to wash off the nematocysts. Urine, fresh water, and rubbing with sand should be avoided.

Should the victim present to the physician's office or emergency department, household vinegar (5% acetic acid)[1] should be liberally applied for 30 minutes or until the pain subsides followed by removal of the nematocysts, usually through use of the gloved hand or with forceps. Another method for removing the nematocysts is to apply

---

[1]Not FDA approved for this indication.

 CURRENT THERAPY

Ingestions
- Avoidance is the best strategy.
- Early decontamination with activated charcoal (Actidose-Aqua) can reduce duration of symptoms.
- Symptomatic care is generally sufficient.

Jellyfish
- Remove visible stingers.
- Acetic acid 5%[1] can be used to denature stingers on skin.
- Control pain with topical analgesia.

Trauma
- Avoiding water at feeding time can help to avoid injury.
- If envenomation is suspected, consider hot water immersion.
- Tetanus status should be checked.
- Antibiotic coverage should take marine pathogens into account.

---

[1]Not FDA approved for this indication.

shaving cream or baking soda slurry to the area and scrape off the nematocysts with a razor. Applications of cold, in the form of an ice pack, and immesion in hot water have variously been shown to improve pain, but because of the self-limited nature of the discomfort it is hard to gauge an optimum therapy. Either is probably acceptable until the patient is comfortable. Meat tenderizer has been found to be ineffective. Local anesthetics, antihistamines, and steroids are all used to control prolonged symptoms based on anecdotal experience. Antibiotics are not generally necessary. In the rare cases of cardiovascular collapse, supportive care and principles of treatment of anaphylaxis should be followed. A delayed hypersensitivity reaction can occur 1 to 3 days out, which will almost certainly be self-limited and can be treated with oral antihistamines and topical steroids if symptoms are severe.

Sea bather's itch is a form of jellyfish sting caused by the larvae of the thimble jellyfish. It is characterized by a painful, itchy rash under the edges of the bathing suit or wet suit. It can occasionally progress to a popular rash. Topical steroids can be used to relieve symptoms.

Prevention

Prevention is mostly a matter of common sense. Staying away from the organism (the tentacles can extend several meters from the body of the organism) and staying out of the water when jellyfish are known to be present are the most effective. There is a commercially available product, (Safe Sea), which has been shown to reduce the number of nematocyst discharges and thus the severity of the sting should a swimmer need to be in the water when jellyfish are present. Wetsuits and other protective gear are ineffective.

ECHINODERMS

The Echinoderm family includes sea urchins. Urchins have toxin-coated spines that break off, leaving calcareous material in the wound, which can potentially cause infection. Symptoms include local pain, burning, and local discoloration. The discoloration is thought to be a temporary tattooing of the skin resulting from dye in the spines; absence of a spine is indicated if the discoloration spontaneously resolves within 48 hours. Theoretically, hot water disables the toxin, although there is no evidence in humans that it is effective. If a spine is present and easily accessible, it should be removed with fingers or forceps. If it is close to a joint or neurovascular structure it should be surgically removed. If the spines do not cause symptoms, retained pieces will likely reabsorb into the skin.

STINGRAYS

Although many fish are venomous, stingrays are the most clinically important, accounting for an estimated 1500 mostly minor injuries in the United States annually. These creatures partially bury themselves in the shallow, sandy bottom of the ocean, leading water enthusiasts to accidentally step on them or grab at what they think is a seashell.

Clinical Features

Stingrays have a spine at the base of their tail, which contains a venom gland. The spine, including the venom gland, is broken off and may be left in the resulting wound. The venom has vasoconstrictive properties that can lead to cyanosis and necrosis with poor wound healing and infection. Symptoms can include immediate and intense pain, salivation, nausea, vomiting, diarrhea, muscle cramps, dyspnea, seizures, headaches, and cardiac arrhythmias. Fatalities are rare and mostly a consequence of exsanguination at the scene or penetration of a vital organ.

Treatment

Home care should include rinsing the area thoroughly with fresh water if available (salt water if not) and removing any foreign body. If the damage is minimal the victim may soak the wound in warm water at home. The victim should watch for signs of infection and seek care for excessive bleeding, retained foreign body, or infection.

For severe wounds that lead the victim to seek medical attention, treatment should include achieving hemostasis followed by submersion of the affected region in hot but not scalding water (42-45°C, 108-113°F) for 30 to 90 minutes or until the pain resolves. Spines and stingers are typically radiopaque, so radiographs or an ultrasound should be obtained if a retained spine is suspected. The wound should be thoroughly cleansed, and delayed closure should be allowed. Tetanus immunization status should be reviewed and updated as appropriate. Surgical exploration may be necessary to remove residual foreign bodies. Prophylactic antibiotics are typically not necessary unless there is a residual foreign body or if the patient is immunosuppressed. If the wound becomes infected, Staphylococcus and Streptococcus species are the most common pathologic organisms. Unique to the marine environment are *Vibrio vulnificus* and *Mycobacterium marinum*, and antibiotic coverage should include coverage for all of these (Table 2).

OTHER VENOMOUS SEA CREATURES

Seasnakes are venomous creatures found most commonly in the Indo-Pacific area. Bites are uncommon (and envenomation is even less common), but should they occur, the toxin is very potent. The care is supportive. There is antivenom, which may be available in areas where the snakes are endemic.

Certain other fish and octopi have been associated with envenomation and occasional death. Most are tropical such as the stonefish, scorpionfish, and rabbitfish and the blue-ringed octopus. Certain varieties of catfish have venom as well. Envenomations, are rare and if they occur, treatment is based on good first-aid principles and antivenom where available (mostly in tropical areas).

Certain cone shells contain a toxin that can be fatal. This toxin is injected by the mollusk into the victim from a proboscis which it extends from the small end of the cone. Treatment is primarily supportive.

Trauma

Abrasions, bites, and lacerations are usually the result of a marine animal's instinct to protect itself against a perceived danger. The most commonly involved marine animals are octopi, sharks, moray eels, and barracuda. The trauma alone creates problems for patients but the trauma can be further complicated by envenomation. It is often difficult to identify the marine animal involved in the attack. Treatment is for the most part symptomatic, with local cleansing and topical dressing usually sufficing. If the wound becomes infected, antibiotics should cover common organisms (see Table 2).

ENVIRONMENTAL HAZARDS

Abrasions from the ambient environment are also common. These wounds should be thoroughly cleansed with soap and water and a topical antibiotic applied, because the wounds can contain toxins and are commonly contaminated with bacteria. Coral contains nematocysts and also has very sharp edges. Scuba divers in particular suffer

TABLE 2 Antibiotic Choices in Marine Injuries

Drug	Dosage Pediatric	Dosage Adult
Outpatient Management		
Ciprofloxacin (Cipro)	20-30 mg/kg/day PO × 14 d[1]	500 mg PO bid × 14 d
Levofloxin (Levaquin)		750 mg PO qd × 14 d
Doxycycline (Vibramycin, Doryx)	>8 y: 2.2 mg/kg PO qd × 14 d	100 mg bid × 14 d
Inpatient Management		
Preferred		
Ceftazidime (Fortaz, Tazicef) *plus*	150 mg/kg/d q8h	1 g IV q8h
PO or IV quinolone or doxycycline	150 mg/kg/d q8h	1 g IV q8h
Alternative		
Gentamicin *plus*	Typically based on institutional protocol and adjusted based on serum levels	Typically based on institutional protocol and adjusted based on serum levels
TMP-SMX (Bactrim, Cotrim, Septra)	8-10 mg/kg/d TMP	8-10 mg/kg (lean body mass)/d TMP

[1] Not FDA approved for this indication.
TMP-SMX = trimethoprim-sulfamethoxazole.

> **BOX 2 Management of Marine Trauma**
>
> Remove the victim from the water.
> Ensure airway control.
> Control bleeding.
> Do not remove the wet suit if the victim is wearing one.
> Attempt to identify the animal involved in the injury.
> If the injury is severe, transport the victim to a hospital.
> If envenomation is suspected, consider hot water immersion.
> Irrigate the wound with normal saline.
> Perform surgical débridement of the wound as appropriate.
> If sutures must be placed, place them loosely and allow drainage. Primary suturing should be avoided in puncture wounds, crush injuries, and wounds in the distal extremities.
> Start appropriate antibiotics if indicated.

from coral cuts in the course of their recreational diving. If these wounds become infected, coverage for *Vibrio* species should be included as well.

SHARKS

Although sharks attacks receive a lot of publicity, there are only around 50 such attacks worldwide annually and they result in fewer than 10 deaths. The majority of the deaths are in South Africa. Typically these attacks involve the tiger, great white, gray reef, and bull sharks. Attacks occur in shallow water within 100 feet of shore during the evening hours when sharks tend to feed. Common sense dictates avoiding areas where aggressive shark feeding has been noted.

Sequelae of a shark attack range from abrasions to death from hemorrhage. Abrasions and lacerations can occur when sharks brush or aggressively investigate humans. Soft tissue damage, fractures, and neurovascular damage result from such attacks. The majority of attacks result in minor injuries that require simple suturing. Morbidity increases in wounds that are greater than 20 cm or where more than one myofascial compartment is lost. General principles of first aid in marine animal injuries are found in Box 2. Although it would seem self-evident, practices such as urinating on the injury, applying oil or gasoline to injuries, and application of any strong oxidizing agents, such as strong bases or acids should be counseled against when doing patient education regarding self-care.

REFERENCES

Centers for Disease Control and Prevention: Management of *Vibrio vulnificus* wound infection. Available at http://www.bt.cdc.gov/disasters/hurricanes/katrina/vibriofaq.asp (accessed June 13, 2008).
Edmonds C: Marine animal injuries. In Bove AA (ed): Bove and Davis' Diving Medicine. 4th ed, Philadelphia. Saunders, 2004, pp 287-318.
Fleming LE: Ciguatera fish poisoning. Miami, FL: National Institute of Environmental Health Sciences, Marine and Freshwater Biomedical Sciences Center; 2006; available at http://www.rsmas.miami.edu/groups/niehs/science/ciguatera.htm (accessed June 14, 2008).
Isbister GK: Venomous fish stings in tropical northern Australia. Am J Emerg Med 2001;19:561-565.
Lahey T: Invasive *Mycobacterium marinum* infections. Emerg Infect Dis [serial online] 2003 November; Available at http://www.cdc.gov/ncidod/EID/vol9no11/03-0192.htm (accessed June 14, 2008).
Lehane L, Olley J: Histamine (scombroid) fish poisoning: A review in a risk-assessment framework. Canberra, Australia, National Office of Animal and Plant Health, 1999.
Lynch PR, Bove AA. Marine poisonings and intoxications. In Bove AA (ed): Bove and Davis' Diving Medicine. 4th ed. Philadelphia. Saunders, 2004, pp 287-318.
Nomura JT: A randomized paired comparison trial of cutaneous treatments for acute jellyfish (*Carybdea alata*) stings. Am J Emerg Med 2002; 20:624-626.
Perkins A, Morgan S: Poisonings, envenomations, and trauma from marine creatures. Am Fam Physician 2004;69:885-890.
Thomas C, Scott SA: All Stings Considered: First Aid and Medical Treatment of Hawaii's Marine Injuries. Honolulu. University of Hawaii Press, 1997.
Thomas CS, Scott SA, Galanis DJ, Goto RS: Box jellyfish *Carybdea alata* in Waikiki. The analgesic effect of Sting-Aid, Adolph's meat tenderizer and fresh water on their stings: A double-blinded, randomized, placebo-controlled clinical trial. Hawaii Med J 2001;60:205-210.
Thomas CS, Scott SA, Galanis DJ, Goto RS: Box jellyfish *Carybdea alata* in Waikiki. Their influx cycle plus the analgesic effect of hot and cold packs on their stings to swimmers at the beach: A randomized, placebo-controlled, clinical trial. Hawaii Med J 2001;60:100-107.

Medical Toxicology: Ingestions, Inhalations, and Dermal and Ocular Absorptions

Method of
Howard C. Mofenson, MD, Thomas R. Caraccio, PharmD, Michael McGuigan, MD, and Joseph Greensher, MD

Introduction and Epidemiology

According to the national Toxic Exposure Surveillance System (TESS), over 2.4 million potentially toxic exposures were reported last year to Poison Control Centers throughout the United States. Poisonings were responsible for 1183 deaths and more than 500,000 hospitalizations. Poisoning accounts for 2% to 5% of pediatric hospital admissions, 10% of adult admissions, 5% of hospital admissions in the elderly (>65 years of age), and 5% of ambulance calls. In one urban hospital, drug-related emergencies accounted for 38% of the emergency department visits. An evaluation of a medical intensive care unit and step-down unit over a 3-month period indicated that poisonings accounted for 19.7% of admissions.

The largest number of fatalities resulting from poisoning reported to the TESS are caused by analgesics. The other principal toxicologic causes of fatalities are antidepressants, sedative hypnotics/antipsychotics, stimulants/street drugs, cardiovascular agents, and alcohols. Less than 1% of overdose cases reaching the hospitals result in fatality. However, patients presenting in deep coma to medical care facilities have a fatality rate of 13% to 35%. The largest single cause of coma of inapparent etiology is drug poisoning.

Pharmaceutical preparations are involved in 50% of poisonings. The number one pharmaceutical agent involved in exposures is acetaminophen. The severity of the manifestations of acute poisoning exposures varies greatly depending on whether the poisoning was intentional or unintentional. Unintentional exposures make up 85% to 90% of all poisoning exposures. The majority of cases are acute, occurring in children younger than 5 years of age, in the home, and resulting in no or minor toxicity. Many are actually ingestions of relatively nontoxic substances that require minimal medical care. Intentional poisonings, such as suicides, constitute 10% to 15% of exposures and may require the highest standards of medical and nursing care and the use of sophisticated equipment for recovery. Intentional ingestions are often of multiple substances and frequently include ethanol, acetaminophen, and aspirin. Suicides make up 54% of the reported fatalities. About 25% of suicides are attempted with drugs. Sixty percent of patients who take a drug overdose use their own medication and 15% use drugs prescribed for close relatives.

The majority of the drug-related suicide attempts involve a central nervous system (CNS) depressant, and coma management is vital to the treatment.

Assessment and Maintenance of the Vital Functions

The initial assessment of all patients in medical emergencies follows the principles of basic and advanced cardiac life support. The adequacy of the patient's airway, degree of ventilation, and circulatory status should be determined. The vital functions should be established and maintained. Vital signs should be measured frequently and should include body core temperature. The assessment of vital functions should include the rate numbers (e.g., respiratory rate) and indications of effectiveness (e.g., depth of respirations and degree of gas exchange). Table 1 gives important measurements and vital signs.

Level of consciousness should be assessed by immediate AVPU (Alert, responds to Verbal stimuli, responds to Painful stimuli, and Unconscious). If the patient is unconscious, one must assess the severity of the unconsciousness by the Glasgow Coma Scale (Table 2).

If the patient is comatose, management requires administering 100% oxygen, establishing vascular access, and obtaining blood for pertinent laboratory studies. The administration of glucose, thiamine, and naloxone, as well as intubation to protect the airway, should be considered. Pertinent laboratory studies include arterial blood gases (ABG), electrocardiography (ECG), determination of blood glucose level, electrolytes, renal and liver tests, and acetaminophen plasma concentration in all cases of intentional ingestions. Radiography of the chest and abdomen may be useful. The severity of a stimulant's effects can also be assessed and should be documented to follow the trend.

The examiner should completely expose the patient by removing clothes and other items that interfere with a full evaluation. One should look for clues to etiology in the clothes and include the hat and shoes.

Prevention of Absorption and Reduction of Local Damage

EXPOSURE

Poisoning exposure routes include ingestion (76.8%), dermal (8%), ophthalmologic (5%), inhalation (6%), insect bites and stings (4%), and parenteral injections (0.5%). The effect of the toxin may be local, systemic, or both.

Local effects (skin, eyes, mucosa of respiratory or gastrointestinal tract) occur where contact is made with the poisonous substance. Local effects are nonspecific chemical reactions that depend on the chemical properties (e.g., pH), concentration, contact time, and type of exposed surface.

Systemic effects occur when the poison is absorbed into the body and depend on the dose, the distribution, and the functional reserve of the organ systems. Shock and hypoxia are part of systemic toxicity.

DELAYED TOXIC ACTION

Therapeutic doses of most pharmaceuticals are absorbed within 90 minutes. However, the patient with exposure to a potential toxin may be asymptomatic at this time because a sufficient amount has not yet been absorbed or metabolized to produce toxicity at the time the patient presents for care.

Absorption can be significantly delayed under the following circumstances:

1. Drugs with anticholinergic properties (e.g., antihistamines, belladonna alkaloids, diphenoxylate with atropine [Lomotil], phenothiazines, and tricyclic antidepressants).
2. Modified release preparations such as sustained-release, enteric-coated, and controlled-release formulations have delayed and prolonged absorption.
3. Concretions may form (e.g., salicylates, iron, glutethimide, and meprobamate [Equanil]) that can delay absorption and prolong the toxic effects. Large quantities of drugs tend to be absorbed more slowly than small quantities.

Some substances must be metabolized into a toxic metabolite (acetaminophen, acetonitrile, ethylene glycol, methanol, methylene chloride, parathion, and paraquat). In some cases, time is required to produce a toxic effect on organ systems (*Amanita phalloides* mushrooms, carbon tetrachloride, colchicine, digoxin [Lanoxin], heavy metals, monoamine oxidase inhibitors, and oral hypoglycemic agents).

Initial Management

1. Stabilization of airway, breathing, and circulation and protection of same.
2. Identification of specific toxin or toxic syndrome.
3. Initial treatment: D50W; consider thiamine, naloxone (Narcan), oxygen, and antidotes if needed.
4. Physical assessment.
5. Decontamination: Gastrointestinal tract, skin, eyes.

DECONTAMINATION

In the asymptomatic patient who has been exposed to a toxic substance, decontamination procedures should be considered if the patient has been exposed to potentially toxic substances in toxic amounts.

Ocular exposure should be immediately treated with water irrigation for 15 to 20 minutes with the eyelids fully retracted. One should not use neutralizing chemicals. All caustic and corrosive injuries should be evaluated with fluorescein dye and by an ophthalmologist.

Dermal exposure is treated immediately with copious water irrigation for 30 minutes, not a forceful flushing. Shampooing the hair, cleansing the fingernails, navel, and perineum, and irrigating the eyes are necessary in the case of an extensive exposure. The clothes should be specially bagged and may have to be discarded. Leather goods can become irreversibly contaminated and must be abandoned. Caustic (alkali) exposures can require hours of irrigation. Dermal absorption can occur with pesticides, hydrocarbons, and cyanide.

Injection exposures (e.g., snake envenomation) can be treated with venom extracts. Venom extractors can be used within minutes of envenomation, and proximal lymphatic constricting bands or elastic wraps can be used to delay lymphatic flow and immobilize the extremity. Cold packs and tourniquets should not be used and incision is generally not recommended. Substances of abuse may be injected intravenously or subcutaneously. In these cases, little decontamination can be done.

Inhalation exposure to toxic substances is managed by immediate removal of the victim from the contaminated environment by protected rescuers.

Gastrointestinal exposure is the most common route of poisoning. Gastrointestinal decontamination historically has been done by gastric emptying: induction of emesis, gastric lavage, administration of activated charcoal, and the use of cathartics or whole bowel irrigation. No procedure is routine; it should be individualized for each case. If no attempt is made to decontaminate the patient, the reason should be clearly documented on the medical record (e.g., time elapsed, past peak of action, ineffectiveness, or risk of procedure).

Gastric Emptying Procedures

The gastric emptying procedure used is influenced by the age of the patient, the effectiveness of the procedure, the time of ingestion (gastric emptying is usually ineffective after 1 hour postingestion), the patient's clinical status (time of peak effect has passed or the patient's condition is too unstable), formulation of the substance ingested (regular release versus modified release), the amount ingested, and

TABLE 1 Important Measurements and Vital Signs

Age	Body Surface Area (m²)	Weight (kg)	Height (cm)	Pulse (bpm) Resting	Hypotension	Hypertension Significant	Hypertension Severe	Respiratory Rate (rpm)
Newborn	0.19	3.5	50	70-190	<60/40	>96	>106	30-60
1 mo-6 mo	0.30	4-7	50-65	80-160	<70/45	>104	>110	30-50
6 mo-1 y	0.38	7-10	65-75	80-160	<70/45	>104	>110	20-40
1-2 y	0.50-0.55	10-12	75-85	80-140	<74/47	>112/74	>118/82	20-40
3-5 y	0.54-0.68	15-20	90-108	80-120	<80/52	>116/76	>124/84	20-40
6-9 y	0.68-0.85	20-28	122-133	75-115	<90/60	>122/82	>130/86	16-25
10-12 y	1.00-1.07	30-40	138-147	70-110	<90/60	>126/82	>134/90	16-25
13-15 y	1.07-1.22	42-50	152-160	60-100	<90/60	>136/86	>144/92	16-20
16-18 y	1.30-1.60	53-60	160-170	60-100	<90/60	>142/92	>150/98	12-16
Adult	1.40-1.70	60-70	160-170	60-100	<90/60	>140/90	>210/120	10-16

Data from Nadas A: Pediatric Cardiology, 3rd ed. Philadelphia, WB Saunders, 1976; Blumer JL (ed): A Practice Guide to Pediatric Intensive Care. St Louis, Mosby, 1990; AAP and ACEP: Respiratory Distress in APLS Pediatric Emergency Medicine Course, 1993; Second Task Force: Blood pressure control in children—1987, Pediatr 79:1, 1987; Linakis JG: Hypertension. In Fliesher GR, Ludwig S (eds); Textbook of Pediatric Emergency Medicine, 3rd ed. Baltimore, Williams & Wilkins, 1993.

TABLE 2 Glasgow Coma Scale

Scale	Adult Response	Score	Pediatric, 0-1 Years
Eye opening	Spontaneous	4	Spontaneous
	To verbal command	3	To shout
	To pain	2	To pain
	None	1	No response
Motor response			
To verbal command	Obeys	6	
To painful stimuli	Localized pain	5	Localized pain
	Flexion withdrawal	4	Flexion withdrawal
	Decorticate flexion	3	Decorticate flexion
	Decerebrate extension	2	Decerebrate flexion
	None	1	None
Verbal response: adult	Oriented and converses	5	Cries, smiles, coos
	Disoriented but converses	4	Cries or screams
	Inappropriate words	3	Inappropriate sounds
	Incomprehensible sounds	2	Grunts
	None	1	Gives no response
Verbal response: child	Oriented	5	
	Words or babbles	4	
	Vocal sounds	3	
	Cries or moans to stimuli	2	
	None	1	

Data from Teasdale G, Jennett B: Assessment of coma impaired consciousness. Lancet 2:83, 1974; Simpson D, Reilly P: Pediatric coma scale. Lancet 2:450, 1982; Seidel J: Preparing for pediatric emergencies. Pediatr Rev 16:470, 1995.

---

the rapidity of onset of CNS depression or stimulation (convulsions). Most studies show that only 30% (range, 19% to 62%) of the ingested toxin is removed by gastric emptying under optimal conditions. It has not been demonstrated that the choice of procedure improved the outcome.

A mnemonic for gathering information is STATS:

S—substance
T—type of formulation
A—amount and age
T—time of ingestion
S—signs and symptoms

The examiner should attempt to obtain AMPLE information about the patient:

A—age and allergies
M—available medications
P—past medical history including pregnancy, psychiatric illnesses, substance abuse, or intentional ingestions
L—time of last meal, which may influence absorption and the onset and peak action
E—events leading to present condition

The intent of the patient should also be determined.

The Regional Poison Center should be consulted for the exact ingredients of the ingested substance and the latest management. The treatment information on the labels of products and in the Physician's Desk Reference are notoriously inaccurate.

Ipecac Syrup

Syrup of ipecac–induced emesis has virtually no use in the emergency department. Although at one time it was considered most useful in young children with a recent witnessed ingestion, it is no longer advised in most cases. Current guidelines from the American Association of Poison Control Centers have significantly limited the indications for inducing emesis because the risk most often exceeds the benefit derived from this procedure. The Poison Control Center should be called if inducting emesis is being considered.

Contraindications or situations in which induction of emesis is inappropriate include the following:

- Ingestion of caustic substance
- Loss of airway protective reflexes because of ingestion of substances that can produce rapid onset of CNS depression (e.g., short-acting benzodiazepines, barbiturates, nonbarbiturate sedative-hypnotics, opioids, tricyclic antidepressants) or convulsions (e.g., camphor [Ponstel], chloroquine [Aralen], codeine, isoniazid [Nydrazid], mefenamic acid, nicotine, propoxyphene [Darvon], organophosphate insecticides, strychnine, and tricyclic antidepressants)
- Ingestion of low-viscosity petroleum distillates (e.g., gasoline, lighter fluid, kerosene)
- Significant vomiting prior to presentation or hematemesis
- Age under 6 months (no established dose, safety, or efficacy data)
- Ingestion of foreign bodies (emesis is ineffective and may lead to aspiration)
- Clinical conditions including neurologic impairment, hemodynamic instability, increased intracranial pressure, and hypertension
- Delay in presentation (more than 1 hour postingestion)

The dose of syrup of ipecac in the 6- to 9-month-old infant is 5 mL; in the 9- to 12-month-old, 10 mL; and in the 1- to 12-year-old, 15 mL. In children older than 12 years and in adults, the dose is 30 mL. The dose can be repeated once if the child does not vomit in 15 to 20 minutes. The vomitus should be inspected for remnants of pills or toxic substances, and the appearance and odor should be documented. When ipecac is not available, 30 mL of mild dishwashing soap (not dishwasher detergent) can be used, although it is less effective.

Complications are very rare but include aspiration, protracted vomiting, rarely cardiac toxicity with long-term abuse, pneumothorax, gastric rupture, diaphragmatic hernia, intracranial hemorrhage, and Mallory-Weiss tears.

Gastric Lavage

Gastric lavage should be considered only when life-threatening amounts of substances were involved, when the benefits outweigh the risks, when it can be performed within 1 hour of the ingestion, and when no contraindications exist.

The contraindications are similar to those for ipecac-induced emesis. However, gastric lavage can be accomplished after the insertion of an endotracheal tube in cases of CNS depression or controlled convulsions. The patient should be placed with the head lower than the hips in a left-lateral decubitus position. The location of the tube should be confirmed by radiography, if necessary, and suctioning equipment should be available.

Contraindications to gastric lavage include the following:

- Ingestion of caustic substances (risk of esophageal perforation)
- Uncontrolled convulsions, because of the danger of aspiration and injury during the procedure
- Ingestion of low-viscosity petroleum distillate products
- CNS depression or absent protective airway reflexes, without endotracheal protection
- Significant cardiac dysrhythmias
- Significant emesis or hematemesis prior to presentation
- Delay in presentation (more than 1 hour postingestion)

Size of Tube

The best results with gastric lavage are obtained with the largest possible orogastric tube that can be reasonably passed (nasogastric tubes are not large enough to remove solid material). In adults, a large-bore orogastric Lavacuator hose or a No. 42 French Ewald tube should be used; in young children, orogastric tubes are generally too small to remove solid material and gastric lavage is not recommended.

The amount of fluid used varies with the patient's age and size. In general, aliquots of 50 to 100 mL per lavage are used in adults. Larger amounts of fluid may force the toxin past the pylorus. Lavage fluid is 0.9% saline.

Complications are rare and may include respiratory depression, aspiration pneumonitis, cardiac dysrhythmias as a result of increased vagal tone, esophageal-gastric tears and perforation, laryngospasm, and mediastinitis.

Activated Charcoal

Oral activated charcoal adsorbs the toxin onto its surface before absorption. According to recent guidelines set forth by the American Academy of Clinical Toxicology, activated charcoal should not be used routinely. Its use is indicated only if a toxic amount of substance has been ingested and is optimally effective within 1 hour of the ingestion. Because of the slow absorption of large quantities of toxin, activated charcoal may be beneficial after 1 hour postingestion.

Activated charcoal does not effectively adsorb small molecules or molecules lacking carbon (Table 3). Activated charcoal adsorption may be diminished by milk, cocoa powder, and ice cream.

There are a few relative contraindications to the use of activated charcoal:

1. Ingestion of caustics and corrosives, which may produce vomiting or cling to the mucosa and falsely appear as a burn on endoscopy.
2. Comatose patient, in whom the airway must be secured prior to activated charcoal administration.
3. Patient without presence of bowel sounds.

Note: Activated charcoal was shown not to interfere with effectiveness of *N*-acetylcysteine in cases of acetaminophen overdose, so it is no longer contraindicated as was thought in the past.

TABLE 3 Substances Poorly Adsorbed by Activated Charcoal

C	Caustics and corrosives
H	Heavy metals (arsenic, iron, lead, mercury)
A	Alcohols (ethanol, methanol, isopropanol) and glycols (ethylene glycols)
R	Rapid onset of absorption (cyanide and strychnine)
C	Chlorine and iodine
O	Others insoluble in water (substances in tablet form)
A	Aliphatic hydrocarbons (petroleum distillates)
L	Laxatives (sodium, magnesium, potassium, and lithium)

The usual initial adult dose is 60 to 100 g and the dose for children is 15 to 30 g. It is administered orally as a slurry mixed with water or by nasogastric or orogastric tube. *Caution:* Be sure the tube is in the stomach. Cathartics are not necessary.

Although repeated dosing with activated charcoal may decrease the half-life and increases the clearance of phenobarbital, dapsone, quinidine, theophylline, and carbamazepine (Tegretol), recent guidelines indicate there is insufficient evidence to support the use of multiple-dose activated charcoal unless a life-threatening amount of one of the substances mentioned is involved. At present there are no controlled studies that demonstrate that multiple-dose activated charcoal or cathartics alter the clinical course of an intoxication. The dose varies from 0.25 to 0.50 g/kg every 1 to 4 hours, and continuous nasogastric tube infusion of 0.25 to 0.5 g/kg/h has been used to decrease vomiting.

Gastrointestinal dialysis is the diffusion of the toxin from the higher concentration in the serum of the mesenteric vessels to the lower levels in the gastrointestinal tract mucosal cell and subsequently into the gastrointestinal lumen, where the concentration has been lowered by intraluminal adsorption of activated charcoal.

Complications of treatment with activated charcoal include vomiting in 50% of cases, desorption (especially with weak acids in intestine), and aspiration (at least a dozen cases of aspiration have been reported). There are many cases of unreported pulmonary aspirations and "charcoal lungs," intestinal obstruction or pseudoobstruction (three case reports with multiple dosing, none with a single dose), empyema following esophageal perforation, and hypermagnesemia and hypernatremia, which have been associated with repeated concurrent doses of activated charcoal and saline cathartics. Catharsis was used to hasten the elimination of any remaining toxin in the gastrointestinal tract. There are no studies to demonstrate the effectiveness of cathartics, and they are no longer recommended as a form of gastrointestinal decontamination.

Whole-Bowel Irrigation

With whole bowel irrigation, solutions of polyethylene glycol (PEG) with balanced electrolytes are used to cleanse the bowel without causing shifts in fluids and electrolytes. The procedure is not approved by the U.S. Food and Drug Administration for this purpose.

Indications

The procedure has been studied and used successfully in cases of iron overdose when abdominal radiographs reveal incomplete emptying of excess iron. There are additional indications for other types of ingestions, such as with body-packing of illicit drugs (e.g., cocaine, heroin).

The procedure is to administer the solution (GoLYTELY or Colyte), orally or by nasogastric tube, in a dose of 0.5 L per hour in children younger than 5 years of age and 2 L per hour in adolescents and adults for 5 hours. The end point is reached when the rectal effluent is clear or radiopaque materials can no longer be seen in the gastrointestinal tract on abdominal radiographs.

Contraindications

These measures should not be used if there is extensive hematemesis, ileus, or signs of bowel obstruction, perforation, or peritonitis. Animal experiments in which PEG was added to activated charcoal indicated that activated charcoal-salicylates and activated charcoal-theophylline combinations resulted in decreased adsorption and desorption of salicylate and theophylline and no therapeutic benefit over activated charcoal alone. Polyethylene solutions are bound by activated charcoal in vitro, decreasing the efficacy of activated charcoal.

Dilutional treatment is indicated for the immediate management of caustic and corrosive poisonings but is otherwise not useful. The administration of diluting fluid above 30 mL in children and 250 mL in adults may produce vomiting, reexposing the vital tissues to the effects of local damage and possible aspiration.

Neutralization is not proven to be either safe or effective.

Endoscopy and surgery have been required in the case of body-packer obstruction, intestinal ischemia produced by cocaine ingestion, and iron local caustic action.

Differential Diagnosis of Poisons on the Basis of Central Nervous System Manifestations

Neurologic parameters help to classify and assess the need for supportive treatment as well as provide diagnostic clues to the etiology. Table 4 lists the effects of CNS depressants, CNS stimulants, hallucinogens, and autonomic nervous system anticholinergics and cholinergics.

Central nervous system depressants are cholinergics, opioids, sedative-hypnotics, and sympatholytic agents. The hallmarks are lethargy, sedation, stupor, and coma. In exception to the manifestations listed in Table 4, (a) barbiturates may produce an initial tachycardia; (b) convulsions are produced by codeine, propoxyphene (Darvon), meperidine (Demerol), glutethimide, phenothiazines, methaqualone, and tricyclic and cyclic antidepressants; (c) benzodiazepines rarely produce coma that will interfere with cardiorespiratory functions; and (d) pulmonary edema is common with opioids and sedative-hypnotics.

The CNS stimulants are anticholinergic, hallucinogenic, sympathomimetic, and withdrawal agents. The hallmarks of CNS stimulants are convulsions and hyperactivity.

There is considerable overlapping of effects among the various hallucinogens, but the major hallmark manifestation is hallucinations.

Guidelines for In-hospital Disposition

Classification of patients as high risk depends on clinical judgment. Any patient who needs cardiorespiratory support or has a persistently altered mental status for 3 hours or more should be considered for intensive care.

Guidelines for admitting patients older than 14 years of age to an intensive care unit, after 2 to 3 hours in the emergency department, include the following:

1. Need for intubation
2. Seizures
3. Unresponsiveness to verbal stimuli
4. Arterial carbon dioxide pressure greater than 45 mm Hg
5. Cardiac conduction or rhythm disturbances (any rhythm except sinus arrhythmia)
6. Close monitoring of vital signs during antidotal therapy or elimination procedures
7. The need for continuous monitoring
8. QRS interval greater than 0.10 second, in cases of tricyclic antidepressant poisoning
9. Systolic blood pressure less than 80 mm Hg
10. Hypoxia, hypercarbia, acid–base imbalance, or metabolic abnormalities
11. Extremes of temperature
12. Progressive deterioration or significant underlying medical disorders

Use of Antidotes

Antidotes are available for only a relatively small number of poisons. An antidote is not a substitute for good supportive care. Table 5 summarizes the commonly used antidotes, their indications, and their methods of administration. The Regional Poison Control Center can give further information on these antidotes.

Enhancement of Elimination

The acceptable methods for elimination of absorbed toxic substances are dialysis, hemoperfusion, exchange transfusion, plasmapheresis, enzyme induction, and inhibition. Methods of increasing urinary excretion of toxic chemicals and drugs have been studied extensively, but the other modalities have not been well evaluated.

In general, these methods are needed in only a minority of cases and should be reserved for life-threatening circumstances when a definite benefit is anticipated.

DIALYSIS

Dialysis is the extrarenal means of removing certain substances from the body, and it can substitute for the kidney when renal failure occurs. Dialysis is not the first measure instituted; however, it may be lifesaving later in the course of a severe intoxication. It is needed in only a minority of intoxicated patients.

Peritoneal dialysis uses the peritoneum as the membrane for dialysis. It is only 1/20 as effective as hemodialysis. It is easier to use and less hazardous to the patient but also less effective in removing the toxin; thus it is rarely used except in small infants.

Hemodialysis is the most effective dialysis method but requires experience with sophisticated equipment. Blood is circulated past a semipermeable extracorporeal membrane. Substances are removed by diffusion down a concentration gradient. Anticoagulation with heparin is necessary. Flow rates of 300 to 500 mL/min can be achieved, and clearance rates may reach 200 or 300 mL/min.

Dialyzable substances easily diffuse across the dialysis membrane and have the following characteristics: (a) a molecular weight less than 500 daltons and preferably less than 350; (b) a volume of distribution less than 1 L/kg; (c) protein binding less than 50%; (d) high water solubility (low lipid solubility); and (e) high plasma concentration and a toxicity that correlates reasonably with the plasma concentration. Considerations for hemodialysis and hemoperfusion are cases of serious ingestions (the nephrologist should be notified immediately), and cases involving a compound that is ingested in a potentially lethal dose and the rapid removal of which may improve the prognosis. Examples of the latter are ethylene glycol 1.4 mL/kg 100% solution or equivalent and methanol 6 mL/kg 100% solution or equivalent. Common dialyzable substances include alcohol, bromides, lithium, and salicylates.

The patient-related criteria for dialysis are (a) anticipated prolonged coma and the likelihood of complications; (b) renal compromise (toxin excreted or metabolized by kidneys and dialyzable chelating agents in heavy metal poisoning); (c) laboratory confirmation of lethal blood concentration; (d) lethal dose poisoning with an agent with delayed toxicity or known to be metabolized into a more toxic metabolite (e.g., ethylene glycol, methanol); and (e) hepatic impairment when the agent is metabolized by the liver, and clinical deterioration despite optimal supportive medical management. Table 6 gives plasma concentrations above which removal by extracorporeal measures should be considered.

The contraindications to hemodialysis include the following: (a) substances are not dialyzable; (b) effective antidotes are available; (c) patient is hemodynamically unstable (e.g., shock); and (d) presence of coagulopathy because heparinization is required.

Hemodialysis also has a role in correcting disturbances that are not amenable to appropriate medical management. These are easily remembered by the "vowel" mnemonic:

A—refractory acid–base disturbances
E—refractory electrolyte disturbances
I—intoxication with dialyzable substances (e.g., ethanol, ethylene glycol, isopropyl alcohol, methanol, lithium, and salicylates)
O—overhydration
U—uremia

Complications of dialysis include hemorrhage, thrombosis, air embolism, hypotension, infections, electrolyte imbalance, thrombocytopenia, and removal of therapeutic medications.

TABLE 4 Agents with Central Nervous System (CNS) Effects

Agents	General Manifestations	Agents	General Manifestations
CNS Depressants Alcohols and glycols (S-H) Anticonvulsants (S-H) Antidysrhythmics (S-H) Antihypertensives (S-H) Barbiturates (S-H) Benzodiazepines (S-H) Butyrophenones (Syly) β-Adrenergic blockers (Syly) Calcium channel blockers (Syly) Digitalis (Syly) Opioids Lithium (mixed) Muscle relaxants Phenothiazines (Syly) Nonbarbiturate/benzodiazepine glutethimide, methaqualone, methyprylon, sedative-hypnotics (chloral hydrate, ethchlorvynol, bromide) Tricyclic antidepressants (late Syly)	Bradycardia Bradypnea Shallow respirations Hypotension Hypothermia Flaccid coma Miosis Hypoactive bowel sounds	**Hallucinogens** Amphetamines[‡] Anticholinergics Cardiac glycosides Cocaine Ethanol withdrawal Hydrocarbon inhalation (abuse) Mescaline (peyote) Mushrooms (psilocybin) Phencyclidine	Tachycardia and dysrhythmias Tachypnea Hypertension Hallucinations, usually visual Disorientation Panic reaction Toxic psychosis Moist skin Mydriasis (reactive) Hyperthermia Flashbacks
		Anticholinergics Antihistamines Antispasmodic gastrointestinal preparations Antiparkinsonian preparations Atropine Cyclobenzaprine (Flexeril) Mydriatic ophthalmologic agents Over-the-counter sleep agents Plants (Datura spp/mushrooms Phenothiazines (early) Scopolamine Tricyclic/cyclic antidepressants (early)	Tachycardia, dysrhythmias (rare) Tachypnea Hypertension (mild) Hyperthermia Hallucinations ("mad as a hatter") Mydriasis (unreactive) ("blind as a bat") Flushed skin ("red as a beet") Dry skin and mouth ("dry as a bone") Hypoactive bowel sounds Urinary retention Lilliputian hallucinations ("little people")
CNS Stimulants Amphetamines (Sy) Anticholinergics* Cocaine (Sy) Camphor (mixed) Ergot alkaloids (Sy) Isoniazid (mixed) Lithium (mixed) Lysergic acid diethylamide (H) Hallucinogens (H) Mescaline and synthetic analogs Metals (arsenic, lead, mercury) Methylphenidate (Ritalin) (Sy) Monoamine oxidase inhibitors (Sy) Pemoline (Cylert) (Sy) Phencyclidine (H)[†] Salicylates (mixed) Strychnine (mixed) Sympathomimetics (Sy) (phenylpropanolamine, theophylline, caffeine, thyroid) Withdrawal from ethanol, β-adrenergic blockers, clonidine, opioids, sedative-hypnotics (W)	Tachycardia Tachypnea and dysrhythmias Hypertension Convulsions Toxic psychosis Mydriasis (reactive) Agitation and restlessness Moist skin Tremors	**Cholinergics** Bethanechol (Urecholine) Carbamate insecticides (Carbaryl) Edrophonium Organophosphate insecticides (Malathion, parathion) Parasympathetic agents (physostigmine, pyridostigmine) Toxic mushrooms (Clitocybe spp.)	Bradycardia (muscarinic) Tachycardia (nicotinic effect) Miosis (muscarinic) Diarrhea (muscarinic) Hypertension (variable) Hyperactive bowel sounds Excess urination (muscarinic) Excess salivation (muscarinic) Lacrimation (muscarinic) Bronchospasm (muscarinic) Muscle fasciculations (nicotinic) Paralysis (nicotinic)

Abbreviations: H = hallucinogen; S-H = sedative–hypnotic; Sy = sympathomimetic; Syly = Sympatholytic; W = withdrawal.

*Anticholinergics produce dry skin and mucosa and decreased bowel sounds.

[†]Phencyclidine may produce miosis.

[‡]The amphetamine hybrids are methylene dioxymethamphetamine (MDMA, ecstasy, "ADAM"), methylene dioxyamphetamine (MDA, "Eve"), which are associated with deaths.

TABLE 5 Initial Doses of Antidotes for Common Poisonings

Antidote	Use	Dose	Route	Adverse Reactions/Comments
N-Acetyl Cysteine (NAC, Mucomyst): Stock level to treat 70 kg adult for 24 h: 25 vials, 20%, 30 mL	Acetaminophen, carbon tetrachloride (experimental)	140/mg/kg loading, followed by 70 mg/kg every 4 h for 17 doses.	PO	Nausea, vomiting. Dilute to 5% with sweet juice or flat cola. useful for those who cannot tolerate oral route
Atropine: Stock level to treat 70 kg adult for 24 h: 1 g (1 mg/mL in 1, 10 mL)	Organophosphate and carbamate pesticides: bradydysrhythmics, β-adrenergics, calcium channel blockers/nerve agents	150 mg/kg in 200 mL of D_5W over 1hr, then 50 mg/kg in 1 liter D_5W over 16 hrs Child: 0.02-0.05 mg/kg repeated q5-10 min to max of 2 mg as necessary until cessation of secretions Adult: 1-2 mg q5-10 min as necessary. Dilute in 1-2 mL of 0.9% saline for ET instillation. IV infusion dose: Place 8 mg of atropine in 100 mL D_5W or saline. Conc. = 0.08 mg/mL; dose range = 0.02-0.08 mg/kg/h or 0.25-1 mL/kg/h. Severe poisoning may require supplemental doses of IV atropine intermittently in doses of 1-5 mg until drying of secretions occurs.	IV IV/ET	Tachycardia, dry mouth, blurred vision, and urinary retention. Ensure adequate ventilation before administration.
Calcium Chloride (10%): Stock level to treat 70 kg adult for 24 h: 10 vials 1 g (1.35 mEq/mL)	Hypocalcemia, fluoride, calcium channel blockers, β-blockers, oxalates, ethylene glycol, hypermagnesemia	0.1-0.2 mL/kg (10-20 mg/kg) slow push every 10 min up to max 10 mL (1 g). Since calcium response lasts 15 minutes, some may require continuous infusion 0.2 mL/kg/h up to maximum of 10 mL/h while monitoring for dysrhythmias and hypotension.	IV	Administer slowly with BP and ECG monitoring and have magnesium available to reverse calcium effects. Tissue irritation, hypotension, dysrhythmias from rapid injection. Contraindications: digitalis glycoside intoxication.
Calcium Gluconate (10%): Stock level to treat 70 kg adult for 24 h: 20 vials 1 g (0.45 mEq/mL)	Hypocalcemia, fluoride, calcium channel blockers, hydrofluoric acid; black widow envenomation	0.3-0.4 mL/kg (30-40 mg/kg) slow push; repeat as needed up to max dose 10-20 mL (1-2 g).	IV	Same comments as calcium chloride.
Infiltration of Calcium Gluconate	Hydrofluoric acid skin exposure	Dose: Infiltrate each square cm of affected dermis/subcutaneous tissue with about 0.5 mL of 10% calcium gluconate using a 30-gauge needle. Repeat as needed to control pain.	Infiltrate	
Intra-arterial Calcium Gluconate	Hydrofluoric acid skin exposure	Infuse 20 mL of 10% calcium gluconate (not chloride) diluted in 250 mL D_5W via the radial or brachial artery proximal to the injury over 3-4 hours.		Alternatively, dilute 10 mL of 10% calcium gluconate with 40-50 mL of D_5W.
Calcium Gluconate Gel: Stock level: 3.5 g	Hydrofluoric acid skin exposure	2.5 g USP powder added to 100 mL water-soluble lubricating jelly, e.g., K-Y Jelly or Lubifax (or 3.5 mg into 150 mL). Some use 6 g of calcium carbonate in 100 g of lubricant. Place injured hand in surgical glove filled with gel. Apply q4h. If pain persists, calcium gluconate injection may be needed (above).	Dermal	Powder is available from Spectrum Pharmaceutical Co. in California: 800-772-8786. Commercial preparation of Ca gluconate gel is available from Pharmascience in Montreal, Quebec: 514-340-1114.

Continued

TABLE 5 Initial Doses of Antidotes for Common Poisonings—cont'd

Antidote	Use	Dose	Route	Adverse Reactions/Comments
Cyanide Antidote Kit: Stock level to treat 70 kg adult for 24 h: 2 Lilly Cyanide Antidote kits	Cyanide Hydrogen sulfide (nitrites are given only) Do not use sodium thiosulfate for hydrogen sulfide Individual portions of the kit can be used in certain circumstances (consult PCC)	Amyl nitrite: 1 crushable ampule for 30 secs of every min. Use new amp q3 min. May omit step if venous access is established.	Inhalation	If methemoglobinemia occurs, do not use methylene blue to correct this because it releases cyanide.
	Cyanide Hydrogen sulfide (nitrites are given only) Do not use sodium thiosulfate for hydrogen sulfide Individual portions of the kit can be used in certain circumstances (consult PCC)	Sodium nitrite: *Child:* 0.33 mL/kg of 3% solution if hemoglobin level is not known, otherwise based on tables with product. *Adult:* up to 300 mg (10 mL). Dilute nitrite in 100 mL 0.9% saline, administer slowly at 5 mL/min. Slow infusion if fall in BP.	IV	If methemoglobinemia occurs, do not use methylene blue to correct this because it releases cyanide.
	Do not use sodium thiosulfate for hydrogen sulfide Individual portions of the Kit can be used in certain circumstances (consult PCC)	Sodium thiosulfate: *Child:* 1.6 mL/kg of 25% solution, may be repeated every 30-60 min to a maximum of 12.5 g or 50 mL in adult. Administer over 20 min.	IV	Nausea, dizziness, headache. Tachycardia, muscle rigidity, and bronchospasm (rapid administration).
Dantrolene Sodium (Dantrium): Stock level to treat 70 kg adult for 24 h: 700 mg, 35 vials (20 mg/vial)	Malignant hyperthermia	2–3 mg/kg IV rapidly. Repeat loading dose every 10 minutes, if necessary up to a maximum total dose of 10 mg/kg. When temperature and heart rate decrease, slow the infusion 1-2 mg/kg every 6 hours for 24-28 h until all evidence of malignant hyperthermia syndrome has subsided. Follow with oral doses 1-2 mg/kg four times a day for 24 h as necessary.	IV/PO	Hepatotoxicity occurs with cumulative dose of 10 mg/kg. Thrombophlebitis (best given in central line). Available as 20 mg lyophilized dantrolene powder for reconstruction, which contains 3 g mannitol and sodium hydroxide in 70-mL vial. Mix with 60 mL sterile distilled water without a bacteriostatic agent and protect from light. Use within 6 hours after reconstituting.
Deferoxamine (Desferal): Stock level to treat 70 kg adult for 24 h: 17 vials (500 mg/amp)	Iron	IV infusion of 15 mg/kg/h (3 mL/kg/h: 500 mg in 100 mL D_5 W) max 6 g/d Rates of >45 µg/kg/h if conc >1000 µg/dL.	Preferred IV: avoid therapy >24 h	Hypotension (minimized by avoiding rapid infusion rates) DFO challenge test 50 mg/kg is unreliable if negative.
Diazepam (Valium): Stock level to treat 70 kg adult for 24 h: 200 mg, 5 mg/mL; 2,10 mL	Any intoxication that provokes seizures when specific therapy is not available, e.g., amphetamines, PCP, barbiturate and alcohol withdrawal.	Adult, 5-10 mg IV (max 20 mg) at a rate of 5 mg/min until seizure is controlled. May be repeated 2 or 3 times. Child, 0.1-0.3 mg/kg up to 10 mg IV slowly over 2 min.	IV	Confusion, somnolence, coma, hypotension. Intramuscular absorption is erratic Establish airway and administer 100% oxygen and glucose.
Digoxin-Specific Fab Antibodies (Digibind): Stock level to treat 70 kg adult for 24 h: 20 vials.	Chloroquine poisoning. Digoxin, digitoxin, oleander tea with the following: (1) Imminent cardiac arrest or shock, (2) hyperkalemia >5.0 mEq/L. (3) serum digoxin >5 ng/mL (child) at 8-12 h post ingestion in adults, (4) digitalis delirium, (5) ingestion over 10 mg in adults or 4 mg in child,	(1) If amount ingested is known total dose × bioavailability (0.8) = body burden. The body burden + 0.6 (0.5 mg of digoxin is bound by 1 vial of 38 mg of FAB) = # vials needed. (2) If amount is unknown but the steady state serum concentration is known in ng/mL: Digoxin: ng/mL: (5.6 L/kg Vd) × (wt kg) = µg body burden.	IV	Allergic reactions (rare), return of condition being treated with digitalis glycoside. Administer by infusion over 30 min through a 0.22-µ filter. If cardiac arrest imminent, may administer by bolus. Consult PCC for more details.

	(6) bradycardia or second- or third-degree heart block unresponsive to atropine, (7) life threatening digitoxin or oleander posioning.	Body burden ÷ 100 = mg body burden/ 0.5 = # vials needed. Digitoxin body burden = ng/mL × (0.56 L/kg Vd) × (wt kg) Body burden ÷ 1000 = mg body burden/ 0.5 = # vials needed. (3) If the amount is not known, it is administered in life-threatening situations as 10 vials (400 mg) IV in saline over 30 min in adults. If cardiac arrest is imminent, administer 20 vials (adult) as a bolus.	
Dimercaprol (BAL in Peanut Oil): Stock level to treat 70 kg adult for 24 h: 1200 mg (4 amps—100 mg/mL 10% in oil in 3 mL amp)	Chelating agent for arsenic, mercury, and lead.	3-5 mg/kg q4th usually for 5-10 d	Deep IM	Local infection site pain and sterile abscess, nausea, vomiting, fever, salivation, hypertension, and nephrotoxicity (alkalinize urine).
2,3 Dimercaptosuccinic Acid (DMSA Succimer): 100 mg/capsule: 20 capsules	Used as a chelating agent for lead, especially blood lead levels >45 μg/dL. May also be used for symptomatic mercury exposure	10 mg/kg 3 × daily for 5 days followed by 10 mg/kg 2 × daily for 14 days.	PO	Precautions: monitor AST/ALT; use with caution in G6PD-deficient patients. Avoid concurrent iron therapy. Relatively safe antidote, rarely severe, uncommon minor skin rashes may occur.
Diphenhydramine (Benadryl): Antiparkinsonian action. Stock level to treat a 70 kg adult for 24 h: 5 vials (10 mg/mL, 10 mL each)	Used to treat extrapyramidal symptoms and dystonia induced by phenothiazines, phencyclidine, and related drugs.	*Children:* 1-2 mg/kg IV slowly over 5 minutes up to maximum 50 mg followed by 5 mg/kg/24 h orally divided every 6 hours up to 300 mg/24h *Adults:* 50 mg IV followed by 50 mg orally four times daily for 5-7 days Note: Symptoms abate within 2-5 min after IV.	IV	Fatal dose: 20-40 mg/kg. Dry mouth, drowsiness.
Ethanol (Ethyl Alcohol): Stock level to treat 70 kg adult for 24 h: 3 bottles 10% (1 L each)	Methanol, ethylene glycol	10 mL/kg loading dose concurrently with 1.4 mL/kg (average) infusion of 10% ethanol (consult PCC for more details)	IV	Nausea, vomiting, sedation. Use 0.22 μm filter if preparing from bulk 100% ethanol.
Flumazenil (Romazicon): Stock level to treat 70 kg adult for 24 h: 4 vials (0.1 mg/mL, 10 mL)	Benzodiazepines (may also be beneficial in the treatment of hepatic encephalopathy)	Administer 0.2 mg (2 mL) IV over 30 sec (pediatric dose not established, 0.01 mg/kg), then wait 3 min for a response, then if desired consciousness is not achieved, administer 0.3 mg (3 mL) over 30 sec, then wait 3 min for response, then if desired consciousness is not achieved, administer 0.5 mg (5 mL) over 30 sec at 60-sec intervals up to a maximum cumulative dose of 3 mg (30 mL) (1 mg in children). Because effects last only 1-5 hours, if patient responds monitor carefully over next 6 hours for resedation. If multiple repeated doses, consider a continuous infusion of 0.2-1 mg/h.	IV	Nausea, vomiting, facial flushing, agitation, headache, dizziness, seizures, and death. It is not recommended to improve ventilation. Its role in CNS depression needs to be clarified. It should not be used routinely in comatose patients. It is **contraindicated** in cyclic antidepressant intoxications, stimulant overdose, long-term benzodiazepine use (may precipitate life-threatening withdrawal), if benzodiazepines are used to control seizures, in head trauma.
Folic Acid (Folvite): Stock level to treat 70 kg adult for 24 h: 4 100-mg vials	Methanol/ethylene glycol (investigational)	1 mg/kg up to 50 mg q4h for 6 doses.	IV	Uncommon

Continued

Medical Toxicology

1169

TABLE 5 Initial Doses of Antidotes for Common Poisonings—cont'd

Antidote	Use	Dose	Route	Adverse Reactions/Comments
Fomepizole (4-MP, Antizol): Stock level to treat 70 kg adult for 24 h: 4 1.5-mL vials (1 g/mL)	Ethylene glycol Methanol	Loading dose: 15 mg/kg (0.015 mL/kg) IV followed by maintenance dose of 10 mg/kg (0.01 mL/kg) every 12h for 4 doses; then 15 mg/kg every 12h until ethylene glycol levels are <20 mg/dL. Fomipazole can be given to patients undergoing hemodialysis (dose q4h).	IV	Suggested: co-administer folate 50 mg IV (child 1 mg/kg), thiamine 100 mg/d (child 50 mg), and pyridoxine 50 mg IV/IM q6h until intoxication is resolved. Monitor for urinary oxalate crystals. Adverse reactions include headache, nausea, and dizziness. Antizole should be diluted in 100 mL 0.9% saline or D_5W and mixed well. Antizole should not be given undiluted.
Glucagon: Stock level to treat 70 kg adult for 24 h: (10 vials, 10 units)	β-Blocker, calcium channel blocker	3-10 mg in adult, then infuse 2-5 mg/h (0.05-0.1 mg/kg in child, then infuse 0.07 mg/kg/h) Large doses up to 100 mg/24h used	IV	Use D_5W, not 0.9% saline, to reconstitute the glucagon (rather than diluent of Eli Lilly, which contains phenol).
Magnesium Sulfate: Stock level to treat 70 kg adult for 24 h: approx 25 g (50 mL of 50% or 200 mL of 12.5%)	Torsades de pointes	Adult: 2 g (20 mL or 20%) over 20 min. If no response in 10 min, repeat and follow by continuous infusion 1 g/h. Children: 25-50 mg/kg initially and maintenance is (30-60 mg/kg/24h) (0.25-0.5 mEq/kg/24h) up to 1000 mg/24h. (Dose not studied in controlled fashion.)	IV	Vomiting precautions. Use with caution if renal impairment is present.
Methylene Blue: Stock level to treat 70 kg adult for 24 h: 5 amps (10 mg/10 mL)	Methemoglobinemia	0.1-0.2 mL/kg of 1% solution, slow infusion, may be repeated every 30-60 min	IV	Nausea, vomiting, headache, dizziness.
Naloxone (Narcan): Stock level to treat 70 kg adult for 24 h: 3 vials (1 mg/mL, 10 mL)	Comatose patient; decreased respirations <12; opioids	In postoperative opioid depression reversal, IV 0.1-0.5 µg/kg every 2 min as needed and may repeat up to a total dose of 1 µg/kg. In **suspected overdose**, administer IV 0.1 mg/kg in a child younger than 5 years of age up to 2 mg, in older children and adults administer 2 mg every 2 min up to a total of 10-20 mg. Can also be administered into the endotracheal tube. If no response by 10 mg, a pure opioid intoxication is unlikely. If **opioid abuse** is suspected, **restraints** should be in place before administration; **initial dose** 0.1 mg to avoid withdrawal and violent behavior. The initial dose is then doubled every minute progressively to a total of 10 mg. A **continuous infusion** has been advocated because many opioids outlast the short halflife of naloxone (30-60 min). The **naloxone infusion hourly rate** to produce a response is	IV, ET	**Larger doses** of naloxone may be required for more poorly antagonized synthetic opioid drugs: buprenorphine (Buprenex), codeine, dextromethorphan, fentanyl, pentazocine (Talwin), propoxyphene (Darvon), diphenoxylate, nalbuphine (Nubain), new potent "designer" drugs, or long-acting opioids such as methadone (Dolophine). **Complications.** Although naloxone is safe and effective, there are rare reports of complications (<1%) of pulmonary edema, seizures, hypertension, cardiac arrest, and sudden death. The infusions are titrated to avoid respiratory depression and opioid withdrawal manifestations. Tapering of infusions can be attempted after 12h and when the is stable.

Physostigmine (Antilirium): Stock level to treat 70 kg adult for 24 h: 2-4 mg (2 mL each)	Anticholinergic agents (not routinely used, only indicated if life-threatening complications).	equal to the effective dose required (improvement in ventilation and arousal). An additional dose may be required in 15-30 min as a bolus. *Child:* 0.02 mg/kg slow push to max 2 mg q30-60 min; *Adult:* 1-2 mg q5 min to max 6 mg.	IV	Bradycardia, asystole, seizures, bronchospasm, vomiting, headaches. Do not use for cyclic antidepressants.
Pralidoxime (2PAM, Protopan): Stock level to treat 70 kg adult for 24 h: 12 vials (1 g per 20 mL)	Organophosphates/nerve agents	*Child* ≤12 y, 25-50 mg/kg max (4 mg/min); >12 y, 1-2 g/dose in 250 mL of 0.9% saline over 5-10 min. Max 200 mg/min. Repeat q6-12h for 24-48h. Max adult 6 g/d. Alternative: Maintenance infusion 1 g in 100 mL, of 0.9% saline at 5-20 mg/kg/h (0.5-12 mL/kg/h) up to max 500 mg/h or 50 mL/h. Titrate to desired response. End point is absence of fasciculations and return of muscle strength.	IV	Nausea, dizziness, headache; tachycardia. muscle rigidity, bronchospasm (rapid administration).
Pyridoxine (Vitamin B₆): Stock level to treat 70 kg adult for 24 h: 100 mg/mL 10% solution. For a 70 kg patient, 10 g = 10 vials	Seizures from isoniazid or *Gyromitra* mushrooms; ethylene glycol	*Isoniazid: Unknown amt ingested:* 5 g (70 mg/kg) in 50 mL D₅W over 5 min + diazepam 0.3 mg/kg IV at rate of 1 mg/min in child or 10 mg dose at rate up to 5 mg/min in adults. Use different site (synergism). May repeat q5–20 min until seizure controlled. Up to 375 mg/kg have been given (52 g). *Known amount:* 1 g for each gram isoniazid ingested over 5 min with diazepam (dose above) *Gyromitra mushroom: Child* 25 mg/kg or 2-5 g, adults IV over 15-30 min to max 20 g.	IV	After seizure is controlled, administer remainder of pyridoxine 1 g/1 g isoniazid total 5 g as infusion over 60 min. Adverse reactions uncommon; do not administer in same bottle as sodium bicarbonate. For *Gyromitra* mushrooms, some use PO 25 mg/kg/d early when mushroom ingestion is suspected.
Sodium Bicarbonate (NaHCO₃): Stock level to treat 70 kg adult for 24 h: 10 ampules or syringes (500 mEq)	Tricyclic antidepressant cardiotoxicity (QRS >0.12 sec; ventricular tachycardia, severe conduction disturbances); metabolic acidosis; phenothiazine toxicity *Salicylate:* to keep blood pH 7.5-7.55 (not >7.55) and urine pH 7.5-8.0. Alkalinization recommended if salicylate conc. >40 mg/dL in acute poisoning and at lower levels if symptomatic in chronic intoxication. 2 mEq/kg will raise blood pH 0.1 unit	*Ethylene glycol:* 100 mg IV daily. 1-2 mEq/kg undiluted as a bolus. If no effect on cardiotoxicity, repeat twice a few minutes apart *Adult with clear physical signs and laboratory findings of acute moderate or severe salicylism:* Bolus 1-2 mEq/kg followed by infusion of 100-150 mEq NaHCO₃ added to 1 L of 5% dextrose at rate of 200-300 mL/h *Child:* Bolus same as adult followed by 1-2 mEq/kg in infusion of 20 mL/kg/h 5% dextrose in 0.45% saline. Add potassium when patient voids. Rate and amount of the initial infusion, if patient is volume depleted: 1 h to achieve urine output of 2 mL/kg/h and urine pH 7-8. In mild cases without acidosis and urine pH >6 administer 5% dextrose in 0.9% saline with 50 mEq/L or 1 mEq/kg NaHCO₃ as maintenance to replace	IV	Monitor sodium, potassium, and blood pH because fatal alkalemia and hyponatremia have been reported. Monitor both urine and blood pH. Do not use the urine pH alone to assess the need for alkalinization because of the paradoxical aciduria that may occur. Adjust the urine pH to 7.5-8 by NaHCO₃ infusion. After urine output established, add potassium 40 mEq/L.

Continued

TABLE 5 Initial Doses of Antidotes for Common Poisonings—cont'd

Antidote	Use	Dose	Route	Adverse Reactions/Comments
		ongoing renal losses. If acidemia is present and pH <7.2, add 2 mEq/kg as loading dose followed by 2 mEq/kg q3 to 4h to keep pH at 7.5-7.55. If acidemia is present, recommend isotonic NaHCO$_3$, 3 ampules to 1 L of D$_5$W @ 10-15 mL/kg/h or sufficient to produce normal urine flow and a urine pH of 7.5 or higher.		
	Long-acting barbiturates: Phenobarbital and primidone (Mysoline) Note: Alkalinization is ineffective for the short- or intermediate-acting barbiturates	NaHCO$_3$: 2 mEq/kg during the first hour or 100 mEq in 1 L of D$_5$W with 40 mEq/L potassium at rate of 100 mL/h in adults. Adequate potassium is necessary to accomplish alkalinization	IV	Additional sodium bicarbonate and potassium chloride may be needed. Adjust the urine pH to 7.5-8 by NaHCO$_3$ infusion.
Thiamine: 100 mg/mL, 2 vials	Thiamine deficiency, ethylene glycol poisoning, alcoholism	100 mg IV followed with 100 mg V/IM for 5-7 days in an alcoholic and followed by 100 mg/d orally.	IV/IM	
Vitamin K$_1$ (Aqua Mephyton): 10 mg/1-5 mL; 5 mg tablets	Warfarin anticoagulant or rodenticide toxicity	Oral 0.4 mg/kg/dose child, 10-25 mg adults. If evidence of bleeding administer vitamin K$_1$ SC, IV 0.6 mg/kg/dose child and up to 25-50 mg adults for 6 hours depending on severity.	PO/SC, IV	Give vitamin K daily until PT/INR are normal. Examine stools and urine for evidence of bleeding.

Abbreviations: ALT = alanine aminotransferase; amp = ampule; AST = aspartate aminotransferase; BAL = British anti-Lewisite; BP = blood pressure; Conc. = concentration; ECG = electrocardiogram; ET = endotracheal; G6PD = glucose-6-phosphate dehydrogenase; IM = intramuscular; IV = intravenous; PCC = poison control center; PO = oral; PT = prothrombin time; SC = subcutaneous.

HEMOPERFUSION

Hemoperfusion is the parenteral form of oral activated charcoal. Heparinization is necessary. The patient's blood is routed extracorporeally through an outflow arterial catheter through a filter-adsorbing cartridge (charcoal or resin) and returned through a venous catheter. Cartridges must be changed every 4 hours. The blood glucose, electrolytes, calcium, and albumin levels; complete blood cell count; platelets; and serum and urine osmolarity must be carefully monitored. This procedure has extended extracorporeal removal to a large range of substances that were formerly either poorly dialyzable or nondialyzable. It is not limited by molecular weight, water solubility, or protein binding, but it is limited by a volume distribution greater than 400 L, plasma concentration, and rate of flow through the filter. Activated charcoal cartridges are the primary type of hemoperfusion that is currently available in the United States.

The patient-related criteria for hemoperfusion are (a) anticipated prolonged coma and the likelihood of complications; (b) laboratory confirmation of lethal blood concentrations; (c) hepatic impairment when an agent is metabolized by the liver; and (d) clinical deterioration despite optimally supportive medical management.

The contraindications are similar to those for hemodialysis.

Limited data are available as to which toxins are best treated with hemoperfusion. Hemoperfusion has proved useful in treating glutethimide intoxication, phenobarbital overdose, and carbamazepine, phenytoin, and theophylline intoxication.

Complications include hemorrhage, thrombocytopenia, hypotension, infection, leukopenia, depressed phagocytic activity of granulocytes, decreased immunoglobulin levels, hypoglycemia, hypothermia, hypocalcemia, pulmonary edema, and air and charcoal embolism.

HEMOFILTRATION

Continuous arteriovenous or venovenous hemodiafiltration (CAVHD or CVVHD, respectively) has been suggested as an alternative to conventional hemodialysis when the need for rapid removal of the drug is less urgent. These procedures, like peritoneal dialysis, are minimally invasive, have no significant impact on hemodynamics, and can be carried out continuously for many hours. Their role in the management of acute poisoning remains uncertain, however.

PLASMAPHERESIS

Plasmapheresis consists of removal of a volume of blood. All the extracted components are returned to the blood except the plasma, which is replaced with a colloid protein solution. There are limited clinical data on guidelines and efficacy in toxicology. Centrifugal and membrane separators of cellular elements are used. It can be as effective as hemodialysis or hemoperfusion for removing toxins that have high protein binding, and it may be useful for toxins not filtered by hemodialysis and hemoperfusion.

Plasmapheresis has been anecdotally used in treating intoxications with the following agents: paraquat (removed 10%), propranolol (removed 30%), quinine (removed 10%), L-thyroxine (removed 30%), and salicylate (removed 10%). It has been shown to remove less than 10% of digoxin, phenobarbital, prednisolone, and tobramycin. Complications include infection; allergic reactions including anaphylaxis; hemorrhagic disorders; thrombocytopenia; embolus and thrombus; hypervolemia and hypovolemia; dysrhythmias; syncope; tetany; paresthesia; pneumothorax; acute respiratory distress syndrome; and seizures.

Supportive Care, Observation, and Therapy for Complications

ALTERED MENTAL STATUS

If airway protective reflexes are absent, endotracheal intubation is indicated for a comatose patient or a patient with altered mental status. If respirations are ineffective, ventilation should be instituted, and if hypoxemia persists, supplemental oxygen is indicated. If a cyanotic patient fails to respond to oxygen, the practitioner should consider methemoglobinemia.

HYPOGLYCEMIA

Hypoglycemia accompanies many poisonings, including with ethanol (especially in children), clonidine (Catapres), insulin, organophosphates, salicylates, sulfonylureas, and the unripe fruit or seed of a Jamaican plant called ackee. If hypoglycemia is present or suspected, glucose should be administered immediately as an intravenous bolus. Doses are as follows: in a neonate, 10% glucose (5 mL/kg); in a child, 25% glucose 0.25 g/kg (2 mL/kg); and in an adult, 50% glucose 0.5 g/kg (1 mL/kg).

A bedside capillary test for blood glucose is performed to detect hypoglycemia, and the sample is sent to the laboratory for confirmation. If the glucose reagent strip visually reads less than 150 mg/dL, one administers glucose. Venous blood should be used rather than capillary blood for the bedside test if the patient is in shock or is hypotensive. Large amounts of glucose given rapidly to nondiabetic patients may cause a transient reactive hypoglycemia and hyperkalemia and may accentuate damage in ischemic cerebrovascular and cardiac tissue. If focal neurologic signs are present, it may be prudent to withhold glucose, because hypoglycemia causes focal signs in less than 10% of cases.

THIAMINE DEFICIENCY ENCEPHALOPATHY

Thiamine is administered to avoid precipitating thiamine deficiency encephalopathy (Wernicke-Korsakoff syndrome) in alcohol abusers and in malnourished patients. The overall incidence of thiamine deficiency in ethanol abusers is 12%. Thiamine 100 mg intravenously should be administered around the time of the glucose administration but not necessarily before the glucose. The clinician should be prepared to manage the anaphylaxis that sometimes is caused by thiamine, although it is extremely rare.

OPIOID REACTIONS

Naloxone (Narcan) reverses CNS and respiratory depression, miosis, bradycardia, and decreased gastrointestinal peristalsis caused by opioids acting through μ, κ, and δ receptors. It also affects endogenous opioid peptides (endorphins and enkephalins), which accounts for the variable responses reported in patients with intoxications from ethanol, benzodiazepines, clonidine (Catapres), captopril (Capoten), and valproic acid (Depakote) and in patients with spinal cord injuries. There is a high sensitivity for predicting a response if pinpoint pupils and circumstantial evidence of opioid abuse (e.g., track marks) are present.

In cases of suspected overdose, naloxone 0.1 mg/kg is administered intravenously initially in a child younger than 5 years of age. The dose can be repeated in 2 minutes, if necessary up to a total dose of 2 mg. In older children and adults, the dose is 2 mg every 2 minutes for five doses up to a total of 10 mg. Naloxone can also be administered into an endotracheal tube if intravenous access is unavailable. If there is no response after 10 mg, a pure opioid intoxication is unlikely. If opioid abuse is suspected, restraints should be in place before the administration of naloxone, and it is recommended that the initial dose be 0.1 to 0.2 mg to avoid withdrawal and violent behavior. The initial dose is then doubled every minute progressively to a total of 10 mg. Naloxone may unmask concomitant sympathomimetic intoxication as well as withdrawal.

Larger doses of naloxone may be required for more poorly antagonized synthetic opioid drugs: buprenorphine (Buprenex), codeine, dextromethorphan, fentanyl and its derivatives, pentazocine (Talwin), propoxyphene (Darvon), diphenoxylate, nalbuphine (Nubain), and long-acting opioids such as methadone (Dolophine).

Indications for a continuous infusion include a second dose for recurrent respiratory depression, exposure to poorly antagonized opioids, a large overdose, and decreased opioid metabolism, as with impaired liver function. A continuous infusion has been

TABLE 6 Plasma Concentrations Above Which Removal by Extracorporeal Measures Should Be Considered

Drug	Plasma Concentration	Protein Binding (%)	Volume Distribution (L/kg)	Method of Choice
Amanitin	NA	25	1.0	HP
Ethanol	500-700 mg/dL	0	0.3	HD
Ethchlorvynol	150 µg/mL	35-50	3-4	HP
Ethylene glycol	25-50 µg/mL	0	0.6	HD
Glutethimide	100 µg/mL	50	2.7	HP
Isopropyl alcohol	400 mg/dL	0	0.7	HD
Lithium	4 mEq/L	0	0.7	HD
Meprobamate (Equanil)	100 µg/mL	0	NA	HP
Methanol	50 mg/dL	0	0.7	HD
Methaqualone	40 µg/dL	20-60	6.0	HP
Other barbiturates	50 µg/dL	50	0-1	HP
Paraquat	0.1 mg/dL	poor	2.8	HP > HD
Phenobarbital	100 µg/dL	50	0.9	HP > HD
Salicylates	80-100 mg/dL	90	0.2	HD > HP
Theophylline		0	0.5	
Chronic	40-60 µg/mL			HP
Acute	80-100 µg/mL			HP
Trichlorethanol	250 µg/mL	70	0.6	HP

Abbreviations: HD = hemodialysis; HP = hemoperfusion; HP > HD hemoperfusion preferred over hemodialysis.
Note: Cartridges for charcoal hemoperfusion are not readily available anymore in most locations, so hemodialysis may be substituted in these situations. In mixed or chronic drug overdoses, extracorporeal measures may be considered at lower drug concentrations.
Data from Winchester JF: Active methods for detoxification. In Haddad LM, Winchester JF (eds). Clinical Management of Poisoning and Drug Overdose, 2nd ed. Philadelphia, WB Saunders, 1990; Balsam L, Cortitsidis GN, Fienfeld DA: Role of hemodialysis and hemoperfusion in the treatment of intoxications. Contemp Manage Crit Care 1:61, 1991.

advocated because many opioids outlast the short half-life of naloxone (30 to 60 minutes). The hourly rate of naloxone infusion is equal to the effective dose required to produce a response (improvement in ventilation and arousal). An additional dose may be required in 15 to 30 minutes as a bolus. The infusions are titrated to avoid respiratory depression and opioid withdrawal manifestations. Tapering of infusions can be attempted after 12 hours and when the patient's condition has been stabilized.

Although naloxone is safe and effective, there are rare reports of complications (less than 1%) of pulmonary edema, seizures, hypertension, cardiac arrest, and sudden death.

AGENTS WHOSE ROLES ARE NOT CLARIFIED

Nalmefene (Revex), a long-acting parenteral opioid antagonist that the Food and Drug Administration has approved, is undergoing investigation, but its role in the treatment of comatose patients and patients with opioid overdose is not clear. It is 16 times more potent than naloxone, and its duration of action is up to 8 hours (half-life 10.8 hours, versus naloxone 1 hour).

Flumazenil (Romazicon) is a pure competitive benzodiazepine antagonist. It has been demonstrated to be safe and effective for reversing benzodiazepine-induced sedation. It is not recommended to improve ventilation. Its role in cases of CNS depression needs to be clarified. It should not be used routinely in comatose patients and is not an essential ingredient of the coma therapeutic regimen. It is contraindicated in cases of co-ingestion of cyclic antidepressant intoxication, stimulant overdose, and long-term benzodiazepine use (may precipitate life-threatening withdrawal) if benzodiazepines are used to control seizures. There is a concern about the potential for seizures and cardiac dysrhythmias that may occur in these settings.

Laboratory and Radiographic Studies

An electrocardiogram (ECG) should be obtained to identify dysrhythmias or conduction delays from cardiotoxic medications. If aspiration pneumonia (history of loss of consciousness, unarousable state, vomiting) or noncardiac pulmonary edema is suspected, a chest radiograph is needed. Electrolyte and glucose concentrations in the blood, the anion gap, acid–base balance, the arterial blood gas (ABG) profile (if patient has respiratory distress or altered mental status), and serum osmolality should be measured if a toxic alcohol ingestion is suspected. Table 7 lists appropriate testing on the basis of clinical toxicologic presentation. All laboratory specimens should be carefully labeled, including time and date. For potential legal cases, a "chain of custody" must be established. Assessment of the laboratory studies may provide a clue to the etiologic agent.

TABLE 7 Patient Condition/Systemic Toxin and Appropriate Tests

Condition	Tests
Comatose	Toxicologic tests (acetaminophen, sedative-hypnotic, ethanol, opioids, benzodiazepine), glucose.
Respiratory toxicity	Spirometry, FEV$_1$, arterial blood gases, chest radiograph, monitor O$_2$ saturation
Cardiac toxicity	ECG 12-lead and monitoring, echocardiogram, serial cardiac enzymes (if evidence or suspicion of a myocardial infarction), hemodynamic monitoring
Hepatic toxicity	Enzymes (AST, ALT, GGT), ammonia, albumin, bilirubin, glucose, PT, PTT, amylase
Nephrotoxicity	BUN, creatinine, electrolytes (Na, F, Mg, Ca, PO$_4$), serum and urine osmolarity, 24-hour urine for heavy metals if suspected, creatine kinase, serum and urine myoglobin, urinalysis and urinary sodium
Bleeding	Platelets, PT, PTT, bleeding time, fibrin split products, fibrinogen, type and match

Abbreviations: ALT = alanine aminotransaminase; AST = aspartate aminotransaminase; BUN = blood urea nitrogen; ECG = electrocardiogram; FEV$_1$ = forced expiratory volume at 1 second; GGT = γ-glutamyltransferase; PT = prothrombin time; PTT = partial thromboplastin time.

TABLE 8 Etiologies of Metabolic Acidosis

Normal Anion Gap Hyperchloremic	Increased Anion Gap Normochloremic	Decreased Anion Gap
Acidifying agents	Methanol	Laboratory error[†]
Adrenal insufficiency	Uremia*	Intoxication—bromine, lithium
Anhydrase inhibitors	Diabetic ketoacidosis*	Protein abnormal
Fistula	Paraldehyde,* phenformin	Sodium low
Osteotomies	Isoniazid	
Obstructive uropathies	Iron	
Renal tubular acidosis	Lactic acidosis[†]	
Diarrhea, uncomplicated*	Ethanol,* ethylene glycol*	
Dilutional	Salicylates, starvation solvents	
Sulfamylon		

*Indicates hyperosmolar situation. Studies have found that the anion gap may be relatively insensitive for determining the presence of toxins.
[†]Lactic acidosis can be produced by intoxications of the following: carbon monoxide, cyanide, hydrogen sulfide, hypoxia, ibuprofen, iron, isoniazid, phenformin, salicylates, seizures, theophylline.

ELECTROLYTE, ACID-BASE, AND OSMOLALITY DISTURBANCES

Electrolyte and acid–base disturbances should be evaluated and corrected. Metabolic acidosis (usually low or normal pH with a low or normal/high $Paco_2$ and low HCO_3) with an increased anion gap is seen with many agents in cases of overdose.

The anion gap is an estimate of those anions other than chloride and HCO_3 necessary to counterbalance the positive charge of sodium. It serves as a clue to causes, compensations, and complications. The anion gap (AG) is calculated from the standard serum electrolytes by subtracting the total CO_2 (which reflects the actual measured bicarbonate) and chloride from the sodium: $(Na - [Cl + HCO_3]) = AG$. The potassium is usually not used in the calculation because it may be hemolyzed and is an intracellular cation. The lack of anion gap does not exclude a toxic etiology.

The normal gap is usually 7 to 11 mEq/L by flame photometer. However, there has been a "lowering" of the normal anion gap to 7 ± 4 mEq/L by the newer techniques (e.g., ion selective electrodes or colorimetric titration). Some studies have found anion gaps to be relatively insensitive for determining the presence of toxins.

It is important to recognize anion gap toxins, such as salicylates, methanol, and ethylene glycol, because they have specific antidotes, and hemodialysis is effective in management of cases of overdose with these agents.

Table 8 lists the reasons for increased anion gap, decreased anion gap, or no gap. The most common cause of a decreased anion gap is laboratory error. Lactic acidosis produces the largest anion gap and can result from any poisoning that results in hypoxia, hypoglycemia, or convulsions.

Table 9 lists other blood chemistry derangements that suggest certain intoxications.

Serum osmolality is a measure of the number of molecules of solute per kilogram of solvent, or mOsm/kg water. The osmolarity is molecules of solute per liter of solution, or mOsm/L water at a specified temperature. Osmolarity is usually the calculated value and osmolality is usually a measured value. They are considered interchangeable where 1 L equals 1 kg. The normal serum osmolality is 280 to 290 mOsm/kg. The freezing point serum osmolarity measurement specimen and the serum electrolyte specimens for calculation should be drawn simultaneously.

The serum osmolal gap is defined as the difference between the measured osmolality determined by the freezing point method and the calculated osmolarity. It is determined by the following formula:

$$(Sodium \times 2) + (BUN/3) + (Glucose/20)$$

(where BUN is blood urea nitrogen).

This gap estimate is normally within 10 mOsm of the simultaneously measured serum osmolality. Ethanol, if present, may be included in the equation to eliminate its influence on the osmolal gap (the ethanol concentration divided by 4.6; Table 10).

The osmolal gap is not valid in cases of shock and postmortem state. Metabolic disorders such as hyperglycemia, uremia, and dehydration increase the osmolarity but usually do not cause gaps greater than 10 mOsm/kg. A gap greater than 10 mOsm/mL suggests that unidentified osmolal-acting substances are present: acetone, ethanol, ethylene glycol, glycerin, isopropyl alcohol, isoniazid, ethanol, mannitol, methanol, and trichloroethane. Alcohols and glycols should be sought when the degree of obtundation exceeds that expected from the blood ethanol concentration or when other clinical conditions exist: visual loss (methanol), metabolic acidosis (methanol and ethylene glycol), or renal failure (ethylene glycol).

A falsely elevated osmolar gap can be produced by other low molecular weight un-ionized substances (dextran, diuretics, sorbitol, ketones), hyperlipidemia, and unmeasured electrolytes (e.g., magnesium).

Note: A normal osmolal gap may be reported in the presence of toxic alcohol or glycol poisoning, if the parent compound is already metabolized. This situation can occur when the osmolar gap is measured after a significant time has elapsed since the ingestion. In cases of alcohol and glycol intoxication, an early osmolar gap is a result of the relatively nontoxic parent drug and delayed metabolic acidosis, and an anion gap is a result of the more toxic metabolites.

The serum concentration is calculated as mg/dL = mOsm gap × MW of substance divided by 10.

TABLE 9 Blood Chemistry Derangements in Toxicology

Derangement	Toxin
Acetonemia without acidosis	Acetone or isopropyl alcohol
Hypomagnesemia	Ethanol, digitalis
Hypocalcemia	Ethylene glycol, oxalate, fluoride
Hyperkalemia	β-Blockers, acute digitalis, renal failure
Hypokalemia	Diuretics, salicylism, sympathomimetics, theophylline, corticosteroids, chronic digitalis
Hyperglycemia	Diazoxide, glucagon, iron, isoniazid, organophosphate insecticides, phenylurea insecticides, phenytoin (Dilantin), salicylates, sympathomimetic agents, thyroid, vasopressors
Hypoglycemia	β-Blockers, ethanol, insulin, isoniazid, oral hypoglycemic agents, salicylates
Rhabdomyolysis	Amphetamines, ethanol, cocaine, or phencyclidine, elevated creatine phosphokinase

TABLE 10 Conversion Factors for Alcohols and Glycols

Alcohols/Glycols	1 mg/dL in Blood Raises Osmolality mOsm/L	Molecular Weight	Conversion Factor
Ethanol	0.228	40	4.6
Methanol	0.327	32	3.2
Ethylene glycol	0.190	62	6.2
Isopropanol	0.176	60	6.0
Acetone	0.182	58	5.8
Propylene glycol	not available	72	7.2

Example: Methanol osmolality. Subtract the calculated osmolality from the measured serum osmolarity (freezing point method) = osmolar gap × 3.2 (one-tenth molecular weight) = estimated serum methanol concentration.
Note: This equation is often not considered very reliable in predicting the actual measured blood concentration of these alcohols or glycols.

RADIOGRAPHIC STUDIES

Chest and neck radiographs are useful for suspected pathologic conditions such as aspiration pneumonia, pulmonary edema, and foreign bodies and to determine the location of the endotracheal tube. Abdominal radiographs can be used to detect radiopaque substances.

The mnemonic for radiopaque substances seen on abdominal radiographs is CHIPES:

C—chlorides and chloral hydrate
H—heavy metals (arsenic, barium, iron, lead, mercury, zinc)
I—iodides
P—PlayDoh, Pepto-Bismol, phenothiazine (inconsistent)
E—enteric-coated tablets
S—sodium, potassium, and other elements in tablet form (bismuth, calcium, potassium) and solvents containing chlorides (e.g., carbon tetrachloride)

TOXICOLOGIC STUDIES

Routine blood and urine screening is of little practical value in the initial care of the poisoned patient. Specific toxicologic analyses and quantitative levels of certain drugs may be extremely helpful. One should always ask oneself the following questions: (a) How will the result of the test alter the management? and (b) Can the result of the test be returned in time to have a positive effect on therapy?

Owing to long turnaround time, lack of availability, factors contributing to unreliability, and the risk of serious morbidity without supportive clinical management, toxicology screening is estimated to affect management in less than 15% of cases of drug overdoses or poisonings. Toxicology screening may look specifically for only 40 to 50 drugs out of more than 10,000 possible drugs or toxins and more than several million chemicals. To detect many different drugs, toxic screens usually include methods with broad specificity, and sensitivity may be poor for some drugs, resulting in false-negative or false-positive findings. On the other hand, some drugs present in therapeutic amounts may be detected on the screen, even though they are causing no clinical symptoms. Because many agents are not sought or detected during a toxicologic screening, a negative result does not always rule out poisonings. The specificity of toxicologic tests is dependent on the method and the laboratory. The presence of other drugs, drug metabolites, disease states, or incorrect sampling may cause erroneous results.

For the average toxicologic laboratory, false-negative results occur at a rate of 10% to 30% and false-positives at a rate of 0% to 10%. The positive screen predictive value is approximately 90%. A negative toxicology screen does not exclude a poisoning. The negative predictive value of toxicologic screening is approximately 70%. For example, the following benzodiazepines may not be detected by some routine immunoassay benzodiazepine screening tests: alprazolam (Xanax), clonazepam (Klonopin), temazepam (Restoril), and triazolam (Halcion).

The "toxic urine screen" is generally a qualitative urine test for several common drugs, usually substances of abuse (cocaine and metabolites, opioids, amphetamines, benzodiazepines, barbiturates, and phencyclidine). Results of these tests are usually available within 2 to 6 hours. Because these tests may vary with each hospital and community, the physician should determine exactly which substances are included in the toxic urine screen of his or her laboratory. Tests for ethylene glycol, red blood cell cholinesterase, and serum cyanide are not readily available.

For cases of ingestion of certain substances, quantitative blood levels should be obtained at specific times after the ingestion to avoid spurious low values in the distribution phase, which result from incomplete absorption. The detection time for drugs is influenced by many variables, such as type of substance, formulation, amount, time since ingestion, duration of exposure, and half-life. For many drugs, the detection time is measured in days after the exposure.

Common Poisons

ACETAMINOPHEN (PARACETAMOL, N-ACETYL-PARAAMINOPHENOL)

Toxic Mechanism

At therapeutic doses of acetaminophen, less than 5% is metabolized by P450-2E1 to a toxic reactive oxidizing metabolite, N-acetyl-p-benzoquinoneimine (NAPQI). In a case of overdose, there is insufficient glutathione available to reduce the excess NAPQI into nontoxic conjugate, so it forms covalent bonds with hepatic intracellular proteins to produce centrilobular necrosis. Renal damage is caused by a similar mechanism.

Toxic Dose

The therapeutic dose of acetaminophen is 10 to 15 mg/kg, with a maximum of five doses in 24 hours for a maximum total daily dose of 4 g. An acute single toxic dose is greater than 140 mg/kg, possibly greater than 200 mg/kg in a child younger than age 5 years. Factors affecting the P450 enzymes include enzyme inducers such as barbiturates and phenytoin (Dilantin), ingestion of isoniazid, and alcoholism. Factors that decrease glutathione stores (alcoholism, malnutrition, and HIV infection) contribute to the toxicity of acetaminophen. Alcoholics ingesting 3 to 4 g/d of acetaminophen for a few days can have depleted glutathione stores and require N-acetylcysteine therapy at 50% below hepatotoxic blood acetaminophen levels on the nomogram.

Kinetics

Peak plasma concentration is usually reached 2 to 4 hours after an overdose. Volume distribution is 0.9 L/kg, and protein binding is less than 50% (albumin).

Route of elimination is by hepatic metabolism to an inactive nontoxic glucuronide conjugate and inactive nontoxic sulfate metabolite by two saturable pathways; less than 5% is metabolized into reactive metabolite NAPQI. In patients younger than 6 years of age, metabolic elimination occurs to a greater degree by conjugation via the sulfate pathway.

The half-life of acetaminophen is 1 to 3 hours.

Manifestations

The four phases of the intoxication's clinical course may overlap, and the absence of a phase does not exclude toxicity.

- Phase I occurs within 0.5 to 24 hours after ingestion and may consist of a few hours of malaise, diaphoresis, nausea, and vomiting or produce no symptoms. CNS depression or coma is not a feature.
- Phase II occurs 24 to 48 hours after ingestion and is a period of diminished symptoms. The liver enzymes, serum aspartate aminotransferase (AST) (earliest), and serum alanine aminotransferase (ALT) may increase as early as 4 hours or as late as 36 hours after ingestion.
- Phase III occurs at 48 to 96 hours, with peak liver function abnormalities at 72 to 96 hours. The degree of elevation of the hepatic enzymes generally correlates with outcome, but not always. Recovery starts at about 4 days unless hepatic failure develops. Less than 1% of patients with a history of overdose develop fulminant hepatotoxicity.
- Phase IV occurs at 4 to 14 days, with hepatic enzyme abnormalities resolving. If extensive liver damage has occurred, sepsis and disseminated intravascular coagulation may ensue.

Transient renal failure may develop at 5 to 7 days with or without evidence of hepatic damage. Rare cases of myocarditis and pancreatitis have been reported. Death can occur at 7 to 14 days.

Laboratory Investigations

The therapeutic reference range is 10 to 20 µg/mL. For toxic levels, see the nomogram presented in Figure 1.

Appropriate and reliable methods for analysis are radioimmunoassay, high-pressure liquid chromatography, and gas chromatography. Spectroscopic assays often give falsely elevated values: bilirubin, salicylate, salicylamide, diflunisal (Dolobid), phenols, and methyldopa (Aldomet) increase the acetaminophen level. Each 1 mg/dL increase in creatinine increases the acetaminophen plasma level 30 µg/mL.

If a toxic acetaminophen level is reached, liver profile (including AST, ALT, bilirubin, and prothrombin time), serum amylase, and blood glucose must be monitored. A complete blood cell count (CBC); platelet count; phosphate, electrolytes, and bicarbonate level measurements; ECG; and urinalysis are indicated.

Management

Gastrointestinal Decontamination

Although ipecac-induced emesis may be useful within 30 minutes of ingestion of the toxic substance, we do not advise it because it could result in vomiting of the activated charcoal. Gastric lavage is not necessary. Studies have indicated that activated charcoal is useful within 1 hour after ingestion. Activated charcoal does adsorb N-acetylcysteine (NAC) if given together, but this is not clinically important. However, if activated charcoal needs to be given along with NAC, separate the administration of activated charcoal from the administration of NAC by 1 to 2 hours to avoid vomiting.

N-Acetylcysteine (Mucomyst)

NAC (Table 11), a derivative of the amino acid cysteine, acts as a sulfhydryl donor for glutathione synthesis, as surrogate glutathione, and may increase the nontoxic sulfation pathway resulting in conjugation of NAPQI. Oral NAC should be administered within the first 8 hours after a toxic amount of acetaminophen has been ingested. NAC can be started while one awaits the results of the blood test for acetaminophen plasma concentration, but there is no advantage to giving it before 8 hours. If the acetaminophen concentration result after 4 hours following ingestion is above the upper line on the modified Rumack-Matthew nomogram (see Figure 1), one should continue with a maintenance course. Repeat blood specimens should be obtained 4 hours after the initial level is measured if it is greater than 20 mg/mL, which is below the therapy line, because of unexpected delays in the peak by food and co-ingestants. Intravenous NAC (see Table 11) is approved in the United States.

There have been a few cases of anaphylactoid reaction and death by the intravenous route.

Variations in Therapy

In patients with chronic alcoholism, it is recommended that NAC treatment be administered at 50% below the upper toxic line on the nomogram.

If emesis occurs within 1 hour after NAC administration, the dose should be repeated. To avoid emesis, the proper dilution from 20% to 5% NAC must be used, and it should be served in a palatable vehicle, in a covered container through a straw. If this administration is unsuccessful, a slow drip over 30 to 60 minutes through a nasogastric tube or a fluoroscopically placed nasoduodenal tube can be used. Antiemetics can be used if necessary: metoclopramide (Reglan) 10 mg per dose intravenously 30 minutes before administration of NAC (in children, 0.1 mg/kg; maximum, 0.5 mg/kg/d) or ondansetron (Zofran) 32 mg (0.15 mg/kg) by infusion over 15 minutes and repeated for three doses if necessary. The side effects of these antiemetics include anaphylaxis and increases in liver enzymes.

Some investigators recommend variable durations of NAC therapy, stopping the therapy if serial acetaminophen blood concentrations become nondetectable and the liver enzyme levels (ALT and AST) remain normal after 24 to 36 hours.

There is a loss of efficacy if NAC is initiated 8 or 10 hours postingestion, but the loss is not complete, and NAC may be initiated 36 hours or more after ingestion. Late treatment (after 24 hours) decreases the rates of morbidity and mortality in patients with fulminant liver failure caused by acetaminophen and other agents.

Extended relief formulations (ER embossed on caplet) contain 325 mg of acetaminophen for immediate release and 325 mg for delayed release. A single 4-hour postingestion serum acetaminophen concentration can underestimate the level because ER formulations can have secondary delayed peaks. In cases of overdose of the ER formulation, it is recommended that additional acetaminophen levels be obtained at 4-hour intervals after the initial level is measured. If any level is in the toxic zone, therapy should be initiated.

It is recommended that pregnant patients with toxic plasma concentrations of acetaminophen be treated with NAC to prevent hepatotoxicity in both fetus and mother. The available data suggest no teratogenicity to NAC or acetaminophen.

Indications for NAC therapy in cases of chronic intoxication are a history of ingestion of 3 to 4 g for several days with elevated liver enzyme levels (AST and ALT). The acetaminophen blood concentration is often low in these cases because of the extended time lapse since ingestion and should not be plotted on the Rumack-Matthew nomogram. Patients with a history of chronic alcoholism or those on chronic enzyme inducers may also present with elevated liver enzyme levels and should be considered for NAC therapy if they have a history of taking acetaminophen on a chronic basis, because they are considered to be at a greater risk for hepatotoxicity despite a low acetaminophen blood concentration.

Specific support care may be needed to treat liver failure, pancreatitis, transient renal failure, and myocarditis.

Liver transplantation has a definite but limited role in patients with acute acetaminophen overdose. A retrospective analysis determined that a continuing rise in the prothrombin time (4-day peak, 180 seconds), a pH of less than 7.3 2 days after the overdose, a serum creatinine level of greater than 3.3 mg/dL, severe hepatic encephalopathy, and disturbed coagulation factor VII/V ratio greater than 30

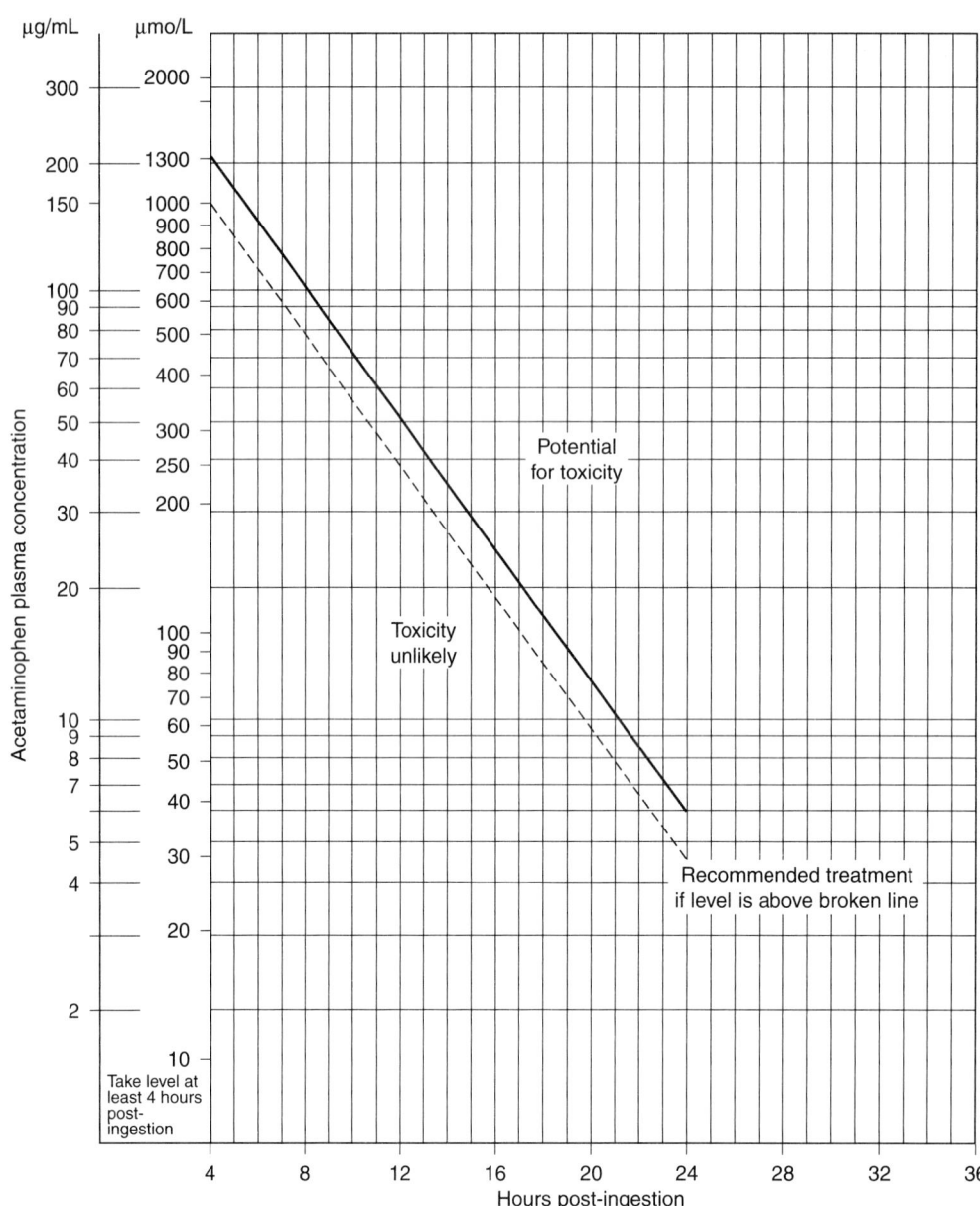

FIGURE 1. Nomogram for acetaminophen intoxication. N-acetylcysteine therapy is started if levels and time coordinates are above the lower line on the nomogram. Continue and complete therapy even if subsequent values fall below the toxic zone. The nomogram is useful only in cases of acute single ingestion. Levels in serum drawn before 4 hours may not represent peak levels. (From Rumack BH, Matthew H: Acetaminophen poisoning and toxicity. Pediatrics 55:871, 1975.)

suggest a poor prognosis and may be indicators for hepatology consultation for consideration of liver transplantation.

Extracorporeal measures are not expected to be of benefit.

Disposition

Adults who have ingested more than 140 mg/kg and children younger than 6 years of age who have ingested more than 200 mg/kg should receive therapy within 8 hours postingestion or until the results of the 4-hour postingestion acetaminophen plasma concentration are known.

AMPHETAMINES

The amphetamines include illicit methamphetamine ("Ice"), diet pills, and formulations under various trade names. Analogues include MDMA (3,4 methylenedioxymethamphetamine, known as "ecstasy," "XTC," "Adam") and MDA (3,4-methylenedioxyamphetamine,

TABLE 11 Protocol for N-Acetylcysteine Administration

Route	Loading Dose	Maintenance Dose	Course	FDA Approval
Oral	140 mg/kg	70 mg/kg every 4 h	72 h	Yes
Intravenous	150 mg/kg over 15 min	50 mg/kg over 4 h followed by 100 mg/kg over 16h	20 h	Yes

known as "Eve"). MDA is a common hallucinogen and euphoriant "club drug" used at "raves," which are all-night dances. Use of methamphetamine and designer analogues is on the rise, especially among young people between the ages of 12 and 25 years. Other similar stimulants are phenylpropanolamine and cocaine.

Toxic Mechanism

Amphetamines have a direct CNS stimulant effect and a sympathetic nervous system effect by releasing catecholamines from α- and β-adrenergic nerve terminals but inhibiting their reuptake.

Hallucinogenic MDMA has an additional hazard of serotonin effect (refer to serotonin syndrome in the SSRI section). MDMA also affect the dopamine system in the brain. Because of its effects on 5-hydroxytryptamine, dopamine, and norepinephrine, MDMA can lead to serotonin syndrome associated with malignant hyperthermia and rhabdomyolysis, which contributes to the potentially life-threatening hyperthermia observed in several patients who have used MDMA.

Phenylpropanolamine stimulates only the β-adrenergic receptors.

Toxic Dose

In children, the toxic dose of dextroamphetamine is 1 mg/kg; in adults, the toxic dose is 5 mg/kg. The potentially fatal dose of dextroamphetamine is 12 mg/kg.

Kinetics

Amphetamine is a weak base with pKa of 8 to 10. Onset of action is 30 to 60 minutes, and peak effects are 2 to 4 hours. The volume distribution is 2 to 3 L/kg.

Through hepatic metabolism, 60% of the substance is metabolized into a hydroxylated metabolite that may be responsible for psychotic effects.

The half-life of amphetamines is pH dependent—8 to 10 hours in acid urine (pH <6.0) and 16 to 31 hours in alkaline urine (pH >7.5). Excretion is by the kidney—30% to 40% at alkaline urine pH and 50% to 70% at acid urine pH.

Manifestations

Effects are seen within 30 to 60 minutes following ingestion.

Neurologic manifestations include restlessness, irritation and agitation, tremors and hyperreflexia, and auditory and visual hallucinations. Hyperpyrexia may precede seizures, convulsions, paranoia, violence, intracranial hemorrhage, psychosis, and self-destructive behavior. Paranoid psychosis and cerebral vasculitis occur with chronic abuse.

MDMA is often adulterated with cocaine, heroin, or ketamine, or a combination of these, to create a variety of mood alterations. This possibility must be taken into consideration when one manages patients with MDMA ingestions, as the symptom complex may reflect both CNS stimulation and CNS depression.

Other manifestations include dilated but reactive pupils, cardiac dysrhythmias (supraventricular and ventricular), tachycardia, hypertension, rhabdomyolysis, and myoglobinuria.

Laboratory Investigations

The clinician should monitor ECG and cardiac readings, ABG and oxygen saturation, electrolytes, blood glucose, BUN, creatinine, creatine kinase, cardiac fraction if there is chest pain, and liver profile. Also, one should evaluate for rhabdomyolysis and check urine for myoglobin, cocaine and metabolites, and other substances of abuse. The peak plasma concentration of amphetamines is 10 to 50 ng/mL 1 to 2 hours after ingestion of 10 to 25 mg. The toxic plasma concentration is 200 ng/mL. When the rapid immunoassays are used, cross-reactions can occur with amphetamine derivatives (e.g., MDA, "ecstasy"), brompheniramine (Dimetane), chlorpromazine (Thorazine), ephedrine, phenylpropanolamine, phentermine (Adipex-P), phenmetrazine, ranitidine (Zantac), and Vicks Inhaler (L-desoxyephedrine). False-positive results may occur.

Management

Management is similar to management for cocaine intoxication. Supportive care includes blood pressure and temperature control, cardiac monitoring, and seizure precautions. Diazepam (Valium) can be administered. Gastrointestinal decontamination can be undertaken with activated charcoal administered up to 1 hour after ingestion.

Anxiety, agitation, and convulsions are treated with diazepam. If diazepam fails to control seizures, neuromuscular blockers can be used and the electroencephalogram (EEG) monitored for nonmotor seizures. One should avoid neuroleptic phenothiazines and butyrophenone, which can lower the seizure threshold.

Hypertension and tachycardia are usually transient and can be managed by titration of diazepam. Nitroprusside can be used for hypertensive crisis at a maximum infusion rate of 10 μg/kg/minute for 10 minutes followed with a lower infusion rate of 0.3 to 2 mg/kg/minute. Myocardial ischemia is managed by oxygen, vascular access, benzodiazepines, and nitroglycerin. Aspirin and thrombolytics are not routinely recommended because of the danger of intracranial hemorrhage. It is important to distinguish between angina and true ischemia. Delayed hypotension can be treated with fluids and vasopressors if needed. Life-threatening tachydysrhythmias may respond to an α-blocker such as phentolamine (Regitine) 5 mg IV for adults or 0.1 mg/kg IV for children and a short-acting β-blocker such as esmolol (Brevibloc) 500 μg/kg IV over 1 minute for adults, or 300 to 500 μg/kg over 1 minute for children. Ventricular dysrhythmias may respond to lidocaine or, in a severely hemodynamically compromised patient, immediate synchronized electrical cardioversion.

Rhabdomyolysis and myoglobinuria are treated with fluids, alkaline diuresis, and diuretics. Hyperthermia is treated with external cooling and cool 100% humidified oxygen. More extensive therapy may be needed in severe cases. If focal neurologic symptoms are present, the possibility of a cerebrovascular accident should be considered and a CT scan of the head should be obtained.

Paranoid ideation and threatening behavior should be treated with rapid tranquilization using a benzodiazepine. One should observe for suicidal depression that may follow intoxication and may require suicide precautions.

Extracorporeal measures are of no benefit.

Disposition

Symptomatic patients should be observed on a monitored unit until the symptoms resolve and then observed for a short time after resolution for relapse.

ANTICHOLINERGIC AGENTS

Drugs with anticholinergic properties include antihistamines (H_1 blockers), neuroleptics (phenothiazines), tricyclic antidepressants, antiparkinsonism drugs (trihexyphenidyl [Artane], benztropine [Cogentin]), ophthalmic products (atropine), and a number of common plants.

The antihistamines are divided into the sedating anticholinergic types, and the nonsedating single daily dose types. The sedating types include ethanolamines (e.g., diphenhydramine [Benadryl], dimenhydrinate [Dramamine], and clemastine [Tavist]), ethylenediamines (e.g., tripelennamine [Pyribenzamine]), alkyl amines (e.g., chlorpheniramine [Chlor-Trimeton], brompheniramine [Dimetane]), piperazines (e.g., cyclizine [Marezine], hydroxyzine [Atarax], and meclizine [Antivert]), and phenothiazine (e.g., Phenergan). The nonsedating types include astemizole (Hismanal), terfenadine (Seldane), loratadine (Claritin), fexofenadine (Allegra), and cetirizine (Zyrtec).

The anticholinergic plants include jimsonweed (*Datura stramonium*), deadly nightshade (*Atropa belladonna*), henbane (*Hyoscyamus niger*), and antispasmodic agents for the bowel (atropine derivatives).

Toxic Mechanism

By competitive inhibition, anticholinergics block the action of acetylcholine on postsynaptic cholinergic receptor sites. The toxic mechanism primarily involves the peripheral and CNS muscarinic receptors. H_1 sedating-type agents also depress or stimulate the CNS, and in large overdoses some have cardiac membrane–depressant effects (e.g., diphenhydramine [Benadryl]) and α-adrenergic receptor blockade effects (e.g., promethazine [Phenergan]). Nonsedating agents produce peripheral H_1 blockade but do not possess anticholinergic or sedating actions. The original agents terfenadine (Seldane) and astemizole (Hismanal) were recently removed from the market because of the severe cardiac dysrhythmias associated with their use, especially when used in combination with macrolide antibiotics and certain antifungal agents such as ketoconazole (Nizoral), which inhibit hepatic metabolism or excretion. The newer nonsedating agents, including loratadine (Claritin), fexofenadine (Allegra), and cetirizine (Zyrtec), have not been reported to cause the severe drug interactions associated with terfenadine and astemizole.

Toxic Dose

The estimated toxic oral dose of atropine is 0.05 mg/kg in children and more than 2 mg in adults. The minimal estimated lethal dose of atropine is more than 10 mg in adults and more than 2 mg in children. Other synthetic anticholinergic agents are less toxic, and the fatal dose varies from 10 to 100 mg.

The estimated toxic oral dose of diphenhydramine (Benadryl) in a child is 15 mg/kg, and the potential lethal amount is 25 mg/kg. In an adult, the potential lethal amount is 2.8 g. Ingestion of five times the single dose of an antihistamine is toxic.

For the nonsedating agents, an overdose of 3360 mg of terfenadine was reported in an adult who developed ventricular tachycardia and fibrillation that responded to lidocaine and defibrillation. A 1500-mg overdose produced hypotension. Cases of delayed serious dysrhythmias (torsades de pointes) have been reported with doses of more than 200 mg of astemizole. The toxic doses of fexofenadine (Allegra), cetirizine, and loratadine (Claritin) need to be established.

Kinetics

The onset of absorption of intravenous atropine is in 2 to 4 minutes. Peak effects on salivation after intravenous or intramuscular administration are at 30 to 60 minutes.

Onset of absorption after oral ingestion is 30 to 60 minutes, peak action is 1 to 3 hours, and duration of action is 4 to 6 hours, but symptoms are prolonged in cases of overdose or with sustained-release preparations.

The onset of absorption of diphenhydramine is in 15 minutes to 1 hour, with a peak of action in 1 to 4 hours. Volume distribution is 3.3 to 6.8 L/kg, and protein binding is 75% to 80%. Ninety-eight percent of diphenhydramine is metabolized via the liver by N-demethylation. Interactions with erythromycin, ketoconazole (Nizoral), and derivatives produce excessive blood levels of the antihistamine and ventricular dysrhythmias.

The half-life of diphenhydramine is 3 to 10 hours.

The chemical structure of nonsedating agents prevents their entry into the CNS. Absorption begins in 1 hour, with peak effects in 4 in 6 hours. The duration of action is greater than 24 hours.

These agents are metabolized in the gastrointestinal tract and liver. Protein binding is greater than 90%. The plasma half-life is 3.5 hours. Only 1% is excreted unchanged; 60% of that is excreted in the feces and 40% in the urine.

Manifestations

Anticholinergic signs are hyperpyrexia ("hot as a hare"), mydriasis ("blind as a bat"), flushing of skin ("red as a beet"), dry mucosa and skin ("dry as a bone"), "Lilliputian type" hallucinations and delirium ("mad as a hatter"), coma, dysphagia, tachycardia, moderate hypertension, and rarely convulsions and urinary retention. Other effects include jaundice (cyproheptadine [Periactin]), dystonia (diphenhydramine [Benadryl]), rhabdomyolysis (doxylamine), and, in large doses, cardiotoxic effects (diphenhydramine).

Overdose with nonsedating agents produces headache and confusion, nausea, and dysrhythmias (e.g., torsades de pointes).

Laboratory Investigations

Monitoring of ABG (in cases of respiratory depression), electrolytes, glucose, and the ECG should be undertaken. Anticholinergic drugs and plants are not routinely included on screens for substances of abuse.

Management

For patients in respiratory failure, intubation and assisted ventilation should be instituted. Gastrointestinal decontamination can be instituted. Caution must be taken with emesis in cases of diphenhydramine (Benadryl) overdose because of the drug's rapid onset of action and risk of seizures. If bowel sounds are present for up to 1 hour after ingestion, activated charcoal can be given. Seizures can be controlled with benzodiazepines (diazepam [Valium] or lorazepam [Ativan]).

The administration of physostigmine (Antilirium) is not routine and is reserved for life-threatening anticholinergic effects that are refractory to conventional treatments. It should be administered with adequate monitoring and resuscitative equipment available. The use of physostigmine should be avoided if a tricyclic antidepressant is present because of increased toxicity. Urinary retention should be relieved by catheterization to avoid reabsorption of the drug and additional toxicity.

Supraventricular tachycardia should be treated only if the patient is hemodynamically unstable. Ventricular dysrhythmias can be controlled with lidocaine or cardioversion. Sodium bicarbonate 1 to 2 mEq/kg IV may be useful for myocardial depression and QRS prolongation. Torsades de pointes, especially when associated with terfenadine and astemizole ingestion, has been treated with magnesium sulfate 4 g or 40 mL 10% solution intravenously over 10 to 20 minutes and countershock if the patient fails to respond.

Hyperpyrexia is controlled by external cooling. Hemodialysis and hemoperfusion are not effective.

Disposition

Antihistamine H_1 Antagonists

Symptomatic patients should be observed on a monitored unit until the symptoms resolve, then observed for a short time (3 to 4 hours) after resolution for relapse.

Nonsedating Agents

All asymptomatic children who acutely ingest more than the maximum adult dose and all symptomatic children should be referred to a health care facility for a minimum of 6 hours' observation as well as cardiac monitoring. Asymptomatic adults who acutely ingest more than twice the maximum adult daily dose should be monitored for a minimum of 6 hours. All symptomatic patients should be monitored for as long as there are symptoms present.

BARBITURATES

Barbiturates have been used as sedatives, anesthetic agents, and anticonvulsants, but their use is declining as safer, more effective drugs become available.

Toxic Mechanism

Barbiturates are γ-aminobutyric acid (GABA) agonists (increasing the chloride flow and inhibiting depolarization). They enhance the CNS depressant effect of GABA and depress the cardiovascular system.

Toxic Dose

The shorter-acting barbiturates (including the intermediate-acting agents) and their hypnotic doses are as follows: amobarbital (Amytal), 100 to 200 mg; aprobarbital (Alurate), 50 to 100 mg; butabarbital (Butisol), 50 to 100 mg; butalbital, 100 to 200 mg; pentobarbital (Nembutal), 100 to 200 mg; secobarbital (Seconal), 100 to 200 mg. They cause toxicity at lower doses than long-acting barbiturates and have a minimum toxic dose of 6 mg/kg; the fatal adult dose is 3 to 6 g.

The long-acting barbiturates and their doses include mephobarbital (Mebaral), 50 to 100 mg, and phenobarbital, 100 to 200 mg. Their minimum toxic dose is greater than 10 mg/kg, and the fatal adult dose is 6 to 10 g. A general rule is that an amount five times the hypnotic dose is toxic and an amount 10 times the hypnotic dose is potentially fatal. Methohexital and thiopental are ultrashort-acting parenteral preparations and are not discussed.

Kinetics

The barbiturates are enzyme inducers. Short-acting barbiturates are highly lipid-soluble, penetrate the brain readily, and have shorter elimination times. Onset of action is in 10 to 30 minutes, with a peak at 1 to 2 hours. Duration of action is 3 to 8 hours. The volume distribution of short-acting barbiturate is 0.8 to 1.5 L/kg; pKa is about 8. Mean half-life varies from 8 to 48 hours.

Long-acting agents have longer elimination times and can be used as anticonvulsants. Onset of action is in 20 to 60 minutes, with a peak at 1 to 6 hours. In cases of overdose, the peak can be at 10 hours. Usual duration of action is 8 to 12 hours. Volume distribution is 0.8 L/kg, and half-life is 11 to 120 hours. The pKa of phenobarbital is 7.2. Alkalinization of urine promotes its excretion.

Manifestations

Mild intoxication resembles alcohol intoxication and includes ataxia, slurred speech, and depressed cognition. Severe intoxication causes slow respirations, coma, and loss of reflexes (except pupillary light reflex).

Other manifestations include hypotension (vasodilation), hypothermia, hypoglycemia, and death by respiratory arrest.

Laboratory Investigations

Most barbiturates are detected on routine drug screens and can be measured in most hospital laboratories. Investigation should include barbiturate level; ABG; toxicology screen, including acetaminophen; glucose, electrolyte, BUN, creatinine, and creatine kinase levels; and urine pH. The minimum toxic plasma levels are greater than 10 μg/mL for short-acting barbiturates and greater than 40 μg/dL for long-acting agents. Fatal levels are 30 μg/mL for short-acting barbiturates and 80 to 150 μg/mL for long-acting agents. Both short-acting and long-acting agents can be detected in urine 24 to 72 hours after ingestion, and long-acting agents can be detected up to 7 days.

Management

Vital functions must be established and maintained. Intensive supportive care including intubation and assisted ventilation should dominate the management. All stuporous and comatose patients should have glucose (for hypoglycemia), thiamine (if chronically alcoholic), and naloxone (Narcan) (in case of an opioid ingestion) intravenously and should be admitted to the intensive care unit. Emesis should be avoided especially in cases of ingestion of the shorter-acting barbiturates. Activated charcoal followed by MDAC (0.5 g/kg) every 2 to 4 hours has been shown to reduce the serum half-life of phenobarbital by 50%, but its effect on clinical course is undetermined.

Fluids should be administered to correct dehydration and hypotension. Vasopressors may be necessary to correct severe hypotension, and hemodynamic monitoring may be needed. The patient must be observed carefully for fluid overload. Alkalinization (ion trapping) is used only for phenobarbital (pKa 7.2) but not for short-acting barbiturates. Sodium bicarbonate, 1 to 2 mEq/kg IV in 500 mL of 5% dextrose in adults or 10 to 15 mL/kg in children during the first hour, followed by sufficient bicarbonate to keep the urinary pH at 7.5 to 8.0, enhances excretion of phenobarbital and shortens the half-life by 50%. Diuresis is not advocated because of the danger of cerebral or pulmonary edema.

Hemodialysis shortens the half-life to 8 to 14 hours, and charcoal hemoperfusion shortens the half-life to 6 to 8 hours for long-acting barbiturates such as phenobarbital. Both procedures may be effective in patients with both long-acting and short-acting barbiturate ingestion. If the patient does not respond to supportive measures or if the phenobarbital plasma concentration is greater than 150 μg/mL, both procedures may be tried to shorten the half-life.

Bullae are treated as a local second-degree skin burn. Hypothermia should be treated.

Disposition

All comatose patients should be admitted to the intensive care unit. Awake and oriented patients with an overdose of short-acting agents should be observed for at least 6 asymptomatic hours; overdose of long-acting agents warrants observation for at least 12 asymptomatic hours because of the potential for delayed absorption. In the case of an intentional overdose, psychiatric clearance is needed before the patient can be discharged. Chronic use can lead to tolerance, physical dependency, and withdrawal and necessitates follow-up.

BENZODIAZEPINES

Benzodiazepines are used as anxiolytics, sedatives, and relaxants.

Toxic Mechanism

The GABA agonists produce CNS depression and increase chloride flow, inhibiting depolarization.

Flunitrazepam (Rohypnol; street name "roofies") is a long-acting benzodiazepine agonist sold by prescription in more than 60 countries worldwide, but it is not legally available in the United States.

Toxic Dose

The long-acting benzodiazepines (half-life >24 hours) and their maximum therapeutic doses are as follows: chlordiazepoxide (Librium), 50 mg; clorazepate (Tranxene), 30 mg; clonazepam (Klonopin), 20 mg; diazepam (Valium), 10 mg in adults or 0.2 mg/kg in children; flurazepam (Dalmane), 30 mg; and prazepam, 20 mg.

The short-acting benzodiazepines (half-life 10 to 24 hours) and their doses include the following: alprazolam (Xanax), 0.5 mg, and lorazepam (Ativan), 4 mg in adults or 0.05 mg/kg in children, which act similar to the long-acting benzodiazepines.

The ultrashort-acting benzodiazepines (half-life <10 hours) are more toxic and include temazepam (Restoril), 30 mg; triazolam (Halcion), 0.5 mg; midazolam (Versed), 0.2 mg/kg; and oxazepam (Serax), 30 mg.

In cases of overdose of short- and long-acting agents, 10 to 20 times the therapeutic dose (>1500 mg diazepam or 2000 mg chlordiazepoxide) have been ingested with resulting mild coma but without respiratory depression. Fatalities are rare, and most patients recover within 24 to 36 hours after overdose. Asymptomatic unintentional overdoses of less than five times the therapeutic dose can be seen. Ultrashort-acting agents have produced respiratory arrest and coma within 1 hour after ingestion of 5 mg of triazolam (Halcion) and death with ingestion of as little as 10 mg. Midazolam (Versed) and diazepam (Valium) by rapid intravenous injection have produced respiratory arrest.

Kinetics

Onset of CNS depression is usually in 30 to 120 minutes; peak action usually occurs within 1 to 3 hours when ingestion is by the oral route.

The volume distribution varies from 0.26 to 6 L/kg (LA, 1.1 L/kg); protein binding is 70% to 99%. For flunitrazepam, the onset of action is in 0.5 to 2 hours, oral peak is in 2 hours, and duration 8 hours or more. The half-life of flunitrazepam is 20 to 30 hours, volume distribution is 3.3 to 5.5 L/kg, and 80% is protein bound. Flunitrazepam can be identified in urine 4 to 30 days after ingestion.

Manifestations

Neurologic manifestations include ataxia, slurred speech, and CNS depression. Deep coma leading to respiratory depression suggests the presence of short-acting benzodiazepines or other CNS depressants. In elderly persons, the therapeutic doses can produce toxicity and can have an additive effect with other CNS depressants. Chronic use can lead to tolerance, physical dependency, and withdrawal.

Laboratory Investigations

Most benzodiazepines can be detected in urine drug screens. Quantitative blood levels are not useful. Some of the immunoassay urinary screens cannot detect all of the new benzodiazepines currently available. A consultation with the laboratory analyst is warranted if a specific case occurs in which the test result is negative but benzodiazepine use is suspected by the patient's history. Situations in which benzodiazepines may not be detected include ingestion of a low dose (e.g., <10 mg), rapid elimination, and a different or no metabolite. Some immunoassay methods can produce a false-positive finding for the benzodiazepines when nonsteroidal anti-inflammatory drugs (tolmetin [Tolectin], naproxen [Aleve], etodolac [Lodine], and fenoprofen [Nalfon]) are used. If this is a concern, the laboratory analyst should be consulted.

In cases in which "date rape" drugs such as flunitrazepam are suspected, a police crime or reference laboratory should be consulted for testing.

Management

Emesis and gastric lavage should be avoided. Activated charcoal can be useful only if given early before the peak time of absorption occurs. Supportive treatment should be instituted but rarely requires intubation or assisted ventilation.

Flumazenil (Romazicon) is a specific benzodiazepine receptor antagonist that blocks the chloride flow and inhibitor of GABA neurotransmitters. It reverses the sedative effects of benzodiazepines, zolpidem (Ambien), and endogenous benzodiazepines associated with hepatic encephalopathy. It is not recommended to reverse benzodiazepine-induced hypoventilation. The manufacturer advises that flumazenil be used with caution in cases of overdose with possible benzodiazepine dependency (because it can precipitate life-threatening withdrawal), if cyclic antidepressant use is suspected, or if a patient has a known seizure disorder.

Disposition

If the patient is comatose, he or she must be admitted to the intensive care unit. If the overdose was intentional, psychiatric clearance is needed before the patient can be discharged.

β-ADRENERGIC BLOCKERS (β-BLOCKERS)

β-Blockers are used in the treatment of hypertension and of a number of systemic and ophthalmologic disorders. Properties of β-blockers include the factors listed in Table 12.

Lipid-soluble drugs have CNS effects, active metabolites, longer duration of action, and interactions (e.g., propranolol). Cardioselectivity is lost in overdose. Intrinsic partial agonist agents (e.g., pindolol) may initially produce tachycardia and hypertension. Cardiac membrane depressive effect (quinidine-like) occurs in cases of overdose but not at therapeutic doses (e.g., with metoprolol or sotalol). α-Blocking effect is weak (e.g., with labetalol or acebutolol).

Toxic Mechanism

β-Blockers compete with the catecholamines for receptor sites and block receptor action in the bronchi, the vascular smooth muscle, and the myocardium.

Toxic Dose

Ingestions of greater than twice the maximum recommended daily therapeutic dose are considered toxic (see Table 12). Ingestion of 1 mg/kg propranolol in a child may produce hypoglycemia. Fatalities have been reported in adults with 7.5 g of metoprolol. The most toxic agent is sotalol, and the least toxic is atenolol.

Kinetics

Regular-release formulations usually cause symptoms within 2 hours. Propranolol's onset of action is 20 to 30 minutes and peak is at 1 to 4 hours, but it may be delayed by co-ingestants. The onset of action with sustained-release preparations may be delayed to 6 hours and the peak to 12 to 16 hours. Volume distribution is 1 to 5.6 L/kg. Protein binding is variable, from 5% to 93%.

Metabolism

Atenolol (Tenormin), nadolol (Corgard), and santalol (Betapace) have enterohepatic recirculation. The duration of action for regular-acting agents is 4 to 6 hours, but in cases of overdose it may be 24 to 48 hours. The duration of action for sustained-release agents is 24 to 48 hours.

The regular preparation with the longest half-life is nadolol, at 12 to 24 hours, and the one with the shortest half-life is esmolol, at 5 to 10 minutes.

Manifestations

See "Toxic Properties" and Table 12.

Highly lipid soluble agents produce coma and seizures. Bradycardia and hypotension are the major cardiac symptoms and may lead to cardiogenic shock. Intrinsic partial agonists initially may cause tachycardia and hypertension. ECG changes include atrioventricular conduction delay or asystole. Membrane-depressant effects produce prolonged QRS and QT interval, which may result in torsades de pointes. Sotalol produces a very prolonged QT interval. Bronchospasm may occur in patients with reactive airway disease with any β-blocker because the selectivity is lost in overdose. Other manifestations include hypoglycemia (because β-blockers block catecholamine counter-regulatory mechanisms) and hyperkalemia.

Laboratory Investigations

Measurements of blood levels are not readily available or useful. ECG and cardiac monitoring should be maintained, and blood glucose and electrolytes, BUN, and creatinine levels should be monitored, as well as ABG if there are respiratory symptoms.

Management

Vital functions must be established and maintained. Vascular access, baseline ECG, and continuous cardiac and blood pressure monitoring should be established. A pacemaker must be available. Gastrointestinal decontamination can be undertaken initially with activated charcoal up to 1 hour after ingestion. MDAC is no longer recommended, based on the latest guidelines. Whole-bowel irrigation can be considered in cases of large overdoses with sustained-release preparations, but there are no studies evaluating the efficacy of intervention.

If there are cardiovascular disturbances, a cardiac consultation should be obtained. Class IA antidysrhythmic agents (procainamide, quinidine) and III (bretylium) are not recommended. Hypotension is treated with fluids initially, although it usually does not respond.

TABLE 12 Pharmacologic and Toxic Properties of β-Blockers

Blocker	Maximum Solubility	Therapeutic Plasma Level	Lipid Solubility	Intrinsic Sympathomimetic Activity (Partial Agonist)	Membrane Stabilizing Effect	Cardiac Selectivity β-Selective β1	β2	α-Selective
Acebutolol (Sectral)	800 mg	200-2000 ng/mL	Moderate	+	+	+	+	
Alprenolol[2]	800 mg	50-200 ng/mL	Moderate	2+	+	−	−	
Atenolol (Tenormin)	100 mg	200-500 ng/mL	Low	−	−	2+	−	
Betaxolol (Kerlone)	20 mg	NA	Low	+	−	+	−	
Carteolol (Cartrol)	10 mg	NA	No	+	−	−	−	
Esmolol (Brevibloc) (Class II antidysrhythmic, IV only)			Low	−	−	+	−	
Labetalol (Trandate)	800 mg	50-500 ng/mL	Low	+	+/−	−	+	
Levobunolol (AKBeta eyedrop) (Eye drops 0.25% and 0.5%)	20 mg	NA	No	−	−	−	−	
Metoprolol (Lopressor)			Moderate	−	−	2+	−	
Nadolol (Corgard)	320 mg	20-40 ng/mL	Low	−	−	−	−	
Oxyprenolol[2]	480 mg	80-100 ng/mL	Moderate	2+	+	−	−	
Pindolol (Visken)	60 mg	50-150 ng/mL	Moderate	3+	+/−	−	−	
Propranolol (Inderal) (Class II antidysrhythmic)	360 mg	50-100 ng/mL	High	−	2+	−	−	
Sotalol (Betapace) (Class II antidysrhythmic)	480 mg	500-4000 ng/mL	Low	−	−	−	−	
Timolol (Blocadren)	60 mg	5-10 ng/mL	Low	−	+/−	−	−	

[2]Not available in the United States.

Frequently, glucagon and cardiac pacing are needed. Bradycardia in asymptomatic, hemodynamically stable patients requires no therapy. It is not predictive of the future course of the disease. If the patient is unstable (has hypotension or a high-degree atrioventricular block), atropine 0.02 mg/kg (up to 2 mg) in adults, glucagon, and a pacemaker can be used. In case of ventricular tachycardia, overdrive pacing can be used. A wide QRS interval may respond to sodium bicarbonate. Torsades de pointes (associated with sotalol) may respond to magnesium sulfate and overdrive pacing. Prophylactic magnesium for prolonged QT interval has been suggested, but there are no data. Epinephrine must not be used because an unopposed α effect may occur.

Hypotension and myocardial depression are managed by correction of dysrhythmias, Trendelenburg position, fluids, glucagon, or amrinone (Inocor), or a combination of these. Hemodynamic monitoring with a Swan-Ganz catheter or arterial line may be necessary to manage fluid therapy.

Glucagon is the initial drug of choice. It works through adenyl cyclase and bypasses catecholamine receptors; therefore, it is not affected by β-blockers. Glucagon increases cardiac contractility and heart rate. It is given as an intravenous bolus of 5 to 10 mg[C] over 1 minute and followed by a continuous infusion of 1 to 5 mg/h (in children, 0.15 mg/kg followed by 0.05 to 0.1 mg/kg/h). In large doses and in infusion therapy D_5W, sterile water, or saline should be used as a dilutant to reconstitute glucagon in place of the 0.2% phenol diluent provided with some drugs. Effects are seen within minutes. It can be used with other agents such as amrinone.

Amrinone (Inocor) inhibits phosphodiesterase enzyme, which metabolizes cyclic AMP. It is administered as a bolus of 0.15 to 2 mg/kg (0.15 to 0.4 mL/kg) intravenously, followed by infusion of 5 to 10 μg/kg/min.

Hypoglycemia should be treated with intravenous glucose. Life-threatening hyperkalemia is treated with calcium (avoid if digoxin is present), bicarbonate, and glucose or insulin. Convulsions can be controlled with diazepam or phenobarbital. If bronchospasm is present, β2 nebulized bronchodilators are given.

Extraordinary measures such as intra-aortic balloon pump support can be instituted. Extracorporeal measures can be undertaken. Hemodialysis for cases of atenolol, acebutolol, nadolol, and sotalol (low volume distribution, low protein binding) ingestion may be helpful, particularly when there is evidence of renal failure. Hemodialysis is not effective for propranolol, metoprolol, and timolol.

Prenalterol[A] has successfully reversed both bradycardia and hypotension but is not currently available in the United States.

Disposition

Asymptomatic patients with history of overdose require baseline ECG and continuous cardiac monitoring for at least 6 hours with regular-release preparations and for 24 hours with sustained-release preparations. Symptomatic patients should be observed with cardiac monitoring for 24 hours. If seizures or abnormal rhythm or vital signs are present, the patient should be admitted to the intensive care unit.

CALCIUM CHANNEL BLOCKERS

Calcium channel blockers are used in the treatment of effort angina, supraventricular tachycardia, and hypertension.

Toxic Mechanism

Calcium channel blockers reduce influx of calcium through the slow channels in membranes of the myocardium, the atrioventricular nodes, and the vascular smooth muscles and result in peripheral, systemic, and coronary vasodilation, impaired cardiac conduction, and depression of cardiac contractility. All calcium channel blockers

[C]Exceeds dosage recommended by the manufacturer.

[A]Not available in the United States.

have vasodilatory action, but only bepridil, diltiazem, and verapamil depress myocardial contractility and cause atrioventricular block.

Toxic Dose

Any ingested amount greater than the maximum daily dose has the potential of severe toxicity. The maximum oral daily doses in adults and toxic doses in children of each are as follows: amlodipine (Norvasc), 10 mg for adults and more than 0.25 mg/kg for children; bepridil (Vascor), 400 mg for adults and more than 5.7 mg/kg for children; diltiazem (Cardizem), 360 mg for adults (toxic dose > 2 g) and more than 6 mg/kg for children; felodipine (Plendil), 40 mg for adults and more than 0.56 mg/kg for children; isradipine (DynaCirc), 40 mg for adults and more than 0.4 mg/kg for children; nicardipine (Cardene), 120 mg for adults and more than 0.85 mg/kg for children; nifedipine (Procardia), 120 mg for adults and more than 2 mg/kg for children; nimodipine (Nimotop), 360 mg for adults and more than 0.85 mg/kg for children; nitrendipine (Baypress),[A] 80 mg for adults and more than 1.14 mg/kg for children; and verapamil (Calan), 480 mg for adults and 15 mg/kg for children.

Kinetics

Onset of action of regular-release preparations varies: for verapamil it is 60 to 120 minutes, for nifedipine 20 minutes, and for diltiazem 15 minutes after ingestion. Peak effect for verapamil is 2 to 4 hours, for nifedipine 60 to 90 minutes, and for diltiazem 30 to 60 minutes, but the peak action may be delayed for 6 to 8 hours. Duration of action is up to 36 hours. The onset of action for sustained-release preparations is usually 4 hours but may be delayed, and peak effect is at 12 to 24 hours. In cases of massive overdose, concretions and prolonged toxicity can develop.

Volume distribution varies from 3 to 7 L/kg. Hepatic elimination half-life varies from 3 to 7 hours. Patients receiving digitalis and calcium channel blockers run the risk of digitalis toxicity, because calcium channel blockers increase digitalis levels.

Manifestations

Cardiac manifestations include hypotension, bradycardia, and conduction disturbances occurring 30 minutes to 5 hours after ingestion. A prolonged PR interval is an early finding and may occur at therapeutic doses. Torsades de pointes has been reported. All degrees of blocks may occur and may be delayed up to 16 hours. Lactic acidosis may be present. Calcium channel blockers do not affect intraventricular conduction, so the QRS interval is usually not affected.

Hypocalcemia is rarely present. Hyperglycemia may be present because of interference in calcium-dependent insulin release. Mental status changes, headaches, seizures, hemiparesis, and CNS depression may occur.

Laboratory Investigations

Specific drug levels are not readily available and are not useful. Monitor blood sugar, electrolytes, calcium, ABG, pulse oximetry, creatinine, and BUN, and also use hemodynamic monitoring, ECG, and cardiac monitoring.

Management

Vital functions must be established and maintained. Baseline ECG readings should be obtained and continuous cardiac and blood pressure monitoring maintained. A pacemaker should be available. Cardiology consultation should be sought.

Gastrointestinal decontamination with activated charcoal is recommended. If a large dose of a sustained-release preparation was ingested, whole-bowel irrigation can be considered, but its effectiveness has not been investigated.

[A]Not available in the United States.

If the patient is symptomatic, immediate cardiology consult must be obtained, because a pacemaker and hemodynamic monitoring may be needed. In the case of heart block, atropine is rarely effective and isoproterenol (Isuprel) may produce vasodilation. The use of a pacemaker should be considered early.

Hypotension and bradycardia can be treated with positioning, fluids, and calcium gluconate or chloride, glucagon, amrinone (Inocor), and ventricular pacing. Calcium salts must be avoided if digoxin is present. Calcium usually reverses depressed myocardial contractility but may not reverse nodal depression or peripheral vasodilation. Calcium chloride can be given in a 10% solution, 0.1 to 0.2 mL/kg up to 10 mL in an adult, or calcium gluconate in a 10% solution 0.3 to 0.4 mL/kg up to 20 mL in an adult. Administration is intravenous, over 5 to 10 minutes. One should monitor for dysrhythmias, hypotension, and the serum ionized calcium. The aim is to increase calcium 4 mg/dL to a maximum of 13 mg/dL. The calcium response lasts 15 minutes and may require repeated doses or a continuous calcium gluconate infusion 0.2 mL/kg/h up to maximum of 10 mL/h.

If calcium fails, glucagon can be tried for its positive inotropic and chronotropic effect, or both. Amrinone (Inocor), an inotropic agent, may reverse the effects of calcium channel blockers. An effective dose is 0.15 mg to 2 mg/kg (0.15 to 0.4 mL/kg) by intravenous bolus followed by infusion of 5 to 10 µg/kg/min.

In case of hypotension, fluids, norepinephrine (Levophed), and epinephrine may be required. Amrinone and glucagon have been tried alone and in combination. Dobutamine and dopamine are often ineffective.

Extracorporeal measures (e.g., hemodialysis and charcoal hemoperfusion) are not useful, but extraordinary measures such as intraaortic balloon pump and cardiopulmonary bypass have been used successfully.

For cases of calcium channel blocker toxicity that fail to respond to aggressive management, recent studies demonstrate that insulin and glucose have therapeutic value. The suggested dose range for insulin is to infuse regular insulin at 0.5 IU/kg/h with a simultaneous infusion of glucose 1 g/kg/h, with glucose monitoring every 30 minutes for at least the first 4 hours of administration and subsequent glucose adjustment to maintain euglycemia (70 to 100 mg/dL). Potassium levels should be monitored regularly, as they may shift in response to the insulin.

Disposition

Patients who have ingested regular-release preparations should be monitored for at least 6 hours and those who have ingested sustained-release preparations should be monitored for 24 hours after the ingestion. Intentional overdose necessitates psychiatric clearance. Symptomatic patients should be admitted to the intensive care unit.

CARBON MONOXIDE

Carbon monoxide is an odorless, colorless gas produced from incomplete combustion; it is also an in vivo metabolic breakdown product of methylene chloride used in paint removers.

Toxic Mechanism

Carbon monoxide's affinity for hemoglobin is 240 times greater than that of oxygen. It shifts the oxygen dissociation curve to the left, which impairs hemoglobin release of oxygen to tissues and inhibits the cytochrome oxidase enzymes.

Toxic Dose and Manifestations

Table 13 describes the manifestations of carbon monoxide toxicity. Exposure to 0.5% for a few minutes is lethal. Sequelae correlate with the patient's level of consciousness at presentation. ECG abnormalities may be noted. Creatine kinase is often elevated, and rhabdomyolysis and myoglobinuria may occur.

The carboxyhemoglobin (CoHB) expresses in percentage the extent to which carbon monoxide has bound with the total

TABLE 13 Carbon Monoxide Exposure and Possible Manifestations

CoHB Saturation (%)	Manifestations
3.5	None
5	Slight headache, decreased exercise tolerance
10	Slight headache, dyspnea on vigorous exertion, may impair driving skills
10-20	Moderate dyspnea on exertion, throbbing, temporal headache
20-30	Severe headache, syncope, dizziness, visual changes, weakness, nausea, vomiting, altered judgment
30-40	Vertigo, ataxia, blurred vision, confusion, loss of consciousness
40-50	Confusion, tachycardia, tachypnea, coma, convulsions
50-60	Cheyne-Stokes, coma, convulsions, shock, apnea
60-70	Coma, convulsions, respiratory and heart failure, death

hemoglobin. This may be misleadingly low in the anemic patient with less hemoglobin than normal. The patient's presentation is a more reliable indicator of severity than the CoHB level. The manifestations listed in Table 13 for each level are in addition to those listed at the level above. The CoHB may not correlate reliably with the severity of the intoxication, and linking symptoms to specific levels of CoHB frequently leads to inaccurate conclusions. A level of carbon monoxide greater than 40% is usually associated with obvious intoxication.

Kinetics

The natural metabolism of the body produces small amounts of CoHB, less than 2% for nonsmokers and 5% to 9% for smokers.

Carbon monoxide is rapidly absorbed through the lungs. The rate of absorption is directly related to alveolar ventilation. Elimination also occurs through the lungs. The half-life of CoHB in room air (21% oxygen) is 5 to 6 hours; in 100% oxygen, it is 90 minutes; in hyperbaric pressure at 3 atmospheres oxygen, it is 20 to 30 minutes.

Laboratory Investigations

An ABG reading may show metabolic acidosis and normal oxygen tension. In cases of significant poisoning, the ABG, electrolytes, blood glucose, serum creatine kinase and cardiac enzymes, renal function tests, and liver function tests should be monitored. A urinalysis and test for myoglobinuria should be obtained. Chest radiograph can be useful in cases of smoke inhalation or if the patient is being considered for hyperbaric chamber. ECG monitoring should be maintained, especially if the patient is older than 40 years, has a history of cardiac disease, or has moderate to severe symptoms. Which toxicology studies are used is based on symptoms and circumstances. CoHB should be monitored during and at the end of therapy. The pulse oximeter has two wavelengths and overestimates oxyhemoglobin saturation in carbon monoxide poisoning. The true oxygen saturation is determined by blood gas analysis, which measures the oxygen bound to hemoglobin. The co-oximeter measures four wavelengths and separates out CoHB and the other hemoglobin binding agents from oxyhemoglobin. Fetal hemoglobin has a greater affinity for carbon monoxide than adult hemoglobin and may falsely elevate the CoHB as much as 4% in young infants.

Management

The first step is to adequately protect the rescuer. The patient must be removed from the contaminated area, and his or her vital functions must be established.

The mainstay of treatment is 100% oxygen via a non-rebreathing mask with an oxygen reservoir or endotracheal tube. All patients receive 100% oxygen until the CoHB level is 5% or less. Assisted ventilation may be necessary. ABG and CoHB should be monitored and the present CoHB level determined. *Note:* A near-normal CoHB level does not exclude significant carbon monoxide poisoning, especially if the measurement is taken several hours after termination of exposure or if oxygen has been administered prior to obtaining the sample.

The exposed pregnant woman should be kept on 100% oxygen for several hours after the CoHB level is almost 0, because carbon monoxide concentrates in the fetus and oxygen is needed longer to ensure elimination of the carbon monoxide from fetal circulation. The fetus must be monitored, because carbon monoxide and hypoxia are potentially teratogenic.

Metabolic acidosis should be treated with sodium bicarbonate only if the pH is below 7.2 after correction of hypoxia and adequate ventilation. Acidosis shifts the oxygen dissociation curve to the right and facilitates oxygen delivery to the tissues.

The decision to use the hyperbaric oxygen chamber must be made on the basis of the ability to handle other acute emergencies that may coexist in the patient and of the severity of the poisoning. The standard of care for persons exposed to carbon monoxide has yet to be determined, but most authorities recommend using the hyperbaric oxygen chamber under any of the following conditions:

- If the patient is in a coma or has a history of loss of consciousness or seizures
- If there is cardiovascular dysfunction (clinical ischemic chest pain or ECG evidence of ischemia)
- If the patient has metabolic acidosis
- If symptoms persist despite 100% oxygen therapy
- In a child, if the initial CoHB is greater than 15%
- In symptomatic patients with preexisting ischemia
- If there are signs of maternal or fetal distress regardless of CoHB level (infants and fetus are a special problem because fetal hemoglobin has greater affinity for carbon monoxide)

Although controversial, a neurologic-cognitive examination has been used to help determine which patients with low carbon monoxide levels should receive more aggressive therapy. Testing should include the following: general orientation memory testing involving address, phone number, date of birth, and present date; and cognitive testing, involving counting by 7s, digit span, and forward and backward spelling of three-letter and four-letter words. Patients with delayed neurologic sequelae or recurrent symptoms up to 3 weeks may benefit from hyperbaric oxygen chamber treatment.

Seizures and cerebral edema must be treated.

Disposition

Patients with no or mild symptoms who become asymptomatic after a few hours of oxygen therapy and have a carbon monoxide level less than 10%, and normal physical and neurologic-cognitive examination findings can be discharged, but they should be instructed to return if any signs of neurologic dysfunction appear. Patients with carbon monoxide poisoning requiring treatment need follow-up neuropsychiatric examinations.

CAUSTICS AND CORROSIVES

The terms *caustic* and *corrosive* are used interchangeably and can be divided into acids and alkalis. The U.S. Consumer Product Safety Commission Labeling Recommendations on containers for acids and alkalis indicate the potential for producing serious damage, as follows:

- Caution—weak irritant
- Warning—strong irritant
- Danger—corrosive

Some common acids with corrosive potential include acetic acid, formic acid, glycolic acid, hydrochloric acid, mercuric chloride, nitric acid, oxalic acid, phosphoric acid, sulfuric acid (battery acid), zinc chloride, and zinc sulfate. Some common alkalis with corrosive potential include ammonia, calcium carbide, calcium hydroxide (dry), calcium oxide, potassium hydroxide (lye), and sodium hydroxide (lye).

Toxic Mechanism

Acids produce mucosal coagulation necrosis and may be absorbed systemically; they do not penetrate deeply. Injury to the gastric mucosa is more likely, although specific sites of injury for acids and alkalis are not clearly defined.

Alkalis produce liquefaction necrosis and saponification and penetrate deeply. The esophageal mucosa is likely to be damaged. Oropharyngeal and esophageal damage is more frequently caused by solids than by liquids. Liquids produce superficial circumferential burns and gastric damage.

Toxic Dose

The toxicity is determined by concentration, contact time, and pH. Significant injury is more likely with a substance that has a pH of less than 2 or greater than 12, with a prolonged contact time, and with large volumes.

Manifestations

The absence of oral burns does not exclude the possibility of esophageal or gastric damage. General clinical findings are stridor; dysphagia; drooling; oropharyngeal, retrosternal, and epigastric pain; and ocular and oral burns. Alkali burns are yellow, soapy, frothy lesions. Acid burns are gray-white and later form an eschar. Abdominal tenderness and guarding may be present if perforation has happened.

Laboratory Investigations

If acid ingestion has taken place, the patient's acid–base balance and electrolyte status should be determined. If pulmonary symptoms are present, a chest radiograph, ABG measurement, and pulse oximetry are called for.

Management

It is recommended that the container be brought to the examination, as the substance must be identified and the pH of the substance, vomitus, tears, or saliva tested.

If the acid or alkali has been ingested, all gastrointestinal decontamination procedures are contraindicated except for immediate rinse, removal of substance from the mouth, and dilution with small amounts (sips) of milk or water. The examiner should check for ocular and dermal involvement. Contraindications to oral dilution are dysphagias, respiratory distress, obtundation, or shock. If there is ocular involvement one should immediately irrigate the eye with tepid water for at least 30 minutes, perform fluorescein stain of eye, and consult an ophthalmologist. If there is dermal involvement, one should immediately remove contaminated clothes and irrigate the skin with tepid water for at least 15 minutes. Consultation with a burn specialist is called for.

In cases of acid ingestion, some authorities advocate a small flexible nasogastric tube and aspiration within 30 minutes after ingestion.

Patients should receive only intravenous fluids following dilution until endoscopic consultation is obtained. Endoscopy is valuable to predict damage and risk of stricture. The indications are controversial, with some authorities recommending it in all cases of caustic ingestions regardless of symptoms, and others selectively using clinical features such as vomiting, stridor, drooling, and oral or facial lesions as criteria. We recommend endoscopy for all symptomatic patients or patients with intentional ingestions. Endoscopy may be performed immediately if the patient is symptomatic, but it is usually done 12 to 48 hours postingestion.

The use of corticosteroids is considered controversial. Some feel they may be useful for patients with second-degree circumferential burns. They recommend starting with hydrocortisone sodium succinate (Solu-Cortef) intravenously 10 to 20 mg/kg/d within 48 hours and changing to oral prednisolone 2 mg/kg/d for 3 weeks before tapering the dose. We do not usually recommend using corticosteroids because they have not been shown to be effective.

Tetanus prophylaxis should be provided if the patient requires it for wound care. Antibiotics are not useful prophylactically. Contrast studies are not useful in the first few days and may interfere with endoscopic evaluation; later, they can be used to assess the severity of damage.

Emergency medical therapy includes agents to inhibit collagen formation and intraluminal stents. Esophageal and gastric outlet dilation may be needed if there is evidence of stricture. Bougienage of the esophagus, however, has been associated with brain abscess. Interposition of the colon may be necessary if dilation fails to provide an adequate-sized passage.

Management of inhalation cases requires immediate removal from the environment, administration of humid supplemental oxygen, and observation for airway obstruction and noncardiac pulmonary edema. Radiographic and ABG evaluation should be obtained when appropriate. Intubation and respiratory support may be required.

Certain caustics produce systemic disturbances. Formaldehyde causes metabolic acidosis, hydrofluoric acid causes hypocalcemia and renal damage, oxalic acid causes hypocalcemia, phenol causes hepatic and renal damage, and picric acid causes renal injury.

Disposition

Infants and small children should be medically evaluated and observed. All symptomatic patients should be admitted. If they have severe symptoms or danger of airway compromise, they should be admitted to the intensive care unit. After endoscopy, if no damage is detected, the patient may be discharged when he or she can tolerate oral feedings. Intentional exposures require psychiatric evaluation before the patient can be discharged.

COCAINE (BENZOYLMETHYLECGONINE)

Cocaine is derived from the leaves of *Erythroxylum coca* and *Truxillo coca*. "Body packing" refers to the placement of many small packages of contraband cocaine for concealment in the gastrointestinal tract or other areas for illicit transport. "Body stuffing" refers to spontaneous ingestion of substances for the purpose of hiding evidence.

Toxic Mechanism

Cocaine directly stimulates the CNS presynaptic sympathetic neurons to release catecholamines and acetylcholine, while it blocks the presynaptic reuptake of the catecholamines; it blocks the sodium channels along neuronal membranes; and it increases platelet aggregation. Long-term use depletes the CNS of dopamine.

Toxic Dose

The maximum mucosal local anesthetic therapeutic dose of cocaine is 200 mg or 2 mL of a 10% solution. Although CNS effects can occur at relatively low local anesthetic doses (50 to 95 mg), they are more common with doses greater than 1 mg/kg; cardiac effects can occur with doses greater than 1 mg/kg. The potential fatal dose is 1200 mg intranasally, but death has occurred with 20 mg parenterally.

Kinetics

Cocaine is well absorbed by all routes, including nasal insufflation, and oral, dermal, and inhalation routes (Table 14). Protein binding is 8.7%, and volume distribution is 1.5 L/kg.

Cocaine is metabolized by plasma and liver cholinesterase to the inactive metabolites ecgonine methyl ester and benzoylecgonine. Plasma pseudocholinesterase is congenitally deficient in 3% of the population and decreased in fetuses, young infants, the elderly,

TABLE 14 The Different Routes and Kinetics of Cocaine

Type	Route	Onset	Peak (min)	Half-life (min)	Duration (min)
Cocaine leaf	Oral, chewing	20-30 min	45-90	NA	240-360
Hydrochloride	Insufflation	1-3 min	5-10	78	60-90
	Ingestion	20-30 min	50-90	54	Sustained
	Intravenous	30-120 sec	5-11	36	60-90
Free base/crack	Smoking	5-10 sec	5-11	—	Up to 20
Coca paste	Smoking	Unknown	—	—	—

pregnant people, and people with liver disease. These enzyme-deficient individuals are at increased risk for life-threatening cocaine toxicity.

Ten percent of cocaine is excreted unchanged. Cocaine and ethanol undergo liver synthesis to form cocaethylene, a metabolite with a half-life three times longer than that of cocaine. It may account for some of cocaine's cardiotoxicity and appears to be more lethal than cocaine or ethanol alone.

Manifestations

The CNS manifestations of cocaine ingestion are euphoria, hyperactivity, agitation, convulsions, and intracranial hemorrhage. Mydriasis and septal perforation can occur, as well as cardiac dysrhythmias, hypertension, and hypotension (with severe overdose). Chest pain is frequent, but only 5.8% of patients have true myocardial ischemia and infarction. Other manifestations include vasoconstriction, hyperthermia (because of increased metabolic rate), ischemic bowel perforation if the substance is ingested, rhabdomyolysis, myoglobinuria, and renal failure. In pregnant users, premature labor and abruptio placentae can occur.

Body cavity packing should be suspected in cases of prolonged toxicity.

Mortality can result from cerebrovascular accidents, coronary artery spasm, myocardial injury, or lethal dysrhythmias.

Laboratory Investigations

Monitoring of the ECG and cardiac rhythms, ABG, oxygen saturation, electrolytes, blood glucose, BUN, creatinine, and creatine kinase levels should be maintained. One should monitor cardiac fraction if the patient has chest pain, as well as the liver profile, and the urine for myoglobin. Intravenous drug users should have HIV and hepatitis virus testing.

Urine should be tested for cocaine and metabolites and other substances of abuse, and abdominal radiographs or ultrasonogram should be ordered for body packers. If the urine sample was collected more than 12 hours after cocaine intake, it will contain little or no cocaine. If cocaine is present, cocaine has been used within the past 12 hours. Cocaine's metabolite benzoylecgonine may be detected within 4 hours after a single nasal insufflation and for up to 114 hours. Cross-reactions with some herbal teas, lidocaine, and droperidol (Inapsine) may give false-positive results by some immunoassay methods.

Management

Supportive care includes blood pressure, cardiac, and thermal monitoring and seizure precautions. Diazepam (Valium) is the drug of choice for treatment of cocaine toxicity agitation, seizures, and dysrhythmias; doses are 10 to 30 mg intravenously at 2.5 mg per minute for adults and 0.2 to 0.5 mg/kg at 1 mg per minute up to 10 mg for a child.

Gastrointestinal decontamination should be instituted, if the cocaine was ingested, by administration of activated charcoal. MDAC may adsorb cocaine leakage in body stuffers or body packers. Whole-bowel irrigation with polyethylene glycol solution (PEG) has been used in body packers and stuffers if the contraband is in a firm container. If the packages are not visible on plain radiographs of the abdomen, a contrast study or CT scan can help to confirm successful passage. Cocaine in the nasal passage can be removed with an applicator dipped in a non–water-soluble product (lubricating jelly) if this is done within a few minutes after application.

In body packers and stuffers, venous access must be secured, and drugs must be readily available for treating life-threatening manifestations until the contraband is passed in the stool. Surgical removal may be indicated if the packet does not pass the pylorus, in an asymptomatic body packer, or in the case of intestinal obstruction.

Hypertension and tachycardia are usually transient and can be managed by careful titration of diazepam. Nitroprusside may be used for severe hypertension. Myocardial ischemia is managed by oxygen, vascular access, benzodiazepines, and nitroglycerin. Aspirin and thrombolysis are not routinely recommended because of the danger of intracranial hemorrhage.

Dysrhythmias are usually supraventricular (SVT) and do not require specific management. Adenosine is ineffective. Life-threatening tachydysrhythmias may respond to phentolamine (Regitine) 5 mg IV bolus in adults or 0.1 mg/kg in children at 5- to 10-minute intervals. Phentolamine also relieves coronary artery spasm and myocardial ischemia. Electrical synchronized cardioversion should be considered for patients with hemodynamically unstable dysrhythmias. Lidocaine is not recommended initially but may be used after 3 hours for ventricular tachycardia. Wide complex QRS ventricular tachycardia may be treated with sodium bicarbonate 2 mEq/kg as a bolus. β-Adrenergic blockers are not recommended.

Anxiety, agitation, and convulsions can be treated with diazepam. If diazepam fails to control seizures, neuromuscular blockers can be used. The EEG should be monitored for nonmotor seizure activity. For hyperthermia, external cooling and cool humidified 100% oxygen should be administered. Neuromuscular paralysis to control seizures will reduce temperature. Dantrolene and antipyretics are not recommended. Rhabdomyolysis and myoglobinuria are treated with fluids, alkaline diuresis, and diuretics.

If the patient is pregnant, the fetus must be monitored and the patient observed for spontaneous abortion.

Paranoid ideation and threatening behavior should be treated with rapid tranquilization. The patient should be observed for suicidal depression that may follow intoxication and may require suicide precautions. If focal neurologic manifestations are present, one should consider the possibility of a cerebrovascular accident and obtain a CT scan.

Extracorporeal clearance techniques are of no benefit.

Disposition

Patients with mild intoxication or a brief seizure that does not require treatment who become asymptomatic may be discharged after 6 hours with appropriate psychosocial follow-up. If cardiac or cerebral ischemic manifestations are present, the patient should be monitored in the intensive care unit. Body packers and stuffers require care in the intensive care unit until passage of the contraband.

CYANIDE

Hydrogen cyanide is a byproduct of burning plastic and wools in residential fires. Hydrocyanic acid is the liquefied form of hydrogen cyanide. Cyanide salts can be found in ore extraction. Nitriles, such as acetonitrile (artificial nail removers) are metabolized in the body to produce cyanide. Cyanogenic glycosides are present in some fruit seeds (such as amygdalin in apricots, peaches, and apples). Sodium nitroprusside, the antihypertensive vasodilator, contains five cyanide groups.

Toxic Mechanism

Cyanide blocks the cellular electron transport mechanism and cellular respiration by inhibiting the mitochondrial ferricytochrome oxidase system and other enzymes. This results in cellular hypoxia and lactic acidosis. *Note:* Citrus fruit seeds form cyanide in the presence of intestinal β-glucosidase (the seeds are harmful only if the capsule is broken).

Toxic Dose

The ingestion of 1 mg/kg or 50 mg of hydrogen cyanide can produce death within 15 minutes. The lethal dose of potassium cyanide is 200 mg. Five to 10 mL of 84% acetonitrile is lethal. Infusions of sodium nitroprusside in rates above 2 µg/kg per minute may cause cyanide to accumulate to toxic concentrations in critically ill patients.

Kinetics

Cyanide is rapidly absorbed by all routes. In the stomach, it forms hydrocyanic acid. Volume distribution is 1.5 L/kg. Protein binding is 60%. Cyanide is detoxified by metabolism in the liver via the mitochondrial thiosulfate-rhodanase pathway, which catalyzes the transfer of sulfur donor to cyanide, forming the less toxic irreversible thiocyanate that is excreted in the urine. Cyanide is also detoxified by reacting with hydroxocobalamin (vitamin B_{12a}) to form cyanocobalamin (vitamin B_{12}).

The cyanide elimination half-life from the blood is 1.2 hours. The elimination route is through the lungs.

Manifestations

Hydrogen cyanide has the distinctive odor of bitter almonds or silver polish. Manifestations of cyanide intoxication include hypertension, cardiac dysrhythmias, various ECG abnormalities, headache, hyperpnea, seizures, stupor, pulmonary edema, and flushing. Cyanosis is absent or appears late.

Laboratory Investigations

The examiner should obtain and monitor ABGs, oxygen saturation, blood lactate, hemoglobin, blood glucose, and electrolytes. Lactic acidemia, a decrease in the arterial-venous oxygen difference, and bright red venous blood occurs. If smoke inhalation is the possible source of cyanide exposure, CoHB and methemoglobin (MetHb) concentrations should be measured.

Cyanide levels in whole blood, red blood cells, or serum are not useful in the acute management because the determinations are not readily available. Specific cyanide blood levels are as follows: smokers have less than 0.5 µg/mL; a patient with flushing and tachycardia has 0.5 to 1.0 µg/mL, one with obtundation has 1.0 to 2.5 µg/mL, and one in coma or who has died has more than 2.5 µg/mL.

Management

If the cyanide was inhaled, the patient must be removed from the contaminated atmosphere. Attendants should not administer mouth-to-mouth resuscitation. Rescuers and attendants must be protected. Immediate administration of 100% oxygen is called for and oxygen should be continued during and after the administration of the antidote. The clinician must decide whether to use any or all components of the cyanide antidote kit.

The mechanism of action of the antidote kit is twofold: to produce methemoglobinemia and to provide a sulfur substrate for the detoxification of cyanide. The nitrites make methemoglobin, which has a greater affinity for cyanide than does the cytochrome oxidase enzymes. The combination of methemoglobin and cyanide forms cyanomethemoglobin. Sodium thiosulfate provides a sulfur substrate for the rhodanese enzyme, which converts cyanide into the relatively nontoxic sodium thiocyanate, which is excreted by the kidney.

The procedure for using the antidote kit is as follows:

Step 1: Amyl nitrite inhalant perles is only a temporizing measure (forms only 2% to 5% methemoglobin) and it can be omitted if venous access is established. Alternate 100% oxygen and the inhalant for 30 seconds each minute. Use a new perle every 3 minutes.

Step 2: Sodium nitrite ampule is indicated for cyanide exposures, except for cases of residential fires, smoke inhalation, and nitroprusside or acetonitrile poisonings. It is administered intravenously to produce methemoglobin of 20% to 30% at 35 to 70 minutes after administration. A dose of 10 mL of 3% solution of sodium nitrite for adults and 0.33 mL/kg of 3% solution for children is diluted to 100 mL 0.9% saline and administered slowly intravenously at 5 mL/min. If hypotension develops, the infusion should be slowed.

Step 3: Sodium thiosulfate is useful alone in cases of smoke inhalation, nitroprusside toxicity, and acetonitrile toxicity and should not be used at all in cases of hydrogen sulfide poisoning. The administration dose is 12.5 g of sodium thiosulfate or 50 mL of 25% solution for adults and 1.65 mL/kg of 25% solution for children intravenously over 10 to 20 minutes.

If cyanide symptoms recur, further treatment with nitrites or the perles is controversial. Some authorities suggest repeating the antidotes in 30 minutes at half of the initial dose, but others do not advise this for lack of efficacy. The child dosage regimen on the package insert must be carefully followed.

One hour after antidotes are administered, the methemoglobin level should be obtained and should not exceed 20%. Methylene blue should not be used to reverse excessive methemoglobin.

Gastrointestinal decontamination of oral ingestion by activated charcoal is recommended but is not very effective because of the rapidity of absorption. Seizures are treated with intravenous diazepam. Acidosis should be treated with sodium bicarbonate if it does not rapidly resolve with therapy. There is no role for hyperbaric oxygen or hemodialysis or hemoperfusion.

Other antidotes include hydroxocobalamin (vitamin B_{12a}) (Cyanokit), which has proven effective when given immediately after exposure in large doses of 4 g (50 mg/kg) or 50 times the amount of cyanide exposure with 8 g of sodium thiosulfate. Hydroxocobalamin has FDA orphan drug approval.

Disposition

Asymptomatic patients should be observed for a minimum of 3 hours. Patients who ingest nitrile compounds must be observed for 24 hours. Patients requiring antidote administration should be admitted to the intensive care unit.

DIGITALIS

Cardiac glycosides are found in cardiac medications, common plants, and the skin of the Bufo toad.

Toxic Mechanism

Cardiac glycosides inhibit the enzyme sodium/potassium-adenosine triphosphatase (NA^+, K^+, ATPase), leading to intracellular potassium loss and increased intracellular sodium, and producing phase 4 depolarization, increased automaticity, and ectopy. There is increased intracellular calcium and potentiation of contractility. Pacemaker cells are inhibited, and the refractory period is prolonged, leading to atrioventricular blocks. There is increased vagal tone.

Toxic Dose

Digoxin total digitalizing dose, the dose required to achieve therapeutic blood levels of 0.6 to 2.0 ng/mL, is 0.75 to 1.25 mg or 10 to 15 µg/kg for patients older than 10 years of age; 40 to 50 µg/kg for patients younger than 2 years of age; and 30 to 40 µg/kg for patients 2 to 10 years of age.

The acute single toxic dose is greater than 0.07 mg/kg or greater than 2 or 3 mg in an adult, but 2 mg in a child or 4 mg in an adult usually produces only mild toxicity. One to 3 mg or more may be found in a few leaves of oleander or foxglove. Serious and fatal overdoses are more than 4 mg in a child and more than 10 mg in an adult.

Acute digitoxin ingestion of 10 to 35 mg has produced severe toxicity and death. Digitoxin therapeutic steady state is 15 to 25 ng/mL. In cases of chronic or acute-on-chronic ingestions in patients with cardiac disease, more than 2 mg may produce toxicity; however, toxicity can develop within therapeutic range on chronic therapy.

Patients at greatest risk of overdose include those with cardiac disease, those with electrolyte abnormalities (low potassium, low magnesium, low T_4, high calcium), those with renal impairment, and those on amiodarone (Cordarone), quinidine, erythromycin, tetracycline, calcium channel blockers, and β-blockers.

Kinetics

Digoxin is a metabolite of digitoxin. In cases of oral overdose, the typical onset is 30 minutes, with peak effects in 3 to 12 hours. Duration is 3 to 4 days. Intravenous onset is in 5 to 30 minutes; peak level is immediate, and peak effect is at 1.5 to 3 hours.

Volume distribution is 5 to 6 L/kg. The cardiac-to-plasma ratio is 30:1. After an acute ingestion overdose, the serum concentration is not reflective of tissue concentration for at least 6 hours or more, and steady state is 12 to 16 hours after last dose.

Sixty percent to 80% of the parent compound is excreted unchanged in the urine. The elimination half-life is 30 to 50 hours.

Manifestations

Onset of manifestations is usually within 2 hours but may be delayed up to 12 hours.

Gastrointestinal effects of nausea and vomiting are frequently present in cases of acute ingestion but may also occur in cases of chronic ingestion. The "digitalis effect" on ECG is scooped ST segments and PR prolongation; in cases of overdose, any dysrhythmia or block is possible but none are characteristic. Bradycardia occurs in patients with acute overdose with healthy hearts; supraventricular tachycardia occurs in patients with existing heart disease or chronic overdose. Ventricular tachycardia is seen only in cases of severe poisoning.

The CNS effects include headaches, visual disturbances, and colored halo vision. Hyperkalemia occurs following acute overdose and correlates with digoxin level and outcome. Among patients with serum potassium levels of less than 5.0 mEq/L, all survive. If the level is 5 to 5.5, 50% survive, and if the level is greater than 5.5, all die. Hypokalemia is commonly seen with chronic intoxication. Patients with normal digitalis levels may have toxicity in the presence of hypokalemia.

Chronic intoxications are more likely to produce scotoma, color perception disturbances, yellow vision, halos, delirium, hallucinations or psychosis, tachycardia, and hypokalemia.

Laboratory Investigations

Continuous monitoring of ECG, pulse, and blood pressure is called for. Blood glucose, electrolytes, calcium, magnesium, BUN, and creatinine levels should also be monitored. An initial digoxin level should be measured on patient presentation and repeated thereafter. Levels should be measured more than 6 hours postingestion because earlier values do not reflect tissue distribution. Digoxin clinical toxicity is usually associated with serum digoxin levels of greater than 3.5 ng/mL in adults.

An endogenous digoxin-like substance cross-reacts in most common immunoassays (not with high-pressure liquid chromatography) and values as high as 4.1 ng/mL have been reported in newborns, patients with chronic renal failure, patients with abnormal immunoglobulins, and women in the third trimester of pregnancy.

Management

A cardiology consult should be obtained and a pacemaker should be readily available.

In undertaking gastrointestinal decontamination, excessive vagal stimulation should be avoided (e.g., emesis and gastric lavage). Activated charcoal should be administered, and if a nasogastric tube is required for the activated charcoal, pretreatment with atropine (0.02 mg/kg in children and 0.5 mg in adults) should be considered.

Digoxin-specific antibody fragments (Fab, Digibind) 38 mg binds 0.5 mg digoxin and then is excreted through the kidneys. The onset of action is within 30 minutes. Problems associated with Fab therapy are mainly from withdrawal of digoxin and worsening heart failure, hypokalemia, decrease in glucose (if the patient has low glycogen stores), and allergic reactions (very rare). Digitalis administered after Fab therapy is bound and may be inactivated for 5 to 7 days.

Absolute indications for Fab therapy include the following:

- Life-threatening malignant (hemodynamically unstable) dysrhythmias
- Ventricular dysrhythmias, unstable severe bradycardia, or second- or third-degree blocks unresponsive to atropine or rapid deterioration in clinical status
- Life-threatening digitoxin and oleander poisonings
- Relative indications for Fab therapy include the following:
- Ingestions greater than 4 mg in a child and 10 mg in an adult
- Serum potassium level greater than 5.0 mEq/L
- Serum digoxin level greater than 10 ng/mL in adults or greater than 5 ng/mL in children 6 hours after an acute ingestion
- Digitalis delirium and thrombocytopenia response

Digoxin-specific Fab fragments therapy can be administered as a bolus through a 22-µm filter if the case is a critical emergency. If the case is less urgent, then it can be administered over 30 minutes. An empiric dose is 10 vials in adults and 5 vials in a child for an unknown amount ingested in a symptomatic patient with history of a digoxin overdose.

To calculate the dose in the case of a known ingestion, the following equation is used:

$$\text{Amount (total mg)} \times (0.8) \text{ body burden}$$

If liquid capsules were taken or the substance was given intravenously the 80% bioavailability figure is not used. Instead, the body burden divided by 0.5 (0.5 mg digoxin is bound by 1 vial of 38 mg of Fab) equals the number of vials needed.

If the amount is unknown but the steady state serum concentration is known, the following equations are used:

For digoxin

$$\text{Digitoxin ng/mL} \times (5.6 \text{ L/kg Vd}) \times (\text{wt kg}) = \text{mg body burden}$$
$$\text{Body burden} \div 1000 = \text{mg body burden}$$
$$\text{Body burden}/0.5 = \text{number of vials needed}$$

For digitoxin

$$\text{Digitoxin ng/mL} \times (0.56 \text{ L/kg Vd}) \times (\text{wt kg}) = \text{mg body burden}$$
$$\text{Body burden} \div 1000 = \text{mg body burden}$$
$$\text{Body burden}/0.5 = \text{number of vials needs}$$

Antidysrhythmic agents or a pacemaker should be used only if Fab therapy fails. For ventricular tachydysrhythmias, electrolyte disturbances should be corrected by the administration of lidocaine or phenytoin. For torsades de pointes, magnesium sulfate 20 mL 20% IV can be given slowly over 20 minutes (or 25 to 50 mg/kg in a child), titrated to control the dysrhythmia. Magnesium should be discontinued if hypotension, heart block, or decreased deep tendon reflexes are present. Magnesium is used with caution if the patient has renal impairment.

Unstable bradycardia and second-degree and third-degree atrioventricular block should be treated by Fab first. A pacemaker should be available if necessary. Isoproterenol should be avoided because it causes dysrhythmias. Cardioversion is used with caution, starting at a setting of 5 to 10 joules. The patient should be pretreated with lidocaine, if possible, because cardioversion may precipitate ventricular fibrillation or asystole.

Potassium disturbances are caused by a shift, not a change, in total body potassium. Hyperkalemia (>5.0 mEq/L) is treated with Fab only. Calcium must never be used, and insulin/glucose and sodium bicarbonate should not be used concomitantly with Fab because they may produce severe life-threatening hypokalemia. Sodium polystyrene sulfonate (Kayexalate) should not be used. Hypokalemia must be treated with caution because it may be cardioprotective. Treatment can be administered if the patient has ventricular dysrhythmias or a serum potassium level less than 3.0 mEq/L and atrioventricular block.

Extracorporeal procedures are ineffective. Hemodialysis is used for severe or refractory hyperkalemia.

One must never use antidysrhythmic types Ia (procainamide, quinidine, disopyramide [Norpace], amiodarone [Cordarone]), Ic (propafenone [Rythmol], flecainide [Tambocor]), II (β-blockers), or IV (calcium channel blockers). Class Ib drugs (lidocaine, phenytoin [Dilantin], mexiletine [Mexitil], and tocainide [Tonocard]) can be used.

Disposition

Consultation with a poison control center and a cardiologist experienced with digoxin-specific Fab fragments is warranted. All patients with significant dysrhythmias, symptoms, elevated serum digoxin concentration, or elevated serum potassium level should be admitted to the intensive care unit.

ETHANOL

Table 15 lists the features of alcohols and glycols.

Toxic Mechanism

Ethanol has CNS depressant and anesthetic effects. Ethanol stimulates the γ-aminobutyric acid (GABA) system. It promotes cutaneous vasodilation (contributes to hypothermia), stimulates secretion of gastric juice (gastritis), inhibits the secretion of the antidiuretic hormone, inhibits gluconeogenesis (hypoglycemia), and influences fat metabolism (lipidemia).

Toxic Dose

A dose of 1 mL/kg of absolute ethanol (100% ethanol, or 200 proof) gives a blood ethanol concentration of 100 mg/dL. A potentially fatal dose is 3 g/kg for children or 6 g/kg for adults. Children are more prone to developing hypoglycemia than adults.

Kinetics

Onset of action is 30 to 60 minutes after ingestion; peak action is 90 minutes on empty stomach. Volume distribution is 0.6 L/kg. The major route of elimination (>90%) is by hepatic oxidative metabolism. The first step is by the enzyme alcohol dehydrogenase, which converts ethanol to acetaldehyde. Alcohol dehydrogenase metabolizes ethanol at a constant rate of 12 to 20 mg/dL/h (12 to 15 mg/dL/h in nondrinkers, 15 to 30 mg/dL/h in social drinkers, 30 to 50 mg/dL/h in heavy drinkers, and 25 to 30 mg/dL/h in children). At very low blood ethanol concentration (>30 mg/dL), the metabolism is by first-order kinetics. In the second step, acetaldehyde is metabolized by acetaldehyde dehydrogenase to acetic acid, which is metabolized by the Krebs cycle to carbon dioxide and water. The enzyme steps are nicotinamide adenine dinucleotide-dependent, which interferes with gluconeogenesis. Less than 10% of ethanol is excreted unchanged by the kidneys. The relationship between blood ethanol concentration (BEC) and dose (amount ingested) can be calculated as follows:

$$BEC\ (mg/dL) = amount\ ingested\ (ml) \times \%\ ethanol\ product \times SG\ (0.79)/Vd\ (0.6\ L/kg) \times body\ wt\ (kg)$$

$$Dose\ (amount\ ingested) = BEC\ (mg/dL) \times Vd\ (0.6) \times body\ wt\ (kg)\ /\ \%\ ethanol \times specjfjc\ gragvity\ (0.79)$$

Manifestations

Table 16 lists the clinical signs of acute ethanol intoxication.

Chronic alcoholic patients tolerate higher blood ethanol concentration, and correlation with manifestations is not valid. Rapid interview for alcoholism is the CAGE questions:

- C—Have you felt the need to Cut down?
- A—Have others Annoyed you by criticism of your drinking?
- G—Have you felt Guilty about your drinking?
- E—Have you ever had a morning Eye-opening drink to steady your nerves or get rid of a hangover?

Two affirmative answers indicate probable alcoholism.

Laboratory Investigations

The blood ethanol concentration should be specifically requested and followed. Gas chromatography or a breathanalyzer test gives rapid reliable results if no belching or vomiting is present. Enzymatic

TABLE 15 Summary of Alcohol and Glycol Features

	Methanol	Isopropanol	Ethanol	Ethylene Glycol
Principal uses	Gas line antifreeze, Sterno, windshield de-icer	Solvent jewelry cleaner, rubbing alcohol	Beverage, solvent	Radiator antifreeze, windshield de-icer
Specific gravity	0.719	0.785	0.789	1.12
Fatal dose	1 mL/Kg 100%	3 mL/kg 100%	5 mL/kg 100%	1.4 mL/kg
Inebriation	±	2+	2+	1+
Metabolic change		Hyperglycemia	Hypoglycemia	Hypocalcemia
Metabolic acidosis	4+	0	1+	2+
Anion gap	4+	±	2+	4+
Ketosis	Ketobutyric	Acetone	Hydroxybutyric	None
Gastrointestinal tract	Pancreatitis	Hemorrhagic gastritis	Gastritis	
Osmolality*	0.337	0.176	0.228	0.190

*1 mL/dL of substances raises freezing point osmolality of serum. The validity of the correlation of osmolality with blood concentrations has been questioned.

TABLE 16 Clinical Signs in the Nontolerant Ethanol Drinker

Ethanol Blood Concentration (mg/dL)*	Manifestations
>25	Euphoria
>47	**Mild incoordination,** sensory and motor impairment
>50	Increased risk of motor vehicle accidents
>100	Ataxia (legal toxic level in many localities)
>150	**Moderate incoordination,** slow reaction time
>200	Drowsiness and confusion
>300	Severe incoordination, stupor, blurred vision
>500	**Flaccid coma,** respiratory failure, hypotension; may be fatal

*Ethanol concentrations sometimes reported in %.
Note: mg% is not equivalent to mg/dL because ethanol weighs less than water (specific gravity 0.79). A 1% ethanol concentration is 790 mg/dL and 0.1% is 79 mg/dL. There is great variation in individual behavior at different blood ethanol levels. Behavior is dependent on tolerance and other factors.

methods do not differentiate between the alcohols. ABG, electrolytes, and glucose should be measured, the anion and osmolar gaps determined (measure by freezing point depression, not vapor pressure), and a check for ketosis made.

Management

The examiner should inquire about trauma and disulfiram use. The patient must be protected from aspiration and hypoxia. Vital functions must be established and maintained. The patient may require intubation and assisted ventilation.

Gastrointestinal decontamination plays no role in the management of ethanol intoxication.

If the patient is comatose, glucose should be administered intravenously, 1 mL/kg 50% glucose in adults and 2 mL/kg 25% glucose in children. Thiamine, 100 mg intravenously, is administered if the patient has a history of chronic alcoholism, malnutrition, or suspected eating disorders to prevent Wernicke-Korsakoff syndrome. Naloxone (Narcan) has produced a partial inconsistent response but is not recommended for known alcoholics.

General supportive care includes administration of fluids to correct hydration and hypotension and correction of electrolyte abnormalities and acid–base imbalance. Vasopressors and plasma expanders may be necessary to correct severe hypotension. Hypomagnesemia is frequent in chronic alcoholics. In case of hypomagnesemia, a loading dose of 2 g magnesium sulfate 10% is administered by intravenous solution over 5 minutes in the intensive care unit with blood pressure and cardiac monitoring and calcium chloride 10% on hand in case of overdose. This is followed with constant infusion of 6 g of 10% solution over 3 to 4 hours. Caution must be taken with the use of magnesium if renal failure is present.

Hypothermic patients should be warmed. See the section on disturbances caused by cold.

Hemodialysis can be used in severe cases when conventional therapy is ineffective (rarely needed).

Repeated or prolonged seizures should be treated with diazepam (Valium). The brief "rum fits" do not need long-term anticonvulsant therapy. Repeated seizures or focal neurologic findings may warrant skull radiographs, lumbar puncture, and CT scan of the head, depending on the clinical findings. Withdrawal is treated with hydration and large doses of chlordiazepoxide (Librium) 50 to 100 mg or diazepam (Valium) 2 to 10 mg intravenously; these doses may be repeated in 2 to 4 hours. Very large doses of benzodiazepines may be required for delirium tremens. Withdrawal can occur in presence of elevated blood ethanol concentration and can be fatal if left untreated.

Chest radiograph is warranted to determine whether aspiration pneumonia is present. Renal and liver function tests and bilirubin level measurement should be made.

Disposition

Clinical severity (e.g., intubation, assisted ventilation, aspiration pneumonia) should determine the level of hospital care needed. Young children with significant unintentional exposure to ethanol (calculated to reach a blood ethanol concentration of 50 mg/dL) should have blood ethanol concentration obtained and blood glucose levels monitored for hypoglycemia frequently for 4 hours after ingestion. Patients with acute ethanol intoxication seldom require admission unless a complication is present. However, intoxicated patients should not be discharged until they are fully functional (can walk, talk, and think independently), have suicide potential evaluated, have proper disposition environment, and have a sober escort.

ETHYLENE GLYCOL

Ethylene glycol is found in solvents, de-icers, radiator antifreeze (95%), and air-conditioning units. Ethylene glycol is a sweet-tasting, colorless, water-soluble liquid with a sweet aromatic fragrance.

Toxic Mechanism

Ethylene glycol is oxidized by alcohol dehydrogenase to glycolaldehyde, which is metabolized to glycolic acid and glyoxylic acid. Glyoxylic acid is metabolized to oxalic acid via a pyridoxine-dependent pathway to glycine and by thiamine and magnesium-dependent pathways to α-hydroxy-ketoadipic acid. The metabolites of ethylene glycol produce a profound metabolic acidosis, increased anion gap, hypocalcemia, and oxalate crystals, which deposit in tissues (particularly the kidney).

Toxic Dose

The ingestion of 0.1 mL/kg 100% ethylene glycol can result in a toxic serum ethylene glycol concentration of 20 mg/dL. Ingestion of 3.0 mL (less than 1 teaspoonful or swallow) of a 100% solution in a 10-kg child or 30 mL of 100% ethylene glycol in an adult produces a serum ethylene glycol concentration of 50 mg/dL, a concentration that requires hemodialysis. The fatal amount is 1.4 mL/kg of 100% solution.

Kinetics

Absorption is via dermal, inhalation, and ingestion routes. Ethylene glycol is rapidly absorbed from the gastrointestinal tract. Onset is usually in 30 minutes but may be delayed by co-ingestion of food and ethanol. The usual peak level is at 2 hours. Volume distribution is 0.65 to 0.8 L/kg.

For metabolism, see *Toxic Mechanism*.

The half-life of ethylene glycol without ethanol is 3 to 8 hours; with ethanol, it is 17 hours, and with hemodialysis it is 2.5 hours. Renal clearance is 3.2 mL/kg/minute. About 20% to 50% is excreted unchanged in the urine. The relationship between serum ethylene glycol concentration (SEGC) and dose (amount ingested) can be calculated as follows:

$$0.12\,\text{mL/kg of } 100\% = \text{SEGC}\,10\,\text{mg/dL}$$

Manifestations

Phase I

The onset of manifestations is 30 minutes to several hours longer after ingestion with concomitant ethanol ingestion. The patient may be inebriated. Hypocalcemia, tetany, and calcium oxalate and hippuric acid crystals in urine can be seen within 4 to 8 hours but are not always present. Early, before metabolism of ethylene glycol, an osmolal gap may be present (see *Laboratory Investigations*). Later, the metabolites of ethylene glycol produce changes starting 4 to 12 hours following ingestion, including an anion gap, metabolic acidosis, coma, convulsions, cardiac disturbances, and pulmonary and cerebral edema. Because fluorescein is added to some antifreeze, the presence of fluorescence may be a clue to ethylene glycol exposure. However, it has been shown that fluorescent urine is not a reliable indicator of ethylene glycol ingestion and should not be used as a screen.

Phase II

After 12 to 36 hours, cardiopulmonary deterioration occurs, with pulmonary edema and congestive heart failure.

Phase III

Phase III occurs 36 to 72 hours after ingestion, with pulmonary edema and oliguric renal failure from oxalate crystal deposition and tubular necrosis predominating.

Phase IV

Neurologic sequelae may occur rarely, especially in patients who fail to receive early antidotal therapy. The onset ranges from 6 to 10 days after ingestion. Findings include facial diplegia, hearing loss, bilateral visual disturbances, elevated cerebrospinal fluid pressure with or without elevated protein levels and pleocytosis, vomiting, hyperreflexia, dysphagia, and ataxia.

Laboratory Investigations

Blood glucose and electrolytes should be monitored. Urinalysis should look for oxalate ("envelope") and monohydrate ("hemp seed") crystals. Urine fluorescence is not reliable as a screen. ABG, ethylene glycol, and ethanol levels, plasma osmolarity (using freezing point depression method), calcium, BUN, and creatinine should be measured. A serum ethylene glycol concentration of 20 mg/dL is toxic (ethylene glycol levels are very difficult to obtain). If possible, a glycolate level should be obtained. Cross-reactions with propylene glycol, a vehicle in many liquids and intravenous medications (phenytoin [Dilantin], diazepam [Valium]), other glycols, and triglycerides may produce spurious ethylene glycol levels. False-positive ethylene glycol values may occur with colorimetric or gas chromatography using an OV-17 column in the presence of propylene glycol.

The following equations can be used to calculate the osmolality, osmolal gap, and ethylene glycol level:

$$2(Na + mEq/L) + (Blood\ glucose\ mg/dL)/20 + (BUN\ mg/dL)/3 = Total\ calculated\ osmolality\ (mOsmL/L)$$

$$Osmolar\ Gap = measured\ osmolality\ (by\ freezing\ point\ depression\ method) - calculate\ osmolality$$

A gap greater than 10 is abnormal. *Note:* if ethanol is involved, add ethanol level/4.6 to the calculated equation.

An increased osmolal gap is produced by the following common substances: acetone, dextran, dimethyl sulfoxide, diuretics, ethanol, ethyl ether, ethylene glycol, isopropanol, paraldehyde, mannitol, methanol, sorbitol, and trichloroethane. Table 10 gives the conversion factors for these substances.

Although a specific blood level of ethylene glycol in milligrams per deciliter can be estimated using the equation below, this is not considered to be a reliable method and should not take the place of obtaining a measured ethylene glycol blood concentration.

$$osmolar\ gap \times conversion\ factor = serum\ concentration$$

Caution: The accuracy of the ethylene glycol estimated decreases as the ethylene glycol levels decrease. The toxic metabolites are not osmotically active, and patients presenting late may show signs of severe toxicity without an elevated osmolar gap.

The anion gap can be calculated using the following equation:

$$Na - (Cl + HCO_3) = anion\ gap$$

The normal gap is 8 to 12. Potassium is not used because it is a small amount and may be hemolyzed. Table 8 lists factors that may account for an increased or a decreased anion gap.

Management

Vital functions should be established and maintained. The airway must be protected, and assisted ventilation can be used, if necessary. Gastrointestinal decontamination has a limited role. Only gastric aspiration can be used within 60 minutes after ingestion. Activated charcoal is not effective.

Baseline measurements of serum electrolytes and calcium, glucose, ABGs, ethanol, serum ethylene glycol concentration (may be difficult to obtain readily in some institutions), and methanol concentrations should be obtained. In the first few hours, the measured serum osmolality should be determined and compared to calculated osmolality (see osmolality equation, earlier). If seizures occur, one should measure serum calcium (preferably ionized calcium) and treat with intravenous diazepam. If the patient has hypocalcemic seizures, he or she should also be treated with 10 to 20 mL 10% calcium gluconate (0.2 to 0.3 mL/kg in children) slowly intravenously, with the dose repeated as needed. Metabolic acidosis should be corrected with intravenous sodium bicarbonate.

Ethanol therapy should be initiated immediately if fomepizole (Antizol) is unavailable (see next paragraph). Alcohol dehydrogenase has a greater affinity for ethanol than ethylene glycol. Therefore, ethanol blocks the metabolism of ethylene glycol. Ethanol therapy is called for if there is a history of ingestion of 0.1 mL/kg of 100% ethylene glycol, serum ethylene glycol concentration is greater than 20 mg/dL, there is an osmolar gap not accounted for by other alcohols or factors (e.g., hyperlipidemia), metabolic acidosis is present with an increased anion gap, or there are oxalate crystals in the urine. Ethanol should be administered intravenously (the oral route is less reliable) to produce a blood ethanol concentration of 100 to 150 mg/dL. The loading dose is 10 mL/kg of 10% ethanol intravenously, administered concomitantly with a maintenance dose of 10% ethanol of 1.0 mL/kg/h. This dose may need to be increased to 2 mL/kg/h in patients who are heavy drinkers. The blood ethanol concentration should be measured hourly and the infusion rate should be adjusted to maintain a blood ethanol concentration of 100 to 150 mg/dL.

Fomepizole (Antizol, 4-methylpyrazole) inhibits alcohol dehydrogenase more reliability than ethanol and it does not require constant monitoring of ethanol levels and adjustment of infusion rates. Fomepizole is available in 1 g/mL vials of 1.5 mL. The loading dose is 15 mg/kg (0.015 mL/kg) IV; maintenance dose is 10 mg/kg (0.01 mL/kg) every 12 hours for four doses, then 15 mg/kg every 12 hours until the ethylene glycol levels are less than 20 mg/dL. The solution is prepared by being mixed with 100 mL of 0.9% saline or D_5W (5% dextrose in water). Fomepizole can be given to patients requiring hemodialysis but should be dosed as follows:

Dose at the beginning of hemodialysis:

- If <6 hours since last Antizol dose, do not administer dose
- If >6 hours since last dose, administer next scheduled dose

Dosing during hemodialysis:

- Dose every 4 hours

Dosing at the time hemodialysis is completed:

- If <1 hour between last dose and end of dialysis, do not administer dose at end of dialysis
- If 1 to 3 hours between last dose and end of dialysis, administer one half of next scheduled dose
- If >3 hours between last dose and end of dialysis, administer next scheduled dose

Maintenance dosing off hemodialysis:
- Give the next scheduled dose 12 hours from the last dose administered

Hemodialysis is indicated if the ingestion was potentially fatal; if the serum ethylene glycol concentration is greater than 50 mg/dL (some recommend at levels of >25 mg/dL); if severe acidosis or electrolyte abnormalities occur despite conventional therapy; or if congestive heart failure or renal failure is present. Hemodialysis reduces the ethylene glycol half-life from 17 hours on ethanol therapy to 3 hours. Therapy (fomepizole and hemodialysis) should be continued until the serum ethylene glycol concentration is less than 10 mg/dL, the glycolate level is nondetectable (not readily available), the acidosis has cleared, there are no mental disturbances, the creatinine level is normal, and the urinary output is adequate. This may require 2 to 5 days.

Adjunct therapy involving thiamine, 100 mg/d (in children, 50 mg), slowly over 5 minutes intravenously or intramuscularly and repeated every 6 hours and pyridoxine, 50 mg IV or IM every 6 hours, has been recommended until intoxication is resolved, but these agents have not been extensively studied. Folate, 50 mg IV (child 1 mg/kg), can be given every 4 hours for 6 doses.

Disposition

All patients who have ingested significant amounts of ethylene glycol (calculated level above 20 mg/dL), have a history of a toxic dose, or are symptomatic should be referred to the emergency department and admitted. If the serum ethylene glycol concentration cannot be obtained, the patient should be followed for 12 hours, with monitoring of the osmolal gap, acid–base parameters, and electrolytes to exclude development of metabolic acidosis with an anion gap. Transfer should be considered for fomepizole therapy or hemodialysis.

HYDROCARBONS

The lower the viscosity and surface tension of hydrocarbons or the greater the volatility, the greater the risk of aspiration. Volatile substance abuse has produced the "Sudden Sniffing's Death Syndrome," most likely caused by dysrhythmias.

Toxicologic Classification and Toxic Mechanism

All systemically absorbed hydrocarbons can lower the threshold of the myocardium to dysrhythmias produced by endogenous and exogenous catecholamines.

Aliphatic hydrocarbons are branched straight chain hydrocarbons. A few aspirated drops are poorly absorbed from the gastrointestinal tract and produce no systemic toxicity by this route. However, aspiration of very small amounts can produce chemical pneumonitis. Examples of aliphatic hydrocarbons are gasoline, kerosene, charcoal lighter fluid, mineral spirits (Stoddard's solvent), and petroleum naphtha. Mineral seal oil (signal oil), found in furniture polishes, is a low-viscosity and low-volatility oil with minimum absorption that never warrants gastric decontamination. It can produce severe pneumonia if aspirated.

Aromatic hydrocarbons are six carbon ring structures that are absorbed through the gastrointestinal tract. Systemic toxicity includes CNS depression and, in cases of chronic abuse, multiple organ effects such as leukemia (benzene) and renal toxicity (toluene). Examples are benzene, toluene, styrene, and xylene. The seriously toxic ingested dose is 20 to 50 mL in adults.

Halogenated hydrocarbons are aliphatic or aromatic hydrocarbons with one or more halogen substitutions (Cl, Br, Fl, or I). They are highly volatile and are abused as inhalants. They are well absorbed from the gastrointestinal tract, produce CNS depression, and have metabolites that can damage the liver and kidneys. Examples include methylene chloride (may be converted into carbon monoxide in the body), dichloroethylene (also causes a disulfiram [Antabuse] reaction known as "degreaser's flush" when associated with consumption of ethanol), and 1,1,1-trichloroethane (Glamorene Spot Remover, Scotchgard, typewriter correction fluid). An acute lethal oral dose is 0.5 to 5 mL/kg.

Dangerous additives to the hydrocarbons can be summed up with the mnemonic CHAMP: C, camphor (demothing agent); H, halogenated hydrocarbons; A, aromatic hydrocarbons; M, metals (heavy); and P, pesticides. Ingestion of these substances may warrant gastric emptying with a small-bore nasogastric tube.

Heavy hydrocarbons have high viscosity, low volatility, and minimal gastrointestinal absorption, so gastric decontamination is not necessary. Examples are asphalt (tar), machine oil, motor oil (lubricating oil, engine oil), home heating oil, and petroleum jelly (mineral oil).

Laboratory Investigations

The ECG, ABG, pulmonary function, serum electrolytes, and serial chest radiographs should be continuously monitored. Liver and renal function should be monitored in cases of inhalation of aromatic hydrocarbons.

Management

Asymptomatic patients who ingested small amounts of aliphatic petroleum distillates can be followed at home by telephone for development of signs of aspiration (cough, wheezing, tachypnea, and dyspnea) for 4 to 6 hours. Inhalation of any hydrocarbon vapors in a closed space can produce intoxication. The victim must be removed from the environment, have oxygen administered, and receive respiratory support.

Gastrointestinal decontamination is not advised in cases of hydrocarbon ingestion that usually do not cause systemic toxicity (aliphatic petroleum distillates, heavy hydrocarbons). In cases of ingestion of hydrocarbons that cause systemic toxicity in small amounts (aromatic hydrocarbons, halogenated hydrocarbons), the clinician should pass a small-bore nasogastric tube and aspirate if the ingestion was within 2 hours and if spontaneous vomiting has not occurred. Some toxicologists advocate ipecac-induced emesis under medical supervision instead of small-bore nasogastric gastric lavage; we do not.

Patients with altered mental status should have their airway protected because of concern about aspiration. The use of activated charcoal has been suggested, but there are no scientific data as to effectiveness and it may produce vomiting. Activated charcoal may, however, be useful in adsorbing toxic additives such as pesticides or co-ingestants.

The symptomatic patient who is coughing, gagging, choking, or wheezing on arrival has probably aspirated. The clinician should provide supportive respiratory care and supplemental oxygen, while monitoring pulse oximetry, ABG, chest radiograph, and ECG. The patient should be admitted to the intensive care unit. A chest radiograph for aspiration may be positive as early as 30 minutes after ingestion, and almost all are positive within 6 hours. Negative chest radiographs within 4 hours do not rule out aspiration.

Bronchospasm is treated with a nebulized β-adrenergic agonist and intravenous aminophylline if necessary. Epinephrine should be avoided because of susceptibility to dysrhythmias. Cyanosis in the presence of a normal arterial Pao$_2$ may be a result of methemoglobinemia that requires therapy with methylene blue. Corticosteroids and prophylactic antimicrobial agents have not been shown to be beneficial. (Fever or leukocytosis may be produced by the chemical pneumonitis.)

Most infiltrations resolve spontaneously in 1 week; lipoid pneumonia may last up to 6 weeks. It is not necessary to surgically treat pneumatoceles that develop because they usually resolve. Dysrhythmias may require α- and β-adrenergic antagonists or cardioversion.

There is no role for enhanced elimination procedures.

Methylene chloride is metabolized over several hours to carbon monoxide. See treatment of carbon monoxide poisoning. Halogenated hydrocarbons are hepatorenal toxins; therefore, hepatorenal function should be monitored. *N*-acetylcysteine therapy may be useful if there is evidence of hepatic damage.

Extracorporal membrane oxygenation (ECMO) has been used successfully for a few patients with life threatening respiratory failure. Surfactant used for hydrocarbon aspiration was found to be detrimental.

Disposition

Asymptomatic patients with small ingestions of petroleum distillates can be managed at home. Symptomatic patients with abnormal chest radiographic, oxygen saturation, or ABG findings should be admitted. Patients who become asymptomatic and have normal oxygenation and a normal repeat radiograph can be discharged.

IRON

There are more than 100 iron over-the-counter preparations for supplementation and treatment of iron deficiency anemia.

Toxic Mechanism

Toxicity depends on the amount of elemental iron available in various salts (gluconate 12%, sulfate 20%, fumarate 33%, lactate 19%, chloride 21% of elemental iron), not the amount of the salt. Locally, iron is corrosive and may cause fluid loss, hypovolemic shock, and perforation. Excessive free unbound iron in the blood is directly toxic to the vasculature and leads to the release of vasoactive substances, which produces vasodilation. In cases of overdose, iron deposits injure mitochondria in the liver, the kidneys, and the myocardium. The exact mechanism of cellular damage is not clear but is thought to be related to free radical formation.

Toxic Dose

The therapeutic dose is 6 mg/kg/d of elemental iron. An elemental iron dose of 20 to 40 mg/kg may produce mild self-limited gastrointestinal symptoms, 40 to 60 mg/kg produces moderate toxicity, more than 60 mg/kg produces severe toxicity and is potentially lethal, and more than 180 mg/kg is usually fatal without treatment. Children's chewable vitamins with iron have between 12 and 18 mg of elemental iron per tablet or 0.6 mL of liquid drops. These preparations rarely produce toxicity unless very large quantities are ingested and have never caused death.

Kinetics

Absorption occurs chiefly in the upper small intestine. Ferrous (+2) iron is absorbed into the mucosal cells, where it is oxidized to the ferric (+3) state and bound to ferritin. Iron is slowly released from ferritin into the plasma, where it binds to transferrin and is transported to specific tissues for production of hemoglobin (70%), myoglobin (5%), and cytochrome. About 25% of iron is stored in the liver and spleen. In cases of overdose, larger amounts of iron are absorbed because of direct mucosal corrosion. There is no mechanism for the elimination of iron (elimination is 1 to 2 mg/d) except through bile, sweat, and blood loss.

Manifestations

Serious toxicity is unlikely if the patient remains asymptomatic for 6 hours and has a negative abdominal radiograph. Iron intoxication can produce five phases of toxicity. The phases may not be distinct from one another.

Phase I

Gastrointestinal mucosal injury occurs 30 minutes to 12 hours postingestion. Vomiting starts within 30 minutes to 1 hour of ingestion and is persistent; hematemesis and bloody diarrhea may occur; abdominal cramps, fever, hyperglycemia, and leukocytosis may occur. Enteric-coated tablets may pass through the stomach without causing symptoms. Acidosis and shock can occur within 6 to 12 hours.

Phase II

A latent period of apparent improvement occurs over 8 to 12 hours postingestion.

Phase III

Systemic toxicity phase occurs 12 to 48 hours postingestion with cardiovascular collapse and severe metabolic acidosis.

Phase IV

Two to 4 days postingestion, hepatic injury associated with jaundice, elevated liver enzymes, and prolonged prothrombin time occur. Kidney injury with proteinuria and hematuria occur. Pulmonary edema, disseminated intravascular coagulation, and *Yersinia enterocolitica* sepsis can occur.

Phase V

Four to 8 weeks postingestion, pyloric outlet or intestinal stricture may cause obstruction or anemia secondary to blood loss.

Laboratory Investigations

Iron poisoning produces anion gap metabolic acidosis. Monitoring should include complete blood cell counts, blood glucose level, serum iron, stools and vomitus for occult blood, electrolytes, acid–base balance, urinalysis and urinary output, liver function tests, and BUN and creatinine levels. Blood type and match should be obtained.

Serum iron measurements taken at the proper time correlate with the clinical findings. The lavender top Vacutainer tube contains EDTA, which falsely lowers serum iron. One must obtain the serum iron measurement before administering deferoxamine. Serum iron levels of less than 350 μg/dL at 2 to 6 hours predict an asymptomatic course; levels of 350 to 500 μg/dL are usually associated with mild gastrointestinal symptoms; those greater than 500 μg/dL have a 20% risk of shock and serious iron toxicity. A follow-up serum iron measurement after 6 hours may not be elevated even in cases of severe poisoning, but a serum iron measurement taken at 8 to 12 hours is useful to exclude delayed absorption from a bezoar or sustained-release preparation. The total iron-binding capacity is not necessary.

Adult iron tablet preparations are radiopaque before they dissolve by 4 hours postingestion. A "negative" abdominal radiograph more than 4 hours postingestion does not exclude iron poisoning.

Patients who develop high fevers and signs of sepsis following iron overdose should have blood and stool cultures checked for *Yersinia enterocolitica*.

Management

Gastrointestinal decontamination should involve immediate induction of emesis in cases of ingestions of elemental iron of greater than 40 mg/kg if vomiting has not already occurred. Activated charcoal is ineffective. An abdominal radiograph should be obtained after emesis to determine the success of gastric emptying. Children's chewable vitamins and liquid iron preparations are not radiopaque. If radiopaque iron is still present, whole-bowel irrigation with polyethylene glycol solution should be considered. In extreme cases, removal by endoscopy or surgery may be necessary because coalesced iron tablets produce hemorrhagic infarction in the bowel and perforation peritonitis.

Deferoxamine (Desferal) in a dose of about 100 mg binds 8.5 to 9.35 mg of free iron in the serum. The deferoxamine infusion should not exceed 15 mg/kg/h or 6 g daily, but faster rates (up to 45 mg/kg) and larger daily amounts have been administered and tolerated in extreme cases of iron poisoning (>1000 mg/dL). The deferoxamine-iron complex is hemodialyzable if renal failure develops.

Indications for chelation therapy are any of the following:

- Very large, symptomatic ingestions
- Serious clinical intoxication (severe vomiting and diarrhea [often bloody], severe abdominal pain, metabolic acidosis, hypotension, or shock)
- Symptoms that persist or progress to more serious toxicity
- Serum iron level greater than 500 mg/dL

Chelation should be performed as early as possible within 12 to 18 hours to be effective. One should start the infusion slowly and gradually increase to avoid hypotension.

Adult respiratory distress syndrome has developed in patients with high doses of deferoxamine for several days; infusions longer than 24 hours should be avoided.

The endpoint of treatment is when the patient is asymptomatic and the urine clears if it was originally a positive "vin rosö" color.

For supportive therapy, intravenous bicarbonate may be needed to correct the metabolic acidosis. Hypotension and shock treatment may require volume expansion, vasopressors, and blood transfusions. The physician should attempt to keep the urinary output at greater than 2 mL/kg/h. Coagulation abnormalities and overt bleeding require blood products or vitamin K. Pregnant patients are treated in a fashion similar to any other patient with iron poisoning.

Hemodialysis and hemoperfusion are ineffective. Exchange transfusion has been used in single cases of massive poisonings in children.

Disposition

The asymptomatic or minimally symptomatic patient should be observed for persistence and progression of symptoms or development of toxicity signs (gastrointestinal bleeding, acidosis, shock, altered mental state). Patients with mild self-limited gastrointestinal symptoms who become asymptomatic or have no signs of toxicity for 6 hours are unlikely to have a serious intoxication and can be discharged after psychiatric clearance, if needed. Patients with moderate or severe toxicity should be admitted to the intensive care unit.

ISONIAZID

Isoniazid is a hydrazide derivative of vitamin B_3 (nicotinamide) and is used as an antituberculosis drug.

Toxic Mechanism

Isoniazid produces pyridoxine deficiency by increasing the excretion of pyridoxine (vitamin B_6) and by inhibiting pyridoxal 5-phosphate (the active form of pyridoxine) from acting with L-glutamic acid decarboxylase to form γ-aminobutyric acid (GABA), the major CNS neurotransmitter inhibitor, resulting in seizures. Isoniazid also blocks the conversion of lactate to pyruvate, resulting in profound and prolonged lactic acidosis.

Toxic Dose

The therapeutic dose is 5 to 10 mg/kg (maximum 300 mg) daily. A single acute dose of 15 mg/kg lowers the seizure threshold; 35 to 40 mg/kg produces spontaneous convulsions; more than 80 mg/kg produces severe toxicity. A fatal dose in adults is 4.5 to 15 g. The malnourished patients, those with a previous seizure disorder, alcoholic patients, and slow acetylators are more susceptible to isoniazid toxicity. In cases of chronic intoxication, 10 mg/kg/d produces hepatitis in 10% to 20% of patients but less than 2% at doses of 3 to 5 mg/kg/d.

Kinetics

Absorption from intestine occurs in 30 to 60 minutes, and onset is in 30 to 120 minutes, with peak levels of 5 to 8 µg/mL within 1 to 2 hours. Volume distribution is 0.6 L/kg, with minimal protein binding.

Elimination is by liver acetylation to a hepatotoxic metabolite, acetyl-isoniazid, which is then hydrolyzed to isonicotinic acid. In slow acetylators, isoniazid has a half-life of 140 to 460 minutes (mean 5 hours), and 10% to 15% is eliminated unchanged in the urine. Most (45% to 75%) whites and 50% of African blacks are slow acetylators, and, with chronic use (without pyridoxine supplements), they may develop peripheral neuropathy. In fast acetylators, isoniazid has a half-life of 35 to 110 minutes (mean 80 minutes), and 25% to 30% is excreted unchanged in the urine. About 90% of Asians and patients with diabetes mellitus are fast acetylators and may develop hepatitis on chronic use.

In patients with overdose and hepatic disease, the serum half-life may increase. Isoniazid inhibits the metabolism of phenytoin (Dilantin), diazepam, phenobarbital, carbamazepine (Tegretol), and prednisone. These drugs also interfere with the metabolism of isoniazid. Ethanol may decrease the half-life of isoniazid but increase its toxicity.

Manifestations

Within 30 to 60 minutes, nausea, vomiting, slurred speech, dizziness, visual disturbances, and ataxia are present. Within 30 to 120 minutes, the major clinical triad of severe overdose includes refractory convulsions (90% of overdose patients have one or more seizures), coma, and resistant severe lactic acidosis (secondary to convulsions), often with a plasma pH of 6.8.

Laboratory Investigations

Isoniazid produces anion gap metabolic acidosis. Therapeutic levels are 5 to 8 µg/mL and acute toxic levels are greater than 20 µg/mL. These levels are not readily available to assist in making decisions in acute overdose situations. One should monitor the blood glucose (often hyperglycemia), electrolytes (often hyperkalemia), bicarbonate, ABGs, liver function tests (elevations occur with chronic exposure), BUN, and creatinine.

Management

Seizures must be controlled. Pyridoxine and diazepam should be administered concomitantly through different IV sites. Pyridoxine (vitamin B_6) is given in a dose of 1 g for each gram of isoniazid ingested. If the dose ingested is unknown, at least 5 g of pyridoxine should be given intravenously. Pyridoxine is administered in 50 mL D_5W or 0.9% saline over 5 minutes intravenously. It must not be administered in the same bottle as sodium bicarbonate. Intravenous pyridoxine is repeated every 5 to 20 minutes until the seizures are controlled. Total doses of pyridoxine up to 52 g have been safely administered; however, patients given 132 and 183 g of pyridoxine have developed a persistent crippling sensory neuropathy.

Diazepam is administered concomitantly with pyridoxine but at a different site. They work synergistically. Diazepam should be administered intravenously slowly, 0.3 mg/kg at a rate of 1 mg/min in children or 10 mg at a rate of 5 mg/min in adults. After the seizures are controlled, the remainder of the pyridoxine is administered (1 g/1 g isoniazid) or a total dose of 5 g.

Phenobarbital or phenytoin is ineffective and should not be used.

In asymptomatic patients or patients without seizures, pyridoxine has been advised by some toxicologists prophylactically in gram-for-gram doses in cases of large overdoses (<80 mg/kg per dose) of isoniazid, although there are no studies to support this recommendation. In comatose patients, pyridoxine administration may result in the patient's rapid regaining of consciousness. Correction of acidosis may occur spontaneously with pyridoxine administration and correction of the seizures. Sodium bicarbonate should be administered if acidosis persists.

Hemodialysis is rarely needed because of antidotal therapy and the short half-life of isoniazid, but it may be used as an adjunct for cases of uncontrollable acidosis and seizures. Hemoperfusion has not been adequately evaluated. Diuresis is ineffective.

Disposition

Asymptomatic or mildly symptomatic patients who become asymptomatic can be observed in the emergency department for 4 to 6 hours. Larger amounts of isoniazid may warrant pyridoxine administration and longer periods of observation. Intentional ingestions necessitate psychiatric evaluation before the patient is discharged. Patients with convulsions or coma should be admitted to the intensive care unit.

ISOPROPANOL (ISOPROPYL ALCOHOL)

Isopropanol can be found in rubbing alcohol, solvents, and lacquer thinner. Coma has occurred in children sponged for fever with isopropanol. See Table 10 for ethanol features of alcohols and glycols.

Toxic Mechanism

Isopropanol is a gastric irritant. It is metabolized to acetone, a CNS and myocardial depressant. It inhibits gluconeogenesis. Normal propyl alcohol is related to isopropyl alcohol but is more toxic.

Toxic Dose

A toxic dose of 0.5 to 1 mg/kg of 70% isopropanol (1 mL/kg of 70%) produces a blood isopropanol plasma concentration of 70 mg/dL. The CNS depressant potency is twice that of ethanol.

Kinetics

Onset of action is within 30 to 60 minutes, and peak is 1 hour postingestion. Volume distribution is 0.6 kg/L. Isopropyl alcohol metabolizes to acetone. Its excretion is renal.

Note: The serum isopropyl concentration and amount ingested can be estimated using the same equation as is used in ethanol kinetics and substituting the specific gravity of 0.785 for isopropyl alcohol.

Manifestations

Ethanol-like inebriation occurs, with an acetone odor to the breath, gastritis, occasionally with hematemesis, acetonuria, and acetonemia without systemic acidosis.

Depression of the CNS occurs: lethargy at blood isopropyl alcohol levels of 50 to 100 mg/dL, coma at levels of 150 to 200 mg/dL, potentially death in adults at levels greater than 240 mg/dL.

Hypoglycemia and seizures may occur.

Laboratory Investigation

Monitoring of blood isopropyl alcohol levels (not readily available in all institutions), acetone, glucose, and ABG should be maintained. The osmolal gap increases 1 mOsm per 5.9 mg/dL of isopropyl alcohol and 1 mOsm per 5.5 mg/dL of acetone. The absence of excess acetone in the blood (normal is 0.3 to 2 mg/dL) within 30 to 60 minutes or excess acetone in the urine within 3 hours excludes the possibility of significant isopropanol exposure.

Management

The airway must be protected with intubation, and assisted ventilation administered if necessary. If the patient is hypoglycemic, glucose should be administered. Supportive treatment is similar to that for ethanol ingestions.

Gastrointestinal decontamination has no role in the treatment of isopropanol ingestion. Hemodialysis is warranted in cases of life-threatening overdose but is rarely needed. A nephrologist should be consulted if the bloodisopropanol plasma concentration is greater than 250 mg/dL.

Disposition

Symptomatic patients with concentrations greater than 100 mg/dL require at least 24 hours of close observation for resolution and should be admitted. If the patient is hypoglycemic, hypotensive, or comatose, he or she should be admitted to the intensive care unit.

LEAD

Acute lead intoxication is rare and usually occurs by inhalation of lead, resulting in severe intoxication and often death. Lead fumes can be produced by burning of lead batteries or use of a heat gun to remove lead paint. Acute lead intoxication also occurs from exposure to high concentrations of organic lead (e.g., tetraethyl lead).

Chronic lead poisoning occurs most often in children 6 months to 6 years of age who are exposed in their environment and in adults in certain occupations (Table 17). In the United States, the prevalence in children aged 1 to 5 years with a venous blood lead greater than 10 µg/dL decreased from 88.2% in a 1976-1980 survey to 8.9% in a 1988-1991 survey as a consequence of measures to reduce lead in the environment, particularly leaded gasoline. However, an estimated 1.7 million children between 1 and 5 years of age and more than 1 million workers in over 100 different occupations still have blood lead levels greater than 10 µg/dL.

Toxic Dose

In cases of chronic lead poisoning, a daily intake of more than 5 µg/kg/d in children or more than 150 µg/d in adults can give a positive lead balance. In 1991, the Centers for Disease Control and Prevention (CDC) recommended routine screening for all children younger than 6 years of age. In children a venous blood level greater than 10 µg/dL was determined to be a threshold of concern. The average venous blood level in the United States is 4 µg/dL. In cases of occupational exposure (see Table 17), a venous blood level greater than 40 µg/dL is indicative of increased lead absorption in adults.

Toxic Mechanism

Lead affects the sulfhydryl enzyme systems, the immature CNS, the enzymes of heme synthesis, vitamin D conversion, the kidneys, the bones, and growth. Lead alters the tertiary structure of cell proteins by denaturing them and causing cell death. Risk factors are mouthing behavior of infants and children and excessive oral behavior (pica), living in the inner city, a poorly maintained home, and poor nutrition (e.g., low calcium and iron). The CDC questionnaire given in Table 18 is recommended at every pediatric visit. If any answers to the CDC questionnaire are "positive," a blood screening test for lead should be administered. To be more accurate, however, identifying lead exposure studies have suggested that the questionnaire will have to be modified for each individual community because it has had poor sensitivity (40%) and specificity (60%) as it stands.

Table 19 lists sources of lead. The number one source is deteriorating lead-based paint, which forms leaded dust. Lead concentrations

TABLE 17 Occupations Associated with Lead Exposure

Lead production or smelting	Demolition of ships and bridges
Production of illicit whiskey	Battery manufacturing
Brass, copper, and lead foundries	Machining/grinding lead alloys
Radiator repair	Welding of old painted metals
Scrap handling	
Sanding of old paint	Thermal paint stripping of old buildings
Lead soldering	
Cable stripping	Ceramic glaze/pottery mixing
Worker or janitor at a firing range	

Modified from Rempel D: The lead-exposed worker. JAMA 262:533, 1989.

TABLE 18 CDC Questionnaire: Priority Groups for Lead Screening

1. Children age 6–72 months (was 12–36 months) who live in or are frequent visitors to older, deteriorated housing built before 1960.
2. Children age 6–72 months who live in housing built prior to 1960 with recent, ongoing, or planned renovation or remodeling.
3. Children age 6–72 months who are siblings, housemates, or playmates of children with known lead poisoning.
4. Children age 6–72 months whose parents or other household members participate in a lead-related industry or hobby.
5. Children age 6–72 months who live near active lead smelters, battery recycling plants, or other industries likely to result in atmospheric lead release.

in indoor paint were not reduced to safer (0.06%) levels until 1978. Lead can also be produced by improper interior or exterior home renovation (scraping or demolition). It is found in pre-1960 built homes. The use of leaded gasoline (limited in 1973) resulted in residue from leaded motor vehicle emissions. Lead persists in the soil near major highways and in deteriorating homes and buildings. Vegetables grown in contaminated soil may contain lead.

Oil refineries and lead-processing smelters produce lead residue. Food cans produced in Mexico contain lead solder (95% do not in United States). Lead water pipes (until 1950) and lead solder (until 1986) deliver lead-containing drinking water (calcium deposits, however, may offer some protection). Water at a consumer's tap should contain less than 15 parts per billion (ppb) of lead (Table 20).

For occupational exposure, see Table 17. The Occupational Safety and Health Administration (OSHA) standards require employers to provide showering and clothes changing facilities for personnel working with lead; however, businesses with fewer than 25 employees are exempt from the regulation. The OSHA lead standard of 1978 set a limit of 60 μg/dL for occupational exposure to lead. At a blood lead level of 60 μg/dL, a worker should be removed from lead exposure and not allowed back until his or her lead level is below 40 μg/dL. Many authorities believe that this level should be lower. The lead residue on the clothes of the workers may represent a hazard to the family. Other occupations that are potential sources of lead exposure include plumbers, pipe fitters, lead miners, auto repairers, shipbuilders, printers, steel welders and cutters, construction workers, and rubber product manufacturers.

Leaded pots to make molds for "kusmusha" tea represent lead exposure. Imported pottery lined with ceramic glaze can leach large amounts of lead into acids (e.g., citrus fruit juices).

Hobbies associated with lead exposure are listed in Box 1. Some "traditional" folk remedies or cosmetics that contain lead include the following:

TABLE 19 Sources of Lead

Product	Lead Content (%) by Dry Weight
Paint	0.06
Solder	0.6
Plastic additives	2.0
Priming inks	2.0
Plumbing fixtures	2.0
Pesticides	0.1
Stained glass cames	0.1
Wine bottle foils	0.1
Construction material	0.1
Fertilizers	0.1
Glazes, enamels	0.06
Toys/recreational games	0.1
Curtain weights	0.1
Fishing weights	0.1

- "Azarcon por empacho" ("Maria Louisa" 90 to 95% lead trioxide): a bright orange powder used in Hispanic culture, especially Mexican, for digestive problems and diarrhea.
- "Greta" (4% to 90% lead): a yellow powder "por empacho" ("empacho" refers to a variety of gastrointestinal symptoms), used in Hispanic cultures, especially Mexican.
- "Pay-loo-ah": an orange-red powder used for rash and fever in Southeast Asian cultures, especially among Northern Laos Hmong immigrants.
- "Alkohl" (Al-kohl, kohl, suma 5% to 92% lead): a black powder used in Middle Eastern, African, and Asian cultures as a cosmetic and an umbilical stump astringent.
- "Farouk": an orange granular powder with lead used in Saudi Arabian culture.
- "Bint Al Zahab": used to treat colic in Saudi Arabian culture.
- "Surma" (23% to 26% lead): a black powder used in India as a cosmetic and to improve eyesight.
- "Bali goli": a round black bean that is dissolved in "grippe water," used by Asian and Indian cultures to aid digestion.

Cases of substance abuse involving lead poisoning have been reported, in which the patient sniffs leaded gasoline or uses improperly synthesized amphetamines.

Kinetics

Absorption of lead is 10% to 15% of the ingested dose in adults; in children, up to 40% is absorbed, especially in cases of iron deficiency anemia. With inhalation of fumes, absorption is rapid and complete. Volume distribution in blood (0.9% of total body burden) is 95% in red blood cells. Lead passes through the placenta to the fetus and is present in breast milk.

Organic lead is metabolized in the liver to inorganic lead. Its half-life is 35 to 40 days in blood; in soft tissue, the half-life is 45 days and in bone (99% of the lead), the half-life is 28 years. The major elimination route is the stool, 80% to 90%, and then renal 10% (80 g/d) and hair, nails, sweat, and saliva. Nine percent of organic lead is excreted in the urine per day.

Manifestations

Adverse health effects are given in Table 21 and include the following.

Hematologic

Lead inhibits γ-aminolevulinic acid dehydratase (early in the synthesis of heme) and ferrochelatase (transfers iron to ferritin for incorporation of iron into protoporphyrin to produce heme). Anemia is a late finding. Decreased heme synthesis starts at >40 μg/dL. Basophilic stippling occurs in 20% of severe lead poisoning.

Neurologic

Segmental demyelination and peripheral neuropathy, usually of the motor type (wrist and ankle drop), occurs in workers. A venous blood level of lead greater than 70 μg/dL (usually >100 μg/dL), produces encephalopathy in children (symptom mnemonic "PAINT": P, persistent forceful vomiting and papilledema; A, ataxia; I, intermittent stupor and lucidity; N, neurologic coma and refractory convulsions; T, tired and lethargic). Decreased cognitive abilities have been reported with a venous blood level of lead greater than 10 μg/dL, including behavioral problems, decreased attention span, and learning disabilities. IQ scores may begin to decrease at 15 μg/dL. Encephalopathy is rare in adults.

Renal

Nephropathy as a result of damaged capillaries and glomerulus can occur at a venous blood level of lead greater than 80 μg/dL, but recent studies show renal damage and hypertension with low venous blood levels. A direct correlation between hypertension and venous blood

TABLE 20 Agency Regulations and Recommendations Concerning Lead Content

Agency	Specimen	Level	Comments
CDC	Blood (child)	10 µg/dL	Investigate community
OSHA	Blood (adult)	60 µg/dL	Medical removal from work
OSHA	Air	50 µg/m^3	PEL*
	Air	0.75 µg/m^3	Tetraethyl or tetramethyl
ACGIH	Air	150 µg/m^3	TWA†
EPA	Air	1.5 µg/m^3	Three-month average
EPA	Water	15 µg/L (ppb)	5 ppb circulating
EPA	Food	100 µg/d	Advisory
FDA	Wine	300 ppm	Plan to reduce to 200 ppm
EPA	Soil/dust	50 ppm	
CPSC	Paint	600 ppm (0.06%) by dry weight	

Abbreviatons: ACGIH = American Conference of Governmental Industrial Hygienists; CDC = Centers for Disease Control and Prevention; CPSC = Consumer Product Safety Commission; EPA = Environmental Protection Agency; FDA = Food and Drug Administration; OSHA = Occupational Safety and Health Administration.
*PEL = permissible exposure limit (highest level over an 8-hour workday).
†TWA = time-weighted average (air concentration for 8-hour workday and 40 hour workweek).

level over 30 µg/dL has been reported. Lead reduces excretion of uric acid, and high-level exposure may be associated with hyperuricemia and "saturnine gout," Fanconi's syndrome (aminoaciduria and renal tubular acidosis), and tubular fibrosis.

Reproductive

Spontaneous abortion, transient delay in the child's development (catch up at age 5 to 6 years), decreased sperm count, and abnormal sperm morphology can occur with lead exposure. Lead crosses the placenta and fetal blood levels reach 75% to 100% of maternal blood levels. Lead is teratogenic.

Metabolic

Decreased cytochrome P450 activity alters the metabolism of medication and endogenously produced substances. Decreased activation of cortisol and decreased growth is caused by interference in vitamin conversion (25-hydroxyvitamin D to 1,25 hydroxyvitamin D) at venous blood levels of 20 to 30 µg/dL.

Other Manifestations

Abnormalities of thyroid, cardiac, and hepatic function occur in adults. Abdominal colic is seen in children at doses greater than 50 µg/dL. "Lead gum lines" at the dental border of the gingiva can occur in cases of chronic lead poisoning.

BOX 1 Hobbies Associated with Lead Exposure

Casting of ammunition
Collecting antique pewter
Collecting/painting lead toys (e.g., soldiers and figures)
Ceramics or glazed pottery
Refinishing furniture
Making fishing weights
Home renovation
Jewelry making, lead solder
Glass blowing, lead glass
Bronze casting
Print making and other fine arts (when lead white, flake white, chrome yellow pigments are involved)
Liquor distillation
Hunting and target shooting
Painting
Car and boat repair
Burning/engraving lead-painted wood
Making stained leaded glass
Copper enameling

TABLE 21 Summary of Lead-Induced Health Effects in Adults and Children

Blood Lead Level (µg/dL)	Age Group	Health Effect
>100	Adult	Encephalopathic signs and symptoms
>80	Adult	Anemia
	Child	Encephalopathy
		Chronic nephropathy (e.g., aminoaciduria)
>70	Adult	Clinically evident peripheral neuropathy
	Child	Colic and other gastrointestinal symptoms
>60	Adult	Female reproductive effects
		CNS disturbance symptoms (i.e., sleep disturbances, mood changes, memory and concentration problems, headaches)
>50	Adult	Decreased hemoglobin production
		Decreased performance on neurobehavioral tests
	Adult	Altered testicular function
		Gastrointestinal symptoms (i.e., abdominal pain, constipation, diarrhea, nausea, anorexia)
	Child	Peripheral neuropathy*
>40	Adult	Decreased peripheral nerve conduction
		Hypertension, age 40–59 years
		Chronic neuropathy*
>25	Adult	Elevated erythrocyte protoporphyrin in males
15-25	Adult	Elevated erythrocyte protoporphyrin in females
>10	Child	Decreased intelligence and growth
		Impaired learning
		Reduced birth weight*
		Impaired mental ability
	Fetus	Preterm delivery

*Controversial.
From Anonymous: Implementation of the Lead Contamination Control Act of 1988. MMWR Morb Mortal Wkly Rep 41:288, 1992.

Laboratory Investigations

Serial venous blood lead measurements are taken on days 3 and 5 during treatment and 7 days after chelation therapy, then every 1 to 2 weeks for 8 weeks, and then every month for 6 months. Intravenous infusion should be stopped at least 1 hour before blood lead levels are measured. Table 22 gives a classification of blood lead concentrations in children.

One should evaluate CBC, serum ferritin, erythrocyte protoporphyrin (>35 μg/dL indicates lead poisoning as well as iron deficiency and other causes), electrolytes, serum calcium and phosphorus, urinalysis, BUN, and creatinine. Abdominal and long bone radiographs may be useful in certain circumstances to identify radiopaque material in bowel and "lead lines" in proximal tibia (which occur after prolonged exposure in association with venous blood lead levels greater than 50 μg/dL).

Neuropsychological tests are difficult to perform in young children but should be considered at the end of treatment, especially to determine auditory dysfunction.

Management

The basis of treatment is removal of the source of lead. Cases of poisoning in children should be reported to local health department and cases of occupational poisoning should be reported to OSHA. The source must be identified and abated, and dust controlled by wet mopping. Cold water should be let to run for 2 minutes before being used for drinking. Planting shrubbery (not vegetables) in contaminated soil will keep children away.

Supportive care should be instituted, including measures to deal with refractory seizures (continued antidotal therapy, diazepam, and possibly neuromuscular blockers), with the hepatic and renal failure, and intravascular hemolysis in severe cases. Seizures are treated with diazepam followed by neuromuscular blockers if needed.

Lead does not bind to activated charcoal. One must not delay chelation therapy for complete gastrointestinal decontamination in severe cases. Whole-bowel irrigation has been used prior to treatment. Some authorities recommend abdominal radiographs followed by gastrointestinal decontamination if necessary before switching to oral therapy. Chelation therapy can be used for patients in whom venous blood level of lead is greater than 45 μg/dL in children and greater than 80 μg/dL in adults or in adults with lower levels who are symptomatic or who have a "positive" lead mobilization test result (not routinely performed at most centers) (Table 23).

Succimer (dimercaptosuccinic acid, DMSA, Chemet), a derivative of British anti-Lewisite (BAL), is an oral agent for chelation in children with a venous blood level of greater than 45 μg/dL. The recommended dose is 10 mg/kg every 8 hours for 5 days, then every 12 hours for 14 days. DMSA is under investigation to determine its role in children with a venous blood level less than 45 μg/dL. Although not approved for adults, it has been used in the same dosage. Monitoring should be maintained by CBC, liver transaminases, and urinalysis for adverse effects.

D-Penicillamine (Cuprimine) is another oral chelator that is given in doses of 20 to 40 mg/kg/d not to exceed 1 g/d. However, it is not FDA approved and has a 10% adverse reaction rate. Nevertheless, D-penicillamine has been used infrequently in adults and children with elevated venous blood lead levels.

Edetate calcium disodium (ethylene diaminetetra-acetic acid or CaNa$_2$EDTA Versenate) is a water-soluble chelator given intramuscularly (with 0.5% procaine) or intravenously. The calcium in the compound is displaced by divalent and trivalent heavy metals, forming a soluble complex, which is stable at physiologic pH (but not at acid pH) and enhances lead clearance in the urine. EDTA usually is administered intravenously, especially in severe cases. It must not be administered until adequate urine flow is established. It may redistribute lead to the brain; therefore, BAL may be given first at a venous blood lead level of greater than 55 μg/dL in children and greater than 100 μg/dL in adults. Phlebitis occurs at a concentration greater than 0.5 mg/mL. Alkalinization of the urine may be helpful. CaNa$_2$EDTA should not be confused with sodium EDTA (disodium edetate), which is used to treat hypercalcemia; inadvertent use may produce severe hypocalcemia.

Dimercaprol (BAL) is a peanut oil–based dithiol (two sulfhydryl molecules) that combines with one atom of lead to form a heterocyclic stable ring complex. It is usually reserved for patients in whom venous blood lead is greater than 70 μg/dL, and it chelates red blood cell lead, enhancing its elimination through the urine and bile. It crosses the blood–brain barrier. Approximately 50% of patients have adverse reactions, including bad metallic taste in the mouth, pain at the injection site, sterile abscesses, and fever.

A venous blood lead level greater than 70 μg/dL or the presence of clinical symptoms suggesting encephalopathy in children is a potentially life-threatening emergency. Management should be accomplished in a medical center with a pediatric intensive care unit by a multidisciplinary team including a critical care specialist, a toxicologist, a neurologist, and a neurosurgeon. Careful monitoring of neurologic status, fluid status, and intracranial pressure should be undertaken if necessary. These patients need close monitoring for hemodynamic instability. Hydration should be maintained to ensure renal excretion of lead. Fluids, renal and hepatic function, and electrolyte levels should be monitored.

While waiting for adequate urine flow, therapy should be initiated with intramuscular dimercaprol (BAL) only (25 mg/kg/d divided into 6 doses). Four hours later, the second dose of BAL should be given intramuscularly, concurrently with CaNa$_2$EDTA 50 mg/kg/d as a single dose infused over several hours or as a continuous infusion. The double therapy is continued until the venous blood level is less than 40 μg/dL.

As long as the venous blood level is greater than 40 μg/dL, therapy is continued for 72 hours and followed by two alternatives: either parenteral therapy with two drugs (CaNa$_2$EDTA and BAL) for 5 days or continuation of therapy with CaNa$_2$EDTA alone if a good response is achieved and the venous blood level of lead is less than 40 μg/dL. If one cannot get the venous blood lead report back, one should continue therapy with both BAL and EDTA for 5 days. In patients with lead encephalopathy, parenteral chelation should be continued with both drugs until the patient is clinically stable before changing

TABLE 22 Classification of Blood Lead Concentrations in Children

Blood Lead (μg/dL)	Recommended Interventions
<9	None
10-14	Community intervention
	Repeat blood lead in 3 months
15-19	Individual case management
	Environmental counseling
	Nutritional counseling
	Repeat blood lead in 3 months
20-44	Medical referral
	Environmental inspection/abatement
	Nutritional counseling
	Repeat blood lead in 3 months
45-69	Environmental inspection/abatement
	Nutritional counseling
	Pharmacologic therapy
	DMSA succimer oral or CaNa$_2$EDTA parenteral
	Repeat every 2 weeks for 6-8 weeks, then monthly for 4-6 months
>70	Hospitalization in intensive care unit
	Environmental inspection/abatement
	Pharmacologic therapy
	Dimercaprol (BAL in oil) IM initial alone
	Dimercaprol IM and CaNa$_2$EDTA together
	Repeat every week

Abbreviations: BAL = British anti-Lewisite; CaNa$_2$EDTA = Edetate calcium disodium; DMS = dimercaptosuccinic acid; IM = intramuscular.

TABLE 23 Pharmacologic Chelation Therapy of Lead Poisoning

Drug	Route	Dose	Duration	Precautions	Monitor
Dimercaprol (BAL in oil)	IM	3-5 mg/kg q4-6h	3-5 days	G6PD deficiency Concurrent iron therapy	AST/ALT enzymes
CaNa$_2$ EDTA (calcium disodium. versenate)	IM/IV	50 mg/kg per day	5 days	Inadequate fluid intake Renal impairment Penicillin allergy	Urinalysis, BUN Creatinine Urinalysis, BUN
D-Penicillamine (Cuprimine)	PO	10 mg/kg per day increase 30 mg/kg over 2 weeks	6-20 weeks	Concurrent iron therapy; lead exposure Renal impairment	Creatinine, CBC
2,3-Dimercaptosuccinic acid (DMSA; succimer)	PO	10 mg/kg per dose 3 times daily 10 mg/kg per dose twice daily for 14 days	19 days	AST/ALT Concurrent iron therapy G6PD deficiency lead exposure	AST/ALT

Abbreviations: ALT = alanine aminotransferase; AST = aspartate transaminase; BAL = British anti-Lewisite; bid = twice daily; BUN = blood urea nitrogen; CBC = complete blood count; G6PD = glucose-6-phosphate dehydrogenase; IM = intramuscular; IV = intravenous; PO = oral; tid = three times daily.

therapy. Mannitol and dexa-methasone can reduce the cerebral edema, but their role in lead encephalopathy is not clear. Surgical decompression is not recommended to reduce cerebral edema in these cases.

If BAL and CaNa$_2$EDTA are used together, a minimum of 2 days with no treatment should elapse before another 5-day course of therapy is considered. The 5-day course is repeated with CaNa$_2$EDTA alone if the blood lead level rebounds to greater than 40 µg/dL or in combination with BAL if the venous blood level is greater than 70 µg/dL. If a third course is required, unless there are compelling reasons, one should wait at least 5 to 7 days before administering the course.

Following chelation therapy, a period of equilibration of 10 to 14 days should be allowed and a repeat venous blood lead concentration should be obtained. If the patient is stable enough for oral intake, oral succimer 30 mg/kg/d in three divided doses for 5 days followed by 20 mg/kg/d in two divided doses for 14 days has been suggested, but there are limited data to support this recommendation. Therapy should be continued until venous blood lead level is less than 20 µg/dL in children or less than 40 µg/dL in adults.

Chelators combined with lead are hemodialyzable in the event of renal failure.

Disposition

All patients with a venous blood lead level of greater than 70 µg/dL or who are symptomatic should be admitted. If a child is hospitalized, all lead hazards must be removed from the home environment before allowing the child to return. The source must be eliminated by environmental and occupational investigations. The local health department should be involved in dealing with children who are lead poisoned, and OSHA should be involved with cases of occupational lead poisoning. Consultation with a poison control center or experienced toxicologist is necessary when chelating patients. Follow-up venous blood lead concentrations should be obtained within 1 to 2 weeks and followed every 2 weeks for 6 to 8 weeks, then monthly for 4 to 6 months if the patient required chelation therapy. All patients with venous blood level greater than 10 µg/dL should be followed at least every 3 months until two venous blood lead concentrations are 10 µg/dL or three are less than 15 µg/dL.

LITHIUM (ESKALITH, LITHANE)

Lithium is an alkali metal used primarily in the treatment of bipolar psychiatric disorders. Most intoxications are cases of chronic overdose. One gram of lithium carbonate contains 189 mg (5.1 mEq) of lithium; a regular tablet contains 300 mg (8.12 mEq) and a sustained-release preparation contains 450 mg or 12.18 mEq.

Toxic Mechanism

The brain is the primary target organ of toxicity, but the mechanism is unclear. Lithium may interfere with physiologic functions by acting as a substitute for cellular cations (sodium and potassium), depressing neural excitation and synaptic transmission.

Toxic Dose

A dose of 1 mEq/kg (40 mg/kg) of lithium will give a peak serum lithium concentration about 1.2 mEq/L. The therapeutic serum lithium concentration in cases of acute mania is 0.6 to 1.2 mEq/L, and for maintenance it is 0.5 to 0.8 mEq/L. Serum lithium concentration levels are usually obtained 12 hours after the last dose. The toxic dose is determined by clinical manifestations and serum levels after the distribution phase.

Acute ingestion of twenty 300-mg tablets (300 mg increases the serum lithium concentration by 0.2 to 0.4 mEq/L) in adults may produce serious intoxication. Chronic intoxication can be produced by conditions listed below that can decrease the elimination of lithium or increase lithium reabsorption in the kidney.

The risk factors that predispose to chronic lithium toxicity are febrile illness, impaired renal function, hyponatremia, advanced age, lithium-induced diabetes insipidus, dehydration, vomiting and diarrhea, and concomitant use of other drugs, such as thiazide and spironolactone diuretics, nonsteroidal anti-inflammatory drugs, salicylates, angiotensin-converting enzyme inhibitors (e.g., captopril), serotonin reuptake inhibitors (e.g., fluoxetine [Prozac]), and phenothiazines.

Kinetics

Gastrointestinal absorption of regular-release preparations is rapid; serum lithium concentration peaks in 2 to 4 hours and is complete by 6 to 8 hours. The onset of toxicity may occur at 1 to 4 hours after acute overdose but usually is delayed because lithium enters the brain slowly. Absorption of sustained-release preparations and the development of toxicity may be delayed 6 to 12 hours.

Volume distribution is 0.5 to 0.9 L/kg. Lithium is not protein bound. The half-life after a single dose is 9 to 13 hours; at steady state, it may be 30 to 58 hours. The renal handling of lithium is similar to that of sodium: glomerular filtration and reabsorption (80%) by the proximal renal tubule. Adequate sodium must be present to prevent lithium reabsorption. More than 90% of lithium is excreted by the kidney, 30% to 60% within 6 to 12 hours.

Manifestations

The examiner must distinguish between side effects, acute intoxication, acute or chronic toxicity, and chronic intoxications. Chronic is the most common and dangerous type of intoxication.

Side effects include fine tremor, gastrointestinal upset, hypothyroidism, polyuria and frank diabetes insipidus, dermatologic manifestations, and cardiac conduction deficits. Lithium is teratogenic.

Patients with acute poisoning may be asymptomatic, with an early high serum lithium concentration of 9 mEq/L, and deteriorate as the serum lithium concentration falls by 50% and the lithium distributes to the brain and the other tissues. Nausea and vomiting may occur within 1 to 4 hours, but the systemic manifestations are usually delayed several more hours. It may take as long as 3 to 5 days for serious symptoms to develop. Acute toxicity and acute on chronic toxicity are manifested by neurologic findings, including weakness, fasciculations, altered mental state, myoclonus, hyperreflexia, rigidity, coma, and convulsions with limbs in hypertension. Cardiovascular effects are nonspecific and occur at therapeutic doses, flat T or inverted T waves, atrioventricular block, and prolonged QT interval. Lithium is not a primary cardiotoxin. Cardiogenic shock occurs secondary to CNS toxicity. Chronic intoxication is associated with manifestations at lower serum lithium concentrations. There is some correlation with manifestations, especially at higher serum lithium concentrations. Although the levels do not always correlate with the manifestations, they are more predictive in cases of severe intoxication. A serum lithium concentration greater than 3.0 mEq/L with chronic intoxication and altered mental state indicates severe toxicity. Permanent neurologic sequelae can result from lithium intoxication.

Laboratory Investigations

Monitoring should include CBC (lithium causes significant leukocytosis), renal function, thyroid function (chronic intoxication), ECG, and electrolytes. Serum lithium concentrations should be determined every 2 to 4 hours until levels are close to therapeutic range. Cross-reactions with green-top Vacutainer specimen tubes containing heparin will spuriously elevate serum lithium concentration 6 to 8 mEq/L.

Management

Vital function must be established and maintained. Seizure precautions should be instituted and seizures, hypotension, and dysrhythmias treated. Evaluation should include examination for rigidity and hyperreflexia signs, hydration, renal function (BUN, creatinine), and electrolytes, especially sodium. The examiner should inquire about diuretic and other drug use that increase serum lithium concentration, and the patient must discontinue the drugs. If the patient is on chronic therapy, the lithium should be discontinued. Serial serum lithium concentrations should be obtained every 4 hours until serum lithium concentration peaks and there is a downward trend toward almost therapeutic range, especially in sustained-release preparations. Vital signs should be monitored, including temperature, and ECG and serial neurologic examinations should be undertaken, including mental status and urinary output. Nephrology consultation is warranted in case of a chronic and elevated serum lithium concentration (>2.5 mEq/L), a large ingestion, or altered mental state.

An intravenous line should be established and hydration and electrolyte balance restored. Serum sodium level should be determined before 0.9% saline fluid is administered in patients with chronic overdose because hypernatremia may be present from diabetes insipidus. Although current evidence supports an initial 0.9% saline infusion (200 mL/h) to enhance excretion of lithium, once hydration, urine output, and normonatremia are established, one should administer 0.45% saline and slow the infusion (100 mL/h) for all patients.

Gastric lavage is often not recommended in cases of acute ingestion because of the large size of the tablets, and it is not necessary after chronic intoxication. Activated charcoal is ineffective. For sustained-release preparations, whole-bowel irrigation may be useful but is not proven. Sodium polystyrene sulfonate (Kayexalate), an ion exchange resin, is difficult to administer and has been used only in uncontrolled studies. Its use is not recommended.

Hemodialysis is the most efficient method for removing lithium from the vascular compartment. It is the treatment of choice for patients with severe intoxication with an altered mental state, those with seizures, and anuric patients. Long runs are used until the serum lithium concentration is less than 1 mEq/L because of extensive re-equilibration. Serum lithium concentration should be monitored every 4 hours after dialysis for rebound. Repeated and prolonged hemodialysis may be necessary. A lag in neurologic recovery can be expected.

Disposition

An acute asymptomatic lithium overdose cannot be medically cleared on the basis of single lithium level. Patients should be admitted if they have any neurologic manifestations (altered mental status, hyperreflexia, stiffness, or tremor). Patients should be admitted to the intensive care unit if they are dehydrated, have renal impairment, or have a high or rising lithium level.

METHANOL (WOOD ALCOHOL, METHYL ALCOHOL)

The concentration of methanol in Sterno fuel is 4% and it contains ethanol, in windshield washer fluid it is 30% to 60%, and in gas-line antifreeze it is 100%.

Toxic Mechanism

Methanol is metabolized by alcohol dehydrogenase to formaldehyde, which is metabolized to formate. Formate inhibits cytochrome oxidase, producing tissue hypoxia, lactic acidosis, and optic nerve edema. Formate is converted by folate-dependent enzymes to carbon dioxide.

Toxic Dose

The minimal toxic amount is approximately 100 mg/kg. Serious toxicity in a young child can be produced by the ingestion of 2.5 to 5.0 mL of 100% methanol. Ingestion of 5-mL 100% methanol by a 10-kg child produces estimated peak blood methanol of 80 mg/dL. Ingestion of 15 mL 40% methanol was lethal for a 2-year-old child in one report. A fatal adult oral dose is 30 to 240 mL 100% (20 to 150 g). Ingestion of 6 to 10 mL 100% causes blindness in adults. The toxic blood concentration is greater than 20 mg/dL; very serious toxicity and potential fatality occur at levels greater than 50 mg/dL.

Kinetics

Onset of action can start within 1 hour but may be delayed up to 12 to 18 hours by metabolism to toxic metabolites. It may be delayed longer if ethanol is ingested concomitantly or in infants. Peak blood methanol concentration is 1 hour. Volume distribution is 0.6 L/kg (total body water).

For metabolism, see *Toxic Mechanism*.

Elimination is through metabolism. The half-life of methanol is 8 hours, with ethanol blocking it is 30 to 35 hours, and with hemodialysis 2.5 hours.

Manifestations

Metabolism creates a delay in onset for 12 to 18 hours or longer if ethanol is ingested concomitantly. Initial findings are as follows:

- 0 to 6 hours: Confusion, ataxia, inebriation, formaldehyde odor on breath, and abdominal pain can be present, but the patient may be asymptomatic. Note: Methanol produces an osmolal gap (early), and its metabolite formate produces the anion gap metabolic acidosis (see later). Absence of osmolar or anion gap does not always exclude methanol intoxication.
- 6 to 12 hours: Malaise, headache, abdominal pain, vomiting, visual symptoms, including hyperemia of optic disc, "snow vision," and blindness can be seen.

- More than 12 hours: Worsening acidosis, hyperglycemia, shock, and multiorgan failure develop, with death from complications of intractable acidosis and cerebral edema.

Laboratory Investigation

Methanol can be detected on some chromatography drug screens if specified. Methanol and ethanol levels, electrolytes, glucose, BUN, creatinine, amylase, and ABG should be monitored every 4 hours. Formate levels correlate more closely than blood methanol concentration with severity of intoxication and should be obtained if possible.

Management

One should protect the airway by intubation to prevent aspiration and administer assisted ventilation as needed. If needed, 100% oxygen can be administered. A nephrologist should be consulted early regarding the need for hemodialysis.

Gastrointestinal decontamination procedures have no role.

Metabolic acidosis should be treated vigorously with sodium bicarbonate 2 to 3 mEq/kg intravenously. Large amounts may be needed.

Antidote therapy is initiated to inhibit metabolism if the patient has a history of ingesting more than 0.4 mL/kg of 100% with the following conditions:

- Blood methanol level is greater than 20 mg/dL
- The patient has osmolar gap not accounted for by other factors
- The patient is symptomatic or acidotic with increased anion gap and/or hyperemia of the optic disc.

The ethanol or fomepizole therapy outlined below can be used.

Ethanol Therapy

Ethanol should be initiated immediately if fomepizole is unavailable (see *Fomepizole Therapy*). Alcohol dehydrogenase has a greater affinity for ethanol than ethylene glycol. Therefore, ethanol blocks the metabolism of ethylene glycol.

Ethanol should be administered intravenously (oral administration is less reliable) to produce a blood ethanol concentration of 100 to 150 mg/dL. The loading dose is 10 mL/kg of 10% ethanol administered intravenously concomitantly with a maintenance dose of 10% ethanol at 1.0 mL/kg/h. This dose may need to be increased to 2 mL/kg/h in patients who are heavy drinkers. The blood ethanol concentration should be measured hourly and the infusion rate should be adjusted to maintain a concentration of 100 to 150 mg/dL.

Fomepizole Therapy

Fomepizole (Antizol, 4-methylpyrazole) inhibits alcohol dehydrogenase more reliably than ethanol and it does not require constant monitoring of ethanol levels and adjustment of infusion rates. Fomepizole is available in 1 g/mL vials of 1.5 mL. The loading dose is 15 mg/kg (0.015 mL/kg) IV, maintenance dose is 10 mg/kg (0.01 mL/kg) every 12 hours for 4 doses, then 15 mg/kg every 12 hours until the ethylene glycol levels are less than 20 mg/dL. The solution is prepared by being mixed with 100 mL of 0.9% saline or D_5W. Fomepizole can be given to patients requiring hemodialysis but should be dosed as follows:

Dose at the beginning of hemodialysis:

- If less than 6 hours since last Antizol dose, do not administer dose
- If more than 6 hours since last dose, administer next scheduled dose

Dosing during hemodialysis:

- Dose every 4 hours

Dosing at the time hemodialysis is completed:

- If less than 1 hour between last dose and end dialysis, do not administer dose at end of dialysis
- If 1 to 3 hours between last dose and end dialysis, administer one half of next scheduled dose
- If more than 3 hours between last dose and end dialysis, administer next scheduled dose

Maintenance dosing off hemodialysis:

- Give the next scheduled dose 12 hours from the last dose administered

Hemodialysis increases the clearance of both methanol and formate 10-fold over renal clearance. A blood methanol concentration greater than 50 mg/dL has been used as an indication for hemodialysis, but recently some toxicologists from the New York City Poison Center recommended early hemodialysis in patients with blood methanol concentration greater than 25 mg/dL because it may be able to shorten the course of intoxication if started early. One should continue to monitor methanol levels and/or formate levels every 4 hours after the procedure for rebound. Other indications for early hemodialysis are significant metabolic acidosis and electrolyte abnormalities despite conventional therapy and if visual or neurologic signs or symptoms are present.

A serum formate level greater than 20 mg/dL has also been used as a criterion for hemodialysis, although this is often not readily available through many laboratories. If hemodialysis is used, the infusion rate of 10% ethanol should be increased 2.0 to 3.5 mL/kg/h. The blood ethanol concentration and glucose level should be obtained every 2 hours.

Therapy is continued with both ethanol and hemodialysis until the blood methanol level is undetectable, there is no acidosis, and the patient has no neurologic or visual disturbances. This may require several days.

Hypoglycemia is treated with intravenous glucose. Doses of folinic acid (Leucovorin) and folic acid have been used successfully in animal investigations to enhance formate metabolism to carbon dioxide and water. Leucovorin 1 mg/kg up to 50 mg IV is administered every 4 hours for several days.

An initial ophthalmologic consultation and follow-up are warranted.

Disposition

All patients who have ingested significant amounts of methanol should be referred to the emergency department for evaluation and blood methanol concentration measurement. Ophthalmologic follow-up of all patients with methanol intoxications should be arranged.

MONOAMINE OXIDASE INHIBITORS

Nonselective monoamine oxidase inhibitors (MAOIs) include the hydrazines phenelzine (Nardil) and isocarboxazid (Marplan), and the nonhydrazine tranylcypromine (Parnate). Furazolidone (Furoxone) and pargyline (Eutonyl)[2] are also considered nonselective MAOIs. Moclobemide,[2] which is available in many countries but not the United States, is a selective MAO-A inhibitor. MAO-B inhibitors include selegiline (Eldepryl), an antiparksonism agent, which does not have similar toxicity to MAO-A and is not discussed. Selectivity is lost in an overdose. MAOIs are used to treat severe depression.

Toxic Mechanism

Monoamine oxidase enzymes are responsible for the oxidative deamination of both endogenous and exogenous catecholamines such as norepinephrine. MAO-A in the intestinal wall also metabolizes tyramine in food. MAOIs permanently inhibit MAO enzymes until a new enzyme is synthesized after 14 days or longer. The toxicity results from the accumulation, potentiation, and prolongation of the catecholamine action followed by profound hypotension and cardiovascular collapse.

---

[2]Not available in the United States.

Toxic Dose

Toxicity begins at 2 to 3 mg/kg and fatalities occur at 4 to 6 mg/kg. Death has occurred after a single dose of 170 mg of tranylcypromine in an adult.

Kinetics

Structurally, MAOIs are related to amphetamines and catecholamines. The hydrazine peak levels are at 1 to 2 hours; metabolism is hepatic acetylation; and inactive metabolites are excreted in the urine. For the nonhydrazines, peak levels occur at 1 to 4 hours, and metabolism is via the liver to active amphetamine-like metabolites.

The onset of symptoms in a case of overdose is delayed 6 to 24 hours after ingestion, peak activity is 8 to 12 hours, and duration is 72 hours or longer. The peak of MAO inhibition is in 5 to 10 days and lasts as long as 5 weeks.

Manifestations

Manifestations of an acute ingestion overdose of MAO-A inhibitors are as follows:

Phase I

An adrenergic crisis occurs, with delayed onset for 6 to 24 hours, and may not reach peak until 24 hours. The crisis starts as hyperthermia, tachycardia, tachypnea, dysarthria, transient hypertension, hyperreflexia, and CNS stimulation.

Phase II

Neuromuscular excitation and sympathetic hyperactivity occur with increased temperature greater than 40°C (104°F), agitation, hyperactivity, confusion, fasciculations, twitching, tremor, masseter spasm, muscle rigidity, acidosis, and electrolyte abnormalities. Seizures and dystonic reactions may occur. The pupils are mydriatic, sometimes nonreactive with "ping-pong gaze."

Phase III

CNS depression and cardiovascular collapse occur in cases of severe overdose as the catecholamines are depleted. Symptoms usually resolve within 5 days but may last 2 weeks.

Phase IV

Secondary complications occur, including rhabdomyolysis, cardiac dysrhythmias, multiorgan failure, and coagulopathies.

Biogenic interactions usually occur while the patient is on therapeutic doses of MAOI or shortly after they are discontinued (30 to 60 minutes), before the new MAO enzyme is synthesized. The following substances have been implicated: indirect acting sympathomimetics such as amphetamines, serotonergic drugs, opioids (e.g., meperidine, dextromethorphan), tricyclic antidepressants, specific serotonin reuptake inhibitors (SSRI; e.g., fluoxetine [Prozac], sertraline [Zoloft], paroxetine [Paxil]), tyramine-containing foods (e.g., wine, beer, avocados, cheese, caviar, chocolate, chicken liver), and L-tryptophan. SSRIs should not be started for at least 5 weeks after MAOIs have been discontinued.

In mild cases, usually caused by foods, headache and hypertension develop and last for several hours. In severe cases, malignant hypertension and severe hyperthermia syndromes consisting of hypertension or hyperthermia, altered mental state, skeletal muscle rigidity, shivering (often beginning in the masseter muscle), and seizures may occur.

The serotonin syndrome, which may be a result of inhibition of serotonin metabolism, has similar clinical findings to those of malignant hyperthermia and may occur with or without hyperthermia or hypertension.

Chronic toxicity clinical findings include tremors, hyperhidrosis, agitation, hallucinations, confusion, and seizures and may be confused with withdrawal syndromes.

Laboratory Investigations

Monitoring of the ECG, cardiac monitoring, CPK, ABG, pulse oximeter, electrolytes, blood glucose, and acid–base balance should be maintained.

Management

In the case of MAOI overdose, ipecac-induced emesis should not be used. Only activated charcoal alone should be used.

If the patient is admitted to the hospital and is well enough to eat, a nontyramine diet should be ordered.

Extreme agitation and seizures can be controlled with benzodiazepines and barbiturates. Phenytoin is ineffective. Nondepolarizing neuromuscular blockers (not depolarizing succinylcholine) may be needed in severe cases of hyperthermia and rigidity. If the patient has severe hypertension (catecholamine mediated), phentolamine (Regitine), a parenteral β-blocking agent, 3 to 5 mg intravenously, or labetalol (Normodyne), a combination of an α-blocking agent and a β-blocker, 20-mg intravenous bolus, should be given. If malignant hypertension with rigidity is present, a short-acting nitroprusside and benzodiazepine can be used. Hypertension is often followed by severe hypotension, which should be managed by fluid and vasopressors. *Caution:* Vasopressor therapy should be administered at lower doses than usual because of exaggerated pharmacologic response. Norepinephrine is preferred to dopamine, which requires release of intracellular amines.

Cardiac dysrhythmias are treated with standard therapy but are often refractory, and cardioversion and pacemakers may be needed.

For malignant hyperthermia, dantrolene (Dantrium), a nonspecific peripheral skeletal relaxing agent, is administered, which inhibits the release of calcium from the sarcoplasm. Dantrolene is reconstituted with 60 mL sterile water without bacteriostatic agents. Glass equipment must not be used, and the drug must be protected from light and used within 6 hours. Loading dose is 2 to 3 mg/kg intravenously as a bolus, and the loading dose is repeated until the signs of malignant hyperthermia (tachycardia, rigidity, increased end-tidal CO_2, and temperature) are controlled. Maximum total dose is 10 mg/kg to avoid hepatotoxicity.

When malignant hyperthermia has subsided, 1 mg/kg IV is given every 6 hours for 24 to 48 hours, then orally 1 mg/kg every 6 hours for 24 hours to prevent recurrence. There is a danger of thrombophlebitis following peripheral dantrolene, and it should be administered through a central line if possible. In addition one should administer external cooling and correct metabolic acidosis and electrolyte disturbances. Benzodiazepine can be used for sedation. Dantrolene does not reverse central dopamine blockade; therefore, bromocriptine mesylate (Parlodel) 2.5 to 10 mg should be given orally or through a nasogastric tube three times a day.

Rhabdomyolysis and myoglobinuria are treated with fluids. Urine alkalinization should also be treated.

Hemodialysis and hemoperfusion are of no proven value.

Biogenic amine interactions are managed symptomatically, similar to cases of overdose. For the serotonin syndrome cyproheptadine (Periactin), a serotonin blocker, 4 mg orally every hour for three doses, or methysergide (Sansert), 2 mg orally every 6 hours for three doses, should be considered. The effectiveness of these drugs has not been proven.

Disposition

All patients who have ingested more than 2 mg/kg of an MAOI should be admitted to the hospital for 24 hours of observation and monitoring in the intensive care unit because the life-threatening manifestations may be delayed. Patients with drug or dietary interactions that are mild may not require admission if symptoms subside within 4 to 6 hours and the patients remain asymptomatic. Patients with symptoms that persist or require active intervention should be admitted to the intensive care unit.

OPIOIDS (NARCOTIC OPIATES)

Opioids are used for analgesia, as antitussives, and as antidiarrheal agents and are illicit agents (heroin, opium) used in substance abuse. Tolerance, physical dependency, and withdrawal may develop.

Toxic Mechanism

At least four main opioid receptors have been identified. The μ receptor is considered the most important for central analgesia and CNS depression. The κ and δ receptors predominate in spinal analgesia. The σ receptors may mediate dysphoria. Death is a consequence of dose-dependent CNS respiratory depression or secondary to pulmonary aspiration or noncardiac pulmonary edema. The mechanism of noncardiac pulmonary edema is unknown.

Dextromethorphan can interact with MAOIs, causing severe hyperthermia, and may cause the serotonin syndrome (see *Selective Serotonin Reuptake Inhibitors*). Dextromethorphan inhibits the metabolism of norepinephrine and serotonin and blocks the reuptake of serotonin. It is found as a component of a large number of nonprescription cough and cold remedies.

Toxic Dose

The toxic dose depends on the specific drug, route of administration, and degree of tolerance. For therapeutic and toxic doses, see Table 24. In children, respiratory depression has been produced by 10 mg of morphine or methadone, 75 mg of meperidine, and 12.5 mg of diphenoxylate. Infants younger than 3 months of age are more susceptible to respiratory depression. The dose should be reduced by 50%.

Kinetics

Oral onset of analgesic effect of morphine is 10 to 15 minutes; the action peaks in 1 hour and lasts 4 to 6 hours. With sustained-release preparations, the duration is 8 to 12 hours. Opioids are 90% metabolized in the liver by hepatic conjugation and 90% excreted in the urine as inactive compounds. Volume distribution is 1 to 4 L/kg. Protein binding is 35% to 75%. The typical plasma half-life of opiates is 2 to 5 hours, but that of methadone is 24 to 36 hours. Morphine metabolites include morphine-3-glucuronide (inactive) and morphine-6-glucuronide (active) and normorphine (active). Meperidine (Demerol) is rapidly hydrolyzed by tissue esterases into the active metabolite normeperidine, which has twice the convulsant activity of meperidine. Heroin (diacetylmorphine) is deacetylated within minutes to 6-monacetylmorphine and morphine. Propoxyphene (Darvon) has a rapid onset of action, and death has occurred within 15 to 30 minutes after a massive overdose. Propoxyphene is metabolized to norpropoxyphene, an active metabolite with convulsive, cardiac dysrhythmic, and heart block properties. Symptoms of diphenoxylate overdose appear within 1 to 4 hours. It is metabolized into the active metabolite difenoxin, which is five times more active as a regular respiratory depressant agent. Death has been reported in children after ingestion of a single tablet.

Manifestations

Initially, mild intoxication produces miosis, dull face, drowsiness, partial ptosis, and "nodding" (head drops to chest then bobs up). Larger amounts produce the classic triad of miotic pupils (exceptions below), respiratory depression, and depressed level of consciousness (flaccid coma). The blood pressure, pulse, and bowel activity are decreased.

Dilated pupils do not exclude opioid intoxication. Some exceptions to the miosis effect include dextromethorphan (paralyzes iris), fentanyl, meperidine, and diphenoxylate (rarely). Physiologic disturbances including acidosis, hypoglycemia, hypoxia, and postictal state, or a co-ingestant may also produce mydriasis.

Usually, the muscles are flaccid, but increased muscle tone can be produced by meperidine and fentanyl (chest rigidity). Seizures are rare but can occur with ingestion of codeine, meperidine, propoxyphene, and dextromethorphan. Hallucinations and agitation have been reported.

Pruritus and urticaria are caused by histamine release by some opioids or by sulfite additives.

Noncardiac pulmonary edema may occur after an overdose, especially with intravenous heroin abuse. Cardiac effects include vasodilation and hypotension. A heart murmur in an intravenous addict suggests endocarditis. Propoxyphene can produce delayed cardiac dysrhythmias.

Fentanyl is 100 times more potent than morphine and can cause chest wall muscle rigidity. Some of its derivatives are 2000 times more potent than morphine.

Laboratory Investigations

For patients with overdose, one should obtain and monitor ABG, blood glucose, and electrolyte levels; chest radiographs; and ECG. For drug abusers, one should consider testing for hepatitis B, syphilis, and HIV antibody (HIV testing usually requires consent). Blood opioid concentrations are not useful. They confirm diagnosis (morphine therapeutic dose, 65 to 80 ng/mL; toxic, <200 ng/mL), but are not useful for making a therapeutic decision. Cross-reactions can occur with Vick's Formula 44, poppy seeds, and other opioids (codeine and heroin are metabolized to morphine). Naloxone 4 mg IV was not associated with a positive enzyme multiplied immunoassay technique urine screen at 60 minutes, 6 hours, or 48 hours.

Management

Supportive care should be instituted, particularly an endotracheal tube and assisted ventilation. Temporary ventilation can be provided by a bag-valve mask with 100% oxygen. The patient should be placed on a cardiac monitor, have intravenous access established, and have specimens for ABG, glucose, electrolytes, BUN, and creatinine levels, CBC, coagulation profile, liver function, toxicology screen, and urinalysis taken.

For gastrointestinal decontamination, emesis should not be induced, but activated charcoal can be administered if bowel sounds are present.

If it is suspected that the patient is an addict, he or she should be restrained first and then 0.1 mg of naloxone (Narcan) should be administered. The dose should be doubled every 2 minutes until the patient responds or 10 to 20 mg has been given. If the patient is not suspected to be an addict, then 2 mg every 2 to 3 minutes to total of 10 to 20 mg is administered.

It is essential to determine whether there is a complete response to naloxone (mydriasis, improvement in ventilation), because it is a diagnostic therapeutic test. A continuous naloxone infusion may be appropriate, using the "response dose" every hour. Repeat doses of naloxone may be necessary because the effects of many opioids can last much longer than naloxone does (30 to 60 minutes). Methadone ingestions may require a naloxone infusion for 24 to 48 hours. Half of the response dose may need to be repeated in 15 to 20 minutes, after the infusion has been started.

Acute iatrogenic withdrawal precipitated by the administration of naloxone to a dependent patient should not be treated with morphine or other opioids. Naloxone's effects are limited to 30 to 60 minutes (shorter than most opioids) and withdrawal will subside in a short time.

Nalmefene (Revex), an FDA-approved long-acting (4 to 8 hours) pure opioid antagonist, is being investigated, but its role in cases of acute intoxication is unclear and it could produce prolonged withdrawal. It may have a role in place of naloxone infusion.

Noncardiac pulmonary edema does not respond to naloxone, and the patient needs intubation, assisted ventilation, positive end-expiratory pressure, and hemodynamic monitoring. Fluids should be given cautiously in patients with opioid overdose because opioids stimulate the antidiuretic hormone.

TABLE 24 Doses and Onset and Duration of Action of Common Opioids

Drug	Adult Oral Dose	Child Oral Dose	Onset of Action	Duration of Action	Adult Fatal Dose
Camphored tincture of opium	25 mL	0.25-0.50 mL/kg (0.4 mg/mL)	15-30 min	4-5 h	NA
Codeine	30-180 mg	0.5-1 mg/kg	15-30 min	4-6 h	800 mg
	>1 mg/kg is toxic in a child, above 200 mg in adult >5 mg/kg fatal in a child				
Dextromethorphan	15 mg	0.25 mg/kg	15-30 min	3-6 h	NA
	10 mg/kg is toxic				
Diacetylmorphine; street heroin is less than 10% pure	60 mg	NA	15-30 min	3-4 h	100 mg
Diphenoxylate natiopine (Lomotil)	5-10 mg	NA	120-240 min	14 h	300 mg
	7.5 mg is toxic in a child, 300 mg is toxic in adult				
Fentanyl (Duragesic)	0.1-0.2 mg	0.001-0.002 mg/kg	7-8 min	Intramuscular: 1/2-2h	1.0 mg
Hydrocodone with APAP (Lortab)	5-30 mg	0.15 mg/kg	30 min	3-4 h	100 mg
Hydromorphone (Dilaudid)	4 mg	0.1 mg/kg	15-30 min	3-4 h	100 mg
Meperidine (Demerol)	100 mg	1-1.5 mg/kg	10-45 min	3-4 h	350 mg
Methadone (Dolophine)	10 mg	0.1 mg/kg	30-60 min	4-12 h	120 mg
Morphine	10-60 mg	0.1-0.2 mg/kg	<20 min	4-6 h	200 mg
	Oral dose is 6 times parenteral dose, MS Contin sustained release prep				
Oxycodone APAP (Percocet)	5 mg	NA	15-30 min	4-5 h	NA
Pentazocine (Talwin)	50-100 mg	NA	15-30 min	3-4 h	NA
Propoxyphene (Darvon)	65-100 mg	NA	30-60 min	2-4 h	700 mg

If the patient is comatose, 50% glucose (3% to 4% of comatose opioid overdose patients have hypoglycemia) and thiamine should be given prior to naloxone. If the patient has seizures that are unresponsive to naloxone, one administers diazepam and examines for metabolic (hypoglycemia, electrolyte disturbances) causes and structural disturbances.

Hypotension is rare and should direct a search for another etiology. If the patient is agitated, hypoxia and hypoglycemia must be excluded before opioid withdrawal is considered as a cause. Complications to consider include urinary retention, constipation, rhabdomyolysis, myoglobinuria, hypoglycemia, and withdrawal.

Disposition

If a patient responds to intravenous naloxone, careful observation for relapse and the development of pulmonary edema is required, with cardiac and respiratory monitoring for 6 to 12 hours. Patients requiring repeated doses of naloxone or an infusion, or those who develop pulmonary edema, require intensive care unit admission and cannot be discharged from the intensive care unit until they are symptom free for 12 hours. Intravenous overdose complications are expected to be present within 20 minutes after injection, and discharge after 4 symptom-free hours has been recommended. Adults with oral overdose have delayed onset of toxicity and require 6 hours of observation. Children with oral opioid overdose should be admitted to the hospital for observation because of delayed toxicity. Some toxicologists advise restraining a patient who attempts to sign out against medical advice after treatment with naloxone, at least until the patient receives psychiatric evaluation.

ORGANOPHOSPHATES AND CARBAMATES

Cholinergic intoxication sources are insecticides (organophosphates or carbamates), some medications, and some mushrooms. Examples of organophosphate insecticides are malathion (low toxicity, median lethal dose [LD_{50}] 2800 mg/kg), chlorpyrifos, which has been removed from market (moderate toxicity), and parathion (high toxicity, LD_{50} 2 mg/kg). Carbamate insecticides include carbaryl (low toxicity, LD_{50} 500 mg/kg), propoxur (moderate toxicity, LD_{50} 95 mg/kg), and aldicarb (high toxicity, LD_{50} 0.9 mg/kg). Pharmaceuticals with carbamate properties include neostigmine (Prostigmin) and physostigmine (Antilirium). Cholinergic compounds also include the "G" nerve war weapons tabun (GA), sarin (GB), soman (GB), and venom X (VX).

Toxic Mechanism

Organophosphates phosphorylate the active site on red cell acetylcholinesterase and pseudocholinesterase in the serum, neuromuscular and parasympathetic neuroeffector junctions, and in the major synapses of the autonomic ganglia, causing irreversible inhibition. There are two types of organophosphate intoxication: (a) direct action by the parent compound (e.g., tetraethylpyrophosphate), or (b) indirect action by the toxic metabolite (e.g., parathoxon or malathoxon).

Carbamates (esters of carbonic acid) cause reversible carbamylation of the active site of the enzymes. When a critical amount, greater than 50%, of cholinesterase is inhibited, acetylcholine accumulates and causes transient stimulation at cholinergic synapses and sympathetic terminals (muscarinic effect), the somatic nerves, the autonomic ganglia (nicotinic effect), and CNS synapses. Stimulation of conduction is followed by inhibition of conduction.

The major differences between the carbamates and the organophosphates are as follows: (a) carbamate toxicity is less and the duration is shorter; (b) carbamates rarely produce overt CNS effects (poor CNS penetration); (c) carbamate inhibition of the acetylcholinesterase enzyme is reversible and activity returns to normal rapidly; (d) pralidoxime, the enzyme regenerator, may not be necessary in the management of mild carbamate intoxication (e.g., carbaryl).

Toxic Dose

Parathion's minimum lethal dose is 2 mg in children and 10 to 20 mg in adults. The lethal dose of malathion is greater than 1375 mg/kg and that of chlorpyrifos is 25 g; the latter compound is unlikely to cause death.

Kinetics

Absorption is by all routes. The onset of acute ingestion toxicity occurs as early as 3 hours, usually before 12 hours and always before 24 hours. Lipid-soluble agents absorbed by the dermal route (e.g., fenthion) may have a delayed onset of more than 24 hours. Inhalation toxicity occurs immediately after exposure. Massive ingestion can produce intoxication within minutes.

Metabolism is via the liver. With some pesticides (e.g., parathion, malathion), the effects are delayed because they undergo hepatic microsomal oxidative metabolism to their toxic metabolites, the -oxons (e.g., paroxon, malaoxon).

The half-life of malathion is 2.89 hours and that of parathion is 2.1 days. The metabolites are eliminated in the urine and the presence of p-nitrophenol in the urine is a clue up to 48 hours after exposure.

Manifestations

Many organophosphates produce a garlic odor on the breath, in the gastric contents, or in the container. Diaphoresis, excessive salivation, miosis, and muscle twitching are helpful clues to diagnosis.

Early, a cholinergic (muscarinic) crisis develops that consists of parasympathetic nervous system activity. DUMBELS is the mnemonic for defecation, cramps, and increased bowel motility; urinary incontinence; miosis (mydriasis may occur in 20%); bronchospasm and bronchorrhea; excess secretion; lacrimation; and seizures. Bradycardia, pulmonary edema, and hypotension may be present.

Later, sympathetic and nicotinic effects occur, consisting of MATCH: muscle weakness and fasciculation (eyelid twitching is often present), adrenal stimulation and hyperglycemia, tachycardia, cramps in muscles, and hypertension. Finally, paralysis of the skeletal muscles ensues.

The CNS effects are headache, blurred vision, anxiety, ataxia, delirium and toxic psychosis, convulsions, coma, and respiratory depression. Cranial nerve palsies have been noted. Delayed hallucinations may occur.

Delayed respiratory paralysis and neurologic and neurobehavioral disorders have been described following certain organophosphate ingestions or dermal exposure. The "intermediate syndrome" is paralysis of proximal and respiratory muscles developing 24 to 96 hours after the successful treatment of organophosphate poisoning. A delayed distal polyneuropathy has been described with ingestion of certain organophosphates, such as triorthocresyl phosphate, bromoleptophos, and methomidophos.

Complications include aspiration, pulmonary edema, and acute respiratory distress syndrome.

Laboratory Investigations

Monitoring should include chest radiograph, blood glucose (nonketotic hyperglycemia is frequent), ABG, pulse oximetry, ECG, blood coagulation status, liver function, hyperamylasemia (pancreatitis reported), and urinalysis for the metabolite alkyl phosphate paranitrophenol. Blood should be drawn for red blood cell cholinesterase determination before pralidoxime is given. The red blood cell cholinesterase activity roughly correlates with clinical severity. Mild poisoning is 20% to 50% of normal, moderate poisoning is 10% to 20% of normal, and severe poisoning is 10% of normal (>90% depressed). A post-exposure rise of 10% to 15% in the cholinesterase level determined at least 10 to 14 days after the exposure confirms the diagnosis.

Management

Protection of health care personnel with clothing (masks, gloves, gowns, goggles) and respiratory equipment or hazardous material suits, as necessary, is called for. General decontamination consists of isolation, bagging, and disposal of contaminated clothing and other articles. Vital functions should be established and maintained. Cardiac and oxygen saturation monitoring are needed. Intubation and assisted ventilation may be needed. Secretions should be suctioned until atropinization drying is achieved.

Dermal decontamination involves prompt removal of clothing and cleansing of all affected areas of skin, hair, and eyes. Ocular decontamination involves irrigation with copious amounts of tepid water or 0.9% saline for at least 15 minutes. Gastrointestinal decontamination, if the ingestion was recent, involves the administration of activated charcoal.

Atropine sulfate can be given as an antidote. It is both a diagnostic and a therapeutic agent. Atropine counteracts the muscarinic effects but is only partially effective for the CNS effects (seizures and coma). Preservative-free atropine (no benzyl alcohol) should be used. If the patient is symptomatic (bradycardia or bronchorrhea), a test dose should be administered, 0.02 mg/kg in children or 1 mg in adults, intravenously. If no signs of atropinization are present (tachycardia, drying of secretions, and mydriasis), atropine should be administered immediately, 0.05 mg/kg in children or 2 mg in adults, every 5 to 10 minutes as needed to dry the secretions and clear the lungs. Beneficial effects are seen within 1 to 4 minutes and maximum effect in 8 minutes. The average dose in the first 24 hours is 40 mg, but 1000 mg or more has been required in severe cases. Glycopyrrolate (Robinul) can be used if atropine is not available. The maximum dose should be maintained for 12 to 24 hours, then tapered and the patient observed for relapse. Poisoning, especially with lipophilic agents (e.g., fenthion, chlorfenthion), may require weeks of atropine therapy. An alternative is a continuous infusion of atropine 8 mg in 100 mL 0.9% saline at rate of 0.02 to 0.08 mg/kg/h (0.25 to 1.0 mL/kg/h) with additional 1 to 5 mg boluses as needed to dry the secretions.

Pralidoxime chloride (Protopam) has both antinicotinic and antimuscarinic effects and possibly also CNS effects. Successful treatment with pralidoxime chloride may allow a reduction in the dose of atropine. Pralidoxime acts to reactivate the phosphorylated cholinesterases by binding the phosphate moiety on the esteritic site and displacing it. It should be given early before "aging" of phosphate bond produces tighter binding. However, recent reports indicate that pralidoxime chloride is beneficial even several days after the poisoning. Improvement is seen within 10 to 40 minutes. The initial dose of pralidoxime chloride is 1 to 2 g in 250 mL 0.89% saline over 5 to 10 minutes, maximum 200 mg/minute, in adults or 25 to 50 mg/kg, maximum 4 mg/kg/minute, in children younger than 12 years of age. The dose can be repeated every 6 to 12 hours for several days. An alternative is a continuous infusion of 1 g in 100 mL 0.89% saline at 5 to 20 mg/kg/h (0.5 to 12 mL/g/h) up to 500 mg/h and titrated to desired response. Maximum adult daily dose is 12 g. Cardiac and blood pressure monitoring are advised during and for several hours after the infusion. The end point is absence of fasciculations and return of muscle strength.

Contraindicated drugs include morphine, aminophylline, barbiturates, opioids, phenothiazine, reserpine-like drugs, parasympathomimetics, and succinylcholine.

Noncardiac pulmonary edema may require respiratory support. Seizures may respond to atropine and pralidoxime chloride but often require anticonvulsants. Cardiac dysrhythmias may require electrical cardioversion or antidysrhythmic therapy if the patient is hemodynamically unstable. Extracorporeal procedures are of no proven value.

Disposition

Asymptomatic patients with normal examination findings after 6 to 8 hours of observation may be discharged. In cases of intentional poisoning, the patients require psychiatric clearance for discharge. Symptomatic patients should be admitted to the intensive care unit. Observation of milder cases of carbamate poisoning, even those requiring atropine, for 6 to 8 hours symptom-free may be sufficient to exclude significant toxicity. In cases of workplace exposure, OSHA should be notified.

PHENCYCLIDINE (ANGEL DUST)

Phencyclidine is an arylcyclohexylamine related to ketamine and chemically related to the phenothiazines. Originally a "dissociative" anesthetic banned in United States since 1979, it is now an illicit substance, with at least 38 analogs. It is inexpensively manufactured by "kitchen chemists" and is mislabeled as other hallucinogens. Improper phencyclidine synthesis may release cyanide when heated or smoked and can cause explosions.

Toxic Mechanism

The mechanism of phencyclidine is complex and not completely understood. It inhibits some neurotransmitters and causes a loss of pain sensation without depressing the CNS respiratory status. It stimulates α-adrenergic receptors and may act as a "false neurotransmitter." The effects are sympathomimetic, cholinergic, and cerebellar.

Toxic Dose

The usual dose of phencyclidine mixed with marijuana joints is 100 to 400 mg of phencyclidine. Joints or leaf mixtures contain 0.24% to 7.9% of PCP, 1 mg of PCP/150 leaves. Tablets contain 5 mg (the usual street dose). CNS effects at doses of 1 to 6 mg include hallucinations and euphoria, 6 to 10 mg produces toxic psychosis and sympathetic stimulation, 10 to 25 mg produces severe toxicity, and more than 100 mg has resulted in fatalities.

Kinetics

Phencyclidine is a lipophilic weak base, with a pKa of 8.5 to 9.5. It is rapidly absorbed when smoked and snorted, poorly absorbed from the acid stomach, and rapidly absorbed from the alkaline middle small intestine. It has an enterogastric secretion and is reabsorbed in the small intestine. The onset of action when smoked is 2 to 5 minutes, with a peak in 15 to 30 minutes. With oral ingestion, the onset is in 30 to 60 minutes and when taken intravenously it is immediate. Most adverse reactions in cases of overdose begin within 1 to 2 hours. Its duration of action at low doses is 4 to 6 hours and normality returns in 24 hours; in large overdoses, fluctuating coma may last 6 to 10 days.

Volume distribution is 6.2 L/kg. Phencyclidine concentrates in brain and adipose tissue. Protein binding is 70%. The route of elimination is by gastric secretion, liver metabolism, and 10% urinary excretion of conjugates and free phencyclidine. Renal excretion may be increased 50% with urinary acidification. The half-life is 1 hour (in cases of overdose, it is 11 to 89 hours).

Manifestations

The classic picture is bursts of horizontal, vertical, and rotary nystagmus, which is a clue to diagnosis (occurs in 50% of cases), miosis, hypertension, and fluctuating altered mental state. There is a wide spectrum of clinical presentations.

Mild intoxication with 1 to 6 mg produces drunken and bizarre behavior, agitation, rotary nystagmus, and blank stare. Violent behavior and sensory anesthesia make these patients insensitive to pain, self-destructive, and dangerous. Most are communicative within 1 to 2 hours, are alert and oriented in 6 to 8 hours, and recover completely in 24 to 48 hours.

Moderate intoxication with 6 to 10 mg produces excess salivation, hypertension, hyperthermia, muscle rigidity, myoclonus, and catatonia. Recovery of consciousness occurs in 24 to 48 hours and complete recovery in 1 week.

Severe intoxication with 10 to 25 mg results in opisthotonus, decerebrate rigidity, convulsions, prolonged fluctuating coma, and respiratory failure. Patients in this category have a high rate of medical complications. Recovery of consciousness occurs in 24 to 48 hours, with complete normality in a month. Medical complications include apnea, aspiration pneumonia, cardiac arrest, hypertensive encephalopathy, hyperthermia, intracerebral hemorrhage, psychosis, rhabdomyolysis and myoglobinuria, and seizures. Loss of memory and "flashbacks" last for months. Phencyclidine-induced depression and suicide have been reported.

Fatalities occur with ingestions of greater than 100 mg and with serum levels greater than 100 to 250 ng/mL.

Laboratory Investigations

Marked elevation of creatine kinase level may occur. Values greater than 20,000 units have been reported. Urinalysis should be monitored and urine tested for myoglobin. One should monitor the blood for creatine kinase, uric acid (an early clue to rhabdomyolysis), BUN, creatinine, electrolytes (hyperkalemia), blood glucose (20% of patients have hypoglycemia), urinary output, liver function tests, ECG, and ABG if the patient has any respiratory manifestations. Measurement of phencyclidine in the gastric juice is called for because concentrations are 10 to 50 times higher than in blood or urine. Phencyclidine blood concentrations are not helpful. Phencyclidine may be detected in the urine of the average user for 10 days to 3 weeks after the last dose. In chronic users, it can be detected for over 1 month. The analogs of phencyclidine may not produce positive test results for phencyclidine in the urine. Cross-reactions with bleach and dextromethorphan may cause false-positive urine test results on immunoassay, and cross-reaction with doxylamine may produce a false-positive finding on gas chromatography.

Management

The patient should be observed for violent, self-destructive, bizarre behavior and paranoid schizophrenia. Patients should be placed in a low sensory environment and dangerous objects should be removed from the area.

Gastrointestinal decontamination is not effective because phencyclidine is rapidly absorbed from intestines. Overtreating the mild intoxication should be avoided. There is insufficient evidence to support the use of MDAC. In cases of severe toxicity (stupor or coma), continuous gastric suction can be tried (with protection of the airway) because the drug is secreted into the gastric juice. The value of this procedure is controversial because of limited data.

The patient must be protected from harming himself or herself or others. Physical restraints may be necessary, but they should be used sparingly and for the shortest time possible because they increase risk of rhabdomyolysis. Metal restraints such as handcuffs should be avoided. For behavioral disorders and toxic psychosis, diazepam is the agent of choice. Pharmacologic intervention includes diazepam (Valium) 10 to 30 mg orally or 2 to 5 mg intravenously initially and titrated upward to 10 mg; however, up to 30 mg may be required. "Talk down" technique is usually ineffective and dangerous. Phenothiazines and butyrophenones should be avoided in the acute phase because they lower the convulsive threshold; however, they may be needed later for psychosis. Haloperidol (Haldol) administration has been reported to produce catatonia.

Seizures and muscle spasm are managed with diazepam, from 2.5 mg up to 10 mg. Hyperthermia (>38.5°C [101.3°F]) is treated with external cooling measures. Hypertension is usually transient and does not require treatment. In the case of emergent hypertensive crisis (blood pressure >200/115 mm Hg) nitroprusside can be used in a dose of 0.3 to 2 μg/kg/min. Maximum infusion rate is 10 μg/kg/min for only 10 minutes.

Acid ion trapping diuresis is not recommended because of the danger of myoglobin precipitation in the renal tubules. Rhabdomyolysis and myoglobinuria are treated by correcting volume depletion and insuring a urinary output of greater than 2 mL/kg/h. Alkalinization is controversial because of reabsorption of phencyclidine.

Hemodialysis is beneficial if renal failure occurs; otherwise, the extracorporeal procedures are not beneficial.

Disposition

All patients with coma, delirium, catatonia, violent behavior, aspiration pneumonia, sustained hypertension greater than 200/115, and significant rhabdomyolysis should be admitted to the intensive care unit until asymptomatic for at least 24 hours. If patients with mild intoxication are mentally and neurologically stable and become asymptomatic (except for nystagmus) for 4 hours, they may be discharged in the company of a responsible adult. All patients must be assessed for suicide risk before discharge. Drug counseling and psychiatric follow-up should be arranged. Patients should be warned that episodes of disorientation and depression may continue intermittently for 4 weeks or more.

PHENOTHIAZINES AND NONPHENOTHIAZINES (NEUROLEPTICS)

Toxic Mechanism

Neuroleptics have complex mechanisms of toxicity, including (a) block of the postsynaptic dopamine receptors; (b) block of peripheral and central α-adrenergic receptors; (c) block of cholinergic muscarinic receptors; (d) quinidine-like antidysrhythmic and myocardial depressant effect in cases of large overdose; (e) lowering of the convulsive threshold; (f) effect on hypothalamic temperature regulation (Table 25).

Toxic Dose

Extrapyramidal reactions, anticholinergic effects, and orthostatic hypotension may occur at therapeutic doses. The toxic amount is not established, but the maximum daily therapeutic dose may result in significant side effects, and twice this amount may be potentially fatal. Chlorpromazine (Thorazine), the prototype, may produce serious hypotension and CNS depression at doses greater than 200 mg (17 mg/kg) in children and 3 to 5 g in an adult. Fatalities have been reported after 2.5 g of loxapine (Loxitane) and mesoridazine (Serentil) and 1.5 g of thioridazine (Mellaril).

Kinetics

These agents are lipophilic and have unpredictable gastrointestinal absorption. Peak levels occur 2 to 6 hours postingestion and have enterohepatic recirculation.

The mean serum half-life in phase 1 is 1 to 2 hours and the biphasic half-life is 20 to 40 hours. Volume distribution is 10 to 40 L/kg; protein binding is 92% to 98%. Chlorpromazine taken orally has an onset of action in 30 to 60 minutes, peak in 2 to 4 hours, and duration of 4 to 6 hours. With sustained-release preparations, the onset is in 30 to 60 minutes and duration is 6 to 12 hours.

Elimination is by hepatic metabolism, which results in multiple metabolites (some are active). Metabolites can be detected in urine months after chronic therapy. Only 1% to 3% is excreted unchanged in the urine.

Manifestations

In cases of phenothiazine overdose, anticholinergic symptoms may be present early but are not life-threatening. Miosis is usually present (80%) if the phenothiazine has strong α-adrenergic blocking effect (e.g., chlorpromazine), but anticholinergic activity mydriasis may occur. Agitation and delirium rapidly progress into coma. Major problems are cardiac toxicity and hypotension. The cardiotoxic effects are seen more commonly with thioridazine and its metabolite mesoridazine. These agents have produced the largest number of fatalities in patients with phenothiazine overdose. Cardiac conduction disturbances include prolonged PR, QRS, and QTc intervals, U- and T-wave abnormalities, and ventricular dysrhythmias, including torsades de pointes. Seizures occur mainly in patients with convulsive disorders or with administration of loxapine. Sudden death in children and adults has been reported.

Idiosyncratic dystonic reactions are most common with the piperidine group. Reactions are not dose-dependent and consist of opisthotonos, torticollis, orolingual dyskinesia, or oculogyric crisis (painful upward gaze). These reactions are more frequent in children and women. Neuroleptic malignant syndrome occurs in patients on chronic therapy and is characterized by hyperthermia, muscle rigidity, autonomic dysfunction, and altered mental state. There is one case reported with acute overdose. The loxapine syndrome consists of seizures, rhabdomyolysis, and renal failure.

Laboratory Investigations

Monitoring should include arterial blood gases, renal and hepatic function, electrolytes, blood glucose, and creatine kinase and myoglobinemia in neurol-eptic malignant syndrome. Most of these agents

TABLE 25 Neuroleptics and Properties

Compound	Antipsychotic	Anticholinergic	Extrapyramidal	Hypotensive and Cardiotoxic	Sedative
Phenothiazine					
Aliphatic	1+	3+	2+	2+	3+
Chlorpromazine (Thorazine)					
Promethazine (Phenergan)					
Piperazine	3+	1+	3+	1+	1+
Fluphenazine (Prolixin)					
Perphenazine (Trilafon)					
Prochlorperazine (Compazine)					
Trifluoperazine (Stelazine)					
Piperidine	1+	2+	1+	3+	3+
Mesoridazine (Serentil)					
Thioridazine (Mellaril)					
Nonphenothiazine					
Butyrophenone	3+	1+	3+	1+	1+
Haloperidol (Haldol)					
Dibenzoxazepine	3+	1+	3+	1+	2+
Loxapine (Loxitane)					
Dihydroindolone	3+	1+	3+	1+	1+
Molindone (Moban)					
Thioxanthenes	3+	1+	3+	3+	1+
Thiothixene (Navane)					
Chlorprothixene (Taractan)					

1+ = very low activity; 2+ = moderate activity; 3+ = very high activity.

are detected on routine screening. Quantitative serum levels are not useful in management. Cross-reactions with enzyme multiplied immunoassay technique tests occur with cyclic antidepressants. Phenothiazines give false-negative results on pregnancy urine tests using human chorionic gonadotropin as an indicator, and give false-positive results for urine porphyrins, indirect Coombs test, urobilinogen, and amylase.

Management

Vital functions must be established and maintained. All overdose patients require venous access, 12-lead ECG (to measure intervals), cardiac and respiratory monitoring, and seizure precautions. One should monitor core temperature to detect poikilothermic effect. If the patient is comatose, intubation and assisted ventilation may be required, as well as 100% oxygen, intravenous glucose, naloxone (Narcan), and thiamine.

Emesis is not recommended. Activated charcoal can be administered if ingestion was within 1 hour. MDAC has not been proven beneficial. A radiograph of the abdomen may be useful, if the phenothiazine is radiopaque. Haloperidol (Haldol) and trifluoperazine (Stelazine) are most likely to be radiopaque. Whole-bowel irrigation may be useful when a large number of pills are visualized on radiograph or if sustained-release preparations were taken, but whole-bowel irrigation has not been evaluated in patients with phenothiazine overdose.

Convulsions are treated with diazepam or lorazepam (Ativan). Loxapine (Loxitane) overdose may result in status epilepticus. If nondepolarizing neuromuscular blockade is required, pancuronium (Pavulon) or vecuronium (Norcuron) should be used (not succinylcholine [Anectine], which may cause malignant hyperthermia), and EEG should be monitored during paralysis.

Patients with dysrhythmias should be monitored with serial ECGs. Unstable rhythms can be treated with electrical cardioversion. Class 1a antidysrhythmics (procainamide, quinidine, and disopyramide [Norpace]) must be avoided.

Hypokalemia predisposes to dysrhythmias and should be corrected aggressively. Supraventricular tachycardia with hemodynamic instability is treated with electrical cardioversion. The role of adenosine has not been defined. Calcium channel and β-blockers should be avoided.

Prolongation of the QRS interval is treated with sodium bicarbonate 1 to 2 mEq/kg by intravenous bolus over a few minutes. Torsades de pointes is treated with magnesium sulfate IV 20% solution 2 g over 2 to 3 minutes. If there is no response in 10 minutes, the dose is repeated and followed by a continuous infusion of 5 to 10 mg/min or given as an infusion of 50 mg/minute for 2 hours followed by 30 mg/minute for 90 minutes twice a day for several days, as needed. The dose in children is 25 to 50 mg/kg initially and maintenance dose is 30 to 60 mg/kg per 24 hours (0.25 to 0.50 mEq/kg per 24 hours) up to 1000 mg per 24 hours. Serum magnesium levels should be monitored.

To treat ventricular tachydysrhythmias in a stable patient, lidocaine is used. If the patient is unstable, electrical cardioversion is used. Patients with heart block with hemodynamic instability should be managed with temporary cardiac pacing.

Hypotension is treated with the Trendelenburg position and 0.9% saline. If the condition is refractory to treatment or there is a danger of fluid overload, vasopressors are administered. The vasopressor of choice is α-adrenergic agonist norepinephrine (Levophed), titrated to response. Epinephrine and dopamine should not be used because β-receptor stimulation in the presence of α-receptor blockade may provoke dysrhythmias and phenothiazines are antidopaminergic.

Hypothermia and hyperthermia are treated with external warming and cooling measures, respectively. Antipyretic drugs must not be used.

Management of the neuroleptic malignant syndrome includes the following actions:

- Immediately discontinuing the offending agent
- Hyperventilating the patient, using 100% humidified, cooled oxygen at high gas flows (at least 10 L/min) because of rapid breathing
- Administering a benzodiazepine to control convulsions and facilitate cooling measures
- Initiating appropriate mechanical cooling measures, which may include intravenous cold saline (not lactated Ringer's), ice baths, cold lavage of the stomach, bladder, and rectum, and a hypothermic blanket
- Correcting acid–base and electrolyte disturbances and treating significant hyperkalemia with hyperventilation, calcium, sodium bicarbonate, intravenous glucose, and insulin; hemodialysis may be necessary

In addition, dysrhythmias usually respond to correction of the underlying acid–base disturbances and hyperkalemia. If antidysrhythmic agents are required, calcium channel blockers must be avoided because they may precipitate hyperkalemia and cardiovascular collapse. Dantrolene sodium (Dantrium), which is a phenytoin derivative, inhibits calcium release from the sarcoplasmic reticulum and results in decreased muscle contraction. Dantrolene acts peripherally and does not reverse the rigidity or psychomotor disturbances resulting from the central dopamine blockade; it therefore is often used in combination with bromocriptine. Bromocriptine mesylate (Parlodel) acts centrally as a dopamine agonist, as does amantadine hydrochloride (Symmetrel). Bromocriptine and dantrolene have been reported to be successful in combination with cooling and good supportive measures in malignant hyperthermia.

Dosing for these agents is as follows: dantrolene sodium at 2 to 3 mg/kg IV as a bolus, then 1 mg/kg/minute to a maximum of 10 mg/kg or until the tachycardia, rigidity, increased end-tidal CO_2, and temperature elevation are controlled. *Note:* Hepatotoxicity occurs with doses greater than 10 mg/kg. To prevent symptom recurrence, 1 mg/kg should be administered every 6 hours for 24 to 48 hours after the episode. After that time, oral dantrolene can be used at a dose of 1 mg/kg every 6 hours for 24 hours as necessary. The patient should be observed for thrombophlebitis following intravenous dantrolene. It is best administered via a central line. Bromocriptine mesylate at 2.5 to 10 mg orally or via a nasogastric tube, three times a day, should be used in combination with dantrolene.

Idiosyncratic dystonic reaction can be treated with diphenhydramine (Benadryl) 1 to 2 mg/kg/dose intravenously over 5 minutes up to maximum of 50 mg intravenously; a response is noted within 2 to 5 minutes. This can be followed with oral doses for 4 to 6 days to prevent recurrence.

Extracorporeal measures (hemodialysis, hemoperfusion) are not effective in removing these agents.

Disposition

Asymptomatic patients should be observed for at least 6 hours after gastric decontamination. Symptomatic patients with cardiotoxicity, hypotension, and convulsions should be admitted to the intensive care unit and monitored for 48 hours.

SALICYLATES (ACETYLSALICYLIC ACID, SALICYLIC ACID)

Toxic Mechanism

The primary toxic mechanisms include (a) direct stimulation of the medullary chemoreceptor trigger zone and respiratory center; (b) uncoupling oxidative phosphorylation; (c) inhibition of the Krebs cycle enzymes; (d) inhibition of vitamin K dependent and independent clotting factors; (e) alteration of platelet function; and (f) inhibition of prostaglandin synthesis.

Toxic Dose

Acute mild intoxication occurs at a dose of 150 to 200 mg/kg, moderate intoxication at 200 to 300 mg/kg, and severe intoxication at 300 to 500 mg/kg. Acute salicylate plasma concentration greater than 30 mg/dL (usually >40 mg/dL) may be associated with clinical toxicity. Chronic intoxication occurs at ingestions greater than 100 mg/kg/d for more than 2 days because of accumulation kinetics. Methyl salicylate (oil of wintergreen) is the most toxic form of salicylate. A dose of 1 mL of 98% contains 1.4 g of salicylate. Fatalities have occurred with ingestion of 1 teaspoonful in children and 1 ounce in adults. It is found in topical ointments and liniments (18% to 30%).

Kinetics

Acetylsalicylic acid and salicylic acid are weak acids with a pKa of 3.5 and 3.0, respectively. Acetylsalicylic acid is absorbed from the stomach, from the small bowel, and dermally. Onset of action is within 30 minutes. Methyl salicylate and effervescent tablets are absorbed more rapidly. Salicylate plasma concentration is detectable within 15 minutes after ingestion and peaks in 30 to 120 minutes. The peak may be delayed 6 to 12 hours in cases of large overdose, overdose with enteric-coated or sustained-release preparations, and development of concretions. The therapeutic duration of action is 3 to 4 hours but is markedly prolonged in cases of overdose.

Volume distribution is 0.13 L/kg for salicylic acid but increases as the salicylate plasma concentration increases. Protein binding is greater than 90% for salicylic acid at pH 7.4 and a salicylate plasma concentration of 20 to 30 mg/dL, 75% at a salicylate plasma concentration greater than 40 mg/dL, 50% at a salicylate plasma concentration of 70 mg/dL, and 30% at a salicylate plasma concentration of 120 mg/dL.

The half-life for salicylic acid is 3 hours after a 300 mg dose, 6 hours after a 1 g overdose, and greater than 10 hours after a 10-g overdose. Elimination includes Michaelis-Menten hepatic metabolism by three saturable pathways: (a) glycine conjugation to salicyluric acid (75%); (b) glucuronyl transferase to salicyl phenol glucuronide (10%); and (c) salicyl aryl glucuronide (4%). Nonsaturable pathways are hydrolysis to gentisic acid (<1%). Ten percent is excreted unchanged.

Acidosis increases the severity of the intoxication by increasing the non-ionized salicylate that can cross membranes and enter the brain cells. In kidneys, the unionized salicylic acid undergoes glomerular filtration, and the ionized portion undergoes tubular secretion in proximal tubules and passive reabsorption in the distal tubules. Renal excretion of salicylate is enhanced by alkaline urine.

Manifestations

The ingestion of concentrated topical salicylic acid preparations (e.g., wart remover) can cause mucosal caustic injury to the gastrointestinal tract. Occult salicylate overdose should be considered in any patient with unexplained acid–base disturbance.

The manifestations of acute overdose of salicylates are as follows:

Minimal Symptoms

Tinnitus, dizziness, and deafness may occur at high therapeutic salicylate plasma concentrations of 20 to 30 mg/dL. Nausea and vomiting may occur immediately because of local gastric irritation.

Phase I. Mild manifestations occur at 1 to 12 hours after ingestion with a 6-hour salicylate plasma concentration of 45 to 70 mg/dL. Nausea and vomiting followed by hyperventilation are usually present within 3 to 8 hours after acute overdose. Hyperventilation, an increase in both rate (tachypnea) and depth (hyperpnea), is present but it may be subtle. It results in a mild respiratory alkalosis with a serum pH greater than 7.4 and urine pH greater than 6.0. Some patients may have lethargy, vertigo, headache, and confusion. Diaphoresis may be noted.

Phase II. Moderate manifestations occur at 12 to 24 hours after ingestion with a 6-hour salicylate plasma concentration of 70 to 90 mg/dL. Serious metabolic disturbances, including a marked respiratory alkalosis with anion gap metabolic acidosis, dehydration, and urine pH less than 6.0, may occur. Other metabolic disturbances include hypoglycemia or hyperglycemia, hypokalemia, decreased ionized calcium, and increased BUN, creatinine, and lactate. Mental disturbances (confusion, disorientation, hallucinations) may occur. Hypotension and convulsions have been reported.

Phase III. Severe intoxication occurs more than 24 hours after ingestion with a 6-hour salicylate plasma concentration of 90 to 130 mg/dL. In addition to the above clinical findings, coma and seizures develop and indicate severe intoxication. Pulmonary edema may occur. Metabolic disturbances include metabolic acidemia (pH <7.4) and aciduria (pH <6.0). In adults, alkalosis may persist until terminal respiratory failure.

In children younger than 4 years of age, a mixed metabolic acidosis and respiratory alkalosis develop earlier (within 4 to 6 hours) than in adults because children have less respiratory reserve and accumulate lactate and other organic acids. Hypoglycemia is more common in children.

Fatalities occur at 6-hour salicylate plasma concentrations greater than 130 to 150 mg/dL and result from CNS depression, cardiovascular collapse, electrolyte imbalance, and cerebral edema.

Chronic salicylism is more serious than acute intoxication and the 6-hour salicylate plasma concentration does not correlate well with the manifestations in both acute and chronic cases of intoxication. Chronic intoxication usually occurs with therapeutic errors in young children or the elderly with underlying illness, and the diagnosis is delayed because it is not recognized. Noncardiac pulmonary edema is a frequent complication in the elderly. The mortality rate is about 25%. Chronic salicylate poisoning in children may mimic Reye syndrome. It is associated with exaggerated CNS findings (hallucinations, delirium, dementia, memory loss, papilledema, bizarre behavior, agitation, encephalopathy, seizures, and coma). Hemorrhagic manifestations, renal failure, and pulmonary and cerebral edema may occur. The metabolic picture is hypoglycemia and mixed acid-base derangements. A chronic salicylate plasma concentration greater than 60 mg/dL with metabolic acidosis and an altered mental state is very serious.

Laboratory Investigations

All patients with intentional salicylate overdoses should have acetaminophen plasma level measured after 4 hours.

One should continuously monitor ECG, urine output, urine pH, and specific gravity. Every 2 to 4 hours in cases of severe intoxication, salicylate plasma concentration, glucose (in a case of salicylism, CNS hypoglycemia may be present despite normal serum glucose), electrolytes, ionized calcium, magnesium and phosphorous, anion gap, ABGs, and pulse oximeter should be monitored. Daily monitoring of BUN, creatinine, liver function tests, and prothrombin time should take place.

The therapeutic salicylate plasma concentration is less than 10 mg/dL for analgesia and 15 to 30 mg/dL for anti-inflammatory effect. Cross-reaction with diflunisal (Dolobid) will give a falsely high salicylate plasma concentration. The Done nomogram is not considered accurate in evaluating acute or chronic salicylate intoxications.

Management

Treatment is based on clinical and metabolic findings, not on salicylate levels. Continuous monitoring of the urine pH is essential for successful alkalinization treatment. One should always obtain an acetaminophen plasma level.

Vital functions must be established and maintained. If the patient is in an altered mental state, glucose, naloxone, and thiamine are administered in standard doses. Depending on the severity, the initial studies include an immediate and a 6-hour postingestion salicylate plasma concentration, ECG and cardiac monitoring, pulse oximeter, urine (analysis, pH, and specific gravity), chest radiograph, ABGs, blood glucose, electrolytes and anion gap calculation, calcium (ionized), magnesium, renal and liver profiles, and prothrombin time. Gastric contents and stool should be tested for occult blood. Bismuth and magnesium salicylate preparations may be radiopaque on radiographs. Consultation with a nephrologist is warranted in cases of moderate, severe, or chronic intoxication.

For gastrointestinal decontamination, activated charcoal is useful (each gram of activated charcoal binds 550 mg of salicylic acid) if a toxic dose was ingested up to 4 hours postingestion. MDAC is not recommended for salicylate intoxication.

Concretions may occur with massive (usually >300 mg/kg) ingestions. If blood levels fail to decline, prompt contrast radiography of the stomach may reveal concretions that have to be removed by repeated lavage, whole-bowel irrigation, endoscopy, or gastrostomy.

Fluids and electrolyte treatment of salicylate poisonings is given in Table 26. For shock, perfusion and vascular volume should be established with 5% dextrose in 0.9% saline, then the treatment can proceed with correction of dehydration and alkalinization.

For cases of acute moderate or severe salicylism (see Table 26), adults should receive a bolus of 1 to 2 mEq/kg of sodium bicarbonate ($NaHCO_3$) followed by an infusion of 100 to 150 mEq $NaHCO_3$ added to 500 to 1000 mL of 5% dextrose and administered over 60 minutes. Children should receive a bolus of 1 to 2 mEq/kg of $NaHCO_3$ followed by an infusion of 1 to 2 mEq/kg added to 20 mL/kg of 5% dextrose administered over 60 minutes. Potassium is added after the patient voids. The goal is to achieve a urine output of greater than 2 mL/kg/hr and a urine pH of greater than 8. The initial infusion is followed by subsequent infusions (two to three times normal maintenance) of 200 to 300 mL/h in adults or 10 mL/kg/h in children. If the patient is acidotic and has a serum pH of less than 7.15, an additional 1 to 2 mEq/kg of $NaHCO_3$ is given over 1 to 2 hours; persistent acidosis may require 1 to 2 mEq/kg of bicarbonate every 2 hours. The infusion rate, the amount of bicarbonate, and the electrolytes should be adjusted to correct serum abnormalities and to maintain the targeted urine output and urinary pH. Diuresis is not as important as the alkalinization. Careful monitoring for fluid overload should take place for patients at risk of pulmonary and cerebral edema (e.g., the elderly) and because of inappropriate secretion of the antidiuretic hormone.

In patients with mild intoxication who are not acidotic and have a urine pH greater than 6, 5% dextrose in 0.45% saline should be administered as maintenance to replace ongoing fluid loss. Some toxicologists may consider adding sodium bicarbonate 50 mEq/L or 1 mEq/kg in some cases.

To achieve alkalinization, sodium bicarbonate is administered to produce a serum pH 7.4 to 7.5 and a urine pH greater than 8. Carbonic anhydrase inhibitors (acetazolamide [Diamox]) should not be used. If the patient is acidotic, additional bicarbonate may be required. About 2 mEq/kg raises the blood pH 0.1. In children, alkalinization may be a difficult problem because of the organic acid production and hypokalemia. Hypokalemic and fluid-depleted patients cannot be adequately alkalinized. Alkalinization is usually discontinued in asymptomatic patients with a salicylate plasma concentration less than 30 to 40 mg/dL but is continued in symptomatic patients regardless of the salicylate plasma concentration. A decreased serum bicarbonate but normal or high blood pH indicates respiratory alkalosis predominating over metabolic acidosis, and the bicarbonate should be administered cautiously. An alkalemic pH of 7.40 to 7.50 is not a contraindication to bicarbonate therapy because these patients have a significant base deficit in spite of elevated blood pH.

Potassium is added, 20 to 40 mEq/L, to the infusion after the patient voids. In cases of severe, late, and chronic salicylism, 60 mEq/L of potassium may be needed. When the serum potassium is below 4.0 mEq/L, 10 mEq/L should be added over the first hour. If the patient has hypokalemia less than 3 mEq/L and flat T waves and U waves, 0.25 to 0.5 mEq/kg up to 10 mEq/h is administered. Potassium should be administered under ECG monitoring. Serum potassium is rechecked after each rapidly administered dose. A paradoxical urine acidosis (alkaline serum pH and acid urine pH) indicates that potassium is probably needed.

Convulsions are treated with diazepam or lorazepam, but hypoglycemia, low ionized calcium, cerebral edema, and hemorrhage should first be excluded with a CT scan. If tetany develops, the $NaHCO_3$ therapy is discontinued and calcium gluconate 0.1 to 0.2 mEq/kg 10% administered.

Pulmonary edema management consists of fluid restriction, high FIO_2, mechanical ventilation, and positive end-expiratory pressure.

Cerebral edema management consists of fluid restriction, elevation of the head, hyperventilation, osmotic diuresis, and administration of dexamethasone. Vitamin K_1 is administered parenterally to correct an increased prothrombin time (>20 seconds) and coagulation abnormalities. If the patient has active bleeding, fresh plasma and platelets are administered as needed. Hyperpyrexia is managed by external cooling measures, not antipyretics.

Hemodialysis is the choice for removal of salicylates because it corrects the acid–base, electrolyte, and fluid disturbances as well. The indications for hemodialysis include the following:

- Acute poisoning with salicylate plasma concentration greater than 100 mg/dL without improvement after 6 hours of appropriate therapy
- Chronic poisoning with cardiopulmonary disease and a salicylate plasma concentration as low as 40 mg/dL with refractory acidosis, severe CNS manifestations (coma and seizures), and progressive deterioration, especially in elderly patients
- Impairment of vital organs of elimination

TABLE 26 Fluid and Electrolyte Treatment of Salicylate Poisoning

Type of Salicylism	Metabolic Disturbance	Blood pH	Urine pH	Hydrating Solution	Amount of NaHCO₃ (mEq/L)	Amount of Potassium (mEq/L)
Mild	Respiratory alkalosis	>7.4	>6.0	5% Dextrose, 0.45% saline	50 (adult) 1 mEq/kg (child)	20
Moderate Chronic Child <4 Years	Respiratory alkalosis Metabolic acidosis	>7.4 or <7.4	<6.0	5% Dextrose in water	100 (adult) 1-2 mEq/kg (child)	40
Severe Chronic Child <4 years	Metabolic acidosis Respiratory alkalosis	<7.4	<6.0	5% Dextrose in water	150 (adult) 2 mEq/kg (child)	60
CNS Depressant Co-ingestant	Respiratory acidosis	<7.4	<6.0	5% Dextrose in water	100-150*	60

*Correct hypoventilation.
Modified from Linden CH, Rumack BH: The legitimate analgesics, aspirin and acetaminophen. In Hansen W Jr (ed): Toxic Emergencies. New York, Churchill Livingstone, 1984.

- Clinical deterioration in spite of good supportive care and alkalinization
- Severe refractory acid–base or electrolyte disturbances despite appropriate corrective measures

Disposition

There are limitations of salicylate plasma levels and patients are treated on the basis of clinical and laboratory findings. Patients who are asymptomatic should be monitored for a minimum of 6 hours, and longer if enteric-coated tablets or massive overdose was taken or if there is suspicion of concretions. Those who remain asymptomatic with a salicylate plasma concentration less than 35 mg/dL may be discharged following psychiatric evaluation, if indicated. Chronic salicylate-intoxicated patients with acidosis and an altered mental state should be admitted to the intensive care unit. Patients with acute ingestion and a salicylate plasma concentration less than 60 mg/dL and mild symptoms may be able to be treated in the emergency department. Patients with moderate and severe intoxications should be admitted to the intensive care unit.

SELECTIVE SEROTONIN REUPTAKE INHIBITORS

Selective serotonin reuptake inhibitors (SSRIs) are primarily prescribed as antidepressants. SSRIs include fluoxetine (Prozac), paroxetine (Paxil), and sertraline (Zoloft).

Toxic Mechanism

The SSRIs interfere with the neuron reuptake of serotonin (5-hydroxytryptamine) at the presynaptic ganglia sites in the brain, increasing the activity of serotonin. SSRIs should not be used within 5 weeks of when a MAOI is given, nor should MAOI therapy be initiated or discontinued within 5 weeks of SSRI therapy.

Toxic Dose

The therapeutic oral dose of fluoxetine is 20 to 80 mg/d. No toxicity is seen in children with up to 3.5 mg/kg/dose orally. A fatal dose for adults is 6 g. The therapeutic dose for paroxetine is 20 to 50 mg/d. In 35 adult patients, none developed serious side effects after the ingestion of 10 to 1000 mg, and a study involving 35 children failed to demonstrate serious adverse effects at doses less than 180 mg. The therapeutic dose for sertraline is 50 mg to 200 mg/d. Patients have ingested up to 2.6 g without serious side effects. Overdose involving children who ingested less than 100 mg failed to cause adverse events.

Kinetics

Fluoxetine is well absorbed from the gastrointestinal tract, and has a peak plasma concentration at 6 to 8 hours. Volume distribution is 20 to 42 L/kg; 95% is protein bound. The half-life is 4 days (for the demethylated active metabolite norfluoxetine, the half-life is 7 to 15 days). Elimination is 80% renal. Fluoxetine and other serotonin inhibitors are inhibitors of the cytochrome P450, CYP 2D6 enzyme. Therefore interactions may occur with many other medications, such as antidysrhythmic class IC drugs (quinidine), phenytoin (Dilantin), haloperidol, lithium, tricyclic antidepressants (TCAs), β-blockers, codeine, and carbamazepine (Tegretol).

Paroxetine is almost completely absorbed from the gastrointestinal tract, with a peak in 2 to 8 hours. Protein binding is greater than 90%; volume distribution is 13 L/kg. Paroxetine undergoes extensive first-pass liver metabolism by oxidation and methylation to inactive metabolites. It inhibits the P450 system (see fluoxetine metabolism). The average half-life is 21 hours.

Sertraline peaks in 8 to 12 hours. Its volume distribution is 20 L/kg and protein binding is 98%. The average half-life of sertraline is 26 hours. It is metabolized to form a less-active metabolite, N-desmethylsertraline (half-life of 62 to 104 hours).

Manifestations

All SSRIs may cause serotonin syndrome, a potentially life-threatening reaction, if they are administered concurrently with an MAOI. Serotonin syndrome is caused by cerebral serotonergic stimulation and can cause severe hyperthermia, myoclonus, rhabdomyolysis, confusion, tremors, and a variety of psychological disturbances. In addition, cardiovascular complications and extrapyramidal side effects, including akathisia, dyskinesia, and Parkinson-like syndromes may occur. Also, increased suicidal ideation, seizures, sexual disorders, and hematologic disorders (platelet serotonin activity blockade leading to prolonged bleeding times) may develop. Inappropriate secretion of antidiuretic hormone resulting in hyponatremia may occur when SSRIs are administered to the elderly. This effect is usually seen within the first week of therapy.

Overdose effects are similar to the serotonin syndrome.

Laboratory Investigations

One should obtain a complete blood count (CBC), electrolytes, glucose levels, a coagulation profile, liver function tests, creatine kinase level, and an ECG.

Management

There is no specific antidote to SSRI intoxication.

Initial management consists of stabilizing vital functions, including thermoregulation. Supportive therapy and anticipation of potential life-threatening manifestations (hypotension, hyperthermia, seizures, coma, disseminated intravascular coagulation, ventricular tachycardia, and metabolic acidosis), are essential. Vital signs, EEG, creatine kinase, and blood chemistry should be monitored.

Benzodiazepines are administered to prevent and control muscle hyperactivity (diazepam [Valium] for seizures, clonazepam [Klonopin] for myoclonus). If benzodiazepine therapy fails to control muscle activity or seizures, anesthesia or nondepolarizing neuromuscular blockade may be necessary.

Electrolyte abnormalities and acid–base balance should be corrected. Fluids are used to maintain a urine output of greater than 2 mL/kg/h if there is a risk of myoglobinuria.

There are no data to support the use of gastrointestinal decontamination, although activated charcoal may be used if an ingestion has occurred within 1 hour. Hemodialysis and charcoal hemoperfusion are unlikely to be beneficial. Haloperidol (Haldol), phenothiazines, and other highly protein-bound drugs are to be avoided.

Benzodiazepine and cooling therapy can be used for hyperthermia. Serotonin antagonists, such as cyproheptadine (Periactin), may be useful in treating serotonin syndrome, although there are no controlled data. Dantrolene (Dantrium) and bromocriptine (Parlodel) are not recommended and may actually precipitate serotonin syndrome.

Disposition

Cases of ingestions in children up to 5 years of age of less than 180 mg of paroxetine (Paxil), less than 3.5 mg/kg of fluoxetine (Prozac), or less than 100 mg of sertraline (Zoloft) can be observed at home. Symptomatic patients should be admitted to the intensive care unit until asymptomatic for 24 hours. Asymptomatic patients should be observed for 6 hours. All patients should be assessed for risk of suicide before discharge. When taken chronically, SSRIs may increase cholesterol and triglycerides and decrease uric acid, so these test results should be followed.

THEOPHYLLINE

Theophylline (Slo-Phyllin) is a methylxanthine alkaloid similar to caffeine and theobromine. Aminophylline is 80% theophylline. Theophylline is used in the acute treatment of asthma, pulmonary edema, chronic obstructive pulmonary disease, and neonatal apnea.

Toxic Mechanism

The proposed mechanisms of action include phosphodiesterase inhibition, adenosine receptor antagonism, inhibition of prostaglandins, and increase in serum catecholamines. Theophylline stimulates the central nervous, respiratory, and emetic centers and reduces the seizure threshold. It has positive cardiac inotropic and chronotropic effects, acts as a diuretic, relaxes smooth muscle, and causes peripheral vasodilation but cerebral vasoconstriction. Gastric secretions, gastrointestinal motility, lipolysis, glycogenolysis, and gluconeogenesis are all increased.

Toxic Dose

A single dose of 1 mg/kg produces a theophylline plasma concentration of approximately 2 μg/mL. The therapeutic range usually is 10 to 20 μg/mL. An acute, single dose greater than 10 mg/kg causes mild toxicity, a dose greater than 20 mg/kg causes moderate toxicity, and a dose greater than 50 mg/kg causes serious, possibly fatal toxicity. Fatalities occur at lower doses in patients with chronic toxicity, especially those with risk factors (see *Kinetics*).

Kinetics

The pKa is 9.5. Absorption from the stomach and upper small intestine is complete and rapid, with onset in 30 to 60 minutes. Peak theophylline plasma concentration occurs within 1 to 2 hours after ingestion of liquid preparations, 2 to 4 hours after ingestion of regular tablets, and 7 to 24 hours after ingestion of slow-release formulations. Volume distribution is 0.3 to 0.7 L/kg. Protein binding is 40% to 60% in adults, mainly to albumin (low albumin increases free active theophylline).

Elimination is 90% by hepatic metabolism to an active metabolite, 2-methyl xanthine. The half-life is 3.5 hours in a child and 4 to 6 hours in an adult. The half-life is shorter in smokers and patients taking enzyme-inducing drugs. Only 8% to 10% of the drug is excreted unchanged in the urine.

Risk factors that produce a longer half-life include age younger than 6 months or older than 60 years, use of enzyme-inhibitor drugs (calcium channel blockers, oral contraceptives, cimetidine [Tagamet], ciprofloxacin [Cipro], erythromycin, macrolide anti-biotics, isoniazid), illness (persistent fever >38.9°C [>102°F]), viral illness, liver impairment, heart failure, chronic obstructive pulmonary disease, and influenza vaccination.

Manifestations

Acute toxicity generally correlates with blood levels; chronic toxicity does not (Table 27).

In the case of an acute, single, regular-release overdose, vomiting and occasionally hematemesis occur at low theophylline plasma concentrations. CNS stimulation includes restlessness, muscle tremors, and protracted tonic–clonic seizures, but coma is rare. Convulsions are a sign of severe toxicity and usually are preceded by gastrointestinal symptoms (except with sustained-release and chronic intoxications). Cardiovascular disturbances include cardiac dysrhythmias (supraventricular tachycardia) and transient hypertension with mild overdoses, but hypotension and ventricular dysrhythmias with severe intoxications. Rhabdomyolysis and renal failure are occasionally seen. Children tolerate higher serum levels, and cardiac dysrhythmias and seizures occur at theophylline plasma concentrations greater than 100 μg/mL. Possible metabolic disturbances include hyperglycemia, pronounced hypokalemia, hypocalcemia, hypomagnesemia, hypophosphatemia, increased serum amylase, and elevation of uric acid.

Chronic intoxication, defined as multiple doses of theophylline over 24 hours, or cases in which interacting drugs or illness interfere with theophylline metabolism are more serious and difficult to treat. Cardiac dysrhythmias and convulsions may occur at theophylline plasma concentrations of 40 to 60 μg/mL and there is no correlation with TPC. The seizures occur without warning and are protracted and repetitive and may produce status epilepticus. Vomiting and typical metabolic disturbances do not occur.

TABLE 27 Theophylline Blood Concentrations and Acute Toxicity

Plasma Concentration (μg/mL)	Toxicity Degree	Manifestations
8-10	None	Bronchodilation
10-20	Mild	Therapeutic range: nausea, vomiting, nervousness, respiratory alkalosis, tachycardia
15-25		35% have mild manifestations of toxicity
20-40	Moderate	Gastrointestinal complaints and central nervous system stimulation Transient hypertension, tachypnea, tachycardia; 80% will have some manifestations of toxicity
60	Severe	Convulsions, dysrhythmias
100		Hypokalemia, hyperglycemia Ventricular dysrhythmias, protracted convulsions, hypotension, acid–base abnormalities

Reprinted and modified from Linden CH, Rumack BH, In Toxic Emergencies (Honser W Jr [ed]): The legitimate analgesics, aspirin and acetaminophen, copyright 1984, with permission from Elsevier.

Differences with slow-release preparations are that few or no gastrointestinal symptoms occur, peak concentrations and convulsions may be delayed 12 to 24 hours postingestion, and convulsions occur without warning.

Laboratory Investigations

Monitoring includes vital signs, pulse oximeter, ABG, hemoglobin, hematocrit (for gastrointestinal hemorrhage), ECG and cardiac monitor, renal and hepatic function, electrolytes, blood glucose, acid–base balance, and serum albumin. Gastric contents and stools should be tested for occult blood. Samples for theophylline plasma concentration measurement should be drawn within 1 to 2 hours after ingestion of liquid preparations, 2 to 4 hours after ingestion of regular-release formulations, and 4 hours after ingestion of slow-release formulations. One should check the serum albumin level because a decrease in albumin levels may cause manifestations of toxicity despite normal theophylline plasma concentration. A single theophylline plasma concentration reading may be misleading; therefore, theophylline plasma concentration measurement should be repeated every 2 to 4 hours to determine the trend until a declining trend is reached and then monitored every 4 to 6 hours until it is below 20 μg/mL.

Management

Vital functions must be established and maintained. If the patient is in a coma or has convulsions or vomiting, he or she should be intubated immediately. The theophylline plasma concentration is obtained and repeated every 2 to 4 hours to determine peak absorption, and a theophylline bezoar should be considered if the theophylline plasma concentration fails to decline. Consultation with a nephrologist about charcoal hemoperfusion is recommended.

Gastrointestinal decontamination is warranted in the case of an acute overdose, but emesis must not be induced. Activated charcoal is the choice decontamination procedure in a dose of 1 g/kg to all patients, followed with MDAC 0.5 g/kg every 2 to 4 hours until the theophylline plasma concentration is less than 20 μg/mL. MDAC is effective in treating acute, chronic, and intravenous overdoses.

Activated charcoal shortens the half-life of theophylline by about 50% and may be indicated up to 24 hours following ingestion.

Whole-bowel irrigation with polyethylene-electrolyte solution has been recommended for cases of massive overdose, possible concretions, and ingestion of sustained-release preparations. If intractable vomiting occurs, the antiemetic metoclopramide (Reglan) (0.1 mg/kg adult dose), droperidol (Inapsine) (2.5 to 10 mg IV), or ondansetron (Zofran) (8 to 32 mg IV) is administered. Ondansetron, however, inhibits metabolism of theophylline after a few doses.

Convulsions are controlled with lorazepam (Ativan) or diazepam (Valium) and phenobarbital. Phenytoin (Dilantin) is ineffective. The convulsions in patients with chronic intoxication are often refractory and may require, in addition to anticonvulsants, neuromuscular paralyzing agents, sedation, assisted ventilation, and EEG monitoring.

Hypotension is treated with fluids and vasopressors, if necessary. Norepinephrine (Levophed) 0.05 µg/kg/min is preferred as the vasopressor over dopamine.

Supraventricular tachycardia with hemodynamic instability requires cardioversion. Low-dose β-blockers may be used but should not be used in patients with reactive airway disease or hypotension. Adenosine (Adenocard) is ineffective. For ventriculardys rhythmias, electrolyte disturbances should be corrected. Lidocaine is the treatment of choice but has the potential to cause seizures at toxic concentrations. Cardioversion may be needed.

Hematemesis is managed with sucralfate (Carafate) 1 g four times daily and/or Maalox TC 30 mL every 2 hours and blood replacement, if necessary. H$_2$ antihistamine blockers that are enzyme inhibitors are not used.

Fluid and metabolic disturbances should be corrected. Hyperglycemia does not require insulin therapy. Hypokalemia should be corrected cautiously, as it may be largely an intracellular shift and not total body loss. Usually adding 40 mEq potassium to a liter of fluid will suffice. The serum potassium level must be monitored closely.

Charcoal hemoperfusion is the management of choice for patients with serious intoxications. Hemoperfusion can increase the clearance twofold to threefold over hemodialysis, but hemodialysis can be used if hemoperfusion is not available. Criteria for charcoal hemoperfusion are as follows:

- Life-threatening events such as convulsions or dysrhythmias
- Intractable vomiting refractory to antiemetics
- Acute intoxications with a theophylline plasma concentration greater than 80 µg/mL or greater than 70 µg/mL 4 hours after overdose with a sustained-release formulation and greater than 40 µg/mL in the case of chronic intoxication
- Acute or chronic overdoses with a theophylline plasma concentration greater than 40 µg/mL, especially if the patient has risk factors that lengthen the half-life of the drug (see Kinetics).

Disposition

Patients with mild symptoms and a theophylline plasma concentration less than 20 µg/mL can be treated in emergency department and discharged when asymptomatic for a few hours. Any patient with acute ingestion and a theophylline plasma concentration greater than 35 µg/mL should be admitted to a monitored bed with seizure precautions and suicide precautions, if needed. If neurologic or cardiotoxic effects or a theophylline plasma concentration greater than 50 µg/mL is present, the patient should be admitted to the intensive care unit. A patient with an overdose of a sustained-release preparation, regardless of symptoms or initial theophylline plasma concentration, requires admission, monitoring, activated charcoal, and MDAC. In patients on chronic therapy, toxicity may occur at a lower theophylline plasma concentration, and these patients should not be discharged until they are asymptomatic for several hours.

TRICYCLIC AND CYCLIC ANTIDEPRESSANTS

Historically, tricyclic antidepressants are an important cause of pharmaceutical overdose fatalities. The mortality rate was reduced from 15% in the 1970s to less than 1% in the 1990s because of a better understanding of the pathophysiology of these agents and improvements in management (Table 28).

Toxic Mechanism

The major mechanisms of toxicity of the tricyclic antidepressants are (a) central and peripheral anticholinergic effects; (b) peripheral α-adrenergic blockade; (c) quinidine-like cardiac membrane stabilizing action blockade of the fast inward sodium channels; and (d) inhibition of synaptic neurotransmitter reuptake in the CNS presynaptic neurons. The tetracyclics, monocyclic aminoketones, and dibenzoxazepines possess convulsive activity and less cardiac toxicity in overdose than the older tricyclic antidepressants. Triazolopyridine has less serious cardiac and CNS toxicity.

Toxic Dose

The therapeutic dose of imipramine (Tofranil) is 1.5 to 5 mg/kg; a dose greater than 5 mg/kg may be mildly toxic; 10 to 20 mg/kg may be life threatening, although less than 20 mg/kg has produced few fatalities; greater than 30 mg/kg carries a 30% mortality rate; and at a dose greater than 70 mg/kg, patients rarely survive. In children 375 mg and in adults as little as 500 mg have been fatal. In adults, five times the maximum daily dose is toxic and 10 times is potentially fatal. Although major overdose symptoms are associated with plasma concentrations greater than 1 µg/mL (>1000 ng/mL), plasma tricyclic levels do not correlate well with toxicity; clinical signs and symptoms should guide therapy.

The relative dosage or potency equivalents are as follows: amitriptyline (Elavil) 100 mg = amoxapine (Asendin) 125 mg = desipramine (Norpramin) 75 mg = doxepin (Sinequan) 100 mg = imipramine (Tofranil) 75 mg = maprotiline (Ludiomil) 75 mg = nortriptyline (Pamelor) 50 mg = trazodone (Desyrel) 200 mg. This allows one to determine an equivalent dosage of an agent compared with another (see Table 28).

Kinetics

The tricyclic and cyclic antidepressants are lipophilic. They are rapidly absorbed from the alkaline small intestine, but absorption may be prolonged and delayed in cases of massive overdose owing to anticholinergic action. Onset varies from less than 1 hour (30 to 40 minutes) to, rarely, 12 hours. The peak serum levels are reached in 2 to 8 hours and the peak effect is in 6 hours but may be delayed 12 hours because of erratic absorption. The clinical effects correlate poorly with plasma levels.

Cyclic antidepressants are highly protein-bound to plasma glycoproteins, 98% at a pH 7.5 and 90% at 7.0. Volume distribution is 10 to 50 L/kg. The elimination route is by hepatic metabolism. The tertiary amines are metabolized into active demethylated secondary amine metabolites. The active secondary amine metabolites undergo a 15% enterohepatic recirculation and are metabolized over a period of days into nonactive metabolites. The intestinal bacterial flora may reconstitute the metabolites, which are active.

The half-life varies from 10 hours for imipramine to 81 hours for amitriptyline and 100 hours for nortriptyline. The active metabolites have longer half-lives.

Only 3% of the ingested dose is excreted in the urine unchanged.

Manifestations

There are reports of asymptomatic patients who, upon arrival to an emergency department, suddenly have a seizure, develop hemodynamically unstable dysrhythmias, and die shortly thereafter from ingestion of a tricyclic antidepressant. Most patients with severe toxicity

TABLE 28 Cyclic Antidepressants, Daily Dose and Their Major Properties

Generic Name	Adult Daily Dose (mg)	Therapeutic Range (ng/mL)	Half-life (hours)	Antichol	CNS	Cardiac
Tertiary Amines						
Amitriptyline (Elavil)	75-300	120-250	31-46	3+	3+	3+
Imipramine (Tofranil)	75-300	125-250	9-24	3+	3+	2+
Doxepin (Sinequan)	75-300	30-150	8-24	3+	3+	2+
Trimipramine (Surmantil)	75-200	10-240	16-18	3+	3+	2+
Secondary Amines						
Nortriptyline (Pamelor)	75-150	50-150	18-93	2+	3+	3+
Desipramine (Norpramin)	75-200	75-160	14-62	1+	3+	3+
Protriptyline (Vivactil)	20-60	70-250	54-198	2+	3+	3+
Newer Cyclic Antidepressants						
Teracyclic			30-60	1+	2+	3+
Maprotiline (Ludiomil)	75-300	—	30-60	1+	2+	3+
Trizolopyridine, a noncyclic, produces less serious cardiac and CNS toxicity						
Trazodone (Desyrel)	50-600	700	4-7	1+	1+	1+
Monocyclic Aminoketones						
Bupropion (Wellbutrin)	200-400	—	8-24	1+	3+	1+
Dibenzazepine						
Clomipramine (Anafranil)	100-250	200-500	21-32	2+	2+	2+
Dibenoxazepine						
Amoxapine (Ascendin)	150-300	200-500	6-10	1+	3+	2+

*Antichol = anticholinergic effect; CNS = central nervous system effect primarily seizures; Cardiac = cardiac effect.
Other drugs with similar structures are cyclobenzaprine, a muscle relaxant (similar to amitriptyline), and carbamazepine, an anticonvulsant (similar to imipramine); however, they cause less cardiac toxicity.

develop symptoms within 1 to 2 hours, but symptoms may be delayed 6 hours after overdose.

Small overdoses produce early anticholinergic effects, agitation, and transient hypertension, which are not life-threatening. Large overdoses produce depression of the CNS and myocardium, convulsions, and hypotension. Death can occur within the first 2 to 6 hours following ingestion.

Some ECG screening tools for predicting cardiac or neurologic toxicity from ingestion of a tricyclic antidepressant have been developed: (a) A QRS greater than 0.10 second may produce seizures, and if greater than 0.16 second, 50% of patients may develop ventricular dysrhythmias (20% of these may be life-threatening) and seizures; (b) a terminal 40 msec of the QRS axis greater than 120 degrees in the right frontal plane may be associated with toxicity; or (c) a large R wave greater than 3 mm in ECG lead aVR may predispose the patient to toxicity. The quinidine cardiac membrane stabilizing effect produces depression of myocardium, conduction, and ECG changes. The peripheral α-adrenergic blockade produces hypotension.

The secondary amines are metabolized to inactive metabolites. The tetracyclics produce a high incidence of cardiovascular disturbances and seizures. Monocyclic aminoketones produce seizures in doses greater than 600 mg. Dibenzoxazepines produce a syndrome of convulsions, rhabdomyolysis, and renal failure.

Laboratory Investigations

If the patient has altered mental status or ECG abnormalities, ABG, ECG, chest radiograph, blood glucose, serum electrolytes, calcium, magnesium, blood urea nitrogen, and creatinine levels, liver profile, creatine kinase level, urine output, and, in severe cases, hemodynamic monitoring are indicated. Levels of the tricyclic and cyclic antidepressants less than 300 ng/mL are therapeutic; levels greater than 500 ng/mL indicate toxicity, and levels greater than 1000 ng/mL indicate serious poisoning and are associated with QRS widening.

Management

Vital functions must be established and maintained. Even if the patient is asymptomatic, intravenous access should be established, vital signs and neurologic status monitored, and baseline 12-lead ECG and continuous cardiac monitoring obtained for at least 6 hours from admission or 8 to 12 hours postingestion. QRS interval should be measured on a limb lead ECG every 15 minutes for 6 hours postingestion.

For gastrointestinal decontamination, emesis should not be induced and gastric lavage should not be used. Activated charcoal is preferable. If the patient is in an altered mental state, the airway must be protected. Activated charcoal 1 g/kg is recommended up to 1 hour postingestion. Benefit from MDAC has not been demonstrated.

Alkalinization does not control seizures; diazepam or lorazepam should be used. Status epilepticus may require high-dose barbiturates or neuromuscular blockers with intravenous diazepam. If not successful, the patient can be paralyzed with short-term nondepolarizing neuromuscular blockers such as vecuronium (Norcuron), intubation, and assisted ventilation. A bolus of sodium bicarbonate is recommended as an adjunct to correct the acidosis produced by the seizures.

Sodium bicarbonate is administered in a dose of 1 to 2 mEq/kg undiluted as a bolus and repeated twice a few minutes apart, if needed, for "sodium loading" and alkalinization, which may increase protein binding from 90% to 98%. The sodium loading overcomes the sodium channel blockage and is more important than the alkalinization. Indications include (a) a QRS complex greater than 0.12 second, (b) ventricular tachycardia, (c) severe conduction disturbances, (d) metabolic acidosis, (e) coma, and (f) seizures. A continuous infusion of sodium bicarbonate is of limited usefulness for controlling dysrhythmias. Bolus therapy should be used as needed.

Hyperventilation alone has been recommended, but the pH elevation is not as instantaneous and there is compensatory renal excretion of bicarbonate; therefore, we do not recommend it. The combination of hyperventilation and sodium bicarbonate has produced fatal alkalemia and is not recommended. One should monitor serum potassium level (the sudden increase in blood pH can aggravate or precipitate hypokalemia), serum sodium, and ionized calcium levels (hypocalcemia may occur with alkalinization) and blood pH.

Specific cardiovascular complications should be treated as follows: Hypotension is treated with norepinephrine, a predominantly α-adrenergic drug, which is preferred over dopamine. Hypertension that occurs early rarely requires treatment. Sinus tachycardia usually does not require treatment. Supraventricular tachycardia in a patient who is hemodynamically unstable requires synchronized electrical cardioversion, starting at 0.25 to 1.0 watt-second per kg, after sedation. Ventricular tachycardia that persists after alkalinization requires intravenous lidocaine or countershock if the patient is hemodynamically unstable. Ventricular fibrillation should be treated with defibrillation. Torsades de pointes is treated with magnesium sulfate IV 20% solution, 2 g over 2 to 3 minutes, followed by a continuous infusion of 1.5 mL 10% solution or 5 to 10 mg per minute. For the treatment of bradydysrhythmias, atropine is contraindicated because of the anticholinergic activity. Isoproterenol 0.1 µg/kg/minute, used with caution, may produce hypotension. If the patient is hemodynamically unstable, a pacemaker is used.

Extraordinary measures, such as aortic balloon pump and cardiopulmonary bypass, have been successful.

Investigational treatments include FAB fragments specific for tricyclic antidepressant, which have been successful in animals. Prophylactic $NaHCO_3$ to prevent dysrhythmias is also being investigated.

Physostigmine has produced asystole, and flumazenil has produced seizures. Both are contraindicated.

Disposition

A patient with an antidepressant overdose who meets any of the following criteria should be admitted to the intensive care unit for 12 to 24 hours: (a) ECG abnormalities except sinus tachycardia, (b) altered mental state, (c) seizures, (d) respiratory depression, and (e) hypotension. Low-risk patients include those in whom the above symptoms are absent at 6 hours postingestion, those who present with minor transient manifestations such as sinus tachycardia who subsequently become and remain asymptomatic for a 6-hour period, and asymptomatic patients who remain asymptomatic for 6 hours. These patients may be discharged if the ECG remains normal, they have normal bowel sounds, and they undergo psychiatric disposition.

Even if the patient is asymptomatic upon presentation to the health care facility, intravenous access should be established, vital signs and neurologic status monitored, a baseline 12-lead ECG obtained, and cardiac monitoring continued for at least 6 hours. *Caution:* in 25% of fatal cases, the patients were initially alert and awake at presentation. However, in most cases of fatality initially deemed as sudden cardiac death, the patient, upon reexamination, actually had symptoms that were missed.

Children younger than 6 years of age with non-intentional (accidental) exposures to amitriptyline (Elavil), desipramine (Norpramin), doxepin (Sinequan), imipramine (Tofranil), or nortriptyline (Aventyl) in a dose less than 5 mg/kg, who are asymptomatic and have what are deemed reliable caregivers, can be observed at home, with close poison control follow-up for 6 hours. Parents or caregivers should be given instructions regarding signs and symptoms to be alert for. Children who are symptomatic, or who ingested greater than 5 mg/kg, should be referred to the emergency department for monitoring, observation, and activated charcoal treatment.

SECTION 19

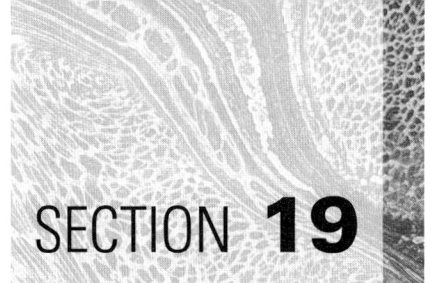

Appendices and Index

Reference Intervals for the Interpretation of Laboratory Tests

Method of
Laura J. McCloskey, PhD

Most of the tests performed in a clinical laboratory are quantitative; that is, the amount of a substance present in blood or serum is measured and reported in terms of concentration, activity (e.g., enzyme activity), or counts (e.g., blood cell counts). The laboratory must provide reference intervals to assist the clinician in the interpretation of laboratory results. These reference intervals represent the physiologic quantities of a substance (concentrations, activities, or counts) to be expected in healthy persons. Deviation above or below the reference range may be associated with a disease process, and the severity of the disease process may be associated with the magnitude of the deviation. Unfortunately, a sharp demarcation rarely exists to distinguish between physiologic and pathologic values, and the time of transition between the two is often gradual as the disease process progresses.

Defining Normal Values

The terms "normal" and "abnormal" have been used to describe laboratory values that fall inside and outside the reference range, respectively. Use of these terms is inappropriate because no good definition of normality exists in the clinical sense, and the term "normal" may be confused with the statistical term "gaussian." Reference ranges are established from statistical studies in groups of healthy volunteers. These study subjects must be free of disease, but they may have lifestyles or habits that result in variations in certain laboratory values. Examples of these variables include diet, body mass, exercise, and geographic location. Age and gender can also affect reference values.

When the data from a large cohort of healthy subjects fit a gaussian distribution, the usual statistical approach is to define the reference limits as 2 standard deviations (SD) above and below the mean. By definition, the reference range excludes the 2.5% of the population with the lowest values and the 2.5% with the highest values. Nongaussian distributions are handled by different statistical methods, but the result is similar, in that the reference range is defined by the central 95% of the population. In other words, the probability that a healthy person has a laboratory result falling outside the reference range is 1 in 20. If 12 laboratory tests are performed, the probability that at least one of the results is outside the reference range increases to about 50%, which means that all healthy persons are likely to have a few laboratory results that are unexpected. The clinician must then integrate these data with other clinical information, such as the history and physical examination, to arrive at an appropriate clinical decision.

The reference intervals for many tests (especially enzyme and immunochemical measurements) vary with the method used. Accordingly, each laboratory must establish its own reference intervals that are appropriate for the methods used.

International System of Units

During the 1980s, a concerted effort was made to introduce the International System of Units (Systéme International d'Unités; SI units). The rationale for conversion to SI units is sound. Laboratory data are scientifically more informative when the units are based on molar concentration rather than on mass concentration. For example, the conversion of glucose to lactate and pyruvate or the binding of a drug to albumin is more easily understood in units of molar concentration. Another example is illustrated as follows:

Conventional Units	SI Units
1.0 g of hemoglobin:	4.0 mmol of hemoglobin:
Combines with 1.37 mL of oxygen	Combines with 4.0 mmol of oxygen
Contains 3.4 mg of iron	Contains 4.0 mmol of iron
Forms 34.9 mg of bilirubin	Forms 4.0 mmol of bilirubin

The use of SI units would also enhance the standardization of nomenclature to facilitate global communication of medical and scientific information. The units, symbols, and prefixes used in the international system are shown in Tables 1, 2, and 3.

TABLE 1 Base SI Units

Property	Unit	Symbol
Length	Meter	m
Mass	Kilogram	kg
Amount of substance	Mole	mol
Time	Second	s
Thermodynamic temperature	Kelvin	K
Electrical current	Ampere	A
Luminous intensity	Candela	cd
Catalytic amount	Katal	kat

Abbreviation: SI = International System of Units.

TABLE 2 Derived SI Units and Non-SI Units Retained for Use with SI Units

Property	Unit	Symbol
Area	Square meter	m^2
Volume	Cubic meter	m^3
	Liter	L
Mass	Kilograms per cubic meter	kg/m^3 concentration
	Grams per liter	g/L
Substance concentration	Moles per cubic meter	mol/m^3
		mol/L
Temperature	Degree Celsius	C = K−273.15
Dynamic viscosity	Pascal-second	$Pa\cdot s = 1\ kg\cdot m^{-1}\cdot s^{-1}$

Abbreviation: SI = International System of Units.

Unfortunately, problems have arisen with the implementation of SI units in the United States. The introduction of this system in 1987 prompted many medical journals to report laboratory values in both SI and conventional units in anticipation of complete conversion to SI units in the early 1990s. The lack of a coordinated effort toward this goal forced a retrenchment on the issue. Physicians continue to think and practice with laboratory results expressed in conventional units, and few, if any, hospitals or clinical laboratories in the United States use SI units exclusively. Complete conversion to SI units is not likely to occur in the foreseeable future, but most medical journals will probably continue to publish both sets of units. For this reason, the values in the tables of reference ranges in this appendix are given in both conventional units and SI units.

Tables of Reference Intervals

Some of the values included in the tables that follow have been established by the Clinical Laboratories at the Thomas Jefferson University Hospital in Philadelphia and have not been published elsewhere. Other values have been compiled from the sources cited in the suggested readings. These tables are provided for information and educational purposes only. Laboratory values must always be interpreted in the context of clinical data derived from other sources, including the medical history and physical examination. One must exercise individual judgment when using the information provided in this appendix.

REFERENCES

American Medical Association: Drug Evaluations Annual, Chicago: American Medical Association, 1994.

Bick RL (ed): Hematology: Clinical and Laboratory Practice, St Louis: Mosby–Year Book, 1993.

Borer WZ: Selection and use of laboratory tests. In Tietz NW, Conn RB, Pruden EL (eds): Applied Laboratory Medicine. Philadelphia: WB Saunders, 1992, pp 1-5.

Campion EW: A retreat from SI units. N Engl J Med 1992;327:49.

Friedman RB, Young DS: Effects of Disease on Clinical Laboratory Tests, 3rd ed. Washington, DC: American Association for Clinical Chemistry Press, 1997.

Henry JB: Clinical Diagnosis and Management by Laboratory Methods, 19th ed. Philadelphia: WB Saunders, 1996.

Hicks JM, Young DS: DORA 97-99: Directory of Rare Analyses, Washington, DC: American Association for Clinical Chemistry Press, 1997.

Jacob DS, Demott WR, Grady HJ, et al (eds): Laboratory Test Handbook, 4th ed. Baltimore: Williams & Wilkins, 1996.

Kaplan LA, Pesce AJ: Clinical Chemistry: Theory, Analysis, and Correlation, 3rd ed. St Louis: Mosby–Year Book, 1996.

Kjeldsberg CR, Knight JA: Body Fluids: Laboratory Examination of Amniotic, Cerebrospinal, Seminal, Serous and Synovial Fluids, 3rd ed. Chicago: ASCP Press, 1993.

Laposata M: SI Unit Conversion Guide, Boston: NEJM Books, 1992.

Scully RE, McNeely WF, Mark EJ, McNeely BU: Normal reference laboratory values. N Engl J Med 1992;327:718-724.

Speicher CE: The Right Test: A Physician's Guide to Laboratory Medicine, 3rd ed. Philadelphia: WB Saunders, 1998.

Tietz NW (ed): Clinical Guide to Laboratory Tests, 3rd ed. Philadelphia: WB Saunders, 1995.

Wallach J: Interpretation of Diagnostic Tests: A Synopsis of Laboratory Medicine, 6th ed. Boston: Little, Brown, 1996.

Young DS: Effects of Preanalytical Variables on Clinical Laboratory Tests, 2nd ed. Washington, DC: American Association for Clinical Chemistry Press, 1997.

Young DS: Effects of Drugs on Clinical Laboratory Tests, 4th ed. Washington, DC: American Association for Clinical Chemistry Press, 1995.

Young DS: Determination and validation of reference intervals. Arch Pathol Lab Med 1992;116:704-709.

Young DS: Implementation of SI units for clinical laboratory data. Ann Intern Med 1987;106:114-129.

TABLE 3 Standard Prefixes

Prefix	Multiplication Factor	Symbol
yocto	10^{-24}	y
zepto	10^{-21}	z
atto	10^{-18}	a
femto	10^{-15}	f
pico	10^{-12}	p
nano	10^{-9}	n
micro	10^{-6}	μ
milli	10^{-3}	m
centi	10^{-2}	c
deci	10^{-1}	d
deca	10^{1}	da
hecto	10^{2}	h
kilo	10^{3}	k
mega	10^{6}	M
giga	10^{9}	G
tera	10^{12}	T

Reference Intervals* for Hematology

Test	Conventional Units	SI Units
Acid hemolysis (Ham test)	No hemolysis	No hemolysis
Alkaline phosphatase, leukocyte	Total score, 14-100	Total score, 14-100
Cell counts		
Erythrocytes		
Males	4.6-6.2 million/mm^3	4.6-6.2 × 10^{12}/L
Females	4.2-5.4 million/mm^3	4.2-5.4 × 10^{12}/L
Children (varies with age)	4.5-5.1 million/mm^3	4.5-5.1 × 10^{12}/L
Leukocytes, total	4500-11,000/mm^3	4.5-11.0 × 10^9/L
Leukocytes, differential counts*		
Myelocytes	0%	0/L
Band neutrophils	3-5%	150-400 × 10^6/L
Segmented neutrophils	54-62%	3000-5800 × 10^6/L
Lymphocytes	25-33%	1500-3000 × 10^6/L
Monocytes	3-7%	300-500 × 10^6/L
Eosinophils	1-3%	50-250 × 10^6/L
Basophils	0-1%	15-50 × 10^6/L
Platelets	150,000-400,000/mm^3	150-400 × 10^9/L
Reticulocytes	25,000-75,000/mm^3 (0.5%-1.5% of erythrocytes)	25-75 × 10^9/L
Coagulation Tests		
Bleeding time (template)	2.75-8.0 min	2.75-8.0 min
Coagulation time (glass tube)	5-15 min	5-15 min
D dimer	<0.5 µg/mL	<0.5 mg/L
Factor VIII and other coagulation factors	50-150% of normal	0.5-1.5 of normal
Fibrin split products (Thrombo-Welco test)	<10 µg/mL	<10 mg/L
Fibrinogen	200-400 mg/dL	2.0-4.0 g/L
Partial thromboplastin time, activated (aPTT)	20-25 s	20-35 s
Prothrombin time (PT)	12.0-14.0 s	12.0-14.0 s
Coombs' Test		
Direct	Negative	Negative
Indirect	Negative	Negative
Corpuscular values of erythrocytes		
Mean corpuscular hemoglobin (MCH)	26-34 pg/cell	26-34 pg/cell
Mean corpuscular volume (MCV)	80-96 µm^3	80-96 fL
Mean corpuscular hemoglobin concentration (MCHC)	32-36 g/dL	320-360 g/L
Haptoglobin	20-165 mg/dL	0.20-1.65 g/L
Hematocrit		
Males	40-54 mL/dL	0.40-0.54 g/L
Females	37-47 mL/dL	0.37-0.47 g/L
Newborns	49-54 mL/dL	0.49-0.54 g/L
Children (varies with age)	35-49 mL/dL	0.35-0.49 g/L
Hemoglobin		
Males	13.0-18.0 g/dL	8.1-11.2 mmol/L
Females	12.0-16.0 g/dL	7.4-9.9 mmol/L
Newborns	16.5-19.5 g/dL	10.2-12.1 mmol/L
Children (varies with age)	11.2-16.5 g/dL	7.0-10.2 mmol/L
Hemoglobin, fetal	<1.0 of total	<0.01 of total
Hemoglobin A1c	3-5% of total	0.03-0.05 of total
Hemoglobin A2	1.5-3.0% of total	0.015-0.03 of total
Hemoglobin, plasma	0.0%-5.0 mg/dL	0.0-3.2 µmol/L
Methemoglobin	30%-130 mg/dL	19-80 µmol/L
Erythrocyte sedimentation rate (ESR)		
Westergren:		
Males	0-15 mm/h	0-15 mm/h
Females	0-20 mm/h	0-20 mm/h
Wintrobe:		
Males	0-5 mm/h	0-5 mm/h
Females	0-15 mm/h	0-15 mm/h

*Conventional units are percentages; SI units are absolute cell counts.
Abbreviation: SI = International System of Units.

Reference Intervals* for Clinical Chemistry (Blood, Serum, and Plasma)

Analyte	Conventional Units	SI Units
Acetoacetate plus acetone		
Qualitative	Negative	Negative
Quantitative	0.3-2.0 mg/dL	30-200 mol/L
Acid phosphatase, serum (thymolphthalein monophosphate substrate)	0.1-0.6 U/L	0.1-0.6 U/L
ACTH (see Corticotropin)		
Alanine aminotransferase (ALT), serum (SGPT)	1-45 U/L	1-45 U/L
Albumin, serum	3.3-5.2 g/dL	33-52 g/L
Aldolase, serum	0.0-7.0 U/L	0.0-7.0 U/L
Aldosterone, plasma		
Standing	5-30 ng/dL	140-830 pmol/L
Recumbent	3-10 ng/dL	80-275 pmol/L
Alkaline, phosphatase (ALP), serum		
Adult	35-150 U/L	35-150 U/L
Adolescent	100-500 U/L	100-500 U/L
Child	100-350 U/L	100-350 U/L
Ammonia nitrogen, plasma	10-50 µmol/L	10-50 µmol/L
Amylase, serum	25-125 U/L	25-125 U/L
Anion gap, serum calculated	8-16 mEq/L	8-16 mmol/L
Ascorbic acid, blood	0.4-1.5 mg/dL	23-85 µmol/L
Aspartate aminotransferase (AST), serum (SGOT)	1-36 U/L	1-36 U/L
Base excess, arterial blood, calculated	0±2 mEq/L	0±2 mmol/L
Bicarbonate		
Venous plasma	23-29 mEq/L	23-29 mmol/L
Arterial blood	21-27 mEq/L	21-27 mmol/L
Bile acids, serum	0.3-3.0 mg/dL	0.8-7.6 mmol/L
Bilirubin, serum		
Conjugated	0.1-0.4 mg/dL	1.7-6.8 µmol/L
Total	0.3-1.1 mg/dL	5.1-19.0 µmol/L
Calcium, serum	8.4-10.6 mg/dL	2.10-2.65 mmol/L
Calcium, ionized, serum	4.25-5.25 mg/dL	1.05-1.30 mmol/L
Carbon dioxide, total, serum or plasma	24-31 mEq/L	24-31 mmol/L
Carbon dioxide tension (P_{CO_2}), blood	35-45 mm Hg	35-45 mm Hg
β-Carotene, serum	60-260 µg/dL	1.1-8.6 µmol/L
Ceruloplasmin, serum	23-44 mg/dL	230-440 mg/L
Chloride, serum or plasma	96-106 mEq/L	96-106 mmol/L
Cholesterol, serum or EDTA plasma		
Desirable range	<200 mg/dL	<5.20 mmol/L
Low-density lipoprotein (LDL) cholesterol	60-180 mg/dL	1.55-4.65 mmol/L
High-density lipoprotein (HDL) cholesterol	30-80 mg/dL	0.80-2.05 mmol/L
Copper	70-140 µg/dL	11-22 µmol/L
Corticotropin (ACTH), plasma, 8 AM	10-80 pg/mL	2-18 pmol/L
Cortisol, plasma		
8:00 AM	6-23 µg/dL	170-630 µmol/L
4:00 PM	3-15 µg/dL	80-410 µmol/L
10:00 PM	<50% of 8:00 AM value	<50% of 8:00 AM value
Creatine, serum		
Males	0.2-0.5 mg/dL	15-40 µmol/L
Females	0.3-0.9 mg/dL	25-70 µmol/L
Creatine kinase (CK), serum		
Males	55-170 U/L	55-170 U/L
Females	30-135 U/L	30-135 U/L
Creatinine kinase MB isoenzyme, serum	<5% of total CK activity	<5% of total CK activity
	<5% of ng/mL by immunoassay	<5% of ng/mL by immunoassay
Creatinine, serum	0.6-1.2 mg/dL	50-110 µmol/L
Erythrocytes	145-540 ng/mL	330-120 nmol/L
Estradiol-17β, adult		
Males	10-65 pg/mL	35-240 pmol/L
Females		
Follicular	30-100 pg/mL	110-370 pmol/L
Ovulatory	200-400 pg/mL	730-1470 pmol/L
Luteal	50-140 pg/mL	180-510 pmol/L
Ferritin, serum	20-200 ng/mL	20-200 µg/L
Fibrinogen, plasma	200-400 mg/dL	2.0-4.0 g/L
Folate, serum	3-18 ng/mL	6.8-4.1 nmol/L
Follicle-stimulating hormone (FSH), plasma		
Males	4-25 mU/mL	4-25 U/L
Females, premenopausal	4-30 mU/mL	4-30 U/L
Females, postmenopausal	40-250 mU/mL	40-250 U/L
Gastrin, fasting, serum	0-100 pg/mL	0-100 mg/L
Glucose, fasting, plasma or serum	70-115 mg/dL	3.9-6.4 nmol/L
γ-Glutamyltransferase (GGT), serum	5-40 U/L	5-40 U/L
Growth hormone (hGH), plasma, adult, fasting	0-6 ng/mL	0-6 µg/L
Haptoglobin, serum	20-165 mg/dL	0.20-1.65 g/L

Reference Intervals* for Clinical Chemistry (Blood, Serum, and Plasma)—cont'd

Analyte	Conventional Units	SI Units
Immunoglobulins, serum (see table, Reference Intervals for Tests of Immunologic Function)		
Iron, serum	75-175 µg/dL	13-31 µmol/L
Iron-binding capacity, serum		
Total	250-410 µg/dL	45-73 µmol/L
Saturation	20-55%	0.20-0.55
Lactate		
Venous whole blood	5.0-20.0 mg/dL	0.6-2.2 mmol/L
Arterial whole blood	5.0-15.0 mg/dL	0.6-1.7 mmol/L
Lactate dehydrogenase (LD), serum	110-220 U/L	110-220 U/L
Lipase, serum	10-140 U/L	10-140 U/L
Lutropin (LH), serum		
Males	1-9 U/L	-9 U/L
Females		
Follicular phase	2-10 U/L	2-10 U/L
Midcycle peak	15-65 U/L	15-65 U/L
Luteal phase	1-12 U/L	1-12 U/L
Postmenopausal	12-65 U/L	12-65 U/L
Magnesium, serum	1.3-2.1 mg/dL	0.65-1.05 mmol/L
Osmolality	275-295 mOsm/kg water	275-295 mOsm/kg water
Oxygen, blood, arterial, room air		
Partial pressure (PaO_2)	80-100 mm Hg	80-100 mm Hg
Saturation (SaO_2)	95-98%	95-98%
pH, arterial blood	7.35-7.45	7.35-7.45
Phosphate, inorganic, serum		
Adult	3.0-4.5 mg/dL	1.0-1.5 mmol/L
Child	4.0-7.0 mg/dL	1.3-2.3 mmol/L
Potassium		
Serum	3.5-5.0 mEq/L	3.5-5.0 mmol/L
Plasma	3.5-4.5 mEq/L	3.5-4.5 mmol/L
Progesterone, serum, adult		
Males	0.0-0.4 ng/mL	0.0-1.3 mmol/L
Females		
Follicular phase	0.1-1.5 ng/mL	0.3-4.8 mmol/L
Luteal phase	2.5-28.0 ng/mL	8.0-89.0 mmol/L
Prolactin, serum		
Males	1.0-15.0 ng/mL	1.0-15.0 µg/L
Females	1.0-20.0 ng/mL	1.0-20.0 µg/L
Protein, serum, electrophoresis		
Total	6.0-8.0 g/dL	60-80 µg/L
Albumin	3.5-5.5 g/dL	35-55 µg/L
Globulins		
α_1	0.2-0.4 g/dL	2.0-4.0 g/L
α_2	0.5-0.9 g/dL	5.0-9.0 g/L
β	0.6-1.1 g/dL	6.0-11.0 g/L
γ	0.7-1.7 g/dL	7.0-17.0 g/L
Pyruvate, blood	0.3-0.9 mg/dL	0.03-0.10 mmol/L
Rheumatoid factor	0.0-30.0 IU/mL	0.0-30.0 kIU/L
Sodium, serum or plasma	135-145 mEq/L	135-145 mmol/L
Testosterone, plasma		
Men	300-1200 ng/dL	10.4-41.6 nmol/L
Women	20-75 ng/dL	0.7-2.6 nmol/L
Pregnant	40-200 ng/dL	1.4-6.9 nmol/L
Thyroglobulin	3-42 ng/mL	3-42 µg/L
Thyrotropin (hTSH), serum	0.4-4.8 µIU/mL	0.4-4.8 mIU/L
Thyrotropin-releasing hormone (TRH)	5-60 pg/mL	5-60 ng/L
Thyroxine, free (FT_4), serum	0.9-2.1 ng/dL	12-27 pmol/L
Thyroxine (T_4), serum	4.5-12.0 µg/mL	58-154 nmol/L
Thyroxine-binding globulin (TBG)	15.0-34.0 µg/mL	15.0-34.0 mg/L
Transferrin	250-430 mg/dL	2.5-4.3 g/L
Triglycerides, serum, after 12-h fast	40-150 mg/dL	0.4-1.5 g/L
Triiodothyronine (T_3), serum	70-190 ng/dL	1.1-2.9 nmol/L
Triiodothyronine uptake, resin (T_3RU)	25-38%	0.25-0.38
Troponin I	0.05-0.50 ng/mL	0.05-0.50 ng/mL
Urate		
(FT_4) Males	2.5-8.0 mg/dL	150-480 µmol/L
(FT_4) Females	2.2-7.0 mg/dL	130-420 µmol/L
Urea, serum or plasma	24-49 mg/dL	4.0-8.2 nmol/L
Urea nitrogen, serum or plasma	11-23 mg/dL	8.0-16.4 nmol/L
Viscosity, serum	1.1-1.8 cP	1.1-1.8 mPas-s
Vitamin A, serum	20-80 µg/dL	0.70-2.80 µmol/L
Vitamin B_{12}, serum	180-900 pg/mL	133-664 pmol/L

*Reference values can vary depending on the method and sample source used.
Abbreviations: EDTA = ethylenediaminetetraacetic acid; SI = International System of Units.

Reference Intervals for Therapeutic Drug Monitoring (Serum or Plasma)*

Analyte	Therapeutic Range	Toxic Concentrations	Proprietary Analyte Name(s)
Analgesics			
Acetaminophen	10-40 µg/mL	>150 µg/mL	Tylenol, Datril
Salicylate	100-250 µg/mL	>300 µg/mL	Aspirin, Bufferin
Antibiotics			
Amikacin	20-30 µg/mL	Peak >35 µg/mL Trough >10 µg/mL	Amkin
Gentamicin	5-10 µg/mL	Peak >10 µg/mL Trough >2 µg/mL	Garamycin
Tobramycin	5-10 µg/mL	Peak >10 µg/mL Trough >2 µg/mL	Nebcin
Vancomycin	5-35 µg/mL	Peak >40 µg/mL Trough >10 µg/mL	Vancocin
Anticonvulsants			
Carbamazepine	5-12 µg/mL	>15 µg/mL	Tegretol
Ethosuximide	40-100 µg/mL	>250 µg/mL	Zarontin
Phenobarbital	15-40 µg/mL	40-100 ng/mL (varies widely)	Luminal
Phenytoin	10-20 µg/mL	>20 µg/mL	Dilantin
Primidone	5-12 µg/mL	>15 µg/mL	Mysoline
Valproic acid	50-100 µg/mL	>100 µg/mL	Depakene
Antineoplastics and Immunosuppressives			
Cyclosporine A	150-350 ng/mL	>400 ng/mL	Sandimmune
Methotrexate, high-dose, 48 h	Variable	>1 µmol/L, 48h after dose	
Sirolimus (within 1 h of 2-mg dose)	4.5-14 ng/mL	Variable	Rapamune
Sirolimus (within 1 h of 5-mg dose)	10-28 ng/mL	Variable	Rapamune
Tacrolimus (FK-506), whole blood	3-20 µg/L	>15 µg/L	Prograf
Bronchodilators and Respiratory Stimulants			
Caffeine	3-15 ng/mL	>30 ng/mL	Elixophyllin
Theophylline (aminophylline)	10-20 µg/mL	>30 µg/mL	Quibron
Cardiovascular Drugs			
Amiodarone (obtain specimen more than 8 h after last dose)	1.0-2.0 µg/mL	>2.0 µg/mL	Cordarone
Digoxin (obtain specimen more than 6 h after last dose)	0.8-2.0 ng/mL	>2.4 ng/mL	Lanoxin
Disopyramide	2-5 µg/mL	>7 µg/mL	Norpace
Flecainide	0.2-1.0 µg/mL	>1 µg/mL	Tambocor
Lidocaine	1.5-5.0 µg/mL	>6 µg/mL	Xylocaine
Mexiletine	0.7-2.0 µg/mL	>2 µg/mL	Mexitil
Procainamide	4-10 µg/mL	>12 µg/mL	Pronestyl
Procainamide plus NAPA (N-acetyl procainamide)	8-30 µg/mL	>30 µg/mL	
Propranolol	50-100 ng/mL	Variable	Inderal
Quinidine	2-5 µg/mL	>6 µg/mL	Cardioquin, Quinaglute
Tocainide	4-10 ng/mL	>10 ng/mL	Tonocard
Psychopharmacologic Drugs			
Amitriptyline	120-150 ng/mL	>500 ng/mL	Elavil, Triavil
Bupropion	25-100 ng/mL	Not applicable	Wellbutrin
Desipramine	150-300 ng/mL	>500 ng/mL	Norpramin
Imipramine	125-250 ng/mL	>400 ng/mL	Tofranil
Lithium (obtain specimen 12 h after last dose)	0.6-1.5 mEq/L	>1.5 mEq/L	Lithobid
Nortriptyline	50-150 ng/mL	>500 ng/mL	Aventyl, Pamelor

*Values can vary depending on the method and sample collection device used. Always consult the reference values provided by the laboratory performing the analysis.

Reference Intervals* for Clinical Chemistry (Urine)

Analyte	Conventional Units	SI Units
Acetone and acetoacetate, qualitative	Negative	Negative
Albumin		
Qualitative	Negative	Negative
Quantitative	10-100 mg/24 h	0.15-1.5 µmol/d
Aldosterone	3-20 µg/24 h	8.3-55 nmol/d
δ-Aminolevulinic acid (δ-ALA)	1.3-7.0 mg/24 h	10-53 µmol/d
Amylase	<17 U/h	<17 U/h
Amylase-to-creatinine clearance ratio	0.01-0.04	0.01-0.04
Bilirubin, qualitative	Negative	Negative
Calcium (regular diet)	<250 mg/24 h	<6.3 nmol/d
Catecholamines		
Epinephrine	<10 µg/24 h	<55 nmol/d
Norepinephrine	<100 µg/24 h	<590 nmol/d
Total free catecholamines	4-126 µg/24 h	24-745 nmol/d
Total metanephrines	0.1-1.6 mg/24 h	0.5-8.1 µmol/d
Chloride (varies with intake)	110-250 mEq/24 h	110-250 mmol/d
Copper	0-50 µg/24 h	0.0-0.80 µmol/d
Cortisol, free	10-100 µg/24 h	27.6-276 nmol/d
Creatine		
Males	0-40 mg/24 h	0.0-0.30 mmol/d
Females	0-80 mg/24 h	0.0-0.60 mmol/d
Creatinine	15-25 mg/kg/24 h	0.13-0.22 mmol/kg/d
Creatinine clearance (endogenous)		
Males	110-150 mL/min/1.73 m2	110-150 mL/min/1.73 m2
Females	105-132 mL/min/1.73 m2	105-132 mL/min/1.73 m2
Cystine or cysteine	Negative	Negative
Dehydroepiandrosterone		
Males	0.2-2.0 mg/24 h	0.7-6.9 µmol/d
Females	0.2-1.8 mg/24 h	0.7-6.2 µmol/d
Estrogens, total		
Males	4-25 µg/24 h	14-90 nmol/d
Females	5-100 µg/24 h	18-360 nmol/d
Glucose (as reducing substance)	<250 mg/24 h	<250 mg/d
Hemoglobin and myoglobin, qualitative	Negative	Negative
Hemogentisic acid, qualitative	Negative	Negative
17-Hydroxycorticosteroids		
Males	3-9 mg/24 h	8.3-25 µmol/d
Females	2-8 mg/24 h	5.5-22 µmol/d
5-Hydroxyindoleacetic acid		
Qualitative	Negative	Negative
Quantitative	2-6 mg/24 h	10-31 µmol/d
17-Ketogenic steroids		
Males	5-23 mg/24 h	17-80 µmol/d
Females	3-15 mg/24 h	10-52 µmol/d
17-Ketosteroids		
Males	8-22 mg/24 h	28-76 µmol/d
Females	6-15 mg/24 h	21-52 µmol/d
Magnesium	6-10 mEq/24 h	3-5 mmol/d
Metanephrines	0.05-1.2 ng/mg creatinine	0.03-0.70 mmol/mmol creatinine
Osmolality	38-1400 mOsm/kg water	38-1400 mOsm/kg water
pH	4.6-8.0	4.6-8.0
Phenylpyruvic acid, qualitative	Negative	Negative
Phosphate	0.4-1.3 g/24 h	13-42 mmol/d
Porphobilinogen		
Qualitative	Negative	Negative
Quantitative	<2 mg/24 h	<9 µmol/d
Porphyrins		
Coproporphyrin	50-250 µg/24 h	77-380 nmol/d
Uroporphyrin	10-30 µg/24 h	12-36 nmol/d
Potassium	25-125 mEq/24 h	25-125 mmol/d
Pregnanediol		
Males	0.0-1.9 mg/24 h	0.0-6.0 µmol/d
Females		
Proliferative phase	0.0-2.6 mg/24 h	0.0-8.0 µmol/d
Luteal phase	2.6-10.6 mg/24 h	8-33 µmol/d
Postmenopausal	0.2-1.0 mg/24 h	0.6-3.1 µmol/d
Pregnanetriol	0.0-2.5 mg/24 h	0.0-7.4 µmol/d
Protein, total		
Qualitative	Negative	Negative
Quantitative	10-150 mg/24 h	10-150 mg/d
Protein-to-creatinine ratio	<0.2	<0.2

Continued

Reference Intervals* for Clinical Chemistry (Urine)—cont'd

Analyte	Conventional Units	SI Units
Sodium (regular diet)	60-260 mEq/24 h	60-260 mmol/d
Specific gravity		
Random specimen	1.003-1.030	1.003-1.030
24-h collection	1.015-1.025	1.015-1.025
Urate (regular diet)	250-750 mg/24 h	1.5-4.4 mmol/d
Urobilinogen	0.5-4.0 mg/24 h	0.6-6.8 µmol/d
Vanillylmandelic acid (VMA)	1.0-8.0 mg/24 h	5-40 µmol/d

*Values can vary depending on the method used.
Abbreviation: SI = International System of Units.

Reference Intervals for Toxic Substances

Analyte	Conventional Units	SI Units
Arsenic, urine	<130 µg/24 h	<1.7 µmol/d
Bromides, serum, inorganic	<100 mg/dL	<10 mmol/L
Toxic symptoms	140-1000 mg/dL	14-100 mmol/L
Carboxyhemoglobin, blood	Saturation, percent	
Urban environment	<5%	<0.05
Smokers	<12%	<0.12
Symptoms		
Headache	>15%	>0.15
Nausea and vomiting	>25%	>0.25
Potentially lethal	>50%	>0.50
Ethanol, blood	<0.05 mg/dL, <0.005%	<1.0 mmol/L
Intoxication	>100 mg/dL, >0.1%	>22 mmol/L
Marked intoxication	300-400 mg/dL, 0.3%-0.4%	65-87 mmol/L
Alcoholic stupor	400-500 mg/dL, 0.4%-0.5%,	87-109 mmol/L
Coma	>500 mg/dL, >0.5%	>109 mmol/L
Lead, blood		
Adults	<20 µg/dL	<1.0 µmol/L
Children	<10 µg/dL	<0.5 µmol/L
Lead, urine	<80 µg/24 h	<0.4 µmol/d
Mercury, urine	<10 µg/24 h	<150 nmol/d

Abbreviation: SI = International System of Units.

Reference Intervals for Tests Performed on Cerebrospinal Fluid

Test	Conventional Units	SI Units
Cells	<5 mm^3; all mononuclear	<5 × 10^6/L, all mononuclear
Protein electrophoresis	Albumin predominant	Albumin predominant
Glucose	50-75 mg/dL (20 mg/dL less than in serum)	2.8-4.2 mmol/L (1.1 mmol/L less than in serum)
IgG		
Children <14 y	<8% of total protein	<0.08 of total protein
Adults	<14% of total protein	<0.14 of total protein
IgG index	0.3-0.6	0.3-0.6
Oligoclonal banding on electrophoresis	Absent	Absent
Pressure, opening	70-180 mm H$_2$O	70-180 mm H$_2$O
Protein, total	15-45 mg/dL	150-450 mg/L

Abbreviations: Ig = immunoglobulin; SI = International System of Units.

Reference Intervals for Tests of Gastrointestinal Function

Test	Conventional Units
Bentiromide	6-h urinary arylamine excretion >57% excludes pancreatic insufficiency
β-Carotene, serum	60-250 ng/dL
Fecal fat estimation	
Qualitative	No fat globules seen by high-power microscope
Quantitative	<6 g/24 h (>95% coefficient of fat absorption)
Gastric acid output	
Basal	
Males	0.0-10.5 mmol/h
Females	0.0-5.6 mmol/h
Maximum (after histamine or pentagastrin)	
Males	9.0-48.0 mmol/h
Females	6.0-31.0 mmol/h
Ratio: basal/maximum	
Males	0.0-0.31
Females	0.0-0.29
Secretin test, pancreatic fluid	
Volume	>1.8 mL/kg/h
Bicarbonate	>80 mEq/L
D-Xylose absorption test, urine	>20% of ingested dose excreted in 5 h

Reference Intervals for Tests of Immunologic Function

Test	Conventional Units	SI Units
Autoantibodies, Serum, Adult		
Anti-CCP antibody	0-19 U	
Anti-dsDNA antibody	0-40 IU	0-40 IU
Antinuclear antibody	<1:40	
Rheumatoid factor (total IgG, IgA, IgM)	0-30 mg/dL	
Complement, Serum		
C3	85-175 mg/dL	0.85-1.75 g/L
C4	15-45 mg/dL	150-450 mg/L
Total hemolytic (CH$_{50}$)	150-250 U/mL	150-250 U/mL
Immunoglobulins, Serum, Adult		
IgA	70-310 mg/dL	0.70-3.1 g/L
IgD	0.0-6.0 mg/dL	0.0-60 mg/L
IgE	0.0-430 ng/dL	0.0-430 mg/L
IgG	640-1350 mg/dL	6.4-13.5 g/L
IgM	90-350 mg/dL	0.90-3.5 g/L

Helper-to-suppressor ratio: 0.8-1.8

Abbreviations: anti-CCP = anticyclic citrullinated peptide; dsDNA = double-stranded DNA; Ig = immunoglobulin; SI = International System of Units.

Reference Intervals for Lymphocyte Subsets, Whole Blood, Heparinized

Antigen(s) Expressed	Cell Type	Percentage	Absolute Cell Count
CD2	E rosette T cells	73-87%	1040-2160
CD3	Total T cells	56-77%	860-1880
CD3 and CD4	Helper-inducer cells	32-54%	550-1190
CD3 and CD8	Suppressor-cytotoxic cells	24-37%	430-1060
CD3 and DR	Activated T cells	5-14%	70-310
CD16 and CD56	Natural killer (NK) cells	8-22%	130-500
CD19	Total B cells	7-17%	140-370

Reference Values for Semen Analysis

Test	Conventional Units	SI Units
Volume	2-5 mL	2-5 mL
Liquefaction	Complete in 15 min	Complete in 15 min
pH	7.2-8.0	7.2-8.0
Leukocytes	Occasional or absent	Occasional or absent
Spermatozoa		
Count	60-150 × 10^6 mL	60-150 × 10^6 mL
Fructose	>150 mg/dL	>8.33 mmol/L
Morphology	80-90% normal forms	>0.80-0.90 normal
Motility	>80% motile	>0.80 motile

Abbreviation: SI = International System of Units.

Toxic Chemical Agents Reference Chart: Symptoms and Treatment

Method of
James J. James, MD, DrPH, MHA, and James M. Lyznicki, MS, MPH

Toxic chemical agents are poisonous vapors, aerosols, gasses, liquids, or solids that have toxic effects on people, animals, or plants. Most of these agents are liquid at room temperature and are disseminated as vapors and aerosols. They may be released as bombs, sprayed from aircraft and boats, or disseminated by other means to intentionally create a hazard to people and the environment. Some of these agents are highly toxic and persistent, features that can render a site uninhabitable and require costly and potentially hazardous decontamination and remediation. Health effects range from irritation and burning of skin and mucous membranes to rapid cardiopulmonary collapse and death.

Efficient deployment of hazardous materials (HazMat) teams is critical to control a chemical agent attack. Although all major cities and emergency medical systems have plans and equipment in place to address this situation, physicians and other health professionals must be aware of principles involved in managing a patient or multiple patients exposed to these agents. Chemical weapon agents have a high potential for secondary contamination from victims to responders. This requires that medical treatment facilities have clearly defined procedures for handling contaminated casualties, many of whom will transport themselves to the facility. Precautions must be used until thorough decontamination has been performed or the specific chemical agent is identified. Health care professionals must first protect themselves (e.g., by using protective suits, respiratory protection, and chemical-resistant gloves) because secondary contamination with even small amounts of these substances (particularly nerve agents such as VX) may be lethal.

Primary detection of exposure to chemical agents will be based on the signs and symptoms of the potential victim (Table 1). Confirmation of a chemical agent, using detection equipment or laboratory analyses, will take considerable time and will not likely contribute to the early management of mass casualty victims. Several patients presenting with the same symptoms should alert physicians and hospital staff to the possibility of a chemical attack. If a chemical attack occurs, most victims will likely arrive within a short time. This situation differentiates a chemical attack from a biological attack involving infectious microorganisms. Additional diagnostic clues include:

- Unusual temporal or geographic clustering of illness
- Any sudden increase in illness in previously healthy persons
- Sudden increase in non-specific syndromes (e.g., sudden unexplained weakness in previously healthy persons; dimmed or blurred vision; hypersecretion, inhalation, or burn-like syndrome)

A coordinated communication network is critical for transmitting reliable information from the incident scene to treatment facilities. Any suspicious or confirmed exposure to a chemical weapons agent should be reported to the local health department, local Federal Bureau of Investigations office, and the Centers for Disease Control and Prevention (1-770-488-7100).

TABLE 1 Quick Reference Chart on Chemical Weapon Agents

Chemical Agent	Diagnostic Considerations	Treatment Considerations*
Cyanides Cyanogen chloride (CK) Hydrogen cyanide (AC)	• Symptom onset: rapid, seconds to minutes • Odor: bitter almond, musty, or chlorine-like • Nonspecific hypoxic and hypoxemic symptoms • Binds cellular cytochrome oxidase causing chemical asphyxia • Respiratory: shortness of breath, chest tightness, hyperventilation, respiratory arrest • GI: nausea, vomiting • Cardiovascular: ventricular arrhythmias, hypotension, cardiac arrest, shock • CNS: anxiety, headache drowsiness, weakness, apnea, convulsions, seizure, coma • CNS effects may be confused with carbon monoxide and hydrogen sulfide poisoning • Metabolic acidosis and increased concentration of venous oxygen (patient also may present with cyanosis) • Laboratory testing: cyanide, thiocyanate, serum lactate levels; venous and arterial partial oxygen pressure	• Immediate treatment of symptomatic patients is critical • Antidote: sodium nitrite and sodium thiosulfate; repeat one-half initial doses of both agents in 30 minutes if there is inadequate clinical response • Amyl nitrate capsules are available for first aid until intravenous access is achieved • Cyanide antidone kits are commercially available • Investigational in the United States, available in Europe: hydroxycobalamin (vitamin B_{12a}) administered with thiosulfate • Activated charcoal[A] for oral exposure • Mechanical ventilation as needed • Circulatory support with crystalloids and vasopressors • Metabolic acidosis corrected with IV sodium bicarbonate • Seizures controlled with benzodiazepines
Incapacitating Agents Agent 15 3-quinuclidinyl benzilate (BZ)	• Symptom onset: hours 0-4 h: parasympathetic blockade and mild CNS effects 4-20 h: stupor with ataxia and hyperthermia 20-96 h: full-blown delirium Resolution phase: paranoia, deep sleep, reawakening, crawling, climbing automatisms, eventual reorientation • Odorless	• Antidote: physostigmine salicylate (Antilirium)[A] • Support, intravenous fluids

[A]Not FDA approved for this indication.
*Different situations may require different treatment and dosage regimens. Please consult other references as well as a regional poison control center (1-800-222-1222), medical toxicologist, clinical pharmacologist, or other drug information specialist for definitive dosage information, especially dosages for pregnant women and children.
Abbreviations: CNS = central nervous system; GI = gastrointestinal.

TABLE 1 Quick Reference Chart on Chemical Weapon Agents—cont'd

Chemical Agent	Diagnostic Considerations	Treatment Considerations*
Nerve Agents Cyclohexyl sarin (GF) Sarin (GB) Soman (GD) Tabun (GA) VX	• Competitive inhibitor of acetylcholine muscarinic receptor • Mydriasis, blurred vision, dry mouth, dry skin, possible atropine-like flush, initial rise in heart rate, decreased level of consciousness, confusion, disorientation, visual hallucinations, impaired memory • Symptom onset: vapor (seconds), liquid (minutes or hours); symptom onset may be delayed up to 18 hours particularly for localized exposures • Odor: none (GB, VX), fruity (GA), camphor-like (GD) • Most toxic of known chemical agents • Irreversible acetylcholinesterase inhibitors • Eyes: excessive lacrimation, miosis may be present • Respiratory: rhinorrhea, bronchospasm, respiratory failure • GI: hypersalivation, nausea, vomiting, diarrhea • Skin: localized sweating • Cardiac: sinus bradycardia • Skeletal muscles: fasciculations followed by weakness, flaccid paralysis • CNS: loss of consciousness, convulsions, apnea, seizures • May be confused with organophosphate and carbamate pesticide poisoning • Laboratory testing: erythrocyte or serum cholinesterase activity to confirm exposure	• Rapid establishment of patent airway • Antidote: Atropine[A] and pralidoxime[A] chloride (Protopam chloride, 2-PAM); additional doses until bronchial secretions are cleared and ventilation improved • Early administration of 2-PAM is critical to minimize permanent agent inactivation of acetylcholinesterase (i.e., "aging") • Benzodiazepines to control nerve agent-induced seizures • Airway and ventilatory support as needed • Atropine,[A] pralidoxime,[A] and diazepam[A] are available in autoinjector kits through the U.S. military
Pulmonary or Choking Agents Acrolein Ammonia (NH3) Chlorine (CL) Choloropicrin (PS) Diphosgene (DP) Nitrogen oxides (NO$_x$) Perflouroisobutylene (PFIB) Phosgene (CG) Sulfur dioxide (SO$_2$)	• Symptom onset: rapid or delayed; 1-24 h (rarely up to 72 h) • Odor (CG): freshly mown hay or grass • Easily absorbed via mucous membranes of eyes, nose, oropharynx. Degree of water solubility of the agent influences onset and severity of respiratory injury. • Eye and airway irritation, dyspnea, chest tightness, rhinorrhea, hypersalivation, cough, wheezing • High dose inhalation may produce laryngospasm, pneumonitis, and acute lung injury with delayed onset (≤48 h) of acute respiratory distress syndrome • Chest radiograph: hyperinflation, noncardiogenic pulmonary edema • May be confused with inhalation exposure to industrial chemicals (e.g., HCl, Cl$_2$, NH$_3$)	• No specific antidote • Supportive measures; specific treatment depends on the agent • IV fluids for hypotension; no diuretics • Ventilation with or without positive airway pressure • Bronchodilators for bronchospasm • Methylprednisolone[A] may be effective in preventing noncardiogenic pulmonary edema
Riot Control Agents Mace (CN) Tear gas (CS)	• Symptom onset: immediate • Odor: apple blossom (CN); pepper (CS) • Metallic taste • SN$_2$ alkylating agents • Burning and pain on mucosal membranes and skin • Eyes: irritation, pain, tearing, blepharospasm • Airways: burning in nose and mouth, respiratory discomfort, bronchospam (may be delayed 36 h) • Skin: tingling, erythema • Nausea and vomiting common • CN can cause corneal opacification • No specific laboratory tests	• Supportive care • Irrigation as necessary • Persons with asthma, emphysema may need oxygen, inhaled bronchodilators, steroids, assisted ventilation • Lotions, such as calamine,[A] for persistent erythema
Vesicant or Blister Agents	• Symptoms onset: immediate (L, CX); delayed 2-48 h (H, HD) • Primary liquid hazard • May be confused with skin exposure to caustic irritants (e.g., sodium hydroxide, ammonia) • Intracellular enzyme and DNA alkylating agents • Clinical effects dependent on extent and route of exposure; effects may be delayed, appearing hours after exposure	• Immediate decontamination • Supportive care • Thermal burn-type treatment • Symptomatic management of lesions
Sulfur mustard (H) Distilled mustard (HD)	• Odor: garlic, horseradish, or mustard • Skin: erythema and blisters (may be delayed ≤8 h), pruritus • Eye: irritation, conjunctivitis, corneal damage, lacrimation, pain, blepharospasm • Respiratory: mild to marked acute airway damage, pneumonitis within 1-3 d, respiratory failure • GI effects (nausea, vomiting diarrhea) may be present • Bone marrow stem cell suppression leading to pancytopenia and increased susceptibility to infection	• No specific antidote • Skin: silver sulfadiazine[A] • Eye: homatropine[A] ophthalmic ointment • Pulmonary: antibiotics, bronchodilators, steroids • Colony stimulating factor may be helpful for leukopenia • Systemic analgesic and antipruritics • Early use of positive-end expiratory pressure or continuous positive airway pressure

Continued

TABLE 1 Quick Reference Chart on Chemical Weapon Agents—cont'd

Chemical Agent	Diagnostic Considerations	Treatment Considerations*
Lewisite (L)	• Fever, sputum production • Combination with Lewisite (called mustard-Lewisite or HL) results in rapid effects of Lewisite and delayed effects of mustard agents • Odor: fruity or geranium • More volatile than mustard • Damages eyes, skin, and airways by direct contact • Skin: gray area of dead skin within 5 min, erythema within 30 min, blistering 2-3 h, immediate irritation or burning pain on contact, severe tissue necrosis • Eye: pain, blepharospasm, conjunctival and lid edema • Airway: pseudomembrane formation, nasal irritation • Intravascular fluid loss, hypovolemia, shock, organ congestion, leukocytosis	• Maintain fluid and electrolyte balance (do not excessively fluid resuscitate as in thermal burns) • Antidote: British Anti-Lewisite (BAL or Dimercaprol)
Phosgene Oxime (CX)	• Odor: freshly mown hay • Urticant, nonvesicant agent • Vapor extremely irritating; vapor and liquid cause tissue damage upon contact • Immediate burning, irritation, wheal-like skin lesions, eye and airway damage, conjunctivitis, lacrimation, lid edema, blepharospasm • No distinctive laboratory findings	• No antidote • Parenteral methylprednisolone[A] may be effective in preventing noncardiogenic pulmonary edema • Experimental: aerosolized dexamethasone[A] and theophylline[A] for pulmonary involvement
Vomiting (Arsine-Based) Agents Adamsite (DM) Diphenylchlorarsine (DA) Diphenylcyanoarsine (DC)	• Symptom onset: All rapidly acting within minutes • Odor: none (DA), garlic (DC), burning fireworks (DM) • Primary route of absorption is through respiratory system • Arsine gas depletes erythrocyte glutathione and causes hemolysis • Eyes: conjunctival irritation, tearing, and blepharospasm • Airways: sneezing, mucosal lung irritation, edema, progressive cough, wheezing • Cardiac: tachypnea, tachycardia • GI: intestinal cramps, emesis, diarrhea • Skin: erythema, edema at the site of dermal contact • CNS: depression, syncope • Chest radiograph to rule out chemical pneumonitis	• Supportive care • Monitor for hemolysis • Wheezing or dyspnea; may need albuterol inhalation • Eye irrigation (water, normal saline, lactated Ringer's solution) in patients sustaining ocular exposure • Treat repetitive emesis with IV hydration and antiemetics • Blood transfusion may be required • Exchange transfusion may be required • Hemodialysis may be useful in decreasing arsenic level and treating renal failure

Biologic Agents Reference Chart—Symptoms, Tests, and Treatment

Method of
James J. James, MD, DrPH, MHA, and James M. Lyznicki, MS, MPH

Biologic weapons are devices used intentionally to cause disease or death through dissemination of microorganisms or toxins in food and water, by insect vectors, or by aerosols. Potential targets include human beings, food crops, livestock, and other resources essential for national security, economy, and defense. Unlike nuclear, chemical, and conventional weapons, the onset of a biological attack will probably be insidious. For some infectious agents, secondary and tertiary transmission may continue for weeks or months after the initial attack.

Initial detection of an unannounced biological attack will likely occur when an astute health professional notices an unusual case or disease cluster and reports his or her concerns to local public health authorities. Physicians and other health professionals should be alert to the following:

- Unusual temporal or geographic clustering of illnesses
- Sudden increase of illness in previously healthy persons
- Sudden increase in non-specific illnesses (e.g., pneumonia, flulike illness; bleeding disorders; unexplained rashes, particularly in adults; neuromuscular illness; diarrhea)

To enhance detection and treatment capabilities, physicians and other health professionals in acute care settings should be familiar with the clinical manifestations, diagnostic techniques, isolation precautions, treatment, and prophylaxis for likely causative agents (e.g., smallpox, pneumonic plague, anthrax, viral hemorrhagic fevers). Table 1 provides a quick summary of diagnostic and treatment considerations for various infectious and toxic biological agents. For some of these agents, delay in medical response could result in a potentially devastating number of casualties. To mitigate such consequences, early identification and intervention are imperative. Front-line physicians must have an increased level of suspicion regarding the possible intentional use of biological agents as well as an increased sensitivity to reporting those suspicious to public health authorities, who, in turn, must be willing to evaluate a predictable increase in false positive reports.

Medical response efforts require coordination and planning with emergency management agencies, law enforcement, health care facilities, and social services agencies. Health care agencies should ensure that physicians know whom to call with reports of suspicious cases and clusters of infectious diseases, and should work to build a good relationship with the local medical community. Resource integration is absolutely necessary to:

- Establish adequate capacity to initiate rapid investigation of an outbreak
- Educate the public
- Begin mass distribution of antibiotics and vaccines
- Ensure mass medical care
- Control public anger and fear

In an epidemic, overwhelming numbers of critically ill patients will require acute and follow-up medical care. Both infected persons and the *worried well* will seek medical attention, with a corresponding need for medical supplies, diagnostic tests, and hospital beds. The impact — or even the threat — of an attack can elicit widespread panic and civil disorder, overwhelm hospital resources, and disrupt social services.

Any suspicious or confirmed exposure to a biological weapons agent should be reported immediately to the local health department, local Federal Bureau of Investigation office, and the Centers of Disease Control and Prevention (1-770-488-7100).

TABLE 1 Quick Reference Chart on Biological Weapon Agents

Disease/Agent	Diagnostic Considerations	Treatment Considerations[1]	Prophylaxis
Bacteria Anthrax *Bacillus anthracis*	Incubation period: 1-5 d (perhaps ≤60 d)[2] *Cutaneous:* • Evolving skin lesion (face, neck, arms), progresses to vesicle, dispressed ulcer, and black necrotic lesions • Lethality: 20% if untreated, otherwise rarely fatal *Gastrointestinal* • Nausea, vomiting, abdominal pain, bloody diarrhea, sepsis • Lethality: approaches 100% if untreated but data are limited; rapid, aggressive treatment may reduce mortality *Inhalational* • Abrupt onset of flu-like symptoms, fever with or without chills, sweats, fatigue or malaise, non- or minimally productive cough, nausea, vomiting, dyspnea, headache, chest pain, followed in 2-5 d by severe respiratory distress, mediastinitis, hemorrhagic meningitis, sepsis, shock.[3] • Widened mediastinum on chest radiograph is characteristic for inhalational and occasionally GI anthrax.[4]	Combination therapy of ciprofloxacin (Cipro) or doxycycline (Vibramycin) plus one or two other antimicrobials should be considered with inhalational anthrax[6] Penicillin[A] should be considered if strain is susceptible and does not possess inducible β-lactamases If meningitis suspected, doxycycline (Vibramycin) may be less optimal because of poor CNS penetration Steroids may be considered for severe edema and for meningitis.	Ciprofloxacin (Cipro) or doxycycline (Vibramycin) with or without vaccination If strain is susceptible, penicillin[A] or amoxicillin[A] (Amoxil) should be considered Inactivated vaccine (licensed but not readily available); six injections and annual booster

Continued

TABLE 1 Quick Reference Chart on Biological Weapon Agents—cont'd

Disease/Agent	Diagnostic Considerations	Treatment Considerations[1]	Prophylaxis
	• Lethality: Once respiratory distress develops, mortality rates may approach 90%; begin treatment when inhalational anthrax is suspected, do not wait for confirmatory testing.[5] Gram stain and culture of blood, pleural fluid, cerebrospinal fluid, ascitic fluid, vesicular fluid or lesion exudate; sputum rarely positive; confirmatory serological and PCR tests available through public health laboratory network		
Brucellosis *B. abortus* *B. canis* *B. mellitensis* *B. suis*	Incubation period: 5-60 d (usually 1-2 mo) • Non-specific flu-like symptoms, fever, headache, profound weakness and fatigue, GI symptoms such as anorexia, nausea, vomiting, diarrhea, or constipation • Osteoarticular complications common • Lethality: less than 5% even if untreated; tends to incapacitate rather than kill. Blood and bone marrow culture (may require 6 wk to grow *Brucella*); confirmatory culture and serological testing available through public health laboratory network	Doxycycline (Vibramycin) plus streptomycin or rifampin[A] (Rifadin) *Alternative therapies:* Ofloxacin (Floxin)[A] plus rifampin[A] (Rifadin) Doxycycline (Vibramycin) plus gentamicin (Garamycin) TMP/SMX (Bactrim,[A] Septra) plus gentamicin (Garamycin)	Doxycycline (Vibramycin) plus streptomycin or rifampin (Rifadin) No approved human vaccine
Inhalational (Pneumonic) Tularemia *Francisella tularensis*	Incubation period: 3-5 d (range of 1-21 d) • Sudden onset of acute febrile illness, weakness, chills, headache, generalized body aches, elevated WBCs • Pulmonary symptoms such as dry cough, chest pain or tightness with or without objective signs of pneumonia • Progressive weakness, malaise, anorexia, and weight loss occurs, potentially leading to sepsis and organ failure • Largely clinical diagnosis • Lethality: ≈30-60% fatal if untreated Culture of blood, sputum, biopsies, pleural fluid, bronchial washings (culture is difficult and potentially dangerous); confirmatory testing available through public health laboratory network	Streptomycin or gentamicin (Garamycin) *Alternative therapies:* Ciprofloxacin (Cipro)[A] Doxycycline (Vibramycin) Chloramphenicol[A] (Chloromycetin)	Tetracycline Doxycycline (Vibramycin) Ciprofloxacin (Cipro)[A] Live attenuated vaccine (USAMRIID, IND) given by scarification; currently under FDA review; limited availability
Pneumonic Plague *Yersinia pestis*	Incubation period: 1-10 d (typically 2-3 d) • Acute onset of flu-like prodrome: fever, myalgia, weakness, headache; within 24 h of prodrome, chest discomfort, cough with bloody sputum, and dyspnea. By day 2 to 4 illness, symptoms progressing to cyanosis, respiratory distress, and hemodynamic instability	Streptomycin; gentamicin (Garamycin) *Alternative therapies:* Doxycycline (Vibramycin) Tetracycline Ciprofloxacin[A] (Cipro) Chloramphenicol[A] (Chloromycetin) is first choice for meningitis except for pregnant women	Tetracycline Doxycycline (Vibramycin) Ciprofloxacin[A] (Cipro) Inactivated whole cell vaccine licensed but not readily available; injection with boosters Vaccine not effective against aerosol exposure

TABLE 1 Quick Reference Chart on Biological Weapon Agents—cont'd

Disease/Agent	Diagnostic Considerations	Treatment Considerations[1]	Prophylaxis
	• Lethality: almost 100% if untreated; 20–60% if appropriately treated within 18-24 h of symptoms; begin treatment when diagnosis of plague is suspected; do not wait for confirmatory testing Gram stain and culture of blood, CSF, sputum, lymph node aspirates, bronchial washings; confirmatory serological and bacteriological tests available through public health laboratory network		
Rickettsia Q-Fever *Coxiella burnetii*	Incubation period: 2-14 d (may be ≤40 days) • Nonspecific febrile disease, chills, cough, weakness and fatigue, pleuritic chest pain, pneumonia possible • Lethality: 1-3%. Fatalities are uncommon even if untreated but relapsing symptoms may occur Isolation of organism may be difficult; confirmatory testing via serology or PCR available through public health laboratory network	Tetracycline Doxycycline (Vibramycin)	Tetracycline Doxycycline (Vibramycin) Inactivated whole cell[B] vaccine (IND) Skin test to determine prior exposure to *C. burnetii* recommended before vaccination
Viruses Smallpox Variola major virus	Incubation period: 7-17 d • Prodrome of high fever, malaise, prostration, headache, vomiting, delirium followed in 2-3 d maculopapular rash uniformly progressing to pustules and scabs, mostly on extremities and face • Requires astute clinical evaluation; may be confused with chickenpox, erythema multiforme with bullae, or allergic contact dermatitis • Lethality: 30% in unvaccinated persons Pharyngeal swab, vesicular fluid, biopsies, scab material for electron microscopy and PCR testing through public health laboratory network Notify CDC Poxvirus Section at 1-404-639-2184	Supportive care Cidofovir (Vistide) shown to be effective in vitro and in experimental animals infected with surrogate orthopox virus	Live attenuated vaccinia vaccine derived from calf lymph; given by scarification (licensed, restricted supply) New vaccine being developed from tissue culture Vaccination given within 3-4 d following exposure can prevent or decrease the severity of disease
Viral Encephalitis Eastern (EEE) Western (WEE) Venezuelan (VEE)	Incubation period: 2-6 d (VEE); 7-14 d (EEE, WEE) • Systemic febrile illness, with encephalitis developing in some populations • Generalized malaise, spiking fevers, headache, myalgia • Incidence of seizures and/or focal neurologic deficits may be higher after biological attack • White blood cell count may show striking leukopenia and lymphopenia • Clinical and epidemiologic diagnosis • Lethality: <10% (VEE); 10% (WEE); 50-75% (EEE)	Supportive care Analgesics, anticonvulsants as needed	Several IND vaccines, poorly immunogenic, highly reactogenic

Continued

TABLE 1 Quick Reference Chart on Biological Weapon Agents—cont'd

Disease/Agent	Diagnostic Considerations	Treatment Considerations[1]	Prophylaxis
Viral Hemorrhagic Fevers (VHFs) Arenaviruses (Lassa, Junin, and related viruses) Bunyaviruses (Hanta, Congo-Crimean, Rift Valley) Filoviruses (Ebola, Marburg) Flaviviruses (yellow fever, dengue, various tick-borne disease viruses)	Confirmatory test and viral isolation available through public health laboratory network Incubation period: 4-21 d • Fever with mucous membrane bleeding, petechiae, thrombocytopenia and hypotension in patients without underlying malignancies • Malaise, myalgias, headache, vomiting, diarrhea possible • Lethality: Variable depending on viral strain; 15-25% with Lassa fever to ≤ 90% with Ebola Confirmatory testing and viral isolation available through public health laboratory network Call CDC Special Pathogens Office at 1-404-639-1115	Supportive therapy Ribavirin (Virazole)A may be effective for Lassa fever, Rift Valley fever, Argentine hemorrhagic fever, and Congo-Crimean hemorrhagic fever	Ribavarin (Virazole)[A] is suggested for Congo-Crimean hemorrhagic fever and Lassa fever Yellow fever vaccine is the only licensed vaccine available Vaccines for some of the other VHFs exist but are for investigational use only
Biological Toxins **Botulism** *Clostridium botulinum* toxin	Symptom onset: 1-5 d (typically 12-36 h) • Blurred vision, diplopia, dry mouth, ptosis, fatigue • As disease progresses, acute bilateral descending flaccid paralysis, respiratory paralysis resulting in death • Clinical diagnosis • Lethality: 60% without ventilatory support Serum and stool should be assayed for toxin by mouse neutralization bioassay, which may require several days	Intensive and prolonged supportive care; ventilation may be necessary Trivalent equine antitoxin (serotypes A, B, E, — licensed, available from the CDC) should be administered immediately after clinical diagnosis Anaphylaxis and serum sickness are potential complications of antitoxin Aminoglycosides and clindamycin (Cleocin)A must not be used	Pentavalent toxoid (A-E), yearly booster (IND, CDC) Not available to the public Antitoxin may be sufficient to prevent illness following exposure but is not recommended until patient is showing symptoms
Enterotoxin B *Staphylococcus aureus*	Symptom onset: 3-12 h • Acute onset of fever, chills headache, nonproductive cough • Normal chest radiograph • Clinical diagnosis • Lethality: probably low (few data available for respiratory exposure) Serology on acute and convalescent serum can confirm diagnosis	Supportive care	No vaccine available
Ricin toxin *Ricinus communis*	Symptom onset: ≤6-24 h • Weakness, nausea, chest tightness, fever, cough, pulmonary edema, respiratory failure, circulatory collapse, hypoxemia resulting in death (usually within 36-72 h) • Clinical and epidemiological diagnosis • Lethality: mortality data not available but is likely to be high with extensive exposure Confirmatory serological testing available through public health laboratory network	Supportive care Treatment for pulmonary edema Gastric decontamination if toxin ingested	No vaccine available
T-2 Mycotoxins *Fusarium* *Myrothecium* *Trichoderma* *Stachybotrys*	Symptom onset: minutes to hours • Abrupt onset of mucocutaneous and airway irritation and pain • May include skin, eyes, and GI tract; systemic toxicity may follow	Clinical support Soap and water washing within 4-6 h reduces dermal toxicity; washing within 1 h may eliminate toxicity entirely	No vaccine available

TABLE 1 Quick Reference Chart on Biological Weapon Agents—cont'd

Disease/Agent	Diagnostic Considerations	Treatment Considerations[1]	Prophylaxis
Other filamentous fungi	• Lethality: severe exposure can cause death in hours to days Consult with local health department regarding specimen collection and diagnostic testing procedures; confirmation requires testing blood, tissue, and environmental samples		

[A]Not FDA approved for this indication.
[B]Not available in the United States.
[1]Different situations may require different dosage and treatment regimens. Please consult other references and an infectious disease specialist for definitive dosage information, especially dosages for pregnant women and children.
[2]Data from 22 patients infected with anthrax in October and November 2001 indicate a median incubation period of 4 d (range 4-7 d) for inhalational anthrax and a mean incubation of 5 d (range 1-10 d) for cutaneous anthrax.
[3]Limited data from the October/November 2001 anthrax infections indicate hemorrhagic pleural effusions to be strongly associated with inhalational anthrax; rhinorrhea was present in only 1/10 patients.
[4]Chest radiograph abnormalities include paratracheal and hilar fullness and may be subtle. Consider chest computed tomography if diagnosis is uncertain.
[5]Limited data from the 2001 terrorist-related anthrax infections indicate that early treatment significantly decreased the mortality rate.
[6]Other agents with in vitro activity suggested for use in conjunction with ciprofloxacin (Cipro) or doxycycline (Vibramycin) for treatment of inhalational anthrax include rifampin (Rifadin), vancomycin (Vancocin), imipenem (Primaxin), chloramphenicol (Chloromycetin), penicillin and ampicillin, clindamycin (Cleocin), and clarithromycin (Biaxin).
Abbreviations: CDC = Centers for Disease Control and Prevention; CNS = central nervous system; CSF = cerebrospinal fluid; GI = gastrointestinal; IND = investigational new drug; PCR = polymerase chain reaction; TMP-SMX = trimethoprim-sulfamethoxazole; USAMRIID, U.S. Army Medical Research Institute of Infectious Diseases; WBC = white blood cell.
Adopted for *Biological Weapons: Quick Reference Guide.* American Medical Association; 2002. Available at http://www.amaassn.org/ama1/pub/upload/mm/415/quickreference0902.pdf.

Some Popular Herbs and Nutritional Supplements

Method of
Miriam M. Chan, BSc, PharmD

Herb/Nutritional Supplement[1]	Common Uses	Reasonable Adult Oral Dosage*	Precautions and Drug Interactions
Bilberry fruit	Often used orally to improve visual acuity and to treat degenerative retinal conditions Also used orally to treat chronic venous insufficiency, varicose veins, and hemorrhoids Approved in Germany to use orally for acute diarrhea and topically for mild inflammation of the mucous membranes of the mouth and throat	For eye conditions and circulation, 80-160 mg tid of the extract standardized to at least 25% anthocyanosides For diarrhea, 20-60 g/d of the dried, ripe berries or as a tea preparation (5-10 g of crushed dried berries in 150 mL water, brought to a boil for 10 min, then strained) For external use, 10% decoction	No known side effects reported with bilberry fruit and extract However, bilberry leaf taken in large quantities or used long-term has been shown to cause wasting, anemia, jaundice, acute excitation, disturbances of tonus, and death in animals The anthocyanidin extracts from bilberry may increase the risk of bleeding in those taking warfarin (Coumadin) or other blood thinners
Black cohosh root	Commonly used to relieve hot flashes and other menopausal symptoms Also used to treat premenstrual discomfort and dysmenorrhea	20 mg bid of the rhizome extract standardized to triterpene glycosides The German guidelines do not recommend its use for >6 mo	Black cohosh may have an estrogen-like effect and should be avoided in women with breast cancer Large doses may induce miscarriage and it is contraindicated during pregnancy It may cause GI disturbances, headache, and hypotension International case reports of liver dysfunction suspected to be associated with its use
Black haw	To relieve uterine cramps and painful periods To prevent miscarriage and ease pain that follows childbirth	For menstrual pain, 5 mL of tincture in water, taken 3-5 times daily For prevention of miscarriage, 1-2 cups of tea per d (1 tsp of dried herb in 1 cup of boiling water, steeped for 10 min)	Black haw should not be used in pregnancy because of its uterine relaxant effects The salicylate constituent in black haw could trigger allergic reactions in persons with aspirin allergies or asthma Black haw can aggravate tinnitus Large doses of black haw can prolong bleeding time The oxalic acid component of black haw can increase kidney stone formation in susceptible persons Black haw can interact with warfarin and increase risk of bleeding
Chamomile flower	Used orally to calm nerves and treat GI spasms and inflammatory diseases of the GI tract Used topically to treat wounds, skin infections, and skin or mucous membrane inflammation	1 cup of freshly made tea 3-4 times daily (1 tbsp or 3 g of dried flower in 150 mL boiling water for 5-10 min)	Chamomile may cause an allergic reaction, especially in people with severe allergies to ragweed or other members of the daisy family (e.g., echinacea, feverfew, and milk thistle) Should not be taken concurrently with other sedatives, such as alcohol or benzodiazepines
Chaste tree berry (Chasteberry, Vitex)	For normalizing irregular menstrual periods and relieving premenstrual complaints For relieving menopausal symptoms For restoring fertility in women For treating acne associated with menstrual cycles	For menstrual irregularities and premenstrual complaints, 30-40 mg/d of the dried berries or an equivalent amount of aqueous-alcoholic extracts (50%-70% v/v) Dried fruit extract, standardized to 0.6%	Chaste tree berry can have uterine stimulant properties and should be avoided in pregnancy Women with hormone-dependent conditions (e.g., breast, uterine, and ovarian cancers, and endometriosis and uterine

Herb/Nutritional Supplement[1]	Common Uses	Reasonable Adult Oral Dosage*	Precautions and Drug Interactions
	Also for increasing breast milk production in lactating women	agnusides, is used in doses of 175-225 mg/d For other conditions, no established dosage documented	fibroids) and men with prostate cancer should avoid chaste tree berry because it contains progestins Side effects include intermenstrual bleeding, dry mouth, headache, nausea, rash, alopecia, and tachycardia High doses (≥480 mg/d extract) can paradoxically decrease lactation Chaste tree berry is thought to have dopaminergic effects and can interact with dopamine antagonists, such as antipsychotics and metoclopramide Chaste tree berry can also decrease the effects of oral contraceptives and hormone replacement therapy
Chondroitin	Orally, often used in combination with glucosamine for osteoarthritis Topically, in combination with sodium hyaluronate, as a viscoelastic agent in cataract surgery	Oral: 200-400 mg tid	Occasional mild side effects include nausea, indigestion, and allergic reactions Chondroitin derived from bovine cartilage carries a potential risk of contamination from diseased animals
Chromium	For diabetes For hypercholesterolemia Commonly found in weight-loss products Also promoted for body building	For diabetes, 100 µg bid for ≤4 mo or 500 µg bid for 2 mo For hypercholesterolemia, 200 µg tid or 500 µg bid for 2-4 mo For body building, 200-400 µg/d Chromium picolinate has been used in most studies, even though the chloride form is also available	Adverse effects are rare, but they may include headaches, insomnia, sleep disturbances, irritability and mood changes. Some patients also experience cognitive, perceptual, and motor dysfunction Long-term use of high doses (600-2400 µg/d) can cause anemia, thrombocytopenia, hemolysis, hepatic dysfunction, and renal failure Two case reports of interstitial nephritis A few studies suggest that chromium can cause DNA damage Chromium competes with iron for binding to transferrin and can cause iron deficiency Antacids, H_2 blockers, and proton pump inhibitors can decrease the absorption of chromium
Coenzyme Q10	As adjunctive treatment for congestive heart failure, angina, hypertension, and diabetes Also used for reducing cardiotoxicity associated with doxorubicin (Adriamycin)	For heart failure, 100 mg/d in two or three divided doses For angina, 50 mg tid For hypertension, 60 mg bid For diabetes, 100-200 mg/d	Mild adverse events include gastric distress, nausea, vomiting, and hypotension Doses >300 mg/d can cause elevated liver enzyme levels Coenzyme Q10 can reduce the anticoagulation effects of warfarin Oral hypoglycemic agents and HMG-CoA reductase inhibitors can reduce serum coenzyme Q10 levels
Cranberry	To prevent and treat UTIs or *Helicobacter pylori* infections that can lead to stomach ulcers To prevent dental plaque As an antioxidant to prevent cardiovascular disease and cancer	For UTIs, 150-600 mL of cranberry juice daily or 300-400 mg of standardized extract bid For other conditions, no dosage determined	Drinking excessive amounts of juice could cause GI upset or diarrhea Prolonged use of cranberry juice in large doses may increase the risk of kidney stone formation due to its high oxalate content Cranberry can interact with warfarin and cause an increase in INR

Herb/Nutritional Supplement[1]	Common Uses	Reasonable Adult Oral Dosage*	Precautions and Drug Interactions
			The effectiveness of proton pump inhibitors may be reduced by cranberry due to its acidity
Creatine	To enhance muscle performance, especially during short-duration, high-intensity exercise	Loading dose of 20 g/d for 5-7 d followed by a maintenance dose of ≥2 g/d An alternative dosing of 3 g/d for 28 d has been suggested	Creatine can cause gastroenteritis, diarrhea, heat intolerance, muscle cramps, and elevated serum creatinine levels Creatine is contraindicated in patients taking diuretics Concurrent use with cimetidine (Tagamet), probenecid, or NSAIDs increases the risk of adverse renal effects Caffeine can decrease creatine's ergogenic effects
Dehydroepi-androsterone (DHEA)	Replace low serum DHEA levels in adrenal insufficiency Treat SLE Reverse aging Used in many other conditions, including Alzheimer's disease, depression, diabetes, menopause, osteoporosis, impotence, and AIDS Used to promote weight loss Used by bodybuilders to increase muscle mass	For replacement therapy, 25-50 mg/d For SLE, 200 mg/d For antiaging and osteoporosis, 50 mg/d For other conditions, no established dosage documented	Most common side effects are androgenic in nature, and include acne, hair loss, hirsutism, and deepening of the voice Cases of hepatitis have been reported When used in high doses, DHEA can cause insomnia, manic symptoms, and palpitations DHEA at physiologic doses increases circulating androgens in women, but not in men; it also increases circulating estrogens in both men and women Should be avoided in persons with a history of sex hormone–dependent malignancy No information on the safety of DHEA in persons <30 y DHEA inhibits the cytochrome P450 3A4 isoenzyme (CYP3A4) and could increase serum concentrations of drugs metabolized by this isozyme, e.g., lovastatin (Mevacor), ketoconazole (Nizoral), itraconzaole (Sporanox), and triazolam (Halcion)
Dong quai root	Commonly used for the relief of premenstrual and menopausal symptoms Also used as a "blood tonic" and a strengthening treatment for the heart, spleen, liver, and kidneys	For premenstrual and menopausal symptoms, 3-4 g/d in three divided doses For other conditions, no established dosage documented	Dong quai should not be used in pregnant women due to its uterine stimulant and relaxant effects Women with hormone-sensitive conditions (e.g., breast, uterine, and ovarian cancers, and endometriosis and uterine fibroids) should avoid dong quai because of its estrogenic effects Drinking the essential oil of dong quai is not recommended because it contains a small amount of carcinogenic constituents Dong quai contains psoralens that can cause photosensitivity and photodermatitis Dong quai contains natural coumarin derivatives that can increase the risk of bleeding in those who are taking anticoagulant or antiplatelet drugs

Herb/Nutritional Supplement[1]	Common Uses	Reasonable Adult Oral Dosage*	Precautions and Drug Interactions
Echinacea	As an immune stimulant, particularly for preventing and treating the common cold and influenza Supportive therapy for lower urinary tract infections Used topically to treat skin disorders and promote wound healing	300 mg tid of *Echinacea pallida* root or 2-3 mL tid of expressed juice of *Echinace purpurea* herb Do not use for >8 wk because echinacea can suppress immunity if used long term	Echinacea should not be used in transplant patients and those with autoimmune disease or liver dysfunction Allergic reactions have been reported Adverse events are rare and can include mild GI effects It should be discontinued as far in advance of surgery as possible Echinacea can decrease the effectiveness of immunosuppressants
Ephedra (ma huang)	For diseases of the respiratory tract with mild bronchospasm Can be found in weight-loss products that are available online Also marketed as a stimulant for performance enhancement	1 tsp or 2 g of dried herb (15-30 mg of ephedrine) in 240 mL boiling water for 10 min In Canada, the maximum allowable dosage of ephedrine is 8 mg per dose or 32 mg per d	Ephedra contains ephedrine, which has sympathomimetic activities; consequently, it should not be used in patients who have cardiovascular disease, diabetes, glaucoma, hypertension, hyperthyroidism, prostate enlargement, psychiatric disorders, or seizures Serious adverse effects, including seizures, arrhythmias, heart attack, stroke, and death, have been associated with the use of ephedra; as a result, the FDA has banned the sale of ephedra products in the United States Because of the cardiovascular effects of ephedrine, patients taking ephedra should discontinue use at least 24 h before surgery Concurrent use of ephedra and digitalis, guanethidine, MAOIs, or other stimulants, including caffeine, is not recommended
Evening primrose oil	For PMS, especially if mastalgia is present For treatment of atopic eczema Also used for other medical conditions, including rheumatoid arthritis, menopausal symptoms, Raynaud's phenomenon, Sjögren's syndrome, and diabetic neuropathy	For PMS, 2-4 g/d For atopic eczema, 6-8 g/d For rheumatoid arthritis, 2.8 g/d These doses are based on products standardized to 9% γ-linolenic acid Daily dose can be given in divided doses	Evening primrose oil can increase the risk of pregnancy complications Side effects can include indigestion, nausea, soft stools, and headache Seizures have been reported in patients with schizophrenia who were taking phenothiazines and evening primrose oil concomitantly Evening primrose oil can interact with anesthesia and cause seizures Concomitant use of evening primrose oil with anticoagulant and antiplatelet drugs can increase the risk of bleeding
Fenugreek seed	For diabetes and hypercholesterolemia Also for constipation, dyspepsia, gastritis, and kidney ailments Approved in Germany for use orally for loss of appetite and topically as a poultice for local inflammation	For loss of appetite, 1-2 g of the seed tid or 1 cup of tea (500 mg seed in 150 mL cold water for 3 h) several times a d Maximum 6 g/d For other conditions, no established dosage documented For topical use, 50 g powdered seed in 250 mL of hot water to form a paste	Fenugreek can cause uterine contractions and should be avoided in pregnancy Persons who have allergies to peanuts or soybeans may also be allergic to fenugreek Fenugreek can cause diarrhea and flatulence; it can also make the urine smell like maple syrup Hypoglycemia can occur if fenugreek is taken in large amounts

Herb/Nutritional Supplement[1]	Common Uses	Reasonable Adult Oral Dosage*	Precautions and Drug Interactions
			Repeated external applications can result in undesirable skin reactions
			Fenugreek contains small amounts of coumarins and can interact with anticoagulants and antiplatelet drugs
			High mucilage content of fenugreek can affect the absorption of oral drugs; therefore, fenugreek should not be taken within 2 h of other drugs
Feverfew	For migraine headache prophylaxis For treatment of fever, menstrual problems, and arthritis	50-125 mg qd of the encapsulated dried leaf extract standardized to at least 0.2% parthenolide	Feverfew can induce menstrual bleeding and is contraindicated in pregnancy Fresh leaves can cause oral ulcers and GI irritation Sudden discontinuation of feverfew can precipitate rebound headache Feverfew can interact with anticoagulants and potentiate the antiplatelet effect of aspirin
Fish oils (omega-3 fatty acids)	Commonly used in treating hypertriglyceridemia Used to prevent CHD and stroke Also used in many noncardiac conditions, including depression, diabetes, dysmenorrhea, rheumatoid arthritis, and IgA nephropathy Used to reduce the risk of developing age-related maculopathy, Alzheimer's disease, and cancer Promotes visual and mental development in children	For hypertriglyceridemia, 3-5 g/d For cardioprotection, 1 g/d for patients with CHD; oily fish at least twice a wk, or about 0.5 g/d for people with no known heart disease For other conditions, no established dosage documented Fish oils are composed of EPA and DHA. Fish oil capsules vary widely in amounts and ratios of EPA and DHA. The most common fish oil capsules in the United States provide 180 mg of EPA and 120 mg DHA per capsule, and three capsules provide about 1 g/d of omega-3 fatty acids	Common side effects include fishy aftertaste, GI disturbances, belching, halitosis, and heartburn. High doses can cause nausea and loose stools Doses >3g/d can inhibit platelet aggregation, suppress immune function, increase blood glucose levels, and raise LDL cholesterol levels Long-term use may be associated with weight gain Less well-controlled preparations can contain appreciable amounts of organochloride contaminants Fish oil can increase the risk of bleeding in patients taking warfarin, an antiplatelet agent, or herbs that have antiplatelet constituents (e.g., garlic, ginkgo, and red clover) Fish oils can lower blood pressure and might have additive effects with antihypertensive agents Oral contraceptives can interfere with the triglyceride-lowering effects of fish oils
Flaxseed	Approved in Germany for chronic constipation, colons damaged by laxative abuse, irritable colon, diverticulitis, gastritis, and enteritis For hypercholesterolemia For hot flushes and breast pain	For constipation, 1 tbsp (10 g) of whole or "bruised" seeds in 150 mL of liquid 2-3 times daily For bowel inflammation, soak 2-3 tbsp of milled flaxseed in 200-300 mL water and strain after 30 min For hypercholesterolemia, 35-50 g of crushed seeds daily For hot flushes, 1-2 tbsp of ground flaxseed daily	Flaxseed should be taken with plenty of water to prevent possible intestinal blockage Patients with ileus should not take flaxseed High mucilage content of flaxseed can delay absorption of other drugs taken at the same time
Garlic	To lower blood pressure and serum cholesterol To prevent atherosclerosis	Fresh clove: one 4-g clove per d Tablet: 300 mg bid to tid standardized to 0.6%-1.3% allicin	Intake of large quantities can lead to stomach complaints Garlic has antiplatelet effects, so patients should discontinue use of garlic at least 7 d before surgery

Herb/Nutritional Supplement[1]	Common Uses	Reasonable Adult Oral Dosage*	Precautions and Drug Interactions
Ginger root	As an antiemetic For prevention of motion sickness	Fresh rhizome: 2-4 g/d Powdered ginger: 250 mg 3 to 4 times daily Tea: 1 cup of tea tid (0.5-1 g dried root in 150 mL boiling water for 5-10 min)	Concomitant use of garlic and anticoagulants can increase the risk of bleeding Ginger should not be used by patients with gallstones because of its cholagogic effect Can inhibit platelet aggregation; cases of postoperative bleeding have been reported Large doses of ginger can increase bleeding time in patients taking antiplatelet agents
Ginkgo biloba leaf	To slow cognitive deterioration in dementia To increase peripheral blood flow in claudication To treat sexual dysfunction associated with the use of SSRIs	60-120 mg bid of extract Egb761 standardized to 24% flavonoids and 6% terpenoids	Adverse effects are rare and include mild stomach or intestinal upset, headache, or allergic skin reaction Ginkgo can inhibit platelet aggregation; reports of spontaneous bleeding have been published Patients should discontinue ginkgo at least 36 h before surgery. Concurrent use of ginkgo and anticoagulants, antiplatelet agents, vitamin E, or garlic can increase the risk of bleeding
Ginseng root	As a tonic during times of stress, fatigue, disability, and convalescence To improve physical performance and stamina	Root: 1-2 g/d Tablet: 100 mg bid of extract standardized to 4%-7% ginsenosides A 2- to 3-wk period of using ginseng followed by a 1- to 2-wk rest period is generally recommended Ginseng is commonly adulterated, especially Siberian ginseng products	Ginseng has a mild stimulant effect and should be avoided in patients with cardiovascular disease Tachycardia and hypertension can occur Overdosages can lead to ginseng abuse syndrome, characterized by insomnia, hypotonia, and edema Ginseng has estrogenic effects and can cause vaginal bleeding and breast tenderness Ginseng has been shown to inhibit platelets, so patients should discontinue ginseng use at least 7 d before surgery Ginseng should not be used with other stimulants Patients taking antidiabetic agents and ginseng should be monitored to avoid the hypoglycemic effects of ginseng Ginseng can interact with warfarin and cause a decreased INR Siberian ginseng can increase digoxin levels Drug interaction between ginseng and phenelzine (an MAOI) resulting in insomnia, headache, tremulousness, and manic-like symptoms have been reported
Glucosamine	For osteoarthritis	500 mg tid with meals Glucosamine is available in the forms of sulfate, hydrochloride, or N-acetyl salt. Glucosamine sulfate	Side effects are generally limited to mild GI symptoms, including stomach upset, heartburn, diarrhea, nausea, and indigestion

Herb/Nutritional Supplement[1]	Common Uses	Reasonable Adult Oral Dosage*	Precautions and Drug Interactions
		is the form that has been used in most clinical studies	Glucosamine derived from marine exoskeletons can cause reactions in people allergic to shellfish Glucosamine can raise blood glucose level in patients with diabetes
Grape seed	For conditions related to the heart and blood vessels, such as atherosclerosis, high blood pressure, high cholesterol, and poor circulation For vision problems, diabetic neuropathy or retinopathy, and swelling after an injury or surgery For cancer prevention and wound healing	For general health purposes, 100-300 mg daily of a standardized extract (95% oligomeric proanthocanidin complexes)	Side effects include headache, dizziness, nausea, and dry, itchy scalp Concomitant use with warfarin or antiplatelet agents can increase risk of bleeding due to the tocopherol content of grape seed oil
Hawthorn leaf with flower	Commonly used in Germany to increase cardiac output in patients with NYHA stages I and II heart failure	160-900 mg water-ethanol extract (30-169 mg procyanidins or 3.5-19.8 mg flavonoids) divided into 2-3 doses	Side effects include GI upset, palpitations, hypotension, headache, dizziness, and insomnia Concomitant use with CNS depressants can have additive CNS effects Hawthorn can potentiate effects of digoxin and vasodilators
Hops	For mood disturbances such as restlessness and anxiety For sleep disturbances Commonly found in combination products with other herbal sedatives	0.5 g of cut or powdered strobile in a single dose; can be taken as tea (0.5 g in 150 mL water), fluid extract 1:1 (0.5 mL), tincture 1:5 (2.5 mL), or dry extract 6-8:1 (60-80 mg) The preparation contains at least 0.35% (v/w) essential oil	Side effects are rare but include drowsiness and allergic reactions Hops is not recommended for use during pregnancy and lactation It can potentiate the sedative effect of CNS depressants (e.g., benzodiazapines, alcohol) and other herbal tranquilizers
Horse chestnut seed	To relieve symptoms of chronic venous insufficiency	250 mg bid of extract standardized to 50 mg aescin in delayed-release form Unsafe to ingest the raw seed, which contains significant amounts of the most toxic constituent, esculin	Mild GI symptoms, headache, dizziness, and pruritus have been reported Ingestion of high doses can cause renal, hepatic, and hematologic toxicities Concomitant use with anticoagulants can increase the risk of bleeding Horse chestnut can potentiate the effects of hypoglycemic drugs
Kava kava	As an anxiolytic for nervous anxiety, stress, and restlessness As a sedative to induce sleep	Herb and preparations equivalent to 60-120 mg/d of kava pyrones Most clinical trials have used 100 mg tid of extract standardized to 70% kava pyrones for anxiety disorders	Kava should not be used by patients with depression Kava should be avoided in pregnant or nursing women Kava can affect motor reflexes and judgment, so it should not be taken while driving or operating heavy machinery Accommodative disturbances have been reported; kava can exacerbate Parkinson's disease Extended use can cause a temporary yellow discoloration of the skin, hair, and nails Reports have linked kava use to at least 25 cases of severe liver toxicity; sale of products containing kava has been banned in Canada and several European countries Kava has been shown to have additive CNS depressant effects with benzodiazapines, alcohol, and herbal tranquilizers

Herb/Nutritional Supplement[1]	Common Uses	Reasonable Adult Oral Dosage*	Precautions and Drug Interactions
			Kava can potentiate the sedative effects of anesthetics, so kava should be discontinued at least 24 h before surgery
Lutein	Commonly used to prevent AMD and cataracts Also used to prevent skin cancer, breast cancer, and colon cancer To protect against cardiovascular disease	For AMD and cataracts, 6-20 mg/d of lutein from diet For other uses, no established dosage documented Foods containing high concentrations of lutein include kale, spinach, broccoli, and romaine lettuce Not known if supplemental lutein is as effective as natural lutein Supplemental lutein in the form of esters might require a higher fat intake for effective absorption than purified lutein	No major adverse effects and drug interactions have been reported
Lycopene	Commonly used to prevent and treat prostate cancer Also used for cancer prevention, arthrosclerosis prevention, and reduction of asthma symptoms	For decreasing the growth of prostate cancer, 15 mg supplement bid For prostate cancer prevention, at least 6 mg/d from tomato products (or ≥ 10 servings/wk) For other uses, no established dosage documented Heat processing converts lycopene in fresh tomatoes from the *trans* to the *cis*-configuration. The *cis* isomer has better bioavailability Lycopene supplements usually do not specify the type and amount of isomers in their product labeling	Lycopene, when consumed in amounts found in foods, is generally considered to be safe Concomitant ingestion of β-carotene can increase lycopene absorption Lycopene might reduce cholesterol levels and potentiate the effects of statins
Melatonin	For jet lag, insomnia, shift-work disorder, and circadian rhythm disorders Also for other medical conditions, including depression, multiple sclerosis, tinnitus, headache, and cancer	For jet lag, 5 mg at bedtime for 2-5 d beginning the d of return For sleep disorders, 0.3-5 mg taken 2 h before bedtime Avoid melatonin from animal pineal gland due to possibility of contamination	Avoid use in pregnancy, because melatonin decreases serum luteinizing hormone concentrations and increases serum prolactin levels The common adverse reactions include headache, transient depressive symptoms, daytime fatigue and drowsiness, dizziness, abdominal cramps, irritability, and reduced alertness Concomitant use of melatonin with alcohol, benzodiazepines, or other CNS depressants can cause additive sedation Melatonin can affect immune function and can interfere with immunosuppressive therapy Concomitant use with other herbs that have sedative properties (e.g., chamomile, goldenseal, hops, kava, valerian) can produce additive CNS-impairing effects
Milk thistle fruit	As a hepatoprotectant and antioxidant, particularly for treatment of hepatitis, cirrhosis, and toxic liver damage	Average daily dose is 12-15 g of crude drug or formulations equivalent to 200-400 mg of silymarin	Adverse effects are rare but include diarrhea and allergic reactions

Herb/Nutritional Supplement[1]	Common Uses	Reasonable Adult Oral Dosage*	Precautions and Drug Interactions
	Used in Europe to treat hepatotoxic mushroom poisoning from *Amanita phalloides*		Milk thistle can potentiate the hypoglycemic effect of antidiabetic agents
Red clover flower	Commonly used for conditions associated with menopause, such as hot flushes, cardiovascular health, and osteoporosis Also used for PMS, BPH, and cancer prevention Used topically to treat psoriasis, eczema, and other rashes	For hot flushes, 40 mg/d of the isoflavones extract (Promensil) For other conditions, no established dosage documented	Red clover has estrogenic activity and should be avoided during pregnancy and lactation Women with hormone-dependent conditions (e.g., breast, uterine, and ovarian cancers; endometriosis; uterine fibroids) and men with prostate cancer should also avoid taking red clover Side effects include headache, myalgia, nausea, and rash Red clover contains coumarin derivatives and can increase the risk of bleeding in those who are taking anticoagulants or antiplatelet drugs Preliminary report suggests that red clover might antagonize the effects of tamoxifen (Nolvadex) Some evidence suggests that red clover can increase the levels of drugs that are metabolized by the cytochrome P450 3A4 isoenzyme, e.g., lovastatin (Mevacor), ketoconazole (Nizoral), itraconzaole (Sporanox), fexofenadine (Allegra), and triazolam (Halcion)
SAMe (*S*-adenosyl-methione)	For treatment of osteoarthritis, depression, fibromyalgia, and liver disease	For osteoarthritis, 200 mg tid For depression and fibromyalgia, 800 mg bid For liver disease, 600-800 mg bid	Common side effects include flatulence, nausea, vomiting, and diarrhea SAMe can cause anxiety in people with depression and hypomania in people with bipolar disorder Concurrent use of SAMe and other antidepressants can cause serotonin syndrome
Saw palmetto berry	To treat symptomatic BPH and irritable bladder	160 mg bid of extract standardized to 85%-95% fatty acids and sterols	Adverse effects are rare but include headache, nausea, and upset stomach High doses can cause diarrhea
Soy	Commonly used for cholesterol reduction in combination with a low-fat diet Also used for menopausal symptoms and for prevention of osteoporosis and cardiovascular disease in postmenopausal women	For lowering cholesterol, 25-50 g/d of soy protein For hot flushes, 20-60 g/d of soy protein For osteoporosis, 40 g/d of soy protein containing 90 mg isoflavones	Soy, when consumed as whole foods (e.g., tofu or soy milk), has minimal adverse effects Consumption of large amounts of soy can cause gastric complaints such as constipation, bloating, and nausea Long-term use of soy tablets containing isoflavones (150 mg/d for 5 y) has been shown to cause endometrial hyperplasia
St. John's wort	Effective for treatment of mild to moderate depression May have antiinflammatory and antiinfective activities	300 mg tid of hypericum extract standardized to 0.3% hypericin	St. John's wort should not be used in pregnancy Side effects include dry mouth, GI upset, dizziness, fatigue, and constipation St. John's wort can induce photosensitivity, especially in fair-skinned persons It can cause serotonin syndrome if used with other antidepressants, including SSRIs, or other serotoninergic drugs It has been shown to induce CYP3A4 and decrease blood levels of many drugs such

Herb/Nutritional Supplement[1]	Common Uses	Reasonable Adult Oral Dosage*	Precautions and Drug Interactions
			as indinavir (Crixivan), nevirapine (Viramune), cyclosporine (Neoral), digoxin, theophylline, simvastatin (Zocor), oral contraceptive pills, and warfarin St. John's wort should be discontinued at least 5 d before surgery to avoid any potential drug interactions
Stinging nettle root	Approved in Germany for difficulty in urination in BPH stages 1 and 2	4-6 g/d of cut root; can be taken as tea (1.5 g in 150 mL boiling water for 10-20 min, tid), fluid extract 1:1 (1.5 mL tid), tincture 1:5 (5-7.5 mL tid), or dry extract 5.4-6.6:1 (0.22-0.33 g tid)	Occasionally, mild GI upsets occur No known interactions with drugs
Valerian root	Used as a mild sedative for insomnia and anxiety	2-3 g of dried root or 1-3 mL of tincture, qd to several times per d Two clinical trials found 400-450 mg of the root extract effective for insomnia	Valerian has a bad odor and can cause morning drowsiness Long-term administration can lead to paradoxical stimulation including restlessness and palpitations Because of the risk of benzodiazepine-like withdrawal, valerian should be tapered over a period of several weeks before surgery It can potentiate the sedative effect of CNS depressants (e.g., benzodiazepines, alcohol) and other herbal tranquilizers

*Doses presented in the table are adapted from the German Commission E Monographs and/or data from clinical trials. Products from different manufacturers vary considerably. A reliable product should have a label clearly stating the botanical name of the herb and milligram amount contained in the product. Standardized extracts should be used whenever possible and are often disclosed on the label of quality products.

AMD = age-related macular degeneration; BPH = benign prostatic hyperplasia; CHD = coronary heart disease; CNS, central nervous system; DHA = docosahexaenoic acid; EPA = eicosapentaenoic acid; FDA = Food and Drug Administration; GI = gastrointestinal; HMG-CoA = 3-hydroxy-3-methylglutaryl coenzyme A; Ig = immunoglobulin; INR = international normalized ratio; LDL = low-density lipoprotein; MAOI = monoamine oxidase inhibitor; NSAID = nonsteroidal antiinflammatory drug; NYHA = New York Heart Association; PMS = premenstrual syndrome; SLE = systemic lupus erythematosus; SSRI = selective serotonin reuptake inhibitor; UTI = urinary tract infection.

[1]Available as dietary supplement

REFERENCES

Ang-Lee MK, Moss J, Yuan C: Herbal medicines and perioperative care. JAMA 2001;286:208-216.

Blumenthal M (ed): Herbal medicines: Expanded Commission E monographs, Austin, TX: American Botanical Council, 2000.

Blumenthal M (ed): Complete German Commission E monographs: Therapeutic guide to herbal medicines. 1st ed. Austin, TX: American Botanical Council, 1998.

Cupp MJ: Herbal remedies: Adverse effects and drug interactions. Am Fam Physician 1999;59(5):1239-1244.

Ernst E: The risk–benefit profile of commonly used herbal therapies: Ginkgo, St John's wort, ginseng, echinacea, saw palmetto, and kava. Ann Intern Med 2002;136:42-53.

Jellin JM, Gregory P, Batz F, et al: Pharmacist's Letter/Prescriber's Letter Natural Medicines Comprehensive Database, 7th ed. Stockton, CA: Therapeutic Research Faculty, 2005.

Klepser TB, Klepser ME: Unsafe and potentially safe herbal therapies. Am J Health-Syst Pharm 1999;56:125-138.

Kronenberg F, Fugh-Berman A: Complementary and alternative medicine for menopausal symptoms: A review of randomized controlled trials. Ann Intern Med 2002;137:805-813.

Mar C, Bent S: An evidence-based review of the 10 most commonly used herbs. West J Med 1999;171(3):168-171.

PDR for herbal medicines. 3rd ed. Montvale, NJ: Medical Economics Co, 2004.

O'Hara MA, Kiefer D, Farrell K, Kemper K: A review of 12 commonly used medicinal herbs. Arch Fam Med 1998;7:523-536.

Rotblatt MD: Cranberry, feverfew, horse chestnut, and kava West J Med 1999;171:195-198.

Smet P: Herbal remedies. N Engl J Med 2002;2046-2056.

New Drugs in 2008 and Agents Pending FDA Approval

Method of
Miriam M. Chan, RPh, PharmD

NEW DRUGS IN 2007

Generic Name	Trade Name (Manufacturer)	Strength	Dosage Form	Normal Dosage Range	Pregnancy Rating*	FDA Approval Date	Indication	Classification
New Molecular Entity								
Aliskiren	Tekturna (Novartis)	150, 300 mg	Tablet	150 mg qd; may increase dose to 300 mg qd as needed	C (first trimester) D (second and third trimesters)	3/5/07	Treatment of hypertension, alone or with other antihypertensives	Antihypertensive, renin inhibitor
Ambrisentan	Letairis (Gilead Sciences)	5, 10 mg	Tablet	5 mg once daily, may increase dose to 10 mg once daily if tolerated	X	6/15/07	Treatment of pulmonary artery hypertension (WHO Group I) in patients with WHO class II or III symptoms to improve exercise capacity and delay clinical worsening	Antihypertensive, endothelin receptor antagonist
Doripenem	Doribax (Johnson & Johnson)	500 mg vial	Injection	500 mg IV in 100 mL NS or D$_5$W infusion over 1 h q8h	B	10/12/07	Treatment of complicated intraabdominal infections; Treatment of complicated urinary tract infections including pyelonephritis	Antibiotic, carbapenem
Eculizumab	Soliris (Alexion)	10 mg/mL, 30-mL vial	Injection	Start at 600 mg IV infusion (120 mL) over 35 min q wk x 4 wk; in wk 5 give 900 mg IV (180 mL), then 900 mg IV q2wk thereafter	C	3/16/07	To reduce hemolysis in patients with paroxysmal nocturnal hemoglobinuria	Complement inhibitor, monoclonal antibody
Ixabepilone	Ixempra (Bristol-Myers Squibb)	15, 45 mg/vial	Injection	40 mg/m² IV infusion (final infusion must be between 0.2 and 0.6 mg/mL) over 3 h q3wk	D	10/16/07	In combination with capecitabine for the treatment of patients with metastatic or locally advanced breast cancer after failure of an anthracycline and a taxane; As monotherapy for the treatment of metastatic or locally advanced breast cancer in patients whose tumors are resistant or refractory to anthracyclines, taxanes, and capecitabine	Antineoplastic, microtubule inhibitor
Lanreotide	Somatuline Depot (Biomeasure)	60, 90, 120 mg prefilled syringe	Injection	90 mg SC once q4wk x 3 mo; adjust dosage based on growth hormone and/or insulin growth factor-1 levels	C	8/30/07	Long-term treatment of acromegalic patients who have had an inadequate response to or cannot be treated	Hormone, somatostatin analogue

Section 19 Appendices and Index

Lapatinib	Tykerb (GlaxoSmithKline)	250 mg	Tablet	1,250 mg once daily on d 1-21 continuously in combination with capecitabine 2000 mg/m²/d (in 2 divided doses q12h) on d 1-14 in a repeating 21-d cycle	D	3/13/07	In combination with capecitabine for advanced or metastatic breast cancer in patients whose tumors overexpress HER2 and who have received treatment with an anthracycline, a taxane, and trastuzumab with surgery and/or radiotherapy	Antineoplastic, kinase inhibitor
Lisdexamfetamine dimesylate	Vyvanse (Shire)	30, 50, 70 mg	Capsule	Children 6-12 y: 30 mg once daily in AM; may increase dose by 20 mg/d and at weekly intervals as needed to a max of 70 mg/d	C	2/23/07	Treatment of ADHD	CNS stimulant, amphetamine
Maraviroc	Selzentry (Pfizer)	150, 300 mg	Tablet	150 mg bid when given with strong CYP 3A inhibitors including protease inhibitors (except tipranavir/ritonavir), delavirdine 300 mg bid when given with NRTIs, tipranavir/ritonavir, nevirapine, and other drugs that are not strong CYP 3A inhibitors or CYP 3A inducers 600 mg bid when given with CYP 3A inducers, such as efavirenz	B	8/6/07	Combination antiretroviral treatment of adults infected with only CCR5-tropic HIV-1 detectable, who have evidence of viral replication and HIV-1 strains resistant to multiple antiretroviral agents	Antiretroviral, CCR5 co-receptor antagonist
Methoxy polyethylene glycol-epoetin beta	Mircera (Hoffman La-Roche)	50, 100, 200, 300, 400, 600, 1000 µg single-use vial 50, 75, 100, 150, 200, 250 µg single-use prefilled syringe	Injection	Patients not currently treated with an erythropoiesis stimulating agent (ESA): 0.6 µg/kg IV or SC once q2wk; may adjust dose to achieve and maintain a hemoglobin level at 10-12 g/dL Patients currently treated with an ESA: give once q2wk or once monthly to patients whose hemoglobin has been stabilized by treatment with an ESA; the starting dose is based on the total ESA dose at the time of conversion	C	11/14/07	Treatment of anemia associated with chronic renal failure, including patients on dialysis and patients not on dialysis	Hematopoietic, ESA
Nebivolol	Bystolic (Mylan Bertek)	2.5, 5, 10 mg	Tablet	5 mg qd; may increase dose at 2-wk intervals, up to 40 mg qd	C	12/17/07	Treatment of hypertension, alone or with other antihypertensives	Antihypertensive, β-blocker
Nilotinib		200 mg	Capsule		D	10/29/07		

Continued

NEW DRUGS IN 2007—cont'd

Generic Name	Trade Name (Manufacturer)	Strength	Dosage Form	Normal Dosage Range	Pregnancy Rating*	FDA Approval Date	Indication	Classification
	Tasigna (Novartis)			400 mg q12h; no food for at least 2 h before or 1 h after the dose			Treatment of chronic phase and accelerated-phase Philadelphia chromosome–positive chronic myelogenous leukemia (CML) in adults resistant to or intolerant to prior therapy that included imatinib (Gleevec)	Antineoplastic, tyrosine kinase inhibitor
Protein C Concentrate (Human)	Ceprotin (Baxter)	500, 1000 IU/vial	Injection	Acute episode/short-term prophylaxis: start at 100-120 units/kg IV, followed by 60-80 units/kg IV q 6 h x 3 doses; then a maintenance dose of 45-60 U/kg IV q6h or q12h Long-term prophylaxis: 45-60 U/kg q12h	C	3/30/07	Prevention and treatment of deep venous thrombosis and purpura fulminans in patients with severe congenital protein C deficiency	Blood product, anticoagulant
Raltegravir	Isentress (Merck)	400 mg	Tablet	400 mg bid	C	10/12/07	In combination with other antiretroviral agents for the treatment of HIV-1 infection in treatment-experienced adults who have evidence of viral replication and HIV-1 strains resistant to multiple antiretroviral agents	Antiretroviral, integrase inhibitor
Retapamulin	Altabax (GlaxoSmithKline)	1% in 5, 10, 15-g tube	Topical ointment	Apply a thin layer of ointment to the affected area bid x 5 d; may cover affected area with sterile dressing; max dose: 100 cm² total area in adults or 2% total BSA in children	B	4/12/07	Topical treatment of impetigo due to methicillin-susceptible Staphylococcus aureus or Streptococcus pyogenes in patients ages ≥9 mo	Antibiotic, pleuromutilin
Rotigotine	Neupro (Schwarz BioSciences)	2, 4, 6 mg/24 h	Transdermal delivery system	Apply 2 mg/24 h patch once daily; may increase dose weekly by 2 mg/24 h up to 6 mg/24 h	C	5/9/07	Treatment of the signs and symptoms of early-stage idiopathic Parkinson's disease	Antiparkinsonian, dopamine agonist
Sapropterin	Kuvan (Biomarin Pharm)	100 mg	Tablet	Start at 10 mg/kg/d once daily with food; may adjust dose in the range of 5-20 mg/kg/d with regular monitoring of blood Phe levels	C	12/13/07	In conjunction with a Phe-restricted diet to reduce blood Phe levels in patients with hyperphenylalaninemia (HPA) due to	Enzyme, PAH cofactor

Temsirolimus	Torisel (Wyeth)	25 mg/mL vial	Injection	Dissolve tablets in 4-8 oz of water or apple juice and take within 15 min 25 mg IV infusion over 30-60 min once a wk until disease progresses or unacceptable toxicity occurs	D	Treatment of advanced renal cell carcinoma	Antineoplastic, mTOR (kinase) inhibitor

New Ester, New Salt, or Other Derivative

Armodafinil	Nuvigil (Cephalon)	50, 150, 250 mg	Tablet	OSAHS, narcolepsy: 150 to 250 mg once daily in AM Shift-work sleep disorder: 150 mg once daily 1 h before start of the work shift	C	To improve wakefulness in patients with excessive sleepiness associated with obstructive sleep apnea/hypopnea syndrome (OSAHS), narcolepsy, and shift-work sleep disorder	CNS stimulant, dopamine reuptake inhibitor
Diclofenac epolamine	Flector Patch	1.3% (180 mg/ 10 cm × 14 cm patch)	Topical patch	1 patch to the most painful area bid	C	Topical treatment of acute pain due to minor strains, sprains, and contusions	Topical, NSAID
Fluticasone furoate	Veramyst (GlaxoSmithKline)	27.5 µg/spray in 120 sprays/ 10 g bottle	Nasal spray	Adults and adolescents ≥12 y: 2 sprays per nostril once daily Children 2-11 y: 1 spray per nostril once daily	C	Treatment of symptoms of seasonal and perennial allergic rhinitis in adults and children ≥2 y	Respiratory inhalant, intranasal steroid
Levocetirizine	Xyzal (Sanofi-Aventis)	5 mg	Tablet	Adults and children ≥12y: 5 mg qd in the evening Children 6-12 y: 2.5 mg qd in the evening	B	Relief of symptoms associated with seasonal and perennial allergic rhinitis Treatment of the uncomplicated skin manifestations of chronic idiopathic urticaria	Antihistamine, H$_1$-receptor antagonist

New Combination

Amlodipine/Olmesartan	Azor (Daiichi Sankyo)	5 mg/20 mg, 10 mg/20 mg, 5 mg/40 mg, 10 mg/40 mg	Tablet	1 tab once daily; may increase dose after 2 wk to a max daily dose of 10 mg amlodipine and 40 mg olmesartan	C (first trimester) D (second and third trimesters)	Treatment of hypertension, alone or with other antihypertensive agents	Antihypertensive, calcium channel blocker, angiotensin II receptor blocker
Amlodipine/Valsartan	Exforge (Novartis)	5 mg/160 mg, 5 mg/320 mg, 10 mg/160 mg, 10 mg/ 320 mg	Tablet	1 tab once daily after patient is stabilized on each of the components	C (first trimester) D (second and third trimesters)	Treatment of hypertension	Antihypertenive, calcium channel blocker, angiotensin II receptor blocker
Brimonidine/timolol	Combigan (Allergan)	0.2%/ 0.5%	Ophthalmic solution	1 drop in affected eye q 12 h	C	To reduce elevated intraocular pressure in patients with glaucoma or ocular hypertension	Antiglaucomic, α-agonist, β-antagonist

Continued

NEW DRUGS IN 2007—cont'd

Generic Name	Trade Name (Manufacturer)	Strength	Dosage Form	Normal Dosage Range	Pregnancy Rating*	FDA Approval Date	Indication	Classification
Sitagliptin/ Metformin	Janumet	50 mg/500 mg, 50 mg/ 1000 mg	Tablet	1 tab bid given with meals; individualize the starting dose based on the patient's current regimen. May increase dose gradually as needed to a max daily dose of 100 mg sitagliptin and 2000 mg metformin	B	3/30/07	As an adjunct to diet and exercise to improve glycemic control in patients whose type 2 diabetes mellitus is not adequately controlled on sitagliptin or metformin alone or in patients already being treated with this combination of drugs	Antidiabetic, DDP-4 inhibitor/ biguanide
New Formulation								
Azithromycin	AzaSite (Inspire)	1%, 2.5 mL in 5-mL bottle	Ophthalmic solution	1 drop bid x 2 d, followed by 1 drop qd x 5 d, for a total of 9 drops per affected eye	B	4/27/07	Treatment of bacterial conjunctivitis	Ophthalmic antibiotic, macrolide
Diclofenac sodium	Voltaren Gel	1%, 100-g tube supplied with dosing cards	Topical gel	Lower extremities: apply 4 g to the affected area qid; max dose 16 g/d. Upper extremities: apply 2 g to the affected area qid; max dose 8 g/d. Total dose should not exceed 32 g/d	C	10/17/07	Relief of the pain of osteoarthritis of joints amenable to topical treatment, such as the knees and those of the hands	Topical, NSAID
Levonorgestrel/ ethinyl estradiol	Lybrel (Wyeth)	90 µg/20 µg	Tablet	1 tab once daily without any tablet-free interval	X	5/22/07	Prevention of pregnancy in women who elect to use oral contraceptives as a method of contraception	Hormones, combination oral contraceptives
Lidocaine hydrochloride monohydrate	Zingo (Anesiva)	0.5 mg powder in a single-use system	Intradermal injection system	Apply one Zingo (0.5 mg) to the site planned for venipuncture or IV cannulation, 1-3 min before needle insertion. Perform the procedure within 10 min after Zingo administration	B	8/16/07	To provide local analgesia prior to venipuncture or peripheral IV cannulation in children 3-18 y	Topical local analgesics, amide

| Rivastigmine transdermal system | Exelon Patch | 4.6 mg/24 h, 9.5 mg/24 h | Transdermal patch | Start at one 4.6 mg/24 h patch once daily; may increase dose after a minimum of 4 wk of treatment to a max dose of one 9.5 mg/24 h patch once daily | B | 7/6/07 | Treatment of mild to moderate dementia of the Alzheimer's type Treatment of mild to moderate dementia associated with Parkinson's disease | CNS agents, acetylcholinesterase inhibitor |

ADHD = attention-deficit/hyperactivity disorder; BSA = body surface area; CCR5 = chemokine (C-C motif) receptor 5; CNS = central nervous system; DDP-4 = dipeptidyl peptidase 4; D_5W = 5% dextrose in water; NRTI = nucleoside reverse transcriptase inhibitor; NS = normal (0.9%) saline; NSAID = nonsteroidal antiinflammatory drug; PAH = phenylalanine hydroxylase; Phe = phenylalanine; WHO = World Health Organization.

FDA PREGNANCY CATEGORIES

A: Adequate studies in pregnant women have not demonstrated a risk to the fetus in the first trimester of pregnancy, and there is no evidence of risk in later trimesters.
B: Animal studies have shown an adverse effect, but adequate studies in pregnant women have not demonstrated a risk to the fetus during the first trimester of pregnancy, and there is no evidence of risk in later trimesters.
C: Animal studies have shown an adverse effect on the fetus, but there are no adequate studies in humans; the benefits from the use of the drug in pregnant women may be acceptable despite its potential risks.
D: There is evidence of human fetal risk, but the potential benefits from the use of the drug in pregnant women may be acceptable despite its potential risks.
X: Adverse reaction reports indicate evidence of fetal risk; the risk of use in a pregnant woman clearly outweighs any possible benefit.
No drug should be administered during pregnancy unless it is clearly needed and the potential benefit outweighs the potential hazard to the fetus, regardless of the pregnancy category.

AGENTS PENDING FDA APPROVAL

Generic Name	Trade Name (Manufacturer)	Indication
ABT-335/Rosuvastatin	No brand name (Abbott & AstraZeneca)	Treatment of mixed dyslipidemia
Anecortave acetate	Retaane (Alcon)	Treatment of wet macular degeneration
Almorexant	No brand name (Actelion)	Treatment of primary insomnia
Apixaban	No brand name (Bristol-Myers Squibb/Pfizer)	Prevention of venous thromboembolism and prevention of stroke
Bazedoxifene	Viviant (Wyeth)	Prevention of postmenopausal osteoporosis
17 alpha-hydroxy-progesterone caproate	Gestiva (Adeza)	Prevention of preterm delivery (before 35 wk) in women with a history of prior preterm delivery
Ceftobiprole	No brand name (Johnson & Johnson)	Treatment of complicated skin and soft tissue infections, including diabetes-related foot infections
Cilomilast	Ariflo (GlaxoSmithKline)	Treatment of patients with COPD who are poorly responsive to albuterol
CI inhibitor	Cinryze (Lev Pharma)	Acute treatment of hereditary angioedema
Clodronate	Bonefos (Berlex Laboratories)	Adjuvant oral treatment for reducing the occurrence of bone metastases in stage II/III breast cancer patients
Dextromethorphan/quinidine	Zenvia (Avanir)	Treatment of involuntary emotional expression disorder Treatment of diabetic peripheral neuropathic pain
Efaproxiral	Efaproxyn (Allos Therapeutics, Inc.)	An adjunct agent to whole-brain radiation therapy for the treatment of brain metastases in patients with breast cancer
Eprodisate	Kiacta (Neurochem)	Treatment of amyloid A amyloidosis
Everolimus	Certican (Novartis)	Prevention of rejection after heart and kidney transplantation
Febuxostat	No brand name (TAP)	For management of hyperuricemia in patients with chronic gout
Fesoterodine	No brand name (Schwarz/Pfizer)	Treatment of overactive bladder
Garenoxacin mesylate	Geninax (Schering)	Treatment of acute bacterial exacerbation of chronic bronchitis, acute bacterial sinusitis, community-acquired pneumonia, complicated and uncomplicated skin and skin-structure infections, and complicated intraabdominal infections
Icatibant	No brand name (Jerini)	Treatment of hereditary angioedema
Iloperidone	Zomaril (Vanda)	Treatment of schizophrenia
Liraglutide	No brand name (Novo Nordisk)	Treatment of type 2 diabetes
Niacin ER/laropiprant	Cordaptive (Merck)	Improvement of HDL-cholesterol levels and reduced flushing
Prasugrel	Effient (Daiichi Sankyo/Eli Lilly)	Treatment of patients with acute coronary syndrome who are managed with percutaneous coronary intervention, including coronary stenting
Rufinamide	No brand name (Eisai)	Adjunctive therapy for Lennox–Gastaut syndrome in children 4 y of age and older and as adjunctive therapy for partial-onset seizures with and without secondary generalization in adults and adolescents 12 y and older
Sitaxsentan sodium	Thelin (Encysive Pharmaceuticals)	Treatment of pulmonary arterial hypertension
SnET2 (tin ethyl etiopurpurin)	No brand name (Miravent Medical Technologies)	Slow the progression of wet age-related macular degeneration
Tedisamil	Pulzium (Solvay Pharmaceuticals)	For conversion of atrial fibrillation or atrial flutter to normal sinus rhythm
Telavancin	No brand name (Theravance Inc)	Treatment of skin and skin-structure infections
Tocilizumab	Actemra (Chugai/Roche)	Treatment of moderate to severe rheumatoid arthritis
Vapreotide	Sanvar IR (H3 Pharma)	Treatment of acute esophageal variceal bleeding secondary to portal hypertension
Venakalant	No brand name (Astellas Pharma)	For conversion of atrial fibrillation to normal sinus rhythm
Vildagliptin	Galvus (Novartis)	Treatment of type 2 diabetes

COPD = chronic obstructive pulmonary disease; HDL = high-density lipoprotein.

Index

Note: Page numbers followed by f, t, and b indicate figures, tables, and boxed material, respectively. Drugs are listed under the generic name.

A

AA. *See* Aplastic anemia (AA).
A–a (alveolar–arterial) O$_2$ gradient, 225, 226t
AAA. *See* Abdominal aortic aneurysm (AAA).
AAT (α_1-antitrypsin) deficiency, 231–232
   cirrhosis due to, 498t, 501
Abacavir (Ziagen), for HIV, 50t, 51t
Abacavir + lamivudine (Epzicom), for HIV, 51t
Abacteriuric cystitis, 682, 683b, 684
Abatacept (Orencia, CTLA-4Ig)
   for arthritis
      juvenile idiopathic, 985–986
      rheumatoid, 981t, 982
   for systemic lupus erythematosus, 809
Abbokinase (urokinase)
   for deep venous thrombosis/pulmonary embolism, 273–274
   for ischemic stroke, 894
Abciximab (Reopro)
   for myocardial infarction, 364, 366
   for unstable angina pectoris, 301, 301t
ABCs. *See* Airway, breathing, and circulation (ABCs).
Abdominal aortic aneurysm (AAA), 291–292, 374–375
   diagnosis of, 291, 293b
   incidence and natural history of, 291
   infrarenal, 292
   rupture of, 291
   screening for, 292
   treatment of, 291–292, 294b
Abelcet. *See* Amphotericin B lipid complex (ABLC, Abelcet).
Abetalipoproteinemia, 543
Abilify (aripiprazole)
   for bipolar disorder, 1127–1128
   for schizophrenia, 1130t
ABLC. *See* Amphotericin B lipid complex (ABLC, Abelcet).
ABO mismatch, 484–485
Abscess(es)
   amebic liver, 563–564
      clinical presentation of, 59–60
      diagnosis of, 60, 60t
      treatment of, 61, 61t
   anorectal, 526–527
      differential diagnosis of, 525, 525t
      evaluation of, 525–527
      history of, 525
      pathogenesis of, 526
      physical examination of, 525, 527
      treatment of, 527
   cutaneous, 836b, 837
   lung, 258
      clinical features of, 258
      diagnosis of, 258–259, 258b
      etiology of, 258
      treatment of, 259, 259b

Abscess(es) *(Continued)*
   Pautrier's micro-, 795
   renal, 683–685
   tubo-ovarian, 1080
Absence seizures
   in adolescents and adults, 900, 901t
   childhood and juvenile, 908–909
Absolute neutrophil count (ANC), 413, 414t
ABT-335. *See* Rosuvastatin (Crestor, ABT-335).
Acalculous cholecystitis, 494
Acamprosate (Campral), for alcohol dependence, 1103
Acanthosis nigricans, acral, 878
Acarbose (Precose), for diabetes, 580t
Accident-related injury, 158, 158b
Accolate (zafirlukast), for asthma
   in adolescents and adults, 767–768t
   in children, 773–774t
Accommodation, 187
Accompanied multidrug therapy (A-MDT), for leprosy, 101
Accuneb. *See* Albuterol (Accuneb, Proventil, Ventolin).
Accutane (isotretinoin)
   for acne, 788
   for rosacea, 789
ACD. *See* Allergic contact dermatitis (ACD).
ACE (angiotensin-converting enzyme), in sarcoidosis, 276
Acebutolol (Sectral)
   for angina pectoris, 299
   intoxication with, 1182–1183, 1183t
ACEIs. *See* Angiotensin-converting enzyme inhibitors (ACEIs).
Acendin (amoxapine), poisoning due to, 1214–1216, 1215t
Acetaminophen (Tylenol)
   for fever, 24
   for high-altitude sickness, 1140–1141
   metabolism of, 1176–1177
   for osteoarthritis, 1000
   for pain, 2
   therapeutic dose of, 1176
   for typhoid fever, 175
Acetaminophen intoxication, 1176–1216
   disposition for, 1178
   kinetics of, 1176–1177
   laboratory investigations of, 1177, 1178f
   management of, 1177, 1178t
   manifestations of, 1177
   mechanism of, 1176
   toxic dose for, 1176
Acetate, in parenteral nutrition, 621, 622t
Acetazolamide (Diamox)
   for glaucoma, 200
   for high-altitude sickness, 1140–1142, 1142b
Acetohydroxamic acid (Lithostat), for renal calculi, 746t
Acetone, and serum osmolality, 1176t

Acetonemia, due to poisoning, 1175t
Acetonitrile, cyanide poisoning due to, 1187–1188
Acetorphan, for acute infectious diarrhea, 19
Acetylcholine receptor (AChR), in myasthenia gravis, 940–942
Acetylcholinesterase (AChE), in myasthenia gravis, 942–943
Acetylsalicylic acid (ASA)
   for ischemic stroke prevention, 894
   poisoning due to, 1209–1212, 1211t
Achalasia, 510–511
Achilles tendinosis, 1009
Achromycin. *See* Tetracycline (Achromycin, Sumycin).
Acid(s)
   burns due to, 1138
   poisoning due to, 1185–1186
   for verrucae, 823
Acid suppression, for gastroesophageal reflux disease, 553–554, 554t
Acid-base disturbances, due to poisoning, 1174–1175, 1175t
Acidosis, metabolic
   in chronic renal failure, 729
      and disease progression, 729
      laboratory values for, 727, 727t
      symptoms of, 727
      treatment of, 730
   with parenteral nutrition, 625t
   due to poisoning, 1175t
ACIP (Advisory Committee on Immunization Practices), 148
Aciphex. *See* Rabeprazole (Aciphex).
ACIS (adenocarcinoma in situ), of cervix, 1090
Acitretin (Soriatane)
   for actinic keratosis, 834
   for psoriasis, 802
ACL (anterior cruciate ligament) tears, 1008
Aclovate (alclometasone), for atopic dermatitis, 860–861
Acne excoriée, 788
Acne keloidalis, 792
Acne vulgaris, 787–788
   behavioral issues with, 788
   clinical features of, 787
   diagnosis of, 789b
   pathogenesis of, 787
   postinflammatory hyperpigmentation due to, 878
   treatment of, 787–788, 789b
Acoustic neuroma, 208
Acquired immunodeficiency syndrome (AIDS). *See* Human immunodeficiency virus (HIV).
ACR (American College of Rheumatology) criteria, for rheumatoid arthritis, 977, 978t
Acral acanthosis nigricans, 878
Acrivastine (Semprex), for allergic rhinitis, 779t

Acrivastine/pseudoephedrine (Semprex-D), for allergic rhinitis, 779**t**
Acrodermatitis chronica atrophicans, 137
Acrolein, as chemical weapon, 1226–1228**t**
Acromegaly, 633
  associated endocrine abnormalities with, 635
  clinical manifestations of, 633–635
  defined, 633
  diagnosis of, 635
    biochemical, 635
    imaging in, 635
  epidemiology of, 633
  etiopathogenesis of, 633
  GH/IGF-1 axis and, 633, 634**f**
  mortality due to, 635
  treatment of, 635–636
Acromioclavicular joint, injuries to, 1009
ACS (acute chest syndrome), in sickle cell disease, 406, 409–410
Actemra (tocilizumab), 1244–1249**t**
ACTH. *See* Adrenocorticotropic hormone (ACTH).
ActHIB. *See Haemophilus influenzae* type b (Hib) vaccine (PedvaxHIB, ActHIB, HibTITER).
Actidose-Aqua. *See* Activated charcoal (Actidose-Aqua).
Actifed Cold & Allergy (triprolidine/pseudoephedrine), for allergic rhinitis, 779**t**
Actigall (ursodiol), for cholestasis, 34**b**
Actinic cheilitis, 833**b**, 834, 834**b**, 850
Actinic keratosis(es) (AK), 833–834
  clinical features of, 793, 833
  diagnosis of, 794**b**, 833**b**
  epidemiology of, 793
  of lips, 833**b**, 834, 834**b**, 850
  treatment of, 794, 794**b**, 833–834, 834**b**
Activase. *See* Tissue plasminogen activator (TPA, rtPA, Activase).
Activase (alteplase), for myocardial infarction, 364**t**
Activated charcoal (Actidose-Aqua), for poisoning, 1164, 1164**t**
  ciguatera, 1157**t**
  due to theophylline, 1213–1214
Active core rewarming, for hypothermia, 1145–1146, 1147**b**
Active external rewarming, for hypothermia, 1145, 1147**b**
Activities of daily living (ADLs), stroke rehabilitation for, 896–897
Activity, in postpartum period, 1028
Actonel. *See* Risedronate (Actonel).
Actos (pioglitazone), for diabetes, 580**t**, 581
Acute bacterial meningitis. *See* Bacterial meningitis.
Acute chest syndrome (ACS), in sickle cell disease, 406, 409–410
Acute coronary syndrome
  with heart block, 319
  unstable angina pectoris due to, 300
    treatment of, 300–301, 301**t**
Acute erosive and hemorrhagic gastropathy, 528–529
Acute hemolytic transfusion reaction (AHTR), 484–486, 484–485**t**
acute infectious diarrhea due to, 15–16, 19–20**t**
Acute intermittent porphyria (AIP), 475**t**, 476**t**
Acute kidney injury. *See* Acute renal failure (ARF).
Acute lung injury (ALI), 229–230
  due to shock, 70
  transfusion-related, 484–485**t**, 487–488
Acute lymphoblastic leukemia (ALL), 444
  in children
    classification of, 450, 450**t**
    epidemiology of, 450–451, 451**f**
    medical emergencies in, 453–454

Acute lymphoblastic leukemia (ALL) *(Continued)*
    molecular pathogenesis of, 452, 452**t**
    predispositions to, 451–452, 452**t**
    prognosis for, 451
    relapse of, 455–456
    risk stratification for, 454
    treatment of, 454–455, 455**t**
  classification of, 446**b**
    in children, 450, 450**t**
  prognostic factors for, 446**b**
    in children, 451
  treatment of, 447**b**, 449
Acute motor and sensory axonal neuropathy (AMSAM), 962
Acute motor axonal neuropathy (AMAN), 962
Acute mountain sickness (AMS), 1141–1142
  clinical course of, 1141
  defined, 1141
  diagnosis of, 1141, 1142**b**
  differential diagnosis of, 1141, 1141**b**
  incidence of, 1140
  prevention of, 158, 1140–1141
  risk factors for, 1140
  symptoms of, 158
  treatment of, 158, 1141–1142, 1142**b**
Acute myeloid leukemia (AML), 444
  in children
    classification of, 450, 450**b**
    epidemiology of, 450–451, 451**f**
    medical emergencies in, 453–454
    molecular pathogenesis of, 452, 452**t**
    predispositions to, 451–452, 452**t**
    prognosis for, 451
    relapse of, 455–456
    risk stratification for, 454
    treatment of, 455, 455**t**
  classification of, 446**b**
    in children, 450, 450**b**
  etiology of, 444
  prognostic factors for, 446**b**
    in children, 451
  treatment of, 445–448, 447**b**
    consolidation chemotherapy for, 446
    induction chemotherapy for, 445–446
    investigational, 448, 448**t**
    maintenance chemotherapy for, 447
    in older patients, 447–448
    stem-cell transplantation for, 446–447
Acute otitis media (AOM)
  clinical guidelines for, 203
  defined, 203
  diagnosis of, 203, 204**b**
  impact of, 203
  treatment of, 203–204, 203**b**
Acute Physiology and Chronic Health Evaluation (APACHE) II, for acute pancreatitis, 547
Acute promyelocytic leukemia (AML-M3)
  disseminated intravascular coagulation in, 429
  treatment of, 446**b**, 448–449
Acute pyelonephritis (APN), 683
  clinical presentation of, 683, 704
  complicated, 704, 704**b**
  vs. cystitis, 682, 683
  defined, 704
  diagnosis of, 683**b**, 704–705, 705**b**
  differential diagnosis of, 705**b**
  epidemiology of, 704
  etiology and pathogenesis of, 683, 704
    microbial, 705
  follow-up for, 706
  imaging of, 706
  treatment of, 684**b**, 685, 705–706, 705**b**, 706**b**
  urinary tract infection due to, 682–683
Acute renal failure (ARF), 721
  classification of, 721–724, 722**b**
  defined, 721
  diagnosis of, 724**b**, 724–725

Acute renal failure (ARF) *(Continued)*
  emerging issues with, 724–725
  epidemiology of, 721
  intrinsic (intrarenal), 722
    due to acute tubular necrosis, 722**b**, 723, 724**t**, 724**b**
    causes of, 722, 722**b**
    due to cholesterol emboli syndrome, 722
    defined, 721
    due to glomerular disease, 722–723
    due to interstitial disease, 722**b**, 723–724
    medication-induced, 722, 722**b**, 723
    due to radiocontrast agents, 723, 725
    due to small vessel vasculitis, 722
  parenteral nutrition with, 623–624
  due to postrenal obstruction, 724
    causes of, 722**b**, 724
    defined, 721
    diagnosis and treatment of, 724, 724**b**
  prerenal azotemia as, 721–722
    causes of, 721, 722**b**, 723**f**
    defined, 721
    laboratory findings in, 721–722, 724**b**
    treatment of, 724, 724**b**
Acute respiratory distress syndrome (ARDS), 229–230
  parenteral nutrition with, 624
  due to shock, 70
Acute respiratory failure, 225
  due to acute lung injury and ARDS, 229–230
  due to cardiogenic pulmonary edema, 230
  clinical presentation of, 225
  in COPD, 228–229
  definitions for, 225–226
  diagnosis of, 229**b**
  hypercapneic, 225–226, 226**b**, 227**b**
  hypoxic/hypoxemic, 225, 226**t**, 226**b**
  pathophysiology of, 225–226, 226**t**
  treatment of, 226–228, 229**b**
    mechanical ventilation for, 227–228, 229**b**
      invasive, 228, 229, 229**b**
      noninvasive, 227–228, 228**t**, 229**b**
    oxygen therapy for, 226–227, 227**t**
Acute tubular necrosis (ATN), 723
  causes of, 722**b**, 723
  ischemic, 723
  laboratory values in, 724**t**, 724**b**
  natural history of, 723
  prerenal azotemia *vs.*, 724**t**
  septic, 723
  toxic, 723
Acyclovir (Zovirax)
  for Bell's palsy, 951–952, 962
  for erythema multiforme, 863–864, 864**b**
  for herpes simplex virus, 841–842, 841**t**, 842
    orolabial, 849
  for neonatal conjunctivitis, 196
  for postherpetic neuralgia, 964
  for varicella, 76–78, 77**b**
  for varicella zoster virus, 841**t**, 842
  for viral meningitis or encephalitis, 931
AD. *See* Alzheimer's disease (AD).
ADACEL. *See* Tetanus and diphtheria toxoids and acellular pertussis vaccine (Tdap, BOOSTRIX, ADACEL).
Adalat. *See* Nifedipine (Adalat, Procardia).
Adalimumab (Humira)
  for ankylosing spondylitis, 987–988
  for arthritis
    juvenile idiopathic, 985–986
    rheumatoid, 980, 981, 981**t**
  for inflammatory bowel disease, 517
  for psoriasis, 803, 803**t**
  for systemic lupus erythematosus, 809
"Adam" (3,4-methylenedioxymethamphetamine)
  abuse of, 1110
  intoxication with, 1178–1179
Adamsite, as chemical weapon, 1226–1228**t**

ADAMTS13, in thrombotic thrombocytopenic purpura, 430–431
Adapalene (Differin), for acne, 787
Adderall (amphetamine salts, mixed), for ADHD, 918t
Addiction, 1105
　defined, 4–5
　to opioids, 4–5
　signs and symptoms of, 4–5
Adefovir (Hepsera), for hepatitis B and C viruses, 536t, 537
Adenocarcinoma
　of bladder, 736
　of cervix, 1090–1091
　　clear cell, 1090
　　in situ, 1090
　　invasive, 1090–1091
　　microinvasive, 1090
　gastric, 556–557
　　classification and epidemiology of, 556
　　diagnosis of, 556–557, 556b
　　Helicobacter pylori–associated, 529, 556
　　risk factors for, 556
　　staging of, 557
　　treatment of, 557, 557b
　vulvar, 1092–1093
Adenocarcinoma in situ (ACIS), of cervix, 1090
Adenoma(s), pituitary
　Cushing's syndrome due to, 642f, 644
　growth hormone–secreting, 633
Adenomatous polyps, 558–559
　due to acromegaly, 635
Adenomyosis, 1054
Adenosine
　for atrial tachycardia, 323
　for atrioventricular reciprocating tachycardia, 322
Adenosis tumor, 1047
Adenosquamous carcinoma, of cervix, 1090
Adenovirus
　keratoconjunctivitis due to, 194–195
　meningitis or encephalitis due to, 928–930t
ADH. *See* Antidiuretic hormone (ADH).
ADH (atypical ductal hyperplasia), 1047
ADHD. *See* Attention-deficit/hyperactivity disorder (ADHD).
Adherence, to HAART, 52–53
Adipsia, diabetes insipidus with, 648
Adjustable laparoscopic band, 610–611, 611f
Adjuvant therapy, for breast cancer, 1052–1053
ADLs (activities of daily living), stroke rehabilitation for, 896–897
Adolescents. *See also* Children.
　ADHD in, 917, 916b
　asthma in, 762
　　aggravating factors for, 763
　　allergic sensitization and, 763, 765
　　assessment for, 763–764
　　　of aggravating factors, 763
　　　of asthma control, 764t
　　　of current status, 763–764
　　　of past severity, 763
　　classification of severity of, 763t
　　diagnosis of, 764
　　differential diagnosis of, 763
　　environmental triggers for, 763, 765, 765b
　　follow-up for, 768–769
　　immunotherapy for, 765
　　impact of, 762
　　long-term management of, 764–768, 769b
　　　comparative daily dosages for inhaled corticosteroids in, 769t
　　　goals of, 764, 765
　　　long-term control medications in, 767–768t
　　　nonpharmacologic therapy in, 764–765, 765b
　　　pharmacologic step therapy in, 765–768, 768t

Adolescents (Continued)
　　　quick-relief medications in, 766t
　　psychosocial factors in, 763, 765
　　treatment of exacerbations of, 769–770, 769b
　bariatric surgery in, 610
　diabetes mellitus in, 583
　　diabetic ketoacidosis due to, 584
　　diagnosis of, 584
　　exercise for, 588
　　goals of therapy for, 586, 586t
　　hypoglycemia with, 588
　　initial management of, 584
　　insulin replacement therapy for, 586–587, 587t
　　initiation of, 584–585, 585f
　　medical nutrition therapy for, 587–588
　　outpatient care for, 585
　　patient education for, 585–586
　　psychosocial support for, 588
　　screening in
　　　for complications, 588–589, 589t
　　　for other autoimmune diseases, 589
　　self-monitoring of, 587
　　sick day management for, 588
　　type 1, 583
　　type 2, 583, 589–590
　　　medications for, 590, 590t
　　　risk factors for, 589t, 590
　dyslipoproteinemia in, 606
　epilepsy in, 901
　　chronic and refractory, 902, 903
　　clinical approach to, 900–902
　　clinical features of, 899
　　defined, 899
　　diagnosis and classification of, 899–902, 900t
　　differential diagnosis of, 900, 901t
　　epidemiology of, 898
　　etiology of, 899, 899t
　　historical background of, 898–899
　　interictal state in, 901
　　new-onset, 901–902
　　status epilepticus in, 906
　　treatment of, 902–906, 904t
Adrenal computed tomography, for aldosteronism, 655
Adrenal cortex, physiology of, 637
Adrenal crisis, 638, 639
　treatment of, 639, 639b
Adrenal disease, Cushing's syndrome due to, 641b, 642f, 643–644
　treatment of, 644–645
Adrenal hyperplasia
　bilateral, 654
　congenital, 637
　primary, 654
Adrenal insufficiency. *See* Adrenocortical insufficiency.
Adrenal vein sampling, for aldosteronism, 655
Adrenalectomy
　for Cushing's syndrome, 644–645
　unilateral laparoscopic, for aldosteronism, 656
Adrenalin. *See* Epinephrine (Adrenalin).
Adrenergic urticaria, 874
Adrenocortical insufficiency, 637
　acute, 638
　biochemical diagnosis of, 638–639, 638b
　chronic, 638
　clinical presentation of, 638–639
　defined, 637
　endocrine physiology and, 637
　etiology of, 637–638, 637b
　primary, 637–639
　relative, 638
　secondary, 637–639
　treatment of, 639–640, 639b

Adrenocorticotropic hormone (ACTH), 637
　in hypopituitarism, 657
　for infantile spasms, 909
Adrenocorticotropic hormone (ACTH)-dependent Cushing's syndrome, 641b, 642f, 643–644
Adrenocorticotropic hormone (ACTH)-independent Cushing's syndrome, 641b, 642f, 643–644
　treatment of, 644–645
Adrenocorticotropic hormone (ACTH) release inhibitors, for Cushing's syndrome, 645t
Adrenocorticotropic hormone (ACTH) stimulation test, 638, 638b
Adrenoleukodystrophy, 637–638
Adriamycin (doxorubicin)
　for multiple myeloma, 469b, 470
　for ovarian cancer, 1096
Adrucil. *See* 5-Fluorouracil (5-FU, Adrucil, Efudex, Carac, Fluoroplex).
Adult inclusion conjunctivitis, 195
Advair (fluticasone/salmeterol). *See* Fluticasone/salmeterol (Advair).
Advanced sleep phase, 888
Adverse drug reactions (ADRs), to HAART, 53, 54–55t, 58t, 784t
Advil. *See* Ibuprofen (Advil, Motrin).
Advisory Committee on Immunization Practices (ACIP), 148
AED (automated external defibrillator), for cardiac arrest, 304–305
Aeroallergens, in allergic rhinitis, 776
AeroBid (flunisolide inhalation), for asthma
　in adolescents and adults, 769t
　in children, 773–774t
Aeromonas hydrophila, necrotizing skin and soft tissue infections due to, 84t, 85t
Aeromonas species, foodborne illness due to, 81
Aerophagia, gaseousness due to, 9–10, 10t
AeroSpan (flunisolide hydrofluoroalkane), for asthma, 769t
AF. *See* Atrial fibrillation (AF).
Affective flattening, in schizophrenia, 1129
AFP. *See* -fetoprotein (AFP).
African plum, for benign prostatic hyperplasia, 715–717
African sleeping sickness, 843, 844t
Afrin. *See* Oxymetazoline (Afrin).
Afterdepolarizations, 320
　delayed, 320, 320f
　early, 320, 320f
AG (anion gap), in poisonings, 1174–1175, 1175t
Agenerase (amprenavir), for HIV, 50t
　drug interactions with, 58t
Agent 15, as chemical weapon, 1226–1228t
Aggrastat (tirofiban)
　for myocardial infarction, 364
　for unstable angina pectoris, 301, 301t
Aggrenox (dipyridamole)
　for ischemic stroke prevention, 894
　for transient ischemic attacks, 208–209
Agitation, due to alcohol withdrawal, 1102–1103b
Agoraphobia, 1131
Agranulocytosis, 413, 414t
　due to thionamide drugs, 668
Agrylin (anagrelide), for polycythemia vera, 474
AH (alcoholic hepatitis), 498–499, 498t
AH (atypical hyperplasia), of breast, 1045, 1045f, 1047
AHI (apnea-hypopnea index), 239–241
AHTR (acute hemolytic transfusion reaction), 484–486, 484–485t
AIDS. *See* Human immunodeficiency virus (HIV).
AIH (autoimmune hepatitis), 498t, 499
AIP (acute intermittent porphyria), 475t, 476t

Air pollutants, and asthma, 765b
Air travel, and venous thrombosis, 158
　epidemiology of, 376
　etiology of, 376–377
　prevention of, 377
　risk factors for, 376, 376b
Airway, breathing
　circulation, drugs (ABCDs), for newborn resuscitation, 970, 1034
　circulation (ABCs)
　　for burns, 1135
　　for traumatic brain injury in children
　　　moderate, 970
　　　severe, 970–971
Airway management
　for cardiac arrest, 303
　in newborn resuscitation, 1031
Airway remodeling, in childhood asthma, 770
Airway surface fluid, hydration of, for cystic fibrosis, 238
AK. See Actinic keratosis(es) (AK).
AKBeta eyedrop (levobunolol)
　for glaucoma, 200
　intoxication with, 1182–1183, 1183t
ALA dehydratase deficiency porphyria, 475t, 476t
Alavert (loratadine)
　for allergic rhinitis, 779t
　for urticaria, 875
Alavert-D (loratadine/pseudoephedrine), for allergic rhinitis, 779t
Albendazole (Albenza)
　for acute infectious diarrhea, 19–20t
　for *Ascaris,* 569, 570t
　for *Encephalocytozoon intestinalis,* 565–566t, 569
　for giardiasis, 63–64, 64t, 64b, 565–566t
　for hookworm, 570t
　for pinworm, 570t
　for strongyloidiasis, 570t
　for trichuriasis, 570t, 571
Albumin, serum, in nutritional assessment, 619
Albumin (Albuminar)
　for hepatorenal syndrome, 503
　for nephrotic syndrome, 701
Albuterol (Accuneb, Proventil, Ventolin)
　for anaphylaxis, 761t
　for asthma, 28b
　　in adolescents and adults, 766t
　　in children, 772b, 774–775, 775t
　for bronchospasm, 28b
　for COPD, 28b
　for high-altitude sickness, 1142b
　for traumatic brain injury, 968
Alclometasone (Aclovate), for atopic dermatitis, 860–861
Alcohol(s)
　features of, 1190t
　and serum osmolality, 1175, 1176t
Alcohol abuse, 1099, 1101t
Alcohol dependence
　diagnostic criteria for, 1099, 1101t
　medication management of, 1103
　psychosocial interventions for, 1103
Alcohol intoxication, 1190–1191
　alcohol and glycol features and, 1190t
　disposition for, 1191
　kinetics of, 1190
　laboratory investigations of, 1190–1191
　management of, 1191
　manifestations of, 1190, 1191t
　mechanism of, 1190
　toxic dose for, 1190
Alcohol Use Disorders Identification test (AUDIT), 1098, 1098t
Alcohol withdrawal
　assessment for, 1100–1101, 1102–1103b
　detoxification for, 1100–1103
　diagnostic criteria for, 1101t

Alcohol withdrawal *(Continued)*
　general principles for, 1106, 1107b
　medications for, 1101–1103, 1107b, 1191
Alcoholic hepatitis (AH), 498–499, 498t
Alcoholic liver disease, cirrhosis due to, 496, 498t
Alcoholism, 1097
　brief intervention for, 1099–1100
　with bulimia nervosa, 1115–1116
　and depression, 1121
　diagnosis of, 1099, 1099b, 1101t
　and drug abuse, 1104
　economic and medical sequelae of, 1097
　in elderly, 1098, 1100b
　epidemiology of, 1097
　mood and anxiety disorders with, 1099
　pancreatitis due to, 546, 549
　risk classification for, 1097b
　screening for, 1097–1099
　　Alcohol Use Disorders Identification test in, 1098, 1098t
　　brief, 1097–1099
　　CAGE questionnaire in, 1098, 1099b, 1190
　　CRAFFT questionnaire in, 1098, 1099b
　　laboratory testing in, 1098–1099
　　rationale for, 1097
　　Short Michigan Alcoholism Screening Test–Geriatric in, 1098, 1100b
　　standard drinks in, 1098b
　　TWEAK questionnaire in, 1098, 1099t
　treatment of, 1100–1103, 1101b
　　Clinical Institute Withdrawal Assessment–Alcohol Revised in, 1100–1101, 1102–1103b
　　detoxification for, 1100–1103, 1102–1103b
　　pharmacologic therapy in
　　　for alcohol dependence, 1103
　　　for withdrawal, 1101–1103
　　psychosocial interventions in, 1103
Aldactone. See Spironolactone (Aldactone).
Aldara. See Imiquimod (Aldara).
Aldicarb, poisoning due to, 1205–1206
Aldomet (methyldopa), for hypertension in pregnancy, 1023t
Aldosterone, 637
　plasma concentration of, 654
Aldosterone antagonists, for hypertension, 356t
Aldosterone-producing adenoma (APA), 654
Aldosteronism, 653
　diagnosis of, 654–655
　glucocorticoid-remediable, 654
　screening for, 654, 654b
　subtypes of, 654, 654b
　　determination of, 655, 655f
　treatment of, 655–656
Alefacept (Amevive), for psoriasis, 803–804, 803t
Alemtuzumab (Campath)
　for chronic lymphocytic leukemia, 462–463
　for lymphoma
　　cutaneous T-cell, 799
　　non-Hodgkin's, 466
Alendronate (Fosamax)
　for hyperparathyroidism, 652
　for osteoporosis, 614–615
　　postmenopausal, 1073b
　for Paget's disease of bone, 617
Alexander's law, 206
Alfuzosin (Uroxatral)
　for benign prostatic hyperplasia, 714–716, 714t
　for prostatitis, 710–711
ALI. See Acute lung injury (ALI).
Alinia (nitazoxanide)
　for cryptosporidiosis, 565–566t, 568
　for giardiasis, 63–64, 64t, 64b, 544, 564–567, 565–566t
Aliphatic hydrocarbons, 1193

Aliphatic phenothiazines, poisoning due to, 1208–1209, 1208t
Aliskiren (Tekturna), 1243
Alkali(s)
　burns due to, 1138–1139
　poisoning due to, 1185–1186
Alkaline phosphatase, elevated serum, with parenteral nutrition, 625t, 626
Alkeran (melphalan), for multiple myeloma, 469b, 470
"Alkohl," lead in, 1197
ALL. See Acute lymphoblastic leukemia (ALL).
Allegra. See Fexofenadine (Allegra).
Allergen(s)
　in allergic rhinitis, 776
　and asthma
　　in adolescents and adults, 765b
　　in children, 771
　atopic dermatitis due to, 860
　for patch testing, 870
Allergen immunotherapy, for allergic rhinitis, 780–781
Allergic conjunctivitis
　drug-induced, 194t
　seasonal, 193–194, 194t
Allergic contact dermatitis (ACD), 30b, 31b
　diagnosis of, 870, 870b
　pathogenesis of, 870
　treatment of, 870–871, 871b
Allergic disease(s)
　allergic reactions to drugs as, 781
　allergic reactions to insect stings as, 784
　allergic rhinitis as, 776
　anaphylaxis and serum sickness as, 759
　asthma as
　　in adolescents and adults, 762
　　in children, 770
Allergic reaction(s), 777
　to drugs, 781
　　desensitization for, 782–783
　　evaluation of, 783–784, 784t
　　graded challenge for, 782–783, 783b
　　pathophysiology of, 782–783, 782f 783b
　　types of, 781–782
　to insect stings, 784
　　diagnosis of, 784–785, 784b
　　epidemiology of, 784
　　localized *vs.* systemic, 784
　　pathogenesis of, 784
　　prevention of, 785–786, 786t
　　risk of future, 785, 785t
　　treatment and avoidance of, 785, 785b
Allergic rhinitis, 214, 776
　classification of, 776–777
　　by severity and frequency, 776–777, 777b
　　by type of aeroallergen, 776
　comorbid conditions with, 777
　cough due to, 28b
　diagnosis of, 778–779
　differential diagnosis of, 777–778, 778b
　epidemiology of, 776
　impact of, 776
　intermittent, 776–777
　pathogenesis of, 777
　persistent, 776–777
　treatment of, 779–781
　　avoidance and environmental controls in, 780
　　pharmacotherapy in, 779–780, 779t, 780t
　　specific allergen immunotherapy for, 780–781
Allergic Rhinitis and Its Impact on Asthma Workshop Group (ARIA), 776–777, 777b
Allergic rhinoconjunctivitis, 777
Allergic salute, 778
Allergic sensitization, and asthma, 763, 765
Allergic shiners, 778
Allergic transfusion reactions, 484–485t, 488–489

Allergy diagnostic testing, 778–779
Allogeneic bone marrow transplantation, for chronic myeloid leukemia, 460
Allogeneic stem-cell transplantation, for multiple myeloma, 470
Alloimmune thrombocytopenia, 426
Alloimmunization
  to RhD antigen, 416
    diagnosis of, 416b
    prevention of, 416
    treatment of, 416–418, 417b
  transfusion-related, 484, 491
Allopurinol (Zyloprim)
  for hyperuricemia, 599–600, 600t
  for leishmaniasis, 96
  for renal calculi, 746t
  for renal failure, due to multiple myeloma, 471
All-*trans*-retinoic acid (ATRA, tretinoin, Vesanoid), for acute promyelocytic leukemia, 448–449
Almorexant, 1244–1249t
Almotriptan (Axert), for migraine headache, 925t, 926
ALND (axillary lymph node dissection), 1052
Aloe vera, for inflammatory bowel disease, 519
Alopecia
  androgenic, 791
  areata, 791–792
  central centrifugal scarring, 792
  frontal fibrosing, 792
  traction, 792
Alosetron (Lotronex), for irritable bowel syndrome, 524–525
α adrenergic agonists, for stress incontinence, 695b, 696
α adrenergic antagonists (α-blockers)
  for pheochromocytomas and paragangliomas, 675
  poisoning due to, 1179–1180
  for prostatitis, 710–711
α₁ adrenergic antagonists (α₁-blockers)
  for benign prostatic hyperplasia, 714–718, 714t
  for hypertension, 358
  for urinary incontinence in children, 691
α₁-antitrypsin (AAT) deficiency, 231–232
  cirrhosis due to, 498t, 501
α₂ adrenergic receptor agonists
  for glaucoma, 200, 200t
  for Tourette's syndrome, 920
α₂-adrenergic stimulants, central, for hypertension, 358–359
α-fetoprotein (AFP)
  in hepatocellular carcinoma, 504
  during pregnancy, 1012
  in testicular cancer, 738
Alphagan (brimonidine), for glaucoma, 200
17-Alpha-hydroxy-progesterone caproate (Gestiva), 1244–1249t
AlphaquinHP (hydroquinone 4% cream with glycolic acids and sunscreens)
  for melasma, 876–877
  for solar lentigines, 877
Alprazolam (Xanax)
  intoxication with, 1181–1182
  for panic disorder, 1132, 1132t
  for premenstrual syndrome, 1069
  for psychiatric dizziness, 209
  for tinnitus, 38
Alprenolol, intoxication with, 1182–1183, 1183t
Alprostadil (Caverject), for erectile dysfunction, 719
ALT (argon laser trabeculoplasty), for glaucoma, 200
Altabax (retapamulin), 1243
Altace (ramipril), for angina pectoris, 297
Alteplase (Activase), for myocardial infarction, 364t

Altitude sickness. See High-altitude sickness.
Altocor (lovastatin)
  for angina pectoris, 298
  for dyslipoproteinemia, 605t
Alupent (metaproterenol), for asthma in children, 775t
Alurate (aprobarbital), intoxication with, 1180–1181
Alveolar process, disorders of, 853–855
Alveolar–arterial (A–a) O₂ gradient, 225, 226t
Alveolitis
  in idiopathic inflammatory myopathy, 813
  in systemic sclerosis, 811
Alzheimer's disease (AD), 881
  clinical presentation of, 881
  defined, 881
  differential diagnosis of, 881, 882t
  epidemiology of, 881–882
  evaluation of, 883t, 886b
  pathology of, 882
  risk factors for, 882
  stages of, 882t
  treatment and management of, 886b
    for behavioral and psychiatric symptoms, 884–887, 885t
    for cognitive symptoms, 882–884, 883t
Amalgam tattoo, 854
AMAN (acute motor axonal neuropathy), 962
Amantadine (Symmetrel)
  for influenza, 260, 260b
    pneumonia due to, 266–267, 267t, 269b
  for multiple sclerosis, 939b
  for neuroleptic intoxication, 1209
  for parkinsonism, 957–958
  after traumatic brain injury, 969
Amaryl (glimepiride), for diabetes, 578, 580t
Ambien (zolpidem), for insomnia, 888, 888t
AmBisome. See Amphotericin B, liposomal (L-AmB, AmBisome).
Ambrisentan (Letairis), 1243
Ambulation, stroke rehabilitation for, 896
A-MDT (accompanied multidrug therapy), for leprosy, 101
Amebiasis, 59, 563–564, 565–566t
  acute infectious diarrhea due to, 16, 19–20t
  cutaneous, 843, 844t
  diagnosis of, 60, 60t
  epidemiology of, 59
  intestinal, 59
  pathogenesis of, 59
  therapy for, 60–61, 61t
Amebic colitis
  clinical presentation of, 59
  diagnosis of, 60, 60t
  treatment of, 60–61, 61t
Amebic dysentery, 563
  acute infectious diarrhea due to, 16
Amebic liver abscess, 563–564
  clinical presentation of, 59–60
  diagnosis of, 60, 60t
  treatment of, 61, 61t
Amegakaryocytic thrombocytopenia, 381t
Amenorrhea, 1062
  classification of, 1062
  defined, 1062
  diagnosis of, 1064–1065, 1064b
  epidemiology of, 1062
  etiology of, 1062–1064, 1062f
    hypothalamic compartment in, 1062–1063, 1064b
    outflow tract compartment in, 1063, 1064b
    ovarian compartment in, 1063, 1064b
    pituitary compartment in, 1063, 1064b
  in normal situations, 1062
  physiologic, 1062
  primary *vs.* secondary, 1062
Amerge (naratriptan), for migraine headache, 925t, 926

American College of Rheumatology (ACR) criteria, for rheumatoid arthritis, 977, 978t
Amevive (alefacept), for psoriasis, 803–804, 803t
Amicar (ε–aminocaproic acid), for hemophilia, 422
Amikacin (Amikin)
  for bacterial meningitis, 115t
  for *Mycobacterium avium intracellulare* complex, 289
  for tuberculosis, 285t
Amiloride (Midamor), for ascites, 501
Amino acid solution, for high-risk neonate, 1035
Amino acid–based infant formula, 1043b
Amino acid–modified infant formula, 1043b
ε–Aminocaproic acid (Amicar), for hemophilia, 422
Aminoglutethimide (Cytadren), for Cushing's syndrome, 645t
Aminoglycosides
  for infective endocarditis, 345
  for pyelonephritis, 685
Aminophylline, for heart block, 318
Aminosalicylates, for inflammatory bowel disease, 515–516, 519
5-Aminosalicylic acid (5-ASA), for inflammatory bowel disease, 515–516, 519–520
Amiodarone (Cordarone)
  for atrial fibrillation, 310, 310b
  for cardiac arrest, 306
  for cardioversion, 311, 311t
  for myocardial infarction, 365
  peripheral neuropathy due to, 963
  for premature ventricular complexes, 314
Amitiza (lubiprostone), for constipation, 10t, 22, 22b
Amitriptyline (Elavil)
  for anogenital pruritus, 872b
  for ciguatera poisoning, 1157t
  for dyspepsia, 528
  for fibromyalgia, 998b
  for gaseousness, 10t
  for multiple sclerosis, 939b
  for neuropathic pain, 964, 964t
  poisoning due to, 1214–1216, 1215t
  for temporomandibular disorder, 992–993
  for tinnitus, 38
AML. See Acute myeloid leukemia (AML).
AML-M3 (acute promyelocytic leukemia)
  disseminated intravascular coagulation in, 429
  treatment of, 446b, 448–449
Amlodipine (Norvasc)
  for angina pectoris, 299t
  intoxication with, 1183–1184
  for systemic sclerosis, 811t
Amlodipine/olmesartan (Azor), 1243
Amlodipine/valsartan (Exforge), 1243
Ammonia (NH₃), as chemical weapon, 1226–1228t
Amniocentesis, 1012
  for Rh-sensitized women, 417, 418
Amobarbital (Amytal), intoxication with, 1180–1181
Amoebae, 563–567, 565–566t
Amoebic. See Amebic.
Amoxapine (Asendin), poisoning due to, 1214–1216, 1215t
Amoxicillin (Amoxil)
  for anthrax, 126t
  for bacterial overgrowth, 10t
  for endocarditis prophylaxis, 347t
  for indigestion, 11t
  for Lyme disease, 138, 139t
  for otitis media, 203–204, 203b
  for peptic ulcer disease, 532t
  for pyelonephritis, 706b
  for relapsing fever, 136t
  for *Salmonella* gastroenteritis, 173
  for urinary tract infections

Amoxicillin (Amoxil) *(Continued)*
    in girls, 687b
    in women
        catheter-associated bacteriuria as, 684–685
        cystitis as, 684, 684b
        pyelonephritis as, 685
        recurrent, 685
Amoxicillin-clavulanate (Augmentin)
    for otitis media, 203–204
    for streptococcal pharyngitis, 223t
    for urinary tract infections in males, 681t
Amoxil. *See* Amoxicillin (Amoxil).
Amphetamine(s)
    abuse of, 1105b, 1109–1110
    intoxication with, 1178–1179
    kinetics of, 1179
Amphetamine salts, mixed (Adderall), for ADHD, 918t
Amphotericin B, liposomal (L-AmB, AmBisome)
    for cryptococcosis in HIV, 56
    for histoplasmosis, 254
    for leishmaniasis, 94b, 95
    for necrotizing skin and soft tissue infections, 85t
Amphotericin B colloidal dispersion (Amphicil, Amphotec), for leishmaniasis, 94–95
Amphotericin B deoxycholate (Fungizone)
    for blastomycosis, 255, 255b
    for coccidioidomycosis, 250b, 250t, 251t
        acute, 250–251
        chronic, 251
    for cryptococcosis in HIV, 56
    for histoplasmosis, 253, 253t, 253b
    for leishmaniasis, 94b, 94–95
    for necrotizing skin and soft tissue infections, 85t
Amphotericin B lipid complex (ABLC, Abelcet)
    for histoplasmosis, 254
    for leishmaniasis, 94–95
    for necrotizing skin and soft tissue infections, 85t
Ampicillin (Omnipen)
    for bacterial meningitis, 115t
    for endocarditis prophylaxis, 346–347t
    for pyelonephritis, 685, 706, 706b
    for rat-bite fever, 132–133
    for *Salmonella* gastroenteritis, 173
Ampicillin/sulbactam (Unasyn)
    for pelvic inflammatory disease, 1080b
    for pyelonephritis, 706, 706b
Amprenavir (Agenerase), for HIV, 50t
    drug interactions with, 58t
Amrinone (Inocor), for poisoning
    due to β-blockers, 1183
    due to calcium channel blockers, 1184
AMS. *See* Acute mountain sickness (AMS).
AMSAM (acute motor and sensory axonal neuropathy), 962
Amylase, serum, in pancreatitis, 546–547
Amylin agonists, for diabetes, 580t, 581
Amyloid precursor protein (APP), in Alzheimer's disease, 882
Amyloidosis, 961
Amyotrophy, diabetic, 962–963
Amytal (amobarbital), intoxication with, 1180–1181
ANA (antinuclear antibodies), in peripheral neuropathy, 961
Anabolic agents
    for osteoporosis, 615
    parenteral nutrition with, 624
Anabolic steroids, abuse of, 1111
Anafranil. *See* Clomipramine (Anafranil).
Anagen effluvium, 791
Anagen phase, of hair growth, 790
Anagrelide (Agrylin), for polycythemia vera, 474

Anakinra (Kineret), for arthritis
    juvenile idiopathic, 985–986
    rheumatoid, 981t, 982
Anal fissures, 526
    defined, 526
    differential diagnosis of, 525, 525t
    evaluation of, 525–526
    history of, 525–526
    physical examination of, 525–526
    symptoms of, 525
    treatment of, 526
Analgesic(s)
    for osteoarthritis, 999–1000
    reference intervals for, 1222t
    for renal calculi, 744–745, 745t
Analgesic staircase, for vasoocclusive pain in sickle cell disease, 407–408, 410f
Anaphylactic reactions, to transfusions, 484–485t
Anaphylaxis, 759–761
    agents that cause, 759–760, 760t
    clinical presentation of, 759, 759b
    defined, 759
    diagnosis of, 759b
    diagnostic criteria for, 759
    differential diagnosis of, 760
    epidemiology of, 759
    idiopathic, 760, 760
    IgE dependent, 760t
    IgE independent, 760t
    management of, 760–761, 761t
    pathophysiology of, 759
    prevention of, 761, 761t
    recurrent (biphasic), 760
Anaplasma species. *See* Anaplasmosis.
Anaplasmosis, 178
    clinical features and diagnosis of, 178
    epidemiology of, 178
    treatment of, 178–179, 179b
Anaplastic thyroid cancers, 672, 673t
Anaprox. *See* Naproxen sodium (Anaprox, Naprelan, Naprosyn).
Anastrozole (Arimidex), for breast cancer, 1053
ANC (absolute neutrophil count), 413, 414t
Ancef (cefazolin)
    for endocarditis prophylaxis, 346–347t
    for osteomyelitis, 1006–1007
Ancobon (flucytosine), for cryptococcosis, 56
Ancylostoma brazilense, 844, 844t
Ancylostoma duodenale, 570t, 571, 844t, 845
Androderm (testosterone patch), for hypopituitarism, 658
AndroGel (testosterone gel), for hypopituitarism, 658
Androgen, for adrenocortical insufficiency, 639b, 640
Androgen deprivation therapy, for prostate cancer, 732
Androgenic alopecia, 791
Androgenic anabolic steroids, abuse of, 1111
Anecortave acetate (Retaane), 1244–1249t
Anemia(s)
    aplastic, 379
        defined, 379
        diagnosis of, 380b
        diagnostic criteria for, 379
        differential diagnosis of, 379, 381t
        severity classification of, 380b
        supportive care for, 379–380
        survival with, 379, 380f
        treatment of, 380–382, 382b
            hematopoietic stem cell transplantation for, 382, 382f
            immunosuppressive therapy for, 380–382
            long-term complications of, 382–383
            triage of, 380, 381f
    in chronic renal failure, 727, 727t, 729–730
    Cooley's
        clinical manifestations of, 398–399

Anemia(s) *(Continued)*
        diagnosis of, 398b
        genetic basis for, 398
        treatment of, 398b
    Fanconi, 381t
        and childhood leukemia, 452t
    hemolytic
        autoimmune, 387
            classification and serology of, 387, 387t
            cold agglutinin syndrome as, 388–389, 388b
            drug-induced, 389, 389b
            paroxysmal cold hemoglobinuria as, 389
            warm, 387–388, 388b
        microangiopathic, 430–431
        nonimmune, 390
            acquired, 393–394
            causes of, 391t
            due to chemical and physical agents, 391t, 394
            congenital, 391–393, 393t
            diagnosis of, 390, 390b
            due to erythrocyte fragmentation, 391t, 394
            due to erythrocyte membrane abnormalities, 391–392, 391t
            due to erythrocyte metabolism abnormalities, 391t, 392–393, 393t
            due to glucose-6-phosphate dehydrogenase deficiency, 392–393, 393t
            due to hemoglobinopathies, 391t, 393
            hereditary elliptocytosis and pyropoikilocytosis as, 392
            hereditary spherocytosis as, 391–392
            hereditary stomatocytosis and xerocytosis as, 392
            due to infection, 391t, 394
            paroxysmal nocturnal hemoglobinuria as, 393–394
            due to pyruvate kinase deficiency, 393
            treatment of, 390–391, 390b
    iron-deficiency, 384t
        pruritus due to, 32b
    due to multiple myeloma, 471
    pernicious and other megaloblastic, 394
        clinical features of, 395
        diagnosis of, 395–396, 395b
        etiology and pathophysiology of, 394b, 395
        malabsorption in, 543
        treatment of, 396–397, 396b
    sickle cell, 404
Anesthetics, and SSRIs, 1122–1123b
Aneurysm
    aortic (*See* Aortic aneurysm)
    defined, 291
    intracranial, orofacial pain due to, 992t
Angel dust. *See* Phencyclidine (PCP, angel dust).
Angina, postinfarction, 366t
Angina pectoris, 295
    clinical features of, 295
    diagnosis of, 295–296
    differential diagnosis of, 296b
    functional classification of, 296
    high-risk, 296, 300, 300b
    management of, 295–300
        for refractory disease, 300
        for stable disease, 296–298, 297b
            antianginal drugs in, 298–299, 299t
            anticoagulants in, 298
            β-blockers in, 299, 299t
            blood pressure in, 296–297
            calcium channel blockers in, 299, 299t
            cholesterol in, 297–298, 298t
            futures therapies in, 299–300
            metabolic syndrome in, 297–298
            weight and diet in, 297
        for unstable disease, 300–301, 300b, 301t

Angina pectoris (Continued)
    stable
        defined, 295
        treatment of, 296–298, 297b
    unstable, 300–301
        biomarkers for, 301
        clinical findings in, 300, 300b
        defined, 295
        treatment of, 300–301, 301t
    in women, 295
Angina pectoris equivalents, 295
Angioedema, 873
    causes of, 873, 874b
    defined, 873
    diagnosis of, 873b
    evaluation of, 874
    hereditary, 876
    of labial mucosa, 850–851
    migratory, 844, 844t
    pathogenesis of, 873
    due to transfusion, 488
    treatment of, 874b, 875–876
Angiomax (bivalirubin), for myocardial infarction, 366
Angiomyolipoma, of kidney, 734, 734b
Angiotensin II, 637
Angiotensin receptor blockers (ARBs)
    for focal and segmental glomerulosclerosis, 701–702
    for glomerular disease, 700–701
    for hypertension, 356t, 358
    for membranoproliferative glomerulonephritis, 703
    for membranous nephropathy, 702
    during pregnancy, 1023
    and SSRIs, 1122–1123
    for systemic sclerosis, 811t
Angiotensin-converting enzyme (ACE), in sarcoidosis, 276
Angiotensin-converting enzyme inhibitors (ACEIs)
    allergy to, 783
    for angina pectoris, 297
    cough due to, 26–27
    for focal and segmental glomerulosclerosis, 701–702
    for glomerular disease, 700–701
    for heart failure, 339t, 340
    for hypertension, 356t, 357–358
    for membranoproliferative glomerulonephritis, 703
    for membranous nephropathy, 702
    for myocardial infarction, 364, 365t
    during pregnancy, 1011–1012, 1023
Angle-closure glaucoma
    acute, 200
    primary, 199, 198b
    secondary, 199
Angular cheilitis, 849
Animal bites, 836b
Animal dander
    allergic rhinitis due to, 776, 780
    and asthma, 765b
Anion gap (AG), in poisonings, 1174–1175, 1175t
Anisaka spp, 570t, 572
Anisakiasis, 570t, 572
Ankle injuries, due to sports, 1009
Ankle sprains, 1009
    high, 1009
Ankylosing spondylitis (AS), 986
    defined, 986
    diagnosis of, 986–987, 987b
        clinical features in, 987
        diagnostic criteria in, 987, 987b
        difficulties and delays in, 986–987
    prognosis and long-term outcomes for, 988
    treatment of, 987–988, 988b

Ann Arbor staging system, for Hodgkin's lymphoma, 434–435, 435t, 440t, 441f
Anogenital pruritus, 31f
    clinical features and diagnosis of, 872, 872b
    defined, 871
    epidemiology of, 871
    etiology of, 871–872
    treatment of, 872–873, 872b, 873b
Anorectal abscess and fistula, 526–527
    differential diagnosis of, 525, 525t
    evaluation of, 525–527
    history of, 525
    pathogenesis of, 526
    physical examination of, 525, 527
    treatment of, 527
Anovulatory bleeding, 1058–1059
Ansamycins, for leprosy, 102b
Antabuse (disulfiram), for alcohol dependence, 1103
Antacids
    for gastroesophageal reflux disease, 554
    for peptic ulcer disease, 531–532
Antepartum care, 1011
    for backache and pelvic discomfort, 1015–1016
    for bleeding, 1013
    for constipation, 1015
    dental, 1016
    diagnosis in, 1015b
    for heartburn, 1014
    high-risk obstetric referrals in, 1011, 1011b
    hospitalization for, 1017
    immunization in, 1016
    for infection, 1014–1015, 1015b
    on intercourse, 1016
    for leg cramps, 1016
    for nausea, 1013–1014
    nutrition and weight gain in, 1014
    preconception counseling in, 1011
    tests of fetal well-being in, 1016–1017, 1016b, 1017t
    therapy in, 1016b
    timeline of, 1011–1013
        at 15 to 18 weeks' gestation, 1012
        at 18 to 20 weeks' gestation, 1012–1013
        at 28 weeks' gestation, 1013, 1013b
        at 36 weeks' gestation, 1013
        first visit and early care in, 1011–1012
        for post-term gestation, 1013
    for upper extremity discomfort, 1015
    for urinary symptoms, 1014
    for varicose veins, 1015
    x-rays, ionizing radiation, and imaging in, 1016
Anterior cruciate ligament (ACL) tears, 1008
Anterior inferior cerebellar artery syndrome, vertigo due to, 209
Anterior knee pain syndrome, 1008
Anterior uveitis, due to sarcoidosis, 275–276
Anthrax, 123
    background of, 123–124
    as biological weapon agent, 1229–1233t
    clinical features of, 124
    cutaneous
        clinical features of, 124
        diagnosis of, 124, 125b
        etiology of, 124
        treatment of, 125–126, 125b, 126t, 127
    diagnosis of, 124–125, 125b
    forms of, 124
    gastrointestinal
        clinical features of, 124
        diagnosis of, 124, 125b
        etiology of, 124
        treatment of, 125–126, 125b, 126t
    historical background of, 123
    inhalational
        clinical features of, 124

Anthrax (Continued)
    diagnosis of, 124–125, 125b
    etiology of, 124
    treatment of, 125–126, 125b, 126t
microbiology of, 123
oropharyngeal
    clinical features of, 124
    diagnosis of, 124, 125b
    etiology of, 124
postexposure prophylaxis for, 126t, 127
treatment of, 125–127, 125b, 126t
Anthrax vaccine (BioThrax), 127
Anti-anginal drug therapy, 298–299, 299t
Antiarrhythmic drugs
    for atrial fibrillation, 310b, 310t
    for myocardial infarction, 365
Antibiotic(s)
    for acute bronchitis, 260
    for acute infectious diarrhea, 18b, 19, 19–20t
    for cystic fibrosis, 239
    for gaseousness, 10t
    for infective endocarditis, 345, 346–347t
    for inflammatory bowel disease, 517–518
    for neutropenia, 414–415
    oral
        for acne, 788
        for rosacea, 789
    for osteomyelitis, 1006–1007, 1006t
        by Cierny-Mader stage, 1007
        suppressive, 1007
    reference intervals for, 1222t
    topical, for rosacea, 789
Antibiotic prophylaxis
    for acute infectious diarrhea, 17
    for infective endocarditis, 345–347
        conditions not needed in, 348t
        indications for, 348t
        preprocedural, 347t
    for surgical site infections, 838
Antibody testing, for myasthenia gravis, 941–942
Anti-c antibodies, 418–419
Anticatabolic agents, for osteoporosis, 614–615
Anticholinergic(s)
    abuse of, 1111
    for asthma
        in adolescents and adults, 766t
        in children, 774–775
    for nausea and vomiting, 8, 8t
    for parkinsonism, 957
    poisoning due to, 1166t, 1179–1180
    topical, for allergic rhinitis, 780
    for urinary incontinence
        in children, 691
        urge, 695, 695b
Anticoagulation
    for angina pectoris, 298
    for atrial fibrillation, 309, 309t
Anticonvulsants. See Antiepileptic drugs (AEDs).
Anticytokine therapy, for inflammatory bowel disease, 517
Antidepressant(s)
    for Alzheimer's disease, 884, 885t
    bupropion as, 1123
    for gaseousness, 10t
    for irritable bowel syndrome, 524t
    for major depression, 1121–1124, 1122–1123b
    MAOIs as, 1124
    for migraine headache, 925
    mirtazipine as, 1124
    nefazodone as, 1124
    for panic disorder, 1132, 1132t
    SNRIs as, 1123
    SSRIs as, 1121–1123, 1122–1123b
    trazodone as, 1124
    tricyclic, 1123–1124
Antidiarrheal medications, 18b, 19
    for irritable bowel syndrome, 524t

Antidiuretic hormone (ADH)
  circulating
    high, 595, 595b, 596–597
    low, 595b
  in hospitalized children, 627
  secretion of inappropriate, 596–597, 597b
Antidotes, for poisonings, 1165, 1167–1172t
Antidromic reciprocating tachycardia (ART), 321–322, 322f
Antiemetic drugs
  for nausea and vomiting, 7–9, 8t
  parkinsonism due to, 954b
  for renal calculi, 745t
  for *Salmonella* gastroenteritis, 172
Antiepileptic drugs (AEDs)
  for alcohol withdrawal, 1103
  for Alzheimer's disease, 885t, 884–886
  for bipolar disorder, 1127
  for elevated intracranial pressure in children, 971
  for epilepsy
    in adolescents in adults, 903–905, 904t
      cost of, 905
      monitoring of, 903–905
      monotherapy with, 903
      for refractory disease, 903
      withdrawal from, 905
    in infants and children, 911–915, 912t, 913t
  for intracerebral hemorrhage, 892
  for migraine headache, 925
  reference intervals for, 1222t
  and SSRIs, 1122–1123b
Antifungal agents, for coccidioidomycosis, 250b, 250t, 251t
Antigenic drift, 90
Antigenic shift, 90
Antihistamines
  abuse of, 1111
  for allergic rhinitis, 779, 779t
  for anaphylaxis, 760
  for motion sickness and vertigo, 206t
  for nausea and vomiting, 8, 8t
  poisoning due to, 1179–1180
  for scombroid poisoning, 1157
  for serum sickness, 762
  and SSRIs, 1122–1123b
  for urticaria, 875
Antihypertensive drugs
  for preeclampsia, 1025
  during pregnancy, 1023, 1023t, 1024
  for Tourette's syndrome, 920b
Anti-IgE (omalizumab), for asthma
  in adolescents and adults, 767–768t
  in children, 775
Antiinflammatory agents
  for cystic fibrosis, 239
  for osteoarthritis, 1000
Antiinflammatory molecules, in sepsis, 67b
Anti-Kell antibodies, 418–419
Antilirium. *See* Physostigmine (Antilirium).
Antimalarial drugs, 107–109, 107b, 108t
  for systemic lupus erythematosus, 806–808, 807t
Antimicrobial agents, topical, for acne, 787–788
Antimitotics, for verrucae, 823
Antimotility agents, for *Salmonella* gastroenteritis, 172
Antimuscarinics, for urge incontinence, 695b
Antinausea medications. *See* Antiemetic drugs.
Antineoplastics, reference intervals for, 1222t
Antinuclear antibodies (ANA), in peripheral neuropathy, 961
Antioxidants, for preeclampsia, 1025
Antiparkinsonism drugs, poisoning due to, 1179–1180
Antipseudomonal penicillin, for pyelonephritis, 685

Antipsychotics
  atypical
    for Alzheimer's disease, 884–886, 885t
    for bipolar disorder, 1127–1128
    for Tourette's syndrome, 920–921, 920b
  conventional, for Tourette's syndrome, 921, 920b
  for delirium, 1119–1120, 1119b
  parkinsonism due to, 954b
  for schizophrenia, 1130–1131, 1129b, 1130t
Antipyretic medications, 24–25
Antirefluxants, for gastroesophageal reflux disease, 554
Antiretroviral therapy, for HIV, 49–50, 48b
  adherence to, 52–53
  adverse drug reactions and drug interactions with, 53, 54–55t, 58t
  currently approved drugs for, 50t
  drug resistance and resistance testing with, 51–52, 52t
  failure of, 52, 52t
  goal of, 49–50
  historical background of, 47
  monitoring response to, 51
  during pregnancy, 58
  regimens for, 49–50, 51t
  when to initiate, 50–51
Antirheumatic drugs, disease-modifying. *See* Disease-modifying antirheumatic drug(s) (DMARDs).
Antisecretory agents, for peptic ulcer disease, 531t
Antiseizure medications. *See* Antiepileptic drugs (AEDs).
Antispasmodic agents
  for gaseousness, 10t
  for irritable bowel syndrome, 524t
Antithymocyte globulin (Atgam, ATG), for aplastic anemia, 380
Antithyroid drug therapy, for hyperthyroidism, 667–668
Antitussive agents, for acute bronchitis, 260
Antivenin, for snakebite, 1153–1155
Antivert (meclizine)
  for motion sickness and vertigo, 206t, 210
  for nausea and vomiting, 8t
Antizol. *See* Fomepizole (4-methylpyrazole, 4-MP, Antizol).
Antrypol (suramin sodium), for African sleeping sickness, 843, 844t
Anturane (sulfinpyrazone), for hyperuricemia, 599
Anus, pruritus of, 31f, 871
  clinical features and diagnosis of, 872, 872b
  defined, 871
  epidemiology of, 871
  etiology of, 871–872
  treatment of, 872–873, 872b, 873b
Anxiety
  due to alcohol withdrawal, 1102–1103b
  in fibromyalgia, 997–998
  organic causes of, 1112, 1112b
Anxiety disorder(s), 1111
  with alcoholism, 1099
  with bulimia nervosa, 1115–1116
  clinical features of, 1112
  diagnosis of, 1112
  differential diagnosis of, 1112, 1112b
  factors contributing to, 1112
  generalized, 1112–1113
    diagnosis of, 1112–1113
    epidemiology of, 1113
    treatment of, 1113, 1113t, 1113b
  helpful resources for, 1113b
  impact of, 1111–1112
  obsessive compulsive disorder as, 1113–1114
    diagnosis of, 1113–1114
    treatment of, 1113b, 1114, 1114t

Anxiety disorder(s) (Continued)
  pharmacologic treatment for, 1112
  psychotherapeutic interventions for, 1112
Anxiolytics
  abuse of, 1105b, 1107–1108, 1108t
  for Alzheimer's disease, 884, 885t
  for premenstrual syndrome, 1069
Anzemet (dolasetron), for nausea and vomiting, 7, 8t
AOM. *See* Acute otitis media (AOM).
Aorta, coarctation of, 328, 329f
  antibiotic prophylaxis with, 345
Aortic aneurysm, 291–292
  abdominal, 291–292, 374–375
    diagnosis of, 291, 293b
    incidence and natural history of, 291
    infrarenal, 292
    rupture of, 291
    screening for, 292
    treatment of, 291–292, 294b
  diagnosis of, 291, 293b
  in familial diseases, 292
  incidence and natural history of, 291
  inflammatory, 291
  mycotic, 291
  risk factors for, 375
  rupture of, 291, 375
  screening for, 292, 374–375
  thoracic, 291
    diagnosis of, 291, 293b
    rupture of, 291
    treatment of, 292, 294b
  treatment of, 291–292, 294b, 375
Aortic dissection, 293
Aortic injury, traumatic, 293–294
Aortic occlusive disease, 292–293
Aortic stenosis, 328
  antibiotic prophylaxis with, 345
APA (aldosterone-producing adenoma), 654
APACHE (Acute Physiology and Chronic Health Evaluation) II, for acute pancreatitis, 547
Aphasia
  acquired epileptic, 910
  after stroke, 897
Apheresis platelets, 482
Aphthous ulcer(s), 850
  herpetiform, 850
  major, 850
Apidra (insulin glulisine), for diabetes
  in adults, 582t
  in children, 587t
Apixaban, 1244–1249t
Aplastic anemia (AA), 379
  defined, 379
  diagnosis of, 380b
  diagnostic criteria for, 379
  differential diagnosis of, 379, 381t
  severity classification of, 380b
  supportive care for, 379–380
  survival with, 379, 380f
  treatment of, 380–382, 382b
    hematopoietic stem cell transplantation for, 382, 382f
    immunosuppressive therapy for, 380–382
    long-term complications of, 382–383
    triage of, 380, 381f
APN. *See* Acute pyelonephritis (APN).
Apnea, in newborn, 1031–1032
Apnea-hypopnea index (AHI), 239–241
Apolipoprotein, in dyslipoproteinemia, 603
Apolipoprotein E (ApoE), in Alzheimer's disease, 882
Apomorphine (Apokyn), for parkinsonism, 956
Apomorphine hydrochloride (Uprima), for erectile dysfunction, 719
APP (amyloid precursor protein), in Alzheimer's disease, 882

Appearex (biotin)
  for brittle nails, 818**b**, 819
  in parenteral nutrition, 621**t**
Apraclonidine (Iopidine), for glaucoma, 200
Apraxias, after stroke, 897
Apresoline (hydralazine)
  for hypertension in pregnancy, 1027
  peripheral neuropathy due to, 963
Aprobarbital (Alurate), intoxication with, 1180–1181
APS (autoimmune polyglandular syndrome) type 1, 637
APS (autoimmune polyglandular syndrome) type 2, 637
Aptivus (tipranavir/ritonavir), for HIV, 50**t**, 51
Aqua Mephyton (vitamin K$_1$), for poisoning, 1167–1172**t**
Aqueous crystalline penicillin G, for syphilis, 755**t**
Ara-C (cytarabine), for leukemia
  acute lymphoblastic, 449
  acute myeloid, 445–446, 448
Arachidonic acid (ARA), in infant formulas, 1042
Aralen. *See* Chloroquine phosphate (Aralen).
Aranesp (darbopoetin), for chronic renal failure, 729–730
Arava (leflunomide)
  for juvenile idiopathic arthritis, 985–986
  for rheumatoid arthritis, 981–982, 981**t**
ARB(s). *See* Angiotensin receptor blockers (ARBs).
Arboviruses, meningitis or encephalitis due to, 928–930**t**
Arcanobacterium haemolyticum, pharyngitis due to, 220
ARDS. *See* Acute respiratory distress syndrome (ARDS).
Aredia (pamidronate), for multiple myeloma, 471–472
Arenaviruses, as biological weapon agents, 1229–1233**t**
ARF. *See* Acute renal failure (ARF).
Argatroban (Novastan), for deep venous thrombosis/pulmonary embolism, 273
L-Arginine, for erectile dysfunction, 719
Arginine vasopressin (AVP, Pitressin), for diabetes insipidus, 647, 647**t**
Argon laser trabeculoplasty (ALT), for glaucoma, 200
ARIA (Allergic Rhinitis and Its Impact on Asthma Workshop Group), 776–777, 777**b**
Aricept (donepezil), for Alzheimer's disease, 882–884, 883**t**
Ariflo (cilomilast), 1244–1249**t**
Arimidex (anastrozole), for breast cancer, 1053
Aripiprazole (Abilify)
  for bipolar disorder, 1127–1128
  for schizophrenia, 1130**t**
Aristocort A cream (triamcinolone acetonide topical)
  for anogenital pruritus, 872–873
  for contact dermatitis, 871, 871**b**
Arixtra (fondaparinux)
  for deep venous thrombosis/pulmonary embolism, 273
  for myocardial infarction, 367
Arm, pruritus of, 31**f**
Armondafinil (Nuvigil), 1243
Aromasin (exemestane), for breast cancer, 1053
Aromatase inhibitors, for breast cancer, 1053
Aromatic hydrocarbons, 1193
Arranon (nelarabine), for acute lymphoblastic leukemia, 449
Arrhythmias
  due to bulimia nervosa, 1116
  due to hypertrophic cardiomyopathy, 333
Arrhythmogenic right ventricular dysplasia or cardiomyopathy (ARVD/C), 323–324

Arsenic, reference intervals for, 1224**t**
Arsenic trioxide (Trisenox)
  for acute myeloid leukemia, 448
  for acute promyelocytic leukemia, 448
Arsine-based agents, as chemical weapons, 1226–1228**t**
ART (antidromic reciprocating tachycardia), 321–322, 322**f**
ART (assisted reproductive technology), 1061, 1061**f**
Artane (trihexphenidyl), poisoning due to, 1179–1180
Artemisinin, for malaria, 109
Arterial carbon dioxide tension (Pa$_{CO_2}$), 226, 226**t**
Arterial hypertension, due to acromegaly, 634
Arterial oxygen saturation (Sa$_{O_2}$), 225
Arterial oxygen tension (Pa$_{O_2}$), 225
Arterial thrombosis, due to polycythemia vera, 472
Artesunate, for malaria, 108**t**, 109
Arthralgia, temporomandibular disorders due to, 991**b**
Arthritis
  gouty (*See* Gout)
  juvenile idiopathic (*See* Juvenile idiopathic arthritis (JIA))
  Lyme, 137, 138
  osteo- (*See* Osteoarthritis (OA))
  psoriatic, 801
  rheumatoid (*See* Rheumatoid arthritis (RA))
  sarcoid, 276
  septic, in sickle cell disease, 406
Arthrocentesis, for temporomandibular disorder, 993
Arthroplasty, for osteoarthritis, 1002
Arthropods, skin infections due to, 844**t**, 845–846
Arthroscopy, for osteoarthritis, 1001
ARVD/C (arrhythmogenic right ventricular dysplasia or cardiomyopathy), 323–324
AS. *See* Ankylosing spondylitis (AS).
as biological weapon agent, 1229–1233**t**
ASA (5-aminosalicylic acid), for inflammatory bowel disease, 515–516, 519–520
ASA (acetylsalicylic acid)
  for ischemic stroke prevention, 894
  poisoning due to, 1209–1212, 1211**t**
Asacol (mesalamine), for inflammatory bowel disease, 516, 520
Asbestos, 278
  exposure to, 278
  permissible exposure limit for, 278
Asbestosis, 278–279, 278**t**
  benign pleural disease due to, 279
  classification (grading) of, 278
  clinical presentation of, 278
  diagnosis of, 278–279, 279**b**
  lung cancer and malignant mesothelioma due to, 279
  treatment of, 279, 279**b**
Ascariasis, 569, 570**t**
Ascaris lubricoides, 569, 570**t**
Ascending aortic aneurysm, 291
  dissection of, 291
  treatment of, 292
Ascites, 497**t**, 501–502, 501**t**
Ascorbic acid
  in parenteral nutrition, 621**t**
  for preeclampsia, 1025
ASCT. *See* Autologous stem-cell transplantation (ASCT).
ASD (atrial septal defect), 327
Ashman phenomenon, 312
Asmanex (mometasone furoate dry powder inhaler), for asthma
  in adolescents and adults, 769**t**
  in children, 773–774**t**

Aspergillus species, necrotizing skin and soft tissue infections due to, 85**t**
Asphyxia, of neonate, 1034, 1034**b**
Aspirin
  allergy to, 783
  for angina pectoris, 298
  for atrial fibrillation, 309, 310**b**
  for fever, 24
  for giant cell arteritis, 1004
  for high-altitude sickness, 1140–1141
  for juvenile idiopathic arthritis, 985
  for myocardial infarction, 362–363, 365**t**, 366
  for pericarditis, 370
  for polycythemia vera, 34**b**
  for polymyalgia rheumatica, 1004
  for preeclampsia, 1025
  for prevention of venous thrombosis during air travel, 377
  for thalassemia, 400**b**
  for transient ischemic attacks, 208–209
Assisted reproductive technology (ART), 1061, 1061**f**
Astatic seizures, 900
Astelin. *See* Azelastine (Astelin).
Asthma
  in adolescents and adults, 762
    aggravating factors for, 763
    allergic sensitization and, 763, 765
    assessment for, 763–764
      of aggravating factors, 763
      of asthma control, 764**t**
      of current status, 763–764
      of past severity, 763
    classification of severity of, 763**t**
    diagnosis of, 762
    differential diagnosis of, 763
    environmental triggers for, 763, 765, 765**b**
    follow-up for, 768–769
    immunotherapy for, 765
    impact of, 762
    long-term management of, 764–768, 769**b**
      comparative daily dosages for inhaled corticosteroids in, 769**t**
      goals of, 764, 765
      long-term control medications in, 767–768**t**
      nonpharmacologic therapy in, 764–765, 765**b**
      pharmacologic step therapy in, 765–768, 768**t**
    quick-relief medications in, 766**t**
    psychosocial factors in, 763, 765
    treatment of exacerbations of, 769–770, 769**b**
  and allergic rhinitis, 777
  in children, 770
    diagnosis of, 771**b**
      history in, 771
      physical examination in, 771–772
    differential diagnosis of, 770–771, 770**t**
    epidemiology of, 770
    hygiene hypothesis of, 770
    key diagnostic points for, 771
    pathophysiology of, 770
    treatment of, 772–774, 772**b**
      education and environmental control in, 776
      medications for, 774–776, 775**t**
      stepwise approach to, 773–774**t**
    triggers for, 771, 771**b**
  cough due to, 26–27, 28**b**
Astigmatism, 188
Astrocytoma(s)
  anaplastic
    epidemiology of, 972
    genetics and etiology of, 972
    outcome with, 975
    pathology of, 972

Astrocytoma(s) (Continued)
  genetics and etiology of, 972
  high-grade, imaging of, 974f
  imaging of, 972, 974f
  low-grade
    chemotherapy for, 974–975
    epidemiology of, 972
    imaging of, 974f
    outcome with, 975
    pathology of, 972, 974f
  pathology of, 973t
  treatment of
    chemotherapy for, 974–975
    surgery for, 973–974
Asystole, cardiac arrest due to, 305–306
AT (atrial tachycardia), 322–323
Atabrine (quinacrine), for giardiasis, 63–64, 64t, 544, 565–566t
Atarax. See Hydroxyzine (Atarax, Vistaril).
Ataxia, familial periodic, 209
Ataxia-telangiectasia, and childhood leukemia, 452t
Atazanavir (Reyataz), for HIV, 50t, 51t
  drug interactions with, 58t
Atelectasis, 230
  acute, 230
  adhesive, 230
  chronic, 230
  cicatrization, 230
  compression, 230
  defined, 230
  diagnosis of, 230–231, 231b
  incidence of, 230, 230t
  lobar, 230
  nonobstructive, 230
  obstructive, 230
  passive, 230
  rounded, 230
    due to asbestosis, 279
  treatment of, 231, 231b
Atenolol (Tenormin)
  for angina pectoris, 299t
  for hyperthyroidism, 666
  intoxication with, 1182–1183, 1183t
  for pheochromocytomas and paragangliomas, 675
  during pregnancy, 1023
ATG (antithymocyte globulin), for aplastic anemia, 380
Atgam (antithymocyte globulin), for aplastic anemia, 380
Atherosclerosis
  of aorta, 292–293
  dyslipoproteinemia with, 606
  erectile dysfunction due to, 716
Athletes
  exertional heat stroke in, 1148
  injuries in (See Sports injuries)
Ativan. See Lorazepam (Ativan).
Atlanta Classification, for acute pancreatitis, 547, 547t
ATN. See Acute tubular necrosis (ATN).
Atomoxetine (Strattera), for ADHD, 918, 918t
Atonic seizures, 900
Atopic dermatitis, 859
  complicating features of, 859
  diagnosis of, 859
  differential diagnosis of, 860
  epidemiology of, 859
  etiology of, 859
  pruritus due to, 30b
  psychosocial aspects of, 859–860
  treatment of, 860–862, 861f
    anti-infective measures in, 861–862
    antipruritic measures in, 862
    hydration and barrier repair in, 860
    identification and elimination of exacerbating factors in, 860

Atopic dermatitis (Continued)
  for recalcitrant disease, 862
  topical inflammatory medications in, 860–861
  triggers of, 860
Atopic keratoconjunctivitis, 859
Atorvastatin (Lipitor)
  for angina pectoris, 297–298
  for dyslipoproteinemia, 605t
  for glomerular disease, 701
Atorvastatin-amlodipine (Caduet), for dyslipoproteinemia, 605t
Atovaquone (Mepron)
  for Pneumocystis jiroveci pneumonia, 55, 56t
  for toxoplasmosis, 166t
    in HIV, 56t
Atovaquone-proguanil (Malarone), for malaria, 108t, 109, 111–112t, 156, 157t
ATRA (all-trans-retinoic acid), for acute promyelocytic leukemia, 448–449
Atrial complexes, premature, 312–313
  blocked, 312
  clinical features of, 312–313
  electrocardiographic features of, 312
  treatment of, 313
Atrial fibrillation (AF), 308
  classification of, 308
  diagnosis of, 308–309, 308b
  epidemiology of, 308
  after myocardial infarction, 366t
  paroxysmal, 308
  permanent, 308
  persistent, 308
  postoperative, 311
  presentation of, 308
  treatment of, 309–311, 309b
    antiarrhythmic drugs for, 310b, 310t
    anticoagulation for, 309, 309t
    cardioversion for, 311, 311t
    catheter ablation for, 310–311
    long-term options for, 310b
    pacing for, 311
    rate vs. rhythm control in, 309–310, 310b, 310t
Atrial flutter, 323
  after myocardial infarction, 366t
Atrial septal defect (ASD), 327
Atrial tachycardia (AT), 322–323
Atrioventricular (AV) block, after myocardial infarction, 366t
Atrioventricular (AV) canal defect, 327–328
Atrioventricular node reentrant tachycardia (AVNRT), 321, 321f, 322b
Atrioventricular reciprocating tachycardia (AVRT), 321–322, 322f
Atropa belladonna, poisoning due to, 1179–1180
Atrophic rhinitis, 216
Atrophie blanche, 855
Atropine (AtroPen)
  for asthma in children, 772b
  for heart block, 317–318
  for poisoning, 1167–1172t
    due to β-blockers, 1182–1183
    due to ciguatera, 1156, 1157t
    due to organophosphates and carbamates, 1206
  poisoning due to, 1179–1180
Atrovent. See Ipratropium bromide (Atrovent).
Attention-deficit/hyperactivity disorder (ADHD), 916
  clinical presentation of, 916, 916b
  co-morbid psychiatric conditions with, 917
  diagnosis of, 916–917, 916b, 917b
    in adults, 917, 916b
    in children and adolescents, 917, 916b
  epidemiology of, 916
  overview of, 916
  resources on, 918b

Attention-deficit/hyperactivity disorder (ADHD) (Continued)
  treatment of, 917–918, 917b, 918t
Attenuvax (measles vaccine), 142–143
Atypical antipsychotics
  for Alzheimer's disease, 884–886, 885t
  for bipolar disorder, 1127–1128
  for Tourette's syndrome, 920–921, 920b
Atypical ductal hyperplasia (ADH), 1047
Atypical hyperplasia (AH), of breast, 1045, 1045f, 1047
Audiometric testing, for Ménière's disease, 211
AUDIT (Alcohol Use Disorders Identification test), 1098, 1098t
Auditory disturbances, due to alcohol withdrawal, 1102–1103b
Augmentin. See Amoxicillin-clavulanate (Augmentin).
Aura, migraine headache with, 923
Auspitz's sign, 801
Autoantibodies, reference intervals for, 1225t
Autoantibody mechanism, of drug-induced hemolytic anemia, 389, 389b
Autoimmune disease, vs. fibromyalgia, 996b
Autoimmune gastritis, 529
Autoimmune hemolytic anemia, 387
  classification and serology of, 387, 387t
  cold agglutinin syndrome as, 388–389
    diagnosis of, 388
    serology of, 387t
    treatment of, 388–389, 388b
  drug-induced, 389, 389b
  paroxysmal cold hemoglobinuria as, 389
    diagnosis of, 389
    serology of, 387t
    treatment of, 389
  warm, 387–388
    diagnosis of, 387
    serology of, 387t
    treatment of, 387–388, 388b
Autoimmune hepatitis (AIH), 498t, 499
Autoimmune hypothyroidism, 662
Autoimmune polyglandular syndrome (APS) type 1, 637
Autoimmune polyglandular syndrome (APS) type 2, 637
Autoimmune thrombocytopenia, 426, 427b
Autoimmune thyroid disease, in diabetic children, 589
Autoimmune thyroiditis, 677–678
Autologous stem-cell transplantation (ASCT)
  for acute myeloid leukemia, 446–447
  for lymphoma
    cutaneous T-cell, 800
    non-Hodgkin's, 466–467
  for multiple myeloma, 470
  for systemic lupus erythematosus, 809
Autolytic débridement, for pressure ulcers, 858
Automated external defibrillator (AED), for cardiac arrest, 304–305
Automaticity, 320
  abnormal, 320
Autonomic dysfunction, in parkinsonism, 953b
Autonomic neuropathy, 959b, 960t
  in diabetes, 962
Autonomic storms, after traumatic brain injury, 969
AV (atrioventricular) block, after myocardial infarction, 366t
AV (atrioventricular) canal defect, 327–328
Avandia (rosiglitazone), for diabetes, 580t, 581
Avascular necrosis, in sickle cell disease, 407, 411
Avastin (bevacizumab), for non–small cell lung cancer, 247, 247t
Avelox. See Moxifloxacin (Avelox).
Avian influenza, 90

Avinza. *See* Morphine sulfate (Avinza, Kadian, MS Contin, Oramorph SR, MSIR).
AVNRT (atrioventricular node reentrant tachycardia), 321, 321f, 322b
Avodart (dutasteride), for benign prostatic hyperplasia, 714–716, 714t
Avonex (interferon-β-1a)
 for multiple sclerosis, 936
 for optic neuritis, 197
AVP (arginine vasopressin), for diabetes insipidus, 647, 647t
AVRT (atrioventricular reciprocating tachycardia), 321–322, 322f
Axert (almotriptan), for migraine headache, 925t, 926
Axial pain, 42–43
Axid (nizatidine)
 for gastroesophageal reflux disease, 553, 554t
 for peptic ulcer disease, 531t
Axillary lymph node dissection (ALND), 1052
Axillary lymph node involvement, in breast cancer, 1050
Axonopathy, 958, 961
Aygestin (norethindrone acetate)
 for anovulatory bleeding, 1058–1059
 for menorrhagia, 1059
Azactam (aztreonam)
 for necrotizing skin and soft tissue infections, 85t
 for pyelonephritis, 685
5-Azacytidine (Vidaza), for acute myeloid leukemia, 448
"Azarcon por empacho," lead in, 1197
AzaSite (azithromycin ophthalmic), 1243
Azathioprine (Imuran, Azasan)
 for autoimmune hepatitis, 499
 for bullous pemphigoid, 867, 868t, 869t
 for crescentic glomerulonephritis, 703–704
 for cutaneous vasculitis, 816t
 for idiopathic inflammatory myopathy, 813
 for IgA nephropathy, 703
 for inflammatory bowel disease, 516–517, 519–520
 for multiple sclerosis, 938
 for myasthenia gravis, 944t, 945
 for neuromyelitis optica, 938–939
 for pemphigus vulgaris, 869
 for rheumatoid arthritis, 981t, 982
 for systemic lupus erythematosus, 807t, 808, 808f
 for warm autoimmune hemolytic anemia, 387
Azelaic acid (Azelex, Finacea)
 for acne, 788
 for melasma, 877
 for postinflammatory hyperpigmentation, 878
 for rosacea, 789
Azelastine (Astelin)
 for allergic rhinitis, 779t, 780t
 for nonallergic rhinitis, 217, 217b
 for postnasal drip syndrome, 28b
Azilect (rasagiline), for parkinsonism, 957
Azithromycin (Zithromax)
 for chancroid, 750
 for *Chlamydia trachomatis,* 1078b, 1078–1079
 for cholera, 80, 80t
 for diarrhea
  acute infectious, 18b, 19t–20t
  traveler's, 156, 156t
 for endocarditis prophylaxis, 347t
 for epididymitis, 697b, 698
 for gonorrhea, 751, 752b
 for granuloma inguinale, 750
 for legionellosis, 271, 271t
 for Lyme disease, 138, 139t
 for *Mycobacterium avium intracellulare,* 289
  in HIV, 56t
 for mycoplasmal pneumonia, 270t
 for nongonococcal urethritis, 753

Azithromycin (Zithromax) *(Continued)*
 for relapsing fever, 136t
 for sinusitis
  acute, 28b
  bacterial, 28b
 for streptococcal pharyngitis, 223t
 for toxoplasmosis, 166t
 for typhoid fever, 176t
Azithromycin ophthalmic (AzaSite), 1243
Azmacort (triamcinolone acetonide inhalation), for asthma
 in adolescents and adults, 769t
 in children, 773–774t
Azoles
 for coccidioidomycosis, 250b, 250t
 for leishmaniasis, 95
Azopt (brinzolamide), for glaucoma, 200
Azor (amlodipine/olmesartan), 1243
Azotemia, prerenal, 721–722
 vs. acute tubular necrosis, 724t
 causes of, 721, 722b, 723f
 defined, 721
 laboratory findings in, 721–722, 724b
 with parenteral nutrition, 625t
 treatment of, 721–722
Aztreonam (Azactam)
 for necrotizing skin and soft tissue infections, 85t
 for pyelonephritis, 685
Azulfidine. *See* Sulfasalazine (Azulfidine).

B

Baby blues, 1029
Bacille Calmette-Guérin (BCG) vaccine, for leprosy, 103
Bacillus anthracis. See Anthrax.
Bacillus cereus, foodborne illness due to, 81
Back, pruritus of, 31f
Back pain, 39
 assessment of, 40
  examination in, 40–41
  history in, 40
 diagnosis of, 41b, 43, 43t
 emergent or urgent conditions with, 41b
 epidemiology of, 39
 management of, 41, 42b
  with axial pain predominating, 42–43
  clinical pearls on, 43t
  nonsurgical or minimally invasive, 43
  with radicular pain predominating, 41–42, 42b
  surgical, 43
 natural course of, 41
 pathophysiology of, 39–40, 40f
 radicular (neuropathic)
  assessment of, 40
  management of, 41–42, 42b
  natural course of, 41
  pathophysiology of, 39–40
 somatic (nociceptive)
  history of, 40
  pathophysiology of, 39–40
Backache, during pregnancy, 1015–1016
Baclofen (Lioresal)
 for multiple sclerosis, 939b
 for traumatic brain injury, 967–968
Bacteremia, due to salmonellosis, 173
 treatment of, 173
Bacteria
 acute infectious diarrhea due to, 14–16, 14b, 15b
 as biological weapon agents, 1229–1233t
Bacterial conjunctivitis, 194t, 195
 in neonate, 195, 196t
Bacterial contamination, of blood products, 484–485t, 487
Bacterial endocarditis. *See* Infective endocarditis.

Bacterial meningitis, 112
 adjunctive therapy for, 114
 antibiotics for, 114b
  dosage of, 115t
  selection of, 113
   by age group and probable pathogen, 113t, 114b
   CSF morphology and, 113t
   in persons with special risks, 114t
   special considerations with, 113–114
 chemoprophylaxis for, 114–115
 in children, 113t, 114b, 115t
 diagnosis of, 112–113, 112b
 drug-resistant, 113
 due to gram-negative bacilli, 113
 monitoring of, 114
 due to *Neisseria meningitidis,* 114
 vaccines for, 115
 with ventriculoatrial and ventriculoperitoneal shunts, 113
Bacterial overgrowth
 diarrhea due to, 17
 gaseousness due to, 10, 10t
Bacterial pericarditis, 368b, 368–369, 371
Bacterial pneumonia, 261
 atypical, 262, 266
 community-acquired, 261–263
  admission criteria for, 262, 262t
  diagnostic criteria for, 261b
  diagnostic testing for, 261–262
  epidemiology of, 261
  etiology of, 262, 262b
  prevention of, 263
  treatment of, 262–263, 263b
 health care–acquired, 263–264
  defined, 263
  diagnosis of, 263–264
  epidemiology of, 263
  etiology of, 263
  prevention of, 264
  treatment of, 264, 264t
Bacterial sinusitis, cough due to, 26–27, 28b
Bacterial skin infection(s), 835
 due to animal bites, 836b
 cellulitis as, 835–836, 836b
 complicated, 835
 cutaneous abscess as, 836b, 837
 diabetic foot infection as, 838
 diagnosis and treatment of, 836b
 erysipelas as, 836, 836b
 furuncles as, 836b, 837, 837f
 hidradenitis suppurativa as, 837–838
 due to human bites, 836b
 impetigo as, 836b, 836–837, 837f
 due to methicillin-resistant *Staphylococcus aureus,* 835–836, 836b, 837f
 necrotizing soft tissue, 836b, 839
 surgical site, 836b, 838–839, 838b
 uncomplicated, 835
Bacterial vaginosis (BV), 1074
 during pregnancy, 1014, 1074, 1074b
Bacteriuria
 benign, of elderly, 682
 catheter-associated, 682, 684–685
 during pregnancy, 1014
Bacteroides fragilis, acute infectious diarrhea due to, 16
Bactocill. *See* Oxacillin (Bactocill, Prostaphlin).
Bactrim. *See* Trimethoprim-sulfamethoxazole (TMP-SMX, Septra, Bactrim, cotrimoxazole, Cotrim).
Bactroban (mupirocin), for atopic dermatitis, 861–862
BAFF (B-cell activating factor), in systemic lupus erythematosus, 809
BAL (British anti-lewisite), for poisoning, 1167–1172t
 due to lead, 1199–1200, 1200t

BAL (bronchoalveolar lavage), for sarcoidosis, 276
Balacet (propoxyphene + acetaminophen)
  for osteoarthritis, 1000
  for pain, 4t
Balance, after menopause, 1071
Balanitis xerotica obliterans, urethral stricture disease due to, 740
Balantidiasis, 565–566t, 567
Balantidium coli, 565–566t, 567
"Bali goli," lead in, 1197
Balsalazide (Colazal), for inflammatory bowel disease, 516
Balthazar Score, for acute pancreatitis, 547
Baraclude (entecavir), for hepatitis B and C viruses, 536t, 537
Barbiturates
  abuse of, 1105b, 1107–1108, 1108t
  for alcohol withdrawal, 1103
  for elevated intracranial pressure in children, 971
  intoxication with, 1180–1181
Bariatric surgery, 610
  in children and adolescents, 610
  contraindications for, 610
  gastric banding and adjustable laparoscopic band as, 610–611, 611f
  indications for, 610
  preoperative evaluation for, 610
  roux-en-Y gastroplasty as, 611, 611f
  surgical assessment for, 610
Barrier methods, of contraception, 757
  in postpartum period, 1029t
Barrier repair, for atopic dermatitis, 860
Bartholin's duct cyst, 1091
Bartonella henselae. See Cat-scratch disease (CSD).
Basal cell carcinoma (BCC)
  clinical features of, 793
  diagnosis of, 794b
  epidemiology of, 793
  morpheaform, 793
  nodular, 793
  prevention and screening for, 794
  superficial, 793
  treatment of, 794, 794b
  of vulva, 1094
Basal metabolic rate (BMR), 620
Basilar meningitis, 208
Bathing trunk nevi, 828
Baypress (nitrendipine), intoxication with, 1183–1184
BayRab (human rabies immune globulin), 131
BayTet (human tetanus immune globulin), 144–145, 144b
Bazedoxifene (Viviant), 1244–1249t
BCC. See Basal cell carcinoma (BCC).
B-cell activating factor (BAFF), in systemic lupus erythematosus, 809
B-cell depletion, for systemic lupus erythematosus, 809
B-cell stimulator (BlyS), in systemic lupus erythematosus, 809
B-cell survival, inhibition of, for systemic lupus erythematosus, 809
BCG (bacille Calmette-Guérin) vaccine, for leprosy, 103
BCR-ABL gene, in chronic myeloid leukemia, 456–457
BCT (breast conservation therapy), 1051–1052
  for ductal carcinoma in situ, 1050
BEC (blood ethanol concentration), 1190
Beck, Aaron, 1124
Beclomethasone (Beconase, Vancenase), for rhinitis
  allergic, 780t
  nonallergic, 217, 217b

Beclomethasone hydrofluoroalkane (QVAR), for asthma
  in adolescents and adults, 769t
  in children, 773–774t
BECTS (benign epilepsy of childhood associated with central-temporal spikes), 909
Behavior modification
  for obesity, 609
  for urinary incontinence in children, 691
Behavioral issues, with acne, 788
Behavioral self-management, for diabetes, 576b, 577–578, 578f
Behavioral symptoms, of Alzheimer's disease, 881
  treatment of, 884–887, 885t
Behavioral therapy, for irritable bowel syndrome, 521, 524t
Belching, 9
Belimumab, for systemic lupus erythematosus, 809
Bell, Charles, 949
Belladonna/ergotamine/phenobarbital (Bellergal), for cluster headache, 926t
Bell's palsy, 949, 962
  clinical evaluation of, 950–951
  defined, 949
  diagnosis of, 950–951, 950b
  differential diagnosis of, 949, 949b
  epidemiology of, 949
  pathogenesis of, 949–950
  scoring system for, 950, 950b
  treatment of, 951–952, 951f, 952b, 962
Benadryl. See Diphenhydramine (Benadryl).
Bence Jones myeloma, 467–468
Benign bacteriuria of the elderly, 682
Benign epilepsy of childhood associated with central-temporal spikes (BECTS), 909
Benign paroxysmal positional vertigo (BPPV), 205–206, 205f, 206f
Benign prostatic hyperplasia (BPH), 712
  diagnosis of, 713–717
  epidemiology of, 712–716
  pathophysiology of, 712–716
  symptoms of, 713–716, 713f
  treatment of, 714–718
    medications for, 714t
      α_1-adrenergic blocking agents as, 714–718, 714t
      efficacy of, 714–720
      5α-reductase inhibitors as, 714–718, 714t
    minimally invasive therapies for, 715–719
    phytotherapy for, 715–718
    watchful waiting for, 714–718
Benign rolandic epilepsy, 909
Bentyl (dicyclomine)
  for dyspepsia, 528
  for gaseousness, 10t
BenzaClin (benzoyl peroxide with clindamycin), for acne, 788
Benzamides, for nausea and vomiting, 8, 8t
Benzamycin (benzoyl peroxide with erythromycin), for acne, 788
Benzathine penicillin G (Bicillin)
  for anthrax, 126t
  for streptococcal pharyngitis, 223, 223t
  for syphilis, 755, 755t
Benzodiazepines
  abuse of, 1105b, 1107–1108, 1108t
  for alcohol withdrawal, 1101–1103
  for Alzheimer's disease, 884, 885t
  for anxiety disorder(s), 1112
    generalized, 1113
  for delirium, 1119b, 1120
  for insomnia, 887–888, 888t
  intoxication with, 1181–1182
  kinetics of, 1181–1182
  for motion sickness and vertigo, 206t
  for nausea and vomiting, 8

Benzodiazepines (Continued)
  for panic disorder, 1132, 1132t
  and SSRIs, 1122–1123b
Benzoquin (hydroquinone 2% cream), for vitiligo, 879
Benzoyl peroxide, for acne, 787–788
Benzoyl peroxide with clindamycin (BenzaClin, Duac), for acne, 788
Benzoyl peroxide with erythromycin (Benzamycin), for acne, 788
Benzoylecgonine, 1187
Benztropine (Cogentin), poisoning due to, 1179–1180
Benzylpenicilloyl-polylysine (PPL, Pre-Pen), 782
Bepridil (Vascor), intoxication with, 1183–1184
Bernard-Soulier syndrome (BSS), 427
β agonists
  for asthma in children, 774–775
  for cystic fibrosis, 238–239
β_2 agonists
  long-acting
    for asthma
      in adolescents and adults, 767–768t
      in children, 773–774t, 775
    for COPD, 234
  short-acting
    for asthma in adolescents and adults, 766t
    for COPD, 234
β-adrenergic antagonists (β-blockers)
  for angina pectoris, 299, 299t
  for atrial fibrillation, 309, 310b
  for esophageal varices, 505, 507
  for glaucoma, 200, 200t
  for heart failure, 339t, 340
  for hypertension, 356t, 357
  for hyperthyroidism, 666–667
  for hypertrophic cardiomyopathy, 332–333
  kinetics of, 1182
  metabolism of, 1182
  for migraine headache, 925
  for myocardial infarction, 364, 365t
  for pheochromocytomas and paragangliomas, 675
  poisoning due to, 1182–1183, 1183t
  and SSRIs, 1122–1123b
  for thyroid storm, 669
β-carotene (Solatene), for protoporphyria, 480
Betagan (levobunolol)
  for glaucoma, 200
  intoxication with, 1182–1183, 1183t
Betahistine (Serc), for tinnitus, 38
Betamethasone dipropionate (Diprolene), for atopic dermatitis, 860–861
Betamethasone syrup (Celestone Syrup), for aphthous ulcers, 850
Betapace (sotalol)
  for atrial fibrillation, 310, 310b
  intoxication with, 1182–1183, 1183t
Betaseron (interferon-β-1b)
  for multiple sclerosis, 936
  for optic neuritis, 197
Betaxolol (Kerlone), intoxication with, 1182–1183, 1183t
Betimol (timolol)
  for glaucoma, 200
  intoxication with, 1182–1183, 1183t
Bevacizumab (Avastin), for non–small cell lung cancer, 247, 247t
Bexarotene (Targretin), for cutaneous T-cell lymphomas, 798–799
  with denileukin, 800
  with phototherapy, 798
Biaxin. See Clarithromycin (Biaxin).
Bicarbonate
  for chronic renal failure, 730
  for diabetic ketoacidosis, 592t, 593–594, 593t
Bichloracetic acid, for verrucae, 823
Bicillin. See Benzathine penicillin G (Bicillin).

Bicyclic fatty acid, for constipation, 22, 22**b**
Bigeminy, 312
Biguanides, for diabetes
    in adults, 580**t**, 580–581
    in children, 590**t**
Bilberry fruit, 1234–1243**t**
Bile acid malabsorption, 541**b**, 542, 545
Bile duct stones. *See* Choledocholithiasis.
Bile reflux gastritis, indigestion due to, 11**t**
Bilevel positive airway pressure (BiPAP), for acute respiratory failure, 227
Biliary cirrhosis, primary, 498**t**, 499
Biliary colic, 496**b**
Biliary pancreatitis, 548–549
Biliary sludge, 495
Biliary tract infections, sepsis due to, 68**t**
Bilirubin, elevated, with parenteral nutrition, 625**t**, 626
Biltricide (praziquantel)
    for schistosomiasis, 570**t**, 844**t**, 845
    for tapeworms, 570**t**
Bimatoprost (Lumigan), for glaucoma, 199–200
Binet staging system, for chronic lymphocytic leukemia, 461, 461**t**
Binge episode, 1115
"Bint Al Zahab," lead in, 1197
Biofeedback
    for stroke rehabilitation, 896**b**
    for urinary incontinence in children, 691
Biogenic amine interactions, due to MAOIs, 1203, 1203
Biological response modifier(s) (BRMs), for rheumatoid arthritis, 978, 978**b**
    abatacept as, 981**t**, 982
    anakinra as, 981**t**, 982
    rituximab as, 981**t**, 982
    TNF-α inhibitors as, 979–981, 981**t**
Biological therapies
    for cutaneous T-cell lymphomas, 797**b**, 799
    for psoriasis, 802–804, 803**t**
Biological weapon agents, 1229
    biological toxins as, 1229–1233**t**
Biomarkers, of pericarditis, 369–370
Biophysical profile, during pregnancy, 1017
Biopsy(ies)
    of breast, 1048
    endometrial, for dysfunctional uterine bleeding, 1058
    of giant cell arteritis, 1002–1003, 1003**b**
    liver, for hemochromatosis, 433
    renal, for chronic renal failure, 726
    sentinel lymph node
        for breast cancer, 1052
        for melanoma, 832
    skin, for leprosy, 100
    of thyroid nodule, 670–671, 671**t**
Bioterrorism
    plague in, 122
    Q fever in, 128–129
    smallpox in, 179, 179
BioThrax (anthrax vaccine), 127
Biotin (vitamin H, vitamin B$_7$, Appearex)
    for brittle nails, 818**b**, 819
    in parenteral nutrition, 621**t**
BiPAP (bilevel positive airway pressure), for acute respiratory failure, 227
Bipolar disorder, 1126–1128
    depression *vs.*, 1121
    diagnosis of, 1126, 1126**b**
    epidemiology of, 1126
    hypomanic episodes in, 1126
    manic episode in, 1126, 1126**b**
    mixed episodes in, 1126
    and suicide, 1126
    treatment of, 1126–1128
Bi-RADS (Breast Imaging Reporting and Data System), 1048, 1049**t**
Birth, assessing response to, 1031

Birth control. *See* Contraception.
Birth control pills. *See* Oral contraceptives (OCs).
Bisacodyl (Dulcolax), for constipation, 10**t**, 22**b**
Bismuth subsalicylate (Pepto-Bismol)
    for diarrhea
        acute infectious, 19
        traveler's, 155–156, 156**t**
    for indigestion, 11**t**
    for peptic ulcer disease, 532**t**
    for *Salmonella* gastroenteritis, 172
Bisphosphonates
    for hyperparathyroidism, 652
    for osteoporosis, 614–615
        postmenopausal, 1072, 1073**b**
    for Paget's disease of bone, 616–617
Bites, infections due to, 836**b**
Bivalirubin (Angiomax), for myocardial infarction, 366
Black cohosh root, 1234–1243**t**
Black haw, 1234–1243**t**
Black widow spider bites, 1151
Bladder
    overactive, 693
    underactive, 691
    unstable, 686
Bladder capacity, 690
Bladder carcinoma, 735–737
    adenocarcinoma as, 736
    bilharzial, 736–737
    diagnosis of, 735, 735**b**
    epidemiology of, 735
    squamous cell, 736–737
    transitional cell, 735
    treatment of, 735–736, 736**b**
Bladder compliance, poor, 693
Bladder control, 690
Bladder injuries, 708
    classification of, 708
    diagnosis of, 707**b**, 708
    extraperitoneal, 708, 708**f**
    intraperitoneal, 708, 708**f**
    treatment of, 708, 708**b**
Bladder irritability, during pregnancy, 1014
Bladder outlet obstruction (BOO)
    acute renal failure due to, 722**b**, 724
    due to benign prostatic hyperplasia, 712–715
Bladder rupture, 708
    imaging of, 708, 708**f**
    treatment of, 708
Blastocystis hominis, 565–566**t**, 567
Blastomycosis, 254
    clinical manifestations of, 254
    CNS infection with, 254–255
    diagnosis of, 254–255, 255**b**
    epidemiology of, 254
    extrapulmonary, 254–255
    pulmonary, 254–255
    treatment of, 255–256, 255**b**
Bleeding. *See also* Hemorrhage.
    dysfunctional uterine, 1058
        anovulatory, 1058–1059
        defined, 1058
        diagnosis of, 1059**b**
            endometrial biopsy in, 1058
            history in, 1058
            imaging in, 1058
            laboratory evaluation in, 1058
        differential diagnosis of, 1058
        etiology of, 1058
        after menopause, 1070–1071
        ovulatory, 1059
        treatment for, 1059**b**
        due to uterine hemorrhage, 1059–1060
    life-threatening, in childhood leukemia, 453
    due to poisoning, 1174**t**
    due to polycythemia vera, 472, 474
    vaginal

Bleeding *(Continued)*
    in late pregnancy, 1019
        hemodynamic compromise due to, 1019–1020
        due to placenta previa, 1020, 1020**b**
        due to placental abruption, 1020–1021, 1021**b**
        due to uterine rupture, 1021, 1021**b**
        due to vasa previa, 1021, 1021**b**
    in pregnancy, 1013
Bleeding disorder(s), 419
    hemophilia as, 419–422
    platelet-mediated, 425
    rare, 424**t**, 425
    von Willebrand's disease as, 422–425
Bleomycin (Blenoxane)
    for keloids, 821
    for verrucae, 823
Blister agents, as chemical weapons, 1226–1228**t**
Bloating, 9–10
    functional, 10**t**
Blocadren (timolol)
    for glaucoma, 200
    intoxication with, 1182–1183, 1183**t**
Blocked milk ducts, 1028
Blood chemistry, reference intervals for, 1220–1221**t**
Blood components, therapeutic uses of, 480
Blood ethanol concentration (BEC), 1190
Blood glucose goals, for diabetes mellitus in children, 586, 586**t**
Blood glucose self-monitoring, for diabetes, 576, 576**b**
Blood pressure (BP)
    and angina pectoris, 296–297
    classification of, 349, 351**t**
    diastolic, 349, 351**t**, 351–352
    goals for, for diabetes, 576**b**
    management of, for intracerebral hemorrhage, 891
    measurement of, 351–353
    monitoring of
        ambulatory, 353
        home, 352–353
    physiologic variability of, 349, 350**f**
    placebo effect for, 352
    with poisonings, 1162**t**
    during pregnancy, 1012, 1022
    systolic, 349, 351**t**, 351–352
Blood products, bacterial contamination of, 484–485**t**, 487
Blood schizonticides, for malaria, 108
Blood transfusion(s), 484
    adverse effect(s) of, 484
        acute lung injury as, 484–485**t**, 487–488
        allergic, 488–489
        alloimmunization as, 484, 491
        due to bacterial contamination of blood products, 487
        febrile, 488
        graft-*versus*-host disease as, 489, 489**b**
        immunomodulation as, 486**t**, 490–491
        infectious, 485**t**, 489–490, 490**b**
        massive transfusion coagulopathy as, 486**t**, 491–492
        purpura as, 486**t**, 491
        refractoriness to platelet transfusions as, 486**t**, 491
        transfusion reactions as, 484–489
            defined, 484
            hemolytic, 484–487, 484–485**t**
            massive, 486**t**
            nonhemolytic, 484–485**t**, 487–489
            volume overload as, 486**t**, 491
    for cold agglutinin syndrome, 389
    of cryoprecipitate, 483
    of granulocytes, 483
    of plasma, 483

Blood transfusion(s) *(Continued)*
   frozen, 483
   indications for, 483
  of platelets, 482–483
   indications for, 482
   irradiated, 482
   leukoreduced, 482
   platelet refractoriness with, 482–483
   washed, 482
  of red blood cells, 480–482
   frozen, 481
   indications for, 481–482
   irradiated, 481
   leukoreduced, 480–481
   packed, 480
   washed, 481
  for sickle cell disease, 412–413, 412**t**
  for thalassemia, 399**t**, 400–401
  for warm autoimmune hemolytic anemia, 388
Blood urea nitrogen (BUN), in chronic renal failure, 730
Bloom's syndrome, and childhood leukemia, 452**t**
Blue nevi, 828–829, 828**b**
Blue-toe syndrome, 292
Blunted affect, in schizophrenia, 1129
BlyS (B-cell stimulator), in systemic lupus erythematosus, 809
BMD (bone mineral density), 612–613
BMR (basal metabolic rate), 620
BMT (bone marrow transplantation)
  for chronic myeloid leukemia, 460
  for non-Hodgkin's lymphoma, 466–467
BNP (brain-natriuretic peptide), in unstable angina pectoris, 301
Bobath neurodevelopmental therapy, for stroke rehabilitation, 896**b**
Body louse, 844**t**, 845
Body mass index (BMI), 607
  clinical use of, 607**t**
  defined, 606, 607**t**
  health risk based on, 608**f**
  and mortality risk, 607, 607**f**
  in nutritional assessment, 619
  during pregnancy, 1012
Body packing, with cocaine, 1186–1187
Body stuffing, with cocaine, 1186–1187
Body temperature, with poisonings, 1162**t**
Boils, 836**b**, 837, 837**f**
Bone, Paget's disease of, 615
  diagnosis of, 615–616
  treatment of, 616–617
  type 1 vs. type 2, 616
Bone disease
  due to hyperparathyroidism, 650
  due to thalassemia, 402
Bone infarcts, in sickle cell disease, 407, 411
Bone lesions, in multiple myeloma, 471–472
Bone marrow transplantation (BMT)
  for chronic myeloid leukemia, 460
  for non-Hodgkin's lymphoma, 466–467
Bone mass measurement, for hyperparathyroidism, 651
Bone metabolism, abnormalities in, due to acromegaly, 635
Bone mineral density (BMD), 612–613
Bone turnover, biochemical markers of, 613
Bonefos (clodronate), 1244–1249**t**
Bone-specific alkaline phosphatase (BSAP) level, 615–616
Bonine (meclizine)
  for motion sickness and vertigo, 206**t**, 210
  for nausea and vomiting, 8**t**
Boniva (ibandronate), for osteoporosis, 614
  postmenopausal, 1073**b**
BOO (bladder outlet obstruction)
  acute renal failure due to, 722**b**, 724
  due to benign prostatic hyperplasia, 712–715

BOOSTRIX. *See* Tetanus and diphtheria toxoids and acellular pertussis vaccine (Tdap, BOOSTRIX, ADACEL).
Borderline personality disorder, with bulimia nervosa, 1116–1117
Bordetella pertussis. See Pertussis.
Borrelia, relapsing fever due to. *See* Relapsing fever.
Borrelia burgdorferi. See Lyme disease.
Borreliosis, Lyme. *See* Lyme disease.
Bortezomib (Velcade, PS-341), for multiple myeloma, 469**b**, 470–471
Bosentan (Tracleer)
  for portopulmonary hypertension, 503–504
  for systemic sclerosis, 811
Botulinum toxin, for dysphagia, 510
Botulism, 82
  as biological weapon agent, 1229–1233**t**
Bovine papular stomatitis, 843
Bowenoid papulosis, 834–835
  diagnosis of, 833**b**
  genital warts and, 824
  treatment of, 834**b**, 835
Bowen's disease, 833**b**, 834, 834**b**
BP. *See* Blood pressure (BP).
BPH. *See* Benign prostatic hyperplasia (BPH).
BPPV (benign paroxysmal positional vertigo), 205–206, 205**f**, 206**f**
Brachoradial pruritus, 32**b**
Brachytherapy
  for endometrial cancer, 1085
  for prostate cancer, 732
Brain metastases, 975–976
  epidemiology of, 975
  treatment of, 975–976
Brain stimulation, for major depression, 1126
Brain tumor(s), 972
  ependymoma as, 975
  epidemiology of, 972
  gliomas as, 972–975
   brainstem, 975
   clinical presentation of, 972
   diagnostic studies for, 972, 974**f**
   genetics and etiology of, 972
   incidence of, 972
   outcome for, 975
   pathology of, 972, 973**t**, 974**f**
   prognostic factors for, 973
   routes of spread of, 972
   staging of, 972–973
   treatment of, 973–975
     chemotherapy for, 974–975
     radiation therapy for, 974
     surgery for, 973–974
  histopathology of, 973**t**
  medulloblastoma as, 975
  metastatic, 975–976
   epidemiology of, 975
   treatment of, 975–976
  primary CNS lymphoma as, 975
Brainerd diarrhea, 17
Brain-natriuretic peptide (BNP), in unstable angina pectoris, 301
Brainstem glioma, 975
BRCA1 gene
  and breast cancer, 1047–1048
  and ovarian cancer, 1094
BRCA2 gene
  and breast cancer, 1047–1048
  and ovarian cancer, 1094
Breakbone fever, 162
Breast(s)
  development of, 1062–1063
  during pregnancy, 1012
Breast biopsy, 1048
Breast cancer
  adjuvant therapy for, 1052–1053
  atypical ductal and lobular hyperplasia and, 1047

Breast cancer *(Continued)*
  epidemiology of, 1050, 1050**t**
  Halsted paradigm *vs.* Fisher paradigm for, 1051
  histology of, 1050
  inflammatory, 1054
  in situ, 1048–1050
  invasive, 1050–1051
  locally advanced, 1051**f**, 1054
  male, 1053
  in pregnancy, 1053–1054
  proliferative benign breast disease and, 1046–1047
  risk factors for, 1047–1048
  screening for, 1048
  staging of, 1050, 1051**f**
  surgical treatment of, 1051
   breast conservation therapy as, 1051–1052
   breast reconstruction after, 1052
   mastectomy as, 1052
  surgical treatment of axilla for, 1052
  surveillance after diagnosis of, 1053
  workup of a breast mass for, 1048, 1049**f**, 1049**t**
Breast conservation therapy (BCT), 1051–1052
  for ductal carcinoma in situ, 1050
Breast cysts, 1045–1046, 1046**f**
Breast disease(s), 1045
  benign, 1045, 1045**t**
   atypical hyperplasia as, 1045, 1045**f**, 1047
   fat necrosis as, 1047
   fibroadenoma as, 1047
   fibrocystic, 1045–1046, 1046**f**
   hamartomas as, 1047
   mastitis and duct ectasia as, 1046
   Mondor's disease as, 1047
   multiple peripheral papillomas as, 1047
   nonproliferative, 1045–1046, 1045**t**, 1045**f**
   proliferative, 1045**t**, 1046–1047
   pseudoangiomatous stromal hyperplasia as, 1047
   radial scars as, 1047
   sclerosing and microglandular adenosis as, 1047
  gynecomastia as, 1053
  malignant (*See* Breast cancer)
  nipple discharge and, 1053
  phyllodes tumor as, 1053
Breast Imaging Reporting and Data System (Bi-RADS), 1048, 1049**t**
Breast mass, workup of, 1048, 1049**f**, 1049**t**
Breast milk, composition of, 1042
Breast reconstruction, 1052
Breast self-examination (BSE), 1048
Breast-feeding, 1041–1042
  contraindications to, 1042
  mastitis during, 1046
  in postpartum period, 1027–1028
  recommendations on, 1041–1042
Breath hydrogen testing, 542
Breath-holding spells, 907
Breathing
  in newborn resuscitation, 1031–1032
  for traumatic brain injury in children
   moderate, 970
   severe, 971
Breathing management, for cardiac arrest, 303
Brethine (terbutaline), for asthma in children, 772**b**, 774–775, 775**t**
Brevibloc. *See* Esmolol (Brevibloc).
Brief intervention, for alcoholism, 1099–1100
Brimonidine (Alphagan), for glaucoma, 200
Brimonidine/timolol (Combigan), 1243
Brinzolamide (Azopt), for glaucoma, 200
Bristol stool chart, 521, 522**f**
British anti-lewisite (BAL), for poisoning, 1167–1172**t**
  due to lead, 1199–1200, 1200**t**

Brittle nails, 817**b**, 818**b**, 818–819
BRMs. *See* Biological response modifier(s) (BRMs).
Bromides, reference intervals for, 1224**t**
Bromocriptine mesylate (Parlodel)
   for Cushing's syndrome, 645**t**
   for hyperprolactinemia, 660, 660**t**
   for neuroleptic intoxication, 1209
   for parkinsonism, 955
   after traumatic brain injury, 969
Brompheniramine (Lodrane XR, LoHist 12 Hours), for allergic rhinitis, 779**t**
Bronchiectasis, cough due to, 28–29
Bronchiolitis, 266
Bronchitis
   acute, 259
      clinical features of, 259
      diagnosis of, 259–260, 260**b**
      etiology of, 259
      pathophysiology of, 260
      treatment of, 259—261, 260**b**
   chronic, 231–232
   eosinophilic, cough due to, 28, 28**b**
Bronchoalveolar lavage (BAL), for sarcoidosis, 276
Bronchoconstriction, in childhood asthma, 770
Bronchodilators
   for acute bronchitis, 260
   for asthma in children, 774–775, 775**t**
   for COPD, 233–234
   for cystic fibrosis, 238–239
   reference intervals for, 1222**t**
Bronchoscopy, for lung cancer, 245
Bronchospasm, cough due to, 28**b**
Brown recluse spider bites, 1150–1151
Brucella. See Brucellosis.
Brucellosis, 72
   as biological weapon agent, 1229–1233**t**
   case definitions and classification of, 73**b**
   clinical features of, 73, 73**b**, 74**t**
   diagnosis of, 73–74, 74**b**, 74**t**, 73**b**
   epidemiology of, 72–73
   etiology of, 72, 72**t**
   pathogenesis of, 73
   prevention of, 75
   treatment of, 74–75, 74**b**, 75**t**
Brugada syndrome, 324–326, 325**f**
Brugia spp, 844, 844**t**
Bruits, in tinnitus, 36
Brunnstrom method, for stroke rehabilitation, 896**b**
Brush border, transport defects at, 543
Bruxism, sleep, 993
BSAP (bone-specific alkaline phosphatase) level, 615–616
BSE (breast self-examination), 1048
BSS (Bernard-Soulier syndrome), 427
Bubble hair deformity, 793
Bubo, 122
Bubonic plague, 122
Buccal mucosa, disorders of, 851
Budd-Chiari syndrome, cirrhosis due to, 498**t**
Budesonide capsules (Entocort EC), for inflammatory bowel disease, 520
Budesonide dry powder inhaler (Pulmicort)
   for asthma, 28**b**
      in adolescents and adults, 769**t**
      in children, 773–774**t**
   for bronchospasm, 28**b**
Budesonide inhalation suspension for nebulization (Pulmicort Respules), for asthma in children, 773–774**t**
Budesonide nasal inhaler (Rhinocort)
   for allergic rhinitis, 780**t**
   for nonallergic rhinitis, 217, 217**b**
Budesonide/formoterol (Symbicort), for asthma
   in adolescents and adults, 767–768**t**
   in children, 773–774**t**

Bulbar signs, of myasthenia gravis, 940, 941**t**
Bulimia nervosa, 1115
   clinical features of, 1115–1116
   comorbid borderline personality disorder with, 1116–1117
   comorbid psychiatric disorders with, 1115–1116
   comorbid substance-use disorders with, 1115–1117
   conditions that resemble, 1115
   diagnosis of, 1115, 1115**b**
   epidemiology of, 1115
   physiologic complications of, 1116–1117
   prognosis for, 1117
   purging *vs.* non-purging, 1115
   treatment of, 1116–1117, 1116**b**
Bulking agents, for irritable bowel syndrome, 524**t**
Bullectomy, for COPD, 236
Bullous disease(s), 866
   bullous pemphigoid as, 866–867
   cicatricial pemphigoid as, 867–869
   diagnosis of, 867**b**
   pemphigus foliaceus as, 869
   pemphigus vulgaris as, 869
   treatment of, 867**b**
Bullous external otitis, 201
Bullous pemphigoid, 30**b**, 866–867
   differential diagnosis of, 866
   pathogenesis of, 866
   treatment of, 866–867
      for aggressive and generalized disease, 867, 869**t**
      for localized and nonaggressive disease, 866–867, 868**t**
BUN (blood urea nitrogen), in chronic renal failure, 730
Bundle branch block
   alternating, 317
   right, 317
Bunyaviruses, as biological weapon agents, 1229–1233**t**
Buprenorphine (Subutex), for opiate withdrawal, 1109
Bupropion (Wellbutrin)
   for major depression, 1123, 1125–1126
   for multiple sclerosis, 939**b**
   poisoning due to, 1214–1216, 1215**t**
Buproprion (Zyban), for smoking cessation, 1107
Burkholderia cepacia, in cystic fibrosis, 237
Burkholderia multivorans, in cystic fibrosis, 237
Burkitt's leukemia, 447**b**, 449
Burkitt's lymphoma, 464, 466
Burn(s), 1135
   chemical, 1138–1139
   in children, 1139
      due to child abuse, 1140
   and concomitant trauma, 1139
   diagnosis of, 1138**b**
   electric, 1138
   estimating extent of, 1135, 1136**f**, 1137**f**
   of eyes, 1136–1137
   facial, 1136–1137
   fluid resuscitation for, 1135–1136
   of hands, 1137
   due to inhalation injury, 1139
   initial management of, 1135
      ABCs in, 1135
      eschariotomies and/or fasciotomies in, 1135
      estimating extent in, 1135, 1136**f**, 1137**f**
      fluid resuscitation in, 1135
      history in, 1135
      referral in, 1135
      universal precautions in, 1135
      wound covering in, 1135
   Lund-Browder Classification of, 1135, 1137**f**
   partial thickness (second-degree), 1135–1136

Burn(s) *(Continued)*
   in patients with preexisting medical disorders, 1139
   referral for, 1135, 1140
   Rule of Nines for, 1135, 1136**f**
   third-degree (full-thickness), 1137–1138
   treatment of, 1138**b**
Burning tongue syndrome, 852–853
Bursitis, 994–995
   causes of, 994, 994**b**
   diagnosis of, 994**b**, 995
   sites of, 994**b**
   symptoms of, 994–995, 994**b**
   treatment of, 995, 997**b**
Buserelin (Suprefact), for premenstrual syndrome, 1069
Buspirone (BuSpar)
   for Alzheimer's disease, 884–886, 885**t**
   for generalized anxiety disorder, 1113, 1113**t**
   for obsessive compulsive disorder, 1114
   for premenstrual syndrome, 1069
Butabarbital (Butisol), intoxication with, 1180–1181
Butalbital, intoxication with, 1180–1181
Butenafine (Mentax) cream, for cutaneous tinea infection, 848**b**
Butoconazole 2% cream (Femstat-3, Mycelex 3), for vulvovaginal candidiasis, 1075**b**, 1075**b**
Butoconazole 2% SR cream (Gynazole-1), for vulvovaginal candidiasis, 1075**b**
Butorphanol (Stadol), for pain, 4**t**
Butyrophenones
   for nausea and vomiting, 8, 8**t**
   poisoning due to, 1208–1209, 1208**t**
BV (bacterial vaginosis), 1074
   during pregnancy, 1014, 1074, 1074**b**
Byetta (exanatide), for diabetes, 580**t**, 581
Bystolic (nebivolol), 1243

C

CA-125, in ovarian cancer, 1094–1095
CAA (cerebral amyloid angiopathy), intracerebral hemorrhage due to, 890
CAB (catheter-associated bacteriuria), 682, 684–685
Cabergoline (Dostinex), for hyperprolactinemia, 660, 660**t**
CAD. *See* Coronary artery disease (CAD).
Caduet (atorvastatin-amlodipine), for dyslipoproteinemia, 605**t**
Caffeine headache, 924–925
CAGE questionnaire, 1098, 1099**b**, 1190
Calabar swellings, 844, 844**t**
Calan. *See* Verapamil (Calan, Isoptin, Verelan).
Calcibind (sodium cellulose phosphate), for renal calculi, 746**t**
Calcimimetic, for hyperparathyroidism, 652
Calcineurin inhibitors
   for atopic dermatitis, 861
   for psoriasis, 802
Calcipotriene (Dovonex), for psoriasis, 801
Calcitonin, for Paget's disease of bone, 616–617
Calcium
   in extremely low birth weight infants, 1039–1040**t**
   for inflammatory bowel disease, 518
   for osteoporosis, 614
      in rheumatoid arthritis, 977**b**
   in parenteral nutrition, 622**t**
   for preeclampsia, 1025
   during pregnancy, 1014
   for premenstrual syndrome, 1069
   for thalassemia, 400**b**
Calcium acetate (PhosLo), for chronic renal failure, 730
Calcium carbonate, for hypoparathyroidism, 653

Calcium channel blockers (CCBs)
  for angina pectoris, 299, 299t
  for atrial fibrillation, 309, 310b
  for hypertension, 356t, 358
  for hypertrophic cardiomyopathy, 333
  intoxication with, 1183–1184
  kinetics of, 1184
  for migraine headache, 925
  for myocardial infarction, 365
  and SSRIs, 1122–1123b
  for systemic sclerosis, 811, 811t
  for tinnitus, 38
Calcium chloride, for poisoning, 1167–1172t
  due to calcium channel blockers, 1184
Calcium citrate (Citrical)
  for chronic renal failure, 730
  for renal calculi, 746t
Calcium gluconate, for poisoning, 1167–1172t
  due to calcium channel blockers, 1184
Calcium metabolism, abnormalities in, due to acromegaly, 635
Calcium pyrophosphate dihydrate disease (CPPD), 1001
Calcium restriction
  for hyperparathyroidism, 651–652
  for renal calculi, 745
Calcium stones, 743, 743t, 744t, 746t
Calcium-phosphate deposition, in chronic renal failure, 729
Calciviruses
  acute infectious diarrhea due to, 16
  foodborne illness due to, 81–82
Calculi, renal. See Renal calculi.
Caloric requirements, 619–620, 620f
  for high-risk neonate, 1035
  of infants, 1044
Calorie-to-nitrogen ratio, 620
Calorimetry, indirect, 620
CAM (confusion assessment method), 1118, 1118b
Campath. See Alemtuzumab (Campath).
Camphorated tincture of opium, intoxication with, 1204–1205, 1205t
Campral (acamprosate), for alcohol dependence, 1103
Camptosar (irinotecan), for small cell lung cancer, 248
Campylobacter jejuni, and Guillain-Barré syndrome, 962
Campylobacter species
  acute infectious diarrhea due to, 15, 19–20t
  foodborne illness due to, 82
CA-MRSA. See Community-acquired methicillin-resistant *Staphylococcus aureus* (CA-MRSA).
CaNa₂ EDTA (edetate calcium disodium), for lead poisoning, 1199–1200, 1200t
Canal of Nuck, cysts of, 1091
Canalith repositioning maneuver, 205, 205f
Canasa (mesalamine suppositories), for inflammatory bowel disease, 516, 519
Candida, onychomycosis due to, 818
Candida albicans
  cutaneous infection with, 846–847, 847b, 848b
  vaginosis due to, during pregnancy, 1014
Candida antigen, for verrucae, 823–824
Candidiasis
  cutaneous, 846–847, 847b, 848b
  vulvovaginal, 1074–1075, 1075b
Canker sore, 850
Cannabinoids, for nausea and vomiting, 8–9, 8t
Cannabis, abuse of, 1110
Canthardin (Cantharone), for verrucae, 823
CaO₂ (carrying capacity of arterialized blood), 225
CAP. See Community-acquired pneumonia (CAP).
Capoten (captopril)
  for myocardial infarction, 365t
  for systemic sclerosis, 812

Capreomycin (Capastat), for tuberculosis, 285t
Capsaicin (Capsin, Zostrix)
  for anogenital pruritus, 873
  for neuropathic pain, 964t, 965
  for osteoarthritis, 1001
  for pain, 3
  for pruritus, 34b
Captopril (Capoten)
  for myocardial infarction, 365t
  for systemic sclerosis, 812
Carac. See 5-Fluorouracil (5-FU, Adrucil, Efudex, Carac, Fluoroplex).
Carafate. See Sucralfate (Carafate).
Carbamate poisoning, 1205–1206
Carbamazepine (Tegretol)
  for alcohol withdrawal, 1103
  for benzodiazepine abuse, 1106b
  for benzodiazepine withdrawal, 1108
  for bipolar disorder, 1127
  for epilepsy
    in adolescents in adults, 904t, 903, 905
    in infants and children, 911, 912t
  for multiple sclerosis, 939b
  for neuropathic pain, 964t, 964–965
  for sedative hypnotic abuse, 1106b
  for tinnitus, 38
  for trigeminal neuralgia, 948
Carbaryl, poisoning due to, 1205–1206
Carbenicillin indanyl sodium (Geocillin), for prostatitis, 681
Carbidopa/levodopa (Parcopa, Sinemet-CR), for parkinsonism, 954–955
Carbidopa/levodopa-entacapone (Stalevo), for parkinsonism, 956–957
Carbohydrate(s), in diabetic diet
  for adults, 577–578, 579b
  for children, 587–588
Carbohydrate intake, for high-risk neonate, 1035
Carbohydrate malabsorption, 541b, 542
Carbohydrate-modified infant formula, 1043b
Carbon monoxide (CO) poisoning, 1139, 1184–1185, 1185t
Carbonic anhydrase inhibitors, for glaucoma, 200, 200t
Carbonyl iron (Feosol Carbonyl Iron tablets, ICAR Pediatric Chewables, ICAR Pediatric Suspension), 385, 385t
Carboplatin (Paraplatin), for non–small cell lung cancer
  advanced and metastatic, 247
  local, 246
  locoregional, 247
Carboprost tromethamine (Hemabate), for postpartum hemorrhage, 1028t
Carboxyhemoglobin (CoHB)
  in carbon monoxide poisoning, 1184–1185
  reference intervals for, 1224t
Carbuncles, 837, 837f
  renal, 679
Carcinoid tumors
  pruritus due to, 32b
  of stomach, 558
Carcinomatous neuropathy, 964
Cardene (nicardipine), intoxication with, 1183–1184
Cardiac arrest, 302
  due to asystole, 305–306
  defined, 302
  epidemiology of, 302
  etiology of, 302, 303t, 304f
  due to hypertrophic cardiomyopathy, 331–333
  initial rhythm in, 302
  management of, 302
    activation of EMS system in, 303
    airway in, 303
    breathing (ventilation) in, 303
    chain of survival in, 302–303
    circulation in, 303

Cardiac arrest *(Continued)*
    defibrillation in, 303–305
    early recognition in, 303
    ILCOR recommendations on, 302, 305f
    pharmacologic treatment in, 306
      alternative routs of administration for, 306
      with drugs used to restore rhythm, 306
      with drugs used to support blood pressure, 306
  prognosis for, 302
  from pulseless electrical activity, 305
  survivors of
    implantable cardiac defibrillators for, 307–308
    management and evaluation of, 306–307
    neurologic assessment of, 307–308
Cardiac arrhythmias
  due to bulimia nervosa, 1116
  due to hypertrophic cardiomyopathy, 333
Cardiac catheterization, for survivor of cardiac arrest, 307
Cardiac conduction disturbances. See Heart block.
Cardiac death, sudden. See Cardiac arrest.
Cardiac disease
  congenital (See Congenital heart disease)
  due to thalassemia, 399t, 402
Cardiac glycosides, intoxication due to, 1188–1190
Cardiac murmurs, 326–327
Cardiac rehabilitation, after myocardial infarction, 367
Cardiac toxicity, 1174t
Cardinal motor signs, of parkinsonism, 952–953, 953b
Cardiogenic pulmonary edema, 230
Cardiogenic shock, myocardial infarction with, 366t, 367
Cardiomyopathy
  hypertrophic (See Hypertrophic cardiomyopathy (HCM))
  peripartum, 1028
Cardiopulmonary bypass, heated, 1146
Cardiopulmonary resuscitation (CPR), for cardiac arrest, 303
Cardiovascular disease
  acquired diseases of the aorta as, 291
  due to acromegaly, 634
  acute myocardial infarction as, 360
  acute pericarditis as, 367
  angina pectoris as, 295
  atrial fibrillation as, 308
  cardiac arrest as, 302
  cardiomyopathy as, 331
  congenital, 326
  in extremely low birth weight infants, 1039–1040t
  heart block as, 315
  heart failure as, 338
  hypertension as, 349
  infective endocarditis as, 342
  mitral valve prolapse as, 334
  peripheral arterial disease as, 373
  premature beats as, 312
  tachycardias as, 320
  venous thrombosis as, 375
Cardiovascular drugs, reference intervals for, 1222t
Cardiovascular risk management, for diabetes
  in adults, 575–576
  in children, 588–589
Cardiovascular sequelae, of hypertension, 350–351, 352f
Cardiovascular system, in hypothermia, 1144, 1146
Cardioversion
  for atrial fibrillation, 311, 311t
  for hypertrophic cardiomyopathy, 333

Carditis, due to Lyme disease, 136–137
Cardizem. *See* Diltiazem (Cardizem).
Cardura. *See* Doxazosin mesylate (Cardura).
Carisbamate, for epilepsy, 904t
Carotid artery stenting, 374
Carotid endarterectomy, 374
Carotid occlusive disease, 374
Carpal tunnel syndrome, 961–962
　during pregnancy, 1015
Carrying capacity of arterialized blood (CaO$_2$), 225
Carteolol (Cartrol), intoxication with, 1182–1183, 1183t
Carteolol ophthalmic (Ocupress), for glaucoma, 200
Carvedilol (Coreg)
　for angina pectoris, 299t
　for heart failure, 339t
Castle, William, 395
Cataflam (diclofenac)
　for juvenile idiopathic arthritis, 985
　for pain, 2t
Catagen phase, of hair growth, 790
Cataplexy, 888
　vs. seizures, 901t
Catapres. *See* Clonidine (Catapres).
Catecholaminergic polymorphic ventricular tachycardia (CPVT), 324
Catechol-*O*-methyl transferase (COMT) inhibitors, for parkinsonism, 956–957
Catheter ablation, for atrial fibrillation, 310–311
Catheter sepsis, with parenteral nutrition, 625–626
Catheter-associated bacteriuria (CAB), 682, 684–685
Cat-scratch disease (CSD), 169
　clinical manifestations of, 169
　diagnosis of, 169–170
　epidemiology of, 169
　prevention of, 170
　treatment of, 170, 169b
Caustics, poisoning due to, 1185–1186
Caverject (alprostadil), for erectile dysfunction, 719
CAVHD (continuous arteriovenous hemodiafiltration), for poisonings, 1173
CBD (corticobasal degeneration), 954
CBT. *See* Cognitive behavioral therapy (CBT).
CC-5013 (lenalidomide)
　for cutaneous T-cell lymphomas, 800
　for multiple myeloma, 469b, 470, 471
CCBs. *See* Calcium channel blockers (CCBs).
CCI (corrected count increment), for platelets, 482, 491
CD. *See* Contact dermatitis (CD); Crohn's disease (CD).
CD (cluster designation) groups, 444
CD4 antibodies, for cutaneous T-cell lymphomas, 800
CD4+ helper T lymphocytes, in HIV, 46, 50–51
CDC (Centers for Disease Control and Prevention), on immunizations, 148
CDH (congenital diaphragmatic hernia), 1039
CEE. *See* Conjugated equine estrogens (CEE, Premarin).
Cefadroxil (Duricef)
　for endocarditis prophylaxis, 347t
　for streptococcal pharyngitis, 223t
Cefazolin (Ancef)
　for endocarditis prophylaxis, 346–347t
　for osteomyelitis, 1006–1007
Cefdinir (Omnicef), for urinary tract infections in girls, 687b
Cefepime (Maxipime)
　for bacterial meningitis, 115t
　for osteomyelitis, 1006–1007

Cefixime (Suprax)
　for acute infectious diarrhea, 19–20t
　for gonorrhea, 751, 752b
　for typhoid fever, 176t
　for urinary tract infections in girls, 687b
Cefizox (ceftizoxime), for pelvic inflammatory disease, 1080b
Cefotan (cefotetan)
　for *Chlamydia trachomatis,* 1078b
　for pelvic inflammatory disease, 1080b
Cefotaxime (Claforan)
　for acute infectious diarrhea, 19–20t
　for bacterial meningitis, 115t
　for bleeding esophageal varices, 506
　for Lyme disease, 138, 139t
　for necrotizing skin and soft tissue infections, 85t
　for neonatal conjunctivitis, 195–196
　for osteomyelitis, 1006–1007
　for pelvic inflammatory disease, 1080b
　for *Salmonella* gastroenteritis, 173
　for spontaneous bacterial peritonitis, 502
　for typhoid fever, 176t
　for urinary tract infections in girls, 687b
Cefotetan (Cefotan)
　for *Chlamydia trachomatis,* 1078b
　for pelvic inflammatory disease, 1080b
Cefoxitin (Mefoxin)
　for *Chlamydia trachomatis,* 1078b
　for pelvic inflammatory disease, 1080b
Cefprofil (Cefzil), for urinary tract infections in girls, 687b
Ceftazidime (Fortaz, Tazicef)
　for bacterial meningitis, 115t
　for marine injuries, 1159t
　for necrotizing skin and soft tissue infections, 85t
　for urinary tract infections in girls, 687b
Ceftin (cefuroxime axetil)
　for Lyme disease, 138, 139t
　for streptococcal pharyngitis, 223t
Ceftizoxime (Cefizox), for pelvic inflammatory disease, 1080b
Ceftobiprole, 1244–1249t
Ceftriaxone (Rocephin)
　for acute infectious diarrhea, 19–20t
　for bacterial meningitis, 115t
　for brucellosis, 74b, 75
　for chancroid, 750
　for *Chlamydia trachomatis,* 1078b
　for endocarditis prophylaxis, 346–347t
　for epididymitis, 697b, 698
　for fever, 24
　for gonorrhea, 751, 752b
　for infective endocarditis, 345
　for Lyme disease, 138, 139t
　for necrotizing skin and soft tissue infections, 85t
　for neonatal conjunctivitis, 195–196
　for pelvic inflammatory disease, 1080b
　for pericarditis, 371
　for pyelonephritis, 706b
　for relapsing fever, 136t
　for *Salmonella* gastroenteritis, 173
　for spontaneous bacterial peritonitis, 502
　for toxic shock syndrome, 89, 89b
　for typhoid fever, 176t
　for urinary tract infections in girls, 687b
Cefuroxime axetil (Ceftin)
　for Lyme disease, 138, 139t
　for streptococcal pharyngitis, 223t
Cefzil (cefprofil), for urinary tract infections in girls, 687b
Celecoxib (Celebrex)
　for arthritis
　　juvenile idiopathic, 985
　　osteo-, 1000
　　rheumatoid, 983

Celecoxib (Celebrex) *(Continued)*
　for dysmenorrhea, 1066t
　for pain, 2–3, 2t
Celestone Syrup (betamethasone syrup), for aphthous ulcers, 850
Celexa. *See* Citalopram (Celexa).
Celiac disease, 541b, 543
　in diabetic children, 589
　gaseousness due to, 10, 10t
CellCept. *See* Mycophenolate mofetil (MMF, CellCept).
Cellulitis, 835–836, 836b
　of scalp, dissecting, 792
Centers for Disease Control and Prevention (CDC), on immunizations, 148
Central α$_2$-stimulants, for hypertension, 358–359
Central centrifugal scarring alopecia, 792
Central nervous system (CNS)
　of extremely low birth weight infants, 1039–1040t
　in hypothermia, 1144
Central nervous system (CNS) complications, of sickle cell disease, 406–407, 410–411
Central nervous system (CNS) depressants, poisoning due to, 1166t
Central nervous system (CNS) disorders, nausea and vomiting due to, 6, 6t
Central nervous system (CNS) hemorrhage, due to hemophilia, 420
Central nervous system (CNS) lymphomas, primary, 975
Central nervous system (CNS) radiation therapy, in children
　for acute lymphoblastic leukemia, 454
　for acute myeloid leukemia, 455
Central nervous system (CNS) stimulants, poisoning due to, 1166t
Central nervous system (CNS) symptoms, due to HAART, 54–55t
Central nervous system (CNS) toxicity, 1165, 1166t
　of lead, 1197
Central venous catheters, for parenteral nutrition, 622
Central venous solutions, composition of, 620–622, 621t, 622t
CEP (congenital erythropoietic porphyria), 475t, 477b, 479
Cephalexin (Keflex)
　for endocarditis prophylaxis, 347t
　for streptococcal pharyngitis, 223t
　for urinary tract infections in girls, 687b
Cephalosporins, allergy to, 782
Cephulac (lactulose), for hepatic encephalopathy, 502–503
Ceprotin (protein C concentrate), 1243
Cerebellar pontine angle tumor, orofacial pain due to, 992t
Cerebral adaptation, to hyponatremia, 597
Cerebral amyloid angiopathy (CAA), intracerebral hemorrhage due to, 890
Cerebral edema
　due to diabetic ketoacidosis, 594–595
　high-altitude, 1141–1142
　　clinical presentation of, 158, 1141
　　diagnosis of, 1141, 1142b
　　differential diagnosis of, 1141b
　　prevention of, 158, 1140–1141
　　treatment of, 1141–1142, 1142b
　due to salicylate poisoning, 1211
Cerebral infarction, vertigo due to, 209
Cerebral perfusion pressure (CPP), with traumatic brain injury, 967
　in children, 970–971
Cerebrospinal fluid (CSF)
　in bacterial meningitis, 112–113, 112b, 113t
　in multiple sclerosis, 933–934
　in viral meningitis or encephalitis, 927, 930

Cerebrospinal fluid (CSF) diversion, for elevated intracranial pressure, 967
Cerebrospinal fluid (CSF) tests, reference intervals for, 1224t
Cerebrovascular complications, of sickle cell disease, 406–407, 410–411
Cerebrovascular disease
 hypertension and, 350, 356t
 ischemic, 893
  diagnosis of, 893–894, 894b
  epidemiology and etiology of, 893
  ischemic stroke due to, 894
  pathophysiology of, 893
  prevention of, 894–895, 897
  risk factors for, 893
  symptoms of, 893
  transient ischemic attacks due to, 893–894
Cerebyx (fosphenytoin)
 for elevated intracranial pressure in children, 971
 for status epilepticus in neonates, 910
Certican (everolimus), 1244–1249t
Certolizumab pegol (Cimzia), 1244–1249t
 for inflammatory bowel disease, 517
Cerubidine. See Daunorubicin (Cerubidine).
Cerumen, 201
Cervarix. See Human papillomavirus (HPV) vaccines (Cervarix, Gardasil).
Cervical cancer, 1086
 adenocarcinoma as, 1090–1091
  clear cell, 1090
  in situ, 1090
  invasive, 1090–1091
  microinvasive, 1090
 adenosquamous carcinoma as, 1090
 of cervical stump, 1090
 chemoprevention and vaccination for, 1091
 epidemiology of, 1086
 etiology and pathogenesis of, 1086
 examination and testing for, 1087, 1087b
 follow-up for, 1089
 glassy cell carcinoma as, 1090–1091
 histopathology of, 1086, 1087b
 after hysterectomy, 1090
 pathophysiology of, 1086
 physical findings in, 1086
 during pregnancy, 1090
 recurrence of, 1089, 1090f
 risk factors for, 1086, 1086b
 small cell carcinoma as, 1091
 spread pattern of, 1086–1087
 staging of, 1086–1087, 1087b
 treatment of, 1087–1089
  chemoradiation therapy for, 1087–1088, 1088t
  chemotherapy for, 1089, 1090f
  complications of, 1089, 1089b
  radiation therapy for, 1087–1088, 1088t, 1089, 1089b
  for recurrence, 1089, 1090f
  by stage, 1088–1089
  surgery for, 1087, 1089, 1089b
Cervical cap (FemCap), 757
 in postpartum period, 1029t
Cervical radiculopathy
 management of, 42–43, 42b
 natural course of, 41
Cervical stump, carcinoma of, 1090
Cervicitis
 due to gonorrhea, 751
 mucopurulent, due to *Chlamydia trachomatis*, 1076, 1078b
Cestodes, 570t, 573
Cetirizine (Zyrtec)
 for allergic rhinitis, 779t
 for urticaria, 875
Cetirizine/pseudoephedrine (Zyrtec-D), for allergic rhinitis, 779t

Cetrorelix (Cetrotide), for uterine leiomyoma, 1082
CF. See Cystic fibrosis (CF).
CF (correction factor), for insulin dose, 586
CFS. See Chronic fatigue syndrome (CFS).
CFTR (cystic fibrosis transmembrane regulator) gene, 236
CGN (crescentic glomerulonephritis)
 diagnosis of, 700b, 700b
 treatment of, 702b, 703–704
CHAD$_2$ score, for atrial fibrillation, 309, 309t
Chagas' disease, 843, 844t
Chagoma, 843
Chain of survival, for cardiac arrest, 302–303
Chamomile flower, 1234–1243t
CHAMPS (Controlled High-Risk Subjects Avonex Multiple Sclerosis Prevention Study), 197
Chancroid, 749–750
Chantix (varenicline), for smoking cessation, 1107
Charcot-Marie-Tooth (CMT) disease, 963
Chaste tree berry, 1234–1243t
Chasteberry, 1234–1243t
CHD. See Coronary heart disease (CHD).
Cheek-chewing, 851
ChEI(s) (cholinesterase inhibitors)
 for Alzheimer's disease, 882–886, 883t
 for myasthenia gravis, 942–943, 942t
Cheilitis
 actinic, 833b, 834, 834b, 850
 angular, 849
 reactive, 850
Cheiracanthium envenomation, 1151
Chelation therapy
 for iron poisoning, 1195
 for lead poisoning, 1199–1200, 1200t
 for thalassemia, 401–402, 403t
Chemet (2,3-dimercaptosuccinic acid), for poisoning, 1167–1172t
 due to lead, 1199, 1200t
Chemical agents, hemolytic anemia due to, 391t, 394
Chemical burns, 1138–1139
Chemical conjunctivitis, in neonate, 195, 196t
Chemical weapon agents, 1226
Chemoimmunotherapy, for chronic lymphocytic leukemia, 463, 463t
Chemoprophylaxis
 for bacterial meningitis, 114–115
 for influenza, 92, 92t
 for malaria, 110–112, 111–112t, 156–157, 157t
 for opportunistic infections in HIV, 53, 56t
 for plague, 123
 for tetanus, 144b, 145, 145t
 for toxic shock syndrome, 90
Chemoradiation therapy, for cervical cancer, 1087–1088, 1088t
Chemotherapy
 for bladder carcinoma, 736
 for brain metastases, 976
 for breast cancer, 1052
 for cervical cancer, 1089, 1090f
 for colorectal cancer, 561–562
 for endometrial cancer, 1085
 for gastric adenocarcinoma, 557
 for gliomas, 974–975
 hair loss due to, 791
 for leukemia
  acute lymphoblastic, 449
   in children, 454–455, 455t
  acute myeloid
   in children, 455, 455t
   consolidation, 446
   induction, 445–446
   maintenance, 447
  acute promyelocytic, 448–449
  chronic lymphocytic, 461–463, 462t

Chemotherapy (Continued)
 for lung cancer
  non–small cell
   advanced and metastatic, 247–248
   local, 245–246
   locoregional, 246–247
  small cell, 248
 for lymphoma
  cutaneous T-cell, 797b, 798–799
  non-Hodgkin's
   diffuse large B-cell, 466
   indolent, 465–466
   lymphoblastic and Burkitt's, 466
 for multiple myeloma
  high-dose, with autologous stem cell transplantation, 470
  novel agents in, 471
  for refractory disease, 471
  regimens of, 469b
  with standard alkylating agent, 470–471
 nausea and vomiting due to, 9
 for ovarian cancer, 1095–1096
 for psoriasis, 802
 for testicular carcinoma, 739
Chest compression
 for cardiac arrest, 303
 in newborn resuscitation, 1032
Chest pain. See also Angina pectoris.
 due to pericarditis, 369
Chest x-ray, of pericarditis, 369
Chickenpox. See Varicella.
Chilblain, 1146–1147, 1147b
Child(ren)
 acute leukemia in, 450
  classification of, 450, 450t, 450b
  clinical presentation of, 452–453, 453b
  differential diagnosis of, 454
  epidemiology of, 450–451, 451f
  etiology of, 451–452, 452t
  medical emergencies in, 453–454
  prognosis for, 451
  relapse of, 455–456
  risk stratification for, 454
  treatment of, 454–455, 455t
   late effects of, 456, 456t
 asthma in, 770
  diagnosis of, 771b
   history in, 771
   physical examination in, 771–772
  differential diagnosis of, 770–771, 770t
  epidemiology of, 770
  hygiene hypothesis of, 770
  key diagnostic points for, 771
  pathophysiology of, 770
  treatment of, 772–774, 772b
   education and environmental control in, 776
   medications for, 774–776, 775t
   stepwise approach to, 773–774t
  triggers for, 771, 771b
 bacterial meningitis in, 113t, 114b, 115t
 bariatric surgery for, 610
 burns in, 1139
  due to child abuse, 1140
 dehydration of, 628–631
  assessment of, 628–630, 628t, 629t
  classification of, 628, 629
  diagnosis of, 630
  fluid management for, 630–631
   indications for, 630
   with intravenous therapy, 630–631
   maintenance requirements in, 631
   with oral rehydration therapy, 630
   rapid rehydration in, 631
   rehydration requirements (deficit therapy) in, 630–631
   replacement requirements in, 631
  due to gastroenteritis, 628

Child(ren) (Continued)
  laboratory tests for, 628–630
    scale for, 629, 629t
    signs of, 628–629, 628t
    weight loss and, 629
  diabetes mellitus in, 583
    diabetic ketoacidosis due to, 584
    diagnosis of, 584
    exercise for, 588
    goals of therapy for, 586, 586t
    hypoglycemia with, 588
    initial management of, 584
    insulin replacement therapy for, 586–587, 587t
      initiation of, 584–585, 585f
    medical nutrition therapy for, 587–588
    outpatient care for, 585
    patient education for, 585–586
    psychosocial support for, 588
    screening in
      for complications, 588–589, 589t
      for other autoimmune diseases, 589
    self-monitoring of, 587
    sick day management for, 588
    type 2, 583, 589–590
      medications for, 590, 590t
      risk factors for, 589t, 590
  dyslipoproteinemia in, 606
  epilepsy in, 907
    absence, 908–909
    assessment of, 910–911
    benign rolandic, 909
    childhood and juvenile, 908–909
    classification of, 907–908, 908b
    defined, 907
    differential diagnosis of, 907–908, 907b
    epidemiology of, 907
    generalized, 908–909, 908b
    localization-related, 909
    myoclonic, 908–909
    syndromes of, 908–910, 908b
    treatment of, 911–915, 912t, 913t
  fever in, 24
  juvenile idiopathic arthritis in, 983
    enthesitis related, 984
    epidemiology of, 983–984
    evaluation of, 984–985, 984b
    oligoarthritis (pauciarthritis) with iridocyclitis as, 984
    polyarthritis forms of, 984
    prognosis for, 985
    psoriatic, 984
    rheumatoid factor in, 984
    subtypes of, 984
    systemic, 984
    treatment of, 985–986, 985b
  malaria in, 108t, 110
  multiple sclerosis in, 939–940
  parenteral fluid therapy for, 626
    for dehydration, 628–631
      assessment of, 628–630, 628t, 629t
      diagnosis of, 630
      fluid management with, 630–631
      indications for, 630
      maintenance requirements in, 631
      rapid rehydration in, 631
      rehydration requirements (deficit therapy) in, 630–631
      replacement requirements in, 631
    maintenance fluids in, 626–628
      electrolyte requirements for, 627, 627t
      fluid requirements for, 626–627, 627t
      glucose in, 627
      method for prescribing, 627–628
      volume of, 628
    monitoring of, 631
  relapsing fever in, 136t
  traumatic brain injury in, 969

Child(ren) (Continued)
  closed, 969
  diagnosis of, 971b
  epidemiology of, 969
  etiology of, 969
  Glasgow Coma Scale for, 970, 970t
  increased intracranial pressure due to, 971
  mild, 970
  moderate, 970
  open, 969
  primary, 969–970
  secondary, 970
  severe, 970–971
  due to shaking-impact syndrome, 970
  subdural hematomas due to, 969–970
  treatment of, 971b
  types and severity of, 969–970
Child abuse, burns due to, 1140
Childhood glaucoma, 199
Child-Pugh score, for cirrhosis, 497, 497t
Chlamydia, cough due to, 28b
Chlamydia pneumoniae
  pharyngitis due to, 220
  pneumonia due to, 269
Chlamydia psittaci. See Psittacosis.
Chlamydia trachomatis, 1076
  clinical presentation of, 1076
  diagnosis and screening for, 1076–1078, 1077b
  dysuria-pyuria syndrome due to, 682, 684
  epididymitis due to, 698
  impact of, 1076
  pelvic inflammatory disease due to, 1078b, 1079–1080
  during pregnancy, 1014
  treatment of, 1078–1079, 1078b
  urethritis due to, 752–753
Chlamydial conjunctivitis, 194t, 195
  in neonate, 196, 196t
Chlamydophila psittaci. See Psittacosis.
Chloasma, 876–877, 877t, 1012
Chlorambucil (Leukeran)
  for cold agglutinin syndrome, 388
  for membranous nephropathy, 702
  for minimal change disease, 701
Chloramphenicol (Chloromycetin)
  for Rocky Mountain spotted fever, 177, 179b
  for Salmonella gastroenteritis, 173
Chlordiazepoxide (Librium)
  for alcohol withdrawal, 1101, 1191
  intoxication with, 1181–1182
  for tinnitus, 38
Chloride, in parenteral nutrition, 621, 622t
Chloride channel activators, for constipation, 10t
Chlorine (Cl), as chemical weapon, 1226–1228t
Chloromycetin (chloramphenicol)
  for Rocky Mountain spotted fever, 177, 179b
  for Salmonella gastroenteritis, 173
Chloropicrin, as chemical weapon, 1226–1228t
Chloroquine phosphate (Aralen)
  for malaria, 108t, 109, 111–112t, 157t
    resistance to, 105t, 107b, 108t, 109–110
    sensitivity to, 107b, 109–110
  for osteoarthritis, 1002
  for porphyria cutanea tarda, 479
  for systemic lupus erythematosus, 806–808, 807t
Chlorpheniramine (Chlor-Trimeton), for allergic rhinitis, 779t
Chlorpromazine (Thorazine)
  for acute porphyria, 476, 477b
  for erectile dysfunction, 720
  for nausea and vomiting, 8t
  poisoning due to, 1208–1209, 1208t
Chlorprothixene (Taractan), poisoning due to, 1208–1209, 1208t
Chlorpyrifos, poisoning due to, 1205–1206
Chlorthalidone (Hygroton), for renal calculi, 746t

Chlor-Trimeton (chlorpheniramine), for allergic rhinitis, 779t
Choking agents, as chemical weapons, 1226–1228t
Cholangiopancreatography, endoscopic retrograde, 495–496, 550
Cholangitis, primary sclerosing, 498t, 499–500
Cholecalciferol, for hypoparathyroidism, 653
Cholecystectomy
  laparoscopic, 494
    and bile duct exploration, 495–496
  mini-laparotomy, 494
Cholecystitis
  acalculous, 494
  acute, 493–495
    clinical manifestations of, 493
    complications of, 494–495
    diagnosis of, 493–494
    etiology of, 493
    in pregnancy, 494–495
    treatment of, 494
  chronic, 495
    gaseousness due to, 10t
  emphysematous, 494
  gangrenous, 494
Choledocholithiasis, 495–496
  diagnosis of, 494b, 495
  differential diagnosis of, 495, 496b
  presentation of, 495
  treatment of, 495–496, 495b
Cholelithiasis, 493
  classification of, 493
  complications of, 493b
  diagnosis of, 494b
  epidemiology of, 493
  indigestion due to, 11t
  risk factors for, 493, 493b
  in sickle cell disease, 407
Cholera, 78
  acute infectious diarrhea due to, 15–16, 19–20t
  complications and prognosis for, 80
  diagnosis of, 78b
  etiology of, 78–79, 79t
  historical background of, 78
  treatment of, 79–80, 78b
    maintenance phase of, 79–80
    pharmacologic, 80, 78b, 80t
    rehydration phase of, 79, 79t, 78b
Cholera vaccine (Dukoral), 18
Cholestasis
  intrahepatic, of pregnancy, pruritus due to, 32b
  pruritus due to, 32b, 34b
Cholestatic liver function tests, 496b
Cholesterol
  and angina pectoris, 297–298, 298t
  screening for, 602
Cholesterol emboli syndrome, acute renal failure due to, 722
Cholesterol Treatment Trialists' (CTT) Collaborators, 297
Cholestyramine (Questran)
  for cholestasis, 34b
  for dyslipoproteinemia, 605, 605t
  for pruritus due to primary biliary cirrhosis, 499
Choline magnesium trisalicylate (Trilisate), for pain, 2t
Cholinergic(s), poisoning due to, 1166t
Cholinergic urticaria, 874
Cholinesterase inhibitors (ChEIs)
  for Alzheimer's disease, 882–884, 883t, 884–886
  for myasthenia gravis, 942–943, 942t
Chondrocyte transplantation, for osteoarthritis, 1002
Chondroitin sulfate, 1234–1243t
  for osteoarthritis, 1002

Choriocarcinoma, 738–739
Chorionic villus sampling (CVS), 1012
Chromium
   as nutritional supplement, 1234–1243t
   in parenteral nutrition, 621, 621t
Chronic fatigue syndrome (CFS), 117
   defined, 117, 118b
   diagnosis of, 117–119, 118b
   epidemiology of, 117
   treatment of, 119–120, 119b
Chronic inflammatory demyelinating polyneuropathy, 962
Chronic kidney disease, hypertension and, 350, 353, 356t, 359
Chronic limb ischemia (CLI), 373–374
Chronic lymphocytic leukemia (CLL), 460–463
   clinical staging and prognostic factors for, 461, 461t
   diagnosis of, 457b, 459b, 461
   differential diagnosis of, 461, 461t
   incidence and risk factors for, 460–461
   treatment of, 459b, 461–463, 462t, 463t
Chronic myeloid leukemia (CML), 456–457
   clinical features and diagnosis of, 456–457, 457b
   initial evaluation of, 457
   natural history of, 457, 458t
   prognostic categories for, 457
   treatment of, 457–460, 459b, 460b, 460t
      allogeneic bone marrow transplantation for, 460
      imatinib mesylate for, 457–460, 459b
         failure of, 458–459, 460t
         monitoring of, 458
         toxicity of, 458, 460b
      objectives for, 457, 458b
      second-line therapy for, 459–460
Chronic obstructive pulmonary disease (COPD), 231
   acute exacerbations of, 228–229, 235–236
   classification of, 232–233, 233f
   cough due to, 26, 28b
   diagnosis of, 232
   epidemiology of, 232
   guidelines for, 231
   management of
      for acute exacerbations, 235–236
      for stable disease, 233–235, 234b
      surgical options for, 236
   pathophysiology of, 231–232
   risk factors for, 232
Chronic pancreatitis (CP), 549–552
   diagnosis of, 549–550, 550b, 550t
   etiology and pathogenesis of, 549, 549t
   incidence of, 549
   treatment of
      endoscopic, 552
      medical, 550
      surgical, 550–551, 551t
Chronic paroxysmal hemicrania, orofacial pain due to, 992t
Chronic pelvic pain syndrome (CPPS), 710–712
   diagnosis of, 710, 711b
   treatment of, 710–712, 711b, 711f
Chronic renal failure (CRF), 725
   anemia in, 727, 727t, 729–730
   calcium-phosphate deposition in, 729
   causes of, 725
   defined, 725
   diagnosis of, 726b
      approach to, 725–726
      clinical and laboratory abnormalities in, 726–727, 727t
      symptoms and signs in, 727
   divalent ion metabolism in, 727, 730
   epidemiology of, 725
   factors causing progression of, 728–729
   glomerular filtration rate in, 725

Chronic renal failure (CRF) (Continued)
      measurement of, 725–726
      and staging, 728
   glomerular hypertrophy in, 728–729
   glomerular prostaglandin production in, 729
   hyperkalemia in, 726–727, 727t, 730
   hyperlipidemia in, 729
   hyperparathyroidism in, 727, 730
   hyperphosphatemia in, 727, 727t, 730
   hypertension in, 727, 727t, 729
      intraglomerular, 728–729
   hyponatremia and hypernatremia in, 726, 727t
   impact of, 725
   metabolic acidosis in
      and disease progression, 729
      laboratory values for, 727, 727t
      symptoms of, 727
      treatment of, 730
   parenteral nutrition with, 624
   proteinuria in, 726, 729
   pruritus due to, 32b
   staging of, 728
   treatment of, 730b
      general approach to, 728
      to reduce rate of progression, 729
      to treat significant laboratory abnormalities, 729–731
   tubulointerstitial disease in, 729
   uremia in, 727, 727t, 730
   vitamin D in, 730
   volume overload in, 727, 730–731
Chvostek sign, 652
CI inhibitor (Cinryze), 1244–1249t
Cialis (tadalafil), for erectile dysfunction, 719
   in multiple sclerosis, 939b
Cicatricial pemphigoid, 867–869
Ciclopirox (Loprox), for onychomycosis, 818
Cidofovir (Vistide)
   for CMV disease in HIV, 57
   for herpes simplex virus, 842
Cierny-Mader staging system, for osteomyelitis, 1005, 1005b
Cigarette smoking
   and asthma
      in adolescents and adults, 765b
      in children, 771
   cessation of, 1106–1107
   and COPD, 232
   cough due to, 26
   erectile dysfunction due to, 716
   and lung cancer, 242
   during pregnancy, 1012
   rhinitis due to, 215–216
Ciguatera poisoning, 1155–1157, 1156b, 1157t
Ciliary body, 187, 188f
Ciliates, 563–567
Cilomilast (Ariflo), 1244–1249t
Cimetidine (Tagamet)
   for gastroesophageal reflux disease, 553, 554t
   for peptic ulcer disease, 531t
   for scombroid poisoning, 1157
CIMT (constraint-induced movement therapy), for stroke rehabilitation, 896b
Cimzia (certolizumab pegol), 1244–1249t
   for inflammatory bowel disease, 517
Cinchonism, 108–109
Cinnamon, oral mucosal reaction to, 851
Cinryze (CI inhibitor), 1244–1249t
Ciprofloxacin (Cipro)
   for anthrax, 126t
   for bacterial meningitis, 114–115
   for brucellosis, 75t
   for carrier state of salmonellosis, 174
   for chancroid, 750
   for cholera, 80t
   for cyclosporiasis, 565–566t, 568
   for diarrhea
      acute infectious, 18b, 19t, 19–20t

Ciprofloxacin (Cipro) (Continued)
      traveler's, 156, 156t
   for enteric fever, 173
   for granuloma inguinale, 750
   for inflammatory bowel disease, 520
   for isosporiasis, 565–566t, 568
   for legionellosis, 271t
   for marine injuries, 1159t
   for necrotizing skin and soft tissue infections, 85t
   for osteomyelitis, 1006t
   for pericarditis, 371
   for plague, 123
   for pyelonephritis, 706b
   for Salmonella gastroenteritis, 173
   for spontaneous bacterial peritonitis, 502
   for typhoid fever, 176t
   for urinary tract infections in males, 681t
Circadian rhythm disorders, 888
Circulation
   for cardiac arrest, 303
   in newborn resuscitation, 1032
   for traumatic brain injury in children
      moderate, 970
      severe, 971
Circumcision, and urinary tract infections, 679
Cirrhosis, 496
   due to alcoholic hepatitis, 498–499, 498t
   due to alpha$_1$-antitrypsin deficiency, 498t, 501
   due to autoimmune hepatitis, 498t, 499
   due to Budd-Chiari syndrome, 498t
   causes of, 497, 498t
   clinical manifestations of, 496, 497t
   complication(s) of, 501–504, 501t
      ascites as, 497t, 501–502, 501t
      esophageal varices as, 497t, 502
      hepatic encephalopathy as, 497t, 501t, 502–503, 503t
      hepatocellular carcinoma as, 497t, 501t, 504
      hepatopulmonary syndrome as, 497t, 501t, 503
      hepatorenal syndrome as, 497t, 501t, 503, 503t
      portopulmonary hypertension as, 497t, 501t, 503–504
      spontaneous bacterial peritonitis as, 497t, 501t, 502
   cryptogenic, 498t
   defined, 496
   diagnosis of, 497, 497t, 497b
   due to hemochromatosis, 500
   laboratory and imaging findings in, 496–497
   liver transplantation for, 504
   due to nonalcoholic steatohepatitis, 498t, 500
   pathogenesis of, 496
   primary biliary, 498t, 499
   due to primary sclerosing cholangitis, 498t, 499–500
   severity of, 497, 497t
   treatment of, 497–498, 498b
   vaccination with, 504
   due to viral hepatitis, 498t
   due to Wilson's disease, 498t, 500–501
Cisplatin (Platinol)
   for lung cancer
      non–small cell
         advanced and metastatic, 247, 247t
         local, 245–246
         locoregional, 246–247
      small cell, 248
   for ovarian cancer, 1096
   peripheral neuropathy due to, 963
Citalopram (Celexa)
   for Alzheimer's disease, 884–886, 885t
   for gaseousness, 10t
   for major depression, 1123, 1125–1126
   for multiple sclerosis, 939b
   for premenstrual syndrome, 1068, 1068b

Citrate toxicity, due to transfusion, 486t
Citrical (calcium citrate)
　　for chronic renal failure, 730
　　for renal calculi, 746t
CIWA-Ar (Clinical Institute Withdrawal Assessment–Alcohol Revised), 1100–1101, 1102–1103b
CJD (Creutzfeldt-Jakob disease), variant, transfusion-associated, 490
CK(s) (cytokeratins), in lung cancer, 243
CK-MB (MB isoforms of creatine kinase)
　　in myocardial infarction, 361
　　in pericarditis, 369–370
Cl (chlorine), as chemical weapon, 1226–1228t
Cladribine (Leustatin), for chronic lymphocytic leukemia, 462
Claforan. *See* Cefotaxime (Claforan).
Clarinex (desloratadine)
　　for allergic rhinitis, 779t
　　for urticaria, 875
Clarithromycin (Biaxin)
　　for Chlamydia, 28b
　　for COPD, 28b
　　for endocarditis prophylaxis, 347t
　　for indigestion, 11t
　　for legionellosis, 271t
　　for leprosy, 101
　　for *Mycobacterium avium intracellulare* complex, 289
　　for *Mycobacterium avium-intracellulare*, in HIV, 56–57, 56t
　　for mycoplasma, 28b
　　for mycoplasmal pneumonia, 270t
　　for peptic ulcer disease, 532t
　　for streptococcal pharyngitis, 223t
　　for toxoplasmosis, 166t
Claritin (loratadine)
　　for allergic rhinitis, 779t
　　for urticaria, 875
Claritin-D (loratadine/pseudoephedrine), for allergic rhinitis, 779t
Clark's nevi, 828b, 829
Claudication, 292, 373
　　with back pain, 40
Clavicle, fractures of, 1009
Clear cell adenocarcinoma, of cervix, 1090
Clemastine (Tavist), for allergic rhinitis, 779t
CLI (chronic limb ischemia), 373–374
Clindamycin (Cleocin, Dalacin)
　　for bacterial vaginosis, 1074b
　　for *Chlamydia trachomatis*, 1078b
　　for endocarditis prophylaxis, 347t
　　for furunculosis, 837
　　for malaria, 108t, 109
　　for necrotizing skin and soft tissue infections, 85t
　　for osteomyelitis, 1006t, 1007
　　for pelvic inflammatory disease, 1080b
　　for *Pneumocystis jiroveci* pneumonia, 55
　　for streptococcal pharyngitis, 223
　　for toxic shock syndrome, 89, 89b
　　for toxoplasmosis, 165t, 167–168
Clindamycin-tretinoin (Ziana), for acne, 788
Clinical chemistry, reference intervals for
　　blood, serum, and plasma, 1220–1221t
　　urine, 1223–1224t
Clinical Institute Withdrawal Assessment–Alcohol Revised (CIWA-Ar), 1100–1101, 1102–1103b
Clinoril (sulindac)
　　for juvenile idiopathic arthritis, 985
　　for osteoarthritis, 1000
CLL. *See* Chronic lymphocytic leukemia (CLL).
Clobetasol propionate (Temovate)
　　for anogenital pruritus, 872b, 873
　　for atopic dermatitis, 860–861
　　for bullous pemphigoid, 866–867

Clobetasol propionate (Temovate) *(Continued)*
　　for lichen planus, 804
　　for vitiligo, 878–879
Clodronate (Bonefos), 1244–1249t
Clofarabine (Clolar), for acute myeloid leukemia, 448
Clofazimine (Lamprene), for leprosy, 101, 101b
Clomiphene citrate (Clomid), for infertility, 1061
Clomipramine (Anafranil)
　　for neuropathic pain, 964
　　for obsessive compulsive disorder, 1114, 1114t
　　poisoning due to, 1214–1216, 1215t
　　for premenstrual syndrome, 1068
　　for psychiatric dizziness, 209
Clonazepam (Klonopin)
　　intoxication with, 1181–1182
　　for motion sickness and vertigo, 206t
　　for multiple sclerosis, 939b
　　for panic disorder, 1132, 1132t
　　for visual vertigo, 210
Clonidine (Catapres)
　　for menopausal symptoms, 1072t
　　for opiate withdrawal, 1108, 1108b
　　for smoking cessation, 1107
　　for Tourette's syndrome, 920
Clopidogrel bisulfate (Plavix)
　　for angina pectoris
　　　　stable, 298
　　　　unstable, 300–301, 301t
　　for myocardial infarction, 363, 366
　　for transient ischemic attacks, 208–209
Clorazepate (Tranxene), intoxication with, 1181–1182
Clostridium botulinum
　　as biological weapon agent, 1229–1233t
　　foodborne illness due to, 82
Clostridium difficile, acute infectious diarrhea due to, 16, 19–20t
Clostridium perfringens
　　acute infectious diarrhea due to, 16
　　foodborne illness due to, 82
　　necrotizing skin and soft tissue infections due to, 84t, 85t
Clostridium septicum, necrotizing skin and soft tissue infections due to, 84t, 85t
Clostridium tetani. *See* Tetanus.
Clotrimazole 100 mg tablet (Mycelex-7 Combo pack), for vulvovaginal candidiasis, 1075b
Clotrimazole 200 mg suppository/vaginal tablet (Gyne-Lotrimin 3), for vulvovaginal candidiasis, 1075b
Clotrimazole (Lotrimin) cream, for cutaneous candidiasis, 847, 848b
Clotrimazole cream (Gyne-Lotrimin 7, Mycelex-7), for vulvovaginal candidiasis, 1075b
Cloxacillin (Cloxapen), for toxic shock syndrome, 89, 89b
Clozapine (Clozaril), for schizophrenia, 1130, 1130t
Cluster designation (CD) groups, 444
Cluster headache
　　clinical features of, 923
　　epidemiology of, 923
　　etiology of, 923
　　evaluation and diagnosis of, 922t, 923
　　orofacial pain due to, 992t
　　treatment of, 924t, 926–927, 926t
CML. *See* Chronic myelogenous leukemia (CML).
CMN (congenital melanocytic nevi), 828, 828b
CMT (Charcot-Marie-Tooth) disease, 963
CMV. *See* Cytomegalovirus (CMV).
CNS. *See* Central nervous system (CNS).
CO (carbon monoxide) poisoning, 1139, 1184–1185, 1185t

Coagulation
　　disseminated intravascular, 428
　　　　acute, 429
　　　　in childhood leukemia, 453
　　　　chronic, 429
　　　　clinical presentation of, 428
　　　　defined, 428
　　　　diagnosis of, 428–429
　　　　differential diagnosis of, 429
　　　　etiology of, 428b
　　　　fulminant, 428
　　　　due to heat stroke, 1150
　　　　pathogenesis of, 428
　　　　during pregnancy, 429
　　　　treatment of, 429
　　factors VIII and IX in, 419
Coagulation tests, reference intervals for, 1219t
Coagulopathy
　　intracerebral hemorrhage due to, 890, 892
　　massive transfusion, 486t, 491–492
Coal tar, for psoriasis, 802
Coal workers' pneumoconiosis, 278t
Coarctation of the aorta, 328, 329f
　　antibiotic prophylaxis with, 345
Coated and hairy tongue, 852
Cobalamin
　　in diet, 396
　　metabolism of, 396
　　in parenteral nutrition, 621t
Cobalamin deficiency, 395
　　clinical features of, 395
　　diagnosis of, 395–396
　　peripheral neuropathy due to, 963
　　physiologic issues relative to, 396
　　treatment of, 396–397
Cobalamin malabsorption, 541b, 542
Cobalt lung, 278t
Cobblestoning, 778
COC(s) (combination oral contraceptives), 756
　　in postpartum period, 1029t
Cocaine, kinetics of, 1186–1187, 1187t
Cocaine abuse, 1105b, 1109
　　bulimia nervosa and, 1117
Cocaine intoxication, 1186–1187
Coccidioidomycosis, 248
　　acute, 249–251, 250t
　　chronic, 249, 251, 250t
　　clinical manifestations of, 249
　　diagnosis of, 249–250, 249b
　　disseminated, 249, 250t
　　epidemiology of, 249
　　historical background of, 248
　　pathogenesis of, 248–249
　　treatment of, 250–251, 250b, 250t
　　　　for acute infections, 250–251, 250t
　　　　antifungal agents in, 250b, 250t, 251t
　　　　for chronic infections, 251, 250t
　　　　for disseminated infections, 250t
Cockroaches
　　allergic rhinitis due to, 776, 780
　　and asthma
　　　　in adolescents and adults, 765b
　　　　in children, 771
Cockroft-Gault formula, for creatinine clearance, 725–726
Codeine, intoxication with, 1204–1205, 1205t
Codeine + acetaminophen, for pain, 4t
Coenzyme Q10, 1234–1243t
Cogentin (benztropine), poisoning due to, 1179–1180
Cognex (tacrine), for Alzheimer's disease, 882–883
Cognitive behavioral therapy (CBT)
　　for anxiety disorders, 1112
　　for bulimia nervosa, 1117
　　for fibromyalgia, 997
　　for major depression, 1124
　　for panic disorder, 1132

Cognitive behavioral therapy (CBT) (Continued)
  for premenstrual syndrome, 1069
  for schizophrenia, 1129–1130
Cognitive deficits, in Alzheimer's disease, 881
  treatment of, 882–884, 883t
Cognitive impairment, mild, of the amnestic type, 881
Cognitive symptoms
  of Alzheimer's disease, treatment of, 884–887, 885t
  of schizophrenia, 1129
Cognitive therapy, for tinnitus, 39
Cognitive-communication impairments, after stroke, 897
CoHB (carboxyhemoglobin)
  in carbon monoxide poisoning, 1184–1185
  reference intervals for, 1224t
Colace (docusate sodium), for constipation, 22b
Colazal (balsalazide), for inflammatory bowel disease, 516
Colchicine
  for gout, 599–600, 600t
  for pericarditis, 370–372
Colchicine for Acute Pericarditis (COPE) trial, 370
Colchicine for Recurrent Pericarditis (CORE) trial, 370
Cold(s), common, 265
  cough due to, 28b
Cold agglutinin syndrome, 388–389
  diagnosis of, 388
  serology of, 387t
  treatment of, 388–389, 388b
Cold injury(ies), 1143
  hypothermia as, 1143–1146
    classification of, 1144
    clinical presentation of, 1144
    defined, 1143
    diagnosis of, 1146b
    drugs and chemicals that cause, 1145b
    effect on drug metabolism or clearance of, 1146b
    emergency department evaluation of, 1144–1145
    epidemiology of, 1143
    pathophysiology of, 1143–1144
    rewarming strategies for, 1145–1146, 1147b
    risk factors for, 1143, 1144b
    therapeutic, 1147–1148
  peripheral, 1146–1147
    chilblain as, 1146–1147, 1147b
    clinical presentation of, 1146–1147
    frostnip and frostbite as, 1146–1147, 1147b
    pathophysiology of, 1146
    sequelae of, 1147
    treatment of, 1147, 1147b
    trench foot and immersion foot as, 1147, 1147b
Cold sores, 1146
Cold stress, in neonate, 1035, 1036f
Cold urticaria, 874
Cold-water immersion, for heat stroke, 1149, 1149b
Colesevelam hydrochloride (Welchol)
  for diabetes, 583
  for dyslipoproteinemia, 605, 605t
Colestipol (Colestid)
  for dyslipoproteinemia, 605, 605t
  for pruritus due to primary biliary cirrhosis, 499
Colic, biliary, 496b
Colitis
  amebic
    clinical presentation of, 59
    diagnosis of, 60, 60t
    treatment of, 60–61, 61t
  ulcerative (See Ulcerative colitis (UC))
Colonic adenomatous polyps, 558–559
  due to acromegaly, 635

Colonic diverticula, 512b, 513b, 514
Colorectal cancer (CRC), 558
  due to acromegaly, 635
  clinical presentation of, 559
  diagnosis and work-up for, 559, 560b, 560f
  epidemiology of, 558
  etiology and risk factors for, 558
  hereditary, 558
  metastatic, 562
  recurrent, 562
  screening for, 558–559, 559b
  staging of, 559, 559t, 559b
  surveillance for, 562, 562t
  with inflammatory bowel disease, 521
  treatment of, 559–562, 560b
    adjuvant and neoadjuvant therapies in, 561–562, 562f
    surgical, 560–561, 561t, 561f
Colovesicular fistulas, 514
Colyte (polyethylene glycol)
  for constipation, 10t, 22b
  for whole-bowel irrigation, 1164–1165
Coma
  Glasgow Coma Scale for, 965, 965t
    for children, 970, 970t
  myxedema, 664
  due to poisoning, 1161, 1163t, 1174t
Combigan (brimonidine/timolol), 1243
Combination oral contraceptives (COCs, Ortho-Evra), 756
  in postpartum period, 1029t
Combivax. See Hepatitis B virus (HBV) vaccine (Recombivax-HB, Engerix-B, Combivax, Pediarix).
Combivent (ipratropium with albuterol), for asthma, 766t
Combivir (zidovudine + lamivudine), for HIV, 51t
Combunox (oxycodone + ibuprofen), for pain, 4t
Comedones, 787
Command hallucinations, in schizophrenia, 1128–1129
Commit (nicotine polacrilex gum), 1107
Common cold(s), 265
  cough due to, 28b
Community-acquired methicillin-resistant Staphylococcus aureus (CA-MRSA)
  cellulitis due to, 835–836, 837f
  necrotizing skin and soft tissue infections due to, 84t, 85t
  toxic shock syndrome due to, 87, 89
Community-acquired pneumonia (CAP), 261–263
  admission criteria for, 262, 262t
  atypical, 262, 266
  diagnostic criteria for, 261b
  diagnostic testing for, 261–262
  epidemiology of, 261
  etiology of, 262, 262b
  due to influenza, 266–267
  mycoplasmal, 266–270
  prevention of, 263
  treatment of, 262–263, 263b
Compazine. See Prochlorperazine (Compazine).
Complement
  reference intervals for, 1225t
  in serum sickness, 762
Complementary and alternative therapies, for epilepsy, 906
Complementary foods, for infants, 1042–1044
Compound W (salicylic acid topical), for verrucae, 823
Compression hosiery, for prevention of venous thrombosis during air travel, 377
Compression therapy, for venous leg ulcers, 856
Compulsions, 1113–1114

Computed tomography (CT), for angina pectoris
  electron beam, 296
  multislice, 296
Computed tomography angiography (CTA), for pulmonary embolism, 272
Computed tomography (CT)-guided percutaneous transthoracic tube drainage, of lung abscess, 259
COMT (catechol-O-methyl transferase) inhibitors, for parkinsonism, 956–957
Comtan (entacapone), for parkinsonism, 956
Conceptrol (nonoxynol-9), 757
Concerta (methylphenidate extended-release tablets), for ADHD, 918t
Concussions, 965, 968–969
  due to sports, 1010
Conditioning, for nocturnal enuresis, 692–693
Condoms, 757
  in postpartum period, 1029t
Condyloma acuminatum, 824
  clinical presentation of, 824
  diagnosis of, 824, 825b
  differential diagnosis of, 824
  etiology and pathogenesis of, 824
  genital skin types and, 824
  morphologic types of, 824
  transmission and prevention of, 826–827
  treatment of, 824, 825b
    choice of, 824–826
    modalities for, 826
    patient-applied, 825b, 826
    provider-administered, 825b, 826
  vulvar, 1092
Condylox (podofilox), for condyloma acuminatum, 825b, 826, 1092
Cone shell toxin, 1159
Confusion assessment method (CAM), 1118, 1118b
Confusional arousals, 889
Congenital adrenal hyperplasia, 637
Congenital diaphragmatic hernia (CDH), 1039
Congenital erythropoietic porphyria (CEP), 475t, 477b, 479
Congenital glaucoma, 199
Congenital heart disease, 326
  acyanotic
    with increased pulmonary blood flow, 327–328
    with obstruction, 328
  aortic stenosis as, 328
  atrial septal defect as, 327
  atrioventricular canal defect as, 327–328
  coarctation of the aorta as, 328, 329f
  cyanotic
    with decreased pulmonary blood flow, 328–330
    with increased pulmonary blood flow, 330–331
  diagnosis of, 326–327, 326b
  etiology of, 326
  hypoplastic left heart as, 331
  management of, 326b
  patent ductus arteriosus as, 328
  prevalence of, 326
  pulmonary stenosis as, 328
  tetralogy of Fallot as, 328–329, 329b
  total anomalous pulmonary venous connection as, 331
  transposition of the great arteries as, 330
  tricuspid atresia as, 329–330, 330f
  truncus arteriosus as, 330–331
  ventricular septal defect as, 327
Congenital melanocytic nevi (CMN), 828, 828b
Congenital rubella syndrome (CRS), 140–141, 1014, 1015b
Congenital toxoplasmosis, 165t, 168–169, 168b
Congo-Crimean virus, as biological weapon agent, 1229–1233t

Conivaptan (Vaprisol), for hyponatremia, 598
Conjugated equine estrogens (CEE, Premarin)
  for anovulatory bleeding, 1059
  for intermenstrual bleeding, 1059
  after menopause, 1071–1072, 1072t
  for uterine hemorrhage, 1059–1060
Conjunctiva, 193
Conjunctivitis, 193
  adult inclusion, 195
  allergic
    drug-induced, 194t
    seasonal, 193–194, 194t
  and allergic rhinitis, 777
  bacterial, 194t, 195
    in neonate, 195, 196t
  chlamydial, 194t, 195
    in neonate, 196, 196t
  defined, 193
  differential diagnosis of, 194t
  in dry eye syndrome, 194t
  gonococcal, 194t, 752b
    in neonate, 195–196, 196t
  neonatal, 195–196, 196t
    bacterial, 195, 196t
    chemical, 195, 196t
    chlamydial, 196, 196t
    gonococcal, 195–196, 196t
    viral, 196, 196t
  viral, 194–195, 194t
    in neonate, 196, 196t
Conn, Jerome, 653–654
Connective tissue disorder(s), 805
  and mitral valve prolapse, 336–337
  polymyositis/dermatomyositis as, 812–813
  scleroderma/systemic sclerosis as, 809–812
  systemic lupus erythematosus as, 805–809
Consciousness level, with poisonings, 1161, 1163t
Consolidation chemotherapy, for acute myeloid leukemia, 446
Constipation, 20
  clinical features and diagnosis of, 21–22, 21b
  defined, 21
  epidemiology and pathophysiology of, 20–21
  gaseousness due to, 10t
  medical causes of, 21b
  due to medications, 21b
  due to multiple sclerosis, 939
  normal transit, 21
  during pregnancy, 1015
  Rome III criteria for, 21, 21b
  secondary causes of, 21, 21b
  slow-transit, 21–22
  treatment of, 22, 22b
Constitutional delay, of puberty, 1063
Constraint-induced movement therapy (CIMT), for stroke rehabilitation, 896b
Contact dermatitis (CD), 870
  allergic, 30b, 31b, 870
  vs. atopic dermatitis, 860
  diagnosis of, 870, 870b
  irritant, 788, 870
  treatment of, 870–871, 871b
Continuity of care, in stroke rehabilitation, 898
Continuous arteriovenous hemodiafiltration (CAVHD), for poisonings, 1173
Continuous positive airway pressure (CPAP)
  for acute respiratory failure, 227
  for obstructive sleep apnea, 240–242, 241b
Continuous renal replacement therapy (CRRT), for acute renal failure, 724
Continuous subcutaneous insulin infusion (CSII), for diabetes mellitus, in children, 586–587
Continuous venovenous hemodiafiltration (CVVHD), for poisonings, 1173
Continuous venovenous hemofiltration, for acute renal failure, 724

Contraception, 755
  barrier methods and spermicides for, 757
  emergency, 758
  historical background of, 755–756
  hormonal methods for, 756–757
    estrogen-progestin combinations as, 756
    progestin only, 756–757
  intrauterine devices for, 757
  lactational amenorrhea method for, 1029t
  natural family planning and fertility awareness methods for, 756
  postpartum, 1028, 1029t
  with sickle cell disease, 411–412
  sterilization for, 757–758
Contraceptive diaphragm, 757
  in postpartum period, 1029t
Contraceptive implant (Norplant), 757
Contraceptive injection, progestin, 757
Contraceptive patch, transdermal, 756
Contraceptive ring, intravaginal, 756
  in postpartum period, 1029t
Contraceptive sponge (Today Sponge), 757
Contraction stress test, during pregnancy, 1016–1017, 1017t
Contrast agents, acute renal failure due to, 723, 725
Controlled High-Risk Subjects Avonex Multiple Sclerosis Prevention Study (CHAMPS), 197
Cooley's anemia
  clinical manifestations of, 398–399
  diagnosis of, 398b
  genetic basis for, 398
  treatment of, 399t
Coombs' test, reference intervals for, 1219t
Copaxone (glatiramer acetate)
  for multiple sclerosis, 936, 937t
  for optic neuritis, 197
COPD. See Chronic obstructive pulmonary disease (COPD).
COPE (Colchicine for Acute Pericarditis) trial, 370
Copegus (ribavirin)
  for bronchiolitis, 266
  for hepatitis B and C viruses, 536t, 538
Coping skills
  for chronic fatigue syndrome, 119
  for diabetes, 578, 580b
Copper, in parenteral nutrition, 621, 621t
Copper IUD (ParaGard), 757
  for emergency contraception, 758
  in postpartum period, 1029t
Coprolalia, 919
Coproporphyria, hereditary, 475t, 476t
Copropraxia, 919
Coral cuts, 1159–1160
Coral snake envenomation, 1152–1153
Cordaptive (niacin ER/laropiprant), 1244–1249t
Cordarone. See Amiodarone (Cordarone).
Core biopsy, of breast, 1048
Core temperature after-drop, 1145
CORE (Colchicine for Recurrent Pericarditis) trial, 370
Coreg (carvedilol)
  for angina pectoris, 299t
  for heart failure, 339t
Corgard (nadolol)
  for hyperthyroidism, 666
  intoxication with, 1182–1183, 1183t
Cornea, 187, 188f
Corneal pachymetry, 190
Corneal thickness, 190
Corneal topography, 190, 192f
Coronary artery disease (CAD)
  cardiac arrest due to, 303t
  chronic limb ischemia as, 373–374
  dyslipoproteinemia and, 601–603, 602b
  obesity and, 608

Coronary heart disease (CHD)
  dyslipoproteinemia and, 603–606, 603t
  hypertension and, 356t
  obesity and, 608
Coronary risk factors, in angina pectoris, 297
Corpuscular value of erythrocytes, reference intervals for, 1219t
Corrected count increment (CCI), for platelets, 482, 491
Correction factor (CF), for insulin dose, 586
Corrosives, poisoning due to, 1185–1186
Cortef (hydrocortisone), for hypopituitarism, 658
Cortical stimulation, for stroke rehabilitation, 896b
Corticobasal degeneration (CBD), 954
Corticosteroids. See also Glucocorticoid(s).
  for allergic rhinitis, 779–780, 780t
  for anaphylaxis, 760
  for aplastic anemia, 380
  for asthma
    in adolescents and adults, 765
      inhaled, 765, 767–768, 769t
      systemic, 765, 766t, 767–768t
    in children
      inhaled, 773–774t, 775
      systemic, 773–774t, 775
  for atopic dermatitis, 860–861
  for bacterial meningitis, 114
  for Bell's palsy, 951, 951f
  for brain metastases, 975–976
  for bullous pemphigoid, 867
  for caustic or corrosive burns, 1186
  for COPD, 234
  for cutaneous vasculitis, 816
  for cystic fibrosis, 239
  for gout, 599
  for hypersensitivity pneumonitis, 281, 281b
  for idiopathic inflammatory myopathy, 812–813
  for idiopathic thrombocytopenic purpura, 427b
  for infectious mononucleosis, 117
  for inflammatory bowel disease, 516, 519–520
  for intracerebral hemorrhage, 892
  for keloids, 821
  for laryngitis, 219
  for multiple sclerosis, 935–936, 937t, 938
  for myasthenia gravis, 943–945
  for nausea and vomiting, 8, 8t
  for optic neuritis, 196–197, 197f
  for osteoarthritis, 1000–1001
  for pain, 3
  for pemphigus vulgaris, 869
  for pericarditis, 370–371, 372
  for rheumatoid arthritis, 977, 980b, 982
  for sarcoidosis, 277
  for septic shock, 71
  for systemic lupus erythematosus, 807t, 808, 808f
  varicella with, 78
  for warm autoimmune hemolytic anemia, 387
Corticotropin (adrenocorticotropic hormone, ACTH, HP Acthar), for infantile spasms, 909
Corticotropin-releasing hormone (CRH) stimulation test, for Cushing's syndrome, 641, 643
Cortisol, 637
  in Cushing's syndrome
    midnight serum or salivary, 643, 643f
    urine-free excretion of, 643, 643f, 644
  in hypopituitarism, 657
Corvert (ibutilide), for atrial fibrillation, 311, 311t
Corynebacterium diphtheriae pharyngitis, 220
Costimulatory interactions, inhibition of, for systemic lupus erythematosus, 809

Cosyntropin stimulation test, 638, 638**b**
Cotrim. *See* Trimethoprim-sulfamethoxazole (TMP-SMX, Septra, Bactrim, cotrimoxazole, Cotrim).
Cotrimoxazole. *See* Trimethoprim-sulfamethoxazole (TMP-SMX, Septra, Bactrim, cotrimoxazole, Cotrim).
Cotswold criteria, for Hodgkin's lymphoma, 434–435, 435**t**
Cough, 25
  acute, 25
    due to acute sinusitis, 28**b**
    due to allergic rhinitis, 28**b**
    due to *Bordetella pertussis*, 27, 28**b**
    causes of, 25, 25**b**
    due to common cold, 28**b**
    due to COPD, 26, 28**b**
    defined, 25
    evaluation of, 26
    treatment of, 28**b**
  chronic, 26
    with abnormal chest radiography, 27
    due to ACE inhibitors, 26–27
    due to asthma, 26–27, 28**b**
    due to bronchiectasis, 28–29
    causes of, 26, 26**b**
    defined, 26
    without definitive etiology, 27, 27**f**
    due to eosinophilic bronchitis, 28, 28**b**
    evaluation of, 26**b**, 27
    due to gastroesophageal reflux, 27, 28**b**
    due to postnasal drip, 26–27, 28**b**
    due to smoking, 26
    treatment of, 28**b**
  diagnosis of, 26–29, 26**b**
  laryngitis due to, 218
  pathogenesis of, 25
  postinfectious, 25–26
    due to bacterial sinusitis, 26–27, 28**b**
    due to *Bordetella pertussis*, 27, 28**b**
    due to bronchospasm, 28**b**
    causes of, 25–26, 25**b**
    due to chlamydia/mycoplasma, 28**b**
    evaluation of, 26–27, 26**b**
    due to postnasal drip, 26–27, 28**b**
    treatment of, 28**b**
  treatment of, 28**b**, 29
Cough reflex, 25
Coumadin. *See* Warfarin (Coumadin).
Couplets, 312
Cow's milk, in infant's diet, 1044
COX. *See* Cyclooxygenase (COX).
Coxibs, for rheumatoid arthritis, 983
Coxiella burnetii. See Q fever.
Cozaar (losartan), for systemic sclerosis, 811**t**
CP. *See* Chronic pancreatitis (CP).
CPAP (continuous positive airway pressure)
  for acute respiratory failure, 227
  for obstructive sleep apnea, 240–242, 241**b**
CPP (cerebral perfusion pressure), with traumatic brain injury, 967
  in children, 970–971
CPPD (calcium pyrophosphate dihydrate disease), 1001
CPPS. *See* Chronic pelvic pain syndrome (CPPS).
CPR (cardiopulmonary resuscitation), for cardiac arrest, 303
CPVT (catecholaminergic polymorphic ventricular tachycardia), 324
Crab louse, 844**t**, 845
CRAFFT questionnaire, 1098, 1099**b**
Cranberry, as nutritional supplement, 1234–1243**t**
Cranial irradiation, in children
  for acute lymphoblastic leukemia, 454
  for acute myeloid leukemia, 455
Craniectomy, decompressive, for elevated intracranial pressure, 967–968

CRC. *See* Colorectal cancer (CRC).
C-reactive protein (CRP)
  in dyslipoproteinemia, 603
  in unstable angina pectoris, 301
Creatine, as nutritional supplement, 1234–1243**t**
Creatine kinase, MB isoforms of
  in myocardial infarction, 361
  in pericarditis, 369–370
Creatinine, serum, hypertension and, 356**b**
Creatinine clearance (CrCl), 725–726
Creeping eruption, 844, 844**t**
Creon (pancrelipase), for cystic fibrosis, 237
Crescentic glomerulonephritis (CGN)
  diagnosis of, 700**b**, 700**b**
  treatment of, 702**b**, 703–704
Crestor. *See* Rosuvastatin (Crestor, ABT-335).
Creutzfeldt-Jakob disease (CJD), variant, transfusion-associated, 490
CRF. *See* Chronic renal failure (CRF).
CRH (corticotropin-releasing hormone) stimulation test, for Cushing's syndrome, 641, 643
Cricopharyngeal myotomy, for dysphagia, 510
Critically ill patients, gout in, 600–601
Crixivan (indinavir/ritonavir), for HIV, 50**t**
  drug interactions with, 58**t**
CroFab (Crotalidae polyvalent immune Fab [ovine] antivenin), 1155
Crohn's disease (CD)
  clinical features of, 515
  colon cancer surveillance with, 521
  diagnosis of, 515, 515**b**
  malabsorption due to, 543
  management strategies for, 520
  mild to moderate, 520
  natural history of, 515
  pathogenesis of, 514–515
  pregnancy with, 520–521
  severe, 520
  treatment of, 515**b**
    alternative therapy in, 519
    nutritional support in, 518
    pharmacologic, 515–518
      aminosalicylates for, 515–516
      antibiotics/probiotics for, 517–518
      anticytokine therapy for, 517
      azathioprine/6-mercaptopurine for, 516–517
      corticosteroids for, 516
      cyclosporine for, 517
      experimental therapies for, 518
      methotrexate for, 517
    surgical, 518–519
Cromolyn sodium inhaler (Intal), for asthma
  in adolescents and adults, 767–768**t**
  in children, 773–774**t**, 775
Cromolyn sodium nasal spray (Nasalcrom), for allergic rhinitis, 780, 780**t**
Crotalidae polyvalent immune Fab (ovine) antivenin (CroFab), 1155
Croup, 265–266
CRP (C-reactive protein)
  in dyslipoproteinemia, 603
  in unstable angina pectoris, 301
CRRT (continuous renal replacement therapy), for acute renal failure, 724
CRS (congenital rubella syndrome), 140–141, 1014, 1015**b**
Crude coal tar, for psoriasis, 802
Crusted scabies, 845–846
Cryoprecipitate, 483
  for disseminated intravascular coagulation, 429
Cryotherapy
  for actinic keratoses, 794
  for condyloma acuminatum, 825**b**, 826
  for prostate cancer, 732
  for solar lentigines, 877

Cryptococcosis, in HIV, 55–56
Cryptosporidiosis, 565–566**t**, 567–568
Cryptosporidium parvum, 565–566**t**, 567–568
Cryptosporidium spp, malabsorption due to, 544
Crystalluria, due to HAART, 54–55**t**
CSA. *See* Cyclosporine (CSA, Neoral, Gengraf, Sandimmune).
CSD. *See* Cat-scratch disease (CSD).
CSF. *See* Cerebrospinal fluid (CSF).
CSII (continuous subcutaneous insulin infusion), for diabetes mellitus, in children, 586–587
CT (computed tomography), for angina pectoris
  electron beam, 296
  multislice, 296
CTA (computed tomography angiography), for pulmonary embolism, 272
CTCL. *See* Cutaneous T-cell lymphomas (CTCL).
CT-guided percutaneous transthoracic tube drainage, of lung abscess, 259
CTLA-4Ig. *See* Abatacept (Orencia, CTLA-4Ig).
CTT (Cholesterol Treatment Trialists') Collaborators, 297
Cubicin. *See* Daptomycin (Cubicin).
Cuprimine. *See* D-penicillamine.
Cushing's disease, 642**f**, 644
Cushing's syndrome, 640
  ACTH-dependent, 641**b**, 642**f**, 643–644
  ACTH-independent, 641**b**, 642**f**, 643–644
    treatment of, 644–645
  clinical presentation of, 640–641, 640**t**
  diagnostic evaluation of, 641–644, 642**f**, 643**f**
  differential diagnosis of, 642**f**
  due to endogenous glucocorticoid production, 641**b**, 641–642, 642**f**
    treatment of, 644–646, 645**t**
  epidemiology of, 640–641
  etiology of, 640–641, 641**b**
  due to exogenous glucocorticoids, 641, 641**b**
    treatment of, 644
  due to pituitary adenoma, 642**f**, 644
  due to primary adrenal disease, 641**b**, 642**f**, 643–644
    treatment of, 644–645
  pseudo-, 641**b**, 643**f**
  subclinical, 641, 641**b**
  therapeutic interventions for, 644–646, 640**t**
Cutaneous abscess, 836**b**, 837
Cutaneous larva migrans, 844, 844**t**
Cutaneous leishmaniasis, 843, 844**t**
  clinical features of, 94
  diffuse, 96
    epidemiology of, 94
    pathogenesis of, 93
  epidemiology of, 93–94
  treatment of, 94**b**, 96, 844**t**
Cutaneous T-cell lymphomas (CTCL), 30**b**, 795
  classification of, 795
  clinical and pathologic features of, 795–796
  diagnosis of, 796**b**
  epidemiology of, 795
  etiology, molecular biology, and molecular genetics of, 795–796
  and related cutaneous lymphomas, 795
  staging and prognostic factors for, 796**b**, 796–797, 797**t**
  treatment of, 797–800, 797**b**
    for advanced-stage disease, 798–800
    biological therapies for, 797**b**, 799
    CD4 antibodies for, 800
    combined therapy for, 797**b**
    denileukin diftitox for, 799–800
    for early-stage disease, 797–798
    extracorporeal photochemotherapy for, 799
    histone deacetylase inhibitors for, 800
    immunomodulatory therapy for, 800
    interferon-α for, 799

Cutaneous T-cell lymphomas (CTCL) (Continued)
  investigational approaches for, 797**b**, 800
  monoclonal antibodies for, 799
  nitrogen mustard for, 798
  peripheral stem cell transplantation for, 797**b**, 800
  phototherapy for, 797–798
  retinoids for, 798–799
  systemic chemotherapy for, 797**b**, 798–799
  targeted modalities for, 799–800
  topical, 797**b**, 798
  total skin electron beam, 798
  vaccine therapy for, 800
Cutaneous ulcers, in returning traveler, 163
Cutaneous vasculitis (CV), 813
  clinical presentation of, 813–814, 814**f**
  diagnosis of, 814**b**
  differential diagnosis of, 814–815
  etiology of, 814
  evaluation of, 815**t**
  histopathology of, 814, 815**t**
  due to serum sickness, 761
  treatment of, 815–816, 815**b**, 816**t**
Cuticle, 816–817, 817**f**
Cutivate (fluticasone topical), for atopic dermatitis, 860–861
CV. *See* Cutaneous vasculitis (CV).
CVS (chorionic villus sampling), 1012
CVVHD (continuous venovenous hemodiafiltration), for poisonings, 1173
Cyanide(s), as chemical weapons, 1226–1228**t**
Cyanide antidote kit, 1167–1172**t**, 1188
Cyanide poisoning, 1167–1172**t**, 1187–1188
Cyanide salts, 1187–1188
Cyanocobalamin
  in parenteral nutrition, 621**t**
  for vitamin B$_{12}$ deficiency, 397
Cyanogen chloride, as chemical weapon, 1226–1228**t**
Cyanogenic glycosides, 1187–1188
Cyanokit (hydroxycobalamin), for cyanide poisoning, 1188
Cyanotic breath-holding spells, 907
Cyclic antidepressants, poisoning due to, 1214–1216, 1215**t**
Cyclobenzaprine (Flexeril)
  for fibromyalgia, 997, 998**b**
  for temporomandibular disorder, 993
Cyclohexyl sarin, as chemical weapon, 1226–1228**t**
Cyclooxygenase (COX) inhibitors, for rheumatoid arthritis, 982–983
Cyclooxygenase-2 (COX-2) selective inhibitors
  for dysmenorrhea, 1066**t**
  for osteoarthritis, 1000
  for pain, 2–3, 2**t**
Cyclophosphamide (Cytoxan)
  for bullous pemphigoid, 868**t**
  for cold agglutinin syndrome, 388
  for cutaneous vasculitis, 816**t**
  for glomerulonephritis
    crescentic, 703–704
    membranoproliferative, 703
  for leukemia
    acute lymphoblastic, 449
    chronic lymphocytic, 462
  for minimal change disease, 701
  for multiple myeloma, 469**b**, 470
  for multiple sclerosis, 938
  for myasthenia gravis, 944**t**, 945
  for nephropathy
    IgA, 703
    membranous, 702
  for ovarian cancer, 1096
  for systemic lupus erythematosus, 807**t**, 808, 808**f**

Cyclophosphamide (Cytoxan) (Continued)
  for systemic sclerosis, 811
  for warm autoimmune hemolytic anemia, 387
Cycloserine (Seromycin), for tuberculosis, 285**t**
Cyclospora cayetanensis, 565–566**t**, 568
Cyclosporiasis, 565–566**t**, 568
Cyclosporine (CSA, Neoral, Gengraf, Sandimmune)
  for aplastic anemia, 380, 381–382
  for arthritis
    juvenile idiopathic, 985–986
    rheumatoid, 981**t**, 982
  for cutaneous vasculitis, 816**t**
  for focal and segmental glomerulosclerosis, 702
  for inflammatory bowel disease, 517, 520
  for membranous nephropathy, 702
  for minimal change disease, 701
  for myasthenia gravis, 944**t**, 945
  for psoriasis, 802
  for urticaria, 875
Cyklokapron (tranexamic acid)
  for hemophilia, 422
  for menorrhagia, 1059
Cylert (pemoline), for multiple sclerosis, 939**b**
Cymbalta. *See* Duloxetine (Cymbalta).
Cynodon nlemfuëisis, for benign prostatic hyperplasia, 715–717
Cyproheptadine hydrochloride (Periactin)
  for allergic rhinitis, 779**t**
  for cluster headache, 926**t**
  for Cushing's syndrome, 645**t**
  for pruritus due to primary biliary cirrhosis, 499
Cyst(s)
  breast, 1045–1046, 1046**f**
  epidermoid, 837
  sebaceous, 837
    of vulva, 1091
  vulvar, 1091
    Bartholin's duct, 1091
    of canal of Nuck, 1091
    epidermal inclusion, 1091
    sebaceous, 1091
    Skene duct, 1091
Cystic fibrosis (CF), 236
  classification of, 236
  clinical presentation of, 236–237, 238**b**
    gastrointestinal, 236–237, 238**b**
    pulmonary, 237, 238**b**
  diagnosis of, 237–238
  epidemiology of, 236
  newborn screening for, 238
  pancreatic insufficient, 236, 237**b**
  pancreatic sufficient, 236, 237**b**
  pathophysiology of, 236
  treatment of, 238**f**
    antibiotics for, 239
    antiinflammatory therapy for, 239
    bronchodilators for, 238–239
    diet for, 237
    gene therapy for, 238
    hydration of airway surface fluid for, 238
    lung transplantation for, 239
    mucolytic therapy for, 239
    oxygen therapy for, 239
    pancreatic enzyme replacement for, 237
    physical therapy for, 238
Cystic fibrosis transmembrane regulator (*CFTR*) gene, 236
Cystine stones, 743, 744**t**
Cystinuria, renal calculi due to, 743, 744**t**, 746**t**
Cystitis, 682, 684
  abacteriuric, 682, 683**b**, 684
  defined, 686**b**
  diagnosis of, 683**b**
  vs. pyelonephritis, 682–683
  recurrent, 684, 684**b**
  treatment of, 684, 684**b**

Cystosarcoma phyllodes, 1053
Cytadren (aminoglutethimide), for Cushing's syndrome, 645**t**
Cytarabine (Ara-C, Cytosar-U), for leukemia
  acute lymphoblastic, 449
  acute myeloid, 445–446, 448
Cytokeratins (CKs), in lung cancer, 243
Cytokine(s), pyrogenic, 23
Cytokine blockade, for systemic lupus erythematosus, 809
Cytomegalovirus (CMV)
  in HIV, 57
  meningitis or encephalitis due to, 928–930**t**
  pharyngitis due to, 220–221
  during pregnancy, 1014
  transfusion-associated, 490, 490**b**
Cytosar-U (cytarabine), for leukemia
  acute lymphoblastic, 449
  acute myeloid, 445–446, 448
Cytotec. *See* Misoprostol (Cytotec).
Cytotoxic agents, for systemic lupus erythematosus, 807**t**, 808–809, 808**f**
Cytovene (ganciclovir), for CMV disease in HIV, 57
Cytoxan. *See* Cyclophosphamide (Cytoxan).

D

DAB389-IL-2 (denileukin diftitox), for cutaneous T-cell lymphomas, 799–800
Dacogen (decitabine), for acute myeloid leukemia, 448
DAI (diffuse axonal injury), 966
Dalacin. *See* Clindamycin (Cleocin, Dalacin).
Dalbavancin, 1244–1249**t**
Dalmane (flurazepam)
  for insomnia, 888**t**
  intoxication with, 1181–1182
Danazol (Danocrine)
  for dysmenorrhea, 1065
  for endometriosis, 1055, 1056–1057, 1057**t**
  for hereditary angioedema, 876
  for menorrhagia, 1059
  for warm autoimmune hemolytic anemia, 388
Dantrolene sodium (Dantrium), for poisoning, 1167–1172**t**
  due to MAOIs, 1203
  due to neuroleptics, 1209
DAP (3,4-diaminopyridine), for Lambert-Eaton myasthenic syndrome, 946–947
Dapsone
  for bullous pemphigoid, 866–867, 868**t**
  for cicatricial pemphigoid, 869
  for cutaneous vasculitis, 816
  for leprosy, 101**b**
  for *Pneumocystis jiroveci* pneumonia, 55, 56**t**
  for toxoplasmosis, 166**t**
    in HIV, 56**t**
Daptacel (pertussis vaccine), 147, 147**t**
Daptomycin (Cubicin)
  for endocarditis prophylaxis, 346–347**t**
  for necrotizing skin and soft tissue infections, 85**t**
  for pyelonephritis, 685
Daraprim. *See* Pyrimethamine (Daraprim).
Darbopoetin (Aranesp), for chronic renal failure, 729–730
Darifenacine (Enablex), for urge incontinence, 695**b**
Darunavir/ritonavir (Preszista), for HIV, 50**t**
Darvocet (propoxyphene + acetaminophen)
  for osteoarthritis, 1000
  for pain, 4**t**
Darvon. *See* Propoxyphene (Darvon).
Darvon Compound 32 (propoxyphene + aspirin + caffeine), for pain, 4**t**
Darvon Compound 65 (propoxyphene + aspirin + caffeine), for pain, 4**t**

Dasatinib (Sprycel), for chronic myeloid leukemia, 459–460
"Date rape" drugs, 1182
Datura stramonium, poisoning due to, 1179–1180
Daunorubicin (Cerubidine), for leukemia
 acute lymphoblastic, 449
 acute myeloid, 445
 acute promyelocytic, 448
DAWN (Drug Abuse Warning Network), 1109
Daypro (oxaprozin), for juvenile idiopathic arthritis, 985
Daytime incontinence, in childhood, 690–692
 continuous, 689–690, 690b
 etiology of, 690–691, 690b
 evaluation of, 691
 intermittent, 689–690, 690b
 treatment of, 691–692, 692t
Daytime sleepiness, excessive, 888
Daytrana (methylphenidate transdermal system), for ADHD, 918t
DBS (deep brain stimulation), for parkinsonism, 958
DBT (dialectical behavior therapy), for bulimia nervosa, 1117
D&C (dilation and curettage), for ectopic pregnancy, 1017–1018
DCIS (ductal carcinoma in situ), 1049–1050
D-dimer assay, for pulmonary embolism, 272
DDVAP. *See* Desmopressin acetate [1-deamino(8-D-arginine) vasopressin, DDAVP].
de Quervain's thyroiditis, 665, 677
Dead space, with osteomyelitis, 1007
Deadly nightshade, poisoning due to, 1179–1180
1-Deamino(8-D-arginine) vasopressin.
 See Desmopressin acetate [1-deamino(8-D-arginine) vasopressin, DDAVP].
Débridement
 for osteomyelitis, 1007
 for pressure ulcers, 858
Decadron. *See* Dexamethasone (Deltasone, Decadron).
Decitabine (Dacogen), for acute myeloid leukemia, 448
Declomycin (demeclocycline), for hyponatremia, 598
Decompressive craniectomy, for elevated intracranial pressure, 967–968
Decongestants, for allergic rhinitis, 780
Decontamination, for poisoning, 1161–1165
 due to acetaminophen, 1177
 activated charcoal for, 1164, 1164t
 gastric emptying procedures for, 1161–1163
 gastric lavage for, 1163–1164
 ipecac syrup for, 1163
 due to theophylline, 1213–1214
 whole-bowel irrigation for, 1164–1165
Deep brain stimulation (DBS), for parkinsonism, 958
Deep venous thrombosis (DVT), 271
 air travel and, 158, 375
  epidemiology of, 376
  etiology of, 376–377
  prevention of, 377
  risk factors for, 376, 376b
 clinical risk of, 271–272
 diagnosis of, 272
 with sepsis, 65–66
 after stroke, 897
 treatment of, 272–274
  alternative agents for initial, 273
  long-term, 273
  low-molecular-weight heparin for, 273, 273b
  thrombolytic therapy for, 273–274
  unfractionated heparin for, 272–273, 273b

Deep venous thrombosis (DVT) *(Continued)*
 venocaval interruption and inferior vena cava filter placement for, 273
 warfarin for, 273, 273b
DEET, for malaria, 157
Defecation, after stroke, 897
Deferasirox (DFS, Exjade), for thalassemia, 402, 403t
Deferiprone (DFP, Ferriprox, Kelfer), for thalassemia, 402, 403t
Deferoxamine (DFO, Desferal)
 for poisoning, 1167–1172t
  due to iron, 1194–1195
 for thalassemia, 402, 403t
Defibrillation, for cardiac arrest, 303–304
Defibrillator(s)
 automated external, 304–305
 implantable cardiac, 307–308
Deficit therapy, for rehydration of infants and children, 630–631
Degenerative joint disease. *See* Osteoarthritis (OA).
Degreaser's flush, 1193
Dehydration
 due to cholera, 79–80, 79t, 78b
 of infants and children, 628–631
  assessment of, 628–630, 628t, 629t
  classification of, 628–629
  diagnosis of, 630
  fluid management for, 630–631
   indications for, 630
   with intravenous therapy, 630–631
   maintenance requirements in, 631
   with oral rehydration therapy, 630
   rapid rehydration in, 631
   rehydration requirements (deficit therapy) in, 630–631
   replacement requirements in, 631
  due to gastroenteritis, 628
  laboratory tests for, 628–630
  scale for, 629, 629t
  signs of, 628–629, 628t
  weight loss and, 629
 in sickle cell disease, 404
Dehydroepiandrosterone (DHEA)
 for adrenocortical insufficiency, 639b, 640
 as nutritional supplement, 1234–1243t
Delatestryl (testosterone enanthate), for hypopituitarism, 658
Delaviridine (Rescriptor), for HIV, 50t
 drug interactions with, 58t
Delayed circadian phase, 888
Delayed hemolytic transfusion reaction (DHTR), 484–485t, 486–487
Delayed pressure urticaria, 874
Delayed-type hypersensitivity, in allergic contact dermatitis, 870
Delirium, 1118
 agitated, 1119–1120
 clinical description of, 1118
 course and prognosis for, 1120
 diagnosis of, 1118, 1118b, 1118b
 hyperactive, 1118
 hypoactive, 1118
 iatrogenic complications of, 1119
 due to infections, 1119
 medication-induced, 1119
 due to metabolic disturbances, 1119
 mixed, 1118
 nonagitated, 1119
 prevention of, 1118–1119
 treatment of, 1118f, 1119–1120, 1119b
Delirium tremens (DTs), 1100, 1105b
Delivery, of high-risk neonate, 1033–1034
Delivery room care, for extremely low birth weight infants, 1039–1040t
Delta wave, on ECG, 322, 322f

Delta-Cortef. *See* Prednisolone (Delta-Cortef, Prelone, Orapred).
δ storage pool disease (δSPD), 427–428
Deltasone. *See* Dexamethasone (Deltasone, Decadron); Prednisone (Deltasone, Orasone, Medrol, Sterapred).
Delusions
 of parasitosis, pruritus due to, 32b
 in schizophrenia, 1129
Demeclocycline (Declomycin), for hyponatremia, 598
Dementia. *See also* Alzheimer's disease (AD).
 causes of, 882t
 evaluation of, 883t
 frontotemporal, 881
 Parkinson's disease, 954
 vascular, 881
Dementia with Lewy bodies (DLB), 881, 954
Demerol. *See* Meperidine (Demerol).
Demyelinating neuropathies, 961, 961b
Denavir (penciclovir), for herpes simplex virus, 841
Dengue, as biological weapon agent, 1229–1233t
Dengue fever, 162
Denileukin diftitox (DAB389-IL-2, Ontak), for cutaneous T-cell lymphomas, 799–800
Dental care, during pregnancy, 1016
Dental procedures, endocarditis prophylaxis for, 347t
Dental sinus tract, 854
Denture epulis, 854
Denture fibroma, 854
Denture papillomatosis, 851–852
Denture stomatitis, 851
Depade. *See* Naltrexone (ReVia, Depade, Vivitrol).
Depakene. *See* Valproic acid (Depakene).
Depakote. *See* Divalproex sodium (Depakote).
Dependence, 5
 pharmacologic, 1105
Depo-Medrol (methylprednisolone acetate), for asthma, 766t
Depo-Provera, Se Medroxyprogesterone acetate, injectable (DMPA, Depo–Provera, Depo–Sub Q Provera)
Depo-Sub Q Provera, Se Medroxyprogesterone acetate, injectable (DMPA, Depo–Provera, Depo–Sub Q Provera)
Depression, 1120–1126
 diagnosis of, 1120–1121, 1120b
 differential diagnosis of, 1121
 epidemiology of, 1120
 in fibromyalgia, 997–998
 in menopause, 1071
 in multiple sclerosis, 939
 postpartum, 1029
 after stroke, 898
 substance abuse and, 1121
 and suicide, 1120–1121
 treatment of, 1121–1126
  antidepressant drugs for, 1121–1124, 1122–1123b
  brain stimulation for, 1126
  phases of, 1121, 1121f
  psychotherapy for, 1124
  treatment-resistant, 1124–1126, 1125f
Dermal exposure, to toxins, 1161
Dermatitis
 atopic (*See* Atopic dermatitis)
 contact
  allergic, 30b, 31b, 870
  vs. atopic dermatitis, 860
  diagnosis of, 870, 870b
  irritant, 788, 870
  treatment of, 870–871, 871b
 herpetiformis, 30b
 seborrheic, 788, 804
 uncinarial, 844t, 845
 venous stasis, 855

Dermatobia hominis, 844t, 845–846
Dermatographism, 874
Dermatologic conditions. *See* Skin disease(s).
Dermatomyositis (DM), 812–813
  clinical characteristics of, 812, 812t
  diagnosis of, 813b
  treatment of, 812–813, 813b
Dermatophyte skin infections, 846
Descending thoracic aortic aneurysm (DTAA), 291
  diagnosis of, 291, 293b
  rupture of, 291
  treatment of, 292, 294b
Desensitization, drug, 782–783
Desferal. *See* Deferoxamine (DFO, Desferal).
Desiccated thyroid preparations, 663
Desiccation and curettage, for verrucae, 823
Desipramine (Norpramin), poisoning due to, 1214–1216, 1215t
Desloratadine (Clarinex)
  for allergic rhinitis, 779t
  for urticaria, 875
Desmopressin acetate [1-deamino(8-D-arginine) vasopressin, DDAVP]
  for diabetes insipidus, 646–648, 647t, 658
  for hemophilia, 421
  for nocturnal enuresis, 692
  for platelet dysfunction of uremia, 427, 427b
  for von Willebrand's disease, 423–425
Desonide (Desonate)
  for atopic dermatitis, 860–861
  for vitiligo, 878–879
Desoximetasone (Topicort), for contact dermatitis, 871, 871b
Desquamative gingivitis, 854–855
Desvenlafaxine succinate (Pristiq), 1244–1249t
Desyrel. *See* Trazodone (Desyrel).
Detrol. *See* Tolterodine (Detrol).
Detrusor overactivity, 693
Developmental care, for high-risk neonate, 1037
Devic's disease, 196–197, 933, 938–939
Dew itch, 844t, 845
Dexamethasone (Deltasone, Decadron)
  for acute lymphoblastic leukemia, 449
  for adrenocortical insufficiency, 638–639, 639b, 640
  for bacterial meningitis, 114
  for high-altitude sickness, 1141–1142, 1142b
  for infectious mononucleosis, 117
  for multiple myeloma, 469b, 470
    with spinal cord compression, 472
  for nausea and vomiting, 8, 8t
  for temporomandibular disorder, 993
Dexamethasone suppression test, for Cushing's syndrome
  high-dose, 644
  overnight, 641, 643
Dexamethasone-suppressed corticotropin-releasing hormone stimulation test, for Cushing's syndrome, 641, 643
Dexamethasone-suppressible hyperaldosteronism, 654
Dexbrompheniramine + pseudoephedrine (Drixoral Cold and Allergy Tablets)
  for bacterial sinusitis, 28b
  for common cold, 28b
  for postnasal drip syndrome, 28b
Dexferrum (iron dextran), 386
Dexmethylphenidate (Focalin), for ADHD, 918t
Dexoxyn (methamphetamine hydrochloride tablets), for ADHD, 918t
Dextroamphetamine (Dexedrine)
  abuse of, 1109–1110
  for ADHD, 918t
  intoxication with, 1178–1179
Dextromethorphan
  intoxication with, 1204–1205, 1205t
  and MAOIs, 1204

Dextromethorphan/quinidine (Zenvia), 1244–1249t
Dextrose
  for diabetic ketoacidosis, 592, 592t, 593t
  for hyperglycemic hyperosmolar state, 592, 594t
  in parenteral fluid therapy for infants and children, 627
  for salicylate poisoning, 1211, 1211t
DFO. *See* Deferoxamine (DFO, Desferal).
DFP (deferiprone), for thalassemia, 402, 403t
DFS (deferasirox), for thalassemia, 402, 403t
DGI (disseminated gonococcal infections), 751, 752b
DHA (docosahexaenoic acid)
  for IgA nephropathy, 703
  in infant formulas, 1042
DHE-45 (dihydroergotamine), for migraine headache, 925
DHEA (dehydroepiandrosterone)
  for adrenocortical insufficiency, 639b, 640
  as nutritional supplement, 1234–1243t
DHTR (delayed hemolytic transfusion reaction), 484–485t, 486–487
Diabetes education, for diabetic children, 585–586
Diabetes insipidus (DI), 646
  central (neurogenic)
    diagnosis of, 646, 657
    preparation for diagnostic tests or therapeutic procedures with, 649
    treatment of
      in alert patient with adipsia, 648
      in alert patient with intact thirst, 648
      in confused, obtunded, or unconscious patient, 647–648
      general principles of, 646–648
      with hypernatremia, 648–649
      with hyponatremia, 647–649
      medications for, 647, 647t, 658
  gestational, 648
  nephrogenic, 649
  postoperative, 648
Diabetes mellitus (DM)
  in adults, 575
    cardiovascular risk management with, 575–576
    complications of, 576
    diagnosis of, 575, 576t, 576
    epidemiology of, 575
    pathophysiology of, 575–576
    screening for, 575, 575
    treatment of, 576–583
      behavioral self-management for, 576b, 577–578, 578f
      colesevelam hydrochloride for, 583
      diet for, 576b, 577–578, 579b
      goals for, 576b
      insulin for, 580t, 581–582, 582t
      oral agents for, 579–581, 580t
      pharmacologic, 578–582
      physical activity for, 576b, 578, 579b
      stress reduction for, 578, 580b
      for type 1 disease, 583
      for type 2 disease, 583
    type 1, 575, 583
    type 2, 575, 583
  in children and adolescents, 583
    diabetic ketoacidosis due to, 584
    diagnosis of, 584
    exercise for, 588
    goals of therapy for, 586, 586t
    hypoglycemia with, 588
    initial management of, 584
    insulin replacement therapy for, 586–587, 587t
      initiation of, 584–585, 585f
    medical nutrition therapy for, 587–588

Diabetes mellitus (DM) *(Continued)*
    outpatient care for, 585
    patient education for, 585–586
    psychosocial support for, 588
    screening in
      for complications, 588–589, 589t
      for other autoimmune diseases, 589
    self-monitoring of, 587
    sick day management for, 588
    type 1, 583
    type 2, 583, 589–590
      medications for, 590, 590t
      risk factors for, 589t, 590
  classification of, 575, 576t, 583, 584t
  erectile dysfunction due to, 716
  etiology of, 584t
  gestational, 1013
    in postpartum period, 1028
  hypertension and, 353, 356t
  maturity-onset, of the young, 575, 583–584
  nausea and vomiting due to, 9
  obesity and, 608
  pre-, 576t
Diabetes nurse educator (DNE), 585
Diabetic amyotrophy, 962–963
Diabetic foot infection, 838
Diabetic ketoacidosis (DKA), 590
  in children, 584
    treatment of, 592t
  complications of, 594–595
  diagnosis of, 591
  monitoring of, 592t, 593t, 594
  with parenteral nutrition, 625t
  precipitating causes of, 591
  treatment of, 591–594
    in adults, 593t
    bicarbonate in, 592t, 593–594, 593t
    in children and adolescents, 592t
    dextrose in, 592, 592t, 593t
    fluids in, 591, 592t, 593t
    insulin in, 591–592, 592t, 593t
    phosphate in, 592–593
    potassium in, 592, 592t, 593t
Diabetic nephropathy, in children, 588
Diabetic neuropathic pain, 2
Diabetic neuropathy, 962–963
Diabetic retinopathy, in children, 589
Diacetylmorphine, intoxication with, 1204–1205, 1205t
Dialectical behavior therapy (DBT), for bulimia nervosa, 1117
Dialysis
  for acute renal failure, 724
  parenteral nutrition with, 624
  for poisonings, 1165, 1174t
3,4-Diaminopyridine (DAP), for Lambert-Eaton myasthenic syndrome, 946–947
Diamox (acetazolamide)
  for glaucoma, 200
  for high-altitude sickness, 1140–1142, 1142b
Diaphragm(s), contraceptive, 757
  in postpartum period, 1029t
Diaphragmatic hernia, congenital, 1039
Diarrhea
  acute infectious, 13
    bacterial, 14–16, 14b, 15b
    differential diagnosis of, 16–17, 16b
    epidemiology of, 14
    etiology of, 14–16, 14b, 15b
    investigation of, 14, 14b, 18b
    prevention of, 17b
    protozoal, 14b, 15b, 16
    treatment of, 18b
      antibiotics for, 18b, 19, 19t, 19–20t
      antidiarrheal medications for, 18b, 19
      empiric, 18b, 19t
      pathogen-specific, 19–20t
      probiotics for, 17–20

Diarrhea (Continued)
    rehydration for, 18b, 18–19
    viral, 14b, 16
  due to bacterial overgrowth, 17
  Brainerd, 17
  defined, 13
  febrile dysenteric, 19t
  in immunocompromised states, 17
  inflammatory, 13, 15b
  persistent, 19t
  secretory, 13
  traveler's, 17, 155–156
    defined, 155
    epidemiology of, 17, 155
    pathogenesis of, 155
    prevention of, 155, 155b
    in returning traveler, 162, 162f
    treatment of, 19t, 155–156, 156t, 156t
  types of, 13
Diazepam (Valium, Diastat)
  for alcohol withdrawal, 1101, 1106b, 1191
  for benzodiazepine abuse, 1106b
  for cannabis intoxication and withdrawal, 1110
  for cocaine abuse, 1109
  for febrile seizures, 910
  for hallucinogen intoxication, 1111
  for heat stroke, 1149–1150
  intoxication with, 1181–1182
  for motion sickness and vertigo, 206t, 210
  for multiple sclerosis, 939b
  for opiate withdrawal, 1108
  for poisoning, 1167–1172t
    due to amphetamines, 1179
    due to cocaine, 1187
    due to ethanol, 1191
    due to isoniazid, 1195
    due to phencyclidine, 1207
  for sedative hypnotic abuse, 1106b
  for temporomandibular disorder, 993
  for tinnitus, 38
Dibenzapine, poisoning due to, 1214–1216, 1215t
Dibenzoxazepine, poisoning due to, 1208–1209, 1208t, 1214–1216, 1215t
Dibenzyline (phenoxybenzamine), for pheochromocytomas and paragangliomas, 675
DIC. See Disseminated intravascular coagulation (DIC).
Diclofenac (Cataflam, Voltaren)
  for juvenile idiopathic arthritis, 985
  for pain, 2t
Diclofenac epolamine (Flector Patch), 1243
Diclofenac sodium gel (Solaraze, Voltaren Gel), 1243
  for actinic keratosis, 834
Dicyclomine (Bentyl)
  for dyspepsia, 528
  for gaseousness, 10t
Didanosine (Videx), for HIV, 50t, 51t
Dientamoeba fragilis, 565–566t, 567
Dientamoebiasis, 565–566t, 567
Diet. See also Nutrition.
  for alcoholic liver disease, 498
  for angina pectoris, 297
  for chronic fatigue syndrome, 120
  for chronic renal failure, 729
  for cirrhosis, 498b
  and colorectal cancer, 558
  for cystic fibrosis, 237
  for diabetes
    in adults, 576b, 577–578, 579b
    in children, 587–588
    and dyslipidemia, 602
  for dyslipoproteinemia, 604, 604b
  for dysmenorrhea, 1066
  for dyspepsia, 528

Diet (Continued)
  for epilepsy
    in adolescents and adults, 906
    in infants and children, 915
  gluten-free, 543
  for hemorrhoids, 526
  for hyperparathyroidism, 651–652
  for inflammatory bowel disease, 519
  iron in, 383–385
  for Lennox-Gastaut Syndrome, 909
  for Ménière's disease, 211
  and migraine headache, 923b
  for nausea and vomiting, 7
    during pregnancy, 1014
  for obesity, 608–609
  and osteoporosis, 612
  and pancreatitis, 549
  for preeclampsia, 1024
  during pregnancy, 1014
    for nausea and vomiting, 1014
  for pressure ulcers, 858
  for renal calculi, 745, 746t
  for thalassemia, 400b, 402
  and thyroid cancer, 670
Dietary supplements, for menopausal symptoms, 1072t
Dietary thermogenesis, 620
Diethylcarbamazine (Hetrazan)
  for loiasis, 844
  for lymphatic filariasis, 844, 844t
Differin. See Tretinoin topical (Retin-A, Renova, Differin, Tazorac).
Differin (adapalene), for acne, 787
Diffuse axonal injury (DAI), 966
Diflucan. See Fluconazole (Diflucan).
Diflunisal (Dolobid), for pain, 2t
Digestive disorder(s)
  bleeding esophageal varices as, 504
  cholelithiasis and cholecystitis as, 493
  cirrhosis as, 496
  diverticula as, 511
  dysphagia and esophageal obstruction as, 508
  gastritis and peptic ulcer disease as, 527
  gastroesophageal reflux disease as, 552
  hemorrhoids, anal fissure, anorectal abscess and fistula as, 525
  hepatitis as, 533
  inflammatory bowel disease as, 514
  intestinal parasites as, 563
  irritable bowel syndrome as, 521
  malabsorption as, 539
  pancreatitis as, 545
  tumors of colon and rectum as, 558
  tumors of stomach as, 556
Digibind (digoxin-specific antibody fragments), 1167–1172t, 1189
Digital ulcers, in systemic sclerosis, 810–811
Digitalis intoxication, 1188–1190
Digitoxin, intoxication due to, 1188–1190
Digoxin (Lanoxin)
  for atrial fibrillation, 309
  for heart failure, 339t, 340
  intoxication due to, 1188–1190
  kinetics of, 1189
Digoxin-specific antibody fragments (digoxin immune Fab, Digibind), 1167–1172t, 1189
Dihydrocodeine + acetaminophen + caffeine (Panlor), for pain, 4t
Dihydrocodeine + aspirin + caffeine (Synalgos-DC), for pain, 4t
Dihydroergotamine (DHE-45, Migranal NS), for migraine headache, 925
Dihydroindolone, poisoning due to, 1208–1209, 1208t
Dihydropyridine, for pheochromocytomas and paragangliomas, 675
1,25-Dihydroxyvitamin D, for hypoparathyroidism, 653

Diiodohydroxyquin. See Iodoquinol (diiodohydroxyquin, Yodoxin).
Dilantin. See Phenytoin (Dilantin).
Dilation and curettage (D&C), for ectopic pregnancy, 1017–1018
Dilaudid (hydromorphone)
  intoxication with, 1204–1205, 1205t
  for pain, 4t
Dilavproex sodium (Depakote)
  for benzodiazepine abuse, 1106b
  for benzodiazepine withdrawal, 1108
  for sedative hypnotic abuse, 1106b
DILI (drug induced liver injury), due to antituberculous agents, 286–287
Diloxanide furoate (Furamide), for amebiasis, 61t, 565–566t
Diltiazem (Cardizem)
  for angina pectoris, 299t
  for atrial fibrillation, 309
  intoxication with, 1183–1184
  for systemic sclerosis, 811t
Dimenhydrinate (Dramamine), for motion sickness and vertigo, 206t
Dimercaprol (British anti-lewisite, BAL), for poisoning, 1167–1172t
  due to lead, 1199–1200, 1200t
2,3-Dimercaptosuccinic acid (DMSA, Succimer, Chemet), for poisoning, 1167–1172t
  due to lead, 1199, 1200t
Dinitrochlorobenzene (DNCB), for verrucae, 823–824
DIOS (distal intestinal obstruction syndrome), due to cystic fibrosis, 236–237
Diovan (valsartan), for systemic sclerosis, 811t
DIP (distal interphalangeal) joint, mallet deformity of, 1010
Dipentum (olsalazine), for inflammatory bowel disease, 516
Dipeptidyl peptidase-4 (DPP-4) inhibitors, for diabetes, 580t, 581
Diphenhydramine (Benadryl)
  for allergic rhinitis, 779t
  for anaphylaxis, 761t
  for nausea and vomiting, 8t
  for poisoning, 1167–1172t
    due to neuroleptics, 1209
  scombroid, 1157
  poisoning due to, 1179–1180
  for urticaria, 875
Diphenoxylate natiopine (Lomotil), intoxication with, 1204–1205, 1205t
Diphenylchlorarsine, as chemical weapon, 1226–1228t
Diphenylcyanoarsine, as chemical weapon, 1226–1228t
Diphosgene, as chemical weapon, 1226–1228t
Diphtheria and tetanus toxoids (DT), 145t
Diphtheria and tetanus toxoids and acellular pertussis vaccine (DTaP), 145t
  schedule for, 149–150t
  catch-up, 151t
Diphyllobothriasis, 570t, 573
Diphyllobothrium latum, 570t, 573
  malabsorption due to, 545
Dipivefrin (Propine), for glaucoma, 200
Diprivan (propofol), for traumatic brain injury, 967–968
Diprolene (betamethasone dipropionate), for atopic dermatitis, 860–861
Dipyridamole (Aggrenox, Persantine)
  for ischemic stroke prevention, 894
  for transient ischemic attacks, 208–209
Direct vasodilators, for hypertension, 359
Direct vision internal urethrotomy (DVIU), for urethral stricture disease, 741–741
Directly observed treatment short-course (DOTS) approach, for tuberculosis, 284
Disaccharidase deficiency, 543

Disease-modifying antirheumatic drug(s) (DMARDs)
  for juvenile idiopathic arthritis, 985–986
  for rheumatoid arthritis, 978, 978b, 980b
    azathioprine as, 981t, 982
    cyclophosphamide as, 982
    cyclosporine as, 981t, 982
    early use of, 977–978
    gold salts as, 982
    hydroxychloroquine as, 981, 981t
    initiation of, 980b
    leflunomide as, 981–982, 981t
    methotrexate as, 978–979, 981t
    monitoring of, 981t
    other, 981–982
    sulfasalazine as, 981t, 982
    tapering of, 980b
Disequilibrium, without vertigo, 205t
Disk displacements, temporomandibular disorders due to, 991b
Disk disruption, back pain due to, 40
Disk herniation, lumbar radicular pain due to, 40
Diskitis, back pain due to, 40
Disopyramide (Norpace), for hypertrophic cardiomyopathy, 333
Disorganized speech and behavior, in schizophrenia, 1129
Disorientation, due to alcohol withdrawal, 1102–1103b
Dissecting cellulitis of the scalp, 792
Disseminated gonococcal infections (DGI), 751, 752b
Disseminated intravascular coagulation (DIC), 428
  acute, 429
  in childhood leukemia, 453
  chronic, 429
  clinical presentation of, 428
  defined, 428
  diagnosis of, 428–429
  differential diagnosis of, 429
  etiology of, 428b
  fulminant, 428
  due to heat stroke, 1150
  pathogenesis of, 428
  during pregnancy, 429
  treatment of, 429
Distal and lateral subungual onychomycosis (DLSO), 818
Distal esophageal spasm, 510–511
Distal interphalangeal (DIP) joint, mallet deformity of, 1010
Distal intestinal obstruction syndrome (DIOS), due to cystic fibrosis, 236–237
Distal symmetric sensory polyneuropathy (DSPN), in diabetes, 962
Distilled mustard, as chemical weapon, 1226–1228t
Disulfiram (Antabuse), for alcohol dependence, 1103
Ditropan. See Oxybutynin chloride (Ditropan, Oxytrol).
Ditropan XL (exybutynin extended release), for urinary incontinence in children, 692t
Diuretics
  for heart failure, 339t
  for hypertension, 356–357, 356t
  for preeclampsia, 1024
Divalent ion metabolism, in chronic renal failure, 727, 730
Divalproex sodium (Depakote)
  for alcohol withdrawal, 1103
  for Alzheimer's disease, 885t, 884–886
  for bipolar disorder, 1127
  for cluster headache, 926t
  for epilepsy in infants and children, 908–909
  for migraine headache, 925

Divalproex sodium (Depakote) (Continued)
  for vestibular migraine, 209
Diverticulum(a), 511
  colonic, 512b, 513b, 514
  defined, 511
  diagnosis of, 512b
  duodenal, 512b, 513, 513b
  gastric, 512–513, 512b, 513b
  jejunoileal, 512b, 513, 513b
  Meckel's, 512b, 513–514, 513b
  midesophageal or epiphrenic, 512, 512b, 513b
  treatment of, 513b
  Zenker's (pharyngoesophageal), 511–512
    clinical features of, 511
    defined, 511
    diagnosis of, 511, 512b
    dysphagia due to, 509–510
    treatment of, 511–512, 513b
Dix-Hallpike maneuver, 205, 205f
Dizziness. See also Vertigo.
  classification of, 204, 205t
  physiologic, 205t, 209–210
  post-traumatic, 209
  psychiatric, 205t, 209
DKA. See Diabetic ketoacidosis (DKA).
DLB (dementia with Lewy bodies), 881, 954
DLSO (distal and lateral subungual onychomycosis), 818
DM. See Dermatomyositis (DM); Diabetes mellitus (DM).
DMARDs. See Disease-modifying antirheumatic drug(s) (DMARDs).
DMN (dysplastic melanocytic nevi), 828b, 829
DMPA, Se Medroxyprogesterone acetate, injectable (DMPA, Depo–Provera, Depo–Sub Q Provera)
DMSA (2,3-dimercaptosuccinic acid), for poisoning, 1167–1172t
  due to lead, 1199, 1200t
DNase (Pulmozyme), for cystic fibrosis, 239
DNCB (dinitrochlorobenzene), for verrucae, 823–824
DNE (diabetes nurse educator), 585
Dobutamine (Dobutrex)
  for heart block, 318
  for shock, 69t
Docetaxel (Taxotere)
  for non–small cell lung cancer, 247–248
  for prostate cancer, 732
Docosahexaenoic acid (DHA)
  for IgA nephropathy, 703
  in infant formulas, 1042
Docusate calcium (Surfak), for constipation, 22b
Docusate sodium (Colace), for constipation, 22b
Dofetilide (Tikosyn), for atrial fibrillation, 310, 310b
Dolasetron (Anzemet), for nausea and vomiting, 7, 8t
Dolobid (diflunisal), for pain, 2t
Dolophine (methadone)
  intoxication with, 1204–1205, 1205t
  for opiate withdrawal, 1108–1109
Domiperidone (Motilium), for gastroparesis, 10t
Donepezil (Aricept), for Alzheimer's disease, 882–884, 883t
Dong quai root, 1234–1243t
Donovanosis, 749–750
Dopamine (Intropin)
  for anaphylaxis, 761, 761t
  for elevated intracranial pressure, 967
  for shock, 69–70, 69t
Dopamine agonists
  for hyperprolactinemia, 660–661, 660t
  for parkinsonism, 955–956
Dopamine antagonists, for nausea and vomiting, 7–8
Dopamine receptors, in schizophrenia, 1129
Doral (quazepam), for insomnia, 888t

Doripenem (Doribax), 1243
Doryx. See Doxycycline (Vibramycin, Vibra-Tabs, Doryx).
Dorzolamide (Trusopt), for glaucoma, 200
Dostinex (cabergoline), for hyperprolactinemia, 660, 660t
DOTS (directly observed treatment short-course) approach, for tuberculosis, 284
Double-voiding, for urinary incontinence in children, 691
Dovonex (calcipotriene), for psoriasis, 801
Down syndrome
  and childhood leukemia, 452t
  prenatal screening for, 1012
Doxazosin mesylate (Cardura)
  for benign prostatic hyperplasia, 714–717, 714t
  for systemic sclerosis, 811t
  for urinary incontinence, in children, 691, 692t
Doxepin (Sinequan)
  for contact dermatitis, 871
  poisoning due to, 1214–1216, 1215t
  for pruritus, 33b
  for urticaria, 875
Doxorubicin, pegylated liposomal (Doxil), for cutaneous T-cell lymphomas, 798
Doxorubicin (Adriamycin)
  for multiple myeloma, 469b, 470
  for ovarian cancer, 1096
Doxycycline, sub-antimicrobial (Oracea), for rosacea, 789
Doxycycline (Vibramycin, Vibra-Tabs, Doryx)
  for acute infectious diarrhea, 19–20t
  for anthrax, 126t, 126t
  for brucellosis, 74–75, 74b, 75t
  for bullous pemphigoid, 867
  for cat-scratch disease, 170, 169b
  for Chlamydia trachomatis, 1078b
  for cholera, 80, 78b, 80t
  for dysuria-pyuria syndrome, 684
  for ehrlichial infections, 178, 179b
  for epididymitis, 697b, 698
  for gonorrhea, 752b
  for granuloma inguinale, 750
  for legionellosis, 271t
  for Lyme disease, 138, 139t
  for malaria, 108t, 111–112t, 156–157, 157t
  for marine injuries, 1159t
  for mycoplasmal pneumonia, 270, 270t
  for nongonococcal urethritis, 753
  for osteoarthritis, 1002
  for pelvic inflammatory disease, 1080b
  for plague, 123
  for psittacosis, 128, 128b
  for pyelonephritis, 685
  for Q fever, 129, 129t
  for relapsing fever, 136t
  for Rocky Mountain spotted fever, 177, 179b
Doxylamine (Unisom), for nausea during pregnancy, 1014
D-penicillamine (Cuprimine)
  for lead poisoning, 1200t
  for renal calculi, 746t
  for Wilson's disease, 500–501
DPP-4 (dipeptidyl peptidase-4) inhibitors, for diabetes, 580t, 581
Dracunculiasis, 844, 844t
Dracunculus medinensis, 844, 844t
Dramamine (dimenhydrinate), for motion sickness and vertigo, 206t
Dressings
  for burns, 1135
  for venous leg ulcers, 857
Driving
  with epilepsy, 902
  by stroke survivors, 896

Drixoral Cold and Allergy Tablets. *See* Dexbrompheniramine + pseudoephedrine (Drixoral Cold and Allergy Tablets).
Dronabinol (Marinol), for nausea and vomiting, 8–9, 8**t**
Drop attacks, 210
Droperidol (Inapsine)
  for nausea and vomiting, 8, 8**t**
  for theophylline intoxication, 1214
Drotrecogin alfa (activated) (Xigris), for sepsis, 71
Drug(s). *See also* Medication(s).
Drug abuse, 1104
  and alcoholism, 1104
  of amphetamines and derivatives, 1105**b**, 1109–1110
  of anabolic steroids, 1111
  of anticholinergics and antihistamines, 1111
  with bulimia nervosa, 1115–1116
  of cannabis, 1110
  clinical features of, 1105–1106
  of cocaine, 1105**b**, 1109
  and depression, 1121
  economic, medical, and treatment costs of, 1104–1105
  evaluation of, 1105–1106
  of hallucinogens and phencyclidine, 1110–1111
  of inhalants, 1111
  intracerebral hemorrhage due to, 891
  morbidity and mortality due to, 1104, 1104**t**
  of nicotine, 1106–1107
  of opiates, 1105**b**, 1108–1109, 1108**b**
  pharmacologic dependence in, 1105
  pharmacologic tolerance in, 1105
  prevalence of, 1104
  of sedative hypnotics and anxiolytics, 1105**b**, 1107–1108, 1108**t**
  seizures due to, 899**t**
  treatment of, 1106–1111, 1106**b**, 1107**b**
  withdrawal with
    characteristics of, 1105, 1105**b**
    treatment of, 1106, 1106**b**
Drug Abuse Warning Network (DAWN), 1109
Drug allergic reaction(s), 781
  desensitization for, 782–783
  evaluation of, 783–784, 784**t**
  graded challenge for, 782–783, 783**b**
  pathophysiology of, 782–783, 782**f** 783**b**
  types of, 781–782
Drug desensitization, 782–783
Drug induced liver injury (DILI), due to antituberculous agents, 286–287
Drug monitoring, reference intervals for, 1222**t**
Drug overdose. *See* Poisoning (s).
Drug poisoning. *See* Poisoning(s).
Drug resistance, in HIV, 51–52, 52**t**
Drug-induced allergic conjunctivitis, 194**t**
Drug-induced autoimmune hemolytic anemia, 389, 389**b**
Drug-induced erectile dysfunction, 717**b**
Drug-induced hyperpigmentation, 877, 877**t**
Drug-induced neuropathies, 963, 963**b**
Drug-induced neutropenia, 413–414
Drug-induced parkinsonism, 954, 954**b**
Drug-induced rhinitis, 215, 215**b**
Drug-induced skin reactions, 783
Drug-induced Stevens-Johnson syndrome, 865, 865**b**
Drug-induced thyroiditis, 678
Drug-induced toxic epidermal necrolysis, 865, 865**b**
Drug-related hypertension, 359, 359**b**
Dry eye syndrome, 194**t**
DSPN (distal symmetric sensory polyneuropathy), in diabetes, 962
DT(s) (delirium tremens), 1100, 1105**b**
DT (diphtheria and tetanus toxoids), 145**t**

DTAA. *See* Descending thoracic aortic aneurysm (DTAA).
DTaP. *See* Diphtheria and tetanus toxoids and acellular pertussis vaccine (DTaP).
Duac (benzoyl peroxide with clindamycin), for acne, 788
Dual-chamber pacing, for hypertrophic cardiomyopathy, 334
Dual-energy x-ray absorptiometry (DXA), 612–613
  for hyperparathyroidism, 651
Duct ectasia, 1046
Duct tape occlusion, for verrucae, 824
Ductal carcinoma in situ (DCIS), 1049–1050
Ductal hyperplasia, atypical, 1047
Ductus arteriosus, patent, 328
  antibiotic prophylaxis with, 345
  in extremely low birth weight infants, 1039–1040**t**
Dukoral (cholera vaccine), 18
Dulcolax (bisacodyl), for constipation, 10**t**, 22**b**
Duloxetine (Cymbalta)
  for major depression, 1123
  for multiple sclerosis, 939**b**
  for radicular pain, 41–42
  for visual vertigo, 210
Duodenal diverticula, 512**b**, 513, 513**b**
DuoNeb (ipratropium with albuterol), for asthma, 766**t**
Duradrin (isometheptene with dichloralphenazone and acetaminophen), for migraine headache, 925
Duragesic (fentanyl)
  intoxication with, 1204–1205, 1205**t**
  for pain, 4**t**
Duricef (cefadroxil)
  for endocarditis prophylaxis, 347**t**
  for streptococcal pharyngitis, 223**t**
during pregnancy, 1015
Dust mites
  in allergic rhinitis, 776
  and asthma
    in adolescents and adults, 765**b**
    in children, 771
Dutasteride (Avodart), for benign prostatic hyperplasia, 714–716, 714**t**
DVIU (direct vision internal urethrotomy), for urethral stricture disease, 741
DVT. *See* Deep venous thrombosis (DVT).
DXA (dual-energy x-ray absorptiometry), 612–613
  for hyperparathyroidism, 651
D-xylose absorption test, 542
Dyazide (hydrochlorothiazide and triamterene), for Ménière's disease, 211
Dynacin. *See* Minocycline (Minocin, Dynacin, Solodyn).
DynaCirc (isradipine), intoxication with, 1183–1184
Dynamic hyperinflation (PEEPi), 229
Dyrenium (triamterene), for ascites, 501
Dysarthrias, after stroke, 897
Dysentery, amoebic, 563
  acute infectious diarrhea due to, 16
Dysfunctional uterine bleeding, 1058
  anovulatory, 1058–1059
  defined, 1058
  diagnosis of, 1059**b**
    endometrial biopsy in, 1058
    history in, 1058
    imaging in, 1058
    laboratory evaluation in, 1058
  differential diagnosis of, 1058
  etiology of, 1058
  after menopause, 1070–1071
  ovulatory, 1059
  treatment of, 1059**b**
  due to uterine hemorrhage, 1059–1060
Dysfunctional voiding, 691

Dyskeratosis congenita, 381**t**
Dyskinesia, due to levodopa, 955
Dyslipidemia
  due to acromegaly, 635
  defined, 601
  in diabetic children, 588–589
Dyslipoproteinemia(s), 601
  and coronary artery disease, 601–603, 602**b**
  defined, 601
  diagnosis of, 602–603, 603**b**
  epidemiology of, 601
  natural history of, 602, 602**b**
  pathogenesis of, 601–602
  screening for, 602
  treatment of, 603–606
    adjunctive measures for, 606
    with atherosclerosis, 606
    in children and adolescents, 606
    in elderly, 606
    goals for, 603–604, 604**t**
    indications for, 603, 603**t**
    lifestyle changes for, 604, 604**b**
    management strategies for, 605–606
    medications for, 604–605, 605**t**
Dysmenorrhea, 1065
  defined, 1065
  epidemiology of, 1065
  pathogenesis of, 1065
  primary, 1065–1066
    clinical features of, 1065
    defined, 1065
    diagnosis of, 1065, 1065**b**
    treatment of, 1065, 1065**b**
      complementary therapies for, 1065–1066
      hormonal therapy for, 1065
      NSAIDs for, 1065, 1066**t**
      suppression of ovarian function for, 1065
  secondary, 1065, 1066
Dyspepsia, 527–528. *See also* Indigestion.
  defined, 527
  etiology and differential diagnosis of, 527–528
  evaluation of, 528, 531**b**
  management of, 528
  prevalence of, 527
Dysphagia, 508
  clinical manifestations of, 508
  defined, 508
  diagnosis of, 508–510, 508**b**, 511**f**
  epidemiology of, 508
  esophageal, 509–510
    causes of, 509, 509**b**
    diagnosis of, 509–510
    treatment of, 510–511
  motility, 509**b**, 510
  oropharyngeal, 508–509
    causes of, 509**b**
    clinical manifestations of, 508–509
    diagnosis of, 508–509
    treatment of, 510
  pathophysiology of, 508
  solid food, 510
  after stroke, 897
  structural, 509**b**, 510
  treatment of, 510–511, 510**b**
Dysphonia, habitual of psychogenic, 220
Dysplastic melanocytic nevi (DMN), 828**b**, 829
Dyssynergic defecation, gaseousness due to, 10**t**
Dysuria, 684, 684**b**
  during pregnancy, 1014
Dysuria-pyuria syndrome, 682, 683**b**, 684

E

EAEC (enteroaggregative *E. coli*), acute infectious diarrhea due to, 15, 19–20**t**
Ear canal
  anatomy and physiology of, 201
  pruritus of, 31**f**

Early Treatment of Multiple Sclerosis (ETOMS), 197
Eastern equine encephalitis (EEE), as biological weapon agent, 1229–1233**t**
E-Base (erythromycin base)
 for *Chlamydia trachomatis*, 1078**b**
 for nongonococcal urethritis, 753
EBNA (Epstein-Barr virus nuclear antigen), 116–117
Ebola virus, as biological weapon agent, 1229–1233**t**
EBV. *See* Epstein-Barr virus (EBV).
Ecamsule (Mexoryl SX), 880
ECG. *See* Electrocardiogram (ECG).
Echinacea, 1234–1243**t**
Echinoderm envenomations, 1158–1159
Echocardiography
 of infective endocarditis, 344
 of pericarditis, 369
 of pulmonary embolism, 272
 for survivor of cardiac arrest, 307
Echolalia, 919
Echopraxia, 919
Eclampsia, 1026**f**
Econazole (Spectazole) cream, for cutaneous tinea infection, 848**b**
Economy class syndrome, 376
ECP (emergency contraceptive pill), 758
ECP (extracorporeal photochemotherapy), for cutaneous T-cell lymphomas, 799
Ecstasy (3,4-methylenedioxymethamphetamine)
 abuse of, 1110
 intoxication with, 1178–1179
ECT (electroconvulsive therapy), for major depression, 1126
Ectasia, 291
Ecthyma contagiosum, 843
Ectopic beat, 312
Ectopic pregnancy, 1017
 diagnosis of, 1017–1019, 1017**b**, 1018**f**
 risk factors for, 1017
 treatment of, 1019, 1019**b**
Eculizumab (Soliris), 1243
Eczema
 herpeticum, 840, 859, 862
 xerotic, 30**b**
ED. *See* Erectile dysfunction (ED).
EDC (estimated date of confinement), 1011
Edecrin (ethacrynic acid), for hypertension, 357
Edema
 cerebral (*See* Cerebral edema)
 pulmonary (*See* Pulmonary edema)
Edetate calcium disodium (ethylene diamine tetra-acetic acid, CaNa$_2$ EDTA, versenate), for lead poisoning, 1199–1200, 1200**t**
EDHs (epidural hematomas), 965–966
Edrophonium chloride (Tensilon), for myasthenia gravis, 942**t**
Edrophonium chloride (Tensilon) test, for myasthenia gravis, 941
EE (ethinyl estradiol), in oral contraceptives, 756
EEE (Eastern equine encephalitis), as biological weapon agent, 1229–1233**t**
EES. *See* Erythromycin ethylsuccinate (EES, E-Mycin).
Efalizumab (Raptiva), for psoriasis, 803–804, 803**t**
Efaproxiral (Efaproxyn), 1244–1249**t**
Efavirenz (Sustiva), for HIV, 49–50, 50**t**, 51**t**
 drug interactions with, 53, 58**t**
Effexor. *See* Venlafaxine (Effexor).
Effient (prasugrel), 1244–1249**t**
Eflornithine (Ornidyl), for African sleeping sickness, 843, 844**t**
Efudex. *See* 5-Fluorouracil (5-FU, Adrucil, Efudex, Carac, Fluoroplex).
EFW (electrolyte-free water), for infants and children, 627, 627**t**

EGFR (epidermal growth factor receptor) antagonists, for non–small cell lung cancer, 248
EHEC (enterohemorrhagic *E. coli*), acute infectious diarrhea due to, 15, 19–20**t**
Ehlers-Danlos syndrome, aortic aneurysm in, 292
Ehrlichia species. *See* Ehrlichiosis.
Ehrlichiosis, 178–179
 clinical features and diagnosis of, 178
 epidemiology of, 178
 pathogenesis of, 178
 treatment of, 178–179, 179**b**
EIA (enzyme immunoassay), for HIV, 48
Eicosapentaenoic acid, for IgA nephropathy, 703
EIEC (enteroinvasive *E. coli*), acute infectious diarrhea due to, 15, 19–20**t**
Elavil. *See* Amitriptyline (Elavil).
Elbow, tennis, 1009
Elbow injuries, due to sports, 1009
ELBW (extremely low birth weight) infant, 1039, 1039–1040**t**
Eldepryl (selegiline), for parkinsonism, 957
Elderly
 acute myeloid leukemia in, 447–448
 alcoholism in, 1098, 1100**b**
 benign bacteriuria of, 682
 dyslipoproteinemia in, 606
 gout in, 600
 Hodgkin's lymphoma in, 438
 multiple sclerosis in, 939–940
Eldisine (vindesine), for non–small cell lung cancer, 245–246
Electrical burns, 1138
Electrical stimulation, for stroke rehabilitation, 896**b**
Electrical testing, for Bell's palsy, 951
Electrocardiogram (ECG)
 of angina pectoris, 296
 of atrial fibrillation, 309
 of heart block, 316–317
 of infective endocarditis, 344
 of myocardial infarction, 361
 of pericarditis, 369
 of premature atrial complexes, 312
 of premature junctional complexes, 313
 of premature ventricular complexes, 313–314
 for survivor of cardiac arrest, 307
Electroconvulsive therapy (ECT), for major depression, 1126
Electrolyte(s), in parenteral nutrition, 621, 622**t**
Electrolyte concentrations, in cholera, 79**t**
Electrolyte disturbances, due to poisoning, 1174–1175, 1175**t**
Electrolyte requirements, for infants and children, 627, 627**t**
Electrolyte-free water (EFW), for infants and children, 627, 627**t**
Electrolyte-modified infant formula, 1043**b**
Electromyography (EMG)
 for myasthenia gravis, 942
 for peripheral neuropathy, 960–961
Electron beam computed tomography, for angina pectoris, 296
Electroneurography (ENog), for Bell's palsy, 950, 950**b**
Electrophysiologic testing
 for myasthenia gravis, 942
 for peripheral neuropathy, 960–961
 for survivor of cardiac arrest, 307
Electrotherapy, for pressure ulcers, 858–859
Elephantiasis, 844, 844**t**
Eletriptan (Relpax), for migraine headache, 925**t**, 926
Elidel. *See* Pimecrolimus (Elidel).
Elimite (permethrin)
 for pediculosis, 844**t**, 845
 for scabies, 844**t**, 846

Elitek (rasburicase), for gout, 601
Elliptocytosis, hereditary, 392
Elmiron (pentosan polysulfate), for prostatitis, 711
Elocon (mometasone topical), for atopic dermatitis, 860–861, 861
Elspar (L-asparaginase), for acute lymphoblastic leukemia, 449
EM (erythema migrans)
 in Lyme disease, 136
 of tongue, 852
Embryonal cell carcinoma, 738–739
Embryonal tumors, of brain, 973**t**
Emergencies
 with back pain, 41**b**
 hypertensive, 360
 pain, 5
Emergency contraception, 758
Emergency contraceptive pill (ECP, Plan B), 758
Emergency department management, of acute exacerbations of asthma, 769–770
Emergency medical system (EMS), for cardiac arrest, 303–304
Emesis. *See also* Nausea and vomiting.
 ipecac-induced, for poisoning, 1163
EMG (electromyography)
 for myasthenia gravis, 942
 for peripheral neuropathy, 960–961
Emmetropia, 187, 188**f**
Emotional stress, atopic dermatitis due to, 860
Emotionally induced rhinitis, 216
Emphysema, 231–232
Emphysematous cholecystitis, 494
Empiric therapy
 for acute infectious diarrhea, 18**b**, 19**t**
 for neutropenia, 414–415
Employment, of stroke survivors, 896–897
Empty sella syndrome, amenorrhea due to, 1063
Empyema, 257–258
EMS (emergency medical system), for cardiac arrest, 303–304
Emtricitabine (Emtriva), for HIV, 50**t**, 51**t**
E-Mycin. *See* Erythromycin ethylsuccinate (EES, E-Mycin).
Enablex (darifenacine), for urge incontinence, 695**b**
Enalapril (Vasotec), for heart failure, 339**t**
Enbrel. *See* Etanercept (Enbrel).
Encephalitis
 HSV, 840
 due to mumps, 121
 toxoplasmic, 163, 166**t**, 167–168, 167**b**
 viral, 927
  as biological weapon agent, 1229–1233**t**
  clinical features of, 927
  diagnosis of, 927–930, 931**b**
  etiology of, 927–930**t**
  treatment of, 930–932, 932**b**
Encephalocytozoon intestinalis, 565–566**t**, 568–569
Encephalomyelitis, acute disseminated, 928–930**t**
Encephalopathy
 hepatic, 497**t**, 501**t**, 502–503, 503**t**
 hypertensive, 350
 thiamine-deficiency, 1173
Endobulin, Intravenous immunoglobulin (IVIg, Endobulin)
Endocarditis
 infective (*See* Infective endocarditis)
 due to Q fever, 129
 subacute bacterial, in sickle cell disease, 410
Endocrine disorder(s)
 acromegaly as, 633
 adrenocortical insufficiency as, 637
 Cushing's syndrome as, 640
 diabetes insipidus as, 646
 erectile dysfunction due to, 717**b**
 hyperprolactinemia as, 659
 hyperthyroidism as, 665

Endocrine disorder(s) *(Continued)*
  hypopituitarism as, 656
  hypothyroidism as, 661
  pheochromocytomas as, 673
  primary aldosteronism as, 653
  primary hyperparathyroidism and hypoparathyroidism as, 649
  due to thalassemia, 399t, 402
  thyroid cancer as, 670
  thyroiditis as, 676
End-of-dose wearing off, with levodopa, 955
Endolymph, 210
Endometrial biopsy, for dysfunctional uterine bleeding, 1058
Endometrial cancer, 1083
  clinical features of, 1083, 1083t
  diagnosis of, 1083, 1084b
  epidemiology of, 1083
  etiology of, 1083
  future directions for, 1085
  histologic classification of, 1083b
  molecular features of, 1083t
  prognosis for, 1083–1084, 1084t
  staging of, 1083–1084, 1084t
  treatment of, 1084–1085, 1084b, 1085f
  type I vs. type II, 1083, 1083t
Endometriosis, 1054
  clinical presentation of, 1055
  defined, 1054
  diagnosis of, 1055, 1055b
  epidemiology of, 1054–1055, 1055b
  etiology of, 1054
  genetics of, 1054
  and infertility, 1061
  pathogenesis of, 1054
  postmenopausal, 1055
  treatment of, 1055–1057, 1056b
    medical, 1055–1056
      and infertility, 1056–1057, 1057f
      results of, 1056–1057, 1057f
    medical and surgical, 1057, 1057t
    surgical, 1056
      results of, 1057
Endometritis, postpartum, 1028
Endosalpingiosis, 1054
Endoscopic retrograde cholangiopancreatography (ERCP), 495–496, 550
Endothelin 1 (ET1) receptor blocker, for systemic sclerosis, 811
Endotracheal intubation
  for cardiac arrest, 303
  laryngitis due to, 219
  in newborn resuscitation, 1031
Endovascular repair
  of aortic aneurysms, 292
  for aortic occlusive disease, 292
  for traumatic aortic injury, 294
Energy expenditure, 619–620
  resting, 620
  total, 620
Energy requirements, 619–620, 620f
  of infants, 1044
Enfuvirtide (Fuzeon), for HIV, 50t
Engerix-B. *See* Hepatitis B virus (HBV) vaccine (Recombivax-HB, Engerix-B, Combivax, Pediarix).
ENL (erythema nodosum leprosum), 102–103
ENog (electroneurography), for Bell's palsy, 950, 950b
Enoxaparin (Lovenox)
  for myocardial infarction, 364, 366
  for unstable angina pectoris, 301t
Entacapone (Comtan), for parkinsonism, 956
Entamoeba histolytica. *See* Amebiasis.
Entecavir (Baraclude), for hepatitis B and C viruses, 536t, 537
Enteral nutrition, for inflammatory bowel disease, 518

Enteric fever, 173
  acute infectious diarrhea due to, 15
  treatment of, 173
Enteritis, necrotic, 82
Enteroaggregative *E. coli* (EAEC), acute infectious diarrhea due to, 15, 19–20t
Enterobacter sakazakii, foodborne illness due to, 82
Enterobiasis, 570t, 572
Enterobius vermicularis, 570t, 572
Enterococcal endocarditis, 345
  antibiotic prophylaxis for, 346–347t
Enterocytozoon bineusi, 565–566t, 568–569
Enterohemorrhagic *E. coli* (EHEC), acute infectious diarrhea due to, 15, 19–20t
Enteroinvasive *E. coli* (EIEC), acute infectious diarrhea due to, 15, 19–20t
Enteropathogenic *E. coli* (EPEC), acute infectious diarrhea due to, 15, 19–20t
Enteropathy, protein-losing, 541–542, 541b
Enterotoxigenic *E. coli* (ETEC), acute infectious diarrhea due to, 15, 18, 19–20t
Enterotoxin B, as biological weapon agent, 1229–1233t
Enteroviruses (EVs), meningitis or encephalitis due to, 927, 930, 928–930t
  treatment of, 931
Enthesitis related juvenile idiopathic arthritis, 984
Entocort EC (budesonide capsules), for inflammatory bowel disease, 520
Entry and fusion inhibitors, for HIV, 49, 50t
Enuresis
  nocturnal, 692–693
    defined, 689–690, 690b, 692
    epidemiology of, 692
    etiology of, 692
    monosymptomatic, 692
    nonmonosymptomatic, 692
    primary, 692
    secondary, 692
    treatment of, 692–693
  in sickle cell disease, 411
Enuresis alarm, 692–693
Envenomations
  marine (*See* Marine envenomations)
  snake (*See* Snakebite)
Environmental controls
  for allergic rhinitis, 780
  for asthma in children, 776
Environmental toxins, peripheral neuropathy due to, 963b
Environmental triggers, for asthma
  in adolescents and adults, 763, 765, 765b
  in children, 771, 771b
Enzymatic débridement, for pressure ulcers, 858
Enzyme immunoassay (EIA), for HIV, 48
Eosinophilic bronchitis, cough due to, 28, 28b
Eosinophilic esophagitis, 510
EPEC (enteropathogenic *E. coli*), acute infectious diarrhea due to, 15, 19–20t
Ependymoma, 975
Ephedra, 1234–1243t
Epidermal growth factor receptor (EGFR) antagonists, for non–small cell lung cancer, 248
Epidermal inclusion cysts, of vulva, 1091
Epidermoid cysts, 837
Epididymitis, 696
  acute, 697
  due to *Chlamydia trachomatis*, 1078b
  clinical presentation of, 696–697
  complications of, 698–699
  defined, 696
  diagnosis of, 697–698, 697b
  differential diagnosis of, 698
  epidemiology of, 696
  due to gonorrhea, 751, 752b

Epididymitis *(Continued)*
  nonspecific bacterial, 697–698
  pathogenesis of, 697
  risk factors for, 697
  sexually transmitted, 698
  treatment of, 697–698, 697b
  tuberculous, 698
  uncommon causes of, 698
Epidural hematomas (EDHs), 965–966
Epifrin (epinephrine ophthalmic), for glaucoma, 200
Epilepsy
  in adolescents and adults, 898
    chronic and refractory, 902, 903
    clinical approach to, 900–902
    clinical features of, 899
    defined, 899
    diagnosis and classification of, 899–902, 900t
    differential diagnosis of, 900, 901t
    epidemiology of, 898–899
    etiology of, 899, 899t
    historical background of, 898–899
    interictal state in, 901
    new-onset, 901–902
    status epilepticus in, 906
    treatment of, 902–906, 904t
  in infants and children, 907
    absence, 908–909
    assessment of, 910–911
    benign rolandic, 909
    childhood and juvenile, 908–909
    classification of, 907–908, 908b
    defined, 907
    differential diagnosis of, 907–908, 907b
    epidemiology of, 907
    generalized, 908–909, 908b
    localization-related, 909
    myoclonic, 908–909
    syndromes of, 908–910, 908b
    treatment of, 911–915, 912t, 913t
  mesial temporal-lobe, 905
Epileptic aphasia, acquired, 910
Epileptic vertigo, 209
Epinephrine (Adrenalin)
  for anaphylaxis, 760, 761t
  for asthma in children, 772b, 775
  for cardiac arrest, 306
  for heart block, 318
  for insect stings, 785
  in newborn resuscitation, 1032
  for shock, 69t
Epinephrine auto-injector (EpiPen, TwinJect)
  for anaphylaxis prevention, 761, 761t
  for angioedema, 875–876
  for insect stings, 785
Epinephrine ophthalmic (Epifrin), for glaucoma, 200
Epiphrenic diverticula, 512, 512b, 513b
EpiQuin Micro (hydroquinone 4% and retinol), for melasma, 876–877
Epithelial migration, 201
Epivir. *See* Lamivudine (Epivir).
Eplerenone (Inspra), for aldosteronism, 656
Epley maneuver, 206
Eponychium, 816–817, 817f
Epoprostenol (Flolan)
  for high-altitude sickness, 1143
  for portopulmonary hypertension, 503–504
  for systemic sclerosis, 811
EPP (erythropoietic porphyria), 475t, 477b, 479–480
  congenital, 475t, 477b, 479
Epratuzumab, for systemic lupus erythematosus, 809
Eprex (recombinant erythropoietin), for anemia, 471
Eprodisate (Kiacta), 1244–1249t

EPS (extrapyramidal symptoms), 1130
Epstein-Barr virus (EBV)
  and chronic fatigue syndrome, 117
  infectious mononucleosis due to (See Infectious mononucleosis)
  meningitis or encephalitis due to, 928–930t
  pharyngitis due to, 220–221
Epstein-Barr virus nuclear antigen (EBNA), 116–117
Eptifibatide (Integrilin)
  for myocardial infarction, 364
  for unstable angina pectoris, 301, 301t
Epulis
  denture, 854
  fissuratum, 854
Epzicom (abacavir + lamivudine), for HIV, 51t
ERCP (endoscopic retrograde cholangiopancreatography), 495–496, 550
Erectile dysfunction (ED), 715
  due to atherosclerosis, 716
  due to cigarette smoking, 716
  defined, 715
  due to diabetes mellitus, 716
  diagnosis of, 720b
    laboratory studies in, 718
    patient history in, 717–718
    physical examination in, 718
  drug-induced, 717b
  due to endocrine disorders, 717b
  epidemiology of, 715–716
  due to hyperlipidemia, 717
  due to hypertension, 716
  multifactorial, 717b
  neurogenic, 717b
  pathophysiology of, 716–717, 717b
  psychogenic, 717b
  quantification of severity of, 717–718, 717b
  treatment of, 718–720, 720b
    alprostadil for, 719
    apomorphine for, 719
    chlorpromazine for, 720
    dietary supplements for, 719
    future trends in, 720
    moxisylyte chlorhydrate for, 720
    papaverine for, 719–720
    penile prostheses for, 720
    phentolamine for, 719
    sildenafil citrate for, 718
    tadalafil for, 719
    testosterone for, 720
    trazodone for, 719
    vacuum constrictive device for, 720
    vardenafil for, 718–719
    vasoactive intestinal peptide for, 720
  vascular causes of, 717b, 717
Erectile function, testosterone and, 716
Erection, physiology of, 716, 716f
Ergocalciferol, for hypoparathyroidism, 653
Ergotamine (Ergocaff PB, Ergomar), for migraine headache, 925
Erlotinib (Tarceva), for non–small cell lung cancer, 247
EryPed (erythromycin suspension oral), for relapsing fever, 136t
Erysipelas, 836, 836b
Ery-Tab. See Erythromycin delayed-release (Ery-Tab).
Erythema infectiosum, 842
  during pregnancy, 1014
Erythema migrans (EM)
  in Lyme disease, 136
  of tongue, 852
Erythema multiforme, 862–864
  classification of, 862–863
  clinical features of, 862
  diagnosis of, 863b
  etiology of, 863, 863b
  minor vs. major, 862–863

Erythema multiforme (Continued)
  vs. Stevens-Johnson syndrome and toxic epidermal necrolysis, 862, 863t
  treatment of, 863–864, 864b
Erythema nodosum, due to sarcoidosis, 276
Erythema nodosum leprosum (ENL), 102–103
Erythrocin. See Erythromycin stearate (Erythrocin).
Erythrocyte cell counts, reference intervals for, 1219t
Erythrocyte fragmentation, hemolytic anemia due to, 391t, 394
Erythrocyte membrane abnormalities, hemolytic anemia due to, 391–392, 391t
Erythrocyte metabolism abnormalities, hemolytic anemia due to, 391t, 392–393, 393t
Erythrocyte sedimentation rate (ESR)
  in peripheral neuropathy, 961
  reference intervals for, 1219t
Erythrocytosis
  hypoxemia-induced, 473
  due to polycythemia vera, 473
  secondary, 473
Erythromycin
  for acute infectious diarrhea, 18b
  for Bordetella pertussis, 28b
  for gastroparesis, 10t
  for mycoplasmal pneumonia, 270t
  for streptococcal pharyngitis, 223
  for systemic sclerosis, 811–812
Erythromycin base (E-Base)
  for Chlamydia trachomatis, 1078b
  for nongonococcal urethritis, 753, 753
Erythromycin delayed-release (Ery-Tab)
  for chancroid, 750
  for legionellosis, 271, 271t
  for neonatal conjunctivitis, 196
Erythromycin ethylsuccinate (EES, E-Mycin)
  for cat-scratch disease, 170, 169b
  for Chlamydia trachomatis, 1078b
  for erythema multiforme, 863
  for Lyme disease, 138, 139t
  for nongonococcal urethritis, 753
Erythromycin lactobionate, for mycoplasmal pneumonia, 270t
Erythromycin stearate (Erythrocin)
  for acute infectious diarrhea, 19–20t
  for erythema multiforme, 863
  for nongonococcal urethritis, 753
  for relapsing fever, 136t
Erythromycin suspension oral (EryPed), for relapsing fever, 136t
Erythroplakia, of floor of mouth, 853
Erythroplasia of Queyrat, 834
Erythropoietic porphyria (EPP), 475t, 477b, 479–480
  congenital, 475t, 477b, 479
Erythropoietin (Procrit), for chronic renal failure, 729–730
Eschariotomies, for burns, 1135
Escherichia coli
  acute infectious diarrhea due to, 14–15, 19–20t
  pyelonephritis due to, 705
  urinary tract infections in girls due to, 686–687
Escherichia coli O157:H7, foodborne illness due to, 82–83
Escitalopram (Lexapro)
  for anxiety disorder(s), 1112
    generalized, 1113, 1113t
  for major depression, 1123
  for premenstrual syndrome, 1068b
  for psychiatric dizziness, 209
Esidrix. See Hydrochlorothiazide (Esidrix, Hydrodiuril).
Eskalith. See Lithium (Lithobid, Eskalith, Lithane).

Esmolol (Brevibloc)
  for amphetamine intoxication, 1179
  for angina pectoris, 299t
  intoxication with, 1182–1183, 1183t
  for myocardial infarction, 365t
Esomeprazole (Nexium)
  for gastroesophageal reflux disease, 554, 554t
  for indigestion, 11t
  for peptic ulcer disease, 531t, 532t
Esophageal cancer, 510
Esophageal dysphagia, 509–510. See also Dysphagia.
  causes of, 509, 509b
  diagnosis of, 509–510
  treatment of, 510–511
Esophageal procedures, endocarditis prophylaxis for, 347t
Esophageal ring, 510
Esophageal spasm, distal, 510–511
Esophageal varices
  bleeding, 504
    diagnosis of, 505b
    prophylaxis of
      primary, 505–506, 506f
      secondary, 506–507, 507f
    rebleeding of, 505–507, 507f
    scope of problem with, 505
    spontaneous control of, 505
    treatment of, 505–507, 506b, 507f
  cirrhosis and, 497t, 502
  diagnosis of, 505b
  epidemiology of, 505
  portal hypertension and, 505
Esophageal web, 510
Esophagitis
  eosinophilic, 510
  pill-induced, 510
  radiation-related, 510
Esophagus, nutcracker, 510–511
ESR (erythrocyte sedimentation rate)
  in peripheral neuropathy, 961
  reference intervals for, 1219t
Essential fatty acid deficiency, with parenteral nutrition, 625t
Essure procedure (female sterilization), 757–758
  in postpartum period, 1029t
Estazolam (ProSom), for insomnia, 888t
Estimated date of confinement (EDC), 1011
Estrace. See Micronized estradiol (Estrace).
Estrace Vaginal (estrogen cream), for urogenital atrophy, 1072b
17-β Estradiol, after menopause, 1072t
Estradiol vaginal tablet (Vagifem), for urogenital atrophy, 1072b
Estring (estrogen-containing vaginal ring), for urogenital atrophy, 1072b
Estrogen breakthrough, 1058
Estrogen cream (Estrace Vaginal, Premarin Vaginal), for urogenital atrophy, 1072b
Estrogen therapy
  for anovulatory bleeding, 1059
  for uterine hemorrhage, 1059–1060
Estrogen-containing vaginal ring (Estring), for urogenital atrophy, 1072b
Estrogen-progestin contraceptives, 756
  for anovulatory bleeding, 1058–1059
  for endometriosis, 1056, 1057t
  for menorrhagia, 1059
  for uterine hemorrhage, 1059–1060
ESWL (extracorporeal shock-wave lithotripsy), for renal calculi, 745
Eszopiclone (Lunesta), for insomnia, 888, 888t
ET1 (endothelin 1) receptor blocker, for systemic sclerosis, 811
Etanercept (Enbrel)
  for ankylosing spondylitis, 987–988
  for arthritis
    juvenile idiopathic, 985–986

Etanercept (Enbrel) *(Continued)*
 rheumatoid, 980–981, 981t
 for pemphigus vulgaris, 869
 for psoriasis, 803, 803t
 for systemic lupus erythematosus, 809
Etavirine (Intelence), for HIV, 50t
ETEC (enterotoxigenic *E. coli*), acute infectious diarrhea due to, 15, 18, 19–20t
Ethambutol (Myambutol)
 for *Mycobacterium avium intracellulare*, 289
 in HIV, 56–57
 for *Mycobacterium kansasii*, 289
 for tuberculosis, 285t, 286t, 287t, 287b
 for tuberculous pericarditis, 371
Ethanol
 blood concentration of, 1190
 features of, 1190t
 kinetics of, 1190
 for poisoning, 1167–1172t
  due to ethylene glycol, 1192
  due to methanol, 1202
 reference intervals for, 1224t
 and serum osmolality, 1175, 1176t
Ethanol intoxication, 1190–1191
 alcohol and glycol features and, 1190t
 disposition for, 1191
 kinetics of, 1190
 laboratory investigations of, 1190–1191
 management of, 1191
 manifestations of, 1190, 1191t
 mechanism of, 1190
 toxic dose for, 1190
Ethinyl estradiol (EE), in oral contraceptives, 756
Ethionamide (Trecator-SC), for tuberculosis, 285t
Ethosuximide (Zarontin), for epilepsy
 in adolescents in adults, 904t
 in infants and children, 908–909, 912t
Ethyl alcohol, for poisoning, 1167–1172t
Ethylene diamine tetra-acetic acid (edetate calcium disodium), for lead poisoning, 1199–1200, 1200t
Ethylene glycol
 features of, 1190t
 intoxication due to, 1191–1193
 kinetics of, 1191
 and serum osmolality, 1176t
 sources of, 1191
Etodolac (Lodine)
 for osteoarthritis, 1000
 for pain, 2–3, 2t
ETOMS (Early Treatment of Multiple Sclerosis), 197
Etoposide (VePesid), for lung cancer
 non–small cell
  local, 245–246
  locoregional, 246
 small cell, 248
Euflexxa (sodium hyaluronate), for osteoarthritis, 1001, 1001t
Euthyroid sick syndrome, 665
EV(s) (enteroviruses), meningitis or encephalitis due to, 927, 930, 928–930t
 treatment of, 931
Evans, Barbara, 395
"Eve" (3,4-methylenedioxyamphetamine), intoxication with, 1178–1179
Evening primrose oil, 1234–1243t
Everolimus (Certican), 1244–1249t
Evista (raloxifene)
 for menopausal symptoms, 1073
 for osteoporosis, 615
Evoked potential studies, for multiple sclerosis, 934
Exanatide (Byetta), for diabetes, 580t, 581
Excessive daytime sleepiness, 888
Excoriations, neurotic, pruritus due to, 32b, 34b

Exelon (rivastigmine), for Alzheimer's disease, 882–884, 883t
Exelon Patch (rivastigmine transdermal system), 1243
Exemestane (Aromasin), for breast cancer, 1053
Exercise
 and asthma in children, 771
 for chronic fatigue syndrome, 119–120
 for diabetes
  in adults, 576b, 578, 579b
  in children, 588
 for dyslipoproteinemia, 604
 exertional heat stroke due to, 1148
 for fibromyalgia, 997
 for obesity, 609
 for osteoarthritis, 999
 for osteoporosis, 614
 thermic effect of, 620
 for venous leg ulcers, 857
Exercise electrocardiogram, for angina pectoris, 296
Exertional heat stroke, 1148
Exforge (amlodipine/valsartan), 1243
Exjade (deferasirox), for thalassemia, 402, 403t
Exostosis(es), mandibular, 854
Exposure-related pruritus, 31b
Extended field irradiation, for Hodgkin's lymphoma, 440, 442f
Extended preparation oral contraceptives (Seasonale, Seasonique), 756
Extensively drug-resistant tuberculosis (XDR-TB), 282, 288
External meatus, furuncles at, 202
External otitis. *See* Otitis externa.
Extracorporeal measures, for poisonings, 1165, 1174t
Extracorporeal photochemotherapy (ECP), for cutaneous T-cell lymphomas, 799
Extracorporeal shock-wave lithotripsy (ESWL), for renal calculi, 745
Extracorporeal warming, 1146
Extrapyramidal symptoms (EPS), 1130
Extremely low birth weight (ELBW) infant, 1039, 1039–1040t
Exybutynin extended release (Ditropan XL), for urinary incontinence in children, 692t
Eye(s)
 anatomy and physiology of, 187, 188f
 burns of, 1136–1137
 pruritus of, 31f
Eye care, for Stevens-Johnson syndrome and toxic epidermal necrolysis, 864b, 866
Eyelids, pruritus of, 31f
Ezetimibe (Zetia), for dyslipoproteinemia, 605

F

Facet joint injuries, back pain due to, 40
Facial burns, 1136–1137
Facial nerve decompression surgery, for Bell's palsy, 952
Facial nerve paralysis, differential diagnosis of, 949, 949b
Facial pain. *See* Orofacial pain.
Facial paralysis, idiopathic acute peripheral. *See* Bell's palsy.
Factive (gemifloxacin), for mycoplasmal pneumonia, 270, 270t
Factor I deficiency, 424t
Factor II deficiency, 424t
Factor V and VIII combined deficiency, 424t
Factor V deficiency, 424t
Factor VII deficiency, 424t
Factor VIII, in coagulation, 419
Factor VIII deficiency, 419
 clinical features of, 421t
 pathophysiology of, 419, 420f
 treatment of, 422t

Factor IX, in coagulation, 419
Factor IX deficiency, 419
 clinical features of, 421t
 pathophysiology of, 419
 treatment of, 422t
Factor X deficiency, 424t
Factor XI deficiency, 424t
Factor XIII deficiency, 424t
Failure to thrive, 1044
Falls, in stroke survivors, 896
Famciclovir (Famvir)
 for erythema multiforme, 863–864, 864b
 for herpes simplex virus, 841–842, 841t
 for varicella, 76–78, 77b
 for varicella zoster virus, 841t, 842
Familial adenomatous polyposis (FAP), 558
Familial hyperaldosteronism (FH)
 type I, 654
 type II, 654
Familial periodic ataxia, vertigo due to, 209
Family counseling, with high-risk neonate, 1033
Famotidine (Pepcid)
 for gastroesophageal reflux disease, 553, 554t
 for indigestion, 11t
 for peptic ulcer disease, 531t
Famvir. *See* Famciclovir (Famvir).
Fanconi anemia, 381t
 and childhood leukemia, 452t
FAP (familial adenomatous polyposis), 558
"Farouk," lead in, 1197
Far-sightedness, 187–188, 188f
Fasciotomies, for burns, 1135
Fat, in diabetic diet, 579b
Fat intake, for high-risk neonate, 1035
Fat malabsorption, 541, 541b
Fat necrosis, of breast, 1047
Fatigue, due to multiple sclerosis, 939
Fat-modified infant formula, 1043b
Fatty liver, due to HAART, 54–55t
Febrile nonhemolytic transfusion reactions (FNHTR), 488
 leukoreduced platelets for, 482
Febrile seizures, 24, 910
Febuxostat, 1244–1249t
 for gout, 601
Fecal incontinence, after stroke, 897
Feet, pruritus of, 31f
Felbamate (Felbatol)
 for epilepsy
  in adolescents in adults, 904t
  in infants and children, 913t
 for Lennox-Gastaut Syndrome, 909
Felodipine (Plendil)
 intoxication with, 1183–1184
 for systemic sclerosis, 811t
Female condom, 757
Female sterilization (Essure procedure), 757–758
 in postpartum period, 1029t
Femara (letrozole), for breast cancer, 1053
FemCap (cervical cap), 757
 in postpartum period, 1029t
Femizol-M (miconazole cream), for vulvovaginal candidiasis, 1075b
Femoral head, osteonecrosis or avascular necrosis of, in sickle cell disease, 407, 411
Femstat-3 (butoconazole 2% cream), for vulvovaginal candidiasis, 1075b
Fenamates, for dysmenorrhea, 1066t
Fenofibrate (Tricor), for dyslipoproteinemia, 605, 605t
Fenoprofen (Nalfon), for juvenile idiopathic arthritis, 985
Fentanyl (Duragesic, Fentora)
 intoxication with, 1204–1205, 1205t
 for pain, 4t
Fenthion, poisoning due to, 1205–1206
Fenugreek seed, 1234–1243t

Feosol Carbonyl Iron tablets (carbonyl iron), 385, 385t
Feosol Ferrous Sulfate Tablets (ferrous sulfate), 385
Ferning, due to lightning burns, 1138
Ferriprox (deferiprone), for thalassemia, 402, 403t
Ferritin, serum, 384, 384t
  in hemochromatosis, 432
  in thalassemia, 401
Ferrlicit (iron gluconate), 386
Ferrous sulfate (Feosol Ferrous Sulfate Tablets), 385
Fertility awareness, 756
Fesoterodine, 1244–1249t
Fetal blood sampling, for Rh-sensitized women, 418
Fetal blood transfusions, for Rh-sensitized women, 418
Fetal hemoglobin augmentation, for thalassemia, 401
Fetal well-being, tests of, 1016–1017, 1015b, 1017t
Fetus, hemolytic disease of, 416
  diagnosis of, 416b
  from non-RhD antibodies, 418–419
  due to RhD antigen, 416
  treatment of, 417b
FEV$_1$ (forced expiratory volume in 1 second), in asthma
  in adolescents and adults, 762–763
  in children, 770–771
FEV$_1$/FVC (forced expiratory volume in 1 second/forced vital capacity)
  for COPD, 232
  normal, 765t
Fever, 23
  in children, 24
  current diagnosis of, 23b
  definitions of, 23, 23b
  measurement of, 23, 23b
  pathogenesis and physiology of, 23
  in returning travelers, 161–162
  risks and benefits of, 23–24
  treatment for, 24–25, 24b
Fever of unknown origin (FUO), 23–24, 23b
Fever of unknown source, 23
Feverfew, 1234–1243t
Fexofenadine (Allegra)
  for allergic rhinitis, 28b, 779t
  for postnasal drip syndrome, 28b
  for urticaria, 875
Fexofenadine/pseudoephedrine (Allegra-D 12), for allergic rhinitis, 779t
FFP (fresh frozen plasma), 483
  for disseminated intravascular coagulation, 429
FH (familial hyperaldosteronism)
  type I, 654
  type II, 654
Fiber, for constipation, 22, 22b
Fibrates, for dyslipoproteinemia, 605, 605t
Fibrinolysis, 428
Fibrinolytic therapy, for myocardial infarction, 361–362, 363b, 364t
Fibroadenoma, 1047
Fibrocystic breast disease, 1045–1046, 1046f
Fibroma
  of buccal mucosa, 851
  denture, 854
  peripheral ossifying, of alveolar process/gingiva, 854
Fibromyalgia syndrome, 996–998
  clinical features of, 994b, 996
  diagnosis of, 994b
    diagnostic criteria for, 996, 996b
    laboratory testing for, 996
    differential diagnosis of, 996, 996b

Fibromyalgia syndrome (Continued)
  disorders associated with, 994b
  epidemiology of, 996
  etiology of, 995–996
  mood disorders in, 997–998
  pain due to, 996
  primary vs. secondary, 996
  tender points in, 996, 996b
  treatment of, 996–997, 997b
    cognitive-behavioral therapy in, 997
    exercise in, 997
    patient education in, 996–997
    pharmacologic, 997, 998b
Fifth disease, 842
  during pregnancy, 1014
FIGO staging system. See International Federation of Gynecology and Obstetrics (FIGO) staging system.
Filamentous fungi, as biological weapon agents, 1229–1233t
Filariasis
  lymphatic, 844, 844t
  pruritus due to, 32b
Filgrastim (Neupogen), for neutropenia, 415
Filoviruses, as biological weapon agents, 1229–1233t
Finacea. See Azelaic acid (Azelex, Finacea).
Finasteride (Propecia, Proscar)
  for androgenic alopecia, 791
  for benign prostatic hyperplasia, 714–717, 714t
Fine needle aspiration (FNA) biopsy, of thyroid nodule, 670–671, 671t
Finger(s), numbness and tingling of, during pregnancy, 1015
Finger injuries, 1010
Fish oil supplements, 1234–1243t
  for dysmenorrhea, 1066
  for IgA nephropathy, 703
Fisher paradigm, for breast cancer, 1051
Fissured tongue, 852
Fistula
  anorectal, 526–527
    differential diagnosis of, 525, 525t
    evaluation of, 525–527
    history of, 525
    pathogenesis of, 526
    physical examination of, 525, 527
    treatment of, 527
  perilymphatic, 208
Fitz-Hugh-Curtis syndrome, due to pelvic inflammatory disease, 1080
Flagellates, 563–567
Flagyl. See Metronidazole (Flagyl).
Flat affect, in schizophrenia, 1129
Flatulence, 10
Flaviviruses
  as biological weapon agents, 1229–1233t
  transfusion-associated, 489–490
Flaxseed, 1234–1243t
Flecainide (Tambocor)
  for atrial fibrillation, 309–310, 310b
  for cardioversion, 311, 311t
Flector Patch (diclofenac epolamine), 1243
Flexeril (cyclobenzaprine)
  for fibromyalgia, 997, 998b
  for temporomandibular disorder, 993
FLG (filaggrin) gene, in atopic dermatitis, 859
Flight socks, for prevention of venous thrombosis during air travel, 377
Flixonase AQ. See Fluticasone propionate (Flonase, Flixonase AQ).
Flolan. See Epoprostenol (Flolan).
Flomax. See Tamsulosin (Flomax).
Flonase. See Fluticasone propionate (Flonase, Flixonase AQ).
Floor of mouth, disorders of, 853
Floppy mitral valve (FMV). See Mitral valve prolapse (MVP).

Floppy valve syndrome, 335
Florinef. See Fludrocortisone (Florinef).
Flovent (fluticasone hydrofluoroalkane), for asthma
  in adolescents and adults, 769t
  in children, 773–774t
Floxin. See Ofloxacin (Floxin, Oflox).
Fluarix. See Influenza vaccine (Fluzone, FluMist, Fluvirin, Fluarix, FluLevel).
Flucinolone acetonide/hydroquinone/tretinoin cream (Tri-Luma cream)
  for postinflammatory hyperpigmentation, 878
  for solar lentigines, 877
Fluconazole (Diflucan)
  for angular cheilitis, 849
  for blastomycosis, 255, 255b
  for candidiasis
    cutaneous, 848b
    vulvovaginal, 1075b, 1075b
  for coccidioidomycosis, 250b, 250t, 251t
    acute, 250–251
    chronic, 251
  for cryptococcosis, 56
  for histoplasmosis, 253t, 253b, 254
  for leishmaniasis, 94b, 95
  for tinea
    corporis, 804
    cutaneous, 848b
Flucytosine (Ancobon), for cryptococcosis, 56
Fludarabine (Fludara)
  for acute myeloid leukemia, 448
  for chronic lymphocytic leukemia, 462
Fludrocortisone (Florinef)
  for adrenocortical insufficiency, 639–640, 639b
  for diabetic neuropathy, 962
  for septic shock, 71
Fludrocortisone (Florinef) acetate suppression, for diagnosis of aldosteronism, 655
Fluent aphasia, after stroke, 897
Fluid and electrolyte therapy
  for extremely low birth weight infants, 1039–1040t
  for salicylate poisoning, 1211, 1211t
  for Salmonella gastroenteritis, 172
Fluid balance, with diabetes insipidus, 648–649
Fluid deficit, in infants and children, 630
Fluid losses, insensible, 627, 627t
Fluid management
  for dehydration in infants and children, 630–631
    indications for, 630
    with intravenous therapy, 630–631
    maintenance requirements in, 631
    with oral rehydration therapy, 630
    rapid rehydration in, 631
    rehydration requirements (deficit therapy) in, 630–631
    replacement requirements in, 631
  for diabetic ketoacidosis, 591, 592t, 593t
  for hyperglycemic hyperosmolar state, 591, 594t
Fluid replacement
  for cholera, 79–80, 79t, 78b
  for high-risk neonate, 1035
  for sepsis, 68–69
Fluid requirements, for infants and children, 626–627, 627t
Fluid restriction, for hyponatremia, 597–598
Fluid resuscitation, for burns, 1135–1136
Fluid therapy, for sickle cell disease, 404
FluLevel. See Influenza vaccine (Fluzone, FluMist, Fluvirin, Fluarix, FluLevel).
Flumadine (rimantadine), for influenza, 260, 260b
  with pneumonia, 266–267, 267t, 269b
Flumazenil (Romazicon), for poisoning, 1167–1172t, 1174
  due to benzodiazepines, 1182
  due to sedative hypnotics, 1107

FluMist. See Influenza vaccine (Fluzone, FluMist, Fluvirin, Fluarix, FluLevel).
Flunarizine (Sibelium), for tinnitus, 38
Flunisolide 0.025% nasal solution (Nasarel Spray), for allergic rhinitis, 780t
Flunisolide hydrofluoroalkane (AeroSpan), for asthma, 769t
Flunisolide inhalation (AeroBid), for asthma
 in adolescents and adults, 769t
 in children, 773–774t
Flunitrazepam (Rohypnol), intoxication with, 1181–1182
Fluocinonide (Lidex, Synalar)
 for atopic dermatitis, 860–861
 for vitiligo, 878–879
Fluorescent treponemal antibody absorption test (FTA-ABS), 755
Fluoride, for infants, 1042
Fluoroplex. See 5-Fluorouracil (5-FU, Adrucil, Efudex, Carac, Fluoroplex).
Fluoroquinolone(s)
 for epididymitis, 698
 for urinary tract infections in males, 681, 681t
Fluoroquinolone-resistant *Neisseria gonorrhoeae* (FQRNG), 751
5-Fluorouracil (5-FU, Adrucil, Efudex, Carac, Fluoroplex)
 for actinic keratoses, 794, 834
 for Bowen's disease, 834
 for condyloma acuminatum, 826, 1092
 for keloids, 821
 for verrucae, 823
 for vulvar intraepithelial neoplasia, 1092
Fluoxetine (Prozac, Serafem)
 for anxiety disorder(s), 1112
  generalized, 1113t
 for bulimia nervosa, 1116b, 1117
 intoxication due to, 1212
 kinetics of, 1212
 for major depression, 1123
 for menopausal symptoms, 1072t
 for multiple sclerosis, 939b
 for obsessive compulsive disorder, 1114, 1114t
 for panic disorder, 1132t
 for premenstrual syndrome, 1068–1069, 1068b
Fluphenazine (Prolixin), poisoning due to, 1208–1209, 1208t
Flurazepam (Dalmane)
 for insomnia, 888t
 intoxication with, 1181–1182
Fluticasone furoate (Veramyst), 1243
 for allergic rhinitis, 780t
Fluticasone hydrofluoroalkane (Flovent), for asthma
 in adolescents and adults, 769t
 in children, 773–774t
Fluticasone propionate (Flonase, Flixonase AQ)
 for eosinophilic bronchitis, 28b
 for postnasal drip syndrome, 28b
 for rhinitis
  allergic, 780t
  nonallergic, 217, 217b
Fluticasone topical (Cutivate), for atopic dermatitis, 860–861
Fluticasone/salmeterol (Advair), for asthma, 28b
 in adolescents and adults, 767–768t
 in children, 773–774t
Fluvastatin (Lescol)
 for angina pectoris, 298
 for dyslipoproteinemia, 605t
Fluvirin. See Influenza vaccine (Fluzone, FluMist, Fluvirin, Fluarix, FluLevel).
Fluvoxamine (Luvox)
 for major depression, 1123
 for obsessive compulsive disorder, 1114, 1114t
Fluzone. See Influenza vaccine (Fluzone, FluMist, Fluvirin, Fluarix, FluLevel).

FMV (floppy mitral valve). See Mitral valve prolapse (MVP).
FNA (fine needle aspiration) biopsy, of thyroid nodule, 670–671, 671t
FNHTR (febrile nonhemolytic transfusion reactions), 488
 leukoreduced platelets for, 482
Focal and segmental glomerulosclerosis (FSGS)
 diagnosis of, 700b, 700b
 treatment of, 701–702, 702b
Focal fibrous hyperplasia, of buccal mucosa, 851
Focalin (dexmethylphenidate), for ADHD, 918t
Folate
 in diet, 396
 metabolism of, 396
 during pregnancy, 1014, 1016b
Folate deficiency, 395
 diagnosis of, 395–396
 physiologic issues relative to, 396
 treatment of, 397
Folic acid (Folvite)
 for alcoholic liver disease, 498
 in parenteral nutrition, 621t
 for poisoning, 1167–1172t
  due to ethylene glycol, 1193
 for tropical sprue, 544
Folinic acid (Leucovorin)
 for acute lymphoblastic leukemia, 449
 for neonatal seizures, 910
 for *Pneumocystis jiroveci* pneumonia, 55
 for *Toxoplasma gondii*, 56t
Folkers, Karl, 395
Follicle-stimulating hormone (FSH), in amenorrhea, 1062, 1064
Follicular thyroid cancer, 671–672
Folliculitis, 30b, 837
 pruritic, of pregnancy, 32b
Folvite. See Folic acid (Folvite).
Fomepizole (4-methylpyrazole, 4-MP, Antizol), for poisoning, 1167–1172t
 due to ethylene glycol, 1192
 due to methanol, 1179
Fomon, Samuel, 1044
Fondaparinux (Arixtra)
 for deep venous thrombosis/pulmonary embolism, 273
 for myocardial infarction, 367
Food allergens, atopic dermatitis due to, 860
Foodborne illness, 81
 due to *Aeromonas* species, 81
 due to *Bacillus cereus*, 81
 due to caliciviruses, 81–82
 due to *Campylobacter* species, 82
 due to *Clostridium botulinum*, 82
 due to *Clostridium perfringens*, 82
 due to *Enterobacter sakazakii*, 82
 due to *Escherichia coli* O157:H7, 82–83
 etiology, diagnosis, and treatment of, 81–83
 history of, 81
 due to *Listeria monocytogenes*, 83
 due to *Staphylococcus aureus*, 83
Food-induced rhinitis, 216
Foradil. See Formoterol (Foradil).
Foramen ovale, patent, and ischemic stroke, 894
Forced expiratory volume in 1 second (FEV$_1$), in asthma
 in adolescents and adults, 762–763
 in children, 770–771
Forced expiratory volume in 1 second/forced vital capacity (FEV$_1$/FVC)
 for COPD, 232
 normal, 765t
Fordyce's granules, 849
Formoterol (Foradil)
 for asthma, 28b
  in adolescents and adults, 767–768t
  in children, 773–774t

Formoterol (Foradil) (Continued)
 for bronchospasm, 28b
 for COPD, 234
Formula, infant, 1042, 1043b
Fortaz. See Ceftazidime (Fortaz, Tazicef).
Forteo (teriparatide), for osteoporosis, 615
Fortovase (saquinavir/ritonavir soft gel), for HIV, 50t
 drug interactions with, 58t
Fosamax. See Alendronate (Fosamax).
Fosamprenavir (Lexiva), for HIV, 50t, 51t
Foscarnet (Foscavir)
 for CMV disease in HIV, 57
 for herpes simplex virus, 842
Fosfomycin (Monurol), for cystitis, 684
Fosphenytoin (Cerebyx)
 for elevated intracranial pressure in children, 971
 for status epilepticus in neonates, 910
Fosrenol (lanthanum), for chronic renal failure, 730
Four-gland hyperplasia, 649–650
Four-pack platelet concentrates, 482
Fovea, 188f
FOXP3 gene, 860
FQRNG (fluoroquinolone-resistant *Neisseria gonorrhoeae*), 751
Fracture(s)
 of clavicle, 1009
 of knee, 1008
 due to osteoporosis
  epidemiology of, 613
  risk factors for, 612
  treatment of, 615
 scaphoid, 1009, 1009–1010
 skull, 965
 tibial stress, 1008–1009
 vertebral compression, back pain due to, 40
Framingham Heart Study, 296–297
Francisella tularensis, as biological weapon agent, 1229–1233t
Fresh frozen plasma (FFP), 483
 for disseminated intravascular coagulation, 429
Frontal fibrosing alopecia, 792
Frontotemporal dementia, 881
Frostbite
 classification of, 1146
 clinical presentation of, 1146–1147
 defined, 1146
 pathophysiology of, 1146
 prognostic factors for, 1146–1147
 sequelae of, 1147
 stages of, 1146
 treatment of, 1147, 1147b
Frostnip, 1146–1147, 1147b
Frovatriptan (Frova), for migraine headache, 925t, 926
Frozen plasma, 483
Frozen red blood cells, 481
Fructans, bloating due to, 9
Fructose intolerance, gaseousness due to, 10
Fructose malabsorption, 543
FSGS (focal and segmental glomerulosclerosis)
 diagnosis of, 700b
 treatment of, 701–702, 702b
FSH (follicle-stimulating hormone), in amenorrhea, 1062, 1064
FTA-ABS (fluorescent treponemal antibody absorption test), 755
5-FU. See 5-Fluorouracil (5-FU, Adrucil, Efudex, Carac, Fluoroplex).
Fumagillin, for *Enterocytozoon bineusi*, 565–566t, 569
Functional rectosigmoid obstruction, 21
Fungal endocarditis, 344–345
Fungal pericarditis, 368b, 369
Fungal rhinosinusitis, invasive, 214

Fungal skin infection(s), 846
 dermatophyte, 846
 diagnosis of, 846, 847b
 in HIV/AIDS patients, 847–849
 nondermatophyte, 846–847
 onychomycosis as, 847
 tinea capitis as, 847
 treatment of, 848b
Fungizone. *See* Amphotericin B deoxycholate (Fungizone).
FUO (fever of unknown origin), 23–24, 23b
Furamide (diloxanide furoate), for amebiasis, 61t, 565–566t
Furazolidone (Furoxone)
 for acute infectious diarrhea, 19–20t
 for cholera, 80t
 for giardiasis, 63, 64t, 64b, 565–566t
Furosemide (Lasix)
 for ascites, 501
 for chronic renal failure, 731
 for elevated intracranial pressure, 967
 for heart failure, 339t
 for heat stroke, 1149b, 1149–1150
 for hyponatremia, 598
 for nephrotic syndrome, 701
 for patent ductus arteriosus, 1039–1040t
Furoxone. *See* Furazolidone (Furoxone).
Furuncles, 836b, 837, 837f
 at external meatus, 202
Furunculosis, 836b, 837
Fusarium, as biological weapon agent, 1229–1233t
Fusarium species, necrotizing skin and soft tissue infections due to, 85t
Fuzeon (enfuvirtide), for HIV, 50t

G

G6PD (glucose-6-phosphate dehydrogenase) deficiency, 392–393, 393t
GABA (γ-aminobutyric acid), in schizophrenia, 1129
Gabapentin (Neurontin)
 for acute porphyria, 477
 for alcohol withdrawal, 1103
 for anogenital pruritus, 872b
 for epilepsy
  in adolescents in adults, 904t, 903
  in infants and children, 914, 913t
 for fibromyalgia, 997
 for hiccups, 13, 13b
 for menopausal symptoms, 1072t
 for multiple sclerosis, 939b
 for pain
  neuropathic, 964–965, 964t
  radicular, 41
 for tinnitus, 38–39
 for trigeminal neuralgia, 948
GABHS pharyngitis. *See* Group A β-hemolytic streptococci (GABHS) pharyngitis.
Gabitril (tiagabine), for epilepsy
 in adolescents in adults, 904t
 in infants and children, 914, 913t
GAD. *See* Generalized anxiety disorder (GAD).
Gadolinium, acute renal failure due to, 725
Gait training, in stroke rehabilitation, 896
Galantamine (Razadyne, Reminyl), for Alzheimer's disease, 882–884, 883t
Gallbladder perforation, 494
Gallium nitrate (Ganite), for Paget's disease of bone, 616
Gallstone(s). *See* Cholelithiasis.
Gallstone pancreatitis, 548–549
Galvus (vildagliptin), 1244–1249t
 for diabetes, 580t
Gamene (lindane)
 for pediculosis, 845
 for scabies, 846

Gametocytocidal activity, by antimalarial drugs, 108
γ-aminobutyric acid (GABA), in schizophrenia, 1129
Gammaglobulin, intravenous (Gammagard), for cutaneous vasculitis, 816t
Gammaglobulin (Gamimune N), for asthma in children, 775
Ganciclovir (Cytovene), for CMV disease in HIV, 57
Ganciclovir intraocular implant (Vitrasert), for CMV disease in HIV, 57
Gangrenous cholecystitis, 494
Ganite (gallium nitrate), for Paget's disease of bone, 616
GAQ (Global Assessment Questions), 717b
Garamycin. *See* Gentamicin (Garamycin).
Gardasil. *See* Human papillomavirus (HPV) vaccines (Cervarix, Gardasil).
Garenoxacin mesylate (Geninax), 1244–1249t
Garlic, 1234–1243t
Garment-type nevi, 828
Gas gangrene, necrotizing skin and soft tissue infections due to, 84t, 85t
Gas-bloat syndrome, gaseousness due to, 10t
Gaseousness, 9–11
 diagnosis for, 10t
 etiology of, 9
 functional, 10t
 pathophysiology of, 9–10, 10t
 signs and symptoms of, 9–10
 treatment of, 10–11, 10t
Gastric adenocarcinoma, 556–557
 classification and epidemiology of, 556
 diagnosis of, 556–557, 556b
 Helicobacter pylori–associated, 529, 556
 risk factors for, 556
 staging of, 557
 treatment of, 557, 557b
Gastric banding, 610, 611f
Gastric diverticula, 512–513, 512b, 513b
Gastric emptying procedures, for poisoning, 1161–1163
Gastric lavage, for poisoning, 1163–1164
Gastric lymphomas, 557b, 558
Gastric tumors, 556
Gastric vascular ectasia, in systemic sclerosis, 811–812
Gastrinomas, 532–533
Gastritis, 528–529
 acute erosive and hemorrhagic gastropathy as, 528–529
 bile reflux, indigestion due to, 11t
 classification of, 529b
 Helicobacter pylori
  chronic, 529
  indigestion due to, 11t, 11–12
 pernicious anemia–associated atrophic (type A, autoimmune), 529
Gastroenteritis
 dehydration due to, 628
 due to salmonellosis, 171–172
 treatment of, 172–173, 172b
Gastroesophageal reflux disease (GERD), 552
 and asthma in children, 771
 cough due to, 27, 28b
 defined, 552
 diagnosis of, 552–553, 553b
 dyspepsia due to, 528
 indigestion due to, 11t, 11–12
 laryngitis due to, 218, 219
 symptoms of, 552
 in systemic sclerosis, 811–812
 treatment of, 553–555, 553b
  endoscopic and surgical, 555
  lifestyle changes for, 553
  long-term (maintenance) therapy for, 554–555
  on-demand therapy for, 554

Gastroesophageal reflux disease (GERD) *(Continued)*
 pharmacologic, 553–555, 554t
 step therapy for, 554
Gastrointestinal (GI) bleeding
 in rheumatoid arthritis, 977b
 with sepsis, 66
Gastrointestinal decontamination, for poisoning, 1161–1165
 due to acetaminophen, 1177
 activated charcoal for, 1164, 1164t
 gastric emptying procedures for, 1161–1163
 gastric lavage for, 1163–1164
 ipecac syrup for, 1163
 due to theophylline, 1213–1214
 whole-bowel irrigation for, 1164–1165
Gastrointestinal dialysis, for poisoning, 1164
Gastrointestinal disorders
 due to bulimia nervosa, 1116
 nausea and vomiting due to, 6, 6t
Gastrointestinal exposure, to toxins, 1161
Gastrointestinal function tests, reference intervals for, 1225t
Gastrointestinal intolerance, due to HAART, 54–55
Gastrointestinal stromal tumors (GISTs), 557–558, 557b
Gastrointestinal tract involvement, in systemic sclerosis, 811–812, 812b
Gastroparesis, gaseousness due to, 10t
Gastropathy, acute erosive and hemorrhagic, 528–529
Gastroplasty
 roux-en-Y, 611, 611f
 vertical-banded, 610, 611f
Gastroschisis, 1038–1039
GAS-TSS. *See* Group A β-hemolytic streptococcus toxic shock syndrome (GAS-TSS).
Gatifloxacin (Tequin)
 for mycoplasmal pneumonia, 270, 270t
 for pyelonephritis, 685
 for tuberculosis, 285t
GBS (Guillain-Barré syndrome), 962
GBS (group B streptococcus), during pregnancy, 1013
GCA. *See* Giant cell arteritis (GCA).
GCS. *See* Glasgow Coma Scale (GCS).
G-CSF (granulocyte colony-stimulating factor), for neutropenia, 415
Gemcitabine (Gemzar), for cutaneous T-cell lymphomas, 798
Gemfibrozil (Lopid), for dyslipoproteinemia, 605, 605t
Gemifloxacin (Factive), for mycoplasmal pneumonia, 270, 270t
Gemtuzumab ozogamycin (Mylotarg)
 for acute myeloid leukemia, 448
 for acute promyelocytic leukemia, 448
Gene therapy
 for cystic fibrosis, 238
 for osteoarthritis, 1002
Generalized anxiety disorder (GAD), 1112–1113
 diagnosis of, 1112–1113
 epidemiology of, 1113
 treatment of, 1113, 1113t, 1113b
Genetic counseling, for pheochromocytomas and paragangliomas, 674–675, 675f
Gengraf. *See* Cyclosporine (CSA, Neoral, Gengraf, Sandimmune).
Geninax (garenoxacin mesylate), 1244–1249t
Genital herpes, 840
 during pregnancy, 1015
Genital ulcer disease (GUD), 749
 due to chancroid, 749
 diagnosis of, 749
 due to granuloma inguinale, 749–750
 therapy for, 750

Genital warts. *See* Condyloma acuminatum.
Genitourinary (GU) disorders. *See* Urogenital disorder(s).
Genitourinary symptoms, of menopause, 1070
    treatment for, 1072b
Genitourinary tract, trauma to, 706, 706b
Genotropin (growth hormone replacement), for hypopituitarism, 658
Gentamicin (Garamycin)
    for bacterial meningitis, 115t
    for brucellosis, 74–75, 74b, 75t
    for *Chlamydia trachomatis*, 1078b
    for endocarditis prophylaxis, 346–347t
    for infective endocarditis, 345
    for marine injuries, 1159t
    for Ménière's disease, 212
    for pelvic inflammatory disease, 1080b
    for plague, 123
    for pyelonephritis, 706b
    for urinary tract infections in girls, 687, 687b
Geocillin (carbenicillin indanyl sodium), for prostatitis, 681
Geodon. *See* Ziprasidone (Geodon).
Geographic tongue, 852
GERD. *See* Gastroesophageal reflux disease (GERD).
Germ cell tumors
    of brain, 973t
    of testis, 738
German measles. *See* Rubella.
Gestational diabetes insipidus, 648
Gestational diabetes mellitus, 1013
    in postpartum period, 1028
Gestational hypertension, 1022t, 1024
Gestive (17-alpha-hydroxy-progesterone caproate), 1244–1249t
GFR. *See* Glomerular filtration rate (GFR).
GH. *See* Growth hormone (GH).
Ghrelin, 633, 634f
GI. *See* Gastrointestinal (GI).
Giant cell arteritis (GCA)
    diagnosis of, 1002–1004, 1003b
        biopsy in, 1002–1003, 1003b
        clinical and laboratory features in, 1003b
        diagnostic criteria in, 1003–1004, 1003t
        ultrasonography in, 1002–1003, 1003b
    treatment of, 1004–1005, 1004b
Giardia duodenalis. *See* Giardiasis.
Giardia intestinalis. *See* Giardiasis.
Giardia lamblia. *See* Giardiasis.
Giardiasis, 61, 564–567, 565–566t
    acute infectious diarrhea due to, 16, 19–20t
    background of, 61
    causative organism of, 61
    clinical features of, 62–63
    diagnosis of, 63, 63f, 63b
    epidemiology of, 61–62, 62f
    follow-up for, 64
    malabsorption due to, 544
    pathogenesis of, 62
    prevention of, 64
    prognosis for, 64
    treatment of, 63–64, 64t
Gigantism, due to acromegaly, 634
Gilles de la Tourette syndrome, 918
    clinical features of, 919
    defined, 919
    differential diagnosis of, 919–920, 920b
    historical background of, 919
    natural history and epidemiology of, 919
    psychiatric disorders associated with, 921
    treatment of, 920–921, 920b, 921b
Ginger root, 1234–1243t
Gingiva, disorders of, 853–855
Gingival hyperplasia, generalized, 854
Gingivitis
    acute necrotizing ulcerative, 854
    desquamative, 854–855

Gingivostomatitis, primary herpetic, 854
Ginkgo biloba, 1234–1243t
    for erectile dysfunction, 719
    for tinnitus, 38
Ginseng root, 1234–1243t
GISTs (gastrointestinal stromal tumors), 557–558, 557b
Glanzmann's thrombasthenia (GT), 427
Glasgow Coma Scale (GCS), 965, 965t
    for children, 970, 970t
    for poisonings, 1161, 1163t
Glassy cell carcinoma, of cervix, 1090–1091
Glatiramer acetate (Copaxone)
    for multiple sclerosis, 936, 937t
    for optic neuritis, 197
Glaucoma, 198
    angle-closure
        acute, 200
        primary, 199, 198b
        secondary, 199
    childhood, 199
    defined, 198
    diagnosis of, 198b
    epidemiology of, 198
    normal-pressure, 198
    open-angle
        primary, 198–199, 198b
        secondary, 199
    treatment of, 199–201, 199b, 200t
        α_2 adrenergic agonists for, 200, 200t
        beta-adrenergic antagonists for, 200, 200t
        carbonic anhydrase inhibitors for, 200, 200t
        laser therapy for, 200
        nonspecific sympathomimetics and parasympathomimetics for, 200
        prostaglandin analogues for, 199–200, 200t
        surgery for, 200–201
    types of, 198–199
Gleevec. *See* Imatinib mesylate (Gleevec).
Glenohumeral articulation, anterior dislocation or subluxation of, 1009
Glimepiride (Amaryl), for diabetes, 578, 580t
Glinides, for diabetes, 580, 580t
Glioblastoma multiforme
    epidemiology of, 972
    genetics and etiology of, 972
    outcome with, 975
    pathology of, 972, 974f
Gliomas, 972–975
    brainstem, 975
    clinical presentation of, 972
    diagnostic studies for, 972, 974f
    genetics and etiology of, 972
    incidence of, 972
    outcome for, 975
    pathology of, 972, 973t, 974f
    prognostic factors for, 973
    routes of spread of, 972
    staging of, 972–973
    treatment of, 973–975
        chemotherapy for, 974–975
        radiation therapy for, 974
        surgery for, 973–974
Glioneuronal tumors, 973t
Glipizide (Glucotrol), for diabetes, 578, 580t
Global aphasia, after stroke, 897
Global Assessment Questions (GAQ), 717b
Global Initiative for Chronic Obstructive Lung Disease (GOLD), 231
Glomerular disease(s), 699
    acute renal failure due to, 722–723
    clinical presentation of, 699, 699b, 700b
    diagnosis of, 699–700, 700b
    focal and segmental glomerulosclerosis as
        diagnosis of, 700b
        treatment of, 701–702, 702b
    glomerulonephritis as
        acute postinfectious (diffuse proliferative)

Glomerular disease(s) *(Continued)*
    diagnosis of, 700b
    treatment of, 702b, 703
crescentic
    diagnosis of, 700b
    treatment of, 702b, 703–704
membranoproliferative
    diagnosis of, 700b
    treatment of, 702b, 703
membranous
    diagnosis of, 700b
    treatment of, 702–703, 702b
histologic findings of, 700b
minimal change disease as
    diagnosis of, 700b
    treatment of, 701, 702b
nephropathy as
    IgA
        diagnosis of, 700b
        treatment of, 702b, 703
    membranous
        diagnosis of, 700b
        treatment of, 702–703, 702b
treatment of, 700–704, 701b, 702b
Glomerular filtration rate (GFR), in chronic renal failure, 725
    measurement of, 725–726
    and staging, 728
Glomerular hypertrophy, in chronic renal failure, 728–729
Glomerular prostaglandin production, in chronic renal failure, 729
Glomerulonephritis
    acute postinfectious (diffuse proliferative)
        diagnosis of, 700b
        treatment of, 702b, 703
    crescentic
        diagnosis of, 700b
        treatment of, 702b, 703–704
    membranoproliferative
        diagnosis of, 700b
        treatment of, 702b, 703
    membranous
        diagnosis of, 700b, 700b
        treatment of, 702–703, 702b
    rapidly progressive, 699b, 723
Glomerulopathy, in sickle cell disease, 407, 411
Glomerulosclerosis, focal and segmental
    diagnosis of, 700b
    treatment of, 701–702, 702b
Glossitis, benign migratory, 852
Glossopharyngeal neuralgia, orofacial pain due to, 992t
Glossopyrosis, idiopathic, 852–853
Glucagon
    for anaphylaxis, 761t
    for hypoglycemia in diabetic children, 588
    for poisoning, 1167–1172t
        due to β-blockers, 1182–1183
        due to calcium channel blockers, 1184
Glucantime (meglumine antimoniate), for leishmaniasis, 94, 94b
Glucocorticoid(s). *See also* Corticosteroids.
    for adrenocortical insufficiency, 639–640, 639b
    excess endogenous production of, Cushing's syndrome due to, 641, 644–646, 642f
        treatment of, 644–646, 645t
    exogenous, Cushing's syndrome due to, 641, 641b
        treatment of, 644
    for giant cell arteritis, 1004–1005, 1004b
    glaucoma due to, 199
    for polymyalgia rheumatica, 1004–1005, 1004b
    for systemic lupus erythematosus, 807t
Glucocorticoid receptor antagonist, for Cushing's syndrome, 645t
Glucocorticoid replacement, for hypopituitarism, 658

Glucocorticoid-remediable aldosteronism (GRA), 654
Glucophage (metformin), for diabetes
  in adults, 578, 580t, 580–581
  in children, 590, 590t
Glucosamine
  as nutritional supplement, 1234–1243t
  for osteoarthritis, 1002
Glucose
  for acute porphyria, 477
  for alcoholic liver disease, 498
  in extremely low birth weight infants, 1039–1040t
  in parenteral fluid therapy for infants and children, 627
  for poisoning
    due to calcium channel blockers, 1184
    due to ethanol, 1191
Glucose intake, for high-risk neonate, 1035
Glucose intolerance
  due to acromegaly, 635
  parenteral nutrition with, 622–623, 623t
  due to thalassemia, 402
Glucose metabolism, abnormalities in, due to acromegaly, 634–635
Glucose monitoring, for diabetes, 576, 576b
Glucose tolerance test, during pregnancy, 1013, 1015b
Glucose-6-phosphate dehydrogenase (G6PD) deficiency, 392–393, 393t
Glucose-galactose malabsorption, 543
α-Glucosidase inhibitors, for diabetes, 580t
Glucotrol (glipizide), for diabetes, 578, 580t
Glutamate, in schizophrenia, 1129
Glutamine, parenteral nutrition with, 625
Gluten-free diet, 543
Glyburide (Glynase), for diabetes, 580t
Glycemic control, for diabetes, 576b, 578
Glycemic targets, for diabetes mellitus in children, 586, 586t
Glycerin (Osmoglyn), for glaucoma, 200
Glycet (miglitol), for diabetes, 580t
Glycol(s), and serum osmolality, 1175, 1176t
Glycolax (polyethylene glycol)
  for constipation, 10t, 22b
  for whole-bowel irrigation, 1164–1165
Glycoprotein (GP) IIb/IIIa inhibitor
  for myocardial infarction, 364, 366
  for unstable angina pectoris, 301, 301t
Glycopyrrolate (Robinul), for organophosphate and carbamate poisoning, 1206
Glycosuria, with parenteral nutrition, 625t
Glynase (glyburide), for diabetes, 580t
Glyquin-XM (hydroquinone 4% cream with hyaluronic acid, glycolic acid, and sunscreens), for postinflammatory hyperpigmentation, 878
GnRH. See Gonadotropin-releasing hormone (GnRH).
Goiter, toxic nodular, 669
Goitrous thyroiditis, 678
Gold, peripheral neuropathy due to, 963
GOLD (Global Initiative for Chronic Obstructive Lung Disease), 231
Gold salts, for rheumatoid arthritis, 982
GoLYTELY (polyethylene glycol)
  for constipation, 10t, 22b
  for whole-bowel irrigation, 1164–1165
Gonadal failure, secondary, 657
Gonadal steroid replacement, for hypopituitarism, 658
Gonadoblastoma, 740
Gonadotropin ovulation induction, for infertility, 1061
Gonadotropin-releasing hormone (GnRH) agonists
  for endometriosis, 1056
  postoperative, 1057t

Gonadotropin-releasing hormone (GnRH) agonists (Continued)
  results of, 1056, 1057f
  for premenstrual syndrome, 1069
Gonadotropin-releasing hormone (GnRH) analogues and antagonists, for uterine leiomyoma, 1082
Gonioscopy, 198
Gonococcal conjunctivitis, 194t, 752b
  in neonate, 195–196, 196t
Gonococcal infection(s)
  disseminated, 751, 752b
  during pregnancy, 1014
  urethral stricture disease due to, 740
Gonococcal ophthalmia neonatorum, 751
Gonorrhea, 750
  antimicrobial resistance and therapy of, 751, 752b
  clinical manifestations of, 750–751
  diagnosis of, 751
  epidemiology of, 750
  etiology of, 750
  in men, 751
  in neonates, 751
  pathogenesis of, 750
  of pharynx, 751, 752b
  prevention of, 752
  rectal, 751
  screening for, 752
  uncomplicated, 752b
  in women, 751
Gonorrheal pharyngitis, 220
Goserelin (Zoladex)
  for endometriosis, 1056
  for uterine leiomyoma, 1082
Gout, 599
  acute, 599
  chronic, 599–600, 600t
  in critically ill patients, 600–601
  diagnosis of, 599–600
  in elderly patients, 600
  epidemiology of, 599
  intercritical, 599
  pain due to, 2
  pathogenesis of, 599
  pseudo-, 1001
  resistant, 600
  in transplant patients, 601
  treatment of, 599–601
    indications for, 599, 600b
    potentially new and alternative, 601
Gouty arthritis. See Gout.
Gouty diathesis, renal calculi due to, 744t, 746t
GP (glycoprotein) IIb/IIIa inhibitor
  for myocardial infarction, 364, 366
  for unstable angina pectoris, 301, 301t
GRA (glucocorticoid-remediable aldosteronism), 654
Graded challenge, 782–783, 783b
Graft-versus-host disease (GVHD), transfusion-associated, 484–485t, 489, 489b
  irradiated platelets for, 482
  irradiated red blood cells for, 481
Gram-negative organisms
  endocarditis due to, 345
  meningitis due to, 113
Granisetron (Kytril), for nausea and vomiting, 7, 8t
Granulation tissue formation, for pressure ulcers, 859
Granulocyte colony-stimulating factor (G-CSF), for neutropenia, 415
Granulocyte transfusions, 483
  for neutropenia, 415
Granuloma
  inguinale, 749, 749–750
  Majocchi's, 846, 847b
  pyogenic (peripheral giant cell), of alveolar process/gingiva, 854

Granulomatous mediastinitis, due to histoplasmosis, 252, 253t
Granulomatous thyroiditis, 665, 677
Grape seed, 1234–1243t
Graves' ophthalmopathy, radioiodine treatment and, 668
Gray platelet syndrome, 427–428
Great arteries, transposition of, 330
Greater auricular nerve thickening, due to leprosy, 99, 100f
Gregg, Norman, 140
"Greta," lead in, 1197
Griseofulvin (Grifulvin V, Gris-PEG)
  for cutaneous tinea infection, 846, 848b
  for tinea capitis, 847, 848b
  for tinea corporis, 804
Groin, pruritus of, 31f
Ground itch, 844t, 845
Group A β-hemolytic streptococci (GABHS) pharyngitis, 220
  clinical manifestations of, 221
  diagnosis of, 221–222, 221b
  epidemiology of, 221
  microbiology of, 220–221
  recurrent, 223, 223t
  treatment of, 222–223
    drugs and dosages for, 223t
    indications for, 222–223, 222t
    strategies for, 222–223, 222t
Group A β-hemolytic streptococcus toxic shock syndrome (GAS-TSS), 86
  diagnosis of, 87b, 88, 88b
  epidemiology of, 87
  pathogenesis of, 87
  treatment of, 89, 89b
Group A streptococci, necrotizing skin and soft tissue infections due to, 84, 84t, 85t
Group B streptococcus (GBS), during pregnancy, 1013
Growth, of infants, 1044–1045, 1044b
Growth factors, parenteral nutrition with, 624–625
Growth hormone (GH)
  consequences of excess of, 634–635
  in hypopituitarism, 657
  measurement of, 635
  parenteral nutrition with, 624
  regulation of, 633, 634f
Growth hormone (GH) deficiency, 657–658
Growth hormone (GH) replacement (Genotropin, Humatrope, Norditropin, Nutropin), for hypopituitarism, 658
Growth hormone (GH)-secreting tumors, etiopathogenesis of, 633
Growth hormone/insulin-like growth factor-1 (GH/IGF-1) axis, physiology, biochemistry, and regulation of, 633, 634f
Growth hormone–releasing hormone (GHRH), 633, 634f
Growth impairment, in sickle cell disease, 407
GSPα mutations, 633
GT (Glanzmann's thrombasthenia), 427
GU. See Genitourinary (GU).
Guanfacine (Tenex), for Tourette's syndrome, 920
GUD. See Genital ulcer disease (GUD).
Guillain-Barré syndrome (GBS), 962
Guinea worm, 844, 844t
Günther's disease, 475t, 477b, 479
Gustatory rhinitis, 216, 777–778
Guttate hypomelanosis, idiopathic, 879
GVHD. See Graft-versus-host disease (GVHD).
Gynazole-1 (butoconazole 2% SR cream), for vulvovaginal candidiasis, 1075b
Gynecology
  amenorrhea in, 1062
  breast diseases in, 1045
  cervical cancer in, 1086

Gynecology (Continued)
  Chlamydia trachomatis in, 1076
  dysfunctional uterine bleeding in, 1058
  dysmenorrhea in, 1065
  endometrial cancer in, 1083
  endometriosis in, 1054
  infertility in, 1060
  menopause in, 1070
  ovarian cancer in, 1094
  pelvic inflammatory disease in, 1079
  premenstrual syndrome in, 1066
  uterine leiomyomas in, 1081
  vulvar neoplasms in, 1091
  vulvovaginitis in, 1074
Gynecomastia, 1053
Gyne-Lotrimin 3 (clotrimazole 200 mg suppository/vaginal tablet), for vulvovaginal candidiasis, 1075b
Gyne-Lotrimin 7 (clotrimazole cream), for vulvovaginal candidiasis, 1075b

H

H₁ receptor antagonists (H₁RAs)
  for allergic rhinitis, 779, 779t
  for anaphylaxis, 760
  poisoning due to, 1179–1180
  for serum sickness, 762
  for urticaria, 875
H₂ receptor antagonists (H₂RAs)
  for anaphylaxis, 760
  for gastroesophageal reflux disease, 553, 554t
  for indigestion, 11t
  for peptic ulcer disease, 531–532, 531t
  for urticaria, 875
HA(s). See Hemolytic anemia(s) (HAs).
HA (hydrofluoric acid), burn injury due to, 1138
HAART. See Highly active antiretroviral therapy (HAART).
Habitual dysphonia, 220
HACE. See High-altitude cerebral edema (HACE).
HACEK group, endocarditis prophylaxis for, 346–347t
Haemophilus ducreyi, chancroid due to, 749
Haemophilus influenzae type b (Hib) vaccine (PedvaxHIB, ActHIB, HibTITER), 115
  schedule for, 149–150t
    catch-up, 151t
Hair(s)
  ethnic variations in, 793
  excessive, 790b, 792–793
  lanugo, 790
  structure of, 790
  whisker, 791
Hair disorder(s), 790
  acne keloidalis as, 792
  alopecia as
    androgenic, 791
    areata, 791–792
    central centrifugal scarring, 792
    frontal fibrosing, 792
    traction, 792
  anagen effluvium as, 791
  classification of, 790b
  dissecting cellulitis of scalp as, 792
  hirsutism as, 793
  due to infections, 792
  lichen planopilaris as, 792
  due to lupus erythematosus, 792
  due to psoriasis, 792
  telogen effluvium as
    acute, 790
    chronic, 790–791
    laboratory studies for, 791b
    medication-induced, 791b
  trichotillomania as, 792
Hair growth, 790, 790

Hair loss
  due to chemotherapy, 791
  evaluation of, 790, 790b
  inflammatory, 790b, 791–792
    nonscarring, 791–792
    scarring, 792
  noninflammatory, 790–791, 790b
  patterned, 791
Hair shaft abnormalities, 790b, 793
Hairy leukoplakia, of tongue, 853
Halcion (triazolam)
  for insomnia, 888t
  intoxication with, 1181–1182
Haldol. See Haloperidol (Haldol).
Hallucinations, in schizophrenia, 1128–1129
Hallucinogens
  abuse of, 1110–1111
  poisoning due to, 1166t
Halo nevi, 827–828, 828b
Halobetasol propionate ointment (Ultravate), for anogenital pruritus, 873
Halogenated hydrocarbons, 1193
Haloperidol (Haldol)
  for alcohol withdrawal, 1103
  for Alzheimer's disease, 885t, 884–886
  for cocaine abuse, 1109
  for delirium, 1119–1120, 1119b
  for hallucinogen intoxication, 1111
  for nausea and vomiting, 8t
  poisoning due to, 1208–1209, 1208t
  for Tourette's syndrome, 921
Halsted paradigm, for breast cancer, 1051
Hamartomas, of breast, 1047
Hand, foot, and mouth disease, 842
Hand(s)
  burns of, 1137
  pruritus of, 31f
Hand injuries, due to sports, 1009–1010
Hansen, Gerhard Armauer, 97
Hansen's disease. See Leprosy.
Hanta virus, as biological weapon agent, 1229–1233t
HAP. See Health care–acquired pneumonia (HCAP).
HAPE. See High-altitude pulmonary edema (HAPE).
Hapten mechanisms, of drug-induced hemolytic anemia, 389, 389b
Hard metal lung disease, 278t
Hard palate, disorders of, 851–852
Hashimoto's thyroiditis, 662, 678
Hashish, abuse of, 1110
HAV. See Hepatitis A virus (HAV).
Haverhill fever, 132
Havrix. See Hepatitis A virus (HAV, HepA) vaccine (Havrix, Vaqta).
Hawthorn leaf with flower, 1234–1243t
Hb. See Hemoglobin (Hb).
HBV. See Hepatitis B virus (HBV).
HC. See Hemochromatosis (HC).
HCAP. See Health care–acquired pneumonia (HCAP).
HCC. See Hepatocellular carcinoma (HCC).
β-hCG. See -Human chorionic gonadotropin (β-hCG).
HCM. See Hypertrophic cardiomyopathy (HCM).
HCP (hereditary coproporphyria), 475t, 476t
HCQ. See Hydroxychloroquine (Plaquenil, HCQ).
Hct. See Hematocrit (Hct).
HCV. See Hepatitis C virus (HCV).
HDAC (histone deacetylase) inhibitors, for cutaneous T-cell lymphomas, 800
HDD (high-dose dexamethasone), for multiple myeloma, 469b, 470
HDL cholesterol. See High-density lipoprotein (HDL) cholesterol.

HDM (high-dose melphalan), for multiple myeloma, 469b, 470
HDT (high-dose therapy), for multiple myeloma, 470
HDV. See Hepatitis D virus (HDV).
HE (hepatic encephalopathy), 497t, 501t, 502–503, 503t
Head and neck disease(s)
  conjunctivitis as, 193
  episodic vertigo as, 204
  glaucoma as, 198
  hoarseness and laryngitis as, 218
  laser vision correction as, 187
  Ménière's disease as, 210
  nonallergic perennial rhinitis as, 214
  optic neuritis as, 196
  otitis externa as, 201
  otitis media as, 203
  sinusitis as, 212
  streptococcal pharyngitis as, 220
Head injuries. See Traumatic brain injury (TBI).
Head louse, 844t, 845
Head shaking, for vestibular neurolabyrinthitis, 207b
Headache, 921
  due to alcohol withdrawal, 1102–1103b
  caffeine, 924–925
  cluster
    clinical features of, 923
    epidemiology of, 923
    etiology of, 923
    evaluation and diagnosis of, 922t, 923
    orofacial pain due to, 992t
    treatment of, 924t, 926–927, 926t
  epidemiology of, 922
  evaluation and diagnosis of, 922–923, 922t
  migraine, 2
    with aura (classic), 923
    without aura (common), 923
    cause of, 923
    epidemiology of, 922, 923
    evaluation and diagnosis of, 922t, 923
    postmenopausal, 1071
    vs. seizures, 901t
    treatment of, 924–926, 924t, 925t
    triggers of, 923b, 924b
    types of, 923
    vestibular, 209
  red flags with, 922
  tension-type
    clinical features of, 923
    etiology of, 923
    evaluation and diagnosis of, 923, 922t
    pathophysiology of, 923
    treatment of, 924, 924t
  treatment of, 923–927, 924t
    abortive vs. prophylactic, 924
    nonpharmacologic vs. pharmacologic, 924
Health care–acquired pneumonia (HCAP, HAP), 263–264
  defined, 263
  diagnosis of, 263–264
  epidemiology of, 263
  etiology of, 263
  prevention of, 264
  treatment of, 264, 264t
Heart block, 315
  with acute myocardial infarction, 319, 319b
  approach to patient with, 318–319
  bundle branch
    alternating, 317
    right, 317
  diagnosis of, 317b
  etiology of, 315–316, 316b
  mechanisms of, 315, 316b
  after myocardial infarction, 366t
  second-degree, 317
  signs and symptoms of, 316–317

Heart block (Continued)
  transient third-degree, 316, 317
  treatment of, 317–318, 318**b**
    pacing for, 318–319, 319**b**
    pharmacologic, 317–318
Heart disease
  congenital (See Congenital heart disease)
  hypertensive, 350–351, 352**f**
  structural, cardiac arrest due to, 303**t**
Heart failure, 338
  chronic, hypertension and, 350, 356**t**
  classification and stages of, 338–339, 339**b**, 340**b**
  defined, 338
  diagnosis of, 339**b**, 339–340
  prognosis for, 340
  treatment of, 339–341, 341**b**
    disease management and other resources in, 341
    emerging approaches for, 341–342
    nonpharmacologic, 340–341, 341**b**
    pharmacologic, 339**t**, 340
    targets for, 340, 341**b**
Heart murmurs, 326–327
Heart Outcomes Prevention Evaluation (HOPE) Trial, 297
Heartburn, during pregnancy, 1014
Heat exposure, pruritus due to, 31**b**
Heat loss, in neonate, 1035, 1036**f**
Heat modalities, for osteoarthritis, 999
Heat production, in neonate, 1035
Heat stroke, 1148
  classic (nonexertional), 1148
  diagnosis of, 1149**b**
  exertional, 1148
  pathophysiology of, 1148–1149
  treatment of, 1149–1150, 1149**b**
Heat urticaria, 874
Heated cardiopulmonary bypass, 1146
Heavy hydrocarbons, 1193
Heberden's nodes, 1001
Helicobacter pylori
  diagnostic tests for, 529, 531**t**
  dyspepsia due to, 528
Helicobacter pylori eradication, for peptic ulcer disease, 532, 532**t**
Helicobacter pylori gastritis
  chronic, 529
  indigestion due to, 11**t**, 11–12
Helicobacter pylori–associated gastric adenocarcinoma, 529, 556
Helicobacter pylori–associated ulcers, 529–530, 530**f**
HELLP syndrome, 1026–1027
  clinical findings in, 1026–1027
  diagnostic criteria for, 1026, 1026**b**
Helminths, 569–573, 570**t**
  skin infections due to, 843–845, 844**t**
Helper T cells (THs)
  in allergic rhinitis, 777
  in cutaneous T-cell lymphomas, 795
Hemabate (carboprost tromethamine), for postpartum hemorrhage, 1028**t**
Hemarthrosis, due to hemophilia, 419–420
Hematin (Panhematin), for acute porphyria, 476–477
Hematocrit (Hct)
  in polycythemia vera, 473–474
  reference intervals for, 1219**t**
  in sickle cell disease, 406**t**
Hematologic disorder(s)
  anemia(s) as
    aplastic, 379
    hemolytic
      autoimmune, 387
      nonimmune, 390
    pernicious and other megaloblastic, 394
  disseminated intravascular coagulation as, 428

Hematologic disorder(s) (Continued)
  due to HAART, 54–55**t**
  hemochromatosis as, 432
  hemolytic disease of the fetus and newborn as, 416
  hemophilia and related bleeding disorders as, 419
  iron deficiency as, 383
  due to lead poisoning, 1197
  leukemias as
    acute
      in adults, 444
      in children, 450
    chronic, 456
  lymphoma as
    Hodgkin's, 434
      radiation therapy for, 439
    non-Hodgkin's, 464
  multiple myeloma as, 467
  neutropenia as, 413
  platelet-mediated bleeding disorders as, 425
  polycythemia vera as, 472
  porphyria as, 475
  sickle cell disease as, 404
  thalassemia as, 397
  thrombotic thrombocytopenic purpura as, 430
Hematology, reference intervals for, 1219**t**
Hematoma(s)
  due to intracerebral hemorrhage, 891
    evacuation of, 891–892
    preventing expansion of, 892
  muscle, due to hemophilia, 420
  subungual, 819
  due to traumatic brain injury
    epidural, 965–966
    intraparenchymal, 966
    subdural, 966
    in children, 969–970
Hematopoietic stem cell transplantation (HSCT)
  for aplastic anemia, 382, 382**f**
  long-term complications of, 382–383
  for sickle cell disease, 412**t**, 413
  for thalassemia, 401
Hematuria
  microscopic, due to *Staphylococcus saprophyticus*, 682
  recurrent macroscopic, 699**b**
  in sickle cell disease, 411
Heme, for acute porphyria, 476–477
Heme arginate (Normosang), for acute porphyria, 477
Heme hydroxide, for acute porphyria, 476
Hemicrania, chronic paroxysmal, 992**t**
Hemochromatosis (HC), 432
  cirrhosis due to, 500
  clinical features of, 432–433
  diagnosis of, 433, 433**b**, 500
  genetic basis for, 432, 500
  and hepatocellular carcinoma, 500
  screening for
    family, 433
    population, 433–434
  treatment of, 433, 433**b**, 500
Hemodialysis, for poisoning, 1165, 1174**t**
  ethylene glycol, 1193
  lithium, 1201
  methanol, 1202
  salicylate, 1211–1212
Hemodynamic compromise, during pregnancy, 1019–1020, 1020
Hemodynamic management, for sepsis, 68–69
Hemofiltration, for poisonings, 1173
Hemoglobin (Hb)
  in polycythemia vera, 473
  reference intervals for, 1219**t**
Hemoglobin A1C goals, for diabetes mellitus in children, 586, 586**t**

Hemoglobin C (HbC), 404
Hemoglobin E/β-thalassemia, 400
Hemoglobin H (HbH) disease, 398, 400
Hemoglobin H–Constant Spring (HbH-CS) disease, 398, 400
Hemoglobin S (HbS), 404, 404
Hemoglobin SC (HbSC), 404
Hemoglobin SS (HbSS), 404
Hemoglobinopathies, hemolytic anemia due to, 391**t**, 393
Hemoglobinuria, paroxysmal
  cold, 389
    diagnosis of, 389
    serology of, 387**t**
    treatment of, 389
  nocturnal, 379, 393–394
Hemolytic anemia(s) (HAs)
  autoimmune, 387
    classification and serology of, 387, 387**t**
    cold agglutinin syndrome as, 388–389
      diagnosis of, 388
      serology of, 387**t**
      treatment of, 388–389, 388**b**
    drug-induced, 389, 389**b**
    paroxysmal cold hemoglobinuria as, 389
      diagnosis of, 389
      serology of, 387**t**
      treatment of, 389
    warm, 387–388
      diagnosis of, 387
      serology of, 387**t**
      treatment of, 387–388, 388**b**
  microangiopathic, 430, 431
  nonimmune, 390
    acquired, 393–394
    causes of, 391**t**
    due to chemical and physical agents, 391**t**, 394
    congenital, 391–393, 393**t**
    diagnosis of, 390, 390**b**
    due to erythrocyte fragmentation, 391**t**, 394
    due to erythrocyte membrane abnormalities, 391–392, 391**t**
    due to erythrocyte metabolism abnormalities, 391**t**, 392–393, 393**t**
    due to glucose-6-phosphate dehydrogenase deficiency, 392–393, 393**t**
    due to hemoglobinopathies, 391**t**, 393
    hereditary elliptocytosis and pyropoikilocytosis as, 392
    hereditary spherocytosis as, 391–392
    hereditary stomatocytosis and xerocytosis as, 392
    due to infection, 391**t**, 394
    paroxysmal nocturnal hemoglobinuria as, 393–394
    due to pyruvate kinase deficiency, 393
    treatment of, 390–391, 390**b**
Hemolytic disease of the fetus and newborn, 416
  diagnosis of, 416**b**
  from non-RhD antibodies, 418–419
  due to RhD antigen, 416
  treatment of, 417**b**
Hemolytic transfusion reactions, 484–487, 484–485**t**
  acute, 484–486, 484–485**t**
  due to bacterial contamination of blood products, 484–485**t**, 487
  delayed, 484–485**t**, 486–487
Hemolytic uremic syndrome (HUS), 426, 431
Hemoperfusion
  for poisonings, 1165–1173
  for theophylline intoxication, 1214
Hemophilia, 419–422
  clinical features of, 419–420, 420**t**
  diagnosis of, 420, 420**b**, 421**t**
  epidemiology of, 419

Hemophilia *(Continued)*
  pathophysiology of,, 419, 420f
  severity of, 419–420, 420t
  treatment of, 420–422, 421b, 422t
    complications of, 422
Hemophilia A, 419
  clinical features of, 421t
  pathophysiology of, 419, 420f
  treatment of, 422t
Hemophilia B, 419
  clinical features of, 421t
  pathophysiology of, 419
  treatment of, 422t
Hemopoietic neoplasms, of brain, 973t
Hemorrhage. *See also* Bleeding.
  in disseminated intravascular coagulation, 428, 428
  intracerebral, 890
    diagnosis of, 891, 891b
    epidemiology and etiology of, 890–891, 890b
    scoring system for, 891, 891t
    treatment of, 891–892, 892t
  intraventricular, in extremely low birth weight infants, 1039–1040t
  due to peptic ulcer disease, 532
  postpartum, 1027
    defined, 1027
    epidemiology of, 1027
    etiology of, 1027, 1027b
    due to placenta previa, 1020
    treatment of, 1027, 1028t
  uterine, 1059–1060
Hemorrhagic stroke, 890
  diagnosis of, 891, 891b
  epidemiology and etiology of, 890–891, 890b
  scoring system for, 891, 891t
  in sickle cell disease, 407
  treatment of, 891–892, 892t
Hemorrhoids, 525–526
  defined, 525
  differential diagnosis of, 525, 525t
  evaluation of, 525, 526
  external, 525–526
    thrombosed, 526
  history of, 525, 526
  internal, 525, 526t
  pathogenesis of, 525
  physical examination of, 525, 526
  treatment of, 526
Hemosiderin, 383
Henbane, poisoning due to, 1179–1180
Henderson-Patterson bodies, 842–843
Henoch, Eduard, 815
Henoch-Schönlein purpura (HSP), 814–815
HEP (hepatoerythropoietic porphyria), 475t, 477b, 479
HepA. *See* Hepatitis A virus (HAV, HepA).
Heparin
  for disseminated intravascular coagulation, 429
  low-molecular-weight
    for deep venous thrombosis/pulmonary embolism, 273, 273b
    for myocardial infarction, 364
  unfractionated
    for deep venous thrombosis/pulmonary embolism, 272–273, 273b
    for myocardial infarction, 363–364
Heparin-induced thrombocytopenia (HIT), 426
Hepatic dysfunction, parenteral nutrition with, 624
Hepatic encephalopathy (HE), 497t, 501t, 502–503, 503t
Hepatic toxicity, 1174t
Hepatitis, 533, 535b
  acute, 533
  alcoholic, 498–499, 498t

Hepatitis *(Continued)*
  autoimmune, 498t, 499
  chronic, 533–534
  cirrhosis due to, 498t
Hepatitis A and B virus vaccine (Twinrix), 534t
  for travelers, 159–160t
Hepatitis A virus (HAV, HepA), 534–535
  characteristics of, 534t
  clinical features of, 534
  diagnosis of, 534–535, 535t
  epidemiology of, 534
  treatment and prevention of, 535
Hepatitis A virus (HAV, HepA) vaccine (Havrix, Vaqta), 534t, 535
  schedule for, 149–150t
    catch-up, 151t
  for travelers, 159–160t, 160, 161
Hepatitis B virus (HBV), 535–537
  characteristics of, 534t
  clinical features of, 535
  diagnosis of, 535–536, 536t
  epidemiology of, 535
  and hepatitis D virus, 538, 538
  and hepatocellular carcinoma, 539
  and HIV coinfection, 539
  prevention of, 537
  transfusion-associated, 489
  treatment of, 536–537, 536t
Hepatitis B virus (HBV) vaccine (Recombivax-HB, Engerix-B, Combivax, Pediarix), 534t, 537
  schedule for, 149–150t
    catch-up, 151t
  for travelers, 159–160t, 161
Hepatitis C virus (HCV)
  characteristics of, 534t
  clinical features of, 537
  diagnosis of, 537–538, 537t
  epidemiology of, 537
  and hepatocellular carcinoma, 539
  and HIV coinfection, 539
  transfusion-associated, 489
  treatment of, 536t, 538
Hepatitis D virus (HDV), 538
  characteristics of, 534t
  diagnosis and treatment of, 538, 538t
  epidemiology and clinical features of, 538
  and hepatitis B virus, 538, 538
Hepatitis E virus (HEV), 538–539
  characteristics of, 534t
  clinical features of, 538
  diagnosis, treatment, and prevention of, 538–539, 539t
  epidemiology of, 538
Hepatitis vaccines, 534t
Hepatocellular carcinoma (HCC)
  cirrhosis and, 497t, 501t, 504
  hemochromatosis and, 500
  hepatitis and, 539
  prevention of, 504
  screening for, 504
  treatment of, 504
Hepatoerythropoietic porphyria (HEP), 475t, 477b, 479
Hepatopulmonary syndrome (HPS), 497t, 501t, 503
Hepatorenal syndrome (HRS), 497t, 501t, 503, 503t
Hepatotoxicity, due to HAART, 54–55t
Hepcidin, 383
Hepsera (adefovir), for hepatitis B and C viruses, 536t, 537
Herald patch, 805
Herbal remedies, 1234
  for chronic fatigue syndrome, 120
  seizures due to, 899t
Hereditary coproporphyria (HCP), 475t, 476t
Hereditary elliptocytosis, 392

Hereditary hemochromatosis (HH), 432
  clinical features of, 432–433
  diagnosis of, 433, 433b
  genetic basis for, 432
  screening for
    family, 433
    population, 433–434
  treatment of, 433, 433b
Hereditary neuropathies, 963
Hereditary neuropathy with liability to pressure palsies (HNPP), 963
Hereditary nonpolyposis colorectal cancer (HNPCC), 558
  and ovarian cancer, 1094
Hereditary pyropoikilocytosis, 392
Hereditary spherocytosis, 391–392
Hereditary stomatocytosis, 392
Hereditary xerocytosis, 392
Hernia, congenital diaphragmatic, 1039
Heroin, intoxication with, 1204–1205, 1205t
Herpes
  genital, 840
    during pregnancy, 1015
  orofacial, 840, 849
Herpes gestationis, pruritus due to, 32b
Herpes gladiatorum, 840
Herpes labialis, 840, 849
Herpes simplex
  recurrent intraoral, 852
  of tongue, 853
Herpes simplex virus (HSV), 839
  clinical features of, 840
  conjunctivitis due to, 195
  diagnosis of, 841
  epidemiology of, 839–840
  erythema multiforme due to, 863, 864
  etiology of, 839
  in HIV patients, 840
  keratitis due to, 840
  meningitis or encephalitis due to, 840, 927, 930, 928–930t
    treatment of, 930, 931
  neonatal, 840, 842
  pathogenesis of, 840
  pathogens related to, 842–843
  treatment of, 841–842, 841t
Herpes zoster
  clinical features of, 840–841
  diagnosis of, 841
  oticus, 202
  peripheral neuropathy due to, 964
  pruritus due to, 32b
  treatment of, 841t, 842
Herpetic gingivostomatitis, primary, 854
Herpetic whitlow, 840
Herpetiform aphthous ulcers, 850
HES (hiccup-evoking site), 12
Hesitancy, urinary, in children, 690
Hetrazan (diethylcarbamazine)
  for loiasis, 844
  for lymphatic filariasis, 844, 844t
HEV. *See* Hepatitis E virus (HEV).
HFE gene, in hemochromatosis, 432, 433
HGA. *See* Human granulocytic anaplasmosis (HGA).
HH. *See* Hereditary hemochromatosis (HH).
HHS. *See* Hyperglycemic hyperosmolar state (HHS).
HHV. *See* Human herpesvirus (HHV).
Hib vaccine. *See Haemophilus influenzae* type b (Hib) vaccine (PedvaxHIB, ActHIB, HibTITER).
HibTITER. *See Haemophilus influenzae* type b (Hib) vaccine (PedvaxHIB, ActHIB, HibTITER).
Hiccup(s), 12
  chronic, 12b, 12
  current diagnosis of, 12b

Hiccup(s) (Continued)
  defined, 12, 12b
  etiology of, 12, 12b
  intractable, 12b, 13
  treatment of, 12–13, 13b
Hiccup-evoking site (HES), 12
Hidradenitis suppurativa, 837–838
High altitude, normal acclimatization to, 1140
High-altitude cerebral edema (HACE), 1141–1142
  clinical presentation of, 158, 1141
  diagnosis of, 1141, 1142b
  differential diagnosis of, 1141b
  incidence of, 1140
  prevention of, 158, 1140–1141
  risk factors for, 1140
  treatment of, 1141–1142, 1142b
High-altitude pulmonary edema (HAPE), 158, 158, 1142–1143
  clinical course of, 1142
  clinical presentation of, 1142
  defined, 1142
  differential diagnosis of, 1141b
  incidence of, 1140
  prevention of, 1140–1141
  risk factors for, 1140
  treatment of, 1142, 1142b, 1143
High-altitude sickness, 158, 1140
  acute mountain sickness as, 158, 1141–1142
    clinical course of, 1141
    defined, 1141
    diagnosis of, 1141, 1142b
    differential diagnosis of, 1141, 1141b
    incidence of, 1140
    prevention of, 1140–1141
    risk factors for, 1140
    treatment of, 1141–1142, 1142b
  defined, 1140
  diagnosis of, 1142b
  high-altitude cerebral edema as (See High-altitude cerebral edema (HACE))
  high-altitude pulmonary edema as (See High-altitude pulmonary edema (HAPE))
  incidence of, 1140
  normal acclimatization vs., 1140
  prevention of, 1140–1141
  reascent after, 1143
  risk factors for, 1140
  treatment of, 1142b
High-density lipoprotein (HDL) cholesterol, 601, 602t
  and coronary artery disease, 602–603
  screening for, 602
High-dose dexamethasone (HDD), for multiple myeloma, 469b, 470, 470
High-dose melphalan (HDM), for multiple myeloma, 469b, 470
High-dose radiation (HDR) therapy, for prostate cancer, 732
High-dose therapy (HDT), for multiple myeloma, 470
Highly active antiretroviral therapy (HAART), 49–50, 48b
  adherence to, 52–53
  adverse drug reactions and drug interactions with, 53, 54–55t, 58t
  currently approved drugs for, 50t
  drug resistance and resistance testing with, 51–52, 52t
  failure of, 52, 52t
  goal of, 49–50
  historical background of, 47
  monitoring response to, 51
  during pregnancy, 58
  regimens for, 49–50, 51t
  when to initiate, 50–51
High-risk neonate, 1033
  due to asphyxia, 1034, 1034b
  due to congenital diaphragmatic hernia, 1039

High-risk neonate (Continued)
  counseling for family of, 1033
  defined, 1033
  delivery management of, 1033–1034
  demographics of, 1033
  developmental care for, 1037
  diagnosis of, 1041b
  due to extremely low birth weight, 1039, 1039–1040t
  due to gastroschisis, 1038–1039
  due to hyaline membrane disease, 1037
  due to meconium aspiration syndrome, 1038
  nutrition for, 1035–1037
  palliative care for, 1039–1041
  parental involvement in care of, 1037
  due to persistent pulmonary hypertension of the newborn, 1038
  postnatal care for, 1034–1037
  prenatal diagnosis of, 1033
  resuscitation of (See Newborn resuscitation)
  thermoregulation with, 1035, 1035t, 1036f, 1036t
  due to transient tachypnea of the newborn, 1037–1038
  treatment of, 1041b
High-volume continuous venovenous hemofiltration, for septic shock, 71
Hirsutism, 793
Hirudin, for deep venous thrombosis/pulmonary embolism, 273
Histamine, in anaphylaxis, 759
Histamine fish poisoning, 1157
Histone deacetylase (HDAC) inhibitors, for cutaneous T-cell lymphomas, 800
Histoplasmosis, 251
  with AIDS, 253t
  clinical manifestations of, 251–253
  diagnosis of, 252, 252b
  disseminated, 252, 253t
  etiology and epidemiology of, 251
  pathogenesis of, 251
  pulmonary
    acute, 252, 253t
    chronic, 252, 253t
    diffuse, 252
    localized, 252
  treatment of, 253–254, 253t, 253b
HIT (heparin-induced thrombocytopenia), 426
HIV. See Human immunodeficiency virus (HIV).
Hivid (zalcitabine), for HIV, 50t
HLH (hypoplastic left heart), 331
HMD (hyaline membrane disease), 1037, 1039–1040t
HME. See Human monocytotropic ehrlichiosis (HME).
HMG-CoA reductase inhibitors. See 3-Hydroxy-3-methyl-glutaryl coenzyme A (HMG-CoA) reductase inhibitors.
HNPCC (hereditary nonpolyposis colorectal cancer), 558
  and ovarian cancer, 1094
HNPP (hereditary neuropathy with liability to pressure palsies), 963
Hoagland sign, in infectious mononucleosis, 116
Hoarseness, 218–219
  acute, 218–219
  chronic, 219–220
  defined, 218
  diagnosis of, 218–219, 218b
  etiology of, 218
  treatment of, 219, 219b
  and voice production, 218, 218b
  when to refer for, 219
Hobbies, associated with lead exposure, 1197, 1198b
Hobo spider bites, 1151
Hodgkin, Thomas, 434

Hodgkin's lymphoma, 434
  clinical presentation and diagnosis of, 435–436, 436b, 439–440, 440b
  epidemiology of, 434
  histologic classification of, 434, 435f
  pruritus due to, 32b
  staging and risk categorization for, 434–435, 435t, 440t, 441f
  survivorship of, 438–439
  treatment of, 436–438, 437b
    for advanced-stage disease, 437, 437b, 443–444
    combined modality therapy for, 442, 443
    with HIV infection, 438
    for limited-stage disease, 436–437, 437b
    for nodular lymphocyte–predominant disease, 438
    in older patients, 438
    during pregnancy, 438
    radiation therapy for, 439
      complications of, 444
      extended field, 440, 442f
      involved field, 440, 443f
      mantle field, 440–441, 442f
      with mediastinal involvement, 442–443
      patient evaluation and staging for, 439–440, 440t, 440b
      recommendations and results of, 442–444, 442b, 443t, 443f
      subdiaphragmatic, 441–443
      subtotal nodal, 440
      techniques of, 440, 441f
      treatment volumes in, 440
    for relapsed or refractory disease, 437–438, 437b, 443–444
Hoerr, Stanley, 203
Home glucose monitoring, 576, 576b
Homocysteine, in dyslipoproteinemia, 603
Hook effect, 660
Hookworm, 570t, 571
Hoover's sign, 228
HOPE (Heart Outcomes Prevention Evaluation) Trial, 297
Hops, 1234–1243t
Hormonal methods, of contraception, 756–757
  estrogen-progestin combinations as, 756
  progestin only, 756–757
Hormonal rhinitis, 215
Hormonal therapy
  for breast cancer, 1052–1053
  for dysmenorrhea, 1065
  for endometrial cancer, 1085
  for osteoporosis, 615
  for prostate cancer, 732, 732
Hormone replacement therapy (HRT), after menopause, 1071–1072, 1072t, 1072b
Horse chestnut seed, 1234–1243t
Hospital-acquired pneumonia. See Health care–acquired pneumonia (HAP).
Hospitalization
  for acute exacerbations of asthma, 769–770
  for atopic dermatitis, 862
  for epididymitis, 698
  for pericarditis, 370, 370b
  for pyelonephritis, 705–706, 705b
  for urinary tract infections in girls, 688b
Hot flushes, 1070
  treatment for, 1072t
Hot tub lung, 288
House-Brackmann scale, for Bell's palsy, 950, 950b
House-dust mites
  in allergic rhinitis, 776
  and asthma
    in adolescents and adults, 765b
    in children, 771
HP Acthar (corticotropin), for infantile spasms, 909

HPS (hepatopulmonary syndrome), 497t, 501t, 503
HPV. See Human papillomavirus (HPV).
HR (high-dose radiation) therapy, for prostate cancer, 732
HRS (hepatorenal syndrome), 497t, 501t, 503, 503t
HRT (hormone replacement therapy), after menopause, 1071–1072, 1072t, 1072b
HSCT. See Hematopoietic stem cell transplantation (HSCT).
HSG (hysterosalpingography), 1060–1061
HSP (Henoch-Schönlein purpura), 814–815
HSV. See Herpes simplex virus (HSV).
5-HT3 (serotonin) antagonists, for nausea and vomiting, 7, 8t
hTIG (human tetanus immune globulin), 144, 144b, 144–145
Humalog (insulin lispro), for diabetes
 in adults, 582t
 in children, 586–587, 587t
Human bites, 836b
β-Human chorionic gonadotropin (β-hCG)
 during pregnancy, 1012
  ectopic, 1017, 1019
 in testicular cancer, 738
Human diploid cell vaccine (Imovax), 131
 for travelers, 159–160t
Human granulocytic anaplasmosis (HGA), 178
 clinical features and diagnosis of, 178
 epidemiology of, 178
 treatment of, 178–179, 179b
Human herpesvirus 3 (HHV-3)
 clinical features of, 840–841
 diagnosis of, 841
 treatment of, 841t, 842
Human herpesvirus 6 (HHV-6)
 meningitis or encephalitis due to, 928–930t
 pharyngitis due to, 220–221
Human immunodeficiency virus (HIV), 45
 acute syndrome of, 46, 46t
 causative agent for, 45
 CD4+ helper T lymphocytes in, 46, 50–51
 chancroid and, 749
 changing face of, 47
 cryptosporidiosis with, 568
 cyclosporiasis with, 568
 diagnosis of, 48, 48b
 epidemiology of, 45
 fungal skin infections with, 847–849
 genital ulcer disease and, 749
 and hepatitis coinfection, 539
 herpes simplex virus with, 840
 histoplasmosis with, 253t
 historical background of, 45
 immune reconstitution inflammatory syndrome in, 53
 intensive care with, 71–72
 isosporiasis with, 568
 latency stage of, 46
 leprosy with, 102
 lymphomas with
  Hodgkin's, 438
  non-Hodgkin's, 466
 management of, 48–53
  antiretroviral therapy in, 49–50, 48b
   adherence to, 52–53
   adverse drug reactions and drug interactions with, 53, 54–55t, 58t, 784t
   currently approved drugs for, 50t
   drug resistance and resistance testing with, 51–52, 52t
   failure of, 52, 52t
   goal of, 49–50
   historical background of, 47
   monitoring response to, 51
   during pregnancy, 58

Human immunodeficiency virus (HIV) (Continued)
   regimens for, 49–50, 51t
   when to initiate, 50–51
  initial evaluation in, 48–49, 49t
  meningitis or encephalitis due to, 928–930t
  opportunistic condition(s) in, 53–58
   chemoprophylaxis for, 53, 56t
   cryptococcosis as, 55–56
   cytomegalovirus disease as, 57
   disseminated Mycobacterium avium infection as, 56–57, 56t
   etiology of, 57t
   general considerations for, 53
   Pneumocystis jiroveci pneumonia (PCP) as, 53–55, 56t
   Toxoplasma gondii as, 56t
   tuberculosis as, 56t, 57–58, 58t, 284b, 287–288
  pathogenesis and natural history of, 46–47, 46t, 47t
  peripheral neuropathy due to, 964
  pharyngitis due to, 220–221
  postexposure prophylaxis of, 58–59
  during pregnancy, 58, 1014, 1016b
  pruritus due to, 32b
  sepsis with, 71–72
  syphilis and, 755
  testing for, 47–48, 49t
  toxoplasmosis in, 166t, 167–168, 167b
  transfusion-associated, 489
  transmission of, 45–46
  varicella with, 77–78
Human immunodeficiency virus (HIV) antivirals, and SSRIs, 1122–1123b
Human milk fortifiers, 1043b
Human monocytotropic ehrlichiosis (HME), 178
 clinical features and diagnosis of, 178
 epidemiology of, 178
 treatment of, 178–179, 179b
Human papillomavirus (HPV)
 and cervical cancer, 1086
 condyloma acuminatum due to, 824, 826
  vulvar, 1092
 verrucae due to, 822
 and vulvar intraepithelial neoplasia, 1092
Human papillomavirus (HPV) vaccines (Cervarix, Gardasil), 822
 and cervical carcinoma, 1091
 schedule for, 149–150t
  catch-up, 151t
Human parvovirus B19, 842
 during pregnancy, 1014
Human rabies immune globulin (Imogam, BayRab), 131
Human tetanus immune globulin (hTIG, BayTet), 144, 144b, 144–145
Humatin. See Paromomycin (Humatin).
Humatrope (growth hormone replacement), for hypopituitarism, 658
HuMax-CD4 (zanolimumab), for cutaneous T-cell lymphomas, 800, 800
Humeral head, osteonecrosis or avascular necrosis of, in sickle cell disease, 407, 411
Humira. See Adalimumab (Humira).
Humulin N (NPH insulin), for diabetes
 in adults, 582, 582t
 in children, 586, 587t
Humulin R (regular insulin), for diabetes
 in adults, 582t
 in children, 587t
Hürthle cell cancer, 671, 672
 follow-up for, 671, 672
HUS (hemolytic uremic syndrome), 426, 431
Hutchinson's sign, 841
Hyalgan (sodium hyaluronate), for osteoarthritis, 1001, 1001t

Hyaline membrane disease (HMD), 1037, 1039–1040t
Hyaluronan, high molecular weight (Orthovisc), for osteoarthritis, 1001t
Hyaluronan(s), intra-articular, for osteoarthritis, 1001, 1001t
Hyaluronate, intra-articular, for osteoarthritis, 1001, 1001t
Hyaluronic acid, intra-articular, for osteoarthritis, 1001, 1001t
Hydralazine (Apresoline)
 for hypertension in pregnancy, 1027
 peripheral neuropathy due to, 963
Hydration
 of airway surface fluid, for cystic fibrosis, 238
 for atopic dermatitis, 860
 for pressure ulcers, 858
Hydrea (hydroxyurea)
 for polycythemia vera, 474
 for sickle cell disease, 412t, 412–413
Hydrocarbon poisoning, 1193–1194
Hydrochlorothiazide (Esidrix, Hydrodiuril)
 for hypertension, 356–357
  in pregnancy, 1023t
 for renal calculi, 746t
Hydrochlorothiazide and triamterene (Dyazide, Maxzide-25), for Ménière's disease, 211
Hydrocodone + acetaminophen (Lortab, Maxidon, Norco, Vicodin, Xodol, Zydone)
 intoxication with, 1204–1205, 1205t
 for pain, 4t
 for renal calculi, 745t
Hydrocodone + ibuprofen (Vicoprofen), for pain, 4t
Hydrocolloid dressings, for pressure ulcers, 858
Hydrocortisone (Cortef), for hypopituitarism, 658
Hydrocortisone ointment (Hytone), for anogenital pruritus, 872–873
Hydrocortisone sodium succinate (Solu-Cortef)
 for adrenocortical insufficiency, 639, 639b, 640
 for caustic or corrosive burns, 1186
 for inflammatory bowel disease, 516, 519–520
 for septic shock, 71
Hydrocortisone valerate cream, for vitiligo, 878–879
Hydrocyanic acid, 1187–1188
Hydrodiuril. See Hydrochlorothiazide (Esidrix, Hydrodiuril).
Hydrofluoric acid (HA), burn injury due to, 1138
Hydrogen cyanide, as chemical weapon, 1226–1228t
Hydrogen cyanide poisoning, 1187–1188
Hydromorphone (Dilaudid)
 intoxication with, 1204–1205, 1205t
 for pain, 4t
Hydroquinone 2% cream (Benzoquin), for vitiligo, 879
Hydroquinone 4% and retinol (EpiQuin Micro), for melasma, 876–877
Hydroquinone 4% cream with glycolic acids and sunscreens (AlphaquinHP)
 for melasma, 876–877
 for solar lentigines, 877
Hydroquinone 4% cream with hyaluronic acid, glycolic acid, and sunscreens (Glyquin-XM), for postinflammatory hyperpigmentation, 878
Hydroquinone 4% cream with sunscreen (Solaquin Forte)
 for melasma, 876–877
 for postinflammatory hyperpigmentation, 878
Hydrothermal endometrial ablation, for uterine leiomyoma, 1082t
3-Hydroxy-3-methyl-glutaryl coenzyme A (HMG-CoA) reductase inhibitors
 for angina pectoris, 297–298
 for chronic renal failure, 729

3-Hydroxy-3-methyl-glutaryl coenzyme A
  (HMG-CoA) reductase inhibitors
  (Continued)
    drugs that interact with, 603**b**, 605
    for dyslipoproteinemia, 604–605, 605**t**
    for myocardial infarction, 364–365, 365**t**
    and SSRIs, 1122–1123**b**
Hydroxychloroquine (Plaquenil, HCQ)
  for arthritis
    juvenile idiopathic, 985–986
    rheumatoid, 981, 981**t**
  for idiopathic inflammatory myopathy, 813
  for malaria prophylaxis, 111–112**t**
  for osteoarthritis, 1002
  for porphyria cutanea tarda, 479
  for Q fever, 129, 129**t**
  for sarcoidosis, 277
  for systemic lupus erythematosus, 806–808, 807**t**
Hydroxycobalamin (vitamin B$_{12a}$, Cyanokit)
  for cyanide poisoning, 1188
  for vitamin B$_{12}$ deficiency, 397
Hydroxyurea (Hydrea)
  for polycythemia vera, 474
  for sickle cell disease, 412**t**, 412–413
Hydroxyzine (Atarax, Vistaril)
  for allergic rhinitis, 779**t**
  for contact dermatitis, 871, 871**b**
  for nausea and vomiting, 8**t**
  for pruritus, 33**b**
    due to primary biliary cirrhosis, 499
  for systemic sclerosis, 810
  for urticaria, 875
Hygiene hypothesis, of asthma, 770
Hygroton (chlorthalidone)
  for hypertension, 356–357
  for renal calculi, 746**t**
Hylan G-F20 (Synvisc), for osteoarthritis, 1001, 1001**t**
Hyoscyamine (Levsin), for urinary incontinence
  in children, 691, 692**t**
  urge, 695**b**
Hyoscyamus niger, poisoning due to, 1179–1180
Hyperacusis, 37
Hyperaldosteronism
  dexamethasone-suppressible, 654
  familial
    type I, 654
    type II, 654
  idiopathic, 654
Hyperalimentation, 619
Hyperbaric oxygen chamber, for carbon
  monoxide poisoning, 1185
Hypercalcemia
  differential diagnosis of, 650, 650**t**
  hypertension and, 356**b**
  due to multiple myeloma, 471
  with parenteral nutrition, 625**t**
Hypercalciuria
  due to acromegaly, 635
  due to hyperparathyroidism, 650
  renal calculi due to, 743, 743**t**, 744**t**, 746**t**
Hypercapnia, pathophysiologic mechanisms of, 225–226, 226**b**
Hypercarbia, with parenteral nutrition, 625**t**
Hyperchloremia, with parenteral nutrition, 625**t**
Hypercholesterolemia
  and angina pectoris, 297–298
  epidemiology of, 601
  hypertension and, 356**b**
Hypercortisolemia, medical management of, 645–646, 645**t**
Hypercortisolism
  endogenous, 641**b**, 644–646, 642**f**
    treatment of, 644–646, 645**t**
  etiologies of, 640–641, 641**b**
  exogenous, 641, 641**b**
    treatment of, 644
  nonpathologic, 641**b**

Hyperemesis gravidarum, 1014
Hyperglycemia
  hypertension and, 356**b**
  with parenteral nutrition, 622–623, 623**t**, 625**t**
  due to poisoning, 1175**t**
Hyperglycemic hyperosmolar state (HHS), 590–591
  diagnosis of, 591
  monitoring of, 594, 594**t**
  precipitating causes of, 591
  treatment of, 591–594, 594**t**
    dextrose in, 592, 594**t**
    fluids in, 591, 594**t**
    insulin in, 591–592, 594**t**
    potassium in, 592, 594**t**
Hypergonadotropic hypogonadism, 1062
Hyper-IgE syndrome, 860
Hyperinfection syndrome, with *Strongyloides,* 571
Hyperkalemia
  in chronic renal failure, 726–727, 727**t**, 730
  in extremely low birth weight infants, 1039–1040**t**
  hypertension and, 356**b**
  with parenteral nutrition, 625**t**
  due to poisoning, 1175**t**
  due to transfusion, 486**t**
Hyperleukocytosis, in childhood leukemia, 453
Hyperlipidemia
  in chronic renal failure, 729
  defined, 601
  erectile dysfunction due to, 717
  in glomerular disease, 701
Hypermagnesemia, with parenteral nutrition, 625**t**
Hypernatremia
  in chronic renal failure, 726, 727**t**
  diabetes insipidus with, 648–649
  in extremely low birth weight infants, 1039–1040**t**
  postoperative, 648
Hyperopia, 187–188, 188**f**
Hyperosmolar nonketotic dehydration or coma, with parenteral nutrition, 625**t**
Hyperoxaluria, renal calculi due to, 744**t**, 746**t**
Hyperparathyroidism, 649–652
  in chronic renal failure, 727, 730
  clinical forms of, 650
  diagnosis and evaluation of, 650–651
    bone mass measurement in, 651
  differential diagnosis of, 650, 650**t**
  incidence and general characteristics of, 649–650
  pathophysiology, molecular genetics, and pathology of, 650
  signs and symptoms of, 650
  treatment of, 651, 651**t**
Hyperphosphatemia
  due to acromegaly, 635
  in chronic renal failure, 727, 727**t**, 730
Hyperpigmentation disorder(s), 876–878
  acral acanthosis nigricans as, 878
  drug-induced, 877, 877**t**
  etiology and pathogenesis of, 876
  melasma as, 876–877, 877**t**
  postinflammatory, 877–878
  solar lentigo as, 877
  treatment of, 876
Hyperprolactinemia, 659
  amenorrhea due to, 1063, 1063
  causes of, 659, 659**b**
  clinical manifestations of, 659
  diagnosis of, 659–660, 659
  epidemiology of, 659
  long-term management of, 661
  treatment of, 660–661, 660**t**, 660
Hypersensitivity pneumonitis, 280
  diagnosis of, 281
  predictors of, 281**b**
  treatment of, 281, 281**b**

Hypersensitivity reaction(s)
  in allergic contact dermatitis, 870
  due to HAART, 54–55**t**
Hypersensitivity vasculitis. *See* Cutaneous vasculitis.
Hypersomnolence disorders, 889
Hypersplenism, thrombocytopenia due to, 427
Hypertension, 349
  accelerated, 353
  arterial, due to acromegaly, 634
  blood pressure goal for, 353
  borderline, 353
  in chronic renal failure, 727, 727**t**, 729
  classification of, 349, 351**t**
  definitions for, 349–353
  in diabetic children, 588, 589**t**
  drug-related, 359, 359**b**
  erectile dysfunction due to, 716
  essential (idiopathic, primary), 353
  evaluation of, 353–355**b**, 356**b**, 359**b**
  in glomerular disease, 700–701
  and intracerebral hemorrhage, 890–891
  intraglomerular, in chronic renal failure, 728–729
  labile, 353
  malignant, 353
  masked, 352
  measurement of, 351–353
  obesity and, 608
  obstructive sleep apnea and, 240
  pathogenesis of, 353
  and physiologic variability of blood pressure, 349, 350**f**
  portal
    and ascites, 501
    and esophageal varices, 505
  portopulmonary, 497**t**, 501**t**, 503–504
  in postpartum period, 1028
  pre-, 349–350, 351**t**, 351**f**
  during pregnancy, 1021
    chronic, 1022–1024
      classification of, 1022–1023
      clinical findings in, 1022**t**
      diagnosis of, 1022–1023, 1022**b**
      epidemiology of, 1022
      low risk *vs.* high risk, 1022
      maternal and fetal risks with, 1023
      primary (essential) *vs.* secondary, 1022
      treatment of, 1023–1024, 1023**t**, 1023**b**
    definitions and classification of, 1022
    epidemiology of, 1021
    gestational, 1022**t**, 1024
    in HELLP syndrome, 1026–1027
      clinical findings in, 1026–1027
      diagnostic criteria for, 1026, 1026**b**
      intrapartum and postpartum management of, 1027
      mode of delivery with, 1027
    preeclampsia as, 1024–1026
      with chronic hypertension, 1023
      classification of, 1024, 1024**b**
      clinical findings in, 1022**t**, 1024**b**
      defined, 1024
      mild, 1024, 1025, 1025**f**
      mode of delivery with, 1027
      pathogenesis and pathophysiology of, 1024
      prevention of, 1024–1025, 1025**b**
      risk factors for, 1025
      severe, 1024, 1024**b**, 1025–1026, 1026**f**
      treatment of, 1025–1027, 1025**f**, 1026**f**
    due to renal disease, 1022**t**
  prevalence of, 349–350, 350**f**, 352**f**
  pseudo-, 351
  pulmonary
    persistent, of newborn, 1038
    in sickle cell disease, 406, 410
    in systemic sclerosis, 811

Hypertension *(Continued)*
  refractory, 353
  renovascular, 359
  resistant, 353, 359
  secondary, 353, 359–360
  treatment of, 353–359, 360b
    lifestyle modification for, 353
    pharmacologic, 353
      ACE inhibitors for, 356t, 357–358
      aldosterone antagonists for, 356t
      α_1-blockers for, 358
      angiotensin receptor blockers for, 356t, 358
      β-blockers for, 356t, 357
      calcium channel blockers for, 356t, 358
      central α_2-stimulants for, 358–359
      direct vasodilators for, 359
      diuretics for, 356–357, 356t
      dosing strategies and drug efficacy in, 355
      drug classes in, 355–359
      drug selection for, 353–355, 356t
  vascular risks of, 350–351, 352f
  venous, 855
  white coat (office), 352
Hypertensive emergencies, 360
Hypertensive encephalopathy, 350
Hyperthermia, 23, 23b
  malignant, due to MAOIs, 1203
Hyperthyroidism, 665
  causes of, 666b
  classification of, 665
  common features of, 665
  diagnosis of, 665–666
  with elevated radioactive iodine uptake, 665, 666b
  with low radioactive iodine uptake, 665, 666b
  physical examination for, 665
  and pregnancy, 669
  relapses of, 668
  subclinical, 666
  treatment of, 666–669, 667
    general measures and patient education for, 666
    initial treatment of symptoms in, 666–667
    radioactive iodine for, 667, 668
    reduction of serum thyroid hormone levels in, 667
    surgery for, 667, 668–669
    thionamide drug therapy for, 667–668, 667
Hypertonic saline, for elevated intracranial pressure, 967
Hypertriglyceridemia
  hypertension and, 356b
  with parenteral nutrition, 625t
Hypertrophic cardiomyopathy (HCM), 331
  clinical manifestations of, 331–332
  defined, 331
  diagnosis of, 331, 331b
  genetic screening for, 332
  molecular genetics of, 332
  pathogenesis of, 332
  prevalence of, 331
  sudden cardiac death due to, 331–332
  treatment of, 332–334, 332b
    for cardiac arrhythmias, 333
    experimental pharmacologic agents in, 334
    for outflow tract obstruction, 333–334
    by risk of sudden cardiac death, 332
    in symptomatic patients, 332–333
    for syncope, 333
Hypertrophic scars, keloids *vs.*, 820
Hyperuricemia, 599
  asymptomatic, and risk of gout, 599
  chronic, 599–600
  hypertension and, 356b
  treatment of, 599, 600b

Hyperuricosuria, renal calculi due to, 743, 744t, 746t
Hyperventilation
  for cyclic antidepressant intoxication, 1215
  for elevated intracranial pressure, 967
  vertigo due to, 210
Hyperviscosity syndrome, due to multiple myeloma, 472
Hypnagogic hallucinations, 888
Hypnosis, for verrucae, 824
Hypnotics
  abuse of, 1105b, 1107–1108, 1108t
  for insomnia, 887–888, 888t
Hypoallergenic formula, for infants, 1043b
Hypoarousal, after traumatic brain injury, 969
Hypocalcemia
  clinical features of, 652
  diagnosis of, 652
  with parenteral nutrition, 625t
  due to poisoning, 1175t
  treatment of, 652–653
Hypocitraturia, renal calculi due to, 744t, 746t
Hypocomplementemia, 699b
Hypoglycemia
  in diabetic children, 588
  insulin-induced test for, 638, 638b
  due to poisoning, 1173, 1175t
  rebound, with parenteral nutrition, 625t
Hypogonadism
  hypergonadotropic, 1062
  hypogonadotropic, 1062
Hypokalemia
  due to bulimia nervosa, 1116
  hypertension and, 356b
  with parenteral nutrition, 625t
  due to poisoning, 1175t
Hypomagnesemia
  with parenteral nutrition, 625t
  due to poisoning, 1175t
  with ethanol, 1191
Hypomagnesuria, renal calculi due to, 744t
Hypomanic episodes, 1126
Hypomelanosis, idiopathic guttate, 879
Hyponatremia, 595
  acute, 597, 598
  asymptomatic, 598
  due to bulimia nervosa, 1116–1117
  causes of, 595b
  cerebral adaptation to, 597
  chronic, 597–598
  in chronic renal failure, 726, 727t
  classification of, 595b
  defined, 595
  diabetes insipidus with, 647–648, 649
  euvolemic, 596–597, 596f
    medications associated with, 596b
    treatment of, 598f
  evaluation of, 595–597
  hyperosmolar, 595, 595b
  hypervolemic, 596, 596f
  hypo-osmolar, 595
    causes of, 595b
    diagnostic approach to, 595–597, 596f
    volume status in, 595–597
  hypovolemic, 596, 596f
  normo-osmolar, 595, 595b
  pathogenesis of, 595
  pseudo-, 595, 595b
  due to SIADH, 596–597, 597b
  symptoms of, 597
  treatment of, 597–598, 598, 598f
Hyponychium, 816–817, 817f
Hypoparathyroidism, 652–653
  clinical features of, 652
  diagnosis of, 651, 652
  etiology of, 652, 652t
  pseudo-, 652
  treatment of, 651, 652–653

Hypophosphatemia, with parenteral nutrition, 625t
Hypopigmentation disorder(s), 878–879
  etiology and pathogenesis of, 876
  idiopathic guttate hypomelanosis as, 879
  pityriasis alba as, 879
  treatment of, 876
  vitiligo as, 878–879
Hypopituitarism, 656
  defined, 656
  diagnosis of, 656–658, 657
  etiology of, 656, 657t
  pan-, 656
  partial, 656
  treatment of, 658
Hypoplastic left heart (HLH), 331
Hypotension
  due to massive pulmonary embolism, 274
  sepsis-induced, 65
Hypothalamic causes, of amenorrhea, 1062–1063, 1064b
Hypothermia, 1143–1146
  classification of, 1144
  clinical presentation of, 1144
  defined, 1143
  diagnosis of, 1146b
  drugs and chemicals that cause, 1145b
  effect on drug metabolism or clearance of, 1146b
  for elevated intracranial pressure in children, 971
  emergency department evaluation of, 1144–1145
  epidemiology of, 1143
  etiology of, 1143
  for newborn, 1033
  pathophysiology of, 1143–1144
  rewarming for, 1145–1146, 1147b
  risk factors for, 1143, 1144b
  therapeutic, 1147–1148
Hypothyroidism, 661–663
  autoimmune, 662
  central, 662b
  diagnosis of, 662
  etiology of, 662, 662b
  medication-induced, 662, 662b
  myxedema coma due to, 664
  during pregnancy, 664–665
  prevalence of, 662
  primary, 662b
  due to primary biliary cirrhosis, 499
  due to radiation therapy for Hodgkin's disease, 444
  screening for, 663
  secondary, 662, 664
  severe, 663b
  signs and symptoms of, 662, 663b
  subclinical, 663–664
  transient, 662, 662b, 665
  treatment for, 662–663
Hypouricemic therapy, 599, 600, 600b
Hypovolemia, in newborn, 1032
Hypovolemic shock, in newborn, 1032
Hypoxemia
  chronic, in sickle cell disease, 406
  pathophysiologic mechanisms of, 225, 226t
Hypoxemia-induced erythrocytosis, 473
Hypoxia, pathophysiologic mechanisms of, 225, 226t
Hysterectomy
  for cervical cancer
    laparoscopic-assisted radical vaginal, 1087
    radical, 1087
      complications of, 1089b
    cervical cancer after, 1090
  for uterine leiomyoma, 1082, 1082t
Hysterosalpingography (HSG), 1060–1061

Hytone (hydrocortisone ointment), for anogenital pruritus, 872–873
Hytrin. *See* Terazosin hydrochloride (Hytrin).

I

IALT (International Adjuvant Lung Trial), 245–246
Ibandronate (Boniva), for osteoporosis, 614
 postmenopausal, 1073b
IBD. *See* Inflammatory bowel disease (IBD).
IBM (inclusion body myositis), 812, 812t
IBMFSs (inherited bone marrow failure syndromes), *vs.* aplastic anemia, 379, 381t
IBS. *See* Irritable bowel syndrome (IBS).
Ibuprofen (Advil, Motrin)
 for cystic fibrosis, 239
 for dysmenorrhea, 1066t
 for fever, 24, 24
 for juvenile idiopathic arthritis, 985
 for migraine headache, 926
 for osteoarthritis, 1000
 for pain, 2t
 for pericarditis, 370–372
 for renal calculi, 745t
Ibutilide (Corvert), for atrial fibrillation, 311, 311t
ICAR Pediatric Chewables/Suspension (carbonyl iron), 385, 385t
Icatibant, 1244–1249t
ICD. *See* Irritant contact dermatitis (ICD).
ICD (implantable cardioverter-defibrillator), 307–308
 for myocardial infarction, 365
ICD (internal cardioverter-defibrillator) implantation, for hypertrophic cardiomyopathy, 332–333
ICH. *See* Intracerebral hemorrhage (ICH).
ICP. *See* Intracranial pressure (ICP).
ICS(s) (inhaled corticosteroids), for COPD, 234
ICSI (intracytoplasmic sperm injection), 1061
Idarubicin (Idamycin), for acute myeloid leukemia, 445
Idiopathic hyperaldosteronism (IHA), 654
Idiopathic inflammatory myopathy (IIM), 812–813
 clinical characteristics of, 812, 812t
 diagnosis of, 813b
 treatment of, 812–813, 813b
Idiopathic rhinitis, 215, 216
Idiopathic thrombocytopenic purpura (ITP), 426, 427b
IDL (intermediate-density lipoprotein), 601
IEED (involuntary emotional expression disorder), after stroke, 898
IFNs. *See* Interferon(s) (IFNs).
Ig(s). *See* Immunoglobulin(s) (Igs).
IGF-1. *See* Insulin-like growth factor-1 (IGF-1).
IGFBPs (insulin-like growth factor biding proteins), 633, 634f
IHA (idiopathic hyperaldosteronism), 654
IIEF (International Index of Erectile Function), 717b
IIM. *See* Idiopathic inflammatory myopathy (IIM).
IL-6 (interleukin 6), for systemic lupus erythematosus, 809
ILAE (International League Against Epilepsy), 899–900
ILCOR (International Liaison Committee on Resuscitation), on management of cardiac arrest, 302–304, 305f
ILCOR (International Liaison Committee on Resuscitation) guidelines, 1030
ILD (interstitial lung disease)
 in idiopathic inflammatory myopathy, 813
 in systemic sclerosis, 811
Ileal pouch–anal anastomosis (IPAA), for inflammatory bowel disease, 518–519

Ileus, meconium, due to cystic fibrosis, 236
Iloperidone (Zomaril), 1244–1249t
Iloprost (Ventavis), for systemic sclerosis, 811
Imaging, during pregnancy, 1016
Imatinib mesylate (Gleevec)
 for gastrointestinal stromal tumors, 558
 for leukemia
  acute lymphoblastic, 449
  chronic myeloid, 457–458, 458–460, 459b
   failure of, 458–459, 460t
   monitoring of, 458
   toxicity of, 458, 460b
Imdur (isosorbide mononitrate), for angina pectoris, 298, 299t
Imipenem-cilastatin (Primaxin), for necrotizing skin and soft tissue infections, 85t
Imipramine (Tofranil)
 for generalized anxiety disorder, 1113
 for neuropathic pain, 964
 poisoning due to, 1214–1216, 1215t
 for psychiatric dizziness, 209
 for urinary incontinence
  in children, 692t
  mixed, 696
  nocturnal enuresis as, 692
  stress, 696
  urge, 695b
 for vestibular migraine, 209
 for visual vertigo, 210
Imiquimod (Aldara)
 for actinic keratoses, 794
 for Bowen's disease, 834
 for condyloma acuminatum, 825b, 826, 1092
 for keloids, 821–822
 for leishmaniasis, 95–96
 for verrucae, 823
 for vulvar intraepithelial neoplasia, 1092
Imitrex (sumatriptan), for migraine headache, 925t, 926
Immediate-type hypersensitivity, in allergic contact dermatitis, 870
Immersion foot, 1147
Immune complex(es), in serum sickness, 761–762
Immune complex mechanism, of drug-induced hemolytic anemia, 389, 389b
Immune dysregulation polyendocrinopathy, enteropathy, X-linked (IPEX) syndrome, 860
Immune modulators, and SSRIs, 1122–1123b
Immune reconstitution inflammatory syndrome (IRIS), 287–288
 in HIV, 53, 53
Immune suppression, lymphomas with, 466
Immune-mediated platelet destruction, 426
Immunization(s), 147. *See also* Vaccine(s).
 assessment of individual needs for, 148, 152b
 assessment of overall process and outcomes of, 152–153
 change-ups of, 154
 with chronic liver disease, 504
 contraindications to, 154
 decisions to do to, 154
 delivery of, 152
 free-of-charge, 153
 locus of responsibility for, 153
 minimizing discomfort of, 152
 missed or delayed, 153–154
 patient education on, 148–152
 during pregnancy, 1016, 1016b
 preparation for, 152
 prevention of needle injury from, 152
 recall reminders and tracking of, 153
 records of, 152
  incomplete, 154
  sharing of, 152
 registries for, 152
 reporting adverse events with, 153

Immunization(s) *(Continued)*
 requirements for, 148
 schedule for, 148, 149–150t
  catch-up, 151t, 152–153
 shortages of vaccines for, 153
 staff education on, 148
 standing orders for, 153
 for travelers, 158–161, 159b
  doses for, 159–160t
  recommended, 160–161
  required, 159–160
  routine, 158–159
 vaccine storage for, 152
 Vaccines for Children program for, 153
 websites on, 148
Immunization Action Coalition, 148–152
Immunoablation, for systemic lupus erythematosus, 809
ImmunoCAP assay, 779
Immunocompromised hosts
 cat-scratch disease in, 170, 169b
 diarrhea in, 17
 toxoplasmosis in, 164b, 165t, 166t, 167–168, 167b
Immunodeficiency
 lymphomas with, 466
 varicella with, 77–78
Immunoglobulin(s) (Igs)
 intravenous (*See* Intravenous immunoglobulin (IVIg, Endobulin))
 reference intervals for, 1225t
Immunoglobulin A (IgA) nephropathy
 diagnosis of, 700b
 treatment of, 702b, 703
Immunoglobulin E (IgE), in allergic rhinitis, 777
Immunologic function tests, reference intervals for, 1225t
Immunomodulation
 for asthma, 767–768t
 for cutaneous T-cell lymphomas, 800
 for optic neuritis, 197
 for Rh-sensitized women, 418
 for toxic shock syndrome, 89–90
 transfusion-related, 486t, 490–491
Immunoreactive trypsinogen (IRT), in cystic fibrosis, 238
Immunosuppressive therapy (IST)
 for aplastic anemia, 380–382
  long-term complications of, 382–383
 for asthma in children, 775
 for myasthenia gravis, 943, 944t, 945
 reference intervals for, 1222t
Immunotherapy
 for allergic rhinitis, 780–781
 for asthma
  in adolescents and adults, 765
  in children, 775–776
 for chronic lymphocytic leukemia, 462–463, 463
 for epilepsy, in infants and children, 915
 for non-Hodgkin's lymphoma, 466
 venom, 785–786, 785t, 786t
IMNs (internal mammary nodes), in breast cancer, 1050
Imodium (loperamide)
 for acute infectious diarrhea, 19
 for traveler's diarrhea, 155–156, 156t
Imogam (human rabies immune globulin), 131
Imovax (rabies vaccine), 131, 131b
 for travelers, 159–160t, 161
Impavido (miltefosine), for leishmaniasis, 95
Impetigo, 836b, 836–837, 837f
Implanon (progesterone implant), for contraception in postpartum period, 1029t
Implantable cardioverter-defibrillator (ICD), 307–308
 for myocardial infarction, 365
Impotence. *See* Erectile dysfunction (ED).

Imuran. *See* Azathioprine (Imuran, Azasan).
In vitro fertilization (IVF), 1061, 1061f
Inactivated poliovirus vaccine (IPV), schedule for, 149–150t
  catch-up, 151t
Inapsine (droperidol)
  for nausea and vomiting, 8, 8t
  for theophylline intoxication, 1214
Incapacitating agents, as chemical weapons, 1226–1228t
Inclusion body myositis (IBM), 812, 812t
Inclusion conjunctivitis, adult, 195
Incontinence, urinary. *See* Urinary incontinence.
Incretin(s), for diabetes, 580t, 581
Incretin agonists, for diabetes, 580t, 581
Incubator, for neonate, 1036t
Inderal. *See* Propranolol (Inderal).
Indigestion, 11–12. *See also* Dyspepsia.
  due to bile reflux gastritis, 11t
  due to cholelithiasis, 11t
  defined, 11
  drug-induced, 11t
  evaluation of, 11, 11t
  functional, 11
  due to gastroesophageal reflux disease, 11t, 11–12
  due to *Helicobacter pylori* gastritis, 11t, 11–12
  pathophysiology of, 11, 11t
  due to peptic ulcer disease, 11t
  treatment of, 11t, 11–12
Indinavir/ritonavir (Crixivan), for HIV, 50t
  drug interactions with, 58t
Indirect calorimetry, 620
Indomethacin (Indocin)
  for cluster headache, 926t
  for gout, 599
  for patent ductus arteriosus, 1039–1040t
Induction chemotherapy, for acute myeloid leukemia, 445–446
Infancy, defined, 1041
Infanrix (pertussis vaccine), 147, 147t
Infant(s). *See also* Child(ren).
  dehydration of, 628–631
    assessment of, 628–630, 628t, 629t
    classification of, 628, 629
    diagnosis of, 630
    fluid management for, 630–631
      indications for, 630
      with intravenous therapy, 630–631
      maintenance requirements in, 631
      with oral rehydration therapy, 630
      rapid rehydration in, 631
      rehydration requirements (deficit therapy) in, 630–631
      replacement requirements in, 631
    due to gastroenteritis, 628
    laboratory tests for, 628–630, 629–630
    scale for, 629, 629t
    signs of, 628–629, 628t
    weight loss and, 629
  epilepsy in, 907
    absence, 908–909
    assessment of, 910–911
    benign rolandic, 909
    childhood and juvenile, 908–909
    classification of, 907–908, 908b
    defined, 907
    differential diagnosis of, 907–908, 907b
    epidemiology of, 907
    generalized, 908–909, 908b
    localization-related, 909
    myoclonic, 908–909
    syndromes of, 908–910, 908b
    treatment of, 911–915, 912t, 913t
  extremely low birth weight, 1039, 1039–1040t
  growth of, 1044–1045, 1044b
  low-birth-weight, 1035–1037
  premature

Infant(s) (Continued)
  classification of, 1039
  infant formula for, 1043b
  nutrition for, 1035–1037
  resuscitation of, 1032
Infant feeding, 1041
  breast-feeding for, 1041–1042
  caloric requirements for, 1044
  fluoride in, 1042
  and growth, 1044–1045, 1044b
  infant formula for, 1042, 1043b
  introduction of complementary foods in, 1042–1044
  iron in, 1042
  nutritional requirements for, 1044
  obesity and, 1044
  overnutrition in, 1044–1045
  potassium requirements in, 627
  protein requirements in, 1044
  sodium requirements in, 627
  and undernutrition, 1044–1045
  vegetarian diets for, 1044
  vitamin and mineral supplementation of, 1042
  and weight gain, 1044
Infant formula, 1042, 1043b
  hypoallergenic, 1043b
Infantile spasms, 909
Infection(s)
  bacterial skin (*See* Bacterial skin infection(s))
  delirium due to, 1119
  vs. fibromyalgia, 996b
  hemolytic anemia due to, 391t, 394
  laryngitis due to, 218
  nausea and vomiting due to, 6, 6t
  in neutropenia, 413
  pleural space, 257–258
  during pregnancy, 1014–1015
  puerperal, 1028
  in rheumatoid arthritis, 977b
  seizures due to, 899t
  in sickle cell disease, 405–406, 409–410
  viral respiratory, 264
    bronchiolitis as, 266
    common colds as, 265
    croup as, 265–266
    diagnosis of, 265b
    etiology of, 264–265
    influenza-like illness due to, 265
    treatment of, 265b
Infection control, for pressure ulcers, 859
Infection stones, 744t, 746t
Infectious agents, atopic dermatitis due to, 860
Infectious complications, of transfusions, 485t, 489–490, 490b
Infectious disease(s)
  amebiasis as, 59
  anthrax as, 123
  bacterial meningitis as, 112
  brucellosis as, 72
  cat-scratch disease as, 169
  cholera as, 78
  chronic fatigue syndrome as, 117
  foodborne illness as, 81
  giardiasis as, 61
  HIV as, 45
  infectious mononucleosis as, 116
  influenza as, 90
  leishmaniasis as, 93
  leprosy as, 97
  Lyme disease as, 136
  malaria as, 103
  measles (rubeola) as, 141
  mumps as, 121
  necrotizing skin and soft tissue infections as, 83
  office-based immunization practices for, 147
  pertussis as, 146
  plague as, 122

Infectious disease(s) (Continued)
  psittacosis as, 127
  Q fever as, 128
  rabies as, 130
  rat bite fever as, 131
  relapsing fever as, 133
  rickettsial and ehrlichial infections as, 176
  rubella and congenital rubella syndrome as, 140
  salmonellosis as, 170
  severe sepsis and septic shock as, 65
  smallpox as, 179
  tetanus as, 143
  toxic shock syndrome as, 86
  toxoplasmosis as, 163
  in travel medicine, 155
  typhoid fever as, 174
  varicella (chickenpox) as, 76
Infectious mononucleosis, 116
  clinical manifestations of, 116
  diagnosis of, 116–117, 116b, 116t
  epidemiology of, 116
  etiology of, 116
  treatment of, 117, 117b
Infectious neuropathies, 963–964
Infective endocarditis, 342
  acute, 342
  antibiotic prophylaxis for, 345–347
    conditions not needed in, 348t
    indications for, 348t
    preprocedural, 347t
  clinical manifestations of, 343
  diagnosis of, 343–345, 345b, 346b
  epidemiologic changes in, 342
  factors predisposing to, 343b
  forms of, 342
  microbiology of, 342–343, 344t
  native valve, 342, 343b
  nosocomial, 342, 343b
  prosthetic valve, 342, 343b
  subacute, 342
  treatment of, 345–347, 349b
    antibiotics for, 345, 346–347t
    surgical, 345
InFeD (iron dextran), 386
Inferior petrosal sinus sampling (IPSS), for Cushing's syndrome, 644, 644
Inferior vena cava (IVC) filter, for deep venous thrombosis/pulmonary embolism, 273
Infertility, 1060
  age and, 1060, 1060f
  assisted reproductive technology for, 1061, 1061f
  clomiphene citrate for, 1061
  defined, 1060
  diagnosis of, 1061b
  endometriosis-associated, 1056–1057, 1057f, 1061
  epidemiology of, 1060
  gonadotropin ovulation induction for, 1061
  hysterosalpingography for, 1060–1061
  in vitro fertilization for, 1061, 1061f
  intracytoplasmic sperm injection for, 1061
  male-factor, 1060
  menstrual cycle and, 1061
  treatment of, 1061b
  uterine factors in, 1060–1061
Infiltrative disorders, malabsorption due to, 543–544
Inflammation, in childhood asthma, 770
Inflammatory back pain, due to ankylosing spondylitis, 987
Inflammatory bowel disease (IBD), 514
  clinical features of, 515
  colon cancer surveillance with, 521
  defined, 514–515
  diagnosis of, 515, 515b
  management strategies for, 519–520

Inflammatory bowel disease (IBD) *(Continued)*
  natural history of, 515
  pathogenesis of, 514–515
  pregnancy with, 520–521
  treatment of, 515**b**
    alternative therapy in, 519
    nutritional support in, 518
    pharmacologic, 515–518
      aminosalicylates for, 515–516
      antibiotics/probiotics for, 517–518
      anticytokine therapy for, 517
      azathioprine/6-mercaptopurine for, 516–517
      corticosteroids for, 516
      cyclosporine for, 517
      experimental therapies for, 518
      methotrexate for, 517
    surgical, 518–519
Inflammatory diseases, malabsorption due to, 543
Inflammatory fibrous hyperplasia, of alveolar process/gingiva, 854
Inflammatory myopathy, idiopathic, 812–813
  clinical characteristics of, 812, 812**t**
  diagnosis of, 813**b**
  treatment of, 812–813, 813**b**
Inflammatory papillary hyperplasia (IPH), of hard palate, 851–852
Infliximab (Remicade)
  for ankylosing spondylitis, 987, 988
  for arthritis
    juvenile idiopathic, 985–986
    rheumatoid, 980, 981, 981**t**
  for inflammatory bowel disease, 517, 520
  for psoriasis, 803, 803**t**
  for systemic lupus erythematosus, 809
Influenza, 90
  acute bronchitis due to, 260, 260**b**
  avian, 90
  chemoprophylaxis for, 92, 92**t**, 266–267
  clinical manifestations of, 267
  complications of, 92
  epidemiology of, 9091, 266
  evaluation of, 91–92, 92**b**
  microbiology of, 90
  pneumonia due to, 266–267
    with bacterial superinfection, 267
    clinical manifestations of, 267
    diagnosis of, 267, 268**b**
    etiology and pathogenesis of, 266
    prevention of, 266–267
    treatment of, 267, 267**t**, 269**b**
  treatment of, 92–93, 92**t**, 93**b**, 267, 267**t**
  types of, 90
Influenza vaccine (Fluzone, FluMist, Fluvirin, Fluarix, FluLevel), 90–91, 91**b**, 91
  for COPD, 234–235
  schedule for, 149–150**t**
Influenza virus, meningitis or encephalitis due to, 928–930**t**, 932
Influenza-like illness, 265
Infrainguinal bypass, for chronic limb ischemia, 373–374
Ingrown nails, 817**b**, 818**b**, 819
INH. *See* Isoniazid (INH, Nydrazid, Laniazid).
Inhalants, abuse of, 1111
Inhalation exposure, to toxins, 1161
Inhalation injury, 1139
Inhalation therapy, laryngitis due to, 219
Inhaled corticosteroids (ICSs), for COPD, 234
Inhaled nitric oxide (INO), for high-altitude sickness, 1143
Inherited bone marrow failure syndromes (IBMFSs), *vs.* aplastic anemia, 379, 381**t**
Inocor (amrinone), for poisoning
  due to β-blockers, 1183
  due to calcium channel blockers, 1184
Insect(s), parasitic skin infections due to, 30**b**

Insect stings, allergic reactions to, 784
  diagnosis of, 784–785, 784**b**
  epidemiology of, 784
  localized *vs.* systemic, 784
  pathogenesis of, 784
  prevention of, 785–786, 786**t**
  risk of future, 785, 785**t**
  treatment and avoidance of, 785, 785**b**
Insecticides, poisoning due to, 1205–1206
Insensible fluid losses, 627, 627**t**
Insomnia, 887–888, 887**t**, 888**t**
Inspra (eplerenone), for aldosteronism, 656
Insulin
  for calcium channel blocker intoxication, 1184
  for diabetes mellitus
    in adults, 581–582, 582**t**
      barriers to use of, 581
      basal, 580**t**, 582, 582**t**
      dosage of, 580**t**
      effects of, 580**t**
      fix the fasting first rule for, 582
      fixed-ratio combined, 582–583, 582**t**
      initiation of, 579, 581–582
      meal, 580**t**, 582, 582**t**
      pattern management for, 582
      preparations of, 582**t**
    in children, 586–587, 586, 587**t**
      initiation of, 584–585, 585**f**
      total daily dose of, 585, 585**f**
  for diabetic ketoacidosis, 591–592, 592**t**, 593**t**
  for hyperglycemic hyperosmolar state, 591–592, 594**t**
Insulin aspart (Novolog), for diabetes
  in adults, 582**t**
  in children, 586–587, 587**t**
Insulin detemir (Levemir), for diabetes
  in adults, 582, 582**t**
  in children, 587**t**
Insulin glargine (Lantus), for diabetes
  in adults, 582, 582**t**
  in children, 586, 587**t**
Insulin glulisine (Apidra), for diabetes
  in adults, 582**t**
  in children, 587**t**
Insulin lispro (Humalog), for diabetes
  in adults, 582**t**
  in children, 586–587, 587**t**
Insulin mixtures, for diabetes mellitus
  in adults, 582–583, 582**t**
  in children, 587**t**
Insulin pump, for diabetes mellitus in children, 586–587
Insulin resistance, 575
  due to acromegaly, 635
  obesity and, 607–608
  obstructive sleep apnea and, 240
Insulin secretagogues, for diabetes, 578–580, 580**t**
Insulin zinc preparation, for diabetes in children, 587**t**
Insulin-induced hypoglycemia test, 638, 638**b**
Insulin-like growth factor biding proteins (IGFBPs), 633, 634**f**
Insulin-like growth factor-1 (IGF-1), 633, 634**f**
  consequences of excess of, 634–635
  measurement of, 635
Insulin-to-carbohydrate ratio, 586
Intal (cromolyn sodium inhaler), for asthma
  in adolescents and adults, 767–768**t**
  in children, 773–774**t**, 775
Integrase inhibitors, for HIV, 49, 50**t**
Integrilin (eptifibatide)
  for myocardial infarction, 364
  for unstable angina pectoris, 301, 301**t**
Intense pulsed light (IPL), for verrucae, 823
Intercourse, during pregnancy, 1016
Interferon(s) (IFNs), for verrucae, 823
Interferon-α (IFN-α) modulation, for systemic lupus erythematosus, 809

Interferon-α-2a (IFN-α-2a, Roferon-A), for cutaneous T-cell lymphomas, 799
Interferon-α-2b (IFN-α-2b, Intron-A)
  for cutaneous T-cell lymphomas, 799
  for hepatitis B and C viruses, 536**t**
  for keloids, 821
  for polycythemia vera, 34**b**
Interferon-β-1 (IFN-β-1), for multiple sclerosis, 936–937, 937**t**
Interferon-β-1a (IFN-β-1a, Avonex, Rebif)
  for multiple sclerosis, 936
  for optic neuritis, 197
Interferon-β-1b (IFN-β-1b, Betaseron)
  for multiple sclerosis, 936
  for optic neuritis, 197
Interferon-γ (IFN-γ) assays (QuantiFERON-TB assays), for tuberculosis, 283
Interictal state, 901
Interleukin 6 (IL-6), for systemic lupus erythematosus, 809
Intermediate-density lipoprotein (IDL), 601
Intermenstrual bleeding, 1059
Internal cardioverter-defibrillator (ICD) implantation, for hypertrophic cardiomyopathy, 332–333
Internal jugular venous sampling, for Cushing's syndrome, 644
Internal mammary nodes (IMNs), in breast cancer, 1050
International Adjuvant Lung Trial (IALT), 245–246
International Federation of Gynecology and Obstetrics (FIGO) staging system
  for cervical cancer, 1087**b**
  for endometrial cancer, 1083, 1084**t**
  for vulvar cancer, 1093**b**
International Index of Erectile Function (IIEF), 717**b**
International League Against Epilepsy (ILAE), 899–900
International Liaison Committee on Resuscitation (ILCOR), on management of cardiac arrest, 302–304, 305**f**
International Liaison Committee on Resuscitation (ILCOR) guidelines, 1030
International Prognostic Index (IPI), for Hodgkin's lymphoma, 434–435, 435**t**
International Prostate Symptom Score (IPSS), 713–716, 713**f**
International Staging System (ISS), for multiple myeloma, 468, 468**t**
International System of Units (SI Units), 1217–1218, 1217**t**, 1218**t**, 1218**t**
Interpersonal psychotherapy (IPT), for major depression, 1124
Interstitial lung disease (ILD)
  in idiopathic inflammatory myopathy, 813
  in systemic sclerosis, 811
Interstitial nephritis, acute renal failure due to, 722**b**, 723–724
Intertrigo, 847–848
Intestinal dysfunction, parenteral nutrition with, 625
Intestinal parasite(s), 563
  amoebae as, 563–567, 565–566**t**
  Anisaka spp as, 570**t**, 572
  Ascaris lumbricoides as, 569, 570**t**
  Balantidium coli as, 565–566**t**, 567
  Blastocystis hominis as, 565–566**t**, 567
  cestodes as, 570**t**, 573
  ciliates as, 563–567
  Cryptosporidium spp as, 565–566**t**, 567–568
  Cyclospora cayetanensis as, 565–566**t**, 568
  diagnosis of, 563, 564**b**
  Dientamoeba fragilis as, 565–566**t**, 567
  Diphyllobothrium latum as, 570**t**, 573
  Encephalocytozoon intestinalis as, 565–566**t**
  Entamoeba histolytica as, 563–564, 565–566**t**

Intestinal parasite(s) *(Continued)*
  Enterobius vermicularis as, 570t, 572
  Enterocytozoon bineusi as, 565–566t
  flagellates as, 563–567
  Giardia lamblia as, 564–567, 565–566t
  helminths as, 569–573, 570t
  hookworm as, 570t, 571
  Isospora belli as, 565–566t, 568
  microsporidia as, 565–566t, 568–569
  nematodes as, 569–572, 570t
  protozoa as, 563–567, 565–566t
    spore-forming, 565–566t, 567–569
  Pseudoterranova decipiens as, 570t, 572
  Schistosoma spp as, 570t, 572–573
  signs and symptoms of, 564b
  Strongyloides as, 570t, 571–572
  Taenia spp as, 570t, 573
  trematodes as, 570t, 572–573
  whipworm as, 569–571, 570t
Intoxication(s). *See* Poisoning(s).
Intraabdominal infections, sepsis due to, 68t
Intra-articular injections, for osteoarthritis, 1000–1001
Intracerebral hemorrhage (ICH), 890
  diagnosis of, 891, 891b
  epidemiology and etiology of, 890–891, 890b
  scoring system for, 891, 891t
  treatment of, 891–892, 892b
Intracerebral hemorrhage (ICH) score, 891, 891t
Intraclavicular nodal involvement, in breast cancer, 1050
Intracranial aneurysm, orofacial pain due to, 992t
Intracranial conditions, orofacial pain due to, 991, 992t
Intracranial hemorrhage, in sickle cell disease, 411
Intracranial pressure (ICP), elevated, due to traumatic brain injury
  in children, 971
  monitoring of, 967
  Monroe-Kellie doctrine for, 966–967
  treatment of, 967–968, 967b
Intracytoplasmic sperm injection (ICSI), 1061
Intradialytic parenteral nutrition, 624
Intraductal carcinoma, 1049, 1050
Intrafascicular ventricular tachycardia, 323
Intrahepatic cholestasis of pregnancy, pruritus due to, 32b
Intraocular pressure (IOP), in glaucoma, 198, 199
Intraoral appliances, for temporomandibular disorder, 993
Intraparenchymal hematomas, 966
Intrapericardial therapy, for pericarditis, 372
Intraperitoneal (IP) chemotherapy, for ovarian cancer, 1096
Intrauterine devices (IUDs), 757
  for emergency contraception, 758
  in postpartum period, 1029t
  progestin-releasing, 757
    for menorrhagia, 1059
    in postpartum period, 1029t
Intravaginal contraceptive ring (NuvaRing), 756
  in postpartum period, 1029t
Intravenous (IV) fluids, for infants and children
  maintenance, 626–628
    electrolyte requirements for, 627, 627t
    fluid requirements for, 626–627, 627t
    glucose in, 627
    method for prescribing, 627–628
    volume of, 628
  for rehydration, 630–631
    deficit therapy in, 630–631
    indications for, 630
    maintenance requirements in, 631
    rapid, 631
    replacement requirements in, 631

Intravenous immunoglobulin (IVIg, Endobulin)
  for bullous pemphigoid, 867
  for chronic inflammatory demyelinating polyneuropathy, 962
  for Guillain-Barré syndrome, 962
  for myasthenia gravis, 945–946
  for pemphigus vulgaris, 869
  for Stevens-Johnson syndrome and toxic epidermal necrolysis, 864b, 865
  for systemic lupus erythematosus, 809
  for toxic shock syndrome, 89–90
  for warm autoimmune hemolytic anemia, 388
Intravenous methylprednisolone (IVMP), for optic neuritis, 197, 197
Intraventricular hemorrhage (IVH), in extremely low birth weight infants, 1039–1040t
Intrinsic sphincter deficiency (ISD), 693, 695b, 696
Intron-A. *See* Interferon-α-2b (IFN-α-2b, Intron-A).
Intropin. *See* Dopamine (Intropin).
Invasive fungal rhinosinusitis, 214
Invirase (saquinavir/ritonavir hard gel), for HIV, 50t, 51t
  drug interactions with, 58t
Involuntary emotional expression disorder (IEED), after stroke, 898
Involved field irradiation, for Hodgkin's lymphoma, 440, 443f
Iodides, exogenous, for thyroid storm, 669
Iodine, radioactive, for hyperthyroidism, 667, 668
Iodoquinol (diiodohydroxyquin, Yodoxin)
  for acute infectious diarrhea, 19–20t
  for balantidiasis, 565–566t
  for cutaneous amebiasis, 843
  for dientamoebiasis, 565–566t, 567
  for *Entamoeba histolytica*, 564, 565–566t
Ion channel abnormality, cardiac arrest due to, 303t
Ionizing radiation, during pregnancy, 1016
IOP (intraocular pressure), in glaucoma, 198, 199
Iopanoic acid, for thyroid storm, 669
IP (intraperitoneal) chemotherapy, for ovarian cancer, 1096, 1096
IPAA (ileal pouch–anal anastomosis), for inflammatory bowel disease, 518–519
Ipecac syrup, for poisoning, 1163
IPEX (immune dysregulation polyendocrinopathy, enteropathy, X-linked) syndrome, 860
IPH (inflammatory papillary hyperplasia), of hard palate, 851–852
IPI (International Prognostic Index), for Hodgkin's lymphoma, 434–435, 435t
IPL (intense pulsed light), for verrucae, 823
Ipratropium bromide (Atrovent)
  for allergic rhinitis, 780, 780t
  for asthma
    in adolescents and adults, 766t
    in children, 772b, 774–775
  for common cold, 28b
  for nonallergic rhinitis, 217b
  for postnasal drip syndrome, 28b
  for traumatic brain injury, 968
Ipratropium bromide with albuterol (Combivent, DuoNeb), for asthma, 766t
IPSS (International Prostate Symptom Score), 713–716, 713f
IPSS (inferior petrosal sinus sampling), for Cushing's syndrome, 644
IPT (interpersonal psychotherapy), for major depression, 1124
IPV (inactivated poliovirus vaccine), schedule for, 149–150t
  catch-up, 151t
Iridocyclitis, juvenile idiopathic arthritis with, 984

Irinotecan (Camptosar), for small cell lung cancer, 248
Iris, 187, 188f
IRIS (immune reconstitution inflammatory syndrome), 287–288
  in HIV, 53
Iris registration, 189, 192f
Iron
  carbonyl, 385, 385t
  for chronic renal failure, 729–730
  dietary, 383–385
  heme *vs.* nonheme, 383
  for infants, 1042, 1042
  kinetics of, 1194
  normal metabolism of, 383
  in parenteral nutrition, 621
  during pregnancy, 1014
  total body, 383
Iron deficiency, 383
  causes of, 383–384
  iron replacement therapy for, 384–386, 386b
    adverse effects of, 385t
    failure of, 386
  laboratory abnormalities with, 384, 384t, 385b
  signs and symptoms of, 384, 385b
Iron deficiency anemia, 384t
  pruritus due to, 32b
Iron dextran (InFeD, Dexferrum), 386
Iron gluconate (Ferrlicit), 386
Iron overload
  in hemochromatosis, 432, 433
  in sickle cell disease, 409, 412
  in thalassemia, 401–402
    assessment of, 401
    chelation therapy for, 401–402, 403t
    complications of, 399t
  due to transfusion, 486t
Iron poisoning, 1194–1195
Iron replacement therapy, 384–386, 386b
  adverse effects of, 385t
  failure of, 386
Iron salts, 385–386, 385t
Iron sucrose (Venofer), 386
Irradiated platelets, 482
Irradiated red blood cells, 481
Irritable bowel syndrome (IBS), 521
  alarm symptoms in, 523, 523b
  Bristol stool chart for, 521, 522f
  defined, 521
  diagnosis of, 522–523, 523b, 523f
  diagnostic criteria for, 521, 522b
  differential diagnosis of, 523
  epidemiology of, 521–522
  pathogenesis of, 522
  prognosis for, 522
  subtypes of, 521, 522b
  treatment of, 523–525, 524b, 524t
Irritant(s), atopic dermatitis due to, 860
Irritant contact dermatitis (ICD), 788
  diagnosis of, 870, 870b
  pathogenesis of, 870
  treatment of, 870–871, 871b
Irritant rhinitis, 777–778
Irritation fibroma, of buccal mucosa, 851
IRT (immunoreactive trypsinogen), in cystic fibrosis, 238
Ischemic cerebrovascular disease, 893
  diagnosis of, 893, 894, 894b
  epidemiology and etiology of, 893
  ischemic stroke due to, 894
  pathophysiology of, 893
  prevention of, 894–895, 897
  risk factors for, 893
  symptoms of, 893
  transient ischemic attacks due to, 893–894
Ischemic heart disease
  hypertension and, 353
  ventricular arrhythmias in, 325–326

Ischemic stroke, 894
  clinical features of, 893.894
  diagnosis of, 893, 894, 894**b**
  epidemiology of, 893
  pathophysiology of, 893, 894
  prevention of, 894–895, 897
  risk factors for, 893
  in sickle cell disease, 407
  treatment of, 894, 895**b**
ISD (intrinsic sphincter deficiency), 693, 695**b**, 696
Isentress (raltegravir), 1243
  for HIV, 50**t**
Isolated tumor cells (ITCs), in breast cancer, 1050
Isometheptene with dichloralphenazone and acetaminophen (Midrin, Duradrin), for migraine headache, 925
Isoniazid (INH, Nydrazid, Laniazid)
  intoxication due to, 1195–1196
  kinetics of, 1195
  for *Mycobacterium kansasii*, 289
  peripheral neuropathy due to, 963
  for tuberculosis, 285**t**, 286**t**, 287**t**, 287**b**, 288**t**
    in HIV, 56**t**
  for tuberculous pericarditis, 371
Isopropanol
  features of, 1190**t**
  kinetics of, 1196
  poisoning due to, 1196
  and serum osmolality, 1176**t**
Isopropyl alcohol poisoning, 1196
Isoproterenol (Isuprel)
  for cyclic antidepressants intoxication, 1215–1216
  for heart block, 318
Isoptin. *See* Verapamil (Calan, Isoptin, Verelan).
Isosorbide dinitrate (Isordil), for angina pectoris, 298, 299**t**
Isosorbide mononitrate (Imdur), for angina pectoris, 298, 299**t**
Isospora belli, 565–566**t**, 568
  malabsorption due to, 544
Isosporiasis, 565–566**t**, 568
Isotretinoin (Accutane, Sotret)
  for acne, 788
  for rosacea, 789
Isradipine (DynaCirc), intoxication with, 1183–1184
ISS (International Staging System), for multiple myeloma, 468, 468**t**
IST. *See* Immunosuppressive therapy (IST).
Istalol (timolol)
  for glaucoma, 200
  intoxication with, 1182–1183, 1183**t**
Isuprel (isoproterenol)
  for cyclic antidepressants intoxication, 1215–1216
  for heart block, 318
Itard, Jean, 919
ITC(s) (isolated tumor cells), in breast cancer, 1050
Itching. *See* Pruritus.
ITP (idiopathic thrombocytopenic purpura), 426, 427**b**
Itraconazole (Sporanox)
  for blastomycosis, 255, 255**b**
  for coccidioidomycosis, 250**b**, 250**t**, 251**t**
    acute, 250–251
    chronic, 251
  for fungal skin infections with HIV, 848–849
  for histoplasmosis, 253, 253**t**, 253**b**, 254
  for leishmaniasis, 95
  for onychomycosis, 818, 818**b**
  for tinea
    cutaneous, 848**b**
    unguium, 847, 848**b**
    versicolor, 805

IUDs. *See* Intrauterine devices (IUDs).
IV fluids. *See* Intravenous (IV) fluids.
IVC (inferior vena cava) filter, for deep venous thrombosis/pulmonary embolism, 273
Ivermectin (Stromectol)
  for *Ascaris*, 565–566**t**
  for cutaneous larva migrans, 844, 844**t**
  for larva currens, 844**t**, 845
  for onchodermatitis, 844**t**, 845
  for scabies, 844**t**, 846
  for strongyloidiasis, 570**t**
  for trichuriasis, 570**t**, 571
IVF (in vitro fertilization), 1061, 1061**f**
IVH (intraventricular hemorrhage), in extremely low birth weight infants, 1039–1040**t**
IVIg. *See* Intravenous immunoglobulin (IVIg, Endobulin).
IVMP (intravenous methylprednisolone), for optic neuritis, 197
Ixabepilone (Ixempra), 1243

J

JAK2 gene, in polycythemia vera, 472, 473
Janumet (sitagliptin/metformin), 1243
Januvia (sitagliptin), for diabetes, 580**t**, 581
Japanese encephalitis vaccine (JE Vax), for travelers, 159–160**t**
Japanese encephalitis virus, 927, 928–930**t**
Jarisch-Herxheimer reaction (JHR), 135, 135**b**
Jaundice
  differential diagnosis of, 496**b**
  in extremely low birth weight infants, 1039–1040**t**
JE Vax (Japanese encephalitis vaccine), for travelers, 159–160**t**
Jejunoileal diverticula, 512**b**, 513, 513**b**
Jellyfish envenomation, 1158, 1158**b**
Jet lag, 158
JHR (Jarisch-Herxheimer reaction), 135, 135**b**
JIA. *See* Juvenile idiopathic arthritis (JIA).
Jimsonweed, poisoning due to, 1179–1180
Joint lavage, for osteoarthritis, 1001
Jumper's knee, 1008
Junctional complexes, premature, 313
Junctional reciprocating tachycardia, permanent form of, 322
Junin virus, as biological weapon agent, 1229–1233**t**
Juvenile idiopathic arthritis (JIA), 983
  enthesitis related, 984
  epidemiology of, 983–984
  evaluation of, 984–985, 984**b**
  oligoarthritis (pauciarthritis) with iridocyclitis as, 984
  polyarthritis forms of, 984
  prognosis for, 985
  psoriatic, 984
  rheumatoid factor in, 984
  subtypes of, 984
  systemic, 984
  treatment of, 985–986, 985**b**

K

Kadian. *See* Morphine sulfate (Avinza, Kadian, MS Contin, Oramorph SR, MSIR).
Kala-azar. *See* Leishmaniasis, visceral.
Kaletra (lopinavir/ritonavir), for HIV, 50**t**, 51**t**
  drug interactions with, 58**t**
Kanamycin (Kantrex), for tuberculosis, 285**t**
Kangaroo care, for high-risk neonate, 1037
Kaposi's varicelliform eruption, 840
Katayama's fever, 572
Kava kava, 1234–1243**t**
Kayser-Fleischer (KF) rings, 500
Keflex. *See* Cephalexin (Keflex).
Kelfer (deferiprone), for thalassemia, 402, 403**t**

Kell antigen system, 418–419
Keloids, 820
  clinical features of, 820
  diagnosis of, 820**b**
  vs. hypertrophic scars, 820
  treatment of, 820–822, 821**b**
Kenalog. *See* Triamcinolone (Kenalog).
Keppra. *See* Levetiracetam (Keppra).
Keratectomy, photorefractive, 189, 191**f**
  complications of, 192**f**, 193
Keratitis, HSV, 840
Keratoconjunctivitis
  adenovirus (epidemic), 194, 195
  atopic, 859
Keratoconus, 192**f**
Keratolytic agents, for psoriasis, 802
Keratomileusis
  laser in situ, 189, 190**f**
    complications of, 190–193, 192**f**
    waverfront-guided, 189, 191**t**
  laser-assisted subepithelial, 189, 191**f**
Keratosis(es), actinic, 833–834
  clinical features of, 793, 833
  diagnosis of, 794**b**, 833**b**
  epidemiology of, 793
  of lips, 833**b**, 834, 834**b**, 850
  treatment of, 794, 794**b**, 833–834, 834**b**
Kerion, 792, 847
Kerlone (betaxolol), intoxication with, 1182–1183, 1183**t**
Ketamine (Ketalar), for asthma in children, 772**b**
Ketek (telithromycin)
  for legionellosis, 271**t**
  for mycoplasmal pneumonia, 270, 270**t**
Ketoacidosis, diabetic. *See* Diabetic ketoacidosis (DKA).
Ketoconazole (Nizoral)
  for blastomycosis, 255, 255**b**
  for coccidioidomycosis, 250**t**, 251**t**
    acute, 250–251
    chronic, 251
  for Cushing's syndrome, 645**t**
  for cutaneous candidiasis, 848**b**
  for histoplasmosis, 254
  for leishmaniasis, 94**b**, 95
  for tinea
    cutaneous, 848**b**
    versicolor, 805, 847, 848**b**
Ketogenic diet
  for epilepsy
    in adolescents and adults, 906
    in infants and children, 915
  for Lennox-Gastaut Syndrome, 909
Ketoprofen (Orudis, Oruvail), for dysmenorrhea, 1066**t**
Ketorolac (Toradol)
  for pain, 2**t**
  for renal calculi, 744–745, 745**t**
KF (Kayser-Fleischer) rings, 500
Kiacta (eprodisate), 1244–1249**t**
Kidney(s)
  myeloma, 471
  trauma to, 706–707
    complications of, 707
    diagnosis of, 707, 707**b**
    grading of, 707, 707**t**, 707**f**
    surgical exploration for, 707
    treatment of, 708**b**
Kidney disease
  chronic, hypertension and, 350, 353, 356**t**, 359
  due to hyperparathyroidism, 650
Kidney injury, acute. *See* Acute renal failure (ARF).
Kidney stones. *See* Renal calculi.
Kineret (anakinra), for arthritis
  juvenile idiopathic, 985–986
  rheumatoid, 981**t**, 982
KKIT, for tinnitus, 39

Klebsiella granulomatis, granuloma inguinale due to, 749–750
Klonopin. *See* Clonazepam (Klonopin).
Knee
 jumper's, 1008
 osteoarthritis of, 1008
  pain due to, 4
  prophylactic measures for, 999, 999b
Knee injuries, due to sports, 1007–1008
Knott and Voss proprioceptive neuromuscular facilitation, for stroke rehabilitation, 896b
Koebner phenomenon, 801, 817, 819, 878
Kohl, lead in, 1197
Koplik's sports, 142
Kostmann's syndrome, and childhood leukemia, 452t
"Kusmusha" teapots, lead in, 1197
Kussmaul breathing, 591
Kuvan (sapropterin), 1243
Kwell (lindane)
 for pediculosis, 845
 for scabies, 846
K-Y Plus (nonoxynol-9), 757
Kytril (granisetron), for nausea and vomiting, 7, 8t

L

La Cross virus, meningitis or encephalitis due to, 928–930t
L-α-acetylmethadol (LAAM), for opiate withdrawal, 1108–1109
LABAs. *See* Long-acting β₂ agonists (LABAs).
LABC (locally advanced breast cancer), 1051f, 1054
Labetalol (Normodyne, Trandate)
 for angina pectoris, 299t
 for hypertension in pregnancy, 1023t, 1027
 intoxication with, 1182–1183, 1183t
 for MAOI intoxication, 1203
Labial mucosa, disorders of, 850–851
Laboratory sleep test, for obstructive sleep apnea, 240
Laboratory tests, reference intervals for. *See* Reference intervals.
Labyrinthectomy, for Ménière's disease, 212
Lacosamide, for epilepsy, 904t
Lactase deficiency, 543
Lactation, leprosy in, 101–102
Lactational amenorrhea method, 1029t
Lactational mastitis, 1046
Lactic acidosis, due to HAART, 54–55t
Lactinol, for hepatic encephalopathy, 502–503
Lactulose (Cephulac), for hepatic encephalopathy, 502–503
LAIV (live, attenuated influenza vaccine), 91
 schedule for, 149–150t
L-AmB. *See* Amphotericin B, liposomal (L-AmB, AmBisome).
Lambert-Eaton myasthenic syndrome (LEMS), 946–947
Lamisil. *See* Terbinafine (Lamisil).
Lamivudine (Epivir)
 for hepatitis B and C viruses, 536t, 537
 for HIV, 50t, 51t
 resistance to, 51
Lamotrigine (Lamictal)
 for bipolar disorder, 1127, 1127
 for epilepsy
  in adolescents in adults, 904t, 903
  in infants and children, 908–909, 914, 913t
 for neuropathic pain, 964t, 964–965
Lampit (nitrofurtimox), for Chagas' disease, 843, 844t
Lamprene (clofazimine), for leprosy, 101, 101b
Landau-Kleffner syndrome, 910
Language disorders, stroke rehabilitation for, 897
Laniazid. *See* Isoniazid (INH, Nydrazid, Laniazid).

Lanoxin. *See* Digoxin (Lanoxin).
Lanreotide (Somatuline), 1243
 for acromegaly, 636
Lansoprazole (Prevacid)
 for gastroesophageal reflux disease, 28b, 553–554, 554t
 for indigestion, 11t
 for peptic ulcer disease, 531t, 532t
Lanthanum (Fosrenol), for chronic renal failure, 730
Lantus (insulin glargine), for diabetes
 in adults, 582, 582t
 in children, 586, 587t
Lanugo hairs, 790
Laparoscopic cholecystectomy, 494
Laparoscopic cholecystectomy and bile duct exploration (LC+BDE), 495–496
Laparoscopic-assisted radical vaginal hysterectomy (LARVH), for cervical cancer, 1087
Lapatinib (Tykerb), 1243
Large artery involvement, in hypertension, 351
Lariam (mefloquine), for malaria, 108t, 109, 111–112t, 157, 157t
Larva currens, 844t, 845
Laryngeal edema, 220
Laryngeal fracture, 219
Laryngeal hemorrhage, 219
Laryngitis, 218–219
 acute, 218–219
 chronic, 219–220
 diagnosis of, 218–219, 218b
 etiology of, 218
 treatment of, 219, 219b
 and voice production, 218, 218b
 when to refer for, 219
Laryngopharyngeal reflux (LPR), 219–220
LASEK (laser-assisted subepithelial keratomileusis), 189, 191f
Laser destruction, of verrucae, 823
Laser in situ keratomileusis (LASIK), 189, 190f
 complications of, 190–193, 192f
 waverfront-guided, 189, 191t
Laser therapy, for keloids, 822
Laser trabeculoplasty, for glaucoma, 200
Laser vision correction (LVC), 187
 anatomy and physiology of eye and, 187, 188f
 assessment of visual function for, 188–189
 background of, 187, 188f
 complications of, 190–193, 192f
 iris registration for, 189, 192f
 laser in situ keratomileusis (LASIK) for, 189, 189, 190f
  complications of, 190–193, 192f
  waverfront-guided, 189, 191t
 laser-assisted subepithelial keratomileusis (LASEK) for, 189, 189, 191f
 photorefractive keratectomy (PRK) for, 189, 191f
  complications of, 192f, 193
 procedure for, 189
 recent advances in, 189, 191t, 192f
 refractive errors and, 187–188, 188f
 screening examinations for, 189–190, 192f
Laser-assisted subepithelial keratomileusis (LASEK), 189, 191f
LASIK. *See* Laser in situ keratomileusis (LASIK).
Lasix. *See* Furosemide (Lasix).
L-asparaginase (Elspar), for acute lymphoblastic leukemia, 449
Lassa virus, as biological weapon agent, 1229–1233t
Latanoprost (Xalatan), for glaucoma, 199–200
Latent tuberculosis infection (LTBI), 282
 diagnosis of, 282–283
 treatment of, 286–287, 288t
Lateral epicondylosis, 1009
Latrodectus envenomation, 1151

Laxatives, for constipation, 10t, 22, 22b
LBRF (louse-borne relapsing fever)
 clinical manifestations of, 133–134, 134
 epidemiology of, 133, 134t
LBW (low-birth-weight) infant, nutrition for, 1035–1037
LC+BDE (laparoscopic cholecystectomy and bile duct exploration), 495–496
LCIS (lobular carcinoma in situ), 1048–1049, 1049–1050
LDL cholesterol. *See* Low-density lipoprotein (LDL) cholesterol.
Lead, reference intervals for, 1224t
Lead poisoning, 1196–1200
 disposition for, 1200
 epidemiology of, 1196
 hobbies associated with, 1197, 1198b
 kinetics of, 1197
 laboratory investigations of, 1198–1199, 1199t
 management of, 1199–1200, 1200t
 manifestations of, 1198t
 due to occupational exposure, 1196t, 1197
 and recommended lead content, 1197, 1198b
 screening for, 1196, 1197t
 sources of, 1196–1197, 1197t
 toxic dose in, 1196
 toxic mechanism in, 1196–1197
 due to traditional folk remedies, 1197
Lea's shield, 757
Leflunomide (Arava)
 for juvenile idiopathic arthritis, 985–986
 for rheumatoid arthritis, 981–982, 981t
Left ventricular (LV) dysfunction
 hypertension and, 353
 after myocardial infarction, 366t
Left ventricular hypertrophy, hypertension and, 350
Left ventricular outflow tract obstruction, due to hypertrophic cardiomyopathy, 333–334
Leg(s), pruritus of, 31f
Leg cramps, during pregnancy, 1016
Leg ulcers, in sickle cell disease, 407, 411
Legionellosis, 270
 clinical features of, 271
 diagnosis of, 261–262, 271
 epidemiology of, 270
 historical background of, 270
 vs. mycoplasmal pneumonia, 269
 pathogenesis of, 270
 treatment of, 271, 271t
Leiomyomas, uterine, 1081
 diagnosis of, 1081, 1081b
 epidemiology of, 1081
 management of, 1081–1082, 1082t, 1082b
 pathophysiology of, 1081
 symptoms and signs of, 1081
Leiomyosarcoma, of vulva, 1094
Leishmania. *See* Leishmaniasis.
Leishmaniasis, 93
 clinical features of, 94
 cutaneous, 843, 844t
  clinical features of, 94
  diffuse, 96
   epidemiology of, 94
   pathogenesis of, 93
  epidemiology of, 93–94
  treatment of, 94b, 96, 844t
 epidemiology of, 93–94
 mucocutaneous
  clinical features of, 94
  epidemiology of, 94
  pathogenesis of, 93
  treatment of, 94b, 96
 pathogenesis of, 93
 treatment of, 94–96, 94b
  amphotericin B for, 94–95
  azoles for, 95
  combination therapy for, 96

Leishmaniasis *(Continued)*
 imiquimod for, 95–96
 miltefosine for, 95
 paromomycin for, 95
 pentamidine for, 95
 pentavalent antimonials for, 94
 physical methods for, 96
 sitamaquine for, 95
 visceral (kala-azar)
  anthroponotic, 96
  clinical features of, 94
  epidemiology of, 93
  pathogenesis of, 93
  treatment of, 94b
  zoonotic, 96
LEMS (Lambert-Eaton myasthenic syndrome), 946–947
Lenalidomide (Revlimid, CC-5013)
 for cutaneous T-cell lymphomas, 800
 for multiple myeloma, 469b, 470, 471
Lennox-Gastaut Syndrome (LGS), 909
Lens, 187, 188f
Lente insulin, for diabetes in children, 587t
Lentigo, solar (senile), 877
Lepirudin (Refludan), for deep venous thrombosis/pulmonary embolism, 273
Lepra bonita, 100
Lepromin test, for leprosy, 100
Leprosy, 97
 borderline borderline (BB), 98–99, 98t, 99f
 borderline lepromatous (BL), 98t, 99, 99f
 borderline tuberculoid (BT), 98, 98t, 98f
 clinical features of, 97–99, 98t
 diagnosis of, 100b
  clinical, 99–100
  laboratory, 100
 epidemiology of, 97
 etiopathogenesis of, 97
 histoid, 100–101, 101f
 with HIV infection, 102
 indeterminate, 97, 98f
 lepromatous (LL), 98t, 99, 99f
 Lucio (LuLp), 100, 103
 nerve involvement in, 99, 100f
 peripheral neuropathy due to, 964
 in pregnancy and lactation, 101–102
 prevention of, 103
 prevention of disabilities and rehabilitation for, 103
 pure neuritic, 100
 rare variants of, 100–101
 reactions in, 102–103
  type 1 (reversal, RR), 102, 102f
  type 2 (erythema nodosum leprosum, ENL), 102–103
 systemic involvement in, 99
 treatment of, 101–102, 102b, 101b0
 tuberculoid (TT), 97–98, 98t
 with tuberculosis, 102
 types of, 97–99, 98t, 100
 WHO strategy for, 103
Leptomeninges, melanosis of, 828
Leriche's syndrome, 292
LES (lower esophageal sphincter), hypertensive, 510, 511
Lescol (fluvastatin)
 for angina pectoris, 298
 for dyslipoproteinemia, 605t
Lesional tachycardias, 323
Letairis (ambrisentan), 1243
Letrozole (Femara), for breast cancer, 1053
Leucovorin. *See* Folinic acid (Leucovorin).
Leukemia(s)
 acute
  in adults, 444
   classification of, 444–445, 446b
   diagnosis of, 444, 445b, 445t
   lymphoblastic, 446b, 447b, 449

Leukemia(s) *(Continued)*
   myeloid, 445–448, 446b, 447b
   prognostic factors for, 445, 446b
   promyelocytic, 429, 448–449
   treatment of, 445–449, 448t
  in children, 450
   classification of, 450, 450t, 450b
   clinical presentation of, 452–453, 453b
   differential diagnosis of, 454
   epidemiology of, 450–451, 451f
   etiology of, 451–452, 452t
   medical emergencies in, 453–454
   prognosis for, 451
   relapse of, 455–456
   risk stratification for, 454
   treatment of, 454–455, 455t, 456, 456t
  lymphoblastic, 444
   classification of, 446b, 450, 450t
   prognostic factors for, 446b
   treatment of, 447b, 449
  myeloid, 444
   classification of, 446b, 450, 450b
   etiology of, 444
   prognostic factors for, 446b
   treatment of, 445–448, 447b
  promyelocytic
   disseminated intravascular coagulation in, 429
   treatment of, 448–449
 Burkitt's, 447b, 449
 chronic, 456
  lymphocytic, 460–463
   clinical staging and prognostic factors for, 461, 461t
   diagnosis of, 457b, 459b, 461
   differential diagnosis of, 461, 461t
   incidence and risk factors for, 460–461
   treatment of, 459b, 461–463, 462t, 463t
  myeloid, 456–457
   clinical features and diagnosis of, 456–457, 457b
   initial evaluation and treatment objectives for, 457, 458b
   natural history of, 457, 458t
   prognostic categories for, 457
   treatment of, 457–460, 460b, 459b, 460t
 classification of, 450
 defined, 450
 lymphoblastic/lymphocytic
  acute, 444
   in children, 450
   classification of, 446b
   prognostic factors for, 446b
  chronic, 460–463
   clinical staging and prognostic factors for, 461, 461t
   diagnosis of, 457b, 459b, 461
   differential diagnosis of, 461, 461t
   incidence and risk factors for, 460–461
   treatment of, 459b, 461–463, 462t, 463t
 minimal residual disease in, 444
 myeloid
  acute, 444
   in children, 450
   classification of, 446b
   etiology of, 444
   prognostic factors for, 446b
   treatment of, 445–448, 447b
  chronic, 456–457
   clinical features and diagnosis of, 456–457, 457b
   initial evaluation and treatment objectives for, 457, 458b
   natural history of, 457, 458t
   prognostic categories for, 457, 457
   treatment of, 457–460, 460b, 459b, 460t
Leukeran. *See* Chlorambucil (Leukeran).
Leukocyte cell counts, reference intervals for, 1219t

Leukocytoclastic vasculitis, 814
Leukocytosis, in sickle cell disease, 404
Leukoedema, of buccal mucosa, 851
Leukoencephalopathy, progressive multifocal, natalizumab and, 935
Leukokeratosis, of lip, 833b, 834, 834b
Leukoplakia
 of floor of mouth, 853
 of lip, 833b, 834, 834b
Leukoreduced platelets, 482
Leukoreduced red blood cells, 480–481
Leukotriene modifiers
 for asthma
  in adolescents and adults, 767–768t
  in children, 773–774t
 for urticaria, 875
Leukotriene receptor antagonists
 for allergic rhinitis, 779
 for asthma
  in adolescents and adults, 767–768t
  in children, 775
Leuprolide acetate (Lupron)
 for acute porphyria, 477–478
 for dysmenorrhea, 1065
 for endometriosis, 1056
 for premenstrual syndrome, 1069
 for uterine leiomyoma, 1082
Leustatin (cladribine), for chronic lymphocytic leukemia, 462
Levalbuterol (R-albuterol, Xopenex), for asthma
 in adolescents and adults, 766t
 in children, 774–775, 775t
Levamisole, for *Ascaris*, 569
Levaquin. *See* Levofloxacin (Levaquin).
Level of consciousness, with poisonings, 1161, 1161, 1163t
Levemir (insulin detemir), for diabetes
 in adults, 582, 582t
 in children, 587t
Levetiracetam (Keppra)
 for epilepsy
  in adolescents in adults, 904t
  in infants and children, 908–909, 914, 913t
 for multiple sclerosis, 939b
Levitra (vardenafil), for erectile dysfunction, 718–719
 in multiple sclerosis, 939b
Levobunolol (AKBeta eyedrop, Betagan)
 for glaucoma, 200
 intoxication with, 1182–1183, 1183t
Levocetirizine (Xyzal), 1243
Levodopa, for parkinsonism, 954–955
Levofloxacin (Levaquin)
 for bacterial overgrowth, 10t
 for *Chlamydia trachomatis*, 1078b
 for diarrhea
  acute infectious, 18b, 19–20t
  traveler's, 156t
 for epididymitis, 697b, 698
 for legionellosis, 271t
 for marine injuries, 1159t
 for mycoplasmal pneumonia, 270, 270t
 for necrotizing skin and soft tissue infections, 85t
 for nongonococcal urethritis, 753
 for pelvic inflammatory disease, 1080b
 for plague, 123
 for pyelonephritis, 685, 706b
 for tuberculosis, 285t
 for urinary tract infections in males, 681t
Levonorgestrel/ethinyl estradiol (Lybrel), 1243
Levonorgestrel-releasing intrauterine device (Mirena), 757
 for menorrhagia, 1059
 in postpartum period, 1029t
Levophed. *See* Norepinephrine (Levophed).

Levothyroxine (L-thyroxine, Synthroid, Levothroid, Levoxyl)
  for hypopituitarism, 658
  for hypothyroidism, 663
    during pregnancy, 664–665
  for myxedema coma, 664
  for thyroiditis
    chronic, 678
    subacute, 677
Levsin (hyoscyamine), for urinary incontinence
  in children, 691, 692t
  urge, 695b
Lewisite, as chemical weapon, 1226–1228t
Lewy bodies, dementia with, 881, 954
Lexapro. See Escitalopram (Lexapro).
Lexipafant, for acute pancreatitis, 548
Lexiva (fosamprenavir), for HIV, 50t, 51t
Leydig cell tumors, 739–740
LGS (Lennox-Gastaut Syndrome), 909
LHRH (luteinizing hormone–releasing hormone) analogues, for prostate cancer, 732
Lialda (multi-matrix mesalamine), for inflammatory bowel disease, 516
Liberatory maneuver, 206, 206f
Librium. See Chlordiazepoxide (Librium).
Lice, 30b, 844t, 845
Lichen planopilaris, 792
Lichen planus, 30b, 804
  of buccal mucosa, 851
  of nails, 804, 817
Lichen sclerosis (LS), 872, 872b
Lichen sclerosis et atrophicus, urethral stricture disease due to, 740
Lichen simplex chronicus (LSC), 30b, 872, 872b
Lidex (fluocinonide)
  for atopic dermatitis, 860–861
  for vitiligo, 878–879
Lidocaine (Xylocaine)
  for cardiac arrest, 306
  for hiccups, 12–13, 13b
  for myocardial infarction, 365
  for neonatal seizures, 910
  for premature ventricular complexes, 314
  for tinnitus, 38, 38, 38, 38
Lidocaine hydrochloride monohydrate (Zingo), 1243
Lidocaine topical (Lidoderm), for pain, 3
Lie to stand, for vestibular neurolabyrinthitis, 207b
Lifestyle changes
  for diabetes, 576b, 577–578, 578f
  for dyslipoproteinemia, 604, 604b
  for gastroesophageal reflux disease, 553
  for hypertension, 353
Lifestyle concerns, in rheumatoid arthritis, 977b
Li-Fraumeni syndrome, and childhood leukemia, 452t
Light chain deposition disease, 471
Light destruction, of verrucae, 823
Light-chain myeloma, 467–468
Lightning injury, 1138
Light's criteria, for pleural effusion, 257, 257t
Lindane (Kwell, Gamene)
  for pediculosis, 845, 845
  for scabies, 846
Linea alba, oral, 851
Linea nigra, 1012
Linezolid (Zyvox)
  for necrotizing skin and soft tissue infections, 85
  for osteomyelitis, 1006–1007
  for pyelonephritis, 685
Lioresal (baclofen)
  for multiple sclerosis, 939b
  for traumatic brain injury, 967, 968
Lip(s)
  disorders of, 849–850
  leukokeratosis or leukoplakia of, 833b, 834, 834b

Lipid(s), categories of, 601, 602t
Lipid disorders
  obesity and, 608
  pathogenesis of, 601–602
Lipid emulsion, for high-risk neonate, 1035
Lipid goals, for diabetes, 576b
Lipid metabolism, abnormalities in, due to acromegaly, 635
Lipid profile, 602
Lipitor. See Atorvastatin (Lipitor).
Lipodermatosclerosis, 855
Lipodystrophy, due to HAART, 54–55t
Lipoprotein(s), categories of, 601, 602t
5-Lipoxygenase inhibitor, for asthma, 767–768t
Liquid diet preparations, 609
Liquid nitrogen
  for keloids, 821
  for solar lentigines, 877
  for verrucae, 822–823
Liraglutide, 1244–1249t
Lisdexamfetamine dimesylate (Vyvanse), 1243
Lisinopril (Prinivil, Zestril), for myocardial infarction, 365t
Listeria monocytogenes, foodborne illness due to, 83
Listeriosis, 83
Lithium (Lithobid, Eskalith, Lithane)
  for bipolar disorder, 1126–1127
  for cluster headache, 926t
  intoxication due to, 1200–1201
  kinetics of, 1200
  nephrogenic diabetes insipidus due to, 649
Lithostat (acetohydroxamic acid), for renal calculi, 746t
Little Leaguers' shoulder, 1009
Live, attenuated influenza vaccine (LAIV, FluMist), 91
  schedule for, 149–150t
Liver abscess, amebic, 563–564
  clinical presentation of, 59–60
  diagnosis of, 60, 60t
  treatment of, 61, 61t
Liver biopsy, for hemochromatosis, 433
Liver disease, due to thalassemia, 399t, 402
Liver dysfunction
  hypertension and, 356b
  due to parenteral nutrition, 626, 626b
Liver failure, parenteral nutrition with, 624
Liver function tests, cholestatic, 496b
Liver injury, antituberculous drug induced, 286–287
Liver spots, 877
Liver transaminases, elevated, with parenteral nutrition, 625t
Liver transplantation (LT)
  for acetaminophen poisoning, 1177–1178
  for chronic liver disease, 504
  for hepatorenal syndrome, 503
LMWH (low-molecular-weight heparin)
  for deep venous thrombosis/pulmonary embolism, 273, 273b
  for myocardial infarction, 364
Loa loa, 844, 844t
Lobular carcinoma in situ (LCIS), 1048–1050
Lobular hyperplasia, atypical, 1047
Locally advanced breast cancer (LABC), 1051f, 1054
Lockjaw, 143
Locomotion, stroke rehabilitation for, 896
Locomotor system disorder(s)
  ankylosing spondylitis as, 986
  bursitis, tendinitis, myofascial pain, and fibromyalgia as, 994
  juvenile idiopathic arthritis as, 983
  osteoarthritis as, 998
  osteomyelitis as, 1005
  polymyalgia rheumatica and giant cell arteritis as, 1002

Locomotor system disorder(s) (Continued)
  rheumatoid arthritis as, 977
  due to sports injuries, 1007
  temporomandibular disorders and orofacial pain as, 988
Lodine (etodolac)
  for osteoarthritis, 1000
  for pain, 2–3, 2t
Lodrane XR (brompheniramine), for allergic rhinitis, 779t
Lofgren's syndrome, 276
LoHist 12 Hours (brompheniramine), for allergic rhinitis, 779t
Loiasis, 844, 844t
Lomefloxacin (Maxaquin), for urinary tract infections in males, 681t
Lomotil (diphenoxylate natiopine), intoxication with, 1204–1205, 1205t
Long QT syndrome (LQTS), 324, 324t
Long-acting β_2 agonists (LABAs)
  for asthma
    in adolescents and adults, 767–768t
    in children, 773–774t, 775
  for COPD, 234
Long-term care patients, male, urinary tract infections in, 681
Loop diuretics
  for heart failure, 339t
  for hypertension, 357
Loose anagen syndrome, 791
Loperamide (Imodium)
  for acute infectious diarrhea, 19
  for traveler's diarrhea, 155–156, 156t
Lopid (gemfibrozil), for dyslipoproteinemia, 605, 605t
Lopinavir/ritonavir (Kaletra), for HIV, 50t, 51t
  drug interactions with, 58t
Lopressor. See Metoprolol (Lopressor).
Loprox (ciclopirox), for onychomycosis, 818
Loratadine (Claritin, Alavert)
  for allergic rhinitis, 779t
  for urticaria, 875
Loratadine/pseudoephedrine (Claritin-D 12, Alavert-D, Claritin-D 24), for allergic rhinitis, 779t
Lorazepam (Ativan)
  for alcohol withdrawal, 1101, 1106b
  for Alzheimer's disease, 884, 885t
  for delirium, 1120
  intoxication with, 1181–1182
  for motion sickness and vertigo, 206t
  for nausea and vomiting, 8t
  for status epilepticus, 906
Lortab. See Hydrocodone + acetaminophen (Lortab, Maxidon, Norco, Vicodin, Xodol, Zydone).
Losartan (Cozaar), for systemic sclerosis, 811t
Losigamone, for epilepsy, 904t
Lotrimin (clotrimazole) cream, for cutaneous candidiasis, 847, 848b
Lotronex (alosetron), for irritable bowel syndrome, 524–525
Louse-borne relapsing fever (LBRF)
  clinical manifestations of, 133–134
  epidemiology of, 133, 134t
Lovastatin (Mevacor, Altocor)
  for angina pectoris, 298
  for dyslipoproteinemia, 605t
Lovenox (enoxaparin)
  for myocardial infarction, 364, 366
  for unstable angina pectoris, 301t
Low-birth-weight (LBW) infant, nutrition for, 1035–1037
Low-carbohydrate ketogenic diets, 609
Low-density lipoprotein (LDL) cholesterol, 601, 602t
  and angina pectoris, 297–298
  and coronary artery disease, 602–603

Low-density lipoprotein (LDL) cholesterol (Continued)
  in diabetic children, 588–589
  screening for, 602
Lower esophageal sphincter (LES), hypertensive, 510, 511
Lower leg pain, due to sports, 1008–1009
Lower urinary tract dysfunction, 690
Lower urinary tract symptoms (LUTS), of benign prostatic hyperplasia, 713–716
Low-molecular-weight heparin (LMWH)
  for deep venous thrombosis/pulmonary embolism, 273, 273**b**
  for myocardial infarction, 364
Low-salt diet, for preeclampsia, 1024
Loxapine (Loxitane), poisoning due to, 1208–1209, 1208**t**
Loxosceles envenomation, 1150–1151
Lozol (indapamide), for hypertension, 356–357
LPR (laryngopharyngeal reflux), 219–220
LQTS (long QT syndrome), 324, 324**t**
LS (lichen sclerosis), 872, 872**b**
LSC (lichen simplex chronicus), 30**b**, 872, 872**b**
LT. *See* Liver transplantation (LT).
LTBI. *See* Latent tuberculosis infection (LTBI).
L-thyroxine. *See* Levothyroxine (L-thyroxine, Synthroid, Levothroid, Levoxyl).
Lubiprostone (Amitiza), for constipation, 10**t**, 22, 22**b**
Lubricants, for constipation, 22, 22**b**
Lucio leprosy (LuLp), 100, 103
Lucio's phenomenon, 103
Ludiomil (maprotiline), poisoning due to, 1214–1216, 1215**t**
Lugol's solution, for thyroid storm, 669
Lumbar radicular pain
  natural course of, 41, 41
  pathophysiology of, 40
Lumigan (bimatoprost), for glaucoma, 199–200
Lumpectomy. *See* Breast conservation therapy (BCT).
Lund-Browder Classification, of burns, 1135, 1137**f**
Lunesta (eszopiclone), for insomnia, 888, 888**t**
Lung abscess, 258
  clinical features of, 258
  diagnosis of, 258–259, 258**b**
  etiology of, 258
  treatment of, 259, 259**b**
Lung cancer, 242
  due to asbestosis, 279
  clinical presentation of, 243
  epidemiology of, 242
  functional evaluation of, 243–245, 245**b**
  non–small cell
    pathology of, 243
    staging of, 243–244
    treatment for, 245–247
      advanced and metastatic, 247–248, 247**t**
      local, 245–246
      locoregional, 246–247
  pathology of, 243
  screening for, 242–243
  small cell
    pathology of, 243
    staging of, 243, 244
    treatment for, 248
  staging of, 243–245, 244**b**, 244**t**
  treatment of, 245–248
    follow-up after, 248
    for non–small cell disease, 245–247
      advanced and metastatic, 247–248, 247**t**
      local, 245–246
      locoregional, 246–247
    for small cell disease, 248
Lung injury, acute, 229–230
Lung transplantation
  for COPD, 236
  for cystic fibrosis, 239

Lung volume reduction surgery (LVRS), for COPD, 236
Lunula, 816–817, 817**f**
Lupron. *See* Leuprolide acetate (Lupron).
Lupus erythematosus
  hair disorders due to, 792
  systemic (*See* Systemic lupus erythematosus (SLE))
Lutein, 1234–1243**t**
Luteinizing hormone–releasing hormone (LHRH) analogues, for prostate cancer, 732
LUTS (lower urinary tract symptoms), of benign prostatic hyperplasia, 713–716
Luvox (fluvoxamine)
  for major depression, 1123
  for obsessive compulsive disorder, 1114, 1114**t**
LV. *See* Left ventricular (LV).
LVC. *See* Laser vision correction (LVC).
LVRS (lung volume reduction surgery), for COPD, 236
Lybrel (levonorgestrel/ethinyl estradiol), 1243
Lycopene, 1234–1243**t**
Lyme arthritis, 137, 138
Lyme disease, 136
  clinical features of, 136–137
  diagnosis of, 137**b**
  early, 136–137
  epidemiology of, 136
  laboratory testing in, 137–138, 137**b**
  late, 137
  peripheral neuropathy due to, 964
  persistent (treatment-resistant), 138
  postexposure prophylaxis for, 139
  post-Lyme disease syndrome after, 138–139
  prevention of, 139
  treatment of, 138–139, 138**b**, 139**t**
Lyme vaccine (LYMErix), 139
Lymphatic filariasis, 844, 844**t**
Lymphatic sac decompression/shunting, for Ménière's disease, 212
Lymphoblastic/lymphocytic leukemia
  acute, 444
    in children, 450
    classification of, 446**b**
    prognostic factors for, 446**b**
  chronic, 460–463
    clinical staging and prognostic factors for, 461, 461**t**
    diagnosis of, 457**b**, 459**b**, 461
    differential diagnosis of, 461, 461**t**
    incidence and risk factors for, 460–461
    treatment of, 459**b**, 461–463, 462**t**, 463**t**
Lymphocyte subsets, whole blood, heparinized, reference intervals for, 1225**t**
Lymphocytic choriomeningitis virus, 928–930**t**
Lymphoma(s)
  B-cell, 464**t**
    diffuse large, 466
  Burkitt's, 464, 466
  cutaneous T cell (*See* Cutaneous T-cell lymphomas (CTCL))
  follicular, 465
  gastric, 557**b**, 558
  Hodgkin's (*See* Hodgkin's lymphoma)
  indolent, 464, 465–466
  lymphoblastic, 464, 466
  non-Hodgkin's, 464
    classification of, 464, 464**t**
    epidemiology and genetics of, 464
    evaluation, staging, and prognosis for, 464–465, 465**b**
    treatment of, 465–466, 465**b**
  primary CNS, 975
  related to immune suppression or deficiency, 466
  related to infectious agents, 466
  small lymphocytic, 465

Lymphoma(s) (Continued)
  T-cell and NK cell, 464**t**
  of testis, 740
Lyrica. *See* Pregabalin (Lyrica).
Lysodren (mitotane), for Cushing's syndrome, 645**t**

M

M protein, in multiple myeloma, 467–468
M2 inhibitors, for influenza, 265
MA (microalbuminemia), in diabetic children, 588, 589**t**
Ma huang, 1234–1243**t**
MAC. *See* Mycobacterium avium intracellulare complex (MAC).
Mace, as chemical weapon, 1226–1228**t**
Macroadenomas, 633
  hyperprolactinemia due to, 661
Macrobid. *See* Nitrofurantoin (Macrobid, Macrodantin).
Macrodantin. *See* Nitrofurantoin (Macrobid, Macrodantin).
Macroglossia, 853
Macrolide antibiotics
  for leprosy, 102**b**
  and SSRIs, 1122–1123**b**
Macula, 188**f**
MADSAM (multifocal acquired demyelinating sensory and motor neuropathy), 962
Magnesium, in parenteral nutrition, 622**t**
Magnesium sulfate
  for acute porphyria, 477
  for asthma in children, 772**b**, 775
  during labor and delivery, with preeclampsia, 1027
  for poisoning, 1167–1172**t**
    due to cyclic antidepressants, 1215–1216
    due to ethanol, 1191
    due to neuroleptics, 1209
Magnetic resonance imaging (MRI), of breast, 1048
Maintenance chemotherapy, for acute myeloid leukemia, 447
Maintenance fluids, for infants and children, 626–628
  electrolyte requirements for, 627, 627**t**
  fluid requirements for, 626–627, 627**t**
  glucose in, 627
  method for prescribing, 627–628
  volume of, 628
Majocchi's granuloma, 846, 847**b**
Major depression, 1120–1126
  diagnosis of, 1120–1121, 1120**b**
  differential diagnosis of, 1121
  epidemiology of, 1120
  substance abuse and, 1121
  and suicide, 1120, 1120–1121
  treatment of, 1121–1126
    antidepressant drugs for, 1121–1124, 1122–1123**b**
    brain stimulation for, 1126
    phases of, 1121, 1121**f**
    psychotherapy for, 1124
    treatment-resistant, 1124–1126, 1125**f**
Malabsorption, 539
  bile acid, 541**b**, 542, 545
  carbohydrate, 541**b**, 542
  causes of, 539, 540**b**
  due to celiac disease, 541**b**, 543
  defined, 539
  diagnosis of, 539–542, 540**b**
  due to disaccharidase deficiency, 543
  evaluation of suspected, 542–543, 542**f**
  fat, 541, 541**b**
  fructose, 543
  gaseousness due to, 10, 10**t**
  generalized (pan-), 539, 543–545

Malabsorption (Continued)
  glucose-galactose, 543
  due to infiltrative disorders, 543–544
  due to inflammatory diseases, 543
  due to *Mycobacterium avium–intracellulare*, 544
  due to pancreatic exocrine insufficiency, 541b, 542, 545
  due to parasitic diseases, 544
  postoperative, 545
  protein, 541–542, 541b
  due to small bowel bacterial overgrowth, 541b, 542, 544
  specific, 539, 543
  symptoms and signs of, 539–540, 540b
  systemic diseases associated with, 540b
  tests for, 540–542, 541b
  due to transport defects at brush border, 543
  treatment of, 541b
  due to tropical sprue, 544
  vitamin B$_{12}$, 541b, 542
  due to Whipple's disease, 544
  due to Zollinger-Ellison syndrome, 545
Malaria, 103
  cerebral, 106
  chemoprophylaxis for, 110–112, 111–112t, 156–157, 157t
  in children, 108t, 110
  clinical features of, 104–106, 106b
  congenital, 110
  diagnosis of, 106–107, 106b
  drug-resistant, 105t, 107–108–110
  epidemiology of, 103–104, 105t, 156
  etiology of, 103, 104, 105f
  imported, 103–104
  locally acquired, 104
  personal protective measures for, 106, 157–158, 157b
  in pregnancy, 107b, 110
  quartan, 104
  relapse of, 104
  severe
    clinical features of, 104–106
    diagnosis of, 106
    treatment of, 107b, 110
  in travel medicine, 103–104
    after return, 162
  treatment of, 107–110, 107b, 108t
Malarone (atovaquone-proguanil), for malaria, 108t, 109, 111–112t, 156, 157t
Malassezia furfur, 804–805, 847
Malassezia sympodialis, 859, 860
Malathion, poisoning due to, 1205–1206
Maldigestion, 539
  evaluation of suspected, 542f
  symptoms and signs of, 540b
  systemic diseases associated with, 540b
Male breast cancer, 1053
Male condoms, 757
  in postpartum period, 1029t
Male sterilization, 758
Malignant hyperthermia, due to MAOIs, 1203, 1203, 1203
Malignant melanoma. *See* Melanoma.
Malignant melanoma in situ (MMIS), 832
Mallet deformity, of distal interphalangeal joint, 1010
Malnutrition, index of, 619
Mammography
  BI-RADS classification for, 1048, 1049t
  screening, 1048, 1048
Mandibular tori/exostoses, 854
Manganese, in parenteral nutrition, 621, 621t
Manic episode, 1126, 1126b
Mannitol (Osmitrol)
  for ciguatera poisoning, 1156, 1157t
  for elevated intracranial pressure, 967
    in children, 971

Mannitol (Osmitrol) (Continued)
  for glaucoma, 200
  for heat stroke, 1149b, 1149–1150
Mantle field irradiation, for Hodgkin's lymphoma, 440–441, 442f
Mantoux method, 282–283
MAO-B (monoamine oxidase B) inhibitors, for parkinsonism, 957
MAOIs. *See* Monoamine oxidase inhibitors (MAOIs).
Maprotiline (Ludiomil), poisoning due to, 1214–1216, 1215t
Maraviroc (Selzentry), 1243
  for HIV, 50t
Marburg virus, as biological weapon agent, 1229–1233t
Marfan syndrome
  aortic aneurysm in, 292
  aortic dissection in, 293
  mitral valve prolapse in, 336
"Maria Louisa," lead in, 1197
Marijuana
  abuse of, 1110
  for nausea and vomiting, 8–9
Marine envenomations, 1158–1159
  due to cone shells, 1159
  diagnosis of, 1156b
  due to echinoderms, 1158–1159
  due to jellyfish, 1158, 1158b
  due to other venous sea creatures, 1159
  due to seasnakes, 1159
  due to stingrays, 1159
  treatment of, 1158b, 1159t
Marine injuries, 1159–1160
  diagnosis of, 1156b
  due to environmental hazards, 1159–1160
  due to sharks, 1160, 1160b
  treatment of, 1158b, 1157t, 1160b
Marine poisonings, 1155–1158
  due to ciguatera, 1155–1157, 1156b, 1157t
  due to contaminated bivalves, 1157
  diagnosis of, 1156b
  due to puffer fish, 1158
  due to scombroid, 1157
  due to shellfish, 1157–1158
  treatment of, 1158b
Marinol (dronabinol), for nausea and vomiting, 8–9, 8t
Mask of pregnancy, 876
Massage therapy, for high-risk neonate, 1037
Massive transfusion coagulopathy, 486t, 491–492
Mast cell(s), in anaphylaxis, 759
Mast cell stabilizer
  for allergic rhinitis, 780, 780t
  for asthma in children, 773–774t
Mastectomy, 1052
  for ductal carcinoma in situ, 1050
Mastitis, 1028, 1046
Mastocytosis, systemic, 760
Maturity-onset diabetes of the young (MODY), 575, 583–584
Maxair (pirbuterol chlorofluorocarbon), for asthma
  in adolescents and adults, 766t
  in children, 774–775, 775t
Maxalt (rizatriptan), for migraine headache, 925t, 926
Maxaquin (lomefloxacin), for urinary tract infections in males, 681t
Maxidon. *See* Hydrocodone + acetaminophen (Lortab, Maxidon, Norco, Vicodin, Xodol, Zydone).
Maxipime (cefepime)
  for bacterial meningitis, 115t
  for osteomyelitis, 1006–1007
Maxzide-25 (hydrochlorothiazide and triamterene), for Ménière's disease, 211

MB isoforms of creatine kinase (CK-MB)
  in myocardial infarction, 361
  in pericarditis, 369–370
MCA-PV (middle cerebral artery peak velocity), for Rh-sensitized women, 417–418
MCD (minimal change disease)
  diagnosis of, 700b, 700b
  treatment of, 701, 702b
MCL (medial collateral ligament) tears, 1008
MCP (metacarpophalangeal) joint, injuries to, 1010
MCV4. *See* Meningococcal polysaccharide diphtheria toxoid conjugate vaccine (MCV4, Menactra).
MDA (3,4-methylenedioxyamphetamine), intoxication with, 1178–1179
MDAC (multiple dose activated charcoal), for theophylline intoxication, 1213–1214
MDMA (3,4-methylenedioxymethamphetamine)
  abuse of, 1110
  intoxication with, 1178–1179
MDR (multidrug-resistant) typhoid fever, 174, 175, 176t
MDRD (Modification of Diet in Renal Disease) formula, for creatinine clearance, 725–726, 726
MDR-TB (multidrug-resistant), 282, 284b, 288
MDT (multidrug therapy), for leprosy, 101, 101b
Measles, 141
  atypical, 142
  clinical features of, 142
  complications of, 142
  diagnosis of, 142, 142b
  epidemiology of, 141–142
  German (*See* Rubella)
  meningitis or encephalitis due to, 928–930t
  mumps
    rubella, and varicella (MMRV) vaccine, 141
    and rubella (MMR) vaccine, 141, 143
      schedule for, 149–150t
      schedule for, catch-up, 151t
  prevention of, 142–143
  treatment of, 142, 142b
  vaccine-modified form of, 142
Measles vaccine (Attenuvax), 142–143
Mebaral (mephobarbital), intoxication with, 1180–1181
Mebendazole (Vermox)
  for *Ascaris*, 569, 570t
  for giardiasis, 63–64
  for hookworm, 570t
  for pinworm, 570t
  for trichuriasis, 570t, 571
  for uncinarial dermatitis, 844t, 845
Mechanical obstruction, gaseousness due to, 10, 10t
Mechanical ventilation
  for acute exacerbations of COPD, 235–236
  for acute respiratory failure, 227–228, 229b
    invasive, 228, 229b
    noninvasive, 227–228, 228t, 229b
  for sepsis, 70
Meckel's diverticula, 512b, 513–514, 513b
Meclizine (Antivert, Bonine)
  for motion sickness and vertigo, 206t, 210
  for nausea and vomiting, 8t
Meclofenamate, for dysmenorrhea, 1066t
Meconium aspiration, 1032, 1038
Meconium ileus, due to cystic fibrosis, 236
Mederma (onion extract), for keloids, 821
Medial collateral ligament (MCL) tears, 1008
Mediastinitis, granulomatous, due to histoplasmosis, 252, 253t
Mediastinoscopy, for lung cancer, 245
Medical conditions, nausea and vomiting due to, 6t

Medical nutrition therapy, for diabetes
    in adults, 576**b**, 577–578, 579**b**
    in children, 587–588
Medical toxicology. *See* Poisoning.
Medicated urethral system for erection (MUSE), 719
Medication(s). *See also* Drug(s).
    constipation due to, 21**b**
    indigestion due to, 11**t**
    nausea and vomiting due to, 6, 6**t**
    new, 1243
    in newborn resuscitation, 1032
    pending approval, 1244–1249**t**
    during pregnancy, 1011–1012
    pruritus due to, 31**b**
Medication-induced acute renal failure, 722, 722**b**, 723
Medication-induced delirium, 1119
Medication-induced hypothyroidism, 662, 662**b**
Medication-induced rhinitis, 215, 215**b**
Medication-induced serum sickness, 761–762, 762**t**
Medication-induced telogen effluvium, 791**b**
Medrol. *See* Methylprednisolone (Medrol, Solu-Medrol); Prednisone (Deltasone, Orasone, Medrol, Sterapred).
Medroxyprogesterone acetate, injectable (DMPA, Depo-Provera, Depo-Sub Q Provera), 757
    for Alzheimer's disease, 884–886
    for anovulatory bleeding, 1058–1059
    for contraception, 757
        in postpartum period, 1029**t**
    for dysmenorrhea, 1065
    for endometriosis, 1055–1056, 1057**t**
Medroxyprogesterone acetate (MPA, Provera)
    for anovulatory bleeding, 1058–1059
    after menopause, 1071–1072, 1072**t**
Medullary thyroid carcinomas (MTCs), 672, 673**t**
    follow-up for, 672, 673**t**
Medulloblastoma, 975
MEE. *See* Middle ear effusion (MEE).
Mefenamic acid (Ponstel)
    for dysmenorrhea, 1066**t**
    for pain, 2**t**
Mefloquine (Lariam), for malaria, 108**t**, 109, 111–112**t**, 157, 157**t**
Megace (megestrol acetate), after menopause, 1072**t**
Megaloblastic anemia, 394
    clinical features of, 395
    defined, 394–395
    diagnosis of, 395–396, 395**b**
    etiology and pathophysiology of, 394**b**, 395
    treatment of, 396–397, 396**b**
Megestrol acetate (Megace), after menopause, 1072**t**
Meglumine antimoniate (Glucantime, Prostib), for leishmaniasis, 94, 94**b**
Melanin, 876
Melanocytic nevi, 827
    acquired, 827, 828**b**
    benign, 828**b**
    blue, 828–829, 828**b**
    compound, 827
    congenital, 828, 828**b**
    defined, 827
    diagnosis of, 828**b**
    dysplastic (Clark's), 828**b**, 829
    halo, 827–828, 828**b**
    intradermal, 827
    junctional, 827
    malignant, 828**b**
    recurrent, 827, 828**b**
    Spitz, 828**b**, 829
    treatment of, 828**b**
Melanoma, 830
    ABCDEs of, 830, 830**b**
    acral lentiginous, 831

Melanoma *(Continued)*
    diagnosis of, 830–831, 830**b**
    epidemiology of, 830
    follow-up for, 832
    in situ, 832
    lentigo maligna, 831
    melanocytic nevi and
        congenital, 828
        dysplastic, 829
    metastatic, 832, 832, 832**b**
    nodular, 831
    risk factors for, 830, 830**b**
    staging and prognosis for, 831, 831**t**
    subtypes of, 831
    superficial spreading, 831
    of vulva, 1093–1094
    work-up and treatment of, 831–832, 832**b**
Melanosis, 876
    of leptomeninges (neurocutaneous), 828
Melanotic macule, 849–850
Melasma, 876–877, 877**t**
Melatonin, as nutritional supplement, 1234–1243**t**
Melatonin receptor agonist, for insomnia, 887–888, 888**t**
MELD (Model for End-stage Liver Disease) score, for cirrhosis, 497, 497**t**
Mellaril (thioridazine), poisoning due to, 1208–1209, 1208**t**
Meloxicam (Mobic)
    for juvenile idiopathic arthritis, 985
    for pain, 2–3
Melphalan (Alkeran), for multiple myeloma, 469**b**, 470, 470
Memantine (Namenda), for Alzheimer's disease, 883**t**, 884
Membranoproliferative glomerulonephritis (MPGN)
    diagnosis of, 700**b**, 700**b**
    treatment of, 702**b**, 703
Membranous glomerulonephritis (MGN)
    diagnosis of, 700**b**
    treatment of, 702–703, 702**b**
Membranous nephropathy
    diagnosis of, 700**b**
    treatment of, 702–703, 702**b**
MEN. *See* Multiple endocrine neoplasia (MEN).
Menactra. *See* Meningococcal polysaccharide diphtheria toxoid conjugate vaccine (MCV4, Menactra).
Menarche, 1062–1063
Ménière's disease, 210
    clinical presentation of, 210–211
    defined, 210
    office evaluation of, 210–211, 211**b**
        audiometric and vestibular testing in, 211
        laboratory and radiologic testing in, 211
    pathophysiology of, 210
    treatment of, 211–212, 211**b**
        Meniett for, 211–212
        ototoxic antibiotics for, 212
        surgical, 212
Meniett, for Ménière's disease, 211–212
Menin, in acromegaly, 633
Meningeal tumors, 973**t**
Meningitis
    due to anthrax, 126**t**
    bacterial (*See* Bacterial meningitis)
    basilar, 208
    due to Lyme disease, 136–137
    Mollaret's, 928–930**t**
    due to mumps, 121
    viral, 927
        clinical features of, 927
        diagnosis of, 927–930, 931**b**
        etiology of, 927–930**t**
        treatment of, 930–932, 932**b**
Meningitis belt, 160

Meningococcal polysaccharide diphtheria toxoid conjugate vaccine (MCV4, Menactra), 115
    schedule for, 149–150**t**
    for travelers, 160, 159–160**t**
Meningococcal polysaccharide vaccine (MPSV4, Menomune), 115
    schedule for, 149–150**t**
    for travelers, 160, 159–160**t**
Meningococcal vaccine, 115
    schedule for, 149–150**t**
    for travelers, 160, 159–160**t**
Meniscal injuries, 1008
Menkes' kinky hair disorder, 793
Menomune (meningococcal polysaccharide vaccine), 115
    schedule for, 149–150**t**
    for travelers, 160, 159–160**t**
Menopause, 1070
    age of, 1070
        factors that influence, 1070**b**
    and balance, 1071
    bleeding after, 1070–1071
    defined, 1070
    diagnosis of, 1070, 1070**b**, 1071**b**
    differential diagnosis of, 1070, 1071**b**
    genitourinary symptoms of, 1070
        treatment for, 1072**b**
    and menstrual migraines, 1071
    mood disturbances in, 1071
    and osteoporosis, 1071, 1071**b**
        treatment for, 1072, 1073**b**
    sleep disturbances in, 1070
    staging system for, 1070, 1070**b**
    systemic manifestations of, 1070–1071
    treatment for, 1071–1073, 1071**b**
        bisphosphonates in, 1072, 1073**b**
        hormone replacement therapy in, 1071–1072, 1072**t**, 1072**b**
        for osteoporosis, 1072, 1073**b**
        SERMS in, 1072–1073, 1073**b**
        SSRIs in, 1072**t**
        for urogenital atrophy, 1072**b**
        for vasomotor symptoms, 1072**t**
    vasomotor symptoms of, 1070
        treatment for, 1072**t**
Menorrhagia, 1059
Menstrual cycle, 1062
    and infertility, 1061
Menstrual history, for dysfunctional uterine bleeding, 1058
Menstrual migraines, after menopause, 1071
Menstruation, retrograde, 1054
Mental status, altered, due to poisoning, 1173
Mental status examination, for Alzheimer's disease, 883**t**
Mentax (butenafine) cream, for cutaneous tinea infection, 848**b**
Meperidine (Demerol)
    for acute porphyria, 476, 477**b**
    intoxication with, 1204–1205, 1205**t**
    kinetics of, 1204
    for pain, 4**t**
Mephobarbital (Mebaral), intoxication with, 1180–1181
Mepron. *See* Atovaquone (Mepron).
Mequinol and tretinoin (Solagé), for solar lentigines, 877
6-Mercaptopurine (6-MP, Purinethol)
    for acute promyelocytic leukemia, 448–449
    for inflammatory bowel disease, 516–517, 519–520
Mercury, reference intervals for, 1224**t**
Meridia (sibutramine), for obesity, 609–610, 610**t**
Meropenem (Merrem)
    for bacterial meningitis, 115**t**
    for necrotizing skin and soft tissue infections, 85**t**
    for pyelonephritis, 685

Meruvax (rubella vaccine), 141
Mesalamine (Asacol, Salofalk), for inflammatory bowel disease, 516, 520
Mesalamine enemas (Rowasa), for inflammatory bowel disease, 516, 519
Mesalamine suppositories (Canasa), for inflammatory bowel disease, 516, 519
Mesial temporal-lobe epilepsy (MTLE), 905
Mesoridazine (Serentil), poisoning due to, 1208–1209, 1208t
Mesothelioma, malignant, due to asbestosis, 279
Mestinon (pyridostigmine bromide), for myasthenia gravis, 942t, 943
Metabolic acidosis
 in chronic renal failure, 729
 and disease progression, 729
 laboratory values for, 727, 727t
 symptoms of, 727
 treatment of, 730
 with parenteral nutrition, 625t
 due to poisoning, 1175t
Metabolic disorder(s)
 cardiac arrest due to, 303t
 delirium due to, 1119
 diabetes mellitus as
  in adults, 575
  in children and adolescents, 583
 diabetic ketoacidosis as, 590
 dyslipoproteinemias as, 601
 vs. fibromyalgia, 996b
 hyperuricemia and gout as, 599
 hyponatremia as, 595
 due to lead poisoning, 1198
 obesity as, 606
 osteoporosis as, 612
 Paget's disease of bone as, 615
 parenteral fluid therapy for
  in adults, 618
  in infants and children, 626
 seizures due to, 899t
Metabolic management, for sepsis, 70–71
Metabolic neuropathies, 963–964
Metabolic rate
 basal, 620
 stress and, 620, 621, 620f
Metabolic syndrome, 575
 and angina pectoris, 298
 obesity and, 607–608
Metacarpophalangeal (MCP) joint, injuries to, 1010
Metadate CD (methylphenidate extended-release capsules), for ADHD, 918t
Metamucil (psyllium hydrophilic mucilloid), for dyslipoproteinemia, 604
Metanephrine (MN), in pheochromocytomas and paragangliomas, 675t
Metaproterenol (Alupent), for asthma in children, 775t
Metastasis(es), to brain, 975–976
 epidemiology of, 975
 treatment of, 975–976
Metastatic melanoma, 832, 832b
Metastatic non–small cell lung cancer, 247–248, 247t
Metastatic prostate carcinoma, 732, 732
Metastatic renal cell carcinoma, 733–734
Metastatic renal tumors, 734, 734
Metastatic testicular carcinoma, 738
Metastatic vulvar cancer, 1092, 1092t, 1093t
Metered-dose inhaler, for asthma, 766t
Metformin (Glucophage), for diabetes
 in adults, 578, 580t, 580–581
 in children, 590, 590t
Methadone (Dolophine)
 intoxication with, 1204–1205, 1205t
 for opiate withdrawal, 1108, 1108–1109
Methamphetamine hydrochloride tablets (Desoxyn), for ADHD, 918t

Methamphetamine intoxication, 1178–1179
Methanol
 features of, 1190t
 kinetics of, 1201
 and serum osmolality, 1176t
Methanol poisoning, 1201–1202
Methazolamide (Neptazane), for glaucoma, 200
Methergine (methylergonovine), for postpartum hemorrhage, 1028t
Methicillin-resistant Staphylococcus aureus (MRSA)
 acute infectious diarrhea due to, 16
 community-acquired pneumonia due to, 262–263
 endocarditis prophylaxis for, 346–347t
 necrotizing skin and soft tissue infections due to, 84t, 85t
 skin infections due to, 835–836, 836b, 837f
 toxic shock syndrome due to, 87, 89
Methicillin-resistant Staphylococcus epidermidis (MRSE), endocarditis prophylaxis for, 346–347t
Methimazole (MMI, Tapazole)
 for hyperthyroidism, 667–668
 for thyroid storm, 669
Methotrexate (MTX, Rheumatrex, Trexall)
 for arthritis
  juvenile idiopathic, 985–986
  rheumatoid, 978–979, 981t
 for asthma in children, 775
 for bullous pemphigoid, 868t
 for ectopic pregnancy, 1019, 1019b
 for inflammatory bowel disease, 517, 520
 for leukemia
  acute lymphoblastic, 449, 449
  acute promyelocytic, 448–449
 for multiple sclerosis, 938
 for psoriasis, 802
 for sarcoidosis, 277
 for systemic lupus erythematosus, 807t, 808
Methoxsalen (Oxsoralen lotion), for vitiligo, 879
Methoxy polyethylene glycol-epoetin beta (Mircera), 1243
Methoxypsoralen, for vitiligo, 879
Methscopolamine (Pamine), for allergic rhinitis, 780
Methyl alcohol poisoning, 1201–1202
Methyldopa (Aldomet), for hypertension in pregnancy, 1023t
Methylene blue, for poisoning, 1167–1172t
3,4-Methylenedioxyamphetamine (MDA, "Eve"), intoxication with, 1178–1179
3,4-Methylenedioxymethamphetamine (MDMA, Ecstasy, XTC, "Adam")
 abuse of, 1110
 intoxication with, 1178–1179
Methylergonovine (Methergine), for postpartum hemorrhage, 1028t
Methylin (methylphenidate chewable tablets and oral solution), for ADHD, 918t
Methylmalonic acid (MMA), 395, 396
Methylphenidate (Ritalin)
 abuse of, 1109–1110
 for ADHD, 918t
 for multiple sclerosis, 939b
Methylphenidate chewable tablets and oral solution (Methylin), for ADHD, 918t
Methylphenidate extended-release capsules (Metadate CD), for ADHD, 918t
Methylphenidate extended-release tablets (Concerta), for ADHD, 918t
Methylphenidate transdermal system (Daytrana), for ADHD, 918t
Methylprednisolone (Medrol, Solu-Medrol)
 for alcoholic liver disease, 498–499
 for anaphylaxis, 761t
 for asthma
  in adolescents and adults, 766t, 767–768t

Methylprednisolone (Medrol, Solu-Medrol) (Continued)
  in children, 772b, 773–774t
 for bursitis, 997b
 for crescentic glomerulonephritis, 703
 for giant cell arteritis, 1004b
 for idiopathic inflammatory myopathy, 812–813
 for idiopathic thrombocytopenic purpura, 427b
 for IgA nephropathy, 703
 for infectious mononucleosis, 117
 for inflammatory bowel disease, 516, 519–520
 for multiple sclerosis, 936
 for optic neuritis, 197
 for systemic lupus erythematosus, 808
 for tendinitis, 997b
 for vertigo due to multiple sclerosis, 209
Methylprednisolone acetate (Depo-Medrol), for asthma, 766t
4-Methylpyrazole (4-MP). See Fomepizole (4-methylpyrazole, 4-MP, Antizol).
Methylxanthines, for asthma
 in adolescents and adults, 767–768t
 in children, 773–774t
Metipranolol (OptiPranolol), for glaucoma, 200
Metoclopramide (Reglan)
 for diabetic neuropathy, 962
 for dyspepsia, 528
 for gastroesophageal reflux, 28b
 for gastroparesis, 10t
 for motion sickness and vertigo, 206t
 with N-acetylcysteine, 1177
 for nausea and vomiting, 8, 8t
 for renal calculi, 745t
 for systemic sclerosis, 811–812
 for theophylline intoxication, 1214
Metolazone (Zaroxolyn)
 for chronic renal failure, 731
 for hypertension, 356–357
Metopirone (metyrapone), for Cushing's syndrome, 645t
Metoprolol (Lopressor)
 for angina pectoris, 299, 299t
 for hyperthyroidism, 666
 intoxication with, 1182–1183, 1183t
 for myocardial infarction, 364, 365t
MetroGel (metronidazole gel), for rosacea, 789
MetroGel-Vaginal (metronidazole vaginal gel)
 for bacterial vaginosis, 1074b
 for trichomoniasis, 1075
MetroLotion (metronidazole lotion), for rosacea, 789
Metronidazole (Flagyl)
 for acute infectious diarrhea, 19t, 19–20t
 for amebiasis, 60–61, 61t, 564, 565–566t
  cutaneous, 843, 844t
 for bacterial overgrowth, 10t
 for bacterial vaginosis, 1074b
 for balantidiasis, 565–566t, 567
 for Chlamydia trachomatis, 1078b
 for dientamoebiasis, 565–566t, 567
 for dracunculiasis, 844
 for giardiasis, 63, 64t, 64b, 544, 564–567, 565–566t
 for hepatic encephalopathy, 502–503
 for indigestion, 11t
 for inflammatory bowel disease, 517–518, 520
 for necrotizing skin and soft tissue infections, 85t
 for nongonococcal urethritis, 753
 for osteomyelitis, 1006t
 for pelvic inflammatory disease, 1080b
 for peptic ulcer disease, 532t
 for systemic sclerosis, 811–812
 for trichomoniasis, 1075, 1075b
Metronidazole cream (Noritate), for rosacea, 789
Metronidazole gel (MetroGel), for rosacea, 789
Metronidazole lotion (MetroLotion), for rosacea, 789

Metronidazole vaginal gel (MetroGel-Vaginal, Vandazole)
 for bacterial vaginosis, 1074**b**
 for trichomoniasis, 1075
Metyrapone (Metopirone), for Cushing's syndrome, 645**t**
Mevacor (lovastatin)
 for angina pectoris, 298
 for dyslipoproteinemia, 605**t**
Mexoryl SX (ecamsule), 880
MF. See Mycosis fungoides (MF).
MG. See Myasthenia gravis (MG).
MGN (membranous glomerulonephritis)
 diagnosis of, 700**b**
 treatment of, 702–703, 702**b**
MGUS (monoclonal gammopathy of undetermined significance), 467, 467**b**, 468
MI. See Myocardial infarction (MI).
Miacalcin (salmon calcitonin nasal spray), for osteoporosis, 615
Miconazole 100 mg suppository (Monistat-7), for vulvovaginal candidiasis, 1075**b**
Miconazole 200 mg suppository (M-zole 3 combo pack), for vulvovaginal candidiasis, 1075**b**
Miconazole 1200 mg suppository (Monistat-1 Combination Pack), for vulvovaginal candidiasis, 1075**b**
Miconazole cream (Femizol-M, Monistat-7), for vulvovaginal candidiasis, 1075**b**
Microabscesses, Pautrier's, 795
Microadenomas, 633
 hyperprolactinemia due to, 660–661
Microalbuminemia (MA), in diabetic children, 588, 589**t**
Microalbuminuria
 in chronic renal failure, 726
 in sickle cell disease, 407
Microangiopathic hemolytic anemia, 430, 431
Microglandular adenosis, of breast, 1047
Micronized estradiol (Estrace)
 for anovulatory bleeding, 1059
 for intermenstrual bleeding, 1059
 for uterine hemorrhage, 1059–1060
Micronor (progestin only pills), 756–757
 in postpartum period, 1029**t**
Micronutrients, in parenteral nutrition, 620, 621, 621**t**
Micropremie, 1039
Microsporidia, 565–566**t**, 568–569
 malabsorption due to, 544–545
Microsporidiosis, 565–566**t**, 568–569
Microsporium canis, 847, 848**b**
Microvascular decompression (MVD), for trigeminal neuralgia, 948–949
Micrurus fulvius envenomation, 1152–1153
Midamor (amiloride)
 for ascites, 501
 for hypertension, 357
Midazolam (Versed)
 for elevated intracranial pressure, 967
 intoxication with, 1181–1182
Middle cerebral artery peak velocity (MCA-PV), for Rh-sensitized women, 417–418
Middle ear effusion (MEE), 203
 diagnosis of, 203
 treatment of, 204, 204
Midesophageal diverticula, 512, 512**b**, 513**b**
Midodrine (ProAmatine), for hepatorenal syndrome, 503
Midrin (isometheptene with dichloralphenazone and acetaminophen), for migraine headache, 925
Midurethral slings, for stress incontinence, 696
Mifepristone (RU-486, Mifeprex), for Cushing's syndrome, 645**t**
Miglitol (Glycet), for diabetes, 580**t**

Migraine headache, 2
 with aura (classic), 923
 without aura (common), 923
 cause of, 923
 epidemiology of, 922, 923
 evaluation and diagnosis of, 922**t**, 923
 postmenopausal, 1071
 vs. seizures, 901**t**
 treatment of, 924–926, 924**t**, 925**t**
 triggers of, 923**b**, 924**b**
 types of, 923
 vestibular, 209
Migraine variant, orofacial pain due to, 992**t**
Migranal NS (dihydroergotamine), for migraine headache, 925
Migratory angioedema, 844, 844**t**
Milk ducts, blocked, 1028
Milk of magnesia, for constipation, 10**t**
Milk thistle fruit, 1234–1243**t**
Milk-based formula, 1043**b**
Milker's nodule, 843
Miltefosine (Miltex, Impavido), for leishmaniasis, 95
Mineral(s), in parenteral nutrition, 620–621, 621**t**
Mineral oil, for constipation, 22**b**
Mineral supplementation, for infants, 1042
Mineralocorticoid(s), for adrenocortical insufficiency, 639, 639**b**, 640
Mineralocorticoid receptor antagonists, for aldosteronism, 656, 656
Mini-laparotomy cholecystectomy, 494
Minimal change disease (MCD)
 diagnosis of, 700**b**
 treatment of, 701, 702**b**
Minimal residual disease (MRD), in leukemia, 444
Minipills, for contraception, 756–757
Minipress (prazosin)
 for pheochromocytomas and paragangliomas, 675
 for systemic sclerosis, 811**t**
Minocycline (Minocin, Dynacin, Solodyn)
 for acne, 788
 for bullous pemphigoid, 867
 for leprosy, 101, 101
 for necrotizing skin and soft tissue infections, 85**t**
 for osteoarthritis, 1002
Minor antigens, hemolytic disease of the fetus and newborn from, 418–419
Minoxidil (Rogaine), for androgenic alopecia, 791
Mintezol (thiabendazole)
 for cutaneous larva migrans, 844, 844**t**
 for strongyloidiasis, 570**t**
MiraLax (polyethylene glycol)
 for constipation, 10**t**, 22**b**
 for whole-bowel irrigation, 1164–1165
Mirapex (pramipexole), for parkinsonism, 955, 956**t**
Mircera (methoxy polyethylene glycol-epoetin beta), 1243
Mirena. See Levonorgestrel-releasing intrauterine device (Mirena).
Mirtazapine (Remeron), for major depression, 1124
Mirtazapine (Remiron), for Alzheimer's disease, 884, 885**t**, 884–886
Misoprostol (Cytotec)
 for osteoarthritis, 1000
 for pain, 2–3
 for peptic ulcer disease, 531**t**, 531–532
Mistransfusion, 484, 486
Mitomycin C (Mutamycin), for keloids, 821
Mitotane (Lysodren), for Cushing's syndrome, 645**t**
Mitoxantrone (Novantrone)
 for acute lymphoblastic leukemia, 449
 for acute myeloid leukemia, 445

Mitoxantrone (Novantrone) *(Continued)*
 for multiple sclerosis, 937, 937**t**
 for prostate cancer, 732
Mitral regurgitation, after myocardial infarction, 366**t**
Mitral valve, floppy. See Mitral valve prolapse (MVP).
Mitral valve prolapse (MVP), 334
 classification of, 336, 337**t**
 clinical observations in, 335–336, 335**f**
 complications and natural history of, 336–337, 337**f**
 diagnostic considerations for, 336, 336**b**, 336**f**
 due to heritable connective tissue disorders, 336–337
 high-risk patients with, 337–338, 337**f**
 historical perspective on, 336
 pathologic observations in, 334–335, 335**f**
 surgical considerations with, 338
 treatment of, 337, 337**b**
Mitral valvular regurgitation (MVR). See Mitral valve prolapse (MVP).
Mixed germ cell tumors, 738–739
Mixed venous O_2 saturation (Mvo_2), 225
MM. See Multiple myeloma (MM).
MMA (methylmalonic acid), 395, 396
MMF. See Mycophenolate mofetil (MMF, CellCept).
MMI (methimazole)
 for hyperthyroidism, 667–668
 for thyroid storm, 669
MMIS (malignant melanoma in situ), 832
MMN (multifocal motor neuropathy), 962
MMR vaccine. See Measles, mumps, and rubella (MMR) vaccine.
MMX (multi-matrix mesalamine), for inflammatory bowel disease, 516
MN (metanephrine), in pheochromocytomas and paragangliomas, 675**t**
Moban (molindone), poisoning due to, 1208–1209, 1208**t**
Mobic (meloxicam)
 for juvenile idiopathic arthritis, 985
 for pain, 2–3
Mobility, stroke rehabilitation for, 896
Modafinil (Provigil)
 for motion sickness, 210
 for multiple sclerosis, 939**b**
Model for End-stage Liver Disease (MELD) score, for cirrhosis, 497, 497**t**
Modification of Diet in Renal Disease (MDRD) formula, for creatinine clearance, 725–726, 726
MODS (multiple organ dysfunction syndrome), 65
MODY (maturity-onset diabetes of the young), 575, 583–584
Mohs' micrographic surgery
 for basal cell carcinoma, 794
 for squamous cell carcinoma, 794
Moist wound environment, for pressure ulcers, 858
Moisture vapor transmission rate (MVTR), of wound dressings, 858
Mold(s)
 in allergic rhinitis, 776
 and asthma
  in adolescents and adults, 765**b**
  in children, 771
Moles. See Melanocytic nevi.
Molindone (Moban), poisoning due to, 1208–1209, 1208**t**
Mollaret's meningitis, 928–930**t**
Molluscum contagiosum, 842–843
Mometasone furoate dry powder inhaler (Asmanex), for asthma
 in adolescents and adults, 769**t**
 in children, 773–774**t**

Mometasone furoate monohydrate (Nasonex), for allergic rhinitis, 28**b**, 780**t**
Mometasone topical (Elocon), for atopic dermatitis, 860–861
Mondor's disease, 1047
Monilethrix, 791
Monistat-1 (tioconazole cream), for vulvovaginal candidiasis, 1075**b**
Monistat-1 Combination Pack (miconazole 1200 mg suppository), for vulvovaginal candidiasis, 1075**b**
Monistat-7 (miconazole vaginal suppository or cream), for vulvovaginal candidiasis, 1075**b**
Monkeypox, *vs.* smallpox, 185**f**
Monoamine oxidase B (MAO-B) inhibitors, for parkinsonism, 957
Monoamine oxidase inhibitors (MAOIs)
 biogenic interactions with, 1203, 1203
 intoxication due to, 1202–1204
 kinetics of, 1203
 for major depression, 1124
 malignant hyperthermia due to, 1203
 for obsessive compulsive disorder, 1114
 serotonin syndrome due to, 1203, 1204
 SSRIs and, 1203, 1212
Monoclonal antibody therapy
 for chronic lymphocytic leukemia, 462–463
 for cutaneous T-cell lymphomas, 799
 for non-Hodgkin's lymphoma, 466
Monoclonal gammopathy of undetermined significance (MGUS), 467, 467**b**, 468
Monocyclic aminoketones, poisoning due to, 1214–1216, 1215**t**
Mononeuritis multiplex, 959
Mononeuropathies, 961–962
Mononucleosis, infectious. *See* Infectious mononucleosis.
Monroe-Kellie doctrine, 966–967
Montelukast (Singulair)
 for allergic rhinitis, 779
 for asthma, 28**b**
  in adolescents and adults, 767–768**t**
  in children, 773–774**t**
 for urticaria, 875
Monurol (fosfomycin), for cystitis, 684
Mood disorder(s), 1120
 with alcoholism, 1099
 bipolar disorder as, 1126–1128
  diagnosis of, 1126, 1126**b**
  epidemiology of, 1126
  treatment of, 1126–1128
 with bulimia nervosa, 1115–1116
 in fibromyalgia, 997–998
 major depression as, 1120–1126
  diagnosis of, 1120–1121, 1120**b**
  differential diagnosis of, 1121
  epidemiology of, 1120
  substance abuse and, 1121
  and suicide, 1120–1121
  treatment of, 1121–1126
   antidepressant drugs for, 1121–1124, 1122–1123**b**
   brain stimulation for, 1126
   phases of, 1121, 1121**f**
   psychotherapy for, 1124
   treatment-resistant, 1124–1126, 1125**f**
 in menopause, 1071
 in postpartum period, 1029
 after stroke, 898
Mood stabilizers, for bipolar disorder, 1126–1128
Morning after pill, 758, 758
Morning sickness, 6, 9, 1013–1014
Morning stiffness, due to rheumatoid arthritis, 978**t**
Morphea, 809–810
Morphine sulfate (Avinza, Kadian, MS Contin, Oramorph SR, MSIR)
 for acute porphyria, 476
 intoxication with, 1204–1205, 1205**t**

Morphine sulfate (Avinza, Kadian, MS Contin, Oramorph SR, MSIR) *(Continued)*
 kinetics of, 1204
 for pain, 4**t**
 for renal calculi, 745**t**
 for traumatic brain injury, 967, 968
Motility disorder, gaseousness due to, 10**t**
Motility therapy, for gastroesophageal reflux disease, 554
Motilium (domperidone), for gastroparesis, 10**t**
Motion sickness, 9, 158
Motor fluctuations, due to levodopa, 955
Motor learning, for stroke rehabilitation, 896**b**
Motor neuropathy(ies)
 multifocal, 962
 pattern of distribution of, 959, 960**t**
 pure, 960**t**
 signs and symptoms of, 959**b**
Motor recovery, after stroke, 895, 896**b**
Motor signs, cardinal, of parkinsonism, 952–953, 953**t**
Motrin. *See* Ibuprofen (Advil, Motrin).
Mouth
 floor of, disorders of, 853
 trench, 854
Mouth care, for Stevens-Johnson syndrome and toxic epidermal necrolysis, 864**b**, 866
Mouth disease(s), 849
 of alveolar process/gingiva, 853–855
 of buccal mucosa, 851
 of floor of mouth, 853
 of hard palate, 851–852
 of labial mucosa, 850–851
 of lips, 849–850
 of soft palate/tonsillar pillars, 852
 of tongue, 852–853
 xerostomia as, 849
Moxifloxacin (Avelox)
 for legionellosis, 271**t**
 for leprosy, 102
 for mycoplasmal pneumonia, 270, 270**t**
 for tuberculosis, 285**t**
Moxisylyte chlorhydrate, for erectile dysfunction, 720
4-MP (4-methylpyrazole). *See* Fomepizole (4-methylpyrazole, 4-MP, Antizol).
6-MP (6-mercaptopurine)
 for acute promyelocytic leukemia, 448–449
 for inflammatory bowel disease, 516–517, 519–520
MPA (medroxyprogesterone acetate)
 for anovulatory bleeding, 1058–1059
 after menopause, 1071–1072, 1072**t**
MPGN (membranoproliferative glomerulonephritis)
 diagnosis of, 700**b**
 treatment of, 702**b**, 703
MPSV4 (meningococcal polysaccharide vaccine), 115
 schedule for, 149–150**t**
 for travelers, 160, 159–160**t**
MRD (minimal residual disease), in leukemia, 444
MRI (magnetic resonance imaging), of breast, 1048
MRSA. *See* Methicillin-resistant *Staphylococcus aureus* (MRSA).
MRSE (methicillin-resistant *Staphylococcus epidermidis*), endocarditis prophylaxis for, 346–347**t**
MS. *See* Multiple sclerosis (MS).
MS Contin. *See* Morphine sulfate (Avinza, Kadian, MS Contin, Oramorph SR, MSIR).
MSA (multiple system atrophy), 953
MSIR. *See* Morphine sulfate (Avinza, Kadian, MS Contin, Oramorph SR, MSIR).
MTCs (medullary thyroid carcinomas), 672, 673**t**
 follow-up for, 672, 673**t**

MTLE (mesial temporal-lobe epilepsy), 905
MTX. *See* Methotrexate (MTX, Rheumatrex, Trexall).
Mucinous cysts, of vulva, 1091
Mucocele, of labial mucosa, 850
Mucocutaneous leishmaniasis
 clinical features of, 94
 epidemiology of, 94
 pathogenesis of, 93
 treatment of, 94**b**, 96
Mucolytic therapy, for cystic fibrosis, 239
Mucomyst (*N*-acetylcysteine), for poisoning, 1167–1172**t**
 due to acetaminophen, 1177–1178, 1178**t**
Mucopurulent cervicitis, due to *Chlamydia trachomatis*, 1076, 1078**b**
Mucormycosis, necrotizing skin and soft tissue infections due to, 85**t**
Mucosal protectants, for peptic ulcer disease, 531**t**
Mucous membrane pemphigoid, 867–869
Multidrug therapy (MDT), for leprosy, 101, 101**b**
Multidrug-resistant (MDR-TB), 282, 284**b**, 288
Multidrug-resistant (MDR) typhoid fever, 174, 175, 176**t**
Multifocal acquired demyelinating sensory and motor neuropathy (MADSAM), 962
Multifocal motor neuropathy (MMN), 962
Multi-Matrix (MMX) mesalamine (Lialda), for inflammatory bowel disease, 516
Multiple dose activated charcoal (MDAC), for theophylline intoxication, 1213–1214
Multiple endocrine neoplasia (MEN)
 hyperparathyroidism in, 649–650, 650
 hypoparathyroidism in, 652
Multiple endocrine neoplasia type 2 (MEN-2), pheochromocytomas and paragangliomas in, 674–675
Multiple myeloma (MM), 467
 clinical features of, 467–468
 complications of, 471–472
 defined, 467
 diagnosis of, 467–468, 468**b**, 467**b**
 diagnostic criteria for, 468
 epidemiology of, 467
 premalignant phase of, 467
 pruritus due to, 32**b**
 smoldering, 467**b**, 468
 staging and prognosis for, 467–469, 468**t**
 treatment of, 469–472, 469**b**
  chemotherapy for
   high-dose, with autologous stem cell transplantation, 470
   novel agents in, 471
   for refractory disease, 471
   regimens of, 469**b**
   with standard alkylating agent, 470–471
  overview of, 469–470
  for refractory disease, 471
  stem-cell transplantation for
   allogeneic, 470
   autologous, 470
  supportive, 471–472
Multiple organ dysfunction syndrome (MODS), 65
Multiple sclerosis (MS), 932
 in children, 939–940
 clinical course of, 932–933, 933**f**
 defined, 932
 diagnosis of, 933–935, 933**b**
  CSF evaluation in, 933–934
  diagnostic criteria for, 933, 934**t**
  evoked potential studies in, 934
  imaging in, 933, 934**f**, 935**f**, 935**f**
 differential diagnosis of, 934–935
 in elderly, 939–940

Multiple sclerosis (MS) (Continued)
  epidemiology of, 932
  monitoring of, 938
  neuromyelitis optica in, 196–197, 933, 938–939
  pathology of, 932
  during pregnancy, 939
  progressive
    primary, 933, 938
    secondary, 933, 933f, 938
  relapse-remitting, 932, 933f, 935–936
  symptoms and classification of, 932–933, 933f
  treatment of, 935–938, 935b
    advanced, 937–938
    corticosteroids for, 935–936, 937t, 938
    glatiramer acetate in, 936, 937t
    interferon-β-1 in, 936–937, 937t
    for long-term disease, 936, 937t
    mitoxantrone in, 937, 937t
    natalizumab in, 937–938, 937t
    optimal initial, 936–937
    other immunomodulatory therapies in, 938
    for relapses, 935–936
    for symptom management, 938, 939b
  vertigo due to, 209
Multiple system atrophy (MSA), 953
Multislice computed tomography, for angina pectoris, 296
Mumps, 121
  clinical manifestations of, 121
  complications of, 121, 121t
  diagnosis of, 121, 121b
  differential diagnosis of, 122b
  epidemiology of, 121
  etiology of, 121
  meningitis or encephalitis due to, 928–930t
  prevention of, 121–122
  treatment of, 121, 121b
Mumps vaccine, 121–122
Mupirocin (Bactroban), for atopic dermatitis, 861–862
Murmurs, 326–327
Muscle hematomas, due to hemophilia, 420
Muscle-specific receptor tyrosine kinase (MuSK), in myasthenia gravis, 942
Musculoskeletal disorders, in acromegaly, 634
MUSE (medicated urethral system for erection), 719
Mustargen (nitrogen mustard), for cutaneous T-cell lymphomas, 798
Mutamycin (mitomycin C), for keloids, 821
MVD (microvascular decompression), for trigeminal neuralgia, 948–949
Mvo$_2$ (mixed venous O$_2$ saturation), 225
MVP. See Mitral valve prolapse (MVP).
MVR (mitral valvular regurgitation). See Mitral valve prolapse (MVP).
MVTR (moisture vapor transmission rate), of wound dressings, 858
Myambutol. See Ethambutol (Myambutol).
Myasthenia, transient neonatal, 946
Myasthenia gravis (MG), 940
  clinical features of, 940, 941t
  diagnosis of, 940–942, 940t
    antibody testing in, 941–942
    edrophonium chloride (Tensilon) test in, 941
    electrophysiologic testing in, 942
  epidemiology of, 940
  medications that exacerbate, 940t
  pathophysiology of, 940
  prognosis for, 942
  treatment of, 942–946, 943b
    cholinesterase inhibitors for, 942–943, 942t
    corticosteroids for, 943–945
    immunosuppressive agents for, 943, 944t, 945
    intravenous immunoglobulin for, 945–946
    for myasthenic crisis, 946
    plasma exchange for, 945

Myasthenia gravis (MG) (Continued)
    for pure ocular disease, 943
    thymectomy for, 946
Myasthenic crisis, 946
Mycelex-3 (butoconazole 2% cream), 1075b, 1075b
Mycelex-7 (clotrimazole cream), for vulvovaginal candidiasis, 1075b
Mycelex-7 Combo pack (clotrimazole 100 mg tablet), for vulvovaginal candidiasis, 1075b
Mycobacteria, nontuberculous, 288–289, 289b
Mycobacterium avium intracellulare complex (MAC), 289
  in HIV, 56–57, 56t
  malabsorption due to, 544
Mycobacterium kansasii, 289
Mycobacterium leprae. See Leprosy.
Mycobacterium tuberculosis. See Tuberculosis (TB).
Mycobutin. See Rifabutin (Mycobutin).
Mycophenolate mofetil (MMF, CellCept)
  for bullous pemphigoid, 867, 868t
  for crescentic glomerulonephritis, 703–704
  for cutaneous vasculitis, 816t
  for focal and segmental glomerulosclerosis, 702
  for minimal change disease, 701
  for multiple sclerosis, 938
  for myasthenia gravis, 944t, 945
  for nephropathy
    IgA, 703
    membranous, 703
  for pemphigus vulgaris, 869
  for systemic lupus erythematosus, 807t, 808–809, 808f
  for urticaria, 875
Mycoplasma(s)
  cough due to, 28b
  genital, 753
Mycoplasma pneumoniae
  erythema multiforme due to, 863
  pharyngitis due to, 220
  pneumonia due to (See Mycoplasmal pneumonia)
Mycoplasmal pneumonia, 266–270
  clinical presentation of, 268
  diagnosis of, 268b, 269
  differential diagnosis of, 268–269
  treatment of, 269–270, 269b, 270t
Mycosis fungoides (MF), 30b, 795
  clinical and pathologic features of, 795–796
  diagnosis of, 796b
  epidemiology of, 795
  etiology, molecular biology, and molecular genetics of, 795, 796
  and related cutaneous lymphomas, 795
  staging and prognostic factors for, 796b, 796–797, 797t
  treatment of, 797–800, 797b
    for advanced-stage disease, 798–800
    for early-stage disease, 797–798
    investigational approaches for, 797b, 800
Myectomy, for hypertrophic cardiomyopathy, 333
Myelinopathy, 958
Myeloid leukemia
  acute, 444
    in children, 450
    classification of, 446b
    etiology of, 444
    prognostic factors for, 446b
    treatment of, 445–448, 447b
  chronic, 456–457
    clinical features and diagnosis of, 456–457, 457b
    initial evaluation of, 457
    natural history of, 457, 458t
    prognostic categories for, 457
    treatment of, 457–460, 459b
      allogeneic bone marrow transplantation for, 460

Myeloid leukemia (Continued)
      imatinib mesylate for, 457–458–460, 460b, 459b, 460t
      objectives for, 457, 458b
      second-line therapy for, 459–460
Myeloma
  light-chain or Bence Jones, 467–468
  multiple (See Multiple myeloma (MM))
  smoldering, 467b, 468
Myeloma kidney, 471
Myiasis, 844t, 845–846
Mylotarg (gemtuzumab ozogamycin)
  for acute myeloid leukemia, 448
  for acute promyelocytic leukemia, 448
Myocardial infarction (MI), 360
  acute, 360
    complications of, 366t, 367
    evaluation of, 361, 362f
    premature ventricular complexes in survivors of, 314
  cardiac rehabilitation and secondary prevention after, 367
  cardiogenic shock with, 367
  clinical presentation of, 361, 361t
  diagnosis of, 360
  dyslipoproteinemia and, 603
  heart block with, 319
  hypertension and, 356t
  incidence of, 360
  non–ST elevation
    adjunct therapy for, 366–367
    evaluation of, 362f
    initial therapy for, 365–366
    pathology of, 365
    risk score for, 365t
  pathophysiology of, 360–361
  right ventricular, 367
  ST elevation
    adjunctive therapy for, 362–365, 365t
    evaluation of, 362f
    fibrinolytic therapy for, 361–362, 363b, 364t
    initial management of, 361
    percutaneous coronary intervention for, 362, 364b
    reperfusion therapy for, 361, 363f
    risk score for, 363t
  ventricular tachycardia after, 325–326
Myocardial rupture, after myocardial infarction, 366t
Myoclonic epilepsy, juvenile, 908, 908–909
Myofascial pain, 991b
  regional, 995–996
Myoglobin, for myocardial infarction, 361
Myolysis, for uterine leiomyoma, 1082, 1082t
Myomectomy
  for hypertrophic cardiomyopathy, 333
  for uterine leiomyoma, 1082, 1082t
Myopathy
  due to HAART, 54–55t
  idiopathic inflammatory, 812–813
    clinical characteristics of, 812, 812t
    diagnosis of, 813b
    treatment of, 812–813, 813b
Myopia, 187, 188f
Myrothecium, as biological weapon agent, 1229–1233b
Mysoline (primidone), for epilepsy
  in adolescents in adults, 904t, 905
  in infants and children, 912t
Myxedema coma, 664
M-zole 3 combo pack (miconazole 200 mg suppository), for vulvovaginal candidiasis, 1075b

N

NAATs (nucleic acid amplification techniques), for *Chlamydia trachomatis*, 1077

Nabumetone (Relafen)
    for juvenile idiopathic arthritis, 985
    for osteoarthritis, 1000
N-acetylcysteine (NAC, Mucomyst), for
        poisoning, 1167–1172t
    due to acetaminophen, 1177–1178, 1178t
N-acetyl-paraaminophenol poisoning,
        1176–1178
N-acetyl-p-benzoquinoneimine (NAPQI), 1176
Nadolol (Corgard)
    for hyperthyroidism, 666
    intoxication with, 1182–1183, 1183t
Nafarelin acetate (Synarel)
    for endometriosis, 1056
    for uterine leiomyoma, 1082
Nafcillin (Unipen)
    for bacterial meningitis, 115t
    for endocarditis prophylaxis, 346–347t
    for osteomyelitis, 1006–1007, 1006t
    for toxic shock syndrome, 89, 89b
Naftifine (Naftin) cream, for cutaneous tinea
        infection, 848b
NaHCO₃. See Sodium bicarbonate (NaHCO₃).
Nail(s)
    anatomy of, 816–817, 817f
    brittle, 817b, 818b, 818–819
    ingrown, 817b, 818b, 819
    in lichen planus, 804, 817
    in psoriasis, 819–820
Nail bed, 816–817
Nail disease(s), 816
    diagnosis of, 817b
    onychomycosis as, 817b, 817–818, 818b
    primary (simple) chronic paronychia as, 817b,
        818b, 820
    primary (simple) onycholysis as, 817b, 818b,
        820
    subungual hematoma as, 819
    treatment of, 818b
Nail folds, 816–817, 817f
Nail matrix, 816–817
Nail plate, 816, 817f
Nalbuphine (Nubain)
    for opioid-induced pruritus, 34b
    for pain, 4t
Nalfon (fenoprofen), for juvenile idiopathic
        arthritis, 985
Nalmefene (Revex), for poisoning, 1174
    due to opioids, 1204
Naloxone (Narcan)
    for cholestasis, 34b
    for opioid overdose, 1173–1174, 1204–1205
    for poisoning, 1167–1172t
Naltrexone (ReVia, Depade, Vivitrol)
    for alcohol dependence, 1103
    for cholestasis, 34b
    for pruritus due to primary biliary cirrhosis, 499
Namenda (memantine), for Alzheimer's disease,
        883t, 884, 884
NAPQI (N-acetyl-p-benzoquinoneimine), 1176
Naproxen sodium (Anaprox, Naprelan,
        Naprosyn)
    for cluster headache, 926t
    for dysmenorrhea, 1066t
    for juvenile idiopathic arthritis, 985
    for pain, 2t
Naratriptan (Amerge), for migraine headache,
        925t, 926
Narcan. See Naloxone (Narcan).
Narcolepsy, 888–889
Narcotic opiates. See Opioid(s).
Nardil (phenelzine), for major depression, 1124
NARES (nonallergic rhinitis with eosinophilia
        syndrome), 215, 778
Narrow-band ultraviolet light B (NB-UVB), for
        cutaneous T-cell lymphomas, 798
Nasacort AQ (triamcinolone acetonide nasal),
        for allergic rhinitis, 780t

Nasal cannula, 227t
Nasal polyps
    and allergic rhinitis, 777
    and asthma in children, 771
Nasalcrom (cromolyn sodium nasal spray), for
        allergic rhinitis, 780, 780t
Nasarel Spray (flunisolide 0.025% nasal
        solution), for allergic rhinitis, 780t
NASH (nonalcoholic steatohepatitis), 498t, 500
Nasonex (mometasone furoate monohydrate),
        for allergic rhinitis, 28b, 780t
Natalizumab (Tysabril), for multiple sclerosis,
        937–938, 937t
Nateglinide (Starlix), for diabetes, 580t
National Childhood Vaccine Injury Act, 148
Native valve endocarditis, 342, 343b
Natural family planning, 756
    in postpartum period, 1029t
Nausea and vomiting, 5
    due to alcohol withdrawal, 1102–1103b
    chemotherapy-induced, 9
    clinical assessment of, 6–7
    due to CNS disorders, 6, 6t
    in diabetes, 9
    diagnostic testing for, 7, 6b
    differential diagnosis of, 5–6, 6t
    due to gastrointestinal disorders, 6, 6t
    idiopathic, 6t
    infectious causes of, 6, 6t
    due to medical conditions, 6t
    medication-induced, 6, 6t
    due to motion sickness, 9
    pathogenesis of, 5
    postoperative, 9
    during pregnancy, 6, 9, 1013–1014
    due to psychological/psychiatric disorders, 6, 6t
    treatment of, 7, 7b, 8t
        antiemetic drugs for, 7, 7–9, 8t
        antihistamines and anticholinergics for, 8, 8t
        benzamides for, 8, 8t
        benzodiazepines for, 8
        butyrophenones for, 8, 8t
        cannabinoids for, 8–9, 8t
        corticosteroids for, 8, 8t
        diet for, 7
        dopamine antagonists for, 7–8
        nonpharmacologic, 9
        phenothiazines for, 8, 8t
        serotonin antagonists for, 7, 8t
Navane (thiothixene), poisoning due to, 1208–
        1209, 1208t
Navelbine (vinorelbine), for non–small cell lung
        cancer, 245–246
NB-UVB (narrow-band ultraviolet light B), for
        cutaneous T-cell lymphomas, 798
NCSs (nerve conduction studies), for peripheral
        neuropathy, 960–961
NDT (neurodevelopmental therapy), for stroke
        rehabilitation, 896b
Near-sightedness, 187, 188f
Nebcin (tobramycin), for bacterial meningitis,
        115t
Nebivolol (Bystolic), 1243
Nebulizer solutions, for asthma, 766t
NebuPent (pentamidine, aerosolized), for
        Pneumocystis jiroveci pneumonia, 56t
Necator americanus, 570t, 571, 844t, 845
Neck pain
    management of, 42–43, 42b
    natural course of, 41
Necrotic arachnidism
    Loxosceles, 1150–1151
    non-Loxosceles, 1151
Necrotic enteritis, 82
Necrotizing skin and soft tissue infections, 83,
        836b, 839
    clinical features of, 84, 84t
    diagnosis of, 84t, 84–85, 86b

Necrotizing skin and soft tissue infections
        (Continued)
    etiology of, 83–84, 84t
    fungal, 84, 85t, 86
    monomicrobial, 84, 85t, 86
    polymicrobial, 83–84, 85t, 86
    treatment of, 85–86, 85t, 86b
Nedocromil (Tilade), for asthma
    in adolescents and adults, 767–768t
    in children, 773–774t, 775
Nefazodone, for major depression, 1124
Negative symptoms, of schizophrenia, 1129
Neisseria gonorrhoeae
    conjunctivitis due to, 194t
        in neonate, 195–196, 196t
    epididymitis due to, 698
    gonorrhea due to, 750
    pelvic inflammatory disease due to, 1079,
        1079–1080
Neisseria meningitidis, meningitis due to, 114
Nelarabine (Arranon), for acute lymphoblastic
        leukemia, 449
Nelfinavir (Viracept), for HIV, 50t
    drug interactions with, 58t
Nematocysts, 1158
Nematocytes, 1158
Nematodes, 569–572, 570t
Nembutal. See Pentobarbital (Nembutal).
Neonatal conjunctivitis, 195–196, 196t
Neonatal herpes simplex virus, 840, 842
Neonatal intensive care unit (NICU)
    care for extremely low birth weight infants in,
        1039–1040t
    developmental care in, 1037
Neonatal seizures, 909–910
Neonatal tetanus, 143
Neonate(s). See also Newborn.
    gonorrhea in, 751
    high-risk, 1033
        due to asphyxia, 1034, 1034b
        due to congenital diaphragmatic hernia, 1039
        counseling for family of, 1033
        defined, 1033
        delivery management of, 1033–1034
        demographics of, 1033
        developmental care for, 1037
        diagnosis of, 1041b
        due to extremely low birth weight, 1039,
            1039–1040t
        due to gastroschisis, 1038–1039
        due to hyaline membrane disease, 1037
        due to meconium aspiration syndrome,
            1038
        nutrition for, 1035–1037
        palliative care for, 1039–1041
        parental involvement in care of, 1037
        due to persistent pulmonary hypertension
            of the newborn, 1038
        postnatal care for, 1034–1037
        prenatal diagnosis of, 1033
        resuscitation of (See Newborn resuscitation)
        thermoregulation with, 1035, 1035t, 1036f,
            1036t
        due to transient tachypnea of the newborn,
            1037–1038
        treatment of, 1041b
Neoplasia, with acromegaly, 635
Neoral. See Cyclosporine (CSA, Neoral, Gengraf,
        Sandimmune).
Neostigmine bromide (Prostigmin)
    for myasthenia gravis, 942t
    poisoning due to, 1205–1206
Neo-Synephrine. See Phenylephrine (Neo-
        Synephrine).
Nephrectomy, for renal cell carcinoma
    partial, 733
    radical, 733
Nephritic syndrome, 699b

Nephritis, interstitial, acute renal failure due to, 722**b**, 723–724
Nephrogenic diabetes insipidus, 649
Nephrolithiasis. *See* Renal calculi.
Nephropathy
 diabetic, 588, 588
 IgA
  diagnosis of, 700**b**
  treatment of, 702**b**, 703
 membranous
  diagnosis of, 700**b**
  treatment of, 702–703, 702**b**
Nephrotic syndrome, 699**b**, 701
Nephrotoxicity, 1174**t**
 due to HAART, 54–55**t**
 of lead, 1197–1198
Neptazane (methazolamide), for glaucoma, 200
Nerve agents, as chemical weapons, 1226–1228**t**
Nerve conduction studies (NCSs), for peripheral neuropathy, 960–961
Neupogen (filgrastim), for neutropenia, 415, 415, 415
Neupro (rotigotine), 1243
 for parkinsonism, 956, 956**t**
Neuralgia
 orofacial pain due to, 992**t**
 postherpetic, 840–842, 964
  orofacial pain due to, 992**t**
 trigeminal (*See* Trigeminal neuralgia (TN))
Neuritis
 optic (*See* Optic neuritis)
 vestibular, 206–207, 207**b**
Neuroborreliosis, 136–137
Neurocutaneous melanosis, 828, 828
Neurodermatitis, pruritus due to, 32**b**
Neurodevelopmental therapy (NDT), for stroke rehabilitation, 896**b**
Neuroendocrine carcinoma, of cervix, 1091
Neurofibromatosis type 1 (NF1)
 and childhood leukemia, 452**t**
 pheochromocytomas and paragangliomas in, 674–675
Neurogenic conditions, orofacial pain due to, 991, 992**t**
Neurolabyrinthitis, vestibular, 206–207, 207**b**
Neuroleptic(s)
 poisoning due to, 1208–1209, 1208**t**
 for Tourette's syndrome, 921, 920**b**
Neuroleptic malignant syndrome (NMS), 1130, 1208, 1209
Neurologic assessment, for survivor of cardiac arrest, 307–308
Neurologic changes, due to traumatic brain injury, 968
Neurologic complications, of sickle cell disease, 406–407, 410–411
Neurologic disorder(s)
 Alzheimer's disease as, 881
 attention-deficit/hyperactivity disorder as, 916
 Bell's palsy as, 949
 brain tumors as, 972
 Gilles de la Tourette syndrome as, 918
 headache as, 921
 intracerebral hemorrhage as, 890
 ischemic cerebrovascular disease as, 893
 multiple sclerosis as, 932
 myasthenia gravis and related disorders as, 940
 parkinsonism as, 952
 peripheral neuropathies as, 958
 rehabilitation of stroke survivor as, 895
 seizures and epilepsy as
  in adolescents and adults, 898
  in infants and children, 907
 sleep disorders as, 887
 traumatic brain injury as
  in adults, 965

Neurologic disorder(s) *(Continued)*
 in children, 969
 trigeminal neuralgia as, 947
 viral meningitis and encephalitis as, 927
Neurologic examination, for Alzheimer's disease, 883**t**
Neuroma, acoustic, 208
Neuromyelitis optica, in multiple sclerosis, 196, 197, 933, 938–939
Neuronal tumors, of brain, 973**t**
Neuronopathy(ies), 958, 960**t**
Neurontin. *See* Gabapentin (Neurontin).
Neuropathic back pain
 assessment of, 40
  examination in, 40–41
  history in, 40
 management of, 41–42, 42**b**
 natural course of, 41
 pathophysiology of, 39–40
Neuropathic pain, 1, 964–965, 964**t**
 diabetic, 2
 due to multiple sclerosis, 939
Neuropathy(ies), peripheral. *See* Peripheral neuropathy(ies).
Neuropsychiatric dysfunction, in parkinsonism, 953**b**
Neurosarcoidosis, 276
Neurosyphilis, 755
Neurotic excoriations, pruritus due to, 32**b**, 34**b**
Neurotoxicity, 1165, 1166**t**
 of lead, 1197
Neurovascular compression, vertigo due to, 208
Neurovascular conditions, orofacial pain due to, 991, 992**t**
Neutral thermal environment (NTE), for neonate, 1035
Neutropenia, 413
 acquired, 413–414, 414**b**
 clinical presentation of, 413
 clinical significance of, 413, 414**t**
 congenital, 414**b**
 defined, 413
 differential diagnosis of, 413, 414**b**
 drug-induced, 413–414
 evaluation of, 413–414, 414**b**, 415**b**
 sepsis with, 68**t**
 treatment of, 414–415, 415**b**
Nevirapine (Viramune), for HIV, 49–50, 50**t**, 51**t**
 drug interactions with, 58**t**
Nevus(i)
 melanocytic (*See* Melanocytic nevi)
 sebaceus, 833**b**, 834**b**, 835
New York Heart Association (NYHA) classification, for heart failure, 338–339, 339**b**
Newborn. *See also* Neonate(s).
 hemolytic disease of, 416
  diagnosis of, 416**b**
  from non-RhD antibodies, 418–419
  due to RhD antigen, 416
  treatment of, 417**b**
 persistent pulmonary hypertension of, 1038
 transient tachypnea of, 1037–1038
Newborn resuscitation, 1029
 ABCDs of, 970, 1034
 airways in, 1031
 algorithm for, 1030**f**
 anticipation of, 1030, 1034
 assessing response to birth in, 1031
 availability of qualified personnel for, 1034
 breathing in, 1031–1032
 care after, 1032–1033
 circulation in, 1032
 demographics of, 1029
 documentation of, 1033
 drugs in, 1032
 endotracheal intubation in, 1031
 guidelines for, 1030

Newborn resuscitation *(Continued)*
 hypothermia in, 1033
 indications for, 1029–1030
 initial stabilization and evaluation in, 1030–1032
 for meconium aspiration, 1032
 oxygen supplementation in, 1031–1032
 preparation for, 1034
 for preterm infants, 1032
 principles of, 1034**t**
 withholding and withdrawing of, 1032
Nexium. *See* Esomeprazole (Nexium).
NF1 (neurofibromatosis type 1)
 and childhood leukemia, 452**t**
 pheochromocytomas and paragangliomas in, 674–675
NGU. *See* Nongonococcal urethritis (NGU).
NH_3 (ammonia), as chemical weapon, 1226–1228**t**
NHL. *See* Non-Hodgkin's lymphoma (NHL).
Niacin (Niaspan)
 for dyslipoproteinemia, 604
 in parenteral nutrition, 621**t**
Niacin ER/laropiprant (Cordaptive), 1244–1249**t**
Niacinamide, for bullous pemphigoid, 867
Nicardipine (Cardene), intoxication with, 1183–1184
Niclosamide (Yomesan), for tapeworms, 570**t**
Nicoderm CQ (nicotine transdermal patch), 1107
Nicotine. *See also* Cigarette smoking.
Nicotine dependence, 1106–1107
Nicotine inhaler (Nicotrol Inhaler), 1107
Nicotine nasal spray (Nicotrol NS), 1107
Nicotine polacrilex gum (Commit), 1107
Nicotine replacement, 1106–1107
Nicotine transdermal patch (Nicoderm CQ), 1107
NICU (neonatal intensive care unit)
 care for extremely low birth weight infants in, 1039–1040**t**
 developmental care in, 1037
Nifedipine (Adalat, Procardia)
 for angina pectoris, 299**t**
 for chilblain, 1147
 for ciguatera poisoning, 1156
 for dysmenorrhea, 1065–1066
 for high-altitude sickness, 1141, 1142**b**, 1143, 1143
 for hypertension in pregnancy, 1023**t**, 1027
 intoxication with, 1183–1184
 for renal calculi, 744–745, 745**t**
 for systemic sclerosis, 811**b**
Niferex Film Coated Tablets (polysaccharide-iron complex), 385
Nightmares, 889–890
Nilotinib (Tasigna), 1243
 for acute lymphoblastic leukemia, 449
 for chronic myeloid leukemia, 460
Nimodipine (Nimotop), intoxication with, 1183–1184
Nipent (pentostatin), for cutaneous T-cell lymphomas, 798
Nipple discharge, 1053
Nit(s), 844**t**, 845
Nitazoxanide (Alinia)
 for cryptosporidiosis, 565–566**t**, 568
 for giardiasis, 63–64, 64**t**, 64**b**, 544, 564–567, 565–566**t**
Nitrates
 for angina pectoris, 298–299, 299**t**
 for myocardial infarction, 365
Nitrendipine (Baypress), intoxication with, 1183–1184
Nitric oxide (NO)
 in erection, 716, 716, 716**f**
 for high-altitude sickness, 1143
Nitriles, cyanide poisoning due to, 1187–1188

NitroDur (nitroglycerin patches), for dysmenorrhea, 1065–1066
Nitrofurantoin (Macrobid, Macrodantin), for urinary tract infections
　in girls, 687b, 688t
　in males, 681, 681, 681t
　in multiple sclerosis, 939b
　in women
　　catheter-associated bacteriuria as, 684–685
　　cystitis as, 684, 684b
　　recurrent, 685
Nitrofurtimox (Lampit), for Chagas' disease, 843, 844t
Nitrogen mustard (Mustargen), for cutaneous T-cell lymphomas, 798
Nitrogen oxides (NO$_x$), as chemical weapon, 1226–1228t
Nitroglycerin (Nitrostat, Nitrolingual, Nitrol, Nitroglyn)
　for angina pectoris, 298, 298, 299t
　for myocardial infarction, 365
　for systemic sclerosis, 811t
Nitroglycerin patches (NitroDur), for dysmenorrhea, 1065–1066
Nitroimidazoles, for amebiasis, 60–61, 61t
Nitroprusside
　for amphetamine intoxication, 1179
　cyanide poisoning due to, 1188
　for phencyclidine intoxication, 1207
Nitrostat. See Nitroglycerin (Nitrostat, Nitrolingual, Nitrol, Nitroglyn).
Nitrous oxide, peripheral neuropathy due to, 963
Nix Cream Rinse (permethrin)
　for pediculosis, 844t, 845
　for scabies, 844t, 846
Nizatidine (Axid)
　for gastroesophageal reflux disease, 553, 554t
　for peptic ulcer disease, 531b
Nizoral. See Ketoconazole (Nizoral).
NLV (Norwalk-like virus), 81–82
N-methyl-D-aspartate (NMDA) receptor, in schizophrenia, 1129
N-methyl-D-aspartate (NMDA) receptor antagonist, for Alzheimer's disease, 883t, 884
NMN (normetanephrine), in pheochromocytomas and paragangliomas, 675t
NMS (neuroleptic malignant syndrome), 1130, 1208, 1209
NNRTIs. See Non-nucleoside reverse transcriptase inhibitors (NNRTIs).
NO (nitric oxide)
　in erection, 716, 716, 716f
　for high-altitude sickness, 1143
Noameba-DS (secnidazole)
　for amebiasis, 60–61
　for giardiasis, 63–64, 64t, 64b
Nociceptive back pain
　history of, 40
　pathophysiology of, 39–40
　referred, 40
Nocturia, during pregnancy, 1014
Nocturnal enuresis, 692–693
　defined, 689–690, 690b, 692
　epidemiology of, 692
　etiology of, 692
　monosymptomatic, 692
　nonmonosymptomatic, 692
　primary, 692
　secondary, 692
　treatment of, 692–693
Noise avoidance, for tinnitus, 37
Nolvadex. See Tamoxifen (Nolvadex).
Nonalcoholic steatohepatitis (NASH), 498t, 500
Nonallergic rhinitis, 214
　atrophic, 216
　classification of, 214

Nonallergic rhinitis (Continued)
　diagnosis of, 214–215, 215b
　differential diagnosis of, 216, 216b
　drug-induced, 215, 215b
　emotionally induced, 216
　food-induced, 216
　hormonal, 215
　management of, 216–217, 215b, 217b
　occupational, 215, 215b
　pathophysiology of, 215
　perennial (vasomotor, idiopathic), 215, 216
　due to physical and chemical factors, 215–216
　prevalence of, 215
Nonallergic rhinitis with eosinophilia syndrome (NARES), 215, 778
Noncompliance, with HAART, 52–53
Nondermatophye skin infections, 846–847
Nondippers, 349
Nonfluent aphasia, after stroke, 897
Nongonococcal urethritis (NGU), 752
　due to Chlamydia trachomatis, 1076, 1078b
　chronic, 753
　clinical presentation of, 752
　complications of, 753
　diagnosis of, 752–753
　etiology of, 752
　follow-up for, 753
　treatment of, 753
Nonhemolytic transfusion reactions, 484, 484–485t, 487–489
　acute lung injury as, 484–485t, 487–488
　allergic, 488–489
　febrile, 488
　　leukoreduced platelets for, 482
　graft-versus-host disease as, 489, 489b
Non-Hodgkin's lymphoma (NHL), 464
　Burkitt's, 464, 466
　classification of, 464, 464t
　diffuse large B-cell, 466
　epidemiology and genetics of, 464
　evaluation, staging, and prognosis for, 464–465, 465b
　indolent, 464, 465–466
　lymphoblastic, 464, 466
　related to immune suppression or deficiency, 466
　related to infectious agents, 466
　treatment of, 465–466, 465b
Nonimmune hemolytic anemia, 390
　acquired, 393–394
　causes of, 391t
　due to chemical and physical agents, 391t, 394
　congenital, 391–393, 393t
　diagnosis of, 390, 390b
　due to erythrocyte fragmentation, 391t, 394
　due to erythrocyte membrane abnormalities, 391–392, 391t
　due to erythrocyte metabolism abnormalities, 391t, 392–393, 393t
　due to glucose-6-phosphate dehydrogenase deficiency, 392–393, 393t
　due to hemoglobinopathies, 391t, 393
　hereditary elliptocytosis and pyropoikilocytosis as, 392
　hereditary spherocytosis as, 391–392
　hereditary stomatocytosis and xerocytosis as, 392
　due to infection, 391t, 394
　paroxysmal nocturnal hemoglobinuria as, 393–394
　due to pyruvate kinase deficiency, 393
　treatment of, 390–391, 390b
Noninvasive positive-pressure ventilation (NPPV), for acute exacerbations of COPD, 235–236
Non-nucleoside reverse transcriptase inhibitors (NNRTIs), for HIV, 49, 49–50, 50t
　adverse drug reactions to, 54–55t
　drug interactions with, 53

Non-nucleoside reverse transcriptase inhibitors (NNRTIs), for HIV (Continued)
　failure of, 52t
　resistance to, 51, 52t
Nonoxynol-9 (Conceptrol, K-Y Plus, Semicid), 757
Nonphenothiazines, poisoning due to, 1208–1209, 1208t
Nonrebreathing oxygen masks, 227t
non-Rh antibodies, hemolytic disease of the fetus and newborn from, 418–419
Nonseminomatous germ cell tumors (NSGCTs), 738, 738–739, 739b
Non–small cell lung cancer (NSCLC)
　pathology of, 243
　staging of, 243–244
　treatment for, 245–247
　　advanced and metastatic, 247–248, 247t
　　local, 245–246
　　locoregional, 246–247
Non–ST elevation myocardial infarction (NSTEMI)
　adjunct therapy for, 366–367
　evaluation of, 362f
　initial therapy for, 365–366
　pathology of, 365
　risk score for, 365t
Nonsteroidal antiinflammatory drug(s) (NSAIDs)
　allergy to, 783
　for ankylosing spondylitis, 987
　for arthritis
　　juvenile idiopathic, 985
　　osteo-, 1000
　　rheumatoid, 977, 980b, 982–983
　for cholecystitis, 494
　for cystic fibrosis, 239
　for dysmenorrhea, 1065, 1066t
　gastropathy due to, 528–529
　for gout, 599, 600
　for menorrhagia, 1059
　for migraine headache, 926
　for pain, 2–3, 2t
　for pericarditis, 370, 372
　for renal calculi, 744–745
　and SSRIs, 1122–1123b
　for systemic lupus erythematosus, 806, 807t
　for temporomandibular disorder, 993
　ulcers due to, 530
　for vasoocclusive pain, in sickle cell disease, 407–408, 408t
Nonstress test, during pregnancy, 1016
Nontuberculous mycobacteria (NTM), 288–289, 289b
Nootropic drugs, for tinnitus, 38
Nootropil (piracetam), for tinnitus, 38
Norco. See Hydrocodone + acetaminophen (Lortab, Maxidon, Norco, Vicodin, Xodol, Zydone).
Norcuron (vecuronium), for asthma in children, 772b
Norditropin (growth hormone replacement), for hypopituitarism, 658
Norepinephrine (Levophed)
　for elevated intracranial pressure, 967
　for shock, 69, 70
　for theophylline intoxication, 1214
Norethindrone acetate (Aygestin)
　for anovulatory bleeding, 1058–1059
　for menorrhagia, 1059
Norfloxacin (Noroxin)
　for bleeding esophageal varices, 506
　for cholera, 80t
　for Salmonella gastroenteritis, 173
　for spontaneous bacterial peritonitis, 502
　for urinary tract infections in males, 681t
Noritate (metronidazole cream), for rosacea, 789
Normabrain (piracetam), for tinnitus, 38

Normal saline, for cholera, 79t, 78b
Normal values, 1217. See also Reference intervals.
Normetanephrine (NMN), in pheochromocytomas and paragangliomas, 675t
Normodyne. See Labetalol (Normodyne, Trandate).
Normosang (heme arginate), for acute porphyria, 477
Norovirus, 81–82
Noroxin. See Norfloxacin (Noroxin).
Norpace (disopyramide), for hypertrophic cardiomyopathy, 333
Norplant (contraceptive implant), 757
Norpramin (desipramine), poisoning due to, 1214–1216, 1215t
Norprolac (quinagolide), for hyperprolactinemia, 660, 660t
Nortriptyline (Pamelor)
  for gaseousness, 10t
  for major depression, 1124
  for multiple sclerosis, 939b
  poisoning due to, 1214–1216, 1215t
  for psychiatric dizziness, 209
  for smoking cessation, 1107
  for temporomandibular disorder, 992–993
Norvasc. See Amlodipine (Norvasc).
Norvir (ritonavir), for HIV, 50t
Norwalk virus, 81–82
  acute infectious diarrhea due to, 16
Norwalk-like virus (NLV), 81–82
Norwegian scabies, 845–846
Nose, pruritus of, 31f
Nosocomial endocarditis, 342, 343b
Notalgia paresthetica, 32b, 34b
Novantrone. See Mitoxantrone (Novantrone).
Novastan (argatroban), for deep venous thrombosis/pulmonary embolism, 273
Novolin N (NPH insulin), for diabetes
  in adults, 582, 582t
  in children, 586, 587t
Novolin R (regular insulin), for diabetes
  in adults, 582t
  in children, 587t
Novolog (insulin aspart), for diabetes
  in adults, 582t
  in children, 586–587, 587t
NO$_x$ (nitrogen oxides), as chemical weapon, 1226–1228t
Noxafil. See Posaconazole (Noxafil).
NPH insulin (Humulin N, Novolin N), for diabetes
  in adults, 582, 582t
  in children, 586, 587t
NPPV (noninvasive positive-pressure ventilation), for acute exacerbations of COPD, 235–236
NRTIs. See Nucleoside/nucleotide reverse transcriptase inhibitors (NRTIs).
NSAIDs. See Nonsteroidal antiinflammatory drug(s) (NSAIDs).
NSCLC. See Non–small cell lung cancer (NSCLC).
NSTEMI. See Non–ST elevation myocardial infarction (NSTEMI).
NTE (neutral thermal environment), for neonate, 1035
NTM (nontuberculous mycobacteria), 288–289, 289b
Nubain (nalbuphine)
  for opioid-induced pruritus, 34b
  for pain, 4t
Nuchal translucency, 1012
Nucleic acid amplification techniques (NAATs), for Chlamydia trachomatis, 1077, 1077, 1077
Nucleoside/nucleotide reverse transcriptase inhibitors (NRTIs), for HIV, 49–50, 50t
  adverse drug reactions to, 54–55t
  failure of, 52t

Nucleoside/nucleotide reverse transcriptase inhibitors (NRTIs), for HIV (Continued)
  resistance to, 51, 52t
Nutcracker esophagus, 510, 511
Nutrient requirements, 620, 621t
Nutrition. See also Diet.
  for extremely low birth weight infants, 1039–1040t
  for high-risk neonate, 1035–1037
  parenteral (See Parenteral nutrition (PN))
  in postpartum period, 1028
  during pregnancy, 1014
  for pressure ulcers, 858
  with sepsis, 70
Nutrition assessment, 618–619, 619b
Nutritional biomarkers, 619
Nutritional disorders, due to thalassemia, 399t
Nutritional neuropathies, 963, 963b
Nutritional requirements
  estimation of, 619–620, 620f, 621t
  of infants, 1044
Nutritional status, assessment of, 618–619, 619b
Nutritional supplements, 1234
Nutritional support, for inflammatory bowel disease, 518
Nutropin (growth hormone replacement), for hypopituitarism, 658
NuvaRing (intravaginal contraceptive ring), 756
  in postpartum period, 1029t
Nuvigil (armondafinil), 1243
Nydrazid. See Isoniazid (INH, Nydrazid, Laniazid).
NYHA (New York Heart Association) classification, for heart failure, 338–339, 339b
Nystatin, for vulvovaginal candidiasis, 1075b

O

OA. See Osteoarthritis (OA).
Obesity, 606
  assessment of, 607
  benefits of modest weight loss for, 611
  BMI and, 606, 607, 607t
  definition of, 606, 607t
  diagnosis of, 607
  energy expenditure with, 620
  epidemiology of, 606
  etiology and pathophysiology of, 607, 607t
  in infants, 1044
  medical consequence(s) of, 607–608
    coronary heart disease as, 608
    diabetes mellitus as, 608
    hypertension as, 608
    insulin resistance and metabolic syndrome as, 607–608
    lipid dyscrasias as, 608
    pulmonary abnormalities as, 608
  medications that promote, 607, 607t
  and mortality risk, 606, 607f
  and obstructive sleep apnea, 240, 241
  overweight vs., 607
  treatment of, 608–610
    bariatric surgery for, 610
      in children and adolescents, 610
      contraindications for, 610
      gastric banding and adjustable laparoscopic band as, 610–611, 611f
      indications for, 610
      preoperative evaluation for, 610
      roux-en-Y gastroplasty as, 611, 611f
      surgical assessment for, 610
    behavior modification in, 609
    diet in, 608–609
    exercise in, 609
    future options for, 611–612
    initial evaluation in, 608, 608f

Obesity (Continued)
  pharmacotherapy in, 609–610, 610t
  and type 2 diabetes in children, 590
  waist circumference and, 607
Obesity hypoventilation syndrome, 608
Obsessions, 1113–1114
Obsessive compulsive disorder (OCD), 1113–1114
  diagnosis of, 1113–1114
  treatment of, 1113b, 1114, 1114t
Obstetrics and gynecology
  amenorrhea in, 1062
  antepartum care in, 1011
  breast diseases in, 1045
  care of the high-risk neonate in, 1033
  cervical cancer in, 1086
  Chlamydia trachomatis in, 1076
  dysfunctional uterine bleeding in, 1058
  dysmenorrhea in, 1065
  ectopic pregnancy in, 1017
  endometrial cancer in, 1083
  endometriosis in, 1054
  hypertensive disorders of pregnancy in, 1021
  infertility in, 1060
  menopause in, 1070
  normal infant feeding in, 1041
  ovarian cancer in, 1094
  pelvic inflammatory disease in, 1079
  postpartum care in, 1027
  premenstrual syndrome in, 1066
  resuscitation of the newborn in, 1029
  uterine leiomyomas in, 1081
  vaginal bleeding in late pregnancy in, 1019
  vulvar neoplasms in, 1091
  vulvovaginitis in, 1074
Obstructive pancreatitis, 549
Obstructive sleep apnea (OSA), 239
  due to acromegaly, 634
  clinical features of, 240
  defined, 239–240
  diagnosis of, 240, 240–241, 241b
  epidemiology of, 240
  and epilepsy, 906
  obesity and, 608
  severity of, 241
  in sickle cell disease, 410
  treatment of, 241–242, 241b
Obstructive sleep apnea syndrome (OSAS). See Obstructive sleep apnea (OSA).
Obstructive uropathy, chronic renal failure due to, 726
OC(s). See Oral contraceptive(s) (OCs).
Occlusal HP (salicylic acid topical), for verrucae, 823
Occlusive dressings, for pressure ulcers, 858, 858, 858
Occupational exposure
  to lead, 1196t, 1197
  pruritus due to, 31b
Occupational rhinitis, 215, 215b
Occupational therapy (OT), for juvenile idiopathic arthritis, 985, 986
OCD. See Obsessive compulsive disorder (OCD).
OCP (oral contraceptive pill). See Oral contraceptive(s) (OCs).
Octreotide (Sandostatin)
  for acromegaly, 636
  for bleeding esophageal varices, 506
  for Cushing's syndrome, 645t
  for hepatorenal syndrome, 503
  for systemic sclerosis, 811–812
Ocular exposure, to toxins, 1161
Ocular Hypertension Treatment Study, 198–199
Ocular manifestations
  of hypertension, 350–351
  of myasthenia gravis, 940, 941t
Ocular toxoplasmosis, 166–167
Ocular trauma, glaucoma due to, 199

Ocupress (carteolol ophthalmic), for glaucoma, 200
Odontogenic pathology, orofacial pain due to, 992t
Odynophagia, 508
Office hypertension, 352
Ofloxacin (Floxin, Oflox)
  for brucellosis, 75t
  for *Chlamydia trachomatis*, 1078b
  for epididymitis, 697b, 698
  for leprosy, 101, 101
  for nongonococcal urethritis, 753
  for pelvic inflammatory disease, 1080b
  for plague, 123
  for Q fever, 129t
  for *Salmonella* gastroenteritis, 173
  for typhoid fever, 176t
  for urinary tract infections in males, 681t
OGTT (oral glucose tolerance test)
  for diabetes mellitus in children, 584
  for peripheral neuropathy, 961
OIs. *See* Opportunistic infection(s) (OIs).
Olanzapine (Zyprexa)
  for Alzheimer's disease, 885t, 884–886
  for bipolar disorder, 1127
  for delirium, 1119–1120, 1119b
  for obsessive compulsive disorder, 1114
  for schizophrenia, 1130, 1130t
  for Tourette's syndrome, 921
Older patients. *See* Elderly patients.
Oligoarthritis, juvenile idiopathic, 984
Oligoastrocytomas
  epidemiology of, 972
  outcome with, 975
Oligodendrogliomas
  epidemiology of, 972
  genetics and etiology of, 972
  pathology of, 972, 973t
Oligomenorrhea, 1062
Olsalazine (Dipentum), for inflammatory bowel disease, 516
Omalizumab (Anti-IgE, Xolair), for asthma
  in adolescents and adults, 767–768t
  in children, 775
Omega-3 fatty acids, 1234–1243t
  for dysmenorrhea, 1066
Omeprazole (Prilosec)
  for gastroesophageal reflux disease, 553–554, 554t
  for indigestion, 11t
  for peptic ulcer disease, 531t, 532t
  for systemic sclerosis, 811–812
Omnicef (cefdinir), for urinary tract infections in girls, 687b
Omnipen. *See* Ampicillin (Omnipen).
Oncaspar (PEG-asparaginase), for acute lymphoblastic leukemia, 449
Onchocerca volvulus, 844t, 844–845
Onchocerciasis, pruritus due to, 32b
Onchodermatitis, 844t, 844–845
Oncotyomas, renal, 734, 734b
Ondansetron (Zofran)
  for cholestasis, 34b
  for motion sickness and vertigo, 206t
  with *N*-acetylcysteine, 1177
  for nausea and vomiting, 7, 8t
  for opioid-induced pruritus, 34b
  for theophylline intoxication, 1214
Onion extract (Mederma), for keloids, 821
Ontak (denileukin diftitox), for cutaneous T-cell lymphomas, 799–800
ONTT (Optic Neuritis Treatment Trial), 196–197
Onychocorneal band, 816–817, 817f
Onychodermal band, 816–817, 817f
Onycholysis
  defined, 820
  due to lichen planus, 817
  primary (simple), 817b, 818b, 820

Onychomycosis, 817–818, 847
  clinical features and diagnosis of, 817b, 818, 847, 847b
  distal and lateral subungual, 818
  proximal subungual, 818
  superficial white, 818
  total dystrophic, 818
  treatment of, 818, 818b, 847, 848b
Onychorrhexis, due to lichen planus, 817
Opana (oxymorphone), for pain, 4t
Open-angle glaucoma
  primary, 198–199, 198b
  secondary, 199
Ophthalmia neonatorum, 195–196, 196t
Ophthalmia nodosa, 1151
Ophthalmopathy, Graves', radioiodine treatment and, 668
Opiates, abuse of, 1105b, 1108–1109, 1108b
Opioid(s)
  addiction to, 4–5, 1109
  increased sensitivity to chronic administration of, 1109
  intolerance to, 3
  kinetics of, 1204
  for pain, 3, 4t
  pruritus due to, 34b
  side effects of, 3
  for vasoocclusive pain, in sickle cell disease, 407–408, 408t
Opioid intoxication, 1173–1174, 1204–1205, 1205t
Opioid reactions, 1173–1174
Opioid receptors, 1204
Opisthotonos, due to tetanus, 143
Opportunistic infection(s) (OIs), in HIV, 53–58
  chemoprophylaxis for, 53, 56t
  cryptococcosis as, 55–56
  cytomegalovirus disease as, 57
  disseminated *Mycobacterium avium* infection as, 56–57
  etiology of, 57t
  general considerations for, 53
  Pneumocystis jiroveci pneumonia (PCP) as, 53–55
  tuberculosis as, 56t, 57–58, 58t
Optic nerve, 187, 188f
Optic neuritis, 196
  diagnosis of, 196, 197b
  in multiple sclerosis, 196, 197, 933, 938–939
  natural history of, 196
  treatment of, 196–197, 197b
    corticosteroids for, 196–197, 197f
    immunomodulation agents for, 197
  typical *vs*. atypical, 196
Optic Neuritis Treatment Trial (ONTT), 196, 197, 197
OptiPranolol (metipranolol), for glaucoma, 200
Oracea (doxycycline, sub-antimicrobial), for rosacea, 789
Oral appliance therapy, for obstructive sleep apnea, 241
Oral azoles, for coccidioidomycosis, 250b, 250t
Oral contraceptive(s) (OCs)
  for acne, 788
  for anovulatory bleeding, 1058–1059
  for dysmenorrhea, 1065
  for endometriosis, 1056, 1057t
  estrogen-progestin combinations in, 756
  extended preparations for, 756
  for menorrhagia, 1059
  in postpartum period, 1029t
  for premenstrual syndrome, 1069
  progestin only, 756–757
  with sickle cell disease, 411–412
  for uterine hemorrhage, 1059–1060
Oral contraceptive pill (OCP). *See* Oral contraceptive(s) (OCs).

Oral disorder(s), 849
  of alveolar process/gingiva, 853–855
  of buccal mucosa, 851
  of floor of mouth, 853
  of hard palate, 851–852
  of labial mucosa, 850–851
  of lips, 849–850
  of soft palate/tonsillar pillars, 852
  of tongue, 852–853
  xerostomia as, 849
Oral glucose tolerance test (OGTT)
  for diabetes mellitus in children, 584
  for peripheral neuropathy, 961
Oral hypoglycemic agents
  for diabetes
    in adults, 578–581, 580t
    in children, 590, 590t
  and SSRIs, 1122–1123b
Oral mucosal cinnamon reaction, 851
Oral procedures, endocarditis prophylaxis for, 347t
Oral rehydration solution (ORS)
  for acute infectious diarrhea, 19
  for cholera, 79, 79t, 78b
  for traveler's diarrhea, 155, 156t
Oral rehydration therapy (ORT), for infants and children, 630
Oral salt loading, for diagnosis of aldosteronism, 654–655
Oramorph SR. *See* Morphine sulfate (Avinza, Kadian, MS Contin, Oramorph SR, MSIR).
Orap (pimozide), for Tourette's syndrome, 921
Orapred. *See* Prednisolone (Delta-Cortef, Prelone, Orapred).
Orasone. *See* Prednisone (Deltasone, Orasone, Medrol, Sterapred).
Orchitis, due to mumps, 121
Orencia. *See* Abatacept (Orencia, CTLA-4Ig).
Orf, 843
Organophosphate poisoning, 1205–1206
Orlistat (Xenical), for obesity, 610, 610t
Ornidazole (Tiberal)
  for amebiasis, 60–61
  for giardiasis, 63–64, 64t, 64b
Ornidyl (eflornithine), for African sleeping sickness, 843, 844t
Orofacial herpes, 840, 849
Orofacial pain, 988
  atypical, 947–948
  classification of, 991, 992t
  clinical features of, 988–989
  defined, 988–989
  diagnosis of, 989–991, 989b
    biobehavioral evaluation in, 989–990, 990b
    biomedical evaluation in, 989
    yellow flags in, 990, 990b
  differential diagnosis of, 991, 992t
  epidemiology of, 989
  treatment of, 991–993, 991b
    biobehavioral, 993
    biomedical, 991–993, 993b
Oropharyngeal dysphagia, 508–509
  causes of, 509b
  clinical manifestations of, 508, 508, 509
  diagnosis of, 508–509
  treatment of, 510
ORS. *See* Oral rehydration solution (ORS).
ORT (oral rehydration therapy), for infants and children, 630
Ortho Evra (transdermal hormonal contraceptive patch), 756
Orthodromic reciprocating tachycardia (ORT), 321, 322, 322f
Ortho-Evra (combination oral contraceptives), 756
  in postpartum period, 1029t
Orthovisc (hyaluronan, high molecular weight), for osteoarthritis, 1001t

Orudis (ketoprofen), for dysmenorrhea, 1066t
Oruvail (ketoprofen), for dysmenorrhea, 1066t
OSA. *See* Obstructive sleep apnea (OSA).
OSAS (obstructive sleep apnea syndrome). *See* Obstructive sleep apnea (OSA).
Oscillopsia, 207
Oseltamivir (Tamiflu), for influenza, 92, 92t, 260, 260b, 265, 267, 267t
Osgood-Schlatter syndrome, 1008
Osler, William, 81
Osler's sign, 351
Osmitrol. *See* Mannitol (Osmitrol).
Osmoglyn (glycerin), for glaucoma, 200
Osmolal gap, with poisoning, 1174–1175, 1176t
Osmolality, serum, with poisoning, 1174–1175, 1176t
Osmotherapy, for elevated intracranial pressure in children, 971
Osmotic laxatives, for constipation, 22, 22b
Osteitis, skull base, 202
Osteitis fibrosa cystica, 650
Osteoarthritis (OA), 998
　clinical features of, 999
　cystic erosive (inflammatory), 1001
　diagnosis of, 999b
　epidemiology of, 998
　factors contributing to, 998–999
　of knee, 1008
　　pain due to, 4
　　prophylactic measures for, 999, 999b
　pathophysiology of, 998, 998
　primary (idiopathic) *vs.* secondary, 998–999
　sites of, 999
　of TMJ, 991b
　treatment of, 999–1002, 1000b
　　chondrocyte transplantation for, 1002
　　comprehensive management program for, 999b
　　for cystic erosive (inflammatory) disease, 1001
　　disease-modifying drugs for, 1001–1002
　　exercise for, 999
　　gene therapy for, 1002
　　general considerations for, 999
　　glucosamine and chondroitin sulfate for, 1002
　　heat modalities for, 999
　　intra-articular injections for, 1000–1001, 1001t
　　joint lavage and arthroscopy for, 1001
　　new approaches to, 1001–1002
　　nonpharmacologic, 999
　　pharmacologic, 999–1000
　　prophylactic measures in, 999, 999b
　　surgery for, 1002
Osteoarthrosis, of TMJ, 991b
Osteomyelitis, 1005
　classification of, 1005
　clinical manifestations of, 1005–1006
　contiguous focus, 1005, 1006
　dead space with, 1007
　diagnosis of, 1005–1006, 1006b
　etiology of, 1005
　hematogenous, 1005, 1005–1006, 1006
　microbiology of, 1006
　radiology of, 1006
　in sickle cell disease, 406, 409
　signs and symptoms of, 1005–1006
　staging of, 1005, 1005b
　treatment of, 1006–1007, 1006t, 1006b
Osteonecrosis, in sickle cell disease, 407, 411
Osteoporosis, 612
　defined, 612
　diagnosis of, 613
　differential diagnosis of, 613, 614b
　epidemiology of, 612–613
　etiology of, 612
　fractures due to

Osteoporosis *(Continued)*
　epidemiology of, 613
　risk factors for, 612
　treatment of, 615
　postmenopausal, 1071, 1071b
　　treatment for, 1072, 1073b
　due to primary biliary cirrhosis, 499
　in rheumatoid arthritis, 977b
　risk factors for, 612–613
　treatment of, 613–615
　　anabolic agents in, 615
　　anticatabolic agents in, 614–615
　　calcium in, 614
　　exercise in, 614
　　for fractures, 615
　　vitamin D in, 614
Osteoradionecrosis, of temporal bone, 202
OT (occupational therapy), for juvenile idiopathic arthritis, 985, 986
Otitis externa, 201
　anatomy and physiology of ear canal and, 201
　bullous, 201
　defined, 201
　diagnosis of, 201, 202b
　differential diagnosis of, 201–202
　treatment of, 201
Otitis media, 203
　acute
　　clinical guidelines for, 203
　　defined, 203
　　diagnosis of, 203, 204b
　　impact of, 203
　　treatment of, 203–204, 203b
　and allergic rhinitis, 777
　classification of, 203
　clinical guidelines for, 203
　definitions for, 203
　diagnosis of, 203, 204b
　with effusion
　　clinical guidelines for, 203
　　defined, 203
　　etiology of, 203
　　impact of, 203
　treatment of, 203–204, 203b
Otolithic vertigo, 207–208
Otomycosis, 201
Ototoxic antibiotics, for Ménière's disease, 212
Outflow tract causes, of amenorrhea, 1063, 1064b
Outflow tract obstruction, due to hypertrophic cardiomyopathy, 333–334
Outflow tract ventricular tachycardia, 323
Ovarian cancer, 1094
　diagnosis of, 1095, 1095b
　epidemiology of, 1094
　genetic basis for, 1094
　histologic subtypes of, 1094
　lifetime risk of, 1094
　median age for, 1094
　screening for, 1094–1095
　treatment of, 1095–1096, 1095b
Ovarian causes, of amenorrhea, 1063, 1064b
Ovarian failure, premature, 1063
Ovarian function, suppression of, for dysmenorrhea, 1065
Overdose. *See* Poisoning(s).
Overfeeding, 619
Overnutrition, of infants, 1044–1045
Overweight, 607
Ovrette (progestin only pills), 756–757
　in postpartum period, 1029t
Ovulation induction, for infertility, 1061
Ovulatory dysfunctional uterine bleeding, 1059
Oxacillin (Bactocill, Prostaphlin)
　for endocarditis prophylaxis, 346–347t
　for osteomyelitis, 1006–1007
　for toxic shock syndrome, 89, 89b

Oxamniquine, for schistosomiasis, 570t
Oxandrolone (Oxandrin), parenteral nutrition with, 624
Oxaprozin (Daypro), for juvenile idiopathic arthritis, 985
Oxazepam (Serax)
　for alcohol withdrawal, 1101
　for Alzheimer's disease, 884, 885t
　for delirium, 1120
　intoxication with, 1181–1182
Oxcarbazepine (Trileptal)
　for epilepsy
　　in adolescents in adults, 904t, 903, 905
　　in infants and children, 911, 913t
　for neuropathic pain, 964–965
　for trigeminal neuralgia, 948
Oxiconazole (Oxistat), for cutaneous tinea infection, 848b
Oxsoralen lotion (methoxsalen), for vitiligo, 879
Oxybutynin chloride (Ditropan, Oxytrol), for urinary incontinence
　in children, 691, 692t
　in multiple sclerosis, 939b
　urge, 695t
Oxycodone (OxyR, OxyContin), for pain, 4t
Oxycodone + acetaminophen (Percocet, Tylox, Roxicet)
　intoxication with, 1204–1205, 1205t
　for pain, 4t
Oxycodone + aspirin (Percodan), for pain, 4t
Oxycodone + ibuprofen (Combunox), for pain, 4t
OxyContin (oxycodone), for pain, 4t
Oxygen delivery (D_{O_2}), 225
Oxygen delivery systems, 227t
Oxygen extraction ratio (O_2ER), 225
Oxygen masks, 227t
Oxygen supplementation, in newborn resuscitation, 1031–1032
Oxygen therapy
　for acute respiratory failure, 226–227, 227t
　for anaphylaxis, 760
　for COPD, 235
　for cystic fibrosis, 239
　for sepsis, 70
Oxymetazoline (Afrin)
　for allergic rhinitis, 780, 780t
　for sinusitis
　　acute, 28b
　　bacterial, 28b
Oxymorphone (Opana), for pain, 4t
Oxyprenolol, intoxication with, 1182–1183, 1183t
OxyR (oxycodone), for pain, 4t
Oxytocin (Pitocin), for postpartum hemorrhage, 1028t
Oxytrol. *See* Oxybutynin chloride (Ditropan, Oxytrol).

P

PAC(s). *See* Premature atrial complexes (PACs).
PAC (plasma aldosterone concentration), 654, 654
Pacemaker
　for atrial fibrillation, 311
　for heart block, 318–319, 319b
Pacemaker-mediated tachycardia, 322
Pacing
　for atrial fibrillation, 311
　dual-chamber, for hypertrophic cardiomyopathy, 334
　for heart block, 318–319, 319b
Packed red blood cells, 480
Paclitaxel (Taxol)
　for non–small cell lung cancer
　　advanced and metastatic, 247
　　local, 246
　peripheral neuropathy due to, 963

Paco$_2$ (arterial carbon dioxide tension), 226, 226t
PAD, Se Peripheral arterial disease (PAD)
PAD (public access defibrillation), 304–305
Paget's disease
　of bone, 615
　　diagnosis of, 615–616
　　treatment of, 616–617
　　type 1 vs. type 2, 616
　of vulva, 1092
PAH (primary adrenal hyperplasia), 654
PAH (pulmonary artery hypertension), in systemic sclerosis, 811
Pain, 1
　acute, 1
　chronic, 1, 3
　classification of, 1
　current diagnosis for, 3b
　emergencies with, 5
　mixed, 1
　myofascial, 991b
　　regional, 995–996
　neuropathic, 1, 964–965, 964t
　　diabetic, 2
　nociceptive, 1
　orofacial (See Orofacial pain)
　somatic (nociceptive), 1
　spine (See Spine pain)
　treatment of, 1–4, 5b
　　goals of, 1
　　issues in, 4–5
　　medication(s) for, 2–3
　　　acetaminophen as, 2
　　　approach to using, 2–3
　　　capsaicin as, 3
　　　choice of, 2
　　　disease-specific, 2
　　　initiation of, 2
　　　lidocaine as, 3
　　　nonopioid, 2t
　　　NSAIDs as, 2–3, 2t
　　　opioid, 3, 4t
　　　reevaluation of, 2
　　　routes of administration of, 3
　　　steroids as, 3
　　　tramadol as, 3
　　nonpharmacologic, 3–4
　　under-, 5
　visceral, 1
　as vital sign, 1
Pain contract, 2
Pain management, for pressure ulcers, 858
Palilalia, 919
Palivizumab (Synagis), for bronchiolitis, 266
Palliative care, for high-risk neonates, 1039–1041
Pallid breath-holding spells, 907
2PAM (pralidoxime chloride), for poisoning, 1167–1172t
　due to organophosphates and carbamates, 1206
Pamelor. See Nortriptyline (Pamelor).
Pamidronate (Aredia), for multiple myeloma, 471, 471–472
Pamine (methscopolamine), for allergic rhinitis, 780
p-aminosalicylic acid (PAS, Paser), for tuberculosis, 285t
PAMPs (pathogen-associated molecular patterns), in sepsis, 66–67
Pancrease (pancrelipase), for cystic fibrosis, 237
Pancreatic enzyme replacement, for cystic fibrosis, 237
Pancreatic exocrine insufficiency, 541b, 542, 545, 550
Pancreatic infection, 548
Pancreatic necrosis, 548
Pancreatic pseudocyst, 551–552
Pancreatic secretory trypsin inhibitor (PSTI), in pancreatitis, 546, 546

Pancreatitis, 545
　acute, 545–549
　　clinical manifestations of, 545–546
　　defined, 545–546
　　diagnosis of, 546–547, 546b
　　etiology of, 546, 546t
　　incidence of, 546
　　management of, 547–548, 548b
　　mild, 547, 547t, 548b
　　necrosis and infection in, 548
　　pathogenesis of, 546
　　quantification of severity of, 547, 547t
　　severe, 547–548, 547t, 548b
　biliary (gallstone), 548–549
　chronic, 549–552
　　diagnosis of, 549–550, 550b, 550t
　　etiology and pathogenesis of, 549, 549t
　　incidence of, 549
　　treatment of
　　　endoscopic, 552
　　　medical, 550
　　　surgical, 550–551, 551t
　differential diagnosis of, 496b
　due to HAART, 54–55t
　obstructive, 549
　parenteral nutrition with, 623
　tropical, 549
Pancrelipase (Creon, Pancrease), for cystic fibrosis, 237
PANDAS hypothesis, 920
Panhematin (hematin), for acute porphyria, 476, 476–477
Panhypopituitarism, 656
Panic attacks
　defined, 1131
　epidemiology of, 1131
　symptoms of, 1131b
Panic disorder, 1131
　and comorbid psychiatric disorders, 1131–1132
　diagnosis of, 1131b, 1132b
　differential diagnosis of, 1131
　epidemiology of, 1131
　etiology and clinical features of, 1131–1132
　treatment of, 1132, 1132b, 1132t
Panlor (dihydrocodeine + acetaminophen + caffeine), for pain, 4t
Panmalabsorption, 539, 543–545
Pantoprazole (Protonix)
　for gastroesophageal reflux disease, 553–554, 554t
　for indigestion, 11t
　for peptic ulcer disease, 531t
Pantothenic acid, in parenteral nutrition, 621t
Pao$_2$ (arterial oxygen tension), 225
Papaverine, for erectile dysfunction, 719, 719–720
Papillary muscle rupture, after myocardial infarction, 366t
Papillary thyroid cancer, 671
　follow-up for, 672–673, 673t
Papilloma(s)
　multiple peripheral, of breast, 1047
　of soft palate/tonsillar pillar region, 852
Papillomatosis, denture, 851–852
PAPP-A (pregnancy-associated plasma protein A), 1012
Papular purpuric stocking-and-glove syndrome, 842
Papules, in returning traveler, 163
Papulosquamous eruption(s), 801
　differential diagnosis of, 801b
　lichen planus as, 804
　pityriasis rosea, 805
　psoriasis as, 801–804, 803t
　seborrheic dermatitis as, 804
　tinea corporis as, 804
　tinea versicolor as, 804–805

Paracentesis, for ascites, 502
Paracetamol poisoning, 1176–1178
Paragangliomas (PGLs), 673
　defined, 673
　diagnosis of, 674, 676
　　algorithm for, 674f
　　imaging for, 674
　　laboratory testing in, 674, 675t
　differential diagnosis of, 674
　epidemiology of, 673
　follow-up of, 675–676
　genetic counseling for, 674–675, 675f
　presentation of, 673–674
　treatment of, 675, 676
ParaGard. See Copper IUD (ParaGard).
Parainfluenza virus, 266
Paraneoplastic syndromes, in lung cancer, 243
Paraplatin. See Carboplatin (Paraplatin).
Parapneumonic effusions, 257
Paraproteinemic neuropathies, 963
Parasitic infection(s)
　intestinal (See Intestinal parasite(s))
　malabsorption due to, 544
　pruritus due to, 32b
　of skin, 30b, 844t
　　due to arthropods, 844t, 845–846
　　due to helminths, 843–845, 844t
　　due to protozoa, 843, 844t
　due to transfusions, 485t, 490
Parasitosis, delusions of, pruritus due to, 32b
Parasomnias, 889–890
　vs. seizures, 901t
Parasympathomimetics, for glaucoma, 200
Parathion, poisoning due to, 1205–1206
Parathyroid adenoma, 650
Parathyroidectomy, for renal calculi, 746t
Parcopa (carbidopa/levodopa), for parkinsonism, 954–955
Parental involvement, in care of high-risk neonates, 1037
Parenteral fluid therapy, for infants and children, 626
　for dehydration, 628–631
　　assessment of, 628–630, 628t, 629t
　　diagnosis of, 630
　　fluid management with, 630–631
　　indications for, 630
　　maintenance requirements in, 631
　　rapid rehydration in, 631
　　rehydration requirements (deficit therapy) in, 630–631
　　replacement requirements in, 631
　maintenance fluids in, 626–628
　　electrolyte requirements for, 627, 627t
　　fluid requirements for, 626–627, 627t
　　glucose in, 627
　　method for prescribing, 627–628
　　volume of, 628
　monitoring of, 631
Parenteral nutrition (PN), 618
　with acute renal failure, 623–624
　with acute respiratory distress syndrome, 624
　administration and venous access for, 622
　with anabolic agents, 624
　with chronic renal failure, 624
　complication(s) of, 625–626, 625t
　　catheter sepsis as, 625–626
　　liver dysfunction as, 626, 626b
　　metabolic, 622
　composition of central and peripheral venous solutions for, 620–622, 621t, 622t
　decision steps prior to initiating, 618, 618b
　estimating nutritional requirements for, 619–620
　　energy requirements in, 619–620, 620f
　　nutrient requirements in, 620, 621t
　for extremely low birth weight infants, 1039–1040t

Parenteral nutrition (PN) (Continued)
  with glucose intolerance, 622–623, 623t
  glutamine-supplemented, 625
  with growth factors, 624–625
  with growth hormone, 624
  with hepatic dysfunction and liver failure, 624
  for high-risk neonate, 1035
  indications and contraindications for, 618, 618f
  for inflammatory bowel disease, 518
  infusion and patient monitoring for, 622
  with intestinal dysfunction, 625
  intradialytic, 624
  nutritional assessment for, 618–619, 619b
  with other conditions and nutritional treatments, 624–625
  with pancreatitis, 623
Paresthesias, due to multiple sclerosis, 939
Parinaud's oculoglandular syndrome (POGS), 169
Parkinsonism, 952
  causes of, 953–954, 953b, 954t
  clinical features of, 952–953
  diagnosis of, 953–954, 953b
  differential diagnosis of, 953–954, 953b, 954t
  drug-induced, 954, 954b
  treatment of, 954–958, 955b
    for advanced disease, 958
    amantadine for, 957–958
    anticholinergics for, 957
    COMT inhibitors for, 956–957
    deep brain stimulation for, 958
    dopamine agonists for, 955–956, 956t
    for early disease, 958
    levodopa for, 954–955
    MAO-B inhibitors for, 957
Parkinson-plus syndromes, 953–954
Parkinson's disease (PD), 953, 953
Parkinson's disease dementia (PDD), 954
Parlodel. See Bromocriptine mesylate (Parlodel).
Parnate (tranylcypromine), for major depression, 1124
Paromomycin (Humatin)
  for acute infectious diarrhea, 19–20t
  for amebiasis, 60–61, 61t
  for dientamoebiasis, 565–566t
  for *Entamoeba histolytica*, 564, 565–566t
  for giardiasis, 63–64, 64t, 64b, 565–566t
  for leishmaniasis, 94b, 95, 96
Paronychia, primary (simple) chronic, 817b, 818b, 820
Parotitis, due to mumps, 121, 122b
Paroxetine (Paxil)
  for anxiety disorder(s), 1112
    generalized, 1113, 1113t
  for gaseousness, 10t
  intoxication due to, 1212
  kinetics of, 1212
  for major depression, 1123
  for menopausal symptoms, 1072t
  for multiple sclerosis, 939b
  for obsessive compulsive disorder, 1114, 1114t
  for panic disorder, 1132t
  for polycythemia vera, 34b
  for premenstrual syndrome, 1068–1069, 1068b
  for pruritus due to primary biliary cirrhosis, 499
  for psychiatric dizziness, 209
Paroxysmal cold hemoglobinuria, 389
  diagnosis of, 389
  serology of, 387t
  treatment of, 389
Paroxysmal hemicrania, chronic, orofacial pain due to, 992t
Paroxysmal nocturnal hemoglobinuria (PNH), 379, 393–394

Paroxysmal spells
  in adolescents and adults, 900, 901t
  in infants and children, 907–908, 907b
Paroxysmal sweats, due to alcohol withdrawal, 1102–1103b
Partial nephrectomy, for renal cell carcinoma, 733
Partial rebreathing oxygen masks, 227t
Partial weight support, for stroke rehabilitation, 896b
Particle repositioning maneuver, 206
Parulis, 854
Parvovirus B19
  pruritus due to, 32b
  in sickle cell disease, 406, 409–410
  transfusion-associated, 490
PAS (p-aminosalicylic acid), for tuberculosis, 285t
Paser (p-aminosalicylic acid), for tuberculosis, 285t
PASH (pseudoangiomatous stromal hyperplasia), 1047
PASI (Psoriasis Area Severity Index), 803
Passive external rewarming, for hypothermia, 1145, 1147b
Patch testing, for delayed-type hypersensitivity, 870
Patella, dislocation or subluxation of, 1008
Patellar tendinosis, 1008
Patellofemoral pain, 1008
Patent ductus arteriosus (PDA), 328
  antibiotic prophylaxis with, 345
  in extremely low birth weight infants, 1039–1040t
Patent foramen ovale (PFO), and ischemic stroke, 894
Pathogen-associated molecular patterns (PAMPs), in sepsis, 66–67
Patient education
  for ADHD, 917
  for asthma
    in adolescents and adults, 764–765
    in children, 776
  for chronic fatigue syndrome, 119
  for contact dermatitis, 871
  for diabetes mellitus in children, 585–586
  for fibromyalgia, 996–997
  for hyperthyroidism, 666
  on immunizations, 148–152
  for Stevens-Johnson syndrome and toxic epidermal necrolysis, 866
Pauciarthritis, juvenile idiopathic, 984
Pautrier's microabscesses, 795
Paxil. See Paroxetine (Paxil).
"Pay-loo-ah," lead in, 1197
PBC (primary biliary cirrhosis), 498t, 499
PBG (porphobilinogen), urinary, 475b
PCI (percutaneous coronary intervention), 362, 364b
PCL (posterior cruciate ligament) tears, 1008
PCNL (percutaneous nephrostolithotomy), for renal calculi, 745
PCNSLs (primary central nervous system lymphomas), 975
PCOS (polycystic ovary syndrome), 1063
PCP (*Pneumocystis jiroveci* pneumonia), 53–55, 56t
PCP (phencyclidine). See Phencyclidine (PCP, angel dust).
PCR (polymerase chain reaction), for leprosy, 100
PCT (porphyria cutanea tarda), 475t, 477b, 479
PCV. See Pneumococcal conjugate vaccine (PCV, Prevnar).
PD (Parkinson's disease), 953
PD (potential difference), in cystic fibrosis, 238, 238
PDA. See Patent ductus arteriosus (PDA).

PDD (Parkinson's disease dementia), 954
PDT (photodynamic therapy)
  for actinic keratoses, 794, 834
  for verrucae, 823
PE. See Pulmonary embolism (PE).
PEA (pulseless electrical activity), cardiac arrest from, 305
Peak expiratory flow (PEF), for asthma, 769, 769, 769
Pediatrix. See Hepatitis B virus (HBV) vaccine (Recombivax-HB, Engerix-B, Combivax, Pediarix).
Pediculosis, 30b, 844t, 845
Pediculosis capitis, 844t, 845
Pediculosis corporis, 844t, 845
Pediculosis pubis, 844t, 845
Pediculus humanus, 844t, 845
PedvaxHIB. See *Haemophilus influenzae* type b (Hib) vaccine (PedvaxHIB, ActHIB, HibTITER).
PEEPi (dynamic hyperinflation), 229
PEF (peak expiratory flow), for asthma, 769, 769, 769
PEG (polyethylene glycol)
  for constipation, 10t, 22b
  for whole-bowel irrigation, 1164–1165
PEG (polyethylene glycol)-modified uricase, for gout, 601
PEG-asparaginase (Oncaspar), for acute lymphoblastic leukemia, 449
PEG-interferon-α-2a (PEG-IFN-α-2a, Pegasys), for hepatitis B and C viruses, 536–537, 536t, 538
PEG-interferon-α-2b (PEG-IFN-α-2b, PEG-Intron), for hepatitis B and C viruses, 536–537, 536t, 538
Pegvisomant, for acromegaly, 636
PEL (permissible exposure limit)
  for asbestos, 278
  for silica, 279
Pelvic discomfort, during pregnancy, 1015–1016
Pelvic examination, during pregnancy, 1012
Pelvic exenteration, for cervical cancer, 1089
Pelvic floor dyssynergia, 21
Pelvic inflammatory disease (PID), 1079
  due to *Chlamydia trachomatis*, 1078b, 1079, 1079–1080
  complications of, 1080
  defined, 1079
  diagnosis of, 1079–1080, 1080b
  epidemiology of, 1079
  due to gonorrhea, 751
  pathophysiology of, 1079
  prevention of, 1080–1081
  treatment of, 1080, 1080b
Pelvic trauma, 707b
Pemoline (Cylert), for multiple sclerosis, 939b
Pemphigoid
  bullous, 30b, 866–867
    differential diagnosis of, 866
    pathogenesis of, 866
    treatment of, 866–867
      for aggressive and generalized disease, 867, 869t
      for localized and nonaggressive disease, 866–867, 868t
  cicatricial (mucous membrane), 867–869
  gestationis, pruritus due to, 32b
Pemphigus foliaceus, 869
Pemphigus vulgaris, 869
  mucocutaneous, 869
  mucosal, 869
  of soft palate/tonsillar pillar region, 852
Penciclovir (Denavir), for herpes simplex virus, 841
Penicillin(s)
  for infective endocarditis, 345
  for osteomyelitis, 1006–1007, 1006t

Penicillin(s) (Continued)
  for streptococcal pharyngitis, 222–223
  for syphilis, 755, 755**t**
  for toxic shock syndrome, 89, 89**b**
Penicillin allergy, 782
  desensitization for, 782
  evaluation of, 782, 782**f**
Penicillin G
  for bacterial meningitis, 115**t**
  for endocarditis prophylaxis, 346–347**t**
  for Lyme disease, 138, 139**t**
  for necrotizing skin and soft tissue infections, 85**t**
  for rat-bite fever, 132–133
  for streptococcal pharyngitis, 222–223
  for syphilis, 755**t**
Penicillin G benzathine (Bicillin)
  for anthrax, 126**t**
  for streptococcal pharyngitis, 223, 223**t**
  for syphilis, 755, 755**t**
Penicillin G parenteral aqueous (Pfizerpen)
  for anthrax, 126**t**
  for relapsing fever, 136**t**
Penicillin V potassium (Pen-Vee K, Veetids)
  for acute necrotizing ulcerative gingivitis, 854
  for anthrax, 126**t**
  for rat-bite fever, 132–133
  for relapsing fever, 136**t**
  for streptococcal pharyngitis, 223**t**
Penile amputation, 709
Penile cancer, 737–738
  diagnosis of, 737, 737**b**
  treatment of, 737**b**, 737–738
Penile fracture, 709
Penile injuries, 709
Penile prostheses, for erectile dysfunction, 720
Penile strictures, 742
Penn-Vee K. See Penicillin V potassium (Penn-Vee K, Veetids).
Pentamidine, aerosolized (NebuPent), for *Pneumocystis jiroveci* pneumonia, 56**t**
Pentamidine (Pentacarinat, Pentam)
  for leishmaniasis, 94**b**, 95
  for *Pneumocystis jiroveci* pneumonia, 55
Pentavalent antimonials (Sb), for leishmaniasis, 94, 96
Pentazocine (Talwin), intoxication with, 1204–1205, 1205**t**
Pentazocine + acetaminophen (Talacen), for pain, 4**t**
Pentazocine + naloxone (Talwin-NX), for pain, 4**t**
Pentobarbital (Nembutal)
  for elevated intracranial pressure, 967
    in children, 971
  intoxication with, 1180–1181
Pentosan polysulfate (Elmiron), for prostatitis, 711
Pentostam (sodium stibogluconate pentavalent antimony), for leishmaniasis, 94, 94**b**
  cutaneous, 843, 844**t**
Pentostatin (Nipent), for cutaneous T-cell lymphomas, 798
Pentoxifylline (Trental)
  for alcoholic liver disease, 498
  for toxic shock syndrome, 89–90
  for venous leg ulcers, 857
PEP. See Postexposure prophylaxis (PEP).
Pepcid. See Famotidine (Pepcid).
Peptic strictures, 510
  radiation-related, 510
Peptic ulcer disease (PUD), 529–532
  clinical features of, 530
  complications of, 532
  defined, 529
  diagnostic work-up for, 530–531, 531**b**, 531**t**
  differential diagnosis of, 531
  dyspepsia due to, 528

Peptic ulcer disease (PUD) (Continued)
  epidemiology of, 529
  etiology of, 529–530
  Helicobacter pylori–associated, 529–530, 530**f**
  idiopathic, 530
  indigestion due to, 11**t**
  NSAID-induced, 530
  prevention of, 532
  treatment of, 531–532, 531**t**, 532**t**, 532**b**
Pepto-Bismol. See Bismuth subsalicylate (Pepto-Bismol).
Percocet (oxycodone + acetaminophen)
  intoxication with, 1204–1205, 1205**t**
  for pain, 4**t**
Percodan (oxycodone + aspirin), for pain, 4**t**
Percutaneous coronary intervention (PCI), 362, 364**b**
Percutaneous nephrostolithotomy (PCNL), for renal calculi, 745
Perennial rhinitis, 215, 216
Perfluoroisobutylene (PFIB), as chemical weapon, 1226–1228**t**
Pergolide (Permax)
  for hyperprolactinemia, 660
  for parkinsonism, 955
Periactin. See Cyproheptadine hydrochloride (Periactin).
Perianal abscess, 526–527
  differential diagnosis of, 525, 525**t**
  evaluation of, 525–527
  history of, 525
  pathogenesis of, 526
  physical examination of, 525, 527
  treatment of, 527
Perianal skin tags, 525–526
Pericardial effusion, due to pericarditis, 369
Pericardial friction rub, 369
Pericardiocentesis, 371
Pericarditis, 367
  bacterial, 368–369, 368**b**, 371
  diagnosis of, 369–370, 371**b**
  etiology of, 368–369, 368**b**
  fungal, 368**b**, 369
  due to histoplasmosis, 252
  hospitalization for, 370, 370**b**
  idiopathic, 368**b**, 370–371
  prognosis for, 371
  purulent, 371
  due to radiation therapy for Hodgkin's disease, 444
  recurrent, 371–372
  treatment of, 370–372, 372**b**
  tuberculous, 369, 371
  viral, 368, 368**b**, 370–371
Pericardium, anatomy and physiology of, 367–368
Perilymph, 210
Perilymphatic fistula, 208
Perimenopause, 1070**b**
Periodic limb movements, 889
Peripheral arterial disease (PAD), 373
  abdominal aortic aneurysm as, 374–375
  carotid occlusive disease as, 374
  chronic limb ischemia as, 373–374
  diagnosis of, 373**b**
  differential diagnosis of, 373
  hypertension and, 351
  impact of, 373
  screening for, 373
  treatment of, 373**b**
Peripheral cold injury(ies), 1146–1147
  chilblain as, 1146–1147, 1147**b**
  clinical presentation of, 1146–1147
  frostnip and frostbite as, 1146–1147, 1147**b**
  pathophysiology of, 1146
  sequelae of, 1147
  treatment of, 1147, 1147**b**
  trench foot and immersion foot as, 1147, 1147**b**

Peripheral giant cell granuloma, of alveolar process/gingiva, 854
Peripheral nervous system (PNS), anatomy of, 958
Peripheral neuropathy(ies), 958
  autonomic, 959**b**, 960**t**
  axonopathy as, 958, 961
  carcinomatous, 964
  classification of, 958–961
    by fiber type, 959, 959**b**
    by key signs, 960, 960**b**
    by pathologic and neuropathologic features, 960–961, 961**b**
    by pattern of distribution, 959, 960**t**
    by temporal course, 959–960
  demyelinating, 961, 961**b**
    chronic inflammatory, 962
  diabetic, 962–963
  diagnosis of, 958–961, 961**b**
  Guillain-Barré syndrome as, 962
  due to HAART, 54–55**t**
  hereditary, 963
  infectious, 963–964
  investigations of, 961
  metabolic, 963–964
  mononeuropathies as, 961–962
  motor
    multifocal, 962
    pattern of distribution of, 959, 960**t**
    pure, 960**t**
    signs and symptoms of, 959**b**
  myelinopathy as, 958
  neuronopathies as, 958, 960**t**
  nutritional, 963, 963**b**
  pain due to, 964–965, 964**t**
  paraproteinemic, 963
  pruritus due to, 32**b**
  sensorimotor, 959, 960**t**
  sensory
    large fiber, 959**b**
    pure, 960**t**
    small fiber, 959**b**
  toxic, 963, 963**b**
  treatment of, 961–964
  vasculitic, 964
Peripheral ossifying fibroma, of alveolar process/gingiva, 854
Peripheral parental nutrition (PPN), 621–622
Peripheral stem cell transplantation, for cutaneous T-cell lymphomas, 797**b**, 800
Peripheral venous solutions, composition of, 620–622, 621**t**, 622**t**
Peripherally inserted central venous catheters (PICC), for parenteral nutrition, 622
Peristalsis
  primary, 508
  secondary, 508
  tertiary, 508
Peritoneal dialysis, for poisonings, 1165
Peritoneal lavage, for rewarming, 1146
Peritonitis, spontaneous bacterial, 497**t**, 501**t**, 502
Permax (pergolide)
  for hyperprolactinemia, 660
  for parkinsonism, 955
Permethrin (Nix Cream Rinse, Elimite)
  for pediculosis, 844**t**, 845
  for scabies, 844**t**, 846
Permethrin 0.5% (Permanone), for malaria, 157–158
Permissible exposure limit (PEL)
  for asbestos, 278
  for silica, 279
Pernicious anemia, 394
  clinical features of, 395
  diagnosis of, 395–396, 395**b**
  etiology and pathophysiology of, 394**b**, 395
  malabsorption in, 543
  treatment of, 396–397, 396**b**

Pernicious anemia–associated atrophic gastritis, 529
Pernio, 1146–1147, 1147**b**
Peroneal neuropathy, 962
Perphenazine (Trilafon), poisoning due to, 1208–1209, 1208**t**
Persantine (dipyridamole)
　for ischemic stroke prevention, 894
　for transient ischemic attacks, 208–209
Persistent pulmonary hypertension of the newborn (PPHN), 1038
Personal protective measures, for malaria, 106, 157–158, 157**b**
Pertussis, 146
　clinical symptoms of, 146
　complications of, 146, 146**t**
　cough due to, 27, 28**b**
　diagnosis of, 146–147, 146**b**
　epidemiology of, 146
　immunity to, 146
　microbiology and pathophysiology of, 146
　prevention of, 147, 147**t**
　treatment of, 147, 147**b**
Pertussis toxoid (PT), 147**t**
Pertussis vaccine (Tripedia, Infanrix, Daptacel), 147, 147**t**
Pesticides, poisoning due to, 1205–1206
PFIB (perfluoroisobutylene), as chemical weapon, 1226–1228**t**
Pfizerpen (penicillin G parenteral aqueous)
　for anthrax, 126**t**
　for relapsing fever, 136**t**
PFO (patent foramen ovale), and ischemic stroke, 894
PGE$_1$ (prostaglandin E1), for erectile dysfunction, 719
PGLs. *See* Paragangliomas (PGLs).
PH(s). *See* Pheochromocytomas (PHs).
Ph (Philadelphia) chromosome, 456–457
Phakic intraocular lens surgery, 187
Pharmacologic dependence, 1105
Pharmacologic tolerance, 1105
Pharyngeal gonorrhea, 751, 752**b**
Pharyngitis
　microbiology of, 220–221, 221**b**
　streptococcal, 220
　　clinical manifestations of, 221
　　diagnosis of, 221–222, 221**b**
　　epidemiology of, 221
　　microbiology of, 220–221
　　recurrent, 223, 223**t**
　　treatment of, 222–223
　　　drugs and dosages for, 223**t**
　　　indications for, 222–223, 222**t**
　　　strategies for, 222–223, 222**t**
Pharyngoesophageal diverticulum(a), 511–512
　clinical features of, 511
　defined, 511
　diagnosis of, 511, 512**b**
　dysphagia due to, 509, 510
　treatment of, 511–512, 513**b**
Phenazopyridine (Pyridium), for dysuria, 684, 684**b**
Phencyclidine (PCP, angel dust)
　abuse of, 1110–1111
　intoxication with, 1206–1208
　kinetics of, 1207
Phenelzine (Nardil), for major depression, 1124
Phenergan. *See* Promethazine hydrochloride (Phenergan).
Phenobarbital
　for alcohol withdrawal, 1103
　for benzodiazepine withdrawal, 1108**t**
　for epilepsy
　　in adolescents in adults, 904**t**, 905
　　in infants and children, 912**t**
　for febrile seizures, 910
　intoxication with, 1180–1181

Phenobarbital *(Continued)*
　for pruritus due to primary biliary cirrhosis, 499
　for status epilepticus in neonates, 910
Phenothiazines
　for alcohol withdrawal, 1103
　for nausea and vomiting, 8, 8**t**
　poisoning due to, 1208–1209, 1208**t**
Phenoxybenzamine (Dibenzyline), for pheochromocytomas and paragangliomas, 675
Phentermine (Ionamin), for obesity, 609, 610**t**
Phentolamine (Regitine)
　for amphetamine intoxication, 1179
　for erectile dysfunction, 719
　for poisoning
　　due to cocaine, 1187
　　due to MAOIs, 1203
Phenylephrine (Neo-Synephrine)
　for allergic rhinitis, 780
　for elevated intracranial pressure, 967
　for shock, 69, 69**t**
Phenylpropanolamine, for stress incontinence, 696
Phenytoin (Dilantin)
　for epilepsy
　　in adolescents in adults, 904**t**, 905
　　in infants and children, 912**t**
　for multiple sclerosis, 939**b**
　for post-traumatic seizures, 968
　for status epilepticus, 906
Pheochromocytomas (PHs), 673
　defined, 673
　diagnosis of, 674, 676
　　algorithm for, 674**f**
　　imaging for, 674
　　laboratory testing in, 674, 675**t**
　differential diagnosis of, 674
　epidemiology of, 673
　follow-up of, 675–676
　genetic counseling for, 674–675, 675**f**
　presentation of, 673–674
　treatment of, 675, 676
Philadelphia (Ph) chromosome, 456–457
Phlebotomy
　for hemochromatosis, 433, 500
　for polycythemia vera, 473–474
Phonation, 218, 218**b**
Phosgene, as chemical weapon, 1226–1228**t**
Phosgene oxime, as chemical weapon, 1226–1228**t**
PhosLo (calcium acetate), for chronic renal failure, 730
Phosphate
　for diabetic ketoacidosis, 592–593
　for hyperparathyroidism, 652
　in parenteral nutrition, 621, 622**t**
Phosphodiesterase type 5 inhibitor, for systemic sclerosis, 811
Photochemotherapy
　extracorporeal, for cutaneous T-cell lymphomas, 799
　for vitiligo, 879
Photodynamic therapy (PDT)
　for actinic keratosis, 794, 834
　for verrucae, 823
Photopheresis, for cutaneous T-cell lymphomas, 799
Photorefractive keratectomy (PRK), 189, 191**f**
　complications of, 192**f**, 193
Phototherapy
　for cutaneous T-cell lymphomas, 797–798
　for psoriasis, 802
PHPT (primary hyperparathyroidism), 649–652
Phthirus pubis, 844**t**, 845
Phyllodes tumor, 1053
Physical activity. *See also* Exercise.
　for diabetes
　　in adults, 576**b**, 578, 579**b**

Physical activity *(Continued)*
　　in children, 588
　for dyslipoproteinemia, 604
　for obesity, 609
Physical agents, hemolytic anemia due to, 391**t**, 394
Physical and chemical injury(ies)
　burns as, 1135
　due to cold, 1143
　drug intoxication as, 1160
　due to heat, 1148
　high-altitude illness as, 1140
　marine poisonings, envenomations, and trauma as, 1155
　snakebite as, 1152
　spider bites and scorpion stings as, 1150
Physical modalities, for dysmenorrhea, 1066
Physical therapy (PT)
　for cystic fibrosis, 238
　for juvenile idiopathic arthritis, 985, 986
　for temporomandibular disorder, 993
　for urinary incontinence in children, 691–692
Physiotherapy, adapted, for tinnitus, 39
Physostigmine (Antilirium)
　for poisoning, 1167–1172**t**
　　due to anticholinergics, 1180
　poisoning due to, 1205–1206
Phytotherapy, for benign prostatic hyperplasia, 715–718
PI(s). *See* Protease inhibitors (PIs).
Pica, 384
PICC (peripherally inserted central venous catheters), for parenteral nutrition, 622
Pick-up exercise, for vestibular neurolabyrinthitis, 207**b**
Pickwickian syndrome, 608
Picovir (pleconaril), for viral meningitis or encephalitis, 931
PID. *See* Pelvic inflammatory disease (PID).
Pigment dispersion syndrome, 199
Pigmentary disorder(s), 876
　acral acanthosis nigricans as, 878
　etiology and pathogenesis of, 876
　hyper-, 876–878
　　drug-induced, 877, 877**t**
　　postinflammatory, 877–878
　hypo-, 878–879
　idiopathic guttate hypomelanosis as, 879
　melasma as, 876–877, 877**t**
　pityriasis alba as, 879
　solar lentigo as, 877
　treatment of, 876
　vitiligo as, 878–879
Pill-induced esophagitis, 510
Pilocarpine (Pilocar), for glaucoma, 200
Pimecrolimus (Elidel)
　for anogenital pruritus, 873
　for atopic dermatitis, 861
　for contact dermatitis, 871, 871**b**
　for psoriasis, 801
Pimozide (Orap), for Tourette's syndrome, 921
Pindolol (Visken)
　for angina pectoris, 299
　intoxication with, 1182–1183, 1183**t**
Pineal parenchymal tumors (PPTs), 973**t**
Pinworm, 570**t**, 572
Pin-X. *See* Pyrantel pamoate (Pin-X).
Pioglitazone (Actos), for diabetes, 580**t**, 581
Piperacillin (Pipracil), for pyelonephritis, 685
Piperacillin/tazobactam (Tazocin, Zosyn), for necrotizing skin and soft tissue infections, 85**t**
Piperazines, poisoning due to, 1208–1209, 1208**t**
Piperidines, poisoning due to, 1208–1209, 1208**t**
Piracetam (Nootropil, Normabrain), for tinnitus, 38

Pirbuterol chlorofluorocarbon (Maxair), for asthma
  in adolescents and adults, 766t
  in children, 774–775, 775t
PIRO staging, of sepsis, 65–66, 66b
Pit viper bite
  clinical characteristics of, 1153, 1153t
  dry, 1153, 1154, 1154t
  etiology of, 1153
  identification of, 1153
  with minimal envenomation, 1154, 1154t
  with moderate envenomation, 1154, 1154t
  with severe envenomation, 1154, 1154t
  severity of, 1154t
  treatment of, 1153–1155
Pitch, 218
Pitocin (oxytocin), for postpartum hemorrhage, 1028t
Pitressin (arginine vasopressin), for diabetes insipidus, 647, 647t
Pitressin (vasopressin)
  for cardiac arrest, 306
  for shock, 69t, 70
Pituitary adenoma(s)
  Cushing's syndrome due to, 642f, 644
  growth hormone–secreting, 633
Pituitary causes, of amenorrhea, 1063, 1064b
Pityriasis alba, 879
Pityriasis rosea, 805
Pityriasis versicolor, 804–805, 847, 847b, 848b
Pityrosporum orbiculare, 804–805
Pityrosporum ovale
  in atopic dermatitis, 859, 860
  in seborrheic dermatitis, 804
PJCs (premature junctional complexes), 313
PK (pyruvate kinase) deficiency, 393
Placenta accreta, 1020
Placenta increta, 1020
Placenta percreta, 1020
Placenta previa, 1020, 1020b
Placental abruption, 1020–1021, 1021b
Placental migration, 1020
Plague, 122
  in bioterrorism, 122, 1229–1233t
  bubonic, 122
  diagnosis of, 123, 123b
  epidemiology of, 122
  etiology of, 122
  historical background of, 122
  pathogenesis and clinical syndromes of, 122–123
  pneumonic, 122
    as biological weapon agent, 1229–1233t
  prevention and control of, 123
  septicemic, 122–123
  transmission of, 122
  treatment of, 123, 123b
Plan B (emergency contraceptive pill), 758
Plaquenil. *See* Hydroxychloroquine (Plaquenil, HCQ).
Plasma aldosterone concentration (PAC), 654, 654
Plasma chemistry, reference intervals for, 1220–1221t
Plasma exchange. *See* Plasmapheresis.
Plasma porphyrin fluorescence pattern, 475b
Plasma renin activity (PRA), 654
Plasma transfusion, 483
  frozen, 483
  indications for, 483
Plasmapheresis
  for cold agglutinin syndrome, 389
  for crescentic glomerulonephritis, 703–704
  for myasthenia gravis, 945
  for poisonings, 1173
  for Rh-sensitized women, 418
  for thrombotic thrombocytopenic purpura, 431

Plasmodium falciparum. See also Malaria.
  chloroquine-resistant, 105t, 109
    during pregnancy, 107b
  uncomplicated chloroquine-sensitive, 107b
Plasmodium malariae
  drug-resistant, 105t
  uncomplicated, 107b
Plasmodium ovale
  drug-resistant, 105t
  uncomplicated, 107b
Plasmodium spp. *See also* Malaria.
  chloroquine-sensitive, 109–110
  transfusion-associated, 490
Plasmodium vivax. See also Malaria.
  chloroquine-resistant, 105t, 107b, 110
  in pregnancy, 107b
  uncomplicated, 107b
Platelet(s)
  apheresis, 482
  random donor, 482
  single-donor, 482
  whole blood–derived, 482
Platelet concentrates, 482
Platelet destruction, increased, 426–427
Platelet function, elements of, 425
Platelet pheresis, 482
Platelet production, decreased, 426–427
Platelet refractoriness, 482–483, 486t, 491
Platelet transfusion(s), 482–483
  indications for, 482
  irradiated, 482
  leukoreduced, 482
  refractoriness to, 482–483, 486t, 491
  washed, 482
Platelet-mediated bleeding disorders, 425
  diagnosis of, 426b
  qualitative, 427–428
    acquired, 427
    hereditary, 427–428
  quantitative, 425–427
  treatment of, 427b
Platinol. *See* Cisplatin (Platinol).
Plavix. *See* Clopidogrel bisulfate (Plavix).
Pleconaril (Picovir), for viral meningitis or encephalitis, 931
Plendil (felodipine)
  intoxication with, 1183–1184
  for systemic sclerosis, 811t
Pleural effusion(s), 256
  due to asbestosis, 279
  diagnosis of, 256–257, 256b
    imaging in, 256–257
    pleural fluid analysis in, 257, 257t, 257b
    thoracentesis in, 257
  etiology of, 256, 256b
  exudative, 256, 256b, 257t
  Light's criteria for, 257, 257t
  transudative, 256, 256b, 257
  treatment of, 257, 257b
Pleural fluid analysis, 257, 257t, 257b
Pleural fluid volume, 256
Pleural irrigation, for rewarming, 1146
Pleural plaques, due to asbestosis, 279
Pleural space infection, 257–258
Pleural thickening, diffuse visceral, due to asbestosis, 279
Pleurodesis, for pleural effusion, 257
Plicamycin, for Paget's disease of bone, 616
PM. *See* Polymyositis (PM).
PMF (progressive massive fibrosis), 280
PML (progressive multifocal leukoencephalopathy), natalzumab and, 935
PMR (polymyalgia rheumatica)
  diagnosis of, 1003b, 1003t, 1004
  treatment of, 1004–1005, 1004b, 1004b
PMS. *See* Premenstrual syndrome (PMS).
PN. *See* Parenteral nutrition (PN).

Pneumococcal conjugate vaccine (PCV, Prevnar), 115
  schedule for, 149–150t
  catch-up, 151t
Pneumococcal polysaccharide vaccine (PPV, Pneumovax 23), 263
  schedule for, 149–150t
Pneumococcal vaccine, 115
  schedule for, 149–150t
  catch-up, 151t
Pneumoconiosis(es), 278, 278t
  asbestosis as, 278–279
  diagnosis of, 279b
  etiology of, 278
  management of, 279
  silicosis as, 279–280
Pneumocystis jiroveci pneumonia (PCP), 53–55, 56t
Pneumonia
  bacterial, 261
    community-acquired, 261–263
      admission criteria for, 262, 262t
      diagnostic criteria for, 261b
      diagnostic testing for, 261–262
      epidemiology of, 261
      etiology of, 262, 262b
      prevention of, 263
      sepsis due to, 68t
      treatment of, 262–263, 263b
    health care–acquired, 263–264
      defined, 263
      diagnosis of, 263–264
      epidemiology of, 263
      etiology of, 263
      prevention of, 264
      sepsis due to, 68t
      treatment of, 264, 264t
    ventilator-associated
      defined, 263
      diagnosis of, 263–264
      epidemiology of, 263
      etiology of, 263
      prevention of, 264
      treatment of, 264, 264t
  due to coccidioidomycosis
    acute, 249
    chronic, 249
  mycoplasmal, 266–270
    clinical presentation of, 268
    diagnosis of, 268b, 269
    differential diagnosis of, 268–269
    treatment of, 269–270, 269b, 270t
  Pneumocystis jiroveci, 53–55, 56t
  in sickle cell disease, 406
  due to viral influenza, 266–267
    with bacterial superinfection, 267
    clinical manifestations of, 267
    diagnosis of, 267, 268b
    etiology and pathogenesis of, 266
    prevention of, 266–267
    treatment of, 267, 267t, 269b
Pneumonia severity index (PSI), 262, 262t
Pneumonic plague, 122
  as biological weapon agent, 1229–1233t
Pneumonitis
  hypersensitivity, 280
    diagnosis of, 281
    predictors of, 281b
    treatment of, 281, 281b
  radiation, in Hodgkin's disease, 444
Pneumovax 23 (pneumococcal polysaccharide vaccine), 263
  schedule for, 149–150t
PNF (proprioceptive neuromuscular facilitation), for stroke rehabilitation, 896b
PNH (paroxysmal nocturnal hemoglobinuria), 379, 393–394

PNS (peripheral nervous system), anatomy of, 958
POAG (primary open-angle glaucoma), 198–199, 198**b**
Podofilox (Condylox), for condyloma acuminatum, 825**b**, 826, 1092
Podophyllin resin (Podofin, Podocon-25, Podofilm), for condyloma acuminatum, 825**b**, 826
POGS (Parinaud's oculoglandular syndrome), 169, 169
Poisoning(s), 1160
  with acetaminophen, 1176–1178, 1178**f**, 1178**t**
  with amphetamines, 1178–1179
  with anticholinergic agents, 1179–1180
  with barbiturates, 1180–1181
  with benzodiazepines, 1181–1182
  with β-adrenergic blockers, 1182–1183, 1183**t**
  with calcium channel blockers, 1183–1184
  with carbon monoxide, 1184–1185, 1185**t**
  cardiac arrest due to, 303**t**
  with caustics and corrosives, 1185–1186
  CNS manifestations of, 1165, 1166**t**
  with cocaine, 1186–1187, 1187**t**
  with cyanide, 1167–1172**t**, 1187–1188
  delayed toxin action in, 1161
  with digitalis, 1188–1190
  epidemiology of, 1160–1161
  with ethanol, 1190–1191, 1190**t**, 1191**t**
  with ethylene glycol, 1191–1193
  with hydrocarbons, 1193–1194
  with iron, 1194–1195
  with isoniazid, 1195–1196
  with isopropanol, 1196
  lead, 1196–1200
    disposition for, 1200
    epidemiology of, 1196
    hobbies associated with, 1197, 1198**b**
    kinetics of, 1197
    laboratory investigations of, 1198–1199, 1199**t**
    management of, 1199–1200, 1200**t**
    manifestations of, 1198**t**
    due to occupational exposure, 1196**t**, 1197
    and recommended lead content, 1197, 1198**t**
    screening for, 1196, 1197**t**
    sources of, 1196–1197, 1197**t**
    toxic dose in, 1196
    toxic mechanism in, 1196–1197
    due to traditional folk remedies, 1197
  with lithium, 1200–1201
  management of
    for altered mental status, 1173
    antidotes in, 1165, 1167–1172**t**
    assessment and maintenance of vital functions in, 1161, 1162**t**, 1163**t**
    decontamination in, 1161–1165
      activated charcoal for, 1164, 1164**t**
      gastric emptying procedures for, 1161–1163
      gastric lavage for, 1163–1164
      ipecac syrup for, 1163
      whole-bowel irrigation for, 1164–1165
    for dermal exposure, 1161
    for electrolyte, acid-base, and osmolality disturbances, 1174–1175, 1175**t**, 1175**t**, 1176**t**
    enhancement of elimination in, 1165–1173
      dialysis for, 1165, 1174**t**
      hemofiltration for, 1173
      hemoperfusion for, 1165–1173
      plasmapheresis for, 1173
    flumazenil in, 1174
    for gastrointestinal exposure, 1161
    for hypoglycemia, 1173
    for inhalation exposure, 1161
    in-hospital disposition in, 1165

Poisoning(s) *(Continued)*
    laboratory studies in, 1174–1176, 1174**t**
    nalmefene in, 1174
    for ocular exposure, 1161
    for opioid reactions, 1173–1174
    prevention of absorption and reduction of local damage in, 1161–1165
    radiographic studies in, 1175–1176
    supportive care, observation, and therapy for complications in, 1173–1174
    for thiamine deficiency encephalopathy, 1173
    toxicologic studies in, 1176
  marine (*See* Marine poisonings)
  with methanol, 1201–1202
  with monoamine oxidase inhibitors, 1202–1204
  with opioids, 1173–1174, 1204–1205, 1205**t**
  with organophosphates and carbamates, 1205–1206
  with phencyclidine, 1206–1208
  with phenothiazines and nonphenothiazines, 1208–1209, 1208**t**
  routes of exposure in, 1161
  with salicylates, 1209–1212, 1211**t**
  due to snakebite (*See* Snakebite)
  with SSRIs, 1212
  with theophylline, 1212–1214, 1213**t**
  with tricyclic and cyclic antidepressants, 1214–1216, 1215**t**
Poliovirus vaccine, schedule for, 149–150**t**
  catch-up, 151**t**
Pollens, and asthma
  in adolescents and adults, 765**b**
  in children, 771
Polyarthritis, juvenile idiopathic, 984
Polycystic ovary syndrome (PCOS), 1063
Polycythemia rubra vera, pruritus due to, 32**b**
Polycythemia vera (PV), 472
  clinical presentation of, 472
  defined, 472
  diagnosis of, 473, 473**b**
  genetic basis for, 472
  natural history of, 472–473
  pruritus due to, 34**b**
  treatment of, 473
Polyethylene glycol (PEG, MiraLax, Glycolax, GoLYTELY, Colyte)
  for constipation, 10**t**, 22**b**
  for whole-bowel irrigation, 1164–1165
Polyethylene glycol (PEG)-modified uricase, for gout, 601
Polymerase chain reaction (PCR), for leprosy, 100
Polymyalgia rheumatica (PMR)
  diagnosis of, 1003**b**, 1003**t**, 1004
  treatment of, 1004–1005, 1004**b**, 1004**b**
Polymyositis (PM), 812–813
  clinical characteristics of, 812, 812**t**
  diagnosis of, 813**b**
  treatment of, 812–813, 813**b**, 813**b**
Polyneuropathy
  chronic inflammatory demyelinating, 962
  distal symmetric sensory, in diabetes, 962
Polysaccharide-iron complex (Niferex Film Coated Tablets), 385
Ponstel (mefenamic acid)
  for dysmenorrhea, 1066**t**
  for pain, 2**t**
POPs (progestin only pills), 756–757
  in postpartum period, 1029**t**
Porokeratosis, 833**b**, 834**b**, 835
Porphobilinogen (PBG), urinary, 475**b**
Porphyria(s), 475
  acute hepatic
    acute attacks of, 476–479
    classification of, 475**t**
    diagnosis of, 476**t**, 476**b**

Porphyria(s) *(Continued)*
    drugs and chemical that exacerbate, 477, 474–478**b**
    frequent recurrent attacks of, 477–478
    prevention of attacks of, 478–479
    seizures in, 477
    treatment of, 476–479, 477**b**
  acute intermittent, 475**t**, 476**t**
  ALA dehydratase deficiency, 475**t**, 476**t**
  chronic cutaneous
    classification of, 475**t**
    diagnosis of, 476**b**
    treatment of, 477**b**, 479–480
  classification of, 475, 475**t**
  diagnosis of, 475–476, 475**b**, 476**t**, 476**b**
  erythropoietic, 475**t**, 477**b**, 479–480
    congenital, 475**t**, 477**b**, 479
  hepatoerythropoietic, 475**t**, 477**b**, 479
  hereditary copro-, 475**t**, 476**t**
  proto-, 475**t**, 477**b**, 479–480
  treatment of, 476–480, 477**b**
  variegate, 475**t**, 476**t**
Porphyria cutanea tarda (PCT), 475**t**, 477**b**, 479
Portal hypertension
  and ascites, 501
  and esophageal varices, 505
Portopulmonary hypertension (PPHTN), 497**t**, 501**t**, 503–504
Posaconazole (Noxafil)
  for blastomycosis, 255–256
  for coccidioidomycosis, 250**t**, 251, 251**t**
  for necrotizing skin and soft tissue infections, 85**t**
Positioning, after stroke, 897
Positive symptoms, of schizophrenia, 1128–1129
Postconcussive syndrome, 965
Posterior cruciate ligament (PCL) tears, 1008
Posterior inferior cerebellar artery syndrome, vertigo due to, 209
Postexposure prophylaxis (PEP)
  for anthrax, 126**t**, 127
  for HIV infection, 58–59
  for Lyme disease, 139
Postherpetic neuralgia, 840–841, 842, 964
  orofacial pain due to, 992**t**
Postinfectious cough, 25–26
  causes of, 25–26, 25**b**
  evaluation of, 26–27, 27, 26**b**
  treatment of, 28**b**
Postinflammatory hyperpigmentation, 877–878
Post-Lyme disease syndrome, 138–139
Postnasal drip
  cough due to, 26–27, 28**b**
  laryngitis due to, 220
Postnatal care, of high-risk neonate, 1034–1037
Postoperative malabsorption, 545
Postoperative nausea and vomiting, 9
Postpartum depression, 1029
Postpartum hemorrhage, 1027
  defined, 1027
  epidemiology of, 1027
  etiology of, 1027, 1027**b**
  due to placenta previa, 1020
  treatment of, 1027, 1028**t**
Postpartum period, 1027
  breast-feeding in, 1027–1028
  contraception in, 1028, 1029**t**
  defined, 1027
  diagnosis in, 1028**b**
  hemorrhage in, 1027, 1027**b**, 1028**t**
  medical complications in, 1028–1029
  mood disorders in, 1029
  nutrition and activity in, 1028
  puerperal infections in, 1028
  treatment in, 1028**b**
Postpartum psychosis, 1029
Postpartum thyroiditis, 665

Postrenal failure, 724
  causes of, 722b, 724
  defined, 721
  diagnosis and treatment of, 724, 724b
Post-stroke central pain syndrome, 897–898
Post-term gestation, 1013
Post-transfusion purpura (PTP), 486t, 491
Post-traumatic seizures, 968
  in children, 970
Postural auscultatory phenomena, in mitral valve prolapse, 335, 335f
Postvoid residual (PVR), 694–695
Potassium
  for diabetic ketoacidosis, 592, 592t, 593t
  for hyperglycemic hyperosmolar state, 592, 594t
  in parenteral nutrition, 621, 622t
  for salicylate poisoning, 1211, 1211t
Potassium citrate (Urocit-K), for renal calculi, 746t
Potassium requirements, for infants and children, 627
Potassium-sparing diuretics, for hypertension, 357
Potential difference (PD), in cystic fibrosis, 238
Poverty of content, in schizophrenia, 1129
Poverty of speech, in schizophrenia, 1129
Poxviruses, 842–843
PP (protoporphyria), 475t, 477b, 479–480
PPHN (persistent pulmonary hypertension of the newborn), 1038
PPHTN (portopulmonary hypertension), 497t, 501t, 503–504
PPIs. See Proton pump inhibitors (PPIs).
PPL (benzylpenicilloyl-polylysine), 782
PPMS (primary progressive multiple sclerosis), 933, 938
PPN (peripheral parental nutrition), 621–622
PPTs (pineal parenchymal tumors), 973t
PPV (pneumococcal polysaccharide vaccine), 263
  schedule for, 149–150t
PRA (plasma renin activity), 654
Pralidoxime chloride (2PAM, Protopam), for poisoning, 1167–1172t
  due to organophosphates and carbamates, 1206
Pramipexole (Mirapex), for parkinsonism, 955, 956t
Pramlinitide (Symlin), for diabetes, 580t, 580t, 581
Prandin (repaglinide), for diabetes, 580t
Prasugrel (Effient), 1244–1249t
Pravastatin (Pravachol)
  for angina pectoris, 297–298, 298
  for dyslipoproteinemia, 605, 605t
Pravastatin-aspirin (Pravigard), for dyslipoproteinemia, 605t
Prazepam, intoxication with, 1181–1182
Praziquantel (Biltricide)
  for schistosomiasis, 570t, 844t, 845
  for tapeworms, 570t
Prazosin (Minipress)
  for pheochromocytomas and paragangliomas, 675
  for systemic sclerosis, 811t
Prealbumin, in nutritional assessment, 619
Preconception counseling, 1011
Precose (acarbose), for diabetes, 580t
Prediabetes, 576t
Prednisolone (Delta-Cortef, Prelone, Orapred)
  for asthma
    in adolescents and adults, 766t, 767–768t
    in children, 772b, 773–774t
  for caustic or corrosive burns, 1186
Prednisone (Deltasone, Orasone, Medrol, Sterapred)
  for acute lymphoblastic leukemia, 449
  for adrenocortical insufficiency, 639
  for alcoholic liver disease, 498–499

Prednisone (Deltasone, Orasone, Medrol, Sterapred) (Continued)
  for asthma
    in adolescents and adults, 766t, 767–768t
    in children, 772b, 773–774t
  for autoimmune hepatitis, 499
  for Bell's palsy, 951, 951f, 962
  for bronchospasm, 28b
  for bullous pemphigoid, 867
  for chronic inflammatory demyelinating polyneuropathy, 962
  for cluster headache, 926t
  for contact dermatitis, 871, 871b
  for COPD, 28b
    with acute exacerbation, 229
  for crescentic glomerulonephritis, 703–704
  for cutaneous vasculitis, 816
  for diabetic neuropathy, 962–963
  for eosinophilic bronchitis, 28b
  for giant cell arteritis, 1004–1005, 1004b, 1004b
  for gout, 599
  for hypersensitivity pneumonitis, 281, 281b
  for hypopituitarism, 658
  for idiopathic inflammatory myopathy, 812–813
  for idiopathic thrombocytopenic purpura, 427b
  for infectious mononucleosis, 117
  for insect stings, 785
  for juvenile idiopathic arthritis, 986
  for multiple myeloma, 469b, 470
    with hypercalcemia, 471
  for myasthenia gravis, 943, 944t
  for nephropathy
    IgA, 703
    membranous, 702
  for optic neuritis, 197
  for pain, 3
  for pemphigus vulgaris, 869
  for pericarditis, 371, 372
  for polymyalgia rheumatica, 1004–1005, 1004b, 1004b
  for systemic lupus erythematosus, 808
  for systemic sclerosis, 810, 811
  for urticaria, 875
  for warm autoimmune hemolytic anemia, 387
Preeclampsia, 1024–1026
  with chronic hypertension, 1023
  classification of, 1024, 1024b
  clinical findings in, 1022t, 1024b
  defined, 1024
  mild, 1024, 1025, 1025f
  mode of delivery with, 1027
  pathogenesis and pathophysiology of, 1024
  in postpartum period, 1028
  prevention of, 1024–1025, 1025b
  risk factors for, 1025b
  severe, 1024, 1024b, 1025–1026, 1026f
  treatment of, 1025–1026, 1025f, 1026f, 1027
Pregabalin (Lyrica)
  for anogenital pruritus, 872b
  for epilepsy, 904t, 903
  for fibromyalgia, 997
  for neuropathic pain, 964–965
  for radicular pain, 42
Pregnancy
  acute cholecystitis in, 494–495
  alpha fetoprotein testing during, 1012
  amniocentesis during, 1012
  antepartum care during, 1011
  backache and pelvic discomfort during, 1015–1016
  bleeding during, 1013
  blood pressure during, 1012
  breast cancer during, 1053–1054
  cervical cancer during, 1090
  constipation during, 1015

Pregnancy (Continued)
  dental care during, 1016
  diabetes insipidus during, 648
  disseminated intravascular coagulation during, 429
  ectopic, 1017
    diagnosis of, 1017, 1017–1019, 1017b, 1018f
    risk factors for, 1017
    treatment of, 1019, 1019b
  folate prophylaxis during, 397
  heartburn during, 1014
  high-risk referrals during, 1011, 1011b
  HIV infection during, 58, 1014, 1016b
  Hodgkin's lymphoma during, 438
  hospitalization during, 1017
  hypertension during, 1021
    chronic, 1022–1024
      classification of, 1022–1023
      clinical findings in, 1022t
      diagnosis of, 1022–1023, 1022b
      epidemiology of, 1022
      low risk vs. high risk, 1022
      maternal and fetal risks with, 1023
      primary (essential) vs. secondary, 1022
      treatment of, 1023–1024, 1023t, 1023b
    definitions and classification of, 1022
    epidemiology of, 1021
    gestational, 1022t, 1024
    in HELLP syndrome, 1026–1027
      clinical findings in, 1026–1027
      diagnostic criteria for, 1026, 1026b
      intrapartum and postpartum management of, 1027
      mode of delivery with, 1027
    preeclampsia as, 1024–1026
      with chronic hypertension, 1023
      classification of, 1024, 1024b
      clinical findings in, 1022t, 1024b
      defined, 1024
      mild, 1024, 1025, 1025f
      mode of delivery with, 1027
      pathogenesis and pathophysiology of, 1024
      prevention of, 1024–1025, 1025b
      risk factors for, 1025b
      severe, 1024, 1024b, 1025–1026, 1026f
      treatment of, 1025–1026, 1025f, 1026f, 1027
    due to renal disease, 1022t
  hyperthyroidism and, 669
  hypothyroidism during, 664–665
  immunization during, 1016, 1016b
  infection during, 1014–1015, 1015b
  inflammatory bowel disease in, 520–521
  intercourse during, 1016
  leg cramps during, 1016
  leprosy in, 101–102
  malaria in, 107b, 110, 110
  mask of, 876
  medications during, 1011–1012
  multiple sclerosis during, 939
  nausea and vomiting in, 6, 9, 1013–1014
  nutrition and weight gain during, 1014
  post-term, 1013
  pruritus in, 32b
  RhD antigen alloimmunization during, 416
    diagnosis of, 416b
    prevention of, 416
    treatment of, 416–418, 417b
  Rocky Mountain spotted fever in, 177, 179b
  rubella exposure during, 140–141
  with sickle cell disease, 411
  smoking during, 1012
  syphilis during, 755
  systemic lupus erythematosus during, 806
  tests of fetal well-being during, 1016–1017, 1016b, 1017t
  thyroiditis after, 677

Pregnancy (Continued)
    toxoplasmosis in, 165t, 168
    ultrasonography during, 1013
    upper extremity discomfort during, 1015
    urinary symptoms during, 1014
    vaginal bleeding in late, 1019
    varicose veins during, 1015
    von Willebrand's disease in, 425
    warning signs and symptoms prompting medical attention during, 1013b
    x-rays, ionizing radiation, and imaging during, 1016
Pregnancy-associated plasma protein A (PAPP-A), 1012
Prehypertension, 349–350, 351t, 351f
Prelone. See Prednisolone (Delta-Cortef, Prelone, Orapred).
Premalignant skin lesion(s), 833
    actinic cheilitis as, 834
    actinic keratosis as, 833–834
    bowenoid papulosis as, 834–835
    Bowen's disease as, 834
    diagnosis of, 833b
    nevus sebaceus as, 835
    porokeratosis as, 835
    risk factors for, 833
    treatment of, 834b
Premarin. See Conjugated equine estrogens (CEE, Premarin).
Premarin Vaginal (estrogen cream), for urogenital atrophy, 1072b
Premature atrial complexes (PACs), 312–313
    blocked, 312
    clinical features of, 312–313
    electrocardiographic features of, 312
    treatment of, 313
Premature beats, 312
    diagnosis of, 312b
    etiology and pathogenesis of, 312
    premature atrial complexes as, 312–313
    premature junctional complexes as, 313
    premature ventricular complexes as, 313–314
    treatment of, 313b
Premature infant(s)
    classification of, 1039
    infant formula for, 1043b
    nutrition for, 1035–1037
    resuscitation of, 1032
Premature junctional complexes (PJCs), 313
Premature ovarian failure, 1063
Premature rupture of membranes (PROM), bacterial vaginosis and, 1074
Premature ventricular complexes (PVCs), 313–314
    classification of, 314
    clinical features of, 314
    electrocardiographic features of, 313–314
    treatment of, 314
Prematurity, rate of, 1033
Premenstrual dysphoric disorder (PMDD), 1067, 1067–1068
Premenstrual syndrome (PMS), 1066
    defined, 1066–1067
    diagnosis of, 1067–1068, 1067b, 1068b
    etiology of, 1067
    morbidity of, 1067
    prevalence of, 1067
    symptoms of, 1067, 1067b
    treatment of, 1068–1069, 1068b
Premonitory symptoms, of tics, 919
Prenalterol, for β-blocker intoxication, 1183
Prenatal care. See Antenatal care.
Prenatal diagnosis, of high-risk neonate, 1033
Preoperative care, with sickle cell disease, 412
Pre-Pen (benzylpenicilloyl-polylysine), 782
Prerenal azotemia, 721–722
    vs. acute tubular necrosis, 724t
    causes of, 721, 722b, 723f

Prerenal azotemia (Continued)
    defined, 721
    laboratory findings in, 721–722, 724b
    with parenteral nutrition, 625t
    treatment of, 721–722
Presbyopia, 188
Presbyphonia, 219
Presenilin, in Alzheimer's disease, 882
Pressure, for keloids, 821
Pressure relief, for pressure ulcers, 857–858
Pressure ulcers, 857
    differential diagnosis of, 857, 857b
    treatment of
        débridement in, 858
        electrotherapy in, 858–859
        granulation tissue formation in, 859
        infection control in, 859
        moist wound environment in, 858
        nutrition and hydration in, 858
        occlusive dressings in, 858
        pain management in, 858
        pressure relief in, 857–858
        principles of, 857, 858b
        vacuum-assisted closure in, 858
        wound fluid in, 859
Presyncope, 205t
Preszista (darunavir/ritonavir), for HIV, 50t
Preterm infants. See Premature infant(s).
Prevacid. See Lansoprazole (Prevacid).
Prevnar. See Pneumococcal conjugate vaccine (PCV, Prevnar).
Priapism, in sickle cell disease, 407, 411
Prick testing, for immediate-type hypersensitivity, 870
Priftin (rifapentine)
    for leprosy, 102
    for tuberculosis, 285t, 287t
Prilosec. See Omeprazole (Prilosec).
Primaquine phosphate
    for malaria, 108t, 109, 111–112t, 157, 157t
    for Pneumocystis jiroveci pneumonia, 55
Primary adrenal hyperplasia (PAH), 654
Primary biliary cirrhosis (PBC), 498t, 499
Primary central nervous system lymphomas (PCNSLs), 975
Primary hyperparathyroidism (PHPT), 649–652
    clinical forms of, 650
    diagnosis and evaluation of, 650–651
        bone mass measurement in, 651
    differential diagnosis of, 650, 650t
    incidence and general characteristics of, 649–650
    pathophysiology, molecular genetics, and pathology of, 650
    signs and symptoms of, 650
    treatment of, 651, 651t
Primary open-angle glaucoma (POAG), 198–199, 198b
Primary progressive multiple sclerosis (PPMS), 933, 938
Primary sclerosing cholangitis (PSC), 498t, 499–500
Primaxin (imipenem-cilastatin), for necrotizing skin and soft tissue infections, 85t
Primidone (Mysoline), for epilepsy
    in adolescents in adults, 904t, 905
    in infants and children, 912t
Primsol Oral Solution (trimethoprim oral solution), for urinary tract infections in girls, 687b, 688t
Prinivil (lisinopril), for myocardial infarction, 365t
Prions, due to transfusions, 485t, 490
Pristiq (desvenlafaxine succinate), 1244–1249t
PRK (photorefractive keratectomy), 189, 191f
    complications of, 192f, 193
ProAmatine (midodrine), for hepatorenal syndrome, 503

Pro-Banthine (propantheline), for urge incontinence, 695b
Probenecid
    for Chlamydia trachomatis, 1078b
    for hyperuricemia, 599
    for pelvic inflammatory disease, 1080b
    for syphilis, 755t
Probiotics
    for acute infectious diarrhea, 17–18
    for inflammatory bowel disease, 518
Procaine penicillin (Wycillin), for syphilis, 755t
Procardia. See Nifedipine (Adalat, Procardia).
Prochlorperazine (Compazine)
    for motion sickness and vertigo, 206t
    for nausea and vomiting, 8t
    poisoning due to, 1208–1209, 1208t
    for renal calculi, 745t
    for Salmonella gastroenteritis, 172
Procrit (erythropoietin), for chronic renal failure, 729–730
Prodelion (quinagolide), for hyperprolactinemia, 660, 660t
Progesterone, in ectopic pregnancy, 1017
Progesterone implant (Implanon), for contraception in postpartum period, 1029t
Progestin(s)
    for anovulatory bleeding, 1058–1059
    for endometrial cancer, 1085
    for menorrhagia, 1059
Progestin injection. See Depot medroxyprogesterone acetate (DMPA, Depo-Provera, Depo-Sub Q Provera).
Progestin only methods, of contraception, 756–757
Progestin only pills (POPs, Micronor, Ovrette), 756–757
    in postpartum period, 1029t
Progestin-releasing intrauterine device (Mirena), 757
    for menorrhagia, 1059
    in postpartum period, 1029t
Progestogens, for endometriosis, 1055–1056, 1057t
Prograf. See Tacrolimus (Prograf).
Progressive massive fibrosis (PMF), 280
Progressive multifocal leukoencephalopathy (PML), natalzumab and, 935
Progressive supranuclear palsy (PSP), 953
Proinflammatory molecules, in sepsis, 67b
Prokinetic drugs
    for constipation, 22, 22b
    for gastroesophageal reflux disease, 554
    for gastroparesis, 10t
Prolactin secretion, normal physiology of, 659
Prolactinomas, 659, 660–661
Prolactin-producing tumor, amenorrhea due to, 1063
Prolixin (fluphenazine), poisoning due to, 1208–1209, 1208t
PROM (premature rupture of membranes), bacterial vaginosis and, 1074
Promethazine hydrochloride (Phenergan)
    for motion sickness and vertigo, 206t, 210
    for nausea and vomiting, 8t
    poisoning due to, 1208–1209, 1208t
    for posterior inferior cerebellar artery syndrome, 209
    for Salmonella gastroenteritis, 172
Propafenone (Rythmol)
    for atrial fibrillation, 309–310, 310b
    for cardioversion, 311, 311t
Propantheline (Pro-Banthine), for urge incontinence, 695b
Propecia (finasteride)
    for androgenic alopecia, 791
    for benign prostatic hyperplasia, 714–717, 714t,
Propine (dipivefrin), for glaucoma, 200

Propionic acids, for dysmenorrhea, 1066t
Propofol (Diprivan), for traumatic brain injury, 967, 968
Propoxur, poisoning due to, 1205–1206
Propoxyphene (Darvon)
    intoxication with, 1204–1205, 1205t
    kinetics of, 1204
    for osteoarthritis, 1000
    for pain, 4t
Propoxyphene + acetaminophen (Balacet, Darvocet)
    for osteoarthritis, 1000
    for pain, 4t
Propoxyphene + aspirin + caffeine (Darvon Compound 32, Darvon Compound 65), for pain, 4t
Propranolol (Inderal)
    for acute porphyria, 476, 477b
    for angina pectoris, 299, 299t
    for cocaine abuse, 1109
    for esophageal varices, 505
    for hyperthyroidism, 666
    intoxication with, 1182–1183, 1183t
    for subacute thyroiditis, 677
    for thyroid storm, 669
    for vestibular migraine, 209
Proprioceptive neuromuscular facilitation (PNF), for stroke rehabilitation, 896b
Propylene glycol, and serum osmolality, 1176t
Propylthiouracil (PTU)
    for hyperthyroidism, 667–668
    for thyroid storm, 669
Proscar (finasteride)
    for androgenic alopecia, 791
    for benign prostatic hyperplasia, 714–717, 714t,
ProSom (estazolam), for insomnia, 888t
Prostacyclin analogues, for systemic sclerosis, 811
Prostaglandin
    in chronic renal failure, 729
    in dysmenorrhea, 1065
Prostaglandin analogues, for glaucoma, 199–200, 200t
Prostaglandin E1 (PGE$_1$), for erectile dysfunction, 719
Prostaphlin. See Oxacillin (Bactocill, Prostaphlin).
Prostate carcinoma, 731–732
    diagnosis of, 731–732, 731b
    epidemiology of, 731
    grading of, 732
    hereditary, 731
    metastatic, 732
    staging of, 732
    treatment of, 732, 732b
Prostatectomy, radical, for prostate cancer, 732
Prostate-specific antigen (PSA), 714–716, 731–732
Prostatic hyperplasia, benign. See Benign prostatic hyperplasia (BPH).
Prostatitis, 709
    asymptomatic inflammatory, 712
    bacterial
        acute, 709–710, 711b
        chronic, 710, 711b
    chronic
        bacterial, 710, 711b
        nonbacterial, 710–712
            diagnosis of, 710, 711b
            treatment of, 710–712, 711b, 711f
    classification of, 709, 710b
    diagnosis of, 711b
    epidemiology of, 709
    treatment of, 711b
    urinary tract infections due to, 680, 681
Prostheses, for obstructive sleep apnea, 241
Prosthetic valve endocarditis (PVE), 342, 343b

Prostib (meglumine antimoniate), for leishmaniasis, 94, 94b
Prostigmin (neostigmine bromide)
    for myasthenia gravis, 942t
    poisoning due to, 1205–1206
Protease inhibitors (PIs), for HIV, 49–50, 50t
    adverse drug reactions to, 54–55t
    drug interactions with, 53
    failure of, 52t
    resistance to, 51, 52t
Protective tanning, 880
Protein C, recombinant human activated, for sepsis, 71
Protein C concentrate (Ceprotin), 1243
Protein hydrolysate with medium-chain triglycerides, in infant formula, 1043b
Protein intake
    for hepatic encephalopathy, 502–503
    for high-risk neonate, 1035
Protein malabsorption, 541–542, 541b
Protein requirements, 620
    of infants, 1044
    during pregnancy, 1014
Protein restriction, for chronic renal failure, 729
Protein-losing enteropathy, 541–542, 541b
Proteinuria, in chronic renal failure, 726, 729
Proton pump inhibitors (PPIs)
    for gastroesophageal reflux disease, 553–554, 554, 554, 554, 554t
    for indigestion, 11t, 11t
    for peptic ulcer disease, 531–532, 531t, 532t
Protonix. See Pantoprazole (Protonix).
Protopam (pralidoxime chloride), for poisoning, 1167–1172t
    due to organophosphates and carbamates, 1206
Protopic. See Tacrolimus ointment (Protopic).
Protoporphyria (PP), 475t, 477b, 479–480
Protozoa, 563–567, 565–566t
    acute infectious diarrhea due to, 14b, 15b, 16
    skin infections due to, 843, 844t
    spore-forming, 565–566t, 567–569
Protriptyline (Vivactil)
    for major depression, 1124
    poisoning due to, 1214–1216, 1215t
Proventil. See Albuterol (Accuneb, Proventil, Ventolin).
Provera (medroxyprogesterone acetate)
    for anovulatory bleeding, 1058–1059
    after menopause, 1071–1072, 1072t
Provigil (modafinil)
    for motion sickness, 210
    for multiple sclerosis, 939b
Proximal diabetic neuropathy, 962–963
Proximal subungual onychomycosis (PSO), 818
Prozac. See Fluoxetine (Prozac).
Prurigo
    nodularis, 30b
    of pregnancy, 32b
Pruritic folliculitis of pregnancy, 32b
Pruritic urticarial papules and plaques of pregnancy, 32b
Pruritus, 29
    ani and vulvae, 31f, 871
        clinical features and diagnosis of, 872, 872b
        defined, 871
        epidemiology of, 871
        etiology of, 871–872
        treatment of, 872–873, 872b, 873b
    brachoradial, 32b
    causes of, 31f
    due to cholestasis, 32b, 34b
    complications of, 33–34
    due to dermatitis, 30b
    diagnosis of, 29–30, 29b, 33t
    exposure-related, 31b
    follow-up for, 34
    due to neurotic excoriation, 32b, 34b

Pruritus (Continued)
    due to notalgia paresthetica, 32b, 34b
    pathogenesis of, 29
    due to polycythemia vera, 34b
    in pregnancy, 32b
    due to primary biliary cirrhosis, 499
    refractory, 33t
    due to spinal opioids, 34b
    due to systemic disease, 29, 32b
    treatment of, 30–33, 30b, 33b, 34b
    due to uremia, 34b
PS-341 (bortezomib), for multiple myeloma, 469b, 470, 471
PSA (prostate-specific antigen), 714–716, 731–732
PSC (primary sclerosing cholangitis), 498t, 499–500
Pseudoangiomatous stromal hyperplasia (PASH), 1047
Pseudo-Cushing's syndrome, 641b, 643f
Pseudocyst, pancreatic, 551–552
Pseudoephedrine (Sudafed), for stress incontinence, 695b, 696
Pseudoexfoliation syndrome, 199
Pseudogout, 1001
Pseudohypertension, 351
Pseudohyponatremia, 595, 595b
Pseudohypoparathyroidism, 652
Pseudomonas aeruginosa
    in cystic fibrosis, 237
    necrotizing skin and soft tissue infections due to, 84t, 85t
Pseudopregnancy regimen, for endometriosis, 1056, 1057b
Pseudoseizures, 900, 901t
Pseudoterranova decipiens, 570t, 572
PSI (pneumonia severity index), 262, 262t
Psittacosis, 127
    clinical features of, 127
    diagnosis of, 127–128, 128b
    epidemiology of, 127
    management of, 128, 128b
    risk factors for, 127
PSO (proximal subungual onychomycosis), 818
Psoralens with ultraviolet light A (PUVA)
    for cutaneous T-cell lymphomas, 797–798
    for psoriasis, 802
    for vitiligo, 879
Psoriasis, 30b, 801–804
    biologicals for, 802–804, 803t
    clinical features of, 801
    epidemiology of, 801
    factors influencing, 801
    guttate, 801
    hair disorders due to, 792
    nails in, 819–820
    phototherapy for, 802
    systemic therapy for, 802
    topical therapy for, 801–802
Psoriasis Area Severity Index (PASI), 803
Psoriatic arthritis, 801, 984
PSP (progressive supranuclear palsy), 953
PSTI (pancreatic secretory trypsin inhibitor), in pancreatitis, 546, 546
Psychiatric disorder(s)
    alcoholism as, 1097
    anxiety disorders as, 1111
    bulimia nervosa as, 1115
    comorbid with bulimia nervosa, 1115–1116
    delirium as, 1118
    drug abuse as, 1104
    mood disorders as, 1120
    nausea and vomiting due to, 6, 6t
    panic disorder as, 1131
    schizophrenia as, 1128
Psychiatric dizziness, 205t, 209
Psychiatric symptoms, of Alzheimer's disease, 881

Psychodynamic psychotherapy, for major depression, 1124
Psychoeducation, for schizophrenia, 1129–1130
Psychogenic dysphonia, 220
Psychogenic nonepileptic spells, 900, 901t
Psychopharmacologic drugs, reference intervals for, 1222t
Psychosis, postpartum, 1029
Psychosocial factors, and asthma, 763, 765
Psychosocial interventions
 for alcohol dependence, 1103
 for schizophrenia, 1129–1130
Psychosocial support
 for diabetes in children, 588
 for thalassemia, 402–404
Psychotherapy
 adapted, for tinnitus, 39
 for major depression, 1124
Psyllium hydrophilic mucilloid (Metamucil), for dyslipoproteinemia, 604
PT (pertussis toxoid), 147t
PT (physical therapy). *See* Physical therapy (PT).
PTP (post-transfusion purpura), 486t, 491
PTU (propylthiouracil)
 for hyperthyroidism, 667–668
 for thyroid storm, 669
Puberty
 constitutional delay of, 1063
 delayed, in sickle cell disease, 407
Pubic louse, 844t, 845
Public access defibrillation (PAD), 304–305
Pubovaginal sling, for stress incontinence, 696
PUD. *See* Peptic ulcer disease (PUD).
Puerperal fever, 1028
Puerperal infections, 1028
Puerperium. *See* Postpartum period.
Puffer fish poisoning, 1158
Pulmicort. *See* Budesonide dry powder inhaler (Pulmicort).
Pulmonary abnormalities, obesity and, 608
Pulmonary agents, as chemical weapons, 1226–1228t
Pulmonary artery hypertension (PAH), in systemic sclerosis, 811
Pulmonary cavities, due to coccidioidomycosis, 249
Pulmonary edema
 cardiogenic, 230
 high-altitude, 158, 1142–1143
  clinical course of, 1142
  clinical presentation of, 1142
  defined, 1142
  differential diagnosis of, 1141b
  treatment of, 1142, 1142b, 1143
 due to salicylate poisoning, 1211
Pulmonary embolism (PE), 271
 during airplane travel, 158
 clinical risk of, 271–272
 diagnosis of, 271–272, 272b
  studies that confirm, 272, 272t
  studies that exclude, 272, 272t
 epidemiology of, 271
 etiology of, 271
 hypotension due to, 274
 treatment of, 272–274, 273b
  alternative agents for initial, 273
  hemodynamic management for, 274
  long-term, 273
  low-molecular-weight heparin for, 273, 273b
  surgical embolectomy for, 274
  thrombolytic therapy for, 273–274
  unfractionated heparin for, 272–273, 273b
  venocaval interruption and inferior vena cava filter placement for, 273
  warfarin for, 273, 273b
Pulmonary fibrosis, in systemic fibrosis, 811
Pulmonary function tests, for COPD, 232

Pulmonary hypertension
 persistent, of newborn, 1038
 in sickle cell disease, 406, 410
 in systemic sclerosis, 811
Pulmonary nodules, due to coccidioidomycosis, 249
Pulmonary rehabilitation, for COPD, 235
Pulmonary stenosis, 328
 antibiotic prophylaxis with, 345
Pulmonary venous connection, total anomalous, 331
Pulmozyme (DNase), for cystic fibrosis, 239
Pulse, with poisonings, 1162t
Pulseless electrical activity (PEA), cardiac arrest from, 305
Pulzium (tedisamil), 1244–1249t
Pupil, 187, 188f
Purified chick embryo cell culture vaccine (RabAvert), 131
 for travelers, 159–160t
Purinethol (6-mercaptopurine)
 for acute promyelocytic leukemia, 448–449
 for inflammatory bowel disease, 516–517, 519–520
Purpura
 Henoch-Schönlein, 814–815
 post-transfusion, 486t, 491
 thrombocytopenic
  idiopathic, 426, 427b
  thrombotic, 430
   classification of, 430, 430b
   clinical presentation of, 430–431
   defined, 430
   diagnosis of, 431, 431b
   etiology of, 430, 430b
   pathogenesis of, 430
   prognosis for, 431–432
   thrombocytopenia due to, 426
   treatment of, 431, 432f
PUVA. *See* Psoralens with ultraviolet light A (PUVA).
PV. *See* Polycythemia vera (PV).
PVCs. *See* Premature ventricular complexes (PVCs).
PVE (prosthetic valve endocarditis), 342, 343b
PVR (postvoid residual), 694–695
Pyelonephritis, 704
 acute, 704
  clinical presentation of, 683, 704
  complicated, 704, 704b
  vs. cystitis, 682, 683
  defined, 704
  diagnosis of, 683b, 704–705, 705b
  differential diagnosis of, 705b
  epidemiology of, 704
  etiology and pathogenesis of, 683, 704
  microbial, 705
  follow-up for, 706
  imaging of, 706
  treatment of, 684b, 685, 705–706, 705b, 706b
  urinary tract infection due to, 682–683
 chronic, 683–684
  diagnosis of, 683–684
  treatment of, 685
 clinical, 686b
 during pregnancy, 1014, 1016b
 proved, 686b
Pygeum africanum, for benign prostatic hyperplasia, 715–717
Pyogenic granuloma, of alveolar process/gingiva, 854
Pyrantel pamoate (Pin-X)
 for *Ascaris*, 569
 for hookworm, 570t
 for pinworm, 570t
Pyrazinamide
 for tuberculosis, 285t, 286t, 287t, 287b
 for tuberculous pericarditis, 371

Pyrethrin piperonyl butoxide liquid (Rid), for pediculosis, 845
Pyridium (phenazopyridine), for dysuria, 684, 684b
Pyridostigmine bromide (Mestinon), for myasthenia gravis, 942t, 943
Pyridoxine
 for alcoholic liver disease, 498
 for *Mycobacterium tuberculosis*, 56t
 for nausea during pregnancy, 1014
 in parenteral nutrition, 621t
 for poisoning, 1167–1172t
  due to isoniazid, 1195, 1195
 for Wilson's disease, 500–501
Pyridoxine challenge, for neonatal seizures, 910
Pyrimethamine (Daraprim)
 for isosporiasis, 568
 for toxoplasmosis, 164, 165t
  in immunocompetent host, 165t, 166
  in immunocompromised host, 56t, 165t, 166t, 167–168
  ocular, 167
  during pregnancy, 165t
Pyrogenic cytokines, 23
Pyropoikilocytosis, hereditary, 392
Pyruvate kinase (PK) deficiency, 393

Q

Q fever, 128
 in bioterrorism, 128–129, 1229–1233t
 clinical features of, 129
 diagnosis of, 129
 endocarditis due to, 129
 etiology of, 128, 128
 prevention of, 129
 treatment of, 129, 129t
QT interval, prolonged, 652
Quadrigeminy, 312
Quadrivalent protein-polysaccharide conjugate vaccine. *See* Meningococcal polysaccharide diphtheria toxoid conjugate vaccine (MCV4, Menactra).
Qualiquin (quinine sulfate), for malaria, 108–109, 108t
QuantiFERON-TB assays (interferon-γ assays), for tuberculosis, 283
Quazepam (Doral), for insomnia, 888t
Questran. *See* Cholestyramine (Questran).
Quetiapine (Seroquel)
 for Alzheimer's disease, 885t, 884–886
 for bipolar disorder, 1127
 for delirium, 1119–1120, 1119b
 for schizophrenia, 1130, 1130t
Quickening, 1012–1013
Quinacrine (Atabrine), for giardiasis, 63–64, 64t, 544, 565–566t
Quinagolide (Norprolac, Prodelion), for hyperprolactinemia, 660, 660t
Quinidine gluconate, for malaria, 108–109, 108t
Quinine sulfate (Qualaquin), for malaria, 108–109, 108t
Quinolone(s)
 for brucellosis, 74–75, 74b
 for cholera, 80
 for leprosy, 102b
 for marine injuries, 1159t
 for pyelonephritis, 685
 for urinary tract infections in males, 681, 681, 681t
3-Quinuclidinyl benzilate, as chemical weapon, 1226–1228t
Quinupristin-dalfopristin (Synercid), for pyelonephritis, 685
QVAR (beclomethasone hydrofluoroalkane), for asthma
 in adolescents and adults, 769t
 in children, 773–774t

R

RA. *See* Rheumatoid arthritis (RA).
RabAvert (purified chick embryo cell culture vaccine), 131
　for travelers, 159–160t
Rabeprazole (Aciphex)
　for gastroesophageal reflux disease, 553–554, 554t
　for indigestion, 11t
　for peptic ulcer disease, 531t, 532t
Rabies, 130
　clinical features of, 130
　diagnosis of, 130, 130b
　encephalitic, 130
　epidemiology of, 130
　management of, 131, 131b
　meningitis or encephalitis due to, 928–930t
　paralytic, 130
　pathogenesis of, 130
　prevention of, 130–131
Rabies vaccine (Imovax), 131, 131b
　for travelers, 159–160t, 161
Rabies vaccine absorbed (RVA), 131
　for travelers, 159–160t
Racecadotril, for acute infectious diarrhea, 19
Radial artery palpation, 351
Radial scars, of breast, 1047
Radiant warmer, for neonate, 1036t
Radiation exposure, during pregnancy, 1016
Radiation pneumonitis, in Hodgkin's disease, 444
Radiation therapy
　for acromegaly, 636
　for acute lymphoblastic leukemia in children, 454
　for acute myeloid leukemia in children, 455
　for brain metastases, 976
　for cervical cancer, 1087–1088, 1088t
　　complications of, 1089b
　　recurrent, 1089
　for ductal carcinoma in situ, 1050
　for endometrial cancer, 1084–1085
　for gliomas, 974
　for Hodgkin's lymphoma, 439
　　complications of, 444
　　extended field, 440, 442f
　　involved field, 440, 443f
　　mantle field, 440–441, 442f
　　with mediastinal involvement, 442–443
　　patient evaluation and staging for, 439–440, 440b, 440t
　　recommendations and results of, 442–444, 442b, 443t, 443f
　　subdiaphragmatic, 441–442, 443
　　subtotal nodal, 440
　　techniques of, 440, 441f
　　treatment volumes in, 440
　for hyperprolactinemia, 661
　for keloids, 822
　for lung cancer
　　non–small cell
　　　local, 246
　　　locoregional, 246–247
　　small cell, 248
　for prostate cancer, 732
　and thyroid cancer, 670
Radiation-related esophagitis, 510
Radiation-related strictures, 510
Radical nephrectomy, for renal cell carcinoma, 733
Radical prostatectomy (RP), for prostate cancer, 732
Radicular pain
　assessment of, 40
　　examination in, 40–41
　　history in, 40
　management of, 41–42, 42b
　natural course of, 41
　pathophysiology of, 39–40

Radioactive iodine, for hyperthyroidism, 667, 668
Radioactive iodine uptake (RAIU), in hyperthyroidism, 665, 666, 666b
Radioallergosorbent tests (RASTs), 779
　for insect stings, 784–785, 785t
Radiographic contrast media (RCM)
　acute renal failure due to, 723, 725
　allergic reactions to, 783
Radioiodine ablation, for hyperthyroidism, 667, 668
Radiosurgery, for trigeminal neuralgia, 948–949
RADTs (rapid antigen detection tests), for streptococcal pharyngitis, 222
Rai classification, for chronic lymphocytic leukemia, 461, 461t
RAIU (radioactive iodine uptake), in hyperthyroidism, 665, 666, 666b
R-albuterol (levalbuterol), for asthma
　in adolescents and adults, 766t
　in children, 774–775, 775t
Raloxifene (Evista)
　for menopausal symptoms, 1073
　for osteoporosis, 615
Raltegravir (Isentress), 1243
　for HIV, 50t
Ramelteon (Rozerem), for insomnia, 887–888, 888t
Ramipril (Altace), for angina pectoris, 297
Ramsay Hunt syndrome, 202
Random donor platelets, 482
Random on/off fluctuations, with levodopa, 955
Ranexa (ranolazine), for angina pectoris, 300
Ranitidine (Zantac)
　for anaphylaxis, 761t
　for gastroesophageal reflux disease, 553, 554t
　for indigestion, 11t
　for peptic ulcer disease, 531t
　for urticaria, 875
Ranolazine (Ranexa), for angina pectoris, 300
Ranson criteria, of severity of acute pancreatitis, 547, 547t
Rapamune (sirolimus), for focal and segmental glomerulosclerosis, 702
Rapid antigen detection tests (RADTs), for streptococcal pharyngitis, 222
Rapid eye movement (REM) sleep behavior disorder, 889–890
Rapid plasma reagin (RPR) test, 754–755
Rapidly progressive glomerulonephritis (RPGN), 699b, 723
Raptiva (efalizumab), for psoriasis, 803–804, 803t
Rasagiline (Azilect), for parkinsonism, 957
Rasburicase (recombinant uricase), for gout, 601
Rasmussen's syndrome, 915
RASTs (radioallergosorbent tests), 779
　for insect stings, 784–785, 785t
Rat-bite fever (RBF), 131
　clinical presentation of, 132
　diagnosis of, 132, 132b
　differential diagnosis of, 132
　epidemiology of, 131–132
　pathogenesis of, 131, 132
　risk factors for, 132
　treatment of, 132–133, 133b
Rate control, for atrial fibrillation, 309, 310b
Rattlesnake bite. *See* Pit viper bite.
Raynaud's phenomenon, in systemic sclerosis, 810–811, 811t
Razadyne (galantamine), for Alzheimer's disease, 883–884, 883t
RBBB (right bundle branch block), 317
RBC transfusion. *See* Red blood cell (RBC) transfusion.
RBF. *See* Rat-bite fever (RBF).
RCC. *See* Renal cell carcinoma (RCC).
RCM (radiographic contrast media)
　acute renal failure due to, 723, 725
　allergic reactions to, 783

Reactive cheilitis, 850
REAL (Revised European American Lymphoma) classification, 434
Rebetro (ribavirin)
　for bronchiolitis, 266
　for hepatitis B and C viruses, 536t, 538
Rebif (interferon-β-1a)
　for multiple sclerosis, 936
　for optic neuritis, 197, 197, 197
Recombinant erythropoietin (Eprex), for anemia, 471
Recombinant plasminogen activator (rPA), for myocardial infarction, 364t
Recombinant uricase (rasburicase, Elitek), for gout, 601
Recombivax-HB. *See* Hepatitis B virus (HBV) vaccine (Recombivax-HB, Engerix-B, Combivax, Pediarix).
Rectosigmoid obstruction, functional, 21
Red blood cell (RBC) transfusion, 480–482
　frozen, 481
　indications for, 481–482
　irradiated, 481
　leukoreduced, 480–481
　packed, 480
　for warm autoimmune hemolytic anemia, 388
　washed, 481
Red cell mass, in polycythemia vera, 473, 473b
Red clover flower, 1234–1243t
Red man syndrome, 783
5α-Reductase inhibitors, for benign prostatic hyperplasia, 714–718, 714t
REE (resting energy expenditure), 620
Reentrant tachycardia, atrioventricular node, 321, 321f, 322b
Reentry, 320, 320f
Reference, delusion of, 1129
Reference intervals, 1217
　for clinical chemistry (blood, serum, plasma), 1220–1221t
　for clinical chemistry (urine), 1223–1224t
　for CSF tests, 1224t
　defining normal values for, 1217
　for GI function tests, 1225t
　for hematology, 1219t
　for immunologic function tests, 1225t
　International System of Units for, 1217–1218, 1217t, 1218t
　for lymphocyte subsets, whole blood, heparinized, 1225t
　for semen analysis, 1225t
　tables of, 1218
　for therapeutic drug monitoring, 1222t
　for toxic substances, 1224t
Referrals
　for burns, 1135, 1140
　for high-risk pregnancy, 1011, 1011b
Referred pain, somatic, 40
Refludan (lepirudin), for deep venous thrombosis/pulmonary embolism, 273
Refractive errors, 187–188, 188f
Refractive lens exchange (RLE), 187
Regional myofascial pain, 995–996
Regitine. *See* Phentolamine (Regitine).
Reglan. *See* Metoclopramide (Reglan).
Regular insulin (Humulin R, Novolin R), for diabetes
　in adults, 582t
　in children, 587t
Regulatory T cells (Tregs), in cutaneous T-cell lymphomas, 795–796
Regurgitation, 6–7
Rehabilitation
　for idiopathic inflammatory myopathy, 813
　after stroke, 895, 898b
　　for activities of daily living, 896–897
　　for common medical complications, 897–898
　　continuity of care in, 898

Rehabilitation (Continued)
    for mobility and locomotion, 896
    research on, 895–896
    for speech and language disorders, 897
    team for, 895
    techniques of, 896b
    after traumatic brain injury, 969
Rehydration
    for cholera, 79–80, 79t, 79t, 78b
    for diarrhea
        acute infectious, 18–19, 18b
        traveler's, 155, 156t
    of infants and children, 628–631
        assessment for, 628–630, 628t, 629t
        with intravenous therapy, 630–631
            deficit therapy in, 630–631
            indications for, 630
            maintenance requirements in, 631
            rapid, 631
            replacement requirements in, 631
        with oral rehydration therapy, 630
        requirements for, 630–631
    for *Salmonella* gastroenteritis, 172
Relafen (nabumetone)
    for juvenile idiopathic arthritis, 985
    for osteoarthritis, 1000
Relapse-remitting multiple sclerosis (RRMS), 932, 933f, 935–936
Relapsing fever, 133
    diagnosis of, 134b
        clinical, 133–134, 135t
        laboratory, 134
    differential diagnosis of, 134
    endemic (tick-borne)
        clinical manifestations of, 133–134, 135t
        epidemiology of, 133, 134t
        prevention of, 135–136
        risk factors for, 133
        treatment of, 136t
    epidemic (louse-borne)
        clinical manifestations of, 133–134
        epidemiology of, 133, 134t
    epidemiology of, 133, 134t
    etiology of, 133, 134t
    outcome of, 135
    prevention of, 135–136
    risk factors for, 133
    treatment of, 134–135, 135b, 136t
        Jarisch-Herxheimer reaction due to, 135, 135b
Relenza (zanamivir), for influenza, 92, 92t, 260, 260b, 265, 267, 267t
Relpax (eletriptan), for migraine headache, 925t, 926
REM (rapid eye movement) sleep behavior disorder, 889–890
Remeron (mitrazipine), for major depression, 1124
Remicade. See Infliximab (Remicade).
Reminyl (galantamine), for Alzheimer's disease, 882–884, 883t
Remiron (mirtazapine), for Alzheimer's disease, 884–886, 885t
Remodulin (treprostinil), for systemic sclerosis, 811
Renagel (sevelamar), for chronic renal failure, 730
Renal abscess, 683–685
Renal biopsy, for chronic renal failure, 726
Renal calculi, 742
    calcium, 743, 743t, 744t, 746t
    classification of, 744t
    cystine, 743, 744t, 746t
    diagnosis of, 743–744, 743b
        history and physical examination in, 743
        imaging studies in, 744
        laboratory studies in, 743–744, 744t
    epidemiology of, 742–743

Renal calculi (Continued)
    follow-up for, 745–747
    due to HAART, 54–55t
    due to hyperparathyroidism, 650
    infection, 744t, 746t
    pathophysiology of, 743, 743t
    recurrent, 743–744, 745
    due to sarcoidosis, 276
    staghorn, 743
    struvite, 743, 744t
    treatment of, 744–745, 745b
        consultations in, 745
        medical, 744–745, 745t, 746t
        surgical, 745
    urate, 743, 744t, 744t, 746t
Renal carbuncle, 679
Renal cell carcinoma (RCC), 733–734
    diagnosis of, 733, 733b
    epidemiology of, 733
    metastatic, 733–734
    pathogenesis of, 733
    risk factors for, 733
    signs and symptoms of, 733
    staging of, 733
    treatment of, 733–734, 733b
Renal complications, of sickle cell disease, 407, 411
Renal crisis, scleroderma, 812
Renal disease
    due to hyperparathyroidism, 650
    hypertension due to, in pregnancy, 1022t
Renal failure
    acute (See Acute renal failure (ARF))
    chronic (See Chronic renal failure (CRF))
    due to multiple myeloma, 471
    platelet dysfunction due to, 427, 427b
Renal injuries, 706–707
    complications of, 707
    diagnosis of, 707, 707b
    grading of, 707, 707t, 707f
    surgical exploration for, 707
    treatment of, 708b
Renal insufficiency, chronic, 699b
Renal involvement, in systemic sclerosis, 812
Renal parenchymal tumors, 732–733
Renal pelvis, tumors of, 734–735
    diagnosis of, 734b, 735
    epidemiology of, 734
    risk factors for, 734, 734–735
    treatment of, 735, 735b
Renal replacement therapy, for acute renal failure, 724
Renal system, in hypothermia, 1144
Renal tubular insufficiency, in sickle cell disease, 404, 407
Renal tumors
    benign, 734, 734b, 734b
    metastatic, 734
Renin activity, plasma, 654
Renova. See Tretinoin topical (Retin-A, Renova, Differin, Tazorac).
Renovascular hypertension, 359
Reopro (abciximab)
    for myocardial infarction, 364, 366
    for unstable angina pectoris, 301, 301t
Repaglinide (Prandin), for diabetes, 580t
Reperfusion therapy, for myocardial infarction, 361, 363f
Repetitive nerve stimulation (RNS), for myasthenia gravis, 942
Reproductive disorders, due to lead poisoning, 1198
Requip (ropinirole), for parkinsonism, 955–956, 956t
RERA (respiratory effort–related arousal), 239–240
Rescriptor (delaviridine), for HIV, 50t
    drug interactions with, 58t

Rescula (unoprostone), for glaucoma, 199–200
Resins, for dyslipoproteinemia, 605, 605t
Respiratory abnormalities, due to acromegaly, 634
Respiratory complications, of sickle cell disease, 406, 410
Respiratory disease(s)
    acute bronchitis as, 259
    acute respiratory failure as, 225
    atelectasis as, 230
    bacterial pneumonia as, 261
    blastomycosis as, 254
    chronic obstructive pulmonary disease as, 231
    coccidioidomycosis as, 248
    cystic fibrosis as, 236
    in extremely low birth weight infants, 1039–1040t
    histoplasmosis as, 251
    hypersensitivity pneumonitis as, 280
    legionellosis as, 270
    lung cancer as, 242
    pleural effusion and empyema thoracis as, 256
    pneumoconiosis as, 278
    primary lung abscess as, 258
    pulmonary embolism as, 271
    sarcoidosis as, 274
    sleep apnea as, 239
    tuberculosis and other mycobacterial diseases as, 282
    viral and mycoplasmal pneumonias as, 266
    viral respiratory infections as, 264
Respiratory distress syndrome, acute, 229–230
Respiratory effort–related arousal (RERA), 239–240
Respiratory failure, acute, 225
    due to acute lung injury and ARDS, 229–230
    due to cardiogenic pulmonary edema, 230
    clinical presentation of, 225
    in COPD, 228–229
    definitions for, 225–226
    diagnosis of, 229b
    hypercapneic, 225–226, 226b, 227b
    hypoxic/hypoxemic, 225, 226t, 226b
    pathophysiology of, 225–226, 226t
    treatment of, 226–228, 229b
        mechanical ventilation for, 227–228, 229b
        oxygen therapy for, 226–227, 227t
Respiratory infection(s), viral, 264
    bronchiolitis as, 266
    common colds as, 265
    croup as, 265–266
    diagnosis of, 265b
    etiology of, 264–265
    influenza-like illness due to, 265
    treatment of, 265b
Respiratory rate, with poisonings, 1162t
Respiratory stimulants, reference intervals for, 1222t
Respiratory syncytial virus (RSV), 266
Respiratory system, in hypothermia, 1144
Respiratory toxicity, 1174t
Respiratory tract procedures, endocarditis prophylaxis for, 347t
Resting energy expenditure (REE), 620
Restless legs syndrome (RLS), 889
Restoril (temazepam)
    for insomnia, 888t
    intoxication with, 1181–1182
Resuscitation, of newborn, 1029
    ABCDs of, 970, 1034
    airways in, 1031
    algorithm for, 1030f
    anticipation of, 1030, 1034
    assessing response to birth in, 1031
    availability of qualified personnel for, 1034
    breathing in, 1031–1032

Resuscitation, of newborn (Continued)
care after, 1032–1033
circulation in, 1032
demographics of, 1029
documentation of, 1033
drugs in, 1032
endotracheal intubation in, 1031
guidelines for, 1030
hypothermia in, 1033
indications for, 1029–1030
initial stabilization and evaluation in, 1030–1032
for meconium aspiration, 1032
oxygen supplementation in, 1031–1032
preparation for, 1034
for preterm infants, 1032
principles of, 1034t
withholding and withdrawing of, 1032
RET gene, in pheochromocytomas and paragangliomas, 674–675
Retaane (anecortave acetate), 1244–1249t
Retapamulin (Altabax), 1243
Retching, 5
Reteplase (Retevase), for myocardial infarction, 364t
Retigabine, for epilepsy, 904t
Retina, 187, 188f
Retin-A. *See* Tretinoin topical (Retin-A, Renova, Differin, Tazorac).
Retinal effects, of hypertension, 350–351
Retinitis, cytomegalovirus, 57
Retinoids
for acne, 787
for cutaneous T-cell lymphomas, 798, 799
for psoriasis, 802
Retinopathy
diabetic, in children, 589
in sickle cell disease, 407
Retrograde menstruation, 1054
Retroperitoneal lymph node dissection (RPLND), for testicular carcinoma, 738–739, 739b
Retrovir (zidovudine), for HIV, 50t, 51t
Revascularization, for chronic limb ischemia, 373–374
Reversal reaction (RR), in leprosy, 102, 102f
Reverse transcriptase inhibitors
non-nucleoside, for HIV, 49–50, 50t
adverse drug reactions to, 54–55t
drug interactions with, 53
failure of, 52t
resistance to, 51, 52t
nucleoside/nucleotide, for HIV, 49–50, 50t
adverse drug reactions to, 54–55t
failure of, 52t
resistance to, 51, 52t
Revex (nalmefene), for poisoning, 1174
due to opioids, 1204
ReVia. *See* Naltrexone (ReVia, Depade, Vivitrol).
Revised European American Lymphoma (REAL) classification, 434
Revlimid (lenalidomide)
for cutaneous T-cell lymphomas, 800
for multiple myeloma, 469b, 470, 471
Rewarming
for frostbite, 1147
for hypothermia, 1145–1146, 1147b
Reyataz (atazanavir), for HIV, 50t, 51t
drug interactions with, 58t
RF (rheumatoid factor), 977–978, 978t
in juvenile idiopathic arthritis, 984
Rh antibody, screening for, 1013
Rh immune globulin (RhoGAM), 417b
postpartum, 416, 417
during pregnancy, 416–417
Rhabdomyolysis, due to poisoning, 1175t
RhD antigen, 416
alloimmunization to, 416
diagnosis of, 416b

RhD antigen (Continued)
prevention of, 416
treatment of, 416–418, 417b
Rheumatic process, pain due to, 2
Rheumatoid arthritis (RA), 977
clinical features of, 977, 977, 978t
criteria for improvement in, 981b
diagnosis of, 977–978, 978t
epidemiology of, 977
general medical concerns in, 977, 977b
GI bleeding in, 977b
infection in, 977b
juvenile (*See* Juvenile idiopathic arthritis (JIA))
lifestyle concerns in, 977b
osteoporosis in, 977b
pathogenesis of, 977, 977
treatment of, 978–983, 980b, 983b
biological response modifier(s) for, 978, 978b
abatecept as, 981t, 982
anakinra as, 981t, 982
rituximab as, 981t, 982
TNF-α inhibitors as, 979–981, 981t
combination therapy for, 982
corticosteroids for, 977, 980b, 982
DMARD(s) for, 978, 978b, 980b
azathioprine as, 981t, 982
cyclophosphamide as, 982
cyclosporine as, 981t, 982
early use of, 977, 978
gold salts as, 982
hydroxychloroquine as, 981, 981t
initiation of, 980b
leflunomide as, 981–982, 981t
methotrexate as, 978–979, 981t
monitoring of, 981t
other, 981–982
sulfasalazine as, 981t, 982
tapering of, 980b
flow diagram for, 979f
goals of, 977, 978
initial, 977
NSAIDs for, 977, 980b, 982–983
Rheumatoid factor (RF), 977–978, 978t
in juvenile idiopathic arthritis, 984
Rheumatoid nodules, 978t
Rheumatrex. *See* Methotrexate (MTX, Rheumatrex, Trexall).
Rhinitis
allergic, 214, 776
classification of, 776–777
by severity and frequency, 776–777, 777b
by type of aeroallergen, 776
comorbid conditions with, 777
cough due to, 28b
diagnosis of, 778–779
differential diagnosis of, 777–778, 778b
epidemiology of, 776
impact of, 776
intermittent, 776–777
pathogenesis of, 777
persistent, 776–777
treatment of, 779–781
avoidance and environmental controls in, 780
pharmacotherapy in, 779–780, 779t, 780t
specific allergen immunotherapy for, 780–781
classification of, 214
defined, 212, 214
gustatory, 216, 777–778
irritant, 777–778
medicamentosa, 778
nonallergic (noninfectious), 214
atrophic, 216
classification of, 214
diagnosis of, 214–215, 215b

Rhinitis (Continued)
differential diagnosis of, 216, 216b
drug-induced, 215, 215b
emotionally induced, 216
with eosinophilia, 215
food-induced, 216
gustatory, 216
hormonal, 215
management of, 216–217, 215b, 217b
occupational, 215, 215b
pathophysiology of, 215
perennial (vasomotor, idiopathic), 215, 216
due to physical and chemical factors, 215–216
prevalence of, 215
vasomotor, 777–778
Rhinoconjunctivitis, allergic, 777
Rhinocort (budesonide nasal inhaler)
for allergic rhinitis, 780t
for nonallergic rhinitis, 217, 217b
Rhinosinusitis, 212
acute, 213b, 214b
cough due to, 28b
bacterial
cough due to, 26–27, 28b
treatment of, 213, 214b
chronic, 213, 214b
classification and etiologic factors for, 212–213
complications of, 213–214
defined, 212
diagnosis of, 213, 213b
epidemiology of, 212
invasive fungal, 214
treatment of, 213, 214b
RhoGAM. *See* Rh immune globulin (RhoGAM).
Rh-sensitized women, management of, 417–418
Rhythm control, for atrial fibrillation, 309–310, 310b, 310t
Ribavirin (Rebetro, Ribasphere, Copegus, Virazole)
for bronchiolitis, 266
for hepatitis B and C viruses, 536t, 538, 538
Riboflavin, in parenteral nutrition, 621t
Rice-water stools, 15–16
Ricin toxin, as biological weapon agent, 1229–1233t
Ricinus communis, as biological weapon agent, 1229–1233t
Rickettsia, 162
as biological weapon agents, 1229–1233t
Rickettsia parkeri, 178
Rickettsia rickettsii. *See* Rocky Mountain spotted fever (RMSF).
Rickettsial infection(s), 176–178
other, 178
Rid (pyrethrin piperonyl butoxide liquid), for pediculosis, 845
Riedel's thyroiditis, 678
Rifabutin (Mycobutin)
for *Mycobacterium avium-intracellulare*, 289, 289
in HIV, 56–57, 56t
for tuberculosis, 285t, 286t
Rifamixin (Xifaxan)
for bacterial overgrowth, 10t
for hepatic encephalopathy, 502–503
for traveler's diarrhea, 156, 156t
Rifampin (Rifadin, Rimactane)
for anthrax, 126t
for bacterial meningitis, 114–115
for brucellosis, 74–75, 74b, 75, 75t
for cholestasis, 34b
for endocarditis prophylaxis, 346–347t
for infective endocarditis, 345, 345
for legionellosis, 271t
for leprosy, 101, 101b
for *Mycobacterium avium intracellulare* complex, 289

Rifampin (Rifadin, Rimactane) *(Continued)*
  for *Mycobacterium kansasii*, 289
  for osteomyelitis, 1006t
  for pruritus, due to primary biliary cirrhosis, 499
  for Q fever, 129
  for tuberculosis, 285t, 286t, 287t, 287b, 288t
    in HIV, 56t, 58t
  for tuberculous pericarditis, 371
Rifapentine (Priftin)
  for leprosy, 102
  for tuberculosis, 285t, 287t
Rift Valley virus, as biological weapon agent, 1229–1233t
Right bundle branch block (RBBB), 317
Right ventricular (RV) infarction, 367
Rimactane. *See* Rifampin (Rifadin, Rimactane).
Rimantadine (Flumadine), for influenza, 260, 260b
  with pneumonia, 266–267, 267t, 269b
Ringer's lactate, for cholera, 79t, 78b
Ringworm, 804, 846, 847b
Riot control agents, as chemical weapons, 1226–1228t
RIPA (ristocetin-induced platelet aggregation) assay, 423, 423t
Risedronate (Actonel)
  for osteoporosis, 614, 614
    postmenopausal, 1073b
  for Paget's disease of bone, 617
Risperidone (Risperdal)
  for Alzheimer's disease, 885t, 884–886
  for bipolar disorder, 1127
  for delirium, 1119–1120, 1119b
  for obsessive compulsive disorder, 1114
  for schizophrenia, 1130, 1130, 1130t
  for Tourette's syndrome, 921
Ristocetin cofactor assay, 423
Ristocetin-induced platelet aggregation (RIPA) assay, 423, 423t
Risus sardonicus, due to tetanus, 143
Ritalin. *See* Methylphenidate (Ritalin).
Ritonavir (Norvir), for HIV, 50t
Rituximab (Rituxan)
  for chronic lymphocytic leukemia, 463
  for membranous nephropathy, 703
  for multiple sclerosis, 938
  for non-Hodgkin's lymphoma, 466
  for rheumatoid arthritis, 981t, 982
  for systemic lupus erythematosus, 809
  for warm autoimmune hemolytic anemia, 387–388
Rivastigmine (Exelon), for Alzheimer's disease, 882–884, 883t
Rivastigmine transdermal system (Exelon Patch), 1243
River blindness, 845
Rizatriptan (Maxalt), for migraine headache, 925t, 926
RLE (refractive lens exchange), 187
RLS (restless legs syndrome), 889
RMSF. *See* Rocky Mountain spotted fever (RMSF).
RNA expression profiling, in lung cancer, 243, 243
RNS (repetitive nerve stimulation), for myasthenia gravis, 942
Robinul (glycopyrrolate), for organophosphate and carbamate poisoning, 1206
Rocephin. *See* Ceftriaxone (Rocephin).
Rocky Mountain spotted fever (RMSF), 176–178
  clinical features and diagnosis of, 177, 177b
  epidemiology of, 177
  pathogenesis of, 177
  in pregnancy, 177, 179b
  prevention of, 177–178
  spotless, 177
  treatment of, 177, 179b

Rofecoxib (Vioxx), for prostatitis, 711
Roferon-A (interferon-α-2a), for cutaneous T-cell lymphomas, 799
Rogaine (minoxidil), for androgenic alopecia, 791
Rohypnol (flunitrazepam), intoxication with, 1181–1182
Rolandic epilepsy, benign, 909
ROM therapy, for leprosy, 101
Romaña's sign, 843
Romazicon. *See* Flumazenil (Romazicon).
Rome criteria, for irritable bowel syndrome, 521, 522b
Rome III criteria, for constipation, 21, 21b
Rood method, for stroke rehabilitation, 896b
Ropinirole (Requip), for parkinsonism, 955–956, 956t
Rosac (sodium sulfacetamide and sulfur compound), for rosacea, 789
Rosacea, 788–789
  classification of, 788
  diagnosis and differential diagnosis of, 788, 789b
  pathogenesis of, 787
  treatment of, 788–789, 789b
Rosenfeld, Richard, 203
Rosiglitazone (Avandia), for diabetes, 580t, 581, 581
Rosuvastatin (Crestor, ABT-335), 1244–1249t
  for angina pectoris, 298
  for dyslipoproteinemia, 605t
Rotavirus, acute infectious diarrhea due to, 16
Rotavirus vaccine (Rota, RotaTeq), 18
  schedule for, 149–150t
  catch-up, 151t
Roth's spots, due to infective endocarditis, 343
Rotigotine (Neupro), 1243
  for parkinsonism, 956, 956t
Roundworms, 569–572, 570t
Roux-en-Y gastroplasty, 611, 611f
Rowasa (mesalamine enemas), for inflammatory bowel disease, 516, 519
Roxicet (oxycodone + acetaminophen)
  intoxication with, 1204–1205, 1205t
  for pain, 4t
Rozerem (ramelteon), for insomnia, 887–888, 888t
RP (radical prostatectomy), for prostate cancer, 732
rPA (recombinant plasminogen activator), for myocardial infarction, 364t
RPGN (rapidly progressive glomerulonephritis), 699b, 723
RPLND (retroperitoneal lymph node dissection), for testicular carcinoma, 738–739, 739b
RPR (rapid plasma reagin) test, 754–755
RR (reversal reaction), in leprosy, 102, 102f
RRMS (relapse-remitting multiple sclerosis), 932, 933f, 935–936
RSV (respiratory syncytial virus), 266
rtPA. *See* Tissue plasminogen activator (TPA, rtPA, Activase).
RU-486 (mifepristone), for Cushing's syndrome, 645t
Rubella, 140
  background and epidemiology of, 140
  clinical features of, 140
  complications of, 140–141
  congenital, 140–141, 1014, 1015b
  diagnosis of, 140, 140b
  meningitis or encephalitis due to, 928–930
  during pregnancy, 140–141, 1014, 1015b
  treatment of, 141, 141b
Rubella vaccine (Meruvax), 141
Rubeola. *See* Measles.
Rufinamide, 1244–1249t
Rule of Nines, for burns, 1135, 1136f
RV (right ventricular) infarction, 367

RVA (rabies vaccine absorbed), 131
  for travelers, 159–160t
Rythmol (propafenone)
  for atrial fibrillation, 309–310, 310b
  for cardioversion, 311, 311t

S

SAAAVE (Screening Abdominal Aortic Aneurysms Very Efficiently) Act, 374–375
SAAG (serum ascites-albumin gradient), 501
SABAs (short-acting β₂ agonists)
  for asthma, 766t
  for COPD, 234
Sabril (vigabatrin)
  for epilepsy, 904t
  for infantile spasms, 909
Sacral nerve stimulation, for urinary incontinence in children, 692
S-adenosylmethionine (SAM-e), 1234–1243t
SAFE (Saline *versus* Albumin Fluid Evaluation) study, 68–69
Safety precautions, for travel, 158, 158b
SAG (superantigen) family, in toxic shock syndrome, 87
SAHA (suberoylanilide hydroxamic acid), for cutaneous T-cell lymphomas, 800
Salicylate(s)
  kinetics of, 1210
  for osteoarthritis, 1000
  for pain, 2–3, 2t
  for systemic lupus erythematosus, 807t
Salicylate poisoning, 1209–1212, 1211t
Salicylic acid
  for fever, 24, 24
  poisoning due to, 1209–1212, 1211t
  for psoriasis, 802
Salicylic acid topical (Compound W, Occlusal HP), for verrucae, 823
Salicylism, 1209–1212, 1211t
Saline infusion, for diagnosis of aldosteronism, 655
Saline nasal washes, for allergic rhinitis, 780
Saline *versus* Albumin Fluid Evaluation (SAFE) study, 68–69
Saliva substitutes, 849
Salivary disease, orofacial pain due to, 992t
Salivary duct stones, 853
Salivary gland tumors, 852
Salmeterol (Serevent)
  for asthma
    in adolescents and adults, 767–768t
    in children, 773–774t
  for COPD, 234
  for high-altitude sickness, 1141, 1142b, 1143
Salmon calcitonin nasal spray (Miacalcin), for osteoporosis, 615
Salmon/Durie staging system, for multiple myeloma, 468
Salmonella enterica typhi, 162
Salmonella paratyphi, 174
Salmonella species, acute infectious diarrhea due to, 15, 18, 19–20t
Salmonella typhi. *See* Typhoid fever.
Salmonellosis, 170
  antibiotic-resistant, 171
  bacteremia and focal infection due to, 173
    treatment of, 173
  carrier state of, 173–174
  clinical presentation of, 170, 171t, 171–172
  diagnosis of, 172b
  enteric fever due to, 173
    treatment of, 173
  epidemiology of, 171
  gastroenteritis due to, 171–172
    treatment of, 172–173, 172b
  microbiology of, 170–171
  nontyphoid, 171, 172b

Salmonellosis *(Continued)*
    pathogenesis of, 171, 171t
    predisposing factors for, 171t
    prevention of, 174
Salofalk (mesalamine), for inflammatory bowel disease, 516, 520
Salt loading, for diagnosis of aldosteronism, 654–655
Salt restriction, for preeclampsia, 1024
SAM-e (*S*-adenosylmethionine), 1234–1243t
Sanctura (trospium), for urge incontinence, 695b
Sandimmune. *See* Cyclosporine (CSA, Neoral, Gengraf, Sandimmune).
Sandostatin. *See* Octreotide (Sandostatin).
Sanger, Margaret, 755–756
Sanvar IR (vapreotide), 1244–1249t
SaO₂ (arterial oxygen saturation), 225
Sapropterin (Kuvan), 1243
Saquinavir/ritonavir hard gel (Invirase), for HIV, 50t, 51t
    drug interactions with, 58t
Saquinavir/ritonavir soft gel (Fortovase), for HIV, 50t
    drug interactions with, 58t
Sarcoidosis, 274
    cardiac, 276
    clinical features and clinical course of, 275–276
    diagnosis and initial workup of, 276–277, 277b, 277b
    epidemiology of, 274–275
    extrapulmonary, 275–276
    factors associated with poor prognosis for, 276b
    hepatic, 276
    immunopathogenesis of, 275
    neuro-, 276
    pulmonary, 275, 275t
    staging of, 275, 275t
    treatment of, 277, 277b
Sarcoma, of vulva, 1094
Sarcoptes scabiei, 844t, 845–846
Sarin
    as chemical weapon, 1226–1228t
    poisoning due to, 1205–1206
SA-TSS. *See Staphylococcus aureus* toxic shock syndrome (SA-TSS).
Saturated solution of potassium iodide, for thyroid storm, 669
Saw palmetto, 1234–1243t
    for benign prostatic hyperplasia, 715–717
Sb (pentavalent antimonials), for leishmaniasis, 94, 96
SBP (spontaneous bacterial peritonitis), 497t, 501t, 502
Scabies, 30b, 844t, 845–846
    vs. atopic dermatitis, 860
    Norwegian or crusted, 845–846
Scalp
    dissecting cellulitis of, 792
    pruritus of, 31f
Scaphoid fractures, 1009–1010
Scar(s), hypertrophic, keloids *vs.*, 820
Scarlet fever, staphylococcal. *See* Toxic shock syndrome (TSS).
SCC. *See* Squamous cell carcinoma (SCC).
SCD. *See* Sickle cell disease (SCD); Sudden cardiac death (SCD).
SCDs (sequential compression devices), for intracerebral hemorrhage, 892
Scedosporium species, necrotizing skin and soft tissue infections due to, 85t
SCFA (short-chain fatty acid) enemas, for inflammatory bowel disease, 519
Schatzki's rings, 510
Schilling test, 542
Schistosoma haematobium, and bladder carcinoma, 736–737

Schistosoma spp, 570t, 572–573, 844t, 845
Schistosomiasis, 570t, 572–573, 844t, 845
    pruritus due to, 32b
Schizophrenia, 1128
    clinical presentation of, 1128
    course and prognosis for, 1128
    diagnosis of, 1128, 1129b
    differential diagnosis of, 1128
    epidemiology of, 1128
    etiology of, 1129
    pathophysiology of, 1129
    symptoms of, 1128–1129
        cognitive, 1129
        negative, 1129
        positive, 1128–1129
    treatment of, 1129–1131, 1130b
        psychopharmacologic, 1130–1131, 1130b, 1130t
        psychosocial, 1129–1130
Schölein, Johann, 815
SCLC. *See* Small cell lung cancer (SCLC).
Scleroderma, 809–812
    clinical features of, 809–810, 810b
    linear, 809–810
    localized, 809–810
    organ involvement in, 809–810, 810b
    pruritus due to, 32b
    treatment of
        general principles of, 810
        for GI tract involvement, 811–812, 812b
        for interstitial lung disease, 811
        organ-based, 810–812
        potentially disease-modifying therapies for, 810, 810b
        for renal involvement, 812
        for skin involvement, 810
        for vascular involvement, 810–811, 811t
Scleroderma renal crisis, 812
Sclerosing adenosis, of breast, 1047
Sclerosing cholangitis, primary, 498t, 499–500
Scombroid poisoning, 1157
Scopolamine (Transderm Scop)
    for motion sickness, 158, 206t
    for nausea and vomiting, 8t
    for vertigo, 206t
Scorpion stings, 1151–1152, 1151b, 1151b
Screening Abdominal Aortic Aneurysms Very Efficiently (SAAAVE) Act, 374–375
Scrotal injuries, 709
SDH(s) (subdural hematomas), 966
    in children, 969–970
SDHB gene, in pheochromocytomas and paragangliomas, 674–675
SDHD gene, in pheochromocytomas and paragangliomas, 674–675
Sea bather's itch, 1158
Sea urchin envenomations, 1158–1159
Seasnake bites, 1159
Seasonal allergens, in allergic rhinitis, 776
Seasonal allergic conjunctivitis, 193–194, 194t
Seasonale (extended preparation oral contraceptives), 756
Seasonique (extended preparation oral contraceptives), 756
Sebaceous cysts, 837
    of vulva, 1091
Seborrheic dermatitis, 788, 804
Secnidazole (Noameba-DS, Secnil)
    for amebiasis, 60–61
    for giardiasis, 63–64, 64t, 64b
Secondary amines, poisoning due to, 1214–1216, 1215t
Secondary progressive multiple sclerosis (SPMS), 933, 933f, 938
Second-generation antipsychotics (SGAs), for schizophrenia, 1130–1131, 1129b, 1130t
Secretagogues, for diabetes, 578, 579–580, 580t

Secretion of inappropriate antidiuretic hormone (SIADH), 596–597, 597b
Sectral (acebutolol)
    for angina pectoris, 299
    intoxication with, 1182–1183, 1183t
Sedative hypnotics
    abuse of, 1105b, 1107–1108, 1108t
    for insomnia, 887–888, 888t
Seizure(s)
    absence
        in adolescents and adults, 900, 901t
        childhood and juvenile, 908–909
    in acute porphyria, 477
    in adolescents and adults, 898
        clinical approach to, 900–902
        defined, 899
        diagnosis and classification of, 899–900, 900t, 901–902
        differential diagnosis of, 900, 901t
        epidemiology of, 898
        etiology of, 899, 899t
        generalized, 900
            absence, 900, 901t
            atonic (astatic), 900
            secondarily, 900, 900t
            tonic, 900
            tonic-clonic, 900, 901t
        historical background of, 898–899
        interictal state in, 901
        new-onset, 901–902
        partial (focal, localization-related), 900, 900t
            complex, 900, 900t, 901t
            simple, 900, 900t
        risk of recurrence of, 902
        treatment of, 902–906, 904t
    due to alcohol withdrawal, 1100
    atonic (astatic), 900
    febrile, 24, 910
    generalized
        in adolescents and adults, 900, 900
            absence, 900, 901t
            atonic (astatic), 900
            secondarily, 900, 900t
            tonic, 900
            tonic-clonic, 900, 901t
        in infants and children, 907–908, 908b
    due to heat stroke, 1149–1150
    in infants and children, 907
        assessment of, 910–911
        classification of, 907–908, 908b
        defined, 907
        differential diagnosis of, 907–908, 907b
        epidemiology of, 907
        febrile, 910
        generalized, 907–908, 908b
        neonatal, 909–910
        partial, 907–908, 908b
            complex, 907–908, 908b
            simple, 907–908, 908b
        post-traumatic, 970
        syndromes of, 908–910, 908b
        treatment of, 911–915, 912t, 913t
    neonatal, 909–910
    partial (focal, localization-related)
        in adolescents and adults, 900, 900t
            complex, 900, 900t, 901t
            simple, 900, 900t
        in infants and children, 907–908, 908b
            complex, 907–908, 908b
            simple, 907–908, 908b
    post-traumatic, 968
        in children, 970
    pseudo-, 900, 901t
    tonic, 900
    tonic-clonic, 900, 901t
Seldane (terfenadine), poisoning due to, 1179–1180

Selective estrogen receptor modulators (SERMs)
for menopausal symptoms, 1072–1073, 1073b
for osteoporosis, 615
Selective laser trabeculoplasty (SLT), for glaucoma, 200
Selective serotonin reuptake inhibitors (SSRIs)
for Alzheimer's disease, 884, 885t, 884–886
for anxiety disorder(s), 1112, 1112
generalized, 1113
drug interactions with, 1122–1123b
hepatic effects of, 1122–1123b
intoxication due to, 1212
kinetics of, 1212
for major depression, 1121–1123
and MAOIs, 1203, 1212
for menopausal symptoms, 1072t
for panic disorder, 1132t
for premenstrual syndrome, 1068–1069, 1068b
side effects of, 1121
and suicide, 1112, 1117
Selegiline, orally disintegrating (Zelapar), for parkinsonism, 957
Selegiline (Eldepryl), for parkinsonism, 957
Selenium, in parenteral nutrition, 621t
Selenium sulfide (Selsun) lotion, for tinea versicolor, 848b
Self-monitoring, for diabetes mellitus in children, 587
Sellar region, tumors of, 973t
Selzentry (maraviroc), 1243
for HIV, 50t
Semen analysis, reference intervals for, 1225t
Semicid (nonoxynol-9), 757
Seminoma, 738, 739b
Semont maneuver, 206, 206f
Semprex (acrivastine), for allergic rhinitis, 779t
Semprex-D (acrivastine/pseudoephedrine), for allergic rhinitis, 779t
Senile lentigines, 877
Sensitivity index (SI), for insulin dose, 586
Sensorimotor neuropathy, 959, 960t
Sensory dysfunction, in parkinsonism, 953b
Sensory neuropathy
large fiber, 959b
pure, 960t
small fiber, 959b
Sentinel lymph node biopsy (SLNB)
for breast cancer, 1052
for melanoma, 832
SEP (Sexual Encounter Profile), 717b
SEPS (subfascial endoscopic perforator vein surgery), for venous leg ulcers, 857
Sepsis, 65
defined, 65, 65
diagnosis of, 66b
epidemiology of, 65
pathogenesis of, 66–67, 67b
PIRO staging of, 65–66, 66b
prognosis for, 72
severe, 65
in sickle cell disease, 405–406, 409
systemic inflammatory response syndrome and, 65–66, 67
treatment of, 67–71, 68b
antithrombotic therapy in, 71
corticosteroid therapy in, 71
hemodynamic management in, 68–69
high-volume continuous venovenous hemofiltration therapy in, 71
with HIV infection, 71–72
source control in, 67–68, 68t
support oxygenation and ventilation in, 70
supportive care for critically ill patient in, 70–71
vasopressor management in, 69–70, 69t
Sepsis-induced hypotension, 65
Septic arthritis, in sickle cell disease, 406

Septic shock
antithrombotic therapy for, 71
corticosteroids for, 71
defined, 65
high-volume continuous venovenous hemofiltration for, 71
support oxygenation and ventilation for, 70
supportive care for, 70–71
vasopressors for, 69, 70
Septicemic plague, 122–123
Septra. *See* Trimethoprim-sulfamethoxazole (TMP-SMX, Septra, Bactrim, cotrimoxazole, Cotrim).
Sequenced Treatment Alternatives to Relieve Depression (STAR*D) study, 1125, 1125f
Sequential compression devices (SCDs), for intracerebral hemorrhage, 892
Serafem. *See* Fluoxetine (Prozac, Serafem).
Serax. *See* Oxazepam (Serax).
Serc (betahistine), for tinnitus, 38
Serenoa repens, for benign prostatic hyperplasia, 715–717
Serentil (mesoridazine), poisoning due to, 1208–1209, 1208t
Serevent. *See* Salmeterol (Serevent).
Serine protease inhibitor Kazal type 1 (SPINK1), in pancreatitis, 546, 546
SERMs (selective estrogen receptor modulators)
for menopausal symptoms, 1072–1073, 1073b
for osteoporosis, 615
Serology, for leprosy, 100
Seromycin (cycloserine), for tuberculosis, 285t
Seroquel. *See* Quetiapine (Seroquel).
Serotonin agonists, for migraine headache, 924–926, 925t
Serotonin (5-HT3) antagonists, for nausea and vomiting, 7, 8t
Serotonin syndrome, 1121
due to MAOIs, 1203, 1204
due to SSRIs, 1212
Serotonin-norepinephrine reuptake inhibitors (SNRIs)
for anxiety disorders, 1112
for irritable bowel syndrome, 524
for major depression, 1123
for panic disorder, 1132t
Sertraline (Zoloft)
for Alzheimer's disease, 884, 885t, 884–886
for gaseousness, 10t
for generalized anxiety disorder, 1113, 1113t
intoxication due to, 1212
kinetics of, 1212
for major depression, 1123, 1125, 1125–1126
for obsessive compulsive disorder, 1114, 1114t
for panic disorder, 1132t
for premenstrual syndrome, 1068–1069, 1068b
for pruritus due to primary biliary cirrhosis, 499
Serum ascites-albumin gradient (SAAG), 501
Serum chemistry, reference intervals for, 1220–1221t
Serum markers, for myocardial infarction, 361
Serum sickness, 761–762
agents that cause, 761–762, 762t
clinical manifestations of, 761
defined, 761
laboratory abnormalities in, 762
pathogenesis of, 762
treatment of, 762
Sevelamar (Renagel), for chronic renal failure, 730
Sexual abuse, and bulimia nervosa, 1115–1116
Sexual dysfunction, due to multiple sclerosis, 939
Sexual Encounter Profile (SEP), 717b
Sexual functioning, after stroke, 898
Sexually transmitted disease(s)
chancroid and granuloma inguinale as, 749
contraception and, 755

Sexually transmitted disease(s) *(Continued)*
gonorrhea as, 750
nongonococcal urethritis as, 752
syphilis as, 754
Sexually transmitted epididymitis, 698
Sézary cells, 795
Sézary's syndrome (SS), 795
clinical and pathologic features of, 795–796
diagnosis of, 796b
epidemiology of, 795
etiology, molecular biology, and molecular genetics of, 795, 796
and related cutaneous lymphomas, 795
staging and prognostic factors for, 796–797, 796b, 797t
treatment of, 797–800, 797b
for advanced-stage disease, 798–800
for early-stage disease, 797–798
investigational approaches for, 797b, 800
SFEMG (single-fiber electromyography), for myasthenia gravis, 942
SGA (subjective global assessment), 619, 619b
SGAs (second-generation antipsychotics), for schizophrenia, 1130–1131, 1129b, 1130t
Shaking-impact syndrome, 970
Shark attacks, 1160, 1160b
Shellfish poisoning, 1157–1158
Shiga-like toxin–producing *E. coli,* acute infectious diarrhea due to, 15
Shigella species, acute infectious diarrhea due to, 15, 19–20t
Shin pain, due to sports, 1008–1009
Shin splints, 1008–1009
Shingles
clinical features of, 840–841
diagnosis of, 841
pruritus due to, 32b
treatment of, 841t, 842
Shock
cardiogenic, myocardial infarction with, 366t, 367
hypovolemic, in newborn, 1032
septic
antithrombotic therapy for, 71
corticosteroids for, 71
defined, 65
high-volume continuous venovenous hemofiltration for, 71
support oxygenation and ventilation for, 70
supportive care for, 70–71
vasopressors for, 69, 70
toxic (*See* Toxic shock syndrome (TSS))
Short bowel syndrome, malabsorption in, 545
Short Michigan Alcoholism Screening Test–Geriatric (S-MAST-G), 1098, 1100b
Short-acting β_2 agonists (SABAs)
for asthma, 766t
for COPD, 234
Short-chain fatty acid (SCFA) enemas, for inflammatory bowel disease, 519
Shoulder, Little Leaguers', 1009
Shoulder injuries, due to sports, 1009
Shoulder pain, after stroke, 897
Shwachman-Diamond syndrome, 381t
SI (sensitivity index), for insulin dose, 586
SI Units (International System of Units), 1217–1218, 1217t, 1218t
SIADH (secretion of inappropriate antidiuretic hormone), 596–597, 597b
Sialolithiasis, 853
Sibelium (flunarizine), for tinnitus, 38
Sibutramine (Meridia), for obesity, 609–610, 610t
Sicca syndrome, due to primary biliary cirrhosis, 499
Sick day management, for diabetes in children, 588
Sickle cell anemia, 404

Sickle cell disease (SCD), 404
  bone infarcts in, 407, 411
  cholelithiasis in, 407
  diagnosis of, 405b, 405b
  fluid therapy for, 404
  genetic basis for, 404
  hematologic disorders in, 404–406, 406t
  impaired growth and delayed puberty in, 407
  infection in, 405–406, 409–410
  iron overload in, 409, 412
  leg ulcers in, 407, 411
  neurologic complications of, 406–407, 410–411
  osteonecrosis or avascular necrosis in, 407, 411
  pregnancy and contraception with, 411–412
  priapism in, 407, 411
  renal complications of, 407, 411
  respiratory complications of, 406, 410
  retinopathy in, 407
  splenic sequestration in, 407
  SS, 404
  subtypes and severity ranking of, 404, 404b
  surgery and preoperative care with, 412
  treatment of, 407–411
    blood transfusion for, 412–413, 412t
    for bone infarcts and avascular necrosis, 411
    comprehensive approach to, 407, 408t
    hydroxyurea for, 412t, 412–413
    for infection, 409–410
    for leg ulcers, 411
    for neurologic complications, 410–411
    for priapism, 411
    for renal complications, 411
    for respiratory complications, 410
    self-care in, 408b
    transplantation for, 412t, 413
    for vasoocclusive pain, 407–409, 409t, 409b, 410f
  vasoocclusive pain in, 405
    differential diagnosis of, 406b
    treatment of, 407–409, 409t, 409b, 410f
Sildenafil citrate (Viagra)
  for diabetic neuropathy, 962
  for erectile dysfunction, 718
    in multiple sclerosis, 939b
  for high-altitude sickness, 1141, 1143
  for systemic sclerosis, 811
Silica, permissible exposure limit for, 279
Silicone, for keloids, 821
Silicoproteinosis, 280
Silicosis, 278t, 279–280
  accelerated, 280
  acute, 280
  chronic, 280
  defined, 279
  diagnosis of, 279b, 280
  etiology of, 279
  radiographic patterns of, 280
  syndromes of, 280
  treatment of, 279b, 280
  and tuberculosis, 280
Silver nitrate drops, neonatal conjunctivitis due to, 195, 196t
Simvastatin (Zocor)
  for angina pectoris, 297–298
  for dyslipoproteinemia, 605t
  for myocardial infarction, 365t
Simvastatin-ezetimibe (Vytorin), for dyslipoproteinemia, 605t
Sinemet-CR (carbidopa/levodopa), for parkinsonism, 954–955
Sinequan. See Doxepin (Sinequan).
Single-donor platelets, 482
Single-fiber electromyography (SFEMG), for myasthenia gravis, 942
Singulair. See Montelukast (Singulair).

Sinus(es), sarcoidosis of, 276
Sinus pathology, orofacial pain due to, 992t
Sinusitis, 212
  acute, 213b, 214b
    cough due to, 28b
    and asthma in children, 771
  bacterial
    cough due to, 26–27, 28b
    treatment of, 213, 214b
  chronic, 213, 214b
  classification and etiologic factors for, 212–213
  complications of, 213–214
  defined, 212
  diagnosis of, 213, 213b
  epidemiology of, 212
  invasive fungal, 214
  treatment of, 213, 214b
Sirolimus (Rapamune), for focal and segmental glomerulosclerosis, 702
SIRS (systemic inflammatory response syndrome), 65–66, 67
Sitagliptin (Januvia), for diabetes, 580t, 581
Sitagliptin/metformin (Janumet), 1243
Sitamaquine (WR 6026), for leishmaniasis, 95
Sitaxsentan sodium (Thelin), 1244–1249t
Sitz marker study, for constipation, 21–22
Six-pack platelet concentrates, 482
SJS. See Stevens-Johnson syndrome (SJS).
Skeletal development, delayed, due to thalassemia, 402
Skeletal disease, due to hyperparathyroidism, 650
Skeletal growth, in acromegaly, 634
Skeletal lesions, in multiple myeloma, 471–472
Skene duct cysts, 1091
Skier's nose, 215–216
Skiers' thumb, 1010
Skin, of extremely low birth weight infants, 1039–1040t
Skin and soft tissue infections (SSTIs), necrotizing, 83, 836b, 839
  clinical features of, 84, 84t
  diagnosis of, 84–85, 84t, 86b
  etiology of, 83–84, 84t
  fungal, 84, 85t, 86
  monomicrobial, 84, 85t, 86
  polymicrobial, 83–84, 85t, 86
  treatment of, 85–86, 85t, 86b
Skin biopsies, for leprosy, 100
Skin cancer
  melanoma as (See Melanoma)
  non-melanoma, 793
    classification of, 793
    clinical features of, 793–794
    diagnosis of, 794b
    epidemiology of, 793
    prevention and screening for, 794
    risk factors for, 793
    treatment of, 794, 794b
Skin disease(s)
  acne vulgaris and rosacea as, 787
  atopic dermatitis as, 859
  bacterial infections as, 835
  bullous, 866
  cancer as, 793
  condyloma acuminatum as, 824
  of connective tissue, 805
  contact dermatitis as, 870
  cutaneous T-cell lymphomas as, 795
  cutaneous vasculitis as, 813
  erythema multiforme, Stevens-Johnson syndrome, and toxic epidermal necrolysis as, 862
  fungal, 846
  of hair, 790
  herpes simplex virus as, 839
  keloids as, 820
  melanocytic nevi as, 827
  melanoma as, 830

Skin disease(s) (Continued)
  of mouth, 849
  of nails, 816
  papulosquamous eruptions as, 801
  parasitic, 843
  pigmentary disorders as, 876
  premalignant lesions as, 833
  pressure ulcers as, 857
  pruritus ani and vulvae as, 871
  in returning traveler, 162–163
  sunburn as, 879
  urticaria and angioedema as, 873
  venous leg ulcers as, 855
  verrucae as, 822
Skin exposure, to toxins, 1161
Skin infection(s)
  bacterial (See Bacterial skin infection(s))
  fungal, 846
    dermatophyte, 846
    diagnosis of, 846, 847b
    in HIV/AIDS patients, 847–849
    nondermatophyte, 846–847
    onychomycosis as, 847
    tinea capitis as, 847, 847b, 848b
    treatment of, 848b
  necrotizing (See Skin and soft tissue infections (SSTIs), necrotizing)
  parasitic, 30b
    due to arthropods, 844t, 845–846
    due to helminths, 843–845, 844t
    due to protozoa, 843, 844t
Skin involvement
  in acromegaly, 634
  in systemic sclerosis, 810
Skin lesions
  in returning traveler, 163
  in sarcoidosis, 276
Skin rash, due to HAART, 54–55t
Skin testing, 779
  for allergic contact dermatitis, 870
  for drug allergies, 783
  for insect stings, 784–785, 785t
Skin-to-skin contact, for high-risk neonate, 1037
Skip lesions, in Crohn's disease, 515
Skull base osteitis, 202
Skull fractures, 965
SLAP (superior labral anterior and posterior) lesions, 1009
SLE. See Systemic lupus erythematosus (SLE).
Sleep, physiology of, 887, 887
Sleep apnea, 239
  due to acromegaly, 634
  clinical features of, 240
  defined, 239–240
  diagnosis of, 240–241, 241b
  epidemiology of, 240
  and epilepsy, 906
  severity of, 241
  in sickle cell disease, 410
  treatment of, 241–242, 241b
Sleep bruxism, 993
Sleep disorder(s), 887
  in allergic rhinitis, 777
  circadian rhythm disorders as, 888
  diagnosis of, 889b
  epidemiology of, 887
  excessive daytime sleepiness as, 888
  hypersomnolence disorders as, 889
  insomnia as, 887–888, 887t, 888t
  in menopause, 1070
  narcolepsy as, 888–889
  parasomnias as, 889–890
  in parkinsonism, 953b
  physiology of sleep and, 887, 887
  restless legs syndrome and periodic limb movements as, 889
  vs. seizures, 901t
  sleep-disordered breathing as, 889

Sleep disorder(s) *(Continued)*
  symptoms of, 887
  treatment of, 889**b**
Sleep hygiene, 887, 887**t**
Sleep paralysis, 888
Sleep terrors, 889
Sleep therapy, for chronic fatigue syndrome, 120
Sleep-disordered breathing, 889
  and heart failure, 340–341
Sleepiness, excessive daytime, 888
Sleep-related eating disorder, 889
Sleepwalking, 889
SLIT (sublingual immunotherapy), for allergic rhinitis, 781
Slit skin smears, for leprosy, 100
SLNB (sentinel lymph node biopsy)
  for breast cancer, 1052
  for melanoma, 832
Slo-Phyllin. *See* Theophylline (Slo-Phyllin, Theobid, TheoDur, Theolair).
Slow brainstem syndrome, tinnitus in, 37
SLT (selective laser trabeculoplasty), for glaucoma, 200
SLUDGE syndrome, 1152
Small bowel bacterial overgrowth, 541**b**, 542, 544
Small cell carcinoma, of cervix, 1091
Small cell lung cancer (SCLC)
  pathology of, 243
  staging of, 243, 244
  treatment for, 248
Small vessel vasculitis, acute renal failure due to, 722
Smallpox, 179
  in bioterrorism, 179, 1229–1233**t**
  clinical course of, 180, 181–183**f**
  clinical features of, 179–180
  diagnosis of, 180, 180**b**, 185**f**
  differential diagnosis of, 180, 184**t**, 184**f**
  treatment of, 180–185, 185**b**
Smallpox vaccine, 179, 180, 185
Small-vessel cutaneous vasculitis. *See* Cutaneous vasculitis (CV).
Small-vessel disease, in sickle cell disease, 406–407
S-MAST-G (Short Michigan Alcoholism Screening Test–Geriatric), 1098, 1100**b**
SMM (smoldering myeloma), 467**b**, 468
Smoke inhalation injury, 1139
Smoking. *See* Cigarette smoking.
Smoking cessation, 1106–1107
  for COPD, 233, 233
Smoldering myeloma (SMM), 467**b**, 468
Snakebite, 1152
  by coral snake, 1152–1153
  diagnosis of, 1152–1153, 1153**b**
  epidemiology of, 1152
  by pit vipers
    clinical characteristics of, 1153, 1153**t**
    dry, 1153, 1154, 1154**t**
    etiology of, 1153
    identification of, 1153
    with minimal envenomation, 1154, 1154**t**
    with moderate envenomation, 1154, 1154**t**
    with severe envenomation, 1154, 1154**t**
    severity of, 1154**t**
    treatment of, 1153–1155
  treatment of, 1153–1155, 1153**t**, 1161
SnET2 (tin ethyl etiopurpurin), 1244–1249**t**
SNRIs. *See* Serotonin-norepinephrine reuptake inhibitors (SNRIs).
SO_2 (sulfur dioxide), as chemical weapon, 1226–1228**t**
Social skills training, for schizophrenia, 1129–1130
Sodium
  in parenteral fluid therapy for infants and children, 628
  in parenteral nutrition, 621, 622**t**

Sodium bicarbonate ($NaHCO_3$), for poisoning, 1167–1172**t**
  due to anticholinergics, 1180
  due to barbiturates, 1181
  due to cyclic antidepressants, 1215
  due to neuroleptics, 1209
  due to salicylates, 1211, 1211**t**
Sodium cellulose phosphate (Calcibind), for renal calculi, 746**t**
Sodium hyaluronate (Hyalgan, Supartz, Euflexxa), for osteoarthritis, 1001, 1001**t**
Sodium nitroprusside
  for amphetamine intoxication, 1179
  cyanide poisoning due to, 1188
  for phencyclidine intoxication, 1207
Sodium requirements, for infants and children, 627
Sodium restriction
  for ascites, 501
  for Ménière's disease, 211
Sodium stibogluconate pentavalent antimony (Pentostam, Solustibosan, Stibanate), for leishmaniasis, 94, 94**b**
  cutaneous, 843, 844**t**
Sodium sulfacetamide and sulfur compound (Rosac), for rosacea, 789
Sodoku, 132
Soft palate, disorders of, 852
Soft tissue infections, necrotizing. *See* Skin and soft tissue infections (SSTIs), necrotizing.
Sokal score, for chronic myeloid leukemia, 457
Solagé (mequinol and tretinoin), for solar lentigines, 877
Solaquin Forte (hydroquinone 4% cream with sunscreen)
  for melasma, 876–877
  for postinflammatory hyperpigmentation, 878
Solar lentigo, 877
Solaraze (diclofenac sodium gel), 1243
  for actinic keratosis, 834
Solatene (β-carotene), for protoporphyria, 480
Solid foods, for infants, 1042–1044
Solifenacin (Vesicare), for urge incontinence, 695**b**
Soliris (eculizumab), 1243
Solodyn. *See* Minocycline (Minocin, Dynacin, Solodyn).
Solu-Cortef. *See* Hydrocortisone sodium succinate (Solu-Cortef).
Solu-Medrol. *See* Methylprednisolone (Medrol, Solu-Medrol).
Solustibosan (sodium stibogluconate pentavalent antimony), for leishmaniasis, 94, 94**b**
  cutaneous, 843, 844**t**
Soman
  as chemical weapon, 1226–1228**t**
  poisoning due to, 1205–1206
Somatic back pain
  history of, 40
  pathogenesis of, 39–40
  referred, 40
Somatization, 990
Somatostatin analogues, for acromegaly, 636
Somatuline (lanreotide), 1243
  for acromegaly, 636
Sonata (zaleplon), for insomnia, 888, 888**t**
Sorbitol, for constipation, 22**b**
Sore throat, due to streptococcal pharyngitis. *See* Streptococcal pharyngitis.
Soriatane (acitretin)
  for actinic keratosis, 834
  for psoriasis, 802
Sotalol (Betapace)
  for atrial fibrillation, 310, 310**b**
  intoxication with, 1182–1183, 1183**t**
Sotret (isotretinoin)
  for acne, 788
  for rosacea, 789

South African star grass, for benign prostatic hyperplasia, 715–717
Soy, as nutritional supplement, 1234–1243**t**
Soy-based formula, 1043**b**
SpA (spondyloarthropathies), 986
Spastic motility disorders, 510, 511
Spasticity
  due to multiple sclerosis, 939
  after stroke, 898
Spectazole (econazole) cream, for cutaneous tinea infection, 848**b**
Spectinomycin, for gonorrhea, 751
Speech disorders, stroke rehabilitation for, 897
Spells of Tumarkin, 210
Spermicides, 757
SPF (sun protection factor), 880
Spherocytosis, hereditary, 391–392
Spider bites, 1150–1151
  diagnosis of, 1151**b**
  by *Latrodectus* species, 1151
  by *Loxosceles* species, 1150–1151
  non-*Loxosceles* necrotic arachnidism due to, 1151
  by tarantulas, 1151
  treatment of, 1151**b**
Spinal cord compression, due to multiple myeloma, 472
Spinal dysraphism, urinary incontinence due to, 690
Spine pain, 39
  assessment of, 40
    examination in, 40–41
    history in, 40
  diagnosis of, 41**b**, 43, 43**t**
  emergent or urgent conditions with, 41**b**
  epidemiology of, 39
  management of, 41, 42**b**
    with axial pain predominating, 42–43
    clinical pearls on, 43**t**
    nonsurgical or minimally invasive, 43
    with radicular pain predominating, 41–42
    surgical, 43, 43
  natural course of, 41
  pathophysiology of, 39–40, 40**f**
  radicular (neuropathic)
    assessment of, 40
    management of, 41–42, 42**b**
    natural course of, 41
    pathophysiology of, 39–40
  somatic (nociceptive), 39–40
    history of, 40
SPINK1 (serine protease inhibitor Kazal type 1), in pancreatitis, 546
Spiramycin, for toxoplasmosis, 165**t**
Spirillum minus, 132
Spiriva (tiotropium), for COPD, 28**b**, 234
Spirometry, for COPD, 232
Spironolactone (Aldactone)
  for aldosteronism, 656
  for androgenic alopecia, 791
  for ascites, 501
  for nephrotic syndrome, 701
Spitz nevi, 828**b**, 829
Splenectomy
  for thalassemia, 401
  for warm autoimmune hemolytic anemia, 388
Splenic sequestration, in sickle cell disease, 407
Split ends, 793
SPMS (secondary progressive multiple sclerosis), 933, 933**f**, 938
Spondylitis, ankylosing. *See* Ankylosing spondylitis (AS).
Spondyloarthropathies (SpA), 986
Spondylolisthesis, back pain due to, 40
Spontaneous bacterial peritonitis (SBP), 497**t**, 501**t**, 502
Spontaneous breathing, trial of, 228, 228**b**
Sporanox. *See* Itraconazole (Sporanox).

Spore-forming protozoa, 565–566t, 567–569
Sports injuries, 1007
　of ankle, 1009
　concussions as, 1010
　diagnosis of, 1008b
　of elbow, 1009
　of head, 968–969
　of knee, 1007–1008
　lower leg pain due to, 1008–1009
　of shoulder, 1009
　treatment of, 1008b
　of wrist and hand, 1009–1010
Sprue
　celiac, 541b, 543
　tropical, 544
Sprycel (dasatinib), for chronic myeloid leukemia, 459, 460
Squamous cell carcinoma (SCC)
　of bladder, 736–737
　of cervix (See Cervical cancer)
　clinical features of, 794
　diagnosis of, 794b
　epidemiology of, 793
　of floor of mouth, 853
　of lips, 850
　of tongue, 853
　treatment of, 794, 794b
　of vulva, 1092–1093, 1093t
Squamous papilloma, of soft palate/tonsillar pillar region, 852
SRS (stereotactic radiosurgery), for brain metastases, 976
SS. See Sézary syndrome (SS).
SSc. See Systemic sclerosis (SSc).
SSRIs. See Selective serotonin reuptake inhibitors (SSRIs).
SSTIs. See Skin and soft tissue infections (SSTIs).
ST elevation myocardial infarction (STEMI)
　adjunctive therapy for, 362–365, 365t
　evaluation of, 362f
　fibrinolytic therapy for, 361–362, 363b, 364t
　initial management of, 361
　percutaneous coronary intervention for, 362, 364b
　reperfusion therapy for, 361, 363f
　risk score for, 363t
St. John's wort, 1234–1243t
St. Louis encephalitis virus, 928–930t
Stachybotrys, as biological weapon agent, 1229–1233t
Stadol (butorphanol), for pain, 4t
Staghorn calculi, 743
Staging of Reproductive Aging Workshop (STRAW) staging system, 1070, 1070b
Stalevo (carbidopa/levodopa-entacapone), for parkinsonism, 956–957
Standby transcutaneous pacing, for heart block, 318, 319b
Standing balance, for vestibular neurolabyrinthitis, 207b
Staphylococcal scarlet fever. See Staphylococcal toxic shock syndrome.
Staphylococcal toxic shock syndrome, 86
　diagnosis of, 87b, 88, 88b
　epidemiology of, 87
　menstrual *vs.* nonmenstrual, 87
　pathogenesis of, 87
　treatment of, 89, 89b
Staphylococcus aureus
　acute infectious diarrhea due to, 16
　and atopic dermatitis, 859, 860
　as biological weapon agent, 1229–1233t
　endocarditis due to, 345
　endocarditis prophylaxis for, 346–347t
　foodborne illness due to, 83
　methicillin-resistant
　　acute infectious diarrhea due to, 16

Staphylococcus aureus (Continued)
　necrotizing skin and soft tissue infections due to, 84t, 85t
　skin infections due to, 835–836, 836b, 837f
　toxic shock syndrome due to, 87, 89
　osteomyelitis due to, 1005
Staphylococcus aureus toxic shock syndrome (SA-TSS), 86
　diagnosis of, 87b, 88, 88b
　epidemiology of, 87
　menstrual *vs.* nonmenstrual, 87
　pathogenesis of, 87
　treatment of, 89, 89b
Staphylococcus epidermidis, endocarditis due to, 345
　prophylaxis for, 346–347t
Staphylococcus saprophyticus, urinary tract infections due to
　in girls, 686–687
　in women, 682, 683b, 684
STAR*D (Sequenced Treatment Alternatives to Relieve Depression) study, 1125, 1125f
Starlix (nateglinide), for diabetes, 580t
Statins
　for angina pectoris, 297–298, 298
　for chronic renal failure, 729
　drugs that interact with, 603b, 605
　for dyslipoproteinemia, 604–605, 605t
　for myocardial infarction, 364–365, 365t
　and SSRIs, 1122–1123b
Status epilepticus, 906
　in neonates, 910
Stavudine (Zerit), for HIV, 50t
Steatohepatitis, nonalcoholic, 498t, 500
Steatorrhea, 539, 542
Stelazine (trifluoperazine), poisoning due to, 1208–1209, 1208t
Stem-cell transplantation
　allogeneic, for multiple myeloma, 470
　autologous
　　for acute myeloid leukemia, 446–447
　　for lymphoma
　　　cutaneous T-cell, 800
　　　non-Hodgkin's, 466–467
　　for multiple myeloma, 470
　　for systemic lupus erythematosus, 809
　hematopoietic
　　for aplastic anemia, 382, 382f
　　long-term complications of, 382–383
　　for sickle cell disease, 412t, 413
　　for thalassemia, 401
STEMI. See ST elevation myocardial infarction (STEMI).
Sterapred. See Prednisone (Deltasone, Orasone, Medrol, Sterapred).
Stereotactic radiosurgery (SRS), for brain metastases, 976
Sterilization, 757–758
　in postpartum period, 1029t
Steroid(s). See Corticosteroids.
　anabolic, abuse of, 1111
Steroid 6β-OH, and SSRIs, 1122–1123b
Steroid biosynthesis inhibitors, for Cushing's syndrome, 645t
Stevens-Johnson syndrome (SJS), 864–866
　clinical presentation of, 864–865
　diagnosis of, 863b
　vs. erythema multiforme and toxic epidermal necrolysis, 862, 863t
　etiology of, 865, 865b
　due to HAART, 54–55t
　treatment of, 864b, 865–866
Stibanate (sodium stibogluconate pentavalent antimony), for leishmaniasis, 94, 94b
　cutaneous, 843, 844t
STICH (Surgical Trial in Intracerebral Hemorrhage) study, 891–892
Stimulant laxatives, for constipation, 22, 22b

Stimulants
　abuse of, 1105b, 1109–1110
　for ADHD, 917–918, 918t
Stinging nettle root, 1234–1243t
Stingray envenomation, 1159
Stomach tumors, 556
Stomatitis
　bovine papular, 843
　denture, 851
Stomatocytosis, hereditary, 392
Stool consistency, 521, 522f
Stool softeners, for constipation, 22, 22b
Storage lesions, 480
Strattera (atomoxetine), for ADHD, 918, 918t
STRAW (Staging of Reproductive Aging Workshop) staging system, 1070, 1070b
Strep throat. See Streptococcal pharyngitis.
Streptase (streptokinase), for deep venous thrombosis/pulmonary embolism, 273–274
Streptobacillus moniliformis. See Rat-bite fever (RBF).
Streptococcal endocarditis, 345
　antibiotic prophylaxis for, 346–347t
Streptococcal pharyngitis, 220
　clinical manifestations of, 221
　diagnosis of, 221–222, 221b
　epidemiology of, 221
　microbiology of, 220–221
　recurrent, 223, 223t
　treatment of, 222–223
　　drugs and dosages for, 223t
　　indications for, 222–223, 222t
　　strategies for, 222–223, 222t
Streptococcal toxic shock syndrome, 86
　diagnosis of, 87b, 88, 88b
　epidemiology of, 87
　pathogenesis of, 87
　treatment of, 89, 89b
Streptococcus durans, endocarditis prophylaxis for, 346–347t
Streptococcus faecalis, endocarditis prophylaxis for, 346–347t
Streptococcus faecium, endocarditis prophylaxis for, 346–347t
Streptococcus pneumoniae, community-acquired pneumonia due to, 261–263
Streptococcus pyogenes
　necrotizing skin and soft tissue infections due to, 84, 84t, 85t
　toxic shock syndrome due to, 86
　diagnosis of, 87b, 88, 88b
　epidemiology of, 87
　pathogenesis of, 87
　treatment of, 89, 89b
Streptococcus viridans, endocarditis prophylaxis for, 346–347t
Streptokinase (Streptase), for deep venous thrombosis/pulmonary embolism, 273–274
Streptomycin
　for brucellosis, 74–75, 74b, 75t
　for infective endocarditis, 345
　for *Mycobacterium avium intracellulare complex*, 289
　for plague, 123
　for tuberculosis, 285t
Stress
　atopic dermatitis due to, 860
　and metabolic rate, 620, 621, 620f
Stress reduction, for diabetes, 578, 580b
Stress testing, for angina pectoris, 296
Stress-diathesis model, for tinnitus, 39
Stretch marks, 1013
Striae, 1013
Striant (testosterone buccal preparation), for hypopituitarism, 658
Striational antibodies, 942
Stricturotomy, for urethral stricture disease, 742

Stroke
　dyslipoproteinemia and, 603
　epidemiology of, 895
　due to intracerebral hemorrhage, 890
　　diagnosis of, 891, 891b
　　epidemiology and etiology of, 890–891, 890b
　　scoring system for, 891, 891t
　　treatment of, 891–892, 892t
　due to ischemic cerebrovascular disease, 893
　　diagnosis of, 893, 894, 894b
　　epidemiology and etiology of, 893
　　pathophysiology of, 893
　　risk factors for, 893
　　symptoms of, 893
　　transient ischemic attacks and, 893–894
　motor recovery after, 895, 896b
　rehabilitation after, 895, 898b
　　for activities of daily living, 896–897
　　for common medical complications, 897–898
　　continuity of care in, 898
　　for mobility and locomotion, 896
　　research on, 895–896
　　for speech and language disorders, 897
　　team for, 895
　　techniques of, 896b
　in sickle cell disease, 407, 410–411
Stromectol. See Ivermectin (Stromectol).
Strongyloides stercoralis, 570t, 571–572, 844t, 845
Strongyloidiasis, 570t, 571–572
Struvite stones, 743, 744t
Stylohyoid process syndrome, orofacial pain due to, 992t
SU(s) (sulfonylureas)
　for diabetes, 579, 579–580, 580t, 580t
　and SSRIs, 1122–1123b
Subacute bacterial endocarditis, in sickle cell disease, 410
Subdiaphragmatic irradiation, for Hodgkin's lymphoma, 441–442, 442, 443
Subdural hematomas (SDHs), 966
　in children, 969–970
Suberoylanilide hydroxamic acid (SAHA), for cutaneous T-cell lymphomas, 800
Subfascial endoscopic perforator vein surgery (SEPS), for venous leg ulcers, 857
Subjective global assessment (SGA), 619, 619b
Sublingual immunotherapy (SLIT), for allergic rhinitis, 781
Substance abuse. See Alcoholism; Drug abuse.
Subtotal nodal irradiation, for Hodgkin's lymphoma, 440
Subungual hematoma, 819
Subutex (buprenorphine), for opiate withdrawal, 1109
Succimer (2,3-dimercaptosuccinic acid), for poisoning, 1167–1172t
　due to lead, 1199, 1200t
Sucralfate (Carafate)
　for indigestion, 11t
　for peptic ulcer disease, 531t, 531–532
　for theophylline intoxication, 1214
Suctioning, of newborn, 1031
Sudafed (pseudoephedrine), for stress incontinence, 695b, 696
Sudden cardiac death (SCD). See also Cardiac arrest.
　aborted, 302
　defined, 302
　due to hypertrophic cardiomyopathy, 331–333
Sudden death, 302
Suicide
　bipolar disorder and, 1126
　depression and, 1120–1121
　SSRIs and, 1112, 1117
　due to toxic ingestion, 1160–1161
Sulfadiazine, for toxoplasmosis, 165t, 166, 167

Sulfasalazine (Azulfidine)
　for inflammatory bowel disease, 515–516, 519–520
　for juvenile idiopathic arthritis, 985–986
　for rheumatoid arthritis, 981t, 982
Sulfinpyrazone (Anturane), for hyperuricemia, 599
Sulfonamides, allergy to, 782–783
Sulfonylureas (SUs)
　for diabetes, 579–580, 580t, 580t
　and SSRIs, 1122–1123b
Sulfur dioxide (SO$_2$), as chemical weapon, 1226–1228t
Sulfur mustard, as chemical weapon, 1226–1228t
Sulindac (Clinoril)
　for juvenile idiopathic arthritis, 985
　for osteoarthritis, 1000
Suma, lead in, 1197
Sumatriptan (Imitrex), for migraine headache, 925t, 926
Sumatriptan/naproxen (Trexima), 1244–1249t
Sumycin. See Tetracycline (Achromycin, Sumycin).
Sun protection factor (SPF), 880
Sunburn, 30b, 879
　diagnosis of, 880b
　grading of, 879
　pathogenesis of, 879
　prevention of, 879–880
　treatment of, 880b
Sunscreens, 880
　for melasma, 877, 877t
Supartz (sodium hyaluronate), for osteoarthritis, 1001, 1001t
Superantigen (SAG) family, in toxic shock syndrome, 87
Superficial white onychomycosis (SWO), 818
Superior canal dehiscence syndrome, 208
Superior labral anterior and posterior (SLAP) lesions, 1009
Superior vena cava syndrome, in childhood leukemia, 453–454
Supportive care
　for aplastic anemia, 379–380
　for neutropenia, 414–415
　for Stevens-Johnson syndrome and toxic epidermal necrolysis, 864b, 865
Suppositories, for constipation, 22b
Supraclavicular nodal involvement, in breast cancer, 1050
Suprax. See Cefixime (Suprax).
Suprefact (buserelin), for premenstrual syndrome, 1069
Suramin sodium (Antrypol), for African sleeping sickness, 843, 844t
Surfactant (Survanta), for extremely low birth weight infants, 1039–1040t
Surfak (docusate calcium), for constipation, 22b
Surgical débridement, for pressure ulcers, 858
Surgical myectomy, for hypertrophic cardiomyopathy, 333
Surgical site infection, 836b, 838–839, 838b
Surgical Trial in Intracerebral Hemorrhage (STICH) study, 891–892
"Surma," lead in, 1197
Surmantil (trimipramine), poisoning due to, 1214–1216, 1215t
Survanta (surfactant), for extremely low birth weight infants, 1039–1040t
Sustiva (efavirenz), for HIV, 49–50, 50t, 51t
　drug interactions with, 53, 58t
Swallowing process, 508, 508
Swallowing rehabilitation, 510
Sweat(s), paroxysmal, due to alcohol withdrawal, 1102–1103b
Sweat test, for cystic fibrosis, 237–238
Swelling, pain due to, 2
SWO (superficial white onychomycosis), 818

Symbicort (budesonide/formoterol), for asthma
　in adolescents and adults, 767–768t
　in children, 773–774t
Symlin (pramlinitide), for diabetes, 580t, 581
Symmetrel. See Amantadine (Symmetrel).
Sympatholytic agents, for systemic sclerosis, 811t
Sympathomimetics, for glaucoma, 200
Symptomatic care
　for acute infectious diarrhea, 13
　for constipation, 20
　for cough, 25
　for fever, 23
　for gaseousness and indigestion, 9
　for hiccups, 12
　for nausea and vomiting, 5
　for pain, 1
　for pruritus, 29
　for spine pain, 39
　for tinnitus, 35
Synacthen (tetracosactide), for membranous nephropathy, 703
Synagis (palivizumab), for bronchiolitis, 266
Synalar (fluocinonide)
　for atopic dermatitis, 860–861
　for vitiligo, 878–879
Synalgos-DC (dihydrocodeine + aspirin + caffeine), for pain, 4t
Synarel (nafarelin acetate)
　for endometriosis, 1056
　for uterine leiomyoma, 1082
Syncope
　due to hypertrophic cardiomyopathy, 333
　vs. seizures, 901t
Synercid (quinupristin-dalfopristin), for pyelonephritis, 685
Synthroid. See Levothyroxine (L-thyroxine, Synthroid, Levothroid, Levoxyl).
Synvisc (hylan G-F20), for osteoarthritis, 1001, 1001t
Syphilis, 754
　clinical manifestations of, 754, 755t
　diagnosis of, 754–755
　epidemiology of, 754, 754
　follow-up for, 755
　and HIV infection, 755
　late (tertiary), 754, 755t
　latent, 754, 755t
　microbiology of, 754
　neuro-, 755
　pathophysiology of, 754
　during pregnancy, 755
　primary, 754, 755t
　secondary, 754, 755t
　treatment of, 755, 755t
Syprine (trientine), for Wilson's disease, 500–501
Syrup of ipecac, for poisoning, 1163
Systemic inflammatory response syndrome (SIRS), 65–66, 67
Systemic lupus erythematosus (SLE), 805–809
　clinical features of, 805, 806, 806
　during pregnancy, 806
　renal, 808f
　treatment of
　　antimalarial agents for, 806–808, 807t
　　B-cell depletion for, 809
　　corticosteroids for, 807t, 808, 808f
　　cytokine blockade for, 809
　　cytotoxic agents for, 807t, 808–809, 808f
　　general principles of, 805–806, 806f
　　immunoablation and autologous stem cell transplantation for, 809
　　inhibition of B-cell survival for, 809
　　inhibition of costimulatory interactions for, 809
　　novel therapies for, 809
　　NSAIDs for, 806, 807t

Systemic sclerosis (SSc), 809–812
  clinical features of, 809–810, 810b
  cutaneous
    diffuse, 809–810, 810b
    limited, 809–810, 810b
  organ involvement in, 809–810, 810b
  pruritus due to, 32b
  treatment of
    general principles of, 810
    for GI tract involvement, 811–812, 812b
    for interstitial lung disease, 811
    organ-based, 810–812
    potentially disease-modifying therapies for, 810, 810b
    for renal involvement, 812
    for skin involvement, 810
    for vascular involvement, 810–811, 811t

T

T SPOT-TB assay, 283
T-2 mycotoxins, as biological weapon agents, 1229–1233t
T₃. See Triiodothyronine (T₃).
T₄. See Thyroxine (T₄).
Tabun
  as chemical weapon, 1226–1228t
  poisoning due to, 1205–1206
Tachyarrhythmia(s)
  mechanisms of, 320, 320f, 320f
  supraventricular, 320–323
  ventricular, 323–324
Tachycardia(s), 320
  atrial, 322–323
  atrioventricular reciprocating, 321–322, 322f, 322f
  defined, 320
  lesional, 323
  mechanisms of, 320, 320f, 320f
  pacemaker-mediated, 322
  reentry, 320, 320f
    atrioventricular nodal, 321, 321f, 321f, 322b
  supraventricular, 320–323
  ventricular, 323–324
    in Brugada's syndrome, 324–326, 325f, 325f
    catecholaminergic polymorphic, 324
    intrafascicular, 323
    in ischemic heart disease, 325–326
    after myocardial infarction, 366t
    outflow tract, 323
Tachypnea, of the newborn, transient, 1037–1038
Tacrine (Cognex), for Alzheimer's disease, 882–883
Tacrolimus (Prograf)
  for focal and segmental glomerulosclerosis, 702
  for membranous nephropathy, 703
  peripheral neuropathy due to, 963
  for psoriasis, 801
Tacrolimus ointment (Protopic)
  for anogenital pruritus, 873
  for atopic dermatitis, 861
  for contact dermatitis, 871, 871b
  for vitiligo, 878–879
Tactile disturbances, due to alcohol withdrawal, 1102–1103b
Tadalafil (Cialis), for erectile dysfunction, 719
  in multiple sclerosis, 939b
Taenia spp, 570t, 573
Taeniasis, 570t, 573
Tagamet. See Cimetidine (Tagamet).
TA-GVHD. See Transfusion-associated graft-versus-host disease (TA-GVHD).
Talacen (pentazocine + acetaminophen), for pain, 4t
Talwin (pentazocine), intoxication with, 1204–1205, 1205t

Talwin-NX (pentazocine + naloxone), for pain, 4t
Tambocor (flecainide)
  for atrial fibrillation, 309–310, 310b
  for cardioversion, 311, 311t
Tamiflu (oseltamivir), for influenza, 92, 92t, 260, 260b, 265, 267, 267t
Tamoxifen (Nolvadex)
  for breast cancer, 1052–1053
  for ductal carcinoma in situ, 1050
  for lobular carcinoma in situ, 1049–1050
  for menopausal symptoms, 1070
Tamsulosin (Flomax)
  for benign prostatic hyperplasia, 714–716, 714t
  for prostatitis, 710–711
  for renal calculi, 744–745, 745t
Tanning, protective, 880
Tapazole (methimazole)
  for hyperthyroidism, 667–668
  for thyroid storm, 669
Tapeworms, 570t, 573
  malabsorption due to, 545
TAPVC (total anomalous pulmonary venous connection), 331
Tar extracts, for psoriasis, 802
Taractan (chlorprothixene), poisoning due to, 1208–1209, 1208t
Tarantula bites, 1151
Tarceva (erlotinib), for non–small cell lung cancer, 247
Tardive dyskinesia (TD), 1130
Target lesion
  in erythema multiforme, 862
  in Stevens-Johnson syndrome, 864–865
Targeted modalities, for cutaneous T-cell lymphomas, 799–800
Targretin. See Bexarotene (Targretin).
Tasigna. See Nilotinib (Tasigna).
Tasmar (tolcapone), for parkinsonism, 956
Tavist (clemastine), for allergic rhinitis, 779t
Taxol. See Paclitaxel (Taxol).
Taxotere (docetaxel)
  for non–small cell lung cancer, 247–248
  for prostate cancer, 732
Tazarotene (Tazorac)
  for acne, 787, 787
  for psoriasis, 801–802
Tazicef. See Ceftazidime (Fortaz, Tazicef).
Tazocin (piperacillin/tazobactam), for necrotizing skin and soft tissue infections, 85t
Tazorac. See Tretinoin topical (Retin-A, Renova, Differin, Tazorac).
TB. See Tuberculosis (TB).
TBI. See Traumatic brain injury (TBI).
TBRF. See Tick-borne relapsing fever (TBRF).
TBSA (total body surface area), of burn, 1135, 1136f, 1137f
TCA(s) (tricyclic antidepressants). See Tricyclic antidepressants (TCAs).
TCA (trichloracetic acid)
  for condyloma acuminatum, 825b, 826, 1092
  for verrucae, 823
T-cell lymphomas, cutaneous. See Cutaneous T-cell lymphomas (CTCL).
TCIs (topical calcineurin inhibitors), for atopic dermatitis, 861
Td. See Tetanus and diphtheria toxoid vaccine (Td).
TD (tardive dyskinesia), 1130
Tdap. See Tetanus and diphtheria toxoids and acellular pertussis vaccine (Tdap, BOOSTRIX, ADACEL).
TDD (total daily dose), of insulin for children, 585, 585f
TDO (total dystrophic onychomycosis), 818
TdP (torsade de pointes), 324, 324
  after myocardial infarction, 366t

TE (toxoplasmic encephalitis), 163, 166t, 167–168, 167b
Tear gas, as chemical weapon, 1226–1228t
Tedisamil (Pulzium), 1244–1249t
TEE (total energy expenditure), 620
TEE (transesophageal echocardiography), for infective endocarditis, 344, 344
Tegaserod (Zelnorm)
  for constipation, 22, 22b
  for irritable bowel syndrome, 524–525
Tegenaria agrestis envenomation, 1151
Tegretol. See Carbamazepine (Tegretol).
Tekturna (aliskiren), 1243
Telangiectasias, of lips, 850
Telavancin, 1244–1249t
Telbivudine (Tyzeka), for hepatitis B and C viruses, 536t, 537
Telithromycin (Ketek)
  for legionellosis, 271t
  for mycoplasmal pneumonia, 270, 270t
Telogen effluvium
  acute, 790
  chronic, 790–791
  laboratory studies for, 791b
  medication-induced, 791b
Telogen phase, of hair growth, 790
Temazepam (Restoril)
  for insomnia, 888t
  intoxication with, 1181–1182
Temovate. See Clobetasol propionate (Temovate).
Temozolomide (Temodal), for cutaneous T-cell lymphomas, 798–799
Temporal arteritis, orofacial pain due to, 992t
Temporal bone, osteoradionecrosis of, 202
Temporary pacing, for heart block, 318, 318, 319, 319f
Temporomandibular disorder(s) (TMDs), 988
  due to arthralgia, arthritis, arthrosis, 991b
  classification of, 990–991, 991b
  clinical features of, 988
  defined, 988
  diagnosis of, 989–991, 989b
    biobehavioral evaluation in, 989–990, 990b
    biomedical evaluation in, 989
    yellow flags in, 990, 990b
  due to disk displacements, 991b
  epidemiology of, 989
  due to muscle disorders, 991b
  treatment of, 991–993, 991b
    biobehavioral, 993
    biomedical, 991–993, 993b
Temporomandibular joint (TMJ)
  osteoarthritis of, 991b
  osteoarthrosis of, 991b
  physical examination of, 989, 989
TEN. See Toxic epidermal necrolysis (TEN).
Tender points, in fibromyalgia, 996, 996b
Tendinitis, 995
  diagnosis of, 994b, 995
  pathogenesis of, 995
  sites of, 994b
  symptoms of, 995
  treatment of, 995, 997b
Tenecteplase (TNKase, TNK), for myocardial infarction, 364t
Tenex (guanfacine), for Tourette's syndrome, 920
Tennis elbow, 1009
Tenofovir (Viread), for HIV, 50t, 51t
Tenofovir + emtricitabine (Truvada), for HIV, 51t
Tenormin. See Atenolol (Tenormin).
Tensilon (edrophonium chloride), for myasthenia gravis, 942t
Tensilon (edrophonium chloride) test, for myasthenia gravis, 941

Tension-type headache (TTHA)
  clinical features of, 923
  etiology of, 923
  evaluation and diagnosis of, 923, 922t
  pathophysiology of, 923
  treatment of, 924, 924t
Tequin. See Gatifloxacin (Tequin).
Teratogens, 1011–1012
Teratoma, 738–739
Terazol (terconazole), for vulvovaginal candidiasis, 1075b
Terazosin hydrochloride (Hytrin)
  for benign prostatic hyperplasia, 714–716, 714t
  for prostatitis, 710–711
  for renal calculi, 745t
  for urinary incontinence in children, 691, 692t
Terbinafine (Lamisil)
  for cutaneous tinea infection, 848b
  for fungal skin infections with HIV, 848–849
  for onychomycosis, 818, 818b
  for tinea capitis, 848b
  for tinea corporis, 804
  for tinea unguium, 847, 848b
Terbutaline (Brethine), for asthma in children, 772b, 774–775, 775t
Terconazole (Terazol), for vulvovaginal candidiasis, 1075b
Terfenadine (Seldane), poisoning due to, 1179–1180
Teriparatide (Forteo), for osteoporosis, 615
Terlipressin, for hepatorenal syndrome, 503
Tertiary amines, poisoning due to, 1214–1216, 1215t
TESS (Toxic Exposure Surveillance System), 1160, 1160
Testicular cancer, 738–740
  diagnosis of, 738, 738b
  metastatic, 738
  treatment of, 738–740, 739b
Testicular injuries, 708b, 709
Testicular rupture, 709
Testis(es), lymphoma of, 740
Testosterone
  for erectile dysfunction, 720
  and erectile function, 716
  for hypopituitarism, 658
  parenteral nutrition with, 624
Testosterone buccal preparation (Striant), for hypopituitarism, 658
Testosterone cypionate, for hypopituitarism, 658
Testosterone enanthate (Delatestryl), for hypopituitarism, 658
Testosterone gel (AndroGel), for hypopituitarism, 658
Testosterone patch (Androderm), for hypopituitarism, 658
Tetanospasmin, 143
Tetanus, 143
  cephalic, 144
  chemoprophylaxis for, 144b, 145, 145t
  clinical features of, 143–144
  diagnosis of, 144, 144b
  differential diagnosis of, 144
  epidemiology of, 143
  etiology of, 143
  forms of, 143–144
  generalized, 143
  local, 144
  neonatal, 144
  prevention of, 144–145, 145t
  treatment of, 144, 144b
Tetanus and diphtheria toxoid vaccine (Td), 145
  for acute wounds, 144b, 151t
  in pregnancy, 145
  schedule for, 145, 145t
    catch-up, 151t

Tetanus and diphtheria toxoids and acellular pertussis vaccine (Tdap, BOOSTRIX, ADACEL), 147, 147t
  schedule for, 149–150t
    catch-up, 151t
Tetanus toxoid (TT), 145, 145
Tetracosactide (Synacthen), for membranous nephropathy, 703
Tetracycline (Achromycin, Sumycin)
  for acute necrotizing ulcerative gingivitis, 854
  for balantidiasis, 565–566t, 567
  for bullous pemphigoid, 867
  for cholera, 80t
  for dientamoebiasis, 565–566t
  for Lyme disease, 138, 139t
  for malaria, 108t, 109
  for osteoarthritis, 1002
  for peptic ulcer disease, 532t
  for psittacosis, 128
  for rat-bite fever, 132–133
  for relapsing fever, 136t
  for rosacea, 789
  for systemic sclerosis, 811–812
  for tropical sprue, 544
Tetrahydrocannabinol (THC), abuse of, 1110
Tetralogy of Fallot, 328–329, 329b
  antibiotic prophylaxis with, 345
TG(s). See Triglycerides (TGs).
TGA (transposition of the great arteries), 330
TH(s) (helper T cells)
  in allergic rhinitis, 777
  in cutaneous T-cell lymphomas, 795
Thalassemia, 397
  carrier state of, 398
  clinical manifestations of, 398–400
  diagnosis of, 398, 398b
  etiology and pathogenesis of, 397, 397–398
  inheritance of, 397–398
  pathophysiology of, 397–398
  treatment of, 399t, 400–404, 400b
    approach to, 400
    for complications, 399t, 402
    for fetal hemoglobin augmentation in, 401
    hematopoietic stem cell transplantation in, 401
    for iron overload, 399t, 401–402, 403t
    psychosocial support in, 402–404
    splenectomy in, 401
    transfusions in, 399t, 400–401
α-Thalassemia
  clinical manifestations of, 400
  diagnosis of, 398b
  genetic basis for, 398
β-Thalassemia intermedia (TI)
  clinical manifestations of, 399–400, 400b
  diagnosis of, 398b
  genetic basis for, 398
  monitoring of, 400b
  treatment, 400b
β-Thalassemia major (TM)
  clinical manifestations of, 398–399
  complications of, 399t, 402
  diagnosis of, 398b
  genetic basis for, 398
  monitoring of, 399t
  treatment of, 399t
Thalassemia trait, 398b
Thalidomide, for multiple myeloma, 469b, 470, 471
THC (tetrahydrocannabinol), abuse of, 1110
Thelarche, 1062–1063
Thelin (sitaxsentan sodium), 1244–1249t
Theophylline (Slo-Phyllin, Theobid, TheoDur, Theolair)
  for asthma
    in adolescents and adults, 767–768t
    in children, 773–774t, 775
  for COPD, 234

Theophylline (Slo-Phyllin, Theobid, TheoDur, Theolair) (Continued)
  intoxication with, 1212–1214, 1213t
Therapeutic drug monitoring, reference intervals for, 1222t
Thermal injury. See Burn(s).
Thermic effect, of exercise, 620
Thermogenesis, dietary, 620
Thermoregulation, of high-risk neonate, 1035, 1035t, 1036f, 1036t
Thermoregulatory responses, 23
Thiabendazole (Mintezol)
  for cutaneous larva migrans, 844, 844t
  for strongyloidiasis, 570t
Thiamine
  for alcohol withdrawal, 1103
  for alcoholic liver disease, 498
  for dysmenorrhea, 1066
  in parenteral nutrition, 621, 621t
  for poisoning, 1167–1172t
    due to ethanol, 1191
    due to ethylene glycol, 1193
Thiamine deficiency
  encephalopathy due to, 1173
  peripheral neuropathy due to, 963
Thiazide diuretics
  for hypertension, 356–357
    in pregnancy, 1023t
  for renal calculi, 746t
Thiazide-like diuretics, for hypertension, 356–357, 357
Thiazolidinediones (TZDs), for diabetes, 580t, 580t, 581
Thiethylperazine (Torecan), for nausea and vomiting, 8t
Thin-layer rapid-use epicutaneous (TRUE) test allergens, 870
Thionamide drugs
  for hyperthyroidism, 667–668, 667
    continuing treatment with, 667
    initial treatment with, 667
    stopping, 668
  side effects of, 667–668
  for thyroid storm, 669
Thiopurine methyltransferase (TPMT) levels, with azathioprine, 867, 869t
Thioridazine (Mellaril), poisoning due to, 1208–1209, 1208t
Thiothixene (Navane), poisoning due to, 1208–1209, 1208t
Thioxanthenes, poisoning due to, 1208–1209, 1208t
Thoracentesis, for pleural effusion, 257
Thoracic aortic aneurysms, 291
  diagnosis of, 291, 293b
  rupture of, 291
  treatment of, 292, 294b
Thoracoabdominal aneurysms, treatment of, 292
Thoracoabdominal paradox, 228
Thorazine. See Chlorpromazine (Thorazine).
Thought blocking, in schizophrenia, 1129
Thought broadcasting, 1129
Thought insertion, 1129
Three-in-one solutions, 621
Throat culture, for streptococcal pharyngitis, 222
Thrombasthenia, Glanzmann's, 427
Thrombin, 428
Thrombin burst, 419
Thrombocytopenia, 425–427
  alloimmune, 426
  amegakaryocytic, 381t
  autoimmune, 426, 427b
  due to decreased platelet production, 426
  diagnosis of, 426b
  heparin-induced, 426
  due to hypersplenism, 427
  due to increased platelet destruction, 426–427
  treatment of, 427b

Thrombolytic therapy, for deep venous thrombosis/pulmonary embolism, 273–274
Thrombosis, due to polycythemia vera, 472–474
Thrombotic manifestations, of disseminated intravascular coagulation, 428, 428
Thrombotic thrombocytopenic purpura (TTP), 430
 classification of, 430, 430b
 clinical presentation of, 430–431
 defined, 430
 diagnosis of, 431, 431b
 etiology of, 430, 430b
 pathogenesis of, 430
 prognosis for, 431–432
 thrombocytopenia due to, 426
 treatment of, 431, 432f
Thumb, gamekeepers' or skiers', 1010
Thumb-tracking exercise, for vestibular neurolabyrinthitis, 207b
Thymectomy, for myasthenia gravis, 946
Thyroid autoantibodies, 662
Thyroid cancer, 670
 anaplastic, 672, 673t
 causes of, 670
 diagnosis of, 670–671, 670b, 671, 671t
 epidemiology of, 670
 follicular, 671–672
  follow-up for, 672, 673t
 follow-up for, 672–673, 673t
 histologic classification of, 670, 671–672
 Hürthle cell, 671, 672
  follow-up for, 672, 673t
 medullary, 672, 673t
 papillary, 671
  follow-up for, 672–673, 673t
 prognosis for, 671–672
 risk factors for, 670, 670b
 signs and symptoms of, 670b
 treatment of, 671–672, 672
 well-differentiated, 672–673, 673t
Thyroid failure, diagnosis of, 662
Thyroid hormone(s)
 normal physiology of, 661–662
 reducing serum levels of, 667
Thyroid hormone bioequivalency, 663
Thyroid hormone replacement, for hypopituitarism, 658
Thyroid nodule, 670–671, 671t
Thyroid preparations, desiccated, 663
Thyroid storm, 669
Thyroidectomy, for hyperthyroidism, 667, 667, 668–669
Thyroiditis, 675
 acute (suppurative), 676–677
 chronic (autoimmune), 677–678
 defined, 676
 diagnosis of, 677
 drug-induced, 678
 Hashimoto's, 662
 Hashimoto's (goitrous), 678, 678
 postpartum, 665, 665, 677
 Riedel's, 678
 silent, 677
 subacute (de Quervain's, viral, granulomatous), 665, 677
 treatment of, 677
Thyroid-stimulating hormone (TSH)
 in hyperthyroidism, 666, 666
 normal physiology of, 661
 normal range for, 662
 in thyroid cancer, 670–671
 in thyroid failure, 662, 662
Thyroxine (T_4)
 for hypothyroidism, 663
  during pregnancy, 664–665
 for myxedema coma, 664
 normal physiology of, 661–662
 reducing serum levels of, 667

TI. See -Thalassemia intermedia (TI).
TIA(s). See Transient ischemic attacks (TIAs).
Tiagabine (Gabitril), for epilepsy
 in adolescents in adults, 904t
 in infants and children, 914, 913t
Tiberal (ornidazole)
 for amebiasis, 60–61
 for giardiasis, 63–64, 64t, 64b
Tibial stress fractures, 1008–1009
Tic(s)
 classification of, 919, 920b
 douloureux (See Trigeminal neuralgia (TN))
 dystonic, 919
 motor
  complex, 919
  simple, 919
 primary, 920
 secondary, 920
 vocal
  complex, 919
  simple, 919
Ticarcillin (Ticar), for pyelonephritis, 685
Ticarcillin-clavulanate (Timentin), for necrotizing skin and soft tissue infections, 85t
Tick-borne relapsing fever (TBRF)
 clinical manifestations of, 133–134, 134, 135t
 epidemiology of, 133, 134t
 prevention of, 135–136
 risk factors for, 133
 treatment of, 136t
Ticlopidine (Ticlid), for angina pectoris, 298
Tigan (trimethobenzamide)
 for nausea and vomiting, 8t
 for Salmonella gastroenteritis, 172
Tightrope exercise, for vestibular neurolabyrinthitis, 207b
Tikosyn (dofetilide), for atrial fibrillation, 310, 310, 310b
Tilade (nedocromil), for asthma
 in adolescents and adults, 767–768t
 in children, 773–774t, 775
Timentin (ticarcillin-clavulanate), for necrotizing skin and soft tissue infections, 85t
Timolol (Timoptic, Betimol, Istalol, Blocadren)
 for glaucoma, 200
 intoxication with, 1182–1183, 1183t
Tin ethyl etiopurpurin (SnET2), 1244–1249t
Tindamax. See Tinidazole (Tindamax).
Tinea barbae, 846, 847b
Tinea capitis, 847, 847b, 848b
Tinea corporis, 804, 846, 847b
Tinea cruris, 846, 847b
Tinea infections
 cutaneous
  complicated, 848b
  diagnosis of, 846, 847b
  treatment of, 846, 848b
  uncomplicated, 846, 848b
 hair loss due to, 792
Tinea pedis, 846, 847b
Tinea unguium, 847, 847b, 848b
Tinea versicolor, 804–805, 847, 847b, 848b
Tinidazole (Tindamax)
 for acute infectious diarrhea, 19–20t
 for amebiasis, 60–61, 61t, 565–566t
 for giardiasis, 63–64, 64t, 64b, 544, 564–567, 565–566t
 for trichomoniasis, 1075, 1075b
Tinnitology, 35, 35
Tinnitus, 35
 bruits in, 36
 clinical types of, 36–37, 36f
 combined endogenous and exogenous, 37
 defined, 35
 and depression, 35
 diagnosis of, 35b
 ear noises in, 35, 35t

Tinnitus (Continued)
 endogenous (maskable), 36–37
 exogenous, 37
 factors of discomfort in, 36t
 general phenomena of, 35–36
 high-frequency, 36, 36
 historical background of, 35
 low-tone, 36, 36
 middle-frequency, 36, 36
 most irritating factors in, 36t
 sleep disturbance due to, 35
 in slow brainstem syndrome, 37
 time/intensity patterns of, 35t
 treatment of, 37–39, 38b
  adapted physiotherapy for, 38
  adapted psychotherapy for, 38
  instrumentation for, 37–38
  noise avoidance in, 37
  pharmacotherapy for, 38–39
Tinnitus retraining therapy (TRT), for tinnitus, 39
Tioconazole cream (Monistat-1, Vagistat-1), for vulvovaginal candidiasis, 1075b
Tiotropium (Spiriva), for COPD, 28b, 234
Tipifarnib (Zarnestra), for acute myeloid leukemia, 448
Tipranavir/ritonavir (Aptivus), for HIV, 50t, 51
TIPSS (transjugular intrahepatic portosystemic stent shunt), for ascites, 502
Tirofiban (Aggrastat)
 for myocardial infarction, 364
 for unstable angina pectoris, 301, 301t
Tissue expander breast implant, 1052
Tissue plasminogen activator (rtPA, Activase), for ischemic stroke, 894
Tissue plasminogen activator (TPA, rtPA, Activase)
 for deep venous thrombosis/pulmonary embolism, 273–274
 for myocardial infarction, 364t
 for posterior inferior cerebellar artery syndrome, 209
Tissue schizonticides, for malaria, 108
TIV (trivalent inactivated influenza vaccine). See Influenza vaccine (Fluzone, FluMist, Fluvirin, Fluarix, FluLevel).
Tizanidine (Zanaflex), for multiple sclerosis, 939b
TLRs (toll-like receptors), in sepsis, 66–67
TLS (tumor lysis syndrome), in childhood leukemia, 453, 453
TM. See -Thalassemia major (TM).
TM (tympanic membrane), 201
TMDs. See Temporomandibular disorder(s) (TMDs).
TMJ. See Temporomandibular joint (TMJ).
TMP-SMX. See Trimethoprim-sulfamethoxazole (TMP-SMX, Septra, Bactrim, cotrimoxazole, Cotrim).
TN. See Trigeminal neuralgia (TN).
TNF-α. See Tumor necrosis factor-α (TNF-α).
TNK (tenecteplase), for myocardial infarction, 364t
TNKase (tenecteplase), for myocardial infarction, 364t
TNM (tumor-node-metastasis) staging, 244b, 244t
 for colorectal cancer, 559, 559t, 559b
TOA (tubo-ovarian abscess), due to pelvic inflammatory disease, 1080
Tobacco. See Cigarette smoking.
Tobramycin (Nebcin), for bacterial meningitis, 115t
Tocilizumab (Actemra), 1244–1249t
Tocopherol, for systemic sclerosis, 811
Today Sponge (contraceptive sponge), 757
Tofranil. See Imipramine (Tofranil).
Tolcapone (Tasmar), for parkinsonism, 956

Tolerance, 5
  pharmacologic, 1105
Toll-like receptors (TLRs), in sepsis, 66–67
Tolmetin sodium (Tolectin), for juvenile idiopathic arthritis, 985
Tolterodine (Detrol), for urinary incontinence
  in children, 691, 692t
  in multiple sclerosis, 939b
  urge, 695b
Tongue
  burning, 852–853
  coated and hairy, 852
  disorders of, 852–853
  fissured, 852
  geographic, 852
Tonic seizures, 900
Tonic spasms, due to multiple sclerosis, 939
Tonic-clonic seizures, 900, 901t
Tonsillar pillars, disorders of, 852
Topamax. *See* Topiramate (Topamax).
Topical azole cream, for vulvovaginal candidiasis, 1075b
Topical calcineurin inhibitors (TCIs), for atopic dermatitis, 861
Topical therapy
  for cutaneous T-cell lymphomas, 797b, 798, 798
  for psoriasis, 801–802
Topicort (desoximetasone), for contact dermatitis, 871, 871b
Topiramate (Topamax)
  for cluster headache, 926t
  for epilepsy
    in adolescents in adults, 904t, 903
    in infants and children, 908–909, 914, 913t
  for migraine headache, 925
  for vestibular migraine, 209
Toradol (ketorolac)
  for pain, 2t
  for renal calculi, 744–745, 745t
Torecan (thiethylperazine), for nausea and vomiting, 8t
Torsade de pointes (TdP), 324
  after myocardial infarction, 366t
Torus(i)
  mandibular, 854
  palatal, 851
Total anomalous pulmonary venous connection (TAPVC), 331
Total body surface area (TBSA), of burn, 1135, 1136f, 1137f
Total daily dose (TDD), of insulin for children, 585, 585f
Total dystrophic onychomycosis (TDO), 818
Total energy expenditure (TEE), 620
Total parenteral nutrition (TPN). *See* Parenteral nutrition (PN).
Total skin electron beam treatment (TSEBT), for cutaneous T-cell lymphomas, 798
Tourette, Gilles de la, 919
Tourette's syndrome, 918
  clinical features of, 919
  defined, 919
  differential diagnosis of, 919–920, 920b, 920b
  historical background of, 919
  natural history and epidemiology of, 919
  psychiatric disorders associated with, 921
  treatment of, 920–921, 920b, 921b
Toxic chemical agents, 1226
Toxic epidermal necrolysis (TEN), 864–866
  clinical presentation of, 865
  diagnosis of, 863b
  vs. erythema multiforme and Stevens-Johnson syndrome, 862, 863t
  due to HAART, 54–55t
  severity of illness score for, 865, 866b
  treatment of, 864b, 865–866, 866b

Toxic Exposure Surveillance System (TESS), 1160, 1160
Toxic neuropathies, 963, 963b
Toxic nodular goiter, 669
Toxic shock syndrome (TSS), 86
  case definitions for, 88b, 88b
  diagnosis of, 87–88, 88b, 88b, 87b
  differential diagnosis of, 88
  epidemiology of, 86–87
  historical background of, 86
  pathogenesis of, 87
  staphylococcal, 86
    diagnosis of, 87b, 88, 88b
    epidemiology of, 87
    menstrual *vs.* nonmenstrual, 87
    pathogenesis of, 87
    treatment of, 89, 89b
  streptococcal, 86
    diagnosis of, 87b, 88, 88b
    epidemiology of, 87
    pathogenesis of, 87
    treatment of, 89, 89b
  treatment of, 88–90, 89b
    antibiotics for, 890, 89b
    chemoprophylaxis for, 90
    immunomodulatory therapy for, 89–90, 89b
Toxic shock syndrome toxin-1 (TSST-1), 87
Toxic substances, reference intervals for, 1224t
Toxic urine screen, 1176
Toxicologic studies, 1176
Toxicology. *See* Poisoning(s).
Toxicology screening, 1176
Toxoplasma gondii. See Toxoplasmosis.
Toxoplasma serologic profile, 164
Toxoplasmic encephalitis (TE), 163, 166t, 167–168, 167b
Toxoplasmosis, 163
  congenital, 165t, 168–169, 168b
  diagnosis of, 164
  etiology and pathogenesis of, 163–164
  in immunocompetent hosts, 164, 164b, 165t, 166
  in immunocompromised hosts, 164b, 165t, 166t, 167–168, 167b
  ocular, 166–167
  during pregnancy, 165t, 168, 1015
  prevalence of, 164
  prevention of, 169
  treatment of, 164–169
    alternative drugs in, 166t
    drugs used in, 164, 165t
    indications for, 164, 164b
TPA. *See* Tissue plasminogen activator (TPA, rtPA, Activase).
TPMT (thiopurine methyltransferase) levels, with azathioprine, 867, 869t
TPN (total parenteral nutrition). *See* Parenteral nutrition (PN).
Trabeculectomy, for glaucoma, 200
Trace elements, in parenteral nutrition, 620, 621, 621t
Tracheal compression, in childhood leukemia, 453–454
Trachelectomy, radical, for cervical cancer, 1087
Tracleer (bosentan)
  for portopulmonary hypertension, 503–504
  for systemic sclerosis, 811
Traction alopecia, 792
TRALI (transfusion-related acute lung injury), 484–485t, 487–488
TRAM (transverse rectus abdominis myocutaneous) flap, 1052
Tramadol (Ultram)
  for osteoarthritis, 1000
  for pain, 3
  neuropathic, 964t, 965
Tramadol plus acetaminophen (Ultracet), for osteoarthritis, 1000

Trandate. *See* Labetalol (Normodyne, Trandate).
Tranexamic acid (Cyklokapron)
  for hemophilia, 422
  for menorrhagia, 1059
Transcoronary septal ablation, for hypertrophic cardiomyopathy, 334
Transcutaneous pacing, for heart block, 318, 319b
Transderm Scop. *See* Scopolamine (Transderm Scop).
Transdermal hormonal contraceptive patch (Ortho Evra), 756
Transepithelial electrical potential difference, in cystic fibrosis, 238
Transesophageal echocardiography (TEE), for infective endocarditis, 344
Transferrin saturation, in hemochromatosis, 432
Transfusion(s). *See* Blood transfusion(s).
Transfusion reaction(s), 484–489
  defined, 484
  hemolytic, 484–487, 484–485t
    acute, 484–486, 484–485t
    due to bacterial contamination of blood products, 484–485t, 487
    delayed, 484–485t, 486–487
    massive, 486t
  nonhemolytic, 484, 484–485t, 487–489
    acute lung injury as, 484–485t, 487–488
    allergic, 484–485t, 488–489
    anaphylactic, 484–485t
    febrile, 488
      leukoreduced platelets for, 482
    graft-*versus*-host disease as, 484–485t, 489, 489b
Transfusion-associated graft-*versus*-host disease (TA-GVHD), 484–485t, 489, 489b
  irradiated platelets for, 482
  irradiated red blood cells for, 481
Transfusion-related acute lung injury (TRALI), 484–485t, 487–488
Transfusion-related complications, 484
  infectious, 485t, 489–490, 490b
  noninfectious, 486t, 490–492
Transfusion-related immunomodulation (TRIM), 486t, 490–491
Transient ischemic attacks (TIAs), 893–894
  due to carotid occlusive disease, 374
  clinical features of, 893–894
  defined, 893
  diagnosis of, 893, 894
  epidemiology of, 893
  pathophysiology of, 893
  vs. seizures, 901t
  and stroke, 893–894
  treatment of, 894
  vertigo due to, 208–209
Transient tachypnea of the newborn (TTN), 1037–1038
Transitional cell carcinoma, of bladder, 735
Transjugular intrahepatic portosystemic stent shunt (TIPSS), for ascites, 502
Transplant patients, gout in, 601
Transposition of the great arteries (TGA), 330
Transrectal ultrasonography (TRUS), of prostate carcinoma, 732
Transsphenoidal adenomectomy, for Cushing's syndrome, 644
  failed, 645
Transurethral incision of the prostate (TUIP), for benign prostatic hyperplasia, 715–718
Transurethral needle ablation (TUNA), for benign prostatic hyperplasia, 715–718
Transurethral resection of the prostate (TURP), for benign prostatic hyperplasia, 715–718
Transvenous pacing, for heart block, 318, 319b
Transverse myelitis, in multiple sclerosis, 933
Transverse rectus abdominis myocutaneous (TRAM) flap, 1052

Index

1341

Tranxene (clorazepate), intoxication with, 1181–1182
Tranylcypromine (Parnate), for major depression, 1124
Trauma
　burns with concomitant, 1139
　to genitourinary tract, 706, 706b
Traumatic brain injury (TBI), 965
　in children, 969
　　closed, 969
　　diagnosis of, 971b
　　epidemiology of, 969
　　etiology of, 969
　　Glasgow Coma Scale for, 970, 970t
　　increased intracranial pressure due to, 971
　　mild, 970
　　moderate, 970
　　open, 969
　　primary, 969–970
　　secondary, 970
　　severe, 970, 970–971
　　due to shaking-impact syndrome, 970
　　subdural hematomas due to, 969–970
　　treatment of, 971b
　　types and severity of, 969–970
　classification of, 965, 966b
　concussion in, 965, 968–969
　diffuse axonal injury due to, 966
　early and delayed neurologic changes due to, 968
　elevated intracranial pressure due to
　　monitoring of, 967
　　Monroe-Kellie doctrine for, 966–967
　　treatment of, 967–968, 967b
　future treatments for, 969
　Glasgow Coma Scale for, 965, 965t
　　in children, 970, 970t
　hematomas due to
　　epidural, 965–966
　　intraparenchymal, 966
　　subdural, 966
　　　in children, 969–970
　mild or moderate, 968
　pathology of, 965–967, 966b
　restorative therapies for, 969
　seizures due to, 968
　severe closed, 967–968
　skull fractures in, 965
　sports-related, 968–969
Traumatic ulcer, of tongue, 852
Travatan (travoprost), for glaucoma, 199–200
Travel kits, 158
Travel medicine, 155
　assessing illness in returning traveler in, 161–163, 161f
　　with dermatologic conditions, 162–163
　　with diarrhea, 162, 162f
　　with fever, 161–162
　deep venous thrombosis in, 158
　epidemiology of, 155, 155b
　high-altitude sickness in, 158
　immunizations in, 158–161, 159b
　　doses for, 159–160t
　　recommended, 160–161
　　required, 159–160
　　routine, 158–159
　infectious illnesses in, 155–158
　jet lag in, 158
　malaria in, 110–112, 156–158
　　chemoprophylaxis for, 111–112t, 156–157, 157t
　　epidemiology of, 103–104, 156
　　personal protective measures for, 106, 157–158, 157b
　　presumptive antirelapse therapy (terminal prophylaxis) for, 110
　motion sickness in, 158
　noninfectious risks in, 158

Travel medicine (Continued)
　pretravel counseling in, 155
　safety precautions in, 158, 158b
　travel kits in, 158
　traveler's diarrhea in (See Traveler's diarrhea)
　websites giving advice on, 163b
Traveler's diarrhea, 17, 155–156
　defined, 155
　epidemiology of, 17, 155
　pathogenesis of, 155
　prevention of, 155, 155b
　in returning traveler, 162, 162f
　treatment of, 19t, 155–156, 156t, 156t
Travoprost (Travatan), for glaucoma, 199–200
Trazodone (Desyrel)
　for Alzheimer's disease, 884, 885t, 884–886
　for erectile dysfunction, 719
　for gaseousness, 10t
　for major depression, 1124
　poisoning due to, 1214–1216, 1215t
　after traumatic brain injury, 969
Trecator-SC (ethionamide), for tuberculosis, 285t
Tregs (regulatory T cells), in cutaneous T-cell lymphomas, 795–796
Trematodes, 570t, 572–573
Tremor
　due to alcohol withdrawal, 1102–1103b
　due to multiple sclerosis, 939
Trench foot, 1147, 1147b
Trench mouth, 854
Trental. See Pentoxifylline (Trental).
Treponema pallidum, syphilis due to, 754
Treprostinil (Remodulin), for systemic sclerosis, 811
Tretinoin (Vesanoid), for acute promyelocytic leukemia, 448–449
Tretinoin topical (Retin-A, Renova, Differin, Tazorac)
　for acne, 787
　for actinic keratosis, 833
　for melasma, 876–877
　for postinflammatory hyperpigmentation, 878
　for solar lentigines, 877
　for verrucae, 823
Trexall. See Methotrexate (MTX, Rheumatrex, Trexall).
Trexima (sumatriptan/naproxen), 1244–1249t
Triamcinolone (Kenalog)
　for alopecia areata, 791–792
　for atopic dermatitis, 860–861
　for bursitis, 997b
　for cicatricial pemphigoid, 869
　for gout, 599
　for lichen planus, 817
　for psoriasis, 801, 819–820
Triamcinolone acetonide inhalation (Azmacort), for asthma
　in adolescents and adults, 769t
　in children, 773–774t
Triamcinolone acetonide nasal (Nasacort AQ), for allergic rhinitis, 780t
Triamcinolone acetonide topical (Aristocort A cream)
　for anogenital pruritus, 872–873
　for contact dermatitis, 871, 871b
Triamterene (Dyrenium), for ascites, 501
Triangle of dysplasia, 323
Triazolam (Halcion)
　for insomnia, 888t
　intoxication with, 1181–1182
Trichinosis, pruritus due to, 32b
Tri-Chlor (trichloracetic acid)
　for condyloma acuminatum, 825b, 826, 1092
　for verrucae, 823
Trichloracetic acid (TCA, Tri-Chlor)
　for condyloma acuminatum, 825b, 826, 1092
　for verrucae, 823

Trichoderma, as biological weapon agent, 1229–1233t
Trichomonas vaginalis, 1075, 1075b
　during pregnancy, 1015, 1075
Trichomonas vaginitis, 1075, 1075b
　during pregnancy, 1015, 1075
Trichomoniasis, 1075, 1075b
　during pregnancy, 1015, 1075
Trichophyton tonsurans, 847, 847
Trichothiodystrophy, 793
Trichotillomania, 792
Trichuriasis, 569–571, 570t
Trichuris trichuria, 569–571, 570t
Tricor (fenofibrate), for dyslipoproteinemia, 605, 605t
Tricuspid atresia, 329–330, 330f
Tricyclic antidepressants (TCAs)
　for major depression, 1123–1124
　for migraine headache, 925
　poisoning due to, 1214–1216, 1215t
Trientine (Syprine), for Wilson's disease, 500–501
Trifluoperazine (Stelazine), poisoning due to, 1208–1209, 1208t
Trifluridine (Viroptic), for neonatal conjunctivitis, 196
Trigeminal neuralgia (TN), 947
　bilateral, 947–948
　clinical features of, 947–948
　diagnosis of, 947–948, 947b
　epidemiology of, 947
　etiology and pathogenesis of, 947
　orofacial pain due to, 992t
　physical examination for, 948
　treatment of, 948–949, 948b
　triggers for, 947–948
Trigger(s), for asthma
　in adolescents and adults, 763, 765, 765b
　in children, 771, 771b
Trigger points
　in regional myofascial pain, 995–996
　for temporomandibular disorder, 993
Triggered activity, 320
Triglycerides (TGs), 601, 602t
　and coronary artery disease, 602–603
　screening for, 602
Trihexyphenidyl (Artane), poisoning due to, 1179–1180
Triiodothyronine (T_3)
　for hypothyroidism, 663
　normal physiology of, 661–662
　reducing serum levels of, 667
　reverse, 661–662
Trilafon (perphenazine), poisoning due to, 1208–1209, 1208t
Trileptal. See Oxacarbazepine (Trileptal).
Trilisate (choline magnesium trisalicylate), for pain, 2t
Tri-Luma cream (fluocinolone acetonide/hydroquinone/tretinoin cream)
　for postinflammatory hyperpigmentation, 878
　for solar lentigines, 877
TRIM (transfusion-related immunomodulation), 486t, 490–491
Trimethobenzamide (Tigan)
　for nausea and vomiting, 8t
　for Salmonella gastroenteritis, 172
Trimethoprim (Trimpex), for Pneumocystis jiroveci pneumonia, 55
Trimethoprim oral solution (Primsol Oral Solution), for urinary tract infections in girls, 687b, 688t
Trimethoprim-sulfamethoxazole (TMP-SMX, Septra, Bactrim, cotrimoxazole, Cotrim)
　for acute infectious diarrhea, 18b, 19t, 19–20t
　for bacterial meningitis, 115t
　for Bordetella pertussis, 28b
　for brucellosis, 74–75, 74b, 75t

Trimethoprim-sulfamethoxazole (TMP-SMX, Septra, Bactrim, cotrimoxazole, Cotrim) *(Continued)*
  for cholera, 80t
  for cyclosporiasis, 565–566t, 568
  for epididymitis, 698
  for granuloma inguinale, 750
  for isosporiasis, 565–566t, 568
  for marine injuries, 1159t
  for membranous nephropathy, 703
  for necrotizing skin and soft tissue infections, 85t
  for *Pneumocystis jiroveci* pneumonia, 55, 56t
  for prostatitis, 681
  for pyelonephritis, 706, 706b
  for Q fever, 129, 129t
  for *Salmonella* gastroenteritis, 173
  for spontaneous bacterial peritonitis, 502
  for toxoplasmosis, 166t, 167–168
    in HIV, 56t
  for urinary tract infections
    in girls, 687b, 688t
    in males, 681, 681t
    in women
      catheter-associated bacteriuria as, 684–685
      cystitis as, 684, 684b
      due to pyelonephritis, 685
      recurrent, 685
Trimipramine (Surmantil), poisoning due to, 1214–1216, 1215t
Trimpex (trimethoprim), for *Pneumocystis jiroveci* pneumonia, 55
Tripedia (pertussis vaccine), 147, 147t
Triple mix solutions, 621
Triplets, 312
Triprolidine/pseudoephedrine (Actifed Cold & Allergy), for allergic rhinitis, 779t
Triptans, for migraine headache, 924–926, 925t
Trisenox (arsenic trioxide)
  for acute myeloid leukemia, 448
  for acute promyelocytic leukemia, 448
Trismus, due to tetanus, 143
Trivalent inactivated influenza vaccine (TIV). *See* Influenza vaccine (Fluzone, FluMist, Fluvirin, Fluarix, FluLevel).
Trizolopyridine, poisoning due to, 1214–1216, 1215t
Tropical pancreatitis, 549
Tropical sprue, 544
Troponins
  in myocardial infarction, 361
  in pericarditis, 369–370
Trospium (Sanctura), for urge incontinence, 695b
Trousseau sign, 652
TRT (tinnitus retraining therapy), for tinnitus, 39
TRUE (thin-layer rapid-use epicutaneous) test allergens, 870
Truncus arteriosus, 330–331
Trunk, pruritus of, 31f
TRUS (transrectal ultrasonography), of prostate carcinoma, 732
Trusopt (dorzolamide), for glaucoma, 200
Truvada (tenofovir + emtricitabine), for HIV, 51t
Trypanosoma bruci, 843, 844t
Trypanosoma cruzi, 843, 844t
  transfusion-associated, 490
Trypanosomiasis, 843
Trypsinogen-activating peptide, in pancreatitis, 546
Tryptase, in anaphylaxis, 759
TSEBT (total skin electron beam treatment), for cutaneous T-cell lymphomas, 798
TSH. *See* Thyroid-stimulating hormone (TSH).
TSS. *See* Toxic shock syndrome (TSS).

TSST-1 (toxic shock syndrome toxin-1), 87
TST (tuberculin skin test), 282
TT (tetanus toxoid), 145
TTHA. *See* Tension-type headache (TTHA).
TTN (transient tachypnea of the newborn), 1037–1038
TTP. *See* Thrombotic thrombocytopenic purpura (TTP).
Tubal ligation, 757
Tube thoracostomy, for empyema, 257–258
Tuberculin skin test (TST), 282
Tuberculosis (TB), 282
  active, 283
  diagnosis of, 282–283, 283b, 282b
  epidemiology of, 282
  extensively drug-resistant, 282, 288
  with HIV coinfection, 56t, 57–58, 58t, 284b, 287–288
  latent, 282
    diagnosis of, 282–283
    treatment of, 286–287, 288t
  leprosy with, 102
  multidrug-resistant, 282, 284b, 288
  natural history of, 282
  pericarditis due to, 369, 371
  silicosis and, 280
  treatment of, 283–288, 284b
    directly observed treatment short-course (DOTS) approach for, 284
    dosage schedule for, 286t
    drugs used for, 285t
    for drug-susceptible disease, 284, 287t
    evaluation prior to, 283–284
    fixed-dose combination preparations for, 287b
    with HIV coinfection, 287–288
    for latent infection, 286–287, 288t
    monitoring during, 284–286
    principles of, 284
    for relapse, treatment failure, and drug-resistant disease, 288
    WHO standard regimens for, 285t
Tuberculous epididymitis, 698
Tuberous sclerosis, renal angiomyolipomas due to, 734, 734b
Tubo-ovarian abscess (TOA), due to pelvic inflammatory disease, 1080
Tubulointerstitial disease, in chronic renal failure, 729
TUIP (transurethral incision of the prostate), for benign prostatic hyperplasia, 715–718
Tularemia, inhalational (pneumonic), as biological weapon agent, 1229–1233t
Tumor lysis syndrome (TLS), in childhood leukemia, 453, 453
Tumor necrosis factor-α (TNF-α blockers/inhibitors/antagonists
  for ankylosing spondylitis, 987–988, 988
  for pemphigus vulgaris, 869
  for psoriasis, 802–804, 803t
  for rheumatoid arthritis, 979–981, 981t
  for systemic lupus erythematosus, 809
Tumor-node-metastasis (TNM) staging, 244b, 244t
  for colorectal cancer, 559, 559t, 559b
TUNA (transurethral needle ablation), for benign prostatic hyperplasia, 715–718
Tunga penetrans, 844t, 846
Tungiasis, 844t, 846
Tunneled catheters, for parenteral nutrition, 622
TURP (transurethral resection of the prostate), for benign prostatic hyperplasia, 715–718
TWEAK questionnaire, 1098, 1099t
TwinJect. *See* Epinephrine auto-injector (EpiPen, TwinJect).
Twinrix (hepatitis A and B virus vaccine), 534t
  for travelers, 159–160t
Tykerb (lapatinib), 1243

Tylenol. *See* Acetaminophen (Tylenol).
Tylox (oxycodone + acetaminophen)
  intoxication with, 1204–1205, 1205t
  for pain, 4t
Tympanic membrane (TM), 201
Tyndall phenomenon, 828–829
Typhim Vi (typhoid vaccine), 18
  for travelers, 159–160t, 161
Typhoid fever, 174
  acute infectious diarrhea due to, 15
  clinical features of, 175
  diagnosis of, 175, 175b
  drug-resistant, 174, 175, 176t
  epidemiology of, 174
  etiology of, 174
  pathogenesis of, 174–175
  preventive strategies for, 175–176
  in returning traveler, 162
  therapy for, 175, 175b, 176t
Typhoid vaccine (Vivotif Berna, Typhim Vi), 18
  for travelers, 159–160t, 161
Tysabril (natalizumab), for multiple sclerosis, 937–938, 937t
Tyzeka (telbivudine), for hepatitis B and C viruses, 536t, 537
TZDs (thiazolidinediones), for diabetes, 580t, 580t, 581

U

UC. *See* Ulcerative colitis (UC).
UCL (ulnar collateral ligament), injuries to, 1009, 1010
UDCA (ursodeoxycholic acid), for primary biliary cirrhosis, 499
UFC (urine-free cortisol), for Cushing's syndrome, 643, 643f, 644
UFH (unfractionated heparin)
  for deep venous thrombosis/pulmonary embolism, 272–273, 273b
  for myocardial infarction, 363–364
UG tumors. *See* Urogenital (UG) tumor(s).
Ugly duckling sign, 830
Ulcer(s)
  aphthous, 850
    herpetiform, 850
    major, 850
  cutaneous, in returning traveler, 163
  leg, in sickle cell disease, 407, 411
  peptic (*See* Peptic ulcer disease (PUD))
  pressure (*See* Pressure ulcers)
  traumatic, of tongue, 852
  venous leg, 855
    background of, 855
    clinical features of, 855
    diagnosis of, 855–856, 855b
    pathophysiology of, 855
    treatment of, 856–857, 856b, 856f
Ulcerative colitis (UC)
  clinical features of, 515
  colon cancer surveillance with, 521
  diagnosis of, 515, 515b
  management strategies for, 519–520
  mild to moderate, 519
  natural history of, 515
  pathogenesis of, 514–515
  pregnancy with, 520–521
  severe, 519–520
  treatment of, 515b
    alternative therapy in, 519
    nutritional support in, 518
    pharmacologic, 515–518
      aminosalicylates for, 515–516
      antibiotics/probiotics for, 517–518
      anticytokine therapy for, 517
      azathioprine/6-mercaptopurine for, 516–517
      corticosteroids for, 516

Ulcerative colitis (UC) *(Continued)*
　　cyclosporine for, 517
　　experimental therapies for, 518
　　methotrexate for, 517
　　surgical, 518–519
Ulnar collateral ligament (UCL), injuries to, 1009, 1010
Ulnar neuropathy, 962
Ultracet (tramadol plus acetaminophen), for osteoarthritis, 1000
Ultralente insulin, for diabetes in children, 587t
Ultram. *See* Tramadol (Ultram).
Ultrasonography, during pregnancy, 1013
　ectopic, 1017
Ultravate (halobetasol propionate ointment), for anogenital pruritus, 873
Ultraviolet light B (UVB), for psoriasis, 802
Ultraviolet (UV)-protective clothing, 880
Ultraviolet protective factor (UPF), 880
Ultraviolet (UV) radiation, sunburn due to, 879
Unasyn (ampicillin/sulbactam)
　for pelvic inflammatory disease, 1080b
　for pyelonephritis, 706, 706b
Uncinarial dermatitis, 844t, 845
Undernutrition, of infants, 1044–1045
Undertreatment, of pain, 5
Unfractionated heparin (UFH)
　for deep venous thrombosis/pulmonary embolism, 272–273, 273b
　for myocardial infarction, 363–364
Unipen. *See* Nafcillin (Unipen).
Unisom (doxylamine), for nausea during pregnancy, 1014
Unoprostone (Rescula), for glaucoma, 199–200
UPF (ultraviolet protective factor), 880
Upper extremity discomfort, during pregnancy, 1015
Uprima (apomorphine hydrochloride), for erectile dysfunction, 719
Urate stones, 743, 744t, 744t, 746t
Urate-lowering therapy, 599, 600, 600b
Urea (Ureaphil)
　for elevated intracranial pressure, 967
　for hyponatremia, 598
　for psoriasis, 802
Uremia
　in chronic renal failure, 727, 727t, 730
　platelet dysfunction of, 427, 427b
　pruritus due to, 34b
Ureteral injuries, 707–708, 707b, 708b
Ureteral obstruction, acute renal failure due to, 722b
Ureteral relaxants, for renal calculi, 744–745, 745t
Ureteral tumors, 734–735
　diagnosis of, 734b, 735
　epidemiology of, 734
　risk factors for, 734, 734–735
　treatment of, 735, 735b
Ureteroscopy, for renal calculi, 745
Urethra, anatomy of, 740
Urethral carcinoma, 737
　diagnosis of, 737, 737b
　treatment of, 737, 737b
Urethral dilation, for urethral stricture disease, 741, 741
Urethral disruption, 708, 709f
Urethral hypermobility, 693
Urethral injuries, 708–709
　anterior, 708
　diagnosis of, 707b, 708, 709f
　female, 708–709
　posterior, 708
　treatment of, 708, 708b
　urethral stricture disease due to, 740
Urethral stents, for urethral stricture disease, 741, 742

Urethral stricture disease, 740
　bulbar, 741, 742
　congenital, 740
　defined, 740
　diagnosis of, 740b, 741, 741f
　etiology of, 740–741
　pathogenesis of, 740
　penile, 742
　posterior *vs.* anterior, 740b
　recurrence of, 742
　treatment of, 741–742, 741b
　　future directions for, 742
Urethritis
　defined, 686b, 752
　gonococcal, 751
　nongonococcal, 752
　　due to *Chlamydia trachomatis,* 1076, 1078b
　chronic, 753
　clinical presentation of, 752
　complications of, 753
　diagnosis of, 752–753
　etiology of, 752
　follow-up for, 755
　treatment of, 753
Urethroplasty, for urethral stricture disease, 741, 741
　anastomotic, 741, 741
　substitution, 742, 742
Urinary abnormalities, persistent asymptomatic, 699b
Urinary diversion, for bladder carcinoma, 736
Urinary frequency
　due to multiple sclerosis, 939
　during pregnancy, 1014
Urinary incontinence, 693
　childhood, 689
　daytime, 690–692
　　anatomic, 690, 690b
　　continuous, 689–690, 690b
　　etiology of, 690–691, 690b
　　evaluation of, 691
　　functional, 690, 690b
　　giggle, 691
　　intermittent, 689–690, 690b
　　neurogenic, 690, 690b
　　stress, 691
　　treatment of, 691–692, 692t
　　urge, 690
　definition and terminology for, 689–690, 690b
　nocturnal enuresis as, 692–693
　　defined, 689–690, 690b, 692
　　epidemiology of, 692
　　etiology of, 692
　　treatment of, 692–693
　normal voiding patterns *vs.,* 690
　etiology of, 693, 693t
　　bladder dysfunction in, 693, 693t
　　transient causes in, 693, 694t
　　urethral-related, 693, 693t
　evaluation of, 693–695, 694b
　mixed
　　diagnosis of, 694b
　　treatment of, 696
　due to multiple sclerosis, 939
　overflow
　　diagnosis of, 694b
　　etiology of, 693
　　treatment of, 695–696
　stress (urethral-related)
　　in children, 691
　　diagnosis of, 694b
　　etiology of, 693
　　treatment of, 695b, 696
　after stroke, 897
　treatment of, 695–696, 696b, 695b
　urge
　　in children, 690

Urinary incontinence *(Continued)*
　　diagnosis of, 694b
　　etiology of, 693
　　treatment of, 695, 695b
Urinary symptoms, during pregnancy, 1014
Urinary tract infection(s) (UTIs)
　defined, 686
　in girls, 686
　　classification of, 686, 686b
　　colony count criteria for, 686, 686b
　　diagnosis of, 686, 687b
　　epidemiology and pathogenesis of, 686
　　prophylaxis for, 687–688, 688t
　　radiologic evaluation for, 688–689, 689f
　　risk factors for, 686
　　treatment of, 686–687, 687b
　　　afebrile, 686–687, 687b
　　　algorithm for, 688f
　　　antibiotic choices for, 687b
　　　febrile, 687
　　　hospitalization for, 688b
　in males, 679
　　complicated, 679, 681, 681t
　　diagnosis and localization of, 680, 680b
　　in long-term care, 681
　　natural history of, 679–680
　　due to prostatitis, 680, 681
　　treatment of, 680–681, 680b
　　　for complicated infections, 681, 681t
　　　for uncomplicated infections, 680–681
　　uncomplicated, 679, 680–681
　due to multiple sclerosis, 939
　sepsis due to, 68t
　upper tract (*See* Pyelonephritis)
　in women, 682
　　benign bacteriuria of elderly as, 682
　　catheter-associated bacteriuria as, 682, 684–685
　　cystitis as, 682, 684
　　diagnosis of, 683b
　　in dysuria-pyuria syndrome, 682, 684
　　overview of, 682
　　during pregnancy, 1014
　　pyelonephritis as
　　　acute, 682–683, 685
　　　chronic, 683–684, 685
　　recurrent, 682, 684b, 685
　　due to renal abscess, 683–685
　　treatment of, 684–685, 684b
Urinary urgency, due to multiple sclerosis, 939
Urine chemistry, reference intervals for, 1220–1221t
Urine volume, low, renal calculi due to, 744t
Urine-free cortisol (UFC), for Cushing's syndrome, 643, 643f, 644
Urocit-K (potassium citrate), for renal calculi, 746t
Urodynamic testing, 695
Urogenital atrophy, postmenopausal, 1070
　treatment for, 1072b
Urogenital disorder(s)
　benign prostatic hyperplasia as, 712
　epididymitis as, 696
　erectile dysfunction as, 715
　glomerular diseases as, 699
　malignancies as, 731
　prostatitis, 709
　pyelonephritis as, 704
　renal calculi as, 742
　renal failure as
　　acute, 721
　　chronic, 725
　due to trauma, 706
　urethral stricture disease as, 740
　urinary incontinence as, 693
　　childhood, 689
　urinary tract infections as

Urogenital disorder(s) (Continued)
  in girls, 686
  in males, 679
  in women, 682
Urogenital (UG) tumor(s), 731
  of bladder, 735–737
  of penis, 737–738
  of prostate, 731–732
  renal
    benign, 734
    metastatic, 734
    renal cell carcinoma as, 733–734
    of renal parenchyma, 732–733
    of renal pelvis, 734–735
  of testicles, 738–740
  of ureter, 734–735
  of urethra, 737
Urokinase (Abbokinase)
  for deep venous thrombosis/pulmonary embolism, 273–274
  for ischemic stroke, 894
Uroxatral (alfuzosin)
  for benign prostatic hyperplasia, 714–716, 714t
  for prostatitis, 710–711
Ursodeoxycholic acid (UDCA), for primary biliary cirrhosis, 499
Ursodiol (Actigall), for cholestasis, 34b
Urticaria, 873
  acute, 873, 874
  adrenergic, 874
  causes of, 873, 874b
  cholinergic, 874
  chronic, 873, 874
  classification of, 873
  cold, 874
  defined, 873
  delayed pressure, 874
  diagnosis of, 873b
  evaluation of, 873–874
  heat, 874
  pathogenesis of, 873
  pruritus due to, 32b
  in serum sickness, 762
  treatment of, 874b, 875, 875f
Urticarial vasculitis, 815, 873
Urticating hairs, of tarantulas, 1151
U.S. Preventative Services Task Force (USPSTF), on screening for alcoholism, 1097
Uterine artery embolization, for uterine leiomyoma, 1082t
Uterine atony, postpartum hemorrhage due to, 1027
Uterine bleeding, dysfunctional, 1058
  anovulatory, 1058–1059
  defined, 1058
  diagnosis of, 1059b
    endometrial biopsy in, 1058
    history in, 1058
    imaging in, 1058
    laboratory evaluation in, 1058
  differential diagnosis of, 1058
  etiology of, 1058
  after menopause, 1070–1071
  ovulatory, 1059
  treatment for, 1059b
  due to uterine hemorrhage, 1059–1060
Uterine hemorrhage, 1059–1060
Uterine infection, postpartum, 1028
Uterine leiomyomas, 1081
  diagnosis of, 1081, 1081b
  epidemiology of, 1081
  management of, 1081–1082, 1082t, 1082b
  pathophysiology of, 1081
  symptoms and signs of, 1081
Uterine rupture, 1021, 1021b
UTIs. See Urinary tract infection(s) (UTIs).
UV (ultraviolet)-protective clothing, 880

UV (ultraviolet) radiation, sunburn due to, 879
UVB (ultraviolet light B), for psoriasis, 802
Uveitis, due to sarcoidosis, 275–276

V

Vaccination. See Immunization(s); Vaccine(s).
Vaccine(s). See also Immunization(s).
  for acute infectious diarrhea, 18
  anthrax, 127
  bacille Calmette-Guérin (BCG), for leprosy, 103
  for bacterial meningitis, 115
  cholera, 18
  contraindications to, 154
  decision not to do, 154
  diphtheria and tetanus toxoids and acellular pertussis, 145t
    schedule for, 149–150t
    catch-up, 151t
  free-of-charge, 153
  Haemophilus influenzae type b (Hib), 115
    schedule for, 149–150t
    catch-up, 151t
  hepatitis A
    schedule for, 149–150t
    catch-up, 151t
    for travelers, 159–160t, 160, 161
  hepatitis A and B, 159–160t
  hepatitis B
    schedule for, 149–150t
    catch-up, 151t
    for travelers, 159–160t, 161
  human diploid cell, 131
    for travelers, 159–160t
  human papillomavirus, schedule for, 149–150t
    catch-up, 151t
  inactivated poliovirus, schedule for, 149–150t
    catch-up, 151t
  influenza, 90–91, 91b
    schedule for, 149–150t
  Japanese encephalitis, 159–160t
  for leprosy, 103
  locus of responsibility for, 153
  Lyme, 139
  measles, 142–143
    mumps
      rubella, and varicella (MMRV), 141
      and rubella (MMR), 141
      and rubella (MMR), schedule for, 149–150t
      and rubella (MMR), schedule for, catch-up, 151t
  meningococcal, 115
    schedule for, 149–150t
    for travelers, 160, 159–160t
  minimizing discomfort of, 152
  missed or delayed, 153
  mumps, 121–122
  pertussis, 147, 147t
  pneumococcal, 115
    conjugate, 115
    polysaccharide, 263
    schedule for, 149–150t
    catch-up, 151t
  prevention of needle injury from, 152
  purified chick embryo cell culture, 131
    for travelers, 159–160t
  rabies, 131, 131b
    for travelers, 159–160t, 161
  recall reminders and tracking of, 153
  reporting adverse events due to, 153
  rotavirus, 18
    schedule for, 149–150t
    catch-up, 151t
  rubella, 141
  schedule for, 148, 149–150t

Vaccine(s) (Continued)
  catch-up, 151t, 152–153
  shortages of, 153
  smallpox, 179, 180, 185
  standing orders for, 153
  storage of, 152
  tetanus and diphtheria toxoid (Td), 145
    for acute wounds, 144b, 151t
    in pregnancy, 145
    schedule for, 145, 145t
    catch-up, 151t
  tetanus and diphtheria toxoids and acellular pertussis (Tdap), schedule for, 149–150t
    catch-up, 151t
  typhoid, 18
    for travelers, 159–160t, 161
  varicella, 76, 77f
    schedule for, 149–150t
    catch-up, 151t
  yellow fever, 160, 159–160t
Vaccine Adverse Events Reporting System (VAERS), 153
vaccine for, 18
Vaccine Information Statements (VISs), 148–152
Vaccine Injury Compensation Program (VICP), 148
Vaccine registries, 152
Vaccine therapy, for cutaneous T-cell lymphomas, 800
Vaccines for Children (VFC), 153
Vacuum constriction device, for erectile dysfunction, 720
Vacuum-assisted closure, for pressure ulcers, 858
VAERS (Vaccine Adverse Events Reporting System), 153
Vagifem (estradiol vaginal tablet), for urogenital atrophy, 1072b
Vaginal atrophy, postmenopausal, 1070
  treatment for, 1072b
Vaginal bleeding
  in late pregnancy, 1019
    hemodynamic compromise due to, 1019–1020
    due to placenta previa, 1020, 1020b
    due to placental abruption, 1020–1021, 1021b
    due to uterine rupture, 1021, 1021b
    due to vasa previa, 1021, 1021b
  in pregnancy, 1013
Vaginal cuff brachytherapy, for endometrial cancer, 1085
Vaginal discharge, during pregnancy, 1013
Vaginal lacerations, 708b
Vaginal ring (NuvaRing), 756
  in postpartum period, 1029t
Vaginitis, Trichomonas, 1075, 1075b
  during pregnancy, 1015
Vaginosis
  bacterial, 1074
    during pregnancy, 1014, 1074, 1074b
  due to Candida albicans, during pregnancy, 1014
Vagistat-1 (tioconazole cream), for vulvovaginal candidiasis, 1075b
Vagus nerve stimulator (VNS), for epilepsy
  in adolescents and adults, 905–906
  in infants and children, 915, 915
Valacyclovir (Valtrex)
  for Bell's palsy, 951f, 951–952
  for erythema multiforme, 863, 864, 864b
  for herpes simplex virus, 841–842, 841t
    orolabial, 849
  for varicella, 76–77, 77b, 78
  for varicella zoster virus, 841t, 842
Valerian root, 1234–1243t
Valganciclovir (Valcyte), for CMV disease in HIV, 57
Valium. See Diazepam (Valium).

Valley fever. See Coccidioidomycosis.
Valproic acid (Depakene)
　for Cushing's syndrome, 645t
　for epilepsy
　　in adolescents in adults, 904t, 903, 905
　　in infants and children, 911–914, 912t
　　for Lennox-Gastaut Syndrome, 909
Valsalva maneuver, laryngitis due to, 219
Valsartan (Diovan), for systemic sclerosis, 811t
Valtrex. See Valacyclovir (Valtrex).
Vancenase (beclomethasone), for rhinitis
　allergic, 780t
　nonallergic, 217, 217b
Vancomycin (Vancocin)
　for acute infectious diarrhea, 19–20t
　allergy to, 783
　for bacterial meningitis, 115t
　for endocarditis prophylaxis, 346–347t, 347t
　for hepatic encephalopathy, 502–503
　for infective endocarditis, 345
　for necrotizing skin and soft tissue
　　infections, 85t
　for osteomyelitis, 1006t, 1006–1007
　for pericarditis, 870
　for toxic shock syndrome, 89, 89b
Vandazole (metronidazole vaginal gel)
　for bacterial vaginosis, 1074b
　for trichomoniasis, 1075
VAP. See Ventilator-associated
　pneumonia (VAP).
Vapreotide (Sanvar IR), 1244–1249t
Vaprisol (conivaptan), for hyponatremia, 598
Vaqta. See Hepatitis A virus (HAV, HepA)
　vaccine (Havrix, Vaqta).
Vardenafil (Levitra), for erectile dysfunction,
　718–719
　in multiple sclerosis, 939b
Varenicline (Chantix), for smoking cessation,
　1107
Variant Creutzfeldt-Jakob disease (vCJD),
　transfusion-associated, 490
Variceal bleeding, esophageal. See Esophageal
　varices, bleeding.
Varicella, 76
　breakthrough, 76
　with corticosteroids, 78
　diagnosis of, 76b
　epidemiology of, 76
　with immunodeficiency, 77–78
　pathogenesis of, 76, 77f
　prophylaxis for, 77b, 78
　vs. smallpox, 184f
　treatment of, 76–78, 77b
Varicella vaccine, 76, 77f
　schedule for, 149–150t
　catch-up, 151t
Varicella zoster immune globulin (VZIG),
　alternatives to, 78
Varicella zoster virus (VZV)
　herpes zoster due to
　　clinical features of, 840–841
　　diagnosis of, 841
　　treatment of, 841t, 842
　meningitis or encephalitis due to, 927,
　　928–930t, 931
　during pregnancy, 1014–1015
　varicella due to (See Varicella)
Varicella zoster virus (VZV) vaccine
　(Zostavax), 842
Varicose veins, during pregnancy, 1015
Variegate porphyria (VP), 475t, 476t
Variola major, 180
　as biological weapon agent, 1229–1233t
Variola minor, 180
Varix(ices)
　esophageal (See Esophageal varices)
　of labial mucosa, 850
Vasa previa, 1021, 1021b

Vascor (bepridil), intoxication with, 1183–1184
Vascular autoregulation, principles of, 721, 723f
Vascular causes, of vertigo, 208–209
Vascular dementia, 881
Vascular disease, erectile dysfunction due to,
　717b, 717
Vascular involvement, in systemic sclerosis,
　810–811, 811t
Vascular malformations, intracerebral
　hemorrhage due to, 890–891
Vascular risks, of hypertension, 350–351, 352f
Vasculitis
　cutaneous (hypersensitivity), 813
　　clinical presentation of, 813–814, 814f
　　diagnosis of, 814b
　　differential diagnosis of, 814–815
　　etiology of, 814
　　evaluation of, 815t
　　histopathology of, 814, 815t
　　due to serum sickness, 761
　　treatment of, 815–816, 815b, 816t
　defined, 813
　leukocytoclastic, 814
　urticarial, 815, 373
Vasculitis neuropathy, 964
Vasectomy, 758
　in postpartum period, 1029t
Vasoactive intestinal peptide (VIP), for erectile
　dysfunction, 720
Vasodepressor reaction, 760
Vasodilators
　direct, for hypertension, 359
　for systemic sclerosis, 811, 811t
Vasomotor rhinitis, 215, 216, 777–778
Vasomotor symptoms, of menopause, 1070
　treatment for, 1072t
Vasoocclusive pain, in sickle cell disease, 405
　differential diagnosis of, 406b
　treatment of, 407–409, 409t, 409b, 410f
Vasopressin (Pitressin)
　for cardiac arrest, 306
　for shock, 69t, 70
Vasopressors
　for anaphylaxis, 761
　for elevated intracranial pressure, 967
　for sepsis, 69–70, 69t
Vasotec (enalapril), for heart failure, 339t
Vasovagal reaction, 760
VATS. See Video-assisted thoracoscopic surgery
　(VATS).
VBG (vertical-banded gastroplasty), 610, 611f
vCJD (variant Creutzfeldt-Jakob disease),
　transfusion-associated, 490
VDRL (Venereal Disease Research Laboratory)
　test, 754–755
Vecuronium (Norcuron), for asthma in
　children, 772b
VEE (Venezuelan equine encephalitis), as
　biological weapon agent, 1229–1233t
Veetids. See Penicillin V potassium (Penn-Vee
　K, Veetids).
Vegetarian diets, for infants, 1044
Velban (vinblastine), for non–small cell lung
　cancer, 245–246
Velcade (bortezomib), for multiple myeloma,
　469b, 470, 471
Venakalant, 1244–1249t
Venereal Disease Research Laboratory (VDRL)
　test, 754–755
Venezuelan equine encephalitis (VEE), as
　biological weapon agent, 1229–1233t
Venlafaxine (Effexor)
　for Alzheimer's disease, 884, 885t
　for anogenital pruritus, 872b
　for anxiety disorder(s), 1112
　　generalized, 1113, 1113t
　for major depression, 1123, 1125, 1125–1126
　for menopausal symptoms, 1072t

Venlafaxine (Effexor) (Continued)
　for multiple sclerosis, 939b
　for obsessive compulsive disorder,
　　1114, 1114t
　for panic disorder, 1132t
　for premenstrual syndrome, 1068, 1068b
　for psychiatric dizziness, 209
　for vestibular migraine, 209
Venocaval interruption, for deep venous
　thrombosis/pulmonary embolism, 273
Venofer (iron sucrose), 386
Venom immunotherapy, 785–786, 785t, 786t
Venom X (VX)
　as chemical weapon, 1226–1228t
　poisoning due to, 1205–1206
Venous access, for parenteral nutrition, 622
Venous hypertension, 855
Venous leg ulcers, 855
　background of, 855
　clinical features of, 855
　diagnosis of, 855–856, 855b
　pathophysiology of, 855
　treatment of, 856–857, 856b, 856f
Venous stasis dermatitis, 855
Venous thrombosis
　air travel and, 375
　　epidemiology of, 376
　　etiology of, 376–377
　　prevention of, 377
　　risk factors for, 376, 376b
　due to polycythemia vera, 472
Ventavis (iloprost), for systemic sclerosis, 811
Ventilation
　for cardiac arrest, 303
　in newborn resuscitation, 1031–1032
Ventilation–perfusion (V/Q) mismatch, 225
Ventilation–perfusion (V/Q) scan, for
　pulmonary embolism, 272
Ventilator-associated pneumonia (VAP)
　defined, 263
　diagnosis of, 263–264
　epidemiology of, 263
　etiology of, 263
　prevention of, 264
　treatment of, 264, 264t
Ventolin. See Albuterol (Accuneb, Proventil,
　Ventolin).
Ventricular arrhythmias, in ischemic heart
　disease, 325–326
Ventricular complexes, premature, 313–314
　classification of, 314
　clinical features of, 314
　electrocardiographic features of, 313–314
　treatment of, 314
Ventricular fibrillation (VF)
　in cardiac arrest, 302, 303–304, 304f
　after myocardial infarction, 366t
Ventricular premature complexes, after
　myocardial infarction, 366t
Ventricular septal defect (VSD), 327
　antibiotic prophylaxis with, 345
　after myocardial infarction, 366t
Ventricular tachyarrhythmias (VTAs), 323–324
　due to heart block, 315
Ventricular tachycardia(s) (VTs), 323–324
　in Brugada's syndrome, 324–326, 325f, 325f
　in cardiac arrest, 302, 303–304, 304f
　catecholaminergic polymorphic, 324
　intrafascicular, 323
　in ischemic heart disease, 325–326
　after myocardial infarction, 366t
　outflow tract, 323
Ventriculoatrial shunt, bacterial meningitis
　with, 113
Ventriculoperitoneal shunt, bacterial
　meningitis with, 113
Venturi masks, 227t
VePesid. See Etoposide (VePesid).

Veramyst (fluticasone furoate), 1243
  for allergic rhinitis, 780t
Verapamil (Calan, Isoptin, Verelan)
  for angina pectoris, 299t
  for atrial fibrillation, 309
  for cluster headache, 926t
  for hypertrophic cardiomyopathy, 333
  intoxication with, 1183–1184
  for vestibular migraine, 209
Vermox. *See* Mebendazole (Vermox).
Verrucae, 822
  contagion and pathophysiology of, 822
  diagnosis of, 822**b**
  plana, 822**b**
  treatment of, 822–824, 823**b**
  vulgaris, 822**b**
Verrucous carcinoma
  of buccal mucosa, 851
  of vulva, 1094
Versed (midazolam)
  for elevated intracranial pressure, 967
  intoxication with, 1181–1182
Versenate (edetate calcium disodium), for lead poisoning, 1199–1200, 1200**t**
Vertebral compression fractures, back pain due to, 40
Vertical-banded gastroplasty (VBG), 610, 611**f**
Vertigo
  due to acoustic neuroma, 208
  due to anterior inferior cerebellar artery syndrome, 209
  due to basilar meningitis, 208
  benign paroxysmal positional, 205–206, 205**f**, 206**f**
  of central origin, 208–209
  due to cerebral infarction, 209
  defined, 204
  description of, 205**t**
  disequilibrium without, 205**t**
  epileptic, 209
  episodic, 204
  examples of, 205**t**
  due to familial periodic ataxia, 209
  due to hyperventilation, 210
  due to motion sickness, 209–210
  due to multiple sclerosis, 209
  due to neurovascular compression, 208
  nonvascular causes of, 209
  otolithic, 207–208
  due to perilymphatic fistula, 208
  of peripheral origin, 205–208
    acute unilateral, 206–207, 206**t**, 207**b**
    bilateral, 207, 207**b**
  physiologic, 205**t**, 209–210
  due to posterior inferior cerebellar artery syndrome, 209
  post-traumatic, 209
  psychiatric, 205**t**, 209
  due to superior canal dehiscence syndrome, 208
  due to transient ischemic attacks, 208–209
  of unknown origin, 209
  vascular causes of, 208–209
  due to vestibular migraine, 209
  visual, 210
Very low calorie diets (VLCDs), 609
Very-low-density lipoprotein (VLDL) cholesterol, 601
Vesanoid (tretinoin), for acute promyelocytic leukemia, 448–449
Vesicant agents, as chemical weapons, 1226–1228**t**
Vesicare (solifenacin), for urge incontinence, 695**b**
Vestibular migraine, 209
Vestibular nerve section, for Ménière's disease, 212
Vestibular neuritis, 206–207, 207**b**

Vestibular neurolabyrinthitis, 206–207, 207**b**
Vestibular testing, for Ménière's disease, 211
VF (ventricular fibrillation)
  in cardiac arrest, 302, 303–304, 304**f**
  after myocardial infarction, 366**t**
VFC (Vaccines for Children), 153
Vfend. *See* Voriconazole (Vfend).
VHFs (viral hemorrhagic fevers), as biological weapon agents, 1229–1233**t**
VHL (von Hippel–Lindau) disease, pheochromocytomas and paragangliomas in, 674–675
VHL gene, in pheochromocytomas and paragangliomas, 674–675
Viagra. *See* Sildenafil citrate (Viagra).
Vibramycin. *See* Doxycycline (Vibramycin, Vibra-Tabs, Doryx).
Vibra-Tabs. *See* Doxycycline (Vibramycin, Vibra-Tabs, Doryx).
Vibrio cholerae. *See* Cholera.
Vibrio parahemolyticus, acute infectious diarrhea due to, 16
Vibrio vulnificus, necrotizing skin and soft tissue infections due to, 84**t**, 85**t**
Vicodin. *See* Hydrocodone + acetaminophen (Lortab, Maxidon, Norco, Vicodin, Xodol, Zydone).
Vicoprofen (hydrocodone + ibuprofen), for pain, 4**t**
VICP (Vaccine Injury Compensation Program), 148
Vidarabine (Vira-A), for neonatal conjunctivitis, 196
Vidaza (5-azacytidine), for acute myeloid leukemia, 448
Video-assisted thoracoscopic surgery (VATS)
  for empyema, 257–258
  for lung cancer, 245
  for pleural effusion, 257
Videx (didanosine), for HIV, 50**t**, 51**t**
Vigabatrin (Sabril)
  for epilepsy, 904**t**
  for infantile spasms, 909
Vildagliptin (Galvus), 1244–1249**t**
  for diabetes, 580**t**
VIN (vulvar intraepithelial neoplasia), 824, 1092, 1092**t**
Vinblastine (Velban), for non–small cell lung cancer, 245–246
Vincent's curtsy, 686
Vincent's infection, 854
Vincristine
  for acute lymphoblastic leukemia, 449
  for multiple myeloma, 469**b**, 470
Vindesine (Eldisine), for non–small cell lung cancer, 245–246
Vinorelbine (Navelbine), for non–small cell lung cancer, 245–246
Vioxx (rofecoxib), for prostatitis, 711
VIP (vasoactive intestinal peptide), for erectile dysfunction, 720
Vira-A (vidarabine), for neonatal conjunctivitis, 196
Viracept (nelfinavir), for HIV, 50**t**
  drug interactions with, 58**t**
Viral agents, acute infectious diarrhea due to, 14**b**, 16
Viral conjunctivitis, 194–195, 194**t**
  in neonate, 196, 196**t**
Viral encephalitis, 927
  as biological weapon agent, 1229–1233**t**
  clinical features of, 927
  diagnosis of, 927–930, 931**b**
  etiology of, 927, 928–930**t**
  treatment of, 930–932, 932**b**
Viral hemorrhagic fevers (VHFs), as biological weapon agents, 1229–1233**t**
Viral hepatitis, cirrhosis due to, 498**t**

Viral infections, due to transfusions, 485**t**, 489–490, 490**b**
Viral influenza pneumonia, 266, 266–267
  with bacterial superinfection, 267
  clinical manifestations of, 267
  diagnosis of, 267, 268**b**
  etiology and pathogenesis of, 266
  prevention of, 266–267
  treatment of, 267, 267**t**, 269**b**
Viral meningitis, 927
  clinical features of, 927
  diagnosis of, 927–930, 931**b**
  etiology of, 927, 928–930**t**
  treatment of, 930–932, 932**b**
Viral pericarditis, 368, 368**b**, 370–371
Viral respiratory infection(s), 264
  bronchiolitis as, 266
  common colds as, 265
  croup as, 265–266
  diagnosis of, 265**b**
  etiology of, 264–265
  influenza-like illness due to, 265
  treatment of, 265**b**
Viramune (nevirapine), for HIV, 49–50, 50**t**, 51**t**
  drug interactions with, 58**t**
Virazole (ribavirin)
  for bronchiolitis, 266
  for hepatitis B and C viruses, 536**t**, 538
Viread (tenofovir), for HIV, 50**t**, 51**t**
Viroptic (trifluridine), for neonatal conjunctivitis, 196
Viruses, as biological weapon agents, 1229–1233**t**
VIS(s) (Vaccine Information Statements), 148–152
Visceral leishmaniasis
  anthroponotic, 96
  clinical features of, 94
  epidemiology of, 93
  pathogenesis of, 93
  treatment of, 94**b**
  zoonotic, 96
Viscosupplementation, 1001
Visken (pindolol)
  for angina pectoris, 299
  intoxication with, 1182–1183, 1183**t**
Vistaril. *See* Hydroxyzine (Atarax, Vistaril).
Vistide (cidofovir)
  for CMV disease in HIV, 57
  for herpes simplex virus, 842
Visual acuity, 188–189
Visual disturbances, due to alcohol withdrawal, 1102–1103**b**
Visual function, assessment of, 188–189
Visual vertigo, 210
Vital capacity, timed, for COPD, 232, 232
Vital functions, assessment and maintenance of, for poisonings, 1161, 1162**t**, 1163**t**
Vital signs, with poisonings, 1161, 1162**t**
Vitamin(s), in parenteral nutrition, 620–621, 621**t**
Vitamin A
  for osteoporosis due to primary biliary cirrhosis, 499
  in parenteral nutrition, 621**t**
Vitamin B_1
  for alcohol withdrawal, 1103
  in parenteral nutrition, 621**t**
Vitamin B_2, in parenteral nutrition, 621**t**
Vitamin B_6
  for nausea during pregnancy, 1014
  in parenteral nutrition, 621**t**
  for poisoning, 1167–1172**t**
    due to isoniazid, 1195, 1195
Vitamin B_7
  for brittle nails, 818**b**, 819
  in parenteral nutrition, 621**t**
Vitamin B_{12}
  in diet, 396
  metabolism of, 396

Vitamin B₁₂ (Continued)
  in parenteral nutrition, 621t
Vitamin B₁₂ deficiency, 395
  clinical features of, 395
  diagnosis of, 395–396
  peripheral neuropathy due to, 963
  physiologic issues relative to, 396
  treatment of, 396–397
Vitamin B₁₂ malabsorption, 541b, 542
Vitamin B₁₂ₐ
  for cyanide poisoning, 1188
  for vitamin B₁₂ deficiency, 397
Vitamin C
  in parenteral nutrition, 621t
  for preeclampsia, 1025
Vitamin D
  in chronic renal failure, 730
  for hypoparathyroidism, 653
  for infants, 1042
  for inflammatory bowel disease, 518
  for osteoporosis, 614
    due to primary biliary cirrhosis, 499
    in rheumatoid arthritis, 977b
  in parenteral nutrition, 621t
  for thalassemia, 400b
Vitamin D₂, for hypoparathyroidism, 653
Vitamin D₃, for hypoparathyroidism, 653
Vitamin deficiencies, peripheral neuropathy due to, 963, 963b
Vitamin E
  for dysmenorrhea, 1066
  for osteoporosis due to primary biliary cirrhosis, 499
  in parenteral nutrition, 621t
  for preeclampsia, 1025
  for systemic sclerosis, 811
Vitamin H
  for brittle nails, 818b, 819
  in parenteral nutrition, 621t
Vitamin K
  for osteoporosis due to primary biliary cirrhosis, 499
  in parenteral nutrition, 621, 621t
Vitamin K₁ (Aqua Mephyton), for poisoning, 1167–1172t
Vitamin K–dependent coagulation factor deficiencies, 424t
Vitamin supplementation, for infants, 1042
Vitasert (ganciclovir intraocular implant), for CMV disease in HIV, 57
Vitex, 1234–1243t
Vitiligo, 878–879
Vitreous humor, 187, 188f
Vivactil (protriptyline)
  for major depression, 1124
  poisoning due to, 1214–1216, 1215t
Viviant (bazedoxifene), 1244–1249t
Vivitrol. See Naltrexone (ReVia, Depade, Vivitrol).
Vivotif Berna (typhoid vaccine), 18
  for travelers, 159–160t, 161
VLCDs (very low calorie diets), 609
VLDL (very-low-density lipoprotein) cholesterol, 601
VNS (vagus nerve stimulator), for epilepsy
  in adolescents and adults, 905–906
  in infants and children, 915
Vocal abuse, laryngitis due to, 218–220
Vocal folds, 218
Vocational rehabilitation, for schizophrenia, 1129–1130
Voice intonation, in schizophrenia, 1129
Voice production, 218, 218b
Voided volume, 690
Voiding, dysfunctional, 691
Voiding disorders, after stroke, 897
Voiding patterns, normal, 690

Voiding postponement, incontinence due to, 690–691
Voltaren (diclofenac)
  for juvenile idiopathic arthritis, 985
  for pain, 2t
Voltaren Gel (diclofenac sodium gel), 1243
  for actinic keratosis, 834
Volume expanders, for hypovolemic shock in newborn, 1032
Volume overload
  in chronic renal failure, 727, 730–731
  due to transfusion, 486t, 491
Volume replacement, for sepsis, 68–69
Vomiting. See also Nausea and vomiting.
  self-induced, 1115
Vomiting agents, as chemical weapons, 1226–1228t
von Hippel–Lindau (VHL) disease, pheochromocytomas and paragangliomas in, 674–675
von Willebrand factor (vWF), 422, 423t
von Willebrand's disease (vWD), 422–425
  acquired, 425
  clinical features of, 421t, 423
  clinical variants of, 423, 423t
  defined, 422
  diagnosis of, 420b, 423
  epidemiology of, 423
  in pregnancy, 425
  treatment of, 421b, 423–425
Voriconazole (Vfend)
  for blastomycosis, 255–256
  for coccidioidomycosis, 250t, 251, 251t
  for necrotizing skin and soft tissue infections, 85t
Vornistat (Zolinza), for cutaneous T-cell lymphomas, 800
VP (variegate porphyria), 475t, 476t
V/Q (ventilation–perfusion) mismatch, 225
V/Q (ventilation–perfusion) scan, for pulmonary embolism, 272
VSD. See Ventricular septal defect (VSD).
VT(s). See Ventricular tachycardia(s) (VTs).
VTAs (ventricular tachyarrhythmias), 323–324
  due to heart block, 315
Vulvar cancer, 1092–1094
  adenocarcinomas as, 1092–1093
  basal cell carcinoma as, 1094
  malignant melanoma as, 1093–1094
  metastasis of
    depth of tumor invasion and, 1092, 1093t
    tumor diameter and, 1092, 1092t
  sarcomas as, 1094
  squamous cell carcinomas as, 1092–1093, 1093t
  staging and classification of, 1092, 1093b, 1093b
  verrucous carcinoma as, 1094
Vulvar intraepithelial neoplasia (VIN), 824, 1092, 1092t
Vulvar neoplasms, 1091
  benign
    condyloma acuminatum as, 1092
    cystic, 1091
    solid, 1091–1092
  diagnosis of, 1093b
  intraepithelial, 1092
    Paget's disease as, 1092
    vulvar intraepithelial neoplasia as, 1092, 1092t
  invasive, 1092–1094
    adenocarcinomas as, 1092–1093
    basal cell carcinoma as, 1094
    malignant melanoma as, 1093–1094
    metastasis of
      depth of tumor invasion and, 1092, 1093t
      tumor diameter and, 1092, 1092t
    sarcomas as, 1094

Vulvar neoplasms (Continued)
    squamous cell carcinomas as, 1092–1093, 1093t
    staging and classification of, 1092, 1093b, 1093b
    verrucous carcinoma as, 1094
  treatment of, 1094b
Vulvovaginal candidiasis, 1074–1075, 1075b, 1075b
Vulvovaginitis, 1074
  due to bacterial vaginosis, 1074
  diagnosis of, 1075b
  impact of, 1074
  symptoms of, 1074
  due to trichomoniasis, 1075, 1075b
  due to vulvovaginal candidiasis, 1074–1075, 1075b
vWD. See Von Willebrand's disease (vWD).
vWF (von Willebrand factor), 422, 423, 423t
VX (venom X)
  as chemical weapon, 1226–1228t
  poisoning due to, 1205–1206
Vytorin (simvastatin-ezetimibe), for dyslipoproteinemia, 605t
Vyvanse (lisdexamfetamine dimesylate), 1243
VZIG (varicella zoster immune globulin), alternatives to, 78
VZV. See Varicella zoster virus (VZV).

W

Waist circumference, 607
Wakana syndrome, 571
Waldvogel classification, of osteomyelitis, 1005
Walk and turn test, for vestibular neurolabyrinthitis, 207b
Walk while turning your head, for vestibular neurolabyrinthitis, 207b
Wallenberg's syndrome, 893
Wallerian degeneration, 958
Warfarin (Coumadin)
  for atrial fibrillation, 309, 310b
  for deep venous thrombosis/pulmonary embolism, 273, 273b
  for thalassemia, 400b
Warfarin (Coumadin)-related intracerebral hemorrhage, 890
Warm autoimmune hemolytic anemia, 387–388
  diagnosis of, 387
  serology of, 387t
  treatment of, 387–388, 388b
Warts, 822
  contagion and pathophysiology of, 822
  diagnosis of, 822b
  flat, 822b
  genital (See Condyloma acuminatum)
  treatment of, 822–824, 823b
Washed platelets, 482
Washed red blood cells, 481
Watchful waiting, for benign prostatic hyperplasia, 714–718
Water exposure, pruritus due to, 31b
Watermelon stomach, in systemic sclerosis, 811–812
Wavefront-guided LASIK, 189, 191t
WD (Wilson's disease), 498t, 500–501
WDTC (well-differentiated thyroid cancers), 672–673, 673t
Weakness
  due to multiple sclerosis, 939
  in myasthenia gravis, 940, 941t
Weapon agents
  biological, 1229
  chemical, 1226
Weather changes, and asthma in children, 771
WEE (Western equine encephalitis), as biological weapon agent, 1229–1233t
Weight, and angina pectoris, 297

Weight gain
    in infants, 1044
    medications that promote, 607, 607t
    during pregnancy, 1014
Weight loss, 619
    for diabetes, 576b, 577–578, 579b
    pruritus due to, 32b
Welchol (colesevelam hydrochloride)
    for diabetes, 583
    for dyslipoproteinemia, 605, 605t
Wellbutrin. See Bupropion (Wellbutrin).
Well-differentiated thyroid cancers (WDTC), 672–673, 673t
Wernicke-Korsakoff syndrome, 1173
West Nile virus
    meningitis or encephalitis due to, 927, 928–930t, 932
    transfusion-associated, 489–490
Western blot assay, for HIV, 48
Western equine encephalitis (WEE), as biological weapon agent, 1229–1233t
Wet-wrap dressings, for atopic dermatitis, 862
Wheelchairs, for stroke survivors, 896
Wheezing, in children, 770–771, 770t
Whiff test, 1074
Whipple's disease, 544
Whipworm, 569–571, 570t
Whisker hairs, 791
White coat hypertension, 352
Whitlow, herpetic, 840
WHO. See World Health Organization (WHO).
Whole blood–derived platelets, 482
Whole-bowel irrigation, for poisoning, 1164–1165
    due to theophylline, 1214
Whole-brain radiation therapy, for brain metastases, 976
Whooping cough. See Pertussis.
Wickham's striae, 804
Widow spider bites, 1151
Wills, Lucy, 395
Wilson's disease (WD), 498t, 500–501
Withdrawal
    from alcohol
        assessment for, 1100–1101, 1102–1103b
        detoxification for, 1100–1103
        diagnostic criteria for, 1101t
        general principles for, 1106, 1107b
        medications for, 1101–1103, 1107b
    from drugs
        characteristics of, 1105, 1105, 1105b
        treatment of, 1106, 1106b
    from opiates
        symptoms of, 1108
        treatment of, 1108–1109, 1108b
Wolff-Parkinson-White (WPW) pattern, 321–322
Wolff-Parkinson-White (WPW) syndrome, 322
Women, angina in, 295
Wood alcohol poisoning, 1201–1202
World Health Organization (WHO)
    classification of acute leukemias by, 445, 446b
    on leprosy, 103
    tuberculosis treatment regimen of, 285t
Wound care, for Stevens-Johnson syndrome and toxic epidermal necrolysis, 864b, 865–866
Wound fluid, for pressure ulcers, 859
WPW (Wolff-Parkinson-White) pattern, 321, 322
WPW (Wolff-Parkinson-White) syndrome, 322
WR 6026 (sitamaquine), for leishmaniasis, 95
Wrist injuries, due to sports, 1009–1010
Wuchereria bancrofti, 844, 844t
Wycillin (procaine penicillin), for syphilis, 755t

X

Xalatan (latanoprost), for glaucoma, 199–200
Xanax. See Alprazolam (Xanax).
XDR-TB (extensively drug-resistant tuberculosis), 282, 288
Xenical (orlistat), for obesity, 610, 610t
Xerocytosis, hereditary, 392
Xerostomia, 849
    due to radiation therapy for Hodgkin's disease, 444
Xerotic eczema, 30b
Xifaxan. See Rifamixin (Xifaxan).
Xigris (drotrecogin alfa [activated]), for sepsis, 71
Xodol. See Hydrocodone + acetaminophen (Lortab, Maxidon, Norco, Vicodin, Xodol, Zydone).
Xolair (omalizumab), for asthma
    in adolescents and adults, 767–768t
    in children, 775
Xopenex (levalbuterol), for asthma
    in adolescents and adults, 766t
    in children, 774–775, 775t
X-rays, during pregnancy, 1016
XTC (3,4-methylenedioxymethamphetamine)
    abuse of, 1110
    intoxication with, 1178–1179
Xylocaine. See Lidocaine (Xylocaine).
Xyzal (levocetirizine), 1243

Y

Yellow fever, as biological weapon agent, 1229–1233t
Yellow fever vaccine (YF-VAX), 160, 159–160t
Yersinia pestis. See Plague.
Yodoxin. See Iodoquinol (diiodohydroxyquin, Yodoxin).
Yohimbine, for erectile dysfunction, 719
Yolk sac carcinoma, 738–739
Yomesan (niclosamide), for tapeworms, 570t
Yo-yo spleen, in sickle cell disease, 407

Z

Zafirlukast (Accolate), for asthma
    in adolescents and adults, 767–768t
    in children, 773–774t
Zalcitabine (Hivid), for HIV, 50t
Zaleplon (Sonata), for insomnia, 888, 888t
Zanaflex (tizanidine), for multiple sclerosis, 939b
Zanamivir (Relenza), for influenza, 92, 92t, 260, 260b, 265, 267, 267t
Zanolimumab (HuMax-CD4), for cutaneous T-cell lymphomas, 800, 800
Zantac. See Ranitidine (Zantac).
Zarnestra (tipifarnib), for acute myeloid leukemia, 448
Zarontin (ethosuximide), for epilepsy
    in adolescents in adults, 904t
    in infants and children, 908–909, 912t
Zaroxolyn (metolazone)
    for chronic renal failure, 731
    for hypertension, 356–357
Zelapar (selegiline, orally disintegrating), for parkinsonism, 957
Zelnorm (tegaserod)
    for constipation, 22, 22b
    for irritable bowel syndrome, 524–525
Zenker's diverticulum(a), 511–512
    clinical features of, 511
    defined, 511
    diagnosis of, 511, 512b
    dysphagia due to, 509, 510
    treatment of, 511–512, 513b
Zenvia (dextromethorphan/quinidine), 1244–1249t
Zerit (stavudine), for HIV, 50t
ZES (Zollinger-Ellison syndrome), 531b, 532–533
    malabsorption due to, 545
Zestril (lisinopril), for myocardial infarction, 365t
Zetia (ezetimibe), for dyslipoproteinemia, 605
Ziagen (abacavir), for HIV, 50t, 51t
Ziana (clindamycin-tretinoin), for acne, 788
Zidovudine (Retrovir), for HIV, 50t, 51t
Zidovudine + lamivudine (Combivir), for HIV, 51t
Zileuton (Zyflo), for asthma, 767–768t
Zinc
    for erectile dysfunction, 719
    in parenteral nutrition, 621, 621t
Zingo (lidocaine hydrochloride monohydrate), 1243
Ziprasidone (Geodon)
    for bipolar disorder, 1127
    for schizophrenia, 1130, 1130t
    for Tourette's syndrome, 921
Zithromax. See Azithromycin (Zithromax).
Zocor. See Simvastatin (Zocor).
Zofran. See Ondansetron (Zofran).
Zoladex (goserelin)
    for endometriosis, 1056
    for uterine leiomyoma, 1082
Zoledronic acid (Zometa)
    for multiple myeloma
        with hypercalcemia, 471
        with skeletal lesions, 471–472
    for osteoporosis, 614
    for Paget's disease of bone, 617
Zolinza (vorinstat), for cutaneous T-cell lymphomas, 800
Zollinger-Ellison syndrome (ZES), 531b, 532–533
    malabsorption due to, 545
Zolmitriptan (Zomig), for migraine headache, 925t, 926
Zoloft. See Sertraline (Zoloft).
Zolpidem (Ambien), for insomnia, 888, 888t
Zomaril (iloperidone), 1244–1249t
Zometa. See Zoledronic acid (Zometa).
Zomig (zolmitriptan), for migraine headache, 925t, 926
Zonisamide (Zonegran), for epilepsy
    in adolescents in adults, 904t, 903
    in infants and children, 914–915, 913t
Zonular fibers, 187
Zostavax (varicella zoster virus vaccine), 842
Zoster, 78
Zostrix. See Capsaicin (Capsin, Zostrix).
Zosyn (piperacillin/tazobactam), for necrotizing skin and soft tissue infections, 85t
Zovirax. See Acyclovir (Zovirax).
Zyban (buproprion), for smoking cessation, 1107
Zydone. See Hydrocodone + acetaminophen (Lortab, Maxidon, Norco, Vicodin, Xodol, Zydone).
Zyflo (zileuton), for asthma, 767–768t
Zygomycetes, necrotizing skin and soft tissue infections due to, 85t
Zyloprim. See Allopurinol (Zyloprim).
Zyprexa. See Olanzapine (Zyprexa).
Zyrtec (cetirizine)
    for allergic rhinitis, 779t
    for urticaria, 875
Zyrtec-D (cetirizine/pseudoephedrine), for allergic rhinitis, 779t
Zyvox. See Linezolid (Zyvox).